NANDA-*Approved* Nursing Diagnoses

Activity Intolerance
Activity Intolerance, High Risk for
Adjustment, Impaired
Airway Clearance, Ineffective
Anxiety
Aspiration, High Risk for
Body Image Disturbance
Body Temperature, High Risk for Altered
Breastfeeding, Effective
Breastfeeding, Ineffective
Breathing Pattern, Ineffective
Communication, Impaired Verbal
Constipation
Constipation, Colonic
Constipation, Perceived
Decisional Conflict (specify)
Decreased Cardiac Output
Defensive Coping
Denial, Ineffective
Diarrhea
Disuse Syndrome, High Risk for
Diversional Activity Deficit
Dysreflexia
Family Coping, Compromised, Ineffective
Family Coping, Disabling, Ineffective
Family Coping: Potential for Growth
Family Processes, Altered
Fatigue
Fear
Fluid Volume Deficit
Fluid Volume Deficit, High Risk for
Fluid Volume Excess
Gas Exchange, Impaired
Grieving, Anticipatory
Grieving, Dysfunctional
Growth and Development, Altered
Health Maintenance, Altered
Health Seeking Behaviors (specify)
Home Maintenance Management, Impaired
Hopelessness
Hyperthermia
Hypothermia
Incontinence, Bowel
Incontinence, Functional
Incontinence, Reflex
Incontinence, Stress
Incontinence, Total
Incontinence, Urge
Individual Coping, Ineffective
Infection, High Risk for
Injury, High Risk for
Knowledge Deficit (specify)
Noncompliance (specify)
Nutrition, Altered: Less than Body Requirements
Nutrition, Altered: More than Body Requirements
Nutrition, Altered: Potential for More than Body Requirements
Oral Mucous Membrane, Altered
Pain
Pain, Chronic
Parental Role Conflict
Parenting, Altered
Parenting, High Risk for Altered
Personal Identity Disturbance
Physical Mobility, Impaired
Poisoning, High Risk for
Post-Trauma Response
Powerlessness
Protection, Altered
Rape-Trauma Syndrome
Rape-Trauma Syndrome: Compound Reaction
Rape-Trauma Syndrome: Silent Reaction
Role Performance, Altered
Self-Care Deficit, Bathing/Hygiene
Self-Care Deficit, Feeding
Self-Care Deficit, Dressing/Grooming
Self-Care Deficit, Toileting
Self-Esteem, Chronic Low
Self-Esteem, Situational Low
Self-Esteem Disturbance
Sensory/Perceptual Alterations (specify) (visual, auditory, kinesthetic, gustatory, tactile, olfactory)
Sexual Dysfunction
Sexuality Patterns, Altered
Skin Integrity, Impaired
Skin Integrity, High Risk for Impaired
Sleep Pattern Disturbance
Social Interaction, Impaired
Social Isolation
Spiritual Distress (Distress of the Human Spirit)
Suffocation, High Risk for
Swallowing, Impaired
Thermoregulation, Ineffective
Thought Processes, Altered
Tissue Integrity, Impaired
Tissue Perfusion, Altered (specify type) (renal, cerebral, cardiopulmonary, gastrointestinal, peripheral)
Trauma, High Risk for
Unilateral Neglect
Urinary Elimination, Altered
Urinary Retention
Violence, High Risk for: Self-directed or Directed at Others

Courtesy of North American Nursing Diagnosis Association, St. Louis, MO.

NURSING CARE OF ADULTS

Frances Donovan Monahan, Ph.D., R.N.
Professor and Chair
Department of Nursing
Rockland Community College
Suffern, New York

Tanya Drake, M.S.N., R.N.
Associate Professor
Department of Nursing
Rockland Community College
Suffern, New York

Marianne Neighbors, Ed.D., R.N.
Associate Professor
Department of Nursing
College of Education
University of Arkansas
Fayetteville, Arkansas

W.B. Saunders Company
A Division of Harcourt Brace & Company
Philadelphia London Toronto Montreal Sydney Tokyo

NURSING CARE OF ADULTS

W.B. SAUNDERS COMPANY
A Division of Harcourt Brace & Company

The Curtis Center
Independence Square West
Philadelphia, Pennsylvania 19106

Library of Congress Cataloging-in-Publication Data

Monahan, Frances Donovan.
Nursing care of adults/France Donovan Monahan, Tanya Drake, Marianne Neighbors.
p. cm.
ISBN 0-7216-1644-5
1. Nursing. I. Drake, Tanya. II. Neighbors, Marianne. III. Title.
[DNLM: 1. Nursing Care. WY 100 M734n 1994]
RT41.M78 1994
610.73—dc20
DNLM/DLC 93-37587

Nursing Care of Adults ISBN 0-7216-1644-5

Printed in the United States of America

Last digit is the print number: 9 8 7 6 5 4 3 2 1

DEDICATED TO OUR STUDENTS, FOR WHOM THIS TEXT WAS WRITTEN;
AND TO OUR COLLEAGUES,
WITH THE DEEPEST RESPECT AND THANKS FOR THEIR INSPIRATION, SUPPORT,
AND ENCOURAGEMENT.

Dedicated with all my love to my husband, William;
my son, Michael;
my daughter, Kerryane;
and to my mother, Isabel Torpey Donovan.

FRAN

Dedicated to my husband, Jay,
and my daughters, Dana *and* Jodi,
for their unflagging love, support, encouragement, and sacrifices;
and to Gloria, *who taught me the true meaning of courage, determination, and perseverance.*

TANYA

Dedicated to my family, especially my parents, Lillian *and* Louis Zadra,
who have always given love, encouragement, and assistance without question,
and my son, Jeremy, *the light of my life;*
and to my friends who are always there when I am in need.

MARIANNE

Reviewers

Elaine L. Ackley, B.S.N., R.N.
Trocaire College
Buffalo, NY

Sandra Lee Anthony, R.N., O.N.C.
Tri County Orthopedic Surgeons, Inc.
Stark Technical College
Massillon, OH

Roberta P. Bartee, M.S., R.N.
Tulane University Medical Center
New Orleans, LA

Joyce M. Black, M.S.N., R.N.,C., C.P.S.N.
University of Nebraska College of Nursing
Omaha, NE

Kathleen Koernig Blais, Ed.D., R.N.
Florida International University, School of Nursing
North Miami, FL

Deanna Mary Bland, B.S., R.N., C.D.E.
University Physicians, Inc.
Tucson, AZ

June Cooper Borden, M.S.N., R.N., E.D.S.
Florida Community College
Jacksonville, FL

Margaret Bowman, M.S.N., R.N.
Wheeling Jesuit College
Wheeling, WV

Bonita E. Broyles, M.A., R.N.
Certified CPR Instructor for ARC
Piedmont Community College
Roxboro, NC

Dorothy A. Calabrese, M.S.N., R.N., C.U.R.N.
Clinical Nurse Specialist–Urology Oncology
Cleveland Clinic Foundation
Cleveland, OH

Kay Lynne Carnegie, M.S., R.N.
Chemeketa Community College
Salem, OR

Kathleen McMahon Casey, M.Ed., M.A., R.N.
National HIV Care Program Clinical Director
Critical Care America
Rhinebeck, NY

Linda M. Coe, M.S.N., R.N., C.D.E.
Clinical Nurse Specialist, Endocrinology
National Institutes of Health Clinical Center
Nursing Department
Bethesda, MD

Ivory C. Coleman, M.S., R.N.
Community College of Philadelphia
Philadelphia, PA

Muriel Sharon Taylor Cooney, M.S.N., R.N.
Watts School of Nursing
Durham Regional Hospital
Durham, NC

Janet Coors Cottingham, R.N.
SOHN (Society of Otolaryngology Head and Neck Nurses)
New Smyrna Beach, FL

Deanna S. Cross, Ph.D., R.N.
Head, Department of Associate Degree Nursing
Armstrong State College
Savannah, GA

Marita G. Donahue, **M.Ed., M.S., R.N.,C., A.N.P.**
Professor, Nurse Education
Massasoit Community College
Brockton, MA

Nancy D. Doolittle, **Ph.D., R.N.**
University of California, San Francisco School of Nursing
San Francisco, CA

Vicki V. Ernest, **M.S., R.N.**
Community College of Denver
Denver, CO

Karen Lee Fahey, **M.S.N., R.N.,C., C.N.M.**
Certified Nurse–Midwife
ANA Certification–Maternal Child Health
Private Practice as CNM
Cleveland, OH
Nursing Instructor, Wheeling Jesuit College
Wheeling, WV

Anne Findeis, **M.S., R.N.**
University of Illinois at Chicago
Chicago Lung Association
Respiratory Nursing Society
American Association of Critical Care Nurses
Chicago, IL

Marcia R. Floyd, **M.S.N., R.N.**
Dunn, NC

Lisa Sheets Glover, **M.N., R.N., C.C.R.N.**
University of California at San Francisco
San Francisco, CA

Patricia Golden, **M.S.N., R.N.**
St. Petersburg Junior College
St. Petersburg, FL

Sybil B. Goulkin, **R.N.**
Nurse Manager
Beth Israel Hospital
Boston, MA

Joanne M. Gordon, **M.A., M.S.N., R.N.**
Southwest Missouri State University
Springfield, MO

Christine Grady, **M.S., R.N., C.S.**
National Center for Nursing Research
National Institutes of Health
Bethesda, MD

Susan Sweat Gunby, **Ph.D., R.N.**
Dean, Georgia Baptist College of Nursing
Atlanta, GA

Jane Hokanson Hawks, **M.S.N., R.N.,C.**
Bishop Clarkson College
Omaha, NE

Phyllis Foster Healy, **Ph.D., R.N.,C.**
University of Southern Maine
School of Nursing
Portland, ME

Marcia Margaret Hegstad, **M.N., R.N., C.S., C.D.E.**
Catherine McAuley Health System
Ann Arbor, MI

Jeanne L. Held, **M.S.N., R.N., C.S.**
Albert Einstein Medical Center
Philadelphia, PA

Renee J. Hinjosa, **M.S., R.N.**
University Hospital and Clinics
Columbia, MO

Marianne Genge Jagmin, **M.S., R.N., C.S., O.N.C.**
Rush-Presbyterian–St. Luke's Medical Center
Chicago, IL

Donna F.M. Jamieson, **M.S., R.N.**
Rush-Presbyterian–St. Luke's Medical Center
Chicago, IL

Elizabeth G. Johnson, **B.S.N., R.N.**
Kentucky Wesleyan College
Owensboro, KY

Marcie Jones, **D.N.Sc., R.N.**
College Misericordia
Dallas, PA

Annabelle M. Keene, **M.S.N., R.N.,C.**
University of Nebraska College of Nursing
Omaha, NE

Nancy J. Kupper, **M.S.N., R.N.**
Associate Professor of Nursing
Tarrant County Junior College
Fort Worth, TX

June C. Larson, **M.S., R.N.**
Department of Nursing
University of South Dakota
Vermillion, SD

Dorothy Lumb Leese, **M.A., R.N., C.D.E.**
Hospital of the Medical College of Pennsylvania
Philadelphia, PA

Laura L. Faires, **B.S.N., R.N., C.N.O.R.**
VA Medical Center
Portland, OR

Jo Ann Maklebust, M.S.N., R.N., C.S.
Clinical Nurse Specialist
Harper Hospital
Detroit Medical Center
Member, Detroit Demonstration Site for Defining and Differentiating
ADN/BSN Nursing Competencies
Detroit, MI

Kimberly J. Mason, M.S.N., R.N., O.N.C.
The Children's Hospital of Philadelphia
Philadelphia, PA

Tracy A. Moran, M.S., R.N.
University of California, San Francisco
San Francisco General Hospital
San Francisco, CA

Carol A. Morris, Ed.D., R.N.
Director Department of Nursing
NEO A & M College
Miami, OK

Carol J. Nelson, M.S.N., R.N.
Spokane Community College
Spokane, WA

Mary N. Parker, Ed.D., R.N.
Cuesta College
San Luis Obispo, CA

Ann Peterson, M.S.N., R.N., C.N.S., C.D.E.
National Institutes of Health Nursing Department
Bethesda, MD

Holly Jane Price, M.S.N., R.N.
Assistant Director
Providence Hospital School of Nursing
Sandusky, OH

Ethel Pruden, M.N., R.N.
Armstrong State College
Savannah, GA

Betty L. Purvis, M.S.N., R.N.
Meridian Community College
Meridian, MS

Neil W. Rheiner, Ed.D., R.N.
Certified Trauma Nurse Specialist
University of Nebraska Medical Center
College of Nursing
Omaha, NE

Karin K. Roberts, M.N., R.N.
Research College of Nursing
Kansas City, MO

Pamela S. Rodrigues, R.N., O.N.C.
Nursing Supervisor
Tri County Orthopedic Surgeons, Inc.
Massillon, OH

Amy Perrin Ross, M.S.N., R.N., C.N.R.N.
Loyola University Medical Center
Chicago, IL

Bernice Rudolph, B.S., R.N., P.H.N.
Casa Loma College
Sylmar, CA

Jean Baloyo Ruiz, M.A., C.C.R.N.
Mercer Medical Center School of Nursing
Trenton, NJ

Patricia L. Ryan, M.S.N., M.A., R.N.
Assistant Professor of Nursing
Gwynedd Mercy College
Gwynedd Valley, PA

Jane Willis Schultz, M.S.N., R.N.
Gwynedd Mercy College
Gwynedd Valley, PA

Rosemary Mimi Clarke Secor, M.Ed., R.N.,C., F.N.P.
Nurse Practitioner Associates
Cambridge, MA

Julie C. Shattuck, M.S., R.N.,C.
Certified Women's Health Nurse Practitioner
Assistant Professor of Clinical Nursing
University of Rochester School of Nursing
Strong Memorial Hospital
Rochester, NY

Patricia Sheer, M.A., R.N.
Phoenix College
Maricopa Community College District
Phoenix, AZ

Janet Lynn Stewart, M.N.Ed., R.N.
The Western Pennsylvania Hospital
Pittsburgh, PA

Anna Mae Tichy, Ed.D., R.N.
Mt. Hood Community College
Gresham, OR

Patricia A. Trangenstein, Ph.D., R.N.
University of Cincinnati
Cincinnati, OH

Evelyn Weiss, M.A., R.N.
Golden West College
Huntington Beach, CA

Contributors

Crestina Adinolfi, B.S.N., R.N., O.C.N.
Montefiore Medical Center,
Bronx, NY
Chapter 9: Knowledge Basic to the Nursing Care of Adults with Immune Dysfunction

Catherine Perry Aievoli, M.S.N., R.N., C.S.
Adjunct Faculty,
Trenton State College;
Director of Medical-Surgical Nursing, Mercer Medical Center,
Trenton, NJ
Chapter 1: Introduction to the Practice of Medical-Surgical Nursing

Margaret S. Argentine, Ph.D., R.N.
Adjunct Clinical Professor, College of Nursing, SUNY Health Science Center;
Education Liaison, Nursing Education and Staff Development,
University Hospital, SUNY Health Science Center,
Syracuse, NY
Chapter 39: Knowledge Basic to the Nursing Care of Adults with Dysfunction of the Eye

Sherry Blankenship, M.S., R.N.
Instructor, Medical-Surgical Nursing, University of Arkansas at Fayetteville,
Fayetteville, AR
Chapter 19: Knowledge Basic to the Nursing Care of Adults with Vascular Dysfunction

Barbara Bodnar, M.S.N., R.N.
Deputy Director of Nursing–Medical-Surgical,
Westchester County Medical Center, Valhalla, NY
Chapter 27: Knowledge Basic to the Nursing Care of Adults with Hepatic Dysfunction
Chapter 28: Nursing Care of Adults with Hepatic Disorders

Ellen K. Boyda, M.S., R.N.
Pulmonary Rehabilitation Program,
Taylor Hospital, Ridley Park, PA
Chapter 3: Knowledge Basic to the Nursing Care of Adults with Fluid, Electrolyte, and Acid-Base Imbalances

Sally A. Brozenec, Ph.D., R.N.

Assistant Professor, Rush University College of Nursing; Practitioner-Teacher, Rush Medical Center, Chicago, IL

Chapter 21: Knowledge Basic to the Nursing Care of Adults with Gastrointestinal Dysfunction
Chapter 22: Nursing Care of Adults with Disorders of the Upper Gastrointestinal System
Chapter 23: Nursing Care of Adults with Disorders of the Lower Gastrointestinal System
Chapter 24: Nursing Care of Adults with Disorders of the Accessory Organs of Digestion

Ellyn Bushkin, M.S., R.N.
(deceased)
Associate Director of Nursing, Mt. Sinai Medical Center, New York, NY

Chapter 11: Nursing Care of Adults with Oncologic Disorders
Chapter 48: Nursing Care of Adults with Breast Disorders

Thomas J. Butler, M.S., R.R.T.

Clinical Coordinator, Respiratory Care, Rockland Community College, Suffern, NY; Kessler Institute for Rehabilitation, East Orange, NJ

Chapter 12: Knowledge Basic to the Nursing Care of Adults with Respiratory Dysfunction

Barbara Clayton, B.S.N., R.N.

Clinical Coordinator, Neurosciences, Hospital for Joint Disease, New York, NY

Chapter 38: Nursing Care of Adults with Nervous System Disorders

Janice R. Close, B.S., R.R.T., C.P.F.T.

Assistant Professor and Program Coordinator, Respiratory Care, Rockland Community College, Suffern, NY; Adjunct Instructor, University of Medicine and Dentistry of New Jersey, Robert Wood Johnson Medical School/EOSHI, Piscataway, NJ

Chapter 12: Knowledge Basic to the Nursing Care of Adults with Respiratory Dysfunction

Patricia A. Cremins, M.S.N., R.N.,C.

Assistant Professor, Department of Nursing, Laboure College, Boston, MA

Chapter 45: Knowledge Basic to the Nursing Care of Men with Reproductive System Dysfunction
Chapter 46: Nursing Care of Men with Disorders of the Reproductive System

Tanya Drake, M.S.N., R.N.

Associate Professor, Department of Nursing, Rockland Community College, Suffern, NY

Chapter 2: Knowledge Basic to the Nursing Care of the Elderly: The Normal Aging Process
Chapter 4: Knowledge Basic to the Nursing Care of Adults Undergoing Surgery
Chapter 8: Nursing Care of Adults with Burn Injuries
Chapter 29: Knowledge Basic to the Nursing Care of Adults with Endocrine Dysfunction
Chapter 30: Nursing Care of Adults with Diabetes Mellitus
Chapter 31: Nursing Care of Adults with Pituitary Disorders
Chapter 32: Nursing Care of Adults with Adrenal Disorders
Chapter 33: Nursing Care of Adults with Thyroid Disorders
Chapter 34: Nursing Care of Adults with Parathyroid Disorders

Sue-Ann Eitches, M.A., R.N.

Assistant Professor, Rockland Community College, Suffern, NY

Chapter 12: Knowledge Basic to the Nursing Care of Adults with Respiratory Dysfunction

Karen S. Emroch, M.S., R.N., O.N.C.

Formerly Clinical Associate, School of Nursing, Virginia Commonwealth University, Medical College of Nursing; formerly Clinical Specialist, Orthopaedics, Medical College of Virginia Hospitals, Richmond, VA

Chapter 35: Knowledge Basic to the Nursing Care of Adults with Musculoskeletal Dysfunction
Chapter 36: Nursing Care of Adults with Musculoskeletal Disorders

Laura L. Faires, B.S.N., R.N., C.N.O.R.

Staff Nurse, Staff Development Coordinator, Operating Room, Veterans Affairs Medical Center, Portland, OR

Chapter 41: Knowledge Basic to the Nursing Care of Adults with Dysfunction of the Ear
Chapter 42: Nursing Care of Adults with Ear Disorders

Sabina Fallon, Ed.D., R.N.,C.

Nursing Quality Improvement Projects Director, St. Mary Hospital, Hoboken, NJ

Chapter 27: Knowledge Basic to the Nursing Care of Adults with Hepatic Dysfunction
Chapter 28: Nursing Care of Adults with Hepatic Disorders

Alayne Araman Fitzpatrick, Ed.D., R.N., C.S.

Associate Professor, Department of Nursing, Mercy College, Dobbs Ferry, NY

Chapter 48: Nursing Care of Adults with Breast Disorders

Judith Anne Flagg, B.S.N., R.N., E.M.T.

Chief Flight Nurse, Assistant Nursing Care Coordinator, STATFLIGHT, Westchester County Medical Center, Valhalla, NY

Chapter 8: Nursing Care of Adults with Burn Injuries

Karen Goodman, M.A., R.N.,C.

Clinical Nurse Specialist, Obstetrics, Beth Israel Medical Center, New York, NY

Chapter 47: Nursing Care of Adults with Sexually Transmitted Diseases

Pauline Laura Guay, M.S.N., R.N.

Associate Chairperson, Level I Nursing, Department of Nursing, Laboure College, Boston, MA
Chapter 45: Knowledge Basic to the Nursing Care of Men with Reproductive System Dysfunction
Chapter 46: Nursing Care of Men with Disorders of the Reproductive System

Pat Heringa, M.S., R.N.,C

Health System Specialist, Office of the Medical Inspector, Department of Veterans Affairs, Washington, DC
Chapter 6: Knowledge Basic to the Nursing Care of Adults with Skin Dysfunction
Chapter 7: Nursing Care of Adults with Skin Disorders

Janet E. Jackson, M.S., R.N.

Instructor, Department of Nursing, Bradley University, Peoria, IL
Chapter 25: Knowledge Basic to the Nursing Care of Adults with Urinary Tract Dysfunction
Chapter 26: Nursing Care of Adults with Urinary Tract Disorders

Paulene Johnson-Hofer, Ed.D., R.N.

Associate Professor of Nursing, Dominican College, Orangeburg, NY
Chapter 24: Nursing Care of Adults with Disorders of the Accessory Organs of Digestion

Joyce LeFever Kee, M.S., R.N.

Associate Professor Emerita, College of Nursing, University of Delaware, Newark, DE; Consultant, VA Medical Center, Wilmington, DE
Chapter 3: Knowledge Basic to the Nursing Care of Adults with Fluid, Electrolyte, and Acid-Base Imbalances

Chestine L. Kurth, Ph.D., R.N., C.C.R.N.

Professor, Central Wyoming College, Riverton, WY
Chapter 17: Knowledge Basic to the Nursing Care of Adults with Cardiac Dysfunction
Chapter 18: Nursing Care of Adults with Cardiac Disorders

Carol A. McAndrews, M.A., R.N.

Nursing Clinical Instructor, North Harris County College, Houston, TX; IMCU, Staff-Resource Nurse, Northeast Medical Center Hospital, Humble, TX
Chapter 21: Knowledge Basic to the Nursing Care of Adults with Gastrointestinal Dysfunction
Chapter 41: Knowledge Basic to the Nursing Care of Adults with Dysfunction of the Ear
Chapter 42: Nursing Care of Adults with Ear Disorders

Maureen McNamara, M.S., C.N.R.N., R.N.,C.

Clinical Nurse II, Neuroscience ICU, Columbia Presbyterian Medical Center, New York, NY
Chapter 37: Knowledge Basic to the Nursing Care of Adults with Neurologic Dysfunction
Chapter 38: Nursing Care of Adults with Nervous System Disorders

Frances D. Monahan, Ph.D., R.N.

Professor and Chair, Department of Nursing, Rockland Community College, Suffern, NY
Chapter 1: Introduction to the Practice of Medical-Surgical Nursing
Chapter 3: Knowledge Basic to the Nursing Care of Adults with Fluid, Electrolyte, and Acid-Base Imbalances
Chapter 5: Death, Dying, Bereavement, and Spiritual Distress
Chapter 6: Knowledge Basic to the Nursing Care of Adults with Skin Dysfunction
Chapter 7: Nursing Care of Adults with Skin Disorders
Chapter 9: Knowledge Basic to the Nursing Care of Adults with Immune Dysfunction
Chapter 10: Nursing Care of Adults with Immunodeficiency and Hypersensitivity Disorders
Chapter 11: Nursing Care of Adults with Oncologic Disorders
Chapter 12: Knowledge Basic to the Nursing Care of Adults with Respiratory Dysfunction
Chapter 13: Nursing Care of Adults with Upper Respiratory Disorders
Chapter 14: Nursing Care of Adults with Lower Respiratory Disorders
Chapter 21: Knowledge Basic to the Nursing Care of Adults with Gastrointestinal Dysfunction
Chapter 22: Nursing Care of Adults with Disorders of the Upper Gastrointestinal System
Chapter 23: Nursing Care of Adults with Disorders of the Lower Gastrointestinal System
Chapter 24: Nursing Care of Adults with Disorders of the Accessory Organs of Digestion
Chapter 37: Knowledge Basic to the Nursing Care of Adults with Neurologic Dysfunction
Chapter 38: Nursing Care of Adults with Nervous System Disorders
Chapter 39: Knowledge Basic to the Nursing Care of Adults with Dysfunction of the Eye
Chapter 40: Nursing Care of Adults with Eye Disorders
Chapter 41: Knowledge Basic to the Nursing Care of Adults with Dysfunction of the Ear
Chapter 42: Nursing Care of Adults with Ear Disorders
Chapter 43: Knowledge Basic to the Nursing Care of Women with Reproductive System Dysfunction
Chapter 44: Nursing Care of Women with Disorders of the Reproductive System
Chapter 45: Knowledge Basic to the Nursing Care of Men with Reproductive System Dysfunction
Chapter 46: Nursing Care of Men with Disorders of the Reproductive System
Chapter 48: Nursing Care of Adults with Breast Disorders

Laurie R. Murray, D.S.N., R.N.

Assistant Dean, Undergraduate Studies, School of Nursing, Widener University, Chester, PA
Chapter 25: Knowledge Basic to the Nursing Care of Adults with Urinary Tract Dysfunction
Chapter 26: Nursing Care of Adults with Urinary Tract Disorders

Mary Nagel, M.S.N., R.N.

Nursing Instructor, California State University, San Marcos, CA; Nursing Instructor, Southwestern College, Otay Mesa, CA
Chapter 15: Knowledge Basic to the Nursing Care of Adults with Dysfunction of the Blood and Blood-Forming Organs
Chapter 16: Nursing Care of Adults with Disorders of the Blood and Blood-Forming Organs
Chapter 19: Knowledge Basic to the Nursing Care of Adults with Vascular Dysfunction
Chapter 20: Nursing Care of Adults with Vascular Disorders

Marianne Neighbors, Ed.D., R.N.

Associate Professor, Department of Nursing, College of Education, University of Arkansas, Fayetteville, AR
Chapter 15: Knowledge Basic to the Nursing Care of Adults with Dysfunction of the Blood and Blood-Forming Organs
Chapter 16: Nursing Care of Adults with Disorders of the Blood and Blood-Forming Organs
Chapter 17: Knowledge Basic to the Nursing Care of Adults with Cardiac Dysfunction
Chapter 18: Nursing Care of Adults with Cardiac Disorders
Chapter 19: Knowledge Basic to the Nursing Care of Adults with Vascular Dysfunction
Chapter 20: Nursing Care of Adults with Vascular Disorders
Chapter 25: Knowledge Basic to the Nursing Care of Adults with Urinary Tract Dysfunction
Chapter 26: Nursing Care of Adults with Urinary Tract Disorders
Chapter 35: Knowledge Basic to the Nursing Care of Adults with Musculoskeletal Dysfunction
Chapter 36: Nursing Care of Adults with Musculoskeletal Disorders

Elizabeth Nykun, M.S.N., R.N.

Staff Nurse, Emergency Department, Morristown Memorial Hospital, Morristown, NJ
Chapter 17: Knowledge Basic to the Nursing Care of Adults with Cardiac Dysfunction
Chapter 18: Nursing Care of Adults with Cardiac Disorders

Joanne Oventhal, M.S.N., R.N.

Instructor, Rockland Community College, Suffern, NY; Clinical Instructor, Nyack Hospital, Nyack, NY; Staff Nurse, Columbia Presbyterian Medical Center, New York, NY
Chapter 21: Knowledge Basic to the Nursing Care of Adults with Gastrointestinal Dysfunction

Angie Z. Patras, M.S., R.N., E.T.

Formerly Nursing Faculty, Rush-Presbyterian-St. Luke's Medical Center, Chicago, IL
Chapter 21: Knowledge Basic to the Nursing Care of Adults with Gastrointestinal Dysfunction
Chapter 22: Nursing Care of Adults with Disorders of the Upper Gastrointestinal System
Chapter 23: Nursing Care of Adults with Disorders of the Lower Gastrointestinal System
Chapter 24: Nursing Care of Adults with Disorders of the Accessory Organs of Digestion

Robert P. Plona, B.S.N., R.N.

Coordinated Care Manager, HIV Program, Visiting Nurse Association and Hospice of Greater Cleveland, Kaiser Permanente–Ohio Region, Cleveland, OH
Chapter 10: Nursing Care of Adults with Immunodeficiency and Hypersensitivity Disorders

Judy Ptak, M.S.N., R.N.

Infectious Disease Nurse Clinician, Infectious Disease Section, Dartmouth-Hitchcock Medical Center, Lebanon, NH
Chapter 9: Knowledge Basic to the Nursing Care of Adults with Immune Dysfunction
Chapter 10: Nursing Care of Adults with Immunodeficiency and Hypersensitivity Disorders

Charlene Wendover Rinne, Ed.D., R.N.

Assistant Professor, Department of Nursing, Mount St. Mary College, Newburgh, NY; Owner, Policy Program Research Consultants, Albany, NY
Chapter 12: Knowledge Basic to the Nursing Care of Adults with Respiratory Dysfunction
Chapter 13: Nursing Care of Adults with Upper Respiratory Disorders
Chapter 14: Nursing Care of Adults with Lower Respiratory Disorders

Pamela S. Schremp, M.S.N., R.N., C.R.N.O.

Clinical Instructor, Francis Payne Bolton School of Nursing, Case Western Reserve University; Director, Department of Risk Management, University Hospitals of Cleveland, Cleveland, OH
Chapter 39: Knowledge Basic to the Nursing Care of Adults with Dysfunction of the Eye
Chapter 40: Nursing Care of Adults with Eye Disorders

Joan C. Stackhouse, M.S., R.N.

Associate Professor, Nursing Counselor, Rockland Community College, Suffern, NY
Chapter 5: Death, Dying, Bereavement, and Spiritual Distress
Chapter 11: Nursing Care of Adults with Oncologic Disorders

Elizabeth Tannhauser, M.S., R.N.

Clinical Instructor, Rockland Community College; Clinical Coordinator, Good Samaritan Hospital Regional Medical Center, Suffern, NY
Chapter 4: Knowledge Basic to the Nursing Care of Adults Undergoing Surgery

Monica Grabois Toll, M.S.N., R.N.,C., C.D.E.

Instructor, Dominican College, Orangeburg, NY; Consultant, Diabetes Education, Nyack Hospital, Nyack, NY
Chapter 30: Nursing Care of Adults with Diabetes Mellitus

Margaret Townsend Warren, Ph.D., R.N.

Professor and Chairperson, Allied Health Department, Rockland Community College, Suffern, NY
Chapter 4: Knowledge Basic to the Nursing Care of Adults Undergoing Surgery

Judy E. White, M.A., M.S.N., R.N.

Associate Professor, Department of Nursing, Rockland Community College, Suffern, NY
Chapter 13: Nursing Care of Adults with Upper Respiratory Disorders
Chapter 14: Nursing Care of Adults with Lower Respiratory Disorders
Chapter 22: Nursing Care of Adults with Disorders of the Upper Gastrointestinal System
Chapter 23: Nursing Care of Adults with Disorders of the Lower Gastrointestinal System
Chapter 44: Nursing Care of Women with Disorders of the Reproductive System
Chapter 46: Nursing Care of Men with Disorders of the Reproductive System
Chapter 48: Nursing Care of Adults with Breast Disorders

Patricia A. Wrobbel, M.A., R.N.

Associate Faculty, Columbia University, School of Nursing, New York, NY; Director, Neurosurgical Patient Services, Department of Neurological Surgery, Montefiore Medical Center, Bronx, NY
Chapter 37: Knowledge Basic to the Nursing Care of Adults with Neurologic Dysfunction
Chapter 38: Nursing Care of Adults with Nervous System Disorders

Preface

The impetus for this text came from our feeling that no medical-surgical book on the market adequately addressed the learning needs of the beginning student. We therefore set out to create a text that would concisely address the important content in a manner that would make it easier for the student to learn and to apply that knowledge to clinical situations. We have designed this text around body systems, an organizing structure that is familar to students from both general life experience and from prerequisite or co-requisite courses in anatomy and physiology. Further, it is an organizational structure that instructors can adapt easily for use with virtually any curricular design. In addition, we have highlighted important aspects of clinical application through features such as Patient Education Charts, Pharmacology Boxes, Nutrition Boxes, and Nursing Care Guides.

The text consists of 14 units, and each unit that deals with a body system begins with a "Knowledge Basic" chapter, which is designed to provide the reader with basic knowledge needed to understand disorders, their medical management, and the appropriate nursing care. Following the Knowledge Basic chapters in the body system units are one or more "Disorders" chapters, which present the disorders that can affect the body system under discussion. At the end of both types of chapters, we present specific information concerning the care of the elderly, a growing segment of our population. In addition, throughout the book, we present nursing care in terms of the five steps of the nursing process.

Our hope in structuring this text was not only to present the necessary content but to promote a method of thinking and learning in the student using it. The thinking pattern the text seeks to teach is that of the nursing process, a form of critical thinking employed in the clinical setting in the design and implementation of nursing care for patients. This method of thinking is logical, and it involves organization of data into categories, identification of relationships, recognition of the norm as well as deviations from it, and constant evaluation. In support of this goal, we present nursing care in terms of the five steps of the nursing process for every disorder, as well as for diagnostic tests and therapeutic modalities that have significant implications for nursing care. The exceptions to this are those disorders or procedures in which there are few implications for nursing care or when the nursing care is essentially identical to that for a disorder or procedure previously discussed, in which case we direct the student to that topic. The reader will find the five steps of the nursing process presented in Nursing Care Guides in many chapters of the book, but the reader will also see them integrated throughout the text in most chapters of the book. Within the text of the chapters, we introduced the steps by the heading "Application of the Nursing Process to the Care of the Patient with . . . ." A brief description of the content presented under that heading follows.

We present assessment data in two sections; first, in terms of patient history information, and second, in terms of physical assessment data to be obtained. In some cases, we provide assessment data for the patient at risk for a disorder, then present a discussion of assessment as it applies to the patient already diagnosed with the disorder. We pair the next two steps of the nursing process, nursing diagnosis and planning, to clearly illustrate their relationship to each other. In order to reinforce this relationship, each nursing diagnosis (diagnostic label and related factors) immediately precedes the expected patient outcomes that reflect successful resolution of the patient problem identified by the diagnosis. All of the nursing diagnoses in this text are from the 1992 NANDA (North American Nursing Diagnosis Association) approved list. The fourth step of the nursing process, presented as nursing interventions in the text, consists of subsections related to each nursing diagnosis identified in the nursing diagnoses and planning section. The diagnostic label serves as a heading, and a discussion of relevant nursing interventions, along with their rationales, follows each. This again reinforces the role of the nursing diagnosis in guiding the selection of appropriate nursing intervention. The use of rationales with each nursing intervention, or group of interventions, identifies the expected response to the intervention and reinforces the concept that nursing care is based on a scientific body of knowledge.

We address the final step of the nursing process, evaluation, each time we present the five-step nursing process. We use a single evaluation statement reminding the student that we evaluate nursing care by comparing the patient's status with the expected outcomes to drill the student visually and verbally on the importance of this step of the nursing process. We take this yet a step further in the nursing care guides, in which the evaluation statement, repeated after each set of assessment findings, nursing diagnoses, patient outcomes, and nursing interventions and rationales, states that if the expected patient outcomes are not met, reassessment and revision of diagnoses, expected outcomes, and interventions are necessary.

"Knowledge Basic" Chapters

The Knowledge Basic chapters begin with a review of the anatomy and physiology of the body system and progress to a description of the common clinical manifestations of a problem, or dysfunction, of the system. These are symptoms that are not unique to one disorder but that reflect the effect of varied pathology on the system. Following the description of common clinical manifestations is a discussion of the assessment of the system.

This assessment section is divided into two parts: patient history and physical examination. Clinical manifestations precede assessment because understanding them is essential to directing the patient history and physical examination.

The chapter next presents the diagnostic tests used in the evaluation and diagnosis of the system under discussion. We include here generally those tests that are nonspecific to a disease but are applicable to the system as a whole.

Each Knowledge Basic chapter also includes a section entitled "Medical Management," which presents (1) noninvasive procedures (Nonsurgical Management) used to manage dysfunction of the system under discussion, and (2) selected surgical procedures (Surgical Management) that are performed on the system under discussion. The surgical procedures selected for inclusion in the Knowledge Basic chapters are those that are common, as well as those that are performed for a variety of treatment reasons. The basis for our decision to include content from the latter group was our belief that students—from the beginning of their studies—need to perceive the breadth and complexity of the field of medical-surgical nursing, and that being familiar with the basics of popular yet not so common topics promotes a sense of professional identity and confidence in the student. We present surgeries done for a variety of reasons in the Knowledge Basic chapters rather than in the Disorders chapters to promote accurate learning and to enable the student to identify the preoperative and postoperative implications of the surgical procedure itself apart from the demands of the underlying disease. This helps the student to identify clearly which changes are necessitated by each specific disorder and thus to better individualize care.

Each Knowledge Basic chapter ends with a section on the elderly, which reviews age-related changes in the system and identifies any specific considerations relating to diagnostic testing or medical management in general.

"Disorders" Chapters

The Disorders chapters move in an orderly fashion through the varied problems (disorders) that can affect the body system under discussion. The following major headings (categories) serve as the organizational framework for presentation of the disorders in the majority of these chapters: Infections and Inflammations, Functional Disorders, Structural Disorders, Trauma, and Neoplasia. To further promote learning, the following topics are discussed for each disorder in a category: definition of the disorder, etiology, pathophysiology, clinical manifestations, medical diagnosis, medical management, and application of the nursing process. These subheadings serve to outline the content presented, thus allowing the student to anticipate the content and attend to the principles and concepts rather than sorting out the sequence. This logical, organized approach to handling information is essential to critical thinking.

Each Disorders chapter ends with a section on the elderly, which includes a review of those disorders most commonly seen in the elderly, with differences in clinical presentation or management highlighted.

Other Points Regarding Organization and Content

We believe that students are under a great deal of pressure and as a result do not always study in the ideal way—i.e., they do not always go back and review related content in another chapter or look back for definitions—often they simply "plow ahead." For these reasons, we include a certain amount of repetition throughout the text, particularly of areas that are sometimes overlooked by students because they are not seen as immediately life-threatening. Thus, in Chapter 4 (which deals with perioperative nursing), we cover in depth preoperative care in relationship to anxiety, patient teaching, preoperative medications, and so on. In addition, in the other chapters, we spell out content in these areas for specific surgeries at least once either in text or in the care guides. This type of repetition occurs not only for the perioperative care of patients but also for the psychosocial and asepsis-related care of all patients. We stress aseptic technique throughout because it is critical to all care, as are the psychosocial aspects of care, which sometimes get relegated to the background since they are usually less concrete and are not seen as life-threatening.

Throughout the text, we attempt to avoid using generalizations such as "teach the patient about perioperative routines," "give instructions for self-care at home," "tell the patient what to expect," and "assess respiratory function." This text provides specifics—what do you tell the patient, what questions do you ask, what do you check. These specifics tie the content to concrete clinical application.

Features of the Text

Learning Objectives help the reader identify the chapter's content.

Chapter Outlines provide a summary of each chapter's topics at a glance, enabling the reader to locate specific content areas quickly.

Nursing Care Guides help the student see the nursing process in action, based on specific patient data and combination problems. Assessment findings are specific—The patient is, does, says, etc.—to parallel findings that nurses collect in the clinical situation; the subsequent nursing diagnoses relate clearly to the findings. Specific and measurable patient outcomes correspond to each nursing diagnosis, and rationales appear for each nursing intervention.

Pharmacology Boxes outline drug classification, action, uses, side effects, interactions, nursing implications, and geriatric considerations.

Patient Education Charts show the reader how to effectively teach patients what to expect, how to adapt, and what (and what not) to do.

Nutrition Boxes provide important information regarding menus, daily nutritional requirements, and specific considerations for patients.

Ancillaries

Accompanying this text are a 400-page Instructor's Manual that includes for each chapter three research abstracts and several case studies, a Student Study Guide, and a Pocket Companion. Additionally, programs adopting the text will receive a 1200-item NCLEX-style computerized testbank and a set of 200 2-color acetate transparencies and transparency masters.

FRANCES D. MONAHAN
TANYA DRAKE
MARIANNE NEIGHBORS

Acknowledgments

Many people have been part of the process of conceptualization, production, and publication of this book. We are pleased to be able to thank them publicly.

For their inspiration, support, and encouragement, we thank the nursing faculty and staff of Rockland Community College: Sr. Marie Peter Buckley; L. Diane Clayton; Ann Dunn; Sue-Ann Eitches; Dorothea Harth; Geraldine Jackson; Marjorie Lopez; Joanne Oventhal; Joan Stackhouse; Mary Ann Swords; Judy White; Irina Mekhlin; Miriam Coyle; Marilyn Ferro; and, especially, Dr. F. Thomas Clark, former president of Rockland Community College.

We were privileged to work with many professionals associated with the W.B. Saunders Company: Martha Tanner, Developmental Editor; Arlene Friday, Copy Editor; Ellen B. Zanolle, Designer; Linda R. Garber, Production Manager; Barbara Nelson Cullen, Acquisitions Editor; and Thomas Eoyang, Editor-in-Chief of Nursing Books. Valuable assistance was also provided by Lauren Shavell, Medical Illustrator, and Patti Maddaloni, Page Layout Artist.

Special thanks to Michael J. Brown, former Acquisitions Editor, and Frances Mues, former Developmental Editor, who started with us and guided us through the initial phases of this project; Dr. Roger Connor, who reviewed Chapters 6 and 7; and Dr. Barbara Murphy, Vice President for Council Affairs of the National League of Nursing, who introduced us to Marianne Neighbors.

FRANCES D. MONAHAN
TANYA DRAKE

I echo my coauthors' sentiments about the W.B. Saunders Company professional staff, with a special thanks to Martha Tanner for her patience and kindness.

In addition, I thank nursing faculty and staff at the University of Arkansas for their continued support, assistance, and interest in the project: Dr. Margaret Sullivan, Dr. Evelyn Eldred, Dr. Kathleen Barta, Trish Watkins, and Judy Stone.

Without friends and family to give inspiration and continuous encouragement, I may have never persevered. I thank each and every one of them, and hope they will continue to be at my side through many more projects: Dr. Melinda Henderson, Gloria Fowlkes, Terri Watts, Bonnie Cooper, Janice Pray, Bonnie Lee, Barbara Talik, Jackie Murphree, Marji Schwickrath, and Gary Hill.

MARIANNE NEIGHBORS

Contents in Brief

Contents in Detail

Chapter Seven

Chapter Eight

Unit Three

Chapter Nine

Chapter Ten

Unit Four

Chapter Twelve

Chapter Thirteen

Chapter Fourteen

Unit Five

Chapter Fifteen

Chapter Sixteen

Chapter Eighteen

Chapter Nineteen

Chapter Twenty

Unit Seven

Chapter Twenty-one

Chapter Twenty-two

Chapter Twenty-three

Unit Nine

Chapter Twenty-seven

Chapter Twenty-eight

Unit Ten

Chapter Twenty-nine

Chapter Thirty

Chapter Thirty-one

Chapter Thirty-eight

Unit Thirteen

Chapter Thirty-nine

Chapter Forty

Chapter Forty-one

Chapter Forty-two

Unit Fourteen

Chapter Forty-three

Chapter Forty-four

Chapter Forty-five

Chapter Forty-six

Chapter Forty-seven

Special Features

Nursing Care Guides

Nursing Guides to Patient Education for Self-Management (Patient Education Charts)

Chapter Thirty

Chapter Thirty-one

Chapter Thirty-two

Chapter Thirty-five

Chapter Thirty-six

Chapter Thirty-eight

Chapter Thirty-nine

Chapter Forty

Chapter Forty-one

Chapter Forty-two

Chapter Forty-three

Chapter Forty-four

Chapter Forty-five

Chapter Forty-six

Chapter Forty-seven

Chapter Forty-eight

Nutrition Boxes

Pharmacology Boxes

Unit One

KNOWLEDGE BASIC TO THE NURSING CARE OF ADULTS

Learning Objectives

AFTER COMPLETING THIS UNIT, THE LEARNER WILL BE ABLE TO:

Chapter One

1. Describe the nature and scope of medical-surgical nursing practice.
2. Define the standards of medical-surgical nursing practice.
3. List types of, and requirements for, certifications in the area of medical-surgical nursing.
4. Identify major trends in the practice of medical-surgical nursing.
5. Explain the steps of the nursing process and their application to the practice of medical-surgical nursing.

Chapter Two

1. Explain the physiologic, psychological, and socio-economic changes commonly associated with the normal aging process.
2. Describe normal assessment findings in the elderly.
3. Identify the nursing implications of altered function and pharmacokinetics in the elderly.
4. State nursing diagnoses and related expected patient outcomes commonly applicable to the elderly.
5. Describe nursing interventions, with their rationales, that promote wellness in the elderly.
6. Describe teaching strategies that promote learning in the elderly.
7. Explain the basis for evaluation of nursing care provided to the elderly.

Chapter Three

1. Explain normal fluid, electrolyte, and acid-base balance physiology, including normal laboratory test values.
2. Define the major fluid, electrolyte, and acid-base imbalances.
3. Describe each of the major fluid, electrolyte, and acid-base imbalances in terms of cause, pathophysiology, clinical manifestations, related diagnostic tests, and medical management.
4. Identify information and physical examination data essential to the assessment of fluid, electrolyte, and acid-base status.
5. State nursing diagnoses and related expected patient outcomes commonly applicable to patients with fluid, electrolyte, or acid-base imbalance.
6. Describe nursing interventions, with their rationales, commonly applicable to patients with fluid, electrolyte or acid-base imbalance.
7. Explain the basis for evaluation of nursing care provided to patients with fluid, electrolyte, or acid-base imbalance.
8. Identify special considerations for the elderly patient with fluid, electrolyte, or acid-base imbalance.

Chapter Four

1. Describe the nature and scope of perioperative nursing practice.
2. Define the standards of perioperative nursing practice.
3. Identify the legal parameters associated with the care of patients undergoing surgery.
4. Describe common preoperative diagnostic procedures and medical management of patients undergoing surgery.
5. Identify information and physical examination data essential to the assessment of preoperative, intraoperative, and postoperative patients.
6. State nursing diagnoses and related expected patient outcomes commonly applicable to patients undergoing surgery.
7. Describe nursing interventions, with their rationales, commonly applicable to patients undergoing surgery.
8. Explain the basis for evaluation of nursing care provided to patients undergoing surgery.
9. Identify special considerations for the patient undergoing ambulatory surgery.
10. Identify special considerations for the elderly patient undergoing surgery.

Chapter Five

1. Explain the stages of dying, including the final tasks toward achieving the acceptance of death.
2. Identify the stages of bereavement, as well as the risk factors and manifestations of dysfunctional grieving.
3. Explain the basic tenets of the world's major religions and their implications for the care of patients who are dying or are in spiritual distress.
4. Identify data essential to the assessment of the psychosocial status of dying patients, bereaved persons, and patients in spiritual distress.
5. State nursing diagnoses and related expected patient outcomes commonly applicable to dying patients, bereaved persons, and patients in spiritual distress.
6. Explain the basis for evaluation of nursing care provided to dying patients, bereaved persons, and patients in spiritual distress.

Chapter One

INTRODUCTION TO THE PRACTICE OF MEDICAL-SURGICAL NURSING

Scope of Medical-Surgical Nursing Practice

Medical-surgical nursing refers to the nursing care of adults who have an actual or potential disorder of physiologic function. Within the broad range of medical-surgical nursing are many specialized areas of practice. These include cardiovascular nursing, emergency nursing, gynecologic nursing, infection control nursing, neurologic nursing, oncologic nursing, orthopedic nursing, and recovery room nursing. There are also medical-surgical nurses whose practice is limited to the care of patients with respiratory disorders, diabetes, burns, eye disorders, ostomies, or wounds.

Medical-surgical nursing is practiced in a variety of settings. These include acute care hospitals, urgent care centers, health maintenance organizations, extended care facilities, clinics, neighborhood health centers, industrial settings, and the home.

Nature of Medical-Surgical Nursing Practice

The practice of medical-surgical nursing is based on the nursing process and is concerned not only with the physiologic component of the patient's response to the health disorder but also with the psychological and social components. It is through the use of the nursing process that nursing care is individualized to meet the unique needs of each patient. Thus, the medical-surgical nurse must understand principles and concepts from the basic biologic, physical, and social sciences; have a basic knowledge of the development, diagnosis, and treatment of disease; and have a firm foundation in nursing theory, nursing skills, and the use of the nursing process.

Preparation for Medical-Surgical Nursing Practice

Medical-surgical nurses are prepared at a variety of educational levels. Some are prepared at the associate or baccalaureate level, others at the master's or doctoral level.

Basic study of nursing prepares a generalist medical-surgical nurse. The generalist has a broad base of knowledge and can function in a variety of settings although the majority of generalist nurses provide bedside care to patients in acute or long-term care facilities. The focus of the generalist is on the use of the nursing process to provide direct care to patients.

Medical-surgical nurse specialists are prepared through advanced study of medical-surgical nursing at the graduate level. Two categories of medical-surgical nurse specialist are nurse practitioner and clinical nurse specialist.

Table 1–1. ELIGIBILITY REQUIREMENTS FOR SELECTED ANCC CERTIFICATION EXAMINATIONS

AREA OF PRACTICE	ELIGIBILITY REQUIREMENTS
Medical-surgical nurse (generalist program)	Active Registered Nurse (RN) license in the United States or its territories. At least 2 years of practice as a licensed RN. At least 1600 hours of medical-surgical nursing practice within 2 of the past 3 years. Currently practice medical-surgical nursing an average of 8 hours per week.
Clinical specialist in medical-surgical nursing	Active RN license in the United States or its territories. Master's degree with a major in nursing. Currently provide direct care to medical-surgical patients an average of at least 4 hours per week. At least 12 months of practice with an active RN license in the United States after completion of the master's degree. 800 hours of post-master's practice giving direct patient care in the past 2 years, or full-time employment as a consultant, administrator, researcher, or educator for 2 of the past 3 years along with at least 400 hours of direct care to medical-surgical patients in the same time period.
Adult nurse practitioner	Active RN license in the United States or its territories. Master's degree with a major in nursing. Preparation as an adult nurse practitioner in an adult nurse or family nurse practitioner master's degree nursing program. *or* Preparation as an adult nurse practitioner in a formal postgraduate adult nurse practitioner or family nurse practitioner track or program in a school of nursing granting graduate credits.

Data from American Nurses Credentialing Center. Certification Catalog. Washington, DC, 1992.

Nurse practitioners function independently in providing patient care. They have advanced skills in physical assessment and diagnose and treat acute and chronic health problems. Nurse practitioners may have a private practice, be in practice with a physician, or be employed in a clinic or other ambulatory care setting.

Clinical nurse specialists are prepared to both provide and promote expert clinical care for a particular group of patients, such as those with diabetes, with renal disease, or with an ostomy. Clinical nurse specialists use the in-depth knowledge of their specialty area to solve patient problems and to develop more effective approaches to patient care. They do this by staying abreast of research and technologic developments affecting their area of practice; serving as consultants to other members of the health care team; engaging in formal and informal teaching with co-workers, patients, and families; and participating in the research process.

Certification

In addition to maintaining their academic credentials, medical-surgical nurses may elect to become certified through the American Nurses Credentialing Center (ANCC).

Nurses who meet the eligibility requirements (Table 1–1) can sit for a certification examination as a generalist medical-surgical nurse, clinical specialist in medical-surgical nursing, or adult nurse practitioner. The examination is based on nationally recognized standards of practice and is designed to demonstrate knowledge and functional expertise beyond that required for basic licensure. Upon passing the examination, the nurse is awarded certification for a period of 5 years, at which time recertification is obtained either by submitting evidence of required continuing education or by retesting.

Standards of Practice

Regardless of level of preparation or certification, all practicing medical-surgical nurses are accountable for meeting the Standards of Clinical Nursing Practice developed by the American Nurses' Association (ANA). These Standards of Clinical Nursing Practice delineate the professional responsibilities of all registered nurses engaged in clinical practice regardless of setting (ANA, 1991, p. 5). The Standards of Clinical Nursing Practice consist of Standards of Care and Standards of Professional Performance. The Standards of Care are built around the steps of the nursing process and define a competent level of nursing care. The Standards of Professional Performance delineate a competent level of professional role behavior in terms of quality of care, performance appraisal, education, collegiality, ethics, collaboration, research, and resource utilization. Each standard (Table 1–2) has accompanying measurement criteria that are considered indicators of competent practice (ANA, 1991, p. 3). Thus, the Standards of Practice address the nursing profession's responsibility to the public and provide a means to measure the outcome of care. It is through these Standards of Practice that nursing maintains professional autonomy and public confidence in its service.

Table 1–2. AMERICAN NURSES' ASSOCIATION STANDARDS OF CLINICAL PRACTICE

STANDARDS OF CARE

STANDARD I. ASSESSMENT
The nurse collects client health data

STANDARD II. DIAGNOSIS
The nurse analyzes the assessment data in determining diagnoses

STANDARD III. OUTCOME IDENTIFICATION
The nurse identifies expected outcomes individualized to the client

STANDARD IV. PLANNING
The nurse develops a plan of care that prescribes interventions to attain expected outcomes

STANDARD V. IMPLEMENTATION
The nurse implements the interventions identified in the plan of care

STANDARD VI. EVALUATION
The nurse evaluates the client's progress toward attainment of outcomes

STANDARDS OF PROFESSIONAL PERFORMANCE

STANDARD I. QUALITY OF CARE
The nurse systematically evaluates the quality and effectiveness of nursing practice

STANDARD II. PERFORMANCE APPRAISAL
The nurse evaluates his/her own nursing practice in relation to professional practice standards and relevant statutes and regulations

STANDARD III. EDUCATION
The nurse acquires and maintains current knowledge in nursing practice

STANDARD IV. COLLEGIALITY
The nurse contributes to the professional development of peers, colleagues, and others

STANDARD V. ETHICS
The nurse's decisions and actions on behalf of clients are determined in an ethical manner

STANDARD VI. COLLABORATION
The nurse collaborates with the client, significant others, and health care providers in providing client care

STANDARD VII. RESEARCH
The nurse uses research findings in practice

STANDARD VIII. RESOURCE UTILIZATION
The nurse considers factors related to safety, effectiveness, and cost in planning and delivering client care

Trends in Medical-Surgical Nursing Practice

Like the profession as a whole, with its intimate relationship to the individual and its broad relationship to society, medical-surgical nursing changes in response to the problems, needs, and issues of the patients it serves.

The aging of the population has brought with it an increase in chronic disease and the challenge of adapting modalities of care to meet the needs of both the well and the frail elderly. Long-term care facilities, home health care agencies, and day care centers and related services for the elderly are integral to the practice of today's medical-surgical nurse either as a primary place of employment or as the facilities from which patients are received or to which they are referred. On another front, the outbreak of acquired immunodeficiency syndrome (AIDS) has given rise to the concept of universal precautions. It has also presented new challenges to practice in terms of patient, family, and public education as well as in the direct care of terminally ill immunodeficient patients.

Medical-surgical nursing practice is also influenced by broad-based societal factors. Development of flexible patterns of education coupled with greater access is bringing into the profession a cadre of individuals with new and varied backgrounds and abilities. The women's movement is responsible for a new focus on women's health and is spawning changes in access and in care. Technologic developments are dramatically altering the diagnosis and management of disease, and computers are rapidly becoming an integral part of patient care management. Also exerting a significant effect on the practice of medical-surgical nursing are the changes in reimbursement patterns, rising health care costs, and cost containment efforts that have altered the financial structure of the health care system. These factors have resulted in treatment of more individuals on an out-patient basis, increased acuity of illness in in-hospital patients, and shorter length of hospital stays, with patients being discharged in need of home care. In terms of practice, these changes have created more opportunities to practice in a variety of settings and have placed a greater emphasis on patient teaching and the use of available family and community support systems in meeting patient needs.

The Nursing Process

Medical-surgical nurses must have a firm foundation in the use of the nursing process in order to provide effective nursing care for medical-surgical patients. Accordingly, a brief review of the nursing process follows.

The nursing process consists of five interrelated, interdependent, somewhat overlapping phases. These are assessment, nursing diagnosis, planning, implementation, and evaluation. These phases form a continuous cycle of thoughts and actions. Each phase is dependent on the accuracy of the previous phase.

Assessment

In the first phase of the nursing process, assessment, the nurse collects and organizes information about the patient in order to identify existing health problems and factors that impact on them. Assessment is the most crucial phase of the nursing process, since the entire plan of care is based on the information gathered. If this information is incorrect, the identification of the problem is incorrect, and incorrect interventions and incorrect expected patient outcomes result.

Data collection is an ongoing process beginning with the initial patient-nurse contact and continuing until the patient is discharged from care. Data collection can be formal, as with a nursing history, or informal, as in conversation and observation during care.

Two basic types of data are collected: historical and current. Historical data are information about past events, such as previous illness, exposure to infections, and prior hospitalizations. Current data are information regarding present events, such as the presence of pain, an elevated temperature, and feelings of anxiety over a scheduled procedure.

The patient is the primary source of data because it is the patient who can most accurately describe symptoms; give a history; share perceptions, problems, and goals; and validate responses to treatment. All other sources of information are secondary.

Data are collected by interview, observation, and physical examination. Data collection varies with the condition and needs of the patient. If the patient is in an urgent situation, such as severe pain or respiratory distress, data collection is limited to evaluation of the priority area and additional information from secondary sources. Patient characteristics such as intellectual development and communication ability also influence data collection.

Once data are gathered, validated, and recorded, they are organized and analyzed for patterns that suggest health problems.

The most common errors of assessment are caused by inaccurate or incomplete data collection, inaccurate interpretation of data (usually the result of using only one clue to make an inference), and lack of clinical knowledge.

Nursing Diagnosis

A nursing diagnosis is a clinical judgment about individual, family, or community responses to actual and potential health problems and life processes. Nursing diagnoses provide the basis for selection of nursing interventions to achieve outcomes for which the nurse is accountable (NANDA, 1992, p 5).

There are three types of nursing diagnoses: actual, high-risk, and wellness. An actual nursing diagnosis is one that currently exists and has been clinically validated by identifiable defining characteristics; that is, at least two signs or symptoms of the diagnosis are present.

A high-risk nursing diagnosis is a diagnosis that indicates an individual, family, or community is more at risk for developing a problem than others in the same or similar situation. It is supported by risk factors that contribute to this increased vulnerability (NANDA, 1992, p 84).

A wellness diagnosis is a clinical judgment that an existing wellness response has a potential for enhancement to a higher state (NANDA, 1992, p 84).

A nursing diagnosis is a one-, two-, or three-part statement formulation that follows from the analysis and interpretation of assessment data. The first part, the diagnostic label or category, represents a pattern of related cues. In the case of actual and high-risk diagnoses, it identifies the alteration being experienced by the patient, or for which the patient is at risk. It provides a clear idea of what needs to change and suggests expected patient outcomes. The second part, the related factors or etiology, is joined to the diagnostic label by the words "related to" (RT) and deals with the reason for the alteration. It describes the physical, psychological, sociocultural, spiritual, or environmental factors that relate to, or contribute to, the health problem. These related factors suggest the type of nursing interventions necessary to eliminate, reduce, or prevent the problem. The nursing diagnosis may be further specified by adding the phrase "secondary to"—for example: Altered nutrition: less than body requirements related to anorexia secondary to chemotherapy.

With the exception of knowledge deficit and rape-trauma syndrome, all actual and high-risk nursing diagnoses have an etiology. In cases in which the etiology cannot be identified, this is noted by the words "related to unknown etiology." Wellness diagnoses also do not contain related factors, but

Table 1–3. NANDA-APPROVED NURSING DIAGNOSES

Activity Intolerance
Activity Intolerance, High Risk for
Adjustment, Impaired
Airway Clearance, Ineffective
Anxiety
Aspiration, High Risk for
Body Image Disturbance
Body Temperature, Altered, High Risk for
Breastfeeding, Effective
Breastfeeding, Ineffective
Breastfeeding, Interrupted
Breathing Pattern, Ineffective
Caregiver Role Strain
Caregiver Role Strain, High Risk for
Communication, Impaired Verbal
Constipation
Constipation, Colonic
Constipation, Perceived
Decisional Conflict (specify)
Decreased Cardiac Output
Defensive Coping
Denial, Ineffective
Diarrhea
Disuse Syndrome, High Risk for
Diversional Activity Deficit
Dysfunctional Ventilatory Weaning Response (DVWR)
Dysreflexia
Family Coping: Compromised, Ineffective
Family Coping: Disabling, Ineffective
Family Coping: Potential for Growth
Family Processes, Altered
Fatigue
Fear
Fluid Volume Deficit
Fluid Volume Deficit, High Risk for
Fluid Volume Excess
Gas Exchange, Impaired
Grieving, Anticipatory
Grieving, Dysfunctional
Growth and Development, Altered
Health Maintenance, Altered
Health Seeking Behaviors (specify)
Home Maintenance Management, Impaired
Hopelessness
Hyperthermia
Hypothermia
Inability to Sustain Spontaneous Ventilation
Incontinence, Bowel
Incontinence, Functional
Incontinence, Reflex
Incontinence, Stress
Incontinence, Total
Incontinence, Urge
Individual Coping, Ineffective
Infant Feeding Pattern, Ineffective
Infection, High Risk for
Injury, High Risk for
Knowledge Deficit (specify)
Noncompliance (specify)
Nutrition, Altered: Less than Body Requirements
Nutrition, Altered: More than Body Requirements
Nutrition, Altered: Potential for More than Body Requirements
Oral Mucous Membrane, Altered
Pain
Pain, Chronic
Parental Role Conflict
Parenting, Altered
Parenting, Altered, High Risk for
Peripheral Neurovascular Dysfunction, High Risk for
Personal Identity Disturbance
Physical Mobility, Impaired
Poisoning, High Risk for
Post-Trauma Response
Powerlessness
Protection, Altered
Rape-Trauma Syndrome
Rape-Trauma Syndrome: Compound Reaction
Rape-Trauma Syndrome: Silent Reaction
Relocation Stress Syndrome
Role Performance, Altered
Self-Care Deficit, Bathing/Hygiene
Self-Care Deficit, Feeding
Self-Care Deficit, Dressing/Grooming
Self-Care Deficit, Toileting
Self-Esteem, Chronic Low
Self-Esteem, Situational Low
Self-Esteem Disturbance
Self-Mutilation, High Risk for
Sensory/Perceptual Alterations (specify) (visual, auditory, kinesthetic, gustatory, tactile, olfactory)
Sexual Dysfunction
Sexuality Patterns, Altered
Skin Integrity, Impaired
Skin Integrity, Impaired, High Risk for
Sleep Pattern Disturbance
Social Interaction, Impaired
Social Isolation
Spiritual Distress (distress of the human spirit)
Suffocation, High Risk for
Swallowing, Impaired
Therapeutic Regimen, Ineffective Management of
Thermoregulation, Ineffective
Thought Processes, Altered
Tissue Integrity, Impaired
Tissue Perfusion, Altered (specify type) (renal, cerebral, cardiopulmonary, gastrointestinal, peripheral)
Trauma, High Risk for
Unilateral Neglect
Urinary Elimination, Altered
Urinary Retention
Violence: Self-directed or directed at others, High Risk for

From North American Nursing Diagnosis Association. NANDA nursing diagnoses: Definitions and classification. St. Louis, MO: North American Nursing Diagnosis Association, 1992, pp 6–9.

simply consist of the diagnostic label preceded by the phrase "Potential for enhanced" (Carpenito, 1993, p 17).

The third component, defining characteristics, specifies the signs and symptoms (identified during assessment) on which the nursing diagnosis is based. When present, the defining characteristics are joined to the related factor by the words "manifested by" (M/B).

Refer to Table 1–3 for the current list of nursing diagnostic categories accepted by the North American Nursing Diagnosis Association (NANDA).

Planning

The third phase of the nursing process is the planning phase. The planning phase consists of four steps: setting priorities, establishing expected patient outcomes, selecting nursing interventions (developing nursing orders), and documenting the plan of care.

Setting priorities serves to organize the delivery of nursing care so that more important problems are considered first. The problem that is given the highest priority is the one that poses the greatest threat to the patient's well-being. Depending on the situation, this may be a problem directly affecting the physical status of the patient or it may be related to a knowledge deficit or to a psychological effect. Setting priorities in other than emergency situations is influenced by the patient's perception of what is important.

Priorities can change day to day, shift to shift, and sometimes minute to minute. Thus the delivery of nursing care must be flexible and geared to the current status of the patient. One problem need not be resolved before another is approached.

Expected outcomes are patient oriented and derived from the nursing diagnosis, specifically from the "related to" portion of the diagnostic statement. They are statements of behaviors that demonstrate the improvement or resolution of a specific problem described by the nursing diagnosis. Each nursing diagnosis must have a specific expected patient outcome. In some cases there may be only one expected patient outcome, whereas in others there may be more than one. In all cases, at least one must relate to the problem statement. Additional expected outcomes may relate to the etiology.

Expected outcomes are patient oriented; that is, they define what the patient will do. Expected patient outcomes may relate to bodily appearance or function, relief or absence of specific symptoms, demonstration of knowledge or psychomotor skills, or psychosocial status. They are set in conjunction with the patient to help ensure their achievement by encouraging patient participation.

Expected patient outcomes must be clearly defined, measurable, and observable. Each expected outcome describes only one behavior and is written as a positive statement. Each must be realistic in terms of the patient's condition and abilities and the resources available.

The third step in the planning phase is selecting the nursing interventions that will best achieve the expected outcomes. They are specific instructions to all nurses caring for the patient based on the etiology component of the nursing diagnosis, and they are aimed at reducing, eliminating, or preventing the cause or contributing factors. All nursing orders must be consistent with the therapeutic approaches of other health professionals involved in the patient's care. All must be individualized to the particular physical and psychological needs of the individual patient, and all must be supported by rationales based on scientific principles. The plan of care is then documented in the patient's record (step four of the planning phase).

Implementation

The fourth phase of the nursing process is the implementation phase. During this phase, the actions are taken that are necessary to enable the patient to achieve the expected outcomes identified in the planning phase.

The implementation phase begins with preparation for care. Nursing interventions to be carried out are reviewed. Time needed for their implementation is estimated, and the time for implementation is selected based on the patient's needs and the other responsibilities of the nurse. The need for assistance from other personnel is evaluated, and if needed, it is arranged before care is begun. The patient's immediate environment is prepared so that it is conducive to efficient care and is supportive of the goals of intervention. The patient is made comfortable physically and psychologically. For example, the patient is pulled up and repositioned in bed and asked if a bedpan is needed prior to the start of a lengthy procedure, and privacy is provided. The patient's rights are considered, and it is ascertained that the patient has given informed consent. When a patient does not consent to a procedure, the right to refuse care is respected.

When preparation is complete, care is given. This may involve performing an action, assisting the patient with an action, supervising the family in performing an action, or teaching the patient and family.

Ongoing assessment is maintained during this phase of care. Such assessment provides the basis for the decision to initiate, continue, modify, or discontinue intervention. It is also used in subsequent evaluation.

Evaluation

The fifth phase of the nursing process is evaluation. This is a judgment of the effectiveness of nursing care. It addresses whether this is the best possible plan of care for this individual patient.

Evaluation consists of two steps. First is the determination of whether the expected patient outcomes have been achieved, and second is a thorough reassessment of the entire plan to identify changes to further improve patient care.

To determine whether expected patient outcomes are achieved, the patient's status is compared with the stated outcomes. Some of the data needed for this comparison may have been collected during the implementation of nursing interventions, whereas other data are collected at the time of evaluation by direct observation, examination, patient interview, pencil and paper tests, and feedback from other staff members. From this comparison, it is determined whether the expected outcomes have been met fully, partially, or not at all. Progress or lack of progress is documented and discussed with the patient.

Reassessment of the entire plan of care is the process of changing, adding, or eliminating previous nursing diagnoses, expected patient outcomes, and nursing interventions based on new patient data. If an expected outcome has been achieved, it is determined whether the problem has been resolved and can be eliminated or whether the problem is ongoing and requires continued nursing interventions. For example, a patient with constipation related to immobility may have achieved the expected outcome of one soft, formed bowel movement per day, but if the patient remains immobilized and the nursing interventions are discontinued, it would be highly likely that the problem would recur. Thus a change in nursing diagnosis to "high risk for constipation related to immobility" and continued nursing intervention would be appropriate.

If the expected outcome is not achieved or only partly achieved, the following questions must be asked:

Was the assessment complete and accurate?
Was the nursing diagnosis correctly identified?
Are the expected outcomes realistic for this patient?
Are the nursing interventions appropriate?
Have priorities changed?
Have new nursing diagnoses arisen?

Depending on the answers to these questions, it may be necessary to reassess the patient, identify new nursing diagnoses, establish new expected outcomes, select new nursing interventions, set new priorities, or establish new dates for evaluation.

Bibliography

American Nurses' Association. Standards of clinical practice. Kansas City, MO: American Nurses' Association, 1991.

American Nurses Credentialing Center. Certification catalog. Washington, DC, 1992.

Carpenito, LJ. Nursing diagnosis application to clinical practice. 5th ed. Philadelphia: JB Lippincott, 1993.

Ellis J, Hartley C. Credentials for nursing practice. In Nursing in today's world. Challenges, issues and trends. 3rd ed. Philadelphia: JB Lippincott, 1988, pp 109–135.

Iyer P, Taptich B, Bernocchi-Losey D. Nursing process and nursing diagnosis. Philadelphia: WB Saunders, 1991, pp 2–18, 84–111.

North American Nursing Diagnosis Association. NANDA nursing diagnoses: Definitions and classification 1992. St. Louis: North American Nursing Diagnosis Association, 1992.

Sparks SM, Taylor CM. Nursing diagnosis reference manual. Springhouse, PA: Springhouse, 1991.

Chapter Two

KNOWLEDGE BASIC TO THE NURSING CARE *of the Elderly: The Normal Aging Process*

In 1989 there were 31 million Americans older than the age of 65. United States Bureau of the Census projections indicate that by the year 2030, 23% of the population in the United States will be older than 65 years of age. The elderly, especially those older than 75 years, represent the fastest-growing segment of the population. Between 1960 and 1980, the population of those older than age 84 increased by 141%.

This spectacular growth in the number of elderly is attributed to many factors. Chief among these are the general rise in health consciousness in the United States and the decline in mortality from chronic diseases, especially cardiovascular disorders, that are common in the elderly. Despite common misconceptions, only 5% of the elderly are institutionalized.

The increase in the number of elderly in the general population has prompted the growth of research and specialized health fields in gerontology and geriatrics. Gerontology is the study of the process of aging and the needs of the elderly. It includes the physiologic, psychological, and socioeconomic changes associated with aging. Geriatrics is a specialized health profession that includes the physiology, pathology, diagnosis, and management of diseases in the elderly. Gerontologic nurses specialize in the care of the elderly in the community and in health care agencies. The goal of persons in the field of aging is to study the aging process and develop a body of knowledge to better meet the needs of the elderly in society and in the health care system.

Numerous changes are associated with the normal aging process. These changes occur at different points in the life span and are affected by the individual's chronologic age, daily activities, nutrition and health history, psychosocial factors and support systems, heredity, and environmental factors. Each person ages at a different rate, and each person adapts to the aging process individually. Although most changes associated with aging occur gradually, events in the life cycle of the individual may accelerate certain changes. Recent life changes can have a major impact on the psychological and physical status of the elderly person.

Knowledge of the changes associated with the aging process enables the nurse to accurately differentiate between normal and abnormal findings in assessing the geriatric patient. This chapter presents a brief overview of the normal changes of aging common in the healthy individual and nursing actions to help the elderly adapt to these changes. The focus of these actions is to provide education, support, and services that enable the individual to maintain optimum function and independence while meeting his or her needs.

Changes Associated with the Normal Aging Process

Psychosocial Aspects

Advanced age is a time when a person must make many social adaptations and complete the final developmental tasks of life. Engaging in activities that contribute to a positive self-image is very important in late adulthood. Personal space and communication and interaction with others are basic human needs. Research has demonstrated that elderly persons have a higher life satisfaction if they have a confidant, someone with whom to share thoughts and feelings. Loneliness, social isolation, depression, low self-esteem, and poor health are major contributing factors to the high rate of alcohol abuse and suicide among the elderly. In the United States, the suicide rate is highest in persons older than 60.

A parent who has spent a lifetime raising a family must adjust when children begin living as independent adults. The impact of decreased responsibilities in the home, or of retirement and its financial and social consequences, can be devastating. Reduced income may make major changes in lifestyle necessary. Advance planning can lessen the impact. Free time can be used to take classes in subjects of interest, start a new career, or participate in hobbies or community activities.

At a time in life when ability to adapt to change is diminished, many elderly persons are faced with voluntary or involuntary relocation and loss of possessions. The stress of relocation is tolerated best by persons who are older than 70, are able to discuss the move with a confidant, have high self-esteem, and are able to take personal possessions to the new environment.

The elderly individual must often cope with the death of a spouse, family members, or friends. It is important for the person to experience the bereavement that follows the loss of a loved one and then be able to go on living and developing new relationships. Religious practices and beliefs often provide elderly persons with a means of coping with loss and also serve as a basis for social support and interaction.

Death of a loved one often triggers reflections on past life experiences that are part of a life review. The process of the life review is an important developmental task of late adulthood. It enables the individual to come to terms with life events and achieve a reasonably positive view of his or her life's worth. For many older adults, preparation for one's own death evolves from the life review. For some, it is important to prepare for the eventuality of death by resolving interpersonal relationships and getting affairs in order. Death need not be imminent for preparations to be made. Indeed, it is usually less stressful if preparations for death are made before they are needed.

Guidelines for Application of the Nursing Process to the Care of the Elderly: Psychosocial Aspects of Aging

Assess for changes in the elderly person's life that are associated with the aging process. Assess the impact recent events have had by questioning the person directly and observing nonverbal cues as events are discussed. Observe verbal and nonverbal cues that indicate self-image during all interactions. Determine participation in social interactions and whether the individual communicates with family, friends, or a confidant. Ask whether the individual has a pet. Pets often supply uninhibited love and emotional gratification for isolated individuals.

Reassure the elderly person that late adulthood can be a productive time of life. Help the individual who has free time to identify activities of interest that contribute to a feeling of self-worth. Suggest ways in which these interests might provide opportunities for socialization. Discuss the fact that social isolation can hasten deterioration of mental processes, reinforce feelings of loneliness, and increase the risk of depression, suicide, and alcohol abuse. Encourage participation in activities for the elderly sponsored by community and religious groups. Free transportation is often available.

Reassure the individual that, as discussed in Chapter 5, grief, anger, and depression over death are a normal part of bereavement. Provide opportunity for verbalization about the death of the deceased person and memories of his or her life. As grieving progresses, help the individual focus first on short-term and then on long-term plans. Encourage socialization to help alleviate loneliness and depression. If grief and depression remain unresolved or interfere with the individual's ability to function, or if suicidal ideation is verbalized, group therapy or individual psychiatric counseling is needed.

Discuss the life review process with older adults. Note that reminiscing about past relationships and life experiences is part of this process. The elderly often enjoy sharing these memories with persons of a younger generation. Provide opportunity for the elderly person to discuss preparations for death. Suggest legal counseling if appropriate.

Body Composition

As a person ages, changes occur in the major components of the body and in their distribution. A gradual decrease in the number of functioning cells in almost all organs of the body begins at about the age of 30. As the person ages, this results in a loss of functional reserve, the ability of organs to meet body needs under conditions of stress or increased demand. Healing processes are also slowed as a result of the loss of functioning cells, slower cell replication, and decreased tissue vascularity.

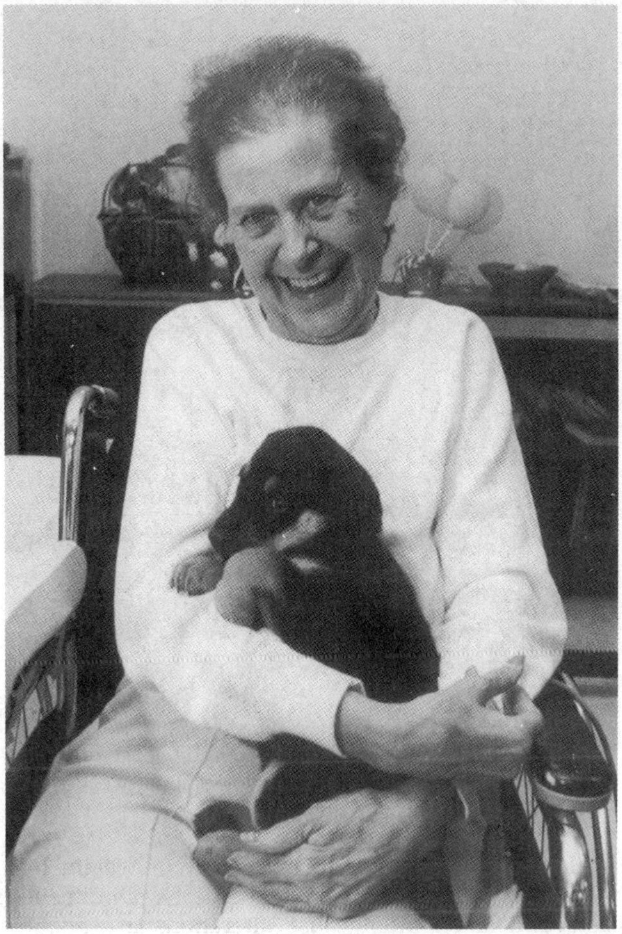

(From Matteson M, McConnell E. Gerontological nursing: Concepts and practice. Philadelphia: WB Saunders, 1988, p 792.)

As the individual ages, total body protein and lean body mass (fat-free tissues of the body) decrease. Distribution of body fat shifts, and fat deposits in and around muscle fibers and the viscera develop. Many elderly persons, regardless of their body weight or build, develop a slightly protuberant abdomen or pot belly and fat deposits on the hips. Because adipose tissue contains little water, the increase in proportion of body fat to lean mass causes a decrease in the proportion of intercellular fluid and total body water to body weight.

Nutritional Needs

Throughout the life cycle, nutrition has a significant effect on physical and emotional well-being. Although lifelong eating habits may be difficult to change in the elderly, the normal changes associated with the aging process can alter individual nutritional requirements. Limited financial resources, physical limitations, and mental changes must be considered as factors that may interfere with the individual's ability to maintain adequate nutrition.

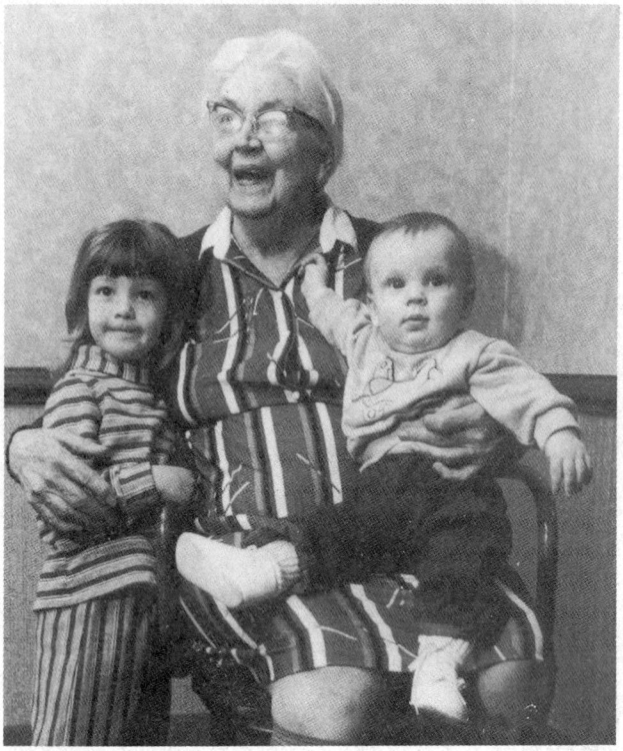

(From Matteson M, McConnell E. Gerontological nursing: Concepts and practice. Philadelphia: WB Saunders, 1988, p 138.)

Malnutrition manifested by obesity or weight loss is a common problem in the elderly. Diminished taste and smell often cause alterations in appetite. Some persons eat less because of loss of sensory stimulation, whereas others eat more in quest of sensory satisfaction. Calcium resorption, which is part of the normal aging process of the bones, can result in tooth deterioration. Vitamin and mineral deficiencies may develop because missing or decayed teeth or ill-fitting dentures cause the individual to avoid certain food groups such as meats, fresh fruits, and vegetables, which are more difficult to chew.

Many elderly people experience depression, loneliness, and lack of motivation to prepare well-balanced meals for one person following the death of a spouse or companion. Referrals to social services, home care agencies, Meals On Wheels, or the local senior citizens center may provide nutritional support. Meals at a community center have the added advantage of providing opportunity for socialization.

Depression, loneliness, and loss are also factors in the incidence of alcoholism in the elderly. The possibility of alcohol abuse should be considered in any malnourished geriatric individual, and if confirmed, a referral to Alcoholics Anonymous should be made.

The recommended dietary allowance (RDA) to meet the nutritional needs of most healthy persons suggests a 10% decrease in calorie intake for persons 51 to 75 years, and a 20% to 25% decrease for persons 76 years or older, because of decreased energy expenditures. Although there is no standard caloric requirement that fits all persons, average calorie intake for a man aged 51 to 75 is approximately 2400 calories, and for a woman, 1800 calories. For a man 76 years or older, average calorie intake is 2050 calories, and for a woman, 1600 calories. Caloric requirements may be further adjusted to allow for activity level and body weight.

Current RDA standards indicate that the diet of all persons, including the elderly, should contain 50% to 55% carbohydrate, 15% to 20% protein, and less than 30% fat. Most of the calories from carbohydrates should be from complex carbohydrates such as breads and grains, with less than 10% coming from simple carbohydrates such as sugar. The RDA also recommends limiting cholesterol by using lean meats and polyunsaturated fats and increasing fiber in the diet.

Vitamin and mineral deficiencies in the elderly are common because of poor dietary habits, limited income, and decreased absorption of nutrients in the intestines as the result of decreased mucosal lubrication. Iron, calcium, and vitamin C are commonly deficient in the diet. Vitamin A deficiency may promote night blindness. There is no consensus on whether the elderly actually have vitamin and mineral requirements different from those of younger adults.

Guidelines for Application of the Nursing Process to the Care of the Elderly: Nutritional Needs

Assess the elderly person's general appearance, height, and weight to establish a baseline for future comparison. Ask whether this is the person's preferred weight. Determine whether there have been any recent unintended weight changes or changes in appetite. Have the individual describe a typical day's nutritional intake. Include snacks, fluids, vitamin or mineral supplements, and alcohol intake. If a nutritional supplement is taken, determine why it is used. Identify foods that are avoided because of difficulty chewing or digestive problems.

Teach the elderly individual to choose varied foods from the basic food groups. Nutrition Box 2–1 identifies guidelines for nutritional requirements in the elderly. Encourage consumption of complex carbohydrates, low-cholesterol protein sources, polyunsaturated fats, and dietary fiber. Suggest food preparation methods such as stewing or braising if chewing is difficult. Encourage use of community resources for nutritional support and increased socialization. If a vitamin or mineral supplement is recommended by the physician, suggest less costly generic brands and review how the preparation is to be taken.

Nutrition Box 2–1.

NUTRITIONAL NEEDS OF THE ELDERLY

Instruct the elderly individual in the following:

Plan a nutritionally sound diet by selecting a variety of familiar foods from the basic food groups.

Group	Servings	Examples of one serving
Bread, Cereal, Rice, and Pasta	6–11	1 slice of bread ½ muffin, bagel ½ cup cooked cereal, pasta, rice, noodles 1 oz dry cereal
Vegetables	3–5	½ cup of most cooked or raw chopped vegetables 1 cup leafy raw vegetables ¾ vegetable juice
Fruit	2–4	½ cup of most fruits 1 small whole fruit 1 melon wedge ½ banana or grapefruit ¾ cup fruit juice
Milk	2–3	1 cup low-fat or skim milk 1 cup low-fat yogurt 1½ oz hard cheese 2 oz processed cheese
Meat, Poultry, Fish, Eggs, and Nuts	2–3	2½ to 3 oz cooked lean meat 3 to 4 oz cooked fish or poultry 1 cup cooked dry beans, peas 2 eggs ($<$3 eggs per week) 4–5 tbsp peanut butter

The minimum number of daily servings provides a caloric intake of approximately 1600 calories if low-fat, lean foods are selected. Add additional servings to achieve desired caloric intake.

Low-fat milk and milk products, canned fish with bones, and dark green leafy vegetables such as broccoli, collard greens, and kale are good sources of calcium.

Citrus fruit or juice, strawberries, cantaloupes, potatoes, tomatoes, and broccoli are good sources of vitamin C. Eat at least one serving daily.

Meat, fish, poultry, grains, legumes, and dark leafy vegetables are good sources of iron and B vitamins.

Dark green and yellow leafy vegetables, dark yellow fruits, liver, and fortified milk products are good sources of vitamin A. Eat at least three servings a week.

Whole-grain breads and cereals, brown rice, dried legumes, fresh fruits with skins, raw or minimally cooked vegetables, nuts, and seeds provide dietary fiber and help prevent constipation.

Apple juice, bananas, citrus fruits and juices, melons, prunes and prune juice, tomatoes and tomato juice, dried beans, white potatoes, sweet potatoes, beef, turkey, and most salt substitutes are good sources of potassium.

Food eaten in five or six small meals daily is generally tolerated and digested better by the elderly.

Chew food thoroughly before swallowing.

Eat soft, chopped, or pureed foods if chewing food well is difficult.

Drink six to eight glasses of fluid a day to help prevent constipation and maintain hydration.

Do not drink fluids within 1 hour before mealtime.

Use fats, oils, and sweets sparingly.

Avoid excessive salt and sodium intake.

Use nonsodium flavor enhancers and spices to season food.

Discuss ideal weight goal and dietary modifications with physician if appropriate.

Weigh weekly to monitor weight maintenance, loss, or gain.

Data from US Department of Agriculture and US Department of Health and Human Services.

Integument

The skin, hair, and nails are the parts of the body most visible to others. Normal aging changes perceived as unattractive by the individual may lower self-esteem and cause the person to avoid contact with others. Provide opportunity for the elderly person to discuss appearance changes and to ventilate feelings about the aging process. Discuss changes in dress or grooming that may help minimize changes in appearance and improve self-esteem. Encourage the individual to continue social activities. Interacting with and being accepted by peers help the person accept his or her own appearance and promote a positive self-image.

SKIN

Changes in the skin of the aging person result from a combination of the aging process, genetics, and environmental factors. Long-term exposure to the sun is the most significant environmental factor, and its effects accentuate the aging process.

With age, cell division slows and replacement of damaged or dead skin cells is diminished. The epithelium thins, collagen fibers stiffen, and elastin formation decreases. The skin becomes thin and less pliable. Decreased activity of the sebaceous and sweat glands causes dryness and itchiness, especially on the extremities. The skin may also become shiny, rough, and flaky. Skin tags on the face and upper extremities are small skin herniations composed of collagen and subcutaneous tissue. They are common in the elderly and can be removed if they become inflamed, cause pain, bleed, or have undergone recent changes.

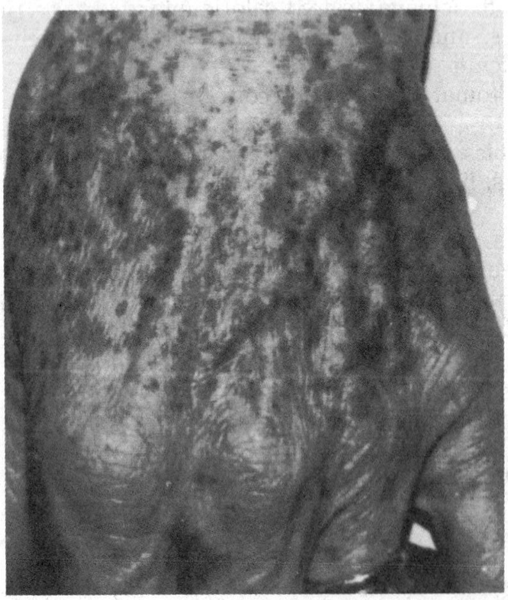

Figure 2–1.

Solar lentigines, or "liver spots," characteristically seen on areas of sun-exposed skin in the elderly. (From Arnold HL, Odom RB, James WD [eds]. Andrews' diseases of the skin. 8th ed. Philadelphia: WB Saunders, 1990, p 809.)

As subcutaneous adipose tissue is lost, the skin becomes wrinkled and, particularly on the arms and legs, loose and flabby. Loss of subcutaneous adipose tissue also makes the tendons, veins, and knuckles of the hands more prominent and exaggerates the bony prominences of the knees, scapulae, and trochanters. Without the cushioning effect of adipose tissue, the skin becomes more susceptible to physical trauma and pressure sores.

The melanocytes, or pigment cells of the skin, become larger but fewer in number in the elderly person. Pigment changes result from diminished melanocyte distribution and function. The skin of white persons not exposed to the sun appears paler and more opaque, whereas skin having long-term sun exposure develops a blotchy appearance with areas of hyperpigmentation mixed with areas of hypopigmentation. Flat brown macules of solar lentigines, commonly called senile lentigo, liver spots, or age spots, develop on sun-exposed areas on the arms, hands, and face as enlarged melanocytes aggregate at the dermoepidermal junction. Solar lentigines are illustrated in Figure 2–1.

Guidelines for Application of the Nursing Process to the Care of the Elderly: Skin Changes

Assess skin for alterations in color, texture, and condition associated with the aging process. Skin assessment is described in detail in Chapter 6. Turgor is difficult to assess in the elderly because of normal wrinkling and tenting of the skin due to loss of subcutaneous tissue. Note signs of scratching, such as inflamed areas or linear scabs, and the presence of lesions. Determine how long lesions have been present and whether they have changed in appearance recently. Ask how long it usually takes for a superficial wound to heal.

Teach the elderly person that frequent applications of nonperfumed lotions and creams that contain lanolin and little or no alcohol help relieve skin dryness. Application of emollients immediately after bathing is very beneficial. Less frequent bathing, using tepid water, bath oils, or superfatted soaps, or using soap only in the genital and axillary areas minimizes dryness. In winter, a furnace humidifier, room humidifier, or pans of water placed near heat sources provide extra moisture in the air and diminish skin dryness. Cosmetic products are available to bleach or cover solar lentigines. Encourage less sun exposure and use of sunscreens to lessen the damaging effects of the sun.

HAIR AND NAILS

The hair of the scalp, trunk, pubis, axillae, and extremities gradually thins, and the thickness of each hair shaft decreases as testosterone production declines and hair follicles die in both sexes. Although the pattern of hair loss and onset of baldness are genetically determined, in general, scalp hair loss occurs primarily in the front and on the top of the head. As estrogen production declines in women after menopause, facial hair becomes more coarse. Hairs in the nostrils and ears also thicken. The onset and pattern of gray hair, which are also genetically determined, occur as the function and number of melanocytes decrease.

Nail growth slows with aging. Nails become dull, dry, brittle, and, in some cases, yellow and thick. They may develop longitudinal ridges and be prone to split into layers.

Guidelines for Application of the Nursing Process to the Care of the Elderly: Hair and Nail Changes

Assess the hair and nails for alterations in color, texture, and distribution associated with the aging process. Assessment of the hair and nails is described in detail in Chapter 6. Ask whether changes occurred gradually or rapidly. Rapid hair loss or change in color, texture, or distribution may be due to a pathologic process. Note the presence of yellow-orange stains on the fingers and nails from smoking.

Discuss the availability of hair coloring products, hairpieces, and wigs with the elderly person who is disturbed by loss and graying of the hair. Facial hair can be bleached or removed by electrolysis to improve appearance. Long ear and nasal hairs can be trimmed. Fingernails should be rounded and smoothed with an emery board to prevent scratching the skin. Toenails should be cut straight across to prevent ingrown toenails. If manual dexterity or vision is impaired, or if the person has a history of diabetes mellitus or peripheral vascular disorders, a podiatrist should cut the toenails to prevent injury.

Thermoregulation

Age-related changes in the skin and its appendages also create problems in regulating body temperature. Decreased sweat production decreases the body's ability to lose heat through evaporation, making the aged prone to heat stroke in hot weather. The elderly are also sensitive to cold because of loss of insulating subcutaneous fat and diminished peripheral circulation. Many elderly persons feel chilled even on temperate days.

Guidelines for Application of the Nursing Process to the Care of the Elderly: Thermoregulation

Question the elderly person about tolerance to environmental temperature fluctuations. Determine whether episodes of weakness, dizziness, or loss of consciousness have occurred in hot weather. Ask whether he or she perspires during physical activity or in hot weather.

Teach the elderly individual to avoid strenuous activity in extreme heat or cold, to increase fluid intake in hot weather, and to avoid high winds, which increase fluid loss, when possible. Lightweight clothing and hats should be worn outdoors on hot days to protect from sun exposure while allowing air to circulate and cool the body. Insulating undergarments, multiple layers, hats, gloves, and scarfs should be worn outdoors in cold temperatures to avoid chills.

Sensory Changes

VISION

Visual accommodation (the ability to focus on near and far objects) decreases with age as a result of weakening of the muscles that control the lens. Most individuals older than 50 need glasses or bifocals to correct presbyopia (far-sightedness) and to compensate for loss in accommodation. With age, color discrimination may deteriorate. Inability to discriminate between blue, violet, and green is common.

Blurred vision, distortion of objects, and a gradual, progressive decrease in visual acuity result from alteration in protein metabolism in the crystalline lens and the lifetime effects of exposure to ultraviolet light. The lens may become discolored and develop opacities. Discoloration of the lens often causes diminished perception of blues and greens. The scattered opacities make the eye sensitive to glare. Degeneration of the lens may progress until the lens is completely opaque and rigid, and the pupil, which is normally black, becomes gray, then milky white. Functional vision is lost. These changes are characteristic of cataract formation, a common eye disorder in the elderly. To restore vision, the opaque lens is removed in an elective surgical procedure, described in Chapter 40.

Gradual fibrosis of the muscular iris causes the pupils to decrease in size. This allows less light to enter the eye and inhibits ability to accommodate to changes in light intensity. Bright, glare-free light is needed for the elderly person to be able to see well. As the blood supply to the oxygen-sensitive cells of the retina decreases, depth perception, peripheral vision, and night vision deteriorate. Loss of peripheral vision must be medically evaluated to rule out glaucoma, a common cause of preventable blindness in the elderly. Glaucoma is discussed in Chapter 40. Decreased function of the lacrimal apparatus may cause dryness and itching of the eyes.

Guidelines for Application of the Nursing Process to the Care of the Elderly: Vision Changes

Assess the vision for loss of acuity and accommodation associated with the aging process. Ask the date of the last eye examination. Test visual fields and pupillary reaction to light. Assessment of the eye and vision is discussed in detail in Chapter 39. Ask about changes in depth perception, loss of color distinction, and difficulty seeing at night. Because visual deterioration occurs gradually, the individual may not be aware that changes have occurred. Look for clues of visual changes such as recent automobile accidents, groping for objects, mismatched socks, or bruises on arms or legs caused by bumping into objects.

Teach the elderly individual to have an annual eye examination and glaucoma screening for early detection and treatment of vision changes. Demonstrate how to turn the head to compensate for loss of peripheral vision to prevent accidents. Suggest use of railings, night-lights, increased home lighting, and removal of environmental hazards such as loose floor coverings to avoid falls. Use of lubricating eye drops helps relieve ocular dryness. Advise the elderly person to allow additional time for the eyes to adjust to changes in light intensity. Also discuss the need to limit driving to daylight hours if night vision is diminished. If vision is impaired to the point of making food preparation tasks dangerous, referral to social services, home care agencies, Meals On Wheels, or a senior citizens center that provides meals may be appropriate. Use red, black, or dark gray in teaching aids instead of blue, violet, or green.

HEARING

The ability to hear high-frequency sounds deteriorates from childhood on, and usually becomes noticeable by late middle age. As the individual continues to age, the ability to differentiate between similar sounds decreases. These changes are caused by increased rigidity of the small bones of the middle ear, degeneration of hair cells in the organ of Corti, atrophy of cochlear capillaries, and reduced sound transmission through a thickened tympanic membrane. In addition to the general loss of hearing acuity, these changes make it especially difficult for the elderly person to participate in group conversations and to hear clearly over the telephone. Sudden loss of hearing is not normal at any age and requires investigation by a physician to rule out a physiologic disorder or obstruction of the external auditory canal by cerumen or foreign object.

Guidelines for Application of the Nursing Process to the Care of the Elderly: Hearing Changes

Assess for diminished hearing acuity associated with the aging process. Ask whether any hearing loss has been noted. Observe for nonverbal cues of impaired hearing such as leaning forward or turning one ear toward the speaker, cupping a hand behind the ear, or frequent misunderstanding of questions. Assessment of the ear and hearing is discussed in detail in Chapter 41. If the person wears a hearing aid, examine the auditory canal for signs of irritation.

Encourage the elderly to have hearing evaluated periodically for early detection and correction of hearing problems. If hearing is impaired, encourage the individual to ask others to face him or her when speaking and to speak clearly in a normal voice. Shouting, which is a high, distorted sound, is more difficult for the hearing impaired to understand than normal speech. One-on-one conversations are easier for the elderly person to follow and understand. Discuss the availability of hearing aids and adaptive devices that modify telephone transmissions for the hearing impaired.

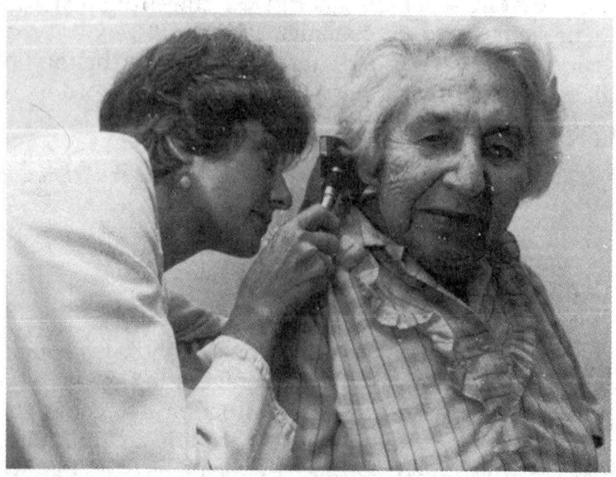

(From Matteson M, McConnell E. Gerontological nursing: Concepts and practice. Philadelphia: WB Saunders, 1988, p 240.)

TASTE AND SMELL

Elderly persons experience a diminished sense of taste and smell as a result of a decrease in the number of taste buds and papillae, decreased saliva flow, and loss of olfactory fibers. Sweet and salty tastes are lost first, followed by bitter and sour.

Guidelines for Application of the Nursing Process to the Care of the Elderly: Altered Taste and Smell

Assess for diminished taste and smell associated with the aging process. Examine the lips and mouth for excessive dryness associated with decreased saliva production. The tongue appears fissured in the elderly. Ask what flavorings the person uses on food.

Teach the elderly person that the taste of food can be improved by increasing the use of non-sodium flavor enhancers and spices. Good oral hygiene with a soft-bristled toothbrush and sucking hard candy may increase saliva production, relieve dry mouth, and help prevent gum disease. A smoke detector should be installed in the living quarters, because the elderly individual may be unable to smell smoke. Some utility companies provide gas detectors.

TACTILE SENSATION

The older person experiences diminished sensitivity to touch, temperature, pressure, and pain as a result of decreased capillary circulation and the death of nerve fibers. Injuries may not be noticed because of increased pain tolerance. As the myelin sheath deteriorates and the nerves degenerate, paresthesias may occur.

Guidelines for Application of the Nursing Process to the Care of the Elderly: Altered Tactile Sensation

Assess for decreased tactile sensitivity associated with the aging process. Examine the hands, feet, and bony prominences for pressure areas, recent injuries, or signs of healed injuries that may have gone undetected. Observe the person's nonverbal behavior to determine response to touch.

Tactile stimulation is important to many elderly, especially as vision and hearing diminish. A gentle touch on the hand, arm, or shoulder during conversations conveys a sense of caring and acceptance to a person for whom touch is important. It is normal for touch to be welcome on some occasions and rejected on others.

Teach the elderly individual to always use potholders to prevent burns when cooking. Demonstrate how to examine the feet and other injury-prone areas to detect wounds and how to test water temperature with the inside of the elbow or a thermometer before washing or bathing to avoid accidental burns. If possible, the thermostat on the hot water heater can be lowered as a further safety measure.

Mental Processes

Thought processes and reaction time often slow with age. Changes in mental processes may be complicated by the changes in sensory function already discussed. Some degree of confusion, forgetfulness, and short-term memory loss occurs in many elderly persons as a result of decreased blood flow and oxygen supply to the brain and a decrease in the number of neurons. No decline in intelligence occurs unless a physical disorder develops. Sudden onset of confusion is usually due to an alteration in physiologic status, such as dehydration or trauma, or to an iatrogenic cause, such as drug toxicity. Relocation to an unfamiliar environment may precipitate relocation stress syndrome, often characterized by confusion, anxiety, dependency, depression, and sleep disturbances. Inability to concentrate or follow directions, deterioration in personal hygiene, and inappropriate behavior, which are not part of the normal aging process, may be due to illness, psychiatric disorders, or the irreversible dementia of Alzheimer's disease and require evaluation by a physician.

Guidelines for Application of the Nursing Process to the Care of the Elderly: Altered Mental Processes

Assess for the alterations in mental processes associated with the aging process. Assessment of mental process is described in detail in Chapter 37. Anticipate that it will take longer for an elderly person to respond. Before identifying an elderly person as confused, determine whether disorientation may be the result of medications, altered sleep pattern, an unfamiliar environment, or a hearing or vision impairment. Provide safety measures for the elderly person in a new environment, especially at night, to prevent injuries.

Written reminders of appointments or tasks to be done help remedy forgetfulness for persons of any age. Reassure the elderly that the ability to learn

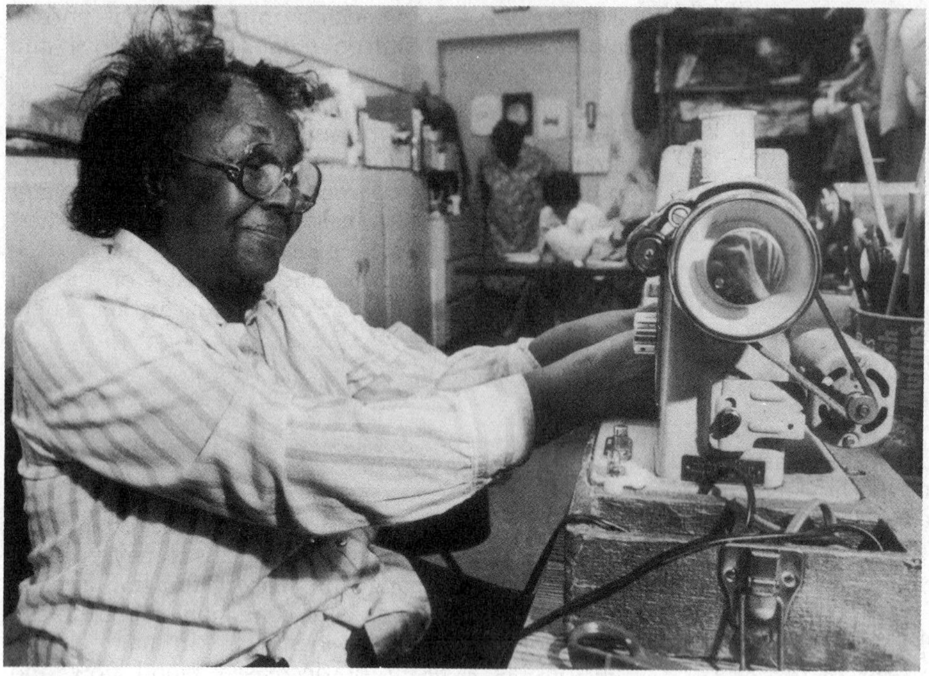

(From Matteson M, McConnell E. Gerontological nursing: Concepts and practice. Philadelphia: WB Saunders, 1988, p 762.)

continues throughout life. Many persons have used the years after retirement to learn new skills or begin a new career. Because mental processes have slowed, learning may take longer and require more repetition of information than at a younger age. Reinforcing new information with written material aids the learning process.

Sleep Patterns

Most adults older than 65 need approximately 6 hours of sleep a night. Normal sleep pattern consists of cycles of the four stages of non–rapid eye movement (non-REM) sleep, followed by REM sleep. Each stage of non-REM sleep is progressively deeper and represents a different stage of relaxation. An elderly person takes longer to move through the stages of non-REM sleep, wakes frequently, and spends less time in the deep sleep of stage 4. A person deprived of stage 4 sleep may become depressed and lethargic. REM sleep, the period when most dreams occur, is a relatively active state characterized by muscle twitching, rapid eye movement, and fluctuations in vital functions. Dreams often review recent events, help relieve tension and anxiety, and often help resolve emotional conflict. Sleep-inducing medications, opiates, and alcohol suppress REM sleep. A person deprived of REM sleep becomes irritable, anxious, and confused.

One or two short naps during the day help maintain energy levels in the elderly and, if integrated into a regular sleep-wake pattern, do not interfere with nighttime sleep. However, frequent or long naps at irregular intervals, usually due to boredom, may interfere with nighttime sleep.

Guidelines for Application of the Nursing Process to the Care of the Elderly: Sleep Patterns

Assess the older person's sleep-wake pattern for alterations associated with the aging process. Determine what time the individual usually retires and awakes and whether he or she awakes during the night. Ask whether he or she feels rested upon awakening. Determine the individual's nap pattern and reasons for taking naps. Observe the elderly person receiving sleep-inducing medications closely for adverse reactions.

Teach the elderly individual that daytime exercise and warm milk, meditation, soft music, or a light carbohydrate snack at bedtime enhance the production of serotonin, a chemical in the brain that plays an important role in sleep induction. Strenuous exercise, alcohol, caffeine, and protein snacks should be avoided for 1 to 2 hours before bedtime because they decrease serotonin production and may slow sleep induction. Assure the person that it is normal for the elderly to take longer to fall asleep and to awake early in the morning. Discuss activities to occupy early morning hours. Night arousals are also normal and do not usually impair the effectiveness of the total sleep period. If the person naps, teach the importance of a regular nap pattern. Encourage participation in activities that interest the individual if boredom is a factor in taking naps.

Cardiovascular Function

In the normal aging process, cardiac output gradually decreases by 30% to 40% as a result of fat infiltration, fibrosis, and hypertrophy of the heart muscle and valves. The ability of the cardiovascular system to respond to fluctuations in body needs diminishes. It also takes longer for the heart to return to a normal heart rate after stress. Slowed response of the autonomic nervous system to position changes may result in episodes of orthostatic hypotension. Calcification and fibrosis of the arterial walls may lead to hypertension, weak peripheral pulses, or arterial insufficiency. Hypertension in the elderly is defined as a systolic pressure of more than 160 mm Hg and a diastolic pressure of more than 90 mm Hg based on the average of two or more readings on two or more occasions. Diminished cerebral circulation may produce episodes of lightheadedness or dizziness. Thickening and fibrosis of the venous walls may lead to varicosities and dependent edema.

Guidelines for Application of the Nursing Process to the Care of the Elderly: Cardiovascular Function

Assess for alterations in cardiovascular function associated with the aging process. Assessment of cardiac function is discussed in detail in Chapter 17, and vascular function in Chapter 19. Obtain blood pressure readings to compare with previous or future readings for the early detection and treatment of hypertension. Determine whether the individual has experienced any episodes of orthostatic hypotension. Ask whether daily activities cause tightness of the chest, unusual fatigue, or dyspnea. Anticipate that the hands and feet may be cool to the touch and peripheral pulses difficult to palpate. Assess for dependent edema and varicosities. Ask whether planned exercise is part of the daily routine.

Teach the elderly person to change position slowly and to rest when tired or short of breath. If varicosities or dependent edema develops, elastic stockings and frequent elevation of the feet during the day may relieve venous pressure and edema. Socks worn to bed at night help relieve the discomfort of cold feet caused by decreased peripheral circulation. A heating pad can be used before retiring to warm the bed sheets. However, it should never be used during sleep because of the danger of fire from electrical malfunction and the possibility of burns because of skin fragility and diminished sensation in the feet.

Encourage participation in a medically approved exercise program to maintain and improve cardiovascular status. Walking is excellent exercise, promotes respiratory and cardiovascular fitness, helps weight maintenance, and provides opportunity for socialization. Many shopping malls open prior to regularly scheduled business hours to accommodate "walkers."

Respiratory Function

Several changes in the normal aging process result in diminished respiratory capacity. Atrophy of the respiratory muscles, combined with kyphosis and an increase in the anteroposterior diameter of the chest, produces a "barrel chest" appearance in many elderly persons and interferes with chest movement and gas exchange. At the same time, loss of elasticity of the respiratory muscles and lungs reduces

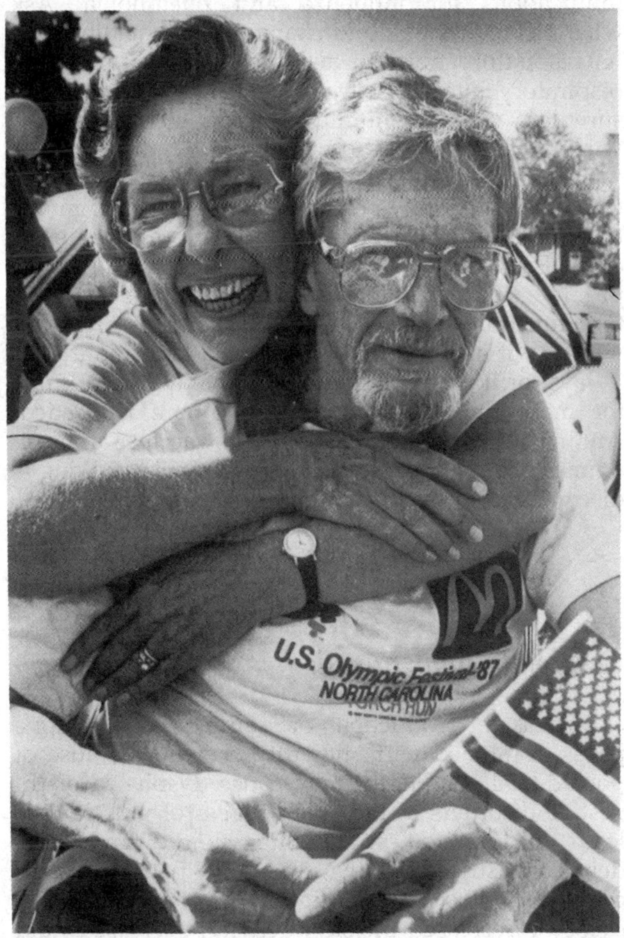

(From Matteson M, McConnell E. Gerontological nursing: Concepts and practice. Philadelphia: WB Saunders, 1988, p 480.)

vital capacity and increases residual volume. Thickening of the walls of the alveolar sacs and capillaries further impairs oxygen–carbon dioxide exchange. The individual is less able to adjust to increased oxygen requirements. As respiratory passages lose muscle tone, mucus secretion and ciliary movement diminish. Changes in respiratory function may result in fatigue, dyspnea on exertion, slowed cough reflex, an ineffective cough, and increased susceptibility to respiratory infections.

Guidelines for Application of the Nursing Process to the Care of the Elderly: Respiratory Function

Assess for alterations in respiratory function associated with the aging process. Assessment of respiratory function is discussed in detail in Chapter 12. Ask whether any changes have been made in daily activities because of respiratory function. Anticipate that older persons will have difficulty holding their breath. Obtain a smoking history and history of immunizations for influenza and pneumonia. Ask what effects weather and changes in air quality have on respiratory function and the frequency of upper respiratory infections. Determine whether any measures are taken to humidify indoor air during the winter.

To help reduce the risk of pulmonary problems, teach the elderly person to use diaphragmatic breathing and to practice pursed lip breathing exercises. Encourage daily exercise such as walking to promote deep breathing and help maximize respiratory function. Also teach that if shortness of breath worsens, if any respiratory infection lasts more than 3 days, or if the individual is unable to retain fluids for more than 24 hours, medical care is needed. Annual influenza and pneumonia vaccines are recommended for all persons older than 65. Smoking is discouraged in persons of all ages.

Gastrointestinal Function

Decreased production of saliva and digestive juices, combined with difficulty chewing because of poor dental conditions, may cause dysphagia or digestive disorders in the elderly. Loss of muscle tone leads to impaired swallowing, slowed peristalsis, delayed gastric emptying, and constipation. The elderly person is also susceptible to constipation because of decreased physical activity, decreased fluid intake, the use of diuretics, decreased secretion of lubricating intestinal mucus, and poor abdominal muscle tone. Diarrhea may develop because of food intolerance, fecal impaction, and loss of sphincter tone. Liver size, hepatic blood flow, enzyme activity, and synthesis of plasma proteins decrease after age 50 as total body mass decreases. Fat intolerance may develop as a result of increased viscosity of the bile and diminished elasticity of the gallbladder.

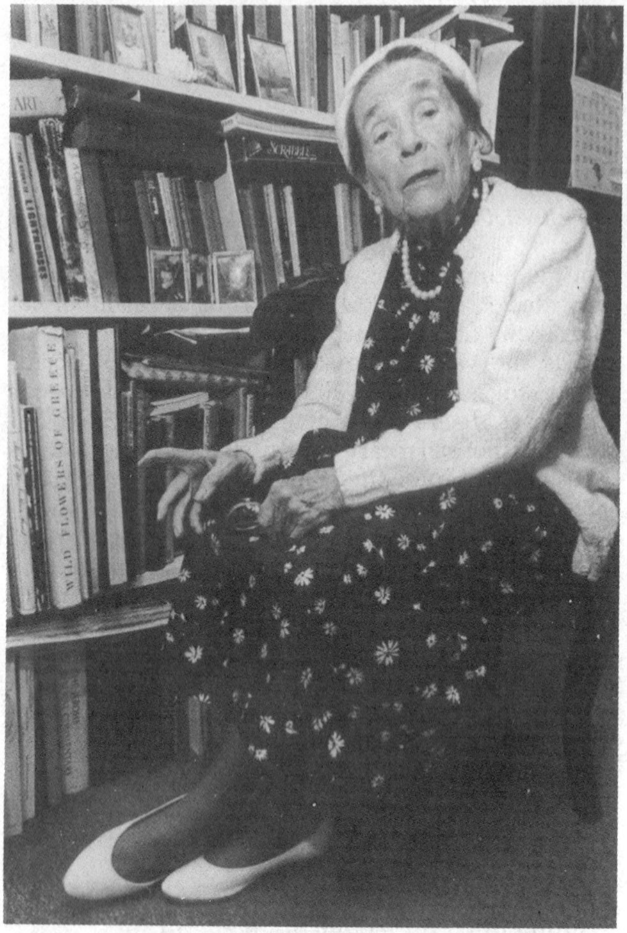

(From Matteson M, McConnell E. Gerontological nursing: Concepts and practice. Philadelphia: WB Saunders, 1988, p 686.)

Guidelines for Application of the Nursing Process to the Care of the Elderly: Gastrointestinal Function

Assess for alterations in gastrointestinal function associated with the aging process. Assessment of gastrointestinal function is discussed in detail in Chapter 21. Determine daily fluid intake. Examine the mouth to assess dental conditions and hydration. Look for inflamed or raw areas indicating poor denture fit. Anticipate that the tongue and lips will appear more fissured and the mouth slightly dryer than in younger adults. Ask how foods are prepared and whether any foods are avoided because of difficulty chewing or swallowing or decreased digestive tolerance. Determine bowel pattern and description of stool, as well as incidence of constipation or diarrhea.

Teach the elderly individual to have a biannual dental examination for tooth and gum evaluation, to chew food thoroughly before swallowing, and to eat soft, chopped, or pureed foods if chewing food is difficult. Because gums shrink with age, denture fit must be evaluated periodically. In general, food eaten in five or six small meals daily that provide a variety of familiar foods from the basic food groups is nutritionally sound and is tolerated and digested better by the elderly person. Provide reassurance that it is not necessary to have a bowel movement daily. Normal bowel patterns vary from several movements a day to one every 3 or 4 days. Teach that increased fluids, fiber, and regular exercise are more effective in preventing constipation than dependence on laxatives.

Urinary Function

Renal blood flow decreases as cardiac output declines in the elderly. Nephrons decrease in size and number, and the number of glomeruli within the nephrons decreases. As the walls of the glomerular capillaries and renal tubules thicken, glomerular filtration rate decreases.

Loss of bladder tone and elasticity, decreased bladder capacity, diminished pelvic muscle tone, and decreased perception of sensory impulses are normal age-related changes in the urinary system. Common complaints of the elderly are urinary frequency and urgency, stress incontinence, and dribbling. It is estimated that between 15% and 30% of non-institutionalized Americans suffer from some degree of loss of control of urination. This problem causes embarrassment and loss of self-esteem and often limits the individual's desire to socialize. Nocturia may interfere with sleep patterns. In men with prostate enlargement, retention and difficulty starting the urinary stream may develop.

Guidelines for Application of the Nursing Process to the Care of the Elderly: Urinary Function

Assess for alterations in urinary pattern associated with the aging process. Assessment of urinary function is discussed in detail in Chapter 25. Determine urinary pattern and character. Ask males especially to describe the urine stream and whether it is difficult starting urination. Determine when the last prostate examination was performed. Inquire specifically about frequency, urgency, dribbling, and stress incontinence, because many people do not volunteer embarrassing information. Ask whether treatment has been sought to correct the problem. Many elderly do not seek treatment because they are embarrassed, do not know treatment is available, or think some degree of loss of urinary control is a normal part of aging. If nocturia is present, determine whether the individual feels that it interferes with a restful night's sleep. Many elderly avoid fluid intake to reduce episodes of nocturia. Dehydration results and further impairs renal blood flow and filtration.

Teach the elderly individual to drink 6 to 8 glasses of fluid during the day to maintain hydration and renal blood flow but to avoid fluid ingestion 3 to 4 hours before bedtime. Encourage pelvic exercises to improve tone of both the pelvic muscles and the urethral sphincter and to help reduce dribbling and stress incontinence in both men and women. Pelvic muscles can be strengthened by tightening the buttocks and pelvic muscles for a count of ten and then relaxing at least three or four times a day, or by stopping the urine stream in midvoiding for a count of ten each time the bladder is emptied. Also teach the individual to void, wait a moment, and then attempt to void again to promote complete emptying of the bladder. Discuss the many commercial products available that can prevent embarrassment if stress incontinence and dribbling occur. Encourage the individual to use measures that enable continued socialization. Referral to a specialized incontinence clinic may be appropriate if the above measures are not effective.

Musculoskeletal Function

MUSCLES

With age, muscles decrease in mass, power, and endurance. They also require more time to recover from a period of exertion. Muscle cells decrease in number, and the remaining cells atrophy. Muscle fibers gradually become infiltrated with fat and fibrotic tissue. Arm and leg muscles in particular become flabby and weak. Movement slows and agility diminishes as a result of loss of sensitivity to neural stimulation and slowed reaction time. Tendons shrink and become sclerotic, further slowing muscle movement. The frequency of muscle cramping increases, especially at night, owing to impaired capillary circulation and accumulation of metabolic wastes during the day. If the person is taking diuretics, cramping may also be due to potassium loss.

BONES AND JOINTS

Bone density decreases with age as a result of increased resorption of bone matrix and minerals. As calcium is resorbed from the bones, the bones become increasingly porous, brittle, and more susceptible to fracture. Although this loss of bone mass, which is called osteoporosis, occurs in all aging persons, it is more severe in women, and because it is closely associated with decreased estrogen secretion, its progression is more rapid following menopause. Osteoporosis is most severe in the long bones and vertebrae.

In the vertebral column, thinning of the intervertebral cartilaginous disks and collapse of the porous vertebral bodies result in kyphosis (dowager's hump). As illustrated in Figure 2–2, kyphosis produces an increase in anteroposterior diameter of the chest and a decrease in height of the trunk. This latter effect is primarily responsible for the decrease in height that occurs in the aged person. Flexion contractures of the hips and knees may also contribute to height loss.

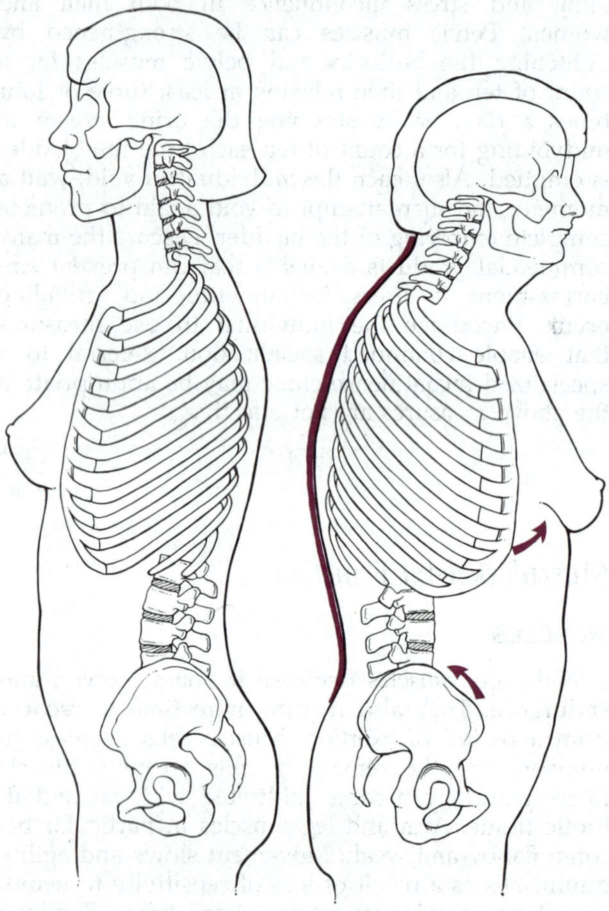

Figure 2–2.

Changes in height and posture due to the effects of aging. Note how deterioration of vertebrae and intervertebral disks causes loss of height, kyphosis of the thoracic spine, straightening of the lumbar curve, slight posterior rotation of the hips, and an increase in anteroposterior diameter of the thorax.

Years of use cause gradual thinning and erosion of joint cartilage. The synovial membrane and synovial fluid thicken. These normal changes of aging result in reduced joint lubrication, stiffness, and crepitation. Ligaments become calcified and lose elasticity. Joints become less stable, and joint swelling and decreased range of motion may result.

Guidelines for Application of the Nursing Process to the Care of the Elderly: Musculoskeletal Function

Assess for alterations in musculoskeletal function associated with the aging process. Assessment of musculoskeletal function is discussed in detail in Chapter 35. Note pattern and stability of gait to identify safety risks. Determine whether the individual participates in daily physical activity or in a daily exercise program. Identify any difficulty performing daily activities. Examine joints for swelling, deformity, crepitation, instability, or decreased function. While assessing range of motion, move limbs gently to avoid pain or injury. Determine intake of calcium-rich foods or calcium supplements.

Teach the elderly individual to avoid using joints and muscles past the point of pain, to rest painful joints, and to use assistive devices for safety as needed. Medically approved walking is an excellent exercise that helps promote a feeling of well-being, aid in weight control, maintain muscle tone and joint mobility, and slow demineralization of the bones. Many elderly people enjoy early morning walks in shopping malls for both the physical and social benefits. To compensate for reduced strength and stamina, the elderly individual should learn to pace activities to correspond to the time of day when energy levels are the highest.

Advise women approaching or in menopause to discuss with their physicians the possible advantages and disadvantages of estrogen replacement therapy to slow bone demineralization. Many research studies have investigated the relationship between calcium and vitamin D intake and the rate of bone demineralization after menopause. Although some studies have been inconclusive, many health care authorities advise adult females that a daily intake of at least 1000 mg of calcium and 400 IU of vitamin D may slow age-related bone deterioration. The RDA of calcium for adults is 800 mg.

Neurologic Function

In the aging person, as neurons die and cannot regenerate, neurologic function gradually deteriorates. Some loss of brain mass, especially parts of the cerebral cortex, occurs. Decreased cardiac output and vascular deterioration impair blood flow and oxygen supply to the brain, which slows mental processes. Slowed reflexes and longer reaction time are also the result of impaired transmission of neuromuscular impulses owing to myelin sheath degeneration and decreased catecholamine production. Muscle tremors may appear at rest and worsen with fatigue.

Guidelines for Application of the Nursing Process to the Care of the Elderly: Neurologic Function

Assess for alterations in neurologic function associated with the aging process. Assessment of neurologic function is discussed in detail in Chapter 37. Inquire about episodes of dizziness, lightheadedness, falls, numbness or tingling, altered speech or behavior patterns, or loss of consciousness, which may indicate severely impaired cerebral blood flow and require evaluation by a physician.

Teach the elderly person that because activity and reactions have slowed, it is normal to require more time to perform daily activities. Special care must be taken to avoid touching surfaces that may be hot or cold, since pain sensitivity and response are impaired. In addition, care must be taken to chew food thoroughly and avoid rushing meals, because the gag reflex may be slow.

Reproductive Function

Both men and women experience reduced sex hormone secretion accompanied by reduction in libido and sexual desire as age advances. Pubic hair thins, reproductive organs atrophy, and secretions diminish. Women may grow coarse facial hair. The breasts atrophy and hang loosely from the chest wall. Nipples become smaller, flatter, and less erective. In men, sperm production decreases. Men experience slow erection and weak ejaculation. Longer stimulation is required before ejaculation. Decreased estrogen levels in women cause the vaginal mucosa to become pale, thin, and dry. Painful intercourse (dyspareunia) may result from slow arousal and decreased vaginal lubrication.

Guidelines for Application of the Nursing Process to the Care of the Elderly: Reproductive Function

Assess for alterations in reproductive function associated with the aging process. Assessment of female reproductive function is discussed in detail in Chapter 43, male reproductive function in Chapter 45. Anticipate that to avoid embarrassment, many individuals will not volunteer information about sexuality and reproductive function because of its intimate nature. Maintain eye contact while asking tactful, direct questions to help put the person at ease and facilitate collection of accurate information.

Assure the elderly that sexual desire and activity are normal and healthy throughout life. Suggest

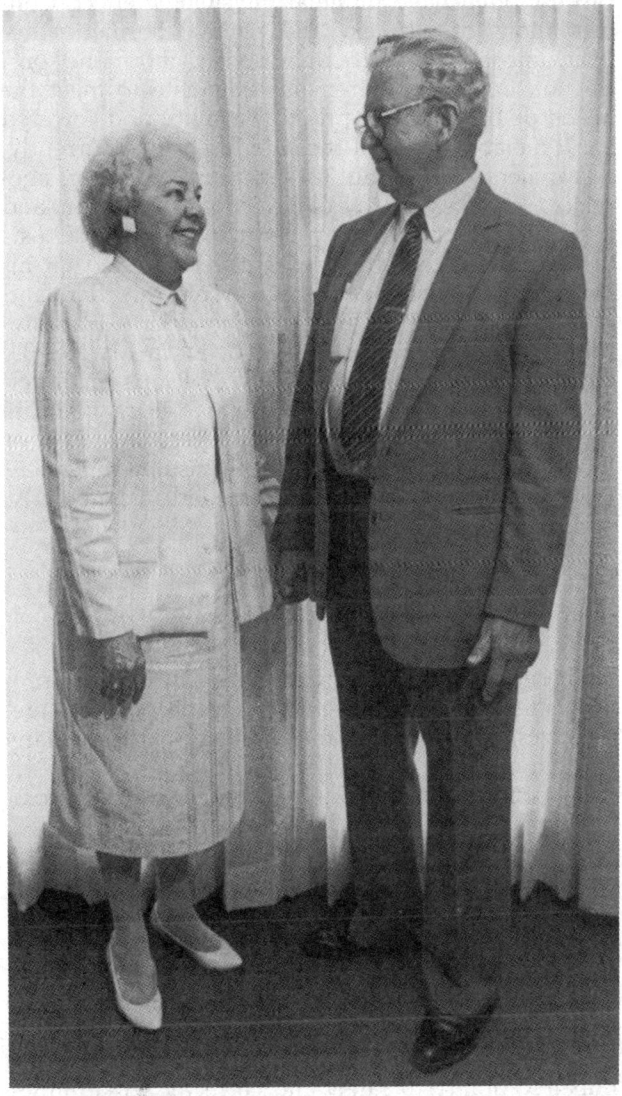

(From Matteson M, McConnell E. Gerontological nursing: Concepts and practice. Philadelphia: WB Saunders, 1988; p 430.)

prolonged foreplay to compensate for slow arousal and lubrication. Discuss delayed ejaculation as an opportunity to increase satisfaction of both partners. A water-soluble lubricant relieves painful intercourse caused by diminished vaginal secretions.

Teach the elderly female to perform monthly breast self-examination as described in Chapter 48 and to be examined by a gynecologist annually. Teach the elderly male to perform monthly breast and testicular self-examination and to have a prostate examination annually.

Endocrine Function

Because the endocrine system has a large functional reserve, changes associated with the aging process often have minimal physiologic effect. Concentrations of pituitary and adrenal hormones appear unchanged. Although thyroid hormone production decreases, it remains adequate to meet the needs of the reduced physical activity and lowered basal metabolic rate of the elderly person. Currently, researchers are trying to determine whether age-related changes in thyroid calcitonin secretion and parathyroid function may be linked to osteoporosis in the elderly. Recent studies have indicated an increase in the incidence of parathyroid disorders and altered calcium metabolism in the elderly. Parathyroid disorders are discussed in detail in Chapter 34. Glucose intolerance occasionally develops in the elderly. The exact cause is unclear, but it may be due to delayed insulin response to glucose ingestion or increased insulin resistance. Non–insulin-dependent diabetes mellitus, a frequent disorder of the elderly, is discussed in Chapter 30.

Pharmacokinetics

The normal physiologic changes of the aging process alter the way the elderly person absorbs, metabolizes, responds to, and eliminates drugs. Many chronic diseases and dietary deficiencies, which are more common in the elderly, also alter pharmacokinetics.

The elderly, who make up 12% of the population, account for almost 50% of all drugs used. Many elderly adults take ten or more prescription drugs, often prescribed by several different physicians, and more than 70% use nonprescription drugs on a daily basis. Each additional drug taken increases the chance of food and drug interactions.

Compounding the problem is the elderly person's impaired ability to safely and correctly self-administer drugs in the presence of musculoskeletal, sensory, and mental changes commonly associated with the aging process. Muscular weakness and stiff joints may inhibit ability to open caps and tempt the elderly to either leave the cap off or pour the medication into another bottle. Visual impairment and decreased tactile sensitivity may cause the elderly person to misread labels or pick up and ingest more than one pill at a time. Many studies have shown that elderly persons who live alone are more prone to medication errors than are younger persons. Some estimates indicate that as many as 60% either forget to take medications or take the wrong dose.

Reduced gastric and intestinal motility increases transit time and drug absorption and increases the opportunity for drug interactions. Lower body temperature, reduced lubrication of mucosa, and diminished vascularity impair absorption of suppositories.

Distribution and binding in body tissues is altered by the decreased amounts of body water, serum albumin, and skeletal muscle in the elderly and the larger amount of adipose tissue and impaired capillary function. Reduced serum albumin levels can result in increased levels of unbound active drugs in the blood. Altered serum concentrations increase the possibility of either toxic or ineffective drug levels in the blood and tissues.

Reduced hepatic blood flow and enzyme production impair drug detoxification, and reduced renal blood flow and filtration impair excretion. Because both these changes alter the body's ability to metabolize and excrete medications, toxic serum levels may occur in the elderly person with what is normally a therapeutic dose.

To further complicate pharmacokinetics, the elderly often respond to drugs differently than younger adults. To decrease the risk of adverse drug reactions in the elderly, the Food and Drug Administration is developing guidelines that will require labeling information for geriatric use on prescription drugs. If the individual is well below normal adult weight, a safe dose may be calculated using a body weight–based formula.

Guidelines for Application of the Nursing Process to the Care of the Elderly: Altered Pharmacokinetics

Assess the elderly person's knowledge about medications currently being taken and their side effects. Specifically ask about nonprescription preparations, because many people do not identify drugs that are not prescribed by a physician as medications. Determine whether each physician caring for the individual is aware of all prescription and nonprescription preparations being taken. Ask how many physicians and pharmacists the person is using. Determine whether the individual is following any special dietary or activity instructions because of medications. Ask what method is used to remember to take all

Table 2–1. NURSING IMPLICATIONS OF THE ALTERED EFFECTS OF DRUGS IN GERIATRIC PATIENTS

DRUG CLASSIFICATION	NURSING IMPLICATIONS SPECIFIC FOR GERIATRIC PATIENTS
All drugs	Many side effects and signs of drug toxicity are common complaints the elderly attribute to aging and therefore may ignore. Provide side effects and signs of toxicity in writing and emphasize the need to report any occurrence lasting more than 24 hours to the physician promptly.
Digitalis glycosides	Decreased renal excretion and increased cardiac sensitivity increase risk of toxicity. Antacids decrease absorption; do not take within 1 hour of digitalis.
Diuretics	Adverse effects more frequent because of sensitivity to fluid loss. Higher risk for postural hypotension, hypokalemia, hyponatremia, muscle cramps, and thrombus formation.
Anti-coagulants	Increased drug activity due to impaired plasma protein binding increases the risk of serious bleeding.
Antihypertensives	Postural hypotension common. Predisposed to bradycardia and respiratory and central nervous system side effects.
Antiarrhythmics	Often treated with lower dose. More sensitive to central nervous system effects.
Calcium channel blockers	Higher risk of adverse reactions, especially orthostatic hypotension. Impaired renal and hepatic function prolong activity.
Anti-inflammatory agents	Adverse reactions with indomethacin extremely high. Increased risk for peptic ulcer, aplastic anemia, and toxic reactions with phenylbutazone.
Oral hypoglycemic agents	Impaired hepatic and renal function impair excretion, prolong activity. Elderly are especially vulnerable to hypoglycemia, and early signs are difficult to detect.
Antianxiety agents	Impaired hepatic and renal function impair excretion, prolong activity. Increased sensitivity to central nervous system effects.
Aminoglycosides	Monitor closely for nephrotoxicity and ototoxicity.
Narcotic analgesics	Increased sensitivity to central nervous system effects. Lower doses usually prescribed.

Chart 2–1.

NURSING GUIDE TO PATIENT EDUCATION FOR SELF-MANAGEMENT: SELF-ADMINISTRATION OF MEDICATIONS FOR THE ELDERLY

Instruct the elderly individual to take medications exactly as prescribed and provide clearly written instructions on the following:

Name, dose, frequency, expected effects, and untoward side effects of each medication.
How to take the medication.
How to open the container and the availability of easy-open, non-childproof caps.
Whether medication is available in liquid or can be crushed and dissolved in fluid or mixed with food.
Methods to ensure accurate self-medication, such as a checkoff calendar or containers labeled with days of the week and medication times during the day.
Method of monitoring effects of medication.
Importance of reporting adverse reactions or absence of desired response to the physician so that the medication or dosage can be changed.
Dietary alterations; include foods or drugs to avoid.
Maintaining a list of current medications to take to each doctor's appointment.
Consulting physician before taking any over-the-counter preparation.
Whom to call for answers about prescribed and over-the-counter medications.
What to do if illness prevents taking medication.

Nursing Care Guide 2–1.

PROMOTING COMPLIANCE WITH MEDICATION REGIMEN BY ELDERLY ADULTS

Assessment Findings: Eighty-one-year-old patient who has a history of congestive heart failure is to be discharged on furosemide (Lasix) and digoxin (Lanoxin) following treatment for exacerbation of symptoms related to failure to follow prescribed medication regimen. When reviewing medications during hospitalization, patient repeatedly confuses medications, forgets when to take them, and cannot remember whether medication was taken.

Nursing Diagnosis: Ineffective management of therapeutic regimen related to insufficient knowledge of medication regimen and inability to differentiate among medications or remember whether medication was taken as prescribed

Patient Outcomes	Nursing Interventions	Rationale
Patient verbalizes understanding of need to follow prescribed medication regimen prior to discharge.	Determine patient's readiness and ability to learn.	Teaching cannot be successful unless the patient is motivated and able to learn.
	Ask patient to identify reasons for current hospitalization. Reinforce with patient failure to take medications as prescribed as reason for hospitalization.	Determines level of knowledge and awareness of cause of hospitalization.
Patient correctly differentiates between a container of digoxin and a container of furosemide 100% of the time.	Assess patient's visual acuity and ability to read medication bottle labels.	Identifies possible cause of noncompliance.
	If patient is unable to read labels, ask the physician to write a note requesting that the patient's pharmacy mark the respective containers with a large "D" or "F" and type labels in all capitals.	Simplifies identification of correct medication. Capital letters are more easily read.
	Review identification method with patient daily.	Repetition reinforces learning.
Patient states the name, dose, frequency, expected actions, and untoward side effects of prescribed medications from memory or by reading printed cards.	Teach patient the name, dose, frequency, expected actions, and untoward side effects of prescribed medications.	Legally all persons must have this information to correctly and safely self-administer medication. Understanding increases compliance.
	Instruct patient to notify physician promptly if condition deteriorates or untoward side effects develop.	Medication or dosage may need to be altered.
	Reinforce verbal information with clearly printed cards.	Repetition reinforces learning.
	Ask patient to read each card.	To be sure lettering is large enough for patient to see.
Patient demonstrates ability to monitor effects of medications:		
a. accurately counts and records pulse	Teach patient how to count the radial or carotid pulse for a full minute and record.	Pulse rate indicates therapeutic effectiveness of digoxin.

(continued)

Nursing Care Guide 2–1. *(continued)*

PROMOTING COMPLIANCE WITH MEDICATION REGIMEN BY ELDERLY ADULTS

Patient Outcomes	**Nursing Interventions**	**Rationale**
b. accurately weighs self and records weight	Teach patient to monitor and record body weight weekly.	Body weight indicates therapeutic effectiveness of furosemide.
	Have patient do return demonstration of ability to correctly monitor and record pulse and weight daily during remainder of hospitalization.	Evaluates learning and identifies need for further teaching and demonstration.
Patient states intent to notify physician if pulse is irregular, below 60 bpm, or above 110 bpm; if weight changes by more than 3 pounds in 1 week; or if ankle edema, nausea, vomiting, muscle weakness, cramps, or visual changes develop.	Instruct patient to notify physician promptly if untoward side effects of medications develop.	Pulse below 60 bpm or above 110 bpm and irregular pulse may indicate digoxin toxicity. Daily weight is the most accurate method of determining change in fluid balance. Each pound represents approximately 500 ml of fluid.
	Reinforce instructions and provide physician's telephone number on clearly printed card.	Repetition reinforces learning. The telephone number will be readily available if needed.
Patient states intent to avoid taking antacid within 1 hour of taking digoxin.	Advise patient that concurrent ingestion of antacids with digoxin inhibits absorption.	Patient must be aware of drug interactions to avoid altered therapeutic response.
Patient states intent to increase dietary intake of potassium-rich foods.	Instruct patient that potassium-rich foods such as bananas, oranges, peaches, and dates must be included in the diet daily to replace potassium lost during furosemide therapy.	Furosemide promotes potassium excretion.
Patient verbalizes intent and demonstrates ability to self-administer medications as prescribed.	Identify and reinforce patient's motivating factors to adhere to medication regimen.	Self-motivation increases learning and compliance.
	Provide method for monitoring self-administration of medication such as checkoff calendar or daily pill boxes.	Ensures therapeutic blood level of medications by preventing extra doses or omitted doses.
	Allow patient to learn at own rate.	Too much information, too fast, causes frustration and interferes with successful learning.
	Provide positive reinforcement.	Positive feedback increases motivation and reinforces learning.
	Have patient use monitoring method for remainder of hospitalization.	Develops familiarity with the method and reduces unexpected problems at home.

Evaluation: Compare the patient's status with the expected patient outcomes. If the outcomes are achieved, evaluate nursing care as successful. If not, reassess the patient, formulate new nursing diagnoses, and revise expected patient outcomes and nursing interventions as appropriate.

medications as prescribed and to remember that a dose was taken.

Always inform the elderly person when a medication is being administered. Name the drug and state its purpose. Repetition reinforces learning. State how many pills or how much liquid must be taken. Administer oral medications with 6 to 8 ounces of water to facilitate swallowing and ensure their passage into the stomach. Have the individual sit upright or stand to reduce the risk of choking or aspiration. It may be necessary to check the person's mouth to be sure pills have been swallowed. Never inject or infuse medication into a paralyzed or immobilized limb, because inactivity and reduced circulation alter drug absorption.

Assess closely for adverse drug reactions. The earliest manifestation of drug toxicity in the elderly is often mental confusion. Any sudden change in condition or mental status could be drug-related. Anticipate that a drug may be given in smaller doses or less frequently to the elderly owing to impaired excretion. Use a body weight formula to confirm safe dosages for frail elderly. Table 2–1 identifies specific geriatric nursing implications for classifications of drugs commonly prescribed for the elderly. Consult with the physician to determine whether a medication can be administered once a day rather than in divided doses, since this may help improve compliance when the individual is at home.

Teach the elderly person to take medications exactly as prescribed and to bring a list of current medications to each doctor's visit. Suggest using one pharmacy to fill all prescriptions, to reduce the risk of drug interactions. Recommend that the pharmacist be asked to use non-childproof caps and to type the label in all capitals to make it easier to read. Reinforce the need to consult the physician before taking any nonprescription preparations and to report any deterioration in condition or unusual sensations that develop after starting a new medication to the physician promptly. Refer to Chart 2–1 for specific guidelines for teaching self-medication to the elderly. Reinforce verbal instructions with clearly written instructions on cards. Nursing Care Guide 2–1 identifies some of the nursing interventions to promote compliance with medication regimen by elderly adults. Initiate a home care referral for individuals who are living alone and who appear unable to safely self-administer medications.

Assessment of the Elderly

In assessing the elderly individual, it is important to remember that each person ages at a different rate and adapts to the aging process differently. Because it takes the elderly longer to process and respond to questions, allow at least 30 minutes for the health interview. If the person uses a hearing aid or glasses, be sure they are worn. Provide bright, glare-free lighting in a comfortably warm environment. Complete assessment of mental processes and neuromuscular coordination early in the examination to avoid inaccurate results due to fatigue.

Patient History

Face the individual, identify yourself, and state questions one at a time in a clear voice. Allow time for the person to answer. If an answer seems inappropriate, do not assume impaired mental processes. The question may have been misunderstood or not heard clearly. Clarify the answer or restate the question.

A complete medication history is essential. Determine whether the individual has brought currently used medications or a list of them with him or her. Because the elderly often have a high tolerance for pain and dismiss many symptoms as being signs of old age, questions must be specific to obtain accurate information. For example, instead of asking about the presence of skin problems, ask specifically about itching, burning, peeling, and visible skin lesions. Ask additional specific questions about findings as they are identified during physical assessment to clarify information collected in the history.

Conclude the interview by asking the individual to review a typical day. This provides the nurse with an opportunity to assess ability to adapt to the aging process and perform self-care activities and activities outside the home. Family members or friends can help clarify information and provide missing information or be used as an alternate source if the individual is unable to communicate.

Physical Examination

Physical assessment of the normal changes associated with the aging process has been identified in each of the preceding sections. Maintain a warm environment and avoid unnecessary or prolonged exposure of body parts during physical examination to prevent excess heat loss. Explain each examination as you proceed. Provide assistance during position changes and maintain safety measures to prevent injury. Palpate and percuss gently to avoid trauma to fragile skin. Palpate and manipulate body parts carefully, and do not move joints beyond the point of pain, to avoid injury.

Accurate assessment of normal versus abnormal findings and early identification of changes in status and responses to therapy are important in the care of the elderly because homeostatic mechanisms are less able to respond to stress and the patient may demonstrate rapid fluctuations in condition. Selected nursing diagnoses with patient outcomes and nursing interventions frequently applicable in the care of geriatric patients are identified in Nursing Care Guide 2–2.

Nursing Care Guide 2–2.

GERIATRIC PATIENTS

Assessment Findings: Geriatric patient complaining of discomfort in right hip and back upon awakening. Examination reveals mild kyphosis and redness over thoracic spine, right scapula, right trochanter, and sacrum. Skin is dry and intact. Patient states difficulty repositioning self in bed.

Nursing Diagnosis: High risk for impaired skin integrity related to prolonged pressure over bony prominences and limited independent mobility in bed

Patient Outcomes	Nursing Interventions	Rationale
Patient identifies lying or sitting in one position for extended periods of time as cause of discomfort and reddened skin.	Inform patient that immobility increases pressure over bony prominences and impairs circulation. Identify impaired circulation as cause of redness, discomfort, and potential skin breakdown.	A simple explanation directly relating the patient's immobility to the skin alterations increases understanding of the need to change positions more frequently.
Patient shifts weight every hour while sitting.	Instruct patient to sit in arm chair with padded seat when possible. Provide egg-crate chair pad.	Use of padded seat and egg-crate cushion reduces pressure over bony prominences and reduces impairment of capillary blood flow.
	Demonstrate how to use chair arms to shift weight, and have patient do return demonstration.	Increases the frequency of position changes by encouraging independence.
Patient verbalizes understanding of need to be repositioned every 2 hours while in bed.	Apply egg-crate mattress or other weight-distributing product to bed.	Reduces pressure over bony prominences and reduces impairment of capillary blood flow.
	Assist patient with repositioning every 2 hours while in bed.	Position changes relieve pressure and allow return of capillary blood flow.
	Consider use of overhead trapeze.	Enables patient to assist with position changes or to move independently.
Patient maintains skin that is clean, dry, and intact.	Examine skin daily to detect potential areas of skin breakdown.	To evaluate effectiveness of care.
	Instruct patient to use nondrying products for bathing and skin care. Gently apply lanolin-based lotions to skin and bony prominences. Encourage intake of six to eight glasses of fluid daily. Keep linens clean, dry, and wrinkle-free.	Adequate hydration and clean, dry, supple skin that is free of irritants reduce the risk of altered skin integrity.

Evaluation: Compare the patient's status with the expected patient outcomes. If the outcomes are achieved, evaluate nursing care as successful. If not, reassess the patient, formulate new nursing diagnoses, and revise expected patient outcomes and nursing interventions as appropriate.

(continued)

Nursing Care Guide 2–2. *(continued)*

GERIATRIC PATIENTS

Assessment Findings: Geriatric female who has recently recovered from a fractured wrist suffered in a fall during a dizzy spell while going to the bathroom at night. Patient identifies occasional lightheadedness when standing from sitting or lying position and difficulty seeing at night. Examination reveals decreased visual acuity, steady gait, mild kyphosis.

Nursing Diagnosis: High risk for trauma related to lack of knowledge of safety precautions needed secondary to orthostatic hypotension, impaired vision, and osteoporosis

Patient Outcomes	Nursing Interventions	Rationale
Patient states intent to use night-light in bedroom, bathroom, and hall.	Inform patient of the visual changes that accompany aging.	To relieve anxiety.
	Advise patient to use bright, glare-free lighting at home. Recommend use of night-lights to lessen danger of falls.	Adequate lighting reduces the risk of falls.
	Suggest that patient keep eyeglasses at bedside and put them on before getting out of bed at night or in the morning.	Poor vision increases the risk of injury.
	Advise patient to allow extra time for eyes to adjust to changes in light intensity.	Adjustment to changes in light is slower in the elderly, and vision is poor until eyes adjust.
Patient demonstrates arising slowly from a sitting position and sitting on the side of the bed before standing.	Explain to patient circulatory changes that accompany the aging process and may cause episodes of orthostatic hypotension.	Understanding increases compliance with safety measures.
	Explain rationale of increased safety with slow position changes. Teach patient to arise slowly from a sitting position and to sit at the edge of the bed for a minute or two before standing.	Changing position slowly allows the peripheral vascular system to adjust to fluctuations in blood pressure and prevents orthostatic hypotension.
	Have patient do return demonstration and continue practice during rest of hospital stay.	Return demonstration allows evaluation of learning.
Patient identifies foods high in calcium that she will include in her diet daily.	Teach patient changes in bone structure that accompany the aging process and the possible benefits of increased calcium intake.	Understanding increases compliance.
	Help patient identify her preferences from a list of high-calcium foods.	Preferred foods are more likely to be eaten.

(continued)

Nursing Care Guide 2–2. *(continued)*

GERIATRIC PATIENTS

Patient Outcomes	Nursing Interventions	Rationale
	Clearly print these foods on a card, with serving size and percentage of daily calcium requirement.	Provides an easily read, handy reference.
	Review menu selections during remainder of hospitalization to reinforce selection of good calcium sources.	Positive feedback increases motivation. Repetition increases learning.

Evaluation: Compare the patient's status with the expected patient outcomes. If the outcomes are achieved, evaluate nursing care as successful. If not, reassess the patient, formulate new nursing diagnoses, and revise expected patient outcomes and nursing interventions as appropriate.

Assessment Findings: Ambulatory geriatric patient identifies irregular bowel pattern during interview: soft, formed stools with periods of infrequent hard stools, treated with laxatives. Last bowel movement was soft, formed, 2 days ago. Examination reveals abdomen soft on palpation, active bowel sounds on auscultation. Passing flatus. Drinks approximately two cups of coffee and two glasses of beverage daily.

Nursing Diagnosis: High risk for colonic constipation related to inadequate fluid intake and laxative abuse

Patient Outcomes	Nursing Interventions	Rationale
Patient identifies nonlaxative measures to prevent constipation.	Teach patient that constipation is a long-term effect of laxative use caused by decreased intestinal muscle tone.	Understanding the undesirable effects of laxatives may encourage reduced use.
	Teach patient that regular exercise, adequate fluids, and high-fiber diet help prevent constipation.	Exercise stimulates peristalsis, fluids soften stool, and fiber increases bulk to promote regular passage of soft, formed stool.
Patient drinks at least eight glasses of fluid daily.	Identify beverage preferences. Teach patient that any beverage counts toward fluid total.	Preferred fluids are more readily consumed.
	Suggest keeping track of intake by marking off numbers 1–8 written on a card each morning.	Accurate recording provides feedback and promotes consumption of desired amount.

(continued)

Nursing Care Guide 2–2. *(continued)*

GERIATRIC PATIENTS

Patient Outcomes	Nursing Interventions	Rationale
Patient chooses high-fiber foods from daily menu selections and states intent to eat high-fiber foods daily at home.	Help patient identify preferences from a list of high-fiber foods.	Preferred foods are more likely to be eaten.
	Clearly print these foods on a card.	Provides an easily read, handy reference.
	Review menu selections during remainder of hospitalization to reinforce selection of good fiber sources.	Positive feedback increases motivation. Repetition increases learning.
Patient has a soft bowel movement within 48 hours and at least one every 3 days thereafter.	Encourage patient to ambulate freely about unit unless contraindicated.	Walking improves abdominal muscle tone and increases peristalsis.
	Identify time of day patient normally defecates. Recommend that a regular time for defecation be part of daily routine.	Identifies patient's regular pattern of elimination and aids in reestablishing regular pattern.
	Advise that urge to defecate often occurs an hour or so after meals. Teach patient to respond to urge to defecate promptly.	Eating stimulates the colorectal reflex to defecate. Failure to respond to urge to defecate suppresses it.
	Provide prune juice or warm beverage 30 minutes before normal defecation time.	Helps stimulate defecation.
	Advise not to hold breath or strain during bowel movement.	Stimulates the vagus nerve and slows the heart rate.

Evaluation: Compare the patient's status with the expected patient outcomes. If the outcomes are achieved, evaluate nursing care as successful. If not, reassess the patient, formulate new nursing diagnoses, and revise expected patient outcomes and nursing interventions as appropriate.

Assessment Findings: Geriatric male patient recovering from fractured hip. Ambulates well with walker but tires easily and cannot climb stairs. Previously lived independently but is to temporarily live with son after discharge. Patient verbalizes frustration over loss of independence, is no longer participating in decision-making, and verbalizes doubts about ability to ever return home.

Nursing Diagnosis: Powerlessness related to loss of independence, decreased stamina, limited mobility, potential loss of home and possessions

Patient Outcomes	Nursing Interventions	Rationale
Patient identifies previous coping mechanisms.	Encourage patient to reminisce about previous successes in solving problems and overcoming obstacles.	Helps patient identify previous coping mechanisms to assist in transferring them to current situation.

(continued)

Nursing Care Guide 2–2. (continued)

GERIATRIC PATIENTS

Patient Outcomes	Nursing Interventions	Rationale
Patient makes decisions in areas over which he has control.	Acknowledge past accomplishments and praise progress since injury.	Positive feedback promotes self-esteem and motivation.
	Help patient identify areas over which he has control.	Promotes independence and a sense of control.
	Provide positive reinforcement when patient participates in decision-making process.	Positive feedback increases participation.
Patient expresses sense of control over events and anticipates future return to own home.	Recognize when patient is seeking information and provide rationale for actions. Encourage patient to verbalize feelings about current status and potential discharge.	Accurate information increases knowledge and understanding and reduces anxiety.
	Schedule health team conference with patient and family to assist patient in formulating realistic goals.	Realistic goals and expectations increase motivation and reduce frustration.

Evaluation: Compare the patient's status with the expected patient outcomes. If the outcomes are achieved, evaluate nursing care as successful. If not, reassess the patient, formulate new nursing diagnoses, and revise expected patient outcomes and nursing interventions as appropriate.

Bibliography

Allen ME. A holistic view of sexuality and the aged. Holistic Nursing Practice 1987; 1(4):76.

Antai-Otong D. Suicidal risk? Geriatr Nurs 1990; 11(5):228.

Antonovsky A, Sagy S. Confronting developmental tasks in the retirement transition. Gerontologist 1990; 30(3):362.

Arnold HL, Odom RB, James WD. Andrews' diseases of the skin. 8th ed. Philadelphia: WB Saunders, 1990.

Bahr RT Sr, Gress L. The 24-hour cycle: Rhythms of healthy sleep. J Gerontol Nurs 1985; 11(4):14.

Bates B. *A* guide to physical examination and history taking. 5th ed. Philadelphia: JB Lippincott, 1991.

Beil AV. Osteoporosis: How to avoid its crippling effects. RN 1986; 49(8):14.

Berliner H. Aging skin. Am J Nurs 1986; 86(10):1138.

Booth DE, Morris CL. Hyperparathyroidism: The overlooked disorder. J Gerontol Nurs 1990; 16(6):16.

Brady PF. Labeling of confusion in the elderly. J Gerontol Nurs 1987; 13(6):29.

Brock AM. Helping the elderly sleep. Nursing 1986; 6(5):122.

Buczny B. Impotence in older men: A newly recognized problem. J Gerontol Nurs 1992; 18(5):25.

Burbank PM. Psychosocial theories of aging: A critical evaluation. ANS 1986; 9(1):73.

Burggraf V, Donlon B. Assessing the elderly: System by system. Am J Nurs 1985; 85(9):974.

Burggraf V, Stanley M. Nursing the elderly: A care plan approach. Philadelphia: JB Lippincott, 1989.

Carpenito LJ. Nursing diagnosis: Application to clinical practice. 4th ed. Philadelphia: JB Lippincott, 1992.

Cassel CK, Walsh JR (eds): Geriatric medicine. New York: Springer-Verlag, 1989.

Clavon A. The black elderly. J Gerontol Nurs 1986; 12(5):6.

Conn VS, Taylor SG, Kelley S. Medication regimen complexity and adherence among older adults. Image J Nurs Sch 1991; 23(4):231.

Cowling WR, Campbell VG. Health concerns of aging men. Nurs Clin North Am 1986; 21(1):75.

de la Cruz LAD. On loneliness and the elderly. J Gerontol Nurs 1986; 12(11):22.

DiIorio C, Price M. Swallowing: An assessment guide. Am J Nurs 1990; 90(7):38.

Doenges M, Moorhouse M. Nurse's pocket guide: Nursing diagnosis with interventions. 3rd ed. Philadelphia: FA Davis, 1990.

Drugay M. Nutritional evaluation: Who needs it? J Gerontol Nurs 1986; 12(4):14.

Dudek SG. Nutrition handbook for nursing practice. Philadelphia: JB Lippincott, 1987.

Eliopoulos C. Gerontological nursing. 3rd ed. Philadelphia: JB Lippincott, 1993.

Ellickson EB. Bowel management plan for the homebound elderly. J Gerontol Nurs 1988; 14(8):16.

Fielo S, Rizzolo MA. The effects of age on pharmacokinetics. Geriatr Nurs 1985; 6(6):328.

Forbis PA. Meeting patients' spiritual needs. Geriatr Nurs 1988; 9(3):158.

Gambert, SR. Handbook of geriatrics. New York: Plenum Publishing, 1986.

Garrett, JE. Multiple losses in older adults. J Gerontol Nurs 1987; 13(8):8.

Gaspar P. What determines how much patients drink? Geriatr Nurs 1988; 9(4):221.

Gibson J. A new approach to better medication compliance. Nursing 1989; 19(4):49.

Goldstein M, Hawthorne ME, Engeberg S, et al. Urinary incontinence: Why people do not seek help. J Gerontol Nurs 1992; 18(4):15.

Gray-Vickrey P. Evaluating Alzheimer's patients. Nursing 1988; 18(12):34.

Gunter LM, Kolanowski AM. Promoting healthy lifestyles in mature women. J Gerontol Nursing 1986; 12(4):6.

Gulino C, Kadin M. Aging and reactive alcoholism. Geriatr Nurs 1986; 7(3):148.

Guyton AG. Texbook of medical physiology. 8th ed. Philadelphia: WB Saunders, 1990.

Haddad AM. Determining competency. J Gerontol Nurs 1988; 14(6):19.

Heim KM. Wandering behavior. J Gerontol Nurs 1986; 12(11):4.

Horwath CC. Nutrition goals for older adults: A review. Gerontologist 1991; 31(6):811.

Hudson MF. Drugs and the older adult. Nursing 1984; 14(8):46.

Iverson-Carpenter M, Haskin D, Maas M, et al. Fulfilling nutritional requirements. J Gerontol Nurs 1988; 14(4):16.

Janelli LM. The realities of body image. J Gerontol Nurs 1986; 12(10):23.

Janz M. Clues to elder abuse. Geriatr Nurs 1990; 11(5):220.

Jess L. Investigating impaired mental status. Nursing 1988; 18(6):42.

Kidd P, Murakami RY. Common pathologic conditions in elderly persons: Nursing assessment and intervention. J Emerg Nurs 1987; 13(1):27.

King KS, Dimond M, McCance KL. Coping with relocation. Geriatr Nurs 1987; 8(5):258.

Kositzke J. A question of balance: Dehydration in the elderly. J Gerontol Nurs 1990; 16(5):4.

Kuhn JK, McGovern M. Respiratory assessment of the elderly. J Gerontol Nurs 1992; 18(5):40.

Loebl S, Spratto GR. The nurse's drug handbook. 5th ed. New York: John Wiley & Sons, 1989.

Longino CF. Who are the oldest Americans? Gerontologist 1988; 28(4):515.

MacIssac A, Rivers R, Adamson CB. Multiple medications: Is your elderly patient caught in the storm? Nursing 1989; 19(7):60.

Madson S. How to reduce the risk of postmenopausal osteoporosis. Gerontol Nurs 1989; 15(9):20.

Malasanos L, et al. Health assessment. 4th ed. St. Louis: CV Mosby, 1990.

Matteson M, McConnell E. Gerontological nursing: Concepts and practice. Philadelphia: WB Saunders, 1988.

McCracken A. Emotional impact of possession loss. J Gerontol 1987; 13(2):14.

McKeon A. Estrogen replacement therapy. J Gerontol Nurs 1990; 16(11):6.

Meis M. Loneliness in the elderly. Orthop Nurs 1985; 4(3):63.

Mion L, Frengley JD, Adams M. Nursing patients 75 years and older. Nurs Manage 1986; 17(9):24.

Mitchell CA. Generalized chronic fatigue in the elderly: Assessment and intervention. J Gerontol Nurs 1986; 12(4):19.

Mull CS, Cox CL, Sullivan JA. Religion's role in the health and well-being of well elders. Public Health Nurs 1987; 4(3):151.

North American Nursing Diagnosis Association. NANDA Nursing Diagnoses: Definitions and Classifications. St. Louis: North American Nursing Diagnosis Association, 1992.

Nesbitt B. Nursing diagnosis in age-related changes. J Gerontol Nurs 1988; 14(7):6.

Newman DK, Lynch K, Smith DA, et al. Restoring urinary continence. Am J Nurs 1991; 91(1):28.

Picariello G. A guide for teaching elders. Geriatr Nurs 1986; 7(1):38.

Powell A, Ptlene M. Alcohol withdrawal syndrome. Am J Nurs 1988; 88(3):312.

Price SA, Wilson LM. Pathophysiology: Clinical concepts of disease processes. St. Louis: Mosby-Year Book, 1992.

Putnam P. Coping in later years: The reconciliation of opposites. Image J Nurs Sch 1987; 19(2):67.

Raffensperger EB. Clinical nursing handbook. Philadelphia: JB Lippincott, 1986.

Ramsey R. Adjusting drug dosages for critically ill elderly patients. Nursing 1988; 18(7):47.

Rapp S, Davis K. Geriatric depression: Physicians' knowledge, perceptions, and diagnostic practices. Gerontologist 1989; 29(2):252.

Robbins SL, Kumar V. Basic pathology. 4th ed. Philadelphia: WB Saunders, 1987.

Santo-Novak DA. Seven keys to assessing the elderly. Nursing 1988; 18(8):60.

Seidel HM, et al. Mosby's guide to physical examination. 2nd ed. St. Louis: CV Mosby, 1991.

Shannon MT, Wilson BA. Govoni and Hayes: Drugs and nursing implications. 7th ed. Norwalk, CT: Appleton & Lange, 1992.

Simon JM. The therapeutic value of humor in aging adults. J Gerontol Nurs 1988; 14(8):8.

Smith JB. The patient who can't remember to take her meds. RN 1986; 49(9):38.

Smith LH, Wyngaarden JB (eds). Cecil review of general internal medicine. 4th ed. Philadelphia: WB Saunders, 1989.

Sowers J, Felicetta J (eds). Endocrinology of aging. New York: Raven Publishing, 1988.

Steffee DR, Suty KA, Delcalzo PV. More than a touch: Communicating with a blind and deaf patient. Nursing 1985; 15(8):36.

Steinke EE. Older adults' knowledge and attitudes about sexuality and aging. Image J Nurs Sch 1988; 20(2):93.

Strumpf NE. A new age for elderly care. Nurs Health Care 1987; 8(8):445.

Sullivan M. Atrophy and exercise. J Gerontol Nurs 1987; 13(7):26.

Taira F. Strategies to promote independence in the elderly. Rehabil Nurs 1988; 13(12):330.

Tariott P, Sunderland T, Murphy D, et al. How memory fails: A theoretical model. Geriatr Nurs 1985; 6(3):144.

Trice LB. Meaningful life experience to the elderly. Image J Nurs Sch 1990; 22(4):248.

Tucker SM, et al. Patient care standards: Nursing process, diagnosis, and outcome. 5th ed. St. Louis: CV Mosby, 1992.

US Department of Agriculture. Human Nutrition Information Service, Home and Garden Bulletin No. 249. Washington, DC: US Government Printing Office, April 1992.

US Department of Agriculture. Human Nutrition Information Service, Leaflet No. 572. Washington, DC: US Government Printing Office, August 1992.

Warner D. Walking to better health. Am J Nurs 1988; 88(1):64.

Webster J. Key to healthy aging. J Gerontol Nurs 1988; 15(12):8.

Weiffenbach JM, Tylenda CA, Baum BJ. Oral sensory changes in aging. J Gerontol 1990; 45(4):M121.

Weiner MB, et al. Working with the aged. 2nd ed. Norwalk, CT: Appleton & Lange, 1987.

Weinrick SP, Boyd M. Education in the elderly: Adapting and evaluating tools. J Gerontol Nurs 1992; 18(1):15.

Williams SR. Nutrition and diet therapy. 6th ed. St. Louis: Times Mirror/Mosby College Publishing, 1989.

Wilson JD, Foster DW (eds). Williams textbook of endocrinology. 8th ed. Philadelphia: WB Saunders, 1992.

Wurtman JJ, Lieberman H, Tsay R, et al. Calorie and nutrient intakes of elderly and young subjects measured under identical conditions. J Gerontol 1988; 43(6):B174.

Yurick AG, et al. The aged person and the nursing process. 3rd ed. Norwalk, CT: Appleton-Century-Crofts, 1989.

Chapter Three

KNOWLEDGE BASIC TO THE NURSING CARE *of Adults with* *Fluid, Electrolyte, and Acid-Base Imbalances*

Fluid, electrolyte, and acid-base imbalances are the three topics presented in this chapter. The four types of fluid imbalance are extracellular fluid volume deficit (ECFVD), extracellular fluid volume excess (ECFVE), extracellular fluid volume shift, and intracellular fluid volume excess. The electrolyte imbalances include potassium, sodium, calcium, and magnesium deficits and excesses. The acid-base imbalances are respiratory acidosis and alkalosis and metabolic acidosis and alkalosis.

Fluid Imbalances

In the adult, water accounts for approximately 60% of the body weight. It is distributed between two major fluid compartments in the body: the intracellular and the extracellular compartments (Fig. 3–1). Intracellular fluid (ICF) is the fluid within cells. Extracellular fluid (ECF) is the fluid between cells, which is called interstitial fluid, and the fluid within the blood vessels, which is called intravascular fluid. Cerebrospinal, synovial, pleural, abdominal, and gastrointestinal (GI) fluids as well as lymph are also classified as ECF. Body fluids shift between these compartments to maintain fluid balance.

Extracellular Fluid Volume Deficit

ECFVD is a loss of fluid from the interstitial and vascular spaces. The loss of fluid can be accompanied by a loss of electrolytes, particularly sodium, which is a major extracellular electrolyte whose primary function is to regulate body fluid. Water loss can also occur without sodium loss. When water and sodium are lost in equal amounts, the fluid loss is referred to as iso-osmolar (isotonic) fluid volume deficit. When the water loss is greater than the sodium loss, the fluid deficit is referred to as hyperosmolar (hypertonic) fluid volume deficit.

The concentration of solutes in body fluid is described as osmolarity or osmolality. The terms *osmolarity* and *osmolality* are used interchangeably. Osmolarity is the osmotic pull exerted by all particles

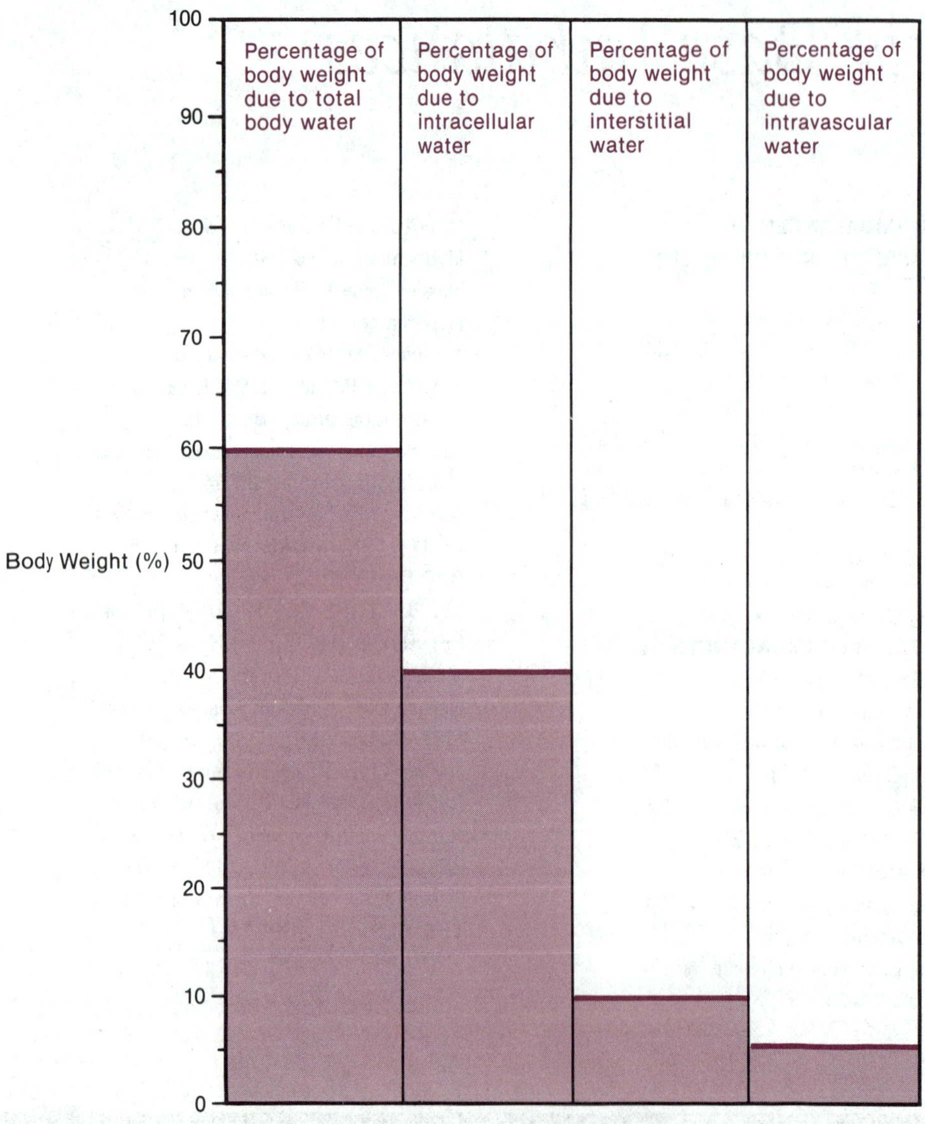

Figure 3–1.

Percentage of body weight due to water.

Table 3–1. CLINICAL MANIFESTATIONS OF BODY FLUID VOLUME DEFICIT

MILD ECFVD	MODERATE ECFVD	SEVERE ECFVD
2% weight loss	5% weight loss	8% weight loss
1–2 L of water loss	3–5 L of water loss	5–10 L of water loss
Thirst	Marked thirst	Marked thirst
Apprehension	Restlessness	Lethargic or irritable, delirium or disorientation
	Flushed skin	Cold, clammy skin
	Dry mucous membranes	Dry mucous membranes
	Poor skin turgor	Poor skin turgor
	Hand veins: slow in filling with hand lowered	Hand veins: slow in filling with hand lowered
	Increased pulse rate	Tachycardia
	Increased respiration	Increased respiration
	Systolic BP drop of 10–15 mm Hg in standing position	Systolic BP (70 mm Hg)
	Urine volume decreased, concentrated urine	Urine volume <25 ml/hr
	Increased BUN, Hgb	Increased BUN, Hgb

Abbreviations: ECFVD, extracellular fluid volume deficit; BP = blood pressure; BUN, blood urea nitrogen; Hgb = hemoglobin.

(solutes) per unit of solution, expressed as osmols or milliosmols per liter of solution. Osmolality is the osmotic pull exerted by all particles (solutes) per unit of water, expressed as osmols or milliosmols per kilogram of water. If there are more particles (sodium, glucose, urea, protein) than water, a hyperosmolar fluid results. If particles and water are of equal proportion, an iso-osmolar fluid results. Hypo-osmolar (hypotonic) fluid has fewer particles than water.

Normal serum osmolality is 275 to 295 mOsm/kg water. If the serum osmolality is less than 275 mOsm/kg water, it is hypo-osmolar (fewer particles and more water); and if the serum osmolality is more than 295 mOsm/kg water, it is hyperosmolar (more particles and less water).

ETIOLOGY

Hyperosmolar fluid volume deficit occurs when the loss of water exceeds the loss of sodium. Another term for this type of fluid volume deficit is dehydration.

Causes of hyperosmolar fluid volume deficit include severe diarrhea, inadequate water intake, diabetic acidosis, and sweating. Hyperosmolar fluid volume deficit may also occur when intake of salt and other solutes occurs without an increase in water intake.

Iso-osmolar fluid volume deficit occurs when water, electrolytes, and other solutes are lost in equal proportion from the ECF space. Profuse diaphoresis, vomiting, diarrhea, GI suction, fistulas, draining abscesses, fever, burns, and hemorrhage can result in iso-osmolar fluid loss. Other causes are diuretic therapy and maintenance on a "nothing by mouth" (NPO) order for a prolonged period of time. Iso-osmolar fluid volume loss is not classified as dehydration, although it is frequently referred to as such.

PATHOPHYSIOLOGY

With hyperosmolar dehydration, the osmotic pressure of the ECF is increased, and as a result, fluid moves quickly out of the ICF into the ECF. This shift maintains relatively normal vascular volume, so symptoms of hypovolemic shock do not occur. However, the shift causes cellular dehydration and imbalances in electrolytes such as potassium and calcium, which result in unstable excitable membranes.

With isotonic fluid loss, ECF osmolality is unchanged; therefore, fluid does not shift from the ICF to ECF, and a decrease in circulatory volume occurs. Compensatory mechanisms begin to function as soon as a decrease in volume occurs, and they are successful in maintaining the perfusion of vital organs until one quarter to one third of the circulating volume is lost. At this point, symptoms of severe hypovolemic shock occur.

CLINICAL MANIFESTATIONS

Whether as a result of water loss in excess of solutes, or water and solute loss in approximately the same proportions, ECFVD can be mild, moderate, or severe. Signs and symptoms vary with the degree of fluid loss, as shown in Table 3–1.

Thirst is a symptom that occurs with mild, moderate, and severe fluid deficit. Both lack of fluid intake and fluid loss lead to thirst. Water intake may correct the fluid deficit before it becomes severe; however, in an elderly person, the thirst mechanism in the medulla may not alert the person to drink fluids. Also the water/fluid container may not be accessible to the person. Thus, a mild type of fluid deficit can lead to moderate fluid deficit. When the fluid loss becomes moderate or severe, shocklike symptoms such as tachycardia, moderate to severe decrease in blood pressure, and increase in respiration become apparent. A fall in systolic blood pressure of 20 mm Hg when a person moves from sitting to standing position, accompanied by an increase in pulse rate by 10 beats per minute (bpm) present 1 minute after position change, indicates that the intravascular fluid volume is decreased (Gettrust & Brabec, 1992). Weight loss also occurs with moderate and severe fluid deficit. A 1-kg change in body weight corresponds to a 1-L net change in fluid balance.

MEDICAL DIAGNOSIS

Laboratory tests such as a general chemistry profile are ordered to determine the type of fluid deficit. An elevated serum osmolality, greater than 295 mOsm/kg, and serum sodium level greater than 146 mEq/L indicate hyperosmolar fluid volume deficit. Other laboratory indicators of fluid volume deficit are blood urea nitrogen (BUN) greater than 30 mg/dl, hemoglobin (Hgb) greater than 18 g/dl, and hematocrit greater than 55%.

Poor skin turgor, cracked gums and tongue, oliguria, decreased central venous pressure (CVP), and decreased pulmonary capillary wedge pressure, less than 6 mm Hg, are additional diagnostic indicators of fluid deficit. Narrowing of pulse pressure (difference between systolic and diastolic pressures) may also suggest fluid loss.

MEDICAL MANAGEMENT

Medical management of fluid volume deficit depends on the severity and the type of fluid deficit. If the fluid loss is mild ECFVD, oral fluid intake is increased if the patient is conscious, not nauseated, and can drink. When hyperosmolar fluid volume deficit is present, intravenous fluids such as dextrose in water or 0.2% saline are ordered. For moderate or severe ECFVD, intravenous fluids such as lactated Ringer's solution or dextrose in 0.45% or 0.9% saline might be prescribed. When hemorrhage is the cause of ECFVD, blood replacement is necessary if blood loss is more than 1 L. Balanced salt solutions such as normal saline and lactated Ringer's solution may be used to replace blood and fluid losses of less than 1 L.

Medical management is also directed at correcting the underlying causes of the fluid volume deficit to decrease or prevent further fluid loss. For example, if the cause is diarrhea, antidiarrheal agents and dietary restrictions are usually ordered.

Application of the Nursing Process to the Care of the Patient with Extracellular Fluid Volume Deficit

Assessment

Obtain a patient history to identify factors that place the patient at risk for ECFVD. Question the patient about any history of renal disease, diabetes mellitus or insipidus, liver disease, burns, or large draining wounds. Also ask about recent surgery, episodes of excessive sweating, salivating, vomiting, diarrhea, fever, or periods of restricted fluid intake. Question also about the use of diuretics, noting brand name, frequency, and dose. Assess the patient's mental status and determine whether any physical limitations exist that would prevent adequate fluid intake (e.g., limited mobility or difficulty swallowing). Obtain a list of fluids (type and amount) ingested in the previous 24 hours and ask whether this represents the usual fluid intake. Also question the patient regarding frequency and amount of urination.

Assess the skin for poor turgor (pinched skin that remains pinched or that only returns slowly to its normal skin surface). Note skin color and temperature. Observe for dry mucous membranes and dry, cracked lips or tongue.

Assess mental status. Observe for apprehension, restlessness, irritability, lethargy, or confusion.

Check pulse rate, respirations, and blood pressure. Remember that as fluid volume deficit occurs, the heart compensates for the fluid loss by increasing the heart rate. If fluid volume continues to be lost, the systolic blood pressure begins to fall. Check blood pressure while the patient is sitting and then standing. A fall in systolic blood pressure of 10 to 15 mm Hg could indicate moderate fluid volume loss.

Assess hand and neck vein filling. A decrease in venous filling in hand veins when the hand is below the heart level and in the jugular vein when the patient is in a low Fowler's position suggests fluid volume deficit.

Measure urinary output and note urine color. An increased urine output as a result of osmotic diuresis from hyperosmolar fluid (diabetic ketoacidosis) suggests fluid volume loss. Keep in mind that decreased urine output may be due to a lack of fluid intake. Review laboratory reports for increased BUN or Hgb.

Nursing Diagnoses and Planning

Nursing diagnoses and related expected patient outcomes most commonly applicable to patients with ECFVD include the following:

NDx: Fluid volume deficit related to insufficient intake, vomiting, diarrhea, or diaphoresis (specify for individual patient)

Planning: Patient outcomes
1. Skin is warm and dry with normal turgor.
2. Capillary refill is within normal limits.
3. Vital signs are within patient's baseline range.
4. Urinary output is at least 50 ml/hour or 1500 ml/day.

NDx: Altered oral mucous membrane related to dehydration

Planning: Patient outcomes
1. Oral mucous membrane is moist and pink.
2. Lips are supple, moist, and free of cracks.
3. Patient denies dryness of the mouth.

Nursing Interventions

NDx: Fluid volume deficit
Monitor vital signs. Compare vital signs with the patient's baseline vital signs. Report marked difference between the present vital signs and the baseline vital signs. Check blood pressure in lying, sitting, and standing positions. Report if the standing (postural) systolic blood pressure falls 20 mm Hg and is accompanied by a pulse rate increase of 10 bpm present 1 minute after position change.

Provide oral fluid intake to replace mild fluid volume loss. Increase oral intake by offering a variety of fluids at frequent intervals between meals. Offer small amounts at one time if the patient has difficulty drinking or is reluctant to drink. Offer both hot and cold fluid unless otherwise contraindicated, and provide assistance as needed. Administer intravenous fluids as ordered for moderate and severe fluid losses.

Monitor skin turgor and mucous membranes for changes, improvement, or deterioration. Also monitor hand and neck vein status. Flattened vein may indicate lack of improvement in fluid status.

Monitor urinary output. Report urine output results and report immediately if urinary output increases or decreases (30 ml/hour).

Monitor body weight. One kilogram, or a 2.2-lb, loss of weight would be equivalent to 1 L (1000 ml) of fluid loss. If the patient lost $7\frac{1}{2}$ lb, the fluid loss would be approximately 3 L; moderate fluid volume deficit would be present.

NDx: Altered oral mucous membranes
Assist the patient in rinsing the mouth frequently and in brushing the teeth after eating. Avoid the use of agents with a drying effect on mucous membranes such as commercial mouthwash or lemon and glycerin. Use a solution of equal parts of hydrogen peroxide and water to remove debris and deodorize the mouth, or use a solution composed of a half teaspoon of sodium bicarbonate and a pint of warm water to cleanse and soothe the mouth. Apply a water-soluble lubricant to the lips to keep them supple and to prevent cracking.

Evaluation

Evaluate the effectiveness of nursing care for a patient with ECFVD by comparing the patient's status with the expected patient outcomes. Examples of specific outcomes for patients with ECFVD have been provided in the Planning section.

Extracellular Fluid Volume Excess

ECFVE is increased fluid in the vascular system and in the interstitial spaces. When sodium and water are retained in the same proportion, the excess is referred to as iso-osmolar (isotonic) fluid volume excess. As a result of hemodilution, the serum sodium level may be within normal range even though the actual sodium level is increased. Because sodium promotes retention of water, both would be increased.

ETIOLOGY

Causes of iso-osmolar fluid volume excess include heart failure, chronic renal disease, cirrhosis, and increased ingestion of sodium products such as packaged foods, salt, and foods with a high sodium content.

PATHOPHYSIOLOGY

Iso-osmolar fluid volume excess is also called hypervolemia or fluid overload. Normally, there is a free exchange of fluid between the intravascular and interstitial spaces to maintain fluid balance in the ECF compartment. Normal fluid exchange is a function of fluid pressure (hydrostatic pressure) and colloid osmotic (oncotic) pressure in the intravascular space and the interstitial space. Fluid pressure (force exerted by intravascular fluid against the walls of the blood vessels) acts to push fluid into the tissue spaces, and the oncotic pressure (colloid osmotic pressure caused by albumin and other proteins) holds fluid in the vessels. When there is volume excess or fluid overload, the fluid pressure is greater than the oncotic pressure in the vessels. Fluid is pushed into the tissue spaces, and peripheral edema results. As the fluid pressure increases, fluid is also pushed across the alveolocapillary membrane of the lungs, causing pulmonary edema.

In congestive heart failure (CHF), when the heart fails to maintain adequate blood flow throughout the circulatory system, the buildup of intravascular fluid pressure causes fluid shifts into the interstitial spaces. Thus, left-sided heart failure can cause pulmonary edema as a result of fluid shifts into the alveolar spaces. Renal disease can cause a decrease in sodium and water excretion, with resultant fluid overload. With cirrhosis of the liver, serum protein and albumin levels are decreased; therefore, the oncotic pressure is decreased in the vascular fluids, causing more fluid to move into tissue spaces. With malnutrition, as with cirrhosis, the serum protein level is decreased, and fluid leaves the vessels because of a low oncotic pressure and shifts into the tissue spaces, causing edema.

CLINICAL MANIFESTATIONS

Weight gain, puffy eyelids, and pitting edema in the extremities occur as a result of excess fluid volume. Pulse is rapid, full, and bounding. Blood pressure is elevated, and pulse pressure is decreased. Hand and neck veins are engorged. Hemorrhoids, if present, enlarge; the liver enlarges; and ascites develops as the condition worsens. Rapid, shallow respirations, dyspnea, moist crackles, and an irritable cough occur as fluid shifts into the alveolar spaces.

MEDICAL DIAGNOSIS

Iso-osmolar ECFVE is diagnosed on the basis of the patient's history, presenting symptoms, and a serum osmolality of less than 275 mOsm/kg. BUN, Hgb, and serum protein may also be decreased. If red blood cells swell as fluid excess occurs, hematocrit can remain unchanged.

MEDICAL MANAGEMENT

The three "Ds" (diuretics, digitalis, and diet) are frequently prescribed for the treatment of iso-osmolar ECFVE. Diuretics are used to promote excretion of sodium and water. The potassium-wasting diuretics, which excrete sodium and potassium, are more potent than the potassium-sparing diuretics, which excrete sodium but not potassium. The thiazide diuretics (hydrochlorothiazide [HydroDIURIL]) and the loop or high-ceiling diuretics (furosemide [Lasix]) are potassium-wasting diuretics used to increase excretion of sodium and water. As water and sodium are lost in the urine, blood volume decreases. This decrease in blood volume lowers fluid pressure in the blood vessels and allows fluid to move from the interstitial space into the intravascular space, from which it can be excreted.

Digoxin, a digitalis preparation, is ordered to decrease the heart rate and increase the force of myocardial contraction. Because hypokalemia can precipitate digitalis toxicity, foods such as vegetables or fruits that are high in potassium or potassium supplements may be suggested for patients also taking thiazide or loop (potassium-wasting) diuretics. A diet low in sodium decreases fluid volume because less sodium is available for water retention. In individuals with low serum albumin caused by malnutrition, dietary protein is increased to enable the liver to manufacture albumin. Because albumin is the major determinant of oncotic pressure in the vascular space, increasing albumin increases the oncotic pressure. As a result, fluid moves out of the tissues into the blood vessels, and edema is decreased.

Application of the Nursing Process to the Care of the Patient with an Iso-osmolar Extracellular Fluid Volume Excess

Assessment

Obtain a patient history to identify factors that place the patient at risk for iso-osmolar ECFVE. Ask about any history of cardiac disease, renal disease, or cirrhosis. Question the patient about recent weight gain, and determine whether the patient is taking any medications. Obtain a diet history to determine both sodium and fluid intake.

Assess vital signs. Take blood pressure, keeping in mind that the pulse pressure narrows as compensatory mechanisms reach their limit. Check the pulse. Expect it to be rapid, bounding, and full, with peripheral pulses difficult to obliterate in the presence of iso-osmolar ECFVE.

Assess respirations. Note rate and depth. Auscultate breath sounds. Note location of crackles in the chest and whether there is difficulty breathing. Observe for a constant irritated cough, because this is an early sign of fluid overload.

Check lower extremities for pitting edema in the morning before the patient arises. Edema present in the morning is not dependent edema (edema caused by gravity), but may be due to a cardiac or renal disorder. If the patient is bedridden, check the sacral area for edema. Weigh the patient daily. Keep in mind that 1 L of fluid retained causes a 1-kg weight gain.

Check hand veins for engorgement. Place the hand below the heart level until the veins are full; raise the hand above the heart level and the veins should flatten in 10 to 20 seconds. If the veins remain engorged after 30 seconds, overhydration or fluid overload is most likely present. Assess for liver enlargement, ascites, and enlarged hemorrhoids.

Nursing Diagnoses and Planning

Nursing diagnoses and related expected patient outcomes most commonly applicable to patients with ECFVE include the following:

NDx: Fluid volume excess related to excessive fluid intake or fluid retention *(specify for individual patient)*

Planning: Patient outcomes
1. Vital signs are within patient's baseline range.
2. Chest sounds are clear.
3. Extremities are free of edema.

NDx: High risk for impaired skin integrity related to peripheral edema

Planning: Patient outcomes
1. Skin is warm.
2. Cyanosis is absent.
3. Skin is intact.

Nursing Interventions

NDx: Fluid volume excess
Monitor vital signs and chest sounds. Report elevated blood pressure and a bounding pulse.

Check for pitting edema in extremities each morning. Press one or two fingers on the edematous area over a bony prominence. If an indentation is present for 15 seconds or more, record the degree of pitting edema as +1 (least severe), +2, +3, or +4 (most severe) according to the depth of the indentation and the length of time it takes for the indentation to disappear.

Check the patient's weight each morning. A weight gain of 1 kg or 2.2 lb is equivalent to 1 L of body fluid. Usually edema does not occur unless there is 3 L or more of excess fluids.

Administer diuretics as ordered, and monitor intake and output. Also monitor for electrolyte and acid-base imbalances during diuretic therapy. Restrict fluid and sodium in the diet as per physician's order. Encourage the patient to drink small amounts of the total fluid allowed at intervals throughout the day to avoid long periods when fluids cannot be taken. In preparation for self-care, teach the patient or significant other about sources of sodium in the diet and provide a list of sodium-rich foods and condiments to be avoided. Make certain it is understood that salt (sodium chloride) is only one source of sodium and that foods containing other sodium compounds such as monosodium glutamate must also be limited.

NDx: High risk for impaired skin integrity
Keep edematous skin areas at risk for breakdown clean, and apply an emollient to prevent dryness and flaking. Apply antiembolic stockings before getting the patient out of bed to minimize the pooling of fluid in the legs and feet as a result of gravity. Assist with repositioning at least every 2 hours as needed to prevent pressure, which will further impair circulation. Remember that prevention of skin breakdown is critical because edema slows the transport of oxygen to the cells and thus impairs healing.

Evaluation

Evaluate the effectiveness of nursing care for a patient with ECFVE by comparing the patient's status with the expected patient outcomes. Examples of specific outcomes for patients with ECFVE have been provided in the Planning section.

Extracellular Third-Space Fluid Volume Shift

Fluid shifts within the ECF compartment are constantly occurring between the intravascular (vascular) and the interstitial spaces for the purpose of maintaining fluid balance. When an abnormal amount of fluid shifts into the interstitial space and remains there, it is referred to as third-space fluid. Third-space fluid is physiologically useless because it does not circulate to provide nutrients to cells.

ETIOLOGY

The common causes of fluid shift from the intravascular to the interstitial spaces are (1) severe inflammation and tissue damage from burns, abdominal surgery, crushing injury, or severe infection; (2) increased hydrostatic fluid pressure resulting from CHF, renal disease, and corticosteroid therapy; and (3) decreased colloid (oncotic) pressure from protein deficit caused by cirrhosis of the liver, malnutrition, or renal disease.

PATHOPHYSIOLOGY

When tissue is injured, increased capillary permeability allows fluid, protein, and other solutes to shift into the interstitial spaces. In cirrhosis, serum albumin levels are frequently decreased because of poor dietary practice. This results in a decreased plasma oncotic pressure, so fluid shifts from the blood vessels to the peritoneal cavity and to the interstitial spaces in the extremities. Ascites and peripheral edema result. CHF can precipitate fluid and sodium overload. This, in turn, increases hydrostatic fluid pressure and pushes fluid into the interstitial spaces of the extremities (peripheral edema) and into the lung tissues (pulmonary edema).

Two phases of fluid shift to the third space usually occur as a result of tissue injury such as burns and abdominal surgery. The first phase is from the intravascular space to the interstitial space, and the second phase is from the interstitial space back to the intravascular space. With the first phase, fluid volume deficit (hypovolemia) results, which may lead to shock. With the second phase, fluid volume excess occurs if the kidneys are unable to excrete excess fluid. Table 3–2 presents the two phases of fluid volume shift.

CLINICAL MANIFESTATIONS

In fluid shifts resulting from tissue injury, it usually takes 24 to 48 hours for the fluid to leave the blood vessels and accumulate in the interstitial spaces at the injured site. Edema may or may not be visible. Vital signs may indicate hypovolemia, with shocklike symptoms of tachycardia, a decrease in systolic pressure, and tachypnea.

Three to 5 days after an injury caused by burns, surgery, or tissue destruction, the fluid shifts from

Table 3–2. FLUID VOLUME SHIFT

PHASE	FLUID SHIFT	TIME	CAUSE
I	Intravascular (vessel) to interstitial (tissue) spaces	24–48 hr	Major: Burns, abdominal surgery, intestinal obstruction, crushing wounds, severe infection Minor: Blister, sprain
II	Interstitial to intravascular spaces	72–120 hr (3–5 days)	

the injured site to the blood vessels. If the kidneys cannot excrete this extra fluid from the vascular compartment, hypervolemia results. Clinical manifestations of hypervolemia include dyspnea, chest crackles, engorgement of the jugular vein, and increased CVP.

In cirrhosis, heart failure, or renal disease, pitting edema (+1 to +4) occurs because of a decreased oncotic pressure and an increased fluid (hydrostatic) pressure. Edema in the extremities occurs when there is an accumulation of approximately 3 L of fluid. Plus one (+1) edema indicates a mild case, whereas +4 edema indicates a large amount of fluid accumulation (severe peripheral edema).

MEDICAL DIAGNOSIS

Serum albumin and electrolytes are some of the laboratory tests used for diagnosing ECF shift. A decreased serum albumin level causes a decreased oncotic pressure and fluid accumulation in the extremities. A decrease in urinary output may indicate a fluid shift to the tissue spaces, and an increase in urinary output can indicate fluid shift back to the intravascular space.

Clinical findings confirm the fluid imbalance. Pitting edema (+1 to +4) indicates fluid shift to the interstitial spaces of the extremities. Crackles, dyspnea, and vein engorgement are signs of hypervolemia caused by fluid shifts into the lung tissues.

MEDICAL MANAGEMENT

Medical management begins with the determination of the cause of the fluid volume shift. Hypovolemia resulting from tissue injury such as burns requires large amounts of intravenous fluid replacement. The amount of fluid infusion may be three times greater than the urinary output. The type of intravenous fluid replacement used is iso-osmolar solution. During the second phase, in which fluid shifts back into the circulation, the urinary output may be three times greater than the fluid intake. Fluid intake is restricted.

Diuretics may be used for peripheral and pulmonary edema. Electrolyte replacement is determined by the serum electrolyte results. A diet rich in protein and low in sodium may increase the serum protein level, thus increasing the oncotic pressure, which pulls fluid back from the third space.

Application of the Nursing Process to the Care of the Patient with an Extracellular Third-Space Fluid Volume Shift

The assessment, nursing diagnoses, expected patient outcomes, nursing interventions, and evaluation for patients with an extracellular third-space fluid volume shift are a combination of those described previously for patients with ECFVD or ECFVE (depending on the stage of the fluid shift) and those that derive from the specific disorder underlying the fluid shift.

Intracellular Fluid Volume Excess

Intracellular fluid volume excess (ICFVE) is not as common a fluid imbalance as ECFVD and ECFVE. ICFVE results from hypo-osmolar fluid in the intravascular system, which can be due to either excess water or a decrease in solutes. The hypo-osmolar fluid moves to the cells that contain iso-osmolar fluid to maintain fluid balance. This movement of fluid is due to osmosis (i.e., fluid moving from an area of lesser concentration of solutes to one of greater concentration). ICFVE caused by hypo-osmolar (hypotonic) fluid is also called water intoxication. Water intoxication is not the same as edema. Edema is the accumulation of water and sodium in the interstitial spaces, and water intoxication is an accumulation of water in the cells. Individuals at greatest risk for water intoxication are the elderly, the malnourished, and the debilitated.

ETIOLOGY

Conditions that cause ICFVE, or water intoxication, are excessive intake of water, solute (electrolytes, protein) deficit, increased secretion of antidiuretic hormone (ADH), and inability of the kidneys to excrete excess water. Specific causes of each of these conditions are presented in Table 3–3.

PATHOPHYSIOLOGY

ICFVE, or water intoxication, causes cellular edema and electrolyte dilution. Within the brain,

Table 3–3. CAUSES OF INTRACELLULAR FLUID VOLUME EXCESS

CONDITION	CAUSES
Excess water	Excessive intake of water or ice chips Psychogenic polydipsia Continuous use of intravenous D_5W Brain injury or tumor with increased ADH production
Solute deficit	Diet low in electrolytes and protein Multiple tap-water enemas Irrigation of nasogastric tube with water and not normal saline
Impaired excretion	Kidney dysfunction; congestive heart failure; syndrome of inappropriate ADH, which can be due to stress, surgery, drugs (narcotics, anesthesia), pain, and tumors (brain, lung)

Abbreviations: D_5W, dextrose 5% in water; ADH, antidiuretic hormone.

edema causes increased intracranial pressure and can either depress or stimulate various nerve centers.

CLINICAL MANIFESTATIONS

Increased fluid in the cerebral cells (cerebral edema) causes headache and behavioral changes such as incoordination, apprehension, irritability, and confusion. Anorexia, nausea, projectile vomiting, blurred vision, and papilledema may also occur. Changes in vital signs, including an increased blood pressure, decreased pulse rate, and increased respirations, also develop. Acute weight gain is evident. Convulsions are common with severe ICFVE.

MEDICAL DIAGNOSIS

The diagnosis of ICFVE is made on the basis of patient history, clinical findings, and laboratory values. A serum osmolality of less than 275 mOsm/kg suggests the possibility of ICFVE, but no one laboratory test is diagnostic.

MEDICAL MANAGEMENT

Medical management begins with water restriction. Diuretics and hypertonic saline solutions may also be prescribed. If the cause is the syndrome of inappropriate ADH (SIADH), in which excessive ADH from the posterior pituitary promotes increased water resorption in the renal tubules, secondary to surgery, anesthesia, narcotic use, or continuous parenteral administration of 5% dextrose in water (D_5W), treatment is to change the intravenous solution to dextrose in normal saline (0.9%) or dextrose in one-half normal saline (0.45%) or lactated Ringer's solution.

Prevention should be the main medical management for ICFVE. Continuous parenteral administration of D_5W and excess oral water intake dilute the vascular fluid, causing ICFVE. This is prevented by making certain that intravenous solutions and oral fluid intake contain solutes such as sodium chloride and other electrolytes.

Application of the Nursing Process to the Care of the Patient with Intracellular Fluid Volume Excess

Assessment

Assess for factors that place the patient at risk for ICFVE. Note the patient's age and explore any history of chronic or debilitating disease. Inquire specifically about any history of renal disease, and ask about current urinary output in terms of frequency and amount. Explore recent medical problems or treatments such as surgery, intravenous therapy, and enemas. Assess the patient's recent fluid intake. Determine the volume and type of both oral and intravenous fluids. Note the intake of hypo-osmolar fluids such as water, ice chips, and D_5W relative to the intake of iso-osmolar or hyperosmolar fluids.

Assess vital signs and compare them with baseline values. Observe for an increase in blood pressure; slow, bounding pulse; and an increased respiratory rate, which are signs of cerebral edema. Assess also for neurologic changes. Assess alertness and orientation, and ask about headache, vision changes, and projectile vomiting.

Check the patient's weight, because with ICFVE there is usually an acute weight gain. Assess for peripheral edema, which is slight with ICFVE.

Nursing Diagnoses and Planning

The nursing diagnoses and related expected patient outcomes most commonly applicable to patients with ICFVE or water intoxication include the following:

NDx: Fluid volume excess: water intoxication related to excess water intake, decrease in solutes, oversecretion of ADH, or renal dysfunction secondary to ICFVE

Planning: Patient outcomes
1. Serum osmolality returns to between 275 and 295 mOsm/kg.
2. Vital signs return to patient's baseline level.
3. Neurologic signs of brain-cell edema are absent.

NDx: High risk for injury related to incoordination, confusion, and convulsion

Planning: Patient outcomes
1. Patient complies with safety measures.
2. Patient remains free of injury.

Nursing Interventions

NDx: Fluid volume excess: water intoxication
Monitor fluid replacement. Keep in mind that if intravenous D_5W is given continuously and oral intake is only water and ice chips, ICFVE is likely to occur because dextrose is a solute that is metabolized quickly, leaving only water, which is a hypo-osmolar fluid. Ensure that several of the intravenous solutions contain saline (0.45% or 0.9%). When clear liquids are ordered, give broth because it contains solutes that increase the serum osmolality.

Monitor urinary output. As output increases, ICFVE should decrease.

NDx: High risk for injury
Protect the patient from falls or other injury that may result from incoordination or confusion. Keep the bedside rails up. Provide assistance and supervision if the patient is out of bed. Keep personal items and the call bell within reach. If the patient is confused, reorient with each interaction.

To decrease central nervous system (CNS) stimulation and the risk of seizures, maintain a quiet environment. Eliminate sources of loud noise and avoid sudden stimuli.

Institute seizure precautions to protect the patient from injury should a seizure occur.

Evaluation

Evaluate the effectiveness of nursing care for a patient with ICFVE by comparing the patient's status with the expected patient outcomes. Examples of specific outcomes for patients with ICFVE have been provided in the Planning section.

Electrolyte Imbalances

Electrolytes, found in ECF and ICF (Fig. 3–2), are compounds that produce an electrical charge when in fluid. These compounds break up into particles known as ions, which carry either a positive charge (cation) or a negative charge (anion). Positively charged electrolytes are potassium, sodium, calcium, and magnesium. Negatively charged electrolytes are chloride, bicarbonate, phosphate, and sulfate. The electrolytes that are most plentiful in the cells (ICF) are potassium and phosphate. Those most plentiful in the ECF are sodium, chloride, and bicarbonate.

The electrolytes that are cations (potassium, sodium, calcium, and magnesium) are discussed in relation to deficits and excesses. Names for these deficits and excesses are hypokalemia and hyperkalemia (potassium deficit and excess), hyponatremia and hypernatremia (sodium deficit and excess), hypocalcemia and hypercalcemia (calcium deficit and excess), and hypomagnesemia and hypermagnesemia (magnesium deficit and excess).

Potassium Imbalance

Potassium, the predominant intracellular cation, is essential for the transmission and conduction of nerve impulses and for contraction of skeletal, smooth, and cardiac muscle. Potassium is absorbed through the GI tract; and 80% to 90% of potassium is excreted by the kidneys. Potassium is not stored in the body, so a daily potassium intake of 40 to 60 mEq is needed. Foods rich in potassium include vegetables, fruits, dry fruits, nuts, and meats. Increased sodium intake promotes potassium loss.

Potassium is continually moving between the ICF and the ECF under control of the sodium-potassium pump. Normal potassium level in the cells (ICF) is 150 mEq/L, whereas the serum potassium level (ECF) is 3.5 to 5.3 mEq/L. Body potassium levels can be obtained only from intravascular (serum) fluid, so actual intracellular potassium levels are unknown. A serum potassium level less than 3.5 mEq/L is called hypokalemia, and a serum potassium level greater than 5.3 mEq/L is called hyperkalemia.

HYPOKALEMIA

ETIOLOGY

Decreased serum potassium is a common disorder that can result from an abnormal loss of potassium from the body, the movement of excessive amounts of potassium into the cells, or, rarely, inadequate intake. The major source of abnormal loss of potassium from the body is the GI tract. Because there are large amounts of potassium in the tract, vomiting, diarrhea (including that from abuse of laxatives), GI suction, and drainage from a fistula or an ostomy all result in loss of potassium. Hypokalemia is worsened if metabolic alkalosis develops, because this causes increased renal excretion of potassium. Other causes of abnormal potassium loss include increased aldosterone secretion (aldosterone promotes sodium retention and potassium excretion), use of steroids, and use of potassium-wasting diuretics such as the thiazides, ethacrynic acid, furosemide, or acetazolamide.

Hypokalemia resulting from the movement of large amounts of potassium from the ECF into the ICF occurs secondary to metabolic alkalosis. It also occurs as a result of excessive amounts of insulin in the blood (hyperinsulinism), as seen in patients receiving hyperalimentation therapy.

Hypokalemia resulting from insufficient intake of potassium is seen in patients maintained on NPO status for several days and in patients who receive

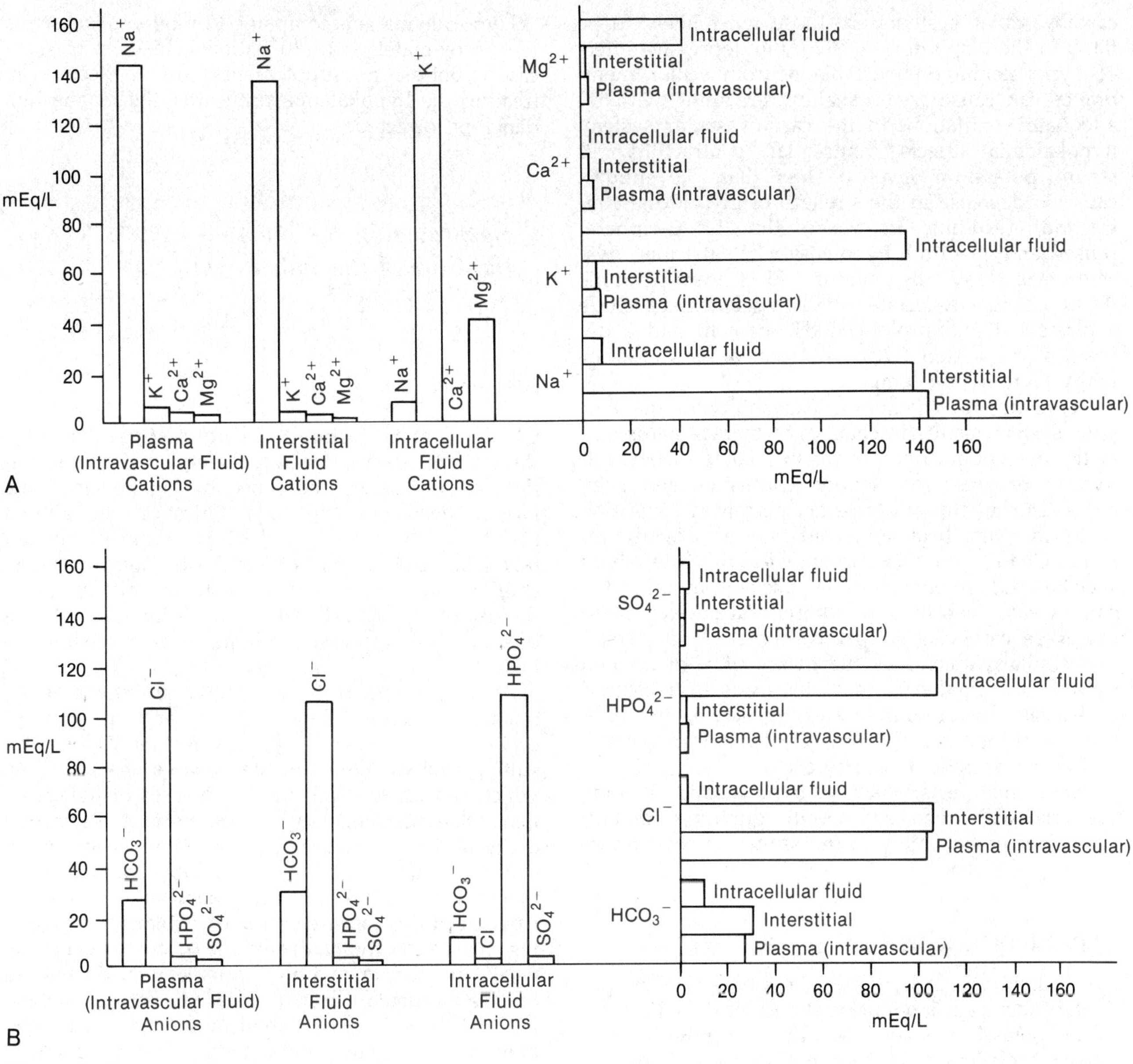

Figure 3–2.

Distribution of major cations (sodium, potassium, calcium, and magnesium) *(A)* and anions (bicarbonate, chloride, phosphate, and sulfate) *(B)* in body fluid compartments. (Na^+, sodium; K^+, potassium; Ca^{2+}, calcium; Mg^{2+}, magnesium; HCO_3^-, bicarbonate; Cl^-, chloride; HPO_4^{2-}, phosphate; SO_4^{2-}, sulfate.)

large volumes of parenteral fluids without a potassium supplement.

PATHOPHYSIOLOGY

Decreased serum potassium levels relative to intracellular potassium levels cause an increased resting potential in nerve and muscle fiber membranes, causing the membranes to be less readily excited. Further, when depolarization does occur, a return to the resting potential is slowed because membrane permeability to potassium is decreased. Thus, both decreased responsiveness to stimuli and slowed impulse transmission manifested as slowed neural response and decreased muscle contractility result from hypokalemia.

The severity of the pathophysiologic effects of hypokalemia is directly proportional to the rapidity with which the hypokalemia occurs.

CLINICAL MANIFESTATIONS

Clinical manifestations of hypokalemia involve most body systems. Effects on the respiratory and cardiovascular systems are those most likely to be fatal. In the respiratory system, the depressive effect of hypokalemia on excitable neuromuscular membranes can cause weak, shallow breathing with inadequate ventilation. In the cardiovascular system, hypokalemia affects ventricular contractility. A serum potassium level of less than 3.0 mEq/L causes a decrease in the strength of myocardial contraction, resulting in weak, thready peripheral pulses and postural hypotension. Ventricular dysrhythmias may also occur. Electrocardiographic (ECG) changes associated with hypokalemia include a depressed and prolonged ST segment and a depressed or inverted T wave. Cardiac arrest can occur with severe hypokalemia.

Depression of membrane excitability in the nervous system results in changes in mental status and tactile perception. Initial signs of anxiety or irritability can progress to lethargy, confusion, and even coma. During this progression, peripheral sensation of touch, pain, heat, and cold may also be diminished. Changes in tissue excitability also affect both skeletal and smooth muscle. Skeletal muscles become weak, deep tendon hyporeflexia develops, and in severe cases flaccid paralysis occurs. Hypokalemia similarly decreases the contractility of smooth muscle, and in the GI tract this leads to decreased peristalsis. Bowel sounds are hypoactive, and nausea, vomiting, constipation, abdominal distention, and even paralytic ileus may occur.

Renal manifestations of hypokalemia include polyuria, with decreased specific gravity secondary to the decreased ability of the kidney to concentrate urine.

MEDICAL DIAGNOSIS

The diagnosis of hypokalemia is based on the patient history and laboratory and clinical findings. A serum potassium level lower than 3.5 mEq/L indicates hypokalemia. It does not indicate, however, whether there is a real deficit of potassium or a shift from ECF to ICF.

MEDICAL MANAGEMENT

Medical management is designed to return the serum potassium level to within normal range and to correct the underlying cause of the hypokalemia to prevent recurrence.

Treatment instituted to return serum potassium to within normal range varies with the severity of the hypokalemia. If the serum potassium level is between 3.0 and 3.5 mEq/L, foods rich in potassium accompanied by an oral or intravenous potassium supplement are prescribed. One hundred to 200 mEq/L of intravenous potassium is needed to raise the serum level by 1 mEq/L. Larger deficits require 200 to 400 mEq/L of intravenous potassium to raise the serum level 1 mEq/L (Pharmacology Box 3–1).

Hypokalemia is accompanied by hypomagnesemia in approximately 4 of 10 patients. In most of these cases, potassium supplements are ineffective in treating the hypokalemia until after the magnesium deficit is corrected.

Application of the Nursing Process to the Care of the Patient with Hypokalemia

Assessment

Obtain a patient history to identify factors that place the patient at risk for hypokalemia. Note the patient's age, because the concentrating power of the kidney decreases with age. Question the patient about any history of renal disease, and obtain detailed information on both prescribed and over-the-counter medications taken. Ask specifically about the use of steroids, diuretics, and laxatives. Obtain a dietary history to assess adequacy of potassium intake.

Assess the patient for signs and symptoms of hypokalemia, noting time of onset and duration of each episode. Assess for respiratory insufficiency resulting from weakness of the muscles of respiration, which can cause death in severe cases of hypokalemia. Observe rate, depth, and effort of respiration every 2 hours. Auscultate for diminished breath sounds. Note the color of the nail beds and mucous membranes. Assess cardiovascular status. Check peripheral pulses for strength and regularity, recognizing that with hypokalemia the pulse is generally weak and thready with a variable rate, depending on the particular dysrhythmia presenting. Review ECG findings. Measure blood pressure while the patient is lying, sitting, and standing to check for postural hypotension. Assess mental status. Obtain baseline information on usual mental status, mood, and personality from a family member or significant other. Assess for tactile sensation (i.e., perception of touch, pain, heat, and cold). Assess for skeletal muscle weakness. Observe the patient's ability to move, stand, ambulate, and perform activities of daily living. Check lifts and grips. Assess GI function. Ask about nausea, vomiting, and constipation. Auscultate bowel sounds in all quadrants, and check for abdominal distention by measuring abdominal girth. Assess renal function. Measure urinary output and check specific gravity. Note color and volume of urine.

Nursing Diagnoses and Planning

Nursing diagnoses and related expected patient outcomes most commonly applicable to patients with

Pharmacology Box 3–1.

POTASSIUM SUPPLEMENTS

Potassium Supplements
Potassium preparations for oral or intravenous administration, designed to increase the amount of potassium, the principal intracellular cation, in the body. Most are in the form of potassium chloride.

Action
Potassium is essential for nerve impulse transmission and muscular contraction, tissue growth and repair, and maintenance of acid-base balance.

Uses
Oral supplements: prevention and treatment of mild hypokalemia.
Intravenous supplements: treatment of moderate to severe hypokalemia.

Side Effects
Nausea, vomiting, abdominal discomfort, diarrhea, ulceration, and gastrointestinal (GI) bleeding, skin rash, and hyperkalemia, which is characterized by paresthesias, muscle weakness progressing to flaccid paralysis, confusion, hypotension, and cardiac dysrhythmias. Intravenous preparations can cause chemical phlebitis and, if extravasated, tissue irritation and necrosis.

Interactions
Severe hyperkalemia can occur when potassium supplements are used concurrently with potassium-sparing diuretics or with salt substitutes containing potassium salts.

Increases in serum potassium decrease both effectiveness and toxicity of digitalis.

Anticholinergic agents increase the risk of GI ulceration resulting from oral potassium supplements because they decrease GI motility and gastric emptying.

Nursing Implications
Check for patient history of renal dysfunction, which would increase risk of hypercalcemia.
Never administer parenteral potassium intramuscularly or subcutaneously.
Always dilute intravenous preparation. Never give as a bolus.
Give slowly because rapid administration can cause severe hyperkalemia with cardiac dysrhythmias and cardiac arrest.
Always use a controller or pump for administration.
Do not mix intravenous potassium in solutions containing calcium or magnesium because precipitation results.
Protect against extravasation because severe irritation and necrosis result.
Monitor for chemical phlebitis at the site of administration because potassium is highly irritating.
Monitor electrolyte levels, electrocardiogram, and urinary output.
Stop potassium infusion if urinary output drops to less than 20 ml/hr for 2 consecutive hr.
Instruct patients on the correct use of oral potassium supplements as presented in Chart 3–1.

Geriatric Considerations
Elderly are at increased risk for hyperkalemia secondary to potassium replacement because of lower lean body mass and total body potassium. Decreased renal function that occurs with age can increase the amount of retained potassium. Elderly are at increased risk for ulcerative GI lesions.

Chart 3–1.

NURSING GUIDE TO PATIENT EDUCATION FOR SELF-MANAGEMENT: USE OF ORAL POTASSIUM SUPPLEMENTS

Instruct the patient in the following:

Dissolve liquid, powder, or effervescent tablets in 4 to 8 oz of cold fruit juice or water.
Measure liquids in drops to avoid overdose.
Wait until effervescent preparations have stopped fizzing before drinking.
Avoid chewing or breaking tablets unless they are specifically designated as "chewable."
Avoid dissolving tablets in the mouth because ulcerations can occur.
Expect a strong, salty taste.
Sip dissolved preparations over 5- to 10-min period.
Take in divided doses over the day as directed to help maintain extracellular fluid levels.
Take with meals to decrease gastrointestinal distress.
Return for scheduled visits and to have serum potassium levels measured.
Report muscle weakness, numbness, tingling, or pulse changes.
Observe for and report tarry or bloody stools.

varying degrees of hypokalemia include the following:

NDx: High risk for decreased cardiac output related to weak or dysrhythmic myocardial contraction

Planning: Patient outcomes
1. Vital signs remain within the individual's normal range.
2. ECG readings indicate a normal sinus rhythm.

NDx: High risk for injury related to muscle weakness and changes in mental status

Planning: Patient outcomes
1. Patient complies with safety precautions.
2. Patient uses assistance as needed.
3. Patient remains free of injury.

NDx: Constipation related to decreased peristalsis

Planning: Patient outcomes
1. Patient passes soft, formed stool at regular intervals.
2. Defecation occurs without undue straining.
3. Defecation occurs without pain.

NDx: High risk for altered health maintenance related to lack of knowledge of measures to prevent hypokalemia

Planning: Patient outcomes
1. Patient defines hypokalemia.
2. Patient lists good dietary sources of potassium.
3. Patient describes factors that can lead to hypokalemia.

Nursing Interventions

NDx: High risk for decreased cardiac output
Monitor cardiovascular status. Measure blood pressure when the patient is lying, sitting, and standing, because postural hypotension develops before a generalized hypotensive state. Report ECG changes such as prolonged, depressed ST segments and flat or inverted T waves, which are indicative of hypokalemia. Be alert for severe bradycardia and the development of heart block, especially in patients taking digitalis, because low serum potassium levels potentiate digitalis toxicity. Monitor serum potassium levels, and administer supplemental potassium according to the guidelines found in Chart 3–1.

NDx: High risk for injury
Protect the patient from accidental falls caused by muscle weakness or confusion. Keep the side rails up when the patient is in bed. Provide assistance and supervision when the patient is out of bed. Ensure that personal items are easily accessible to limit the need for reaching or for getting out of the bed or chair. Also keep the call bell within reach. Assist with self-care as necessary. If the patient is experiencing mental status changes, reorient to time and place with each interaction. Also restate who you are, what you are going to do, and what is expected of the patient.

NDx: Constipation
Explain the role of low serum potassium level in causing constipation. Reassure the patient that as the serum potassium level returns to normal range bowel function will begin to normalize. Within the

limits of any dietary restrictions, ensure that the patient is placed on a high-fiber diet and consumes 2500 ml of fluid per day. When possible, have the patient use a toilet or commode rather than a bedpan, and also provide privacy.

Encourage physical activity, whether it be bed exercises or ambulation, to promote bowel function. Administer drugs such as metoclopramide hydrochloride (Reglan), which stimulate GI activity, per physician's order.

NDx: High risk for altered health maintenance

Explain to the patient what hypokalemia is and how it can be prevented. Provide the patient with a list of foods high in potassium (bananas; oranges; cantaloupe; dates; raisins; avocado; apricots; dried fruits; green, leafy vegetables; broccoli; carrots; potatoes; beans; meats; nuts; coffee; cocoa; and cola beverages).

Stress the importance of including potassium-containing foods in the daily diet, especially if the patient is also taking drugs such as potassium-wasting diuretics, cortisone, laxatives, or lithium carbonate. Explain that cooking foods by prolonged boiling in water causes a loss of potassium, and suggest steaming or broiling as alternative preparation techniques. If the patient uses a salt substitute, explain that some contain potassium salts and, therefore, may provide all the extra dietary potassium needed. If oral potassium supplements are ordered, instruct the patient in correct administration, as presented in Pharmacology Box 3–1. If the patient is very weak, lethargic, or confused, instruct a family member or significant other in correct administration. Teach the correct use of laxatives and diuretics, and stress the importance of having blood for serum potassium levels drawn as scheduled. Tell the patient to report signs of hypokalemia: slow or irregular heartbeat, muscle cramps, numbness or tingling in the hands or the feet, weakness, difficulty concentrating, forgetfulness or confusion, constipation, abdominal distention, and nausea.

Additional Interventions

Chop or purée foods and assist the patient with eating if muscle weakness necessitated. Give small, frequent meals. If a GI tube is in place, irrigate the tube with normal saline to avoid electrolyte loss. Measure and record intake and output. Record and report signs and symptoms of progressive hypokalemia, and remember that immediate medical intervention is needed if the serum potassium level is lower than 3.0 mEq/L.

Evaluation

Evaluate the effectiveness of nursing care for a patient with hypokalemia by comparing the patient's status with the expected patient outcomes. Examples of specific outcomes for patients with hypokalemia have been provided in the Planning section.

HYPERKALEMIA

ETIOLOGY

Hyperkalemia occurs less often than hypokalemia and rarely in persons with normal renal function, because potassium is not stored in the body but is continuously excreted by the kidneys. When it does occur, it may be due to impaired potassium excretion, movement from ICF to ECF, or excessive intake. Impaired excretion can occur in kidney failure with oliguria; as a result of hypoaldosteronism secondary to adrenalectomy, adrenal insufficiency, or Addison's disease; or as an effect of potassium-sparing diuretics such as spironolactone (Aldactone) and amiloride (Midamor). Movement from ICF to ECF occurs secondary to starvation, surgery, burns, and crushing tissue injuries. It also occurs secondary to metabolic acidosis because, in the acidotic state, hydrogen ions are taken into the cells and potassium is released. Hyperkalemia resulting from excessive intake can develop as a result of overuse of potassium supplements or salt substitutes, rapid administration of intravenous potassium, or transfusion with blood in which cell damage has occurred. The last instance may result from blood storage for longer than 48 hours or from physical disruption of cells caused by improper handling or administration through a small access device.

PATHOPHYSIOLOGY

Increased serum potassium levels relative to the ICF level cause a decreased resting membrane potential, resulting in increased excitability of the membrane. However, repolarization is slow, and thus the additional time taken for return to resting membrane potential limits the speed of, and eventually prevents, response to stimuli. Of all excitable membranes, cardiac muscle is the most sensitive to hyperkalemia. As with hypokalemia, severity of pathophysiologic changes varies directly with the speed of onset of the increased serum potassium level.

CLINICAL MANIFESTATIONS

The cardiovascular system is most seriously affected by hyperkalemia. Hypotension and bradycardia occur sometimes preceded by tachycardia as well as ectopic beats. As the hyperkalemia worsens, ECG changes, a tall, peaked T wave, a prolonged PR interval, and a wide QRS complex, occur. There is risk of ventricular fibrillation and cardiac arrest as the serum potassium approaches 7 mEq/L. Neurologic symptoms associated with mild hyperkalemia are due to membrane hyperexcitability and include muscle twitching, cramps, and paresthesias. As hyperkalemia persists or worsens, neural responses to stimuli are slowed or blocked because of prolonged membrane repolarization time, and weakness progressing to flaccid paralysis in the muscles of the upper and lower extremities results. This begins in the hands and feet and progresses medially.

GI effects of hyperkalemia relate to increased GI motility. Bowel sounds are hyperactive, and nausea, abdominal cramping, and diarrhea occur.

MEDICAL DIAGNOSIS

The diagnosis of hyperkalemia is confirmed by a serum potassium level higher than 5.3 mEq/L.

MEDICAL MANAGEMENT

The treatment of hyperkalemia varies with its severity. With a slight elevation of serum potassium level, 5.3 to 5.6 mEq/L, potassium intake is restricted. A low-potassium diet is instituted, and all potassium supplements, parenteral solutions containing potassium, and drugs containing potassium, such as potassium penicillin, are eliminated. Blood transfusions are avoided whenever possible, but if required, only blood stored for fewer than 48 hours is used. For severe hyperkalemia, sodium polystyrene (Kayexalate) is administered to increase the excretion of potassium. This drug is a cation-exchange resin. It is nondigestible and in the GI tract releases sodium (Na^+) and absorbs potassium (K^+) before being excreted in the feces. It may be administered orally or rectally. Because time is required for the desired effect of the drug to be achieved in cases in which the potassium level is critically high, dialysis or ultrafiltration may be used to rid the body of the excess.

Measures designed to lower serum potassium level by promoting the movement of potassium from the ECF to the ICF can also be used. Glucose (10%–50%) with insulin may be given, because potassium moves with glucose into the cells. If acidosis is present, sodium bicarbonate may also be given to elevate the pH and further promote the movement of potassium into the cells. Calcium gluconate (10%) may be used to decrease the irritability of the myocardium.

Application of the Nursing Process to the Care of the Patient with Hyperkalemia

Assessment

Obtain a patient history to identify factors that place the patient at risk for hyperkalemia. Ask about any history of renal or adrenal disorders, and explore any recent medical or surgical problems and their treatment. If the patient denies any history of renal disease, ask specific questions about urinary output such as frequency, amount, and appearance of the urine. Question the patient about the use of prescribed and over-the-counter medications. Ask specifically about potassium-sparing diuretics. Review the patient's diet. Explore the intake of potassium-rich foods and use of salt substitutes containing potassium salts.

Assess the patient for signs and symptoms of hyperkalemia, noting time of onset and duration of each episode. Begin with cardiovascular status. Check pulse and blood pressure, and question the patient about palpitations and skipped beats. Review ECG results. Assess neuromuscular status. Ask about and observe for muscle twitching, cramping, and paresthesias. Assess for muscle weakness in the extremities: check lifts and grips. In regard to GI function, auscultate for hyperactive bowel sounds and ask about cramping and diarrhea.

Nursing Diagnoses and Planning

Nursing diagnoses and related expected patient outcomes most commonly applicable to patients with hyperkalemia include the following:

NDx: High risk for decreased cardiac output related to dysrhythmia secondary to the effect of hyperkalemia on the myocardium

Planning: Patient outcomes
1. Vital signs remain within the individual's normal range.
2. ECG readings indicate a normal sinus rhythm.

NDx: Diarrhea related to increased peristalsis

Planning: Patient outcomes
1. Stool is formed.
2. Frequency of defecation is consistent with patient's normal pattern.
3. Perianal skin remains free of irritation.

NDx: Altered health maintenance related to lack of knowledge of potassium restriction

Planning: Patient outcomes
1. Patient describes need to restrict potassium.
2. Patient identifies sources of potassium.
3. Patient describes plan for avoiding excessive potassium.

Nursing Interventions

Eliminate all external sources of potassium. In accordance with the physician's orders, discontinue parenteral infusions containing potassium, oral potassium supplements, and medications containing potassium. Also place the patient on a potassium-restricted diet. If the patient must have a blood transfusion, check that the blood has been stored for no longer than 48 hours; longer storage is associated with blood cell damage and release of intracellular potassium. Monitor urinary output to check renal function. Output should be at least 25 ml/hour or 600 ml/day.

NDx: High risk for decreased cardiac output
Monitor cardiovascular status. Be alert for hypotension, tachycardia or bradycardia, and ECG changes such as QRS spread and peaked T waves that occur as the serum potassium drops. Monitor serum potassium levels and report those greater than 5.3 mEq/L. Remember that levels greater than 7.0 mEq/L can cause cardiac arrest.

NDx: Diarrhea
Record the time, amount, and characteristics of stool passed. Administer medications prescribed to decrease intestinal motility. Provide a diet low in fiber residue and milk products to avoid stimulating peristalsis. Record intake and output. Increase fluid intake as necessary to maintain normal urine specific gravity. Provide fluids such as water and flat ginger ale, which are low in potassium and do not further stimulate peristalsis. For the latter reason, do not serve very hot or very cold liquids.

NDx: Altered health maintenance
Explain the risk of hyperkalemia to patients with renal dysfunction and to those taking potassium-sparing diuretics (spironolactone and amiloride). Stress the importance of adhering to a potassium-restricted diet. Provide patients with both a list of high-potassium foods to be avoided and a list of low-potassium foods, which may be ingested at will. Such low-potassium foods include cranberry juice, cranberry sauce, ginger ale, root beer, sugar, honey, jelly, beans, gumdrops, butter, and margarine. Caution patients that many salt substitutes contain potassium salts, and these should be used sparingly, if at all.

If the episode of hyperkalemia is related to the incorrect use of diuretics or potassium supplements, review the correct administration procedure and stress its importance.

Evaluation

Evaluate the effectiveness of nursing care for a patient with hyperkalemia by comparing the patient's status with the expected patient outcomes. Examples of specific outcomes for patients with hyperkalemia have been provided in the Planning section.

Sodium Imbalance

Sodium, the principal cation in the ECF, is essential for the conduction and transmission of nerve impulses, contraction of muscles, regulation of body fluid volumes, and regulation of the distribution and concentration of other electrolytes. The sodium-potassium pump keeps the concentration of sodium low in the ICF and high in the ECF.

Sodium, like potassium, is plentiful in the GI tract. The daily sodium requirement is 2 to 4 g; however, most Americans consume 5 to 15 g per day (1 teaspoon of salt contains 2.3 g of sodium). Sodium levels in the body are regulated by the kidney, which can excrete excess sodium or conserve sodium under the influence of aldosterone. When sodium levels decrease, serum osmolality decreases, and secretion of ADH by the posterior pituitary is inhibited. The subsequent decrease in ADH increases the excretion of water by the kidney. This results in less dilution of the sodium in the body fluids and therefore increases its concentration.

Decreases in sodium concentration are also picked up by sensors in the renal afferent arteriole. When this occurs, a series of reactions are initiated through the renin-angiotensin mechanism, resulting in increased secretion of aldosterone, which increases renal reabsorption of both sodium and water. The normal serum sodium level is 135 mEq/L. A serum sodium level less than 135 mEq/L is called hyponatremia, and a serum sodium level higher than 145 mEq/L is known as hypernatremia.

HYPONATREMIA

ETIOLOGY

Decreased serum sodium can result from dilution caused by excessive gain of water or by excessive loss of sodium. Hyponatremia from dilution is associated with an increase in ECF volume. Causes of this dilution-induced hyponatremia include the following: cardiac, renal, or hepatic failure; excessive irrigation of body cavities with water or other hypotonic fluids; and near-drowning in fresh water.

Excessive loss of sodium can occur in the presence of either normal or decreased ECF volume. Causes of hyponatremia with a normal ECF volume include diaphoresis with water but not electrolyte replacement, hyperglycemia, long-term use of drugs such as morphine sulfate or vincristine, and SIADH. In SIADH, excessive amounts of ADH are released from the posterior pituitary gland, which promotes increased water reabsorption in the renal tubules. The reabsorbed water dilutes the sodium concentration and causes hyponatremia. SIADH is seen in patients with head injuries and cerebrovascular accidents and for 1 or 2 days after surgery.

Hyponatremia with decreased ECF volume occurs secondary to hemorrhage, excessive wound drainage, vomiting, diarrhea, adrenal insufficiency, and use of diuretics.

PATHOPHYSIOLOGY

The pathophysiologic effects of hyponatremia are most pronounced on excitable membranes because the movement of sodium from the ECF across the membrane to the ICF is a primary trigger of depolarization. The most common effect of hyponatremia on excitable membranes is to depress them (i.e., make them less responsive to stimuli). The excitable membranes most sensitive to hyponatremia are those in the CNS, the neuromuscular tissues, and the smooth muscle of the GI system. Tissues such as cardiac muscle that autoinitiate depolarization are basically unaffected by a decrease in serum sodium.

In some cases, CNS hyperexcitability occurs instead of or in conjunction with depression. This happens if fluid shifts into the nerve cells secondary to decreased ECF osmolality and osmotic pressure caused by the decrease in sodium. This swelling of the brain can cause increased intracranial pressure, which depresses some nerve centers and stimulates others.

CLINICAL MANIFESTATIONS

The severity of the clinical manifestations of hyponatremia varies with the speed of onset and the extent of the sodium decrease. Of these two factors, however, speed is more critical, and a patient with mild to moderate rapid-onset hyponatremia has clinical manifestations of greater severity than a patient with more severe hyponatremia of gradual onset.

The most common CNS manifestations of hyponatremia include headache, decreased attention span, drowsiness, and confusion. Less commonly, signs of hyperexcitability such as apprehension, agitation, and seizures occur.

Neuromuscular symptoms include generalized muscular weakness with decreased muscle tone and deep tendon hyporeflexia. Motility of the GI smooth muscle is increased, and nausea, abdominal cramping, and frequent, explosive passage of watery stool result.

When hyponatremia is accompanied by a fluid volume change, cardiovascular symptoms also occur. If hypovolemia coexists, the pulse is rapid, weak, and thready; peripheral pulses are easily obliterated; and an orthostatic progression to generalized hypotension develops. If hypervolemia coexists, pulses are full and strong, and blood pressure is normal or elevated.

Urinary specific gravity in hyponatremia is less than 1.008. Other renal manifestations vary with ECF volume and underlying disease. In SIADH, urinary output is decreased, accompanied by weight gain without peripheral edema.

MEDICAL DIAGNOSIS

History of the health problem, laboratory findings (serum sodium and serum osmolality), and clinical findings are used in the medical diagnosis of a sodium imbalance.

The osmolality of the plasma or serum is determined mainly by the concentration of sodium. When the serum sodium level is decreased, the plasma/serum osmolality is also decreased. Normal serum osmolality is 275 to 295 mOsm/kg. Serum osmolality of less than 275 mOsm/kg indicates hypo-osmolality, fluid volume excess, or hyponatremia.

MEDICAL MANAGEMENT

Oral sodium replacement is usually prescribed for mild hyponatremia resulting from excessive loss of sodium. For moderate hyponatremia, 125 mEq/L, intravenous solutions of normal saline (0.9% sodium chloride) or lactated Ringer's solution may be ordered. With severe hyponatremia, 115 mEq/L, concentrated saline solutions (3% sodium chloride) are generally indicated.

If the hyponatremia is due to dilution secondary to fluid volume excess, sodium may not need to be replaced. In such cases, sodium-conserving water-excreting diuretics such as the osmotic diuretics, water restriction, and the treatment of the underlying disorder may return the serum sodium level to normal.

In the treatment of hyponatremia caused by SIADH, ADH receptor blockers or ADH antagonists may be used.

Application of the Nursing Process to the Care of the Patient with Hyponatremia

Assessment

Obtain a patient history to identify factors that place the patient at risk for hyponatremia. Note the patient's age, and question the patient about any history of renal, cardiac, or hepatic disorders. Ask about any recent episodes of vomiting, diarrhea, or fever. Ascertain what prescribed or over-the-counter medications the patient uses, making certain to specifically inquire about diuretics, morphine, and chemotherapeutic agents. Explore the patient's usual diet. Determine whether the patient purposefully limits salt and, if so, how. For example, determine whether the patient avoids the use of table salt, avoids cooking with salt, limits high-salt foods, or uses a salt substitute. Question the patient about recent activities, especially strenuous activities in a hot, humid environment in which marked diaphoresis can be expected.

Assess the patient for signs and symptoms of hyponatremia, noting time of onset of each episode. Assess neuromuscular status. Obtain baseline information on the patient's usual mental status from a family member or significant other, and inquire whether any changes have been noted. Assess the patient's current orientation and alertness. Ask about headaches, drowsiness, and lethargy. Check lifts and grips to assess muscle tone. Check patellar and Achilles tendon reflexes. Auscultate for hyperactive bowel sounds, and ask about nausea, cramping, and diarrhea. Question the patient about the frequency and amount of urination. Observe the color of urine and measure its specific gravity. Assess cardiovascular status. Check apical rate, blood pressure, peripheral pulses, and venous filling capacity. Observe for edema.

Nursing Diagnoses and Planning

Nursing diagnoses and related expected patient outcomes most commonly applicable to patients with varying degrees of hyponatremia include the following:

NDx: Diarrhea related to increased GI motility

Planning: Patient outcomes
1. Stool is formed.
2. Frequency of defecation is consistent with patient's normal pattern.
3. Perianal area remains free of irritation.

NDx: High risk for injury related to potential altered thought processes and muscle weakness

Planning: Patient outcomes
1. Patient complies with safety precautions.
2. Patient remains free of injury.

NDx: Pain (headache) related to increased intracranial pressure secondary to intracellular edema

Planning: Patient outcomes
1. Patient complies with position restrictions.
2. Patient reports relief of headache.

NDx: High risk for altered health maintenance related to lack of knowledge of dietary sodium and water requirements

Planning: Patient outcomes
1. Patient describes need for increased dietary sodium.
2. Patient identifies food high in sodium.
3. Patient affirms plan to ingest needed daily sodium.

Nursing Interventions

Administer saline infusions per physician's order. Use a controller or a pump to control rate because too rapid administration can cause serious problems as a result of overresponse of excitable membranes. A general principle is that the rate of replacement of sodium should parallel the rate of loss.

Monitor the patient for signs and symptoms of fluid volume excess when the patient is receiving saline solutions, especially concentrated saline solutions.

Administer diuretics as ordered. Record intake and output, and monitor the patient closely for signs and symptoms of excessive loss of fluid or potassium. Also monitor for signs and symptoms of too rapid or excessive sodium increase.

NDx: Diarrhea
Explain to the patient or significant other that diarrhea will be relieved as sodium is replaced. Assist patient onto the bedpan or to the bathroom promptly. Protect the perianal skin by gentle washing with mild soap and warm water. Apply a skin-barrier ointment. If perianal irritation develops despite precautions, apply witch hazel compresses or topical anesthetic ointment. Record the time, amount, and characteristics of stool passed.

NDx: High risk for injury
Protect the patient from injury that may result from muscle weakness or confusion. Keep the side rails up when the patient is in bed. Provide assistance and supervision when the patient is out of bed. Keep the call bell within reach. Also keep personal items within reach to limit the need for reaching or getting out of the bed or chair. Provide a quiet environment free of unnecessary stimuli, because the patient with hyponatremia is abnormally sensitive to sensory input. Remove the telephone and eliminate loud noise from the television, radio, and the like. Reorient the patient to time and place with each interaction if needed.

NDx: Pain
Administer analgesics for headache as ordered. Keep in mind that morphine aggravates SIADH and should be avoided if this is the cause of the hyponatremia. Keep the head of the bed elevated to promote venous return from the brain. Also instruct the patient to avoid bending over, because this causes an increase in intracranial pressure.

NDx: High risk for altered health maintenance
The patient who is losing abnormal amounts of sodium but on a regular diet should be instructed

about the need to ingest daily fluids and foods high in sodium. Provide a list of dietary sources of sodium, including condiments. Suggest nutritious, sodium-rich snacks that are easy to prepare and ingest, such as tomato juice and beef bouillon. Advise the patient against drinking plain water.

If fluids are also restricted, explain the reason to the patient. Encourage the patient to plan a spaced pattern of fluid intake over each 24-hour period to avoid ingesting the entire amount of fluids permitted early in the day, thus leaving a period of thirst. Teach patients to monitor intake and output.

Evaluation

Evaluate the effectiveness of nursing care for a patient with hyponatremia by comparing the patient's status with the expected patient outcomes. Examples of specific outcomes for patients with hyponatremia have been provided in the Planning section.

HYPERNATREMIA

ETIOLOGY

Hypernatremia develops as a result of either excessive sodium in the body or concentration of normal amounts of sodium because of the loss of water. Excessive sodium in the body can be due to excessive intake or to decreased renal excretion. Sources of excessive intake include sodium chloride in foods, sodium bicarbonate preparations, and sodium-containing parenteral fluids. Causes of decreased renal excretion include renal insufficiency, hyperaldosteronism, Cushing's disease, and the use of cortical steroids. Hypernatremia from concentration of sodium resulting from the loss of water can be caused by decreased fluid intake or increased water loss. Causes of increased water loss include excessive diaphoresis, hyperventilation, pyrexia, diarrhea, and osmotic diuresis.

PATHOPHYSIOLOGY

An increase in serum sodium results in a greater concentration gradient for sodium between the ECF and the ICF. This means that sodium passes more easily across excitable membranes and thus initiates depolarization more quickly and in response to less intense stimuli (i.e., the excitable membranes become irritable). As hypernatremia worsens, however, the opposite effect sets in. Water moves out of the cells into the ECF in an attempt to dilute the sodium concentration, and this leaves the cells dehydrated and excitable membranes nonresponsive to stimuli. The excitable membranes most sensitive to these changes are those of the brain, skeletal muscle, cardiac muscle, and, last, smooth muscle.

CLINICAL MANIFESTATIONS

Symptoms of hypernatremia depend on the severity and speed of the sodium increase and the presence or absence of a coexisting volume imbalance. Mental status changes that occur with hypernatremia in the presence of normal or decreased fluid volumes include shortened attention span, lack of concentration, hypersensitivity to sensory stimuli, agitation, confusion, and even convulsions.

When hypernatremia is accompanied by increased fluid volume, mental activity is depressed, and lethargy, drowsiness, stupor, and coma can occur. Changes in skeletal muscles proceed from twitching and spasms with mild levels of hypernatremia to weakness with hyporeflexia and even rigid paralysis as the hypernatremia worsens.

The effect of hypernatremia on cardiac muscle is generally depressive, manifested by decreased contractility and decreased cardiac output. Pulse and blood pressure vary with fluid volume changes as described under Hyponatremia. Changes in the skin that occur with hypernatremia also vary with fluid volume status. When ECF volume is decreased, the skin is pale and has poor turgor. With increased ECF volume, color ranges from pale to flushed and turgor is increased (i.e., skin does not pinch up and pressure leaves depressions that are very slow to disappear). In all cases, the skin is dry and flaky.

Renal changes also occur as a result of hypernatremia. Urinary output is decreased, and the urine is concentrated (specific gravity >1.025) and is marked by a strong odor.

MEDICAL DIAGNOSIS

History, clinical findings, serum sodium, and serum osmolality all contribute to the diagnosis of hypernatremia. Serum sodium levels higher than 145 mEq/L are indicative of hypernatremia. A serum osmolality higher than 295 mOsml/kg indicates hyperosmolality, fluid volume deficit, and hypernatremia.

MEDICAL MANAGEMENT

Management of hypernatremia depends on its severity as well as the underlying cause. Dietary restriction of sodium, often in conjunction with water restriction, can prevent hypernatremia when renal excretion of sodium is impaired and can prevent existing hypernatremia from worsening. It cannot rapidly lower serum sodium levels. Loop diuretics (furosemide and ethacrynic acid), which are sodium excreting, are used to increase the renal excretion of sodium and therefore lower serum levels if renal function allows. If hypernatremia is due to fluid loss, parenteral administration of glucose and water is used to restore volume, thus diluting sodium concentration and returning serum sodium level to normal range.

Application of the Nursing Process to the Care of the Patient with Hypernatremia

Assessment

Obtain a patient history to identify factors that place the patient at risk for hypernatremia. Question the patient about any history of renal disease, adrenal disease, or recent episodes of fever, vomiting, diarrhea, or diaphoresis. Assess for factors that might indicate that the patient has difficulty maintaining oral fluid intake. Note the patient's age and mental and mobility status. Ascertain what prescribed or over-the-counter medications the patient takes. Specifically, explore the use of osmotic diuretics as well as drugs that contain sodium, such as cortisone preparations, certain antibiotics, cough syrups, and cold medications. Explore also the patient's dietary intake of sodium. Identify usual intake of high-sodium foods, including processed and canned foods, fluids, and condiments. Establish fluid intake for the past 24 hours, noting both the type and the amount of ingested fluids. Also establish the frequency and amount of urinary output.

Assess the patient for signs and symptoms of hypernatremia, noting the time of onset of each episode. Assess neuromuscular status. Ask about the presence of insomnia, irritability, agitation, muscle twitches, or convulsions. Observe for signs of confusion or inability to maintain attention. Assess for signs of late or severe hypernatremia and hyperkalemia: Check for hypoactive, deep tendon reflexes; check lifts and grips to assess muscle weakness; and observe for lethargy.

Assess cardiovascular status: Measure blood pressure and heart rate. Check the quality of peripheral pulses. Observe the neck veins for distention. Observe for dry, flaky skin, and inspect the oral mucous membranes for dryness. Check skin turgor and note skin color. Measure urinary output, and note the color and odor of the urine.

Review serum sodium and osmolality values. Remember that doubling the serum sodium level gives an estimate of the serum osmolality value.

Nursing Diagnoses and Planning

Nursing diagnoses and related expected patient outcomes most commonly applicable to patients with varying degrees of hypernatremia include the following:

NDx: High risk for injury related to CNS irritability

Planning: Patient outcomes

1. Patient complies with safety measures
2. Patient remains free of injury.

NDx: Altered nutrition: more than body requirements related to excessive sodium intake

Planning: Patient outcomes

1. Patient states reason for sodium-restricted diet.
2. Patient identifies sources of dietary sodium to be avoided.
3. Patient selects and plans low-sodium meals and snacks.

Nursing Interventions

NDx: High risk for injury

Protect the patient from injury that may be caused by muscle weakness, confusion, or convulsions. Keep the side rails up, the bed low, and the call bell within reach. Provide assistance with moving and self-care activities. If the patient is confused, reorient at each interaction. To decrease CNS stimulation and the risk of seizures, maintain a calm, quiet environment. Eliminate bright lights, loud noises, and sudden movement. Pad the side rails of the bed to guard against injury if a seizure occurs.

NDx: Altered nutrition: more than body requirements

Explain the role of dietary sodium in hypernatremia. Stress the importance of adhering to a sodium-restricted diet. Discuss sources of ingested sodium with the patient, and provide a list of high-sodium foods to be avoided. These include canned foods, lunch meats, ham, pork, pickles, potato chips, and pretzels. Caution the patient to avoid using salt when cooking or eating. See Charts 20–2 and 20–3 for additional information on sodium restriction.

Evaluation

Evaluate the effectiveness of nursing care for a patient with hypernatremia by comparing the patient's status with the expected patient outcomes. Examples of specific outcomes for patients with hypernatremia have been provided in the Planning section.

Calcium Imbalance

Calcium, an extracellular and intracellular electrolyte, has many functions. It is essential for (1) transmission of nerve impulses and contraction of the skeletal, smooth, and cardiac muscles; (2) maintenance of cellular permeability; (3) formation of teeth and bones; and (4) coagulation of blood. Approximately 55% of serum calcium is bound to albumin, and 45% is free ionized calcium. It is the free calcium that is physiologically active and is affected by pH. During acidosis (decreased pH), more calcium is ionized even if the serum calcium level is decreased, and during alkalosis (increased pH), there is a decrease in free ionized calcium.

The normal total serum calcium level is 4.5 to 5.5 mEq/L or 9 to 11 mg/dl, and the ionized calcium level is 2.2 to 2.5 mEq/L or 4.5 to 5.0 mg/dl. The serum calcium result given in laboratory reports is the combined ionized and non-ionized calcium. A decreased serum calcium level, less than 4.5 mEq/L, is called hypocalcemia, and an increased serum calcium level, more than 5.5 mEq/L, is known as hypercalcemia.

Vitamin D promotes calcium absorption from the GI tract, and phosphorus inhibits calcium absorption. The physiologic relationship of calcium and phosphorus is inverse. Both calcium and phosphorus are stored in bone and excreted by the kidneys. When the serum calcium level is increased, the serum phosphorus is decreased. Parathyroid hormone (PTH) maintains the serum calcium level; however, PTH and vitamin D promote calcium movement from the bone to the vascular fluid, causing an increase in the serum calcium level. Phosphorus and calcitonin (from the thyroid gland) promote calcium return to the bone, causing a decrease in serum calcium level.

HYPOCALCEMIA

ETIOLOGY

Calcium deficit or hypocalcemia usually occurs when there is a decreased absorption of calcium from the GI tract, a decreased release of calcium from the bone, an increase in calcium binding to albumin (less free calcium), and an increased loss of calcium by urine excretion. With renal failure, the serum calcium level is decreased and the serum phosphorus level is increased.

Decreased absorption from the GI tract can be due to inadequate intake of calcium or vitamin D, lactase deficiency, Crohn's disease, or other malabsorption disorders. A decrease in the release of calcium from the bone may be due to a lack of PTH. This can occur as a result of a loss of parathyroid tissue secondary to thyroidectomy or radiation. It can also be the result of neck injuries. An increase in protein-bound calcium, and therefore a decrease in the ionized fraction of calcium, can be the result of hyperproteinemia, alkalosis, calcium chelates or binders such as citrate, and acute pancreatitis. Because citrate is a chelating agent (binds ionized calcium), temporary hypocalcemia may occur as a result of the massive administration of citrated blood. Calcium can also be lost through diarrhea, steatorrhea, wound drainage, and the action of loop diuretics such as furosemide.

PATHOPHYSIOLOGY

Calcium normally acts as a sedative on nervous tissue; therefore, hypocalcemia leads to nervous irritability. Decreased serum calcium levels increase permeability of excitable membranes to sodium. As a result, the membrane is more readily depolarized and an action potential is easily generated. Tissues most affected by hypocalcemia are peripheral nerves, skeletal muscles, and GI smooth muscle, whose actions are stimulated, and cardiac muscle, the contraction of which is depressed. Prolonged hypocalcemia leads to osteoporosis, and a very marked or prolonged decrease in serum calcium can interfere with the conversion of prothrombin to thrombin and thus impair clotting.

CLINICAL MANIFESTATIONS

The most common clinical manifestation of hypocalcemia (decreased ionized calcium) is tetany. This is a condition resulting from the excitability of peripheral nerves and muscles characterized by tingling and numbness of the extremities, muscle twitching, cramps, carpopedal spasm, laryngeal spasm, and convulsions. Typically, the onset of tetany is heralded by paresthesias (numbness and tingling) of the hands and feet. As the condition progresses, carpopedal spasm, twitching of the mouth, and sustained contraction of individual muscle groups ensure and can lead to convulsions, respiratory paralysis, and death. Tetany does not occur with metabolic acidosis, even when the serum calcium level is decreased, because more albumin-bound calcium is freed as the pH is decreased. It is when the acidotic state is corrected and calcium rebinds with protein that tetany symptoms might occur.

Other clinical manifestations of hypocalcemia include diarrhea resulting from increased intestinal motility, restlessness, and lack of concentration. Marked hypocalcemia may also result in a weak, slightly more rapid heartbeat.

MEDICAL DIAGNOSIS

The diagnosis of hypocalcemia is based on history, laboratory results, and clinical findings. A serum calcium level less than 4.5 mEq/L and 9 mg/dl indicates hypocalcemia.

Tetany resulting from a decrease in free ionized calcium can be confirmed by a positive Chvostek test and positive Trousseau's test. For the Chvostek test, the patient's face is tapped over the facial nerve (2 cm anterior to the ear lobe). If the facial muscle twitches, the test is positive (Fig. 3–3*A*). The Trousseau test is performed by inflating a blood pressure cuff on the upper arm to slightly above the systolic presence to constrict circulation. If carpal spasm (palmar flexion) of the hand occurs after 1 to 5 minutes, the test is positive (Fig. 3–3*B*).

MEDICAL MANAGEMENT

Acute hypocalcemia requires immediate medical intervention. Calcium gluconate or calcium chloride

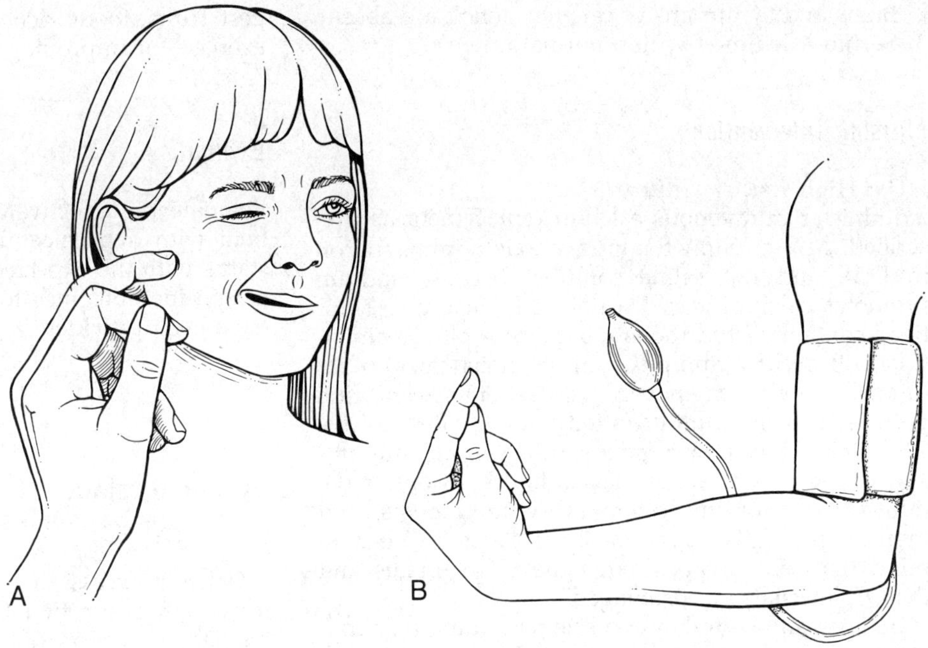

Figure 3–3.

Manifestations of hypocalcemia. *A,* Positive Chvostek's sign. A tap on the facial nerve anterior to the ear lobe below the zygomatic process causes a spasm in muscles supplied by the facial nerve. *B,* Positive Trousseau's sign. Carpal spasm occurs when compression of the upper arm causes ischemia to the distal nerves.

is given intravenously to correct acute hypocalcemia. Calcium chloride provides more ionized calcium than calcium gluconate. However, it is more irritating to the subcutaneous tissue; and if calcium chloride infiltrates, sloughing of the tissue results.

In cases of mild hypocalcemia, oral calcium supplements (calcium carbonate, calcium gluconate, or calcium lactate) are prescribed. For best absorption, these supplements are taken a half-hour before meals.

Aluminum hydroxide is sometimes used to treat hypocalcemia because it decreases serum phosphorus, which in turn increases serum calcium. Magnesium preparations are also used because an increase in serum magnesium results in an increase in serum calcium. Vitamin D may be prescribed in an effort to increase the absorption of calcium from the GI tract.

Application of the Nursing Process to the Care of the Patient with Hypocalcemia

Assessment

Question the patient about any history of health problems that can cause hypocalcemia. Ask about hypoparathyroidism, previous thyroidectomy, radiation, or injury to the neck. Question the patient about any chronic diarrhea, and check for overuse of laxatives or antacids. Obtain a dietary history to assess intake of calcium and vitamin D. Question the patient about usual intake of dairy products, legumes, and other foods rich in calcium and vitamin D. Also question the patient about the use of calcium and vitamin D supplements. Determine the patient's activity level and the usual amount of exposure of the skin to sunlight.

Assess for signs and symptoms of hypocalcemia such as numbness and tingling in the hands or feet; carpopedal spasm; twitching of the mouth; laryngeal spasm; abdominal cramping; hyperactive bowel sounds; diarrhea; rapid, weak pulse; and bleeding tendencies. Check for positive Chvostek's and Trousseau's signs. Review serum calcium levels.

Nursing Diagnoses and Planning

The nursing diagnoses and related expected patient outcomes most commonly applicable to patients with acute hypocalcemia include the following:

NDx: High risk for injury related to tetany secondary to hypocalcemia

Planning: Patient outcomes
1. Serum calcium level returns to normal range.
2. Signs of skeletal muscle hyperexcitability are absent.

The nursing diagnosis and related expected patient outcomes most commonly applicable to patients with chronic hypocalcemia are as follows:

NDx: Altered nutrition: less than body requirements related to inadequate intake of calcium or vitamin D

Planning: Patient outcomes
1. Patient reports adequate dietary intake of calcium.

2. Signs and symptoms of calcium deficit are absent.
3. Serum calcium is within normal range.

Nursing Interventions

NDx: High risk for injury
Administer intravenous calcium replacement as prescribed. Mix calcium for intravenous administration in D_5W and not saline solution, because sodium promotes calcium loss. Do not add calcium to solutions containing bicarbonate because rapid precipitation will occur. Administer intravenous calcium solutions slowly whenever the patient's condition permits. During administration, monitor for positive Chvostek's and Trousseau's signs every 15 minutes and check serum calcium levels hourly. Monitor the infusion site for infiltration every 15 minutes, and monitor the ECG continuously if possible. Keep in mind that with hypocalcemia the ST segments and the QT intervals are prolonged.

Because any stimulation of the neuromuscular condition can worsen the tetanic condition, control environmental stimuli. If Chvostek's and Trousseau's signs are positive, maintain the patient on complete bed rest in a quiet, darkened room. Avoid unnecessarily touching the patient, and protect against loud noises, bright lights, and sudden position changes. Avoid accidentally bumping the patient's bed, turn off the ringer on the telephone, eliminate access to television, and limit visitors. Maintain seizure precautions: Keep the side rails up and padded, and keep the bed in its lowest position. Have oxygen, suction, ventilation (Ambu) bag, and tracheostomy tray readily available at the patient's bedside.

NDx: Altered nutrition: less than body requirements
Suggest that the patient consume foods high in calcium, such as milk, milk products, and protein. Protein is needed to enhance calcium absorption. Administer oral calcium supplements before or after meals.

Monitor the pulse regularly if the patient is receiving a digitalis preparation as well as calcium supplements. Calcium excess enhances the action of digitalis and can cause digitalis toxicity, which is characterized by nausea, vomiting, anorexia, bradycardia, cardiac dysrhythmias, and visual changes.

Additional Interventions
Instruct the patient to avoid overuse of antacids and to avoid the chronic laxative habit. Excessive use of certain antacids can cause alkalosis, decreasing calcium ionization. In addition, many antacids contain magnesium, which can lower the serum calcium level. Many laxatives contain phosphates (phosphorus), which have an opposing effect on calcium, causing calcium loss. Chronic use of laxatives decreases calcium absorption from the GI tract. Suggest fruits, foods rich in fiber, plenty of fluids, and exercise for improving bowel elimination.

Evaluation

Evaluate the effectiveness of nursing care for a patient with hypocalcemia by comparing the patient's status with the expected patient outcomes. Examples of specific outcomes for patients with hypocalcemia have been provided in the Planning section.

HYPERCALCEMIA

ETIOLOGY

Calcium excess, or hypercalcemia, can result from increased absorption, decreased excretion, or increased resorption of calcium from bone. Increased absorption can occur secondary to excessive oral intake of either calcium or vitamin D. Decreased excretion can be due to renal failure or the use of thiazide diuretics (hydrochlorothiazide [HydroDIURIL]). Increased resorption from bone can be caused by prolonged immobilization, cancer that causes bone destruction, hyperparathyroidism, and use of glucocorticoids. Fractures also cause a release of calcium into the vascular fluid, thus increasing the serum calcium level.

PATHOPHYSIOLOGY

Increased levels of calcium in ECF (hypercalcemia) decrease the permeability of excitable membranes to sodium. This means that the membranes are less easily depolarized, and action potentials are less easily generated. Depression or decreased irritability of the excitable membrane is the result. Excitable membranes most sensitive to this effect of hypercalcemia are found in cardiac muscle, skeletal muscle, smooth muscle of the GI tract, and peripheral and CNS tissue.

Hypercalcemia also affects many enzyme systems within the body, including those involved in blood clotting. The effect of hypercalcemia on the latter is to decrease clotting time, thus predisposing to excessive clot formation, particularly in areas of slow blood flow.

CLINICAL MANIFESTATIONS

The clinical manifestations of hypercalcemia are most pronounced in systems containing excitable membranes easily depressed by the increase in calcium. The severity of the clinical manifestations is generally a function of both the amount of calcium increase and the speed with which it occurs (i.e., the greater the increase and the faster it develops, the more severe the symptoms). Rapid onset of mild hypercalcemia may present with more serious clinical manifestations than the gradual onset of a more marked hypercalcemia.

Clinical manifestations of hypercalcemia related to the GI tract include anorexia, nausea, constipation, abdominal distention, and decreased bowel sounds. Effects of hypercalcemia on neuromuscular function include weak, flabby muscles; diminished or absent deep tendon reflexes; lack of coordination; slurred speech; lethargy; memory lapses; and depression. In severe cases, confusion, psychotic behavior, or coma may also occur. In the heart, effects on both muscle function and electrical conduction occur. These result in tachycardia; elevated blood pressure; full, bounding peripheral pulses; and a shortened QT interval on ECG. With severe hypercalcemia, bradycardia and even cardiac standstill can occur. Hypercalcemia also affects renal function. The increased extracellular calcium results in polyuria, which in turn can lead to dehydration. Renal calculi or kidney stones characterized by flank pain can also develop as a result of the precipitation of excess calcium.

Hypercalcemic crisis occurs when the serum calcium levels are 16 to 17 mg/dl. Clinical manifestations include severe thirst, polyuria, altered levels of consciousness (confusion to coma), nausea, vomiting, and severe abdominal pain. Correction of a hypercalcemic crisis state is a medical emergency.

MEDICAL DIAGNOSIS

The diagnosis of hypercalcemia is suggested by history and clinical findings. The diagnosis is confirmed by a serum calcium level higher than 5.5 mEq/L and 11 mg/dl.

MEDICAL MANAGEMENT

Medical management of hypercalcemia is aimed at promoting calcium excretion while limiting sources of external calcium. No intravenous fluids containing calcium (e.g., calcium gluconate) are administered. All thiazide diuretics, antacids containing calcium, calcium supplements, and vitamin supplements are discontinued. To promote calcium excretion, intravenous isotonic saline may be given both to dilute the ECF and to provide sodium, which inhibits the tubular (resorption of calcium. Loop diuretics such as furosemide (Lasix), which enhance calcium excretion, may be given, as can calcium binders or chelates such as the cytotoxic antibiotic mithramycin (plicamycin). Drugs such as calcitonin (Calcimar) and prostaglandin inhibitors (acetylsalicylic acid and nonsteroidal anti-inflammatory drugs), which inhibit calcium resorption from bone, may also be administered. In acute cases of hypercalcemia in which immediate lowering of the serum calcium level is necessary, dialysis may be performed.

Application of the Nursing Process to the Care of the Patient with Hypercalcemia

Assessment

Question the patient about any history of health problems associated with hypercalcemia: cancer, parathyroidism, immobility, hyperthyroidism, and renal failure. Ask about the patient's use of medications with the potential for affecting calcium levels; glucocorticoids, thiazide diuretics, calcium or vitamin D supplements, and antacids. Explore the usual daily intake of milk and other dairy products.

Assess for signs and symptoms of hypercalcemia. Review serum calcium levels. Ask the patient about anorexia, nausea, and constipation. Assess for abdominal distention and listen to bowel sounds. Assess muscle tone, strength, and deep tendon reflexes. Observe for coordination and check orientation. Question a family member or significant other about the patient's usual level of alertness, interest, and activity to establish a basis for assessment of mental status changes. Assess cardiac status. Observe for changes in heart rate and rhythm, and review ECG strips for changes in the QT interval. Measure urinary output, and question the patient about symptoms of renal calculi. Assess for factors leading to slow or impaired blood flow, because the patient with hyperglycemia is prone to the development of blood clots. Note the time of onset of all reported symptoms.

Nursing Diagnoses and Planning

Nursing diagnoses and related expected patient outcomes most commonly applicable to patients with hypercalcemia include the following:

NDx: Constipation related to decreased intestinal motility

Planning: Patient outcomes
1. Patient defecates at regular intervals.
2. Stool is soft and moist.
3. Patient defecates without straining.

NDx: High risk for injury related to muscle weakness, incoordination, memory lapses, and confusion

Planning: Patient outcomes
1. Patient complies with safety precautions.
2. Patient remains free of injury.

Nursing Interventions

Discontinue all calcium-containing parenteral fluids and oral medications per physician's order. Administer diuretics that enhance calcium excretion or drugs that inhibit calcium resorption from bone as ordered. Promote active and passive exercises for the bedridden patient to decrease calcium loss from the bone. Instruct the patient to avoid foods high in calcium and to increase fluid intake to dilute calcium in the serum and to decrease the risk of urinary calculi.

NDx: Constipation
Explain the role of elevated serum calcium in causing constipation. Reassure the patient that, as serum calcium returns to normal, bowel function will also begin to normalize. Within the limits of any dietary restrictions, encourage a high-fiber diet and the consumption of 2500 ml of fluid or more per day. When possible, have the patient use a toilet or commode rather than a bedpan, and always provide for privacy.

Encourage physical activity, whether it be bed exercises or ambulation, to promote bowel function. Administer drugs to stimulate GI activity as ordered.

NDx: High risk for injury
Institute measures to protect the patient from falls or other injuries that may result from muscle weakness, incoordination, or mental status changes. Keep the side rails of the bed up and the call bell within easy reach. Provide assistance and supervision when the patient is out of bed. Keep personal or other items the patient may want within reach to discourage leaning over the side rails and attempting to get up without assistance. If the patient is confused, reorient him or her at each interaction.

Evaluation

Evaluate the effectiveness of nursing care for a patient with hypercalcemia by comparing the patient's status with the expected patient outcomes. Examples of specific outcomes for patients with hypercalcemia have been provided in the Planning section.

Magnesium Imbalance

Magnesium is the second most plentiful intracellular cation. Like other cations, magnesium promotes the transmission and conduction of nerve impulses and the contraction of skeletal, smooth, and cardiac muscle. Additional functions of magnesium include activating enzymes for carbohydrate and protein metabolism; influencing utilization of potassium, calcium, and protein; exerting a sedative action on the CNS; and directly affecting peripheral arteries by producing vasodilation.

The normal serum magnesium level is 1.5 to 2.5 mEq/L or 1.8 to 3.0 mg/dl. One third of the serum magnesium is bound to protein, and the remaining two thirds is free ionized circulating magnesium (physiologically active magnesium). A serum magnesium level less than 1.5 mEq/L is called hypomagnesemia (magnesium deficit), and a serum magnesium level more than 2.5 mEq/L is known as hypermagnesemia (magnesium excess). Magnesium is absorbed primarily from the distal small intestine and is excreted by the kidneys. A decreased serum calcium level promotes magnesium absorption while the kidneys conserve magnesium when intake is decreased.

The minimum daily adult requirement for magnesium is an average of 250 mg (200–300 mg); for an infant, it is 150 mg. Foods rich in magnesium include green vegetables, seafood, fish, whole grains, beans, and nuts.

HYPOMAGNESEMIA

ETIOLOGY

Hypomagnesemia can result from decreased absorption of dietary magnesium or from an increase in the amount of magnesium excreted by the kidneys. Causes of decreased absorption of magnesium include inadequate intake, chronic alcoholism, prolonged gastric suction, severe diarrhea, prolonged intravenous or hyperalimentation therapy without magnesium replacement, and loss of absorbing surface resulting from distal small-bowel resection or destruction of the distal mucosa, as in ileitis. Excessive phosphorus in the GI tract can also interfere with the absorption of magnesium. Hypomagnesemia resulting from an increase in renal excretion of magnesium can be due to the effect of drugs such as loop diuretics, osmotic diuretics, aminoglycosides, and some antineoplastic agents. It can also occur with diabetic ketoacidosis because of diuresis resulting from concentrated blood glucose, hypoparathyroidism, and primary aldosteronism.

PATHOPHYSIOLOGY

Decreased magnesium in the ECF results in an increased release of acetylcholine from the presynaptic membrane. This increases impulse transmission from nerve to nerve or nerve to muscle and thus increases neuromuscular irritability.

CLINICAL MANIFESTATIONS

Neuromuscular clinical manifestations of hypomagnesemia and related changes in calcium and potassium levels include hyperactive reflexes, tremors, muscle spasms, positive Chvostek's and Trousseau's signs, tetany, generalized tonic-clonic seizures, and in some cases depression, agitation, or confusion. Hypomagnesemia is also associated with hypertension and cardiac dysrhythmias such as premature ventricular contractions and ventricular fibrillation. ECG changes are similar to those found with hypokalemia: The T wave is flat or inverted, and the ST segment is depressed. Hypomagnesemia also enhances the action of digitalis, which can lead to digitalis toxicity. Symptoms of hypomagnesemia usually do not occur until the serum level drops to 1.0 mEq/L or below.

MEDICAL DIAGNOSIS

Hypomagnesemia is often unrecognized because a serum magnesium test is rarely ordered and symptoms usually do not occur until the serum level drops to 1.0 mEq/L. ECG changes suggest hypomagnesemia when combined with other findings.

MEDICAL MANAGEMENT

Mild hypomagnesemia can be corrected by a diet high in magnesium-containing foods such as green vegetables, nuts, legumes, chocolate, bananas, oranges, and grapefruit. Supplementary oral magnesium sulfate is also available. If the deficiency is severe, intravenous magnesium salts are given.

Application of the Nursing Process to the Care of the Patient with Hypomagnesemia

Assessment

Assess the patient for risk factors for hypomagnesemia. Be certain to check dietary intake of magnesium. If the patient has been receiving prolonged intravenous or hyperalimentation therapy, determine whether magnesium supplements have been provided. Also assess for symptoms of hypomagnesemia: muscle tumors, twitching, spasms, hyperreflexia, and cardiac dysrhythmias. Check the ECG for flat or inverted T waves, which are associated with both hypomagnesemia and hypokalemia.

Nursing Diagnoses and Planning

Nursing diagnoses and related expected patient outcomes most commonly applicable to patients with hypomagnesemia include the following:

NDx: High risk for injury related to neuromuscular excitability

Planning: Patient outcomes
1. Patient remains free of injury.

NDx: Altered nutrition: less than body requirements related to intake of magnesium

Planning: Patient outcomes
1. Patient describes importance of adequate dietary magnesium for health.
2. Patient identifies foods rich in magnesium.
3. Patient states intent to incorporate recommended amounts of these foods into the daily diet.

Nursing Interventions

NDx: High risk for injury
If the patient is confused, institute safety precautions as for the patient with hypernatremia. Institute seizure precautions if the magnesium deficit is marked.

NDx: Altered nutrition: less than body requirements
Administer oral or intravenous magnesium sulfate as ordered. If the oral drug is given, monitor the patient for diarrhea, which is a common side effect and which can exacerbate a magnesium deficit. If the intravenous drug is ordered, administer the drug slowly to prevent a hot or flushed feeling. Also monitor vital signs.

Explain to the patient the need for magnesium in the daily diet. Identify foods that are rich in magnesium, such as meat, green vegetables, seafood, whole grains, and nuts. Provide the patient with a list of these foods, and assist him or her in planning how to incorporate adequate amounts of them into the daily diet.

Additional Interventions
Because the patient with a magnesium deficit is at risk for dysphagia, use water to check the patient's ability to swallow before giving other oral fluids, medications, or foods. If the patient is taking digitalis, assess for symptoms of toxicity (bradycardia, nausea, vomiting, and visual disturbances), because hypomagnesemia enhances the action of digitalis.

Evaluation

Evaluate the effectiveness of nursing care for a patient with hypomagnesemia by comparing the patient's status with the expected patient outcomes. Examples of specific outcomes for patients with hypomagnesemia have been provided in the Planning section.

HYPERMAGNESEMIA

ETIOLOGY

Hypermagnesemia is most often due to renal insufficiency. It can also occur as a result of severe dehydration, untreated diabetic ketoacidosis, and excessive use of magnesium-containing laxatives (magnesium sulfate, milk of magnesia, and citrate solutions) or antacids (Maalox, Mylanta, Di-Gel, Aludrox).

PATHOPHYSIOLOGY

Increased serum magnesium inhibits the release of acetylcholine at the neuromuscular junction and depresses the excitability of nerve fibers.

CLINICAL MANIFESTATIONS

Mild hypermagnesemia is characterized by vasodilatation and resultant hypotension. Bradycardia and ECG changes consisting of a peaked T wave, prolonged PR intervals, and broad QRS complex also develop.

Other symptoms that develop as the magnesium level continues to increase include drowsiness, lethargy, muscle weakness, loss of deep tendon reflexes, and paralysis. Respiratory depression, coma, and cardiac standstill can ultimately occur.

MEDICAL DIAGNOSIS

A serum magnesium level higher than 2.5 mEq/L or 3.0 mg/dl is diagnostic of hypermagnesemia. In the absence of serum levels, characteristic ECG changes suggest the diagnosis when combined with other findings.

MEDICAL MANAGEMENT

When possible, medical management of hypermagnesemia is directed at correcting the underlying cause, thereby decreasing the serum magnesium level and preventing further increases. When renal failure is the underlying problem, dialysis may be necessary to return the serum magnesium to normal levels. In acute situations, intravenous calcium, which is an antagonist to magnesium, may be given to control symptoms.

Application of the Nursing Process to the Care of the Patient with Hypermagnesemia

Assessment

Assess the patient for risk factors of hypermagnesemia. Be certain to check for a history of renal insufficiency or failure and for the chronic use of laxatives or antacids containing magnesium salts. Also assess for symptoms of hypermagnesemia: change in level of consciousness, hyporeflexia, shallow respirations, bradycardia, and hypotension.

Nursing Diagnoses and Planning

The nursing diagnosis and related expected patient outcomes most commonly applicable to patients with hypermagnesemia are as follows:

NDx: Altered nutrition: more than body requirements related to intake of magnesium

Planning: Patient outcomes

1. Patient describes need to limit dietary magnesium.
2. Patient identifies foods rich in magnesium to be restricted.
3. Patient states intent to restrict dietary magnesium as recommended.

Nursing Interventions

Discontinue administration of magnesium-containing drugs and parenteral fluids per physician's order. Monitor urinary output, because an output of more than 750 ml per day is necessary to allow for the excretion of magnesium. If not contraindicated, increase fluid intake to dilute serum magnesium and increase urinary output. Administer loop diuretics as prescribed to increase renal excretion of magnesium further.

NDx: Altered nutrition: more than body requirements

Explain to the patient the need to restrict intake of magnesium. Instruct the patient to limit intake of magnesium-rich foods such as meat, seafood, nuts, green vegetables, and whole grains. Assist the patient in planning and selecting meals low in magnesium and refer to the dietitian if needed. Also instruct the patient to avoid over-the-counter drugs such as laxatives and antacids that contain large amounts of magnesium. Show the patient how to read drug labels to ascertain magnesium content.

Evaluation

Evaluate the effectiveness of nursing care for a patient with hypermagnesemia by comparing the patient's status with the expected patient outcomes. Examples of specific outcomes for patients with hypermagnesemia have been provided in the Planning section.

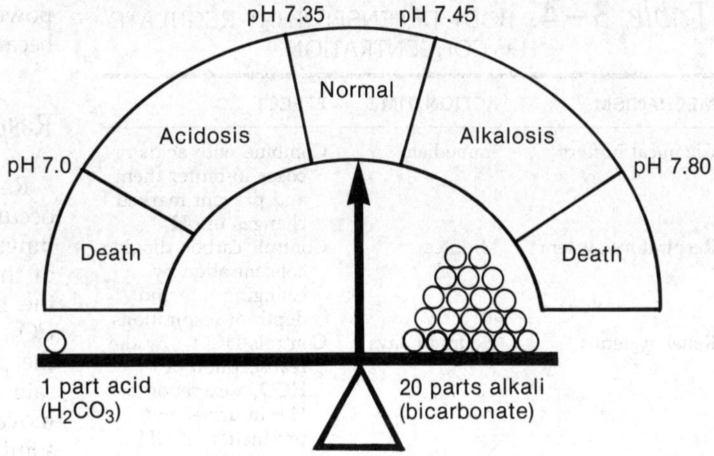

Figure 3–4.

Limits of pH and bicarbonate–carbonic acid balance. The relationship of 20 parts bicarbonate to one part carbonic acid maintains H^+ and pH within normal limits. An increase in acid or a decrease in base causes acidosis; a decrease in acid or increase in base causes alkalosis. (Redrawn from Abbott Laboratories: Fluid and electrolytes. North Chicago, IL: Abbott Laboratories, 1970.)

Acid-Base Imbalance

Hydrogen ions (H^+) are vital to life and health. Although hydrogen ions exist in far lower concentrations in body fluids than other ions (e.g., chloride [Cl^-] and K^+), they play a major role in the regulation of biochemical and metabolic activities necessary for proper cellular function.

The H^+ concentration determines the acidity or alkalinity of solution. The greater the H^+ concentration in a solution, the more acidic is the solution. The lower the H^+ concentration, the more alkaline it is.

pH is the symbol used to indicate the H^+ concentration in a solution or the acidity or alkalinity of that solution. Neutral pH is 7.0. The higher the pH, the lower the H^+ concentration in the solution and vice versa. The normal pH range of the blood is 7.35 to 7.45. A blood pH below 7.35 indicates acidosis (which is high H^+ concentration). A pH above 7.45 indicates alkalosis (which is a low H^+ concentration). pH limits compatible with life are 6.9 to 7.9 (Fig. 3–4).

Hydrogen circulates through the body fluids in two forms: first as the volatile H^+ of carbonic acid (H_2CO_3), and second as the nonvolatile hydrogen ions of metabolic acids. Volatile hydrogen ions are found in the form of carbon dioxide (CO_2) and water and must be excreted in gaseous form by the lungs. Nonvolatile hydrogen ions are derived from acids such as sulfuric, pyruvic, phosphoric, and lactic acids. Nonvolatile hydrogen ions are eliminated by the kidneys.

Maintaining a proper H^+ concentration and normal pH is the key to acid-base balance. This balance between acids and bases in the blood is best expressed by the relationship between bicarbonate ion (HCO_3^-) and H_2CO_3. This relationship is represented as follows:

$$pH = pk + \log \frac{HCO_3^-}{H_2CO_3}$$

The ratio of bicarbonate to carbonic acid is 20:1 (see Fig. 3–4). The body strives to maintain this ratio at all times. This is done by retaining or blowing off CO_2 by the lungs or by retaining or excreting HCO_3^- by the kidneys. The relationship is expressed in Figure 3–5.

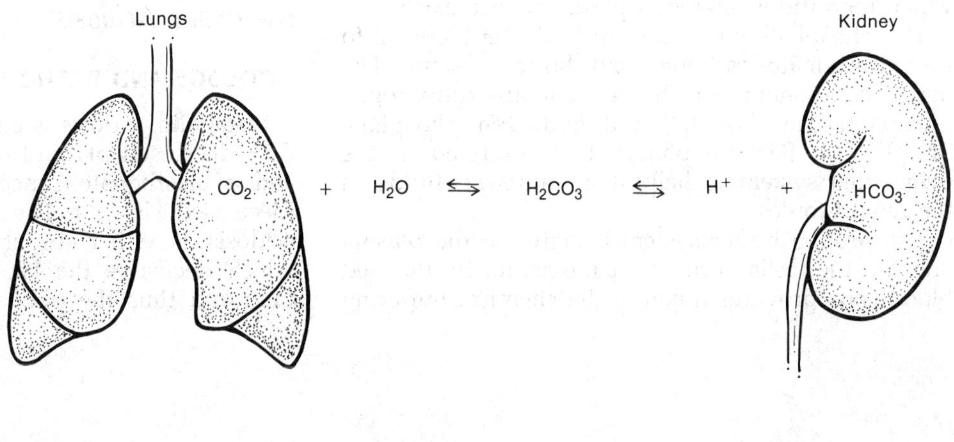

Figure 3–5.

The lungs help control acid-base balance by blowing off or retaining CO_2; the kidneys help regulate acid-base balance by excreting or retaining HCO_3^-.

Table 3–4. BODY DEFENSES THAT REGULATE H+ CONCENTRATION

MECHANISM	ACTION TIME	EFFECT
Chemical buffers	Immediate	Combine with acids or bases to buffer them and prevent marked changes in pH
Respiratory system	Minutes	Controls carbon dioxide concentration by changing rate and depth of respirations
Renal system	Hours to days	Controls HCO_3^- by the reabsorption of HCO_3^-; excretion of H+ in urine; and production of NH_3.

Abbreviations: H+, hydrogen ion; HCO_3^-, bicarbonate ion; NH_3, ammonia.

The body has three main defenses that regulate the H^+ concentration in the body and, therefore, acid-base balance. They are the chemical buffer systems, the respiratory system, and the kidneys (Table 3–4).

Buffer System

A buffer is a substance that can act as a chemical sponge by either releasing or soaking up H^+. This is an immediate process that functions to keep the pH at 7.40. This system works by adding a buffered solution to a strong acid (or base), which results in a weak acid (or base) and a salt. A weak acid (or base) does not ionize in solution as much as a strong acid (or base), so there is less free H^+ to alter the pH. The pH of the solution then remains within the normal range. The main buffer systems are the bicarbonate–carbonic acid system, the phosphate system, and protein. The bicarbonate–carbonic acid system is the one that is monitored clinically. If this buffer system is stable, the others are stable also. Within the body fluids, HCO_3^- and H_2CO_3 operate together, buffering and protecting the body from large amounts of acid. H_2CO_3 is a weak acid, and sodium HCO_3 ($NaHCO_3$) is its salt, which ionizes into Na^+ and HCO_3^-. Again, it is not absolute values that regulate acid-base balance but the ratio of HCO_3 to H_2CO_3 that is crucial to H^+ balance. When the ratio is altered, a pH imbalance exists.

The phosphate buffer system is almost identical to the bicarbonate–carbonic acid buffer system. The major components of this system are dihydrogen phosphate ion ($H_2PO_4^-$) and hydrogen phosphate ion (HPO_4). Because phosphate is excreted in the urine, this system is helpful in buffering fluids in the renal tubules.

The protein buffer system is active in the plasma and in the cells. Protein hemoglobin in the red blood cells provides much of the chemical buffering power of body fluids. Proteins are important buffers because they are found throughout the body.

Respiratory Control of pH

Respiratory control of H^+ levels in the body occurs by varying the rate of CO_2 removal in the lungs. The respiratory control center in the medulla of the brain responds to changes of CO_2 and H^+ in the body. A rise in the partial pressure of arterial CO_2 ($PaCO_2$) is a strong stimulus for breathing. In the presence of a low pH (acidosis), the respiratory rate and depth are increased, causing a greater removal of CO_2, which reduces the amount of acid in solution, thereby raising the pH. Conversely, when the pH is high (alkalosis), the respiratory rate is decreased, causing CO_2 to be retained, which raises the amount of acid in solution and lowers the pH. This response occurs within minutes to maintain acid-base balance within the body.

Renal Control of pH

Renal control of H^+ is accomplished by regulating bicarbonate via the bicarbonate–carbonic acid buffer system and eliminating nonvolatile H^+. This response is slow—it takes hours to days—but the renal system is powerful and complete in its acid-base regulation. To correct H^+ imbalance, the kidneys alter the rate of excretion of metabolic acids by three major processes: the reabsorption of HCO_3^-; the secretion of H^+ by the proximal and distal tubules; and the production of ammonia (NH_3).

Maintenance of acid-base balance depends on the healthy functioning of the kidneys, lungs, and buffer systems. These systems normally respond swiftly and efficiently to changes in H^+ concentration. However, when there is an excessive amount of acid or HCO_3^- in the body fluids, or in the presence of certain diseases, H^+ regulation fails and imbalances result. There are two major types of imbalances: acidosis and alkalosis. There are two types of acidosis (respiratory and metabolic) and two types of alkalosis (respiratory and metabolic). Figure 3–6 summarizes four types of imbalances that occur. Table 3–5 lists the laboratory values for the four imbalances.

Metabolic Acidosis

ETIOLOGY AND PATHOPHYSIOLOGY

Metabolic acidosis is characterized by a pH below 7.35 (decreased pH and increased H^+ concentration) and a bicarbonate concentration below 22 mEq/L (decreased HCO_3^-). The general cause of metabolic acidosis is either an abnormal loss of $NaHCO_3$, which decreases the HCO_3^- in the HCO_3^-/H_2CO_3 ratio and thus the pH, or an excess of nonvolatile

Figure 3–6.

Four major acid-base (H^+) imbalances. (From Luckmann J, Sorensen KC. Medical-surgical nursing. 3rd ed. Philadelphia: WB Saunders, 1987, p 154.)

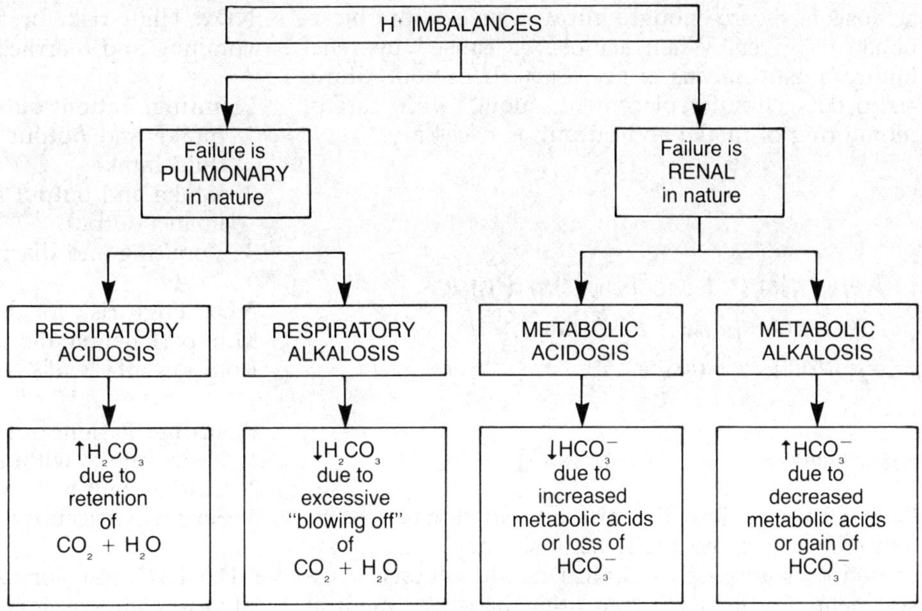

acid, which is more carbonic acid than the kidney is able to handle. Metabolic acidosis occurs in diabetic ketoacidosis, lactic acidosis, starvation, high fever, hypothyroidism, trauma, salicylate poisoning (and other poisons), oliguric renal disease, and diarrhea (Table 3–6).

CLINICAL MANIFESTATIONS

As in all acidotic states, a decreased pH produces CNS depression, which may include apathy, headache, disorientation, weakness, stupor, and coma. The skin is often warm and flushed because skin vessels become less responsive to sympathetic nervous system vasoconstrictor input. Skin is often dry and skin turgor poor when fluid deficit accompanies acidosis. The hyperventilation of Kussmaul's respiration occurs as a compensatory attempt to blow off CO_2, thereby correcting the acidosis. Hyperkalemia may occur from the movement of potassium out of the cells as hydrogen ions move in and from retention of potassium by the kidneys. In addition, when the pH falls below 7.0, cardiac dysrhythmias develop, and heart rate and cardiac output decrease.

MEDICAL DIAGNOSIS

Arterial blood gas measurements are essential in the diagnosis of all acid-base disturbances. In metabolic acidosis, there is a low arterial blood gas pH (<7.35) and a low blood gas bicarbonate level (<22 mEq/L). High serum potassium (hyperkalemia) may also occur as potassium leaves the cell. Compensatory hyperventilation decreases blood gas CO_2 levels (<40 mm Hg). Diagnosis is made by correlating the arterial blood gas findings to other known abnormal conditions.

MEDICAL MANAGEMENT

Management of metabolic acidosis is directed toward treating the underlying cause and correcting the electrolyte imbalance. Through supportive intervention, the renal and respiratory systems can help correct and compensate for the imbalance. If the

Table 3–5. LABORATORY VALUES FOR ACID-BASE DISTURBANCES

IMBALANCE	pH	$Paco_2$	HCO_3^-
Metabolic acidosis			
Uncompensated	↓	Normal	↓
Partially compensated	↓ or normal	↓	↓
Metabolic alkalosis			
Uncompensated	↑	Normal	↑
Partially compensated	↑ or normal	↑	↑
Respiratory acidosis			
Uncompensated	↓	↑	Normal
Partially compensated	↓ or normal	↑	↑
Respiratory alkalosis			
Uncompensated	↑	↓	Normal
Partially compensated	↑ or normal	↓	↓

Abbreviations: $Paco_2$, partial pressure of arterial carbon dioxide; HCO_3^-, bicarbonate ion. *Symbols:* ↓, decreased; ↑, increased.

Table 3–6. CAUSES OF METABOLIC ACIDOSIS

Diabetic ketoacidosis	Hypothyroidism
Lactic acidosis	Trauma
Starvation	Salicylate poisoning
Renal failure	Diarrhea
Fever	Alcoholic ketoacidosis

acidosis is severe enough, intravenous sodium bicarbonate is given. When acidosis is caused by renal failure, renal dialysis is necessary. If osmotic diuresis occurs, fluid replacement, along with careful monitoring of intake and output, is necessary.

Application of the Nursing Process to the Care of the Patient with Metabolic Acidosis

Assessment

Obtain and review the arterial blood gas results. Remember that metabolic acidosis may exist in the presence or absence of clinical manifestations or assessment findings. Review the patient's medical problems, because they can suggest the possible development of metabolic acidosis (i.e., the cause of metabolic acidosis). Ask specifically about renal problems, diabetes mellitus, and persistent diarrhea. Also ask about the use of prescribed and over-the-counter medications. Note those medications that may affect acid, base, fluid, and electrolyte balance. Assess for apathy, decreased alertness, disorientation, weakness, stupor, and coma, which can occur in acidosis as a result of CNS depression. If necessary, obtain or confirm this information with a family member or significant other. Acidosis, if severe enough, also affects cardiac muscle function, so assess for cardiac dysrhythmias, low heart rate, and low cardiac output. Assess fluid status to determine whether a volume deficit exists. Obtain a detailed dietary history. Review serum electrolytes for abnormal findings that may cause or be a result of metabolic acidosis. Observe for Kussmaul's respiration, which is present if the patient is having a compensatory reaction by the lung. Keep in mind that skin and mucous membranes are pink, warm, and dry as a result of the increased gas exchange and vasodilatation.

Nursing Diagnoses and Planning

Nursing diagnoses and related expected patient outcomes most commonly applicable to patients with metabolic acidosis include the following:

NDx: High risk for altered thought processes related to CNS depression

Planning: Patient outcomes
1. Patient is alert.
2. Patient is coherent.
3. Patient responds appropriately to questions and commands.

NDx: High risk for fluid volume deficit related to vomiting and diarrhea

Planning: Patient outcomes
1. Intake and output record demonstrates adequate fluid intake.
2. Intake and output record indicates intake approximates output.
3. Vomiting and diarrhea are absent.

NDx: High risk for decreased cardiac output related to hyperkalemia and altered cardiac muscle function from low pH levels

Planning: Patient outcomes
1. Heart rate is within normal limits.
2. Cardiac output is within normal limits.
3. Serum potassium is within normal limits.

NDx: High risk for ineffective breathing pattern related to compensatory mechanism by lungs

Planning: Patient outcomes
1. Respiratory rate remains within normal limits.
2. Patient verbalizes that breathing is easy and not labored or hard.

NDx: High risk for injury related to disorientation, weakness, or stupor

Planning: Patient outcomes
1. Patient remains free of injury.

Nursing Interventions

NDx: High risk for altered thought processes
For the patient with metabolic acidosis, intervention directed toward returning the pH to normal also corrects the change in thought process. Implement the medical plan designed to correct the pH. If dialysis is necessary, provide nursing care as described in Chapter 26.

If the patient has diabetic ketoacidosis, administer insulin as ordered by the physician. Administer replacement fluids, bicarbonate, and other medical treatments per physician orders. Monitor patient's mental status throughout care to detect improvement. Orient patient to time and place, and restate who you are and what you are going to do at each interaction. When feasible, have the patient use his or her eyeglasses or hearing aid if applicable.

NDx: High risk for fluid volume deficit
Monitor and record accurate fluid intake and output. Administer fluid replacement as ordered. Support patient if vomiting occurs. Document the amount and provide a description of vomitus. If diarrhea is present, provide adequate skin care and provide bedpan or commode (if needed) for easy

access. Document the amount, color, consistency, and frequency of diarrheal stool.

NDx: High risk for decreased cardiac output
Place the patient on a cardiac monitor if severe acidosis is present. Monitor heart rate closely and be alert for dysrhythmias. Measure the cardiac output if ordered. Measure arterial blood pressure regularly. Review relevant laboratory data including K^+ and Cl^-. Reassure and comfort the patient to alleviate anxiety that may arise from cardiac symptoms.

NDx: High risk for ineffective breathing pattern
Maintain good pulmonary function to facilitate the compensatory excretion of CO_2. Encourage airway clearance through deep breathing and incentive spirometry. Facilitate rest, which is essential for sufficient energy to maintain a higher level of ventilation. Remember that as the primary disorder is treated, the level of ventilation will return to normal.

NDx: High risk for injury
Keep side rails raised and maintain the bed in a low position. Keep the call bell within easy reach. Assist the patient in meeting physical needs until he or she is capable of self-care. Closely observe and assist the patient if he or she is out of bed. Keep the environment adequately lighted for safety.

Evaluation

Evaluate the effectiveness of nursing care for a patient with metabolic acidosis by comparing the patient's status with the expected patient outcomes. Examples of specific outcomes for patients with metabolic acidosis have been provided in the Planning section.

Metabolic Alkalosis

ETIOLOGY AND PATHOPHYSIOLOGY

Metabolic alkalosis is characterized by a pH higher than 7.45 (increased pH and decreased H^+) and a bicarbonate concentration greater than 28 mEq/L (increased HCO_3^-). It is produced when there is an excess amount of bicarbonate or a loss of H^+. This disturbance does not occur often, but when it does, its most common cause is vomiting or prolonged nasogastric suctioning, which results in a loss of hydrochloric acid with gastric contents. Other causes include those associated with the loss of K^+, such as drainage from an intestinal fistula, diarrhea, and use of potassium-losing diuretics (e.g., thiazides, furosemides, and ethacrynic acid), and those associated with excessive adrenocorticoid hormones, as in hyperaldosteronism and Cushing's disease. Hypokalemia produces metabolic alkalosis by the conservation of potassium in the kidneys, creating an increased excretion of H^+ and by cellular potassium moving out of the cells into the ECF in an attempt to achieve a near-normal serum level. Other causes of metabolic alkalosis include excessive alkali ingestion (e.g., antacids, baking soda) to alleviate acid indigestion or ulcer symptoms and the administration of intravenous sodium bicarbonate during cardiopulmonary resuscitation (Table 3–7).

Table 3–7. CAUSES OF METABOLIC ALKALOSIS

Vomiting	Hypokalemia
Nasogastric suctioning	Hyperaldosteronism
Intestinal fistulas	Cushing's disease
Diuretic therapy (thiazides, furosemides, and ethacrynic acid)	Alkali ingestion
	Sodium bicarbonate during cardiopulmonary resuscitation

CLINICAL MANIFESTATIONS

In metabolic alkalosis, as in all alkalotic conditions, an elevated pH results in a CNS excitation, which produces such neurologic symptoms as belligerence, irritability, mental confusion, tingling of the fingers and toes, dizziness, hyperactive reflexes, tetany, and convulsions. These neurologic findings usually occur only with acute and severe metabolic alkalosis. Metabolic alkalosis also leads to compensatory hypoventilation (which results in retention of CO_2 by not blowing it off, thereby increasing the carbonic acid and H^+ content). This is manifested by shallow, slow respirations with decreased thoracic movements (limited by the body's need for oxygen). In some cases, hypokalemia, hypochloremia, or fluid volume deficit may also occur.

MEDICAL DIAGNOSIS

The diagnosis of metabolic alkalosis is made on the basis of the results of arterial blood gas evaluation displaying a pH higher than 7.45 and an HCO_3^- level higher than 28 mEq/L. Hypokalemia may occur when the body attempts to conserve H^+, thereby excreting K^+, or when diuretics producing a potassium loss are given. Hypochloremia exists in the presence of metabolic alkalosis when Cl^- is lost in the gastric contents (through vomiting or nasogastric suction). Compensation by the lungs is apparent when the $PaCO_2$ increases. Hypoventilation may be more pronounced in the unconscious and debilitated patient, and hypoxemia may occur as a result of the hypoventilation. Diagnosis is made by correlating the arterial blood gas findings to the underlying cause or medical condition.

MEDICAL MANAGEMENT

The treatment of metabolic alkalosis is directed at correcting the underlying cause or condition. Nasogastric suction or vomiting should be controlled when possible. Administration of alkali is discontinued, as is the administration of diuretics when those therapies are contributing to the metabolic alkalosis. Fluid-volume deficit as well as chloride depletion is usually corrected with lactated Ringer's solution (which contains chloride) or normal saline. In severe cases, ammonium chloride or hydrochloric acid may be administered intravenously to replace the H^+ and Cl^- loss. To correct a K^+ loss, potassium chloride is administered. Diamox, a carbonic anhydrase inhibitor, is a diuretic that relieves alkalosis by increasing the excretion of bicarbonate by the kidneys.

Application of the Nursing Process to the Care of the Patient with Metabolic Alkalosis

Assessment

Because the patient with metabolic alkalosis has few symptoms, anticipating and assessing for the conditions that cause metabolic alkalosis are essential. Review results of laboratory tests for depletion of chloride and potassium.

Check arterial blood gas results for elevated pH and HCO_3^- values. Assess fluid intake and output for volume deficit. Measure the amount of nasogastric drainage or vomiting when applicable. Assess the neurologic status of the patient; look for symptoms of alkalosis such as dizziness, irritability, numbness in fingers and toes, mental confusion, tetany, and convulsions. If the patient has a history of ulcers or acid indigestion, question him or her as to the amount of antacids or baking soda ingested. Assess the patient's respiratory status for decreased rate and depth of ventilation.

Nursing Diagnoses and Planning

Nursing diagnoses and related expected patient outcomes most commonly applicable to patients with metabolic alkalosis include the following:

NDx: High risk for fluid volume deficit related to vomiting or nasogastric suction and K^+ or Cl^- loss

Planning: Patient outcomes
1. Vomiting has ceased.
2. Nasogastric suction is discontinued.
3. Fluid intake is greater than output.
4. K^+ and Cl^- values are normal.

NDx: High risk for altered thought processes related to increased excitability of the nervous system secondary to increased pH and bicarbonate level, resulting in irritability, dizziness, and mental confusion

Planning: Patient outcomes
1. Patient is alert and responsive.
2. Patient is cooperative.
3. Patient follows directions.
4. Patient denies dizziness.

NDx: High risk for ineffective breathing pattern related to the compensatory mechanism of decreased rate and depth of ventilation

Planning: Patient outcomes
1. Labored breathing is absent.
2. Ventilation is of normal rate and depth.
3. Hypoxemia is absent.
4. Patient is alert and cooperative.

NDx: High risk for injury related to belligerence, mental confusion, dizziness, tetany, and convulsions secondary to CNS excitement

Planning: Patient outcomes
1. Patient complies with safety precautions.
2. Patient remains free of injury.

Nursing Interventions

NDx: High risk for fluid volume deficit
For the person with metabolic alkalosis resulting from prolonged vomiting or nasogastric suctioning, record and report the amount of emesis or drainage if excessive. Encourage fluid intake as ordered. Monitor laboratory values for alterations in K^+ or Cl^-. If K^+ or Cl^- replacement is ordered, give oral or intravenous medication as prescribed. Administer intravenous fluids carefully and in appropriate time intervals as ordered by the physician.

NDx: High risk for altered thought processes
Be aware that a change in the patient's mood or personality to one of irritability or belligerence may be due to a chemical excitability of the CNS from alkalosis. Treat the patient with understanding and support until the underlying cause is treated and the mental confusion subsides. By appropriate conversation, keep the patient oriented to time and place and to what is going on. Protect the patient from harm by keeping the bedside rails up while in bed and assist with ambulation when needed.

NDx: High risk for ineffective breathing pattern
Encourage deep breathing, coughing, and the use of incentive spirometry to keep the airways clear and

to prevent atelectasis. Support the patient in a semi-Fowler's position if necessary to aid chest expansion and ease of breathing. Administer oxygen therapy as ordered by the doctor if hypoxemia is present. Explain to the patient the reason for the change in breathing pattern and reassure him or her that breathing will return to normal once the cause of the alkalosis is treated.

NDx: High risk for injury
Because the patient with severe metabolic alkalosis may become confused or dizzy and has the potential to develop convulsions, institute precautions for the patient's protection. Keep side rails up when the patient is in bed. Stay with the patient or assist with ambulation if the alkalosis is severe. Explain the importance of safety precautions to the patient, and enlist his or her cooperation while the alkalosis is present.

Evaluation

Evaluate the effectiveness of nursing care for a patient with metabolic alkalosis by comparing the patient's status with the expected patient outcomes. Examples of specific outcomes for patients with metabolic alkalosis have been provided in the Planning section.

Respiratory Acidosis

ETIOLOGY AND PATHOPHYSIOLOGY

Respiratory acidosis is characterized by a pH less than 7.35 (pH and H^+) and a $PaCO_2$ higher than 45 mm Hg. Any condition that decreases the rate of pulmonary ventilation increases the concentration of CO_2, which increases carbonic acid and H^+ concentration. In addition to an elevated $PaCO_2$, which causes hypoventilation, hypoxemia (partial pressure of arterial oxygen, or PaO_2) usually exists. Respiratory acidosis may be either acute or chronic.

The causes of respiratory acidosis include any condition that impairs gas exchange. Acute respiratory acidosis can result from impaired function of the medullary center (narcotic overdose, head injury, oversedation, and anesthesia); from chest injuries; from weakness of the respiratory muscles (paralysis of respiratory muscles as in Guillain-Barré syndrome); or from airway obstruction (pneumonia, pulmonary edema, respiratory distress syndrome, extreme obesity, and upper airway obstruction). Chronic respiratory acidosis is most commonly caused by chronic obstructive pulmonary disease (emphysema, chronic bronchitis, asthma, and bronchiectasis (Table 3–8). Because renal compensation

Table 3–8. CAUSES OF RESPIRATORY ACIDOSIS

Acute	Chronic
Drug overdose	Chronic obstructive pulmonary disease
Head injury	Emphysema
Oversedation	Chronic bronchitis
Postanesthesia	Asthma
Chest injuries	Bronchiectasis
Paralysis of the respiratory muscles	Kyphoscoliosis
Pneumonia	Extreme obesity

(retention of bicarbonate) takes hours to days to stabilize the pH, the pH can drop severely in patients with acute respiratory acidosis. Respiratory acidosis is often accompanied by hypoxemia. Signs of hypoxemia often develop before those of respiratory acidosis because CO_2 diffuses 20 times faster than oxygen (O_2) across the alveolar-capillary membrane. When CO_2 accumulates in the blood, ventilation increases and eliminates a portion of the CO_2, but the O_2 uptake moves more slowly.

Acute respiratory acidosis can occur in patients with chronic lung disease who have chronically elevated $PaCO_2$ levels. This is often called CO_2 narcosis. In this situation, the medullary respiratory center has become insensitive to elevated levels of CO_2 and no longer responds to increases in $PaCO_2$. Rather, the oxygen level in the blood now becomes the major stimulus for breathing. If oxygen is administered at a level that suppresses this stimulus, the rate and depth of respiration decrease, $PaCO_2$ rises, and respiratory distress ensues.

CLINICAL MANIFESTATIONS

The signs and symptoms of respiratory acidosis are variable and depend on whether the condition is acute or chronic. Because respiratory acidosis is often accompanied by hypoxemia, the manifestations of each are often intermixed. Acute onset of hypercapnia (increased $PaCO_2$) can cause an increased pulse, respiration, and blood pressure; mental cloudiness; and feeling of fullness in the head. An increased $PaCO_2$ can cause cerebral vasodilatation and increased cerebral blood flow. If the condition is severe and prolonged, it can cause such signs and symptoms as papilledema, dull headache, blurred vision, behavioral changes (e.g., depression, paranoia, and hallucinations), weakness, paralysis, stupor, and coma. In less severe cases, warm, flushed skin, weakness, and tachycardia may be present. Ventricular fibrillation may be the first sign of respiratory acidosis in anesthetized patients.

MEDICAL DIAGNOSIS

The diagnosis of respiratory acidosis is based on arterial blood gases with a pH less than 7.35 and a

Pa_{CO_2} level higher than 45 mm Hg. When compensation (the kidney's retention of bicarbonate) has occurred, the pH may return to within the lower limits of normal.

The patient's underlying pulmonary dysfunction or medical condition often suggests the possibility of respiratory acidosis. Hypoventilation and hypoxemia strongly suggest respiratory acidosis as well. The diagnosis is made by correlating the arterial blood gas findings to the underlying cause or medical condition.

MEDICAL MANAGEMENT

Management of respiratory acidosis is directed at treating the underlying condition and improving ventilation so that the exchange of CO_2 and O_2 improves. This is accomplished by using respiratory care techniques such as bronchodilators to help reduce bronchospasm; postural drainage and percussion to loosen and raise thickened mucus; suctioning to rid the airway of secretions; humidity to loosen secretions; and antibiotics for respiratory infections. Low-flow oxygen (1–3 L/minute) is given to a hypoxemic patient who has a chronically high Pa_{CO_2}. In severe cases, mechanical ventilation may be necessary to correct the hypoxemia or the acidosis and hypercapnia adequately. In such cases, the elevated Pa_{CO_2} must be brought down slowly. If the acidosis is severe enough, intravenous sodium bicarbonate may be administered to bring the pH to within a safe range quickly. Close monitoring and frequent arterial blood gases are necessary in this case to avoid a severe alkalosis from overcompensation.

Application of the Nursing Process to the Care of the Patient with Respiratory Acidosis

Assessment

Assessment of the patient with respiratory acidosis reveals mainly cardiopulmonary findings. Question the patient about and observe for dyspnea on exertion, because this is often the patient's prominent symptom. Also assess for indications of cerebral vasodilatation caused by hypercapnia. These include blurred vision, headache, papilledema, behavioral changes such as depression, paranoia, hallucinations, weakness, paralysis, stupor, and coma. Be aware that a patient's moodiness, belligerence, anxiety, irritability, or paranoia may be a result of chemical changes in the blood such as hypercapnia and hypoxemia. Review and relate the arterial blood gas values to the patient's medical problems. Auscultate lung sounds for crackles (rales), rhonchi, wheezes, and decreased breath sounds, which suggest impaired gas exchange or airway clearance. Check vital signs regularly for tachycardia, tachypnea, and elevated blood pressure. Monitor for cardiac dysrhythmias. Examine the skin condition to determine whether the skin is warm and flushed.

Nursing Diagnoses and Planning

Nursing diagnoses and related expected patient outcomes most commonly applicable to patients with respiratory acidosis include the following:

NDx: Impaired gas exchange related to inadequate ventilation

Planning: Patient outcomes
1. pH is within normal limits.
2. Respiratory rate is within patient's normal limits.
3. Heart rate returns to within patient's normal limits.
4. Patient is alert and oriented without being agitated.
5. Color of skin and mucous membranes is normal for patient.

NDx: Ineffective airway clearance related to inadequate ventilation and lung condition

Planning: Patient outcomes
1. Crackles and wheezes are absent.
2. Patient coughs and raises secretions effectively.
3. Patient describes the need to increase fluids to keep secretions loose.
4. Vital signs are within patient's normal limits.

NDx: Ineffective breathing pattern related to inadequate ventilation and underlying lung condition

Planning: Patient outcomes
1. Respiratory rate, depth, and rhythm return to within patient's normal limits.
2. Patient demonstrates effective diaphragmatic breathing pattern.
3. Adventitious breath sounds return to within patient's normal limits.
4. Patient demonstrates correct use of prescribed respiratory drugs and equipment.

NDx: Decreased cardiac output related to poor gas exchange of O_2 and CO_2

Planning: Patient outcomes
1. Heart rate is within patient's normal limits.
2. Serious dysrhythmias are absent.
3. Blood pressure is within patient's normal limits.

NDx: Activity intolerance related to dyspnea on exertion and ineffective breathing patterns

Planning: Patient outcomes
1. Patient verbalizes need to pace activity.
2. Activity level returns to patient's normal level.

3. Patient verbalizes plan to engage in regular exercise.
4. Patient describes need for effective breathing with activity.

NDx: Anxiety related to dyspnea

Planning: Patient outcomes
1. Patient expresses fear of breathlessness.
2. Patient demonstrates effective breathing pattern.
3. Patient verbalizes ability to deal with anxiety level.

Nursing Interventions

NDx: Impaired gas exchange
When hypoventilation is present, interventions to improve the level of ventilation also improve the respiratory acidosis. Perform bronchial hygiene measures such as nebulizer treatments, postural drainage, and percussion as ordered. Coordinate the patient's plan of care to ensure that all aspects of care are implemented. If oxygen therapy is ordered for hypoxemia, frequently assess both proper function of the oxygen administration equipment and patient compliance. Administer antibiotics to treat respiratory infection and bronchodilators to open the airways as prescribed. If chronic lung disease is present, teach the patient to use an effective breathing pattern. If the level of ventilation is very poor and the respiratory acidosis suggests respiratory failure, maintain mechanical ventilation as ordered. In this event, assess the patient's respiratory status and function of the ventilator closely. Throughout care, monitor the patient's respiratory status for changes in gas-exchange status.

NDx: Ineffective airway clearance
With many pulmonary disorders, increased secretions develop as a result of the primary lung problem or a secondary lung infection. Implement measures to loosen and raise secretions such as effective coughing, increased fluids, and postural drainage. Teach the patient effective breathing and coughing techniques as well as the need to drink six to eight glasses of liquid a day. Administer medication to loosen secretions or antibiotics to treat an infection as prescribed. If large amounts of secretions are present, use nasotracheal suctioning as necessary. Throughout the patient's care, monitor respiratory status periodically to detect changes in respiratory status.

NDx: Ineffective breathing pattern
Implement nursing interventions as described for impaired gas exchange and ineffective airway clearance. As the patient's method of breathing, clearing of secretions, and stabilization of oxygenation all improve, gas exchange and breathing pattern also improve. If the patient has a chronic breathing problem, instruct him or her in breathing techniques, methods to maintain a patent airway, and use of medication to improve ventilation.

NDx: Decreased cardiac output
Hypoxemia affects cardiac status, causing an increased heart rate, dysrhythmias, and changes in blood pressure. Closely monitor heart rate and cardiac rhythm during the unstable phase of hypoventilation. Administer cardiac medication as ordered. Maintain accurate record of intake and output.

NDx: Activity intolerance
When dyspnea occurs as a result of an ineffective breathing pattern and poor gas exchange, the patient's activity level is affected. Provide assistance as needed with bathing, shaving, getting out of bed, and eating. Take care to pace activities, and plan care so that severe dyspnea does not occur. Teach the patient the importance of self-pacing activity so that the respiratory condition is not aggravated. If the patient has a chronic lung condition, teach him or her the importance of regular, planned exercise as well as how to coordinate breathing with exercise. Encourage attendance at a pulmonary rehabilitation program.

NDx: Anxiety
Dyspnea, whether acute or chronic, causes anxiety. Explain to the patient, in simple terms, what is happening. Also explain the plan of care. Part of the anxiety may be due to impaired gas exchange, so interventions previously mentioned to correct hypoxemia and hypoventilation will reduce the anxiety. If the patient has a chronic lung condition, teach proper breathing techniques and methods to control breathlessness.

Evaluation

Evaluate the effectiveness of nursing care for a patient with respiratory acidosis by comparing the patient's status with the expected patient outcomes. Examples of specific outcomes for patients with respiratory acidosis have been provided in the Planning section.

Respiratory Alkalosis

ETIOLOGY AND PATHOPHYSIOLOGY

Respiratory alkalosis is characterized by a pH greater than 7.45 and a Pa_{CO_2} less than 35 mm Hg. Respiratory alkalosis is always due to hyperventilation, which is the excessive exhaling of CO_2. This causes a decrease in Pa_{CO_2}, which causes a decrease in carbonic acid and consequently a rise in pH. Hyperventilation means that the respiratory rate and depth are greater than needed to maintain a normal $PaCO_2$ and should not be confused with the hyperpnea of exercise. One of the most common cause of hyperventilation is anxiety. Other causes include pain, hypoxemia, and overventilation of patients with mechanical ventilators. Respiratory alkalosis can occur from overstimulation of the respiratory center in the brain and is caused by fever, gram-negative sepsis, CNS diseases such as meningitis, encephalitis, brain tumors, early salicylate poisoning, and hyperthyroidism. Respiratory alkalosis can be caused by voluntary hyperventilation and is often the result of psychological and environmental factors or diseases that are not necessarily respiratory in nature. Renal compensation exists when the HCO_3^- decreases until it restores the 20:1 ratio of HCO_3^- to H_2CO_3. The kidney is slow in the reabsorption of HCO_3^- and the decrease of H^+ secretion as well as the decrease in NH_3 production. If respiratory alkalosis is self-limited, renal compensation will not have time to develop.

CLINICAL MANIFESTATIONS

The major characteristics of respiratory alkalosis are those associated with hyperexcitability of the nervous system and a decrease in cerebral blood flow. They include an inability to concentrate, lightheadedness, numbness and tingling of the fingers and toes, hyperreflexia, and positive Chvostek's and Trousseau's signs. There may also be associated sweating, palpitations, panic, and air hunger. If respiratory alkalosis becomes severe, tetany and convulsions may occur. Cardiac dysrhythmias caused by a decreased serum potassium level also develop.

MEDICAL DIAGNOSIS

Diagnosis of respiratory alkalosis is made by analyzing the arterial blood gases. Respiratory alkalosis is present when the pH is greater than 7.45 and the $PaCO_2$ is less than 35 mm Hg. If the situation is compensated, the kidneys lower the bicarbonate level to lower the pH to normal. The kidneys cannot do this quickly, however.

MEDICAL MANAGEMENT

Management of respiratory alkalosis is directed toward treatment of the underlying cause. People who are hyperventilating can inhale their own exhaled CO_2 from a paper bag, thus lowering the $PaCO_2$ and increasing H_2CO_3 in their blood. This is especially useful when anxiety or pain is the cause of the respiratory alkalosis. If the patient is on a mechanical ventilator and the $PaCO_2$ is less than 35 mm Hg, it is likely that the level of ventilation is too great, and the respiratory rate of the machine should be decreased. If the alkalosis is severe and tetany is present, calcium gluconate is given intravenously. Renal function is maintained to allow for adequate compensation of the disturbance.

Application of the Nursing Process to the Care of the Patient with Respiratory Alkalosis

Assessment

Obtain a history of the patient. Determine when the onset of symptoms occurred, and identify a precipitating event if possible. Ask about prior similar episodes. Assess current status. Ask about lightheadedness and numbness or tingling of the fingers and toes. Examine the patient for the presence of hyperreflexia, Chvostek's and Trousseau's signs, muscular twitching, or tetany. Also observe for convulsions because they sometimes occur. Review arterial blood gas results to identify the presence of respiratory alkalosis. Check the patient's temperature routinely because fever may be the cause of the hyperventilation. Assess the patient for anxiety. Observe for associated symptoms such as sweating, palpitations, panic, air hunger, and dyspnea. If the patient is on a ventilator, perform routine ventilator checks to identify inappropriate settings that may cause hyperventilation.

Nursing Diagnoses and Planning

Nursing diagnoses and related expected patient outcomes most commonly applicable to patients with respiratory alkalosis include the following:

NDx: Anxiety related to the symptoms of respiratory alkalosis and the precipitating event

Planning: Patient outcomes
1. Hyperventilation is absent.
2. Patient states anxiety has decreased.
3. Patient expresses confidence in ability to cope.

NDx: Ineffective breathing pattern resulting from hyperventilation or an incorrectly adjusted respiratory rate on mechanical ventilator

Planning: Patient outcomes
1. Breathing pattern is slow and easy.
2. Eupnea is present (normal respiratory rate and depth).

NDx: High risk for injury related to nervous system hyperexcitability

Planning: Patient outcomes
1. Patient complies with safety precautions.
2. Patient remains free of injury.

Nursing Interventions

NDx: Anxiety. Listen to the patient who is emotionally upset. Encourage expression of feelings and help to work through anxiety. Administer sedation as ordered if the patient is extremely anxious.

NDx: Ineffective breathing pattern
Demonstrate the slow, relaxed breathing pattern necessary to help reduce the symptoms caused by hyperventilation and alkalosis (panic, dizziness, tingling, hyperreflexia, and lightheadedness). Encourage slow, even breaths. When indicated, assist patient in blowing into a paper bag to reinhale CO_2 to arrest the hyperventilation.

NDx: High risk for injury
If the patient is in danger of developing the serious consequences of alkalosis, institute precautions to ensure the patient's safety. Keep side rails up while the patient is in bed. Assist with moving and walking if dizziness or lightheadedness is present. Routinely monitor for mental alertness throughout the course of the patient's stay in the hospital.

Evaluation

Evaluate the effectiveness of nursing care for a patient with respiratory alkalosis by comparing the patient's status with the expected patient outcomes. Examples of specific outcomes for patients with respiratory alkalosis have been provided in the Planning section.

The Elderly: Special Considerations

The elderly are at greater risk for fluid imbalance than are younger individuals. Of all the imbalances, dehydration (hyperosmolar ECFVD) is the most common. There are numerous reasons for this. First, with advancing age, lean body mass is increasingly replaced with fat tissue. This results in a decrease in total body fluid because fat tissue has a lower volume of ICF. Second, the kidney's ability to concentrate urine decreases with advancing age. This is due to decreased sensitivity of the renal tubules to ADH, with progressive loss of renal mass and a decrease in renal perfusion. By 80 years of age, renal mass has decreased by approximately 30% and renal perfusion by 50%. The third factor predisposing the elderly to dehydration is insufficient intake. This is the result of decreased thirst sensation or impaired mobility, which limits access to fluids, intentional restriction of fluids in an attempt to control incontinence, or the presence of a health problem that makes the ingestion of fluids difficult or increases the need for fluids because of excessive loss. Examples of such health problems are dysphagia, vomiting, and diarrhea. Elderly persons also have decreased taste perception of salt. This can lead to excessive use of table salt, which, without an associated increase in water intake, can lead to dehydration and hyperosmolality.

Identifying signs of dehydration is more difficult in the elderly than in younger persons. Skin turgor is generally poor in the elderly because of a loss of skin elasticity and, therefore, is not always a good indicator of hydration status. Similarly, because many elderly experience decreased production of saliva, dry oral mucous membranes and a furrowed, furry tongue do not always indicate dehydration. Often the first change noted in the patient is altered cognitive function such as the development of mild confusion. Other signs are the development of constipation and episodes of orthostatic hypotension.

Dehydration is a particularly dangerous problem to the patient with a respiratory infection. It contributes to the development of very thick, very tenacious sputum, which the elderly person with a weakened cough reflex cannot raise. This can both prolong the existing infection and contribute to reinfection.

Just as there is impaired ability to concentrate urine and conserve water on the part of the aged kidney, there is also an impaired ability to dilute urine. Excretion of excess water by the aged kidney is slow. Intravenous solutions containing sodium are given to the elderly with caution because they can lead to hypervolemia and precipitate CHF.

The elderly are also at increased risk for electrolyte imbalance. As with the fluid imbalances, this increased risk is related to a loss of adaptive capacity. For example, it takes the aged kidney half again as long as the younger kidney to decrease the amount of sodium excreted in the urine in response to a decreased sodium intake. Because the aged kidney is also less sensitive to the effects of aldosterone, the elderly are also at risk for hyperkalemia, especially if experiencing GI bleeding or receiving intravenous potassium.

Bibliography

Ames SW, Kneisel CR. Essentials of adult health nursing. Menlo Park, CA: Addison-Wesley, 1988.

Atkinson DE, Bourke E. Metabolic aspects of regulation of systemic pH. Am J Physiol 1987;252:F947.

Bidani A. Electrolyte and acid-base disorders. Med Clin North Am 1986;70(5):1013.
Boyda EB. Respiratory assessment–Nursing assessment series. Oradell, NJ: Medical Economics, 1985.
Buddle N. Arterial blood gases: A simple method for interpretation. J Post Anesth Nurs 1987;2(4):227.
Carroll HJ, Oh MS. Water, electrolyte and acid-base metabolism. 2nd ed. Philadelphia: JB Lippincott, 1989.
Chernow B, Bamberger S, Stoiko M, et al. Hypomagnesemia inpatients in postoperative intensive care. Chest 1989;95(2):391.
Cormack D (ed). Geriatric nursing: A conceptual approach. Oxford, England: Blackwell Scientific, 1985.
Esberger KK, Hughes ST Jr. Nursing care of the aped. Norwalk, CT: Appleton & Lange, 1989.
Fischbach F. Laboratory diagnostic tests. 3rd ed. Philadelphia: JB Lippincott, 1988.
Gambert SR (ed). Handbook of geriatrics. New York: Plenum Press, 1987.
German K. Fluid and electrolyte problems associated with diabetes insipidus and syndrome of inappropriate antidiuretic hormone. Nurs Clin North Am 1987;22(4):785.
Gershan JA, Freeman CM, Ross MC, et al. Fluid volume deficit: Validating the indicators. Heart Lung 1990;19(2):152.
Gettrust KV, Brabec PD. Nursing diagnosis. Albany, NY: Delmar, 1992.
Guyton AC. Textbook of medical physiology. 8th ed. Philadelphia: WB Saunders, 1991.
Ham RJ, Sloane PD. Primary care geriatrics. 2nd ed. St. Louis: Mosby-Year book, 1991.
Heitkemper MM, Bond E. Fluid and electrolytes: Assessment and interventions. J Enterostomal Ther 1988;15(1):18.
Kee JL. Fluids and electrolytes with clinical applications. 4th ed. New York: John Wiley & Sons, 1986.
Kee JL. Laboratory and diagnostic tests with nursing implications. 3rd ed. Norwalk, CT: Appleton & Lange, 1991.
Kee JL. Potassium imbalances. Nursing 87 1987;17(9):32K.
Konlen J. Interpreting acid-base problems through arterial blood gases. Crit Care Nurse 1983;3(5):34.
Kositzke JA. A question of balance dehydration in the elderly. J Gerontol Nurs 1990;16(5):4.
Lewis EM, Collier IC. Medical surgical nursing. 2nd ed. New York: McGraw-Hill, 1987.
Luckmann J, Sorensen KC. Medical surgical nursing—A psychophysiologic approach. 3rd ed. Philadelphia: WB Saunders, 1987.
Lye M (ed). Acute geriatric medicine. Lancashire, England: MTP Press, 1985.
Mathewson M, Mathewson RE: Establishing acid-base balance. Crit Care Nurse 1987;7(5):82.
Mecca RS. Acid-base disorders in the postoperative period. Curr Rev Nurse Anesthetists 1987;9(25):202.
Metheny NM. Fluid and electrolyte balance. Philadelphia: JB Lippincott, 1987.
Pfister SM, Bullas JB. Arterial blood gas equilibrium: Metabolic acidemia. Crit Care Nurs 1989;9(1):70.
Porth CM. Pathophysiology. 3rd ed. Philadelphia: JB Lippincott, 1990.
Stein JH. Hypokalemia: Common and uncommon causes. Hosp Pract 1988;23:55.
Urrows S (ed). Symposium on fluid, electrolytes, and acid-base balance. Nurs Clin North Am 1980;15:535.
Valle GA, Lemberg L. Electrolyte imbalances in cardiovascular disease: The forgotten factor. Heart Lung 1987;22(4):797.
Watson JE. Fluid and electrolyte disorders in cardiovascular patients. Nurs Clin North Am 1987;22(4):797.
York K. The lung and fluid-electrolyte and acid-base imbalances, Nurs Clin North Am. 1987;22(4):805.
Young ME, Flynn KT. Third-spacing: When the body conceals fluid loss. RN 1988;51:46.

Chapter Four

KNOWLEDGE BASIC TO THE NURSING CARE *of Adults Undergoing Surgery*

Surgery is any procedure performed on the human body that uses instruments to alter the integrity of tissues or organs. The purpose of the surgical procedure may be diagnostic (e.g., excision of tissue for biopsy), corrective (e.g., repair of a defective heart valve), reconstructive (e.g., skin grafts after a burn injury), or palliative (e.g., debulking an inoperative tumor to relieve pain or to temporarily restore function).

Nursing care of the patient undergoing surgery requires clinical expertise based on sound understanding of anatomy and physiology, the planned surgical procedure, and the effects of surgery on the body's homeostatic mechanisms. The patient and loved ones depend on the nurse's knowledge, understanding, compassion, and technical expertise to allay their concerns, demystify the surgical experience, and help the patient through a smooth, successful surgery and recovery. The nurse's roles as educator and patient advocate are a primary focus throughout the perioperative period. This chapter presents physiologic and psychological factors that affect the patient undergoing surgery and perioperative nursing activities to promote a successful surgical experience.

Perioperative Nursing

Perioperative nursing is nursing care of the patient who requires surgical intervention. Perioperative nursing is divided into three phases: preoperative, intraoperative, and postoperative. The Association of Operating Room Nurses, Inc. (AORN) has established standards and recommended practices for perioperative nursing. These standards, which are represented by the examples of nursing activities presented in Table 4–1, help define the scope of nursing practice during the perioperative period.

Legal Parameters

INFORMED CONSENT

Written permission must be obtained from the patient before any surgical procedure, any procedure during which anesthesia is administered or the physician plans to enter a body cavity, any procedure that carries a high risk, and diagnostic tests with potentially sensitive outcomes (e.g., human immunodeficiency virus [HIV] antibody testing). Informed

Table 4–1. EXAMPLES OF NURSING ACTIVITIES IN PERIOPERATIVE NURSING PRACTICE

PREOPERATIVE PHASE	INTRAOPERATIVE PHASE	POSTOPERATIVE PHASE
PREOPERATIVE ASSESSMENT Home/clinic 1. initiates initial preoperative assessment 2. plans teaching methods appropriate to patient's needs 3. involves family in interview Surgical unit 1. completes preoperative assessment 2. coordinates patient teaching with other nursing staff 3. explains phases in perioperative period and expectations 4. develops a plan of care Surgical suite 1. assesses patient's level of consciousness 2. reviews chart 3. identifies patient 4. verifies surgical site PLANNING 1. determines a plan of care PSYCHOLOGICAL SUPPORT 1. tells patient what is happening 2. determines psychological status 3. gives prior warning of noxious stimuli 4. communicates patient's emotional status to other appropriate members of the health care team	MAINTENANCE OF SAFETY 1. assures that the sponge, needle, and instrument counts are correct 2. positions the patient a. functional alignment b. exposure of surgical site c. maintenance of position throughout procedure 3. applies grounding device to patient 4. provides physical support PHYSIOLOGICAL MONITORING 1. calculates effects on patient of excessive fluid loss 2. distinguishes normal from abnormal cardiopulmonary data 3. reports changes in patient's pulse, respirations, temperature, and blood pressure PSYCHOLOGICAL MONITORING (prior to induction and if patient conscious) 1. provides emotional support to patient 2. stands near/touches patient during procedures/induction 3. continues to assess patient's emotional status 4. communicates patient's emotional status to other appropriate members of the health care team NURSING MANAGEMENT 1. provides physical safety for the patient 2. maintains aseptic, controlled environment 3. effectively manages human resources	COMMUNICATION OF INTRAOPERATIVE INFORMATION 1. gives patient's name 2. states type of surgery performed 3. provides contributing intraoperative factors, ie, drain, catheters 4. states physical limitations 5. states impairments resulting from surgery 6. reports patient's preoperative level of consciousness 7. communicates necessary equipment needs POSTOPERATIVE EVALUATION Recovery area 1. determines patient's immediate response to surgical intervention Surgical unit 1. evaluates effectiveness of nursing care in the OR 2. determines patient's level of satisfaction with care given during perioperative period 3. evaluates products used on patient in the OR 4. determines patient's psychological status 5. assists with discharge planning Home/clinic 1. seeks patient's perception of surgery in terms of the effects of anesthetic agents, impact on body image, distortion, immobilization 2. determines family's perceptions of surgery

Reprinted with permission from AORN Standards and Recommended Practices for Perioperative Nursing, 1991, pp I:1–4. Copyright © AORN Inc, 10170 East Mississippi Avenue, Denver, CO 80231.

consent protects the patient's right to make an informed decision about his or her medical treatment and protects the health care facility and staff from legal action should the patient or significant other claim the procedure was performed without the person's permission or knowledge.

Competent adults 18 years of age may consent to their own treatment. Minors may consent if they are "emancipated," that is, living without parents or guardians and managing their own financial affairs; on active duty with the United States armed forces; pregnant; or married, whether or not the marriage has been dissolved. Consent is obtained from a parent or legal guardian if the patient is a minor or an incompetent adult. Incompetent adults are individuals who are unconscious or mentally incompetent regarding their actions.

Consent for treatment must be an "informed" consent given voluntarily, without coercion, by the patient or legal substitute. Informed consent implies that the patient or legal guardian has been informed by the physician of the nature, risks, desired results, and possible complications associated with the planned procedure and that alternative treatments were discussed. The explanation must be given in terminology and a language understood by the person signing the consent and must include information that any reasonably prudent person would need in order to make an intelligent decision about the proposed procedure or treatment. Consent cannot be obtained from an individual under the influence of a potentially mind-altering substance.

In nonemergency situations when the patient's health is at risk but consent is not obtainable from the patient or legal guardian or if consent is refused, the hospital may obtain a court order for treatment such as blood transfusions or necessary surgery. Implied consent refers to emergency treatment or surgery that is performed without written permission when it is believed that the patient would have given permission if competent, able to understand the situation, and able to do so.

Each agency has a form that must be signed, dated, and witnessed indicating informed consent. It specifies the patient, the surgery or procedure, and the physician performing the surgery or procedure. The agency defines in its procedure policies the role of he nurse in obtaining consent forms and in witnessing such forms. As a witness, the nurse is verifying that the patient has signed the form voluntarily and understands the procedure to which he or she is consenting. The physician is responsible for explaining both the benefits and the risks to the patient before the patient gives a valid informed consent. If a patient indicates lack of understanding, confusion, or ambivalence regarding the consent, the physician is notified immediately and consent is not obtained.

Finally, remember that a patient can revoke consent at any time before the procedure. Document the patient's unwillingness to proceed with the procedure and notify the physician immediately.

ADVANCE DIRECTIVE FOR TREATMENT

Laws have been passed by various legislative bodies to ensure patients' rights to direct their treatment. The Federal Patient Self Determination Act requires that health care provider agencies receiving Medicare payments must inform all patients 18 years or older of their right to plan in advance for their care. Failure to comply with this law can result in loss of Medicare payments. If patients so desire, they can indicate the life-sustaining treatments they do and do not want or designate an individual to make decisions on their behalf if they become unable to make their wishes known. This individual is referred to as the patient's health care agent or surrogate. The documents for recording these decisions are defined as advance directives and are commonly referred to as a living will or health care proxy. Instructions in the advance directive should be as specific as possible to ensure compliance with patients' wishes. For example, a phrase such as "no heroic measures" may be interpreted different ways. Instead, the directive should state which specific treatments are to be refused and under what circumstances, for example, "If I become terminally ill, with no hope of recovery, I do not want to receive chemotherapy, cardiopulmonary resuscitation, artificial respiration, or nutrition and hydration through a feeding tube." Each agency determines who is responsible for advising patients of their rights under this law and how this communication is to be documented. In-service education must be provided for all agency personnel involved in this process.

In addition to the Federal Patient Self Determination Act, many states have enacted laws regulating "Do Not Resuscitate" (DNR) orders. A DNR order means that no attempt will be made to revive heart or lung function if these activities stop. Although the specifics of the laws vary from state to state, in general, a DNR request must be made by the patient or the patient's family or health care agent. For it to be valid, the DNR order must be documented in the patient record by the physician. The DNR protocol usually requires completion of a DNR request form by the patient, the family or surrogate, and the physician. Agency policy or state law may require renewal of a DNR order at periodic intervals. A DNR decision may be revoked at any time by the requesting party.

ORGAN DONATION

Federal required request laws mandate that all health care provider institutions who receive Medicare reimbursements establish a written policy and procedure to identify potential organ donors and refer them to certified organ procurement organizations. Failure to comply with this law can result in loss of Medicare payments. The procedure must specify who is to identify the potential donor, of whom the request can legally be made, whom to notify of the donation, and how to document the request and response. In-service education must be provided for all agency personnel named in the policy.

Classification of Conditions Requiring Surgery

Surgical procedures are classified in many different ways. The most common classifications are based on the extent of surgery, the urgency of surgery, and the surgical approach used.

EXTENT OF SURGERY

Procedures are described as major or minor on the basis of risk involved and extent of surgery. Minor surgical procedures involve a limited body area and a short period of time to complete the procedure and constitute minimal risk to the patient. An example is the removal of a benign skin lesion that could be performed in a hospital ambulatory setting or in a physician's office.

Major surgical procedures involve an extended body area or a longer period of surgical time and present an increased risk to the patient. These procedures are performed in an operating room and require a surgical team. Examples of major surgery are an abdominal bowel resection (opening into the abdominal cavity to excise a portion of the bowel) or a craniotomy (an opening into the skull to operate on a portion of the brain).

URGENCY OF SURGERY

Another method of classifying surgical procedures is based on the degree of urgency for the procedure to be performed. Emergency surgery must be performed immediately to save the patient's life, to maintain organ or limb function, to remove a damaged organ or limb that endangers the patient's life, or to stop hemorrhage. A gunshot or stab wound lacerating a large blood vessel would require emergency surgery.

Urgent surgery requires surgical intervention within 24 to 48 hours and includes procedures such as removal of kidney or ureteral stones. Required surgery denotes a surgical procedure that needs to be performed but can be scheduled a few weeks or months ahead. Cataract removal or a tonsillectomy are examples.

Elective surgery involves a condition for which surgery is recommended, but if the procedure was delayed or not done there would be no adverse effects. A vaginal repair or a scar removal are examples of elective surgical procedures. To ensure the necessity of elective surgical procedures, many insurance companies are requiring the opinion of a second surgeon. Optional surgery is performed on the basis of the patient's personal choice. Cosmetic surgery in most instances is optional.

SURGICAL APPROACH

The surgical approach and location of the surgical incision are influenced by many factors, including the patient's diagnosis, expected pathology, provision for maximum exposure of the operative area, ease of increasing the size of the incision if necessary, ease of closure, minimum postoperative discomfort, and maximum provision for wound healing and aesthetic effect. Examples of surgical procedures classified by approach include vaginal hysterectomy (removal of the uterus by way of the vagina), abdominal hysterectomy (removal of the uterus through an abdominal incision), transurethral prostatectomy (removal of the prostate gland by way of the urethra), and perineal prostatectomy (removal of the prostate gland through an incision in the perineum).

Some surgery can also be performed through straight or flexible fiberoptic/endoscopic tubes inserted into the body through external orifices or small surgical incisions. These tubes allow instruments for cutting, applying clips, electrical cauterization, and laser light to be guided into the body and manipulated by the surgeon, who visualizes the procedure either through an optical scope in the tube or on a visual display monitor attached to a camera on the end of the tube. Surgery of the gastrointestinal tract, the urinary tract, the respiratory tract, the circulatory system, and reproductive organs can be performed through fiberoptic/endoscopic tubes.

Other surgical techniques include application of chemical agents to superficial skin lesions to damage the tissue and cause it to die and slough off. Electric current may be applied to a lesion to cauterize it or its vascular supply and base of attachment to underlying structures. The lesion is then manually removed or allowed to die and slough off. Laser light can be used to vaporize lesions or cauterize blood vessels supplying a lesion. Surgical approaches and the nursing care specific to each are discussed in detail in the appropriate chapters throughout the text.

Assessment of Factors Affecting Surgical Risk

Every surgical procedure involves certain risk. The amount of risk depends on the patient's overall physical and mental health status, the presence of certain factors that are known to increase surgical risk, the nature and extent of the disease being treated, and the location and extent of the planned procedure. To determine surgical risk, the patient history, physical examination, and diagnostic evaluation are completed by the surgeon. The patient's present condition and any other concurrent physical conditions that might affect the ability to tolerate surgery or alter the outcome of the surgical intervention are identified. If the risks of surgery are determined to be greater than the benefits to the patient, surgery may be delayed until the patient is in better condition, or it may be canceled altogether.

HISTORY AND PHYSICAL EXAMINATION

A thorough medical history and physical examination are essential to a successful surgical outcome. Each agency has a patient history form to guide data collection and to facilitate documentation. Common symptoms that require special emphasis during data collection include pain, vomiting, change in bowel habits, hematemesis, passage of blood through the rectum, and trauma. Obtain information about the present illness, family history, and the patient's history and emotional background. Detailed discussion of interview techniques and data collection are presented in nursing fundamentals texts.

PSYCHOSOCIAL ASSESSMENT

Regardless of the extent or urgency of the surgical procedure, it is a stressful event and has an emotional and well as physical impact on the patient. It is common to experience many fears on learning of the necessity for surgery. Fear of the unknown, fear of an altered body image, fear of a change in lifestyle, fear of separation, fear of cancer, fear of pain, and fear of death are common responses. At the same time, a patient may experience or verbalize feelings of relief that a course of action has been decided on to diagnose or treat a disorder through surgery. It is common for responses of fear and relief to be present simultaneously.

Stress elicits a physical as well as an emotional response depending on the degree of stress experienced. Age, physical condition, and experience with stressful situations and surgery affect the patient's response. Patients under stress may be overly anxious or appear deceptively calm and relaxed. They may have difficulty concentrating and be easily distracted or may focus exclusively on one detail. The patient may become withdrawn, agitated, angry, hostile, or demanding. Stimulation of the sympathetic nervous system and neuroendocrine response to stress is manifested by decreased urinary output, increased heart rate and cardiac output, increased blood pressure, and increased physical activity such as pacing.

During the perioperative period, the patient requires psychological and emotional support. Explain the surgical procedure and what can be expected during the perioperative period in understandable terminology to alleviate anxiety. Diagrams and pictures frequently help patients understand the surgical procedure. Cultural influences vary, and an individual's family can be an important support system during the perioperative phase. Include family members or significant others in the discussion when possible. Offer spiritual support through clergy. Preoperative teaching, tailored to the patient's cultural and educational background, provides psychological and emotional support and alleviates anxiety.

ECONOMIC FACTORS

Financial implications of surgery are dependent on the type and extent of the procedure as well as the patient's recovery. Extensive surgery requires a longer recuperation than a minor surgical procedure. The impact of the hospitalization, surgery, and recovery may add to the patient's stress and alter postsurgical lifestyle and independence.

At the least, surgery may require time lost from work and responsibilities at home. The individual may lose income while unable to work and may be concerned about job loss. Surgery may render the person unable to continue in his or her former occupation, further altering income and socioeconomic status. Many individuals have no insurance to cover health care costs or may be undergoing treatments that are not covered by insurance. Referral to resources for financial assistance, often coordinated by the agency's social workers, helps the patient cope with the economic impact of surgery, increases the patient's sense of control over the situation, and reduces stress.

NUTRITIONAL STATUS

Both malnutrition and obesity increase the surgical patient's risk. Nutritional deficits increase the risk for poor wound healing, inadequate hemostasis, and postoperative infection. Nutritional deficits are found primarily in elderly patients or in those with chronic illnesses, cancer, or intestinal disease. They are also common among the homeless and alcohol and drug abusers. Malnourished patients might require nutritional support with oral supplements, enteral feedings, or parenteral hyperalimentation therapy before surgery.

Obesity increases surgical risk because of a higher incidence of postoperative wound complications and concomitant disease in the obese. Poor wound healing and infection are common in obese individuals because fat tissue has a poor blood supply, and nutrients and antibodies do not reach the operative area in the needed quantities. Pulmonary complications are also more likely to occur in the obese because (1) ventilatory expansion may be compromised by abdominal fat; (2) these individuals have greater difficulty moving, coughing, and deep breathing postoperatively; and (3) postanesthetic recovery is prolonged because fat cells retain anesthetic agents longer than other cells. To decrease risks, a nutritionally sound weight-loss program is undertaken before elective surgery.

FLUID AND ELECTROLYTE BALANCE

Fluid and electrolyte disturbances increase surgical risk by altering the body's ability to adjust to, and recover from, the stress and trauma of surgery. Fluid and electrolyte imbalances are more common in the elderly because of reduced renal function, decreased cardiovascular and respiratory function, altered hormonal regulatory functions, and decreased total body fluids as a result of the aging process. Fluid excess increases the risk of cardiovascular and respiratory complications. It may be caused by acute or chronic cardiac, renal, and liver disorders, overadministration of parenteral fluids, and hypernatremia. Fluid volume deficit may be caused by fluid loss from vomiting, diarrhea, hemorrhage, or inadequate fluid intake. Additional fluids are lost during surgery from evaporation and blood loss. Fluid volume deficit increases risk of altered tissue perfusion, cardiovascular complications, and hypovolemic shock. Electrolyte imbalance may develop in many acute and chronic conditions. They are most commonly the result of altered electrolyte intake or absorption, altered electrolyte excretion, or electrolyte shift between the cells and extracellular fluid. A loss or gain of sodium is usually associated with a loss or gain of water. Electrolyte imbalance places the patient at risk for fluid imbalance, acid-base imbalance, and disturbances in neuromuscular impulse transmission and response. In nonemergency situations, fluid and electrolyte imbalances are corrected before surgery. Fluid and electrolyte imbalances are discussed in detail in Chapter 3.

IMMUNE STATUS

An infection anywhere in the body can affect the outcome of a surgical procedure. The body's normal defenses are involved in fighting the infection; therefore, the ability to withstand the stress of surgery is compromised. For this reason, elective surgery may be postponed if any signs or symptoms of infection such as an elevated temperature, skin lesions, sore throat, coughing, or sneezing are present.

When an immunodeficiency disorder exists, the patient's risk for postoperative complications and even death is greatly increased.

A strong personal or family history of allergic disorders might be indicative of hypersensitivity to drugs and needs to be considered by the surgeon and anesthesiologist because drug allergies, sensitivities, and incompatibilities as well as adverse drug reactions may be fatal. Chapters 9 and 10 discuss the immune system and its disorders in detail.

CARDIOVASCULAR STATUS

Concurrent cardiac disease increases the risk associated with surgery because of altered or exaggerated myocardial responses to anesthetic agents, electrolyte imbalance, and catecholamine release stimulated by the stress and trauma of surgery. Prior cardiovascular disorders compromise the patient's ability to adjust to alterations in fluid balance and tissue perfusion and to recover from the effects of blood loss and shock. Recent or unstable anginal pain, signs of a recent myocardial infarction, cardiac dysrhythmia, valvular heart disease, and cardiac failure are evaluated, treated, or controlled before surgery. An electrocardiogram is often done for adults who will undergo major surgery. Surgery, if not an emergency or urgent in nature, is postponed for 6 months after a myocardial infarction. Cardiac function and disorders are discussed in detail in Chapters 17 and 18.

Peripheral vascular disease and hypertension increase the risk of clot and emboli formation postoperatively. The patient's current status is evaluated and, if needed, treatment is initiated to control the problem and reduce surgical risk. The vascular system and its disorders are discussed in detail in Chapters 19 and 20.

RESPIRATORY STATUS

Smoking and the presence of pulmonary disease greatly increase the surgical patient's risk. Smoking irritates the respiratory passages, destroys cilia, and decreases vital capacity. The individual is less able to cough effectively to clear pulmonary secretions and is, therefore, at increased risk for pulmonary tract infections, atelectasis, and impaired clearance of inhaled anesthetic agents. In addition, heavy smokers may become restless or agitated postoperatively because of nicotine withdrawal if unable to smoke, may be noncompliant with activity restrictions in order to smoke, or may create a fire hazard by smoking while confined to bed.

Upper and lower respiratory tract infections are contraindications for elective surgery because of the increased risk of airway obstruction and postoperative atelectasis. The presence of chronic obstructive pulmonary disease (COPD), bronchial asthma, and restrictive lung disease increases the number and severity of postoperative complications as a result of inadequate exchange of respiratory gases. During the history and physical examination, the finding of any pulmonary disease or assessments indicative of pulmonary disease, such as exertional dyspnea, exercise intolerance, cough, production of sputum, or history of smoking, may necessitate further evaluation and pulmonary function tests. A radiologic chest examination may be done to rule out active pulmonary disease. Respiratory functions and disorders are discussed in detail in Chapters 12, 13, and 14.

RENAL FUNCTION

Impaired renal function places the patient at risk for fluid and electrolyte imbalances because of altered excretion of catabolic waste products and fluid retention. Renal function is evaluated by a complete

urinalysis and measurement of serum creatinine, albumin, and blood urea nitrogen. Renal patients receiving dialysis treatments require dialysis the day before surgery and as soon as possible postoperatively to decrease excessive accumulation of toxic metabolites.

Many medications commonly used during the perioperative period are toxic to the kidney, and dosages are modified in patients with renal disease. These include antibiotics, antituberculosis agents, anti-inflammatory agents, hypoglycemic agents, analgesics, anesthetics, hypnotics, and antineoplastic drugs. Renal function and urinary tract disorders are discussed in detail in Chapter 25 and 26.

HEPATIC FUNCTION

Liver disease is associated with increased surgical risk because adequate liver function is important for biotransformation and detoxification of drugs and anesthetic agents and the production of clotting factors. If the history and physical reveal the possibility of liver disease, chronic malnutrition, alcoholism, or drug abuse, further hepatic studies are indicated. Hepatic function and disorders are discussed in detail in Chapters 27 and 28.

ENDOCRINE STATUS

Endocrine abnormalities must be recognized and treated preoperatively to prevent acute hormone imbalances triggered by stress or anesthetic agents. Diabetes mellitus and chronic thyroid, adrenal, or other endocrine disorders increase the patient's risk for infections, impaired wound healing, and cardiovascular complications. Endocrine disorders require evaluation, treatment, and control before elective surgery to minimize perioperative risk. Endocrine gland functions and disorders are discussed in detail in Chapters 29, 30 (diabetes mellitus), 31 (pituitary), 32 (adrenal), 33 (thyroid), and 34 (parathyroid).

NEUROLOGIC STATUS

Neurologic disorders increase the risk for impaired respiratory function and altered response to anesthetic and analgesic agents because of altered neurologic function. Anesthesia and the stress of surgery may exacerbate a chronic neurologic disorder such as epilepsy, multiple sclerosis, or myasthenia gravis, increasing the risk for injury and poor wound healing. Chronic neurologic conditions are stabilized before elective surgery. A preoperative neurologic examination for all surgical candidates provides baseline data for postoperative reference and evaluation. Neurologic function and disorders are discussed in detail in Chapters 37 and 38.

HEMATOLOGIC STATUS

In general, moderate anemia does not increase the hazards of surgery, although the recovery period may be prolonged. Ideally, moderate anemia and deficiencies of iron, folic acid, and vitamin B_{12} are corrected before elective surgery. Elective surgery is postponed for severe anemia. Anticoagulants are usually discontinued before surgery to prevent delayed clotting.

Sickle-cell disease is usually accompanied by chronic anemia and increased risk of thrombosis formation because the stress of surgery causes sickling of the red blood cells. Before surgery, hydration is increased and blood transfusions may be administered to increase the hemoglobin to normal levels. The hematologic system and its disorders are discussed in detail in Chapters 15 and 16.

PREGNANCY

The need for surgery arises in the pregnant woman just as often as in the nonpregnant woman of the same age. When the maternal need for surgery arises, fetal risk must be considered. Only emergency and urgent operations are performed during pregnancy. Elective operations are postponed until the postpartum period. In addition, radiologic examinations of the lower abdomen and pelvis are avoided, if possible, especially during the first 6 weeks of pregnancy.

The more common disease entities that require surgical intervention during pregnancy include appendicitis, hiatal hernia, and cholecystitis. Less frequently, intestinal obstruction, breast cancer, and ovarian tumor require surgery during pregnancy. Perioperative care during pregnancy is presented in obstetric textbooks.

THERAPEUTIC DRUGS

Many prescription and nonprescription medications can alter a person's response to surgery or anesthetic agents. Antihypertensives, antiarrhythmics, antibiotics, and anticonvulsants can interact adversely with anesthetic agents. Corticosteroids generally diminish the patient's ability to withstand the stress of surgery. Aspirin and other anticoagulants increase the chance of hemorrhage. Diuretics increase the risk for postoperative electrolyte imbalance. For these reasons, all medications that the patient takes routinely are evaluated, and discontinuation or dosage adjustment may be ordered.

ALCOHOLISM

Alcohol is a central nervous system depressant that can interact with medications given during the perioperative period and result in unexpected and often dangerous reactions. Patients tend to understate their alcohol consumption and deny symptoms that might be associated with alcoholism.

Chronic alcoholism leads to malnutrition and clotting disorders. Cirrhosis of the liver leads to a reduction of the clotting factors II (prothrombin), V, VII, and X. Platelets may be severely reduced in

acute alcoholism and may be responsible for bleeding problems. Bleeding from the gastrointestinal tract is usually caused by esophageal varices, gastritis, or hemorrhoids. Bleeding further compromises the patient's condition and increases the risk of complications. Liver disorders related to alcohol abuse are discussed in Chapter 28.

SUBSTANCE ABUSE

Patients who abuse substances such as caffeine, drugs, and alcohol are at increased surgical risk. Caffeine withdrawal can lead to jitteriness, tremors, insomnia, or agitation. Specific responses of drug withdrawal depend on the substance abused by the patient. Withdrawal from alcohol can lead to delirium tremens and unexpected gastrointestinal bleeding. In most instances, the surgeon, anesthesiologist, and nurse are unaware of the substance abuse and become knowledgeable because of the effects of withdrawal during the postoperative period.

Preoperative Period

The preoperative period begins at the time it is determined that surgery is the best course of treat-

Table 4–2. COMMON PREOPERATIVE DIAGNOSTIC STUDIES

STUDY	PURPOSE AND PROCEDURE	NURSING IMPLICATIONS
BLOOD STUDIES		
CBC	Examination of venous blood sample to evaluate Hgb concentration, Hct, RBC, and WBC; white cell differential identifies percentages of each type of leukocyte	No special preparation needed; there is slight discomfort during needle insertion; the arm is elevated without bending elbow, and pressure applied until bleeding stops
Platelet count and coagulation studies	Evaluation of venous blood sample for platelet level and PT, PTT; used to evaluate homeostatic function and identify patients at risk for prolonged bleeding or coagulation abnormalities during and after surgery	Same as CBC; assess skin and mucous membranes for petechiae and ecchymoses; ask about bleeding from gums, rectum to identify patients at risk
Serum test profile (SMA 12)	Automated electronic system examines venous serum sample for multiple diagnostic studies; 12 determinations include glucose, cholesterol, albumin, and total protein (nutrition status); bilirubin level (liver function); BUN and uric acid levels (renal function); AST (tissue injury); alkaline phosphatase (bone-tissue injury); and calcium and phosphate levels (parathyroid function)	Instruct the patient to maintain NPO status except for water 4 hr before test; venous blood sample per CBC
Serum electrolytes	Sodium, potassium, chloride, calcium are measured; magnesium may be included	Abnormal electrolyte values are immediately reported to physician; no special preparation; venous blood sample per CBC
RENAL FUNCTION		
Urinalysis	Screening test for urinary tract and renal disease as well as some metabolic and systemic disorders	No preparation; send random sample of at least 15 ml fresh urine for analysis immediately or refrigerate; first-morning urine preferred; collect specimen in clean, dry container; indicate current medications on laboratory requisition
CARDIAC FUNCTION		
ECG	Evaluate cardiac status, provide baseline data. Electrodes are placed on the four extremities and the chest	Male patients may need some chest hair shaved to permit proper adhesion of the leads; test involves no preparation or discomfort
RADIOLOGIC STUDIES		
Radiography (x-ray examination)	Shadow image of the contour and density of a part of the body produced by roentgen rays; used to visualize size, position, foreign objects, or injury	Determine date of LMP; radiographic studies are avoided during pregnancy, especially in first trimester; patient preparation depends on examination; jewelry in the area to be examined must be removed
Chest roentgenogram (chest x-ray examination)	Assess pulmonary status and determine location and size of pulmonary lesions	Instruct patient that it is necessary to hold breath on inhalation while the films are taken; patient preparation per view

(continued)

ment and concludes with admission of the patient to the operative suite. Diagnostic studies are completed, preoperative teaching is initiated, body system disorders are stabilized, and the consent for treatment is obtained. The preoperative period can be very short, as with emergency surgery, or extended in length, as with elective or optional surgery.

Diagnostic Procedures

Depending on the planned surgical procedure and the age and condition of the patient, a variety of diagnostic procedures may be completed before surgery. The purposes of these procedures are as follows:

1. Establish baseline values for intraoperative and postoperative comparison.
2. Screen for diseases or conditions that may affect the surgical result (e.g., infectious processes).
3. Identify diseases that may contraindicate elective surgery or require treatment before surgery (e.g., diabetes mellitus or respiratory disorders). If elective surgery is being contemplated, surgery could be delayed by low blood counts, infection, or fluid and electrolyte imbalance.

Table 4–2. COMMON PREOPERATIVE DIAGNOSTIC STUDIES (*continued*)

STUDY	PURPOSE AND PROCEDURE	NURSING IMPLICATIONS
RADIOLOGIC STUDIES		
CT (or CAT) scan	An x-ray system that produces detailed cross-section images of body tissues and organs not clearly seen with regular x-ray films; a contrast agent may be injected to improve visualization; used to detect organ dysfunction and to determine size and volume of tumor	Patient preparation per area examined; if contrast agent is to be used, NPO for 3 hr before examination; oral medications may be taken with sip of water; determine whether patient is claustrophobic and explain that he or she will be positioned flat on narrow table that slides into center of donut-shaped scanner; table moves every few seconds; examination may take 15–60 min depending on body part being examined
MRI	Uses a strong magnetic field and radiowaves to produce precise images of the body's internal organs and tissues; a contrast agent may be injected to improve visualization; used to detect organ and tissue dysfunction not visible by x-ray film or CT scan	All metal objects and jewelry are removed; all items with metal clips and parts, including hearing aids, are removed; patients with pacemakers, neurostimulators, or any type of metal implants, clips, prostheses, or metal shrapnel or fragments cannot have MRI scans because of strong magnetic fields created; determine date of LMP; not recommended during pregnancy; NPO for 3 hr before scan if contrast agent to be used; oral medications may be taken with sips of water; determine whether patient is claustrophobic and explain that he or she will be positioned flat on a narrow table that slides into center of donut-shaped magnet; examination may take 15–90 min depending on body part being examined
ULTRASOUND IMAGING		
Ultrasonography (ultrasound examination)	Produces image of deep body structures by measuring and recording reflection of pulsed or continuous high-frequency sound waves; used to visualize organs	Patient preparation depends on body organ being examined; electrode jelly applied over body surface to facilitate movement of transmitter/receiver
NUCLEAR MEDICINE	Patient receives radioactive compound that circulates through body; gamma rays given off by compound are detected in tissues and organs by gamma scanners and imagers and in blood and urine by gamma counters; used to evaluate organ function and extent of certain diseases	Patient preparation and participation depends on study; reassure patient that radioactive dose is very low; agents lose most of their activity in hours or days and are usually quickly eliminated from body; refer to facility procedure manual for specific precautions; determine date of LMP; not done during pregnancy

Abbreviations: CBC, complete blood count; BUN, blood urea nitrogen; AST, aspartate aminotransferase (formerly SGOT); LDH, lactic dehydrogenase; LMP, last menstrual period; Hgb, hemoglobin; Hct, hematocrit; RBC, red blood cell; WBC, white blood cell; PT, prothrombin; PTT, partial thromboplastin time; CT, computed tomography; NPO, nothing by mouth; MRI, magnetic resonance imaging; CAT, computed axial tomography; ECG, electrocardiogram.

4. Initially diagnose or further evaluate conditions that require surgery (e.g., appendicitis, fractures).
5. Evaluate the extent and nature of preexisting medical conditions (e.g., heart disease, renal disease).

Diagnostic examinations depend on the planned surgical procedure and the condition of the patient. A complete blood count, serum electrolytes and chemistries, and urinalysis are the most common preoperative diagnostic procedures. Completion of blood coagulation studies, radiologic studies of the chest, and an electrocardiogram are dependent on the age, condition, diagnosis, and medical history of the patient as well as agency policy and physician preference.

Additional diagnostic studies may be required to clarify results of these examinations or to further aid the surgeon in determining the patient's diagnosis or the extent of the area involved in the planned surgery. Radiologic studies of specific body parts or organs, computed tomography, magnetic resonance imaging, ultrasonography, and nuclear medicine studies are examples of these types of diagnostic procedures. Table 4–2 describes common preoperative diagnostic studies and their nursing implications.

Preoperative Medical Management

Patients who have an extensive medical history or who have been treated medically before surgical intervention are examined by their medical physician before surgery and their progress followed throughout recovery to ensure consistent, ongoing management of concurrent medical conditions. The surgeon, during a final preoperative examination and evaluation, reviews diagnostic findings with the patient as well as the anticipated plan for surgery, answers questions to clarify areas of concern, and writes specific orders for preoperative restrictions and final preparation of the patient for surgery.

FOOD AND FLUID RESTRICTIONS

Dietary modifications depend on the scheduled time of surgery, the type of anesthesia to be used, and the surgical procedure. Solid food intake is restricted for a minimum of 7 hours preoperatively, and fluids for at least 4 hours, to prevent regurgitation or vomiting, which could result in airway obstruction, aspiration pneumonia, or atelectasis.

If surgery is scheduled in the morning, the patient usually receives a light diet the evening before and then nothing by mouth (NPO) after midnight. If surgery is scheduled for the afternoon and it does not involve the gastrointestinal tract, the patient may receive a soft or liquid diet for breakfast, then be on NPO status. Administration of intravenous fluids may be initiated the day or night before surgery to prevent dehydration in the elderly and other patients at risk for dehydration during fluid restriction.

ELIMINATION

All patients are instructed to void and defecate before administration of preoperative medications. Preoperative laxatives and cleansing enemas are not routinely ordered, except in the instance of bowel or gastrointestinal surgery. In those situations, multiple cleansing enemas as well as cathartics might be ordered to reduce microorganisms in the operative area and the risk of contamination of the abdomen with stool. Gastric or intestinal suction tubes to remove gastrointestinal contents and to prevent aspiration and abdominal distention may be inserted preoperatively or in the operating room.

For abdominal surgery or surgery of the genitourinary or reproductive tract, an indwelling urinary catheter is often inserted to lessen the risk of accidental bladder injury by maintaining bladder decompression. It may be inserted preoperatively or in the operating room.

SKIN PREPARATION

The purpose of skin preparation is to reduce the risk of postoperative wound infection by reducing the number of microorganisms on the skin to a minimum. In most instances, it is begun on the unit and is completed in the operating room. If possible, the patient bathes or showers the evening before or the morning of surgery.

Hair removal at and surrounding the operative site may be requested before an operative procedure. Some institutions remove hair only if it interferes with the surgical procedure (e.g., craniotomy) because of the risk of nicks, cuts, rash, and infection. Hair removal is completed the morning of surgery. Depending on agency policy and surgeon preference, hair can be removed with an electric clipper, a depilatory, or a sharp, disposable razor. An antimicrobial agent is used to cleanse the area. The anatomic area to be prepared, the type of solution, and the length of scrub time after hair removal varies with each surgery and with agency policy.

If a rash is present or develops after skin preparation, or if skin integrity is broken during hair removal, the surgeon is notified immediately. Altered skin integrity increases the risk of infection and may necessitate a delay in surgery. Document skin preparation in the patient record.

Preanesthesia Management

Patients scheduled for surgery are assessed by the anesthesiologist either the day before or the day of surgery. The anesthesiologist reviews the medical history and current diagnostic findings and obtains

a history of anesthetic experiences, current and past medication use, drug reactions, and allergies. A physical examination emphasizing the areas of the head, neck, chest, back, and arms is completed to identify potential intravenous access sites and difficulties with intubation and airway management. Anesthesia and operating room procedures are explained. The anesthesiologist writes orders for preanesthesia medication and decides the type of anesthesia to be administered.

PREANESTHESIA MEDICATION

The major goal of preoperative medication is to promote sedation and to reduce anxiety and apprehension. Additional goals depend on the specific medications used. The preanesthetic medication regimen usually consists of a sedative given at the hour of sleep on the evening before surgery and various combinations of narcotics, barbiturates, tranquilizers, antihistamines, and anticholinergic medications given approximately 1 hour before surgery.

Narcotic analgesics (morphine, meperidine) minimize the perception of pain and supplement the action of general anesthesia. However, narcotics depress the respiratory and cardiovascular systems and decrease gastric motility, which may predispose the patient to nausea and vomiting. The narcotic antagonist naloxone hydrochloride rapidly reverses respiratory depression and should be readily available.

Barbiturates (pentobarbital, secobarbital) and tranquilizers (diazepam) provide sedation with minimal respiratory or circulatory depression and rarely cause postoperative nausea or vomiting. They also reduce anxiety and apprehension.

Antihistamines (promethazine, hydroxyzine pamoate) provide sedation. They potentiate the action of other medications; therefore, a decreased dose of analgesic can be administered with the same effect.

Anticholinergics (atropine, scopolamine) reduce oral, respiratory, and gastric secretions to facilitate intubation and also prevent reflex bradycardia caused by surgical manipulation.

Application of the Nursing Process to the Care of the Preoperative Patient

Assessment

Assessment of the surgical patient begins with the first encounter, whether in the physician's office, the clinic, or the emergency room or on admission to the hospital. Obtain a history of hospitalizations and surgical experience. Determine the patient's understanding of the diagnosis, diagnostic procedures, planned surgery, expected outcome of surgery, sequence of recovery, and impact of surgery and recovery on lifestyle to identify areas of concern and teaching needs. Assess the patient's ability to understand and cooperate with diagnostic procedures. Review the medical history and therapeutic drug use, and assess physical status to identify factors that increase surgical risk or the risk of postoperative complications. Specifically ask about current and past alcohol consumption, drug use, smoking habits, and allergies. Ask female patients whether they might be pregnant and determine the date of the last menstrual period (LMP). Determine how the patient copes with stress, and identify family members or significant others who provide emotional support and encouragement.

Nursing Diagnoses and Planning

Nursing diagnoses and related expected patient outcomes most commonly applicable to preoperative patients include the following:

NDx: Anxiety related to hospitalization, surgery, outcome of surgery, and impact on lifestyle

Planning: Patient outcomes

1. Patient asks questions and verbalizes concerns.
2. Patient states that feelings of apprehension have decreased.

NDx: Knowledge deficit: diagnosis, diagnostic procedures, planned surgery, expected outcome of surgery, admission procedures

Planning: Patient outcomes

1. Patient states diagnosis and verbalizes an understanding of the diagnosis.
2. Patient verbalizes understanding of diagnostic procedures and cooperates in their timely completion.
3. Patient identifies planned surgery and states the reason it was chosen as treatment.
4. Patient verbalizes realistic expectations of surgery.
5. Patient arrives at the hospital or ambulatory surgery unit and is admitted as scheduled.

NDx: High risk for altered health maintenance related to insufficient knowledge of postoperative activities and exercises to promote respiratory and circulatory function

Planning: Patient outcomes

1. Patient verbalizes understanding of the benefits of each exercise.
2. Patient demonstrates each exercise.
3. Patient states intent to perform each exercise hourly as instructed.

NDx: Knowledge deficit: preoperative preparations and postoperative routines

Planning: Patient outcomes

1. Patient verbalizes understanding of preoperative preparations and postoperative routines.
2. Patient participates in preoperative preparations and postoperative routines.

Nursing Interventions

The primary goal of preoperative nursing care is to ensure that the patient is prepared physically and mentally for surgery to the fullest extent possible given the specific circumstances. Preoperative teaching is a major focus of patient preparation and preoperative nursing care. It facilitates recovery and decreases length of hospital stay. Studies have documented that patients who receive preoperative teaching have a smoother induction into anesthesia, fewer postoperative complications, more rapid recovery, less anxiety, and a better feeling about themselves than patients who do not receive preoperative instruction. Chart 4–1: Nursing Guide to Preoperative Patient Preparation and Patient Teaching summarizes important points to include in the patient's preoperative preparation. Nursing Care Guide 4–1 presents a general plan of care for a preoperative patient scheduled for surgery.

NDx: Anxiety

Provide ample opportunity for the patient and significant others to express thoughts and concerns about diagnosis, planned treatment, hospitalization, and their possible impact on current lifestyle and financial situation. Encourage questions to demonstrate interest and concern. Answer honestly in terms the patient can understand. Do not offer false reassurance. Reinforce the physician's explanations of the planned surgery and its expected outcome to increase understanding. Refer questions you cannot answer to an appropriate resource. Offer social service and clergy referral if a need is indicated.

NDx: Knowledge deficit: diagnosis, diagnostic procedures, hospitalization procedures, planned surgery, expected outcome of surgery, admission procedures

Depending on the patient's diagnosis, condition, and urgency of the planned surgery, diagnostic procedures may be completed before or after hospitalization. Explain the diagnostic procedures, their purpose, patient preparation and participation, and expected sensations during the procedure. When possible, provide written as well as verbal instructions. Answer questions and provide necessary assistance to ensure timely and accurate completion of diagnostic evaluation. Once diagnosis is confirmed and surgery is planned, answer questions and reinforce the physicians' explanations of the diagnosis, planned surgery, and its expected outcome to correct misconceptions and reduce anxiety. Encourage the patient to telephone if he or she has any further questions. New questions frequently come to mind after the patient has had time to think about the planned surgery.

Review hospital admission procedures and how and when the patient will be advised of the date of surgery and admission date and time. Remind the patient to bring all hospitalization and medical insurance information to the admitting office.

NDx: High risk for altered health maintenance

Teach and reinforce postoperative activities that promote respiratory and circulatory function and help prevent postoperative complications. Explain the benefit of each activity or exercise. Tell the patient that he or she will be encouraged and assisted to perform exercises hourly on the day of surgery and the first postoperative day. Frequency thereafter depends on the patient's condition, risk factors, and ability to ambulate. Place the patient in a semi- to high Fowler's position to promote maximum lung expansion during respiratory exercises. Document teaching, return demonstration, and independent performance of exercises in the patient record. Many agencies use a checklist for each teaching topic and for documenting demonstration of learning by the patient.

Deep Breathing Exercises: Teach the patient to take deep breaths using the diaphragm, as illustrated in Figure 4–1. Instruct the patient to exhale completely and then place a fist high up on the abdomen, just below the breast bone, and inhale gently and deeply through the nose, making the fist move outward without making the shoulders rise. Hold the breath 3 seconds and then exhale slowly and gently through pursed lips, as if whistling. Repeat the cycle three to five times and perform each hour. This exercise dilates the respiratory passages and alveoli, increases gas exchange, helps prevent atelectasis, and enables the patient to get more air into the lungs with less effort.

Coughing Exercises: Teach the patient to sit upright and lean slightly forward, or to bend the knees while seated in a high Fowler's position in bed, and breathe in and out deeply, using the diaphragm as just described. Repeat the procedure. Take a third deep breath and then, with the mouth open, give three short, shallow coughs with short breaths in between. Keeping the mouth open, inhale quickly and immediately cough forcibly once or twice from below the diaphragm where the fist is pressed, using the abdominal muscles. Inhale deeply to reinflate collapsed alveoli. If abdominal surgery is scheduled, teach the patient to splint the incision with both hands and interlaced fingers or a folded blanket or sheet to decrease discomfort when

Chart 4–1.

NURSING GUIDE TO PREOPERATIVE PATIENT PREPARATION AND PATIENT TEACHING

Instruct the patient and provide written instructions when possible in the following:

Prior to Admission

Review physician's explanation of scheduled surgical procedure, anticipated location of incision, possibility of surgical drains, anticipated surgical outcome, and recovery to clarify information, answer questions, and identify teaching needs.

Anticipated sequence of events from preadmission diagnostic procedures through admission, preoperative preparation, intraoperative procedures, and postoperative care.

Diagnostic procedures to be completed before admission, their scheduled date, time, location, patient preparation, and participation.

Date and time of admission, location of the hospital and admitting office.

Food and fluid restrictions and skin preparation to be performed at home if surgery is scheduled the day of admission.

Documents and personal items to bring to the hospital and what to leave at home for safekeeping.

What to wear and who must accompany the patient if ambulatory or day surgery is scheduled.

Prior to Surgery

Diagnostic procedures, patient preparation, and participation.

Review, again, the physician's explanation of scheduled surgical procedure, anticipated location of incision, possibility of surgical drains, anticipated surgical outcome, and recovery to clarify information, answer questions, and identify teaching needs.

Review the informed consent form to ensure signatures have been obtained.

Review patient's wishes for advance directive for treatment and organ donation.

Time surgery is scheduled.

Increased fluid intake the day and evening before surgery.

Food and fluid restrictions after predetermined time.

Preoperative skin preparation, bowel and bladder preparation.

Removal of jewelry, nail polish, dental appliances, contact lenses, and prostheses, and ensure safekeeping of belongings during surgery.

Changing into hospital gown, removing underwear, and emptying the bowel and bladder before premedication.

Preoperative medications, parenteral fluids.

Transport to the operating room or preanesthesia holding area.

Positioning on the operating table, skin preparation, expected sensations, cool environment.

Induction of anesthesia, expected sensations.

Postanesthesia care unit procedures, expected sensations.

Transport to postsurgical unit.

Postoperative positioning, movement, respiratory exercises, circulatory exercises, splinting techniques, pain management, and early ambulation.

coughing, as illustrated in Figure 4–2. This exercise mobilizes secretions to clear the lungs of mucus.

Incentive Spirometer: This is a device designed to motivate the patient to get more air into the lungs. The exact apparatus varies with each institution, but all measure the amount of inhaled air and display the amount clearly to the patient. Teach the patient to place the mouthpiece between the lips and take slow, deep breaths through the mouth, moving the spirometer indicator. Repeat 5 to 10 times every hour. Encourage the patient to use the spirometer before surgery to increase vital capacity and to promote alveolar inflation. Mark the preoperative inspiratory level to provide a postoperative comparison.

Nursing Care Guide 4–1.

PREOPERATIVE PREPARATION OF THE PATIENT SCHEDULED FOR SURGERY

Assessment Findings: Patient scheduled for surgery is tense and restless and complains of dry mouth and sweaty palms. Pulse rate and blood pressure are slightly above patient's baseline levels. Patient expresses concern over upcoming surgery, its outcome, and impact on lifestyle.

Nursing Diagnosis: Anxiety related to scheduled surgery, outcome of surgery, and impact on lifestyle

Patient Outcomes	Nursing Interventions	Rationale
Patient asks questions and verbalizes concerns.	Assure patient that some anxiety before surgery is expected. Provide ample opportunity for the patient to express thoughts and concerns.	Provides emotional support and reassures patient that feelings are normal.
	Provide a calm, restful environment. Orient patient to surroundings.	Calm environment helps reduce anxiety by reducing stressful stimuli.
	Encourage questions and expression of thoughts and concerns. Ask whether the patient wishes to see a member of the clergy.	Provides opportunity for patient to express concerns, demonstrates interest and concern for patient's well-being and spiritual beliefs.
Patient verbalizes realistic expectations of planned surgery, expected outcome, recovery, and impact on lifestyle.	Ask the patient what he or she was told by the surgeon.	Determines patient's level of knowledge.
	Answer questions honestly in terms the patient can understand. Reinforce the physician's explanations of the planned surgery, expected outcome, recovery, and impact on lifestyle. Do not give false reassurance. Refer questions you cannot answer to appropriate resources.	Accurate information corrects misunderstandings, increases the patient's knowledge, and helps reduce anxiety.
Patient states feelings of apprehension have decreased. Pulse and blood pressure are within patient's normal range.	Ask what methods patient has successfully used in the past to reduce stress. Encourage use of stress-reduction techniques: slow, deep breathing; guided imagery; back rub; low lighting; distraction; presence of significant other.	Use of previously successful coping techniques promotes a sense of control and reduces anxiety.

(continued)

Nursing Care Guide 4–1. *(continued)*

PREOPERATIVE PREPARATION OF THE PATIENT SCHEDULED FOR SURGERY

Evaluation: Compare the patient's status with the expected patient outcomes. If the outcomes are achieved, evaluate nursing care as successful. If not, reassess the patient, formulate new nursing diagnoses, and revise expected patient outcomes and nursing interventions as appropriate.

Assessment Findings: Patient is scheduled for surgery. When questioned, patient verbalizes no knowledge of preoperative preparations or postoperative exercises.

Nursing Diagnosis: High risk for altered health maintenance related to insufficient knowledge of preoperative preparations and postoperative exercises

Patient Outcomes	Nursing Interventions	Rationale
Patient verbalizes understanding of and participates in preoperative preparations.	Explain preoperative preparations, the purpose of each, and its importance. Include the information identified in Chart 4–1.	Adequate preoperative preparation increases patient understanding, reduces anxiety, minimizes the risk of intra- and postoperative complications, and promotes recovery.
Patient demonstrates postoperative exercises.	Provide preoperative teaching in activities and exercises to promote respiratory and circulatory function during the postoperative period.	Teaching postoperative exercises and activities before surgery improves patient learning and provides an opportunity for return demonstration and practice.
	Teach deep breathing, coughing, use of incentive spirometer, leg exercises, frequent turning and positioning, and early ambulation as discussed in the text and illustrated in Figures 4–1, 4–2, 4–3.	These activities promote rapid recovery from anesthesia and minimize the risk of postoperative respiratory and circulatory complications.
Patient states reasons for each activity/exercise.	Explain the purpose of each activity/exercise and how it will benefit the patient.	Understanding of benefit to self increases motivation and compliance.

Evaluation: Compare the patient's status with the expected patient outcomes. If the outcomes are achieved, evaluate nursing care as successful. If not, reassess the patient, formulate new nursing diagnoses, and revise expected patient outcomes and nursing interventions as appropriate.

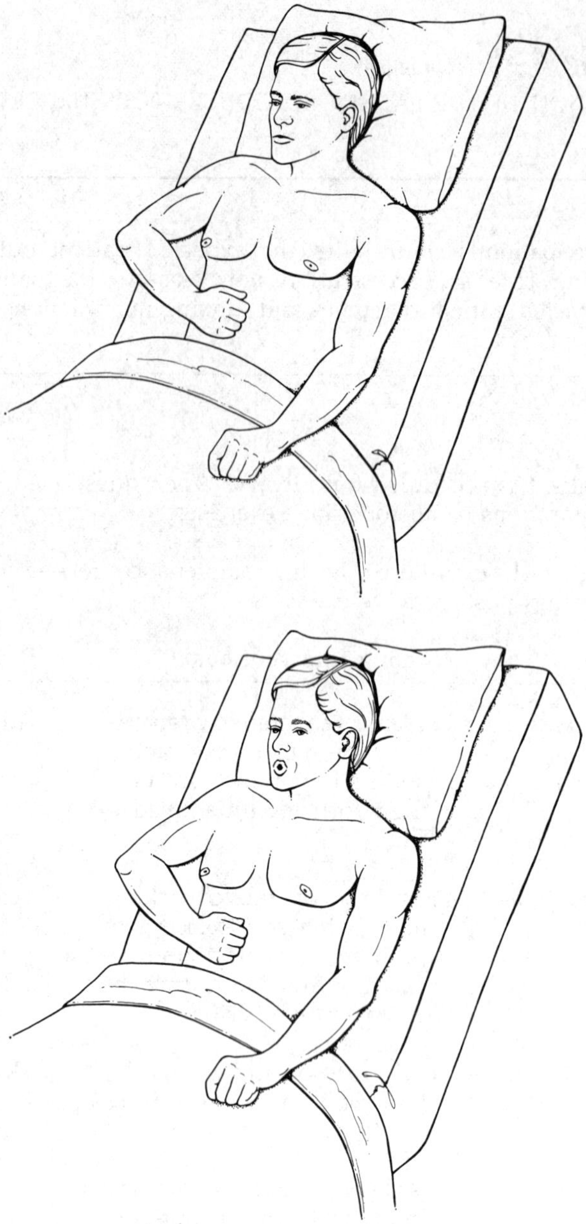

Figure 4–1.

Instructions for deep breathing exercise.

A. Elevate head of bed.
B. Exhale completely.
C. Place fist midway between umbilicus and sternum. (See top figure, right.)
D. Inhale deeply through the nose, making fist move outward.
E. Hold the breath for 3 seconds.
F. Exhale slowly and gently through pursed lips. (See bottom figure, right.)
G. Repeat cycle three to five times each hour.

Turning and Positioning: Teach the patient to use the side rails to turn and change position at least every 2 hours. A patient unable to move independently is assisted in changing position at least every 2 hours. Active movement stimulates circulation, promotes venous return, and prevents thrombus formation by minimizing venous stasis. Repositioning promotes comfort, helps maintain skin integrity, and mobilizes respiratory secretions.

Leg Exercises: These strengthen the muscles and improve blood circulation in the feet and legs. As illustrated in Figure 4–3, teach the patient to flex the foot toward the head, stretching the toes upward, and then point the feet toward the bottom of the bed, curling the toes downward. Trace circles with the feet by rotating the ankle in a circle in one direction and then in the opposite direction. Flex the leg by bending the knee, sliding the foot along the mattress as far back as possible, lift the foot, and then stretch the leg out completely. Exercise the quadriceps by tightening the buttocks for a count of 10 and releasing. Repeat each exercise 5 to 10 times every hour.

NDx: Knowledge deficit: preoperative preparations and postoperative routines

Ideally, preoperative teaching begins at the point that surgery is recommended. In elective surgery, the surgeon's office nurse begins the instruction. Information, especially written, presented to the patient before admission to the hospital is often retained better than information presented the day or evening before surgery. Concrete, factual informa-

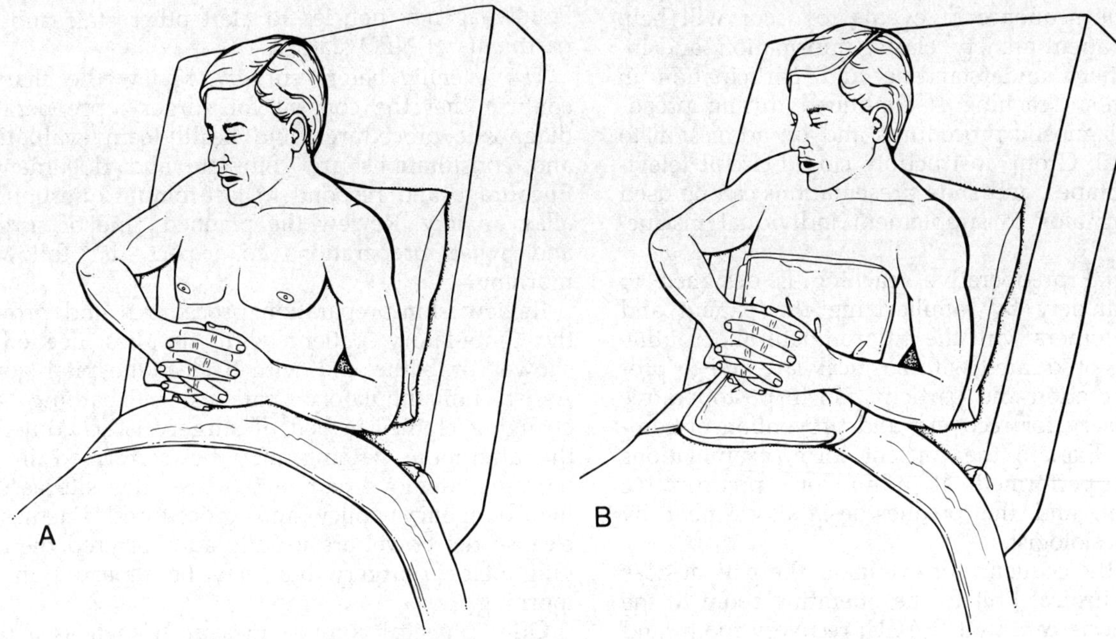

Figure 4–2.

Splint an abdominal incision with both hands and interlaced fingers (A) or with a folded sheet or blanket (B) to decrease discomfort while coughing.

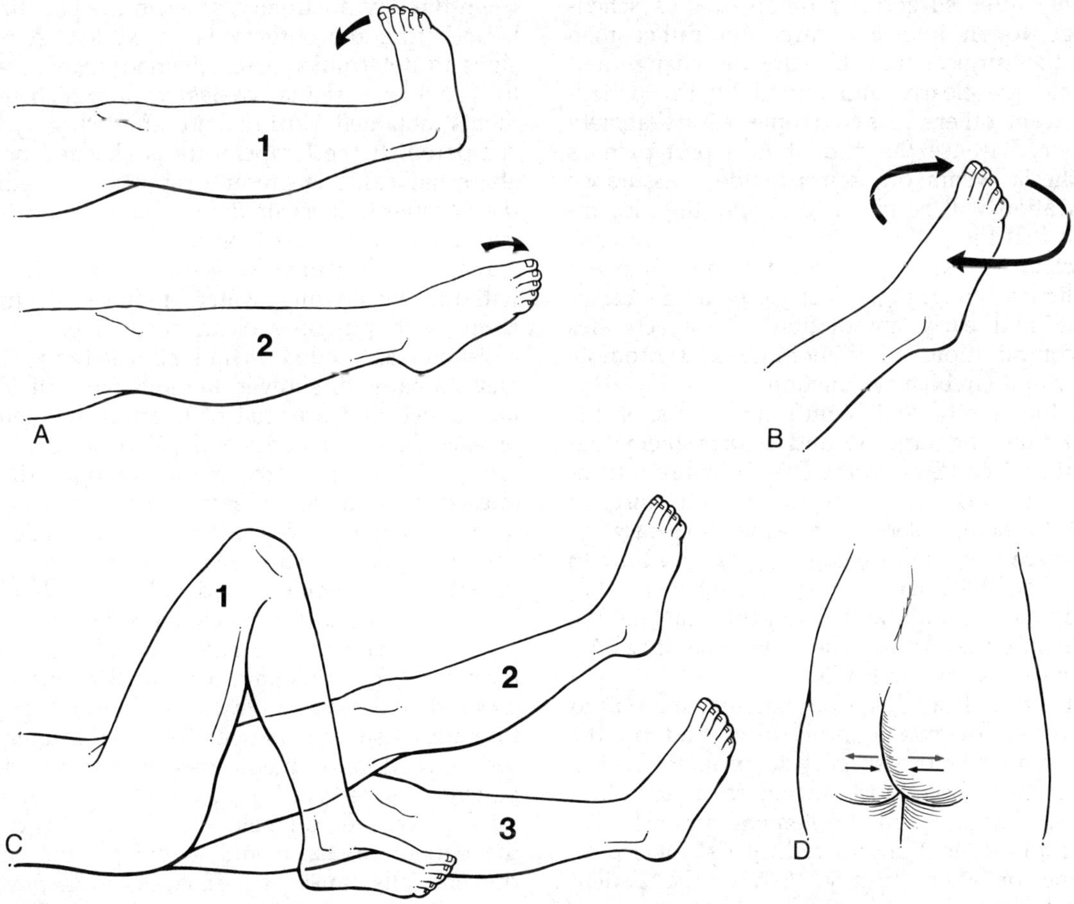

Figure 4–3.

Exercises to strengthen muscles and improve circulation in the feet and legs. A, Flex (1) and extend (2) the feet. B, Make circles with the feet. C, Bend the knee (1), raise the foot and extend the leg (2), then relax (3). D, Tighten and relax the buttocks.

tion on the sequence of events to occur will help decrease patient anxiety, clarify information, and increase patient understanding and participation in these events. Teaching is continued during preadmission diagnostic procedures and on admission to the hospital. Group instruction, closed-circuit television, videotapes, and slide presentations can be used as teaching aids to supplement individual instruction.

In-hospital preoperative teaching is designed to decrease anxiety by familiarizing the patient and significant others with the environment and routine procedures associated with surgical care and to promote cooperation and participation in postoperative care necessary for recovery and prevention of complications. Explain the consent form, examinations and tests performed at admission, preoperative preparation, and the preanesthesia assessment by the anesthesiologist.

Review the sequence of events as the patient goes from the surgical unit to the operating room to the postanesthesia care unit (PACU; recovery room) and back to the surgical unit so the patient knows what to expect. Describe the PACU and its routines, including the fact that male and female patients and, in some cases, children are cared for in the unit immediately after surgery. If the patient is scheduled to go to an intensive care unit rather than return to the surgical unit, be sure the change and its rationale are clearly understood by the patient and significant others to avoid unnecessary anxiety after surgery. Advise the patient to expect pain as the anesthesia wears off, but provide reassurance that medication will be given to relieve the discomfort. Stress that the patient should not hesitate to ask for medication because pain relief reduces anxiety and facilitates coughing, deep breathing, easier movement, and early ambulation. These activities prevent complications of immobility and promote respiratory and circulatory function.

Advise the family and significant others of the scheduled time for surgery, and inform them that the patient will be taken to the PACU before returning to the nursing unit. Explain that the surgeon will speak to them as soon as possible after surgery. Explain where they wait during surgery and how to find out when the operation is over, when the patient returns to the unit, and when they can see the patient. Be sure they know where the patient will go after he or she leaves the PACU.

If not contraindicated, encourage increased fluid intake between diagnostic procedures and on the day and evening before surgery to promote hydration and reduce discomfort during food and fluid restrictions. Explain and implement preoperative food and fluid restrictions to reduce risk of aspiration during or after surgery. Advise the patient what time bedside food and fluids will be removed, and reinforce instructions not to eat or drink afterward. Notify oncoming staff and document the NPO status in the chart and on the patient care plan. Follow agency policies to alert other staff and departments of NPO status.

The evening before surgery, review the chart to confirm that the consent for surgery, preoperative diagnostic procedures, and health-team evaluations and consultations are complete and documented. Encourage and respond to last-minute questions to allay anxiety. Review the planned time of surgery and what preparations to expect the following morning.

Review skin-preparation procedures and provide the ambulatory patient with supplies needed to shower or bathe and with a clean hospital gown. Assist nonambulatory patients in bathing and changing clothes in bed. If surgery is scheduled in the afternoon, bathing may be performed in the morning. Remove hair in the operative site according to agency policy and procedures. Enemas to cleanse the bowel are usually administered the evening before surgery but may be repeated in the morning.

Offer physical comfort measures, such as a back rub or warm, noncaffeinated beverage, and provide a quiet atmosphere to increase comfort, help reduce anxiety, and promote sleep. Offer a sedative if one is ordered by the surgeon or anesthesiologist.

On the day of surgery, awaken the patient about 1 hour before the surgery is scheduled. Assess vital signs to determine current hemodynamic status and to provide baseline values with which measurements obtained during and after surgery will be compared. If the temperature is elevated or another abnormal value is present, report it immediately to the anesthesiologist or the surgeon because the surgery may have to be delayed.

Instruct the patient to cleanse the mouth and teeth without swallowing water, remove all undergarments, and put on a clean hospital gown. Provide assistance as needed. If time allows, the patient may wish to bathe or shower. Remove facial makeup and nail polish and artificial nails on at least one finger of each hand so peripheral perfusion can be accurately evaluated by the anesthesiologist during the operation. Remove all jewelry, prostheses, and wigs to prevent injury, loss, or damage. A wedding ring, tied or taped in place, may be worn, but all other valuables are removed and either sent home or labeled and placed in the hospital safe.

Ask the patient to urinate and defecate just before receiving the preoperative medications. Double-check that the operative consent form is signed before administering preoperative medications. A consent signed after medicating is invalid. After the patient has received premedication, raise the side rails, place the call bell within reach, and instruct the patient to use it and to not get out of bed to prevent falls caused by dizziness from the medications. Reinforce that the medication promotes relaxation but does not necessarily induce sleep. A quiet, darkened room enhances the effect of preoperative medication. Assess the patient every 15 minutes for

30 minutes after he or she receives premedication to evaluate response and detect untoward side effects from the medications.

Document preoperative preparations and premedication in the patient record. In most agencies, a preoperative checklist on the front of the chart is completed before transporting the patient to the operating room. Although the form varies with the institution, Figure 4–4 illustrates possible contents.

Transport the surgical patient to the operating room on a stretcher, with the side rails elevated and safety belt in place. The surgical floor nurse confirms the patient's identity with the operating room nurse, reviews the chart and preoperative checklist, and reports on vital signs, general condition, surgical risk factors, alterations in mobility or neurologic function, parenteral infusions, preoperative preparations, and medications to ensure continuity of care. Advise the surgical nurse if the patient is wearing a prosthesis or jewelry and if family members are present.

Stamp with identification plate

Date ____ Age ____
Allergies ____ Language ____
LOC ____ Hearing ____
Speech: Distinct ____ Other: ____
Vision: No aids __ Glasses __ Contacts __ Blind: R __ L __
Skin: Intact: ____ Other: ____

On Chart:
Consent ____
History and Physical ____ Consults ____
Test results: CBC __ UA __ CXR __ ECG __ Lytes __
Type and crossmatch ____ # of units ____
Medication Record: ____
Nursing Care Plan: ____
Indentification Plate: ____

Patient Preparation:
Preoperative teaching: Group ____ Individual ____
Skin Prep: Area ____
Bowel Prep: ____ Douche ____
Voided ____ Foley ____ Date inserted ____
Antiembolic Stockings ____
Dentures/Bridge removed ____ Loose teeth ____
Prostheses: Type and removed ____
Nail polish removed ____ Jewelry removed ____
Makeup removed ____ Hair pins removed ____
Hospital gown ____
IV ____
NPO ____
Identification band ____
Comments ____

Preoperative medications:
____ Time: ____
____ Time: ____
____ Time: ____

Vital Sign: T ____ P ____ R ____ BP ____
Cardiac Rhythm: Reg ____ Irreg ____ Pacemaker ____
Respiratory Rhythm: Reg ____ Irreg ____ Labored ____
Unlabored ____ Orthopneic ____

Nurse's Note Completed: ____
Signature: ____

Figure 4–4.

Example of a preoperative checklist.

Evaluation

Evaluate the effectiveness of nursing care for a preoperative patient by comparing the patient's status with the expected patient outcomes. Examples of specific outcomes for preoperative patients have been provided in the Planning section.

Intraoperative Period

The intraoperative period is the time during which the patient is transported to the operating room, receives anesthesia, undergoes surgical intervention, and is transferred to the recovery room. The patient is sedated and anesthetized during the intraoperative period and is, therefore, unable to prevent injury or make needs known. The nurse, as part of the surgical team, is the patient's advocate. The nurse monitors patient safety, maintains asepsis, and initiates activities that facilitate completion of the surgical procedure with minimal anesthesia time and patient trauma. Nursing interventions reduce the risk of intraoperative complications and promote optimum recovery.

Surgical Team

The surgical team is composed of a group of specialized individuals working together for the welfare and safety of the patient. It includes the surgeon, assistants to the surgeon, anesthesiologist, scrub assistant, and circulating nurse.

The surgeon is the physician whose primary responsibility is to perform the operative procedure. The surgeon may assist with positioning, preparing, and draping the patient or may delegate these duties to the first assistant or to a perioperative nurse.

The assistant to the surgeon may be another surgeon, resident, intern, physician's assistant, or nurse. The assistant's responsibilities include preparation of the operative site, exposure of the operative field with the use of retractors, and sponging and suctioning blood and fluid that might obscure visual exposure of the operative field.

The anesthesiologist is a physician who specializes in the administration of anesthesia to relieve pain and relax muscles. An anesthetist is a nurse, dentist, or anesthesia assistant who is specially trained in the administration of anesthesia. The person who administers anesthesia is also responsible for airway insertion and for maintaining a patent airway and adequate exchange of respiratory gases. He or she monitors fluid and blood loss, provides intravenous fluid replacement, and monitors respiratory and cardiac function.

The scrub assistant may be a nurse or a surgical technician. The scrub assistant is responsible for maintaining a sterile environment and preparing sterile instruments and supplies that will be needed during surgery. The scrub assistant and circulating nurse count the instruments, needles, and sponges before the surgery and again before closure of the wound to ensure that all instruments have been removed from the patient. The scrub assistant prepares and hands surgical instruments to the surgeon and assistant, advises the circulating nurse when additional supplies are needed, and ensures that all team members adhere to the principles of surgical asepsis.

The circulating nurse is a registered nurse who manages and coordinates the activities in the operating room, brings needed supplies and medications, and removes used or contaminated items. The circulating nurse implements the nursing care plan, provides emotional support before anesthesia and during emergence from anesthesia, assists the anesthesiologist with induction, monitors patient safety and positioning, monitors the patient's fluid losses and general condition, and documents assessments and interventions throughout the surgical procedure. At the conclusion of surgery, the circulating nurse supervises, confirms, and records the final sponge and instrument count with the scrub assistant and then accompanies the anesthesiologist and patient to the PACU and reports to the PACU nurse.

Positioning

Position for surgery is determined by the site of the operation, type of anesthesia, maintenance of respiratory and cardiac function, age and size of the patient, and preexisting physical limitations or disease conditions. Regardless of the selected position, basic principles mut be observed to maintain the patient's dignity and safety and to prevent neuromuscular and peripheral vascular complications despite depression of normal responses to pain and pressure by preoperative medications and anesthesia. These principles are as follows: Expose only the operative area, use a safety belt, maintain normal body alignment, pad all equipment used for positioning, do not cross the legs, and do not allow extremities to rest on body surfaces or to hang off the table.

Common surgical positions are illustrated in Figure 4–5. These include supine or dorsal recumbent,

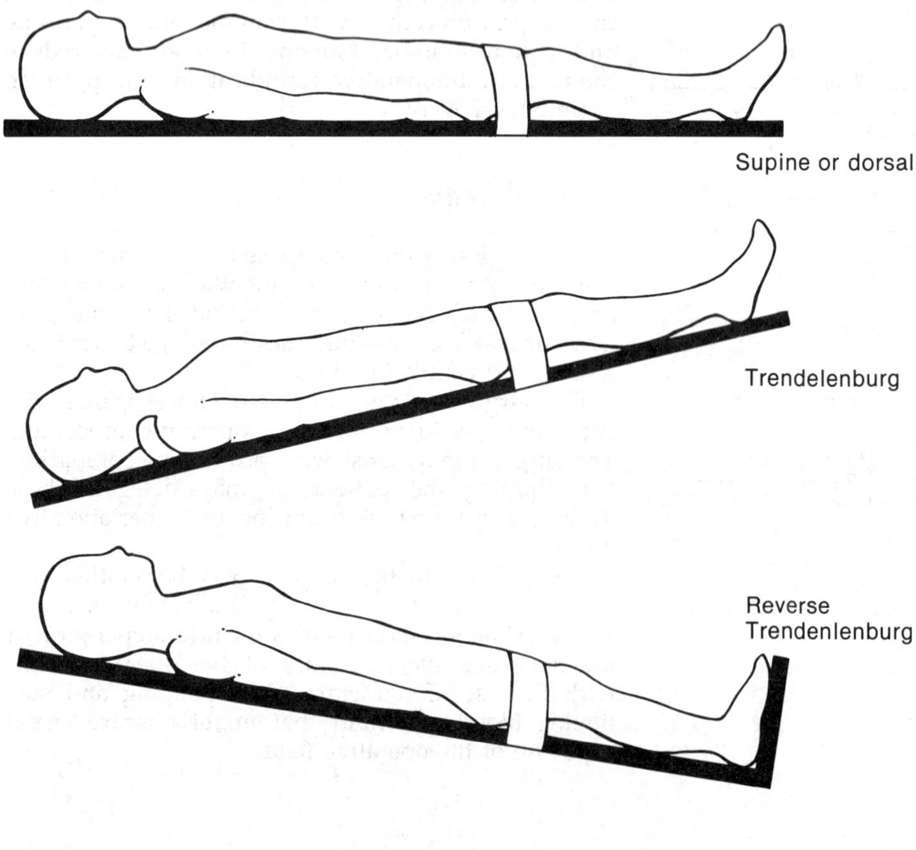

Figure 4–5.

Common surgical positions.

Figure 4–5. (continued)

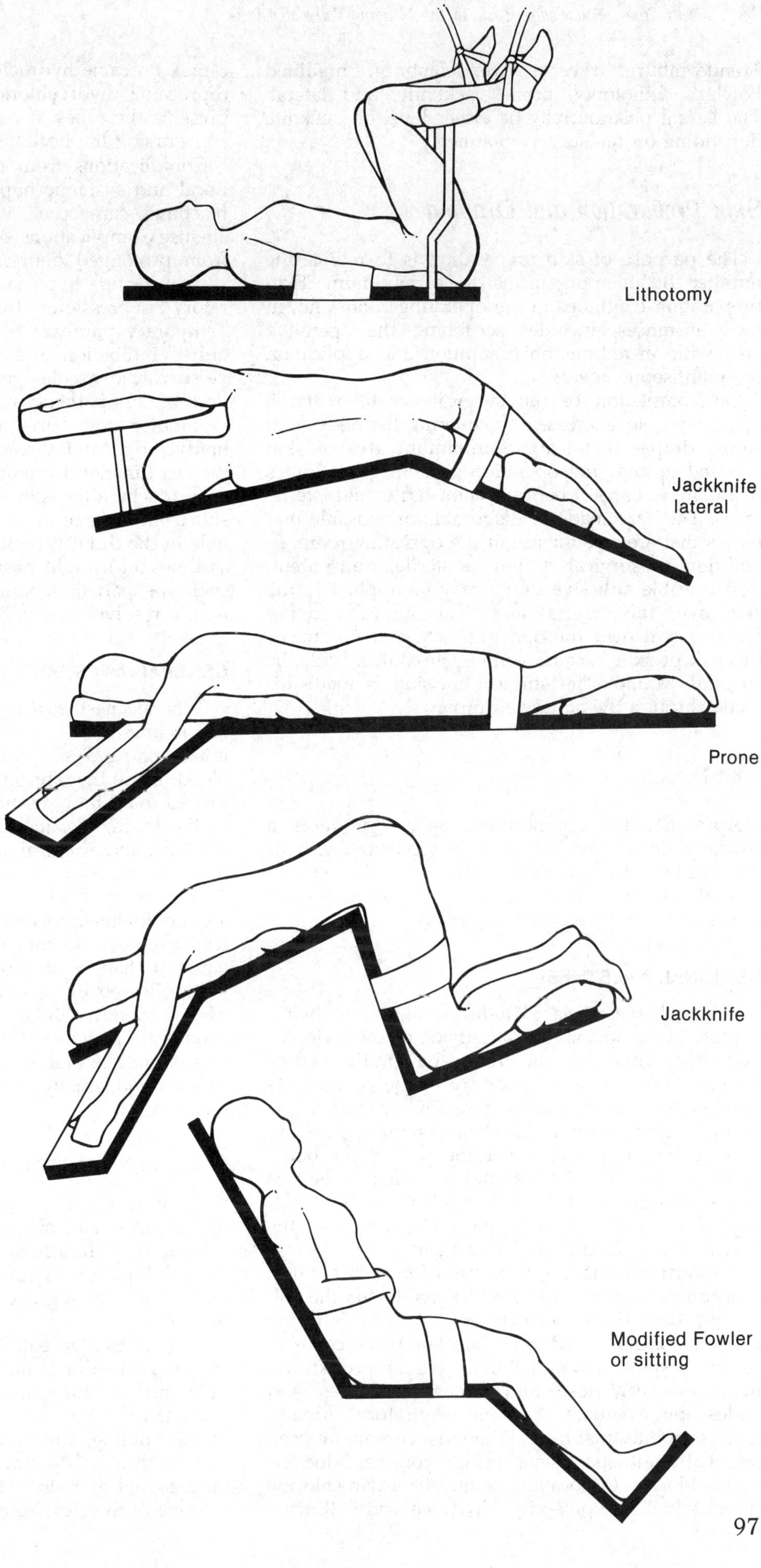

Trendelenburg, reverse Trendelenburg, modified Fowler's, lithotomy, prone, jackknife, and lateral. The lateral position may be either level or jackknife depending on the surgery planned.

Skin Preparation and Draping

The purpose of skin preparation is to reduce the number of microorganisms to a minimum. Skin preparation continues in the operating room and, in most instances, includes scrubbing the operative area with an antimicrobial solution and application of an antiseptic agent.

On completion of the surgical scrub, a sterile operating field is created by covering the body with sterile drapes that leave a minimum area of skin exposed around the operative site. Surgical drapes maintain a barrier between nonsterile and sterile areas. They are made of disposable or reusable materials that are safe for use in the operating room. In addition to surgical drapes, a sterile, transparent, impermeable adhesive drape may be applied to the skin over the surgical area. This adhesive drape forms a seal over the operative site and minimizes the risk of skin bacteria coming in contact with the surgical wound. The surgical incision is made directly through the adhesive drape.

Anesthesia

Administration of anesthetic agents produces a partial or complete loss of pain sensation with or without loss of consciousness, muscle relaxation, and loss of reflexes. The two major types of anesthesia are regional and general anesthesia.

REGIONAL ANESTHESIA

Regional anesthesia includes local, nerve block, epidural, and spinal. The anesthetic agent is deposited either directly in the area to be anesthetized or along a nerve or nerve pathway to the central nervous system that transmits the pain stimulus to the brain. It temporarily blocks transmission of pain and sensory impulses from a specific part of the body. Motor function may or may not be affected. The size of the anesthetized field is dependent on the site of application, the amount of anesthetic used, and the specific effects of the anesthetic agent.

Regional anesthesia can be used for most surgical procedures and is particularly suitable for the following operations: cosmetic procedures; biopsies; excisions of moles and cysts; hernia repairs; cesarean sections; some abdominal and pelvic procedures; many eye, ear, nose, and throat procedures; and endoscopic examination of the respiratory, urinary, and gastrointestinal tracts. The most commonly used regional anesthetic agents include cocaine, lidocaine hydrochloride (Xylocaine), tetracaine hydrochloride (Pontocaine), mepivacaine hydrochloride (Carbocaine), procaine hydrochloride (Novocain), and chloroprocaine hydrochloride (Nesacaine). Table 4–3 presents the types of regional anesthesia, their uses, and nursing implications.

Complications from regional anesthesia are rare. Local and systemic hypersensitivity or idiosyncratic reactions can occur with all regional anesthetic agents. Complications of spinal anesthesia resulting from prolonged depression of the central nervous system include hypoxia, irregular respirations, respiratory depression, drowsiness, and convulsions. Temporary paralysis of the respiratory muscles requires intubation and mechanical ventilation. Adverse cardiovascular reactions caused by interruption of sympathetic nerve pathways and loss of vasomotor tone are manifested by hypotension, bradycardia, and thready pulse. Bladder control is the last function to return after spinal anesthesia.

Headache after spinal anesthesia is thought to result from leakage of cerebrospinal fluid through the hole in the dura. It typically occurs when the patient assumes an upright position but is unrelated to how soon the patient ambulates. With adequate hydration, it resolves in 1 to 3 days.

GENERAL ANESTHESIA

General anesthesia is produced either by injection of an anesthetic agent directly into a vein or by inhalation and absorption of the agent into the blood from the alveoli. The anesthetic agents are carried to all body tissues via the circulatory system. In the brain, the anesthetic agent interrupts nerve-cell activity. Central nervous system alterations begin at the cortex and work down the brain stem. As the patient loses consciousness, sensory messages are no longer processed by the brain and motor responses are no longer issued to body parts. Behavioral changes and loss of social inhibitions occur first, followed by loss of memory, loss of consciousness, loss of voluntary muscle control, loss of response to pain, loss of body temperature control, loss of muscle and vascular tone, loss of protective reflexes and, finally, loss of respiratory and circulatory control.

STAGES OF GENERAL ANESTHESIA

Administration of general anesthesia produces four characteristic stages.

Stage 1: Relaxation. This is the period of induction. The patient is drowsy and dizzy and appears inebriated. Hearing is exaggerated; pain sensation is decreased.

Stage 2: Excitement. This stage is characterized by irregular breathing, increased muscle tone, and involuntary motor movements of all extremities. Movement, touch, or noise may trigger vomiting, breath holding, and thrashing about. Avoid stimulation, be sure safety straps are properly applied, and be prepared to assist with patient restraint.

Stage 3: Surgical Anesthesia. This period is char-

Table 4–3. TYPES OF REGIONAL ANESTHESIA

TYPE	ADMINISTRATION	USE	POSSIBLE COMPLICATIONS	NURSING INTERVENTION
Topical	Spray, gargle, or application of packs soaked with anesthetic agent to surface area to be anesthetized	Anesthesia of respiratory passage to facilitate intubation; diagnostic procedures of larynx, bronchus, vagina, rectum, or urinary bladder	Cardiovascular collapse when applied to respiratory tract	Monitor vital signs frequently
Local infiltration	Injection of agent into subcutaneous tissue with needle and syringe	Minor operations of short duration; before administration of spinal anesthesia		
Nerve block	Injection of agent into and around nerve or group of nerves supplying a specific region	Common nerve blocks: digital, radial, ulnar, intercostal, sciatic, femoral, brachial plexus, cervical plexus. Also used to identify cause of pain, to increase circulation in some vascular diseases, and for relief of chronic pain	Nerve damage	Monitor neuromuscular function
Caudal and epidural blocks	Injection of agent into epidural space through sacral hiatus (caudal) or into epidural space between vertebrae (epidural)	Anorectal, vaginal, and perineal procedures	Nerve damage	Monitor vital signs frequently
Spinal anesthesia	Injection of agent into subarachnoid space (most frequently the interspace between third and fourth lumbar vertebrae); to achieve level of anesthesia, patient's head is immediately lowered after injection of anesthetic agent until desired height of anesthesia is realized; after 15–20 min, level is set and cannot be altered by positional changes		Hypotension, spinal headache (up to 48 hr) postoperatively caused by dura mater not sealing off after removal of needle and resultant leakage of CSF into epidural space and decreased CSF pressure; nausea and vomiting; respiratory paralysis; paresthesia or paralysis of legs	Maintain client flat in bed for 12–24 hr as ordered Monitor vital signs frequently Monitor neuromuscular function
Low spinal (saddle block)	Involves sacral nerves (S-1–S-5)	Perineal and anal region procedures		
Midspinal	Thoracic nerves (T-10)	Procedures below umbilicus		
High spinal	Thoracic nerves (T-4)	Procedures below nipple line		

Abbreviation: CSF, cerebrospinal fluid.

acterized by quiet regular breathing, a relaxed jaw, constricted pupils that still respond to light, loss of auditory and pain sensation, absence of eyelid reflex, and decreased muscle tone.

Plane 1. Muscle tone decreases. Eyelid, gag, cough, and swallow reflexes are lost. Type of surgery: craniotomy, mastectomy, reduction of small-bone fractures.

Plane 2. Muscle tone further decreases; pause between respirations increases; there is a slight increase in pupil size. Type of surgery: amputation, large-bone surgery, thoracic.

Plane 3. Muscle tone markedly decreased; pupils are more dilated. Type of surgery: upper abdominal, hernioplasties, rectal procedures, cesarean section.

Plane 4. Anesthesia should not reach this level. Pupils are widely dilated and do not react to light; intercostal muscles are paralyzed; diaphragm maintains respirations. Blood pressure and pulse decrease.

Stage 4: Danger. The patient is near death with fixed, dilated pupils; absence of respirations; rapid, thready pulse; and all reflex activity is absent. Vital organs are compromised during this stage, and respiratory failure and cardiac arrest can occur if the patient is not returned to the appropriate surgical anesthesia plane.

Table 4–4. INHALATION ANESTHETIC AGENTS

AGENT	USE	POTENTIAL COMPLICATIONS	NURSING IMPLICATIONS	COMMENTS
Nitrous oxide	Short procedures	Hypertension, tachycardia	Monitor vital signs frequently	Used in combination with other agents because of minimal anesthetic potency
Halothane (Fluothane)	Not recommended for individuals who might require multiple surgeries (hepatototxicity may result)	Cardiovascular depression Hypothalamus depression, shivering immediately postoperatively Liver damage in some individuals	Monitor vital signs frequently Maintain warm environment; provide warmed blankets Liver function screening pre- and postoperatively	Provides smooth induction and rapid emergence with minimal excitement
Enflurane (Ethrane)	Intraabdominal surgical procedures	With increased depth of anesthesia, ventilation decreases and blood pressure is lowered Liver damage	Monitor vital signs frequently Liver function screening pre- and postoperatively	Provides abdominal muscle relaxation; rapid and smooth induction Associated with seizures and renal failure
Methoxyflurane (Penthrane)	Surgical procedures of short duration	Some nausea and vomiting Kidney toxicity	Monitor kidney function pre- and postoperatively	Slow induction and long emergence Excellent muscle relaxation and good analgesia at low concentration
Isoflurane (Forane)	Appears to be most ideal inhalation agent	Mild respiratory depression	Monitor vital signs frequently	Cardiac output and myocardial contractility well maintained Agent of choice for diminished renal or liver function

INHALATION ANESTHESIA

Anesthetic agents that are inhaled are either in gaseous form (nitrous oxide) or liquid form that can easily be vaporized (halothane, enflurane) and then inhaled. Table 4–4 lists the most common inhalation agents and their nursing implications. All these agents produce rapid induction. The principal advantage of inhalation anesthetics is the ability to control the depth of anesthesia by controlling the rate at which the agent enters and exits the lungs. Another advantage is that the rate of recovery from inhaled anesthesia with adequate alveolar ventilation is quite predictable.

Inhalation anesthetics are administered by a mask placed over the nose and mouth or by endotracheal tube. Use of an endotracheal tube allows anesthetic gases and oxygen to flow directly into the tracheobronchial tree, as illustrated in Figure 4–6. The anesthesiologist inserts the endotracheal tube after the patient is anesthetized sufficiently by intravenous or mask inhalation anesthesia to be unaware of the procedure. Postoperatively, many patients who have been intubated complain of a sore throat caused by irritation.

Inhalation anesthetics are primarily eliminated from the body through the respiratory system. Unless surgery lasts more than a few hours, the inhalation agent is almost completely excreted by the time the patient returns to the postoperative surgical unit.

INTRAVENOUS ANESTHESIA

General anesthesia can also be produced by the intravenous administration of one or more central nervous system depressants, narcotic analgesics, and neuromuscular blocking agents. Intravenous agents may be administered alone or in combination with an inhalation agent. Intravenous anesthetics cause a rapid onset of unconsciousness and are often used to initiate anesthesia. Their disadvantage is that they must be metabolized by the liver before they are excreted by the kidneys. Therefore, they are not rapidly removed from the body, and their action cannot be stopped once they are injected. Table 4–5 lists the most common intravenous anesthetic agents.

COMPLICATIONS OF GENERAL ANESTHESIA

Hypothermia, hypotension, hypoxia due to inadequate ventilation or oxygen administration, and unexpected individual variations of response to anesthetic agents are the most common complications of general anesthesia. Complications are most likely to occur at the time of induction or of emergence.

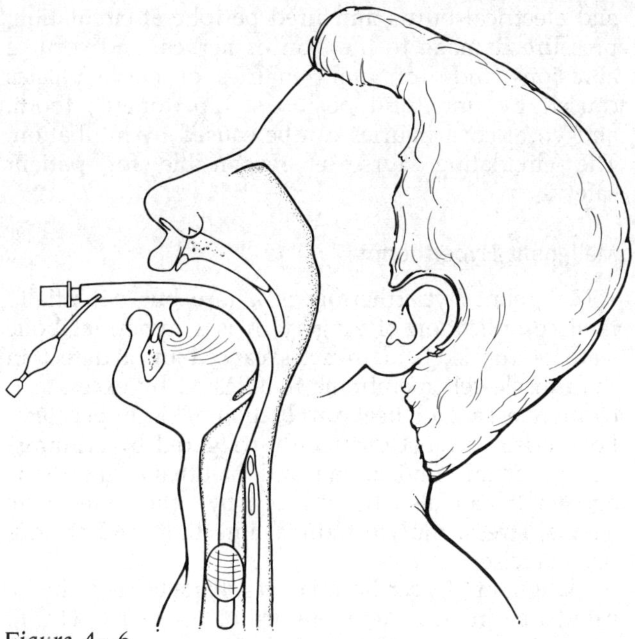

Figure 4–6.

Endotracheal tube in position for ventilation.

Transient decreased urinary output after general anesthesia is common. It is caused by reduced renal perfusion during surgery and release of antidiuretic hormone in response to the stress of surgery. Slow return of bladder tone may cause transient postoperative urinary retention.

Hypothermia

The operating room is a cool, air-conditioned environment. Evaporation of skin-preparation solutions and exposure of internal organs and blood vessels in air-conditioned operating rooms cause excessive loss of body heat and a decrease in body temperature during surgery. In some instances, hypothermia is induced to lower cellular metabolism and thereby reduce oxygen requirements. Shivering is an attempt by the body to raise core temperature, but it increases oxygen consumption and energy expenditure and could compromise myocardial and peripheral tissue perfusion. Shivering that occurs on emergence from anesthesia is a side effect of inhalation anesthetic agents. Hypothermia is reduced by minimizing exposure of nonsurgical body parts,

Table 4–5. INTRAVENOUS ANESTHETIC AGENTS

AGENT	USE	POTENTIAL COMPLICATIONS	NURSING IMPLICATIONS	COMMENTS
BARBITURATES (thiopental sodium [Pentothal] is principal agent)	To induce surgical anesthesia	Large doses can cause respiratory and cardiac depression	Anesthetic machine available to control or assist ventilation; monitor vital signs frequently	Onset of action is 30 sec, and duration is ultrashort
NARCOTICS	Used as adjunct to anesthesia to improve analgesia	Cardiac and respiratory depression	Monitor vital signs frequently; have naloxone (Narcan) or nalbuphine (Nubain) available	Given in small, repeated doses to provide more intense analgesia
Fentanyl citrate (Sublimaze)				Synthetic narcotic with potency 80–100 times greater than morphine
Innovar				Produces excellent analgesia with little postoperative nausea and vomiting
Ketamine hydrochloride (Ketalar)	Superficial operations not requiring muscle relaxation			Administered IV or IM
NEUROMUSCULAR BLOCKERS	Provide profound muscle relaxation without deep levels of anesthesia	Profound respiratory depression	Must monitor respirations carefully for at least 1 hr after effects of drug appear to have worn off; monitor ability to lift and hold head up for 10 sec; monitor for firm handgrip	Must be provided with artificial ventilation
Tubocurarine chloride (curare) (Tubarine)		Hypotension, bronchospasm		Produces muscle relaxation in 3–5 min, and duration is 20–60 min
Pancuronium bromide (Pavulon)		Hypertension, tachycardia		Longer acting than Curare
Succinylcholine chloride (Anectine)	Frequently used for intubation			Rapid acting, duration 3–5 min

Abbreviations: IV, intravenously; IM, intramuscularly.

minimizing exposure time between skin preparation and application of surgical drapes, use of a head covering and blankets, and administration of warmed intravenous fluids and anesthetic agents during surgery.

Respiratory Complications

Hypoxia is a major concern during general anesthesia. Aspiration of secretions or vomitus can occur with loss of pharyngeal and cough reflexes. Gaseous exchange is affected by inhaled anesthetic agents that alter pulmonary ventilation percentages of oxygen and carbon dioxide and, along with the preanesthetic medications, cause respiratory depression. Neuromuscular relaxants weaken or paralyze respiratory muscles. Lung expansion may be further compromised by the patient's position on the operating table. Anesthesia-induced vasodilation reduces cardiac output and pulmonary tissue perfusion. The anesthesiologist is responsible for maintaining a patent airway. Perfusion of the patient's skin, conjunctivae, mucous membranes, and fingers are monitored by the anesthesiologist and circulating nurse. A pulse oximeter applied to a finger, toe, or ear lobe constantly monitors blood-oxygen saturation.

Peripheral Vascular Complications

Effective peripheral perfusion requires adequate blood volume as well as sufficient stroke volume and heart rate to maintain cardiac output. Anesthetic agents decrease the heart rate or the force of contractions and cause vasodilation and pooling of blood, which reduces venous return to the heart. These actions combine to reduce cardiac output and are manifested by a rapid drop in blood pressure during induction and hypotension during anesthesia. Adequate fluid and blood replacement helps to minimize hypotension.

Reduced peripheral perfusion increases the risk of compromised blood flow, tissue ischemia, and nerve damage caused by direct pressure, hyperextension, flexion, or twisting of body parts. In many surgical positions, body weight is supported over bony prominences, increasing the risk of pressure sores and decubitus ulcers. Impaired peripheral perfusion and nerve and tissue damage are prevented by avoiding extreme surgical positions, by anatomic positioning of uninvolved body parts, and by padding potential pressure areas and instruments used in positioning.

Bodily Injury

General anesthesia interferes with the body's protective mechanisms for maintenance of homeostasis. The patient is unconscious, and pain sensation and reflexes are abolished as the central nervous system is depressed by anesthetic agents. The patient must be protected from injury caused by trauma, thermal and electrical burns, impaired peripheral circulation, pressure damage to the skin or nerves, and corneal abrasions and from joint injuries or nerve palsies caused by unnatural positions. Lip, tongue, tooth, and vocal cord injuries can be caused by intubation. The circulating nurse is responsible for patient safety.

Malignant Hyperthermia

Malignant hyperthermia is a rare but potentially fatal complication of surgery. It is a hypermetabolic state of the skeletal muscles caused by a defect in the muscle-cell membrane manifested by excess calcium release and heat production. This hypermetabolic crisis is most commonly triggered by administration of succinylcholine and halothane anesthetic agents. It can also be induced by other anesthetic agents, stress, muscle trauma, infection, and strenuous exercise.

Malignant hyperthermia is characterized by a rapid rise in body temperature of up to 1°C (1.8°F) every 5 minutes. Other clinical manifestations include muscle contraction and rigidity, tachycardia, tachypnea, cardiac dysrhythmias, and respiratory and metabolic acidosis. The patient's skin first has a flushed, rosy color from dilated peripheral vessels and then a mottled, cyanotic appearance caused by hypoxia. Surgery and anesthesia are stopped immediately, and intravenous dantrolene sodium, a skeletal muscle relaxant, is administered. The patient is ventilated with 100% oxygen, cooling blankets and ice packs are used to reduce body temperature, and cardiac dysrhythmias and acidosis are corrected.

Malignant hyperthermia is a genetically transmitted autosomal dominant trait more common in male children and adolescents. It is associated with inherited skeletal muscle disorders and dystrophies, although most individuals are not aware a disorder exists. Individuals with scoliosis, a large bulky muscular build, a family history of malignant hyperthermia or skeletal muscle disorders, or a history of muscle or joint injuries preceded by minimal trauma are at risk for malignant hyperthermia. Regional or spinal anesthesia is preferred for surgery. Body temperature is monitored continually by a probe if general anesthesia is used. Dantrolene sodium is administered as prophylaxis to individuals with a known history of malignant hyperthermia if general anesthesia is required.

Application of the Nursing Process to the Care of the Intraoperative Patient

Assessment

In some instances, assessment of the intraoperative patient begins with a preanesthesia visit by the operating room nurse. In most instances, the patient's admission to the operating suite is the initial contact.

Greet the patient and identify yourself. Confirm the patient's identity with the surgical floor nurse by checking the identification band and chart and ask, "What is your name?" Review the chart, consent, advance directive for treatment, general condition, surgical risk factors, location and types of permanent prostheses, alterations in mobility or neurologic function, special needs, preoperative checklist, and preoperative vital signs to ensure continuity of care and compliance with legal requirements. Confirm food and fluid restrictions, parenteral infusions, preoperative preparations, removal of prostheses and jewelry, and the time preoperative medications were administered. Assess the patient's emotional state and general condition, vital signs, and response to preanesthetic medications.

Nursing Diagnoses and Planning

Nursing diagnoses and related expected patient outcomes most commonly applicable to intraoperative patients include the following:

NDx: High risk for injury related to loss of independent defense mechanisms secondary to anesthesia

Planning: Patient outcomes

1. Patient remains free from injury.

NDx: High risk for infection related to contamination of wound during surgical procedure

Planning: Patient outcomes

1. Patient remains free from infection the first 48 hours after surgery as evidenced by absence of the following:
   a. Fever
   b. Purulent or malodorous wound drainage
   c. Increasing redness or edema around the incision

Nursing Interventions

The primary goals of intraoperative nursing care are to maintain patient safety, maintain asepsis, prevent intraoperative complications, and promote optimum recovery. The circulating nurse coordinates the activities of all individuals who enter the operating room and documents nursing care provided during the intraoperative period in the patient's chart. Many agencies have a special surgical record form for perioperative documentation.

NDx: High risk for injury
Throughout the intraoperative period, the circulating nurse functions as the patient advocate to prevent injury. Because the patient has received premedication and might be drowsy or disoriented, maintain safety measures and remain with the patient, if possible, before transfer to the operating table. An agitated or confused patient cannot be left alone. Speak in a calm, reassuring voice, explaining procedures and anticipated sensations to reduce anxiety.

Confirm patient identity, diagnosis, and planned surgery with the scrub assistant and anesthesiologist on transfer to the operating room and with the surgeon before surgery. Assist patient transfer to and from the operating table and positioning for surgery. Avoid extreme surgical positions when possible to prevent injury from hyperextension of joints and muscles that are atonic from anesthesia. Maintain functional anatomic position of uninvolved body parts to prevent injury to nerves, vessels, and muscles. Pad all instruments used for positioning and potential pressure areas to prevent compromise of peripheral circulation. Determine the presence of peripheral pulses and assess skin color and temperature after positioning and throughout surgery. Attach safety straps to prevent falls and injury from uncontrolled movement during induction and recovery from anesthesia. Assist with draping to ensure maximum access to the surgical site for the surgeon and access for the anesthesiologist while maintaining dignity for the patient. Minimize exposure of uninvolved body parts to reduce heat loss.

Confirm and document instrument, needle, and sponge count before surgery begins and before wound closure. Ensure that electrical grounding plates are covered with conductive gel and applied away from pressure points but as close to the operative site as possible to prevent electrical injury. Monitor fluid loss and replacement, body temperature, and cardiovascular status to prevent hemodynamic disequilibrium.

NDx: High risk for infection
The circulating nurse is responsible for maintenance of surgical asepsis. Assist with surgical skin scrub and draping to minimize risk of wound contamination. Assist surgeons and scrub assistant in putting on sterile gloves and gowns. Monitor sterile supplies, and provide additional supplies as needed. Remove specimens and used or contaminated supplies from the operating area. Assist in the application of dressings to protect the wound. Document skin preparation, wound drains, and irrigation devices and dressings.

Evaluation

Evaluate the effectiveness of nursing care for an intraoperative patient by comparing the patient's status with the expected patient outcomes. Examples of specific outcomes for intraoperative patients have been provided in the Planning section.

Postoperative Period

The postoperative period begins when the surgical procedure is complete and the patient is transferred to either the PACU or the surgical floor. It ends with recovery from surgery and the stresses associated with surgical intervention.

The surgical team transfers the patient from the operating room table to a stretcher by lifting or using a roller. Apply safety straps and raise the side rails to prevent injury. Protect the incision and any drainage tubes, intravenous tubing, and airway to prevent trauma and dislodgement. The anesthesiologist and circulating nurse accompany the patient to the PACU, confirm the patient's identity with the PACU nurse, give a report, and review postoperative orders. The report includes name, age, language spoken, allergies, type and extent of the surgical procedure, preoperative and intraoperative vital signs, position during surgery, type of anesthetic agent, estimated blood loss, drugs and intravenous solutions administered, complications, location and type of catheters, drains or packs, altered sensory or motor functions, and intraoperative events that might affect the postoperative course.

The PACU is an area, usually adjacent to the operating room, staffed by nurses and personnel specially trained to assess and care for the surgical patient who has received general or regional anesthesia. To meet the patient's needs during recovery and to respond to emergencies, the PACU is equipped with oxygen and suction outlets; bedside cardiac monitors; emergency cart with defibrillator, endotracheal equipment, and emergency drugs; equipment for drawing arterial and venous blood samples; chest tube equipment; ventilators; cutdown infusion equipment; blanket warmer; various medications; and intravenous solutions and supplies.

The patient remains in the unit until the effects of general anesthesia have worn off. Criteria for discharge from the PACU include the following:

1. The patient must be sufficiently awake or easily aroused to respond to simple questions.
2. Vital signs must be stable with patent airway and spontaneous respirations.
3. The gag reflex must be present.
4. The peripheral pulses distal to the operative site must be present.
5. Pain must be minimal.
6. Postoperative complications must be resolved or under control.

If regional anesthesia was administered, the patient must have return of motor function and partial sensory return to all anesthetized parts. The patient is discharged from the PACU by the anesthesiologist and is usually transferred to a general surgical unit. However, if the surgery was major, if concurrent illnesses may complicate recovery, or if the operative or anesthetic course was complicated, the patient might be transferred to an intensive care unit.

Application of the Nursing Process to the Care of the Patient in a Postanesthesia Care Unit

Assessment

On the patient's admission to the PACU, confirm patient identity. Listen to breath sounds, and assess blood pressure, pulse quality and rhythm, and respiratory status immediately on arrival. Receive report and review postoperative orders with the anesthesiologist and circulating nurse. Complete a head-to-toe assessment of the patient, including blood pressure, apical pulse, temperature, respiratory status and breath sounds, skin color and temperature, level of consciousness, and response to commands. Determine the rate of flow of parenteral infusions and the solution being infused and compare with the doctor's orders. Assess the infusion site for signs of infiltration or inflammation. Examine dressings to ensure placement and adherence, and note drainage. Check beneath the patient for wound drainage or bleeding. Determine the placement of drains or irrigating devices, connect drains to appropriate receptacles and irrigating devices to solutions, and ensure proper function. Note the amount and characteristics of all drainage. Examine bony prominences and pressure areas for redness or unusual pallor and for signs of altered perfusion caused by pressure from the operating table or instruments used for positioning during surgery.

Nursing Diagnoses and Planning

Nursing diagnoses and related expected patient outcomes most commonly applicable to patients in a PACU include the following:

NDx: High risk for ineffective airway clearance related to tracheobronchial obstruction by tongue or secretions, depressed cough and gag reflexes, impaired swallowing, possible regurgitation, or vomiting secondary to general anesthesia.

Planning: Patient outcomes
1. Patient maintains clear, open airway as evidenced by normal breath sounds.

NDx: High risk for ineffective breathing pattern related to hypoventilation secondary to the effects of general anesthesia, pain, and positioning

Planning: Patient outcomes

1. Patient maintains spontaneous, unlabored respirations of more than 10/minute and fewer than 30/minute.
2. Patient remains free of dyspnea and cyanosis.

NDx: High risk for altered tissue perfusion: systemic related to hypovolemia, peripheral vasodilation and blood pooling, hypothermia

Planning: Patient outcomes

1. Patient maintains adequate tissue perfusion as evidenced by the following:
   a. Pulse greater than 60 beats per minute (bpm) but less than 100 bpm, with regular rhythm
   b. Blood pressure stable, more than 90 mmHg systolic
   c. Capillary refill less than 3 seconds
   d. Urine output greater than 30 ml/hour
   e. Is easily aroused, oriented

NDx: High risk for injury related to restlessness during recovery from anesthesia and diminished awareness of, and responses to, internal and external stimuli

Planning: Patient outcomes

1. Patient remains free of injury.

Nursing Interventions

The goals of nursing care of a patient in a PACU are to support hemodynamic stabilization after anesthesia and surgery, promote recovery from anesthesia, promote physical comfort and wound healing, and prevent injury and postoperative complications. Table 4–6 describes common postoperative complications and their management.

Patient status is monitored and documented on admission, at least every 15 minutes for the first hour, and then every 30 minutes until stable. Many agencies have a special PACU documentation form for use during the immediate postoperative period.

NDx: High risk for ineffective airway clearance

Maintenance of a patent airway and adequate respiratory exchange are nursing priorities for the postoperative patient. On admission to the PACU, the patient's reflexes, including the pharyngeal cough and gag reflex, may be absent because of the effects of general anesthesia. Many patients feel nauseated and retch within the first 5 to 10 minutes after waking from anesthesia. Airway obstruction most commonly occurs as a result of the tongue, which is relaxed from anesthesia, falling back against the pharynx or from secretions or gastric fluids collecting in the oropharynx. Keep the bed flat and, unless contraindicated, position the patient to the side to allow drainage of secretions until the patient is conscious and swallowing occurs. Monitor breath sounds to detect airway obstruction. Noisy respirations, snoring, wheezes, and gurgling indicate partial airway obstruction. Suction to remove vomitus or mucus that may be obstructing the airway. An oropharyngeal airway to prevent obstruction by the tongue is often in place on transfer to the PACU.

Table 4–6. COMMON POSTOPERATIVE COMPLICATIONS

COMPLICATION	CAUSES	MAJOR CLINICAL MANIFESTATIONS	TREATMENT	PREVENTATIVE NURSING INTERVENTIONS
Atelectasis (collapse of alveoli with retained mucous secretions)	Obstruction of airway by secretions; closure of bronchioles because of shallow breathing or failure to periodically hyperventilate lungs	Fever, tachypnea, tachycardia; decreased breath sounds, scattered rales	Chest percussion, coughing, suctioning; bronchodilators and mucolytics via nebulizer	Early ambulation, coughing and deep breathing, incentive spirometry
Aspiration	Depression of gastroesophageal and pharyngoesophageal sphincter reflexes resulting from drugs and irritation from endotracheal or nasogastric tubes; food in stomach when given general anesthesia; improper positioning of the patient	Signs of airway obstruction, atelectasis, pulmonary abscess, pneumonitis, pneumonia, or shock	Establish a patent airway by endotracheal suctioning or bronchoscopy	Avoid general anesthesia for patients who have recently eaten; position patient correctly before intubation; use pressure cuffs when prolonged intubation is required
Pneumonia	Atelectasis, aspiration, copious secretions as found in a heavy smoker or patient with chronic obstructive lung disease	Fever, tachypnea, increased secretions	Antibiotics on basis of sputum culture and sensitivity, chest physiotherapy	Coughing and deep breathing, frequent position changes, early ambulation

(continued)

Table 4–6. COMMON POSTOPERATIVE COMPLICATIONS (continued)

COMPLICATION	CAUSES	MAJOR CLINICAL MANIFESTATIONS	TREATMENT	PREVENTATIVE NURSING INTERVENTIONS
Thrombophlebitis	Venous stasis caused by prolonged immobilization or pressure on vein walls from leg straps in the OR, leg holders for lithotomy position	Redness, heat, pain, swelling in calf	Anticoagulation, bed rest, moist heat on affected area	Antiembolic stockings, postoperative leg exercises, early ambulation
Pulmonary embolism	Formed from venous thrombus; usually originating in legs, pelvis, or right side of heart, then traveling to and being trapped in pulmonary circulation	Sudden severe chest pain or tightness, tachycardia, hypotension, pallor or cyanosis, restlessness, anxiety	Oxygen administration, Fowler's position, anticoagulant therapy, analgesics	Passive and active range-of-motion exercises, antiembolic stockings, low-dose heparin administration if predisposing factors present, early ambulation
Shock	Two most common causes: hemorrhage and sepsis	Decreased blood pressure; elevated pulse; cold, clammy skin; decreased urinary output	If hemorrhage, ligate bleeder and give blood; if septic, antibiotics on basis of blood culture sensitivity.	
Wound infection	Break in aseptic technique or a dirty wound; predisposing factors: inadequate preoperative screening and preparation, coexistent conditions such as diabetes mellitus or uremia, obesity, malnutrition, corticosteroid therapy	Fever; foul-smelling, greenish-white drainage from wound; persistent edema, redness	Antibiotics on basis of culture and sensitivity of wound	Strict aseptic technique in OR and during postoperative dressing changes
Wound dehiscence (opening of the wound) and wound evisceration (protrusion of viscera through opening)	Inadequate surgical closure; increased intra-abdominal pressure from coughing, vomiting, or straining at stool; poor wound healing caused by malnutrition, poor circulation, old age, or preoperative radiation	Discharge of serosanguineous drainage from the wound; sensation that "something gave or let go"	Lay patient down, cover wound with sterile saline-soaked gauze or towels; return to OR for repair, monitor for shock	Splint wound when coughing, medicate for nausea and vomiting; highest risk during 5th to 8th postoperative days
Delayed wound healing	Inadequate supplies of protein, vitamin C, and trace minerals ferrous iron and zinc manganese; inadequate oxygen supply; administration of steroids; wound infections; additional injuries	Edges of wound are not approximated; granulation is not evident	High-protein, high-vitamin, high-calorie diet; splint and support wound during activity	Provide adequate dietary intake; maintain aseptic technique; promote rest for adequate healing
Wound infection with abscess	Poorly nourished individual; surgical contamination; wound drains create entrance site for bacteria; deep wounds more prone to abscess	Temperature elevation; inflammation and edema around wound; malaise; persistent pain	High-protein, high-vitamin, high-calorie diet; antibiotics on basis of wound culture and sensitivity; aseptic technique with dressing changes; abscess treated with incision and drainage	Aseptic technique throughout perioperative period; improve nutritional status preoperatively
Hematoma (collection of blood and clots in wound)	Imperfect hemostasis, use of anticoagulants, coagulation disorders	Elevation and discoloration of wound edges	If small, may reabsorb; otherwise surgical evacuation	

(continued)

Table 4–6. (continued) COMMON POSTOPERATIVE COMPLICATIONS

COMPLICATION	CAUSES	MAJOR CLINICAL MANIFESTATIONS	TREATMENT	PREVENTATIVE NURSING INTERVENTIONS
Seroma (collection of fluid other than blood or pus in the wound)	Inadequate drainage from incisional area	Elevation of wound edges	Needle aspiration or surgical drainage	
Adhesions after abdominal surgery (fibrous bands that form between abdominal wall and viscera or between viscera)	Unknown; represents overhealing of tissue and is more extensive if inflammatory process present	Bowel obstruction, pain	Surgery for lysis of adhesions	Aseptic technique in operating room; aseptic dressing changes
Paralytic ileus	Anesthetic agents, manipulation of the bowel, wound infection, electrolyte imbalance	Absent bowel sounds, no passage of flatus or feces, abdominal distention	Nasogastric suction, IV fluids, rectal tube, ambulate	Early ambulation
Bowel obstruction	Intestinal adhesions	Similar to paralytic ileus although BM may occur before obstruction	Bowel decompression with a Miller-Abbott tube, surgical correction	
Urinary retention	Lack of urge to void because of anesthetics, narcotic, or anticholinergic drugs; surgery of pelvic or perineal area resulting in edema in area of bladder	Little or no output; palpably distended bladder, restlessness, discomfort	Measures to promote voiding (privacy, run water, sit patient up); catheterization if above methods fail	Adequate hydration; early ambulation
Urinary tract infection	Urinary retention, catheterization, contamination of urinary tract	Mild fever, dysuria, hematuria, malaise	Adequate hydration, maintenance of good bladder drainage, antibiotics on basis of urine culture and sensitivity	Encourage fluid intake, early ambulation; avoid catheterization
Gastric erosion and stress ulcer	Intense physical or emotional stress resulting in increased secretion of adrenocorticotropic hormone from pituitary and cortisol from adrenal cortex	Bleeding often first symptom, epigastric pain	Antacids; small, frequent meals; emotional support	Identification of patients at risk: gram-negative sepsis, acute renal failure, central nervous system lesions, severe injuries
Temperature elevation	Infection, dehydration, response to stress and trauma, prolonged hypotension, transfusion reaction, respiratory congestion, thrombophlebitis	Temperature elevated above 99.5°F (37.5°C); elevated pulse and respiratory rates; diaphoresis; lethargy	Antipyretics; cooling sponge baths; increasing fluids	Dependent on cause
Parotitis (inflammation of parotid glands)	Poor oral hygiene, malnutrition	Mild fever, edema anterior to the ear lobe, discomfort	Antibiotics; incision and drainage	Frequent oral hygiene, adequate fluid intake
Hiccups (singultus)	Idiopathic; irritation of phrenic nerve	Periodic release of air through glottis, emanating noise; abdominal distention	Breathe in and out of paper bag for 5-min intervals; administration of 5% carbon dioxide in oxygen mix for few minutes	None
Sore throat	Intubation; presence of oral or nasopharyngeal airways, nasogastric tubes; dry, irritating nature of inhalants	Pain in throat	Mouthwash; ice chips; throat lozenges; warm beverages if allowed oral fluids	None

Abbreviations: OR, operating room; IV, intravenous; BM, bowel movement.

The patient usually pushes the airway out on regaining consciousness. If the tongue obstructs the airway because no oropharyngeal airway is in place, and a side-lying position is contraindicated, tilt the head back slightly and thrust the jaw forward by lifting at the angle of the jaw or lift the jaw under the chin to move the tongue forward and reopen the airway.

NDx: High risk for ineffective breathing pattern
Monitor the quality and rate of respirations at least every 15 minutes until breathing is regular and unlabored and then every 30 minutes until the patient is discharged from the PACU. Administer continuous humidified oxygen and encourage deep breathing and coughing every 5 to 15 minutes to promote gaseous exchange and removal of inhaled anesthetic agents. Reposition the patient side to side every 15 minutes to promote lung expansion and to prevent atelectasis. Administer analgesics to promote pain relief and participation in respiratory exercises. Because of the potential side effect of respiratory depression, narcotic analgesics are often administered in reduced dosages in the PACU. Attach a pulse oximeter to a finger, a toe, or an ear lobe to monitor arterial oxygen saturation. Note the color of the skin, lips, mucous membranes, and nail beds to detect cyanosis caused by hypoxia. If an endotracheal tube is in place, maintain patency and mechanical ventilation or oxygen administration as prescribed. Monitor the patient's ability to follow commands, to lift the head or a limb and hold it steady for 5 seconds, and to maintain spontaneous respirations of more than 10/minute and fewer than 30/minute with pulse oximeter readings of greater than 95%, which are criteria for extubation by the anesthesiologist. Arterial blood gas levels to confirm adequate oxygenation are usually determined before extubation.

NDx: High risk for altered tissue perfusion: systemic
Hypoxemia and respiratory acidosis are common causes of cardiac dysrhythmias in the immediate postoperative period. Attach the patient to a cardiac monitor to monitor heart rate and rhythm continuously. Monitor vital signs, heart sounds, the quality and rate of peripheral pulses, and capillary refill every 5 to 15 minutes until stable and then every 30 minutes and compare with preoperative and intraoperative assessments to detect changes in cardiac output and cardiovascular function. Monitor temperature and urine output every hour. A rapid, thready pulse and a drop in blood pressure is reported immediately, because these changes may indicate shock. Other clinical manifestations of shock include the following: rapid, shallow respirations; restlessness or slowed responses; pallor; cold, moist skin; cyanosis; decreased urine output; and decreased temperature. Possible causes of shock include untoward reaction to the anesthetic or other medications, fluid or blood loss, and bacterial infection.

Administer intravenous infusions to replace intraoperative fluid losses. Monitor the type of solution, flow rate, and infusion site to prevent fluid overload or infiltration. Auscultation of crackles with breath sounds indicates fluid overload. If the patient has lost an excessive amount of blood during surgery, a transfusion may be administered. Ensure blood compatibility according to agency policies, regulate infusion flow rate to complete transfusion within 4 hours, and monitor for signs of a transfusion reaction. Chapter 15 discusses administration of blood products in detail.

Examine dressings and check behind the patient every 15 to 30 minutes for bleeding or drainage. Report rapid saturation of the dressing or frank bleeding to the surgeon immediately. Circle a small amount of drainage on the dressing, and record the time and date on the dressing so the amount of subsequent drainage in a given period of time can be monitored. The operative dressing can usually be reinforced as necessary, although the original dressing is not removed without the surgeon's order. Check placement of drains or irrigating devices, gastrointestinal tubes, indwelling urinary catheters, and monitoring devices every 15 minutes to ensure proper function. Note the color, odor, amount, and consistency of all drainage.

Reposition the patient every 10 to 15 minutes to prevent venous stasis and to promote return of vasculomotor function. Examine bony prominences each time the patient is repositioned for early detection and prevention of pressure areas. Gently massage bony prominences and pressure areas to promote capillary circulation. The risk of rapid development of pressure areas remains high until full vasculomotor function returns. Provide blankets to promote warming and to prevent vasoconstriction associated with shivering. Apply antiembolic stockings, if not already in use, and remind the patient not to cross the legs or ankles to prevent venous impairment. Do not massage the feet or legs; massage can cause dislodgement of a thrombus. As the patient becomes more alert, encourage independent movement of feet and legs and position changes per preoperative teaching to promote circulation and vascular tone.

NDx: High risk for injury
Keep the side rails of the stretcher raised and the wheels locked. Monitor level of consciousness frequently. Stimulate verbal interaction and reorient the patient to surroundings each time vital signs are assessed. Speak in a calm, reassuring manner and explain all procedures to reduce anxiety. The first responses that the patient will make are reflex motor responses. These are followed by spontaneous movements or movement in response to a command. The patient will at first be drowsy and then be more alert and talkative and oriented to time and

place. Some patients become temporarily combative or disoriented. Determine the cause of agitation or restlessness. Although it is a common response to recovery from anesthesia, it may also be caused by pain, hypoxia, cardiac ischemia, hemorrhage, urinary retention, lying too long in one position, and impaired circulation or limb constriction caused by bandages or casts. If restlessness or agitation persists despite interventions, the patient may need to be restrained to prevent injury. Restraints are always a last resort because restriction of movement increases the risk of circulatory impairment and may aggravate the patient's emotional status.

Evaluation

Evaluate the effectiveness of nursing care for a patient in a PACU by comparing the patient's status with the expected patient outcomes. Examples of specific outcomes for patients in a PACU have been provided in the Planning section.

Application of the Nursing Process to the Care of the Postsurgical Patient

The postsurgical unit is notified when the patient has met the discharge criteria and is ready to be released. The PACU nurse accompanies the patient to the unit, gives a report to the receiving nurse, and reviews postoperative medical orders. The report includes the following: the name, age, language spoken, and status of the patient; allergies; surgery performed; type of anesthetic agent; estimated blood loss; drugs and intravenous solutions administered; intraoperative and postoperative complications and treatment; summary of stay in PACU; location and type of dressings, catheters, drains, irrigation tubes, or packing; altered sensory or motor functions; and any special instructions. The patient is transferred to the bed in the postsurgical unit. Family members or significant others are notified of the patient's return and told when they may visit.

Assessment

On patient transfer from the PACU, confirm patient identity and assist transfer into bed. Listen to breath sounds and assess blood pressure, pulse quality and rhythm, and respiratory status immediately on the patient's arrival. Receive the report and review postoperative orders with the PACU nurse. Complete a head-to-toe assessment of the patient, including blood pressure, apical pulse, temperature, respiratory status, skin color and temperature, level of consciousness, response to commands, and independent movement. Examine dressings to ensure placement and adherence, and note drainage. Check beneath the patient for wound drainage or bleeding. Determine placement of drains or tubes, connect to appropriate receptacles, and ensure proper function. Note the amount and characteristics of all drainage. Determine the rate of flow of parenteral infusions and the solution being infused and compare with the physician's orders. Assess the infusion site for signs of infiltration or inflammation.

Nursing Diagnoses and Planning

Nursing diagnoses and related expected patient outcomes most commonly applicable to postsurgical patients include the following:

NDx: High risk for ineffective breathing pattern related to tracheobronchial obstruction by secretions or hypoventilation secondary to the effects of general anesthesia, postoperative analgesics, pain, and positioning

Planning: Patient outcomes

1. Patient maintains patent airway as evidenced by normal breath sounds.
2. Patient maintains spontaneous, unlabored respirations of more than 10/minute and fewer than 30/minute.
3. Patient remains free of dyspnea and cyanosis.

NDx: High risk for fluid volume deficit related to NPO status and inadequate replacement of fluid loss in surgery, or from gastrointestinal tract and/or wound drainage

Planning: Patient outcomes

1. Patient maintains adequate hydration as evidenced by the following:
   a. Pulse greater than 60 bpm but less than 100 bpm, with regular rhythm
   b. Blood pressure stable, more than 90 mm Hg systolic
   c. Capillary refill less than 3 seconds
   d. Urine output more than 30 ml/hour
   e. Is easily aroused, oriented
   f. Moist mucous membranes
   g. Skin supple with good turgor

NDx: Pain related to surgical incision, manipulation of internal structures during surgical procedure

Planning: Patient outcomes

1. Patient verbalizes relief of pain to tolerable levels.

NDx: High risk for injury related to diminished awareness of, and responses to, internal and external stimuli secondary to postoperative analgesics

Planning: Patient outcomes
1. Patient remains free of injury.

NDx: High risk for infection related to presence of surgical incision and wound drains

Planning: Patient outcomes
1. Patient remains free from infection as evidenced by absence of the following:
   a. Fever
   b. Purulent or malodorus wound drainage
   c. Increasing redness or edema around the incision

NDx: Impaired physical mobility related to pain, surgical procedure, and side effects of narcotic analgesics

Planning: Patient outcomes
1. Patient resumes independent ambulation and physical care activities within physical limitations by the third postoperative day.

NDx: High risk for altered urinary elimination related to decreased bladder tone secondary to effects of general or spinal anesthesia

Planning: Patient outcomes
1. Patient voids within 8 hours of surgery.

NDx: High risk for altered nutrition: less than body requirements related to nausea or absence of peristalsis secondary to general anesthesia

Planning: Patient outcomes
1. Patient has return of peristalsis as evidenced by presence of bowel sounds by the third postoperative day.
2. Patient ingests and retains 75% of prescribed diet within 24 hours of return of peristalsis.

NDx: High risk for body image disturbance related to surgical procedure, surgical incision, presence of wound drains, loss of independence

Planning: Patient outcomes
1. Patient verbalizes acceptance of permanent changes in appearance and physical status.
2. Patient assumes as much independence as able.
3. Patient makes positive statements about self.

NDx: High risk for altered health maintenance related to insufficient knowledge of postoperative self-management after discharge

Planning: Patient outcomes
1. Patient verbalizes understanding of wound-care procedures and postoperative instructions.
2. Patient demonstrates correct technique in wound-care management, if appropriate.

Nursing Interventions

The goals of nursing care of the postsurgical patient are to promote physical comfort and wound healing, to prevent injury and postoperative complications, and to prepare the patient for discharge. The risk of altered tissue perfusion as a result of postoperative hemorrhage is highest in the first 48 hours postoperatively. Expected outcomes and nursing interventions for this nursing diagnosis continue as previously discussed in PACU care.

Cardiovascular and respiratory status, level of consciousness, and the condition of all infusions, wounds, drains, and dressings are monitored and documented at least every 15 minutes for the first hour, every 30 minutes for the next hour, every hour for 4 hours, and every 4 hours for a minimum of 24 hours after the patient's transfer to the postsurgical unit. Status is monitored more frequently if the patient's condition indicates the need.

As the patient progresses through the postoperative period, some assessments, such as frequent determination of level of consciousness or vital signs, may no longer be necessary, whereas other assessments, such as auscultation of bowel sounds, ability to perform self-care procedures, and understanding of discharge instructions, become more significant. Nursing Care Guide 4–2 includes a general plan of care for a patient after surgery.

NDx: High risk for ineffective breathing pattern

Position the patient side to side every hour until fully conscious, and then every 2 hours, to prevent aspiration and stasis of secretions. Auscultate breath sounds, and monitor rate and depth of respirations to detect accumulation of secretions or reduced ventilation. Manifestations of compromised respiratory status include rapid, thready pulse; restlessness; apprehension; rapid, shallow breathing; confusion; and cyanosis. Arouse the patient every time status is monitored, and encourage deep breathing and coughing to expel residual anesthetic agents and to promote gaseous exchange and respiratory function. As the patient becomes more alert, elevate the head of the bed to promote chest expansion and diaphragmatic excursion. Encourage the patient to perform respiratory exercises and to use the incentive spirometer every hour the day of surgery then at least every 2 hours as taught preoperatively to mobilize secretions and to prevent atelectasis. Administer prescribed analgesics, and assist the patient in sitting upright and in splinting abdominal incisions when coughing and deep breathing to reduce incisional pain. Monitor respiratory rate and depth before analgesic administration to avoid respiratory depression from narcotic agents. Early ambulation and mobility are major factors in the prevention of postoperative respiratory complications. Assist the patient in getting out of bed to a chair and in am-

Nursing Care Guide 4–2.
POSTOPERATIVE PATIENT CARE

Assessment Findings: Patient returns to surgical unit after discharge from postanesthesia care unit after surgery under general anesthesia. Patient is asleep but awakens to touch and name. Respirations are deep and regular (10/min).

Nursing Diagnosis: High risk for ineffective breathing pattern related to effects of general anesthesia, postoperative pain.

Patient Outcomes	Nursing Interventions	Rationale
Patient maintains patent airway as evidenced by normal breath sounds, spontaneous respirations that are regular and unlabored (>10/min).	Position patient side to side every hour until fully conscious. Arouse patient every 15–30 min and encourage deep breathing, coughing, use of incentive spirometer. Auscultate for abnormal breath sounds.	Frequent position changes, coughing, and deep breathing help expel residual anesthetic agents, prevent stasis of secretions, promote lung expansion, and improve gaseous exchange.
	Elevate head of bed as patient becomes more alert. Assist patient to sit upright when coughing and deep breathing. Encourage early ambulation.	Upright position and ambulation promote chest expansion and diaphragmatic excursion to improve ventilation.
	Offer analgesic medication at prescribed intervals.	Acute pain and increased incisional pain when coughing and deep breathing reduce patient's participation in respiratory exercises.

Evaluation: Compare the patient's status with the expected patient outcomes. If the outcomes are achieved, evaluate nursing care as successful. If not, reassess the patient, formulate new nursing diagnoses, and revise expected patient outcomes and nursing interventions as appropriate.

(continued)

bulating short distances within 24 hours after surgery to minimize the risk of respiratory complications.

NDx: High risk for fluid volume deficit

Adequate circulating fluid volume is necessary for tissue oxygenation and repair and for reduction of the risk of postoperative circulatory complications such as thrombophlebitis. Monitor heart rate and quality of pulse, blood pressure, level of consciousness, capillary refill, and urine output to detect changes in cardiovascular function and fluid balance. Inspect mucous membranes and skin turgor to detect dryness. An increase in heart rate, drop in blood pressure, decrease in level of consciousness, slow capillary refill, decreased urine output, dry mucous membranes, and poor skin turgor are manifestations of fluid volume deficit. Monitor and maintain intravenous infusions to replace intraoperative and postoperative fluid losses as discussed in altered tissue perfusion in PACU care. Document all fluid intake and output, including wound drainage, catheters, urine, emesis, gastrointestinal tubes, and liquid stool, to monitor fluid balance. Encourage oral fluid intake to 3000 ml daily, unless contraindicated, when oral intake is resumed to promote and maintain good hydration.

Text continued on page 116

Nursing Care Guide 4–2. *(continued)*

POSTOPERATIVE PATIENT CARE

Assessment Findings: Six hours after surgery performed under general anesthesia, patient has not voided. Intravenous solution is infusing at 100 ml/hour. Patient is sleepy, easily aroused, denies urge to void.

Nursing Diagnosis: High risk for altered urinary elimination related to decreased bladder tone secondary to effects of general anesthesia

Patient Outcomes	Nursing Interventions	Rationale
Patient voids within 8 hours of surgery.	Palpate abdomen for distended bladder.	Distended bladder indicates urinary retention.
	Review pre-, intra-, and postoperative fluid loss and intake, especially if bladder is not palpable. Assess for signs of dehydration: dry mucous membranes, poor skin turgor, lethargy.	Determine whether intake was sufficient to adequately hydrate patient. Dehydration is a possible cause of decreased urine production.
	Assist female patient to upright position on bedpan or to bedside commode or bathroom to void. Assist a male patient to stand to void. Provide privacy.	Comfortable position and privacy promote sphincter relaxation and voiding.
	Run water in the room or place patient's hand in warm water.	Association with water often stimulates voiding.
	Perform sterile straight catheterization of bladder if patient is unable to void despite these interventions.	Overdistention of the bladder causes further loss of bladder tone. Stasis of urine increases risk of bladder infection.
Patient voids within 8 hours of straight catheterization and four or more times per day thereafter.	Continue to monitor patient for adequate hydration and return of spontaneous voiding within 8 hours of catheterization. Monitor voiding pattern for 48 hours thereafter.	Close monitoring identifies return of bladder function and normal pattern of urinary elimination.

Evaluation: Compare the patient's status with the expected patient outcomes. If the outcomes are achieved, evaluate nursing care as successful. If not, reassess the patient, formulate new nursing diagnoses, and revise expected patient outcomes and nursing interventions as appropriate.

(continued)

Nursing Care Guide 4–2. *(continued)*

POSTOPERATIVE PATIENT CARE

Assessment Findings: Postsurgical patient is reluctant to change position. Patient complains of pain on movement and guards incision and grimaces when moving.

Nursing Diagnosis: Pain related to surgical incision

Patient Outcomes	Nursing Interventions	Rationale
Patient states relief of pain to tolerable level.	Determine location, duration, and intensity of pain (on a scale of 1 to 10) before administration of medication.	Cause of pain must be identified. It is unsafe to assume all postoperative pain is related to surgery.
	Encourage patient to request analgesic before pain becomes severe. Offer analgesic at prescribed intervals the first 48 hours after surgery if patient demonstrates nonverbal signs of discomfort but does not request medication.	Administration of analgesics before pain becomes severe maintains better pain control and reduces fear of acute episodes of pain. Adequate pain management promotes patient participation in postoperative exercises and encourages independent movement and early ambulation.
	Assist patient to assume comfortable position. Provide comfort measures such as smooth bedding, back rub, and position change. Encourage guided imagery and distraction.	These measures promote relaxation and enhance pain relief by reducing anxiety.
	Elevate side rails and instruct patient to call for assistance before getting out of bed after administration of analgesics.	Analgesics can alter awareness of environment, reduce protective instincts, alter judgment, and increase risk of injury.
	Ask the patient whether the pain is relieved or reduced to a tolerable level. Ask the patient to again rate the pain on a scale of 1 to 10. Monitor for nonverbal signs of pain relief or failure of analgesic to relieve pain.	Evaluates effectiveness of pain management.
	Advise the surgeon if pain is not relieved or reduced to a tolerable level.	Analgesic medication, dosage, or frequency may need to be adjusted.

Evaluation: Compare the patient's status with the expected patient outcomes. If the outcomes are achieved, evaluate nursing care as successful. If not, reassess the patient, formulate new nursing diagnoses, and revise expected patient outcomes and nursing interventions as appropriate.

(continued)

Nursing Care Guide 4–2. *(continued)*

POSTOPERATIVE PATIENT CARE

Assessment Findings: Second-day postsurgical patient with an abdominal incision closed with staples and with drain in place. The dressing is saturated with serosanguineous drainage. Incision is free of redness, purulent drainage. There is minimal edema along staple line.

Nursing Diagnosis: High risk for infection related to surgical incision and wound drain

Patient Outcomes	Nursing Interventions	Rationale
Patient remains free of the manifestations of wound infection: a. is afebrile b. absence of redness, increasing edema around incision c. absence of purulent, malodorous drainage from wound.	Wash hands before and after patient contact. Teach patient good hand-washing practices also. Use aseptic technique in all wound care.	Prevents contamination of wound and cross-contamination from staff or other patients.
	Change moist dressings promptly. Expect copious drainage from wounds with drains in place. Cleanse wound and area around the wound.	Soiled, warm, moist dressings provide excellent environment for the growth of pathogens. Cleansing removes drainage and pathogens.
	Examine wound with each dressing change for signs of delayed healing or infection: increasing redness, warmth, or edema around the incision and purulent or malodorous drainage. Obtain culture if wound appears infected.	Early detection and diagnosis of infection ensures prompt treatment.
	Encourage high-protein diet with increased vitamins B and C.	These nutrients are necessary for tissue repair.
Patient demonstrates proper wound-care technique and states signs and symptoms of wound infection before discharge.	Teach patient wound care and the signs and symptoms of wound infection to report to physician in preparation for discharge. Provide written instructions. Have patient demonstrate wound care.	Many patients are discharged before wound heals completely. Written instructions reinforce teaching, avoid confusion, and reduce anxiety when the patient is discharged. Demonstration evaluates learning.

Evaluation: Compare the patient's status with the expected patient outcomes. If the outcomes are achieved, evaluate nursing care as successful. If not, reassess the patient, formulate new nursing diagnoses, and revise expected patient outcomes and nursing interventions as appropriate.

(continued)

Nursing Care Guide 4–2. *(continued)*

POSTOPERATIVE PATIENT CARE

Assessment Findings: Three days after abdominal surgery, the patient is unable to tolerate clear liquid diet and complains of nausea and "gas pains." He states he passed flatus once. Bowel sounds are diminished in frequency and intensity.

Nursing Diagnosis: High risk for altered nutrition: less than body requirements related to nausea and diminished peristalsis secondary to manipulation of gastrointestinal organs during surgery

Patient Outcomes	Nursing Interventions	Rationale
Patient has return of peristalsis by third day after surgery as evidenced by presence of active bowel sounds.	Auscultate for bowel sounds in all four quadrants. Listen for 2 min at a point midway between the umbilicus and the anterior iliac crest before documenting absence of bowel sounds. Ask if patient has passed flatus or is experiencing gas pain.	Bowel sounds and passage of flatus indicate return of peristalsis. Gas pains are caused when air accumulates in the intestine and causes distention.
	Encourage ambulation. Teach patient that walking is the best method to relieve gas pains.	Walking stimulates peristalsis and helps relieve distention caused by air in the intestine.
	Monitor for increased frequency of bowel sounds.	Increased frequency of bowel sounds indicates return to normal peristalsis.
	Report continued absence of active bowel sounds on the third day after surgery.	Absence of active bowel sounds may indicate paralytic ileus.
Patient tolerates prescribed diet.	Administer antiemetic as prescribed. Encourage patient to request antiemetic at the first sign of nausea.	Antiemetics relieve nausea more effectively if administered as soon as nausea develops.
	Progress diet as tolerated. Monitor for nausea and vomiting after ingesting food or fluids.	Patient should be able to tolerate food and fluids with return of peristalsis.
	Report continued inability to tolerate food or fluids to the physician.	Postoperative nausea may be caused by something other than food intolerance.

Evaluation: Compare the patient's status with the expected patient outcomes. If the outcomes are achieved, evaluate nursing care as successful. If not, reassess the patient, formulate new nursing diagnoses, and revise expected patient outcomes and nursing interventions as appropriate.

Promotion of good blood flow is also supported by measures that prevent venous stasis. Apply antiembolic stockings if ordered by the physician, encourage the patient to perform leg exercises at least every hour while awake, assist with early ambulation, and elevate the patient's legs when he or she is sitting in a chair to promote venous return. Do not raise the knee support of the bed unless the foot of the bed is also elevated or place anything under the knees, to avoid pressure on the popliteal space. Teach the patient to avoid crossing the legs or ankles to prevent impaired venous flow.

NDx: Pain

Remind the patient that postoperative pain is expected. Offer and administer prescribed analgesics to provide relief. Explain that analgesics should reduce pain to a tolerable level, but not necessarily eliminate it altogether. Do not assume that all pain after surgery is related to the surgical procedure. Determine the location, type, and characteristics of pain to rule out other causes. Ask the patient to rate the pain on a scale of 1 (minimal) to 10 (excruciating) to quantify the severity of pain. Administer the analgesic and document the patient's stated or apparent (e.g., patient asleep) degree of pain relief. Use other comfort measures such as distraction, imagery, a quiet environment, position changes, and back massage to enhance the effect of analgesics. Advise the surgeon if pain is not relieved. Adequate analgesia promotes not only patient comfort but also independent movement and position changes and early ambulation and improves patient participation in exercises to promote respiratory and circulatory function. Pain relief reduces anxiety and fear of movement and promotes recovery.

Patient-Controlled Analgesia: Patient-controlled analgesia (PCA) allows the patient to control the amount and frequency of self-administered narcotic analgesic within predetermined safe limitations. Intravenous morphine sulfate (Duramorph) is the most commonly used drug. The patient usually receives a loading dose of narcotic, and then the PCA pump delivers an additional bolus dose when the patient pushes a button. The PCA pump may also deliver a set basal dose independent of the patient's control. For safety, the PCA pump has a set lock-out time to maintain a minimum interval between bolus doses and a maximum number of bolus doses per hour. The patient must be able to operate the PCA control button and understand the instructions. PCA promotes patient independence through optimal pain relief and minimizes patient's fear of severe pain by avoiding peaks and troughs of serum drug levels.

Document the programming mode each shift or when the program is altered. Monitor and document respiratory rate, blood pressure, pulse, level of consciousness, pain relief, and infusion site every hour for 4 hours when PCA is initiated and at least every 4 hours throughout PCA therapy. Notify the physician if respirations are less than 10/minute and prepare for administration of a narcotic antagonist. A narcotic antagonist such as naloxone hydrochloride (Narcan) must be available on the postsurgical unit throughout PCA therapy.

Spinal Administration of Analgesics: Administration of narcotic analgesics, usually morphine, via catheter into the epidural or subarachnoid space is another alternative method of postoperative pain relief. Postoperative use is usually limited to 48 to 72 hours to reduce the risk of central nervous system infection. The physician or anesthesiologist administers a loading dose of narcotic and may administer additional bolus doses at 12- to 36-hour intervals depending on patient comfort. Respiratory depression, sedation, nausea and vomiting, urinary retention, and pruritus are possible side effects. A pulse oximeter or apnea monitor is used to continuously monitor oxygenation and respiratory function. Monitor for side effects of analgesic, and document monitor readings, respiratory rate, level of consciousness, and pain relief every hour or per agency policy to detect respiratory depression. Notify the physician if respirations are less than 10/minute and have Narcan available for rapid treatment. Continue to monitor the patient for residual respiratory depression for 24 hours after the last dose of narcotic. Be sure the catheter is securely taped and protected by a dressing to prevent dislodgement. Examine the catheter insertion site every 4 hours for redness, swelling, and discomfort to detect early signs of irritation or infection.

NDx: High risk for injury

Anesthesia and postoperative analgesics can alter patient awareness of the environment, reduce protective reflexes, cause confusion and disorientation, and increase the risk of injury. Keep side rails elevated until the patient is fully alert, oriented, and recovered from anesthesia. Elevate the side rails after administration of narcotic analgesic. Keep one side rail elevated to assist the patient in independent movement and position changes. Encourage the patient to use the call bell and to ask for assistance when getting out of bed. Assist the patient when getting out of bed and ambulating until his or her gait is steady to prevent injury. Demonstrate how to get out of and into bed safely and how to manage intravenous infusion lines and poles, drains, and catheters to prevent dislodgement.

NDx: High risk for infection

Wash hands before and after patient contact, and use aseptic technique in all wound care to prevent contamination. Examine dressings for excess drainage and change saturated dressings to prevent contamination of the wound by capillary action. Soiled, warm, moist dressings provide an excellent environment for the growth of pathogens. Ensure proper function of wound drains to promote tissue approximation and healing. Examine wounds for early signs of infection or delayed healing. Wound edges should be approximated, or touch, in wounds healing by primary intention, or granulation tissue should be present in wounds healing by secondary intention. Inflammation, edema, and bloody or serosanguineous drainage are normal the first 3 days postoperatively. Redness and edema should gradually subside, and the drainage should cease as healing progresses. Increasing inflammation or edema, purulent drainage, foul odor, persistent pain, delayed healing, and fever are signs of wound infection.

Wound healing may also be delayed by dehiscence (partial or complete separation of the wound edges) and evisceration (protrusion of internal organs through a dehisced wound). Infection, fluid accumulation in the wound, obesity, malnutrition, fragile skin in the aged, cancer, and excessive coughing increase the risk of dehiscence and evisceration. Immediately examine any wound if a sudden increase in drainage or bleeding occurs or if the patient reports a sensation that something "popped" or "gave way." Notify the surgeon immediately if wound disruption has occurred, and instruct the patient to avoid coughing or moving. Position the patient to prevent further stress on the wound. Wound dehiscence may or may not require surgical repair. Wound evisceration requires emergency surgery to prevent impaired perfusion and possible gangrene of protruding organs. Cover protruding internal organs with sterile gauze moistened with sterile saline to prevent drying. Place the patient on NPO status, and initiate preparations for surgery as ordered by the surgeon. Prophylactic antibiotics are usually administered to minimize the risk of peritonitis. Explain all procedures and provide emotional support to reduce patient anxiety.

Most patients are discharged from the hospital before wounds are completely healed. Advise the patient to wear loose-fitting clothes to avoid irritation of the incision. Describe the expected appearance of the wound as it heals and the signs of infection to promote early detection of altered healing. Teach the patient to wash hands before and after wound care. Determine whether the patient can bathe or shower. Teach the patient how to remove and apply the dressing without contaminating the wound and how to cleanse the wound. Provide written instructions to reinforce teaching. Observe return demonstration to evaluate learning. If the wound is large or requires irrigation or if the dressing is complicated, a home-care referral may be appropriate. If sutures or staples are in place, confirm with the patient when to return to the surgeon for their removal.

NDx: Impaired physical mobility

Physical mobility promotes positive self-esteem and is essential to the optimal function of all body systems. The stress of surgery and limitation of nutritional intake can leave the patient weak and unsteady. Encourage and assist the patient to turn, change position, and perform leg exercises to begin physical activity immediately after surgery. Assist the patient out of bed as soon as possible after surgery to promote respiratory and circulatory function. Most patients should be able to sit in a chair the evening of surgery and ambulate short distances by the end of the first postoperative day. Monitor activity tolerance by changes in pulse rate. A rise or drop of more than 10 bpm indicates poor tolerance and the patient is returned to bed. Gradually increase activity based on the patient's response. Encourage the patient to sit or stand upright when out of bed to prevent pressure on internal organs from poor posture. Adequate pain relief encourages patient willingness to ambulate.

NDx: High risk for altered urinary elimination

The urge to void may be reduced postoperatively because of reduced bladder tone from the effects of general anesthesia. Bladder distention and urinary retention are possible up to 24 hours after spinal anesthesia as a result of blocked bladder innervation. More men than women suffer from urinary retention postoperatively. Review intraoperative, PACU, and postoperative intake and output records and compare fluid loss and intake to determine whether failure to void may be due to inadequate fluid replacement. If hydration is adequate, the patient should void within 6 to 8 hours after surgery. Ask if discomfort or an urge to void is present. Palpate the abdomen to detect a distended bladder. Offer a bedpan or urinal, assist a male patient to stand to void or assist a female patient to a bedside commode, and provide privacy to facilitate relaxation and voiding. Run water or place the patient's hand in a basin of warm water to stimulate voiding. Encourage voiding before administration of analgesic medications, which may promote further muscle relaxation or have a sedating or antimicturition effect on the patient. If the patient is unable to void and the bladder is distended, straight catheterization may be necessary. Acute postoperative urinary retention usually resolves spontaneously within 48 hours. Straight catheterization is repeated every 6 to 8 hours as necessary during this period to prevent bladder distention. An indwelling catheter may delay return of bladder tone and is not recommended.

NDx: High risk for altered nutrition: less than body requirements

General anesthesia causes temporary loss of gastrointestinal muscle tone and interruption of peristaltic function. Patients who had surgery that does not involve gastrointestinal organs can often begin taking oral fluids as soon as they are fully awake and free of nausea. Manipulation of gastrointestinal organs delays the return of peristalsis. To prevent vomiting and abdominal distention, patients who had surgery that involved manipulation of the gastrointestinal tract are allowed nothing by mouth until gastrointestinal function returns. Gastrointesti-

Chart 4–2.

NURSING GUIDE TO PATIENT EDUCATION FOR SELF-MANAGEMENT: POSTOPERATIVE DISCHARGE INSTRUCTIONS

Instruct the patient and provide written instructions in the following:

Follow physician's instructions for cleansing and dressing the wound. Demonstrate and explain aseptic technique if it is required for wound care. Observe patient performing wound care.
Allow for additional rest during the recovery period.
Resume previous activities of daily living gradually per physician's instructions. *(Specify schedule.)*
Take medications as prescribed. Be sure to take *all* of the doses of antibiotic.
Modify or restrict diet as specified by physician. Prescribed diet: ______________________
Return for follow-up appointment on *(specify date).*

nal function should resume by the third day postoperatively. Auscultate bowel sounds to detect return of peristalsis. Listen for 2 minutes at a point midway between the umbilicus and the anterior iliac crest before documenting absence of bowel sounds. Determine whether the patient has passed flatus or is experiencing gas pains. Patients swallow air while on NPO status. The air accumulates in the stomach while peristalsis is absent and may cause abdominal distention. As peristalsis returns, the air moves slowly along the intestinal tract and gas pains are common. The passage of flatus and then a bowel movement usually follow. Encourage ambulation to promote peristalsis and relief of gas pains.

Paralytic ileus is the absence of peristalsis beyond the third day of surgery. Abdominal distention, nausea, and a feeling of fullness may also be present. The patient is allowed nothing by mouth, and a nasogastric tube may be inserted to decompress the stomach until peristalsis returns.

The patient is maintained on intravenous dextrose and electrolyte solutions until oral intake is adequate to prevent dehydration and electrolyte imbalance. Begin oral intake with clear fluids in small amounts to avoid distention and vomiting once positive bowel sounds indicate return of gastrointestinal function. Progress the diet as tolerated to full fluids, then a soft diet, and finally a regular diet or diet prescribed by the physician. Monitor for nausea or vomiting to determine whether the diet is being tolerated. Administer antiemetics at the onset of nausea to prevent vomiting and withhold solid food for several hours. Document dietary tolerance. Encourage a diet high in vitamins and protein to promote wound healing.

NDx: High risk for body image disturbance

The body image of a surgical patient may be threatened by the appearance of the wound, dressings, drainage, dependence on others for self-care activities, impaired mobility, changes in body function, and loss of body parts. Encourage the patient to look at the surgical site to ensure realistic knowledge of its appearance and the extent of surgery. Encourage as much independence as possible in hygiene and grooming but provide necessary assistance to prevent fatigue. Assist the patient in getting out of bed and ambulating to promote return to independence. Encourage the patient to wear his or her own clothing when feasible and to use light cosmetics if usually worn to foster a positive self-image. Keep the bedside unit neat and orderly and provide privacy for all treatments and dressing changes to promote a sense of self-worth. Allow the patient to make decisions about care, clothing, and activities whenever possible to promote a sense of control. Provide opportunities for the patient and family members or significant others to discuss feelings, fears, or concerns about appearance, self-care, and activities after discharge. Provide information on community support services if appropriate.

NDx: High risk for altered health maintenance

Patients who have an uncomplicated postoperative course are often discharged before complete wound healing. Early discharge minimizes exposure to nosocomial (hospital-based) infections, promotes recovery, and helps to minimize hospital costs. Provide all discharge information in writing to reinforce instructions, minimize errors, and reduce anxiety. Chart 4–2 summarizes topics to include in discharge teaching.

If dressings are still in place, determine the patient's ability to change the dressing and care for the wound. Teach the patient and a caregiver how to remove and dispose of the old dressing, how to examine the wound for healing and infection, what changes in the wound or patient's condition are reported to the physician immediately, how to care for and prevent dislodgement of drains, and how to cleanse the wound and apply a fresh dressing. Observe wound care to evaluate technique. Identify sources for the purchase of wound-care supplies. A visiting nurse or home care referral may be necessary if the patient or caregiver is unable to care for the wound.

Review activity restrictions to prevent injury to the operative site that may delay healing. Stress the need for planned rest periods to avoid fatigue and to promote recovery. Specify when the patient can expect to resume household chores, lifting, work, driving, sexual intercourse, and leisure activities. Review prescribed medications, administration schedule, expected action, and possible side effects to prevent self-medication errors that may complicate recovery. Review dietary modifications or restrictions and the effect of proper nutrition on recovery. Protein and vitamins B and C promote tissue repair and wound healing. Reinforce the need for follow-up care and identify when the patient is to return to the physician, hospital, or clinic for reevaluation of recovery progress.

Evaluation

Evaluate the effectiveness of nursing care for a postsurgical patient by comparing the patient's status with the expected patient outcomes. Examples of specific outcomes for postsurgical patients have been provided in the Planning section.

Ambulatory Surgery

Significant technologic advances in surgery and anesthesiology permit many surgical procedures that once required a hospital stay to be performed on an outpatient basis in an ambulatory surgical unit. These units may be based within the hospital itself or may be an independent health facility. It is estimated that as many as 60% of all operations can be performed safely and at a much lower cost in an ambulatory unit. The surgical procedures are usually elective procedures of short duration (less than 90 minutes) that present minimal risk for perioperative complications, do not require an overnight stay, and are associated with minimal postoperative nausea, vomiting, and pain. Examples of surgical procedures that can be performed in an ambulatory unit are listed in Table 4–7. Regional or general anesthesia can be used if the facility has a PACU.

Patients who are candidates for this form of surgery are screened to ensure general good health. Preoperative diagnostic procedures are completed before the day of surgery. Any chronic health problems must be well controlled and present minimal risk for perioperative complications. The patient must be capable of understanding and following preoperative and postoperative instructions. Depending on the surgery, it may also be necessary for someone to be available to assist with self-care in the immediate postoperative period.

Guidelines for Application of the Nursing Process to the Care of the Patient in Ambulatory Surgery

Nursing care of the patient in ambulatory surgery includes all of the aspects of care of the patient undergoing in-hospital surgery already discussed, except he extended recovery period on a postsurgical unit. The goals of nursing care of a patient in an ambulatory surgical unit are to provide safe, well-organized, cost-effective care; promote patient participation through education; minimize patient anxiety; promote rapid recovery; and reduce the risk of postoperative complications.

PREOPERATIVE PERIOD

In most instances, the office nurse initiates nursing care of the ambulatory surgical patient. Collect data to develop an individualized plan of care. Initiate preoperative teaching, and provide information booklets or written instructions to reinforce verbal

Table 4–7. EXAMPLES OF AMBULATORY SURGERY PROCEDURES

SPECIALTY	AMBULATORY SURGERY PROCEDURES
General surgery	Hernia repair; hemorrhoidectomy; laser procedures; excision and biopsy of small masses, lesions, cysts, tumors
Ear, nose, and throat	Tonsillectomy, adenoidectomy, myringotomy, nasal polypectomy, oral surgery
Gynecology	Laparoscopy, tubal ligation, dilation and curettage, abortion, and cervical laparoscopy, biopsy, and conization
Urology	Cystoscopy, vasectomy, circumcision
Ophthalmology	Cataract excision and lens implant, laser surgery
Orthopedics	Arthroscopy, fracture reduction, tendon repair, carpal tunnel surgery, bunionectomy
Neurology	Hand surgery, ganglionectomy, nerve repair
Plastic surgery	Face lift, rhinoplasty, eyelid surgery, breast augmentation

instructions. Describe and discuss the preoperative preparations and intraoperative and postoperative course to reinforce the surgeon's explanation and increase understanding of perioperative routines. Encourage questions and correct any misconceptions to reduce anxiety and to promote realistic expectations. Instruct the patient to make arrangements for transportation home after the procedure if driving will be prohibited. Review discharge instructions and home care to promote uncomplicated recovery. Advise the patient of the need for preadmission diagnostic evaluation and how he or she will be notified of the date and time to report for the tests. Review the date and time to report to the facility for surgery.

On the day of surgery, review the preadmission documents and assess the physical and psychological status of the patient to ensure readiness for surgery. Obtain baseline vital signs and complete the preoperative checklist. Review the anticipated sequence of events, and answer questions to reduce anxiety. Accompany the patient to the dressing area and give instructions on how to secure personal possessions and where to go after changing.

POSTOPERATIVE PERIOD

The recovery period is divided into two steps. Step 1 involves those patients who have received general anesthesia or local or regional anesthesia with sedation. The nursing care for these patients parallels that for PACU in-patients.

Patients in Step 2 have received only local or regional anesthesia without sedation or have progressed from Step 1 and are now conscious. Monitor vital signs every 30 minutes to detect changes in hemodynamic status and vital functions. Transfer the patient to a reclining chair and encourage him or her to awaken, cough and deep breathe, move about, and get ready to ambulate to promote recovery from anesthesia. Monitor closely for disorientation, and maintain safety measures to prevent injury. Gradually adjust the recliner to the sitting position as the patient recovers. Offer oral fluids as tolerated. Administer oral analgesics for pain control.

DISCHARGE

Review the written discharge instructions received before surgery to ensure understanding. Criteria for discharge from the ambulatory surgery unit include stable vital signs; presence of swallow, cough, and gag reflexes; ability to ambulate; minimal nausea, vomiting, and dizziness; no respiratory distress; and that patient is alert and oriented. Determine how the patient is returning home. In most instances, a follow-up telephone call is made during the 24-hour period after discharge to review home-care instructions, answer questions, determine whether there are any problems or complications, and reconfirm the first follow-up appointment.

The Elderly: Special Considerations

Surgical mortality and morbidity of the geriatric patient are higher than for the rest of the adult population. The physiologic changes of aging discussed in Chapter 2 and concurrent health problems common in the elderly (e.g., diabetes, COPD, cardiovascular disease, impaired renal or hepatic function, altered mental status) can compromise the individual's ability to respond to surgery and can slow recovery. Except in emergency situations, concurrent health problems are corrected or brought under control before elective surgery to minimize risk.

In general, the elderly individual has less tolerance for the stresses of surgery and less physiologic reserves to aid in recuperation from the trauma of surgery. Patients who are bedridden have a higher risk than those who are active. The risks of surgery increase with age, the number and severity of coexisting health problems, the extent of physiologic derangement from surgery, and the duration of anesthesia. The incidence of postoperative and life-threatening complications is three times higher in patients 75 years of age and older compared with those 65 to 74 years of age. However, because each individual's physical and psychological response to the aging process and management of chronic health problems is different, chronologic age alone is not the best determinant of surgical risk. Many times it is ethically difficult to determine the benefit and necessity for surgical intervention. When weighing surgical risk against potential benefits, it is important that the surgeon, patient, and significant others explore whether the proposed elective surgery will improve the quality of life as well as prolong survival.

Guidelines for Application of the Nursing Process to the Care of the Elderly Patient in Surgery

The increasing numbers of elderly patients undergoing surgery present a challenge in perioperative nursing care. The goals of nursing care are the same as for a younger patient. The nurse must understand the impact of age-related changes on the patient's response to surgery to develop a comprehensive care plan to minimize surgical risks and postoperative complications. Early activity is vital after surgery to prevent complications and permanent disability from immobility despite successful surgical intervention.

PREOPERATIVE PERIOD

Obtain a complete health history to identify potential surgical risks. Allow adequate time for the interview so the patient will not feel rushed and omit information. Identify drug allergies, previous response to surgical anesthetics, and current use of over-the-counter and prescribed medications. Document all prosthetic and assistive devices used. Tell the patient how and where they will be secured. Be alert to nonverbal cues and ask specific questions, such as "Have you recently experienced . . ." to elicit information the patient may omit. Elderly people may omit information or not report symptoms because they do not consider it important, consider it a normal part of aging, fear a serious illness will be diagnosed, or are afraid of losing their independence or autonomy. Older persons experiencing severe depression are considered high risk for surgery because psychological response and motivation for recovery are unpredictable. Mental function, physical status and coexisting health problems, social support system, ability to perform activities of daily living, previous experience coping with illness and stress, and economic resources all impact on the individual's short-term and long-term recovery from surgery.

Complete physical examination includes assessment of fluid balance, cardiovascular status, pulmonary function, and hepatic and renal function. Diagnostic studies further evaluate physical status, concurrent health problems, and potential risk factors. Studies that require the patient to be on NPO status are scheduled as early in the day as possible to avoid dehydration and hypoglycemia. Review required oral intake restrictions for diagnostic procedures before placing the patient on NPO status. Often fluids are permitted, whereas solid foods are restricted. An intravenous infusion may be necessary to maintain hydration during fluid restrictions for multiple diagnostic procedures and before surgery.

Dehydration, anemia, malnutrition, and constipation are common in the elderly and are corrected before surgery by fluid intake, dietary support, and stool softeners or enemas. If enemas are required to correct constipation or to prepare for diagnostic examinations, assess the patient between irrigations for fatigue, excess fluid loss, bradycardia, or cardiac dysrhythmias.

Assess and document range of motion and condition of teeth and skin. Stiff neck or loose teeth may interfere with intubation. Fragile skin, stiff joints, and loss of subcutaneous tissue over bony prominences require special precautions during intraoperative positioning and additional padding. Encourage ambulation, frequent position changes, and joint exercises to maintain mobility and muscle tone. Maintain a safe environment to prevent injury from unfamiliar surroundings and diminished sight, vision, and tactile sensitivity.

Allow extra time for preoperative teaching and reinforce instructions frequently. Preoperative medications are frequently omitted or dosages are reduced to prevent suppression of vital functions and possible disorientation caused by their sedative effect. Elevate side rails, and monitor the patient closely after administration of preoperative medication to detect untoward reactions and to prevent injury.

INTRAOPERATIVE PERIOD

Operating time is minimized to reduce exposure to anesthetic agents. The elderly require less anesthetic agents and are at high risk for toxicity and untoward reactions from anesthesia as well as from the cumulative effects of anesthesia and preoperative medications because of impaired hepatic, renal, and pulmonary function and dehydration. When possible, regional or local anesthesia is used. Monitor for rapid onset of hypotension with all anesthetic agents.

Hypothermia is a higher risk in the elderly because of lower basal metabolism and loss of subcutaneous fat. Minimize exposure and use a head covering, blankets, and warmed intravenous and irrigating solutions to prevent hypothermia. Decreased joint mobility, impaired peripheral circulation, loss of subcutaneous fat, prolonged immobilization, and hard operating room surfaces increase the risk of tissue ischemia. Risk increases with the length of time the operation requires. Handle body parts gently, use care in positioning, provide extra padding of pressure areas, and monitor peripheral circulation frequently to prevent injury.

POSTOPERATIVE PERIOD

Immediate postoperative care of the elderly patient is similar to the care of a younger patient, but recovery from anesthesia is slower. Closely monitor cardiovascular, respiratory, and renal function to ensure early detection and treatment of complications. Ability to compensate for fluctuations in blood pressure and fluid volume status is impaired by reduced cardiac output, impaired peripheral circulation, and diminished vasculomotor response. Impaired peripheral circulation increases the risk for pressure sores and thrombus formation. Change position slowly, to prevent rapid fluctuations in blood pressure, but frequently, to prevent tissue ischemia and circulatory stasis. Encourage early ambulation, foot exercises, and movement of limbs to promote circulation and improve muscle tone. Antiembolic stockings and low-dose prophylactic subcutaneous heparin reduce the risk of deep vein thrombosis. Monitor for signs of fluid overload, and regulate intravenous infusions to prevent congestive heart failure caused by diminished cardiac efficiency. Monitor urine output to detect fluid volume deficit or inadequate renal perfusion.

The elderly are at increased risk of atelectasis and pneumonia because of decreased ciliary action, loss of lung elasticity, reduced vital capacity, and weakened respiratory muscles. A decrease in lean body mass and relative increase in body fat content delay excretion of fat-soluble anesthetic agents. Monitor for restlessness, an early sign of cerebral hypoxia. Encourage deep breaths and coughing to stimulate respiratory function, to mobilize secretions, and to promote excretion of inhaled anesthetic gases. Low concentrations of humidified oxygen improve oxygenation and reduce the risk of hypoxia. The elderly are also at high risk of aspirating gastric contents because of decreased intestinal motility. Withhold oral intake until bowel sounds return, position the patient upright before oral intake, and maintain the patient in a semi-Fowler's position immediately after intake to prevent aspiration.

Postoperative confusion after general anesthesia or heavy sedation with regional anesthesia is common and sometimes lasts several days. It occurs more frequently in elderly patients who have experienced hypothermia or excess blood loss during surgery and may be associated with cerebral hypoxia. Assess the patient to rule out pain, hypoxia, cerebral vascular accident, and adverse medication reaction as a cause of disorientation. Speak in short phrases to communicate and reorient the patient. Be sure that hearing aids, if worn, are inserted properly and are turned on. Maintain safety measures to prevent injury but avoid restraints, which often increase disorientation and anxiety. Administer analgesics to promote comfort but monitor closely for increased confusion, toxic, and cumulative effects, which occur more frequently in the elderly.

Wounds heal more slowly in the elderly and risk of infection is greater because of impaired immune response and peripheral circulation. Use strict aseptic technique in wound care to avoid contamination. Remove tape gently by pulling toward the wound to avoid tension on the edges of the wound. Apply countertraction while removing the tape to prevent tearing fragile skin. If the patient is disoriented protect the incision with fluffed gauze or a gauze wrap over the dressing, to prevent trauma.

Discharge planning requires collaboration among the patient, family, nurses, physicians, and home care or discharge-planning staff. Placement in an extended-care or rehabilitation facility may be necessary before discharge home. Discharge teaching begins as soon as possible and should include family members or the caregiver. Reinforce instructions with large-lettered, printed information. A follow-up telephone call 1 or 2 days after discharge to answer questions and reinforce instructions helps reduce anxiety and prevent errors.

Bibliography

Abrams AC. Clinical drug therapy: Rationales for nursing practice. 3rd ed. Philadelphia: JB Lippincott, 1991.

Adkins RB Jr, Scott HW. Surgical care for the elderly. Baltimore: Williams & Wilkins, 1988.

American Association of Operating Room Nurses, Inc: Examples of nursing activities in perioperative nursing practice. In AORN standards and recommended practices for perioperative nursing. Denver, CO: AORN, Inc, 1991, pp I: 1–4.

American Association of Operating Room Nurses, Inc: Recommended practices: preoperative skin preparation. AORN J 1988;48(5):950.

Bailes BK. Perioperative nursing research: Part IV. Intraoperative phase. AORN J 1989;49(5):1397.

Ball KA. The basics of laser technology. Nurs Clin North Am 1990;25(3):619.

Barash PG, et al. Clinical anesthesia. Philadelphia: JB Lippincott, 1989.

Barret JB, Deehan RM. Preoperative patient teaching. AORN J 1989;50(3):602.

Bland DS. Pulse oximetry: Monitoring arterial hemoglobin oxygen saturation. AORN J 1987;45(4)L964.

Brenner ZR. Diagnostic tests and procedures: Applying the nursing process. Norwalk, CT: Appleton & Lange, 1987.

Bullock BL, Rosendahl PP. Pathophysiology: Adaptations and alterations in function. 2nd ed. Boston: Little, Brown, 1988.

Burden N. Regional anesthesia: What patients and nurses need to know. RN 1988;51(5):56.

Cahill-Wright C. Managing postoperative pain. Nursing 1991; 21(12):42.

Campbell A, Johnston CA. OR-PACU reports: What they should tell you about your postoperative patient. Nursing 1991;21(10):49.

Carpenito LJ. Nursing diagnosis: Application to clinical practice. 4th ed. Philadelphia: JB Lippincott, 1992.

Cassel CK, Walsh JR (eds). Geriatric medicine. New York: Springer-Verlag, 1989.

Cella JH, Watson J. Nurse's manual of laboratory tests. Philadelphia: FA Davis, 1989.

Chenevy B. Overview of fluids and electrolytes. Nurs Clin North Am 1987;22(4):749.

Chitwood LB. Unveiling the mysteries of anesthesia. Nursing 1987;17(2):52.

Cover BM, Overcase TD (eds). Organ procurement and transplantation manual: Laws, regulations, and guidelines. Owings Mills, MD: Rynd Communications, 1987.

Dunajcik L. Controlling the dangers of epidural analgesia. RN 1988;51(1):40.

Edel EM, Johnson PR, Tiller SG. Perioperative documentation: Incorporating nursing diagnoses into the intraoperative record. AORN J 1989;50(3):596.

Ehrhardt BS, Graham M. Pulse oximetry: An easy way to check oxygen saturation. Nursing 1990;20(3):50.

Eliopoulos C. Gerontological nursing. 3rd ed. Philadelphia: JB Lippincott, 1993.

Federle MP, Brant-Zavadzki M (eds). Computed tomography in the evaluation of trauma. 2nd ed. Baltimore: Williams & Wilkins, 1986.

Felver L, Pendarvis JH. Electrolyte imbalances: Intraoperative risk factors. AORN J 1989;49(4):992.

Fishbach F. A manual of laboratory and diagnostic tests. 4th ed. Philadelphia: JB Lippincott, 1992.
Fraulini KE. After anesthesia: A guide for PACU, ICU and medical-surgical nurses. Norwalk, CT: Appleton & Lange, 1987.
Frost EAM, Goldiner PL. Postanesthetic care. Norwalk, CT: Appleton & Lange, 1990.
Gallagher M, Kahn C. Lasers: Scalpels of light. RN 1990;53(5):46.
Gordon M. Nursing diagnosis: Process and application. St. Louis: CV Mosby, 1991.
Greenfield LJ (ed). Complications in surgery and trauma. 2nd ed. Philadelphia: JB Lippincott, 1990.
Gruendemann BJ, Meeker MH. Alexander's care of the patient in surgery. 8th ed. St. Louis: CV Mosby, 1987.
Hall LT. Cardiovascular lasers—A look into the future. Am J Nurs 1990;90(7):27.
Hardy JD. Hardy's textbook of surgery. 2nd ed. Philadelphia: JB Lippincott, 1988.
Hill GJ. Outpatient surgery. 3rd ed. Philadelphia: WB Saunders, 1988.
Jackson MF. Elder care: Implications of surgery in very elderly patients. AORN J 1989;50(4):859.
Jaffee SN (ed). Lasers in general surgery. Baltimore: Williams & Wilkins, 1989.
Kleinbeck S. Developing nursing diagnosis for a perioperative care plan. AORN J 1989;49(6):1613.
Kositske J. A question of balance: Dehydration in the elderly. J Gerontol Nurs 1990;18(10):34.
Kyba FN, Ogburn-Russell L, Rutledge NJ. Magnetic resonance imaging: The latest in diagnostic technology. Nursing 1987; 17(1):44.
Lancaster LE. Renal and endocrine regulation of water and electrolyte balance. Nurs Clin North Am 1987;22(4):761.
Lawler M. Preventing postop complications: Managing other complications. Nursing 1991;21(11):40.
Leckrone L. Preparing your patient for surgery. Nursing 1991;21(7):46.
Lehne RA. Pharmacology for nursing care. Philadelphia: WB Saunders, 1990.
Litwack K. Managing postanesthetic emergencies. Nursing 1991;21(9):49.
Malseed RT, Harrigan G. Textbook of pharmacology and nursing care: The nursing process. 2nd ed. Philadelphia: JB Lippincott, 1989.
Martin JT. Positioning in anesthesia and surgery. 2nd ed. Philadelphia: WB Saunders, 1987.
Matteson MA, McConnell ES. Gerontological nursing: Concepts and practice. Philadelphia: WB Saunders, 1988.
McConnell EA. Fluid and electrolyte concerns in intestinal surgical patients. Nurs Clin North Am 1987;22(4):853.
McConnell EA. Preventing postop complications: Minimizing respiratory problems. Nursing 1991;21(11):34.
McDonagh A. Getting your patient ready for a nuclear medicine scan. Nursing 1991;21(2):53.
Monroe D. Patient teaching for x-ray and other diagnostics. RN 1989;52(9):50.
Mullooly VM, Levin RF, Feldman HR. Music for postoperative pain and anxiety. J NY State Nurses Assoc 1988;19(3):4.
Noriega L, Mudd DL. Perioperative nursing research: Part VII. Postoperative care. AORN J 1989;50(2):379.
Norris MKG. Action stat: Malignant hyperthermia. Nursing 1990;20(6):33.
North American Nursing Diagnosis Association. NANDA Nursing diagnoses: Definitions and classifications. St. Louis: North American Nursing Diagnosis Association, 1992.
Poyss AS. Assessment and nursing diagnosis in fluid and electrolyte disorders. Nurs Clin North Am 1987;22(4):773.
Robbins SL, Kumar V. Basic pathology. 4th ed. Philadelphia: WB Saunders 1987.
Rothrock JC. Perioperative nursing research: Part I. Preoperative psychoeducational interventions. AORN J 1989;49(2):597.
Rowland MA. Myths and facts about postop discomfort. Am J Nurs 1990;90(5):60.
Schultheis AH. When and how to extubate in the recovery room. Am J Nurs 1989;89(8):1040.
Schwartz MW. Potassium imbalance. Am J Nurs 1987;87(10):1292.
Silo HM. Perioperative nursing research: Part V. Intraoperative recommended practices. AORN J 1989;49(6):1627.
Siskind J. Handling hemorrhage wisely. Nursing 1990;20(3):50.
Snyder LA, Peter NK. How to manage organ donation. Am J Nurs 1989;89(10):1294.
Sweeney ML. Legally speaking: Your role in informed consent. RN 1991;54(8):55.
Tucker SM, et al. Patient care standards: Nursing process, diagnosis, and outcome. 5th ed. St. Louis: CV Mosby, 1992.
Ulrich SP, Canale SW, Wendell SA. Nursing care planning guides: A nursing diagnosis approach. 2nd ed. Philadelphia: WB Saunders, 1990.
Way LW. Current surgical diagnosis and treatment. Norwalk, CT: Appleton & Lange, 1988.
Weber BB. Timely tips on adhesive tape. Nursing 1991;21(10):52.
Welter ER, Reiff PA. Transferring patients from the OR: What the postanesthesia room nurse needs to know. AORN J 1989;50(6):1248.
Wild L, Coyne C. Epidural analgesia: The basics and beyond. Am J Nurs 1992;92(4):26.
Wlody GS. Malignant hyperthermia: Potential crisis in patient care. AORN J 1989;50(2):286.
Wyngaarden JB, Smith LH (eds). Cecil textbook of medicine. 18th ed. Philadelphia: WB Saunders, 1988.
York K. The lung and fluid-electrolyte and acid-base imbalances. Nurs Clin North Am 1987;22(4):805.

Chapter Five

DEATH, DYING, BEREAVEMENT, AND SPIRITUAL DISTRESS

Nurses devote a great deal of time to taking care of those who are dying or who are grieving the loss of others. This chapter discusses death, dying, bereavement, and spiritual distress and presents ways in which the nurse can assist patients experiencing these states. Although called upon to support others in these situations, nurses must also learn to cope with the emotional stress created by providing such support. Nurses must support each other in this process.

In assisting others who are facing death or experiencing bereavement, some familiarity with the person's spiritual orientation is helpful. To this end, this chapter presents a summary of various religious beliefs and practices regarding death. The chapter also covers hospices and home care assistance, which provide alternatives to hospitalization for dying patients and their families. Nurses and patients involved in death and dying face a number of ethical issues, such as euthanasia and organ donation, which are discussed at the end of the chapter.

"In the last analysis, it is our conception of death which decides our answer to all questions that life puts before us."

DAG HAMMARSKJÖLD

Death

Personal Awareness of Death

Death is a fact of life. Regardless of all our efforts to ignore, evade, or deny our death, it is inevitable for each one of us. It is a paradox that death is so universal and yet so unique.

Try to imagine that you have been informed that you have only a short while to live. After the initial shock, you would value every moment you have left. That crisis, like many crises, would carry some positive potential.

To live fully and freely, we must really understand that we will die. Knowing that gives us the awareness to try to live in the "here and now." We stop wasting time. We start to focus on things that have meaning. Our appreciation of beauty deepens, and we cherish and enrich our relationships. We ignore or give up much of the pettiness, greed, and manipulation that clutters our lives. We are less dominated by conventional expectations or stereotypes. The uniqueness of our death deepens personal awareness and respect. The universality of our death deepens regard for our common humanity and helps us feel at one with others who suffer. Our impending death usually deepens our awareness of God and of our spiritual nature as well.

Kubler-Ross called death the final stage of growth, and, as quoted in Beauchamp and Perlin (1978), said

"It is the denial of death that is partially responsible for people living empty, purposeless lives; for when you live as if you'll live forever, it becomes too easy to postpone the things you know you must do. You live your life for preparation for tomorrow or in remembrance of yesterday, and meanwhile, each today is lost. In contrast, when you fully understand that each day you awaken could be the last you have, you take the time that day to grow, to become more of who you really are, to reach out to other human beings."

When they care for dying persons, nurses expose themselves to an awareness of their own mortality as well as to their patients' grief and sadness. It is very important that nurses examine their philosophy about death in order to live more fully and freely. Also, nurses need to prepare themselves for those times when they are suddenly confronted by death in their professional and personal lives. A few questions follow regarding personal beliefs about death that nurses might examine and attempt to work through early in their career:

Do you equate death with termination, loss, and failure to survive? Do you see death as closure, conclusion, completion, fulfillment, and graduation? Is death actually a *death-birth* into richer, fuller existence, similar to the fetal *death-birth* from the security of the womb into this more complex, wondrous existence? Or is it the end of our existence? As health professionals, is the care of the dying basically a battle to be fought with death, the enemy? Can we be powerful, positive agents of healing even in death?

Everyone should develop his or her own philosophy and theology of death.

Death as a Developmental Stage of Life

"When John Quincy Adams was eighty years old he met on the streets of Boston an old friend who shook his trembling hand, and said, 'Good morning, and how is John Quincy Adams today?' 'Thank you,' replied the former President, 'John Quincy Adams is quite well, sir, but the house in which he lives at present is becoming dilapidated. It is tottering upon its foundations. Time and the seasons have nearly destroyed it. Its roof is pretty well worn out. Its walls are much shattered, and it trembles with every wind. The old tenement is becoming almost uninhabitable, and I think John Quincy Adams will have to move out of it soon; but he himself is quite well, sir, quite well.' "

SOURCE UNKNOWN

Dying is the final developmental stage of life. With ever-lengthening life expectancies, the majority of deaths occur in the elderly during the seventh decade of life. Erikson suggests that ego-integrity versus despair is the developmental task of old age. Death can be viewed as a meaningful conclusion to life if one feels satisfied with one's life as it is reviewed. Despair results from the realization that there is no more time to fulfill missed opportunities or correct mistakes or failures. Expectation of death is deeply resented.

Robert Peck identifies three developmental tasks for the elderly, all of which are preparation for death. The grieved loss of role in retirement is called work preoccupation. Many persons define their identity in terms of their work or role. In response to the question "Who are you?", they say, "I am a nurse," "I am a mother," "I was a policeman," or "I was a teacher." Successful adjustment and reinvestment in many roles and in being, rather than in doing, is called ego differentiation by Peck. The physical effects of aging bring diminished speed, strength, and sensory acuity along with various physical discomforts and annoying malfunctions such as chronic constipation. The ability to continue to enjoy life rather than be dominated by these disabilities is called body transcendence versus body preoccupation. Calm acceptance and peaceful preparation for one's death as closure to one's life is called ego transcendence. Peck labels failure of this stage of development ego preoccupation and describes it as frequent, fearful, resentful thoughts of death.

Erikson and Peck both suggest that successful mastery of each developmental task is built upon mastery of earlier developmental tasks. Therefore, it is no surprise that people usually face death the way they faced earlier life crises. We experience many small losses on an almost daily basis in life as we develop and adjust to the many changes required of us. Each loss is a small death. We learn that struggle and suffering along with pleasure and beauty are an integral part of life. As we struggle to cope and adjust to these small deaths, we prepare for our final death.

Dying

Stages of Dying

Much has been written and discussed about the five stages of grief and dying identified by Elisabeth Kubler-Ross. In her interviews with hundreds of dying persons, she witnessed them passing through five emotional or subjective stages.

DENIAL

Denial is an initial normal reaction, which helps push away the shock in order to cope with the reality bit by bit while the full impact settles into our consciousness. It has been characterized as the "No, not me" stage.

ANGER

Anger often follows denial. The rage can seem overwhelming. Fury is often displaced upon health professionals, who are accused of being incompetent and uncaring. Spiritual distress occurs when belief systems are challenged as one rages at God, asking "Why did you permit this to happen?" or "Why me!"

BARGAINING

Bargaining is the "Yes, me, but" stage, in which the person makes a promise, usually to God, or to do a particular thing to become a better person in exchange for longer time to live. Often the request is to be present at a special event like a wedding or a graduation or to be able to complete a specific project that is currently in process.

DEPRESSION

Depression occurs when the reality of the impending loss has registered. The enormity of what is happening is fully faced. This depression of mourning is normal, healthy behavior when one is dying. One grieves what has already been lost, such as health, attractiveness, independence, one's role in life. One also grieves future losses, such as separation from loved ones and from life itself. This is the resigned "Yes, me" stage.

ACCEPTANCE

Acceptance occurs when one has been allowed to work through the depression of mourning. Initially there are brief episodes of acceptance, which occur with greater and greater frequency. One has a sense of "Yes, me, and I am ready." The emotional tone of this stage fully realized is peaceful, calm acceptance. It is a quiet stage and is more positive than mere resignation. It occurs when one has been able to resolve the earlier stages to complete one's grief work. Acceptance, the final stage of dying, is not fully experienced by many persons. In some cases, the death is sudden and the dying person does not have time to complete the necessary tasks to achieve acceptance.

It is very important to note that the stages do not necessarily, or even usually, occur separately or in sequence as listed here. It is sometimes possible to identify indications of all five stages during one session when interviewing a dying patient. There are fluctuations in all emotions in humans on a daily, even an hourly, basis. Nor do all dying persons manifest all these stages. Any grief, regardless of the source of loss—whether life, object, person, or function—has been found to manifest these same five emotional stages.

Kubler-Ross made a significant contribution in the identification of these stages of dying and grief. She, more than any other individual, is responsible for bringing awareness and discussion of death issues out of the closet during the past 20 years. Some persons do not want to talk about their death, but many do. Their distress is compounded by loneliness and isolation when there is a conspiracy of silence by their loved ones and medical caregivers.

Tolstoy described this very movingly in *The Death of Ivan Ilych:*

"What tormented Ivan Ilych most was the deception, the lie, which for some reason all accepted, that he was not dying but was simply ill. . . . The deception tortured him. . . . This falsity around him and within him did more than anything else to poison his last days."

LEO TOLSTOY

Final Tasks Toward Achieving Acceptance of Death

For the stage of acceptance to be reached, there are certain tasks that a dying person must accomplish. These are the things that must be done to prepare for death. Each of the subjective stages of denial, anger, bargaining, and depression is experienced and resolved. Although we prepare for our death throughout our life, the final period requires completion of these tasks in order to accept death with peace and calm, that is, to reach Kubler-Ross's fifth stage of acceptance. Some of these tasks may have been completed earlier in life by some patients. All of them blend together, overlap, and assume greater or lesser importance at different periods during the dying process. They often occur, more or less, in the following sequence.

DEVELOPING AWARENESS OF IMPENDING DEATH

Initially, this awareness may be only a suspicion, or it may be maintained for only brief periods as denial is worked through. Initial lack of awareness may be due to factors outside of the patient's control, such as a pact of silence by family and caregivers. Persons whose life patterns have included a great deal of denial and patterns of avoidance and fear have difficulty working through denial and completing this task.

BALANCING HOPE AND FEAR

Fear is always a part of dying. Death itself is often less feared than a prolonged, suffering dying process. Fears include pain, uncertainty, helplessness, loss and deprivation, isolation, alienation, abandonment, disfigurement, indignity, and judgment. Fear can be conquered only when hope is allowed to balance each fear whenever it emerges.

Nurses can do much to help provide hope. Patients must never be left without hope, because it is the antidote to fear. We need to listen as the patient's hope changes. An early expression might be "I hope there is nothing wrong," followed by "I hope there is a cure," then "I hope I am not a burden," then "I hope I will not have pain," and finally, "I hope I will die soon."

RELINQUISHING THE WILL TO LIVE

Relinquishing the will to live is another final task necessary to arrive at acceptance of one's death. Reversal of the physical struggle for survival seems to be a conscious decision on the part of many patients near death, unless they are comatose or heavily sedated. Family and caregivers often notice the changes as withdrawal and diversion of energy away from the physical struggle. This fight for survival is so basic to life that a conflict and then a reversal of the will to live seems to be taking place in order to initiate the actual acceptance of death. Often a patient manages to "hang on" and to continue the physical struggle in order to be alive for special family events like the birth of a grandchild, a homecoming, a graduation, or a wedding. Shortly thereafter, the patient relinquishes the struggle and dies peacefully. Sometimes loved ones need to be helped to give permission to the dying patient to cease a heroic fight to remain alive.

LETTING GO OF AUTONOMOUS CONTROL

Letting go of autonomous control also occurs as the will to live is reversed. This is not the same loss of control experienced earlier in illness when one struggles to cope with the adjustment to debilitating illness. Rather, it is a positive "countercontrol" in which one puts oneself peacefully into the hands of others for safe passage to death.

DETACHING FROM FORMER EXPERIENCES AND RELATIONSHIPS

Detachment from former experiences and relationships can cause loved ones misunderstanding and pain if they are not aware that this is a natural part of the final dying process. This liberating detachment enables an emotionless, peaceful preparation for impending death.

ACHIEVING SPIRITUAL PREPARATION AND INTEGRATION

Spiritual preparation and integration are easiest for those who are devout or have actively practiced their faith and for those who believe in eternal life. Various patient surveys support what caregivers frequently observe, namely that persons with religious faith have an easier time achieving acceptance of their death.

Persons who are nonreligious should be supported in the review and integration of their life experiences and their search for meaning in life. This search is explained by Cicely Saunders, the founder of St. Christopher's Hospice near London, upon which many hospices have been modeled. Regardless of persons' beliefs, she often sees in them something that could be called "reaching out trustfully." "They come to remember things from the past, things that they have been too busy to listen to before, and as death approaches, they find that things begin to make sense. They bring a new attention to the old truths. This is something entirely different from plucking at straws, and is an extremely personal matter for each patient" (Doyle, 1972). Saunders feels that attending to individual spiritual needs is an important aspect of total care.

Dying is a very difficult process, full of fear and sadness. It requires great fortitude. Those fortunate ones who have completed these tasks report a sense of achievement and peace. They are observed to die with dignity, self-respect, and acceptance.

Application of the Nursing Process to the Psychosocial Care of the Dying Patient

Assessment

Information regarding the prognosis, diagnosis, and expected clinical cause of death is needed to deliver quality nursing care to the person who is grieving his or her impending death. Assess the patient's understanding of the illness, the desire or lack of desire to talk about dying, the subjective stages of the dying experience, and the communication patterns of patient and family. Review the patient's medical history, medical treatments, and past crises. Investigate the patient's religious and philosophical beliefs and practices as they relate to life and death. Assess resources available to help the patient and significant others deal with the crisis of death. Potential resources include family, friends, religious faith and advisors, financial resources, and personal coping patterns.

Nursing Diagnoses and Planning

The nursing diagnosis and related expected patient outcomes most commonly applicable to the dying patient include the following:

NDx: Anticipatory grieving related to impending death

Planning: Patient outcomes

1. Patient demonstrates awareness of dying by talking about it, reviewing his or her life; putting affairs in order, such as drawing up a will; expressing farewells; giving keepsakes to significant others; and planning his or her funeral.
2. Patient identifies feelings of denial, anger, bargaining, depression, and acceptance as normal phases of dying, not as signs of weakness.
3. Patient demonstrates control of fear and expresses realistic and appropriate aspects of hope in the situation.
4. Patient communicates his or her decision to relinquish the will to live by ceasing the physical struggle to survive, by letting go of autonomous control, and by emotional detachment.
5. Patient prepares spiritually for death by examining beliefs and expressing a desire or lack of desire to have a religious leader visit for comfort, counseling, and religious rituals.
6. Patient expresses satisfaction with completion of his or her lifework.

Nursing Interventions

NDx: Anticipatory grieving

To aid the dying person in working through the stages of grief, to accept death and to die with dignity, provide the opportunity to talk about feelings and to learn that it is permissible, normal, and even healthy to grieve. Remember that there are many anticipated losses to be mourned: unfulfilled future plans and dreams, roles that were enjoyed, beloved family and friends, the beauty of this earth, former physical attractiveness, abilities and health, sense of a meaningful life, and hope of continuation of life on earth. Offer frequent, regular opportunities for the patient to talk out these feelings. Some patients may not wish to talk about their death. If so, respect this wish, but continue to gently provide occasional openers from time to time in case they change their mind. Some patients feel that they must act strong for their loved ones and should not burden them with their own suffering. They fear dragging the beloved downward by allowing them to see the extent of their own despair. Nurses and other helping persons can provide crucial opportunities for the patient to ventilate feelings, using therapeutic communication techniques. Encourage visitors and other social contacts as desired by the patient to reduce loneliness and isolation.

Display authentic respect for the person and consistent regard for his or her experience. To help bolster bruised self-esteem, the sense of unreality, and the fear of breakdown, let it be known that crying and other expressions of grief are not cowardly signs of weakness but healthy, normal aspects of the grief work. Tears can release feelings of helplessness in the face of tragedy. Keep advice to a minimum, but use nonverbal expressions of comfort to the maximum, since they carry the most potent messages.

Make every effort to combat hopelessness. Keep appointments and commitments with the patient faithfully, and only make promises that can be fulfilled. Be open to communication, because everyone in this situation needs at least one person in whom to freely and honestly confide. Remember that pretense stifles hope. Do not pretend to be overly cheery, but be honest and genuine regarding one's own feelings, without projecting them onto patients. Do not minimize or negate feelings, because this increases the patient's guilt and dependency. Structure for their success by dividing patient goals and tasks into short-term attainable units. Provide satisfying aesthetic experiences with music, nature, and art, to help inspire hope.

Keep hope alive when fear threatens, because hope is the antidote for fear and despair. Do not encourage hope that the death is not real. This is dishonest and inappropriate. Rather by word and deed assure the patient that he or she will be comfortable and well cared for and that the bereaved family will be helped. Provide opportunities to speak with peers who have worked through the earlier stages of the process if appropriate.

Sensitively offer opportunities to discuss life after death or the patient's religious beliefs. Offer to share experiences of prayer, because this often can bring comfort and kindle the hope that a loving God is in control. Arrange visits by chaplains or other spiritual leaders of the patient's choice. Clergy visits can inspire a sense that God's blessing is being conveyed and can be deeply comforting. Do not proselytize. Convey respect for the patient's beliefs or lack of belief by learning and discussing the basic tenets of his or her religious or personal belief system.

Evaluation

Evaluate the effectiveness of nursing care for a patient grieving for his or her impending death by comparing the patient's status with the expected patient outcomes. Examples of specific outcomes for patients grieving for impending death have been provided in the Planning section.

Bereavement

Stages of Bereavement

DENIAL

The first emotion felt by the bereaved after the death of a relative or friend is shock, even when the death is expected and invited. Denial is a useful buffer. Feelings of numbness, or of being in an unreal dream world, are experienced for several days or weeks. These feelings are followed by episodes of emotional pain and extremes of behavior in which a person becomes either hyperactive or almost inert. Various somatic complaints and mood swings are experienced. Physical symptoms include choking, sighing, shortness of breath, insomnia, and various gastrointestinal complaints, like anorexia and inability to taste the flavor of food. The bereaved person is preoccupied with thoughts of the deceased. Episodes of denial continue to resurface from time to time right up to final acceptance of the death and resolution of the grief.

ANGER

Manifestations of anger in the bereaved can be observed during the acute period also. Rage is felt against God for permitting the suffering. Anger is felt toward health care providers for failing to save the loved one. Resentment is felt toward the loved one for the desertion. Resentment is felt toward others who are happy and are not suffering a loss. Rage at oneself is felt for not being the one who died. During the entire mourning period, strong feelings of anger can suddenly occur, gradually diminishing in intensity with time. Spiritual distress commonly occurs during this stage as beliefs are challenged by anger regarding the suffering.

BARGAINING

Manifestations of bargaining in the bereaved are noted throughout the process by the "If only" thoughts and comments. They are attempts to negotiate, delay, and reduce the reality of the loss. They begin during the anticipatory grief prior to death, with prayers like "Lord, if only you will spare her, I will be a good person and will serve you the rest of my life." After death, there is a great deal of daydreaming about the deceased. Often the bereaved imagines the close presence of the deceased or suddenly seems to see him or her in a crowd of people. Magical thinking, like that of children, occurs frequently, in thoughts like "If only I pretend that he is here with me now, maybe it will happen." Restless searching for the beloved is a defense against recognition that the loss is final. Such seeking sometimes leads the bereaved to dabble in spiritualism and become fixated at this stage, unable to complete their grief work to resolution.

DEPRESSION

Manifestations of depression in the bereaved indicate that this is the most difficult stage of all and occurs as the permanence of the death becomes real. It becomes very difficult for the bereaved to concentrate and to make decisions. Life seems out of control and seems to lose all meaning. A sense of hopelessness often pervades, as indicated by comments such as

"It's no use."
"Why bother?"
"It will never work out now . . ."

"Nothing can be done anyway."
"It's too late."
"Everything's going down the drain."
"It's all senseless anyway."
"There's no hope."

Apathy, withdrawal, and passive acquiescence are noted. Motivation is lacking and there is little energy to invest in things and persons outside of oneself. Depression saps initiative, and the bereaved drifts along in seeming purposelessness. Guilt, remorse, and regret are common feelings and contribute to a decreased sense of self-worth. Withdrawal into isolation can occur, with frequent complaints of loneliness. Haunting fears are almost overwhelming regarding security or health. There are excessive fears concerning the health or welfare and safety of family and friends. Complaints are usually irrational, and the bereaved fears that he or she is having a mental breakdown. A few transient episodes might occur in which one hears the voice or senses the presence of the one who has died. This may either heighten the fear of losing one's sanity or it may be very comforting to the bereaved persons.

ACCEPTANCE

Manifestations of acceptance in the bereaved occur some months after the death, when the bereaved begins to note a gradual reduction in the periods f depression with increased times of well-being. The confusion fades, and things begin to take on meaning again. The bereaved is finally able to experience real sources of comfort. Thoughts of the dead loved one find easier expression and are less and less idealized. The bad is remembered along with the good, and increasing calm acceptance is felt. The old pain of loss is always there, especially on anniversaries and holidays, but the former fears, remorse, anger, and guilt have diminished. Energy increases. The bereaved begins to reorder life. The grief work is over. Life starts to seem interesting and even to be fun again. Other people begin to capture the bereaved's attention, and gradually he or she is able to invest in new relationships.

Those who lose a loved one may engage in anticipatory grieving during the dying. This is thought to aid and to shorten the grief process afterwards. Nonetheless the final reality of death almost always comes as a shock.

Resolution of grief is vital for one's future mental and physical health. Dysfunctional grieving can cause crippling emotional problems. Death of a spouse rates highest on the scale of life stress events. A strong correlation exists between significant loss and subsequent deteriorating health, including cancer, of the survivors. Premature deaths of the bereaved often occur.

Cathexis, a term developed by Freud, refers to one's investment of emotional energy. Mourning is the process of gradual decathecting or "letting go" of the dead loved one. Decathexis is an intense emotional process and cannot be rushed. Acceptance is attained when the earlier stages have been completed.

Especially Difficult Deaths

DEATH OF A CHILD

It is generally agreed that it is easiest to cope with the deaths of the elderly, particularly if they have lived full and satisfactory lives. The deaths of children and young adults are more difficult to accept, causing great suffering for the survivors as well as the patients. Their unfulfilled potential and missed opportunities are greatly grieved by all.

After the death of a child, the process of mourning is usually more painful and complicated and seems to take longer than other bereavements. It is compounded by the guilt of failure to keep one's child safe and secure. Parents brood about the things they did or did not do with their child. Parents feel that their future is gone, particularly if an only child dies. Opportunities to talk with others who have had similar experiences and negotiated them adequately are often helpful. Referral should be made to self-help groups or other counseling services. Only other parents who have lost a child can understand what they have experienced. Compassionate Friends is a self-help group of such parents, which has chapters in many cities in the United States and other countries. (See address in resource list at end of this chapter.)

Frequent opportunities to review and talk out the details of the death are extremely important. Children should be included, with the understanding that children's magical thinking may cause them to carry unexpressed feelings of responsibility for the death if they had previously quarreled with the dying person or briefly wished him or her dead.

STIGMATIZED OR VIOLENT DEATH

Stigmatized or violent deaths are particularly traumatic for the survivors. Humiliation and alienation are added to the anguish. Deaths due to acquired immunodeficiency syndrome (AIDS), suicide, murder, or substance abuse are examples. Advising the dying and their survivors that their guilt and shame are inappropriate and unwarranted does not really help. Owing to the isolating and alienating aspects of these deaths, it is imperative that counseling be available to those who are closely involved. Opportunities to talk out the grief over and over agains are needed. If grief is buried, it festers and sooner or later erupts in an inappropriate manner. Health professionals must be sensitive to the lack of frequent opportunities to talk about the anguish faced by these survivors of stigmatized deaths. Nurses and others must not become so preoccupied with physical care that they fail to address these tremendous psychosocial needs.

SUDDEN DEATH

Sudden, unexpected deaths and deaths about which there are ambivalent feelings also cause particular distress for survivors. In the former cases, opportunities for closure and anticipatory grief are denied. Too many things are left unsaid and undone, and too many questions remain unanswered. In the latter, relief is felt that the difficult person is gone, but it may be mixed with heavy guilt, which plays a major role in complicating and compounding the grief process.

TEENAGE SUICIDE

The suicides of troubled teenagers include all these problems. They are the sudden, ambivalent, violent, stigmatized death of youth. It is no wonder that their effect is catastrophic. Public education is desperately needed to help prevent teenage suicides and to equip others in assisting survivors to deal with the disaster. Publicity about teenage suicide creates a dilemma because of the contagious nature of the phenomenon. When a teenage suicide is publicized, a tragic rash of teenage suicide often follows.

Application of the Nursing Process to the Care of the Patient Suffering Bereavement

Assessment

Assess manifestations of each of the five stages of grief in the bereaved.

Assess for signs of denial and for associated mood swings and physical symptoms. Observe for sighing or choking, and note complaints of shortness of breath. Ask about insomnia and anorexia and other gastrointestinal complaints. Listen for expressions of anger or resentment toward God, health care workers, the deceased, or survivors. Listen also for "if only" statements indicative of bargaining, and note daydreaming or magical thinking. Observe for signs of depression, such as apathy, withdrawal, and statements reflecting guilt or a sense of life's being out of control or lacking in meaning. Observe also for signs of acceptance, such as acknowledging the deceased person's weaknesses as well as strengths and expressions of interest in resuming personal and social activities.

Nursing Diagnoses and Planning

The nursing diagnosis and related expected patient outcomes most commonly applicable to patients suffering bereavement include the following:

NDx: Grieving related to the recent death of a loved one

Planning: Patient outcomes

1. Patient exhibits signs of shock for several days after the death and reaches out appropriately to others for comfort, support, and assistance.
2. Patient openly ventilates, projects, and displaces feelings of anger and guilt for several weeks after the death.
3. Patient gradually demonstrates acceptance of the death by talking freely and appropriately about it and expressing increasing themes of satisfaction and pleasure, by demonstrating increased interest in new aspects of life, by emotionally investing oneself in new relationships, and by manifesting ability to solve problems and make major decisions again.

Nursing Interventions

NDx: Grieving

To help the bereaved to complete the grief work, provide an opportunity for the family to say farewells with visual and tactile contact as desired during the immediate postdeath experience. Keep in mind that some families assume total responsibility for care of the body based on the ritual practices of their religion. Resolution of the denial stage of grief is aided by such physical contact. Survivors who never have a chance to see their dead have difficulty progressing beyond denial. Provide strong support and protection of the bereaved during this traumatic, vulnerable period. Should the survivors develop physical complaints, check them out with honest concern and gentle reassurance.

Help the bereaved through the anger phase by demonstrating empathy, patience, and tolerance, especially when anger is directed at the health professionals. Explain that anger at the dead or rage at God is common and normal to help reduce guilt. Encourage contact with self-help organizations in the community, such as groups for widows and widowers or bereaved parents. Arrange exposure to peers who are able to express feelings openly, to stimulate the bereaved to openly express what is being experienced. Provide frequent, regularly scheduled opportunities to ventilate, to sort out ambivalence, and to express resentments. Engage in frequent conversations with the bereaved about the deceased and description of their experiences together. Always be authentic and considerate in order to promote the bereaved's self-esteem. Reinforce reality with gentle reminders to help correct misperceptions and misinterpretations regarding the cause of death, because blame is nonproductive. Be patient with constant negative expressions and attitudes, and avoid the counterproductive tendency to advise the mourner to "Try to change your attitude and think more positively." Encourage participation in religious ceremonies and rituals, prayer, or counseling for spiritual support if appropriate to the patient's belief. Be honest in communicating about anger, doubt, or disbelief, which often occur during this phase.

To intervene during this painful time, listen actively and patiently when the bereaved repeat accounts or thoughts over and over again about the death and the deceased. This enables the loss to become real and eventually accepted. Engage in frequent conversations with the bereaved, but keep in mind that the bereaved also need time by themselves. Be alert to signs of excessive apathy and withdrawal.

Avoid suppressing the symptoms of grief with the use of tranquilizers and sedatives, which tend to mask reactions and delay the grief work. Be aware, however, that acute anxiety attacks or constant insomnia that persists may need drug therapy for a while. Counsel the bereaved to avoid major changes and decisions, because bereaved persons are too fragile to cope with added unnecessary stress at this time or may make reactive decisions that they may later regret. Encourage the bereaved to continue working unless the job is terribly stressful, since work provides valuable structure, organization, and socialization during this chaotic period when life often seems out of control.

Make family and friends aware of the importance of being patient with petty, irrational anxieties, fears, and phobias, and explain that the strange feelings and compulsive behaviors the bereaved are experiencing are part of normal grieving. Encourage family and friends to take a positive approach with the grieving person rather than posing a question that is likely to be answered in the negative by a depressed person. For example, it is better to say, "Plans have been made for us to have lunch together," rather than "Would you like to go?"

Do not try to rush acceptance of the loss. It usually takes 6 months to a year to achieve and can take as long as 2 years. Feelings of acceptance occur gradually with increased frequency and duration as the other phases are resolved. Assist the bereaved at this stage by continuing to encourage talk about the deceased but without a "halo" idealizing effect, remembering the annoying, troublesome aspects of the relationship along with the joyous, satisfactory aspects. Support the learning of new or rediscovered coping strategies. Encourage problem-solving with a neutral, objective, compassionate person to help in making major decisions and with life changes like selling one's home or moving to another community or into the home of one's son or daughter.

Evaluation

Evaluate the effectiveness of nursing care for a patient suffering bereavement by comparing the patient's status with the expected patient outcomes. Examples of specific outcomes for patients suffering bereavement have been provided in the Planning section.

Dysfunctional Grieving

Destructive, pathologic patterns of grief can sometimes be predicted. High-risk factors include a history of emotional problems with ineffective coping and frequent conflict between the dying person and the survivors during their life together. Repression of feelings as manifested by total lack of expressed emotion serves only to delay normal mourning, which is apt to occur and haunt one at some unexpected time in the future.

The usual pattern is that dysfunctional grieving lasts beyond the normal 1- to 2-year period and becomes fixated at any of the stages leading up to acceptance or resolution. Acute grief continues well beyond the normal 6- to 8-week period. Months after a death, the bereaved still manifest a dreamlike state of shock as if the death had occurred the previous day. Psychosomatic symptoms result in serious illnesses or hypochondria or conversion hysteria. Severe anxiety reactions or an agitated depression can be easily triggered, and long-lasting phobias may develop. The bereaved may regress to childlike dependency for a prolonged period and be unable to carry responsibility. Severe egocentricity may alienate others. Prolonged self-deprecation and self-blame result from unresolved guilt. Sometimes there is continued rage at health professionals or God or deep resentment at feeling abandoned by the deceased. Idealization of the deceased is frequently and inappropriately expressed. Persistent refusal to discuss feelings regarding the death feeds dysfunctional patterns. Chronic hostility toward everyone and everything may be openly expressed but is more apt to be manifested as passive-aggression or the super-sweetness of reaction-formation, which makes others uncomfortable because of the underlying hostility. Prolonged envy of others' happiness and security feeds this hostility and bitterness. Suicidal ideation and activity are not uncommon. Self-destructive activities that induce pain and discomfort or are dangerous to health and well-being occur subconsciously. Deliberate suicide attempts may also occur and be successful.

Application of the Nursing Process to the Care of the Patient with Dysfunctional Grieving

Assessment

Take a careful nursing history regarding past emotional problems. Try to accurately assess the quality of the relationship of the griever with the dead person, realizing the possibility of an increased need to maintain a halo effect, excessively glorifying the dead if the relationship was troubled. Learn the length of time since the occurrence of the death to determine whether the grieving has exceeded the normal 1- to 2-year period. Listen for expressions of the various stages of normal grieving. Ask about situations that may have prevented the bereaved from freely expressing grief at the appropriate time. Assess the quality of life since the death in terms of sleep and eating patterns, social isolation or dependency, emotional repression or lability, and psychosomatic manifestations. Assess the griever's ability to talk freely and honestly about the death, and listen for themes of guilt or anger. It is especially important to ask about suicidal ideation and to consider the possibility of past or present suicide attempts.

Nursing Diagnoses and Planning

The nursing diagnosis and related expected patient outcomes most commonly applicable to patients with dysfunctional grieving include the following:

NDx: Dysfunctional grieving related to inability to express feelings as needed to complete the mourning process or ambivalent feelings resulting from chronic, unresolved conflict with the deceased

Planning: Patient outcomes

1. Patient expresses awareness of the necessity to complete all the phases of the grief work and a desire to emotionally accept the death.
2. Patient identifies some of the unresolved aspects of the grief process in his or her experience.
3. Patient openly and frequently expresses impacted or unresolved feelings of denial, anger, guilt, and despair and actively seeks constructive ways to complete the mourning.
4. Patient actively demonstrates efforts to change nonproductive behaviors and dysfunctional feelings by altering old patterns and adapting new ones.
5. Patient seeks and carries through on psychiatric consultations or psychotherapy as indicated.
6. Patient demonstrates healthy detachment from the deceased by talking freely of strengths and weaknesses of the relationship without pain and by reinvesting appropriately in new friendships of both sexes or relationships with the opposite sex.

Nursing Interventions

NDx: Dysfunctional grieving

Employ the interventions for normal mourning to help an individual correct and resolve maladaptive responses to death and complete the grieving process. These are usually effective since dysfunctional grieving often occurs because assistance needed to enable the bereaved person to satisfactorily complete a phase of the normal process was lacking. Perhaps empathetic listeners were unavailable to enable expression of the anger and despair. Perhaps the help of a caretaker was not there during the fragile, vulnerable period immediately post death. Sometimes the bereaved have had to be so brave and pretend to be so strong that they have suppressed or repressed their grief to the point that it has become impacted and later haunts them. Give information and assist with referrals for counseling when basic interventions are not successful. Role play with an experienced counselor can help relieve such impacted pain so that the person can go on to complete the process and resolve the crisis. This can also help in reworking other unresolved feelings. Initiate immediate referral for psychiatric consultation if evidence of deep depression with suicide potential, continuing hallucinations, or delusional thinking develops.

Evaluation

Evaluate the effectiveness of nursing care for a patient with dysfunctional grieving by comparing the patient's status with the expected patient outcomes. Examples of specific outcomes for patients with dysfunctional grieving have been provided in the Planning section.

Spiritual Distress

Spiritual Needs

One's spiritual nature is the very ground of one's being. Regardless of whether or not a person adheres to a conscious or an organized religion, all people have a spiritual nature. The self, or the soul, distinguishes humanity from other animals. It transcends our body, our mind, our emotion, our relationships with other persons, and our relatedness to the environment.

A basic human drive that motivates all of us, consciously or not, is the desire to immortalize ourselves. We yearn to extend ourselves beyond the bounds of finitude, to achieve victory over our creatureliness, to be more than just an animal, more than just grass of the field that passes away. This is the basic human urge—to be unique, to matter, to count—not just for a little while or a few days, but for eternity. The terror of death is that the self will be extinct, our bodies will decay, our lives will be in vain, and we will be forgotten (Becker, 1973).

The comfort of most major religions is that god is at the very center of our existence and that the meaning and goal of human experience is to achieve perfect communion with God and to have eternal life.

Spiritual needs, when met, can be a powerful force in transcending illness and suffering. Spiritual distress can also be all-pervasive in its disruptive force. Recognition of patients' spirituality and attention to those needs demand high priority from nursing. Spiritual beliefs are so private and personal that nurses generally avoid them. Fortunately, more nurses are coming to grips with the importance of this aspect of care and are taking steps to learn about and to deal with spiritual distress.

To meet the spiritual needs of patients, the nurse must know core beliefs of the patient's religion and practices that relate to issues of death and dying. The nurse must respect the patient's beliefs and not impose personal values and beliefs. Honest sharing of personal faith by the nurse may be helpful in small amounts when it is done to help sustain the patient and is not an effort to boost the nurse's ego.

The best way to learn about a patient's religious beliefs is to go to the primary source. Ask the patient: Are you a religious person? Would you like to tell me about your spiritual beliefs and how they affect your life? Spirituality is a very private matter for many, but most are willing and even eager to discuss these matters with an open-minded, nonjudgmental, sincerely interested listener. This is never more true than near the time of death. Bereaved family members usually need to be able to talk about life after death as well.

Another important reason for asking the person is that personal beliefs and practices sometimes vary greatly from those of one's official religious affiliation. Most often one's religious affiliation develops historically and culturally. It is derived from the early influences of family and community. Personal choice, commitment, and inspiration may follow later in life, but these things usually affect the degree of religious practice more than the choice of religious affiliation. Therefore, some personal beliefs and practices may not be totally consistent with one's religious "label." Presuppositions should not be made.

Religious Beliefs and Practices Regarding Death

The five major world religions in alphabetical order are

1. Buddhism
2. Christianity
3. Hinduism
4. Islam
5. Judaism

Geographically most Buddhists live in Asia; most Christians live in Europe, North and South America, and Africa; most Hindus live in India; most Muslims live in the Middle East and northern Africa; and most Jews live in Israel, Europe, and North America. The last group, in particular, demonstrate what is happening worldwide as people move from place to place. One often hears it said that there are more Jews living in New York City than in Jerusalem. Immigration worldwide means that most nurses will care for members of each of these world religions in the course of their career.

Additionally, in the modern world, many people do not adhere to any religion but prefer to call themselves secular humanists, agnostics, or atheists. The first term applies to belief in mankind and human ability to practice goodness and justice. Agnostics believe that we cannot know whether or not God exists. Atheists feel sure that God does not exist. All these labels refer to individuals whose behavior is guided by moral values rather than belief in divine guidance or fear of divine judgment.

A brief description of the beliefs and practices of each major religious group with emphasis on death and dying issues follows.

BUDDHISM

Buddhists refer to the deity as Gautama Buddha and refer to their belief as a religion of enlightenment. The goal of life is to reach Nirvana, which is considered the state of enlightenment or ultimate reality. Buddhists strive to reach Nirvana by the eight "rights" or paths: concentration, knowledge, mindfulness, effort, intentions, conduct, speech, and livelihood. Considerable time is spent in meditation and contemplation toward this end.

Buddhists believe in reincarnation. Death is defined as the total nonfunctioning of the body and mind or life force. The true self is reborn almost immediately after death in another form. Rebirth can occur as a lesser being, even as a pig or snake or turtle if one's life has been evil and lived with no effort toward enlightenment. One might be reborn as a higher, more enlightened being, such as a buddhist monk, if one has lived an exemplary life. Eventually one becomes so enlightened that one reaches Nirvana and no longer needs to be reborn. The importance of cleanliness, goodness, and beauty is stressed in this religion.

Buddhism grew out of Hinduism, and variations or subgroups evolved culturally in different parts of Asia. Various Buddhist subgroups emphasize different values and rituals of worship. In Shintoism, the dominant religion of Japan, ancestors, heroes, and the emperor are worshiped. Since it is believed that ancestor spirits exist in nature, there is a tremendous regard and appreciation of all of nature and a strong emphasis on beauty, aesthetics, personal cleanliness, and joy in life and nature. Shintoists believe in prayer healing. It is important to them to have family present when one is dying in order to provide physical care and emotional support.

Zen, another subgroup of Buddhism, stresses simplicity in all of life, seeking truth and honesty via long hours of meditation in the lotus, or cross-legged, position. Zen Buddhists may ask to have the Zen master visit when a member is dying, to help the patient remain calm and concentrate on dying.

All Buddhists value the body far less than the soul. Belief in karma, or destiny, helps them accept things that happen to them. Because of their belief in reincarnation, they want to remain alert, calm, and quiet as death approaches. Buddhist patients may deny pain and refuse medications. Treatments may also be refused on holy days, which occur once or twice almost every month. Use of alcohol, tobacco, and drugs is discouraged. A Buddhist monk traditionally chants last rites at the bedside when one is dying, and monks (priests) may be requested to visit for consultation at various times. The family is traditionally present, physically and emotionally caring for the dying person. Cremation is usually practiced, and there is seldom opposition to autopsy or organ donation and transplantation.

CHRISTIANITY

Christian practices vary widely around the world among various groups and individuals. The three main branches of Christianity are, in alphabetical order, Eastern Orthodoxy, Protestantism, and Roman Catholicism. Many subgroups with varied modifications in culture, government, forms of worship (liturgy), and beliefs (theology) exist in the first two major divisions. Roman Catholics remain united worldwide under the authority of the Vatican in Rome.

Core beliefs that Christians hold in common relate to their Judeo-Christian heritage. They all believe in an omnipotent, merciful, caring, and ethical God who created persons in His own image and imbued them with goodness and freedom of will. People rebel against God and sometimes choose evil. Jesus Christ is a perfect aspect or expression of God. He became a historical person, experiencing the limitations and sufferings of humankind in order to identify and communicate with us and to save us from the eternal consequences of our evil. His resurrection from death and promise of eternal life provide comfort and hope for Christians who face suffering and death. Christian teaching stresses that eternal life is available now, in this life, through faith in Jesus Christ. Holy Scripture for all Christians is the Old and New Testament Bible.

EASTERN ORTHODOXY

Some Eastern Orthodox Christian churches stem historically from the earliest communities of believers of the eastern Mediterranean region. Major subgroups include Armenian, Coptic (Egyptian), Greek, Syrian, and Russian Orthodox churches. Liturgy is greatly stressed in all groups. The authority of the Pope in Rome is not recognized, and priests marry. The veneration of Mary and the saints is practiced. Use of pictures of Jesus, Mary, and the saints, called icons, is very important in assisting with worship and as a source of comfort to Orthodox Church believers. An ancient calendar is used to establish holy days that often fall at slightly different times than the holy days of other Christian groups. Easter is more elaborately celebrated than Christmas.

Eastern Orthodox believers often fast, avoiding meat and dairy products, although they are exempt from fasting when seriously ill. They believe that every effort should be made to prolong life, with termination of life left in God's hands only. Patients and families may request that an Orthodox priest visit for Holy Communion, anointing the sick, and administering holy unction. Last rites are mandatory for the dying. Autopsy, embalming, and cremation are often opposed.

Russian Orthodox followers usually wear a cross necklace, which should never be removed except in emergencies. Males remain unshaven unless absolutely necessary. Hands are placed in the form of a cross at death. Strong belief in eternal life is emphasized by these believers.

Abortion is opposed. Infant baptism is not practiced by most Orthodox groups. However, the Greek Orthodox stress infant baptism and will want a nurse or anyone else to baptize infants in danger of death, saying "I baptize thee in the name of the Father, Son, and Holy Spirit," while touching the infant's forehead three times with water.

PROTESTANTISM

Christian Protestant churches can be classified into four major categories:

1. Mainline denominations
2. Evangelicals
3. Fundamentlists
4. Other

The category "other" includes groups whose special practices and beliefs about illness and death have important implications for health care workers. There are many Protestant groups of churches.

Mainline Denominations

The major mainline Protestant denominations predominantly found in the United States are the following:

Baptists*
Disciples of Christ (Christian Churches)
Episcopalians (Anglicans in Britain and Canada)
Lutherans (most subgroups are now reunited)
Methodists (most subgroups are now reunited; African-Methodist-Episcopal and A.M.E. Zion are two large separate denominations of black churches)
Presbyterians (Church of Scotland in Britain)
Reformed (Protestant Churches of Holland, France, Hungary, Germany, Switzerland, England, and South Africa)
United Church of Christ (includes churches formerly known as Congregationalist)

All mainline Protestant churches hold traditional Christian beliefs about everlasting life and the Trinitarian understanding of the nature of God as Father, Son, and Holy Spirit. Worship of Jesus Christ as the perfect expression of God is an essential belief. Mary and the saints are respected but not venerated. The Bible is authoritative but not literally interpreted. Most of these churches derive historically from the 16th century Reformation in Europe when they separated from Roman Catholicism. Their worship is formal. Lutherans and Episcopalians stress liturgy more than the other denominations. All clergy are ordained after several years of postgraduate education. Most ministers (clergy) have extensive training in pastoral counseling. These churches work cooperatively and emphasize service to mankind as a basic mission and means of expressing love and gratitude to God.

Beliefs and practices in these churches are much less dogmatic than in other Christian groups. Most believe that God continues to reveal truth. There is strong emphasis on individual conscience and responsibility with individual differences of belief.

Dying members and family may request clergy visits for counseling, comfort, Holy Communion, prayers of healing, or confession. There are no formal or mandated last rite ceremonies. Some denominations practice special healing services and anointing of the sick.

After death, the body is removed for embalming by a funeral director. Closed casket funerals in the churches are encouraged, or memorial services may be conducted, at which the body is not present. Eternal life with resurrection of the spiritual body (immortal soul) is a basic belief but is not adhered to by all members. Plain crosses that do not contain images of the body of Christ are sometimes used in order to emphasize belief in Christ's resurrection.

Organ donation and transplantation are permitted and encouraged as needed. Autopsies are acceptable, as is cremation, which is performed with increasing frequency. Passive euthanasia, that is, removal of all extraordinary measures to sustain life, is sanctioned when severe brain damage is irreversible.

Evangelical Churches

Evangelical Protestant churches are categorized together because of their common concern for sharing the "good news of the Gospel," or proselytizing. They are generally more conservative than mainline denominations, and most have a shorter history and are liturgically less formal. Billy Graham is the most famous representative of this group. Some individuals within mainline denominations would also describe themselves as Evangelicals. Major Evangelical churches in alphabetical order include

Christian and Missionary Alliance
Christian Reformed Church
Church of Christ
Church of the Brethren
Evangelical Free Church
Missouri Synod Lutherans
Nazarenes
Salvation Army
Southern Baptists

Frequent strong emphasis is made on making a personal decision of commitment of one's life to Christ's service.

These Christians generally accept organ donation and transplantation, autopsy, cremation, and passive euthanasia. Infant baptism is not generally practiced. Many members are strong opponents of abortion.

Fundamentalist Churches

Fundamentalist churches are more dogmatic and conservative in practice and belief, with emphasis on the literal interpretation of the Bible. Their lifestyle is closely knit within their Christian community. Alcohol, tobacco, and dancing are prohibited. Many churches exist as separate, independent congregations. Worship is usually liturgically free, and some churches have no sacraments. Clergy are ordained as they feel called by God, and special education is not required. Jerry Falwell is a well-known representative of this group. Some examples of churches in this group are

Bible Churches
Gospel Tabernacles
Independent churches
Many Baptist churches

* The vast majority of Baptist churches would be classified as fundamentalist, evangelical, or pentecostal. See descriptions to follow.

Practices among these groups vary greatly and in general are more conservative and restrictive about medical and nursing issues as well as other aspects of life. Emphasis on the resurrection of the body may preclude cremation, autopsy, and organ donation among some groups. Most fundamentalists actively oppose abortion and do not practice infant baptism.

Other

Churches listed under the heading of "Other" have varied aspects of belief and practice with important implications for health care workers. They are listed alphabetically. They differ considerably from each other and must be described separately. Some do not adhere to core Christian beliefs.

Church of Christ, Scientist

Christian Science (Church of Christ, Scientist) defines God as Divine Mind. Only things of the spirit are considered to be real and eternal. Matter is believed to be merely an illusion, as is pain, illness, and evil. Christian Science leaders are called practitioners and readers of their authoritative book, *Science and Health with Key to the Scriptures* by Mary Baker Eddy.

Medical treatment including immunizations is avoided by Christian Scientists unless required by law. All psychotherapy and physical and medical testing are avoided. Sometimes Christian Scientists enter hospitals or seek medical care because of family pressure, self-doubt, or the desperation of pain. Sometimes they later suffer intense guilt or regret, which should be dealt with compassionately. Free hospital visitation of Christian Science practitioners should be allowed as desired by patients.

Nondrug measures to control pain are preferred by these believers. Medications, intravenous lines, and transfusions are often refused. Patients prefer to die at home. No last rites are practiced, and autopsies are avoided. Names of Christian Science nurses and leaders are listed in the *Christian Science Journal* if a patient or family seeks assistance for home care.

Jehovah's Witnesses

Jehovah's Witnesses emphasize Bible texts in Leviticus and Acts, which they interpret as prohibiting the intake of blood. There is mandatory opposition to organ transplantation and artificial insemination as well as blood transfusion. Informed consent for any procedures possibly requiring blood transfusions in an emergency cannot be signed by these believers. Those who need transfusions to survive and cannot make their own choice, such as children, may be temporarily appointed to the guardianship of the courts for the needed treatment. Foods to which blood products are added, such as luncheon meats and sausage, are also prohibited.

Jehovah Witnesses practice pacifism. They do not participate in national holidays or the oath of allegiance, and all are conscientious objectors in wartime. They practice no last rites or other rituals surrounding death and are opposed to abortions.

Mennonites

Mennonites (including the Amish) are divided into several subgroups whose lifestyles differ with varying degrees of strictness. Historically, Mennonites developed from Protestant churches primarily in Switzerland, and they hold traditional Protestant Christian beliefs similar to those of other churches included in the Evangelical category. It is their religious practice and culture that differentiate them.

Many Mennonites, like the Amish, live mid–19th century lifestyles, rejecting modern machinery and dress codes. Their most honored vocation is farming, because they believe that work on the land, with all the uncertainties of nature, keeps one in constant close touch with God. Handicrafts are also highly respected. Higher education is not encouraged. Modern technology and materialism are felt to provide too many distractions and influences away from their simple, pious lifestyle. They use horse and buggies instead of automobiles and avoid telephones and electricity, and they dress in simple, plain clothing. Strong community ties help them maintain clean, moral, hard-working lifestyles.

Mennonites are pacifists. They feel that allegiance should be to God only. Therefore they take no national oath and do not serve in the military. They do finance and volunteer to do relief work to help the suffering in times of war and disaster. They do not believe in insurance, including health insurance, but are noted for responsibly paying all their medical bills, often with contributions from Mennonite neighbors and friends. They generally practice home remedies to heal the sick but will use modern medical and surgical therapies and hospitals as needed. They have no formally educated clergy but nominate their religious leaders, who are then chosen by lot on a rotating basis. These men serve by preaching on Sundays and visiting the sick. They continue to work their farms while doing so.

Mennonites do not believe in using extraordinary measures to keep a person alive and practice passive euthanasia when the patient is in a vegetative state. Clergy may anoint the sick and dying or baptize them if they request it. Infant baptism is not practiced. They prefer not to have autopsies performed but do not resist if necessary. Organ donation and transplantation is accepted but seldom practiced. Mennonites do not believe in cremation. After death, the embalmed body is brought by the undertaker to the family home for the "viewing" for several hours while the community comes to pay their respects to the dead and to comfort the bereaved. Afterward the body is taken to the church for burial.

Mormons

Mormons (members of the Church of Jesus Christ of Latter-day Saints and the Reorganized Church) supplement the Bible with the Book of Mormon, both of which are sources of inspiration for them. Mormon high priests are authoritative leaders. Places of worship are called temples and tabernacles. Each Mormon male is considered an official missionary and is expected to donate 2 years of full-time service to this work.

Mormons call the body the temple of God and believe that faith keeps one well. Health promotion is highly valued. Illness results from breaking health laws and disobeying God. No coffee, tea, or other caffeine beverages, alcohol, or tobacco are used. Moderation in eating is practiced, particularly with meat.

The community is closely knit and supportive during illness. Marriage in a Mormon temple is believed to be sealed in eternity. Infant baptism is not practiced; Mormons believe that the unbaptized dead can be baptized with a living person as proxy. Some may also preach to the dead, believing that they can still receive eternal salvation in the afterlife.

Belief in divine healing is practiced by laying hands on the sick during a ritual of healing. Special white garments are worn, which should not be removed by the nurse. The sacrament of the Last Supper may be administered by Mormon clergy to a dying person. This church opposes cremation.

New Age Movement

The New Age Movement has been growing in numbers since the 1970s. It is not a formal, organized religion. It is more a philosophy and way of life than a theology. Based primarily in the United States, many followers come from the Christian tradition, although some adhere to other religions or no religion. There is a very strong emphasis on the mystical practices of Hinduism and Buddhism within the New Age Movement led by various Eastern gurus. The Maharishi Mahesh Yogi, founder of transcendental mediation, is one example. A Jewish-born, Harvard psychology professor named Richard Alpert went to India to study under a guru and emerged as a guru in his own right, was renamed Ram Das, and is another major person in the Movement.

An early precursor of the New Age Movement is the Theosophical Society, dating back to the late 19th century. It emphasizes the integration of Eastern thought into Western life and stresses the unity of all religions, an essential concept of the New Age perspective. Other large subgroups within the movement include the Sufi order of Islam and the Unity School of Christianity. Acceptance of specific beliefs is not a criterion for acceptance in the movement, and some New Age followers do not practice any religion.

Common practices include daily meditation, use of natural foods, vegetarianism, and emphasis on non-traditional healing methods. These are usually referred to as holistic health practices. New Age health food stores, bookstores, and retreat and healing centers are examples of places where New Age precepts are practiced. Promotion of ecology, humanizing technology, and world peace are major concerns and efforts of these followers. Psychic and metaphysical beliefs and practices of New Agers can include astrology and use of Tarot cards and crystals. They tend to avoid other occult practices associated with spiritualism, such as mediums who supposedly consult the dead.

Some New Age adherents believe that the body should remain untouched for several hours after death while the soul passes. This might eliminate the possibility of organ donation for some individuals. New Agers tend to respect natural death and passive euthanasia. Cremation is their preferred practice, and autopsy is not generally resisted.

Pentecostal Churches

Pentecostal churches vary widely among charismatics, who all emphasize the aspect of God known as the Holy Spirit. There are many independent Pentecostal churches. Major groups include the Assemblies of God and the Four Square Gospel Churches, which are evangelical or fundamentalist. There is also a charismatic movement within the Roman Catholic church and several mainline Protestant denominations. This is a rapidly growing movement.

The emphasis of Pentecostalism is on the gifts of the Holy Spirit, including healing and speaking in tongues (glossolalia). Most of these groups do not reject traditional medical treatments, but some prohibit them. Some Pentecostal fundamentalist groups believe that illness is due to divine punishment or demon possession. Fasting is practiced by some, and alcohol is prohibited. Belief in eternal life is stressed. Rituals surrounding death vary from group to group, as do regulations regarding cremation, abortion, infant baptism, passive euthanasia, autopsy, and organ transplants.

Quakers

Quakers (Society of Friends), as they call themselves, are associated theologically with mainline Protestant denominations because they do not stress strict theological dogma. However, their practices distinguish them. Guidance by the Holy Spirit is emphasized because of their central belief that God is present in each person. Authority and inspiration come from within. They do not practice glossolalia. They have no appointed clergy, but learning and a disciplined life among all members are emphasized. Each member ministers to others with consistent practice as well as stated beliefs in the worth and equality of all people. Quakers are noted for their honesty and compassion.

Quakers have a long illustrious history of effective social action for the downtrodden, leading such movements as the abolition of slavery, child labor, and disenfranchisement of women. They are antiwar and are currently active in the peace movement. At times Quakers have been reviled for their socially unpopular stands, such as pacifism. There is less emphasis on the afterlife among Quakers and more emphasis on improving the "here and now" for everyone.

Quaker religious services are free of liturgy. Worshiping in a simple plain room, Friends share thoughts as inspired by God, spending long periods meditating together silently. Infant baptism is not observed. Cremation is preferred. Quakers visit each other to lend support in sickness and death but practice no deathbed rituals. Quakers are not apt to resist autopsy, passive euthanasia, or organ donation. They diligently seek information about treatments and actively participate in care and decisions during crisis periods of illness and death.

Seventh Day Adventists

Seventh Day Adventists place greater emphasis on Old Testament beliefs and teachings than do other Christian groups. Otherwise they closely resemble Evangelical churches. The Ten Commandments are stressed. There is strong emphasis on the belief that the dead are asleep until the Second Coming of Christ, when judgment will take place.

These Christians highly value health education and preventive measures. They do not use tobacco, alcohol, coffee, tea, meat (especially pork), and shellfish. They are strict about keeping the Sabbath holy and worship on Saturday instead of Sunday. They oppose infant baptism.

Nurses should prepare to use nonmedication pain control measures with Seventh Day Adventists. Narcotics and stimulants are usually refused. Believers are likely to request Holy Communion while ill as well as anointment with oil and healing prayers by the clergy.

Unitarians/Universalists

Unitarians/Universalists are closely identified with mainline Protestant denominations. They are also close in belief to many Reformed Jews. They worship God the Creator but recognize Jesus Christ only as a highly respected person or prophet. They are liberal in theology and religious practice. Worship is dignified, with strong emphasis on knowledge, education, and rational belief. Study and individual responsibility are important. Infant baptism and eternal life are not stressed. Cremation is preferred. Autopsy, organ transplantation, and passive euthanasia are encouraged as individual decisions. Some members also are active in the Hemlock Society, which supports justifiable suicides and active euthanasia in certain circumstances.

Roman Catholicism

Roman Catholicism is the largest Christian group. It exists worldwide with central authority in Rome, which is believed to date back to the Apostle Peter. Catholics believe that authority for beliefs and practices also derive from the Bible, the bishops, and Church tradition. God is worshiped as Father, Son, and Holy Spirit. The Virgin Mary and the saints are venerated as holy. Roman Catholics believe in heaven, hell, and purgatory as an intermediate state of judgment and cleansing. In common with most other Christians, they believe that the soul lives on after life. Christ is expected to come again, when His will will prevail on earth and suffering will cease. God is aware and saddened by our suffering. Suffering is not His personal judgment, but God is believed to allow suffering for reasons beyond man's understanding. The Roman Catholic Church believes that this life begins at conception, so abortion is strongly opposed. Abortion is not permitted in Catholic hospitals.

Liturgy is stressed within the Catholic Church, and seven sacraments are practiced. They are baptism, confirmation, Holy Eucharist (Communion), reconciliation (confession), matrimony, holy orders (ordination), and anointment of the sick (last rites). The term "last rites" is now discouraged because that term became associated only with death and was feared and avoided by many Catholics. Anointment of the sick is encouraged at any time during any illness and is no longer mandatory when death is impending.

In addition to priests, laypeople who are appointed Eucharistic ministers, as well as ordained, married deacons may administer Holy Communion to the sick. Catholics often ask for the consolation of Communion and prayers when sick. Requests for a priest to hear confession and confer forgiveness prior to death are traditional.

Fasting and abstaining from meat is practiced on Ash Wednesday and Good Friday, although the elderly and sick are exempted. Attendance at Mass is required on Sundays or late Saturdays and on holy days, with exemptions for the frail and ill.

Catholics do not believe that extraordinary measures must be sustained to prolong life when the chance for a meaningful life is gone. Donation and transplantation of organs is approved and encouraged if the donor's possible harm is no greater than the recipient's benefit.

Baptism is mandatory when death threatens newborns and live fetuses. Anyone present can baptize in an emergency, provided one does so "In the name of the Father, Son, and Holy Spirit" when sprinkling water on the infant's forehead.

Autopsy is permitted. Cremation is now allowed. Roman Catholics may now be buried in vaults and mausoleums as well as consecrated grounds. Catholics who commit suicide are allowed to be buried in Catholic cemeteries because they believe that only God can understand and judge the reasons people take their own lives.

HINDUISM

Hinduism developed in India and is a very old, complex religion dating back to 3000 B.C. Hinduism historically has a pantheon of Gods with three major ones: creator (Brahma), preserver (Vishnu), and destroyer (Shiva). The life goal and greatest desire of Hindus is mystical union with the Absolute (Brahman). Theirs is a religion abundant with mythology. Life is a continuous process, with death and birth thought to be one and the same because of belief in reincarnation. The soul (atman) does not change but is continuously reborn. The status of each rebirth or reincarnation depends upon past deeds, knowledge, and experience. Ways to train to reach God are via worship (puja) or via yoga exercises, or meditations, repeating sacred formulas (mantras), or via scripture reading such as the Upanishads or the bhagavad-Gita. Fasting, vegetarianism, and abstinence from alcohol are practiced by devout Hindus. Prayers for freedom from bodily desires are considered the highest form of prayer, since Hindus attempt to withdraw from mundane life. Prayer for healing is considered a low form of prayer. Hindus are generally stoic in the face of suffering and do not seek medical care except as a last resort. Some Hindus view illness, injury, or amputation as punishment.

When death is imminent, a Hindu will strive to stay alert. Priests confer the death rites and tie a cord around the wrist or neck, which should not be removed from the body. After death, only family and special friends should be allowed to touch the body. Cremation is the preferred practice. There are no special prohibitions regarding passive euthanasia or autopsy. Hindus who still believe in the ancient caste system, which is now outlawed but still influential in India, may have problems with organ transplantation. The need to remove donor organs within an hour after death may rule out those Hindus or Buddhists who believe that the soul is not reborn until several hours after death. Most believe that rebirth occurs immediately, however.

ISLAM

Islam is a complete way of life as well as a formal religion. Major subgroups within Islam include the Sunnis and the Shi'ites. Islam is the youngest of the world's major religions. Muslims worship Allah as the One Divine Being and revere Mohammed as His last and greatest prophet. Jesus and Abraham are also highly revered by Muslims. They believe in eternal life, heaven, hell, and judgment. Muslims feel that each believer has a direct relationship to Allah and that there are no special intermediaries needed. They find the use of all images of God to be blasphemous. Reading Scriptures (the Koran) is strongly emphasized for daily guidance, and Muslims pray, wherever they are located at the appointed time, five times daily, facing Mecca.

Muslims stress cleanliness and moderation, especially in eating and drinking. Eating pork, drinking alcohol, and gambling are prohibited. No eating or drinking of any kind is permitted from sunrise to sunset during the month of Ramadan, which varies on the Western calendar.

Women generally lead strictly segregated lives, desiring care from only female nurses and doctors. In most Muslim cultures, the rights and opportunities of women are very limited.

Muslim believers are fatalistic about sickness and death, although they believe that life should be prolonged as long as possible. Confessing and seeking forgiveness are a traditional ritual of dying. Only family and close friends are permitted to touch the body after death. The family ritually washes it and turns it toward Mecca. No body part is to be removed, although organ donation and transplantation may be practiced by some liberal Muslims. Autopsy is generally opposed unless mandated by law, and cremation is not allowed by Islamic teaching.

The Nation of Islam, or "Black Muslims," is a relatively recent movement of black people in the United States and elsewhere seeking to reestablish their African roots and traditions. Members of the Nation of Islam stress morality, self-discipline, and moderation in all things. Americans use personal names that are traditionally Muslim to highlight their Islamic identity. They reject traditional African-American foods such as pork chitterlings and other foods prepared with pork (e.g., collard greens and corn bread). They generally seek to identify with Muslim instead of traditional African-American cultural patterns.

JUDAISM

Judaism is practiced worldwide owing to the historical dispersion of Jewish people. God (Jehovah) is worshiped as just, merciful, ethical, and omnipotent. Humans are believed to derive innate worth and dignity from being God's creation and from one's reaction to one's personal life experiences. Humans are immortal. The Jewish scholar Maimonides considered belief in the afterlife to be one of the basic truths that every Jew is commanded to hold.

There are three major subgroups in Judaism: the Orthodox, the Conservative, and the Reformed. Hasidism is one very strict from of orthodoxy, which emphasizes mysticism and a separate, strict lifestyle. Orthodox Jewish believers generally stress literal interpretation of the Torah, Talmud, and other sacred writings. They are legalistically strict regarding such practices as dietary and Sabbath rules as well as other customs. Conservative Jewish congregations are less literal and more optional about strict adherence to regulations. Reformed Jews are the most liberal and varied in their beliefs and practices. A kosher home is not likely to be kept by Reformed Jews. The home may or may not be kept kosher in a Conservative Jewish family, and a strict kosher home is always kept in an Orthodox Jewish family. Kosher dietary laws include abstinence from certain foods like pork and shellfish, with care not to mix dairy products and meat at the same meal. Use of separate dishes and strict preparation regulations are also included in kosher practices.

Jews generally value education and family ties. They respect and emphasize medical treatment. They see no value in suffering and readily report pain and discomfort and actively seek relief and treatment. Rabbinical consultation and exemptions can be obtained from religious obligations when they endanger health. Very Orthodox Jewish men believe that head and feet should remain covered, and they will insist on wearing socks and yarmulkes on the head in the hospital. It is taboo for them to touch a menstruating female, so they may be uneasy about contact with female nurses.

According to strict tradition, after death of a devout Jew, the body is ritually cleansed and prepared for burial by a Chevra Kadisha, or burial society. Watchers (shomrim) stay with the body until burial. Autopsy and cremation are strictly opposed by the Orthodox, and the sanctity of corpses and cremeteries is maintained because of belief in later resurrection of the body with the soul for all righteous men at some future time ordained by God. After death, Jewish families "sit shiva" at home for 7 days while friends pay their respects and offer sympathy to the bereaved. In Judaism there is an official mourning period of 12 months after death. Embalming is resisted.

Jews do not believe in artificially prolonging life when there is no hope of recovery. Rabbinical permission may be granted for organ donation or transplantation.

Application of the Nursing Process to the Care of the Dying Patient in Spiritual Distress

Assessment

Observe patients for evidence of religious practices such as scripture reading, use of religious pictures, jewelry, medals, special clothing, visits from clergy, prayer, and speaking about religious topics.

Make direct assessments with questions to the patient or family such as the following:

- "Would you like to talk about religion?"
- "What are your spiritual beliefs?"
- "How does your religion influence your life?"
- "Do your recent experiences affect your spiritual life in any way?"
- "Would you like your own spiritual advisor or a hospital chaplain to come to see you?"
- "What are the religious practices or ceremonies that comfort and strengthen you the most?"
- "What can I do to be helpful to you spiritually?"

Assess for distress at being unable to attend religious services of their faith, maintain dietary practices or prayer routines, read Scriptures, or confer with clergy of their own faith.

Assess for more subtle signs of spiritual distress related to a crisis of challenged beliefs. Note whether persons speak of feeling all alone or feeling empty and missing God's presence, whose daily presence they previously experienced. Be alert to expressions about the meaninglessness of life, the pervasiveness of suffering, the ethical dilemmas of treatments, or other complaints of hopelessness and despair such as lack of the will to live. Note their occurrence and further explore them. Be aware that sometimes spiritual distress takes the form of cynical criticisms of religious persons, institutions, and practices; crude jokes about heaven and hell; or angry, questioning comments about a God who "doesn't care." Note incongruities such as use of religious medals, pictures, and other artifacts along with firm refusal to talk with their clergy, attend ceremonies, or have rituals performed such as anointing of the sick.

Blaming God for causing the suffering or indications that the patient feels punished justly or unjustly for past omissions or wrongdoing may occur, even among highly educated people who might not be expected to hold primitive beliefs.

Assess for physical signs of distress such as restlessness, sighing, dry mouth, frequent swallowing, insomnia, gastrointestinal upset, and a general appearance of unhappiness.

Make no presuppositions when it comes to religion. Private, personal beliefs are not necessarily those held by one's official religious affiliation, and these comparisons and contrasts need to be understood by the nurse and religious advisors as they seek to minister to the patient's spiritual needs. Understand that human beings are very complex creatures as they work through the emotional stages of dying or bereavement.

Nursing Diagnoses and Planning

Nursing diagnoses and related expected patient outcomes most commonly applicable to dying patients in spiritual distress include the following:

NDx: Spiritual distress related to separation and inability to engage in usual religious practices secondary to the confinement of severe illness

Planning: Patient outcomes
1. Patient participates in religious practices with clergy when available.
2. Patient discusses religious dispensations related to illness with visiting clergy.
3. Patient verbalizes feeling better because of opportunity to practice religion.
4. Patient describes feeling less powerlessness and loneliness.

NDx: Spiritual distress related to beliefs challenged by intense suffering and impending death

Planning: Patient outcomes
1. Patient openly expresses religious doubts and seeks answers from clergy, nurses, and other members of his or her faith.
2. Patient resumes practices like prayer, Scripture reading, and attendance at worship.
3. Patient states that he or she feels less angry or more at peace with God.

Nursing Interventions

NDx: Spiritual distress
Act as an advocate in regard to religious practices, especially in hospitals where an active chaplaincy program is nonexistent, so that the patient can experience spiritual comfort and strength by participating in practices of his or her religion. Prayer with and for the patient brings comfort to many but can be embarrassing to others. Sensitively explore the possibility of praying with the patient.

Encourage religious practices and rituals at the bedside, or arrange for the patient to be transported to the chapel. Enable the patient to keep religious symbols nearby. Request that the hospital chaplain or other spiritual advisor visit the patient. Inform them about the patient's spiritual distress and physical disabilities so that they can counsel the patient regarding allowed dispensations. Remember that the patient is apt to accept such counsel only from leaders of his or her own religion. Arrange for privacy for the patient and clergy and carefully maintain it, because interruptions during religious ceremonies can be extremely upsetting.

To lessen the patient's spiritual distress and help resolve challenges to his or her belief system, engage in open, nonjudgmental, empathetic communication. Avoid quickly formulated pat answers that stifle communication and are alienating. Remind the patient that the quest for the meaning of suffering is universal and has no easy answers. It takes time. Comply with requests for privacy for prayer and life review whenever possible in the busy hospital routine. Listen carefully and share personal faith and concept of God as loving and caring, if appropriate. Respectful treatment of the patient communicates the message that his or her life and soul have meaning and value regardless of the seeming meaninglessness of the present suffering. Encourage frequent visits by loved ones and other members of the religious community to help sustain and strengthen faith.

Do not leave patients without hope. Do not promote hope for a cure when the prognosis is terminal, but do strengthen the hope that he or she will be well cared for, will have pain controlled, will be supported, will not be abandoned, will be appreciated for courageous efforts, and will leave loved ones who are coping adequately. When the prognosis is uncertain, encourage hope for remission or recovery. Thoughts that no one cares or can do anything to alleviate the suffering result in despair. To provide comfort and courage to cope, give reassurance that God continues to love, is aware of the suffering, and cares.

Evaluation

Evaluate the effectiveness of nursing care for a dying patient in spiritual distress by comparing the patient's status with the expected patient outcomes. Examples of specific outcomes for dying patients in spiritual distress have been provided in the Planning section.

Other Aspects of Death and Dying

Hospices and Home Care

Hospice is essentially a nursing care concept. Historically, it is an ancient concept. The name dates back to the days of the Roman Empire and refers to service and refuge for guests or nonfamily. The words *hospitality* and *hospital* are derived from the same root.

A terminal prognosis, estimated as 6 months or less left to live, is required to be eligible for hospice service. Since no one can really predict the moment of death, this is only an estimate. Hospice patients must prefer to receive supportive care rather than hospital care during their final months of life.

Cicely Saunders, a nurse-physician in England, is the pioneer of the modern hospice movement. She founded St. Christopher's Hospice near London in 1967. Her work grew out of a deep concern that the legitimate needs of the dying are seldom met in busy, acute care hospitals committed to healing and maintaining life. Modeled after St. Christopher's, the first hospice in the United States was established in New Haven, Connecticut, in 1974. The movement has grown rapidly in the United States and elsewhere. There are now several hundred hospices worldwide.

AN IDEAL HOSPICE

Hospices vary greatly. Ideally a hospice has certain characteristics and components. It is an autonomous hospice administration and offers a comprehensive program of care by a health team educated in thanatology (the study of death and dying) in both in-patient and home care settings. Family, patients, volunteers, and staff should work closely as colleagues to control symptoms and enable the individual to complete his or her lifework and die in peace and dignity.

St. Columba's Hospice in Edinburgh, Scotland, embodies these ideals. It is located on a lovely campus overlooking the blue water of the Firth of Forth. The patients' attractive rooms have large, low windows and sliding glass doors to enable patients to enjoy the views. Luxuriant, vividly colored flower beds and lawns are carefully maintained by many volunteers. A children's playground is within view. Day care for hospice workers is deliberately located nearby so that patients can continue to watch and enjoy children and pets on the grounds.

Everything is planned for the well-being of the dying and the bereaved. Detailed attention goes into the selection of furnishings and equipment. For example, lamps at the bedsides have a pinkish glow to offset the sallow appearance of the dying when family members visit. Visitors are graciously received and encouraged, served tea, and provided accommodations when they wish to spend the night or have a private time together with their loved one. A number of special bathtubs for invalids are available because the majority of patients derive more enjoyment from tub baths and are too weak to arise from conventional bathtubs. Dietary preferences are given a great deal of attention. Nurses, physicians, and other health care workers conduct workshops in thanatology. There is a relaxed atmosphere of good-humored camaraderie among staff and patients. A nonsectarian chapel, made beautiful by volunteer artists, is available for prayer and farewells. It accommodates a hospital bed so that patients can be wheeled there, if they desire, when death is approaching. A private entrance and exit was planned with sensitivity to the needs of the bereaved.

Until death occurs, the in-patient unit has a swinging door policy encouraging home care when patients' needs can best be met there and providing respite with in-patient care for a weary family from time to time. An active home care unit at St. Columba's is staffed by nurses and aides. Most hospice nurses are trained and experienced in sophisticated pain control measures. In Edinburgh, the hospice nurses work as close consultants with the district community health nurses to meet the special needs of the dying in the community.

A third unit at St. Columba's is the Day Program. This is another area that utilizes a large staff of active volunteers from the Church of Scotland. Transportation is provided to bring patients from home to hospice for several hours, several days a week. A wide variety of programs and activities are available as needed and physically tolerated. The goal is to offset patients' sense of loneliness, isolation, sensory deprivation, and fear. Nurses also work in this unit counseling, administering medications, providing treatments, and sometimes bathing patients or offering other services of personal care.

Sponsored by the Church of Scotland, St. Columba's also receives private donations and reimbursement funds from insurance companies and the National Health Service. Patients of all religions, socioeconomic levels, and medical diagnoses are admitted. St. Columba's provides seminars and professional education programs for visiting nurses, doctors, and other health professionals. An active training program for their large staff of volunteers has the added benefit of helping to educate the general public about death and dying issues. The persons involved are helped to cease denying the reality of their own death in order to live their lives with greater freedom and fullness.

Full-service hospices such as St. Columba's now exist in some communities in the United States. In state-approved, certified hospice programs, Medicare covers 100% of the cost of approved services in the hospice and at home. Not all hospices are certified. Some certified hospices may not have their own buildings and grounds. Sometimes they contract for beds within a chronic disease hospital or a long-term care facility. It is best when separate units are set up with special staff trained in thanatology. Home care services are crucial to most hospices. Those hospices without their own community nursing staff have contracts or make referrals to other home care agencies within the community.

Many noncertified hospices are run by concerned persons who volunteer their time. A valuable service is provided by helping patients locate sources of help in the community and by visiting patients an hour or so weekly to ease their fears or loneliness. Hospice programs require volunteers to attend training sessions to help them talk with the dying and bereaved comfortably and competently. Full-service hospices like St. Columba's often evolve from the work of such volunteer beginnings. A large proportion of hospice volunteers are nurses who donate their time to this valuable service.

HOME CARE ASSISTANCE

Most people voice a preference to die in their own homes, yet few do so despite the fact that home care is clearly more cost-effective than in-patient care. Many elderly persons live alone or with a feeble spouse, and children often live in a distant city or have demanding careers that take them out of the home daily. This means that supplemental care must be provided, which can be extremely expensive over a period of weeks and months. This situation is worsened by the fact that there is an acute shortage of home health aides available for hire because their hourly pay scale is so low in comparison with that of other workers.

Third party reimbursement for these services is available, with Blue Cross incurance or Medicare as the major provider for people older than 65. However, the criteria for need are strict and are basically as follows:

First, patients must be essentially homebound, meaning they are so sick that they can leave only occasionally and with someone's assistance to go to the doctor's office or to attend to other important matters. They also must need more than custodial care. Their condition must be acute or in an acute phase, needing short-term, *skilled* professional services. Examples of skilled nursing care include catheter care, injections, dressing changes, intravenous infusions, monitoring cardiorespiratory or neurologic status, and teaching colostomy and diabetic or other care to patient and family. Bathing or oral medication administration is not considered skilled care. A home health aide needed to bathe a dying patient and change bed linens will only be paid by Medicare when the aide is extending the service of a skilled nurse, physical or speech therapist, or social worker. Even then, Medicare normally pays for an aide only a couple of hours, two or three times a week. All these services are provided for only a few weeks while the patient's condition is changing. Once a plateau is reached or the condition is chronic, services must be discontinued.

Another of Medicare's strict criteria is that these services must be provided by a certified home health agency. Certified agencies can hire only registered professional nurses, and aides must complete an approved course of training to be certified. Periodic inspections by Medicare and state Health Department officials ensure that high standards are maintained. Many visiting nurse associations are certified agencies as well as many local Departments of Health. In recent years, many acute care hospitals have opened their own Home Care Departments to become certified home health agencies. Certified home health agencies must be nonprofit.

An abundance of proprietary home care agencies are being established around the country. The telephone directory yellow pages in any community usually lists several of these agencies under "Nursing." They differ from certified agencies in that they are profit-making, private businesses and vary greatly in quality. Many of them offer fine service to meet the needs of patients. Nurses, aides, and homemakers can sign up to work for them to take private duty cases on a full-time or part-time basis. They are not under the same strict regulatory requirements that govern certified agencies. Patients are billed for the services they receive and are sometimes reimbursed by their insurance companies. Medicare pays directly only for service secured from a certified agency.

It is sometimes best that a patient not spend the last days at home. In some cases there is inadequate pain control. In other cases, families are so traumatized by their loved one's suffering or so depleted from the responsibility of the care that it is impossible for them to keep the dying at home. Sometimes there is no family available. There are also cases in which the patients' stage of emotional detachment or comatose state makes their setting immaterial to them.

Afterlife or Near-Death Experiences

In recent years, increasing numbers of persons have reported afterlife experiences. They usually occur during cardiac arrest, attempted suicide, severe traumas, or near-drownings. Moody first investigated these experiences and published his findings of 150 near-death experiences in 1976. Osis and Haraldsson (1977) also published the results of their cross-cultural research on more than 1000 afterlife experiences of Hindus and Christians in India and the United States.

The phenomenon has come to be called near-death experience, or NDE. A remarkable similarity of experiences has been described by people of widely varied cultural and religious backgrounds. Most of them report the following, which are called the core experiences of NDE:

- a sense of peace, overwhelming joy, and happiness free of all pain or other previously felt discomforts is experienced.
- Subsequent awareness of leaving the physical body and serenely looking down upon it and other persons who may be present, attempting resuscitation.
- A sense of the soul floating and then moving rapidly through a tunnel-like darkness as a lovely sound resembling ringing, humming, or buzzing is heard. Perception of other beings warmly welcoming and guiding the patient.
- Awesome awareness of a beautiful radiance or brilliance. This light is filled with a Presence that is otherworldly, exuding love, and engulfing the patient in a sense of cosmic oneness, wisdom, and bliss.
- Finally, the sense of viewing one's life in a non-critical way. Questions are presented nonverbally and lovingly by the Presence. Deceased loved ones are present also and are warm and welcoming. The euphoria continues until a barrier or border is reached with sudden awareness that a decision must be made. A yearning is felt to remain, but a compulsion to decide to return to the body is also felt. The decision to return may seem unpleasant, and there is a sudden awareness of being back in the body.

Following publicity on Moody's findings, hundreds of persons who had been reluctant to talk about their NDEs or lacked the descriptive vocabulary reported similar experiences. In many instances, these had occurred 10 to 20 years prior but had never been shared because of their otherworldly quality.

In 1980, Ring conducted the first scientific study of NDEs with a sample of 102 people who nearly died. Forty-nine of them described NDEs with at least one of the five core experiences. In 1982, Seborn studied 116 cardiac arrest patients, with 49 of them having NDEs. According to a Gallup poll, 35% of Americans who approached death have had NDEs (Papowitz, 1986).

The scientific community has not yet endorsed the validity of these experiences. It has not been determined whether NDEs have a physiologic, a psychic, or a spiritual basis.

After the NDE, nurses, more than other persons, are chosen by these patients as confidants if the nurse is perceived as receptive and able to be trusted to respect the awesomeness and reality of the experience. Reassurance as well as information about the International Association of Near-Death Studies (IANDS) should be offered. (See Resources list at the end of this chapter.)

Ethical Issues in Death and Dying

The number and complexity of ethical issues facing nursing are growing at a rapid rate owing to advanced technology and the expanded role of the nurse. Nowhere are moral dilemmas more poignant and pressing than in the area of death and dying. Before the advent of modern medicine, death was usually caused by infections and was not a prolonged process. Pneumonia was known as "an old man's friend." Today medical technology such as mechanical ventilators, artificial feedings, and sophisticated medications makes it possible to keep someone alive in a vegetative state for a very long time.

TERMINATION OF LIFE-SUSTAINING TREATMENT: THE QUINLAN CASE

The case of Karen Quinlan publicized the plight of such persons and led to legislative action affecting treatment of the dying. Karen was maintained on a respirator for months after irreversible brain damage occurred, caused initially by a prolonged episode of respiratory arrest. As time passed, Karen's family wished her removed from life-support systems. Devout Roman Catholics, they first sought the counsel of their church and were advised that their wishes were permissible within the tenets of Roman Catholic teaching. However, expert neurologists asserted with medical certainty that Karen was not brain dead. Yet her comatose condition rendered her grossly incompetent to express her own wishes. The case was brought to court. At length, the first judge ruled that by legal and medical definition, Karen was alive regardless of her irreversible, comatose state. She therefore had a constitutional right to life that others could not deny her, and she could not be removed from the respirator.

Karen's parents appealed the case to the Supreme Court of New Jersey. That court defined the act of ceasing life-saving measures to be a distinctly different act than homicide. Karen's father was eventually appointed her guardian with authority to withdraw the life-sustaining mechanisms that were prolonging her existence. This was done, and she was transferred to a nursing home where she continued to breathe on her own for some time before expiring. The long ordeal of the Quinlan family resulted in a landmark case helping to establish a legal basis for passive euthanasia or the removal of artificial life-sustaining measures to allow a natural death.

EUTHANASIA: KILLING OR ALLOWING DEATH?

The word *euthanasia* is much misunderstood and often fraught with terror. It simply means "a good death." The prefix *eu* means good, or painless, and the suffix *thanatos* comes from the Greek word meaning death. The word *euthanasia* was horribly corrupted by the Nazis and erroneously came to be associated with genocide and legalized mass murder. Most people still think of the term as "mercy killing," which more appropriately applies to the definition of active euthanasia only.

Some people argue that active euthanasia on a voluntary basis is more humane and has its place for patients suffering from incurable, intractable pain who want assistance in dying. The subject is loaded with ethical dilemmas and dangers.

Years before Hitler had the power to legalize and mandate euthanasia and genocide, German doctors and nurses were participating in active euthanasia. They began with mercy killings by assisting the suffering to die when they requested release from their world of pain. Soon influential persons in the health care field began talking and writing about the need for euthanasia for others whose lives were "devoid of value." Mentally retarded, psychiatric, and chronically ill patients were gradually added to the list, and the concept of voluntary choice was soon forgotten. As early as 1920, a book was published by two prominent German scientists, Hoche and Binding, advocating legal permission to kill "worthless people." It was popular enough to warrant a second printing (Wertham, 1980). The killings increased in number in Germany. The purpose soon shifted to perfection of the race by killing off those who were physically, emotionally, or mentally defective.

"In 1941 the psychiatric institution Hadamar celebrated the cremation of the ten thousandth mental patient in a special ceremony. Psychiatrists, nurses, attendants and secretaries all participated. Everyone received a bottle of beer for the occasion."

FREDRIC WERTHAM

There are very important lessons to be learned from the German euthanasia program. The first is that it was conceived and voluntarily carried out by doctors and nurses long before Hitler's mandated programs of genocide. The second is that what started somewhat altruistically and innocently in a climate of social acceptance soon developed into a notorious program of killing the sick and defenseless.

Passive euthanasia, although morally more acceptable, also presents many dilemmas that directly affect nurses. These dilemmas pose such questions as the following: When should life be prolonged and who should be resuscitated? Who should make the decision to begin extraordinary measures such as a feeding tube or a respirator, and who should discontinue them when the patient is unable to make the decision? When the family has various reasons for wishing an end to the ordeal, should they be forced to make the decision and bear the guilt of their decision? Should the decision rest with medical personnel, who may fear criticism for negligence or threat of malpractice suits if all possible measures to promote and prolong life are not used? Should such intimately personal and private matters of a profound nature become the domain of the courts and be impersonally decided legally for all of us?

At the forefront of attempts to clarify and resolve some of these issues is the work of the Hastings Center and the Euthanasia Education Council, now known as Choice in Dying, Inc. The latter developed The Living Will and has distributed thousands of Box 5-1 gives an example of a living will. This document is not legally binding everywhere. Nevertheless it offers individuals an opportunity prior to the crisis to express an opinion and decision about the use of heroic measures to prolong their lives. It provides guidance to family, physicians, clergymen, and lawyers in their decisions on behalf of patients if they become incompetent to decide for themselves. Many states have health care proxy legislation to permit a designated agent to make decisions to withhold or withdraw life support.

The Hastings Center, or the Institute of Society, Ethics and the Life Sciences, is a nonprofit organization that was founded in 1969 and is staffed by experts from various fields. The Hastings Center seeks to examine ethical issues in the life sciences with research, development of guidelines for care, and professional education seminars. Of all the ethical issues to be addressed, care of the dying has been at the forefront of their work.

DEFINITION OF DEATH

Not so long ago, in developed nations, and today in most of the world, death is determined and pronounced by simple measures: finding no palpable pulse; no signs of breathing; and no moisture seen on a mirror held in front of the mouth and nose. Death is not so simply defined by modern medicine. Even a flat electroencephalogram is not an adequate criterion in itself for a definition of death.

In 1967, a group at Harvard University Medical School developed six criteria for the definition of brain death, which have become quite widely accepted, especially in North America. The criteria are

1. Unreceptivity and unresponsiveness—no response even to painful stimuli like strong pinching.
2. No movements after observation by a physician for an hour continuously, and no breathing after 3 minutes off the respirator.
3. No reflexes, including brain stem reflexes. Pupils are fixed and dilated.
4. A flat electroencephalogram (EEG). This is considered of great confirmatory value if technically adequate.
5. All these tests repeated at least 24 hours later with no change.
6. Two conditions must be excluded: hypothermia and central nervous system depression by drugs such as barbiturates.

In 1972, the Hastings Center studied these criteria and substantially supported them, emphasizing the danger of sole reliance on flat EEG findings.

DO NOT RESUSCITATE POLICIES

Do not resuscitate (DNR) policy decisions are also needed to help doctors and nurses with the ethical dilemmas they face. It is often the nurse who is present when the patient goes into cardiac arrest. Unless a clear decision has been communicated—which often is *not* the case—it is the nurse who initiates cardiopulmonary resuscitation (CPR) or basic life support (BLS) which, once begun, is continued until and unless death has been clearly determined.

A Committee on Policy for Do Not Resuscitate Decisions was appointed in 1978 at Yale-New Haven Hospital and outlines, as an ideal, management plans from which several decisions about terminating treatment can follow. An outline of a DNR policy is found in Box 5–2. New York State now requires all hospitals to have DNR policies as of April 1988. Guidelines developed by the Hastings Center for the termination of treatment were published in September 1987. They were derived from examination of these issues, including DNR, living wills, and definition of death. Included are procedural guidelines, a collection of case studies, and recommendations for curriculum development for health care providers. Copies of the Guidelines for Termination of Care can be secured by contacting the Hastings Center. The address is listed at the end of this chapter.

ORGAN DONATIONS

Another major issue currently involving nurses is organ donation for transplantation. The Uniform Anatomical Gift Act governs various aspects of donation, such as when, how, and who will decide that the donor's life has ceased. Organs must be

Box 5–1.

A LIVING WILL

"Living Will."*
Declaration

Declaration made this ________________ day of ________________ 19 ____ .

I, ________________________________ , being of sound mind, willfully and voluntarily make known my desires that my dying shall not be artificially prolonged under the circumstances set forth below, and do declare:

If at any time I should have an incurable injury, disease, or illness certified to be a terminal condition by two (2) physicians who have personally examined me, one of whom shall be my attending physician, and the physicians have determined that my death will occur whether or not life-sustaining procedures are utilized and where the application of life-sustaining procedures would serve only to artificially prolong the dying process, I direct that such procedures be withheld or withdrawn, and that I be permitted to die naturally with only the administration of medication or the performance of any medical procedure deemed necessary to provide me with comfort or care or to alleviate pain.

In the absence of my ability to give directions regarding the use of such life-sustaining procedures, it is my intention that this declaration shall be honored by my family and physician(s) as the final expression of my legal right to refuse medical or surgical treatment and accept the consequences of such refusal.

I understand the full import of this declaration and I am emotionally and mentally competent to make this declaration.

Signed ________________________________

Address ________________________________

____

I believe the declarant to be of sound mind. I did not sign the declarant's signature above for or at the direction of the declarant. I am at least 18 years of age and am not related to the declarant by blood or marriage, entitled to any portion of the estate of the declarant according to the laws of intestate succession of the ________________ ________________ or under any will of the declarant or codicil thereto, or directly financially responsible for declarant's medical care. I am not the declarant's attending physician, an employee of the attending physician, or an employee of the health facility in which the declarant is a patient.

Witness ________________________________

Address ________________________________

____

Witness ________________________________

Address ________________________________

____

ss.:

Before me, the undersigned authority, on this ____________ day of ________________ , 19 ____ , personally appeared ________________________ , and ________________________ , known to me to be the Declarant and the witnesses, respectively, whose names are signed to the foregoing instrument, and who, in the presence of each other, did subscribe their names to the attached Declaration (Living Will) on this date, and that said Declarant at the time of execution of said Declaration was over the age of eighteen (18) years and of sound mind.

[SEAL]
My commission expires:

____
Notary Public

* Check requirements of individual state statute.

(President's Commission for the Study of Ethical Problems in Medicine and Biobehavioral Research. *Deciding to forego life-sustaining treatment* [pp. 314–315]. Washington, D.C.: U.S. Government Printing Office.)

removed within an hour after death. The patient's attending physician pronounces death but cannot participate in the organ removal process or the transplantation. Because of a critical shortage of needed organs, some states have passed laws requiring "routine requests" for organs by hospital administrators or their designees, who are often nurses. It is usually a nurse on duty at the time of death who is designated to approach the family for a signed release requesting the family to donate organs if the patient's wishes were not made clear in advance. Many states now request that individuals record their decision in advance when applying for driver's licenses. In cases of brain death, plans for organ donations are made before ventilators and other equipment are removed. The protocol encourages discretion and sensitivity to the survivors' suffering and respect for religious beliefs as well as

Box 5–2.

GUIDELINES CONCERNING DO NOT RESUSCITATE ORDERS

The purpose of cardiopulmonary resuscitation (CPR) is to prevent sudden, unexpected death. Initiation of CPR on patients who are irreversibly and terminally ill, and whose death is not unexpected, may be both medically unsound and contrary to the patient's wishes and expectations. Since, in hospital practice, all patients who cease to breathe and/or suffer arrest of heart action are subject to CPR, it is necessary to anticipate and prevent these measures when they are not in the best interest of the patient. The attending physician has the responsibility to address the question of a Do Not Resuscitate (DNR) order when the patient's circumstances so warrant. The possibility of a DNR order may be raised with the attending physician by the patient, the patient's family, or any member of the health care team. Physicians and other health care professionals should make every effort to ensure that patients and their families understand the nature of CPR and are comfortable with a decision to undertake or forgo CPR.

Procedures

When, in the opinion of the attending physician, a patient's condition is irreversible, death is not unexpected, and CPR should not be initiated, the following procedures shall be followed:

1. If the patient is competent,* the relevant facts shall be discussed with the patient to determine the patient's preference with respect to a DNR order.
2. If the patient is incompetent, the attending physician shall consult at a minimum with the next of kin and any legally appointed conservator of the person or guardian of the patient, since there are no definitive legal guidelines concerning the rights of the patient's immediate family.
3. A DNR order should not be written unless the patient, or in the case of an incompetent patient, the next of kin, any legal representative, and all adult members consulted, approve of the order.
4. The responsible attending physician shall write the DNR order, unabbreviated, in the physician's order sheet. Supporting clinical information, documentation of consultations with other physicians, if any, and a record of discussions with the patient, next of kin, other family members, and legal representative shall be included in the patient's chart.
5. The attending physician shall ensure that the DNR order and its meaning are discussed with appropriate members of the hospital staff.
6. DNr orders are compatible with maximal therapeutic care. A patient may receive vigorous support in all other therapeutic modalities.
7. The DNR order shall be subject to ongoing review by all concerned parties and may be rescinded at any time.
8. Members of the health care team who have questions about these guidelines or individual patient cases should contact their supervisor, department chairperson, or director of the relevant special care unit, as appropriate.

*A competent patient is (1) an adult (18 years or older or an emancipated minor); (2) conscious and able to understand the nature and severity of his or her illness and to make informed choices about treatment; and (3) a patient for whom a conservator of the person has not been appointed. If a patient satisfies (1) and (2), but not (3), that is, the adult patient is lucid, but a conservator of the person has been appointed, the appropriate department chairperson or director of special care should be consulted prior to making decision with respect to a DNR order.

obvious nonsuitability for organ and tissue donations. The American Nurses' Association encourages nurses to support organ procurement measures.

Resources

Compassionate Friends
P.O. Box 3696
Oak Brook, IL 60522

Choice in Dying, Inc.
200 Varick Street
New York, NY 10014-4810

The Foundation of Thantology
630 West 168th Street
New York, NY 10032

The Hastings Center
Institute of Society, Ethics and the Life Sciences
255 Elm Road
Briarcliff Manor, NY 10510

International Association of Near-Death Studies
P.O. Box 7767
Philadelphia, PA 19101

Hemlock Society, U.S.A.
P.O. Box 11830
Eugene, Oregon 97440

OMEGA: The Journal of Death and Dying
Baywood Publishing Company
26 Austin Ave.
P.O. Box 337
Amityville, NY 11701

Bibliography

Adam J. What about the relatives? Prof Nurse 1990; 5(5):260.

Bane JD, Kutscher A, Neale R, Reeves B. Death and ministry—Pastoral care of the dying and the bereaved. New York: Seaburg Press, 1975.

Beauchamp TL, Perlin S. Ethical issues in death and dying. Englewood Cliffs, NJ: Prentice-Hall, 1978.

Becker E. The denial of death. New York: The Free Press, Macmillan Publishing, 1973.

Bourne E. What a dying patient needs from you—Helping your patient die at home. RN 1987; 50(6):65.

Carpenito L. The nursing diagnosis: Application to clinical practice. 3rd ed. New York: JB Lippincott, 1990.

Caswell D, Omery A. The dying patient in the critical care setting: Making the critical difference. AACN Clin Issues Crit Care Nurs 1990; 1(1):178.

Childress J, Macquarrie J. The Westminister dictionary of Christian Ethics. Louisville, KY: Westminster John Knox Press, 1986.

Coco P. When would I use the nursing diagnosis of "impaired social interactions related to grief and loss" and how should I intervene? Adv Clin Care 1990; 5(3):45.

Corcoran DK. Helping patients who've had near-death experiences. Nursing 1988; 18(11):34.

Cox HB. The valley of the shadow. Point View 1990; 27(1):12.

Crinn K. Abington dictionary of living religions. Nashville: Abington Press, 1981.

Doyle N. The dying person and the family. Public Affairs Pamphlet No. 485. New York; 1972, p 7.

DuFresne F. Home care: An alternative to the nursing home. Elgin, IL: Bethlehem Press, 1983.

Erikson E. Childhood and Society. 2nd ed. New York: Norton, 1963, pp 263–269.

Ethical, legal and policy issues pertaining to solid organ. Report of the Hastings Center Project on Organ Transplantations. New York: Briarcliff Manor, October 1985.

Frankl V. Man's search for meaning. New York: Washington Square Press, 1963.

Groat M. Helping bereaved parents. Nurs RSA Verpleging 1990; 5(1):12.

Haber J, Hoskens P, Leach A, Sedeleau B. Comprehensive psychiatric nursing. New York: McGraw-Hill, 1987.

Hammarskjöld D. Markings. New York: Alfred A. Knopf, 1964.

Herth K. Relationship of hope, coping styles, concurrent losses, and setting to grief resolution in the elderly widow(er). Res Nurs Health 1990; 13(2): 109.

Hick J. Death and eternal life. New York: Harper and Row, 1980.

Highfield M, Cason C. Spiritual needs of patients: Are they recognized? Cancer Nurs 1983; 6(3): 187.

Johnson B. Adaptation and growth: Psychiatric mental health nursing. 2nd ed. New York: JB Lippincott, 1989.

Kubler-Ross, E. On death and dying. New York: Macmillan Publishing, 1969.

Kubler-Ross, E. Death: The final stage of growth. Englewood Cliffs, NJ: Prentice-Hall 1975.

Kutscher A, et al. Hospice USA. New York: Columbia University Press, 1983.

Lamm M. The Jewish way in death and mourning. New York: Jonathan David Publishers, 1969.

Lewis CS. A grief observed. New York: Harcourt Brace Jovanovich, 1958.

Lewis SL, Collier IC. Medical-surgical nursing. New York: McGraw-Hill, 1987.

Loader S. Heaven can wait: Near death experiences. Prof Nurse 1990; 5(9):458.

Madison DC, Viola A. The health of widows the year following bereavement. J Psychosom Med Res 1968; 12:297.

McFarland G, Thomas M. Psychiatric mental health nursing. New York: JB Lippincott, 1991, pp 450–456.

McFarland G, Wasli E. Nursing diagnosis and process in psychiatric mental health nursing. Philadelphia: JB Lippincott, 1986.

Mead FS. Handbook of denominations in the United States. Nashville: Abington Press, 1970.

Melton J. Cults in America. New York: Garland Publishing, 1986.

Mian P. Sudden bereavement: Nursing interventions in the ED. Crit Care Nurse 1990; 10(1):30.

Mitford J. The American way of death. Greenwich, CT: Fawcett Publications, 1963.

Moody RA. Life after life. Harrisburg, PA: Stackpole Books, 1976.

Moody RA. Reflections on life after life. New York: Bantam Books, 1977.

Murray R, Huelskoetter MM. Psychiatric/mental health nursing: Giving emotional care. Norwalk, CT: Appleton & Lange, 1987.

Muyskens J. Moral problems in nursing: A philosophical investigation. Totowa, NJ: Rowan and Littlefield, 1982.

Osis K, Haraldsson E. At the hour of death. New York: Abon Publishers, 1977.

Papowitz L. The NDE phenomenon verified. Am J Nurs 1986; 86(4):419.

Pasquali E, Alesi E, Arnold H, DeBasio N. Mental health nursing: A holistic approach. 3rd ed. St. Louis: CV Mosby, 1989.

Peck RC. Psychological developments in the second half of life. In Neugarten BL (ed). Middle-age and aging: A reader in social psychology. Chicago: University of Chicago Press, pp 88–92.

Poss S. How the terminal patient accepts dying. Based on a paper given as part of the "Doctors' Course" of the International Terminal Care Teaching Programme, St. Christopher's Hospice, London, June 1978. Patient Couns Health Educ Second Quarter, 1980; p 72.

Potter P, Perry A. Basic nursing theory and practice. St. Louis: CV Mosby, 1987.

Saunders, C. The last stages of life. Am J Nurs 1965; 65:70.

Scruby LS, Sloan JA. Evaluation of bereavement intervention. Can J Public health 1989; 80(6):394.

Sheard T. In memoriam. Focus Crit Care 1990; 17(3):238.

Steeves RH, Kahn, DL. Experience of meaning in suffering. Image Nurs Sch 1987; 19:113.

Stickney, SK, Gardner ER. Companions in suffering . . . families need help. Am J Nurs 1984; 84:1491.

Stiles MK. The shining stranger: A phenomenological investigation of the nurse-family spiritual relationship [Ph.D. thesis]. Denver: University of Colorado Health Sciences Center, 1988.

Strom-Paikin J. Studying the NDE phenomenon. Near-death experiences. Am J Nurs 1986; 86(4):420.

Thompson I, Melia K, Boyde K. Nursing ethics. Edinburgh: Churchill Livingstone, 1983.

Tolstoy L. Death and the meaning of life. In A confession. New York: Thomas Crowell, 1899.

Tolstoy L. The death of Ivan Ilych. New York: The New American Library, 1960, pp 137–138.

Trevelyan J. Near death experiences. Nurs Times 1989; 85(28):39.

Twycross R. Continuing and terminal care—Overview of analgesia. Excerpt from address delivered May 1978 at the Venice Conference on Pain. Arch of the Foundation of Thanatology 1988; 6(4):90.

Ufema J. Death and dying. Nursing 90 1990: 20:90.

Ufema J. Insights on death and dying. Nursing 90 1990; 20:94.

Ufema J. Meeting the challenge of a dying patient [interview]. Nursing 91 1991; 21:42.

Veatch R. Death, dying and the biological revolution. New Haven, CT: Yale University Press, 1976.

Weisman A. On dying and denying: A psychiatric study of terminality. New York: Behavioral Publications, 1972, pp 121, 151.

Wertham F. The German euthanasia program. Cincinnati, OH: Hayes Publishing, 1980.

Unit Two

ADULTS WITH INTEGUMENTARY DYSFUNCTION

Chapter Six: Knowledge Basic to the Nursing Care of Adults with Skin Dysfunction

Chapter Seven: Nursing Care of Adults with Skin Disorders

Chapter Eight: Nursing Care of Adults with Burn Injuries

Learning Objectives

AFTER COMPLETING THIS UNIT, THE LEARNER WILL BE ABLE TO:

Chapter Six

1. Explain the normal anatomy and physiology of the skin and related structures.
2. Describe common clinical manifestations of skin disease.
3. Identify information and physical examination data essential to the assessment of the skin.
4. Describe basic diagnostic tests and modalities of medical management (pharmacologic therapy, topical therapy, radiation therapy) used in the treatment of patients with skin disorders.
5. Describe basic surgical procedures and techniques (curettage and desiccation, cryosurgery, laser surgery, skin grafting, and cosmetic procedures) used in the treatment of patients with skin disorders.
6. Identify data essential to the assessment of patients undergoing treatment of skin disorders.
7. State nursing diagnoses and related expected patient outcomes commonly applicable to patients undergoing treatment of skin disorders.
8. Describe nursing interventions, with their rationales, commonly applicable to patients undergoing treatment of skin disorders.
9. Explain the basis for evaluation of nursing care provided to patients undergoing treatment of skin disorders.
10. Identify special considerations for the elderly patient with altered skin function.

Chapter Seven

1. Describe common skin disorders in terms of etiology, pathophysiology, clinical manifestations, diagnostic procedures, and medical management.
2. Identify information and physical examination data essential to the assessment of patients with common skin disorders.
3. State nursing diagnoses and related expected patient outcomes commonly applicable to patients with skin disorders.
4. Describe nursing interventions, with their rationales, commonly applicable to patients with skin disorders.
5. Explain the basis for evaluation of nursing care provided to patients with common skin disorders.
6. Identify special considerations for the elderly patient with a skin disorder.

Chapter Eight

1. Describe thermal, chemical, and electrical burn injuries in terms of etiology, pathophysiology, clinical manifestations, diagnostic procedures, and medical and surgical management.
2. Identify information and physical examination data essential to the assessment of patients with burn injuries.
3. State nursing diagnoses and related expected patient outcomes commonly applicable to patients with burn injuries.
4. Describe nursing interventions, with their rationales, commonly applicable during the immediate, emergent, acute, and rehabilitation phases of care of patients with burn injuries.
5. Explain the basis for evaluation of nursing care provided to patients with burn injuries.
6. Identify special considerations for the pregnant patient with burn injuries.
7. Identify special considerations for the elderly patient with burn injuries.

Chapter Six

KNOWLEDGE BASIC TO THE NURSING CARE *of Adults with Skin Dysfunction*

The skin is the largest organ in the body. It accounts for 15% of the body's weight and varies in thickness from $\frac{1}{50}$ to $\frac{1}{4}$ of an inch. The skin is durable and pliable. It absorbs, reflects, cushions, and limits the effects of environmental factors on the body. It provides a barrier against invasion of microorganisms; aids in the regulation of temperature, fluid, and electrolytes; serves as a sense organ for touch, pain, heat, cold, and pressure; and is a source of vitamin D through the action of ultraviolet light on cholesterol compounds in the skin. It is also the interface between the self and society, because it affects how an individual is perceived by others.

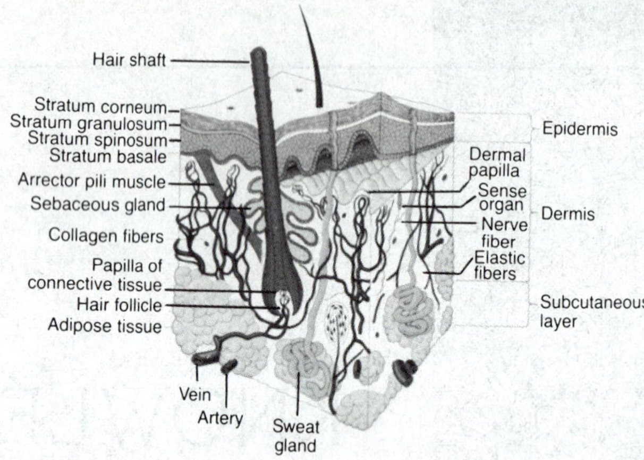

Figure 6–1.

Anatomy of the skin. The stratum corneum, the outermost layer of the epidermis, provides the skin's protective barrier to penetration of water and electrolytes. The dermis acts as a support for the skin's appendages, blood vessels, and nerves. (From O'Toole M. Miller-Keane encyclopedia and dictionary of medicine, nursing, and allied health. 5th ed. Philadelphia. WB Saunders, 1992, color plate 18.)

Anatomy and Physiology

Skin is composed of the epidermis, dermis, subcutaneous fat, and skin appendages, such as the glands and hair follicles (Fig. 6–1).

Epidermis

The epidermis is the outer layer of skin. Its four layers, as illustrated in Figure 6–2, are as follows: the basal layer, or stratum germinativum; prickle cell layer, or stratum spinosum; stratum granulosum; and the stratum corneum, which is the outer, protective horny layer. The epidermis is composed of stratified squamous epithelial cells. Ninety-five percent of these cells are keratinocytes. Five percent consists of melanocytes, the pigment cells that produce melanin and thus give the skin its color.

The stratum corneum is the skin's protective barrier. It is made up of many layers of thick or keratinized squamous cells that lack nuclei and cy-

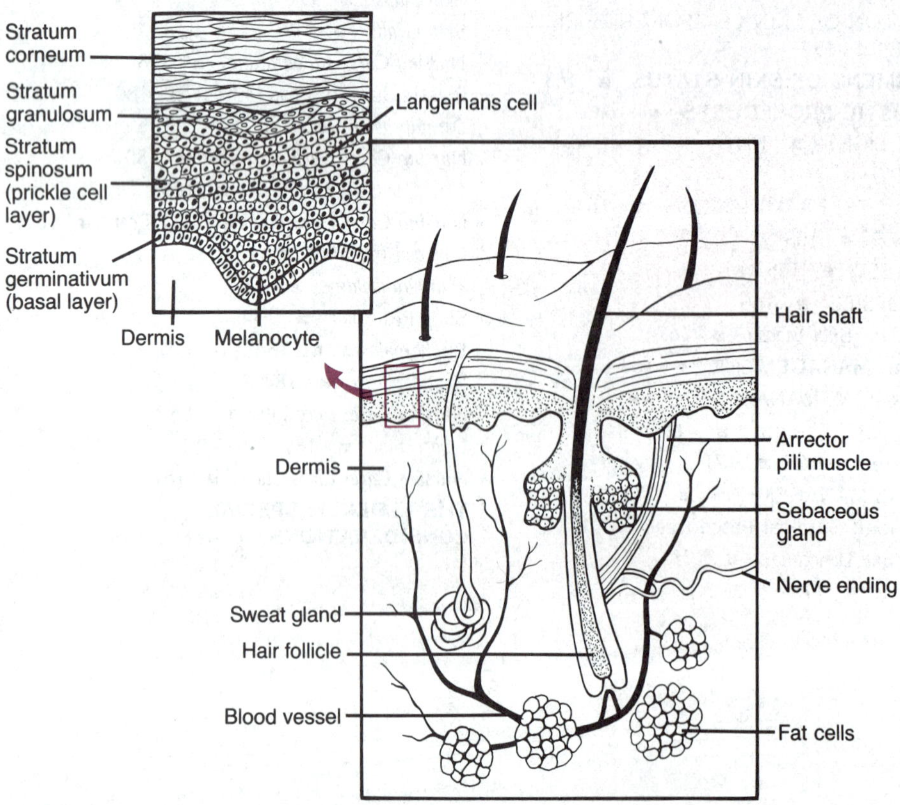

Figure 6–2.

Layers of the epidermis.

toplasm. Ten percent of the stratum corneum is water. Lipids that hold the water in keratin make up 7% to 9%. Mucous membrane structures, such as the lips and labia, lack stratum corneum. Skin lacking stratum corneum is freely permeable. Minor disruptions of the skin, such as paper cuts, stripping with tape, or extensive hand washing, weaken the barrier.

The basal cell layer, which is the innermost layer of the epidermis, is the site where new cells are produced to replace those that are sloughed or damaged. After being produced, new cells migrate upward and undergo keratinization as they pass through the succeeding layers. Cell migration from the basal layer to the top of the stratum granulosum takes approximately 2 weeks. These cells form the protective stratum corneum for about another 14 days, after which they reach the surface and are shed.

Basal cells also line the hair follicles and the sweat and sebaceous glands, which are located in the dermis.

The rete ridges anchor the epidermis to the dermis at the dermoepidermal junction.

Dermis

The dermis is thick and gives bulk to the skin. It is made up of connective tissue, cellular elements, and ground substance.

Connective tissues in the form of collagen fibers, elastin fibers, and reticular fibers provide support and give elasticity to the skin.

The cellular elements of the dermis include reticulohistiocytes, myeloid cells, and lymphoid cells. The reticulohistiocytes include the following: fibroblasts, which are migrating cells that continually break down and re-form collagen fibers and are important in wound healing; histiocytes, which are active in phagocytosis; mast cells, which release histamine and heparin when injured and are increased in itching dermatoses; and reticulum cells, which may cause increased plasma cells in chronic inflammation. The myeloid cells are the polymorphonuclear leukocytes and eosinophilic leukocytes found especially in allergic dermatosis. Lymphoid cells are found in inflammatory lesions.

Ground substance is gel-like and contains proteins, mucopolysaccharides, soluble collagens, enzymes, immune bodies, metabolites, and other substances. It surrounds the cells of the dermis and contributes to the turgor and suppleness of the skin.

The dermis contains blood vessels, which provide nourishment and temperature regulation. The epidermis has no intrinsic blood supply and depends on diffusion from the vessels in the papillary dermis for nutrients and oxygen.

In the dermis, two horizontal plexuses, or vascular beds, are interconnected via shunts. The deep plexus is in the reticular dermis. The superficial plexus is in the papillary dermis. Increased blood flow in the superficial plexus allows heat loss. Heat is conserved by shunting blood to the deep plexus.

The dermis also contains widespread free nerve endings and receptors, which allow detecting of the sensations of touch, temperature, and pain.

Subcutaneous Fat

The subcutaneous fat (subcutis, subcorium, adipose tissue) is a layer of loose connective tissue containing lipocytes, which are cells that manufacture and store fat. There is a wide variation in individual fat distribution. Some individuals store enormous quantities of fat, whereas others store little. Some areas of the body such as the eyelids have little. Subcutaneous fat supports the upper skin layers, serves as a caloric reservoir, and insulates the body against heat loss.

Glands

The sebaceous, apocrine, and eccrine sweat glands originate in the epidermis and extend into the dermis. The sebaceous glands are the oil-producing glands of the skin. They secrete sebum, a complex lipoidal mixture that has a role in vitamin D synthesis. Sebaceous glands are most abundant on the face, scalp, scrotum, and upper trunk. They are absent on the palms and soles.

Apocrine sweat glands, the largest glands of the skin, are found in the axillae, the areolae of the nipples, and the periumbilical, perianal, and genital regions. The apocrine sweat glands begin to function as a result of hormonal influences at puberty. They secrete minute quantities of a sterile, odorless, milky-white fluid that is unnoticed on the skin. Bacterial changes account for distinctive body odors characteristic of the apocrine glands. The apocrine and sebaceous glands usually have a common excretory path through a hair follicle.

The eccrine sweat glands are distributed over the entire surface of the body. By secreting sweat through the pores of the skin, the eccrine glands provide thermoregulation. The hypothalamus regulates eccrine sweating in response to heat. Emotional stress also produces sweating, especially of the forehead, axillae, palms, and soles. Eccrine sweat glands also excrete lactate ion, urea, ammonia, and sodium chloride in varying quantities.

Hair

A hair follicle is an invagination of the epidermis, extending at an angle into the dermis. Hair cells form the hair matrix in the bulb. They divide, differentiate, and form a keratinized hair shaft, pushing hair outward at an average rate of 1 cm per month. Melanocytes in the matrix determine hair color.

Tiny, light-colored vellus hairs grow over most body surfaces. Terminal hairs acquire special characteristics at different sites, including the scalp, eyebrow, eyelash, beard, axilla, trunk, extremities, and pubis. Terminal hair, especially scalp hair, contributes to cosmetic appearance and self-image.

Individual hair follicles grow in cycles with an anagen, or growth, phase and telogen, or resting phase. In scalp hair, the anagen phase lasts approximately 6 years and the telogen phase lasts approximately 4 months. Normally 50 to 100 hairs are shed from the scalp each day, with 80% to 90% of scalp hair in the anagen phase and 10% to 20% in the telogen phase. Diffuse hair loss may not be noticed until 50% of the hair is lost.

Testosterone influences hair growth in males and females in curious ways. It stimulates beard growth in males and hair growth in the axillae and groin in both sexes at puberty; yet testosterone also causes scalp baldness.

Nails

Nails form from a matirx of dividing epidermal cells (keratin). The matrix lies under the proximal nail fold, extending under the nail plate and appearing as the lunula. The nail bed produces keratin, which adheres to the nail plate. Blood vessels in the dermis cause the pink color in the nail bed. The stratum corneum at the proximal nail fold (eponychium) forms the cuticle. The hyponychium lies under the free distal edge of the nail plate, producing stratum corneum that forms a cuticle at the distal nail bed and plate.

Fingernails grow at a rate of approximately 0.1 mm per day. Toenails grow more slowly. Nails range in thickness from 0.3 mm to 0.65 mm.

Nails reflect local stresses. Persistent occupational trauma thickens nails. Nail biting doubles the growth rate.

The specific function of each skin component is presented in Table 6–1.

Table 6–1. FUNCTIONS OF SPECIFIC SKIN STRUCTURES

STRUCTURE	FUNCTION
Epidermis	Barrier
Stratum corneum	Physical
Melanocytes	Light
Langerhans' cells	Immunologic
Dermis	
Connective tissue	Support and elasticity
Cellular elements	Forms collagen, immunologic
Subcutaneous fat	
Connective tissue	Support
Lipocyte	Manufactures and stores fat energy
Fat	Insulation from cold and trauma
Glands	
Sebaceous gland	Forms sebum
Apocrine gland	Unknown except mammary glands
Eccrine sweat gland	Temperature regulation
Hair	Decorative
Nails	Grasp
Blood vessels	Nourishment, temperature regulation
Nerves	Sensation

Data from Lookingbill D, Marks JG Jr. Principles of dermatology. Philadelphia: WB Saunders, 1986.

Clinical Manifestations of Skin Disease

Alteration of Skin Color

The normal components of skin color are brown, yellow, red, and blue.

Generalized hyperpigmentation is the term for a generalized increase in the brown component of skin color. Generalized hyperpigmentation resulting from increased production of melanin-stimulating hormone is sometimes seen as a bronzing of the skin in Addison's disease.

Generalized erythroderma is caused by vasodilation of the arterioles and capillaries in the papillary dermis and increased oxyhemoglobin, the red component of skin color. The red color of oxyhemoglobin is more readily apparent in areas such as the lips where the stratum corneum is absent.

Vasoconstriction decreases capillary blood flow, resulting in a pale or ashen skin color. Pallor is more apparent in the palms, soles, head, and neck areas, where the cutaneous arterial flow and capillary perfusion is high.

Cyanosis gives the skin a blue appearance. It occurs when the blood contains 5 g/100 ml or more of reduced hemoglobin. The more brown pigment in the skin, the less apparent the reduced hemoglobin or blue color.

Alteration of Skin Turgor

Skin turgor is the resiliency of the skin caused by the outward pressure of cells and intercellular fluid. Alteration in skin turgor can be determined by gently pinching the skin. If it does not return to normal position immediately, then skin turgor is decreased. Causes of decreased turgor include dehydration, edema, and normal aging. Skin with decreased turgor is at greater risk for breakdown than skin with normal turgor.

Alteration of Skin Temperature

Surface temperature varies over different parts of the body. Normally, skin temperature is between that of the body core (temperature of the internal organs) and the temperature of the surrounding environment, or approximately 95°F (35°C). Body-surface temperature can vary as much as 20° to 40°C without damage. A local skin temperature of 65°F (18°C) or lower or 113°F (45°C) or higher is associated with body pain or injury.

Cooler skin results from evaporation of sweat. Vasoconstriction can also lower the skin temperature, especially in the extremities. Warmer skin temperature can result from heat, stress, and vasodilation.

The actual temperature of the skin is rarely recorded. In most patient-care situations, it is sufficient to document assessment of skin temperature by describing it as warm to touch or cool to touch, by comparing the temperature of symmetric body parts, and by noting whether this temperature is generalized or localized.

Alteration of Skin Sensation

Alteration in skin sensation is a subjective assessment of skin integrity. It involves asking the patient how the skin feels. Descriptive terms include itching, burning, pain, decreased sensation, numbness, tingling, and hot or cold.

The most common symptom by far in dermatology is itching, or pruritus.

Pruritus results from stimulation of itch receptors located at the junction of the epidermis and the dermis. It can be caused by skin disease or internal disease, or it may be idiopathic. Systemic diseases that can cause pruritus include diabetes mellitus; renal, liver, and thyroid disorders; and anemia. It can also be caused by cancer, and there are theories that symptoms of itching may precede a malignancy by 2 years. Pruritus may also be due to medications; contact with perfumes, soaps, wool, and other substances; radiation therapy; or dry skin. When the cause is unknown, a medical workup is sometimes performed to rule out internal disease and malignancy.

Pruritus, which is often worse at night, leads to scratching, which in turn can result in redness, excoriations, infection, and changes in pigment.

Alteration of Skin Components: Skin Lesions

TYPES OF LESIONS

MACULE

A macule is a flat lesion characterized by a change in skin color resulting from either a change in the pigment-forming cells (melanocytes) or a change in vascularity. There is no change in the texture of the skin surface (Fig. 6–3*A*). A depigmented lesion appears white because there are no melanocytes. Hypopigmented lesions are lighter than normal skin because of a decreased production of melanin.

Hyperpigmented lesions such as ephelides (freckles) contain fewer melanocytes than adjacent pale skin, but these melanocytes have the capacity to form melanin faster than nonfreckled areas. The hyperpigmentation in a café au lait spot results from melanocytes lying nearer to the surface of the skin than the basal layer. In the blue hyperpigmentation of a mongolian spot, the melanocytes are deeper than normal, lying within the dermis. The blue color is due to the scattering of light as it passes through the dermis and is called the Tyndall phenomenon.

Erythematous macules are flat, red lesions caused by a temporary dilation of capillaries or by a permanent vascular disorder. They blanch with pressure and on diascopy (p. 164). Drug eruptions and viral exanthems, such as measles, are common causes of transitory capillary dilation. Capillary hemangiomas are vascular abnormalities that appear as macular patches (nevus flammeus). Strawberry hemangiomas are bright red, rapidly expanding capillary hemangiomas, the majority of which subsequently undergo complete regression.

Petechiae, purpura, and ecchymoses are skin lesions caused by red blood cells that have extravasated or leaked out into the tissue. These lesions do not blanch with pressure or on diascopy. Size is the distinguishing characteristic of these lesions. Petechiae are pinpoint red lesions that are smaller than purpura. An ecchymosis (black and blue mark) is larger than purpura.

Telangiectasias are small, permanently dilated blood vessels. They may appear alone or as part of another lesion (Fig. 6–3*B*). Telangiectasias blanch with pressure and on diascopy.

PAPULE

A papule is a raised palpable lesion that is less than 1 cm in breadth (Fig. 6–3*C*). It may involve the epidermis, dermis, or both. Pathophysiologic changes resulting in papular lesions include inflammation, vascular changes, accumulation of epidermal cells in the dermis, thickening of the stratum corneum, and destruction of cells with accumulation of cell remnants. Warts and raised moles are examples of papules.

PLAQUE

A plaque (Fig. 6–3*D*) is a raised lesion that is larger in diameter than a papule but not deeper. Because it is superficial, plaque is usually considered to be formed by an epidermal process. Plaques occur in disorders such as psoriasis and seborrheic keratosis.

NODULE

A nodule (Fig. 6–3*E*) is a raised, solid mass. It is deeper than a papule and is due either to changes in the epidermis or to proliferative events in the dermis.

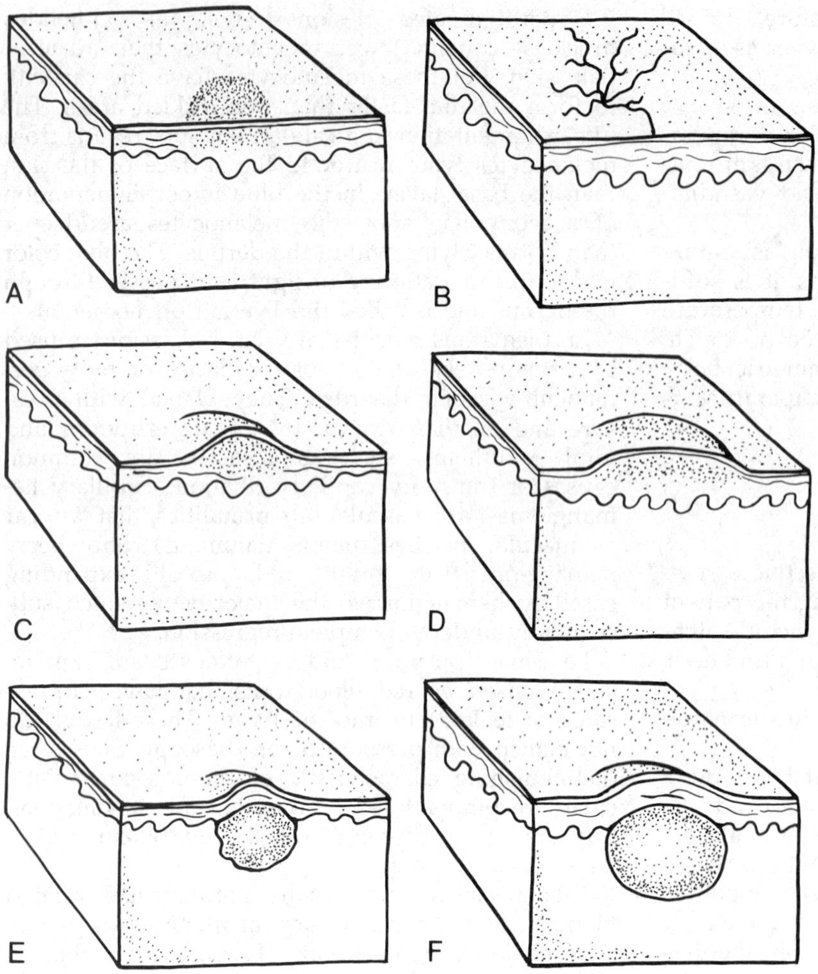

Figure 6–3.

Types of skin lesions. *A,* Macule; *B,* telangiectasia; *C,* papule; *D,* plaque; *E,* nodule; *F,* cyst.

CYST

A cyst is similar to a nodule, but, instead of being solid, it is filled with liquid or semisolid expressible material (Fig. 6–3*F*). A sebaceous cyst is filled with material from the sebaceous glands and hair follicles.

TUMOR

A tumor is larger than a nodule and can be benign or malignant. Tumors of the skin are composed of cells having the same origin as the cells that make up the different structures and tissues of normal skin. For example, a basal cell skin tumor originates in the basal cells of the epidermis. A melanoma arises from melanocytes. Some tumors on the skin result from metastases of internal malignancies.

PUSTULE

A pustule (Fig. 6–3*G*) is a cavity filled with pus (white cells, debris, and microorganisms and their products). Pustules are usually caused by infection, but some may be sterile. Pustules are common in acne.

ABSCESS

An abscess is a circumscribed, walled-off cavity filled with various proportions of pus and serosanguineous fluid. A skin abscess is usually caused by a staphylococcal infection. It can be superficial or deep.

WHEAL

A wheal (hive, urticaria) is a transient, irregularly shaped elevation of the skin. It is caused by a vascular reaction in which vasodilation causes erythema or redness (Fig. 6–3*H*). Fluid leaks diffusely out of the blood vessels into the tissue, causing edema in the dermis. The fluid contains no red blood cells, and there is no free fluid. Wheals may look like tiny papules or giant erythematous plaques.

VESICLES AND BULLAE

Vesicles (Fig. 6–3*I*) and bullae (blisters) (Fig. 6–3*J*) are lesions with cavities that contain free fluid. The fluid flows out when the cavity wall is ruptured. A bulla is larger than a vesicle.

Vesicles or bullae may arise just below the stra-

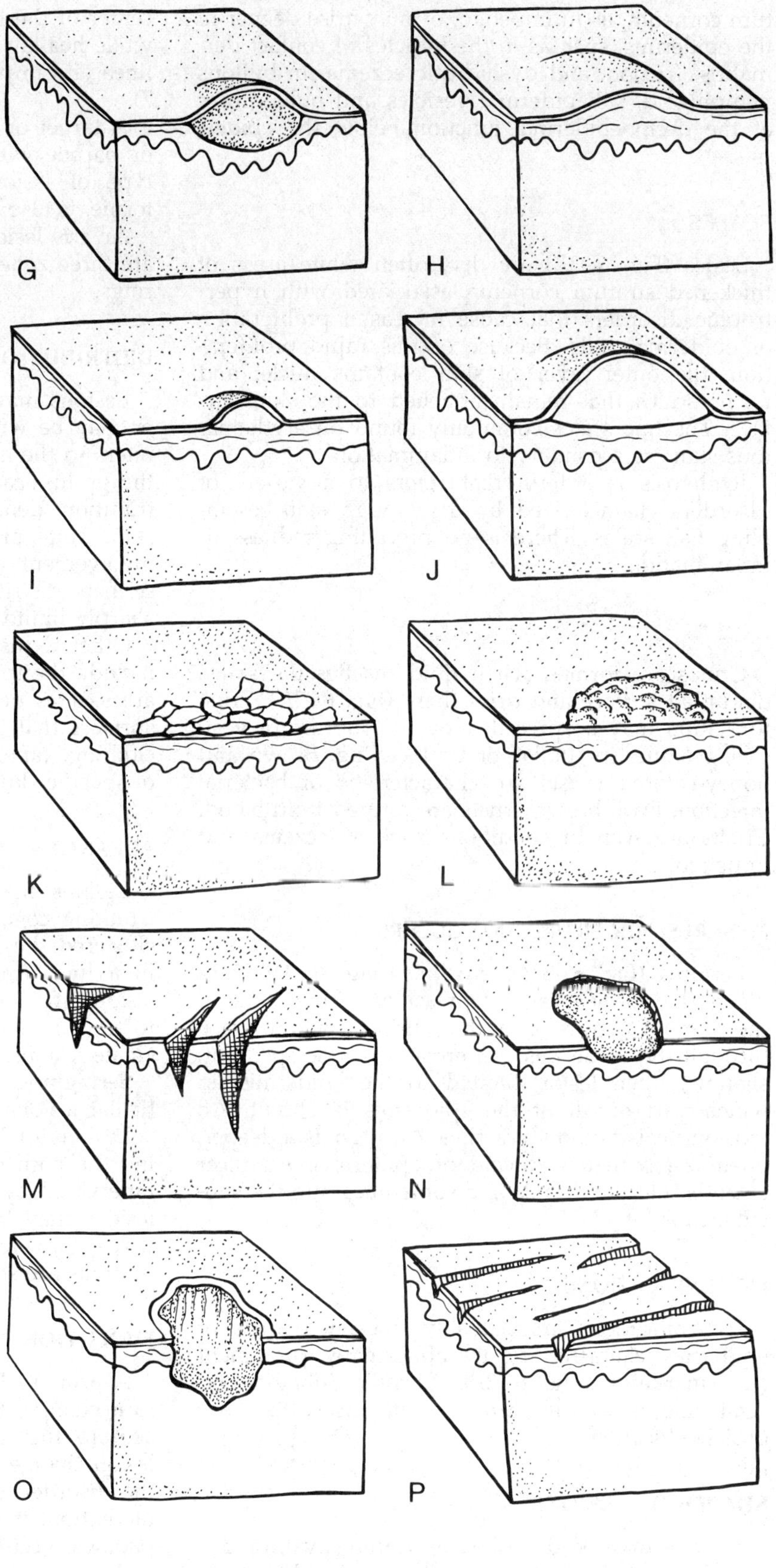

Figure 6–3 (continued).

G, pustule; *H*, wheal; *I*, vesicle; *J*, bulla; *K*, scales; *L*, crust; *M*, fissures; *N*, erosion; *O*, ulcer; *P*, lichenification.

tum corneum, as in impetigo, or may arise deeper in the epidermis, such as in the vesicles of contact dermatitis, friction, and dyshidrotic eczema. In bullous pemphigoid, subepidermal vesicles and bullae form at the dermoepidermal junction below the epidermis.

SCALES

Scales (Fig. 6–3*K*) are dry, often white areas of thickened stratum corneum associated with hypertrophic disorders that cause increased proliferation of epidermal cells. Because of this rapid proliferation, the outer layer of skin contains nuclei and forms scales that remain attached to the skin surface. The fine scales commonly found on erythematous skin are secondary to inflammation.

Ichthyosis is a term that refers to a variety of disorders characterized by dry, rough skin resembling fish scales. There is no preceding redness or inflammation.

CRUSTS

Crusts are formed when fluid reaches the skin's disrupted surface and dries there (Fig. 6–3*L*). Crust formation may be preceded by the rupture of vesicles, pustules, or bullae or by bleeding. Brown and honey-colored crusts are characteristic of bacterial infection. Dark brown crusts are formed from blood. Crusts are seen in conditions such as eczema and impetigo.

FISSURES, EROSIONS, AND ULCERS

Fissures (Fig. 6–3*M*), erosions (Fig. 6–3*N*), and ulcers (Fig. 6–3*O*) leave depressions in the plane of the skin. A fissure is a thin, linear rent or crack through the epidermis. An erosion is a scraped-out, shallow, open lesion limited to the epidermis, in which part or all of the epidermis is absent. An erosion heals without scarring. An ulcer is a deeper, open lesion that is devoid of epidermis. An ulcer extends into the dermis and sometimes into the subcutaneous fat.

LICHENIFICATIONS

Lichenifications are palpably thickened areas of epidermis characterized by abnormally prominent skin markings (Fig. 6–3*P*). Chronic rubbing and scratching as seen in chronic dermatitis is the cause of lichenifications.

SHAPES OF LESIONS

Lesions may be described as round, oval, or discoid, elongated or tubular, and irregular. There are also ring-shaped lesions that are described as annular. An annular lesion begins to develop in the center of the ring and then spreads to the periphery while healing in the center. These lesions are seen in tinea and impetigo infections (see figures in Chapter 7).

A target or bull's-eye lesion is an annular macule or papule with a purplish or vesicular center. This type of lesion, which occurs in erythema multiforme, is also illustrated in Chapter 7.

An iris lesion resembles the iris of the eye. There are three zones of color change present in concentric rings.

DISTRIBUTION OF LESIONS

Lesions may be localized to one area of the body or may be widely distributed. Regional distribution refers to the area of the body being affected such as the groin, scalp, palms, and soles. Generalized distribution denotes widespread involvement of the skin. Total or universal distribution denotes entire involvement of the hair, skin, and nails. Circumscribed distribution refers to involvement that is sharply limited to a specific area by clean borders.

Other terms used to describe distribution patterns include the following: scattered, symmetric, exposed areas; sites of pressure; intertriginous areas or skin surfaces that touch; areas that are occluded by tight clothing, tape, or dressings; and characteristic sites of specific skin ailments.

ARRANGEMENT OF LESIONS

Lesions may be discrete (separate) or confluent (running together). They may also be grouped or clustered. Lesions described as linear are arranged in a line. Arciform lesions form an arc. Circinate lesions are annular lesions that have grown together to form larger lesions. Polycyclic denotes many circinate lesions.

Serpiginous lesions wind like snakes, whereas reticular lesions are netlike, such as a telangiectasia.

Lesions of herpes zoster are described as following the path of a dermatome (i.e., the area of skin innervated by a single nerve root). Herpes simplex lesions may be described as grouped, clustered, or herpetiform lesions. Lesions with geographic configurations are sometimes seen in psoriasis.

EVOLUTION OF LESIONS

A primary lesion develops without any preceding skin change; that is, it is the initial reaction of the skin to the underlying disorder. When a primary lesion changes in character by natural progression of the disorder, scratching, rubbing, or therapeutic intervention, it becomes a secondary lesion. Macules, papules, nodules, vesicles, bullae, pustules, wheals, plaques, and cysts are primary lesions. Scales, crusts, fissures, ulcers, and excoriations are secondary lesions.

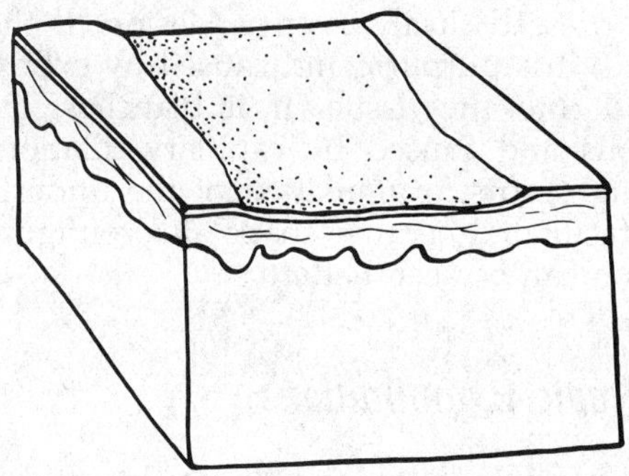

Figure 6–4.

Atrophy.

SCARS

Scars are an alteration in appearance of the skin after repair of an injury with fibrous tissue. In an atrophic, depressed scar, there is too little tissue to fill the healed area completely. Acne is a common cause of atrophic scar formation. Hypertrophic scars contain excess fibrous tissue. They are raised and are usually caused by an injury.

ATROPHY

Skin atrophy results when there is loss of subcutaneous tissue (Fig. 6–4). In epidermal atrophy, there is a decrease in the number of epidermal cells, resulting in an alteration of surface appearance. Although the skin may or may not retain its normal skin lines, they are usually absent. Atrophied skin may be bluish and look like wrinkled cigarette paper.

Dermal atrophy results in a clinically detectable depression in the skin caused by a decrease in the papillary or reticular dermal connective tissue. Dermal atrophy is usually caused by inflammation or injury. If dermal atrophy occurs without epidermal atrophy, the skin is normal in color and markings.

Striae commonly result from stretching of the skin, such as during pregnancy or from obesity. The overstretching results in epidermal and dermal atrophy, with a crinkled appearance of the affected skin and blood vessels seen through it.

Assessment of Skin Status

Patient History

Ask the patient whether he or she is currently experiencing any skin problem; if so, obtain a description. Determine where on the body it began and when and whether it is associated with any other symptoms such as itching, burning, stinging, numbness, fever, sore throat, nausea, vomiting, or diarrhea. Determine what, if any, treatment measures the patient has used and whether the condition has worsened or improved.

Because factors in both the external and internal environment may contribute to dermatologic disorders, explore any factors associated with the onset or worsening of the problem, such as exposure to the sun, heat, cold, stress, or menstruation. Take special care to question the patient about recent changes in laundry products, use of hand and body lotions, and use of birth control pills, contraceptive creams, foams, vaginal tablets, vaginal sponges, and condoms. Explore dietary patterns, and identify any new or rarely eaten foods that have been recently ingested. Review the climates and environments in which the patient has lived and traveled, and explore any possible exposure to chemicals, amount of time spent outdoors exposed to ultraviolet light, and exposure to ionizing radiation therapy. Question the patient as to present and past medical problems, including any known allergies. Identify any prescribed or over-the-counter medication or topical preparation currently used or used in the recent past. Note when any medication was begun, dosage and frequency of administration, and when the last dose was taken.

Determine whether any member of the patient's family has a history of dermatologic disorders. If so, note the type of problem and the relationship of the affected individuals to the patient.

Physical Examination

Physical assessment of the skin includes examination of the skin on all body surfaces, hair, nails, and mucous membrane.

Inspect in good light all areas of the skin and mucous membrane. Observe for color, vascular changes, and breaks or other lesions. Be certain to examine areas between skin folds carefully. If local areas of color variation are present, note the size and location.

Keep in mind that areas of the skin exposed to the sun are generally deeper in color than nonexposed areas. If assessing color in a dark-skinned individual, increase the light to make the reddish hue to undertone characteristic of healthy dark skin more visible. Remember that erythema of dark skin manifests as a purplish to gray tone, that pallor appears as ashen gray to yellow-brown because of the absence of underlying red tones, and that the conjunctivae of dark-skinned people are normally yellow, so the hard palate must be checked for evidence of jaundice. If vascular changes are evident, note location and distribution. Also note their color and size, and palpate for the presence of pulsation. Describe any marks on the skin in terms of location, size, and type of break (e.g., tear, erosion, or ulcer). Note the amount and color of any drainage and any signs of infection. Describe any rashes, papules, nodules, or other lesions in terms of location and appearance. Note the color, size, shape, and distribution of lesions. Palpate to determine whether lesions are flat or elevated and hard or soft. Use a metric ruler to measure size.

Place the back of your hand on the skin surface to check skin temperature. Describe any local variations in temperature, and note affected areas. When palpating, also note skin texture, mobility, and moisture. Note areas of dry, flaky skin or water-logged, macerated skin. Observe for edema, which can make the skin appear taut, shiny, and pale. Check skin turgor, and observe for needle tracks, which can indicate a substance abuse problem.

Assess hair and nails. Note the hair color and distribution. Also note whether the hair is thick or thin and shiny or dull. Observe for dandruff, nits, and other hair or scalp alteration. Inspect the nails, noting configuration, color, and consistency. Remember that the angle between the nail and the base should be 160 degrees and that the base of the nails should be firm on palpation.

Throughout the assessment, note the patient's general hygiene. If hygiene appears to be lacking in one or more areas, observe the patient for mobility or other problems that could indicate a self-care deficit.

Diagnostic Procedures

Diagnostic procedures that aid in the diagnosis of skin disorders include direct examination of the lesions, microscopic examinations, cultures, biopsies, and patch tests. The nurse wears gloves or uses aseptic technique, or both, when collecting specimens for dermatologic examination. Blood tests, urine tests, and x-ray films may be ordered for patients suspected of having a systemic disorder with dermatologic manifestations.

Wood's Light

Wood's light, a hand-held, long-wave, ultraviolet light or black light used in a darkened room occasionally helps in the diagnosis of skin disease. It is used to accentuate pigment changes, especially in fair-skinned persons. It can also demonstrate the presence of certain skin infections that are associated with areas of blue-green or red fluorescence when viewed under the light.

Diascopy

Diascopy helps determine whether a macular or papular lesion is due to either capillary dilation or extravasation of blood into the tissue. A microscope slide is pressed firmly over the lesion. If the lesion stays red, it is purpuric and caused by extravasation of blood into the tissue. If it blanches, it is erythematous and caused by capillary dilation. When blanching occurs, examination of the underlying lesion is facilitated because shape and configuration of the lesion can be seen better.

Microscopic Examinations

Because of the risk of self-contamination or contamination of the lesion, gloves are always worn when collecting specimens for microscopic examination. The patient is advised of the purpose of the examination and of the collection procedure.

POTASSIUM HYDROXIDE MOUNT FOR FUNGAL INFECTIONS

The potassium hydroxide (KOH) mount for fungal infections is a simple office procedure done on most scaling lesions to rule out fungal infection. It may be performed by the physician or an experienced dermatology nurse trained in the technique.

To collect the specimen, scales are scraped from the edge of the lesion onto a glass slide with another glass slide or a scalpel. The scrapings are then treated with KOH and examined under low power with a microscope. The presence of hyphae, characteristic fungal filaments, is diagnostic for fungal infections. The results are documented as KOH (−) or KOH (+).

TZANCK TEST

A Tzanck test is diagnostic for herpes viral infections. A vesicle is opened with a blade, and the fluid contents are scraped onto a glass slide. The specimen is air-dried, fixed with methanol, and stained with Giemsa, Wright's, or toluidine blue stain. The finding of multinucleated giant cells under the microscope is immediately diagnostic for herpes simplex or herpes zoster virus.

OIL MOUNT OF SKIN SCRAPING

An oil mount of skin scraping is done when scabies is suspected but definite burrows cannot be found. Small papules or questionable burrows are scraped vigorously with a blade moistened with mineral oil so that the skin adheres to it. The skin is then transferred to a drop of oil on a glass slide, covered with a coverglass, and examined under the microscope for a scabies mite.

DARKFIELD EXAMINATION

A darkfield microscopic examination is done to diagnose an active syphilis infection. Serous fluid is collected from a suspected chancre or secondary

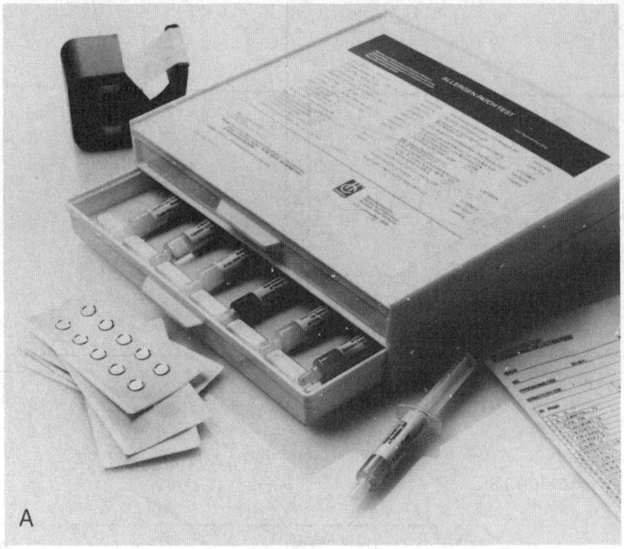

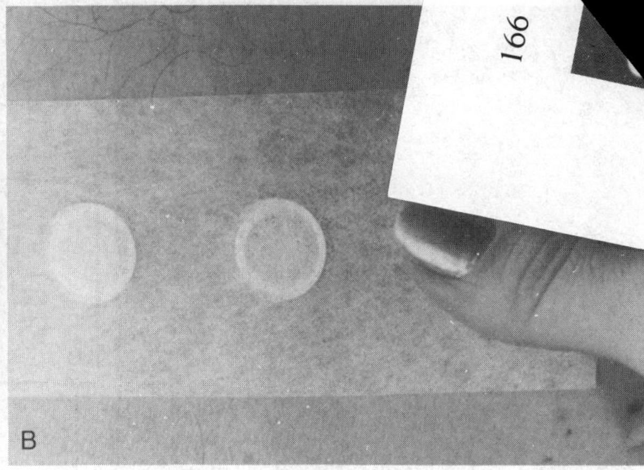

Figure 6–5.

A, Patch test. *B*, Patch test being applied to patient's back. (Courtesy of Hermal Pharmaceutical Laboratories, Delmar, NY.)

syphilis lesion and examined under the microscope. Because a dry specimen cannot be interpreted, it is often collected in the immediate proximity of the laboratory. The darkfield examination is most often performed in venereal clinics.

GRAM'S STAIN

A Gram's stain is done to diagnose bacterial infections. The fluid contents of an intact bulla are examined to diagnose bullous impetigo, and an intact pustule is examined to determine whether the cause of a lesion is bacterial. An intact bulla or pustule can be ruptured to swab contents that have not been contaminated by surface bacteria.

Cultures

Fungal and bacterial cultures confirm and further characterize pathogens.

For fungal cultures, skin scrapings are collected from the surface of a lesion. The scrapings are cultured in a fungal media bottle for 1 to 2 weeks. The growth is then examined grossly and microscopically to identify the fungus.

Bacterial cultures are collected from intact bullae, vesicles, and pustules. The lesion is aseptically punctured, and the exudate is swabbed with a culturette for transport to the microbiology laboratory, where it is cultured and examined.

Patch Test

The patch test identifies allergens responsible for allergic contact dermatitis. It tests delayed Type IV hypersensitivity response to contact allergens. Patch testing is done when the dermatitis persists despite avoidance of likely causative agents and institution of appropriate topical therapy.

The three types of patch test are use, open, and closed. In a use test, the suspected causative agent such as a cream or a cosmetic is applied to an area of the skin distant from the affected area. This is done twice a day for at least 7 days unless a reaction occurs, in which case the test is stopped.

In an open patch test, a suspected allergen is simply applied to the skin on the upper, outer arm twice a day for 2 days.

In a closed patch test, suspected allergenic materials are applied to the skin and covered with an adhesive bandage for 48 hours. Solid materials such as rubber as well as topical medications, cosmetics, and the like can be tested in this way. Results of open and closed patch tests are read as described later.

If the allergen evades identification, a standard patch test series may be performed. For this, a kit that contains 20 allergens in nonirritating concentrations packaged in syringe dispensers is used. Each of the allergens to be tested (may be some or all of the 20) is applied to a patch or other holding device (Fig. 6–5). It is then taped to the skin, preferably on the patient's back, and the perimeter of the test site is outlined with 0.5% gentian violet. The test strips are removed in 48 hours, and an initial reading is done at that time. A second reading is done in 3 to 7 days to check for a delayed reaction. Test reactions are read as follows:

+	Weak, positive reaction characterized by erythema, infiltration, and sometimes papules
++	Strong, positive reaction characterized by edema and vesicles
+++	Extreme positive reaction characterized by spreading bullae and ulcers
–	Negative reaction

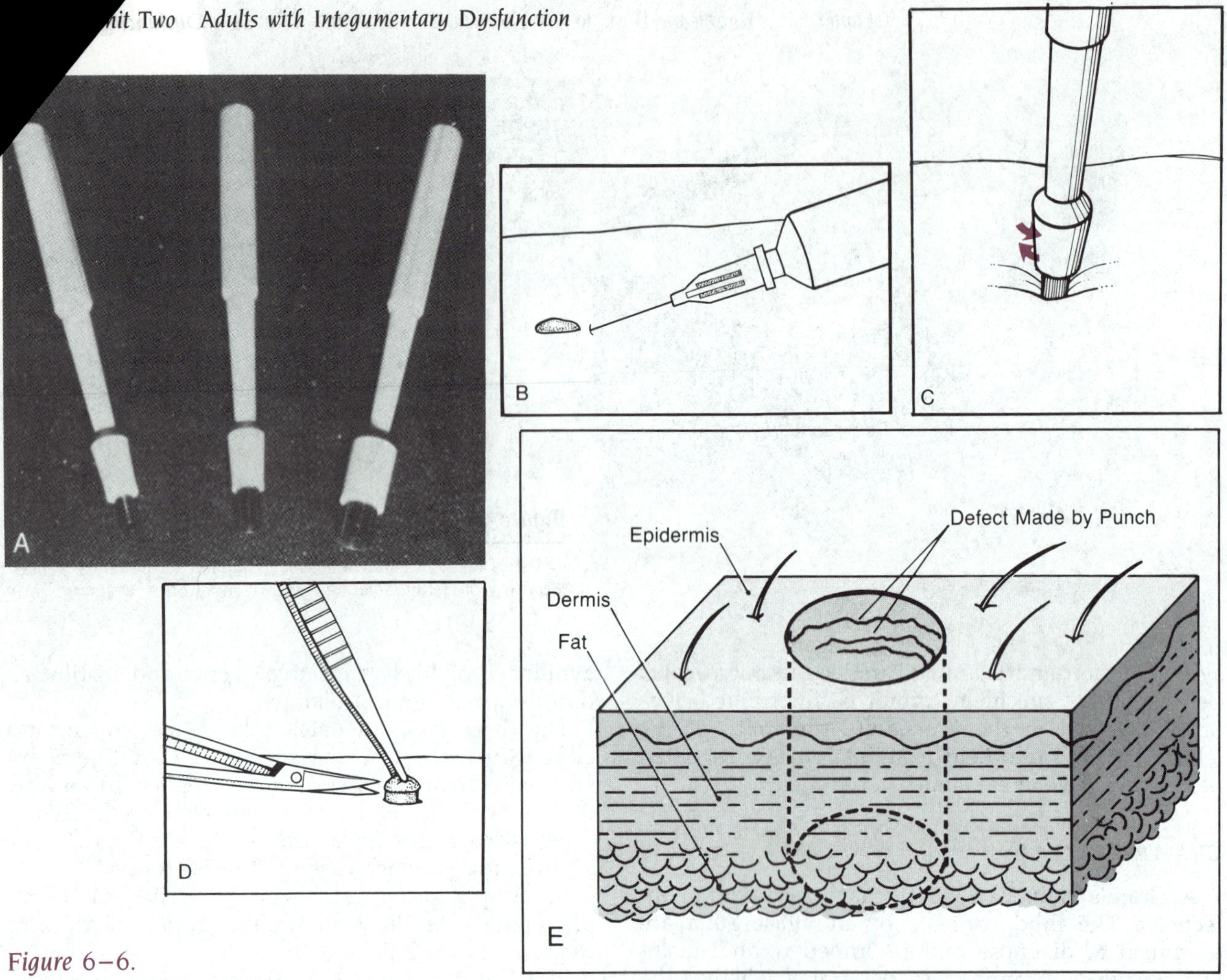

Figure 6–6.

Punch biopsy. *A*, Disposable punch biopsy instruments come in 3 mm, 4 mm, and 6 mm sizes. A #8 nondisposable punch biopsy instrument can be used for larger lesions. *B*, Infiltration of local anesthesia. *C*, Punch biopsy obtained using a pressing, back and forth twisting motion. *D*, Specimen is removed using a forceps and a scissors. *E*, Schematic drawing of the defect made by the punch. (A, from Moschella SL, Hurley HJ. Dermatology. 2nd ed. Philadelphia: WB Saunders, 1985, p 198. E, reprinted with permission, Heilman ER, Friedman RJ, et al: Skin biopsy: Key to diagnosis but beware of pitfalls. Mediguide to Dermatology 1988; 3[1]:4. Copyright © 1988 Lawrence DellaCorte Publications, Inc.)

Skin Biopsies

USES

Skin biopsies are done to obtain skin specimens for microscopic examination and diagnosis of a skin disorder and to determine the stage of a disease process. Biopsies are obtained from fully developed lesions. Primary lesions are preferred.

TYPES OF SKIN BIOPSY

The types of biopsies commonly done in dermatology are punch biopsies, shave biopsies, and excision biopsies. The type of biopsy is determined by the physician's preference and by the location and type of lesion. An excision biopsy is done whenever malignant melanoma or deep inflammatory disease is suspected. Shave biopsies are done on raised, superficial lesions other than malignant melanoma, and punch biopsies are appropriate for any superficial lesion, whether inflammatory, bullous, or neoplastic, with the exception of melanoma.

PROCEDURE

Biopsy procedures may be performed in the physician's office or in an ambulatory surgery clinic.

In all biopsy procedures, the area around the lesion is cleansed with an appropriate antibacterial agent, and the site is marked with a skin-marking pen. Hair may also be shaved from the area. A 30-gauge needle is used to inject local anesthetic around the site

PUNCH BIOPSY

A punch biopsy is illustrated in Figure 6–6. To obtain the specimen, a skin punch, which looks like a very-large-bore needle, is pressed into the skin at a 90-degree angle using a rotary motion. The specimen is lifted gently and snipped off at the level of the subcutaneous fat. Hemostasis is achieved with absorbable gelatin sponge (Gelfoam) packing, electrodesiccation, or aluminum chloride 35% in isopropyl alcohol 50% applied with a cotton-tipped applicator. The wound from a punch biopsy has smooth,

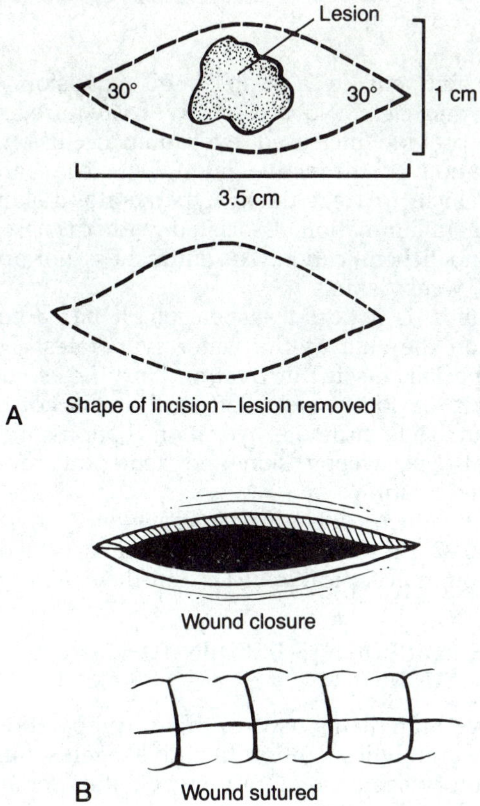

Figure 6–7.

A, The design of the standard ellipsoidal scalpel excision with a length-to-width ratio of axes of 3.5:1. The apical angles should be 30 degrees. B, Wound closure with suture (side-to-side approximation).

round edges and heals well by secondary intention, leaving a slightly depressed scar that is cosmetically acceptable. A punch-biopsy wound may be sutured, but, although healing is faster than by secondary intention, the wound margins do not approximate well.

SHAVE BIOPSY

To obtain a specimen by shave biopsy, a wheal is first raised in the skin by injecting local anesthetic intradermally under the lesion. The lesion is then shaved with a no. 15 blade to obtain the specimen.

EXCISION BIOPSY

An excision biopsy is obtained under local anesthesia by the physician, who uses a scalpel to remove an elliptic section of involved skin (Fig. 6–7). The surgical wound is sutured closed.

Guidelines for Application of the Nursing Process to the Care of the Patient Having a Skin Biopsy

Before the procedure, question the patient regarding allergies to local anesthetics, topical anesthetics, or topical skin preparations. Assess the patient's understanding of the procedure and anxiety level concerning it. Allow the patient to express concerns and ask questions. Clarify the patient's understanding of the purpose of the biopsy and the procedure involved. Reassure the patient that skin biopsy is a minor procedure, complications are rare, and scarring is minimal. Instruct the patient in self-care as presented in Chart 6–1. Make provisions for the patient to obtain biopsy results: Make certain he or she knows whether to call, to expect a telephone call, or to return for a follow-up visit. Also explain when and by whom the patient will be informed of the results.

Chart 6–1.

NURSING GUIDE TO PATIENT EDUCATION FOR SELF-MANAGEMENT: SELF-CARE AFTER SKIN BIOPSY

Instruct the patient to:

Keep dressing dry and intact for at least 8 hours.
Leave site open to air after initial dressing is removed unless cover is needed for cosmetic appearance or if located in area prone to contamination.
Clean biopsy site three times per day with cotton-tipped applicator and hydrogen peroxide after removal of initial dressing.
Apply topical antibiotic ointment as ordered by physician.
Report erythema or excessive drainage.
Return for suture removal on *(specify date if needed).*

Medical Management

Nonsurgical Management

PHARMACOLOGIC THERAPY

Pharmacologic therapy in dermatology may be topical, intralesional, or systemic, or a combination of these. Topical administration is the most widely used. Topical preparations deliver medication directly to the involved area of the skin. They are safer than systemic therapy but are often time-consuming, expensive, and aesthetically unpleasant and may require a large volume of medication.

Topical medications must be absorbed percutaneously to be effective. Absorption is influenced by the active ingredient, the concentration of the active ingredient, the vehicle or substance that contains the active ingredient, and the condition of the integument to which the topical agent is applied. The active ingredient in a topical preparation is the chemical substance that is responsible for its effects.

VEHICLES USED IN TOPICAL PREPARATIONS

Vehicles used in topical agents are therapeutically inactive substances that contain the active ingredient. The most common vehicles are emollients, creams, ointments, and lotions.

Emollients are skin softeners such as mineral oil, white petrolatum, lanolin, paraffins, glycerin, and urea. They increase hydration of the stratum corneum by trapping water particles on the skin. Emollients allow scales to fall off the skin by decreasing the binding forces within the horny layers. Emollients are used in the treatment of dry skin, psoriasis, eczema, and pruritus. They can cause folliculitis by occluding hair follicles.

A cream is an oil-in-water emulsion. It is white and nongreasy and vanishes when rubbed into the skin. Parabens and formaldehyde preservatives are added to creams to prevent the growth of bacteria and fungi. The preservatives can cause allergic-contact dermatitis. Creams are used to treat subacute inflammation. They are usually the preferred vehicle for applying steroids to the face, underarms, and groin.

An ointment is a water-in-oil emulsion. It is greasy and clear. No preservative is required. Ointments provide increased hydration, occlusion, and penetration of the active ingredient. They are the best vehicle to treat thick, hyperkeratotic skin and chronic inflammation associated with dryness, scaling, and lichenification. An ointment is not applied to wet, weepy skin.

A lotion is a liquid suspension. It has a cooling effect on the skin as the water evaporates. Lotions are especially useful in treating hairy areas such as the scalp. A lotion wears off easily. It is not useful as a barrier to promote hydration. Lotions are used to treat wet, weepy skin and acute inflammation with vesiculation.

Other vehicles include gels, powders, and pastes. Table 6–2 presents a summary comparison of the most common topical vehicles and their uses.

ACTIVE INGREDIENTS USED IN TOPICAL PREPARATIONS

Active ingredients used in topical preparations include keratolytics; antiproliferative agents; anti-inflammatory agents; and antifungal, antibacterial, and antiviral agents.

Keratolytics soften and remove the horny layer of the skin. Salicylic acid 2% to 20% is the most commonly used keratolytic agent. Lactic acid is also keratolytic. These agents can be added to any vehicle and combined with other active ingredients. They are used to treat acne, psoriasis, warts, corns, and calluses.

Crude coal tar (CCT) is an antiproliferative agent that also has antipruritic, astringent, vasoconstrictive, and disinfective properties. It suppresses epidermal deoxyribonucleic acid (DNA) synthesis and enhances ultraviolet B therapy. CCT is dark in color and smells like tar. It stains clothes and linens and can cause scarring of the skin. Lqiuid carbonic detergens (LCD) is a 20% solution of CCT that also stains and scars. Coal tars are used to treat psoriasis, eczemas, and pruritus.

Anthralin is a synthetic coal tar used to treat psoriatic plaques. It is an antiproliferative agent that affects mitochondrial DNA. Low concentrations of 0.01% to 0.05% can be applied and left on the skin. High-dose, short-contact anthralin therapy is effec-

Table 6–2. COMPARISON OF VEHICLES FOR APPLICATION OF TOPICAL MEDICINE

VEHICLE	DESCRIPTION	USE	ADVANTAGES	DISADVANTAGES
Lotion	Oil in water (liquid emulsion)	Acute inflammation; wet, weepy skin with vesiculation; hairy areas, scalp	Cooling effect	Wears off easily; not a barrier; does not promote hydration
Cream	Oil in water (semisolid emulsion)	Subacute inflammation; preferred for face, underarms, groin	Nongreasy	Antibacterial preservatives added; may cause contact dermatitis
Ointment	Water in oil	Chronic inflammation; thick hyperkeratotic skin; dryness, scaling, and lichenification	Provides the most hydration, occlusion, and penetration of active ingredient	Greasy; cannot be used on wet, weepy skin

Table 6–3. TOPICAL CORTICOSTEROID POTENCY

POTENCY	PROPRIETARY NAME	GENERIC NAME	PERCENTAGE
Strong	Temovate	Clobetasol propionate	0.05
	Halog	Halcinonide	0.1
	Lidex	Fluocinonide	0.5
	Diprosone	Betamethasone dipropionate	0.5
	Topicort	Desoximetasone	0.25
Medium	Valisone	Betamethasone valerate	0.1
	Aristocort, Kenalog	Triamcinolone acetonide	0.1
	Synalar	Fluocinolone acetonide	0.025
	Westcort	Hydrocortisone valerate	0.2
Weak	Hytone, Carmol HC	Hydrocortisone	1.0

Adapted from Lookingbill D, Marks JG Jr. Principles of dermatology. Philadelphia: WB Saunders, 1986, p 50.

tive in treating thick plaques. High-dose anthralin is applied in 1% to 3% concentrations to the plaques and removed after 30 minutes to 1 hour.

Anthralin causes irritation to normal skin. Caution must be used to ensure that the medicine is applied only to the area being treated. White petrolatum applied to the normal skin around the plaques before applying anthralin protects uninvolved skin. Anthralin stains clothes and the bathtub. Anthralin treatment is usually administered in in-patient settings or in psoriasis treatment centers, but it can be self-administered at home if the patient understands how to apply the medicine and the implications of staining and damage to normal skin.

TOPICAL AND SYSTEMIC PREPARATIONS

Corticosteroids

Topical steroid preparations are antiproliferative and anti-inflammatory. They provide high therapeutic benefit with little toxicity. However, most potent steroids can cause significant local and systemic side effects. Systemic side effects can occur when a strong preparation of a topical steroid is absorbed into the system through the skin or mucous membrane. Weak topical steroid preparations rarely cause systemic or local side effects. Table 6–3 lists topical steroids in categories by potency.

The vehicle affects the potency of the steroid. The vehicle is selected on the basis of its occlusive property and according to the presenting condition of the skin. The vehicle is changed as the skin condition progresses from acute to chronic.

Topical steroids are usually applied twice daily. Because the stratum corneum becomes a reservoir for the steroid and continues to release it into the skin after initial application, a thin application provides the same benefit as a thick application.

Topical steroids are absorbed more readily when applied to the mucous membrane, mouth, scrotum, eyelids, and face. Penetration is decreased on the lower arms and legs and dorsa of the hands and feet. The nails, palms, and soles do not readily absorb the drug. The topical steroid must penetrate into the dermis to be effective.

Side effects can be avoided by using no more than 50 g (20 oz) of a potent steroid per week. Side effects include skin atrophy, striae, telangiectasis, glaucoma and cataracts when applied around the eyes, and perioral dermatitis (acne eruption around the mouth). Cushing's syndrome is rare but has been reported as a side effect with chronic, excessive use of potent topical steroids applied over large areas of skin and usually covered by an occlusive substance such as plastic wrap.

Hydrocortisone cream 0.5% has no side effects and can be purchased over the counter. Hydrocortisone cream 1% is also safe and can also be purchased over the counter.

Intralesional corticosteroid therapy is used to treat keloids and to provide prolonged anti-inflammatory effects in a localized lesion. The corticosteroid is injected into the lesion by the physician with a 30-gauge, half-inch needle or with a pressure jet. The patient may have some pain at the injection site similar to that felt on injection of a local anesthetic by the dentist.

Systemic corticosteroids may be administered orally, intramuscularly, or intravenously for acute dermatitis.

Antibacterials

Systemic antibiotics are used to treat bacterial skin infections. Tetracycline and erythromycin are the most common antibiotics used in dermatology.

Local antibiotics are applied two to four times daily to treat minor local infections or to prevent wound infections. Their efficacy in treating existing infections is questionable.

Chlorhexidine gluconate (Hibiclens) is an antiseptic, antimicrobial skin cleanser with bactericidal activity. It is the preferred anti-infective agent to treat skin infections. It is effective against gram-negative and gram-positive bacteria.

Povidone-iodine (Betadine) is also effective against gram-negative and gram-positive bacteria, but local skin sensitivity is more common than with Hibiclens.

Hexachlorophene (pHisoHex) is effective against

gram-positive bacteria. It has been found to cause neurotoxicity and cannot be applied to mucous membrane or to any open-skin lesions.

Antifungals

Most cutaneous dermatophyte and yeast infections can be treated with topical antifungal agents such as imidazole carboxamide creams applied twice daily until 2 weeks after the infection is clinically clear. Nystatin and nystatin with corticosteroids (Mycolog) are effective in treating yeast infections but not dermatophytes.

Griseofulvin is a systemic fungistatic antibiotic used to treat dermatophyte infections of the scalp and nails and, sometimes, generalized skin infections. It is administered in daily doses of 500 mg orally for 4 to 6 weeks to treat tinea capitis and 1 g daily for 12 months or more to treat toenail infections. Griseofulvin may cause hematologic, renal, and hepatic toxicity. Periodic blood studies and evaluation of renal and hepatic function are recommended.

Antivirals

Acyclovir is used in the treatment of herpes simplex virus (HSV) infections. Acyclovir 5% ointment is applied topically in initial herpes infections and to genital and localized, cutaneous HSV infections in immunocompromised patients to decrease healing time, viral shedding, and duration of pain. It may also decrease viral shedding in recurrent HSV infections. Intravenous acyclovir is indicated in the treatment of severe primary herpes simplex, neonatal herpes, and herpes simplex and herpes zoster infections in immunocompromised patients. Oral acyclovir is effective against primary and recurrent HSV infections.

Retinoids

Retinoids are derivatives of vitamin A. They have a direct effect on the growth and differentiation of keratinizing epithelium. Retinoids are used primarily to treat cystic acne and psoriasis.

Isotretinoin (Accutane) is a highly toxic retinoid administered orally for the treatment of severe recalcitrant cystic acne. It inhibits sebaceous gland function and keratinization. A course of therapy consists of 0.5 to 2 mg/kg body weight divided into two doses daily for 15 to 20 weeks.

Isotretinoin is teratogenic. It must not be given to pregnant females because major human fetal abnormalities have been reported. Patients are advised not to become pregnant for at least 3 months after discontinuing therapy. Pregnancy tests are required in women of childbearing age before initiating therapy, and birth-control measures should be adhered to during treatment. Other significant adverse effects include intracranial hypertension, corneal opacities, inflammatory bowel disease, hypertriglyceridemia, musculoskeletal symptoms, and cheilitis (dermatitis of the lip). Isotretinoin should be prescribed only by dermatologists. Transient exacerbation of acne sometimes occurs in the early treatment period.

Etretinate is an oral systemic retinoid that is effective in treating pustular, joint, palmar-plantar, and erythrodermic psoriasis. Studies in Europe have shown it to be effective in combination with psoralen plus ultraviolet A (PUVA) treatments (p. 172) for plaque psoriasis. Etretinate is teratogenic and hepatotoxic. No safe time has been established for pregnancy after discontinuing the drug.

Tretinoin (Retin-A) is a topical retinoid used in the treatment of acne vulgaris and comedones (blackheads). It is available as a cream, gel, or solution. Tretinoin stimulates mitotic activity and increases turnover of follicular epithelial cells, causing extrusion of comedones. It is applied once daily at bedtime. Patients may experience a temporary exacerbation of their condition because of the action of the medication on deep, unseen lesions. Inform patients that erythema and desquamation (peeling) are expected during the first 1 to 3 weeks of therapy. Patients should stay out of sunlight or use a sun protection factor (SPF) 15 sunscreen during treatment because of increased sensitivity to ultraviolet rays.

Antimetabolites

Antimetabolites inhibit DNA synthesis in cells and are used as antiproliferative agents in treating dermatologic conditions. Methotrexate is used to treat psoriasis. It is usually given by mouth in three divided doses over 2 days weekly. Laboratory studies to determine the effect of methotrexate on lymphocytes and renal and liver function are done frequently during the course of treatment. Liver biopsies are also done before initiating treatment and periodically while undergoing treatment. The patient must abstain from alcohol to prevent liver damage.

Fluorouracil is an antimetabolite used to treat multiple actinic keratosis and superficial basal cell carcinoma. It is available in a cream or solution. Clinically apparent lesions and subclinical lesions undergo selective inflammatory response during treatment. Normal skin does not become inflamed as a result of application of topical fluorouracil. The inflammatory response progresses through stages of erythema, vesiculation, erosion, ulceration, and necrosis if the medication is continued. A course of therapy for actinic keratosis is usually 2 to 4 weeks or until the response reaches the erythema stage. The arms may require 6 to 8 weeks of treatment.

The patient is closely monitored to assess when an adequate response is achieved. Gloves are worn to apply fluorouracil, and caution is used when applying it around the eyes, nose, and mouth.

Antihistamines

Hydroxyzine hydrochloride (Atarax) is a systemic antihistamine used to treat pruritus. As much as 25 to 50 mg by mouth four times daily or 25 to 50 mg at bedtime, or both, is administered to treat severe itching. The patient can take another dose during the night if he or she becomes uncomfortable. Precautions must be taken so the patient is not oversedated, and the patient should not take the medicine during the day if driving or working.

Hydroxyzine hydrochloride (Atarax) and diphenhydramine hydrochloride (Benadryl) are prescribed for histamine-mediated allergic skin disorders such as urticaria. Benadryl is not as effective as Atarax in treating pruritus.

Sun Sensitizers

Methoxsalen, a psoralen derivative, is used to increase skin sensitivity to ultraviolet A (UVA) light in the treatment of vitiligo and psoriasis. It is taken in 30- to 60-mg doses 2 hours before PUVA therapy. The patient is instructed to wear UVA-blocking glasses indoors and outdoors for 24 hours after ingesting psoralen and to avoid sun exposure.

Psoralen is sometimes used to treat vitiligo in natural sunlight.

Sunscreens

A sunscreen blocks out the sun's burning ultraviolet rays and allows the skin to tan gradually. It is applied to sun-exposed areas of the skin before going outdoors and reapplied after swimming or heavy perspiration. The ratio between the amount of sun exposure to cause redness with and without a sunscreen is the SPF. SPF is always listed on the sunscreen bottle. The Skin Cancer Foundation grants its seal of acceptance to products of SPF 15, which meet the criteria to aid in the prevention of sun-induced damage to the skin. SPF 15 is appropriate for all skin types. Table 6–4 lists the sun-reactive skin types used in dermatology practice.

Table 6–4. CLASSIFICATION OF SUN-REACTIVE SKIN TYPES USED IN DERMATOLOGY PRACTICE

TYPE	DESCRIPTION
I	Always burn, never tan (often have red hair, blue eyes, of Irish ancestry)
II	Always burn, sometimes tan (blonde, brunette; blue or brown eyes)
III	Always tan, rarely burn
IV	Always tan, never burn (Mediterranean)
V	Asian
VI	Black

Note: To assess skin type, ask patients if they burned or tanned as a child on the first day they spent outdoors in the sun each summer.

TOPICAL TREATMENTS

Water is one of the most important therapeutic agents in dermatology. Dry skin is due to a lack of water in the stratum corneum. The keratinocytes in the stratum corneum are capable of absorbing vast amounts of water.

BATHS

Therapeutic baths are soothing, antipruritic, cleansing, relaxing, hydrating, debriding, and anti-inflammatory. Topical medicines and ultraviolet therapies penetrate the skin more deeply if the skin is hydrated and debrided before treatment.

To hydrate the skin, the patient soaks in plain, warm water of approximately 96° to 103°F (35°–39°C) for 20 minutes once or twice daily. The entire body, up to the neck, is immersed. Underarms, groin, and feet can be washed with soap and water at the end of the bath. After the bath, pat the skin dry. An ointment such as white petrolatum is applied to damp, dry skin to hold the water in the skin.

A similar procedure is used to debride scaling skin. After 20 to 30 minutes in the bath, the patient uses a soft cloth to gently debride the buildup of scales. The water temperature may be as high as 103°F (30°C) for patients with psoriasis.

Cool-water baths are antipruritic. The same procedure is followed for antipruritic baths as for hydrating baths. For patients with acute dermatitis, the water temperature should be 96°F (35°C).

CCT baths are antieczematous and antipruritic and increase photosensitivity. Two capfuls of CCT are added to 6 to 8 inches of bath water or as prescribed.

Starch baths and Aveeno Colloidal Oatmeal are soothing and antipruritic for generalized itching, dry skin, winter itching, and urticaria.

Bath oils may relieve itching and dryness. They should be added to the bath after 20 minutes of soaking in plain water. If added earlier, the oil may prevent the stratum corneum from absorbing water but, when added after 20 minutes, it acts as a barrier to hold the water in the stratum corneum. The patient is cautioned to use care not to slip in the bathtub.

WET DRESSINGS

Wet dressings are prescribed to treat acute inflammation, oozing, crusting, and itching. They may be prescribed for psoriasis, eczematous dermatitis, and sunburn.

Water is the most important agent used in wet dressings. Active ingredients used in wet dressings include potassium permanganate, Burow's solution, and silver nitrate. Gauze pads, wraparound gauze, cotton sheets torn into smaller sizes, towels, or old T-shirts can be used to apply wet dressings. The fabric is soaked in water or other prescribed agent and then applied to the skin for 15 to 30 minutes. An occlusive wrap is never applied over a wet dressing. Special masks, gloves, and cotton socks to treat the face, hands, and feet can be purchased or improvised.

OCCLUSIVE DRESSINGS

Occlusive dressings may be prescribed to enhance the action of keratolytics and, occasionally, other topical preparations. An occlusive dressing, such as plastic wrap, placed over a topical preparation may enhance penetration of the medication 10 to 100 times. Although deeper penetration of the topical preparation is usually beneficial to the patient, occlusive dressings increase the risk of skin irritation and toxic side effects. This is especially true with topical corticosteroids. Occlusive dressings also interfere with heat exchange and increase the risk of infection and folliculitis. Occlusive dressings should be used only with an order from a dermatologist. The patient and his or her skin condition are frequently monitored for untoward side effects of therapy.

SCALP TREATMENTS

Keratolytic agents are applied to the scalp to debride the scales of psoriasis. The scalp is hydrated under running water for a few minutes before applying the keratolytic agent. Baker's P&S (2% salicylic acid) is an over-the-counter preparation that is keratolytic and can be applied to the scalp to debride scales. Salicylic acid 2% to 10% is also available in an oil base. The oil softens the scales, and the salicylic acid loosens them. The scales can then be gently debrided by lifting them with a soft-tooth comb. This procedure can be repeated for a severe, neglected buildup of scales in psoriasis.

Corticosteroids are applied in a lotion base to erythematous psoriatic lesions on the scalp. Corticosteroids are also indicated in treating eczematous dermatitis and seborrheic dermatitis of the scalp.

RADIATION

Ionizing Radiation

Ionizing radiation therapy is effective in treating basal cell and squamous cell skin cancer. However, it is time-consuming and requires multiple visits over a period of 1 to 2 months. Radiation therapy is a good alternative to surgery for patients unable or unwilling to undergo a surgical procedure and for lesions located in anatomic sites that are difficult to treat surgically. It should not be used in children because of increased risk of future skin cancer from the radiation. The side effects of radiation therapy are discussed in Chapter 11.

Total-body electron-beam radiation is effective in treating the skin lesions of mycosis fungoides. Electron-beam therapy uses electrons instead of photons. The electrons have limited penetration through the skin, so internal organ damage is avoided.

Ultraviolet Radiation

Ultraviolet radiation is effective in treating psoriasis, eczema, uremic pruritus, vitiligo, and mycosis fungoides. Its primary use is the treatment of psoriasis.

Artificial light sources have been developed that emit ultraviolet radiation in the UVB (ultraviolet B) middle-wave spectrum and in the UVA (ultraviolet A) long-wave ultraviolet-light spectrum. These bulbs are arranged in ultraviolet phototherapy cabinets with 12 to 60 bulbs per cabinet. An ultraviolet cabinet may have UVB bulbs, UVA bulbs, or both.

UVB treatment may be combined with tar, anthralin, white petrolatum, or steroid therapy, or a combination of these. A nurse or specially trained phototherapist administers the treatment. The patient wears UVB-blocking goggles during the treatment and keeps the eyes closed. The eyelids do not provide adequate protection from the UVB rays. The patient stands nude in the cabinet and is treated with gradually increasing doses of UVB radiation. Treatments range from a minimum of 30 seconds to a maximum of 20 minutes, with 30- to 60-second increments determined by the individual's response to treatment. Treatments are administered daily or three times weekly until improvement is noted. The nurse inspects the patient before each treatment for untoward reactions such as sunburn, itching, or increased psoriasis. Sunburn-sensitive areas can be covered during treatment, and no treatment is given to sunburned areas. Many patients have a quick response, with remission of as long as 18 months.

PUVA consists of exposure to long-range UVA rays 2 hours after administration of psoralen, a photosensitizing drug. UVA rays promote tanning and are the type of rays used in commercial tanning booths. However, in a tanning booth, patients would not achieve a therapeutic dose because no photosensitizing drug is administered to increase UVA penetration into the skin.

PUVA treatment is administered according to established protocols, with gradual increments at each treatment until the patient shows improvement. When the patient achieves an acceptable clearing of lesions (80%–100%), the number of treatments is tapered to achieve a monthly maintenance schedule. PUVA therapy has improved the quality of life for many psoriasis patients over the past 10 years.

Patients must wear wraparound UVA-blocking glasses indoors and outdoors during daylight hours for 24 to 48 hours after psoralen ingestion to prevent cataract formation. Wraparound UVA-blocking goggles are also worn during the treatment. Patients who have received PUVA therapy are at increased risk for squamous cell carcinoma in sun-exposed areas and are instructed to have periodic skin examinations. Other risks associated with PUVA treatment include itching, pain, blistering sunburn, freckles over the entire body, and hyperpigmentation or total-body tan.

When administering ultraviolet light therapy, consideration is given to the patient's skin type (see Table 6–4). Caution and a conservative approach are used in administering ultraviolet therapy to patients with Type I and Type II skin, who are at higher risk for skin cancer.

Surgical Management

Common surgical procedures in dermatology are the ellipsoidal scalpel excision described previously, curettage and desiccation, cryosurgery, and Mohs' micrographic surgery.

DERMATOLOGIC SURGICAL PROCEDURES

CURETTAGE AND DESICCATION

Uses

Curettage and desiccation (C&D) is the most common procedure used for the removal of early basal cell and squamous cell skin cancers. It is also a valuable treatment in the destruction of the lesions of Bowen's disease, actinic keratosis, skin tags, seborrheic keratosis, nevi, and hemangiomas.

Procedure

Curettage consists of using a sharp curet to remove material from the skin lesion for a biopsy. Curettage is followed by desiccation (electrosurgery or surgical diathermy), which coagulates and destroys tissue through the use of electric current. Electrocoagulation controls bleeding by creating instantaneous dehydration, which generates heat in the tissue adjacent to the needle point. Cellular fluids evaporate, blanching the area. Tissue destruction results from the conversion of electric energy emitted by an electrode into heat in a warm body.

The type and location of a lesion are more important than its size in determining the suitability of C&D for removal. Local anesthesia (lidocaine 1%) is infiltrated around and under the lesions to be removed. No dressing is required for all lesions. The physician may prescribe topical antibiotics and dressings for larger wounds.

Postoperative Course

Healing usually takes place in 1 to 3 weeks by granulation. A crust forms and sloughs in 7 to 10 days. If the lesion was large, two or three successive crusts may form and slough off. Premature removal of the crust should be prevented. Areas with good blood supply and abundant subcutaneous fat heal fastest.

The cure rate of primary early small basal cell and squamous cell skin cancers with this procedure is excellent (approximately 96%). The procedure is simple and convenient and leaves a cosmetically acceptable scar in most sites.

CRYOSURGERY

Uses

Cryosurgery uses liquid nitrogen applications to destroy lesions such as warts, actinic keratosis, seborrheic keratosis, and benign lentigo.

Procedure

Liquid nitrogen (−195.6°C) is applied to the lesion with either a cotton swab or a cryospray unit. An ice ball develops at the site of freezing. A blister forms within 24 hours and dries in several days, and then the skin with the lesion peels off. Cryosurgery does not require local anesthesia. If needed, the procedure may be repeated at 2- to 3-week intervals until the lesion disappears.

Postoperative Course

Immediately after cryosurgery, the operative area swells, and within hours, redness, throbbing, and mild pain occur. This is usually followed by the development of a blister filled with clear or blood-tinged fluid in 24 to 48 hours. Oozing occurs at the site for several days, after which the swelling begins to decrease. A scab forms in 7 to 10 days and falls off in 3 to 4 weeks. Healing time is longer for lesions on the neck, trunk, and extremities. Complications are rare, and the cosmetic result is excellent.

Guidelines for Application of the Nursing Process to the Care of the Patient Having Dermatologic Cryosurgery

Confirm the patient's understanding of the procedure. Question the patient about any history of cryoglobulinemia, cold urticaria, or other inability to tolerate the procedure. When the procedure is completed, instruct the patient in self-care, as presented in Chart 6–2.

Chart 6–2.

NURSING GUIDE TO PATIENT EDUCATION FOR SELF-MANAGEMENT: SELF-CARE AFTER DERMATOLOGIC CRYOSURGERY

Instruct the patient to:

Take two acetaminophen tablets every 4 to 6 hours or apply warm soaks for 10 to 15 minutes every 2 to 3 hours to relieve discomfort, or both.
Expect swelling of the area, followed in 1 to 2 days by the development of a blister filled with clear or blood-tinged fluid, subsequent oozing, and then formation of a scab in 7 to 10 days.
Keep the affected area elevated to decrease swelling by supporting an affected arm on pillows or a leg on a chair or by sleeping in a semi-upright position with three or four pillows supporting the back.
Avoid breaking the blister.
Keep the affected area clean by washing with mild soap and water or cleansing with cotton or gauze and hydrogen peroxide. Apply a thin film of antibiotic ointment if ordered and cover with a Band-Aid, Telfa-pad, or other dressing.
Leave the area open to the air once the scab forms to promote dryness. If you feel you must cover the area for aesthetic reasons, do so for the shortest time possible, leaving it uncovered at home and at night.
Let the scab fall off by itself, usually in about 1 month.
Report fever or increasing redness around the affected area because this can indicate infection.
Return for a follow-up appointment on *(specify date)*.

Chart 6–3.

NURSING GUIDE TO PATIENT EDUCATION FOR SELF-MANAGEMENT: SELF-CARE AFTER DERMATOLOGIC CARBON DIOXIDE LASER SURGERY

Instruct the patient who has had a carbon dioxide laser procedure to:

Leave the initial pressure dressing in place for 24 hours.
Keep the site dry for 48 hours.
Cleanse the wound with hydrogen peroxide, and apply a thin layer of antibiotic ointment three times a day beginning 48 hours after surgery.
Keep the wound covered with a dry, sterile dressing, or cover only when the potential for exposure to contaminants exists as directed by the physician's preference.
Take nonnarcotic analgesics and apply 5% lidocaine ointment as directed for discomfort, which may occur 3 to 7 days postoperatively.
Accept as a normal occurrence spontaneous bleeding from the healing site from 1 to 3 weeks after surgery.
Apply direct pressure to control minor, spontaneous bleeding.
Recognize that clear, yellow drainage is normal and not a sign of infection.
Protect the wound from friction, which may cause blister formation until healing is complete in several months.
Inspect the healed area regularly to ensure early detection of recurrence.

MOHS' MICROGRAPHIC SURGERY

Uses

Mohs' micrographic surgery is used to treat recurrent basal cell epithelioma, primary and recurrent squamous cell skin cancer, morphea (fibrosing, sclerosing), basal cell epithelioma, and basal cell epitheliomas of the ala nasi and other facial sites. It has a 99% cure rate for primary and recurrent skin cancer while minimizing damage to healthy tissue.

Procedure

The lesion is removed after the area is prepped and anesthetized. The wound is covered with a dressing, and the patient waits in a waiting room while the specimen is prepared for microscopic examination. The undersurface and borders are examined. If malignant cells are still present, then more tissue is removed but only in the areas of cancer involvement seen under the microscope. The process is repeated until a cancer-free plane is reached. The surgery is usually completed in a few hours but can take more than 1 day. Wound closure varies according to the extent and location of surgery. Flap or graft procedures may be done for large wounds; a smaller wound is sutured or allowed to granulate.

Postoperative Course

The postoperative course varies with the extent of the wound and the type of closure. Small wounds are simply kept clean and dry. Large wounds with grafts require care, as described later in this chapter.

LASER SURGERY

Uses

The carbon dioxide (CO_2) laser is used in dermatology for removal of warts, tattoos, and selected types of skin cancer. Port-wine stains, telangiectasias, and cherry angiomas are treated with the argon laser.

The Q-switched ruby laser, which emits a deep-red beam, is used to remove tattoos made of dark carbon-based pigment.

The CO_2 laser beam is absorbed by water and hence by body cells, most of which are composed of approximately 85% water. When the CO_2 laser beam is absorbed by the intracellular water, it causes the water to boil. This, in turn, causes the cells to swell and burst, releasing water vapor, carbon, and cell fragments. Put another way, the CO_2 laser vaporized tissues instantly. It does no damage to surrounding structures and has a maximum penetration depth of 0.1 mm.

The argon laser penetrates 1.0 mm. It is selective for hemoglobin and pigmented tissue. It can coagulate surface vessels precisely and safely.

The neodymium:yttrium-aluminum-garnet (Nd: YAG) laser, which penetrates up to 6 mm, is used in dermatology to treat deep cavernous hemangiomas. It passes through water and is absorbed in tissue protein, resulting in deep coagulation.

There are no restrictions on undergoing laser surgery for the elderly or during pregnancy. Because laser wavelengths are non-ionizing forms of radiation, laser light does not accumulate or cause cellular changes. Laser treatment has not been found to cause cancer.

Procedure

Local anesthesia is used for most laser procedures. Some procedures are performed after the operative area is numbed with ice.

Postoperative Course

After CO_2 laser surgery, the wound is cleansed with hydrogen peroxide, and antibiotic ointment and a pressure dressing are applied. Discomfort, usually treated effectively with non-narcotic analgesics or topical lidocaine, may occur 3 to 5 days postoperatively. Reepithelialization of the wound begins at the periphery and proceeds centrally, taking anywhere from 1 to 2 months, depending on size and location. During the first 1 to 3 weeks of this process, as blood vessels regrow, spontaneous bleeding may occur. This is usually controlled easily by direct pressure.

The postoperative course after other types of laser surgery varies with the specific laser. For example, after surgery with a yellow laser, which does not create an open wound, healing can occur in as few as 2 days. After tattoo removal, a scar similar to a burn scar remains.

Guidelines for Application of the Nursing Process to the Care of the Patient Having Dermatologic Laser Surgery

Be certain to assess the patient's expectations of the outcomes of surgery; if expectations are unrealistic, alert the surgeon and provide for additional information and discussion. Keep in mind that comprehensive preoperative teaching is essential to promote patient compliance with safety procedures and to prevent undue anxiety. Prepare the patient for expected sights and sounds. Clearly explain the need to wear protective goggles, the need to remain still, and the reason for the "DANGER" signs posted on the doors.

After the procedure, instruct the patient in self-care as presented in Chart 6–3.

CLOSURE OF SKIN WOUNDS

Skin wounds can be closed in a variety of ways: simple side-by-side approximation, granulation, skin grafting, or use of skin flaps. The method of closure used varies with the size, type, and location of the wound as well as the patient's general condition.

SIDE-TO-SIDE APPROXIMATION

Suturing the edges of a wound together is the simplest method of closing a skin wound. The result is best when the wound is elliptic in shape, the edges of the wound are perpendicular, and the skin lines were followed in making the incision. An elliptic excision is illustrated in Figure 6–7.

Wounds closed by side-to-side approximation are dressed with Band-Aids or gauze dressings. The patient is instructed to keep the wound dry for 24 hours and to return to the clinic if problems arise with bleeding, purulent drainage, or excessive pain. Acetaminophen is recommended for pain. Suture removal depends on the site and wound tension. Generally, facial sutures are removed in 5 to 7 days.

GRANULATION

Sometimes a wound is allowed to granulate in from the edges and heal by secondary intention. Healing by secondary intention is slower. Its use depends on the size and anatomic location of the wound and patient preference.

SKIN FLAPS

A flap is tissue raised from one area of the body and transferred either to an adjacent area with its blood supply intact or to a distant site where the blood supply is reestablished. The indications for flaps include replacing full-thickness tissue loss; covering densely scarred areas that have a compromised blood supply; covering exposed tendon, bone, or nerve; providing protection for delicate structures (e.g., vascular grafts in the groin); and providing coverage to reduce infection until final surgery can be performed.

Flaps can be classified according to blood supply, location of donor tissue in relation to the defect, or anatomic composition. Flaps based on blood supply are classified as random-pattern or axial-pattern flaps. Random-pattern flaps consist of skin and subcutaneous tissue supplied with blood from random vessels. Axial-pattern flaps have a known arterial and venous blood supply.

Flaps based on location of the donor tissue in relation to the defect are described as local or distant. Local flaps are created from tissue adjacent to the defect. Distant flaps are designed in one area of the body and transferred to a defect in another area. Free flaps are a type of distant flap that are completely detached from the donor site and moved into a defect where a new blood supply is created

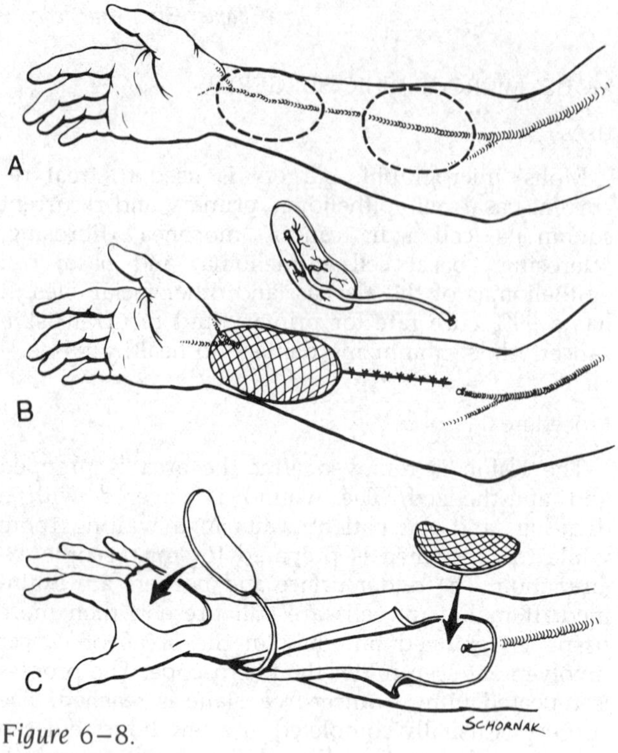

Figure 6–8.

The radial forearm fasciocutaneous flap. *A,* Potential donor sites for flap to cover defect on back of hand. *B,* Flap elevated as a free flap from the selected donor site. *C,* Flap ready to be placed in the defect; crosshatching indicates skin grafting of donor site. (From McCarthy JG [ed]. Plastic Surgery. Vol. 1, General principles. Philadelphia: WB Saunders, 1990, p 297.)

by attaching vessels in the flap to vessels in the defect (Fig. 6–8).

Flaps based on anatomic composition are classified as skin, muscle, bone, fascia, omentum, or composite grafts. A musculocutaneous flap is composed of skin and the underlying muscle.

Sometimes the word "pedicle" is used to describe the tissue that houses the blood supply for a flap. In the past, flaps were transferred with long pedicles to cover defects. For example, the nose was reconstructed with tissue from the underside of the arm. A long pedicle flap was raised and the tissue sutured to the nose. Thus, the patient had the arm attached to the nose until a blood supply was reestablished from local vessels. Today, the pedicle is seldom visible. It is tunneled through other tissues. For example, to reconstruct the breast, a surgeon may use a flap from the abdomen or back. The pedicle supplying blood to the tissue is located in the abdomen or axilla. It is imperative to understand where the blood supply is coming from for a flap, because no amount of pressure can be applied to the flap without risking necrosis of the tissues. Free flaps do not have a pedicle, because the surgeon has created a new blood supply for the tissues.

SKIN GRAFTS

Skin grafting transplants skin that has been totally detached from its blood supply in a donor site to a recipient site. This is done to cover defects that re-

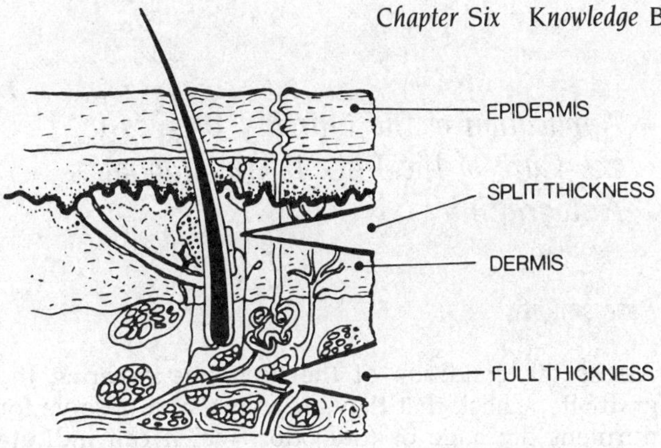

Figure 6–9.

Diagram of a cross section of the skin, demonstrating split-thickness and full-thickness skin grafts. (From Roberts JR, Hedges JR. Clinical procedures in emergency medicine. 2nd ed. Philadelphia: WB Saunders, 1991, p 573.)

sult from skin loss caused by trauma, burns, or excision of a cutaneous malignancy.

For a graft to "take"—that is, attach and revascularize—the "bed," or recipient site, must have a good blood supply and the grafted tissue must be immobilized because shearing of the graft from the bed destroys any ingrowth of capillaries. Both the bed and the graft must also be free of infection.

Classification of Skin Grafts According to Source

Skin grafts are classified according to source into autografts, homografts or allografts, and heterografts or xenografts.

An autograft is skin transferred from a donor site to a recipient site on the same person. The donor site is the area of healthy, intact skin on the body from which the graft is taken. Although grafts are thin, the donor site is an open wound. Donor sites heal in approximately 2 weeks and can be used over and over. Only an autograft can supply permanent skin coverage.

A homograft is skin transplanted from one person to another. Most homografts come from cadavers because no advantages have been found in the use of living donors. Homografts generally remain attached for 3 to 10 weeks before sloughing off.

A heterograft is skin transferred from an animal to a human. Heterografts are used to limit fluid loss, control temperature, decrease the risk of infection, and stimulate epithelialization. Most heterografts are porcine (i.e., consist of pigskin). Because it is a foreign protein, the heterograft does not grow and is sloughed off in 3 to 7 days. A heterograft is replaced on a regular basis until the wound is healed or autografting is complete.

Because homografts and heterografts provide only temporary emergency cover for burns or other trauma, they are referred to as biologic dressings.

Types of Skin Grafts on the Basis of Thickness

Skin grafts consist of epidermis and varying thicknesses of dermis (Fig. 6–9). Thus, they are divided into full-thickness and split-thickness grafts, depending on the number of skin layers taken from the donor site. The type of skin graft used is determined by the location of the defect, its size, and the desired cosmetic and functional result.

Full-thickness skin grafts are used to repair defects extending into the subcutaneous tissue, especially when the skin loss is on the face. Donor sites for full-thickness grafts include the retroauricular area, supraclavicular area, eyelids, abdomen, and thigh. The donor site is selected to best match skin color, texture, and hair growth on the recipient area. Because all skin layers are removed, donor sites must be sutured closed or covered with split-thickness skin grafts.

A full-thickness graft has less tendency to contract or to become hyperpigmented postoperatively and is functionally superior to a split-thickness graft in that it is more resistant to trauma.

Split-thickness skin grafts are used to cover large areas of denuded skin from burns and other trauma. Closure of wounds after excision of large, pigmented nevi or burn scars may also require a split-thickness skin graft. In some instances, a primary defect is covered with a flap and the secondary defect is covered with a split-thickness skin graft. The split-thickness graft revascularizes more rapidly and requires shorter immobilization to survive than a full-thickness skin graft. However, it is less resistant to trauma, tends to contract, lacks sensation, has impaired sweating ability, and has a poor cosmetic appearance.

The anterior thigh is the most common donor site for split-thickness skin grafts.

Mesh grafts are thin split-thickness grafts with many tiny slits cut into the graft. The slits allow the graft to be stretched or expanded in two directions to 1.5 to 9 times its original size. Mesh grafts are used to cover extensive wounds or irregular surfaces such as the ankle that could not have otherwise been covered because of a lack of available donor sites (Fig. 6–10). Once the graft takes, the epidermal

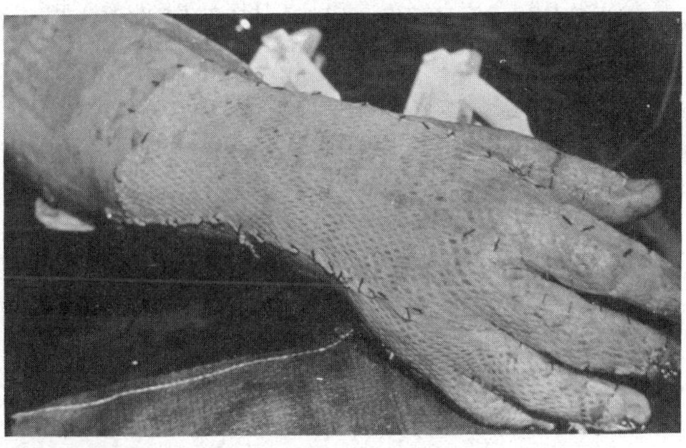

Figure 6–10.

Mesh graft used to cover an extensive defect of the upper extremity.

cells grow into the spaces until the interstices have completely filled in. Use of a mesh graft also allows rapid closure of the wound and decreases the risk of infection. The graft may be held in place with sutures, staples, sterile tape, or dressings.

Autografting Procedure

A donor site is selected on the basis of the healthy condition of the skin; the match to the recipient site in terms of color, texture, and hair growth; and the inconspicuousness of its location. The graft is removed from the donor site with a dermatome or razor blade. It is then prepared and fitted to the recipient site, where it may or may not be sutured into place. The completed graft is usually covered with petrolatum-impregnated dressings and wrapped in several layers of Kerlix to protect it and to keep it from drying out because a dry graft will lift off the wound or curl at the edges and will not take. Depending on location, the graft site may also be splinted to keep adjacent joints from moving and dislodging the graft.

The donor site, which heals by reepithelialization, may be covered with a synthetic dressing such as Op-Site for moist healing or covered with a single layer of nonadherent gauze for dry healing. Both types of dressing are covered with a pressure dressing for 24 to 48 hours to control bleeding.

Postgrafting Course

The surgeon performs the first dressing change of the graft site approximately 3 days after the grafting procedure. By this time, a successful graft or a take will appear pink and be attached to the bed of the wound. If the graft was meshed, the interstices will show beginning signs of new epithelial cell growth. Revascularization is indicated by a pink color to the graft (Fig. 6–11).

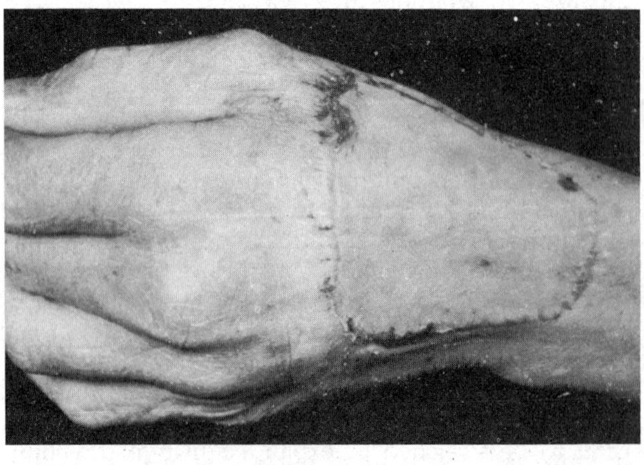

Figure 6–11.

Typical appearance of a skin graft at 5 days when take has been completed. (From Peacock EE. Wound repair. 3rd ed. Philadelphia: WB Saunders, 1984, p 223.)

Application of the Nursing Process to the Care of the Patient Undergoing Autografting

Assessment

Assess the condition of the dressings covering the graft site. Check that they are intact, and observe for purulent drainage or foul odor, which can indicate infection. Check peripheral circulation, and inspect any splints in use for proper application and placement. During dressing changes, assess the graft for adherence to the bed. Look for signs of epithelialization, vascularization, and new granulation. Also be alert for signs of infection, including redness of the skin surrounding the graft site. Inspect the donor site for signs of both healing and infection.

Assess the patient's compliance with instructions regarding care of the graft and donor sites (e.g., maintaining immobility, preventing pressure on the sites, keeping sites free of contamination).

Assess the patient's general physical and psychological response to the procedure. Keep in mind that immobility can impact all body systems and that patients undergoing grafting are coping not simply with the stress of the procedure itself but with the stress of the trauma or disease that necessitated grafting. Thus, it is critical to assess the patient's anxiety level, coping skills, and sources of support.

Nursing Diagnoses and Planning

Nursing diagnoses and related expected patient outcomes most commonly applicable to patients who have had skin grafting include the following:

NDx: High risk for infection related to multiple routes of possible invasion by microorganisms secondary to breaks in the skin

Planning: Patient outcomes

1. Spreading erythema around the graft is absent.
2. Purulent drainage is absent.
3. Foul odor from the graft site is absent.

NDx: High risk for altered peripheral tissue perfusion: graft related to trauma to the graft site

Planning: Patient outcomes

1. Patient observes precautions, such as keeping the part elevated and free from pressure, designed to protect the graft.
2. Graft remains in close contact with its bed.
3. Graft is pink.

NDx: Pain related to surgical trauma at newly created donor sites

Chart 6–4.

NURSING GUIDE TO PATIENT EDUCATION FOR SELF-MANAGEMENT: SELF-CARE OF GRAFTS AND PROTECTION OF NEW SKIN

Instruct the patient to:

Wear pressure garments as directed over recipient site.
Elevate involved extremities.
Wear layers of clothing as needed to prevent cold injury.
Massage graft and donor sites with lanolin or cocoa butter to soften the skin, decrease itching, and increase circulation. Do this at least once per day for 2 to 18 months once the area is healed in 2 to 3 weeks.
Avoid exposure of the graft sites to sunlight, heat, or other potential sources of trauma because there is a loss of feeling in the area and, as a result, risk of injury is increased.
Avoid exposure of the donor site to sunlight because the new skin has increased sensitivity.
Return for a follow-up visit on *(specify date)*.

Planning: Patient outcomes
1. Patient accepts medication and other comfort measured for pain.
2. Patient sleeps.
3. Patient states pain is manageable or relieved.

NDx: High risk for altered health maintenance related to insufficient knowledge of self-care of grafts and protection of new skin

Planning: Patient outcomes
1. Patient describes self-care as presented in Chart 6–4.
2. Patient demonstrates care of the graft.
3. Patient verbalizes willingness and ability to perform required self-care.

When grafts or flaps are necessary because of extensive traumatic wounds or disfiguring surgery for cancer, many additional nursing diagnoses are likely to apply.

Nursing Interventions

NDx: High risk for infection
Use strict aseptic technique during graft care until the graft has taken. Wear cap, mask, gown, and sterile gloves. After the initial dressing change by the surgeon, remove dressings, gently cleanse the graft, and reapply dressings as per the surgeon's orders.

NDx: High risk for altered peripheral tissue perfusion: graft
Maintain the patient on bed rest. Elevate the graft site to promote drainage from the area, thus decreasing the risk of increased intravascular pressure rupturing fragile new capillaries in the graft.

Do not disturb the dressing, and take precautions to ensure that the dressing is not moved.

Position the patient off the graft and donor sites, and prevent any movement at these sites. Use prescribed splints to immobilize joints adjacent to the graft.

Use a bed cradle or other device to prevent sheets from lying on the graft or donor sites. If the patient has been undergoing physical therapy and tank or tubbing treatments before grafting, such therapy is discontinued until ordered resumed by the physician. It is resumed as soon as possible to maintain joint function and mobility.

NDx: Pain
Administer prescribed analgesics as needed. Remember that new donor sites are more painful than graft sites. Enhance the effect of analgesics by maintaining a restful atmosphere, offering comfort measures such as a back rub and washing of mouth, face, and hands and providing distraction such as light music if desired by the patient. Do not change the patient's position for comfort unless it can be done without moving or putting pressure on the graft site.

NDx: High risk for altered health maintenance
Instruct the patient on care of the graft and in protection of the new skin as it grows, as presented in Chart 6–4.

Additional Interventions
Preoperatively protect the selected donor site from injury and infection if the site is known.

Evaluation

Evaluate the effectiveness of nursing care for a patient undergoing skin grafting by comparing the patient's status with the expected patient outcomes. Examples of specific outcomes for patients undergoing skin grafting have been provided in the Planning section.

PLASTIC SURGERY PROCEDURES

Plastic or reconstructive surgery is surgery done to reconstruct defects from congenital or acquired disorders or to improve appearance or function. It can involve bone, muscles, cartilage, and nerves as well as skin. Plastic surgery performed primarily for aesthetic effect is often referred to as cosmetic surgery.

DERMABRASION

Dermabrasion is surgical planing or sanding of the epidermis, which leaves a smoother surface.

Uses

Dermabrasion is done to smooth the skin and correct acne scars, scars from trauma, and disfiguring marks. Acne scars on the face are the most common reason for dermabrasion.

Physical Preparation of the Patient

The operative area is washed daily with a germicidal cleansing agent for several days before the procedure.

Procedure

Dermabrasion is usually done as an ambulatory procedure under local or general anesthesia. Gentian violet is applied to the operative area to stain and accentuate the depth of the scars so the areas to be planed are visible. A high-speed abrasive rotary instrument is used to remove the epidermis and upper dermis. Subsequently, basal cells in the remaining sweat glands and hair follicles proliferate and reepithelialize the abraded surface in 7 to 21 days.

To achieve the optimum result, dermabrasion may be repeated, with at least 2 weeks between procedures.

Although dermabrasion removes the epidermis and the upper dermis, it is not deep enough to correct pitted acne scars or other defects that penetrate to the dermis. Pitted acne scars can be removed by punch biopsy or can be filled with collagen before dermabrasion.

Postprocedure Course

Lidocaine-soaked gauze relieves the pain immediately after dermabrasion.

Vaseline gauze or N-interface dressing covered with a pressure dressing is applied to the face for 24 hours after dermabrasion to control oozing. This dressing is removed in 24 hours either in the physician's office or by the patient at home. In some cases, warm-water soaks followed by drying with a hair blow-dryer are started on the first postoperative day to remove the fine-mesh gauze over a period of several days. There is a sensation of deep warmth and throbbing after the procedure, which is usually relieved with bandaging. It requires 7 to 21 days for the face to reepithelialize.

Complications

The complications of dermabrasion include infection, milia, pigment changes, and scarring. Erythema and edema resolve as the site heals. There is also a risk of herpes infection in patients prone to outbreaks.

Dermabrasion is used with caution in patients with darkly pigmented skin, which may repigment unevenly or form keloid scars. These patients can have a test dermabrasion, which is done several months before dermabrasion.

Guidelines for Application of the Nursing Process to the Care of the Patient Undergoing Dermabrasion

Review the procedure with the patient, and encourage the patient to ask questions. Use photographs of past procedures to prepare the patient for the postoperative dressing and the appearance of the face at various stages of healing. Reassure the patient that pain is controlled during and immediately after the procedure by local anesthesia. Instruct the patient in self-care after dermabrasion, as presented in Chart 6–5.

DEEP CHEMICAL FACE PEELS

Chemical peeling consists of the application of an irritant chemical solution (phenol and trichloroacetic acid) to the skin to soften and dissolve the horny layer of the epidermis and to destroy the keratin cells. A light peel involves the epidermis; a medium peel involves the lower papillary and upper reticular dermis; and a deep peel penetrates to the deep

Chart 6–5.

NURSING GUIDE TO PATIENT EDUCATION FOR SELF-MANAGEMENT: SELF-CARE AFTER DERMABRASION

Instruct the patient to:

Expect edema for 48 hours.
Elevate head of bed to facilitate drainage.
Remove dressing or return for physician to remove dressing in 24 hours.
Apply warm-water compresses for 15 to 20 minutes four times per day for 2 days to prevent drying and crusting of the dermabraded area.
Take frequent, gentle, warm showers to further prevent drying and crusting.
Apply bacitracin ointment to dermabraded area for 5 days between soaks and showers.
Use newly purchased, nonallergenic makeup if desired after 5 days and if no open areas exist.
Resume shaving after 10 days.
Expect erythema, which typically fades in 3 to 6 weeks but may persist to some degree for months.
Avoid sun exposure for at least 4 months.
Apply sunscreen with sun protection factor 15 or higher, and wear a hat when outside in the sun.
Avoid straining, heavy lifting, and exposure to extreme heat or cold to prevent damage to new capillaries.
Avoid taking aspirin.

reticular dermis. A phenol-based solution is most often used because the resultant burn is both controlled and predictable.

Uses

Deep peels are done to remove fine, crosshatched wrinkles (rhytides), lentigines, and xanthelasma. They are also used to remove multiple squamous cell carcinomas and actinic keratoses and to treat acne scars. Deep peels are most effective when used on fair, thin skin with few sebaceous glands.

Procedure

Intravenous fluids are given to ensure adequate hydration and thus promote excretion of any absorbed phenol. Intravenous sedatives such as meperidine and diazepam are given for relaxation, and a local nerve block is done to anesthetize the face. The facial skin is cleaned and then thoroughly degreased with acetone to allow penetration of the peel solution. Subsequently, a small area (approximately 2 inches) of the skin is painted with the solution every 15 minutes until the face is completely covered. This spaced application of the peel solution is designed to prevent toxic levels of absorbed phenol. An occlusive dressing composed of layers of ½-inch-wide adhesive tape may be applied to the entire face, except for the eyes and mouth, to increase phenol penetration and to cause a deeper peel. In other cases, a moisturizer of the physician's choice is applied immediately, and the facial surface is left exposed to the air. A cardiac monitor is used throughout the procedure because of the risk of cardiac dysrhythmia from phenol. Blood pressure is checked every 15 minutes.

Postprocedure Course

Postoperative care varies somewhat according to the preferences of the attending physician. A typical plan of care is now discussed.

Occlusive dressings are removed in 48 hours, and antibacterial thymol iodide powder is sprinkled over the face twice a day for 3 days. This forms a thick crust, which begins to itch, peel, and crack on about day 6. At this time, tepid water soaks and application of a moisturizer such as Eucerin cream or Crisco (providing it is a new can) is begun to promote sloughing. In approximately 2 weeks, the crusts are gone and the face is smooth and red. If an occlusive dressing is not used, moisturizers are applied three times per day for 2 weeks.

Moderate to severe pain and burning during the first night after the peel can be controlled with one or two doses of an analgesic such as acetaminophen with codeine. A 10-day course of erythromycin and acyclovir may be ordered as prophylaxis against bacterial infection and herpetic flares. Patients sleep with the head elevated to decrease edema and return for a follow-up visit in 2 weeks. Postoperative erythema usually disappears in 10 to 12 weeks but may persist for 6 months.

Complications

Potential complications of a deep peel are many. They include cardiac dysrhythmias, laryngeal edema, infection, keloid formation, pigment changes, telangiectasia, milia, and ectropion of the lower eyelid.

Guidelines for Application of the Nursing Process to the Care of the Patient Having a Deep Chemical Face Peel

Use photographs of patients who have had a deep peel to prepare the patient for the postoperative bandage and appearance of the face at various stages of the healing process. Instruct the patient in self-care after the deep peel, as presented in Chart 6–6.

COLLAGEN IMPLANTS

Uses

Collagen implants are used to treat soft-tissue defects such as fine rhytides (wrinkles), atrophy, traumatic scars, surgical scars, and pitted scars caused by acne and pox virus.

Procedure

Zyderm I and II are semisolid gels containing purified bovine (cattle) collagen. The gel is placed in the upper dermis to correct superficial wrinkles. Zyplast is a cross-linked bovine collagen product that is placed deeper into the dermis to correct acne scars, deep nasolabial folds, and other defects.

A test for allergic reaction is done before initial treatment. A small amount of collagen product is injected into the forearm, which is then checked for any untoward reaction in 72 hours and at the end of 4 weeks. The treatment is a simple out-patient procedure. The area is iced, and collagen is injected into the defect. This is repeated at 2- to 3-week intervals until no further correction is noted on two subsequent treatments or until there is 100% correction.

Chart 6–6.

NURSING GUIDE TO PATIENT EDUCATION FOR SELF-MANAGEMENT: SELF-CARE AFTER DEEP CHEMICAL FACE PEEL

Instruct the patient to:

Take acetaminophen with codeine or other analgesic as ordered for burning and throbbing the night after the peel.
Sleep with the head elevated.
Expect swelling and serous drainage.
Ingest liquids through a straw for 24 to 48 hours, and progress to soft food as comfort permits.
Move the mouth as little as possible if an occlusive mask is in place to avoid loosening the tape.
Return for removal of an occlusive mask on *(specify date).*
Wash hands thoroughly before touching face.
Sprinkle thymol iodide powder over the face twice a day for 3 days to form a thick crust.
Avoid picking crusts.
Soak face with tepid water, and apply moisturizer when crusts begin to peel on approximately Day 6.
Apply moisturizers three times per day for 2 weeks beginning the day after the peel if an occlusive mask is not used.
Use sunscreen continually when crusts slough off because the skin will never tan evenly.
Avoid taking aspirin.
Avoid all deliberate exposure to the sun.
Wear a protective hat when outside in sunny weather.
Take oral anti-infective medication as ordered.
Return for a follow-up visit in 2 weeks.
Expect erythema to fade gradually over a period of up to 6 months.
Use makeup as desired when given permission by the physician, usually in 3 to 4 weeks. Select blue-purple hues for the best effect.

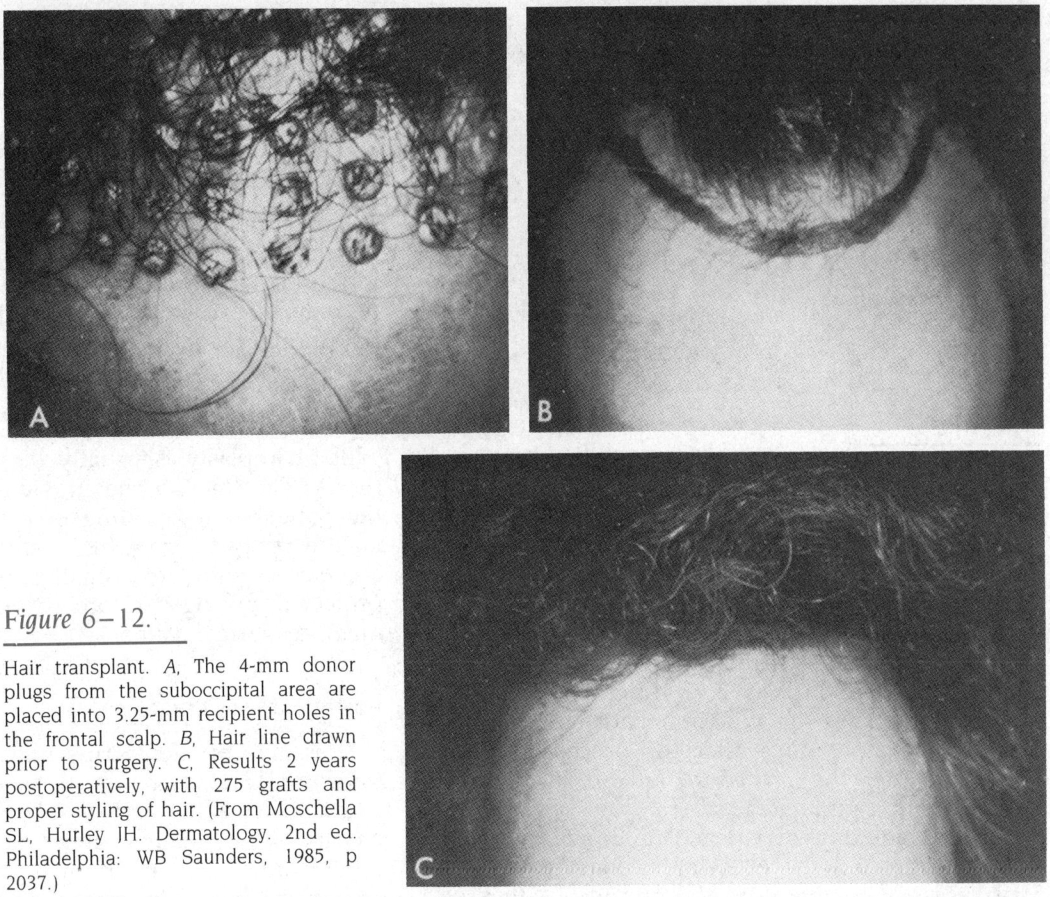

Figure 6–12.

Hair transplant. *A*, The 4-mm donor plugs from the suboccipital area are placed into 3.25-mm recipient holes in the frontal scalp. *B*, Hair line drawn prior to surgery. *C*, Results 2 years postoperatively, with 275 grafts and proper styling of hair. (From Moschella SL, Hurley JH. Dermatology. 2nd ed. Philadelphia: WB Saunders, 1985, p 2037.)

Injections may be somewhat uncomfortable, especially around the nose and mouth. The collagen implant softens indurated scars and remains pliable. Accidental overcorrection is not permanent. Correction lasts 3 to 9 months, and then periodic touchups are required.

Immediately after the implant, puffiness, blushing, slight bruising, and tenderness may occur at the treatment sites. These symptoms are normal and disappear in a few days.

Contraindications

Contraindications to collagen-implant treatment are a positive skin test to Zyderm, history of autoimmune or collagen-vascular disease, and history of anaphylaxis. A new collagen preparation, Fibrel, which is mixed with the patient's plasma just before use, effectively corrects depressed cutaneous scars for a year or more with few adverse reactions.

HAIR TRANSPLANTS

Hair transplants replace hair permanently lost as a result of male pattern baldness, trauma, or other conditions.

Hair transplants are done in four or more sessions, 3 weeks apart, with 60 to 70 plugs transplanted per session.

Physical Preparation of the Patient

The patient is instructed to wash the hair the night before the procedure.

Procedure

Hair transplants are done as an ambulatory procedure, with a local anesthetic of lidocaine 1% with epinephrine. Both the recipient and the donor sites are anesthetized. Donor plugs, 3.5 to 4 mm in diameter, are usually taken from the lower posterior scalp using a hand-held power punch. Normal saline is injected into the donor site before removal of plugs to tense the skin. This decreases bleeding and results in neater grafts. Pressure is applied over the donor site while preparing the recipient site. The donor site may heal by secondary intention or may be sutured, depending on physician preference.

The donor plugs are placed in a sterile container and rinsed with normal saline. Blood and loose hair are removed. Donor plugs are placed into recipient sites after recipient plugs are removed. No sutures are used. The plugs are positioned so that the hair from the plug goes in the same direction as the surrounding hair (Fig. 6–12). Antibiotic ointment is applied to recipient and donor sites, and a pressure dressing is applied for 24 hours.

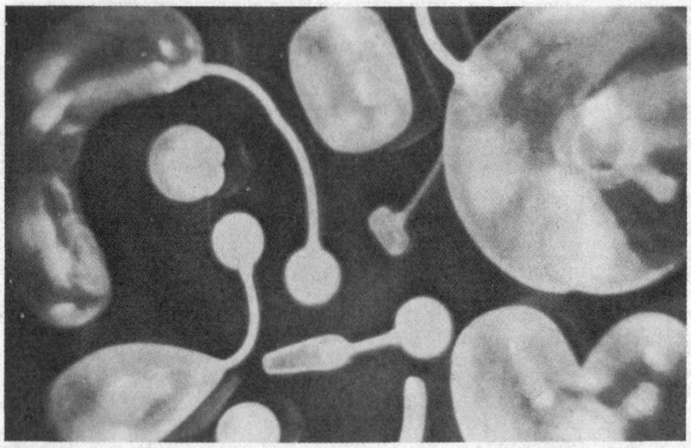

Figure 6–13.

Various shapes of implants used for skin expansion. (Courtesy of Cox-Uphoff International.)

Postoperative Course

Once planted, the hair sheds in 3 to 6 weeks and regrows in approximately 2 to 4 months. The transplanted hair grows for a lifetime. Patients can gently wash their hair 3 days after the procedure. Scabs that form after the procedure fall off in 10 to 20 days, leaving a pink circle.

The patient may experience mild edema of the scalp and around the eyes for as long as 1 week. Hairpieces cannot be worn the first week after surgery and only for short periods during the second week.

SCALP REDUCTION

Scalp reduction is a procedure to remove areas of alopecia or thinning hair. The result is immediate.

Procedure

Local anesthesia is injected into the scalp. The affected area is removed, and the two edges of skin are approximated and sutured together. Scalp reduction is sometimes done in stages to minimize tension on the suture line, which can lead to infection and necrosis. During the procedure, bleeding is controlled with sutures, cautery, and suction.

Postoperative Course

A pressure dressing is worn for 48 hours. The patient can apply ice for 24 hours for discomfort and bleeding. Acetaminophen with codeine may be prescribed for pain for the first 48 hours. Strenuous activity is avoided. Once healed, the suture line is a fine hair scar.

A new development in scalp reduction in the use of a tissue expander. This is a balloon-type implant placed under the skin and gradually inflated intraoperatively or over a number of weeks to stretch the skin (Fig. 6–13.). When the skin is sufficiently stretched, the tissue expander is removed and the stretched tissue is used to create local flaps to cover adjacent defects.

BLEPHAROPLASTY

Blepharoplasty is a procedure to correct sagging, wrinkled, baggy eyelids caused by the protrusion of intraorbital fat or the aging process. It is also done to remove excess tissue in patients with a visual-field impairment.

Procedure

Blepharoplasty is usually done under local anesthesia. The lines of the incisions are marked while the patient is in a sitting position. Excess skin and fat are removed from the eyelids, and the incisions are closed with very small sutures. The cornea is protected during the procedure with drops, ointment, or normal saline.

Postoperative Course

Dressings or Steri-Strips may be omitted or applied for 12 to 24 hours. Iced compresses are used to reduce swelling and discoloring around the eyes. Neosporin ophthalmic ointment (polymyxin B sulfate, neomycin sulfate, bacitracin) may be applied to the suture lines. Sutures are removed in 3 to 7 days. Blindness caused by intraoperative or postoperative hemorrhage is a rare complication of blepharoplasty.

RHYTIDOPLASTY

Rhytidoplasty/rhytidectomy is an operation to remove wrinkles. Also called a face lift, rhytidoplasty corrects the effects of aging skin such as redundancy of the upper eyelids, fullness of the lower eyelids, prominence of the nasolabial fold, and sagging neck tissue. The term *rhytid* means wrinkle; therefore, rhytidectomy indicates excision of wrinkles.

Procedure

Rhytidoplasty is performed under local or general anesthesia and often in an out-patient setting. Incisions are concealed in natural skin folds and within the hairline (Fig. 6–14). Loose skin, separated from muscle, is pulled up and back, and the excess is removed. In some cases, fat is suctioned simultaneously from the area of the neckline.

Postoperative Course

Postoperatively, analgesics are prescribed for facial tightness and discomfort. The patient rests for 24 hours and is instructed to keep the head elevated and to avoid flexing the neck to optimize circulation and to decrease edema and the risk of bleeding.

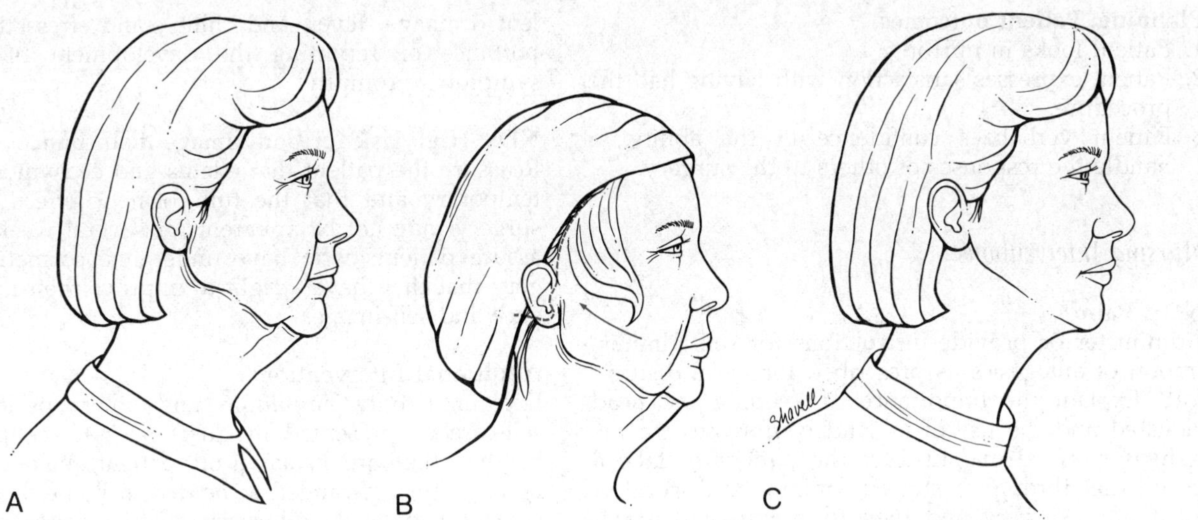

Figure 6–14.

A, Appearance before face lift. B, The face lift procedure. C, Appearance after face lift. (Redrawn courtesy of American Society of Plastic and Reconstructive Surgeons Arlington Heights, IL.)

Dressings are removed between the third and fifth day, the face is cleansed of crusted drainage, and a thin layer of antibiotic ointment may be applied. Diet is progressed from liquids taken through a straw to a regular diet as the ability to chew permits. Swelling and bruising gradually subside over several weeks.

Surgery on the aging face does not provide a permanent result because the aging process continues. Improvement usually lasts up to 10 years. Younger patients have better results than older patients. Some patients desire more than one operation.

Potential complications of rhytidoplasty include sloughing skin, head and neck deformity, and facial paralysis.

Application of the Nursing Process to the Care of the Patient Having a Face Lift

PREOPERATIVE NURSING CARE

Assessments, nursing diagnoses, expected patient outcomes, nursing interventions, and evaluation for the patient scheduled for a face lift are similar to those for any preoperative patient, with several considerations. If the patient is to be awake under local anesthesia during the procedure, be sure he or she is aware of this. Explain that photographs are often taken before and after any cosmetic or reconstructive procedure. Obtain consent if necessary, and inform the patient that these pictures become part of the medical record.

POSTOPERATIVE NURSING CARE

Assessment

Assess response to surgery as for any surgical patient. Further assess the patient's understanding of, and ability to comply with, the postoperative instructions for wound care and limitations in activity to achieve the best possible cosmetic result.

Nursing Diagnoses and Planning

Nursing diagnoses and related expected patient outcomes most commonly applicable to patients who have had a face lift include the following:

NDx: Pain related to tissue trauma during surgery

Planning: Patient outcomes
1. Patient follows instructions designed to limit discomfort.
2. Patient states that discomfort is manageable.

NDx: High risk for infection related to surgical wound

Planning: Patient outcomes
1. Spreading erythema is absent from the wound.
2. Purulent drainage is absent from the wound.
3. Patient is afebrile.

NDx: High risk for body image disturbance related to the patient's concern with appearance and others' reaction to his or her attempt to look and feel better through cosmetic surgery

Planning: Patient outcomes
1. Patient looks in mirror.
2. Patient expresses satisfaction with having had the procedure.
3. Patient verbalizes confidence in the ability to handle the responses of others to the surgery.

Nursing Interventions

NDx: Pain
Administer or provide instructions for self-administration of analgesics as prescribed for facial discomfort. Explain the importance of keeping the head elevated and the use of ice and compresses for the reduction of edema. Instruct the patient to take a liquid diet through a straw to minimize discomfort right after surgery and then to progress to a soft diet as chewing comfort allows.

NDx: High risk for infection
Review instructions on wound care after the procedure or before the patient is discharged.

Describe the amount of edema, discoloration, and bleeding to be expected. Specify the length of time to leave the dressing in place and how to reinforce it with tape should it come loose. Also specify when the patient can allow the wound to get wet and how and when to apply antibiotic ointment if prescribed. Instruct the patient in how to remove crusts with hydrogen peroxide if ordered by the surgeon. Teach the patient the signs and symptoms of wound infection—redness, increased pain, warmth, purulent drainage, fever, and chills—and stress the importance of reporting the development of these symptoms promptly.

NDx: High risk for body image disturbance
Reassure the patient that edema and ecchymosis are temporary and that the full cosmetic effect of the surgery may not be apparent for several weeks. Reassure patients who have undergone cosmetic surgery that they have a right to improve their appearance and self-image.

Additional Interventions
Explain activity limitations and other specifics of self-care as presented in Chart 6–7. If the patient has had the surgery as an out-patient, make certain he or she has arranged to be driven home. Also the clinic nurse or the physician's office nurse should call out-patients at home 1 to 2 days after the procedure to check on their condition.

Evaluation

Evaluate the effectiveness of nursing care for a patient who has had a rhytidoplasty by comparing the patient's status with the expected patient outcomes. Examples of specific outcomes for patients who have had a rhytidoplasty have been provided in the Planning section.

Chart 6–7.

NURSING GUIDE TO PATIENT EDUCATION FOR SELF-MANAGEMENT: SELF-CARE AFTER RHYTIDOPLASTY

Instruct the patient to:

Rest for 48 hours and then gradually resume activities.
Avoid taking aspirin.
Avoid lifting and bending for 10 days because these actions encourage edema and bleeding.
Keep the head elevated when in bed, and avoid flexing the neck to prevent impaired circulation to the face.
Expect tightness in the face and take non-narcotic analgesics as directed for discomfort.
Ingest liquids through a straw, progressing to a soft and then a regular diet when able to chew comfortably.
Shampoo hair when all sutures have been removed.
Use hair blow-dryer on warm only, because ears remain numb for some time and can be burned.
Expect face to appear swollen and bruised for several weeks.
Report signs of infection immediately: redness, increased pain, warmth, purulent drainage, fever, and chills.
Return for follow-up visit on *(specify date)*.

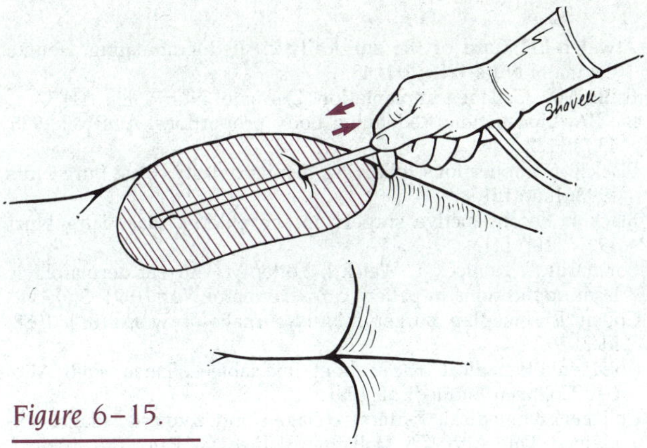

Figure 6–15.

Liposuction technique.

LIPOSUCTION

Liposuction is the surgical removal of diet-resistant fat in the body to improve contour. It is currently one of the most popular cosmetic surgeries. Many areas can be treated: submental neck and chin, nasolabial fold, abdomen, lateral thigh, buttocks, ankles, medial knees, flanks, and male breasts. Patients who maintain a stable weight, who are not obese, and who have good skin tone have the best result with liposuction. Liposuction is not a method of weight reduction.

Procedure

Liposuction may be done under local or general anesthesia and on either an in-patient or an outpatient basis. A small incision, 4 to 5 mm, is made in an inconspicuous location in areas of the body to be treated. A cannula is advanced under the skin into the fat, as illustrated in Figure 6–15. Suction is applied as the cannula moves back and forth along the axial plane parallel to the skin. The fat removed is a yellow-white semisolid. About 1 L of fat can be removed without depletion of body fluids. If more fat is removed, body fluids must be replaced intravenously. The incisions are sutured, and a pressure garment or adhesive pressure tape is applied.

The amount of fat in the collection bottle is monitored and documented so that the same amount is removed in symmetric areas.

Postoperative Course

The patient leaves the compression garment or tape in place as directed by the surgeon. This can range from 7 to 10 days, with removal before the return visit up to 6 weeks. Anticoagulants are contraindicated because of the risk of bleeding.

Because of edema, change in body contour may not be noticeable for 2 to 4 months. Patients are encouraged to use dietary discretion to maximize the effect of liposuction.

Complications

Complications of liposuction include contour irregularity, hematoma formation, and fat embolism. Excessive blood loss and shock can also occur.

Contraindications

Liposuction is contraindicated in patients who are obese and who have wrinkled or inelastic skin.

Application of the Nursing Process to the Care of the Patient Having Liposuction

The assessment, nursing diagnoses, expected patient outcomes, nursing interventions, and evaluation for

Chart 6–8.

NURSING GUIDE TO PATIENT EDUCATION FOR SELF-MANAGEMENT: SELF-CARE AFTER LIPOSUCTION

Instruct the patient to:

Rest for 12 hours and then gradually resume activities.
Remove the compression garment or tape in 7 to 10 days as directed by the surgeon.
Apply ice packs to affected area to reduce swelling.
Take nonaspirin pain relievers for discomfort.
Avoid consumption of alcohol and aspirin.
Return for follow-up visit and suture removal in 5 to 7 days.
Use discretion in eating to avoid weight gain.

patients having liposuction surgery are similar to those for patients having any cosmetic surgery procedure. Postoperative instructions do vary, however, so instruct the patient in self-care after liposuction, as presented in Chart 6–8.

The Elderly: Special Considerations

Skin changes throughout life result from aging, heredity, and environmental exposure. As the individual ages, the epidermis becomes thinner and has less water content. This results in dry skin. The activity of the sebaceous and apocrine glands decreases, which adds to the dry-skin problem.

The dermis becomes less flexible and loses elasticity. Some of the fatty cushion is lost. These changes cause wrinkles. Fingernails and toenails become tough and brittle.

Almost all men experience some baldness as they age. Women's hair also becomes thinner. The degree of baldness one experiences and the changes in hair color are genetically determined. After 45 years of age, facial hair sometimes increases in women.

Blood vessels become more fragile with aging, and this results in ecchymosis and petechiae from minimal trauma. Common lesions that appear on the aging skin are described in Chapter 7.

Benign clinical features on the aging face resulting from actinic (sun) damage include actinic keratosis, xerosis (dry skin), solar lentigines, telangiectasia, follicular cysts, and open comedones. Loss of elasticity, wrinkles, diffuse erythema, freckles, and diffuse brown pigmentation also result from the cumulative effects of sun exposure.

Skin changes associated with sun exposure can be minimized by protecting the skin during youth. Measures to protect the skin are avoiding sunlight exposure between 10 A.M. and 3 P.M., wearing protective clothing and hats, and using sunscreens.

Skin changes associated with smoking include lines or wrinkles on the face radiating at right angles from the upper and lower lips and corners of the eyes. There may be deep lines on the cheeks or numerous shallow lines on the cheeks and lower jaw. Facial features develop a subtle gauntness with a prominence of bony contours. "Smoker's face" has a leathery, worn, and rugged appearance.

Bibliography

Arndt KA. Manual of dermatologic therapeutics. 4th ed. Boston: Little, Brown, 1988.

Atwater EE. Care of the surgically created granulating wound. Dermatol Nurs 1989; 1(1):43.

Bailin MD. Collagen implantation. Dermatol Nurs 1989; 1(1):37.

Baj PA. Liposuction: Redefining body proportions. AORN J 1986; 43(5):1127.

Black J. Complications following blepharoplasty. Plast Surg Nurs 1990; 10(4):151.

Black J. Reconstructive surgery in the elderly. Plast Surg Nurs 1991; 11(4):141.

Borchardt C, Konicek T, Weick J, Yotter M. Current dermatologic laser applications in patient care. Dermatol Nurs 1991; 3(6):411.

Cohen L. Free-flap surgery: Nurses make it work. RN 1988; 51(3):26.

Collagen Biomedical. Facts about injectable collagen. Palo Alto, CA: Collagen Biomedical, 1991.

Collagen Biomedical. Zyderm collagen and Zyplast collagen explained. Palo Alto, CA: Collagen Biomedical, Palo Alto, 1991.

Converse J. Reconstructive plastic surgery. Philadelphia: WB Saunders, 1990.

Eisenbaum S, Black J. Melanoma. Plast Surg Nurs 1988; 8(2):42.

Evey P. Patch test. Dermatology Nurses Association FOCUS 1986; 5(1):5.

Goodman T. Flaps and grafts in plastic surgery. AORN J 1988; 48(4):650.

Graham D. Managing malignant melanoma. Plast Surg Nurs 1989; 9(1):9.

Habif TP. Clinical dermatology. 2nd ed. St. Louis: CV Mosby, 1990.

Johnson TM, Brown MD, Swanson NA. Use of tissue expanders in dermatology. Mediguide to Dermatology 1991; 4(1):1.

Karel-Brant R. Healing by second intention: Its use in Mohs micrographic surgery. Dermatol Nurs 1990; 2(2):69.

Kim M, McFarland G, McLane A. Pocket guide to nursing diagnosis. No. 3. St. Louis: CV Mosby, 1989.

Laudano JB, Leach EE, Armstrong RB. Acne: Therapeutic perspectives with an emphasis on the role of isotretinoin. Dermatol Nurs 1990; 2(6):328.

Lookingbill DP, Marks, JG Jr. Principles of dermatology. Philadelphia: WB Saunders, 1986.

McKeown A. Pulsed-dye laser treatment of vascular lesions. Dermatol Nurs 1991; 3(5):330.

Meusch R, Lillis PJ. Liposuction: The tumescent technique. Dermatol Nurs 1991; 3(4):255.

Moschella S, Herley HJ. Dermatology. Philadelphia: WB Saunders, 1985.

Oregon Health Service University. Carbon dioxide laser surgery (patient information sheet). Portland, OR: Oregon Health Sciences University, Department of Dermatology, 1990.

Rumsfield J. Sunscreens: What you and your patients should know. Dermatol Nurs 1990; 2(3):139.

Russell B, Russell R. The role of the plastic surgery nurse collagen specialist. Plast Surg Nurs 1990; 10(2):51.

Salisbury C, Kaye B. Complications following rhytidectomy. Plast Surg Nurs 1987; 7(3):76.

Sheppard M, Fowler M. Anesthesia in plastic surgery. Plast Surg Nurs 1989; 9(4):151.

Smalley PJ. Laser technology: A nursing perspective. Dermatol Nurs 1991; 3(4):241.

Stark RB (ed). Plastic surgery of the head and neck. New York: Churchill Livingstone, 1987.

Storck L. Deep peels: What the nurse does. Dermatol Nurs 1991; 3(3):164.

Vander Kam V, Achauer B. Lasers in plastic surgery: Applications and nursing interventions. Plast Surg Nurs 1990; 10(3):107.

Vargo N. Reconstructive surgery and flaps. Lecture presented at Nursing Perspectives in Dermatology Surgery, Hines, IL, 1986.

Westlake C. Committment to function: Microsurgical flaps. Plast Surg Nurs 1991; 11(3):95.

Whyte A. Cryosurgery for the dermatology nurse. Dermatol Nurs 1990; 2(5):271.

Zacheri A. Perioperative CO_2 laser nursing responsibilities. Laser Nurs 1988; 2(1):5.

Chapter Seven

NURSING CARE *of Adults with Skin Disorders*

Skin disorders are a major cause of disability, disfigurement, and discomfort; most of the population will suffer from some type of skin disorder during their lifetime. Skin disorders may be localized or disseminated, asymptomatic, or accompanied by severely distressing symptoms such as itching, burning, or weeping. They may be infectious in origin or caused by exposure to sunlight, an allergen, or an irritant. For many disorders, the cause is unknown. Skin changes also accompany a variety of systemic disorders and often are the first manifestation of the internal problem. Because many skin disorders are chronic in nature, patients require not only good physical care but consistent encouragement and emotional support.

Infections

Most pathogenic organisms that cause skin infections reach the skin by an external route. The stratum corneum usually provides a barrier to invading organisms. When this barrier is altered and invading organisms enter, the body's secondary immunologic barrier localizes the infection and prevents systemic invasion. Most individuals recover completely from acute infectious skin ailments. However, some individuals suffer from chronic skin infections. This can be due to poor hygiene, chronic irritation that alters the physical barrier, or an immunologic defect.

Bacterial Infections

Pyodermas are bacterial skin infections. They are most often caused by staphylococci or streptococci. They do not always produce pus, as the term *pyoderma* suggests.

FOLLICULITIS

Folliculitis is a common, relatively superficial infection of the hair follicle frequently seen in young adults.

ETIOLOGY

Folliculitis is usually caused by *Staphylococcus aureus*. Open wounds, maceration, dirt, friction, tight-fitting clothing, occlusive cosmetics, and ointments are predisposing factors. Some patients with chronic folliculitis are nose and throat carriers of *S. aureus*.

PATHOPHYSIOLOGY

Bacteria enter the skin through the hair follicle and infect the epidermal lining. As illustrated in Figure 7–1, pustules form in the hair follicle just below the stratum corneum. The inflammation spreads to the surrounding epidermis. Spread to new areas of the body may occur secondary to inoculation by the fingernails.

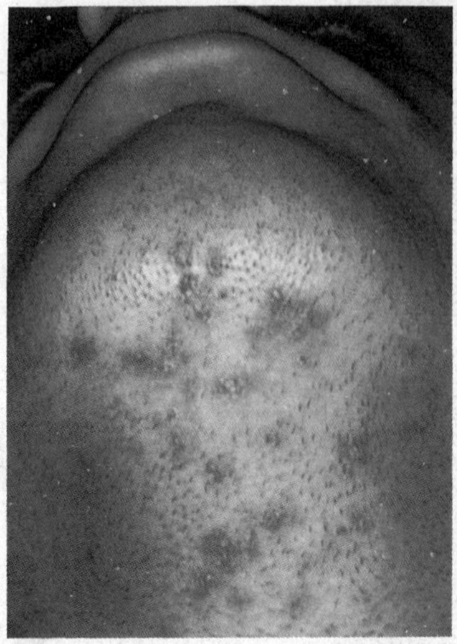

Figure 7–1.

Tiny follicular pustules characteristic of folliculitis. (From Jarvis C. Physical examination and health assessment. Philadelphia: WB Saunders, 1992, p. 270.)

CLINICAL MANIFESTATIONS

Single or multiple papules or pustules with centrally located hairs are the presenting lesions. In some cases, furuncles or carbuncles may subsequently develop.

MEDICAL DIAGNOSIS

Diagnosis is made on the basis of the appearance of the lesions. A Gram stain or bacterial culture confirms the presence of *S. aureus*.

MEDICAL MANAGEMENT

Treatment consists of daily cleansing with chlorhexidine gluconate (Hibiclens) or povidone-iodine (Betadine) for several weeks.

Systemic antibiotics, such as erythromycin or dicloxacillin, are given for 7 to 10 days for extensive involvement.

Prolonged use of antiseptic cleansers is indicated for patients with chronic folliculitis.

FURUNCLE

A furuncle, or boil, is a deep folliculitis. Although furuncles occur in healthy individuals, they are more common in the presence of predisposing factors such as poor hygiene, obesity, diabetes, poor nutrition, and immunosuppression.

ETIOLOGY

A furuncle is usually caused by infection of the hair follicle by *S. aureus.* It is a single, deep-seated nodule. Predisposing factors include repeated irritation, pressure, friction, and heavy perspiration.

PATHOPHYSIOLOGY

When a furuncle develops, initial bacterial invasion of the hair follicle has extended into the surrounding dermis, causing intense inflammation and destroying the entire hair follicle.

When multiple or recurrent furuncles exist, the condition is referred to as furunculosis.

CLINICAL MANIFESTATIONS

Furuncles are most commonly found on the back of the neck, in the axillae, or on the buttocks. A furuncle first appears as a small, red, elevated, tender nodule. As the infection spreads, the surrounding tissues become red, indurated, and painful. Involved tissues undergo necrotic changes, and in a few days the furuncle "points" or "comes to a head."

MEDICAL DIAGNOSIS

Diagnosis is made clinically by the appearance of the lesion. It can be confirmed by culture of the exudate or of material obtained by an incision and drainage (I&D).

MEDICAL MANAGEMENT

Treatment includes the application of hot, wet compresses using a clean cotton washcloth soaked in hot tap water four times daily. The furuncle can be gently nicked when it comes to a head to promote drainage, or it may heal on its own. Surgical I&D may be performed for painful lesions.

Squeezing a furuncle can force pathogens deeper into the surrounding tissues and is not recommended.

Systemic antibiotics are sometimes administered. For multiple, simultaneous, and recurrent furuncles, systemic antibiotics are prescribed, and the routine use of antiseptic topical agents is indicated. In chronic furunculosis, the physician may also prescribe cleansing the entire body every other day with antiseptic cleansers and applying antibiotic ointment to the nares twice daily.

CARBUNCLE

A carbuncle is a collection of furuncles. It is deeper than a furuncle and drains purulent exudate through a number of points to the surface. Before the discovery of antibiotics, carbuncles could be fatal because of intracranial extension.

ETIOLOGY

Carbuncles are generally caused by *S. aureus.* They occur most often in areas where the skin is thick and inelastic, such as the back of the neck and the buttocks. In the presence of immunosuppression, gram-negative bacilli may be the infecting organisms.

PATHOPHYSIOLOGY

Carbuncles are formed when furuncles develop in adjoining hair follicles and then coalesce in the dermis to form a large, pus-filled mass. This mass produces increased pressure on the nerve endings and thus severe pain.

CLINICAL MANIFESTATIONS

The patient complains of extreme tenderness and pain in the involved area. The area is red and edematous, with multiple pustules present. Fever and malaise are common.

MEDICAL DIAGNOSIS

Diagnosis is made by clinical appearance and is confirmed by bacterial cultures. The patient may have mild leukocytosis.

MEDICAL MANAGEMENT

Medical treatment includes immobilizing and avoiding manipulation of the affected area and systemic antibiotic therapy such as penicillin.

To avoid spreading the infection, a carbuncle is never incised. Extreme care is needed with lesions around the upper lip and nose because of possible intracranial extension and fatal cerebral thrombophlebitis.

ABSCESS

ETIOLOGY

An abscess is similar to a furuncle except that it usually results from traumatic inoculation of bacteria into the skin by a puncture wound, laceration, or surgical incision.

PATHOPHYSIOLOGY

The sudden inoculation of many bacteria into the dermis causes a vigorous inflammatory response followed by a collection of inflammatory cells. The abscess develops in the dermis and sometimes penetrates the subcutaneous fat. As it forms, it creates a painful, pus-filled nodule.

CLINICAL MANIFESTATIONS

The clinical manifestations of an abscess include tender, red nodules that enlarge and become more painful as the abscess grows. Regional lymph node enlargement is common.

MEDICAL DIAGNOSIS AND MEDICAL MANAGEMENT

The medical diagnosis and medical management are the same for an abscess as for a furuncle.

IMPETIGO

Impetigo is a superficial skin infection that can occur at any age but is most commonly seen in children. Preexisting conditions such as poor health and poor hygiene increase its chance of occurrence.

ETIOLOGY

Impetigo is caused either by *S. aureus* or group A streptococci.

PATHOPHYSIOLOGY

Impetigo involves only the epidermis, but there may be mild erythema resulting from an inflammatory reaction in the dermis. Bacteria enter the epidermis at an area of minor trauma and cause an inflammatory response. A pustule forms below the stratum corneum. When the pustule breaks, a crusted lesion is formed. Healing occurs without scarring.

CLINICAL MANIFESTATIONS

Honey-colored crusts on an erythematous base are characteristic presenting lesions of impetigo. Initially, a red macule forms, which becomes vesicular and then fills with a thin, yellow pus. When the lesions break, crusts are formed. There is glistening, weeping, and erosion under the crusts. Impetigo usually occurs on the face (Fig. 7–2) but can develop anywhere on the body.

MEDICAL DIAGNOSIS

Diagnosis is made on the basis of clinical findings. A Gram stain shows gram-positive cocci. A bacterial culture typically grows *S. aureus.* Culture specimens are obtained from the weeping erosion after removing the crust.

MEDICAL MANAGEMENT

Treatment consists of oral antibiotics for 7 to 10 days, usually erythromycin or dicloxacillin. Topical antibiotics are ineffective in treating impetigo. Crusts are removed by scrubbing gently with chlorhexadine, and an antiseptic ointment is applied to the erosion. If the causative organism is streptococcus, the patient is closely monitored for glomerulonephritis, which is a rare complication of streptococcal infection.

CELLULITIS

Cellulitis is a deep infection of the skin and subcutaneous tissue.

ETIOLOGY

Cellulitis is usually caused by group A streptococci and *S. aureus. Cryptococcus neoformans* can cause cellulitis in patients who are immunosuppressed.

PATHOPHYSIOLOGY

The pathogen enters the dermis via an external route typically near a surgical wound or a cutaneous ulcer or through the blood stream. Bacterial proliferation triggers an inflammatory response with tissue edema, as shown in Figure 7–3. The inflammation spreads horizontally through the tissues. Impaired lymphatic circulation may result from damage to the local lymphatic vessels and predisposes the patient to recurrent episodes of cellulitis, as do lymphatic changes caused by lymph node resection or radiation therapy.

CLINICAL MANIFESTATIONS

The involved skin is inflamed, and the classic signs of inflammation are evident: warmth, redness,

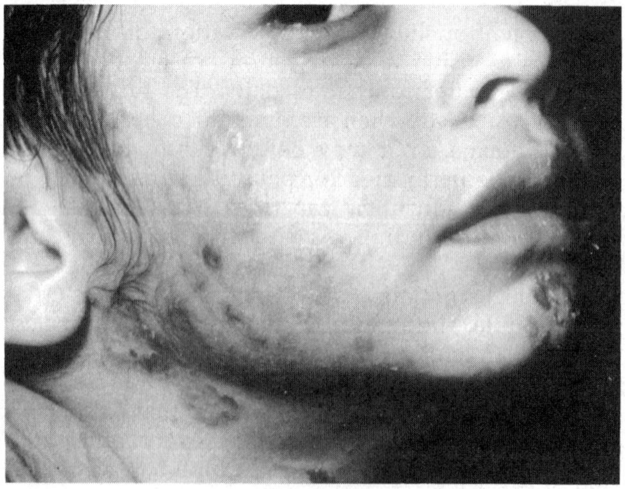

Figure 7–2.

Vesicular impetigo characterized by a thick, honey-yellow adherent crust covering the eroded surface. (Courtesy of Dr. WE Farrar, from Infectious Diseases, Farrar et al., Gower Medical Publishing, London, UK, 1984.)

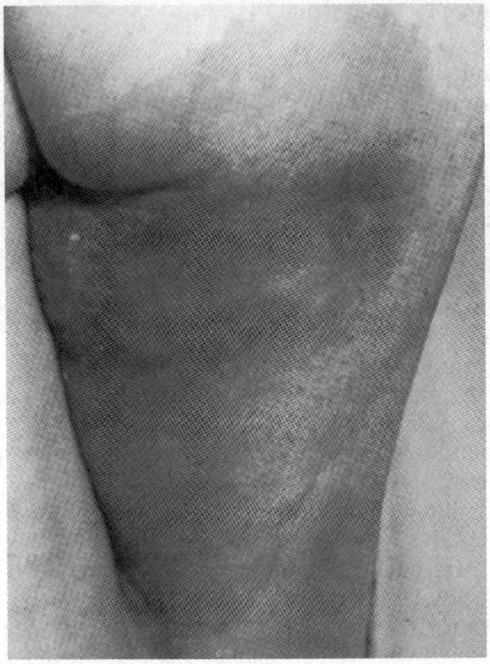

Figure 7–3.

Deep red, swollen, tender area characteristic of cellulitis. (From Lookingbill DP, Marks JG. Principles of dermatology. Philadelphia: WB Saunders, 1986, p. 189.)

swelling, and pain. This is accompanied by fever, malaise, and chills. Leukocytosis with a left shift (increased number of white blood cells with immature granulocytes prominent in the differential count) and a slightly elevated sedimentation rate may also occur. Cellulitis is most common in the lower legs.

MEDICAL DIAGNOSIS

Diagnosis is made on the basis of clinical appearance and laboratory findings. Skin and blood cultures may be obtained, but the bacterial pathogen is not always found.

MEDICAL MANAGEMENT

The treatment of cellulitis consists of bed rest, elevation of the affected area, and administration of parenteral antibiotics such as erythromycin, dicloxacillin, or cephalosporin. Mild cases of cellulitis on an extremity can be treated with oral antibiotics and with close, out-patient follow-up. Driving is contraindicated if the legs are affected.

Complete recovery is expected with antibiotic therapy. The fever usually subsides within 48 hours. Skin inflammation may take 2 weeks to resolve. Prophylactic antibiotics may be given for months or years in cases of recurrent disease. Before the advent of antibiotics, cellulitis was potentially life threatening.

ERYSIPELAS

Erysipelas is an acute inflammatory form of cellulitis that is characterized by significant lymphatic involvement. It can produce subcutaneous abscess and widespread infection.

ETIOLOGY

Erysipelas is usually caused by group A beta-hemolytic streptococci.

PATHOPHYSIOLOGY

Erysipelas occurs most often in apparently normal areas of the skin with no identifiable portal of entry. The infectious process is similar to cellulitis but with prominent lymphangitis. As the infection spreads, vesicles and bullae may form over a large area. Erysipelas is most common on the lower legs, face, and ears.

CLINICAL MANIFESTATIONS

The clinical manifestations of erysipelas are similar to those of cellulitis. It presents with a red, hot, shiny, indurated, tender area of skin. In contrast to cellulitis, erysipelas has a sharp advancing border (the involved area is clearly demarcated from the surrounding normal skin) and streaking (red lines along lymphatic vessels in the direction of the lymph nodes).

MEDICAL DIAGNOSIS AND MEDICAL MANAGEMENT

The medical diagnosis and medical management of erysipelas are the same as for cellulitis.

PARONYCHIA

Paronychia is an infection of the nail fold. It may be acute or chronic.

ETIOLOGY AND PATHOPHYSIOLOGY

Acute paronychia may develop spontaneously or occur after trauma to the nail fold. It is usually caused by infection with *S. aureus.* Chronic paronychia develops slowly and is common among dishwashers, dentists, and others whose hands are repeatedly exposed to moisture. In chronic paronychia, the cuticle separates from the nail plate, creating a portal of entry for a wide variety of infecting organisms.

CLINICAL MANIFESTATIONS

The onset of acute paronychia is sudden. It can affect any finger or toe, but the second and third fingers are most commonly involved. Edema is present. The nail throbs with pain and is red and swollen. An abscess or cellulitis may develop.

The onset of chronic paronychia is characterized by mild swelling and tenderness of the nail fold, with all or several fingers involved. The skin surrounding the nail becomes pale red, and sometimes a small amount of pus can be expressed from under the proximal nail fold.

MEDICAL DIAGNOSIS

Acute paronychia can be mistaken for herpetic whitlow. A Tzanck preparation and culture provide confirmation of the diagnosis. If the acute bacterial infection is unresponsive to antibiotics, x-ray films are taken to rule out osteomyelitis.

In chronic paronychia, a culture may be done on debris under the cuticle to identify the causative organisms.

MEDICAL MANAGEMENT

Medical treatment of acute paronychia consists of I&D and administration of systemic antibiotics such as erythromycin and dicloxacillin. Treatment of chronic paronychia begins with keeping the hands as dry as possible. Topical application of a thymol solution until the cuticle regrows is the most effective treatment.

Application of the Nursing Process to the Care of the Patient with a Bacterial Infection of the Skin

Assessment

In assessing the patient with a bacterial skin infection, obtain a complete history, including duration of the lesions and personal and family history of similar lesions. Ask about associated subjective symptoms such as tenderness or pruritus, and determine whether trauma or insect bites preceded the inflammation. Review personal hygiene practices.

Examine the patient to assess and document objective symptoms: the types of lesions present, the extent of involvement of the primary disorder, and the presence of secondary infection. Note the appearance of lesions and their number, configuration, and distribution.

Determine the patient's understanding of the disease process, the prescribed treatment, and factors that may contribute to the disease process, such as tight-fitting clothing, maceration caused by obesity, and occlusive cosmetics.

Assess the patient's ability for self-care or the presence of a significant other to help with care.

Nursing Diagnoses and Planning

Nursing diagnoses and related expected patient outcomes most commonly applicable to patients with a bacterial skin infection include the following:

NDx: Impaired skin integrity related to the presence of lesions

Planning: Patient outcomes
1. Skin lesions clear.

NDx: High risk for infection related to spread

Planning: Patient outcomes
1. Patient describes measures to reduce the risk of spread.
2. Infection remains localized.

NDx: Altered health maintenance related to insufficient knowledge of prevention of and early intervention for recurrence

Planning: Patient outcomes
1. Patient describes measures to reduce risk of recurrence.
2. Patient has few recurrences.
3. Patient recognizes recurrence and seeks early treatment.

Nursing Interventions

NDx: Impaired skin integrity
Instruct the patient to apply warm, moist compresses for 20 minutes three times per day to increase circulation and to hasten healing. Substitute astringent compresses made with aluminum acetate (Burow's) solution to promote crusting. Stress the importance of allowing the area to dry thoroughly between compresses by wearing loose-fitting clothing and by proper positioning to allow good air circulation to the area. Instruct in self-administration of prescribed systemic and topical antibiotics.

NDx: High risk for infection
Instruct the patient in self-care to prevent the spread of infection, as presented in Chart 7–1. Advise the patient to notify the physician if the infection does not heal within the expected time frame (24 hours to 3 weeks, depending on the infection) or if it becomes worse.

NDx: Altered health maintenance
Instruct the patient to shower and shampoo daily with an antibacterial soap to eliminate the causative pathogen from the skin. Review the medical prescription and instructions for prophylactic antibiotic therapy. Teach the patient to avoid contributing factors such as overuse of bath or hair oils, occlusive cosmetics, tight-fitting clothing, and obesity.

Chart 7–1.

NURSING GUIDE TO PATIENT EDUCATION FOR SELF-MANAGEMENT: PREVENTION OF SPREAD OF BACTERIAL SKIN INFECTIONS

Instruct the patient to:

Refrain from squeezing or otherwise manipulating skin lesions because this can rupture the wall of tissue formed in the body's effort to localize the infection.
Wash hands thoroughly before and after treating the infected area.
Cleanse surrounding skin with an antibacterial soap.
Apply a thin layer of any ordered antibiotic ointment to the surrounding skin.
Wash all clothing and linens that come in contact with the lesion after each use.
Keep wounds covered with a dry dressing after incision and drainage.
Dispose of soiled dressings by wrapping in paper and burning, if possible.

Instruct the patient in the early recognition of recurrence of infection, and stress the importance of seeking immediate treatment.

Additional Interventions
Instruct the patient regarding immobilizing affected areas, bed rest, and limits on activity. Refer for home care if the patient needs frequent evaluation or does not have the knowledge or ability to manage the condition at home.

Evaluation

Evaluate the effectiveness of nursing care for a patient with a bacterial skin infection by comparing the patient's status against the expected patient outcomes. Examples of specific outcomes for patients with a bacterial skin infection have been provided in the Planning section.

Fungal Infections

Fungal infections are classified as dermatophyte (tinea) and nondermatophyte (yeast) infections.

DERMATOPHYTE INFECTIONS

ETIOLOGY

Dermatophytes cause superficial fungal infections of the skin and its appendages. These dermatophytes produce keratinase, an enzyme that breaks down keratin. They live only on dead keratin, the main constitutent of the hair, nails, and outer horny layer of the skin. Dermatophyte infections, referred to in lay language as ringworm, are classified according to the area of the body involved (Table 7–1).

The source of the infecting organism may be another person, an animal, or the soil. Dermatophytes that grow only on humans are called anthropophilic; those that grow on animals, zoophilic; and those that live in the soil, geophilic. Both zoophilic and

Table 7–1. CLASSIFICATION OF DERMATOPHYTE INFECTIONS BY SITE AND THE RELATED CLINICAL MANIFESTATIONS

INFECTION	SITE	CLINICAL MANIFESTATIONS
Tinea capitis	Scalp	Noninflammatory tinea capitis: scaling area with broken hair shafts; inflammatory tinea capitis: plaques, pustules, lymphadenopathy, possible scarring, and possible permanent hair loss.
Tinea corporis	Body, arms, legs	Elevated, scaling, erythematous, serpiginous border with central clearing
Tinea cruris	Groin	Sharply demarcated area with elevated, scaling, serpiginous borders.
Tinea pedis	Feet	Interdigital maceration or diffuse scaling on soles and sides of feet or vesicles and pustules on instep.
Tinea manuum	Hand	Dry, scaling hyperkeratotic lesions, usually only on one palm
Tinea unguium (onychomycosis)	Nails	Separation from the nail bed with debris under the nail.

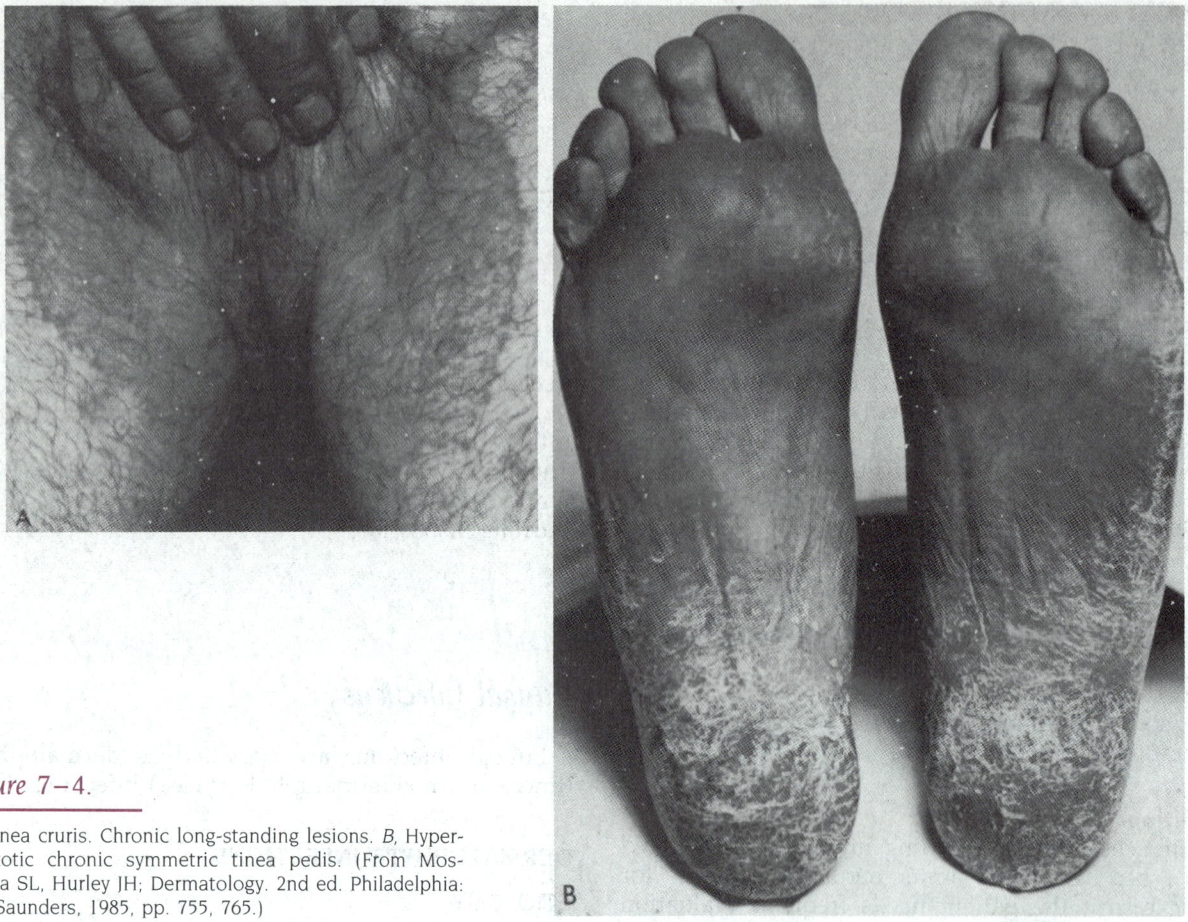

Figure 7–4.

A, Tinea cruris. Chronic long-standing lesions. *B*, Hyperkeratotic chronic symmetric tinea pedis. (From Moschella SL, Hurley JH; Dermatology. 2nd ed. Philadelphia: WB Saunders, 1985, pp. 755, 765.)

Chart 7–2.

NURSING GUIDE TO PATIENT EDUCATION FOR SELF-MANAGEMENT: PREVENTION OF RECURRENCE OF DERMATOPHYTE (TINEA) INFECTIONS

Instruct the patient to take the following measures to keep skin clean and dry:

Bathe daily, preferably after activities causing exertion and sweating.
Dry skin thoroughly, with particular attention to intertriginous and interdigital areas.
Apply talc or antifungal powder once a day if needed to control moisture.
Place cotton wads between toes at night if needed to absorb moisture and to prevent maceration.
Avoid tight-fitting clothing, which decreases air circulation and creates a warm, moist environment.
Wear cotton underwear and socks to promote air circulation and absorption of moisture.
Change clothes frequently.
Launder clothing and linens in hot water.
Change clothes frequently.
Avoid wearing a wet bathing suit for a prolonged period of time.
Wear leather sandals or other "breathable" footwear.
Avoid wearing the same shoes 2 days in a row.
Avoid plastic shoes, sneakers, or other footwear that hold moisture.
Avoid sharing combs, brushes, hats, clothing, or personal linens.

geophilic dermatophytes may infect humans. Dermatophyte infections are most often spread by direct contact, although spread via fomites such as combs and bed linens also occurs. Factors that increase susceptibility to dermatophyte infection include a warm, humid environment and a break in the stratum corneum.

PATHOPHYSIOLOGY

The stratum corneum is thickened and infiltrated with fungal hyphae (threadlike elements of the mycelium of the fungus). There may be inflammation in the dermis. Slow-growing dermatophytes affect only the stratum corneum, with no dermal inflammation. Zoophilic dermatophytes cause more skin inflammation than anthropophilic dermatophytes. Dermatophyte infections do not invade beyond the epidermis because they depend on keratin and because human serum is fungistatic.

CLINICAL MANIFESTATIONS

A major characteristic of tinea infections is the "active border," which is red, scaly, and slightly elevated, and a central area, which is often paler in color than adjacent nonaffected skin.

Table 7–1 describes clinical manifestations by site of infection on the body. Figure 7–4 illustrates different dermatophyte infections at different sites.

MEDICAL DIAGNOSIS

The finding of hyphae on a potassium hydroxide (KOH) preparation is diagnostic for tinea. A KOH preparation is performed on all scaling lesions to rule out fungal infection.

MEDICAL MANAGEMENT

Topical agents are prescribed to treat most tinea infections. The imidazole creams are antifungal agents that can be applied twice daily for 1 to 2 weeks after cleaning of the area with soap and water. If the area is severely inflamed, with vesicles or bullae present, wet soaks may be used. Four to 6 weeks of treatment, or longer, may be required.

Systemic antifungal agents such as griseofulvin are prescribed for widespread fungal disease, tinea capitis, and tinea unguium (onychomycosis).

Application of the Nursing Process to the Care of the Patient with a Dermatophyte Infection

Assessment

Inspect the involved areas. Note appearance, number, and location of the lesions. Ask about any associated symptoms su
describe when and ho
question about at-home
of over-the-counter prepa
any household member or
a similar infection and whet
or has recently been expos
When the affected area is th
explore the type and frequency o

Nursing Diagnoses and Planning

Nursing diagnoses and related expected
comes most commonly applicable to patie
dermatophyte infection include the followin

NDx: Impaired skin integrity related to prese
open lesions secondary to dermatophyte infectio

Planning: Patient outcomes

1. Patient describes or demonstrates prescribed therapeutic measures.
2. Lesions heal.

NDx: Altered health maintenance related to insufficient knowledge of prevention of spread and recurrence of tinea infection

Planning: Patient outcomes

1. Patient lists basic precautions to be taken to prevent spread to others.
2. Patient describes preventive measures, as presented in Chart 7–2.

Nursing Interventions

NDx: Impaired skin integrity

Explain the importance of keeping the area clean, dry, and free from irritation. Instruct the patient to use a clean washcloth and towel daily and to pat the skin dry thoroughly, paying particular attention to skin-fold areas. Encourage exposure of the affected areas to air as often as possible. Also instruct the patient to apply the prescribed topical agent twice daily until the skin is clear and then for 2 additional weeks. Stress that it may take 6 to 8 weeks for the lesions to clear, and caution the patient against becoming discouraged and stopping the treatment.

NDx: Altered health maintenance

To prevent spread of the infection, instruct the patient to wash hands thoroughly after touching the affected area. Instruct the patient to avoid tight-fitting clothing that causes chafing and occlusion. Clothes should be absorbent (cotton) rather than synthetic. Powders should not be allowed to cake in skin folds.

Instruct the patient in measures to prevent recurrence, as presented in Chart 7–2.

ɪal Interventions

.g is a problem, suggest application of cool .sses. Suggest sitz baths for tinea cruris.

ɪation

.luate the effectiveness of nursing care for a pa-.ɪt with a dermatophyte infection by comparing ɐ patient's status with the expected patient out-ɔmes. Examples of specific outcomes for patients vith dermatophyte infection have been provided in the Planning section.

NONDERMATOPHYTE FUNGAL INFECTIONS

Infections caused by nondermatophytes, or yeast fungal infections, are candidiasis and tinea versicolor.

CANDIDIASIS

Candidiasis (moniliasis) is an inflammatory reaction caused by *Candida albicans* infection in the epidermis.

Etiology

C. albicans is normally present on the skin and in the gastrointestinal tract, mouth, and vagina. When it penetrates and colonizes the surface of the skin or mucous membrane, it becomes pathogenic. Factors that predispose to the developing of candidiasis include pregnancy, use of oral contraceptives, diabetes, depression of cell-mediated immunity as in acquired immunodeficiency syndrome (AIDS) or chemotherapy, and antibiotic or topical steroid therapy. The elderly and patients with cancer, particularly leukemia, appear to be at increased risk.

Pathophysiology

C. albicans penetrates only the outer layers of the skin or mucous membrane. The toxins that are released cause an acute inflammatory response. The primary lesion is a pustule, whose contents spread under the stratum corneum and peel it away.

Clinical Manifestations

The infected skin area appears glistening, fiery red, or moist pink and may be surrounded by erythematous papules, a border fringe of white scale and pustules outside the area of opposing skin (Fig. 7–5). Severe itching and burning are present.

Skin-fold areas, which provide the warm, moist environment that yeast need to grow, are most often affected. These include the perianal area, groin, toe

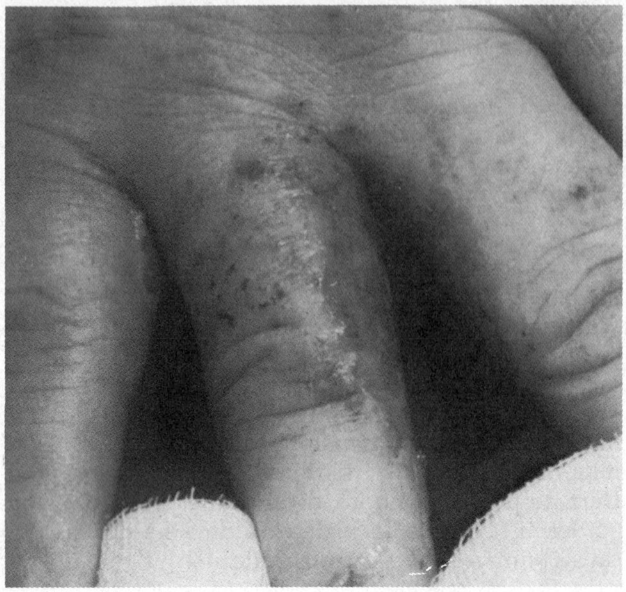

Figure 7–5.

Interdigital candidiasis. Note fringe of scale at edges of lesion. (From Moschella SL, Hurley JH. Dermatology. 2nd ed. Philadelphia: WB Saunders, 1985, p. 800.)

webs, and areas under pendulous breasts or between abdominal folds. This is referred to as *Candida* intertrigo. In acute oral candidiasis, the mucosa is typically red and sore with a white, creamy exudate or adherent white plaques, although a variety of presentations can occur. The tongue is almost always involved. Candidiasis can also cause chronic paronychia (nail infection).

Medical Diagnosis

Candidiasis is diagnosed by the presenting symptoms and a KOH preparation.

Medical Management

Most intertriginous candidal infections are treated with topical agents, including the imidazole derivatives and nystatin. They are applied sparingly, twice daily.

Application of the Nursing Process to the Care of the Patient with Candidiasis

The assessment, nursing diagnoses, expected patient outcomes, nursing interventions, and evaluation for patients with candidiasis are similar to those described previously for patients with a dermatophyte infection, with several additional considerations. Assess carefully for factors that decrease host resistance, because candidiasis can be an opportunistic infection. These factors include immunosuppressive drug therapy, antibiotic therapy, diabetes, cancer, and nutritional problems. If the patient with candidiasis has limited mobility, position the patient to maintain good air circulation to the affected and at-risk areas. For example, place a pillow between the patient's knees or under each arm to support them away from the chest walls and to allow air circulation to the axillae.

TINEA VERSICOLOR

Tinea versicolor is a common, chronic disorder that results in hypopigmentation or loss of skin color. It is seen worldwide but is most common in hot, tropical climates. It is chronic. Tinea versicolor is not known to be contagious.

Etiology

The term *tinea* is a misnomer because tinea versicolor is a nondermatophyte infection. It is caused by the yeast *Pityrosporum orbiculare,* which is part of the normal skin flora, and occurs in greatest numbers in areas of sebaceous glands. Factors that may predispose to infection include high heat and humidity, malnutrition, burns, corticosteroid therapy, pregnancy, and oral contraception.

Pathophysiology

The spores of the yeast proliferate in the outer layers of the stratum corneum. Infection occurs when the spores are transformed to hyphae, which penetrate deeper in the stratum corneum, resulting in thickening and scaling of the stratum corneum. It is not known whether hypopigmentation occurs as a result of the thickened infected stratum corneum, which may block out ultraviolet (UV) rays or whether it is a result of enzymes acting on surface lipids, thus inhibiting the enzyme responsible for melanin production.

Clinical Manifestations

The lesions of tinea versicolor are macular and vary in size, shape, and color. Typically, they begin as multiple, small, round macules that enlarge radially to become confluent patches. They may cover the upper trunk, lower abdomen, and proximal portions of the extremities. After sun exposure, the infected skin does not tan.

Medical Diagnosis

The finding of hyphae on a KOH preparation is diagnostic for tinea versicolor.

Medical Management

Tinea versicolor is primarily treated for cosmetic reasons. Antifungal creams are effective, but the lesion recurs as soon as treatment is stopped. If the infection is widespread, it is more economical to treat with selenium sulfide shampoo. The shampoo is applied in the shower to all affected areas and is left on for 10 minutes. The shampoo is initially applied three nights in a row, then weekly, and then every 3 months.

Guidelines for Application of the Nursing Process to the Care of the Patient with Tinea Versicolor

Assess the patient's knowledge of the skin condition. Determine how long the lesions have been present. Examine the entire skin to determine the extent of the lesions. Ask the patient whether any past treatments have been successful or unsuccessful. Determine the patient's ability and interest in self-management of this skin condition.

Explain that, although tinea versicolor is caused by a fungus, it is not contagious and can be controlled. Teach the patient how to apply antifungal creams and use selenium sulfide shampoo:

1. Apply selenium sulfide shampoo to the trunk, arms, and thighs in the shower; leave it on for 10 minutes and then rinse off.
2. Apply antifungal creams in a thin layer to the affected areas of the skin. Because the entire trunk may be affected, explain that the cream may be applied using the palms of the hands and downward strokes. Inform the patient that applicators to reach the back can be purchased in drug stores specializing in skin-care products.

Explain that it may take several months for hypopigmented areas to clear.

Viral Infections

Viral infections of the skin are caused by papovavirus, poxvirus, and herpes virus.

WARTS

Warts, or verrucae, are benign epidermal neoplasms. Warts are one of the most common skin ailments. They most frequently occur between the ages of 12 and 16 years.

Table 7–2. CLINICAL MANIFESTATIONS, COMMON LOCATIONS, AND TREATMENT OF WARTS

TYPE	APPEARANCE	COMMON LOCATIONS	TREATMENT
Common (verruca vulgaris)	Flesh-colored or brownish-gray scaling, vegetative papule or nodule.	Hands	Cryosurgery, desiccation and curettage, and cantharidin
Plantar	Solitary, grouped, or mosaic scaling papules	Feet	Chemical destruction (salicylic acid and lactic acid in flexible collodion)
Flat	Flesh colored or tan, soft, 1–3 mm	Face, neck, and sometimes forearms, hands	Cryosurgery, tretinoin (Retin-A)
Filiform	Soft, finger-like growth	Face and neck	Desiccation and curettage; cryosurgery
Condyloma acuminatum (moist)	Soft, vegetative	Mucocutaneous skin in anogenital area	Cryosurgery; podophyllin 25% in benzoin tincture; 5-fluorouracil; laser surgery

ETIOLOGY

Warts are caused by infection with human papillomavirus (HPV). Different HPV strains are responsible for different types of lesions.

Warts are transmitted by touch. Plantar warts are frequently transmitted between young adults using common showers. A single primary wart may develop numerous warts around it through autoinoculation. Warts are commonly found on the hands secondary to nail biting or other trauma.

PATHOPHYSIOLOGY

HPV is a deoxyribonucleic acid (DNA) virus that replicates in the epidermis. The altered DNA stimulates epidermal thickening and hyperkeratosis.

CLINICAL MANIFESTATIONS

Warts are characterized by epidermal thickening and hyperkeratosis. They interrupt normal skin lines and may have small, red dots from thrombosed capillaries or small black dots, hemosiderin, on their surfaces. The clinical manifestations of the different types of warts and most common locations are listed in Table 7–2. Figure 7–6 illustrates multiple plantar warts.

MEDICAL DIAGNOSIS

Most warts are diagnosed by appearance. They undergo biopsy only if there is suspicion of squamous cell cancer. A darkfield examination and serology tests may be done if the lesions are suspected to be condylomata lata associated with secondary syphilis. HPV has not been cultured, and HPV typing is experimental at this time.

MEDICAL MANAGEMENT

Medical treatment involves destruction of the infected keratinocytes and is about 80% effective. Although two thirds of all warts disappear in 2 years without treatment, their unsightly appearance and awkward locations prompt people to seek treatment. Painless plantar warts are often best left to resolve spontaneously rather than subjecting the patient to a prolonged program of treatment.

Cryosurgery is the most common method of treatment (see Chapter 6), but chemical destruction (keratolytic therapy) is preferred in children and patients with numerous warts. For chemical destruction, the lesion is first soaked in water, then salycylic acid and lactic acid in varying strengths in flexible collodion are applied to the wart. The area is covered with tape for 6 to 8 hours. The tape is removed, and the dead tissue is rubbed off with an emery board or pumice stone. This treatment can be repeated once or twice daily. The acid solution is caustic to normal skin.

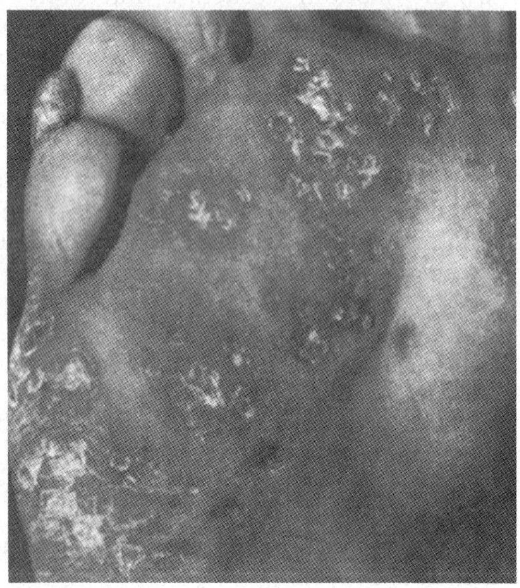

Figure 7–6.

Plantar warts. (From Moschella SL, Hurley JH. Dermatology. 2nd ed. Philadelphia: WB Saunders, 1985, p. 691.)

Podophyllin 25% in benzoin tincture is a cytotoxic agent used to treat condylomata acuminata (genital warts) in moist areas. It is applied carefully to the lesion during an outpatient visit and is washed off by the patient in 6 to 8 hours. Treatment is repeated weekly in the clinic or office until warts are resolved. Severe systemic reactions can occur from absorption of podophyllin, including renal toxicity, polyneuritis, and shock. It is not used during pregnancy.

Cantharidin is a vesicant or blistering agent applied to the wart after paring with a scalpel. The wart is then occluded for 24 hours or until it starts to hurt. The blister crusts and falls off in 7 to 14 days. The wart is re-treated if necessary.

Desiccation followed by curettage of dead tissue is most effective for common and filiform warts. Tretinoin has been found useful in treating flat warts. Recalcitrant warts have been treated intradermally with topical 5-fluorouracil and bleomycin. Laser surgery is used to treat condylomata acuminata extending into the vagina.

There are no vaccines to treat warts, and biologic treatments are not recommended to induce immune responses.

Guidelines for Application of the Nursing Process to the Care of the Patient with Warts

When caring for a patient with warts, note the number, appearance, and location. Ask whether the warts are frequently rubbed or irritated during daily activities and whether they cause discomfort or pain because of their location. Determine when they appeared and what, if any, measures have been used to treat them. Additional assessments as well as nursing diagnoses, expected outcomes, and nursing interventions relate to the selected mode of treatment. When chemical destruction is selected, carefully instruct the patient in the correct application of the topical medication. Also provide written instructions because package-insert directions may vary. Caution the patient against overtreating the warts, that is, using the medication more often than prescribed.

MOLLUSCUM CONTAGIOSUM

Molluscum contagiosum is a viral infection of the epidermis. It is more common in children than in adults. It is spread by autoinoculation, by scratching, or by touching a lesion. Venereal transmission occurs in adults.

ETIOLOGY AND PATHOPHYSIOLOGY

Molluscum contagiosum is caused by a DNA poxvirus that infects the epidermis. The virus replicates in the cytoplasm of a keratin cell, resulting in proliferation of the epidermis and in eosinophilic cytoplasmic inclusion bodies.

CLINICAL MANIFESTATIONS

The lesion of molluscum contagiosum appears as a flesh-colored, dome-shaped papule with a cheesy core. In children, the lesions appear on the face, trunk, and extremities. In sexually active adults, they are most common on the genitalia.

MEDICAL DIAGNOSIS

Diagnosis is made on the basis of clinical observation. It can be confirmed with Wright's stain.

MEDICAL MANAGEMENT

Curettage and cryosurgery are reliable methods of treatment. Spontaneous remission often occurs within 6 to 9 months.

Application of the Nursing Process to the Care of the Patient with Molluscum Contagiosum

The assessment, nursing diagnoses, expected patient outcomes, nursing interventions, and evaluation for patients with molluscum contagiosum vary with the treatment mode selected. See Chapter 6 for specific information on the care of patients having curettage or cryosurgery.

HERPES SIMPLEX

Herpes simplex virus (HSV) is one of the most common viruses found in humans. Although most of the adult population has been infected with HSV, not all infected individuals have experienced a clinically active eruption.

There are two types of herpes simplex virus: HSV 1 and HSV 2. HSV 1 is generally associated with oral infections (fever blisters or cold sores [Fig. 7–7]) and HSV 2 with genital infections. However,

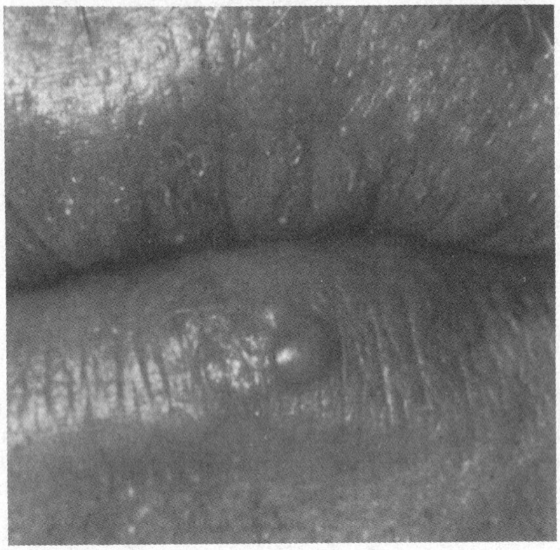

Figure 7–7.

Herpes simplex labialis, an early lesion at the mucocutaneous margin appears as a localized swelling that subsequently reveals itself to be a group of vesicles. (From Moschella SL, Hurley JH. Dermatology. 2nd ed. Philadelphia: WB Saunders, 1985, p. 1847.)

HSV 1 genital infections and HSV 2 oral infections do occur and, in fact, are increasing in frequency. HSV 1 may also infect the eye (herpes keratitis) and the brain (herpes encephalitis).

See Chapter 47 for a discussion of the etiology, pathophysiology, clinical manifestations, medical diagnosis, and treatment of herpes simplex.

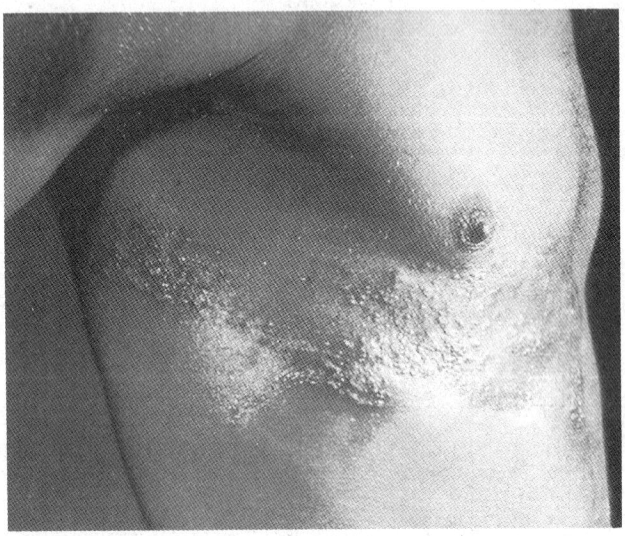

Figure 7–8.

Herpes zoster affecting a single thoracic dermatome. Note that vesicles vary in size. (Courtesy of Dr. WE Farrar, from Infectious Diseases, Farrar et al., Gower Medical Publishing, London, UK, 1984.)

Application of the Nursing Process to the Care of the Patient with HSV 1 Oral Infection

Refer to Chapter 22 for the assessment, nursing diagnoses, expected outcomes, nursing interventions, and evaluation commonly applicable to patients with oral infections. Be certain to explain to patients with herpes simplex of the lip that the lesion can be spread by kissing, by oral-genital sexual contact, or by any contact of the lesion with impaired skin (e.g., the patient's own finger with a paper cut, macerated skin from excessive hand washing).

Because the virus can be shed even when lesions are not apparent, protect self and others by routinely wearing gloves when performing oral or tracheal suctioning. When coming into direct contact with herpetic lesions or secretions, wear gown and gloves, and wash hands carefully on completing care.

HERPES ZOSTER

Herpes zoster (shingles) is a viral infection generally involving the skin of a single dermatone. It occurs in 10% to 20% of the population (Habif, 1990, p. 290). Its incidence has increased among the elderly and immunosuppressed individuals. It is also seen in patients with AIDS and is equally common in men and women.

ETIOLOGY

Herpes zoster is caused by activation of the latent varicella-zoster virus in persons who have had varicella (chickenpox) or by exposure to the varicella virus in persons with no immunity to it.

PATHOPHYSIOLOGY

The varicella-zoster virus enters the cutaneous nerves during an episode of chickenpox and travels to the dorsal root ganglia, where it becomes latent. It later reactivates, replicates, and travels back down the sensory nerve to the skin. The epidermis becomes inflamed, and bullae and multinucleated giant cells develop, along with perivascular inflammation in the dermis. Factors associated with reactivation of the virus include advancing age, immunosuppressive drugs, fatigue, emotional upset, and radiation therapy.

CLINICAL MANIFESTATIONS

The lesions appear as grouped vesicles in a linear pattern on an erythematous base. As shown in Figure 7–8, they follow the course of a peripheral sensory nerve, are usually unilateral, and do not cross the midline. Although individual lesions crust and drop off in about 10 days, one episode may produce continuous eruptions over a prolonged period of time.

Severe itching, burning, and pain occur 4 to 5 days before the appearance of the eruption. Fever, headache, and malaise may also precede the eruption by several days, and lymphadenopathy may be present. These symptoms gradually subside as the eruption appears. The course of herpes zoster can be long and drawn out over a year and is very exasperating and demoralizing for the patient. Secondary infection is always a concern.

For the elderly and immunosuppressed patients, herpes zoster infection can be very serious. One third of patients older than 60 years infected with herpes zoster acquire postherpetic neuralgia (pain persisting in a dermatome for months or years after the eruption has disappeared). This pain is often severe, accentuated by tactile stimuli, and exhausting.

Disseminated zoster occurs only in patients with severe immunosuppression. It occurs 5 to 7 days after the initial eruption. Symptoms include fever, malaise, and generalized vesicular eruptions. The liver, lungs, and central nervous system may be involved.

MEDICAL DIAGNOSIS

The characteristic lesions distributed along the dermatome are diagnostic for herpes zoster infection.

MEDICAL MANAGEMENT

Treatment of localized herpes zoster lesions includes cool compresses, Burow's compresses, zinc oxide lotion, and analgesics and antipruritics, such as hydroxyzine, that are strong enough to relieve the patient's pain and itching. Because discomfort and itching are especially severe at night, antipruritics are administered before sleep.

Oral steroids can effectively reduce acute pain and, when given within several days of disease onset to patients older than 50 years, may decrease the incidence of postherpetic neuralgia. Lidocaine (Xylocaine) injected subcutaneously every 4 to 5 days at the most painful sites also effectively relieves pain. Sympathetic blocks are also used to control acute pain.

Disseminated zoster is treated with intravenous acyclovir, which reduces pain and stops dissemination and vesicle formation.

Topical acyclovir applied four times per day for 10 days shortens healing time in immunocompromised patients.

Application of the Nursing Process to the Care of the Patient with Herpes Zoster

Assessment

Inspect the affected area. Note appearance and distribution of lesions. Question the patient as to when the lesions developed, and ask about associated pain, itching, headache, and malaise. Check for elevated temperature. Because the incidence of herpes zoster is increased in immunosuppressed individuals, review the patient's medical history and current health status. Similarly, explore the patient's status relative to stress and fatigue because these factors are also implicated in reactivation of the varicella virus. Assess for signs of secondary infection.

Nursing Diagnoses and Planning

Nursing diagnoses and related expected patient outcomes most commonly applicable to patients with herpes zoster include the following:

NDx: Impaired skin integrity related to presence of lesions secondary to herpes zoster infection

Planning: Patient outcomes
1. Patient explains or demonstrates skin-care regimen.
2. Lesions heal without secondary infection.

NDx: Pain related to inflammation secondary to herpes zoster infection

Planning: Patient outcomes
1. Patient uses a variety of pain-control techniques.
2. Patient reports increased comfort.

NDx: High risk for ineffective individual coping related to prolonged, severe discomfort and change in appearance

Planning: Patient outcomes
1. Patient verbalizes concerns about the herpes zoster infection and its symptoms.
2. Patient identifies plans for coping with the effects of the herpes zoster infection.
3. Patient expresses confidence in ability to cope with the herpes zoster infection.

Nursing Interventions

Adhere to wound and skin precautions for hospitalized patients with localized herpes zoster. Follow strict isolation procedures for patients with disseminated herpes zoster. Instruct patients at home on wound and skin precautions, and stress the importance of avoiding contact with pregnant women to avoid transmitting the disease to the mother and fetus.

NDx: Impaired skin integrity
Keep the affected area clean, dry, and free from irritation. Wash with mild soap and warm water. Rinse and pat dry thoroughly. If a dressing is used, change it frequently, making certain it does not rub or otherwise irritate the lesions.

Review with the patient the importance of adequate rest and good nutrition, including the need for vitamin C, to the healing process.

Instruct the patient to avoid scratching the lesions to avert further tissue damage and to decrease the risk of secondary infection. Instruct the patient to notify the physician if purulent drainage, fever, or severe malaise develops.

NDx: Pain
Acknowledge that the pain and itch can be excruciating, and reassure the patient that a variety of pain-control methods can be used to provide relief.

Administer or teach self-administration of prescribed analgesics and antipruritics. Explain the importance of taking the medication at bedtime because both pain and itching tend to be worse at night. Because pain and itch are not always satisfactorily relieved with medication, encourage the use of showers and cool compresses. Also guide the patient in the use of pain-control techniques such as progressive relaxation, imaging, and distraction.

Assist the patient in selecting clothing that is loose and that does not trigger pain through tactile stimulation of the affected area. If needed, plan for a bed cradle to keep the pressure of bed linens from stimulating the area.

NDx: High risk for ineffective individual coping
Recognize that patients with herpes zoster are at risk for ineffective individual coping for a variety of reasons that include the experience of prolonged severe pain, lack of adequate rest and sleep because of the pain, interference with usual activities, inability to dress in usual style because of the need for loose clothing, and disfigurement, particularly when the affected area is the face. Encourage the patient to verbalize concerns and feelings, and acknowledge their validity. When necessary, correct any misinformation, and guide the patient in realistically assessing the problems and in identifying methods of coping and sources of support.

Evaluation

Evaluate the effectiveness of nursing care for a patient with herpes zoster infection by comparing the patient's status with the expected patient outcomes. Examples of specific outcomes for patients with herpes zoster infection have been provided in the Planning section.

Inflammations

Eczematous Dermatitis (Eczema)

Eczematous dermatitis (eczema) is a common superficial inflammation of the skin characterized by itching, erythema, and edema of the involved area. Papules, vesicles, crusts, scales, and fissures may also develop.

NONSPECIFIC ECZEMATOUS DERMATITIS

ETIOLOGY

Nonspecific idiopathic eczematous dermatitis is a self-perpetuating epidermal eruption. It may be acute or chronic, localized or generalized. Its cause is unknown.

PATHOPHYSIOLOGY

A papulovesicular eruption develops with intense itching. Scratching results in histamine release, which causes more itching and worsens the dermatitis. In chronic eczematous eruptions, the epidermis becomes hyperkeratotic or thickened. Perivascular inflammation is present in both acute and chronic eczema.

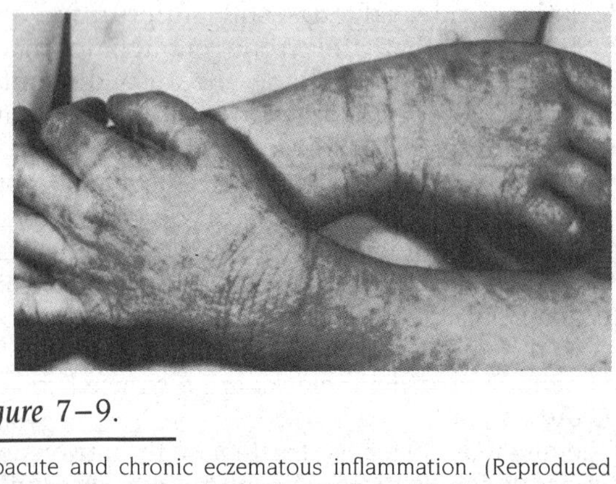

Figure 7–9.

Subacute and chronic eczematous inflammation. (Reproduced with permission from Fitzpatrick TB, Freedberg IM. Dermatology in general medicine. 3rd ed. New York: McGraw-Hill, 1987, p. 1368.)

Table 7–3. IDIOPATHIC ECZEMAS CLASSIFIED BY PRESENTING LESION, SITE, AND CONTRIBUTING FACTORS

IDIOPATHIC ECZEMA	SUGGESTED CONTRIBUTING FACTORS	PRESENTING LESION	SITE
Dyshidrotic	Excessive hand washing; "housewives' eczema"	Deep-seated vesicles	Palms, soles, sides of fingers
Autosensitization (intradermal eruption)	Hypersensitivity reaction to substance produced by acute dermatitis of hands or feet	Subacute dermatitis	Face, neck, arms, and thighs
Xerotic	Low humidity, dry skin	Dry, fissured skin	Trunk, extremities, especially lower legs
Nummular	Biopsychosocial factors	Oval patches with crusted papulovesicles	Trunk, extremities

CLINICAL MANIFESTATIONS

Severe itching that interferes with sleep and activities of daily living is characteristic of nonspecific eczematous dermatitis. Acute presenting symptoms include vesicles, weeping, and crusted patches. Oozing papules are the presenting lesions in subacute eczema. Chronic eczema is characterized by lichenified, scaling plaques. Secondary lesions seen in eczemas are crusts, scales, and fissures. An indistinct border between normal and eczematous skin is characteristic. Figure 7–9 illustrates acute and chronic nonspecific eczema.

Idiopathic eczemas that have been classified by presenting lesions, common sites, and possible causes are identified in Table 7–3.

MEDICAL DIAGNOSIS

History, KOH, patch tests, and skin biopsy help differentiate chronic eczematous dermatitis from contact dermatitis, psoriasis, drug eruption, and fungal infection.

Presenting lesions, Tzanck preparation, KOH, and Gram's stain differentiate acute eczematous dermatitis from contact dermatitis, herpes, fungal infection, and impetigo.

MEDICAL MANAGEMENT

Eczematous dermatitis is treated with topical, systemic, or intralesional corticosteroids. Oral prednisone in tapering doses is given for acute and subacute eczema.

Triamcinolone, 40 mg intramuscularly, can be given for acute eczema. It can help for up to 4 weeks.

Wet dressings and baths soothe the skin, reduce inflammation, and remove crusts and scales. Antihistamines are prescribed for itching, especially at bedtime.

Erythromycin and dicloxacillin are antibiotics prescribed for secondary bacterial infections.

Application of the Nursing Process to the Care of the Patient with Eczema

Assessment

Assess the patient's knowledge of the condition. Determine the onset, duration, and previous treatments, including self-remedies and over-the-counter drugs. Assess the extent of the lesions and the discomfort caused by itching. Also assess the impact of the condition on the patient's self-esteem and lifestyle.

Nursing Diagnoses and Planning

Nursing diagnoses and related expected patient outcomes most commonly applicable to patients with nonspecific eczematous dermatitis include the following:

NDx: Impaired skin integrity related to presence of acute or chronic eruption

Planning: Patient outcomes
1. Eruption clears.
2. Frequency and severity of recurrences decrease.

NDx: High risk for body image disturbance related to presence of skin lesions

Planning: Patient outcomes
1. Patient verbalizes positive, realistic perception of self.
2. Patient expresses confidence in own coping ability.
3. Patient participates in social activities.

Nursing Interventions

NDx: Impaired skin integrity
Instruct the patient in self-administration of prescribed steroid therapy and in the application of wet dressings and the use of therapeutic baths. Explain the importance of taking antihistamines, especially at bedtime, to prevent unintentional scratching, which perpetuates the eczema. During waking hours, encourage cool baths and the use of skin moisturizers such as petrolatum to decrease itching and dryness. Stress that seeking immediate treatment for acute eczema and control of the itch-scratch cycle is essential to the control and prevention of chronic eczema.

NDx: High risk for body image disturbance
Encourage the patient to express feelings about the eczema and its impact on personal appearance. Be alert for behaviors or verbalizations indicating negative feelings about self. Explore with the patient how to use clothing to conceal affected areas and to enhance overall appearance.

Evaluation

Evaluate the effectiveness of nursing care for a patient with eczema by comparing the patient's status with the expected patient outcomes. Examples of specific outcomes for patients with eczema have been provided in the Planning section.

CONTACT DERMATITIS

Contact dermatitis is a common inflammatory skin ailment caused by an exogenous chemical. Statistics show that contact dermatitis causes more than 50% of occupational illnesses, excluding injuries, accounts for 25% of lost work time, and costs millions of dollars per year.

There are two types of contact dermatitis: irritant dermatitis and allergic contact dermatitis.

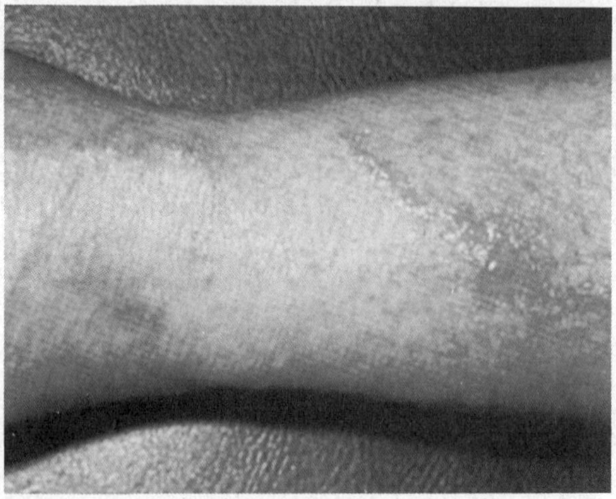

Figure 7–10.

Linear streaks of papulovesicles characteristic of contact dermatitis caused by poison ivy or other plants. (From Lookingbill DP, Marks JG. Principles of dermatology. Philadelphia: WB Saunders, 1985, p. 38.)

ETIOLOGY

Irritant dermatitis is caused by substances that are toxic to the skin such as acids, alkalis, solvents, and detergents.

Allergic contact dermatitis is a tissue inflammation caused by an immunologic reaction to chemicals such as plants, rubber, metals, and medicines. The most common causes of allergic contact dermatitis are listed in Table 7–4.

PATHOPHYSIOLOGY

Irritant dermatitis is an inflammatory skin reaction to a toxic substance. It usually occurs within a few hours after contact but may develop after days of multiple applications with a weaker irritant.

Allergic contact dermatitis is caused by a cell-mediated, Type IV immunologic reaction. The sensitization phase occurs when a chemical on the skin combines with an epidermal protein. A hapten-protein complex is formed, and the antigen stimulates the T lymphocytes to produce effector memory and suppressor lymphocytes in the lymph nodes.

Table 7–4. COMMON CAUSES OF ALLERGIC-CONTACT DERMATITIS

ALLERGY	SOURCE	CROSS-SENSITIVITY
Rhus (plant)	Poison ivy, poison oak, poison sumac	Cashews, mangoes, lacquer trees, ginkgo trees, smoke of burning plants
Paraphenylenediamine	Hair dye	Aso and aniline dyes, benzocaine, procaine, hydrochlorothiazide, sulfonamides
Nickel	Garters; all jewelry; earrings, including hypoallergenic	
Rubber	Clothing, foot gear, dress shields, gloves, breast pads, condoms, contraceptive diaphragms, eyelash curlers	
Ethylenediamine	Mycolog cream, dyes, insecticides, rubber accelerators, synthetic waxes, resins	Aminophylline, paraphenylenediamine

This phase takes 7 days. On reexposure to the antigen, the elicitation phase occurs, resulting in the inflammation of allergic contact dermatitis. The allergic response is later suppressed by the suppressor T cells.

Contact dermatitis, like other eczematous dermatitis conditions, is characterized by perivascular inflammation of the dermis, with vesicle formation and spongiosis in the epidermis.

CLINICAL MANIFESTATIONS

Clinical manifestations of irritant contact dermatitis are vesicles, fluid-filled papules, and lichenified plaques with sharp margins. Contact with the irritant may precede the eruption by hours or days.

In allergic contact dermatitis, the eruption occurs 1 to 4 days after exposure to the irritant. A vesicular, papular eruption occurs in the area of contact. The configuration varies. Linear streaks of papulovesicles are characteristic for contact dermatitis caused by poison ivy or other plants (Fig. 7–10).

MEDICAL DIAGNOSIS

There is no standard method for diagnosing irritant contact dermatitis. Patch testing is done for allergic contact dermatitis (see Chapter 6).

MEDICAL MANAGEMENT

Acute, severe, and generalized contact dermatitis is treated with a 10-day course of systemic steroids and baths or wet dressing. If a secondary infection occurs, it is treated with systemic antibiotics because topical antibiotics can aggravate contact dermatitis. Topical steroids and systemic antihistamines are prescribed for less severe cases. Acute contact dermatitis subsides within 3 weeks.

Chronic eczematous dermatitis develops with repeated exposure to the irritant or allergen. It is treated as chronic eczema.

Application of the Nursing Process to the Care of the Patient with Contact Dermatitis

Assessment

Obtain a patient and family history of skin disease. Ask the patient about recent use of prescribed and over-the-counter oral and topical medications and preparations. Include medications the patient is preparing for use by someone else.

Obtain a work history. Does the patient handle chemicals? Is the work environment hot and humid or very dry? Obtain a home and recreation history.

Document the location, course, and appearance of the lesions. Determine what the patient has used to treat the condition.

Nursing Diagnoses and Planning

The nursing diagnosis and related expected patient outcomes most commonly applicable to patients with contact dermatitis are as follows:

NDx: Altered health maintenance related to insufficient knowledge of the cause and prevention of contact dermatitis

Planning: Patient outcomes

1. Patient identifies causative factors.
2. Patient describes ways to avoid causative factors.

Nursing Interventions

NDx: Altered health maintenance

Explain that avoiding the causative irritant or allergen is the best way to prevent recurrence. Teach about sources of the irritant or allergen and cross-sensitivities to allergies (see Table 7–4). Be certain to explain that allergens may be transmitted via the hands. Acknowledge that avoidance of the causative factor may be difficult and in some cases may require changes in lifestyle and occupation. Explore with the patient what changes may be necessary and how they might best be instituted. Explain that protective clothing rarely helps. Advise the patient to avoid factors that increase sensitivity such as perspiration and tight-fitting clothing.

For nickel dermatitis, instruct the patient to purchase a kit to test jewelry for nickel. If jewelry is found to contain nickel, cover jewelry with four coats of nail polish.

Additional Interventions

Assist the physician and the patient in identifying etiologic factors by history and patch testing.

Instruct the patient in the use of prescribed topical therapies to treat contact dermatitis. These may include wet dressings of cool water; aluminum acetate solution; soothing, tepid baths; and colloidal oatmeal (Aveeno) baths.

Teach the patient the correct method of applying topical steroids.

Evaluation

Evaluate the effectiveness of nursing care for a patient with contact dermatitis by comparing the patient's status with the expected patient outcomes. Examples of specific outcomes for patients with contact dermatitis have been provided in the Planning section.

SEBORRHEIC DERMATITIS

Seborrheic dermatitis is a common, chronic inflammatory condition that affects the hairy areas of the body, mainly the scalp, eyebrows, and face.

ETIOLOGY AND PATHOPHYSIOLOGY

Seborrheic dermatitis is characterized by hyperkeratosis in the epidermis and perivascular inflammation in the dermis. Its cause is unknown.

CLINICAL MANIFESTATIONS

Seborrheic dermatitis occurs in the hairy regions of the body where there are many sebaceous glands. These areas include the scalp, eyebrows, eyelids, nasolabial folds, ears, chest, and intertriginous areas (axilla, groin, buttocks, inframammary folds). The patches and plaques of seborrhea are bilateral, symmetric, and erythematous, with indistinct borders and greasy, yellowish scales (Fig. 7–11).

Dandruff, a mild form of seborrheic dermatitis, presents as fine, white scales with no erythema.

MEDICAL DIAGNOSIS

The diagnosis of seborrheic dermatitis is made on the basis of clinical presentation.

MEDICAL MANAGEMENT

Treatment of seborrheic dermatitis consists of shampoos that contain any of the following keratolytic ingredients: sulfur, salicylic acid, coal tar, selenium sulfide, or zinc pyrithione. These preparations remove scales and soften the horny layer.

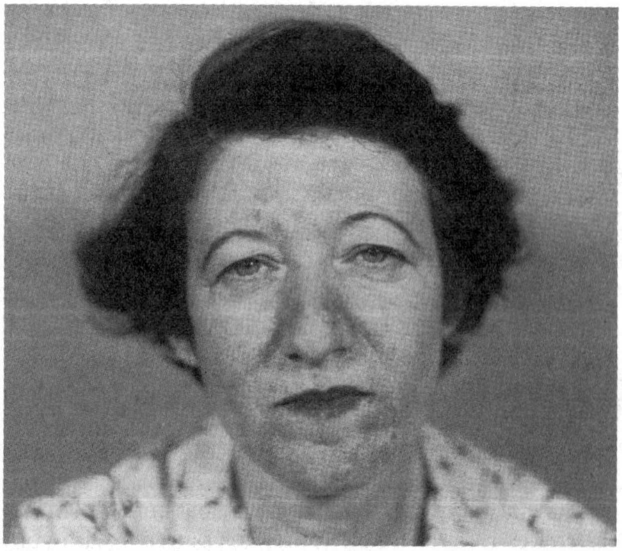

Figure 7–11.

Seborrheic dermatitis. Characteristic involvement of forehead, eyebrows, nasal folds, and chin. (From Pillsbury DM, Heaton CL. A manual of dermatology. Philadelphia: WB Saunders, 1980, p. 64.)

Topical steroid lotion is applied to hairy areas that do not respond to treatment or that are highly inflamed. Hydrocortisone cream 1% can be used to control seborrhea in nonhairy areas. High-potency steroid creams are contraindicated because, although they are initially effective, recurrent episodes of seborrheic dermatitis cease to respond and the treated skin develops atrophic changes.

Guidelines for Application of the Nursing Process to the Care of the Patient with Seborrheic Dermatitis

Assess the extent, onset, and duration of the seborrhea. Instruct the patient to wash hair with an antiseborrheic shampoo as follows: shampoo, rinse, shampoo again, leave in scalp 10 minutes, and rinse again. Also instruct the patient to apply hydrocortisone lotion 1% sparingly to the involved area of the scalp two times daily. If areas of the face are affected, instruct the patient to apply a thin layer of hydrocortisone 1% cream to the face twice daily as ordered by the physician. Remind the patient that a corticosteroid cream is readily absorbed on the face, and a thin layer provides the same therapeutic effect as a thick layer. Advise the patient to discontinue the hydrocortisone when the condition clears and to reapply at first sign of recurrence of seborrhea.

STASIS DERMATITIS

Stasis dermatisis is an eczematous eruption of the lower legs. The lower leg above the medial malleolus is the most common site.

ETIOLOGY AND PATHOPHYSIOLOGY

Stasis dermatitis is a complication of peripheral vascular disease. Venous incompetence causes increased hydrostatic pressure, swelling, and edema. Capillary proliferation and extravasation of red blood cells and vascular fluid causes the inflammatory eczematous dermatitis. Skin changes are similar to those seen in chronic, nonspecific dermatitis.

CLINICAL MANIFESTATIONS

The clinical manifestations of stasis dermatitis are edema, brown pigmentation, dull erythema, petechiae, thickened skin, scaling, and weeping of the skin (Fig. 7–12). Varicose veins may be present. Peripheral pulses are present. Dusky erythema precedes ulceration.

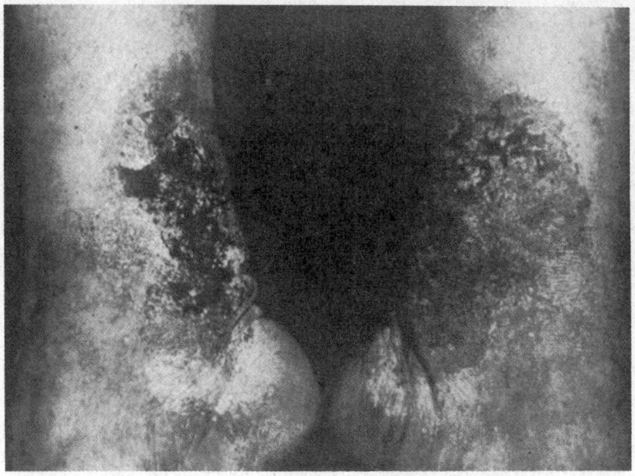

Figure 7–12.

Bilateral stasis dermatitis. (From Moschella SL, Hurley JH. Dermatology. 2nd ed. Philadelphia: WB Saunders, 1985, p. 369.)

MEDICAL DIAGNOSIS

The diagnosis of stasis dermatitis is made clinically. Cellulitis, contact dermatitis with a recent history of topical medication, fungal infection, and arterial disease may need to be ruled out.

MEDICAL MANAGEMENT

Medical treatment consists of the use of support hose or restrictive boots to prevent venous stasis and edema. Standing for long periods is discouraged. Weight reduction is necessary if the patient is obese. Frequent rest periods with leg elevation promote venous return.

Wet dressings are applied to the skin if oozing or crusting is present. Topical steroids may also be prescribed.

If ulceration occurs, Unna's boot is recommended for ambulation and bed rest with leg elevation is encouraged. Skin grafts may be required for deep ulcers. Antiseptic cleansing is important to prevent infection. Antibiotics are not helpful in the healing process unless cellulitis is present. Topical antibiotics are contraindicated because they can cause contact dermatitis as a result of the compromised epidermal barrier. This occurs in more than one half of patients with stasis dermatitis.

Application of the Nursing Process to the Care of the Patient with Stasis Dermatitis

The assessment, nursing diagnoses, expected patient outcomes, nursing interventions, and evaluation for patients with stasis dermatitis are similar to those described for patients with peripheral vascular disease and to those concerning symptomatic relief for patients with eczematous dermatitis. If grafting is necessary because of ulceration, nursing care is as described in Chapter 6.

LICHEN SIMPLEX CHRONICUS

Lichen simplex chronicus, or neurodermatitis, is a chronic eczematous eruption caused by scratching.

ETIOLOGY

The etiology of lichen simplex chronicus is not well understood. The patient experiences severe pruritus, which causes the scratching. The itching may be preceded by frustration, depression, or stress.

PATHOPHYSIOLOGY

Scratching causes lichenification and starts the itch-scratch cycle. The epidermis becomes thickened, with perivascular inflammation in the dermis. The skin changes are similar to those seen in stasis dermatitis and chronic nonspecific eczematous dermatitis.

CLINICAL MANIFESTATIONS

Lichen simplex chronicus is characterized by an erythematous, lichenified plaque on an area of skin within reach of scratching fingers (Fig. 7–13).

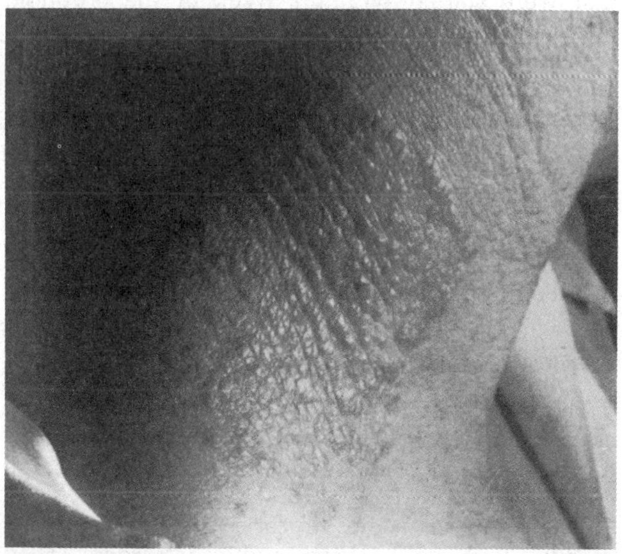

Figure 7–13.

Lichen simplex chronicus (neurodermatitis) affecting the side of the neck. (From Moschella SL, Hurley JH. Dermatology. 2nd ed. Philadelphia: WB Saunders, 1985, p. 367.)

MEDICAL DIAGNOSIS

Medical diagnosis is made by clinical appearance.

MEDICAL MANAGEMENT

Treatment includes administration of topical steroids and wet dressings. Tranquilizers and antidepressants may be indicated to control the itching.

Application of the Nursing Process to the Care of the Patient with Lichen Simplex Chronicus

The assessment, nursing diagnoses, expected patient outcomes, nursing interventions, and evaluation for patients with lichen simplex chronicus are similar to those described previously for patients with other eczematous eruptions, with emphasis on methods of controlling itching.

Drug Eruptions

Drug eruptions are the most common cause of generalized erythematous eruptions.

ETIOLOGY AND PATHOPHYSIOLOGY

Drug eruptions are usually caused by new drugs that were started within 1 week of the eruption. Three common types are morbilliform eruption (generalized, measles-like erythema), acute urticaria, and erythema multiforme (a skin and mucous membrane reaction characterized by the sudden onset of an erythematous eruption of which the characteristic lesion is the bull's eye or target lesion). Toxic epidermal necrolysis (TEN) is a rare reaction in which the epidermis peels away from the dermis. The involved area resembles a severe burn and, if large, may be life-threatening.

CLINICAL MANIFESTATIONS

The most common drug-related reaction is a generalized, itchy, macular/papular, bright-red morbilliform eruption with confluent lesions over large areas, as illustrated in Figure 7–14*A*.

The hives of acute urticaria are erythematous plaques with pale centers and red borders. They may be confluent and have a geographic configuration. Distribution may be generalized or localized on specific areas of the body. Individual hives last less than 24 hours, but new hives may continue to develop after the initial eruption. There is severe itching (Fig. 7–14*B*).

Target lesions are diagnostic for erythema multiforme. Three zones of color must be present in the lesions to diagnose erythema multiforme. The lesions have a central, dark area surrounded by pale edema, with a peripheral rim of erythema (Fig. 7–14C). The distribution is often symmetric and is frequently found on the palms and soles.

MEDICAL DIAGNOSIS

Patient history of recent new drug use and clinical manifestations help to diagnose a drug reaction. The only skin test helpful in diagnosing a drug reaction is a penicillin test for immediate hypersensitivity reaction in hives.

MEDICAL MANAGEMENT

The offending drug is discontinued. If the patient is taking several drugs and the offender is not apparent, the number of drugs administered is reduced to a minimum. Possible offenders should be changed to alternatives if feasible. Table 7–5 lists drugs that frequently cause dermatologic drug eruptions.

Symptomatic treatment may include antihistamines; soothing baths; cool, wet dressings; antipruritic lotions such as calamine; body lotions with menthol; and topical steroids. Systemic steroids are rarely required, but severe reactions may necessitate hospitalization and intravenous steroid therapy.

Patients with hives should not take aspirin or salicylates, which may exacerbate the condition.

Table 7–5. COMMON DRUGS ASSOCIATED WITH ALLERGIC SKIN REACTIONS

MOST COMMON OFFENDING DRUGS IN THE BOSTON COLLABORATIVE DRUG SURVEILLANCE PROGRAM	REACTION RATE (REACTIONS/100 RECIPIENTS)
Trimethoprim-sulfamethoxazole	5.9
(Septra, Bactrim)	5.2
Ampicillin	
Semisynthetic penicillins	3.6
Blood, whole human	3.5
Blood platelets	2.8
Erythromycin	2.3
Sulfisoxazole	1.7
Penicillin G	1.6
Gentamicin sulfate	1.6
Cephalosporins	1.3
Quinidine	1.2

Data from Arndt KA, Jick H. Rates of cutaneous reactions to drugs. A report from the Boston Collaborative Drug Surveillance Program. JAMA 1976; 235:918.

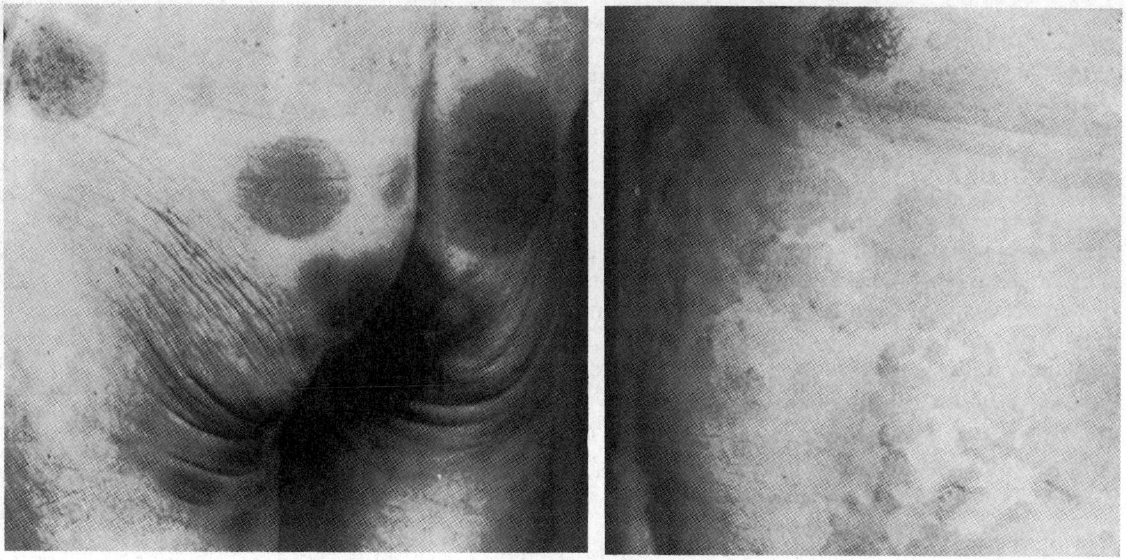

A B

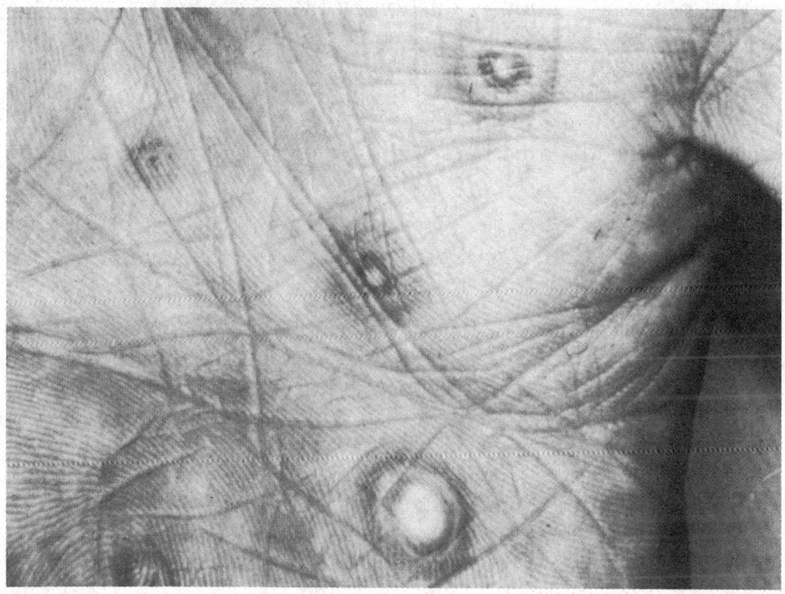

C

Figure 7–14.

Drug eruptions. *A*, Maculopapular lesions. (Reproduced with permission from Fitzpatrick TB, Freedberg IM. Dermatology in general medicine. 3rd ed. New York: McGraw-Hill, 1987. p. 1361.) *B*, Urticarial reaction to aspirin. (From Moschella SL, Hurley JH. Dermatology. 2nd ed. Philadelphia, WB Saunders, 1985, p. 436.) *C*, Target lesions. (From Price SA, Wilson LM. Pathophysiology. 4th ed. St. Louis: Mosby–Year Book, 1992, p. 1018.)

Guidelines for Application of the Nursing Process to the Care of the Patient with a Drug Eruption

Assess extent and characteristics of the eruption. Ask the patient whether any new drugs or over-the-counter preparations have been started 7 to 10 days before eruption. Specifically ask about acetylsalicylic acid (ASA), penicillin, other antibiotics, and quinidine, which frequently cause drug eruptions.

When a drug eruption is suspected, withhold the possible offender and notify the physician. Advise outpatients to discontinue the drug and to see or call the physician when a drug eruption is suspected.

Once a drug eruption is diagnosed and the causative agent identified, instruct the patient in methods of symptomatic relief as prescribed, and explain that the drug eruption may worsen over the next few days before it improves, with total clearing taking 1 to 2 weeks. Also explain the importance of alerting health care providers and pharmacists to the allergy and carrying medical alert information with him or her at all times.

Acne

Acne is a skin disorder of multifactoral origin affecting the sebaceous glands.

ACNE VULGARIS

Acne vulgaris is the most common skin disease seen by dermatologists. It can affect people of all ages but is most commonly seen among adolescents. In one survey, 85% of high school students indicated that they had acne. Although acne vulgaris is more prevalent and usually more severe in males, in females it may continue into the third and fourth decades of life.

ETIOLOGY AND PATHOPHYSIOLOGY

Etiologic factors associated with acne vulgaris include androgenic hormone stimulation, which causes increased sebum production by the sebaceous glands, obstruction of the sebaceous glands caused by keratinous impaction, and proliferation of anaerobic bacteria. The contents of the dilated sebaceous unit extravasate into the dermis, causing inflammation and comedo formation, as illustrated in Figure 7–15.

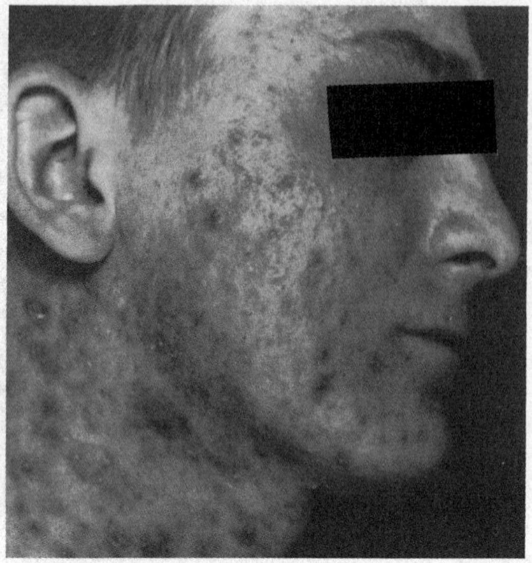

Figure 7–15.

Inflammatory acne with lesions spreading off the face. There are extensive comedones and small and large papules and cysts. (From Moschella SL, Hurley JH. Dermatology, 3rd ed. Philadelphia: WB Saunders, 1992, p. 1479.)

CLINICAL MANIFESTATIONS

The open comedo consists of a dilated pore filled with black keratinous material (blackhead). The closed comedo is a small, skin-colored, dome-shaped papule (whitehead). These lesions are not inflamed.

The inflammatory lesions are papules, pustules, nodules, and cysts, often surrounded by erythema. The face and upper trunk are the most common sites for both comedones and the inflammatory lesions of acne vulgaris. Cystic acne is characterized by nodules that have suppurated and by large deep cysts that often cause permanent scarring.

MEDICAL DIAGNOSIS

Diagnosis of acne vulgaris is made clinically by appearance of the lesions.

MEDICAL MANAGEMENT

Treatment includes use of topical keratolytic agents such as benzoyl peroxide, topical comedolytic agents such as tretinoin (Retin-A), topical antibiotics such as clindamycin (Cleocin T), systemic antibiotics such as tetracycline and erythromycin, and, for severe recalcitrant acne, systemic retinoids. Suppression of androgen secretion may be attempted by administration of low-dose glucocorticoids to males and estrogen-dominant oral contraceptives to females.

Collagen injections and dermabrasion (see Chapter 6) are used to treat severe acne scarring.

Application of the Nursing Process to the Care of the Patient with Acne Vulgaris

Assessment

Determine the patient's concept of the severity of his or her acne condition, and assess the psychosocial response to it. Keep in mind that most often the individual's acne occurs in teenage years, when self-consciousness is greatest, and individual psychosocial responses will vary greatly. Assess the actual extent of the acne, presence or absence of excoriations, and tissue damage.

Question the patient regarding over-the-counter preparations or other remedies that have been used to treat the acne and the degree of success of these remedies.

Obtain a history regarding any other possible diseases present such as endocrine disorders, medicines the patient may be taking (i.e., corticosteroids) that can cause steroid-induced acne, and use of cosmetics that might aggravate acne, especially in late-onset acne in women.

Assess the patient's interest in treatment and the ability to comply with the prescribed regimen.

The nurse working for a dermatologist in office practice or with a dermatologist in a clinic setting is also responsible for follow-up assessments on the effectiveness of treatments, patient compliance, and psychosocial effects of the disease and treatment.

Nursing Diagnoses and Planning

Nursing diagnoses and related expected patient outcomes most commonly applicable to patients with acne vulgaris include the following:

NDx: High risk for body image disturbance related to the presence of facial lesions

Planning: Patient outcomes
1. Patient verbalizes positive feelings about self.
2. Patient expresses confidence in ability to treat and control the acne.

NDx: Altered health maintenance related to insufficient knowledge of the cause and treatment of acne vulgaris

Planning: Patient outcomes
1. Patient lists basic principles of skin care.
2. Patient explains the prescribed medical treatment, including the name, frequency, method of use, and precautions related to prescribed medications.
3. Patient ascribes to importance of consistent daily treatment.

Table 7–6. TOPICAL AND SYSTEMIC MEDICATIONS USED IN THE TREATMENT OF ACNE VULGARIS

MEDICATION	ACTION	ADMINISTRATION	PATIENT TEACHING
TOPICAL PREPARATIONS			
Benzoyl peroxide	Antibacterial and keratolytic agent decreases inflammatory lesions, decreases sebum production, promotes breakdown of comedo plugs	Lotion, cream, or gel applied to affected area once a day initially may go to 4 times daily as tolerance permits	Available over the counter and by prescription; redness and scaling may occur when first used; avoid contact with eyes, mouth, mucous membrane, denuded skin areas.
Tretinoin (vitamin A acid)	Speeds turnover of epithelial cells, forcing out comedones and suppressing formation of new plugs; enhances penetration of other antiacne drugs	Cream, gel, or liquid applied at bedtime after skin is washed, toweled dry, and left to dry further for 15–30 min	Stop use of abrasive soaps or keratolytics before using tretinoin; may cause blistering, peeling, crusting, burning, or edema; do not apply to open areas or to areas of sun-or windburn; avoid contact with eyes, nose, and mouth.
Antibiotics (erythromycin, tetracycline, clindamycin)	Suppresses growth of *Propionibacterium acnes*; decreases skin surface free fatty acid levels; decreases comedones, pustules, papules	Apply thin layer to clean, dry skin	No systemic side effects
SYSTEMIC PREPARATIONS			
Antibiotics (tetracycline, erythromycin)	Anti-infective agents used in moderate to severe inflammatory acne characterized by pustules, abscesses, scarring	Small doses given over months to years	Take tetracycline 2 hr before meals; stop if become pregnant to avoid potential altered tooth formation in the fetus as result of effect of tetracycline on calcium metabolism; potential side effects include photosensitivity, nausea, diarrhea, vaginitis
Isotretinoin (vitamin A derivative)	Decreases sebum production, inflammation, keratinization, and secondarily the number of *P. acnes*; used for severe, recalcitrant acne.	0.5–1 mg/kg/day in 2 divided doses for 15 to 20 weeks.	Teratogenic causing hydrocephalus, microcephalus, cleft palate, facial and external ear deformities, and cardiovascular defects; pregnancy test done and contraception begun 1 month before therapy; contraception continued until 4–8 weeks after treatment ends; cheilitis, dryness or itching of the skin, nose, and mouth, and nosebleeds are almost universal side effects; blood triglycerides are measured before and during treatment to check for elevation; supplementary vitamin A and alcohol should be avoided.

Nursing Interventions

NDx: High risk for body image disturbance

Encourage the patient to express feelings about the acne and its impact on self. Monitor the patient for expression of negative feelings about his or her body. Be alert to behaviors or verbalizations indicating feelings of powerlessness, fear of negative reactions or rejection by others, or unwillingness to look at or touch affected skin areas.

Listen to the patient's complaints, and avoid giving soothing advice that minimizes the seriousness of the acne. Offer encouragement regarding the patient's ability to control the condition.

Dispel myths about acne (e.g., it is caused by uncleanliness, masturbation, or sexual activity). Stress that it is caused by factors beyond individual control such as heredity and large sebaceous glands.

NDx: Altered health maintenance

Instruct the patient in the basic principles of skin care. Caution the patient to void overdrying the skin with soaps and cleansers, which may exacerbate the condition. Recommend washing the face with a mild soap twice a day to remove surface oil. If an oily feeling is a problem, recommend a mild abrasive soap or a drying agent. Advise the patient to keep the hair off the face and to shampoo daily if necessary. Stress the importance of not touching affected areas and not "picking" or squeezing the lesions.

Instruct the patient in the prescribed medical treatment and associated precautions (Table 7–6). Explore with the patient how he or she will incorporate the prescribed regimen into his or her daily activities. Stress that improvement requires consistent daily treatment, and it will be 4 to 6 weeks before obvious improvement is seen. Encourage a healthy diet, which may reduce the severity of the condition. Explain that, although stress or the ingestion of chocolate and fatty foods may cause exacerbation of the condition in some individuals, no etiologic connection has been proven.

Additional Interventions

Reevaluate the patient on return visits. If there is no improvement in 2 months, the physician needs to reevaluate the patient for more intensive treatment.

Evaluation

Evaluate the effectiveness of nursing care for a patient with acne vulgaris by comparing the patient's status with the expected patient outcomes. Examples of specific outcomes for patients with acne vulgaris have been provided in the Planning section.

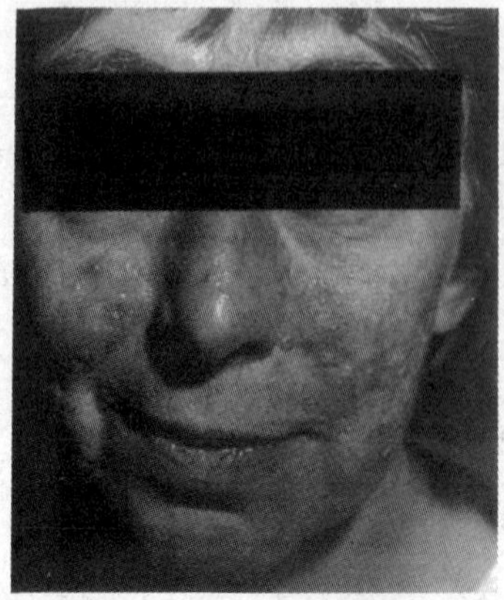

Figure 7–16.

Severe rosacea. Note "butterfly distribution" of acne-like pustules over the nose and cheeks. (From Lookingbill DB, Marks JG. Principles of dermatology. Philadelphia: WB Saunders, 1986, p. 159.)

ACNE ROSACEA

Acne rosacea is a chronic inflammatory disorder of adulthood that affects the blood vessels and pilosebaceous units of the face. It is most common in women between 30 and 50 years of age. Acne rosacea is most severe in men and increases in severity if untreated.

ETIOLOGY AND PATHOPHYSIOLOGY

Acne rosacea is a fairly common disorder of unknown etiology. It is characterized by intrafollicular pustules in the epidermis and telangiectasia with perivascular inflammation. Sun exposure, hot, spicy foods, alcohol, and caffeine have been suggested as causes of the vascular component of rosacea.

CLINICAL MANIFESTATIONS

Acne rosacea begins as an erythematous eruption over the nose and central part of the face (butterfly distribution). Papules and pustules develop. Telangiectasias are also present (Fig. 7–16).

MEDICAL DIAGNOSIS

Diagnosis of acne rosacea is made on the basis of clinical appearance.

MEDICAL MANAGEMENT

Metronidazole 0.75% topical gel (MetroGel) is used to treat the inflammatory papules, pustules, and erythema of acne rosacea. It is applied twice daily to the affected area, with improvment generally seen in 3 weeks. Pustules and papules may also be treated with oral antibiotics, and hydrocortisone 1% cream may be used to help decrease erythema. The condition may recur once treatment is discontinued.

Guidelines for Application of the Nursing Process to the Care of the Patient with Acne Rosacea

Explore the patient's lifestyle to check for factors that might contribute to the acne rosacea. Inquire specifically about exposure to the sun, ingestion of spicy foods, and alcohol and caffeine intake.

Advise the patient that antibiotics may be needed for months or years to treat rosacea and to prevent recurrences and complications. Explain that most individuals show improvment with antibiotics within weeks, although the telangiectasias persist.

Instruct the patient for whom MetroGel is prescribed to perform the following:

Wash the area thoroughly before applying the medication to the affected area.
Apply a thin film twice a day.
Use cosmetics, if desired, after the application of metronidazole.

Psoriasis

Psoriasis is a chronic disorder with a wide variation in severity and distribution of skin lesions. Its course is unpredictable and is marked by remissions and exacerbations. It occurs equally among males and females and is more frequent among light-skinned races. It can occur at any age; the average age of onset is in the late twenties. Psoriasis can be economically, socially, psychologically, and physically disabling.

ETIOLOGY

The multifactorial genetic and environmental stimuli responsible for the clinical expression of psoriasis are unclear. Approximately one third of affected individuals have a positive family history for psoriasis, and 80% of identical twins are affected concurrently. Among environmental factors that appear to trigger its expression are skin injury such as from surgery or sunburn; infections such as a cold, sinusitis, or sore throat; hormonal changes; stress; and drugs such as beta-blockers, indomethacin, and antimalarials.

PATHOPHYSIOLOGY

The normal epidermis has a cell turnover rate of 28 days. The psoriatic cell turnover rate can be as fast as 4 days. This results in hyperkeratosis, acanthosis (increased thickness of prickle cell layer) with elongated rete pegs, infiltration by neutrophils, and an accumulation of scales. There is perivascular inflammation in the dermis.

CLINICAL MANIFESTATIONS

The lesions of psoriasis are erythematous plaques with a sharp, well-defined border and silver-white scales. If the scale is removed, bleeding may occur because of the proximity of dilated blood vessels to the surface. Lesions are usually symmetric and may be few in number or may cover the total surface of a part (Fig. 7–17).

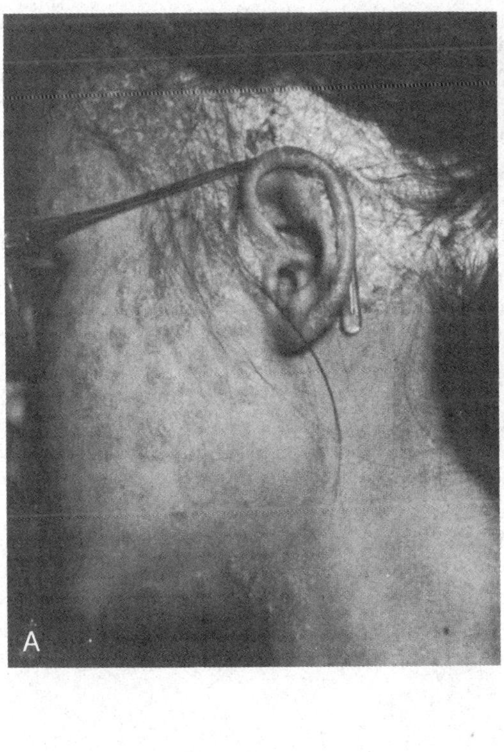

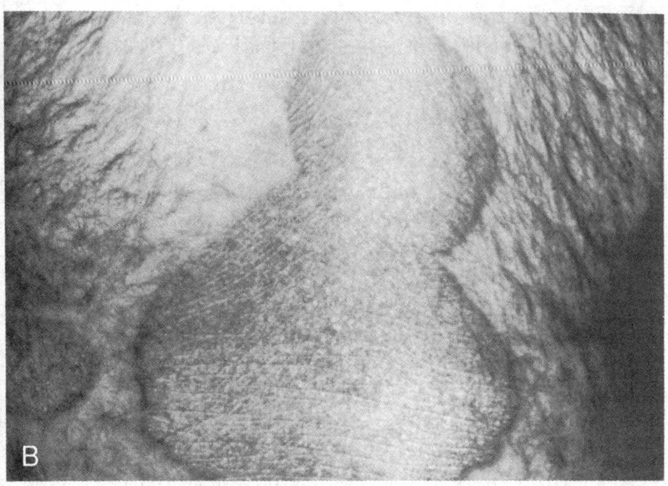

Figure 7–17.

A, Distribution of skin lesions in psoriasis. Commonest sites affected are the elbows, knees, lumbosacral skin, and scalp. *B*, Morphology of psoriatic skin lesions. Note sharply marginated border and white scales. (From Moschella SL, Hurley JH. Dermatology. 2nd ed. Philadelphia: WB Saunders, 1985, pp. 508, 509.)

Table 7–7. TYPES OF PSORIASIS

TYPE	LESIONS	CHARACTERISTICS	SITES
Plaque (nummular, common)	Round, oval plaques that may be small or very large and confluent, serpiginous, or geographic; silvery-white scales present on plaques in untreated psoriasis		Elbows, knees, scalp, trunk
Inverse	Red, sharply defined, less scaling because of maceration	May exclusively inverse or appear with plaque psoriasis	Intertriginous folds of axillae, inguinal, intergluteal, perianal skin
Guttate	Small, droplike psoriasis lesions with minimal scaling	Appears abruptly, often after streptococcal infections	Trunk and proximal extremities
Palmar	Hyperkeratosis and thick scales on the palms and fingers	May be due to trauma to the area; often occurs with elbow and knee lesions	Volar surfaces of fingers and palms
Erythrodermic (exfoliative)	Generalized redness, little scaling	Can result from overaggressive treatment such as tar and ultraviolet light; requires cautious, nonirritating treatment and hospitalization	Generalized
Acute generalized pustular psoriasis (von Zumbusch)	Skin becomes red and tender: tiny pustules appear at edges of lesions and coalesce to form lakes of pus	Plaque psoriasis irritated by drugs, pregnancy, or infections; if patient is very ill, hospitalization necessary; there is fluid, albumin, and heat loss	Generalized

The most common sites of psoriasis are the elbows, knees, scalp, and lumbosacral skin, but it can occur on all skin surfaces. It affects the nails in 30% of patients. Pitting of the nails is the classic nail change in psoriasis. Other nail changes are yellowish discoloration, onycholysis (separation of the nail from the bed), thickening, grooving, splitting, and subungual hyperkeratosis.

Table 7–7 presents the various types of psoriasis.

MEDICAL DIAGNOSIS

Psoriasis is diagnosed by the characteristic lesions. Uncharacteristic lesions and lesions that do not respond to treatment undergo biopsy.

MEDICAL MANAGEMENT

The goal of medical management is to decrease epidermal proliferation and dermal inflammation. Treatment includes application of emollients, keratolytics, coal tar, anthralin, and topical steroids. Phototherapy (ultraviolet B light, or UVB) and photochemotherapy (psoralen-ultraviolet light, or PUVA) are treatments for generalized and difficult cases of psoriasis. Retinoids, antimetabolites, and occasionally systemic steroids are used for severe, acute, and recalcitrant psoriasis. Refer to Chapter 6 for an in-depth discussion of pharmacologic therapy and topical treatment including ultraviolet radiation.

Patients with pustular von Zumbusch psoriasis or erythroderma require hospitalization, rest, and conservative skin care. They must be observed for congestive heart failure, pulmonary embolus, exhaustion, pneumonia, and sepsis.

Application of the Nursing Process to the Care of the Patient with Psoriasis

Assessment

Obtain a history of the current condition. Ask when it began, what area of the body was first affected, how it progressed, whether there were any identifiable precipitating factors, what treatments have been used, and whether or not they were effective. Question the patient about any family history of psoriasis, noting age of onset in family members and a description of the course of the disease in terms of remissions and exacerbations.

Inspect the skin. Examine all areas of the skin for involvement, including scalp, ears, trunk, groin, buttocks, perianal area, arms, legs, intertriginous areas under the arms and breasts, hands, feet, and nails.

Compare the actual extent of the psoriasis with the patient's perception. Question the patient about associated symptoms such as fever and pruritus. Remember that some patients with psoriasis do not itch, whereas others will be scratching during the interview.

Explore the psychosocial impact of the disease on the patient. Ask the patient to describe how the condition affects comfort, lifestyle, body image, employment, and social relationships.

Assess for factors that will make some treatment plans unrealistic for individual patients. For example, some patients may be unable or unwilling to apply corticosteroids or tar preparations three times daily. In particular, patients who are in frequent contact with the public may be unwilling to apply tar preparations that will cause them to smell like tar.

Nursing Diagnoses and Planning

Nursing diagnoses and related expected patient outcomes most commonly applicable to patients with psoriasis include the following:

NDx: Impaired skin integrity related to skin lesions secondary to psoriasis

Planning: Patient outcomes
1. Patient performs skin care correctly.
2. Skin lesions clear.

NDx: Pain related to itching

Planning: Patient outcomes
1. Patient lists basic self-care measures to reduce or control pruritus.
2. Patient states pruritus is relieved or controlled.

NDx: High risk for body image disturbance related to unsightly or extensive psoriatic lesions with dry, flaky scales

Planning: Patient outcomes
1. Patient verbalizes positive feelings about self.
2. Patient maintains good grooming.
3. Patient interacts with staff members, family, and friends.

NDx: High risk for ineffective individual coping related to presence of a chronic disease and the demands of the treatment regimen

Planning: Patient outcomes
1. Patient identifies potential precipitating factors.
2. Patient discusses ways to avoid precipitating stressors.
3. Patient describes available support sources.
4. Patient expresses confidence in ability to cope.

Nursing Interventions

NDx: Impaired skin integrity
Teach the patient with psoriasis about the disease. Advise the patient to avoid factors that may aggravate psoriasis such as obesity, consumption of alcoholic beverages, sunburn, trauma to the skin, scratching, dry skin, stress, infection, and shaving with a razor.

Instruct the patient in the prescribed therapy. Provide verbal and written instructions on the sequence of therapy, application of therapeutic agents, and the frequency of treatment.

Teach the patient to use topical steroids sparingly for acute lesions to decrease the potency of the steroid and then to use an emollient. Review the side effects (skin atrophy, striae, telangiectasia) of aggressive topical steroid therapy. Explain that side effects are insidious and can be irreversible, but they usually occur only with long-term therapy.

Instruct the patient in self-administration of prescribed tar therapy and over-the-counter topical preparations as discussed in Chapter 6. Encourage patients with extensive psoriasis to make treatment a priority.

When therapeutic baths are ordered, instruct the patient to use a circular motion and to gently rub lesions to remove loose scales and to pat, not rub, the skin dry. When UV light treatments are ordered, instruct the patient to report any burning or tenderness of the skin, which can indicate overexposure. Also explain the use of sunscreens and how to shield sunburned areas.

Teach the patient with a history of extensive psoriasis to seek treatment during the early signs of exacerbation of the condition.

NDx: Pain
Instruct the patient in measures to reduce pruritus, as presented in Chart 7–3.

Chart 7–3.

NURSING GUIDE TO PATIENT EDUCATION FOR SELF-MANAGEMENT: MEASURES TO REDUCE PRURITUS ASSOCIATED WITH PSORIASIS

Instruct the patient to:

Avoid scratching itchy areas because this creates the scratch-itch cycle and can cause excoriation.
Use a room humidifier for moisture if the environment is dry.
Use warm, not hot, water for bathing.
Avoid use of strong soaps.
Lubricate the skin with petrolatum when it is free of topical therapeutic agents.
Take antihistamines as prescribed.

NDx: High risk for body image disturbance
Be sensitive to the patient's feelings about appearance, and encourage expression of them. Take care to avoid any inadvertent expressions of distaste when treating the affected areas. Use touch as appropriate to indicate acceptance. Stress that the disease is not contagious and that the skin returns to normal with effective treatment. Encourage good grooming, interaction with others, and participation in self-care.

NDx: High risk for ineffective individual coping
Provide encouragement and emotional support. This is a chronic, frustrating condition for the patient to deal with because of frequent exacerbations and remissions. Foster verbalization of concerns and feelings, which may involve anger, revulsion, inadequacy, powerlessness, anxiety, and depression. Guide the patient toward a realistic view of the problem, acknowledging its negative aspects but also focusing on treatment and control. Discuss the role of stress and emotional factors in flare-ups of the disease, and explore with the patient ways to minimize stress. Stress-reducing measures to be considered include a program of physical exercise, relaxation therapy, and counseling.

Provide the patient with information about support services for psoriasis patients in the community. Tell the patient about nurse-managed psoriasis day care treatment centers, which are found in all major metropolitan areas in the United States, Canada, and Europe. These centers provide acute care for exacerbations of psoriasis, patient education, follow-up, and maintenance of chronic psoriasis. Support services of dietitians, social workers, psychiatrists, psychologists, podiatrists, and self-help groups are offered at some centers. The centers are usually affiliated with a university medical center dermatology program or owned and operated by a board-certified dermatologist. Registered nurses usually manage the patient care as ordered by the physician.

Nursing care in these centers includes PUVA, UVB, combination PUVA and UVB, full day-care treatment programs hand and foot UV treatments, hot quartz-lamp therapy, Goekerman treatment (tar and UV), Ingram treatments (anthralin and UV), modified Goekerman treatments, administration of and follow-up for patients on chemotherapy, and a great deal of encouragement.

Also inform the patient about voluntary psoriasis organizations such as the Psoriasis Foundation in Portland, Oregon, and the Psoriasis Research Institute at Stanford University, Stanford, California. These organizations publish newsletters that have practical information for patients. Information on the disease process and new products and letters from psoriasis patients are commonly found in these newsletters.

Evaluation

Evaluate the effectiveness of nursing care for a patient with psoriasis by comparing the patient's status with the expected patient outcomes. Examples of specific outcomes for patients with psoriasis have been provided in the Planning section.

Bullous Diseases

PEMPHIGUS VULGARIS

Pemphigus vulgaris is the most common and severe form of pemphigus. It is characterized by flaccid, easily ruptured bullae, which develop on apparently normal skin and mucous membranes. Pemphigus vulgaris usually occurs during middle or old age. It occurs among all races and ethnic groups. There may be increased prevalence in Jews (Moschella & Hurley, 1985). Before corticosteroid therapy, 50% of patients with pemphigus vulgaris died within 12 months.

ETIOLOGY AND PATHOPHYSIOLOGY

Pemphigus vulgaris is an autoimmune disease. The bullae of pemphigus vulgaris are intradermal. They form below the basal layer of the skin resulting from a loss of cohesion between epidermal cells. There is little inflammation associated with the condition unless the ruptured bullae become infected.

CLINICAL MANIFESTATIONS

The flaccid bullae usually develop on noninflamed skin. As the bullae rupture, they leave a large denuded, bleeding, weeping crusted erosion (Fig. 7–18). Although the bullae may develop anywhere on the body, the oral mucosa is often the initial site. The bullae extend laterally when pressure is applied (Nikolsky's sign).

MEDICAL DIAGNOSIS

A skin biopsy is performed for direct immunofluorescent studies of the perilesional skin to detect characteristic changes such as the presence of immunoglobulin G (IgG) in the epidermal intercellular space. Serum antibody studies may demonstrate the presence of IgG pemphigus antibody.

MEDICAL MANAGEMENT

The goal of medical treatment is to administer enough steroids, along or in combination with a cytotoxic agent such as azathioprine, cycloposphamide, or methotrexate, to suppress the clinical manifestations of the disease. Gold is another treatment for pemphigus.

Figure 7–18.

Flaccid bullae of pemphigus vulgaris forming on noninflamed skin. (From Moschella SL, Hurley SL, Dermatology. 2nd ed. Philadelphia: WB Saunders, 1985, p. 558.)

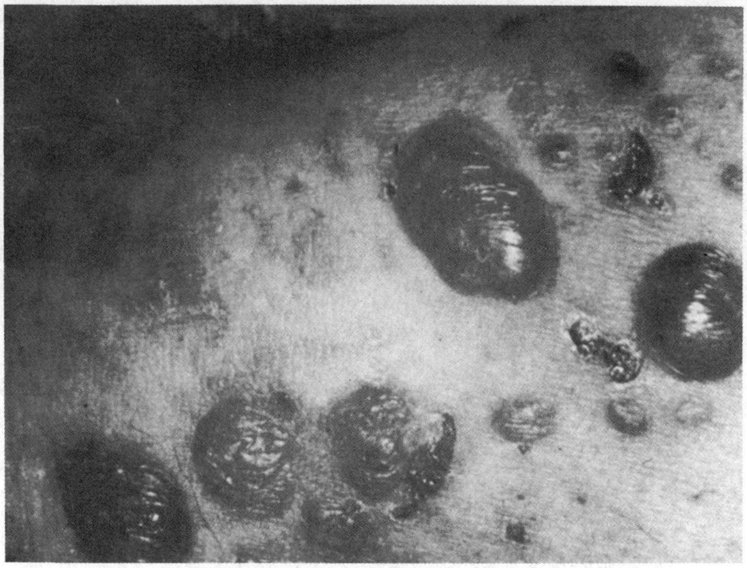

The patient is hospitalized and monitored closely while high doses of intravenous corticosteroids are administered to control acute pemphigus. As the condition begins to resolve, oral corticosteroid therapy is begun and the dosage gradually reduced.

The patient can be weaned off all medicine when there are no clinical manifestations or pemphigus antibodies present in the serum. The patient is followed closely, and treatment is resumed if symptoms return or if pemphigus antibody is found in the serum.

Wet dressings for 15 minutes, four times daily, help to remove debris from the lesions and prevent infection. Potent topical fluorinated steroids may be prescribed for localized occurrences.

Systemic corticosteroids prevent death in pemphigus vulgaris from bronchopneumonia, metabolic changes, exhaustion, septicemia, and renal failure. Today the major cause of death is from complications of long-term corticosteroid therapy (Lookingbill & Marks, 1986).

Application of the Nursing Process to the Care of the Patient with Pemphigus Vulgaris

The assessment, nursing diagnoses, expected patient outcomes, nursing interventions, and evaluation for patients with pemphigus vulgaris are a combination of those for patients with a chronic, life-threatening disease, those for patients with open-skin lesions, and those for patients whose treatment involves steroids and cytotoxic agents.

BULLOUS PEMPHIGOID

The blisters of bullous pemphigoid arise from erythematous or urticarial plaque. It has been reported in all age groups but occurs mainly in individuals older than 60 years. Although the disease is serious because it occurs in the elderly, mortality is low.

ETIOLOGY AND PATHOPHYSIOLOGY

Bullous pemphigoid is another autoimmune disease. The blister in bullous pemphigoid forms below the epidermis at the dermoepidermal junction. Perivascular inflammation develops in the dermis.

CLINICAL MANIFESTATIONS

Localized bullous pemphigoid is most common on the lower extremities. Other sites include the groin, axillae, and other flexural areas. The bullae are large and tense (Fig. 7–19). They do not extend laterally when pressure is applied. Healing usually occurs without scarring.

MEDICAL DIAGNOSIS

Biopsy specimens for direct and indirect immunofluorescence reveal a linear band of IgG and complement when the blister forms.

MEDICAL MANAGEMENT

The disease may subside spontaneously within months or years. Localized pemphigoid can be treated with wet dressings and potent topical fluorinated steroids. Widespread bullae require treatment with systemic steroids and immunosuppressive agents.

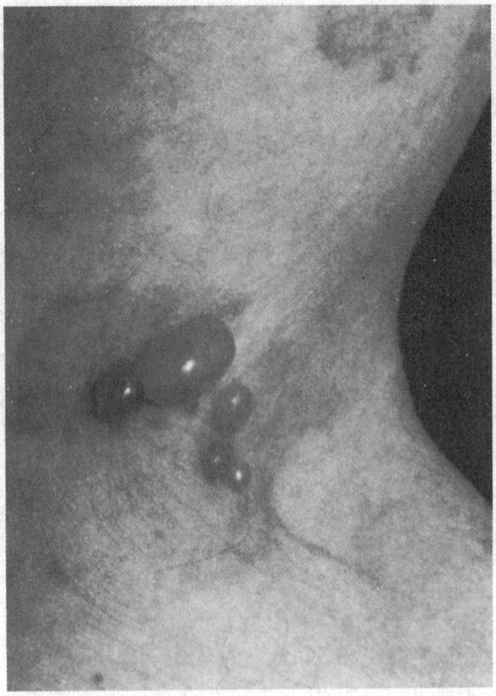

Figure 7–19.

Tense blister of bullous pemphigoid in flexural area. (Courtesy of Leonard J. Swinyer, M.D.)

Application of the Nursing Process to the Care of the Patient with Bullous Pemphigoid

The assessment, nursing diagnoses, expected patient outcomes, nursing interventions, and evaluation for patients with bullous pemphigoid are similar to those described for patients with any chronic disease characterized by skin lesions. Because bullous pemphigoid is common in the elderly, pay particular attention to the patient's ability to perform the prescribed treatments and to obtain needed supplies. Support the patient's spirits by emphasizing that bullous pemphigoid is generally not fatal and that it may spontaneously subside in months or even years.

Stings

Hymenoptera stings cause approximately 30 deaths per year in the United States. These insects sting for defense and offense. Hymenoptera include the honeybee, bumblebee, wasps, hornets, yellow jackets, mud daubers, and fire ants.

ETIOLOGY

The venoms of the Hymenoptera are a mixture of allergens and active amines and peptides. Any of the components of the venom may cause an allergic reaction. Cross-sensitization to Hymenoptera venom may occur.

PATHOPHYSIOLOGY

The reaction to the sting is a combination of local and systemic effects of the peptides and amines in the venom and individual hypersensitivity to the allergens of the venom.

CLINICAL MANIFESTATIONS

Reactions to Hymenoptera venom may be immediate or delayed (after 2 hours). Immediate nonallergic reactions are characterized by local edema, erythema, pain, and itching, which subside within a few hours. Multiple stings may cause malaise, nausea, and fever and can be fatal. Patients with hypersensitivity have more severe and prolonged local reactions and may also develop generalized urticaria and pruritus, severe bronchospasm, and laryngeal edema, leading to shock and death. Such anaphylactic reactions usually occur within 10 to 30 minutes after the sting.

The sting of fire ants produces a cluster of cutaneous lesions. Two hemorrhagic puncta at the site of attachment are surrounded by a circle of pustules from multiple stings. Immediate pain subsides quickly and a 2 to 10-mm wheal forms. A vesicle forms in approximately 4 hours. After 24 hours, the lesion becomes a pustule on an erythematous base.

MEDICAL DIAGNOSIS

Patients are usually aware of a bee or ant sting, and the reaction is diagnosed by the symptoms.

The most sensitive test for Hymenoptera allergy is the venom test, but it is still imperfect.

MEDICAL MANAGEMENT

The honeybee is the only stinging insect that leaves the stinger in the skin. It is removed carefully by scraping with a flat blade to avoid breaking or squeezing the venom sac and spreading the venom.

Treatment for mild, local reactions includes ice, elevation, and antihistamines. For a delayed local reaction after 24 hours, systemic steroids may be prescribed for 5 days.

There is no effective treatment for the local reaction to a fire ant sting except to keep it clean to prevent secondary infection.

To protect against anaphylaxis in the allergic individual, epinephrine, 0.1 to 0.5 ml of 1:1000 solution, is given subcutaneously and repeated every 5 to 15 minutes as needed. Maintenance of an airway and administration of intravenous fluids, vasopressors, and oxygen are emergency measures instituted if anaphylaxis occurs.

Hyposensitization (venom immunotherapy) is conducted on patients with a history of severe systemic reaction and a positive venom skin test.

Application of the Nursing Process to the Care of the Patient with a Sting

Assessment

Determine the number of stings, their location, the time of occurrence, and whether the causative insect is known. Keep in mind that multiple stings and stings on the head and neck have the most serious potential and that anaphylactic reactions usually occur within 10 to 20 minutes after a sting.

Determine whether there is a known allergy to Hymenoptera. Ask about any previous stings and reaction to them.

Assess for both systemic and local reactions. Observe for signs of respiratory distress and question about nausea. Inspect the area of the sting for edema and erythema, and question the patient about pain and itch.

Nursing Diagnoses and Planning

Nursing diagnoses and related expected patient outcomes most commonly applicable to patients with a sting include the following:

NDx: High risk for ineffective breathing pattern related to bronchoconstriction and laryngeal edema

Planning: Patient outcomes

1. Respiratory rate and depth are within normal limits.
2. Respirations are easy and silent.
3. Cyanosis is absent.

NDx: Altered health maintenance related to insufficient knowledge of prevention of stings and self-care measures for individuals allergic to Hymenoptera venom

Chart 7–4.

NURSING GUIDE TO PATIENT EDUCATION FOR SELF-MANAGEMENT: INSTRUCTIONS FOR PATIENTS ALLERGIC TO HYMENOPTERA VENOM

Instruct the patient to:

Carry MedicAlert identification indicating allergy to Hymenoptera at all times.

Keep available at all times a commercially available bee-sting kit containing a tourniquet, syringe, epinephrine, and antihistamine tablets. In the event of a sting

- Inject self with epinephrine immediately.
- If stung by a honeybee, scrape the site swiftly with the fingernail to remove the stinger.
- If stung on an extremity, apply a tourniquet above the sting.
- Cleanse the area of the sting with soap and water.
- Apply ice to the area of the sting.
- Proceed to the nearest health care facility.

Explore the need for hyposensitization therapy with the physician.

Decrease exposure to bees by

- Avoiding feeding areas such as flower gardens, orchards, areas of clover, garbage cans, picnic sites, and other areas with food refuse.
- Wearing shoes outdoors because yellow jackets and fire ants are found in the ground.
- Wearing dark colors when outside because bees are attracted to bright colors.
- Avoiding use of perfumes and scented soaps, deodorants, or hair sprays when going outside because these attract bees.
- Remaining still if a bee is buzzing around because movement increases the risk of being stung.
- Keeping home area free of bees by keeping garbage cans covered, eliminating decorative fruit trees such as crab apple, and having nests or hives removed by an exterminator.

Planning: Patient outcomes

1. Patient lists ways to limit exposure to Hymenoptera.
2. Allergic patient explains importance of carrying Medic Alert identification and a bee-sting kit.
3. Allergic patient states protocol to be followed in the event of a bee sting.
4. Allergic patient describes importance of discussing hyposensitization therapy with the physician.

Nursing Interventions

NDx: High risk for ineffective breathing pattern

Administer epinephrine as ordered to protect the allergic patient from anaphylaxis. Hasten absorption of the epinephrine by massaging the injection site to increase circulation. Monitor respiratory and cardiovascular status. If anaphylaxis occurs, maintain an airway, administer oxygen and intravenous fluids, and support cardiovascular status as discussed in Chapter 10.

NDx: Altered health maintenance

Instruct the patient allergic to Hymenoptera venom in self-care as presented in Chart 7–4.

Evaluation

Evaluate the effectiveness of nursing care for a patient with a bee sting by comparing the patient's status with the expected patient outcomes. Examples of specific outcomes for patients with a bee sting have been provided in the Planning section.

Alopecia

Alopecia means loss of hair. It is most commonly used to refer to the loss of terminal hair on the scalp. However, hair can be lost from any other part of the body such as the beard area, the chest, or the extremities.

The etiology, pathophysiology, clinical mainifestations, and medical management of the various types of alopecia are described in Table 7–8. Diagnosis is made on the basis of clinical findings.

Guidelines for Application of the Nursing Process to the Care of the Patient with Alopecia

Question the patient about the onset of hair loss and family history of baldness or hair disorders. Ask the patient whether he or she is taking any prescribed or over-the-counter medications. Determine whether the patient has been under any unusual emotional or physical stress within the past few months.

Table 7–8. TYPES OF ALOPECIA (HAIR LOSS)

TYPE OF ALOPECIA	ETIOLOGY AND PATHOPHYSIOLOGY	CLINICAL MANIFESTATIONS	MEDICAL MANAGEMENT
Stress induced	Caused by physical or emotional stress such as high fever, childbirth, chronic illness, major surgery, severe emotional disorder, crash diets, hypothyroidism, and drugs (i.e., heparin, indomethacin [Indocin], vitamin A); greater than 25% of hair is in the telogen, or resting, phase	Diffuse hair loss not readily apparent until 50% or more is lost	Usually resolves within 2–6 months
Androgenic	Genetic alopecia in which the finer depigmented vellus hairs replace the coarse, dark terminal hairs in bald areas	Bitemporal hair recession with female pattern baldness over the crown of the head; scalp is normal; most evident from age 20–40	Hair transplant; scalp reduction; topical minoxidil is investigational treatment
Alopecia areata	Autoimmune disorder in which lymphocytes surround the hair bulb in the dermis and hair follicle is dystrophic and lacks hair shaft	Round and oval well-circumscribed patches of hair loss 2–3 cm in diameter	Topical, intralesional, and oral corticosteroids; topical minoxidil (investigational) psoralen-ultraviolet A light; topical anthralin; majority of patients recover spontaneously, but hair loss of more than 1 year has poor prognosis for regrowth.
Alopecia totalis	Autoimmune disorder	Loss of all scalp hair	None
Alopecia universalis	Autoimmune disorder	Loss of all scalp, face, and body hair, including underarms and groin	None

Assess the extent and pattern of hair loss. Is it patchy? Is it diffuse? Does it involve only the scalp? Are eyebrows and eyelashes affected?

Discuss treatments, and be honest with the patient regarding the percentage of patients who experience hair regrowth.

Explore the effect of the hair loss on the individual's self-image. Keep in mind that hair loss can have a devastating impact on self-image, even though humans can live normal lives without hair. A new hair style or hair color causes self-consciousness, and individuals will spend hundreds of dollars to correct their mistakes if the hair is too curly or too straight or if the hair dye turns the hair purple. Some individuals miss work and stay indoors until their hair satisfies their self-image.

Inform patients about the National Alopecia Areata Foundation, Mill Valley, California, which is a patient-support organization.

Neoplasia

Neoplasms of the skin are very common; most individuals have one or more types during their lifetime. In addition to being classified as benign or malignant, neoplasms of the skin are further classified according to the skin structure from which they arise: epidermal lesions, dermal and subcutaneous lesions, and pigmented lesions.

Pigmented lesions are derived from the pigment-forming cells, the dendritic melanocytes in the epidermis, and the nevus cells arranged in nests in the dermis. Some lesions are further identified as premalignant because of a high incidence of malignant transformation (change to a malignant tumor).

Benign Neoplasms

The majority of cutaneous neoplasms are benign. Information on common benign neoplasms of the skin is presented in Table 7–9.

Application of the Nursing Process to the Care of the Patient with a Benign Neoplasm of the skin

Assessment

Assess the lesion, noting and documenting location, size, color, symmetry, and characteristics of the border. Observe for crusting, bleeding, and areas of erosion.

Determine when the lesion first appeared, and ask the patient to describe any changes in the lesion that have occurred. Specifically ask whether the lesion has changed in size. Is it larger? Is it smaller? Has it changed in depth? Ask whether there has been any bleeding, crusting, or ulceration. Has there been a color change? Is it darker? Is it lighter? Is itching or pain present?

Question the patient regarding any previous similar lesions, history of sun exposure, exposure to occupational hazards, and any coexisting medical problems.

Assess the patient's psychological response to the skin lesion. Be alert for signs of anxiety over possible malignancy. Also be attuned to indications of undue embarrassment, fear of others' reactions, fear of rejection, or negative feelings about the body.

Nursing Diagnoses and Planning

Nursing diagnoses and related expected patient outcomes most commonly applicable to patients with a benign neoplasm of the skin include the following:

NDx: Anxiety related to procedures to be done and the perceived possibility of skin cancer

Planning: Patient outcomes
1. Patient verbalizes concerns about procedures to be done.
2. Patient discusses fear of malignancy.
3. Patient states that anxiety is reduced.

NDx: Altered health maintenance related to insufficient knowledge of follow-up care, self-examination of the skin, changes in lesion to be reported to physician

Planning: Patient outcomes
1. Patient states instructions for follow-up self-care.
2. Patient describes technique of self-examination of the skin.
3. Patient lists changes in lesions to be reported to the physician.

NDx: High risk for body image disturbance related to presence of cosmetically unacceptable lesions

Planning: Patient outcomes
1. Patient identifies ways in which lesions can be camouflaged.
2. Patient realistically discusses the effect of the lesion on appearance.
3. Patient verbalizes positive feelings about self.

Nursing Interventions

NDx: Anxiety
Support the patient during diagnostic and surgical procedures by reinforcing the physician's explana-

Table 7–9. BENIGN NEOPLASMS OF THE SKIN

TYPE	DESCRIPTION
EPIDERMAL	
Skin tags	Soft, flesh-colored 1–10-mm pedunculated papules of unknown cause; occur most often on neck, eyelids, axilla, and inframammary areas of adults older than age 50; removed with scissors or frozen nitrogen if irritated or cosmetically unacceptable; specimen sent to pathology if necrotic, crusted, or otherwise suspicious looking
Seborrheic keratosis	Flesh-colored, tan, brown, and black, round or oval 2-mm to 2-mm papules or plaques that appear greasy and pasted to the skin; develop in middle age or later and most frequently on head, neck, trunk, and extremities; may resemble pigmented basal cell epithelioma, malignant melanoma, or actinic keratosis; an excisional or shave biopsy is performed for diagnosis; if irritated or cosmetically unacceptable, may be removed by liquid nitrogen, C&D, or excision
Corns	Painful area of hyperkeratosis (overgrowth of horny layer) appearing as a whitish-gray or yellowish-brown with a translucent core and normal skin lines; caused by pressure from poor-fitting shoes or skeletal deformity; treated by use of proper-fitting footwear, orthotic devices, rings or pads to reduce mechanical trauma, paring down by a podiatrist, or surgical correction of any underlying deformity
DERMAL AND SUBCUTANEOUS NEOPLASMS	
Epidermal cyst	Sebaceous cyst whose wall is lined with keratin-secreting epithelial cells and which is connected to the skin surface by narrow channel, opening of which may be imperceptible or blocked with keratin plug; presents as round, smooth, protruding movable mass common on face, back, or base of ears, chest, or back; may remain small or grow until rupture into dermis, initiating inflammatory response; inflamed cysts may require incision and drainage; large cysts may be excised for comfort and appearance
Cherry (senile) hemangioma	Proliferation of blood vessels in the dermis presenting as multiple red-to-purple raised flat or dome-shaped papules on the trunk that bleed slightly with trauma; commonly occur after age 30; can be removed by scissor excision or C&D
Xanthoma	Accumulation of lipid-laden histiocytes in the dermis associated with chronic hyperlipoproteinemia (persistent elevated serum cholesterol or triglycerides); xanthelasma (yellowish plaques on the eyelids); eruptive xanthoma (crops of yellow papules on erythematous base found on buttocks and extensor aspects of elbows and knees, which clear when serum triglycerides return to normal); tuberous xanthoma (plaquelike or nodular lipid deposit on elbows and knees); tendenous xanthomas (hard nodules on the tendons, usually the Achilles or the extensor tendons of the fingers); xanthomas may be excised if problematic cosmetically or otherwise; may recur unless the hyperlipoproteinemia is controlled
Neurofibroma	Collection of neural fibers in the dermis caused by overgrowth of cells from neural crest; presents as soft, skin-colored papules or nodules that evaginate into skin on compression (buttonhole sign); neurofibromatosis (von Recklinghausen's disease or elephant man disease); characterized by multiple lesions, café au lait spots, axillary freckles, and disfiguring skeletal and CNS involvement; is inherited as autosomal dominant
Dermatofibroma	Area of dermal fibrosis usually on legs that presents most often as a solitary, firm, slightly elevated lesion ranging in color from light tan to dark brown; "dimpling sign" is characteristic of the lesion (i.e., pinching the lesion results in simple dimple); enlarging or atypically covered lesions may undergo biopsy; otherwise treatment is unnecessary; common in women
Keloid	Excessive proliferation of scar tissue in response to trauma; presents as shiny, firm, protuberant mass with irregular border extending beyond area of original trauma; pink in light-skinned persons and dark brown in dark-skinned; occurs most often on ear lobes, shoulders, upper chest, and back in blacks; best treatment is prevention (i.e., avoid surgery or other trauma); intralesional steroid injections over months result in some decrease in size; laser and radiation therapy also used with some success

(continued)

Table 7–9. *(continued)* BENIGN NEOPLASMS OF THE SKIN

TYPE	DESCRIPTION
DERMAL AND SUBCUTANEOUS NEOPLASMS *(continued)*	
Lipoma	Subcutaneous fat tumor of unknown cause that presents as 1–10 cm soft, elevated mass under normal skin on the trunk, neck, and upper extremities; most common in 40–50-year-old women; excision biopsy sometimes performed to rule out malignancy; otherwise no treatment needed
PIGMENTED LESIONS	
Ephelis (freckle)	Irregularly shaped 1–6-mm discrete brown macule caused by increased melanin production in basal layer; develops during childhood on sun-exposed skin and darkens with ultraviolet exposure
Lentigo	Brown-black macule caused by increase in number of melanocytes and resultant increased melanin; actinic lentigo or liver spot has indistinct border, occurs in sun-exposed areas, and develops in later life; if cosmetically unacceptable, may be removed with liquid nitrogen or bleached with hydroquinone. Porcelana is a 2% preparation available over the counter
Melasma	Symmetric macular hyperpigmented lesions on the cheeks and forehead with a well-defined border; occurs in women secondary to sunlight exposure, pregnancy (known as chloasma), and use of oral contraceptives; lesions, which may be bleached with hydroquinone, fade slowly when precipitating factor is eliminated; sunscreens with SPF 15 may aid in prevention
Pigmented nevi (moles)	Benign tumors composed of nevus cells, which are derived from melanocytes; individuals average 30 to 40 nevi; biopsy is done if changes occur in color, size, border, if there is bleeding, crusting, or persistent itching, or if a new mole occurs after age 40; repeatedly irritated or unsightly nevi can be removed by shave, punch, or excisional biopsy; all are sent for pathologic examination regardless of clinical appearance
PREMALIGNANT LESIONS	
Actinic keratosis (senile or solar keratosis)	Most common precancerous lesions; excessive exposure to ultraviolet rays results in atypical keratinocytes and hyperkeratosis of epidermis and chronic inflammation in dermis; lesions are well defined, round, or irregularly shaped red to brownish to grayish papules covered by dry adherent scale that feels like sandpaper when fingers run over it; occurs most often on face, ears, neck, and dorsal hand or forearm. Surrounding skin is often dry, leathery, and wrinkled, with freckles and other signs of chronic sun exposure; treatment consists of removal by liquid nitrogen, curettage and electrodesiccation, or simple excision, especially if malignant change is suspected; multiple lesions are treated with 5FU (Efudex); without treatment, lesions enlarge, and 25% develop into squamous cell carcinoma; occurs more often in women than men
Bowen's lesion	Intraepidermal squamous cell carcinoma or cancer in situ found in older, light-skinned males; risk factors are exposure to environmental chemical carcinogen and chronic sunlight exposure; lesion is a well-defined erythematous eczematous plaque covered with yellow to yellow-brown crust; diagnosis is via punch biopsy, and treatment is surgical excision; periodic follow-up skin evaluation is required
Cutaneous horn	Hard keratotic protrusion developing from normal skin; horns are removed and measured because base of horn may have squamous cell cancer
Leukoplakia	White plaque on the mucous membrane of mouth or vagina
Dysplastic nevus	Flat atypical nevus about 10 mm in diameter with irregular border and palpable dermal component; in dysplastic nevus syndrome, 10–100 or more nevi occur on all areas of the body: scalp, axilla, trunk, groin; diagnosed by biopsy; treated by removal or monthly self-examination and examination by physician every 3–6 months, and medical photography to detect change

Abbreviations: C & D, curettage amd desiccation; CNS, central nervous system; SPF, sun protection factor; 5FU, 5-fluorouracil.

tion of the purpose and protocol of the procedures. Answer the patient's questions and correct any misconceptions. If a biopsy has been done, inform the patient of when and from whom he or she will receive a pathology report.

NDx: Altered health maintenance
Instruct the patient in self-examination of the skin, as shown in Figure 7–20. Explain why and how often it should be performed. Teach the early warning signs of a nevus transforming into a malignant melanoma. Use the ABCD acronym:

*A*symmetry
*B*order irregularity
*C*hange in color, surface, or sensation in a mole
*D*iameter more than 6 mm

Stress the importance of seeing a dermatologist for evaluation and biopsy if any signs of malignancy occur.

Stress the importance of follow-up care after diagnostic and surgical procedures, and provide the patient with written instructions related to care of any wound, use of topical or systemic medications, and time, date, and place of follow-up visit.

NDx: High risk for body image disturbance
Explore the patient's perception of the effect of the lesion on his or her appearance, and provide a realistic perspective when necessary. Discuss cosmetic camouflage for lesions on exposed areas of the body.

Evaluation

Evaluate the effectiveness of nursing care for a patient with a benign skin neoplasm by comparing the patient's status with the expected patient outcomes. Examples of specific outcomes for patients with a benign neoplasm of the skin have been provided in the Planning section.

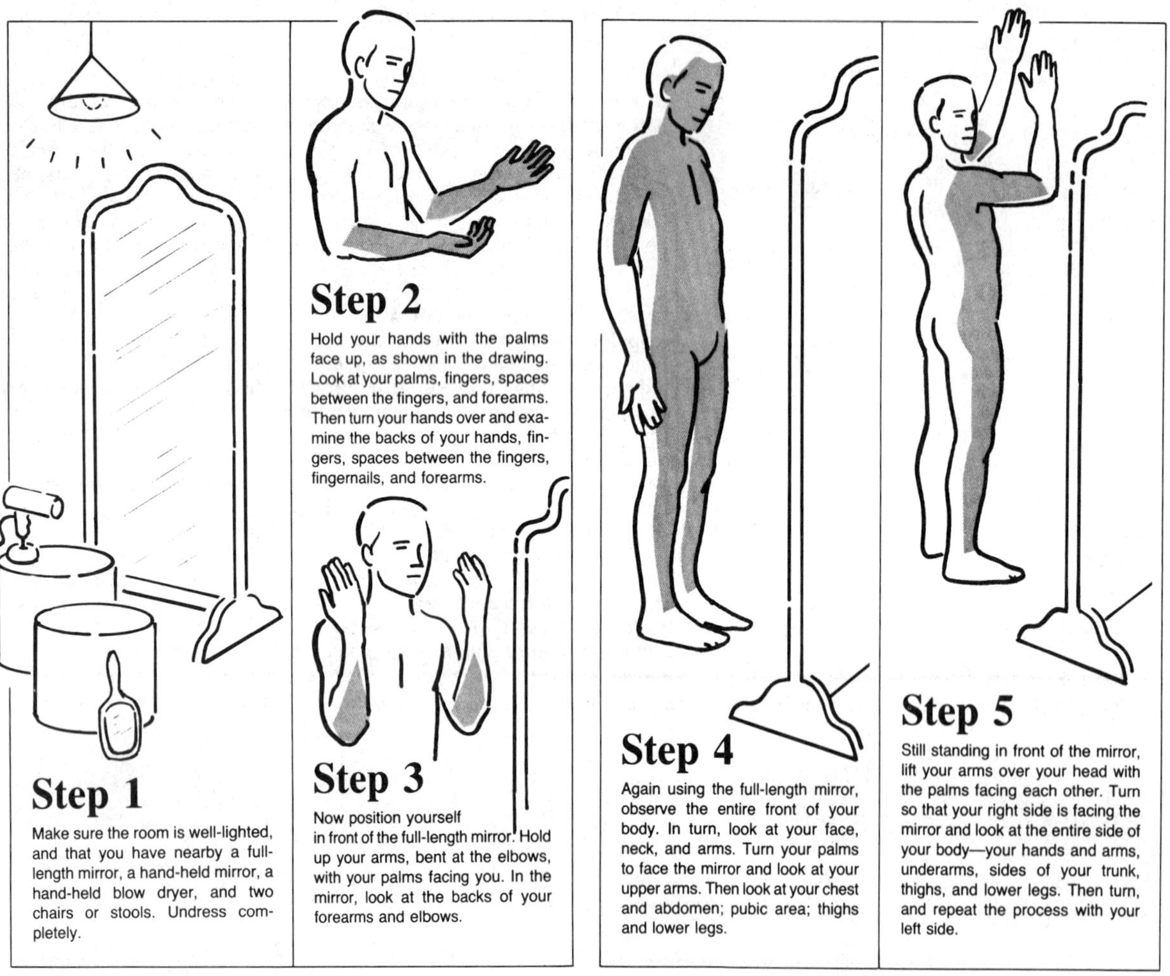

Figure 7–20.

Technique for self-examination of the skin. (Courtesy of the American Cancer Society.)

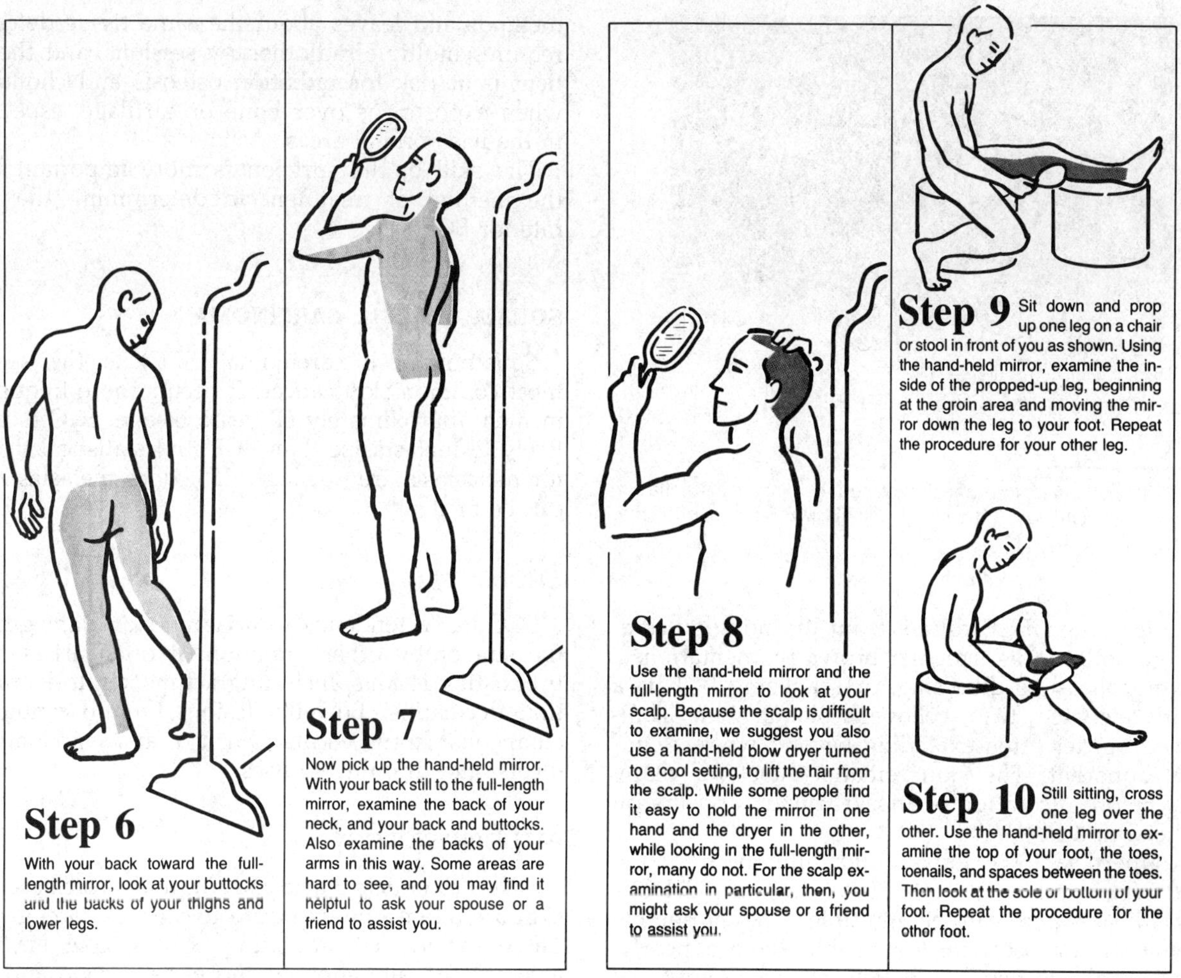

Figure 7–20. (*Continued*)

Malignant Neoplasms

Basal cell epithelioma (BCE), squamous cell skin cancer, and malignant melanoma are the three types of skin cancer. They each arise from the epidermis.

BASAL CELL EPITHELIOMA

BCE (basal cell carcinoma) is probably the most common of all human cancers. It is most common in blue-eyed men older than age 40 with blond or red hair and fair skin. BCE is rare in blacks and Asians. BCE rarely, if ever, metastasizes, but it can spread locally, destroying all the tissue, cartilage, and bone in the area.

ETIOLOGY

BCEs usually develop in sun-exposed areas of the skin. The longer the exposure to the sun, the higher the risk. These areas include the face, scalp, neck, forearms, hands, and back. Arsenic in drinking water, ionizing radiation, burn scars and vaccinations may also increase the risk of the development of BCE.

PATHOPHYSIOLOGY

BCEs contain cells that resemble the elongated, palisaded basal cells of the epidermis. The epidermis becomes thickened. The invasive buds and lobules of basaloid cells spread through the dermis.

CLINICAL MANIFESTATIONS

BCEs present in many different sizes and forms. A pearly, translucent border and telangiectasias (dilated blood vessels) are highly characteristic. The tumor may show no signs of tissue invasion for years or may be rapidly destructive.

A noduloulcerative BCE, the most common form, has a central ulceration and pearly, nodular border (Fig. 7–21). The nodule may have a gelatinous appearance. It begins as a small, waxy nodule, often with a few small telangiectasias on its surface. The lesion increases slowly in size and undergoes central ulceration. It is commonly found on the face.

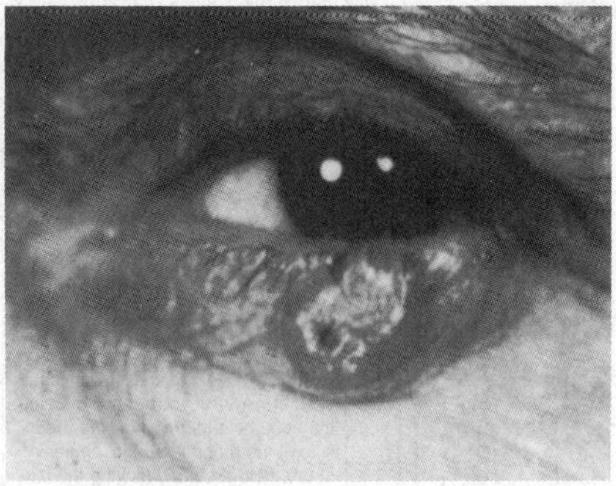

Figure 7–21.

Basal cell carcinoma. Note translucent nodule. (From Moschella SL, Hurley JH. Dermatology. 3rd ed. Philadelphia: WB Saunders, 1992, p. 1747.)

A pigmented BCE differs from the noduloulcerative type only in its irregular brown pigmentation.

A morphea-like, fibrosing, or sclerosing BCE is a slightly elevated, firm, yellowish plaque with an ill-defined border often extending beyond what is clinically apparent. The skin remains intact for many years before ulceration occurs. It usually appears on the head and neck.

A superficial BCE looks quite different from the other types and is less aggressive. Superficial BCEs vary in size and can be multiple. They resemble eczematous or psoriatic lesions but have a pearly, rolled border. Superficial BCEs occur predominantly on the trunk.

MEDICAL DIAGNOSIS

Diagnosis of BCE is made on the basis of histologic examination of shave, punch, or excisional biopsies.

MEDICAL MANAGEMENT

Curettage and desiccation (C&D) is the most common method of treating BCEs. It is 96% to 100% effective in appropriate lesions. The lesions best treated by C&D are in areas of increased subcutaneous fat such as the cheek, forehead, and trunk. It is not recommended for lesions larger than 2 cm, those over bone or cartilage, tumors bordering mucosa or eyelids, or morphea-like BCEs.

Surgical excision has a high cure rate in the same locations amenable to treatment with C&D. The resulting tissue defect is similar, but healing time is shorter.

Mohs' micrographic surgery is done in cases of recurrent BCE, sclerosing BCE, and tumors in the nasolabial fold.

Radiation therapy is noninvasive, less painful to the debilitated patient, and equally effective as other methods and leaves about the same tissue defect. It requires multiple radiotherapy sessions, and the patient is at risk for radiation osteosis and chondritis when exposure is over bone or cartilage, especially in the naso-orbital areas.

The skill of the surgeon is more important than the method of treatment in determining the cure rate for BCE.

SQUAMOUS CELL CARCINOMA

Squamous cell carcinoma (SCC) is the second most common skin cancer. It occurs more frequently in men approximately 60 years of age. SCC is more likely to metastasize than BCE, but statistical figures for metastasis are not high. If it does metastasize, it can be fatal.

ETIOLOGY

SCC has a tendency to arise on skin damaged by the sun or by other radiation. It often arises from preexisting lesions, including actinic keratosis, radiation dermatitis, Bowen's lesions, keratoacanthoma, cutaneous horns, scars, burn scars, vaccinations, ulcers, and draining sinuses.

PATHOPHYSIOLOGY

DNA, ribonucleic acid (RNA), and proteins in the skin are altered by exposure to various carcinogens. These include UV radiation, x-rays, coal tar, and arsenic. The alteration in the genetic code and cell structure results in epidermal hyperkeratosis and atypical keratinocytes. An invasive tumor and inflammation develop in the dermis.

CLINICAL MANIFESTATIONS

Change from a precancerous lesion is often heralded by induration of the lesion and surrounding inflammatory changes. In early stages, SCC may appear to be a thickened actinic keratosis. Arising from normal skin, it appears as a solitary, slowly enlarging nodule with an indurated base. The nodule is firm and develops a central crust that ultimately ulcerates (Fig. 7–22).

SCC may clinically resemble a BCE, but it tends to enlarge more rapidly and usually is firmer, with greater induration and inflammation.

MEDICAL DIAGNOSIS

Diagnosis of SSC is confirmed by biopsy and histologic examination.

MEDICAL MANAGEMENT

Treatments for SCC include C&D for smaller lesions, surgical excision, radiation therapy for elderly

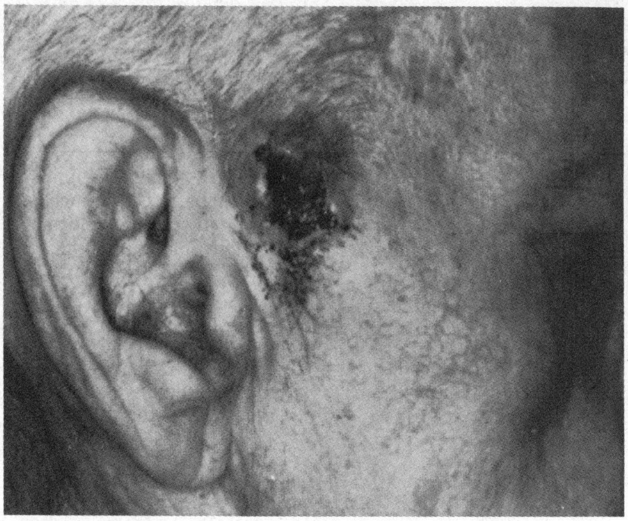

Figure 7–22.

Squamous cell carcinoma. Ulcerated lesion. (From Moschella SL, Hurley JH. Dermatology. 3rd ed. Philadelphia: WB Saunders, 1992, p. 1736.)

and debilitated patients who cannot tolerate a surgical procedure, and Mohs' micrographic surgery for difficult and recurrent lesions or lesions without a well-defined border.

CUTANEOUS MALIGNANT MELANOMA

Cutaneous malignant melanoma, or malignant melanoma, is a neoplasm of pigment-forming cells (melanocytes). Although it is the least common form of skin cancer, it is the most common fatal illness seen by dermatologists. The disease is not life-threatening when recognized and treated early.

The incidence of malignant melanoma has been increasing. It occurs most frequently in white males.

ETIOLOGY

Exposure to environmental carcinogens, recurrent sunburn, sun exposure, and immunosuppression are believed to be the primary etiologic factors in malignant melanoma. Hereditary tendencies and periods of increased hormonal activity may also be factors.

PATHOPHYSIOLOGY

Atypical pigmented melanoma cells are seen in the epidermis. There are various-sized nests of atypical melanoma cells in the dermis.

Malignant melanoma can metastasize. It requires more aggressive treatment than SCC and BCE. If malignant melanoma is diagnosed early, the patient can be cured.

CLINICAL MANIFESTATIONS

The positive signs for malignant melanoma, in order of significance, are a lesion with variegated color, irregular border, and irregular surface (Fig. 7–23).

The variegated colors include shades of blue, white, and red in a brown or black lesion. Bluish-black, bluish-red, or bluish-gray melanomas may be uniform in color.

The clinical features and characteristics of the four types of melanoma are listed in Table 7–10. Lesions develop most frequently on the head and neck, back, chest, abdomen, forearms, and in females, on the legs.

MEDICAL DIAGNOSIS

The only method of diagnosing cutaneous malignant melanoma is biopsy of the lesion.

The diagnosis is established by an excisional biopsy with a 2- to 4-mm margin. Incisional biopsy is done on a large lesion. If the lesion is confirmed to be a malignant melanoma, then more extensive surgery is done.

After diagnosis of a primary melanoma, a clinical staging work-up, which includes chest x-ray film, complete blood count, blood chemistry, and liver function tests, is completed. Liver, brain, and bone scans do not detect metastasis in asymptomatic patients but are performed as base studies for later comparison.

Clinically, Stage I melanomas are localized, Stage II melanomas have regional node disease, and Stage III melanomas are disseminated melanomas. Patients with Stages II and III melanomas usually die within

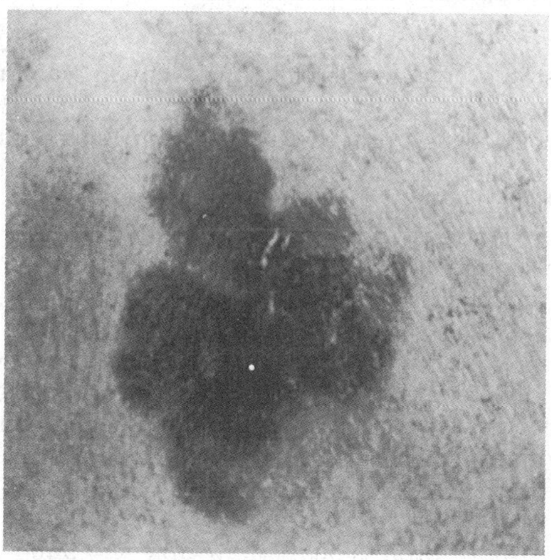

Figure 7–23.

Malignant melanoma. Irregular lesion with varying pigmentation and early central thickening. (From Moschella SL, Hurley JH. Dermatology. 2nd ed. Philadelphia: WB Saunders, 1985, p. 1576.)

Table 7–10. CHARACTERISTICS OF THE FOUR MAJOR TYPES OF CUTANEOUS MALIGNANT MELANOMA

TYPE	APPEARANCE	% OF ALL MELANOMAS	INCIDENCE	MALIGNANT SPREAD VERTICAL
Lentigo maligna melanoma (LMM)	Multicolored with dark brown, red, white, and blue nevus, elevated in areas; face is most common site	5–10	Affects females 2–3 times more often than males; usually occurs after age 70	Preceded by lentigo maligna (melanoma in epidermis); change in size and color is insidious; malignant transformation takes 15 months–40 years (average, 9 years); it is not as aggressive as other types of melanoma
Superficial spreading melanoma (SSM)	Irregular in color and surface, and has notched border; variety of colors in the lesion can be tan-black, brown, blue-gray to violaceous pink; lesions occur anywhere on body but are most common on lower extremities and back	70–75	Affects males and females equally; most common between ages 40 and 50	Lateral growth phase is prolonged, often 5–7 years, with lesion having diameter of approximately 2.5 cm
Nodular melanoma (NM)	Characterized by rapid growth; surface lesion may be smaller than 0.5 cm; can be blue, blue-gray, or reddish-blue and smooth or eroded.	10–15	Affects males twice as often as females; most common between ages 40 and 50	Lateral spread is absent with immediate dermal invasion
Acral lentiginous melanoma	Presents as spreading pigmented patch with varying degrees of pigment intensity; occurs on palms soles, finger, toes	<10		Lesion starts as spreading pigmented patch; vertical growth is difficult to notice because of location on thickened palms or soles

Chart 7–5.

NURSING GUIDE TO PATIENT EDUCATION FOR SELF-MANAGEMENT: PREVENTION AND EARLY DETECTION OF RECURRENT SKIN CANCER

Instruct the patient to take the following measures to minimize exposure to ultraviolet radiation:

Avoid being out in the sun between 10 a.m. and 3 p.m., when ultraviolet radiation light is most intense.
Start with short (15–20 minutes) exposures in early morning or late afternoon when sun exposure cannot be avoided.
Apply a sunscreen with 15 or higher sun protection factor (SPF) every day all year when out in the sun if light complexioned or if skin burns easily.
Reapply even water-resistant sunscreens after swimming, strenuous exercise, or prolonged sunbathing.
Apply a lip balm with an SPF of 15 or higher.
Wear protective clothing such as a hat and long sleeves when out in the sun.
Remember that ultraviolet rays penetrate clouds.
Avoid use of tanning lamps or commercial tanning booths.
Monitor for skin changes possibly indicating malignancy.
Perform monthly self-evaluation of skin. Pair with breast self-examination or testicular self-examination when possible.
Return for professional follow-up every 3 months for a year and then every 6 months for life.
Report changes in color, shape, size, occurrence of crusting, scaling, itching, bleeding, and redness or swellling of skin around the lesion.
Report development of any new lesions.

10 years of diagnosis. The best prognosis is with melanoma less than 1.7 mm thick.

MEDICAL MANAGEMENT

Wide excision with a 2 to 3-cm margin on all sides is the treatment for Stage I melanoma. A wide excision includes removal of skin, fat, and muscle and leaves a large defect that often requires grafting.

Patients with Stage II melanoma and clinically abnormal regional lymph nodes should have excision of the primary tumor, as with Stage I, and radical regional lymph node dissection.

The role of immunotherapy for patients with Stage III melanoma is being investigated. Regional hyperthermic limb perfusion is considered as an alternative to radical amputation for recurrent melanoma with intransigent metastases in an extremity.

Application of the Nursing Process to the Care of the Patient with Skin Cancer

Assessment

Perform a complete skin assessment and note the size, location, appearance, and duration of the lesion for which treatment is being sought. Assess the skin for additional lesions. Question the patient about any concurrent physical problems. Assess the patient's emotional response to the problem as well as his or her understanding of it. Be particularly alert for signs of anxiety out of proportion to the diagnosis.

After medical treatment, make assessments required by the type of treatment used. For example, after wide excision for malignant melanoma done under general anesthesia, make postoperative assessments as described in Chapter 3.

Nursing Diagnoses and Planning

Nursing diagnoses and related expected patient outcomes most commonly applicable to patients with skin cancer include the following:

NDx: Anxiety related to treatment, cosmetic result of treatment, prognosis, recurrence

Planning: Patient outcomes

1. Patient verbalizes concerns.
2. Patient realistically describes expected cosmetic result of treatment and prognosis.
3. Signs of undue anxiety are absent.

NDx: Altered health maintenance related to insufficient knowledge of follow-up care for prevention and early detection of recurrence

Planning: Patient outcomes

1. Patient identifies ways to decrease risk of skin cancer.
2. Patient explains the procedure for and importance of monthly self-screening of skin.
3. Patient lists skin changes to be reported to the physician.
4. Patient explains need for follow-up care.

NDx: Impaired skin integrity related to removal of a skin cancer

Planning: Patient outcomes

1. Patient describes care of the wound as ordered by the physician.
2. Wound heals without excessive scarring or infection.

Nursing Interventions

NDx: Anxiety

Encourage the patient to ask questions and express concerns and feelings about the disease, treatment, and prognosis. Allay unnecessary anxiety by clarifying and reinforcing information provided by the physician as needed. Acknowledge anxiety as normal. Provide emotional support by listening, being understanding, and providing encouragement. Because recurrence is a major source of anxiety, be certain to emphasize the high rate of cure. For patients with basal cell carcinoma, stress the rarity of metastasis. For patients with SCC, stress that metastasis is rare. Reassure patients with Stage I or Stage II malignant melanoma that the prognosis for cure is excellent with early removal.

NDx: Altered health maintenance

Instruct the patient in follow-up care needed for prevention and early detection of recurrence, as presented in Chart 7–5.

NDx: Impaired skin integrity

Instruct the patient in the care of the wound. Keep in mind that instructions will vary with the type of surgery performed and with the physician's preference. For example, cleansing of the wound with hydrogen peroxide, application of a topical antibiotic as prophylaxis against infection, and use of a dressing to protect against trauma and contamination may be ordered.

Be certain the patient knows what solution, medication, and types of dressing to use, how often to use them, and how to care for the wound aseptically. Have the patient demonstrate wound care when possible.

Provide specific instructions as needed on the basis of the location and extent of the wound. For example, for surgery around the mouth, instruct the patient to drink with a straw and to avoid unnecessary movement from chewing and talking. Instruct patients who have had excision and suturing of the thigh to avoid running, jumping, and other activities that exert strain on the suture line, causing disruption and less than optimal healing. If wide excision with grafting is performed for malignant melanoma, provide instructions on wound care, as discussed in Chapter 6.

Additional Interventions
When a diagnosis of malignant melanoma is first suspected, reinforce to the patient that biopsy and excision are urgent.

Evaluation

Evaluate the effectiveness of nursing care for a patient with a cancer of the skin by comparing the patient's status with the expected patient outcomes. Examples of specific outcomes for patients with a cancer of the skin have been provided in the Planning section.

The Elderly: Special Considerations

It is estimated that 1 of every 10 elderly persons has a skin disorder (Matteson & McConnell, 1988, p. 156). As in any age group, the disorder may be limited to the skin or may be a manifestation of systemic disease. The most common skin lesions found in the elderly are keratoses, SCCs, and basal cell carcinomas, all of which are associated to some degree with long-term exposure to sunlight. Seborrheic dermatitis is also common in the elderly. It is characterized by scaling, with erythema on the nasolabial fold, eyebrows, and forehead. It is more severe and resistant to treatment in persons with Parkinson's disease and in the immunosuppressed.

Fungal infections are also frequently seen because warm, moist areas between skin folds provide good conditions for fungal growth. These conditions are present in many elderly as a result of obesity, impaired mobility, or weakness, which interfere with adequate cleansing and drying of skin-fold areas such as under the breast, the axilla, the perineum, and the groin.

Xerotic eczema, however, is by far the most common of all skin problems in the elderly, affecting virtually everyone older than 70 years to some degree. It is characterized by pruritus and dry, scaly skin. It is most marked on the lower arms and legs, hands and feet, skin-fold areas, and anoperineal area. It results from decreased sebum production in the elderly and is worsened by exposure to cold, dry weather, soaps, and other drying agents. Treatment of xerotic eczema involves decreasing bathing to once or twice a week, avoiding use of deodorant soaps, and use of emollients such as Eucerin or Intensive Care Lotion. Antihistamines such as Benadryl may also be prescribed.

The elderly are also at high risk for drug-related skin reactions and pressure sores.

Systemic diseases frequently associated with skin disorders in the elderly include diabetes, gout, and other metabolic disturbances; cancer in organs other than the skin; and neurologic and vascular disorders.

Bibliography

Arndt KA. Manual of dermatologic therapeutics. 4th ed. Boston: Little, Brown, 1988.
Atwater EE. Care of the surgically created granulating wound. Dermatol Nurs 1989; 1(1):43.
Bailin MD. Collagen implantation. Dermatol Nurs 1989, 1(1):37.
Bailin MD. Zyderm collagen implants. Dermatology Nurses Association FOCUS 1990; 3(2):2.
Baj PA. Liposuction—Redefining body proportions. AORN J 1986; 43(5):1127.
Balch CM, Houghton A, Milton G, et al. Cutaneous melanoma. 2nd ed. Philadelphia: JB Lippincott, 1992.
Bielan B. An overview of AIDS and its dermatologic manifestations. Dermatol Nurs 1989; 1(1):31.
Cohen L. Free-flap surgery: Nurses make it work. RN 1988; 51(3):26.
Collagen Biomedical. Facts about injectable collagen. Palo Alto, CA: Collagen Biomedical, 1991.
Converse J. Reconstructive plastic surgery. Philadelphia: WB Saunders, 1990.
Evey P. Patch test. Dermatology Nurses Association FOCUS 1986; 5(1):5.
Fitzpatrick TB, Eisen AZ, Wolff K, et al. Dermatology in general medicine. 3rd ed. New York: McGraw-Hill, 1987.
Grizzard D. Understanding the pathophysiology of psoriasis: A nursing perspective. Dermatol Nurs 1991; 3(5):305.
Habif TP. Clinical dermatology. 2nd ed. St. Louis: CV Mosby, 1990
Hanno DM. Accutane: An update for dermatology nurses. Dermatol Nurs 1989; 1(1):27.
Johnson TM, Brown MD, Swanson NA. Use of tissue expanders in dermatology. In Mediguide to dermatology. New York: Hoechst-Roussel Pharmaceuticals, 1991, 1–6.
Karel-Brant R. Healing by second intention: Its use in Moh's micrographic surgery. Dermatol Nurs 1990; 2(2):69.
Kim M, McFarland G, McLane A. Pocket guide to nursing diagnosis. No. 13. St. Louis: CV Mosby, 1989.
Laudano JB, Leach EE, Armstrong RB. Acne: Therapeutic perspectives with an emphasis on the role of isotretinoin. Dermatol Nurs 1990; 2(6):328.
Lookingbill DP, Marks JG Jr. Principles of dermatology. Philadelphia: WB Saunders, 1986.
Matteson MA, McConnell ES. Gerontological nursing: Concepts and practice. Philadelphia: WB Saunders, 1988.
McKeown A. Pulsed-dye laser treatment of vascular lesions. Dermatol Nurs 1991; 3(5):330.
Meusch R, Lillis PJ. Liposuction: The tumescent technique. Dermatol Nurs 1991; 3(4):255.

Moschella S, Hurley HJ. Dermatology. Philadelphia: WB Saunders, 1985.

Oregon Health Services University. Carbon dioxide laser surgery (patient information sheet). Portland, OR: Oregon Health Science University, Department of Dermatology, 1990.

Pillsbury DM, Heaton CL. A manual of dermatology. 2nd ed. Philadelphia: WB Saunders, 1980.

Rumsfield J. Sunscreens: What you and your patients should know. Dermatol Nurs 1990; 2(3):139.

Sauer GC. Manual of skin diseases. 6th ed. Philadelphia: JB Lippincott, 1991.

Shelk JL. Phototherapy: A nursing overview. Dermatol Nurs 1991; 3(6):401.

Smalley PJ. Laser technology: A nursing perspective. Dermatol Nurs 1991; 3(4):241.

Soter NA, Baden HP. Pathophysiology of dermatologic disease. 2nd ed. Philadelphia: JB Lippincott, 1991.

Storck L. Deep peels: What the nurse does. Dermatol Nurs 1991; 3(3):164.

Vargo N. Reconstructive surgery and flaps. Lecture presented at Nursing Perspectives in Dermatology Surgery Symposium, Hines, IL, 1986.

Whyte A. Cryosurgery for the dermatology nurse. Dermatol Nurs 1990; 2(5):271.

Yotter M. Contact dermatitis: Nursing intervention. Dermatol Nurs 1990; 2(5):267.

Chapter Eight

NURSING CARE *of Adults with Burn Injuries*

Each year between 2 and 3 million Americans sustain a burn injury. Approximately 300,000 of them require hospitalization, and 12,000 eventually die from their injuries.

A burn is one of the most devastating injuries that can occur to the human body. It affects almost every organ system of the body and is one of the most severe injuries that the body can endure and still survive.

In addition to the physical injury, the patient may also endure psychological, social, and economic problems. The patient may suffer loss of home, loss of ability to return to previous employment, and possibly loss of family members. The patient may have even been the victim of a crime. The burn affects not only the patient who sustains the injury but everyone associated with the patient.

A team approach is absolutely essential for successful care of the burn patient. The burn team consists of surgeons, internists, nurses, physical and occupational therapists, social workers, nutritionists, psychiatrists, skin bank personnel, epidemiologists, various technicians, and clergy. This team not only must work together but must communicate continually. Frequent team conferences are required to allow all members of the team to formulate a care plan. One goal of the team is to keep the family and, when possible, the patient aware of the plan of care. The nurse is the one who coordinates the team, because she or he spends the most time at the patient's bedside. Burn patients are one of nursing's toughest challenges as well as one of its greatest rewards.

Assessment of the Burn Injury

As discussed in Chapter 6, the skin has many functions. It protects against infection, prevents loss of body fluids, helps regulate body temperature, acts as an excretory organ, produces vitamin D, and contributes to individual identity. Depending on the depth and size of the burn injury, these functions will be either altered or eliminated. Although all of these functions are important, the loss of the first three functions as a result of a major burn injury must be dealt with immediately to prevent loss of life.

History of the Burn Injury

A brief history of the cause and circumstances of the injury is extremely valuable in the management of the burn patient.

1. At what time did the injury occur? This information is needed to calculate the patient's fluid requirements.
2. Was the victim in an enclosed space? This information alerts the burn center personnel to the possibility of inhalation injury and acute airway obstruction.
3. How did the accident occur?
   a. Water-heater explosions, propane-gas explosions, and other explosions that result in burn injuries frequently throw the patient some distance and may result in internal injuries and fractures. Enclosed areas such as tunnels, tanks, and furnaces affect the patient's ability to ventilate, leading to asphyxiation, carbon monoxide (CO) poisoning, and pulmonary injury.
   b. If a chemical burn occurred, what type of agent caused the injury?
4. Did the patient lose consciousness?
5. Does the patient have any chronic illnesses (e.g., diabetes mellitus; hypertension; cardiac, pulmonary, renal diseases; or alcohol/drug addiction)? Is the patient taking any medications?
6. Does the patient have any allergies or sensitivities?
7. What is the patient's tetanus immunization status?

Factors Determining the Severity of the Burn Injury

To classify the severity of a burn injury, many factors must be considered: depth of the burn, size of the burned area, part of the body burned, age of the patient, medical history, and additional injuries acquired at the time of the incident.

SIZE OF THE AREA BURNED

After a burn injury, fluid moves out of the blood stream and into body tissues for approximately 48 to 72 hours. This fluid shift causes widespread edema, even in small burns, and results in reduced circulating blood volume. To maintain perfusion of vital organs, the fluid must be replaced until it is reabsorbed from the tissues in 48 to 72 hours. The size of the body area burned is important in determining the amount of parenteral fluid replacement the patient will require in the first hours after a burn injury and is part of the consideration in calculating the probability of survival.

The size of the burn is expressed as the percentage of total body surface area (TBSA). The quickest and easiest method of estimating the size of the area burned is the "rule of nines," which is illustrated in Figure 8–1. Using this method, different body parts are assigned percentages that are multiples of nine: head, 9%; each anterior arm, 4.5%; each posterior arm, 4.5%; each anterior leg, 9%; each posterior leg, 9%; anterior thorax, 18%; posterior thorax, 18%; and perineum, 1%. The rule of nines is a good method to use for rapid assessment at the scene of an injury or in the emergency room. It does not, however, pro-

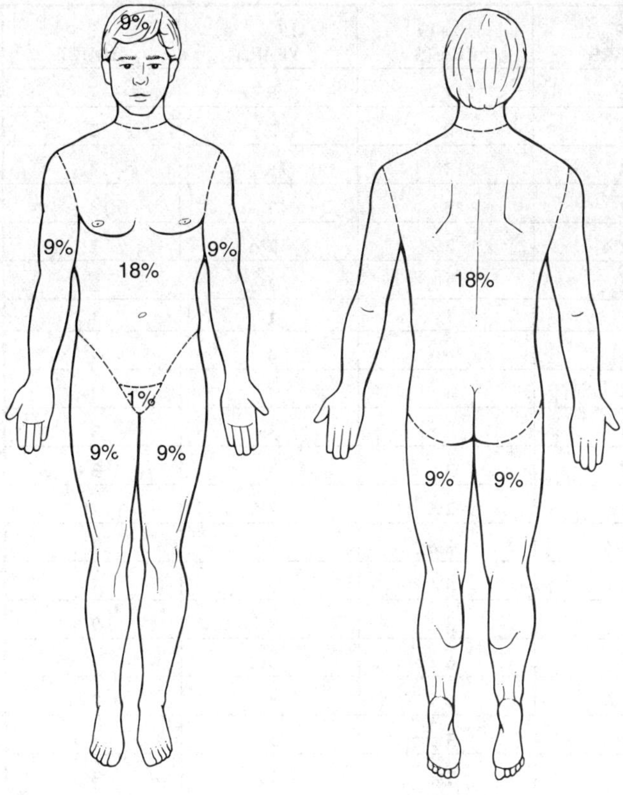

Figure 8–1.

The "rule of nines" used to estimate the size of a burned area. Head and neck = 9%, each arm = 9%, anterior torso = 18%, posterior torso = 18%, anterior leg = 9%, posterior leg = 9%, perineum = 1%.

vide the accurate calculation of percentages necessary for intensive in-hospital care.

The Lund and Browder chart is another method of estimating TBSA burned. This method takes into account the changes in body proportion that occur with age. Its greater accuracy is of benefit in determining exact fluid replacement requirements after a burn injury. Figure 8–2 illustrates a modified Lund and Browder method developed by Berkow, which is commonly used.

PART OF THE BODY AFFECTED

The part of the body burned is an important factor in determining the severity of the injury. Certain areas of the body present serious potential complications. Burns that involve the face, neck, and chest are associated with a greater possibility of pulmonary complications. Burns of the hands, feet, or major joints require intense physical and occupational rehabilitation, whereas burns of the perineum have a high rate of infection. Because of the high incidence of complications, any burn involving the hands, face, eyes, ears, feet, or perineum is considered to be a major burn injury regardless of the total size of the burned area.

DEPTH OF THE BURN

Determining the depth of the burn injury identifies which skin layers have been damaged or destroyed and provides the burn team with important information that aids in developing treatment plans for the patient.

The severity of damage to the innermost layer of the epidermis, the stratum germinativum or basal cell layer, has significant impact on burn care. This layer is the site where new cells are produced to replace destroyed or damaged cells. Basal cells are also found in the dermis lining the hair follicles and the sweat and sebaceous glands. It is the presence of adequate numbers of basal cells that determines whether a burn wound heals spontaneously by regenerating new skin or whether it requires skin grafting to heal (transplanting living tissue from one area of the body to another).

Burn depth, as summarized in Table 8–1, is classified as either partial thickness or full thickness. Partial-thickness injuries are subdivided into superficial injuries or deep injuries.

PARTIAL-THICKNESS BURNS

Superficial Partial-Thickness Burns

Superficial partial-thickness burn injuries (previously called first degree burns) are commonly caused by brief contact with a hot object, low-voltage electricity, a spatter scald, or, most commonly, ultraviolet light (sunburn). They involve only the epidermis of the skin; therefore, skin functions are minimally affected.

These burn wounds are typically pink to red in color, with a dry surface, no vesicles present, and absent or minimal edema. They are painful, blanch with application of pressure, and demonstrate quick capillary refill. The burn area may blister and peel after 24 hours. Superficial partial-thickness burns heal spontaneously, without scarring, in 3 to 5 days. An example of a superficial partial-thickness burn can be seen in Figure 8–3.

Deep Partial-Thickness Burns

Deep partial-thickness burn injuries (previously called second degree burns) are caused by more prolonged contact with flame, hot objects, hot liquids, or chemicals. These burns involve all of the epidermis and part of the dermis but do not completely destroy the sweat glands, the hair follicles, or the basal cells lining them.

Deep partial-thickness burns are red, mottled, or waxy white in color. Fluid-filled surface vesicles or bullae form rapidly and may or may not be intact on the patient's arrival at the hospital. An important characteristic is that these burns are always wet and glistening in appearance, and hairs that are present in the wound will remain firmly in place if pulled. The patient usually experiences a great deal of pain from a deep partial-thickness burn because of the

Body Area	0–1 YEAR	1–4 YEARS	5–9 YEARS	10–14 YEARS	15 YEARS	ADULT
Head	19	17	13	11	9	7
Neck	2	2	2	2	2	2
Ant. Trunk	13	13	13	13	13	13
Post. Trunk	13	13	13	13	13	13
R. Buttock	2½	2½	2½	2½	2½	2½
L. Buttock	2½	2½	2½	2½	2½	2½
Genitalia	1	1	1	1	1	1
R. U. Arm	4	4	4	4	4	4
L. U. Arm	4	4	4	4	4	4
R. L. Arm	3	3	3	3	3	3
L. L. Arm	3	3	3	3	3	3
R. Hand	2½	2½	2½	2½	2½	2½
L. Hand	2½	2½	2½	2½	2½	2½
R. Thigh	5½	6½	8	8½	9	9½
L. Thigh	5½	6½	8	8½	9	9½
R. L. Leg	5	5	5½	6	6½	7
L. L. Leg	5	5	5½	6	6½	7
R. Foot	3½	3½	3½	3½	3½	3½
L. Foot	3½	3½	3½	3½	3½	3½

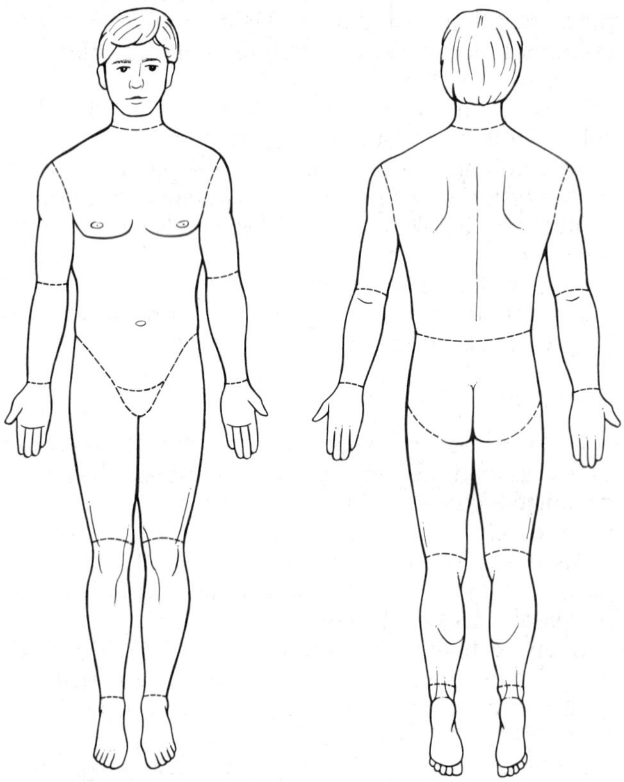

Figure 8–2.

The above chart explains Berkow's formula of Lund and Browder's method of calculation of total body surface area (TBSA) burned. This method reflects changes in TBSA that occur with normal growth patterns.

damaged nerve endings. Blanching and capillary refill will occur but not as rapidly as with the more superficial injury. Edema is present and varies from moderate to severe. An example of a deep partial-thickness burn can be seen in Figure 8–4.

In the care of partial-thickness burns, it is important to prevent conversion of the wound to a full-thickness injury as a result of further trauma, infection, poor tissue perfusion, prolonged pressure, or inadequate nutrition. Partial-thickness burns can heal spontaneously by regeneration from the basal cells. However, the burn team may opt to graft wounds that will take more than 2 to 3 weeks to heal to minimize functional loss and scarring. In some patients, original skin color may not return because melanoblasts have been destroyed. These are cells located primarily in the deepest layer of the epidermis, which produce the melanin that determines skin pigmentation.

FULL-THICKNESS BURNS

A full-thickness burn injury (previously called third degree burn), as seen in Figure 8–5, involves total destruction of the epidermis and dermis. These injuries are commonly caused by prolonged contact with flames, electricity, chemicals, hot liquids (immersion), and hot objects. Brief contact with high-voltage electricity can also result in a full-thickness burn injury.

A full-thickness burn injury may be black, waxy white, cherry red, or tan. It is leathery, dry, and hard. The capillary bed is destroyed, and throm-

Table 8-1. DEPTH OF BURN

CLASSIFICATION	SKIN LAYERS DAMAGED	CLINICAL MANIFESTATIONS	SENSATION	HEALING TIME	TIME
Superficial partial-thickness (first degree)	Epidermis	Pink to red; no blisters, bullae; skin dry; minimal to little edema	Painful for short duration	3–5 days	No scarring
Deep partial-thickness (second degree)	Entire epidermis, partial dermis	Red to ivory white; blisters, bullae; wet, glistening surface; edema formation; slow blanching and capillary refill	Very painful	14–28 days	Scarring varies
Full-thickness (third degree)	Entire epidermis, entire dermis, and sometimes fat, muscle, bone	White, black, cherry red, tan; thrombosed vessels; no blister formation; dry, leathery surface; no elasticity; massive edema	Painless	Requires grafting	Scarring

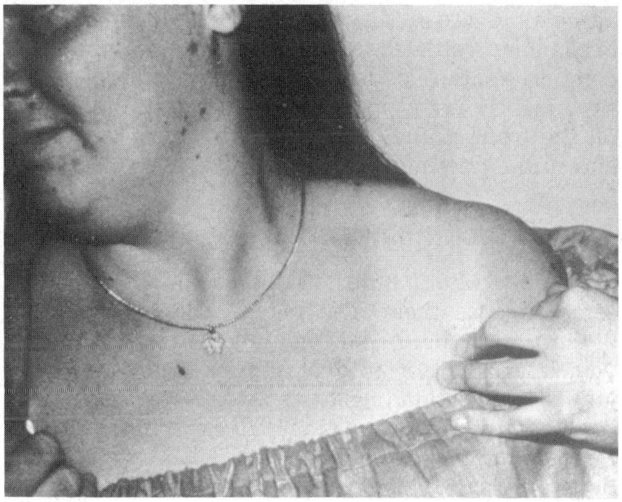

Figure 8–3.

Sunburn is the most common example of a superficial partial-thickness burn injury.

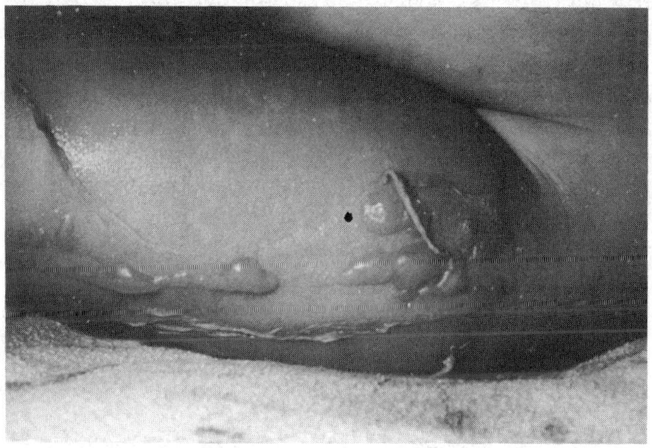

Figure 8–4.

Glistening wet surface, thick peeling skin, and fluid-filled vesicles typical of a deep partial-thickness burn injury.

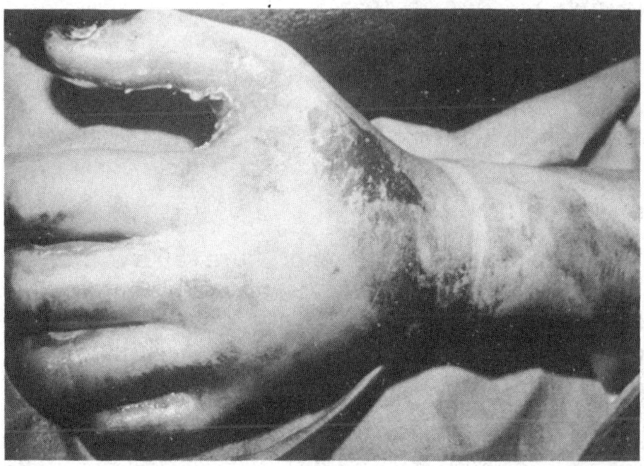

Figure 8–5.

Dry, leathery white, taut skin and severe edema in a full-thickness burn injury.

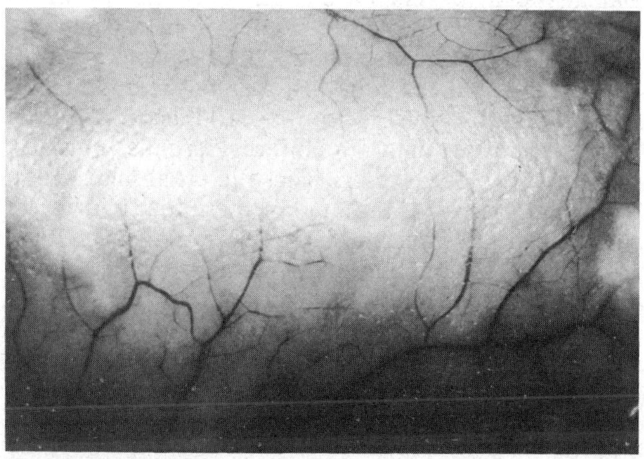

Figure 8–6.

Thrombosed vessels with hemolyzed blood seen beneath the surface of a full-thickness burn injury. Note the taut skin from severe edema.

bosed vessels, as illustrated in Figure 8–6, may sometimes be seen within the wound. Blanching does not occur. Any hairs remaining in the wound can be easily pulled out. Although full-thickness burns are painless because of destruction of the nerves, any surrounding areas of partial-thickness burn injury will still be very painful. Surface edema may not appear as severe in a full-thickness burn as with a partial-thickness burn because the loss of the skin's elasticity does not allow for expansion. However, it is important to remember that edema develops within the deeper tissues and can cause serious problems because of increased pressure on blood vessels and internal structures.

Because both the epidermal and dermal skin layers, with the basal cells, are destroyed, spontaneous healing will not occur by primary granulation. If the wound is the size of a half dollar or smaller, doctors may elect to allow the wound to cover itself with the granulating wound edges. This will leave a small scar and is commonly referred to as allowing the wound to "scar in." Larger wounds must receive skin grafts to heal.

It should be noted that initial assessment of the depth of a burn injury is not always accurate. Even after initial debridement of the wound, it may take 2 or 3 days for the full extent of the injury to become apparent. In addition, extensive burns usually present with several depths of tissue injury. It is therefore important to take into consideration the history and cause of the burn injury when initially assessing the patient and determining treatment.

TYPE OF AGENT CAUSING THE BURN

Burns are classified as thermal (heat, hot liquids, radiation), chemical, and electrical. The depth of the injury caused by hot liquids is dependent on the temperature of the liquid and the length of exposure. Generally, oil burns are deeper because oil reaches higher temperatures and adheres to the skin. Management of chemical and electrical burns is complicated by the nature of the agent causing the burn. Chemical burns require dilution and neutralization and will continue to cause tissue destruction until neutralization is complete. Electrical burns create extensive injury to internal organs, muscles, nerves, and blood vessels. These internal injuries are difficult to assess at the time of the initial injury, yet may greatly complicate care. Some may even take months or years to become apparent. In addition, electrical arcing may cause clothing to ignite, resulting in a thermal burn in addition to the electrical injury. A complete history of the circumstances of the injury assists the burn team's ability to anticipate problems.

AGE OF THE PATIENT

The child younger than 10 years and the adult older than 50 years with a burn injury are considered at high risk during treatment. The dermis of both the very young and elderly is thinner, allowing a deeper burn from exposure to the heat source. Diminished blood supply to the skin in the elderly lengthens healing time, while a weaker immune response increases the risk of infection. Recovery of the elderly patient may be further complicated by preexisting health problems that compromise cardiovascular, respiratory, and nutritional status and increase the risk of complications. Because of higher mortality, any burn to a person in these age groups is considered a potentially serious burn injury and should be evaluated in an emergency room.

MEDICAL HISTORY

It is extremely important to obtain a medical history from the patient, a family member, or a significant other. Any preexisting conditions (e.g., cardiovascular disease, diabetes, seizure disorder) may become exacerbated after a burn injury and may complicate the patient's recovery. Allergies are prominently noted in the patient record and posted on the front of the chart, on the medication record, and in the nursing care plan.

ASSOCIATED INJURIES

Patients often suffer additional injuries at the same time as their burn injury. These occur most often when the patient is involved in a motor-vehicle accident or an explosion or when the victim jumps from a building to escape fire or smoke. Associated injuries can range from minor to life-threatening and can include internal injuries, lacerations, fractures, spinal cord injury, and head trauma. Any additional injury will further complicate the patient's recovery.

Categorizing the Severity of a Burn Injury

The American Burn Association has established criteria for categorizing the severity of a burn injury and protocols for treatment.

MINOR BURN INJURY

The patient with a minor burn injury may be cared for in an emergency room with complete facilities for initial burn care and then treated as an outpatient. A minor burn is one in which there is

1. Partial-thickness injury of less than 15% TBSA in adults or 10% TBSA in persons younger than 10 years or older than 50 years.
2. Full-thickness injury of less than 2% TBSA.
3. No burn involving the hands, face, eyes, ears, feet, perineum, or major joints.
4. No other complication present.

MODERATE BURN INJURY

A moderate burn injury is one in which there is

1. Partial-thickness injury of 15% to 25% TBSA in adults or 10% to 20% TBSA in persons younger than 10 years or older than 50 years.
2. Full-thickness injury of less than 5% TBSA.
3. No burn involving the hands, face, eyes, ears, feet, perineum, or major joints.
4. No other complication present.

MAJOR BURN INJURY

A major burn injury is one in which there is

1. Partial-thickness injury of more than 25% TBSA in adults or 20% TBSA in persons younger than 10 years or older than 50 years.
2. Full-thickness injury of 5% TBSA or more.
3. Burns involving the hands, face, eyes, ears, feet, perineum, or major joints.
4. Inhalation injury.
5. Associated injuries.
6. Electrical burn.
7. Chemical burn.
8. Preexisting health problems.

CRITERIA FOR TRANSPORT TO A BURN CENTER

The following includes the injuries that the American Burn Association has identified as those for which the patient should be transported to a burn center after initial assessment and treatment at an emergency department.

1. Deep partial-thickness and full-thickness burns of 10% or more of the body surface in patients younger than 10 years or older than 50 years.
2. Deep partial-thickness and full-thickness burns of more than 20% of the body surface in other age groups.
3. Full-thickness burns of more than 5% of the body surface area in any age group.
4. Deep partial-thickness and full-thickness burns that involve the face, hands, feet, genitalia, perineum, or major joints.
5. Electrical burns, including lightning injury.
6. Chemical burns.
7. Inhalation injury with burn injury.
8. Circumferential burns of the extremity and chest.
9. Lesser burns in patients with preexisting medical problems that could complicate management.
10. Associated injuries or pregnancy.

If trauma injuries pose a far greater immediate risk than the burn injury, the patient may initially be treated in a trauma center until stable before being transferred to a burn center. This decision is made by the trauma physician in consultation with the regional burn center.

Care of the Patient with a Burn Injury

Care of the patient with a burn injury is determined in part by the time elapsed since the burn injury occurred. The four phases of burn care are: immediate care, or care at the scene of the injury; emergent phase, or care given during the first 48 to 72 hours; acute phase, or period of time that begins with the reabsorption of interstitial fluid at the end of the emergent period and ends with the closure of the wound; and rehabilitation phase.

Although for clarity of presentation each of the phases of burn care are discussed individually, it is important to remember that, to provide continuity of care, many aspects of patient care in each phase of burn management overlap with other phases. For example, wound care, which is presented as a primary focus of the acute phase, begins with immediate care at the scene of the accident and continues through the rehabilitation phase; and rehabilitation, discussed as the final phase of burn care, begins on first contact with health care professionals and continues through all phases of burn care. Nursing Care Guide 8–1 illustrates this necessary overlap of aspects of patient care among the four phases.

Immediate Care

The priority of immediate care at the scene, as summarized in Table 8–2, is to stop the burning process, prevent further injury, and maintain vital functions until the ambulance arrives with monitoring and life-support equipment. The nurse at the scene must first determine the safest access to the victim. Next, the victim must be moved to a safe area before treating. Successful treatment cannot be given in a smoke-filled area, nor can the nurse be of help if he or she is overcome from inhaling smoke or is injured from falling debris.

STOP THE BURNING PROCESS

The first step in treating the victim is to stop the burning process to halt the penetration of heat to deeper tissue, causing greater damage. First, remove the heat source. If the victim is still on fire, roll him or her immediately on the ground, smother the flames in a blanket, or douse the flames with low-pressure water until they are extinguished. Next, remove all clothing in contact with the burn. Synthetic fabrics ignite, burn rapidly at high temperatures, and melt into hot plastic residue, which continues to burn the victim and creates later problems in removing the material from the skin. If the material is embedded in the burn, do not remove it. It will be removed later by the burn team. Finally, flush the burns with low-pressure cool water. Do not apply ice because it may deepen the injury as a result of vasoconstriction.

Text continued on page 249

Nursing Care Guide 8–1.

PATIENTS WITH THERMAL BURN INJURIES

Assessment Findings: Patient is 1 hour post–thermal burn injury of the anterior torso, neck, chin, and upper arms. Fire occurred in the patient's small bedroom. Patient is alert and oriented. Nasal hairs are singed, external nares blistered. Oral mucous membranes are pink, moist. Breath sounds: clear and unlabored; respiratory rate: 16, regular and unlabored.

Nursing Diagnosis: High risk for ineffective airway clearance related to possible upper airway edema secondary to inhalation of superheated air

Patient Outcomes	Nursing Interventions	Rationale
Patient maintains patent airway with regular, unlabored respirations between 12 and 20 per minute.	Identify body surface areas burned. Determine the circumstances of the burn injury.	Risk of upper airway injury is greater in burns of the face, neck, or upper chest and if the fire occurred in a confined space.
	Examine the patient for singed nasal hairs; soot on the tongue, pharynx, or in the sputum; redness or blistering of the lips, face, or buccal mucosa.	These manifestations indicate possible upper airway burn injury.
	Auscultate breath sounds, and assess rate, depth, rhythm of respirations, level of consciousness, and voice quality at least hourly.	Edema narrows respiratory passages, causing frequent cough, wheezing, crackles (rales), stridor, or hoarseness. Restlessness, increasing respiratory rate, altered respiratory depth, irregular respiratory rhythm, and decreasing level of consciousness (LOC) indicate impaired respiratory function.

(continued)

Nursing Care Guide 8–1. *(continued)*

PATIENTS WITH THERMAL BURN INJURIES

Patient Outcomes	Nursing Interventions	Rationale
	Elevate the head of the bed.	Elevation promotes venous drainage to reduce edema and promotes chest expansion and diaphragmatic excursion to ease breathing.
	Provide humidified oxygen.	Prevents drying of respiratory tissues and improves oxygenation.
	Administer intravenous narcotic analgesics as needed and before wound care.	Pain increases anxiety and oxygen requirements.
	Encourage position changes, deep breathing, coughing, and use of incentive spirometer.	Prevents stasis of secretions and promotes respiratory function.
	Monitor arterial blood gases.	An increasing partial pressure of carbon dioxide ($Paco_2$) and a decreasing partial pressure of oxygen (Pao_2) indicate respiratory compromise.
	Notify physician promptly of any indication of deteriorating respiratory status.	Intubation may be necessary to maintain patent airway. Early intervention prevents further deterioration in status and the risk of hypoxia.

Evaluation: Compare the patient's status with the expected patient outcomes. If the outcomes are achieved, evaluate nursing care as successful. If not, reassess the patient, formulate new nursing diagnoses, and revise expected patient outcomes and nursing interventions as appropriate.

(continued)

Nursing Care Guide 8–1. *(continued)*

PATIENTS WITH THERMAL BURN INJURIES

Assessment Findings: Patient is 2 hours post–thermal burn injury with partial-thickness burns over 40% of total body surface area (TBSA). Burned areas are edematous and blistered, with open areas weeping serous fluid. Patient is lethargic, urine output is 25 ml/hour via indwelling urinary catheter, blood pressure (BP) is 90/60, pulse rate is 100 bpm, central venous pressure (CVP) is 5 cm of water (H_2O), intravenous (IV) lactated Ringer's solution infusing 600 ml/hour via large-bore IV catheter. Patient is to receive 9600 ml of IV fluid resuscitation over 24 hours from time of the burn injury.

Nursing Diagnosis: High risk for fluid volume deficit related to inadequate replacement of fluids lost through evaporation from the burn wound and fluid shift into interstitial spaces

Patient Outcomes	Nursing Interventions	Rationale
Patient maintains adequate hydration as evidenced by: 1. Being mentally alert 2. Urine output > 30 ml/hour 3. BP > 90/60 4. Heart rate > 60 but < 100 bpm 5. CVP 4–15 mm H_2O 6. Moist mucous membranes 7. Capillary refill < 3 seconds	Weigh patient and obtain vital signs on admission. Monitor vital signs, LOC, CVP, urine output, and capillary refill at least hourly.	Changes in these parameters indicate the adequacy of fluid resuscitation. Hypovolemia is indicated by decreasing LOC, urine output < 30 ml/hour, BP < 90/60, heart rate > 100 bpm, dry mucous membranes, delayed capillary refill.
	Maintain IV infusion for fluid resuscitation. Calculate flow rate to ensure that 50% of the total fluid volume prescribed for the initial 24-hour period from the time of the injury will infuse over the first 8 hours. The remaining 50% infuses over the next 16 hours. Assess infusion sites hourly.	Infusion of large volumes of fluids and electrolytes is necessary to maintain perfusion of vital organs and tissues during the emergent period when fluids shift into interstitial spaces and are lost through the burn wound.
	Auscultate breath sounds hourly. Notify physician immediately if dyspnea, orthopnea, crackles (rales), cough, or pink, frothy sputum develops.	Fluid overload from too rapid fluid infusion may cause pulmonary edema.

Evaluation: Compare the patient's status with the expected patient outcomes. If the outcomes are achieved, evaluate nursing care as successful. If not, reassess the patient, formulate new nursing diagnoses, and revise expected patient outcomes and nursing interventions as appropriate.

(continued)

Nursing Care Guide 8–1. *(continued)*

PATIENTS WITH THERMAL BURN INJURIES

Assessment Findings: Patient with burn injury is restless, moans when touched, complains of pain. Patient states pain is intolerable.

Nursing Diagnosis: Pain related to burn injury

Patient Outcomes	Nursing Interventions	Rationale
Patient states pain is within tolerable limits.	Administer intravenous morphine or other narcotic analgesic in small, frequent doses or continuous infusion during the emergent phase and fluid mobilization in the acute phase.	Subcutaneous or intramuscular medication is poorly absorbed during the emergent and fluid mobilization phases because of fluid imbalances. Small, frequent doses or continuous infusion provide better pain management.
	Administer bolus dose of analgesic before wound care.	Minimizes pain during painful procedures and reduces fear of the procedure.
	Monitor respirations, LOC.	Narcotics are a central nervous system (CNS) depressant.
	Assist patient to assume comfortable position within limits of injury. Provide emotional support and comfort measures. Encourage distraction and relaxation exercises. Allow patient to assist with wound care.	These measures promote relaxation and enhance pain relief by reducing anxiety. Patient participation provides a sense of control.

Evaluation: Compare the patient's status with the expected patient outcomes. If the outcomes are achieved, evaluate nursing care as successful. If not, reassess the patient, formulate new nursing diagnoses, and revise expected patient outcomes and nursing interventions as appropriate.

(continued)

Nursing Care Guide 8–1. *(continued)*
PATIENTS WITH THERMAL BURN INJURIES

Assessment Findings: Patient has partial- and full-thickness burn wounds.

Nursing Diagnosis: High risk for infection related to open burn wounds, suppressed immune response

Patient Outcomes	Nursing Interventions	Rationale
Patient remains free from infection as evidenced by: 1. Absence of fever 2. Daily increase in wound granulation and healing 3. Wound free of increasing edema, foul odor, purulent drainage 4. <100,000 bacteria per gram of wound tissue	Maintain good hand-washing technique for all persons entering patient's room. Use aseptic technique, and wear cap, mask, gown, and sterile gloves during wound care. Change gloves between wounds.	Minimizes risk of wound contamination and cross contamination between wounds.
	Cleanse wounds one to two times daily or as prescribed.	Cleansing removes exudates, eschar, and necrotic tissue, which inhibit healing and provide a medium for the growth of microorganisms.
	Assess wounds after cleansing for signs of healing or infection. Small blood vessels, bleeding, shiny-pink granulation tissue indicate healing. Foul odor, purulent drainage, expanding redness, or edema indicates infection. Notify physician if wound is not healing or if signs of infection are present.	Infection is the most common cause of death in the acute phase of burn care. Wounds that fail to heal may be infected. Burn wounds with manifestations of surface infection must undergo biopsy for tissue culture to diagnose infection because surface colonization is common but does not necessarily indicate tissue infection.
	Gently apply topical agent and cover with gauze dressings as prescribed. Be sure dressings do not constrict blood flow.	Antimicrobial topical agents minimize risk of infection. Gentle handling of the wound prevents disruption of fragile granulation tissue and new blood vessels.
	Provide care of graft and donor sites as discussed in Chapter 6.	Proper care prevents disruption of the graft, which will inhibit wound healing and closure. Donor sites are a new wound and potential site for infection.
	Maintain a warm environment and minimize patient exposure during wound care.	Prevents hypothermia.
Patient demonstrates correct wound-care technique before discharge.	Teach patient how to cleanse and re-dress open wounds, as presented in Chart 8–1.	Correct wound-care technique minimizes the risk of infection and promotes healing.

(continued)

Nursing Care Guide 8–1. (continued)
PATIENTS WITH THERMAL BURN INJURIES

Patient Outcomes	Nursing Interventions	Rationale
Patient verbalizes care of newly healed skin.	Teach patient to take precautions to prevent trauma to newly healed skin and to protect it from exposure to ultraviolet light and hot objects.	Newly healed skin is fragile and sensitive to ultraviolet light and heat.
	Teach patient to massage emollient moisturizers into skin.	Restores moisture and suppleness, stimulates circulation, and reduces flaking and itching.
Patient puts on pressure garment correctly and verbalizes intent to wear it at least 23 hours a day.	Teach patient the purpose of pressure garment. Stress that it must be worn at least 23 hours a day to be effective.	Pressure garments minimize the risk of hypertrophic scarring if worn at least 23 hours daily.
	Be sure the patient has two garments before discharge. Review garment care as presented in Chart 8–1.	Garment must be washed and air-dried daily.

Evaluation: Compare the patient's status with the expected patient outcomes. If the outcomes are achieved, evaluate nursing care as successful. If not, reassess the patient, formulate new nursing diagnoses, and revise expected patient outcomes and nursing interventions as appropriate.

Assessment Findings: Family preparing to visit loved one 8 hours post–thermal burn injury of 60% of TBSA. Patient is intubated; severe edema has distorted physical features and has closed eyes. Bulky dressings cover most burned areas.

Nursing Diagnosis: Anxiety related to appearance of loved one, unknown outcome of treatment

Patient Outcomes	Nursing Interventions	Rationale
Family is prepared for the appearance of the patient.	Discuss the patient's appearance with the family before they see the patient.	Preparation for what they will see will lessen the shock.
	Explain the need for the endotracheal tube and how it is helping the patient. Explain why the patient's features are distorted.	Understanding what they see will lessen their anxiety.
	Encourage family to speak to the patient and touch unburned areas. Assure them that the patient can still hear and understand.	Communication and touch can provide emotional support for patient and family.

(continued)

Nursing Care Guide 8–1. *(continued)*

PATIENTS WITH THERMAL BURN INJURIES

Patient Outcomes	Nursing Interventions	Rationale
Family asks questions and verbalizes concerns.	Encourage questions and expression of thoughts and concerns both before and after visits.	Provides emotional support and opportunity for family to express concerns.
	Offer pastoral services to family and patient.	Demonstrates concern for spiritual needs.
Family verbalizes understanding that the outcome of treatment is uncertain because of the severity of the burn injury.	Answer questions honestly in terms the family can understand. Reinforce the physician's explanations of the desired outcome and prognosis of treatment. Do not give false assurances. Refer questions you cannot answer to appropriate resources.	Accurate information provides assurance that everything possible is being done for the patient.

Evaluation: Compare the patient's status with the expected patient outcomes. If the outcomes are achieved, evaluate nursing care as successful. If not, reassess the patient, formulate new nursing diagnoses, and revise expected patient outcomes and nursing interventions as appropriate.

Assessment Findings: Patient is 54 hours post–thermal burn injury of 40% of TBSA. Urine output has been > 100 ml/hour for 2 hours.

Nursing Diagnosis: High risk for fluid volume excess related to mobilization of fluids from interstitial spaces into the intravascular circulation

Patient Outcomes	Nursing Interventions	Rationale
Patient maintains fluid balance as evidenced by the following: 1. Urine output > 30 but < 100 ml/hour 2. Blood pressure > 90/60 but < 140/90 3. Heart rate > 60 but < 100 bpm, regular rhythm 4. Central venous pressure > 4 but < 15 mm of water 5. Lungs clear to auscultation 6. Body weight within 5% of preinjury weight	Assess for respiratory distress, auscultate breath sounds, monitor urine output and vital signs at least hourly. Weigh patient daily. Compare with patient's baseline values.	Diuresis, with corresponding loss in body weight, is an expected manifestation of fluid mobilization. The rapid shift of fluid into the vascular circulation may result in left ventricular failure or pulmonary edema.
	Monitor electrolyte levels. Auscultate heart and bowel sounds.	Diuresis may cause rapid shift in serum electrolytes.
	Maintain intravenous infusion. Offer oral fluids if bowel sounds are present and patient is free of nausea and able to drink.	Fluid intake will prevent dehydration.

Evaluation: Compare the patient's status with the expected patient outcomes. If the outcomes are achieved, evaluate nursing care as successful. If not reassess the patient, formulate new nursing diagnoses, and revise expected patient outcomes and nursing interventions as appropriate.

Table 8–2. PRIORITIES OF CARE AT THE SCENE OF A THERMAL BURN INJURY

PRIORITY	INTERVENTION
PRIMARY SURVEY AND MANAGEMENT	
Assess scene safety	Do not attempt to treat unless Patient has been removed from smoke-filled or unsafe area. Double gloves have been applied if chemicals were involved. Electric current has been turned off, or patient has been moved from the current with nonconductive tools.
Stop the burning process	Roll the victim, or douse with water. Remove clothing that does not stick. Flush burn with cool-to-tepid water.
Manage airway distress	Assess respiratory status. Maintain patent airway. Perform rescue breathing.
Treat associated life-threatening injuries	Assess circulatory status. Perform CPR, if needed. Assess for bleeding. Apply direct pressure to control bleeding. Maintain cervical alignment.
Maintain peripheral circulation	Remove rings, bracelets, anklets, and so on. Open shirts, pants, skirts; remove belts.
Maintain body temperature	Cover victim with a clean sheet and blankets.
Initiate fluid resuscitation, if possible	Start an intravenous line with a large-bore needle. Administer Ringer's lactate solution at 500 ml/hr (for patients older than 15 years of age).
SECONDARY SURVEY AND MANAGEMENT	
Assess level of consciousness	Determine patient's level of consciousness using AVPU method: A = alert V = responds to verbal stimuli P = responds only to painful stimuli U = unresponsive
Maintain airway	Assist ventilation. Closely monitor for need to intubate.
Identify associated injuries	Stabilize fractures. Cover open wounds with dressings.
Obtain patient history	Determine characteristics of injury: Cause of burn Possibility of inhalation: Fire in an enclosed space Patient unconscious Chemicals involved Time of injury Obtain patient-related factors: age, illnesses, medications, allergies, etc.
Monitor patient	Monitor vital signs and ventilatory status.

Abbreviation: CPR, Cardiopulmonary resuscitation.

If the injury has been caused by a chemical, use caution in approaching the scene to prevent contact with the chemical, particularly when the accident has occurred as a result of a spill or explosion. All persons who touch the patient should first put on a double set of rubber gloves to prevent contact with any chemical on the patient's skin or clothing. Protective clothing and eye covering is also desirable. Do not waste time in determining the correct neutralizing agent if identification of the chemical is not immediately available. The priority is to remove any chemical in contact with the patient. First, rapidly remove the patient's garments, which will retain the chemical agent. Next, brush any chemical in powdered or visible form from the skin. Flush the chemical with large amounts of water for at least 20 to 30 minutes to dilute and wash away the chemical. Use a shower or hose if available. Flush chemical burns of the eyes from the inner canthus, next to the nose, toward the outer canthus to avoid washing the chemical from one eye into the other. Remove contact lenses, and continue eye irrigation throughout transport to the hospital.

It is extremely important that anyone assisting at the scene of an electrical burn take precautions in approaching the victim to prevent becoming a second victim. Make sure the electrical current has been turned off before touching the victim. Use a long pole made of dry wood or dry rubber to remove the victim from the electrical source if the current cannot be turned off.

MAINTAIN PATENT AIRWAY

Proper airway management is imperative. Assess the victim's breathing. The airway must be open and free of debris. Establish a patent airway, if needed, by tilting the victim's head back or use the chin lift if there is a possibility of neck or spinal injury. If the victim is not breathing, perform rescue breathing.

TREAT ASSOCIATED LIFE-THREATENING INJURIES

Very often, these victims have life-threatening injuries in addition to the burn injury. Associated injuries occur when the victim is burned in an accident (e.g., airplane or motor vehicle), an explosion, or a fall or jump from a burning building. Assess circulatory status, and perform cardiopulmonary resuscitation if needed. Apply direct pressure to control bleeding, and maintain body and spinal alignment to stabilize skeletal injuries.

MAINTAIN PERIPHERAL CIRCULATION

Remove rings, bracelets, necklaces, ankle bracelets, and anything the patient is wearing that is potentially constrictive. As edema develops, these objects will compress the blood vessels and impair circulation to the distal portion of the extremity. Assess the

Table 8–3. RESPIRATORY ALTERATIONS ASSOCIATED WITH THERMAL BURN INJURIES

TYPE	CAUSE	CLINICAL MANIFESTATIONS	MEDICAL MANAGEMENT	NURSING IMPLICATIONS
Carbon monoxide poisoning	Mild exposure (10%–20% COHb)	Headache, decreased visual acuity, possible breathlessness, irritability	Inhalation of 100% oxygen Monitor arterial blood gases Monitor COHb level	Administer 100% oxygen. Observe patient color. Monitor arterial blood gases. Monitor COHb levels. Monitor vital signs.
	Moderate exposure (20%–40% COHb)	Decreased blood pressure, increased pulse, Cheyne-Stokes respirations, dilated pupils, confusion, headache, irritability, vertigo, nausea and vomiting, decreased visual acuity, reddish skin color	Same Intubation for ventilation may be necessary	Same
	Major exposure (40%–60% COHb)	Dysrhythmias, convulsions, coma	Same	Same
	Extreme exposure (>60% COHb)	Usually respiratory arrest and death	Same	Same
Inhalation injury above the glottis	Inhalation of superheated air	Early: soot on tongue, pharynx, or sputum; singed nasal hairs; dry, red buccal mucosa; burns of face, neck, upper chest Late: dyspnea, coughing, wheezing, hoarseness, inability to control secretions	Early intubation Mechanical respiratory support Baseline arterial blood gases Baseline chest x-ray examination	Administer prescribed oxygen. Observe for increased cough and hoarseness. Auscultate lung fields. Observe lung expansion. Monitor vital signs. Monitor arterial blood gases.
Inhalation injury below the glottis	Inhalation of smoke and chemicals of combustion	Fever, dyspnea, wheezing, rales, decreased tidal volume, poor gas exchange, productive cough	Administration of oxygen Intubation, if required Baseline arterial blood gases Baseline chest x-ray examination	Administer prescribed oxygen. Suction hourly. Monitor vital signs and oxygen saturation. Monitor arterial blood gases. Turn patient every 1–2 hr.
Restrictive disease	Decreased vital capacity	Anxiety, restlessness, decreased level of consciousness, labored breathing	Administration of oxygen Intubation, if required Baseline arterial blood gases Baseline chest x-ray examination	Administer prescribed oxygen. Monitor vital signs. Monitor arterial blood gas results and oxygen saturation.

Abbreviation: COHb, carboxyhemoglobin.

status of the distal circulation, checking for cyanosis, impaired capillary refill, paresthesias, and deep-tissue pain.

MAINTAIN BODY TEMPERATURE

Cover the victim with a clean sheet and enough blankets to prevent heat loss caused by loss of the protective heat-regulating function of the skin. If the victim's temperature is not maintained at the scene and during transport, the victim may be dangerously hypothermic by the time he or she arrives in the emergency room or burn center.

Emergent Phase

The emergent phase, sometimes referred to as the fluid resuscitation stage, is the first 2 to 3 days after a burn injury. The focus of medical and nursing management during this phase of burn care is identification and treatment of life-threatening alterations in respiratory function, fluid and electrolyte balance, and peripheral vascular circulation. Although pain management and intensive care of the burn wound itself begin in the emergent period, they are primary focuses of the acute period and are discussed in detail later.

RESPIRATORY FUNCTION

Respiratory failure is a major cause of death from a burn injury in the emergent phase. As many as 60% to 70% of the patients who die in a burn center have an inhalation injury.

As illustrated in Table 8–3, several types of airway problems may develop in burn patients depending on the circumstances of the burn accident.

Many patients with severe respiratory involvement from a burn injury die before reaching the hospital. Death from respiratory compromise during the early postburn period can be attributed to inhalation of carbon monoxide, smoke, or noxious chemicals; acute airway obstruction caused by inhalation of superheated air; or pulmonary complications caused by decreased vital capacity.

CARBON MONOXIDE POISONING

Carbon monoxide (CO) is a colorless, odorless, and tasteless gas that is nonirritating to the mucous membranes. It is produced by the incomplete combustion of carbon-containing materials. Carbon monoxide poisoning is most likely to occur when a fire occurs in an enclosed space.

Pathophysiology

Carbon monoxide has an affinity for hemoglobin that is 200 times stronger than that of oxygen. When carbon monoxide is introduced into the blood stream, it binds with hemoglobin and forms carboxyhemoglobin by displacing oxygen molecules. Hypoxemia results from decreased oxygen transport to the tissues. Even when low levels of carbon monoxide are present, blood levels of carboxyhemoglobin are elevated.

Clinical Manifestations

The severity of the clinical manifestations of carbon monoxide poisoning directly correlates with the concentration of carbon monoxide present in the blood. Cerebral hypoxia is the earliest manifestation of carbon monoxide poisoning. Symptoms include intense headache, restlessness, impaired judgment, slowed thought processes, irritability, confusion, and slight breathlessness. Visual acuity may be impaired. Although the skin color may be either pale or cyanotic, it often has a pink flush caused by vasodilation in response to tissue hypoxia. A unique indicator of carbon monoxide poisoning is a cherry-red appearance of the mucous membranes.

Later symptoms include drowsiness or stupor, vertigo, muscular rigidity of the jaw, convulsions, dilated pupils, respiratory stridor, and a rapid, bounding pulse. A carboxyhemoglobin level of 50% or greater is usually associated with loss of consciousness or coma.

INHALATION INJURY ABOVE THE GLOTTIS

Inhalation injury is seen more commonly above the glottis than below it. It is usually caused by inhalation of superheated air (>300°F, 149°C), but may also be caused by steam inhalation, aspiration of scalding liquids, and explosions. These inhalation injuries result in a thermal burn and edema of the tissues of the upper airway. Acute airway obstruction usually occurs within the first 30 minutes to 48 hours after the burn.

Pathophysiology

Thermal damage to tissues of the respiratory tract is usually confined to the upper airway because the lower airway is protected from heat by the tremendous ability of the tracheobronchial tract to cool airborne particles. As the damaged tissue in the upper airway becomes edematous, the airway narrows and eventually closes.

Clinical Manifestations

Upper respiratory tract injury should be suspected if the patient was in a confined space during the fire. Acute airway obstruction can be prevented if a thorough history is obtained and accurate observations are made that allow early detection and intervention. The patient is usually able to breathe until final obstruction occurs. However, early intubation, when the edema is minimal, is indicated if upper airway injury is suspected.

Early manifestations of upper respiratory tract injury include soot present on the tongue, on the pharynx, or in the sputum; singed nasal hairs; a burn involving the face, neck, or upper chest; a dry, red buccal mucosa. Deterioration in mental status or loss of consciousness is often due to progressing anoxia.

Late signs include dyspnea, use of accessory muscles, coughing, wheezing, inability to cough up secretions, a change in the voice, and increasing hoarseness. If any of the late signs are noted, the patient must be intubated immediately.

INHALATION INJURY BELOW THE GLOTTIS

Smoke contains many noxious and potentially toxic chemicals in addition to carbon monoxide. These chemicals result from combustion of various substances and can cause damage to the lower respiratory tract and pulmonary tissue when inhaled.

Pathophysiology

Inhalation of smoke and noxious chemicals damages the mucosa lining the alveoli and lower respiratory passages, causing inflammation, edema, and increased secretions from the inflamed mucosa. Edema inhibits oxygen and carbon dioxide exchange, and progressive hypoxia develops. Pulmonary edema or bronchiolitis with subsequent atelectasis, pneumonia, and adult respiratory distress syndrome are common.

Clinical Manifestations

Symptoms of damage from inhalation of noxious or toxic substances may not occur for several days after the burn injury. The symptoms include fever, dyspnea, wheezing, crackles (rales), decreased tidal volume, poor gas exchange, productive cough, pleuritic pain, and densities on chest x-ray examinations. When obtaining the history from a burn patient or fire department personnel, it is important to determine whether burning chemicals were involved in the fire.

RESTRICTIVE DISEASE

Patients with burns of more than 40% TBSA often have decreased vital capacity and increased pulmonary resistance known as restrictive disease. The etiology and pathophysiology of restrictive disease are poorly understood. They are, however, associated with increased risk of pulmonary complications such as atelectasis and pneumonia.

Clinical manifestations of restrictive disease include increasing anxiety and restlessness followed by decreasing level of consciousness, labored breathing with use of accessory muscles, and cyanosis.

MEDICAL DIAGNOSIS OF ALTERED RESPIRATORY FUNCTION

Medical diagnosis of carbon monoxide poisoning is based on the patient's history, clinical manifestations, and laboratory determination of carboxyhemoglobin levels and arterial blood gases. Pulse oximetry is used as an adjunct but, because the oximeter is not sensitive to the presence of carbon monoxide-bound hemoglobin but only indicates the saturation of oxygen-bound hemoglobin, oximetry does not eliminate the need for arterial carbon monoxide measurements. A carboxyhemoglobin level of more than 20% is considered toxic. It is important to determine whether the patient received oxygen during transport to the hospital, because this will lower the carboxyhemoglobin levels, yet the patient may still be at high risk for carbon monoxide poisoning.

Arterial blood gases (ABGs) are measured on admission for any burn victim with burns of the upper chest, neck, and face; evidence of burns of the upper airway; suspected exposure to superheated air; risk of inhalation of noxious fumes; or history of chronic respiratory disorder. The initial values are used as a baseline to compare with repeat arterial blood gas determinations every 4 to 6 hours to monitor the patient's respiratory function. An increasing partial pressure of carbon dioxide ($PaCO_2$) and a decreasing partial pressure of oxygen (PaO_2) are indicative of impending airway obstruction or respiratory failure resulting from inhalation injury or restrictive disease.

Diagnosis of acute airway obstruction is made on the basis of the patient's history, clinical manifestations, and arterial blood gas values or on direct visualization of the respiratory passages with a fiberoptic bronchoscope. Depending on the severity of the upper airway injury, the patient may be either prophylactically intubated or reexamined by bronchoscope every 4 to 6 hours for the first 24 to 36 hours.

Diagnosis of lower airway injury is made on the basis of the patient's history of inhalation of noxious chemicals and clinical manifestations and examination with the fiberoptic bronchoscope. A very sophisticated method of diagnosing lower airway injury is by use of the xenon 133 lung scan. This, however, is a very expensive procedure and requires transport of the patient to the nuclear medicine department. A chest x-ray examination, usually done at the patient's bedside, aids in the diagnosis of lower airway injury and provides a baseline for comparison with later pulmonary changes.

MEDICAL MANAGEMENT OF ALTERED RESPIRATORY FUNCTION

The medical treatment of alterations in respiratory function associated with thermal burn injuries depends on the type and severity of the respiratory dysfunction. All patients are treated with humidified oxygen and aggressive pulmonary hygiene, as discussed in Chapter 12. Those with carbon monoxide poisoning receive inhalation of 100% oxygen to shorten the half-life of the carbon monoxide molecules and to increase the oxygen saturation of the blood.

Respiratory status and arterial blood gas results are monitored frequently. The patient is intubated at the first indication of deteriorating respiratory status. Patients with confirmed upper airway injury may be intubated prophylactically. Early intubation prevents the risk of hypoxia and is less traumatic to the tissues if performed before edema becomes severe. If the patient is intubated for upper airway obstruction with no lower airway pulmonary involvement, mechanical ventilation is rarely necessary. Intubation is usually necessary only until the edema resolves in 2 or 3 days. Care of the intubated patient and the patient with altered respiratory function are discussed in detail in Unit IV.

Application of the Nursing Process to the Care of the Patient with Altered Respiratory Function After a Burn Injury

Assessment

Obtain as accurate a description as possible of the circumstances surrounding the incident. Determine the cause of the burn injury (thermal, chemical, or electrical) and whether there was exposure to smoke, superheated air, or noxious chemicals to determine the risk of respiratory involvement. Ask where the patient was found and whether he or she was in an enclosed space. Determine whether the patient was unconscious. Unless the patient also has head trauma, loss of consciousness indicates probable hypoxia from inhalation of carbon monoxide, smoke, or noxious chemicals. Ask whether the patient stopped breathing at any time prior to arrival at the hospital and if so, for how long.

Assess for flushed skin, pallor, cyanosis, and cherry-red mucous membranes. These signs are indicative of carbon monoxide poisoning but may be difficult to see on a dark-complexioned person or on a patient who has been burned. Observe for burns of the face, neck, and upper chest. Burns in these areas increase the possibility of respiratory injury. Assess for soot on the tongue, on the pharynx, or in the sputum and the presence of singed nasal hairs, which indicate possible inhalation injury.

Use pulse oximetry to determine the patient's oxygen saturation. Assess vital signs and voice quality to provide a baseline to facilitate early detection of altered respiratory function. Observe the patient's breathing pattern, rate, and depth for difficulty in breathing and use of accessory muscles. Auscultate for wheezes, stridor, or crackles (rales), which indicate upper airway edema or accumulation of secretions. Breath sounds may be distant or difficult to hear if the thorax is edematous as a result of burns. Assess for general signs of hypoxia. Agitation, restlessness, and anxiety are early signs of hypoxia. Hoarseness, change in voice quality, persistent cough, and decreasing level of orientation or consciousness are late signs of upper airway edema and hypoxia.

Nursing Diagnoses and Planning

Nursing diagnoses and related expected patient outcomes most commonly applicable to patients with altered respiratory function after a major burn injury include the following:

NDx: Impaired gas exchange related to decreased level of consciousness secondary to hypoxia from inhalation of carbon monoxide

Planning: Patient outcomes

1. Patient is alert, oriented, and able to follow simple commands.
2. Patient's skin and mucous membrane color are normal for race.

NDx: High risk for ineffective airway clearance related to edema of respiratory airway secondary to inhalation of superheated air, smoke, or noxious chemicals

Planning: Patient outcomes

1. Patient is alert and oriented.
2. Patient's respirations remain clear and unlabored, more than 12 and fewer than 20 per minute.
3. Patient speaks without hoarseness or persistent cough.

Nursing Interventions

The primary goal of the nursing care of a patient with respiratory dysfunction after a burn injury is to ensure that the patient maintains adequate ventilation and oxygenation.

NDx: Impaired gas exchange

Encourage deep breathing and administer 100% humidified oxygen to displace the carbon monoxide, which binds with hemoglobin in the blood stream. Observe for decreasing level of consciousness and inability to follow simple commands, which indicate cerebral hypoxia. Monitor laboratory results of carboxyhemoglobin levels and arterial blood gases. Decreasing levels of carboxyhemoglobin are a reliable indicator of the effectiveness of treatment. Limit patient activity to decrease oxygen requirements.

NDx: High risk for ineffective airway clearance

Administer humidified oxygen to increase oxygen saturation and tissue oxygenation. Elevate the head of the bed, if not contraindicated by associated injuries, to ease diaphragmatic excursion, promote venous drainage, and reduce edema. Encourage coughing and deep breathing, and turn the patient hourly to promote lung expansion and to prevent stasis of secretions. Patients with an inhalation injury have copious amounts of secretions. Suction as necessary to maintain patent airway, but avoid unnecessary suctioning, which can increase edema. Talk to the patient frequently, explaining procedures and treatments to allay anxiety, decrease oxygen requirements, and encourage verbalization of concerns.

Monitor respiratory status and auscultate breath sounds at least hourly to detect deterioration in condition. Note the rate and rhythm of respirations and the use of accessory muscles. Monitor the quality of the patient's voice every hour by asking a question that requires a brief, multiple-word answer to detect laryngeal edema. Report deterioration in arterial blood gas values, pulse oximeter saturation, increasing restlessness, anxiety, respiratory stridor, wheezes, crackles, frequent cough, hoarseness, or decreasing level of consciousness to the physician immediately and prepare for intubation.

Evaluation

Evaluate the effectiveness of nursing care for a patient with altered respiratory function after a burn injury by comparing the patient's status with the expected patient outcomes. Examples of specific outcomes for patients with altered respiratory function after a burn injury have been provided in the Planning section.

HYPOVOLEMIA AND ELECTROLYTE IMBALANCE

Severe hypovolemia and electrolyte imbalance, commonly referred to as burn shock, occur after a major burn injury because large volumes of plasma and proteins are lost through the burn wound and shift from the vascular system into the interstitial spaces, where they cause severe edema. Burn shock differs from hemorrhagic shock in that the blood volume lost is plasma, not whole blood. Although the plasma is effectively removed from the intravascular circulation, much of it remains in the body to be reabsorbed or remobilized in 3 to 14 days. Despite these differences, the physiologic effects of burn shock and hemorrhagic shock are the same.

PATHOPHYSIOLOGY

Several factors contribute to the fluid shift from the intravascular to the interstitial spaces, which leads to edema and burn shock:

1. Capillaries at the site of the burn injury, and to a lesser extent throughout the body, become more permeable and allow leakage of large amounts of water, electrolytes, albumin, and globulin into the interstitial spaces.
2. Histamine is released from the damaged cells, causing vasodilation and engorgement. This, in turn, increases hydrostatic pressure within the vessels, pushing more fluid out of the highly permeable vessels and into the interstitial spaces.
3. Large protein molecules leak through the permeable capillaries into the interstitial spaces. These molecules, which normally pull fluid into the intravascular circulation, now pull it into the interstitial spaces.
4. The lymphatic system, which normally drains excess interstitial fluid and returns it to the general circulation, becomes overwhelmed by the amount of interstitial edema. In addition, because the lymphatic vessels have very thin walls, they are the first to be compressed by burn-wound edema, further inhibiting their ability to drain fluid.

The decrease in the volume of circulating intravascular fluid results in decreased venous return, decreased cardiac output, and decreased perfusion and function of vital organs, especially the brain, kidney, and heart. Hypovolemia and decreased cardiac output may cause myocardial hypoxemia and further compromise cardiac function. Decreased perfusion results in tissue hypoxia and anaerobic metabolism with the production of lactic acid. The release of catecholamines in response to trauma and stress alters glucose metabolism, promoting the breakdown of body fats and protein into glucose and acid end products. The acid end products and lactic acid accumulate in the blood because decreased renal perfusion impairs renal function. Metabolic acidosis results.

Along with this massive fluid shift and hypovolemia, electrolyte imbalance occurs with a major burn injury. Aldosterone, which promotes sodium and water reabsorption in the renal tubules, is secreted in response to the reduction in circulating intravascular fluid. The retained sodium quickly accumulates in the interstitial spaces as fluid continues to shift out of the vascular system. Additionally, the sodium pump fails; normally it pumps sodium out of the cell in exchange for potassium. Sodium accumulates within the cells of the tissues, bringing water with it, as potassium is released. Additional potassium is released into the intravascular spaces from tissue cells and hemolysis of red blood cells damaged by the burn. Urinary excretion of potassium is impaired because of decreased renal perfusion and function. As a result of these processes, serum sodium levels decrease as serum potassium levels increase. The physiologic events that cause hypovolemia and electrolyte imbalance after a major burn injury are illustrated in Figure 8–7.

After the first 24 hours, the hydrostatic pressure in the interstitial spaces begins to resist the flow of fluid out of the capillaries. Normal capillary membrane permeability is gradually restored and fluid loss slows. Edema continues to increase, but more slowly, until approximately 48 hours after injury, at which time it stabilizes and then begins to decrease.

CLINICAL MANIFESTATIONS

The clinical manifestations of burn shock include those common in hypovolemic shock: dehydration, decreased urine output, hematuria, hypotension, tachycardia, weak pulse, decreased central venous pressure, decreased cardiac output, decreased pulmonary artery wedge pressure, decreasing level of consciousness, and dry mucous membranes. Cardiac dysrhythmias may result from the hyperkalemia and decreased peristalsis from the hyponatremia.

MEDICAL DIAGNOSIS

Medical diagnosis is made on the basis of the clinical manifestations and the results of laboratory studies. These studies include serum electrolytes and proteins, serum and urine osmolality, urine specific gravity, hematocrit, blood urea nitrogen (BUN), and arterial blood gas analysis. Results will show increasing serum and urine osmolality, increased specific gravity, hemoconcentration, hyponatremia, hyperkalemia, hypoproteinemia, elevated BUN, and metabolic acidosis. The patient is in negative nitrogen balance because of excess tissue catabolism and protein loss through the burn.

MEDICAL MANAGEMENT

Treatment of the hypovolemia and electrolyte imbalances associated with burn shock is an immediate priority if rapid deterioration and death of the pa-

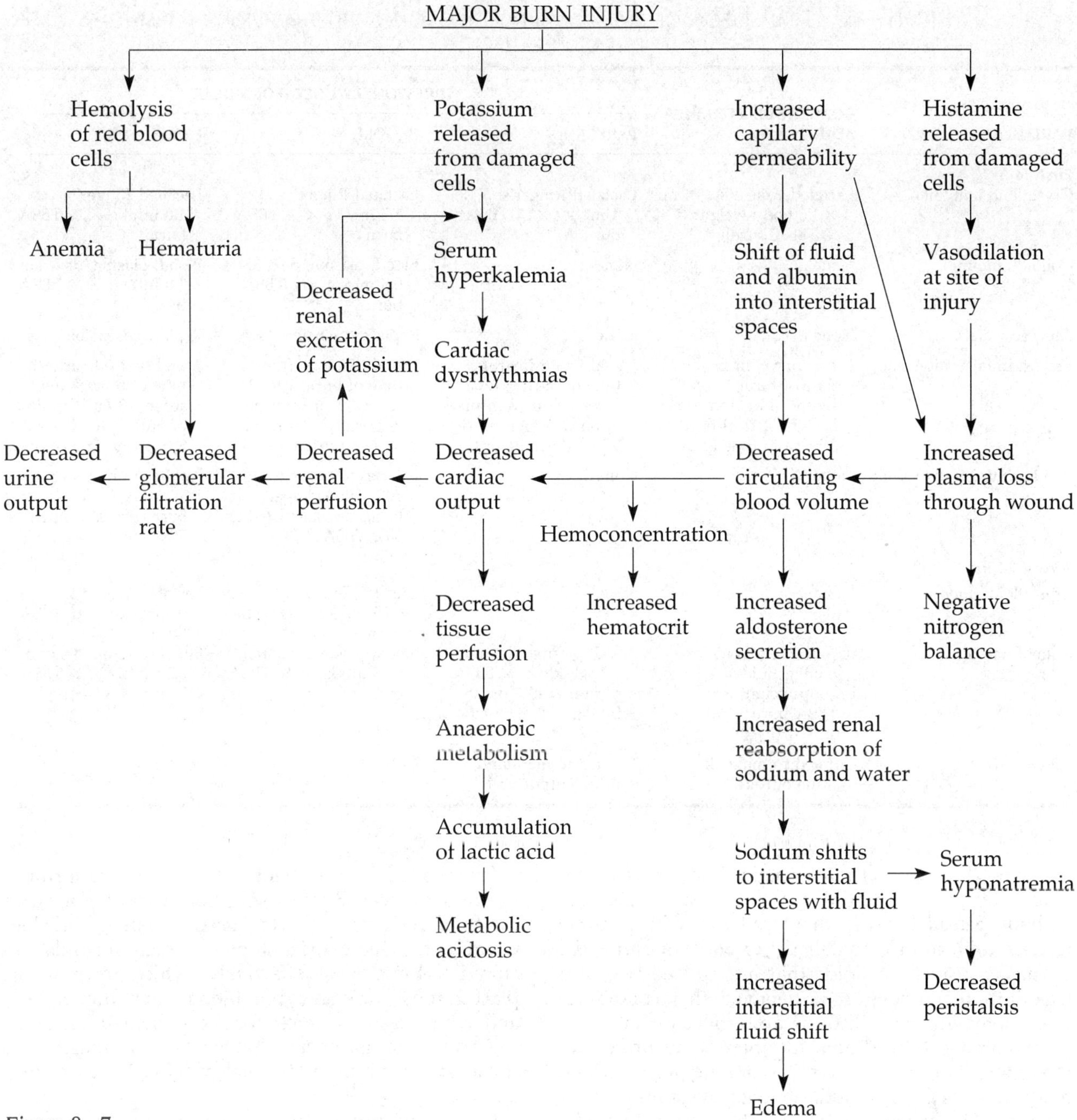

Figure 8–7.

The physiologic events that lead to hypovolemia, electrolyte imbalance, and metabolic acidosis following a major burn injury.

tient are to be prevented. Adequate fluid replacement in burn shock is so vital that it is commonly referred to as fluid resuscitation. To maintain cardiac output, perfusion of vital organs, and renal function, the patient must receive fluids in adequate volumes to replace fluids lost through the burn wound and interstitial edema. All burns of greater than 20% and burns involving the very young and the elderly require parenteral fluid resuscitation.

The goal of fluid resuscitation is to replace the fluid lost through injured tissue and sequestered in the interstitial spaces in a manner that closely approximates the amount and type of fluid lost as well as the rapidity of the loss. A few studies indicate that the entire fluid loss may occur within 12 to 18 hours after the burn, but most indicate continued fluid loss for as long as 36 to 48 hours.

Owing to increased capillary permeability and the need to replace electrolytes, Ringer's lactate (crystalloid fluid) is the choice for the fluid resuscitation. Hypertonic saline is not advocated because it may precipitate severe hypernatremia in some patients.

Table 8–4. COMPARISON OF THE CONSENSUS FORMULA WITH PREVIOUS FORMULAS FOR FLUID RESUSCITATION

VARIABLE	CONSENSUS FORMULA ADULT	PREVIOUSLY USED FORMULAS: PARKLAND	BROOKE	EVANS
First 24 hr				
Crystalloid amount	Lactated Ringer's 2–4 ml × kg body weight × % TBSA burn	Lactated Ringer's: 4 ml/kg × % TBSA burn	Lactated Ringer's: 1.5 ml/kg × % TBSA burn	Lactated Ringer's: 1.0 ml/kg × % TBSA burn
Colloid amount	None	None	Blood, plasma, dextran: 0.5 ml/kg ×% TBSA burn	Blood, plasma, dextran: 1.0 ml/kg × % TBSA burn
Glucose water	None	None	Replace insensible loss	Replace insensible loss
Fluid administration rate	½ total first 8 hr from time of burn; ¼ total second 8 hr from time of burn; ¼ total third 8 hr from time of burn	½ total first 8 hr from time of burn; ¼ total second 8 hr from time of burn; ¼ total third 8 hr from time or burn	½ total first 8 hr from time of burn; ¼ total second 8 hr from time of burn; ¼ total third 8 hr from time of burn	½ total first 8 hr from time of burn; ¼ total second 8 hr from time of burn; ¼ total third 8 hr from time of burn
Fluid administration limit	None	None	Applies to burns up to 50% TBSA; larger burns are calculated as 50% TBSA	Applies to burns up to 50% TBSA; larger burns are calculated as 50% TBSA
Second 24 hr				
Crystalloid amount	None	None	Lactated Ringer's: 0.75 ml/kg × % TBSA burn	Lactated Ringer's: 0.5 ml/kg × % TBSA burn
Colloid amount	0.3–0.5 ml colloid-containing fluid × kg body weight × % TBSA burn	Blood, plasma, dextran: 0.3 ml/kg × % TBSA burn if <40% or 0.5 ml/kg × % TBSA burn if >40%	Blood, plasma, dextran: 0.25 ml/kg × % TBSA burn	Blood, plasma, dextran: 0.5 ml/kg × % TBSA burn
Glucose water	Titrated to maintain urine output	Titrated to maintain urine output	2000 ml	2000 ml

Colloids (human plasma protein fraction [Plasmanate], salt-poor albumin) are not used in the first 24-hour period because the capillaries will continue to leak until approximately 30 to 36 hours after the burn. Because the colloids that are infused will also leak into the tissues, it is believed that colloid replacement will have little if any effect on intravascular volume. In addition, the increase in protein in the interstitial spaces exerts a pulling force, which tends to increase interstitial edema by pulling water with it. Many burn care specialists support the view that colloid administration in this early period does not significantly increase intravascular volume. The amount of Ringer's lactate to be given is determined by the consensus formula and varies slightly according to whether the patient is an adult or a child. The adult formula, based on the age, weight, and TBSA burned, is: 2 to 4 ml Ringer's lactate × kg body weight × percentage burn.

The rate of fluid administration is calculated from the time the burn injury occurred. One half of the calculated volume is replaced in the first 8 hours from the time of injury. The capillary permeability and the intravascular loss are the greatest during this time. The remaining fluid is administered over the next 16 hours.

Prior to the endorsement of the consensus formula by the American Burn Association, various formulas for fluid resuscitation were used in burn medicine. Great controversy existed over which formula restored volume most effectively, which formula replaced most precisely the blood constituents lost, and which was the safest for the patient in terms of electrolyte replacement. Table 8–4 compares the consensus formula with the previously used formulas.

It is very important to keep in mind that the consensus formula is just a guide to fluid replacement. In the face of obvious hypo- or hypervolemia, the infusion rate must be adjusted regardless of what requirements have been calculated. There are some specific cases in which it can be predicted that the calculated replacement will be insufficient to meet the patient's resuscitation needs. Examples of this are (1) pulmonary injury, in which great fluid losses occur in the lungs secondary to increased alveolar capillary permeability, which is not measured in the TBSA burned and therefore not accounted for in the formulas; (2) electrical burns, in which internal injury cannot be accurately measured; (3) patients in whom resuscitation is delayed; (4) and patients burned while intoxicated. The usual causes for overresuscitation are overestimation of burn percentage and overly aggressive fluid replacement in the field.

After the first 24 hours, the fluid lost is free water, an electrolyte-free solution that is lost as evaporative water loss through the burned skin. Evaporative loss, which is normally 10 ml/kg a day, may increase to 2.5 to 12 L a day and must be replaced. Capillary permeability gradually returns toward normal by the end of the second postburn day. Colloids can be effective at this time to keep the amount of fluid administered to a minimum. The fluid therapy of choice, for adults, after the first 24 hours postburn is to infuse 0.3 to 0.5 ml × kg body weight × percentage TBSA burn of a colloid-containing fluid in addition to enough electrolyte-free fluid to maintain adequate urinary output and a serum sodium of 140 mEq/L.

Monitoring the serum sodium is an important tool in determining whether the patient is hypernatremic and dehydrated or hyponatremic and overhydrated. Depending on the severity of the burn and the patient's gastrointestinal status, parenteral fluid replacement may no longer be required after 48 hours. Patients with small burns may never require parenteral replacement if they can tolerate adequate amounts of electrolyte solutions and nutritionally balanced fluids by mouth.

Diuretics are avoided in the early postburn period because the decreased urine output is due to hypovolemia, which would be further aggravated by increasing the amount of fluid excreted.

Application of the Nursing Process to the Care of the Patient with Hypovolemia and Electrolyte Imbalance After a Major Burn Injury

Assessment

Obtain baseline vital signs and weight on admission for later comparison and evaluation of fluid replacement. Remove any clothes the patient was wearing at the time of the accident before weighing to obtain an accurate body weight. Use a bed scale if the patient is unable to stand. Ask the patient, significant other, emergency personnel, or transferring agency what time the burn injury occurred. Examine the patient to locate all burned areas. Assist in determining the size of the injury by using the agency's chart to calculate TBSA burned. Data regarding accurate weight, time of the injury, and TBSA burned are essential in calculating the amount of fluid to be administered during fluid resuscitation.

Assess the patient's level of consciousness. Talk to the patient to determine awareness of person, place, and time. Level of consciousness and orientation are indicators of cerebral perfusion. Be sure someone has told the patient where he or she is and what has happened. Many patients are not initially aware of exactly what has occurred or what hospital they have been taken to, especially if the burn center is not in a local facility.

Auscultate bowel sounds and obtain specimens for baseline serum chemistries (sodium [Na], potassium [K], chloride [Cl], bicarbonate [HCO_3], BUN, glucose) and arterial blood gases for later comparison and evaluation of electrolyte and acid-base balance.

Nursing Diagnoses and Planning

Nursing diagnoses and related expected patient outcomes most commonly applicable to patients with hypovolemia and electrolyte imbalance after a major burn injury include the following:

NDx: High risk for fluid volume deficit related to inadequate replacement of fluids lost through evaporation from the burn wound and fluid shift into interstitial spaces

Planning: Patient outcomes
1. Patient is alert and oriented.
2. Patient maintains adequate hydration as evidenced by the following:
   a. Heart rate regular and more than 60 but fewer than 100 bpm.
   b. Blood pressure stable and higher than 90/60.
   c. Urine output more than 30 ml per hour.
   d. Central venous pressure 4 to 12 mm of water.
   e. Capillary refill less than 3 seconds.
   f. Moist mucous membranes.
3. Patient's weight increases by 15% to 20%.
4. Patient has bowel sounds and is free of nausea.

Nursing Interventions

The primary goal of the nursing care of a patient with hypovolemia and electrolyte imbalance after a major burn injury is to minimize burn shock by providing adequate fluid resuscitation and electrolyte replacement. Determination of the adequacy of fluid resuscitation is based on the premise that adequate fluid replacement ensures perfusion and function of vital organs.

NDx: High risk for fluid volume deficit
Establish intravenous access as soon as possible using at least an 18-gauge intravenous catheter to facilitate rapid fluid infusion. Administer and document fluid replacement to ensure that the patient is receiving prescribed fluids within the appropriate time frame. Monitor intravenous administration and infusion sites at least hourly to detect altered flow rate, leakage, or infiltration. The risk of problems

with parenteral infusions is greater with rapid infusion of high volumes of fluid. Auscultate breath sounds hourly to detect crackles, which may indicate pulmonary edema and fluid overload from rapid fluid infusion. Report inability to maintain prescribed flow rate or any infusion-related problems to the physician immediately.

Insert an indwelling urinary catheter with a low-volume graduate to measure urine output accurately. Monitor heart rate, blood pressure, capillary refill, level of consciousness, and urine output hourly to evaluate the adequacy of fluid replacement and perfusion of vital organs. Tachycardia may be present even though fluid resuscitation is adequate as a result of trauma, pain, and anxiety. The heart rate should return to normal range within 18 to 24 hours. Blood pressure should be within low-normal limits for the patient by history and age. Capillary refill of less than 3 seconds and a clear sensorium indicate adequate peripheral and cerebral perfusion. Urine output greater than 30 ml/hour in adults (or 0.5 ml/kg/hour) is an indication of adequate renal perfusion. A central venous catheter may be inserted for more accurate hourly measurement of hemodynamic status and fluid balance. Occasionally, a Swan-Ganz catheter is inserted to monitor cardiac output and pulmonary wedge pressure. It is not uncommon for initial central pressures and cardiac output to be low and then return to normal range in 18 to 24 hours. Care of the patient with a central line is discussed in Chapter 17.

Weigh the patient at the same time daily with the same scale and the same amount of clothing to monitor fluid balance. Accuracy is improved if the patient can be weighed without dressings or topical creams covering the burn wounds. Note on the flow sheet or chart whether dressings were removed. An increase in body weight of 15% to 20% is expected with successful fluid resuscitation.

Auscultate the abdomen every 4 hours to determine the presence of bowel sounds. Hyponatremia and poor bowel perfusion may cause hypoperistalsis. The presence of bowel sounds and the absence of nausea indicate good bowel perfusion and adequate serum sodium levels. Attach the patient to a cardiac monitor to detect dysrhythmias caused by hyperkalemia. Review serum electrolyte and arterial blood gas values daily to monitor electrolyte balance and metabolic acidosis.

Evaluation

Evaluate the effectiveness of nursing care for a patient with hypovolemia and electrolyte imbalance after a major burn injury by comparing the patient's status with the expected patient outcomes. Examples of specific outcomes for patients with hypovolemia and electrolyte imbalance after a burn injury have been provided in the Planning section.

CIRCUMFERENTIAL BURNS

Impaired peripheral circulation and compromised respiratory movement may occur with a full-thickness burn that involves the entire circumference of a limb or the thorax.

PATHOPHYSIOLOGY

In a full-thickness burn injury, elastin is destroyed and the tissues cannot expand to accommodate increasing edema. The wound becomes covered by an eschar, a dry, tight, inelastic covering that forms from dead tissue and wound exudate. If the eschar forms completely around the circumference of a limb, it acts like a tourniquet, compressing lymphatic vessels and impairing arterial blood flow and venous return. Circulation may be so compromised that the viability of the limb is impaired. If the circumferential burn involves the upper torso, chest expansion for respiration may be impaired.

CLINICAL MANIFESTATIONS

The clinical manifestations of impaired peripheral circulation caused by a circumferential burn of an extremity include cyanosis distal to the burn wound, loss of the distal pulse measured by Doppler ultrasound, delayed capillary refill, and paresthesias or decreased sensation. The clinical manifestations of compromised respiratory function resulting from a circumferential burn of the torso are decreased tidal volume and respiratory excursion with increasing signs of respiratory distress and hypoxia.

MEDICAL DIAGNOSIS

A medical diagnosis of impaired peripheral circulation or respiratory compromise caused by circumferential burn is based on the presence of the clinical manifestations. Hypoxia is confirmed by decreasing oxygen saturation on pulse oximetry or arterial blood gases.

MEDICAL MANAGEMENT

Treatment for circulatory impairment in an extremity or restriction of chest expansion is an escharotomy, a shallow incision made through the eschar with a scalpel or using electrocautery. The incision is made lengthwise, only along the lateral and medial aspects of the extremity and never inside the fingers. Hand and finger escharotomies do not improve local circulation but do increase the risk of loss of function. If performed on the torso, commonly preferred incisions are clavicle to costal margin, bilaterally, and incisions along the anterior axillary lines joined by transverse incisions. An escharotomy immediately releases pressure on underlying tissues to restore blood flow to the extremity or to allow expansion of the chest.

An escharotomy is performed at the bedside. Because it involves only the dead eschar in a full-

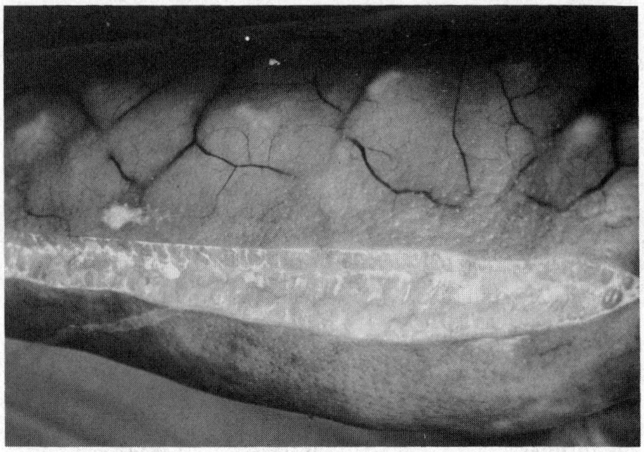

Figure 8–8.

This escharotomy into the dead tissue of a full-thickness burn was done to relieve pressure from edema on underlying deep tissues and blood vessels.

thickness burn injury, no analgesia other than what the patient is already receiving is required. The incision is generally covered by the same topical agent as is used on the patient's burn wounds. An escharotomy can be seen in Figure 8–8.

Application of the Nursing Process to the Care of the Patient with Circumferential Burns

Assessment

Assess the depth of the wound to identify possible areas of full-thickness injury and eschar formation. Assess pulses, color, temperature, sensation, and capillary refill in extremities with circumferential full-thickness burns immediately on admission to determine baseline neurovascular status. Use a Doppler ultrasound instrument to assess nonpalpable pulses. To assess capillary refill, press on the skin or nail bed distal to the injury and note how long it takes for the color to return. Color should return in less than 3 seconds.

If the circumferential injury involves the torso, assess respiratory status and chest expansion with each respiration. Auscultate breath sounds. The patient should be able to fully expand the chest with each respiration, and breath sounds should be present in all lobes.

Nursing Diagnoses and Planning

Nursing diagnoses and related expected patient outcomes most commonly applicable to patients with circumferential burns include the following:

NDx: High risk for peripheral neurovascular dysfunction related to edema and circulatory impairment secondary to circumferential full-thickness burn injury of the extremity

Planning: Patient outcomes

1. Patient maintains peripheral circulation distal to circumferential full-thickness burn injury as evidenced by the following:
   a. Distal pulses present.
   b. Normal sensation distal to the injury.
   c. Capillary refill less than 3 seconds.

NDx: High risk for ineffective breathing pattern related to impaired chest expansion secondary to circumferential full-thickness burn injury of the torso

Planning: Patient outcomes

1. Patient is able to expand chest fully with each respiration.
2. Patient breathes with regular, unlabored respirations.

Nursing Interventions

The primary goal of nursing care of a patient with circumferential burns is to maintain adequate peripheral circulation and adequate chest expansion.

NDx: High risk for peripheral neurovascular dysfunction

Remove all clothing and rings, necklaces, bracelets, anklets, and any other jewelry or item that could occlude peripheral circulation with edema formation. Elevate burned extremities above the level of the heart to promote venous return and to minimize edema.

Monitor neurovascular status of extremities and digits distal to circumferential full-thickness burns at least hourly to ensure early detection of impaired peripheral circulation. Report inability to obtain pulse by Doppler ultrasound, cyanotic or pale skin or nail beds, cool temperature, loss of sensation or paresthesias, or capillary refill longer than 3 seconds to the physician immediately.

Prepare the patient for an escharotomy by reinforcing the surgeon's explanation of how and why the procedure is performed. Provide reassurance that the procedure is painless. Obtain signed consent. Assemble sterile supplies for the procedure: scalpel, gauze sponges, drapes, gloves, and waterproof covering to protect the bed. Assist during the escharotomy, and apply prescribed antibacterial agent over the incisions to prevent infection.

Continue to assess the extremities distal to the escharotomy hourly for circulatory impairment. In some cases, the escharotomy requires revision.

NDx: High risk for ineffective breathing pattern

Monitor respiratory status of the patient with a circumferential full-thickness burn of the thorax at least hourly to ensure early detection of compromised respiratory function. Chest expansion and breath sounds should remain equal bilaterally. Monitor oxygen saturation with pulse oximeter. Pulse oximetry cannot be used if all digits and both ear lobes have full-thickness burns. Review arterial blood gas results for decreasing oxygen saturation and increasing carbon dioxide levels. Report increasing anxiety or restlessness, dyspnea, labored or shallow respirations, absent or diminished breath sounds, unequal chest expansion, or deterioration of arterial blood gases to the physician immediately. If necessary, prepare the patient for escharotomy as described previously. Continue to monitor respiratory status and chest expansion hourly after torso escharotomy to ensure adequate respiratory function.

Evaluation

Evaluate the effectiveness of nursing care for a patient with circumferential burns by comparing the patient's status with the expected patient outcomes. Examples of specific outcomes for patients with circumferential burns have been provided in the Planning section.

Acute Phase

The acute phase of burn care immediately follows the emergent phase. It is sometimes referred to as the postemergent phase, the fluid mobilization phase, or the diuretic phase.

The acute phase begins with reabsorption of fluid from the interstitial spaces and its mobilization into the intravascular circulation. It continues until the wound is closed either by spontaneous healing or by successful skin grafts. During the acute phase, the focus of the health team is fluid and electrolyte balance, pain management, care of the wound to prevent infection, meeting metabolic requirements, and supporting the patient and family's psychological adjustment. Rehabilitation and physical therapy continue through acute care.

FLUID MOBILIZATION AND ELECTROLYTE IMBALANCE

PATHOPHYSIOLOGY

After the first 24 hours, the hydrostatic pressure in the interstitial spaces begins to resist the flow of fluid out of the capillaries and the capillaries begin to return to their preburn function. Edema continues to increase, but more slowly, until approximately 48 hours after injury, at which time it stabilizes and then begins to decrease.

Table 8.5. COMPARISON OF FLUID AND ELECTROLYTE SHIFT IN THE EMERGENT AND DIURETIC ACUTE PHASES

	PHASE	
	Emergent	Acute (diuretic)
Capillary permeability	Increases	Returns to normal
Interstitial edema	Increases	Decreases
Intracellular sodium	Increases	Decreases
Intracellular potassium	Decreases	Increases
Extracellular sodium	Decreases	Increases
Extracellular potassium	Increases	Decreases
Vasodilation	Increases	Decreases
Cardiac output	Decreases	Increases
Venous return	Decreases	Increases

As capillary permeability decreases, the leakage of large protein molecules and fluid into the interstitial spaces stops. Slowly at first and then more rapidly, fluid is pulled out of the tissues and into the intravascular system. As edema decreases, the lymphatic system is able to drain excess interstitial fluid and return it to the general circulation. The increased volume of intravascular fluid results in increased venous return, increased cardiac output, and increased perfusion and function of vital organs. During fluid mobilization, as large volumes of fluid are reabsorbed back into the circulation, the patient is at risk for rapid onset of left ventricular failure and pulmonary edema from fluid overload.

With improved systemic perfusion and fluid mobilization, the cellular sodium pump resumes normal function, pumping sodium out of the cell in exchange for potassium. Fluid leaves the cells with the sodium, decreasing intracellular edema. A comparison of the fluid and electrolyte shifts in burn shock in the emergent phase and fluid mobilization in the acute phase is presented in Table 8–5.

CLINICAL MANIFESTATIONS

The earliest clinical manifestation of the onset of fluid remobilization in the acute phase is a rapid increase in urine output. The blood pressure and heart rate return to the patient's normal limits as the central venous pressure, cardiac output, and pulmonary artery wedge pressure increase.

MEDICAL MANAGEMENT

Fluid loss in the acute phase is vastly reduced and is mainly due to evaporative loss of free water through the burned skin. The larger the size of the burn wound, the greater the evaporative loss. This fluid is primarily replaced with 5% dextrose in water to maintain fluid balance, urine output, and a serum sodium of 140 mEq/L. In addition, colloids are administered to replace protein loss and to pull fluid from the interstitial space back into the vascular system. Fluid replacement in the acute phase is at a much slower rate, and lesser volume, than in the emergent phase.

Application of the Nursing Process to the Care of the Patient During Fluid Mobilization After a Major Burn Injury

Fluid mobilization in the acute phase of burn care represents a continuation of care as the patient experiences a physiologic shift from a state of circulatory hypovolemia to a state of potential fluid overload. With fluid mobilization, the focus of care changes from treating hypovolemia to replacing evaporative fluid loss and maintaining electrolyte balance. As illustrated in Nursing Care Guide 8–1, nursing care during fluid mobilization is similar to, and a continuation of, the care of the burn patient presented in the emergent phase.

Assessment

The initial indication of fluid mobilization is an increase in urine output to greater than 50 ml/hour. Document the precise time of increased urine output, and notify the physician so the infusion rate of parenteral fluids can be decreased.

Nursing Diagnoses and Planning

Nursing diagnoses and related expected patient outcomes most commonly applicable to patients during fluid mobilization after a major burn injury include the following:

NDx: High risk for fluid volume excess related to overreplacement of fluids lost through evaporation from the burn wound during mobilization of fluid from the interstitial spaces into the circulatory system

Planning: Patient outcomes

1. Patient remains free of manifestations of fluid overload as evidenced by:
   a. Heart rate regular and more than 60 but fewer than 100 bpm.
   b. Blood pressure stable and higher than 90/60 but lower than 140/90.
   c. Respirations clear and unlabored.
   d. Central venous pressure 4 to 12 mm H_2O.
   e. Capillary refill less than 3 seconds.
   f. Moist mucous membranes.
2. Patient's urine output is more than 30 ml/hour but less than 100 ml/hour after initial diuresis.
3. Patient's weight is within 5% of preburn weight after diuresis.
4. Patient has bowel sounds and is free of nausea.

Nursing Interventions

NDx: High risk for fluid volume excess

Monitor parenteral infusions hourly to ensure correct rate of flow and to prevent fluid overload. Continue to auscultate bowel sounds every 4 hours to detect hypoperistalsis or paralytic ileus caused by dilutional hyponatremia. The intravenous infusion may be discontinued or changed to a heparin lock if bowel sounds are present and the patient is free of nausea and able to ingest adequate amounts of fluids.

Urine measurement can usually be decreased to every 4 hours for 24 hours when output is greater than 50 ml/hour for 4 consecutive hours. Expect output to be greater than 100 ml/hour during initial diuresis. Be sure the urine-collection container can hold the increased urine volume. The indwelling urinary catheter may be removed if the patient is able to use the bedpan or urinal without contaminating the burn wound. Urine specific gravity decreases as the urine becomes more dilute. Diuresis is complete when urine specific gravity returns to normal and output is less than 100 ml/hour for 4 hours.

Continue hourly measurements of hemodynamic parameters until diuresis is complete. Vital signs, central venous pressure, and pulmonary artery wedge pressures should remain within normal limits. An increase in heart rate or peripheral or central blood pressure or a change in heart rhythm may indicate left ventricular failure. Continue electrocardiogram monitoring for early detection of cardiac dysrhythmias caused by rapid shift in serum potassium levels. Review results of electrolyte studies to evaluate electrolyte balance.

Observe for increased restlessness, anxiety, or dyspnea, and auscultate breath sounds for crackles (rales) and wheezes, which indicate pulmonary edema from fluid overload. Elevate the head of the bed to promote pulmonary venous drainage and to ease diaphragmatic excursion if not contraindicated by the location of injuries. Because of the generalized interstitial edema, assessment of dependent edema and distended neck veins is not clinically useful in detecting fluid overload in the burn patient.

Report deterioration in the patient's circulatory or respiratory status to the physician immediately. Continue to weigh the patient daily to monitor fluid balance. Expect rapid weight loss during diuresis. Fluid replacement is successful if the patient is within 5% of preburn weight at the end of diuresis.

Evaluation

Evaluate the effectiveness of nursing care for a patient during fluid mobilization after a major burn injury by comparing the patient's status with the expected patient outcomes. Examples of specific outcomes for patients during fluid mobilization after a major burn injury have been provided in the Planning section.

PAIN MANAGEMENT

Burn patients are in pain 24 hours a day because of unprotected nerve endings until the wound heals or is grafted. Wound care and physical therapy add to the already intense pain. Burn patients may undergo repeated surgical procedures during hospitalization and after discharge. Often the surgeries will follow each other in rapid succession. After these procedures, the patient usually experiences a temporary increase in pain and discomfort.

Narcotic analgesics are used for pain management. Intravenous morphine sulfate administered in frequent, small doses or by continuous low-dose infusion or by patient-controlled analgesia, combined with a bolus dose before painful procedures, is most effective for pain management during the emergent phase and fluid remobilization. Oral, subcutaneous, and intramuscular routes are contraindicated at this time because of poor absorption. When fluid balance is stabilized, oral narcotic agents can be used. The addition of psychotropic agents and the use of guided imagery and relaxation techniques may increase the effectiveness of pain control for some patients. The use of inhalation of a preset mixture of oxygen and nitrous oxide immediately before extremely painful procedures as part of pain management is being evaluated.

Application of the Nursing Process to the Care of the Patient with Pain After a Burn Injury

Assessment

Assess the need for pain medication. Burn injuries are extremely painful and remain so until grafting is completed or until the wound closes spontaneously. Pain is intensified by movement and wound-care procedures. The patient may verbalize pain or demonstrate pain by facial grimacing, refusal to move, stiffness, guarding, or refusing treatments. Anorexia, dilated pupils, elevated blood pressure, and increased pulse or respiratory rate may also indicate pain. Ask the patient to identify the location and type of pain to confirm that the patient's wounds, treatments, or associated injuries are the cause of the pain.

Nursing Diagnoses and Planning

Nursing diagnoses and related expected patient outcomes most commonly applicable to patients with pain after a burn injury include the following:

NDx: Pain related to open burn wounds, treatments, and dressing changes

Planning: Patient outcomes
1. Patient expresses relief from analgesics and is adequately medicated to tolerate painful procedures.
2. Pain from open burn wounds decreases in intensity daily as healing occurs.
3. Patient talks about, participates in, and tolerates wound care.

Nursing Interventions

Pain assessment and management are critical to the recovery of the burn patient. Almost every procedure and intervention, whose goal is to promote wound healing, causes pain. People have different degrees of tolerance and response to pain; therefore, administration of analgesics must be adjusted for each patient. General nursing interventions in pain management are discussed in detail in the care of the postoperative patient in Chapter 4.

NDx: Pain
Administer narcotic analgesics as needed. Monitor the patient's response to determine the need for additional medication or increased or decreased dosage. Administer parenteral narcotic 20 minutes, or intravenous narcotic analgesic 5 minutes, before dressing changes, debridement, and other painful procedures to allow enough time for the medication to take effect.

Acknowledge the patient's pain and fear of procedures that increase pain. Assure the patient that feelings of fear, anger, hostility, and frustration are normal. Explain the cause of the pain and the goals of pain management to correct misconceptions and fears of drug addiction. Explain procedures, and allow the patient to make decisions and participate in his or her care as much as possible. Encourage verbalization, keep the patient informed, and give the patient a degree of control to reduce anxiety and fear and promote pain management by reducing feelings of helplessness. Explore with the patient the use of distraction, deep breathing, and other relaxation techniques to reduce anxiety and enhance pain relief.

Table 8–6. COMPARISON OF OPEN AND CLOSED METHODS OF WOUND CARE

METHOD	DESCRIPTION	ADVANTAGES	DISADVANTAGES
Open	Wounds covered with topical agent; gauze dressings not used	Wound easily visualized and assessed; avoids dark, warm, moist environment conducive to growth of microorganisms; wound care takes less time	Topical antibacterial agent is easily rubbed off onto equipment or falls onto the floor, becoming cleaning problem, safety hazard, and source of cross-contamination; must be reapplied frequently to maintain wound coverage and provide a barrier against infection
Closed	Wounds covered with topical agent and covered with gauze dressing	Wound always covered, providing a constant barrier against infection; topical agent does not contaminate equipment or fall onto the floor	Dressings provide dark, warm, moist environment conducive to the growth of microorganisms; visual assessment of the wound is difficult; dressings become stuck to wound if not enough agent applied or if too much time elapsed making it difficult to remove, thus causing bleeding, increased pain, and damage to healing skin

Evaluation

Evaluate the effectiveness of nursing care for a patient with pain after a burn injury by comparing the patient's status with the expected patient outcomes. Examples of specific outcomes for patients with pain after a burn injury have been provided in the Planning section.

WOUND CARE

Although wound care begins at the scene of the injury and continues throughout the emergent, acute, and rehabilitation periods, it is a primary focus of the acute period. The two most common methods of wound care are the open method and the closed method. Table 8–6 summarizes their characteristics, advantages, and disadvantages. The goals of wound care are:

1. Minimize wound and systemic infection.
2. Prevent conversion of a partial-thickness wound to a full-thickness wound.
3. Debride the injury to remove all dead tissue to prepare healthy granulation tissue for grafting.
4. Complete wound closure as soon as possible, using grafts when necessary.
5. Minimize scar and contracture formation to maximize appearance and function.

Although no burn wound is sterile, it is important to keep the wound as clean and as free from microorganisms as possible. Risk of burn-wound infection is high for two reasons. First, the body's primary line of defense, the skin, is extensively damaged, disrupting natural protection against invasion by microorganisms. Second, the body's immune system is suppressed after a major burn injury. The patient's normal flora become a source of infection as well as nosocomial bacteria from the hospital environment. The most common organisms in burn-wound infection are *Pseudomonas, Klebsiella, Staphylococcus aureus, Streptococcus,* and *Staphylococcus* resistant to methicillin (MRSA).

Protein exudate in the burn wound provides an ideal medium for microorganism growth. Wound infection places the patient at risk for sepsis, and, as the infectious process destroys healthy tissue, necrosis deepens the wound and a partial-thickness burn can convert to a full-thickness burn wound. An infected wound will not heal.

The surface of most burn wounds is contaminated by a small number of organisms. This is referred to as colonization of the wound and is not considered a wound infection. Wound infection occurs when microorganisms have penetrated the surface of the wound and invaded the eschar or underlying viable tissue. Because of the eschar covering the wound, colonization of the surface of the wound, and the body's inflammatory response to the injury, an infected burn wound may be difficult to identify by inspection. Increasing localized edema, increasing redness and warmth along the wound edges, purulent drainage, or foul odor when dressings are removed indicates infection. Figure 8–9 illustrates the difference in appearance between a clean, noninfected wound and an infected wound.

Penetration of the surface of the wound by microorganisms is determined by biopsy. A small piece of eschar or tissue is excised, microscopically examined, and cultured for determination of the types of organisms present, the number per gram of tissue, and the antibiotics to which the organisms are sensitive. Once bacteria exceed 100,000 per gram of tissue with invasion of subadjacent unburned tissue, the wound is defined as infected. A topical or systemic antibiotic to which the pathogen is sensitive is

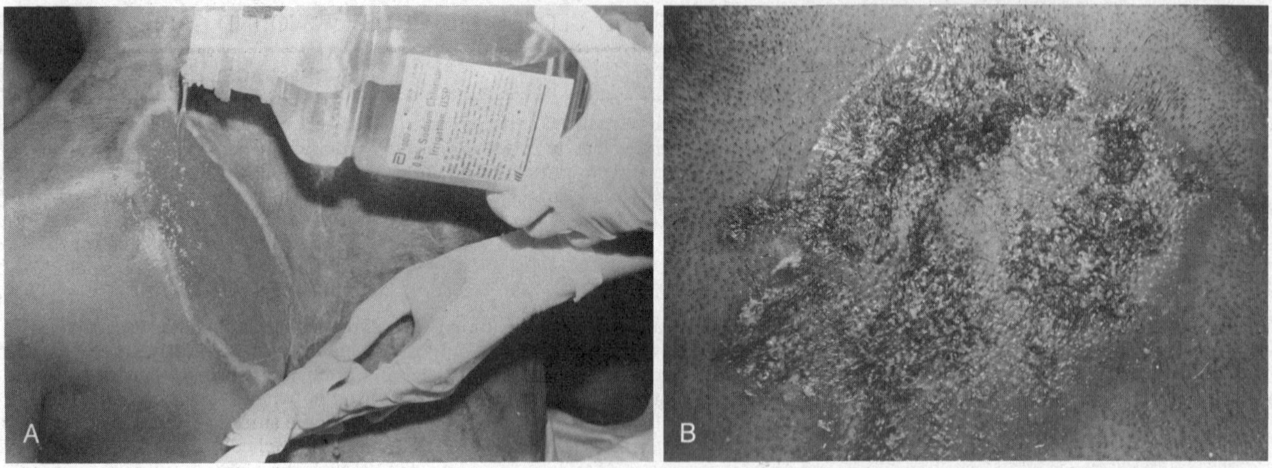

Figure 8–9.

A, A clean, noninfected burn wound with new tissue growth around the edges of the wound. *B*, An infected burn wound with black necrotic tissue in the bed of the wound.

prescribed, and the wound is evaluated for debridement.

Sepsis from burn-wound infection is the leading cause of death in the acute period of burn care. It may occur at any time until the burn wounds are completely closed. Clinical manifestations of sepsis include anorexia, malaise, headache, confusion, elevated or subnormal temperature, chills, increased pulse and respirations, decreased blood pressure, and decreased urine output. Blood cultures confirm septicemia. Wound, urine, and all invasive access sites may be cultured to identify the primary source of infection. Broad-spectrum intravenous antibiotics effective against gram-negative bacteria are started immediately. Once sensitivity studies are complete, antibiotic therapy and the topical agent may be changed to increase effectiveness against the identified microorganism. The patient may require aggressive supportive interventions to prevent or to treat septic shock.

DEBRIDEMENT

On admission to the hospital or burn unit, the burn wound is cleansed, and all loose, dead tissue is removed or debrided. Once the wound is initially debrided, the depth of the burn is reassessed. Debridement is repeated many times during the healing process to remove dead tissue and eschar. If not removed by debridement, the eschar will separate from the wound in 16 to 20 days. The eschar provides an excellent medium for the growth of microorganisms and, as long as it remains on the wound, the chances of wound infection are increased. Early removal of the eschar and necrotic tissue also promotes growth of epithelial tissue and exposes the clean, viable granulation tissue, which can then heal or accept a graft.

Several methods are commonly used to debride the wound. Mechanical debridement removes small sections of the eschar and necrotic tissue with sterile scissors, forceps, or scalpel during dressing changes. It may be done at the bedside, in the shower, or in a hydrotherapy tank. Debridement is a painful procedure, and the patient is premedicated with a narcotic analgesic. Early excision of the entire wound or debridement of large sections, usually followed by grafting, is performed in the operating room under general anesthesia.

Enzymatic debridement uses a commercially prepared enzyme agent applied to the eschar and covered with sterile gauze dressings. The enzyme breaks down the eschar, speeds natural separation of the eschar, and makes mechanical removal easier. The use of these agents is controversial because of variations in effectiveness and possible degradation of viable tissue.

HYDROTHERAPY

Hydrotherapy can be used daily or several times weekly to remove topical agents and dressings and to cleanse and debride the wounds. Medicate the patient before hydrotherapy. Many burn centers have showers that allow the patient to lie down, sit, or stand during hydrotherapy. The shower head is adjusted to different heights or is hand held. Wounds can be easily visualized and treated in the shower, and cross-contamination of wounds is minimized. Adjust and maintain water temperature to prevent excess heat loss. The shower enables the patient to participate in wound care and gives the patient a greater feeling of control over the situation.

Hydrotherapy can also be done in hydrotherapy tubs with liners of disposable plastic sheeting that is changed after each use. Physical therapy may be performed at the same time. The tubbing procedure has several disadvantages. Cross-contamination from

Table 8–7. COMMONLY USED TOPICAL AGENTS

AGENT	DESCRIPTION	ACTION	ADVANTAGES	DISADVANTAGES	NURSING IMPLICATIONS
Silver sulfadiazine	White, soluble cream	Broad-spectrum antimicrobial sulfonamide effective against gram-negative and gram-positive bacteria and yeast	Soothing to wound Easily applied Does not affect acid-base balance Dressings not required	May not completely penetrate eschar Transient leukopenia may occur in first 4 days Gram-negative bacilli may become resistant after prolonged use	Cleanse wound to remove old cream and loose necrotic tissue. Use sterile glove, tongue blade, or gauze pad to aseptically apply $\frac{1}{16}$-inch thick layer 2–3 times daily. Additional cream is applied between scheduled applications to areas rubbed off.
Mafenide acetate (Sulfamylon)	Thick, white, water-soluble cream	Broad-spectrum bacteriostatic sulfonamide agent effective against many gram-negative and gram-positive organisms and certain anaerobes	Excellent penetration of the eschar Not inactivated by pus or serum or affected by pH changes	May cause burning or stinging upon application Inhibits carbonic anhydrase, resulting in alkaline urine and metabolic acidosis Leukopenia may occur Hypersensitivity reactions may occur as late as 10–14 days	Application is the same as for silver sulfadiazine. Dressings are optional.
Silver nitrate	0.5% aqueous solution	Wide-spectrum bactericidal agent	Painless upon application High degree of effectiveness; prevents cross-contamination of burn wounds	Poor penetration of eschar, allowing subeschar infection & sepsis Caustic to skin if allowed to dry Heat loss through wet dressings Joint mobility may be impaired Hyponatremia and hypochloremia possible Time consuming, messy dressings Leaves brown or black stains on skin, clothing, equipment	Apply bulky dressings soaked in silver nitrate solution. Rewet dressings at least every 2 hr using a bulb syringe or catheters imbedded in the dressing. Apply petrolatum to unburned skin bordering burn to prevent skin staining. Silver nitrate is most commonly used in patients with neutropenic reaction to silver sulfadiazine until neutropenia resolves.
Bacitracin	Ointment	Minimal antibiotic effect	Painless on application Prevents drying of wound Keeps eschar soft	No major antibiotic effect	Apply to clean wound twice daily. Cover with petrolatum gauze and bandage. Bacitracin is used for small burns and facial burns.

Table 8–8. COMPARISON OF GRAFT TYPES

VARIABLE	HETEROGRAFT	HOMOGRAFT	AUTOGRAFT SHEET	AUTOGRAFT MESHED 1.5:1	AUTOGRAFT MESHED 3:1	ALLOGRAFT
Biologic dressing	Yes	Yes	Yes	Yes	Yes	Yes
Permanent	No	No	Yes	Yes	Yes	Yes
Cosmetic results	N/A	N/A	Superior	Moderate	Poor	Good*
Maximal skin coverage	Yes	Yes	Poor	Moderate	Superior	*
Source	Pig	Cadaver	Patient	Patient	Patient	Cadaver
Fragility	N/A	N/A	Minimal	Moderate	Maximal	*

Abbreviation: N/A, not applicable.
* This technique is still in the research phase.

infected to clean wounds may occur, the patient may lose sodium from the wounds into the tub water, resulting in hyponatremia, and getting the patient into and out of the tub may be difficult.

Both methods are currently in use, and preferences for each vary among burn centers.

TOPICAL AGENTS

Many topical agents are available for use in burn care. They provide a physical barrier against the invasion of microorganisms and inhibit the growth of microorganisms in the wound and eschar. Each agent has its advantages and disadvantages. The three most widely used agents are silver sulfadiazine, mafenide acetate, and silver nitrate. The pharmacokinetics and nursing implications of topical agents commonly used in burn-wound care are described in Table 8–7.

TETANUS PROPHYLAXIS

Tetanus toxoid is administered as soon as possible in all burn injuries in which dead tissue is present and in those associated with penetrating injuries. Patients receive a tetanus booster if already immunized against tetanus but with more than 5 years elapsed since the last booster. Patients who have never been immunized against tetanus should receive hyperimmune human tetanus globulin as well as the tetanus immunization series.

GRAFTING PROCEDURES IN BURN-WOUND CARE

As discussed in Chapter 6 and summarized in Table 8–8, there are three common types of skin grafts by source: homograft, heterograft, and autograft. Application of a graft slows evaporative loss through the wound, reduces pain, and reduces the risk of infection.

Homografts and heterografts are used as a temporary biologic dressing either to protect the wound bed while small adherent bits of eschar separate or to provide temporary wound coverage until the bed is ready to accept a permanent graft. Figure 8–10 shows the use of porcine heterografts as a temporary biologic dressing on the bed of a full-thickness burn injury.

Autografts are used in burn-wound care to permanently cover a full-thickness burn, which is incapable of regenerating skin, or deep partial-thickness burns that will require more than 2 weeks to heal. Split-thickness skin grafts and mesh grafts are most commonly used. Solid sheets of split-thickness grafts are preferred for closing wounds on the face because scarring is minimal. Sheet grafting is not possible when the availability of donor sites is limited by a massive burn injury. It is important that the patient understand that the grafted skin will retain properties of the area of the body from which it was grafted.

Once a graft is applied, it is covered with petrolatum-impregnated dressings and wrapped in a bulky gauze dressing to protect it from trauma and to keep it from drying out. A dry graft will lift off the wound or curl up at the edges and will not take (adhere and grow on the wound). The graft site may also be splinted to keep adjacent joints from moving and dislodging the graft.

The first dressing change is done approximately 3 days after the grafting procedure. By this time, a successful autograft will be pink and appear as

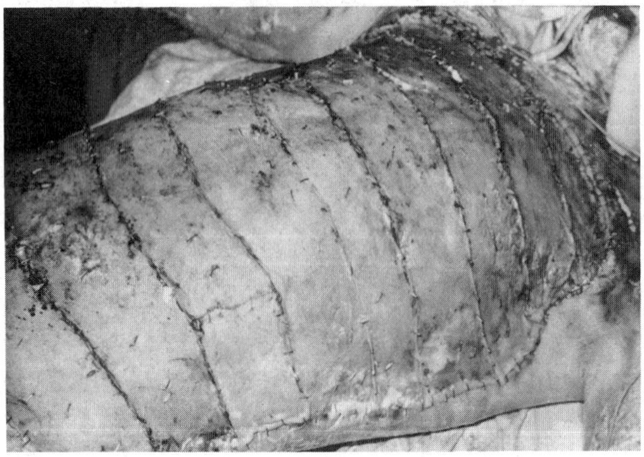

Figure 8–10.

Solid sheets of porcine heterograft used to temporarily cover a full-thickness burn wound of the anterior torso.

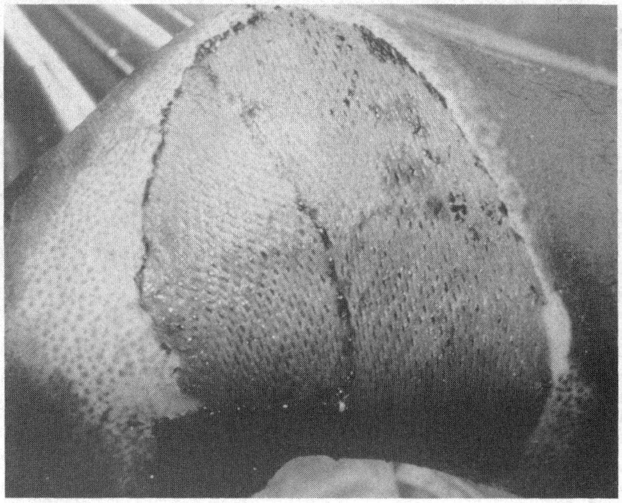

Figure 8–11.

Successful mesh graft with new epithelial cell growth in the interstitial spaces.

though it is attached to the bed of the wound. If the graft was meshed, the interstices usually show signs of new epithelial cell growth in 5 to 7 days. The interstices will continue to fill in until the spaces disappear completely. The meshed appearance of the skin will eventually disappear. Figure 8–11 shows a successful mesh graft, with new epithelial cell growth beginning to fill in the interstitial spaces.

As discussed in Chapter 6, the donor sites for skin grafts heal in approximately 2 weeks and can be reused. Although donor sites heal quickly, each one is a new open wound in an immunocompromised patient and increases the burn patient's morbidity risk. As illustrated in Figure 8–12, a donor site has the wet appearance of a deep partial-thickness burn

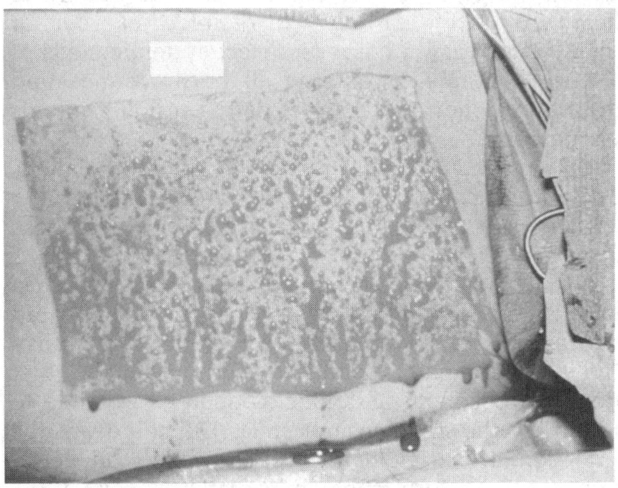

Figure 8–12.

A newly harvested donor site has the wet appearance of a deep partial-thickness burn wound.

wound and can be as painful. An infected donor site can become a full-thickness wound and place the patient at risk for sepsis. Because blood and serum are lost through the donor site, its area is added to the TBSA when calculating the patient's fluid and nutritional requirements.

Allografts

Lack of available donor sites in a massive burn injury presents a major problem in burn care. Recent development of an epidermal skin equivalent grown from cultured keratinocytes holds great promise for resolving this problem.

In this process, the epidermal layer is removed from the dermal layer of donated skin (usually cadaver). The epidermal cells are then grown in a culture that prevents antigen development. The cultured epidermis is grafted onto the wound. Because allografts from cultured epidermal cells are free of antigens that trigger the immune response, tissue rejection and sloughing of the graft do not occur. The use of allografts is still in the research phase and has limited clinical application.

Application of the Nursing Process to the Care of the Patient with a Burn-Wound Injury

Assessment

Assess burn wounds for signs of healing or infection. A clean wound is free of redness, edema, and purulent or foul-smelling drainage and is the same temperature to the touch as other parts of the body. A partial-thickness wound heals by reepithelialization as skin buds and new patches of epithelial cells develop. Healthy granulation tissue in a full-thickness wound is moist and pink to red in color and looks like fleshy bumps or masses emerging from the bed and edges of the wound. Granulation tissue indicates adequate revascularization of the wound bed and readiness to receive a graft. Figure 8–13 illustrates the appearance of healthy epithelial and granulation tissue.

After a grafting procedure, examine the dressings to ensure that they are intact, that peripheral circulation is adequate, and that splints are properly applied. Assess dressings over donor sites for bleeding and excessive drainage.

Nursing Diagnoses and Planning

Nursing diagnoses and related expected patient outcomes most commonly applicable to patients being treated for burn wound injuries include the following:

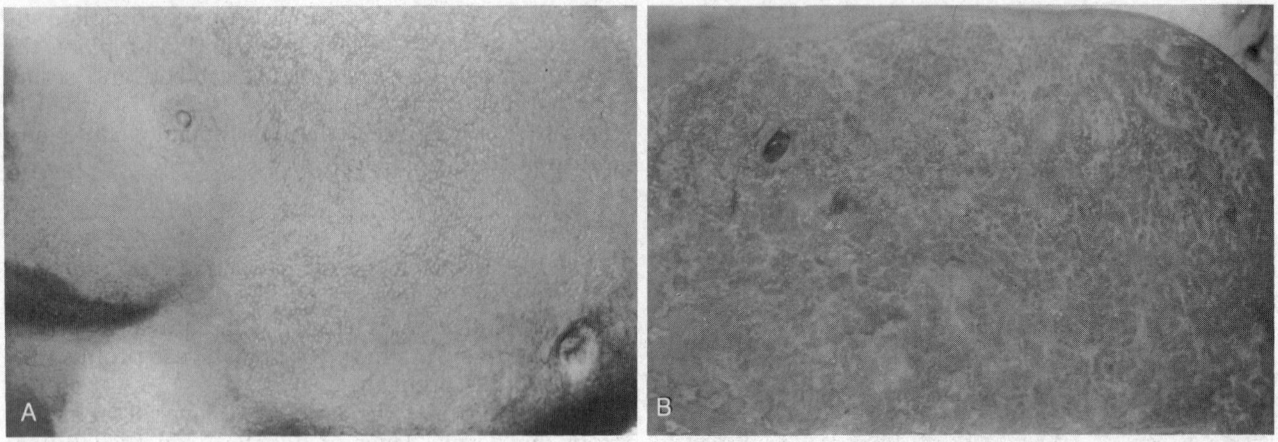

Figure 8–13.

A, Skin buds and patches of epithelial tissue growing in a partial-thickness burn wound. *B*, Fleshy masses of granulation tissue growing in the bed of a full-thickness burn wound.

NDx: High risk for infection related to burn wounds, donor site wounds, and multiple routes of possible invasion by microorganisms

Planning: Patient outcomes

1. Patient's debrided wounds show daily evidence of healing by increased granulation tissue or reduced area or depth.
2. Patient remains free from infection as evidenced by the following:
   a. Patient is afebrile.
   b. Skin around wounds is the same temperature as other parts of the body.
   c. Wounds are free of increasing edema or redness, foul odor, purulent drainage.
   d. There are fewer than 100,000 bacteria per gram of wound tissue.

NDx: Impaired physical mobility related to pain from burn wounds and donor sites and application of splints after grafting procedures

Planning: Patient outcomes

1. Patient expresses relief of pain to tolerable level.
2. Patient maintains function and mobility of all joints.

Nursing Interventions

The focus of the nursing care of a patient with burn-wound injuries is to keep the wounds, grafts, and donor sites clean and free from infection to maximize comfort, minimize scarring, and promote graft adherence and growth.

NDx: High risk for infection

Wash hands before and after all patient care. Improper hand washing is the biggest cause of nosocomial infections. A single room with equipment used only for the patient, and with specialized airflow and filtration system, further reduces the risk of cross-contamination.

Use aseptic technique, and wear cap, mask, gown, and sterile gloves during wound care to prevent contamination. Remove all of the topical agent and dressings from the wound, cleanse the wound, and re-dress daily or as prescribed to minimize growth of microorganisms. Keep the wound covered at all times with a topical agent to promote healing and provide a physical barrier against invasion by microorganisms. Wounds should not be uncovered for longer than necessary during wound care to minimize invasion of bacteria. Bulky dressings provide protection from trauma, which can delay healing.

Shave all hair growing within 2 inches of the wound to remove a possible source of microorganisms. Examine the wound with each dressing change for signs of healing or infection. Failure to heal is often the earliest sign of infection. Monitor vital signs every 4 hours to detect systemic signs of sepsis. Continue to observe all burn wounds and graft and donor sites at least daily until all wounds have closed.

Use aseptic technique in caring for all catheters, infusion sites, and invasive monitoring devices. Any access site is a potential route of entry for pathogens into the body.

Notify the physician immediately of any manifestations of wound infection or sepsis to ensure rapid treatment. Obtain specimens for culture and sensitivity to facilitate diagnosis. Administer the first dose of parenteral antibiotic as soon as possible to minimize the risk of septicemia. Do not delay the initiation of antibiotic therapy to collect all specimens if they cannot be immediately obtained because pathogens will continue to grow. Document any antibiotic administered before specimen collection on the laboratory requisition.

Once all wounds and donor sites have healed, the

risk of wound infection is eliminated. Nursing interventions to promote adherence and growth of skin grafts and the care of donor sites are presented in Chapter 6.

NDx: Impaired physical mobility

Consult with the physician and physical and occupational therapists to determine whether splints will be applied after grafting. Splints immobilize joints adjacent to the grafts to prevent skin movement, which could dislodge the grafts. Discuss the use and benefits of the splints with the patient and family. Advise them to expect bulky dressings that may further limit movement and pain from the donor sites. Knowledge of anticipated sensations reduces fear of the unknown. Understanding of postoperative procedures and restrictions promotes participation and compliance, which promote healing.

After surgery, administer prescribed analgesics as needed. New donor sites are as painful as partial-thickness burn injuries, inhibiting the patient's desire and ability to move. Assure the patient that donor site pain will decrease as it heals. Reepithelialization occurs more rapidly in donor sites covered with occlusive dressings than with fine-mesh gauze. Table 8–9 compares healing time and characteristics of three commonly used donor-site dressings.

Maintain bed rest and examine splints to ensure that they are secure and correctly positioned. Elevate the limb to reduce edema. Monitor temperature and capillary refill distal to the splint to confirm adequate peripheral circulation. Position the patient off the graft and donor sites to reduce pain and to promote blood flow and healing. Use a bed cradle or other device to prevent sheets from lying on the graft or donor sites. Discontinue physical therapy to involved limbs for 3 to 5 days to prevent dislodging the graft. The surgeon will resume physical therapy as soon as possible to maintain joint function and mobility. If possible, continue exercises to noninvolved joints throughout the postoperative period to maintain muscle tone and joint flexibility.

Evaluation

Evaluate the effectiveness of nursing care for a patient with a burn wound injury by comparing the patient's status with the expected patient outcomes. Examples of specific outcomes for patients with burn-wound injuries have been provided in the Planning section.

METABOLIC NEEDS

The body's metabolic needs remain at near-normal levels during fluid resuscitation in the emergent period after a burn injury. Then, in direct proportion to the extent of the burn injury, the metabolic rate rises rapidly and continues to rise until it peaks between the sixth and tenth days after the burn. Metabolic requirements during the acute period can increase 150% to 200% as the metabolic rate rises. After peaking, metabolism slowly decreases until it returns to near-normal levels with closure of the wound.

PATHOPHYSIOLOGY

The metabolic response to a burn injury can be attributed to many factors. Most significant of these are hypermetabolism, to compensate for heat loss, and severe protein wasting.

A major burn injury destroys the ability of the skin to conserve heat and to regulate body temperature. As large amounts of fluid evaporate through the open wound, body heat is lost. Use of wet silver nitrate dressings and hydrotherapy may accelerate heat loss. The basal metabolic rate rises to compensate for the heat loss. High caloric intake is necessary to provide fuel to meet hypermetabolic requirements and prevent catabolism of body tissues for energy.

Protein wasting results from the loss of protein in wound exudate and the catabolism of skeletal mus-

Table 8–9. COMPARISON OF DONOR SITE CARE

VARIABLE	DUODERM	BIOBRANE	FINE MESH GAUZE
Healing time	7–10 days	10–14 days	12–16 days
Mobility	Moderate	Moderate	Poor
Risk of conversion to deeper wounds	Minimal	Moderate	Significant
Pain management	Minimal to no pain	Moderate pain	Severe pain
Special considerations	Wound becomes exudative. Reinforce dressing for moderate leakage. Replace if only exudate causes nonadherence.	Pressure dressing is applied to Biobrane for the first 24 hr to promote adherence. As donor site heals, if pockets of bloody or serous drainage form, the Biobrane is trimmed at that spot.	Heat lamps may be used over donor sites for the first 24 hr to dry sites. As the donor site heals, the fine mesh gauze is trimmed. If donor site becomes "soupy," the fine mesh gauze is trimmed and an antimicrobial agent is applied.

cle to meet metabolic needs. Protein loss through wound exudate is maximum in the early postburn period and then gradually decreases until closure of the wound. Protein is used for tissue repair and wound healing and may be oxidized as fuel to replace heat loss. In the absence of adequate protein intake to replace protein losses and to meet metabolic needs, the body breaks down muscle tissue.

Protein loss and muscle wasting also contribute to excess nitrogen loss. The burn patient may lose 30 g of nitrogen a day as opposed to 6 to 7 g of nitrogen lost daily by postsurgical patients. This loss results in a severe negative nitrogen balance, which further impairs the body's ability to repair tissue.

Failure to maintain sufficient caloric and protein intake to meet metabolic needs results in weight loss, decreased resistance to infection, impaired wound healing, and loss of body tissues. The burn patient can lose as much as 1 kg of body mass a day. Weight loss for a patient with a 40% TBSA burn can be as much as 20% of the patient's preburn weight.

CLINICAL MANIFESTATIONS

Current body weight compared with the preburn weight is the most reliable factor in determining nutritional status. In addition to weight loss, signs of malnutrition include sunken and dull eyes, dry lips, sparse and brittle hair, pale and swollen tongue, inflamed gums, and a distended abdomen. A low serum albumin level confirms a decrease in body proteins and the need for increasing protein in the patient's diet.

MEDICAL MANAGEMENT

Bowel function returns, and the burn patient is usually able to tolerate oral nourishment 48 to 72 hours after injury. Several formulas have been developed to calculate approximate caloric need. One of the more widely used is the Curreri formula:

$$(25 \text{ kcal} \times \text{kg preburn weight}) + (40 \text{ kcal} \times \% \text{ TBSA burned}) \text{ daily}$$

Caloric requirements can exceed 5000 calories a day in patients with major burn injuries.

Patients with a burn of less than 20% TBSA without complications receive a high-protein, high-calorie diet with multivitamin supplements. Patients with larger burns or those who have complications may require enteral feedings. Parenteral hyperalimentation (intravenous infusion of amino acid, fat, and dextrose solutions) may be required by patients who have extensive burns, severe complications, or a persistent paralytic ileus.

Even in the absence of complications, it may be difficult to provide sufficient dietary intake to meet the patient's increased caloric and nutritional needs. Sometimes it becomes necessary to use several methods of feeding to provide adequate nutrition.

Gastrointestinal Complications

Paralytic ileus and acute stress (Curling's) ulcer are the most common gastrointestinal complications that occur in the burn patient. Paralytic ileus is more common. It usually develops in the emergent or early acute period of recovery. Causative factors include hyponatremia, hypovolemia, and stress. Sepsis may also be a contributing factor. Paralytic ileus is detected by the absence of bowel sounds. It is usually treated by withholding food and oral fluids until gastrointestinal function returns. Nasogastric intubation for gastric decompression may be necessary.

The exact cause of Curling's ulcer is not known. Physical and psychological stress, caused by the initial injury and later by surgical procedures or sepsis, and the release of massive amounts of histamine from damaged tissues appear to be major factors. Other contributing factors include elevated steroid, epinephrine, and norepinephrine levels caused by stress; decreased gastroduodenal blood flow caused by shock; slowed peristalsis resulting from hyponatremia; and changes in the gastric mucosa caused by hypovolemia.

Prophylactic use of antacids or histamine blockers begun during the emergent period and continued into the acute period has greatly reduced the incidence of Curling's ulcer in the burn patient. Chapter 22 presents a detailed discussion of the diagnosis and medical and nursing management of acute stress (Curling's) ulcer.

Application of the Nursing Process to the Care of the Patient with Increased Metabolic Needs After a Burn Injury

Assessment

Weigh the patient on admission to establish a baseline for comparison with later weights. If significant fluid resuscitation has already occurred, question the patient, family, or friends to determine preburn weight. Determine food allergies, preferences, eating habits, and cultural and religious influences. Auscultate the patient's abdomen for bowel sounds, which indicate the presence of peristalsis.

Nursing Diagnoses and Planning

Nursing diagnoses and related expected patient outcomes most commonly applicable to patients with increased metabolic needs after a burn injury include the following:

NDx: Altered nutrition: less than body requirements related to hypermetabolism and protein wasting as manifested by weight loss

Planning: Patient outcomes

1. Patient consumes an adequate amount of food to meet calculated nutritional requirements.
2. Patient weight loss is less than 10% of preburn weight.

Nursing Interventions

The goal of nursing care of a patient with increased metabolic needs after a burn injury is to assist the patient to meet increased nutritional requirements necessary to prevent body wasting during wound healing and tissue repair.

NDx: Altered nutrition: less than body requirements

Weigh the patient at the same time daily with the same scale and the same amount of clothing to monitor weight loss. Accuracy is improved if the patient can be weighed without dressings or topical creams covering the burn wounds. Note on the flow sheet or chart whether dressings were removed.

Maintain a warm environment to reduce heat loss. Use heat shields, radiant warmers, heat-reflecting blankets, or regular blankets to maintain the patient's body temperature between 37° and 38°C (98.6° and 100.4°F). Reducing heat loss reduces metabolic caloric requirements. Monitor the patient's temperature, and adjust the warming devices accordingly.

Patients with greater than 15% TBSA burn should not be fed during the first 24 hours because of potential impairment of gastrointestinal function as a result of stress and trauma. Most patients with major burn injuries remain on nothing by mouth (NPO) status for at least 72 hours. Auscultate the abdomen every 4 hours to identify the presence of bowel sounds, which indicate return of gastrointestinal function. Feedings are started when bowel function returns, usually 2 or 3 days after the burn. Gradually progress the diet to the desired nutritional intake to evaluate tolerance and to reduce the risk of nausea. Intravenous hyperalimentation is initiated if the patient loses greater than 10% of the preburn weight despite oral intake, is in a malnourished state at the time of injury, or if prolonged wound closure is anticipated.

Review the approximate nutritional requirements calculated by the dietitian or physician. Consult with the dietitian, physician, and patient to formulate a plan to meet the patient's nutritional needs. Review nutritional needs with the patient to increase understanding and cooperation. Stress that adequate nutrition is necessary for burn wounds to heal properly. The ability to eat regular food is psychologically important to most people. Six or more small meals are better tolerated than three large meals. Provide nutritional supplements and snacks to meet high-calorie, high-protein requirements. Encourage significant others to bring food to the patient from home. Avoid unpleasant procedures, sights, or odors immediately before and at mealtime to provide an environment conducive to eating. Encourage oral hygiene before meals to freshen the mouth. Assist the patient to sit up or assume a comfortable position for meals if not contraindicated. Assist with eating if necessary, but allow the patient as much independence as possible to restore self-image.

Maintain daily calorie count to monitor nutritional intake. Document the amount of all food and fluid ingested, and submit totals to the dietitian daily for calculation.

Monitor the patient's energy level daily, and observe for manifestations of deterioration in nutritional status. Report sunken, dull eyes; dry, cracked lips or mucous membranes; sparse, brittle hair; pale, swollen tongue; inflamed gums; distended abdomen; or impaired wound healing to the physician for reevaluation of nutritional intake.

Evaluation

Evaluate the effectiveness of nursing care for a patient with increased metabolic needs after a major burn injury by comparing the patient's status with the expected patient outcomes. Examples of specific outcomes for patients with increased metabolic needs after a burn injury have been provided in the Planning section.

PSYCHOSOCIAL NEEDS

The adult patient with a major burn injury presents with many psychosocial needs. The implications of the injury involve not just the patient but also family, close friends, associates, and employer. In addition to sustaining a life-threatening injury, the patient may have family members or friends who were injured or who perished in the fire. It is not uncommon for the survivors of an accident to feel guilty that they survived when others did not. The individual must deal with the reality that he or she may not survive. These patients are aware not only of their own condition but also of patients around them who do or do not survive. If intubation is required, the patient will be unable to speak until the endotracheal tube is removed and may not be able to write because of burns of the hands. At a time when anxiety is highest, the individual is unable to ask questions, communicate, or make needs easily known.

The burn patient may also be anxious about the survival of family or friends who were also injured. If several members of the same household are injured, they may be hospitalized in different agencies. It is not uncommon for patients to be hospitalized in burn centers that are long distances from home and loved ones. In addition, the home and all possessions may have been lost.

Patients who have sustained burns of the head, face, neck, or hands may be concerned about the possibility of permanent disfigurement or disability. It is important to realize that patients who have sustained burns over less visible parts of their bodies will also be concerned about scars and disfigurement. The patient may fear rejection by family, friends, loved ones, and strangers because of appearance or because of limitations in ability to function.

The patient may resent or be ashamed of dependency on others during hospitalization and may fear the possibility of still being dependent on, or a burden to, others after discharge. Long convalescence, financial hardship, and possible permanent deformities may force the postponement or cancellation of previous plans for the future.

The cost of extended hospital and outpatient care is often a major concern to patients, especially those who have no medical insurance or whose insurance does not cover all expenses. Although most patients are discharged once their wounds heal, extended convalescence, rehabilitation, and further surgery will continue for many months or years. During this time, the patient may not be able to work, resulting in further financial hardship. The injury may prevent return to previous employment, increasing concern over future employment and long-term financial responsibilities.

Because the psychosocial needs of the burn patient can be so involved, it is important that the burn team include mental health specialists, social workers, and clergy. These specialists provide psychosocial support, which is needed by the patient, family, loved ones, and other members of the burn team. Therapeutic support may include discussions with the patient and loved ones, medications to reduce anxiety, hypnosis, and biofeedback training. Many burn centers include staff support in the responsibilities of the mental health specialists.

Application of the Nursing Process to the Care of the Patient with Psychosocial Needs After a Burn Injury

Assessment

Assess psychosocial needs during conversations and therapeutic interactions with the patient, family, and visitors. Determine the circumstances of the accident, other persons injured or killed, and their relationship with the patient. Ask the patient to identify ways he or she has coped with stressful situations in the past. Observe nonverbal cues of emotional status, and encourage the patient to verbalize feelings. Decreased compliance with therapies, persistent hostility or anger, decreased appetite, poor sleep patterns at night, poor eye contact, refusal to look at self, a monotone or sharp voice, refusal to discuss care or injuries, conflict with family or staff, refusal to see visitors, denial of having any worries or concerns, or any marked change in the patient's outlook or behavior pattern may indicate need for aggressive psychological support.

Nursing Diagnoses and Planning

A burn injury may affect any aspect of an individual's life and emotional health. Because similar burn injuries affect individuals differently, all psychosocial nursing diagnoses are potentially applicable. Nursing diagnoses and related expected patient outcomes most commonly applicable to patients with psychosocial needs after a burn injury include the following:

NDx: Post-trauma response related to major burn injury as evidenced by recurrent nightmares, sleep-pattern disturbances, survival guilt, angry outbursts

Planning: Patient outcomes

1. Patient acknowledges the impact of the circumstances of the burn injury on self.
2. Patient talks about the event.
3. Patient verbalizes fear, anger, guilt.
4. Patient reports lessening of frequency of re-experiencing the event.
5. Patient sleeps through the night.

NDx: Body image disturbance related to change in appearance, fear of loss of ability to function independently and to fulfill role performance because of burn injuries

Planning: Patient outcomes

1. Patient grieves and expresses feelings of loss.
2. Patient verbalizes realistic perceptions of appearance.
3. Patient states realistic expectations of long-term ability to function independently and to fulfill role expectations.
4. Patient expresses desire to be discharged.

Nursing Interventions

The goal of nursing care of the patient with psychosocial needs after a burn injury is to assist the patient to cope with the short- and long-term effects of the injuries, hospitalization, treatment, and convalescence.

NDx: Post-trauma response

Provide continuity of nursing care so the patient can develop a positive relationship with primary caregivers. Share information at multidiciplinary conference to determine which member of the health team, clergy, or family can offer the best support for the patient at any given time during recovery.

Spend time talking with the patient when no painful procedures are being performed to provide an opportunity to express feelings and ask questions. Be an active, nonjudgmental listener. Talking about a traumatic event can often help the person come to terms with it. As discussed in Chapter 5, expect the patient to respond to the accident and subsequent injury and losses with denial, shock, anger, guilt, and depression. Assure the patient these feelings are normal after a traumatic event and loss. Assist the patient to understand what happened and the reality of personal involvement. Stay with a patient who has awakened from a nightmare to provide reassurance of safety and to lessen anxiety.

NDx: Body image disturbance
Prepare the patient and visitors for the patient's appearance, especially if facial burns and edema are present. Preparation for what they will see lessens the shock. Explain that edema severely alters initial appearance. Encourage the patient with burns of the head, face, and neck to look in a mirror once the edema has receded. Often the imagined image is worse than reality. Encourage the patient to discuss anticipated results of healing, reconstructive surgery, and rehabilitation with the health team so long-term expectations are realistic. Reassure the patient that the appearance of suture lines of sheet grafts and interstices of mesh grafts usually normalize over time.

Encourage visits by family and friends to prevent feelings of rejection and social isolation. Encourage the patient to leave the sheltered environment of the burn unit for brief excursions to hospital corridors, the cafeteria, or hospital grounds to prepare for the reaction of strangers to the burn scars.

Encourage full participation in the planned program of rehabilitation and wound care to promote full recovery and to minimize the risk of long-term disability. Answer questions honestly. Do not give false reassurances. Refer questions you cannot answer to appropriate resources. Explain procedures, and prepare the patient for anticipated events and sensations to reduce feelings of powerlessness. Give choices when possible to provide a sense control and increase self-esteem. Consult with the patient, family, and health team to develop a plan to provide emotional and financial support for the patient and family throughout hospitalization and postdischarge rehabilitation.

Evaluation

Evaluate the effectiveness of nursing care for a patient with psychosocial needs after a burn injury by comparing the patient's status with the expected patient outcomes. Examples of specific outcomes for patients with psychosocial needs after a burn injury have been provided in the Planning section.

Rehabilitation Phase

Rehabilitation is a process of treatment and education through physical and occupational therapy that enables the patient to restore and maintain maximum function of injured body parts and to achieve maximum independence in activities of daily living. Rehabilitation begins on admission to the hospital or burn unit, continues throughout the healing process and discharge, and culminates in the individual's return to maximum function in society.

In conjunction with nursing and medical management, the goal of rehabilitation is to promote optimum wound healing with minimum contracture and scar formation. While physicians and nurses stabilize the patient in the emergent period, physical and occupational therapists develop care plans to prevent cosmetic and functional deformities that would leave the patient physically impaired or require needless surgery to correct. These initial plans are revised as the patient's physical condition and wound status change throughout the acute period and into the rehabilitation phase. Therapy sessions are scheduled at least daily and may ultimately include retraining in activities of daily living or job rehabilitation to adapt to loss of function or limb loss. Burn patients usually require long-term rehabilitation, and therapy continues on an outpatient basis after discharge.

CONTRACTURES

As burn wounds heal, scar tissue forms. As the healing process continues, connective fibers in the scar tissue contract or shorten. Contraction of scar tissue over a joint can cause deformity and loss of function and mobility of the joint.

Contractures and joint deformities are prevented by exercise, positioning, and splinting throughout the healing process. All patients with deep partial- or full-thickness burns of the joints and burns of the hands, feet, or neck require physical therapy. Early excision and grafting allow earlier resumption of exercises and help minimize contracture formation and loss of function. Therapy begins with range-of-motion exercises to prevent contractures and then progresses to strengthening exercises and activities of daily living to maintain function. If involved joints are unable to be exercised because of associated injury or recent grafting, splints are applied to maintain functional anatomic position of the joints. Splints may be worn at night throughout the

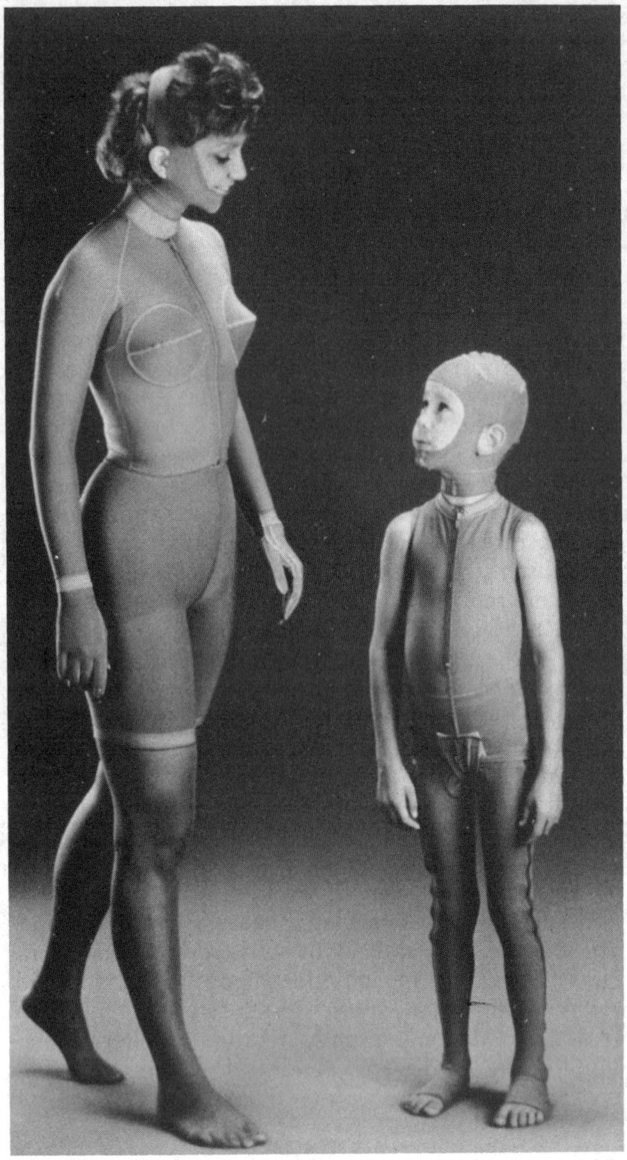

Figure 8–14.

Models wearing Jobskin™ Positive Pressure System garments. Pressure garments have been proved effective in preventing or reducing hypertrophic scarring. (Courtesy of Jobst Institute, Inc., Charlotte, NC.)

healing process to prevent flexion contractures as scar tissue contracts. If contractures do form, surgical release is required to return function to the joint.

HYPERTROPHIC SCARRING

Deep burn wounds initially appear flat and pink as they heal. In some patients with deep partial- or full-thickness burns, excess collagen deposits form in the scar tissue. In these cases, approximately a month after initial healing, the skin becomes raised, is very firm, and lacks moisture. Hyperactive collagen formation continues for approximately 1 year before growth slows, and the scarred skin again becomes supple.

Elastic pressure garments prevent or reduce hypertrophic scarring. Pressure garments, such as those shown in Figure 8–14, are custom-made to conform to body areas burned. By exerting constant uniform pressure over the healed wound, they minimize the proliferation of scar tissue. Pressure garments are applied after the burn wounds have healed or have been grafted, are removed only to bathe, and are worn until the scar matures and softens, which takes approximately 1 year. To be effective, they must be worn at least 23 hours a day and refitted frequently to maintain pressure. Emollients are used in conjunction with pressure garments to soften the skin.

Cosmetic surgery to excise hypertrophic scar tissue cannot be performed for 18 months to 2 years after the initial closure of the wound. Continued hyperactive growth of the scar tissue during this time would result in unsatisfactory cosmetic results.

Application of the Nursing Process to the Care of the Patient Requiring Rehabilitation After a Burn Injury

Assessment

Assess the severity and location of burn injuries to identify patients at risk for contractures and hypertrophic scarring. Patients with full-thickness or deep partial-thickness burns around joints and on the hands, feet, or neck are at high risk for contractures. Examine old scars and determine the healing pattern of old wounds to identify persons at risk for hypertrophic scarring. Hypertrophic scarring occurs more frequently in individuals of African and Mediterranean ancestry. Question the patient and family about specific home- and work-related mobility and dexterity requirements.

Nursing Diagnoses and Planning

Nursing diagnoses and related expected patient outcomes most commonly applicable to patients requiring rehabilitation after a burn injury include the following:

NDx: High risk for impaired physical mobility related to contractures

Planning: Patient outcomes
1. Patient performs active and passive range-of-motion exercises as prescribed.
2. Patient remains free of contractures.
3. Patient performs activities of daily living independently.

Table 8–10. NURSING INTERVENTIONS TO PREVENT CONTRACTURES

AREA BURNED	NURSING INTERVENTIONS
Anterior neck	Hyperextend the neck. Place a rolled towel under the back of the neck, or position the patient at the top of one mattress with the head hanging over and resting on a second mattress underneath. Do not use a pillow under the head at any time.
Posterior neck	Flex the neck. Use no pillow or only a small pillow under the head, and encourage frequent side-to-side and turning motion.
Ears	Do not use a pillow. Place gauze between auricle and head to prevent adhesions.
Upper chest and anterior shoulder	Place a rolled or folded towel parallel to the spine between the scapulae with arms on mattress. Do not use a pillow under the head.
Axilla	Extend arm up over head.
Antecubital fossa, popliteal fossa	Maintain elbow or knee in extension. Hyperextend knee by pressing it into the mattress several times a day.
Hand, ankle, foot	Splint in anatomic position, with digits separated by gauze.
Groin	Maintain hip in extension. If possible, avoid elevating head of bed and hyperextend hip several times a day by placing the patient in a prone position. Place gauze between burned surfaces of the genitalia.

NDx: High risk for altered health maintenance related to insufficient knowledge of physical therapy exercises, use of pressure garments, self-management of grafts and burn scars

Planning: Patient outcomes

1. Patient demonstrates wound care.
2. Patient performs active and passive range-of-motion exercises at home as prescribed.
3. Patient wears pressure garment at least 23 hours a day.
4. Patient remains free of contractures and hypertrophic scarring.
5. Patient resumes social and employment activities.

Nursing Interventions

The goal of nursing care of the patient requiring rehabilitation after a burn injury is to assist the patient to maintain mobility and function of involved joints and limbs and to minimize scarring.

NDx: High risk for impaired physical mobility

Consult with the patient, family, physicians, and therapists to develop a plan for rehabilitation. Reinforce the therapists' explanation of the purpose of splints and exercises. Active patient participation in the planning stages and understanding of the benefits of physical therapy increase compliance and give the patient a sense of control over a stressful situation.

Always keep burned skin surfaces separated by gauze dressings to prevent adhesions and contractures. Unless contraindicated by multiple burned areas or associated injuries, position the patient as described in Table 8–10 to reduce the risk of contracture formation. Position per physician's orders if contraindications to standard positions are present. Apply splints to burned joints at night or as prescribed to prevent flexion contractures. Assess circulation distal to the splints every 2 hours to ensure tissue perfusion.

Administer prescribed analgesic before physical therapy sessions to minimize pain and to maximize compliance. Resume physical therapy to immobilized joints as soon as possible after grafting procedures to minimize the risk of contractures. Encourage, assist, and remind the patient to perform prescribed independent exercises as often as possible between therapy sessions to maintain joint mobility. Document how often the patient does independent exercises and how much assistance is needed. Early, active exercise reduces the risk of contractures and increases strength. Ambulate the patient as soon as possible to promote strength and inhibit bone decalcification.

NDx: High risk for altered health maintenance

Many patients are discharged before burn wounds are completely healed. Teach the patient and a caregiver how to cleanse the wound, reapply topical agent, and redress the wound to promote healing and to minimize the risk of infection. A hand-held shower can be used for cleansing the wound. Observe the patient or caregiver performing wound care to evaluate learning, and answer questions on technique. Review, and provide in writing, the signs of infection and instructions on what to do if they occur.

Newly healed skin burns easily and is sensitive to ultraviolet light, yet until nerve regeneration occurs, it is hyposensitive to heat, cold, and touch. Teach the patient to use a thermometer or an area of unburned skin to test the temperature of water before use to prevent scalding. Instruct the patient to remain out of the sun for at least 1 year, to use sunscreen, and to always wear a hat to prevent sunburn. Newly healed skin is fragile and must be protected from friction and trauma. Examine the skin daily to detect injury or blisters from splints or pressure garments. As new epithelial cells grow, grafts and donor sites flake and itch. Teach the patient to massage in an emollient moisturizer daily to soften the skin, to relieve itching, and to increase circulation. Lubriderm, Nivea, lanolin, and cocoa butter are commonly used.

Reinforce the therapist's instructions to the patient in the purpose, use, and care of splints and pressure garments for the prevention of contractures and hypertrophic scarring. Schedule a time when the pa-

Chart 8–1.

NURSING GUIDE TO PATIENT EDUCATION FOR SELF-MANAGEMENT: DISCHARGE INSTRUCTIONS FOR BURN CARE

Instruct the patient to perform the following:

Wound Care

Wash hands before and after wound care.

Wash the wound gently once a day with a mild, nondetergent, nondeodorant soap (e.g., Ivory) to remove all old topical preparation and wound drainage. The wound may be cleansed in the shower.

Apply a thin layer of prescribed antibacterial cream or ointment and cover with dressing.

Examine wound and surrounding area for redness, swelling, purulent drainage, warmth, or foul odor. Report any of these observations to physician immediately.

Return for follow-up appointment on *(specify date)*.

Use and Care of Pressure Garments

Wear pressure garments at least 23 hours a day. Remove only for shower or bath.

Examine skin under garment for blisters or irritation. If found, call for an appointment and do not wear the garment until seen by the physician.

Wash the garment in a mild nondetergent, nondeodorant soap (e.g., Ivory Snow) and hang to air dry.

Care of Newly Healed Skin

Take precautions to avoid bumps, bruises, or trauma to the fragile newly healed skin.

Rub emollient moisturizer (e.g., Lubriderm, Nivea, lanolin, cocoa butter) into the new skin several times a day.

Apply moisturizer under pressure garment as a protective emollient.

Test the temperature of kitchen, bath, or shower water with a thermometer or an area of nonburned skin to prevent scalds.

Always apply sunscreen with a minimum sun protection factor (SPF) of 15 before leaving the house, and cover healed skin with loose-fitting clothing, hat, socks, or gloves to prevent sunburn. Pressure garments alone do not protect the skin from ultraviolet light. Always wear clothing over the garments. Skin must be protected for a minimum of 1 year.

Wear loose-fitting cotton clothes to prevent rubbing of the skin. Do not wear belts or other constricting items over newly healed skin.

Proper Diet and Exercise

Eat foods rich in protein and high in calories.

Weigh yourself at least twice a week.

Report any weight loss to the physician.

After skin has healed, continue to weigh yourself once a week and maintain even weight to prevent pressure garments from becoming too loose.

Perform prescribed exercises to increase joint mobility and muscle strength.

Walk each day and climb stairs a few times a day to improve health and stamina.

tient is rested and relatively free of pain to be measured for prescribed pressure garments. Observe the patient or caregiver in the application and removal of splints and pressure garments to ensure proper usage. Review, and provide in writing, time of application and removal and care instructions. The patient needs two pressure garments so a clean one can be put on each day after bathing. Instruct the patient to wash the soiled one in a nondetergent, nondeodorant mild soap, such as Ivory Snow, to rinse well, and to hang the garment to dry. Reinforce the need to wear the pressure garment at least 23 hours a day to achieve desired results.

Patient education for self-management after a burn injury is summarized in Chart 8–1.

Evaluation

Evaluate the effectiveness of nursing care for a patient requiring rehabilitation after a burn injury by comparing the patient's status with the expected patient outcomes. Examples of specific outcomes for patients requiring rehabilitation after a burn injury have been provided in the Planning section.

Care of the Patient with a Chemical Burn Injury

There are more than 25,000 products on the market today that are capable of resulting in a chemical burn injury. These products, available for home, industrial, agricultural, and military use, are the cause of more than 3000 deaths a year in the United States. It is estimated that more than 60,000 individuals require medical attention for chemical injuries annually.

Chemicals are broadly classified as acids, alkalis, and vesicants. They are more precisely grouped by their local and systemic actions, as summarized in Table 8–11.

In general, chemical agents do not "burn" or destroy tissue by heat. Instead, they cause destruction of cellular protein by coagulation, a solidification of the protein into a gelatinous mass. A chemical will continue to destroy tissue for up to 72 hours after exposure. Incomplete removal, dilution, or neutralization of the chemical can result in further tissue damage by residual chemicals.

Characteristics of Chemical Burn Injuries

Body tissues are damaged by chemical agents on skin contact and penetration, ingestion, and inhalation. The extent of tissue damage depends on several factors. The greater the quantity of chemical agent that comes in contact with the tissues, the stronger or more concentrated the agent, and the

Table 8–11. CLASSIFICATION OF CHEMICAL AGENTS

CLASSIFICATION	EFFECT ON TISSUE	SYSTEMIC EFFECT	METHOD OF NEUTRALIZATION	EXAMPLES	PRODUCTS COMMONLY FOUND IN
Oxidizing agents	Blisters, ulcerations	Diarrhea, gastrointestinal bleeding, seizures, death	Water	Sodium hypochloride Chromic acid Potassium permanganate	Clorox Metal cleaners Disinfectants
Reducing agents	Eschar formation		Water	Nitric acid Hydrochloric acid Alkyl mercuric acid	Industry Metal cleaning
Corrosive agents	Rapidly penetrate Thick eschar	Central nervous system depression, hypotension, pulmonary edema, hepatic necrosis, nephrotoxicity, death	Brush off powder first		
			Ethyl alcohol or cooking oil followed by copious water	Phenols	Sanitizers, plastic
			1% copper sulfate/water	White phosphorus	Explosives, insecticides
			Water	Dichromate salts Sodium metals Lye Calcium oxide Lime	Cleaning agents Drain cleaners Portland cement Agriculture
Protoplasmic poisons	Eschar formation	Hepatic necrosis, nephrotoxicity, binds calcium	Water	Picric acid Tannic acid Sulfosalicylic acid Acetic acid Formic acid	Industry
			Water/intravenous calcium	Oxalic acid	
	Local vasoconstriction	Bone decalcification	Water/subcutaneous calcium	Hydrofluoric acid	Glass etching
Desiccants	Produce excessive heat; cause severe cell dehydration		Water	Sulfuric acid Muriatic acid	
Vesicants	Blisters, edema Ischemic and anoxic necrosis		Water	Cantharides Dimethyl sulfoxide Dichlorodiethyl sulfide (mustard gas) Chlorovinyldichloroarsine	Veterinary uses Military uses

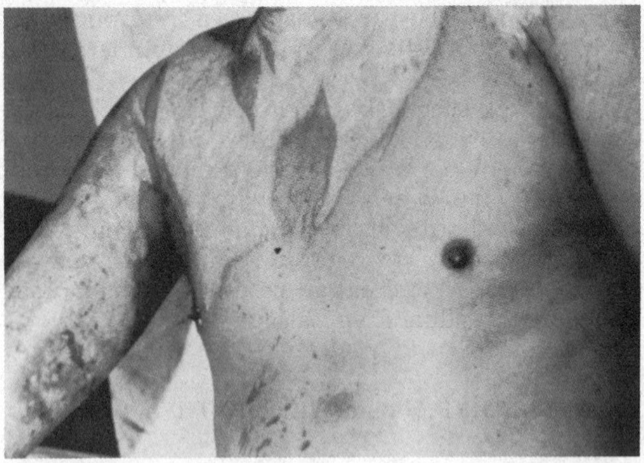

Figure 8–15.

Skin discoloration characteristic of a chemical burn injury. (From Artz CP, Moncrief JA, Pruitt BA [eds]. Burns: A team approach. Philadelphia: WB Saunders, 1979, p 365.)

longer the duration of contact, the more severe the damage. An agent that rapidly penetrates to underlying tissues can cause extensive deep injury. Some chemical agents not only cause contact tissue damage but are also toxins that can cause systemic effects or poisoning.

Clinical manifestations of chemical burns are dependent on the area of contact. A chemical skin burn will have the same appearance as any burn of the same depth. Full-thickness chemical burns are often red, yellow, or brown in color. Contact with the eyes produces initial tearing, blepharospasm, inflammation of the conjunctiva and sclera, and an uncontrollable urge to rub the eyes. Ingestion of a chemical results in esophageal, tracheobronchial, or gastric injuries as well as the risk of systemic poisoning and death. Inhalation of toxic gases or powdered chemicals can cause burns of the upper respiratory tract, respiratory distress, and the risk of systemic poisoning from absorption through respiratory mucosa.

Determination of the depth of the burn and TBSA involved is often difficult. Chemical burns initially appear less severe than they actually are. Additional tissue destruction as a result of continued chemical penetration into deeper tissues may occur for 72 hours after the initial contact. These expanded areas of tissue destruction often appear as yellow-brown or mildly discolored marks rather than burns. An untreated chemical burn is illustrated in Figure 8–15.

Medical Management

Rapid intervention is of prime importance to limit tissue destruction in a chemical injury. Initial emergency treatment was discussed earlier in this chapter under Immediate Care. Flushing the wound with copious amounts of water cannot be overemphasized. Water has been shown to dilute and physically remove the agent, decrease the rate of chemical reaction, decrease inflammatory reaction by decreasing tissue metabolism, reduce hygroscopic action, and restore wound pH levels toward normal in chemical injuries caused by some concentrated acids and alkalis. The use of copious amounts of water also dissipates the heat that is produced when some chemical agents are mixed with water.

Irrigation of chemical eye injuries continues with normal saline for up to 48 hours to minimize the risk of permanent damage and vision loss. The ophthalmologist may apply a Morgan lens to the eye to

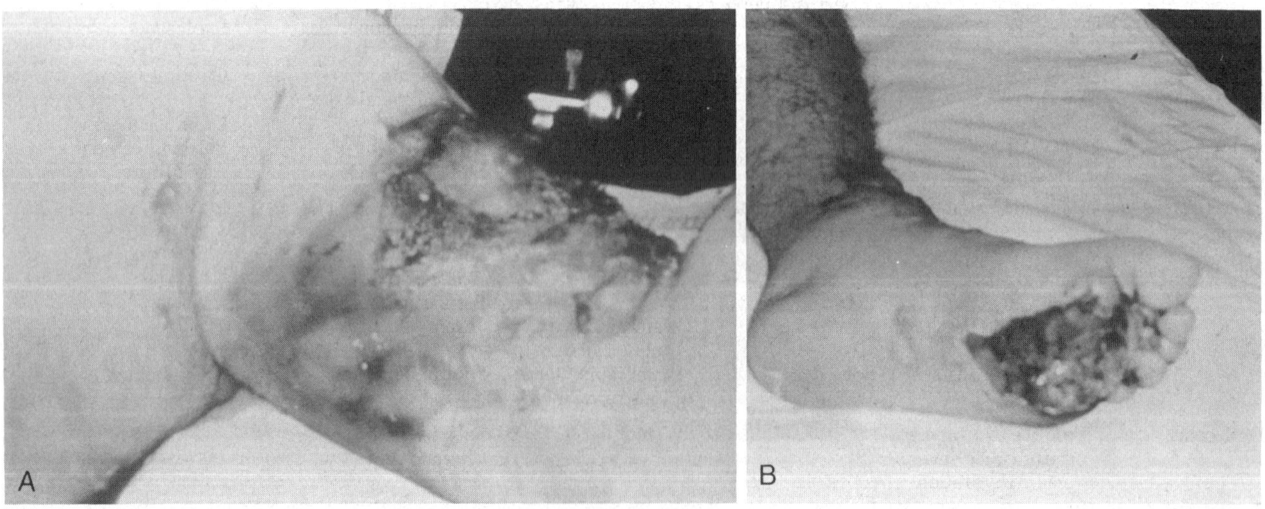

Figure 8–16.

Electrical burn injury. The entrance wound *(A)* is often charred and resembles a full-thickness burn wound. The exit wound *(B)* appears as though something exploded out of it.

facilitate continuous irrigation. Ophthalmic steroid, antibiotic, and anesthetic preparations reduce inflammation and scarring, prevent infection, and increase patient comfort.

Some chemical injuries require further treatment after irrigation and dilution to completely neutralize the agent and to stop tissue destruction. Neutralizing agents for each classification of chemical are included in Table 8–11.

Any patient who has ingested chemicals is evaluated for esophageal and gastric injuries by esophagoscopy within 12 hours of admission. Systemic steroids and antibiotics reduce inflammation, scarring, and infection. Reconstructive surgery or a temporary or permanent gastrostomy for feeding may be required in cases of extensive esophageal damage. Psychiatric evaluation to determine immediate risk to self and others is required if the ingestion of chemicals was a suicide attempt. Suicidal patients are monitored continously to prevent additional attempts and require long-term psychiatric follow-up.

The extent of respiratory injury after inhalation of chemical agents is evaluated by bronchoscopy. Injury to the trachea and bronchi has also been reported after ingestion of chemicals. Treatment with steroids, antibiotics, bronchodilators, and intubation and ventilator support is implemented as needed.

Fluid resuscitation and wound care in chemical injuries are similar to methods used for other burn injuries. However, because of the difficulty in initially determining the full extent and depth of the injury, standard fluid resuscitation calculation is used only as a guideline. Closely monitor the patient for signs of inadequate fluid resuscitation to prevent hypovolemic shock and acute tubular necrosis.

Guidelines for Application of the Nursing Process to the Care of the Patient with a Chemical Burn Injury

Nursing care of patients with chemical burn injuries is similar to that described earlier in this chapter for patients with burn injuries. The goals of the nursing care plan for patients with chemical burn injuries are to assist the patient to limit tissue destruction, avoid or minimize burn shock, keep the wounds clean and free from infection, maximize comfort, meet nutritional needs, maintain mobility and function, minimize scarring, provide psychosocial support, and maintain vision if the eyes are involved.

Identify the area of contact, type of chemical agent, method and duration of contact, and treatment administered at the scene of the accident. Specifically ask whether any of the agent came in contact with the eyes or was swallowed or inhaled. If possible, obtain the container of the agent to ensure accurate identification. The label of many chemical containers gives information on treatment for exposure and ingestion and how to neutralize the agent.

Examine the involved area and surrounding tissue to determine the severity of damage. Remember that chemical penetration and tissue destruction continue for as long as 72 hours, so initial assessment may not reflect the final severity of the injury. Monitor the wound every hour during the irrigation and then every 4 hours after the irrigation. Changes in skin color, additional skin loss, or blistering indicate an increase in the extent or depth of injury.

If the chemical was ingested, monitor for manifestations of gastrointestinal damage and respiratory involvement from aspiration. If the chemical or its fumes were inhaled, auscultate lung sounds and monitor for manifestations of respiratory injury. Report difficulty swallowing, vomiting, and signs of respiratory distress to the physician immediately. Administer enteral or gastrostomy feedings to meet nutritional needs if the patient is receiving nothing by mouth.

Care of the Patient with an Electrical Burn Injury

More than 1000 deaths in the United States each year are caused by electrical shock. Even nonfatal electrical injuries can cause extensive deep muscle, bone, and tissue damage along the path of the current through the body. The stronger the current and the longer the contact, the more severe the internal damage. High-voltage current and lightning can generate temperatures in body tissues as high as 2500°C (4500°F). Different body tissues vary in their resistance to the flow of current. Denser tissues have greater resistance. The slower passage of the current generates more heat and tissue damage.

Characteristics of Electrical Burn Injuries

An entrance-exit wound is the most common visible characteristic of an electrical burn injury. An entrance wound is created at the point of contact as the current enters the body. It has a charred appearance and resembles a full-thickness thermal burn injury. An entrance wound is usually located on an extremity, the most common point of contact with the electrical source. The exit wound, or point at which the current leaves the body, may be located anywhere on the body. It has dry, open edges and looks as though something exploded out through it. Figure 8–16 illustrates the appearance of entrance and exit wounds. Electrical current may enter and

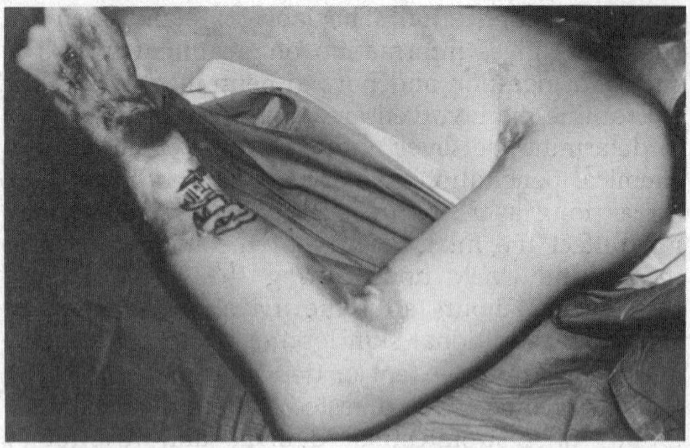

Figure 8–17.

Multiple entrance and exit wounds caused as the electric current exited and re-entered the body.

exit the patient more than once, resulting in multiple sets of entrance and exit wounds, as shown in Figure 8–17. If contact with an electrical flash ignites clothing, the patient may suffer a thermal burn injury as well as an electrical injury.

If the current crosses the heart, cardiac dysrhythmias including extrasystoles, ventricular fibrillation, and cardiac standstill can occur. Fractures may be caused by the sudden, forceful contraction of muscles stimulated by the passage of electric current. Decortication of bone may be caused by the force of the current. Extensive, deep bone, muscle, and tissue necrosis may require amputation. Paralysis may result from permanent nerve damage.

Acute tubular necrosis caused by obstruction of the renal tubules by hemoglobin, which is released from damaged red blood cells, and by myoglobin, which is released from damaged muscle tissue, may develop. Although acute tubular necrosis occurs in full-thickness thermal burns, it is much more common in electrical injury because of extensive muscle damage. The risk of acute tubular necrosis is highest in patients with myoglobinuria or hematuria, signs that the by-products of muscle damage and hemocoagulation are being excreted in the urine.

Late complications of electrical injury may not be apparent for months after the initial injury. These include cataracts, meningitis, progressive spinal cord damage, motor dysfunction, pain syndromes, bacterial endocarditis, and osteomyelitis.

Medical Management

If the patient is in ventricular fibrillation or cardiac standstill, cardiopulmonary resuscitation is initiated at the scene of the accident and continued during transport to the hospital. Advanced cardiac life-support measures, including defibrillation, are implemented on admission to the hospital or as soon as trained personnel are available at the scene.

FLUID REPLACEMENT

Patients with electrical injuries caused by brief contact with low-voltage electricity can usually be resuscitated with the volume calculated for standard fluid-replacement. High-voltage or prolonged-contact electrical injuries, however, involve extensive internal damage along the path of the electric current. Although surface wounds may appear small, the patient requires large-volume fluid resuscitation to replace the rapid loss of fluids into damaged internal tissues and to prevent acute tubular necrosis. Standard fluid-replacement calculation based on TBSA is used only as a rough guideline for fluid resuscitation because the internal tissue destruction is much greater than visible surface injuries. The adequacy of fluid resuscitation is determined by the criteria for successful fluid resuscitation presented earlier in this chapter.

Intravenous mannitol may be administered to promote excretion of myoglobins and to decrease the chance of acute tubular necrosis. Mannitol is administered only if hematuria is present and urine output is greater than 50 ml/hour to avoid dehydrating a hypovolemic patient. Sodium bicarbonate is administered if metabolic acidosis results from the myoglobinemia and altered renal function.

WOUND MANAGEMENT

Low-voltage and brief-contact injuries with minimal internal damage are treated similarly to thermal burns with a topical antibacterial agent. The wound is allowed to slough and heal by granulation or may be excised and grafted. To assess the extent of muscle damage and the possible need for amputation in high-voltage injuries, deep incisions to the muscle fascia, called fasciotomies, are made near the entrance of the wound. The exposed tissues are examined for damage and necrosis. If the tissues are viable, the fasciotomy may be extended along the muscle to relieve pressure from edema within the muscle compartment, thereby preventing further tissue damage from impaired circulation. If the fasciotomy reveals extensively damaged or necrotic muscle, the wound is surgically debrided and grafted. If tissue damage is too extensive for revitalization, the limb is amputated. High-voltage electrical injuries may also result in the loss of internal organs.

The patient with a major electrical injury requires intensive rehabilitation because of extensive tissue, muscle, and skeletal damage. Even if amputation of a limb is not required, the damaged nerves and muscles require retraining and exercise. If a limb is amputated, prosthetic devices and training in their use are needed.

Guidelines for Application of the Nursing Process to the Care of the Patient with an Electrical Burn Injury

Nursing care of patients with electrical burn injuries is similar to that described earlier in this chapter for patients with burn injuries. The goals of the nursing care plan for patients with electrical burn injuries are to assist the patient to salvage viable tissue, avoid or minimize burn shock, keep the wounds clean and free from infection, maximize comfort, meet nutritional needs, maintain mobility and function, minimize scarring, provide psychosocial support, and adapt to limb loss and use of a prosthesis if amputation was necessary.

Question the patient or the persons accompanying the patient to determine the type of current, voltage, amperage, and duration of contact. Determine whether the patient lost consciousness, had a cardiac arrest, or was defibrillated before arrival at the hospital. Examine the entire body for entrance and exit wounds because the current can re-enter the body after exiting. Assess the size and depth of external burn injuries. Determine the presence of associated injuries such as thermal burns, lacerations, and fractures. Obtain baseline electrocardiogram readings and cardiac enzyme levels to evaluate cardiac muscle damage or conduction disorders.

Administer parenteral fluid resuscitation to minimize burn shock and the risk of acute tubular necrosis. Monitor the patient hourly to evaluate fluid replacement. The risk of hypovolemia is high in electrical injuries because the extent of internal tissue damage cannot be accurately determined. If hematuria or myoglobinuria are present, increase the rate of parenteral fluid administration to maintain urine output at 75 to 100 ml/hour until the urine clears. The physician may also order 44 to 50 mEq of sodium bicarbonate per liter of lactated Ringer's solution to produce an alkaline urine and to reverse metabolic acidosis. Myoglobin and hemoglobin are more readily excreted in an alkaline urine. Mannitol is administered to aid in the prevention of tubular necrosis if the urine does not clear.

Prepare the patient for fasciotomy and wound debridement, reinforcing the physician's explanation of the procedure and its purpose. If amputation is necessary, reinforce the physician's explanation of the need for it, and provide emotional support while preparing the patient for surgery. Care of a patient after a fasciotomy, amputation, or other orthopedic injury that may be associated with an electrical burn injury is described in Unit XI.

Monitor the patient daily for peripheral and central nervous system damage. The extent of nerve damage may slowly progress for an extended period of time after the initial injury, and early manifestations may be masked by associated tissue injury. Teach the patient, and provide in writing, the manifestations of the long-term complications of electrical injury to aid in early detection and treatment. Explain that they often are not apparent for months after the injury.

Care of the Pregnant Patient with a Burn Injury

The possibility of pregnancy in any female of childbearing age must be considered and is a complication in burn management. A pregnant female with TBSA burns of 60% or more or who has suffered an inhalation injury is at high risk for loss of that pregnancy.

As with all burn patients, airway stabilization and management are the first and most important concerns. Hypoxia is not tolerated by the fetus and will cause premature labor or abortion, or both.

Constant fetal monitoring is important, particularly in the second or third trimester, to determine fetal distress. Early consultation with both an obstetrician and a burn center physician is imperative.

Delayed or inadequate fluid resuscitation may also cause premature labor or loss of the pregnancy, or both. Response to fluid resuscitation must be closely monitored because fluid needs may exceed calculated amounts. Electrolyte disturbances, alterations in clotting factors, and depletion of fibrinogen and platelets are common complications in pregnant burn patients.

Pregnant patients require that there be no delay in assessment, management, and consultation to ensure viability of the fetus. Transfer to a burn center is recommended.

The Elderly: Special Considerations

The elderly individual is at an increased risk both for getting burned and for experiencing delayed recovery and complications after a burn injury. Many of the elderly live alone. Diminished vision may affect perceptual judgment and cause injuries while working around heaters, stoves, open flames, hot water, and electricity. Visual impairment may also make it impossible for an elderly person to read labels and may lead to a chemical injury. Short-term memory may be impaired and cause an elderly person to forget about lighted cigarettes or to forget the stove is on. Decreased skin sensation may lead to severe burns from bathing in water that is too hot or from a malfunctioning heating pad. Decreased mobility may prevent rapid evacuation once a fire starts.

The possibility that an elderly burn patient may have been a victim of abuse exists. Examine the patient's entire body for wounds, bruises, and scars. Question the patient, family members, or individuals who accompanied the patient to the hospital to determine how the injury occurred. Consult with other members of the health team if the injury does not fit the explanation of the incident, if conflicting explanations are given, or if the explanation of the incident keeps changing. Report incidents of abuse to the proper authorities.

Patients older than 50 years are considered to be at high risk after even a minor burn injury. Pruitt showed a 75% mortality rate for patients older than 60 years with a burn as small as 25% to 30% TBSA. Many factors increase mortality in the elderly. Because of the aging process, the skin is thinner and has less elasticity. This increases the susceptibility of the patient to a deeper burn injury because the muscle tissues and bone are closer to the body surface. The geriatric patient may also be malnourished, which slows wound healing and increases the risk of infection.

Preexisting disorders affect the individual's ability to survive a burn injury. Chronic diseases of the heart, lungs, kidney, and liver are more common in the elderly because of physiologic deterioration associated with the aging process. Elderly patients very often have histories of congestive heart failure, coronary artery disease, diabetes, and chronic respiratory disorders that complicate their recovery from the burn injury. Impaired function of these vital organs is a significant factor in the high mortality rate.

Special care must be taken in the fluid resuscitation of the geriatric patient because of decreased ability of the aging cardiovascular system to adjust to fluctuations in circulating fluid volume. Pruitt noted that, despite careful management, 15% of the patients in his geriatric study died within the first 5 days after burn from either over- or under-fluid resuscitation. Very often these patients experience pulmonary edema and cardiac failure during fluid resuscitation. Monitor vital signs, urine output, electrocardiogram, and cardiac output for signs of cardiac failure. Ambulate the elderly patient as soon as possible, and provide frequent pulmonary hygiene to minimize the risk of circulatory and respiratory complications and the hazards of immobility.

A major concern in burn-wound management is delayed eschar separation in a full-thickness injury as a result of decreased peripheral blood flow common in the elderly. Delayed separation increases susceptibility to infection and slows wound healing. Impaired blood flow also delays revascularization and the growth of granulation tissue. Skin grafting may be delayed, and the risk of graft failure is greater. Handle all burned areas gently to prevent further trauma. Maintain meticulous aseptic wound care to prevent infection and to promote wound closure.

Finally, many times the geriatric patient loses his or her determination to survive. Loss of the will to live and depression are especially common in elderly patients who have lost their home and possessions in the fire. Personal possessions are often memories of a lifetime. Elderly patients may associate hospitals with death or become disoriented in unfamiliar surroundings. It is necessary to use the resources of the entire burn team to support the patient in this crisis. A sympathetic ear or conversations with a social worker, psychiatrist, or clergy might prove more beneficial than use of antidepressant or tranquilizing medications, which may alter the patient's sensorium and worsen the problem.

Successful treatment of the geriatric burn patient is one of the most difficult challenges in all of burn care.

Bibliography

Agee RN, et al. Xenon 133 lung scan for early diagnosis of inhalation injury. Paper presented at the American Burn Association Conference, March 1975.

Arturson MG. The pathophysiology of severe thermal injury. J Burn Care Rehabil 1985; 6(2):129.

Artz CP. Changing concept of electrical injury. A J Surg 1974; 128:600.

Artz CP. Electrical injury. In Artz CP, Moncrief JA, Pruitt BA (eds). Burns: A team approach, Philadelphia; WB Saunders, 1979, pp. 351–362.

Artz CP, Gibson T. Current concepts, management of burns. Mili Med 1976; 141:673.

Artz CP, Moncrief JA. Treatment of burns. 2nd ed. Philadelphia: WB Saunders, 1969.

Asch MJ, Moylan JA Jr, Bruck HM, et al. Ocular complications associated with burns: Review of a 5 year experience including 104 patients. J Trauma 1971; 11:857.

Baxter CR. Present concepts in the management of major electrical injuries. Surg Clin North Am 1970; 50:1401.

Baxter CR. Crystalloid resuscitation of burn shock. In Polk HC, Stone HH (eds). Contemporary burn management. Boston: Little, Brown, 1971.

Baxter CR. Response to initial fluid and electrolyte therapy of burn shock. In Lynch JB, Lewis SR (eds). Symposium on treatment of burns. St. Louis: CV Mosby, 1973.

Baxter CR, Marvin JA, Curreri PW. Early management of thermal burns. Postgrad Med 1974; 55:131.

Blunt CP. Treatment of hydrofluoric acid skin burns by injection with calcium gluconate. Ind Med Surg 1964; 33:869.

Bromberg BE, Song IC, Walden RH. Hydrotherapy of chemical burns. Plast Reconstr Surg 1965; 35:85.

Burgraff V, Stanley M. Nursing the elderly: A care plan approach. Philadelphia: JB Lippincott, 1989.

Caldwell FT. Etiology and control of postburn hypermetabolism. J Burn Care Rehabil 1991; 12(5):385.

Carpenito LJ. Nursing diagnosis: Application to practice. 4th ed. Philadelphia: JB Lippincott, 1992.

Curreri PW. Chemical burns. In Artz CP, Moncrief JA, Pruitt BA (eds). Burns: A team approach. Philadelphia: WB Saunders, 1979, pp 363–369.

Curreri PW, Asch MJ, Pruitt BA. The treatment of chemical burns: Specialized diagnostic, therapeutic and prognostic considerations. J Trauma 1970; 10:634.

Demling RH. Symposium on burns: Fluid and electrolyte management. Crit Care Clin 1985; 1(1):27.

Doenges ME, Moorhouse MF. Nurse's pocket guide: Nursing diagnoses with interventions. 4th ed. Philadelphia: FA Davis, 1993.

Dolan JT. Critical care nursing: Clinical management through the nursing process. Philadelphia: FA Davis, 1991.

Duncan DJ, Driscoll DM. Burn wound management. Crit Care Nurs Clin North Am 1991; 3(2):199.

Eliopoulos C. Gerontological nursing. 3rd ed. Philadelphia: JB Lippincott, 1993.

Farrell J. Nursing care of the older person. Philadelphia: JB Lippincott, 1990.

Fishbach F. A manual of laboratory & diagnostic tests. 4th ed. Philadelphia: JB Lippincott, 1992.

Flack AN, Scofield PD. Hydrofluoric acid burn. In Med 1947; 16:17.

Gerding RL, et al. Outpatient management of partial thickness burns: Biobrane versus 1% silver sulfadiazine. J Burn Care Rehabil 1990; 19(2):121.

Goff DR, Purdue GE, Hunt JL, et al. Cardiac disease and the patient with burns. J Burn Care Rehabil 1990; 11(4):3[illegible].

Goodwin CW, Pruitt BA Jr. The massive burn with sepsis and Curling's ulcer. In Hardy JD (ed). Critical surgical illness. 2nd ed. Philadelphia: WB Saunders, 1980, pp 211–233.

Gordon M. Nursing diagnosis: Process and application. St. Louis: CV Mosby, 1991.

Haller JA, et al. Pathophysiology and management of acute corrosive burns of the esophagus: Results of treatment in 285 children. J Pediatr Surg 1971; 6:578.

Hefton JM, Madden MR, Finkelstein JL, Shires GT. [illegible]fting of burn patients with allografts of cultured epidermal [illegible] Lancet 1983; 2:428.

Hunt JL, et al. Fiberoptic bronchoscopy in acute inhalation injury. J Trauma 1975; 15:641.

Jelenko C. Chemicals that burn. J Trauma 1974; 14:65.

Jones RJ, Samson PC. Esophageal injury. Ann Thorac Surg 1975; 19:216.

Karb VB, et al. Handbook of drugs for nursing practice. St. Louis: CV Mosby, 1989.

Kouwenhoven WB. Effects of electricity on the human body. Electrical Engineering 1949; 68:199.

Kravitz M. Thermal injuries. In Cardona VD, Hurn PD, Mason PJB, et al (eds). Trauma nursing: From resuscitation through rehabilitation. Philadelphia: WB Saunders, 1988, 707–745.

Lewis BK. Chemical burns. A J Surg 1959; 8:928.

Long JM. Burns in geriatric patients. In Artz CP, Moncrief JA, Pruitt BA (eds). Burns: A team approach. Philadelphia: WB Saunders, 1979, pp 334–340.

Lund CC, Browder NC. Estimation of areas of burns. Surg Gynecol Obstet 1944; 79:352.

Luterman A, et al. Treatment of chemical burns. Emerg Med Serv 1988; 17(9):36.

Martin LM. Nursing implications of today's burn care techniques. RN 1989; 52(5):26.

Merell SW, et al. Increased survival after major thermal injury. Am J Surg 1987; 154(12):623.

Miller SF, et al. Burn size estimate reliability: A study. J Burn Care Rehabil 1991; 12(6):546.

Moritz AR, et al. The effects of inhaled heat on the air passages and lungs; An experimental investigation. Am J Pathol 1945; 21:311.

Moylan JA, et al. Fiberoptic bronchoscopy following thermal injuries. Surg Gynecol Obstet 1975; 140:541.

NANDA nursing diagnoses: Definitions and classifications. St. Louis, North American Nursing Diagnosis Association, 1992.

Nebraska Burn Institute, St. Elizabeth Community Health Center, Lincoln Medical Educational Foundation. Advanced burn life support course: Instructor's manual. Lincoln, NE: Nebraska Burn Institute, 1990.

Nebraska Burn Institute, St. Elizabeth Community Health Center, Lincoln Medical Educational Foundation. Pre-hospital advanced burn life support course manual. Lincoln, NE: Nebraska Burn Institute, 1991.

Petroff PA, Pruitt, BA Jr. Pulmonary disease in the burn patient. In Artz CP, Moncrief JA, Pruitt BA (eds). Burns: A team approach. Philadelphia: WB Saunders, 1979, pp 95–106.

Pruitt BA Jr. Management of burns in the multiple injury patient. Surg Clin North Am 1970; 50:1283.

Pruitt BA Jr. Other complications of burn injury. In Artz CP, Moncrief JA, Pruitt BA (eds). A team approach. Philadelphia: WB Saunders, 1979, pp 523–552.

Pruitt BA Jr, et al. Burn injury in the aged or high-risk patient. In Siegel JH, Chadoff PD (eds). The aged and high risk surgical patient. New York: Grune & Stratton, 1976, p 523.

Robins EV. Burn shock. Crit Care Nurs Clin North Am 1990; 2(2):299.

Saffle JR, et al. The continuing challenge of burn care in the elderly. Surgery 1990; 108(3):534.

Shannon MT, Wilson BA. Govoni & Hayes drugs and nursing implications. 7th ed. Norwalk, CT: Appleton & Lange, 1992.

Smith GA, Savinski-Bozinko G. Giving emergency care for burns. Nursing 1989; 19(9):55.

Sommers M. Rapid fluid resuscitation: How to correct dangerous deficits. Nursing 1990; 20(1):52.

Sommers MS. Fluid resuscitation following multiple trauma. Crit Care Nurse 1990; 10(10):74.

Summers TM. Psychosocial support of the burned patient. Crit Care Nurs Clin North Am 1991; 3(2):237.

Taddonio TE, et al. A survey of wound monitoring and topical antimicrobial therapy practices in the treatment of burn injury. J Burn Care Rehabil 1990; 11(5):423.

Thompson P, et al. Effect of early excision on patients with major thermal injury. J Trauma 1987; 27(2):205.

Wilkinson AW. Limited volume therapy with colloids. In Polk HC, Stone HH (eds). Contemporary burn management. Boston: Little, Brown, 1971.

Wilmore DW. Nutrition and metabolism following thermal injury. Clin Plast Surg 1974; 1:603.

Wilmore DW, et al. Effects of ambient temperatures on heat production and heat loss in burn patients. J Appl Physiol 1975; 38:575.

Unit Three

ADULTS WITH IMMUNE DYSFUNCTION

Learning Objectives

AFTER COMPLETING THIS UNIT, THE LEARNER WILL BE ABLE TO:

Chapter Nine

1. Explain the normal anatomy and physiology of the immune system.
2. Identify information and physical examination data essential to the assessment of immune status.
3. Describe basic diagnostic tests and modalities of medical management (immunizations, immunosuppressive therapy) used in the treatment of patients with immune disorders.
4. Describe bone marrow aspiration and bone marrow transplantation.
5. Identify data essential to the assessment of patients undergoing bone marrow aspiration and transplantation.
6. State nursing diagnoses and related expected patient outcomes commonly applicable to patients undergoing bone marrow aspiration and transplantation.
7. Describe nursing interventions, with their rationales, commonly applicable to patients undergoing bone marrow aspiration and transplantation.
8. Explain the basis for evaluation of nursing care provided to patients undergoing bone marrow aspiration and transplantation.
9. Identify special considerations for the elderly patient with altered immune function.

Chapter Ten

1. Describe common immune disorders in terms of etiology, pathophysiology, clinical manifestations, diagnostic procedures, and medical management.
2. Identify information and physical examination data essential to the assessment of patients with common immune disorders.
3. State nursing diagnoses and related expected patient outcomes commonly applicable to patients with immune disorders.
4. Describe nursing interventions, with their rationales, commonly applicable to patients with immune disorders.
5. Explain the basis for evaluation of nursing care provided to patients with common immune disorders.
6. Identify special considerations for the elderly patient with an immune disorder.

Chapter Eleven

1. Explain the normal anatomy and physiology of the cell.
2. Describe cancer in terms of etiology, pathophysiology, clinical manifestations, diagnostic procedures, and medical management (surgery, radiation, chemotherapy).
3. Identify information and physical examination data essential to the assessment of patients with cancer.
4. State nursing diagnoses and related expected patient outcomes commonly applicable to patients with cancer.
5. Describe nursing interventions with their rationales commonly applicable to patients with cancer.
6. Explain the basis for evaluation of nursing care provided to patients with cancer.
7. Identify special considerations for the elderly patient with cancer.

Chapter Nine

KNOWLEDGE BASIC TO THE NURSING CARE *of Adults with Immune Dysfunction*

Immunity is controlled by a very elaborate, highly sophisticated system—the immune system. The classic use of the term *immunity* referred only to the body's resistance to reinfection by a specific microorganism. As knowledge of immunity and the immune system expanded, the meaning of the term *immunity* has also been expanded. A contemporary definition of immunity is the ability of the body to distinguish between self and non-self and to neutralize or eliminate foreign materials without injuring its own tissues. The immune system is a complex defense system that protects the body from exogenous and endogenous agents that are capable of causing disease. A properly functioning immune system is essential for the smooth functioning of all the other body systems. The immune system protects the body by destroying foreign materials. This destruction must be precise and well-controlled or it can result in damage to normal tissues.

The immune system has three primary functions: defense, surveillance, and homeostasis (Table 9–1). Defense provides protection against external "foreign invaders," primarily microorganisms that try to gain entry to the body. Surveillance provides protection from internal "foreign invaders" such as malignant cells. Homeostasis provides the body with "cleanup operations." Cells of the immune system remove dead and damaged cells from all parts of the body.

The immune system's ability to carry out these functions depends on two key factors. One of these factors is the ability of the immune system to recognize and react to a wide variety of foreign substances without reacting to its own normal tissues. This ability is referred to as recognition of non-self and self-tolerance. During embryonic development the immune system learns which antigens (substances that produce a detectable immune response when introduced into a host) belong to it and comes to recognize these antigens as being self. After birth it does not normally respond to these self-antigens. Breakdown of this self-tolerance is thought to be the basic pathologic mechanism of the autoimmune diseases (conditions in which the body reacts against itself and causes damage). The ability of the body not to respond to self must be as specific as its ability to respond to foreign antigens.

Table 9–1. FUNCTIONS OF THE IMMUNE SYSTEM

FUNCTIONAL CATEGORY	PHYSIOLOGIC EFFECT
Defense	Provides protection against invaders from outside the body, such as microorganisms.
Surveillance	Protects the body from internal threats, such as malignant cells.
Homeostasis	Maintains the internal environment by removing dead or damaged cells.

The immune system's other key feature is memory. The immune system is able to "remember" things it has learned. During the first exposure to an antigen, some of the immunologically active cells become memory cells. These cells are programmed to respond to that specific antigen. Upon encountering that antigen again, these memory cells initiate the immunologic responses that are appropriate for that antigen. Unfortunately this memory cannot be passed on from parent to child.

Anatomy and Physiology

Lymphoid Organs

The immune system has no one specific anatomic site. It consists of a complex network of organs and cells that are dispersed throughout the body. The organs of the immune system are connected with each other by lymphatic ducts and blood vessels. Several organs, such as the liver and spleen, have immune functions as well as other functions.

The organs that function in the immune system are often referred to as lymphoid organs and are classified as generative (central or primary) and peripheral (or secondary) organs. The generative lymphoid organs are those in which lymphocytes arise and mature. The two generative lymphoid organs in the human are the thymus and the bone marrow. The peripheral lymphoid organs include the lymph nodes, spleen, liver, tonsils, and Peyer's patches of the intestine. Peripheral lymph organs filter foreign particles and microorganisms from blood and lymph. They also serve as the location in which the mature cells of the immune system interact with each other and react with antigens.

GENERATIVE LYMPHOID ORGANS

THYMUS GLAND

The thymus gland is located in the mediastinal cavity, anterior to and above the heart. The thymus grows from birth to puberty. At puberty, the thymus weighs approximately 40 g. Undifferentiated stem cells from the bone marrow migrate to and enter the thymus gland. In 2 to 3 days these cells acquire a new function and new surface markers as they mature into T lymphocytes (T cells). The mature T cells enter the blood stream via the postcapillary venules of the thymus and then travel to the peripheral lymph organs (Fig. 9–1). T cells are responsible for cell-mediated immunity. The thymus gland also produces a hormone that increases the number of lymphocytes in the peripheral lymphoid organs.

After puberty, the thymus begins to atrophy, and in the mature adult it is a relatively functionless, shriveled mass of fatty tissue. This loss of thymic

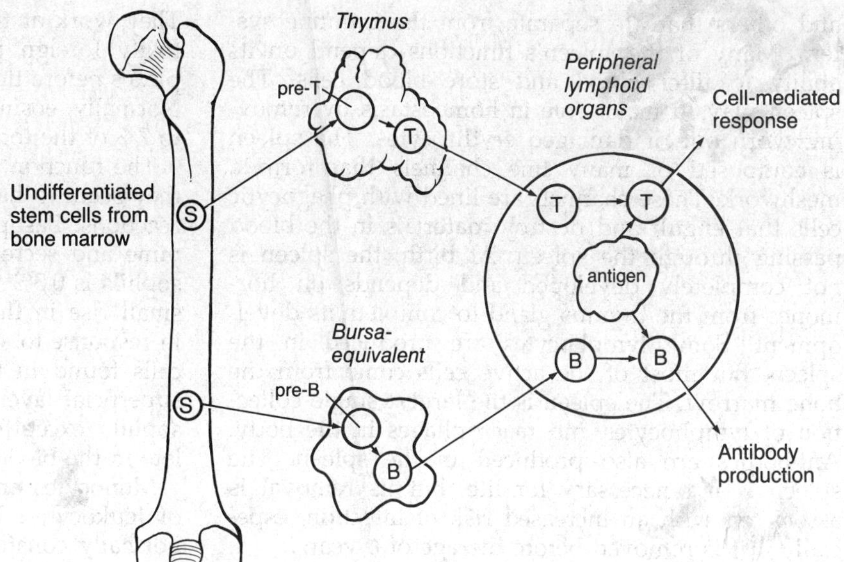

Figure 9–1.

Undifferentiated stem cells move from the bone marrow to either the thymus gland or the bursa-equivalent, where they are transformed into T cells or B cells. They then move to one of the secondary lymphoid organs, where they may contact an antigen and become activated.

function is thought to be responsible for some of the immune deficiencies seen in the elderly. As thymic function decreases with age, the incidence of malignancies and autoimmune diseases increases.

BONE MARROW

The bone marrow is the area of the body where undifferentiated stem cells are transformed into mature B lymphocytes (B cells).

The bone marrow is a highly vascular, sinusoidal tissue that is dispersed within the bones of the body. If it was put all together, its total weight and volume would be about that of the liver. In the adult, active bone marrow is found in the bones of the ribs, sternum, pelvis, skull, femur, and humerus. Active bone marrow is essential for life.

PERIPHERAL LYMPHOID ORGANS

LYMPH NODES

The lymph nodes and other peripheral lymphoid organs are strategically clustered in areas of the body where contact with external antigens is most likely, that is, around areas of the body exposed to the external environment—the respiratory, gastrointestinal, and genitourinary tracts. In addition, the vascular connections of the liver and spleen make them likely to contact internal antigens. This helps increase the chances that an antigen whether external or internal will quickly encounter the active cells of the immune system and be destroyed before disease occurs.

There are more than 500 lymph nodes in the body, varying from the size of a pinhead to that of a lima bean. Lymph nodes contain lymphocytes, plasma cells, macrophages, granulocytes, and a few erythrocytes. The lymph nodes have several important functions. One of these is to filter lymph and remove foreign material and other particulate matter from it. Another is to provide a place where immunologically active cells and antigens can come together and interact with each other. As a result of this interaction with antigen, antibody is produced and phagocytic cells are stimulated. These antibodies and phagocytic cells are released into the general circulation via lymph leaving the lymph node. Lymph nodes containing B cells and T cells that have been antigenically stimulated may increase in size and become palpable. Enlarged lymph nodes are an important clinical sign that an immune response is occurring somewhere in the region of the body that drains into the enlarged node.

Lymph nodes are connected by the lymphatic system, which, in addition to the nodes, is composed of a network of capillaries, vessels, and ducts. Each lymph node drains a distinct region of the body. This region is determined by the location of the lymphatic vessels that flow to the node. The walls of these lymphatic capillaries and vessels are only one cell thick, so substances such as plasma proteins can be picked up from the interstitial spaces of the connective tissues. Capillaries join to form vessels along which the lymph nodes are located. The lymph vessels eventually unite to form the thoracic duct, which joins the venous system at the juncture of the left internal jugular vein and the subclavian vein. Lymph from the right side of the head and neck, the right arm, and the thorax flows to the right lymph duct, which joins the venous system at the juncture of the right subclavian vein and the internal jugular vein.

SPLEEN

The spleen, a peripheral lymphoid organ, has many functions, some of which are immunologic and others that are separate from the immune system. Many of the spleen's functions depend on its ability to filter blood and store blood cells. The spleen plays a major role in homeostasis by removing worn out or damaged erythrocytes. The spleen is composed of many fine channels that form a meshwork. These channels are lined with phagocytic cells that engulf and destroy materials in the blood passing through the spleen. At birth, the spleen is not completely developed and depends on hormones from the thymus gland to complete its development. Some lymphocytes are produced in the spleen, but most of the active cells come from the bone marrow. The spleen is the largest single collection of lymphocytes and macrophages in the body. Antibodies are also produced in the spleen. The spleen is not necessary for life, but its removal is associated with an increased risk of infection, especially if it is removed before the age of 6 years.

TONSILS AND PEYER'S PATCHES

The tonsils of the oropharynx and Peyer's patches of the small intestine contain collections of lymphocytes and macrophages as well as memory cells. These organs are most important in the secondary immune response and may play a role in the primary immune response. These organs may enlarge in size as they become very active in the immune response.

LIVER

The liver contains a large number of fixed macrophages called Kupffer's cells. These Kupffer's cells help filter blood by phagocytizing microorganisms and other foreign particles passing through the liver.

Cells of the Immune System

The white blood cells, or leukocytes, are the cells responsible for immune functions. There are five kinds of leukocytes: polymorphonuclear leukocytes, monocytes, macrophages, lymphocytes, and plasma cells. Each type of cell has a specialized role in the body's defense system.

The polymorphonuclear leukocytes (also called granulocytes) are primarily involved in the acute inflammatory process. Three types of polymorphonuclear leukocytes are neutrophils, eosinophils, and basophils.

Neutrophils make up 50% to 75% of the total white blood cell count. These cells are able to quickly phagocytize large numbers of bacteria and are one of the first lines of defense against infection. The number of neutrophils frequently rises during an infection.

Eosinophils are also phagocytic but respond primarily in allergic reactions, rather than to infection. They work at the site of tissue inflammation to detoxify foreign proteins and antigen-antibody complexes before these substances can damage the body. Normally, eosinophils constitute approximately 0.3% to 7% of the total white cell count.

The function of basophils is not entirely clear, but they seem to have a role in mediating inflammatory reactions. Basophils contain large amounts of histamine and secrete heparin. The normal value of basophils is 0.3% to 2% of the total white cell count. A small rise in the number of basophils may be seen in response to stress and chronic inflammation. Mast cells found in the lungs, gastrointestinal tract, and superficial layers of the skin are very similar to basophils, except they are immobile and do not circulate in the blood.

Monocytes and macrophages are two other types of leukocytes. Monocytes are found in blood and normally constitute 0.6% to 9.6% of the total white cell count. Monocytes migrate into tissue and become macrophages. Both monocytes and macrophages have great phagocytic ability and are able to ingest large numbers of microorganisms and other foreign materials. Some macrophages, called fixed macrophages or histiocytes, remain in one place in body tissues and do not travel around in the blood. Areas where these fixed macrophages are found are the spleen, Kupffer cells of the liver, pulmonary alveoli, and the gastrointestinal tract. Other monocytes circulate freely in the blood, leaving the blood vessels when needed to localize and contain invaders at the site of an injury.

Lymphocytes and plasma cells are the leukocytes responsible for the specific immune response. Lymphocytes normally make up approximately 25% of the total white cell count. There are two types of lymphocytes: T lymphocytes (T cells) and B lymphocytes (B cells). T cells are responsible for cellular immunity, and B cells are responsible for humoral immunity. T cells and B cells have distinct functions but are dependent on each other for proper functioning. The lymphocytes are the immunologic cells that have the important properties of specificity and memory (Table 9–2).

T LYMPHOCYTES (T CELLS)

T cells are responsible for the cellular or cell-mediated response. The cellular response involves tissue reactions that do not require antibodies produced by B cells. Cellular immunity is thought to primarily protect against infection caused by intracellular microorganisms, viruses, and slow-growing bacteria as well as being responsible for the rejection of allografts and malignantly transformed cells. T cells normally constitute 80% to 90% of the total circulating lymphocyte population. From the thymus, where they are produced, T cells travel to the peripheral lymphoid organs, take up residence and carry out their immunologic functions. The functions

Table 9–2. CLASSIFICATION OF LEUKOCYTES

TYPE OF LEUKOCYTE	ROLE IN IMMUNE FUNCTION
POLYMORPHONUCLEAR LEUKOCYTES	Primarily involved in the acute inflammatory response
Neutrophils	Phagocytic cells that are important in defense against infections
Eosinophils	Phagocytic cells that are important in allergic reactions and helminthic infections
Basophils	Release chemical mediators of the allergic reaction
MONOCYTES	Phagocytic cells that attract other cells to the area
MACROPHAGES	Phagocytes that are able to ingest large numbers of microorganisms
LYMPHOCYTES	Responsible for the specific immune response
T cells	Responsible for cellular immunity
B cells	Responsible for humoral immunity
PLASMA CELLS	Fully differentiated B cells that have been stimulated by an antigen and are actively producing antibodies
NATURAL KILLER CELLS	Nonselectively attack unhealthy or abnormal self cells as well as nonself cells

of the T cells include the following: mediation of delayed hypersensitivity reactions through the release of lymphokines (substances produced by T cells that alter the physiology of other cells); destruction of other cells (cytolytic reactions) such as virus-infected cells and tumor cells; and regulation of the type and intensity of virtually all aspects of the specific immune response.

There are several functionally distinct subsets of T cells. Each T cell has one specific function, they are not multifunctional cells. The subsets of T cells are named for the function they perform. They include helper cells, suppressor cells, cytotoxic (killer) cells, and memory cells (Table 9–3). These cells all function in controlling the specific immune response.

Helper T cells (also called inducer cells, T4 cells, or $CD4^+$ [because they carry the most CD4 surface molecule] T cells) usually constitute approximately 60% of the total circulating T cells. Helper T cells interact with B cells to induce antibody production. Some antigens, especially those of low molecular weight, are unable to induce antibody production by themselves. Most antigens interact with the helper T cells, and the helper T cells then induce antibody production by the B cells. Helper T cells also induce other types of T cells and macrophages to become active.

Suppressor T cells (also called T8 Cells) inhibit the activities of other T cells and B cells. They turn the immune response off. The usual ratio of helper T cells to suppressor T cells is 2:1. This ratio is reversed in some diseases, for example, acquired immunodeficiency syndrome (AIDS).

Table 9–3. T-CELL SUBSETS

TYPE OF T CELL	FUNCTION
Helper T cells	Stimulate activity of other immunologically active cells.
Suppressor T cells	Turn off activity of other immunologically active cells.
Cytotoxic (killer) T cells	Kill cells targeted by IgG antibody bound to the cell's surface.
Memory T cells	Remember antigen and respond immediately on succeeding exposures to it.

Cytotoxic (killer) T cells (K cells) are able to kill cells that have been targeted by immunoglobulin G (IgG) antibody bound to the cells' surface. The killer T cells are dependent on the presence of specific IgG antibody.

Memory T cells are another important subset of T cells. Once T cells have been stimulated by an antigen, some T cells become memory cells. These cells appear in the blood approximately 5 days after the primary exposure to an antigen. They continually travel through the blood to every anatomic site that has a blood supply. This allows the memory T cells to come in contact with the antigen wherever it should enter the body in the future. The next time a memory T cell contacts its specific antigen, it undergoes proliferation and differentiation to effector cell in a matter of hours. These effector cells are then able to stimulate other immune cells to respond to the antigen, and the immune response is quickly set into motion.

Natural killer cells (NK cells), although similar to T cells, are not considered a true T-cell subset. Natural killer cells are cytotoxic to targeted cells. Their action is unique in that prior sensitization to the targeted cell is not necessary and it occurs independently of other leukocytes. The cytotoxic action of NK cells seems to be most effective against self cells that are either infected by a virus or that have undergone malignant transformation. NK cells also destroy foreign cells and thus play a role in the rejection of grafts and transplanted organs.

B LYMPHOCYTES (B CELLS)

B cells are responsible for the production of antibodies. The protection that results from the presence of these antibodies in blood and body fluids is referred to as humoral immunity. Humoral immunity is important in the defense against pyogenic infections and in combating the effects of toxins produced by microorganisms. Stem cells are transformed into B cells in the bone marrow. Unstimulated B cells are stimulated either directly by an antigen or by lymphokines from a T cell that has recognized an antigen. Once stimulated, the B cell enlarges, divides, and is transformed into plasma cells and memory B cells. The plasma cells are the cells that actually produce and secrete antibody. Plasma cells are predominantly located in the peripheral lymphoid tissues and are seldom found in peripheral blood. Plasma cells may be found in the peripheral blood in multiple myeloma, scarlet fever, measles, chickenpox, or other severe infection.

B cells are controlled and regulated by the helper and suppressor T cells. The helper T cells turn on or increase antibody production in B cells; suppressor T cells decrease the amount of antibody produced by the B cells. A delicate balance between T-cell subsets and B cells is required to maintain immunologic balance. If this balance is disrupted, disease may result because of either too little antibody production or too much antibody production.

Immune Response

There are two types of immune responses: nonspecific and specific. The nonspecific responses are considered the body's first line of defense. They are primarily responsible for defense against outside invaders, and their importance is frequently underestimated. Intact nonspecific responses present a formidable barrier to the microorganisms that are constantly trying to invade the host. The nonspecific responses can differentiate self from non-self but cannot identify the specific invader. Nonspecific responses are functioning at birth, do not need to be learned, and respond in the same way to all invaders (Table 9–4).

NONSPECIFIC IMMUNE RESPONSE

The nonspecific responses can be grouped into five categories: physical barriers, chemical barriers, interferon, inflammation, and phagocytosis.

Table 9–4. DIFFERENCES BETWEEN SPECIFIC AND NONSPECIFIC IMMUNITY

SPECIFIC IMMUNITY	NONSPECIFIC IMMUNITY
Second line of defense against infections.	First line of defense against infections.
Able to identify specific antigens.	Unable to identify specific antigens.
Reacts differently to different antigens.	Reacts the same to all antigens.
Response needs to be learned and developed.	Present and functioning at birth.

PHYSICAL BARRIERS

Physical barriers help keep microorganisms out of the body. Intact skin and mucous membranes are very effective at keeping most microorganisms out. Coughing and sneezing help expel microorganisms from the respiratory tract. The action of the cilia lining the respiratory tract also helps remove microorganisms before they can get into the lungs. The flushing action of fluids such as urine and tears helps remove microorganisms from their respective body openings.

CHEMICAL BARRIERS

Chemical barriers include various acids and enzymes found in body fluids. Sebaceous secretions contain lactic acid and unsaturated fatty acids, which are active against both bacteria and fungi. Areas of the body with no sebaceous glands, such as between the toes, are frequently the sites of fungal infections. Lysozyme, found in tears, nasal secretions, saliva, and urine, is an enzyme that destroys the cell wall of gram-positive bacteria and to a lesser extent gram-negative bacteria. The highly acid pH of the stomach is very effective at eliminating most of the microorganisms present in food and swallowed from the nose and mouth.

INTERFERON

Interferon is a protein produced by macrophages or lymphocytes, often in response to a viral infection. It protects cells that have not yet been infected by the virus by inducing the production of another protein in these cells, which in turn inhibits viral replication within them. This action does not appear to be virus specific, that is, the interferon produced in response to one type of virus protects cells against other types of viruses. However, interferon does appear to be species specific, in that the interferon produced by a rabbit is not effective in a mouse or a human. Interferon also has some immunoregulatory functions, in that it increases production of natural killer cells.

Interferon differs from antibody in several ways. Interferon is produced by several types of cells, whereas antibody is produced only by B lymphocytes. Interferon is effective against a wide variety of viruses; antibody is only effective against the one specific virus that stimulated its formation. Interferon works on the host's cells to induce protection, whereas antibody inactivates viruses outside the cells.

The lymphocytes in the spleen, liver, and lungs are important sites of interferon production. Synthesis of interferon begins almost immediately after a virus enters the cell. Blood levels of interferon are detectable in approximately 2 hours and persist for several days. Virus-neutralizing antibody appears in the blood about the time interferon levels are decreasing. Interferon is not constantly present in the blood or body fluids. It is found only immediately after an exposure to a virus.

Currently, there is much research on the therapeutic use of interferon. Interferon is being investigated in the treatment of some malignant diseases, the treatment of viral infections (especially chronic viral infections such as hepatitis), and as an aid in reducing the severity of viral infections, such as cytomegalovirus, in persons who are immunosuppressed (such as organ transplant recipients).

INFLAMMATION

Inflammation is a complex nonspecific response that occurs when tissue is injured by any means (physical, chemical, tissue anoxia, damage from microorganisms or their toxins). Inflammation is an attempt by the body to maintain homeostasis and repair the injured tissues. It is a protective response and normally not a harmful reaction. The classic signs of inflammation are redness, swelling, heat, and pain in the area of the injury.

The inflammatory reaction can be divided into three stages. During the first stage, the blood vessels in the area of the injury dilate and become more permeable in response to chemical mediators (histamine, serotonin, kinins, and complement proteins) that are released by the injured cells. This increases the flow of blood and lymph to the injured area and also increases the amount of fluid and cells that is released from the blood vessels. This increased fluid helps dilute and flush out any toxic materials that may be in the area. Neutrophils appear in the area in 30 to 60 minutes. Their prime purpose is to phagocytize (ingest and destroy) any potentially harmful agents such as microorganisms. In a few hours lymphocytes and monocytes arrive in the area. The monocytes also phagocytize any harmful agent. These cells all migrate to the area in response to chemotactic factors that have been released by the injured cells. Phagocytosis and exudate formation occur during the second stage. The exudate is composed of fluid and cells that have been drawn to the area. During the third stage, repair and regeneration of the injured tissue occur (Fig. 9–2).

PHAGOCYTOSIS

Phagocytosis, an important nonspecific immune response, is a process by which a particle is ingested and digested by a cell. Several types of leukocytes (monocytes, macrophages, neutrophils, and eosinophils) have phagocytic abilities. The goal of phagocytosis is to remove foreign substances such as microorganisms. To accomplish this, the phagocytic cell must travel to the area where the substance is, it must then ingest the substance, and finally destroy it. Phagocytes are attracted to the area by chemicals, called chemotactic factors, that are released from bacteria and other host cells, and components of complement (complement is a series of proteins found in the blood that can destroy bacteria when combined with antigen and antibody). Once a phagocyte encounters a microorganism, it attaches to the surface of the microorganism. The external membrane of the phagocyte then engulfs the organism and encloses it in a vesicle. This vesicle separates from the rest of the outer membrane and is internalized within the phagocytic cell, at which point it is called a phagosome (Fig. 9–3). Once internalized, most microorganisms are killed by the acid pH, lysozyme from other granules within the phagocyte, a reaction with a superoxide anion (an oxygen molecule that has had an electron removed, making it highly reactive), or most importantly by a reaction with hydrogen peroxide. However, some microorganisms are not killed once they are ingested by a phagocytic cell. *Mycobacterium tuberculosis*, for example, resists intracellular killing and may survive for long periods of time in macrophages. These viable organisms may spread to other areas of the body via the macrophages and then cause disease where they are deposited when the macrophage finally dies.

Some microorganisms are resistant to phagocytosis, especially those covered by a capsule, such as *Streptococcus pneumoniae* and *Cryptococcus neoformans*. Opsonization helps overcome this barrier to phagocytosis. Opsonization is the coating of the exterior of a microorganism or other foreign particle with a substance that makes the foreign particle more attractive to phagocytes. It is like putting frosting on a cake to make the cake more attractive and appetizing. Complement protein and antibody are the substances that usually serve as opsonins. Some microorganisms require more opsonization than others. "Rough" strains of bacteria may need only the complement factors, whereas the smooth or encapsulated strains need both the complement factors and antibody before they can be phagocytized.

Defects that may leave the host more susceptible to infections can occur at any step in the phagocytic process. For instance there may not be enough phagocytic cells in the body (neutropenia). This may be caused by an inherited disorder, such as congenital agranulocytosis or cyclic neutropenia, but is much more frequently seen as a result of a neoplastic disease or chemotherapy. Almost any medication has the potential to reduce the number of phagocytic cells either by direct cytotoxic effect on the cells or indirectly through immunologic mechanisms. Chemotherapeutic agents used to treat malignancies, sulfa drugs, and chloramphenicol are commonly used drugs that reduce the number of phagocytes.

When the number of polymorphonuclear neutrophils (PMNs) drops below $1000/mm^3$ of blood, the risk of infection rises. This risk of acquiring an infection rises even more if the number of PMNs falls below $500/mm^3$ of blood. Special precautions to protect the patient from infection may be instituted when the number of PMNs drops to these levels.

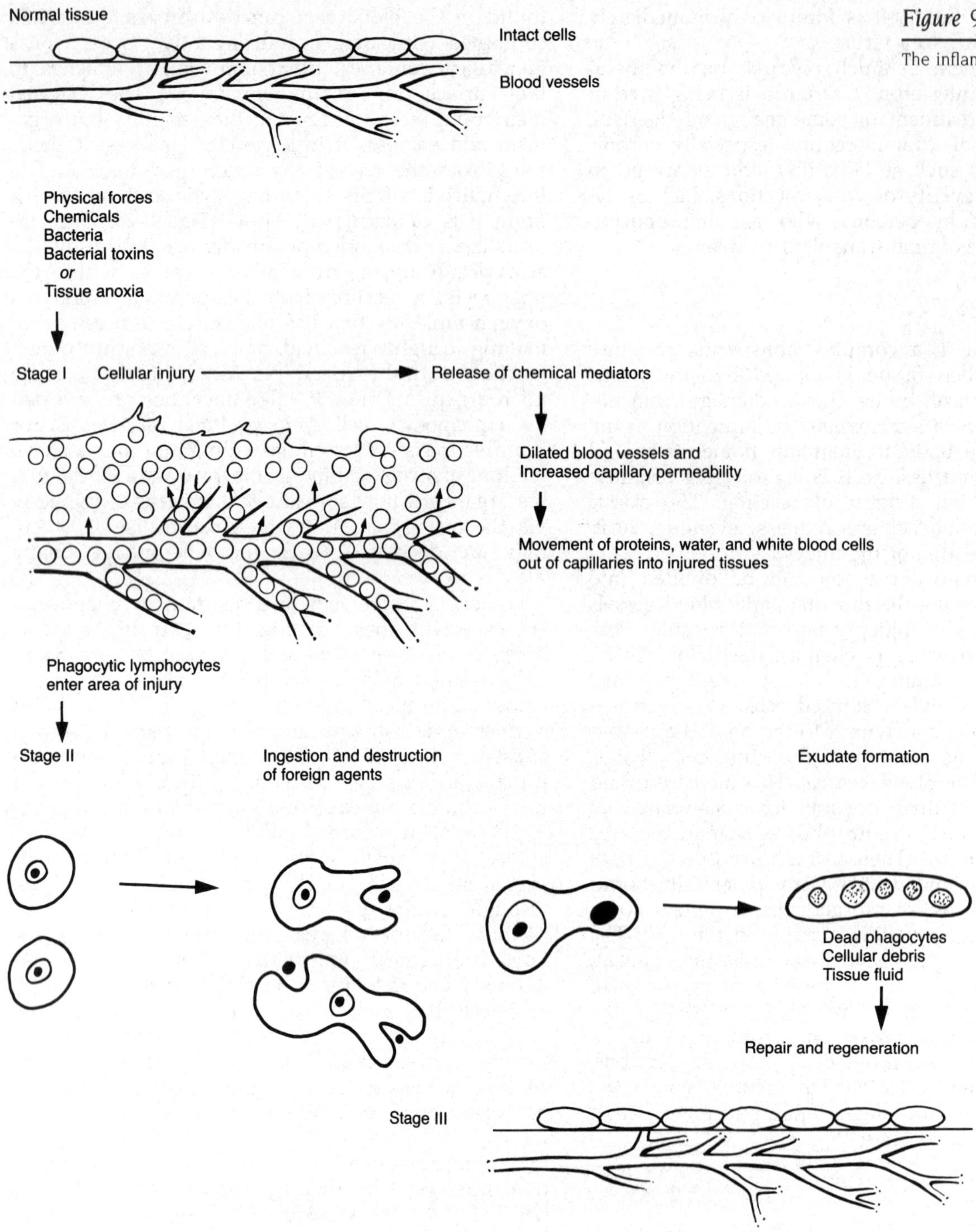

Figure 9–2.

The inflammatory response.

Patients with PMNs lower than 500/mm^3 are generally infected by their own organisms.

Phagocytosis may also be impaired by defects in the ability of the phagocytic cells to emigrate from the blood vessels to tissues or to adhere to tissues. Ingestion of large quantities of alcohol and the use of corticosteroids can decrease these abilities, thus impairing the host's phagocytic functions. Defects in the motility of the phagocytes have also been discovered. The defect can be either intrinsic in the cells, such as in rare disorders like Chediak-Higashi syndrome and juvenile periodontitis, or a defect in the chemotactic factors. Inactivation or inhibition of the chemotactic factors is seen in premature infants and patients with cirrhosis of the liver, Hodgkin's disease, systemic lupus erythematosus, or sarcoidosis.

Opsonization defects can also occur. Splenectomy may cause a defect in the ability to produce the opsonin for *Streptococcus pneumoniae.* This may contribute to the development of the severe pneumococcal infections to which these patients are prone. Pneumovax (a vaccine for several of the common strains of *S. pneumoniae*) can help reduce this susceptibility but should be given at least 1 month before splenectomy to be most effective.

The ability of the phagocyte to kill organisms that it has ingested may be defective. This is the basic pathologic mechanism in chronic granulomatous disease, which is an inherited disorder seen in children characterized by recurrent infections of the skin, lungs, bones, and lymph nodes.

Abnormal phagocytosis is usually manifested by recurrent bacterial infections with such organisms as staphylococci, gram-negative enteric bacteria, *Candida*, or *Aspergillus*. Infection may be found in any part of the body, but the most frequently infected sites are the skin and the respiratory tract. Medical evaluation of patients suspected of having defective phagocytosis involves a complete history and physical examination, complete blood count, bone marrow biopsy, and frequently a number of tests available only at special reference laboratories to evaluate all aspects of phagocytic function. Treatment for defects in phagocytosis is very limited. The most important aspect of care of these patients is early detection and prompt, proper treatment of infections.

SPECIFIC IMMUNE RESPONSE

The specific immune response is the body's surveillance system that recognizes foreign substances in the body and then selectively eliminates them through a complex series of immunologic responses. The specific immune response, both humoral and cellular, is initiated when an antigen makes its way past all the nonspecific defenses of the body and comes in contact with cells of the immune system. This response is highly specific in that it is effective against only the antigen that initiated it.

ANTIGEN

An antigen is a substance that produces a detectable immune response when introduced into a host. There are several factors that determine whether a substance (usually a molecule) is antigenic. One important factor is the size of the molecule. Generally, molecules with a molecular weight of less than 10,000 are only weak antigens or not antigenic at all. Molecules with a molecular weight over 100,000 are generally very potent antigens. Small molecules such as amino acids and monosaccharides are not antigenic, but large protein molecules are good antigens. A second factor is the chemical complexity of the molecule. Very simple molecules are poor antigens. More chemically complex molecules are better antigens. In addition, the host must be genetically able to respond to the substance, and the substance must be administered by the proper route and in an adequate dose. Too much or too little antigen may fail to cause an immune response.

Only a very small part of the antigen molecule is responsible for its immunologic activity and actual binding with antibody. This small part, which has the specific structure that makes it a unique antigen, is called the antigenic determinant or epitope.

Haptens are small molecules that alone are not antigenic but that may bind to another molecule and become antigenic. The antibody that is produced is specific for an antigenic determinant on the hapten not on the molecule to which the hapten is bound. Drugs (particularly penicillin) may act as haptens, becoming antigenic when bound to proteins in the body.

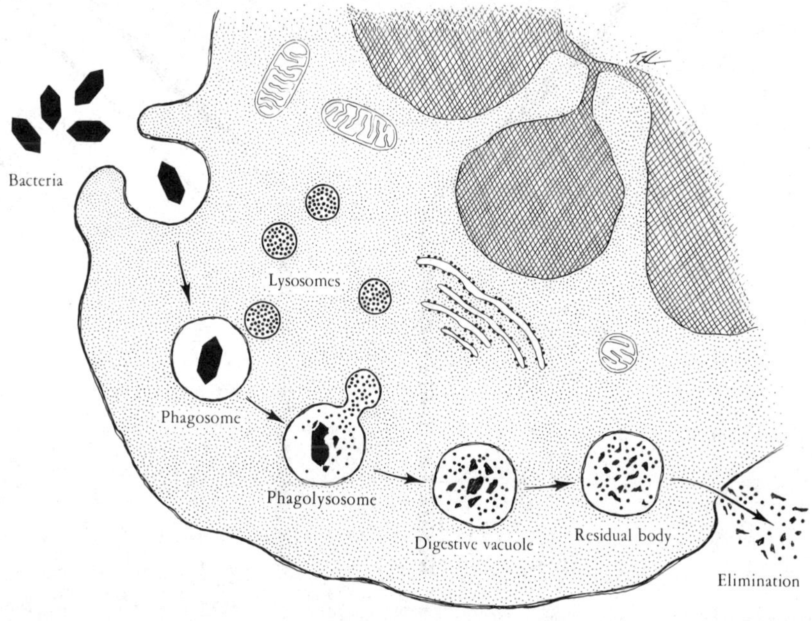

Figure 9–3.

Schematic representation of phagocytosis, showing ingestion process and intracellular digestion. (From Bellanti JA. Immunology III. Philadelphia: WB Saunders, 1985, p 18.)

ANTIBODIES

Antibodies, also called immunoglobulins (Ig), are specialized proteins. They are formed in response to an antigen and react specifically with that antigen. The function of antibody is to provide a specific and efficient mechanism to protect the body from foreign invaders. B cells are responsible for the production of antibodies.

The B cells are stimulated either directly by the antigen binding with the receptors on its surface or indirectly by T cells. Each B cell has a specific receptor site on the surface that reacts only with one specific antigen or a few very closely related antigens. In the lymph nodes, antigens that have been phagocytized by macrophages are presented to the B cell on the surface of the macrophage. This mechanism requires far less antigen than is required if the antigen directly stimulates the B cell. Some antigens cannot directly stimulate B cells and require the assistance of T cells to induce antibody production. Once the B cell is stimulated, it enlarges, divides, and transforms into plasma cells. The plasma cells mature and secrete antibody. Each plasma cell produces only one specific type of antibody.

There are five different classes of human antibodies (Table 9–5). They all have a similar structure, but each has a different role. The basic antibody molecule is composed of four polypeptide chains that are arranged in a Y-shape. There are two heavy chains and two light chains. Each chain has a constant region and on one end a variable region. The antigen-binding sites are found in the variable regions (Fig. 9–4).

Table 9–5. PROPERTIES OF ANTIBODY CLASSES

	IgG	IgA	IgM	IgD	IgE
Percentage of total circulating antibodies	70	21	7	≤0.2	≤0.5
Number of component molecules	1	2	5	1	1
Able to cross the placenta	Yes	No	No	No	No
Able to bind complement	Yes	No	Yes	No	No
Found in body secretions	?	Yes	No	No	No
Has a role in allergic reactions	Yes	?	No	?	Yes

The major serum antibody is IgG, constituting approximately 70% of the total circulating antibodies. IgG is antiviral, antibacterial, and effective against toxins. It can move into all body fluids and is the only antibody that crosses the placenta. It has a half-life of approximately 28 days.

IgA makes up approximately 21% of the total circulating antibodies. It is the main antibody found in external secretions such as tears, saliva, bronchial secretions, and colostrum. It is able to neutralize viruses and inhibit the attachment of bacteria to epithelial surfaces.

IgM is the first antibody produced in response to an antigen. Approximately 7% of the total serum

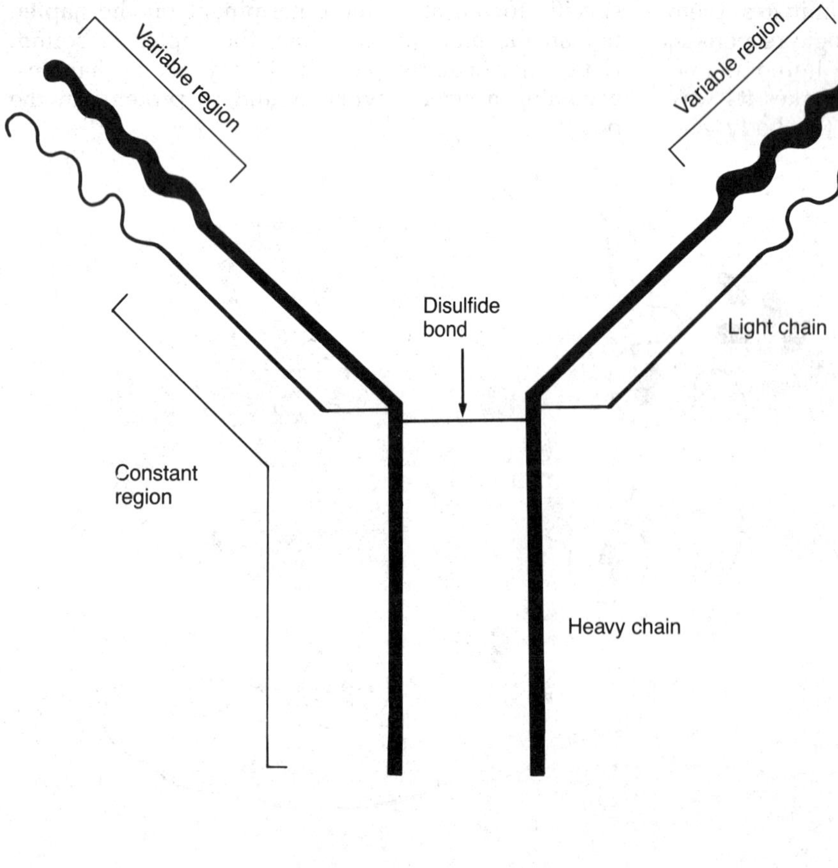

Figure 9–4.

Structure of the basic antibody molecule. The basic antibody molecule is a Y-shaped unit composed of two heavy chains and two light chains. Each chain has a constant region and a variable region that contains the specific antigen-binding site.

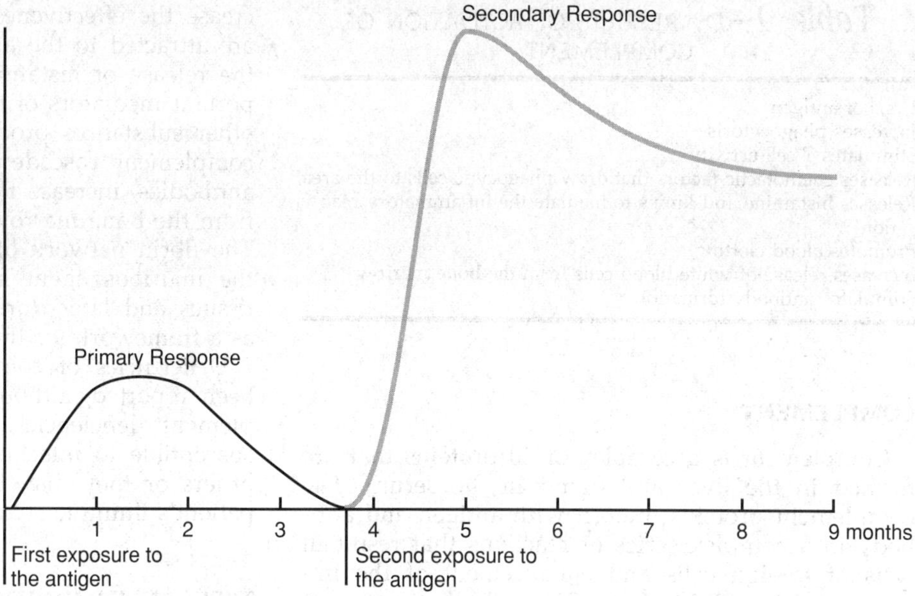

Figure 9–5.

Antibody levels of the primary and secondary responses. Antibody levels produced after the first exposure to an antigen are much lower than the levels produced after succeeding exposures. Antibody production occurs much sooner after the succeeding exposures and lasts much longer.

antibodies are of the IgM class. Owing to size, these antibodies are confined to the blood stream.

IgE antibody is present only in minute quantities in the normal human, accounting for only approximately 0.5% of the total antibody level in the blood. IgE mediates hypersensitivity type I reactions such as hay fever, asthma, and atopic allergies. The constant region of the IgE molecules binds to the surface of mast cells and basophils (see Fig. 9–4). When the appropriate antigen binds to the variable region of the mast cell–bound IgE molecule, the mast cell degranulates, releasing histamine and other chemical substances that play a role in the allergic reaction. Increased levels of IgE can be found in patients infected with intestinal parasites such as roundworms.

IgD is also normally present only in minute quantities in the blood, constituting approximately 0.2% of the total circulating antibodies. The immune function of IgD is unknown. It appears to function only on the surface of B cells, where it may have a regulatory role.

The primary antibody response follows the first exposure to an antigen. Detectable levels of antibodies are not present in the serum until approximately 4 to 10 days after entry of an antigen. During this lag period, the host's defenses are not up to par, and the antigen may have time to produce disease. The antibody levels produced during the primary response are not high, and they do not last for a long time. They peak in 1 to 10 weeks and then drop off to very low levels. The first and most abundant antibody produced during the primary response is IgM.

It is during the initial exposure to an antigen that long-lived memory B cells are programmed.

The second and succeeding encounters with an antigen produce the secondary antibody response. This is a faster, more efficient response, which seems to produce better quality antibodies (Fig. 9–5) than the primary response. Antibody from the secondary response is detectable within 1 to 2 days after exposure to the antigen and lasts much longer, and antibody titers are much higher than that following the primary response. The most abundant antibody of the secondary response is IgG.

Antibodies work in several different ways to protect the host. The antibody may neutralize or block the action of toxins or other substances produced by microorganisms. The microorganism may be killed by the antibody, or antibodies may block the infective ability of the microorganism. The latter mechanism is especially important in protection against viruses in the blood stream. Antibodies may also agglutinate microorganisms, that is, cause them to clump and stick together, making it easier for the phagocytic cells to attack the microorganisms. Another mechanism used by antibodies is opsonization of the microorganism. This occurs when the antibody alters the surface of the microorganism so that phagocytes are more attracted to it.

CELLULAR IMMUNE RESPONSE

The T cells that are responsible for cellular immunity are also activated by the presence of an antigen. Lymphokines produced by helper T cells stimulate B cells to produce antibodies. Suppressor T cells produce lymphokines to regulate the immune response so that it does not overreact to an antigen. They inhibit antibody formation. Suppressor T cells are thought to play an important role in tolerance and in autoimmune reactions. Cytotoxic (killer) T cells are stimulated to kill the appropriate foreign cells. This is especially important when the antigen is a tumor cell, a cell grafted from another host, or a virus-infected cell.

Table 9–6. RESULTS OF ACTIVATION OF COMPLEMENT

Lysis of antigen
Increases phagocytosis
Stimulates T-cell activity
Releases chemotactic factors that draw phagocytic cells to the area
Releases histamine and kinins to mediate the inflammatory reaction
Promotes blood clotting
Increases release of white blood cells from the bone marrow
Stimulates antibody formation

COMPLEMENT

Complement is a complex of 20 proteins that are formed in the liver and found in the serum. The complement proteins interact with antigen and antibody in a complex series of reactions that result in lysis of foreign cells and enhancement of the immune reaction (Table 9–6). The cells that are most susceptible to complement-mediated lysis are gram-negative bacteria, white blood cells, and red blood cells. Complement in conjunction with the appropriate antibody is able to neutralize free virus in the blood and therefore is an important defense against viruses as well as bacteria. Many gram-positive bacteria and fungi resist complement-mediated lysis. There are nine major proteins that make up complement and many minor ones. The nine major proteins are sequentially numbered C1 through C9.

The combination of an antigen with an antibody of the IgG or IgM class is capable of activating C1 and the classic complement pathway. C1 working in conjunction with C2, C3, and C4 acts as the activation unit for the rest of the components. C5 through C9 actually attack the membrane of the antigen and bring about its lysis.

The complement system may also be activated by an alternate pathway called the properdin pathway or amplification loop. Properdin is a serum globulin that in conjunction with some initiating factors starts the complement system at the C3 level. This alternate pathway does not require an antigen-antibody reaction to initiate the complement system. Complex antigens such as polysaccharides, lipopolysaccharides (found in the cell wall of gram-negative bacteria), and glycoproteins (from the capsules of some yeast and bacteria) are capable of activating the alternate pathway.

As a result of the activation of the various components of the complement cascade, several biologically active complement split products are produced. These substances are important in mediating the inflammatory process as well as the immune response. The effects of these substances are varied. Several of the substances are strong chemotactic agents that attract phagocytic cells to the area to participate in the inflammatory reaction. Some components of complement, especially C36, in combination with antibody act as opsonins, helping to increase the effectiveness of the phagocytic cells that are attracted to the area. Other substances promote the release of histamine and kinins, which are important mediators of the inflammatory reaction. Still other substances produced during activation of the complement cascade stimulate B cells to produce antibodies, increase the release of white blood cells from the bone marrow, and promote blood clotting. The fibrin network of the blood clot helps prevent the injurious agent from spreading further in the tissues and later during the healing process serves as a framework for the new tissue.

Deficiencies of components of complement have been reported, although they are rare. These complement deficiencies may leave the patient more susceptible to infections and immune complex disorders or they may have little or no effect on the patient's immune status.

TYPES OF IMMUNITY

Immunity is frequently referred to in terms of the method by which an individual came to possess that immunity. When discussed in this way, immunity is described in terms of natural versus acquired immunity and passive versus active immunity.

NATURAL RESISTANCE

Natural resistance (also called innate or inherited immunity) is that immunity with which a person is born. The nonspecific defense mechanisms (such as the chemical and physical barriers) play a role in natural resistance. Some natural resistance is conferred by virtue of the individual's species. Some microorganisms are pathogenic for one species but not another. Humans are immune to the microorganisms that cause distemper, dog tapeworm, fowl malaria, and fowl typhoid, but dogs, cats, and birds are not. In contrast, humans are susceptible to the virus that causes mumps, whereas dogs and cats are immune to it. Race also plays a role in natural resistance. When differences in economic and social conditions are taken into account, it appears that blacks are more susceptible to tuberculosis than whites, but whites are more susceptible to diphtheria and influenza than blacks. Other factors that play a role in natural resistance are the individual's sex, age (the very young and the elderly are more susceptible to infections), and nutritional status (the phagocytic cells of a malnourished individual are only one tenth to one third as effective as those of a well-nourished individual).

Even though natural resistance is often called natural immunity, the term *resistance* is preferred since much of this phenomenon does not have the precise antigen specificity that is usually associated with immunity. Natural resistance does not require prior exposure to the antigen and is not a learned response.

Table 9–7. ACQUIRED IMMUNITY

Acquired Immunity can be
1. Actively acquired
   a. Naturally by actually having the disease
   b. Artificially by vaccination
2. Passively acquired
   a. Naturally from antibodies (e.g., maternal IgG)
   b. Artificially by injection of antibodies (e.g., immune serum globulin)

ACQUIRED IMMUNITY

Acquired immunity includes all antigen-specific immunities that a person develops during a lifetime. It develops after exposure to an antigen. Acquired immunity can vary widely from person to person, depending on which antigens they have previously been exposed to. Acquired immunity can be actively acquired or passively acquired (Table 9–7). With actively acquired immunity, the individual produces antibodies or sensitized T cells, or both, after being exposed to the antigen. Exposure to the antigen may be either a natural exposure or an artificial one. Natural exposure occurs by chance during the course of an individual's life and may result in overt infection or a subclinical illness. In either case, the exposure to the antigen is sufficient to stimulate the immune response. The resulting immunity is termed naturally acquired active immunity. Artificially acquired active immunity is developed after the individual is purposefully exposed to the antigen in the form of a vaccine or toxoid. Vaccines contain either killed or attenuated (weak but viable organisms) bacteria or viruses. Toxoids are the toxins produced by bacteria that have been altered so that they are no longer toxic but their important antigenic receptor sites remain intact, enabling antibodies to be produced to the antigen-producing toxin.

Passively acquired immunity occurs when the antibodies are produced in one individual and then given to another individual. These passively acquired antibodies are usually given by injection (e.g., immune serum globulin), except in the case of the transfer of maternal antibodies either across the placenta to the fetus or via colostrum and breast milk. When the antibodies are given by injection, it is referred to as artifically acquired passive immunity. The transfer of maternal antibodies to the fetus or newborn infant is said to be naturally acquired passive immunity. Only IgG antibody crosses the placenta. Colostrum and breast milk contain secretory IgA and IgM. These antibodies are absorbed from the infant's gastrointestinal tract, and they also coat it to help prevent intestinal infections.

Although both active and passive immunity provide protection against infections, there are differences between the two. Active immunity lasts much longer and is more effective at preventing subsequent infections than passive immunity. Active immunity lasts for years, as a result of the presence of memory T and B lymphocytes, and can be easily reactivated by a booster dose of antigen. Passively received human antibodies have a half-life of approximately 30 days. (Half-life is the amount of time it takes to metabolize or inactivate half the amount given.) Protection from active immunity takes 5 to 14 days to develop after the first exposure to the antigen and 1 to 3 days after subsequent exposures. Passive immunity provides protection immediately.

Artifically acquired active immunity is primarily used prophylactically before exposure to the antigen is anticipated. Since the incubation period for most infections is less than the time required to develop antibodies, the vaccines must be given at least 2 weeks before exposure to the antigen. (An exception is the live measles vaccine, which prevents disease if given less than 48 hours after exposure.) Passively acquired immunity can be used prophylactically if given before an exposure or immediately after an exposure. It may prevent infection from the exposure but does not provide protection for future exposures. Hepatitis B immune globulin (HBIG) and varicella-zoster immune globulin (VZIG) are two preparations used to help prevent disease following an exposure to hepatitis B and chickenpox, respectively. Passively acquired immunity is sometimes used therapeutically to help treat an infection that has already been established. It is hoped that these antibodies will be able to decrease the duration and severity of the infection.

Assessment of Immune Status

Patient History

Assessment of immune status begins with a health history that includes detailed information related to occurrence of infections, neoplastic disease, and autoimmune disorders; allergies; immunizations; and the condition of nonspecific defenses and factors that can affect them.

In regard to infections, obtain information about usual childhood diseases and infections the patient has had, including the location of infection, date of occurrence, whether any are recurrent, and if so, how often and what treatment was used. Ask the patient about exposure to tuberculosis, when he or she last had a purified protein derivative (PPD) test and chest x-ray examination done, and what the results were. Question all patients about any recent exposure to infections that could currently be in the incubation stage. Obtain information about immunization status and note type and date of all immunizations.

In terms of malignant disease, ask the patient whether any family members have had cancer and, if so, the type, age at onset, and the relationship of the affected individual to the patient. (In cases of grandparents and others, the relationship to the maternal or paternal side of the family is noted.) Also determine whether the patient has ever had a malignancy diagnosed and, if so, the date of diagnosis, the type of tumor, and the type of treatment. Be certain to find out whether chemotherapy or radiation therapy was received by the patient because of the effects of these treatments on the immune system. Whether or not the individual has had a malignancy, determine the date of the last complete physical, rectal, breast, and pelvic or prostate examinations and question the patient about the presence of any symptoms that are warning signs of cancer (see Chapter 11).

Ask about any history of autoimmune disease such as rheumatoid arthritis, psoriasis, and lupus erythematosus. Also question the patient about allergies. If the patient has known allergies, obtain data on what the patient is allergic to (e.g., pollen, dust, bee stings, contact substances, foods, medications); what symptoms are experienced; any seasonal variations in occurrence or severity; and what medications or other treatment measures are used and how effective they are.

Finally, ask the patient about factors related to the function of the body's nonspecific defense mechanisms. For example, ask about smoking (how much and for how long), exposure to air pollutants through occupation or living location, presence of cough, and occurrence of skin problems.

Physical Examination

On physical examination, observe the patient for signs of infection anywhere in the body and for breaks or lesions of the skin or mucous membranes. Palpate anterior and posterior cervical, axillary, and inguinal lymph nodes, and if any are felt, note the size, consistency, and tenderness or lack thereof.

Diagnostic Procedures

Bone Marrow Aspiration and Biopsy

Bone marrow aspiration is done to obtain a small sample of cells from the bone marrow. Bone marrow biopsy is done to obtain a core of tissue from the bone marrow so that the structure can be studied. The procedures, which are usually done at the same time, help diagnose many conditions that have hematologic or immunologic abnormalities. The pathologist studies the bone marrow samples to determine the types and number of cells present, the phase of cellular maturation, the presence of any abnormal cells, and information about the iron stores.

A special large-gauge needle with a stylet is used to aspirate a small amount of bone marrow, usually from the iliac crest or the sternum. The skin is prepared with an antiseptic, and a local anesthetic is infiltrated at the site of aspiration, first into the skin and then deeper into the periosteum. The large-gauge needle is then inserted through the skin, tissues, and bone into the marrow cavity. The stylet is removed, allowing cells to be aspirated through the needle into a sterile syringe. The biopsy device is then inserted and the biopsy sample taken. The needle is removed and the site dressed with a small sterile dressing. The procedure is not very painful if the skin and periosteum have been properly anesthetized. Most patients feel pressure while the needle is being inserted and then a somewhat painful sensation during the actual aspiration of material. Complications include soreness at the puncture site, bleeding, and infection. The latter two may be life-threatening.

Application of the Nursing Process to the Care of the Patient Having a Bone Marrow Aspiration and Biopsy

Assessment

Assess patients undergoing a bone marrow aspiration for level of apprehension about the test and its results, ability to lie in the required position, knowledge of what to expect, and allergy to the local anesthetic that will be used. Also check that the appropriate consent form for the procedure has been signed.

Nursing Diagnoses and Planning

Nursing diagnoses and related expected patient outcomes most commonly applicable to patients undergoing bone marrow aspiration include the following:

NDx: Knowledge deficit: procedure

Planning: Patient outcomes
1. Patient states why the test is being done.
2. Patient states where the test will be done and what staff will be involved.
3. Patient describes the usual sensations associated with the procedure.
4. Patient states the approximate length of the procedure.

NDx: Anxiety related to the procedure or its outcome

Planning: Patient outcomes
1. Patient expresses feelings about the procedure and its outcomes.
2. Patient verbalizes feeling less anxious.
3. Patient attends to directions.

NDx: Pain related to tissue trauma at the site of aspiration

Planning: Patient outcomes

1. Patient states pain is manageable or absent.
2. Patient moves about without signs of excessive distress.

NDx: High risk for decreased cardiac output related to blood loss

Planning: Patient outcomes

1. Evidence of bleeding at the site of aspiration is absent.
2. Vital signs are within the patient's normal limits.

NDx: High risk for infection related to the invasive procedure

Planning: Patient outcomes

1. Redness and swelling at the site of aspiration are absent.
2. Drainage is absent from the site of aspiration.
3. Patient is afebrile.

Nursing Interventions

NDx: Knowledge deficit: procedure
Explain the procedure to the patient in language the individual can understand. Include the reason for the test, sensations the patient is likely to feel, persons who will be in the room and what their roles are, what equipment will be used, the position that the patient will be in, the fact that the procedure will take 5 to 10 minutes, and how long it is expected to take before the results are known. Be sure to allow time for the patient to ask questions.

Additional Preprocedure Interventions
At least 30 minutes before the procedure, obtain baseline vital signs and administer any premedications (such as a sedative) that have been ordered.

Just prior to the procedure, position the patient with pillows to support the arms, legs, and head as needed. Provide a blanket or other cover for warmth and to maintain the patient's modesty.

NDx: Anxiety
Offer support during the procedure by remaining next to the patient, holding the patient's hand if indicated, giving verbal reassurance, and telling the patient what is happening. When the results of the test come back and the physician has informed the patient of them, provide the opportunity for the patient to express his or her reaction and to ask any additional questions. This support is necessary whether the results of the test were normal or abnormal, because it is as necessary to express feelings of happiness and relief as well as anxiety and sadness.

NDx: Pain
Reassure the patient that discomfort will gradually subside in 24 to 48 hours. Position the patient off the site of aspiration for comfort when in bed. Administer prescribed analgesics such as Tylenol every 4 hours as needed.

NDx: High risk for decreased cardiac output
Monitor the site of aspiration for bleeding, and monitor pulse and blood pressure. If a pressure dressing is in place, as following multiple aspirations for harvest of bone marrow for transplant, leave in place until the day after the procedure.

NDx: High risk for infection
Instruct the patient not to take a bath or shower or otherwise wet the aspiration site for 24 hours. After this time, remove the bandage; wash the site with Betadine; apply vitamins A & D ointment; and cover with a Band-Aid. Repeat daily for 3 days if the patient is, or is at risk of being, immunologically impaired.

Check for temperature elevation, and observe the site of the aspiration for redness, swelling, and foul drainage. If the patient is discharged, stress the importance of reporting any of these symptoms.

Evaluation

Evaluate the effectiveness of nursing care for a patient having a bone marrow aspiration by comparing the patient's status with the expected patient outcomes. Examples of specific outcomes for patients undergoing bone marrow aspiration have been provided in the Planning section.

Laboratory Tests Utilizing Antigens and Antibodies

The antigen-antibody reaction is used as the basis of several common laboratory techniques. These techniques use antigen or antibody as a sensitive and highly specific reagent to detect, identify, and quantify proteins and other small molecules such as drugs in blood, body fluids, and tissues. These tests can be used to help diagnose specific infections, some forms of cancer, and immune dysfunctions. The tests involve taking a sample of peripheral venous blood or other body fluid (urine, sputum, cerebrospinal fluid) or tissue for laboratory analysis.

ELECTROPHORESIS

Electrophoresis is a technique that uses an electric current to separate electrically charged particles in a solution. It is frequently used to separate serum proteins (albumin and the different globulins) so that they can be identified and quantified. Electrophoresis is used in the diagnosis of hypogammaglobulinemia and multiple myeloma. Electrophoresis can also be done on cerebrospinal fluid and urine.

RADIOIMMUNOASSAY

Radioimmunoassay is a very sensitive and specific laboratory procedure that can be used to detect very small amounts of a substance in the blood. The test uses antibody specific for the antigen in question and a small amount of antigen that has been labeled with a radiolabeled material. It is commonly used to detect hormones, proteins, and drugs such as digoxin, digitoxin, vitamin B_{12}, folic acid, barbiturates, and members of the opiate family.

IMMUNOFLUORESCENCE

Immunofluorescence is a technique that allows identification of specific antigens. This technique uses antibodies that have been chemically bound to a fluorescent molecule. The specimen with the unknown antigen is fixed to a glass slide, and then the fluorescent antibody is applied to the specimen. If the antibody is specific for the antigen on the slide, the antibody binds with it and remains on the slide. The slide is examined under a special microscope, and any antibody remaining on the slide will fluoresce. Because it is difficult to accurately quantify the amount of antigen that is present with this technique, the results are usually given as positive or negative. Immunofluorescence provides relatively rapid results and is used to identify a wide variety of bacteria, viruses, fungi, and protozoa. Specific organisms that can be identified by immunofluorescence include *Candida albicans,* group A streptococci, *Haemophilus influenzae,* herpes virus, influenza virus, *Mycoplasma pneumoniae, Neisseria gonorrhoeae, Neisseria meningitidis,* rabies virus, *Staphylococcus aureus,* and *Streptococcus pneumoniae.* This technique can be modified to identify antibody by using fluorescent antigens.

AGGLUTINATION

Agglutination refers to the clumping together of microorganisms or other particles. Infection with some organisms causes the body to produce agglutinins (immunoglobulins that cause clumping of the invading organism) specific for that organism. Agglutinins provide a valuable tool to help detect these organisms. The serum of the patient is mixed with a suspension of the organisms. If the agglutinin is present in the serum, it causes the organisms to clump together and the test is positive. The serum is then diluted until agglutination no longer occurs. This dilution process determines the titer (quantity of a substance required to react with or to correspond to a given amount of another substance) of the agglutinin. Diseases that may be diagnosed by this method include typhoid fever, tularemia, typhus fever, and undulant fever. Antigens may be attached to very small latex particles. If the appropriate agglutinin is present in the serum, these antigen-coated latex particles clump together, allowing the reaction to be seen. Tests for rheumatoid factor, hepatitis B, and some urine pregnancy tests use latex particles.

COMPLEMENT FIXATION TEST

Complement fixation is a two-step test usually used to detect the presence of a specific antibody. In the first step, serum from the patient is mixed with an identified antigen and a known amount of complement. If the serum contains antibody specific for the antigen, the antibody and antigen react with each other and consume or "fix" the complement in the process. This is an invisible reaction. In the second step, an indicator is added to determine whether complement is still present. If complement is present, the test result is negative, because the patient's serum did not contain antibody specific for the antigen and no reaction took place. If no complement is present, the test result is positive. The test can also be done to determine whether the patient's serum contains a specific antigen by using a known antibody. The Wassermann test for syphilis is an example of a complement fixation test.

Allergy Tests

Allergy tests are done to help determine the specific antigens to which the patient is allergic. Four types of allergy tests are available: scratch, prick intradermal, and radioallergosorbent tests. The scratch, prick, and intradermal tests all involve administration of a very small amount of various dilute antigens to the skin and observation for a local reaction, usually redness, swelling, and itching. A rare but possible risk with any of these tests is the development of a generalized allergic reaction or anaphylaxis. The radioallergosorbent (RAST) test determines the presence of specific IgE antibodies in a blood sample. The results of these tests are used in conjunction with the patient's allergic history to help determine which antigens cause the patient's allergic symptoms.

SCRATCH TEST

The scratch test is somewhat less sensitive than the other tests, but it is easiest and safest. More antigens can be tested at one time with the scratch test than with the other methods. Scratch tests are usually done on the back or forearms. The skin in the area to be used is cleansed with alcohol. Areas that have abnormal or damaged skin should not be used. After the alcohol has dried, very small super-

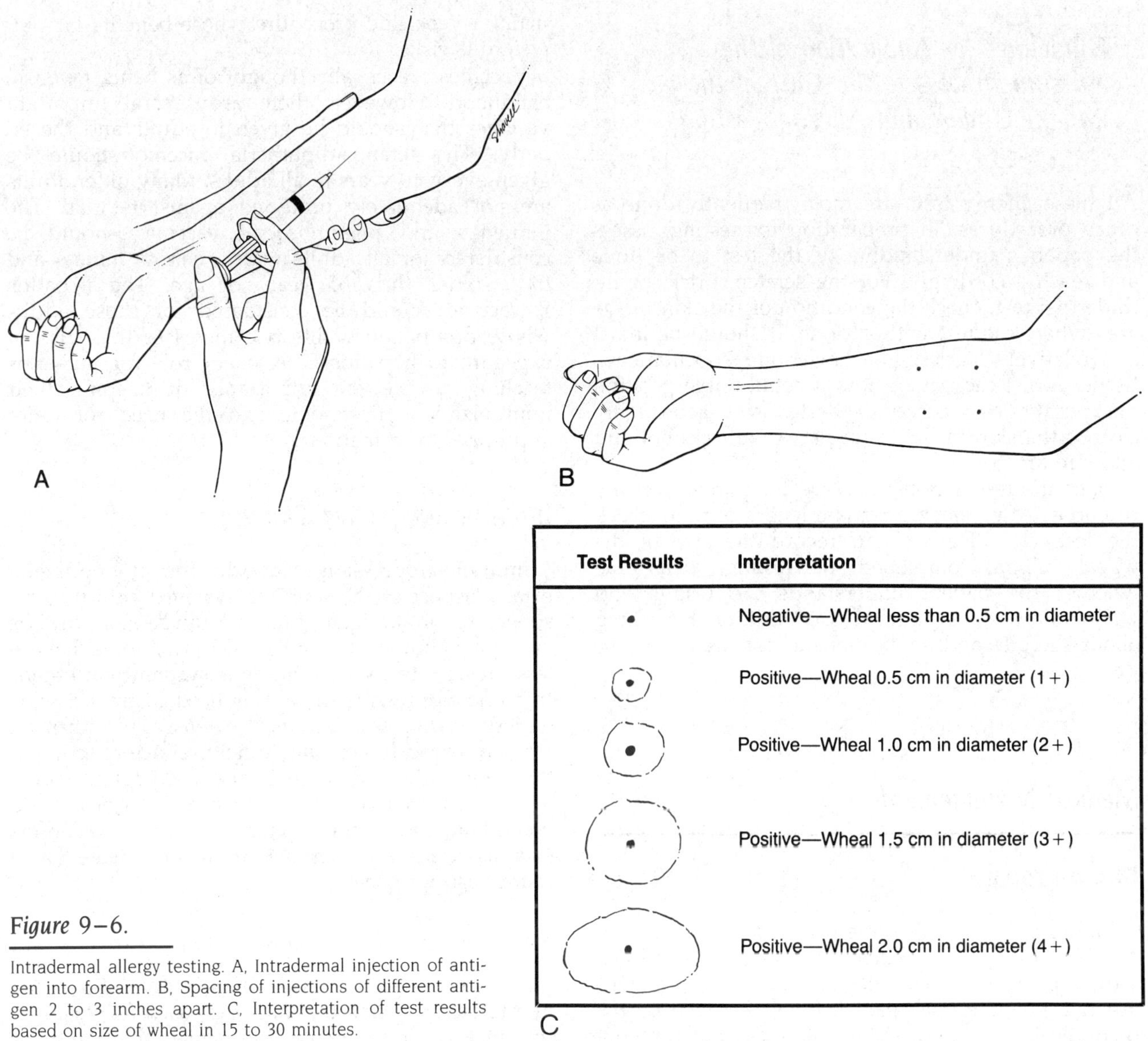

Figure 9–6.

Intradermal allergy testing. A, Intradermal injection of antigen into forearm. B, Spacing of injections of different antigen 2 to 3 inches apart. C, Interpretation of test results based on size of wheal in 15 to 30 minutes.

ficial scratches are made on the skin. These scratches should not bleed. A drop of a dilute antigen solution is applied to one scratch. A different antigen is applied to each scratch. Some redness and swelling at a scratch is a positive result. The results are read in 5 to 30 minutes.

PRICK TEST

The prick test is similar to the scratch test, but is a little more sensitive. A drop of antigen is placed on the skin and then the skin is pricked with a 26-gauge needle through the drop of antigen. Some redness and swelling at the site is a positive test result. The results are read in 15 to 30 minutes.

INTRADERMAL TEST

For the intradermal test, a very small amount of antigen is injected intradermally. It is more painful than the scratch or the prick test, and only a few antigens can be tested at one time, because more space (2 to 3 inches) is needed between each test site. The results are read in 15 to 30 minutes (Fig. 9–6). Some redness and swelling at the site is a positive test result.

RADIOALLERGOSORBENT TEST

Radioallergosorbent test (RAST) determines the presence of allergen-specific IgE antibodies in a blood sample. The RAST test is no more sensitive than the other tests and is more expensive. However, it is useful when the other tests cannot be used, such as when the patient has extensive skin lesions and there is not enough normal skin area available. The RAST test is easier for the patient, and the only risk to the patient is that associated with a simple venipuncture.

Guidelines for Application of the Nursing Process to the Care of the Patient Undergoing Allergy Testing

All these allergy tests are most frequently done as office procedures. In preparation for testing, assess the patient's understanding of the test to be done and teach accordingly. For the scratch, prick, or intradermal test, check the condition of the skin in the area where the test will be done. It should be intact and relatively hairless and have some subcutaneous tissue. Assist the patient into a comfortable position that permits easy access to the test site. Thoroughly cleanse the skin in the testing area with alcohol and allow to air dry.

Once the test is done, observe the patient for any reactions. After the appropriate length of time, check the test site. Measure and record the size of the wheal. Upon completion of testing, determine whether the patient understands the results and what follow-up is planned. Do additional teaching about allergies and medications as required.

Medical Management

Immunizations

Immunizations have served to increase the quality of life and have made some diseases (e.g., smallpox) a thing of the past. Vaccines containing live antigens are not given to pregnant women because of the theoretical risk to the fetus. Live vaccines are not given to immunosuppressed individuals (those receiving corticosteroids, cancer chemotherapy, radiation therapy, or other immunosuppressive agents) or to individuals who have a defect in their cellular, immunity such as patients with leukemia, lymphoma, and Hodgkin's disease. Even though the antigen has been weakened during production of the vaccine, it may be able to overcome the incompetent immune system and cause a serious or fatal disease. Multiple antigens can be administered simultaneously and a good response obtained to each antigen. The preferred site for injection of vaccines in adults is the deltoid muscle or the anterolateral thigh, because injections in the buttocks may deposit the vaccine in fat tissue, where it is not as effective. To maintain their maximum effectiveness, vaccines must be properly stored. Vaccine failures have been caused by improper storage. Some vaccines are produced in eggs and may contain some egg protein. These vaccines should not be administered to patients who are allergic to eggs. Vaccination is normally a very safe procedure whose benefits far outweigh its risks.

Vaccines are usually thought of as being given in childhood. However, there are several important vaccines that should be given to adults and the elderly. The tetanus-diphtheria vaccine should be given every 10 years to all adults. Many older adults are not adequately protected against tetanus. The influenza and pneumococcal vaccines should be considered for all adults with a chronic illness and those older than 65 years of age. The hepatitis B vaccine should be considered for those adults whose occupation or lifestyle increases their risk of exposure to hepatitis B. A major role for nurses is teaching people the importance of keeping their immunizations up-to-date and the need for other appropriate vaccinations.

Immunosuppressive Therapy

Immunosuppression is a reduction or depression in any aspect of the immune system's ability to respond to an antigen. Immunosuppression can be brought about in a number of ways; some have a less severe effect on the immune system than others. Immunosuppressive therapy is used to treat a wide variety of diseases. It is used extensively with most types of organ transplants to help reduce rejection of the transplanted tissue. It is also used for immunologically mediated diseases such as allergies, rheumatoid arthritis, and vasculitis. Collagen disorders such as scleroderma are also frequently treated with immunosuppressives.

ANTIGEN-SPECIFIC IMMUNOSUPPRESSION

Allergy desensitization is one example of induced immunosuppression that has been used for years. In this method, the antigen that causes the allergy is used to suppress the body's response to it. Small amounts of the antigen are injected into the body in an attempt to get the body to produce antibodies of a class other than IgE that are specific to that antigen. Once this occurs, the antigen on entering the body reacts with these non-IgE antibodies before it makes its way to the IgE antibodies on the mast cells. This method is not always successful and in some cases may increase hypersensitivity to the antigen.

Another commonly used method of immune suppression is to administer antibody produced in one individual to another individual who has been exposed to the antigen specific to that antibody. The antibody binds with the antigen, rendering it nonantigenic, before it has a chance to stimulate the immune response in the host. In a sense, the preformed antibody hides the antigen from the immune system. RhoGAM is given to prevent an immune response in Rh-negative individuals who have been exposed to Rh-positive blood cells. A woman who is

Rh negative can receive such an exposure during the termination or delivery of a pregnancy. The antibodies in the RhoGAM bind with antigens on the fetal red blood cells and prevent them from stimulating the woman's immune system.

The two methods just discussed are very specific and induce immunosuppression only to selected antigens. The remaining immunosuppressive methods produce a generalized nonspecific immunosuppression to many antigens.

NONSPECIFIC IMMUNOSUPPRESSION

ANTILYMPHOCYTE SERUM

Antilymphocyte serum (ALS) produces a nonspecific immunosuppression. ALS is produced by injecting animals with human lymphocytes. The animal then produces antibodies against the human lymphocytes. These antibodies are harvested from the animal and purified to make ALS. When ALS is injected into a human, these antibodies destroy the human lymphocytes, causing a transient lymphopenia. Functioning of both T cells and B cells is decreased. ALS tends to have many other unwanted side effects, such as febrile reactions, serum sickness, and sometimes anaphylaxis.

Monoclonal antibodies are a new and much more selective variation of ALS. Monoclonal antibodies consist of identical copies of an antibody molecule that reacts with only a single very specific part of the antigenic determinant. Most antigenic determinants have more than one area that stimulates antibody formation, so several antibodies are produced in response to the antigen. A cell that produces the single desired antibody is combined with a continuously replicating cell line, and a clone of cells develops that produce only that specific antibody. A monoclonal antibody can be produced that reacts with almost any antigen.

The use of monoclonal antibodies to detect as well as to treat cancers is under investigation. To detect cancers, a radioisotope is combined with a monoclonal antibody that binds to tumor antigen. This combination is injected into the patient. The patient is then scanned to determine whether there are areas where the radioisotope is concentrated. To treat cancers, anticancer drugs or toxins are bound to a monoclonal antibody specific for the tumor. The monoclonal antibody brings the drug directly to the tumor. Monoclonal antibodies have opened up many new diagnostic and treatment possibilities. They have also revolutionized laboratory testing procedures and appear to have a very promising future.

PHARMACOLOGIC IMMUNOSUPPRESSION

The most commonly used method of inducing immunosuppression is with drugs. There are many drugs that can cause some degree of immunosuppression ranging from mild to quite profound. Drugs do not affect all aspects of the immune response equally. It is much easier to suppress the primary immune response than it is to depress the secondary immune response. Once memory cells have been formed, it is almost impossible to inhibit the immune response. Some drugs affect T cells more than B cells and vice versa. The timing of the administration of the immunosuppressant in relation to exposure to the antigen is often critical in determining how effective the agent is. Some immunosuppressant agents such as corticosteroids and irradiation must be given just before exposure to the antigen for them to be most effective. Other agents such as mercaptopurine and azathioprine must be given immediately after exposure to the antigen for them to be most effective. Immunosuppressants work either by their effect on T cells and B cells or by their effect on the neutrophils and monocytes. The anti-inflammatory properties of a drug can also produce a degree of immunosuppression. The most important agents used to induce immunosuppression are briefly discussed here.

Corticosteroids

Corticosteroids are extremely useful immunosuppressants and are used in the treatment of a wide variety of diseases. Corticosteroids affect several parts of the immune system; however, their mechanism of action is not completely understood. A single high dose of corticosteroids causes a prompt reduction in the number of lymphocytes. Both T cells and B cells are affected; however, T cells are more affected than B cells, and helper T cells are more affected than suppressor T cells. The lymphocytes are not destroyed but are thought to be redistributed and possibly sequestered in the bone marrow. Within 24 hours, the number of lymphocytes returns to normal.

Corticosteroids also impair the ability of the lymphocytes to synthesize antibodies and lymphokines and decrease the number of functioning monocytes and eosinophils. When corticosteroids are given for several days, there is a decrease in the amount of antibody present. Cell-mediated immunity is inhibited by corticosteroids. All these effects leave the patient who is taking corticosteroids more susceptible to infection. Corticosteroids also stabilize the mast cells and basophils, inhibiting their ability to release histamine and other chemical mediators of the allergic reaction.

Cytotoxic Drugs

Cytotoxic drugs bring about immunosuppression by killing immunologically competent cells. These agents are able to kill any cell that is replicating. Prior to stimulation by an antigen, the immune cells are in a dormant state. Once stimulated by an antigen, the cells begin to divide and are then susceptible to the cytotoxic drugs. Frequently used cytotoxic drugs are azathioprine (Imuran), cyclophosphamide (Cytoxan), cyclosporine, and methotrexate. Azathioprine is also a potent anti-inflammatory agent. It is frequently used in combination with corticosteroids to help prevent rejection of organ transplants and is used to treat disorders with an autoimmune component.

Cyclophosphamide is a potent immunosuppressant affecting both T cells and B cells. It is used to treat disorders with an autoimmune component and those resulting from an aberrant immune response, such as Wegener's granulomatosis and severe rheumatoid arthritis.

Cyclosporine appears to be very selective, destroying only helper T cells. It is very useful in suppressing the rejection of allografts (graft from a genetically different donor of the same species) and is used in many transplant protocols.

Methotrexate inhibits both the humoral and cellular immune responses by inhibiting folate metabolism.

The major side effects of cytotoxic drugs are bone marrow depression, nausea, vomiting, diarrhea, gastrointestinal bleeding, nephrotoxicity, sterility, infection, and an increased risk of cancer.

RADIATION

Radiation can decrease the number of lymphocytes in the general circulation and in lymphoid tissues. It also suppresses the functioning of most immunocompetent cells. Total body radiation and total nodal radiation (administration of the radiation to the major lymph node areas) are used as part of transplant protocols.

SURGERY

The surgical removal of lymphoid tissue can also induce immunosuppression. The removal of the spleen or thymus gland, especially if done at an early age, can produce a type of immunosuppression.

Guidelines for Application of the Nursing Process to the Care of the Patient Undergoing Immunosuppressive Therapy

Nursing care for patients undergoing immunosuppressive therapy varies with the degree of immunosuppression and the length of time that it is expected to persist. Ensure that all patients know why the immunosuppression is needed, what the expected effect of immunosuppression is, and what side effects or complications may occur. In cases of antigen-specific immunotherapy, such teaching may constitute the majority of the nursing role. However, when extensive nonspecific immunosuppression is involved, nursing care becomes very complex. It includes protection from infection, care required for side effects or complications of the specific therapy used, and care related to any underlying disease.

Bone Marrow Transplantation

Bone marrow transplantation (BMT) is a high-risk procedure performed on patients who have exhausted all other treatment options without success. The object of a bone marrow transplant is to replace defective marrow with healthy marrow from a donor, thereby reestablishing normal marrow function in the recipient.

TYPES OF BONE MARROW TRANSPLANT

There are three types of bone marrow transplant: allogeneic, syngeneic, and autologous.

In an allogeneic transplant, bone marrow is harvested from a human leukocyte antigen (HLA) matched donor and infused into the recipient after cytoreduction therapy. A critical difficulty in this type of transplant is the location of a donor who is HLA- and mixed lymphocyte culture (MLC)-compatible. HLA is found on the surface of all nucleated cells in the body. This antigen can induce an immune response if cells are transplanted into a recipient who does not have the same antigen. HLA antigens are considered to be tissue antigens and are different from the ABO antigens on the surface of red blood cells. The immune response that the recipient mounts against these HLA antigens can cause rejection of the grafted tissue.

An in vitro test for MLC is used to help predict the success of the transplant. In this test, peripheral lymphocytes from the donor and the recipient are mixed together in cell culture and observed to determine whether the lymphocytes of the recipient are reacting by proliferation to the lymphocytes of the donor.

The second type of bone marrow transplant, the syngeneic, is one in which bone marrow is harvested from an identical twin. The advantage of a syngeneic graft over an allogeneic graft is that both donor and recipient are identically HLA-matched, so an immune response based on recognition of foreign cells does not occur.

The third type of transplant is an autologous transplant. This is the ideal transplant, because the donor and the recipient are the same. In an autologous transplant, bone marrow is harvested from the patient when healthy, in remission, or when the bone marrow is microscopically free of malignancy. It is then stored for future use.

USES

Bone marrow transplantation is an accepted modality of treatment for severe aplastic anemia, acute leukemia, chronic myelogenous leukemia, refractory non-Hodgkin's lymphoma, relapsed Hodgkin's disease, neuroblastoma, and severe combined immunodeficiency disorder. Autologous bone marrow transplant (ABMT) is also being used in the treatment of selected solid tumors, including melanoma, refractory sarcoma, and refractory malignancies of the stomach, colon, liver, ovary, and breast.

HARVESTING THE TRANSPLANT

Bone marrow is harvested from the donor via multiple bone marrow aspirations. The goal of the harvest is to obtain a sufficient number of stem cells to reestablish a hematopoietic system in the recipient. To this end, from 600 to 2500 ml of marrow mixed with peripheral blood is obtained from an adult donor, usually from the posterior iliac crest, although the anterior iliac crest and sternum can also be used. Harvesting is done in the operating room under local or general anesthesia. Once aspirated, the marrow is filtered and heparinized. For allogeneic or syngeneic transplants, the marrow is then taken to the patient for infusion. In autologous transplants, the marrow is frozen until needed. If there is a possibility that malignant cells might be present in the marrow, it may be purged prior to freezing by physical procedures that separate normal from malignant cells based on density, by immunologic procedures involving immunotoxic or monoclonal antibodies, or by chemotherapy.

PHYSICAL PREPARATION OF THE PATIENT

Prior to starting the transplant procedure, patients are scheduled for a dental examination and any needed dental work, including fluoride and plaque treatments, is completed. This is to avert the need for dental intervention when the patient's platelet count is low and to decrease the risk of abscesses or gum disease, which can seed infection into the vascular space while the patient is neutropenic. Women may have menstruation suppressed pharmacologically to prevent menstrual bleeding during the period of thrombocytopenia. Upon admission, most patients have a permanent venous access device such as a Hickman or Broviac catheter inserted. This makes the administration of the many drugs, blood products, and total parenteral nutrition easier for the patient, because not as many venipunctures are needed. Many of the required blood samples can also be drawn from these lines.

Before the transplant, the patient undergoes a cytoreduction protocol designed to destroy any abnormal cells and suppress the immune system if needed. These protocols typically consist of a combination of chemotherapeutic agents and irradiation. All are immunosuppressive or ablative and leave the patient pancytopenic and at risk for fatal infection or bleeding. Patients are therefore placed on protective isolation, and thrombocytopenic precautions are taken. These protocols also cause severe mucositis, which places the patient at risk for airway obstruction due to swelling of the oral pharyngeal tissues, necessitates parenteral nutrition, and may require opiates for the pain. Additional side effects include sterility, temporary loss of sexual desire in males secondary to low testosterone levels, amenorrhea in females due to decreased estrogen production by the ovary, and hair loss. (Refer to Chapter 11 for a complete discussion of the many other side effects that occur with these modes of treatment.)

PROCEDURE

The transplant is similar to a blood transfusion. The marrow is infused into the patient's blood stream through the venous access. The cells then migrate to the bone marrow cavities of the recipient, where the stem cells from the new marrow mature and should begin to function in 10 to 20 days.

POSTPROCEDURE COURSE

Pancytopenia persists for at least the first 3 to 4 weeks after transplant, and severe immunologic impairment may last for as long as 1 year. During this time, the ratio of helper to suppressor T-cells may be abnormal, T cells may not respond well to antigens, and antibody production is abnormal. Completely normal immune function may not be regained for 12 to 18 months, because it takes time for the transplanted immune system to mature and develop normal function.

As a result of the pancytopenia following the transplant, patients remain on protective isolation and receive broad-spectrum prophylactic antibiotics. Thrombocytopenic precautions are observed until the platelet count returns to normal. Since thrombocytopenia lasts weeks to months, repeated transfusions of irradiated platelets may be required. Discharge from the hospital generally occurs approximately 4 weeks after transplant.

COMPLICATIONS

Major complications of bone marrow transplant include infection and bleeding. In fact, viral infections such as cytomegalovirus pneumonia, fungal infections, hemorrhage, and marrow failure are the chief causes of death in bone marrow transplant patients.

Bone marrow transplant patients are also at risk for veno-occlusive disease (VOD) of the liver. This complication is apparently related to the amount of chemotherapy and radiation the patient has had prior to transplant. VOD is characterized by blocking of the hepatic venules by deposits of collagen and fibrin. This results in obstructed blood flow, liver engorgement, and the development of ascites due to the "weeping" of sodium- and albumin-rich fluid from the liver's surface. Renal perfusion is also decreased secondary to a decrease in intravascular fluid volume. Clinical manifestations of VOD include weight gain and impaired liver function as indicated by jaundice, increased serum alanine aminotransferase (ALT, formerly SGPT) and alkaline phosphatase levels, and coagulation defects. Treatment is supportive and focuses on maintenance of intravascular fluid volume to support renal blood flow. VOD spontaneously resolves in 2 to 3 weeks in approximately half of those affected.

A complication unique to patients who have received allogeneic transplants is graft-versus-host disease (GVHD). In GVHD, cells of the graft mount an immunologic attack against the cells of the recipient. The effects of GVHD are primarily seen in the skin, liver, gastrointestinal tract, and lymphoid tissues. The skin manifestations range from a mild rash occurring on the palms of the hands, soles of the feet, the trunk, and the ears to severe desquamation of the skin. Rises in the levels of serum bilirubin, aspartate aminotransferase, and alkaline phosphatase are seen as the liver becomes involved and in severe cases can lead to liver failure. Involvement of the gastrointestinal tract is characterized by green, watery diarrhea and abdominal cramping that can lead to GI bleeding.

Approximately 30% of allogeneic bone marrow transplant patients experience fatal GVHD, whereas another 30% to 60% experience a lesser degree of the disease. Once the disease process is under way, there is little effective treatment, and in its chronic form it can be very debilitating, causing changes in physical appearance and body image.

Application of the Nursing Process to the Care of the Patient Undergoing Bone Marrow Transplantation

Assessment

Before the transplant, assess how well the patient and significant others understand the underlying disease, the transplant protocol, potential side effects of the protocol, and therapeutic goals of the procedure, as well as the patient's emotional response to the underlying problem and to the scheduled transplant.

Assess the patient's physical condition, giving special attention to nutritional status, because adequate nutrition is essential to the avoidance of postprocedure complications. Adequate nutrition may be compromised either by the underlying disease or by the chemotherapy and irradiation given prior to the transplant. Obtain detailed information about the patient's eating patterns and food preferences for use in encouraging good nutritional intake following the transplant.

Collect information about the patient's living conditions, financial situation, and available sources of emotional and physical support, because the recovery period is long and ongoing care is required. When the pretransplant chemotherapy and irradiation are begun, make ongoing assessments of the patient's physical and psychological responses to the therapy (see Chapter 11).

Both before and after the transplant, make ongoing observations for signs of inflammation and infection. Monitor temperature regularly throughout the day. Always take the patient's temperature by the same method—either oral or axillary; do not take rectal temperatures. Be sure that the thermometer is placed correctly and left for an adequate time. If the patient is taking medications with an antipyretic effect, do not take temperature when the action of the medication is peaking. The patient's temperature may appear to be normal because of the medication's effect. Also be aware that even slight temperature elevations are significant.

Closely observe the patient for nosebleeds, petechiae, conjunctival hemorrhage, and symptoms of cerebral hemorrhage, because bleeding is a potential complication of the procedure. Also check stool and emesis for signs of blood.

Nursing Diagnoses and Planning

Nursing diagnoses and related expected patient outcomes most commonly applicable to patients undergoing a bone marrow transplant include the following:

NDx: Altered nutrition: less than body requirements related to mucositis and esophageal ulceration secondary to chemotherapy and/or radiation

Planning: Patient outcomes

1. Serum albumin is within normal range.
2. Patient's daily nutritional intake is equal to the recommended daily allowance or is as prescribed.

NDx: High risk for altered tissue perfusion related to abnormal bleeding secondary to platelet obliteration

Planning: Patient outcomes
1. Nosebleeds and conjunctival hemorrhages are absent.
2. Signs of cerebral hemorrhage or other internal bleeding are absent.

NDx: High risk for infection related to suppression of the immune system

Planning: Patient outcomes
1. Skin and mucous membranes are intact.
2. Lungs are clear to auscultation.
3. Monilial or herpetic lesions are absent from the mouth.
4. Vaginal itching and discharge are absent.
5. Patient describes sources of potentially infectious organisms and how to avoid them.

NDx: Knowledge deficit: transplant protocol, potential side effects, and/or therapeutic goals

Planning: Patient outcomes
1. Patient describes in sequence the major components of his or her treatment plan; for example, chemotherapy, irradiation, duration of the transplant, and postoperative care.
2. Patient describes potential side effects, both long-term and short-term.
3. Patient states why the transplant is being done and what effect it is expected to have on his or her health status.

NDx: Anxiety related to the procedure and its outcome

Planning: Patient outcomes
1. Patient discusses concerns about the procedure and its outcomes.
2. Signs of anxiety such as pacing, trembling, tachycardia, or inability to focus attention are absent.

NDx: High risk for body image disturbance related to transplant or occurrence of graft-versus-host disease

Planning: Patient outcomes
1. Patient discusses his or her condition or asks questions about it.
2. Patient makes decisions when asked; for example, what to eat, what to wear, when to get up.
3. Patient maintains social contact with staff, family, and others.

NDx: High risk for diversional activity deficit related to extended length of treatment

Planning: Patient outcomes
1. Patient pursues some diversional activity, such as reading, watching television, or writing letters.
2. Patient denies that boredom is a problem.

NDx: High risk for altered health maintenance related to insufficient knowledge of self-care following discharge

Planning: Patient outcomes
1. Patient describes self-care as presented in Chart 9–1.
2. Patient and significant others verbalize ability and willingness to comply with self-care instructions.
3. Patient identifies person and method of contact in the event of questions or problems.

Other nursing diagnoses and patient outcomes that may apply are related to chemotherapy and irradiation given before the procedure. These are discussed in Chapter 11. Since bone marrow transplant is in essence the last hope of a dying patient, nursing diagnoses and patient outcomes related to grieving and death, presented in Chapter 5, also apply.

Nursing Interventions

NDx: Altered nutrition: less than body requirements
Give the patient small, frequent meals that have been planned in accordance with the patient's stated food preferences. Offer between-meal supplements as needed. Avoid performing offensive or distressing procedures immediately before meals. Administer antiemetics so that peak action occurs at mealtime. Maintain a calm, relaxed atmosphere at mealtime, and provide companionship when possible.

In most cases a nutritional assessment should be done by a dietitian and the resulting recommendations followed as to how the patient's nutritional needs can best be met. If parenteral nutrition is necessary, administer it according to hospital procedure.

Weigh the patient daily, using the same scale. Record food and fluid intake for calorie counts periodically.

NDx: High risk for altered tissue perfusion
Apply pressure for several minutes to any puncture sites, as from injections or venipunctures, to help lessen the risk of bleeding. Administer blood products as ordered to maintain adequate levels of platelets and red blood cells.

NDx: High risk for infection
Place the patient in a private room, and help ensure that all personnel wash their hands thoroughly before entering so that the patient is protected from exposure to potentially pathogenic organisms.

Check arrangement of staff assignments so that individuals caring for the patient are healthy, free of communicable diseases such as colds and flu, without active herpetic lesions, and not caring for another patient with an infectious process.

Screen visitors for the presence of communicable diseases. Persons who are ill are not allowed to visit the patient. However, if a visit is essential to the psychological well-being of the patient, instruct the visitor in the appropriate precautions.

Discourage live plants and cut flowers in the room, as they harbor many bacteria and molds that can be very dangerous to the patient during neutropenic episodes. Personnel frequently touch the flowers while admiring, smelling, or moving them. This can contaminate their hands and thus provide a means of spread to the patient.

Institute nursing measures to maintain intact nonspecific defense mechanisms, thus decreasing the opportunity for pathogens to enter the body. The following measures prevent damage to the skin:

Turn and position the patient to relieve pressure on the skin areas prone to breakdown.
When moving the patient, take care to avoid shearing forces and abrasions.
Use lotions, bath oil, and skin moisturizers as necessary to prevent dry, chapped skin.
If the patient's skin is delicate, avoid using tape if possible.
Provide good oral hygiene to prevent damage to the mucous membranes.
Use gentle, nontraumatic techniques, such as soft sponges, gauze, or a Water Pik to clean the teeth and gums.
Rinse the mouth frequently with a nonirritating, nonalcohol-based solution such as normal saline from a container that is changed daily.
Keep the lips moist and soft with vitamins A & D ointment or similar substance.

Promote normal bowel function to avoid possible rectal lacerations or irritation and bleeding or hemorrhoids due to the passage of hard stool. Keep stools soft and avoid constipation by increasing the bulk in the diet, providing plenty of fluids, encouraging as much exercise as possible, and giving stool softeners such as Colace as needed. Avoid taking rectal temperatures, rectal examinations, enemas, and anything else that may injure the intestinal mucosa.

Perform invasive therapies such as intravenous catheterization, insertion of nasogastric tubes, and insertion of Foley catheters only if absolutely necessary. Discontinue them as soon as possible. These therapies are used only for medically indicated reasons, never for the convenience of the staff. Use sterile technique at all times when invasive therapy is necessary.

Encourage the patient to cough and breathe deeply, use an incentive spirometer, maintain good hydration, and get out of bed and walk. Good pulmonary toilet is essential to prevent pulmonary infection.

NDx: Knowledge deficit: transplant protocol, potential side effects, and/or therapeutic goals

Begin teaching during the pretransplant outpatient phase. Use a bone marrow transplant teaching booklet or other patient education materials such as those available from the National Institutes of Health. Review with the patient information related to the procedure, its therapeutic goals, and its potential side effects. Be alert to any patient comments or behaviors that indicate lack of knowledge. Clarify information, and if necessary, notify the physician of the patient's need for further explanation of the medical treatment.

NDx: Anxiety

Ensure that the patient is kept informed of what to expect during all stages of care. Provide the opportunity for both the patient and significant others to express concerns and ask questions. Involve a psychiatric nurse clinician, social workers, and clergy in patient care early in the hospitalization. Plan care so that the patient has private time in which to speak with family members or members of the clergy.

NDx: High risk for body image disturbance

Whenever possible, encourage the patient to make decisions about care, including how to structure the day's activities, what to eat, and what to wear. Encourage the patient to perform as much self-care as possible and to maintain good grooming. Arrange a visit with a former BMT recipient if the patient so desires.

NDx: High risk for diversional activity deficit

Provide appropriate diversional activities such as prescheduled telephone calls, prescheduled video movie showings, television, books, music, games, hobbies, or puzzles to prevent boredom. Also be certain to spend time with the patient. Consult the occupational or recreational therapist to arrange for additional activities for the patient.

NDx: High risk for altered health maintenance

Instruct the patient in self-care following discharge as presented in Chart 9–1. Include significant others in the teaching, because self-care requirements impact the entire household. Provide all instructions in writing for easy reference. Give clear directions as to whom should be contacted should questions or problems occur.

Evaluation

Evaluate the effectiveness of nursing care for a patient undergoing a BMT by comparing the patient's status with the expected patient outcomes. Examples

Chart 9–1.

NURSING GUIDE TO PATIENT EDUCATION FOR SELF-MANAGEMENT: ESSENTIALS OF SELF-CARE AFTER BONE MARROW TRANSPLANTATION

Instruct the patient to:

Expect to tire easily.
Plan for frequent rest periods or naps.
Resume pretransplant activities gradually as tolerance allows.
Take prophylactic antibiotics as prescribed.
Monitor for and report nosebleeds, blood in the stool, bleeding gums, hemoptysis, and the appearance of new bruises until platelet count returns to normal.
Avoid forceful nose blowing until platelet count is normal.
Use an electric razor until platelet count is normal.
Avoid contact sports and other activities with a high risk of injury until platelet count is normal.
Avoid ingestion of irritating or difficult-to-digest foods until platelet count is normal, then progress to usual diet as tolerated.
Avoid use of aspirin and aspirin-containing drugs, cough medicines containing guaifenesin, laxatives containing phenolphthalein, and non-steroidal anti-inflammatory drugs until platelet count is normal.
Postpone sexual activity until platelet count is at least 50,000.
Expect vaginal dryness and dyspareunia, and use a vaginal lubricant when intercourse is resumed.
Monitor for and report signs and symptoms of infection until blood count returns to normal: persistant temperature over 100.4°F (38°C) or temperature over 101°F (38.4°C), shaking chills, sweating, diarrhea of more than 2 day's duration, rectal pain, cough, runny nose, shortness of breath, chest discomfort, painful urination, areas of inflammation (redness, swelling, pain) or an open sore, or vision change.
Practice meticulous personal oral and body hygiene: take daily bath or shower; use mild soap; take particular care in cleansing underarms and perineal area; do not share towels or washcloths with others; use soft nylon toothbrush, and floss daily unless platelet count is less than 50,000 or WBC is less than 15,000 (1.5), in which case use soft toothettes only.
Use mouth rinse of $\frac{1}{2}$ tsp of salt and $\frac{1}{2}$ tsp of baking soda in 8 ounces of water rather than commercial mouthwashes or hydrogen peroxide, which dry and irritate mucous membranes.
Avoid crowds and contact with persons known to have a cold or other contagious disease until blood count returns to normal.
Walk outside regularly.
Wear sunscreen (SP 15 or higher) if in direct sun for more than 20 minutes, because sun exposure can aggravate GVHD or activate a viral infection.
Avoid swimming in lakes or crowded pools for at least 6 months.
Keep home as free of dust and dirt as possible: Get air conditioning or heating units cleaned before return home; use a disinfectant such as ammonia or bleach to clean the bathroom fixtures; wash all dishes in hot water and detergent; launder bath linens twice a week and bed linens once a week.
Avoid handling water and soil from flowers and houseplants for a few months, because they can harbor bacteria.
Have household cats and dogs treated for parasites and toxoplasmosis prior to return home.
Avoid close contact with all animals, and do not clean cages, litter boxes, aquariums, or the like for 12 to 18 months.
Monitor for and report signs of graft-versus-host disease: rash or itching especially on the palms of the hands or the soles of the feet, frequent liquid bowel movements, clay-colored stool, dark urine, and jaundice.
Return for weekly blood tests (CBC with platelets and differential count) until counts return to normal range.
Return for biweekly platelet infusions if needed.
Comply with follow-up schedule of monthly visits to the transplant surgeon, with repeat scans and blood counts for 1 year and every 2 months thereafter.

of specific outcomes for patients undergoing BMT have been provided in the Planning section.

The Elderly: Special Considerations

The immune system is complex, and age-related effects on its structure and function are just beginning to be delineated through research. With advancing age, the cortex of the thymus becomes thinner, and a slow decrease in overall thymic size occurs. Since T cells originate from the thymic cortical cells, these changes suggest that the number of T cells in the peripheral lymphatic tissues declines with age, but this is difficult to document. No atrophy of the lymph nodes or a decrease in B cells in the blood has been found.

Functionally, it appears that a gradual decrease in immunologic competence occurs during senescence, apparently as a result of defects in aged lymphoid cells. There appears to be some decrease in delayed-type hypersensitivity with aging. Studies in this area suggest that in senescence, T memory cells can respond to a booster skin test involving an antigen to which the T cells had been exposed at a young age but are unable to react to an antigen seen for the first time because of thymic hypofunction.

In relationship to humoral immunity, numbers of B cells in the peripheral blood and levels of IgM have been found to be unchanged in the aged. However, total serum IgG and IgA levels increase after age 70 and suggest an enhanced response to antigens or a defect in control of the system. The occurrence of an abnormality in regulation of immune function with age is further suggested by the fact that there is an increased incidence of autoantibodies in the aged. This increased incidence of autoantibodies, which is found even without associated disease, is suggested by some research to be the result of a loss of tolerance to self-antigens (e.g., DNA).

In terms of rapid antibody production in the aged in response to antigens, some studies indicate a diminished response and some a normal response. In any case, a response does occur, and thus immunizations have some positive effect.

Bibliography

Adams A. External barriers to infection. Nurs Clin North Am 1985; 20(1):145.

Adler WH, Nagel JE. Clinical immunology. In Principles of geriatric medicine and gerontology. WR Hazzard (ed). NY: McGraw-Hill, 1989, p 60.

Barber JS. Immunologic responses to trauma. CCQ 1986; 9(1):57.

Barrett JT. Textbook of immunology. St. Louis: CV Mosby, 1988.

Bellanti JA (ed). Immunology III. Philadelphia: WB Saunders, 1985.

Berk SL, Smith JK. Infectious diseases in the elderly. Med Clin North Am 1983; 67(2):273.

Blume KG, Petz LD (eds). Clinical bone marrow transplantation. New York: Churchill Livingstone, 1983.

Bone marrow transplantation teaching plan. New York: Bone Marrow Transplant Service, Division of Nursing, Memorial Sloan-Kettering Cancer Center, 1991.

Busby J, Caranasos GJ. Immune function, autoimmunity and selective immunoprophylaxis in the aged. Med Clin North Am 1985; 69(3):465.

Corman LC, Katz P (eds). Clinical immunology I. Med Clin North Am 1985; 69(3).

Corman LC, Katz P (eds). Clinical immunology II. Med Clin North Am 1985; 69(4).

Delafuente JC. Immunosenescence clinical and pharmacologic considerations. Med Clin North Am 1985; 69(3):475.

Edelson RL, Fink JM. The immunologic function of skin. Sci Am 1985; 252(6):46.

Espersen S. Nursing support of host defenses. CCQ 1986; 9(1):51.

Graziano FM, Bell CL. The normal immune response and what can go wrong: A classification of immunologic disorders. Med Clin North Am 1985; 69(3):439.

Griffin JP. Nursing care of the immunosuppressed patient in an intensive care unit. Heart Lung 1986; 15(2):179.

Gurevich I. The competent internal immune system. Nurs Clin North Am 1985; 20(1):151.

Kemp D. Development of the immune system. CCQ 1986; 9(1):1.

Middleton E, et al. Allergy—Principles and practice. 3rd ed. Vol. 1. St. Louis: CV Mosby, 1988.

The new immunology helping the body heal itself. Am J Nurs 1987; 87(4):455.

Paul WE. Fundamental immunology. 2nd ed. New York: Raven Press, 1989.

Returning home after your bone marrow transplant. New York: Bone Marrow Transplant Service, Division of Nursing/Department of Social Work, Memorial Sloan-Kettering Cancer Center, 1991.

Roitt IM, Brostoff J, Male DK. Immunology. St. Louis: CV Mosby, Gower Medical Publishing, 1989.

Samter M. Immunological diseases. 4th ed. Boston: Little, Brown, 1988.

Smith SL. Immunosuppressive drugs used in clinical practice. CCQ 1986; 9(1)19.

Smith SL. Physiology of the immune system. CCQ 1986; 9(1):7.

Stites DP, Stobo JD, Wells JV (eds). Basic and clinical immunology. 6th ed. Norwalk, CT: Appleton & Lange, 1987

Wells JV, Nelson DS (eds). Clinical immunology illustrated. Baltimore. Williams & Wilkins, 1985.

Chapter Ten

NURSING CARE *of Adults with Immunodeficiency and Hypersensitivity Disorders*

There are many different ways in which disorders of immunity are classified. This chapter basically divides them into immunodeficiency disorders, hypersensitivity disorders, and autoimmune disorders. Immunodeficiency disorders are characterized by the failure of the immune system to respond in a normal manner. Hypersensitivity disorders are those in which the immune system overreacts and tissue damage occurs. Autoimmune disorders are those in which the body reacts immunologically against itself.

Immunodeficiencies

When the immune system fails to produce an adequate response to an antigen, an immunodeficiency exists.

Immunodeficiencies may be caused by a defect or deficiency in B cells, T cells, phagocytes, or complement. The symptoms of immunodeficiencies depend on the components of the immune system that have been affected and the degree to which their function has been impaired. Symptoms seen with many immunodeficiency diseases include chronic or frequently occurring infections, infections caused by unusual organisms or organisms that are normal body flora, poor response to the treatment of the infection, chronic diarrhea, skin rash, abscesses, osteomyelitis, hepatosplenomegaly, and failure to grow and thrive. The deficiency may be present at birth or it may be acquired later in life as a result of a disease or an exposure to a toxic agent or other unknown cause. The ability to diagnose immunodeficiencies is expanding as more is learned about the immune system and laboratory techniques improve.

Primary Immunodeficiencies

Stem-cell deficiency, DiGeorge's syndrome, and agammaglobulinemia are examples of primary immunodeficiencies that are predominantly pediatric problems, because individuals with these diseases seldom live to adulthood. The most severe of these is stem-cell deficiency, also called severe combined immunodeficiency (SCID). This is an inherited trait and is characterized by absence of both T-cell and B-cell function. In DiGeorge's syndrome, there is lack of thymic development and subsequent lack of T cells, resulting in impaired cell-mediated immunity. Agammaglobulinemia is an inherited disorder in which there are no B cells or antibodies. Symptoms of primary immunodeficiencies usually develop very early in life, at about the time protection from maternal antibodies is lost. Treatment consists of aggressive antibiotic therapy for infections and possibly prophylactic antibiotics to help prevent infections. Administration of gamma globulin may be helpful in stem-cell deficiency and agammaglobulinemia. Bone marrow transplants and fetal liver and fetal thymic transplants may be helpful in stem-cell deficiency and DiGeorge's syndrome.

The most common primary immunodeficiency is selective IgA deficiency, which affects approximately 1 in 600 people. Its cause is unknown. It is defined as a serum IgA level of less than 5 mg/dl with normal or increased levels of the other immunoglobulins and normal T-cell function.

Many patients with selective IgA deficiency have no symptoms and remain relatively healthy. Other patients seem to be more susceptible to respiratory tract and gastrointestinal tract infections. Selective IgA deficiency has also been associated with an increased incidence of allergies and autoimmune disorders. When symptoms do occur, it is usually within the first 10 years of life.

Treatment consists of combating infections with the appropriate antibiotics, because no safe effective method is available for replacing just the missing IgA. Gamma globulin is not given, because these patients can produce normal amounts of the other four classes of antibodies. In addition, their immune system can recognize the injected IgA as foreign and produce antibodies against it. These anti-IgA antibodies then increase the patient's risk of developing a transfusion reaction if blood is ever needed, because anti-IgA antibodies would react with the IgA in the transfused blood. With proper treatment of infections and other associated conditions, the prognosis for a normal life span is good.

Secondary Immunodeficiencies

ETIOLOGY AND PATHOPHYSIOLOGY

Secondary immunodeficiencies are caused by a vast array of diseases and drugs and exhibit a wide range of degree and duration of immunosuppression. In addition to the major immunosuppressant drugs discussed in Chapter 9, many other drugs have the potential to cause immunosuppression as a rare side effect. Some infectious diseases also cause a degree of immunosuppression. These include tuberculosis, leprosy, measles, cytomegalovirus, congenital rubella, and acquired immunodeficiency syndrome (AIDS). Immunosuppression is also characteristic of malignant disease. Immunosuppression may be the result of malignancies such as leukemias and lymphomas, which directly involve the cells of the immune system and alter their function, or it may be due to the malnutrition and protein depletion that is frequently associated with malignant diseases. Severe immunosuppression may also result from chemotherapy and radiation therapy used to treat malignant disease.

Patients with severe burns develop some degree of immunosuppression, because their intact skin, a very important defense mechanism, is gone, and antibodies are lost along with the serum in the exudate. Diabetics may have less-efficient phagocytic cells, which combined with high levels of glucose and vascular disease increases their risk of infection.

Alcoholics may experience immunosuppression as a result of the malnutrition often associated with the disease and the liver damage that occurs. Chronic lung diseases tend to destroy the defense mechanisms of the respiratory tract, leaving the patient more susceptible to respiratory infections. Some degree of immunosuppression may also be seen for several weeks after anesthesia and surgery as well as following trauma, emotional and physical stress, and pregnancy.

CLINICAL MANIFESTATIONS

The clinical manifestations vary greatly, depending on the degree and duration of the immunosuppression. Some patients do not develop any infections, whereas others develop one or more fulminating infections. Ultimately, the symptoms depend on what type of infection develops. Infections with opportunistic organisms, such as *Staphylococcus epidermidis* and *Candida albicans,* are much more likely to occur in patients with immunosuppression.

MEDICAL DIAGNOSIS

Diagnosis of secondary immunodeficiency is often based on the patient's clinical picture and history. Frequent infections, infections with unusual organisms, or minor infections that do not heal are clues that the patient may have an immunodeficiency. Laboratory tests can be done to determine T-cell and B-cell function as well as determine levels of antibodies in the blood. Skin tests with common antigens can be done to determine whether cell-mediated immunity is intact, although a small percentage of the population are anergic (i.e., have a diminished reactivity to specific antigens).

MEDICAL MANAGEMENT

The specific medical management depends on the underlying cause of the immunodeficiency. If possible, this cause is eliminated. Infections are treated with antimicrobials effective against the causative organism.

Guidelines for Application of the Nursing Process to the Care of the Patient with an Immunodeficiency

Nursing care of the patient with an immunodeficiency depends on the type, degree, and expected duration of the deficiency. If the person is being treated as an outpatient, teach the patient how to minimize the risk of infection. Explain the importance of good personal hygiene, the need to avoid crowds and contact with persons who are known to be ill, and the necessity of seeking medical care at the first sign of an infection rather than making attempts at self-treatment.

Acquired Immunodeficiency Syndrome

Infection with human immunodeficiency virus (HIV) causes progressive deterioration and dysfunction in cell-mediated immunity and in its most severe manifestation results in the disease syndrome known as acquired immunodeficiency syndrome (AIDS). HIV infection is currently epidemic in the United States and throughout the world.

ETIOLOGY

AIDS results from infection with the human immunodeficiency virus (HIV), of which two strains have been identified. HIV-1 is the prototype virus and is responsible for most cases of AIDS. HIV-2 is found chiefly in West Africa and appears to be less easily transmitted and to have a longer incubation period than HIV-1.

It is not clear what role cofactors may play in susceptibility to infection, transmission of the virus, or the progressive immune deficiency the virus causes. The presence of other sexually transmitted diseases, especially those causing genital ulcers, such as herpes simplex or syphilis, may influence susceptibility either by facilitating viral entry or by increasing the number of activated lymphocytes or monocytes (target cells) for HIV to infect. Susceptibility may also be increased by other infections such as those caused by cytomegalovirus (CMV) and Epstein-Barr virus (EBV), which also activate target cells. Infectivity potential appears to vary with the disease state of the person infected. Transmission has been found to be more frequent after the infected person has been diagnosed with AIDS as opposed to having only minor symptoms or being asymptomatic. This may be due to a higher viral load with declining immune status.

PATHOPHYSIOLOGY

HIV is a retrovirus containing RNA and reverse transcriptase (an enzyme) that primarily infects $CD4^+$ (helper) T cells. The virus enters the $CD4^+$ (helper) T cell after binding to a specific site on the surface of the cell. Once inside the cell, the reverse transcriptase transforms the RNA into DNA. This viral DNA is incorporated into the genome of the $CD4^+$ T cell. Once the $CD4^+$ T cell is activated or stimulated by exposure to other antigens, viral replication occurs. The $CD4^+$ T cell is destroyed when HIV replication occurs. As the cells are destroyed, more HIV is released, which infects more $CD4^+$ T cells, and the cycle repeats. The depletion of $CD4^+$ T cells subsequently causes a wide range of immunologic abnormalities and results in the clinical development of a variety of opportunistic infections and malignancies.

These immunologic abnormalities do not occur all at once, but tend to progress in both number and severity over time. The most important defect is a decrease in the number of $CD4^{+}$ T cells as well as a decrease in the functioning of the ones that remain. Other immunologic abnormalities that may occur include impaired delayed hypersensitivity reactions, decreased primary antibody response, lymphopenia, decreased production of interleukin-2, decreased cytotoxicity, impaired function of natural killer cells, impaired monocyte chemotaxis, increased production of some antibodies, and increased formation of immune complexes. These leave the patient susceptible to a wide variety of opportunistic infections and unusual neoplasms.

Monocytes and macrophages can also be infected by HIV, and this is believed to be the mechanism by which HIV is transported into the central nervous system. Once HIV is inside the central nervous system, damage to neural tissue can occur, producing subacute encephalitis (AIDS dementia complex, also known as HIV encephalopathy or HIV encephalitis).

TRANSMISSION

HIV is transmitted from one person to another by deposition of a body fluid containing HIV from an infected person into a body cavity or the vascular system of an uninfected person. Probability of transmission increases with concentration of HIV. Body fluids that have been shown to transmit the virus are blood, semen, cerebrospinal fluid, vaginal secretions, and breast milk. HIV has been isolated from many other body fuids, such as tears, saliva, and urine, but the amount present is not believed to be significant enough to cause infection.

The three routes of transmission are intimate sexual contact involving the exchange of body fluids; parenteral, by inoculation with infected blood, blood products, or body fluids; and perinatal, from infected mother to fetus or infant. There is no evidence that HIV is spread during casual contact with an infected person or through air, water, or food. HIV is not transmitted via fomites or insect or animal vectors. HIV cannot move independently.

In the United States, transmission of HIV most frequently occurs through intimate sexual activity and intravenous drug use. Transmission of HIV occurs during both heterosexual and homosexual sexual activity. It can be transmitted from male to male, male to female, female to male, and female to female. At this time, the risk of acquiring HIV from a single sexual encounter with an infected person is not known, although it appears to be less easily transmitted than other sexually transmitted diseases such as gonorrhea and syphilis.

Certain sexual practices increase the risk of exposure to body fluids and thereby increase the chance of infection. Those practices that pose a risk of transmission include anal, vaginal, and oral intercourse without the use of a latex barrier. The risk of transmission exists owing to potential tears in the mucous membrane, resulting in direct viral access to the vascular system. In the case of anal intercourse, mucosal damage may not even be necessary, because the high rate of fluid absorption in this part of the digestive system may result in the movement of virus through the mucous membrane. Sexual practices such as insertion of large objects or fists into the anal or vaginal cavities, or those that involve the piercing of various body parts that expose a person to the blood of his or her partner, pose a greater risk of HIV transmission. The portal of entry in these situations may be breaks in the skin or mucous membrane of the active partner.

The use of latex barriers such as gloves, condoms, and vaginal dams reduces the chance of exposure and thereby reduces the risk of infection. It is important that latex be used, because HIV is unable to permeate it. This is not true of animal skin condoms. Water-soluble lubricants or a spermicide containing nonoxynol 9 may be used with condoms. Oil-based lubricants, such as hand lotion, baby oil, or Vaseline, should not be used, because they dissolve latex and cause condom or glove breakage. Avoidance of high-risk sexual practices, especially anal intercourse, should also be encouraged. Limiting the number of sexual partners decreases the number of possible exposures but does not prevent the transmission of this infection.

Transmission by inoculation of infected blood can occur in several ways. The most frequent is through the sharing of blood-contaminated needles and syringes by intravenous drug users. Although the amount of blood present in the needle and syringe may be very small, the frequent, repeated exposure to contaminated blood increases the chance of becoming infected with HIV. Infected intravenous drug users play an important role in transmitting the virus to children and to the heterosexual community that does not engage in intravenous drug use.

HIV can also be transmitted through transfusion of blood or blood products that contain the virus and via organ transplant from an infected donor. Only a small proportion of the patients with AIDS, approximately 3%, have become infected by this route. Since April 1985, all units of blood donated in the United States are screened for antibody to HIV. If antibodies to HIV are present, the unit of blood is not used. Blood products such as clotting-factor concentrates are now being prepared in such a way that the virus, if present, is inactivated. The screening of blood and treating blood products have almost, but not completely, eliminated this route of transmission.

Women infected with HIV may pass the virus to their infants during the perinatal period. This transmission may occur by one of the following routes: from the maternal circulation to the fetus while it is in utero, from exposure of the infant to maternal blood and body fluids during labor and delivery, and through infected breast milk. The risk of transmission from an HIV-infected mother to her child ranges from 20% to 50%.

Health care workers may be exposed to HIV while providing patient care; however, routine care activities do not facilitate transmission of HIV. Accidental transmission of HIV can occur if the health care worker has contact with the blood or body fluids of an HIV-infected patient, especially through percutaneous exposure. To minimize risk of accidental infection with HIV, all health care workers should avoid contact with blood and body fluids of patients. Gloves should be worn whenever contact with blood or body fluids is likely. If blood or body fluids are likely to be splashed, spattered, or aerosolized, masks and goggles should be worn to prevent contact with the mucous membranes of the eyes, nose, and mouth. Gowns should also be worn whenever there is the possibility of blood or body fluids contacting the arms or body. When using needles or other sharp items, health care workers must use extreme care to avoid injuring themselves. Needles should *never* be bent, broken, or recapped. Needles and other sharps should be immediately disposed of in a puncture-resistant container. If a health care worker is exposed to any body fluid, he or she should immediately wash the area with soap and water. All needle-stick injuries, lacerations, or abrasions with body fluid–contaminated materials or instruments should be reported, and if deemed a significant exposure, follow-up testing should be instituted. HIV testing should be performed immediately, and at 3 months, 6 months, and 1 year. The health care worker should be instructed in preventing transmission to sexual partners.

CLINICAL MANIFESTATIONS

HIV infection results in a spectrum of disease manifestations, with four relatively distinct stages (Barrick, 1990). These are an acute infection described as flulike or mononucleosis-like, with a high level of viral replication; an asymptomatic period lasting from 2 months to possibly 15 years, characterized by continuous low-level viral replication and $CD4^+$ T cell loss and, in some cases, the presence of persistent generalized lymphadenopathy; a transitional period or symptomatic disease characterized by mild to moderate immune deficiency; and finally a period marked by the development of a number of opportunistic infections or malignancies.

The acute infection, which not every person infected with HIV develops, is associated with seroconversion. It is characterized by the sudden development of fever, sweats, sore throat, malaise, myalgias, arthralgias, photophobia, diarrhea, anorexia, nausea, vomiting, or headache. There may be generalized lymphadenopathy, enlarged spleen, and a transient maculopapular rash on the chest and trunk, which may also involve the extremities. These symptoms may develop from 6 days to 12 weeks after infection with HIV and resolve spontaneously in 2 to 3 weeks. Aseptic meningitis may also occur during this time. The clinical manifestations include confusion, mood changes, seizures, and changes in mental status. Many patients become completely asymptomatic after these symptoms subside. Others may develop persistent generalized lymphadenopathy (PGL). This is defined as the presence of lymph nodes larger than 1 cm in diameter in two or more extrainguinal sites lasting for more than 3 months. Many patients have no other symptoms and are not aware of their enlarged lymph nodes.

Because HIV causes progressive immunodeficiency, patients enter the transitional period of symptomatic disease. During this phase of the illness, any of the following symptoms or conditions may initially develop: fevers, night sweats, severe malaise and fatigue, mild weight loss, intermittent diarrhea, oral or dermatologic disorders, PGL, and splenomegaly. Frequently seen hematologic abnormalities include neutropenia, lymphopenia, thrombocytopenia, anemia, and decreased number of $CD4^+$ T cells and a reversal of the normal $CD4^+$:T8 ratio. The final stage of HIV disease (AIDS) is characterized by severe immunodeficiency (less than 200 mm^3 $CD4^+$ T cells), which gives rise to the development of a variety of opportunistic infections or malignancies. Any body system or organ can be affected.

Oral manifestations occur in the great majority of patients with HIV infection. Among the most common are oral candidiasis, oral hairy leukoplakia, and recurrent herpes simplex lesions.

Dermatologic manifestations are also very common in patients with AIDS. These include varicella, herpes zoster, molluscum contagiosum, eczema, seborrheic dermatitis, and folliculitis. Kaposi's sarcoma, a vascular neoplasm, may also occur. The lesions of Kaposi's sarcoma may occur anywhere on the body surface as well as on the oral mucosa and internal organs. Lesions begin as pink, red, or purple nodules or plaques. They are usually firm to palpation and nontender, do not blanch when pressure is applied, and do not itch (Fig. 10–1). Visceral and lymphatic involvement may result in pain if the tumor presses against nerves or organs.

The gastrointestinal (GI) tract may be affected by a variety of problems with HIV disease. More than 60% of patients are affected by diarrhea. The diarrhea may be caused by any number of enteric pathogens, such as *Giardia lamblia, Entamoeba histolytica,* and species of *Salmonella, Shigella,* and *Campylobacter.* Organisms only recently recognized as causing human disease, such as the protozoa *Cryptosporidium* spp. and *Isospora belli,* have been found to be common pathogens in AIDS patients. Often a specific cause of the diarrhea is not identified. Kaposi's sarcoma and non-Hodgkin's lymphoma may also affect the GI tract and cause diarrhea or obstruction.

Esophagitis caused by *Candida,* cytomegalovirus, or herpes virus is another common GI problem for

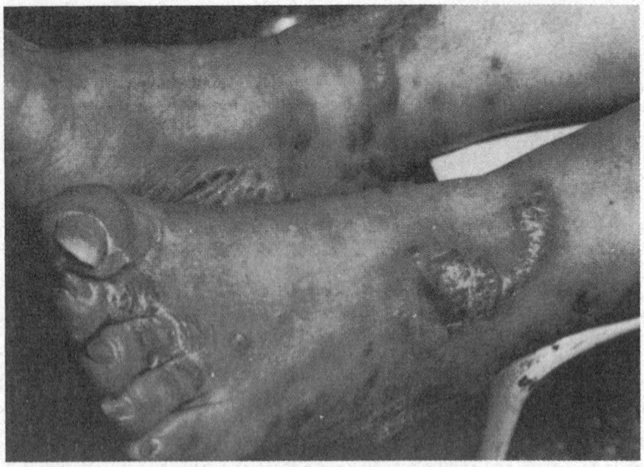

Figure 10–1.

Kaposi's sarcoma. (From Moschella SL, Hurley JH (eds). Dermatology. 3rd ed, Vol 2. Philadelphia: WB Saunders, 1992, p 1785.)

patients with AIDS and can cause severe difficulty swallowing. Chronic, recurrent aphthous ulcers may also contribute to dysphagia. A chronic malabsorption syndrome with no identifiable infectious agent may also occur. This syndrome is characterized by weight loss and diarrhea. Liver dysfunction from hepatitis and infection of the liver by cytomegalovirus or *Mycobacterium avium-intracellulare* is also a problem for some patients with AIDS.

The most frequent pulmonary manifestation of AIDS is pneumonia caused by the protozoa *Pneumocystis carinii.* The common symptoms of *P. carinii* pneumonia (PCP) include fever, dyspnea, tachypnea, and dry cough. These are sometimes accompanied by chills and chest pain. Lung sounds and chest x-ray films may be normal or more often reveal diffuse interstitial infiltrates. Arterial blood gases show a variable degree of hypoxia. A gallium scan may be used in the diagnosis of PCP. Other pulmonary infections that may be seen in persons with AIDS are those caused by cytomegalovirus and *Mycobacterium avium-intracellulare;* Kaposi's sarcoma can also involve the lungs. Other pulmonary conditions that may develop during the symptomatic stages include *Haemophilus influenzae* infection, pneumococcal pneumonia, streptococcal pneumonia, and reactivated *Mycobacterium tuberculosis.*

Neurologic problems are common in patients with progressive HIV infection and cover a wide range of symptoms that involve both the central and peripheral nervous systems. These problems may result from infection of the nervous system with HIV or from opportunistic infections such as cytomegalovirus infection, toxoplasmosis, cryptococcosis and tuberculosis. Lymphoma also frequently affects the central nervous system.

The most common neurologic disorder is a nonfocal encephalopathy that is known as AIDS-dementia complex, which results in cognitive, motor, and behavioral changes. Initially subtle changes such as forgetfulness, poor concentration, decreased spontaneity, poor cognitive flexibility, and psychomotor slowing may occur. A flat affect and apathy similar to that seen with depression and anxiety are also common. Later the patient may exhibit an unsteady gait and incoordination, and loss of libido and withdrawal may occur. Advanced symptoms include confusion, vacant staring, disorientation, organic psychosis, seizures, mutism, urinary and fecal incontinence, hemiparesis, paraparesis, blindness, delirium, and coma.

Patients with AIDS may develop ophthalmologic problems resulting from opportunistic infections of the eye with bacterial, fungal, and viral pathogens. The symptoms are usually blurred vision or loss of vision. Cytomegalovirus retinitis is a common problem.

The heart, kidneys, and endocrine glands are less frequently involved in AIDS. A few patients have been found to have myocarditis or pericarditis caused by a variety of infectious agents. Renal involvement has included proteinuria, azotemia, and renal failure. Some patients with invasive cytomegalovirus infection have been found to have adrenal insufficiency requiring supplemental steroid therapy, and others have developed hypercalcemia suggesting involvement of the parathyroid glands.

In women, there is a high incidence of vaginal candidal infection even in early stages of HIV disease. In HIV-infected women with pelvic inflammatory disease, there is an increased incidence of ovarian abscess. Among all HIV-infected women, there is an increased incidence, severity, and rate of progression of cancer of the cervix (Rubin, 1993, p. 4).

MEDICAL DIAGNOSIS

The diagnosis of AIDS is made when the patient meets the clinical criteria that have been established by the Centers for Disease Control (CDC) (Table 10–1).

AIDS cannot be diagnosed simply by laboratory test, because the test for antibodies to HIV does not determine whether a person does or does not have AIDS. The test merely indicates whether antibodies to HIV are present in the person's blood. If the antibody test is positive, it is presumed that the person was infected with HIV at some time in the past, continues to be infected, and is capable of transmitting the virus to others.

When testing for HIV antibodies, two tests are usually done. The first is an enzyme-linked immunosorbent assay (ELISA). If the ELISA test for antibodies is repeatedly positive, then a confirmatory test for proteins specific to HIV is done by the Western blot method.

The tests for HIV antibodies can have false-negative and false-positive results. False-negative results occur because there is a gap between infection with the virus and appearance of antibodies (called the

Table 10–1. CDC SURVEILLANCE CASE DEFINITION FOR AIDS

I. *HIV status of patient is unknown or inconclusive*
If laboratory tests for HIV infection were not performed or gave inconclusive results and the patient had no other cause of immunodeficiency listed in *IA* (see below), a definitive diagnosis of any disease listed in *IB* (see below) indicates AIDS.

A. *Causes of immunodeficiency that disqualify a disease as an indication of AIDS in the absence of laboratory evidence of HIV infection*
1. The use of high-dose or long-term systemic corticosteroid therapy or other immunosuppressive/cytotoxic therapy within 3 months before the onset of the indicator disease.
2. A diagnosis of any of the following diseases within 3 months after diagnosis of the indicator disease: Hodgkin's disease, non-Hodgkin's lymphoma (other than primary brain lymphoma), lymphocytic leukemia, multiple myeloma, any other cancer of lymphoreticular or histiocytic tissue, or angioimmunoblastic lymphadenopathy.
3. A genetic (congenital) immunodeficiency syndrome or an acquired immunodeficiency syndrome or an acquired immunodeficiency syndrome that is atypical of HIV infection, such as one involving hypogammaglobulinemia.

B. *Diseases that indicate AIDS (requires definitive diagnosis)*
1. Candidiasis of the esophagus, trachea, bronchi, or lungs.
2. Cryptococcosis, extrapulmonary.
3. Cryptosporidiosis with diarrhea persisting for more than 1 month.
4. Cytomegalovirus disease of an organ other than the liver, spleen, or lymph nodes in a patient older than 1 month.
5. Herpes simplex virus infection causing a mucocutaneous ulcer that persists longer than 1 month; or herpes simplex virus infection causing bronchitis, pneumonitis, or esophagitis for any duration in a patient older than 1 month.
6. Kaposi's sarcoma in a patient younger than 60 years.
7. Lymphoid interstitial pneumonia or pulmonary lymphoid hyperplasia (LIP/PLH complex) in a patient younger than 13 years.
8. Lymphoma of the brain (primary) affecting a patient younger than 60 years.
9. *Mycobacterium avium* complex or *M. kansasii* disease, disseminated (at a site other than or in addition to the lungs, skin, or cervical or hilar lymph nodes).
10. *Pneumocystis carinii* pneumonia.
11. Progressive multifocal leukoencephalopathy.
12. Toxoplasmosis of the brain in a patient older than 1 month.

II. *Patient is HIV positive*
Regardless of the presence of other causes of immunodeficiency (see *IA*, above), in the presence of laboratory evidence of HIV infection, any disease listed in *IB* (see above) or in *IIA* or *IIB* (see below) indicates a diagnosis of AIDS. In addition, beginning in 1993, all HIV-positive adults and adolescents with $CD4^+$ T cell counts less than 200/mm^3 or with pulmonary tuberculosis, recurrent pneumonia, or invasive cervical carcinoma should also be included in the AIDS case definition.

A. *Diseases that indicate AIDS (requires definitive diagnosis)*
1. Bacterial infections, multiple or recurrent (any combination of at least two within a 2- to 4-year period), of the following types in a patient younger than 13 years: septicemia, pneumonia, meningitis, bone or joint infection, or abscess of an internal organ or body cavity (excluding otitis media or superficial skin or mucosal abscesses) caused by *Haemophilus*, *Streptococcus* (including pneumococcus), or other pyogenic bacteria.
2. Coccidioidomycosis, disseminated (at a site other than or in addition to the lungs or cervical or hilar lymph nodes).
3. Histoplasmosis, disseminated (at a site other than or in addition to the lungs or cervical or hilar lymph nodes).
4. HIV encephalopathy.
5. HIV wasting syndrome.
6. Isoporiasis with diarrhea persisting for more than 1 month.
7. Kaposi's sarcoma at any age.
8. Lymphoma of the brain (primary) at any age.
9. *M. tuberculosis* disease, extrapulmonary (involving at least one site outside the lungs, regardless of whether there is concurrent pulmonary involvement).
10. Mycobacterial disease caused by mycobacteria other than *M. tuberculosis*, disseminated (at a site other than or in addition to the lungs, skin, or cervical or hilar lymph nodes).
11. Non-Hodgkin's lymphoma of B-cell or unknown immunologic phenotype and the following histologic types: small noncleaved lymphoma (Burkitt's or non-Burkitt's) or immunoblastic sarcoma.
12. *Salmonella* (nontyphoidal) septicemia, recurrent.

B. *Diseases that indicate AIDS (presumptive diagnosis)*
1. Candidiasis of the esophagus.
2. Cytomegalovirus retinitis, with loss of vision.
3. Kaposi's sarcoma.
4. Lymphoid interstitial pneumonia or pulmonary lymphoid hyperplasia (LIP/PLH complex) in a patient younger than 13 years.
5. Mycobacterial disease (acid-fast bacilli with species not identified by culture), disseminated (involving at least one site other than or in addition to the lungs, skin, or cervical or hilar lymph nodes).
6. *P. carinii* pneumonia.
7. Toxoplasmosis of the brain in a patient older than 1 month.

III. *Patient is HIV negative*
With laboratory test results negative for HIV infection, a diagnosis of AIDS for surveillance purposes is ruled out *unless*

A. All the other causes of immunodeficiency listed in *IA* (see above) are excluded; and
B. The patient has had either of the following:
1. *P. carinii* pneumonia diagnosed by a definitive method.
2. A definitive diagnosis of any of the other diseases indicative of AIDS listed in *IB* (see above) and a $CD4^+$ helper-inducer T cell count of less than 400/mm.[3]

Table 10–2. CLASSIFICATION SYSTEM FOR HIV INFECTION

	CLINICAL CATEGORIES		
CD4+ T CELL CATEGORIES	A Asymptomatic, persistent, generalized lymphadenopathy, or acute (primary) HIV infection	B Symptomatic but not included in category C	C AIDS-indicator conditions included in the surveillance case definition (*see Table 10–1*)
1 ≥500/mm³	A1	B1	C1
2 200–499/mm³	A2	B2	C2
3 <200/mm³	A3	B3	C3

window period). For most people, it is 6 to 8 weeks until antibodies develop, but some people may take several months. False-positives can occur for a variety of biologic and technical reasons. For example, infants younger than 6 months of age may have maternal antibodies that cause a positive test when in fact the infant is not infected with HIV.

Serial measures of the level of circulating CD4+ T cells are used to assess disease progression. Levels lower than 200/mm³ are correlated with advancing disease and a worsening prognosis. CD4+ T cell levels also serve as the basis for the CDC proposed classification system for HIV-infected adolescents and adults. The system is based on three ranges of CD4+ T cell counts and three clinical categories, the interface of which produces nine mutually exclusive categories (Table 10–2).

MEDICAL MANAGEMENT

There is no known cure for AIDS. Current medical management primarily consists of treatment of infections and malignancies that develop and antiretroviral therapy with zidovudine (Retrovir, AZT), dideoxyinosine (Videx, ddI), and zalcitabine (Hivid, formerly ddC). These drugs block HIV replication by inhibiting HIV reverse transcriptase. They reduce the spread of HIV to uninfected cells but do not inhibit virus production in chronically infected cells and decrease concentration of HIV in semen only to a limited degree.

The effectiveness of zidovudine therapy decreases over time. Treatment given early in the course of HIV infection delays progression to full-blown AIDS but does not result in an overall increase in survival time. Development of drug resistance is believed to cause the decrease in effectiveness, and combination therapy (use of more than one drug alternatively or simultaneously) is becoming standard practice.

Infections are treated early and aggressively because this usually produces a better outcome than delaying treatment until the infection becomes severe. Prophylactic anti-infectives are often given to prevent recurrence of PCP, lesions caused by the herpes simplex virus, and candidal infections.

Application of the Nursing Process to the Care of the Patient with AIDS

Assessment

The nursing assessment of the patient with AIDS is very complex because there are many physical, psychological, and social issues confronting the patient. In addition, the patient's status may change frequently and very quickly as new infections and problems develop.

Perform a head-to-toe physical assessment, and obtain a detailed description of current symptoms and their severity.

Inspect the patient's skin and mouth for lesions and signs of infection. In the mouth look specifically for the white patches indicative of candidal infection or hairy leukoplakia and for herpes simplex lesions, because these are common causes of oral infections in persons with HIV infection. Question the patient about soreness of the mouth, bleeding gums, and difficulty chewing or swallowing.

Ask the patient about any weight loss, change in appetite, abdominal pain, and diarrhea. If diarrhea is a problem, determine remedies that have been tried and their effectiveness. Assess for signs of dehydration. Also obtain a dietary history to determine the adequacy of the patient's nutritional intake and to determine whether foods are being eaten that are known to contribute to hyperactivity of the bowel.

Carefully assess respiratory status, because persons with AIDS are at risk of developing respiratory difficulties. Check pulse and respirations, color, and lung sounds. Question the patient about cough, chest pain, and sputum production. Review arterial blood gas values.

Because many patients with AIDS have an impairment of mental status caused by the disease itself, opportunistic infections of the central nervous system, metabolic abnormalities caused by other problems, or the adverse effects of drugs, determine the patient's baseline mental status so that changes can be identified. As part of the neurologic assessment, determine the patient's ability to pay attention, to concentrate, and to follow commands. Also assess memory, speech, judgment, and mood. Ask family or significant others whether changes have been observed in these parameters.

Assess the patient's emotional status and coping ability. Explore the patient's current ability for self-care, including for out-patients areas of home management such as food preparation, shopping, getting to and from medical facilities, and so on. Ask about existing support for psychosocial as well as physical needs from family and friends.

Explore the patient's understanding of the disease and its transmission, infections that may develop, available treatment methods, self-care, and available community resources.

Nursing Diagnoses and Planning

Nursing diagnoses and related expected patient outcomes most commonly applicable to patients with AIDS include the following:

NDx: High risk for altered health maintenance related to lack of knowledge of etiology and transmission of the disease, clinical course, treatment, and self-care

Planning: Patient outcomes

1. Patient explains that AIDS is caused by a virus that weakens the immune system and its ability to fight off infections or prevent the development of certain malignancies.
2. Patient explains stages of HIV infection.
3. Patient describes types of available medical therapy and their goals.
4. Patient describes ways HIV is transmitted to others.
5. Patient identifies ways to reduce the risk of spreading the virus to others or acquiring additional sexually transmitted diseases, including "safer sex" and not sharing needles.
6. Patient lists symptoms that require immediate medical evaluation (see Chart 10–1).
7. Patient states where to go for medical evaluation.
8. Patient states name, use, dose, route, frequency, and reportable side effects of all prescribed drugs.
9. Patient describes health habits that promote healthy immune function, including stress reduction, exercise, and good nutrition.

NDx: Pain related to the effects of HIV infection on various tissues and organs.

Planning: Patient outcomes

1. Patient describes correct use of prescribed analgesics.
2. Patient describes nonpharmacologic comfort measures specific to the problem.
3. Patient reports that therapeutic measures result in decreased pain.

NDx: Diarrhea related to GI infection or irritation

Planning: Patient outcomes

1. Patient describes prescribed antidiarrheal regimen accurately.
2. Patient describes signs and symptoms of dehydration and means of treating or preventing its development.
3. Patient lists foods to be avoided because of their irritating or stimulating effect on the GI tract.
4. Patient is free of incontinence due to diarrhea.
5. Limitations on usual activities caused by diarrhea are absent.
6. Patient's fluid and electrolyte values are within normal limits.
7. Patient is free of anal or perineal skin irritation due to diarrhea.

NDs: Altered oral mucous membrane related to *Candida*, herpes simplex, or other infection

Planning: Patient outcomes

1. Patient cares for the mouth as specified in Chart 10–2.
2. Number of lesions decreases.
3. Patient chews and swallows soft foods with minimal discomfort.

NDx: Ineffective breathing pattern related to alteration in respiratory function secondary to infectious and/or neoplastic processes

Planning: Patient outcomes

1. Respirations are easy and quiet.
2. Nail beds and mucous membranes are pink.
3. Arterial blood gas values are within normal limits.
4. Shortness of breath during normal daily activities is absent.

NDx: Social isolation related to social stigma, people's fear of contracting the disease, lack of strength, or lack of motivation to maintain normal social activities

Planning: Patient outcomes

1. Patient initiates conversation with professional staff, other patients, or social acquaintances.
2. Patient maintains contact with family or friends on a regular basis.
3. Patient identifies support persons he or she can rely on in the community.
4. Patient describes available support groups and their meeting times and places.
5. Patient participates in social activities consistent with physical condition.

NDx: Ineffective individual coping related to a contagious life-threatening disease with a degree of social stigma

Planning: Patient outcomes
1. Patient verbalizes feelings and concerns.
2. Patient identifies sources of support.
3. Patient discusses feelings about death and dying.
4. Patient prepares for death (e.g., makes a will, plans funeral arrangements, gives advance directives for health care).

NDx: High risk for impaired home maintenance management related to incapacitating weakness

Planning: Patient outcomes
1. Patient or caregiver identifies areas of home maintenance in which help is or will be needed.
2. Patient or caregiver identifies sources of assistance in the community.
3. Patient lives at home safely with medical as well as basic human needs met.
4. Patient utilizes assistive devices when appropriate.

Nursing Interventions

The nursing care of patients with HIV infection varies greatly from patient to patient depending on which infections develop and the severity of the disease. Care becomes increasingly complex as more problems develop and the patient becomes weaker.

NDx: High risk for altered health maintenance

Explain to the patient what causes the disease, how it affects the body, the stages of disease progression, and the available treatment possibilities both standard and experimental. Carefully explain how the disease is transmitted, and instruct the patient on precautions to take to avoid transmitting the disease to others. Include a discussion of safer sexual practices. Also instruct significant others and people caring for the patient in how to reduce their risk of exposure to the virus (Table 10–3).

Instruct the patient in self-care. Stress the importance of nutritious diet, exercise if possible, rest, and following orders for prescribed treatments conscientiously. Be certain that the patient understands basic information about any prescribed medications, including the name of the drug, the dose, when to take it, how to take it, any side effects that should be reported, and what the drug is for. Also instruct the patient on when to seek additional medical attention for symptoms that develop as specified in Chart 10–1.

NDx: Pain

Pain and discomfort from a wide variety of causes can be a major problem for the patient with AIDS.

Give analgesics as ordered, keeping in mind that they are often more effective when given on a regular schedule than on an as-needed basis. Be sure the patient's basic comfort needs are met. These include proper environmental temperature, a comfortable place to lie or sit, ability to reposition frequently, and good personal hygiene. Teach and encourage the use of nonpharmacologic pain therapies such as relaxation therapies and cutaneous therapies.

Table 10–3. INFECTION CONTROL GUIDELINES FOR CARE OF AIDS PATIENTS AT HOME

Wash hands thoroughly with soap and water before and after giving direct care and preparing foods and in between preparing different food items.

Wear latex gloves when handling blood or body fluids. Rubber gloves made for household cleaning should also be used when cleaning up body fluid spills. These can be disinfected and reused.

Cover any cuts or broken skin that may come into contact with blood or body fluids with Band-Aids.

When using needles, be very careful to avoid needle sticks. Place used needles in a puncture-proof container such as a coffee can immediately after use. Never recap, bend, or break a needle. A puncture-proof container should be in every room in which needles are used and discarded.

Wash dishes used by the patient in hot soapy water. Patients with HIV infection do not require separate dishes or eating utensils.

Use usual cleansers for normal household cleaning. Clean the bathroom regularly using a household disinfectant. Clean up blood spills with a diluted bleach solution (1 part bleach mixed with 10 parts water) and wear gloves for this task. A new bleach solution should be made every 24 hours, because old solutions are less effective.

Allow the patient to prepare food for others provided that he or she does not have any open lesions on the hands or arms and does not have diarrhea.

Do not share personal items such as a toothbrush or razor with the patient.

Wash clothing and linen in the usual manner with soap or detergent in either hot or cold water. It is not necessary to add bleach to kill the virus.

Prevent exposure of the neutropenic patient to people with active infections.

Protect patients with HIV invection from pathogens found in foods:

- Avoid use of raw or undercooked meat, poultry, fish, shellfish, or eggs as well as raw (unpasteurized) milk.
- Wash utensils before reusing with other foods that are being prepared.
- Do not mix raw foods or their juices with other foods.
- Use a plastic rather than a wooden cutting board, because plastic ones are easier to clean.
- Wash fruit and vegetables thoroughly.

NDx: Diarrhea

Diarrhea is one of the most severe problems that affects patients with HIV infection. It can be very debilitating and can force the patient to limit activities. Because it can have so many different causes, there is no one specific plan of medical management. Identifiable infections are treated if a treatment is available and an antidiarrhea regimen found that is effective for the patient. Ensure that the patient has easy access to a bathroom, or if unable to get to the bathroom, that a bedside commode or bedpan is readily available. If needed, provide assistance without delay. Be certain that the anal and perineal areas are kept meticulously clean and apply emollient or other topical preparations to protect the skin from irritation by stool. For patients with peri-

Chart 10–1.

NURSING GUIDE TO PATIENT EDUCATION FOR SELF-MANAGEMENT: SYMPTOMS THAT REQUIRE IMMEDIATE MEDICAL EVALUATION IN THE AIDS PATIENT

Instruct the patient to seek prompt medical attention for any of the following symptoms:

- New cough with or without sputum production
- Shortness of breath or dyspnea on exertion
- Increased fatigue or malaise
- Fever
- Night sweats
- Headache
- Stiff neck
- Visual changes such as floaters, blurred vision, loss of visual field(s), and sensitivity to light
- Change in mental status, such as loss of consciousness, loss of memory, forgetfulness, mood swings, and depression
- Development of skin lesions
- Pain
- New or increased diarrhea with or without abdominal cramping
- Sudden, unintended weight loss
- Increased size or painful lymph node(s)

rectal lesions, a rectal tube can provide relief from the discomfort of stool on the lesions, although in some cases it irritates the bowel, causing discomfort of a different sort.

Instruct the patient to avoid substances that are irritating or stimulating to the bowel. These include fatty foods, lactose-containing foods, caffeine, sugar, and black licorice.

Severe diarrhea can precipitate fluid and electrolyte imbalances and cause a severe nutritional deficit. Patients may require hyperalimentation and fluid replacement if absorption is significantly altered. Record fluid intake and output, replace fluids as needed, and monitor results of laboratory tests such as serum electrolytes.

NDx: Altered oral mucous membrane

Since the majority of patients with AIDS develop infections of the oral mucous membranes, which cause a great deal of pain and discomfort, frequent, thorough oral hygiene is essential. Instruct the patient in care of the mouth as specified in Chart 10–2. Carry out treatments for specific infections as prescribed.

Chart 10–2.

NURSING GUIDE TO PATIENT EDUCATION FOR SELF-MANAGEMENT: CARE OF THE MOUTH FOR THE PATIENT WITH HIV INFECTION

Instruct the patient experiencing oral infections or conditions associated with HIV infection to:

Clean the teeth and gums with a soft gauze pad instead of a brush.
Use mouthwash that does not contain alcohol or other astringent agents.
Lubricate the lips.
Avoid irritating foods such as those that are spicy, contain a lot of acid, are very hot, or are difficult to chew.
Use a local anesthetic such as viscous Xylocaine for discomfort.
Obtain treatment for oral infections such as those caused by *Candida* and herpes simplex virus.

NDx: Ineffective breathing pattern
Monitor for changes in respiratory status by checking vital signs, color, breath sounds, sputum production, and when indicated, pulse oximetry and arterial blood gas values. Arrange for prompt medical evaluation if changes occur.

Encourage coughing and deep breathing and the use of an incentive spirometer. Perform suctioning, administer supplemental oxygen, and maintain the patient on mechanical ventilation as ordered.

NDx: Social isolation
Many patients with HIV infection complain of feeling isolated and alone. These feelings may result from the patient's being afraid to acknowledge the diagnosis and share feelings about it with others or from the withdrawal of family, friends, or acquaintances when the diagnosis is known. Keep in mind that in some cases in which the patient is homosexual, bisexual, or an intravenous drug user, family and friends may have been unaware of the fact until the time AIDS is diagnosed, and this can contribute to withdrawal. Patients who were infected by a sexual partner may also feel betrayed.

To help the patient combat the sense of isolation and aloneness, provide the environment and the opportunity for the patient to discuss the diagnosis and his or her reactions to it. Remember, too, that the patient has a need for physical contact. Giving back rubs, holding the patient's hand, or hugging the patient not only meets this need but encourages others working with the patient to also provide appropriate physical contact. Monitor the patient for suicidal ideation, and refer him or her to a psychologist or psychiatrist if indicated.

In line with the patient's ability, encourage social interaction with other patients or with friends or members of a support group in the community. If the patient is bedridden and at home, arrange for contact with an organization that provides volunteer "friends" or other assistance to persons with HIV infection.

NDx: Ineffective individual coping
Anxiety, anger, and depression are feelings experienced by virtually all patients with HIV infection at some time. Allow the patient to express these feelings by providing a nonjudgmental, accepting atmosphere. Involve other support persons such as chaplains, social workers, and psychiatrists. Encourage the patient's significant others to stay involved, and provide support and help to them in dealing with their feelings. Refer significant others to support groups and other resources for ongoing help in dealing with the problem.

Administer medications to control anxiety and depression as ordered.

Help the patient to deal with death and dying, because HIV infection is a life-threatening disease. For emotional support, put the patient in contact with the local hospice organization. Explore with the patient preparations for death and dying, such as writing a will, making arrangements for power of attorney should the patient become unable to make decisions, making funeral arrangements, and providing advance directives for health care. Support the patient in these endeavors, and if involvement of significant others is desired, support them also, because it is equally difficult for them to deal with these issues.

NDx: High risk for impaired home maintenance management
Much of the patient's care can be provided in an out-patient or home setting, with hospitalization necessary only when serious problems develop that cannot be managed medically otherwise. In order for care at home to be successful, ensure that the patient has needed support services at home. These services may include help with transportation, meals, shopping, and household chores; assistance with medication administration; and financial help. Refer patients to volunteer groups devoted to this kind of help for persons with HIV infection or to hospice organizations or other community resources.

Early assessment to determine the status of the patient's physical, financial, psychosocial, and home environment is vital to developing and implementing the plan of care. Social service referrals should begin as soon as a patient's HIV status is determined, preferably in the out-patient setting.

Additional Interventions
If the patient's mental status deteriorates, ensure a safe environment. Provide additional supervision and assistance with normal activities as needed. Keep changes to a minimum, because the patient functions best in an environment that is familiar. Establish a daily routine, and be as consistent as possible with staff assignments. Orient the patient as needed, and avoid giving central nervous system–depressant drugs when possible. When giving care, give simple explanations and clear directions, one at a time. When possible, involve the family and significant others in daily care. Inform the caregivers about changes that need to be brought to the attention of the patient's health care providers (see Chart 10–1). Be sure written information is provided for medications, dressing changes, access to the health care system in an emergency, and so forth.

Evaluation

Evaluate the effectiveness of nursing care for a patient with HIV infection by comparing the patient's status with the expected patient outcomes. Examples of specific outcomes for patients with HIV infection have been provided in the Planning section.

Hypersensitivity Disorders

Hypersensitivity disorders result when the immune system overreacts to an antigen and tissue damage occurs. There are four basic types of hypersensitivity disorders:

Immediate, or Type I, hypersensitivity reaction
Cytotoxic, or Type II, hypersensitivity reaction
Immune complex, or Type III, hypersensitivity reaction
Cell-mediated, or Type IV, hypersensitivity reaction

Hypersensitivity and allergy are often used synonymously, but they are slightly different variations of the immune response. As the word suggests, hypersensitivity is an overreaction or inappropriate reaction of the normal immune response to an antigen that results in tissue damage. Allergy or atopy is an altered or unusual reaction to an antigen that causes a deviation from the expected immune response. Hypersensitivity reactions may occur in any member of the species. Allergic reactions are seen only in those members who are genetically predisposed to them.

Immediate Hypersensitivity Reactions (Type I)

Immediate hypersensitivity is an immunologic response that occurs within minutes of the antigen's combining with the IgE antibody. Allergic reactions are included with the immediate hypersensitivity disorders. The most severe reaction in the group of immediate hypersensitivity reactions is anaphylaxis.

ANAPHYLAXIS

ETIOLOGY AND PATHOPHYSIOLOGY

Anaphylaxis is a sudden, life-threatening overreaction to an antigen. It is mediated by IgE antibody. IgE is produced following the first exposure to the antigen. It binds to the surface of mast cells and basophils. During subsequent exposures, the antigen binds with the cell-bound IgE molecules. The binding of the antigen and antibody causes the mast cell or basophil to immediately release several chemical mediators, which cause widespread tissue responses. These chemical mediators include

- Histamine, which causes bronchial constriction, vasodilation, and increased capillary permeability
- Serotonin, which has the same effects as histamine
- Slow reacting substance of anaphylaxis (SRS-A), which is a potent bronchoconstrictor that also causes spasm of the smooth muscles of the internal organs and dilation and increased permeability of the venules
- Bradykinin, which causes vasodilation and increases capillary permeability

The bronchoconstriction, vasodilation, and increased capillary permeability caused by these chemical mediators produce most of the clinical manifestations of anaphylaxis. The severe hypotension and shock that can result are what make anaphylaxis a potentially life-threatening event.

CLINICAL MANIFESTATIONS

Early recognition of anaphylaxis is crucial, because within a matter of minutes it can progress to respiratory arrest and shock. The very first signs of systemic anaphylaxis include feelings of anxiety and uneasiness, flushing, diaphoresis, sneezing, and weakness. These are very quickly followed by nausea, dizziness, itching, and sometimes edema, especially of the face, hands, and feet. Severe respiratory distress from bronchospasm and laryngeal edema and severe hypotension from the vasodilation and capillary permeability quickly follow.

MEDICAL DIAGNOSIS

Diagnosis of anaphylaxis needs to be made rapidly on the basis of the patient's signs and symptoms. There is virtually no time for laboratory tests because emergency interventions must be initiated immediately if death is to be prevented.

MEDICAL MANAGEMENT

Medical management consists of drug therapy to help reverse the effects of the chemical mediators, fluid replacement, and airway maintenance. Epinephrine is usually the first drug given. It helps raise the patient's blood pressure by causing vasoconstriction. Epinephrine also helps stop bronchospasm by causing bronchodilation. Diphenhydramine HCl (Benadryl), an antihistamine, is usually given to help stop the effects of the histamine. Steroids may be given to help reduce capillary permeability, thus helping to maintain the intravascular volume. Steroids also help stabilize the mast cells so that they do not release any more chemical mediators. Pressure agents (dopamine, isoproterenol) may be needed to help maintain the patient's blood pressure. Intravenous aminophylline may be required to help relieve the respiratory symptoms. Intravenous fluid replacement with normal saline or Ringer's lactate is used to help maintain the patient's blood pressure. Endotracheal intubation or tracheostomy may be necessary to maintain a patent airway. The patient may require additional oxygen to help maintain normal blood gas levels.

Application of the Nursing Process to the Care of the Patient with Anaphylaxis

Assessment

Assess the patient's physiologic status by monitoring blood pressure, pulse, respirations, color, and level of consciousness. Note the presence of symptoms such as diaphoresis, weakness, sneezing, nausea, dizziness, itching, and edema. Assess the need for emergency measures because edema can compromise the patient's airway. Attempt to identify the factor that triggered the reaction (Table 10–4), and if able, determine whether the patient has any other allergies.

Nursing Diagnoses and Planning

Nursing diagnoses and related expected patient outcomes most commonly applicable to patients with an anaphylactic reaction include the following:

NDx: Ineffective breathing pattern related to bronchoconstriction and laryngeal edema

Planning: Patient outcomes
1. Respiratory rate and depth return to patient's baseline range.
2. Respiratory stridor and wheeze are absent.
3. Cyanosis is absent.
4. Blood gases are within normal limits.

NDx: Altered tissue perfusion related to vasodilation and increased capillary permeability

Planning: Patient outcomes
1. Blood pressure returns to the patient's baseline range.
2. Pulse returns to the patient's baseline range.
3. Patient is alert and oriented.

NDx: High risk for altered health maintenance related to lack of knowledge of causative antigen, the anaphylactic response, preventive measures

Planning: Patient outcomes
1. Patient names the precipitating factor.
2. Patient describes what happens when contact occurs with the precipitating factor.
3. Patient identifies related substances that may cause a similar response.
4. Patient explains how precipitating factors can be avoided.
5. Patient obtains a MedicAlert tag or bracelet.

Table 10–4. EXAMPLES OF SPECIFIC ANTIGENIC SUBSTANCES

CATEGORY OF ANTIGEN	EXAMPLES OF SPECIFIC ANTIGENIC SUBSTANCES
Drugs	ACTH, local anesthetics, antibiotics (especially penicillin and cephalosporins), antitoxins, cocaine, dextran, gamma globulin, insulin, iodides, iron, IVP dye, radiographic contrast media, telepaque, vaccines
Foods	Citrus fruits, eggs, milk, nuts, seafood, strawberries
Insect venom	Bee venom, fire ant venom, hornet venom, wasp venom

Abbreviations: ACTH, adrenocorticotropic hormone; IVP, intravenous pyelography.

Nursing Interventions

Immediate nursing actions are aimed at limiting exposure to the antigen and supporting respiratory and cardiovascular status. If the cause of the anaphylactic reaction has been identified, take action immediately to prevent the patient from receiving more of the antigen. For example, if an intravenous medication is suspected, stop the infusion. Obtain help as soon as the anaphylactic reaction is identified, and get emergency equipment to the scene. If at all possible, do not leave the patient alone.

NDx: Ineffective breathing pattern
Monitor the patient's respiratory status. If needed, use suction to clear secretions from the airway and administer oxygen. Because intubation or emergency tracheostomy may be necessary to maintain a patent airway, keep the equipment needed for these procedures readily available.

NDx: Altered tissue perfusion
Monitor the patient's pulse and blood pressure. If blood pressure is low, lay the patient flat and elevate the legs. If an intravenous line is not already in place, establish one to allow for the administration of medications and fluids.

NDx: High risk for altered health maintenance
Following the incident, provide information and instruct the patient as specified in Chart 10–3.

Additional Interventions
Once the patient is out of danger, document the incident in the patient's record. Include symptoms and their time of onset, vital signs, and all fluids, medications, and treatments given, as well as the patient's response to them. If the cause of the reaction is known, mark this information clearly on the patient's chart, on the medication sheets, and at the bedside.

Chart 10–3.

NURSING GUIDE TO PATIENT EDUCATION FOR SELF-MANAGEMENT: PREVENTION OF ANAPHYLAXIS

Explain to the patient:

What the precipitating factor was.
What happens in the body when exposure to the precipitating antigen occurs.

Identify with the patient:

Related substances that may cause a similar reaction.
Ways to avoid the antigen and related substances in the future.

Instruct the patient to:

Inform all health care providers of the problem.
Carry or wear a MedicAlert tag or other identification that indicates the causative antigen and the response.

If the anaphylactic reaction was precipitated by a bee sting or other known allergen, also instruct the patient to keep an emergency kit containing Adrenalin available at all times and teach the patient or family how to administer the medication.

Evaluation

Evaluate the effectiveness of nursing care for a patient with anaphylaxis by comparing the patient's status with the expected patient outcomes. Examples of specific outcomes for patients with anaphylaxis have been provided in the Planning section.

ALLERGY

As previously stated, allergic or atopic reactions are considered a type of immediate hypersensitivity reaction. They occur in individuals who are genetically susceptible to developing this type of reaction. Approximately 10% of the population has some type of allergy. Allergic rhinitis, popularly called hay fever, is the most common form of allergy. Less common forms are bronchial asthma, atopic dermatitis, GI food allergies, and drug allergies. The symptoms of allergy may first occur at any age, but most people develop symptoms during childhood.

The pathologic mechanism of allergy is basically the same mechanism as that of anaphylaxis, except that the target organs are different. IgE antibody is produced after the first exposure to the antigen, and it binds to the mast cells in the target organ (nasal mucosa, bronchi, skin, or GI tract). During subsequent exposures, the antigen binds with the mast cell–bound IgE, and this triggers the release of the chemical mediators.

ALLERGIC RHINITIS

Etiology and Pathophysiology

Allergic rhinitis is a Type I hypersensitivity reaction that occurs in response to inhaled antigens, with the symptoms being localized to the nasal mucosa and conjunctiva.

Clinical Manifestations

Typical symptoms of allergic rhinitis are a profuse watery nasal discharge, sneezing, swelling of the nasal mucosa (which can cause nasal obstruction), and itching of the nose and palate. These symptoms may be accompanied by intense itching and swelling of the conjunctiva, although conjunctivitis may also occur without the nasal symptoms. The patient may experience some general malaise but no fever. The intense sneezing may cause sore muscles in the chest.

Medical Diagnosis

Allergic rhinitis is primarily diagnosed by history and physical findings during an attack. Nasal secre-

Pharmacology Box 10–1.
ANTIHISTAMINES

Antihistamines:
Class of synthetic drugs that inhibit the effects of histamine.

Action:
Attach to the histamine receptor sites on effector cells and thus prevent histamine from occupying them and exerting its effects. Also inhibit acetylcholine by a similar mechanism.

Uses:
Treatment of allergic disorders such as hay fever, urticaria, and drug, food, and cosmetic allergies.

Side Effects:
Dizziness, drowsiness, impaired coordination, inability to concentrate, dry mouth and throat, occasional nausea and vomiting, and insomnia.

Interactions:
Increase the central nervous system (CNS) depressant effect of alcohol, narcotics, hypnotics, analgesics, anesthetics, tranquilizers, reserpine, bromine, and scopolamine. Have an additive effect with anticholinergic drugs, which can result in urinary retention or constipation. Decrease effects of corticosteroids, estradiol, progesterone, and testosterone. Erythromycin and the antifungal agent aketaconazole slow the metabolism of Seldane and can lead to toxic effects on the heart. Warning signs of a Seldane reaction are faintness, dizziness, and heart palpitations.

Nursing Implications:
Caution patient against drinking alcoholic beverages or taking other depressant drugs while taking antihistamines, except on specific order of a physician.
Caution patient against driving or performing other tasks that are dangerous if not completely alert.
Instruct patient to take medication with food or milk if gastrointestinal distress occurs.
Suggest sugarless gum, sour hard candy, or ice chips for relief of dry mouth.
Suggest coffee or tea to combat drowsiness.
Instruct patient to discontinue use of antihistamines 4 days prior to scheduled allergy testing.

Geriatric Considerations:
Since elderly persons are particularly prone to CNS side effects of antihistamines, interventions to prevent falls or other accidental injuries are essential.

tions may be examined for eosinophils, which will be numerous; however, the number of eosinophils in the peripheral blood may be normal or only slightly increased. IgE levels may range from normal to somewhat elevated.

To determine which specific antigens the patient is allergic to, skin tests are done as described in Chapter 9.

Medical Management

The ideal treatment of allergic rhinitis is for the patient to avoid the antigen. Unfortunately this is not always possible, and medical treatment involving pharmacologic therapy or desensitization is needed to control the allergic response.

The most useful drugs in the treatment of allergic rhinitis are antihistamines. These drugs, which are presented in Pharmacology Box 10–1, have several side effects that tend to limit their use, such as their tendency to cause sedation, dry mouth, dizziness, blurred vision, and nausea. Antihistamines must be taken regularly to be most effective.

Systemic corticosteroids are also very effective at controlling the symptoms of allergic rhinitis, but serious side effects such as increased susceptibility to infection, hypertension, and glaucoma limit their usefulness in treating what is essentially a benign condition. However, corticosteroids and cromolyn sodium in a nasal spray can be helpful in controlling allergic rhinitis symptoms with few side effects because there does not appear to be much, if any, absorption of these drugs from the nasal mucosa.

Desensitization is used for patients whose symptoms cannot be controlled with drugs and environmental controls. It is a form of immunotherapy in which the patient is injected with extracts of the pollen or mold spores to which he or she is allergic. These injections are given weekly in gradually increasing amounts until the maximum dose that the patient can tolerate is reached. Maintenance doses are then given every 2 to 4 weeks. This therapy may be given for the 2 to 3 months prior to the onset of seasonal symptoms or may be given throughout the year. In either case, several years are required before the maximal effectiveness of the therapy is achieved.

Desensitization is not a cure; rather, it allows control of symptoms. How it does this is not specifically known, although it is suggested that it stimulates the production of a new antibody (probably IgG) that prevents the allergen from initiating an allergic response. Because with each injection in the desensitization program there is a risk of a systemic reaction such as hives, an asthma attack, or even anaphylactic shock, all injections should be given by a health care professional who has epinephrine available if needed to counteract a reaction. For this reason too, the patient is observed for approximately 20 minutes following the injection. Desensitization is not effective in every patient.

Application of the Nursing Process to the Care of the Patient with Allergic Rhinitis

Assessment

Determine what symptoms the patient experiences during an attack. Ask about itching, burning, redness, or swelling of the eyes; itching, fullness, or popping of the ears; sneezing; runny nose; itchiness of the nose; mouth breathing; sore throat; postnasal drip; cough; pain; dyspnea; sore chest or abdominal muscles; dermatitis; urticaria; and eczema. Obtain information about any family history of allergy, prior testing for or treatment of allergy, and the patient's usual daily environment in terms of exposure to dust, chemicals, plants, or animals on a regular basis. Also determine whether symptoms occur year round or only in a particular season. Ask whether there are times when the symptoms are more pronounced, such as certain times of the year or month, weekdays or weekends, day or night; whether symptoms occur more often under certain weather conditions such as heat, humidity, cold, or rain; or whether symptoms occur after particular activities such as eating specific foods; mowing the lawn; using perfume, hair spray, or other toiletries; or exposure to animals, flowers, smoking, or paint.

Nursing Diagnoses and Planning

Nursing diagnoses and related expected patient outcomes most commonly applicable to patients with allergic rhinitis include the following:

NDx: High risk for altered health maintenance related to lack of knowledge of the disease, environmental control, use of medications, or desensitization therapy

Planning: Patient outcomes
1. Patient names the antigen(s).
2. Patient briefly explains how the symptoms are produced.
3. Patient describes different treatment options.
4. Patient describes the expected effects of treatment prescribed.
5. Patient lists ways in which exposure to the antigen can be avoided or minimized.
6. Patient describes a specific plan as to how to incorporate the identified measures in his or her lifestyle.
7. Patient names each drug and states the dose, frequency, and route of administration.
8. Patient describes the side effects of each drug.
9. Patient lists things that are contraindicated when taking each drug, such as certain foods, activities, or other medications.

NDx: Pain related to itchy eyes, itchy nose, itchy oral mucous membranes, irritation from nasal secretions, and sore muscles secondary to repeated sneezing

Planning: Patient outcomes
1. Patient avoids rubbing eyes or nose.
2. Patient describes use of measures to relieve discomfort.
3. Complaints of itching of the eyes, nose, or oral mucous membranes are absent.
4. Nasal passages are clear.
5. Patient is free of sneezing.
6. Skin around the nose is free of redness and excoriation.

Nursing Interventions

NDx: High risk for altered health maintenance
Explain the disease process so that the patient understands what triggers the symptoms and what happens in the eyes, nose, and throat to cause the symptoms. Explain that allergic rhinitis often occurs

only during a particular time of year and that it is not a contagious disease and therefore cannot be given to others.

Help the patient identify ways in which the antigen in the environment can be avoided. These will vary with the antigen involved and the ability and willingness of the patient to make changes. If the antigen is an airborne pollen, explore the possibility of an air conditioner to help remove it so that the air inside the house is pollen-free. If the antigen is house dust and dust mites, instruct the patient to "dustproof" the home environment by eliminating furnishings that collect dust, such as drapes, rugs, and overstuffed furniture, by washing all bedding in hot water, zipping mattresses in vinyl, damp mopping floors, and dusting with a damp cloth. Make certain to instruct the patient to wear a dust mask if he or she is doing the cleaning. If the allergy is to animal dander, suggest eliminating the use of down quilts or pillows to help reduce symptoms. Also suggest that household pets be bathed frequently or, if necessary, removed from the home.

Teach about prescribed medications so that the patient knows the name of the drug, how much to take, when to take it, how to take it, how to use it if it is an inhaler or spray, and common side effects. Teach patients that antihistamines can cause drowsiness and so they should avoid driving or participating in other potentially dangerous activities when taking these medications. Also warn them not to take alcohol or other over-the-counter drugs along with the antihistamines.

NDx: Pain
Instruct the patient in measures that can be used to minimize discomfort from symptoms that do occur. Discuss the use of gargles for sore throat and postnasal drip, the use of cold compresses to the eyes to sooth itching, and the need to avoid rubbing eyes.

Evaluation

Evaluate the effectiveness of nursing care for a patient with allergic rhinitis by comparing the patient's status with the expected patient outcomes. Examples of specific outcomes for patients with allergic rhinitis have been provided in the Planning section.

ASTHMA

Asthma is an immunologic allergic disease characterized by chronic inflammation of the lower airways, the end result of which can be permanent structural damage in the lungs. The incidence of asthma is increasing, especially among children and adolescents. It occurs slightly more often among blacks than among whites and tends to run in families. It is estimated that 1 of every 20 people experiences symptoms of asthma at some time, and most have a history of allergies. The severity of the disease varies from person to person and ranges from mild, for which no treatment is needed, to disease so severe that hospitalization with intensive, aggressive therapy is required. Death from asthma is uncommon. However, since 1980 the fatality rate from asthma has begun to increase, with the highest death rate occurring among the elderly.

Etiology

The exact cause of asthma is not known. Neither is the reason for its increasing incidence, although deteriorating air quality, increase in environmental allergens, and increased occupational exposure to allergens have been identified as potential causal factors. Asthma is believed to be basically an allergic response in which airways sensitized by allergens become more reactive to a variety of stimuli that trigger an attack. Some triggers are never identified, but common, well-recognized ones include cold or dry air; air pollutants such as cigarette and industrial smoke, ozone, sulfur dioxide, and formaldehyde; perfumes; allergens such as feathers, animal danders, molds, pollens, dust mites, and cockroaches; enzymes such as those in laundry detergents; chemicals such as those found in solvents, paints, rubber, and plastic; wood dust; vegetable dusts such as flour, coffee, and tea; alcoholic beverages; and foods such as eggs and those containing sulfates (e.g., wine, beer, salads, fresh and dried fruits, fruit juices, molasses, wine vinegar, instant potatoes, shellfish, and snack foods). Asthma attacks can also be triggered by upper respiratory viral infection, stress, exercise, and the act of lying down. In terms of the last factor, it is theorized that lying down may result in gastroesophageal reflux. This in turn results in stimulation of the vagus nerve by gastric acid initiating reflex bronchoconstriction.

Pathophysiology

The pathophysiologic events in the airway that accompany an asthma attack can be divided into the early response and the late response. The early response, which typically lasts 90 minutes or less, is characterized by bronchospasm. This occurs when an inhaled substance, an emotional reaction, or a reflex stimulates mast cells to release histamine and related substances, which in turn trigger contraction of the smooth muscle of the bronchi, edema of the bronchial mucous membrane, and secretion of large amounts of mucus into the bronchi.

The late response occurs 3 to 4 hours later and lasts up to 12 hours. The lungs' immune defense system is activated, and eosinophils moving to the membrane secrete prostaglandins, leukotrienes, major basic protein, and other substances that produce inflammation and promote immunity. Simulta-

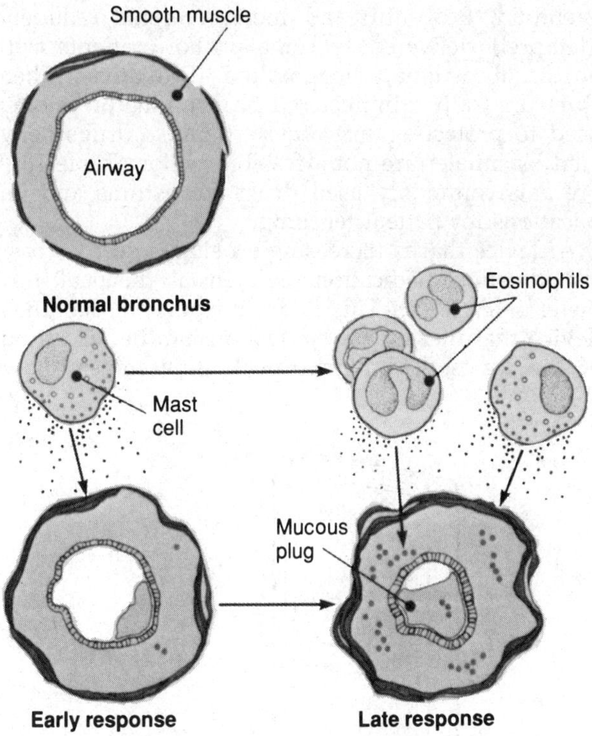

Figure 10–2.

Cross section of normal and asthmatic bronchi. Note that the asthmatic bronchus has a narrowed, thickened muscular wall invaded by inflammatory cells and a collection of mucus in the lumen. (From Hoffman S. Asthma. Part I. Harvard Health Letter. 1991; 16(7):6.)

neously, sensory nerves in the lungs produce substance P, neurokinin A, and calcitonin. The result is sustained inflammation of the bronchial mucosa and a hyperresponsiveness to the original trigger substance. Thus, with the next exposure to a trigger, both the early and late responses are magnified, creating a vicious circle resulting ultimately in structural change in the lung (Fig. 10–2).

Clinical Manifestations

The classic symptoms of asthma are dyspnea, paroxysmal attacks of cough, wheezing, and tightness in the chest. In addition, thick tenacious mucus may be produced. A patient with uncomplicated asthma often has no symptoms between attacks, and in approximately one fourth of all cases beginning in childhood, the attacks cease spontaneously after adolescence. A large number of other patients, however, remain in a chronic state of mild asthma, with symptoms exacerbated during periods of exertion or emotional excitement. On physical examination, the signs are similar to those of diffuse partial airway obstruction. The lungs are hyperinflated, with a resulting hyperresonant sound on percussion, and breath sounds are distant. Expiration is prolonged, with high-pitched wheezes throughout the lung, sometimes audible at a distance.

During an asthma attack, perspiration is common, and cyanosis is sometimes present. If the attack is severe, tachycardia, a respiratory rate of more than 30 per minute, and use of accessory muscles of respiration may occur.

There is wide variation in the duration and the severity of asthma attacks. Symptoms range from mild respiratory discomfort to life-threatening respiratory failure, and for the same patient each attack may be quite different. In "cough variant" asthma, a chronic cough that worsens on exertion or exposure to cold dry air, smoke, or perfume is the presenting symptom.

Asthmatics frequently have other atopic diseases such as allergic rhinitis or eczema and also have a family history of them.

Medical Diagnosis

Diagnosis of asthma depends primarily on a history of recurrent, episodic attacks of wheezing and shortness of breath with symptom-free intervals. Other findings supportive of the diagnosis include decreased flow rates on pulmonary function tests that improve following the administration of aerosolized bronchodilators and an elevated eosinophil count.

Arterial blood gases or pulse oximetry are used to help determine whether hospitalization is required and to monitor the progress of the treatment plan. Any asthmatic seeking medical assistance who has been taking theophylline should have a baseline theophylline level drawn and levels checked subsequently at regular intervals.

Medical Management

Medical management aimed at prevention of attacks begins with skin testing to try to identify specific precipitating allergens. If allergens to which the patient is sensitive are identified, then desensitization may be tried. Desensitization is not a cure, but an attempt to control the symptoms induced by specific antigens. It is of no value if an asthma attack is induced by infection, stress, exercise, or other factors not related to allergy. Results of skin tests cannot be considered absolute, however, because they do not provide an accurate measurement of sensitivity and hyperactivity of the bronchi in most patients.

Current pharmacologic treatment of asthma is designed to suppress inflammation as well as to dilate the bronchi. This reflects the new awareness of chronic inflammation as the underlying disease process and represents a change from past therapy, which focused almost solely on bronchodilation.

Steroids, which are effective anti-inflammatory agents, are being increasingly used, with the goal of not only relieving symptoms in the present but also preventing long-term structural damage. To decrease the risk of side effects of long-term steroid therapy, such as osteoporosis, weight gain, peptic ulcers, dia-

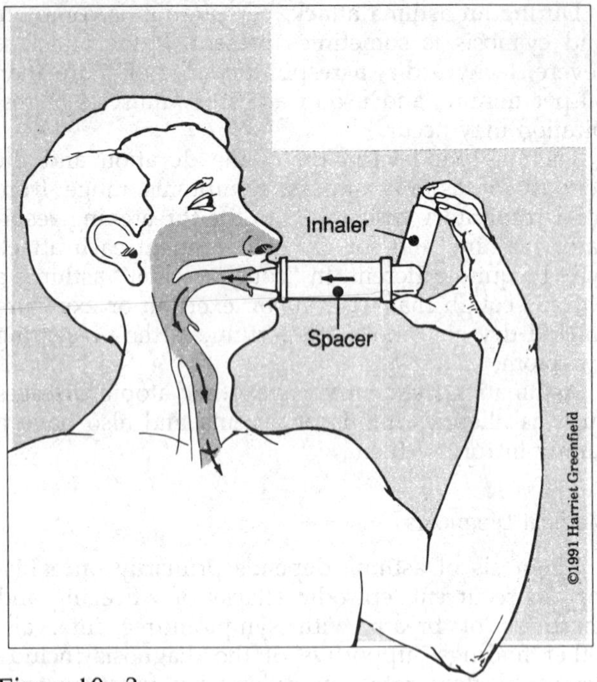

Figure 10–3.

Inhaler with attached spacer. Spacer is a molded plastic chamber attached to the inhaler and held in the mouth. (From Hoffman S. Asthma. Part 2. Harvard Health Letter. 1991; 16(8):3.)

betes, and infections, the steroids are administered directly to the airways by an inhaler with an attached spacer (Fig. 10–3). The spacer (1) prevents large droplets of medication from landing on the mucous membranes of the mouth or on the vocal cords, thus decreasing the chance of yeast infection; (2) dispenses the medication more uniformly and more deeply within the airways; (3) reduces the importance of coordinating use of the inhaler with breathing; and (4) decreases the amount of medication used by reducing the required number and volume of puffs.

Cromolyn sodium (Intal) is another pharmacologic agent used to prevent asthma attacks. It prevents the mast cells in the mucosa of the airways from releasing chemical mediators underlying bronchospasm. Cromolyn sodium is not a bronchodilator and is not always effective. It must be given before exposure to the asthmatic trigger occurs and seems to work best for mild or exercise-induced asthma. For the latter, it is administered 15 minutes before the planned exercise.

Oral steroids, with their many side effects, are used only in severe cases of asthma not controlled by inhaled steroids or cromolyn sodium.

Bronchodilators remain a major mode of therapy for patients with mild or intermittent asthma as well as for the treatment of attacks not prevented by other therapy. The most commonly used bronchodilators are beta$_2$-adrenergic agents such as albuterol (Ventolin, Proventil) and metaproterenal (Alupent, Metaprel) delivered by inhaler. For patients with nocturnal asthma, theophylline (Primatene, Theo-Dur), an orally administered bronchodilator, is often used to protect against attacks because drugs delivered by inhaler are not a feasible option. Table 10–5 presents commonly used drugs for asthma and implications for patient teaching.

A device that is increasingly being used as a basis for adjusting medication regimens is the peak flow meter (Fig. 10–4). This is an inexpensive, handheld device that measures how fast air can be blown out of the lungs. Use of the peak flow meter allows

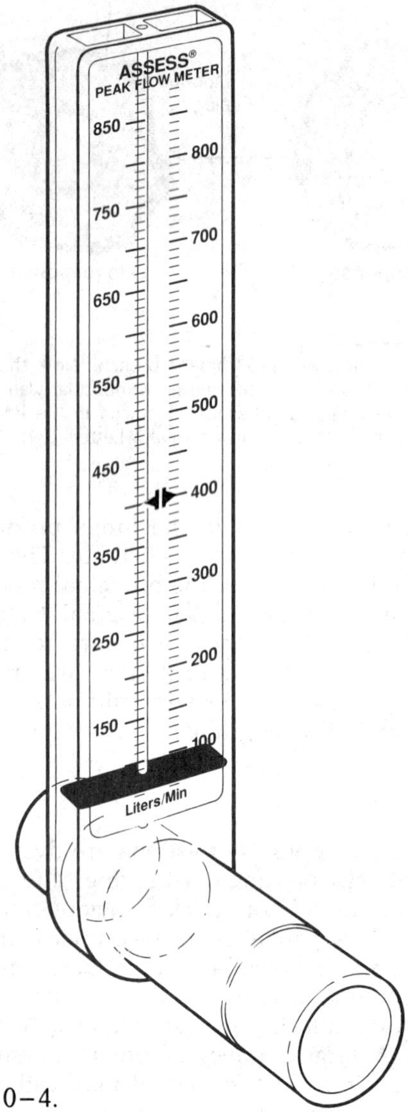

Figure 10–4.

Peak flow meter, which provides an objective measure of peak expiratory flow (PEF). Patient (1) inhales as deeply as possible; (2) places mouth firmly around the mouthpiece so the lips form a tight seal; (3) blows out as hard and fast as possible, causing the red indicator to move up the scale; and (4) records value at the final position of the red indicator. (Courtesy of HealthScan Products Inc., Cedar Grove, NJ.)

changes in the airways to be detected before clinically apparent signs occur. Because decrease in flow rate indicates an attack is impending, early identification of the change allows for pharmacologic intervention designed to avert the attack. For example, patients may be instructed to increase inhaled steroids if peak flow drops to less than 70% of normal, begin oral steroids if peak flow drops to less than 50%, and to seek emergency treatment at 30% (Hoffman, 1991, p. 3).

In addition to anti-inflammatory agents and bronchodilators, sedatives or tranquilizers may be ordered to calm the anxious patient, and antibiotics may be prescribed for a secondary infection.

Patients seeking emergency medical help for severe asthmatic attacks that interfere with the ability to eat, sleep, and perform normal daily activities usually require oxygen because hypoxemia is most often the underlying factor that sends them to the physician or hospital. Intravenous aminophylline or theophylline along with intravenous steroids is usually required to relieve bronchospasm, and hydration is frequently needed because asthmatics are often dehydrated by diaphoresis, hyperventilation, and the inability to drink.

Breathing exercises, postural drainage, and aerosol therapy may be ordered to assist the patient in removing retained secretions.

Application of the Nursing Process to the Care of the Patient with Asthma

Assessment

Obtain a nursing history that includes information about any family or personal history of allergy; previous asthmatic episodes, including precipitating factors and treatment received; the patient's understanding of the disease, prescribed medications, and factors known to precipitate an attack; the patient's emotional responses to the disease; and the effect of the disease on the patient's lifestyle and activities. Obtain information about any coexisting medical problems and medications routinely taken. Assess respirations, including breath sounds, and observe the patient for signs of hypoxia, which include restlessness, tachycardia, confusion, hypotension, and cyanosis. Review results of laboratory tests such as blood gas values.

If the patient is in acute distress, limit the history to immediately needed information. Determine the time of onset of the attack, any identifiable precipitating factor, and the name, dose, and time of any drug taken prior to admission. Obtain additional information from a significant other, or from the patient once symptoms are under control.

Nursing Diagnosis and Planning

Nursing diagnoses and related expected patient outcomes most commonly applicable to patients with asthma include the following:

NDx: Ineffective breathing pattern related to bronchial spasm and hypersecretion of mucus

Planning: Patient outcomes
1. Respiratory rate returns to baseline.
2. Complaints of dyspnea are absent.
3. Audible expiratory wheeze is absent.
4. Cyanosis is absent.
5. Pulse oximeter values are within normal range.

NDx: Anxiety related to shortness of breath and recurrence of attacks

Planning: Patient outcomes
1. Patient attends to what is being said.
2. Patient follows directions.
3. Behaviors such as screaming, crying, or grabbing on to people are absent.

NDx: High risk for altered health maintenance related to insufficient knowledge of disease process; ways to avoid allergens; contributing factors such as smoking, lack of sleep, and stress; medication regimen; and other self-care measures

Planning: Patient outcomes
1. Patient identifies trigger factors.
2. Patient lists ways to eliminate or reduce exposure to trigger factors.
3. Patient states name, dose, route, time of administration, and use of prescribed medication.
4. Patient demonstrates correct use of inhalation medications.
5. Patient demonstrates use of peak flow meter.
6. Patient wears a MedicAlert tag or similar device.
7. Patient describes the importance of informing health care workers of the asthmatic condition.

Nursing Interventions

NDx: Ineffective breathing pattern
Administer medications as ordered to assist the patient in obtaining relief from respiratory distress. Observe the patient for side effects, which include cardiac dysrhythmias, tremor, nervousness, nausea, and headaches. Assist the patient into a position that allows the greatest ease of respiration. Often this is a sitting position with the upper part of the body bent slightly forward. If so, use the over-bed table to provide necessary comfort and support. Keep the environment quiet, and protect the patient from drafts and chills. If diaphoresis is present, change damp linens frequently.

Table 10–5. DRUGS COMMONLY USED FOR ASTHMA AND RELATED PATIENT TEACHING

SYMPATHOMIMETIC DRUGS

DRUG	ACTION/RATIONALE
Metaproterenol (Alupent, Metaprel), available as oral preparation, metered-dose inhaler, and inhalant solution Terbutaline (Brethine, Bricanyl), available in oral and subcutaneous preparations Isoetharine, available in inhalant solution (Bronkosol) and metered-dose inhaler (Bronkometer) Albuterol (Proventil, Ventolin), available as metered-dose inhaler Isoproterenol (Isuprel), available in both metered-dose inhaler and solution for inhalation Epinephrine (Adrenalin), available in injectable preparation	Sympathomimetic drugs reverse chronic airway obstruction by stimulating beta$_2$-receptor sites, increasing the level of cyclic adenosine monophosphate and thus relaxing smooth muscles. Some sympathomimetic drugs exert most of their action by stimulating beta$_2$-receptor sites. Others stimulate beta$_1$-receptors in the myocardium and alpha-receptors. Tachycardia is the result of beta$_1$ stimulation, and vasoconstriction results from alpha stimulation. Beta$_2$-receptor stimulators are preferred because they cause fewer adverse reactions than drugs that stimulate alpha- and beta$_1$-receptor sites as well. Thus, beta$_2$-selective drugs have largely replaced the less selective sympathomimetics.

PATIENT TEACHING:

1. Teach patient correct use and cleaning of metered-dose inhaler or home nebulizer.
2. Instruct patient that inhaled drugs are very effective, but overuse and incorrect use can result in tachycardia, headaches, restlessness, and insomnia. Do not take maintenance doses at bedtime to help prevent insomnia. Discard any discolored solutions.
3. Advise patient to avoid over-the-counter metered-dose inhalers that contain epinephrine. Relief from bronchospasm is brief, and side effects (palpitations, tachycardia) are increased.
4. Instruct patient to call a physician or nurse if the bronchodilator is needed more than q4h, if more than three aerosol treatments are needed in a 24-hr period, or if use of the bronchodilator causes dizziness or chest pain.
5. Instruct patient about expected side effects: shakiness and tremors that decrease with continued use.
6. Space administration times if the patient is taking both xanthine and sympathomimetic drugs. This helps reduce side effects and allows for more constant bronchodilation.

METHYL XANTHINE COMPOUNDS

DRUG	ACTION/RATIONALE

IV Preparations (used for severe bronchoconstriction)
Aminophylline
Theophylline
 	
Oral Preparations
Short acting—4 hr
  Theophylline (Bronkodyl, Elixophyllin)
  Oxtriphylline (Choledyl)
Sustained release—8–12 hr
  Aminophylline (Phyllocontin)
  Theophylline (Sustaire, Theo-Dur)
	Bronchodilator
	Methyl xanthine compounds are believed to reverse airway obstruction by increasing the level of cyclic adenosine monophosphate, a substance that relaxes smooth muscle.

PATIENT TEACHING:

1. Space administration of drugs evenly throughout the day.
2. Teach patient the importance of regular monitoring of serum concentrations until dose response has been stabilized.

Serum level	*Response*
4–5 μg/ml	Bronchodilation begins
10–20 μg/ml	Optimal bronchodilation
>20 μg/ml	Adverse reaction common

3. Instruct patient to take medication even when feeling well.
4. Methyl xanthine compounds should be taken with an antacid or milk and crackers.
5. Instruct the patient to report adverse reactions but not to stop medications unless symptoms are severe. Adverse reactions are
   CNS: headache, irritability, restlessness, insomnia
   CV: palpitation, tachycardia, extrasystoles, flushing, hypotension
   GI: nausea, vomiting, epigastric pain, diarrhea, activation of peptic ulcer
6. Instruct patient to report early signs of possible toxicity that are usually CNS or CV symptoms: irritability, nervousness, palpitation, dizziness, shakiness, marked hypotension, cardiac arrhythmias, and later, seizures. Also report anorexia, nausea, vomiting, and abdominal discomfort.
7. Instruct the patient about smoking. Smoking is not only deleterious to lungs, but the half-life of xanthine compounds is shortened by smoking.
8. Instruct the patient about food and drug interactions: Charcoal-broiled foods decrease half-life of xanthines; coffee, tea, and chocolate affect the metabolism of the drug; certain drugs (e.g., erythromycin, tetracyclines, and cimetidine) prolong the half-life.

(continued)

Table 10–5. *(continued)* DRUGS COMMONLY USED FOR ASTHMA AND RELATED PATIENT TEACHING

ADRENAL CORTICOSTEROIDS

DRUG	ACTION/RATIONALE
Oral Preparations Prednisone (Deltasone, Paracort) ***Inhaled Preparations*** Beclomethasone (Beclovent, Vanceril)	Steroids have anti-inflammatory action. They also enhance the formation of cyclic adenosine monophosphate, which promotes bronchodilation. A short course of steroid therapy may help relieve acute asthma attacks. Some patients require long-term therapy with steroids. These are usually taken daily. A few patients can take a double dose on an alternating-day schedule. The alternating-day schedule lessens adrenal suppression and thus the side effects. Inhaled preparations are a major advance in treatment today since they have minimal or no systemic side effects.

PATIENT TEACHING:

For Oral Steroids:

1. Never abruptly discontinue after long-term use. Decrease slowly over 7 days.
2. Wear MedicAlert bracelet.
3. Take entire dose at one time in the early morning with food or antacids, or both, to help decrease side effects.
4. Side effects of steroids:

CNS:	depression, euphoria, rapid mood swings
GI:	gastric irritation, peptic ulcer
Metabolic:	Cushing's syndrome, hypernatremia, hypokalemia
Skin:	petechiae, ecchymoses, increased facial hair

For Inhaled Steroids:

1. Switch from oral to inhaled steroids gradually. Instruct the patient to report any wheezing during this period.
2. Promote adaption to inhaled steroids by inhaling a bronchodilator before the steroid.
3. Instruct patient on use and cleaning of metered-dose inhaler.
4. After inhaling steroids, gargle with water to prevent systemic absorption and oral fungal infections.
5. Do not use inhaled steroids during an asthma attack. They are supplied in powder form and may make the attack more severe.
6. Instruct patient to report any ongoing stressful situations, (e.g., infection, trauma), which may produce a need for dose adjustment.

For Long-term Therapy:

1. Instruct patient to report sudden or slow weight gains.
2. A low-salt, high potassium, high-protein diet is prescribed.
3. Instruct patient to report persistent low back or chest pain, which may indicate compression fractures, rib fractures, or spontaneous fractures from twisting, turning, or spasmodic coughing.
4. Caution patient about the use of over-the-counter drugs, especially those containing aspirin.

CROMOLYN SODIUM

DRUG	ACTION/RATIONALE
Cromolyn sodium (Intal), available in solution for inhalation and in capsules containing 20 mg of cromolyn sodium mixed with lactose. The contents of each capsule are inhaled through a turbo-inhaler, supplied by the manufacturer.	Cromolyn inhibits the secretion of substances that mediate the allergic response and therefore helps prevent bronchospasm. Some patients respond well to this drug, whereas others show no response. Those who respond best are usually teenagers or younger children with allergic-type asthma or adults with exercise-induced asthma.

PATIENT TEACHING:

1. Instruct the patient that this drug does not relieve symptoms once an attack has begun.
2. Instruct the patient on the use and cleansing procedures of the turbo-inhaler.
3. Explain that optimum response may not occur before 2 months of daily use.

Abbreviations: CNS, central nervous system; CV, cardiovascular; GI, gastrointestinal.

Assist the patient with bronchial toilet as needed. This includes breathing exercises, postural drainage, and suctioning. Note and document color, odor, quantity, and consistency of expectorated sputum.

Monitor fluid intake and output. If tolerated, give a minimum of 2 to 3 L per day of fluid to liquefy secretions. Avoid ingestion of milk products because these thicken secretions.

NDx: Anxiety

Because most patients are anxious and exhausted during an acute asthma attack, treat them with a calm, caring manner. Assure them that they will not be left unattended, and carefully explain each aspect of care. Since moderate to severe anxiety decreases the ability to comprehend, give explanations and instructions very slowly and repeat as necessary.

NDx: High risk for altered health maintenance

Health teaching is done to inform the patient about all aspects of this chronic disease. Explain what triggers the symptoms and what is happening in the lungs to cause the symptoms. Help the patient identify ways to avoid the antigen known to cause an attack. Once avoidance measures are identified, assist the patient in planning how to incorporate them into daily living. To make implementation of these measures more acceptable to the patient, suggest that they be tried on a trial basis for a month or so and then reevaluated. This allows the patient time to see the benefit of the measures and begin to accept the need for them.

If assessment data indicate that emotional stress is a frequent cause of the patient's asthma attacks, recommend a stress management program to assist the patient in identifying ways to prevent a stressor from disrupting life or to lessen the degree of reaction. Relaxation training is one of the methods used in a stress management program. If the patient smokes, also recommend a smoking cessation program.

With regard to medications, teach patients the name of each medication, how much to take, when to take it, and how to take it. When medications are taken by inhaler, have the patient demonstrate its use. Caution the patient not to exceed 4 to 6 inhalation treatments per day. Stress the importance of not discontinuing, increasing, or taking newly prescribed or over-the-counter medications without consulting the physician treating the asthma. This is critical because, for example, if steroids are discontinued abruptly, adrenal crisis from adrenal insufficiency can occur. Propranolol (Inderal) is not given to patients with asthma because of its potential to cause bronchoconstriction. Antihistamines and decongestants are to be avoided because of their drying effect on airway secretions, making expectoration more difficult. (See Table 10-6 for medications to be avoided by the asthmatic.)

If self-management is to be based on peak flow meter values, instruct the patient in the use of the peak flow meter and have the patient demonstrate it (see Fig. 10-4). Review the physician's orders for changes in medication regimen based on peak flow values.

Table 10-6. DRUGS TO BE AVOIDED OR USED CAUTIOUSLY BY INDIVIDUALS WITH ASTHMA

DRUG	REASON FOR CAUTION
Antihistamines	Dry secretions and make expectoration difficult.
Sedatives	Depress respirations and aggravate hypoventilation.
Cough suppressants	Impair clearance of secretions from the airways.
Propranolol	Beta-blocker that causes significant bronchospasm.

Discuss the importance of a good diet with plenty of fluids, avoidance of cigarette smoking, and follow-up for other medical problems. Explain the need to inform all health care providers about the asthma and the name and dose of medications currently being taken. Suggest the use of Medic-Alert or similar identification.

Additional Interventions

If the patient is unable to maintain an adequate nutritional intake because of shortness of breath, high-nutrient supplemental feedings may be necessary.

Encourage asthmatic patients to lead as normal lives as possible. Stress that activities should not be restricted. Encourage participation in exercise and sports. Explain that aerobic activities such as swimming, running, and brisk walking actually increase the efficiency of the body's use of oxygen. Stress that only those activities that precipitate an attack need to be avoided and that often a prophylactic dose of medication will allow participation in almost any activity. Explain that fatigue makes it more difficult for the asthmatic patient to handle stress, and assist the patient in planning for sufficient rest.

Refer patients or families desirous of additional information on asthma to organizations such as the Asthma and Allergy Foundation of America (800-7-ASTHMA), the National Asthma Education Program (301-951-3260), the National Jewish Center for Immunology and Respiratory Medicine (800-222-LUNG), and the National Institute of Allergy and Infectious Diseases (Office of Communications, Bldg. 31, Room 7A32, 9000 Rockville Pike, Bethesda, MD 20892).

Evaluation

Evaluate the effectiveness of nursing care for a patient with asthma by comparing the patient's status with the expected patient outcomes. Examples of specific outcomes for patients with asthma have been provided in the Planning section.

STATUS ASTHMATICUS

Status asthmaticus is a severe asthma attack that lasts for hours or days and that does not respond to the usual forms of treatment. It can progress to respiratory failure and is a life-threatening emergency. In status asthmaticus, severe bronchospasm, mucus plugging, and inflammation of the airways cause increased airway resistance, greatly increasing the amount of work required to breathe. This results in increased oxygen consumption and a build-up of carbon dioxide. As alveolar ventilation decreases, hypoxemia occurs. The end result is carbon dioxide retention, respiratory alkalosis, and hypoxemia. This can cause cardiac dysrhythmias and respiratory failure. Signs and symptoms vary but usually include an audible wheeze, tachycardia, severely labored respirations, and diaphoresis.

Status asthmaticus requires aggressive treatment with epinephrine, aminophylline, and steroids. Careful hydration is usually required, and sodium bicarbonate may be used to correct acidosis. In some cases, mechanical ventilation may be necessary.

Cytotoxic Hypersensitivity Reactions (Type II)

Cytotoxic reactions produce cell damage. IgG or IgM antibody binds with an antigen on the cell surface. This antigen-antibody combination either triggers the complement cascade, which results in cell damage or cell lysis, or may act as an opsonin and attract phagocytic cells, which then cause the damage.

Cytotoxic reactions are the basis of several disorders, of which hemolytic anemia associated with penicillin is one. In this disorder, a drug bound to the surface of the red blood cells acts as an antigen. Antidrug antibody then binds with the drug on the cell and initiates the complement cascade, which in turn destroys the red blood cells. Common drugs known to cause this reaction are penicillin, quinine, and quinidine.

This type of reaction is also responsible for the hemolysis of incompatible red blood cells following a blood transfusion and for the destruction of other blood components such as platelets, polymorphonuclear leukocytes, and lymphocytes. This reaction, when involving antibodies specific for the basement membrane of the skin, results in the blisters and bubbles on the skin characteristic of pemphigoid disorders.

Immune Complex Hypersensitivity Reactions (Type III)

Immune complex, or Type III, hypersensitivity reactions occur when soluble antigens react with antibodies, usually IgG, and form an immune complex that precipitates.

SERUM SICKNESS

ETIOLOGY

Serum sickness is considered the characteristic manifestation of the immune complex hypersensitivity reaction. It was frequently seen in the early part of this century, when antiserum from horses was used to treat diphtheria, tetanus, gas gangrene, and other diseases involving toxins. (A toxin was injected into a horse to induce the production of antibodies. Serum from the horse containing antibodies was then injected into the patient in the hope that the antibodies would inactivate the toxin present in the patient's system.) Now serum sickness is primarily induced by drugs such as penicillin, cephalosporins, sulfonamide, and dextrans and by antilymphocyte serum.

PATHOPHYSIOLOGY

Several days after the injection of an antigen the body begins to produce antibodies specific for that antigen. These antibodies combine with the antigen, and immune complexes are formed. These immune complexes are deposited in various tissues throughout the body. The complement cascade is activated by these immune complexes. This activation of complement results in tissue damage and inflammation at the site of the immune complexes. This tissue damage and inflammation produce the symptoms of the immune complex hypersensitivity reaction.

CLINICAL MANIFESTATIONS

The symptoms of serum sickness develop several days to 3 weeks after the administration of the antigen. Symptoms include fever; malaise; rash or hives; extensive edema of the face, neck, and joints; arthralgia; lymphadenopathy; and splenomegaly. These symptoms last for 1 to 2 weeks and then gradually subside. If the patient has been previously exposed to the antigen, the symptoms appear within 2 to 5 days because antibodies are produced much more quickly during a secondary immune response.

MEDICAL DIAGNOSIS

Diagnosis of serum sickness is primarily based on the clinical symptoms and history.

MEDICAL MANAGEMENT

Medical management is directed at relieving symptoms. Antihistamines and analgesics are usually enough to make the patient comfortable. If they do not relieve the patient's symptoms, corticosteroids may be used.

Application of the Nursing Process to the Care of the Patient with Serum Sickness

Assessment

Assess the patient's symptoms, determining their severity and their impact on overall well-being. Observe for hives or rash. Question the patient regarding itch, and note if the patient is scratching. Also observe for edema and, if present, note location, extent, and any effect on function (e.g., does edema of the face and neck interfere with keeping the eyes open and seeing, with speaking clearly, or with swallowing). Question the patient about the presence of joint pain and note ability to move, walk, and carry out activities of daily living. Take temperature and other vital signs, and assess for enlarged lymph nodes. Assess the patient's understanding of the cause of the reaction, the expected course of the disease, prescribed treatment, and the need to avoid reexposure to the antigen.

Nursing Diagnoses and Planning

Nursing diagnoses and related expected outcomes most commonly applicable to patients with serum sickness include the following:

NDx: High risk for altered health maintenance related to insufficient knowledge of cause, expected course, prescribed treatment, and need to avoid reexposure to the antigen

Planning: Patient outcomes
1. Patient describes what caused the disease.
2. Patient states the expected action and common side effects of prescribed medications.
3. Patient explains importance of avoiding reexposure to the antigen.

NDx: Pain related to inflammation and tissue damage

Planning: Patient outcomes
1. Complaints of joint pain are absent.
2. Patient is able to turn, sit up, walk, and perform the activities of daily living.
3. Patient refrains from scratching.
4. Patient states he or she is comfortable.

Nursing Interventions

NDx: High risk for altered health maintenance
To enable the patient to understand the disease and its treatment and to avoid reexposure to the antigen, explain what serum sickness is, what antigen caused the reaction, the 7- to 14-day duration of the disease, the gradual disappearance of the symptoms, and the need in the future to inform all health care professionals about the reaction. In addition, explain the purpose and expected effects of all treatments and describe the reason for use and common side effects of prescribed medications. If the patient will be responsible for medications and treatments at home, teach dose, route, time, and frequency of medications as well as the correct method of carrying out any treatments.

NDx: Pain
Administer medications and treatments as ordered, and institute palliative nursing measures. Examples of the latter include positioning and use of supporting pillows for the patient with arthralgia and cool compresses for the patient with itchy hives.

Evaluation

Evaluate the effectiveness of nursing care for a patient with serum sickness by comparing the patient's status with the expected patient outcomes. Examples of specific outcomes for patients with serum sickness have been provided in the Planning section.

ARTHUS REACTION

The Arthus reaction is another form of immune complex hypersensitivity. It is primarily an experimental phenomenon. It is produced by repeatedly immunizing an animal until a high level of antibody has been produced. The antigen is then injected intradermally. The circulating antibody reacts with the antigen, and the immune response produces local tissue damage. The first symptoms are extreme edema and erythema around the injection site. Several hours later the center of the area becomes purplish-black. Over the next few days, tissue in the area dies. The area heals in 1 to 2 weeks.

HYPERSENSITIVITY PNEUMONITIDES

Etiology and Pathophysiology

The hypersensitivity pneumonitides are human diseases that result from the Arthus reaction mechanism. After repeated exposures to an inhaled antigen, the patient produces antibodies specific to that antigen. Later when the antigen is again inhaled, it reacts with the previously produced antibody, forming antigen-antibody complexes in the interstitial spaces of the lung. These complexes activate the complement cascade, which results in inflammation and tissue damage in the lungs. Farmer's lung caused by the inhalation of spores from moldy hay is an example of this type of hypersensitivity pneumonitis. Other hypersensitivity pneumonitides and their related antigens are listed in Table 10–7.

Clinical Manifestations

Symptoms of hypersensitivity pneumonitis include a dry cough, shortness of breath, fever, chills, myalgia, and malaise. These symptoms develop 4 to 8 hours after exposure and last up to 18 hours. The patient then feels healthy until the next exposure triggers the onset of symptoms. Pulmonary function tests and the chest x-ray film may be abnormal during the acute attack but are within normal limits in between attacks.

Medical Diagnosis

Diagnosis is usually made by a careful and detailed history of the symptoms and physical findings during the actual attack. A test may be done in which the suspected antigen is inhaled and the patient is observed to see whether the symptoms can be replicated.

Medical Management

The ideal treatment is avoidance of the antigen. When this is not possible, orally administered corticosteroids are used to help control the symptoms. Antihistamines and bronchodilators are not of much benefit in controlling the symptoms of hypersensitivity pneumonitides because histamine and bronchospasm are not the primary cause of symptoms.

Application of the Nursing Process to the Care of the Patient with a Hypersensitivity Pneumonitis

Assessment

Obtain a description of the symptoms the patient is experiencing and their time of onset. Also obtain a history of previous attacks, including when they occurred, how severe they were, how long they lasted, and the type and effectiveness of treatment employed.

Take vital signs and note the depth, sound, and effort of respiration along with the patient's color and any complaints of shortness of breath or chills.

Table 10–7. TYPES OF HYPERSENSITIVITY PNEUMONITIS AND RELATED ANTIGENS

TYPE OF PNEUMONITIS	CAUSATIVE ANTIGEN
Bird (or pigeon)-breeder's lung	Dry bird excreta
Cheese worker's lung	Cheese mold or casings
Farmer's lung	Moldy hay
Laundry worker's lung	Detergent
Malt worker's lung	Moldy malt or barley
Mushroom worker's lung	Moldy compost
Painter's lung	Paint
Plastic worker's lung	Plastic
Woodworker's lung	Moldy wood dust

Assess the patient's understanding of the disorder, the offending antigen, and treatment. Assess the impact of the disorder on lifestyle.

Nursing Diagnoses and Planning

The nursing diagnosis and related expected patient outcomes most commonly applicable to patients with a hypersensitivity pneumonitis are as follows:

NDx: High risk for altered health maintenance related to insufficient knowledge of cause and treatment of the disorder

Planning: Patient outcomes

1. Patient describes the relationship of the antigen to the symptoms.
2. Patient states the correct use of prescribed medications.

Nursing Interventions

NDx: High risk for altered health maintenance

Teach the patient about the disease, the correct use of medications prescribed for the relief of symptoms, the antigen causing the symptoms, and ways to avoid reexposure to it. For example, in many cases, the patient may be able to wear a mask when in the area where the antigen is prevalent. Sometimes a filter on the air handling system or a different type of system helps eliminate the antigen from the air. Some antigens are so prevalent in the environment that avoidance is not feasible for some patients. In these cases, it may be necessary for the patient to change jobs or lifestyle or give up a particular hobby in order to avoid the antigen.

Evaluation

Evaluate the effectiveness of nursing care for a patient with hypersensitivity pneumonitis by comparing the patient's status with the expected patient outcomes. Examples of specific outcomes for patients with hypersensitivity pneumonitis have been provided in the Planning section.

Cell-Mediated Hypersensitivity Reactions (Type IV)

The Type IV, or cell-mediated, hypersensitivity reactions are also referred to as delayed hypersensitivity reactions. This reaction does not depend on antibody or complement, but is mediated by sensitized T cells and the lymphokines they release. When the sensitized T cells are stimulated by exposure to antigen, they release lymphokines, one function of which is to initiate the inflammatory reaction and attract phagocytic cells to the area. This type of response takes at least 24 hours to develop. Contact dermatitis is an example of a human disease that is caused by this mechanism.

Skin tests to detect delayed hypersensitivity are a valuable diagnostic aid. These tests involve the intradermal injection of an antigen. If the patient has been previously exposed to the antigen, erythema and induration (abnormal hardness of the tissue) occur at the injection site in 24 to 48 hours. The induration indicates that cells and plasma have entered the area, and this must be present for the response to be positive.

Skin tests are used to help determine whether the patient has been exposed to a specific disease. An example of such a test is the purified protein derivative (PPD) test used to determine exposure to tuberculosis. A positive skin test result indicates only that the patient has at some point been exposed to that specific antigen. It does not mean that the patient presently has active disease.

Several skin tests can be done at once to determine whether the patient is anergic. Anergy is an impaired or absent delayed hypersensitivity response to an antigen to which the patient has been previously exposed. Anergy to several antigens indicates that the patient's cell-mediated immune responses may be generally impaired. This is not a good prognostic sign because anergic patients are more prone to infection, especially by viruses and fungi.

T cells and the cell-mediated immune response are primarily responsible for the rejection of grafted tissues. T cells detect the foreign antigens on grafted tissues, become sensitized, and then set the immune response into motion. Phagocytic cells are attracted to the graft by T-cell–produced lymphokines. The inner lining of the small blood vessels in the graft is damaged. This causes thrombosis of the vessels, resulting in tissue ischemia and eventual death of the graft. The graft appears to be doing fine for 1 or 2 weeks before the signs of acute rejection and failure become evident. Immunosuppressive drugs are used to decrease or stop rejection of the graft.

There are two other types of graft rejection. Late or chronic rejection of the graft occurring months or years after the transplant appears to be due to immune complexes of IgM and complement forming in the blood vessels of the graft. Immunosuppression does not stop this type of rejection. Hyperacute rejection, characterized by ischemia and necrosis of the graft, occurs within minutes of transplanting the graft. It may be caused by antibodies present in the recipient that respond to tissue antigens on the donor organ.

The four types of hypersensitivity reactions with their related disorders are summarized in Table 10–8.

AUTOIMMUNE REACTION

Autoimmunity is a condition in which the body is reacting immunologically against itself. The body has lost some of its "self-tolerance" and is no longer able to precisely distinguish self from non-self. Autoimmunity may involve T cells or B cells, or both. An autoantibody is one that the body has produced in response to one of its own antigens. The mere presence of an autoantibody does not necessarily mean that an autoimmune disease is present. In fact, more than half the people older than 70 years of age have at least one autoantibody.

Table 10–8. HYPERSENSITIVITY REACTIONS AND RESULTANT DISORDERS

TYPE OF HYPERSENSITIVITY	PATHOPHYSIOLOGY	RESULTING DISORDERS
Type I Immediate	Antigen combines with IgE, triggering release of chemical mediators from mast cells	Anaphylaxis, allergic rhinitis, asthma
Type II Cytotoxic	IgC or IgM binds with antigen on cell surface, resulting in cell damage	Acute hemolytic transfusion reaction, auto immune hemolytic anemia
Type III Immune Complex	Antigen-antibody complexes are deposited in body tissues and complement is activated, causing tissue damage at the site of antigen-antibody complexes	Serum sickness, vasculitis, hypersensitivity pneumonitis, systemic lupus erythematosus
Type IV Cell-mediated	Sensitized T cells cause cell damage	Graft rejection, tuberculosis, sarcoidosis, leprosy, poison ivy

The exact mechanism by which autoimmunity develops is not completely understood, although it is generally felt that suppressor T cells are important in helping to prevent the formation of autoantibodies. Several mechanisms for the development of autoantibodies have been proposed:

- A defect in the suppressor T cells.
- An alteration in a host antigen due to a factor such as a viral disease, causing a change in the surface of the cell or in the haptens that bind to the cell.
- Exposure to a foreign antigen that is so similar to a self-antigen that the antibody reacts with either one (a cross-reaction). This is thought to be the mechanism of rheumatic fever (i.e., the antibodies formed to the beta-hemolytic group A streptococci are thought to cross-react with self-antigens on the heart muscle).
- Abnormal stimulation of helper T cells.
- Exposure of self-antigens that are usually hidden from the immune system, such as when tissue trauma occurs. Specific examples of this are the production of autoantibodies against heart muscle following a myocardial infarction, against the lens after an eye injury, and against sperm after a vasectomy.

The variety of diseases that may have an autoimmune component is extensive and involves all body systems. The following are common characteristics of autoimmune diseases:

- They occur more frequently in women than in men.
- There are usually other family members with the disease or healthy members with detectable autoantibodies.
- The disease improves with immunosuppressive therapy.

Selected autoimmune disorders are presented here. Others, such as rheumatoid arthritis, are discussed under the disorders of the specific body system involved.

SYSTEMIC LUPUS ERYTHEMATOSUS

Systemic lupus erythematosus (SLE) is frequently considered the classic autoimmune disease. It is a chronic disorder characterized by alternating periods of exacerbation and remission. It involves most organ systems and occurs most frequently in women of childbearing age.

ETIOLOGY

The exact etiology of SLE is not yet known, but several causes or triggering mechanisms have been identified. These include drugs such as sulfur, penicillin, and other antibiotics as well as some oral contraceptives; viral infections; ultraviolet light rays; stress; and environmental pollutants. It appears that a combination of one or more of these factors along with a defect in the immune system and possibly a genetic predisposition is needed in order for SLE to develop.

PATHOPHYSIOLOGY

The basic dysfunction in SLE is an imbalance in the immune system with depression of T-cell activity and greatly increased antibody production. Antibodies to DNA and RNA are produced as well as anti-erythrocyte and anti-platelet antibodies. Other immunologic abnormalities that are found with SLE are decreased amounts of complement, positive rheumatoid factor, and false-positive results in serologic tests for syphilis.

The most important of the immunologic abnormalities in SLE is the presence of antinuclear antibodies (ANA) in the serum. These antibodies are responsible for the formation of LE cells and the formation of immune complexes. LE cells are polymorphonuclear leukocytes that have ingested immune complexes composed of ANA and complement combined with nuclear material from damaged cells. These LE cells are present in more than 80% of patients with SLE. A Type III hypersensitivity reaction occurs when the immune complexes formed from the ANA, complement, and DNA are deposited in veins and arteries initiating the inflammatory process in these locations (vasculitis). The clinical symptoms of SLE result from this vasculitis, which causes pain, swelling, and tissue damage in any area of the body.

CLINICAL MANIFESTATIONS

SLE is a very variable disease with no typical presentation. A whole complex of symptoms may develop suddenly, or they may develop slowly one at a time. Any organ or tissue may be affected at any time. In fact, SLE seems to randomly affect different organs, and symptoms depend on which organs and tissues are involved. Organs commonly affected at one time or another during the course of the disease are the joints, skin, pleura, pericardium, heart, kidney, central nervous system, eye, and blood. The course of the disease also varies but generally seems to be most active in the first few years and then to gradually decline. As previously stated, SLE is characterized by periods of exacerbation that are triggered by a variety of factors including emotional or physical stress, infections, fatigue, pregnancy, and exposure to ultraviolet light.

If SLE can be said to have any typical symptoms, they would include the following:

Fever and malaise that tend to occur before and during exacerbations but may be present to some degree all of the time

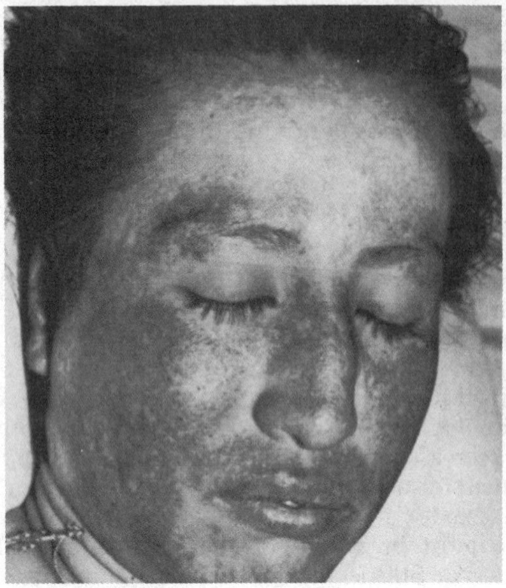

Figure 10–5.

Butterfly rash of lupus erythematosus. (From Moschella SL, Hurley JH (eds). Dermatology. 3rd ed, Vol 1. Philadelphia: WB Saunders, 1992, p 1226.)

Migratory joint pain and stiffness
Skin lesions, particularly an erythematous "butterfly" rash on the face across the bridge of the nose and on the cheeks, composed of discoid (round) or diffuse maculopapular lesions (Fig. 10–5)
Pleurisy, pericarditis, myocarditis, noninfectious endocarditis, and hypertension
Glomerulonephritis, renal dysfunction, and renal failure, which are the most serious problems to SLE patients and account for many of the fatalities
Almost any type of central nervous system pathology, such as impaired cognitive function, psychosis, depression, seizures, peripheral neuropathies, cerebrovascular accidents, and organic brain syndrome
Anemia, leukopenia, and thrombocytopenia
Anorexia, nausea, vomiting, and weight loss
Hepatomegaly and splenomegaly

MEDICAL DIAGNOSIS

Diagnosis of SLE is based on an evaluation of the patient's history, findings on physical examination, and laboratory data.

Specific laboratory tests used in evaluating a patient for SLE include the antinuclear antibody (ANA) test, the LE cell test, and the anti-DNA test. A positive result on any of these tests is suggestive of SLE but is not the basis for a conclusive diagnosis. This is because some people who have SLE have negative test results, whereas some people with disorders other than SLE have positive results. Examples of such disorders are rheumatoid arthritis, scleroderma, carcinoma, tuberculosis, hepatitis, and mononucleosis.

Because of the great variability of the symptoms of SLE and the lack of conclusive laboratory tests, the diagnosis can be very difficult, and the patient may in fact go undiagnosed for years.

MEDICAL MANAGEMENT

Management of SLE is aimed at controlling inflammation and relieving symptoms. It involves ongoing good medical care and avoidance of factors that cause exacerbations.

Drug therapy is individualized and depends on the type and severity of present symptoms. During periods of remission, no drug therapy may be required, whereas in mild phases of the disease, aspirin and other nonsteroidal anti-inflammatory drugs are used to relieve pain and control inflammation. When symptoms are not effectively controlled by these drugs, as during periods of acute exacerbation, corticosteroids and immunosuppressants are used. Antimalarial drugs such as hydroxychloroquine sulfate are also sometimes used, particularly for patients with severe skin lesions. When all other treatment fails or the patient develops life-threatening complications, cytotoxic drugs may be tried. These are used with great care because of serious side effects such as increased risk of infection and renal damage.

Application of the Nursing Process to the Care of the Patient with Systemic Lupus Erythematosus

Assessment

Obtain a detailed patient history. Determine when the disease began, when it was diagnosed, what symptoms have occurred, what types of treatment have been used, and how effective they have been. Ask what symptoms are currently being experienced, what medications are being taken, and whether the medications are adequately controlling symptoms. Explore the patient's understanding of the disease and its treatment, the effect it has had on the patient's lifestyle and personal and family relationships, and how the patient is coping with this chronic, incurable disease.

Because the effects of SLE are so varied, perform a head-to-toe physical assessment. Assess carefully for any signs of respiratory, circulatory, or renal dysfunction. Take the patient's temperature and observe for any signs of infection, because the patient with neutropenia or who is taking steroids is at increased risk. Observe for skin lesions and alopecia. Do a complete neurologic assessment. Check muscle strength and note joint deformity, stiffness, or pain. Review the patient's usual daily diet, and ask about anorexia, nausea, and vomiting.

Nursing Diagnoses and Planning

Because of the chronic, incurable nature of SLE and its varied effects on different organs and systems, almost all nursing diagnoses are at some time applicable to patients with the disease. Nursing diagnoses and related expected patient outcomes most commonly applicable to patients with SLE include the following:

NDx: Pain related to joint inflammation or skin lesions

Planning: Patient outcomes
1. Patient reports joint pain or discomfort from skin lesions is relieved.
2. Patient performs activities of daily living without signs of pain such as moaning or grimacing.

NDx: Activity intolerance related to fatigue

Planning: Patient outcomes
1. Patient describes importance of remaining active while avoiding overexertion and fatigue.
2. Patient describes how daily activities can be planned so that needed rest periods are included.

NDx: High risk for infection related to skin lesions, neutropenia, and steroid therapy

Planning: Patient outcomes
1. Patient is afebrile.
2. Signs and symptoms of infection are absent.

NDx: High risk for ineffective individual coping related to the presence of a chronic, incurable disease and the need for lifestyle restrictions

Planning: Patient outcomes
1. Patient expresses feelings and fears.
2. Patient participates in decisions regarding care.
3. Patient identifies sources of support.
4. Patient maintains contact with family and friends.
5. Patient continues usual participation in social activities.

NDx: High risk for altered health maintenance related to insufficient knowledge of disease, treatment, and self-care

Planning: Patient outcomes
1. Patient describes disease process of SLE.
2. Patient lists factors that are related to exacerbations.
3. Patient identifies ways to avoid exacerbating factors.
4. Patient names prescribed medications and states the purpose of each.
5. Patient states how much of each medication to take and how and when to take it.
6. Patient lists side effects of medications that need to be reported.

Nursing Interventions

Nursing interventions have to be individualized for each patient. They must take into account the symptoms the patient is experiencing, the severity of the disease, and the medications that have been prescribed.

NDx: Pain
Administer analgesic and anti-inflammatory drugs as ordered. When muscle or joint pain is severe, maintain bed rest and support affected joints with pillows.

During periods of remission, do active or passive range-of-motion exercises to maintain joint mobility and, in the case of active exercise, to maintain muscle strength.

Keep skin lesions clean and dry. Encourage the patient to avoid touching, rubbing, or scratching lesions because these activities increase irritation and the risk of infection. Apply local preparations as ordered to control itching and decrease inflammation.

NDx: Activity intolerance
Help the patient structure daily activities to allow for frequent periods of rest so that fatigue and overwork are avoided. Caution the patient against inactivity, which can contribute to feelings of fatigue, muscle weakness, and joint stiffness.

NDx: High risk for infection
Instruct the patient to guard against exposure to infection by staying away from persons with colds, flu, and other infections. Teach the importance of good hygiene, balanced diet, and adequate rest in the prevention of infection.

In the hospital, monitor temperature, and if elevated, obtain blood, sputum, urine, and other cultures as ordered. Initiate protective isolation if severe neutropenia develops.

NDx: High risk for ineffective individual coping
Allow the patient to express feelings and fears and accept the patient's mood swings. Encourage the patient to make as many decisions regarding care as possible to foster a sense of self-worth and control. Focus the patient on the idea that she or he can learn to deal with the disease rather than be controlled by it.

Help the patient identify available support systems and refer the patient to social services or support groups as needed.

NDx: High risk for altered health maintenance
Teach the patient about SLE: what is known about the cause of the disease, its symptoms, how it is treated, and what course can be expected. Also teach about prescribed medications: name of each medication, what it is for, how much to take, when

Chart 10–4.

NURSING GUIDE TO PATIENT EDUCATION FOR SELF-MANAGEMENT: PROTECTION FROM ULTRAVIOLET LIGHT RAYS

Instruct the patient to:

Always wear an effective high–protection factor sunscreen.
Wear protective clothing (hat with a brim, long sleeves, pants, or long skirt) when outside.
Plan outdoor activities for early morning or late afternoon, when the sun is low in the sky.
Avoid indoor sources of ultraviolet rays, such as fluorescent lights, copy machines, and sunlight filtered through windows.

it is to be taken, and what side effects need to be reported. If the patient is taking anti-inflammatory drugs, stress the importance of taking the drugs exactly as prescribed, because abrupt discontinuation of the drug may trigger an exacerbation of symptoms.

Help the patient identify factors that can cause an exacerbation of the disease and ways to avoid them. For example, teach the patient to avoid exposure to ultraviolet light rays, as specified in Chart 10–4. Other exacerbating factors are fatigue and overwork, emotional stress, injuries, and pregnancy.

Evaluation

Evaluate the effectiveness of nursing care for a patient with SLE by comparing the patient's status with the expected patient outcomes. Examples of specific outcomes for patients with SLE have been provided in the Planning section.

SCLERODERMA

Scleroderma, is an autoimmune collagen disorder. It is uncommon and affects women two to three times more frequently than men. Scleroderma occurs in people of all races.

ETIOLOGY

The etiology of scleroderma is unknown.

PATHOPHYSIOLOGY

Scleroderma occurs in both systemic and localized forms. The two types of the systemic form are diffuse scleroderma (progressive systemic sclerosis, or PSS) and the CREST syndrome.

Diffuse scleroderma, which can progress rapidly and be potentially fatal, is characterized by diffuse fibrosis in the skin and thickening of the blood vessel walls with narrowing of the lumen and ischemic effects in affected internal organs. The fingers, joints, esophagus, intestine, kidney, and heart are especially affected. Edema and inflammation of the involved tissue result from the ischemic effects and lead to fibrosis and excessive collagen deposit in the tissues.

In contrast to diffuse scleroderma, the CREST syndrome is more localized and more slowly progressive. It is characterized by calcinosis cutis (calcium deposits on tips of fingers and over bony prominences), Raynaud's phenomenon, sclerodactyly, telagiectasia, and changes in the esophagus.

Morphea is the most common form of localized scleroderma. It is restricted to the skin and is characterized by asymmetric lesions. The epidermis is normal. The dermis is thickened, with an increased number of fibroblasts and collagen bundles.

CLINICAL MANIFESTATIONS

Diffuse scleroderma most often begins with thickening of the skin on the hands or Raynaud's phenomenon. The skin becomes thick, smooth, shiny, and taut (Fig. 10–6). Telangiectases may be prominent, and hyperpigmentation in a speckled light-and-dark pattern may be present. These changes are also common in the face.

The fingers become thick and edematous from the ischemic changes caused by the vasospasm of Raynaud's phenomenon. Ischemic ulcers in the fingertips produce characteristic pitted scars.

As the condition progresses, movement of the hands, face, mouth, and chest become limited. Respirations may be impaired, and contractures and atrophy develop. Esophageal stricture and decreased movement may make swallowing difficult.

Renal failure with severe hypertension is a frequent cause of death with systemic scleroderma.

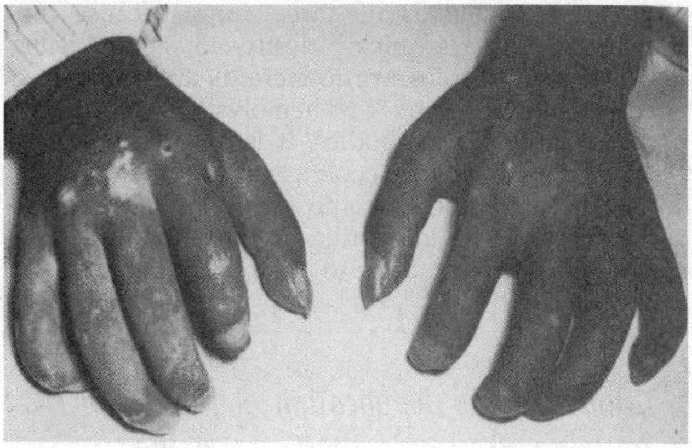

Figure 10–6.

Appearance of the skin in a patient with diffuse scleroderma. (From Moschella SL, Hurley JH (eds). Dermatology. 3rd ed, Vol 1. Philadelphia: WB Saunders, 1992, p 1238.)

Pericarditis, conduction defects, and heart failure are cardiac complications. Pulmonary fibrosis occurs, as does weight loss and malnutrition, secondary to esophageal strictures.

Morphea initially presents as one or more areas of purplish induration. Over time, the center of the plaque becomes thick, firm, hairless, and dull white with a lilac-colored active inflammatory border (Fig. 10–7). Inactive lesions are brown or yellow-brown, and much of the thickening and induration may disappear. Morphea usually occurs on the trunk, although the linear variant is found on the head or extremities. Raynaud's phenomenon is not characteristic of morphea, and the skin does not appear "bound down."

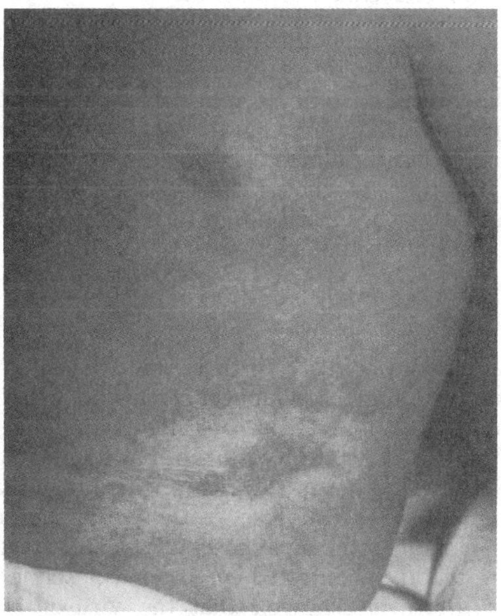

Figure 10–7.

Morphea. Note that the center of the plaque is thick, firm, hairless and dull white, whereas the active inflammatory border is lilac colored. (From Moschella SL, Hurley JH (eds). Dermatology. 3rd ed, Vol 1. Philadelphia: WB Saunders, p 1241.)

MEDICAL DIAGNOSIS

Both systemic scleroderma and morphea are diagnosed by the presenting lesions. A skin biopsy confirms the diagnosis if it is questionable.

Laboratory tests used in the diagnosis of diffuse systemic scleroderma are complete blood count, urinalysis, renal function tests, chest x-ray films, antinuclear antibodies, pulmonary function tests, and barium swallow.

MEDICAL MANAGEMENT

Progressive systemic sclerosis is resistant to treatment.

Penicillamine, which prevents cross-linking of collagen fibers, and colchicine, which inhibits collagen synthesis, as well as immunosuppressive drugs like prednisone and azathioprine may be prescribed but usually are ineffective. Salicylates and nonsteroidal anti-inflammatory drugs may provide relief from musculoskeletal discomfort. Vasodilators may help reduce vasospasm in the hands.

Physical therapy for patients with sclerodactyly prevents flexion contractures. Cold exposure should be avoided, and patients should have insulated gloves to prevent vasospasm in the digits.

There is no truly effective treatment for morphea, although topical steroids and occlusion may result in some slight improvement. In most patients, it is a benign disease, and plaques resolve spontaneously.

Guidelines for Application of the Nursing Process to the Care of the Patient with Scleroderma

Because systemic forms of scleroderma can affect many different parts of the body, a complete assessment with emphasis on the skin and other commonly affected organs, such as the esophagus, kidney, and lungs, is necessary. Nursing diagnoses, expected patient outcomes, and nursing interventions are based on the assessment. Depending on the extent of involvement, they will be similar to those for the patient with Raynaud's disease, rheumatoid arthritis, dysphagia, or kidney failure as well as a chronic skin disease with high risk for impaired skin integrity. Be certain to reinforce the physician's assurance that the prognosis is good with most systemic forms of scleroderma because the disease progresses very slowly. For the patient with a localized form, stress that localized disease rarely progresses to generalized disease.

Inform all patients that the Scleroderma Foundation in Watsanville, CA (408-728-2202) is a source of information and support for individuals with scleroderma.

AUTOIMMUNE HEMOLYTIC ANEMIA

Autoimmune hemolytic anemia refers to a variety of disorders that are characterized by the increased destruction of red blood cells associated with the presence of antibodies specific for the red blood cell.

ETIOLOGY

In more than half the cases, the cause is unknown, and these are referred to as idiopathic autoimmune hemolytic anemia. In the remaining cases, the cause is secondary to some event such as a viral illness, a malignant disease, or use of a drug.

PATHOPHYSIOLOGY

The antibodies responsible for this disease, which may be either acute or chronic, are classified as warm or cold depending on the temperature at which they are most active.

The warm antibodies are the most common type. They are usually IgG class antibodies that are directed at the Rh antigen on the red blood cell. These antibodies are not very active and tend to cause only a very mild anemia.

The cold antibodies are most active at a temperture below 37°C (98.6°F), being almost inactive at this temperature. They are usually an IgM class antibody.

CLINICAL MANIFESTATIONS

Symptoms vary depending on the extent of the anemia and may include fever, malaise, jaundice, and splenomegaly. The red blood cells are usually normal, but indirect serum bilirubin as well as the urobilinogen levels in urine and stool are often elevated. Patients with cold antibodies experience a hemolytic episode after being chilled.

MEDICAL DIAGNOSIS

The diagnosis of autoimmune hemolytic anemia is usually based on the demonstration of immunoglobulins or components of complement on the patient's red blood cells.

MEDICAL MANAGEMENT

If the anemia is secondary to some other disease process, that disease must be treated in order to resolve the anemia. Blood transfusions are given only if the anemia is life-threatening, because the transfused cells are quickly destroyed. For patients with warm antibodies, corticosteroids are sometimes effective in controlling the hemolysis, whereas for patients with cold antibodies, it is essential to keep them warm to prevent cooling to a temperature at which the antibodies become active. In some cases, particularly of the idiopathic, warm antibody type, splenectomy may be done to control the hemolysis.

Guidelines for Application of the Nursing Process to the Care of the Patient with Autoimmune Hemolytic Anemia

Nursing care of the patient with autoimmune hemolytic anemia combines the care required by any patient with anemia with that required by a patient with the underlying disease. It must be remembered, however, that patients with idiopathic hemolytic anemia are often frustrated by the fact that the cause of their problem is unknown and by the lack of definitive treatment. Thus, it is important to allow the patient as much control as possible over his or her care, keep the patient well informed as to the therapeutic plan, and provide an opportunity for the patient to express feelings and reactions.

CHRONIC FATIGUE SYNDROME

Chronic fatigue syndrome (CFS) or chronic fatigue immune dysfunction syndrome (CFIDS), previously called "yuppie flu" or Epstein-Barr virus syndrome, is a nonfatal disorder characterized by unrelenting fatigue. It occurs almost exclusively in whites, and three quarters of those affected are women. The syndrome has been diagnosed in persons of all ages, from children to the elderly.

ETIOLOGY

The etiology of CFS is uncertain. Chronic viral infection, immunoregulatory defect, and depression all have been suggested as possible etiologic agents.

In the late 1980s, CFS was thought to be linked to the Epstein-Barr virus (the main cause of infectious mononucleosis) because several common herpes viruses, including the Epstein-Barr virus, were found in the blood of infected persons. Subsequent research, however, showed that the viruses become reactivated when the immune system is impaired, and it is now believed that Epstein-Barr virus is a result rather than a cause of CFS. A current theory under investigation is that CFS is caused by a retrovirus (a virus composed of RNA that can translate itself into DNA and add its genetic program directly to the genetic program of the affected cell rather than simply "taking charge and overriding" the cell's genetic program as other viruses do). Retroviruses are particularly destructive because they strike specific cells that control immune function, and they are difficult to kill because they become such an integral part of the affected cells.

It is theorized that the retrovirus responsible for CFS could be an entirely new virus or a cousin to the previously identified human T-cell lymphotropic virus (HTLV) and HTLV-2 retroviruses, which affect T cells. It is also hypothesized that the immune system may need to be vulnerable owing to a genetic predisposition, environmental factors such as exposure to toxins, or by stress in order to be susceptible to the causative agent.

The role of depression in CFS also continues to be debated. Some clinicians believe that depression causes CFS. However, most believe that even though persons with CFS often have symptoms of depression, CSF and depression are two separate diseases, although those susceptible to depression could be more susceptible to CFS.

PATHOPHYSIOLOGY

In CFS, the function of the immune system is disrupted, and abnormalities in cell-mediated immunity occur. The number of natural killer (NK) cells is increased while their cytotoxicity is decreased. Production of interleukin-2 is increased, and lymphoproliferative responses and the production of gamma interferon following an appropriate stimulus are decreased. Various abnormalities of peripheral blood lymphocytes have also been found, including an increase in the percentage of suppressor cytotoxic T lymphocytes. None of these findings are unique to CFS, however. In addition to the immune system abnormalities, CFS patients have been found to have an abnormally low blood flow to one of the temporal lobes of the brain.

CLINICAL MANIFESTATIONS

CFS typically begins with flulike symptoms—fever, sore throat, body aches, and listlessness. Rather than disappearing, as in flu, the symptoms worsen. Persistent overwhelming fatigue or easy fatigability disrupts routines of daily living, and additional symptoms such as muscle weakness, headaches, joint pain, memory loss, insomnia, and problems with vision, balance, and concentration develop. Physical findings are essentially normal, and because of the differential effect of the disease on various parts of the immune system, patients typically do not suffer from flus, colds, or other common illnesses, but may complain of acne, monilial infection, or shingles. Symptoms persist for an average of $3\frac{1}{2}$ to 4 years, with many individuals showing improvement after a year. Approximately one in five people are estimated to fully recover, whereas 1 in 20 remain so ill that they are homebound or bedridden.

Table 10–9. CRITERIA OF THE CENTERS FOR DISEASE CONTROL FOR THE DIAGNOSIS OF CHRONIC FATIGUE SYNDROME

1. Symptoms develop over a few hours to a few days.
   - Temperature of 37.5° to 38.6°C (99.5° to 101.5°F) or chills
   - Painful cervical or axillary lymphadenopathy
   - Unexplained generalized muscle weakness
   - Muscle discomfort or pain
   - Prolonged (24 hours or more) generalized fatigue after levels of exercise that would have been easily tolerated previously
   - Headaches different in type, severity, or pattern from any previously experienced
   - Arthralgia without edema or erythema
   - Mental disturbances such as confusion, forgetfulness, irritability, inability to concentrate or reason, painful reaction to bright light, or depression
   - Sleep disturbance—too little or too much
2. Symptoms persist or recur over at least 6 months.
3. The persistent fatigue or easy fatigability must be
   - New to the patient (i.e., patient has no history of this)
   - Unrelieved by bed rest
   - Severe enough to cause the patient's activities to be decreased by more than 50%
4. Other potential causes have been ruled out.

MEDICAL DIAGNOSIS

CFS is diagnosed on the basis of criteria developed by the Centers for Disease Control (Table 10–9). There is no definitive diagnostic test available.

MEDICAL MANAGEMENT

There is no generally accepted treatment for CFS. Immunoregulatory therapy in the form of high doses of intravenous immunoglobulin G has been reported to effectively reduce symptoms in some patients (Lloyd et al, 1990), but the effect of such therapy remains debatable. Also currently under study is the effect of interleukin-2 given to patients in a therapeutic gamma globulin program (Bosse & Ades, 1989). Initial studies on the experimental antivirus drug Ampligen have shown it to relieve extreme fatigue and memory loss in patients severely ill with CFS.

Application of the Nursing Process to the Care of the Patient with Chronic Fatigue Syndrome

Assessment

Obtain a history of the patient's symptoms. Determine what the symptoms are, when they began, and how they have affected the patient's daily function and overall lifestyle. Explore their effects on occupation, role responsibilities, family, and finances.

Nursing Diagnoses and Planning

Nursing diagnoses and related expected patient outcomes most commonly applicable to patients with CSF include the following:

NDx: Fatigue related to chronic fatigue syndrome

Planning: Patient outcomes

1. Patient expresses feelings and concerns about the effects of fatigue on his or her life.
2. Patient sets priorities for daily, weekly, and monthly activities.
3. Patient schedules activities and periods of rest according to individual tolerance.
4. Patient participates as tolerated in a balance of activities that contribute to physical and psychosocial well-being.

NDx: High risk for altered family processes related to difficulties adjusting to changes in patient, roles, routines, and the like

Planning: Patient outcomes

1. Family members verbalize feelings regarding the illness of the patient and the resultant changes in patterns of daily living and lifestyle.
2. Family members support the ill person in attempts to cope.
3. Family members maintain a supportive relationship with one another.
4. Family members use available external resources as needed.

NDx: High risk for situational low self-esteem related to inability to carry out usual activities and responsibilities secondary to the clinical manifestations of chronic fatigue syndrome

Planning: Patient outcomes

1. Patient identifies positive aspects of self.
2. Patient expresses optimism about the future.
3. Patient describes ways to maintain a sense of control.

Nursing Interventions

NDx: Fatigue

Focus on helping the individual to adapt to the fatigued state. Encourage the patient to express feelings, fears, and concerns regarding the impact of fatigue on daily activities and general lifestyle. Explore with the patient which activities are difficult and the manner and extent to which the fatigue interferes with role activities. Guide the patient in the identification of energy patterns and in scheduling activities in relationship to them. Do this by asking the patient to record fatigue level as well as activities engaged in each hour. Provide the patient with directions for recording fatigue, such as use of the Phoben scale of 0 (not tired) to 10 (total exhaustion). Analyze the record with the patient to identify times of peak energy, times of lower energy, and the activities that are related to increasing fatigue. Stress careful, consistent planning as the key to living as normal a life as possible. Explain the importance of conserving energy in preparation for active or stressful events, and encourage the patient to plan daily and weekly schedules accordingly. Stress the importance of adequate sleep, naps, and a daily balance of activities such that more restful activities alternate with more demanding ones.

Analyze routines and the home environment and make necessary changes for work simplification and efficient conservation of energy. Classify activities as essential or nonessential, and identify those that may be performed by others.

Explain that stress depletes energy, and explore with the patient sources of stress in his or her daily life. Help the patient identify how the sources of stress might be reduced or eliminated, as well as methods for controlling the effects of stressful situations on self.

Refer to community resources for household, child care, transportation, or other assistance needed.

NDx: High risk for altered family processes

Involve family members in planning conferences. Provide accurate information, and encourage questions to promote realistic changes in the family's expectations of the patient. Encourage open discussion of individuals' reactions to the effects of the patient's illness and resulting tensions on the family. Allow expressions of anger and anxiety, and acknowledge these feelings as normal. Explore with the family how role responsibilities in the home can be reorganized to foster family function and decrease stress. Assist the family to set priorities, and refer to sources of help as needed. Encourage open discussion of secondary gains associated with the sick role, which can contribute to delay in the patient's resumption of the well role.

NDx: High risk for situational low self-esteem

Promote expression of feelings. Do this by reflecting the patient's feelings both positive and negative and by maintaining an empathetic, nonjudgmental attitude. Help the patient identify positive self-attributes, and recognize and praise positive decisions, activities, and coping strategies. Encourage the patient to structure situations for success through appropriate timing and by allowing adequate time for preparation and rest. Teach cognitive therapy, that is, correction of negative, defeatist thoughts or overgeneralizations, and encourage use of relaxation and guided imagery. Inform the patient about sources of support such as the National CFS Association (3521 Broadway, Suite 222, Kansas City, MO 64111, 816-931-4777), the Chronic Fatigue and Immune Dysfunction Syndrome Association (P.O. Box 220398, Charlotte, NC 28222-0398, 704-362-CFID), and the Chronic Fatigue Immune Dysfunction Syndrome Society (P.O. Box 230108, Portland, OR 97223, 503-684-5261).

Evaluation

Evaluate effectiveness of nursing care for a patient with CFS by comparing the patient's status with the expected patient outcomes. Examples of specific outcomes for patients with CFS have been provided in the Planning section.

The Elderly: Special Considerations

Cancer and infection are the two major disorders that have an increased incidence in the aged and are postulated to be due, at least in part, to age-related changes in the immune system.

Cancer in the Aged

The "immunologic surveillance" theory is that malignant cells are marked by antigens that are identified as foreign by T cells or NK cells. The malignant cell carrying the foreign antigen is then destroyed by the T cell in the properly functioning immune system. According to this theory, the increase in cancer seen in the aged is due to a decrease in effective surveillance by the immune system. This interpretation is supported by the fact that there is also an increase of cancer in younger persons who are immunosuppressed. However, it is also true that aged persons have had a longer time to be exposed to environmental carcinogens and to acquire mutations in the genes, which also contribute to the risk of cancer.

Infection in the Aged

The increased incidence of infection among geriatric patients is due to changes in the immune system as well as to age-related changes in the body's other defenses. For example, decreased skin turgor with its associated decreased resistance to friction damage is a normal effect of aging. Aging also takes its toll on the many nonspecific defense mechanisms of the respiratory tract. The respiratory muscles become weak, and the thoracic cage stiffens. The cilia may have been damaged and their effectiveness decreased by cigarette smoking or other forms of air pollution. Aspiration becomes a problem as the gag and cough reflexes decrease and problems with swallowing develop. These factors may make it difficult for the elderly person to cough and effectively remove foreign materials from the lungs and thus increase susceptibility to influenza and pneumonia.

Changes in the cardiovascular system also contribute to the increasing risk of infection in the elderly. Calcification of the heart valves makes it easier for bacteria to attach and cause endocarditis. The blood supply to peripheral areas of the body may be decreased as the cardiac output decreases and resistance in the arteries increases. This leaves peripheral areas of the body more prone to infections and decreases their ability to heal injured tissues.

The GI tract becomes more prone to infection as its acidity and motility decrease. Normally the acidity of the stomach destroys most ingested microorganisms. Without this protective acidity, organisms can gain access to the GI tract and, because motility has decreased, remain long enough to multiply and cause gastroenteritis and diarrhea.

As renal function decreases, the urinary tract is also more prone to infections. Similarly, structural changes that commonly occur with age, such as urethral stricture and enlargement of the prostate gland, also increase the risk of infection.

Chronic illnesses such as congestive heart failure, diabetes mellitus, alcoholism, lung disease, and cancer seem to make the individual more susceptible to infection. The elderly frequently have one or more of these chronic illnesses, often in addition to other risk factors like dehydration and malnutrition.

CLINICAL MANIFESTATIONS

The geriatric patient with an infection may not exhibit the usual signs and symptoms of infection. Fever is often absent. Many elderly have a normally low body temperature, and a rise of a degree or more is not identified as an elevation in temperature. Other signs, such as an increase in the white blood cell count, cough, pain, and inflammation, may not be present. Often the only clues that an infection is occurring are subtle changes in behavior, such as a decrease in alertness, fatigue, apathy, irritability, and confusion.

MEDICAL MANAGEMENT

Antibiotics are used to treat the infection in doses adjusted as needed based on age and renal function. In addition, supportive treatment is used to maintain optimal function of all body systems. This is of critical importance because, if present, fever increases the basal metabolic rate, thus increasing the heart rate, respiratory rate, blood pressure, and the need for fluids, oxygen, and energy. This stress may cause the geriatric patient with marginal functioning of body systems to begin to decompensate. For example, cardiac dysrhythmias may develop as a result of the increased demand, and renal function may be impaired. Additional oxygen may be required, especially if the patient has preexisting lung disease. If the patient is an insulin-dependent diabetic, the need for insulin is increased.

Measures to lower the temperature (antipyretic medications or cooling techniques) are not instituted unless the patient is at risk of delirium, which is likely at a temperature of 40.5°C (105°F) or higher. Temperature is not lowered, because fever inhibits the growth of pathogens and also provides a clinical indication of the response of the infection to prescribed antibiotics.

Application of the Nursing Process to the Care of the Geriatric Patient with an Infection

Assessment

Assessment of the aged patient with an infection involves observations specific to the type of infection (e.g., if a wound infection, inspect the wound for redness, swelling, and type and amount of drainage; if a respiratory infection, note the presence of cough and type and amount of expectoration, as well as rate, depth, sound, and ease of respiration); observations related to the status of essential body needs and functions; and observation for side effects of the treatments being used.

Take the patient's temperature every 4 hours. Monitor pulse and blood pressure for signs of cardiac dysrhythmias and congestive heart failure, which is a risk during fluid replacement in elderly patients. Monitor respiratory rate and depth, the patient's color, and arterial blood gas values to check for adequate ventilation and oxygenation. Measure and record fluid intake and output to ascertain that the patient is not dehydrated and that the kidneys are functioning.

Assess nutritional status in terms of the additional demands made by the infection. Observe the patient for side effects of prescribed medications and, if the patient is on bed rest, for skin breakdown, constipation, confusion, and other effects of immobility.

Nursing Diagnoses and Planning

Because infection can impact on all aspects of the aged person's functioning, many nursing diagnoses and related expected patient outcomes apply.

Nursing Interventions

Specific nursing interventions depend on the type and extent of infection and the physician's orders. In all cases, however, provide care in a manner that conserves the patient's energy for fighting the infection while preventing loss of functional ability. To keep the patient oriented, keep a clock, a calendar, and selected personal items near the bedside and use a radio or television to provide sensory stimulation.

If the patient is receiving antibiotic therapy, monitor for diarrhea, which can cause severe fluid and electrolyte imbalance. If diarrhea occurs, notify the physician before administering the next dose. If the patient is taking an aminoglycoside, monitor for hearing loss and for elevated blood urea nitrogen and creatinine levels indicative of nephrotoxicity. Also record fluid intake and output, and ensure adequate hydration.

Evaluation

Evaluate the effectiveness of nursing care for a geriatric patient with an infection by comparing the patient's status with the expected patient outcomes.

Specific outcomes depend on the patient, the type of infection, and the nursing diagnosis. Examples might include the following:

Temperature is within patient's normal range.
Lungs are clear on auscultation.
Vital signs are within patient's normal range.
Urinary output is between 1200 and 1500 ml daily.
Skin turgor is good.
Blood gas values are within normal range.
Skin and mucous membranes are intact.
Patient is oriented to person, place, and time.

Bibliography

Ames ME. Learning to live with Epstein-Barr virus. Science 1985; 6:89.
Barrett JT. Textbook of immunology. St. Louis: CV Mosby, 1988.
Barrick B. Light at the end of a decade. AJN 1990; 90(11):37.
Bellanti JA. Immunology III. Philadelphia: WB Saunders, 1985.
Bosse D, Ades EW. Immunotherapy and enhanced antibody-dependent cell-mediated cytotoxicity using virally-infected target cells. J Clin Lab Immunol 1989; 29(3):109.
Brown ML. AIDS and ethics. Oncol Nurs Forum 1987; 14(1):69.
Brown BL, Brown JW. The third international conference on AIDS: Risk of AIDS in healthcare workers. Nurs Manage 1988; 19(3):33.
Cassel W, Archer-Duste H. The new epidemic: Chronic fatigue syndrome. Calif Nurse 1989; 85(4):6.

Centers for Disease Control. The chronic fatigue syndrome [information pamphlet]. Washington, DC: Public Health Service, Department of Health and Human Services, January 1990.

Centers for Disease Control. Caring for someone with AIDS [brochure]. Washington, DC: Public Health Service, Department of Health and Human Services, April 1991.

Cohen PT, Sande MA, Volberding PA (eds). The AIDS knowledge base. Waltham, MA: The Medical Publishing Group, 1990.

Cowley G, Hager M, Joseph N. Chronic fatigue syndrome. Newsweek November 12, 1990:62.

Durham JD, Cohen FL (eds). The person with AIDS: Nursing perspectives. New York: Springer Publishing, 1991.

Ellis NK, Krch-Cole E. Providing a therapeutic milieu experience for a patient diagnosed with AIDS. Arch Psychiatr Nurs 1987; 1(6):436.

Executive Summary: Guidelines for the Diagnosis and Management of Asthma. Publication No. 91-3042A. National Asthma Education Program, Office of Prevention, Education, and Control, National Heart, Lung, and Blood Institute, National Institutes of Health, Bethesda, MD, June 1991.

Flaskerud JH. AIDS: Neuropsychiatric complications. J Psychosoc Nurs Ment Health Serv 1987; 25(12):17.

Gantz NM, Holmes GP. Treatment of patients with chronic fatigue syndrome. Drugs 1989; 38(6):855.

Gee G, Moran TA. AIDS: Concepts in nursing practice. Baltimore: Williams & Wilkins, 1988.

Greenberg DB. Neurasthenia in the 1980's: Chronic mononucleosis, chronic fatigue syndrome and depressive disorders. Psychosomatics 1990; 31(2):129.

Grierson H, Holmes GP, Strauss SE. Coping with chronic fatigue syndrome. Patient Care 1987; 21(18):79.

Habif TP. Clinical dermatology. 2nd ed. St. Louis: CV Mosby, 1990.

Hoffman S. Asthma, Part 1. Harvard Health Letter 1991; 16(7):5.

Hoffman S. Asthma, Part 2. Harvard Health Letter 1991; 16(8):1.

Holmes GP, Kaplan JE, Gantz NM, et al. Chronic fatigue syndrome: A working case definition. Ann Intern Med 1988; 108.387.

Klimos NG, et al. Immunologic abnormalities in chronic fatigue syndrome. J Clin Microbiol 1990; 28(6):1403.

Lloyd A, Hickie I, Wakefield D, et al. A double-blind, placebo-controlled trial of intravenous immunoglobulin therapy in patients with chronic fatigue syndrome. Am J Med 1990; 89(5):561.

Mansmann HC (ed). Guidelines for the diagnosis and management of asthma. National Heart, Lung, and Blood Institute, National Asthma Education Program Expert Panel Report. Pediatric Asthma Allergy and Immunology. 1991; 5(2).

McArthur J. AIDS dementia. RN 1990; 53(3):36.

Middleton E, et al. Allergy principles and practice. 3rd ed. Vol. 1. St. Louis: CV Mosby, 1988.

Paul WE. Fundamental immunology. 2nd ed. New York: Raven Press, 1989.

Peterson PK, Shepard J, Macres M, et al. A controlled trial of intravenous immunoglobulin G in chronic fatigue syndrome. Am J Med 1990; 89(5):551.

Portwood MF. Chronic fatigue syndrome—a diagnosis for consideration. Nurse Pract Am J Primary Health Care. 1988; 13(2):15.

Powell MA. Epstein-Barr antibody titer and chronic fatigue syndrome. J Am Acad Nurse Pract 1990; 2(1):33.

Pritchard V. Preventing and treating geriatric infections. RN 1988; 51(3):36.

Pritchard V. Geriatric infections: The impact of diet. RN 1988; 51(7):54.

Reinke LF, Hoffman LA. Breathing space: How to teach asthma co-management. Am J Nurs 1992; 92(10):40.

Roit IM, Brostoff J, Male DK. Immunology. St. Louis: CV Mosby, Gower Medical Publishing, 1989.

Rubin, RH. Acquired immunodeficiency syndrome. Sci Am 1993; 269:1.

Samter M. Immunological diseases. 4th ed. Boston: Little, Brown, 1988.

Sipes C. AIDS: The haunting facts, the human care. NursingLife 1988; 8(2):33.

Spracklen FH. The chronic fatigue syndrome (myalgic encephalomyelitis)—myth or mystery? S Afr Med J 1988; 74(9):448.

Stites DP, Stobo JD, Wells JV (eds). Basic and clinical immunology. 6th ed. Norwalk, CT: Appleton & Lange, 1987.

Tichy AM, Taloshek ML. Older women. Sexually transmitted diseases and acquired immunodeficiency syndrome. Nurs Clin North Am 1992; 27(4):937.

Tierney LM. Chronic fatigue syndrome: Current recommendations for diagnosis and management. Consultant 1989; 29(3):25.

Chapter Eleven

NURSING CARE of Adults with Oncologic Disorders

In the United States, more than one million people are diagnosed with cancer each year. Cancer occurs among all age groups, although its incidence is greatest in the elderly. It can affect virtually any body system, and despite the many advances in diagnosis and treatment, much of the population still considers a diagnosis of cancer to mean suffering and death. Thus, caring for patients with cancer requires an understanding of the normal physiology and pathophysiology of body systems as well as an understanding of the etiology and pathophysiology of malignant tumors, diagnostic and therapeutic measures in current use, and the related nursing care. Because of the psychological toll of cancer, the nurse also must be sensitive to the needs of both patient and significant others for support, involved in patient and family education in regard to care and prevention, and knowledgeable about available community resources so that appropriate referrals can be made.

Anatomy and Physiology of the Cell

The cell is the basic unit of all living things, and an understanding of its normal structure and function is essential in the study of diseases caused by malignant cells. The human body is composed of more than 75 trillion cells. The majority of these cells reproduce continually in an effort to maintain the body's pattern of growth and to replace damaged tissue and dead cells. Figure 11–1 illustrates the major cellular components and describes their function.

Each cell is surrounded by a membrane that is composed of proteins and lipids. Within the cell are a nucleus and cytoplasm. The nucleus, which is surrounded by a nuclear membrane, contains the cell's genetic controlling material in the form of deoxyribonucleic acid (DNA). Within the nucleus is the nucleolus, which contains additional genetic controlling material in the form of ribonucleic acid (RNA). The cytoplasm surrounds the nucleus and provides a complex microtubule system that transports substances within the cell. The cytoplasm gives the cell its shape and serves as the medium that supports all cell structures. Several highly specialized organelles within the cytoplasm perform functions that allow the cell to carry out metabolism, excretion, and reproduction.

The cell cycle describes the life of a cell. It begins at the midpoint of the mitosis, which results in the formation of a particular cell, and ends at the midpoint of the mitosis, which results in that cell dividing into two daughter cells. The cell cycle (Fig. 11–2) is a dynamic process that is divided into five phases: G_1, G_0, S, G_2, and M.

Phase G_1 is a postmitotic period of cell growth characterized by the development of RNA and pro-

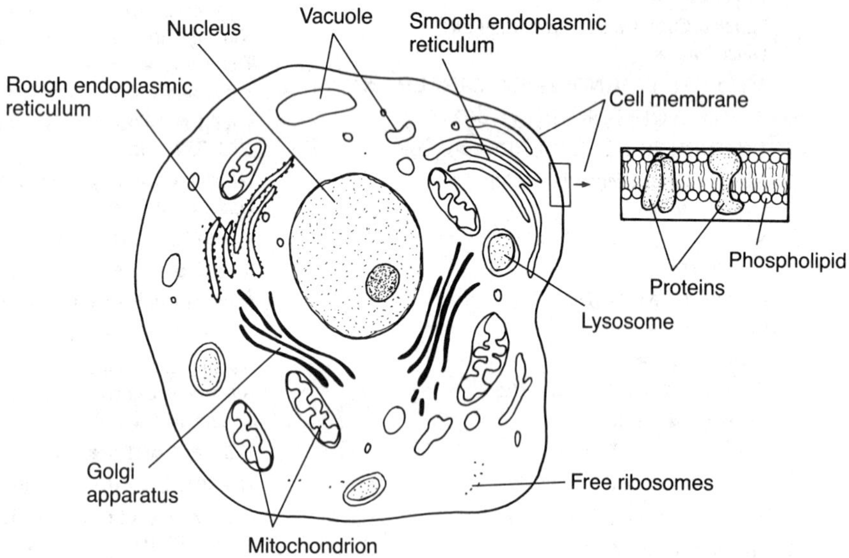

Figure 11–1.

Major cellular components and their functions. The *cell membrane* controls movement of substances in and out of the cell. Small pores allow passage of small molecules. Other substances move in or out by active transport. The *nucleus* directs and controls all cellular activities via the genes, which are located on the chromosomes. The *rough endoplasmic reticulum* is endoplasmic reticulum with ribosomes on its surface. It synthesizes proteins that combine with fats or carbohydrates. *Smooth endoplasmic reticulum* has no ribosomes on its surface. It is part of the intracellular transport system, with a role in fat metabolism, biotransformation, and Ca^{2+} storage. *Free ribosomes* synthesize proteins for intracellular enzymes and structures. A *vacuole* is a clear space in the cytoplasm filled with fluid or air. The *Golgi apparatus* concentrates and packages chemical products into secretion granules that float to the cell membrane for excretion into the extracellular fluid. A *lysosome* is an intracellular digestive system capable of breaking down proteins and carbohydrates. It destroys foreign proteins by phagocytosis. A *mitochondrion* manufactures adenosine triphosphate, which supplies the cell with energy.

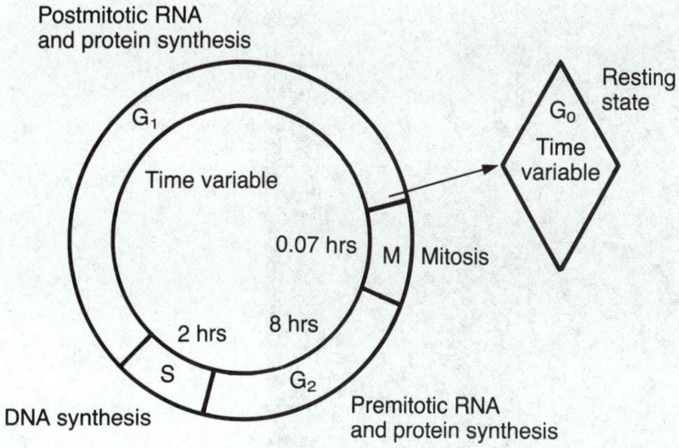

Figure 11–2.

The cell cycle.

tein. Cells may leave phase G_1 and enter G_0 or go on to phase S. Phase G_0 is a dormant or resting stage in which the cell performs all normal functions but does not replicate. Phase S, in contrast, is an active period of DNA synthesis that results in two separate sets of chromosomes in the nucleus. Following phase S is phase G_2, which is a premitotic interval of RNA and protein synthesis similar to G_1. M, or mitosis, is the final phase, during which the cell splits into two daughter cells.

The length of the cell cycle varies from tissue to tissue. It may be as short as 16 hours or extend to 400 hours, as with liver cells. Since the time spent in phases G_2 (8 hours), S (2 hours), and M (0.07 hours) is about the same for all cells, the variability is due to different times spent in phases G_1 and G_0. One factor contributing to this variability is that not all cells enter the G_0 phase. The number that do enter G_0 varies, depending on the type of tissue.

Highly differentiated cells such as neurons never enter the cell cycle because in the process of developing a highly specialized function they have lost the ability to replicate.

Pathophysiology

The term neoplasm (new growth) is used to describe a group of cells that has an abnormal growth pattern. Neoplasms are classified as either benign or malignant. A benign neoplasm is composed of cells that resemble the tissue of origin; is usually encapsulated; grows slowly and by expansion; does not recur or metastasize; does not destroy tissue unless it interferes with blood flow; and does not cause systemic symptoms or death unless it interferes with vital functions owing to its location, as with a brain tumor.

A malignant neoplasm, or cancer, is composed of undifferentiated (immature) cells that have little resemblance to the tissue of origin. The malignant neoplasm tends to grow rapidly, expanding at the periphery and invading and destroying surrounding tissues (Fig. 11–3). It also tends to recur when removed and spreads by way of the blood and lymph to distant areas of the body. It causes systemic manifestations such as alteration in taste, anorexia, weight loss, weakness, and ultimately causes death if not controlled.

Malignant cells in epithelial tissue are called carcinomas. Malignant cells of connective tissue, muscle, or bone are called sarcomas. All these are classified as solid tumors because initially they are confined to a specific tissue or organ. Malignant cells of blood and the lymphatics are called leukemias, myelomas, and lymphomas. These are classified as hematologic cancers, which are disseminated from their beginning.

When a normal cell undergoes transformation to a malignant cell, a number of changes occur in the cell membrane and intracellular structures.

The cell membrane loses its contact inhibition, continuing to grow even when another cell is touched. It also develops a strong negative surface charge and does not form intercellular connections; and its antigens may be altered.

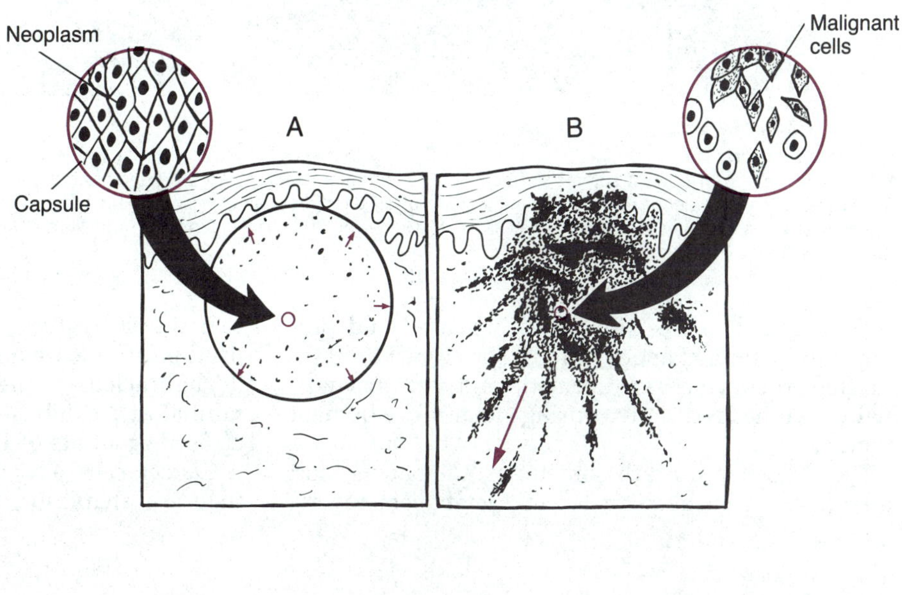

Figure 11–3.

A, Benign encapsulated neoplasm. *B*, Malignant neoplasm showing multiple projections from its periphery into the surrounding tissue.

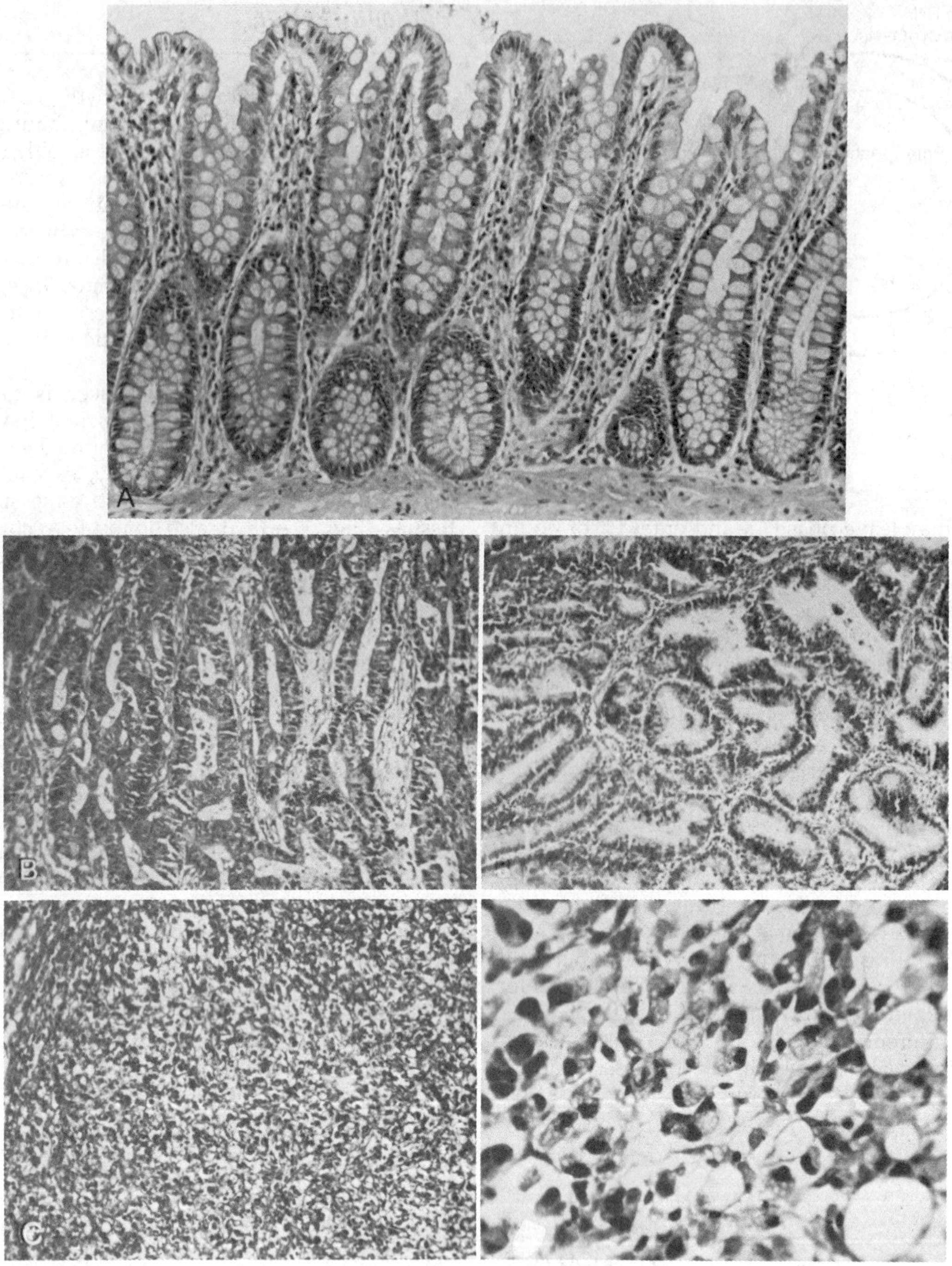

Figure 11–4.

A, Photomicrograph of normal colonic epithelium. *B*, Photomicrograph of a well-differentiated adenocarcinoma that resembles parent tissue in that glands can be identified. *C*, Photomicrograph of an undifferentiated or anaplastic adenocarcinoma. (*A* from Price S, Wilson L. Clinical concepts of disease processes. 3rd ed. New York: McGraw-Hill, 1986, p 73. *B* and *C* from Perez-Tamayo R. Mechanisms of disease. Philadelphia: WB Saunders, 1961, p 205.)

The number of free ribosomes increases, and protein production changes. More structural proteins but fewer enzymes are formed, and proteins normally synthesized only during fetal development appear.

The mitochondria are sometimes edematous, and alterations in metabolism occur. Metabolism reverts to a simpler pattern, generally involving greater utilization of glucose and more anaerobic pathways.

The nucleus of the cell is significantly larger than normal and exhibits abnormal chromosomes and increased amounts of DNA.

Cancer cells also differ from normal cells in that they are anaplastic, that is, they are primitive, undifferentiated cells that no longer resemble the original cells from which the tumor began (Fig. 11–4). Anaplastic cells replicate much more quickly than normal cells and are unable to perform the functions of the tissues from which they are derived. They also do not "age" normally or die "on time."

Growth rate of a tumor is described in terms of doubling time, that is, the time it takes for the total mass of cells in the tumor to double. The growth rate of each malignant tumor depends on how many cells are actively dividing, cell cycle time, and how many cells are dying. Since many cancer cells appear unable to enter the resting G_0 phase of the cell cycle and simply continue to divide until blood and nutrient supply is insufficient, there are generally a greater number of malignant cells replicating at any point in time than there would be in normal tissue.

Malignant tumors spread or metastasize through both a direct and an indirect process. Direct extension involves the infiltration of malignant cells into adjacent tissues. This occurs in an irregular way, with many projections invading surrounding tissues from different areas on the periphery of the tumor. Depending on the tissues affected, hemorrhage, ulceration, necrosis, or fibrosis can occur. Direct extension can also result in seeding of cancer cells into a body cavity. This occurs when a malignant tumor penetrates into a body cavity and cells drop off and implant on the serosal surface.

Indirect spread involves invasion of vascular or lymphatic channels, in which malignant cells break away from the tumor and travel to distant areas of the body, where they implant and develop into secondary tumors. When spread is by way of the lymphatics, malignant cells first lodge in the lymph nodes that drain the tumor site. They may remain there for some time before again breaking away and traveling to more distant nodes and eventually reaching the thoracic duct and entering the blood stream.

Incidence of Cancer

Cancer, which is a general term used to encompass a group of more than 100 malignant disorders, is second only to heart disease as a cause of human death. The disease can occur throughout a person's life span, and any organ of the body can be a target for metastasis of malignant cells.

Currently there are more than 7 million people in the United States who have a history of cancer, and more than 5 million have been alive for more than 5 years after diagnosis.

Statistics compiled by the American Cancer Society indicate that three of every four families in the United States will experience a family member's being diagnosed with an oncologic disorder. One of every three individuals will be diagnosed with cancer at some time during his or her lifetime. Whereas the death rate from other diseases over the last 30 years has gone down, the death rate from cancer has shown an increase, most of which is attributed to the increased incidence of lung cancer (Fig. 11–5).

Gender and Age

In general, the incidence of cancer is the same in both males and females; however, the age distribution is different. Between the ages of 20 and 60, the incidence is higher in females, which may reflect the high rates of breast and cervical cancer during these years. After age 60, males have a marked increase in cancer rates over females.

Race

The incidence of cancer is almost the same for blacks and whites in the United States, although some differences occur related to specific cancer sites. As the social and economic living standards become similar for black and white populations, so do the incidence and death rates from cancer.

Geography

Cancer occurs more frequently in westernized countries where the life span is estimated to be longer. Exposure to environmental carcinogens may be geographically related.

Etiology of Cancer

Although the exact etiology of all oncologic disorders is unknown, epidemiologic research has assisted in identifying risk factors that may influence the development of an oncologic disorder.

The process that causes the uncontrolled and undisciplined growth of cells is thought to involve many steps that may be enhanced by external stimuli. Genetic, environmental, immunologic, and viral factors may individually or as cofactors play an important role in changing normal cells into malignant cells; this process is called carcinogenesis.

Genetic Factors

An important clue to the cause of a malignant disease may actually be hidden in the chromosomal characteristics of the individual as well as in the tumor itself. It has been shown that the cells of nearly all human malignant tumors and most animal tumors contain chromosomal abnormalities. There is evidence that individuals with specific genetic characteristics may have an increased risk of certain cancers.

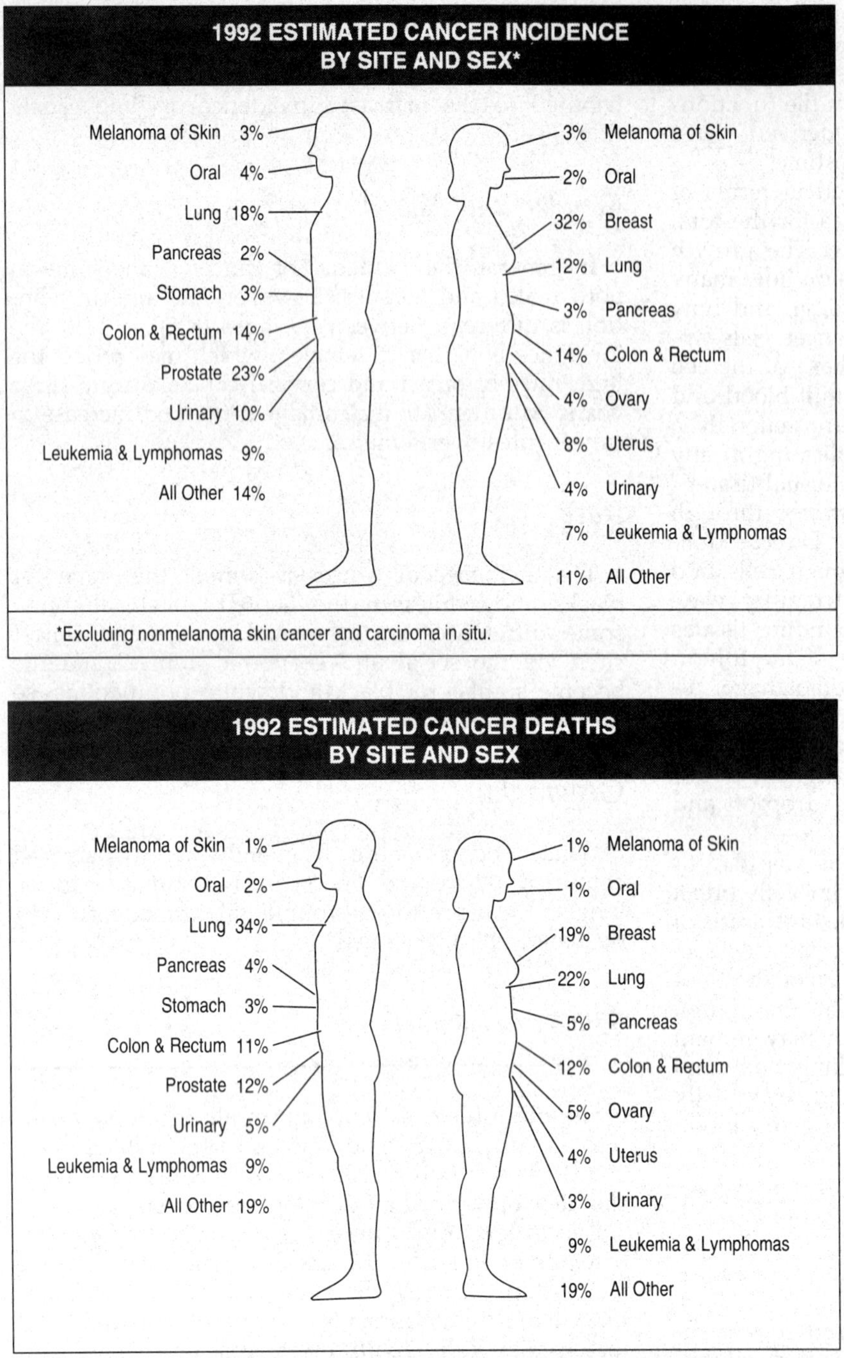

Figure 11–5.

Estimated cancer incidence and deaths by site and sex. (From CA 1992; 42:21.)

Individuals with chromosome disorders such as Bloom's, Fanconi's, Down's, and Klinefelter's syndromes have an increased risk of developing leukemia. The Philadelphia chromosomal alteration (a translocation of the long arm of chromosome 22) is found in 90% of patients diagnosed with chronic myelogenous leukemia.

The high incidence of cancer in members of the same family may indicate a genetic predisposition. Cancers of the breast, gastrointestinal tract, and thyroid and retinoblastomas are known to occur more frequently in patients with a family history of these cancers. Familial cancers may be related to the combined influence of genetics and environment.

Environmental Factors

CHEMICALS AND TOXIC SUBSTANCES

Chemicals and substances in our environment have been identified as significantly contributing to the development of certain oncologic disorders. Certain chemicals have the ability to directly or indirectly alter the structure of DNA within cells.

Chemical carcinogenesis can be divided into a two-step process of initiation and promotion. A chemical initiator is capable of permanently and irreversibly altering cells. A chemical promoter has the ability to temporarily and reversibly change cells. Carcinogenesis is thought to occur when a cell has undergone a permanent change due to the action of an initiating agent and is then repeatedly exposed to a chemical promoter. This two-step process results in cellular oncogenous transformation.

The high incidence of scrotal cancer seen in chimney sweeps more than 150 years ago was perhaps the first recognition of an occupational cause of cancer. The relationship between soldiers exposed to nitrogen mustard gas during World War I and their subsequent development of cancer was another clue to the dangers of exposure to carcinogenic substances. Many chemical compounds have been shown to produce tumors in animals, and several hundred are suspected to be carcinogenic. The majority of these produce cancer in animals and not humans. Examples of agents that exhibit carcinogenic risk to humans include arsenic, asbestos, aromatic amines, benzene, vinyl chloride, aflatoxins. Individuals may be exposed to chemical carcinogens as part of their lifestyle, occupation, and medical history. Asbestos, a mineral fiber used in insulation, as a fire retardant, and in a number of manufacturing applications, is associated with pleural and abdominal mesothelioma after repeated exposure. Medical therapies that utilize certain drugs such as hormones, antitumor drugs, and antibiotics may also cause oncologic disorders.

A variety of federal and state governmental agencies regulate those chemicals that have been proved to be carcinogenic and furnish updated lists of these agents to the public and individuals in the workplace. The lists include new information on carcinogenic chemicals in the workplace, in medicinal agents, in foods, and in the environment. In 1986, the federal government mandated that employees who, in the course of their work, are exposed to hazardous substances, including carcinogens, be trained by employers in correct handling and use of protective clothing.

TOBACCO

Cigarette smoking is the single most preventable cause of disease and death in the United States. It is estimated that more than 30% of all cancer is related to smoking, including cancers of the lung, mouth, throat, larynx, esophagus, and bladder. Eighty-three percent of all lung cancer is related to smoking. As increasing numbers of women began to smoke, their rate of smoking-related cancers also increased.

The relationship between smoking and cancer is well documented, as is evidence that increased risk may be a function of the length of time and number of cigarettes an individual has smoked. In addition, a smoker who also consumes large quantities of alcohol has a substantially increased risk of developing an oral cancer. Chemicals that are known tumor promoters and initiators have been detected in both tobacco and cigarette smoke. Researchers continue to study the effect of cigarette smoke that is inhaled by nonsmokers. This "second-hand smoke" has been found to be a potent carcinogen as well as a significant factor in the development of a variety of other disorders.

ALCOHOL

A relationship has been established between consumption of large amounts of alcohol and the subsequent development of cancers of the head, neck, and esophagus. Heavy consumption of beer may increase the risk of colorectal cancer.

DIET

The relationship between dietary intake and cancer is being closely studied. Dietary intake may be responsible for approximately one third of all oncologic disorders in the United States. Dietary intake may be an environmental promoter and initiator, based on the time periods during which the individual is exposed to certain dietary practices. Epidemiologic studies and animal studies have pointed to the role that dietary fat, nitrites, and chemical food additives may play in the development of certain cancers.

Dietary fat has the ability to cause an increase in the secretion of bile, and it is postulated that the by-products of bile salts may act as promoting agents in the development of colon cancer. Fats also affect the endocrine system and cause increased production of hormones. There may be a relationship between high fat intake and the hormone-dependent tumors of the breast and prostate.

In animal studies, vitamins A and C, riboflavin, and selenium possess a mechanism that appears to have an unexplained ability to protect against the development of cancer. The American Cancer Society suggests a diet that may guard against the development of cancer, which includes fresh vegetables, high fiber, fruits, and foods that contain vitamins A and C.

RADIATION

Ionizing and electromagnetic radiation has the ability to interfere with the structure and function of DNA within cells. Radiation is one of the major therapies used to kill cancerous cells. The relationship between the ultraviolet rays of the sun and inducement of skin cancer was documented more than a century ago. Individuals exposed to atomic radiation have a marked increased risk for breast cancer, leukemia, and lung and thyroid cancer. Radiologists in the early 1900s, before protective methods were employed, had a high incidence of leukemia.

Viruses

The viral etiology theory of cancer suggests that certain viruses have the ability to change the genetic makeup of cells, thus initiating the process of transforming normal cells into malignant cells (oncogenesis). The oncogene has the ability to directly affect cellular DNA. The presence of the virus may be just one factor in the subsequent development of cancer. Several specific viruses have been implicated in the development of certain oncologic diseases. The human T-cell leukemia virus known as HTLV, is associated with hematologic and lymphatic cancers. The Epstein-Barr virus is associated with the development of Burkitt's lymphoma and tumors of the nasopharynx. Cytomegalovirus is associated with the development of carcinoma of the cervix and Kaposi's sarcoma.

Immunologic Defects

The body's immunologic system serves as a surveillance mechanism to assist in the recognition and destruction of foreign agents. The immunologic etiology of cancer purports that this system may play an essential role in regulating the presence of neoplastic cells. When the system fails, tumors are somehow allowed to grow and spread. Individuals with immunologic disorders have a higher risk of developing certain kinds of malignant disorders. This fact is evident in the high incidence of cancer seen in individuals with acquired immunodeficiency syndrome (AIDS). Individuals who have received immunosuppressive therapy for neoplastic and nonneoplastic disorders also have an increased incidence of neoplastic diseases.

Psychosocial Factors

Research demonstrates a strong relationship between psychological stress and the onset of illness as well as its outcome. This seems particularly true following major loss and depression. It is impossible, however, to determine whether or not a direct cause-effect relationship exists, because of inadequate research tools to measure data of a psychosocial nature.

A group of leukemia and lymphoma patients were studied by Green (1966), who noted a strong relationship between loss of significant persons and the subsequent onset of cancer. Not merely major loss, but poor adjustment to loss was reported, resulting in ongoing feelings of helplessness, powerlessness, and depression. LeShan (1966) came to similar conclusions about loss and cancer using interviews and questionnaires in several studies over a 21-year period with approximately 1000 cancer patients and a cancer-free control group. Another group was studied for 20 years by Engel (1967), who also found that the onset of various illnesses coincided with strong feelings of hopelessness following significant losses. Seeman and Seeman (1983) studied 1000 subjects over a 1-year period and determined that a sense of having personal control in their lives was a crucial factor in maintaining their health status. Those who are engaged in counseling cancer patients also report recurrent, almost universal themes of helplessness and powerlessness with lowered self-esteem. These emotions are a predominant effect if not a contributing causative agent of cancer.

Certain personal attributes have been described as making one "cancer-prone." LeShan found in one study (Haber et al, 1987, p. 871) that 95% of the patients with cancer, compared with only 10% without cancer in the control group, exhibited a characteristic profile. This profile describes a person with low self-esteem who sees himself or herself as a victim and harbors resentments that, along with anger and aggression, cannot be expressed. This personality type lacks resiliency, values conformity, and has a narrow range of personal relationships and interests. The person also appears to be dominated by feelings of loss and helplessness. These characteristics existed prior to the onset of cancer. Once cancer is diagnosed, these individuals have a poorer prognosis, with more rapid progression of the disease. Dysfunctional profiles of their families of origin have also been described.

Conversely, a very different personality profile has been associated with above-average remission rates in cancer (Haber et al, 1987, p. 872). These individuals demonstrate a sound sense of self-esteem. They are described as being creative, intelligent, successful, confident, vital, open, and flexible people. They are the "fighters" who seek, expect, and demand the best possible treatments. They have an internal locus of control, that is, they believe that they can directly affect and control the outcome of their situation and do not feel at the mercy of external controls.

A major danger in emphasizing cancer-prone personality profiles is that patients, especially those prone to self-blame, may feel that their attitude is primarily to blame for the onset, the recurrence, or the poor course and prognosis of their cancer. The self-guilt this generates increases depression, which in turn negatively affects prognosis, resulting in a cycle of self-fulfilling prophecy. Persons with significant external locus of control can become more internally controlled. However, this requires significant supportive, long-term counseling to help raise consciousness and self-confidence. Observation of newborns indicates that some persons are constitutionally programmed to be more passive. It is unrealistic and unfair to teach such persons that the de-

Table 11–1. RISK FACTORS AND SYMPTOMS OF COMMON CANCERS

SITE	RISK FACTORS	SYMPTOMS
Lung	Cigarette smoking Exposure to airborne carcinogens Family history	Persistent cough Hemoptysis Recurrent lung infections
Colon	Family or personal history of colon cancer; polyps Inflammatory bowel disease	Bleeding from rectum Blood in stool Change in bowel habits
Breast	Older than age 50	Breast changes: lump, thickening, swelling, dimpling, nipple retraction, nipple discharge, pain, tenderness
Skin	Excessive sun exposure Fair complexion Exposure to carcinogens –coal tar –arsenic	Change in size or color of mole; darkly pigmented lesion; ulcerated lesions, lesion that bleeds easily
Cervix	Early sexual activity Multiple sexual partners Genital herpes History of diethylstilbestrol use by mother	"Contact bleeding"—painless bleeding following intercourse or douching
Prostate	Older than age 50	Hard, nodular, fixed prostate Difficulty initiating urination Weak stream with dribbling Urinary frequency and urgency Nocturia Urinary retention

velopment of a "fighting spirit" is essential to conquer their cancer. In spite of the validity of that "fighting" personality profile, one must use this approach with caution with some patients.

Clinical Manifestations of Cancer

The clinical manifestations of cancer are numerous. Each variant of the disease has its unique symptoms and sequence. Symptoms range from vague complaints of unexplained fatigue, weight loss, and elevated body temperature to severe symptoms of pain, inability to function, and life-threatening medical emergencies.

The signs and symptoms of the more commonly occurring cancers are outlined in Table 11–1.

Application of the Nursing Process to Cancer Prevention and Detection

Assessment

Cancer screening serves to detect cancer at an early stage and assists in identifying high-risk individuals.

When screening a patient for cancer, assess general health status. Be certain to determine whether any of the seven warning signs of cancer are present. These warning signs are

C–Change in bowel or bladder habits
A–A sore that does not heal
U–Unusual bleeding or discharge
T–Thickening or lump in breast or elsewhere
I–Indigestion or difficulty swallowing
O–Obvious change in wart or mole
N–Nagging cough or hoarseness

Assess the patient's knowledge of cancer. Specifically determine understanding of risk factors, self-examination techniques, recommended schedule of screening procedures by health professionals, and symptoms to be reported. Explore the patient's current health practices to determine where change is indicated if risk of cancer is to be reduced.

Nursing Diagnoses and Planning

The nursing diagnosis and related expected patient outcomes most commonly applicable to patients undergoing screening for cancer are as follows:

NDx: High risk for altered health maintenance related to insufficient knowledge of risk factors for cancer, signs and symptoms of cancer, self-detection methods, recommended schedule of screening examinations, or risk-reducing behaviors

Planning: Patient outcomes

1. Patient identifies general factors that have been found to be associated with an increased risk of cancer.

2. Patient identifies factors in family history or lifestyle that predispose to development of cancer.
3. Patient identifies measures that can decrease the risk of cancer.
4. Patient describes the seven warning signs of cancer.
5. Patient performs correctly appropriate self-examinations for detection of cancer.
6. Patient states action to be taken if a warning sign is discovered.
7. Patient states how often screening examinations for particular types of cancer should be done given age, family history, existence of predisposing factors, and so on.

Nursing Interventions

NDx: High risk for altered health maintenance

Review with the patient the common types of cancers and their respective risk factors, signs, and symptoms (see Table 11–1). Discuss health practices that may reduce the risk of cancer (Table 11–2), and teach self-examination techniques such as breast self-examination, skin inspection, or testicular examination. (The details of these examinations are reviewed in related chapters of this textbook.) Explore with the patient how new health behaviors can best be incorporated into his or her lifestyle, and be certain to allow ample time for patient questions and concerns.

Table 11–2. HEALTH PRACTICES THAT MAY REDUCE THE RISK OF CANCER

Eat a diet that includes:
- Vegetables and food high in vitamins A and C
- High fiber foods: whole grain cereal, fruits, and vegetables

Limit:
- Consumption of salt-cured, smoked, and nitrite-cured foods
- Fat intake
- Alcohol consumption

Avoid:
- Smoking
- Obesity
- Sunlight

Have regular physical examinations

Participate in screening for common types of cancer:
- Baseline mammography between ages 35 and 40, every 1 to 2 years between ages 40 and 49, annually after age 50
- Monthly breast self-examination after age 20
- Annual professional breast examination after age 40, every third year between ages 20 and 40
- Annual rectal examination for prostatic cancer
- Monthly testicular self-examination
- Annual digital rectal examination after age 40
- Annual test for occult blood in the stool after age 50
- Skin inspection
- Papanicolaou smear after two negative examination results 1 year apart, every third year between ages 20 (or when sexually active, whichever comes first) and 65
- Pelvic examination every third year between ages 20 and 40, annually after age 40

Evaluation

Evaluate the effectiveness of nursing care for a patient undergoing cancer screening by comparing the patient's status with the expected patient outcomes. Examples of specific outcomes for patients undergoing cancer screening have been provided in the Planning section.

Medical Diagnosis of Cancer

Medical diagnosis requires obtaining a complete patient history and physical examination. Based on patient symptoms, results of the examination, and the type of cancer that is suspected, appropriate diagnostic procedures are scheduled. The only definitive way to diagnose cancer is to obtain a specimen of the suspect tissue through biopsy for pathologic study.

Tumors are further classified based on their histiologic characteristics. The pathologist grades the tissue specimen based on the similarity of tumor cells to normal cells of that tissue as follows:

Grade 1–Well-differentiated (i.e., looks like normal cells)
Grade 2–Moderately well differentiated
Grade 3–Poorly differentiated
Grade 4–Anaplastic

Higher grade tumors (more immature cells) are considered more malignant and possess a higher likelihood of growth and spread.

Staging of Cancer

Staging of cancer is a method of identifying the extent of the disease. The TNM staging system is an internationally accepted method for tumor staging. Each anatomic site (e.g., breast, lung, colon) is classified based on three components: tumor size (T), characteristics of regional lymph nodes and the presence or absence of malignant cells in the lymph nodes (N), and presence or absence of metastatic disease (M).

Diagnostic Procedures

BLOOD TESTS

Blood tests are scheduled to detect abnormalities. A complete blood count (CBC) is done to review the status of the patient's white blood cells, red blood cells, and platelets. Serum chemicals are monitored to assess the patient's metabolic functions. Serum chemical levels can be elevated as part of the oncologic process of organ destruction in metastatic cancer. For example, serum alkaline phosphatase, which is produced in the liver and bone, might be elevated if cancer cells are present and destroying cells of the liver or bone. Other serum chemicals that are monitored to assess for organ destruction include calcium, serum glutamic-oxaloacetic transaminase (SGOT), and serum glutamate pyruvate transaminase (SGPT).

Highly specialized blood tests are done by radioimmunoassays to detect tumor markers. Tumor markers are proteins and hormones that are produced by certain tumors. These proteins and hormones are usually produced only during fetal development and are called oncofetal proteins and ectopic hormones, respectively. The highly immature nature of the cancer cells makes them capable of producing oncofetal proteins and ectopic hormones, which can be measured in the blood. As tumors increase in size, these tumor marker levels increase. As tumor size declines, the levels decrease. An example of an oncofetal protein is carcinoembryonic antigen (CEA), which is produced by several tumors of the gastrointestinal tract. It has also been reported in lung, breast, and ovarian tumors. An example of an ectopic hormone is human chorionic gonadotropin (hCG), which is produced by tumors of the testicle, ovary, and pancreas.

STOOL TESTS

The patient's stool is tested for occult blood. This is an important test for the early detection of colorectal cancer.

Prior to this test, the patient is instructed to refrain from eating red meat for at least 24 hours before a specimen is obtained. This helps reduce false-positive results. If stool specimen cards are given to the patient for feces sampling over a period of a few days, the patient is instructed to use a disposable glove and place a small smear of the fecal material onto the card. The card is then returned to the doctor for testing.

CYTOLOGIC TESTS

Cytology is the study of the structure and function of cells. Specimens of body fluid may be obtained to detect the presence of cancerous cells. Sputum, cervical scrapings, or fluid aspirated from a tumor are examples of tissue fluid that are examined for the presence of cancerous cells.

Sputum cytology is used in the detection of lung cancer. An early morning specimen is usually submitted.

For this test, the patient is instructed to rinse the mouth with saline to reduce the amount of oral bacteria and food particles in the specimen. The patient then takes several deep breaths and expectorates the sputum into a sterile receptacle. If needed, production of sputum can be assisted by use of a nebulizer to inhale a saline solution. Endotracheal suction can also be utilized to obtain a sputum specimen.

A Papanicolaou (Pap) test is performed by obtaining a scraping sample of cells from the cervix, endometrium, and vagina. The cells are obtained using a swab or the like during an internal examination, and the scraping is transferred to a glass slide. The cells are reviewed by a pathologist and classified based on the presence or absence of abnormal cells. One classification system is as follows:

Class 1–Absence of abnormal cells
Class 2–Suggestive, but inconclusive for malignant cells
Class 3–Presence of malignant cells

The American Cancer Society recommends a Pap test every 3 years for women between the ages of 20 and 65 who have had two negative tests a year apart and are not in a high-risk group. The American College of Obstetricians and Gynecologists recommends that the test be done yearly. For further discussion of this procedure, see Chapter 43.

Fluid from a suspicious tumor mass may be obtained through an aspiration needle. The fluid from a breast cyst, lymph node, or palpable organ can be examined for the presence of abnormal cells, as can cerebrospinal fluid and washings of cells from the bronchus, esophagus, and stomach.

Patient preparation depends on how and where the fluid specimen will be obtained. The aspiration of fluid from a breast cyst can be performed in an out-patient setting, whereas a cavital washing such as in the case of obtaining bronchial fluid requires that the patient undergo a bronchoscopy and be sedated (see Chapter 12).

RADIOGRAPHIC AND IMAGING TESTS

CHEST X-RAY FILMS

X-rays are a form of electromagnetic radiation that have the ability to pass through the body and define internal structures. An x-ray film of the chest is obtained to survey the status of the lungs, mediastinum, heart, and thorax by providing a picture of these structures. The x-ray film may reveal the location and size of a primary or metastatic chest tumor.

BODY X-RAY FILMS

Radiographic pictures can be obtained to survey the bones and internal organs. These include contrast x-ray films of the upper gastrointestinal tract (UGI) and small bowel studies. Barium is swallowed for the UGI and given via enema for the small bowel x-ray examination (see Chapter 21).

MAMMOGRAPHY

Mammography is an x-ray examination of the breasts used to detect abnormal breast tissue (see Chapter 48).

TOMOGRAPHY

Tomography uses higher radiation doses than plain x-ray films to visual body structures in linear planes. In this way, sections of the body can be seen without other organs obstructing the field.

ULTRASONOGRAPHY

Ultrasonography uses high frequency sound waves that are directed into the body over a specific organ or body part. The sound echoes that are created reveal external features of the organ. Tumor masses can be localized and measured using this non–radiation-producing imaging method. Ultrasonographic pictures are also used to guide the surgeon during a biopsy.

For ultrasonography of the abdomen and pelvis, the patient is required not to urinate for 1 hour before the examination. The patient is also instructed to drink three to four full glasses of water before the examination. This preparation causes the bladder to fill and assists in pushing the bowel out of the way of the ultrasound waves. In addition, the urine in the bladder improves the transmission of the ultrasound waves. Before the examination, the patient is instructed to remove clothing and is given a hospital gown. The patient is positioned on a table either face up or face down, depending on the type of examination. An oil or gel is applied over the area that is surveyed. This lubrication prevents air from getting between the sound source and the skin. A transducer that resembles a microphone is passed over the area in different directions. The physician or technician is able to view the results of the sound waves on a monitor, and photographs are taken of the images through a camera attached to the ultrasound equipment.

RADIONUCLIDE SCANNING

A radionuclide is a small amount of radioactive material that can be given intravenously, carried through the blood stream, and traced in the body using a scanning machine. Areas of increased blood supply such as tumors can be detected. Scanning is used to evaluate structures in the brain, bones, liver, gallbladder, lungs, spleen, heart, kidney, pancreas, and thyroid. Scanning is begun when the radionuclide is distributed, which can take minutes or hours, depending on the material used and the area to be scanned. For example, a liver scan begins approximately 30 minutes after the injection, whereas a bone scan begins 2 to 3 hours after the injection. The patient is positioned on a table and asked to lie still during the procedure. The patient may also be asked to change positions during the procedure. Scanning times may vary from 15 minutes to 1 hour, based on the organ being surveyed; for example, a bone scan takes longer to perform than a liver scan. A scanning machine moves back and forth over the area to be surveyed. The amount of radiation exposure for nuclide scanning is equal to that of one x-ray film.

COMPUTED TOMOGRAPHY (CT) SCANNING

This radiographic procedure produces a detailed, cross-sectional, three-dimensional image utilizing information analyzed by computer and reconstructed as a series of cross-sectional views. A ring encircling the body contains rotating x-ray tubes that survey the body at varying levels. Intravenous or oral contrast material is sometimes used to enhance the computer-produced images of certain organs.

The patient is instructed to drink only clear fluids for the meal preceding the scan. At the time of the scan, the patient, in a hospital gown, is positioned on the table lying face up. The patient is instructed to lie still and told that the table will slowly move through the x-ray scanner and that the sound of gears and motors in the x-ray ring may be heard. The procedure can take as long as 1 hour to complete.

MAGNETIC RESONANCE IMAGING

Magnetic resonance imaging utilizes magnetic fields and radio waves that are analyzed by a computer to produce two- and three-dimensional, cross-sectional images of the body. This imaging technique does not expose the patient to any radiation or contrast materials. The patient is placed on a nonmagnetic stretcher that slides into a narrow tunnel-like space in the large magnetic resonance machine. The procedure takes between 30 and 90 minutes to complete.

There are no food or fluid restrictions for the examination. The patient is given a gown and asked to remove clothing and metallic objects such as hair pins, glasses, jewelry, and nonpermanent dentures. Patients with cardiac pacemakers or other metallic implant devices cannot be scanned using this method. A patient history is taken, and the patient is checked with a metal detector before the procedure. The patient is informed that a variety of noises from the machine may be heard during the procedure.

ENDOSCOPY TESTS

Endoscopy is the use of fiberoptic instruments to visualize, and in some cases obtain biopsies from, inside the body. Through these instruments, physicians are able to examine the entire gastrointestinal tract, the mediastinum, the bronchial tubes, the bladder, and the abdominal cavity. The specific details of these tests and respective patient preparation and nursing care are detailed in other chapters of this textbook.

Guidelines for Application of the Nursing Process to the Care of the Patient Undergoing Diagnostic Testing for Cancer

Nursing care for patients who undergo radiographic and imaging diagnostic tests involves preparing the patient for the procedure, allaying anxiety, and providing the patient with information related to the test. Explain what the procedure entails, establish a supportive relationship with the patient, and provide time for patient questions. Since the tests may be ordered by a physician as part of a diagnostic workup for cancer, be sensitive to the extreme anxiety and apprehension that the patients and family may be experiencing. In addition, make certain that the patient knows who will give him or her the results of the tests and when they can be expected.

Application of the Nursing Process to the Care of the Patient Newly Diagnosed with Cancer

Assessment

Assess the patient and the family for any misunderstandings related to cause, prognosis, or treatment modes of cancer. This is important since popular myths, such as cancer is contagious and cancer of the breast can be caused by accidentally hitting the breast, are still prevalent. The patient and the family should have a realistic view of the prognosis. Cancer is no longer always and immediately fatal, as believed in the past; rather, some types of cancer respond well to treatment, and patients go on to live a long, full life. The patient and family should also understand that there are many different types of treatment such as surgery, radiation, chemotherapy, and immunotherapy used to treat cancer, and that which is selected for a particular patient depends on the type and stage of the disease.

Assess the patient's and family's emotional response to the diagnosis, with particular attention to the patient's readiness to follow through with treatment and make any decisions that are necessary. Also assess the patient's support systems and coping skills. Gather information about the availability of a person with whom the patient is able to openly share feelings and concerns and about resources available to help the patient carry out the plan of therapy. The latter includes determining factors such as the ability to pay not only for the treatment itself but for help in the home, if needed, and to obtain transportation and assistance to out-patient radiation or chemotherapy treatments and subsequent visits to the physician.

Nursing Diagnoses and Planning

Nursing diagnoses and related expected patient outcomes most commonly applicable to patients diagnosed with cancer include the following:

NDx: High risk for ineffective individual coping related to dealing with the diagnosis of cancer and making adjustments in lifestyle necessitated by diagnosis and plan of treatment

Planning: Patient outcomes
1. Patient openly discusses fears and anxiety.
2. Patient asks questions relevant to the diagnosis, prognosis, and treatment plan.
3. Patient identifies realistic problems.
4. Patient identifies sources of support and how to use them.

NDx: Knowledge deficit: cause, prognosis, and type of malignancy, and treatment methods

Planning: Patient outcomes
1. Patient describes available options, citing the major advantages and disadvantages of each.
2. Patient describes the agreed upon plan of treatment in terms of time frame, side effects, and expected effect on prognosis.

Nursing Interventions

NDx: High risk for ineffective individual coping

Based on assessment data, plan interventions to assist with effective coping. Refer the patient and family to community agencies, community resources, and other professionals if indicated. (See the list of National Resources for Cancer Patients at the end of this chapter.) Many patients benefit from self-help support groups in which groups of persons with cancer share their experiences, problems, and concerns.

NDx: Knowledge deficit: cause, prognosis, and type of malignancy, and treatment methods

Clarify and reinforce information given to the patient and the family by the physician about the disease and its treatment. Because the emotional stress associated with a diagnosis of cancer can interfere with teaching and learning, provide information in writing and allow opportunities for questions. Repeat information as often as necessary.

Evaluation

Evaluate the effectiveness of nursing care for a patient newly diagnosed with cancer by comparing the patient's status with the expected patient outcomes. Examples of specific outcomes for patients newly diagnosed with cancer have been provided in the Planning section.

Medical Management of Cancer

The complex nature of oncologic disorders dictates that there is no single treatment. The major treatment modalities of surgery, radiotherapy, and chemotherapy have been used alone and in combination for preventing, controlling, and eliminating cancerous tumors. Immunotherapy is a newer form of therapy currently being investigated. Treatment selection is based on several individual patient variables, which include the patient's age, type and classification of tumor, stage of disease, response to previous therapies, concomitant medical illnesses, and general health status.

Surgery

Surgery is the oldest and most frequently used treatment for cancer. Since a definitive diagnosis of cancer requires a biopsy specimen, patients may undergo surgical procedures early in the course of treatment. Surgery has many applications in the treatment of cancer. Surgical procedures are performed for cancer prevention, tissue biopsy, primary tumor removal, disease staging, tumor debulking, hormonal ablation, disease palliation, and reconstruction. (See appropriate chapters for nursing care of the surgical patient and related procedures.)

PREVENTIVE SURGERY

Preventive surgery involves the surgical removal of premalignant tumors. Many individuals are predisposed to developing certain tumors because of genetic, congenital, or other health reasons. An example is the high incidence of colon cancer in individuals with multiple colon polyps. For these persons, a prophylactic colectomy may be indicated. Males with cryptorchidism (undescended testicles) have a high incidence of cancer of the testicles. The incidence is decreased when surgery to descend the testicles is performed before the age of 6. Other surgical interventions for cancer prevention include the removal of premalignant skin tumors and benign colon polyps.

BIOPSY

If a suspicious mass is palpated or revealed by a diagnostic procedure, the definitive method for diagnosis is to obtain a biopsy of the mass for examination by a pathologist. Based on the clinical situation, different types of biopsy techniques may be used:

Needle biopsy–The insertion of a needle into a tumor to withdraw fluid or tissue
Incisional biopsy–Removal of a piece of the tumor
Excisional biopsy–Removal of the entire tumor

Closed biopsies are obtained via endoscopy. They are performed on deep lesions that are revealed on imaging tests. The surgeon may use the picture from a CT scan image to locate a lesion for biopsy.

TUMOR REMOVAL

Surgical removal of a malignant tumor may be the only treatment for some tumor types. Early-stage, localized tumors with low incidence of metastasis can be treated by removal of the primary tumor. Surgical removal generally includes removal of the tumor mass, part of the surrounding tissue, and the regional lymph nodes.

STAGING

Staging surgery reveals the extent of disease spread by sampling regional and distant lymph nodes and sampling and viewing other organs for tumor. An example of tumor staging is the removal of axillary lymph nodes during surgery for breast cancer.

TUMOR DEBULKING

In some cases, cancer surgery involves reducing or debulking the amount of tumor. When the entire tumor cannot be removed, or in cases of widespread metastases, the surgeon removes as much tumor as possible. The remaining tumor is then treated with other therapies such as radiation and chemotherapy.

HORMONAL ABLATION

Certain tumor types, such as cancer of the breast and prostate, respond to hormonal manipulation. Removal of hormone-producing organs, such as the ovaries, testicles, or adrenal glands, may be indicated for some patients.

SURGICAL PALLIATION

Surgery may be indicated in advanced cancer for pain relief or to alleviate organ obstruction. Palliative surgery can improve the quality of a patient's life by relieving the physical symptoms caused by tumors.

RECONSTRUCTION AND REHABILITATION

Surgical procedures in the area of reconstruction and rehabilitation have improved in the last decade. Major advances in the field of breast and head and neck reconstruction have made it an important component in cancer treatment. Surgical procedures can be used to return functional losses that may have resulted from prior radiation therapy or surgery.

Guidelines for Application of the Nursing Process to the Care of the Patient Undergoing Surgery for Cancer

Nursing care of the patient undergoing surgery for cancer does not essentially differ from that given to any surgical patient. However, certain problems and related nursing activities may have greater significance as a result of the nature of the diagnosis. For example, the psychological impact of cancer surgery is great. The patient and family may experience a wide range of emotions and reactions to the diagnosis of cancer and the need for surgery. In addition, many types of cancer surgery involve change or loss of body function, limitations of mobility, and change in physical appearance, which can be potentially devastating to the patient.

Radiation

Radiation therapy utilizes the effects of ionization to damage and kill cancer cells. The exact mechanism is unknown; however, it is believed that as radiation waves are absorbed by cells, energy within the cells increases. This energy results in the release of electrons from atomic orbits, causing the atom to become ionized, a process called ionization, which causes damage to cellular DNA and damage to the cell membrane.

Electromagnetic waves and particle waves are the two types of ionizing radiation. Electromagnetic waves are divided into two types: gamma radiation and roentgen radiation (x-rays). Because of the high energy and penetrating capability, gamma rays are used to treat malignant cells. Gamma rays can be produced from radioactive sources such as radium or cobalt or from mechanical sources utilizing electrostatic machines. X-rays are similar to gamma rays but have less energy and are generally produced artificially. X-rays are used in diagnostic procedures rather than the actual treatment of malignant cells.

Particle radiation uses high-energy beams of atomic particles such as neutrons, protons, and alpha and negative pi mesons to destabilize atoms and cause ionization. The principal difference between each type of particle is the size and charge. Negatively charged particles, such as beta, have higher tissue-penetrating power.

Radioactive energy is released during the decay process of radioactive substances that are also known as radioactive isotopes. The length of time that these isotopes emit radiation is called their active life. The half-life is a measurement of the time it takes for the isotope to lose 50% of its radioactive activity. This time can vary from milliseconds to several days to thousands of years depending on the element.

The amount of radiation that is delivered to tissues is measured as the *r*adiation *a*bsorbed *d*ose, known as the rad. The amount of ionizing radiation that has the same biologic effect as one rad is called the *r*oentgen *e*quivalent *m*an dose, known as the rem measurement.

Radiation damages rapidly growing cells so that they are unable to reproduce. A cell is most sensitive to the effects of radiation during the G_2 and mitosis phases of the cell cycle. Some cells lose their ability to reproduce immediately, whereas others may be able to reproduce for only a short time after their initial radiation exposure. In a third group of cells, radiation may cause minor changes within the cell, but not enough to destroy the reproductive process. Since both malignant and normal cells can be damaged during radiation therapy, the goal of radiation therapy is to deliver a lethal dose of radiation to the malignant cells while minimizing the amount of radiation to which normal cells are subjected. There is a direct relationship between the presence of molecular oxygen within tissues and the success of radiation on cancer cells. Hypoxic and anoxic cells are more resistant to ionizing radiation. Pharmacologic agents, including chemotherapy, are being studied for their possible value in increasing cellular oxygen levels and are called radiosensitizers. In addition, agents called radioprotectors that may protect normal tissue from the effects of radiation are being studied.

Radiosensitivity is a measure of susceptibility to radiation-induced damage and cell death. Some tumors are known to be more radiosensitive than others and may be categorized based on the kind of organ tissue that is producing the tumor. Tumors of germinal, epithelial, and skin origin are the most radiosensitive. Radioresistant malignant cells are less sensitive to the effects of ionizing radiation and require extremely high doses of radiation to be destroyed. The amount of radiation required for destruction of radioresistant tumors results in irreversible damage to the normal tissue surrounding the tumor.

THERAPEUTIC USES OF RADIATION

Radiation therapy performs many roles in the treatment of early stage and advanced cancer and is often used as a component of a treatment plan that may include surgery and chemotherapy.

Radiation therapy can result in the total eradication of many tumor types, and in these cases the goal of treatment is cure. Radiation may be used to shrink a tumor that is too large to be surgically removed, allowing for surgical removal of the tumor after the radiation is completed. For certain tumors, such as breast cancer, radiation may be administered to regional lymph nodes after the primary tumor has been surgically excised or chemotherapeutically eradicated. Depending on the type and extent of the tumor, radiation is often prescribed along with surgery and chemotherapy. Radiation is used for palliative treatment in advanced cancer to provide relief from tumor symptoms such as pain or organ obstruction, to prevent further complications from the tumor, and to treat many oncologic emergencies such as superior vena cava syndrome and spinal cord compression.

MODES OF RADIATION THERAPY

Radiation therapy given by external beam is called teletherapy; when given internally, it is called brachytherapy.

EXTERNAL RADIATION THERAPY

External beam equipment delivers radiation to a designated area of the body. Dosimetry is the method used to calculate the size of the area or port to be radiated and the amount of radiation necessary based on tumor type, size, and depth. The radiation port is demarcated using a special marking ink on the skin. The markings remain throughout the treatment course, and patients are told not to remove them. Occasionally small tattoos rather than ink markings are used to demarcate the area.

The radiation is delivered in divided dose increments over a period of several weeks, depending on the amount of radiation required and the size and depth of the tumor. This process of divided doses, called dose fractionation, allows time for normal cellular repair and increased tumor kill. For example, a patient may receive 300 rad per day for 5 days a week over a period of 5 weeks for a total radiation dose of 6000 rad. The radioactive energy that is generated is measured in units of electron volts (eV). Some machines deliver low energy levels that are measured in thousands of volts (kilo electron volts [keV]), also called orthovoltage, whereas other more widely used machines such as the cobalt-60 and the linear accelerator can deliver greater levels that are measured in millions of volts (MeV), called megavoltage. The cobalt-60 equipment can release as much as 3 MeV, as compared with the linear accelerator, which can release as much as 25 MeV. Megavoltage radiation has several advantages over the classic orthovoltage method: deeper tissue penetration; less radiation scattered to normal tissues; less radiation absorption by bone, resulting in more uniform dosage to the tumor; and decreased skin toxicity. External beam radiotherapy is usually performed in an out-patient setting unless the patient's medical condition requires hospitalization.

The patient receives external radiation in a special room that houses the radiation equipment. The patient is positioned on a table, and positioning usually takes longer than the actual radiation treatment. Immobilization devices may be used to ensure that there is no movement during the treatment. Protective shields may also be placed near the radiation site to protect other body parts from the radiation beams. The patient is alone in the room during the treatment; however, the radiation technologist views the patient through a window and can communicate with the patient.

INTERNAL RADIATION THERAPY

Brachytherapy is the technique of implanting sealed or unsealed radioactive material directly adjacent to or within the targeted tumor. Here the tumor is subjected to radioactive activity over a longer period of time as compared with external beam therapy. Sealed isotopes such as iridium (^{192}Ir) and cesium (^{137}Cs) are contained in tubes, needles, capsules, wires, or seeds. The sealed containers are then placed inside the body cavity. In the treatment of many gynecologic cancers, for example, the source is placed vaginally. In the treatment of pleural effusions, the radioactive material is injected into the pleural space. Interstitial placement of sealed radioactive material involves the direct placement of the material into the body tissues, such as the breast, tongue, floor of the mouth, and oropharynx.

Preloading refers to the process of placing the containers with the radioactive material already inside, whereas afterloading refers to the process of first placing the containers within the tissues and then inserting the radioactive material into the containers. Afterloading requires that the needles or tubes be placed into the treatment area and tunneled out of the skin (Fig. 11–6). The procedure is done under local or general anesthesia in the operating room. The radioactive substance is later inserted into the tubes in the patient's hospital room. The patient requires a private room during the procedure, and visitors and staff must limit the amount of time spent in the patient's room. Unsealed isotopes, such as phosphorus (^{32}P) used in the treat-

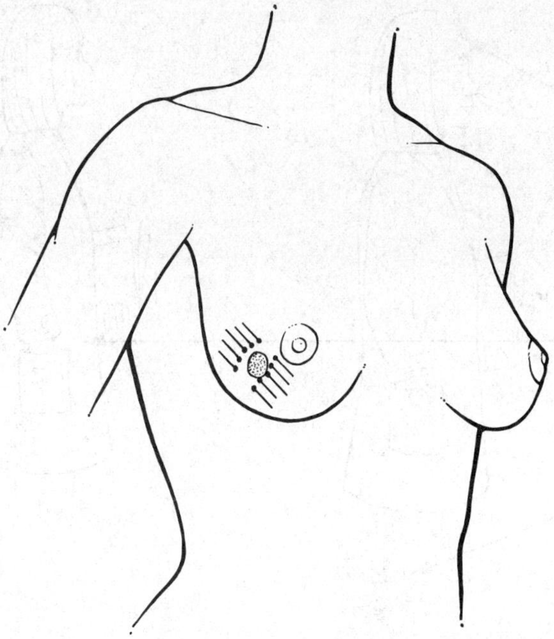

Figure 11–6.

Needles in place in the breast, through which iridium seeds in a plastic tube are passed.

ment of prostatic cancer and iodine (^{131}I) used in the treatment of thyroid cancer, are administered without a protective container. For unsealed isotopes, the risk of radiation contamination is high. Table 11–3 reviews the precautions taken for both sealed and unsealed isotopes.

Table 11–3. INTERNAL RADIATION THERAPY PRECAUTIONS

Wear dosimetry badge.
Keep telephone number of radiation safety officer available.
Place a sign on door of the patient's room warning, CAUTION, RADIOACTIVE MATERIAL.
Indicate on patient's chart that radioactive implant is in place.
Provide patient with private room and private bath.
Limit visitors: no children younger than 16 years of age, no pregnant women.
Instruct visitors to remain at a distance of 6 feet from the radiation source and to limit visit to no more than 30 minutes.
Place lead shield at bedside.
Pregnant nurses should not provide patient care.
For sealed sources, there is no special treatment of body fluids, excrement, or bed linen.
Lead containers and long-handled tongs are placed in patient room in case the sealed source becomes dislodged.

Additional precautions for unsealed radioactive sources:
Keep patient in bed.
Serve meals on disposable materials.
Place linen, bandages, trash, and laundry in labeled bags and keep in room until disposal.
Handle body fluid samples for testing with gloves, and label "radioactive."
Ensure that room is monitored by radiation safety officer during hospitalization, in case of accidental spill or dislodging of source, and after patient discharge.
Contact radiation safety officer as needed.

The radioactive implant may remain in place for several days. In some cases, if the amount of radioactivity is small and the half-life of the isotope is very short, the implant remains permanently.

SAFETY PRECAUTIONS

The Nuclear Regulatory Commission has developed guidelines for occupational exposure to radiation. Every hospital must have a radiation safety officer who is responsible for ensuring compliance with standards. Hospital personnel who care for patients receiving radiation are given special dosimetry badges to wear on their clothing. The badges contain film that measures radiation exposure and are collected monthly and tested for radiation absorption. A permanent record of radiation exposure is kept for all personnel. The results of the dosimetry readings are reviewed on a regular basis by the radiation safety officer. Federal regulations stipulate the maximum permissible annual exposure.

The patient who is receiving external beam radiation is not radioactive and poses no risk to the hospital staff. Radiation precautions must be followed, however, when caring for a patient with a radioactive implant. Radiation safety is based on three important factors: time, distance, and shielding.

Time spent in the patient's room is limited to a total of 30 minutes per 8 hours. The amount of radiation emitted decreases by the inverse square of the distance from the source. This means that working twice as far from the radiation source reduces the amount of radiation by one fourth (Fig. 11–7). It is important to maintain maximum physical distance from the patient whenever possible. Lead shielding provides some additional protection; however, lead shields and lead aprons have a significant disadvantage. They are cumbersome to use and work with and may actually induce a nurse to remain in the room for longer time periods. The nurse should consistently adhere to principles of time and distance while caring for the patient.

SIDE EFFECTS OF RADIATION THERAPY

During radiation therapy, cells of normal tissue are subjected to the ionizing beams. Any tissue near the radiation port can be damaged or destroyed. The side effects of treatment are related to the impact of radiation on normal tissue. Some side effects are acute and temporary, whereas other side effects develop over time and may be irreversible.

SKIN

External radiation must pass through the skin to reach the tumor target. The use of megavoltage therapy has decreased the amount and severity of skin reactions, because here the beams are targeted to become active at greater tissue depth. The most common skin effect is a change in skin color over

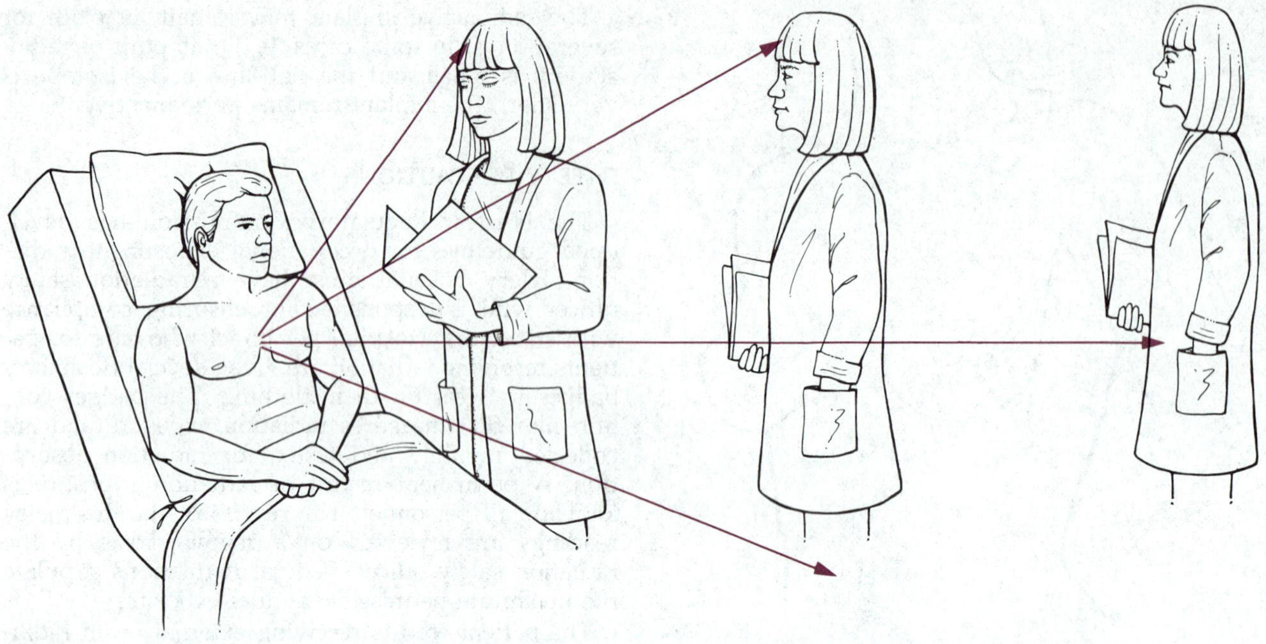

Figure 11–7.

Exposure to radioactivity is a function of distance: As distance from a radiation source increases, exposure decreases by the square of that distance. The nurse nearest the source (the patient) is exposed the most. The nurse at 2 feet receives more than 15 times the radiation that the nurse at 8 feet receives.

the radiation port. The skin may appear to be tanned or red. A tanning reaction is caused by the increased production of pigment. Reddening of skin color is called erythema, which is caused by dermal capillary engorgement. The erythema may cause varying degrees of itching sensations over the area. Dry desquamation, which is flaking of the skin, is caused by the accumulation of dead skin cells. In cases in which the basal cells of the skin are destroyed, the dermal level is exposed, which results in the leakage of serum, called moist desquamation.

Skin reactions are usually temporary. However, in cases of severe skin reaction, long-term effects can include scarring, changes in skin texture, and necrosis. Radiation recall is a delayed skin side effect in which the skin of the radiation port becomes irritated after the patient receives certain chemotherapy drugs. Depending on the severity of the recall reaction, vesicles and wet desquamation can develop.

ORAL CAVITY

Radiation can be given through external beam therapy or interstitial placement of radioactive isotopes to treat tumors of the head and neck region. As the radiation destroys the cancerous cells, healthy cells of the oral cavity are also destroyed. This alters and potentially injures the lining of the oral cavity, the teeth, and the salivary glands.

The rapidly growing cells of the mucous membrane provide a protective lining of cells in the oral cavity. Irritation of the membrane can cause an inflammation of the mucous membrane, known as mucositis or stomatitis. Varying degrees of stomatitis can result from injury to the oral mucosa. Severe stomatitis can cause oral pain and infection and can further complicate the nutritional and hydration status of the patient. Teeth can indirectly be affected by radiation as a result of periodontal membrane damage and the presence of more acidic saliva, which allows for an increased amount of oral bacteria. Injury to the salivary glands can cause a decreased production of saliva, resulting in a condition known as xerostomia or mouth dryness. Saliva is important for lubricating and cleansing the oral cavity, diluting food, and keeping an alkaline environment, which limits bacterial buildup. Salivary secretions may become thick and difficult to expectorate.

Hypogeusia is the term used to describe an alteration or loss of taste sensation, which is related to the effect of radiation on the patient's taste buds. Dysgeusia is the term used to describe the presence of unpleasant tastes sometimes described as metallic; aguesia is the absence of taste sensation. The oral toxicities of radiation therapy can potentially undermine the hydration and nutrition status of the patient.

HEAD

Radiation therapy to the brain can cause cerebral edema. To prevent this, patients are given steroids to combat the inflammatory process.

Patients may also experience nausea and vomiting resulting from the effects of radiation on the chemoreceptor trigger zone in the brain. Since hair follicles are destroyed by radiation, patients receiving radiation to the head experience hair loss called alopecia. Hair may be lost or hair growth totally arrested, depending on the amount of radiation received and the hair follicles' response to the radiation. Possible long-term and often delayed side effects include brain cell necrosis and infarction.

CHEST

Primary or metastatic lung tumors can be treated with radiation therapy. Side effects include esophagitis, pneumonitis, and as a delayed side effect pulmonary fibrosis. The epithelium of the lungs, trachea, and esophagus can be affected by radiation, resulting in inflammation, infection, and obstruction due to narrowing of these structures. Thus, the patient is at risk for negative effects on hydration and nutritional status and respiratory function.

ABDOMEN

Radiation can damage the rapidly growing cells of the gastrointestinal tract. When the upper abdomen receives radiation, the patient may experience nausea and vomiting. This is the result of the mechanical irritation and inflammation of the cells that make up the lining of the stomach. When the lower gastrointestinal tract receives radiation, the patient may experience diarrhea and abdominal cramping.

PELVIS

Cancers of the cervix, endometrium, prostate, bladder, and rectum are sometimes treated with radiation therapy by external beam and internal implants. Patients may experience side effects that include diarrhea; cystitis; vaginal, urethral, and rectal stenosis; and sexual dysfunction as a result of bowel, bladder, and gonad irritation.

SEXUAL FUNCTION

Radiation to the pelvis by external beam or internal implant technique can cause narrowing of the walls of the vagina, decreased secretion of vaginal lubrication, and inflammation and scarring of the vaginal tissue. Patients should be informed of these possible side effects and shown how to use a vaginal dilator or encouraged to continue sexual intercourse as a means to keep the vaginal walls open and flexible. Artificial lubrication can be provided through the use of commercially available creams and lubricants. Radiation to the pelvis and gonads can result in partial and permanent sterility in males. In females, ovarian function can be totally eradicated when high levels of radiation are given to the ovaries. Radiation to the pelvis may result in premature menopause and loss of libido. When possible, the reproductive organs are shielded from radiation. Patients should be informed of the possibility of temporary or permanent sterility, and males should be advised about the availability of sperm banks.

Sexual function may also be altered by fatigue and weakness, along with the multiple side effects of the disease and treatment.

HEMATOPOIETIC SYSTEM

Radiation can affect the production of blood cell components in the bone marrow. The bone marrow is composed of rapidly proliferating cells that include white cells, red cells, and platelets. Radiation to large areas of the body over bony structures such as the pelvis is most likely to produce bone marrow suppression. The patient's blood count should be monitored during the treatment course and through follow-up care. Depression of the red blood cells is called anemia. Depression of the white blood cells, called leukopenia, can compromise the immune system and result in the patient's inability to fight infections. Depression of the platelet count, called thrombocytopenia, can result in an increased susceptibility to bleeding.

Application of the Nursing Process to the Care of the Patient Receiving Radiation Therapy

Assessment

Assess the patient's understanding of the program of radiation therapy, its goals, and its potential side effects.

When external beam therapy is given, assess for changes in skin color, for the presence of dry or moist desquamation, and for pain or other discomfort at the radiation sites. For patients receiving radiation to the head and neck region, observe the mouth for signs of inflammation, infection, and ulceration. Also assess and note the patient's dental status. Determine the patient's ability to eat, take fluids, and swallow. Note the consistency of the saliva. Question the patient in regard to alterations in taste.

If the patient is receiving radiation to the chest or back, side effects often mimic the symptoms of the underlying disease. Observe for symptoms such as sore throat, dysphagia, and upper chest pain related to esophagitis, as well as for dyspnea, dry cough, hemoptysis, and elevation in body temperature. Also assess the patient's need for supplemental oxygen, cough suppressants, analgesics, and nutritional supplements.

Nursing Diagnoses and Planning

The nursing diagnosis and related expected patient outcomes most commonly applicable to patients receiving radiation therapy are as follows:

NDx: High risk for altered health maintenance related to insufficient knowledge of treatment, side effects, self-care measures, and required follow-up

Planning: Patient outcomes

1. Patient describes expected effects of radiation.
2. Patient states the symptoms of side effects most likely to occur given the type of radiation administered.
3. Patient describes the relationship of symptoms to the radiation therapy, noting that specific symptoms will disappear when the radiation therapy is completed.
4. Patient receiving external radiation describes or demonstrates appropriate interventions to control specific side effects.
5. Patient receiving external radiation accurately states symptoms that should be reported to the health care professional.
6. Patient having internal radiation states how the radioactive substance will be placed in the body, where the procedure will be done, and how long the radioactive substance will remain in the body.
7. Patient having internal radiation describes the need for a private room, and the influence of time, distance, and shielding on the effects of radiation.
8. Patient having internal radiation describes the precautions to be observed, given in Table 11–3.
9. Patient having internal radiation describes limitations on movement necessitated by the radiation.
10. Patient having internal radiation identifies self-care activities that are possible despite the limitation on movement, describing how they will be carried out.

In addition, the nursing diagnosis and related expected patient outcomes most commonly applicable to patients receiving internal radiation therapy are as follows:

NDx: Pain related to the presence of a radiation implant and temporary limitation of movement

Planning: Patient outcomes

1. Patient accepts analgesics.
2. Patient participates in relaxation exercises.
3. Patient reports lessened discomfort.

Nursing Interventions

NDx: High risk for altered health maintenance

For all patients having radiation therapy, reinforce explanations of the purpose of the radiation, the treatment procedure, and possible side effects. Instruct patients receiving external radiation therapy in self-care and comfort measures as specified in Chart 11–1. Explain the radiation precautions described in Table 11–3 to patients receiving internal radiation therapy and their families before the implant is done. After the implant is in place, be certain that the patient understands the limitations on movement necessitated by the implant, as well as what self-care activities are possible and expected.

NDx: Pain

Encourage frequent position changes, provide an alternating pressure mattress, and support body parts with pillows. Assist the patient with relaxation exercises, and provide diversionary activities such as reading, watching television, and listening to the radio. Administer analgesics and muscle relaxants as needed in accord with the physician's orders.

Evaluation

Evaluate the effectiveness of nursing care for a patient receiving radiation therapy by comparing the patient's status with the expected patient outcomes. Examples of specific outcomes for patients having radiation therapy have been provided in the Planning section.

Chemotherapy

The use of drugs to kill cancer cells has its origin in chemical warfare. After World War I, scientists noted bone marrow suppression in soldiers exposed to nitrogen mustard gas. This led to the hypothesis that the chemical was able to destroy rapidly growing cells. During the 1950s, several drugs of the same class were successfully used to shrink lymphatic tumors. By the 1980s, chemotherapy was considered the major intervention to treat and cure more than 12 kinds of tumors, including cancer of the testicle or ovary, Hodgkin's disease, leukemia, and several types of lymphoma. The federal government set up an organized system to evaluate new chemotherapeutic drugs under the direction of the National Institutes of Health at the National Cancer Institute. The National Cancer Institute is responsible for overseeing all clinical trials of cancer treatments, including chemotherapy.

Chemotherapeutic drugs are cytotoxic because they have the ability to disrupt the development and reproduction of cells. As with radiation, both normal and malignant cells are affected, and this is a major limiting factor in the use of chemotherapy. The multiple side effects of chemotherapy range from minor patient discomfort to life-threatening occurrences. This treatment modality has become quite complex as new drugs are developed and new combinations of drugs are formulated and tested. More

Chart 11–1.

NURSING GUIDE TO PATIENT EDUCATION FOR SELF-MANAGEMENT: SELF-CARE DURING EXTERNAL RADIATION THERAPY

Care of the Skin Affected by Radiation

Instruct the patient to:
Wear loosely fitting clothing.
Gently wash the affected area with a mild soap and pat dry.
Avoid the use of lotion, perfume, and deodorants.
Avoid pressure on the irritated area.
Avoid exposure to the sun.
Avoid swimming in saltwater or chlorinated water.
Avoid applications of heat or cold to irritated areas.
Use a water-soluble lubricant for dry desquamation.
Use either the open or partially open treatment for moist desquamation.
 Open treatment: Keep area clean, dry, uncovered, and exposed to the air.
 Partially open treatment: Keep area clean and covered with a nonadhering dressing. Change dressing *frequently* to keep wound surface clean and dry.
Use cool, moist compresses or water-soluble lubricants for itching.
Take antihistamines and use topical antipruretic lotions as ordered by the physician.

Care of the Mouth Affected by Radiation

Instruct the patient to:
Perform good oral hygiene after eating and at bedtime using a soft toothbrush, nonabrasive toothpaste, and dental floss.
Increase fluids to at least 2500 ml/day unless otherwise restricted.
Decrease smoking.
Do a daily self-examination of the mouth and report any changes.
Rinse the mouth frequently with mouthwash for xerostomia. Use a mouthwash that does not contain a drying agent such as alcohol.
Breathe through the nose to avoid the drying effect of mouth breathing.
Suck sour, hard candies to help stimulate saliva and create a pleasant taste.
Remove thick oral secretions with a swab, and use an oral gavage bag to irrigate the mouth.
Eat a liquid or blenderized, high-protein diet at room temperature if dysphagia or esophagitis is a problem.

Prevention of Infection

Instruct the patient to:
Wash hands properly.
Keep the fingernails clean and short.
Identify and immediately report any sign of infection, such as fever, severe fatigue, or purulent skin drainage.

than fifty different chemotherapy agents are used to treat cancer. One or several drugs may be prescribed, depending on the tumor type and stage, previous treatment course, and physical status of the patient.

Chemotherapy can be combined with radiation, surgery, or immunotherapy in the treatment of cancer. Chemotherapy is often used before surgery to shrink large tumors and inhibit the microscopic spread of tumor cells. Chemotherapy is used after the surgical removal of a tumor to similarly inhibit the microscopic spread of tumor cells. This method of chemotherapy, called adjuvant therapy, has been successfully used in the postsurgical treatment of breast, colon, lung, and bone tumors. The treatment goal of chemotherapy can be cure, control, or palliation of tumor. It can be given topically, orally, intravenously, intramuscularly, subcutaneously, intrathecally, intraarterially, intrapleurally, and intraperitoneally.

Chemotherapeutic agents are grouped by their activity during the cell cycle. Drugs that affect the cell during certain phases of the cell cycle are considered to be cell cycle–specific. Drugs that do not require the cell to be in a specific phase to be effective are called cell cycle–nonspecific.

CLASSIFICATION OF CHEMOTHERAPEUTIC AGENTS

Chemotherapeutic agents can be classified into six categories: alkylating agents, antimetabolites, antitumor antibiotics, steroids and hormones, alkaloids, and a miscellaneous group. Table 11–4 describes the common drugs in each classification.

Alkylating agents interfere with the structure, synthesis, and function of DNA, which results in cell death. They are active in all phases of the cell cycle and are considered cell cycle–nonspecific agents. An exception is the drug cyclophosphamide, whose cellular activity appears to take place in the S phase. A subclassification in this group includes the nitrosoureas such as carmustine (BCNU), lomustine (CCNU), and streptozocin. The action and cytotoxic effects of these drugs resemble those of the alkylating agents; however, they are also effective against cells in the resting phase and have the ability to cross the blood-brain barrier. This feature makes them valuable in the treatment of central nervous system tumors.

Antimetabolites interfere with normal biochemical processes that cells need to complete the synthesis of DNA and RNA. These agents are cell cycle–specific because their activity takes place during the S phase of the cell cycle. Antimetabolites are more effective against tumors with increased metabolic rates.

Antitumor antibiotics interfere with DNA and RNA synthesis. Their cytotoxic effect results in physical changes to the DNA strands, causing chromosome damage. They are active in all phases of the cell cycle and are considered cell cycle–nonspecific.

Hormones and steroids have a wide range of use in cancer treatment. Some tumors require the presence of hormones on their cell surface to grow and have specific areas on the cell membrane where they attach, known as hormone receptors. The antitumor action of hormones is dependent on the tumor type and the presence of hormonal receptors. Some breast tumors require estrogen for growth, and reducing the availability of estrogen through the administration of male hormones such as androgens or the administration of antiestrogens such as tamoxifen

Table 11–4. DRUG CLASSIFICATION OF CHEMOTHERAPEUTIC AGENTS

CLASSIFICATION	CHEMOTHERAPEUTIC AGENTS
Alkylating Agents	Cyclophosphamide Chlorambucil Melphalan Busulfan Thiotepa
Antimetabolites	Methotrexate 5-Fluorouracil 6-Thioguanine 6-Mercaptopurine Arabinosyl/cytosine
Antitumor Antibiotics	Doxorubicin Daunorubicin Dactinomycin Mitomycin

Steroids and Hormones	Androgens
	  Testosterone
	  Fluoxymesterone
	Estrogens
	  Diethylstilbestrol
	  Ethinyl estradiol
	Progestins
	  Hydroxyprogesterone
	  Medroxyprogesterone
	  Megestrol
	Antiestrogens
	  Tamoxifen
	Corticosteroids
	  Prednisone
	  Methylprednisone
	  Cortisone
	  Dexamethasone

Alkaloids	Vincristine Vinblastine Podophyllins Etoposide
Miscellaneous Agents	L-Asparaginase Streptozocin Hydroxyurea Cisplatin Procarbazine

can retard tumor growth. Prostatic cancer requires the presence of male hormones to grow and is treated by the administration of estrogen or the surgical removal of the testicles, or both, which halts the body's production of the male hormone testosterone. The complex actions of steroids result in an environment that retards tumor growth. Steroids such as prednisone are often used in combination with other chemotherapeutic agents. Steroids do not cause bone marrow suppression and in some cases can actually stimulate blood cell production.

Plant alkaloids are drugs that are derived from plants. They are cell cycle–specific agents, and are active during the mitosis phase of the cell cycle. They inhibit the formation of the spindle fibers, thus preventing the lining up of chromosomes during the mitosis phase. They also have some activity in the G_2 and S phases, during which they inhibit DNA

Table 11–5. STANDARD CHEMOTHERAPY COMBINATIONS

COMBINATION	TREATMENT APPLICATION
*C*yclophosphamide* *M*ethothrexate *F*luorouracil	Breast cancer
*M*ustard (nitrogen mustard) *O*ncovin (vincristine) *P*rednisone *P*rocarbazine	Hodgkin's disease
Doxorubicin Cisplatin	Ovarian cancer
Doxorubicin Bleomycin Vincristine Dactinomycin	Lymphoma

* Italicized letters signify how the particular drug combination is referred to in everyday usage (i.e., CMF regimen and MOPP regimen).

and protein synthesis. Vincristine and vinblastine, which are derived from the periwinkle plant, are two of the most commonly used alkaloids.

Miscellaneous chemotherapeutic agents are those whose action is not fully understood and whose cytotoxic activity does not fit into the other classifications.

COMBINATION CHEMOTHERAPY

Using more than one type of chemotherapy to treat malignant tumors is based on years of research and an increased understanding of the growth, repair, and reproduction of the cancer cell. By combining drugs of different classes, there is an increased chance of being effective at varying times in the cell's reproductive cycle. In many instances the dosage of one drug used alone would be too high; however, combinations of drugs allow for the administration of more drugs at lesser dosages. Drugs with varying side effects can be used together.

Chemotherapy combinations have been tested for their effectiveness on several tumors. New drug combinations continue to be tested. Table 11–5 pairs tumors with their respective standard chemotherapy combinations.

DOSAGE

The amount of chemotherapy that is prescribed for a patient is based on several factors, including the type of tumor to be treated; the patient's past chemotherapy and radiation therapy history; bone marrow, kidney, and liver function; age; physical status; and concomitant medical illnesses.

The dosage of most chemotherapeutic agents is determined by a measurement known as the total body surface area. A special measurement tool called a nomogram (Fig. 11–8) calculates the patient's body surface area per square meter (m^2) as a function of the patient's height and weight. For example, if the dosage of doxorubicin is 30 mg per square meter of body surface area and the patient's body surface area is 1.5 m^2 based on height and weight measurements, the dosage of the drug will be 45 mg (30 mg $\times$ 1.5 m^2 = 45).

TREATMENT SCHEDULES

Chemotherapy is given in time intervals that allow for drug effectiveness and recovery from side effects. For example, in a treatment cycle that consists of 28 days, the patient may receive chemotherapy for the first 14 days and no therapy for 14 days. At the end of 28 days, a new cycle begins. The length of time that treatment is prescribed is based on the tumor type, tumor response, and toxicities, along with other factors. Chemotherapy is usually prescribed by a medical oncologist, a physician who specializes in the diagnosis and treatment of oncologic disorders.

Continuous intravenous infusion of chemotherapy over several hours, days, or weeks is based on the premise that constant exposure of a tumor to small amounts of drugs is effective while less toxic to normal tissues. The use of continuous infusion chemotherapy in gastrointestinal and head and neck tumors is considered standard therapy. Continuous intraperitoneal and intracavital therapy is also being investigated.

CHEMOTHERAPY DELIVERY

The intravenous use of chemotherapy agents over continuous time intervals and the use of agents that are potentially irritating to veins and surrounding tissues, known as vesicant agents (see Skin Toxicity section), led to the development of alternative venous access devices. Venous access devices include the central venous catheter, the implantable venous port, and the Ommaya reservoir. Continuous chemotherapy infusion pumps can be portable or implanted under the skin.

CATHETERS

A central venous catheter is surgically placed near the right atrium, tunneled under the skin of the chest, and exits with an external catheter that is anchored to the skin (Fig. 11–9). The externally placed catheter can be used to obtain blood specimens; administer chemotherapy or other intravenous medications, blood, and blood products; and for total parenteral nutrition.

Catheters can also be placed intraarterially and intraperitoneally for the administration of chemotherapy. Intraarterial catheters are used when chemotherapy is to be delivered directly into an

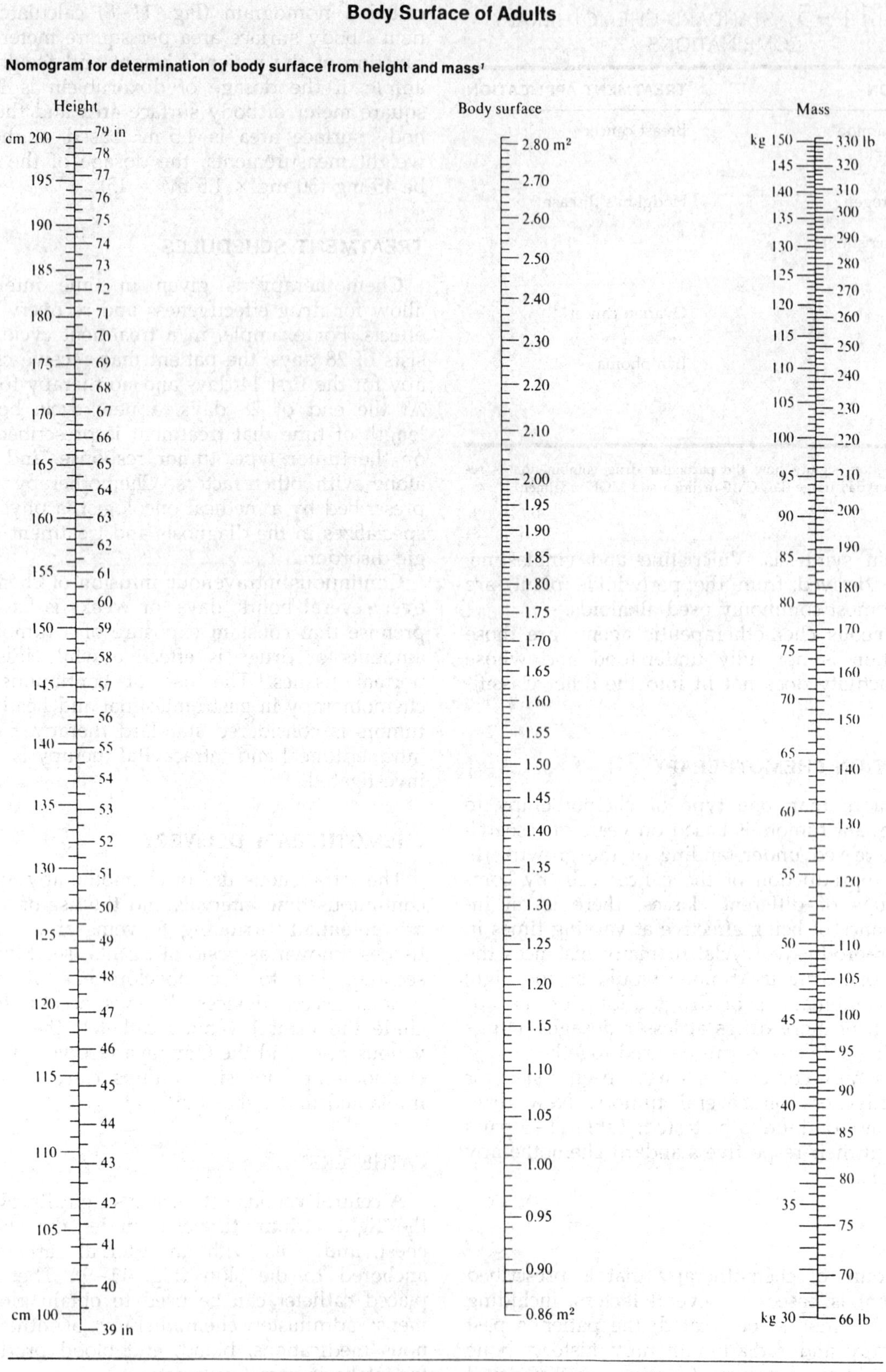

[1] From the formula of Du Bois and Du Bois, *Arch. intern. Med.*, 17, 863 (1916): $S = M^{0.425} \times H^{0.725} \times 71.84$, or $\log S = \log M \times 0.425 + \log H \times 0.725 + 1.8564$ (*S*: body surface in cm², *M*: mass in kg, *H*: height in cm).

Figure 11–8.

Nomogram. (From Lentner C [ed]. Geigy scientific tables. 8th ed, Vol 1. Basel, Switzerland: Ciba-Geigy, 1981, p 227.)

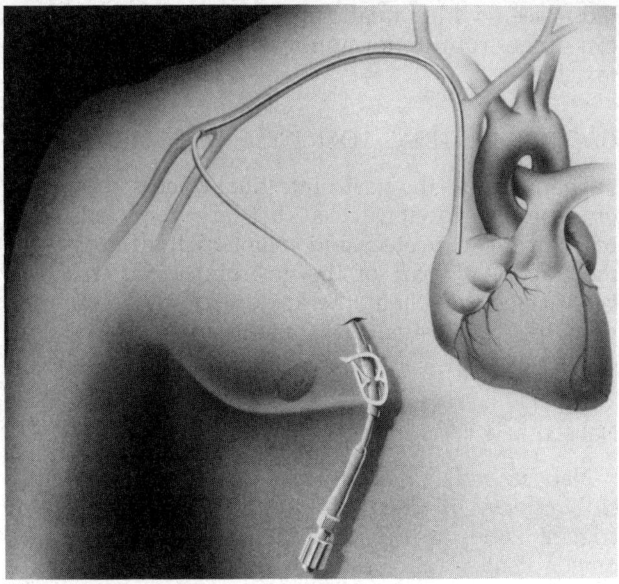

Figure 11–9.

Central venous catheter in place.

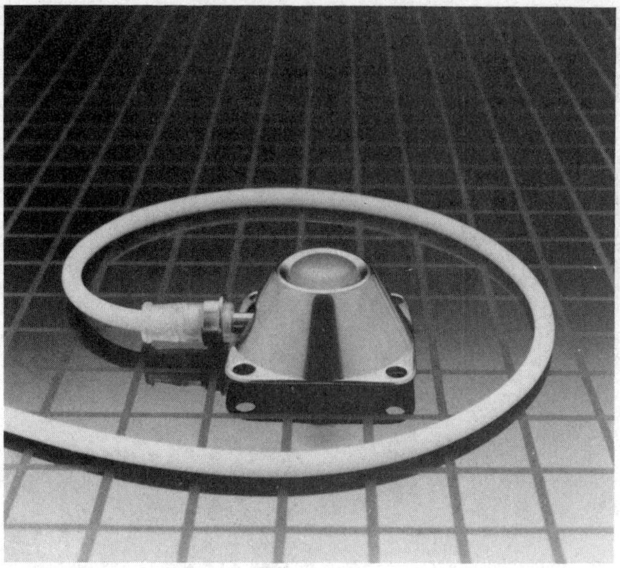

Figure 11–10.

Port-A-Cath Low Profile implantable access system. (Courtesy of Pharmacia Deltec Inc., St. Paul, MN.)

organ, such as the liver. Intraperitoneal catheters are used to bathe the peritoneum with chemotherapy. Chemotherapy can also be instilled into the lungs via an intrapleural catheter.

IMPLANTED VENOUS PORT

An implanted venous port (Fig. 11–10) is similar to the central venous catheter, with the exception that there is no external catheter. A steel septum with a plastic resealing port is implanted under the skin (Fig. 11–11). A special noncoring needle is used to access the port. Dressing changes and frequent flushing are not required. The port is flushed by the nurse after treatment or monthly. Patients can be taught to access the port for self-administration of medications and heparinization.

The Ommaya reservoir is a subcutaneous port that is implanted in the scalp and attached to a catheter that is threaded into the lateral ventricle for the administration of chemotherapy to the brain.

INFUSION PUMPS

Continuous intravenous administration of chemotherapy is given over time intervals that span several hours to several days or weeks. To provide continuous infusion therapy, specialized pumps have been developed. Some of the pumps are portable and can be attached to a waist belt. The patient can be fully ambulatory and active while receiving continuous chemotherapy. The pump (Fig. 11–12) is filled with the chemotherapeutic agent and attached to a central venous line. Some pumps are implanted under the skin and externally filled with the chemotherapeutic agent. The pumps are programmed to deliver small amounts of drug continuously over a given time period.

SAFE HANDLING OF CHEMOTHERAPEUTIC DRUGS

The cytotoxic nature of chemotherapeutic agents requires that personnel who prepare and administer

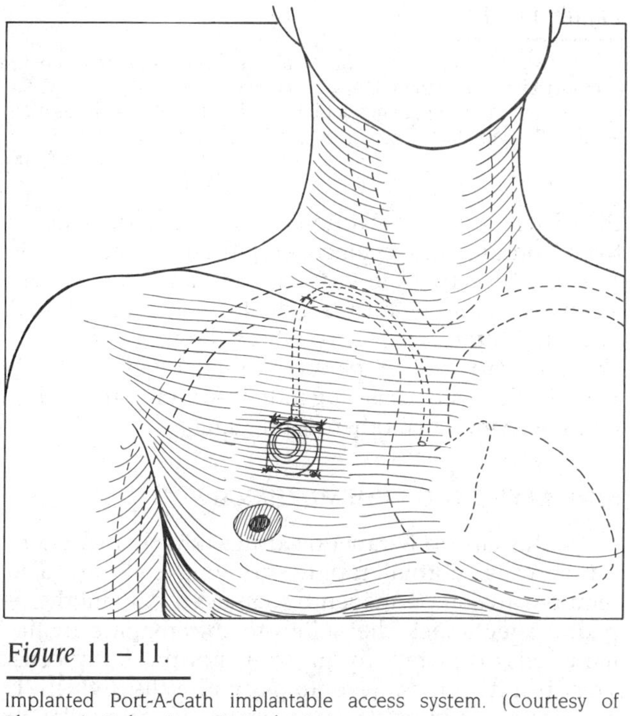

Figure 11–11.

Implanted Port-A-Cath implantable access system. (Courtesy of Pharmacia Deltec Inc., St. Paul, MN.)

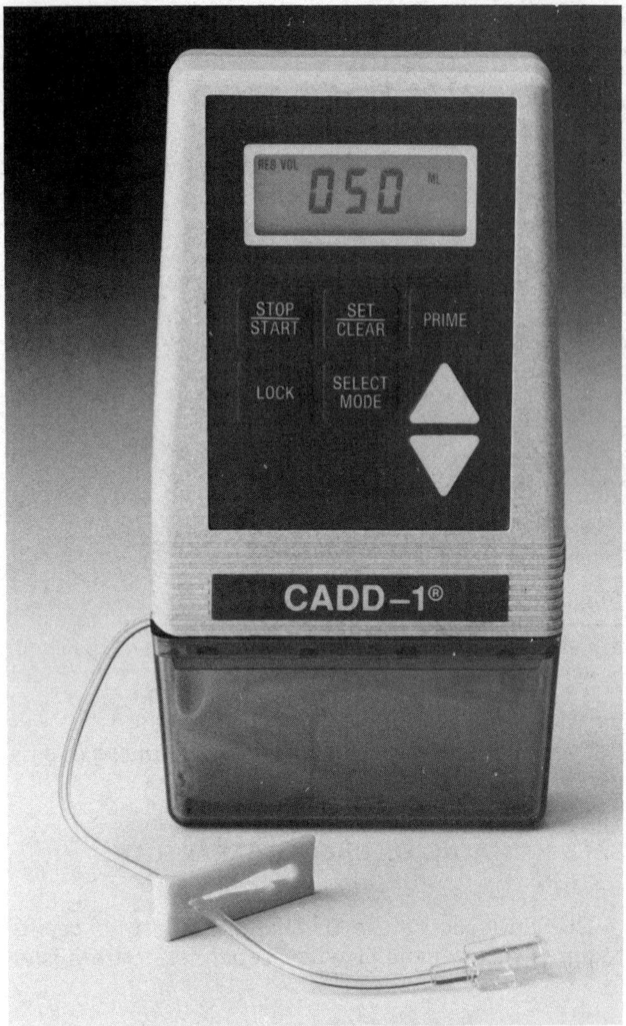

Figure 11–12.

Ambulatory infusion pump, which allows continuous intravenous administration of chemotherapy over several hours, days, or weeks without limiting the patient's mobility. (Courtesy of Pharmacia Deltec Inc., St. Paul, MN.)

the drugs take precautions to protect themselves from coming into contact with these agents (Table 11–6). Protective gloves, gowns, and masks are worn to guard against accidental skin contact and airborne fumes. In areas where large volumes of chemotherapy are prepared, a biologic vertical laminar air flow hood is suggested for preparing and administering chemotherapeutic agents.

SIDE EFFECTS OF CHEMOTHERAPY

As the chemotherapeutic drugs attack malignant tumor cells, normal rapidly growing cells are also temporarily or permanently damaged. Chemotherapeutic agents lack the ability to differentiate malignant cells from rapidly growing normal body cells. This results in damage to normal cells, which is manifested as side effects or drug effects similar to those seen with radiation therapy. The side effects can range from minor annoyances to life-threatening toxicities.

GASTROINTESTINAL TOXICITY

The lining of the gastrointestinal tract is composed of rapidly growing cells that are renewed as a mechanism to protect and maintain the integrity of the tract. Any part of the gastrointestinal tract can be affected by chemotherapy, resulting in nausea, vomiting, mucositis, taste alteratons, diarrhea, and constipation.

Nausea and Vomiting

Nausea and vomiting are the most common early side effects of chemotherapy. The chemoreceptor trigger zone of the medulla is located near the emetic center and is stimulated by the presence of chemicals in the blood. It is believed that this zone in turn stimulates the emetic center. Some drugs such as cisplatin and the nitrosoureas cause severe vomiting. Nausea and vomiting may also result from the actual irritation of the lining of the gastrointestinal tract.

Several antiemetic drugs are used to minimize nausea and vomiting with varying results. The antiemetic agents in the phenothiazine class, such as prochlorperazine, are used because they block stimulation of the chemoreceptor trigger zone and the emetic center. Phenothiazines offer only mild relief, and studies indicate that when the more emetic types of chemotherapy such as the alkylating

Table 11–6. PRECAUTIONS FOR HANDLING CHEMOTHERAPEUTIC AGENTS

Wear:
Disposable latex gloves
Mask to cover nose and mouth
Eye protectors, especially if biologic hood is not available

Use:
Biologic air flow hood if mixing chemotherapeutic agents on a regular basis
Soap and water for skin contact

Avoid:
Spills
Aerosolization when drawing up from a vial
Expelling excess drug from syringes into the air

Dispose of:
Needles and syringes in impervious containers
Chemotherapy bottles and tubing as per hospital policy
Body excretions and fluids as per hospital policy

Always:
Read package inserts
Be familiar with the drugs to be administered
Prepare drugs in a quiet area
Wash hands before and after preparation and administration
Review physician's written chemotherapy order
Double-check drug and drug dosage with another colleague before administering

agents and antimetabolites are used, effectiveness is minimal.

The antiemetic effects of tetrahydrocannabinol (THC), the active ingredient of marijuana, and nabilone, a synthetic form of THC, have been studied with varying results. Most reports suggest that they are more effective for younger patient populations and that the patient must experience a "high" feeling in order for the drug to work. It is hypothesized that THC may suppress the chemoreceptor trigger zone. Metoclopramide, a derivative of the procainamide class of drugs, has been shown to be an effective antiemetic agent. It blocks the chemoreceptor trigger zone, increases gastrointestinal motility, and causes gastric emptying. In high intravenous doses, metoclopramide is effective against nausea and vomiting; however, the extrapyramidal effects may result in patients' experiencing adverse side effects. Antihistamines can be given with the drug to eliminate these side effects. Antihistamines and steroids have some antiemetic action and are also used to enhance the effectiveness of other antiemetic agents. Anxiolytic drugs, such as lorazepam, have been used alone or in combination with other antiemetics for their amnesic and sedative effect.

The psychogenic aspects of nausea and vomiting and behavioral interventions continue to be studied. Many patients benefit from relaxation exercises; biofeedback tapes; hypnosis; diversionary activities such as music, reading, or television; desensitization; and mental imaging. Behavioral therapies provide the patients with something that they can do to actively participate in their care. Any of these techniques can be used in conjunction with administration of the pharmacologic antiemetics.

Mucositis

The cytotoxic action of chemotherapy can damage or destroy the cells of the lining of the oral cavity, resulting in varying degrees of mucositis. Mucositis in the oral cavity is also called stomatitis, and mucositis in the esophagus is called esophagitis.

Patients may develop painful oral and esophageal ulcers as the cells of the mucosa are damaged and cellular repair is decreased. Stomatitis and esophagitis can also occur if the patient is immunosuppressed from the disease or treatment or from malnutrition or dehydration. Mucositis can cause an alteration in the patient's nutritional and hydration status as a result of inhibiting consumption of food and fluids. It also predisposes the patient to development of an infection in the mouth or esophagus. The intensity and degree of inflammation varies, depending on the physical status of the patient and the type, dosage, and scheduling of the chemotherapy or radiotherapy prescribed. Severe stomatitis can cause oral pain and infection and can further complicate the patient's nutrition and hydration status.

Oral topical analgesics, antibiotics, and antifungal pharmacologic agents may be prescribed by the physician.

Xerostomia and Taste Alterations

The cytotoxic effects of chemotherapy on the salivary glands can cause decreased production of saliva, resulting in xerostomia, or mouth dryness. Injury to the taste buds can cause hypogeusia (decrease in taste sensation), dysgeusia (presence of unpleasant tastes sometimes described as metallic), or ageusia (absence of taste sensation). These side effects can further compromise the patient's nutrition and hydration status.

Diarrhea

Destruction of the intestinal lining by chemotherapy results in inflammation and inability of the intestine to produce digestive enzymes. Intestinal motility is stimulated, which results in diarrhea. Along with frequent loose bowel movements, patients can also experience abdominal cramping, flatulence, bloating, and irritation of the rectal mucosa. Diarrhea may also be related to the patient's anxieties and fears. The incidence of diarrhea related to chemotherapy is high, occurring with many of the antimetabolites and antitumor antibiotics. Potential alterations in nutrition and fluid and electrolyte balance result from inadequate digestion and a decrease in nutrient absorption. Pharmacologic agents, such as diphenoxylate with atropine (Lomotil), that slow intestinal peristalsis may be indicated along with nutritional interventions.

Constipation

Chemotherapy-related constipation is a side effect of the vinca alkaloid drugs. The neurotoxicity of vincristine and vinblastine can cause a decrease in intestinal peristalsis, resulting in constipation. Bowel status must be assessed before and during treatment to avoid constipation and possible paralytic ileus. Older patients are especially susceptible to constipation caused by the vinca alkaloids. Constipation may be further aggravated by a decrease in fluid intake and a decrease in physical activity. Severe constipation may require manual disimpaction.

SKIN TOXICITY

Skin side effects include hyperpigmentation, photosensitivity, erythematous skin rashes, radiation recall, alopecia, and chemical tissue infiltration.

Hyperpigmentation of the skin and nail beds is caused by an increased stimulation of the melanin cells in the basal level of the dermis. Skin darkening can be localized in small areas, such as over the veins, or more widespread over the face and trunk. Several agents cause photosensitivity, an acceleration of the tanning process caused by the sun's ultraviolet rays that results in marked hyperpigmentation, deeply tanned skin, and severe sunburn. Hyperpigmentation and photosensitivity are known side effects of fluorouracil, methrotrexate, and bleomycin.

Erythematous skin rashes are caused by a dilation of blood vessels in the skin. These transient rashes sometimes occur after the administration of chemotherapy near the injection site or over other areas of the body and may remain for several hours. The rashes are sometimes accompanied by urticaria, skin flaking, and skin dryness. A hypersensitive reaction to chemotherapy may first be evidenced as a skin rash and quickly progress to an allergic reaction requiring immediate medical intervention.

Radiation recall is a term used to describe the effect that chemotherapy may have on areas of the skin that have been previously or concomitantly exposed to radiation therapy. This can result in erythema, ulceration, wet desquamation, and permanent hyperpigmentation.

Alopecia, which is the term used to describe hair loss, can be an extremely devastating side effect because hair is a significant part of an individual's self-image. Chemotherapy causes alopecia by damaging the rapidly growing and renewing hair follicles. Hair is weakened at the shaft and easily removed from the scalp. The amount of hair loss is dependent on the drug dosage and treatment duration. Some chemotherapy agents do not cause alopecia. Hair loss can range from mild thinning on the scalp to total loss of all scalp hair.

Facial and body hair are less frequently affected by chemotherapy because the growth and renewal rate is slower; nevertheless, patients may experience a loss of facial and body hair. Alopecia may cause the scalp to become irritated and sensitive, with flaking of dry skin. Hair loss is almost always temporary, and complete regrowth can be expected after treatment is stopped. Regrowth time varies, and hair may have a changed color and texture. Hair regrowth is slower in the geriatric population.

Patient preparation must be emphasized as an important component of adaptation to alopecia. Wigs, hairpieces, and hats can be suggested. Scalp hypothermia refers to application of ice to the scalp to decrease blood circulation during chemotherapy administration. This technique has been studied as a means to minimize hair loss. Its use remains controversial on the basis that reducing chemotherapy distribution to the scalp could theoretically create a safe area for cancer cells. Scalp hypothermia is contraindicated in cancers that are known to spread to the brain and soft tissues of the scalp.

Tissue extravasation is defined as the localized tissue damage caused by the infiltration of chemotherapy into the tissues that surround the intravenous administration site. Chemotherapy drugs that produce tissue damage if they are given directly into the tissues or that leak out of veins are called vesicants. Vesicant and irritant chemotherapeutic agents are

Nitrogen mustard	Dactinomycin
Daunorubicin	Vincristine
Doxorubicin	Vinblastine
Mitomycin C	BCNU

Tissue extravasation can cause local pain, induration, erythema, and necrosis. The medical and nursing intervention for tissue extravasation remains controversial, and institutional protocols vary. Studies report the use of subcutaneously and intravenously administered antidotes at the infiltration site, to attempt to neutralize and inactivate the infiltrated drug or limit tissue absorption. The Oncology Nursing Society recommends the following general interventions for chemotherapy-induced tissue extravasation:

- Stop chemotherapy administration.
- Keep intravenous needle in place and try to aspirate residual chemotherapeutic agent from the intravenous tubing, the needle, and the infiltration site.
- Instill antidote as per hospital protocol and/or physician order.
- Antidotes include hydrocortisone, hyaluronidase, and sodium bicarbonate.
- Apply cold or warm compress to area, based on kind of agent and hospital policy.
- Elevate arm.
- Observe area at regular intervals.
- Arrange follow-up visit.

Document the following:

- Time and date
- Needle size and type
- Name of chemotherapy agent and approximate amount of drug volume infiltrated
- Drug administration technique and sequence of administration of multiple drugs
- Immediate interventions taken
- Photograph site, if possible
- Description of infiltration site
- Patient symptoms

Venous access devices are used for the administration of vesicants because they limit the occurrence of tissue infiltration.

HEMATOLOGIC TOXICITY

The action of chemotherapy can directly affect the blood-producing mechanism. Blood components (red blood cells, white blood cells, and platelets) are continually being made by the rapidly growing cells of the bone marrow. The cytotoxic action of chemotherapy inhibits this production. Since red blood cells, also called erythrocytes, carry oxygen to tissues and carbon dioxide away from tissues, a decrease in their number in circulation causes anemia. White blood cells, also called leukocytes, are an integral component of the immune system. A decrease in the production of leukocytes reduces the system's ability to recognize and defend against foreign microorganisms, leading to increased susceptibility to infection. Platelets are blood components that assist with clot formation and blood coagulation. A decrease in the number of platelets in circulation can cause an increased susceptibility to bleeding.

Peripheral blood counts are monitored regularly and are always evaluated before the beginning of a chemotherapy treatment cycle. Based on blood count values, therapy is sometimes modified or delayed. (See Table 11–7 for normal blood count ranges.) Hematologic toxicity from chemotherapy can result in life-threatening anemia, infection, and bleeding. Hematologic status can also be concomitantly compromised by invasion of the primary tumor into the bone marrow, other hematologic disorders, and malnutrition.

RENAL TOXICITY

Renal toxicity is a less common side effect. Impaired renal function has been documented with chemotherapy agents such as cisplatin, methotrexate, and mitomycin C. These drugs are known to be toxic to the renal tubule system and the glomeruli. Renal calculi can form as a result of rapid tumor destruction. Hemorrhagic cystitis caused by bladder irritation is associated with cyclophosphamide.

PULMONARY TOXICITY

Pulmonary toxicity related to chemotherapy is manifested as pulmonary fibrosis and inflammation and is associated with methotrexate and bleomycin. Bleomycin can cause pulmonary fibrosis, which appears to be related to cumulative doses over 400 units. The geriatric population may be at increased risk of pulmonary fibrosis related to changes in respiratory muscles and air capacity of the lungs.

NEUROTOXICITY

Sensory and perceptual alterations result from the effects of chemotherapy on nerve conduction fibers. Neurotoxicity is most often associated with the vinca alkaloid agents (vincristine, vinblastine) and is manifested by peripheral neuropathy. The symptoms are lack of body coordination; feeling of numbness and tingling in the hands and feet; loss of feeling sensation in extremities; loss of deep tendon reflexes; generalized motor weakness; and in severe cases, atonia of the bowel and bladder. Cisplatin can cause motor and sensory neuropathy, tinnitus, and hearing losses. Procarbazine causes peripheral neuropathy and altered levels of consciousness.

Table 11–7. NORMAL BLOOD VALUES

LABORATORY TEST	NORMAL VALUE	
Hematocrit	Male: 40–54% Female: 37–47%	
Hemoglobin	Male: 13.5–18.0 g/dl Female: 12.0–16.0 g/dl	
White blood cell count	4.5–11.0 × 10	
White blood cell differential count (calculated as a percentage of total white blood cell count)	Segmented neutrophils: Bands: Eosinophils: Basophils: Lymphocytes: Monocytes:	56% 3% 3% 0.3% 34% 4%
Platelet count	150,000–400,000	

CARDIOTOXICITY

Cardiotoxicity is a major dose-limiting factor for the antitumor antibiotics doxorubicin and daunorubicin. Cardiotoxicity has been documented after patients receive a total cumulative dose of these agents that ranges from 450 to 550 mg/m^2 of body surface area. Cardiotoxic effects include dysrhythmia and congestive heart failure.

Other risk factors for cardiotoxicity include increasing age, preexisting cardiac disease, and a history of radiation therapy to the mediastinum. Patients who receive the anthracycline antitumor antibiotics are closely monitored for signs and symptoms of congestive heart failure.

Application of the Nursing Process to the Care of the Patient Receiving Chemotherapy

Assessment

Assess the patient's understanding of the disease and the treatment, anxiety level, and coping skills. Also assess the patient's physical and nutritional status. Once therapy has begun, do a complete assessment to identify all side effects (Table 11–8).

Nursing Diagnoses and Planning

The nursing diagnosis and related expected patient outcomes most commonly applicable to patients receiving chemotherapy for cancer are as follows:

NDx: High risk for altered health maintenance related to insufficient knowledge of prescribed treatment, side effects, and their management

Text continued on page 390

Table 11–8. SIDE EFFECTS OF CHEMOTHERAPY WITH RELATED ASSESSMENTS, NURSING DIAGNOSES, EXPECTED PATIENT OUTCOMES, AND NURSING INTERVENTIONS

SIDE EFFECT	ASSESSMENT	NURSING DIAGNOSIS	EXPECTED PATIENT OUTCOMES	NURSING INTERVENTIONS
PULMONARY TOXICITY Patients with preexisting pulmonary disease or previous treatment with lung radiation therapy are at risk for pulmonary fibrosis and inflammation.	Obtain pretreatment pulmonary function studies. Obtain pretreatment chest x-ray film. Assess for: –Cough –Elevated body temperature –Tachycardia –Dyspnea on exertion –Weakness Auscultate lungs. Obtain vital signs. Ascertain activity status. Check blood gas values. Monitor cumulative dose of bleomycin.	High risk for ineffective breathing pattern related to inflammation and decreased lung expansion	Lung sounds are normal. Arterial blood gases are within the patient's normal range.	To alleviate pulmonary fibrosis and inflammation: Medicate with antibiotics, steroids, and bronchodilators as prescribed. Adjust patient to comfortable sitting position. Administer use of respiratory therapy machines as ordered. Administer and monitor effects of oxygen therapy if indicated. Refer patient to visiting nurse service for continued home follow-up. Provide support by explaining all procedures and interventions to patient.
CARDIOTOXICITY	Ascertain cardiac history. Check vital signs. Obtain and monitor pretreatment and at intervals: –Electrocardiogram –Echocardiogram –Cardiac scan Observe for signs of congestive heart failure: –Tachycardia –Moist cough –Shortness of breath –Dyspnea on exertion –Distended neck veins –Cardiomegaly –Hepatomegaly –Pedal edema –Orthopnea Ascertain whether patient has previously received radiation therapy. Assess patient's activity level.	High risk for decreased cardiac output related to toxic effects of chemotherapeutic agents on the heart	Signs and symptoms of congestive heart failure are absent.	Teach signs and symptoms of congestive heart failure, and encourage the patient to report all symptoms. Record cumulative doses of doxorubicin and daunorubicin. Monitor and report changes in interval physical assessments and interval cardiac test results to physician.
NEUROTOXICITY	Ascertain symptoms of peripheral neuropathy: –Paresthesias of hands and feet –Numbness and tingling sensations of extremities –Muscle pain –Loss of Achilles tendon reflex –Falls, loss of balance	High risk for injury related to paresthesias, loss of balance, or other symptoms of peripheral neuropathy	Patient remains free of injury.	Explain to the patient that: Symptoms may be related to chemotherapy Reporting of symptoms is important Instruct the patient to: Avoid use of heating pads to areas with reduced feeling.

	–Bone and joint pain –Changes in gait –Bowel and bladder habits Assess effects of neurotoxocity on physical activity.			Test bath water temperature to avoid scalding. Use gloves for washing dishes and gardening, and protect hands when cooking. Assist with and teach range-of-joint-motion exercises. Use foot board if indicated for foot drop. Use pillows to correct body alignment. Refer patient to visiting nurse service for follow-up care if indicated.
HEMATOLOGIC TOXICITY	Observe for signs and symptoms of infection. Be aware that patients with a low white blood cell count may not exhibit the normal signs of infection such as productive cough, elevated body temperature, redness of skin, edema, and pain due to the absence of neutrophils. Check the white blood cell count. Obtain vital signs. Inspect all body orifices and skin for infection. Ascertain patient complaints. Obtain blood; urine; skin; sputum; and vaginal, rectal, or other cultures as indicated. Obtain history of medication schedule. Assess fluid intake and output. Assess mental status.	High risk for infection related to chemotherapy-induced leukopenia	Patient is afebrile. Signs of specific localized infections are absent. Patient describes measures to reduce the risk of infection.	Implement measures to prevent infection: Restrict visitors. Protect the patient from people with known infections. Provide a private room. Instruct the patient, family, and visitors in hand washing technique. Encourage fluid if not contraindicated by other medical disorders. Suggest a low bacteria diet: –Avoid fresh fruits and vegetables. –All foods should be cooked. To maintain skin integrity: –Bathe daily with antiseptic soap, include nail care. –Change intravenous tubing every 24 hours. –Avoid injections. –Avoid skin breakdown. –Monitor exit sites of central venous catheters, intravenous lines or other venous access devices. Prevent respiratory infection: –Encourage: Ambulation Coughing and deep breathing Fluid intake –Avoid smoking Prevent urinary infections: –Avoid indwelling urinary catheters. –Encourage: Fluid intake Good hygienic measures after bowel movements Provide care for skin breakage.

(continued)

Table 11–8. *(continued)* SIDE EFFECTS OF CHEMOTHERAPY WITH RELATED ASSESSMENTS, NURSING DIAGNOSES, EXPECTED PATIENT OUTCOMES, AND NURSING INTERVENTIONS

SIDE EFFECT	ASSESSMENT	NURSING DIAGNOSIS	EXPECTED PATIENT OUTCOMES	NURSING INTERVENTIONS
HEMATOLOGIC TOXICITY *(continued)*				Avoid enemas and rectal suppositories. Avoid rectal temperatures. Administer antibiotics and antifungal agents as prescribed by physician. Teach the patient and family signs and symptoms of infection. Explain to the patient and family how to notify medical personnel if signs of infection appear.
	Inspect patients for signs and symptoms of bleeding –Inspect skin for petechiae, ecchymoses, and hematomas. –Observe neurologic status for changes associated with intracranial bleeding. –Inspect for bleeding into joints. –Measure abdominal girth. –Inspect and test all body secretions and fluid for blood. Check platelet count. Ascertain chemotherapy regimen. Ascertain whether the patient is currently taking steroids or products that contain aspirin. Ascertain whether the patient has experienced: –Hemoptysis –Hematuria –Epistaxis –Wound bleeding –Hematemesis –Melena –Menometrorrhagia Check: –Vital signs. Include blood pressure in reclining, sitting, and standing positions to assess for postural hypotension.	High risk for decreased cardiac output related to bleeding secondary to chemotherapy-induced thrombocytopenia	Signs and symptoms of bleeding are absent. Patient describes self-care measures to decrease the risk of bleeding.	Implement measures to prevent and control bleeding: Limit injections and venipunctures. Use small-gauge needles, and apply pressure after all skin punctures. Avoid: –Shaving with straight-edge razor. –Using toothbrush and dental floss. –Straining during bowel movements. –Taking any medication that contains aspirin. –Nasotracheal suctioning. –Vomiting. Eliminate objects in patient's environment that may cause bruising due to falls. Suggest: –Mouth care with sponges or gauze –Increased fluid intake and stool softeners, if indicated –Antiemetics, if indicated –For menstruating females: estrogen-progesterone agents can be given to stop menses, if indicated –Soft diet high in fiber and protein –Limited physical activity –If indicated, pad side rails, prevent falls –Use of humidifier if oxygen therapy is indicated to prevent mucosal drying

				For nosebleeding: –Place patient in a high Fowler's position. –Apply ice packs and pressure to bridge of nose. –Notify physician. Administer and monitor platelet transfusions. Administer antacids and ice water lavages for gastric bleeding if ordered.
	Check: –Hemoglobin, hematocrit Ask about symptoms of syncope, drowsiness, dyspnea, diaphoresis, and chest pain. Ask about feelings of fatigue. Ascertain ability to carry out usual activities. Review usual schedule and type of activities.	Fatigue related to chemotherapy-induced anemia	Patient identifies a plan for limiting activity and providing frequent rest periods. Patient reports that he or she is able to carry out basic activities of daily living.	Instruct patient to: –Report symptoms. –Limit physical activity. –Plan frequent rest periods. –Take soft diet high in protein, vitamins, and iron. Administer red blood cell transfusion as ordered by physician.
SEXUAL DYSFUNCTION	Explore questions and concerns related to sexual functioning. Determine current methods of birth control.	Sexual dysfunction related to physiologic and psychological effects of chemotherapy	Patient describes potential effects of chemotherapy on sexual function. Patient verbalizes concerns about sex role and desirability as a sexual partner. Patient identifies measures supportive of sexual function.	Inform females about: –Possible amenorrhea –Possible onset of early menopause with symptoms of "hot flashes," vaginal dryness, and dyspareunia –Use of birth control methods if premenopausal –Possible dyspareunia related to decreased lubrication of vaginal walls. Use water-soluble lubricant or steroid cream if indicated. –Possible decreased libido related to fatigue and hormonal changes Inform males about: –Possible temporary or permanent sterility –Possible impotence related to therapy, anxiety, and fatigue Suggest penile prosthesis implantation, if indicated. Suggest sperm banking before therapy begins, if indicated. Refer patients and partners to appropriate professionals, if indicated. Allow time for discussion of sexual dysfunction. Provide written information regarding contraception methods.

(continued)

Table 11–8. *(continued)* SIDE EFFECTS OF CHEMOTHERAPY WITH RELATED ASSESSMENTS, NURSING DIAGNOSES, EXPECTED PATIENT OUTCOMES, AND NURSING INTERVENTIONS

SIDE EFFECT	ASSESSMENT	NURSING DIAGNOSIS	EXPECTED PATIENT OUTCOMES	NURSING INTERVENTIONS
SKIN TOXICITY Photosensitivity	Inspect skin for erythema, blisters, and other lesions.	High risk for impaired skin integrity related to sunburn	Skin is intact. Skin is free of erythema and lesions.	Teach patient to: –Avoid the rays of the sun by wearing protective clothing and applying sunscreen (SPF 15) if exposed to the sun. –Report signs and symptoms. –Follow topical medication schedules if ordered.
Alopecia Skin Hyperpigmentation	Inspect skin for: –Increased pigmentation –Dark veins near chemotherapy injection sites –Areas of increased pigmentation in mouth and nailbeds –Rashes Assess: –Patient feelings about hair loss –Patient knowledge related to hair loss	High risk for body image disturbance related to skin hyperpigmentation and loss of hair	Patient verbalizes acceptance of self with skin and hair changes. Patient identifies positive aspects of self. Patient expresses pleasure at visits from family or friends.	Explain: –Skin reactions are expected and related to the chemotherapy. –Nail growth may be slowed. –Skin changes and vein and nail darkening are usually temporary. Implement measures to assist the patient in adapting to a change in physical appearance. Explain: –Hair loss is almost always temporary (except with high doses of radiotherapy to the scalp). –Timing of hair loss—will start approximately 14 days after treatment. –Hair sometimes grows back while the patient is still receiving treatment and that it can fall out again. –Hair will start to permanently grow after treatment is withdrawn. –New hair may be different in color and texture. –Facial and body hair can also be affected. –The scalp may become irritated with skin flaking. Suggest: –Purchasing a wig or hairpiece before alopecia begins. –Cutting long hair to decrease the anxiety associated with losing large amounts of hair. –Using a mild shampoo to alleviate scalp irritation. –Using hats and scarves.

				–Methods to reduce the rate of hair loss: Limit hair brushing. Avoid using harsh shampoos. Wear a hair net to sleep at night. Review hypothermia technique if indicated and with physician approval. Inform the patient that the cost of wigs and hairpieces is covered by most third-party health insurance companies. Local units of the American Cancer Society will lend patients wigs free of charge.
GASTROINTESTINAL TOXICITY Nausea and vomiting	Assess: –General appearance –Skin color and turgor Obtain vital signs: temperature, pulse, respiration, and blood pressure. Determine: –Time, frequency, and amount of emesis –Diet history –Medication schedules Examine abdomen; auscultate for bowel sounds (intestinal obstruction). Evaluate level of serum electrolytes and chemistries (hypercalcemia, hyponatremia, uremia, dehydration).	High risk for fluid volume deficit related to inadequate fluid intake and excessive fluid loss secondary to nausea and vomiting	Skin turgor is firm. Mucous membranes are moist. Fluid intake approximates output.	Instruct in measures that provide relief. Advise patient to: –Eat salty foods. –Try dry foods such as toast or crackers. –Drink clear, cool liquids. –Eat small portions of low-fat foods. –Report symptoms and severity. –Limit physical activity after meals. Administer antiemetics as prescribed. Suggest taking antiemetics before receiving chemotherapy and using antiemetics in suppository form. Offer support by: –Explaining that nausea and vomiting are expected side effects. –Explaining relaxation techniques. –Suggesting diversionary activity. –Being available for questions and follow-up.
Stomatitis Xerostomia	Inspect oral cavity for: –Moisture, color, ulceration, inflammation, and fungus –Quality, color, and amount of saliva Assess for symptoms: pain, dysphagia, inability to open mouth, inability to eat and take fluids, taste changes, voice changes. Observe condition of teeth. Ask about patient-initiated comfort measures. Ask about usual regimen for oral hygiene.	Altered oral mucous membrane related to effects of chemotherapeutic agents on the mucosal cells	Oral mucous membrane are intact. Oral mucous membranes are pink and moist. Patient is able to ingest foods and fluids without oral discomfort.	Implement measures to alleviate symptoms: Encourage and assist with mouth care. Rinse mouth with alkaline solutions every hour (1 tsp of baking soda in 8 oz of warm water). Use soft sponge or gauze instead of toothbrush. Remove thick saliva with gauze; irrigate mouth with sodium bicarbonate solution or diluted solution of hydrogen peroxide.

(continued)

Table 11–8. *(continued)* SIDE EFFECTS OF CHEMOTHERAPY WITH RELATED ASSESSMENTS, NURSING DIAGNOSES, EXPECTED PATIENT OUTCOMES, AND NURSING INTERVENTIONS

SIDE EFFECT	ASSESSMENT	NURSING DIAGNOSIS	EXPECTED PATIENT OUTCOMES	NURSING INTERVENTIONS
GASTROINTESTINAL TOXICITY *(continued)* Stomatitis and Xerostomia *(continued)*				Remove dentures for cleaning, keep dentures in place only if comfortable and not causing irritation. Suggest and evaluate effects of topical analgesics, artificial saliva, and lip lubricant. Instruct patient to avoid alcohol, smoking, commercial mouthwashes, and hot, spicy and acidic foods and fluids. Encourage: –Fluids –Ice popsicles –Soft bland diet –Using a straw to sip soups and beverages –Frequent oral irrigation
Diarrhea	Determine frequency and character of bowel movements. Obtain nutrition history. Obtain height, weight, and vital signs. Assess hydration status: tissue turgor, condition of mucous membranes, and serum electrolyte values. Patient knowledge and symptoms related to diarrhea. Determine: –Patient-initiated measures to control diarrhea. –Previous methods used to control diarrhea	Diarrhea related to effects of chemotherapeutic agents on the intestinal mucosa	Stool is formed. Stool is evacuated at intervals normal for the individual patient.	Implement measures to control and prevent diarrhea: Avoid: –Bowel-irritating foods –Gas-forming foods –Fatty foods –Lactose- and caffeine-containing products –Smoking Suggest: –Diet low in residue, high in protein and carbohydrates –Small, frequent meals Teach perianal hygiene: –Cleanse with water and mild soap after bowel movement. –Use sitz baths, if indicated. –Apply topical anesthetics to rectal area, if indicated. Administer and monitor the effects of medications to control diarrhea. –Antidiarrheal agents –Antispasmodics –Opiates and opiate substitutes
Constipation	Determine: –Usual bowel habits. –Patient knowledge related to constipation. –Patient symptoms (e.g., cramping, pain, abdominal distention). –Schedule of all medications (chemotherapy, vinca alkaloids, narcotics).	Constipation related to the effects of chemotherapeutic agents on the bowel	Stool is soft and formed. Stool is evacuated at regular intervals without straining.	Implement measures to prevent and alleviate constipation: Suggest: –Diet high in fiber, roughage, fluid –Drinking warm fluids to stimulate intestinal motility –Increase in physical activity to increase intestinal motility

- Previous medications and interventions used to treat constipation.
- Bowel sound patterns.

- Using toilet or bedside commode instead of bedpan

If patient has past history of constipation and will receive vinca alkaloid agents, suggest all the above to start after first chemotherapy dose.

Avoid using enemas or suppositories without consulting physician.

Administer and monitor the effects of medications prescribed to relieve constipation.
- Stool softeners: dioctyl sodium sulfosuccinate, mineral oil
- Bulk producers: psyllium, calcium, polycarbophil
- Osmotic and saline laxatives: sodium, potassium, and magnesium salts
- Lactulose is especially effective for constipation caused by vinca alkaloids
- Cathartics: castor oil, senna, cascara, bisacodyl

OTHER ASSESSMENTS AND INTERVENTIONS

RENAL TOXICITY

Renal toxicity is caused by specific chemotherapy agents:
- Cisplatin—damage to renal tubules
- Methotrexate—renal tubule necrosis with high doses
- Cyclophosphamide—hemorrhagic cystitis

Hyperuricemia due to rapid tumor destruction or tumor lysis in which tumor cells enter the circulatory system and pass through the renal system.

Review renal function studies: serum creatinine, creatinine clearance, and blood urea nitrogen.

Review urinalysis.

Check past history of renal disease.

Ask about symptoms of dysuria, hematuria (for cyclophosphamide).

For cisplatin:
- Hydrate before therapy as per institutional protocol.
- Measure and record urine output.
- Administer diuretics as ordered by physician.
- Monitor renal function regularly.

For methotrexate:
- Hydrate before therapy as per institutional protocol.
- Measure and record urine output.
- Administer sodium bicarbonate to alkalinize urine.
- Monitor urine pH, must be >7 before treatment.
- Monitor renal function regularly.

For cyclophosphamide:
- Hydrate with intravenous therapy.
- Advise increase in oral fluids.
- Institute measures to prevent hyperuricemia
- Increase oral and intravenous fluids as indicated.
- Alkalinize urine.
- Administer allopurinol (Zyloprim) before and during therapy to break down urates.
- Monitor serum and urine uric acid levels.

Planning: Patient outcomes

1. Patient states what the chemotherapy is expected to accomplish (e.g., shrink tumor in preparation for surgery, eliminate cancer cells remaining after surgery).
2. Patient describes schedule of treatments (i.e., interval at which treatments are given, when oral chemotherapeutic drugs are to be taken, and so on).
3. Patient describes expected side effects of chemotherapy.
4. Patient accurately describes palliative measures that may be used to assist in managing side effects.
5. Patient lists symptoms that should be reported to a health care professional.
6. Patient identifies telephone number at which a health care professional can be reached.
7. Patient states date and time of next appointment.

See Table 11–8 for other nursing diagnoses that are likely to occur in individual patients.

Nursing Interventions

Nursing interventions involve preparing the patient and family for the chemotherapy treatments and their potential side effects, administering prescribed chemotherapy, monitoring side effects, and teaching comfort and other support measures.

NDx: High risk for altered health maintenance

Using language the patient can understand, explain the action and effects of the chemotherapy to the patient and family. Review the treatment regimen and possible side effects of the drugs, stressing that each person's response is individual, so all of the side effects will not necessarily be experienced. Identify for the patient symptoms that should be immediately reported, and give instructions as to how to contact the appropriate health care professional.

Additional interventions are dependent on the specific body system affected by the chemotherapy (see Table 11–8). Keep in mind that each patient will experience one, several, or no side effects, based on multiple factors. Always review the chemotherapy treatment plan to evaluate potential common side effects for each patient's treatment.

When indicated, refer patients and families to other professionals and community programs and agencies. A list of patient resources is provided in the patient resources section of this chapter.

Evaluation

Evaluate the effectiveness of nursing care for a patient having chemotherapy for cancer by comparing the patient's status with the expected patient outcomes. Examples of specific outcomes for patients on chemotherapy have been provided in the Planning section.

Immunotherapy

Immunotherapy can be defined as treatment with chemical or biologic agents that are intended to assist the immune system in destroying cancerous cells. The immune system, which is discussed in Chapter 9, consists of protective mechanisms that recognize and defend against foreign matter, such as bacteria, viruses, and tumors. The immunologic approach in the treatment of cancerous cells is still experimental and is predicated on the assumption that certain parts of the immune system can be enhanced as a means to recognize and destroy tumor cells.

TYPES OF IMMUNOTHERAPY

Historically, immunotherapy has been classified as passive, active, or adaptive. Passive immunotherapy involves the administration of antitumor antibodies that have been sensitized to a specific antigen. Active immunotherapy involves the use of agents that are vaccines prepared from tumor cells, to stimulate both cellular and hormonal immunity. Active immunotherapy can be either specific for a certain kind of tumor cell or nonspecific to stimulate general immunity. An example of active nonspecific immunotherapy is the use of bacille Calmette-Guérin (BCG), an extract of tuberculosis bacilli. An example of active specific immunotherapy would involve the use of a vaccine derived from specific tumor cells, given to treat the same tumor. Adaptive methods are those that involve the stimulation of the immune system through the administration of chemically treated white blood cells. An example of adaptive immunotherapy is the use of interferons and interleukins. Interferons are a group of proteins that are naturally produced by the body in response to viral infections and other inducers. Interferons may have clinical value because of their ability to stimulate the immune system and inhibit cell growth.

Interleukins are natural substances produced by lymphocytes and monocytes, which are currently being studied for their antitumor properties. Currently, extensive research is being carried out to determine the therapeutic value of interferons and interleukins.

Immunotherapy agents are now called biologic response modifiers because they exhibit antitumor effects through mediation of the individual's immune response and, in some cases, directly kill tumor cells. Immunotherapy agents are divided into categories based on how they affect the tumor and the immune response. The classifications include agents that modulate or stimulate the immune system, agents that have the ability to directly kill cancer cells, and agents whose action is as yet unknown. Some immunotherapy agents fall into more than one category. Immunomodulators include interleukins, interferons, and specific and nonspecific vaccines. Immunotherapy is often used in conjunction with other forms of cancer therapies such as chemotherapy, radiotherapy, and surgery.

SIDE EFFECTS

The side effects that patients experience from immunotherapy vary depending upon the type and mode of administration. Intradermal, subcutaneous, and intralesional vaccines can cause localized skin irritation and systemic side effects of elevated body temperature, body chills, diaphoresis, and fatigue. Intravenous administration of immunomodulators has a wider range of systemic side effects, which include elevated body temperature, chills, diaphoresis, fluid retention, nausea, vomiting, and fatigue. Patients receiving investigational forms of immunotherapy are closely monitored for unknown side effects and adverse systemic reactions.

Unconventional Therapies

The very success of medical research and treatment in eradicating such diseases as polio and smallpox has inculcated a general expectation that there must be a definitive "cure" for cancer. The search for a "miracle" cure for oncologic diseases has led patients to investigate and participate in a wide range of therapies such as diet programs, vitamin therapies, and unproven and potentially unsafe biologic vaccines. These unproven methods are often costly and, if used instead of generally accepted treatments, can prevent timely treatment and restoration of health.

An example of a psychological approach to cancer cure that has become quite well known is that developed by the Simontons, a radiation oncologist and psychotherapist team. Their program is based on research that has shown that stress reduces antibody response; immunoglobulin levels change in response to psychological stimuli, and protective "killer cell" lymphocytes become less effective; and stress significantly lowers proliferation of T lymphocytes.

They, and others, teach patients to use mental imagery and other stress reduction techniques to fortify the immune system against cancer. These techniques are valuable adjuncts to traditional treatment regimens when used with appropriate patients. However, they should never be promoted as a substitute for traditional treatment modalities like surgery, radiation, and chemotherapy. The Simontons have developed a step-by-step, self-help program for patient and family participation in the treatment of cancer. Their program includes daily practice of progressive relaxation and mental imagery, daily reading assignments to overcome knowledge deficit on cancer, and self-study meditation to strengthen or correct coping behaviors.

The imagery includes visualization of lymphocytes overpowering and destroying cancer cells, tumors shrinking, and improved general health status and well-being.

Patients may request information related to alternative therapies as a means to ensure that they are reviewing all treatment alternatives. Respond to such requests by providing accurate information related to these therapies, while listening to and exploring the reasons for seeking unproven methods. If the response is unsatisfactory to the patient, provide referrals to educational materials or other professionals who can provide additional and current information regarding the health hazards and risks of unproven cancer treatments. Among sources of information are publications of the Food and Drug Administration, the National Cancer Institute, and the American Cancer Society. These agencies have literature that reviews and assesses unproven drugs, substances, and treatment centers.

Guidelines for Application of the Nursing Process to the Care of the Patient Interested in Unconventional Cancer Therapies

Be sensitive to the fact that many patients and families who seek unconventional therapy may have exhausted all conventional therapy without regression of disease. A patient's inclination to explore unproven therapies may be founded in desperation and not in reason. Remain objective and present patients with information that will assist in their understanding of the risks and implications of unproven cancer therapies. Accept the patient's right to choose whatever therapy he or she finds most desirable, even if in your judgment, it is not the correct choice.

Psychosocial Problems of the Patient Receiving Treatment for Cancer

Cancer presents a complexity of psychosocial problems that vary with individual patients. Nevertheless, certain themes emerge that are noted and reported by cancer patients with frequent regularity:

Anxiety and fear
Threats to self-concept

Altered sexuality
Profound loss and helplessness
Isolation and alienation
Family stress

Anxiety and Fear

Anxiety and fear are universally experienced with cancer. Patients report that one of the most difficult things they experience is the uncertainty that cancer produces. The resultant anxiety induced by that uncertainty promotes a sense of powerlessness to control their lives. Adjustments and changes in role and lifestyle are real and ongoing. Therefore, uncertainty is a constant threat, and the degree of anxiety is increased by threatened self-esteem and actual or anticipated loss.

Fear of recurrence of malignancy, of effects of chemotherapy, and of metastasis and death are frequently reported. A death that is lingering and painful is most feared.

Threats to Self-Concept

Disturbance in self-concept results when one is forced to perceive oneself differently. Forced changes in self-concept may result from lowered self-esteem, difference in role performance, or changes in body image. All these frequently occur in cancer patients. Surgical interventions to remove and hopefully cure the cancer such as a colostomy or ileal conduit may leave the patient with major changes in body function and image. A laryngectomy requires major adjustments to new communication patterns. An amputation or mastectomy may induce feelings of mutilation. Chronic pain produces feelings of vulnerability and lowers self-confidence. These few examples illustrate the profound abrupt changes in body image and threats to self-esteem that cancer engenders. No wonder that patients often feel betrayed by their body when they develop cancer.

Role performance alterations are also common and can lower self-esteem. Effects of surgery and chemotherapy or of the illness itself may prevent the breadwinner from working, prevent the homemaker from caring for the household, or make childbearing impossible. Even when the ability to continue at a satisfying job is not cut off, the demands of chemotherapy and the uncertainty of the outcome may prevent a promotion or inhibit challenging assignments.

Altered Sexuality

Changes in sexual activity may be due to alterations in body functions caused by the disease or by surgical treatments such as excision of the vulva. More commonly noted is potential sexual dysfunction due to altered self-concept.

The presence of a stoma or loss of a breast may induce fears of disgust or rejection by the sexual mate. Males may become impotent as a result of enforced changed role performance and dependency. Chemotherapy agents can also induce temporary sexual dysfunction.

Profound Loss and Helplessness

Profound loss and helplessness have been identified as major factors that often precede illness. These feelings are also experienced during the treatment of cancer. Cancer treatments, to be successful, must be intrusive. This can result in fear, anger, and resentment that one must willingly succumb to "torture." Helplessness to resist the necessity for mutilating surgery or distressingly toxic chemicals results in profound feelings of powerlessness. Depression commonly results from the sense of loss and may be accompanied by spiritual distress, deep hopelessness, and suicidal thoughts or actions.

Certain losses have profound symbolic meaning. Hair or breast loss for some women is deeply disturbing because they are strongly symbolic of feminine attractiveness.

Isolation and Alienation

Isolation commonly occurs in cancer because the disease or treatments produce weakness and difficulty in socializing. Patients are often homebound. Friends may stop visiting because of uneasiness, fear of catching cancer, sadness, or embarrassment at not knowing what to say. This results in feelings of alienation. Isolation is sometimes self-induced if patients are unwilling to be seen in public because of hair and weight loss or other changes in appearance. The loneliness is compounded if they feel unable to talk freely with loved ones about their feelings and worries. Satisfying jobs are very therapeutic in maintaining a sense of structure in their new "world of turmoil." Continuing to work should be encouraged, even on a part-time basis. Disability leaves, when necessary, should be as short-term as possible to reduce feelings of isolation.

Family Stress

Family stress is always experienced when a member develops cancer. Alterations in family processes cannot be avoided because of changes in routines and schedules. Financial strains occur. Family members must watch helplessly as a loved one suffers and must adapt to changes in a loved one who has cancer.

Families that have had various difficulties coping

in the past face additional stress. Invariably the crisis of cancer causes old conflicts to resurface. Unresolved issues or poor relationships can no longer be ignored or left dormant. Superficially healed emotional wounds often are exacerbated and become raw. Cancer, which is a family problem, exposes inadequacies that are present in a family system. The coping styles of patients and their families range from effective to ineffective as the patient adjusts to the diagnosis and required therapies. Coping effectiveness depends on the ability to seek information, follow through on treatment, and talk freely about feelings and concerns, as well as the availability of an adequate support system.

Type of cancer, extent of the disease, forced changes in body image, age at onset, degree of debilitating symptoms, previous experiences with cancer, and financial means to seek and pay for needed care also have a direct effect upon coping abilities.

Application of the Nursing Process to the Psychosocial Needs of the Patient Undergoing Cancer Treatment

The focus of treatment of cancer patients and their ability to cope vary with the prognosis. This focus can be summarized as cure, control, or comfort. Each category of care as well as the specific type of cancer experienced presents different psychosocial problems.

Cure: Coping strategies often focus around needed adjustments to body image due to curative surgery that can result in major body changes. Efforts should be made to reduce anxiety, to ventilate feelings, to maintain a fighting spirit, and to resume a normal lifestyle. Even easily cured types of skin cancer generate fear, which needs to be addressed.

Control: Major adjustments to long-term radiation and chemotherapy deal with profound feelings of vulnerability, dependency, and helplessness. Fear, isolation, and threats to self-esteem are common themes. Family stress and knowledge deficit are additional problems frequently noted.

Comfort: Patients with a terminal prognosis need to be helped to cope and to be spared as much pain, depression, and alienation as possible. A profound sense of loss is often reported and can result in hopelessness or spiritual distress as well as grief.

Assessment

When assessing the psychosocial dimension, keep in mind that careful observation and attentive listening to patients and their families provide the basis for identifying reactions and needs. Promote honest communication by expressing empathy and projecting an attitude of calm acceptance. Use clarifying questions to validate perceptions and broad opening questions to permit the patient's priorities to surface. Paraphrase and reflect feelings to mirror reactions and enable the patients to look more clearly at their response to what they are experiencing.

Remember that sometimes patients are unable to identify the nature of their feelings directly and need to initially address them peripherally by discussing and focusing on persons or happenings around them. Other times they need to use symbolic language or gestures. Always remember that all behavior has meaning. Rude, petty demands may be expressions of feelings of powerlessness, loss, and anger. Passive compliance may indicate problems of low self-esteem or depression. Compare currently observed coping mechanisms with premorbid behavior patterns through discussion with patients, families, or trusted others.

Identify major strengths as well as weaknesses as a basis for planning care. These include the ability to relate and communicate effectively with others, to recognize and express feelings, to effectively seek and request help as needed, to make sound decisions, and to follow instructions with consistency.

Assess important resources such as the quality of medical care, religious faith, supporting family and friends, and adequate finances. Also assess ethnic and cultural influences, past experiences with cancer, the presence of other major problems or burdens in their life, and most importantly, present understanding of condition and prognosis.

Nursing Diagnoses and Planning

Nursing diagnoses and related expected patient outcomes most commonly applicable to the psychosocial needs of patients undergoing cancer treatment include the following:

NDx: Anxiety related to uncertain outcomes and effects of cancer treatment

Planning: Patient outcomes

1. Patient asks relevant questions.
2. Patient reads information about treatments.
3. Patient expresses anxieties and fears openly to nurse and significant others.
4. Patient utilizes self-identified effective coping mechanisms to reduce stress.
5. Patient attempts to limit self-identified counterproductive coping mechanisms.
6. Patient sets realistic goals, breaking them down to small, attainable units.
7. Patient focuses on the present, attempting "to live one day at a time."

8. Patient practices progressive relaxation and mental imagery on a daily basis.
9. Patient keeps as active as possible, performing at least a few simple exercises daily and taking brief, daily walks.
10. Patient attends self-help group or keeps scheduled appointments with cancer support counselor.
11. Patient utilizes problem-solving techniques to reduce fears and uncertainties.

NDx: Body image disturbance related to loss of a body part or to major structural or functional changes (e.g., stoma, immobility, alopecia, inability to speak)

Planning: Patient outcomes
1. Patient talks about feelings of loss, crying appropriately.
2. Patient assumes responsibility for care of altered body part.
3. Patient speaks calmly and naturally about new body part, function, or role.
4. Patient states he or she feels comfortable with self.
5. Patient utilizes effective coping mechanisms to plan rehabilitation.
6. Patient takes steps to secure, adjust, and care for adequate adaptive devices.
7. Patient maintains or resumes social contact with equanimity.
8. Patient participates in physical activities, relaxation exercises, contact with well-adjusted patients, and other techniques that promote adjustment.
9. Patient plans for future with family and significant others.

NDx: Altered role performance related to inability to continue working or dependence upon others, secondary to effects of disease, radiation, and chemotherapy

Planning: Patient outcomes
1. Patient talks about feelings regarding role change.
2. Patient describes new role requirements accurately.
3. Patient assertively defines new role with acceptance and satisfaction.

NDx: Sexual dysfunction related to perceived disfigurement and mutilation, loss of role and self-esteem, presence of appliance, fears, or effects of chemotherapy

Planning: Patient outcomes
1. Patient talks openly and freely to nurse and mate regarding sexual problems.
2. Patient actively seeks ways to reduce stress and cope with problems including willingness to participate in sex counseling as needed.
3. Patient discusses alternative techniques for sexual expression with spouse.

NDx: Powerlessness related to hospitalization, need to participate in undesirable treatment, or overprotectiveness by family

Planning: Patient outcomes
1. Patient, identifying sense of powerlessness, takes steps to avoid preventable insecurities.
2. Patient assertively expresses legitimate complaints and need for independence and control.
3. Patient actively participates in decision-making.
4. Patient, realistically identifying what he or she can continue to do, functions as independently as condition allows.

NDx: Social isolation related to decreased contact with friends or need to stop working

Planning: Patient outcomes
1. Patient describes feelings of isolation and alienation as common to the cancer experience.
2. Patient shares feelings freely with trusted others.
3. Patient maintains work and social schedule with adaptations for physical disability.

NDx: Altered family processes related to difficulties adjusting to changes in the patient, hospitalization of the patient, and disruption of routines, or to the financial burden of treatment

Planning: Patient outcomes
1. Family members verbalize thoughts and feelings regarding effects of cancer to each other and with appropriate health professionals.
2. Family makes positive affirmations by words and deeds of patient as a valued member.
3. Individual members of family weather crisis without long-term psychological disability or alienation.
4. Members work together to attack problems and share responsibilities constructively.
5. Family utilizes community services and referrals appropriately as needed.

Nursing Interventions

Interventions vary with the prognosis and the treatment focus of cure, control, or comfort.

NDx: Anxiety
Therapeutic communication is the priority intervention in the prevention and reduction of anxiety.

Give the patient information in clear, simple terms regarding anticipated treatments and their effects. Stress individual variations of response to chemotherapy and other treatments in order to avoid suggesting or conditioning the patient to expect unpleasant side effects. Schedule regular opportunities for the patient to discuss and ventilate anxieties and fears in an unhurried, empathetic manner. Avoid false reassurances, because these belittle the patient's concerns. Often, encouraging patients to describe anticipated death or other fears in segmented details helps break down and reduce their terror.

Help the patient identify and initiate steps to reduce anxiety: Encourage realistic goal setting, that is, small, easily attainable short-term goals for immediate attention and maximum success. Action reduces anxiety, so to focus on the "here and now" with small, immediate goals helps reduce the anxiety produced by situations about which one feels presently helpless. Teach and guide the patient through progressive relaxation techniques, because when muscles are no longer tense, the person does not feel tense, and total relaxation can result from training in muscle relaxation. Also guide the patient in the use of mental imagery, which is thought to have a positive effect in stimulating and enhancing the body's immune system. Encourage regular daily exercise and activities as valuable means of discharging tensions and dissipating fear and anxiety.

Teach problem-solving techniques such as assessment, analysis, planning, interventions, and evaluation as a means of reducing any uncertainties that can be resolved. Identify and reinforce patients' strengths to help structure for success. Identify and accept other coping mechanisms such as hostility, withdrawal, distraction, or demanding behaviors as manifestations of stress, while helping the patient to set limits on these behaviors.

Counsel and help patients to structure life and environment to avoid extra stress and to keep unnecessary changes and decisions to a minimum.

Arrange for patients to meet with cancer patients who have had successful outcomes to their treatment to reduce anxiety and promote hope. Encourage or assist patients in joining a support group, because others who have come through similar crises understand the patient's distress and may offer the best help in dealing with it on an ongoing basis. When necessary, administer antianxiety medications as ordered.

NDx: Body image disturbance

To help the patient adjust to an alteration in body parts or function, explain the stages of grief and reassure the patient that grief is a normal reaction to loss of body parts and functions. This helps prevent guilt about the feelings associated with the different stages of grief and promotes self-acceptance. Involve the patient gradually in the care of the altered part to avoid overwhelming him or her. Recognize that the patient's first perception of his or her altered appearance is derived from the response of the nurse, whether it be calm acceptance or revulsion. Since better understanding promotes quality care, identify the patient's areas of concern and his or her symbolic meaning of the lost part or function (e.g., mastectomy equals loss of femininity for some women).

Provide reliable resource information regarding quality wigs, prostheses, or adaptive devices to allow for practical steps to improve the patient's well-being. Arrange fittings for prostheses or use of adaptive devices as soon as possible to avoid development of negative habits, resistance, or apathy.

Discuss social situations that are dreaded because of altered body parts or function. Role-play these situations with the patient, because rehearsal in a safe setting builds confidence and structures for later success in real situations. Arrange peer visits or involvement with persons from self-help groups like the Ostomy Association, Reach for Recovery, or the Lost Chord Society, because these people understand the patient's situation better than anyone and therefore can teach and motivate most effectively.

NDx: Altered role performance

To help the patient adjust to role change without excessive dependency patterns, explore and utilize the patient's strengths to plan care and rehabilitation. Facilitate honest expression of feelings, which communicates respect and promotes self-esteem and acceptance. Explore with and assist the patient in techniques of biofeedback, behavior modification, hypnosis, imagery, and relaxation, which increase ability to cope with stress and build self-esteem. Encourage as much physical movement as possible to enable the patient to redefine body space and to build self-confidence.

Be certain to involve the family and patient in planning and problem-solving because patients do not function in isolation. Identify and discuss role changes, role confusion, or role conflicts (e.g., breadwinner versus dependent sick role versus active participant in rehabilitative decisions), so that frustration can be ventilated and areas of confusion corrected. Also identify and discuss stressors that promote role disturbance (e.g., financial stress, changes in sexual performance, changes in appearance, and changes in physical capabilities), because better understanding promotes acceptance and successful adjustment. Assist the patient in sorting out options and identifying ways to structure for success to encourage autonomy and sound decision-making. Explore gender role expectations and needed adaptions for realistic preparation for future demands. Identify family patterns of shielding or dependency on the patient, because these can promote feelings of inadequacy.

NDx: Sexual dysfunction

Gently introduce information about the relationship of stress to sexual interest and performance to promote understanding and acknowledgment of the problem. Differentiate between intrapsychic conflicts and organic factors such as effects of medication. With the patient's permission, explore the mate's reactions to sexual problems. Identify and discuss myths regarding cancer and sexual disability to restore hope and confidence, and explore their willingness to discuss alternative techniques to stimulate and satisfy sexual needs (e.g., body massage, mutual masturbation, and use of erotic routines and materials as aids to sexual stimulation). Make referrals for counseling or sex therapy as needed. If patients desire to have children in the future, give information about sperm banks for freezing and preserving sperm prior to surgery or treatments that potentially sterilize.

NDx: Powerlessness

To enable the patient to make decisions and actively participate in planning for the future, first respect the patient's need to grieve loss of independence, power, and control, as well as body changes and role. Recognize that hospitalization promotes powerlessness and make all possible efforts to offset that effect. Orient the patient to the hospital environment and personnel in order to reduce confusion and feelings of being a stranger. Within the confines and demands of the hospital setting, give the patient as much control as possible. Involve the patient in regulation of temperature, lighting, ventilation, television and radio noise, and furniture placement. Encourage decision-making in terms of scheduling. Keep inconveniences, irritations, and sensory overload to a minimum, because they increase feelings of inadequacy when the patient is helpless to do anything about them. Avoid reinforcing dependency patterns, which in turn reinforce feelings of powerlessness. Teach the family about factors that promote helplessness (e.g., overprotection and isolating the patient) so that members will avoid these destructive tendencies. Also stress that helplessness is a learned response, which can be unlearned and replaced with more responsible responses. Make available reference books such as *The American Cancer Society Cancer Book*, *Coping With Chemotherapy*, or *The Cancer Patient's Handbook* to promote learning and feelings of control. Encourage assertiveness on the part of the patient, and recognize patient demands as coping mechanisms. Be sure to respect legitimate complaints, because to ignore them negates all sense of worth and control.

Explore and encourage spiritual supports. Prayer and meditation, Scripture readings, attendance at religious services, and chaplains' visits can enable patients to relate to God's power and reduce their own sense of powerlessness. If expressions of hopelessness and other signs of despair and depression appear, initiate a referral for counseling.

NDx: Social isolation

To promote patient participation in constructive social and diversional activities, encourage the patient to continue working at a satisfactory job as long as possible. When the patient is unable to work, help identify ways to increase or maintain meaningful social contacts (e.g., regularly scheduled telephone calls, tape recordings, visits, or written correspondence) to prevent isolation. Approach significant family members and friends regarding the importance of continued visits and calls to prevent isolation and alienation. Teach the family to respect privacy but firmly maintain some social involvement if the patient tends to withdraw. Most often, one-to-one and small group contacts are less threatening and therefore more acceptable to the patient. If the patient seems religious, visits from pastor, rabbi, or other spiritual advisor may be desired to encourage hope and a sense of receiving God's blessing and presence with them in their loneliness.

When appropriate, provide specific information or referrals for social involvement (e.g., senior citizen centers, adult education classes, self-help groups, volunteer visitors, and home health aides) because the patient may lack the motivation or energy to seek out and pursue needed information. If transportation is a problem, provide information on what is available in the community (e.g., ambulettes, senior citizen vans). Explore diversional activities appropriate to physical abilities, and make occupational therapy referrals as needed so that the patient gains confidence with mastering new small motor skills and is stimulated by new activities.

Empathize with the patient, and validate that feelings of isolation and alienation are a common component of the cancer experience. Encourage the patient to confide and discuss feelings of isolation and alienation openly with significant others. If needed, role-play interactions with significant others to help the patient communicate on a more intimate, meaningful level. Avoid pat phrases and false reassurances and minimization or disrespect of the patient's feelings, which increase a sense of isolation and loneliness, and teach the family to do likewise. Do not lie to a patient; rather, teach the truth in a supportive manner when the patient provides cues that he or she is ready to learn. Take extra time to promote alternative means of significant communication with a patient who has lost speaking ability in order to prevent loneliness, isolation, and alienation, so characteristic of this disability.

NDx: Altered family processes

To enable the family to maintain mutual support while coping positively with changes caused by cancer and the financial strains of treatment, first recognize that cancer is a family disease. The family's suffering can be as great or greater than that of their loved one because families usually function as integral units. Take time to speak with each family member regarding his or her own stress, and make referrals as needed to cancer support groups or individual counseling. Because reactions of each family member affect the other members, discuss constructive family coping—use of humor, respect of individuality, mutual reliance and support, sharing thoughts and feelings, shared decision-making and planning—because these behaviors promote health and well-being. Identify and discuss potentially destructive family coping tendencies such as denial, separation and withdrawal, exploitation and overdependency, authoritarian approach to problems, and substance abuse by stressed members as a form of escape, because awareness can help decrease these dysfunctional patterns. Teach families that old problems tend to resurface in times of stress, and make referrals as needed for marriage and individual counseling, family therapy, substance abuse interventions (e.g., Al-Anon, Al-Ateen, and Alcoholics Anonymous). Always stress that crises carry potential for positive change and that it is possible to emerge from a crisis as a stronger unit. Avoid giving advice and using appeals to logic because these rarely produce changed behavior. Do provide genuine expressions of empathy to each member, but avoid taking sides in disputes and disagreements because to do so dilutes and negates the nurse's influence and ability to help the family as a whole unit. Facilitate freer family communication patterns by clarifying ambiguous messages and identifying destructive "double bind" patterns to be avoided. Make referrals as needed for financial or other assistance to departments of social services, Medicare, Medicaid, American Cancer Society, hospice, home care agencies, and self-help groups because information about various community services may be unknown to the family.

Evaluation

Evaluate the effectiveness of nursing care in meeting the psychosocial needs of the patient undergoing cancer treatment by comparing the patient's status with the expected patient outcomes. Examples of specific outcomes for patients with psychosocial problems related to cancer treatment have been provided in the Planning section.

Complications of Cancer

Pain

A major factor in advanced cancer is pain. The International Association for the Study of Pain has defined pain as "an unpleasant sensory and emotional experience associated with actual or potential tissue damage or described in terms of such damage." The subjective nature of pain is evidenced by the unique psychological and physiologic responses to pain.

Cancer pain is most often associated with tissue damage and tissue infiltration. As malignant tumors grow within a body part, they stretch normal boundaries of the organ, causing severe pain (Fig. 11–13). As tumors grow and occupy additional space, other organs and structures are affected. Tumor growth and tissue invasion can result in nerve compression, organ and bone invasion, organ obstruction, and organ stretching. Primary or metastatic bone tumors cause pain related to pressure, periosteal irritation, and pathologic fractures. Pain can be experienced as an acute or chronic event. Unrelieved pain can affect a patient's lifestyle, treatment, and ability to cope with his or her disease status.

PHYSIOLOGY OF PAIN

According to the gate control theory, pain is a subjective individualized event that represents several interrelated sensory, affective, and personal factors. Gate control theory demonstrates the relationship between the central nervous system and the peripheral nervous system in the recognition and control of pain. This theory is predicated on the physiologic structure of small, slow conducting afferent nerve fibers of the peripheral nervous system that merge in the dorsal root of the spinal cord. This area, called the substantia gelatinosa, consists of a layer of cells that cover the spinal cord on both sides and provide a "gate" for pain signals to pass. As pain builds, the fibers of the gate open and pain is experienced. Larger nerve fibers have the capacity to inhibit the transmission of pain and cause the gate to close. Afferent nerve impulses, such as memory, attention, and emotions, can either reduce or enhance the pain because they too can stimulate the gate mechanism.

Neurotransmitters are chemicals, such as endorphins and enkephalins, that are produced by the body in response to pain. These chemicals modify and block the transmission of pain impulses and function as opiate receptors throughout the nervous system. Drug therapy with narcotics is used to relieve pain through activating opiate receptors in the central and peripheral nervous system.

PAIN MANAGEMENT

The primary method to relieve tumor-related pain is to destroy the tumor that is the cause. The surgical removal of a tumor mass or chemotherapy used to shrink a tumor mass can relieve pain. Radiation therapy can be directed to localized areas to treat organ and vessel obstructions and to directly treat bone pain. Surgical manipulation of the central nervous system can also relieve pain symptoms.

PHARMACOLOGIC AGENTS

Analgesics, anti-inflammatory agents, and psychotropic agents are used in the treatment of pain as single agents or in combination. These agents control the symptoms of pain, with the goal of improving the patient's comfort. Non-narcotic analgesics control pain by acting on the peripheral nervous system. Non-narcotic analgesics include aspirin, acetaminophen, and the nonsteroidal anti-inflammatory agents such as ibuprofen. Narcotics control pain

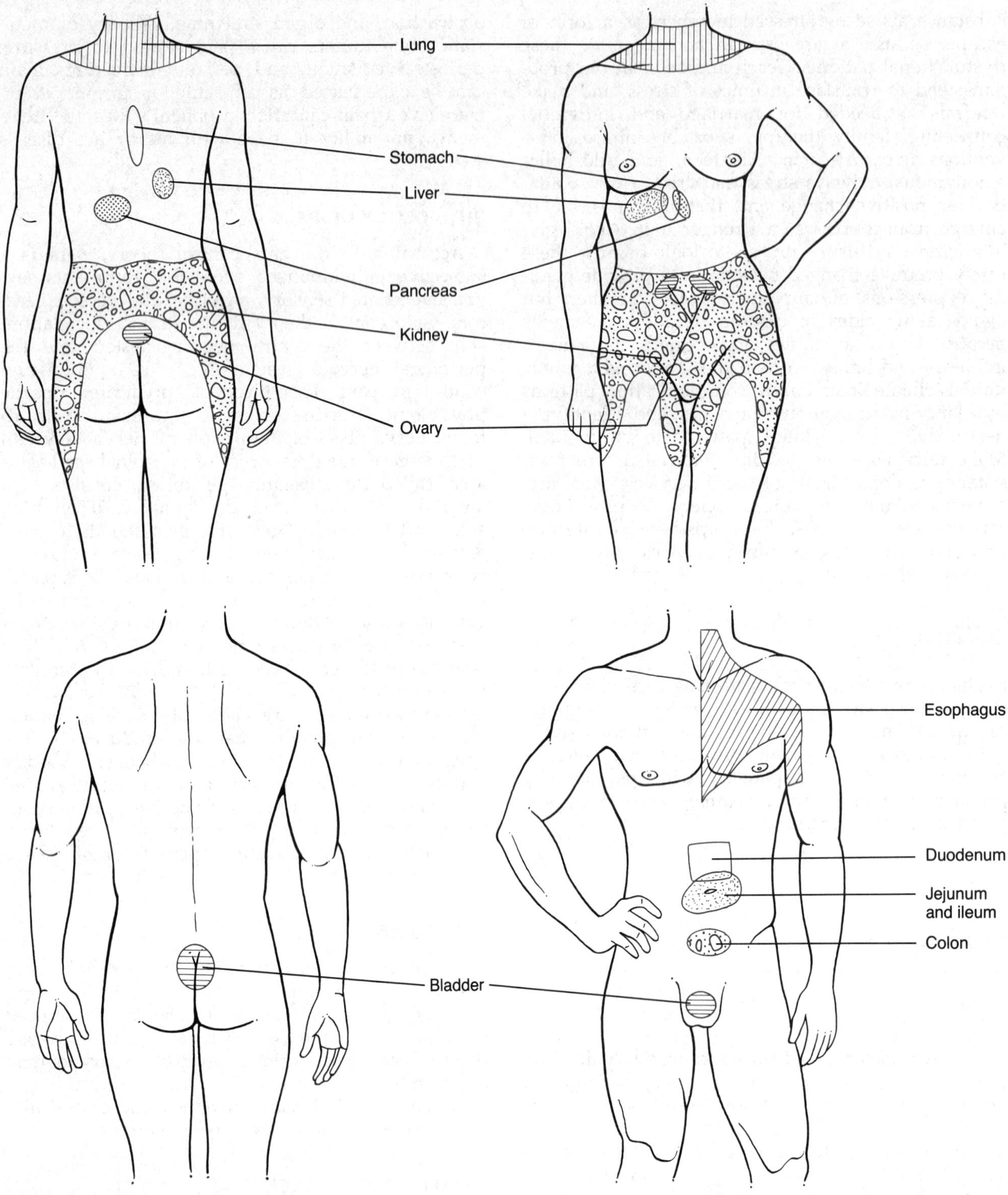

Figure 11–13.

Body surface areas where pain is felt from visceral organs that are frequently the site of cancer.

by acting on the central nervous system and include codeine, morphine, meperidine, and oxycodone. Non-narcotics and narcotics are often prescribed together.

Side effects from narcotics include drowsiness, constipation, nausea and vomiting, and drying of the oral mucosa. Non-narcotics such as aspirin can cause mild drowsiness and gastrointestinal bleeding and can interfere with platelet functioning.

Coanalgesic agents such as steroids, antipsychotic agents, muscle relaxants, and sedatives are also used to control pain-related symptoms. Pharmacologic agents can be given orally or parentally, on intermittent or continuous dosing schedules. The use of oral morphine on an around-the-clock schedule has been shown to be effective in the control of severe pain, as has the use of patient-controlled analgesia. The selection of pharmacologic agents and method of administration is based on patient pain control history, patient preference, and patient response.

The side effects of pharmacologic agents must also be considered. Narcotics can depress the function of the central nervous system.

BEHAVIORAL THERAPIES

Behavioral therapies can be used in conjunction with pharmacologic therapies as a means to promote patient participation in care. Behavioral therapies, which vary in approach, are intended to decrease tension and increase muscle relaxation. They can potentially assist with pain control while ameliorating nausea and vomiting related to other therapy. Further, they can also reduce general anxiety.

Behavioral therapies include

- Diversionary activities such as exercise, hobbies or reading, which assist in the redirection of pain sensation and perceptions.
- Relaxation therapy such as exercises, yoga, meditation, and progressive muscle relaxation. Advanced relaxation techniques involve hypnosis and guided imagery. These therapies can be learned and self-induced as a means to provide deep relaxation.
- Biofeedback, which assists the patient with self-regulation of physiologic activities such as pulse and blood pressure, can result in decreased tension and increased muscle relaxation.

CUTANEOUS THERAPIES

Cutaneous therapies—such as skin massage; application of heat, cold, and lotion; acupuncture; and transcutaneous electrical nerve stimulation (TENS)—can offer additional and temporary pain relief.

Transcutaneous electric nerve stimulation is based on the gate control theory and is accomplished through the use of a small electrical device, powered by a battery pack, which may be worn by the patient and which provides electrical stimulation to the skin. The large fibers of the peripheral nervous system are stimulated in an attempt to override pain stimuli and close the gate that controls pain perception (Fig. 11–14).

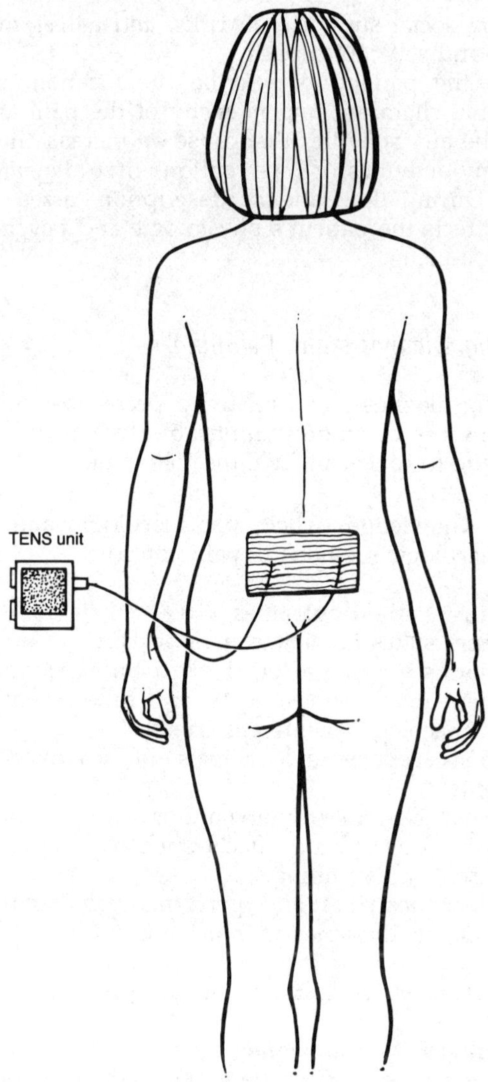

Figure 11–14.

Transcutaneous electrical nerve stimulation (TENS) used for relief of low back pain. Electrodes in place on surface of lower back.

Application of the Nursing Process to the Care of the Patient with Pain Caused by Cancer

Assessment

Review the patient's medical history, previous pain history, and previous and present pain control interventions and their outcomes. Obtain information regarding social support networks, and assess mental status and self-care capacity.

Ask the patient to describe the location, onset, duration, character, and intensity of the pain and to describe any activities that cause an increase in pain and any activities or interventions that alleviate the pain. During the patient's description, assess how pain affects the patient's physiologic and psychological well-being.

Nursing Diagnoses and Planning

Nursing diagnoses and related expected patient outcomes most commonly applicable to patients with pain due to cancer include the following:

NDx: Knowledge deficit: pharmacologic and nonpharmacologic methods of pain control

Planning: Patient outcomes

1. Patient states possible causes of pain.
2. Patient states characteristics of pain experienced.
3. Patient states names, doses, and time schedule of pharmacologic agents prescribed.
4. Patient reports side effects of pharmacologic agents.
5. Patient describes interventions to alleviate the most common side effects such as constipation, nausea, and vomiting.
6. Patient describes and performs behavioral and cutaneous therapies as indicated.

NDx: Pain related to the malignant process

Planning: Patient outcomes

1. Patient uses appropriate methods of pain control.
2. Patient states pain is controlled or alleviated.
3. Signs of pain (noticeable grimacing, splinting of a body part, groaning, and so on) are absent.

Nursing Interventions

NDx: Knowledge deficit: pharmacologic and nonpharmacologic methods of pain control

Explain in language the patient and family can understand the cause of pain and how the various types of interventions affect the pain experience. With regard to pharmacologic therapy, teach the name of prescribed drugs, the dosage schedule, and side effects. Instruct the patient in the use of behavioral therapies and cutaneous therapies such as massage, vibration, and the use of heat, cold, lotions or a TENS device as indicated.

NDx: Pain

Implement measures to control and alleviate pain and administer drug therapy based on individual patient needs and as prescribed by the physician. Note the effectiveness of drugs administered. Monitor for side effects, including changes in mental and cognitive ability, respiratory status, and bowel function. Assist the patient with behavioral or cutaneous therapies as needed.

Collaborate with the physician regarding effectiveness and side effects of therapy, and initiate consults or referrals to other professionals as needed.

If the patient is not hospitalized, ensure that the patient has a follow-up appointment and that the patient and family know how to contact medical personnel in case of an emergency.

Evaluation

Evaluate the effectiveness of nursing care for a patient with pain due to cancer by comparing the patient's status with the expected patient outcomes. Examples of specific outcomes for patients with pain due to cancer have been provided in the Planning section.

Malnutrition

The nutritional status and well-being of the cancer patient can be affected by several interrelated factors: the physical and biologic characteristics of the tumor, the side effects of cancer treatment, and the patient's dietary intake and emotional state. Loss of appetite and weight loss are common symptoms of advanced cancer. Research suggests that patients who suffer from malnutrition have an inferior prognosis as measured by their response and tolerance to treatment and their length of survival. Nutritional assessment and support should be part of the patient's total treatment plan. Food preferences, past dietary patterns, and physical symptoms caused by the disease process and related therapy should be considered. The nurse should suggest small frequent meals served in a pleasant environment.

CACHEXIA

Cachexia is a term used to describe the complex nutritional alterations that result from the disease process, which are further complicated by cancer treatments. Cachexia is characterized by marked anorexia, feeling of abdominal fullness after small amounts of food, marked weight loss (>10% of body weight), and loss of adipose tissue, visceral protein, and skeletal muscle. Cachectic patients complain of fatigue and decreased motor and mental skills. The patient appears physically emaciated as a result of muscle wasting.

The exact cause of cachexia remains unknown, although it has been associated with an imbalanced dietary intake, impaired digestion or absorption, increased use of body nutrients by the tumor, increased metabolic rate, and increased energy expenditure related to the tumor's rapid growth. The treatment of cachexia largely depends on the ability of anticancer therapies to destroy tumors.

FACTORS CONTRIBUTING TO CACHEXIA

Tumor Characteristics

Malignant tumors utilize body nutrients, thereby depriving the individual of necessary nutrients. Tumors can secrete substances that impair the normal metabolic processes and negatively influence the appetite control center in the hypothalamus. This results in a state of nutrient competition between malignant and normal tissues. The malignant tissues become nourished, leaving the normal tissues to absorb nutrients through catabolism as normal tissues such as skeletal muscle break down to provide amino acids.

The physical presence of a tumor mass in the abdomen or gastrointestinal tract can mechanically impair digestion and interrupt the normal feedback system that controls hunger.

Cancer Therapy

The gastrointestinal side effects associated with radiation therapy and chemotherapy can alter the patient's nutritional status. Symptoms of nausea, vomiting, taste alterations, mucositis, taste changes, and diarrhea can impair dietary intake. Surgical interventions to treat tumors of the head and neck region and gastrointestinal tract can affect dietary intake and digestion.

Patient Variables

Reduced dietary intake may be a consequence of the patient's psychological condition. Anorexia may be a direct consequence of psychological stress induced by the diagnosis or required therapies. Patients may experience loss of appetite as a consequence of feelings of depression, anger, fear, anxiety, and hopelessness.

NUTRITIONAL SUPPORT

Nutritional assessment and dietary counseling should be part of the patient's total care in all phases of cancer prevention, treatment, and follow-up. Development of a dietary support program should consider the patient's symptoms related to the disease process, treatment side effects, concomitant medical illnesses, and social support networks. Support with oral, enteral, or parenteral nutrition may be indicated.

Application of the Nursing Process to the Care of the Patient at Risk for Nutritional Alterations Caused by Cancer and Its Treatment

Assessment

Review the patient's medical history, including type and schedule of treatments and side effects experienced. Determine the patient's knowledge about the effect of cancer and cancer treatments on nutritional status.

Assess current nutritional status by measuring the patient's height and weight, mid-arm muscle circumference (MAMC), and triceps skinfold to determine external tissue mass. Also review pertinent laboratory data such as levels of hemoglobin, hematocrit, serum albumin, and blood urea nitrogen. Obtain information on current dietary intake, and calculate the patient's protein, carbohydrate, fat, vitamin, mineral, and fluid needs considering age, activity, and pathology.

Explore the patient's food preferences and patterns of eating. Identify any strategies the patient has initiated to increase dietary intake, and question him or her about their success.

Nursing Diagnoses and Planning

The nursing diagnosis and related expected patient outcomes most commonly applicable to patients at risk for nutritional alterations due to cancer are as follows:

NDx: High risk for altered nutrition: less than body requirements related to the malignant disease process and side effects of cancer therapy

Planning: Patient outcomes
1. Patient describes dietary interventions.
2. Patient maintains weight or limits weight loss.
3. Measurements of serum protein and albumin levels are within normal limits.
4. Measurements of hemoglobin and hematocrit levels are within normal limits.
5. Signs of dehydration are absent.
6. Patient participates in physical activities.

Nutrition Box 11–1.

NUTRITION: SPECIAL CONSIDERATIONS FOR PATIENTS WITH CANCER

Instruct patients with cancer to:
Eat small, frequent meals.
Avoid strong-smelling foods.
Increase caloric and nutrient intake:
- Add wine, beer, or milk to soups and sauces.
- Combine ice cream with soda, milk shakes, or yogurt.
- Drink liquid protein supplements.

Increase intake of lean protein.
Serve foods that are cold or at room temperature.
Take advantage of times when feeling "well" to prepare food and freeze for later use.
Dine in an environment conducive to eating.
Rinse mouth before eating to wash away bad tastes.
Plan meals that meet fluid and caloric needs.
Keep a food diary.

Nursing Interventions

NDx: High risk for altered nutrition: less than body requirements

Discuss aspects of the disease process and treatments that can affect nutritional status with the patient and the family. Teach the basic food groups and instruct the patient as specified in Nutrition Box 11–1 on ways to improve appetite and meet nutritional needs.

Monitor nutritional status on a regular basis, but always avoid statements that may make the patient feel guilty about anorexia, and instruct the family likewise.

If indicated, consult with the physician regarding enteral and parenteral nutritional supplementation, use of oral liquid supplements, and antiemetic or antidiarrheal medications. Initiate referrals to the dietitian and to community agencies that assist with meal preparation as needed.

Evaluation

Evaluate the effectiveness of nursing care for a patient at risk for nutritional alteration due to cancer by comparing the patient's status with the expected patient outcomes. Examples of specific outcomes for patients at risk for nutritional alterations due to cancer have been provided in the Planning section.

Home Care

The diagnosis and treatment of oncologic disorders often do not require extensive hospitalization. Many patients undergoing radiation therapy, chemotherapy, and immunotherapy may safely be treated and monitored on an ambulatory basis. In addition, patients who are in the terminal phases of the disease process may wish to remain at home. Home care should be planned during the patient's hospitalization. Family members and home health professionals can provide needed home care; however, family members will require support and instruction in basic patient care skills. The patient should be referred to the hospital's home care department and a referral made to the local visiting nurse service.

Hospice Care

For the terminally ill, a familiar environment with family members and friends can be a comforting experience during the final stage of cancer. Hospice care is a philosophy of comprehensive psychological, physical, and spiritual support for terminally ill patients and their families. Care is provided by interdisciplinary professionals and community volunteers, either within an institution such as a hospital or within the home. The hospice approach, which started in England in the 1960s, is becoming an integral part of terminal care in the United States. Nurses should familiarize patients and their families with hospice services available in their communities.

The Elderly: Special Considerations

Incidence

The incidence of cancer increases as age increases, with the result that there are more cases of cancer among the elderly than among any other age group. As in the population as a whole, the majority of cancers found in the elderly affect the prostate, the breast, the lung, or the lower GI tract. However, other cancers, although fewer in number, occur almost exclusively among the aged. These include cancers of the skin, the urinary bladder, the vulva, vagina, and uterine endometrium. Multiple myeloma and leukemia, especially chronic lymphocytic leukemia, although not exclusively diseases of the aged, are predominantly so.

Etiology

The reasons for the relationship between advancing age and the development of malignant disease are not fully clear, but at least two factors appear to contribute to it.

The first factor is the defective repair of DNA that has been found in the elderly. Because chromosomes break at all ages, particularly in response to exposure to carcinogens, radiation, and some viruses, it is theorized that the decrease in ability of the elderly to repair DNA results in an accumulation of chromosomal abnormalities that allow uncontrolled cell growth.

The second factor is the decreased effectiveness of the immune system in the elderly, particularly in the identification and destruction of cells carrying foreign antigens.

Pathophysiology

Just as the incidence and the occurrence of specific types of cancer is different in the elderly, so are the characteristics of particular tumors. For example, papillary cancer of the thyroid, which is highly treatable in young women, is very aggressive and highly metastatic in older women. Similarly, malignant melanoma is more aggressive in the elderly, particularly women. In contrast, cancer of the breast has a better prognosis in the elderly because it grows more slowly and tends to metastasize to bone and soft tissue rather than to liver and lungs in this group.

Medical Diagnosis

Early diagnosis is as important in the elderly as in any other age group. Yet in many cases, disease is advanced when the diagnosis is made, because early signs of cancer have been interpreted as normal concomitants of advancing age or symptoms related to coexisting diseases.

Medical Management

Medical treatment is made on the basis of the overall condition of the patient, the type of malignancy, and the presenting symptoms. For example, if the tumor is a very slow growing one and the patient, because of age or the presence of another severe disease, is unlikely to survive long enough to die of the cancer, palliative treatment may be the choice. In other cases, an all-out program of the most aggressive treatment available may be selected. Whatever the circumstances, however, the patient must have informed input into the decision.

Guidelines for Application of the Nursing Process to the Care of the Elderly Patient with Cancer

Stress the importance of cancer screening tests for the elderly at every opportunity. Since many women do not see a gynecologist after the childbearing years, there is a particular need to stress the importance of annual pelvic examinations. Inform elderly women of the increasing risk of endometrial and vaginal cancer. Explain that although noticeable symptoms do not occur until the disease is far advanced, diagnosis in an early, most curable stage can be made by pelvic examination.

Also stress to elderly patients that any new symptoms should be reported to the health care provider and not assumed to be "normal aging" or due to an already diagnosed disease.

When caring for an elderly person who is undergoing diagnostic testing for cancer or who has been diagnosed, be aware that the patient may associate cancer with the past, when the prognosis was more grim. This heightens the need for the patient to talk about the illness and to receive empathy and support. Because some elderly have developed such long-standing fears that they cannot bring themselves to speak or hear the word cancer, referring only to my "tumor," "growth," "sickness" or even using a nonverbal expression to indicate the problem, be alert to the patient's symbolic terminology and use it rather than force a confrontation with fearful words like "cancer" or "malignancy." Quite often, a simple expression of empathy like "It must feel very lonely to be seriously ill" releases a flood of pent-up feelings. Be certain to also correct patient misconceptions and provide current information based on the patient's emotional readiness to hear.

Resources

NATIONAL RESOURCES FOR CANCER PATIENTS

American Cancer Society*
1599 Clifton Road NE
Atlanta, GA 30329
(404) 320-3333

Leukemia Society of America
733 Third Avenue
New York, NY 10017

United Cancer Council
1803 N. Meridian Street
Indianapolis, IN 46202

United Ostomy Association
2001 West Beverly Boulevard
Los Angeles, CA 90057

The National Hospice Organization
1901 N. Fort Myer Drive
Arlington, VA 22209

Office of Cancer Communications
National Cancer Institute
Bethesda, MD 20205

Cancer Information Service
Nationwide toll-free telephone information service
1-800-4-CANCER

National Institutes of Health
Office of Clinical Center Communications
Building 10, Room 1C255
9000 Rockville Pike
Bethesda, MD 20892

International Association of Enterostomal Therapy
2081 Business Center Drive
Irvine, CA 92715

PROFESSIONAL ORGANIZATIONS

Oncology Nursing Society
501 Holiday Drive
Pittsburgh, PA 15220

Association of Pediatric Oncology Nurses
11508 Allecingie Parkway
Richmond, VA 23235

* Most states have local divisions. Refer to telephone book for current locations and telephone numbers.

PROFESSIONAL CANCER NURSING JOURNALS

Oncology Nursing Forum
The Oncology Nursing Press
501 Holiday Drive
Pittsburgh, PA 15220

Cancer Nursing
Raven Press
P.O. 2046
Mahopac, NY 10541

Seminars in Oncology Nursing
Grune & Stratton, Inc.
P.O. Box 6280
Duluth, MN 55806

Bibliography

American Cancer Society. 1990 facts and figures. New York: The American Cancer Society, 1989.

American Nurses' Association and the Oncology Nursing Society. Standards of oncology nursing practice. Kansas City, MO: American Nurses' Association, 1987.

Baird SB, McCorkle R, Grant M (eds). Cancer Nursing. Philadelphia: WB Saunders, 1991.

Barkas G, Duafala ME. Advances in cancer pain management: A review of patient-controlled analgesia. J Pain Symptom Manage 1988; 3(3):150.

Bavier AR. Nursing management of acute oral complications of cancer. NCI Monogr 1990; (9):123.

CA: Cancer J Clin 1992; 42(1).

Carnevali D, Reiner AC. The cancer experience: Nursing diagnosis and management. Philadelphia: JB Lippincott, 1990.

Carpenito LJ: Cancer update 90. Nursing 90 1990; 20(4):61.

Carter P, Engel King C, Rumsey K, Vincent B. Biological response modifier guidelines. Recommendations for nursing education and practice. Pittsburgh PA: Oncology Nursing Society, 1989.

Casciato DA, Lowitz BB (eds). Principles of cancer management: Manual of clinical oncology. Boston: Little, Brown, 1988, pp. 3–89.

Chernecky CC, Ramsey PW. Critical nursing care of the client with cancer. Norwalk, CT: Appleton-Century-Crofts, 1984.

Clark JC, McGee RF (eds). Oncology Nursing Society: Core curriculum for oncology nursing. 2nd ed. Philadelphia: WB Saunders, 1992.

Daeffler RJ, Petrosino B (ed). Manual of oncology nursing practice. Gaithersburg, MD: Aspen, 1990.

Department of Health and Human Services. Coping with cancer. NIH Publication No. 80-2080. Bethesda, MD: National Institutes of Health, 1980.

Department of Health and Human Services. Eating hints, recipes and tips for better nutrition during cancer treatment. NIH Publication No. 91-2079. Bethesda, MD: National Institutes of Health, 1990.

Devita VT. Principles of chemotherapy. In Devita VT, Hellman S, Rosenberg SA (eds). Cancer: Principles and practice of oncology. 2nd ed. Philadelphia: JB Lippincott, 1983.

Division of Cancer Prevention and Control. Screening. In Greenwald P, Sondik E (eds). Cancer control objectives for the nation: 1985–2000. NCI Monograph, NIH Publication No. 86-2880. Bethesda, MD: National Institutes of Health, 1986.

Dodd MJ. Managing side effects of chemotherapy and radiation therapy: A guide for patients and nurses. Norwalk, CT: Appleton & Lange, 1987.

Engel G. A psychological setting of somatic disease: the giving up–given up complex. Proc Roy Soc Med 1967; 60(6):553.

Ganz PA. Current issues in cancer rehabilitation. Cancer 1990; 65(3 suppl):742.

Govani LE, Hayes JE. Drugs and nursing implications. 6th ed. Norwalk, CT: Appleton and Lange, 1988.

Green WA. The psychosocial setting of the development of leukemia and lymphoma. Ann NY Acad Sci 1966; 125:794.

Groenwald SL, Frogge MH, Goodman M, Yarboro CH (eds). Cancer nursing principles and practice. 2nd ed. Boston: Jones and Bartlett, 1990.

Haber J, et al. Comprehensive psychiatric nursing. New York: McGraw-Hill, 1987.

Hellman S. Principles of radiation therapy. In Devita VT, Hellman S, Rosenberg SA (eds). Cancer: Principles and practice of oncology. 3rd ed. Philadelphia: JB Lippincott, 1991.

Holland JC, Rowland JH (eds). Handbook of psychooncology: Psychological care of the patient with cancer. New York: Oxford University Press, 1989.

Holland JF, Frei E. Cancer medicine. 3rd ed. Philadelphia: Lea & Febiger, 1992.

Holler AI. The American Cancer Society cancer book. Garden City, NY: Doubleday, 1988.

Johnson BL, Gross J (eds). Handbook of oncology nursing. New York: John Wiley & Sons, 1985.

Knobf MK, Fisher DS. Cancer chemotherapy treatment and care. 3rd ed. Boston: G.K. Hall Medical Publishers, 1989.

Lentner C (ed). Geigy scientific tables. 8th ed. Vol. 1. Basel, Switzerland: Ciba-Geigy, 1981.

LeShan L. An emotional life-history pattern associated with neoplastic disease. Ann NY Acad Sci 1966; 125:780.

Letter. RN 1990; 53(9):9.

Murray R, Huelskoetter M. Psychiatric mental-health nursing: Giving emotional care. 2nd ed. Norwalk, CT: Appleton & Lange, 1987.

National Cancer Institute. Chemotherapy and you: A guide to self help during treatment. NIH Publication No. 88-1136. Bethesda, MD: Department of Health and Human Services, 1987.

National Institute of Health Consensus Development Conference Statement: Oral complications of cancer therapies: Diagnosis, prevention, and treatment. J Am Dent Assoc 1989; 119(1):179.

Oncology Nursing Society. Access device guidelines, Modules I–III. Pittsburgh, PA: Oncology Nursing Press, 1989–1990.

Oncology Nursing Society. Cancer chemotherapy: Guidelines and recommendations for nursing education and practice. Pittsburgh, PA: Oncology Nursing Press, 1989.

Oncology Nursing Society. Fiscus JA, Hayes NA, Rostad ME, Whedon MA. Safe handling of cytotoxic drugs. Independent study module. Pittsburgh, PA: Oncology Nursing Press, 1989, pp. 3–9.

Oncology Nursing Society and American Nurses' Association Division of Medical Surgical Nursing Practice. Outcome standards for cancer nursing practice. Kansas City, MO: American Nurses' Association, 1989.

Papalia F, O'Hara DM, Larson RL. Cancer update 90. Pain management—up the ladder. How chemotherapy stops cancer cell growth. Nursing 1990; 20(4):61.

Rosenberg S. Principles of surgical oncology. In Devita VT, Hellman S, Rosenberg SA. Cancer: Principles and practice of oncology. 3rd ed. Philadelphia: JB Lippincott, 1991.

Seeman M, Seeman T. Health behavior and personal autonomy: A longitudinal study of the sense of control in illness. J Health Soc Behav 1983; 24(6):144.

Siegel ME. The cancer patient's handbook. New York: Walker, 1986.

Simonton OC, Simonton S. Getting well again. Toronto: Bantam Books, 1980.

Tenenbaum L (ed). Cancer chemotherapy: A reference guide. Philadelphia: WB Saunders, 1989.

U.S. Department of Health and Human Services, Public Health Services. Eating hints, recipes and tips for better nutrition during cancer treatment. NIH Publication No. 81-2079. Bethesda, MD: National Institutes of Health, 1981.

U.S. Department of Health and Human Services, Public Health Services. Radiation therapy and you: A guide to self-help during treatment. NIH Publication No. 88-2227. Bethesda, MD: National Institutes of Health, 1988.

U.S. Department of Labor, Office of Occupational Medicine, Occupational Safety and Health Administration. Work Practice Guidelines for personnel dealing with cytotoxic (antineoplastic) drugs, Publication # 8.1.1., Washington D.C.: Author, 1986.

Weisman DE, et al. Handbook of cancer pain management. Madison, WI: The Wisconsin Pain Institute, 1988.

Welch-McCaffrey D (ed). Nursing considerations in geriatric oncology. Columbus, OH: Adriamycin Laboratories, 1986.

Unit Four

ADULTS WITH RESPIRATORY DYSFUNCTION

Learning Objectives

AFTER COMPLETING THIS UNIT, THE LEARNER WILL BE ABLE TO:

Chapter Twelve

1. Explain the normal anatomy and physiology of the respiratory system.
2. Describe common clinical manifestations of respiratory dysfunction.
3. Identify information and physical examination data essential to the assessment of respiratory status.
4. Describe basic diagnostic tests and modalities of medical management (respiratory therapy, oxygen therapy, artificial airways, mechanical ventilation) used in the treatment of patients with respiratory disorders.
5. Describe basic surgical procedures (pneumonectomy and lobectomy) used in the treatment of patients with respiratory disorders.
6. Identify data essential to the assessment of patients undergoing treatment of respiratory disorders.
7. State nursing diagnoses and related expected patient outcomes commonly applicable to patients undergoing treatment of respiratory disorders.
8. Describe nursing interventions, with their rationales, commonly applicable to patients undergoing treatment of respiratory disorders.
9. Explain the basis for evaluation of nursing care provided to patients undergoing treatment of respiratory disorders.
10. Identify special considerations for the elderly patient with altered respiratory function.

Chapter Thirteen

1. Describe common upper respiratory disorders in terms of etiology, pathophysiology, clinical manifestations, diagnostic procedures, and medical management.
2. Identify information and physical examination data essential to the assessment of patients with common upper respiratory disorders.
3. State nursing diagnoses and related expected patient outcomes commonly applicable to patients with upper respiratory disorders.
4. Describe nursing interventions, with their rationales, commonly applicable to patients with upper respiratory disorders.
5. Explain the basis for evaluation of nursing care provided to patients with common upper respiratory disorders.
6. Identify special considerations for the elderly patient with an upper respiratory tract disorder.

Chapter Fourteen

1. Describe common lower respiratory disorders in terms of etiology, pathophysiology, clinical manifestations, diagnostic procedures, and medical management.
2. Identify information and physical examination data essential to the assessment of patients with common lower respiratory disorders.
3. State nursing diagnoses and related expected patient outcomes commonly applicable to patients with lower respiratory disorders.
4. Describe nursing interventions, with their rationales, commonly applicable to patients with lower respiratory disorders.
5. Explain the basis for evaluation of nursing care provided to patients with common lower respiratory disorders.
6. Identify special considerations for the elderly patient with a lower respiratory tract disorder.

Chapter Twelve

KNOWLEDGE BASIC TO THE NURSING CARE *of Adults with Respiratory Dysfunction*

Respiratory function is complex and integral to the function of all other body systems. It is also directly related to the overall quality of an individual's life. To provide a foundation for studying the nursing care of patients with respiratory disorders, this chapter reviews the basic anatomy and physiology of the respiratory system and presents the major clinical manifestations of respiratory disease. It discusses assessment of respiratory status, diagnostic tests specific to problems of respiratory function, and surgical and nonsurgical modes of treatment that are common to the management of many different respiratory disorders.

Anatomy and Physiology

The respiratory system has several complex functions. The primary function is gas exchange: the delivery of oxygen to the tissues and the removal of carbon dioxide waste. Other functions include chemical synthesis of substances such as surfactant, metabolism and detoxification of drugs and toxins, and defense against infection.

Traditionally, the respiratory system is divided into two parts: the upper respiratory system, which consists of the nasal cavity, sinuses, mouth, pharynx, and larynx (Fig. 12–1), and the lower respiratory system, consisting of the trachea and the lungs, which lie within the thoracic cavity. An alternate division is made on the basis of function. Functionally, the respiratory system has three main divisions: the conducting airways, the respiratory zone, and the accessory structures such as the interstitium of the lung and the bones and muscles of the thorax.

Thorax

The bony thorax houses the lungs and the mediastinum, which contains the heart and the major blood vessels. It is primarily composed of the sternum, the thoracic portion of the vertebral column, and 12 pairs of ribs. The first seven pairs of ribs are called "true" ribs because they attach posteriorly to the vertebral column and anteriorly to the sternum via the costal cartilages. Ribs 8 to 10 are called "false" ribs because they attach to the rib above them rather than directly to the sternum. Ribs 11 and 12 are referred to as "floating" ribs because they have no direct skeletal attachment anteriorly. The spaces between the ribs are called the intercostal spaces. The angle between the xiphoid process of the sternum and the costal cartilages is the costal angle.

The diaphragm, which is the major muscle of respiration, separates the thoracic cavity from the abdominal cavity. Muscles of the thoracic wall, which also play a role in respiration, include the external intercostal muscles, which elevate the ribs and thus facilitate inspiration, and the internal intercostal muscles, which are accessory muscles of expiration. The thorax as a whole has a natural compliance that tends to cause it to spring outward and expand.

Lungs

The lungs, the chief organs of respiration, are paired, spongy, and cone shaped. The right lung, which is thicker, wider, and shorter (because of the height of the liver, which lies beneath the diaphragm on the right side) than the left lung, is di-

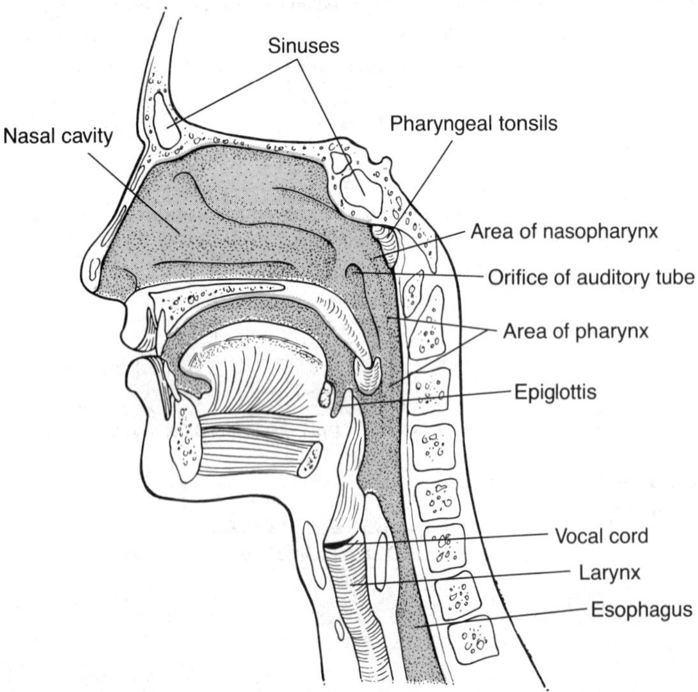

Figure 12–1.

Structure of the upper airway.

vided into three lobes: upper, middle, and lower. These lobes further subdivide into 10 segments. The left lung, which is long and narrow (because of space in the left thorax occupied by the heart) compared with the right lung, is divided into two lobes: upper and lower. These two lobes in turn are divided into eight segments.

The rounded, superior part of each lung is called the apex (plural: apexes or apices), and the concave inferior portion is called the base. The surface of the lung adjoining the thoracic cage is the costal surface, whereas that facing the mediastinum is the mediastinal surface. The cardiac notch is a concavity in the mediastinal surface that accommodates the heart. The major bronchi, blood vessels, nerves, and lymphatic vessels enter each lung through the hilum.

The lungs are lined with two thin but tough layers of serous membrane. The inner layer, which follows the contour of the lung and is virtually inseparable from it, is the visceral pleura. The outer layer, which lines the thoracic wall, covers the diaphragm, and is reflected over mediastinal structures, is called the parietal pleura. There is a small amount of lubricating fluid between the two layers in an airtight region known as the pleural space. This is a potential space and can be seen only when air or fluid collects in it, such as occurs with a pneumothorax or hemothorax. Normally the two layers are in constant, immediate contact during all phases of respiration.

Conducting Airways

The conducting airways extend from the nose to the terminal bronchioles and are primarily tubes that transport air to its ultimate destination: the respiratory units. The conducting airways can be divided into two principal parts: the upper airways and the lower airways.

UPPER AIRWAYS

The upper airways, like the traditional definition of the upper respiratory system, include the nasal cavity, sinuses, mouth, pharynx, and larynx (see Fig. 12–1).

Air in the atmosphere consists of approximately 21% oxygen and 78% nitrogen, with a small amount of other trace gases. When it is inhaled, it must be heated to body temperature and completely saturated with water vapor to prevent drying of the respiratory mucosa. Air that is at body temperature and pressure and that is saturated with water vapor is referred to as body temperature pressure saturated (BTPS). It is primarily the function of the nasal cavity to warm, filter, and humidify the air.

The pharynx consists of three sections: the nasopharynx, the oropharynx, and the laryngopharynx. The nasopharynx contains the adenoids and the openings of the eustachian tubes. These tubes connect the pharynx to the middle ear and are why middle-ear infections are common complications of upper respiratory tract infections. The oral cavity and oropharynx or throat contain the tongue. The tongue is the most common cause of airway obstruction in an unconscious person because, as a person loses muscle tone, the tongue can fall back on the oropharynx. The palatine tonsils are also located in the oropharynx.

The larynx, which connects the pharynx to the trachea, consists of nine cartilages. The epiglottis is a leaf-shaped, flexible cartilage that sits above the opening to the vocal cords. It closes over the larynx during swallowing and prevents aspiration of foreign bodies into the lower airway. Although phonation is its chief function, the larynx is also responsible for a strong cough and spasm reflex to protect against foreign substances entering the lower airways.

LOWER AIRWAYS

The lower airways consist of the trachea, bronchi, and bronchioles (Fig. 12–2) and are normally sterile. The trachea, which sits directly in front of the esophagus, consists of 16 to 20 C-shaped cartilage rings opened to the posterior. At about the level of the space between the second and third ribs, it splits at the carina into right and left main-stem bronchi. The main-stem bronchi lead to each lung. The right main-stem bronchus is shorter, wider, and at a straighter angle than the left. Consequently, any aspirated foreign material usually enters the right lung. The main bronchi divide into the lobar bronchi, which branch into segmental bronchi and then subsegmental bronchi. The conducting airways continue to branch into smaller and smaller divisions, resembling an inverted tree, hence the term *tracheobronchial tree*. Airways smaller than 2 mm in diameter are referred to as bronchioles. The terminal bronchioles are the last of the purely conducting airways. The lower airways, which expand and contract with inspiration and expiration, are referred to as anatomic dead space because they contain about 150 ml of air that never reaches the respiratory zone where gas exchange occurs.

The lower airways are lined with a specialized mucous membrane sometimes referred to as the mucociliary escalator. This respiratory mucosa is composed of pseudostratified columnar epithelium lined with small hairlike structures known as cilia. A layer of mucus sits on top of the cilia to trap dirt and debris. The cilia beat in a constant upward motion and transport the mucus to the pharynx, where it is swallowed. This mechanism is normally highly effective in keeping the lungs clear. The ciliated mucosa is, however, very sensitive to a variety of substances, such as smoke and pollutants, which can paralyze the cilia and erode the mucous membrane, rendering it nonfunctional. Anesthesia, alcohol, administration of high oxygen concentrations, poor tis-

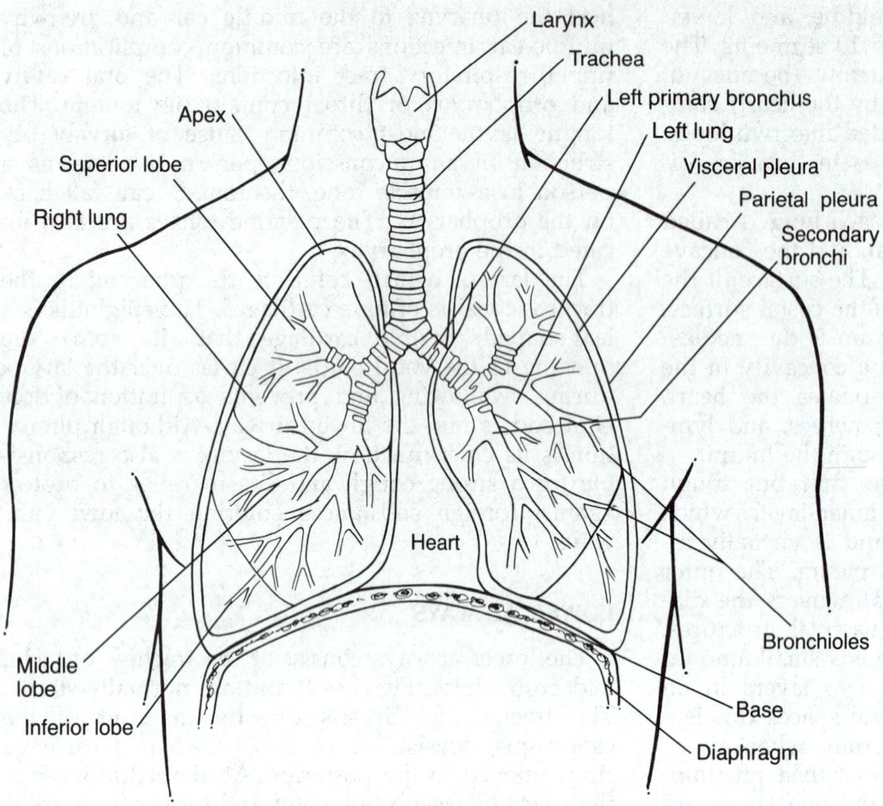

Figure 12–2.

Structure of the lower airways. Note that the right lung has three lobes and the left has two. Note also that the right main bronchus is shorter, wider, and more in line with the trachea than is the left main bronchus.

sue oxygenation, dehydration, and infection are some of the other irritants that can similarly impair the protective function of the respiratory mucosa.

Under the mucosal layer is smooth muscle, which gives the airway tone, and cartilage, which provides support. As the branches become progressively smaller, the smooth muscle, the supporting cartilage, and other tissues of the airway wall thin out.

Respiratory Zone

The respiratory bronchioles mark the transition from the conducting airways to the respiratory zone. Gas exchange begins with the respiratory bronchioles, which lead into the alveolar ducts, alveolar sacs, and ultimately the alveoli, the lumens of which are called alveolar spaces (Fig. 12–3). Adult lungs

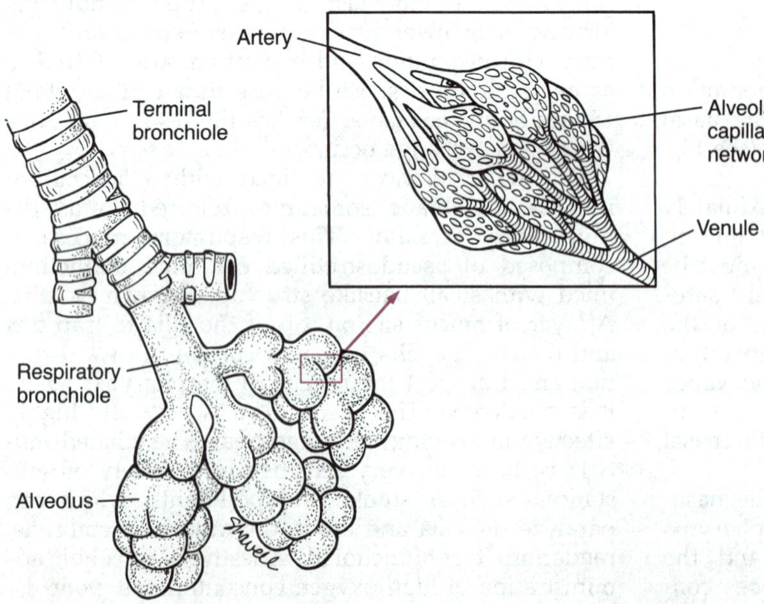

Figure 12–3.

The respiratory bronchiole feeds the alveolar sac, which is surrounded by a capillary plexus. It is here that oxygen diffuses into the blood that returns to the heart through the pulmonary artery.

contain approximately 300 million alveoli, which are surrounded by a vast network of pulmonary capillaries, providing an extremely large and effective surface area for gas exchange. The alveolar epithelium consists of several types of cells. Type I cells line most of the alveolar surface. Type II cells produce surfactant, a phospholipid that alters surface tension to provide mechanical stability to the alveoli. On expiration, it reduces surface tension and prevents alveolar collapse, and on inspiration, it decreases surface tension and helps limit expansion. Alveolar macrophages are phagocytic cells that destroy any bacteria or other foreign particles that get past the mucociliary escalator.

Between the alveoli lies the interstitium, which contains pulmonary capillaries, lymphatic channels, and nerves. The interstitium also contains elastic connective tissue, which gives the lungs their elastic recoil (i.e., the ability to return to resting position after stretching). Elastic and collagen fibers also enable the lung to expand or distend, a property known as compliance. In diseases such as emphysema, the walls between the alveoli break down, decreasing the surface area for gas exchange. The lung loses its elastic recoil and becomes hyperinflated. In pulmonary fibrosis, the connective tissue becomes replaced with scar tissue, making the lung stiff, noncompliant, and difficult to expand.

Mechanics of Ventilation

Ventilation is the bulk movement of air in and out of the respiratory tract. Effective ventilation requires air to reach the alveoli so gas exchange can occur. To accomplish this, the airway must be patent, and the thoracic cage, lung, and muscles of respiration must be intact and functioning. Respiration is the exchange of gases. External respiration occurs in the respiratory units of the lung; internal respiration occurs at the tissue level throughout the body. Effective respiration requires adequate ventilation.

The process of ventilation takes place as a result of pressure gradients between the alveoli and atmospheric air. Atmospheric pressure is normally about 760 mm Hg. The intrathoracic pressure, and consequently the intrapleural pressure, is always slightly below atmospheric pressure. The natural compliance of the lungs and thorax results from opposing forces that are balanced to create these normal resting pressures. Inspiration is the active phase of ventilation. As the diaphragm contracts, it flattens and moves downward and out, expanding the thoracic cage in both the anteroposterior and transverse diameters (Fig. 12–4). As the volume in the chest increases, the pressure in the thoracic cavity decreases even further. This is a function of the physical principle known as Boyle's law, which states that pres-

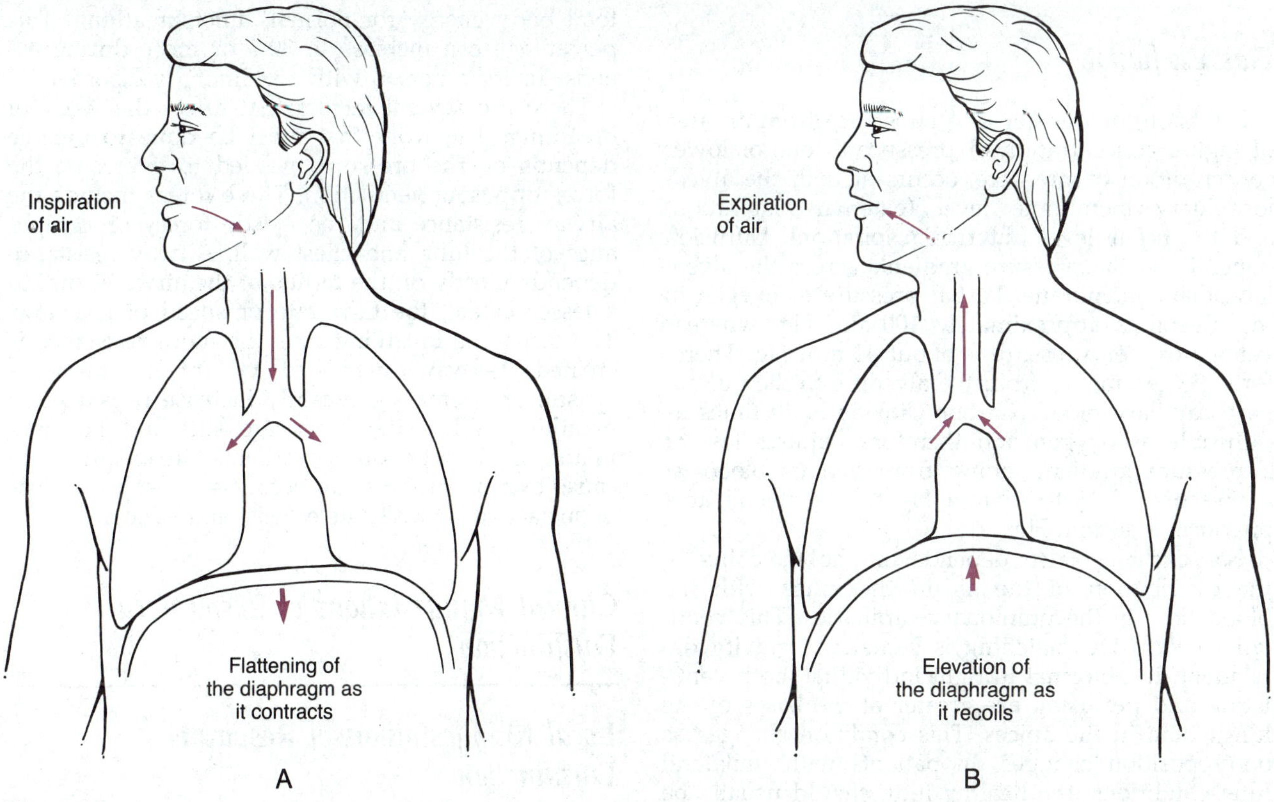

Figure 12–4.

A, During inspiration, the diaphragm flattens as it contracts, and the chest cavity is lengthened. *B*, During expiration, the diaphragm recoils, and the chest cavity shrinks.

sure and volume are inversely proportional. As the airway pressure decreases below atmospheric pressure, air moves into the lungs.

Expiration is normally passive. As the muscles relax and the lung recoils to its normal position, the volume decreases. In turn, the airway pressure increases above atmospheric pressure, causing air to move out.

Ventilation is controlled by several mechanisms. The respiratory centers are located in the medulla. These central chemoreceptors are sensitive to carbon dioxide and hydrogen ion concentrations in the cerebrospinal fluid. Slight increases in either substance stimulate an increase in ventilation. Arterial carbon dioxide tension is the primary stimulus to breathe in a normal person. To a lesser extent, oxygen deficiency can also affect ventilation. The peripheral chemoreceptors located in the carotid and aortic bodies are stimulated when the partial pressure of oxygen in the arterial blood (PaO_2) falls below the normal of 100 mm Hg, with maximal response at a PaO_2 of less than 50 to 60 mm Hg. This serves as a back-up emergency system in a patient with respiratory dysfunction. Several types of lung receptors such as pulmonary stretch receptors (Hering-Breuer reflex), irritant receptors, and J receptors also play a role, although one not completely understood, in controlling ventilation and may be responsible for the sensation of dyspnea or labored breathing.

Gas Exchange

Diffusion, or transfer of a substance from an area of higher concentration or pressure to one of lower concentration or pressure, occurs at both the alveolocapillary membrane level (external respiration) and the tissue level (internal respiration). Diffusion depends on the pressure gradients across the alveolocapillary membrane. Partial pressure of oxygen in the alveoli is approximately 100 mm Hg, whereas venous oxygen pressure is about 40 mm Hg. Therefore, oxygen moves from the alveoli into the pulmonary capillary blood. Carbon dioxide is 20 times as diffusible as oxygen and therefore requires less of a pressure gradient, going from venous blood at a pressure of 46 to 48 mm Hg to the alveoli at a pressure of 40 mm Hg.

Gas exchange also depends on the matching of the distribution of the air in the lungs with the blood flow in the pulmonary capillaries. This ventilation/perfusion matching is somewhat gravity dependent. In a normal upright individual, both ventilation and perfusion are greater at the bases of the lungs than in the apices. This condition changes as body position changes. In patients with unilateral lung conditions, the healthy lung should usually be placed in the gravity-dependent position to maximize ventilation/perfusion matching. If ventilation is present without perfusion, no gas exchange can occur. This condition is referred to as dead space. In the conducting airways where no pulmonary capillaries exist, anatomic dead space is normally present. In disorders such as pulmonary embolism and emphysema, physiologic dead space is created. Conversely, if capillaries are perfused but no ventilation is present, gas exchange cannot take place. This condition is referred to as a shunt. Atelectasis, pneumonia, and adult respiratory distress syndrome (ARDS) are examples of shunt-producing conditions.

Transport of Gases

Oxygen is transported in the blood in two ways. A small portion is carried in dissolved form in the plasma; the major portion is chemically combined with hemoglobin in the red blood cell. Normal arterial oxygen saturation of hemoglobin is 94% to 100%. It can be less than 100% because of several anatomic shunts that dump unoxygenated blood directly back into the arterial system. As the oxygen is released to the tissues, carbon dioxide diffuses into the plasma and eventually into the red blood cells for transport back to the lungs, where it is eliminated. Refer to page 74 for further discussion of gas exchange and transport.

Work of Breathing

Normally a healthy person uses less than 5% of total body energy for normal, quiet breathing. This percentage can increase to 30% or more during exercise or for a person with a pulmonary disorder.

There are several factors that affect the work of breathing. The work that must be done to breathe depends on the pressures needed to overcome the forces opposing ventilation. These forces include the airway resistance and the elastic forces or compliance of the lung and chest wall. Airway resistance depends mostly on the radius of the airways and, to a lesser extent, the flow rate or speed of gas flow. The faster the breathing rate, the more resistance is created. Airways narrowed by mucus, bronchospasm, or edema significantly increase resistance to breathing. When the lungs are stiff and noncompliant, greater pressure gradients are required to cause expansion. This can occur as a result of a loss of surfactant, fibrosis, atelectasis, and edema.

Clinical Manifestations of Respiratory Dysfunction

Local Manifestations of Respiratory Dysfunction

COUGH

Cough is a protective mechanism for clearing the lower airways. When persistent (lasting longer than

2 to 3 weeks), it may indicate the presence of a serious pulmonary disease.

A cough can be described as chronic, paroxysmal, and dry or productive. A chronic cough is commonly associated with irritation of the airway. Smoking is the most common cause, although allergies, sinus infections, chronic upper respiratory tract infections, and inhalation of polluted air can also produce a chronic cough. A paroxysmal cough is a spasmodic type that is difficult to stop. It is commonly observed in patients with asthma or chronic bronchitis. A dry cough is one not accompanied by the production of sputum, whereas a productive cough is associated with the expectoration of sputum.

EXCESSIVE NASAL SECRETIONS

Infection of the upper respiratory tract, irritants, or allergens that induce an allergic response produce congestion of the nasal mucosa. Allergic states produce a pale mucosa with a thin, watery discharge. With infection, the nasal mucosa is very reddened (hyperemic) and the discharge is purulent.

Excessive nasal secretions are common in persons exposed to very dry air in artificially heated environments or to smoke, dust, or fumes. Excessive nasal secretions drain into the back of the throat as a postnasal drip. This may produce coughing, frequent throat clearing, or, in extreme cases, gagging (the vomit reflex).

EXPECTORATION OF SPUTUM

Sputum production is related to irritation of the lower respiratory tract. This irritation stimulates the mucous glands to produce increased amounts of mucus, which is coughed up as sputum. Normally the respiratory tract produces 100 ml of mucus each day. When respiratory passages are irritated, this amount can be increased to as much as 1000 ml each day.

Sputum is described as mucoid, purulent, mucopurulent, rusty, or blood-tinged. Mucoid sputum is white and clear. Purulent sputum may be yellow or greenish as a result of the presence of mucus and pus. Mucopurulent means there is more mucus than pus in the sputum. Rusty sputum is exudate containing blood from capillary destruction. Blood-tinged mucus occurs in certain diseases such as bronchiectasis, tuberculosis, pulmonary infarct, and carcinoma. Blood in the sputum (hemoptysis) may be a presenting sign of either tuberculosis or carcinoma. It is frequently bright red and frothy and has an alkaline pH reaction.

Thick sputum may indicate a need for hydration because mucus is normally 95% water.

PAIN

The lung tissue itself is insensitive to pain. Pain occurs when the muscles of the chest wall or the pleura are affected by disease. Three different types of chest pain—pleuritic, intercostal, and generalized—can occur as a result of respiratory dysfunction. Pleuritic pain is a catching, transient type produced when the thorax is moved. It is usually intensified when breathing deeply and is felt unilaterally. There is often tenderness in the area of the pain. Intercostal pain is produced when coughing or straining causes compression of the intercostal muscles.

DYSPNEA

Labored or difficult breathing (dyspnea) is a common clinical manifestation of respiratory dysfunction. The patient may present with rapid, audible, labored breathing; marked use of the accessory muscles of respiration; dilated nostrils; tachycardia; anxious expression; gasping; and a bluish or gray color to the skin (cyanosis).

Systemic Manifestations of Respiratory Dysfunction

The main function of the lungs is the regulation of arterial oxygenation and carbon dioxide removal. Because of its significant functional reserve, the respiratory system is capable of regulating and maintaining the arterial blood gases (ABGs) despite the presence of pathologic conditions. When the functional reserve is exceeded, however, impairment of oxygenation and carbon dioxide elimination results in systemic manifestations of respiratory dysfunction because of a lack of oxygen in the tissues or the accumulation of carbon dioxide.

HYPOXEMIA AND HYPOXIA

Hypoxemia is insufficient oxygenation of the blood and commonly refers to decreased PaO_2 or saturation below normal levels. Hypoxia is inadequate tissue oxygenation. Anoxia or the absence of oxygen is an extreme degree of hypoxia. Ventilation/perfusion mismatching is the most common cause of hypoxemia and hypoxia. Other causes are high altitude, inadequate oxygen in inspired air, anemia or abnormal types of hemoglobin preventing normal transport, circulatory impairment such as hypotension or low cardiac output, and inability of the cells to use oxygen such as with cyanide poisoning. ABGs are the most reliable indicator of hypoxemia. Most symptoms of hypoxemia are not present unless it is severe.

Cyanosis is the commonly accepted sign of hypoxemia. The slightly blue-gray discoloration of the skin and mucous membranes is due to the presence of abnormal amounts of reduced hemoglobin or other hemoglobin compounds in the capillary blood. True cyanosis can be differentiated from deposition of certain pigments by pressing over the discolored area. Cyanotic skin blanches; pigmented skin does not.

The presence of other hemoglobin compounds in the capillary blood is an uncommon cause of cyanosis, whereas cyanosis caused by unoxygenated blood in the capillaries is a common occurrence.

The presence of cyanosis does not necessarily mean there is arterial hypoxemia. Capillary blood flow and extraction of oxygen by the tissues determine how much more hemoglobin is deoxygenated while in the capillaries. For example, a marked decrease in capillary blood flow permits enough oxygen extraction by the tissues for cyanosis to appear despite adequate arterial oxygenation. This is observed in the finger tips during very cold weather.

Conversely, anemic patients may have a very low arterial blood oxygen level without cyanosis, because they do not have enough reduced hemoglobin to become visible.

The most common clinical manifestations of hypoxemia and hypoxia are tachypnea, tachycardia, and change in cerebral functions. The brain is the organ most sensitive to the lack of oxygen. Acute cerebral hypoxia results in clumsiness, impaired judgment, and a decreased level of consciousness. If severe and continued, cerebral hypoxia will lead to confusion, coma, and death. Chronic hypoxia results in fatigue, apathy, drowsiness, and muscular twitching.

Hypoxemia affects the cardiac system by increasing the heart rate and cardiac output. Cardiac arrhythmias are commonly observed in severe hypoxemia.

Hypoxemia is also an important respiratory stimulant through its effect on the peripheral chemoreceptors in the body. If a patient has a condition of long-standing carbon dioxide retention, the administration of inappropriate amounts of oxygen may result in respiratory depression by removing the hypoxemic ventilatory drive.

Severe hypoxemia causes metabolic acidosis. Because of the inadequate tissue oxygenation, anaerobic metabolism, or metabolism in the absence of oxygen, takes place. The end products of such metabolism include lactic acid, the accumulation of which results in metabolic acidosis.

HYPERCAPNIA

Hypercapnia, or hypercarbia, is the the state of increased (above the normal limit) amounts of carbon dioxide in the arterial blood. Hypercapnia indicates that alveolar ventilation is inadequate for proper elimination of carbon dioxide.

Severe hypercapnia may result in loss of consciousness. Carbon dioxide dilates cerebral blood vessels, with a resultant increase in blood flow to the brain. It has a constricting effect on the pulmonary vessels. As carbon dioxide accumulates, there is an increased hydrogen ion concentration (acidosis), and increased pulse rate, blood pressure, dizziness, headaches, and mental clouding occur.

HYPOCAPNIA

Hypocapnia is a low (below the normal limit) amount of carbon dioxide in the arterial blood. It occurs when ventilation increases out of proportion to the metabolic production of carbon dioxide (blowing off too much carbon dioxide). This excessive alveolar ventilation is known as hyperventilation. Clinically, hypocapnia can be determined only by ABG studies.

Hypocapnia can result in respiratory alkalosis. The clinical symptoms include lightheadedness, fatigue, inability to concentrate, irritability, tingling, muscle twitching, and impaired consciousness. The most common cause of hyperventilation is an anxiety reaction.

Respiratory Failure

Respiratory failure is a nonspecific clinical diagnosis denoting the inability of the respiratory system to supply the body with needed oxygen and rid it of carbon dioxide waste. In terms of ABG values, it can be arbitrarily defined as a PaO_2 of less than 60 mm Hg or a $PaCO_2$ of greater than 45 mm Hg (Murray & Nadel, 1988, p. 1973). Respiratory failure may be acute or chronic and, depending on its cause, can be classified as ventilatory failure or oxygenation failure.

Ventilatory failure, the chief characteristic of which is alveolar hypoventilation with resultant hypoxemia, has many causes. These include upper airway obstruction, depression of the respiratory center in the medulla, impaired transmission of nervous impulses from the respiratory center to the muscles of respiration, and mechanical abnormalities of the lung or the chest wall. Depression of the respiratory center may occur after drug overdose, anesthesia, head trauma, specific types of cerebrovascular accidents, brain tumors, meningitis, encephalitis, hypoxia, or hypercapnia. Impaired transmission of nervous impulses to the muscles of respiration may be due to a lesion at the cervical level of the spinal cord or to a disorder of the involved nerves or neuromuscular junctions. Thus, ventilatory failure is seen in patients with polyneuritis, poliomyelitis, muscular dystrophy, Guillain-Barré syndrome, multiple sclerosis, and myasthenia gravis. Conditions that interfere with lung expansion include pleural effusion, pneumothorax, hemothorax, and flail chest.

Ventilatory failure is also a risk after surgery, particularly after upper abdominal or thoracic procedures and after extensive trauma.

In oxygenation failure, hypoxemia is most often the result of ventilation/perfusion mismatching or physiologic shunting. Disorders associated with oxygenation failure include pneumonia, atelectasis, severe pulmonary edema, and pulmonary embolism.

Management of respiratory failure consists of oxygenation or ventilation, or both, along with treatment of the underlying disorder.

Assessment of Respiratory Status

Patient History

Obtain a thorough patient history as a basis for individualizing care. Question the patient about the predominant complaint. It is usually this complaint that has caused the patient to seek medical attention, and by dealing with it initially a sense of acceptance and understanding is conveyed, which helps establish a trusting relationship. Use open-ended questions to determine the onset of the present problem and the patient's perception of it.

Review the patient's health history, including illnesses since birth. Elicit information about the frequency of illnesses and treatments, with particular attention to colds, pneumonia, allergies, sinus problems, tuberculosis, and asthma. Note the date of the last chest film, tuberculin skin test, and any pulmonary function tests.

Review the family history. Include information about the health status or causes of death of immediate family members. If the patient has reported any hereditary diseases, review the family history for similar problems.

As part of the history, obtain information about smoking and the occupational and geographic environment. Ascertain how long the patient has smoked and how many packs per day. If the patient states he or she does not smoke, follow up by asking whether he or she has ever smoked. Some people will say they do not smoke or have stopped, when in fact they just stopped 2 days ago.

Because many respiratory dysfunctions are associated with occupational pollutants such as chemicals, fumes, asbestos, beryllium, coal, magnesium silicate, and organic dust materials such as moldy wheat and hay, question about type of employment and location of home to provide clues as to possible exposure to these hazards. If the patient was in the armed forces, ask about possible exposure to Agent Orange or other carcinogens.

Direct the interview toward specific clinical manifestations of respiratory dysfunction: cough, nasal secretions, pain, dyspnea, and fatigue.

Question about cough. If cough is present, determine its frequency and duration; coughs lasting longer than 2 to 3 weeks may indicate serious respiratory dysfunction. Ask the patient to describe the type of cough; productive, nonproductive, or paroxysmal. If the cough is productive, ascertain the quantity, color, consistency, and odor of the expectorate.

If nasal secretions are present, ask about frequency and duration. Ask whether they are present when indoors or outdoors. Question the patient about the environment as it relates to the presence or absence of secretions.

Ask about pain. If present, is it associated with deep breathing or coughing? Is it transient or steady? Carefully assess respiratory rate and depth when a patient is experiencing painful breathing because this is often associated with shallow respirations as a result of an attempt to limit movement of the chest.

Question about dyspnea. Remember that persons with normal respiratory function experience dyspnea with strenuous activity such as running upstairs. Determine the level of activity that brings on the dyspnea. For example, can the patient do light housework or mow the lawn without experiencing dyspnea? Question the patient about other related symptoms such as cough. Ask whether the dyspnea occurs at night or during the day. Does the patient use one or two pillows for sleeping?

Ask about fatigue, and correlate it with the level of activity. The patient who experiences fatigue after light activity such as personal grooming or light housework might be hypoxic.

Do a general review of other body systems to assist the patient to remember all signs and symptoms. Record all pertinent information.

Physical Examination

The next step of the nursing respiratory assessment is the physical examination. Proceed in a stepwise manner through inspection, palpation, percussion, and auscultation (Table 12–1). Draw standard imaginary lines through the thorax to localize and record assessment findings (Fig. 12–5). Perform the physical examination in a private, warm, well-lit, and quiet room. Absence of background noise makes it easier to hear breath sounds.

INSPECTION

Begin this part of the physical examination with a general observation of the patient during the inter-

Table 12–1. RESPIRATORY PHYSICAL ASSESSMENT

Inspection:	Posture, contour, movement, dimensions of chest, flared nostrils, use of accessory muscles, skin color, and rate, depth, and rhythm of respirations
Palpation:	Respiratory excursion, tactile fremitus, masses, and tenderness
Percussion:	Flat, dull, tympanic, resonant, and hyperresonant sounds; diaphragmatic excursion
Auscultation:	Breath sounds (vesicular, bronchial, bronchovesicular), voice sounds (bronchophony, egophony, whispered pectoriloquy), adventitious sounds (crackles, wheezing)

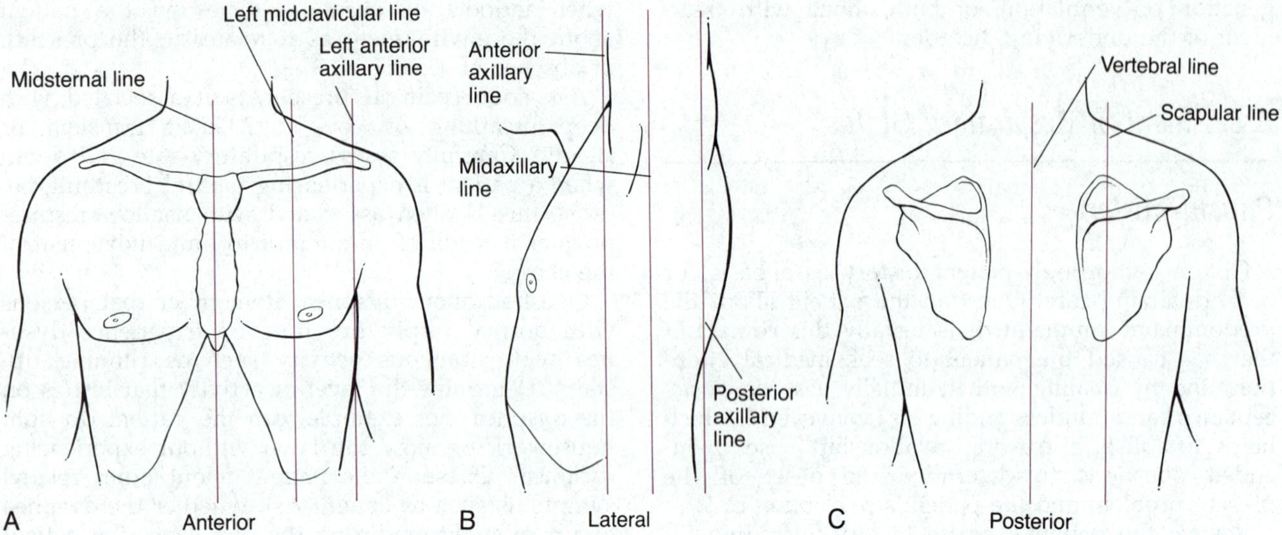

Figure 12–5.

When examining the chest, draw the imaginary lines shown here, and localize and record findings in relationship to them.

view. Note the patient's overall condition, including nutritional status. Observe the patient's posture to obtain clues to the general respiratory condition. Persons with respiratory problems frequently assume positions that help facilitate their breathing, such as sitting upright with arms supported on a table. During the interview, observe whether the patient is able to speak a full sentence without pausing to take a breath.

Ask the patient to disrobe to the waist and sit upright. Observe for flared nostrils, gasping, open mouth, pursed lip breathing, and the use of accessory muscles. These signs indicate respiratory distress. Inspect the skin for lesions, color, and evidence of loss of subcutaneous tissue.

Assess the respiratory rate, depth, and rhythm during inspection. Do this without the patient's awareness because it may alter the normal respiratory pattern. Keep in mind that the normal respiratory rate in adults is 14 to 20 per minute. An increased respiratory rate (tachypnea) may indicate hypoxia. A decreased rate (bradypnea) may be seen when the respiratory center in the medulla is depressed, such as with head injury or drug overdose.

Observe the depth of respirations to obtain important information concerning alveolar ventilation.

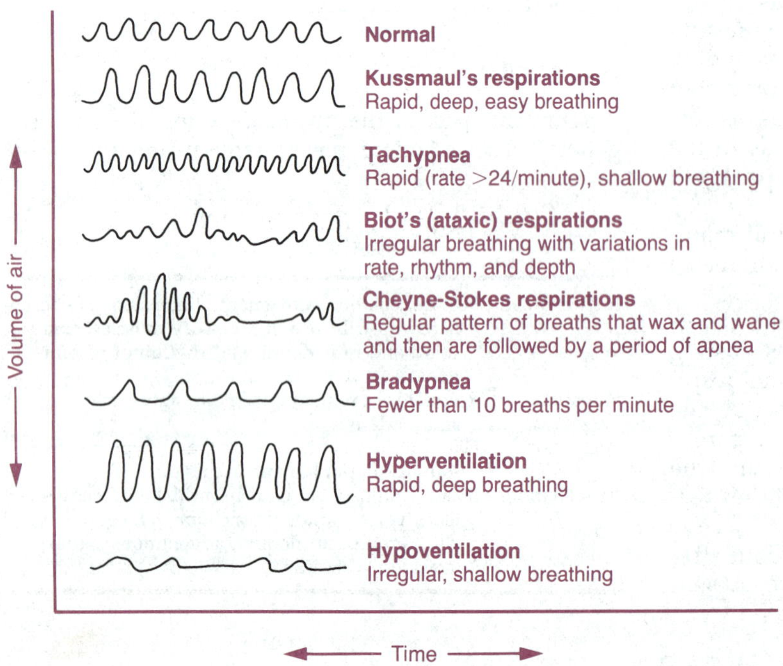

Figure 12–6.

Schematic representation of abnormal breathing patterns.

An increase in the depth of respirations is called hyperpnea. An increase in both the depth and rate is known as hyperventilation. An extreme of hyperventilation, or a rapid, deep breathing, is known as Kussmaul's respiration and is seen in metabolic acidosis. A shallow breathing pattern does not provide air to the alveoli and carbon dioxide is not removed from the lungs. This pattern can result in hypercapnia, hypoxemia, and eventually hypoxia. Patients experiencing painful breathing frequently have this pattern.

Respiratory rhythm usually indicates the status of neurologic control of breathing. In the presence of brain damage, Biot's breathing may occur. These are respirations that vary in depth with irregular periods of apnea (cessation of breathing). Cheyne-Stokes respiration is a cycle of apnea and hyperpnea. See Figure 12–6 for schematic representations of these and other common breathing patterns.

Observe the duration of inspiration and expiration. Expiration, the passive process, is normally 1.5 times as long as inspiration, which requires energy. Prolonged expiration is associated with emphysema resulting from air trapping, which makes it difficult to move air out of the lungs.

Assess the muscles used for breathing. In thin persons, a slight retraction (drawing in of the spaces between the ribs) is normal during quiet breathing. More than slight retraction, however, indicates the use of accessory muscles. In the presence of difficult breathing, the accessory muscles of respiration, such as the neck and shoulder muscles, the scalenes, the sternocleidomastoids, and the trapezius, may be used to assist ventilation. Marked retraction during inspiration, particularly if asymmetric, may indicate blockage of a branch of the respiratory tree. Bulging during expiration implies obstruction of airflow, as in emphysema or pleural effusion.

Note symmetry of the chest wall. Inspect the slope of the ribs and the costal angle. Normally the ribs are curved at an oblique angle of about 45 degrees. In chronic obstructive diseases, they may be fixed in a more rigid, linear position and appear horizontal.

Observe the contour of the chest wall closely. Normally the lateral diameter of the thorax is twice as large as the anteroposterior diameter, or a ratio of 1:2 (Fig. 12–7*A*). In infants and patients with emphysema, this ratio may be 1:1. Some of the abnormalities commonly seen on inspection of the thorax include the following:

Funnel chest (pectus excavatum): a congenital condition in which the sternum is abnormally depressed and the anteroposterior diameter is decreased (see Fig. 12–7*B*).

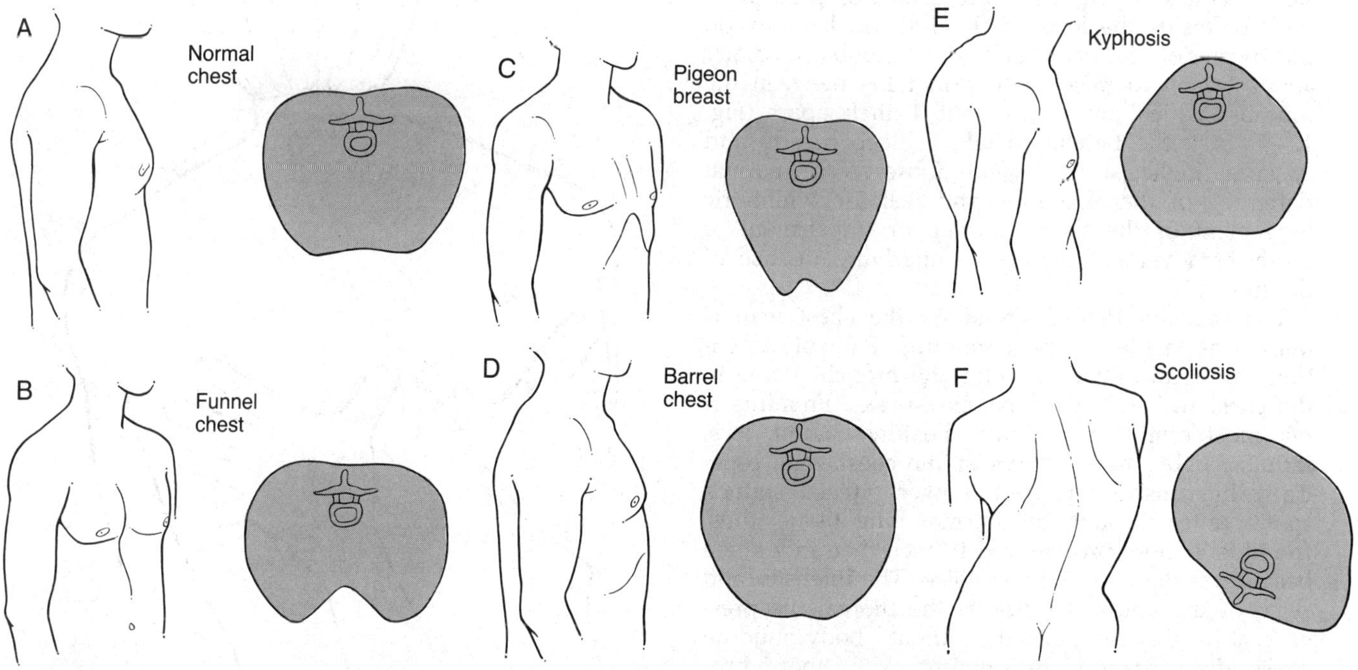

Figure 12–7.

Common abnormalities of the chest. *A*, Normal chest. Elliptic shape with anteroposterior diameter roughly half of the transverse diameter. *B*, Funnel chest. Depression of the sternum starting at second intercostal space and most marked at the xiphoid process. Exaggerated on inspiration. *C*, Pigeon breast. Protrusion of the sternum with depressions at the costochondral junctions and backward sloping of the ribs. *D*, Barrel chest. Anteroposterior diameter enlarged to equal the transverse diameter. Ribs are horizontal rather than downward-sloped. *E*, Kyphosis. Exaggerated posterior curvature of the thoracic spine. *F*, Scoliosis. Lateral S-shaped curvature of the thoracic and lumbar spine.

Pigeon breast (pectus carinatum): abnormal prominence of the sternum with an increase in the anteroposterior diameter (see Fig. 12–7*C*).
Barrel chest: chest appears rounded, with the sternum pulled forward; is associated with emphysema or normal aging (see Fig. 12–7*D*).
Kyphosis (hunchback): an exaggerated curvature of the thoracic spine (see Fig. 12–7*E*).
Scoliosis: a lateral deformity of the spine, frequently identified in early adolescence (see Fig. 12–7*F*).

Observe for finger clubbing, which is a significant finding. Inspect the angle between the nail bed and the digit (Fig. 12–8). Normally this angle is 20 degrees. A flattened angle is an indication of early clubbing. In advanced clubbing, the nail is rounded over the end of the finger and the distal phalange appears bulbous. The nail bed feels soft and spongy. Clubbing occurs when the body attempts to compensate for chronic hypoxia and develops collateral circulation to areas of impaired oxygenation. Clubbing is associated with pulmonary disease, particularly chronic obstructive pulmonary disease (COPD). It is also seen in patients with congenital heart conditions and heart disease.

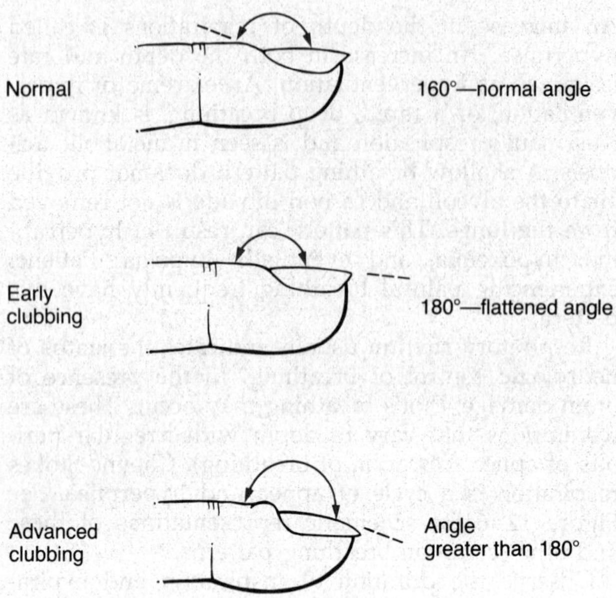

Figure 12–8.

Clubbing of the fingers.

PALPATION

With the pads of your fingers, palpate the anterior, posterior, and lateral portions of the chest for pain, tenderness, and masses. Also palpate to assess respiratory excursion (estimation of thoracic expansion). With your thumbs about 2 inches apart, place your palms at the level of the 10th rib laterally on the posterior thorax. Slide the thumbs medially about 1 inch to raise loose skin folds between the thumbs, which are now about 1 inch apart (Fig. 12–9). Ask the patient to take a deep breath, and observe the chest movement. Observe for normal flattening of the skin fold, and feel for symmetric movement of the thorax. A lag or impairment of thoracic movement indicates underlying disease of the lung.

The capacity to feel sound on the chest wall is known as tactile or vocal fremitus. Palpable vibrations are transmitted through the bronchial tree to the chest wall when the patient speaks. Fremitus is felt most easily over a thin, healthy patient. It is influenced by the thickness of the chest wall, especially by muscle thickness. Lower pitched sounds travel better through the normal lung tissue; thus, fremitus is more pronounced in men than in women because of the deeper male voice. The intensity and pitch of the voice, the size of the thorax, the presence of lung disease, and the patient's body build all cause the vibrations in fremitus. It is more pronounced over the large bronchi and becomes less so over the periphery of the lungs. Fremitus can be increased in conditions in which lung consolidation is exaggerated, such as lobar pneumonia in which the sound waves hit a dense surface. Fremitus is

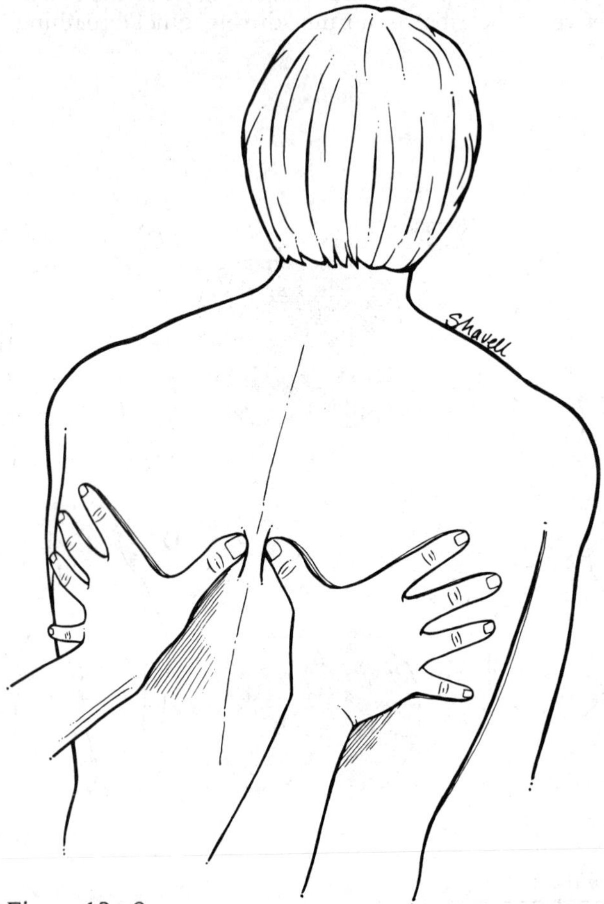

Figure 12–9.

Palpating to assess respiratory excursion. Note skin folds approximately 1 inch apart between the thumbs.

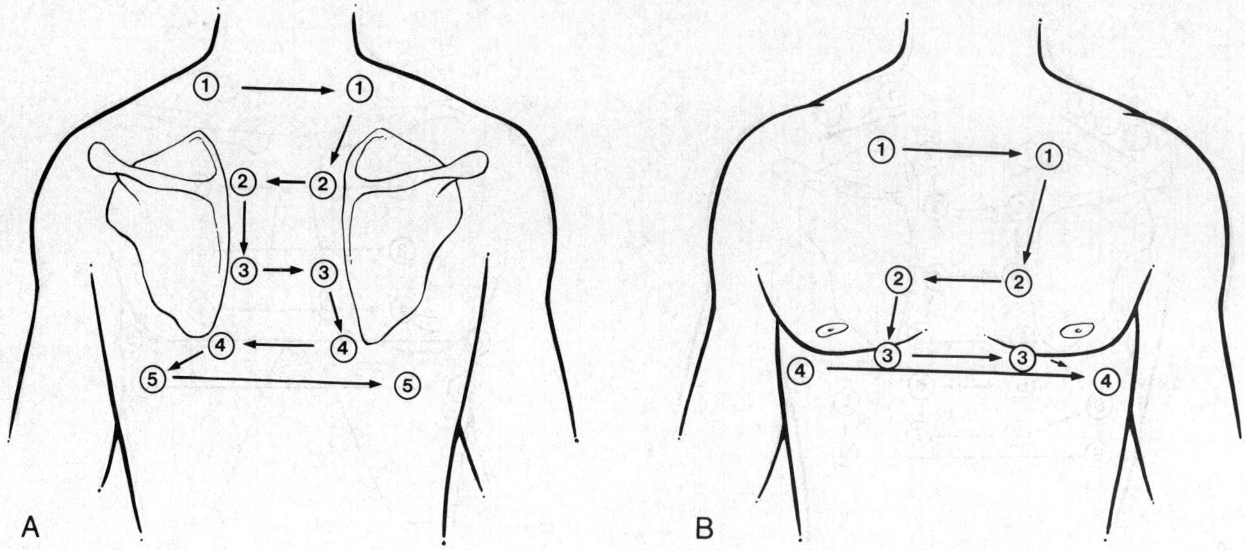

Figure 12–10.

Sequence of palpation for vocal fremitus.

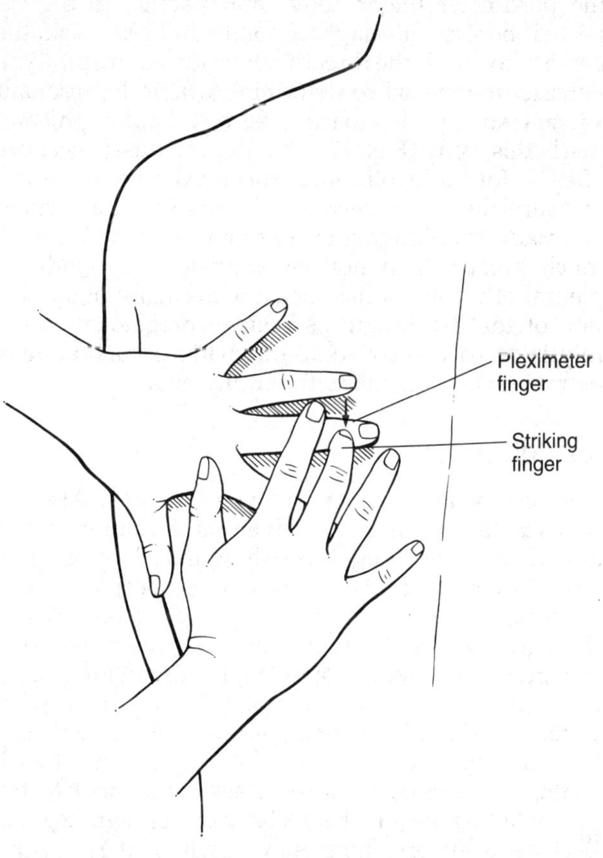

Figure 12–11.

To perform percussion, place the index or middle finger of one hand on the chest wall (this is the pleximeter finger). Strike the pleximeter finger with the middle finger of the other hand (this is the striking finger) near the interphalangeal joint.

decreased or absent when the voice is decreased, the bronchus is obstructed, or the pleural space is occupied by fluid, air, or solid mass.

Use the palmar surface of the fingers and hands or the ulnar aspect of the extended hands placed on the thorax to elicit vocal fremitus. Figure 12–10 demonstrates the sequence of the examination. Use only one hand to facilitate comparison. Ask the patient to repeat the word *ninety-nine* with each movement of the hands.

PERCUSSION

Percussion involves listening to the sounds produced by gently striking the chest wall. This technique sets the chest wall and underlying tissue into motion, producing audible sounds and palpable vibrations. Percussion helps to determine whether underlying tissues are air filled, fluid filled, or solid. Place the index or middle finger of one hand on the chest wall, and strike the stationary finger with the middle finger of the other hand close to the tip near the distal interphalangeal joint (Fig. 12–11).

Describe the quality of percussed sounds in relation to their pitch, intensity, and duration. The pitch is the number of vibrations per second. Intensity is the amplitude of the sound wave, and the duration is the length of time the sound is heard. The five types of sounds detected by percussion are flat, dull, tympanic, resonant, and hyperresonant. A flat (high pitch, very little intensity, decreased duration) sound is heard when a solid area is percussed. This sound may imply the presence of a pleural effusion or mass. Dull (higher pitch, low intensity, very short duration) sounds are heard when there is no air or fluid in the lung such as with consolidation or com-

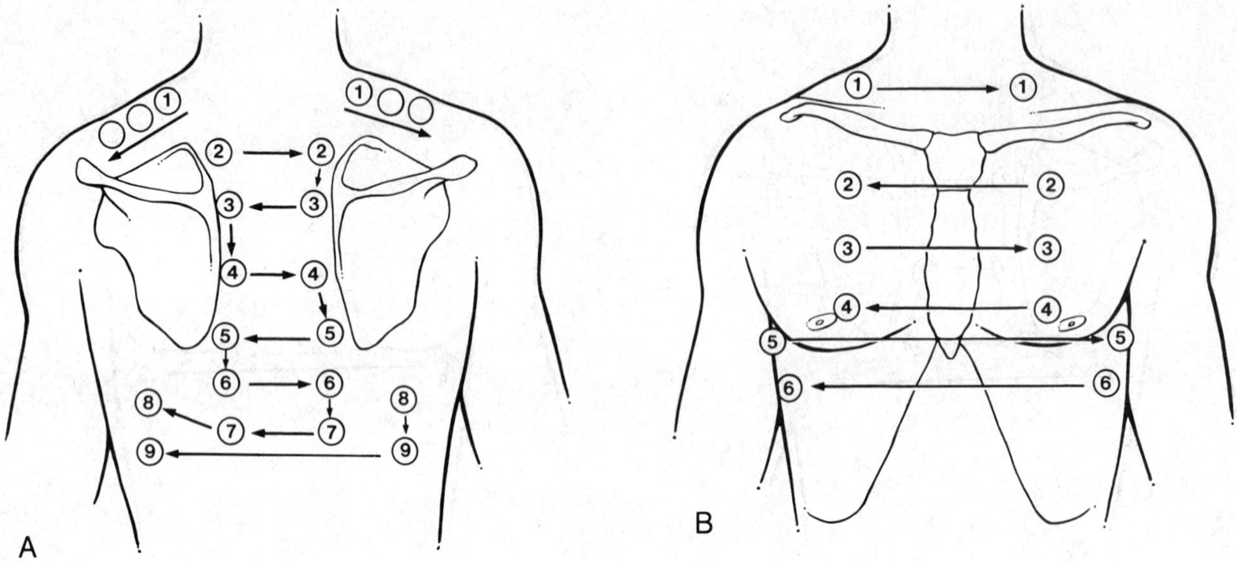

Figure 12–12.

Sequence of percussion and auscultation.

pression atelectasis. Tympanic (high pitch, loud intensity, long duration) sounds are normally heard over the stomach and bowel and below the left hemidiaphragm. Tympany over the chest is considered abnormal. Resonant (low pitch, hollow, moderately loud) sounds are normal. They are produced over the greater part of the lung and are usually of long duration. Hyperresonant (low pitch, booming) sounds are abnormal. They occur when there is free air in the thoracic cavity such as in emphysema. Perform percussion, like palpation, in an organized manner, as shown in Figure 12–12.

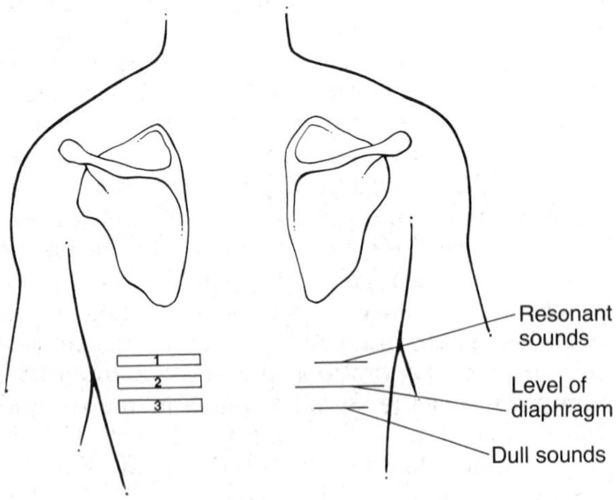

Figure 12–13.

Determine diaphragmatic excursion by holding the pleximeter finger above and parallel to the expected border of diaphragmatic dullness and percuss downward. Measure and mark the distance between the levels of dullness during inspiration and expiration. Normally it is 5 to 7 cm.

Determine the excursion of the diaphragm. Hold the pleximeter finger above and parallel to the expected border of diaphragmatic dullness. Ask the patient to hold the breath after forced inspiration. Percuss downward to determine where the resonant sounds end at the margin of the diaphragm, and mark this spot (Fig. 12–13). Repeat this procedure after a forced expiration. For maximum accuracy, measure the space between the marks with a ruler. Normally diaphragmatic excursion is 5 to 7 cm. A much greater than normal excursion may indicate pleural effusion, ascites, or an abnormally high location of the diaphragm as seen in pregnancy or paralysis. A decreased diaphragmatic excursion may be present in patients with emphysema.

AUSCULTATION

Assess breath sounds and voice sounds. Also assess for the presence of adventitious sounds when auscultating the lungs. Breath sounds have characteristic changes that are related to specific disease processes. Ask the patient to take deep breaths through the mouth while listening with the diaphragm of the stethoscope. While auscultating, keep in mind the pulmonary anatomy to determine what portion of the lung is being assessed. Because it may be necessary to listen to two full respirations at each anatomic location, be sure to ask the patient to tell you whether he or she feels dizzy or lightheaded. Because deep breathing may result in these symptoms of hyperventilation, allow the patient to rest and breathe normally once or twice during the respiratory examination if needed.

Breath sounds are heard as a result of the transmission of vibrations produced by the movement of air in the respiratory passages from the larynx to the alveoli. Voice sounds are heard as a result of vibrations produced by sound waves from the larnyx. Adventitious sounds are abnormal sounds superimposed over the breath sounds.

Normal breath sounds are described as vesicular, bronchial, and bronchovesicular. Keep in mind during the examination the locations at which each sound is normal. Vesicular breath sounds are heard as quiet, low-pitched sounds with a long inspiratory phase and a short expiratory phase. They are heard over most of the lung field except over the sternum and between the scapulae. Vesicular sounds are produced by the movement of air in the bronchioles and alveoli.

Bronchial breath sounds are high-pitched, very loud, and normally heard over the trachea. Bronchial breath sounds have a louder and longer expiratory phase. Make careful note of any bronchial sounds heard over any other portion of the lung, because this indicates respiratory dysfunction.

Bronchovesicular sounds are of medium pitch and are heard between the trachea and peripheral lung. Decreased breath sounds are present when there is fluid, air, or increased tissue in the pleural space that interferes with the transfer of the vibrations to the chest wall. Diminished breath sounds are present when there is obstruction. Patients with severe barrel chest have diminished breath sounds because of torso configuration.

Voice sounds are vibrations produced by the spoken voice that are transmitted to the chest wall via the tracheobronchial tree. During this process, the sounds are diminished in intensity so that syllables are no longer distinguishable. There are three abnormal voice sounds: bronchophony, egophony, and whispered pectoriloquy.

With bronchophony, vocal resonance is increased in intensity and clarity. Place the diaphragm of the stethoscope over various sites on the chest wall, and ask the patient to speak in a normal voice, repeating the word *ninety-nine.*

Egophony is a condition in which the spoken voice has a nasal or bleating sound. Ask the patient to repeat the letter *e* as you listen with the stethoscope. If you hear an *a* sound rather than an *e* sound, the presence of consolidation, usually pleural effusion, is indicated.

To auscultate whispered pectoriloquy, ask the patient to whisper "one, two, three" repeatedly. Normally, these sounds are very muffled. In the presence of very dense consolidation, transmission of high-frequency components of sounds are so enhanced that even whispered words are heard with unusual clarity.

Bronchophony, egophony, bronchial breathing sounds, and an increase in vocal fremitus all indicate an airless or solid consolidation. Therefore, any abnormality detected during percussion or palpation should be more fully assessed during auscultation. Conversely, if normal breath sounds are auscultated in all lung fields, voice sounds need not be routinely assessed.

Adventitious breath sounds, or superimposed sounds in the lungs, indicate the presence of an abnormal condition that affects the bronchial tree and alveoli. In the past, there has been a wide variety of terms used to describe these added lung sounds. Today there are two classifications for adventitious breath sounds: discrete, noncontinuous sounds called crackles and continuous musical sounds of greater duration called wheezes.

Crackles, previously referred to as rales or crepitations, are discrete, noncontinuous sounds that are the result of delayed reopening of deflated airways. They are heard during inspiration as a series of tiny explosions as these deflated airways are reinflated. Fine crackles are heard at the end of inspiration and originate from the alveoli. This sound can be reproduced by rubbing together several strands of hair next to one's ear. Coarse crackles are audible early during inspiration and have a gross, moist sound. The presence of crackles may indicate pneumonia, bronchitis, bronchiectasis, or congestive heart failure. Loud gurgling sounds during inspiration and expiration are produced by secretions in the trachea and large bronchi. They are heard in association with fulminating pulmonary edema and in moribund patients who cannot cough up their secretions. This sound is sometimes referred to as the "death rattle."

Friction rub (pleural rub) is heard during inspiration and expiration over a relatively small portion of the chest wall. It is a crackling, grating sound caused by the jerky movement of pleural surfaces that are inflamed. Friction rubs resemble crackles acoustically. This sound can be imitated by rubbing the thumb and index finger together next to one's ear.

Wheezes, formally called rhonchi, are a continuous musical sound of greater duration. These sounds are produced by air flowing through airways that are narrowed or practically filled with fluid or mucus. Wheezing is most typical during expiration but may occur in both inspiration and expiration. When recording these findings, note whether it was an inspiratory or expiratory wheeze, or both. If the obstruction causing the wheeze is secretion, the wheezing may be cleared with coughing.

When wheezes originate in the smaller bronchi and bronchioles, they may be high pitched. Obstruction in the larger bronchi produces a lower pitched, sonorous sound. Wheezing is most common in patients with emphysema and asthma.

Diagnostic Procedures

Pulmonary Function Studies

Pulmonary function studies measure the functional ability of the lungs by comparing the patient's

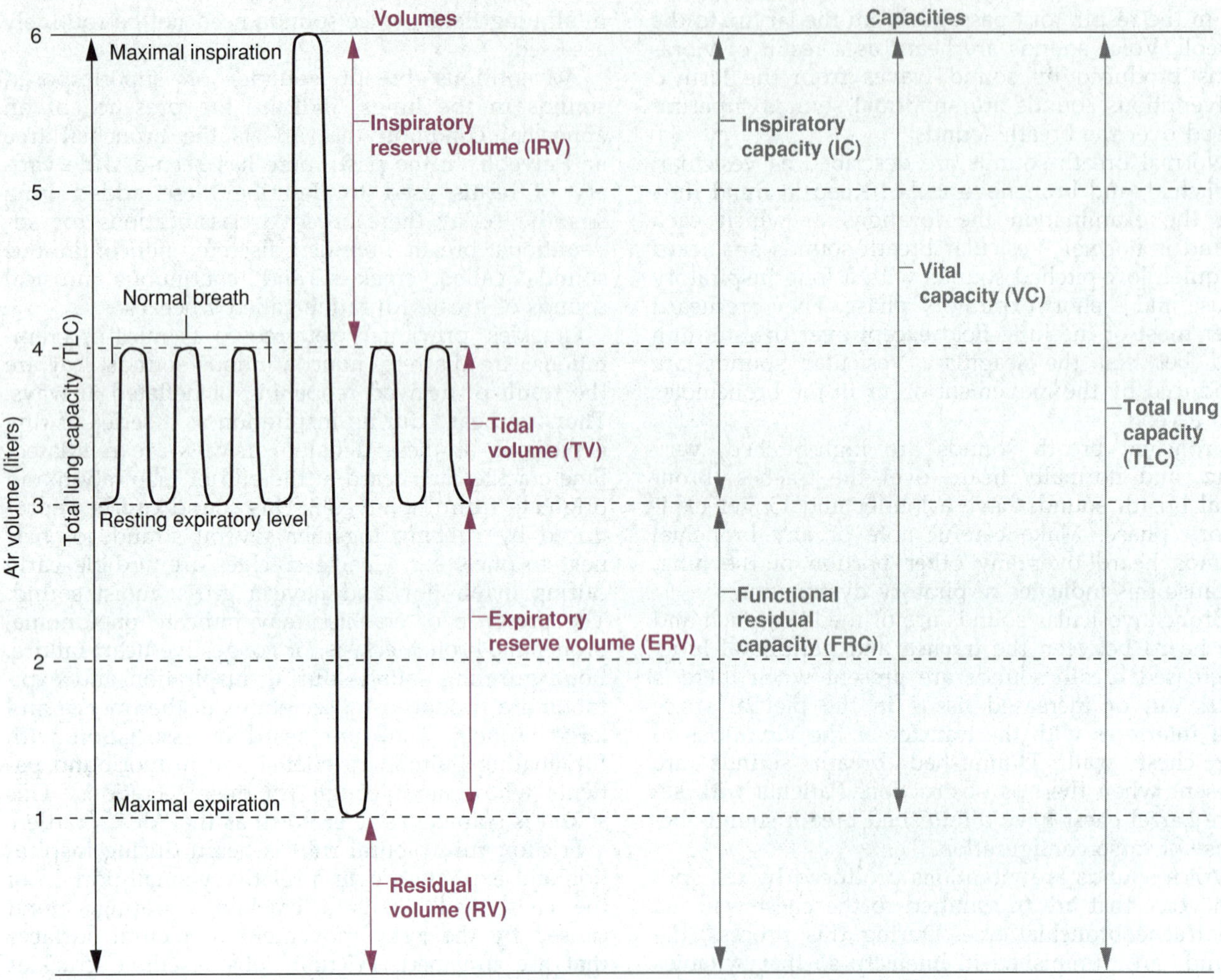

Figure 12–14.

Schematic representation of pulmonary volumes and capacities.

lung volumes and capacities with those of other people of the same age, sex, height, and race.

There are four basic lung volumes: inspiratory reserve volume, tidal volume, expiratory reserve volume, and residual volume. Together, these volumes represent the maximum volume to which the lungs can be expanded.

When evaluating the pulmonary cycle, it is sometimes necessary to consider two or more volumes together. These combinations are called pulmonary capacities (Fig. 12–14).

Lung volumes and capacities can vary with age, sex, height, and weight. They can also vary with the position of the body. Most volumes and capacities decrease when a patient lies down and increase when a patient stands. This is caused by two factors. First, when in the supine position, there is a tendency for the abdominal contents to press upward against the diaphragm. Second, there is an increase in the pulmonary blood volume in the supine position, which correspondingly decreases the space available for air.

Volumes and capacities used in pulmonary function studies are described in Table 12–2.

USES

Pulmonary function tests are used to diagnose specific types of lung abnormalities and to assess the risk of respiratory complications in surgical patients. They are also used to monitor the course of pulmonary diseases over time, to evaluate the effectiveness of prescribed medications, and to determine the need for mechanical ventilation.

PROCEDURE

Pulmonary function studies may be performed in a pulmonary function laboratory, in a physician's office, or at the patient's bedside. They should not be done immediately after a meal, when the stomach is distended and pressing on the diaphragm, and medications such as sedatives, narcotics, and bronchodilators, which may affect respiration, are omitted unless specifically ordered to be given. A spirometer with an attached recording device (kymograph) that produces a graphic record is used for all pulmonary function tests.

The patient, while either sitting or standing, seals the lips around the mouthpiece of the spirometer. A nose clip to prevent air leakage is put in place, and the patient is instructed to breathe normally through the mouth. When the patient is comfortable breathing through the mouthpiece, testing begins. The patient is directed to perform various inspiratory and expiratory maneuvers.

Some spirometric tests may be done during exercise. Methods of exercise include using a bicycle ergometer or stepping up and down a raised platform for several minutes. ABG values may also be measured with the patient at rest and after exercise.

A primary nursing responsibility is to provide the patient with information about the procedures to allay anxiety and promote cooperation. The patient should know the following:

The array of complex equipment used in the pulmonary function laboratory may appear frightening, but the test itself is relatively simple.

Extensive testing can cause fatigue.

For those patients with compromised pulmonary function, feelings of suffocation may occur when the nose clips are in place.

Loose clothing should be worn.

Usual measures aimed at mobilizing and removing secretions are performed before the tests. If this includes intermittent positive pressure breathing (IPPB) treatment, bronchodilators will be withheld for 4 hours before testing so that the test results reflect the usual status of the patient.

Blood Studies

ARTERIAL BLOOD GASES

ABG analysis determines the actual levels of oxygen and carbon dioxide circulating in a sample of arterial blood. It provides direct information about ventilation and diffusion of gases between the alveoli and the blood. Interpretation of ABGs also provides data about the overall acid-base balance of the individual.

An ABG analysis includes determination of the partial pressure of oxygen in arterial blood ($Pa{O_2}$), the oxygen saturation level of hemoglobin in arterial blood ($Sa{O_2}$), the partial pressure of carbon dioxide in arterial blood ($Pa{CO_2}$), the degree to which arterial blood is acid or alkaline (pH), and the level of bicarbonate present in arterial blood (HCO_3^-). (See Table 12–3 for normal values.)

Table 12–2. PULMONARY FUNCTION TESTS

TERM	SYMBOL	DESCRIPTION
LUNG VOLUMES		
Tidal volume	TV or V_t	Volume of air inspired and expired with a normal breath
Inspiratory reserve volume	IRV	Maximum volume that can be inspired from the end of a normal inspiration
Expiratory reserve volume	ERV	Maximum volume that can be exhaled by forced expiration after a normal respiration
Residual volume	RV	Volume of air left in lung after maximal expiration
Minute ventilation	MV or V_e	Volume of air inspired and expired in 1 minute of normal breathing
LUNG CAPACITIES		
Vital capacity	VC	Maximum amount of air that can be expired after a maximal inspiration
Forced vital capacity	FVC	Vital capacity performed with a maximally forced expiration
Forced expiratory volume	FEV_1 (subscript indicates the time interval in seconds)	Amount of air expelled in a specified time of the FVC maneuver
Ratio of timed forced expiratory volume to FVC	FEV_1/FVC	Amount of air forcefully expelled in 1 second compared with total amount forcefully expelled
Maximum expiratory flow rate	$FEF_{200-1200}$	Mean forced expiratory flow after the first 200 ml
Maximum midexpiratory flow	$FEF_{25-75\%}$	Average rate of flow during middle half of FVC
Maximal voluntary ventilation	MVV	Amount of air exchanged per minute with maximal rate and depth of respiration
Inspiratory capacity	IC	Maximum amount of air that can be inhaled after a normal respiration
Functional residual capacity	FRC	Amount of air left in the lungs after a normal expiration
Total lung capacity	TLC	Maximum amount of air the lungs and respiratory passages can hold after a forced inspiration

Table 12–3. ARTERIAL BLOOD GASES

SYMBOL	DESCRIPTION	NORMAL VALUES
pH	Expression of hydrogen ion concentration; represents acidity or alkalinity of the blood	7.35–7.45
Pa_{O_2}	Partial pressure of oxygen in arterial blood	75–100 mm Hg
Pa_{CO_2}	Partial pressure of carbon dioxide in arterial blood	35–45 mm Hg or 38–42 mm Hg
HCO_3^-	Bicarbonate	23–29 mEq/L
Sa_{O_2}	Percentage of oxygen carried in hemoglobin	>94%

USES

ABGs are used to evaluate respiratory functioning in an individual and to help determine the need for and the effectiveness of therapeutic interventions such as the administration of supplemental oxygen.

ABG assessment can indicate the presence of hypoxemia (inadequate oxygen in the arterial blood as measured by Pa_{O_2}), hypoxia (inadequate oxygenation at the cellular level), hypercapnia (excessive carbon dioxide in the arterial blood as measured by Pa_{CO_2}), acidosis or alkalosis (as measured by the pH), and the presence of the body's compensatory efforts to reduce an acid-base imbalance.

PHYSIOLOGIC BASIS OF ABG USE AND INTERPRETATION

Diffusion of Oxygen and Carbon Dioxide

Oxygen and carbon dioxide are gases that diffuse from areas of greater concentration to areas of lesser concentration. For example, oxygen diffuses from the alveoli into the blood when the concentration of oxygen in the alveoli is greater than the concentration of oxygen in the blood. The partial pressure of a gas is defined as the pressure exerted by a particular gas when it is in a mixture of gases.

Inspired air is composed of 21% oxygen, and the partial pressure of atmospheric oxygen is 160 mm Hg (total pressure of atmospheric air is 760 mm Hg at sea level). The partial pressure of oxygen falls to approximately 100 mm Hg in the alveoli after its exposure to vapors and air occupying dead spaces in the lung. After normal ventilation with inspired air, the oxygen concentration in the deoxygenated blood circulating to the lung from the right side of the heart (partial pressure of 40 mm Hg) is significantly lower than the concentration of oxygen in the alveoli (approximately 100 mm Hg). Oxygen therefore diffuses into the blood before it returns to the left side of the heart. The partial pressure of well-oxygenated blood ranges from 75 to 100 mm Hg. Oxygen also diffuses from arterial blood into the tissues through the peripheral capillaries, where oxygen tension is significantly lower (partial pressure of 40 mm Hg).

Carbon dioxide diffuses from deoxygenated blood brought from the right side of the heart (partial pressure of carbon dioxide is 46 to 48 mm Hg) into the alveoli (partial pressure of carbon dioxide is 40 mm Hg). The Pa_{CO_2} falls within the range of 35 to 45 mm Hg. At the cellular level, carbon dioxide diffuses from the tissues into the blood, which contains a lower concentration of this gas.

Oxygen Transport

Oxygen is transported throughout the body in two forms. Approximately 2% of the total oxygen in the blood exists in an unbound, dissolved form. This dissolved gas is the only oxygen that is available for immediate utilization in cell metabolism because it is the only form capable of crossing the cell membrane. The amount of oxygen that exists in the blood in this dissolved form is reflected by, and is directly proportional to, the partial pressure of oxygen (oxygen tension). The partial pressure of oxygen exerted in arterial blood is, therefore, a measurement of the amount of dissolved oxygen in arterial blood and is represented by the Pa_{O_2}.

Approximately 98% of the oxygen circulating and transported in the blood exists in a bound form and is not available for immediate utilization. This oxygen is chemically bound to the hemoglobin molecule within the red blood cells. This union of oxygen and hemoglobin forms the oxyhemoglobin molecule. The Sa_{O_2} is a measurement of the amount of available hemoglobin that is actually bound with oxygen compared with the total capacity of the available hemoglobin for binding. It is expressed as a percentage. The oxygen saturation level of well-oxygenated arterial blood ranges from 94% to 100%.

Oxyhemoglobin Dissociation Curve

The amount of oxygen that exists in the dissolved state is approximately 0.3 ml/100 ml of blood. On the basis of an average hemoglobin level of 15 g/100 ml of blood, the average amount of oxygen carried in the bound state is 20.1 ml of oxygen per 100 ml when oxygen saturation is 100%. (Each gram of hemoglobin is capable of carrying 1.34 ml of oxygen.)

The amount of oxygen that exists in the dissolved state is insufficient to meet the metabolic needs of the body and must therefore be continuously replenished. The chemical bond between oxygen and hemoglobin is a loose one and is easily reversible. The hemoglobin molecule releases oxygen into the plasma in response to cellular metabolic requirements. This released oxygen quickly dissolves and becomes available for utilization by the cells. As dissolved oxygen is used, PaO_2 levels decrease. Hemoglobin molecules respond by releasing oxygen, which in turn decreases SaO_2 levels. The hemoglobin molecule is capable of releasing all of its oxygen; however, hemoglobin saturation usually falls only from a range of 94% to 100% in arterial blood leaving the heart to approximately 75% in the peripheral capillaries.

A definite and complex relationship exists between the partial pressure of oxygen in arterial blood (dissolved oxygen or PaO_2) and the volume of oxygen that will combine with hemoglobin (SaO_2). Oxygen's affinity for hemoglobin and its ability to be released vary. Higher SaO_2 levels reflect a greater affinity of oxygen for hemoglobin, with greater ease of binding and greater difficulty with being released. Lower SaO_2 levels reflect less of an affinity of oxygen for hemoglobin, with less binding capacity and greater ease in being released. The PaO_2 is the critical determinant of oxygen's affinity for hemoglobin and, therefore, of SaO_2 levels. The greater the PaO_2 levels are, the greater the SaO_2 (hemoglobin saturation percentage). In other words, the more oxygen that is dissolved and available for use (PaO_2), the more oxygen one can "store" and bind with hemoglobin (SaO_2). With decreased levels of dissolved oxygen available, less oxygen is bound to hemoglobin, and oxygen is more readily released for consumption. The uptake of oxygen by the blood in the lungs and the release of oxygen to the tissues in the peripheral capillaries depend on this relationship.

The graphic representation of this relationship between the percentage of hemoglobin saturation (SaO_2) and the PaO_2 is known as the oxyhemoglobin dissociation curve (Fig. 12–15). This curve demonstrates the binding capacity of oxygen and hemoglobin, and the ease with which they separate, as the partial pressure of oxygen in arterial blood (PaO_2) varies. Greater or lesser quantities of oxygen become available for consumption by the tissues as the hemoglobin saturation levels (SaO_2) vary. Because the hemoglobin saturation levels vary in relation to the PaO_2, more oxygen is made available (less is bound) when PaO_2 levels are lower, and less oxygen is released (more is bound) when PaO_2 levels are high. A low PaO_2 of 40 mm Hg, such as that encountered in the peripheral capillaries, is accompanied by a hemoglobin saturation level of approximately 75%. Oxygen is readily released by hemoglobin molecules for tissue consumption at this point. A PaO_2 of 75 to 100 mm Hg, such as that encountered in the lungs, is accompanied by a high hemoglobin saturation level of approximately 94% to 100%. Minimal oxygen is released from hemoglobin molecules at this point because adequate dissolved oxygen exists. These relationships are represented by the following formulas:

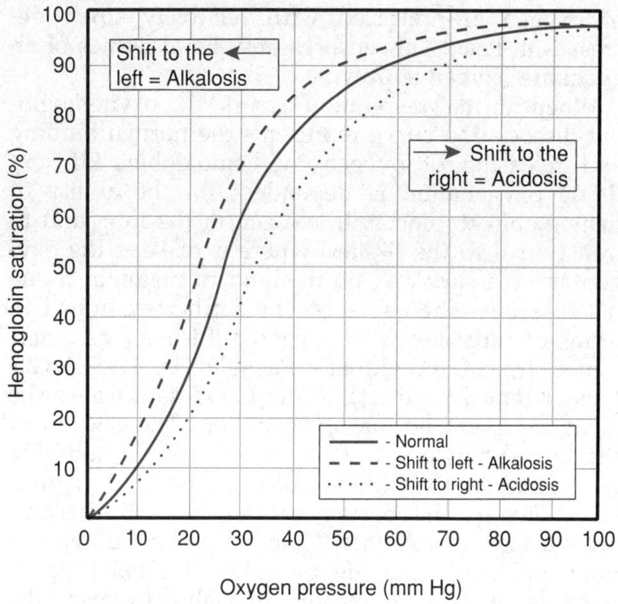

Figure 12–15.

Oxyhemoglobin dissociation curve.

This relationship is not, however, linear, nor is it unlimited. The relationship is depicted by a diphasic, or S, curve rather than a straight line and exists only up to a PaO_2 of 150 mm Hg (above normal). At this level, hemoglobin is 100% saturated and is not capable of combining with any more oxygen. A PaO_2 of greater than 150 mm Hg would not result in a greater saturation of hemoglobin. A PaO_2 of less than 150 mm Hg lowers the hemoglobin saturation percentage. The normal PaO_2 of 75 to 100 mm Hg results in an SaO_2 of 94% to 100%.

Changes in the PaO_2 are not accompanied by equivalent or proportional changes in SaO_2. Examination of the flat portion of the curve reveals that relatively large decreases in PaO_2 levels result in only a small drop in SaO_2 levels. This portion of the curve reflects oxygen uptake in the pulmonary capillaries, where normal PaO_2 levels of 75 to 100 mm Hg result in high SaO_2 levels. A large drop in PaO_2 is required in this portion of the curve before a significant drop in SaO_2 occurs. This serves to protect the individual because it ensures the availability of adequate oxygen to the tissues even if mild hypoxemia exists. The steep portion of the curve, on the other hand, illustrates sharp drops in SaO_2 as the PaO_2 decreases. This portion of the curve reflects PaO_2 levels encountered in the peripheral tissue capillaries. The lower levels of dissolved oxygen found here promote the extraction of oxygen from hemoglobin molecules as SaO_2 levels fall. Large amounts

$$\uparrow PaO_2 \longrightarrow \uparrow SaO_2 \longrightarrow \uparrow O_2 \text{ binding} + \downarrow O_2 \text{ release}$$
$$\downarrow PaO_2 \longrightarrow \downarrow SaO_2 \longrightarrow \downarrow O_2 \text{ binding} + \uparrow O_2 \text{ release}$$

of oxygen are released with relatively small decreases in PaO_2. This ensures peripheral tissues of an adequate oxygen supply.

When normal respiration occurs, the oxyhemoglobin dissociation curve represents the normal binding and releasing of oxygen by hemoglobin. Efficient tissue oxygenation is dependent on the ability of hemoglobin to bind with oxygen in the lung and to transport it to the tissues, where it releases the oxygen as necessary and on demand to maintain tissue oxygenation. The curve can be further examined in terms of three levels of oxygen sufficiency as determined by an individual's PaO_2 levels. PaO_2 levels greater than 75 mm Hg in the blood as it leaves the heart represent normal oxygenation. The portion of the curve between a PaO_2 of 45 and 75 mm Hg represents relative safety (mild to moderate hypoxemia). Finally, the portion of the curve that represents a PaO_2 of less then 45 mm Hg (severe hypoxemia) endangers the life of the individual because there is inadequate oxygen available to meet the needs of the tissues (hypoxia).

A number of factors other than the PaO_2 affect hemoglobin's affinity to bind with oxygen. Certain conditions shift the entire oxyhemoglobin dissociation curve to the right or to the left. Acidosis, hypercapnia, and an elevated temperature shift the curve to the right. A shift in this direction reduces hemoglobin's affinity to bind with oxygen and facilitates the release of oxygen from the oxyhemoglobin molecule to the tissues. These conditions represent an increase in tissue metabolism and a concomitant increase in the need for oxygen. An individual with an altered pH that falls within the acidotic range releases more oxygen for tissue consumption, and maintains a lower SaO_2 than an individual with the same PaO_2 and a normal arterial blood pH. An increase in 2,3-diphosphoglycerate (2,3-DPG), which is found in red blood cells and may be seen in individuals with anemia and prolonged hypoxia, also causes a shift to the right.

Alkalosis, hypocapnia, and decreased temperature shift the curve to the left. A shift in this direction increases hemoglobin's affinity for oxygen and makes it more difficult to release oxygen to the tissues. These conditions represent a decrease in tissue metabolism. An individual with an altered pH that falls within the alkalotic range releases less oxygen and maintains a higher SaO_2 than an individual with the same PaO_2 and a normal pH.

The influence of arterial blood pH on hemoglobin's affinity to bind with oxygen is further illustrated by changes in carbon dioxide levels at various points of the respiratory cycle. Carbon dioxide levels play a major role in determining the pH of the blood, with elevated carbon dioxide levels resulting in acidosis and below-normal levels of carbon dioxide resulting in alkalosis. As blood circulates through the pulmonary capillaries, excess carbon dioxide is released from the blood to the lungs. This raises the pH of the blood and produces a more alkaline environment. This in turn facilitates the formation of oxyhemoglobin in the lungs and results in high SaO_2 levels. In the peripheral tissue capillaries, an increase in carbon dioxide levels exists, as carbon dioxide resulting from cellular metabolism enters the blood. This increase in carbon dioxide levels lowers the pH of the blood and creates an acidic environment. This in turn facilitates the release of oxygen from the blood to the tissues and promotes adequate oxygenation at this level. The following formulas represent the shifts created by these various factors:

$$\left.\begin{matrix}\downarrow \text{pH}\\ \uparrow CO_2\\ \uparrow \text{temperature}\end{matrix}\right\} \longrightarrow \downarrow O_2 \text{ binding} + \uparrow O_2 \text{ release}$$

$$\left.\begin{matrix}\uparrow \text{pH}\\ \downarrow CO_2\\ \downarrow \text{temperature}\end{matrix}\right\} \longrightarrow \uparrow O_2 \text{ binding} + \downarrow O_2 \text{ release}$$

Two additional factors that affect oxygen transport are the individual's hemoglobin level and cardiac output. Hemoglobin levels must fall within normal limits to ensure adequate oxygen transport. Individuals who are anemic may have inadequate tissue oxygen delivery despite normal PaO_2 and SaO_2 levels. Individuals with decreased cardiac output are at risk of inadequate tissue oxygenation despite normal PaO_2 and SaO_2 levels as well.

Carbon Dioxide Transport

Carbon dioxide is transported from the tissues back to the lungs in three forms. The majority of carbon dioxide enters the red blood cells, where approximately 23% combines with hemoglobin to form carbaminohemoglobin (CO_2HHb). The remainder of the carbon dioxide that enters the red blood cells (70%) combines with water within the cells and then exits and is carried as bicarbonate ions (HCO_3^-) in the plasma ($CO_2 + H_2O \rightarrow H^+ \; HCO_3^-$). A very small percentage (7%) of carbon dioxide remains in a dissolved form in the plasma. ABGs measure this dissolved form of carbon dioxide as the $PaCO_2$. This value gives information about cellular production of carbon dioxide through metabolic processes and the removal of it from the body via the lungs. Normal levels of $PaCO_2$ range from 35 to 45 mm Hg. Changes in the $PaCO_2$ are regulated by the respiratory system. Hyperventilation is the term used when an individual is exhaling greater than normal amounts of carbon dioxide, resulting in a $PaCO_2$ of less than 35 mm Hg. Alveolar ventilation that exceeds the body's metabolic activity results in hypocapnia ($PaCO_2 < 35$ mm Hg). Hypoventilation refers to the retention of greater than normal amounts of carbon dioxide, resulting in a $PaCO_2$ of greater than 45 mm Hg. Alveolar ventilation in this case is insufficient to meet the body's metabolic needs and results in hypercapnia ($PaCO_2 > 45$ mm Hg).

The dissolved carbon dioxide becomes a source of carbonic acid in the blood. Because carbon dioxide combines with water to form carbonic acid, with resultant hydrogen ions (H^+), an increase in $PaCO_2$, as in hypoventilation, increases the formation of carbonic acid and in turn increases blood acidity. If more carbon dioxide is blown off, as in hyperventilation, there is a decrease in carbonic acid formation and the blood tends toward alkalinity. The $PaCO_2$ levels thus play a major role in determining the acid-base balance of an individual.

Acid-Base Balance

The pH of the blood reflects the degree of acidity or alkalinity of the blood. It is a measurement of hydrogen ion concentration, with increased hydrogen ions resulting in increased acidity. ABGs measure the pH of arterial blood and express it as a negative logarithm (i.e., as the hydrogen ion concentration rises, the pH decreases, and vice versa). Under normal circumstances, an individual's acid-base balance must be maintained within a very narrow range (7.35–7.45). Deviations above 7.45 (alkalemia) and below 7.35 (acidemia) represent conditions that endanger an individual's life.

Regulation of acid-base balance refers to the maintenance of hydrogen ion concentration in the body within the normal range. This is accomplished by maintaining the proper ratio of bicarbonate to dissolved carbon dioxide, which is 20:1 (see Chapter 3 for detailed discussion of acid-base balance). The respiratory system and kidneys function together to maintain the concentration of hydrogen ions, and therefore the pH, within normal limits.

The lungs adjust ventilation according to metabolic needs by increasing or decreasing the rate of respiration. This in turn increases or decreases the $PaCO_2$ levels and the resulting hydrogen ion levels. The kidneys regulate the bicarbonate concentration in the body by retaining or excreting HCO_3^-. Bicarbonate is a base that plays a major role in the buffering system and therefore in acid-base balance. ABGs measure the amount of bicarbonate in the blood, with normal values ranging between 23 and 29 mEq/L.

When respiratory, kidney, or buffering mechanisms are unable to maintain acid-base balance, abnormal conditions of acidosis ($pH < 7.35$) or alkalosis ($pH > 7.45$) arise. If the increase or decrease in pH is due to a respiratory problem, the imbalance is considered to be respiratory in origin. All other acid-based imbalances are considered to be metabolic in origin.

Accurate interpretation of ABGs can quickly reveal the source of the imbalance. In addition, ABGs can reflect the presence of any compensatory measures initiated by the body, which are aimed at reversing the imbalance.

Acidosis of respiratory origin is a result of hypoventilation (i.e., insufficient carbon dioxide is blown off). This can be secondary to numerous respiratory diseases, infection, obstructive lung disease, drug overdose, neuromuscular diseases, and cardiopulmonary diseases. With hypoventilation, $PaCO_2$ levels increase above 45 mm Hg and acidosis results. Metabolic responsibility for acidosis results from an imbalance of any of the body's metabolic acids or bases with the exception of carbon dioxide. There is either a loss of bases or an excess of acids. It can be due to diabetic ketoacidosis, diarrhea, or renal failure and is reflected by a decreased level of HCO_3^- (below 23 mEq/L).

Respiratory alkalosis develops as a result of hyperventilation (i.e., too much carbon dioxide is blown off). This can be secondary to anxiety, sepsis, or improper management of a patient on a ventilator. ABGs in respiratory alkalosis reflect a $PaCO_2$ level below 35 mm Hg. Metabolic alkalosis stems from an imbalance of the body's acids and bases with the exception of carbon dioxide. A loss of acids or a gain of bases occurs. It can be secondary to sodium bicarbonate ingestion, vomiting, or nasogastric suctioning. ABG values in metabolic alkalosis reflect HCO_3^- levels above 29 mEq/L.

When respiratory acidosis occurs, the kidneys attempt to compensate by retaining bicarbonate to balance the excessive hydrogen ions. With such attempts at compensation, ABGs reflect an elevated HCO_3^- (compensatory) along with the elevated $PaCO_2$ (causative). When respiratory alkalosis occurs, the kidneys excrete above-average amounts of bicarbonate to compensate for the lack of hydrogen ions. In an individual with respiratory alkalosis with compensation, ABGs reflect lowered levels of HCO_3^- (compensatory) along with below-normal levels of $PaCO_2$ (causative).

Metabolic acidosis is compensated for by the respiratory system. Respirations increase in rate and depth in an attempt to blow off carbon dioxide and to reduce the individual's acidotic state. Compensation of this type is reflected in the ABGs by a lowered level of $PaCO_2$ (compensatory) along with a below-normal level of HCO_3^- (causative). In metabolic alkalosis, the lungs compensate for the imbalance by decreasing ventilatory efforts. This retains carbon dioxide in an attempt to replace the metabolic acid lost or to balance the excess metabolic base. ABG interpretation in metabolic alkalosis with compensation reveals an increased $PaCO_2$ (compensatory) along with an increased bicarbonate level (causative).

The procedure for interpretation of ABGs relative to acid-base balance is presented in Table 12–4.

Procedure

Blood specimens used for ABG analysis may be obtained from an arterial catheter or from percutaneous puncture of the femoral, radial, or brachial arteries. The specimen must be collected in a heparinized syringe, placed on ice, and sent to the labora-

Table 12–4. PROCEDURE FOR INTERPRETATION OF ARTERIAL BLOOD GASES RELATIVE TO ACID-BASE BALANCE

1. First examine the pH and determine whether it is normal, above normal, or below normal.
   a. If it falls between 7.35 and 7.45, the patient is within normal limits.
   b. If it is below 7.35, the patient is acidotic.
   c. If it is above 7.45, the patient is alkalotic.
2. Next, determine the origin of the imbalance by examining the partial pressure of arterial carbon dioxide ($Paco_2$).
   a. If the patient is acidotic and the $Paco_2$ level is above normal (above 45 mm Hg), the origin of the acidosis is respiratory. If the $Paco_2$ is normal or below 35 mm Hg, the lungs could not possibly be the source of the excess acid; the origin must therefore be metabolic.
   b. If the patient is alkalotic and the $Paco_2$ is below normal (below 35 mm Hg), the origin of the alkalosis is respiratory. If the $Paco_2$ is normal or above 45 mm Hg, the lungs could not possibly be responsible for the deficiency of acid; the origin must therefore be metabolic.
3. Finally, look for evidence of compensation by examining the bicarbonate ion (HCO_3^-) along with the $Paco_2$. When compensation has occurred, the value that is causing the imbalance and the value that is compensating for the imbalance will both be abnormal in the same direction (i.e., both will be elevated or both will be below normal levels).
   a. A patient with respiratory acidosis with compensatory efforts will have elevated $Paco_2$ levels and elevated HCO_3^- levels as well.
   b. A patient with respiratory alkalosis with compensatory efforts will have decreased $Paco_2$ levels and decreased HCO_3^- levels as well.
   c. A patient with metabolic acidosis with compensatory efforts will have decreased HCO_3^- levels and decreased $Paco_2$ levels as well.
   d. A patient with metabolic alkalosis with compensatory efforts will have elevated HCO_3^- levels and elevated $Paco_2$ levels as well.

Hint: When arrows are used to reflect the direction of deviation for each value including the pH, $Paco_2$, and HCO_3^-, the following rules apply:
   a. Examine the pH to determine whether the patient is acidotic or alkalotic.
   b. When the pH and $Paco_2$ point in opposite directions, the origin of the imbalance is respiratory.
   c. When the pH and $Paco_2$ point in the same direction, the origin of the imbalance is metabolic.
   d. When compensatory efforts are present, the $Paco_2$ and the HCO_3^- will always point in the same direction.

pH $\downarrow$ $Paco_2$ $\uparrow$ HCO_3^- $\uparrow$ = respiratory acidosis
pH $\uparrow$ $Paco_2$ $\downarrow$ HCO_3^- $\downarrow$ = respiratory alkalosis
pH $\downarrow$ $Paco_2$ $\downarrow$ HCO_3^- $\downarrow$ = metabolic acidosis
pH $\uparrow$ $Paco_2$ $\uparrow$ HCO_3^- $\uparrow$ = metabolic alkalosis

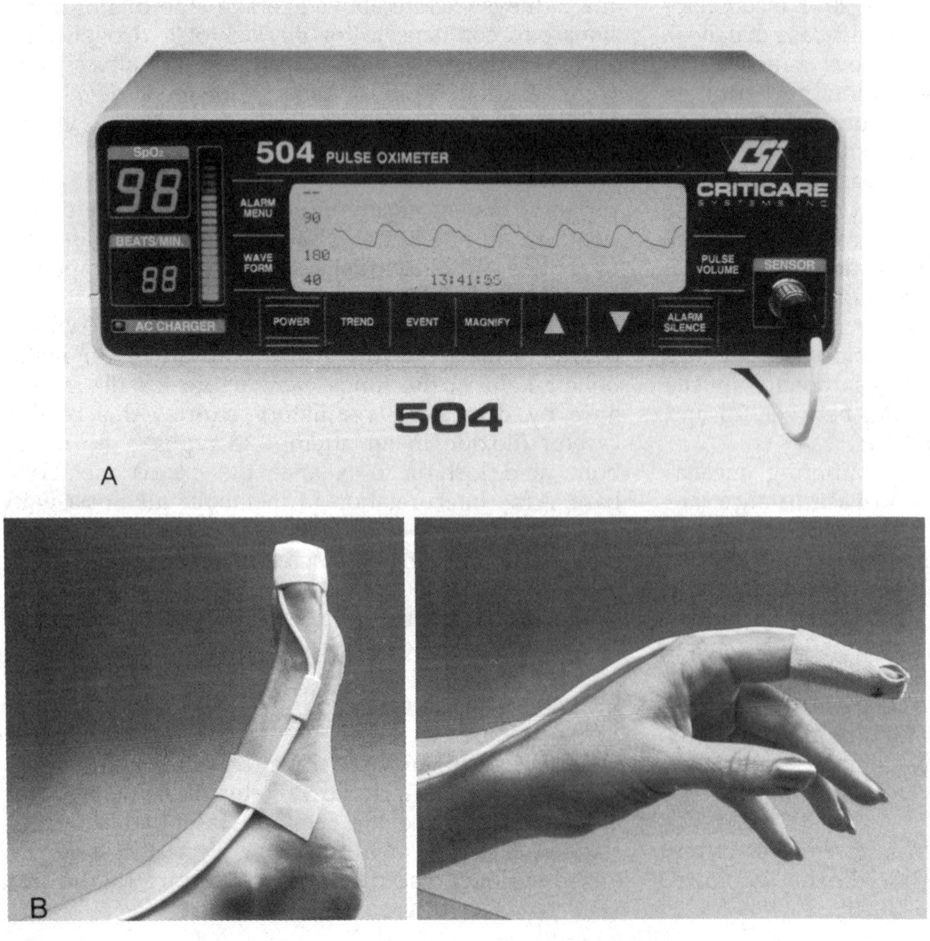

Figure 12–16.

A, Pulse oximeter. *B*, Reusable sensor in place on toe, disposable sensor in place on finger. (Courtesy of Criticare Systems, Waukesha, WI.)

tory immediately. Precautions must be taken to prevent contamination of the specimen with room air. The sample should be appropriately labeled and should include information regarding the time of collection, the patient's temperature, whether the patient was breathing room air or receiving oxygen therapy, whether or not mechanical ventilation was used, and, if yes, the ventilator settings.

Postprocedure Course

After the procedure, manual pressure is applied to the puncture site for at least 5 minutes, or longer if alterations in coagulation exist. This is followed by the application of a sterile dressing. The patient is monitored for bleeding and hematoma formation and for adequate peripheral circulation in the extremity.

PULSE OXIMETRY

Pulse oximetry is the measurement of SaO_2 with a device called a pulse oximeter. It is a painless, noninvasive procedure that requires no calibration and allows continuous monitoring even during patient transport because the oximeter can be operated by battery. The oximeter is frequently used during the perioperative period; in intensive care units, emergency rooms, and obstetrics; in patients undergoing pulmonary function tests; and in the case of patients with chronic respiratory problems and sleep apnea.

The pulse oximeter measures the amount of infrared light absorbed by oxyhemoglobin compared with the amount of red light absorbed by reduced hemoglobin. A probe is attached to the patient over a pulsating vascular bed such as that found in the fingers, toes, nose, ear lobes, and forehead. One side of this probe has two light-emitting diodes that transmit the infrared and red light through the pulsating arterial blood to a photodetector on the other side. The photodetector receives the nonabsorbed light and converts it to an electrical signal. This signal is then sent to a microprocessor, and a digital display of the percentage of oxyhemoglobin compared with total functional hemoglobin (SaO_2) is produced (Fig. 12–16).

Placement of the probe over a pulsating vascular bed is critical to the functioning of the oximeter. During systole, there is an influx of oxyhemoglobin, which results in an increase in the absorption of infrared light; during diastole, there is a decrease in the amount of oxyhemoglobin and hence in the absorption of infrared light. The amount of light absorbed by venous blood, bone, and fat, on the other hand, is the same at all times. The signal resulting from the latter serves as the baseline with which the signal generated from the arterial blood is compared. Thus, inaccurate oximeter readings may result when the pulsatile signal is poor. This can occur as a result of inappropriate placement of the probe, hypotension, presence of a blood pressure cuff, administration of vasoconstricting drugs, or any other factor that causes hypoperfusion. Intravascular dyes, jaundice, patient movement, elevated carboxyhemoglobin levels (carbon monoxide bound to hemoglobin), and hypothermia are additional factors that may interfere with accurate results. There is also the possibility of inaccurate readings caused by the effect of bright external light such as fluorescent or surgical lights, sunlight, and bilirubin lights. For this reason, covering the probe with an opaque material is often recommended. A discrepancy of 2% to 3% between pulse oximetry readings and laboratory-reported SaO_2 levels may occur. Thus, pulse oximetry is better for monitoring changes in oxyhemoglobin levels than for determining baseline oxyhemoglobin levels.

Pulse oximetry is used to provide continuous monitoring and to decrease the need for blood gas analysis. Therapeutic interventions may be implemented and evaluated based on this continuous assessment.

OTHER BLOOD STUDIES

A venous specimen may be drawn for a complete blood count (CBC). An excess of red blood cells, polycythemia, an abnormal finding, may indicate respiratory dysfunction because chronic hypoxemia causes stimulation of red blood cell production. Chronically elevated blood carboxyhemoglobin levels, as seen in heavy smokers of cigarettes and cigars, are also known to cause secondary polycythemia.

Sputum Studies

Sputum may be examined for the presence of malignant cells and for organisms that cause infection. Sputum culture and sensitivity studies are done to identify the causative organism and the corresponding antibiotics to which the organism is susceptible. A "cytologic" examination of sputum is done if carcinoma is suspected.

COLLECTION OF A SPUTUM SPECIMEN

STANDARD METHOD

Sputum specimens are best collected as soon as the patient awakens in the morning because secretions accumulate in the bronchi during the night and a few deep coughs usually bring this sputum to the back of the throat. In addition, the first sputum in the morning is usually the most productive of organisms. Provide the patient with a wide-mouth container, and instruct him or her to take several deep breaths, cough, and expectorate into the container provided. Remember that, when not properly instructed, patients often expectorate saliva rather than sputum.

Collect initial specimens for culture and sensitivity before antibiotic treatment is started. Send speci-

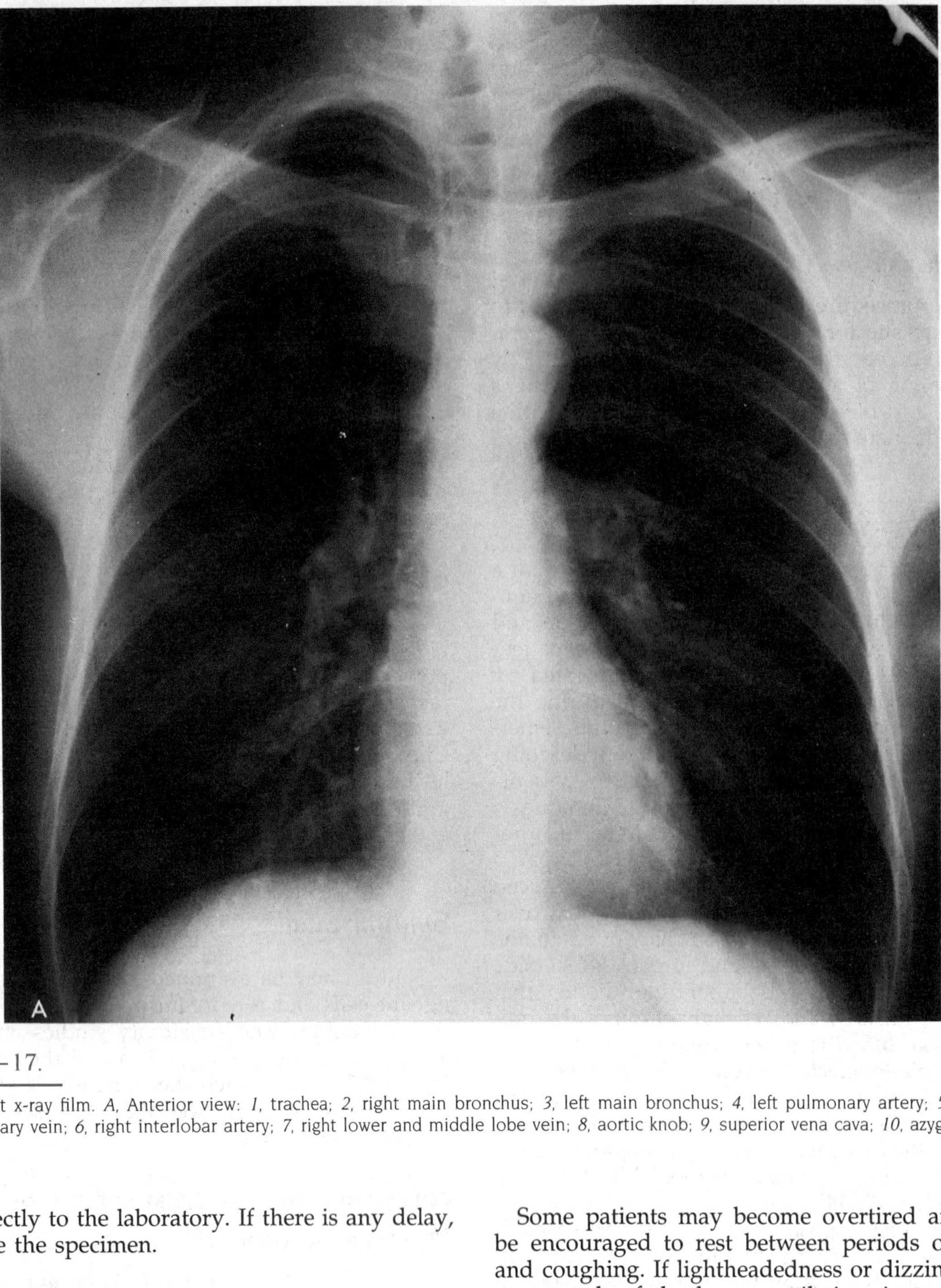

Figure 12–17.

Normal chest x-ray film. *A*, Anterior view: *1*, trachea; *2*, right main bronchus; *3*, left main bronchus; *4*, left pulmonary artery; *5*, right upper lobe pulmonary vein; *6*, right interlobar artery; *7*, right lower and middle lobe vein; *8*, aortic knob; *9*, superior vena cava; *10*, azygos vein.

mens directly to the laboratory. If there is any delay, refrigerate the specimen.

SALINE-INHALATION METHOD

The saline-inhalation method of collecting sputum is used for patients having difficulty raising secretions. Inhalation of a heated saline solution causes the heated vapor to condense on the surface of the tracheobronchial mucosa and thus stimulates production of secretions. Instruct the patient to breathe deeply and cough before the procedure. The mouth is then placed over, but not sealed around, the nebulizer. The vapor is inhaled for a few minutes until coughing is stimulated.

Some patients may become overtired and should be encouraged to rest between periods of inhaling and coughing. If lightheadedness or dizziness occurs as a result of the hyperventilation, instruct the patient to relax and breathe normally for a few minutes. If the patient complains of nausea, discontinue the procedure.

GASTRIC WASHING METHOD

Many patients swallow sputum when coughing in the morning or during sleep. In the gastric washing method, gastric aspiration is used to collect gastric contents that contain this swallowed sputum.

A nasogastric tube is inserted, and a large syringe

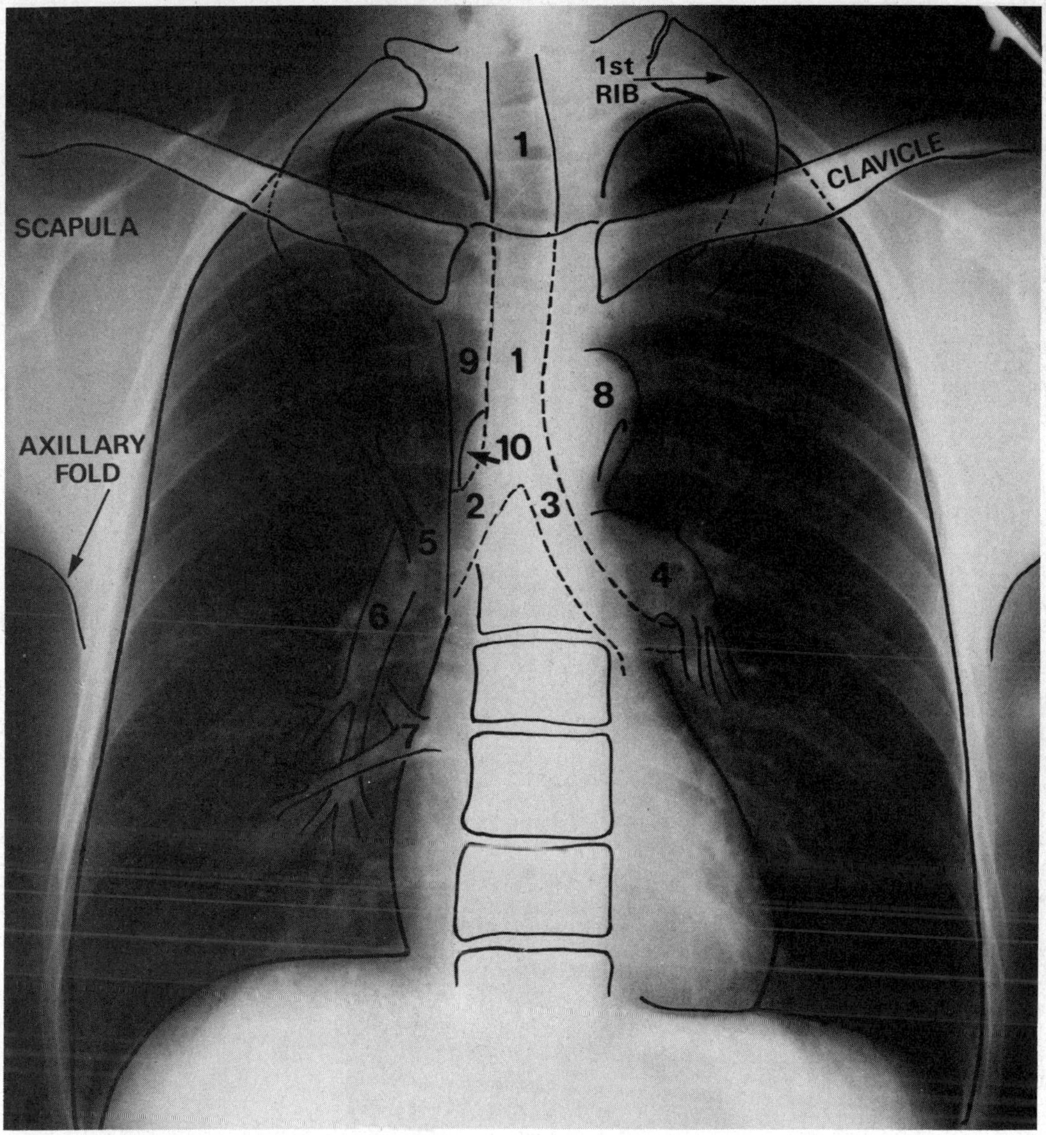

Figure 12–17. *(continued)*

See legend on opposite page. Illustration continued on following page.

is used to gently withdraw a specimen of stomach contents. The nasogastric tube is then removed. The specimen is obtained early in the morning, and breakfast is withheld until after the procedure. A microscopic examination and culture media test are done by the laboratory, just as they are done with other sputum samples. A gastric washing is usually done when the suspected diagnosis is tuberculosis.

Radiographic Studies

CHEST X-RAY FILMS

Chest x-ray films show the size, shape, position, and symmetry of the lungs, heart, diaphragm, and rib cage. Usually posterior and anterior views are taken; however, lateral or oblique views may be obtained from either the left or the right side (Fig. 12–17). Chest x-ray films can be used for screening or diagnosis. Comparison of previous and current x-ray films also assists in determining the progress and development of disease.

There is no special preparation for flat films of the chest, and there is no discomfort during the procedure. The patient is asked to remove clothing from the waist up and any jewelry worn around the neck. The patient is also asked to hold his or her breath briefly while the x-ray film is taken. Female patients who are pregnant or who suspect they may be should be instructed to inform the technician. Children and adult patients who are required to have repeated x-ray films should be shielded with a lead apron as a precautionary measure.

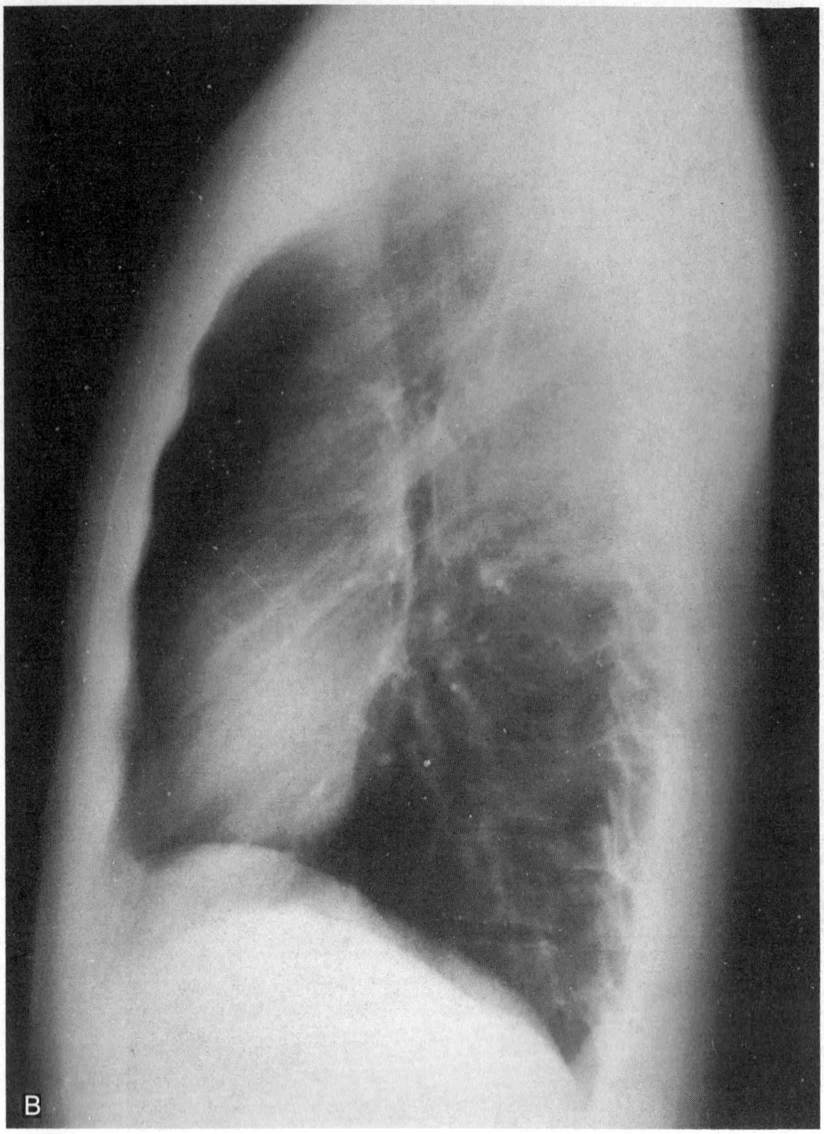

Figure 12–17. *(continued)*

B Lateral view: *1*, tracheal air column; *2*, right intermediate bronchus; *3*, left upper lobe bronchus; *4*, right upper lobe bronchus; *5*, left interlobar artery; *6* right interlobar artery; *7*, confluence of pulmonary veins; *8*, aortic arch; *9*, brachiocephalic vessels. (From Fraser RG, Paré JAP, Paré PD, Fraser RS. Diagnosis of diseases of the chest. 3rd ed, Vol 1. Philadelphia: WB Saunders, 1988, pp 287–290.)

FLUOROSCOPY

Fluoroscopy is an x-ray technique in which the image of internal structures is projected on a screen, allowing movement to be viewed and evaluated.

Fluoroscopy allows expansion and contraction of the lungs and the diaphragm to be observed. It is used to diagnose the location of a tumor or a lesion more precisely than can be done with x-ray film. Fluoroscopy is also used as an adjunct to other procedures to allow visualization of catheters or needles as they are advanced to various areas in the body.

TOMOGRAPHY

Tomograms, or planigrams, are sequential films of the lungs taken in horizontal or vertical planes at different measured depths. These films allow detailed visualization of thoracic structures, including the trachea, bronchi, and hilar lymph nodes. They are valuable in the identification and evaluation of solid lesions, vascularity surrounding a lesion, and changes within a lesion.

When tomography is done, two x-ray tubes suspended over the x-ray table swing rapidly and abruptly in converging and then diverging paths above the patient. This rapid swooping action of the x-ray machine must be described before the test or the patient may be frightened.

LUNG SCAN

There are two types of lung scans: ventilation and perfusion. A ventilation scan uses a radioisotope and a scanning machine to demonstrate patterns of air movement and air distribution in the lungs (Fig. 12–18*A*). A perfusion scan uses a radioisotope and a

Figure 12–17. *(continued)*

See legend on opposite page.

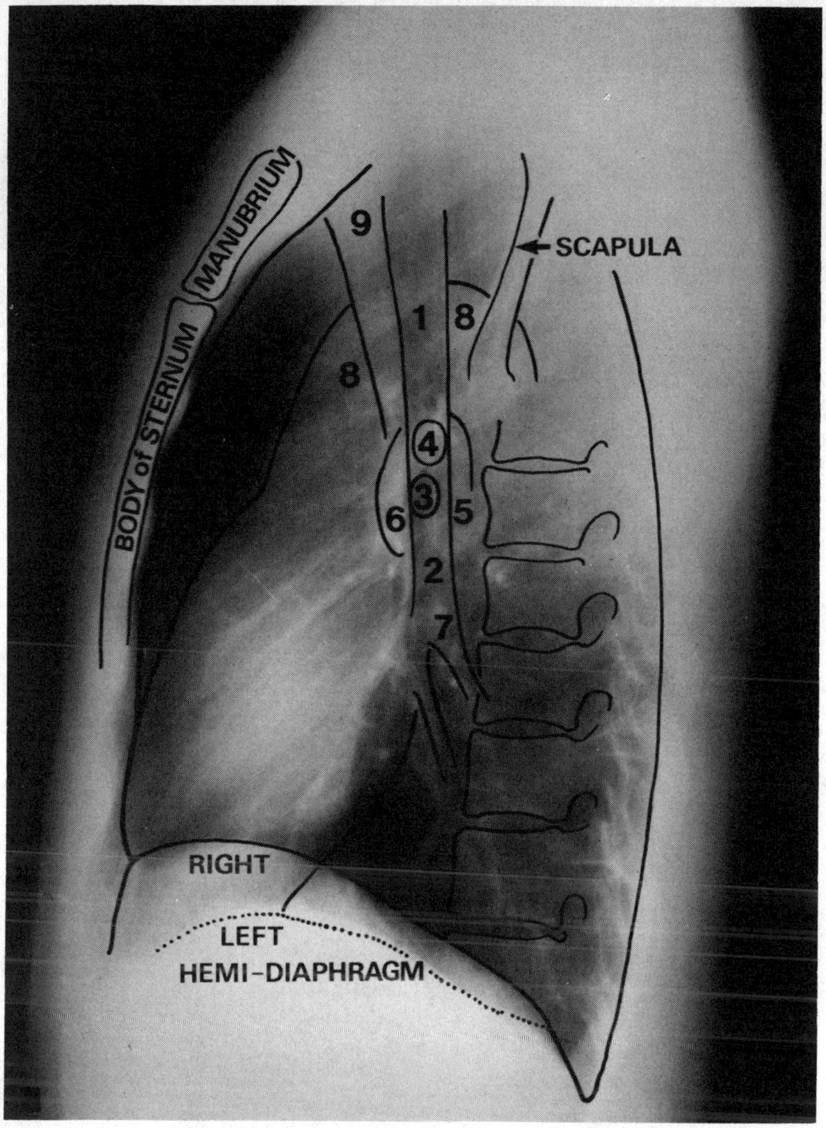

scanning machine to determine patterns of blood flow through the lungs (Fig. 12–18*B*).

USES

The primary use of ventilation and perfusion scans is in the diagnosis of pulmonary embolism. They are also used in the diagnosis of lung cancer, COPD, and pulmonary edema. They are valuable diagnostic tools because they can demonstrate abnormalities in a specific region of the lung before results of other measures of respiratory function are affected.

PROCEDURE

When both ventilation and perfusion scans are ordered, the perfusion scan is done first. With the patient in a supine position and breathing normally, a radionuclide is administered intravenously. Shortly therafter, scanning of the thorax is begun. During scanning, the patient is directed to assume various positions and otherwise to remain still and quiet. An outline results of the pulmonary blood vessels through which the radionuclide passes.

For a ventilation scan, the patient inhales a radioactive gas such as a mixture of xenon 133 and oxygen through a spirometer, which assists in delivering the gas to all areas of the lung. Scanning is then done, and an outline of alveoli into which the radioactive gas entered is obtained.

Radiation exposure is less during a lung scan than during the usual x-ray examination.

PULMONARY ANGIOGRAPHY

Pulmonary angiography is the x-ray visualization of the pulmonary vasculature after injection of a contrast medium.

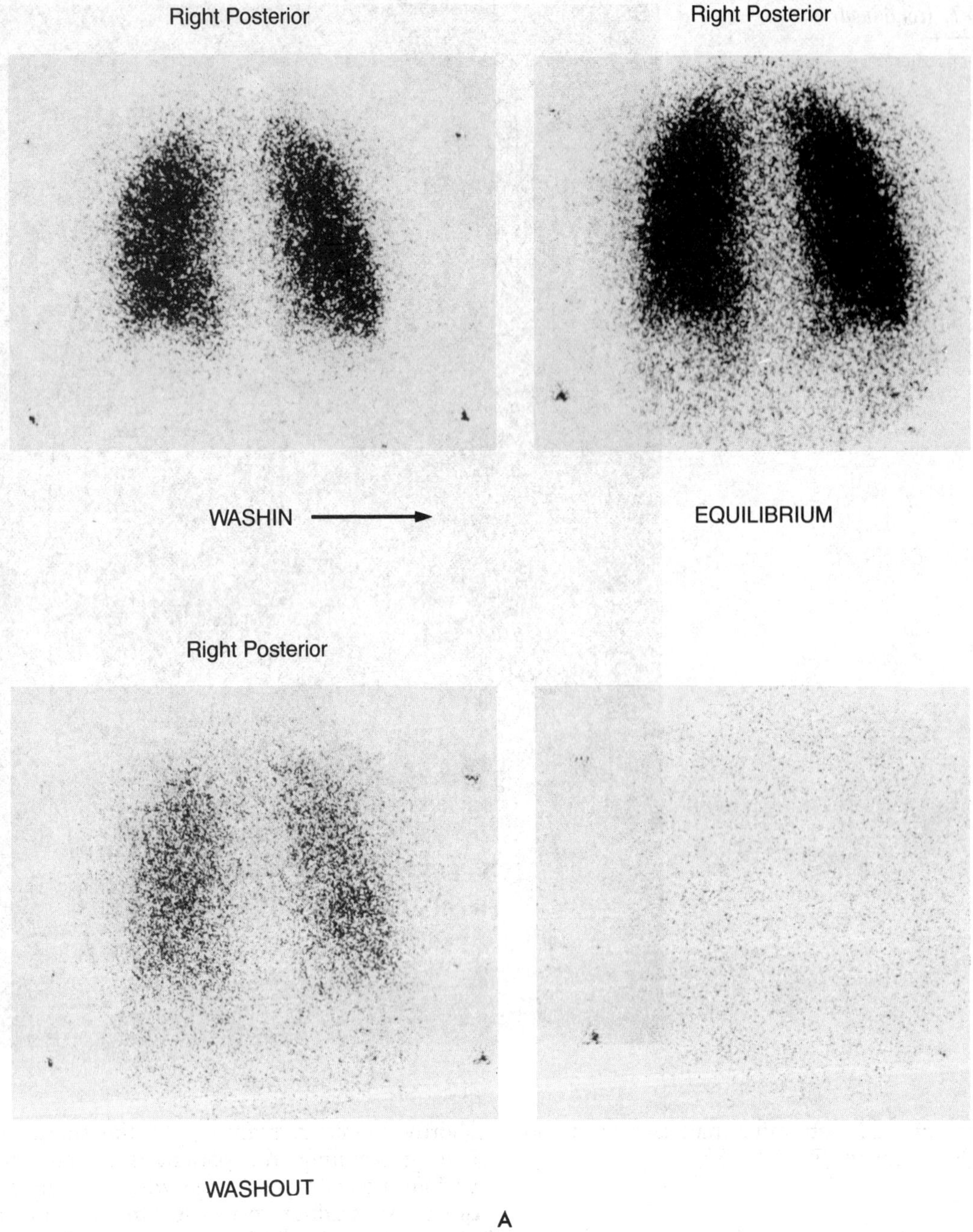

Figure 12–18.

A, Normal posterior ventilation lung scan. *B*, Posterior perfusion lung scan in same patient showing segmental filling defects (*arrowheads*) consistent with pulmonary thromboembolism. *C*, Normal posterior perfusion lung scan provided here for comparison. (From Fraser RG, Paré JAP, Paré PD, Fraser RS. Diagnosis of diseases of the chest. 3rd ed, Vol 1. Philadelphia: WB Saunders, 1988, pp 344, 347, 348.)

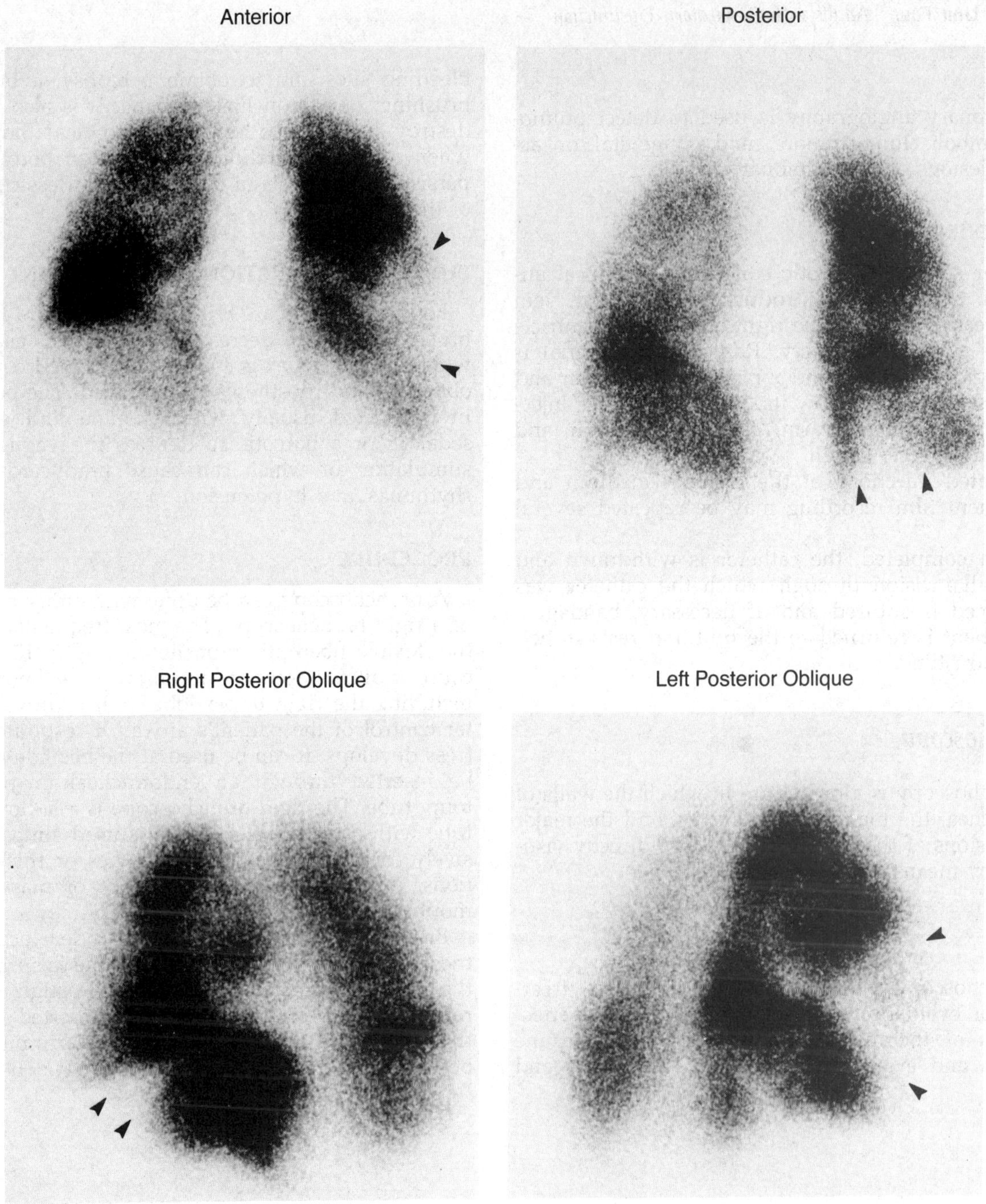

B

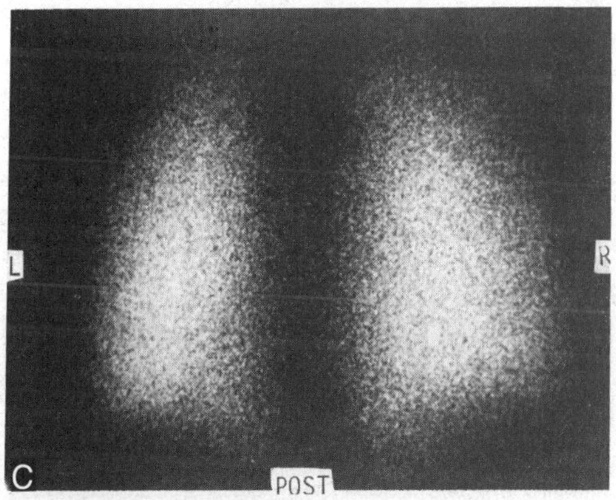

Figure 12–18. *(continued)*

See legend on opposite page.

USES

Pulmonary angiography is used to detect pulmonary emboli, lung tumors, and congenital or acquired lesions of the pulmonary vessels.

PROCEDURE

Under surgically aseptic conditions and local anesthesia, a catheter is introduced into an arm vein and threaded through the right atrium and ventricle into the pulmonary artery. Radiopaque material is then rapidly injected, and x-ray films are taken and recorded on film to show its distribution. This injection may cause a warm, flushed sensation and evoke the urge to cough.

Repeated injections of the contrast medium and subsequent film recording may be repeated several times.

When completed, the catheter is withdrawn and the small incision through which the catheter was introduced is sutured and, if necessary, bandaged. The patient is returned to the unit and rests in bed for a short time.

Bronchoscopy

Bronchoscopy is a procedure in which the walls of the trachea, the main-stem bronchus, and the major subdivisions of the bronchial tubes are directly visualized by means of a bronchoscope.

USES

Bronchoscopy may be done for diagnosis, treatment, or evaluation of disease progression or effectiveness of therapy. It can be used to determine location and extent of lesions such as tumors and bleeding sites and to obtain a biopsy, a bronchial brushing, or a bronchial washing. It is also used to destroy and remove lesions and to clear the airway when retained secretions or a foreign body causes persistent atelectasis (a collapsed or airless condition of the lung).

PHYSICAL PREPARATION OF THE PATIENT

Food and fluids are withheld for 6 hours before a bronchoscopy to decrease the risk of aspiration while the gag reflex is suppressed. Signed consent is obtained, and prostheses are removed. The patient is premedicated usually with atropine and either a sedative or a narcotic to depress the vagus nerve, stimulation of which can cause bradycardia, dysrhythmias, and hypotension.

PROCEDURE

A bronchoscopy can be done with either a flexible or a rigid bronchoscope. The most frequently used is the flexible fiberoptic bronchoscope (Fig. 12–19) because it allows access to more areas of the airways, including the right upper lobe. It also provides better control of the patient's airway if respiratory distress develops. It can be used at the bedside and can be inserted through an endotracheal or tracheostomy tube. The rigid bronchoscope is a hollow metal tube with a light at the end. It is used almost exclusively for removal of foreign bodies or thick secretions, examination in the presence of massive hemoptysis, and endobronchial surgery.

Bronchoscopy is usually done under local anesthesia. An anesthetic such as lidocaine is sprayed on the patient's pharynx to suppress the cough and gag reflexes. The bronchoscope is then inserted through the mouth and into the airways, and examination is begun. When a flexible bronchoscope is used, the

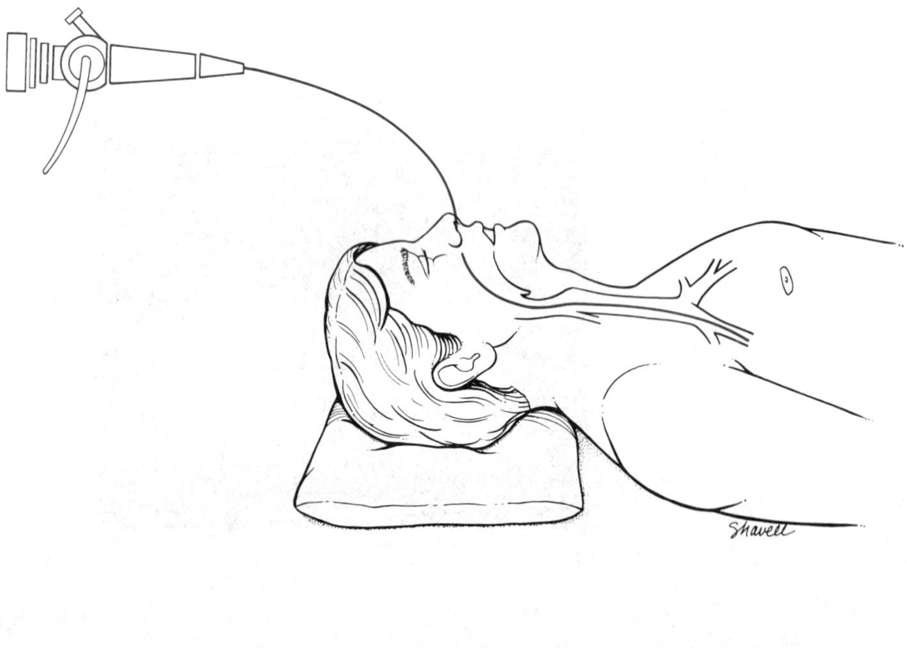

Figure 12–19.

Bronchoscopy using a flexible fiberoptic bronchoscope.

patient may remain in a sitting position if the physician so chooses, and insertion may be through the nose.

COMPLICATIONS

Complications that can occur as a result of bronchoscopy include bronchospasm, hypoxemia, bleeding, perforation, aspiration, and infection. When local anesthesia is used, a reaction to it may also occur.

Application of the Nursing Process to the Care of the Patient Having a Bronchoscopy

Assessment

Prior to a bronchoscopy, assess the patient's understanding of the procedure. Also assess the patient's anxiety level and ability to cooperate with instructions if local anesthesia is used. Monitor the patient's pulse during the procedure. When completed, check for return of the swallow and cough reflexes. Also check for signs of complications: cyanosis, dyspnea, stridor, hemoptysis, hypotension, tachycardia, and dysrhythmias.

Remember that if a biopsy was performed, blood-streaked sputum is expected for several hours, but frank blood is indicative of hemorrhage. Assess elderly patients for confusion and lethargy if lidocaine was used for local anesthesia.

Nursing Diagnoses and Planning

Nursing diagnoses and related expected patient outcomes most commonly applicable to patients undergoing a bronchoscopy include the following:

NDx: Anxiety related to the impending procedure and its outcome

Planning: Patient outcomes
1. Patient's facial expression and body movements appear relaxed.
2. Patient attends to information and directions.
3. Patient verbalizes an understanding of the procedure.

NDx: High risk for aspiration related to suppression of swallow and cough reflexes

Planning: Patient outcomes
1. Respirations are quiet and easy.
2. Respiratory rate is within patient's normal range.
3. Breath sounds are clear.

NDx: Pain related to throat irritation secondary to passage of the bronchoscope

Planning: Patient outcomes
1. Patient swallows saliva and orally ingested liquids.
2. Patient states that throat discomfort is relieved.

Nursing Interventions

NDx: Anxiety
Tell the patient what to expect before, during, and after the bronchoscopy. Include information on food and fluid restrictions and the expected effect of premedications. Stress that premedications may cause feelings of drowsiness, euphoria, or floating but do not induce sleep. If local anesthesia is to be used, acknowledge that some discomfort may be felt, including a transient sense of gagging and being unable to breathe when the local anesthetic is applied. Explain that during the procedure he or she will be asked to keep hands at the sides and to breathe through the nose. Explain also that vital signs will be taken frequently after the procedure and that a sore throat is to be expected. Allow the patient to verbalize concerns, and encourage the use of relaxation techniques.

NDx: High risk for aspiration
Position the patient who is not fully conscious in a flat side-lying position to prevent aspiration.

Position the conscious patient in a flat or semi-Fowler's side-lying position, and instruct him or her to let saliva drain out of the corner of the mouth into a basin or tissues.

Keep the patient on a nothing by mouth (NPO) order until the swallow and cough reflexes return, usually in 2 to 8 hours.

NDx: Pain
Discourage talking, clearing the throat, coughing, and smoking to avoid further irritation of the throat. Apply an ice collar to ease discomfort. When the swallow and cough reflexes have returned, give warm, soothing liquids, gargles, and throat lozenges. When tolerated, provide a soft diet, with return to the patient's regular diet in 24 hours.

Additional Interventions
Make certain that any specific preprocedure laboratory data required (e.g., hematocrit, coagulation studies, or platelet studies) are complete and that results are recorded in the patient's chart.

Evaluation

Evaluate the effectiveness of nursing care for a patient undergoing a bronchoscopy by comparing the patient's status with the expected patient outcomes.

Examples of specific outcomes for patients having a bronchoscopy have been provided in the Planning section.

Bronchogram

A bronchogram is a procedure in which a radiopaque material is inserted into the tracheobronchial tree to coat the mucosa, allowing airways to be visualized on x-ray film. Bronchoscopy is almost always done in conjunction with a bronchogram.

USES

Bronchograms are primarily used in the diagnosis of bronchiectasis. Their use is gradually decreasing because the flexible fiberoptic bronchoscope now allows direct visualization of small, previously inaccessible airways and noninvasive computed tomography (CT) and magnetic resonance imaging (MRI) scans demonstrate detailed lung structure.

PHYSICAL PREPARATION OF THE PATIENT

The patient is maintained on NPO status for 6 or more hours before the procedure to decrease the risk of aspiration of gastric contents. If secretions are copious, postural drainage is done 1 or several days before the procedure to drain secretions from the smaller bronchi so that the radiopaque substance will reach them. Premedication is given to decrease anxiety, suppress coughing, and control secretions.

PROCEDURE

There are various methods of introducing the radiopaque dye used in a bronchogram. In the commonly used transglottic catheterization method, the pharynx, hypopharynx, tonsil area, and epiglottis are sprayed with an anesthetic agent. After a brief wait, additional anesthetic is dropped through the glottis by means of a cannula and syringe. When anesthesia is achieved, a soft, pliable catheter is inserted via the nose or mouth through the larynx to the bifurcation of the trachea. This is done under fluoroscopy with the patient in a high Fowler's or semi-Fowler's position on the x-ray table. Next, the catheter is advanced into the bronchus on the side being studied, and contrast material is then injected through the catheter during the expiratory phase of respiration. The patient is tilted into various positions and is asked to breathe deeply to distribute the radiopaque dye uniformly to the bronchi and bronchioles. A series of x-ray films is then taken.

POSTPROCEDURE COURSE

Foods and fluids are withheld until the cough and swallow reflexes have returned. To clear the lungs of the contrast substance, coughing and deep breathing are encouraged and, in some cases, chest physical therapy and postural drainage are required. A slight temperature elevation is a common occurrence because pneumonitis (inflammation of the lung) can result from the contrast medium.

Application of the Nursing Process to the Care of the Patient Having a Bronchogram

The assessment, nursing diagnoses, expected patient outcomes, nursing interventions, and evaluation for patients having a bronchogram are similar to those described previously for patients having a bronchoscopy. The following additional interventions also apply. Before a bronchogram, institute postural drainage as ordered to clear the airways of secretions. Check for any known allergy to iodine or dye. Prepare the patient for the fact that the gag and cough reflexes are stimulated by the procedure and can cause vigorous retching and coughing. Also explain that the tongue and throat will feel swollen because of the local anesthetic, and panting will help to suppress the urge to cough.

Monitor temperature for 24 hours after the procedure, and institute measures to clear the contrast material from the airways.

Laryngoscopy

Laryngoscopy is direct visualization of the larynx via a laryngoscope for diagnostic or therapeutic purposes. Diagnostically, it is used to obtain tissue for biopsy, to evaluate laryngeal function (e.g., to check for vocal cord paralysis), and to detect the presence of inflammation. Therapeutically, it is used to remove lesions or foreign bodies and to dilate laryngeal strictures.

Laryngoscopy is usually performed under local anesthetic because vocal cord motility can be viewed only when the patient is awake and able to phonate (make a voiced sound).

Before the procedure, a medication such as atropine may be given to reduce secretions.

Application of the Nursing Process to the Care of the Patient Having a Laryngoscopy

The assessment, nursing diagnoses, expected patient outcomes, nursing interventions, and evaluation for patients having a laryngoscopy are similar to those described previously for patients having a bronchoscopy.

Mediastinoscopy

Mediastinoscopy is performed by passing a mediastinoscope through an incision made between the laryngeal prominence and the sternum under local or general anesthesia. It allows for visualization and biopsy of lymph nodes.

Mediastinoscopy is commonly used to detect metastasis of carcinoma of the lung or related structures to the lymph nodes. This procedure is done in an operating room equipped to deal with potential complications that include cardiac arrhythmias, myocardial infarction, bleeding, pneumothorax, and vocal cord paralysis.

Thoracentesis

Thoracentesis is the aspiration of fluid or air from the pleural space (Fig. 12–20).

USES

Thoracentesis may be done for diagnostic or therapeutic purposes. As a diagnostic procedure, it is used to obtain a specimen of fluid from the pleural space (normally there is no fluid in this space) for examination.

When fluid is aspirated for diagnostic purposes, it can be subjected to a variety of examinations. Its gross appearance—that is, bloody (associated with pleural trauma or advanced malignancy), serous (associated with malignancy, inflammatory disorders, or congestive heart failure), or purulent (associated with infection)—is noted, and specific gravity is measured. It can be biochemically analyzed for glucose, amylase, protein, and lactic dehydrogenase. Cytologic and bacteriologic studies, including smears and cultures for acid-fast bacilli, can also be done.

Therapeutically, thoracentesis may be done to relieve respiratory distress or to instill medication into the pleural space. When fluid is drained, the amount is usually limited to 1 to 2 L at one time to avoid mediastinal shift and impaired venous return.

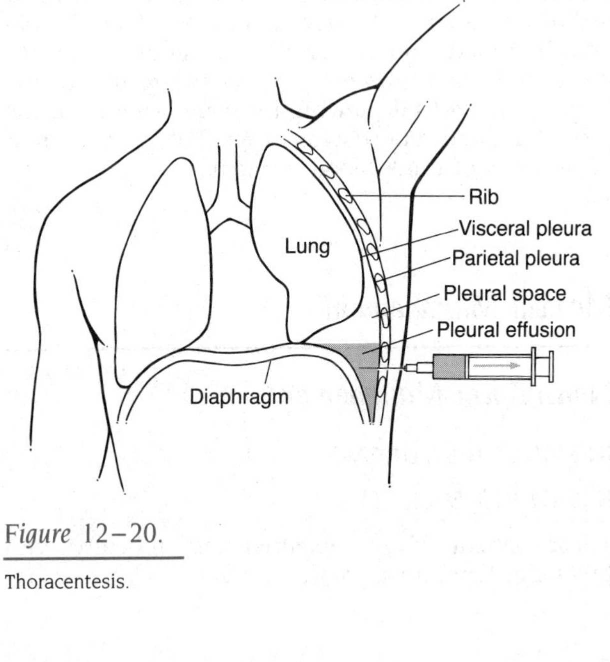

Figure 12–20.

Thoracentesis.

PROCEDURE

A thoracentesis is done at the bedside or in a treatment room. A specialized needle, three-way stopcock, sterile specimen containers, and large sterile receptacle are used. The patient is assisted to a comfortable sitting position, with the feet dangling over the side of the bed or examining table. A pillow is placed on an over-bed table on which the patient can rest his or her arms and head. The arms may be crossed to allow maximal exposure of the intercostal spaces. The site of thoracentesis, which is determined by x-ray examination and percussion, is disinfected, and a local anesthetic is injected. The thoracentesis needle is then introduced, and fluid is removed with a syringe or via a tube connected to a sterile drainage container. When drainage of fluid is completed, an adhesive strip is placed over the needle insertion site and the patient is placed on bed rest. A chest x-ray film is taken after the procedure to check for pneumothorax.

Application of the Nursing Process to the Care of the Patient Having a Thoracentesis

Assessment

Assess the patient's understanding of the thoracentesis procedure and anxiety level regarding it. Assess ability to assume the required position and comply with directions. Obtain baseline vital signs.

Nursing Diagnoses and Planning

The nursing diagnosis and related expected patient outcomes most commonly applicable to patients having a thoracentesis are as follows:

NDx: Anxiety related to discomfort during thoracentesis

Planning: Patient outcomes
1. Patient verbalizes that feelings of anxiety are diminished.
2. Facial expression and posture appear relaxed.

Nursing Interventions

NDx: Anxiety
Briefly describe the thoracentesis procedure to the patient so he or she will know what to expect. Include the following information on sensations that normally occur during the procedure:

- A mild burning sensation occurs as the local anesthetic is injected into the skin.
- A sharp but quickly passing pain occurs as the parietal pleura is infiltrated with the anesthetic.
- A feeling of pressure occurs as the needle is inserted.
- A pulling sensation or desire to cough is felt as the needle is withdrawn and the lung responds.

Reassure the patient, and provide support through touch and eye contact.

Additional Interventions
Obtain an informed consent before the procedure is begun. During the procedure, monitor pulse and respirations. Instruct the patient to sit still and not talk during the procedure to avoid displacement of the needle or perforation of the pleura. Direct the patient to avoid sudden movements, deep breathing, and coughing and to pant if an urge to cough is felt.

On completion, record the total amount of fluid withdrawn, noting its color and viscosity.

Monitor the patient for signs and symptoms of hemorrhage and pneumothorax, which are rare but potential complications. Check blood pressure, pulse, and respirations, and check the insertion site for swelling, which could be due to bleeding. Also be alert for faintness, vertigo, tightness in the chest, uncontrollable cough, and blood-tinged, frothy mucus.

Evaluation

Evaluate the effectiveness of nursing care for a patient having a thoracentesis by comparing the patient's status with the expected patient outcomes. Examples of specific outcomes for patients having a thoracentesis have been provided in the Planning section.

Lung Biopsy

A lung biopsy, like any other biopsy, is done to obtain a specimen for examination and definitive diagnosis. The majority of lung biopsies are done to distinguish benign from malignant lesions.

There are several nonoperative closed techniques used to obtain a lung biopsy. These include transcatheter bronchial brushing, percutaneous needle biopsy, and transbronchial lung biopsy.

A transcatheter bronchial brushing is done with a fiber-optic bronchoscope under fluoroscopy. A small brush is attached to the end of a flexible wire, which is inserted through the bronchoscope to the area under suspicion. It is then brushed back and forth. This causes cells to slough off and adhere to the brush. The brush is removed from the bronchoscope, and a slide is made for cytologic study. This allows for examination of a lung lesion and specific identification of pathogenic organisms.

A percutaneous (through the skin) biopsy uses a cutting or aspiration needle with local anesthesia. The lesion is located under fluoroscopy, and the needle is inserted through the skin into the pleura while the patient holds the breath in midexpiration. The needle is then guided into the lesion, and the biopsy is obtained. The aspiration needle permits syringe aspiration of a small tissue sample. A larger core of tissue is obtained with a cutting needle.

A transbronchial lung biopsy uses cutting forceps introduced via a fiberoptic bronchoscope. This procedure is done when a lung lesion is suspected and sputum samples and bronchoscopic washings are negative. Potential complications of closed-lung biopsy include pneumothorax, hemorrhage, and air embolism.

Application of the Nursing Process to the Care of the Patient Having a Closed-Lung Biopsy

The assessment, nursing diagnoses, expected patient outcomes, nursing interventions, and evaluation for patients having a closed-lung biopsy are similar to those described previously for patients having a bronchoscopy. In addition, when caring for any patient undergoing a lung biopsy, recognize that biopsy has a connotation of cancer for most people. Expect the patient to be anxious regarding this possibility, and encourage verbalization of concerns and use of relaxation techniques if needed. Keep the patient informed, and be certain that he or she knows when and from whom to expect the results of the biopsy. Monitor all patients for complications of the procedure, and report signs of respiratory distress or hemoptysis of frank blood immediately.

Medical Management

Nonsurgical Management

RESPIRATORY THERAPY

BREATHING EXERCISES

The patient who is experiencing difficulty with breathing tends to increase respiratory rate and use the accessory muscles of respiration. This is a counterproductive response because it increases the work of respiration and hence the demand for oxygen. Controlled breathing techniques limit this response and enable the patient to breathe more efficiently to conserve energy. When used in combination with postural drainage, vibration, and percussion, they increase aeration and assist in the movement of secretions. The two main types of controlled breathing are pursed-lip breathing and diaphragmatic breathing.

Pursed-Lip Breathing

Pursed-lip breathing prolongs expiration and increases pressure in the lower airways, preventing collapse of bronchioles. This allows for more complete emptying of air rich in carbon dioxide from the alveoli on exhalation and permits more fresh air to enter the lungs with each inhalation. For this breathing technique, air is inhaled through the nose and exhaled slowly against lips pursed as though ready to whistle. To be effective, exhalation should be twice as long as inspiration. This technique can be practiced by blowing through a straw to make small bubbles in a glass of water, by blowing a Ping-Pong ball steadily across the table, or by blowing at a candle flame to bend it rather than extinguish it.

Diaphragmatic Breathing

Diaphragmatic breathing assists the patient in using the diaphragm rather than the accessory muscles to breathe. Because smaller muscles use more oxygen than large ones, this decreases the work of breathing. Diaphragmatic breathing also increases the volume of air exchanged with a normal breathing effort and enhances the distribution of the inhaled air.

To practice diaphragmatic breathing, the patient is asked to lie down and place the left hand on the rib cage just below the collarbone so that any motion of the rib cage can be felt. The right hand is placed in the area above the navel and just below the rib cage, with the palm down, the smallest finger reaching the navel, and the thumb resting on the sternum. The patient then takes deep breaths through the nose and at the same time allows the area under the palm of the right hand to rise. Pursed-lip breathing is used on expiration and timed to be twice as long as inhalation.

If diaphragmatic breathing is being done properly, the rib cage under the left hand does not move and the abdominal wall below the navel does not rise higher than the area under the right hand. If it does rise higher, the patient is using extra-abdominal muscles, which is unnecessary.

If needed, patients can be helped to master this breathing technique by placing a book on the upper abdomen and watching it rise and fall with inspiration and expiration.

Once the basic technique is learned, it should be practiced in the sitting position to lower the abdominal contents and allow easy descent of the diaphragm.

Diaphragmatic breathing requires more work than pursed-lip breathing alone, so acutely ill patients may be instructed to use pursed-lip breathing only. Otherwise, the combination of diaphragmatic breathing and pursed-lip breathing should be used while performing activities of daily living (ADL) such as walking, standing, or climbing stairs. These techniques of controlled breathing should be practiced often so they are used automatically during acute episodes of breathlessness.

POSTURAL DRAINAGE

Postural drainage is a technique that uses gravity to assist in draining secretions from the lung. The various positions used relate to the entry angle of each segmental bronchus (Fig. 12–21). As specific segments of the lung are drained into the major bronchi and trachea, the patient is more likely to cough effectively and expectorate the excess secretions. Position depends on location of retained secretions, and duration of treatment depends on the patient's tolerance. Generally, this ranges from 5 to 15 minutes and is done two to four times per day, although in acute situations frequency may be as often as every 1 to 2 hours. Postural drainage should not be done for at least 1 hour after a liquid meal and 2 hours after a solid meal. Scheduling postural therapy an hour before meals and at bedtime has the advantage of easing breathing for eating and sleeping.

Lung sounds are auscultated before and after the procedure to determine the areas that need drainage and the effectiveness of therapy. If prescribed, bronchodilators, saline, or water may be nebulized and inhaled before the procedure to reduce bronchospasm, decrease the viscosity of mucus, and combat edema of the bronchial walls. The patient is made as comfortable as possible and, if the prescribed position cannot be tolerated, a modified position is used. Each time position is changed, the patient is instructed to inhale slowly through the nose and exhale through pursed lips several times and then cough and expectorate.

Postural drainage is contraindicated in patients with increased intracranial pressure, such as after head injury or craniotomy. It should also be avoided in patients with hypertension, cardiovascular compromise, and orthopnea.

PERCUSSION

Percussion (also known as "cupping" or "clapping") is a manual technique used in conjunction with postural drainage to loosen secretions in the respiratory tract. The patient is placed in the appropriate postural drainage position for treatment of the affected lung area. The skin is protected by a

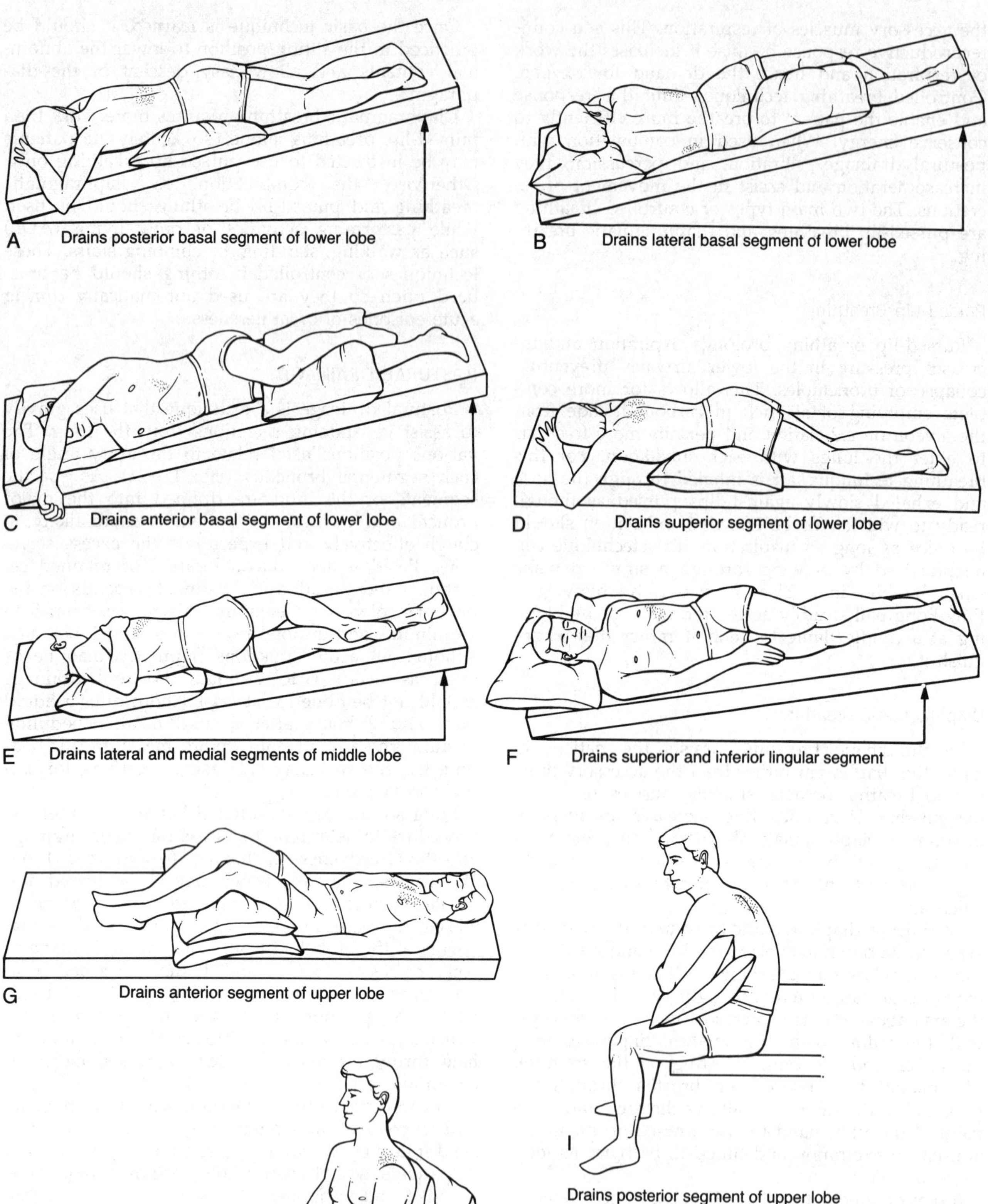

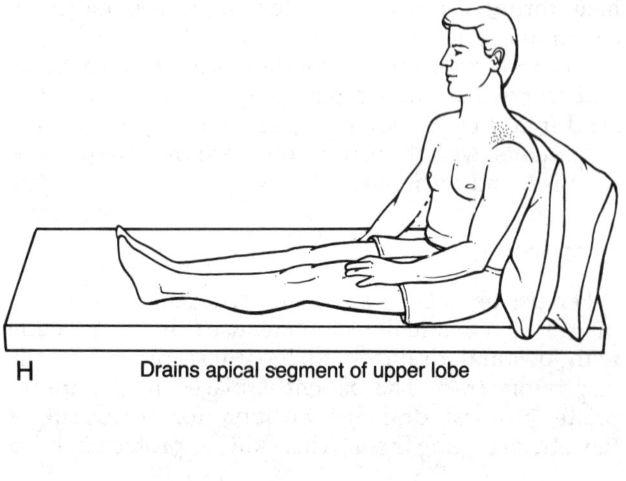

Figure 12–21.

Postural drainage. The patient assumes various positions to facilitate the flow of secretions from various portions of the lung into the bronchi, trachea, and throat so that they can be expectorated. The drawing shows the various positions used to drain each segment of the lung.

thin covering, such as a patient gown or a sheet. The nurse's hands are slightly cupped and facing downward with the fingers and thumbs together. Flexion and extension of the wrists are performed in a rhythmic manner, with a steady, even percussion maintained for 3 to 5 minutes over the affected area.

Percussion should not be done on bare skin, below the ribs, on the spine or scapulae, or over breast tissue. Areas of incision should be avoided. Percussion is contraindicated in patients with hemoptysis, rib fractures, osteoporosis, pulmonary embolism, tuberculosis, and operable lung cancer. Possible complications include fractured ribs and hemoptysis.

If percussion is contraindicated, postural drainage may still be performed effectively.

VIBRATION

Vibration is the technique of applying manual compression and tremor to the chest wall during exhalation. This technique applies little or no pressure to the chest and is useful when other techniques are contraindicated. The nurse's hands are placed over the affected are
The nurse then contracts h
tremities isometrically. T
sion, which produces a
mitted through the che
pulmonary tissue. This proc
to 10 deep breaths or until sec
and cleared by coughing.

The precautions for and hazards of
the same as for percussion.

OXYGEN THERAPY

Supplemental oxygen is administered when the patient has or is at risk for hypoxemia (i.e., when the oxygen transport to body tissues is insufficient or likely to become so). Specific conditions that may require oxygen therapy include pneumonia, COPD, lung cancer, myocardial infarction, shock, and central nervous system disorders in which the respiratory center is depressed.

A variety of methods are used to administer oxygen (Table 12–5). The method used for a specific patient depends on the required concentration of

Table 12–5. COMMON METHODS OF OXYGEN (O_2) ADMINISTRATION AND APPROXIMATE LITER FLOWS AND FRACTION OF INSPIRED OXYGEN (FIO_2)

METHOD	O_2 DELIVERY	ADVANTAGES	DISADVANTAGES
Nasal cannula (nasal prongs)	Low concentrations dependent on rate and depth of breathing FLOWS 1 L = 24% O_2 2 L = 28% O_2 3 L = 32% O_2 4 L = 36% O_2 5 L = 40% O_2 6 L = 44% O_2	Patient can move, talk, and eat without disrupting delivery of O_2	Easily dislodged; risk of necrosis to nostrils, cheeks, and ears; irritation of nasal mucosa; cannot be used for more than 6 L/min; must be humidified if used more than 4 L/min
Simple mask	Low to medium concentrations, 40%–60%; must use liter flow greater than 5 L/min	Higher delivery of O_2 than with a cannula	Discomfort and risk of pressure necrosis caused by tight seal between face and mask; must be removed for eating, drinking, and oral medication
Partial rebreathing mask	Higher concentrations, 60%–80%; must keep reservoir bag inflated at all times		Risk of pressure necrosis; not for long-term use
Non-rebreathing mask	Highest concentrations, 80%–95%; must keep reservoir bag inflated at all times	Useful in emergency situations	Discomfort and risk of necrosis from snug fit; not for long-term use
Venturi mask	Delivers consistent FIO_2 regardless of breathing pattern; concentration and liter flow marked on apparatus; 24%–50% masks available	Useful when accuracy of delivery is essential	Discomfort and risk of skin irritation; must be removed for eating and oral medication
Tracheostomy collar	Delivers O_2 and humidification via tracheostomy; must be connected to a nebulizer; FIO_2 is set on the nebulizer 24%–100%	Adds humidity to liquefy secretions	Must drain condensation often; risk of nosocomial respiratory infection
T-bar (Brigg's adapter)	Delivers O_2 and humidification via tracheostomy; must be connected to a nebulizer; FIO_2 is set on the nebulizer 24%–100%	Adds humidity to liquefy secretions	Must drain condensation often; risk of nosocomial respiratory infection

Table 12–6. GUIDELINES FOR SAFE, EFFECTIVE ADMINISTRATION OF OXYGEN

...CIPLE	IMPLICATIONS FOR OXYGEN ADMINISTRATION
...xiety activates the sympathetic nervous system and increases the body's need for oxygen.	Explain equipment and purpose of therapy to minimize anxiety.
Oxygen supports combustion. Combustion is extremely rapid in the presence of high concentrations of oxygen.	Prevent fire hazards where oxygen is in use. Avoid open flames. Post "no smoking" signs. Check for faulty electrical equipment. Avoid wearing or using synthetic fibers, which build up static electricity. Avoid use of oil, which can ignite spontaneously in the presence of oxygen.
Oxygen is a dry gas and can remove normal moisture from respiratory passages.	Provide needed humidity through use of bubble humidifier (bottle of water attached to oxygen source) or nebulizer.
Correct concentration of oxygen is necessary to maintain effective therapy and to prevent complications.	Check every 8 hours that the prescribed concentration of oxygen is being delivered.
Warm, moist environments support growth of microorganisms.	Change masks and tubes daily.
Oxygen flow and pressure from a mask or cannula are irritating to the skin or nares. Aspiration of oil-based lubricant can cause oil pneumonia.	Wash and dry affected area thoroughly and gently, and apply water-soluble lubricant on skin and nares.
High oxygen concentrations over a prolonged time can cause loss of elastic recoil and airway irritation.	Monitor for signs of oxygen toxicity: nausea and vomiting, substernal pain, dyspnea, cough, rales.

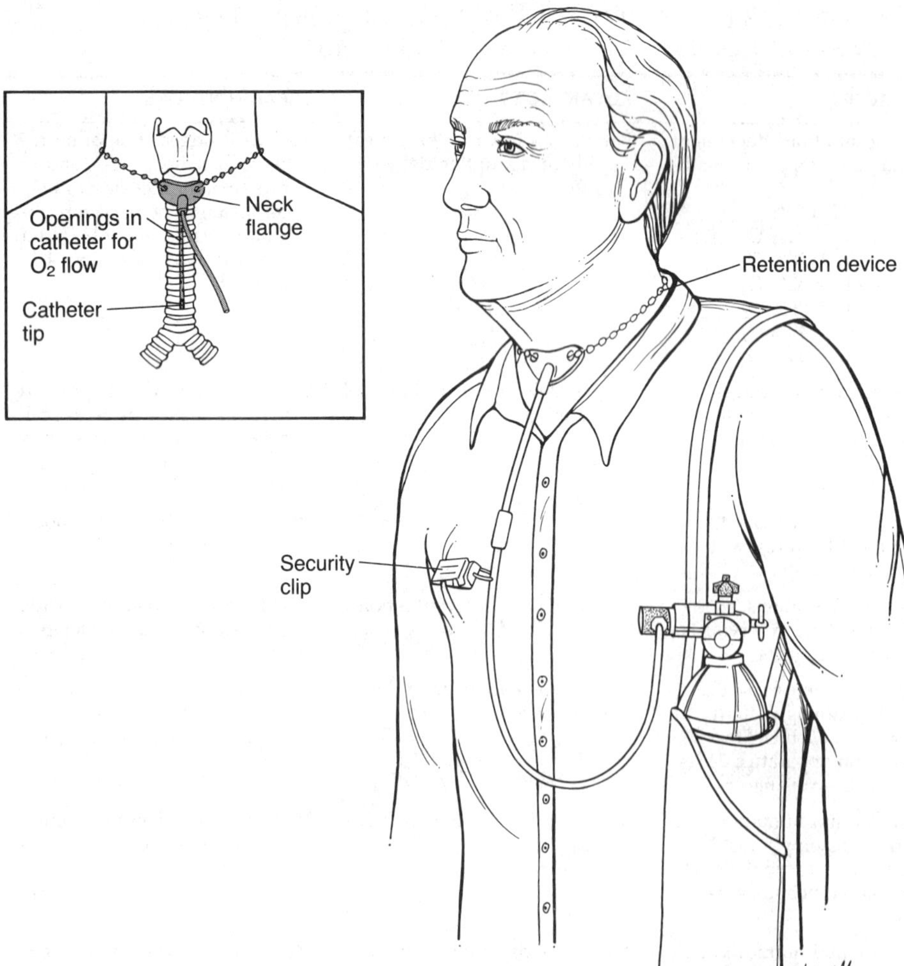

Figure 12–22.

Transtracheal oxygen.

inspired oxygen, the amount of humidification required, and the mental and physical conditions of the patient.

The flow rate at which oxygen is delivered is measured in liters per minute via a flowmeter. This rate varies depending on the condition of the patient and the route being used to administer the oxygen. More precise dosages are prescribed in percentage of inspired oxygen.

Oxygen is a medication, and its characteristics present a variety of hazards to the patient. Principles related to oxygen therapy and their implications for oxygen administration are presented in Table 12–6.

TRANSTRACHEAL OXYGEN

In transtracheal oxygen (TTO_2) therapy, which is used for patients requiring long-term home oxygen therapy, oxygen is administered through a small catheter inserted directly into the trachea through the lower neck. This catheter, which is held in place via a flange, is attached to a tubing that runs under the clothing to a lightweight oxygen tank carried as an over-the-shoulder bag (Fig. 12–22).

There are many advantages of transtracheal oxygen over oxygen via nasal cannula or tracheostomy for the patient requiring long-term continuous therapy. Transtracheal oxygen is more efficient because oxygen is not lost to the environment and it decreases the work of breathing, thereby reducing dyspnea. Further, it does not interfere with coughing, speaking, eating, and shaving, and it does not cause nasal dryness, nosebleeds, sore throat, or changes in taste and smell, which lead to anorexia.

Transtracheal Catheters

Two types of transtracheal oxygen administration sets in use are the Heimlich Microtrach and the SCOOP. Both are inserted over a removable needle and guide wire, but the SCOOP, being a longer, wider catheter, requires a small incision, whereas the Microtrach is inserted through a needle puncture. Oxygen administration can be started immediately after insertion of a Microtrach, but in some cases the wound is first allowed to heal for a week to decrease the risk of subcutaneous emphysema (presence of air in subcutaneous tissue). With the SCOOP, a stent is inserted initially and is replaced with a SCOOP1 catheter at the end of 1 week. This catheter is suitable for low-flow oxygen administration of up to 2 L/minute. If the patient requires a higher flow, a SCOOP2 is inserted at 6 to 8 weeks.

Procedure

Insertion of a transtracheal catheter is an out-patient procedure. The patient is maintained on NPO status for 6 to 8 hours and receives a sedative, a prophylactic antibiotic, and usually a cough suppressant. During the procedure, the patient sits with the head back or lies with a pillow under the shoulders to extend the neck; oxygen is administered by nasal catheter; and electrocardiogram (ECG) and pulse oximetry monitoring are maintained. Once the skin is prepared, a local anesthetic is injected and the catheter is inserted according to the protocol for the type selected. A chest film is then obtained to verify the correct position of the catheter in the trachea and to rule out an accidental pneumothorax.

Transtracheal oxygen cannot be used for patients with respiratory failure or pleural herniation at the insertion site. It is used with caution in those with cardiac arrhythmias, bleeding disorders, or poor mechanical pulmonary reserve.

Application of the Nursing Process to the Care of the Patient Receiving Transtracheal Oxygen

Assessment

Assess for signs of respiratory distress for 2 to 3 hours after insertion of the catheter. Check ABGs and pulse oximetry readings. Inspect the insertion site for displacement of the catheter or for more than a few drops of bloody drainage. Note frequency and depth of coughing. Observe for large amounts of blood-stained sputum, which can be indicative of hemorrhage. Assess for pain and hoarseness.

Nursing Diagnoses and Planning

The nursing diagnosis and related expected patient outcome most commonly applicable to patients receiving transtracheal oxygen are as follows:

NDx: High risk for altered health maintenance related to insufficient knowledge of self-care after transtracheal catheter insertion

Planning: Patient outcomes

1. Patient describes self-care relevant to transtracheal oxygen therapy.

Nursing Interventions

NDx: High risk for altered health maintenance

Instruct the patient and significant others in self-care, as presented in Chart 12–1.

Chart 12–1.

NURSING GUIDE TO PATIENT EDUCATION FOR SELF-MANAGEMENT: TRANSTRACHEAL OXYGEN (O_2) THERAPY

Instruct the patient to:

Adjust flow rate on basis of pulse oximetry readings when on transtracheal O_2.

Schedule follow-up for arterial blood gases to check adequacy of ventilation and oxygenation.

Cleanse skin surrounding catheter at least twice a day:
- Use cotton swab, water, and a soap such as Ivory if desired.
- Rinse thoroughly.
- Pat dry with a tissue.

Avoid use of skin products unless specifically prescribed.

Perform catheter care as appropriate for the type of catheter in use:
- Heimlich Micro-Trach
  - Instill 0.5 to 1 ml sterile normal saline 2 to 3 times per day to stimulate cough and to clear the lungs. Cleaning of Micro-Trach itself is unnecessary.
  - If the Micro-Trach is accidentally dislodged with coughing, wipe with an alcohol swab and reinsert it. If difficult to reinsert, begin nasal O_2 and call physician.
  - Replace in 6 months.
- SCOOP
  - Clean twice a day:
    - For 6 to 8 weeks, clean SCOOP in place using sterile saline and a special rod. Once track is mature, remove and insert a new catheter. Wash the dirty catheter with the cleaning rod and antibacterial soap.
    - Store in clean, dry place.
    - Replace every 3 months.

Take temperature orally twice a day for 7 days after insertion.

Report the following symptoms of complications immediately:
- Cough unrelieved by cough suppressant
- Increased sputum
- Increased dyspnea
- Cyanosis of the lips or nail beds
- Edema of the face or neck
- Marked pain or bleeding at catheter site
- Fever of 37.5°C (99.5° F)

Additional Interventions

Give acetaminophen for pain and cough suppressants as ordered. Reassure the patient that coughing is a normal response to the presence of the catheter in the trachea but that the urge to cough will lessen in a few days. Also reassure the patient that hoarseness experienced right after the insertion procedure will disappear as the local anesthetic wears off.

Evaluation

Evaluate the effectiveness of nursing care for a patient receiving transtracheal oxygen by comparing the patient's status with the expected patient outcomes. Examples of specific outcomes for patients receiving transtracheal oxygen have been provided in the Planning section.

ARTIFICIAL AIRWAYS

In a healthy patient, who has been breathing room air, total airway obstruction will cause death from hypoxia within 5 to 10 minutes. To ensure adequate ventilation when a patient is threatened by an airway obstruction, an artificial airway may be necessary. Various types of artificial airways are depicted in Figure 12–23.

OROPHARYNGEAL AIRWAY

An oral airway holds the tongue away from the pharynx. It is easily inserted and is used when there is nasal obstruction or predisposition to epistaxis (bleeding from the nose). Selection of the correct size is critical, however, because obstruction may occur if the airway is too large.

An oropharyngeal airway is inserted by pointing the tip toward the roof of the mouth and gently advancing it by rotating it 180 degrees. Another method is to hold down the tongue with a tongue depressor and guide the airway over the back of the tongue until it is in place. When the airway is in place, the top and bottom may be taped to the cheeks.

NASOPHARYNGEAL AIRWAY

Nasopharyngeal airways are used to prevent airway obstruction after trauma to the lower face or after oral surgery. Use is contraindicated when a patient has nasal obstruction or predisposition to epistaxis.

Nasopharyngeal airways are easily inserted and allow for suctioning without displacing the patient's nasal turbinates. On the negative side, they may kink or clog, obstructing the airway, or may cause pressure necrosis of the nasal mucosa. Selection of proper size is important because, like the oral airway, a size too large may cause obstruction.

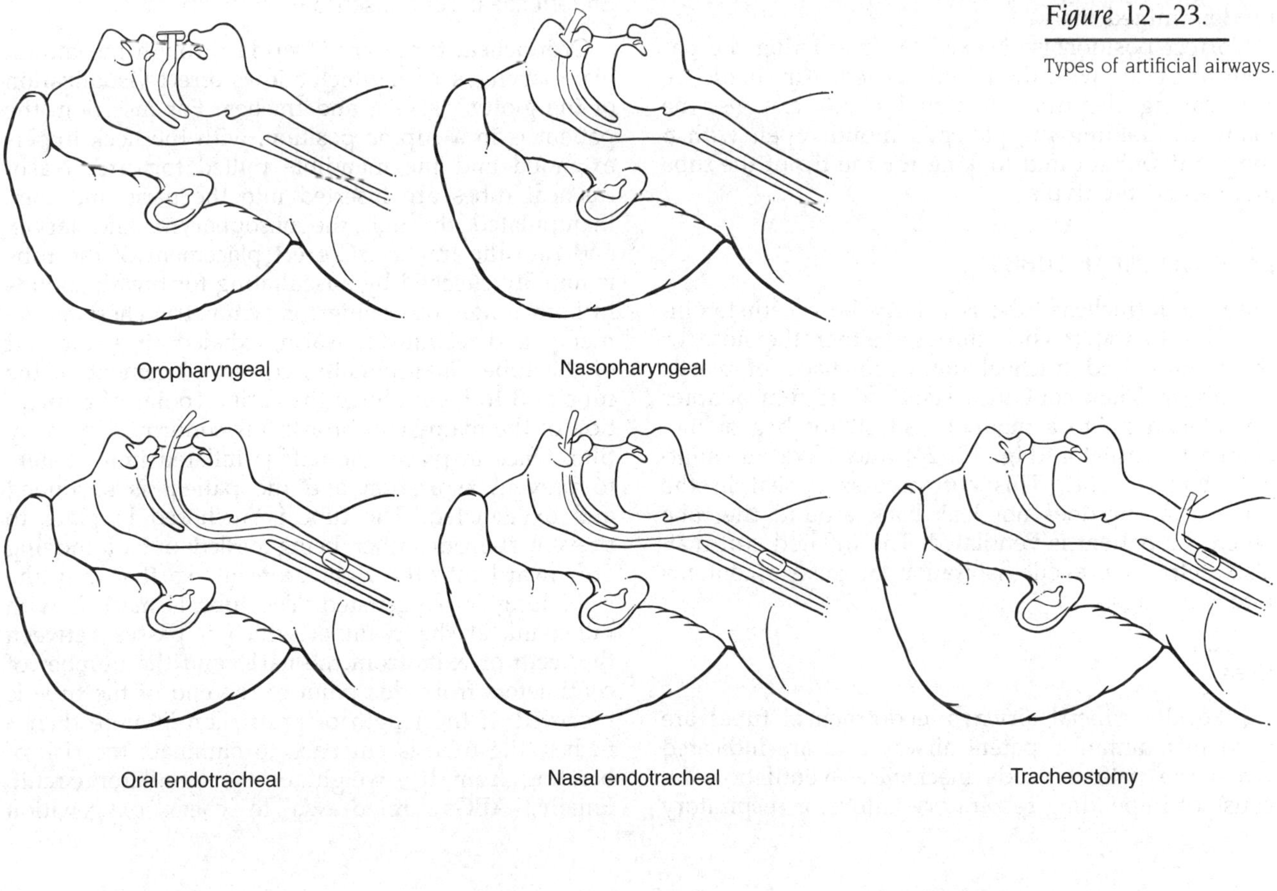

Figure 12–23.

Types of artificial airways.

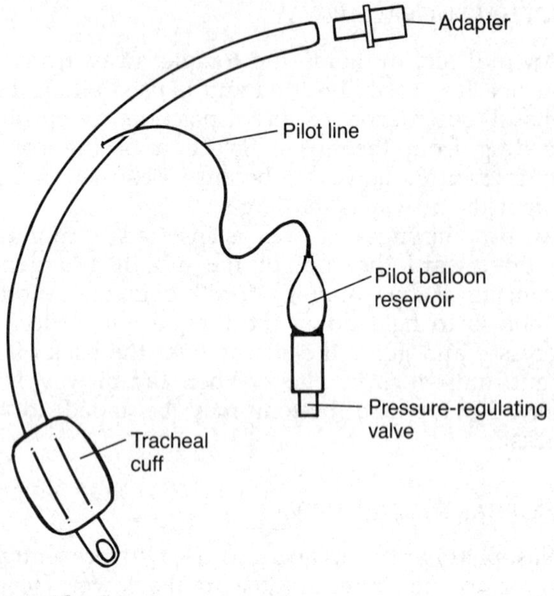

Figure 12–24.

Components of an endotracheal tube.

The correct length of nasopharyngeal airway is determined by measuring from the tip of the nose to the ear lobe and marking the distance on the tube to indicate the depth of insertion. The tube is lubricated with a water-soluble lubricant. The patient is placed in a supine position, and the tip of the nose is pushed up. The airway is then advanced to the predetermined mark.

Correct position is checked by instructing the patient to exhale with the mouth closed. Air should be felt leaving the tube. A visual check can also be made by holding the patient's mouth open with a tongue depressor and looking for the tip of the tube just behind the uvula.

ENDOTRACHEAL TUBES

An endotracheal tube is a large-bore catheter inserted into the trachea through either the nose or the mouth. Endotracheal tubes are made of plastic or rubber. They contain a standard 15-mm adapter for attachment to a manual resuscitator bag or mechanical ventilator (Fig. 12–24) and have an inflatable balloon cuff. This cuff creates a seal in the trachea so air does not leak back around the tube when the patient is ventilated. The inflated cuff may also help to prevent aspiration of gastric contents into the lungs.

Uses

Like all artificial airways, endotracheal tubes are used to maintain a patent airway and are indicated when the patient needs mechanical ventilation because of impending respiratory failure or respiratory arrest. An endotracheal tube isolates the airway, provides access for suctioning secretions from the large airways of the pulmonary tree, and allows delivery of specific concentrations of oxygen up to 100%.

Types of Endotracheal Tubes

Orotracheal tubes are easily inserted and so are used in most emergency situations. They are also used for short-term intubation and mechanical ventilation when the patient has nasal obstruction or a predisposition to epistaxis. These tubes are often inserted with an oropharyngeal airway or bite block to protect them against being bitten or chewed. They increase oropharyngeal secretions and cannot be easily secured in place.

Nasotracheal tubes are more comfortable for the patient than orotracheal tubes, can be more securely held in place, allow for good oral hygiene, and cannot be bitten or chewed. However, they are more difficult to insert and cannot be used if the patient has a nasal obstruction, fractured nose, sinusitis, or predisposition to epistaxis. They also result in increased airway resistance and difficulty suctioning because of the small lumen size needed to fit nasal passages, and they may lacerate pharyngeal mucosa or the larynx during insertion. Pressure necrosis of the nasal mucosa, bleeding on removal, and maxillary sinusitis can also develop when a nasotracheal tube is used.

Endotracheal Tube Insertion

Orotracheal tubes are inserted through the mouth via a laryngoscope, which allows direct visualization of the glottis, larynx, and trachea. For insertion, the patient is in a supine position, with the neck hyperextended and the mandible pulled forward. Nasotracheal tubes are inserted into the naris and then manipulated through the nasopharynx and larynx and into the trachea. Correct placement of the tube is initially checked by auscultating for breath sounds in both lungs, observing for symmetric chest movements, and feeling for warm, exhaled air at the end of the tube. Subsequently, correct placement of the tube at 3 to 5 cm above the carina (point of bifurcation of the main-stem bronchi) is confirmed by x-ray film. Once in place, the cuff is inflated immediately to prevent aspiration and the patient is suctioned and oxygenated. The tube is anchored in place to prevent it from either being pulled out or moving downward into the right bronchus so that only the right lung is oxygenated. The tube is marked with index ink at the point at which it passes between the teeth or exits from the naris, and the number of centimeters from this point to the end of the tube is recorded. If the length of protrusion is more than 3 inches, the tube is cut back to eliminate the risk of bending from the weight of the ventilator circuit. Finally, ABGs are drawn to check oxygenation status. An endotracheal tube can be left in place for 5 to 7 days. If a patient continues to need an airway or mechanical ventilation, a tracheostomy is performed.

Application of the Nursing Process to the Care of the Patient with an Endotracheal Tube

Assessment

Prior to intubation, perform a complete respiratory assessment. If the patient is conscious and the situation permits, also assess the patient's level of anxiety and understanding of the procedure.

When the endotracheal tube is in place, check its placement each shift and after adjusting or changing the tape or plastic anchoring device. This is done by auscultating for breath sounds in both lungs and checking the length of tube protrusion. Be alert for symptoms of partial obstruction such as choking, gagging, dyspnea, cough, wheezing, or stridor. Keep in mind that, when obstruction is minor, symptoms may be slight but that prompt attention is necessary because partial obstruction can become complete obstruction very rapidly.

Observe the sides of the mouth for signs of irritation from orotracheal tubes and the naris for irritation from a nasotracheal tube. Inspect the underlying skin each time the anchoring tape is replaced for irritation or rash. If a ventilator is in use, check periodically that all connections to it remain secure.

Nursing Diagnoses and Planning

Nursing diagnoses and related expected patient outcomes most commonly applicable to patients with an endotracheal tube include the following:

NDx: Anxiety related to the experience of intubation and the effect on other normal functions such as eating and speaking

Planning: Patient outcomes
1. Facial expression and body posture are relaxed.
2. Patient attends to explanations and directions.

NDx: High risk for impaired tissue integrity related to pressure of the endotracheal tube on the trachea and mouth or naris

Planning: Patient outcomes
1. Pressure in tube cuff is maintained at less than 20 mm Hg.
2. Tissues at the corners of the mouth or the naris are nonerythematous and intact.

Nursing Interventions

NDx: Anxiety
In nonemergency situations, prepare the patient for endotracheal intubation by providing brief factual information about the procedure. Explain the need for intubation. Tell the patient that sensations of gagging or suffocating may occur, but provide reassurance that these sensations are normal and pass quickly. Explain that speaking will not be possible once the tube is in place, and plan with the patient some alternate means of communication such as blinking, paper and pencil, Magic Slate, or word, picture, or alphabet charts. Reassure the patient that close observation will be provided and the call bell will be within reach at all times. Explain also that nourishment will be provided intravenously or by tube feeding because nothing can be taken by mouth.

NDx: High risk for impaired tissue integrity
Decrease the risk of erosion and necrosis of tracheal tissue and the development of a tracheoesophageal fistula by preventing traction on the endotracheal tube and carefully following guidelines for proper cuff inflation.

Keep the tube securely anchored, and ascertain that swivel connectors and flexible tubing are used to connect it to the ventilator to prevent traction on it. Avoid unnecessary movement of the patient's head, and, when turning the patient, support both the head and the tube.

When inflating the endotracheal tube, a "minimal leak technique" is normally used. Inflate the cuff until a seal is established, that is, until no harsh sound is heard on inspiration through a stethoscope placed over the trachea but a slight leak on peak inspiration is present; the patient cannot make a sound and no air is felt coming out of the patient's mouth. An alternate technique is known as "minimal occluding volume." Follow the procedure as just described but allow no air leak, even at peak inspiration. Keep in mind that the amount of air needed to inflate the cuff to the point of creating a seal varies with the size of the tube and the size of the patient's trachea. This amount is usually between 5 and 10 ml. If more air is required, it may indicate that a larger size tube is necessary or that the trachea is becoming dilated. Never overinflate the cuff. Maintain the pressure within the cuff at less than 20 mm Hg so as not to exceed the capillary perfusion pressure in the tissues of the trachea. Pressures higher than this impair blood flow and cause tissue damage. When inflating a cuff, document both the volume of air used and the pressure needed to obtain a seal. Check pressure at the end of inspiration if a pressure-limiting cuff is not used.

Periodic deflation of the cuff for 5 to 10 minutes has sometimes been suggested as a method to reduce potential tissue damage. However, the use of this method is of questionable value (Scanlan et al,

Nutrition Box 12–1.

SPECIAL CONSIDERATIONS FOR PATIENTS WITH ENDOTRACHEAL TUBES AND TRACHEOSTOMY TUBES OR WHO ARE ON MECHANICAL VENTILATION

Weigh patient daily, and maintain record of intake and output.
Provide frequent and meticulous mouth care because patient may experience loss of taste and decreased sense of smell.
Evaluate patient's ability to swallow.
Monitor closely for signs of dehydration and report same.
If patient is receiving tube feedings, follow established guidelines, being sure to check for tube placement in the stomach and residual before each feeding.
Replace residual and hold feedings if residual is greater than 100 ml.
If patient is eating, and has a cuffed tracheostomy tube, inflate the cuff.
Provide high-calorie snacks.
Consult with nutritionist for planning of adequate calorie intake, serving of attractive meals to enhance appetite, and provision of some of patient's favorite foods. Remember carbohydrate intake is limited when carbon dioxide retention is a problem.
Always feed patient with head of bed elevated.
Assess and document patient's bowel sounds and activity.

1990) and may in fact be hazardous because of the risk of aspiration and improper ventilation while the cuff is deflated.

Institute measures to protect against tissue damage to the mouth or naris. Apply water-soluble lubricant to the corners of the mouth and lips, and provide good oral hygiene. Reposition orotracheal tubes in alternate sides of the mouth daily. Take extreme care to prevent inadvertent extubation. If scissors are used to cut the tape holding the tube in place, use caution to prevent accidentally cutting the pilot tube. Use of endotracheal tube holders may prevent pressure necrosis and facilitate mouth care.

If a nasotracheal tube is in place, wash the naris gently and apply a water-soluble lubricant. Remove all anchoring tapes gently to avoid abrading the skin. Use hypoallergenic tape if rash or irritation appears.

Additional Interventions
If intubation is done at the bedside, make certain an oxygen source is available because, if intubation is not completed in a reasonable amount of time, the patient may need to be oxygenated with a manual resuscitator using 100% oxygen. Also make certain that a suction source and equipment are at the bedside.

Once intubation is accomplished, monitor equipment to ensure that the prescribed quantities of both oxygen and humidity are being delivered. Keep an extra endotracheal tube of the same size, a 10-cc syringe, and a manual resuscitator at the bedside at all times. If the patient is on a T-piece (provides oxygen and humidity, not mechanical ventilation), hyperinflate or "sigh" the patient every hour to open up atelectatic alveoli. This is not necessary if the patient is on a mechanical ventilator, because mechanical ventilators have a built-in sigh mechanism.

See Nutrition Box 12–1 for nutritional guidelines in the care of the patient with an endotracheal tube.

Evaluation

Evaluate the effectiveness of nursing care for a patient undergoing endotracheal intubation by comparing the patient's status with the expected patient outcomes. Examples of specific outcomes for patients undergoing endotracheal intubation have been provided in the Planning section.

Extubation of an Endotracheal Tube

The patient is extubated when clinical signs, ventilation tests, and ABGs indicate that a patent airway can be maintained and the patient can assume the work of breathing.

Endotracheal tubes are removed with the patient in a sitting position. The patient is hyperoxygenated, the trachea and oropharynx are suctioned, and the cuff is deflated. The patient is then instructed to take a deep breath, the tube is withdrawn, and oxygen is given via a high-humidity face mask. The patient is observed for signs of hemorrhage, laryngeal spasm, and laryngeal edema. Respiratory rate,

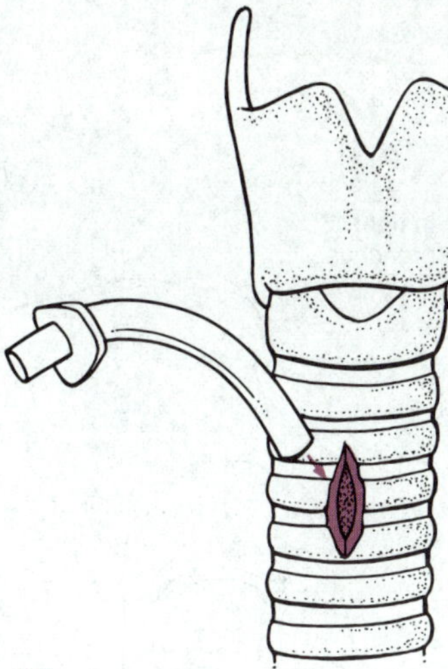

Figure 12–25.

Tracheostomy. The diagram shows a vertical incision through tracheal rings two, three, and four. As illustrated, the tracheostomy tube will be inserted through the incision.

breath sounds, and chest excursion are monitored, and the patient is observed for stridor, pallor or cyanosis, and change in mental status. ABGs and pulse oximetry readings are also monitored to evaluate ventilation and oxygenation.

TRACHEOSTOMY

A tracheostomy is an artificial opening into the trachea created to establish an airway (Fig. 12–25). It may be temporary or permanent.

Uses

Tracheostomies are done to provide a patent airway by by-passing complete upper airway obstruction as from pharyngeal tumors or laryngeal edema by facilitating the removal of secretions or by preventing aspiration of gastric contents. They are also used to allow for long-term mechanical ventilation and to decrease the work of breathing in paralyzed, weak, or critically ill patients by reducing the dead space in the respiratory tract.

Tracheostomy Tubes

Tracheostomy tubes are short, curved tubes with a flange (Fig. 12–26). They are made of silver, stainless steel, or synthetic material and may be cuffed or uncuffed. As with endotracheal tubes, the cuff creates a seal in the trachea, preventing back-leaking of air during mechanical ventilation and aspiration of gastric contents. Most also have a removable inner cannula to facilitate cleaning the inside of the tube. Tracheostomy tubes are held in place by twill tape, which is attached to each side of the tube's flange and tied securely at the side of the neck.

Modifications of the basic tracheostomy tube include the fenestrated tube, cuffed speech-facilitating tubes, and the tracheostomy button. A fenestrated tracheostomy tube allows for air exchange between the lungs and the upper airway through an opening between the flange and the distal end of the tube. It permits the patient to talk when the tracheostomy tube is plugged or to be weaned from a mechanical ventilator.

Also available are cuffed tracheostomy tubes, which facilitate speech. These tubes work by directing an external air supply into the upper airway while the cuff is inflated.

The tracheostomy button fits into the tracheostomy opening extending from the opening to just inside the tracheal wall. It is used with uncuffed or fenestrated tracheostomy tubes and with cuffed tubes when cuffs are deflated. It facilitates talking, coughing, and normal breathing. It is often used in preparation for decannulation.

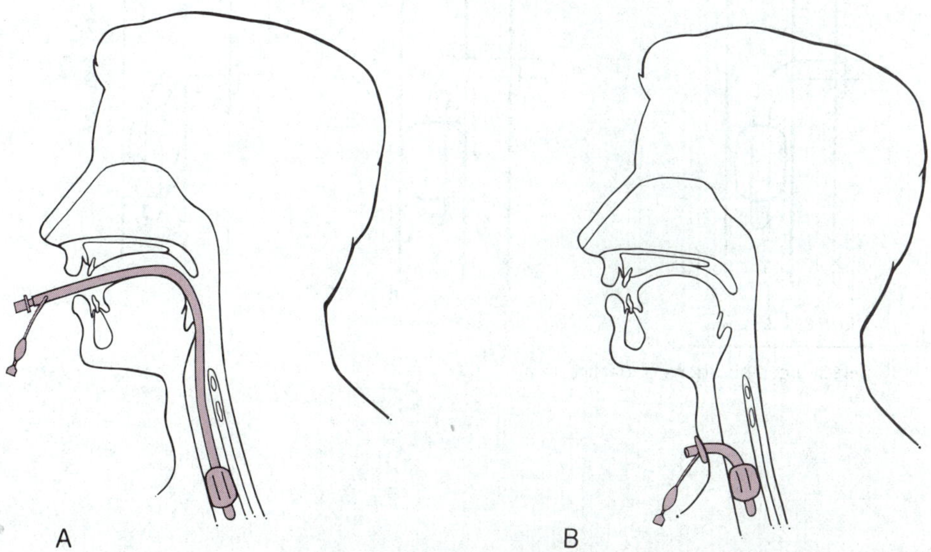

Figure 12–26.

Tracheostomy tube compared with an endotracheal tube. *A*, Endotracheal tube. *B*, Tracheostomy tube.

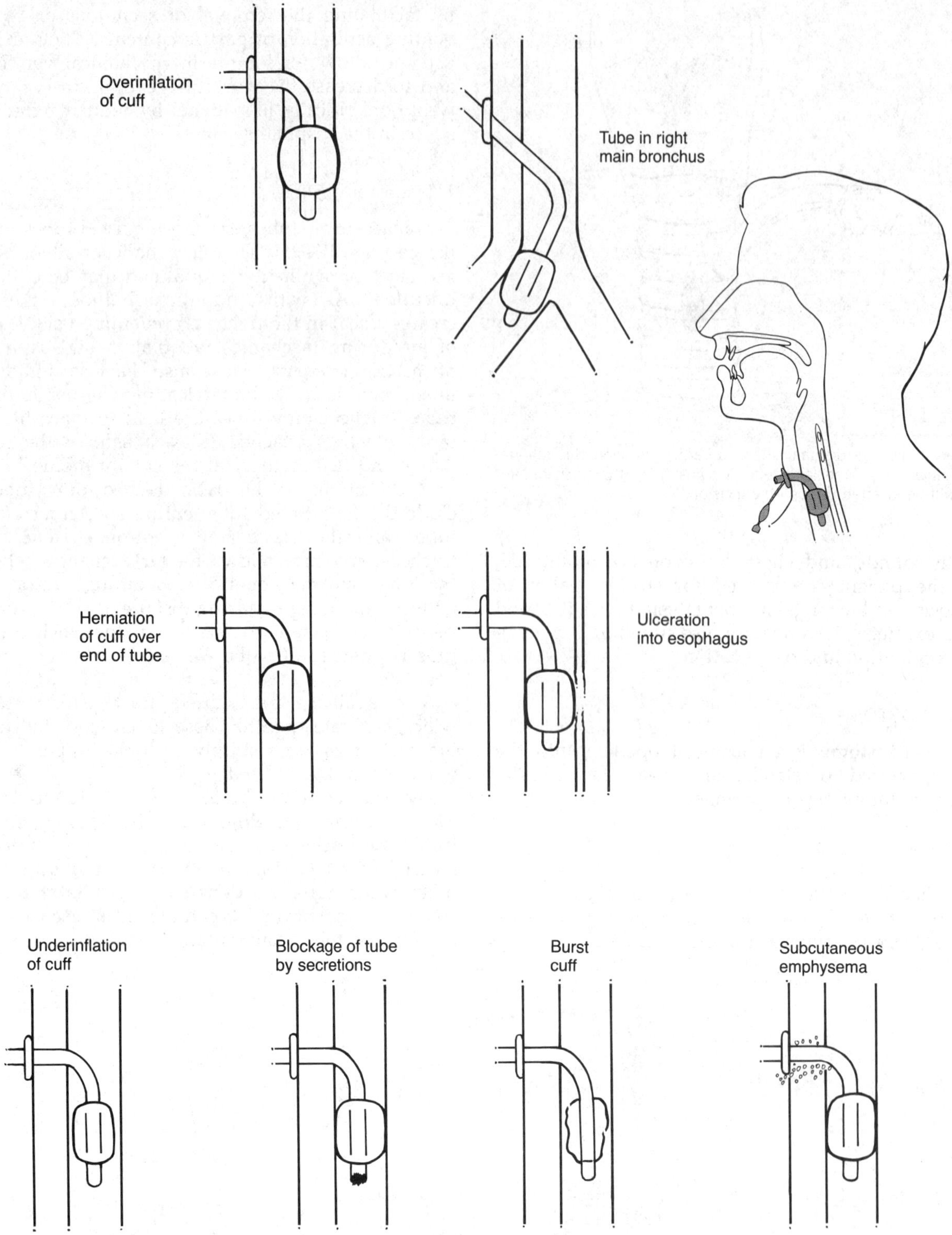

Figure 12–27.

Selected complications of tracheostomy.

Tracheostomy tubes have significant advantages over endotracheal tubes. They are less traumatic because of their length and where and how they are inserted (see Fig. 12–26). Tracheostomy tubes are easier to suction, are more comfortable, and allow the patient to swallow and eat.

Procedure

Elective tracheostomy is a controlled procedure performed in an operating room. Under local anesthesia and with the neck hyperextended, a vertical incision is made in the trachea through the second and third tracheal rings. The trachea is incised, brought to the skin surface, and sutured. Then a tracheostomy tube of appropriate size is inserted with the aid of an obturator. The obturator is removed, and correct placement of the tube is confirmed by chest x-ray film.

Complications

Complications that can occur as a result of tracheostomy surgery include left recurrent laryngeal nerve damage, hemorrhage, pneumothorax, and infection. There is also the risk of technical problems with the tube. These include airway obstruction caused by accidental displacement of the tube, underinflation or overinflation of the cuff, herniation of the cuff over the end of the tube, burst cuff, and blockage of the tube by secretions (Fig. 12–27). Long-term problems that can occur include tracheal stenosis or necrosis and tracheoesophageal fistula.

Application of the Nursing Process to the Care of the Patient with a Tracheostomy

Assessment

Prior to the procedure, perform a complete respiratory assessment. If the situation permits, assess the patient's hearing, language ability, and writing ability in preparation for selecting alternate methods of communication after surgery. Determine the patient's understanding of the procedure, and assess level of anxiety.

After the procedure, note rate, rhythm, and depth of respirations. Note chest excursion, cough, amount and appearance of tracheal secretions, and frequency of the need for suctioning. Review ABG values if available. Check the placement of the tracheostomy tube, and monitor the pressure in the cuff every shift by attaching a manometer to the cuff port. Note whether minimal occlusive volume is increased or decreased. Every 2 to 4 hours, check that the cuff is creating a good seal. Place a stethoscope over the trachea, and listen for a harsh or gurgling sound during expiration; feel for warm air from the mouth during expiration; and check the patient's ability to make sounds. Suspect a leak if any of these occur.

Observe the condition of the dressing and the tapes, and assess for signs of infection. Inspect the surgical site for bleeding, swelling, and purulent drainage. Check for fever, and review laboratory reports for leukocytosis.

Assess also for the development of pneumothorax, pneumomediastinum, and cardiac tamponade. Be alert for cough, sharp chest pain, and tachycardia, which are indicative of pneumothorax, as well as for dyspnea, crepitus, and edema of the face and neck, which are indicative of pneumomediastinum. Check for increased central venous pressure (CVP), narrowed pulse pressure, paradoxical pulse, hypotension, dyspnea, or decreased level of consciousness, which are symptoms of cardiac tamponade.

Nursing Diagnoses and Planning

Nursing diagnoses and related expected patient outcomes most commonly applicable to patients with a tracheostomy include the following:

NDx: Anxiety related to the tracheostomy procedure and its effects on body function

Planning: Patient outcomes
1. Facial expression and body posture are relaxed.
2. Patient is able to rest quietly.
3. Patient attends to explanations and directions.

NDx: High risk for ineffective breathing pattern related to tracheal obstruction

Planning: Patient outcomes
1. Respiratory rate is 14 to 20 per minute.
2. Chest movement is smooth, symmetric, and of normal depth.
3. Breath sounds are clear.
4. Cyanosis is absent.

NDx: High risk for infection related to bacterial contamination of the tracheal wound

Planning: Patient outcomes
1. Tracheostomy site is intact and without redness, edema, or drainage.
2. Purulent tracheal secretions are absent.
3. Patient is afebrile.

NDx: Impaired verbal communication related to interrupted flow of air between the lungs and the upper airway secondary to tracheostomy

Planning: Patient outcomes
1. Patient uses nonverbal methods of communication.
2. Patient communicates needs effectively.

Nursing Interventions

NDx: Anxiety
Prepare the patient and the family for the tracheostomy by listening to their concerns, providing factual information, and answering questions. Ordinarily, the physician has provided an initial explanation of the procedure, so the focus is on reinforcing information. Be certain it is understood that slight discomfort is normal despite the local anesthesia, that speaking will not be possible with the basic tube in place, and that the tracheostomy will have to be suctioned because of the accumulation of secretions. Recognize that patients are often afraid of accidental suffocation when dependent on a tracheostomy to breathe. Reassure the patient in this regard. Remind the patient that tracheostomies are common, that close observation will be provided, and that a call bell will be readily available. Keep the patient physically comfortable, and guide in the use of relaxation exercises if needed.

NDx: High risk for ineffective breathing pattern
If the tracheostomy tube is dislodged after surgery, the opening can close over, leaving the patient unable to breathe. Therefore, keep a replacement tube and obturator at the bedside along with a curved hemostat that could be used to hold the trachea open. Do not change the tapes on the tracheostomy tube or deflate the cuff for the first 24 hours because of the risk of accidental dislodgement. Similarly, do not change the tube for at least a week.

Using strict sterile technique, suction the airway as often as needed to keep it patent. This may be every 5 to 10 minutes immediately after the procedure and later every 2 to 3 hours. Avoid suctioning unnecessarily because it can increase secretions and cause mechanical trauma to the tissues. Suction patients who are sensitive to decreased oxygen levels more frequently but for a shorter time to avoid hypoxemia or hypercapnia. Be sure to document time of suctioning, characteristics of secretions, respiratory status, and patient's response.

Keep a pair of scissors at the bedside to snip the tapes in the event the tracheostomy tube should become dislodged and the tapes tighten around the neck. Also keep a manual resuscitation bag with an adaptor mask at the bedside.

NDx: High risk for infection
Treat the tracheostomy as a surgical wound. Use all sterile equipment (e.g., suction apparatus, gloves, dressings), and maintain strict sterile technique.

Cleanse the tracheostomy and the surrounding area to keep them free of secretions and bacterial contamination. Put on sterile gloves. Use sterile gauze to remove the inner cannula, and soak it in half-strength hydrogen peroxide solution. Suction the outer cannula, and follow with deep breathing either by the patient or via an Ambu bag. Remove the soiled tracheostomy dressing, and use gauze and peroxide solution to remove secretions and crusts from around the tube. Use peroxide-soaked swabs to cleanse under the neck plate and the openings in its sides. Using a new pair of sterile gloves, thoroughly cleanse the inner cannula with a brush and pipe cleaners; rinse in sterile saline or water. Dry thoroughly and replace in the outer cannula. Proceed to change the tracheostomy tapes. Prepare the clean tapes before removing the soiled ones. To prepare, cut the tape, with about two thirds left on one side and one third on the other. Make a horizontal slit 1 inch from each end. Insert this slit end of the tie through the side opening of the outer cannula. Pull the opposite end through the slit and draw securely. Repeat this procedure and secure the other one-third piece to the opposite side of the cannula. Hold the tube while this is being done because the patient could easily cough the tube out, resulting in airway obstruction. Tie the tapes on the side of the neck to eliminate a knot at the back of the neck. Finally, slip a 3 × 3-inch gauze pad folded into a V shape or a factory-made split sponge between the neck and the tracheostomy tube to provide padding and to absorb secretions. Never cut a gauze pad for this use because frayed threads can be aspirated.

NDx: High risk for impaired communication
Before the tracheostomy, if possible, plan a method of communication for the patient to use once the tube is in place. Depending on the patient's physical and mental capacities, consider use of paper and pencil, Magic Slate, pictures, or an adjunct device such as the Passy-Muir valve, Olympic Trach-Talk, the Pitt speaking tube, and the Cyberset tone generator. Keep in mind that the selection of one of these devices depends on individual patient tolerance. Orient significant others to the planned method of communication to avoid creating confusion and frustration.

Evaluation

Evaluate the effectiveness of nursing care for a patient having a tracheostomy by comparing the patient's status with the expected patient outcomes. Examples of specific outcomes for patients having a tracheostomy have been provided in the Planning section.

Removal of a Tracheostomy Tube

Removal of a tracheostomy tube is similar to that of an endotracheal tube. The patient is ventilated, oxygenated, and suctioned. The cuff is deflated, suctioning is repeated, and the tube is removed. A moist gauze pad is placed over the wound, which closes spontaneously in about 5 days.

MECHANICAL VENTILATION THERAPY

Mechanical ventilation therapy is used to overcome the patient's inability to ventilate or oxygenate adequately. It may be intermittent or continuous and short term or long term.

INTERMITTENT POSITIVE PRESSURE BREATHING

IPPB is a mode of therapy used to deliver air or oxygen under a pressure greater than atmospheric pressure until a preset limit is reached. It improves the inspiratory phase of ventilation and promotes the flow of air to the alveoli. This form of therapy is both intermittent and short term.

Uses

The primary use of IPPB is to deliver aerosol medications into the lower respiratory tract for patients unable to take a deep breath. It also promotes alveolar ventilation and removal of secretions and decreases the work of breathing. It may be used in the treatment of restrictive lung disease, COPD, and acute pulmonary edema as well as in the prevention of postoperative atelectasis. Recently, its value has been disputed, and some studies have shown that it is no more effective than good deep breathing and may, in fact, increase air trapping in COPD.

Procedure

Treatments are usually administered for 15 to 20 minutes three to four times per day. The patient is instructed to maintain a slow respiratory rate and to use diaphragmatic breathing during the treatment. Coughing is encouraged every few minutes. If a bronchodilator is administered as part of the treatment, vital signs, breath sounds, and simple bedside pulmonary function measures such as peak flow and vital capacity are recorded before and after it.

Complications

Complications of IPPB therapy are dizziness related to hyperventilation, which lowers carbon dioxide levels, exacerbation of hemoptysis, ruptured alveoli and pneumothorax, increased intracranial pressure, and cardiovascular problems. It may also cause nausea and vomiting if administered too soon after meals. Infection secondary to cross-contamination is another risk because medication or water left in the equipment serves as a medium for bacterial growth. To prevent this, careful cleansing techniques are followed and individual tubing, nebulizers, masks, mouthpieces, and filters are used. IPPB is contraindicated in the presence of untreated pneumothorax, impaired glottis function, and wound dehiscence. It is also contraindicated if the patient experiences a fall in blood pressure of greater than 30 mm Hg during therapy.

MECHANICAL VENTILATION

If a patient is unable to ventilate adequately enough to maintain proper levels of oxygen and carbon dioxide in the blood, mechanical ventilation by a respirator may be indicated.

Types of Ventilators

There are many different types of ventilator models (Table 12–7). The models fall into two cate-

Table 12–7. TYPES OF VENTILATORS

CLASSIFICATION	REMARKS	MODES	ACCESSORY MODES
NEGATIVE PRESSURE VENTILATORS			
Drinker respirator tank (iron lung)	No intubation required; reliable but cumbersome		
Body wrap (raincoat or poncho ventilator)	Consists of rigid cage with a nylon wrap around abdomen and thorax; portable; prone to leaks; causes musculoskeletal pain		
Chest cuirass	Rigid shell over chest; can be used in wheelchair; hard to fit; causes back pain		
POSITIVE PRESSURE VENTILATORS			
Pressure-cycled	Inspiration is terminated when a predetermined pressure is reached; volumes are inconsistent; used short term, such as in the PACU (Bird, PRII)	Control: assist/control	
Volume-cycled	Inspiration terminated when a preset volume is achieved regardless of pressure required; several modes available; most commonly used are the Ma-1, Bear, PB7200, and Servo*	Control: assist/control; IMV/SIMV; CPAP; pressure support	PEEP, sighs
Time-cycled	Inspiration is terminated at a predetermined time; this type is used chiefly in infants (Bear Cub)	Control: assist/control; IMV; CPAP	PEEP

Abbreviations: PACU, postanesthesia care unit; IMV, intermittent mandatory ventilation; SIMV, synchronized intermittent mandatory ventilation; CPAP, continuous positive airway pressure; PEEP, positive end-expiratory pressure.

* The classification of ventilators has been complicated by microprocessor technology. Several ventilators can be classified in different ways, and the distinction is not always readily apparent.

gories: negative pressure ventilators and positive pressure ventilators. Negative pressure ventilators exert negative pressure on the chest and lung to expand them during inspiration. They are used in the care of patients with neuromuscular disorders, such as myasthenia gravis, multiple sclerosis, and muscular dystrophy. Positive pressure ventilators exert positive pressure on airways to inflate alveoli during inspiration. They are used in the care of patients with chest and lung disorders, such as flail chest, chronic bronchitis, emphysema, and ARDS. The most widely used types today are pressure cycled and volume cycled, both positive pressure ventilators.

The pressure-cycled ventilator is set to deliver a preset positive pressure for a specified length of time or until the preset pressure is reached. When the pressure is reached, the machine turns off and normal exhalation begins. The tidal volume (volume of gas) delivered is not necessarily constant because it depends on the resistance of the entire system, including the lung. Change in compliance or airway resistance, or both, can be caused by atelectasis, bronchospasm, mucous plug, or change in the patient's position. As a result, the pressure-cycled ventilators cannot be relied on to deliver consistent volumes for long-term mechanical ventilation. They are generally used for short-term, closely monitored situations, such as in a recovery room.

A volume-cycled ventilator delivers a constant volume of air with each breath regardless of the positive pressure necessary to attain that volume. There is a preset pressure-limiting valve that causes release of excessive pressure if the preset limit is reached. These pressure-limiting valves usually have an audible alarm. The limit can be set just slightly above the pressure required to ventilate the patient. The alarm then sounds when secretions accumulate or when the patient coughs or resists the machine.

Ventilation Modes

Whatever type of ventilator is used, various ventilator modes are adjusted to the individual patient's needs. They are as follows:

1. Assist: This pattern means that the patient's respiratory effort triggers the machine. The negative pressure required to trigger an assist breath is set on the machine. When the patient's inspiratory effort equals or exceeds this preset negative pressure, the machine responds with a positive pressure breath. Both a pressure-cycled or volume-cycled ventilator can be set with the assist mode.
2. Control: This is inflation of the patient's lungs at a set interval regardless of patient effort or breathing pattern. This is used if the patient is apneic or the respiratory rate is too low or if the patient is sedated with neuromuscular paralyzing agents.
3. Assist-control: This is basically the assist pattern with a back-up control rate from the ventilator for minimum ventilation. The ventilator responds with a positive pressure breath to every patient effort, and if the patient stops breathing, the machine automatically takes over ventilation at a preset rate. Hyperventilation is a complication of this pattern.
4. Synchronized intermittent mandatory ventilation (SIMV): This mode allows the patient to breathe spontaneously but also delivers a mandatory positive pressure breath at a predetermined rate. The patient's own breaths are without positive pressure, and inspired oxygen is the same as with the ventilator-delivered breaths. This mode is used to wean patients from ventilators by gradually decreasing the number of breaths by the machine. The patient assumes a larger portion of the minute volume as the ventilator support is gradually removed.
5. Continuous positive airway pressure (CPAP): In this mode, the patient breathes spontaneously while the pressure in the airways is maintained above atmospheric pressure. This may be used as an alternate to T-piece weaning. When this continuous positive pressure on expiration is applied in combination with a mandatory ventilator breath, it is known as positive end-expiratory pressure (PEEP).
6. Pressure support ventilation (PSV): The patient's spontaneous breath is augmented with a preset pressure. It does not provide the entire volume. The rate is not set by the machine but rather by the patient's spontaneous efforts. There are other methods of manipulating or adjusting inspiration or expiration that are accessory modes, which may be used in conjunction with any of the primary modes previously mentioned. These include the following:

- PEEP: In this accessory mode, a positive pressure is maintained in the lungs at the end of exhalation. Its use increases the volume of air left in the lungs at the end of a passive expiration. Its primary purpose is to keep airways and alveoli from collapsing. The positive pressure allows more oxygen to diffuse across the alveolocapillary membrane, thereby improving oxygenation with decreasing oxygen supplementation. Possible complications of PEEP include decreased cardiac output, hypotension, pneumothorax and other barotrauma, and fluid retention caused by inappropriate antidiuretic hormone (ADH) secretion.
- Sighs: A normal person sighs 6 to 10 times per hour. Monotonous tidal volumes on mechanical ventilation can lead to microatelectasis. Although sighs are not always used, strong consideration should be given to providing a deeper than normal breath several times per hour. Some mechanical ventilators sigh the patient automatically or can be adjusted to do so. If the type used does not have this ability, the patient may be sighed manually with a bag-valve resuscitator to prevent atelectasis.

The ventilator used should have a regulator-controlled flow rate at which gas is delivered. It should also have the ability to regulate inspired concentrations of oxygen from 21% to 100%. An oxygen analyzer should always be used to ensure the accuracy of the delivered fraction of inspired oxygen (FIO_2). Basic ventilator characteristics necessary to ensure patient safety are as follows:

- Provision for heating (90–100°F, 32.2–37.7°C) and humidifying the inspired air.
- A reliable visible and audible alarm that sounds if there is a rise or fall in circuit pressure or if a patient disconnects within 15 seconds. *Note: Alarms should never be shut off.*
- Provisions for measurement of expired volumes to determine tidal and minute ventilations.
- Plugs and switches that are insulated and grounded.
- Breathing tubing and parts that are easily removed for sterilization or replacement.
- A fail-safe valve that opens at a few centimeters negative pressure. If there is electrical failure or machine malfunction, this allows the patient to draw in air to prevent suffocation.

Application of the Nursing Process to the Care of the Patient on a Mechanical Ventilator

Assessment

Auscultate lung sounds every 2 hours, and observe for symmetric chest expansion to determine whether both lungs are being ventilated. Assess need for suctioning because secretions increase with the use of mechanical ventilation. Check vital signs every 2 to 4 hours.

Assess the patient for signs of hypoxia, hypercapnia, and hypocapnia. Symptoms of hypoxia are restlessness, anxiety, tachycardia, increased respiratory rate, increased work of breathing, cyanosis, and confusion. Symptoms of hypercapnia are somnolence, lethargy, tachycardia, confusion, and headache. Symptoms of hypocapnia are muscle spasm, tetany, diaphoresis, light headedness, tachypnea, and cardiac dysrhythmia. Assess the patient's synchrony with the ventilator. Check ABG values at regular intervals and whenever ventilator settings are changed.

In patients on PEEP, observe for signs of decreased cardiac output, which is a risk caused by the effect of positive pressure on the thoracic vessels. Be alert for weak peripheral pulses, narrowed pulse pressure, slow capillary refill, decreased urinary output, restlessness, decreasing level of consciousness, pallor, fatigue, and chest pain, all of which are symptoms of decreased cardiac output. If settings for PEEP are decreased, assess for signs of cardiac overload and pulmonary edema. If CVP or pulmonary capillary wedge pressures (PCWP) are required, obtain all readings either with the patient connected or disconnected from the ventilator because the positive pressure alters the readings.

Assess nasogastric drainage or stool for frank and occult blood, because stress ulcers are a potential complication of mechanical ventilation. Review hematocrit values.

Observe the skin for redness and breakdown, because mobility of the patient on a respirator is limited. Also assess joint mobility and nutritional status. Determine the patient's emotional response to the ventilator. Be alert to signs of anxiety and to feelings of powerlessness.

Nursing Diagnoses and Planning

Nursing diagnoses and related expected patient outcomes most commonly applicable to patients on a mechanical ventilator include the following:

NDx: Ineffective breathing pattern related to *(specify)*

or (depending on the specific patient situation)

NDx: Inability to sustain spontaneous ventilation related to *(specify)*

Planning: Patient outcomes
1. ABG values are within normal range.

NDx: High risk for ineffective airway clearance related to excessive secretions

Planning: Patient outcomes
1. Breath sounds are normal.
2. ABG values are within patient's normal range.

NDx: High risk for fluid volume excess related to blocked insensible water loss

Planning: Patient outcomes
1. Chest sounds are clear.
2. Extremities are free of edema.
3. Vital signs are within patient's baseline range.

NDx: Impaired physical mobility related to mechanical ventilation

Planning: Patient outcomes
1. Joints have patient's normal range of motion.
2. Patient moves as directed.

NDx: Anxiety related to being on a mechanical ventilator

Planning: Patient outcomes
1. Body posture appears relaxed.
2. Facial expression appears relaxed.

NDx: High risk for altered thought processes related to change in sensory input secondary to limited mobility

Planning: Patient outcomes
1. Patient is oriented to time, place, and person.

Nursing Interventions

NDx: Ineffective breathing pattern
Maintain ventilator closed-circuit system. Prevent accidental disconnection of the patient from the ventilator by leaving the alarm on at all times, even during suctioning. Keep a manual resuscitator bag at the bedside, and manually ventilate the patient if power fails or the ventilator malfunctions. Respond immediately to any alarm; if the problem cannot be immediately identified and corrected, disconnect the patient and ventilate by hand while the problem is further investigated. Check settings on the ventilator every hour. Also check tubing for condensation, and drain collected water to prevent aspiration.

If a patient is "fighting the ventilator," promote synchronization by slowly ventilating by bag for three to six breaths or by verbally coaching the patient as to when to inhale and exhale. Administer ordered analgesics or sedatives if pain or anxiety is the causative factor.

NDx: High risk for ineffective airway clearance
Direct the patient to cough and deep breathe every 2 hours. Change the patient's position at least every 2 hours. If only one lung is affected, position the patient on the unaffected side or the back. Suction as needed. Maintain humidification, making certain that the water level is maintained in the ventilator reservoir. Also perform chest physiotherapy as ordered to help mobilize secretions. Administer prescribed intravenous or inhaled bronchodilators.

NDx: High risk for fluid volume excess
Measure intake and output. When interpreting these values, adjust for the fact that insensible water loss is blocked by the closed humidification system of the ventilator. Weigh patient daily to check for weight gain, which is indicative of fluid retention. Also monitor for edema, crackles, hyponatremia, and decreased hematocrit, which are additional symptoms of overload.

NDx: Impaired physical mobility
Change the patient's position, and provide skin care every 2 hours. Perform active or passive range-of-motion exercises every 8 hours. Maintain the patient's position of function while the patient is on bed rest to prevent contractures and external hip rotation. Use a footboard, and have the patient wear tie-up shoes or high-top sneakers while in bed to prevent foot drop. Sit the patient up in a chair as soon as his or her condition allows. When permitted, walk the patient while ventilating with oxygen via a bag or while pushing the ventilator along.

NDx: Anxiety
Explain procedures and equipment to the patient and the family. Reassure them regarding the dependability of the machine and its built-in malfunction-detection system. Further reassure them that close supervision is provided by nursing and other health team personnel. Do not leave the patient unattended until he or she has anxiety under control and is comfortable with the ventilator.

Whenever possible, involve the patient in decision-making regarding care to provide a sense of having some control. Also encourage the use of relaxation exercises and tape-recordings as well as other stress-reduction techniques. Provide diversion suited to the patient's conditon and personal preferences.

Remember that significant others are often as anxious as the patient, so facilitate discussion of concerns and provide information as needed. Also make certain to promote communication between the patient and the family.

NDx: High risk for altered thought processes
Speak frequently to the patient even though he or she cannot talk back. Call the patient by name and orient to day, date, time, and place as a part of routine care. Place a calendar and a clock within the patient's view. Dim lighting at bedtime to help distinguish day from night. Ask family members to bring in pictures or other personal items that can be placed in the patient's environment. If possible, provide the patient with a window view for light and sensory stimulation. Encourage diversionary activities and visits by significant others. To the extent possible, plan uninterrupted periods of rest and sleep.

Additional Interventions
Provide oral hygiene every 8 hours to increase comfort and to decrease the likelihood of bacterial contamination of the lower respiratory tract. Give antacids or other medication ordered to combat stress ulcers. Administer tube feedings or total parenteral nutrition (TPN) solutions as ordered. Monitor bowel function.

Evaluation

Evaluate the effectiveness of nursing care for a patient on mechanical ventilation by comparing the patient's status with the expected patient outcomes. Examples of specific outcomes for patients on mechanical ventilation have been provided in the Planning section.

WEANING FROM MECHANICAL VENTILATION

Patients are weaned from dependence on a ventilator gradually over a period of time. Patients are judged ready to be weaned when their conditions are stable and the following criteria are met:

Condition requiring mechanical ventilation has resolved or stabilized.
Airway is patent.
Chest wall is stable.
Respiratory rate is between 12 and 20 per minute.
PEEP is no higher than 5 cm of water.
Vital capacity is greater than 15 ml/kg of body weight.
Inspiratory pressure is at least −25 to −30 cm of water.
Cough is strong and effective.
Lungs are acceptably clear on auscultation and x-ray film.
ABG values are within normal range.
Cardiac output is adequate.
Patient is afebrile.
Nutritional status is satisfactory.

Weaning can be accomplished by several techniques used individually or in combination. These techniques include synchronized IMV (SIMV), pressure support, and use of a T-piece. When SIMV is used, the number of breaths delivered by the ventilator is gradually decreased, thus increasing the amount of spontaneous breathing done by the patient. Pressure support may be used to augment the spontaneous breaths. The positive pressure with this method is also gradually reduced until the patient is weaned from the ventilator. When a T-piece is used, the patient is disconnected from the ventilator and placed on the T-piece with humidified oxygen at an FIO_2 5% to 10% higher than when on the ventilator.

Pharmacology Box 12–1.

DECONGESTANTS

Decongestants:
Drugs that reduce swelling of mucous membranes and relieve congestion.

Action:
Directly stimulate α-adrenergic receptors in the nasal mucosa and cause the release of norepinephrine, which in turn causes vasoconstriction with shrinking of the swollen mucous membranes and nasal drainage.

Uses:
Symptomatic relief of nasal congestion caused by rhinitis, coryza, and sinusitis.

Side Effects:
Nervousness, irritability, restlessness, and insomnia caused by central nervous system (CNS) stimulation; occasional nausea; palpitations; difficulty urinating; and dose-related hypertension caused by vasoconstriction and rebound congestion with repeated use. Side effects more likely with oral use as opposed to topical use.

Interactions:
Systemic decongestants (e.g., ephedrine and phenylpropanolamine) interact with other sympathomimetics, resulting in increased CNS stimulation; inhibit action of adrenergic blocking agents; and interact with monoamine oxidase (MAO) inhibitors and can cause severe hypertension.

Nursing Implications:
Counsel the elderly and those with hypertension, hyperthyroidism, cardiovascular disease, and prostatic hypertrophy to take with caution.
Caution patients not to use topical preparations for longer than 5 days because of rebound.
Instruct patients using drops to instill with the head back and down to decrease the amount swallowed and to allow the solution to spread slowly over the nasal mucosa.
Suggest taking systemic decongestants a few hours before bedtime to decrease risk of insomnia.
Caution patients not to break, cut, crush, or chew timed-release preparations.

Time spent off the ventilator begins with 5- to 10-minute intervals and is gradually increased on the basis of patient tolerance.

Whichever technique is used, the patient should be placed in a high Fowler's position and monitored carefully. Vital signs, vital capacity and negative inspiratory force, pulse oximetry readings, and ABGs should be obtained as often as necessary. Signs of intolerance to the weaning procedure may include tachypnea, dyspnea, tachycardia, arrhythmia, diaphoresis, and change in mental status.

PHARMACOLOGIC THERAPY

Drug therapy plays an important role in the medical management of disorders of the respiratory system. Major categories of drugs specific to the treatment of respiratory problems are nasal decongestants, antihistamines, antitussives, expectorants, mucolytics, and bronchodilators.

Nasal decongestants (Pharmacology Box 12–1) are drugs that reduce swelling of the mucosa and thereby promote drainage and relieve congestion. They are primarily over-the-counter drugs and are used to treat both allergic and nonallergic rhinitis (common cold).

Antihistamines (Pharmacology Box 10–1) are used to relieve sneezing, rhinorrhea, and nasal itching associated with allergic rhinitis. They are most effective when taken prophylactically.

Antitussives (Pharmacology Box 12–2) are cough suppressants. They are used to control nonproductive cough and allow the patient to rest. Antitussives should not be used indiscriminately because cough is a protective mechanism designed to remove excessive secretions and foreign matter from the respiratory tract. The most commonly used nonnarcotic antitussive is dextromethorphan, which is an over-the-counter drug with few side effects.

Expectorants (e.g., terpin hydrate) are medications that make cough more productive by stimulating the flow of secretions, thus making them more liquid

Pharmacology Box 12–2.
ANTITUSSIVES

Antitussives:
Medications that suppress cough; two major groups: opioids (e.g., codeine) and nonopioids (e.g., dextromethorphan).

Action:
Decrease the frequency and intensity of cough by directly inhibiting the response of the cough center in the medulla.

Uses:
Suppress cough that has no therapeutic purpose, such as raising secretions, and is causing throat irritation, discomfort, and loss of sleep.

Side Effects:
Side effects are rare at doses used in antitussives. Low risk of addiction and respiratory depression with codeine preparations, none with dextromethorphan. Toxic effects of opioid antitussives include miosis, bradycardia, tachycardia, hypotension, narcosis, seizures, circulatory collapse, respiratory arrest. Toxic effects of dextromethorphan include euphoria, hyperactivity, staggering gait, lethargy, uncoordinated movements, stupor, and shallow breathing.

Interactions:
Opioid antitussives potentiate the depressant effect of monoamine oxidase (MAO) inhibitors, alcohol, and other central nervous system (CNS) depressants. Dextromethorphan can interact with MAO inhibitors to cause excitation and hyperpyrexia.

Nursing Implications:
Caution patient not to exceed recommended dose and not to mix with CNS depressants.
Instruct patient to report cough lasting longer than 1 week or changing from nonproductive to productive.
Give with caution to patients with a decreased respiratory reserve.

Pharmacology Box 12–3.
BRONCHODILATORS

Bronchodilators:
Medications that relax constricted airways; two groups: β_2-adrenergic agonists (e.g., terbutaline [Brethine]) and methylxanthines (e.g., theophylline).

Action:
β_2-adrenergic agonists are selective sympathomimetic drugs that relax the bronchial smooth muscle and result in bronchial dilation. Methylxanthines also relax bronchial smooth muscle, possibly by blocking the receptors for adenosine.

Uses:
β_2-adrenergic agonists are given by metered dose inhaler or nebulizer to relieve mild to moderate asthma attacks or to prevent exercise-induced attacks. They are given orally if inhaler cannot be used and by injection in emergency situations. Oral theophylline is given as maintenance therapy to decrease the frequency and severity of asthma attacks and the need for other medication. It is given intravenously in emergency situations.

Side Effects:
β_2-adrenergic agonists have minimal side effects when given by inhaler. With oral or parenteral administration, tremor, angina pectoris, and tachydysrhythmias can occur. Theophylline has few side effects at plasma levels below 20 mg/ml. At 20 to 25 mg/ml, nausea, vomiting, diarrhea, insomnia, and restlessness can develop, whereas at levels greater than 30 mg/ml, severe dysrhythmias, convulsions, and death can occur.

Interactions:
β_2-adrenergic agonist effects can be inhibited by β-adrenergic blocking agents such as propranolol. Theophylline levels can be lowered by marijuana, tobacco, and phenobarbital. They can be increased by oral contraceptives, cimetidine, erythromycin, and caffeine.

Nursing Implications:
β_2-adrenergic agonist:
- Teach proper use of metered dose inhaler or nebulizer.
- Instruct the patient to wait at least 1 minute between puffs if two puffs or inhales are needed.
- Warn patient against exceeding recommended dosage.

Systemic preparation:
- Instruct patient to report chest pain or changes in heart rate or rhythm.
- Administer with caution to patients with diabetes, hyperthyroidism, organic heart disease, hypertension or angina pectoris.

Theophylline:
- Instruct the patient not to break, crush, or chew enteric or timed-release preparations.
- Monitor plasma drug levels.
- Caution the patient to avoid ingestion of caffeine-containing food or beverages.

and easier to expectorate. It is questionable whether these drugs are any more effective than fluids, deep-breathing exercises, and position changes in promoting expectoration.

Mucolytics are medications that react with mucus to make it more watery and more easily expectorated. Two solutions used for this purpose are hypertonic saline and acetylcysteine. Both are administered by inhalation, and both can cause reflex bronchospasm.

Bronchodilators (Pharmacology Box 12–3) are medications that relax constricted airways. The two major groups of drugs used for their bronchodilator effects are the β_2-adrenergic agonists and the methylxanthines, also referred to simply as xanthines. Theophylline is the major xanthine used in the treatment of asthma. Aminophylline is a theophylline salt. It has identical pharmacologic actions to theophylline but is more soluble and is most often given intravenously.

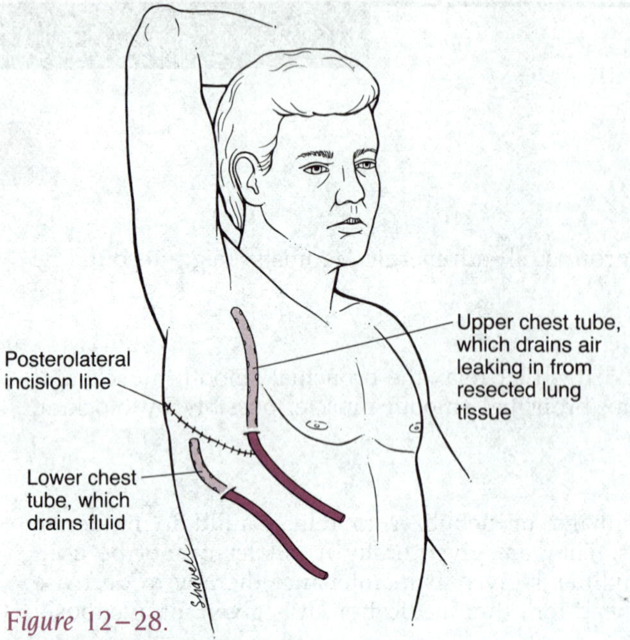

Figure 12–28.

Placement of chest tubes for air and fluid drainage.

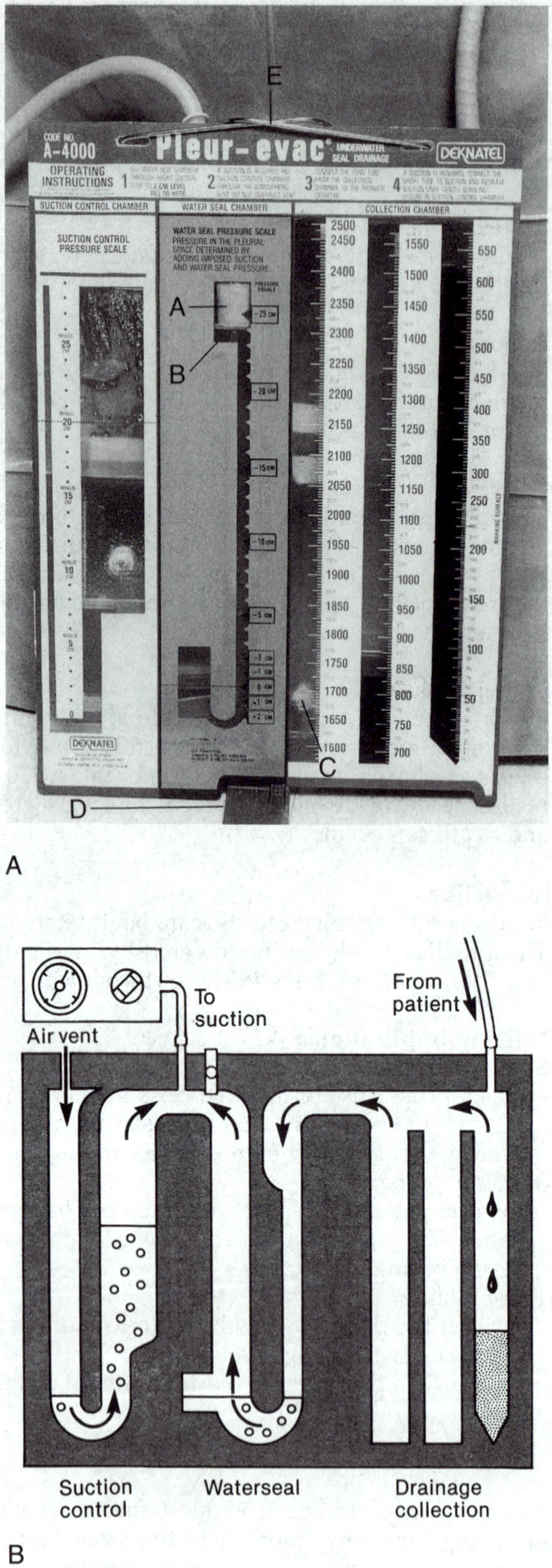

Figure 12–29.

Pleur-evac disposable chest drainage system. (*A*, from Kersten LD. Comprehensive respiratory nursing: A decision making approach. Philadelphia: WB Saunders, 1989, pp 776 and 777. *B*, adapted from Luce J, Tyler M, Pierson D. Intensive respiratory care. Philadelphia: WB Saunders, 1984.)

CHEST DRAINAGE

USES

The lungs are surrounded by the pleura. Under normal conditions, a negative pressure exists within the pleural space, which creates a vacuum that keeps the lungs adherent to the chest wall and permits expansion of the lung as the thorax expands during inspiration. If the integrity of the pleural membranes is disrupted, as in penetrating trauma to the chest wall, thoracic surgery, or open communication with alveoli (e.g., ruptured emphysematous bleb), air enters the pleural space and the negative pressure is lost. This results in lung collapse. To remove air or fluid from the chest and thus restore negative pressure to reexpand the lung, a chest tube is inserted. A single chest tube is placed in the pleural space to remove air. To remove air and fluid, two tubes are placed; one anteriorly through the second intercostal space and the other posteriorly through the eighth or ninth intercostal space in the midaxillary line to drain blood or fluid (Fig. 12–28).

TYPES OF CHEST-DRAINAGE APPARATUS

A chest-drainage system consists of a chest tube attached to a valve mechanism designed to allow air or fluid to drain out of, but not into, the chest cavity. The chest tube is a large-bore catheter, usually a no. 34 F or no. 36 F. The valve mechanism may be a one-way valve, a water-seal drainage system, or a water-seal drainage system with suction. A one-way valve is a simple unidirectional system in which the chest tube is made of soft material that collapses on inspiration and opens on expiration. Thus, the valve is open only when the pressure within the chest exceeds atmospheric pressure so air and fluid are removed from the chest.

The water-seal drainage system is the most common type in use. In this type of system, the chest tube is connected to another tube or glass rod, which remains under water, with the water acting as a seal. Because the tube remains under water and the pressure within the intrapleural space is negative, water rises in the tube. It is important that the underwater seal valve remain at a level far enough below the chest to prevent the column of water from reentering the pleural space. The pressure in the valve is determined by the depth the tube extends under the water. Bottle systems as such are not widely used today. The most common type of water-seal drainage systems used are the Pleur-Evac (Fig. 12–29) and Thorodrain. These are disposable chest-drainage units used for individual patients and then discarded. They represent a three-bottle-system principle. The one-, two-, and three-bottle water-seal systems are described next to illustrate the principles of underwater-seal drainage.

One-Bottle Water-Seal Drainage

One-bottle water-seal drainage provides no suction but effects drainage by gravity. The chest tube is connected to a long underwater-seal glass tube in a transparent water-seal drainage bottle. The short tube serves as an air vent. The tip of the tube under water is submerged about 2 cm below the water surface. If positive pressure in the pleural space is greater than 2 cm, air or fluid will be expelled into the bottle, where the air will escape through the vent. If the tip of the long tube were submerged further into the water, the intrapleural pressure would have to be greater for air to escape. If the tip of the long tube were placed just below the water surface, evaporation of water may cause loss of water seal and air could be sucked into the pleural cavity. In a properly functioning system, the water should oscillate (move up as the patient inhales and move down as the patient exhales) in the underwater-seal tube. Bubbling indicates an air leak from the lung or bronchus. The water level is marked by a tape or other means so the quantity of drainage can be measured (Fig. 12–30*A*).

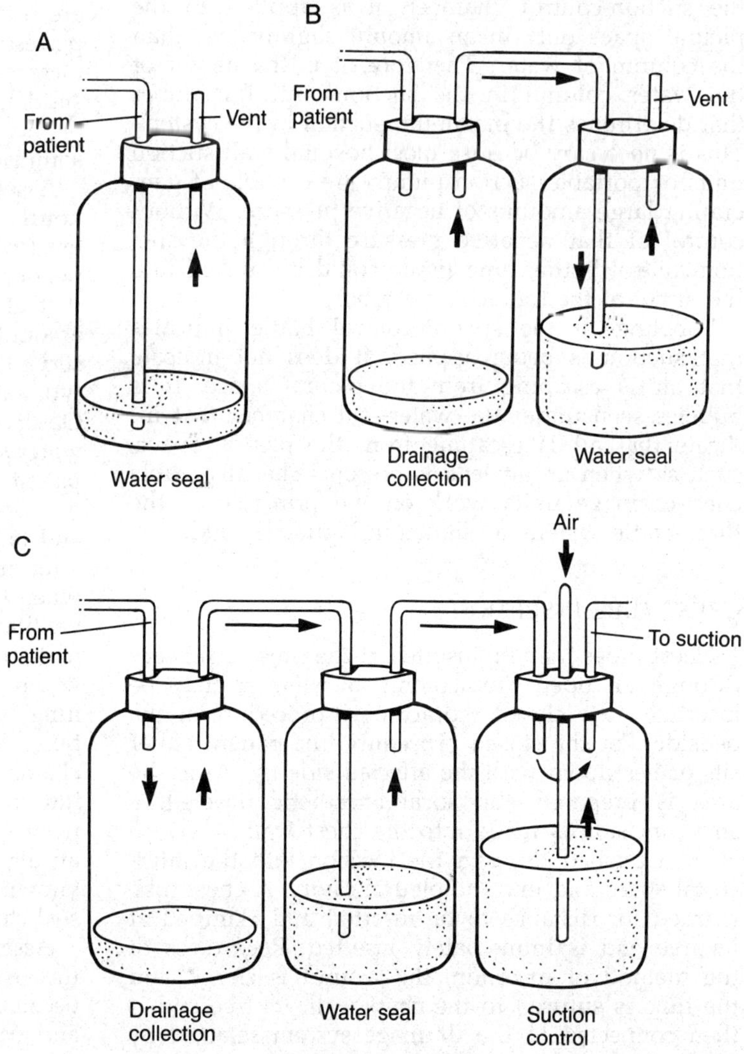

Figure 12–30.

A, One-bottle chest drainage. *B*, Two-bottle chest drainage. *C*, Three-bottle chest drainage.

Two-Bottle Water-Seal Drainage

The two-bottle water-seal drainage consists of a bottle that acts as a collection chamber that traps the fluid drained from the pleural space plus a second bottle, which is the water-seal chamber with an air vent. The open air vent at the top makes it a simple drainage system (Fig. 12–30*B*).

Three-Bottle Water-Seal Drainage

The three-bottle water-seal drainage adds controlled suction to apply negative pressure to the chest. This suction may be necessary when there is a large air leak or large amounts of fluid or when negative intrathoracic pressure must be reestablished. The first bottle is the drainage-collection chamber, the second is the water seal, and the third is the suction control (Fig. 12–30*C*).

The suction-control bottle has the air vent and outlet attached to suction. Suction is maintained between 15 and 20 cm of water pressure. The suction-control chamber contains a long tube with one end open to air and the other under a column of water 10 to 25 cm high. As negative pressure is applied to the suction-control chamber, it is applied to the pleural space only in an amount slightly less than the column of water. Therefore, it is the height of the water column in the suction-control chamber that determines the maximum suction in the system. This is necessary because most hospital wall suction units or portable suction pumps are capable of generating large amounts of negative pressure. Without control of that negative pressure through the suction-control bottle, lung tissue could be sucked into the outlet of the thoracotomy tube.

Bubbling in the suction-control bottle indicates that suction is being applied. It does not indicate that air is escaping from the pleural space. It is bubbles seen under the water-seal chamber that indicate that air is escaping from the pleural space, such as when an air leak is present. The disposable chest-drainage units work on the principle of the three-bottle system, as shown in Figure 12–30*C*.

CHEST TUBE INSERTION

Chest tubes may be inserted at the time of surgery through an open thoracotomy incision or may be inserted via a closed thoracotomy procedure at the bedside. For the closed procedure, the patient either sits or lies down with the affected side up. After the area is prepared and local anesthetic injected, a small incision is made into the chest wall. A clamp is then pushed through the incision into the intercostal space and into the pleural cavity. A chest tube marked for distance to be inserted and clamped at its free end is immediately inserted. Regardless of the method of insertion, the wound is closed and the tube is sutured to the chest wall. Its free end is then connected to the drainage system selected by the physician. All connections are securely taped to maintain an airtight system that reestablishes negative intrapleural pressure. An occlusive sterile dressing is applied to the insertion site, the first layer of which is usually a petrolatum jelly gauze. A chest x-ray film is done to check the position of the tube and to determine whether the lung has reexpanded.

Application of the Nursing Process to the Care of the Patient with Chest Drainage

Assessment

Assess the patient's respiratory status. Auscultate the lungs every 2 hours. Take vital signs every 4 hours. Note the quality of respirations, observe for abnormal chest movements, and check for cyanosis. Be alert to the possibility of an extended pneumothorax or hemothorax resulting from chest-drainage malfunction. Symptoms of extended pneumothorax are increased area of absent breath sounds and hyperresonant percussion note, increased tachycardia, increased respiratory distress, cyanosis, restlessness, sudden sharp chest pain, and confusion. Symptoms of hemothorax are diminished or absent breath sounds, dyspnea, and cyanosis.

Assess the function of the chest drainage system hourly. Check that the drainage system is below the level of the patient's chest and is free of kinks, dependent loops, or other external obstruction. Check that all connections are secure. Note the color and amount of drainage since the previous check. Observe the chest-tube dressing. Note the amount and type of drainage and whether the tape seal is intact. Observe for fluctuation of the fluid level in the water-seal chamber, because its presence indicates a patent drainage system. Remember that, with normal breathing, the water level rises with inspiration and falls with expiration, whereas the opposite (falls with inspiration and rises with expiration) occurs when the patient is on positive pressure mechanical ventilation. Keep in mind too that fluctuation stops if the tube is obstructed, if a dependent loop exists, if the suction is not working properly, and if the lung has reexpanded. When observing for fluctuation, also look for bubbling in the water-seal chamber. If the patient has a known pneumothorax, intermittent bubbling is expected as air is drained from the chest, but constant bubbling is indicative of an air leak in the system. In the patient without a known pneumothorax, any bubbling in the water-seal chamber is suggestive of an air leak.

Assess the patient's anxiety level and his or her understanding of chest drainage. This is important because anxiety can increase the need for oxygen, and patients with conditions affecting the lungs are prone to anxiety because breathing is so essential to life. Be alert to verbal expressions of excessive anxiety as well as nonverbal indicators such as reluctance to move, frequent requests to check the drainage system, and inability to attend to information and directions.

Nursing Diagnoses and Planning

Nursing diagnoses and related expected patient outcomes most commonly applicable to patients with chest drainage include the following:

NDx: Ineffective breathing pattern related to decreased lung expansion

Planning: Patient outcomes
1. Breath sounds are normal.
2. Respirations are unlabored and occur at a rate of 16 to 20 per minute.
3. ABG values are approaching normal.
4. Lung reexpansion is seen on chest x-ray film.

NDx: Anxiety related to perceived risk of chest tube dislodgement, system disruption, inability to breathe

Planning: Patient outcomes
1. Patient realistically describes precautions to be observed relative to the chest-drainage system.
2. Patient describes expected drainage in terms of color and amount, and normal fluctuation and bubbling in the system.

Nursing Interventions

NDx: Ineffective breathing pattern
Maintain an airtight, patent, functioning chest-drainage system. Retape all connections as needed. Retape chest-tube dressing if tape is loose. If the dressing becomes saturated with drainage, reinforce and tape securely or, if allowed, remove and replace wet gauze, being certain not to disrupt the petrolatum gauze seal. Keep the tubing free of loops, kinks, or other external pressure that could interfere with drainage or even force drainage back into the pleural space. Place a rolled towel under the chest tube when the patient is lying on the affected side to protect it from the body's weight.

Encourage the patient to cough and deep breathe frequently. This increases intrapleural pressure and promotes outflow of air and fluid through the chest tube and hence re-expansion of the lung. Change the patient's position frequently to promote both drainage and ventilation. When fluid is being drained from the chest, milk the tube in the direction of the drainage chamber every 2 hours to prevent blockage by clots or fibrin. To do this, take hold of the tube close to the chest, squeezing it between the fingers and the palm of the hand. Place the other hand around the tube just under the first hand and squeeze (Fig. 12–31). Release the first hand, place it under the second hand, and squeeze. Repeat for the length of tube. This action briefly increases the negative pressure applied to the intrapleural space and moves drainage toward the drainage system. Thus, it prevents stasis of drainage and decreases the risk of clotting and tube obstruction. Do not milk a tube if an air leak exists unless specifically directed to do so by the physician.

If fluctuation in the water-seal chamber ceases and the tubing is not kinked or otherwise obstructed, immediately ask the patient to cough or change position. If fluctuation does not begin, milk the tube. If fluctuation is still not restored, "strip" the tube if this is permitted by agency policy and by the attending physician. To strip the tube, lubricate the fingers of one hand and pinch the chest tube closed close to the chest wall with the fingers of the other hand. With the lubricated fingers, squeeze the tube below the pinch and slide them down the tube

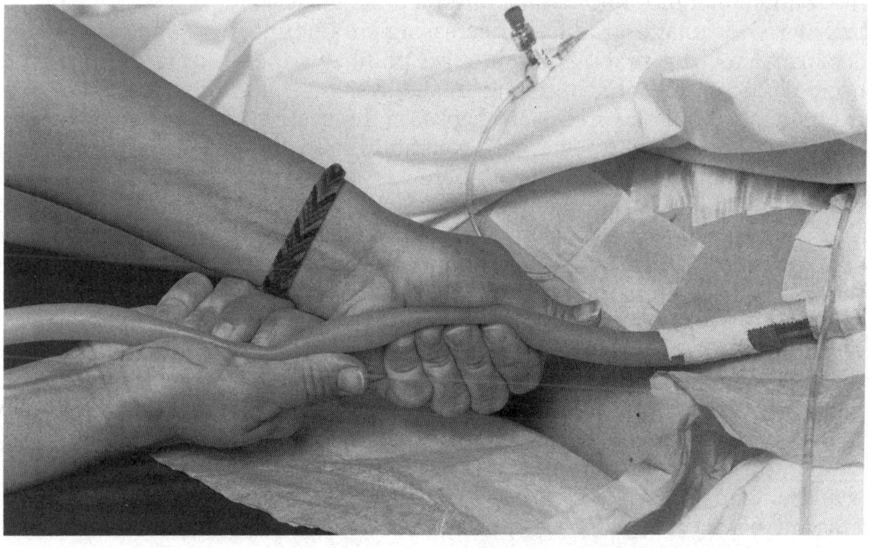

Figure 12–31.

Squeezing the chest tube between fingers and palms to ensure chest tube patency. (From Kersten LD. Comprehensive respiratory nursing: A decision making approach. Philadelphia: WB Saunders, 1989, p 781.)

toward the drainage system. Slowly release the pinch and then release the squeeze of the lubricated fingers. Repeat once or twice. Stripping causes high negative pressure up to 400 mm Hg within the system and is done with great caution and only when fresh bleeding has occurred. It can cause severe pain and injury to the lung. If fluctuation and free drainage still do not occur, notify the physician because tube replacement may be necessary.

If the drainage system is broken or interrupted, clamp the tube or place the end of the tube in a bottle of sterile saline held below the level of the chest and immediately replace the system. Remember that a chest tube can be clamped only momentarily if air can enter the pleural cavity with inspiration. This is because the air entering with each breath has no way to escape if the tube is clamped; therefore, it accumulates in the chest cavity and collapses the lung (a tension pneumothorax). Some institutional protocols require that a clamp be kept at the bedside at all times in case the system is interrupted.

If the chest tube is accidentally dislodged, immediately cover the opening in the chest wall with an occlusive, petrolatum gauze dressing, one of which should be kept at the bedside at all times. Tape this dressing in place on three sides. Leave the fourth side untaped so that if there is air leaking into the chest it can escape rather than causing a tension pneumothorax.

NDx: Anxiety
Provide the patient with basic information about the chest-drainage system to allay anxiety. Explain that, although care must be taken not to exert pull on the tube, it is sutured in place at the chest wall and therefore moving in bed, sitting up, and walking will not cause it to be displaced. Do stress, however, that it is important that the tube not be kinked or compressed and that the drainage apparatus must be kept below chest level. Prepare the patient for the type and amount of drainage expected. For example, the patient should know that, after chest surgery, bright red drainage gradually decreasing in amount is normal for the first 72 hours. Also point out the normal fluctuation and bubbling in the system. Tell the patient about the frequent checks of the system so he or she is aware that this constitutes routine care and is not led to believe there is something wrong. Provide time for the patient to ask questions and express concerns. Reassure the patient that a staff member is nearby and provide easy access to the call bell or intercom.

Additional Interventions
Mark the amount of chest drainage in the collection container at 1- to 4-hour intervals. Do this by placing a piece of tape vertically on the container and drawing a line with date and hour noted each time the drainage is checked. This allows the change in amount of drainage to be evaluated over time and, if the drainage is bloody, serves as a basis for blood replacement.

Notify the physician if there is constant bubbling in the water-seal chamber or if drainage becomes bright red or increases suddenly.

Evaluation

Evaluate the effectiveness of nursing care for a patient with chest drainage by comparing the patient's status with the expected patient outcomes. Examples of specific outcomes for patients with chest drainage have been provided in the Planning section.

CHEST TUBE REMOVAL

Chest tubes are removed when x-ray films confirm the full reexpansion of the lung or when there is no fluctuation of fluid in the tubing. Thirty minutes before removal, the patient is usually given pain medication. When the medication has taken effect, the sutures are cut. A petrolatum gauze dressing is placed at the chest wall ready to occlude the opening so air does not enter the chest; the patient is asked to perform the Valsalva maneuver (take a deep breath, exhale, and bear down), the tube is quickly withdrawn, and an airtight dressing is taped in place. The pleura seals itself off, and the wound heals in less than a week.

After removal, the patient is monitored for respiratory distress and the dressing is checked for drainage.

Surgical Management

OVERVIEW OF THORACIC SURGERY

Thoracic surgery refers to any operative procedure performed on a structure within the chest cavity or on the chest wall. It includes surgery on the heart, esophagus, and mediastinum as well as a variety of surgical procedures performed to maintain respiratory function and to treat lower respiratory tract disorders (Table 12–8).

There are three basic incisions used in thoracic surgery: median sternotomy, anterolateral thoracotomy, and posterolateral thoracotomy. A median sternotomy incision is used primarily for cardiac and other surgery involving the mediastinum. An anterolateral thoracotomy incision is used for relatively simple thoracic procedures such as a lung biopsy. The third type of incision, the posterolateral thoracotomy, is used for the majority of complex procedures involving the lung because it allows good visualization and easy access.

Table 12–8. THORACIC SURGICAL PROCEDURES USED IN THE MANAGEMENT OF RESPIRATORY DISORDERS

PROCEDURE	DESCRIPTION	USUAL INCISION	USES
Pneumonectomy	Removal of an entire lung	Posterolateral	Primarily for cancer; sometimes for lung abscess, bronchiectasis, extensive unilateral tuberculosis
Radical pneumonectomy	Removal of a lung and anterior and posterior mediastinal and tracheobronchial nodes on affected side	Posterolateral	Lung cancer
Lobectomy	Removal of one lobe of lung	Posterolateral or anterolateral	Cancer, bronchiectasis, emphysematous bleb
Wedge resection	Removal of a small section of the lung	Anterolateral for upper and middle lobes, posterolateral for lower lobe	Used to remove small lesions located near the surface
Open-lung biopsy	Removal of small specimen of lung tissue	Anterolateral	Diagnostic tissue examination
Closed thoracotomy (thoracostomy)	Percutaneous insertion of chest tube through intercostal space into pleural cavity	Small incision in midclavicular line: over 2nd to 5th intercostal spaces to remove air; 6th to 8th intercostal spaces posteriorly to remove fluid	To remove blood, fluid, or air in cases of hemothorax, pleural effusion, pneumothorax, or acute empyema
Open thoracotomy (thoracostomy or partial rib resection)	Removal of part of rib(s) to establish continuous drainage	Posterolateral	Acute empyema

After most thoracic surgery, one or more chest tubes are placed in the pleural space to drain air, blood, or other fluid; restore negative pressure; and allow reexpansion of the lung, which would have collapsed as a result of the change in intrathoracic pressure when the chest was opened. Chest tubes are not used after a pneumonectomy because there is no lung to reinflate, and fluid that ultimately solidifies is allowed to fill the remaining space in the thorax.

PATIENT PREPARATION FOR THORACIC SURGERY

The respiratory and cardiac status of the patient is carefully assessed preoperatively because the success of the surgery is largely dependent on the function of these systems. Chest x-ray films, lung scans, and an ECG are obtained. Pulmonary function tests are done to determine whether the proposed surgery will leave sufficient functioning lung tissue. ABGs are determined to provide an additional measure of pulmonary reserve and to provide baseline data for postoperative assessment. An exercise tolerance test may also be done preoperatively, especially when a pneumonectomy is being considered.

Other preoperative laboratory studies include blood sugar, electrolytes, and serum protein studies as well as a CBC.

Patients who smoke are encouraged to stop or at least cut down preoperatively to decrease secretions and to increase oxygen saturation. Antibiotics may be ordered to combat existing infection, and postural drainage may be used to remove excessive secretions.

COMPLICATIONS OF THORACIC SURGERY

Complications after thoracic surgery include atelectasis (most often caused by retained bronchial secretions), pneumonia, hemorrhage, cardiac dysrhythmia, and pulmonary edema secondary to hypervolemia from overinfusion of fluids. Other complications unique to surgery on the lung include bronchopleural fistula, empyema, persistent air leak, and subcutaneous emphysema.

A bronchopleural fistula is an abnormal opening between a bronchus and the pleural space. Symptoms of these fistulas that may develop during the first postoperative week are hemoptysis, fever, subcutaneous emphysema, and a severe air leak. Management usually involves surgical reclosure of the bronchial stump, although occasionally a pneumonectomy may be required.

Empyema is the presence of pus in the pleural cavity. It is characterized by fever, pleuritic pain, and dullness on percussion over the affected area. It is treated with chest drainage and systemic antibiotics.

A persistent air leak occurs when openings in the lung tissue fail to close spontaneously within 72 hours of surgery. An air leak is indicated by bubbling in the underwater-seal chamber of the chest-drainage apparatus. A persistent air leak may be treated by the injection of a sclerosing agent into the pleural cavity or by surgery.

Subcutaneous emphysema is the presence of air under the skin resulting from its escape from the respiratory tract. Subcutaneous emphysema can be due to a persistent air leak or a blocked chest tube.

Symptoms are puffiness of the skin and crepitation (presence of a crackling sound like that produced by crumpling cellophane) when the area is palpated.

Respiratory failure and hypotension are also potential complications of thoracic surgery.

PNEUMONECTOMY

Pneumonectomy is the surgical removal of an entire lung.

USES

Pneumonectomy is performed to treat bronchogenic carcinoma, lung abscess, bronchiectasis, or extensive unilateral tuberculosis. It is done only when disease is so extensive that all involved tissue cannot be removed by a lobectomy.

PROCEDURE

Most pneumonectomies are done through a posterolateral thoracotomy incision. Once the incision is made, the ribs are spread with a retractor, the pleura is entered, and the affected lung collapses because of the change in pressure that occurs when the pleura is opened. The bronchus is transected, the pulmonary artery and veins are ligated and severed, the lung is removed, and the bronchial stump is stapled. The phrenic nerve is severed or crushed. This paralyzes the diaphragm in an elevated position and decreases the size of the chest cavity on the operative side. During the procedure, the remaining lung is ventilated by means of an endotracheal tube and a mechanical ventilator. A chest tube is not generally inserted during a pneumonectomy; rather, the space is left to fill with serosanguineous fluid, which eventually solidifies.

Because pain after a thoracotomy is severe, a nerve block with a long-acting oral anesthetic may be performed just before the incision is closed.

POSTOPERATIVE COURSE

After a pneumonectomy, there is relatively severe pain in the chest and shoulder because of the retraction of the ribs, transection of muscles and other tissues, and irritation of the intercostal nerves. This results in guarding of the operative area and a predisposition to hypoventilation and atelectasis. To prevent impaired mobility and its effects, breathing exercises and arm and shoulder exercises are begun in the immediate postoperative period. The patient is dangled on the evening of surgery and is ambulated on the first postoperative day. Oxygen is generally administered for the first 24 hours.

Intravenous fluids are administered until the patient is stable and oral intake is well established. The rate of administration may be as low as 10 ml per hour because of the risk of pulmonary edema resulting from the decrease in pulmonary vasculature. Oral fluids are begun as soon as the patient is alert provided the abdomen has not been opened and bowel sounds are present. Intake is then increased as tolerated, with a return to a normal diet by the third postoperative day.

The wound is covered with a light dressing at the time of surgery. Because little drainage is expected, it may be left open to the air after 24 hours. Sutures are removed in 1 week, but altered sensation, numbness, or tenderness may persist for months in the area surrounding the incision.

Application of the Nursing Process to the Care of the Patient Having a Pneumonectomy

PREOPERATIVE NURSING CARE

Assessment

Perform a complete respiratory assessment. Question about signs and symptoms related to the patient's respiratory problem. Ask about cough, expectoration, hemoptysis, chest pain, and dyspnea. Assess breathing pattern and determine the amount of exertion needed to produce dyspnea. Assess the patient's respiratory status while performing ADL. Question about exposure to respiratory irritants, and obtain a smoking history. Determine whether the patient currently smokes and how much. If the patient previously smoked, ask how much, for how long, and when he or she stopped.

Assess the patient's general physical status. Note general appearance, mental alertness, and apparent nutritional status. Question about any coexisting medical problems that may have implications for pre- and postoperative care. List all medications taken by the patient, noting purpose and frequency of use, dose, and perceived effectiveness.

Observe the patient for signs of anxiety, and assess the patient's understanding of the planned surgery and its expected outcome.

Nursing Diagnoses and Planning

Nursing diagnoses and related expected patient outcomes most commonly applicable to patients scheduled for a pneumonectomy include the following:

NDx: Anxiety related to the surgical procedure and the postoperative course

Planning: Patient outcomes

1. Patient verbalizes that feelings of anxiety are decreased.

2. Patient verbalizes an understanding of perioperative events.
3. Facial expression and body posture appear relaxed.
4. Vital signs are stable.

NDx: High risk for altered health maintenance related to insufficient knowledge of breathing exercises, effective coughing, wound splinting, arm and shoulder exercises

Planning: Patient outcomes
1. Patient describes the role of breathing exercises, coughing, and arm and shoulder exercises in recovery.
2. Patient demonstrates breathing exercises and effective coughing.
3. Patient demonstrates methods of splinting the incision.
4. Patient demonstrates arm and shoulder exercises to be initiated in the early postoperative period.

Nursing Interventions

NDx: Anxiety
Provide the patient with basic information about the operative experience, such as preoperative preparation, the location of the incision, and what happens in the postanesthesia care unit (PACU). Prepare the patient for the presence of a CVP catheter, arterial catheter, pulmonary artery catheter, urinary bladder catheter, and oxygen equipment. Avoid providing unnecessary detail that could add to the patient's anxiety rather than allay it. If the patient will be going to an intensive care unit, explain the environment or arrange a visit if possible.

Because one of the most common concerns of patients facing a pneumonectomy relates to the ability to breathe after surgery, explain the functional reserve of the respiratory system and reinforce that one of the purposes of many of the preoperative tests is to ensure that he or she is able to tolerate the removal of a lung. Also acknowledge pain as a concern, and reassure the patient that, although significant pain is normal, analgesics will be given to control it.

Remember that significant others are often as anxious as the patient; therefore, provide the opportunity for them as well as the patient to ask questions and express their concerns.

NDx: High risk for altered health maintenance
Explain that deep breathing and coughing help to clear secretions from the airways and facilitate good ventilation of the remaining lung. Acknowledge that it is not easy to cough and deep breathe immediately after surgery but stress their importance. Reassure that discomfort will be minimized by splinting the incision and by the administration of pain medication. Explain, demonstrate, and have the patient practice diaphragmatic and pursed-lip breathing as described on page 91. Help the patient practice effective coughing as follows:

Sit the patient upright with slightly flexed knees. If the patient is unable to sit upright, position him or her on the side with hips and knees flexed.
Splint the incision with the flat of your hands.
Ask the patient to take two or three short breaths followed by a deep inspiration.
Instruct the patient to contract (pull in) the abdominal muscles and cough forcefully with the mouth open.

Explain that a folded blanket or sheet or a pillow can also be used to splint the incision, and demonstrate their use (Fig. 12–32).

Provide the patient with an incentive spirometer. Describe its use, and encourage the patient to try it in preparation for postoperative use.

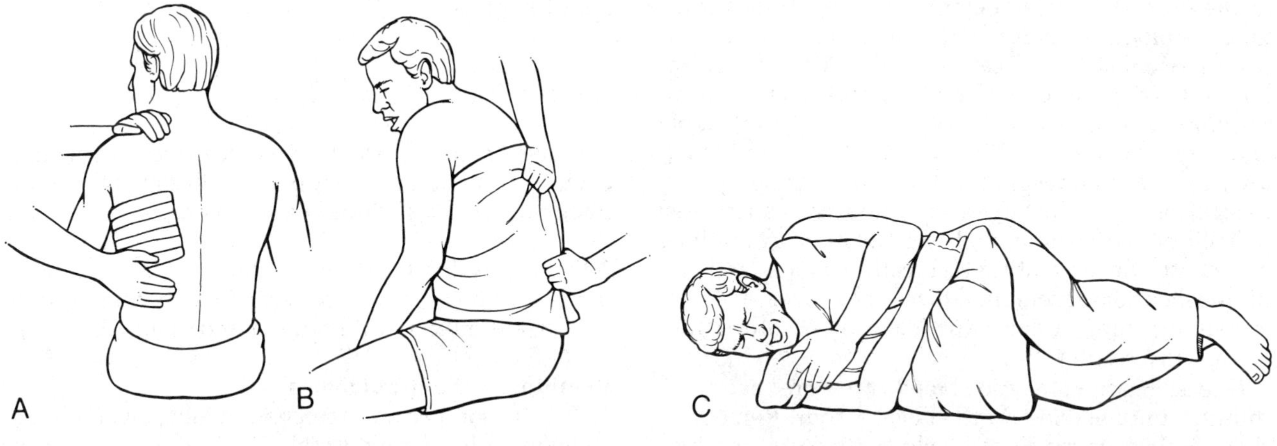

Figure 12–32.

Methods of splinting a thoracotomy incision: *A*, with the flat of the hands; *B*, with a folded blanket; *C*, with a pillow.

Describe to the patient the effect of the surgery on the movement of the chest and shoulder. Explain that passive range-of-motion exercises to the shoulder will be started immediately after surgery to prevent the development of stiffening, limited motion, and ultimately greater discomfort. Familiarize the patient with the range-of-motion exercises by performing them on his or her shoulder. Tell the patient that additional active exercises will be started as he or she progresses in the postoperative period. Explain that they help regain muscle strength as well as maintain free movement of the joint and will have to be continued after return home.

Additional Interventions
Prepare the patient for preoperative diagnostic tests, and institute measures to remove secretions and improve alveolar ventilation. Depending on the patient's condition and the physician's orders, these measures may include forced fluids, humidification to loosen secretions, administration of bronchodilators, chest percussion, and postural drainage.

Instruct all patients on the importance of avoiding exposure to cigarette smoke and other bronchial irritants. Ensure that the preoperative preparation is completed according to the surgeon's directions and that preoperative medications are given as ordered.

Evaluation

Evaluate the effectiveness of nursing care for a patient scheduled for a pneumonectomy by comparing the patient's status with the expected patient outcomes. Examples of specific outcomes for patients scheduled for a pneumonectomy have been provided in the Planning section.

POSTOPERATIVE NURSING CARE

Assessment

In the immediate postoperative period, assess return to physiologic stability. Pay particular attention to respiratory status and cardiac status. Check respiratory rate, and observe for signs and symptoms of respiratory dysfunction every 15 minutes until stable and then every hour. Observe for slow, rapid, shallow, or irregular respirations; use of accessory muscles; orthopnea; duskiness or cyanosis; restlessness; irritability; confusion; and somnolence. Auscultate the chest for adventitious breath sounds and for diminished or absent breath sounds over areas of remaining lung tissue. Review ABG values and chest x-ray results.

Check heart rate and blood pressure every 15 minutes until stable and then every hour. Remember that continuous readings of blood pressure and pulmonary artery pressures are presented on oscilloscopes attached to a Swan-Ganz catheter. Take CVP readings every hour to assess right ventricular function. Measure PCWPs every 1 to 2 hours if ordered to assess left ventricular function.

Take the patient's temperature every hour, because change in temperature alters the metabolism and hence cardiac output.

Assess fluid and electrolyte status. Measure intake and output, and observe for signs of over- or underhydration. Remember that a CVP reading below the normal range of 5 to 12 cm of water is suggestive of hypovolemia, whereas an elevated CVP reading is suggestive of hypervolemia. Keep in mind that at least 30 ml of urine should be excreted per hour.

While a dressing is in place, check it for drainage, noting color and amount. Remember that bloody drainage is not expected. When the dressing is removed, assess the incision every 8 hours. Observe for signs of infection: redness, heat, induration, swelling, lack of approximation, and drainage.

Assess for signs of developing complications. Observe continuous ECG for dysrhythmias because patients who have had a pneumonectomy are at particular risk. Keep in mind that the dysrhythmias most likely to occur are atrial fibrillation and atrial flutter. Observe for signs of pulmonary edema because the decrease in the pulmonary vascular bed places the patient who has had a pneumonectomy at high risk. Be alert for symptoms of pulmonary edema: severe dyspnea, tachycardia, dull percussion note over unoperated areas, adventitious breath sounds, persistent cough with frothy or blood-tinged sputum, cyanosis, and apprehension. Also observe for signs and symptoms of mediastinal shift, which is the movement of the mediastinum including the heart, trachea, esophagus, and great vessels to one side of the thorax and which is a risk after pneumonectomy because one side of the thorax is no longer occupied by a lung. Symptoms of mediastinal shift include severe dyspnea, restlessness, agitation, rapid or irregular pulse, cyanosis, displacement of the trachea from the midline, and a change in the point of apical impulse.

Nursing Diagnoses and Planning

Nursing diagnoses and related expected patient outcomes most commonly applicable to patients after a pneumonectomy include the following:

NDx: Ineffective breathing pattern related to unwillingness to breathe deeply secondary to pain and the depressant effects of anesthesia and analgesia

Planning: Patient outcomes
1. Breath sounds and percussion note over the remaining lung are normal.
2. ABG values are within normal range.

Chart 12–2.

NURSING GUIDE TO PATIENT EDUCATION FOR SELF-MANAGEMENT: DISCHARGE INSTRUCTIONS AFTER PNEUMONECTOMY

Instruct the patient to:

Perform breathing exercises as taught for the first 3 weeks at home.
Perform arm and shoulder exercises five times a day.
Practice standing fully erect in front of a mirror until normal posture is restored.
Expect soreness in the chest and shoulder for several weeks.
Use hot soaks or a heating pad to relieve chest or shoulder pain.
Take prescribed or recommended over-the-counter oral analgesics if additional relief is needed.
Expect altered sensation around the incision for several weeks.
Expect feelings of weakness and fatigue for the first 3 weeks after surgery.
Space activities to allow for frequent rest periods.
Avoid heavy lifting (more than 20 pounds) until muscles of the chest wall have healed completely in 3 to 6 months.
Build up tolerance to walking by using a moderate pace and by gradually increasing distance and duration.
Stop any activity that causes chest pain, shortness of breath, or excessive fatigue.
Stop or decrease smoking if a smoker.
Avoid exposure to smoke, fumes, aerosol sprays, and other respiratory tract irritants.
Avoid exposure to colds and other respiratory infections.
Obtain annual influenza vaccine and pneumonia vaccine as recommended by physician.
Report signs of respiratory infection: persistent fever, increased sputum production, shortness of breath, or increased discomfort or decreased mobility in affected arm and shoulder.
Return for follow-up evaluation of wound healing and respiratory function on *(specify date and time).*

NDx: Ineffective airway clearance related to increased secretions secondary to respiratory tract irritation and poor cough effort secondary to pain and the depressant effects of anesthesia and analgesia

Planning: Patient outcomes
1. Respirations are easy and quiet at a rate of 16 to 20 per minute.
2. Breath sounds and percussion note over remaining lung are normal.
3. ABG values are within normal range.

NDx: Pain (chest and shoulder) related to surgical trauma to muscles, nerves, and other tissues

Planning: Patient outcomes
1. Patient states pain is relieved.
2. Patient exhibits a relaxed body posture.
3. Facial expression is relaxed.
4. Patient coughs effectively.
5. Patient moves easily.

NDx: Impaired physical mobility related to transection of chest muscles, which move shoulder, and severe pain in the chest and shoulder

Planning: Patient outcomes
1. Patient moves shoulder on affected side through usual active range of motion.
2. Patient uses affected arm in performing ADL.
3. Patient exhibits an erect posture.

NDx: Body image disturbance related to loss of a lung and the accompanying change in respiratory function

Planning: Patient outcomes
1. Patient realistically describes change in physical status related to loss of a lung.
2. Patient realistically identifies changes in lifestyle required by altered respiratory status.
3. Patient verbalizes acceptance of the change in respiratory status.

NDx: High risk for altered health maintenance related to insufficient knowledge of self-care after pneumonectomy

Planning: Patient outcomes
1. Patient describes self-care after discharge as presented in Chart 12–2.

2. Patient demonstrates arm and shoulder exercises to be done at home to regain muscle strength.

Nursing Interventions

NDx: Ineffective breathing pattern

Position the patient on the back or with the unoperated side up to promote maximum ventilation of the remaining lung and to help the fluid that accumulates in the pleural space remain below the level of the bronchial stump. Direct the patient in diaphragmatic and pursed-lip breathing and use of an incentive spirometer every 1 to 2 hours to prevent atelectasis. Assist the patient to splint the incision during these breathing exercises, and coordinate them with the time when analgesic medications are exerting their peak effect.

Administer oxygen as ordered, and monitor ABG values. Space patient care activities to provide for frequent rest periods and thus decrease demand on the respiratory system.

NDx: Ineffective airway clearance

Assist the patient to cough and deep breathe and turn every 1 to 2 hours. For maximum effectiveness, assist the patient to a sitting position with the knees slightly flexed. If the patient is unable to sit upright, position the patient on the side with hips and knees flexed. Also assist the patient to splint the incision, and time the activity to correspond with the action of analgesic medications. Monitor breath sounds before and after each coughing and deep-breathing exercise. Record auscultatory finding as well as the amount, color, and viscosity of the expectorate. If the patient is unable to cough, use huffing rather than coughing to promote ventilation and raise secretions. Tell the patient to take a deep diaphragmatic breath and exhale forcefully in a rapid, distinct pant or huff. The effectiveness of huffing is enhanced if it is accompanied by a chest compression technique. To compress the chest, ask the patient to move the upper arms outward to a position midway between the shoulders and the chest. Then instruct the patient to move both upper arms briskly and firmly toward the chest as he or she exhales (Fig. 12–33). Guide the patient in diaphragmatic breathing exercises, and perform percussion, vibration, or postural drainage if ordered to facilitate the removal of copious secretions. Do not percuss or vibrate over the operative site. Administer humidification and mininebulizer therapy if ordered to moisten and thin secretions and to facilitate expectoration. Suction if secretions are present and are not being raised.

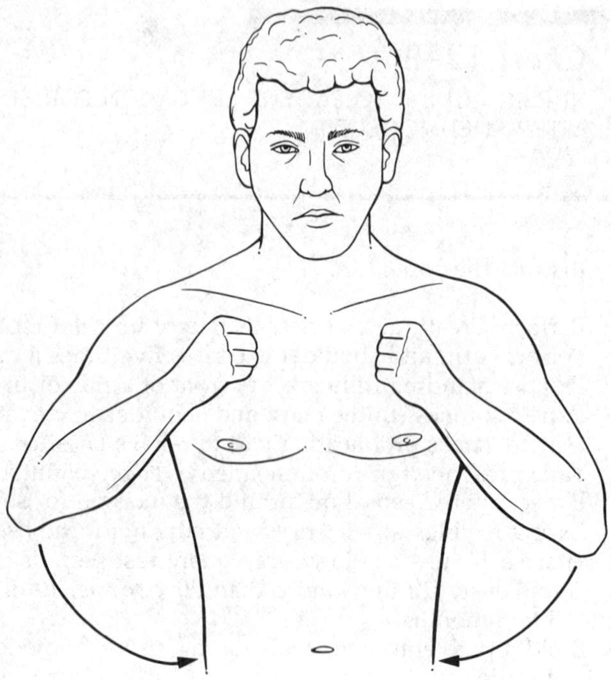

Figure 12–33.

Chest compression technique used to enhance the effectiveness of huffing.

NDx: Pain

Administer prescribed narcotic analgesics as needed to keep the patient comfortable, to enable him or her to deep breathe and cough effectively, and to keep the patient willing to turn, ambulate, and perform arm and shoulder exercises. Effective coughing, deep breathing, turning, and moving are essential to good ventilation in the remaining lung. Arm and shoulder exercises are essential to return of full range of motion and use of the extremity. Administer analgesics before the pain becomes severe or 30 to 40 minutes before painful exercises are done. Be careful not to medicate the patient to the point at which respirations are depressed or the patient is too somnolent to effectively cough and deep breathe, because this leads to poor ventilation and an increased risk of complications. After 48 to 72 hours, give oral analgesics such as codeine or acetaminophen as ordered to control pain.

To prevent unnecessary pain, assist the patient to splint the incision with hands, folded sheet, or pillow when moving, coughing, or deep breathing to reduce pull on inflamed tissues at the incision line. Similarly, support the affected arm and shoulder with pillows or a sling to reduce pull on transected muscles. Promote comfort and the use of relaxation exercises or guided imagery. Maintain a calm, quiet environment and provide diversions such as the radio or television in accordance with the patient's condition and preferences.

NDx: Impaired physical mobility

Perform passive range-of-motion exercises to the affected shoulder a minimum of two times every 4 to 6 hours for the first 24 hours postoperatively. Subsequently, instruct and guide the patient in active arm and shoulder exercises 10 to 20 times every 2 hours. There are many different active exercises that can be used, and some surgeons have a prepared regimen. Examples of exercises used are shoulder shrugs; wall climbing; reaching behind the back with the affected arm and trying to touch the opposite scapula; reaching over the chest and touching the opposite acromial process; extending the arm up and back, out to the side, and back and down at the side; and placing the hands in the small of the back and pushing the elbows as far back as possible.

In addition to scheduled exercises, structure the environment to encourage the use of the affected arm. Place frequently used articles to the patient's operative side to encourage reaching with the affected arm. Attach a rope to the foot of the bed, and encourage the patient to pull on it with the affected arm to raise up to sitting position. Also encourage use of the affected arm in self-care activities. Recognize that use will vary depending on whether the patient's dominant side is involved. Be alert to the patient's posture, and remind the patient as necessary to assume a fully erect position with the affected shoulder back and level with the unaffected one. Guide the patient in diaphragmatic breathing to mobilize the thorax.

NDx: Body image disturbance

Encourage the patient to verbalize feelings about the loss of a lung because confronting these feelings is the first step in coping. Recognize that the patient may feel angry, fearful, sad, or helpless, and acknowledge the feelings as real and valid. Assist the patient to realistically identify the effect of the loss of the lung on respiratory status, physical stamina, and function. Review usual activities and lifestyle patterns with the patient, and encourage identification of areas that will be unaffected by the surgery. Also help the patient to determine changes that are needed and to identify viable options. Facilitate discussion of changes and options between the patient and significant others, and encourage sharing of mutual concerns. Make referrals to appropriate support groups or community resources such as the American Lung Association.

NDx: High risk for altered health maintenance

Instruct the patient in self-care after discharge as presented in Chart 12–2.

Additional Interventions

Give fluids by mouth as soon as the patient is alert, and advance the patient to the regular prescribed diet as tolerated. Weigh the patient daily.

Report temperature of 102°F (38.8°C) or greater to the physician. Also report temperature of less than 98°F (36.6°C). Variation in temperature alters metabolism and increases the demand on the respiratory system. To protect the patient from this physiologic stress, antipyretics are given for temperatures of 102°F (38.8°C) or greater, a cooling mattress is used for temperatures of 104°F (40°C) or greater, and blankets and heating pads are used for hypothermia.

Notify the physician immediately if sputum is excessive or if it contains bright red blood.

Evaluation

Evaluate the effectiveness of nursing care for a patient who has had a pneumonectomy by comparing the patient's status with the expected patient outcomes. Examples of specific outcomes for patients who have had a pneumonectomy have been provided in the Planning section.

LOBECTOMY

A lobectomy is a surgical procedure in which a lobe of a lung is removed.

USES

Lobectomy is performed to treat lung cancer and bronchiectasis or to remove emphysematous blebs. It is done when disease is limited to one lobe of the lung. It is preferred to pneumonectomy because it conserves the unaffected lobes of the lung and thus has a less profound effect on the patient's respiratory status.

PROCEDURE

Depending on the lobe to be removed, either a posterolateral or an anterolateral thoracotomy incision is made and the ribs are spread with a retractor. The pleura is entered, and the lung on the affected side collapses. The bronchus is transected, the blood vessels to the lobe are ligated and severed, and the lobe is removed. Two chest tubes connected to water-seal drainage systems are placed for postoperative removal of air and fluid from the chest cavity. The upper tube drains air, whereas the lower tube drains the serosanguineous fluid that accumulates as a result of the operative procedure.

POSTOPERATIVE COURSE

The postoperative course is essentially the same as that after a pneumonectomy.

Application of the Nursing Process to the Care of the Patient Having a Lobectomy

See Nursing Care Guide 12–1 for nursing care applicable to the patient having a lobectomy.

Text continued on page 484

Nursing Care Guide 12–1.

PATIENTS HAVING A LOBECTOMY

Preoperative Care

Assessment Findings: Restlessness, tense facial expression, occasional trembling. Patient states, "I can't concentrate on anything. I'm just so worried about this whole thing."

Nursing Diagnosis: Anxiety related to the surgical procedure and the postoperative course

Patient Outcomes	Nursing Interventions	Rationale
Patient describes routine perioperative events. Patient verbalizes that feelings of anxiety are decreased. Facial expression and body posture are relaxed. Vital signs are stable.	Provide basic information about the operative experience: preparation, location of incision, function of chest tubes, postanesthesia care unit (PACU) routines, expected presence of a central venous pressure (CVP) catheter, urinary bladder catheter, oxygen.	Familiarity with routines and equipment reduces anxiety.
	Arrange a preoperative visit to the intensive care unit (ICU) if the patient will be admitted there after surgery. If this is not possible, describe the unit to the patient.	
	Encourage patient and significant others to verbalize concerns and ask questions.	Identifies areas of concern, provides perspective, permits a supportive relationship, and allows for clarification.
	Reassure about the ability to breathe postoperatively by explaining the functional reserve of the respiratory system and the role of preoperative tests in determining ability to tolerate the removal of lung tissue.	Reassures the patient of the continued capability to perform the essential life function of breathing.
	Acknowledge that there is significant pain after surgery but that analgesics will be given to control it.	Helps patient accept concerns as appropriate and provides positive facts on which to focus.

Evaluation: Compare the patient's status with the expected patient outcomes. If the outcomes are achieved, evaluate nursing care as successful. If not, reassess the patient, formulate new nursing diagnoses, and revise expected patient outcomes and nursing interventions as appropriate.

(continued)

Nursing Care Guide 12–1. *(continued)*
PATIENTS HAVING A LOBECTOMY

Assessment Findings: Patient is scheduled for a lobectomy and has no prior knowledge of or experience with lung surgery.

Nursing Diagnosis: Knowledge deficit: breathing exercises, effective coughing, wound splinting, arm and shoulder exercises

Patient Outcomes	Nursing Interventions	Rationale
Patient describes the role of breathing exercises, coughing, and arm and shoulder exercises in recovery.	Describe importance of breathing exercises and effective coughing in clearing the airway and allowing for good ventilation.	Provides rationale which promotes compliance.
	Explain the effect of chest surgery on chest and shoulder muscles.	Understanding the reason for interventions promotes cooperation.
	Use the patient's arm to demonstrate the passive range-of-motion (ROM) exercises that will be done after surgery.	Learning is facilitated by involvement of the learner.
	Explain that additional active exercises will be taught postoperatively to maintain full ROM and to regain muscle strength.	Prepares the patient for the acceptance of new exercises during the postoperative period.
Patient demonstrates breathing exercises, effective coughing, and use of incentive spirometer.	Teach patient diaphragmatic and pursed-lip breathing, effective coughing technique, methods of splinting the incision, and use of an incentive spirometer	The best time to learn is when the patient is free from pain and distraction. Teaching before surgery is more effective than teaching in the postoperative period.
	Encourage practice, and obtain return demonstrations of those skills.	Practice improves technique, and return demonstration provides evidence that the patient can perform the required skills.

Evaluation: Compare the patient's status with the expected patient outcomes. If the outcomes are achieved, evaluate nursing care as successful. If not, reassess the patient, formulate new nursing diagnoses, and revise expected patient outcomes and nursing interventions as appropriate.

(continued)

Nursing Care Guide 12–1. *(continued)*
PATIENTS HAVING A LOBECTOMY

Postoperative Care

Assessment Findings: Respirations are shallow at a rate of 28 per minute. Patient is guarding thoracotomy incision with both hands and states, "I can't let my chest move."

Nursing Diagnosis: Ineffective breathing pattern related to unwillingness to breathe deeply secondary to pain, fear of displacing chest tubes, or depressant effects of anesthesia and analgesics

Patient Outcomes	Nursing Interventions	Rationale
Breath sounds and percussion note over remaining lung tissue are normal within 4 postoperative days.	Monitor respiratory rate every 1 to 2 hours.	Allows for early recognition of respiratory distress and provides information about effectiveness of interventions.
Blood gases are within normal range. Lung reexpansion is evident on x-ray film.	Auscultate lungs every 2 to 3 hours.	Allows for early recognition of respiratory distress and provides information about effectiveness of interventions.
	Position patient on the back or with the operated side up for the first 48 hours.	Promotes expansion of remaining lung tissue.
	Monitor chest-tube drainage every 15 minutes immediately postoperatively and then at progressively longer intervals.	Promotes early recognition of tube blockage or bleeding.
	Report persistent chest drainage of more than 200 ml/hour.	Indicates bleeding and thus allows for medical intervention.
	Maintain chest drainage.	Removal of fluids and air from the pleural space allows for reexpansion of the lung.
	Keep patient elevated in semi-Fowler's position.	Facilitates coughing and allows air to rise and escape through the upper chest tube.
	Keep the chest-drainage system below the level of the patient's chest, free of leaks, dependent loops, and external pressure.	Maintains free gravity drainage.
	Monitor fluctuation of the fluid level in the water-seal chamber.	Fluid level should fluctuate with respirations if tube is not blocked.
	Monitor for excessive bubbling in the water-seal chamber.	Excessive bubbling can indicate an air leak within the set.
	Retape all connections in the system as needed to keep it airtight.	Negative pressure in the chest is required for reexpansion of the lung.
	Retape chest-tube dressing if needed to keep it airtight.	Prevents loss of negative pressure by air entering the chest.

(continued)

Nursing Care Guide 12–1. *(continued)*

PATIENTS HAVING A LOBECTOMY

Patient Outcomes	Nursing Interventions	Rationale
	Reinforce or change gauze (not petrolatum gauze seal) of chest-tube dressing if saturated with drainage.	Maintains effectiveness of occlusive dressing.
	Place a rolled towel under the chest tube when patient is lying on the affected side.	Prevents pressure of body weight from occluding chest tube.
	Milk the tube in the direction of the drainage chamber every 2 hours.	Prevents clots or fibrin from blocking tube.
	Direct patient in diaphragmatic and pursed-lip breathing every 1 to 2 hours.	Promotes reexpansion of alveoli.
	Coordinate breathing exercises with time when pain medication is at peak effectiveness.	Patient is more likely to cooperate with deep breathing when pain is eliminated or reduced.
	Instruct and assist patient in splinting the incision anteriorly and posteriorly to facilitate deep breathing.	Reduces strain on suture line and reassures patient that deep breathing will not damage suture line.
	Direct the patient in the use of the incentive spirometer every 2 to 3 hours.	Promotes ventilation.
	Administer oxygen (O_2) if ordered.	Improves oxygenation by providing greater amounts of O_2 in inspired air.
	Plan frequent rest periods.	Diminishes O_2 requirements of the body.
	Monitor arterial blood gas values.	Documents abnormalities and helps identify the need for and effectiveness of interventions.

Evaluation: Compare the patient's status with the expected patient outcomes. If the outcomes are achieved, evaluate nursing care as successful. If not, reassess the patient, formulate new nursing diagnoses, and revise expected patient outcomes and nursing interventions as appropriate.

Assessment Findings: Respirations are shallow and noisy at a rate of 26 per minute. Wheezes are heard on auscultation of the chest. Patient coughs but does not raise and expectorate sputum.

Nursing Diagnosis: Ineffective airway clearance related to increased secretions secondary to respiratory tract irritation and poor cough effort secondary to pain and the depressant effects of anesthesia and analgesia

(continued)

Nursing Care Guide 12–1. *(continued)*

PATIENTS HAVING A LOBECTOMY

Patient Outcomes	Nursing Interventions	Rationale
Respirations are easy and quiet at a rate of 16 to 20 per minute. Breath sounds and percussion note over remaining lobes are normal within 4 postoperative days. Blood gas values are within normal range.	Assist patient to cough and deep breathe every 1 to 2 hours. For most efficient coughing, have patient in a sitting position.	Helps clear secretions from the respiratory tract, allowing better gas exchange. Upright position allows better chest expansion and more forceful cough.
	Assist patient to turn every 1 to 2 hours because remaining in one position fosters retention of secretions in the lower areas of the lung.	Changes the area of the chest wall that is splinted, allowing better aeration of the lung and promoting drainage of secretions.
	Coordinate coughing, deep breathing, and turning with times when pain medication is at its peak effectiveness.	When pain-free or in reduced pain states, the patient is more likely to cooperate in effective deep breathing and coughing exercises.
	Instruct and assist the patient in splinting the incision anteriorly and posteriorly when coughing and moving.	Decreases strain on the incision, thus limiting discomfort and increasing patient willingness to cough and move.
	Monitor amount, color, and viscosity of expectorate.	Allows for early recognition of changes in amounts or types of respiratory secretions.
	Monitor breath sounds before and after each deep breathing and coughing exercise.	Evaluates the effectiveness of coughing and deep breathing.
	Monitor arterial blood gas values.	Evaluates effectiveness of interventions.
	Assist with diaphragmatic breathing and percussion, vibration, and postural drainage if ordered because of copious secretions. Do not percuss or vibrate over the operative site.	Helps aerate all lung tissue by removing secretions.
	Administer humidification and mininebulizer therapy as ordered.	Moistens and thins secretions to facilitate expectoration.
	Suction if secretions are present and are not being raised.	Mechanically removes respiratory secretions.
	Report immediately if expectorate is excessive or contains bright red blood.	Allows early medical intervention for complications.

Evaluation: Compare the patient's status with the expected patient outcomes. If the outcomes are achieved, evaluate nursing care as successful. If not, reassess the patient, formulate new nursing diagnoses, and revise expected patient outcomes and nursing interventions as appropriate.

(continued)

Nursing Care Guide 12–1. *(continued)*

PATIENTS HAVING A LOBECTOMY

Assessment Findings: Patient is lying rigidly in bed with arms pressed against the area of the thoracic incision. Facial expression is drawn, and patient occasionally moans. Patient states, "I can't breathe it hurts so much."

Nursing Diagnosis: Pain (chest and shoulder) related to surgical trauma to muscles, nerves, and other tissues

Patient Outcomes	Nursing Interventions	Rationale
Patient states pain is relieved. Patient exhibits a relaxed body posture. Facial expression is relaxed. Patient coughs effectively. Patient moves easily.	Administer narcotic analgesics as ordered every 2 to 4 hours as occasion requires (PRN) for 48 to 72 hours after surgery.	Narcotics alter awareness of pain.
	Give before the pain becomes severe or 30 to 40 minutes before painful exercises.	Administration before pain becomes severe increases effectiveness of drug. Pain relief promotes coughing, deep breathing, and turning.
	Avoid medicating to the point of inability to cough effectively or respiratory depression.	Overmedication suppresses respirations and diminishes the effectiveness of the cough.
	Administer oral analgesics as ordered after the first 48 to 72 hours.	Controls pain with decreased risk of suppressing respirations.
	Anchor chest tubes.	Minimizes movement of chest tubes, which is very painful.
	Assist the patient in splinting the incision with flat of hands, folded sheet or blanket, or a pillow when moving, coughing, or deep breathing.	Minimizes painful pull on the incision.
	Support the affected arm and shoulder with pillows or a sling.	Prevents painful pull on the surgically traumatized tissues.
	Promote comfort and relaxation with frequent position change, backrubs, use of relaxation exercises, guided imagery, and diversional activities.	Reduces tension and promotes rest, which is conducive to healing.
	Maintain a calm, quiet environment.	Reduces stress and tension, allowing for rest and relaxation.

Evaluation: Compare the patient's status with the expected patient outcomes. If the outcomes are achieved, evaluate nursing care as successful. If not, reassess the patient, formulate new nursing diagnoses, and revise expected patient outcomes and nursing interventions as appropriate.

(continued)

Nursing Care Guide 12–1. *(continued)*

PATIENTS HAVING A LOBECTOMY

Assessment Findings: Patient has a thoracotomy incision that required transection of muscles involved in shoulder movement.

Nursing Diagnosis: Impaired physical mobility related to transection of chest muscles affecting shoulder movement and severe pain in the chest and shoulder secondary to surgery

Patient Outcomes	Nursing Interventions	Rationale
Patient moves shoulder on affected side through usual active range of motion (ROM).	Perform ROM exercises to affected arm at least two times every 4 to 6 hours for 24 hours postoperatively.	Maintains ROM of affected arm.
	Instruct and guide patient in active arm and shoulder exercises 10 to 20 times every 2 hours thereafter.	Prevents atrophy of muscles from disuse.
Patient uses affected arm in performing activities of daily living.	Encourage use of affected arm in self-care activities (keep in mind whether patient is right- or left-handed).	Provides ROM exercises and maintains function of affected arm.
	Structure environment to foster use of affected arm (e.g., place frequently used articles on affected side to encourage reaching with the affected arm).	Promotes movement of affected arm needed to maintain free range of joint motion and muscle strength.
	Guide patient in diaphragmatic breathing.	Mobilizes thorax.
Patient assumes an erect position.	Encourage patient to assume a fully erect position with the affected shoulder back and level with the unaffected one.	Prevents drooping of affected side.
	Suggest patient use a mirror to aid in correcting posture.	Allows patient to visualize posture to guide in positioning.

Evaluation: Compare the patient's status with the expected patient outcomes. If the outcomes are achieved, evaluate nursing care as successful. If not, reassess the patient, formulate new nursing diagnoses, and revise expected patient outcomes and nursing interventions as appropriate.

(continued)

Nursing Care Guide 12–1. *(continued)*
PATIENTS HAVING A LOBECTOMY

Assessment Findings: Two days after a left lower lobectomy, patient verbalizes negative feelings about his or her body and feelings of helplessness and hopelessness and is preoccupied with the loss of part of a lung.

Nursing Diagnosis: Body image disturbance related to loss of part of a lung and the accompanying change in respiratory function

Patient Outcomes	Nursing Interventions	Rationale
Patient realistically describes changes in physical status caused by removal of a lung.	Encourage patient to verbalize perceptions and feelings about the altered respiratory status.	Allows any misconceptions to be identified and corrected.
	Acknowledge feelings of anger, fear, sadness, and helplessness as real and valid.	Communicates understanding and acceptance and encourages verbalization and "working through" of feelings.
	Assist the patient in identifying the effect on respiratory status, physical stamina, and function.	Facilitates realistic self-assessment.
Patient realistically identifies changes in lifestyle required by altered respiratory status.	Encourage patient to review patterns of usual activities, identifying those unaffected by the surgery.	Provides a positive perspective to balance perception of negative changes.
	Help the patient identify areas of lifestyle in which change may be needed and to list available options.	Promotes change in lifestyle to meet health needs. Identification of options provides a sense of control and increases the likelihood that changes will be made.
Patient verbalizes acceptance of the change in respiratory status.	Facilitate discussion of changes and options between the patient and significant others.	Support and encouragement from significant others increase the likelihood of compliance with lifestyle changes.
	Encourage sharing of mutual concerns between patient and significant others.	Changes affect significant others as well as patient.

Evaluation: Compare the patient's status with the expected patient outcomes. If the outcomes are achieved, evaluate nursing care as successful. If not, reassess the patient, formulate new nursing diagnoses, and revise expected patient outcomes and nursing interventions as appropriate.

(continued)

Nursing Care Guide 12–1. *(continued)*

PATIENTS HAVING A LOBECTOMY

Assessment Findings: Patient has no prior knowledge of self-care after lobectomy.

Nursing Diagnosis: High risk for altered health maintenance related to insufficient knowledge of self-care after lobectomy

Patient Outcomes	Nursing Interventions	Rationale
Patient describes self-care after discharge as presented in Chart 12–1. Patient demonstrates arm and shoulder exercises to be done at home to regain muscle strength.	Instruct the patient as described in Chart 12–1.	Provides information necessary for self-care in the postdischarge period.

Evaluation: Compare the patient's status with the expected patient outcomes. If the outcomes are achieved, evaluate nursing care as successful. If not, reassess the patient, formulate new nursing diagnoses, and revise expected patient outcomes and nursing interventions as appropriate.

Additional Assessments and Interventions

Prepare the patient for preoperative diagnostic tests.

Ensure that prescribed measures to minimize secretions and promote alveolar ventilation are carried out. These measures may include increasing fluids and providing humidification, administration of bronchodilators, chest percussion, and postural drainage.

Prepare the patient for surgery according to the surgeon's orders.

Give oral fluids as soon as patient is alert, and progress to regular prescribed diet as tolerated.

Report temperature of 102°F (38.8°C) or higher or lower than 98°F (36.6°C).

Monitor for signs of complications, such as pneumothorax, hemothorax, pulmonary edema, cardiac dysrhythmias, and mediastinal shift.

The Elderly: Special Considerations

Age-related changes make the respiratory system less efficient, with less reserve capacity and tolerance for exercise and stress.

There is a loss of elastic tissue surrounding the alveoli and alveolar ducts. Skeletal changes associated with aging frequently accentuate the dorsal curve of the thoracic spine, producing kyphosis, or a "stooped posture" with an increased anteroposterior diameter of the chest. The respiratory muscles are weaker and the rib cage more rigid, and the elderly patient may not be able to cough or deep breathe as well as a younger patient.

As the lungs undergo fibrosis, they inflate more easily but lose the ability to recoil; thus, a greater residual volume and less tidal volume result. As alveolar membranes become thicker and larger, expiration requires more effort and is less automatic. The thickened alveolar membranes do not diffuse oxygen as quickly. Ventilation and oxygenation usually remain adequate to meet the demands of normal activity.

Bibliography

Anderson S. ABGs: Six easy steps for interpreting blood gases. Am J Nurs 1990; 90(8):42.

Applefeld JJ, Lindberg SE (eds). Acute respiratory care. Cambridge, MA: Blackwell Scientific, 1988.

Barnes C, Kirchhoff K. Minimizing hypoxemia due to endotracheal suctioning: A literature review. Heart Lung 1985; 2:164.

Bates B, Hoeckelman RA. A guide to physical examination and history taking. 4th ed. Philadelphia: JB Lippincott, 1991.

Bates DW. Respiratory function in disease. 3rd ed. Philadelphia: WB Saunders, 1989.

Bernstein B. Breaking the vicious circle of non-compliance. Nursing 1989; 19(1):74.
Bolgiano CS, Bunting K, Shoenberger MM. Administering oxygen therapy: What you need to know. Nursing 1990; 20(6):47.
Brandstetter R. Pulmonary medicine. Oradell, NJ: Medical Economics, 1989.
Brewis RAA, Gibson GJ, Geddes DM. Respiratory medicine. Philadelphia: WB Saunders, 1990.
Burton G, Hodgkin J, Ward JJ. Respiratory care: A guide to clinical practice. 3rd ed. Philadelphia: JB Lippincott, 1991.
Carnevali D. Nursing management for the elderly. 2nd ed. Philadelphia: JB Lippincott, 1988.
Carpenito LJ. Nursing diagnosis: Application to clinical practice. 4th ed. Philadelphia: JB Lippincott, 1992.
Carroll P. Artificial airways: Real risks. Nursing 1986; 8:57.
Carroll P. Nursing the thoracotomy patient. RN 1992; 55(6):34.
Carroll P. Cyanosis: The sign you can't count on. Nursing 1988; 18(3):50.
Carroll PF. Clinical insights: ARDS. Nursing 1988; 18(5):74.
Chatburn RL, Lough MD. Handbook of respiratory care. Chicago: Year Book Medical Publishers, 1990.
Cherniack R, Cherniack L. Respiration in health and disease. 3rd ed. Philadelphia: WB Saunders, 1983.
Donner C, Cooper K. The critical difference: Pulmonary edema. Am J Nurs 1988; 88(1):59.
Engelking C. Teaching, counseling, caring. Am J Nurs 1987; 87(11):1439.
Finucane BT, Santora AH. Principles of airway management. In Lowenthal DT (editor in chief). Essentials of medical education series. Philadelphia: FA Davis, 1988.
Flenley DC. Respiratory medicine. 2nd ed. Philadelphia: WB Saunders, 1990.
Fraser RG, Paré JAP, Paré PD, et al. Diagnosis of diseases of the chest. 3rd ed. Vol. 1. Philadelphia: WB Saunders, 1988.
Fraser RG, Paré JAP, Paré PD, et al. Diagnosis of diseases of the chest. 3rd ed. Vol. 2. Philadelphia: WB Saunders, 1989.
Fraser RG, Paré JAP, Paré PD, et al. Diagnosis of diseases of the chest. 3rd ed. Vol. 3. Philadelphia: WB Saunders, 1990.
Gallo J. Handbook of geriatric assessment. Rockville, MD: Aspen Publishers, 1988.
Goodnough SKC. Reducing tracheal injury and aspiration. DCCN 1988; 7(6):324.
Gorback, MS. Emergency airway management. Philadelphia, BC Decker Inc., 1990.
Grandstrom D, Wierzbicki L. A better way to deliver long term oxygen therapy. RN 1989; 52(9):58.
Guyton AC. A textbook of medical physiology. 8th ed. Philadelphia: WB Saunders, 1991.
Hayden, RA. What keeps oxygenation on track? Am J Nurs 1992; 92(12):32.
Handerhan B, Allegrezza N. Getting your patient off a ventilator. RN 1989; 52(12):60.
Hoffman LA, Mazzocco MC, Roth JE. Fine tuning your chest PT. Am J Nurs 1987; 87(12):1566.
Jablonski RAS. Remember the person attached to the ventilator. Nursing 1992; 22(4):67.
Johnson AP. The elderly and COPD. J Gerontol Nurs 1988; 14(12):20.
Karlinsky JB. Decision making in pulmonary medicine. St. Louis: CV Mosby, 1991.
Kenner C, Guzzetta C, Dossey B. Critical care nursing: Mind, body, spirit. Boston: Little Brown, 1985.
Kersten LD. Comprehensive respiratory nursing—A decision making approach. Philadelphia: WB Saunders, 1989.
Larson M, Kim M. Respiratory muscle training with the incentive spirometer resistive breathing device. Heart Lung 1984; 13(4):341.
Luce J, Tyler M, Pierson D. Intensive respiratory care. Philadelphia: WB Saunders, 1984.
Lush MT, Janson-Bjerklie S, Carrieri VK, Lovejoy N. Dyspnea in the ventilator-assisted patient. Heart Lung 1988; 17(5):528.
Majors M. Nutritional support of the mechanically ventilated patient. Crit Care Nurs Q 1988; 11(3):50.
Maran J, Gray M. Pulmonary laser therapy. Am J Nurs 1988; 88(6):828.
May DF. Rehabilitation and continuity of care in respiratory disease. In Youtsey JW (ed). Faculty lecture series in respiratory disease. St. Louis: Mosby–Year Book, 1991.
McCauley MD, Von Rueden KT. Noninvasive monitoring of the mechanically ventilated patient. Crit Care Nurs Q 1988; 11(3):50.
Mims B. The risks of oxygen therapy. RN 1987; 50(7):20.
Mims BC. Interpreting ABG's. RN 1991; 54(3):42.
Montanari J, Spearing C. The fine art of measuring tracheal cuff pressure. Nursing 1986; 7:46.
Murray JF, Nadel JA. Textbook of respiratory medicine: Vols. 1 and 2. Philadelphia: WB Saunders, 1988.
Palau D, Jones S. Test your skill at trouble shooting chest tubes. RN 1986; 10:43.
Plowman PN. Respiratory medicine. New York: Elsevier, 1987.
Reischman RR. Review of ventilation and perfusion physiology. Crit Care Nurse 1988; 8(7):24.
Ruiz J, et al (eds). Clinical atlas of respiratory diseases. Chicago: Year Book Medical Publishers, 1988.
Rutherford KA. Principles and application of oximetry. Crit Care Nurs Clin North Am 1989; 1(4):649.
Sabiston DC Jr. Textbook of surgery: The biological basis of modern surgical practice. 14th ed. Philadelphia: WB Saunders, 1991.
Sabiston DC Jr, Spencer FC. Surgery of the chest. 5th ed. Philadelphia: WB Saunders, 1990.
Santo-Novak D. Seven keys to assessing the elderly. Nursing 1988; 18(8):60.
Sawisku E, Branthwaite M. Respiratory emergencies. Stoneham, MA: Butterworth, 1988.
Scanlan C, Spearman C, Sheldon R, Egan D (eds). Egan's fundamentals of respiratory therapy. St. Louis: CV Mosby, 1990.
Schafer S. Relieving pain, an analgesic guide. Am J Nurs 1988; 88(6):815.
Shelhamer J, Pizzo PA, Parrillo JE, Masur H. Respiratory disease in the immunosuppressed host. Philadelphia: JB Lippincott, 1991.
Spyr J, Preach MA. Pulse oximetry. RN 1990; 53(5):38.
Sutton PR. Adult respiratory distress syndrome. In Cardiopulmonary emergencies. Springhouse, PA: Springhouse, 1991.
Toben BP, Lewandowski V. Nontraditional and new ventilatory techniques. Crit Care Nurs Q 1988; 11(3):12.
Vasbinder-Dillon D. Understanding mechanical ventilation. Crit Care Nurse 1988; 8(7):42.
Weinberger SE. Principles of pulmonary medicine. Philadelphia: WB Saunders, 1986.
Wesmiller SW, Hoffman LA. Understanding transtracheal oxygen delivery. Nursing 1989; 19(12):43.
Winters C. Monitoring ventilator patients for complications. Nursing 1988; 18(6):38.
Yeaw EMJ. How position affects oxygenation. Good lung down? Am J Nurs 1992; 92(3):27.
Zahourek R (ed). Relaxation and imagery: Tools for therapeutic communication and intervention. Philadelphia: WB Saunders, 1988.

Chapter Thirteen

NURSING CARE *of Adults with* Upper Respiratory Disorders

Upper respiratory tract diseases range in severity from a simple cold to life-threatening cancer of the larynx. The most common upper respiratory tract diseases are inflammations and infections, which include rhinitis, sinusitis, pharyngitis, and laryngitis. These inflammations and infections affect virtually everyone regardless of age. They rarely require hospitalization and, in fact, are often self-treated with over-the-counter preparations. Thus, a major nursing role in relation to these disorders is health education to ensure safe use of over-the-counter preparations and prompt medical attention if needed. At the opposite end of the continuum is nursing care of patients with upper respiratory tract trauma or neoplasia. These patients can be critically ill with severe problems related to airway maintenance, nutrition, risk for infection, communication, and body-image disturbance.

Infections

Upper respiratory tract infections are among the most common forms of human illness. In most cases, they result in discomfort that is more annoying than disabling. Although they may interfere with the normal activities of daily living, they are not life threatening, do not require hospitalization, and do not usually lead to serious chronic disabilities. The focus of therapy is generally on the symptoms. In many instances, the symptoms disappear spontaneously; however, repeated infections may lead to tissue damage, which can alter respiratory function.

Upper respiratory tract infections are responsible for roughly 50% of the total time lost from work by adults and approximately 70% of the time lost from school by children. Studies indicate that the average person among the general population has between three and five episodes of respiratory infection each year. The frequency of occurrence, the economic loss, and the large number of people affected are sound reasons why even uncomplicated upper respiratory tract disorders deserve serious attention by health personnel.

Common Cold

ETIOLOGY AND PATHOPHYSIOLOGY

The common cold or coryza syndrome is an infectious process of the upper respiratory tract, which can be caused by any of 80 to 100 different viruses. Colds are highly communicable by droplet nuclei, particularly at their onset. By themselves, they rarely require hospitalization; however, many other more serious illnesses begin with a cold or symptoms closely resembling those of a cold. Generally, the use of such terms as chest cold, head cold, rhinitis, or pharyngitis refer to the sites of the major symptoms of the cold.

CLINICAL MANIFESTATIONS

Colds can produce a wide variety of symptoms that include nasal discharge with obstruction, sneezing, watery eyes, coughing, fever, chills, and a dry or sore throat. Symptoms usually appear suddenly, and full-blown infection may occur within 48 hours. Often as the cough develops it becomes productive. Other complaints such as lethargy and vague pains in various limbs may be reported. The major symptoms last 5 to 14 days. If a significant temperature elevation occurs with the cold, it may indicate the presence of a concurrent infection such as sinusitis or otitis media. These particular infections may also follow the common cold.

MEDICAL MANAGEMENT

Generally, medical management is neither sought nor required for the common cold. If visited, the physician may prescribe nose drops for nasal congestion and an antitussive for cough. Antibiotics are not generally prescribed because they are not effective against viruses.

Guidelines for Application of the Nursing Process to the Care of the Patient with a Common Cold

Nurses are not usually involved in the direct care of patients with a common cold. Most often, the nurse is simply asked informally for advice. When this occurs, first determine the type of cough, how long it has persisted, whether it is productive, and, if so, the amount and appearance of the expectorate and whether it is associated with any other symptoms. If the cough has been of long duration and is associated with a high fever, purulent or blood-tinged sputum, or other symptoms suggestive of serious disease, refer the patient to a physician or nurse practitioner. If no symptoms exist other than those suggestive of a common cold, instruct or assist the person with care as specified in Chart 13–1.

Sinusitis

Sinusitis—inflammation of a sinus (Fig. 13–1)—may be a primary disorder or a complication of an upper respiratory tract viral infection. It may be either acute or chronic.

Chart 13–1.

NURSING GUIDE TO PATIENT EDUCATION FOR SELF-MANAGEMENT: COMMON COLD

Instruct the patient to:

Rest to conserve energy for the body to use in fighting the infection.

Increase fluid intake to help liquefy secretions.

Eat a balanced diet to provide energy and nutrients needed to fight infection.

Use a vaporizer to soothe mucous membranes and liquefy secretions.

Blow nose by opening the mouth slightly and blowing through both nostrils to equalize pressure.

Use over-the-counter medications carefully:
- Check dosages and follow them exactly: "More is not better."
- Read instructions and do not take if any of the chronic conditions listed as contraindications exist.
- Be alert to side effects and possible interactions with other medications, foods, or alcohol.

Administer nose drops correctly:
- Sit in a chair with the head tilted well back, or lie down with a pillow under the shoulders and the head tilted back.
- Instill no more than three drops (unless otherwise ordered) of solution into each nostril at a time.
- Remain in position with the head tilted back for 5 minutes to permit the solution to reach the posterior nares.
- Use nose drops only as directed.

Control the spread of disease:
- Cover mouth when sneezing or coughing.
- Properly dispose of used tissues.
- Avoid crowded areas.

See a physician if the cough or cold is persistent and does not respond to simple remedies.

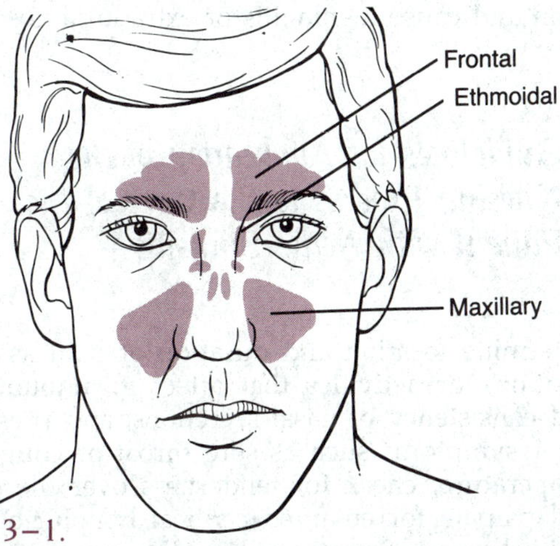

Figure 13–1.
Paranasal sinuses: frontal, ethmoidal, and maxillary.

ACUTE SINUSITIS

ETIOLOGY AND PATHOPHYSIOLOGY

Acute sinusitis is the result of an obstruction of the normal routes of sinus drainage. Abscesses of the upper bicuspid or molar teeth that rupture into the maxillary sinuses, swimming, diving, or the direct trauma associated with fractures may also cause sinusitis. Sinusitis may also occur as a complication of nasogastric tube placement.

CLINICAL MANIFESTATIONS

Basic symptoms of sinusitis result from obstruction of drainage. When all the sinuses are involved, the condition is called pansinusitis. Clinical symptoms include fever, chills, nasal obstruction, pain

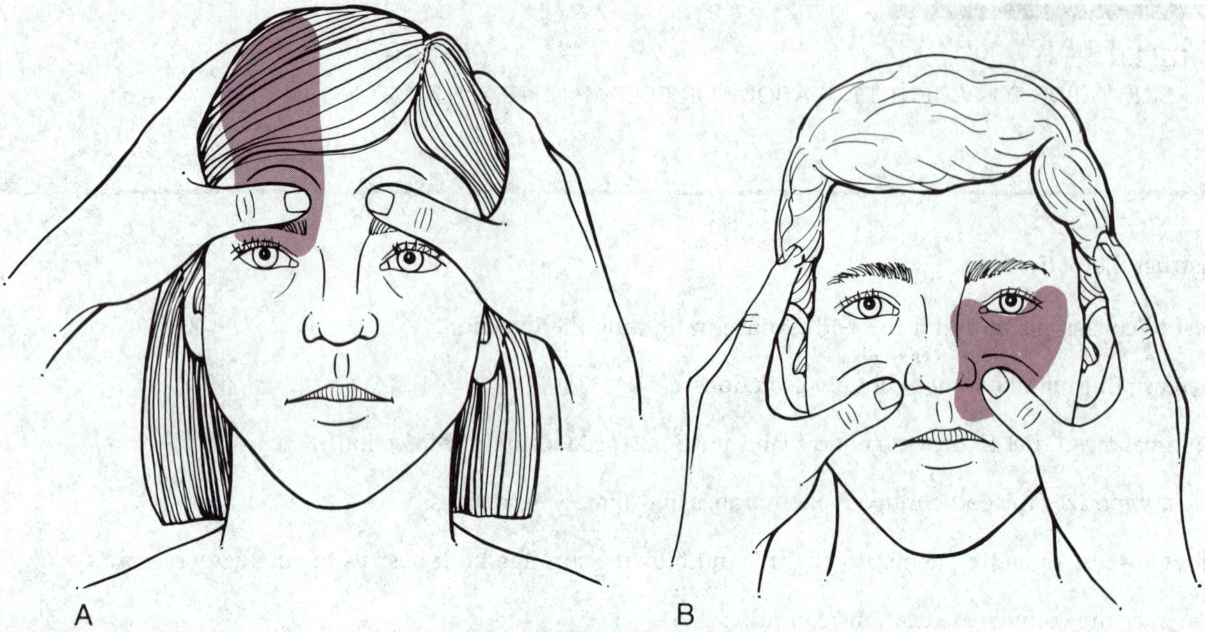

Figure 13–2.

Palpating the frontal and maxillary sinuses for tenderness. *A*, Pressure applied to orbital ridge to check for frontal sinus tenderness. (Color indicates area of frontal sinus pain.) *B*, Pressure applied lateral to the naris to check for maxillary sinus tenderness. (Color indicates area of maxillary sinus pain.)

and tenderness over the involved sinuses, and recurrent headaches that change in intensity with position and disappear shortly after getting out of bed. Frontal sinusitis is characterized by pain in the forehead when pressure is applied over the sinuses or on the lateral edge of the orbital ridges. Swelling and tenderness in the anterior portions of the maxillae are the common clinical manifestations of maxillary sinusitis (Fig. 13–2). If the infection is severe, referred pain may occur in the upper teeth. Ethmoid sinusitis is characterized by pain in and around the eyes, whereas sphenoidal sinusitis causes pain over the mastoid bones and the occipital portion of the head. The fever associated with sinusitis is related to the amount of obstruction present and the virulence of the infection. Temperature may be as high as 104°F (40°C).

MEDICAL DIAGNOSIS

Medical diagnosis is made on the basis of the history and physical findings. Radiologic study of the sinuses may be ordered to identify the specific sinus involved and, if nasal secretions are present, a culture and sensitivity may be done.

MEDICAL MANAGEMENT

Medical management consists of a series of broad-spectrum antibiotics such as penicillin or erythromycin. Vasoconstrictors such as phenylephrine (Neo-Synephrine) 0.25% and ephedrine sulfate 0.25% to 3% may be prescribed to promote drainage. Analgesics such as codeine are prescribed for pain. In some cases, surgical intervention in the form of antral puncture and lavage may be elected.

COMPLICATIONS

Complications of sinusitis are related to the specific sinuses infected as they involve adjacent or contiguous structures. Rhinitis, pharyngitis, laryngitis, bronchitis, and bronchiectasis may all be associated with sinusitis. An acute suppurative infection (empyema) of a sinus may be present. If this empyema ruptures posteriorly, a brain abscess occurs, which constitutes a serious complication. Infection may also travel through the venous supply to the brain and cause meningitis or extradural abscess.

Guidelines for Application of the Nursing Process to the Care of the Patient with Acute Sinusitis

Determine location and duration of pain as well as positions or activities that affect it; amount, color, and consistency of nasal secretions; and presence of other symptoms such as sore throat or cough. Take temperature; check for tenderness over the sinuses; and palpate for enlarged cervical lymph nodes. Explain the use of prescribed medications and instruct the patient as specified in Chart 13–2 about nonpharmacologic measures that promote sinus drainage, comfort, and resolution of the infection.

CHRONIC SINUSITIS

ETIOLOGY AND PATHOPHYSIOLOGY

Chronic sinusitis is characterized by thickened mucous membranes and thickened sinuses as a result of prolonged, repeated irritation and infection. Although some cases of chronic sinusitis are known to be related to persistent or repeated infection as evidenced by repeated isolation of a pathogenic organism, many cases have also been found to be related to other factors such as irritating dusts, gases, or excessive exposure to tobacco smoke.

CLINICAL MANIFESTATIONS

Chronic sinusitis is characterized by a chronic, purulent nasal discharge, chronic cough related to the postnasal drainage, and persistent headaches, which are more pronounced on awakening in the morning. Fatigue, nasal stuffiness, and mental dullness are common symptoms.

MEDICAL DIAGNOSIS

Diagnosis of chronic sinusitis is made on the basis of the patient's history of symptoms, findings on physical examination, and radiologic examination of the sinuses, which show thickening of the mucous membranes as well as diffuse cloudiness.

MEDICAL MANAGEMENT

Treatment for chronic sinusitis includes antibiotics if a causative organism is identified by culture and sensitivity, antiallergic measures, and interventions aimed at promoting drainage. As stated earlier, vasoconstrictive drugs may be prescribed, but the patient should be cautioned regarding overuse.

If these interventions are not successful in the management of chronic sinusitis, surgical treatment may be necessary. Surgery may be done to correct a structural factor contributing to the problem such as a deviated septum, hypertrophied turbinate bones, or nasal polyps. In other cases, surgery may be done to drain the sinuses or to remove the diseased mucous membrane.

Application of the Nursing Process to the Care of the Patient with Chronic Sinusitis

The assessment, nursing diagnoses, expected patient outcomes, nursing interventions, and evaluation for patients treated nonsurgically for chronic sinusitis are similar to those described previously for patients with acute sinusitis. If sinus surgery is performed, nursing care is as follows.

PREOPERATIVE NURSING CARE

Basic preoperative nursing care is given as described in Chapter 4.

POSTOPERATIVE NURSING CARE

Assessment

In addition to the assessments that are standard for any postanesthesia patient, immediately after sinus

Chart 13–2.

NURSING GUIDE TO PATIENT EDUCATION FOR SELF-MANAGEMENT: NONPHARMACOLOGIC TREATMENT MEASURES FOR SINUSITIS

To promote sinus drainage, comfort, and resolution of the infection, instruct the patient to:

Apply heat in the form of hot, wet packs over the affected sinuses to promote comfort and resolution of the infection.
Use a cool-steam vaporizer to provide moisture to liquefy secretions and ease drainage.
Drink large amounts of fluids to help keep secretions liquid.
Keep room temperature constant, because significant changes in environmental temperature aggravate sinusitis.

surgery, observe for repeated swallowing because this may be the first indication of hemorrhage. Also make a gross check of visual acuity to assess for damage to the optic nerve, which is a risk with sinus surgery. Do this by simply holding up one or two fingers in front of the patient and asking how many fingers are seen. Take the patient's temperature every 4 hours, and check for pain over the involved sinus to detect signs of postoperative infection or inadequate drainage.

Nursing Diagnoses and Planning

Nursing diagnoses and related expected patient outcomes most commonly applicable to patients who have had surgery for chronic sinusitis include the following:

NDx: High risk for aspiration related to effects of anesthesia and presence of bloody drainage from the sinuses

Planning: Patient outcomes
1. Respiratory secretions are clear.
2. Respiratory secretions are odorless.
3. Adventitious breath sounds are absent.

NDx: Pain related to surgical trauma

Planning: Patient outcomes
1. Patient states pain is relieved.
2. Patient experiences pain relief as shown by relaxed facial expression and body positioning.

NDx: High risk for altered oral mucous membrane related to drying secondary to mouth breathing

Planning: Patient outcomes
1. Oral mucous membrane is moist and intact.
2. Patient performs frequent mouth care, avoiding use of drying agents.

NDx: High risk for altered health maintenance related to insufficient knowledge of factors that exacerbate sinusitis

Planning: Patient outcomes
1. Patient lists factors that aggravate sinusitis.
2. Patient describes ways to avoid exacerbating factors.

Nursing Interventions

NDx: High risk for aspiration
Immediately after surgery, position the patient well to the side to prevent aspiration of bloody drainage from the nose or throat. When awake and alert, help the patient into a mid-Fowler's position to promote drainage and to decrease edema.

NDx: Pain
Apply ice compresses to the operative area to limit edema and relieve pain. Administer analgesics as prescribed.

NDx: High risk for altered oral mucous membrane
Because the patient will have packing in the nose for 48 hours after surgery and therefore will be breathing by mouth, there is the potential for drying and cracking of the oral mucous membrane. To prevent this, provide ice chips or sips of water frequently. Assist with oral hygiene as often as needed, avoiding the use of products such as lemon-glycerine swabs, which exert a drying effect. Keep the patient's lips lubricated with K-Y jelly or other water-soluble lubricant. Advance oral intake as soon as permitted and tolerated to improve hydration and stimulate salivation.

NDx: High risk for altered health maintenance
Explain that cold and dampness aggravate sinusitis and are therefore best avoided. This means turning on home heat, staying inside on cold, damp days, and avoiding air-conditioned environments. Also explain the irritating effects of tobacco smoke and the importance of avoiding poorly ventilated areas.

Additional Interventions
Change nasal drip pads (piece of gauze folded and taped under the nose) as necessary, and report excessive bloody drainage.

When the nasal packing is removed in 48 hours, instruct the patient not to blow the nose, because this can cause trauma to the operative site, increase local blood pressure, and cause bleeding.

Evaluation

Evaluate the effectiveness of nursing care for a patient undergoing surgery for chronic sinusitis by comparing the patient's status with the expected patient outcomes. Examples of specific outcomes for patients having surgery for chronic sinusitis have been provided in the Planning section.

Pharyngitis

ETIOLOGY AND PATHOPHYSIOLOGY

Pharyngitis, which is an inflammation of the throat, often accompanies other upper respiratory tract infections. It can be caused by several different viruses and bacteria; however, those episodes caused by group A beta-hemolytic streptococcus are most serious because of the potential for dangerous cardiac and renal complications. This organism may normally reside in the upper respiratory tract passages of some people without causing any symptoms of disease. These people are carriers and sources of spread of the organism.

CLINICAL MANIFESTATIONS

Streptococcal pharyngitis, the most commonly occurring upper respiratory tract infection of the streptococcal type, has a 3- to 5-day incubation period. This is followed by a sudden onset of sore throat accompanied by chills, high temperature, headache, and frequently severe dysphagia. A white or yellow patchy exudate may cover the tonsillar area. Acute pharyngitis may precede other communicable diseases.

MEDICAL DIAGNOSIS

Most often a throat culture is obtained to make an exact determination of the microorganism involved. This is very important because of the potential for serious complications such as glomerular nephritis, rheumatic fever, otitis media, cervical adenitis, and mastoiditis. An alternative to the traditional culture is a newer test called Biostar, which allows identification of streptococcus in 15 minutes.

MEDICAL MANAGEMENT

Early antibiotic treatment helps prevent the serious complications related to hemolytic streptococcal infections. Penicillin is the drug of choice, but penicillin-sensitive patients may be treated with other antibiotics (e.g., tetracycline or cephalosporin). Antibiotics are continued for 24 to 48 hours after visible throat inflammation subsides, which usually occurs after 7 to 10 days.

Application of the Nursing Process to the Care of the Patient with Pharyngitis

Assessment

Inspect the throat. Observe for redness, swelling, drainage, and lesions. Be certain to note presence of white patches characteristic of infection with group A beta-hemolytic streptococcus. Palpate cervical lymph nodes for enlargement and tenderness.

Assess the location and extent of the patient's discomfort by asking the patient to describe the pain and noting whether the patient is able to swallow saliva, fluids, and soft foods without indications of distress. If swallowing difficulty exists, also check for signs of dehydration, which could result from decreased fluid intake and fluid loss related to fever. Take the patient's temperature, and if ordered, obtain a throat culture (Fig. 13–3). Check for any other symptoms, such as rash, that could indicate disease other than simple pharyngitis.

If group A beta-hemolytic streptococcus is the causative agent, assess the patient's understanding of the need to take all antibiotics prescribed and to have a follow-up culture.

Nursing Diagnoses and Planning

Nursing diagnoses and related expected patient outcomes most commonly applicable to patients with streptococcal pharyngitis include the following:

NDx: Pain related to inflammation of the pharynx

Planning: Patient outcomes
1. Patient reports acceptable level of comfort.
2. Patient is able to swallow saliva, fluids, and soft foods without statements or facial expressions of discomfort.

NDx: High risk for fluid volume deficit related to decreased fluid intake secondary to pain on swallowing

Planning: Patient outcomes
1. Patient denies thirst.
2. Mucous membranes are moist.
3. Skin turgor is normal.

NDx: High risk for altered health maintenance related to insufficient knowledge of prescribed antibiotic therapy, complications of "strep throat," and follow-up care

Planning: Patient outcomes
1. Patient states dose, time, route, and frequency with which antibiotics are to be taken.
2. Patient explains role of antibiotics in preventing complications and the need to take all the doses prescribed even if symptoms have disappeared.
3. Patient explains the need for a follow-up throat culture to determine whether the infection has been eradicated and thus the risk of complications reduced.
4. Patient describes need to report worsening or recurrence of symptoms.

Nursing Interventions

Patients are not hospitalized for pharyngitis. Thus, the primary mode of nursing intervention is most often giving directions to the patient for self-care rather than the direct administration of physical care.

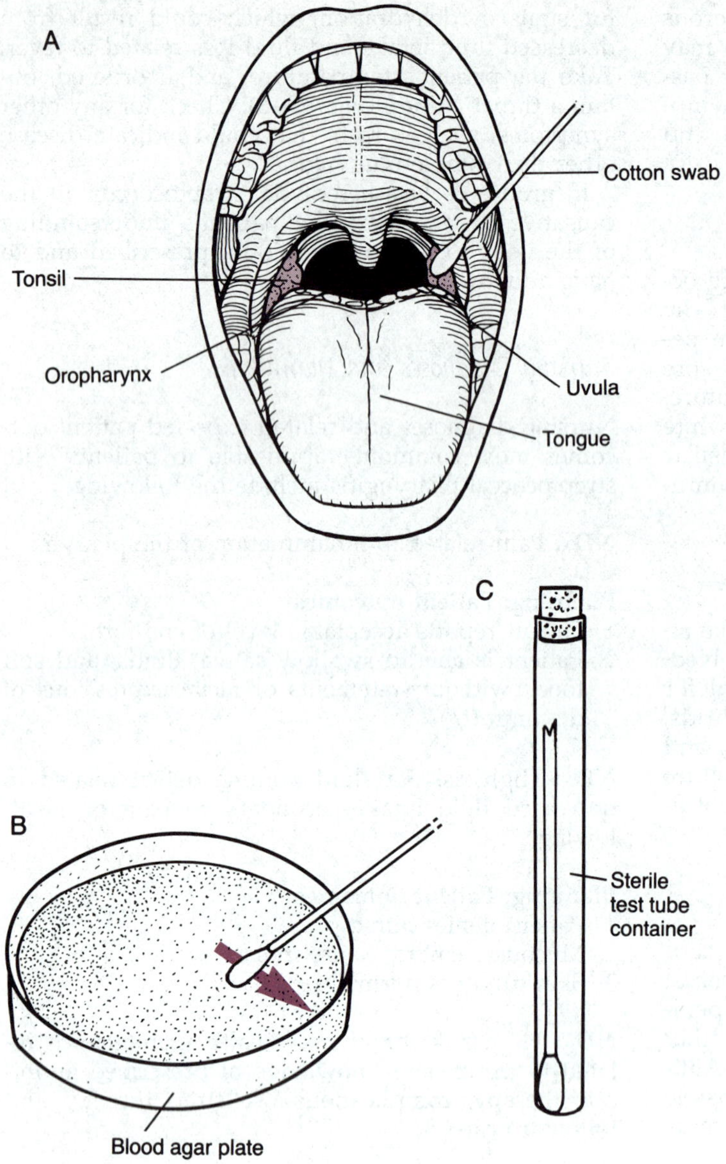

Figure 13–3.

Throat culture. *A,* Run a sterile cotton swab over areas of redness or exudate on the oropharynx to obtain a throat culture. *B,* Streak the swab across a blood agar plate, or insert the swab in a sterile test tube, with the end of the stick broken. *C,* Cap for delivery to the laboratory.

Nutrition Box 13–1.

NUTRITION: SPECIAL CONSIDERATIONS FOR PATIENTS WITH PHARYNGITIS OR TONSILLITIS

Instruct patients with pharyngitis or tonsillitis to:

- Consume cool, clear fluids or ice to soothe the painful throat during the acute stage of the disease.
- Follow clear liquids with milk products such as ice cream and pudding that coat the throat.
- Avoid citrus juices because they tend to irritate.
- Adjust diet from clear liquids to full liquids to a puréed or soft diet depending on individual tolerance.
- Avoid foods that are highly seasoned or irritating to the throat.
- Drink 2000 to 3000 ml of fluid per day.

NDx: Pain
Instruct the patient in the correct administration of prescribed analgesics. Also instruct in the use of moist inhalations to relieve dryness of the throat and in the use of an ice collar for comfort. Encourage warm saline gargles every hour while awake to soothe the mucous membrane and remove irritating secretions. Advise the patient to avoid irritating foodstuffs as outlined in Nutrition Box 13–1.

NDx: High risk for fluid volume deficit
Direct the patient to force fluids to a minimum of 2.5 L per day during the febrile stage of the disease. Advise that very hot or tart fluids that may cause additional discomfort should be avoided.

NDx: High risk for altered health maintenance
Review with the patient the dose, route, time, and frequency of the prescribed antibiotic. Stress that it must be taken as prescribed until the course is completed, even if all symptoms have disappeared. Explain that if only part of the antibiotic is taken, some group A streptococci may remain in the pharynx and reinfection or other complication may occur. Explain the need for a follow-up throat culture and its importance in the prevention of complications. Also be certain the patient understands that worsening of symptoms or occurrence of new symptoms should be reported.

Additional Interventions
Instruct the patient to take his or her temperature in the morning and evening, and advise bed rest while the temperature is elevated. Explain the importance of maintaining a balanced nutritional intake, and suggest that nutritious liquids such as eggnog, cream soups, and farina be substituted for the regular diet if dysphagia is a problem.

Evaluation

Evaluate the effectiveness of nursing care for a patient with pharyngitis by comparing the patient's status with the expected patient outcomes. Examples of specific outcomes for patients with pharyngitis have been provided in the Planning section.

Tonsillitis

Tonsillitis is an inflammation of a tonsil. It most often affects the palatine tonsils, which are masses of lymphoid tissue located in depressions of the mucous membrane of the pharynx (Fig. 13–4).

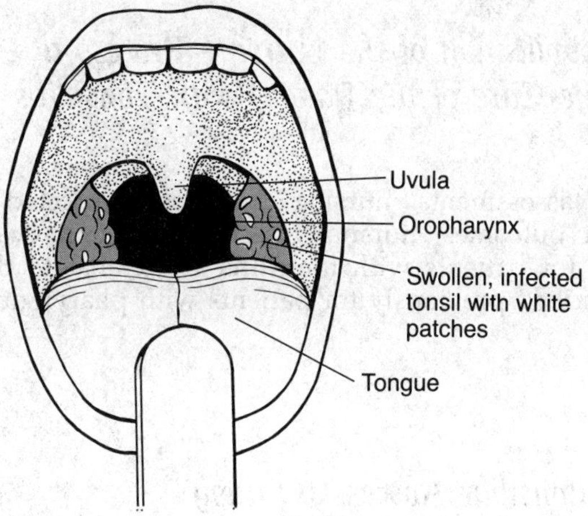

Figure 13–4.
Swollen, infected tonsils.

ETIOLOGY AND PATHOPHYSIOLOGY

Tonsillitis can occur either as a primary bacterial infection or secondary to an upper respiratory tract viral infection. It can be caused by a variety of organisms. A frequent causative agent, and also one of the most important because of the associated risk of cardiac or renal sequelae, is group A beta-hemolytic streptococcus.

CLINICAL MANIFESTATIONS

The patient with tonsillitis has a severe, dry, scratchy sore throat often accompanied by fever, chills, headache, muscle aches, and general malaise. On examination, the tonsils appear reddened and swollen; if the infection is due to group A beta-hemolytic streptococcus, white patches are present. Cervical lymph nodes are tender and swollen.

MEDICAL DIAGNOSIS

A careful history is taken to rule out related conditions such as allergy, asthma, and sinusitis. A culture is obtained from the tonsillar area to determine the presence of pathogens and the antibiotics to which they are most sensitive.

MEDICAL MANAGEMENT

Treatment of tonsillitis is primarily antibiotic therapy on the basis of results of the tonsillar culture and sensitivity. If the causative organism is group A beta-hemolytic streptococcus, a full 10-day course of penicillin is prescribed and follow-up care is required. When other bacteria are the cause, erythromycin, 250 mg, is given four times per day for 10 days. For relief of throat discomfort, analgesics and throat irrigations may be ordered.

Application of the Nursing Process to the Care of the Patient with Tonsillitis

The assessments, nursing diagnoses, expected patient outcomes, nursing interventions, and evaluation for patients with tonsillitis are similar to those described previously for patients with pharyngitis.

Peritonsillar Abscess (Quinsy)

ETIOLOGY AND PATHOPHYSIOLOGY

Peritonsillar abscess is a secondary infection related to tonsillitis. It is an abscess that develops above the tonsil in the tissues of the anterior pillar and soft palate.

CLINICAL MANIFESTATIONS

Peritonsillar abscess is manifested by sore throat, unilateral pain radiating to the ear on swallowing, and enlargement of the tonsil, with redness and swelling of the adjacent soft palate. This swelling, which may occlude the pharynx, is the most serious symptom. In addition, the patient holds the head stiffly toward the side of the abscess and is obviously in pain.

MEDICAL DIAGNOSIS

Medical diagnosis is made on the basis of symptomatology and physical findings.

MEDICAL MANAGEMENT

Medical treatment consists of antibiotics to fight the infection and warm saline irrigations to provide relief from pain. If antibiotics and irrigations are not completely effective, surgical drainage may be necessary. A tonsillectomy (removal of the palatine tonsils) is done approximately 1 month after the infection is resolved to prevent recurrence.

TONSILLECTOMY

Tonsillectomy is one of the most common operations performed despite an ongoing debate over the indications for its use. For this procedure, the patient is admitted to the hospital either the day before or the morning of surgery, is maintained on a nothing by mouth order from midnight the night before, and is discharged the evening of surgery or the day after. For adult patients, the procedure is usually done in a semisitting position under local anesthesia (procaine hydrochloride [Novocaine] 1% or lidocaine hydrochloride [Xylocaine] 1% with epinephrine, 1:100,000).

A major complication of tonsillectomy is immediate or delayed bleeding (5 to 10 days after surgery). Most often this can be controlled by local pressure or vasoconstrictive drugs. Occasionally, resuturing is required to control early bleeding and evacuation of a clot from the tonsillar depression to control late bleeding.

Application of the Nursing Process to the Care of the Patient with a Peritonsillar Abscess

The assessment, nursing diagnoses, expected patient outcomes, nursing interventions, and evaluation for patients treated nonsurgically for peritonsillar abscess are similar to those for patients with pharyngitis. If a tonsillectomy is performed, nursing care is as follows.

PREOPERATIVE NURSING CARE

Basic preoperative assessments, nursing diagnoses, expected patient outcomes, nursing interventions, and evaluation discussed in Chapter 4 apply to the care of a patient scheduled for a tonsillectomy. In addition, because a major risk associated with this procedure is hemorrhage, be certain to assess laboratory reports such as platelet count, clotting time, and hematocrit, and report any abnormalities to the surgeon.

POSTOPERATIVE NURSING CARE

Assessment

After a tonsillectomy, assess blood pressure and pulse every 15 minutes and then every 30 minutes for several hours. Take the patient's temperature every 4 hours, and use the rectal rather than the oral route to avoid possible trauma to the operative site. Carefully observe the patient for signs of postoperative hemorrhage. These signs include frequent swallowing, large amounts of bloody drainage, vomiting large amounts of bright red blood, gradually increasing pulse rate, restlessness, pallor, and ultimately falling blood pressure.

Nursing Diagnoses and Planning

Nursing diagnoses and related expected patient outcomes most commonly applicable to the patient who has had a tonsillectomy include the following:

Chart 13–3.

NURSING GUIDE TO PATIENT EDUCATION FOR SELF-MANAGEMENT: DISCHARGE INSTRUCTIONS AFTER TONSILLECTOMY

Instruct the patient to:

Add soft foods to the diet as tolerated.
Avoid rough foods such as salad and acidic foods such as orange juice for 10 days to protect the scab over the operative area and to prevent bleeding.
Rest in bed or on a couch for 24 hours after the operation and then gradually resume full activity.
Report any heavy bleeding or temperature greater than 100.4°F. (38°C).
Return for check-up in 1 week.

NDx: High risk for aspiration related to loss of the gag reflex as a result of the anesthesia

Planning: Patient outcomes
1. Respiratory secretions are clear.
2. Respiratory secretions are odorless.
3. Adventitious breath sounds are absent.

NDx: Pain related to surgical trauma of the throat

Planning: Patient outcomes
1. Patient states the throat is less sore.
2. Patient swallows liquids without difficulty.

NDx: High risk for trauma: tissue related to mechanical, thermal, or chemical stress to the suture line

Planning: Patient outcomes
1. Patient avoids coughing or clearing throat in the immediate postoperative period.
2. Patient avoids irritating foods.
3. Excessive bleeding from the operative site is absent.

NDx: Anxiety related to bloody drainage or swallowing fluid and foods

Planning: Patient outcomes
1. Patient states that bloody drainage is normal.
2. Patient demonstrates relaxed body posture and facial expressions.
3. Patient takes fluids and soft foods as directed.

NDx: High risk for altered health maintenance related to insufficient knowledge of discharge instructions

Planning: Patient outcomes
1. Patient explains discharge instructions (Chart 13–3).

Nursing Interventions

NDx: High risk for aspiration
Immediately after surgery, place the patient in a side-lying position with an emesis basin placed to catch drainage and secretions until he or she is fully alert. Once fully conscious, elevate the head of the bed to 45 degrees.

NDx: Pain
Give analgesics according to the physician's order, and apply an ice collar if allowed. To relieve pain, encourage warm gargles of saline or dilute hydrogen peroxide every 1 or 2 hours for 24 to 36 hours to promote comfort, remove viscous mucus, and help eliminate foul breath odor.

NDx: High risk for trauma: tissue
To avoid trauma to the operative area, instruct the patient not to cough or clear the throat.

Begin oral intake with ice chips and cool fluids as soon as the patient is alert. If these are tolerated well, give ice cream and add other soft, nonirritating foods such as custards and mashed potatoes as tolerated.

NDx: Anxiety
Reassure the patient that some anxiety is normal, and encourage the patient to verbalize concerns. Reassure the patient that some bloody drainage may be expected and that nonirritating soft foods and fluids will not disrupt the wound.

NDx: High risk for altered health maintenance
Instruct the patient in self-care after tonsillectomy, as specified in Chart 13–3.

Evaluation

Evaluate the effectiveness of nursing care for a patient undergoing a tonsillectomy by comparing the patient's status with the expected patient outcomes. Examples of specific outcomes for patients after tonsillectomy have been provided in the Planning section.

Inflammations

Rhinitis

Rhinitis is an inflammation of the mucous membrane of the nose. Depending on cause and duration, it is classified as acute rhinitis or coryza, allergic rhinitis, vasomotor rhinitis, rhinitis medicamentosa, or chronic rhinitis.

ALLERGIC RHINITIS

Allergic rhinitis, sometimes called hay fever, may be acute and seasonal when caused by flowers and grasses or chronic and perennial when associated with a variety of allergens such as dust, wool, foods, industrial chemicals, or animal dander. The factor responsible can sometimes be identified through a careful and detailed history. Symptoms commonly include nasal obstruction, sneezing, watery eyes, recurring thin, watery nasal discharge, itchy eyes and nose, and headache. On physical examination, the turbinates appear pale and edematous.

Management of allergic rhinitis may include removing the offending antigen, hyposensitization, antihistamine therapy, and suppression of the immune response (see Chapters 9 and 10 for a complete discussion of hay fever).

Persons with both seasonal and perennial rhinitis often develop polyps, which are pale, soft, edematous outpouchings of the nasal or sinus mucosa. Generally, polyps are bilateral and may cause obstruction of the airway. If multiple polyps are involved, severe nasal obstruction may occur. Polypectomy, or surgical removal of the polyps, may be necessary.

VASOMOTOR RHINITIS

The term *vasomotor rhinitis* refers to a symptom complex similar to perennial rhinitis but without any established allergic basis. Although the exact cause is unknown, it is thought to be the result of an instability in the autonomic nervous system resulting from stress, tension, or some endocrine disorder. Treatment is symptomatic.

RHINITIS MEDICAMENTOSA

Rhinitis medicamentosa is a common condition caused by the overuse of nose drops. The same agent used to shrink the nasal membranes and decrease secretions has the disadvantages of possible rebound vasodilation and increased secretion. Treatment of rhinitis medicamentosa consists of discontinuing the use of nose drops completely.

CHRONIC RHINITIS

Chronic rhinitis refers to a chronic inflammation of the nasal mucous membranes caused by repeated infections, by allergy, or by vasomotor rhinitis.

Clinically, chronic rhinitis presents with nasal obstruction and feelings of stuffiness and pressure in the nose. A nasal discharge, which may be serous, mucopurulent, or purulent, is always present. The patient may also complain of frontal headaches, sneezing, and vertigo.

The chronicity of the condition leads to the deposition of large amounts of connective tissue in the nasal mucosa, with resulting hypertrophy. Polyp formation frequently occurs. Eventually, a wasting or atrophy of the mucous membranes, the cartilage, and the bones lining the nasal passages may occur. This creates a large, empty cavern in which an abundant exudate builds up on the walls, causing a very offensive odor. This condition is known as atrophic rhinitis or ozena.

Laryngitis

Laryngitis is an inflammation of the mucosa of the larynx, which occurs in both acute and chronic forms.

The larynx, or voice box, is a short passageway that connects the pharynx with the trachea. The mucous membranes of the larynx are arranged into two pairs of folds: an upper pair called false vocal cords, and a lower pair called true vocal cords (Fig. 13–5). The exhalation of air through the larynx causes vibration of the vocal cords, with resulting sounds. If anything but air passes into the larynx, a cough reflex is triggered.

ETIOLOGY AND PATHOPHYSIOLOGY

Acute laryngitis is most often caused by an upper respiratory tract infection or by abuse of the voice. Chronic laryngitis is usually the result of multiple factors, including irritation from smoking, repeated

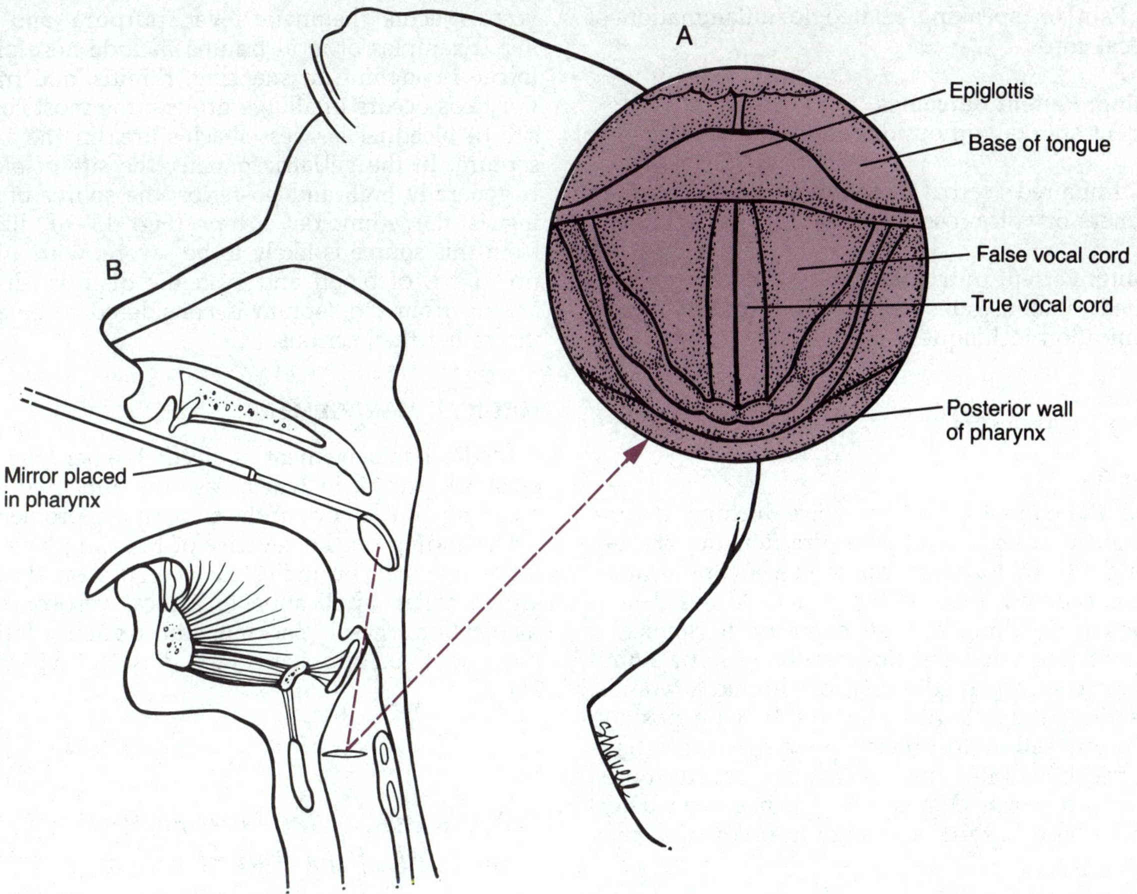

Figure 13–5.

View of the vocal cords and adjacent structures at rest *(A)*, as seen in a mirror placed in the pharynx (indirect laryngoscopy) *(B)*.

episodes of acute laryngitis, sinusitis, prolonged voice abuse, and allergies.

CLINICAL MANIFESTATIONS

Clinical symptoms of acute laryngitis vary from slight hoarseness to complete loss of voice (aphonia), dry cough, and tenacious sputum. Chronic laryngitis is marked by a persistent hoarseness, which can leave the patient unable to speak for hours at a time.

MEDICAL DIAGNOSIS

Diagnosis of laryngitis is made on the basis of history, presenting symptoms, and visual examination of the larynx.

MEDICAL MANAGEMENT

Antibiotics are prescribed to treat any accompanying upper respiratory tract infection. Topical anesthetics in the form of throat lozenges and steam or aerosol inhalations are used to relieve laryngeal pain and irritation.

Application of the Nursing Process to the Care of the Patient with Laryngitis

Assessment

Obtain information regarding onset and duration of hoarseness or voice loss, pain on speaking, and presence of symptoms of an upper respiratory tract infection such as fever, nasal congestion, postnasal drip, and cough. If severe hoarseness or pain is present or if there is total voice loss, obtain these data by having the patient write answers to specific questions or by having a significant other, knowledgeable about the problem, answer in the presence of the patient, thus allowing the patient to confirm or contradict answers with a shake of the head.

Nursing Diagnoses and Planning

Nursing diagnoses and related expected patient outcomes most commonly applicable to patients with laryngitis include the following:

NDx: Pain on speaking related to inflammation of the vocal cords

Planning: Patient outcomes
1. Patient speaks without discomfort.

NDx: Impaired verbal communication related to hoarseness or voice loss

Planning: Patient outcomes
1. Patient demonstrates ability to use alternate communication techniques.

Nursing Interventions

NDx: Pain
Instruct the patient to rest the voice during the acute phase of the disease, and give directions for the use of analgesics or lozenges containing a topical anesthetic as ordered. Instruct the patient to avoid nonproductive coughing and all exposure to smoke or other irritating inhalants. Suggest the use of a humidifier for comfort. In the case of chronic laryngitis, advise the patient to sleep in a side-lying position using a low pillow to prevent pharyngeal secretions from trickling into the larynx. In severe cases, change to a warm climate or, if it has been determined to be a hazard, a change in occupation may be necessary.

NDx: Impaired verbal communication
Suggest alternate methods of communication such as a Magic Slate and a bell for attracting attention. Explain to significant others the need for the patient to avoid speaking, and encourage them to phrase questions so that they can be answered by a shake of the head or a point of a finger whenever possible.

Evaluation

Evaluate the effectiveness of nursing care for a patient with laryngitis by comparing the patient's status with the expected patient outcomes. Examples of specific outcomes for patients with laryngitis have been provided in the Planning section.

Structural Disorders

Epistaxis

ETIOLOGY AND PATHOPHYSIOLOGY

Nosebleed may result from disease or trauma. Some of the diseases associated with epistaxis include arterial hypertension, sclerosis of the blood vessels, acute rheumatic fever, purpura, and leukemia. Examples of local trauma include nose picking, forceful coughing or sneezing, rhinitis, and fracture. Epistaxis occurs in all age groups; the most common site of bleeding is Kiesselbach's area in the anterior septum. In the geriatric patient, the site of bleeding is generally high and posterior; the source of bleeding is the ethmoidal artery (Fig. 13–6). Bleeding from this source is likely to be severe, with a loss of up to 1 L of blood and systemic distress. Epistaxis arising from the septum is considered to be annoying rather than serious.

MEDICAL MANAGEMENT

Medical management is needed when significant epistaxis occurs, in which case the aim is to control bleeding and to correct the underlying problem.

Depending on the severity of bleeding, any of the following may be indicated: pressure on the nares, an ice collar, application of a local vasoconstrictive medication, nasal packing, intravenous fluid replacement, or supplementary doses of vitamins K and C.

Application of the Nursing Process to the Care of the Patient with Epistaxis

Assessment

Determine the amount and location of the bleeding (high or low in the right or left naris). Take vital signs, and note the patient's color.

Question the patient to determine whether this is the first episode of bleeding. If nosebleeds have occurred before, determine their frequency and duration. Ask the patient about any history of trauma to the nose, any recent oral or nasal surgery, allergies, hypertension, or blood disorders. Ask the patient about any medications taken—prescription or over-the-counter—to determine whether a drug affecting the clotting mechanism could be responsible for the bleeding. Also ask the patient what, if anything, has been done to try and stop the bleeding.

Nursing Diagnoses and Planning

Nursing diagnoses and related expected patient outcomes most commonly applicable to patients with epistaxis include the following:

NDx: Anxiety related to bleeding and its cause

Planning: Patient outcomes
1. Patient denies excessive anxiety.
2. Patient's body posture and facial expressions are relaxed.

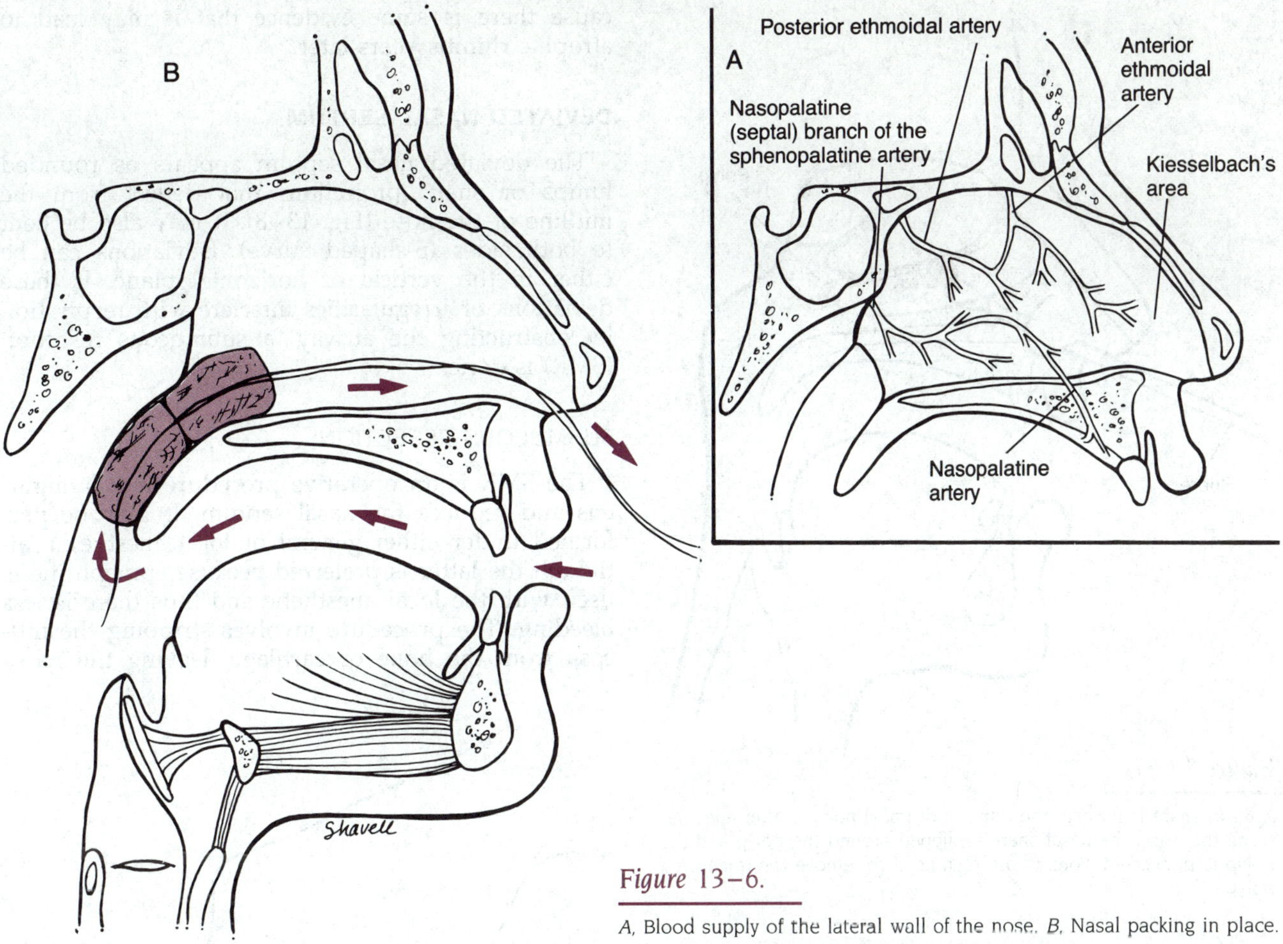

Figure 13–6.

A, Blood supply of the lateral wall of the nose. *B*, Nasal packing in place.

NDx: High risk for altered health maintenance related to insufficient knowledge of cause of bleeding, follow-up care

Planning: Patient outcomes

1. Patient states probable cause of bleeding episode.
2. Patient states the type of follow-up care required and the reason for its need.
3. Patient describes self-care measures that help prevent bleeding caused by blood vessels that are close to the surface and trauma to the nasal mucous membrane.

Nursing Interventions

Loosen clothing around the neck to prevent pressure on the carotid arteries. Assist the patient to a sitting position, with the head tilted slightly forward, and apply pressure to the nares for 10 minutes. If this is not successful in controlling the bleeding, apply an ice collar, administer a local vasoconstrictive drug, or pack the nostrils, depending on the physician's orders.

In case of severe blood loss, administer intravenous fluids and vitamins A and C as ordered.

NDx: Anxiety

Reassure the patient and encourage relaxation. Explain all procedures and measures taken to stop the bleeding. Maintain a quiet, calm environment.

NDx: High risk for altered health maintenance

Explain the cause of bleeding to the patient. If underlying disease is suspected, explain the need for further medical care and make certain the patient knows where and how to obtain it. If the cause of bleeding is simply drying and cracking of the nasal mucosa that has blood vessels close to the surface, suggest the use of a humidifier to keep the membrane moist. Also instruct the patient to avoid hard nose blowing, picking the nose, and other nasal trauma.

Evaluation

Evaluate the effectiveness of nursing care for a patient with epistaxis by comparing the patient's status with the expected patient outcomes. Examples of specific outcomes for patients with epistaxis have been provided in the Planning section.

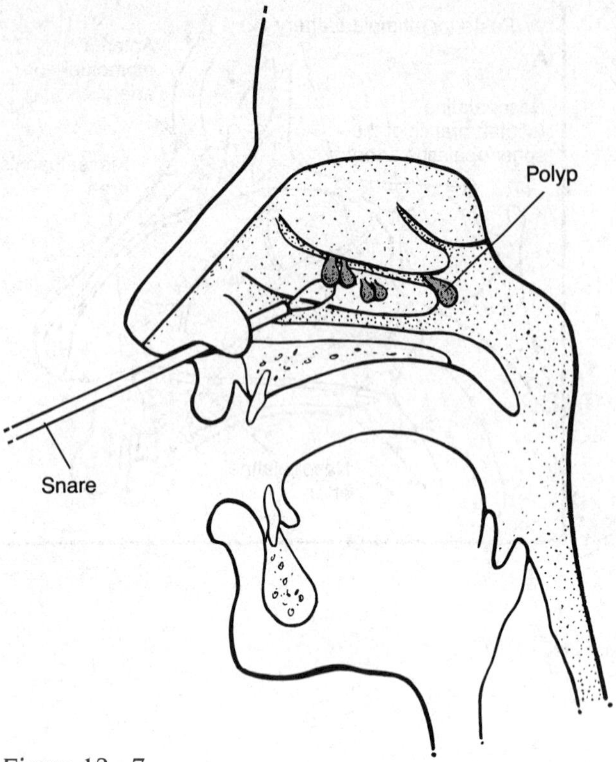

Figure 13–7.

A nasal snare is used in the removal of nasal polyps. After anesthetizing the nose, the nasal snare is slipped around the polyp and the polyp is transected. Forceps are then used to remove the transected polyp.

Nasal Obstruction

NASAL POLYPS

Nasal polyps occur in the nasal or sinus mucosa. They are smooth, pale, benign tumors that are freely movable. Nasal polyps are a frequent complication of allergic rhinitis. The presence of polyps may cause great anxiety for the patient who fears they are malignant. As the polyps develop and mature, symptoms of nasal obstruction occur. Treatment may consist of injection of steroids directly into the polyp or surgical removal called polypectomy (Fig. 13–7). The polypectomy is performed under local anesthesia. Polyps are known to recur if the underlying allergy cannot be controlled.

HYPERTROPHIED TURBINATES

Hypertrophy of the turbinates is a complication related to chronic forms of rhinitis. The enlarged turbinates (three bony projections lined with mucous membrane) interfere with drainage and air passage, thereby contributing to nasal obstruction. Generally, astringent solutions are used to shrink the turbinates back against the side of the nose. A turbinectomy (removal of one of the turbinates) may be performed. However, surgeons are very cautious and selective in recommending this type of surgery because there is some evidence that it may lead to atrophic rhinitis years later.

DEVIATED NASAL SEPTUM

The deviated nasal septum appears as rounded lumps or sharp projections that deflect from the midline of the nose (Fig. 13–8). It may also be bent to both sides (S-shaped curve). Deviations can be either in the vertical or horizontal plane. If these deviations or irregularities interfere with respiration by obstructing the airway, a submucous resection (SMR) is done.

SUBMUCOUS RESECTION

The SMR is an operative procedure that straightens and reduces the nasal septum. It may be performed under either general or local anesthesia, although the latter is preferred because epinephrine is used with the local anesthetic and thus there is less bleeding. The procedure involves stripping the mucosa from the bone or cartilage, leaving the nares

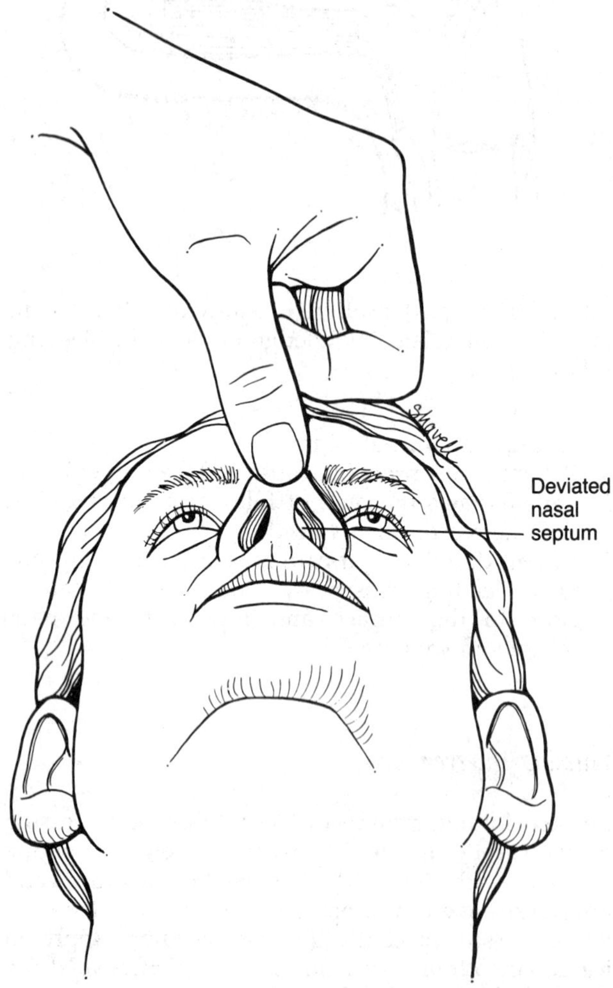

Figure 13–8.

Deviated nasal septum seen protruding into the left naris and obstructing the airway.

Nursing Care Guide 13–1.
PATIENTS HAVING NASAL SURGERY

Preoperative Care

Assessment Findings: Patient asks questions about the surgical experience and aftercare. Patient makes incorrect statements about the surgery and its outcomes.

Nursing Diagnosis: Knowledge deficit: surgical procedure and its effects and perioperative care

Patient Outcomes	Nursing Interventions	Rationale
Patient describes surgery to be done and its expected effects accurately at a level appropriate to his or her background.	Clarify or reinforce surgeon's explanation of the procedure, its purpose, and expected result. If surgery is cosmetic, be sure patient understands that result will not be seen until swelling disappears, which can take several weeks.	Allows identification of concerns and fears, which is essential to provision of information, clarification, and emotional support.
Patient states type of anesthesia to be used and what can be expected in operating room.	If procedure is to be done under local anesthesia, explain this to patient. Describe people, equipment, and routines that will be seen in operating room.	Helps control anxiety for patient. Although some anxiety can be beneficial in preparing the body for the stress of surgery, excessive anxiety is detrimental.

(continued)

separated only by the mucoperichondrium. Both nares are then packed with gauze to discourage bleeding and to hold the remaining mucoperichondrial tissues together in the midline.

Complications after this procedure include tearing of the septum and saddle deformity. The saddle deformity occurs when the bridge of the nose is pulled down by scar formation or falls after the excess cartilaginous or bony support tissue is removed.

RHINOPLASTY

An operative procedure often done along with a repair of a deviated septum is a rhinoplasty. Rhinoplasty is the surgical reconstruction of the nose using local or distal tissues supplemented with alloplasty (use of inert plastic material) as needed. The purpose of this procedure is to cosmetically improve the patient's appearance, but it may also be done to remove an obstruction in the nasal airway resulting from a traumatic or developmental deformity.

Rhinoplasty, usually performed under local anesthesia, is done in a variety of ways, but all involve restructuring the nasal bone and cartilage through an incision made at the end of the nose inside the nostril so that it will not be conspicuous. At the end of the procedure, the nares are packed, the nose secured with tape, and a nose splint applied. This maintains the shape of the nose, limits edema, and provides protection. The splint is left in place for approximately 1 week, at which time more tape may be applied to maintain the shape of the nose. Postoperative swelling and ecchymosis occur around the eyes and the nose.

Complications of this procedure are hemorrhage and infection.

Application of the Nursing Process to the Care of the Patient Having Nasal Surgery

Nursing care of the patient having nasal surgery is presented in Nursing Care Guide 13–1.

Text continued on page 508

Nursing Care Guide 13–1. *(continued)*

PATIENTS HAVING NASAL SURGERY

Patient Outcomes	Nursing Interventions	Rationale
Patient describes typical postoperative events for patients recovering from nasal surgery.	Prepare patient for postoperative routine. Explain the following: ▪ Nasal packing will be in place so breathing by mouth will be necessary. ▪ Nasal pack and back of the throat will be inspected frequently and vital signs monitored. ▪ There is only mild discomfort associated with nasal surgery, but pain medication will be administered as needed. ▪ He or she will be on bed rest, with head elevated for about 6 hours and then will be up and about. ▪ A sucking noise may be heard on swallowing after surgery, but it will disappear when nasal pack is removed. ▪ Oral intake will be resumed in 6–8 hours.	Prepares patient for perioperative events, thus involving patient in plan of care, promoting cooperation, and decreasing risk of anxiety over routine measures.

Evaluation: Compare the patient's status with the expected patient outcomes. If the outcomes are achieved, evaluate nursing care as successful. If not, reassess the patient, formulate new nursing diagnoses, and revise expected patient outcomes and nursing interventions as appropriate.

Assessment Findings: Patient states he or she feels apprehensive; is afraid of the operation; and has a "dry mouth and pounding heart." Patient is unable to sit still and is wringing the hands.

Nursing Diagnosis: Anxiety related to scheduled surgery

Patient Outcomes	Nursing Interventions	Rationale
Patient asks questions about the surgery. Patient attends to information and directions. Verbalization of feelings of overwhelming anxiety is absent.	Encourage patient to verbalize concerns by providing time, private environment, and an opening such as "Tell me how you feel about tomorrow's surgery."	Encourages the patient to share feelings and thus receive support.

(continued)

Nursing Care Guide 13–1. *(continued)*

PATIENTS HAVING NASAL SURGERY

Patient Outcomes	Nursing Interventions	Rationale
Nonverbal signs of excessive anxiety such as pacing and hand wringing are absent.	Acknowledge that anxiety is normal before surgery.	Provides emotional support and reassures patient that feelings are normal.
	Answer questions simply and clearly.	Provides and clarifies information in a manner easily understood by patient.

Evaluation: Compare the patient's status with the expected patient outcomes. If the outcomes are achieved, evaluate nursing care as successful. If not, reassess the patient, formulate new nursing diagnoses, and revise expected patient outcomes and nursing interventions as appropriate.

Postoperative Care

Assessment Findings: Patient has nasal packing and external dressing in place. Patient complains of difficulty breathing by mouth and feels that he or she "can't get enough air."

Nursing Diagnosis: High risk for ineffective breathing pattern related to nasal obstruction secondary to nasal packing, external dressing, and swelling

Patient Outcomes	Nursing Interventions	Rationale
Respirations are of normal rate and depth.	Assist patient into Fowler's position.	Promotes lymphatic and venous drainage, decreases edema, and aids ventilation.
Complaints of dyspnea are absent.	Apply ice to the nasal area.	Decreases edema.
Blood gas values are within normal range.	Remove constricting clothing or bedding to make patient feel it is easier to breathe.	Restrictive clothing and bed covers interfere with chest expansion and increase the sense of difficulty breathing.
	Encourage slow, rhythmic breathing and use of relaxation techniques.	Increases gas exchange and decreases basal metabolic rate, thereby decreasing rate of oxygen utilization.
	Encourage diversions such as soft music or television.	Helps reduce oxygen requirements by reducing stress, thereby slowing heart and respiratory rates.

Evaluation: Compare the patient's status with the expected patient outcomes. If the outcomes are achieved, evaluate nursing care as successful. If not, reassess the patient, formulate new nursing diagnoses, and revise expected patient outcomes and nursing interventions as appropriate.

(continued)

Nursing Care Guide 13–1. *(continued)*

PATIENTS HAVING NASAL SURGERY

Assessment Findings: Patient is breathing by mouth, oral mucous membrane appears dry, and tongue is caked. Patient complains of a "dry, cracky feeling" in the mouth.

Nursing Diagnosis: Altered oral mucous membrane related to dryness secondary to breathing by mouth

Patient Outcomes	Nursing Interventions	Rationale
Oral mucous membranes are moist and smooth. Patient states mouth feels better.	Give frequent, gentle oral hygiene. Irrigate mouth with sterile water, normal saline, or diluted hydrogen peroxide.	Keeps mucous membranes moist, thereby reducing risk of cracking.
	Avoid use of lemon-glycerin swabs or other drying agents.	Dries mucous membranes and increases risk of cracking.
	Lubricate lips with water-soluble lubricant.	Adds to comfort and reduces cracking by maintaining tissue moisture.
	Force fluids.	Prevents dehydration and reduces drying and cracking of oral mucous membranes.

Evaluation: Compare the patient's status with the expected patient outcomes. If the outcomes are achieved, evaluate nursing care as successful. If not, reassess the patient, formulate new nursing diagnoses, and revise expected patient outcomes and nursing interventions as appropriate.

Assessment Findings: Patient has no previous experience with nasal surgery and asks questions about precautions to be taken and self-care in general.

Nursing Diagnosis: High risk for altered health maintenance related to insufficient knowledge of precautions to prevent new nasal bleeding, normal and abnormal signs and symptoms.

Patient Outcomes	Nursing Interventions	Rationale
Patient lists precautions to be taken to prevent new nasal bleeding.	To prevent initiating new bleeding from the nose, instruct patient in the following:	Provides information necessary for self-management after discharge.
	Avoid touching the nose with hands, tissues, or any other objects.	

(continued)

Nursing Care Guide 13–1. *(continued)*

PATIENTS HAVING NASAL SURGERY

Patient Outcomes	Nursing Interventions	Rationale
	Avoid increasing pressure in the nose by doing the following: ■ Using an extra pillow when lying down to keep the head elevated. ■ Not bending over. ■ Not blowing the nose, and, if sneezing cannot be avoided, keeping the mouth open during the sneeze. ■ Not straining during bowel movement ■ Avoiding heavy lifting Avoid external pressure on the nose from eyeglasses. Avoid alcohol, aspirin, and cigarettes.	
Patient states that edema and discoloration are normal and will disappear with time and that final result of cosmetic surgery may not be judged for several weeks.	Reinforce that edema and discoloration are normal and will disappear with time and that the final cosmetic result of surgery cannot be judged for several weeks.	Helps control anxiety by increasing awareness of expected events during course of recovery.
Patient states tarry stools may occur as a result of swallowed blood.	Explain that stools may appear tarry because of swallowed blood.	Helps prevent unnecessary anxiety over normal aspects of recovery course.
Patient lists symptoms to be reported to the surgeon.	Instruct patient to call the surgeon immediately if bleeding from nose or throat, vomiting, or a temperature of greater than 101°F (38.3°C) occurs.	Provides information necessary to recognize postoperative complications as well as appropriate patient responses

Evaluation: Compare the patient's status with the expected patient outcomes. If the outcomes are achieved, evaluate nursing care as successful. If not, reassess the patient, formulate new nursing diagnoses, and revise expected patient outcomes and nursing interventions as appropriate.

Additional Assessments and Interventions:

Inspect the nasal packing and use a flashlight to observe the back of the throat for bleeding.

Inspect and change the gauze pad (mustache dressing) beneath the nares as needed. Note the amount and color of drainage (amount should gradually decrease and the drainage turn from red to brown-tinged).

Trauma

Nasal Fracture

ETIOLOGY AND PATHOPHYSIOLOGY

Fractures are secondary to a blow of some kind to the nasal area. Fractures of the nasal bones or septum may be more common than generally supposed because if there is no displacement of the nose or nasal obstruction the person frequently does not seek medical attention.

CLINICAL MANIFESTATIONS

Nasal fractures can result in nasal pain, edema of the soft tissues, nasal obstruction, and epistaxis. In some cases, bleeding may be copious both from the nostrils and back into the pharynx. In extensive fractures, cerebrospinal fluid, a thin, colorless liquid, may drain from the nares.

MEDICAL DIAGNOSIS

Medical diagnosis is based on the history of trauma and the physical findings. Skull x-ray films are taken to rule out skull fractures and to identify and locate any bone fragments.

MEDICAL MANAGEMENT

If the patient seeks medical care before the edema occurs, the fracture may be set at that time. Nasal fractures that are simple lateral displacements may be reduced by firm pressure on the convex side of the nose (Fig. 13–9). If the nasal fracture requires repair of the bony structure and septum, general anesthesia is used. The fracture cannot be reduced until after the swelling has subsided (usually 2 or 3 days). After reduction, splinting may be used to stabilize the reduction until healing occurs.

If a nasal fracture causing misalignment is not set, deformity, obstruction, chronic rhinitis, or chronic sinusitis can occur.

Guidelines for Application of the Nursing Process to the Care of the Patient with a Nasal Fracture

Nursing care of the patient with a nasal fracture is aimed at preventing complications and providing relief of discomfort. Use alternate hot and cold soaks to relieve pain and swelling. If rhinorrhea (thin, watery discharge from the nose) occurs, instruct the patient not to blow the nose to prevent possible neurologic complications.

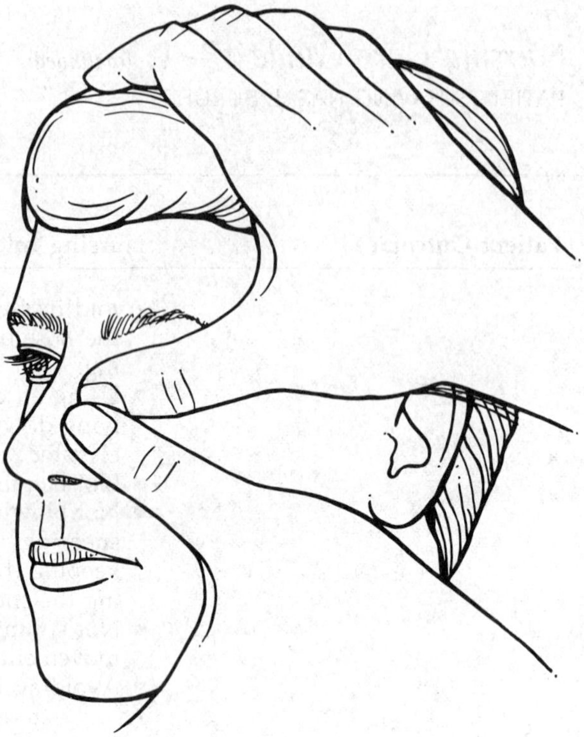

Figure 13–9.

Pressure being applied to the convex side of the nose to reduce a simple nasal fracture.

If surgical reduction is necessary, prepare the patient for surgery as described in Chapter 4. Postoperatively, elevate the head of the bed and apply ice compresses to minimize swelling.

Laryngeal Trauma

ETIOLOGY AND PATHOPHYSIOLOGY

The most common cause of laryngeal trauma is when the neck strikes the steering wheel during an automobile accident. Other causes are iatrogenic and include endoscopy and endotracheal intubation.

Severe laryngeal trauma can cause death from respiratory obstruction unless a tracheostomy is performed immediately. Fracture of the thyroid cartilage can cause the mucosa and other soft tissue inside the larynx to be torn or a hematoma to form.

CLINICAL MANIFESTATIONS

The patient with laryngeal trauma has a tender, swollen, ecchymotic neck. Stridor may also be present because of swelling of the airway tissues. Hoarseness, dysphagia, cyanosis, and hemoptysis may also occur.

MEDICAL MANAGEMENT

An emergency tracheostomy is done, if necessary, to maintain a patent airway, followed by surgical restoration of the larynx and trachea.

Guidelines for Application of the Nursing Process to the Care of the Patient with Laryngeal Trauma

Symptoms of laryngeal injury may not be immediately present after neck trauma; therefore, ongoing, frequent assessment is necessary. Keep instruments for a tracheostomy immediately available because edema or hematoma can develop rapidly. (See Chapter 12, Application of the Nursing Process to the Care of the Patient Undergoing Tracheostomy.)

Neoplasia

Cancer of the Larynx

ETIOLOGY

Cancer of the larynx is the most common upper respiratory tract malignancy. It occurs 5 times more often in men than in women. Heavy cigarette smoking and ingestion of alcohol are believed to be major factors in the development of this type of cancer. Recent statistics indicate that the incidence of laryngeal cancer is rising in the female population.

PATHOPHYSIOLOGY

Cancer of the larynx is classified according to the site of the growth. Intrinsic tumors develop inside the larynx. They generally arise from the true vocal cords and grow slowly. Extrinsic tumors develop outside the larynx on the epiglottis or the piriform fossa. Their growth is more rapid, and there is usually early lymphatic involvement. These tumors are more difficult to treat.

CLINICAL MANIFESTATIONS

The symptoms of intrinsic and extrinsic tumors are clearly different. Hoarseness occurs with tumors of the true cords (intrinsic) because accurate approximation of the cords during phonation is not possible when a space-occupying tumor is present. Hoarseness is the only symptom initially. As the growth spreads to the opposite cord, there is pain and cough. Unchecked, the tumor growth continues and becomes extrinsic.

The symptoms of extrinsic tumors do not occur until late in the disease. Initially, the patient may complain of feeling "something in the throat" or pain or burning of the throat when drinking hot liquids or orange juice. In some cases, an enlarged lymph node in the neck may be the first indication of disease. Late symptoms include dysphagia (difficulty swallowing), dyspnea, hoarseness, weight loss, foul breath, and general disability.

MEDICAL DIAGNOSIS

Tumors on and above the true vocal cords can be visualized by direct laryngoscopy, and tumors below the glottis can be visualized by indirect laryngoscopy. Diagnosis of malignancy is confirmed by biopsy, and specialized radiologic procedures are done to determine the extent of the disease.

MEDICAL MANAGEMENT

Medical management is linked to the classification of the tumor. Early intrinsic cancer of the larynx can be treated successfully by either surgery or irradiation therapy. With more advanced tumors, surgery is the more effective treatment.

LARYNGECTOMY

There are three basic surgical procedures used to treat cancer of the larynx: partial laryngectomy, conservation laryngectomy, which is often accompanied by a radical neck dissection (Nursing Care Guide 13–2), and total laryngectomy.

Partial Laryngectomy

A partial laryngectomy is used to treat early cancers of the true vocal cords or the anterior larynx. In this procedure, the malignant lesion is excised along with a surrounding lip of normal tissue. At surgery, a tracheostomy is also done to protect the patient from postoperative airway obstruction caused by edema or hemorrhage. Once this danger has passed, however, the tracheostomy tube is removed, usually in 2 or 3 days. After this, the patient is allowed to begin to whisper and then gradually to resume full use of the voice. Thus, after a partial laryngectomy, the patient has a normal airway and also retains the ability to speak.

Complications of this procedure include aspiration, bleeding, and subcutaneous emphysema.

Conservation Laryngectomy

A conservation laryngectomy is used to treat selected extrinsic lesions located on the epiglottis or other nearby structures above the true vocal cords.

Text continued on page 518

Nursing Care Guide 13–2.

PATIENTS UNDERGOING CONSERVATION (SUPRAGLOTTIC) LARYNGECTOMY AND RADICAL NECK DISSECTION

Preoperative Care

Assessment Findings: Patient verbalizes fear of surgery, worry about the diagnosis of cancer, and apprehension about being able to breathe, eat, and speak postoperatively. Patient complains of dry mouth, trembling hands, and "heart palpitations." Patient is restless and unable to concentrate.

Nursing Diagnosis: Anxiety related to the diagnosis of cancer, the surgical experience, the effects of surgery on eating, breathing, speaking, appearance, work, and social activities

Patient Outcomes	Nursing Interventions	Rationale
Patient expresses concerns and fears. Patient attends to information given about the surgery and postoperative care. Patient asks questions about the surgery and its effects. Verbalization of feelings of overwhelming anxiety is absent. Nonverbal signs of excessive anxiety such as constant pacing, hand wringing, and trembling are absent.	Provide opportunity and environment conducive to expression of concerns and fears.	Encourages patient to share feelings and thus receive support.
	Acknowledge that anxiety before this surgery is normal.	Encourages patient to share feelings and thus receive support by allaying fears of being perceived negatively because of anxiety.
	Explain postoperative course and routines (i.e., recovery room, suctioning, humidification, coughing and deep breathing, intravenous [IV] fluids, tube feedings, and drains).	Prepares patient for postoperative events, thus promoting cooperation and decreasing the risk of anxiety over routine measures.
	Carefully describe how breathing will occur after surgery.	Helps control anxiety by providing patient with reassurance that breathing, which is essential to life, will be maintained despite the anatomic changes resulting from surgery.
	Discuss alternate modes of communication and, with patient, select the mode that will be used.	Reassures patient that communication of needs will be possible and allows selection of a means acceptable and suitable to the patient, thus increasing probability of its successful use.
	Reassure patient that assistance will be available at all times.	Reassures patient that he or she will not be alone, thus allaying anxiety and providing emotional support.
	Answer all questions clearly and simply.	Provides and clarifies information in a manner easily understood by patient.
	Discuss patient's concerns about body image and also hopes for the future.	Verbalization provides perspective as well as the opportunity for clarification.

(continued)

Nursing Care Guide 13–2. *(continued)*

PATIENTS UNDERGOING CONSERVATION (SUPRAGLOTTIC) LARYNGECTOMY AND RADICAL NECK DISSECTION

Evaluation: Compare the patient's status with the expected patient outcomes. If the outcomes are achieved, evaluate nursing care as successful. If not, reassess the patient, formulate new nursing diagnoses, and revise expected patient outcomes and nursing interventions as appropriate.

Assessment Findings: Patient verbalizes fear of not being able to cope with the tracheostomy, temporary voice loss, difficulty swallowing, and changes in physical appearance that will result from surgery.

Nursing Diagnosis: High risk for ineffective individual coping related to loss of normal breathing and swallowing patterns, inability to speak, and change in physical appearance

Patient Outcomes	Nursing Interventions	Rationale
Patient identifies sources of support that will be available postoperatively.	Assist patient in identifying available sources of support.	Provides objective evidence that assistance is available and thus helps build the patient's confidence in ability to deal successfully with the surgery and its outcomes.
Patient identifies effective coping patterns.	Explore with patient ways of coping that were effective in the past.	Because different people cope best in different ways, identification of coping methods encourages use of strategies proven effective for this individual
Patient expresses confidence in ability to cooperate and participate in postoperative care.	Work with patient to develop a plan for coping with current stress.	Provides patient with sense of control and promotes development of acceptable plan with which patient will cooperate, thus increasing its probability for success.
Patient expresses hope about the future.	Reassure patient that nursing staff and other health care personnel will work with him or her toward recovery.	Provides patient with positive facts on which to focus and base hope for a successful surgical outcome.
	Arrange for meeting with a successfully rehabilitated laryngectomee.	Provides the patient with a positive role model at a time most likely to be acceptable to the patient.

Evaluation: Compare the patient's status with the expected patient outcomes. If the outcomes are achieved, evaluate nursing care as successful. If not, reassess the patient, formulate new nursing diagnoses, and revise expected patient outcomes and nursing interventions as appropriate.

(continued)

Nursing Care Guide 13–2. *(continued)*

PATIENTS UNDERGOING CONSERVATION (SUPRAGLOTTIC) LARYNGECTOMY AND RADICAL NECK DISSECTION

Postoperative Care

Assessment Findings: Patient has difficulty coughing and expectorating secretions. Secretions are heard during respiration and can occasionally be seen bubbling at tracheostomy stoma.

Nursing Diagnosis: Ineffective airway clearance related to increased secretions, impaired cough, and loss of humidification of air by upper airway

Patient Outcomes	Nursing Interventions	Rationale
Airway is cleared of secretions by coughing or suctioning as they accumulate. Respirations are easy and quiet. Respiratory rate is within normal range. Complaints of dyspnea are absent. Lungs are clear on auscultation.	Maintain patient in mid-Fowler's position.	Decreases edema in neck and promotes ventilation because gravity pulls abdominal contents away from diaphragm, thus allowing greater chest expansion.
	Encourage patient to turn, cough, and deep breathe every hour.	Promotes expansion of airway and removal of secretions to allow for maximum gas exchange.
	Splint patient's neck by placing hands behind it when turning and coughing.	Decreases pull on incision line.
	Have patient lean forward when coughing.	Promotes raising and expectoration of airway secretions.
	Suction the tracheostomy as occasion requires (PRN) to prevent obstruction of airflow.	Artificial means of secretion removal may be necessary to maintain a clear airway.
	Insert a few drops of saline into the stoma before suctioning if secretions are viscous and difficult to remove.	Thins secretions and thus aids their removal.
	Administer humidified air or oxygen as ordered.	Moisture liquefies secretions, thus facilitating airway clearance.

Evaluation: Compare the patient's status with the expected patient outcomes. If the outcomes are achieved, evaluate nursing care as successful. If not, reassess the patient, formulate new nursing diagnoses, and revise expected patient outcomes and nursing interventions as appropriate.

(continued)

Nursing Care Guide 13–2. *(continued)*

PATIENTS UNDERGOING CONSERVATION (SUPRAGLOTTIC) LARYNGECTOMY AND RADICAL NECK DISSECTION

Assessment Findings: Patient complains of neck, chest, and shoulder pain. Patient grimaces on moving.

Nursing Diagnosis: Pain: neck, shoulder, and chest related to surgical trauma

Patient Outcomes	Nursing Interventions	Rationale
Patient states pain is relieved. Patient moves and turns easily without groans, grimaces, or other nonverbal indications of pain.	Administer analgesics as ordered, remembering that narcotics are to be avoided because they depress respiration.	Provides pain relief by action specific to drug ordered.
	Keep the head of the bed elevated.	Decreases edema, thereby reducing pressure on surrounding tissues.
	Splint patient's neck when turning or moving.	Decreases pull on incision line.
	Maintain a quiet, restful environment.	Promotes relaxation, rest, and action of analgesic and sedative medications.
	Encourage use of relaxation techniques.	Reduces tension level of body, thereby decreasing strain on body tissues.
	Provide diversion such as soft music.	Promotes relaxation, rest, and action of analgesic and sedative medications.

Evaluation: Compare the patient's status with the expected patient outcomes. If the outcomes are achieved, evaluate nursing care as successful. If not, reassess the patient, formulate new nursing diagnoses, and revise expected patient outcomes and nursing interventions as appropriate.

(continued)

Nursing Care Guide 13–2. *(continued)*

PATIENTS UNDERGOING CONSERVATION (SUPRAGLOTTIC) LARYNGECTOMY AND RADICAL NECK DISSECTION

Assessment Findings: Patient unable to speak because of temporary tracheostomy (about 1 week).

Nursing Diagnosis: Impaired verbal communication related to temporary inability to speak secondary to diversion of air passing in and out of lungs through a tracheostomy

Patient Outcomes	Nursing Interventions	Rationale
Patient uses alternative modes of communication such as a Magic Slate, flash cards, mouthing of words for others to lip-read, and gesture.	Keep call bell within easy reach of patient at all times.	Provides a nonverbal means of communication with individuals not in sight.
Patient successfully communicates wants, needs, and essential information.	Visit patient frequently and assure him or her that help is close by to meet needs.	Reduces sense of isolation.
	Provide equipment for alternate mode of communication such as Magic Slate, pencil and paper, flash cards.	Allows a means of communication.
	Ask questions that require only a short answer or yes or no signal. Do not ask patient to signal with nod or shake or the head because this is painful. Instruct in eye blink, hand, or finger signals instead.	Decreases patient frustration by reducing need for lengthy responses while maintaining communication.
	Allow time for patient to communicate. Do not complete patient's thoughts, and do not "put words in the patient's mouth."	Allows patient to accurately communicate needs and feelings and to feel comfortable in attempts to communicate.
	Post a sign on the door and on the intercom at nurses' station to remind personnel that patient is unable to speak.	Decreases patient frustration and reassures patient that health care workers are aware of his or her needs.
	Try to anticipate needs.	Decreases patient frustration with impaired communication.
	Inform other health care personnel and significant others of the communication systems being used by patient.	Maximizes effective communication through consistent use of one system, decreases patient frustration, and reminds patient that health care workers are aware of his or her needs.

Evaluation: Compare the patient's status with the expected patient outcomes. If the outcomes are achieved, evaluate nursing care as successful. If not, reassess the patient, formulate new nursing diagnoses, and revise expected patient outcomes and nursing interventions as appropriate.

(continued)

Nursing Care Guide 13–2. *(continued)*

PATIENTS UNDERGOING CONSERVATION (SUPRAGLOTTIC) LARYNGECTOMY AND RADICAL NECK DISSECTION

Assessment Findings: Patient is observed having difficulty swallowing. Attempts to swallow are accompanied by coughing and choking.

Nursing Diagnosis: Impaired swallowing related to surgical trauma and removal of the epiglottis and false vocal cords

Patient Outcomes	Nursing Interventions	Rationale
Patient allows saliva to drain from mouth in early postoperative period.	Instruct patient to expectorate or allow saliva to drain out of mouth, not swallow it.	Prevents coughing, choking, and further injury to traumatized tissues.
	Keep patient's head turned to the side.	Promotes drainage of saliva out side of mouth.
	Provide basin and wipes for oral secretions.	Promotes cleanliness and comfort despite need to allow saliva to drain out of side of mouth.
	When patient is resting, place a wick with one end in corner of patient's mouth and the other in emesis basin.	Removes oral secretions and maintains cleanliness and comfort without active participation of patient.
Patient practices swallowing food as directed when tube feedings are discontinued. Patient swallows soft foods and viscous fluids.	When tube feedings are discontinued and oral intake is begun (about 2 weeks postoperatively), start patient on soft, formed foods such as ice cream, custard, Jell-O, and mashed potatoes. Instruct patient to ingest them as follows: ■ Hold the breath. ■ Keep head flexed (chin on chest) and tilted to unaffected side. ■ Place small amount of soft food on back of tongue. ■ Swallow. ■ Cough to expel any foodstuff that may have entered trachea.	Reduces risk of aspiration and facilitates patient in relearning how to swallow foods and fluids.
	Provide privacy for eating to decrease embarrassment and stress.	Fear of others' reactions may decrease nutritional intake.
Patient eats a nutritionally balanced daily diet.	As patient relearns to swallow, add viscous fluids and other soft foods to the diet. Progress to other foods and fluids as tolerated.	Increases variety of food ingested to provide more appetizing and nutritionally balanced diet.

Evaluation: Compare the patient's status with the expected patient outcomes. If the outcomes are achieved, evaluate nursing care as successful. If not, reassess the patient, formulate new nursing diagnoses, and revise expected patient outcomes and nursing interventions as appropriate.

(continued)

Nursing Care Guide 13–2. *(continued)*

PATIENTS UNDERGOING CONSERVATION (SUPRAGLOTTIC) LARYNGECTOMY AND RADICAL NECK DISSECTION

Assessment Findings: Patient has large, disfiguring wound in neck, a shoulder that droops and is painful, and difficulty swallowing food and fluids.

Nursing Diagnosis: High risk for body image disturbance related to changes in body appearance and alteration in body function

Patient Outcomes	Nursing Interventions	Rationale
Patient looks at wound. Patient communicates feelings about body changes. Patient participates in self-care. Patient interacts with others using available means of communication. Patient demonstrates an active interest in personal appearance. Patient maintains relationship with significant others.	Be sensitive to patient's need for acceptance.	Body image is closely tied to self-concept.
	Take care not to indicate shock or distaste in regard to patient's condition by expression or comment.	Body image is derived in part from responses and opinions of others.
	Do not force patient to look at the wound; wait until he or she is ready.	Allows time for acceptance of body-image changes.
	Explain that redness or swelling will decrease with time and then physical changes will not be as severe.	Provides realistic, positive expectations and promotes acceptance of appearance.
	Answer questions about changes in body and appearance honestly.	Promotes trust and provides realistic, positive expectations.
	Involve patient in self-care.	Promotes sense of control, self-confidence, and self-esteem.
	Encourage attention to personal hygiene.	Promotes self-esteem.
	Encourage interaction with family and friends.	Prevents isolation, demonstrates that social interaction and acceptance are still possible, and provides source of emotional support.

Evaluation: Compare the patient's status with the expected patient outcomes. If the outcomes are achieved, evaluate nursing care as successful. If not, reassess the patient, formulate new nursing diagnoses, and revise expected patient outcomes and nursing interventions as appropriate.

(continued)

Nursing Care Guide 13–2. *(continued)*

PATIENTS UNDERGOING CONSERVATION (SUPRAGLOTTIC) LARYNGECTOMY AND RADICAL NECK DISSECTION

Assessment Findings: Patient asks questions about activities, limitations, and precautions to be taken after discharge.

Nursing Diagnosis: High risk for altered health maintenance related to insufficient knowledge of self-care after discharge

Patient Outcomes	Nursing Interventions	Rationale
Patient describes pain in shoulder over a period of months as expected and identifies measures to provide relief.	Explain the following to patient: ■ Pain in shoulder, neck, and chest is expected to persist for months. Use heat, massage, and liniment for relief.	Provides information about normal sequence of recovery and appropriate patient responses.
Patient describes need for precautions because of sensory loss in large area of chest, back, and shoulders.	■ Precautions must be taken to guard against accidental injury because a large area of the shoulder, chest, and back will be numb.	Provides information necessary for self-management after discharge.
Patient describes and demonstrates neck, shoulder, and arm exercises to be done after radical neck dissection.	Teach patient neck, shoulder, and arm exercises.	Increases range of motion in affected side.
Patient explains importance of avoiding exposure to smoke and, if a smoker, identifies plan of action designed to stop smoking.	Reinforce importance of not smoking.	Smoking decreases gas exchange by altering lung structure and function.
Patient lists symptoms to be reported to physician.	Instruct patient to report signs of aspiration pneumonia to physician: dyspnea; cough; wheezing; pink, frothy sputum; and fever.	Provides information necessary to recognize postoperative complications after discharge.

Evaluation: Compare the patient's status with the expected patient outcomes. If the outcomes are achieved, evaluate nursing care as successful. If not, reassess the patient, formulate new nursing diagnoses, and revise expected patient outcomes and nursing interventions as appropriate.

Additional Assessments and Interventions:

Monitor vital signs every 15 minutes until stable, every 1 to 2 hours for the first 24 hours, and then every 4 hours.

Monitor breath sounds.

Check for pooling of blood behind the neck.

Assess for lower facial paralysis, which can occur because of injury of the facial nerve.

Monitor wound drainage, noting amount, color, and odor. Drainage is normally serosanguineous, with up to 120 ml expected in the first 24 hours and gradually decreasing amounts thereafter.

Check function of portable wound suction system and empty as needed.

Assess wound for swelling, which could indicate inadequate drainage and hematoma formation.

Monitor for signs of infection: redness, swelling, purulent drainage from the wound, and fever.

Administer intravenous fluids and tube feedings as ordered.

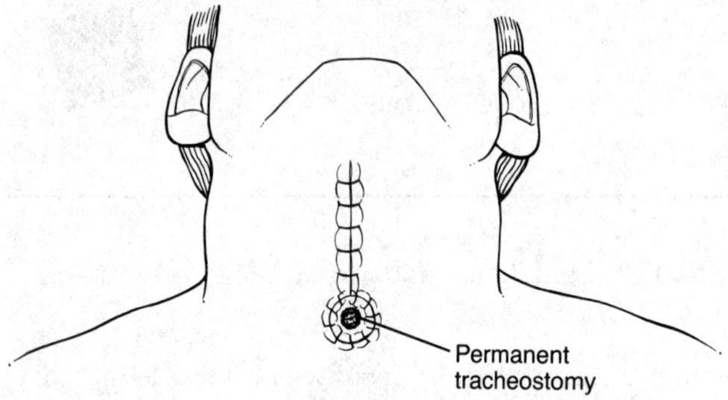

Figure 13–10.

Appearance of wound after total laryngectomy.

The diseased portion of the larynx is removed, and a temporary tracheotomy is performed to protect against postoperative airway obstruction. As with a partial laryngectomy, the patient has a normal airway and normal speech after healing.

A major postoperative risk associated with this procedure is aspiration, because the epiglottis or other protective structures have been removed. The patient has to relearn to swallow, and intravenous therapy or nasogastric tube feedings are not unusual for the first 2 or 3 weeks postoperatively.

There is also a risk of bleeding, carotid rupture, or development of a fistula between the pharyngeal suture line and the skin. These latter problems are most likely to occur if a radical neck dissection has been done along with the laryngectomy and if the

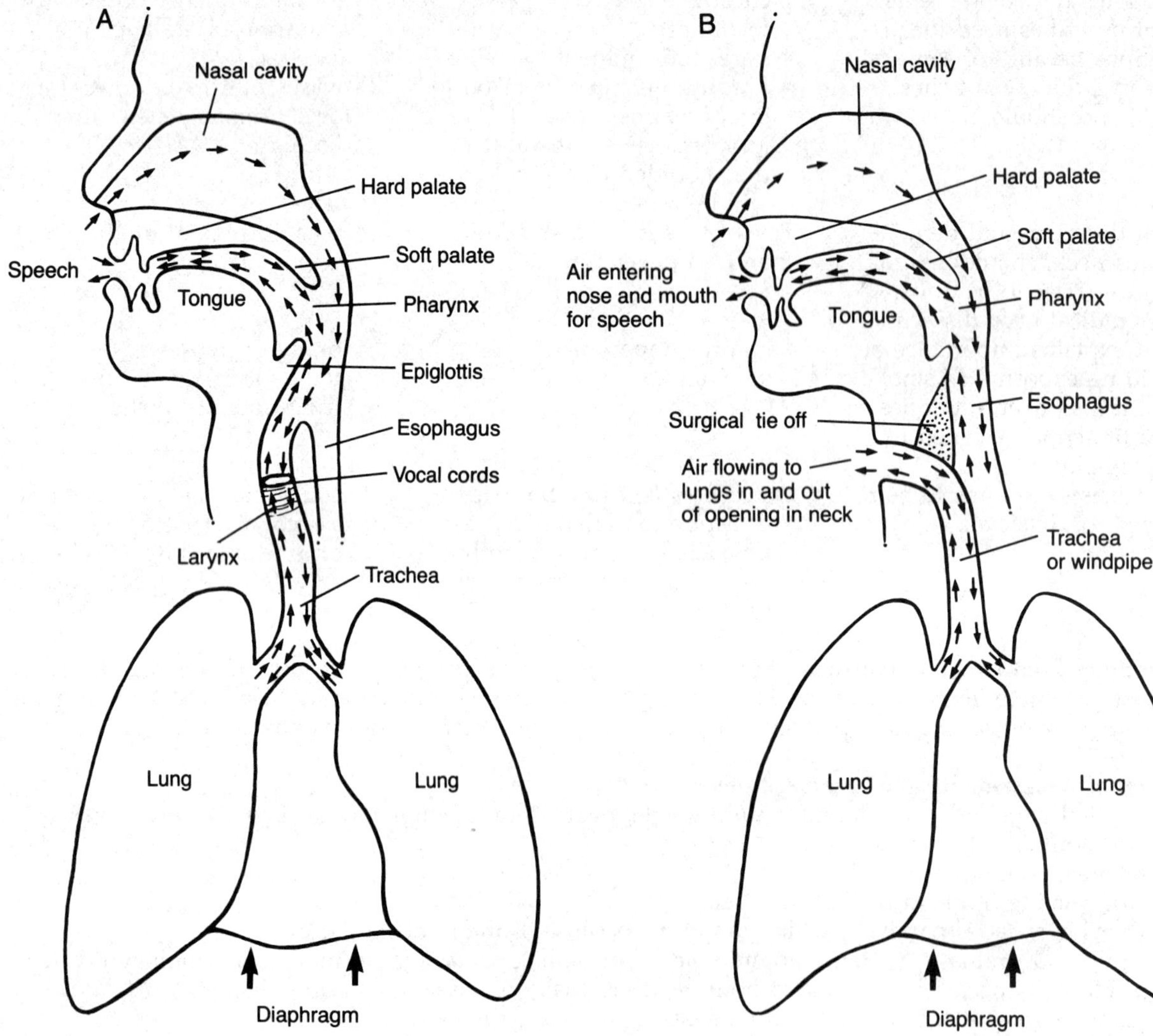

Figure 13–11.

Pattern of air flow for respiration and for speech before and after total laryngectomy. *A*, Before the laryngectomy, air passes in and out of the lungs through the nose and mouth, and speech is created as exhaled air passes through the larynx. *B*, After total laryngectomy, air passes in and out of the lungs through a permanent tracheostomy. Air taken in through the nose or mouth passes through the pharynx and enters the esophagus and may be expelled as a belch to create "esophageal speech."

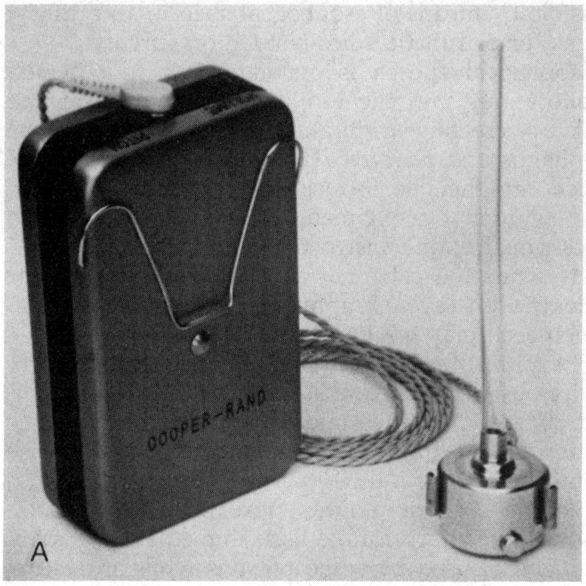

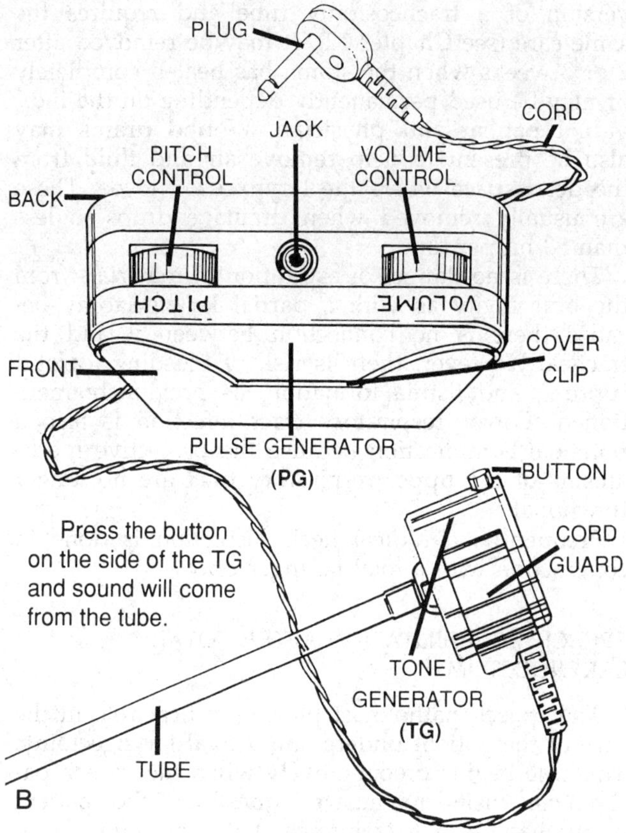

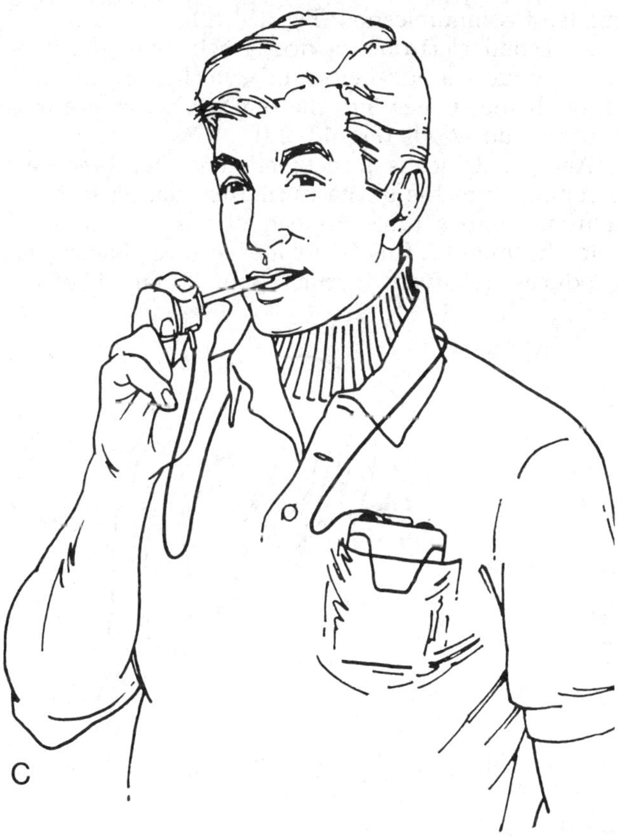

Figure 13–12.

A, Cooper-Rand Electronic Speech Aid. This device provides the vocal tone necessary for speech. Immediate speech is possible for most laryngectomees with this device. *B,* Diagram of Cooper-Rand Electronic Speech Aid, with parts labeled. *C,* Cooper-Rand Electronic Speech Aid in use. Approximately 1 to 2 inches of the plastic tube is inserted into the corner of the mouth. The tip should be above the tongue and pointed toward the roof of the mouth to keep the end from being closed by the tongue. The button on the tone generator is pressed and the patient speaks. Patients are instructed to speak slowly and distinctly, using the tongue and lips to form sounds just as before the loss of the larynx. (Courtesy of Luminaud, Inc., Mentor, OH.)

patient has had previous irradiation therapy to the area.

Total Laryngectomy

A total laryngectomy is done for far-advanced lesions. In this procedure, the entire larynx, the hyoid bone, pre-epiglottic space, strap muscles, and one or more of the tracheal rings are removed. The trachea's pharyngeal opening is closed, and the distal portion of the trachea is formed into a permanent tracheostomy (Fig. 13–10). After this procedure, there is loss of normal speech, loss of normal respiration through the nose and mouth, and olfactory changes secondary to the fact that air is no longer inhaled and exhaled through the nose and mouth (Fig. 13–11). Postoperatively, most patients have a laryngectomy tube in place. This is a wider, shorter version of a tracheostomy tube and requires the same care (see Chapter 12). It may be removed after 2 or 3 weeks when the stoma has healed completely or may be used permanently depending on the individual patient and physician. Wound drains may also be present to help remove air and fluid from the dead space where the larynx used to be. These are usually removed when drainage drops to less than 50 ml per day.

There is no danger of aspiration of materials from the oral cavity as with a partial laryngectomy because there is no connection between it and the trachea. However, there is risk of bleeding, carotid rupture, and fistula formation, as previously mentioned. Lower respiratory tract infection is also a potential complication because the protective mechanisms of the upper respiratory tract are no longer functional.

Frequently, a radical neck dissection is done in conjunction with a total laryngectomy.

SPEECH REHABILITATION AFTER TOTAL LARYNGECTOMY

The speech pathologist plays a critical role in the care of the patient undergoing a total laryngectomy. This role begins preoperatively when the speech pathologist visits to answer questions the patient might have and to reinforce that oral communication is possible after the surgery.

Oral communication after total laryngectomy is possible by means of esophageal speech, an artificial larynx, or prosthetic voice-restoration surgery.

Esophageal speech is generated when a person swallows air into the esophagus and "belches" it back up, creating a vibration at the junction of the esophagus and pharynx. This results in a deep tone, which can then be formed into easily understandable words. Development of esophageal speech takes practice, and instruction may begin preoperatively when the patient is able to ask questions. For patients with severe emphysema or asthma, esophageal speech may not be possible.

The phrase *artificial larynx* describes a variety of devices used to generate sound, which can be modified by oral structures into speech. One such device sends an electronically generated tone into the mouth by way of a tube that the patient inserts into the corner of the mouth approximately 2 inches. This device, which can be used immediately postoperatively, is used by some persons while mastering esophageal speech and by others as the continuing mode of communication (Fig. 13–12).

A second electronic device is held over the neck and produces a buzzing sound, which is transmitted through the tissues into the oral cavity, where it is formed into words (Fig. 13–13).

Another device is a pneumatic one that directs air escaping from the stoma during exhalation through a funnel into a tube, the end of which is inserted into the mouth. This is an inexpensive device that produces relatively normal sound but, like the

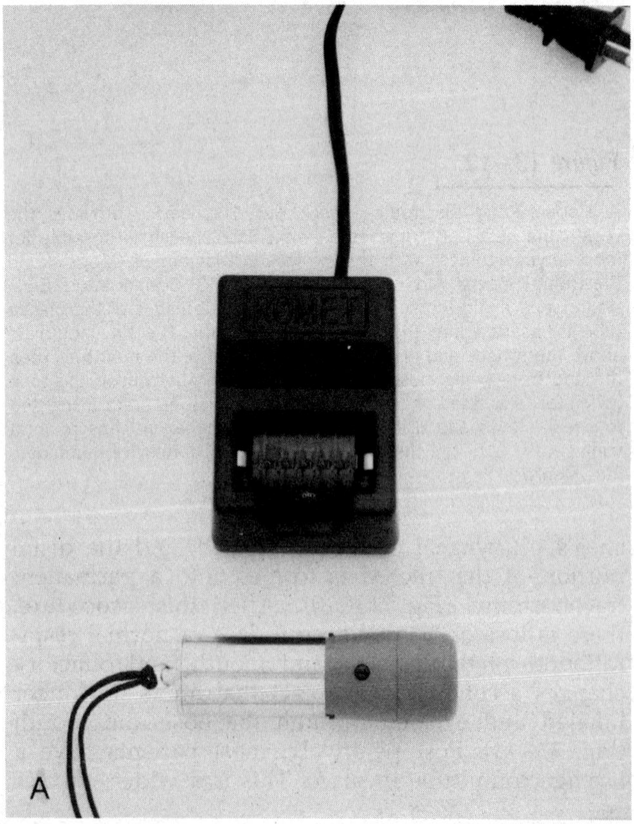

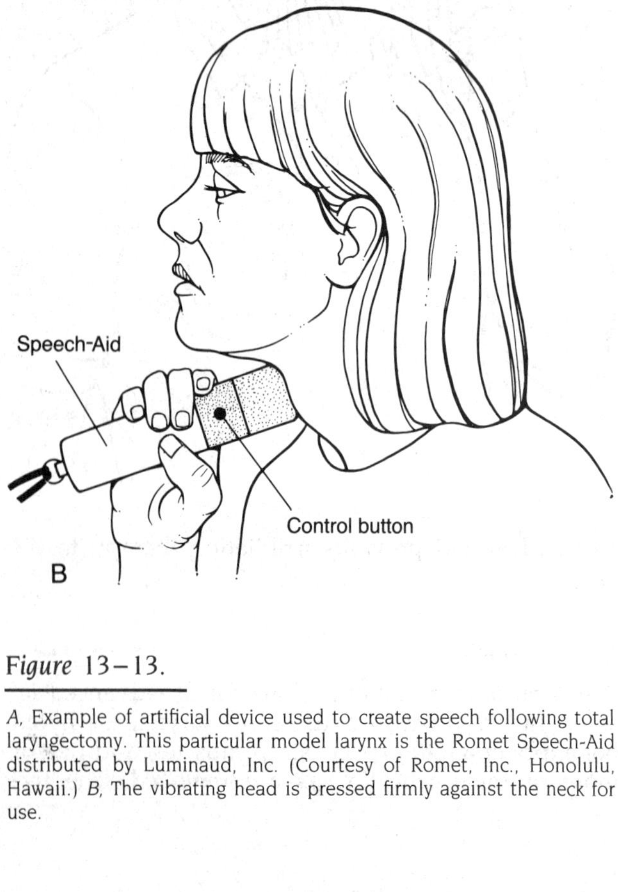

Figure 13–13.

A, Example of artificial device used to create speech following total laryngectomy. This particular model larynx is the Romet Speech-Aid distributed by Luminaud, Inc. (Courtesy of Romet, Inc., Honolulu, Hawaii.) *B*, The vibrating head is pressed firmly against the neck for use.

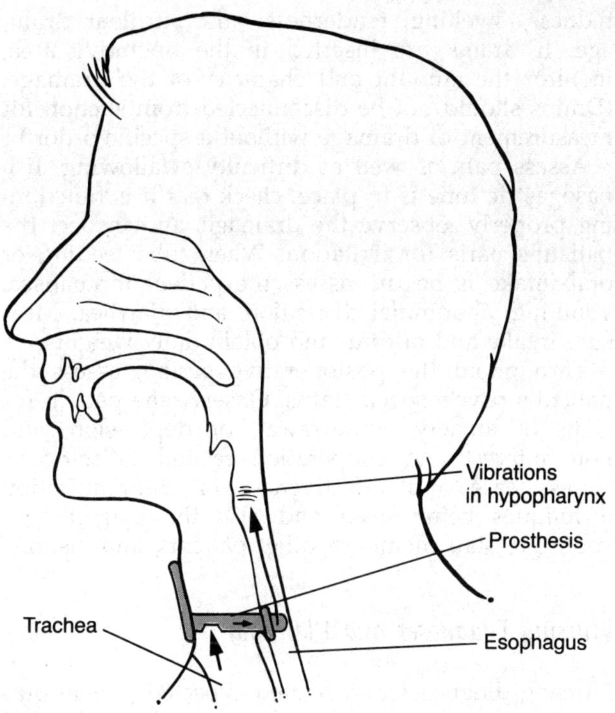

Figure 13–14.

Tracheoesophageal opening with prosthesis in place. Exhaled air from the lungs moves through the trachea, prosthesis, and esophagus to create vibrations in the hypopharynx that allow production of sound.

previous instrument, has the disadvantage of being obvious and requiring one hand to hold it.

Surgical procedures designed to allow speech production include creation of an opening between the esophagus and the trachea with insertion of a one-way valve prosthesis to prevent aspiration. This allows air exhaled from the lungs to pass from the trachea through the prosthesis into the esophagus. This air causes vibrations in the hypopharynx, which allow sound to be produced (Fig. 13–14). Laryngeal reconstruction using arm or leg tendons or rib cartilage has also been attempted.

Application of the Nursing Process to the Care of the Patient Having a Laryngectomy

PREOPERATIVE NURSING CARE

Assessment

The basic assessment required by any preoperative patient (see Chapter 4), as well as that required by any patient diagnosed with cancer (see Chapter 11), applies also to the patient scheduled for a laryngectomy for cancer of the larynx. In addition, be certain to assess the patient's and significant other's understanding of, and emotional response to, the effects of surgery on breathing, swallowing, speech, and appearance.

Because speech will be impossible for some interval after surgery, assess the patient to determine which alternative forms of communication (e.g., pad and pencil, flash cards, or gestures) appear to be most suited to the patient's capabilities and temperament. For example, a Magic Slate would not be appropriate for a patient unable to write in English or one with tremors or paresis of the dominant hand that interferes with motor function.

If the patient is scheduled for a total laryngectomy, assess his or her ability to learn and physically manage self-care postoperatively including tracheostomy care, availability of support systems, and awareness of alternative methods of producing speech.

Nursing Diagnoses and Planning

Nursing diagnoses and related expected patient outcomes most commonly applicable to patients scheduled for laryngectomy include the following:

NDx: Anxiety related to the diagnosis of cancer, the surgical experience, the effects of the surgery on eating, breathing, speaking, appearance, work, and social activities

Planning: Patient outcomes
1. Patient attends to information given about the disease and surgery.
2. Patient asks questions about the surgery and its effect.
3. Patient denies feelings of overwhelming anxiety.
4. Nonverbal signs of excessive anxiety such as constant pacing, refusing to let significant others leave, and so on are absent.

NDx: Anticipatory grieving related to alteration in speech

Planning: Patient outcomes
1. Patient acknowledges that feelings of grief are normal.
2. Patient expresses feelings of grief.

NDx: High risk for ineffective individual coping related to the diagnosis of cancer, the surgical experience, the effects of surgery on speech, appearance, interpersonal relationships, and employment

Planning: Patient outcomes
1. Patient identifies effective and ineffective coping patterns.
2. Patient participates in the decision-making process.

3. Patient reacts with appropriate verbal and nonverbal responses applicable to the situation.

Nursing Interventions

NDx: Anxiety
Acknowledge that anxiety is normal before a laryngectomy, and encourage the patient to verbalize concerns. Answer questions simply but clearly, and describe the postoperative care routine. Tell the patient what tubes and dressings to expect and the reason for each. Be certain to carefully explain how breathing occurs after surgery. Discuss the fact that the patient will begin learning self-care on the day after surgery. Reassure the patient that support and assistance will be available when needed.

NDx: Anticipatory grieving
Allow opportunities for the patient to express grief, and encourage this expression. Provide a calm, private environment to facilitate patient and family grieving. Discuss with the patient and family the impact of this loss on the family unit and its functioning.

NDx: High risk for ineffective individual coping
Depending on the assessment of the individual patient's coping style, a visit from a well-adjusted laryngectomee (a person with a laryngectomy) may be arranged. Encourage the patient to express concerns about surgery, appearance, interpersonal relationships, and employment. Assist the patient in exploring available resources.

Evaluation

Evaluate effectiveness of nursing care for a patient who is scheduled for laryngectomy by comparing the patient's status with the expected patient outcomes. Examples of specific outcomes for patients scheduled for laryngectomy have been provided in the Planning section.

POSTOPERATIVE NURSING CARE

Assessment

Priority assessments are those related to the effectiveness of respiration. Take vital signs, and note depth and effort of breathing as well as the color of nail beds and mucous membranes. Assess the effectiveness of coughing, and observe the amount, color, and viscosity of secretions. Review arterial blood gas values.

Observe the suture line and the tracheostomy for bleeding and later for signs of infection such as redness, swelling, tenderness, and purulent drainage. If drains are inserted in the operative area, monitor the amount and character of the drainage. (Drains should not be disconnected from suction for measurement of drainage without a specific order.)

Assess pain as well as difficulty swallowing. If a nasogastric tube is in place, check that it is functioning properly, observe the drainage, and inspect the patient's naris for irritation. When tube feeding or oral intake is begun, assess the patient for nausea, vomiting, abdominal distention, and diarrhea. Measure intake and output, and obtain daily weights.

Throughout the postoperative period, assess the patient's psychosocial status. Observe the patient for signs of anxiety, withdrawal, or depression, and note interest and cooperation related to self-care. Assess ease and effectiveness of communication techniques being used and also the patient's response to staff members, other patients, and visitors.

Nursing Diagnoses and Planning

Nursing diagnoses and related expected patient outcomes most commonly applicable to patients after laryngectomy include the following:

NDx: Ineffective airway clearance related to increased secretions, impaired cough, and loss of humidification and filtration of inhaled air by the upper airway

Planning: Patient outcomes
1. Secretions are removed from the airway by suctioning or coughing.
2. No dust or other foreign matter enters the tracheostomy.
3. Respirations are easy and quiet.
4. Respiratory rate is within patient's normal range.
5. Complaints of dyspnea are absent.
6. Lungs are clear on auscultation.

NDx: Impaired verbal communication related to inability to speak secondary to diversion of air passing in and out of the lungs through a tracheostomy

Planning: Patient outcomes
1. Patient uses alternative modes of communication such as Magic Slate, flash cards, and gestures.
2. Patient successfully communicates wants, needs, and essential information.

NDx: Pain related to surgical trauma

Planning: Patient outcomes
1. Patient reports pain is relieved.
2. Nonverbal indications of pain are absent.

NDx: Impaired swallowing related to surgical trauma and alteration or loss of the larynx and related structures

Planning: Patient outcomes
1. Patient practices swallowing as directed.
2. Patient swallows soft foods and viscous fluids.
3. Patient gradually adds solid foods to the diet.

NDx: High risk for body image disturbance related to presence of tracheostomy and loss of voice

Planning: Patient outcomes
1. Patient looks at tracheostomy.
2. Patient or significant other participates in care of tracheostomy.
3. Patient interacts with others using available means of communication.
4. Patients with a subtotal laryngectomy practice speaking as directed.
5. Patients with a permanent voice loss actively participate with the speech therapist in learning esophageal speech or the use of a speech device.

NDx: High risk for altered health maintenance related to insufficient knowledge of self-care

Planning: Patient outcomes
1. Patient or significant other demonstrates stoma care, suctioning, and oral hygiene.
2. Patient describes precautions to be observed in regard to the tracheostomy.
3. Patient lists signs and symptoms that need to be reported to a health care professional
4. Patient identifies community resources that can assist with home maintenance and adjustments to effects of surgery and how to contact them.

Nursing Interventions

NDx: Ineffective airway clearance
Encourage the patient to turn, cough, and breathe deeply every 2 hours and more often if excessively large amounts of mucus are produced. Use a lint-free wipe to collect secretions discharged from the stoma during coughing. Have the patient lean forward to assist in expelling secretions. Remember that coughing can be difficult at first when the glottis is removed because the ability to increase intrathoracic pressure is impaired.

Suction the tracheostomy as needed to prevent obstruction of airflow. If secretions are viscous and not easily removed, insert a few drops of saline into the stoma before suctioning.

During the initial postoperative period, administer humidified air or oxygen as ordered to help loosen secretions because normal humidification by the upper airways is lost.

While the laryngectomy tube is in place, clean and change it, as described in Chapter 12 in the discussion of tracheostomy care. When the tube is removed, keep a thin covering over the stoma to allow passage of air but to prevent dust or other foreign matter from accidentally entering the tracheostomy. If dryness is a problem, saturate this cover with normal saline to provide some humidification.

NDx: Impaired verbal communication
For the patient who is unable to speak, it is of critical importance to feel that help is available at all times. Therefore, keep the call bell always within reach and frequently check on the patient's needs.

On the basis of the plan developed preoperatively, encourage the patient to use alternative methods of communication. Be certain to provide sufficient time for the patient to communicate needs and concerns by gesture, notes, beginning esophageal speech, or artificial device. Avoid acting hurriedly, and do not put words into the patient's mouth or complete what the patient appears to be trying to say.

Explain to significant others the importance of allowing the patient the time needed to communicate by an alternative method if the method is to be used with increasing facility and confidence.

NDx: Pain
Give medication for pain if needed. Remember that opiates are contraindicated because of their potential for respiratory depression. However, this is generally not a problem because there is relatively little postoperative pain, and medications with the strength of the opiates are not required.

Enhance the effectiveness of nonopiate drugs by maintaining a quiet environment, making certain the patient is physically comfortable and promoting the use of relaxation techniques and diversionary measures.

NDx: Impaired swallowing
Problems with swallowing vary in degree with the type of laryngectomy performed. Swallowing is least problematic for the patient with a total laryngectomy because there is no longer a connection between the trachea and esophagus, so there is no risk of aspirating ingested food unless a fistula has developed. After a partial laryngectomy, swallowing can be difficult and aspiration can occur, but the greatest problem occurs after a conservation (supraglottic) laryngectomy; aspiration occurs in approximately half of the patients having this procedure.

Patients with a partial laryngectomy usually receive intravenous fluids for 2 or 3 days, and then oral intake is begun. Start the patient on soft foods such as ice cream, custard, and mashed potatoes first because there is less chance of these spilling over into the trachea. As dysphagia diminishes, add viscous fluids and other soft foods to the diet. Instruct the patient to gradually add solid foods as tolerated.

After a conservation laryngectomy with its great risk of aspiration, the patient is maintained on intravenous fluids and tube feedings for 2 or 3 weeks until the suture lines are well healed. At this time, oral intake is resumed, but the patient must relearn

Chart 13–4.

NURSING GUIDE TO PATIENT EDUCATION FOR SELF-MANAGEMENT: DISCHARGE INSTRUCTIONS AFTER TOTAL LARYNGECTOMY

Instruct the patient to:

Wash hands thoroughly before touching the stoma.
Wash the stoma daily with a well-wrung warm washcloth.
Do not use soap, cotton swabs, or tissue, which may obstruct the airway.
Do not use undiluted alcohol on the stoma because it is both drying and irritating.
Apply a thin layer of petrolatum to the skin surrounding the stoma to prevent cracking.
Wear a stoma guard or a light scarf or clothing with a high collar to protect the tracheostomy from cold, drying, and foreign bodies and to eliminate its visibility.
Protect the stoma from water: Cover when bathing, keep showers below neck level, wash hair by hanging the head over a tub or sink, and avoid water sports.
Keep powders, sprays used on the upper body such as hair spray, deodorant sprays, and perfume well away from the tracheostomy.
Place a guard and a towel over the stoma when shaving or having a haircut to prevent hairs from entering the stoma.
Use a nonaerosol type of shaving cream.
Use a humidifier in the home if excessive dryness is a problem.
Avoid air conditioning to protect from excessive coldness.
Check stoma daily for redness, swelling, and purulent drainage, and report to physician if present.
Clean teeth and mouth three times a day because halitosis may go undetected because of loss of smell.
Wear a medical alert bracelet or chain indicating the presence of a tracheostomy and giving instructions to follow in an emergency.

to swallow and this can be difficult. To help the patient relearn to swallow, instruct him or her to place a small amount of a soft food on the back of the tongue while holding the breath and keeping the head flexed; swallow; and then cough to expel any foodstuff that may have entered the trachea. As swallowing becomes easier, add fluids and other foods as described previously.

After a total laryngectomy, patients may receive tube feedings for an interval or may begin taking fluids on the first postoperative day. When fluids are initiated, check the patient's tolerance for both thin and thick fluids, because many patients are able to handle thick fluids more easily than thin fluids. Once fluids are handled well, progress to a normal diet as tolerated.

Provide reassurance and emotional support as oral intake is resumed; because swallowing is no longer an automatic procedure to which no thought needs to be given, patients are often both frustrated and afraid of choking.

NDx: High risk for body-image disturbance

Provide an accepting, nonthreatening environment. Be sensitive to the patient's feelings, and avoid comments or actions that could be construed by the patient as indicating distaste or pity for his or her condition. Be aware that, without speech, verbal expression of feelings is inhibited and may contribute to frustration manifested in nonverbal, angry behavior.

Acknowledge the patient's feelings, and do not force the patient to look at the tracheostomy. When the patient does look at it, explain that the redness and swelling will decrease with time, and provide other additional information needed to correct misconceptions.

Assist the patient as needed to maintain good grooming. Be certain the patient's hair is combed and that male patients are shaved. Encourage female patients to apply makeup, if usually worn. Help all patients to get out of bed and to dress as soon as they are able.

NDx: High risk for altered health maintenance

Health teaching, both for the patient and significant others, is also an integral part of care. Beginning on the first postoperative day, begin teaching about suctioning and care of the tracheostomy, and help the patient perform these tasks with the aid of a mirror. Later teach the patient and significant others about self-care after discharge, as specified in Chart 13–4. As part of this teaching, be sure to show the patient the variety of stoma guards available (i.e. metal, plastic, nylon bibs).

Inform the patient and significant others about community support groups such as the Lost Chord Club and the Nu Voice Club and the availability of equipment and informational materials through the American Cancer Society. Provide telephone numbers and names of contact persons.

Additional Interventions
Position the patient with the head elevated to decrease edema, to limit pull on the suture line, and to promote pulmonary ventilation.

Provide frequent mouth care, and suction oral secretions until the patient is able to swallow. Also suction the nares if needed because the patient is unable to blow the nose.

If wound drains are in place, observe and measure drainage. Record color and amount. Bring drainage of less than 50 ml per day to the attention of the surgeon, because it may be appropriate to remove the drain.

Evaluation

Evaluate the effectiveness of nursing care for a patient after laryngectomy by comparing the patient's status with the expected patient outcomes. Examples of specific outcomes for patients after laryngectomy have been provided in the Planning section.

The Elderly: Special Considerations

Any upper respiratory tract infection or inflammation places the geriatric patient at risk for complications. Atrophy and weakness of respiratory muscles, with resulting thoracic wall rigidity coupled with decreased ciliary movement, make the cough reflex slower and less effective, thus interfering with airway clearance. The immune function of the older person declines, possibly because of T-cell changes; thus, the susceptibility to infection is increased. Often there is coexisting chronic illness, which further predisposes to complications. Older persons should be referred to a physician within 2 to 3 days if cold or other symptoms of upper respiratory tract disease do not start to clear.

Bibliography

Adams GL, Boies LR Jr, Hilger PA (eds). Boies fundamentals of otolaryngology: A textbook of ear, nose, and throat diseases. 6th ed. Philadelphia: WB Saunders, 1989.

Albanese AJ, Toplitz AD. A hassle-free guide to suctioning a tracheostomy. RN 1982; 45(4):24.

American Cancer Society. 1992 cancer facts and figures. New York: American Cancer Society, 1992.

Ballenger JJ. Diseases of the nose, throat, ear, head and neck. 13th ed. Philadelphia: Lea & Febiger, 1985.

Bates B. A guide to physical examination. 5th ed. Philadelphia: JB Lippincott, 1991.

Blackwood S. Back to basics, the pre-op exam. Am J Nurs 1986; 88:39.

Carroll P. Action stat, dislodged trach tube. Nursing 1985; 15(1):46.

Chernechy C, Ramsey P. Critical nursing care of the client with cancer. Norwalk, CT: Appleton-Century-Crofts, 1984.

Colton JJ, Beckhuis GJ. Management of nasal fractures. Otolaryngol Clin North Am 1986; 19(1):73.

Davis RK (ed). Lasers in otolaryngology. Philadelphia: WB Saunders, 1990.

Dennison R. Managing the patient with upper airway obstruction. Nursing 1987; 17(10):34.

DeWeese D, Saunders W. Textbook of otolaryngology. 7th ed. St. Louis: CV Mosby, 1987.

Gorback MS. Emergency airway management. Philadelphia: BC Decker, 1990.

Hogan R. Human sexuality, a nursing perspective. Norwalk, CT: Appleton-Century-Crofts, 1985.

Hutchinson R. The common cold primer. Nursing 1979; 9:57.

Ingram NM. Stanching nosebleeds: Your guide to all the measures available. RN 1982; 45(9):50.

Jarvis C. Physical examination and health assessment. Philadelphia: WB Saunders, 1992.

Lee KJ, Stewart C. Ambulatory surgery and office procedures in head and neck surgery. Philadelphia: WB Saunders, 1986.

Lockhart J, Griffin C. Epistaxis. Nursing 1986; 16(11):33.

Lockhart JS, Bryce J. Restoring speech with tracheoesophageal puncture. Nursing 1993; 23(1):59.

Lore JM Jr. An atlas of head and neck surgery. 3rd ed. Philadelphia: WB Saunders, 1988.

Lucente FE, Sobol SM. Essentials of otolaryngology. 2nd ed. New York: Raven Press, 1988.

Malsanos L, Barkauskas V, Moss M, Stoltenberg AK. Health assessment. 4th ed. St. Louis: Mosby-Year Book, 1989.

Montgomery WW. Surgery of the upper respiratory system, Vol. 2. 2nd ed. Philadelphia: Lea & Febiger, 1989.

Paparella MM, Shumrick DA, Gluckman JL, Meyerhoff WL (eds). Otolaryngology. Vol. 3. Head and neck. 3rd ed. Philadelphia: WB Saunders, 1991.

Patry-Lahey R. Helping a laryngectomy patient go home. Nursing 1985; 15(3):63.

Peterson P. Action stat! Respiratory distress after facial trauma. Nursing 1988; 18(1):33.

Price S, Wilson L. Pathophysiology: Clinical concepts of disease processes. 3rd ed. New York: McGraw-Hill, 1986.

Reichel W, Gallo JJ. Handbook of geriatric assessment. Rockville, MD: Aspen, 1988.

Riley M. Nursing care of the client with ear, nose and throat disorders. New York: Springer Publishing, 1987.

Romm S. Cancer of the larynx: Current concepts of diagnosis and treatment. Surg Clin North Am 1986; 66(1):109.

Shah JP. Color atlas of head and neck surgery: Vol. 2. Mouth, pharynx, larynx, thyroid, parotid, soft tissues and reconstructive surgery. Philadelphia: WB Saunders, 1990.

Stevens S, Becker K. How to perform picture perfect respiratory assessment. Nursing 1988; 18(1):57.

Chapter Fourteen

NURSING CARE *of Adults with Lower Respiratory Disorders*

Lower respiratory tract disease is a major cause of morbidity and mortality in the United States. Infectious diseases caused by opportunistic organisms are on the rise secondary to immunosuppression resulting from chemotherapy for cancer, drug therapy after organ transplantation, and human immunodeficiency virus (HIV) infection. This includes a dramatic increase in the incidence of tuberculosis, which can change from a quiescent state to active disease with only a moderate deficit in immunity. The incidence of chronic obstructive diseases such as chronic bronchitis, emphysema, and asthma (discussed under immune disorders in Chapter 10) is also rising. This is due in part to the aging of the population, but environmental pollution is also believed to be a contributing factor. Similarly, the incidence of lung cancer—the leading cause of cancer deaths in the United States—is on the rise. However, when incidence is examined in relationship to gender, lung cancer is in fact decreasing among men and increasing among women only.

Infections and Inflammations

Acute Bronchitis

Acute bronchitis is an inflammation of the larger bronchi in patients whose airways are otherwise normal. (Chronic bronchitis is discussed under Obstructive Disorders.)

ETIOLOGY AND PATHOPHYSIOLOGY

In acute bronchitis, there is diffuse inflammation of the bronchial tree and an excess production of mucus. Infectious agents such as viruses, especially influenza virus, or pyogenic organisms such as various species of *Streptococcus, Pneumococcus, Staphylococcus,* and *Haemophilus* cause acute bronchitis. Infection is often preceded by the common cold. It may also occur as a primary manifestation during the course of such infectious diseases as measles and typhoid fever or may result from inhalation of pollutants such as smoke, dust, or chemical irritants. Predisposing factors are exposure, chilling, fatigue, and malnutrition. Acute bronchitis is moderately common and usually leads to little permanent disability, although pneumonia is a potential complication.

CLINICAL MANIFESTATIONS

Symptoms of acute bronchitis include fever, which rarely exceeds 101°F (38.3°C), substernal burning discomfort caused by an associated tracheitis, and a cough that is at first dry and painful and later productive of mucopurulent sputum. Paroxysmal attacks of cough and wheezing may be precipitated by inhalation of irritants such as cigarette smoke or by exposure to very cold air.

MEDICAL DIAGNOSIS

Physical findings may not be distinctive, although chest auscultation may reveal wheezes or crackles. If a sputum culture is done, normal mouth flora abound, but no predominant pathogen is evident.

MEDICAL MANAGEMENT

Medical management is generally supportive because bronchitis is self-limiting. Bed rest, and even hospitalization for a severely debilitated patient, may be ordered initially. Hot- or cold-steam inhalations may be ordered to help loosen and liquefy the secretions, as well as antipyretics for any accompanying fever and expectorants to loosen secretions or antitussives to quiet a chronic, nonproductive cough. Antibiotics are not routinely given unless sputum cultures indicate a suprainfection with a bacterial agent or the patient requires prophylaxis against a secondary infection because of a chronic respiratory disease or general debilitation.

Application of the Nursing Process to the Care of the Patient with Acute Bronchitis

Assessment

Review the patient's history for factors placing him or her at risk for other than an uncomplicated, self-limiting episode of acute bronchitis (e.g., asthma, emphysema, or cardiac disease).

Assess current respiratory status. Check rate and depth of respirations. Auscultate breath sounds. Question the patient regarding cough and amount and color of expectoration. Take the patient's temperature.

As a basis for teaching, determine the patient's understanding of the therapeutic regimen. Also assess the patient's knowledge of how to prevent recurrence and spread of the disease.

Nursing Diagnoses and Planning

The nursing diagnosis and related expected patient outcomes most commonly applicable to patients with acute bronchitis are as follows:

Chart 14–1.

NURSING GUIDE TO PATIENT EDUCATION FOR SELF-MANAGEMENT: ACUTE BRONCHITIS

To provide relief of respiratory symptoms, instruct the patient to:

Use hot or cold inhalations to loosen and liquefy secretions.
Increase fluids to help keep secretions liquid.
Expectorate to clear the airways.
Cough and deep breathe to mobilize secretions.

To promote uncomplicated resolution of the infections, instruct the patient to:

Take medication in the correct dose, route, and frequency and for the prescribed length of time.
Report any symptoms of extension of the infection such as persistent fever or dyspnea.

To prevent recurrent infection, instruct the patient to:

Avoid exposure to people with colds and flu.
Avoid exposure to environmental irritants such as cigarrette smoke and pollutants.
Dress warmly.
Eat a well-balanced diet.

To prevent spread of infection, instruct the patient to:

Wash hands thoroughly and often, particularly after coughing, sneezing, or handling soiled tissues, and before handling food.
Cover mouth when coughing or sneezing.
Dispose of soiled tissues properly.
Avoid sharing drinking glasses or towels.

NDx: High risk for altered health maintenance related to insufficient knowledge of self-care

Planning: Patient outcomes
1. Patient lists measures to be used to relieve respiratory symptoms.
2. Patient describes measures to promote uncomplicated resolution of the infection.
3. Patient lists actions to prevent recurrent infection.
4. Patient identifies precautions to be taken to prevent the spread of the infection to others.

Nursing Interventions

NDx: High risk for altered health maintenance
Because most persons with acute bronchitis are outpatients, the primary nursing intervention is health teaching. Instruct the patient in self-care as specified in Chart 14–1.

Evaluation

Evaluate the effectiveness of nursing care for a patient with acute bronchitis by comparing the patient's status with the expected patient outcomes. Examples of specific outcomes for patients with acute bronchitis have been provided in the Planning section.

Pneumonia

Pneumonia is an acute inflammation of the gas-exchanging units of the lungs, which include respiratory bronchioles, alveolar ducts, alveolar sacs, and alveoli. Pneumonia may result from noninfectious causes; however, the term usually applies to acute infection unless otherwise specified.

ETIOLOGY

Pneumonia may be a primary infection of viral, bacterial, or nonbacterial origin. Nonbacterial pneumonias include aspiration pneumonia and atypical pneumonia caused by *Mycoplasma pneumoniae* and *Legionella pneumophila.*

Some conditions that predispose one to pneumonia are chronic lung disease, alcoholism, malnutrition, seizure disorders and other causes of altered consciousness, immunologic disorders, malignant conditions and their treatments, major surgical procedures, and old age.

VIRAL PNEUMONIA

The majority of pneumonias are viral in origin, and many of these remain undiagnosed because the infection is usually mild.

BACTERIAL PNEUMONIA

Less frequent but more serious in nature are the bacterial pneumonias. Ninety percent of these are pneumococcal pneumonias so called because they are caused by *Streptococcus pneumoniae* (group A hemolytic streptococci). This infection, which results in extensive consolidation of part or all of the parenchyma of the involved lobe, is frequently seen in infants, in the elderly, and in patients with sickle-cell disease, congestive heart failure, alcoholism, and diabetes mellitus.

Staphylococcus aureus, a gram-positive coccus, can cause pneumonia as a primary disease in infants but in adults most often develops as a secondary infection in debilitated patients or as a complication of influenza or measles.

Haemophilus influenzae (Type B), a gram-negative bacillus, can also cause pneumonia. In adults, it is usually secondary to viral influenza, measles, or bacterial pneumonitis.

NONBACTERIAL PNEUMONIA

Mycoplasma pneumoniae is the most frequent cause of nonbacterial atypical pneumonia in the civilian population. This organism shares both viral and bacterial characteristics; its particle size is similar to that of viruses, but its enzyme systems are similar to those of bacteria. Transmission is thought to be by contact with infected respiratory secretions.

A second type of nonbacterial, atypical pneumonia is caused by *Legionella pneumophila.* This is a weakly organized gram-negative organism that was identified after a convention of the American Legion, where an outbreak of severe pneumonia occurred. In addition to its effect on the lungs, this organism can cause multisystem illness. It affects males three times more often than females and occurs most frequently in older adults, smokers, and persons who have predisposing chronic illnesses.

ASPIRATION PNEUMONIA SYNDROME

Aspiration pneumonia is the result of aspiration of stomach contents, toxic materials, or a foreign body into the lower respiratory tract. It occurs most frequently when the patient is in an altered state of consciousness as a result of seizures, drugs, alcohol, anesthesia, acute infection, or shock. It also occurs in the presence of nasogastric tubes and tracheostomy tubes.

PATHOPHYSIOLOGY

The host factor is important in the development of pneumonia. When there is significant impairment of the lungs' first line of defense mechanisms (filtration action of upper airways, reflexes closing the epiglottis and glottis, coughing, and mucociliary action), the distal airways and alveoli are at increased risk for contamination by pathogenic organisms. Further, impairment of blood supply, abnormally low numbers of phagocytic cells and other cells involved in cellular immunity, lack of proper antibodies, and any alteration of other elements of the immunologic system can deprive the lungs of their second line of defense, thus placing the person at greater risk for pneumonia.

When pathogenic organisms reach the distal airways, an intense tissue reaction results. This reaction causes an outpouring of inflammatory exudates and cells. Interstitial tissue and alveolar spaces may become involved in this inflammatory process. White blood cells actively phagocytize the organisms and release their enzymes and immunologic mediators. This, in turn, causes further inflammation. Depending on other host factors, the body may or may not be able to ward off further progression at this time. If not, then the infection may continue to involve adjacent lung tissue and interalveolar openings. As a portion of the lung fills with exudate and inflammatory cells, it becomes consolidated. If both the airways and the lung parenchyma are infected, the condition is referred to as bronchopneumonia. If the adjacent pleura is inflamed, a pleural effusion may result. The growth of bacteria capable of causing loss of lung tissue or significant destruction results in necrotizing pneumonia.

Inflammations caused by viruses and mycoplasmas are predominantly in the interstitial tissue. Mycoplasmal and viral pneumonia produces interstitial inflammation, with an accumulation of an infiltrate in the alveolar walls. Therefore, little or no consolidation or exudate occurs.

The physiologic changes associated with pneumonia are the result of reduced functional lung volume and alteration of ventilation and blood flow. The arterial hypoxemia commonly seen in pneumonia is caused by the mismatching of ventilation with perfusion and intrapulmonary shunting. Lung tissue typically returns to normal function after an infection unless there have been significant destructive changes. In these cases, healing proceeds slowly by

Table 14–1. CLINICAL MANIFESTATIONS OF DIFFERENT TYPES OF PNEUMONIA

TYPE	SYMPTOMS
Streptococcal, pneumococcal	Sudden onset, chills, fever, headache, cough with rust-colored sputum, dyspnea, cyanosis, crackles, friction rub, hypoxemia as blood is shunted away from consolidated area, consolidated area visible on x-ray film
Staphylococcal	Gradual onset with a progressive, increasingly severe cough and purulent, copious sputum; high, swinging temperature; shaking chills; and pleuritic chest pain
Klebsiella	Begins abruptly without preceding upper respiratory infection; high temperature, severe cough with thick, tenacious, purulent sputum that is frequently blood stained; lung abscess is common complication, with frank blood expectorated; early treatment is necessary to prevent gram-negative bacteremia with high mortality rate
Pseudomonas aeruginosa	Fever, chills, dyspnea, cyanosis, productive cough of copious amounts of foul-smelling yellow or green sputum; apprehension and confusion
Mycoplasma pneumoniae	Gradual onset of severe headache; irritating, nonproductive cough; anorexia; malaise; low-grade fever; sore throat
Legionella pneumophila	Prodromal period of abdominal pain and diarrhea; breathlessness progresses, and rigors and confusion lead to well-recognized encephalopathic picture
Viral (adenovirus, syncytial virus, varicella, coxsackievirus, echoviruses, influenza viruses, and parainfluenza virus)	Cough, fever, malaise; similar to *Mycoplasma*
Pneumocystis carinii	Insidious onset of nonproductive cough with increasing breathlessness; central cyanosis (low arterial oxygen tension); fever (in 50% only)
Aspergillus fumigatus	Fever, productive cough, hemoptysis, chest pain
Aspiration pneumonia	Patient at risk (comatose, impaired lower cranial nerves, dysphagia, protracted vomiting, presence of nasogastric or endotracheal tubes) in whom fever or leukocytosis develops; may not be able to raise mucus; chest x-ray films show patchy infiltration in lower lobes

deposition of fibrous scar tissue, which results in a measurable loss of lung function.

In aspiration pneumonia, the aspirated substance triggers the development of chemical injury within 48 to 72 hours. The injurious effect depends on the pH of the aspirated substance. If the pH is 2.5 or below, there is little necrotizing of lung tissue. If the pH is above 2.5, atelectasis can occur, followed by pulmonary edema, hemorrhage, and Type II cell necrosis. In severe cases, adult respiratory distress syndrome (ARDS) occurs.

CLINICAL MANIFESTATIONS

General signs and symptoms of pneumonia are fever, chills, productive cough, and general malaise. However, the exact clinical manifestations vary somewhat with the type of pneumonia, as described in Table 14–1.

In the older patient, the symptoms may appear very gradually, and purulent sputum may be the only indication of disease.

MEDICAL DIAGNOSIS

Diagnosis of pneumonia depends on a careful history, with special attention to recent respiratory infections, physical examination, and chest x-ray films. The causative organism is suggested by a Gram's stain of the sputum and confirmed by a sputum culture. Blood cultures may also be done because in many cases the causative organism can be found in the circulation. Identification of the causative agent by culture may not be possible if antimicrobial agents have already been used.

MEDICAL MANAGEMENT

The treatment for pneumonia includes adequate hydration, proper nutrition, supplemental oxygen, analgesics, and antibiotics when appropriate. The choice of antibiotics is determined by bacterial studies. Table 14–2 lists primary and alternative antibiotics used in the treatment of the various pneumo-

Table 14–2. COMMON ANTIBIOTIC TREATMENT OF PNEUMONIAS

CAUSATIVE AGENT	PRIMARY/ALTERNATIVE ANTIBIOTICS
Streptococcus pneumoniae	Penicillin/erythromycin
Staphylococcus aureus	Oxacillin or nafcillin/cephalosporin, vancomycin
Mycoplasma pneumoniae	Erythromycin/tetracycline
Legionella pneumophila	Erythromycin
Pneumocystis carini	Trimethoprim/sulfamethoxazole
Anaerobic organisms	Penicillin/cefoxitin, clindamycin

nias. Bed rest is frequently required because of the debilitating nature of pneumonia. Intermittent positive pressure breathing (IPPB) and chest physiotherapy may be ordered if the patient is producing a large volume of secretions (more than 30 ml/day) and is unable to clear them from the airway.

Patients requiring hospitalization also frequently receive intravenous therapy to replace fluid loss resulting from the elevated temperature. Electrolytes are assessed and replaced as necessary. Diets designed to meet metabolic requirements are ordered to help fight the infection. If respiratory failure occurs, the patient is intubated and placed on mechanical ventilation.

Application of the Nursing Process to the Care of the Patient with Pneumonia

Assessment

Assessment of the patient with pneumonia focuses on four major areas: factors that place the patient at risk for pneumonia and contribute to the severity of the disease, effects of the disease on respiration and other body functions, correct implementation and effectiveness of treatment measures, and the patient's understanding of health measures related to the prevention and cure of the disease.

Because development of pneumonia is associated with impaired first-line defenses in the respiratory system and aspiration of bacteria from the mouth, gather information about recent upper respiratory tract infections, smoking, alcohol use, patterns of oral hygiene, and existence of any predisposing illness.

Take vital signs, and assess the characteristics of the patient's breathing. Include rate, depth, use of accessory muscles, splinting of the chest, presence of nasal flaring, and complaints of dyspnea. Assess lung sounds and laboratory values of arterial blood gases. Observe the patient for cyanosis, and question about chest pain. If the latter is present, determine the type of pain, its location, and association with inspiration or expiration. Assess for cough and expectoration. If a cough is present, note characteristics, such as shallow or deep, dry or loose. If a loose cough exists, observe whether secretions are raised and whether they are expectorated. Check color, odor, amount, and consistency of any expectorate. Table 14–3 lists common findings associated with certain colors of sputum. Because fever predisposes to excessive loss of body water through sweating, assess the patient's state of hydration. Check intake and output, skin turgor, and serum sodium levels. Also assess for anorexia, because an increase in caloric intake is needed to counteract the catabolism associated with the infection.

Ongoing assessments related to treatment measures are also necessary. For example, if the patient is receiving oxygen, check the flow rate, and observe for proper position of the cannula or mask.

In regard to the patient's understanding of general health measures, assess the patient's understanding of control of disease spread by noting whether the patient covers the mouth when coughing, expectorates rather than swallows raised secretions, and properly disposes of used tissues. Further assess the patient's understanding of a balanced diet, the need for increased fluid intake to keep secretions liquid, and the need for rest to foster the body's ability to combat the infection.

Observe for signs of complications of pneumonia such as lung abscess, empyema, pulmonary edema, and pleural effusion to ensure early recognition and treatment.

Nursing Diagnoses and Planning

Nursing diagnoses and related expected patient outcomes most commonly applicable to patients with pneumonia include the following:

NDx: Impaired gas exchange related to inflammatory exudate in the alveolar spaces

Planning: Patient outcomes
1. Patient states dyspnea is absent.
2. Respiratory rate and depth are within normal limits.
3. Lungs are clear on auscultation.
4. Arterial blood gas values are within normal limits.

NDx: Pain related to chest and lung expansion secondary to infection in the lung

Planning: Patient outcomes
1. Patient coughs and breathes deeply as directed.
2. Patient states pain is relieved.

NDx: Hyperthermia related to infection

Planning: Patient outcomes
1. Patient rests.
2. Patient avoids chilling.

Table 14–3. SPUTUM COLORS ASSOCIATED WITH SPECIFIC PNEUMONIAS

COLOR	PNEUMONIA TYPE
Colorless/clear mucoid	Noninfectious process
Creamy yellow	Staphylococcal pneumonia
Green	*Pseudomonas* pneumonia
"Currant jelly"	*Klebsiella* pneumonia
Rusty	Pneumococcal pneumonia

3. Temperature returns to normal range with resolution of the infection.

NDx: High risk for fluid volume deficit related to increased insensible fluid loss secondary to fever and rapid respirations

Planning: Patient outcomes
1. Patient drinks 3 to 4 L of fluid per day (if not contraindicated by a coexistent medical condition).
2. Mucous membranes are moist.
3. Skin turgor is firm.
4. Urinary output is adequate.

NDx: Anxiety related to dyspnea, blood-tinged sputum, chest pain

Planning: Patient outcomes
1. Patient denies being overly anxious.
2. Behavioral signs of excessive anxiety such as hand wringing, trembling, and the like are absent.

NDx: High risk for altered health maintenance related to insufficient knowledge of discharge instructions, risk of smoking, value of influenza vaccine

Planning: Patient outcomes
1. Patient explains instructions for self-care after discharge.
2. Patient identifies risks of smoking and availability of smoking cessation programs.
3. Patient describes need for and benefit of influenza vaccine.

Nursing Interventions

Although the symptoms of the various types of pneumonia vary, the general nursing interventions are similar.

NDx: Impaired gas exchange
Turn the patient, and encourage coughing and deep breathing every 2 hours. If the patient is unable to effectively raise secretions, suction as necessary to provide adequate respiratory toilet. This is best done after bronchodilator treatments and postural drainage. Teach the patient (and family) breathing techniques and exercises to promote maximal ventilation and raise secretions.

NDx: Pain
Give analgesics as needed and ordered for pain relief. Make certain, however, to first assess the patient for restlessness, confusion, aggression, and other signs of cerebral hypoxemia before administering a central nervous system depressant.

Position the patient comfortably, and assist him or her to splint the chest during coughing and deep breathing (Fig. 14–1). If pain is associated with ab-

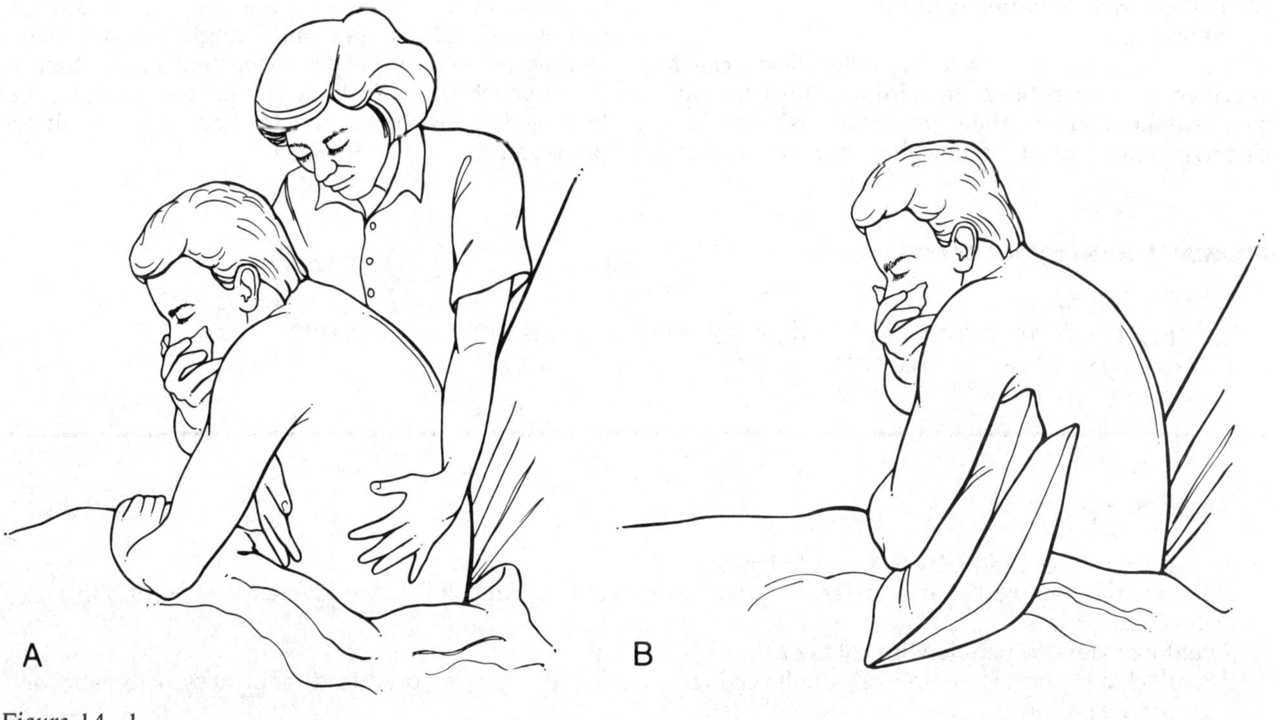

Figure 14–1.

Splinting painful areas during coughing. *A*, Nurse using hands to splint the patient's chest. *B*, Patient using own hand and pillow to splint chest.

dominal distention from swallowing air during intervals of severe dyspnea, encourage ambulation or pass a nasogastric tube if ordered.

NDx: Hyperthermia

Although fever is a positive force in resolving infection, it does make energy demands on the body. Therefore, limit the patient's activity while temperature is elevated. Promote bed rest, and specifically plan for uninterrupted rest periods between times of turning, coughing, deep breathing, and other treatments. Give tepid baths, and provide frequent linen changes to keep the patient comfortable and to prevent chilling in the presence of elevated temperature and diaphoresis.

NDx: High risk for fluid volume deficit

Monitor fluid intake closely. Force fluids up to 3 to 4 L per day (if not contraindicated) to keep the patient well hydrated and to loosen secretions. Keep an accurate record of intake and output to document fluid intake and to aid in preventing fluid deficit or overload.

NDx: Anxiety

Because the patient with pneumonia is often anxious about feeling short of breath, about the presence of chest pain, or about blood-streaked sputum, provide time for the patient to ask questions and express concerns. Explain expected symptoms, treatments, and procedures, and reassure the patient as appropriate in regard to his or her condition.

NDx: High risk for altered health maintenance

Instruct the patient in self-care after discharge as specified in Chart 14–2. In addition, instruct cigarette smokers about their increased risk for lung disorders, and inform them about American Lung Association or American Cancer Society smoking cessation programs. Teach high-risk patients about the benefits of the influenza vaccine, and encourage them to get it at the prescribed times, because influenza increases susceptibility to secondary bacterial pneumonia.

Additional Interventions

If the patient is receiving oxygen, monitor him or her frequently. Closely check the quantity of oxygen being delivered, because a high concentration of oxygen delivered inappropriately to the patient with chronic obstructive pulmonary disease (COPD) blunts the patient's only remaining ventilatory drive and leads to respiratory crisis.

Meet nutritional needs of patients with pneumonia as specified in Nutrition Box 14–1.

Collect sputum specimens from the patient as ordered. To obtain a satisfactory specimen, instruct the patient to perform the following:

Rinse the mouth with water to minimize possible contamination with normal flora.

Breathe deeply several times, and then cough and expectorate into a sterile container.

For aspiration pneumonia, prevention is the best intervention. Place any high-risk patient in a side-lying position with proper pillow supports behind the back, between the knees, and in front of the chest. Give frequent mouth care, and remove secretions as often as needed to prevent aspiration of organisms into the lower respiratory tract. When tube feedings are given, elevate the head of the bed at least 30 degrees during the feeding and for 1 hour after its completion. Check gag and cough reflexes before feeding as well as proper placement of the tube in the stomach. If more than 100 ml are aspirated before feeding, withhold the feeding and consult the physician.

Chart 14–2.

NURSING GUIDE TO PATIENT EDUCATION FOR SELF-MANAGEMENT: DISCHARGE INSTRUCTIONS AFTER PNEUMONIA

Instruct the patient to:

Increase activities gradually to avoid fatigue.

Obtain sufficient rest, eat a balanced diet, and avoid getting chilled to decrease susceptibility to infection.

Avoid exposure to people with colds or flu.

Report change or worsening of cough, change in color or sputum produced, shortness of breath, or recurrence of fever.

Nutrition Box 14–1.

NUTRITION: COMMON NUTRITIONAL PROBLEMS AND INTERVENTIONS FOR PATIENTS WITH PNEUMONIA

Problem	Nutritional Interventions
Increased risk of fluid deficit secondary to fever, insensible loss	Provide 3 L fluids daily. Keep water available at bedside. If oral intake cannot be maintained, intravenous administration may be necessary.
Increased metabolic demands secondary to infection and increased respiratory rate	Provide an intake of at least 1500 calories daily. Ensure diet rich in protein. Aim for nitrogen balance for maintenance or a positive nitrogen balance to replete body tissue. A liquid or blenderized diet may be better tolerated in the beginning.
Dyspnea	Small, frequent feedings.
Anorexia secondary to decreased taste sensation caused by expectoration of sputum	Oral hygiene prior to meals.

Evaluation

Evaluate the effectiveness of nursing care for a patient with pneumonia by comparing the patient's status with the expected patient outcomes. Examples of specific outcomes for patients with pneumonia have been provided in the Planning section.

Lung Abscess

A lung abscess is defined as a collection of pus within the substance of the lung.

ETIOLOGY AND PATHOPHYSIOLOGY

Development of a lung abscess is a pathologic process that develops during the course of any number of different inflammatory conditions of the lung and is caused by a combination of suppuration (the process of pus formation) and necrosis (death of areas of tissue) of lung tissue. Lung abscesses are classified by cause, the most common being a necrotizing infection. This is an infection of the parenchyma by a microorganism capable of destroying the lung tissue. Examples of such organisms are staphylococci, Friedländer's bacillus, tubercle bacillus, and certain fungal infections such as blastomycosis.

Another cause is cavitary infarction. A pulmonary infarct is defined as a dead or devitalized area of lung tissue. Generally, these infarcts heal by fibrosis and scarring, but occasionally the area becomes necrotic and excavates, forming an abscess cavity. Pulmonary emboli, septic pulmonary infarction, and vasculitis are all possible causes of this type of lung abscess.

Cavitary malignancy abscess develops within the substance of a pulmonary neoplasm, which may be primary or secondary. The mechanism of development of this type of lung abscess is not fully understood. Theory suggests that certain malignancies grow faster than their blood supply, thus leading to necrosis of cells and an abscess in the center of the lesion.

Aspiration into the bronchi can also be followed by a lung abscess. Normally, the bronchial defenses are able to deal with nasopharyngeal and oral secretions that may be aspirated into the tracheobronchial tree during sleep. However, during anesthesia, traumatic shock, alcoholic stupor, coma, or postoperative shock, these defenses are impaired. Aspiration of vomitus, which is an irritating fluid, results in a diffuse lobular pneumonia with multiple abscesses. Aspiration of solid matter causes a localized abscess.

Abscesses in general are spherical in shape because of the pull of the surrounding healthy elastic parenchyma.

CLINICAL MANIFESTATIONS

Cough, sputum production, and fever are present in all types of lung abscesses. The duration of the episode and severity of clinical manifestations differ widely. If a febrile respiratory illness develops suddenly in a patient who has recently undergone a surgical procedure, especially involving the mouth, nose, or throat, a lung abscess is suspected. Rupture of an abscess into a bronchus is associated with expectoration of a large quantity of foul-smelling, green or brown sputum. The physical signs associated with lung abscess depend on the size of the abscess cavity, the degree of surrounding pneumonitis, and the distance from the chest wall.

MEDICAL DIAGNOSIS

A careful history seeking information about occupational exposure, preexisting lung conditions, recent episodes of unconsciousness, or presence of periodontal disease provides important clues to the diagnosis of lung abscess. Lung abscess is diagnosed by chest x-ray film. The particular cause of the abscess can usually be established by evaluating the results of laboratory tests, clinical tests, and x-ray films. Sputum examination by Gram's stain and acid-fast stain is important to identify the microorganism for the initial antimicrobial therapy.

MEDICAL MANAGEMENT

The medical regimen has a twofold goal: first to eradicate the underlying cause and second to alleviate the adverse consequences. Pyogenic bacterial infections are treated with specific antibiotics. High intravenous doses are required for the antibiotic to penetrate the necrotic tissue and abscess fluid. Oral antibiotics may be ordered in place of intravenous antibiotics when the patient shows signs of improvement. The entire course of antibiotic therapy may extend from 6 to 12 weeks.

Postural drainage aided by percussion, coughing, and breathing exercises is ordered to provide adequate drainage of the abscess. If these measures are ineffective, a bronchoscopy may be done to drain it.

Surgical intervention may be necessary if the abscess fails to respond to more conservative treatment or when a major hemoptysis occurs. Tube thoracotomy or some other form of surgical drainage may be used to treat the patient who cannot tolerate thoracic surgery.

Application of the Nursing Process to the Care of the Patient with a Lung Abscess

Assessment

Assess rate and depth of respirations, symmetry of chest expansion, characteristics of cough and expectorate, lung sounds, and pulse every 2 hours during the initial phase of the hospitalization. Note the characteristics and amount of purulent drainage from the pleural cavity resulting from postural drainage, and observe the patient for response to antibiotic therapy.

Nursing Diagnoses and Planning

Nursing diagnoses and related expected patient outcomes most commonly applicable to patients with lung abscess include the following:

NDx: High risk for ineffective airway clearance related to pain and ineffective coughing

Planning: Patient outcomes
1. Sputum is expectorated.
2. Breath sounds are normal.
3. Chest expansion is symmetric.

NDx: High risk for altered health maintenance related to insufficient knowledge of self-care

Planning: Patient outcomes
1. Patient states name, dose, route, and frequency of prescribed antibiotics.
2. Patient explains importance of taking antibiotic as prescribed.
3. Patient lists symptoms to be reported.

Nursing Interventions

NDx: High risk for ineffective airway clearance

Position the patient with abscess area up to promote drainage. Teach coughing and deep-breathing exercises to mobilize secretions. Do postural drainage and percussion as ordered. Give analgesics if needed and prescribed beforehand to promote comfort. Force fluids to keep secretions liquid, and stress the importance of expectoration. Ensure that the patient has easy access to tissues and a waste container.

NDx: High risk for altered health maintenance

Teach the patient about prescribed antibiotics, stressing name, dose, route, and frequency. Explain the risk of a relapse if all the antibiotic is not taken. Also explain that suprainfection can occur, and instruct patients to report any diarrhea, vaginal discharge, recurrent fever, or the like.

Additional Interventions

Provide a high-calorie diet, because chronic infection is associated with a catabolic state. Administer antibiotics as prescribed, and monitor the patient's response by observing for signs of drug allergy, suprainfection, and failure to respond to medication.

If surgery was done, change dressings frequently

to prevent excoriation of the skin and an offensive odor. It may also be necessary to teach the family to change simple dressings because of the prolonged period of drainage before the wound closes completely.

Evaluation

Evaluate the effectiveness of nursing care for a patient with lung abscess by comparing the patient's status with the expected patient outcomes. Examples of specific outcomes for patients with lung abscess have been provided in the Planning section.

Empyema

Empyema is a collection of pus in the pleural cavity.

ETIOLOGY

The most common cause of an accumulation of pus in the pleural cavity is direct extension from adjacent structures such as in pneumonia, tuberculosis, pulmonary abscess, bronchiectasis, or esophageal rupture. Empyema may also follow thoracic surgery or penetrating chest wounds.

PATHOPHYSIOLOGY

Empyema is generally situated in the dependent part of the pleural space, usually in the lateral or posterior aspects. If a large empyema remains untreated, septicemia frequently develops. Spontaneous evacuation of the pus may occur either by rupture through the lung into a bronchus (bronchopleural fistula) or by extension through the thoracic wall (empyema necessitatis). Treatment of chronic empyema (recurrent infection) is difficult because the pleura becomes thickened and fibrous and the lung may adhere to the chest wall. The retracted lung and the displaced mediastinum are anchored, and the overlying thoracic cage is retracted and immobile. The multiloculated cavities within the pleural space fill with pus and are difficult to drain.

CLINICAL MANIFESTATIONS

Clinical manifestations include fever, unilateral pleuritic chest pain, dyspnea, and anorexia. Physical examination discloses foul-smelling sputum, pleural friction rub, dullness to percussion, decreased lung sounds over the area of the pus, decreased vocal fremitus, and unequal chest expansion. With chronic empyema, weight loss, low-grade fever, and malaise may be present.

MEDICAL DIAGNOSIS

Diagnosis is made on the basis of history, physical examination, chest x-ray films (usually unilateral pleural fluid with associated lung lesion), and laboratory examination including culture and sensitivity of pleural exudate obtained by thoracentesis. Of special diagnostic value is the pH of the exudate; a pH less than 7.20 is suggestive of empyema that necessitates chest-tube drainage.

MEDICAL MANAGEMENT

Treatment includes thoracentesis to drain the area if it is small and localized, thoracic drainage, thoracotomy (for those patients not responding to tube drainage), antibiotic therapy, oxygen support, bed rest, and breathing and coughing exercises to maintain maximal ventilation and decrease congestion.

Application of the Nursing Process to the Care of the Patient with Empyema

The assessment, nursing diagnoses, expected patient outcomes, nursing interventions, and evaluation for patients with empyema are similar to those described previously for patients with lung abscess. Specific implications for care arise in relation to the long-term, sometimes recurrent nature of empyema and when chest drainage is required.

In regard to the long recovery period associated with empyema, inform the patient and family that the healing process may be slow and that repeated treatments, drainage, irrigation, and follow-up chest x-ray films may be necessary. If empyema is a recurrent problem, teach the patient and family signs and symptoms that should be reported for early treatment: elevated temperature, shortness of breath, increased or foul-smelling sputum, painful breathing, and loss of appetite.

If the patient has chest tubes, provide care as described in Chapter 12, with special attention to monitoring patency of the tubes, because purulent drainage can readily obstruct them.

Influenza

Influenza virus infections cause a nondistinctive syndrome that occurs in characteristic epidemic or pandemic patterns usually in late fall, winter, or early spring. Because of these recognizable patterns, identifiable outbreaks of influenza have been noted as early as the year 1510.

ETIOLOGY

Influenza is caused by viruses that are divided into three major groups: A, B, C, and their variants. These viruses frequently undergo changes in their chemical makeup, and infection with one type of influenza virus offers no immunity to subsequent infections with other types.

Currently, influenza is the only epidemic disease in the United States that can affect a large enough proportion of the population to produce more deaths than otherwise expected (excess mortality). It has been estimated that more than 200,000 deaths in excess of the number normally expected occurred in association with influenza epidemics in the United States from 1968 through 1981. These were due mainly to the Type A virus strain.

PATHOPHYSIOLOGY

Type A virus causes pandemics and local epidemics, whereas Type B strains cause localized outbreaks and sporadic cases. Influenza is able to infect most surface epithelial cells of the respiratory tract and is transmitted principally by the aerosol route. Because it may infect the nasal mucosa, transmission by fomites is also possible.

Complications of influenza include primary influenza virus pneumonia, bacterial pneumonia, or both. Neurologic complications such as Guillain-Barré syndrome or encephalitis as well as acute sinusitis or exacerbation of preexisting respiratory insufficiency may also occur. Complications occur most often in the geriatric population; in patients with cardiovascular disease, pulmonary disease, diabetes mellitus, cirrhosis, or chronic renal disease; in pregnant women; and in patients with conditions that compromise the immune mechanisms.

CLINICAL MANIFESTATIONS

After an incubation period of 1 to 3 days, illness starts with an abrupt onset of fever, sweating, headache, muscular aches, and pains. A nonproductive cough associated with conjunctival irritation and nasal obstruction quickly follows. The fever and cough are essential features of influenza, and a clinical diagnosis of influenza cannot be made if they are not present.

MEDICAL DIAGNOSIS

During periods of a local outbreak, medical diagnosis of influenza may be based on clinical findings. It is also possible to identify Types A, B, and C in complement fixation and hemagglutination inhibition antibody tests. Serologic diagnosis is made on the basis of evidence of a fourfold rise in antibody titers when the acute and convalescent periods are compared 2 weeks apart.

MEDICAL MANAGEMENT

Uncomplicated influenza requires no treatment, although relief of symptoms may be obtained through the prescription of decongestants, expectorants, antitussives, and analgesics. The patient is also advised to rest and force fluids. For patients with known underlying chronic respiratory or cardiac disease, close observation for extensive pulmonary involvement is needed, with supportive respiratory care as necessary. If a bacterial superinfection is documented by sputum Gram's stain, appropriate antibiotic treatment is initiated.

Amantadine hydrochloride (Symmetrel) may be used to treat diagnosed cases of Type A virus. However, it is effective only when begun within 1 to 2 days of onset of infection. Because very few patients are known to have laboratory-diagnosed Type A until after the illness has subsided, it is not widely used.

The Immunization Practices Advisory Committee of the U.S. Public Health Service recommends annual influenza vaccination for all persons older than 65 years and for those with chronic underlying illnesses. The effectiveness of the influenza vaccines has been variable. Problems include short duration of immunity, strain specificity, ineffectiveness against respiratory illnesses, increased incidence of Guillain-Barré syndrome (documented during the 1976–1977 swine influenza program), and long lead time from production to distribution, making the inactivated vaccines useless for controlling epidemics resulting from novel serotypes. Despite these problems, active immunization is the most effective prophylaxis against the influenza virus. After vaccination, people are less likely to be infected and, if infected, have milder courses of illness and shed less virus in their nasal secretions. The vaccine is a preparation of inactivated antigens that represent the influenza virus prevalent in a specific year.

Guidelines for Application of the Nursing Process to the Care of the Patient with Influenza

Nursing care of the patient with influenza is primarily supportive. Assess the patient for the existence of any factors such as a history of cardiac or respiratory disease that predispose to complications of influenza. Then assess the patient's symptom complex on an ongoing basis to determine whether the disease is resolving or worsening and to identify signs of complications as early as possible.

Encourage the patient to rest, force fluids, and eat nutritious, appetizing foods as able. Depending on the situation, administer medications prescribed for symptomatic relief or instruct the patient in their correct use.

Nursing also has an important role in the prevention of influenza. Assess for persons at risk (i.e., those older than 65 years and those with chronic diseases), and, when identified, assess their knowledge of the disease, its mode of transmission, and the immunizations available against it. When a knowledge deficit is found, instruct the patient as needed. Explain the relation of crowding and close contact with groups of individuals to the spread of influenza and thus the importance of avoiding theaters, shopping malls, and so on during an outbreak of influenza.

Provide information on the advantages of immunization and when and where immunizations may be obtained.

Within health care facilities, monitor visitors closely during epidemics to minimize the spread of influenza to patients.

Tuberculosis

Tuberculosis is a chronic pulmonary and extrapulmonary infectious disease primarily acquired by inhalation of droplet nuclei containing tubercle bacilli into the alveolar structure of the lung. It is characterized by stages of early infection, latency, and a potential for recurrent postprimary disease. Tuberculosis occurs most often in crowded, inner-city, economically disadvantaged environments. All suspected and diagnosed cases of tuberculosis are reportable to the local health department.

Tuberculosis was a major health problem in the early part of the 20th century. It was a disease for which there was no real treatment, and it led to isolation, disability, and in many cases death. The advent of effective antibiotic therapy combined with aggressive programs of prevention, detection, and treatment brought the disease under control, and the percentage of the population in developed countries infected with *Mycobacterium tuberculosis* fell from approximately 60% in 1940 to 25% in 1975. This decline led to the projection that by the year 2000 only 5% of these populations would ever be infected. Contrary to this projection, however, tuberculosis reemerged as a threat in the 1980s, with the number of cases in the United States rising by 16% between 1984 and 1990. In 1991, more than 26,000 new cases were diagnosed, and new strains of multi-drug resistant tuberculosis (MDR-TB) were identified throughout the United States. Factors contributing to the resurgence of tuberculosis include social problems such as homelessness, poverty, and drug use as well as an increase in human immunodeficiency virus infection and lack of adequate health programs.

ETIOLOGY

Tuberculosis is caused by infection with *M. tuberculosis,* of which three types exist; human, bovine, and avian. Humans may become infected with any of the three types; however, in the United States, the human type predominates. *M. tuberculosis* is an acid-fast aerobic organism, which, wherever it lodges, causes focal inflammatory reactions called granulomas, whose centers often undergo necrosis. *M. tuberculosis* multiplies slowly and can be killed by heat, sunshine, and ultraviolet light. It is resistant to drying, being able to remain viable for weeks in particles of dried sputum but is not a highly contagious organism in that it requires close, frequent, prolonged contact for transmission.

PATHOPHYSIOLOGY

With respiratory transmission, the primary tuberculosis infection occurs when tubercle bacilli are inhaled into the lungs of a susceptible individual in the form of droplet nuclei, which are released into the air when an infected person talks, coughs, sneezes, or laughs (Fig. 14–2). The inhaled bacilli lodge in the alveoli and give rise to a small area of gray-white inflammatory consolidation, called the primary or Ghon lesion. The tubercle bacilli multiply at this primary site, spread to the hilar lymph nodes, from which they can drain into the lymph, and then enter the blood stream to be carried throughout the body. The phrase Ghon complex is used to refer to the combination of primary lesion and lymph node involvement.

The process of multiplication and spread is interrupted when, in approximately 2 weeks, the body's immune system begins to respond. Mycobacterium-specific lymphocytes attract macrophages to the foci of infection. Some of the macrophages are stimulated to a heightened mycobactericidal state, whereas others are stimulated to differentiate into fibroblasts, which surround the primary lesion with a dense connective tissue enclosure. The resultant granuloma is the characteristic lesion of tuberculosis.

In the majority of people, no symptoms are present during this initial infection, and the granulomatous lesion becomes fibrotic and calcified, leaving them tuberculin positive but without clinical disease. They then enter the latent stage so called because, although there are no symptoms of disease, the tubercle bacilli are not necessarily eliminated and thus there is the potential for reactivation if specific and nonspecific resistance decreases for any reason.

In the approximate 10% of patients whose defenses are not capable of controlling the growth and spread of *M. tuberculosis,* initial infection can progress directly to a granulomatous consolidation of multiple, patchy lung areas. If the wall of a blood vessel is eroded, it can also progress to miliary (ex-

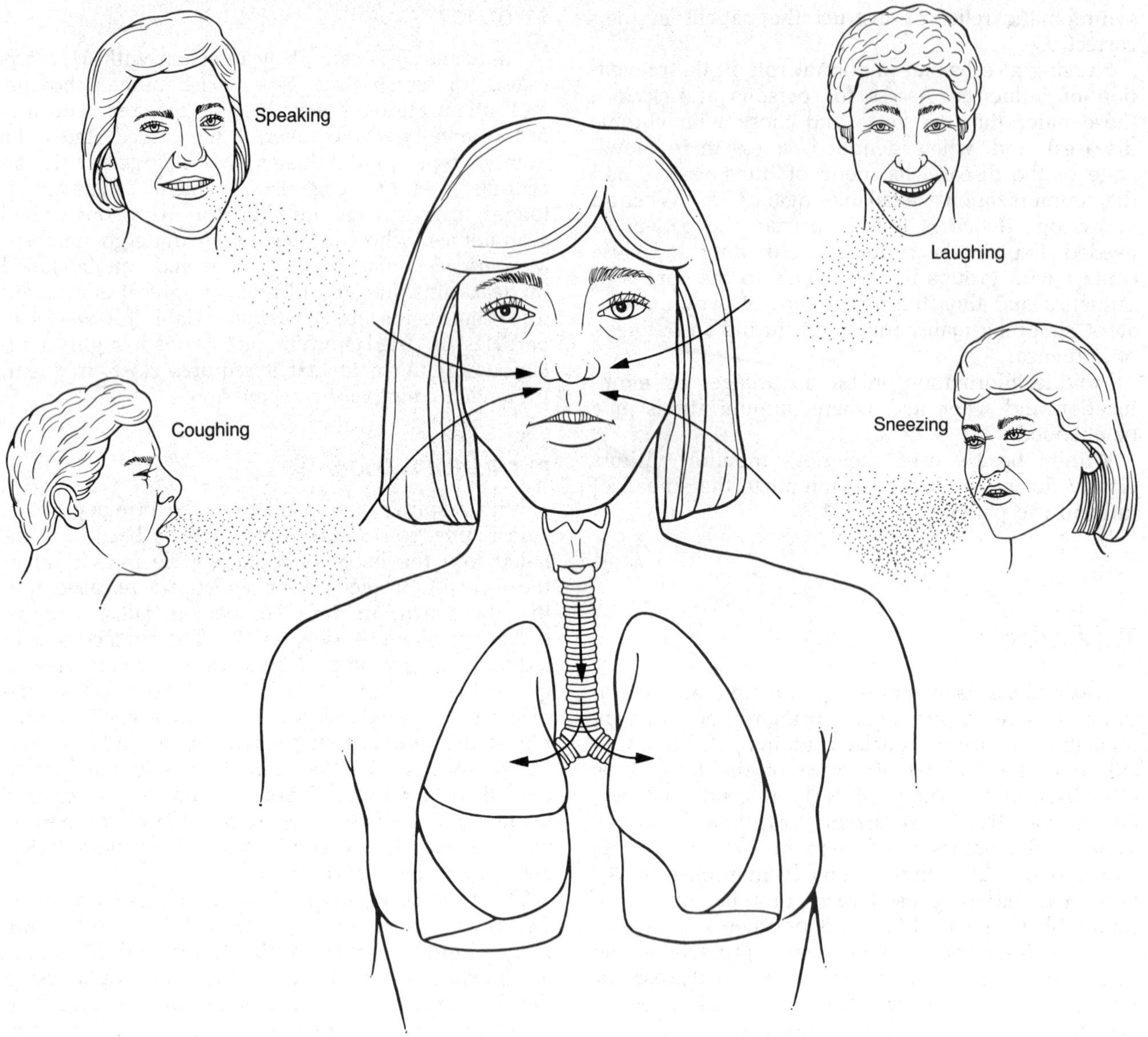

Figure 14–2.

Droplet nuclei containing the tubercle bacilli released into the air by the coughing, sneezing, speaking, or laughing of infected individuals can be inhaled by an unsuspecting person.

tensive dissemination of the tubercle bacillus via the blood stream) tuberculosis or tuberculous meningitis.

Secondary tuberculosis is infection in a person who has already had a primary lesion and an immune reaction to it. It may be due to new infection, although in most cases it involves reactivation of the initial infection. Because the person is already sensitized to the bacillus, the course of secondary tuberculosis is different from the relatively silent, primary infection. On the positive side, the lesions of secondary tuberculosis occur most often in the apices of the lung and tend to remain localized in the lung and the regional lymph nodes because of rapid phagocytosis and destruction of bacilli by activated macrophages. On the negative side, there is an acute local tissue inflammation complicated by necrosis, with resulting ulceration of the infected lung tissue. As a result of developed sensitivity, local clusters of tubercles become surrounded by zones of inflammatory reaction. The surrounding alveoli become filled with exudate, and tuberculous bronchopneumonia develops. The tuberculous tissue gradually becomes caseous and ulcerates into a bronchus, causing a cavity (Fig. 14–3). The ulcerations heal, leaving considerable local scar tissue around the cavity. The pleura over the infected lobe, usually the upper lobe, becomes inflamed and then thickened and retracted by scar tissue. This cyclic process—inflammatory bronchopneumonia, ulceration, cavita-

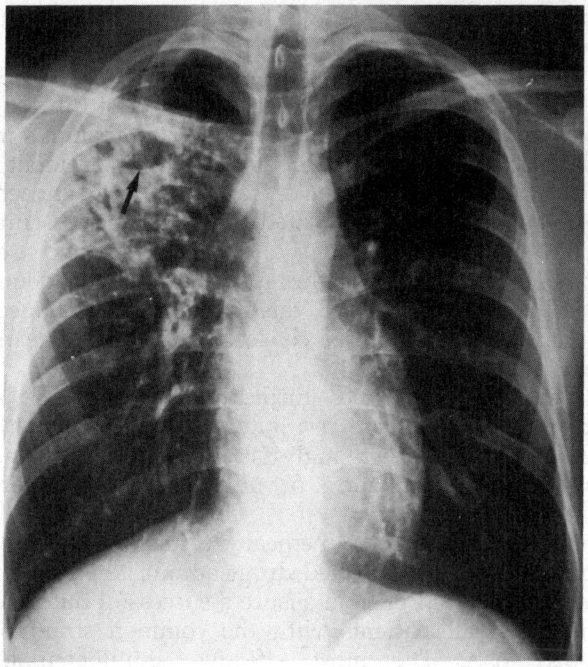

Figure 14–3.

Cavitation in tuberculosis. (From Kersten LD. Comprehensive respiratory nursing: A decision making approach. Philadelphia: WB Saunders, 1989, p 146.)

tion, and scarring—unless arrested spreads slowly downward toward the hilum and may later extend into adjacent lobes. This cavitation makes possible spread to other areas of the respiratory tract as well as spread via the lymphatic vessels to other organs such as the kidney and the bone. There may be long remissions followed by periods of renewed activity.

CLINICAL MANIFESTATIONS

Clinical manifestations of the pulmonary adult form of tuberculosis are insidious in onset, with nonspecific constitutional symptoms developing before symptoms specific to lung disease. Constitutional symptoms include low-grade fever in the afternoon, pallor, chills, night sweats, generalized weakness, fatigue, anorexia, and weight loss. The first symptoms to develop related to pulmonary inflammation are a slight cough occurring first as a "clearing" of the throat each morning or a feeling that a cold is "hanging on" and the expectoration of a scanty amount of mucoid sputum. If cavitation develops as the disease progresses, hemoptysis or expectoration of purulent or blood-stained sputum occurs. Chest pain or pleurisy may also appear late in the disease.

MEDICAL DIAGNOSIS

Presumptive diagnosis is made on the basis of a tuberculin skin test, sputum smear positive for acid-fast bacteria, chest x-ray film, and histologic evidence of granulomatous disease on biopsy. Definitive diagnosis is confirmed through culture and isolation of *M. tuberculosis.*

MANTOUX TEST (TUBERCULIN SKIN TEST OR PURIFIED PROTEIN DERIVATIVE)

Purified protein derivative (PPD) is a product derived from the protein fraction of the tubercle bacilli. For a tuberculin skin test, a small amount of this material is injected intradermally (Fig. 14–4). In sensitized individuals, this results in a reaction manifested by an induration mainly from cellular infiltra-

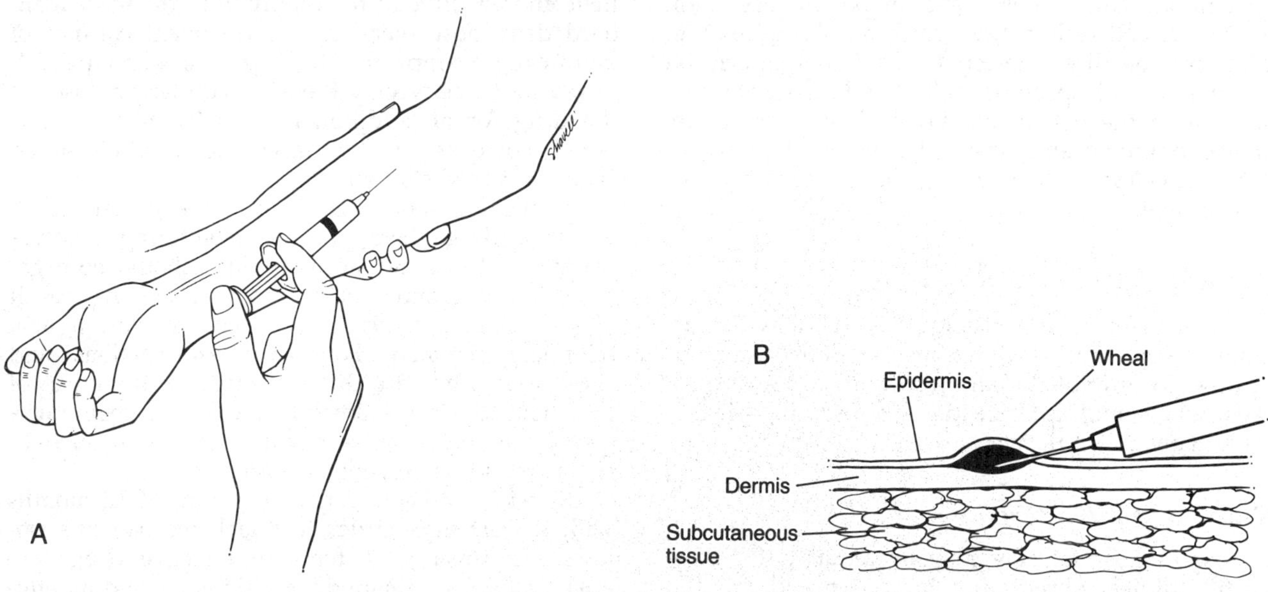

Figure 14–4.

Purified protein derivative (PPD) testing for tuberculosis. *A,* The angle of insertion is almost parallel with the patient's skin. *B,* Intradermal injection results in a small wheal.

tion. This reaction takes place within 48 to 72 hours. The Mantoux test must be intracutaneous, as indicated by the appearance of a definite pale wheal at the site of injection. A small, slender, sharp needle and a syringe graduated in 0.01-ml units (tuberculin syringe) is used. The usual dose is 0.01 ml of PPD solution containing five tuberculin units. The test is positive if a palpable and usually visible area of induration of 10 mm in diameter or greater is present 48 to 72 hours after injection. The intracutaneous Mantoux test is the standard and preferred method of determining tuberculin sensitivity. Other tests have been devised but are used principally in surveys of large populations (tine test, Heaf test, and jet injection gun methods).

BACTERIOLOGIC STUDIES

Diagnosis of tuberculosis is never certain without bacteriologic confirmation. Examination of sputum for acid-fast bacilli is the most important laboratory study in pulmonary tuberculosis. Tubercle bacilli have specific staining characteristics. If not seen in a direct smear, the organisms can be demonstrated after sputum or other suspected material is concentrated by one of several available methods. On the basis of positive smear for acid-fast bacilli, chemotherapy is initiated and the patient's contacts are examined. A culture is done to differentiate *M. tuberculosis* from other acid-fast organisms; it may also reveal their presence when the number of bacilli is small. Sputum cultures are positive within 2 to 3 weeks of active disease and are not positive during a latent period.

The Tuberculosis Stat Test allows detection of *M. tuberculosis* in sputum or respiratory aspirate within 48 hours, as opposed to the 3 to 6 weeks required for culture. This test is based on polymerase chain reaction (PCR) technology, which amplifies DNA to allow for the direct detection of microorganisms. It requires a 5-ml specimen collected in a sterile container after the patient has brushed the teeth or removed dentures and rinsed the mouth with water. After collection, the container must be tightly sealed and refrigerated.

PLEURAL NEEDLE BIOPSY

Tissue samples for histologic study may be obtained by pleural needle biopsy. However, even if positive for granuloma and for the presence of giant cells, which indicate caseation necrosis, the diagnosis remains presumptive.

MEDICAL MANAGEMENT

A short hospital stay may be required for diagnostic studies, observation for effect and possible side effects of drugs, isolation of the patient from family members during the infective stage of disease, and patient instruction regarding the illness, how to cope with it, and how to cooperate with long-term therapy.

In accord with Centers for Disease Control (CDC) 1990 guidelines for preventing outbreaks of tuberculosis and MDR-TB in the hospital setting, patients in high-risk groups for tuberculosis with an unidentified pulmonary problem as well as those diagnosed with tuberculosis are isolated in a negative-pressure room with air ventilated directly outside and exchanged at least six times per hour. For patients with confirmed MDR-TB, this isolation is maintained until the results of three consecutive sputum smears are negative.

The CDC guidelines further recommend that a disposable particulate respirator be worn by health care providers when high-risk procedures such as endotracheal intubation or bronchoscopy are performed.

The cornerstone of medical treatment is chemotherapy. Properly selected drugs administered for an adequate period of time ensure a successful outcome in almost all patients with the common strain of tuberculosis. The most effective antituberculous drug is considered to be isoniazid (INH). It is used in combination with one or sometimes two other drugs. The most common companion drug is rifampin. Both INH and rifampin are bactericidal. The duration of drug therapy with this combination is approximately 9 months. Other effective adjuncts are ethambutol, streptomycin, and pyrazinamide. Chemotherapy involving these other combinations necessitates a longer duration of treatment, usually 18 to 24 months. Table 14–4 presents an overview of some of the drugs used and their most common side effects.

Intermittent drug therapy is another effective means for treatment of tuberculosis when the patient finds it difficult to comply with the more standard daily dose therapy. The treatment consists of daily drug therapy for the first 1 to 4 months followed by twice weekly therapy with larger doses of the drug for an additional 18 to 24 months. It is noted, however, that the larger doses administered cause increased side effects.

Patients are monitored during the course of all types of drug therapy. This monitoring involves sputum cultures and smears, which should be negative after 2 months of therapy. A positive result after 2 months indicates the need to start a new treatment regimen. Follow-up examinations and chest x-ray films are done to evaluate the effect of treatment. Since the advent of effective chemotherapy for tuberculosis, surgical intervention such as thoracoplasty or resection is rare.

MDR-TB is treated for a minimum of 12 months with at least three drugs to which the patient's isolates are sensitive. Potentially effective drugs are ethambutol, pyrazinamide, a quinolone, and an aminoglycoside.

Preventive measures for tuberculosis are the most effective "treatment." They include diagnosis and

Table 14–4. DRUG THERAPY IN THE TREATMENT OF TUBERCULOSIS

DRUG	DOSE AND ROUTE	SIDE EFFECTS	PATIENT MANAGEMENT CONSIDERATIONS
FIRST-LINE TREATMENT			
Isoniazid	300 mg PO OD or 15 mg/kg (900 mg max) PO BIW	Peripheral neuritis: tingling, numbness, burning, or pain of the hands and feet, clumsiness, unsteadiness	Is used alone as prophylaxis against tuberculosis but must be used in combination with another drug such as rifampin or ethambutol when used as treatment; pyridoxine effective as prophylaxis and treatment against isoniazid-induced paresthesias; daily ingestion of alcohol increases risk of liver toxicity
Rifampin	600 mg PO OD	Hepatitis	Always used in combination with another drug because resistance occurs quickly if used alone; negates effect of oral contraceptives; also reduces effectiveness of coumarin derivatives, digitoxin, glucocorticoids, and methadone; liver toxicity most likely in alcoholics and in cases of preexisting liver disease; colors urine, sweat, saliva, and tears orange
Pyrazinamide	15–40 mg/kg PO OD or 50–70 mg/kg PO BIW	Hepatotoxicity	AST and ALT levels obtained before start of treatment and every 2 to 4 weeks thereafter because elevation of these enzymes is first sign of liver damage; must be taken in combination with one or more other antituberculous drugs
Ethambutol	15 mg/kg PO OD or 50 mg/kg PO BIW	Optic neuritis: blurred vision, narrowed visual fields, impaired red-green color discrimination	Always used in combination with other antituberculous drugs; generally effective agianst isoniazid- and rifampin-resistant organisms; baseline vision test at start of treatment; instruct patient to report any vision changes
Streptomycin	15 mg/kg IM OD or 25–30 mg/kg IM BIW	Eighth cranial nerve damage, nephrotoxicity, facial paresthesias, rash	Risk of hearing loss is increased in the elderly; used with caution in presence of renal disease
SECOND-LINE TREATMENT			
PAS	200 mg/kg PO OD in 4 equal doses	GI upset: nausea, vomiting, diarrhea; hepatotoxicity; hypersensitivity	Given as a sodium salt so can produce significant sodium load
Ethionamide	7–15 mg/kg PO OD in 4 equal doses	GI disturbance: anorexia, nausea, vomiting, diarrhea, metallic taste; hepatoxicity; hypersensitivity	Baseline AST and ALT levels before start of treatment and periodically thereafter
Cycloserine	10–15 mg/kg PO OD in 4 equal doses	Anxiety, depression, confusion, psychoses, convulsions, rash	Used with caution in patients with impaired renal function
Capreomycin	15 mg/kg IM OD	Nephrotoxicity; eighth cranial nerve damage: hearing loss, tinnitus, impaired balance	Give deep IM
Kanamycin	15 mg/kg IM OD	Nephrotoxicity, eighth cranial nerve damage	

Abbreviations: PO, by mouth; OD, once a day; BIW, twice weekly; AST, aspartate aminotransferase (formerly SGOT, serum glutamic-oxaloacetic transaminase); ALT, alanine aminotransferase (formerly SGPT, serum glutamic pyruvic transaminase); PAS, para-aminosalicylate; GI, gastrointestinal; IM, intramuscular.

proper therapy of infectious individuals, thus rendering them noninfectious, and identification and treatment of infected persons, thus preventing them from becoming infectious. For persons with a high risk of exposure to tuberculosis, prevention includes regular skin testing, which may be as often as every 3 months for persons in regular contact with MDR-TB patients.

BCG VACCINE

Vaccination with BCG (bacille Calmette-Guérin) derived from an attenuated strain of *Mycobacterium bovis* confers cellular immunity, as seen in naturally infected individuals, against tuberculosis with little danger of reactivation. Its predominant use is to protect people in groups with a high incidence of infection (>20%).

BCG vaccine is rarely used in the United States, where the risk factor for contagion is extremely low because the vaccination produces a positive tuberculin skin test and thus negates the value of the skin test as a method of case finding.

CHEMOPROPHYLAXIS

Because of close proximity and hence ease of transmission, chemoprophylaxis is prescribed for all members of a household of a person newly diagnosed with active tuberculosis regardless of their tuberculin status (positive or negative reactors). Chemoprophylaxis is also used for tuberculin-positive patients who are at risk for reactivation of the tubercle infection because of another health problem or its treatment. These include patients with severe, poorly controlled diabetes, neoplastic disease of the lung, and myeloid or lymphoid systems and those being treated with greater than physiologic doses of corticosteroids or with other immunosuppressive drugs.

For the adult, chemoprophylaxis against tuberculosis consists of INH, 300 mg every day for 1 year. A chemoprophylactic protocol for immunocompromised close contacts of individuals with MDR-TB consists of pyrazinamide with either ethambutol or a quinolone.

Application of the Nursing Process to the Care of the Patient with Tuberculosis

Assessment

When caring for the tuberculosis patient with clinical disease, check the temperature for slight, continued elevation with chills and night sweats, and assess lung sounds, cough, recent weight patterns, and eating habits.

Thoroughly assess the patient's understanding of the disease and its prognosis and the patient's emotional reaction to it. This is important because of the recent increase in the disease and the development of drug resistant strains and because the common strain of tuberculosis still carries a social stigma and is perceived as a dread disease leading to isolation, disability, and death by many people, particularly the older groups who saw relatives and friends die before the development of antimicrobial treatment.

Determine the patient's understanding of the transmission of the disease and methods of preventing spread. This is necessary if spread of the disease before control by antituberculosis drugs is to be prevented and to ensure that misconceptions concerning infectiousness do not result in unnecessary precautions that interfere with the quality of life.

Once a chemotherapeutic regimen has been prescribed, assess the patient's understanding of self-administration of the drugs and the need for consistent long-term therapy.

Nursing Diagnoses and Planning

Nursing diagnoses and related expected patient outcomes most commonly applicable to patients with active pulmonary tuberculosis include the following:

NDx: High risk for infection (transmission) related to lack of understanding of mode of spread or inadequate precautionary measures

Planning: Patient outcomes

1. Patient states when the disease is infectious.
2. Patient explains the mode of spread.
3. Patient describes precautions to be taken to prevent spread to other people.
4. Contacts are free of conversion to a positive tuberculin reaction.

NDx: Anxiety related to the disease, its prognosis, reaction of friends and relatives, effect on employment status, and/or possibility of transmitting it to others

Planning: Patient outcomes

1. Patient expresses belief that drug therapy will effectively control the infection.
2. Patient verbalizes confidence in ability to carry out precautionary measures to prevent transmission to others.
3. Patient is realistic in discussing import of the disease on social and work relationships.

NDx: High risk for noncompliance: drug therapy related to duration, cost, or lack of perceived importance

Planning: Patient outcomes

1. Patient describes a plan for remembering to take the medication.
2. Patient states how and where he or she is able to obtain the medication.
3. Patient verbalizes importance of taking medication as prescribed and intent to comply.
4. On follow-up examination, sputum cultures are negative and chest x-ray films improved.

NDx: High risk for altered health maintenance related to insufficient knowledge of disease, drug therapy, follow-up care

Planning: Patient outcomes

1. Patient describes cause, treatment, and prognosis of tuberculosis.
2. Patient states name, dose, route, and frequency of prescribed medication.
3. Patient explains importance of taking medication consistently for as long as ordered.
4. Patient describes supportive self-care measures, need for medical follow-up, and symptoms that require prompt reporting.

Nursing Interventions

NDx: High risk for infection (transmission)

Teach the patient how tuberculosis is spread and how to protect others from it during the infectious period, which is before and during the first 2 weeks of drug therapy. Explain the importance of careful hand washing, avoidance of direct face-to-face contact, covering the nose and mouth when coughing or sneezing, with double-thickness tissue to block small droplets, and use of a paper bag for disposal of contaminated tissues.

If hospitalization is required, maintain the patient in isolation according to CDC guidelines. Always be fastidious about hand washing, and wear a mask when caring for a patient who is acutely ill and unable to cover the mouth.

NDx: Anxiety
Provide opportunity and encouragement for the patient to discuss feelings about the diagnosis. Recognize that in some circles today tuberculosis is associated with a degree of social stigma because of its prevalence among the socially and economically deprived. Recognize also that tuberculosis still creates a great deal of fear because of publicity about its increase and the development of drug-resistant strains and because many people remember when tuberculosis was a disease basically without treatment that devastated families and often caused early death. Distinguish between tuberculosis and MDR-TB, and explain the effectiveness of drug therapy in controlling the disease and in preventing spread to both the patient and significant others. Encourage them to ask questions, and always answer honestly and clearly.

NDx: High risk for noncompliance
Because the medication schedule must be strictly adhered to if the tuberculosis is to be cured, stress the importance of this aspect of the treatment plan to both patient and family. Compliance can be difficult because of the duration and cost of treatment; therefore, assist the patient to devise a way of remembering to take the medication, such as a monthly check-off chart of scheduled doses to be hung in a corner of the bathroom mirror. Also inform the patient that antituberculosis drugs are available free of charge from most health departments throughout the country so that financial concerns do not interfere with treatment. Instruct the patient in the importance of returning for follow up tests as scheduled to protect both self and others.

NDx: High risk for altered health maintenance
Teach the patient and family about the disease and its treatment. Use teaching aids such as those available from the American Lung Association to facilitate learning. Explain prescribed drug therapy, making certain the patient knows the name, dose, route, and frequency of medication to be taken. Tell the patient that side effects to medication may occur, but stress that the drug should not be discontinued. Tell the patient to report side effects promptly so the medication regimen can be adjusted. Provide written instructions so the patient can refer to them later if needed.

Counsel the patient on the importance of plenty of rest and a nutritious diet high in protein and vitamins in supporting recuperation. Explain the importance of follow-up sputum cultures to determine that the medication is effective. Be certain that the patient understands that recurrence of symptoms or the development of hemoptysis or pleuritic pain should be immediately reported.

Additional Interventions
Collect sputum specimens in the morning as required. Have the patient cleanse the mouth and deeply cough up at least 1 teaspoon of mucus into a sterile, wide-mouthed cup. Replace the lid, and put the container in a sealed plastic bag to avoid contamination of health care workers. Specimens may be refrigerated for several hours if necessary.

Evaluation

Evaluate effectiveness of nursing care for a patient with tuberculosis by comparing the patient's status with the expected patient outcomes. Examples of specific outcomes for patients with tuberculosis have been provided in the Planning section.

Pleurisy

Pleurisy is an acute inflammation of the pleural surfaces. A synonym for pleurisy is pleuritis.

ETIOLOGY

Inflammation of the pleura is almost always a secondary effect of underlying disease. Pulmonary inflammations associated with pleurisy include tuberculosis, pneumonia, lung abscess, pulmonary embolism, and bronchiectasis. Nonpulmonary causes include rheumatic fever, disseminated lupus erythematosus, uremia, and systemic infections caused by bacteria or fungi.

PATHOPHYSIOLOGY

In the acute stage of inflammation, the pleura is red, swollen, and covered with exudate composed of fibrin, lymph, and cellular elements. Pain occurs when the parietal pleura, which contains sensory receptors for pain, touch, and temperature, rubs against the visceral pleura during respiration.

If the exudative reaction is profuse, fluid accumulates in the pleural cavity. This is called "wet" pleurisy or pleurisy with effusion.

Lung expansion in pleurisy is inhibited because of the pain on respiration and the pressure of effusion if present. If not corrected, this reduced lung expansion predisposes the patient both to atelectasis (collapse of lung tissue) and to further infection.

CLINICAL MANIFESTATIONS

The most distinctive symptom of pleurisy is chest pain, which is usually unilateral, well localized along intercostal nerve zones, and related to respiratory movements. The pain is variously described as achy, sharp, burning, a "catch," or a "stitch." It is aggravated by deep breathing, coughing, sneezing, and body movements such as turning or stooping. If the inflammation involves the diaphragmatic pleura, pain is referred to the shoulder and the throat via the phrenic nerve.

Movement of the chest on the affected side may be reduced, and the patient may hold the area or lie still on that side. If a pleural effusion is present, dyspnea may occur. However, patients with "dry" pleurisy may also complain of a feeling of difficulty breathing because the pain calls attention to a process that normally occurs unnoticed.

When the chest is auscultated, a friction rub can be heard over the inflamed area.

MEDICAL DIAGNOSIS

Diagnosis of pleurisy is made on the basis of history and clinical findings such as characteristics of the pain and presence of a friction rub on auscultation of the chest. Because pleurisy is usually not a primary disease, the underlying problem must also be identified. The speed of onset of the pleurisy is suggestive of the causative disease. Acute, immediate onset is associated with pulmonary embolism or pneumothorax; onset over a few hours, especially in the presence of fever and cough, is associated with pneumonia; and onset over a period of weeks is associated with tuberculosis or malignancy.

MEDICAL MANAGEMENT

Analgesics or intercostal blocks may be ordered for the pleuritic pain, but the main thrust of treatment is resolution of the primary disease.

Guidelines for Application of the Nursing Process to the Care of the Patient with Pleurisy

Observe breathing patterns. Note rate, depth, and symmetry of respiration. Auscultate the chest to check for presence of a friction rub. Assess for chest pain. Note the type of pain, its location, and its relation to breathing and other body movement.

Because breathing is so closely associated with life itself (e.g., the breath of life), interference with the process of breathing can produce great anxiety, so also assess the patient's emotional state.

Encourage the patient to breathe deeply every 1 to 2 hours. Change the patient's position every 2 hours, and encourage high Fowler's position when awake to facilitate chest expansion.

As diagnostic tests are done to determine the disease process causing the pleurisy, be certain the patient knows the purpose of each and when and from whom to expect the results. Reassure the patient that anxiety is normal, and encourage expression of concerns and questions. Recognize that the patient's anxiety may be compounded by feelings of not being able to breathe because of the pain, and reassure the patient regarding adequacy of respiration to meet basic needs.

Chronic Obstructive Pulmonary Disease

Millions of people in the United States suffer from some degree of chronic obstructive pulmonary disease (COPD), which can be defined as a permanent or minimally reversible degree of expiratory airflow obstruction. Such obstruction can be due to many causes. The most common are chronic bronchitis and emphysema, which almost always coexist. Regardless of specific cause, the immediate effect of COPD is that alveoli beyond the site of obstruction are insufficiently ventilated. This results in failure of the alveoli to meet the body's oxygen requirements and to rid the blood of carbon dioxide. The result is chronic hypoxemia, hypoxia, and hypercapnia.

Chronic airway obstruction primarily affects expiration, which is a passive process dependent on the inward elastic recoil of the lungs. The strength of the inspiratory muscles is sufficient to pull air past most obstructions, but lung recoil is not as powerful; therefore, the air forced in by inspiratory muscles has difficulty getting out. The result is that the expiratory phase of respiration is noticeably longer than the inspiratory phase.

Chronic obstruction directly leads to hypercapnia by impairing expiration, which causes carbon dioxide retention. It also indirectly compounds the problem of hypoxemia. The hypoxemia exists because inspiration, although not as severely blocked as expiration, is also affected. Some of the air that can be forced in by inspiration is trapped in the alveoli by expiratory difficulty. As breathing continues, this oxygen-depleted air takes up room, limits the amount of oxygen-rich fresh air that can be inspired, and dilutes whatever is inspired.

The increased work of breathing results in a paradoxical problem. The inspiratory muscles, which are working harder to get air into the lungs, require help from the accessory muscles. When lung recoil is unable to move the air out, muscular assistance is again required to force expiration. All of this additional muscular activity uses up oxygen; thus, the very process that provides oxygen also consumes more than the normal requirement. The net effect is that breathing efficiency (oxygen provided by breathing compared with oxygen consumed by the act of breathing) is significantly reduced in the patient who so desperately needs oxygen.

Compensatory processes take place in the body in the presence of chronic obstructive airflow. The heart compensates for hypoxemia by increasing its output to make up for the blood's oxygen deficit. Further, pulmonary capillaries constrict around the insufficiently ventilated alveoli, diverting the blood to more normal areas of the lung. As this chronic condition progresses, the area of involved lung increases so constriction becomes widespread. This forces the right side of the heart to pump harder to push blood through a vasculature blocked by constriction.

Prolonged hypoxemia causes the body to produce more red blood cells (polycythemia), which creates a blood that is more viscous than normal, making it more difficult to move through the blood vessels and again increasing the work for the right side of the heart. The increased work of pumping more and thicker blood through and around constricted vessels results in pulmonary hypertension (high blood pressure in the pulmonary circulation). Over time, the pulmonary hypertension, coupled with the failure to receive adequate oxygen, results in cor pulmonale (disease of the right side of the heart secondary to disease of the lungs; see Chapter 18).

Chronic Bronchitis

Chronic bronchitis is clinically defined as an excess secretion of mucus, which is a consequence of an increase in the size and number of the seromucus-secreting structures in the bronchi.

ETIOLOGY

Chronic bronchitis is usually caused by prolonged exposure to bronchial irritants such as smoking, air pollution, toxic fumes, and dust in the work place. It is more prevalent in males than in females, occurs more frequently in whites than nonwhites, and is more common in city dwellers than those who live in the country. Cigarette smoking is the most consistently important factor in the development of chronic bronchitis.

PATHOPHYSIOLOGY

In chronic bronchitis, inflammation of the bronchi with enlargement and hypersecretion of the mucous glands causes obstruction of expiratory airflow and results in the characteristic changes of COPD. Ventilation-perfusion mismatching develops because areas of inflammation and retained secretions do not occur uniformly throughout the lungs. Repeated infections with persistent obstruction can lead to scarring, necrosis, and destruction of small bronchioles.

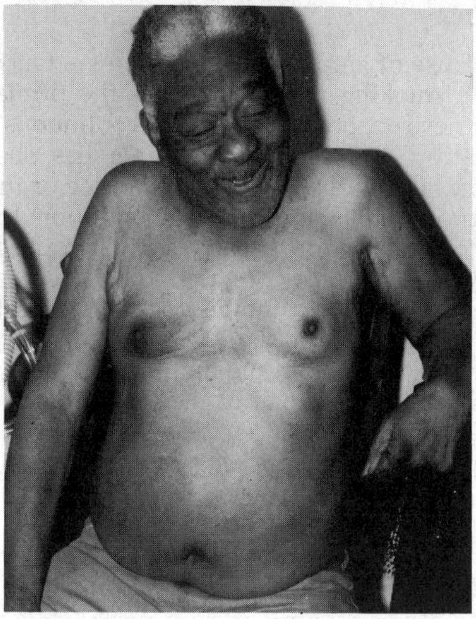

Figure 14–5.

Individual with chronic bronchitis and all the classic findings of the "blue bloater": stocky body build, no history of marked weight loss, onset of symptoms between ages 40 and 50, main complaint of sputum production, low PaO_2, high $PaCO_2$, cyanotic, dependent edema, episodes of right-sided heart failure, and variable clinical course. (From Kersten LD. Comprehensive respiratory nursing: A decision making approach. Philadelphia: WB Saunders, 1989, p 109.)

CLINICAL MANIFESTATIONS

Chronic bronchitis is characterized by repeated episodes of bronchial inflammation with a heavy, productive cough, particularly at night. These episodes persist for months at a time and are generally worse during the cold, damp weather.

The onset of chronic bronchitis is gradual, with the patient frequently describing a "smoker's cough." As the disease progresses, the cough becomes continuous. Dyspnea becomes more severe. Cyanosis is common secondary to the chronic hypoxemia, hypoxia, and hypercapnia caused by the airway obstruction. Generalized edema is also often present, and this swollen appearance, together with the cyanosis, gives rise to the phrase "blue bloater" (Fig. 14–5) used to describe these patients. Other clinical manifestations are those mentioned previously as effects of COPD and include clubbing of the fingers as a result of secondary polycythemia (see Fig. 12–8).

Emphysema

Pulmonary emphysema is defined as a chronically progressive disease in which there is enlargement of the air spaces distal to the terminal nonrespiratory bronchioles with destruction of the alveolar walls.

ETIOLOGY

The cause of emphysema is unknown. Once again, cigarette smoking is implicated as the primary reason for destruction, although any continuous irritant can destroy alveoli. Some research has shown an apparent failure of the connective tissue of the lungs to be protected against protein digestion from enzymes released from the alveolar macrophages and leukocytes. The theory suggests that when there are not enough enzyme inhibitors to control the enzymes released from the macrophages and leukocytes, tissue damage in the lung occurs. A deficiency of alpha-antitrypsin, one of the main agents inhibiting the action of these enzymes, may be a genetic factor related to the incidence of emphysema, which occurs in the third or fourth decade of life.

PATHOPHYSIOLOGY

The changes in the lung parenchyma involve the loss of elasticity. The elastic structure around the alveoli dissolves, resulting in stiffening of the lungs and decreased compliance. The loss of alveolar function diminishes lung recoil. Normally, each of the tiny alveolar walls offers resistance to stretching. As the lung expands during inspiration, these walls are stretched like tiny springs and each pulls back against the stretching. During relaxation of the inspiratory muscles at the end of inspiration, these combined pulls lower intrapleural pressure and draw the chest wall inward, forcing expiration. At the end of expiration, the conflicting pulls of the lung inward and the chest wall outward balance each other, thus producing the normal configuration of the chest at rest.

In the presence of emphysema, many of these inward pulls are lost. Expiration is weakened by the loss of lung recoil. Because less opposition is offered to the outward pull of the chest wall, the chest is partly expanded at the end of expiration, producing a visible "barrel chest" over time.

Emphysema, like chronic bronchitis, may result in pulmonary hypertension and cor pulmonale, as discussed earlier. Also, like chronic bronchitis, it results in a hypoxic drive to respiration; that is, because of gradually increasing levels of carbon dioxide in the blood over a long period of time, the primary stimulus to breathe comes from a decrease in oxygen rather than from an increase in carbon dioxide, as in persons with normal respiratory function. Therefore, the borderline or diminishing ventilatory drive may be further suppressed by increasing the arterial oxygen pressure (PaO_2).

Emphysema is classified into two main types: centrilobular emphysema and panlobular emphysema.

Centrilobular emphysema affects the central portion of the lung lobule close to the respiratory bronchiole. This type of emphysema is localized, and there may be unaffected units of lung tissue surrounding the affected areas. Centrilobular is the more common type and is more prevalent in males than in females. It is usually associated with chronic bronchitis and is very seldom found in nonsmokers.

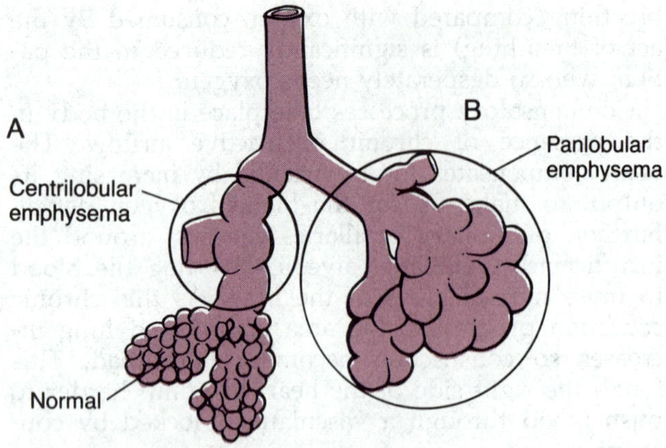

Figure 14–6.

A, Centrilobular emphysema. The center of the pulmonary lobule at the level of the respiratory bronchiole is destroyed. *B*, Panlobular emphysema. Tends to be more diffuse, with the entire primary lobule involved and destruction and distention distal to the respiratory bronchioles.

Panlobular emphysema is the destruction and dilatation of the bronchioles and alveoli within a lobule in which the entire acinus is involved. This type tends to be diffuse and is more severe in the lower lung areas. Panlobular emphysema occurs equally among males and females but is more frequent in older patients who do not have chronic bronchitis or clinical impairment of lung function. Panlobular and centrilobular emphysema, which are compared in Figure 14–6, may occur together or separately.

CLINICAL MANIFESTATIONS

Emphysema unaccompanied by chronic bronchitis, bronchiectasis, or the like causes the insidious development of the following symptoms:

- Dyspnea (the hallmark of emphysema), which worsens over time, may be present at rest and is severe on exertion
- Pursed-lip breathing with prolonged expiration
- Increased anteroposterior diameter of the chest, or barrel chest
- Use of accessory muscles of respiration, especially the sternocleidomastoid and the pectoral muscles
- Hyperresonance of the chest to percussion
- Breath sounds and heart sounds that are distant, absent, or dull
- Anorexia
- Weakness

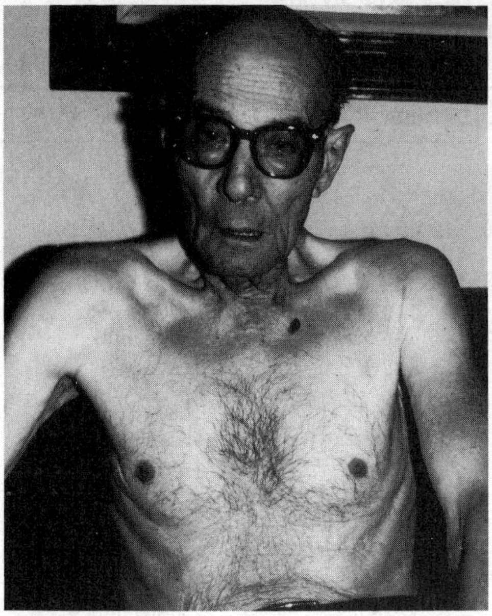

Figure 14–7.

Individual with emphysema and all the classic findings of the "pink puffer": cachectic appearance, history of weight loss, onset of symptoms between ages 50 and 75, main complaint of shortness of breath and cough, normal PaO_2 and $PaCO_2$, normal skin coloration, no edema, no history of right-sided heart failure, and persistent downhill course. Use of accessory muscles of respiration (intercostal, neck, and shoulder muscles) and the cachectic appearance reflect the patient's shortness of breath and the tremendously increased work of breathing necessary to increase minute ventilation and maintain normal arterial blood gas levels. (From Kersten LD. Comprehensive respiratory nursing: A decision making approach. Philadelphia: WB Saunders, 1989, p 109.)

- Decreased muscle mass
- Weight loss

The patient's color is normal until very late in the disease because, in uncomplicated emphysema, compensatory mechanisms are able to provide for adequate oxygenation for an extended length of time. Thus, emphysema patients are referred to as "pink puffers" (Fig. 14–7) as opposed to the oxygen-starved "blue bloaters" with chronic bronchitis.

During the later stages of emphysema, so much carbon dioxide can be retained that it acts as an anesthetic and causes carbon dioxide narcosis. This results in the neurologic symptoms of late emphysema, which include occipital headache, decreased ability to concentrate, and drowsiness. The hands are warm, the pulse is bounding, and the arterial carbon dioxide pressure ($PaCO_2$) levels are found to be greater than 75 mm Hg. Asterixis (flapping tremor), confusion, and coma can result.

In reality, this clinical picture of emphysema is usually complicated by symptoms of coexisting disease of the bronchial airways such as chronic bronchitis because emphysema rarely occurs alone (Table 14–5). Thus, the patient with emphysema generally has a history of cigarette smoking, chronic cough with expectoration, wheezing, and frequent respiratory infections and inspirational coarse crackles heard at the base of the lungs.

MEDICAL DIAGNOSIS

COPD is diagnosed, and severity of disease is determined, on the basis of pulmonary function studies. Characteristic findings include the following: decreased forced expiratory volume (FEV), prolonged expiration, decreased maximum voluntary ventilation (MVV), decreased forced vital capacity (FVC), increased total lung capacity (TLC), and increased residual volume (RV).

Diagnosis is rarely made on the basis of chest x-ray films, although characteristic changes can be identified as the disease progresses. These include an enlarged thoracic cage; a flattened, low diaphragm; the appearance of the heart as elongated and narrow; wider than normal intercostal spaces; blebs and bullae in the lung apices and bases; and dilated bronchioles.

MEDICAL MANAGEMENT

Medical management of COPD is designed to control symptoms and to prevent further deterioration of respiratory status.

Table 14–5. CLINICAL MANIFESTATIONS OF COPD: PREDOMINANT CHRONIC BRONCHITIS VERSUS PREDOMINANT PULMONARY EMPHYSEMA

MANIFESTATION	PREDOMINANT CHRONIC BRONCHITIS (BLUE BLOATER)	PREDOMINANT PULMONARY EMPHYSEMA (PINK PUFFER)
Cough	Early, before onset of dyspnea	Occurs late, after onset of dyspnea
Sputum	Copious, purulent	Scanty, mucoid
Weight loss	Absent or slight	Often marked
Dyspnea	Mild	Usually chief complaint
Chest X-ray films	Enlarged heart, bronchoalveolar markings, normal diaphragm position	Low, flat diaphragm; long, narrow cardiac silhouette
Carbon dioxide retention	Common	Uncommon
Cor pulmonale	Common	Rare

Table 14–6. SPEED OF ONSET AND DURATION OF ACTION OF BRONCHODILATORS USED TO TREAT CHRONIC OBSTRUCTIVE PULMONARY DISEASE

BRONCHODILATOR	DURATION	SPEED OF ONSET
FAST ACTING		
Beta-Antagonists* (metered dose inhalers)		
Albuterol (Proventil, Ventolin)	4–6 hr	1–3 min
Bitolterol (Tornalate)	4–8 hr	1–3 min
Isoetharine (Bronkometer, Bronkosol)	2–4 hr	1–3 min
Isoproterenol (Isuprel)	1–2 hr	1–3 min
Metaproterenol (Alupent, Metaprel)	4–6 hr	1–3 min
Terbutaline (Brethaire)	4–6 hr	1–3 min
SHORT ACTING		
Theophylline (Elixophyllin)	4–8 hr	30–60 min
Aminophyline (Aminophyllin)	4–8 hr	30–60 min
Oxtriphylline (Choledyl, Brondecon)	6–10 hr	30–60 min
SUSTAINED RELEASE		
Theophylline (Slo-bid, Theo-Dur)	8–14 hr	30–60 min
ULTRA-LONG SUSTAINED RELEASE		
Anhydrous theophylline (Theo-24, Uniphyl)	14–24 hr	30–60 min
ANTICHOLINERGIC		
Ipratropium (Atrovent)	3–4 hr	15 min

*Oral beta-antagonists often take 1 hr to begin working, and the action of the drug does not last as long as the inhaled beta-antagonist. Taken orally, they also produce more side effects because of systemic absorption.

Bronchodilators (Table 14–6 and Pharmacology Box 12–3) are prescribed to treat bronchospasm. Initially they are given in the largest doses that can be tolerated by the patient to relieve any reversible bronchospasm present. Subsequently, theophyllines are prescribed in doses necessary to maintain blood levels of 10 to 20 mEq/ml to prevent future episodes of bronchospasm. These maintenance doses are often given in conjunction with β-adrenergic drugs.

In some cases, a trial series of corticosteroids such as prednisone, 20 to 40 mg per day, may be given for 3 to 4 weeks. If improvement is seen on pulmonary function tests, the drug is slowly decreased to the lowest effective maintenance dose. If no improvement occurs, the steroids are discontinued gradually over 1 to 2 weeks.

Antibiotics are ordered for secondary infections. If the sputum becomes purulent, the patient is given a course of 1 g per day of ampicillin or tetracycline. If infection is recurrent, 0.5 to 1 g of tetracycline may be given daily or the patient may be given tetracycline and instructed to take it for 7 to 10 days if purulent sputum or other signs of lower respiratory tract infection develop.

Influenza and pneumonia vaccines are given to protect against these infections. During influenza epidemics when type-specific vaccines are not available, amantadine given prophylactically is considered.

Measures are also prescribed as needed to remove secretions from the airways which interfere with ventilation and predispose to infection. Measures used depend on the patient's response and include inhalation of bronchodilator aerosols followed by bland-mist inhalations, deep breathing, coughing, chest percussion and vibration, and postural drainage.

For the critically ill patient, bronchoscopic removal of secretions, endotracheal intubation, or tracheostomy may be necessary to effectively remove secretions, prevent mucous plugging, and provide ventilatory assistance. These patients most generally are in acute respiratory failure.

Oxygen therapy is administered to maintain a PaO_2 between 50 and 60 mm Hg at a flow rate not exceeding 1 to 3 L/minute. If mechanical ventilation is necessary, the intermittent mandatory ventilation (IMV) technique is used. IMV allows the patient to breathe spontaneously, with the exact amount of additional minute ventilation required to be delivered by the machine. Long-term treatment may include low-flow oxygen for a period of 12 to 15 hours per day. This low-flow oxygen relieves pulmonary hypertension and polycythemia, increases exercise tolerance, and improves mental function by correcting hypoxemia. Research indicates that low-flow oxygen does not prolong the life of patients with COPD; however, it does decrease the number of hospitalizations, which is a great benefit to the patient both psychologically and economically.

A program of exercise is prescribed unless a cardiac or other problem exists that contraindicates it. Exercise does not directly affect the underlying disease, but it does train the skeletal muscles to work more effectively and can increase the patient's ability for self-care and participation in household and social activities.

Other important aspects of treatment are instruction in breathing techniques to maximize ventilation and to control dyspnea, avoidance of smoke and other pollutants and irritants, and psychosocial counseling and vocational rehabilitation.

Application of the Nursing Process to the Care of the Patient with Chronic Obstructive Pulmonary Disease

Assessment

Obtain a thorough history. Include information about the patient's environment, work history, exercise patterns, smoking habits, and the onset and development of symptoms.

Ask whether the symptoms are worse at any particular time of the year or whether they are aggravated by any particular activities (symptoms of chronic bronchitis are usually worse in the cold weather, after intake of alcohol, or after talking for an extended time).

Question the patient about sleeping positions. This helps to differentiate cardiac dysfunction from emphysema. Because persons with cardiac disease have a greater total vital capacity in the sitting or standing position, they are more comfortable sleeping with the head of the bed elevated, whereas those with emphysema are more comfortable sleeping in a flat position because their total vital capacity is greater in the supine position.

Also question the patient about signs and symptoms of peptic ulcer and inguinal hernia, because these two problems are frequently associated with emphysema. Hernia is frequent because of increased pressure and strain created by the frequent hacking cough of emphysema. The factors contributing to concurrent peptic ulcers are cigarette smoking, prolonged hypoxia, and the emotional factors that are related to the occurrence of both emphysema and peptic ulcers.

Review results of all diagnostic studies such as arterial blood gases, pulmonary function tests, and x-ray films.

On physical examination, assess for signs of heavy smoking such as tobacco-stained fingers. Observe for clubbing, distended neck veins on expiration, the presence of a barrel chest with its abnormally large anteroposterior diameter, and a characteristic sinking of the tissues around the neck and supraclavicular spaces. Look for enlargement and active use of the sternocleidomastoid and pectoral muscles. Note any outward flaring motion of the lower rib margins and widening of the subcostal angle. Observe for abdominal breathing, the use of pursed-lip breathing, and chest movements that are singular movements rather than rhythmic. Auscultate the chest, and listen for musical wheezes characteristic of chronic bronchitis and for distant, dull, or absent heart sounds that are associated with moderately severe or severe emphysema.

Assess general physical status, because patients with advanced emphysema are often thin or even emaciated.

Assess the patient's emotional response to the illness as well as available support systems such as significant others and financial and community resources.

Nursing Diagnoses and Planning

Nursing diagnoses and related expected patient outcomes most commonly applicable to patients with COPD include the following:

NDx: Ineffective airway clearance related to excessive, viscous secretions

Planning: Patient outcomes

1. Patient uses nebulizer and medication as ordered.
2. Patient uses breathing exercise techniques during treatments.
3. Patient coughs productively after treatments.
4. Patient uses positioning techniques to help drain lungs after treatments.

NDx: Impaired gas exchange related to impaired expiration and carbon dioxide retention

Planning: Patient outcomes

1. Patient uses oxygen therapy equipment correctly.
2. Patient describes precautions necessary with use of oxygen.
3. Patient lists signs of hypoxia and hypercapnia to be reported.

NDx: Ineffective breathing pattern related to increased work of breathing and associated increased need for oxygen

Planning: Patient outcomes

1. Patient practices consciously controlling the inspiratory-expiratory (I:E) ratio, particularly when shortness of breath occurs.
2. Patient uses diaphragmatic breathing to control dyspnea.
3. Patient exhales through pursed lips.
4. Patient uses relaxation therapy techniques.

NDx: Activity intolerance related to inadequate oxygenation

Planning: Patient outcomes

1. Patient participates in a program of aerobic exercise.
2. Patient describes four basic techniques of energy conservation.

NDx: High risk for ineffective individual coping related to chronic disease, its effects, and its treatments

Planning: Patient outcomes
1. Patient verbalizes anxieties and fears.
2. Patient identifies changes in lifestyle necessitated by the disease.
3. Patient describes a realistic plan for introducing lifestyle changes.

NDx: High risk for altered health maintenance related to insufficient knowledge of prevention, identification, and treatment of respiratory complications of COPD

Planning: Patient outcomes
1. Patient lists ways to avoid irritation of the respiratory tract.
2. Patient identifies methods of avoiding respiratory tract infection.
3. Patient describes use of prophylactic antibiotics correctly.
4. Patient lists symptoms to be reported.

Nursing Interventions

NDx: Ineffective airway clearance
Essential to the improvement of ventilation and ease of the work of breathing are dilatation of the bronchi and removal of obstructing secretions.

Administer bronchodilator drugs as ordered. They may be given orally, subcutaneously, intravenously, or rectally or may be given by nebulization. Nebulized aerosols relieve bronchospasm, decrease mucosal edema, and liquefy bronchial secretions and thus improve ventilatory function. Because nebulized drugs can be delivered by pressurized aerosols, hand-bulb nebulizers, compressor-driven and ultrasonic nebulizers (Fig. 14–8), or IPPB and are used in the home as well as the hospital, teach the patient how to self-administer the drug and how to obtain the needed equipment. Instruct the patient to follow inhalation of bronchodilator aerosols with postural drainage, coughing, and moist inhalations as ordered to promote expectoration and to end the treatment with thorough oral hygiene. Instruct the patient to use the nebulizer before meals to improve lung ventilation and to reduce fatigue associated with eating. Also instruct the patient to use it before events known to precipitate symptoms.

Be certain to monitor the therapeutic effect of the bronchodilator drugs and for side effects such as tachycardia, cardiac dysrhythmias, and central nervous system excitation. The latter is particularly important because a guiding principle of bronchodilator therapy is to administer the maximum dose tolerated by the patient.

Increase fluids to 2 to 3 L/day (unless contraindicated) to replace fluid lost through mouth breathing and thus help to keep secretions liquid. If needed, administer water via a nebulizer to humidify the bronchial tree and add water to the viscous sputum to make expectoration easier.

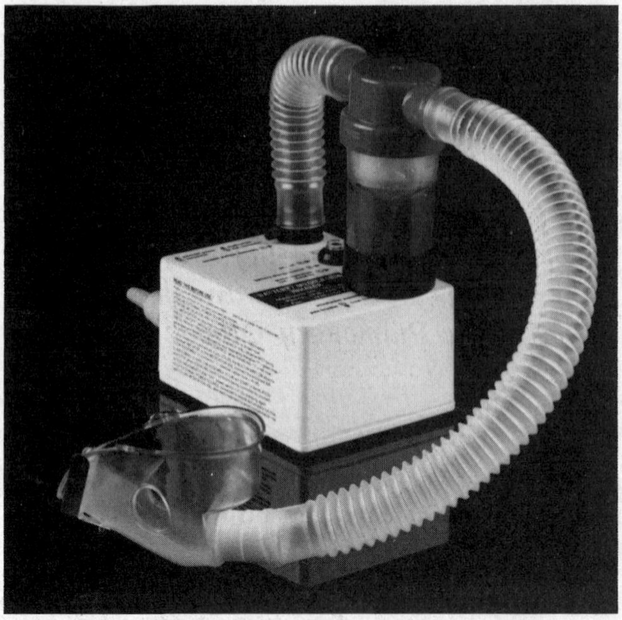

Figure 14–8.

Spiral 3612 portable ultrasonic drug inhaler. (Courtesy of Medisonic USA, Inc., Clarence, NY.)

NDx: Impaired gas exchange
Administer oxygen as ordered, and teach appropriate safety measures. If it has been determined during hospitalization that the patient has a low arterial oxygen level and continuous home oxygen therapy is required, explain the need for regular measurement of arterial blood gas levels to the patient and significant others. Also explain the hypoxic drive to breathe in both chronic bronchitis and emphysema, and caution about using the oxygen only as ordered by the physician, never increasing the flow.

Review the signs and symptoms of hypoxia and hypercapnia with the patient and significant others, and stress the need to report them at once to the responsible health professional, because the appearance of these symptoms may indicate impending respiratory failure. They are increased shortness of breath, restlessness, lethargy, headache, and confusion.

NDx: Ineffective breathing pattern
Three breathing techniques promote good ventilation, ease the work of breathing, and assist in the control of dyspnea: I:E ratio control, diaphragmatic breathing, and pursed-lip breathing.

Inspiratory-Expiratory Ratio Control
I:E ratio control is used to decrease the work of breathing and to control dyspnea during stress and activity.

During quiet breathing, the I:E ratio represents

the efficiency of the breathing pattern. Normally, the exhalation phase of the breathing cycle is passive and longer than the inspiratory phase. In the patient with COPD, however, expiration requires active muscular work because of the resistance to airflow. As demand on the respiratory system increases with activity or stress, the rate and depth of respiration increase and inspiration begins to take more time than expiration. This leaves the patient feeling short of breath as he or she struggles to draw more air in without leaving sufficient time for the air to be exhaled.

Severe uncontrolled dyspnea can be prevented if the patient is able to control the I:E ratio so that expiration is three to four times longer than inspiration. To accomplish this, instruct the patient to practice timing the inhalation and exhalation portions of breathing patterns at rest. When the patient is able to do this easily at rest, have the patient practice consciously controlling the I:E ratio in various situations, particularly when shortness of breath is noticed. This type of practice not only allows the patient to prevent severe uncontrolled shortness of breath but also aids the patient in regaining control of breathing patterns when shortness of breath does occur.

Diaphragmatic Breathing

Diaphragmatic breathing assists the patient in using the diaphragm rather than the accessory muscles to breathe. Because smaller muscles use more oxygen than large ones, using the diaphragm decreases the work of breathing. Diaphragmatic breathing also increases the volume of air exchanged during a normal breathing effort and enhances the distribution of the inhaled air. Several similar techniques for practicing diaphragmatic breathing are available. One of these methods is described here.

To practice diaphragmatic breathing, instruct the patient to lie down and place the left hand on the chest just below the collar bone to feel any motion of the rib cage. The right hand is placed on the area above the navel and just below the rib cage, with the palm down and the smallest finger reaching the navel and the thumb resting on the sternum (Fig. 14–9). Next, tell the patient to take deep breaths through the nose and at the same time allow the area under the palm of the right hand to rise. Instruct the patient to use pursed-lip breathing on expiration, which should be timed to be twice as long as inhalation.

If diaphragmatic breathing is being done properly, the rib cage under the left hand does not move and the abdominal wall below the navel does not rise higher than the area under the right hand. If it does rise higher, the patient is using unnecessary abdominal muscles.

If needed, help patients master this breathing technique by placing a book on the upper abdomen and watching it rise and fall with inspiration and expiration.

Once the technique is perfected, it can be practiced when sitting, standing, walking, and running or during any activity that induces dyspnea. It is unlikely that the patient will ever use diaphragmatic breathing continuously; however, with practice it can be used to control dyspnea without fear.

Pursed-Lip Breathing

Pursing the lips creates resistance to airflow, thereby slowing expiration and increasing pressure in the airways. This results in pressure greater than that in the alveoli and so the airways are supported in their open position. This allows for more complete emptying of the alveoli on exhalation, leaving less trapped air and allowing more fresh air to enter the lungs with each breath.

Instruct the patient to assume conscious control of the I:E ratio, use diaphragmatic breathing, and exhale through pursed lips (as if to whistle), maintaining a relaxed exhalation. Have the patient practice slow, relaxed, pursed-lip exhalations by blowing bubbles in a glass of water with a straw or by blowing a ping-pong ball steadily across a table.

NDx: Activity intolerance

A program of gradually increasing aerobic exercises (exercises that require a prolonged muscular effort and depend on inspired oxygen for energy) is used to train the skeletal muscles to work more efficiently and to increase the patient's tolerance for physical activity. The type and amount of exercise are recommended by the physician, and the program is carried out by the physical therapist or nurse, or both. Common aerobic exercises used for COPD patients include treadmill or walking, stationary bicycle, stair climbing, and bouncing on a minitrampoline. Typical exercise plans are 10 minutes a day four to five times a week. It may take from 2 to 6 weeks on an exercise program for the muscles to increase endurance and produce more work with

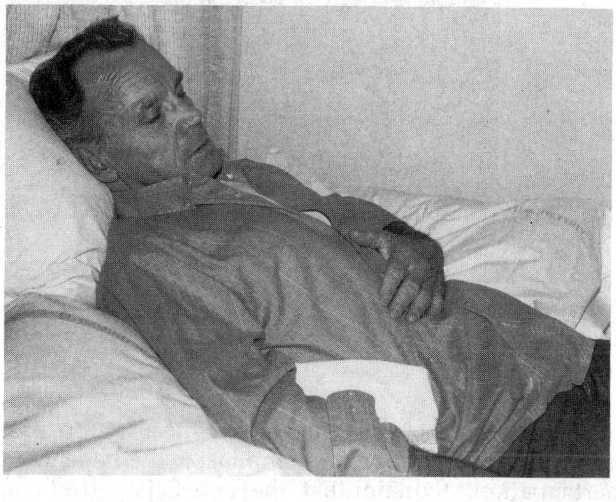

Figure 14–9.

Position of patient practicing diaphragmatic breathing. (From Kersten LD. Comprehensive respiratory nursing: A decision making approach. Philadelphia: WB Saunders, 1989, p 532.)

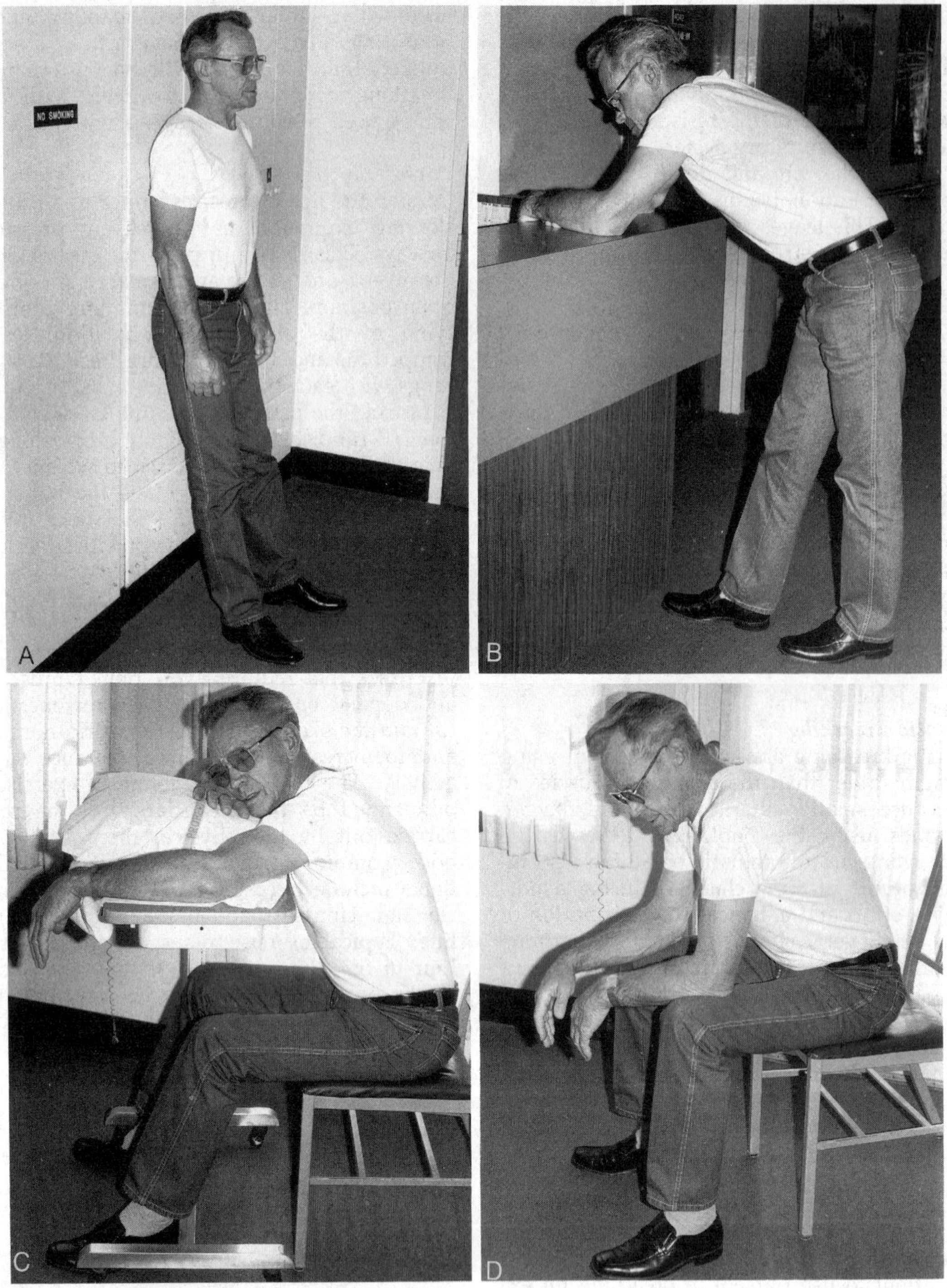

Figure 14–10.

Basic positions of rest to avoid fatigue and dyspnea. (From Kersten LD. Comprehensive respiratory nursing: A decision making approach. Philadelphia: WB Saunders, 1989, p 518.)

less effort. Review the purpose of the exercise program with the patient, and emphasize the benefits of participation. Explain that the beneficial effects of the exercise program last only as long as the program is continued. Point out that, within 6 weeks of not exercising, more than 50% of the gains are lost. Stress that exercise plans are progressive—small steps and at a speed that allows comfortable breathing.

Because patients with COPD need assistance with conserving energy, explore methods of energy conservation with them. Review stress-management techniques, and help eliminate possible sources of tension in daily life. Teach physical and mental relaxation techniques for use in stress-producing situations. Assist the patient to identify work-simplification strategies (i.e., ways to perform tasks at minimal energy costs) and measures to promote restful sleep. Overall, encourage the patient to consciously adopt a slower pace of living, to periodically assume a basic resting position (Fig. 14–10), and to space activities around these periods of rest.

NDx: High risk for ineffective individual coping

Although some patients adjust to chronic disease and cooperate with all modalities of treatment, many display denial and repression, resentment, anger, and anxiety. Depression is common and, in many instances, the psychological and emotional problems affect the patient's response to the overall treatment program. Be aware of these responses, and acknowledge the feelings of these patients. Answer all questions honestly, listen to the patient attentively, and provide clear, concise information about the condition. Through understanding of the condition and management of symptoms, the patient will be better able to cope with chronic respiratory disease.

If a change in job status is necessitated, refer the patient to a vocational counselor. In some instances, it may not be necessary to change jobs: It may be possible simply to alter the job description to accommodate the new level of functioning. If it is not possible for the patient to return to gainful employment, it is important that the health team launch a major effort aimed at achieving maximal self-care and minimizing dependence on the patient's family and the community.

NDx: High risk for altered health maintenance

Instruct the patient in the prevention and treatment of respiratory irritation and infection, as specified in Chart 14–3.

If the patient is a smoker, explain the importance of changing the habit. Provide information on readily available smoking cessation programs, and if possible, arrange for a meeting with another person with COPD who has successfully stopped smoking.

If patients have antibiotics on hand that the physician has instructed them to take at the first sign of a cold, review their proper use, including dose and frequency of administration.

To monitor for the onset of right-sided heart failure, instruct the patient to weigh himself or herself daily and to report a gain of 5.5 lb (2.5 kg) or more because this could be due to fluid retention.

Additional Interventions

A nutritional program designed to meet the needs of the particular patient is necessary if systemic complications are to be avoided. See Nutrition Box 14–2 for specific guidelines for meeting nutritional needs of patients with chronic obstructive lung disease.

Chart 14–3.

NURSING GUIDE TO PATIENT EDUCATION FOR SELF-MANAGEMENT: PREVENTION AND TREATMENT OF RESPIRATORY IRRITATION AND INFECTION IN PATIENTS WITH COPD

To prevent irritation and infection of the airways, instruct the patient to:

Avoid exposure to cigarette, pipe, and cigar smoke as well as to dusts and powders.
Avoid use of aerosol sprays.
Stay indoors when the pollen count is high.
Stay indoors when temperature and humidity are both high.
Use air conditioning to help decrease pollutants and control temperature.
Avoid exposure to persons known to have colds or other respiratory tract infections.
Avoid enclosed, crowded areas during cold and flu season.
Obtain immunization against influenza and streptococcal pneumonia.

To ensure prompt, effective treatment of a developing respiratory infection, instruct the patient to do the following:

Report any change in sputum color or character, increased tightness of the chest, increased dyspnea, or fatigue.
Call the physician if ordered antibiotics do not relieve symptoms within 24 hours.

Nutrition Box 14–2.

NUTRITION: SPECIAL CONSIDERATIONS FOR PATIENTS WITH CHRONIC OBSTRUCTIVE PULMONARY DISEASE (COPD)

Instruct patients with COPD to:

Use microwave oven to help decrease preparation time and conserve energy.
Sit at a table with elbows supported when preparing food to help conserve energy.
Use convenience foods, if appropriate. (Note: Some patients require sodium restrictions and must be instructed to read labels carefully.)
Plan rest periods for 30 minutes before eating to decrease dyspnea.
Avoid exercise and treatments at least 1 hour before and after eating.
Consume liquid, blenderized, or commercial foods to help decrease a "full" stomach, because a full stomach puts pressure on the diaphragm and decreases lung movement.
Avoid large meals and gas-forming foods, which contribute to abdominal distention.
Plan for fluid intake of at least 3 L/day unless contraindicated.
Space fluid intake between meals to prevent abdominal distention.
Maintain ideal weight or a weight slightly below ideal, because restricted activity limits calories required and extra weight may aggravate condition.

Instruct patients on theophylline or antipyrine therapy to:

Maintain regular eating patterns, because high-protein intake decreases half-lives of these drugs and high-carbohydrate intake increases the half-life.
Avoid use of caffeine-containing products (coffee, tea, soft drinks), because they may compound effects of theophylline-like derivatives in them.
Use caution with charcoal-broiled foods, which increase theophylline elimination (may reduce half-life as much as 50%).

Because patients with "pink puffer" COPD require more protein and calories than normal, instruct them to:

Divide their high-protein, high-calorie diet into several small meals.

Evaluation

Evaluate the effectiveness of nursing care for a patient with COPD by comparing the patient's status with the expected patient outcomes. Examples of specific outcomes for patients with COPD have been provided in the Planning section.

Bronchiectasis

Bronchiectasis is a disease in which there is permanent abnormal dilatation and distortion of the bronchi or the bronchioles (Fig. 14–11). This structural change may be in an isolated segment or widespread throughout the bronchial tubes.

ETIOLOGY

Bronchiectasis may be congenital or acquired. It is associated with various hereditary immunodeficiency diseases and with Kartagener's and other immotile cilia syndromes. Diffuse bronchiectasis is seen in patients with cystic fibrosis, asthma, and bronchitis, whereas localized disease is seen in patients with lung tumors and foreign bodies in the respiratory tree. In most cases, it appears that an obstruction in the lung prevents clearance of the airway and leads to infection, which in turn results in the structural changes of bronchiectasis.

PATHOPHYSIOLOGY

Infection in the wall of a bronchus or bronchiole causes changes in normal tissue structure. Smooth muscle and elastic tissue are impaired, and ciliated columnar epithelium is replaced with nonciliated cuboidal epithelium or fibrous tissue. These changes result in dilated, distorted areas of the bronchial tree, which in turn make airway clearance even more difficult and thus predispose to more infection, which can cause further structural damage.

CLINICAL MANIFESTATIONS

There are no clinical manifestations caused by bronchial dilatation itself; rather, symptoms result from associated recurrent infection and hypersecretion of mucus.

A cough productive of large amounts of mucopurulent sputum, particularly in the morning, is characteristic of bronchiectasis. The sputum is unique in two ways. First, it has a rather sickeningly sweet odor from being caught and stagnating in the dilated areas of the bronchial passages where microorganisms grow freely. Second, on standing in a container, it visibly settles into three distinct layers: cloudy on top, clear saliva in the center, and heavy, thick, purulent matter at the bottom.

Other symptoms that may occur are hemoptysis, which may be profuse, malaise, fatigue, and exertional dyspnea, which in advanced disease may progress to cor pulmonale.

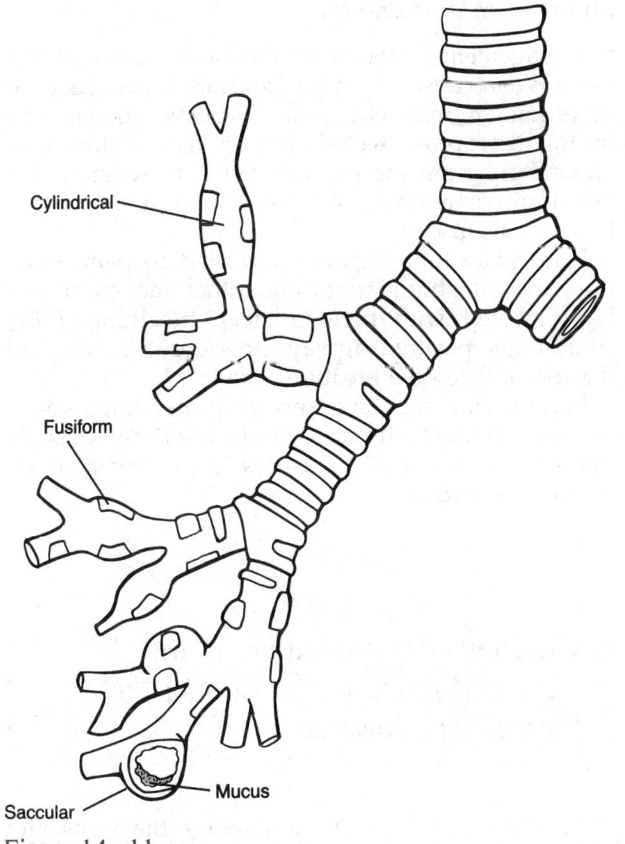

Figure 14–11.

Varieties of bronchiectasis based on type of dilatation of the bronchi. In the saccular form of bronchiectasis, secretions are caught and remain stagnant.

MEDICAL DIAGNOSIS

Diagnosis of bronchiectasis is suggested by a history of persistent cough with copious expectoration and presence of moist, coarse crackles over the affected area. Diagnosis is confirmed by bronchography, which demonstrates the dilated airways.

MEDICAL MANAGEMENT

Management of bronchiectasis is aimed at control of infection, removal of secretions, and avoidance of irritants. Antimicrobial drugs are used to control infection. Because *Haemophilus*, pneumococci, and various anaerobes are the most common causative organisms, ampicillin is usually the drug of choice unless the patient is allergic to penicillin, in which case tetracycline is prescribed. Postural therapy and adequate hydration are used to promote removal of secretions, and oxygen is given as needed.

Application of the Nursing Process to the Care of the Patient with Bronchiectasis

The assessment, nursing diagnoses, expected patient outcomes, nursing interventions, and evaluation for patients with bronchiectasis are similar to those described previously for patients with chronic bronchitis and emphysema. Assess respiratory function carefully, and determine the extent to which it is capable of supporting the patient in carrying out usual activities. Be certain to observe for hemoptysis. In terms of intervention, a major focus is patient education. Stress the importance of avoiding respiratory irritants and sources of infection and the need for vaccination against influenza and pneumonia.

Atelectasis

Atelectasis (localized hypoaeration) is a partial or complete collapse of lung tissue that has previously been expanded (Fig. 14–12). It commonly occurs in

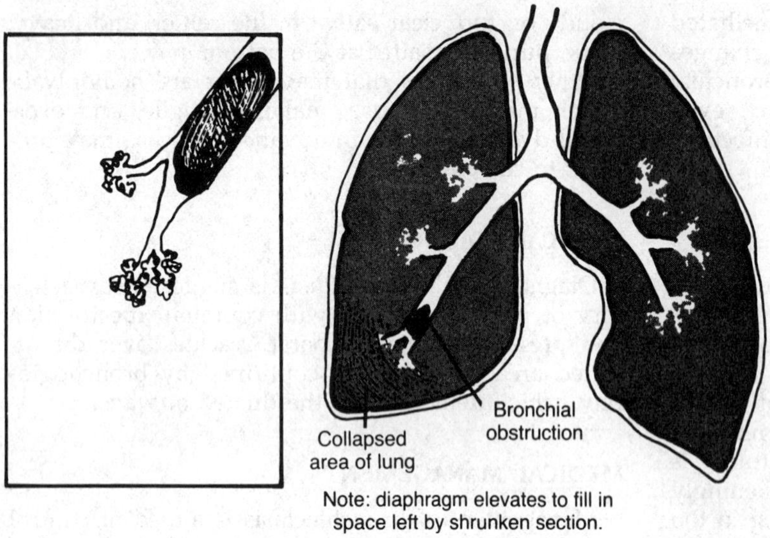

Figure 14–12.

Atelectasis of the right lower lobe due to bronchial obstruction. (From Jarvis C. Physical examination and health assessment. Philadelphia: WB Saunders, 1992, p 520.)

association with many different diseases of the lower respiratory system.

ETIOLOGY AND PATHOPHYSIOLOGY

A major cause of atelectasis is obstruction in the bronchi or lower air passages, which blocks the movement of air in and out of the distal area of the lung. This may be due to a mucous plug or aspiration of a foreign body. Regardless of the cause, the result is that the air trapped in the affected portion of the lung is absorbed into the blood stream over a period of a few hours and the lung segment collapses.

Atelectasis may also result from compression of the lung by a marked elevation of the diaphragm, a large pneumothorax, a pleural effusion, or other space-occupying lesions. In each of these cases, lung volume is reduced to the point at which airway closure occurs, air is then reabsorbed, alveolar size is reduced, and finally complete emptying and collapse occur. In other cases, atelectasis is associated with alveolar instability, as in respiratory distress syndrome, or with fibrotic changes in an area of lung tissue, which cause a decrease in the normal elastic recoil of the tissue and result in shrinkage of the area rather than complete airlessness.

CLINICAL MANIFESTATIONS

If atelectasis occurs rapidly and a large area of lung tissue is involved, then marked dyspnea and signs of hypoxemia are present. With mild to moderate amounts of slowly developing atelectasis, there are few symptoms except those of the underlying disease. After major surgery, dyspnea, cough, fever, and chest discomfort may indicate atelectasis. For patients on mechanical ventilation, an increasing requirement for oxygen is a major indicator of advancing atelectasis.

MEDICAL DIAGNOSIS

Atelectasis is diagnosed by chest x-ray film. If it appears to be due to an obstruction in the airway, a bronchoscopy may be done to identify the specific cause.

MEDICAL MANAGEMENT

Management depends on the cause of the atelectasis. When caused by a foreign object, neoplasm, or other known obstruction, the obstruction is removed by the appropriate technique such as withdrawal of air or fluid from the pleural cavity, resection of the neoplasm, or removal of secretions by bronchial toilet or bronchoscopy.

Inadequate lung expansion related to pain, sedation, mental obtundation, and other factors should be combated with periodic deep breathing, IPPB, continuous positive airway pressure (CPAP), and the use of incentive breathing devices.

Encouraging coughing and deep breathing, assisting with postural drainage, and providing adequate humidification are all measures to prevent atelectasis from occurring.

Guidelines for Application of the Nursing Process to the Care of the Patient with Atelectasis

Carefully assess patients at risk for the signs and symptoms of atelectasis. When atelectasis has occurred, institute measures to improve ventilation and remove secretions. If bronchial obstruction is the cause, encourage coughing and deep breathing.

Use an aerosol ultrasonic nebulizer, postural drainage, and chest percussion as ordered.

Turn patients on bed rest frequently, and position them to support maximal chest expansion to assist in mobilizing secretions. Encourage ambulation as soon as it is permitted.

Disorders of the Pulmonary Circulation

Pulmonary Embolism

Pulmonary embolism is defined as the occlusion of the pulmonary artery or one or more of its branches by matter carried by the blood stream from a vein or the right side of the heart to the lung.

ETIOLOGY

The most common type of pulmonary emboli are detached portions of venous thrombi originating in the deep veins of the lower extremities or pelvis. Such thrombi also occasionally originate in the right atrium. Other types of emboli consist of amniotic fluid, fat, air, bone spicules, or fragments of organs. These latter types constitute a very small percentage of all pulmonary emboli.

Venous stasis, vascular damage, and increased blood coagulability as a result of increased platelets or the release of tissue thromboplastin after surgery or other injury predispose to venous thrombosis and resulting pulmonary emboli. Hence, persons at greatest risk are bedridden patients, particularly those with cardiac disease and congestive heart failure or those immobilized for prolonged periods of time as with multiple injuries.

Other factors that place a patient at risk for venous thrombosis are pregnancy, use of oral contraceptives, varicose veins, carcinoma, obesity, polycythemia vera, and other blood diseases such as sickle cell anemia.

PATHOPHYSIOLOGY

A pulmonary embolism obstructs the flow of blood to the area of the lung beyond it. This, along with vasoconstrictive substances released from the clot, results in a ventilation-perfusion ($\dot{V}/\dot{Q}$) mismatch because ventilation is essentially normal. The $\dot{V}/\dot{Q}$ mismatch, with its concomitant hypoxemia, stimulates an increase in respiratory rate so PCO_2 drops as large amounts of carbon dioxide are exhaled. This drop in turn causes increased vasoconstriction and bronchoconstriction and so compounds the problem rather than solves it.

Occurring simultaneously with these respiratory changes are changes in the circulatory system. Because of the obstruction to blood flow in the lung, pressure in the pulmonary artery and in the right side of the heart increases. This leads to a decrease in cardiac output, a drop in blood pressure, and shock as the pressure exceeds that which the right side of the heart can overcome.

CLINICAL MANIFESTATIONS

The clinical manifestations of pulmonary embolism are extremely variable, ranging from none at all to a virtually instantaneous death.

Most common symptoms are chest pain, tachypnea, dyspnea, apprehension, cough, and hemoptysis. There may also be low-grade fever, signs of pulmonary hypertension, and, if the embolus is massive, rapid, weak pulse and systemic hypotension. The severity of the symptoms is directly related to the size of the embolus, although an atypical presentation with few signs or symptoms is possible.

MEDICAL DIAGNOSIS

Diagnosis of pulmonary embolism is difficult. Blood gas values show marked hypoxemia, with PO_2 levels ranging from 60 to 65 mm Hg and normal or decreased PCO_2, but because these findings are not unique to pulmonary embolism they are not diagnostic. A normal perfusion lung scan rules out the possibility of pulmonary embolus; however, an abnormal one does not necessarily indicate the presence of an embolus. A combination of ventilation and perfusion lung scanning is used to differentiate pulmonary emboli from other lung conditions.

A definite diagnosis can be made by pulmonary angiography, but this is done only if certain potentially risky therapeutic procedures must be performed.

MEDICAL MANAGEMENT

Prevention is the best treatment. Pharmacologic prophylaxis may be based on aspirin to prevent platelet aggregation or on low-dose heparin therapy. For patients older than 40 years having thoracic or abdominal surgery, the latter involves heparin given in a dose of 5000 units subcutaneously 2 hours preoperatively, and the same dose 12 hours postoperatively and thereafter two or three times daily until the patient is fully ambulatory.

Because stasis is a major factor in the development of deep vein thrombosis, measures that increase venous return from the legs are instituted. These include early ambulation, leg elevation and physiotherapy, elastic stockings, and graduated pressure stockings as well as more sophisticated methods such as electrical calf muscle stimulation

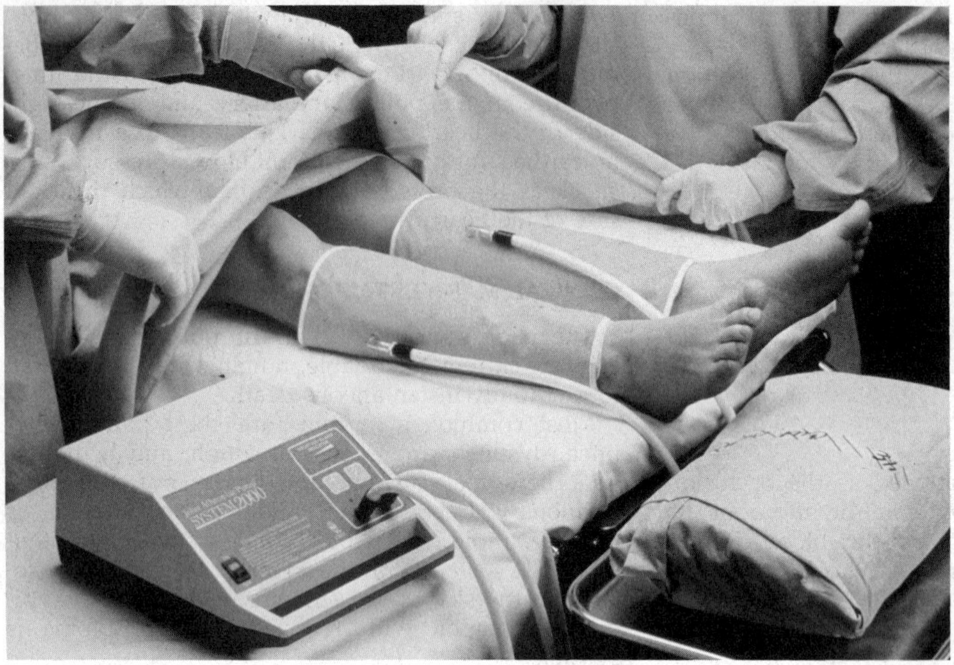

Figure 14–13.

Intermittent calf compression. The application of pneumatic compression to the lower extremities using different cycle times and pressures. This technique empties the deep calf veins of blood and increases pulsatile flow in the femoral veins. (Courtesy of Jobst, Toledo, Ohio—A Beiersdorf Company.)

and intermittent pneumatic calf compression (Fig. 14–13). The patient is also kept well hydrated because dehydration predisposes to clotting.

If embolism occurs, management is aimed at immediate stabilization of cardiorespiratory status because most deaths occur within 2 hours. Oxygen is given for hypoxemia and intravenous isoproterenol or dopamine for hypotension. Depending on condition and arterial blood gas values, the patient may also be placed on a volume-controlled ventilator. Additional medications such as sodium bicarbonate to combat metabolic acidosis, digitalis to strengthen heart contraction, and morphine for pain are given as needed.

Treatment is also initiated to return pulmonary blood flow to normal and to prevent recurrence. To accomplish this, heparin is given for 7 to 10 days in the dose needed to keep the activated partial thromboplastin time (APTT) between 60 and 80 seconds. This is followed by 12 weeks of warfarin therapy. Thrombolytic agents such as streptokinase or urokinase, which hasten the lysis of clots in peripheral veins or pulmonary arteries, may be given, but they are not a substitute for anticoagulation therapy. Occasionally, surgical intervention is used in the management of the patient with pulmonary embolism. If initial stabilization of the patient is not possible because of massive obstruction of pulmonary blood flow, an embolectomy may be done. In other cases when emboli recur despite medical therapy, blood flow through the vena cava may be surgically interrupted to prevent thrombi from the legs or pelvis from reaching the lung. This can be done by ligating the vena cava, using clips to divide it into smaller channels, or inserting a filtering device.

Application of the Nursing Process to the Care of the Patient with Pulmonary Embolism

Assessment

Be alert to the possibility of pulmonary embolism, and carefully assess at-risk patients for dyspnea, chest pain, tachypnea, cough, hemoptysis, and apprehension.

When an embolism has occurred, make ongoing assessments of cardiorespiratory status. Take vital signs, noting characteristics of both pulse and respirations. Observe for cyanosis, cough, and hemoptysis. Question the patient regarding chest pain. Review blood gas values and electrocardiogram (ECG) readings. Assess anxiety level and understanding of the problem and its treatments.

Nursing Diagnoses and Planning

Nursing diagnoses and related expected patient outcomes most commonly applicable to patients with pulmonary emboli include the following:

NDx: Impaired gas exchange related to loss of effective lung tissue secondary to lack of blood circulation

Planning: Patient outcomes

1. Respirations are of normal rate and depth.
2. Complaints of dyspnea are absent.

3. Cyanosis is absent.
4. Blood gas values are within normal range.

NDx: Anxiety related to outcome of the embolism, anticoagulation, and/or recurrence

Planning: Patient outcomes
1. Signs of excessive anxiety such as trembling or crying are absent.
2. Patient rests quietly.
3. Patient accepts being left alone without protest.
4. Patient expresses confidence in the outcome of therapy.

NDx: High risk for impaired skin integrity related to bed rest

Planning: Patient outcomes
1. Skin is free of reddened areas.
2. Skin is intact.

NDx: High risk for altered health maintenance related to insufficient knowledge of anticoagulant therapy, prevention of recurrence

Planning: Patient outcomes
1. Patient states name, dose, route, and frequency of prescribed medications.
2. Patient explains precautions required by anticoagulant therapy.
3. Patient states importance of promptly reporting bruising, prolonged or excessive bleeding, and tarry stools.
4. Patient describes measures to prevent venous stasis.
5. Patient explains importance of follow-up care.

Nursing Interventions

Carry out the prescribed medical regimen of anticoagulant or thrombolytic therapy, intermittent calf compression, or electrical calf stimulation. Apply antiembolic stockings, and perform range-of-motion exercises as prescribed. Monitor respiratory status, including lung sounds, arterial blood gases, prothrombin time, and partial thromboplastin time. Check the patient for signs of bleeding.

NDx: Impaired gas exchange
Place the patient in a semi-Fowler's position to facilitate breathing, and administer oxygen as ordered. Because pain accompanying pulmonary embolism is usually pleuritic, give analgesics as ordered to foster good ventilation.

NDx: Anxiety
Acknowledge that anxiety is normal, and indicate understanding and willingness to help the patient deal with it. Stay with the patient during periods of severe dyspnea. At other times, reassure the patient that someone is close by and will respond quickly if called.

Keep the patient informed about his or her condition as well as about prescribed tests and treatments.

NDx: High risk for impaired skin integrity
Assist the patient to turn every 1 to 2 hours while on bed rest. Keep the bed linens smooth and the patient's skin dry. Massage the back and other areas of pressure to stimulate circulation. Protect bony prominences where skin breakdown is likely to occur using pillows, sheepskin pads, a flotation pad, or the like.

NDx: High risk for altered health maintenance
Instruct the patient in the self-administration of prescribed anticoagulant medications, related precautions, symptoms to be reported, and prevention of recurrences.

Evaluation

Evaluate the effectiveness of nursing care for a patient with pulmonary embolism by comparing the patient's status with the expected patient outcomes. Examples of specific outcomes for patients with pulmonary embolism have been provided in the Planning section.

Pulmonary Hypertension

Pulmonary hypertension is defined as any condition that raises the resistance to blood flow in the pulmonary vascular bed, thereby increasing the systolic blood pressure in the pulmonary artery above normal. In the resting, healthy adult, the systolic blood pressure in the pulmonary artery averages approximately 24 mm Hg and the diastolic approximately 10 mm Hg. Pulmonary hypertension is said to exist when pressure is higher than 30/16 mm Hg.

ETIOLOGY AND PATHOPHYSIOLOGY

There are a number of causes of pulmonary hypertension. Primary involvement of the pulmonary artery by conditions such as pulmonary vasculitis or occlusion by pulmonary emboli can result in pulmonary hypertension. Elevation of left atrial pressure, increased pulmonary blood flow as with ventricular septal defects, and mitral valve disease are examples of disorders that cause "postcapillary" pulmonary hypertension. However, the most common causes of pulmonary hypertension are the conditions in which there is sustained hypoxemia such as emphysema and chronic bronchitis. In these cases, the reduced vascular bed and increased pulmonary artery resistance caused by hypoxemia contribute to the pulmonary hypertension.

CLINICAL MANIFESTATIONS

Dyspnea is the cardinal symptom of pulmonary hypertension. Other symptoms vary depending on the underlying disease.

MEDICAL DIAGNOSIS

Differential diagnosis is made by establishing the presence of lung disease through pulmonary function studies. Cardiac catheterization studies are used to determine the presence of any cardiac defects. Lung scanning and angiography may be done to detect pulmonary emboli.

MEDICAL MANAGEMENT

Management is aimed at the specific underlying disorder once it has been determined.

Guidelines for Application of the Nursing Process to the Care of the Patient with Pulmonary Hypertension

The immediate aim of nursing care for the patient with pulmonary hypertension is provision of adequate oxygenation for respiratory needs. Specific nursing interventions vary with the cause of the hypertension.

Adult Respiratory Distress Syndrome

Adult respiratory distress syndrome (ARDS) is noncardiogenic pulmonary edema, that is, pulmonary edema not due to heart failure. The incidence of ARDS appears to be increasing as technologic advances enable the survival of more critically ill individuals. The mortality rate associated with ARDS is estimated to be 50% to 60% (Shekleton & Litwack, 1991, p. 119).

ETIOLOGY AND PATHOPHYSIOLOGY

Typically, ARDS occurs after a catastrophic physiologic event in individuals with no history of pulmonary disease. Such events include direct injuries to the lung such as aspiration of gastric contents, radiation, near-drowning, inhalation of toxic gases, and pulmonary infection. Other precipitating factors include shock, drug overdose, multiple blood transfusions, hemolytic disorders, cerebrovascular accident, brain tumors, sudden increase in intracranial pressure, and extensive trauma.

ARDS is characterized by damage to the alveolar capillary membrane, which results in the movement of protein, cellular elements, and fluid into the interstitial tissues of the lung. Terminal airways become compressed and obliterated, and there is decreased lung volume and decreased compliance. Gas exchange is impaired, and extensive shunting of blood in the lung occurs.

CLINICAL MANIFESTATIONS

The clinical presentation of ARDS can be divided into three distinct phases. Phase I, also called the latent stage, is characterized by hyperventilation and hypocapnia accompanied by a slight increase in the work of breathing. This period of relative stability lasts 6 to 48 hours. In Phase II, respiratory insufficiency is evident. Tachypnea, dyspnea, and crackles throughout the lung fields are present, with diffuse infiltrates apparent on chest x-ray film. Phase III is the terminal phase. This phase is marked by severe hypoxemia unresponsive to oxygen therapy and by hypercapnia and resulting respiratory and metabolic acidosis.

MEDICAL DIAGNOSIS

Medical diagnosis is based on the patient's history, clinical signs of respiratory failure, a PaO_2 of less than 50 mm Hg, fraction of inspired oxygen (FIO_2) greater than 0.6, and a pulmonary artery wedge pressure greater than 18 mm Hg.

MEDICAL MANAGEMENT

Medical management is aimed at supporting the patient's vital functions while identifying and treating the precipitating problem. Early in the disease process, adequate respiration may be maintained through the administration of supplemental oxygen. Later, intubation and mechanical ventilation with a higher than normal airway pressure are necessary. Adequate circulation is maintained through the administration of intravenous fluids to combat hypovolemia, which can result from the loss of fluid into the interstitial spaces of the lung and through the use of inotropic or vasopressor drugs. Swan-Ganz readings are used to guide fluid administration, because it is critical but difficult to maintain volume without contributing to overload. Nutritional needs are met via enteral or parenteral nutrition.

Guidelines for Application of the Nursing Process to the Care of the Patient with ARDS

Nursing care for patients with ARDS varies on the basis of the precipitating disorder and its care, the phase of ARDS, and the respiratory treatment modalities used.

Occupational Lung Diseases

Pneumoconiosis refers to a fibrous inflammation or chronic induration of the lungs resulting from inhalation of dust. It is a general term used in relation to occupational lung diseases such as silicosis, asbestosis, or coal workers' pneumoconiosis.

Silicosis

The term silicosis refers to one specific disease that is produced by exposure to silica. Occupations involved with quarrying, chipping, grinding, and polishing silica-containing rock are factors in the development of this disease. Coal miners often contract this disease as a result of mining and tunneling in rock such as quartz and sandstone, which are almost pure silica.

The chief symptom of silicosis is shortness of breath. The characteristic pathologic changes in silicosis are silicotic nodules, which are densely packed fibrotic lesions scattered unevenly throughout the lungs, mostly in the upper lobes. Such lesions have been frequently attributed to concurrent tuberculosis.

Asbestosis

Asbestos is a generic name applied to a family of fibrous hydrated silicates widely used in industry. Asbestos has been used for more than 100 years; however, the potential risk was recognized only in the 1960s. The mining and milling of asbestos are obvious sources of asbestos-related disease. Occupational exposure to asbestos also occurs in insulation work, construction, ship building, and building demolition.

The parenchymal reaction to the inhalation of asbestos is the production of pleuropulmonary lesions involving mostly the lower part of the lung fields accompanied by fibrous pleural thickening. Pulmonary fibrosis, bronchogenic carcinoma, pleural effusion, and pleural fibrosis are some of the common pulmonary complications of asbestosis.

Symptoms vary from none in early and mild cases to severe respiratory incapacity in advanced disease. Frequently, 20 to 30 years may elapse before clinical symptoms occur, of which dyspnea is the most common.

Coal Workers' Pneumoconiosis

Coal workers' pneumoconiosis is commonly referred to as "black lung." Unlike silicosis, this specific disease is a result of prolonged exposure to coal dust. In essence, the clearance mechanisms of the lung are overwhelmed, and the coal dust accumulates in terminal air spaces. Severity and duration of exposure are the major factors determining the pathologic changes caused by the coal dust. The area at which coal is cut, known as the coal face, is the dustiest part of the mine for workers. These particular workers are therefore exposed to the highest concentration of coal dust and are at greatest risk for the disease.

In simple coal workers' pneumoconiosis, the coal macule is the characteristic lesion. Coal macules, which appear as black dots on the lung, consist of macrophages filled with coal dust, fibroblasts, and cellular debris. Sometimes there is also a dilatation of the respiratory bronchioles called focal centrilobular emphysema.

The complicated form of coal workers' pneumoconiosis is characterized by large, black areas of fibrotic tissue with cores of dust, collagen, and other insoluble proteins.

Simple coal workers' pneumoconiosis is symptom free, but the complicated form is characterized by dyspnea on exertion and may progress to severe respiratory insufficiency with obstructive lung disease, cor pulmonale, and pulmonary hypertension.

Clinically, evidence of small airway obstruction is demonstrated on pulmonary function studies. Chest x-ray films may show nodules that are small and not well defined. Large shadows of 1 cm or more in diameter are indicators of complicated pneumoconiosis.

Application of the Nursing Process to the Care of the Patient with an Occupational Lung Disease

Assessment

Begin assessment with a detailed occupational and environmental history, which includes information on type and duration of exposure to dust and the development of symptoms in relationship to the work pattern. Obtain information about the patient's smoking habits, activity tolerance, and recent respiratory infections. Auscultate all lung fields, and observe the patient for dyspnea, cough, and expectoration.

Because occupational lung diseases are chronic disorders associated with permanent disability, determine the patient's understanding of the disease course and its outcomes, and assess available support systems.

Nursing Diagnoses and Planning

Nursing diagnoses and related expected patient outcomes most commonly applicable to patients with occupational lung disease include the following:

NDx: Impaired gas exchange related to ineffective ventilation secondary to fibrosis of the lungs

Planning: Patient outcomes
1. Patient describes measures to facilitate ventilation.
2. Patient uses oxygen correctly.
3. Cyanosis is absent.
4. Arterial blood gas values are within normal limits.

NDx: Activity intolerance related to decreased oxygenation

Planning: Patient outcomes
1. Patient describes how to avoid excessive demands on the respiratory system by spacing activities to allow for rest and recuperation of energy.
2. Patient demonstrates use of relaxation techniques.

NDx: Anxiety related to shortness of breath, outcome of the disease, inability to work

Planning: Patient outcomes
1. Patient verbalizes feelings and concerns.
2. Patient demonstrates use of relaxation techniques.
3. Patient expresses confidence in own ability to adapt to lifestyle changes necessitated by the disease.

NDx: High risk for altered health maintenance related to insufficient knowledge of disease, its progress, and its treatment

Planning: Patient outcomes
1. Patient describes ways to avoid further airway irritants, such as wearing a protective mask, hood, or respirator.
2. Patient describes ways of limiting exposure to respiratory infections.
3. Patient with asbestosis explains importance of routine physical examinations.
4. Patient with asbestosis lists the warning signs of cancer.

Nursing Interventions

NDx: Impaired gas exchange
Explain measures that facilitate ventilation, such as use of Fowler's or semi-Fowler's position, avoidance of clothing that constricts the trunk, as well as coughing, deep breathing, and adequate hydration to keep secretions liquid and movable. Instruct the patient and significant others in the use of oxygen and related precautions if needed.

NDx: Activity intolerance
Help the patient to plan activities so that time is provided between activities for energy to be restored. Discuss work-simplification techniques, and assist the patient in implementing them.

NDx: Anxiety
Remain with the patient during episodes of shortness of breath. Provide a calm, quiet environment, and guide the patient in the use of relaxation exercises.

Allow the patient to discuss concerns, and provide reassurance and information on available resources as appropriate.

NDx: High risk for altered health maintenance
Teach patients and the general public about the hazards associated with exposure to industrial products such as silica, coal dust, and asbestos. Teach about the critical need for proper ventilation of work areas, use of wet techniques, and the use of protective masks, hoods, and respirators.

Explain to patients with an occupational lung disease the need to avoid environmental airway irritants outside the work place, to take measures to protect themselves from respiratory infections, and to seek prompt medical treatment if an infection should occur.

Because patients with asbestosis have been found to be at increased risk for cancer, stress the need for routine physical examination and teach the warning symptoms of cancer.

Evaluation

Evaluate the effectiveness of nursing care for a patient with occupational lung disease by comparing the patient's status with the expected patient outcomes. Examples of specific outcomes for patients with occupational lung disease have been provided in the Planning section.

Trauma

Thoracic trauma is injury resulting from penetrating, crushing, or blunt force to the chest. Penetrating or open-chest trauma occurs as a result of gunshot wounds, stab wounds, or other penetrating objects. Traffic accidents are responsible for the majority of blunt or crushing chest trauma. In the United States, trauma is a leading cause of death, and approximately 75% of traumatic deaths involve chest injury.

Chest injuries are always considered serious because of the potential for acute respiratory failure from damage to the chest wall or lower respiratory tract structures and for shock caused by damage to the great vessels. Thus, a priority of treatment is to establish a patent airway and support cardiopulmonary function as needed.

Fractured Ribs

ETIOLOGY AND PATHOPHYSIOLOGY

Rib fractures, the most common type of chest injury, occur primarily as a result of blunt or crushing injury to the chest. Those most often fractured are ribs 5 through 9, which are least protected and therefore more open to trauma.

Fractures can range in severity from a simple crack to a splintered, displaced bony segment. If the broken edge of the bony segment is driven inward, injury to lungs or other underlying structures may result. Thus, complications with rib fractures include hemothorax, pneumothorax, and lacerations of the lung, liver, or spleen

CLINICAL MANIFESTATIONS

Basic symptoms of an uncomplicated rib fracture are pain, which increases with coughing, deep breathing, or movement; point tenderness at the site of the break; and muscle spasm on the affected side of the chest. Splinting and shallow breathing secondary to the pain also occur.

MEDICAL DIAGNOSIS

Rib fracture is suggested on the basis of a history of chest trauma and the symptoms presented by the patient. It is confirmed by chest x-ray film.

Serial blood gas values are obtained to check for lung injury.

MEDICAL MANAGEMENT

Medical management of an uncomplicated rib fracture is aimed at relieving pain to promote effective ventilation. Narcotics are avoided whenever possible because of their depressive effect on respirations and cough. In some cases, an intercostal nerve block may be done to decrease pain and muscle spasm. Healing generally takes 3 to 6 weeks.

Application of the Nursing Process to the Care of the Patient with Fractured Ribs

Assessment

Take vital signs, paying particular attention to rate, depth, and symmetry of respiration. Note the patient's color, and assess pain level. Closely observe the patient for signs of any other injury.

Nursing Diagnoses and Planning

Nursing diagnoses and related expected patient outcomes most commonly applicable to patients with uncomplicated fractured ribs include the following:

NDx: Pain related to movement of the chest secondary to tissue trauma

Planning: Patient outcomes
1. Patient states pain is relieved.
2. Patient's respirations are of normal rate and depth.
3. Patient states name, dose, route, and frequency of medication to be taken at home for pain.

NDx: High risk for ineffective breathing pattern related to pain on chest movement

Planning: Patient outcomes
1. Respirations are of normal rate and depth.
2. Blood gas values are within normal limits.
3. Patient explains need for coughing and deep-breathing exercises.
4. Patient demonstrates coughing and deep breathing correctly.

Nursing Interventions

Because the patient with an uncomplicated fractured rib is not hospitalized, the primary nursing intervention is patient teaching.

NDx: Pain
Give the patient medication for pain as ordered. Then teach the patient the name, dose, route, and frequency of medication to be taken at home for pain relief. Be certain to specify when the first dose may be taken relative to the medication just given.

NDx: High risk for ineffective breathing pattern
Explain the importance of coughing and deep breathing in maintaining good ventilation and preventing complications such as pneumonia. Instruct the patient in effective coughing and deep-breathing techniques, and ask the patient to demonstrate them.

Additional Interventions
If the patient has past knowledge of treatment of a fractured rib, explain, if necessary, that the chest is no longer tightly wrapped or strapped, because it has been found that these interventions inhibit chest expansion and increase the risk of complications.

Evaluation

Evaluate the effectiveness of nursing care for a patient with fractured ribs by comparing the patient's status with the expected patient outcomes. Examples of specific outcomes for patients with fractured ribs have been provided in the Planning section.

Flail Chest

ETIOLOGY

Flail chest is said to exist when there is paradoxic movement of the chest resulting from the action of several floating segments of ribs that have been fractured in two or more places.

PATHOPHYSIOLOGY

The floating ribs move inward during inspiration and outward with expiration. This action negates some of the chest expansion brought about by the anteroposterior and diaphragmatic movement, thus abolishing the pressure gradients essential for inspiration. Movement of air is diminished. Respiratory depth is decreased, and the patient cannot cough effectively. The result is increased secretions and fatigue.

CLINICAL MANIFESTATIONS

Because of intense spasm of the chest wall musculature overlying the fractures, the flail segment may not be immediately obvious. However, as the muscles tire, the paradoxical movement of the affected chest wall segment presents itself (Fig. 14–14). The patient is in respiratory distress with hypoxemia, marked overbreathing, asymmetric chest movements, tachypnea, restlessness, and cyanosis.

MEDICAL DIAGNOSIS

Diagnosis is made on the basis of current history of trauma, observation of the chest, and chest x-ray films.

MEDICAL MANAGEMENT

Management of severe cases of flail chest consists of stabilizing the chest wall. Initially this is done by exerting firm but gentle pressure on the segment with either the palm of the hand or sandbags. Supplemental oxygen and pain medication, if not contraindicated by the presence of a concurrent head injury, are given.

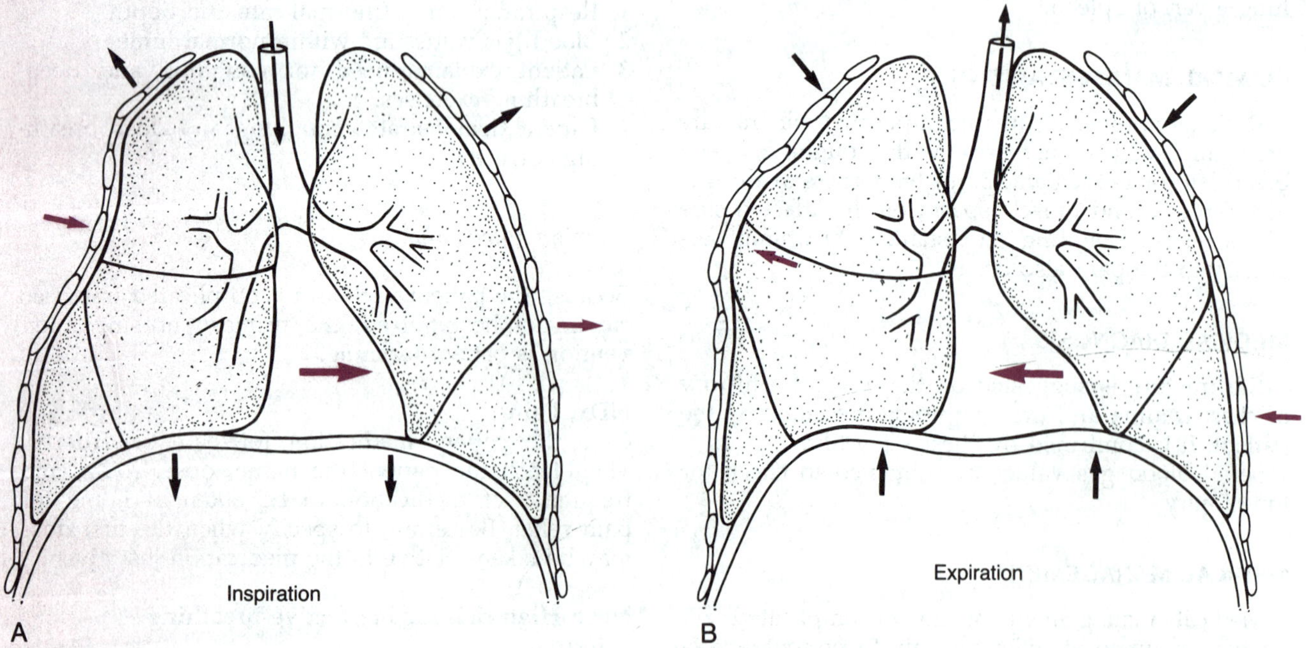

Figure 14–14.

Flail chest. *A,* Flail area of the chest wall sucks in on inspiration. Note that air flows from the lung on the affected side into the opposite lung, thus compromising ventilation of the lung on the flail side. Note also the movement of the mediastinum to the side opposite the flail. *B,* Flail area of the chest wall balloons outward on expiration, and a portion of exhaled air from the lung on the unaffected side passes into the lung on the flail side, again impairing ventilation.

Subsequently, the chest is more effectively stabilized by endotracheal intubation and the use of a volume-controlled mechanical ventilator (internal stabilization) or by operative intervention. There are two approaches to operative stabilization. One uses intramedullary pinning of the ribs, sternum, and costal cartilages. The second uses a stainless steel wire, one end of which is attached to the ribs through a small incision and the other to a rope and pulley with about 5 lb of weight to pull the chest outward.

Regardless of method, it is important that treatment be started as early as possible to prevent changes in the lung from compression such as pulmonary congestion, atelectasis, and pulmonary hemorrhage.

Less severe cases of flail chest may be treated with fluid restriction, diuretics, steroids, colloids, good pulmonary hygiene, and relief of chest pain.

Application of the Nursing Process to the Care of the Patient with Flail Chest

Assessment

All patients with multiple rib fractures should be admitted to a trauma unit or critical care unit, where continued close observation is possible. This is important because patients with chest trauma of this magnitude are likely to have significant injuries of other organs that may or not have been obvious initially. Therefore, make repeated assessments of the abdomen, the extremities, and neurologic function as well as respiratory status.

Nursing Diagnoses and Planning

Nursing diagnoses and related expected patient outcomes most commonly applicable to patients with flail chest include the following:

NDx: Ineffective breathing pattern related to changes in intrathoracic pressure secondary to the flail

Planning: Patient outcomes

1. Restlessness, cyanosis, and dyspnea are absent.
2. Arterial blood gas values are within normal limits.

NDx: High risk for ineffective airway clearance related to ineffective coughing and pain

Planning: Patient outcomes

1. Patient removes secretions from the respiratory tree by coughing or undergoing suctioning.
2. Lungs are clear on auscultation.

Nursing Interventions

NDx: Ineffective breathing pattern

Administer oxygen, and give analgesics as ordered to relieve pain and encourage greater chest expansion. Be reassuring, and keep the environment calm to quiet the patient's anxiety and to lower the demand for oxygen.

NDx: High risk for ineffective airway clearance

Encourage the patient to cough and deep breathe, if able, to mobilize secretions from the respiratory tract. If unable to move secretions in this way, suction as needed. Be sure the patient is always well hydrated to keep secretions liquid.

Additional Interventions

Other nursing interventions depend in part on the type of medical treatment prescribed. Nursing care of the patient who is intubated and on mechanical ventilation is discussed in Chapter 12 and is applicable to the patient whose chest is stabilized in this way. Note, however, that the patient who is being ventilated for flail chest is on controlled, not assisted, ventilation. Administer paralyzing agents as ordered to prevent the patient from "fighting" the respirator and to decrease the overall body oxygen consumption by blocking neuromuscular activity.

Evaluation

Evaluate the effectiveness of nursing care for a patient with flail chest by comparing the patient's status with the expected patient outcomes. Examples of specific outcomes for patients with flail chest have been provided in the Planning section.

Pneumothorax, Hemothorax, and Hemopneumothorax

Pneumothorax is a condition in which there is gas in the pleural space. The presence of blood in the pleural space is a hemothorax. Frequently, with trauma, patients have a combination of pneumothorax and hemothorax, and the term hemopneumothorax is used.

ETIOLOGY AND PATHOPHYSIOLOGY

There are two major types of pneumothorax: open and closed. An open pneumothorax is one in which a hole in the chest wall allows atmospheric air to flow into the pleural space (Fig. 14–15*A*). This may result from a penetrating injury such as a stab or gunshot wound or from a therapeutic procedure such as a thoracotomy or thoracentesis or insertion

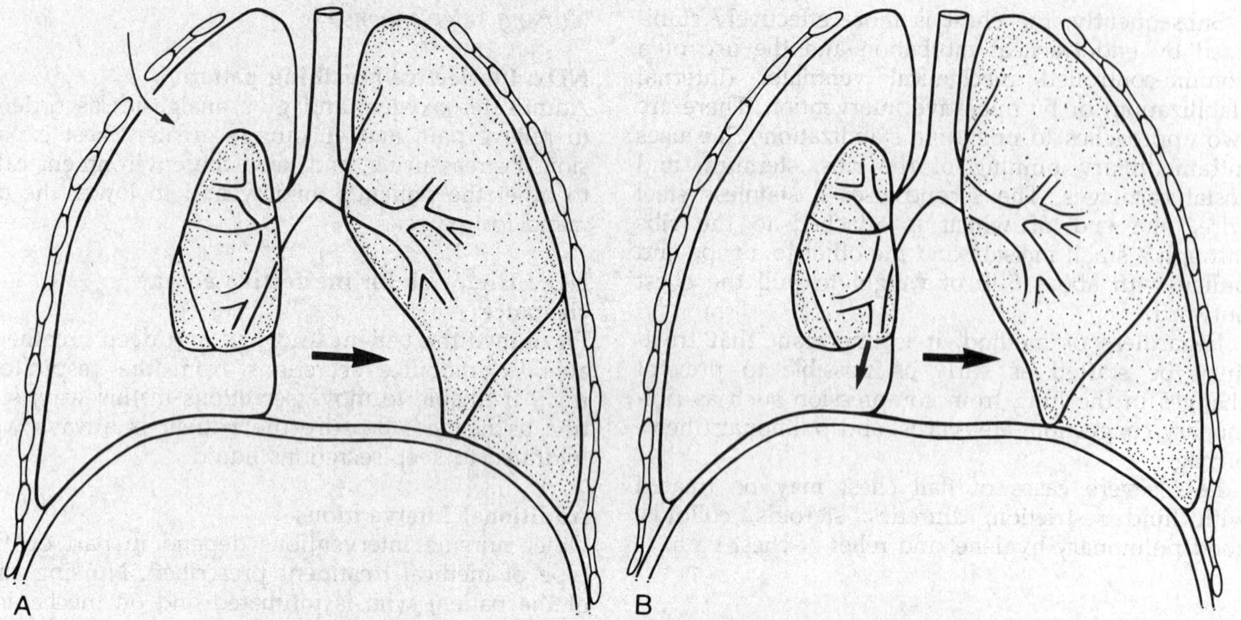

Figure 14–15.

A, Open pneumothorax. Note opening in chest wall through which air enters the pleural space on inspiration. *B*, Closed pneumothorax. Note the tear in the lung through which air enters the pleural space during inspiration.

of a central venous catheter or a Swan-Ganz catheter.

In a closed, or spontaneous, pneumothorax, air enters the pleural space from the lung (Fig. 14–15*B*). If this occurs in the absence of disease, it is called a simple, spontaneous pneumothorax. This type occurs most often in men between the ages of 20 and 40 years and is due to the rupture of blebs on the apex of the lung (small vesicles of unknown cause). If a closed pneumothorax occurs as a result of trauma or pulmonary disease, it is referred to as secondary, or complicated, pneumothorax. Trauma that causes secondary pneumothorax consists of blunt injuries to the chest, such as sudden compression of the thoracic cavity at the height of inspiration with the glottis closed, causing rupture of the alveoli from excessive pressure and perforation of the lung by the end of a fractured rib. The disease most often associated with secondary pneumothorax is widespread emphysema.

In each of these types of pneumothorax, the air in the pleural space causes increased intrapleural pressure, resulting in partial or total collapse of the lung.

A unique type of pneumothorax is a tension pneumothorax. This occurs when injury allows air to leak into the pleural space during inspiration, but it is prevented from leaking out during expiration (Fig. 14–16). With each inspiration, then, the amount of air continues to increase, causing pressure within the pleural space to rise above atmospheric pressure. This results not only in collapse of the lung but also in a shift of the mediastinum to the opposite side. This shift in turn causes pressure on the great vessels returning blood to the heart and impairs venous return.

A hemothorax is an accumulation of blood in the pleural space usually caused by bleeding of the pulmonary parenchyma and vessels, the intercostal and internal mammary arteries, the heart, the aorta, or great vessels. The bleeding is generally self-limiting, but if it persists, respiratory and cardiac impairments as well as hypovolemic shock ensue because a large amount of blood is lost. The total accumulation of blood can range from 300 ml to a much more severe hemothorax with the loss of 1500 ml of blood.

CLINICAL MANIFESTATIONS

The patient with an open pneumothorax has a history of some event that has caused penetration of the chest wall. A sucking sound is audible on inspiration as the chest wall rises, and varying degrees of respiratory distress are present depending on the size of the pneumothorax.

The basic symptoms of a closed pneumothorax are shortness of breath and chest pain; however, the exact clinical signs depend on the size of the pneumothorax. A larger pneumothorax may present with tachypnea, cyanosis, diminished breath sounds, and subcutaneous emphysema. There may also be hyperresonance on the affected side.

A tension pneumothorax presents with clinical signs only as the positive pressure on the affected side increases. There is neck vein engorgement secondary to the pressure on the superior vena cava, progressive dyspnea, paradoxical movement of the chest, deviated trachea, cyanosis, distant breath sounds, hyperresonance on the affected side, and cardiogenic shock.

The clinical findings for hemothorax are the same as for open or tension pneumothorax with the addition of tachycardia, hypotension, dullness on chest percussion, pallor, and anxiety.

MEDICAL DIAGNOSIS

Diagnosis of all types of pneumothorax or hemothorax is made on the basis of chest x-ray film and arterial blood gas values.

MEDICAL MANAGEMENT

Medical management consists of insertion of a chest tube to reestablish the intrapleural pressure (refer to Chapter 12 for chest tube insertion and care). In the case of a tension pneumothorax, which always requires immediate intervention, a large-bore needle (16 to 18 gauge) is inserted either anteriorly at the midclavicular line between the second and third intercostal spaces or at the midlateral line between the fifth and sixth intercostal spaces.

The patient's condition improves markedly once the needle is inserted.

An open pneumothorax should be immediately covered to prevent further entry of air into the chest. In an emergency, anything available is used, but in the hospital petroleum jelly gauze is used. Three sides are taped, and the fourth is left open to permit exhale ventilation and to prevent a tension pneumothorax.

The treatment for hemothorax may require a thoracotomy if the initial chest-tube drainage is greater than 1500 ml, persistent bleeding occurs at a rate greater than 500 ml per hour, increasing hemothorax is identified on chest x-ray film, or the patient's condition remains unstable despite adequate blood replacement.

Other modes of treatment may be required depending on the severity of the initial trauma and complications. They include pain medication, adrenergic agents such as dopamine to maintain blood pressure, oxygen therapy, and mechanical ventilation if there is evidence of respiratory failure.

Application of the Nursing Process to the Care of the Patient with Pneumothorax or Hemothorax

Assessment

A comprehensive respiratory assessment is important for patients with a pneumothorax or hemothorax. Observe for dyspnea, tachypnea, retractions, labored breathing, nasal flaring, cyanosis, asymmetry

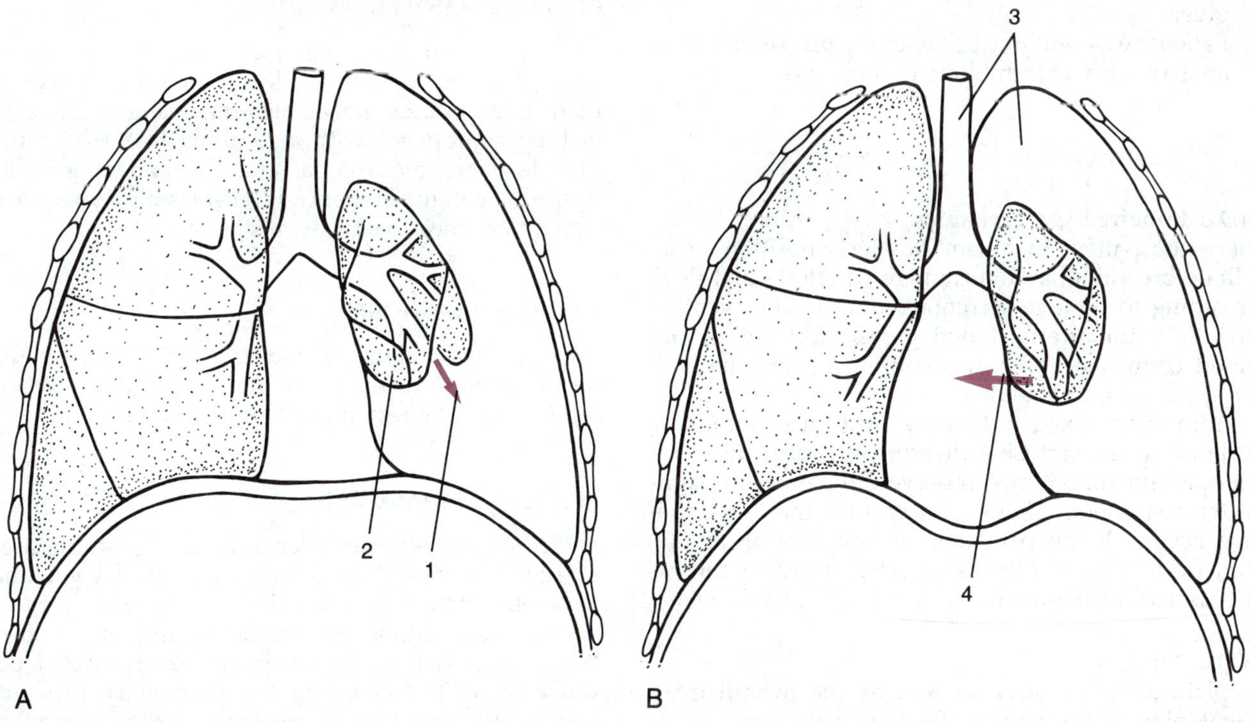

Figure 14–16.

Tension pneumothorax. *A*, On the side of the damaged lung, air accumulates with each respiratory cycle (1), causing the injured lung to collapse as the pressure builds up (2). *B*, There is tracheal deviation (3) and mediastinal shift (4), which compresses the opposite lung.

of the chest wall, and restlessness and confusion. Auscultate the chest for distant or diminished breath sounds and for vocal fremitus or hyperresonance on the affected side. Palpate for tracheal deviation and subcutaneous emphysema, and note the characteristics of any cough or sputum. Assess cardiac status by checking blood pressure and heart rate, auscultating the quality of the heartbeat, and observing the patient's color. Measure urinary output to check renal function.

Nursing Diagnoses and Planning

Nursing diagnoses and related expected patient outcomes most commonly applicable to patients with a pneumothorax or a hemothorax include the following:

NDx: Impaired gas exchange related to collapse of an area of the lung

Planning: Patient outcomes
1. Dyspnea is absent.
2. Cyanosis is absent.
3. Arterial blood gas values are within normal range.

NDx: Anxiety related to dyspnea and/or treatment

Planning: Patient outcomes
1. Patient attends to information and directions given.
2. Patient rests without behavioral signs of excessive anxiety such as trembling, crying, and agitation.

Nursing Interventions

NDx: Impaired gas exchange
Place the patient in a semi-Fowler's position to facilitate breathing, and encourage coughing and deep breathing to remove secretions and enhance ventilation. Monitor arterial blood gases, electrolytes, and blood counts to assist in identifying problems with oxygenation and bleeding.

Administer oxygen therapy and medications as ordered. If an occlusive dressing has been used for an open pneumothorax, observe the patient for signs of tension pneumothorax and remove the dressing if this occurs. If the patient is on mechanical ventilation or if a chest tube is inserted, provide care as discussed in Chapter 12.

NDx: Anxiety
Explain all procedures as well as the overall treatment plan to the patient. Be calm and reassure the patient regarding his or her condition as appropriate.

Additional Interventions
If a hemothorax is present, place special emphasis on monitoring for hypovolemic shock and carrying out fluid- and blood-replacement therapy.

Evaluation

Evaluate the effectiveness of nursing care for a patient with pneumothorax or hemothorax by comparing the patient's status with the expected patient outcomes. Examples of specific outcomes for patients with pneumothorax or hemothorax have been provided in the Planning section.

Pulmonary Contusion

ETIOLOGY AND PATHOPHYSIOLOGY

The crushing and bruising of the lung is known as contusion. It can result from a severe blow to the chest with or without rib or sternal fracture. Because of the damage to the alveolar structures, lung contusion leads to atelectasis and airway obstruction because bronchioles become plugged with blood and edema fluid. Ventilation is also impaired as a result of the reduction in lung compliance.

CLINICAL MANIFESTATIONS

With a mild contusion there may be no symptoms. With more extensive lung contusion, however, there is a progression of atelectasis and a decrease in lung compliance with a resulting low $\dot{V}/\dot{Q}$ ratio. This leads to hypoxemia, and the patient exhibits dyspnea, cough, hemoptysis, increasing hyperpnea, tachypnea, chest pain, and restlessness.

MEDICAL DIAGNOSIS

Diagnosis is made on the basis of a current history of a blow to the chest. As complications occur, x-ray films may reveal areas of atelectasis.

MEDICAL MANAGEMENT

Medical management depends largely on the area affected. In mild cases, supplemental oxygen and close observation may be all that is needed. In more severe cases, fluids are restricted and broad-spectrum antibiotics are given. Fluids are restricted because there is damage to the pulmonary capillary bed, which can lead to pulmonary fluid overload. Antibiotics are given to prevent septicemia, which is a complication of lung contusion.

Guidelines for Application of the Nursing Process to the Care of the Patient with a Pulmonary Contusion

Carefully assess respiratory status and vital signs to monitor for any impending complications.

Whenever possible, place the patient in a high Fowler's position to facilitate breathing. Suction if the patient is unable to raise secretions because of pain. Give oxygen and pain medication as ordered, and have the patient do deep breathing exercises every 1 to 2 hours.

Subcutaneous Emphysema

Subcutaneous emphysema is a potential complication of any injury affecting the integrity of the lower respiratory system. In this condition, air that has escaped from the lung has entered the subcutaneous tissue. Because the air can travel quite a distance, it may be present in the neck, thorax, and face. It can also involve the abdomen, the scrotum, and even the lower extremities. It is easily recognized by the classic crepitations (crackling sounds) heard when palpating the skin.

The presence of subcutaneous emphysema suggests the need for thorough x-ray examination and close observation to determine the extent of the intrathoracic injury. Once the underlying problem is resolved, the air is spontaneously resorbed, a process that can be hastened by the administration of high concentrations of oxygen. In very severe cases of subcutaneous emphysema, a tracheotomy may be needed to keep the airway patent until the air has been resorbed.

Neoplasia

Lung Cancer

ETIOLOGY

The exact cause and pathogenesis of cancer in general remain unknown; however, there is strong evidence to suggest a relation between prolonged inhalation of air pollutants and the occurrence of lung cancer. Smoking is the most common of these pollutants. Ninety percent of all patients with lung cancer are cigarette smokers. The risk of the development of lung cancer diminishes with the cessation of smoking. In fact, some authorities believe that 15 years of abstention from smoking places the former smoker in the same risk category as a person who has never smoked.

Other factors associated with lung cancer are industrial exposure to certain inorganic and synthetic substances, asbestos dust, and radioactive substances. The presence of scars or other chronic lung lesions and, according to a Minnesota study, drinking more than five cups of coffee per day also appear to predispose to lung cancer.

PATHOPHYSIOLOGY

The four major types of lung cancer are squamous cell carcinoma (also referred to as epidermoid), adenocarcinoma, large-cell carcinoma, and small-cell carcinoma.

Squamous cell carcinomas are central in origin; that is, they arise from the major bronchi or their immediate subdivisions. These tumors grow slowly, often into the lumen, thus obstructing the airways. They sometimes cavitate. Poorly differentiated squamous cell carcinomas of the lung tend to metastasize to the small bowel, whereas well-differentiated lesions primarily spread within the thorax. Prognosis is poorest for this type of lung cancer.

Adenocarcinoma, the most common type of lung cancer, tends to arise in the lung periphery. They are often quite large when discovered, having spread in a patchy distribution resembling an infectious process throughout one lobe or an entire lung. Adenocarcinomas frequently invade the pleura, resulting in a pleural effusion containing malignant cells. They metastasize early most often to the brain, although the other lung, the liver, the adrenal glands, and the bone may also be sites of metastases.

Bronchioalveolar carcinomas are a subtype of adenocarcinoma that originate in the terminal bronchioloalveolar regions. They tend to grow on the surfaces of the airways and are associated with copious sputum production. They do not tend to spread by invasion of local tissues but rather by dissemination through the airways.

Large-cell carcinomas tend to arise in peripheral bronchi and do not exhibit the well-defined patterns of other cell types. They generally present as a bulky tumor mass and metastasize early, usually to the central nervous system.

Small-cell carcinomas are the most malignant of all lung cancers. They generally arise centrally and metastasize through the blood stream and lymphatic vessels early in the disease process. Common metastatic sites are the mediastinum, liver, bone and bone marrow, central nervous system, adrenal glands, pancreas, and other endocrine organs.

The main sites of metastases from all primary lung tumors are the liver, brain, bone, kidney, and adrenal glands.

CLINICAL MANIFESTATIONS

Signs and symptoms depend on the location and size of the tumor mass. Localized symptoms include cough (usually mistaken for smoker's cough), dyspnea, hemoptysis, stridor or wheeze, and signs of obstructive pneumonitis. The expectoration of blood-tinged sputum is common. This is caused by the sputum becoming streaked with blood as it passes over the ulcerated tumor surface. Recurring fever may also be present because of an area of persistent pneumonitis.

In some cases, symptoms do not occur until the tumor has spread to adjacent thoracic structures and is putting pressure on nerves or until it has invaded the chest wall or mediastinum. Symptoms then depend on the area of spread and organs and nerves affected.

As the tumor spreads to the outside surface of the lung, there is an accumulation of fluid with resulting pleural effusion. This causes chest pain and difficulty breathing. If the tumor invades the mediastinum, there is obstruction of the superior vena cava, with resulting head and neck edema and possible pericardial effusion with cardiac tamponade. If the left recurrent laryngeal nerve is involved, hoarseness or left vocal cord paralysis may be the presenting symptom. Late in the course of the disease, weakness, anorexia, weight loss, and anemia appear as well as symptoms caused by any distant metastases.

MEDICAL DIAGNOSIS

The diagnosis of bronchogenic carcinoma is suggested by the patient's clinical history and the findings on physical examination and chest x-ray film. The diagnosis is confirmed by sputum cytology or by biopsy obtained during bronchoscopy.

If metastasis is suggested by presenting symptoms, physical examination or results of standard blood chemistries, additional tests such as bone, liver, and brain scans are done.

If surgery is considered, tests of cardiac function and pulmonary function are done to determine the patient's ability to tolerate the physiologic stress of surgery.

MEDICAL MANAGEMENT

Management of lung cancer depends on the type of cancer, the stage of the cancer, and the overall general condition of the patient.

There are three basic forms of treatment: surgery, radiation therapy, and chemotherapy. One or all three methods may be used.

Surgery is usually performed when the tumor is localized with no evidence of metastasis. The surgery may be a lobectomy or a pneumonectomy with resection of involved mediastinal lymph nodes. Palliative surgery is not advisable because symptoms can be alleviated by other forms of treatment (e.g., a thoracentesis may be done to alleviate pain or shortness of breath caused by pleural effusion).

Radiation therapy is used as a definitive treatment for localized intrathoracic lung cancers. It is also used for small-cell and epidermoid tumors that cannot be resected. It is used to decrease the tumor size and relieve the pressure on vital organs and nerves. Relief of symptoms can last from a few weeks to many months and helps to improve the quality of life for these patients.

Because metastasis occurs in 90% of patients with lung cancer, chemotherapy is widely used. The small-cell cancers have been shown to be the most responsive to this form of therapy. The choice of drug depends on the growth of the tumor cell and the specificity of the drug for a cell cycle phase. The chemotherapeutic regimen usually involves administration of cyclophosphamide, methotrexate, vincristine, doxorubicin hydrochloride, and procarbazine in varying three- or four-drug combinations concurrently.

Management of syndrome of inappropriate antidiuretic hormone secretion (SIADH), if present, is aimed at restoring normal fluid balance and osmolality. Restrictions of fluid alone may be useful. If this is unsuccessful, 5% saline solution may be given intravenously. If cardiac problems such as congestive heart failure develop, diuretics are used to promote diuresis followed with potassium supplements. This form of SIADH is chronic in nature when associated with tumors. In some cases, demeclocycline, 900 to 1200 mg daily, may be given, which causes a nephrogenic diabetes insipidus.

Application of the Nursing Process to the Care of the Patient with Lung Cancer

Assessment

Carefully assess the patient's respiratory function. Obtain information about cough patterns, wheezing, chest tightness, hemoptysis, blood-tinged sputum, dyspnea, and hoarseness. Question the patient in regard to shoulder and arm pain, headache, unsteady gait, fatigue, weight loss, edema of the head and neck, and anorexia. Note time of onset and pattern of progression as well as current status of each.

Appraise overall physical condition, noting whether the patient appears nourished or emaciated. Review the patient's history to identify concurrent medical problems, and obtain information on any medications being taken.

Once the diagnosis is made, assess the emotional response of the patient and family as well as their understanding of the diagnosis, diagnostic procedures, and therapeutic interventions.

Nursing Diagnoses and Planning

Nursing diagnoses and related expected patient outcomes most commonly applicable to patients with lung cancer include the following:

NDx: Impaired gas exchange related to decreased functional lung tissue secondary to tumor growth

Planning: Patient outcomes
1. Dyspnea is absent.
2. Cyanosis is absent.
3. Arterial blood gas values are within normal limits.

NDx: Ineffective breathing pattern related to chest pain and/or depressant effects of narcotic analgesics

Planning: Patient outcomes
1. Respirations are of normal rate and depth.
2. Arterial blood gas values are within normal limits.

NDx: High risk for fluid volume excess related to chronic SIADH

Planning: Patient outcomes
1. Patient's weight is stable.
2. Intake and output are balanced.
3. Serum sodium and osmolality levels are within normal limits.

NDx: Anxiety related to diagnosis, its treatment, and its outcomes

Planning: Patient outcomes
1. Patient freely expresses anxiety about the diagnosis.
2. Patient discusses concerns and feelings with family or significant other.
3. Patient practices relaxation techniques daily.
4. Patient identifies available support systems.
5. Patient states home and telephone number of a mental health professional or support group representative to contact if needed.

NDx: High risk for altered health maintenance related to insufficient knowledge of lung cancer, its treatment and prognosis, and self-care

Planning: Patient outcomes
1. Patient verbalizes realistic perceptions about diagnosis and treatments.
2. Patient describes plan of follow-up care.
3. Patient lists general goals of self-care, describing methods of achieving them.

Nursing Interventions

NDx: Impaired gas exchange
Place the patient in high Fowler's position to facilitate chest expansion. Administer oxygen as ordered. Because anxiety increases the oxygen demands of the body, act to put the patient at ease. Keep the environment calm and quiet, reassure the patient that you are available when needed, and prepare the patient well for all aspects of care.

NDx: Ineffective breathing pattern
Give analgesics for chest pain to make the patient comfortable and to eliminate the need to splint the chest and take shallow breaths. Instruct the patient to breathe deeply, cough, and use an incentive spirometer every 2 hours. Assist with postural drainage, percussion, and vibration if ordered.

NDx: High risk for fluid volume excess
Monitor for and report signs and symptoms of SIADH: sudden weight gain, intake greater than output, irritability, lethargy, confusion, peripheral edema, headache, weakness, nausea, abdominal cramping, and seizures.

NDx: Anxiety
Provide frequent, private opportunities for the patient to express anxieties. If the patient indicates inability or reluctance to discuss concerns with significant others, promote discussion of these feelings and, if deemed appropriate, assist the patient to find the right words and approach through role playing.

Guide the patient in the use of relaxation techniques and provide diversion of the patient's choice.

Work with the patient to identify available support systems, and provide the patient with information needed to contact a support group or mental health professional if needed.

NDx: High risk for altered health maintenance
Clarify and reinforce information given by the physician to the patient and the family. Review information on chemotherapy or radiation therapy if planned. Answer questions clearly, and refer to additional sources of informational material as appropriate.

Explain rationale, side effects, and dosage schedules of prescribed medications. Review chest physiotherapy techniques such as postural drainage, percussion, and vibration. Teach the use of any prescribed equipment such as oxygen, IPPB, incentive spirometer, or humidifier, and obtain a return demonstration.

Include the family or significant other in the teaching sessions to promote compliance, and provide a written summary of treatments, procedures, diet, medications, and follow-up appointments.

Provide information about community resources

Chart 14–4.

NURSING GUIDE TO PATIENT EDUCATION FOR SELF-MANAGEMENT: LUNG CANCER

To promote maximum respiratory efficiency, instruct the patient to:

Avoid respiratory irritants:
- Stop smoking.
- Avoid smoke-filled rooms.
- Avoid fumes from household chemicals.
- Avoid extremes of hot and cold temperatures.

Decrease risks of respiratory infection:
- Avoid persons with respiratory infections.
- Avoid crowds.
- Maintain good oral hygiene.
- Carefully cleanse all respiratory equipment.
- Drink at least 10 glasses of liquid daily.

Follow prescribed chest physical therapy routines.

Take medications as ordered.

To control chronic syndrome of inappropriate antidiuretic hormone (SIADH), instruct the patient to:

Take medications as prescribed.

Follow prescribed dietary modifications:
- Increased sodium intake
- Increased potassium intake

Report any new or worsened symptoms of SIADH:
- Lethargy, confusion
- Weakness
- Headache
- Sudden weight gain
- Nausea
- Abdominal cramping
- Intake consistently more than output
- Seizures

(*continued*)

available to assist with home management, such as the American Cancer Society, Visiting Nurse Association, Meals on Wheels, Hospice, and I Can Cope.

Instruct the patient in self-care as specified in Chart 14–4.

Additional Interventions

Other nursing interventions relate directly to the type of medical treatment the patient is receiving. For example, if the patient is undergoing surgery, nursing care of the patient having chest surgery (see Chapter 12 and Nursing Care Guide 14–1) applies, and if the patient is having radiation or chemotherapy, the care related to these respective treatments applies (see Chapter 11).

Evaluation

Evaluate the effectiveness of nursing care for a patient with lung cancer by comparing the patient's status with the expected patient outcomes. Examples of specific outcomes for patients with lung cancer have been provided in the Planning section.

Chart 14–4. *(continued)*

NURSING GUIDE TO PATIENT EDUCATION FOR SELF-MANAGEMENT: LUNG CANCER

To promote adequate nutrition, instruct the patient to:

For loss of appetite:
- Eat small meals frequently.
- Keep snacks handy for nibbling.
- Rely on favorite foods during not-hungry times.
- Prepare foods attractively (e.g., garnished, varied colors).
- Snack at bedtime.
- Try milk shakes, frozen yogurt, eggnog, or ice cream mixed with favorite soft drinks.

For change in taste:
- Try chicken, turkey, fish (avoid strong-smelling fish; cook on barbeque), cheese, eggs
- Add bacon bits, sliced almonds, or ham strips to vegetables for added flavor
- Use tart foods to enhance flavors (e.g., vinegar, lemon or orange juice, pickles)
- Try marinating meats
- Use more and stronger seasonings, such as basil, oregano, rosemary, tarragon
- Try eliminating strange taste in the mouth by drinking more liquids, such as water, tea, and ginger ale, or eating foods that leave their own tastes, such as fresh fruits or hard candies
- Be sure to have dental checkup to rule out dental problems as the source of the change in taste

For feeling of fullness after eating only a little:
- Chew foods slowly.
- Limit greasy foods, butter, and rich sauces.
- Eat smaller meals more often.
- Be sure liquids taken have nutritional content.
- Limit fluids at mealtime.

For feeling too tired to eat:
- Rely on frozen meals made during "well" times.
- Use convenience foods.
- Try canned cream soups with fish or chicken and fresh fruit to make well-balanced and quickly prepared meals.
- Accept offers of help from family and friends.
- Contact community service groups (e.g., Meals on Wheels).

To allow for continuing care as needed, instruct the patient to:

Report the following symptoms:
- Increased symptoms of SIADH (see earlier section)
- Difficulty swallowing
- Increased fatigue, weakness, or shortness of breath
- Pain in shoulder, arm, or neck
- Swollen, painful joints
- Signs and symptoms of hypercalcemia: nausea, vomiting, muscle weakness, confusion, and increased thirst and urination
- Fever that persists
- Increasing productive cough (purulent, foul-smelling, blood-stained sputum)
- Excessive depression or difficulty coping with the diagnosis

Tumors of the Mediastinum

Mediastinal tumors are found adjacent to vital structures and have an unpredictable manner of growth. Lesions of the mediastinum are usually classified according to their location in the anterior, middle, or posterior mediastinal compartments. Some of the more common types are thymic tumor, mesodermal tumors, neurogenic tumors, and endocrine tumors.

ETIOLOGY AND PATHOPHYSIOLOGY

The exact cause of the various mediastinal tumors is unknown. They are usually neoplastic but may be congenital, traumatic, infectious, or degenerative in nature. Tumors that originate in the neck, chest wall, or diaphragm may extend or grow into the mediastinum and simulate a primary mediastinal mass.

CLINICAL MANIFESTATIONS

Symptoms vary depending on which area of the intrathoracic region the tumor is exerting pressure. They include chest pain, orthopnea, cardiac palpitation, anginal attacks, cyanosis, superior vena caval syndromes (swelling of the face, neck, and upper extremities), distention of the neck veins, and dysphagia caused by the pressure on the esophagus.

MEDICAL DIAGNOSIS

X-ray films of the chest and mediastinal region, and computed tomography scanning are used to detect and define mediastinal masses. Sputum examinations to rule out tuberculosis are also routinely done.

MEDICAL MANAGEMENT

The management of mediastinal tumors includes surgery, radiotherapy, and chemotherapy. If the tumor is benign and operable, surgery may be the only treatment necessary.

Application of the Nursing Process to the Care of the Patient with a Mediastinal Tumor

The assessment, nursing diagnoses, expected patient outcomes, nursing interventions, and evaluation for patients with mediastinal tumors are similar to those described for patients with tumors elsewhere in the chest who are treated with surgery, radiation, or chemotherapy (see Chapters 11 and 12).

The Elderly: Special Considerations

All types of lower respiratory tract disease occur in the elderly; COPD, influenza, and pneumonia are among the most common. Lower respiratory tract diseases differ in the elderly in that they are superimposed on normal age-related changes in the structure and function of the respiratory system and often on coexisting disease and medication regimens. This results in highly variable presentation and course of lower respiratory tract diseases, greater severity, and increased risk of complications.

Pneumonia in the elderly is a very serious illness and, with influenza, is the leading infectious cause of death among this age group. Placing the patient at risk for pneumonia is the loss of elasticity in the lung, weakened muscles of respiration, decreased effectiveness of the mucociliary escalator, decreased forced vital capacity (FVC), decreased effectiveness of immune function, and, in many cases, the coexistence of chronic pulmonary disease. Although the potential causative organisms are the same as in other age groups, there is a greater incidence of gram-negative disease, which is associated with a higher mortality rate. The clinical presentation of pneumonia is frequently atypical; an insidious deterioration in overall health status and mental confusion often are the first manifestations. In some cases, an unexplained delayed recovery from another health problem or the sudden worsening of a coexistent problem constitutes the initial sign of the disease. Fever, cough, and purulent sputum—the classic signs of pneumonia—may be absent, although increased respiratory rate and leukocytosis with a left shift are commonly seen. Other symptoms that may be present are chills, vomiting, dyspnea, stabbing chest pain, and lethargy. Thus, the early recognition of pneumonia in the elderly requires astute observation and a high degree of clinical suspicion. Obtaining a sputum specimen for identification of the causative organism can also present problems in the elderly. Because of weakened cough and frequency of dehydration, raising a specimen can be difficult.

Tuberculosis is another disease for which the elderly, particularly those in an institutional setting, are at risk. Many of today's elderly were exposed to family members or friends with active tuberculosis during childhood at a time when tuberculosis was rampant. Because prophylactic medication was not available until the 1950s, many of the elderly who were exposed are now at risk for granuloma breakdown and the development of active disease, particularly in light of impairments in immunity that appear to occur with age. Like pneumonia, the presentation of tuberculosis in the elderly is frequently atypical. Thus, it should be considered a possibility in any patient with unexplained cough or low-grade fever, and information on past exposure as well as current PPD status should be included in all patient histories.

Nursing Care Guide 14–1.

PATIENTS UNDERGOING PNEUMONECTOMY FOR CANCER OF THE LUNG

Preoperative Care

Assessment Findings: Patient states "I'm afraid of anesthesia, I'm afraid of the surgery, and I'm afraid the cancer has spread, so there is nothing that can be done." Patient paces in room and wrings hands. Patient seems "lost in own world."

Nursing Diagnosis: Anxiety related to the diagnosis of cancer and the surgical experience

Patient Outcomes	Nursing Interventions	Rationale
Patient expresses concerns freely.	Provide opportunity and environment conducive to expression of anxiety.	Allows for feedback, provides perspective, and permits a supportive relationship.
Patient attends to information and directions.	Acknowledge that anxiety over the diagnosis of lung cancer and surgery is normal.	Allays patient concerns about being judged negatively because of anxiety.
Pacing, hand wringing, and other behaviors indicative of excessive anxiety are absent.	Reassure patient regarding safety of modern anesthetic and surgical techniques and the ability and concern of all the people involved in his or her care. Describe the close supervision given during each stage of the operative experience.	Provides the patient with positive facts about the operative procedure on which to focus and base hope for a successful surgical outcome.

Evaluation: Compare the patient's status with the expected patient outcomes. If the outcomes are achieved, evaluate nursing care as successful. If not, reassess the patient, formulate new nursing diagnoses, and revise expected patient outcomes and nursing interventions as appropriate.

(continued)

Nursing Care Guide 14–1. *(continued)*

PATIENTS UNDERGOING PNEUMONECTOMY FOR CANCER OF THE LUNG

Assessment Findings: Patient has no prior experience with surgery. Patient asks questions about perioperative care.

Nursing Diagnosis: Knowledge deficit: perioperative care

Patient Outcomes	Nursing Interventions	Rationale
Patient describes preoperative preparations, postanesthesia care unit (PACU) routines, and expected postoperative course and treatments.	Explain perioperative care. Provide information on preparation for and transport to the operating room, the PACU and its routines, and the expected postoperative apparatus such as chest tubes (if used by the surgeon), intravenous fluids, oxygen, central venous pressure catheter, pulmonary artery catheter, and urinary and surgical dressing.	Prepares patient for perioperative events; promotes compliance with perioperative care; and decreases the risk of anxiety over routine perioperative events.
	Tell the patient that chest pain is expected after surgery, that medication will be available, and that he or she should not hesitate to ask for it.	Provides information about normal experiences as well as appropriate patient response.
Patient explains importance of turning, coughing, and deep breathing postoperatively. Patient demonstrates coughing and deep-breathing techniques.	Instruct the patient in the importance and technique of turning, coughing, and deep breathing.	Learning is best accomplished when patient is in a pain-free, low-anxiety state before surgery.
Patient demonstrates use of a pillow or folded towel to splint the area of the incision.	Show the patient how the incision will be splinted with the nurse's hands or pillow or folded towel during turning, coughing, and deep breathing.	Familiarity with procedures promotes cooperation.
Patient demonstrates exercises to maintain full range of motion in the affected shoulder.	Instruct the patient in exercises to maintain range of motion in the shoulders: ■ Reach behind head and neck with affected arm and hand, and try to touch top of shoulder blade on affected side. ■ Reach across chest with affected arm and hand and touch outer edge of unaffected shoulder. ■ Reach behind the middle of the back with affected arm and hand, and touch lower edge of the shoulder blade on unaffected side.	Provides information that will be needed in the postoperative period at a time conducive to learning.

(continued)

Nursing Care Guide 14–1. *(continued)*

PATIENTS UNDERGOING PNEUMONECTOMY FOR CANCER OF THE LUNG

Evaluation: Compare the patient's status with the expected patient outcomes. If the outcomes are achieved, evaluate nursing care as successful. If not, reassess the patient, formulate new nursing diagnoses, and revise expected patient outcomes and nursing interventions as appropriate.

Postoperative Care

Assessment Findings: Rapid, noisy respirations, crackles audible on auscultation, complaints of dyspnea, cough without expectoration

Nursing Diagnosis: Ineffective airway clearance related to excessive secretions and shallow breathing

Patient Outcomes	Nursing Interventions	Rationale
Airway is cleared of secretions by coughing or suctioning. Respirations are quiet and easy. Crackles are absent on auscultation.	Change position every 1 to 2 hours.	Position in bed splints the chest wall, decreasing aeration of tissues. Changing positions changes the section of lung tissue splinted. Position changes also help drain secretions so that they can be removed from the lungs.
	Turn patient on back and to operative side only.	Keeps fluid in pleural space below the bronchial stump.
	Elevate head of bed approximately 30 degrees when blood pressure is stable to promote ventilation.	Gravity pulls the intestines away from the diaphragm, facilitating increased lung expansion.
	Instruct the patient to cough and deep breathe every hour for the first 24 hours after surgery.	Promotes good ventilation and airway clearance.
	Splint the incision to limit discomfort.	Pain decreases patient willingness to cough and breathe deeply.
	Assist with postural drainage if ordered.	Assists in removal of secretions to maintain oxygenation.
	Encourage fluids to 1500–2000 ml per day unless contraindicated.	Fluids thin respiratory secretions so that they can be cleared from the respiratory tract more easily.
	Perform nasotracheal suction if needed.	Removes secretions and maintains gas exchange.

Evaluation: Compare the patient's status with the expected patient outcomes. If the outcomes are achieved, evaluate nursing care as successful. If not, reassess the patient, formulate new nursing diagnoses, and revise expected patient outcomes and nursing interventions as appropriate.

(continued)

Nursing Care Guide 14–1. *(continued)*

PATIENTS UNDERGOING PNEUMONECTOMY FOR CANCER OF THE LUNG

Assessment Findings: Complaints of dyspnea, elevated pulse and respiratory rate, restlessness

Nursing Diagnosis: Impaired gas exchange related to decreased functional lung tissue and hypoventilation

Patient Outcomes	Nursing Interventions	Rationale
Vital signs are within normal range. Cyanosis is absent. Arterial blood gas values are within normal range.	Administer humidified oxygen as ordered.	Increases/maintains Po_2 despite diminished lung tissue.
	Do not position patient on unoperated side.	Prevents bed from splinting the chest, interfering with maximal ventilation of the remaining lung tissue.
	If the patient does not have a chest tube or if it is clamped most of the time, monitor for mediastinal shift with decreased ventilation secondary to compression of the remaining lung and decreased cardiac output secondary to impaired venous return to the heart. This is manifested by dyspnea, cyanosis, nasal flaring and intercostal retraction, severe chest pain, agitation, and tachycardia.	Accumulation of blood or fluid increases pressure on operative side, causing mediastinal shift and compromise of functioning tissue.

Evaluation: Compare the patient's status with the expected patient outcomes. If the outcomes are achieved, evaluate nursing care as successful. If not, reassess the patient, formulate new nursing diagnoses, and revise expected patient outcomes and nursing interventions as appropriate.

(continued)

Nursing Care Guide 14–1. *(continued)*

PATIENTS UNDERGOING PNEUMONECTOMY FOR CANCER OF THE LUNG

Assessment Findings: Patient complains of chest pain. Patient occasionally moans. Patient grimaces and groans on moving.

Nursing Diagnosis: Pain related to chest surgery

Patient Outcomes	Nursing Interventions	Rationale
Patient states pain is relieved. Patient moves and turns easily without grimacing, groaning, or other behavioral indications of pain.	Administer narcotic analgesics as ordered and needed in the early postoperative period, often every 3 hours. Observe for resultant respiratory depression. Later, give analgesics such as acetylsalicylic acid (ASA) or acetaminophen as ordered. Be certain to give pain medication a half-hour or so before exercises or other painful treatments.	Early analgesic administration provides more effective pain relief. Pain relief encourages compliance with postoperative procedures such as coughing, deep breathing, and turning, which improve oxygenation. Because narcotics have a depressant effect on respirations, care should be taken in their administration to the patient whose respiratory status is compromised. Administration 30 minutes before exercise allows medication to reach its maximum effectiveness.
	Splint patient's chest and avoid moving the chest tube when turning or moving.	Reduces pain and increases compliance with turning or moving.
	Maintain a calm, quiet environment.	Tension-reducing environment promotes relaxation and rest.
	Give back care, and reposition frequently.	Reduces muscle tension and promotes rest and relaxation.
	Encourage the use of relaxation techniques.	Reduces tension level and diverts attention from pain.
	Provide diversion such as soft music in accordance with the patient's wishes.	Reduces muscle tension, promoting rest and relaxation.

Evaluation: Compare the patient's status against the expected patient outcomes. If the outcomes are achieved, evaluate nursing care as successful. If not, reassess the patient, formulate new nursing diagnoses, and revise expected patient outcomes and nursing interventions as appropriate.

(continued)

Nursing Care Guide 14–1. *(continued)*

PATIENTS UNDERGOING PNEUMONECTOMY FOR CANCER OF THE LUNG

Assessment Findings: Patient states "I feel like I'm tied up in knots. I feel like something awful is going to happen." Patient also complains of dry mouth and heart palpitations. Voice is tremulous, and patient cries easily. Patient has obvious restlessness and difficulty concentrating.

Nursing Diagnosis: Anxiety related to outcome of treatment, effects of cancer on family and lifestyle, possible recurrence, and death

Patient Outcomes	Nursing Interventions	Rationale
Patient expresses anxieties openly to nurse and significant other.	Schedule regular opportunities for the patient to discuss and ventilate anxieties in an unhurried manner.	Demonstrates concern, facilitates a supportive relationship, and promotes open communication.
Patient asks relevant questions about prognosis, treatments, and self-care.	Give the patient information in clear, simple terms regarding anticipated treatments and their effects.	Promotes effective communication.
	Encourage the patient to ask questions. Avoid false reassurances.	Encouraging the patient to ask questions and avoiding false reassurances promotes a positive interpersonal relationship and provides an environment conducive to sharing of feelings.
Patient expresses confidence in ability to cope.	Arrange for patients to meet with a cancer patient who has had successful surgery for cancer of the lung.	Provides a credible source of hope and information.
	Encourage the patient to join a support group and facilitate contact with the group.	Support groups provide an environment conducive to sharing of feelings as well as resources and problem-solving actions..
Signs of excessive anxiety such as inability to attend to directions or conversation, shaking, and hand wringing are absent.	If needed and ordered, administer antianxiety medications.	Pharmacologically reduces anxiety, allowing patient to focus on positive feelings and actions.

Evaluation: Compare the patient's status with the expected patient outcomes. If the outcomes are achieved, evaluate nursing care as successful. If not, reassess the patient, formulate new nursing diagnoses, and revise expected patient outcomes and nursing interventions as appropriate.

(continued)

Nursing Care Guide 14–1. *(continued)*

PATIENTS UNDERGOING PNEUMONECTOMY FOR CANCER OF THE LUNG

Assessment Findings: Patient has a thoracotomy incision, which affects the trapezius, rhomboideus major, serratus anterior, and latissimus dorsi muscles. Spontaneous movements of the arm on the operative side are limited.

Nursing Diagnosis: High risk for impaired physical mobility related to surgical trauma affecting muscles that control shoulder movement

Patient Outcomes	Nursing Interventions	Rationale
Patient participates in arm and shoulder exercises as directed.	Give passive range-of-motion exercise to the affected shoulder during the early postoperative period.	Maintains free range of joint motion.
Patient regains usual range of motion in the shoulder on the operative side.	Once the patient is out of bed, begin active range-of-motion and arm and shoulder exercises, taught preoperatively, four times per day.	Maintains free range of joint motion, increases muscle strength, and promotes muscle tone.
	Continue to stress the importance of following the exercise routine if shoulder stiffness, limitation of movement, and loss of muscle strength are to be prevented.	Provides incentive to maintain exercise regimen.

Evaluation: Compare the patient's status against the expected patient outcomes. If the outcomes are achieved, evaluate nursing care as successful. If not, reassess the patient, formulate new nursing diagnoses, and revise expected patient outcomes and nursing interventions as appropriate.

(continued)

Nursing Care Guide 14–1. *(continued)*

PATIENTS UNDERGOING PNEUMONECTOMY FOR CANCER OF THE LUNG

Assessment Findings: Patient and various family members describe the family as normally working well as a unit and supportive of its members. The patient's illness is described as creating a great deal of stress for family members.

Nursing Diagnosis: High risk for altered family processes related to one of its members being diagnosed with cancer of the lung and having surgery

Patient Outcomes	Nursing Interventions	Rationale
Family members express thoughts and feelings regarding effects of cancer to each other and to health professional.	Speak with each family member regarding his or her own stress.	Allows each individual to realize that his or her feelings are important, reducing individual stress and promoting family interaction.
Family affirms by words and deeds that the patient is a valued family member. Family members work together to attack problems and share responsibility.	Discuss ways of constructive coping with the family such as use of humor, respect of individuality, mutual reliance and support, sharing thoughts and feelings, and shared decision making.	Promotes use of constructive coping techniques.
	Facilitate freer family communication patterns by clarifying ambiguous messages.	Reduces miscommunication, thereby improving relationship among family members.
	Stress that crises carry potential for positive change.	Helps individual family members recognize the positive as well as the negative sides of a crisis and helps them mobilize for effective coping.
	Encourage family members to help plan posthospital care.	Promotes a sense of control and helpfulness and contributes to the development of a realistic plan of postdischarge care.
	Provide privacy for family visits.	Allows communication at a personal level.
Family uses community services and referrals as needed.	Make referrals as needed to community research groups such as the American Cancer Society.	Community resources help individuals and families meet their needs.

Evaluation: Compare the patient's status against the expected patient outcomes. If the outcomes are achieved, evaluate nursing care as successful. If not, reassess the patient, formulate new nursing diagnoses, and revise expected patient outcomes and nursing interventions as appropriate.

(continued)

Nursing Care Guide 14–1. *(continued)*

PATIENTS UNDERGOING PNEUMONECTOMY FOR CANCER OF THE LUNG

Assessment Findings: Patient has no previous experience with chest surgery and asks questions about self-care after discharge.

Nursing Diagnosis: High risk for altered health maintenance related to insufficient knowledge of self-care after discharge

Patient Outcomes	Nursing Interventions	Rationale
Patient explains need to regularly perform arm and shoulder exercises to prevent a limitation of mobility.	Review the importance of regular arm and shoulder exercises as done in the hospital to prevent limitations of mobility.	Reminds the patient of the need for continued exercise to improve range of motion and strength.
Patient demonstrates ability to perform arm and shoulder exercises without ongoing direction. Patient explains instructions for self-care after discharge.	Instruct the patient to: ■ Continue with coughing exercises, deep breathing, and other breathing exercises for 3 to 4 weeks after discharge. ■ Apply heat, and take oral analgesics as ordered for pain in the chest wall ■ Expect muscle weakness in affected side, and avoid lifting heavy objects for at least 3 months. ■ Expect easy fatigue in the first few weeks after discharge, and plan for frequent rest periods during the day. ■ Avoid respiratory irritants. ■ Report any signs of respiratory infection such as fever, increased secretions, or dyspnea.	Provides information necessary for self-maintenance in the postdischarge period.
Patient describes need for follow-up care. Patient states date and location of next scheduled health care visit.	Explain the importance of follow-up care. Inform patient of the purpose and date of the next health care appointment. Be certain the patient knows the category and location of health care practitioner to be seen.	Promotes compliance by providing rationale for follow-up care and information necessary to comply.

Evaluation: Compare the patient's status against the expected patient outcomes. If the outcomes are achieved, evaluate nursing care as successful. If not, reassess the patient, formulate new nursing diagnoses, and revise expected patient outcomes and nursing interventions as appropriate.

(continued)

Nursing Care Guide 14–1. *(continued)*

PATIENTS UNDERGOING PNEUMONECTOMY FOR CANCER OF THE LUNG

Additional Assessments and Interventions

Take vital signs every 15 minutes for 2 hours and then every hour. Decrease frequency as the patient stabilizes and progresses through the postoperative period.

Assess carefully for cardiac dysrhythmias, which are common after pneumonectomy and are most likely to occur from the second to the sixth postoperative days in patients older than age 50.

Check chest dressing for bleeding. Report bleeding if present because drainage on thoracic dressings is not expected.

Monitor fluid and electrolyte status. Obtain daily weights, and check central venous pressure every hour for indication of hypervolemia (more than 12) or hypovolemia (less than 5). Check that urinary output is at least 30 ml/hour.

Give fluids by mouth when alert, and progress to the patient's usual diet over 72 hours.

Bibliography

Allen MA, Ownby KK. Tuberculosis: The other epidemic. J Assoc Nurses AIDS Care 1991; 2(4):9.

Bates DV. Respiratory function in disease. 3rd ed. Philadelphia: WB Saunders, 1989.

Brewis RAA, Gibson GJ, Geddes DM. Respiratory medicine. Philadelphia: WB Saunders, 1990.

Carroll P. Nursing the thoracotomy patient. RN 1992; 55(6):34.

Caruthers DD. Infectious pneumonia in the elderly. Am J Nurs 1990; 90(2):56.

Centers for Disease Control. Stressing TB control after outbreaks of resistant strains. Hosp Infect Control 1991; 18(10):137.

Colby TV, Lombard C, Yousem SA, Masanori K. Atlas of pulmonary surgical pathology, Philadelphia: WB Saunders, 1991.

Dickinson SP, Bury GM. Pulmonary embolism—Anatomy of a crisis. Nursing 1989, 19(4):34.

DuBois RM, Clarke SW. Fiberoptic bronchoscopy in diagnosis and management. Philadelphia: WB Saunders, 1988.

Esberger KK. Nursing care of the aged. Norwalk, CT: Appleton & Lange, 1989.

Flenley DC. Respiratory medicine. 2nd ed. Philadelphia: WB Saunders, 1990.

Fraser RG, Paré JAP, Paré PD, et al. Diagnosis of diseases of the chest. 3rd ed. Philadelphia: WB Saunders, Vol. 1, 1988; Vol. 2, 1989; Vol. 3, 1990; Vol. 4, 1991.

Gambert SR. (Ed). Handbook of geriatrics. New York: Plenum Press, 1987.

Gift AG, Cahill CA. Psychophysiologic aspects of dyspnea in COPD. Heart Lung 1990; 19(3):252.

Hodgkin JE, Petty TL. Chronic obstructive pulmonary disease: Current concepts. Philadelphia: WB Saunders, 1987.

Hood RM. Techniques in general thoracic surgery. Philadelphia: WB Saunders, 1985.

Hood RM. Surgical diseases of the pleura and chest wall. Philadelphia: WB Saunders, 1986.

Hood RM, Boyd A, Culliford AT. Thoracic trauma. Philadelphia: WB Saunders, 1989.

Jess LW. Chronic bronchitis and emphysema: Airing the differences. Nursing 1992; 22(3):34.

Johnson AP. The elderly and COPD. J Gerontol Nurs 1988; 14(12):20.

Karlinsky JB. Decision making in pulmonary medicine. St. Louis: CV Mosby, 1991.

Larear S, Larson JL. Ineffective breathing pattern related to air flow limitation. Nurs Clin North Am 1987; 22(1):179.

May DF. Rehabilitation and care in pulmonary disorders. St. Louis: CV Mosby, 1991.

Murray JF, Nadel JA. Textbook of respiratory medicine. Vols. 1 and 2. Philadelphia: WB Saunders, 1988.

Petty T, Nett L. Enjoying life with emphysema. 2nd ed. Philadelphia: Lea & Febiger, 1987.

Reichel W, Gallo JJ. Handbook of geriatric assessment. Gaithersburg, MD: Aspen, 1988.

Ruiz J, et al (eds). Clinical atlas of respiratory diseases. Chicago: Year Book Medical, 1988.

Sabiston DC Jr. Textbook of surgery: The biological basis of modern surgical practice. 14th ed. Philadelphia: WB Saunders, 1991.

Sabiston DC Jr, Spencer FC. Surgery of the chest. 5th ed. Philadelphia: WB Saunders, 1990.

Schrier RW. Geriatric medicine. Philadelphia: WB Saunders, 1990.

Schroeder SA. Current medical diagnosis and treatment. 30th ed. Norwalk, CT: Appleton & Lange, 1991.

Sexton DL. Nursing care of the respiratory patient. Norwalk, CT: Appleton & Lange, 1989.

Shekleton ME, Litwack K. Critical care nursing of the surgical patient. Philadelphia: WB Saunders, 1991.

Shelhamer J. Respiratory disease in the immunosuppressed host. Philadelphia: JB Lippincott, 1991.

Stein JH. Internal medicine: Diagnosis and therapy. 2nd ed. Norwalk, CT: Appleton & Lange, 1991.

Thompson J, McFarland G, Hirsch J, et al. Manual of clinical nursing. St. Louis: CV Mosby, 1986.

Tuberculosis takes a turn for the worse. Infect Control Hosp Epidemiol 1991; 12(8):506.

Way LW. Current surgical diagnosis and treatment. 9th ed. Norwalk, CT: Appleton & Lange, 1991.

Yeaw EMJ. How position affects oxygenation good lung down? Am J Nurs 1992; 92(3):27.

Unit Five

ADULTS WITH DYSFUNCTION OF THE BLOOD AND BLOOD-FORMING ORGANS

Learning Objectives

AFTER COMPLETING THIS UNIT, THE LEARNER WILL BE ABLE TO:

Chapter Fifteen

1. Explain the normal anatomy and physiology of the blood and blood-forming organs.
2. Describe common clinical manifestations of dysfunction of the blood and blood-forming organs.
3. Describe the common laboratory tests used to confirm diagnoses of hematologic disorders.
4. Describe medical management and surgical procedures commonly used in the treatment of patients with hematologic disorders.
5. Identify disorders of the blood and blood-forming organs that have a genetic base.
6. Compare and contrast the use of blood and/or blood products for specific disorders.
7. Identify data essential to the assessment of patients undergoing treatment of hematologic disorders.
8. State nursing diagnoses and related expected patient outcomes commonly applicable to patients undergoing treatment of hematologic disorders.
9. Describe nursing interventions, with their rationales, commonly applicable to patients undergoing treatment of hematologic disorders.
10. Explain the basis for evaluation of nursing care provided to patients undergoing treatment of hematologic disorders.
11. Identify special considerations for the elderly patient with altered function of the blood and blood-forming organs.

Chapter Sixteen

1. Describe common hematologic disorders in terms of etiology, pathophysiology, clinical manifestations, diagnostic procedures, and medical management.
2. Analyze the pharmacologic therapies for the anemias and leukemias.
3. Identify information and physical examination data essential to the assessment of patients with common hematologic disorders.
4. State nursing diagnoses and related expected patient outcomes commonly applicable to patients with hematologic disorders.
5. Describe nursing interventions, with their rationales, commonly applicable to patients with hematologic disorders.
6. Explain the basis for evaluation of nursing care provided to patients with hematologic disorders.
7. Identify special considerations for the elderly patient with a hematologic disorder.

Chapter Fifteen

KNOWLEDGE BASIC TO THE NURSING CARE *of Adults with Dysfunction of the Blood and Blood-Forming Organs*

The blood and blood-forming organs constitute the hematologic system. The blood-forming organs include the lymph nodes, bone marrow, spleen, and liver. Dysfunction in the system has profound effect on most other body systems because of the nature of the structure and function of the blood and the blood-forming organs. Diseases, dietary deficiencies, and toxic drugs that affect the hematologic system, in turn, affect the respiratory, circulatory, integumentary, digestive, neurologic, and urinary systems.

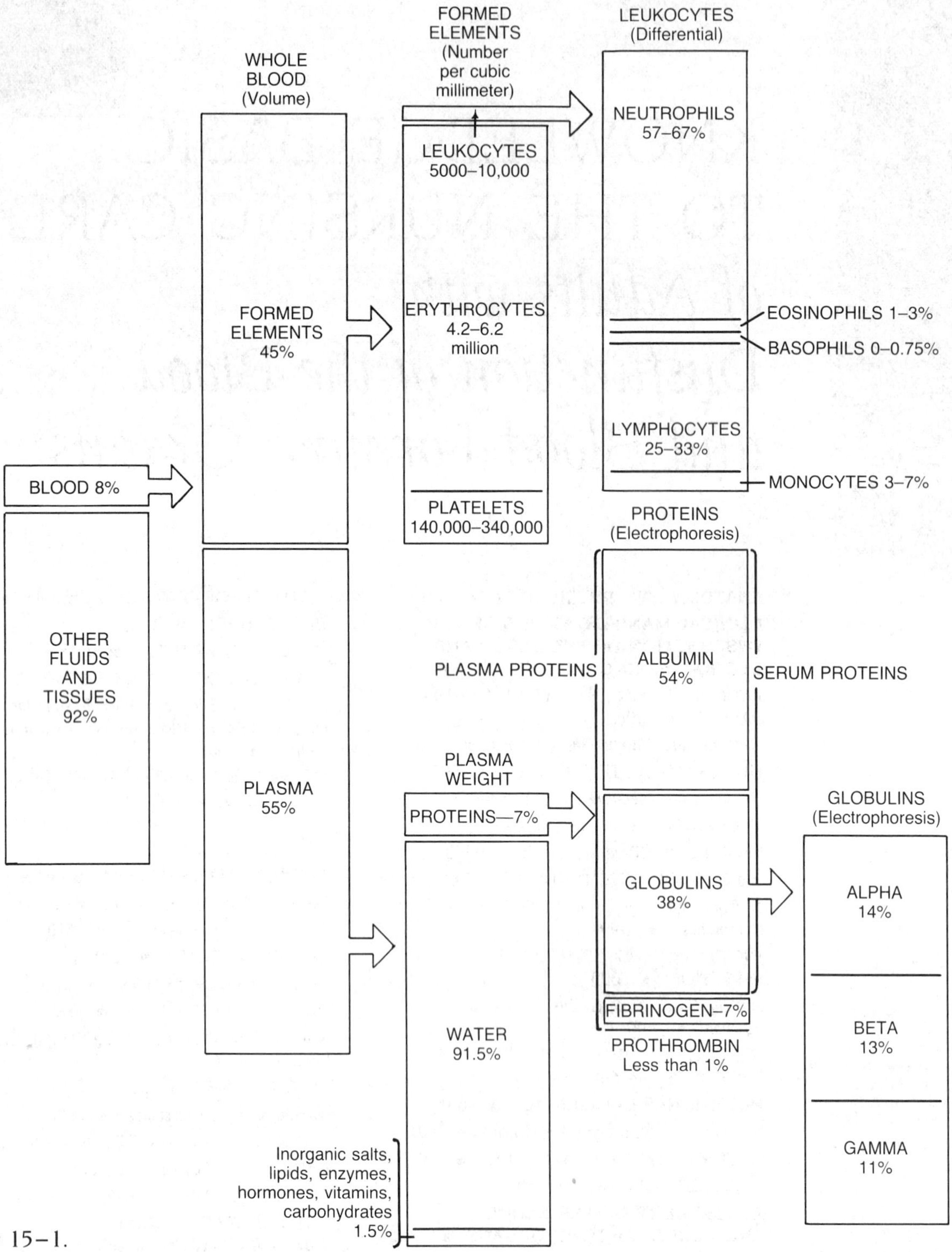

Figure 15–1.

Composition of blood. (From Jacob SW, Francone CA. Elements of anatomy and physiology. 2nd ed. Philadelphia: WB Saunders, 1989, p 164.)

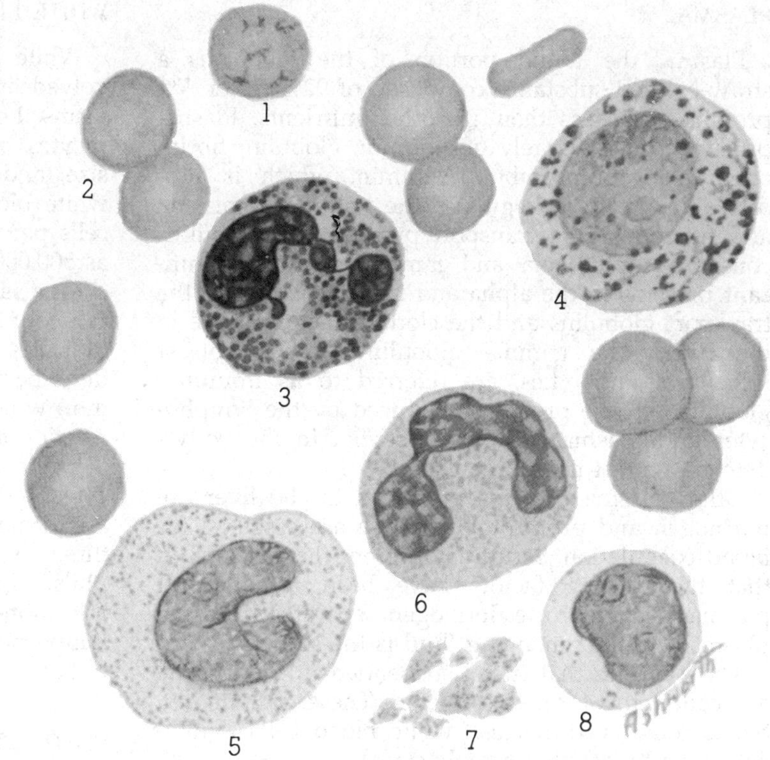

Figure 15–2.

Blood cells: 1, reticulocyte; 2, erythrocyte; 3, eosinophil; 4, basophil; 5, monocyte; 6, neutrophil; 7, platelets; 8, lymphocyte. (From Jacob SW, Francone CA. Elements of anatomy and physiology. 2nd ed. Philadelphia: WB Saunders, 1989, p 165.)

Anatomy and Physiology

Blood

Blood transports oxygen to the cells and carries carbon dioxide from the cells to the lungs for removal from the body. It also has the task of carrying nutrients from the gastointestinal tract to the tissues, while removing waste products from tissues and transporting them to the lungs, kidney, liver, and skin for excretion. The blood transports hormones from the endocrine glands to other parts of the body and protects the body from harmful microorganisms by transporting leukocytes and antibodies to the site of infection, injury, or inflammation. Finally, the blood is responsible for regulating body temperature by transferring heat from within the body to the small vessels supplying the skin, where it can be released into the surrounding environment.

Major characteristics of blood include

- Color: Arterial blood is bright red, as a result of the oxygen and hemoglobin in the red blood cells. Venous blood is dark red because of the loss of oxygen from reduced hemoglobin.
- Volume: An adult has approximately 70 to 75 ml of blood per kg of body weight, which is a total of approximately 5 to 6 L.
- Viscosity: Blood is three to four times more dense than water.
- Reaction: Blood has a slightly salty taste and an alkaline reaction of pH 7.35 to 7.45.

BLOOD COMPONENTS

Blood is composed of straw-colored fluid, the plasma, which accounts for 55% of the blood; cellular suspended particles, the erythrocytes and leukocytes; and non-nucleated cell fragments, the platelets, which constitute the other 45% of the blood. The hematocrit (Hct) is the percentage of total blood volume that is composed of erythrocytes (Figs. 15–1 and 15–2).

The blood cells arise from undifferentiated mesenchymal cells, the hemocytoblasts. During the early intrauterine life, the liver is the dominant blood-forming organ; but by the fifth month, the spleen becomes the dominant producer of blood cells. At birth, neither organ is involved in the production of blood cells.

The bone marrow begins to produce blood cells during the fifth month of intrauterine life and continues the process throughout life. The blood-producing area in the marrow begins in the center of bone and gradually expands through the entire bone marrow up to the time of puberty. At this developmental time, the marrow in the long bones becomes more fatty. The active areas of production of blood cells in the adult are in the skull, ribs, sternum, vertebrae, humerus, femur, and pelvis. In the older adult, increased areas of fat are found in the bones, so blood cell production decreases significantly.

PLASMA

Plasma, the liquid portion of the blood, is a straw-colored substance composed of 92% water, 7% proteins, and less than 1% other nutrients. Plasma proteins consist largely of albumin, globulin, fibrinogen, and prothrombin. Albumin, which is produced in the liver, regulates the volume of plasma and functions as a transport protein. The globulins consist of alpha, beta, and gamma fractions. Significant proteins in the alpha and beta fractions are the transport globulins and the clotting factors made in the liver. The gamma globulins, which consist largely of antibodies, are referred to as immunoglobulins. These proteins, produced by the lymphocytes and plasma cells, are essential in the body's defense against microorganisms.

Other plasma proteins produced in the liver are fibrinogen and prothrombin. These are essential for blood coagulation. Serum is different than plasma in that the clotting factors have been removed. If plasma is clotted, the fibrinogen separates from the plasma and the remaining fluid is the serum.

The particles that travel suspended in the plasma are called the formed elements. These include red blood cells (erythrocytes), white blood cells (leukocytes), and platelets (thrombocytes).

RED BLOOD CELLS

Red blood cells (RBCs), or erythrocytes, are involved in transporting oxygen from the lungs to the tissues. Red blood cells are formed in the red marrow of bone. This process is called erythropoiesis. Prior to the development of a fully mature red blood cell, the nucleus is extruded. The size of the red blood cell is approximately 7μ, but this increases as the pH of the blood decreases. Since the pH of the blood is lower in venous blood, the red blood cell is larger in venous blood than in arterial blood.

The life span of a red blood cell is approximately 120 days. The normal red blood cell count ranges from 4.5 to 5 million cells in 1 cu mm of blood. It is slightly higher in adult men than in adult women. Red blood cell production increases when oxygen to the tissues decreases. Likewise, red blood cell production decreases when oxygen concentration to tissues increases.

Hemoglobin, a part of the red blood cells, is important in transporting oxygen to the tissues. Hemoglobin is formed with the red blood cells in the red marrow of bone. It contains both iron and a globin fraction. The normal level of hemoglobin in males is 15 g/100 ml and 12 to 14 g/100 ml in females.

Red blood cells are broken down and engulfed by macrophages. Two to ten million are destroyed and replaced each second, leaving the total count constant in the healthy individual. When the red blood cells are broken down, hemoglobin is released. This is further broken down to bilirubin and iron. The bilirubin is excreted by the liver with bile, and the iron is used for continued production of red blood cells.

WHITE BLOOD CELLS

White blood cells (WBCs), or leukocytes, are involved in protecting the body against microorganisms. Leukocytes can be differentiated from erythrocytes by the presence of a nucleus, their larger size, and different staining properties. The normal white blood cell count ranges from 5000 to 10,000 cells per cu mm of blood, but it often rises as high as 500,000/cu mm in diseases like leukemia. Leukocytosis is the term used to describe a white blood cell count higher than 10,000/cu mm, which usually indicates infection. Leukopenia is the term used to describe a white blood cell count below 5000/cu mm, which occurs in some viral disorders and as a reaction to certain drugs.

White blood cells are made up of 60% granulocytes and 40% mononuclear cells. The granulocytes are formed in the bone marrow and are divided into three types—neutrophils, eosinophils, and basophils. Mononuclear cells are 30% lymphocytes and 5% monocytes. Lymphocytes are formed in the lymph nodes and the spleen. Monocytes are formed in bone marrow.

PLATELETS

Platelets (thrombocytes) are small particles in the blood plasma. Their numbers vary between 150,000 and 500,000/cu mm of blood. The platelets are formed in the red bone marrow. The platelets provide thrombokinase, a substance that is important in the blood-clotting process.

BLOOD COAGULATION

Blood coagulation is the process of platelet agglutination, blood vessel contraction, and blood components meshing to form a fibrin clot. Fibrin is formed from proteins in the plasma. The mechanisms of fibrin clot formation are shown diagrammatically in Figure 15–3.

Coagulation occurs when the blood vessels are injured or when blood is removed from a vessel. It involves the formation of thromboplastin, the conversion of prothrombin to thrombin, and the conversion of fibrinogen to fibrin. There are four progressive stages of clotting in which coagulation factors are involved. The clotting factors and their associated names are listed in Table 15–1. The first phase of stage 1 lasts 3 to 5 minutes and involves platelet activity. Platelet counts of less than 1,000,000/cu mm indicate moderate interference with stage 1 activity. Ninety percent of all coagulation disorders are due to defects in stage 1. The second phase of stage 1 is the formation of thromboplastin. Stage 2, which lasts 8 to 15 seconds, involves the conversion of prothrombin (Factor II) in the presence of calcium. Stage 3, which lasts 1 second, involves the interaction of thrombin with fibrinogen to form a clot. At the end of this stage, Factor XIII interacts to stabilize the clot. Stage 4 is the removal of the clot through fibrinolysis. Plas-

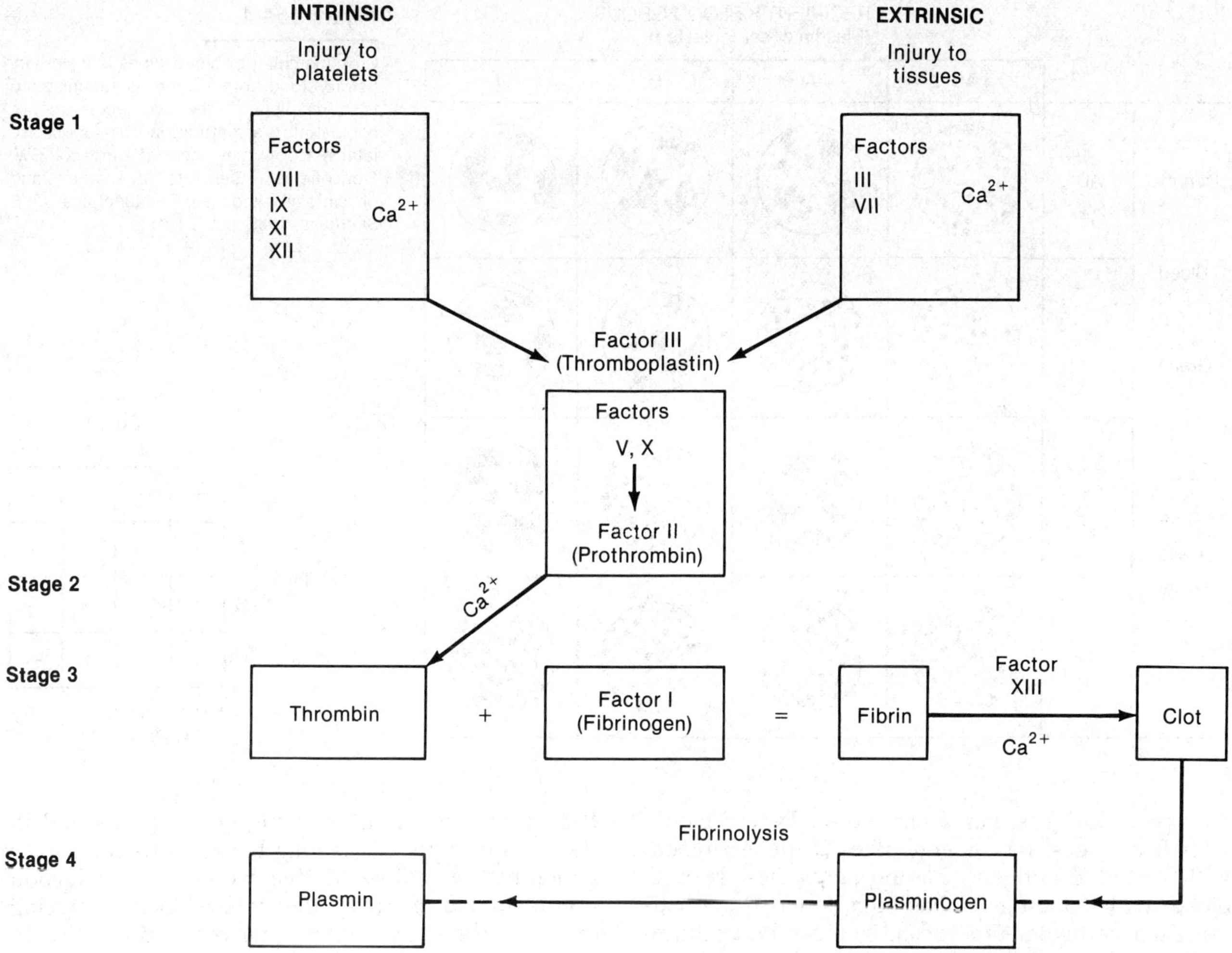

Figure 15–3.

The blood clotting process. This diagram represents the factors necessary to change blood into a solid clot and then dissolve it. The entire chain of reactions occurs at the site of injury. (Adapted from Fischbach F. A manual of laboratory diagnostic tests. Philadelphia: JB Lippincott, 1984, p 85.)

Table 15–1. CLOTTING FACTORS AND NAMES*

FACTOR NUMBER	NAMES
I	Fibrinogen
II	Prothrombin
III	Tissue thromboplastin
IV	Calcium
V	Proaccelerin
VII	Proconvertin
VIII	Antihemophilic globulin (AHG) Antihemophilic factor (AHF)
IX	Plasma thromboplastin component (Christmas factor)
X	Stuart factor
XI	Plasma thromboplastin antecedent (PTA)
XII	Hageman factor
XIII	Fibrin stabilizing factor (FSF)

* The factor numbers and names designate each clotting factor. The numbers indicate the order in which they were discovered. NOTE: There is no Factor VI, which is no longer considered to be a distinct part of coagulation.

minogen is converted to plasmin, which breaks the clot into fibrin split products.

ANTICOAGULATION

Coagulation in the absence of bleeding is prevented by antithrombins and heparin within the vessels. These are anticoagulation factors. The antithrombins prevent the release of thromboplastic substances unless there is injury present. Heparin is produced by mast cells within the body and is used to prevent thrombosis after normal clotting has occurred.

BLOOD GROUPING

Blood classifications are designated by the antigen contained in red blood cells and the specific antibodies in the plasma. The major groups are ABO and Rh. Blood is typed as A, B, AB, and O. For each of these, there are specific antibodies present. Type

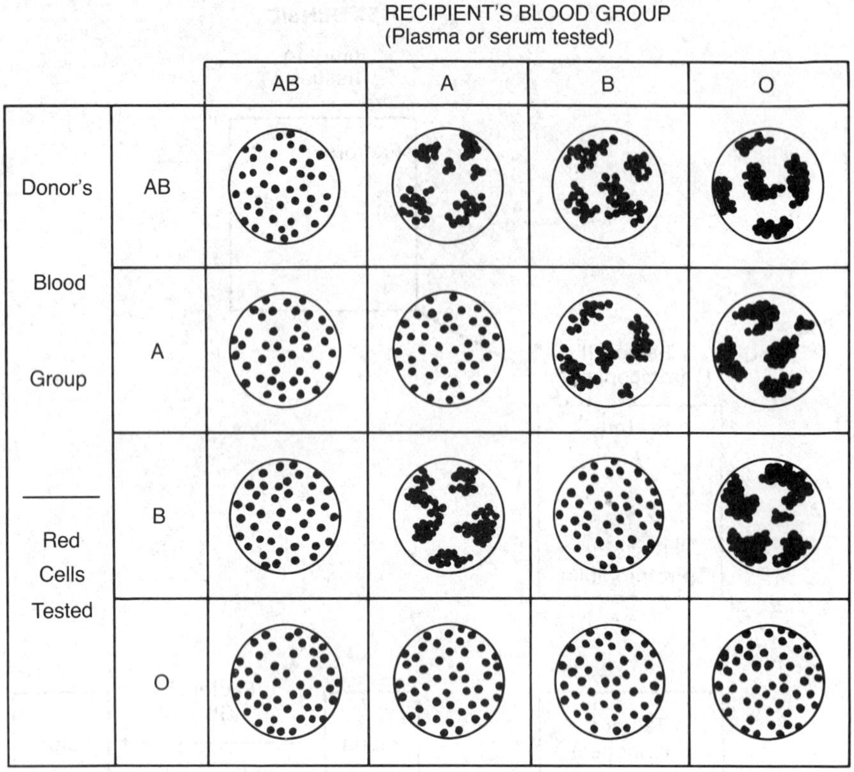

Recipient \ Donor	O	A	B	AB
O	+	−	−	−
A	+	+	−	−
B	+	−	+	−
AB	+	+	+	+

+ = successful
− = agglutination

Figure 15–4.

Crossmatching of blood types is necessary before blood from a donor is administered to a recipient. If the two types are not compatible, agglutination, a serious or fatal reaction, may occur. (From Jacob SW, Francone CA. Elements of anatomy and physiology. 2nd ed. Philadelphia: WB Saunders, 1989, p 171.)

A, with A antigens, has B antibodies. Type B blood, with B antigens, has A antibodies. Type AB blood, with A and B antigens, has no antibodies. Type O blood, with no antigens, has both A and B antibodies. Each particular type of antigen can be agglutinated or clumped by the corresponding antibody (also called the anti-agglutinin) (Fig. 15–4).

The Rh grouping is based on 12 antigens. Of these, D is the most active antigen. Rh-positive blood refers to the presence of antigen D. Rh-negative blood does not contain the antigen D.

Blood-Forming Organs

LYMPH NODES

Lymph nodes are small, rounded bodies located along the lymph vessels throughout the body. Lymph nodes serve as filters for the passing lymph and may fight off pathogenic organisms draining from an infected part of the body. They produce lymphocytes and antibodies, which are added to the lymph fluid. In the adult, the only palpable lymph nodes are in the inguinal and the axillary regions. The cervical and supraclavicular nodes may be palpable during the presence of disease processes (Fig. 15–5).

BONE MARROW

Bone marrow is one of the larger organs of the body, accounting for 4% to 5% of total body weight. It is located in the interior of spongy bones and in the central cavity of the long bones. Bone marrow is either red or yellow. Active blood cell production occurs in red marrow, the major blood-producing organ in the body. Yellow marrow is not active in the production of blood elements and consists primarily of fat cells.

During childhood, the majority of marrow is red and is actively producing blood cells. With age, most of the marrow in the long bones changes into yellow marrow, retaining the ability to convert back to blood-producing tissue if necessary. In the adult, the red marrow is found mainly in flat bones such as the ribs, skull, and parts of the pelvis.

SPLEEN

The spleen is the largest of the lymphatic organs. It is a soft, oval structure approximately 3 inches wide and 5 inches long, weighing about 7 ounces. It is a highly vascular organ located in the upper left quadrant of the abdominal cavity. The spleen stores large quantities of blood; produces lymphocytes, plasma cells, and antibodies; removes old or injured red blood cells and platelets; and filters microorganisms from the blood. The spleen performs a vital function in protecting the body from various stressors through the purification process (Fig. 15–6).

LIVER

The liver is the largest gland of the body and an extremely complex organ. It is located in the upper

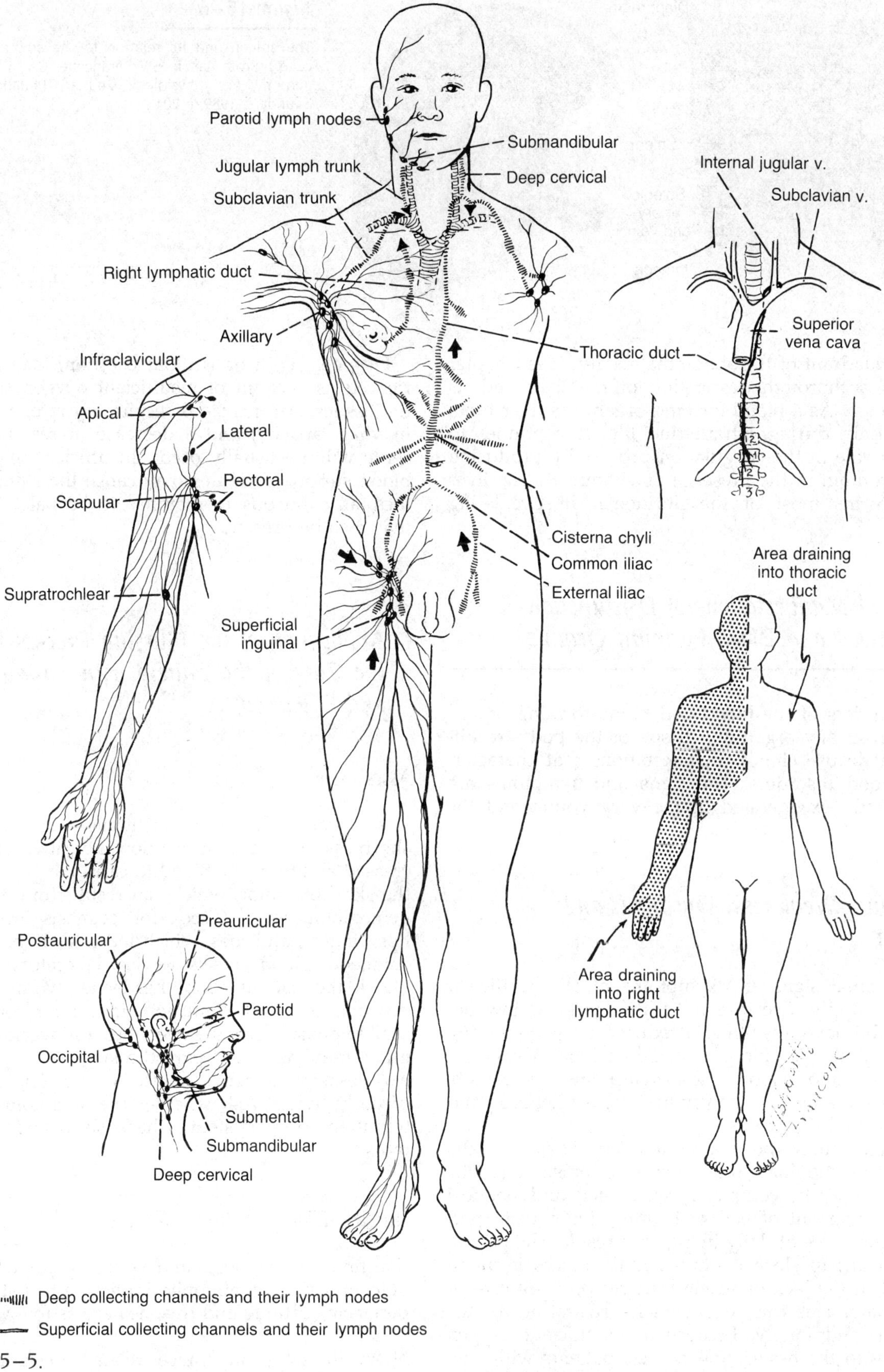

Figure 15–5.

The lymphatic system and drainage. (From Jacob SW, Francone CA. Elements of anatomy and physiology. 2nd ed. Philadelphia: WB Saunders, 1989, p 202.)

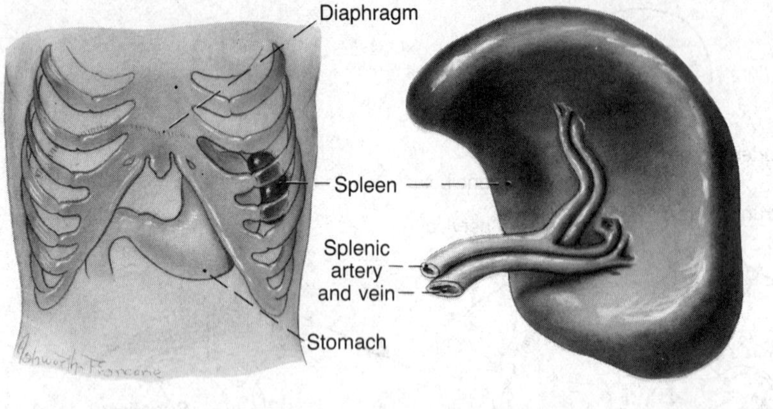

Figure 15–6.

The spleen and its relation to the stomach and rib cage. (From Jacob SW, Francone CA. Elements of anatomy and physiology. 2nd ed. Philadelphia: WB Saunders, 1989, p 204.)

right quadrant of the abdominal cavity. (See Chapter 27 for a thorough description of the liver and its functions.) As a blood-forming organ, the liver functions only during intrauterine life. It continues to play a role in the coagulation process by producing prothrombin in the presence of vitamin K. The liver also forms most of the fibrinogen in circulating blood.

Clinical Manifestations of Dysfunction of the Blood and Blood-Forming Organs

Disorders of the blood and blood-forming organs can affect any organ and tissue of the body, resulting in diffuse clinical manifestations that characterize blood disorders. The signs and symptoms are frequently exaggerated in the very young and the aged.

Fatigue, Weakness, Dyspnea, and Pallor

Common signs and symptoms of an insufficient blood supply, decrease in erythrocytes, or low hemoglobin level resulting in reduced oxygen-carrying capacity of the blood include fatigue, weakness, dyspnea, and pallor. These symptoms are usually found in anemias, polycythemias, leukemias, and hemorrhagic disorders.

Fatigue may be manifested by a slow walk, drooping shoulders, and increased pulse rate. The patient may be completely exhausted and not feel like getting out of bed or bathing. Inability to perform activities of daily living may result. The patient may want to sleep continually. Weakness is manifested in the lack of strength to perform self-care or ambulate. This can be extremely frustrating for the patient and family. Because of insufficient oxygen supply to the tissues and nerves, patients with anemias may experience paresthesia or tingling of the extremities.

Dyspnea, with or without exertion, may be experienced as a result of insufficient oxygen supply to the tissues. An increased respiratory rate, a decrease in vital capacity, and a decrease in respiratory reserve volume usually occur. Insufficient oxygenated blood supply to tissues may cause the skin, fingers, toes, and mucous membranes to be pale. Cyanosis may also be present.

Application of the Nursing Process to the Care of the Patient with Fatigue and Dyspnea

Assessment

Assess for tachycardia, tachypnea, and increased shortness of breath on exertion indicative of the decreased ability of the blood to carry oxygen. Observe the skin for pallor, which can result from decreased hemoglobin level. Check for cyanosis around the lips, fingers, and toes, which indicates hypoxemia in cutaneous blood vessels. Review laboratory results.

Ask the patient about headaches, vertigo, visual disturbances, and confusion, indicating some cerebral hypoxia. Assess extremities for weakness, tingling, numbness, and paresthesia.

Assess the patient's ability to complete activities of daily living. Ask whether the symptoms are intermittent or persistent. Check sleep and rest patterns.

Nursing Diagnoses and Planning

The nursing diagnosis and related expected patient outcomes most commonly applicable to patients experiencing fatigue and dyspnea are as follows:

NDx: Activity intolerance related to fatigue and dyspnea secondary to decreased oxygen-carrying capacity of the blood

Planning: Patient outcomes

1. Patient follows regimen of planned activities and rest periods each day.
2. Patient verbalizes decreased feelings of fatigue and demonstrates increased activity level.
3. Patient completes activities of daily living without signs of fatigue and dyspnea such as tachycardia, tachypnea, shortness of breath, and cyanosis.
4. Patient's vital signs are within the normal ranges for the patient.

Nursing Interventions

NDx: Activity intolerance

Instruct the patient to develop a regimen of activity with frequent rest periods throughout the day. Encourage the patient to do range-of-motion exercises frequently while lying in bed to maintain muscle tone and strength. Note at what times during the day the patient seems the most tired and allow for rest periods at that time.

Tell the patient to avoid sudden movements, such as getting out of bed quickly, since this decreases the blood supply to the brain, aggravating vertigo and disorientation. Have the patient practice deep breathing exercises to increase oxygen and blood to the brain. Provide oxygen therapy if appropriate.

Teach the patient to practice energy-saving techniques to reduce fatigue and shortness of breath. Place frequently used articles within the patient's reach.

Provide and encourage frequent rest periods while delivering patient care. Prevent interruptions during rest periods and at night, whenever possible. Reduce any disturbing noises, and limit visitors as necessary.

Encourage good nutrition to increase the patient's energy level. Offer four to six meals per day. This is less tiring for the patient and prevents gastric overdistention. Assist the patient with feeding if necessary.

Evaluation

Evaluate the effectiveness of nursing care for a patient with fatigue and dyspnea by comparing the patient's status with the expected patient outcomes. Examples of specific outcomes for patients with fatigue and dyspnea have been provided in the Planning section.

Hemorrhagic Tendencies

Hemorrhage, slow bleeding into tissues and joints (hemarthrosis), and minor bleeding from mucous membranes are common problems in hematologic disorders. Hemorrhage results from a decrease in platelet count as seen in the purpuras, or from absence of one or more of the clotting factors, as found in hemophilia. Slow bleeding into tissues or joints may also occur in leukemia, polycythemia, and disseminated intravascular coagulation.

Application of the Nursing Process to the Care of the Patient with Hemorrhagic Tendencies

Assessment

Assess for bruising, ecchymoses, petechiae, and purpura. Check the patient's oral cavity for bleeding in the mucous membranes. Look for retinal hemorrhages, which may occur in patients with severe anemia and decreased platelets. Assess for bleeding in the gastrointestional tract by noting any blood in vomitus and in stools. Check for blood in urine. Review laboratory results of coagulation times. Assess for pain in joints, which may indicate hemarthrosis.

Also assess the patient's respiratory status. Look for cyanosis, shortness of breath on exertion, and inability to complete tasks of daily living. Assess for tachypnea, tachycardia, dyspnea, and orthopnea, and auscultate the chest for adventitious sounds.

Nursing Diagnoses and Planning

Nursing diagnoses and related expected patient outcomes most commonly applicable to patients with hemorrhagic tendencies include the following:

NDx: Knowledge deficit: nature of disease and prevention of complication of hemorrhage

Planning: Patient outcomes

1. Patient states accurate information about the nature of the disease and the resulting complication of hemorrhage.
2. Patient states the signs of bleeding and when to seek medical intervention.
3. Patient relates the measures necessary to lessen the risk of hemorrhage.
4. Patient shows no evidence of bleeding, such as petechiae, purpura, bruising, dark stools, and so forth.

NDx: Altered tissue perfusion, cardiopulmonary, peripheral, and cerebral, related to destruction of platelets or absence of clotting factors causing excessive bleeding

Planning: Patient outcomes

1. Patient's extremities are warm, color is adequate, and pulses are present.
2. Patient's laboratory studies are within normal ranges for the patient.
3. Patient denies headaches, confusion, or nausea.
4. Patient is able to perform activities of daily living without tachypnea, tachycardia, and dyspnea.

Nursing Interventions

NDx: Knowledge deficit: nature of disease and prevention of complication of hemorrhage

Instruct the patient about the clinical course of the disease and the complication of hemorrhage. Teach the patient the signs of bleeding to observe for and when to seek medical assistance. Explain the need for avoiding sharp objects, straight razors, contact sports, and injections and venipuncture whenever possible. Tell the patient to watch for discoloration of urine or stools.

Explain proper oral hygiene methods necessary to prevent further irritation and ulceration of mucous membranes. Instruct the patient to use a soft toothbrush and to use mouthrinse frequently. Show how to inspect the oral cavity, checking the tongue and gums for early signs of irritation. Teach the patient to avoid extremely hot, spicy foods and acidic drinks to lessen oral and gastrointestinal irritation.

Tell the patient to carry an identification card containing the blood disorder, patient's name and address, name of physician, blood type, and a family member to call in an emergency.

Check the laboratory data for the bleeding times and platelet count. Be prepared for an emergency episode of bleeding. Tell the patient not to take aspirin because it may extend the bleeding time.

NDx: Altered tissue perfusion, cardiopulmonary, peripheral, and cerebral

Help the patient conserve oxygen needs by encouraging rest and limiting activities. Assist the patient with meals if needed. Administer oxygen if appropriate. Elevate the head of the bed to aid in chest expansion.

Keep the patient in a comfortable position and reposition frequently to release pressure. Utilize range-of-motion exercises to stimulate circulation. Monitor vital signs and laboratory studies to assess for changes and improvements in status. Encourage ambulation as tolerated, but provide for frequent rest periods to decrease cardiac workload. Assist the patient when ambulating because decreased cerebral circulation may cause disorientaion and vertigo.

Discourage smoking to avoid vasoconstriction. Remove constricting clothing and keep heavy bed linen from restricting peripheral circulation. Keep the patient's legs in a nondependent position when not ambulating. Prevent any bleeding episodes if possible.

Evaluation

Evaluate the effectiveness of nursing care for a patient with hemorrhagic tendencies by comparing the patient's status with the expected patient outcomes. Examples of specific outcomes for patients with hemorrhagic tendencies have been provided in the Planning section.

Ulcerative Lesions

Ulcerative lesions of the tongue, gums, or mucous membranes may occur as a result of abnormal changes in mucous membrane cells, poor nutrition, the use of chemotherapeutic agents, and from a decrease in gastric secretions. These lesions may be found in any of the hematologic disorders but are more common in the severe anemias and leukemias. Bleeding from the lesions in the mouth causes a foul taste, which may exacerbate poor nutrition and leads to halitosis. This may be further aggravated if the patient is receiving oxygen or is a mouth breather, which dries the mucous membranes.

Ulcerative lesions may also occur in the legs in patients with sickle cell anemia as a result of poor circulation from the accumulation of sickled cells in the peripheral circulation.

Application of the Nursing Process to the Care of the Patient with Ulcerative Lesions

Assessment

Examine the oral cavity carefully. Note any bleeding, lesions, discolorations, and sore spots. Assess the tongue for coating, color, and lesions. Check the lips for dryness and cracks.

Palpate the patient's peripheral pulses to assess circulatory status. Note the color of the legs. Check for early signs of breakdown, such as reddened areas and discolorations. Look for shearing, petechiae, cyanosis, and lesions.

Nursing Diagnoses and Planning

The nursing diagnosis and related expected patient outcomes most commonly applicable to patients with ulcerative lesions from hematologic disorders are as follows:

NDx: Impaired skin integrity related to abnormal changes in mucous membranes, effects of therapy, or insufficient peripheral circulation

Planning: Patient Outcomes

1. Patient states causes of ulcerative lesions and measures to prevent the occurrence or recurrence.
2. Patient demonstrates appropriate care of the ulcerative lesions.
3. Patient's oral cavity and legs are free of ulcerative lesions.

Nursing Interventions

NDx: Impaired skin integrity

Teach the patient measures to prevent ulcerative lesions from developing. Avoid irritating the mouth with hot, spicy or acidic foods and fluids. Provide soft or bland foods, especially when lesions are present. Keep the patient well hydrated. Use petrolatum on the lips to prevent cracking. Teach the patient good oral hygiene techniques. Have the patient use a mouthrinse of hydrogen peroxide and water or a commercial preparation frequently. Use a soft toothbrush to prevent irritation to the gums and mucous membranes. Have the patient inspect the oral cavity frequently and to seek medical assistance if any breakdown or soreness is noted.

Teach the patient to exercise, as tolerated, to promote good circulation. Range-of-motion exercises should be done while on bed rest. Turn the patient frequently, and inspect pressure areas for early signs of breakdown. Keep heavy linen from constricting the peripheral circulation by using a bed cradle. Elevate the patient's legs when sitting in a chair. If ulcerations are present, use aseptic technique to cleanse them. Wear gloves during the dressing changes. Teach the patient and family members the proper technique for dressing the legs.

Evaluation

Evaluate the effectiveness of nursing care for a patient with ulcerative lesions by comparing the patient's status with the expected patient outcomes. Examples of specific outcomes for patients with ulcerative lesions have been provided in the Planning section.

Bone and Joint Pain and Deformities

Bone and joint pain and deformities may be the result of bleeding into the joints, hyperactivity of bone marrow, gout, pathologic fractures, and invasion of malignancies into bone. Pain in the knees, wrist, or hands may indicate hemarthrosis, which frequently occurs in sickle cell anemia and hemophilia. Aching bones often result from the pressure of expanding bone marrow as seen in multiple myeloma and leukemias. In multiple myeloma, infiltration of malignancy into the bone causes both pain and fractures.

Application of the Nursing Process to the Care of the Patient with Bone or Joint Pain and Deformities

Assessment

Assess the patient for the extent of the pain; its location, duration, severity, and frequency; and for joint deformities. Look for swelling, redness, and warmth at the site of the pain. Assess for tenderness or pain with pressure applied to the area over the bone or joint. Check the range of motion of the involved joint and the amount of flexibility or stiffness present. Notice the activity level of the patient and whether the pain restricts the patient's movements or ability to do self-care or to ambulate.

Nursing Diagnoses and Planning

The nursing diagnosis and related expected patient outcomes most commonly applicable to patients with bone or joint pain are as follows:

NDx: Pain related to bleeding into joints, invasion of malignancies into bone, and other effects of the hematologic disorder

Planning: Patient outcomes

1. Patient reports that pain is controlled with analgesics.
2. Patient states comfort measures to help relieve pain.
3. Patient states coping measures to help relieve or tolerate pain.

Nursing Interventions

NDx: Pain

Place the patient in comfortable positions and reposition frequently. Use pillows to support bony prominences. Determine when the pain is most severe, and allow the patient to rest during those periods. Give pain medications as ordered prior to activity periods so that the patient can better tolerate the movement.

Help the patient find alternative methods to alleviate or be able to tolerate the pain. Show the patient and family relaxation techniques and how to perform massage. Teach the patient the use of patient-controlled analgesia (PCA), if ordered.

Evaluation

Evaluate the effectiveness of nursing care for a patient with bone or joint pain and deformities by comparing the patient's status with the expected patient outcomes. Examples of specific outcomes for patients with bone and joint pain and deformities have been provided in the Planning section.

Increased Susceptibility to Infection

Patients with disorders involving leukocytes, such as leukemia, leukopenia, and lymphomas, are especially prone to developing local and systemic infections. Patients with depressed immunity caused by treatments such as chemotherapy for malignancies of the hematologic system are also extremely susceptible to infections. When the tissues are hypoxic and there is a reduction in mature circulating leukocytes, there is a reduction in the number of cells available to effectively fight invading microorganisms and produce antibodies. Inadequate nutritional support may also contribute to the patient's overall poor health status, thus increasing the risk for infection.

Application of the Nursing Process to the Care of the Patient with Increased Susceptibility to Infection

Assessment

Assess the patient frequently for signs of respiratory infection. Look for increased respiratory rate, cough, dyspnea, fever, chills, and shortness of breath. Auscultate lungs for adventitious sounds. Check laboratory results, especially the white blood cell count and urinalysis.

Determine whether the patient experiences any pain or burning on urination or low back pain indicative of a urinary tract infection. Note the color and consistency of the urine.

Assess the patient's mouth, looking for signs of infection from lesions. Note any ulcerative lesions on the patient's legs. Look for purulent drainage from the lesions.

Nursing Diagnoses and Planning

The nursing diagnosis and related expected patient outcomes most commonly applicable to patients with increased susceptibility to infection are as follows:

NDx: High risk for infection related to increased susceptibility secondary to compromised immunity

Planning: Patient outcomes
1. Patient's vital signs are within normal ranges for the patient.
2. Patient displays no signs of infection, such as fever, chills, tachycardia, tachypnea, or pain or burning on urination.
3. Patient identifies early signs of infection and measures to prevent infections.

Nursing Interventions

NDx: High risk for infection
Keep the patient warm, and avoid extreme changes in temperature in the room. Restrict visitors to prevent exposure to infections. Use protective isolation if appropriate.

Monitor the patient's vital signs frequently, observing subtle changes that may indicate early signs of infection. Report any changes noted.

Promote good nutrition by serving the meals in a relaxed, attractive atmosphere. Encourage a high-protein, high-vitamin diet. Provide oral hygiene frequently to prevent infection and promote better eating habits.

Encourage mouth cleansing every 2 hours with a nonirritating substance. Keep the patient's lips well-lubricated to prevent skin breakdown. Have the patient use a mixture of hydrogen peroxide and water, especially when bleeding is present, to help prevent the growth of organisms.

Because early identification and treatment may limit the severity of the infection, teach the patient and family to continually observe for signs of developing infection and to notify the physician if such signs appear.

Evaluation

Evaluate the effectiveness of nursing care for a patient with increased susceptibility to infection by comparing the patient's status with the expected patient outcomes. Examples of specific outcomes for patients with increased susceptibility to infection have been provided in the Planning section.

Jaundice, Pruritus, and Skin Problems

Owing to the hemolysis of red blood cells, patients with hematologic disorders may become jaundiced. Pruritus is a common manifestation of jaundice, which can cause extreme discomfort for the patient. If the patient scratches the affected areas, skin breakdown may occur, leading to increased discomfort and infection.

Nursing care for the patient with jaundice includes promoting good skin care. Use nonirritating soaps for bathing, and apply lotion frequently to prevent dry skin. Cut the patient's fingernails short to prevent skin breaks if the patient scratches. Have the patient soak in an oatmeal bath or commercially prepared bath additive to reduce pruritus. Dress area of skin breakdown with aseptic dressings to prevent infection.

Nutritional Deficiencies

Nutritional deficiencies are common problems seen in dysfunctions of the hematologic system. The deficiencies may be the primary cause of the disorder, as in iron deficiency anemia or folic acid deficiency, or they may be secondary to the major disorder, as found in leukemia and multiple myeloma. In these disorders, the nutritional deficiencies are usually related to the effects of the treatment instituted for the disorder.

Ulcerations of the mouth, nausea, and vomiting are common side effects of chemotherapy that interfere with the patient's ability to eat well. Other disorders cause gastrointestinal symptoms that may contribute to poor dietary intake. The extreme fatigue the patient experiences can also affect eating habits. Lack of knowledge about dietary deficiencies and proper diet planning may be a contributing factor to the nutritional deficiency.

Application of the Nursing Process to the Care of the Patient with Nutritional Deficiencies

Assessment

Assess the patient's typical dietary pattern. Note the type and amount of foods consumed and the protein, vitamin, and caloric value. Assess for weight loss. Check for nausea, mouth soreness, diarrhea, constipation, vomiting, and gastric distention. Look for signs of dehydration. Assess the patient's energy level at meal times.

Nursing Diagnoses and Planning

The nursing diagnosis and related expected patient outcomes most commonly applicable to patients with nutritional needs due to hematologic disorders are as follows:

NDx: Altered nutrition: less than body requirements, related to disease process, dietary deficiencies, inability to eat, and complications of treatments

Planning: Patient outcomes

1. Patient chooses appropriate foods to maintain a therapeutic nutritional status, replace deficiencies, and prevent gastrointestinal symptoms.
2. Patient tolerates the food served.
3. Patient relates accurate information about the disease and dietary deficiencies related to the disease or complications of treatments.

Nursing Interventions

NDx: Altered nutrition: less than body requirements

Help the patient maintain good nutritional status by providing high-protein and high-vitamin foods in an attractive atmosphere. Provide six to eight small meals per day to prevent distention, decrease gastric irritability, and increase the amount the patient can eat. Offer bland, soft foods if the patient has mouth lesions.

Assist the patient with meals if extreme fatigue is present. Allow the patient to rest before meals. Encourage increased fluid intake. Avoid foods and fluids which are hot, spicy, acidic, or gas-producing to decrease mouth and gastric irritation.

Provide good oral hygiene after meals and between meals. Teach the patient to cleanse the mouth frequently with a soft toothbrush and to use mouthrinse.

Teach the patient about good nutritional habits. Provide examples of menus for the patient and family. If the patient has a specific dietary deficiency, such as iron deficiency anemia, provide specific instructions about foods high in the deficient nutrient.

Evaluation

Evaluate the effectiveness of nursing care for a patient with nutritional needs by comparing the patient's status with the expected patient outcomes. Examples of specific outcomes for patients with nutritional needs have been provided in the Planning section.

Gastrointestinal Symptoms

Several factors contribute to the gastrointestinal symptoms experienced by the patient with hematologic disorders. Abnormal changes in mucous membranes may result from the disorder or from treatments such as chemotherapy. A decrease in gastric secretions is found in pernicious anemia, causing an irritable stomach.

Ulcerations in the mouth and extreme fatigue may cause the lack of desire to eat properly or the inability to eat. These factors may manifest in symptoms such as anorexia, nausea, vomiting, diarrhea, abdominal distention, flatulence, dehydration, and weight loss.

Nursing care for the patient with gastrointestinal symptoms is similar to that previously discussed under nutritional needs.

Enlarged Organs

Hepatomegaly, splenomegaly, and hypertrophy of bone marrow may occur as a result of congestion in the tissue from overproduction of cells as seen in polycythemia and leukemia. Splenomegaly may also occur from increased demand on the organ to destroy defective cells, as seen in hemolytic anemia.

Nursing care for the patient with enlarged organs includes assessing for symptoms resulting from the organ changes, such as increased bleeding tendency, decreased detoxification ability, abdominal discomfort, and ascites (see Chapter 27).

Assessment of the Blood and Blood-Forming Organs

Assessment of the blood and blood-forming organs (hematologic system) includes a thorough review of laboratory and radiologic studies and presenting symptoms. Each of the structures of the hematologic system is also a component of another body system and is usually evaluated with that particular system. The nursing assessment focuses on the clinical manifestations of the disorders of the blood and blood-forming organs previously described in the chapter.

Diagnostic Procedures

To diagnose disorders of blood and blood-forming organs, a variety of diagnostic procedures may be used. Examination of the blood cells is important for all patients, regardless of the disorder, but it is even more significant in determining dysfunction of the hematologic system. Abnormalities most commonly detected include anemia and leukocyte changes. Since hemostasis may be the primary problem or may be affected by disorders of the hematologic system, coagulation studies are also necessary. Other tests used to evaluate function of blood-forming organs include biopsies, sonograms, and scans.

Methods of Obtaining Blood

Methods of obtaining blood for examination include finger stick, venipuncture, and arterial puncture. The finger stick method is used to obtain capillary blood for peripheral blood smears. Venipuncture is used to obtain venous blood for most hematologic studies. Venous blood is usually drawn from the antecubital vein. Arterial puncture is used to obtain arterial blood for blood gas studies. Arterial blood is usually drawn from the radial or femoral artery.

Because many of the patients with disorders of the hematologic system have hemorrhagic tendencies, bleeding episodes and hematomas (after venous or arterial sticks) are prevented by applying direct pressure with a sterile dressing to the site of the puncture. Pressure is applied for at least 5 minutes after arterial sticks.

Blood Tests

COMPLETE BLOOD COUNT

The complete blood count is the basic screening test for white blood cell (leukocyte) count, red blood cell (erythrocyte) count, differential white blood cell count, hematocrit, hemoglobin, red blood cell indices, stained red cell examination, and platelet count. Abnormal values in any of these may indicate dysfunction in the blood or blood-forming organs. Only disorders of the hematologic system related to each test are discussed in this chapter. It is important to keep in mind that laboratory values vary according to individual laboratory standards (Table 15–2).

WHITE BLOOD CELL COUNT

The white blood cell count (WBC) is the total number of circulating white blood cells. Disease may be associated with either an increase or decrease of white blood cells. The normal range for the white blood cell count is 5000 to 10,000/cu mm.

Leukocytosis is the term used to refer to a white blood cell count higher than 10,000/cu mm. This occurs in infections, malignancies, tissue necrosis, hemorrhage, trauma, tissue injury, circulatory disease, and steroid therapy. Emotional stress, pain, moderate physical exercise, fever, prolonged exposure to cold, convulsions, and paroxysmal tachycardia may cause slight increases in the white blood cell count.

Leukopenia is the term used to refer to a white blood cell count lower than 4000/cu mm. This occurs in some viral infections, hypersplenism, bone marrow depression, radiation therapy, acute leukemia, agranulocytosis, pernicious anemia, aplastic anemia, and multiple myeloma.

Table 15–2. COMMON LABORATORY TESTS FOR DIAGNOSING DYSFUNCTION OF BLOOD OR BLOOD-FORMING ORGANS

TEST	NORMAL RESULTS*	MEASURES
Complete Blood Count (CBC)		
White blood cells (WBC)	5000–10,000/cu mm	Total number
Red blood cells (RBC)	4.2–5.4 million/cu mm (male) 3.6–5.0 million/cu mm (female)	Total number
Hematocrit (Hct)	40–54% (male) 37–47% (female)	Percentage of red blood cells in whole blood
Hemoglobin (Hgb)	14–16.5 g/100 ml (male) 12–15 g/100 ml (female)	Amount of hemoglobin oxygen-carrying capacity in whole blood
Platelet count	150,000–350,000/cu mm	Total number of platelets in whole blood
Coagulation Studies		
Platelet aggregation	< 5 min	Rate of adherence of platelets to one another
Prothrombin time (PT)	12–14 sec	Time for clotting to occur
Partial thromboplasin time (PTT)	30–45 sec	Detects stage 2 clotting deficiences
Activated partial thromboplastin time (APTT)	16–25 sec	Detects stage 2 clotting deficiencies (a more sensitive test and less time consuming)
Leukocyte Alkaline Phosphatase (LAP) Stain	30–130	Amount of enzyme alkaline phosphatase present in WBCs
Direct Coombs' Test	Negative	Presence of antibody on red blood cells or RBC sensitization
Serum iron	100–150 mg/100 ml	Iron transported in blood serum
Total iron-binding capacity (TIBC)	300–400 mg/100 ml	Total iron binding to transfer in protein in blood serum
Serum folic acid	5–21 mg/ml	Amount of folic acid in blood
Bone Marrow Aspiration	Normal percentage of cells and cell substances in bone marrow	A biopsy smear to determine whether bone marrow is producing normal RBCs, WBCs, and platelets
Urine Studies		
Schilling	> 7% excretion in urine	24% urine test to evaluate absorption of ingested vitamin B_{12} from GI tract
Urobilinogen	0–4 mg in 24 hr excreted in urine 50–300 mg in 24 hr excreted in feces	Amount of urobilinogen excreted in urine and feces
Bleeding Time (Ivy method)	2–9.5 minutes	Quality and quantity of platelets and ability of blood vessels to constrict
Hemoglobin Studies		
Sickle cell	Absence of sickle-shaped cells	Detects presence of normal hemoglobin vs. abnormal hemoglobins in red blood cells
Heinz body	Occasional presence only when red blood cell ages	Detects presence of serrated granules containing denatured hemoglobin
Red Blood Cell Studies		
Erythrocyte fragility	Hemolysis begins at 0.45–0.29% Hemolysis ends at 0.33–0.30%	Rate at which red blood cells become fragile and rupture (hemolysis) in saline solution
Erythrocyte sedimentation	0–15 mm/hr (male) 0–20 mm/hr (female) (results vary greatly depending on test used)	Rate at which red blood cells settle in uncoagulated blood
Reticulocyte count	0.5–1.5% of total RBCs	Percentage of immature, non-nucleated red blood cells

*Values vary depending on which laboratory method is used.

RED BLOOD CELL COUNT

The red blood cell count (RBC) reflects the total number of erythrocytes per cubic millimeter of blood. The normal red blood cell count for men is 4.2 to 5.4 million/cu mm and for women is 3.6 to 5.0 million/cu mm.

Increased red blood cell counts are seen with decreased cardiac output, impaired pulmonary gas exchange, steroid therapy, polycythemia vera, severe diarrhea, and dehydration. The higher the altitude, the greater the red blood cell increase. The decreased oxygen content of the air stimulates the production of red blood cells. Extreme exercise or excitement may produce a higher red blood cell count than in basal conditions.

Decreased red blood cell counts occur in B_6 and B_{12} vitamin deficiencies, iron deficiency, chronic in-

Table 15–3. AVERAGE VALUES AND IMPLICATIONS OF DIFFERENTIAL WBC COUNT

LEUKOCYTE CELLS	DIFFERENTIAL COUNT	NUMBER PER cu mm	CLINICAL IMPLICATIONS
Neutrophils	60–70%	3000–7000	Bacterial infections, appendicitis, stress, metabolic or drug intoxication
Eosinophils	1–4%	50–400	Allergic disorders, parasitic infestations, stress, some leukemias, Hodgkin's disease, polycythemia, blood dyscrasias, myeloproliferative diseases
Lymphocytes	20–40%	1000–4000	Viral infections, bacterial infections, infectious mononucleosis
Monocytes	2–6%	100–600	Tuberculosis, monocytic leukemia, subacute bacterial endocarditis, collagen disease, ulcerative colitis

Adapted from Fischbach F. A manual of laboratory diagnostic tests. Philadelphia: JB Lippincott, 1984, p 14.

fections, bone marrow depression, multiple myeloma, leukemia, hemolytic anemia, and pernicious anemia. There is a gradual decrease in the red blood cell count in the aged.

DIFFERENTIAL

The differential white blood cell count (diff) is the leukocyte count differentiated according to the type of cell and its functions, as described in Table 15–3. There are five types of white blood cells: neutrophils, eosinophils, basophils, lymphocytes, and monocytes. The differential count reflects a percentage of the total number of white blood cells. The number and type of cell and degree of change are important in diagnosing leukocyte disorders and other diseases.

HEMATOCRIT

The hematocrit (Hct) measures the percentage of red blood cells in a volume of whole blood. The hematocrit value is approximately three times the hemoglobin value. The hematocrit value can be affected by changes in blood volume. The normal hematocrit value for men is 40% to 54% and for women is 37% to 47%. The hematocrit value continues to decrease slightly after age 50.

Elevated hematocrit levels are seen in dehydration, pernicious anemia, and polycythemia. Immediately after an acute hemorrhage, the hematocrit may be high because of the lower blood volume. A higher than normal hematocrit level is also seen in individuals living in high altitudes.

A hematocrit level of 30% or less indicates moderate to severe anemia. Decreased values may also occur in leukemia, acute hemorrhage, iron deficiency anemia, and hemolytic anemias. The hematocrit can be as much as 10% lower in the evening than in the morning.

HEMOGLOBIN

The hemoglobin level (Hgb) is the amount of hemoglobin per 100 ml of blood. A normal hemoglobin level is necessary for the transport of appropriate amounts of oxygen to the tissues of the body. The normal hemoglobin level for males is 14.0 to 16.5 g/100 ml and for women is 12.0 to 15.0 g/100 ml. Hemoglobin measurements are significant in evaluating anemias.

Increased hemoglobin values occur with increased red blood cell volume, dehydration, impaired pulmonary gas exchange, decreased cardiac output, and severe hemolysis. Drugs that may cause increased hemoglobin levels include gentamicin and methyldopa. The hemoglobin level may be elevated or normal immediately after acute hemorrhage. The hemoglobin level may also be elevated in individuals living in high altitudes.

Decreased hemoglobin values occur with decreased red blood cell volume, severe hemorrhage, decreased red blood cell oxygenation, malnutrition, iron deficiency anemia, and hemolytic anemia.

RED BLOOD CELL INDICES

The red blood cell indices are used to define the red blood cell size and hemoglobin content of the red blood cell. The three red blood cell indices include the mean corpuscular volume (MCV), mean corpuscular hemoglobin (MCH), and mean corpuscular hemoglobin concentration (MCHC). These tests are determined from the same blood sample used for hemoglobin, hematocrit, and red blood cell count.

The red blood cell indices assist in differentiating anemias and in determining whether red blood cells are normal in volume and hemoglobin content. Table 15–4 further describes the red blood cell indices and distinguishes anemias according to high and low values of the red blood cell indices.

The mean corpuscular volume is the most significant index for classifying anemias. The mean corpuscular hemoglobin concentration is the most helpful index in evaluation of appropriate therapy for anemia because the two most accurate hematologic determinations, hematocrit and hemoglobin, are used in the calculation of this test. The mean corpuscular hemoglobin index is important in the diagnosis of severe anemia but not as useful as the mean corpuscular hemoglobin concentration, because the test uses the red cell count in its calculation, which is not always accurate.

Table 15–4. RED BLOOD CELL INDICES

MEASURE		RATIO	VALUE	DISORDERS INDICATED: HIGH VALUES	DISORDERS INDICATED: LOW VALUES
Mean corpuscular volume (MCV)	Red blood cell size	Hematocrit (Hct) / Red blood cell (RBC)	80–94 cm μ/RBC	Liver disease Alcoholism Antimetabolite therapy Macrocytic anemia: Folic acid deficiency (infants) Pernicious anemia	Microcytic anemia: Iron deficiency anemias Thalassemia major from: Spherocytic anemia Pernicious anemia Anemia from chronic blood loss
Mean corpuscular hemoglobin (MCH)	Hemoglobin per red blood cell	Hemoglobin (Hgb) / Red blood cell (RBC)	27–33 pg/RBC	Macrocytic anemias (infants)	Microcytic anemias Pernicious anemia
Mean corpuscular hemoglobin concentration (MCHC)	Hemoglobin per 100 ml of each red blood cell	Hemoglobin (Hgb) / Hematocrit (Hct)	30–38 g/100 ml packed RBC	Spherocytosis	Macrocytic anemias

STAINED RED CELL EXAMINATION

A stained red cell examination is a peripheral blood smear studied under a microscope to determine the characteristics of the red blood cells. This is the best method of determining abnormalities in red blood cell size, shape, structure, hemoglobin content, and staining properties. The examination is useful in diagnosing blood disorders such as anemia, thalassemia, and leukemia. It also serves as a guide to therapy and reveals harmful effects of chemotherapy and radiation treatments. Table 15–5 elaborates on the characteristics and disorders of abnormal red blood cells.

PLATELET COUNT

The platelet count is useful in diagnosing and assessing the extent of bleeding disorders. It is also beneficial in evaluating the effects of anticoagulant therapy and in following the progress of disorders associated with bone marrow failure. The normal range for platelets is 150,000 to 350,000/cu mm.

An increased platelet count (thrombocythemia) occurs in cancer, some leukemias, polycythemia vera, iron deficiency anemia, posthemorrhagic anemia, acute infections, and hemolytic disorders and after splenectomy. Platelets may also be increased at high altitudes, during cold weather, and after strenuous exercise.

Table 15–5. RBC ABNORMALITIES

CELL	CHARACTERISTICS	DISORDERS
Poikilocytosis	Abnormal shape	Anemias
Target	Thin shape, small Hgb in center	Chronic anemias Thalassemia major Hgb C disease
Spherocyte	Small, round shape	Hereditary spherocytosis Congenital hemolytic anemia
Sickle	Crescent or sickle-shaped Hgb S present	Hemolytic anemia Sickle cell anemia
Schistocyte	Fragmented with bizarre shapes	Hemolytic anemia
Hypochromic	Pale from decreased Hgb	Anemias
Basophilic stippling	Immature, non-nucleated	Pernicious anemia Leukemia
Polychromatophilia	Immature, non-nucleated	Hemolytic anemia Acute blood loss
Metarubricyte	Nucleated	Severe anemia
Megaloblasts	Nucleated, large with increased Hgb	Pernicious anemia
Anisocytosis	Abnormal size	Anemias
Microcyte	Small	Microcytic anemias: Iron deficiency anemia Thalassemia major Spherocytic anemia
Macrocyte	Large	Macrocytic anemias Pernicious anemia Folic acid deficiency

A decreased platelet count (thrombocytopenia) occurs in idiopathic thrombocytopenia purpura, pernicious anemia, aplastic anemia, hemolytic anemia, and some leukemias and after several blood transfusions. It may also occur after chemotherapy and in bone marrow depression disorders. A platelet count of 20,000/cu mm or lower may be associated with a tendency for spontaneous bleeding, a prolonged bleeding time, petechiae, and ecchymoses.

Coagulation Tests

PLATELET AGGREGATION

The adherence of platelets to one another is defined as platelet aggregation. This test determines abnormalities in the rate and percentage of platelet aggregation. Platelets usually aggregate in less than 5 minutes. Increased platelet aggregation may occur after surgery, acute illness, venous thrombosis, and pulmonary embolism. Decreased platelet aggregation may occur in infectious mononucleosis, idiopathic thrombocytopenic purpura, acute leukemia, and von Willebrand's disease.

PROTHROMBIN TIME

Prothrombin, a protein formed in the liver, is also known as clotting Factor II. Sufficient intake and absorption of vitamin K is necessary for the formation of prothrombin. The prothrombin time (pro time or PT) detects a defect in Stage II of the clotting mechanism and is a useful screening test for deficiencies of Factors I, II, V, VII, and X. It is also used to monitor the effects of coumarin-derivative anticoagulant therapy. The normal range for prothrombin time is 12 to 14 seconds.

The prothrombin time is elongated in prothrombin deficiency, vitamin K deficiency, anticoagulant therapy, hypervitaminosis A, malabsorption of fats, hyperprothrombinemia, disseminated intravascular coagulation, and liver disease. An elongated prothrombin time may be considered therapeutic for the patient on anticoagulant therapy to prevent clotting, such as is used after myocardial infarction. For this patient, a prothrombin time of one and one-half to two and one-half times the normal may be considered appropriate.

PARTIAL THROMBOPLASTIN TIME AND ACTIVATED PARTIAL THROMBOPLASTIN TIME

The partial thromboplastin time (PTT) is a screening test for coagulations disorders that detects Stage II clotting deficiencies. Thromboplastin is clotting Factor III and is present in both blood and tissue. The PTT measures the time required for blood to clot after a reagent is added to the blood. The normal range for the PTT is 30 to 45 seconds. The PTT is prolonged in heparin anticoagulant therapy and by defects in clotting Factors I (fibrinogen), II (prothrombin), V, VII, IX, X, XI, and XII. The therapeutic range for patients on anticoagulant therapy is two and one-half to three times the normal range.

The activated partial thromboplastin time (APTT) is essentially the same as the PTT but is considered to be slightly more sensitive and takes less time to perform. The APTT is indicated for the same conditions as the PTT, which includes the monitoring of heparin therapy. The normal APTT is 16 to 25 seconds. The APPT is elongated in defects of the same factors as the PTT.

BLEEDING TIME (IVY METHOD)

The bleeding time is a screening method used to differentiate disorders of primary hemostasis from disorders of coagulation defects. The duration of bleeding depends on the quality and quantity of platelets and the ability of the blood vessel wall to constrict. The Ivy method bleeding time is useful in diagnosing platelet disorders and von Willebrand's disease.

Procedure. To evaluate the bleeding time by this method, a blood pressure cuff is applied to the upper arm and inflated to 40 mm Hg. Three small puncture wounds are made on the forearm. These areas are blotted with filter paper every 15 seconds until the bleeding stops. The time it takes for the bleeding to stop is recorded, and the time it takes a platelet clot to form is also noted. If the sites are still bleeding after 15 minutes, the test is discontinued and direct pressure is applied. The normal range for the test is 3 to 6 minutes.

The bleeding time is prolonged when platelets are decreased or abnormal, as in thrombocytopenia, leukemia, aplastic anemia, von Willebrand's disease, and disseminated intravascular coagulation. Alcohol and many drugs also extend the bleeding time (Table 15–6).

COAGULANT FACTOR ASSAYS

The coagulant factor assays determine genetic and acquired bleeding disorders. Deficiencies of all factors except III, IV, and XII are related to hemorrhagic disorders.

Other Blood Component Tests

HEMOGLOBIN ELECTROPHORESIS

The hemoglobin electrophoresis test detects the types of hemoglobin present in the red blood cells and whether they are normal or abnormal. Abnormal hemoglobins may be found in several rare hematologic disorders and in sickle cell anemia. Abnormal hemoglobins include Hgb S, Hgb C, Hgb H, Hgb D, and Hgb E. Hemoglobin electrophoresis is beneficial in diagnosing the exact problem in a Hgb S disorder. The test determines whether only sickled

Table 15–6. DRUGS THAT DELAY COAGULATION

DRUG	CLASS OR USAGE
Alcohol	Nonmedicinal
Allopurinol	Hyperuricemia
Aspirin	Analgesic
Corticosteroids	Anti-inflammatory
Dextran	Plasma expander
Dipyridamole	Angina
Ibuprofen	Analgesic
Indomethacin	Anti-inflammatory
Methyldopa	Antihypertensive
Neomycin	Antibiotic
Phenylbutazone	Anti-inflammatory
Quinidine	Antiarrhythmic

hemoglobin is present, indicating sickle cell anemia, or whether both sickled hemoglobin and normal hemoglobin are present, indicating sickle cell trait.

SICKLE CELL TEST

The sickle cell test, also called hemoglobin S test or Sickledex, is routinely used as a screening test for sickle cell disorder. The test detects Hgb S, an inherited, recessive gene. The erythrocytes are examined for the presence of sickle-shaped forms characteristic of the sickle cell trait or sickle cell anemia.

The test involves oxygen removal from the red blood cells. In the normal red blood cell, the shape is retained, but in the red blood cell with Hgb S, the shape becomes sickled. The difference between sickle cell trait and sickle cell anemia is determined by hemoglobin electrophoresis.

A positive test indicates that large numbers of erythrocytes have assumed the typical sickle cell look or crescent shape. The test is 99% accurate. False-negative results may occur in patients with polycythemias, protein abnormalities, and after transfusions of blood with sickled cells.

HEINZ BODY TEST

Heinz bodies are serrated granules that contain precipitated denatured hemoglobin. They may be found in hemolytic anemias and glucose-6-phosphate dehydrogenase (G6PD) deficiency. G6PD deficiency is diagnosed if 40% or more of the cells contain five or more Heinz bodies. Some drugs may also interfere with the normal functioning of hemoglobin.

Heinz bodies are present in individuals post splenectomy who had unstable hemoglobin syndromes or thalassemia prior to the surgery. Heinz bodies may also be present when the red blood cells undergo normal aging.

ERYTHROCYTE FRAGILITY TEST

The erythrocyte fragility test measures the rate at which erythrocytes become progressively fragile and finally rupture when suspended in hypotonic solutions of saline. Increased erythrocyte fragility is present in congenital hemolytic anemia and hereditary spherocytosis. Decreased erythrocyte fragility is present in thalassemia, sickle cell anemia, iron deficiency anemia, and polycythemia vera and post splenectomy. Erythrocyte fragility is normal in acquired hemolytic anemias.

ERYTHROCYTE SEDIMENTATION RATE

The erythrocyte sedimentation rate (ESR) determines the rate at which red blood cells settle in uncoagulated blood. The erythrocyte sedimentation rate is considered a nonspecific test, which means it is not diagnostic of a specific disorder. It is, however, useful as a screening measure for determining whether there is a problem present.

An elevated ESR occurs in tissue or cell injury, inflammation, carcinoma, and severe anemia. The ESR is extremely elevated in malignant diseases such as multiple myeloma, lymphoma, and metastatic cancer. The presence of fibrinogen, globulins, and cholesterol may increase the ESR value.

RETICULOCYTE COUNT

The reticulocyte count indicates the percentage of immature, non-nucleated red blood cells. Normally, reticulocytes make up 0.5% to 1.5% of the total erythrocytes in males and 0.5% to 2.5% in females.

A reticulocyte count is used to distinguish between anemias related to bone marrow failure resulting from hemorrhage and anemias caused by erythrocyte destruction. The count is also used to determine the effectiveness of treatment in iron deficiency anemia, pernicious anemia, and the recovery of bone marrow function in aplastic anemia. It may be used to monitor the effects of radioactive substances on exposed individuals.

An elevated reticulocyte count indicates an increased rate of erythrocyte production with a premature destruction of mature red blood cells. Increased reticulocyte levels occur in hemolytic anemias, sickle cell disease, metastatic carcinoma, leukemia, hereditary spherocytosis, post hemorrhage (3 to 4 days), post splenectomy, and after treatment of anemias.

A decreased reticulocyte count indicates a reduction in erythrocyte production by the bone marrow. Decreased levels occur in iron deficiency anemia, aplastic anemia, untreated pernicious anemia, chronic infections, and radiation therapy.

LEUKOCYTE ALKALINE PHOSPHATASE STAIN

The enzyme alkaline phosphatase is present in leukocytes located in the bone and liver. Abnormal values in leukocyte alkaline phosphatase (LAP) are associated with disease states that affect bone and liver functions.

Table 15–7. DRUGS THAT CAUSE A FALSE-POSITIVE RESULT ON THE DIRECT COOMBS' TEST

Cephaloridine	Penicillin
Cephalothin	Procainamide
Chlorpromazine	Quinidine
Diphenylhydantoin	Rifampin
Isoniazid	Streptomycin
Levodopa	Sulfonamides
Methyldopa	Tetracycline

An elevated LAP level may be seen in polycythemia vera, thrombocytopenia, and primary bone malignancies. Allopurinol and anticonvulsants may also increase the LAP value.

Decreased values may occur in acute and chronic granulocytic leukemia, paroxysmal nocturnal hemoglobinuria, aplastic anemia, hereditary hypophosphatasia, and idiopathic thrombocytopenia purpura. Some medications such as oral contraceptives and fluorides may also decrease the LAP value.

DIRECT COOMBS' TEST

The direct Coombs' test, or direct antiglobulin test, detects the presence of antibodies against red blood cells, which increases the cell fragility or causes other cellular damage. The normal test result should be negative.

Positive results are reported on a +1 to +4 range. A positive direct Coombs' test result is seen in transfusion reactions and autoimmune hemolytic anemia and may also be found in individuals receiving cephalothin therapy, penicillin, and some other drugs. Drug therapy may also cause a false-positive reading (Table 15–7).

SERUM IRON

The blood levels of iron are measured to determine iron deficiency. The normal range for serum iron is 80 to 160 μg/dl for males and 50 to 150 μg/dl for females.

Serum iron levels are elevated in untreated drug-induced bone marrow failure, hereditary iron-loading anemia, pernicious anemia, and hemolytic anemia. Iron values may also be increased in excessive iron intake, impairment of utilization of iron, and abnormal destruction of red blood cells.

Decreased levels of serum iron are found in dietary iron deficiency, absorption impairment, and hemorrhage. Low iron levels may also be seen in pregnant women, after prolonged heavy menstruation, and in the elderly.

Table 15–8. FOLIC ACID ANTAGONISTS*

Ampicillin	Para-aminosalicylic acid
Chloramphenicol	Phenobarbital
Estrogens	Phenytoin
Erythromycin	Tetracycline
Oral contraceptives	

*Drugs that may lower serum folic acid levels.

TOTAL IRON-BINDING CAPACITY

Iron-binding capacity reflects the transferrin protein content of the serum and the total amount of iron that can bind to the transferrin present in the blood. The normal range for the total iron-binding capacity (TIBC) is 250 to 450 μg/dl.

Increased TIBC values are seen in iron deficiency anemia due to hemorrhage or inadequate intake, bone marrow damage, erythropoiesis, and polycythemia. When serum iron levels are low, the TIBC is increased because there are more transferrin sites to bind with.

Decreased total iron-binding capacity values are seen in iron overload, pernicious anemia, thalassemia, sickle cell anemia, chronic infections, hepatic dysfunction, and cancer. Some interfering factors include altered protein balance, estrogen therapy, hormonal imbalance, hydroxyurea, and adrenocorticotropic hormone therapy. When serum iron levels are high, the TIBC is decreased because the capacity of the transferrin to bind with iron is already saturated. Approximately 30% of the total capacity of transferrin is usually bound to serum iron.

SERUM FOLIC ACID

Folic acid is one of the B vitamins necessary for DNA and red blood cell production and growth. It is synthesized by bacteria in the small intestine and stored in the liver. Folic acid deficiency is frequently associated with dietary inadequacies because only a small amount of folic acid can be stored for future use. The normal range for serum folic acid is 5 to 21 mg/ml.

Other than dietary deficiency, decreased serum folic acid levels may be associated with magaloblastic anemia, hemolytic disorders, liver disease, alcohol ingestion, and carcinomas. Several drugs may also decrease folic acid values. These are listed in Table 15–8.

Guidelines for Application of the Nursing Process to the Care of the Patient Undergoing Diagnostic Blood Testing for Dysfunction of the Blood and Blood-Forming Organs

Review the findings of the studies and the interpretation of the results. Assess the hydration level of the patient, because hypervolemia may decrease the hematocrit and hemoglobin results, whereas hypovolemia may cause increased values.

Assess the oxygenation of the patient with low hemoglobin and hematocrit levels. Look for cyanosis, tachypnea, tachycardia, dyspnea, pallor, and fatigue. If these symptoms are present, allow for frequent rest periods throughout the day while delivering care to the patient. Administer oxygen as needed. Keep the patient warm and prevent drafts.

Assess the nutritional pattern of the patient with a dietary deficiency. Provide patient education about foods containing the needed nutrients and meal planning strategies to replace and maintain the level necessary.

Assess the patient's bleeding potential, because many of the patients subjected to the previously discussed tests may be diagnosed with a coagulation disorder. Look for petechiae, ecchymoses, bruising, and blood in the urine or stools. Teach the patient signs of bleeding and measures to prevent bleeding episodes.

The nursing diagnoses, expected patient outcomes, nursing interventions, and evaluation for patients undergoing diagnostic blood testing are specific to the disorder. Refer to Chapter 16 for application of the nursing process to specific hematologic system disorders. The following additional interventions also apply to the care of patients undergoing diagnostic blood testing. Explain the diagnostic blood studies to be completed to the patient. Apply pressure to the site of the finger stick, venipuncture, or arterial puncture as needed. If it is suspected that the patient has a bleeding disorder, it is extremely important to apply direct pressure to the puncture site for several minutes. For some studies, it may be necessary to withhold food and fluids from the patient after midnight on the test day. Check the institution's laboratory procedure manual for specific preparations.

Other Tests Specific to Hematologic Disorders

SCHILLING TEST

The Schilling test is a 24-hour urine study that indirectly measures intrinsic factor deficiency. It evaluates the body's ability to absorb ingested vitamin B_{12} from the gastrointestinal tract by determining the amount of elimination of radioactive vitamin B_{12}. Normally, individuals absorb and excrete a large proportion of the radioactive vitamin B_{12}. An abnormally low excretion value, less than 7%, indicates the absence of the intrinsic factor.

The Schilling test is used to diagnose macrocytic and pernicious anemia. Some factors that may interfere with the test results include diabetes, hypothyroidism, enteritis, decreased renal function, and incontinence. Ingestion of laxatives during the test time is contraindicated.

Procedure. The patient is instructed to refrain from food or fluid intake, except for water, 12 hours prior to the test. A tasteless capsule of radioactive vitamin B_{12} is given orally. One hour later, the patient is given an intramuscular injection of vitamin B_{12}. Food and fluid intake is resumed at this time. The 24-hour urine collection is started using the appropriate collection container. The patient should drink increased fluids during the test periods to aid in the excretion of urine. The patient collects all urine excreted during the 24 hours in the appropriate receptacle until informed that the test has ended.

UROBILINOGEN TEST

The urinary and fecal urobilinogen test determines the amount of urobilinogen excreted in urine or feces. Urobilinogen is produced when bilirubin is broken down by intestinal tract bacteria. Normally there is a small amount (1%, or 0 to 4 mg in 24 hours) of urobilinogen excreted in urine by the kidneys. Most of the urobilinogen (99%, or 50 to 300 mg) is excreted in the feces. Urinary and fecal urobilinogen both are elevated in hemolytic anemia and pernicious anemia as a result of excessive destruction of red blood cells and hemoglobin. Antibiotics and antibacterials may alter the results of the test.

Tests to Evaluate Blood-Forming Organs

BONE MARROW ASPIRATION AND BIOPSY

A bone marrow aspiration and biopsy determines the ability of the bone marrow to produce normal red blood cells, white blood cells, and platelets. It is an extremely important diagnostic tool for hematologic disorders. The results of the bone marrow smear indicate the cell ratios present. More than 25% lymphocytes or more than 15% monocytes is an abnormal finding. Abnormal cell ratio findings indicate specific diseases.

A bone marrow aspiration is useful in diagnosing aplastic anemia, pernicious anemia, leukemia, purpura, and agranulocytosis. A bone marrow study may also reveal deficiency states of vitamin B_{12}, folic acid, iron, and pyroxidine; bone marrow depression or destruction; and neoplastic disease. It is usually contraindicated in patients with hemophilia and other bleeding disorders. A bone marrow biopsy can be diagnostic for multiple myeloma. Refer to Chapter 9 for a description of the procedure and the application of the nursing process to the care of the patient having a bone marrow aspiration and biopsy.

LYMPH NODE BIOPSY

A biopsy of lymph node tissue may be performed to diagnose Hodgkin's disease or leukemia. The most common sites for the biopsy are cervical, supraclavicular, or axillary nodes. The biopsy is usually performed by needle aspiration. The procedure and nursing care interventions are similar to those applicable to a bone marrow aspiration.

ULTRASONOGRAPHY

Ultrasonography is a noninvasive procedure for visualizing soft tissue structures of the body by monitoring the reflection of ultrasonic waves directed into the tissues. It is useful in determining spleen size and volume when splenomegaly is suspected, as in thrombocytopenic purpura. It may also be used to identify lymph node masses. Only when lymph nodes are enlarged, as in tumor invasion, are they visible on the ultrasonogram. The procedure takes only a few minutes to an hour and causes little, if any, discomfort.

Procedure. Food and fluids are withheld, except water, for 12 hours prior to the test, if necessary. The purpose of the test is explained to the patient, usually by the radiologist. The patient is reassured that the test is noninvasive, is not painful, and is easily tolerated.

COMPUTED TOMOGRAPHY

Computed tomography (CT) scan (also called computerized axial tomography [CAT] scan) provides three-dimensional views of soft body tissues with solid organs and bony structures that are projected onto film. The machine rotates around the body as small beams of x-rays pass through the organs. Photographs are taken of tissue density, and depth images are printed out by a computer. Total body scanning is useful in diagnosing Hodgkin's disease and other lymphomas.

CT scanning is relatively safe for the individual but is often frightening because of the size and complexity of the machine. It delivers no more radiation than a conventional x-ray machine.

Procedure. The procedure is explained to the patient. The patient may be cautioned not to eat or drink fluids 3 to 6 hours prior to the examination to prevent nausea if contrast medium is to be used for the specific test. Although the scanning does not cause discomfort, some individuals are uncomfortable lying on the table for lengthy periods of time. The patient is reassured that it is a safe, noninvasive procedure.

NUCLEAR MAGNETIC RESONANCE AND MAGNETIC RESONANCE IMAGING

The radiation-free nuclear magnetic resonance (NMR) and the magnetic resonance imaging (MRI) procedures produce images of the body similar to those of computed tomography, but with greater sophistication and refined accuracy. The patient is enclosed in a donut-shaped magnet. The surrounding magnetic field causes hydrogen atoms within the body to align in a position to emit radiosignals that are received by an imaging system. The signals are converted by a computer into two-dimensional images that are portrayed on film or the video screen of the system's console. The images can be stored, recalled, and manipulated in a variety of ways, enabling detailed examination of the internal organs. It is a noninvasive diagnostic technique used in the hematologic system to analyze blood flow, detect malignant growths, and distinguish organ size.

Medical Management

Therapeutic goals for patients experiencing dysfunction of the blood or blood-forming organs are focused on diagnosing and correcting the underlying cause of the hematologic disorder. Medical treatment is either palliative or curative and may consist of bed rest with a prescribed regimen of exercise, nutritional support, oxygen therapy, protective isolation, blood and blood component transfusions, radiation therapy, and chemotherapy or other pharmacologic therapy. Surgical interventions include bone marrow transplants, tumor excision, and splenectomy.

Nonsurgical Management

BED REST AND EXERCISE

Bed rest may be recommended to help lower oxygen requirements and reduce the strain on the circulatory and respiratory systems. If the patient is allowed to ambulate and perform activities of daily living, frequent periods of rest are necessary to avoid extreme fatigue and respiratory distress. If the patient cannot actively exercise, passive range-of-motion exercises are performed to promote circulation, enhance joint mobility, and prevent skin breakdown. Application of the nursing process to the care of the patient with activity intolerance was discussed earlier in the chapter.

NUTRITIONAL SUPPORT

A diet high in protein, iron, and vitamins is ordered to promote adequate red blood cell production and to prevent debilitation. Additional iron or vitamin supplements may also be ordered if the diet therapy is inadequate. Application of the nursing process to the care of the patient with nutritional deficiencies was discussed earlier in the chapter.

In cases in which complications of the disorder or treatments interfere with ingestion or digestion, enteral or parenteral support may be required. For the care of the patient receiving enteral or parenteral therapy, see Chapter 21.

OXYGEN THERAPY

The patient may require oxygen owing to the deficiency of oxygen-carrying hemoglobin. Administration of oxygen helps prevent tissue hypoxia and decreases the workload on the heart.

PROTECTIVE ISOLATION

Protective isolation may be ordered to prevent exposing the patient with compromised immunity to microorganisms. This is frequently used for the patient with leukemia or bone marrow depression from a hematologic disorder or from treatment complications. The laminar air flow environment or similar system that uses sterilized air flow and sterile equipment may be used to protect the patient from infection.

BLOOD TRANSFUSIONS

Many components of blood are available for transfusion to patients with specific needs. A patient may receive whole blood, packed red cells, frozen red cells, platelets, granulocytes, plasma, albumin, coagulation factor concentrates, prothrombin complex, cryoprecipitate, or immune serum globulins. Blood for transfusion may be collected from donors (homologous blood), from the intended recipient (autologous blood), or from a donor designated by the recipient (designated [directed] blood).

Blood collected from a donor for transfusion to another individual is the most frequently used blood. Most of this blood is from volunteer donors. Some risks associated with homologous blood transfusions include hemolytic and anaphylactic transfusion reactions, malaria, hepatitis, syphilis, and acquired immunodeficiency syndrome (AIDS).

Blood collected from the intended recipient, or self-donation, is becoming a common procedure prior to elective surgery. Autologous red blood cells can also be salvaged during surgery by the use of automated cell saver equipment or manual suction equipment. Postoperatively, autotransfusion can be instituted using a system designed for collection of drainage from the operative site and reinfusion to the patient with filtration of the blood. This procedure usually takes place while the patient is in an intensive care unit after extensive surgeries such as cardiothoracic surgery or a total hip replacement (Nursing Care Guide 15–1).

Autologous blood transfusions have become more widely used since the public awareness of risks associated with transfusions that was initiated by the AIDS crisis. Autologous transfusions eliminate the risks of immune transfusion reactions and transmission of viral diseases.

Designated (directed) blood is collected from a named donor who has been designated by the recipient. Compatibility testing must be completed prior to the transfusion. The designated blood must be compatible with the recipient's blood in order to be used. Risks are still high with this type of transfusion, because compatibility is a factor, and viral disease may be present in the donor.

WHOLE BLOOD

Whole blood contains both cellular and noncellular plasma components. This includes red blood cells, plasma proteins, stable clotting factors, and an anticoagulant/preservative. It is used to treat acute hemorrhage, requiring the oxygen-carrying properties of red blood cells, and hypovolemic shock resulting from blood loss, requiring plasma expansion.

A unit of blood contains approximately 450 ml of blood with 63 ml of anticoagulant added. The adult dose varies with the patient's needs and symptoms. One unit of whole blood should raise the patient's hematocrit 3 percentage points and the hemoglobin 1 g/dl, providing the patient is no longer hemorrhaging. Other than incompatibility, the major complication of whole blood transfusion is circulatory overload.

PACKED RED CELLS

Transfusions of packed red cells are usually preferred over whole blood because they are more economical and reduce the risk of fluid overload. Packed red cells are indicated for patients requiring an increase in the oxygen-carrying capacity of blood but without the need for volume expansion. Transfusions of packed red cells are ordered for patients with anemia, acute leukemia, or acute or chronic hemorrhage and prior to, during, and after surgical interventions. It is also the treatment of choice for patients with thalassemia major and may relieve the symptoms of sickle cell anemia. In these disorders, monthly or bimonthly transfusions of packed red cells may be ordered if the hemoglobin level falls below 4 g/100 ml. Prophylactically, packed red cells may be administered every 15 days to maintain a hemoglobin level of 12 to 15 g/100 ml.

A unit of packed red cells contains approximately 250 to 300 ml. It is infused for 1 to 3 hours. The adult dose varies with patient need and symptoms or disease process. One unit of packed red cells should increase the hematocrit by 3 percentage points and the hemoglobin by 1 g/dl. Complications are generally a result from incompatibility reactions.

FROZEN RED CELLS

When red blood cells are frozen, they can be stored for as long as 2 years but must be used within 24 hours after thawing. Frozen red cells are less likely to cause an antigen reaction, because antigens are removed. Frozen red cells are very expensive, and their use is therefore usually limited to patients with rare blood types or patients sensitized by previous transfusions.

Nursing Care Guide 15–1.

PATIENTS RECEIVING AN AUTOLOGOUS BLOOD TRANSFUSION

Assessment Findings: Patient presents symptoms of increased temperature, inflammation at wound site, and tachycardia; WBC is elevated.

Nursing Diagnosis: High risk for infection related to surgical intervention, open wound, and intravenous lines

Patient Outcomes	Nursing Interventions	Rationale
Patient's vital signs remain within normal limits for the patient.	Monitor vital signs every 2 hours. Notify physician if significant changes occur.	Vital sign changes may be indicative of complications.
Patient presents no symptoms of an infection such as drainage at site, inflammation, pain at site, and so on.	Maintain aseptic technique when handling transfusion system, changing dressings, or changing tubings. Monitor laboratory values. Check for early signs of infection. Culture any drainage.	Aseptic cleansing at the site and proper handling of the equipment prevents pyogenic infiltration.

Evaluation: Compare the patient's status with the expected patient outcomes. If the outcomes are achieved, evaluate nursing care as successful. If not, reassess the patient, formulate new nursing diagnoses, and revise expected patient outcomes and nursing interventions as appropriate.

Assessment Findings: Patient displays signs of anxiety: tachycardia, increased blood pressure, nervousness, inability to rest; patient asks questions about the intensive care unit (ICU) and blood transfusion.

Nursing Diagnosis: Anxiety related to fear and uncertainty about autologous transfusion and the ICU environment

Patient Outcomes	Nursing Interventions	Rationale
Patient verbalizes fears and concerns.	Allow the patient to verbalize fears and concerns and ask questions.	An understanding of the necessity for the interventions reassures the patient and reduces anxiety.
Patient relates accurate information about the transfusion.	Explain equipment, procedure, and necessity for the transfusion and the ICU environment.	

(continued)

Nursing Care Guide 15–1. *(continued)*

PATIENTS RECEIVING AN AUTOLOGOUS BLOOD TRANSFUSION

Patient Outcomes	Nursing Interventions	Rationale
Patient's anxiety decreases as evidenced by normal vital signs, patient's ability to rest and relax, and verbalization of less fear and concern.	Provide periods of undisturbed quiet and rest for the patient. Monitor vital signs and observe for other signs of anxiety.	Periods of quiet or rest may alleviate some of the patient's anxiety. Vital sign changes such as increased pulse and respiratory rate may indicate increasing anxiety.

Evaluation: Compare the patient's status with the expected patient outcomes. If the outcomes are achieved, evaluate nursing care as successful. If not, reassess the patient, formulate new nursing diagnoses, and revise expected patient outcomes and nursing interventions as appropriate.

Assessment Findings: Patient presents signs of hypovolemia such as decreased blood pressure, dry skin, decreased urine output, and thirst; patient is still losing blood from surgical intervention.

Nursing Diagnosis: High risk for fluid volume deficit related to blood loss

Patient Outcomes	Nursing Interventions	Rationale
Patient's laboratory values are within normal limits for the patient.	Maintain system for autologous transfusion as required to keep adding blood volume as it is lost. Check laboratory values.	Replacement of deficient fluid returns the body to a homeostatic state.
Patient does not have any further blood loss.	Observe for signs of continued bleeding.	Although the nurse may not be able to prevent further blood loss, assessing for early signs of complications of the loss reduces trauma to the patient.
Patient presents no clinical signs of hypovolemia such as vital sign changes, dry skin, and oliguria.	Observe for early signs of hypovolemia. Notify physician if bleeding is greater than expected or if vital sign changes occur.	Vital sign changes may be indicative of continued fluid losses.

Evaluation: Compare the patient's status with the expected patient outcomes. If the outcomes are achieved, evaluate nursing care as successful. If not, reassess the patient, formulate new nursing diagnoses, and revise expected patient outcomes and nursing interventions as appropriate.

PLATELETS

Plasma is first removed from whole blood, and then platelets are separated and pooled together in a collection bag. The patient may receive platelets from several different donors in one unit. Single donor platelet transfusions are available for patients who have developed antibodies to all except transplantation antigen-matched blood products.

Platelets are indicated to control or prevent bleeding episodes in patients with platelet deficiencies associated with low number or dysfunction. They are also used prophylactically for platelet counts below 10,000 to 20,000/cu mm. Platelet transfusions are not recommended for patients with immune thrombocytopenic purpura.

Platelets are stored at room temperature and administered as rapidly as tolerated by the patient. The adult dose varies with the clinical situation. Transfused platelets may function effectively for as long as 5 to 6 days. The transfusions are given according to blood type, but cross-matching is not necessary because platelet concentrates contain few red blood cells. The patient's platelet count is increased by 5000 to 10,000/cu mm for each unit of platelets transfused. One unit of platelets is 50 to 70 ml.

When a patient receives platelet transfusions over an extended period of time, antibodies to the platelets usually develop. If 1 hour after the transfusion is complete the patient's platelet count does not increase, then antibodies are present. If this situation occurs, platelets must be perfectly matched between the donor and recipient to provide adequate transfusions for therapeutic management of the patient's disorder. Adverse reactions to platelet transfusions are usually allergic in nature and treated with an antihistamine.

GRANULOCYTES

A unit of granulocytes contains mostly granulocytes, with less than 10% lymphocytes, 30 to 50 ml red blood cells plasma, and platelets. A unit is approximately 200 to 400 ml. Granulocyte transfusions are indicated for patients with acquired neutropenia, congenital leukocyte dysfunction, leukemia, or bone marrow depression from chemotherapy.

Granulocytes have a short survival time and must be administered rapidly, within 1 to 4 hours per unit. The adult dose is 1 unit daily. The expected outcome is a resolution in infections or prevention of infections. The transfusion does not improve the leukocyte count in adults. Adverse reactions include fever and mild nonhemolytic allergic reactions.

PLASMA

Fresh frozen plasma (FFP) contains approximately 91% water, 7% protein, and 2% carbohydrate. It contains all the clotting factors, which are then preserved by the freezing. Plasma transfusions are used to restore deficient coagulation factors in acquired or inherited bleeding disorders and to replace clotting factors in patient's during hemorrhage. To permanently stop bleeding in patients with hemophilia, plasma is transfused to supply the antihemophilic factor (AHF) to the patient's plasma. The blood must be given within 6 hours after withdrawal from the donor, because AHF deteriorates rapidly.

One unit of plasma is approximately 200 to 250 ml. It should be infused quickly, for 30 to 45 minutes unless otherwise contraindicated. The adult dose is determined by the patient's clinical problem and symptoms. The effect of the transfusion is measured by monitoring coagulation times.

The plasma contains no red blood cells, so cross-matching is not necessary, but ABO typing is usually done. Plasma carries the same complications and risks as whole blood. Sensitization to AHF and the development of autoimmune anticoagulants occur in some cases.

In lieu of plasma, plasma substitutes may be ordered. These substitutes are not blood products but are used to expand plasma volume in emergency situations of massive blood loss. Refer to Pharmacology Box 15–1 for a list of plasma substitutes.

ALBUMIN

Plasma albumin is a large protein molecule considered free of all viral contaminants including hepatitis. Albumin is used for patients in shock as a result of burns, trauma, infection, or surgery to restore blood volume and protein. It is not used for a particular hematologic disorder.

COAGULATION FACTOR CONCENTRATES

Factor VIII concentrate is prepared from donor plasma but does not carry the risk of disease of the plasma owing to the process used to separate the factor. It is used to treat moderate Factor VIII deficiency (hemophilia A). It may also be used for patients lacking fibrinogen or Factor XIII and those with von Willebrand's disease. The adult dose is calculated according to body weight and the level of anticoagulant activity desired. A level of 30% to 50% is the usual goal of the therapy. It is given as an intravenous push.

Factor IX concentrate is also prepared from donor plasma and does not carry risk of disease. It contains Factor IX in large quantities and small amounts of Factors II, VIII, and X. Factor IX concentrate is used to treat a Factor IX deficiency (hemophilia B), congenital Factor VIII deficiency, or Factor X deficiency and to treat hemophiliacs with Factor VIII inhibitors. The adult dose is calculated according to body weight and level of factor activity desired.

PROTHROMBIN COMPLEX

The prothrombin complex blood component contains prothrombin; Factors VII, IX, and X; and part

Pharmacology Box 15–1.

PLASMA SUBSTITUTES

Plasma Substitutes:
Dextran 70 (Gentran 75, Macrodex)
Dextran 40 (Gentran 40, 10% LMD, Rheomacrodex)
6% Hetastarch (Hespan)

Action:
Dextran 70—High molecular weight, expands plasma volume.
Dextran 40—Low molecular weight, reduces blood viscosity.
Hetastarch—Expands plasma volume.

Uses:
Expand plasma volume in massive hemorrhage, fluid loss, and burns.

Side Effects:
Urticaria, fluid overload, nausea, vomiting, wheezing, increased bleeding time, and antigen-antibody reaction.

Interactions:
None

Nursing Implications:
Observe for fluid overload causing respiratory and cardiac distress, bleeding, dehydration, or other side effects. Check renal function. Assess for therapeutic results. Use aseptic technique in handling intravenous equipment and intravenous fluid (plasma substitute).

of Factor XI. Transfusions of prothrombin complex are useful for treating bleeding disorders in patients with congenital or acquired deficiencies of these factors.

CRYOPRECIPITATE

Cryoprecipitate is prepared from whole blood and contains 80 to 120 units of Factor VIII, von Willebrand's factor, fibrinogen, and Factor XIII. Each unit contains approximately 5 to 20 ml. Cryoprecipitate is indicated for deficiencies of Factor VIII, Factor XIII, or fibrinogen and for von Willebrand's disease. The average adult dose is calculated by plasma volume. Eight to ten bags of cryoprecipitate supply enough fibrinogen for hemostasis, approximately 2 g. It is transfused at a rate of 1 to 2 ml/minute. Since cryoprecipitate contains no red blood cells, crossmatching is not required, but ABO compatibility is checked.

IMMUNE SERUM GLOBULINS

Immune serum globulins (ISG) are concentrated aqueous solutions of gamma globulin. Nonspecific ISG is indicated for passive immune protection and to treat hypogammaglobulinemia. Specific ISG is prepared from donors who have a high antibody titer. Some examples of specific ISG include the hepatitis B immune globulin, Rh immune globulin, and varicella-zoster immune globulin. The adult dose varies by the type of ISG. Patients with a history of allergic reactions to plasma should not receive immune globulins. It is given intramuscularly in most instances, but some preparations may be given intravenously. ISG is not generally used for hematologic disorders.

Application of the Nursing Process to the Care of the Patient Receiving Blood or Blood Products

PRETRANSFUSION NURSING CARE

Assessment

Assess the patient prior to the administration of the blood or blood products. Be sure an informed consent is obtained. Check baseline vital signs and record them. Notify the physician if the patient's temperature is elevated. Ask the patient about a history of transfusion reactions. Assess the patient's level of understanding about the procedure.

Nursing Diagnoses and Planning

The nursing diagnosis and related expected patient outcomes most commonly applicable to the care of patients receiving blood transfusions are as follows:

NDx: Knowledge deficit: nature of procedure and signs of potential complications

Planning: Patient outcomes
1. Patient relates accurate information about transfusions and the symptoms of a reaction.
2. Patient reports any unusual symptoms immediately.

Nursing Interventions

NDx: Knowledge deficit: nature of procedure and signs of potential complications
Describe the procedure, length of transfusion, potential for future transfusions, and expected outcomes in terms that are understandable to the patient. Explain the symptoms of a blood reaction, and instruct the patient to report any unusual feeling immediately. Allow time for questions and expression of concerns.

Additional Interventions
Prior to administration of the blood, check that it has been typed and crossmatched and that the ABO group and Rh match that of the patient. The patient's information is usually on a special page in the chart. Observe for abnormal color or cloudiness, indicating hemolysis. Check for the presence of gas bubbles, indicating bacterial growth.

Confirm the patient's name, blood type, Rh factor, and identification number and that which is listed on the blood bag with another nurse before administering the transfusion. Document this confirmation with both nurses' signatures. Check the same data with the patient's identification bracelet. Many institutions use a separate identification band for blood recipients. Verify this information and document the time, date, and confirmation of the match of data. Do not remove any identification information on the blood container until the transfusion is completed. Most institutions require that the blood container be returned to the laboratory upon completion of the transfusion.

Once the blood is unrefrigerated, administer it within 1 hour to prevent hemolysis and bacterial growth. The rate of administration may vary based on the patient's medical history and need, but it is generally administered as rapidly as possible, especially in cases of hemorrhage. It should not take longer than 3 hours to administer one unit of blood.

Follow body substance precautions at all times when performing the venipuncture or handling blood products or blood equipment. Start the primary intravenous line with a 19-gauge or larger needle for adults. Use a Y-tubing blood administration set or other equipment as designated by hospital policy. Usually this intravenous tubing has a blood filter attached to screen out fibrin clots or other particles. It is common to use normal saline as the primary solution. The blood may be given without a primary solution, but in the case of a blood reaction, it is helpful to have a vein open when the blood is discontinued. Document the date and time the infusion is started and any immediate reaction, if noted.

An electronic infusion device should be used only if recommended by the manufacturer. Follow the instructions for appropriate use. Blood warmers may be indicated to decrease the risk of arrhythmias or cardiac arrest associated with rapid transfusion of cold blood in situations of acute massive blood loss. Follow hospital policy and equipment directions when using the blood warmer.

Keep the recording sheet at the bedside for continued noting of the vital signs and symptoms throughout the transfusions. Check the values of the baseline data and compare for changes.

Evaluation

Evaluate the effectiveness of nursing care for a patient receiving a blood transfusion by comparing the patient's status with the expected patient outcomes. Examples of specific outcomes for patients receiving a blood transfusion have been provided in the Planning section.

NURSING CARE DURING TRANSFUSION

Continue to assess the patient during the administration of the blood. Look for early signs of a reaction in the respiratory system, such as tachypnea, apnea, dyspnea, cough, wheezing, or rales. Check for elevated temperature, chills, chest pain, muscle aches, headache, tingling, and numbness.

Assess the cardiovascular system for bradycardia, tachycardia, change in blood pressure, cyanosis, skin temperature changes, and edema. Check the urine output. Look for urticaria, signs of itching, and diaphoresis. Note the vital signs on the record sheet every 15 minutes.

Check the flow rate frequently during administration to be sure the blood is being infused as ordered. Tell the patient to notify the nurse if any unusual symptoms appear. The donor blood may contain viruses, bacteria, or parasites, which is rare, or the patient may be sensitive to leukocytes or platelets. If the blood is contaminated with microorganisms, fever and chills usually develop within 30 minutes after the start of the transfusion. Shock may ensue immediately. Sensitivity to leukocytes or platelets is common, especially in adults who have had previous transfusions or in women who have delivered infants. In sensitivity episodes, fever occurs, but not chills. This reaction is the most common blood transfusion reaction and is usually treated with an antipyretic.

The patient may be sensitive to plasma protein in the blood or to an allergen passed from the donor. To prevent this, donors with multiple allergies are usually disqualified as donors. If the patient reacts to an allergen in the blood, the reaction is usually mild and is treated with an antihistamine. Note any symptoms of a reaction the patient presents, even if it is very mild.

Severe respiratory distress or cardiac distress usually indicates that the patient has received incompatible blood from the donor. Incompatibility occurs when the red blood cells received from the donor blood clump together in the plasma of the recipient. Enzymes quickly break down the red blood cells, exceeding the liver's ability to detoxify the products of this process, resulting in damage to renal tubules. Although this type of reaction usually occurs within 10 minutes of the initiation of the transfusion, observe the patient throughout the transfusion time for such signs of a severe reaction. Interventions must be started immediately.

In an unconscious patient, also take vital signs every 15 minutes, but observe the patient frequently, because the patient cannot warn the nurse of untoward symptoms. Look carefully for signs of a reaction in the unconscious patient, which might include a weak pulse, fever, tachycardia or bradycardia, hypotension, and oliguria. Refer to Nursing Care Guide 15–2 for the care of the patient with a blood transfusion reaction.

POSTTRANSFUSION NURSING CARE

Assessment

When the transfusion is completed, assess the patient's vital signs and record them along with the date and time. Look for any signs of a latent reaction. Document all pertinent information about the patient's symptoms during the transfusion and at the terminal point of the transfusion. Remove the equipment, using body fluid precautions, and dispose of the transfusion equipment appropriately according to the institution's policy. Return the blood container to the blood bank.

Assess the knowledge level of the patient about the signs and symptoms of a delayed blood reaction and when to seek medical attention.

Nursing Diagnoses and Planning

The nursing diagnosis and related expected patient outcomes most commonly applicable to patients after blood transfusions are as follows:

NDx: Knowledge deficit: nature of delayed transfusion reaction, signs, and symptoms, and when to seek medical intervention

Planning: Patient outcomes

1. Patient relates accurate information about delayed transfusion reactions, the signs and symptoms, and when to seek medical intervention.
2. Patient observes for signs and symptoms of a blood reaction after discharge and seeks medical assistance if symptoms are evident.

Nursing Interventions

NDx: Knowledge deficit: nature of delayed transfusion reaction, signs, symptoms, and when to seek medical intervention

Teach the patient to observe for signs of infection such as chills, fever, cough, respiratory distress, or circulatory changes. Explain to the patient that any symptoms of respiratory distress should be reported immediately to the physician. An anaphylactic reaction could be life-threatening, and the patient needs to seek assistance at the first signs of a reaction. Tell the patient that signs of a mild reaction may include a rash, itching, low-grade fever, or headache.

Allow the patient and family to ask questions and voice concerns. Have the patient verbalize the sign and symptoms of a reaction to be certain that there is an understanding of the teaching. Write the signs on a list for the patient or family to take home with them. Inform them that a reaction may not occur until 2 weeks after transfusion.

Evaluation

Evaluate the effectiveness of nursing care for a patient after a blood transfusion by comparing the patient's status with the expected patient outcomes. Examples of specific outcomes for patients after a blood transfusion have been provided in the Planning section.

Text continued on page 622

Nursing Care Guide 15–2.

PATIENTS WITH A BLOOD TRANSFUSION REACTION

Assessment Findings: Patient experiences dyspnea, chest pain, feeling of tightness in chest, increased pulse and respiration, hypertension, chills, fever, facial burning within 15 minutes after transfusion begins, low back pain, headache or full feeling in the head, hematuria, anorexia, oliguria, apprehension, neck vein distention, and shock.

Nursing Diagnosis: High risk for injury related to antigen-antibody incompatibility

Patient Outcomes	Nursing Interventions	Rationale
Patient's vital signs are within normal range for patient. Patient indicates chills, back pain, and headache are absent.	Monitor vital signs. If vital signs change or other untoward symptoms appear, discontinue blood transfusion. Also complete the following: Notify physician stat. Keep intravenous line open with saline.	Although the nurse may not prevent a transfusion reaction, appropriate nursing interventions are important to minimize the trauma of the reaction to the patient.
	Draw client's blood for Hgb, culture, and retyping; obtain urinalysis; and observe voidings. Return remaining blood and tubing to blood bank for repeat typing and culture. Reassure patient. Cover patient with blanket. Administer diuretics and colloids as ordered. If there is a history of previous reactions, may administer Benadryl prophylactically.	The blood is rechecked for errors in typing and cross-matching.

Evaluation: Compare the patient's status with the expected patient outcomes. If the outcomes are achieved, evaluate nursing care as successful. If not, reassess the patient, formulate new nursing diagnoses, and revise expected patient outcomes and nursing interventions as appropriate.

(continued)

Nursing Care Guide 15–2. *(continued)*

PATIENTS WITH A BLOOD TRANSFUSION REACTION

Assessment Findings: Patient experiences weakness, fatigue 1 to 2 weeks post transfusion, decreased Hgb, and positive Coombs' test results.

Nursing Diagnosis: Altered health maintenance related to lack of knowledge of delayed antigen-antibody incompatibility

Patient Outcomes	Nursing Interventions	Rationale
Patient states accurate information about the reaction and potential for a delayed reaction.	Inform patient that this reaction is not dangerous and that subsequent transfusions may cause an acute hemolytic reaction.	Knowledge of the expectations of a reaction alerts the patient to watch for early signs of problems.
Patient states the signs and sympotms of a delayed reaction.	Instruct patient in signs and symptoms of a delayed reaction.	A reaction to the transfusion can be delayed for as long as 2 weeks postinfusion.
Patient verbalizes the necessity to contact medical personnel if symptoms of a reaction become apparent.	Instruct patient to notify the nurse or physician if signs or symptoms are evident. Check Hgb levels if patient experiences signs or symptoms.	Immediate intervention reduces risk of complications.

Evaluation: Compare the patient's status with the expected patient outcomes. If the outcomes are achieved, evaluate nursing care as successful. If not, reassess the patient, formulate new nursing diagnoses, and revise expected patient outcomes and nursing interventions as appropriate.

Assessment Findings: Patient is experiencing fever, chills, headache, flushing, tachycardia, palpitations, nausea, vomiting, diarrhea, malaise, and lumbar pain.

Nursing Diagnosis: High risk for infection related to bacterial pyogens transfused through blood

Patient Outcomes	Nursing Interventions	Rationale
Patient remains free of signs and symptoms of a pyrogenic reaction.	Discontinue blood transfusion. Notify physician stat. Keep vein open with saline.	Appropriate nursing interventions reduce risk of further complications.
Patient's vital signs are within normal ranges for the patient.	Monitor vital signs. Reassure patient and family. Premedicate with antipyretic.	Changes in vital signs may indicate complications.

Evaluation: Compare the patient's status against the expected patient outcomes. If the outcomes are achieved, evaluate nursing care as successful. If not, reassess the patient, formulate new nursing diagnoses, and revise expected patient outcomes and nursing interventions as appropriate.

(continued)

Nursing Care Guide 15–2. *(continued)*

PATIENTS WITH A BLOOD TRANSFUSION REACTION

Assessment Findings: Patient is experiencing dyspnea, nausea, vomiting, urticaria, rash, itching, hives, facial flushing, wheezing, hypotension, shock, diarrhea, tight chest, and anxiety, but no fever.

Nursing Diagnosis: High risk for injury related to allergic reaction

Patient Outcomes	Nursing Interventions	Rationale
Patient remains free of signs and symptoms of an allergic reaction.	Discontinue transfusion. Keep vein open with saline. Notify physician stat. If only symptoms are itching, hives, urticaria, rash, and anxiety, resume transfusion slowly.	Although the nurse may not prevent an allergic reaction, appropriate nursing interventions are important to minimize the trauma of the reaction to the patient.
Vital signs remain within normal range for patient.	Administer antihistamines and monitor vital signs.	Vital sign changes may indicate complications.
Patient indicates that symptoms of a reaction are absent.	If symptoms progress, discontinue transfusion, obtain urinalysis, draw client's blood, notify blood bank, and return remaining blood and tubing. Administer Benadryl 15 to 20 minutes prior to transfusion as ordered if the patient is suspected to have allergies. Give epinephrine, vasopressors, and crystalloids, if ordered.	The blood is rechecked for proper typing and crossmatching if the reaction continues.

Evaluation: Compare the patient's status with the expected patient outcomes. If the outcomes are achieved, evaluate nursing care as successful. If not, reassess the patient, formulate new nursing diagnoses, and revise expected patient outcomes and nursing interventions as appropriate.

(continued)

Nursing Care Guide 15–2. *(continued)*

PATIENTS WITH A BLOOD TRANSFUSION REACTION

Assessment Findings: Patient is experiencing dyspnea; dry cough; rales in lungs; crackles at base of lungs; tightness in chest; bounding pulse; increased blood pressure; orthopnea; cyanosis; tachycardia; neck vein distention; anxiety; coughing of pink, frothy sputum; cold, clammy skin; and restlessness.

Nursing Diagnosis: Fluid volume excess related to circulatory overload from blood transfusion

Patient Outcomes	Nursing Interventions	Rationale
Patient's skin color remains pink, and skin is dry to touch.	Position patient upright. Check the skin for edema, color, and integrity, especially in the extremities.	Signs of fluid pooling, especially in the extremities, is a sign of fluid overload.
Patient's vital signs remain within normal range for patient. Patient's lungs remain clear upon auscultation. Patient denies respiratory or circulatory distress. Patient presents no evidence of peripheral or pulmonary edema.	Monitor vital signs and venous pressure. Monitor lung sounds. Apply rotating tourniquets if ordered. Administer diuretics, oxygen, morphine, vasodilators, and aminophylline if ordered.	Vital sign changes such as increasing pulse rate and blood pressure may be indicative of a fluid overload. Adventitious breath sounds may be the result of pulmonary edema from the fluid overload.

Evaluation: Compare the patient's status with the expected patient outcomes. If the outcomes are achieved, evaluate nursing care as successful. If not, reassess the patient, formulate new nursing diagnoses, and revise expected patient outcomes and nursing interventions as appropriate.

Chart 15–1.

NURSING GUIDE TO PATIENT EDUCATION FOR SELF-MANAGEMENT: SIGNS AND SYMPTOMS OF DELAYED TRANSFUSION REACTIONS

Teach the patient and family to observe for:

Respiratory system symptoms: tachypnea, dyspnea, apnea, wheezing, cyanosis, and rales.
Circulatory system symptoms: tachycardia, chest pain, palpitations, muscle aches, headache, chills, tingling, numbness, weakness, and fever.
Urinary system symptoms: oliguria, and pain or burning with urination.
Integumentary system symptoms: itching, edema, cyanosis, rashes, and excessive perspiration.

TYPES OF TRANSFUSION REACTIONS

There are several types of transfusion reactions that a patient receiving donor blood may experience. An acute hemolytic reaction is caused by infusion of ABO-incompatible blood. This may occur in transfusions of whole blood, packed red cells, or blood components containing red blood cells (10 ml or more). Antigens from the donor's red blood cells react with the patient's antibodies, causing the clinical manifestations. This reaction may cause some of the most severe symptoms.

A febrile, nonhemolytic reaction is the most common type that blood recipients experience. It is caused by sensitization to the donor's platelets, proteins, or white blood cells. The reaction is usually treated symptomatically and the transfusion discontinued. Rarely is the reaction life-threatening.

A mild allergic reaction is caused by sensitivity only to the plasma proteins. The patient may experience a rash, some itching, and a low grade fever. Antihistamines are given, if needed.

An anaphylactic reaction is caused by the infusion of a specific protein to a patient deficient in the protein but who has developed antibodies to it. The patient may experience mild to severe symptoms.

A circulatory overload is a rare transfusion reaction. It is caused by rapid fluid administration in a patient with a circulatory system unable to accommodate the volume. This may occur in the patient with a history of previous cardiac problems.

A septic reaction occurs when contaminated blood is transfused into the patient. The onset of symptoms is usually immediate. The patient experiences fever, chills, hypotension, and shock. It is treated with intravenous antibiotics and symptomatically.

A delayed transfusion reaction may occur in the patient several days to 2 weeks after the transfusions. Prior to discharge, the patient should be taught symptoms of a delayed transfusion reaction (Chart 15–1) and told to seek medical intervention if any of the symptoms are evident. Delayed reactions may be caused by hemolytic reactions, hepatitis B, hepatitis C, human immunodeficiency virus infection, iron overload, or other infectious diseases in the donor blood. Refer to Nursing Care Guide 15–2.

MEDICAL MANAGEMENT FOR TRANSFUSION REACTIONS

Treatment instituted for a transfusion depends on the severity of the reaction. Blood is usually discontinued, but in cases of very mild reactions, blood administration may be continued with careful, continual monitoring of the patient's status. In life-threatening situations, emergency care is instituted immediately. Shock, respiratory distress, or cardiac arrhythmias are reversed with a variety of drugs and support interventions. Hypotension is treated with vasoconstrictors. Renal damage is prevented by administering intravenous colloids. Mannitol may be ordered as an osmotic diuretic. An indwelling catheter may be inserted to monitor urine output. If urine output is not adequate, acute renal tubular necrosis may have developed, and mannitol is contraindicated. The patient is then placed on fluid restriction, and dialysis may be necessary. In cases of mild reactions, antihistamines or antipyretics may be ordered.

NURSING INTERVENTIONS FOR TRANSFUSION REACTIONS

When a transfusion reaction occurs, follow the steps as listed below:

- Stop the transfusion.
- Keep the vein open with the primary solution.
- Take vital signs, have a nurse stay with the patient, and document the symptoms.
- Institute appropriate interventions if life-threatening symptoms appear.
- Report the reaction to the physician and the blood bank.
- Institute medical orders.

- Send the blood container with attached labels to the blood bank.
- Collect urine and blood samples and send to the laboratory.
- Document the symptoms, treatment instituted, patient reaction, and follow-up care.
- Explain the situation to the patient and family, reassure them, make the patient comfortable, and continue to observe for further symptoms.

Surgical Management

SPLENECTOMY

The removal of the spleen can be performed without further complications to the adult, despite its important functions in the hematologic system. After a splenectomy, the role of the spleen is taken over by the liver, lymph nodes, and bone marrow.

USES

A splenectomy is performed for dysfunction of the organ as seen in many hematologic diseases, for rupture of the spleen due to trauma, and for tearing of the organ during abdominal surgery. Hypersplenism, a condition in which the spleen excessively destroys blood components, is another indication for a splenectomy. Splenomegaly, anemia, leukopenia, and compensatory increase in blood cell production by the bone marrow all are signs of hypersplenism. Primary hypersplenism relates to overactivity of the spleen of unknown cause. Secondary hypersplenism indicates overactivity of the spleen due to another disease. Primary hypersplenism is found in idiopathic thrombocytopenia purpura and congenital spherocytosis. Secondary hypersplenism is present in leukemia, lymphoma, and Hodgkin's disease.

The treatment of choice for primary hypersplenism is a splenectomy, which alleviates the disease in 60% to 80% of patients. In secondary hypersplenism, a splenectomy is only a palliative treatment for some of the symptoms of the disease. It does not change the major course of the disorder.

PROCEDURE

A splenectomy is performed much like other abdominal surgeries under general anesthesia. Because the organ is very vascular and may be extremely enlarged as a result of overactivity, the surgery carries the risk of hemorrhage and can be quite difficult to perform. However, in most cases, the prognosis is excellent and the mortality is very low.

PHYSICAL PREPARATION OF THE PATIENT

Preoperatively, the patient is informed about the procedure, risks, and postoperative course. After an operative permit is endorsed by the patient, the physical preparation is instituted. The patient's abdomen is prepped as designated by hospital procedure. A preoperative checklist is completed, and preoperative medication is administered.

POSTOPERATIVE COURSE

If the patient does not have other disease complications, the postoperative course after a splenectomy is usually uneventful. Most patients are discharged in a few days with instructions for home care. Postoperatively, the patient is maintained on intravenous fluids until vital signs are stable and gastrointestinal function returns. A nasogastric tube may be instilled prior to or during surgery. The patient has a sterile dressing on the abdomen which is changed as needed. Prophylactic antibiotic therapy and analgesics may be ordered. Providing there are no other complicating factors, the patient is instructed about signs of bleeding and infection, how to change dressings, activity restrictions for a couple weeks, and when to return to the physician for follow-up care. The patient with other interfering factors, such as a hematologic disease like leukemia, may be hospitalized for several days to weeks and may experience many other treatment modalities instituted for the primary disease problem.

COMPLICATIONS

If the spleen is extremely enlarged, the surgery may be very difficult. Since it is a highly vascular organ, hemorrhage is the major risk during surgery. Postoperatively, the most common complications include infection, bleeding, and interference with healing from other complicating factors from the primary disease.

Application of the Nursing Process to the Care of the Patient Having a Splenectomy

PREOPERATIVE NURSING CARE

Assessment

Complete a physical assessment of the patient. Look for signs of respiratory distress, circulatory problems, nutritional deficits, and general health status to prepare for potential problems in the postoperative period. Assess the patient's understanding of the surgery, the postoperative course, and the self-care responsibilities after discharge.

Nursing Diagnoses and Planning

The nursing diagnosis and related expected patient outcomes most commonly applicable to patients scheduled for a splenectomy are as follows:

NDx: Knowledge deficit: surgical procedure and postoperative course

Planning: Patient outcomes

1. Patient states accurate information about the surgical procedure and expected results.
2. Patient describes the typical postoperative course.

Nursing Interventions

NDx: Knowledge deficit: surgical procedure and postoperative course
Explain to the patient about the surgical procedure, the recovery period, and the postoperative care required. Tell the patient about intravenous therapy that is typically used, what discomforts to expect, and the preventive methods used to arrest respiratory problems after surgery. Allow time for questions and verbalization of concerns from the patient or family.

Evaluation

Evaluate the effectiveness of nursing care for a patient scheduled for a splenectomy by comparing the patient's status with the expected patient outcomes. Examples of specific outcomes for patients having a splenectomy have been provided in the Planning section.

POSTOPERATIVE NURSING CARE

Assessment

Assess the patient's vital signs, orientation, dressings, and intravenous solutions. Check for signs of discomfort and medicate accordingly. Check the respiratory status and the patient's ability to cough and breathe deeply, and auscultate the chest. Assess for voiding within a reasonable time postoperatively. Look for abdominal swelling and drainage on or around the dressing.

Nursing Diagnoses and Planning

Nursing diagnoses and related expected patient outcomes most commonly applicable to the patient after a splenectomy include the following:

NDx: Pain related to surgical incision and manipulation

Planning: Patient outcomes

1. Patient states pain is relieved.
2. Patient moves freely and is able to turn, cough, and breathe deeply without extreme discomfort.

NDx: High risk for infection related to abdominal wound, intravenous lines, and respiratory status

Planning: Patient outcomes

1. Patient's vital signs are within normal range for the patient.
2. Patient's wound shows no signs of infection such as purulent drainage or inflammation.

NDx: Knowledge deficit: self-care after discharge

Planning: Patient outcomes

1. Patient relates accurate information about care needed after discharge.
2. Patient states the need for follow-up medical care.
3. Patient identifies signs of complications and the need to seek medical assistance if signs are evident.

Nursing Interventions

NDx: Pain
Administer ordered analgesics as needed. Encourage the patient to move frequently, to splint the abdomen when turning and coughing, and to request medication when necessary before pain becomes intolerable.

NDx: High risk for infection
Have the patient frequently turn, cough, and breathe deeply. Explain the reason for this intervention, and encourage the patient to perform the routine often while lying in bed. Get the patient up as soon as allowed. Encourage frequent position changes. Use aseptic technique when changing the abdominal dressing and when handling the IV equipment.

NDx: Knowledge deficit: self-care after discharge
Teach the patient about the care of the surgical wound and how to complete an aseptic dressing change. Explain the signs and symptoms of complications and when to seek medical intervention. Tell the patient about any physical restrictions the physician has ordered and when to visit the physician's office for follow-up care.

Evaluation

Evaluate the effectiveness of nursing care for a patient who has had a splenectomy by comparing the patient's status with the expected patient outcomes. Examples of specific outcomes for patients after a splenectomy have been provided in the Planning section.

Other Surgical Procedures and Medical Treatments for Patients with Dysfunction of the Blood and Blood-Forming Organs

BONE MARROW TRANSPLANT

Bone marrow transplantation is used to treat hematologic disorders such as aplastic anemia and leukemia and to treat severe bone marrow depression resulting from other therapeutic interventions. Refer to Chapter 9 for a description of bone marrow transplantation and nursing care applicable to the patient receiving a bone marrow transplant.

RADIATION THERAPY

The goal of radiation therapy for the patient with a hematologic disorder is usually to destroy malignant tissue growth with minimal damage to the normal tissue. Tissue cells more susceptible to radiation include hematopoietic cells of the bone marrow and lymphocytes. Radiation therapy is used to treat Hodgkin's disease, localized non-Hodgkin's disease, some leukemias, and multiple myeloma. Radioactive isotopes may be implanted internally to deliver direct radiation in polycythemia vera. Agranulocytosis is a major complication of radiation therapy. Refer to Chapter 11 for nursing care of the patient receiving radiation therapy.

CHEMOTHERAPY

Chemotherapy is the primary treatment used for patients with leukemia, multiple myeloma, and Hodgkin's disease. Chemotherapy may also be used to treat patients with polycythemia vera and nonlocalized Hodgkin's disease. The choice of chemotherapy, combinations of drugs, and frequency of therapy depends on the specific hematologic disease, its severity, and patient response to treatment. Refer to Chapter 11 for a description of chemotherapeutic agents and nursing care of the patient receiving chemotherapy. See Chapter 16 for the chemotherapeutic agents used for each specific hematologic disease.

The Elderly: Special Considerations

The older adult is prone to developing certain blood disorders as a result of several factors. Aged individuals experience a decrease in the immunologic defense system, which lowers the body's ability to protect against infections and malignancies.

In the elderly, the course of diseases, signs, and symptoms and responses to treatment may be altered because of age-related physiologic changes and drug interactions. Drug toxicity is common in the older adult as a result of reduced renal blood flow from decreased cardiac output, diminished glomerular filtration rate, and tubular reabsorption. Reduced gastric motility in the elderly increases drug absorption; a decreased blood flow to the liver decreases detoxification.

If the older adult undergoes surgery for a hematologic disorder, the risk is significantly increased compared with the risk for the young or middle-aged adult. The elderly adult's coping ability may be reduced by additional stressors, sensory deficits, chronic disease, and limited mobility. The aged usually do not tolerate chemotherapy and radiation therapy as well as a younger adult. Complications of these treatment modalities are more profound in the older adult and require more complicated medical and nursing interventions.

The aging process decreases the recovery and proliferation of normal cells. Tissue tolerance is significantly lessened, which exacerbates the side effects of therapies. The older adult experiences a dry mouth from decreased saliva production, further aggravating problems with mucous membranes.

Older adults with nutritional deficits resulting in hematologic disorders require additional nutritional supplements because vitamin and mineral absorption is diminished. An increased risk of pressure sores is associated with vitamin C, caloric, and protein deficiencies.

Bruising may be caused by hematologic problems as well as normal senile purpura. Delayed wound healing, associated with anemia, may be enhanced in the elderly as a result of reduced vascularity from increased capillary fragility.

When assessing the older adult for hematologic disorders, observe for signs of confusion related to both senility and the decreased oxygen-carrying capacity of the blood. The baseline temperature of the elderly is usually subnormal, so when assessing for infection, a slight increase in temperature may be significant. The white blood count is not as elevated in the aged in the presence of infection as is typical in the younger adult. Fatigue may be a symptom of a blood disorder rather than due to the advanced age of the patient. Fatigue may also be due to the decreased vital capacity of the older adult and increased residual volume leading to inefficient oxygen and carbon dioxide exchange.

It is common for the elderly to lose weight as a result of decreased appetite, fewer taste buds, and gastrointestinal changes. The older patient may become dehydrated and malnourished, resulting in anemia. Dental problems, reduced enzyme secretion, and diminished peristalsis also contribute to the nutritional problems in the elderly.

When planning care for the older adult with a hematologic disorder, consider the patient's lifestyle, living arrangement, transportation, education, financial status, nutritional patterns, support systems, and particularly the individual desires of the patient.

Bibliography

Beare P, Rahr, VA. Quick reference to nursing implications of diagnostic tests. Philadelphia: JB Lippincott, 1982.

Bouchard-Kurtz R, Speese-Owens N. Nursing care of the cancer patient. 4th ed. St. Louis: CV Mosby, 1981.

Brown S. Behind the numbers on the CBC. RN 1990; 53(2):46.

Bume KG, Petz LD. Clinical bone marrow transplantation. New York: Churchill Livingstone, 1983.

Burns N. Nursing and cancer. Philadelphia: WB Saunders, 1982.

Butler S. Current trends in autologous transfusion. RN 1989; 52(11):44.

Campbell C. Nursing diagnoses and intervention in nursing practice. New York: John Wiley & Sons, 1984.

DeVita VT Jr. Principles of chemotherapy. In DeVita VT Jr, Hellman S, Rosenberg SA (eds). Cancer: Principles and practice of oncology. Philadelphia: JB Lippincott, 1982.

Ellerbe S. Massive blood transfusion in fluid and blood component therapy in the critically ill and injured. New York: Churchill Livingstone, 1981.

Fischbach F. A manual of laboratory diagnostic tests. 3rd ed. Philadelphia: JB Lippincott, 1988.

Gunz F, Henderson E. Leukemia. 4th ed. Orlando, FL: Grune & Stratton, 1983.

Hillman R, Finch C. Red cell manual. 5th ed. Philadelphia: FA Davis, 1985.

Illustrated manual of nursing practice. Springhouse, PA: Springhouse Publishing, 1991.

Jarvis C. Physical examination and health assessment. Philadelphia: WB Saunders, 1992.

Judd JW, Barnes A. Clinical and serological aspects of transfusion reactions: a technical workshop. Presented by the Committee on Technical Workshops. Anaheim, CA: American Association of Blood Banks, 1982.

Krause JR (ed). Bone marrow biopsy. New York: Churchill Livingstone, 1981.

Maas M, Buckwalter KC, Hardy M. Nursing diagnoses and interventions for the elderly. Redwood City, CA: Addison-Wesley, 1991.

Malanden DE. Diseases of the lymphatic system: Diagnosis and therapy. New York: Springer-Verlag, 1983.

Masoorli ST. A step-by-step guide to trouble-free transfusions. RN, 1984; 47(5):34.

Miller CA. Nursing care of older adults. Glenville, IL: Scott, Foresman, 1990.

Monroe D. Patient teaching for x-ray and other diagnostics. RN 1989; 52(9):50.

Murphy S, Gilbert J (eds). Leukemia research: Advances in cell biology and treatment. New York: Elsevier Science Publishing, 1983.

National Blood Resource Education Program's Nursing Education Working Group. Transfusion nursing: Trends and practices for the 90's. Am J Nurs 1991; 91(6):42.

Nuscher R, Baltzer L, Repinec DA, et al. Bone marrow transplantation: A lifesaving option. Am J Nurs 1984; 84(6):764.

Perry M, Yarbro J. Toxicity of chemotherapy. Orlando, FL: Grune & Stratton, 1984.

Petz L, Garratty G. Acquired immune hemolytic anemias. New York: Churchill Livingstone, 1980.

Querin JJ, Stahl LD. 12 simple, sensible steps for successful blood transfusions. Nursing '83 1983; 13(11):34.

Ratnoff O, Forbes C. Disorders of hemostasis. Orlando, FL: Grune & Stratton, 1984.

Ristuccia A. Hematolgic effects of cancer chemotherapy. Nurs Clin North Am 1985; 20(1):235.

Rutman RC, Miller WV. Transfusion therapy: Principles and procedures. 2nd ed. Rockville, MD: Aspen Publications, 1985.

Salinger JH. If your patient gets a bone marrow transplant. RN 1984; 47(5):62.

Smith L. Reactions to blood transfusions. Am J Nurs 1984; 84(9):1096.

Snyder C. Oncology nursing. Boston: Little, Brown, 1986.

Snyder EL, Kennedy MS. Blood transfusion therapy: A physician's handbook. Anaheim, CA: American Association of Blood Banks, 1983.

Spivak JL. Fundamentals of clinical hematology. 2nd ed. Philadelphia: JB Lippincott, 1983.

Sympson GM. CATR: A new generation of autologous blood transfusion. Crit Care Nurse 1991; 11(4):60.

Tietz NW. Clinical guide to laboratory tests. Philadelphia: WB Saunders, 1983.

Umlas J, Silvergleid A. Transfusion for the patient with selected clinical problems: A technical workshop. Presented by the Committee on Technical Workshops. Anaheim, CA: American Association of Blood Banks, 1982.

Ungaro PC, Canaday BR. Hematologic diseases: New directions in therapy. 3rd ed. New York: Medical Examination Publishing, 1984.

Vredevoe DL, Brainerd, CA. Concepts of oncology nursing. Englewood Cliffs, NJ: Prentice-Hall, 1981.

Williams WJ, Beutler E, Ersler AJ, Lichtman MA. Hematology. 4th ed. New York: McGraw-Hill, 1990.

Wintrobe M. Clinical hematology. 8th ed. Philadelphia: Lea & Febiger, 1981.

Chapter Sixteen

NURSING CARE *of Adults with Disorders of the Blood and Blood-Forming Organs*

Disorders of the blood and blood-forming organs can affect all other body systems. The disorders range from mild anemias to malignant diseases. All hematologic disorders have many things in common, and this generates some similarities in nursing assessments and interventions. A thorough multisystem assessment and patient history are critical to effective nursing care.

Long-term care is necessary in many hematologic disorders because of the chronicity of the disease. Patient and family education is important for continuing health maintenance. Referrals to other health professionals, such as home health nurses, psychologists, or nutritionists, may be required.

Erythrocyte-Related Disorders

Anemias

Etiology and Pathophysiology. The medical term anemia implies a low red blood cell (RBC) count and a low hemoglobin (Hgb) or hematocrit (Hct) level. Anemia occurs as a result of bone marrow failure or excessive red cell loss, or both. Marrow failure may be caused by nutritional deficiency, toxic exposure, or tumor invasion or may be of unknown causes. Red cell loss may be caused by hemorrhage, decreased red cell production, or increased destruction of red cells. Red cell lysis occurs predominantly in the liver and spleen.

Anemias are classified according to their etiology:

1. Anemias associated with blood loss. In hemorrhagic anemias, a rapid loss of large numbers of erythrocytes occurs, resulting in a severe decrease in blood volume and oxygen in the blood.

   Prognosis depends on the rate and location of bleeding and the volume of blood lost. It is usually less traumatic to the system to slowly lose a large volume of blood than to rapidly lose even a small volume of blood. In the latter situation, the quick change in volume is a major shock to the system. Acute hemorrhage may be caused by a severed blood vessel as a result of trauma, rupture of an aneurysm, or tearing or erosion of an artery.
2. Anemias associated with decreased red blood cell production (hypoproliferative anemias). In the hypoproliferative anemias the marrow is unable to produce adequate numbers of cells, which decreases the red blood cell count. This results from marrow damage by drugs or chemicals, lack of erythropoietin as in renal disease, or the lack of iron, vitamin B_{12}, or folic acid.
3. Anemias associated with red blood cell destruction (hemolytic anemias). Anemia resulting from hemolysis may be indicative of red cell abnormality, as occurs in inherited hemolytic anemias like spherocytosis, sickle cell anemia, thalassemia, and glucose-6-phosphate dehydrogenase (G6PD) deficiency. If the abnormality occurs in the plasma, it may be indicative of an acquired hemolytic anemia, such as immune hemolytic anemia.

Clinical Manifestations. Clinical manifestations of anemia include disorientation resulting from cerebral anoxia and fever. Mucous membranes may become pale or edematous or may bleed because of the low oxyhemoglobin level. As red blood cells are broken down, bilirubin is released. Discoloration of the skin and sclerae occurs when the levels of bilirubin are 1.5 mg/100 ml in the blood stream. Free hemoglobin appears in the plasma and diffuses through the renal glomeruli into the urine. Cloudy or bloody urine and tarry stools may indicate bleeding from within. Clubbing of the nails may occur as a result of chronic hypoxia.

The individual with severe anemia usually experiences dyspnea, palpitations, fatigue, anorexia, and other gastrointestinal disturbances related to tissue hypoxia from red cell loss or marrow failure. Following exercise, these symptoms become more pronounced.

Chills may occur if blood is shunted to major vessels or to areas of greater need. Thermoreceptors in the tissue may be dulled as a result of oxygen deprivation. Elimination patterns may change because of atrophy of the gastrointestinal mucosa.

Medical Diagnosis. The medical diagnosis of anemia is made on the basis of the medical and social history, physical assessment, and laboratory studies of RBC count, RBC indices, Hgb, Hct, and bone marrow. Blood gases may be obtained if the patient exhibits symptoms of anoxia.

Medical Management. Medical management for anemia depends on the cause and may include oxygen therapy, intravenous lines, and blood transfusions, depending on laboratory results. Antipyretic medications are used to reduce fever. Analgesics and joint immobilization are used to reduce pain. Medications such as stool softeners, laxatives, and antidiarrheals may be used according to the patient's needs. Nutritional supplements to provide additional proteins, iron, vitamins, and calories may be used.

Application of the Nursing Process to the Care of the Patient with Anemia

Assessment

Obtain the patient's medical history, and conduct a physical examination. Because fatigue is one of the most common signs of anemia, assess the patient's level of physical activity, ability to perform the usual activities of daily living, and sleep and rest patterns. Check vital signs and observe for shortness of breath on exertion.

Check for signs of bleeding such as bruising, petechiae, and ecchymoses. Assess for bloody urine or tarry stools.

Inspect the mouth, tongue, and gums for redness or pallor, soreness, and ulcers. Observe for disorientation, cyanosis, and pallor in the face, conjunctivae, mouth, and nails caused by decreased hemoglobin levels.

Evaluate hydration by noting skin turgor, weight loss, sunken eyes, and dry skin. Check for pruritus by observing for sign of scratching, redness, lesions, and scabs. Ask the client information about daily food and fluid intake. A dietary deficiency may be the major cause of the anemia.

Assess for abdominal distention, diarrhea, constipation, or flatus, which may be caused by the anemia, drug treatment, or fluid loss. Check for splenomegaly and hepatomegaly, because red blood cell lysis occurs in the spleen and liver.

Assess the patient's level of knowledge about the disorder, treatment, and care needed and instruct accordingly. Allow the patient to ask questions and verbalize concerns. Invite the family to participate when appropriate.

Nursing Diagnoses and Planning

Nursing diagnoses and related expected patient outcomes most commonly applicable to patients with anemia include the following:

NDx: Activity intolerance; fatigue related to decreased oxygen-carrying capacity of the blood

Planning: Patient outcomes

1. Patient follows a regimen of planned activities and rest periods each day.
2. Patient states that he or she is feeling less fatigued and demonstrates signs of increased activity.
3. Patient is able to perform activities of daily living.
4. Patient's vital signs are within normal ranges for the patient.
5. Patient denies shortness of breath on mild exertion.

NDx: Knowledge deficit: nature of the disease, nutritional needs, treatment, and measures to prevent recurrence

Planning: Patient outcomes

1. Patient describes cause, effects, and clinical course of anemia.
2. Patient lists symptoms of anemia and treatments.
3. Patient relates the nutritional therapy for anemia.
4. Patient states the self-care needed to prevent recurrence or complications of anemia.

Nursing Interventions

NDx: Activity intolerance

Instruct the patient to develop a regimen of activity with frequent rest periods throughout the day. Encourage the patient to do range-of-motion exercises frequently while lying in bed to maintain muscle tone and strength. Tell the patient to avoid sudden movements, such as getting out of bed quickly, because this decreases the blood supply to the brain, aggravating vertigo and disorientation. Have the patient practice deep breathing exercises to increase oxygen and blood to the brain.

Teach the patient to practice energy-saving techniques to reduce fatigue and shortness of breath. Place frequently used articles within the patient's reach.

Provide and encourage frequent rest periods while delivering patient care. Prevent interruptions during rest periods and at night, whenever possible. Reduce any disturbing noises and limit visitors as necessary.

Provide warm clothes and blankets to prevent chilling. Avoid unnecessary exposure to drafts or extreme changes in temperature.

Encourage good nutrition to increase the patient's energy level. Offer four to six meals per day. This is less tiring for the patient and prevents gastric overdistention. Ask for consultation with the dietitian.

NDx: Knowledge deficit: nature of the disease, nutritional needs, treatment, and measures to prevent recurrence

Explain the cause, effects, and clinical course of the disorder to the patient. Allow for questions from the patient at any time. Provide appropriate literature about anemia for the patient and family to review. Allow patient to verbalize concerns and fears. Evaluate discharge needs of the patient and family.

Alert the patient to signs and symptoms of anemia, such as fatigue and disorientation from low levels of oxygen. Teach the patient to use safety measures or ask for assistance when out of bed or when ambulating. Stress the need for uninterrupted rest periods and 6 to 10 hours of sleep every night.

Instruct the patient about dietary modifications needed to reduce symptoms or prevent recurrence of the disorder. Explain the need for increases in dietary nutrients specific to the type of anemia present. Initiate counseling with a dietitian to assist with meal planning if needed.

Teach the patient signs of bleeding to observe for and when to seek medical assistance. Explain the need for avoiding sharp objects, straight razors, contact sports, and injections and venipuncture whenever possible (Chart 16–1).

Explain proper oral hygiene methods necessary to prevent further irritation and ulceration of mucous membranes. Instruct the patient to use a soft toothbrush and to use mouthrinse frequently. Show how to inspect the oral cavity, checking the tongue and

Chart 16–1.

NURSING GUIDE TO PATIENT EDUCATION FOR SELF-MANAGEMENT: SELF-CARE FOR A BLEEDING DISORDER

Instruct the patient with a bleeding disorder to:

Exercise caution when using sharp objects.
Brush teeth with a soft toothbrush to prevent gingival irritation.
Use an electric razor rather than a razor blade for shaving.
Observe for signs of bleeding such as bruising, petechiae, and black stools.
Ask for assistance, if needed, to avoid falls.
Avoid contact sports.
Apply direct pressure at the site of active bleeding.
Avoid intramuscular injections.
Take only medications that have been approved by the patient's physician.
Carry identification stating the blood disorder, physician's name and phone number, the patient's blood type, and a significant other to notify in an emergency situation.

gums for early signs of irritation. Teach the patient to avoid extremely hot, spicy foods and acidic drinks to lessen oral and gastrointestinal irritation.

Teach the patient how to achieve comfort by frequent repositioning and padding bony prominences. Show family members how to massage the patient with lotion to promote circulation and prevent skin breakdown. Tell the patient to avoid using heating pads, because thermoreceptors in the tissue may be dulled from oxygen deprivation. Explain the use of a bed cradle to prevent pressure on joints and sensitive areas.

Teach the patient the dosage, route, time, frequency, side effects, and toxic effects of any medication prescribed. Explain the diagnostic studies completed and the need for any follow-up studies after discharge. Include the family in any of the teaching sessions when applicable.

Evaluation

Evaluate the effectiveness of nursing care for a patient with anemia by comparing the patient's status with the expected patient outcomes. Examples of specific outcomes for patients with anemia have been provided in the Planning section.

ANEMIA FROM BLOOD LOSS

Etiology and Pathophysiology. Anemia may result from an acute or chronic blood loss. During massive hemorrhaging, plasma and red blood cells decrease significantly in number and volume. Consequently, oxygen and iron stores in the blood are reduced.

Vasoconstriction occurs with a decrease in the volume of plasma, resulting in the accumulation of red blood cells. The laboratory values may show a falsely high red blood cell count within the first 48 hours post hemorrhage. Normal blood volume is restored by the movement of fluid into the circulating blood from interstitial compartments. The remaining dilute blood is deficient in red blood cells, and thus the oxygen-carrying capacity of the blood is reduced. This stimulates the bone marrow to increase production of red blood cells.

Clinical Manifestations. Clinical manifestations include changes in respirations, dyspnea, vertigo, rapid thready pulse, hypotension, pale skin, headache, restlessness, and disorientation resulting from the lack of oxygen supply to the tissues and major organs of the heart and brain. Bleeding causes the tissues to become edematous, which can be very painful.

Medical Diagnosis. The medical diagnosis is made on the basis of history, physical findings, and laboratory studies. The red blood cell count and hemoglobin and hematrocrit levels may demonstrate falsely high levels within the first 48 hours post hemorrhage before becoming significantly decreased.

Medical Management. Immediate medical management includes replacing the blood that is lost with blood transfusions, administering intravenous fluids to increase the plasma volume, and treating for shock. Sedatives may be ordered if the patient is restless. Complications arise if immediate treatment does not ensue, resulting in death.

Application of the Nursing Process to the Care of the Patient with Anemia from Blood Loss

Assessment

Review the patient's history and medical management. Assess the patient for vital sign changes such as rapid deep respirations, rapid thready pulse, hypotension, and fever, which may indicate continued bleeding or hypovolemia. Assess for changes in consciousness and orientation, skin pallor, and cyanosis. Excessive thirst and diaphoresis may be due to hypovolemia.

Observe for signs of bleeding such as bruising, petechiae, ecchymoses, and edema. Ask the patient about fatigue, urine and stool color changes, and headaches.

Nursing Diagnoses and Planning

Nursing diagnoses and related expected patient outcomes most commonly applicable to patients with anemia from blood loss include those previously described under Anemias and the following:

NDx: Decreased cardiac output related to increased cardiac workload caused by reduced level of red blood cells and hemoglobin from hemorrhage

Planning: Patient outcomes

1. Patient's vital signs and laboratory studies are within normal ranges for the patient.
2. Patient reports decreased fatigue, nonlabored respirations, and increased activity tolerance, all indicative of increased cardiac output without increased workload.

Nursing Interventions

NDx: Decreased cardiac output

Nursing interventions for the patient with anemia from blood loss should focus on replacing fluid loss with intravenous fluids as prescribed. Also offer oral fluids as tolerated. Monitor vital signs and assess circulating fluid volume by arterial or venous pressures, urine output, and signs of overhydration or dehydration. Monitor laboratory studies and observe for signs of continued bleeding.

Since initially the patient may be hypovolemic, look for dry skin, sunken eyes, anuria, and decreased blood pressure. The symptoms vary with the type, location, and rapidity of the blood loss. Also assess for hypervolemia, which may occur after fluid replacement therapy. Look for edema, increasing blood pressure, distention, pulmonary congestion, and scanty urine.

After the patient is stabilized medically, promote a diet of high iron, protein, vitamins, and fluids to replace losses and regain strength (Nutrition Boxes 16–1 and 16–2). Assist the patient in conserving energy to reduce cardiac workload. Keep the patient warm by applying blankets and avoiding cold fluids and drafts.

Additional Interventions

In acute hemorrhagic anemia, continuing blood loss must be arrested. Nursing care focuses on replacing fluids lost and preventing recurrence (Nursing Care Guide 16–1).

Text continued on page 636

Nutrition Box 16–1.

NUTRITION: SPECIAL CONSIDERATIONS FOR PATIENTS WITH IRON DEFICIENCY ANEMIA

Instruct patients with iron deficiency anemia to:

Increase dietary iron intake by eating foods such as meats, fish, and poultry.
Add fortified breads and cereals, dark green vegetables, and fruits such as raisins, prunes, and apricots to the diet.
Take iron supplements with food *only* if intolerable without food. Take iron with orange juice, because it may promote the absorption of iron. Refrain from taking iron supplements with milk or antacids, because they may reduce the absorption of the iron.
Eat some fiber foods to prevent constipation, especially if taking iron supplements along with increased dietary iron. However, because fiber aids in moving food through the intestine quickly, a high-fiber diet may reduce the iron absorption.
Drink an increased amount of fluids daily to prevent constipation.

Nutrition Box 16–2.

FOOD SOURCES FOR HIGH-PROTEIN, HIGH-VITAMIN DIETS

Two food groups contribute large amounts of protein to the daily diet: meat and milk. Examples include:

Food	Serving Size	Approximate Grams of Protein
*Meat Group:**		
Beef	3 oz	21
Ham	3 oz	18
Lamb	3 oz	22
Pork	2 oz	17
Veal	3 oz	23
Chicken	3 oz	26
Duck	3 oz	24
Turkey	3 oz	26
Clams	3 oz	7
Oysters	1 cup	20
Shrimp	3 oz	21
Tuna	3 oz	24
American cheese	1 oz	6
Swiss cheese	1 oz	7
Cottage cheese (2%)	1 cup	31
Peanut butter	2 tbsp	9
Milk Group:		
Whole milk, skim milk, or buttermilk	1 cup	8
Evaporated milk, whole	1 cup	17

Good food sources for high-vitamin diets include:

Vitamin A	Liver Whole milk Butter Cod liver oil Green, leafy vegetables Yellow or orange fruit
Vitamin B complex	Meat Milk Eggs Grains Green vegetables
Vitamin C	Citrus fruits Broccoli Potatoes Tomatoes
Vitamin D	Milk Eggs

*Figures are approximate; vary with cut of meat used.
Adapted from US Department of Agriculture Bulletin: Nutritive Value of Foods, 1986.

Nursing Care Guide 16–1.
PATIENTS WITH ACUTE HEMORRHAGIC ANEMIA

Assessment Findings: Patient experiences restlessness; dyspnea; and rapid, deep respirations followed by shallow respirations. Presence of cyanosis and pallor; clubbing nails; and hypotension.

Nursing Diagnosis: Ineffective breathing pattern related to a reduction in the oxygen-carrying capacity of the blood; a decrease in RBCs

Patient Outcomes	Nursing Interventions	Rationale
Patient exhibits a decrease in labored respirations, signs of cyanosis, and pallor.	Elevate head of bed and maintain the patient in this position as much as possible. Monitor vital signs.	This promotes expanded breathing by pulling diaphragm down and allows for better expansion of the diaphragm.
Patient's chest is fully expanded with respirations maintained between 12 and 16 per minute.	Tell the patient to breathe deeply, slow the respiratory pattern, and try to maintain a steady rate. Instruct patient to avoid gas-forming foods.	A relaxed, deep, full respiratory pattern is more efficient than a shallow, rapid pattern for good oxygen intake and exchange. Some foods produce large amounts of gas, which can lead to abdominal distention, interfering with respirations.
Patient completes activities of daily living without complaints of fatigue.	Plan rest periods throughout day for patient, and provide quiet environment. Place frequently used objects within reach of patient.	Frequent, planned rest periods help conserve strength and reduce oxygen needs.
Patient ambulates at least once every 8 hours for 5 to 15 minutes without respiratory distress.	Encourage ambulation on each shift for 5 to 15 minutes. Monitor blood levels. Administer oxygen as ordered.	Short, frequent periods of ambulation use less energy and oxygen.

Evaluation: Compare the patient's status with the expected patient outcomes. If the outcomes are achieved, evaluate nursing care as successful. If not, reassess the patient, formulate new nursing diagnoses, and revise expected patient outcomes and nursing interventions as appropriate.

(continued)

Nursing Care Guide 16–1. *(continued)*

PATIENTS WITH ACUTE HEMORRHAGIC ANEMIA

Assessment Findings: Patient experiences hypotension; weak, rapid, thready pulse; palpitations; fever; chills; cyanosis and pallor of face, skin, and nails; poor skin turgor; pruritus; and clubbing nails.

Nursing Diagnosis: Fluid volume deficit related to excessive blood loss

Patient Outcomes	Nursing Interventions	Rationale
Patient remains free of fever and exhibits regular strong pulse rate and normal blood pressure.	Check vital signs frequently. Observe skin turgor. Check temperature.	Adequate replacement of fluids may be evident in stability of vital signs and good skin turgor.
Patient maintains adequate blood volume with minimal blood loss as noted by normal results of blood studies.	Administer blood transfusion as ordered. Initiate intravenous therapy. Monitor vital signs and laboratory data.	Fluid replacement reduces the effects of the blood volume deficit.
Patient complies with directions and information given.	Plan rest periods throughout day for patient. Instruct patient to avoid using heating pads. Instruct patient to avoid aspirin products.	Reduced circulation to the peripheral skin surfaces, with low blood volume, may decrease sensations, causing high risk for burns. Aspirin products may increase risk of bleeding, further aggravating blood volume deficit.

Evaluation: Compare the patient's status with the expected patient outcomes. If the outcomes are achieved, evaluate nursing care as successful. If not, reassess the patient, formulate new nursing diagnoses, and revise expected patient outcomes and nursing interventions as appropriate.

Assessment Findings: Patient complains of disorientation, experiencing falls, bruises, extreme hot and cold sensations, vertigo, fever, and headache.

Nursing Diagnosis: High risk for injury related to changes in mental status and sensory perceptions

Patient Outcomes	Nursing Interventions	Rationale
Patient remains alert and oriented to time, place, and person. Patient denies vertigo, headaches, and disorientation.	Orient patient to time, place, and person. Assess patient's alertness. Assist patient when ambulating.	Checking the patient's orientation, reorienting the patient frequently, and assisting the unsure patient may decrease risk for injury due to decreased sensory perceptions.
Patient remains free of injury.	Instruct patient to take deep breaths when moving from supine to sitting position and to sit for a few minutes prior to rising.	Vertigo may be exacerbated by sudden movements such as rising rapidly from a lying position.

(continued)

Nursing Care Guide 16–1. *(continued)*

PATIENTS WITH ACUTE HEMORRHAGIC ANEMIA

Patient Outcomes	Nursing Interventions	Rationale
	Instruct patient to avoid heating pads or extreme cold.	Decreased sensation to skin surfaces may increase risk for burns.

Evaluation: Compare the patient's status with the expected patient outcomes. If the outcomes are achieved, evaluate nursing care as successful. If not, reassess the patient, formulate new nursing diagnoses, and revise expected patient outcomes and nursing interventions as appropriate.

Assessment Findings: Patient complains of nausea and vomiting; red, sore tongue; mouth ulcers; bleeding gums; diarrhea; constipation; abdominal distention; flatus; thirst; poor hydration; and anorexia.

Nursing Diagnosis: Altered nutrition: less than body requirements, related to pain, mouth soreness, and fluid volume deficit

Patient Outcomes	Nursing Interventions	Rationale
Patient's elimination patterns are adequate, without diarrhea or constipation.	Provide bland diet, low in roughage (with diarrhea) or high in roughage (with constipation).	A proper diet is essential to maintain normal intestinal function.
Patient's appetite improves.	Serve patient six to eight small meals per day. Serve foods the patient likes in an attractive manner free from offending odors.	The patient's appetite may improve with foods of choice served in an appealing way.
Patient's mouth remains free of ulcerations.	Offer bland, nonirritating foods	Bland foods may eliminate some of the irritation of the oral mucosa.
Patient states which foods to consume and which to avoid.	Encourage 3000 ml fluid per day. Teach the patient about a nutritious diet, giving examples of meal plans. Administer diet high in proteins, vitamins, and calories. Avoid hot, spicy, and acid foods.	Increased fluids help replace previous losses from diarrhea and increase motility of the intestinal tract. A high-protein, high-vitamin diet with increased calories helps replace deficiencies and prevent further nutritional disorders.
	Provide oral hygiene before and after meals.	Food is more palatable with proper oral hygiene. It also prevents further mouth problems.

Evaluation: Compare the patient's status with the expected patient outcomes. If the outcomes are achieved, evaluate nursing care as successful. If not, reassess the patient, formulate new nursing diagnoses, and revise expected patient outcomes and nursing interventions as appropriate.

(continued)

Nursing Care Guide 16–1. *(continued)*

PATIENTS WITH ACUTE HEMORRHAGIC ANEMIA

Assessment Findings: Patient and family ask questions about the disorder and the needs of the patient.

Nursing Diagnosis: Knowledge deficit: nature of illness, treatment, and prevention

Patient Outcomes	Nursing Interventions	Rationale
Patient verbalizes accurate information about diet, medications, and changes in activities of daily living.	Explain diagnostic tests and treatments to patient to allay anxiety and provide cooperation. Review all medications with patient. Explain dietary changes and provide meal planning guides. Provide information on alterations in activities of daily living to promote adequate rest and relieve fatigue.	The more the patient understands about the disorder and the necessary treatment, the greater the chance for compliance with the prescribed care regimen.
Patient and family express confidence in their ability to cope with the health problems.	Allow time for questions and concerns from the patient and family. Correct any misunderstandings.	Explanation about diet, medications, and changes in lifestyle helps the patient cope with the disorder and eliminates misconceptions about the condition and health care needs.

Evaluation: Compare the patient's status with the expected patient outcomes. If the outcomes are achieved, evaluate nursing care as successful. If not, reassess the patient, formulate new nursing diagnoses, and revise expected patient outcomes and nursing interventions as appropriate.

Evaluation

Evaluate the effectiveness of nursing care for a patient with anemia from blood loss by comparing the patient's status with the expected patient outcomes. Examples of specific outcomes for patients with anemia from blood loss have been provided in the Planning section.

HYPOPROLIFERATIVE ANEMIAS

The hypoproliferative anemias are those that are manifested by a defect in production of red blood cells. This may be caused by lack of iron, vitamin B_{12}, or folic acid; chemical or drug interference; or renal disease.

IRON DEFICIENCY ANEMIA

Etiology and Pathophysiology. Iron deficiency anemia is a depletion of iron stores in the body, resulting in deficient hemoglobin synthesis as a result of impaired absorption, loss, or low intake of iron. The red blood cells are small and pale owing to a hemoglobin deficit. This anemia is the most prevalent type. It occurs most frequently in women between 15 and 45 years of age as a result of blood loss during menstruation. Pregnant women and children are the most vulnerable to iron deficiency anemia owing to increased need for iron and poor dietary supply.

Inadequate iron absorption may also occur in

chronic diarrhea states, in malabsorption syndromes, with a low intake of foods containing iron, and following a gastrectomy.

Excessive blood loss due to trauma, excessive menses, gastrointestinal bleeding, or blood donation can also result in iron depletion in the body.

Clinical Manifestations. Clinical manifestations include fatigue and weakness resulting from decreased oxygen supply from hemoglobin deficit. In severe cases of iron deficiency anemia, palpitations, vertigo, sensitivity to cold, brittle hair and nails, clubbing of the nails (spoon nails characterized by concave curves), dysphagia, mouth ulcerations, and inflamed but smooth red tongue may be evident.

Medical Diagnosis. The medical diagnosis of iron deficiency anemia is made on the basis of the patient's nutritional assessment, social history, and laboratory findings. Diagnostic laboratory tests would include bone marrow examination, platelet count, serum iron, total iron-binding capacity, red blood cell count, red blood cell indices, and hemoglobin level to detect defective red blood cell production and hemoglobin deficiency. A stained red cell examination is used to detect abnormally small red blood cells indicative of iron deficiency anemia.

Medical Management. Medical management includes ferrous sulfate or ferrous gluconate, initially administered orally with food to decrease gastric irritation. After the patient develops a tolerance to the iron, it should be taken between meals. Iron is best absorbed on an empty stomach. Undiluted liquid preparations of iron salts are given through a straw to prevent staining of teeth and gums. Encouraging good oral hygiene is necessary. Ferrous salts may be given with orange juice to promote absorption of the iron. Oral iron preparations are taken for as long as 2 to 3 months after the hemoglobin returns to normal. Iron may also be administered as an injection, called iron dextran.

Application of the Nursing Process to the Care of the Patient with Iron Deficiency Anemia

Assessment

Obtain a social and diet history from the patient to evaluate the environmental and nutritional status. Review the medical history. Ask for a detailed typical daily diet plan. Note whether any of the foods on the list are high in iron. Ask whether the patient takes any dietary supplements.

Look for signs of general malaise, dyspnea, weakness, or vertigo, because the decreased oxygen level may precipitate these symptoms. Inquire about the patient's ability to perform activities of daily living.

Inquire about sensitivity to cold. Look for pallor, nail clubbing, and cyanosis. Assess vital signs and any laboratory studies completed.

Check specifically for mouth irritation and ulceration. Review the patient's oral hygiene practices. Inquire about changes in the diet that were necessitated by the mouth problems, if any.

Nursing Diagnoses and Planning

Nursing diagnoses and related expected patient outcomes most commonly applicable to patients with iron deficiency anemia include those previously described under Anemias and the following:

NDx: Altered nutrition, less than body requirements related to inability to provide for, or lack of knowledge about, needed dietary planning or to mucous membrane soreness and irritation

Planning: Patient Outcomes

1. Patient chooses foods appropriate to replace dietary deficiencies as presented in Nutrition Boxes 16–1 and 16–2.
2. Patient avoids irritating foods and fluids.

Nursing Interventions

NDx: Altered nutrition, less than body requirements

Help the patient maintain adequate nutrition by providing an attractive meal in a pleasant atmosphere. Encourage the patient to eat foods high in iron, protein, and vitamins, such as red meat, liver, oysters, egg yolks, green leafy vegetables, carrots, whole wheat bread, dried fruits, raisins, and molasses. If these foods are taken with vitamin C, absorption will be enhanced. Provide six to eight small meals to prevent distention and reduce fatigue.

Instruct the patient to avoid foods that are gas-forming, because they cause abdominal distention, which may decrease the appetite and also interfere with respiratory efforts. Provide a diet low in roughage. Avoid hot, spicy foods and acidic fluids to decrease gastrointestinal irritation. Encourage increased fluid intake to prevent constipation and promote adequate hydration. Monitor the patient's intake and output.

If the patient is taking iron injections in addition to using specific dietary alterations to increase iron stores, observe and report any adverse reactions, such as pain at injection site, headache, urticaria, and changes in vital signs. If the patient is taking oral iron supplements, instruct the patient to take iron on an empty stomach or with orange juice to enhance absorption (Pharmacology Box 16–1).

Review the cause, symptoms, nutritional implications, treatment, and prevention of iron deficiency with the patient and family. Allow time for ques-

Pharmacology Box 16–1.

HEMATINICS

Hematinics:
Iron salts used for replacement therapy in iron deficiency anemias. Available in oral, parenteral, and intravenous preparations.

Oral iron preparations:	Ferrous sulfate
	Ferrous fumarate
	Ferrous gluconate
Parenteral intravenous iron:	Iron dextran

Action:
Absorbed in the proximal portion of the small intestine. Important in the synthesis of hemoglobin.

Uses:
Replaces or supplements iron stores, which may be low as a result of blood loss, poor diet, pregnancy, or lactation.

Side Effects:
Nausea, constipation, diarrhea, and anorexia. May stain mouth and teeth or color stools dark green or black. If given intramuscularly, pain at injection site, skin staining. If given intravenously, fever, rash, and local phlebitis.

Interactions:
Decreased absorption of tetracycline or penicillamine. Vitamin E may interfere with the effect of the iron therapy.

Nursing Implications:
Dilute liquid preparations in water or orange juice; use a straw with liquid iron preparations to avoid staining teeth.
Take oral iron tablets with orange juice to promote absorption.
Avoid giving iron with food because it slows absorption.
Check patient for constipation, nausea, and diarrhea.
Tell patient that iron supplements may turn stool black.
Do not give more than 2 ml in one intramuscular site because it may be painful or cause hematomas.
Use Z-track injection method.
After intravenous administration of iron, flush vein with saline solution.
Instruct patient not to take oral iron preparations with milk or antacids because they may reduce the absorption rate of the iron.

Geriatric Considerations:
Because iron preparations can be constipating, especially in the older adult, tell the patient to include more bulk in the diet and drink increased amounts of fluids.

tions and verbalization of concerns and misunderstandings.

Evaluation

Evaluate the effectiveness of nursing care for a patient with iron deficiency anemia by comparing the patient's status with the expected patient outcomes. Examples of specific outcomes for patients with iron deficiency anemia have been provided in the Planning section.

PERNICIOUS ANEMIA

Etiology and Pathophysiology. Pernicious anemia is caused by impaired vitamin B_{12} absorption through the small intestine as a result of deficiency of the intrinsic factor, which results from gastric fundus atrophy. Vitamin B_{12} deficiency alters the synthesis of DNA, resulting in defective red blood cells, white blood cells, and platelets.

Only 0.1% of the population develops pernicious anemia. It is found primarily in individuals older than 50 who have a family history of the disorder, and most commonly occurs in blue-eyed Scandinavians.

Clinical Manifestations. Clinical manifestations include changes in activity and strength resulting from decreased oxygen in the blood caused by red blood cell reduction. Jaundice may be present as a result of rupture of large red blood cells in the blood and bone marrow.

Gastrointestinal disturbances and changes in elimination patterns occur because of atrophy of the glandular mucosa of the fundus, resulting in decreased hydrochloric acid secretion. Gastrointestinal bleeding or obstruction from tumors may be present. The incidence of gastric carcinoma and benign gastric polyps is high in patients with pernicious anemia. Papillary atrophy and inflammation of the oral mucous membranes may occur.

Neurologic disturbances may be present from impaired vitamin B_{12} absorption and DNA synthesis and defective red blood cells, white blood cells, and platelets. Hypokalemia may result from initial vitamin B_{12} therapy. Patients are very sensitive to temperature changes and to pain from neurologic changes.

Medical Diagnosis. The medical diagnosis of pernicious anemia is made on the basis of medical and social history, physical assessment, and laboratory findings. Laboratory studies include red blood cell count, stained red cell examination, red blood cell indices, hemoglobin count, white blood cell count, platelet count, glucose-6-phosphate dehydrogenase (G6PD) level, serum iron level, lactate dehydrogenase level, bone marrow examination, bilirubin count, and gastric fluid analysis. A Schilling test is done to differentiate between dietary vitamin B_{12} deficiency and vitamin B_{12} malabsorption.

Medical Management. Medical management includes parenteral vitamin B_{12} therapy, which must be continued for life. It is imperative that the individual continue therapy even when asymptomatic.

Injections of vitamin B_{12} are initially administered daily and tapered to monthly. Most symptoms recede with treatment; however, any spinal cord or brain damage is usually permanent. If the individual continues with adequate treatment for life, anemia does not recur.

Oral iron supplements may be ordered in addition to folic acid. Blood transfusions may be necessary in severe cases.

Diagnostic tests are done to determine the presence of gastrointestinal polyps and carcinoma, because there is a high correlation between these disorders and pernicious anemia.

Delayed treatment in the elderly can result in congestive heart failure and angina. Without treatment, death occurs.

Application of the Nursing Process to the Care of the Patient with Pernicious Anemia

Assessment

Review medical history and complete a nutritional history. Strict vegetarians may suffer from a diet-based vitamin B_{12} deficiency.

Observe for changes in oral mucous membranes; red, smooth tongue, sore mouth, anorexia, and weight loss, indicating disturbances in the gastrointestinal tract. Assess for nausea and vomiting and restlessness, which may indicate gastric bleeding or obstruction from a tumor. Observe for constipation and diarrhea due to atrophy of the gastrointestinal mucosa.

Note any neurologic disturbances, including sensitivity to heat and pain, tingling, numbness of hands and feet, symptoms of gout, ataxia, vision changes, irritability, depression, and psychotic behavior caused by degeneration of the spinal cord and peripheral nerves.

Assess for clinical manifestations of diminished oxygen in the blood as evidenced by dyspnea, weakness, fatigue, palpitations, and pallor. Assess skin color for jaundice resulting from hemolysis.

Identify the patient's knowledge level regarding pernicious anemia and vitamin B_{12} treatment. During initial vitamin B_{12} therapy, observe for signs of hypokalemia as evidenced by muscle weakness, apathy, abdominal distention, paralytic ileus, anorexia, nausea, vomiting, thirst, arrhythmias, diminished tendon reflexes, and mental depression. Observe for signs of anxiety such as inability to follow instructions, crying, trembling, hyperventilation, tachycardia, and cold perspiration.

Nursing Diagnoses and Planning

Nursing diagnoses and related expected patient outcomes most commonly applicable to patients with pernicious anemia include those previously described under Anemias and the following:

NDx: Constipation or diarrhea related to changes in the gastrointestinal mucosa

Planning: Patient outcomes

1. Patient reports normal stool consistency without diarrhea or constipation.
2. Patient eats foods that promote adequate bowel elimination.
3. Patient eats small, frequent meals to prevent digestive problems.
4. Patient drinks adequate fluids to promote proper elimination.

NDx: Knowledge deficit: nature of disease, diet, and use of prescribed medications

Planning: Patient outcomes

1. Patient states accurate information about relationship of vitamin B_{12} to symptoms of disorder.
2. Patient states dose, time, frequency, side effects, and toxic effects of prescribed medications.

Nursing Interventions

NDx: Constipation or diarrhea

Help the patient maintain adequate bowel elimination. Encourage intake of eight glasses of water or other nonirritating fluids daily. Promote frequent moderate exercise and at least 8 hours of sleep per night.

Instruct the patient regarding a balanced diet high in protein, vitamins, and iron, including foods such as fish, red meat, milk, and eggs, to increase intake of vitamin B_{12}. Provide six to eight small meals, if tolerated, to conserve energy and decrease gastrointestinal distress.

Monitor the patient's bowel movements, noting the color, consistency, and amount. Provide stool softeners or antidiarrheal agents as prescribed.

NDx: Knowledge deficit: nature of disease, diet, and use of prescribed medications

Help the patient attain knowledge regarding the disorder by explaining signs, symptoms, causes, and lifelong treatment necessary to prevent complications. Discuss the complications with the patient and family. Explain the signs of hypokalemia and when to seek medical intervention.

Encourage the patient and family to ask questions and express their concerns. Teach the patient about prescribed medications, including the dose, route, time, frequency, side effects, and toxic effects. Encourage the patient to continue with follow-up physician's office visits at least twice per year.

Help the patient decrease stress levels so that coping mechanisms can be effective. Explain that irritability and depression are part of the disease process. Allow the patient and family to express feelings and concerns about lifelong therapy. Encourage relaxation exercises with deep, diaphragmatic breathing.

Evaluation

Evaluate the effectiveness of nursing care for a patient with pernicious anemia by comparing the patient's status with the expected patient outcomes. Examples of specific outcomes for patients with pernicious anemia have been provided in the Planning section.

FOLIC ACID DEFICIENCY

Etiology and Pathophysiology. A deficiency in folic acid results in defective red blood cell production. Folic acid deficiency is an extremely common disorder with an insidious onset. Increased metabolic needs, chronic malnourishment, and intestinal malabsorption can lead to folic acid deficiency.

Ingestion of anticonvulsants, antimetabolites, and certain oral contraceptives can impede the absorption of folic acid. Alcoholics often manifest a deficiency of folic acid, because alcohol interferes with red blood cell production.

Alcoholics and the elderly living alone are more prone to develop folic acid deficiency as a result of dietary deficiencies and ingestion impairment. Folic acid deficiency may also develop in patients on prolonged intravenous feeding or hyperalimentation unless folic acid is given intramuscularly.

Clinical Manifestations. Clinical manifestations of folic acid deficiency are similar to those of pernicious anemia. Symptoms include those associated with anemia combined with gastrointestinal disturbances and a beefy, red tongue. Absence of neurologic symptoms is important in differentiating folic acid deficiency from pernicious anemia.

Medical Diagnosis. The medical diagnosis of folic acid deficiency is made on the basis of history of dietary intake and laboratory studies of red blood cell count and red blood cell indices, serum folic acid level, and bone marrow examination.

Medical Management. Daily oral doses of folic acid are prescribed. Parenteral doses are ordered if the patient has a malabsorption syndrome. Vitamin C may be ordered with folic acid to promote erythropoiesis.

Guidelines for Application of the Nursing Process to the Care of the Patient with Folic Acid Deficiency

Review the patient's history and medical management. Assess for smooth, reddened tongue, chills, and gastrointestinal disturbances. Note any fatigue, dyspnea, and weakness from oxygen deprivation. Check vital signs, auscultate the chest, and note any cardiac arrhythmias.

Ask about the patient's typical daily food intake. Look for dietary deficiencies. Monitor intake and output. Ask whether the patient is taking any anticonvulsants, antimetabolites, or oral contraceptives. Question the patient about alcohol ingestion.

The nursing diagnoses, expected patient outcomes, nursing interventions, and evaluation for patients with a folic acid deficiency include those described previously under Anemias. The following additional interventions also apply to the care of patients with a folic acid deficiency. Help the patient achieve a balanced diet. Promote foods high in calories, proteins, and vitamins based on the patient's food preferences (see Nutrition Box 16–2). Encourage the patient to eat foods high in folic acid, such as green and yellow vegetables, liver, citrus fruits, whole grains, yeast, and legumes. Discourage alcohol consumption. Provide six to eight small meals per day. Teach the patient good oral hygiene techniques to prevent mouth problems.

Maintain activity as tolerated. Use special safety measures if weakness is present. Provide periods of rest between activities. Keep the patient warm and comfortable, free from chilling and drafts. Teach the patient and family the importance of treatment and prevention of recurrence of the disorder.

APLASTIC ANEMIA

Etiology and Pathophysiology. Aplastic anemia is a deficiency of circulating red blood cells, thus indicating an impairment of red blood cell development within the bone marrow. Bone marrow failure may also result in concurrent agranulocytosis and thrombocytopenia. When all three conditions exist simultaneously, pancytopenia or deficiency of all blood elements results.

The onset of aplastic anemia may be insidious, as in hereditary cases, or rapid, when bone marrow failure occurs following myelotoxic drug therapy. A tumor of the thymus is also associated with this disorder.

The cause of aplastic anemia is unknown in half of all affected individuals. More than 50% of individuals with pancytopenia die from hemorrhage or infection. Death occurs within a few months after the onset of anemia. Twenty-five percent of the 40% to 50% who survive die by the end of the third year after onset. The remaining 25% either completely recover or remain invalids for years.

Clinical Manifestations. Clinical manifestations include decreased red blood cell and white blood cell counts with the presence of decreased platelets (thrombocytopenia). Infections and hemorrhage may result from pancytopenia and bone marrow failure. Prevalent symptoms include progressive weakness, fatigue, headache, dyspnea, hemorrhaging, and infections.

Medical Diagnosis. The medical diagnosis of aplastic anemia is made on the basis of history, physical assessment, and laboratory findings. Laboratory studies include white blood cell count, especially granulocytes, red blood cell count, platelet count, and bone marrow examination. Tests are used to confirm whether the patient has been exposed to myelotoxic drugs. Prior use of myelotoxic drugs such as antitumor agents, antimetabolites, antimicrobials, anticonvulsants, antithyroid drugs, antidiabetic agents, antihistamines, analgesics, sedatives, and insecticides can predispose an individual to aplastic anemia.

Medical Management. Medical management includes transfusions of red blood cells and platelets, which may prevent symptoms from recurring. It is important to note that repeated transfusions may result in increased iron in the tissues and splenomegaly.

When patients are receiving myelotoxic drugs, blood cell counts are monitored to evaluate bone marrow function.

Bone marrow transplants and a splenectomy may be indicated. Care of the patient undergoing a bone marrow transplant is discussed in Chapter 9, and care of the patient undergoing a splenectomy is discussed in Chapter 15.

Application of the Nursing Process to the Care of the Patient with Aplastic Anemia

Assessment

Review the medical history for cause of the anemia, such as drug-induced aplastic anemia, and conduct a physical examination. Note any dyspnea on exertion, fever, sore throat, pallor, weakness, and anorexia indicative of a respiratory infection. Assess for pain and burning on urination, which may indicate the presence of a urinary tract infection. Note the patient's urinary output for color, consistency, and amount.

Assess for abnormal bleeding, wounds, and abrasions. Look for irritation or ulcers of the mucous membranes, which could be potential sites of infection.

Review the patient's nutritional intake. Check for recent weight loss. Observe the oral cavity for lesions, because mouth soreness may affect the patient's ability to eat well. Note the patient's bowel movements, checking for regularity and absence of constipation. Check for irritation or bleeding from hemorrhoids. Palpate for splenomegaly.

Allow the patient and family time to voice their concerns and fears about the disorder and treatment. Help the patient find appropriate coping mechanisms.

Nursing Diagnoses and Planning

Nursing diagnoses and related expected patient outcomes most commonly applicable to patients with aplastic anemia include those previously described under Anemias and the following:

NDx: Anxiety related to poor prognosis, fear of death, or vulnerability to complications and prolonged therapy

Planning: Patient outcomes
1. Patient relates concerns about illness to the nurse or other appropriate member of the health care team.
2. Patient and family verbalize accurate information about the disorder, complications, and therapy.
3. Patient expresses feelings of reduced anxiety and fear.
4. Patient displays physical signs of decreased anxiety; vital signs are within normal ranges, and patient is resting well, appears calm, and eats well.

NDx: High risk for infection related to decreased body defenses against microorganisms

Planning: Patient outcomes
1. Patient's vital signs are within normal ranges for the patient.
2. Patient's laboratory studies are within normal ranges for the patient.
3. Patient denies chills, sore throat, cough, shortness of breath, anorexia, or pain or burning on urination.

NDx: Knowledge deficit: nature of disease and prevention of complications

Planning: Patient outcomes
1. Patient states accurate information about the nature of the disease.
2. Patient verbalizes the complications of aplastic anemia, such as bleeding, infection, and poor nutrition, and notes the signs and symptoms of each.
3. Patient relates strategies to avoid complications of the disease.
4. Patient states when it is appropriate to seek medical attention after observing signs of a complication of the disorder.

Nursing Interventions

NDx: Anxiety

Allow patient to verbalize concerns about the disease, its effects on the patient and family, and fears about death. Help the patient and family find coping strategies that are effective to deal with their anxiety level. Allow time for questions from the patient and the family.

Seek assistance from clergy or other professional counselors when appropriate. Make referrals as needed to social service agencies.

NDx: High risk for infection

Keep the patient warm, and avoid extreme changes in temperature in the room. Restrict visitors to prevent exposure to infections. Use protective isolation if appropriate.

Monitor the patient's vital signs frequently, observing subtle changes that may indicate early signs of infection. Report any changes noted.

Promote good nutrition by serving meals in a relaxed, attractive atmosphere. Encourage a high-protein, high-vitamin diet. Provide oral hygiene frequently to prevent infection and promote better eating habits.

NDx: Knowledge deficit: nature of the disease and prevention of complications

Explain the causes, complications, treatment, and prevention of aplastic anemia to the patient and family. Allow the patient to ventilate feelings and ask questions regarding the information presented. Give the patient and family literature about aplastic anemia when appropriate. Use terminology that the patient can comprehend.

Teach the patient signs of bleeding to observe for and when to seek medical assistance. Explain the need for avoiding sharp objects, straight razors, contact sports, and injections and venipuncture whenever possible (see Chart 16–1).

Explain proper oral hygiene methods necessary to prevent further irritation and ulceration of mucous membranes. Instruct the patient to use a soft toothbrush and to use mouthrinse frequently. Show how to inspect the oral cavity, checking the tongue and gums for early signs of irritation. Teach the patient to avoid extremely hot, spicy foods and acidic drinks to lessen oral and gastrointestinal irritation.

Teach the patient to avoid constipation, because hard stools and straining can damage the rectal mucosa and cause bleeding. Obtain an order for a stool softener or laxative when needed.

Help the patient understand the signs of infection and how to prevent them. Tell the patient to stay warm and dry, avoiding extreme changes in temperature. Encourage a diet high in protein and vitamins. Assist with oral care as needed to prevent mucous membrane breakdown, which would increase the potential for infection. Tell family members to avoid contact with the patient when they have colds or other active infections.

Evaluation

Evaluate the effectiveness of nursing care for a patient with aplastic anemia by comparing the patient's status with the expected patient outcomes. Examples of specific outcomes for patients with aplastic anemia have been provided in the Planning section.

HEMOLYTIC ANEMIAS

The hemolytic anemias result from a shortened red blood cell life span caused by intrinsic or extrinsic factors. The hemolysis of red blood cells in these disorders occurs more rapidly than erythropoiesis. If the erythrocyte life span is less than 20 days, a hemolytic anemia is usually present.

HEREDITARY SPHEROCYTOSIS

Etiology and Pathophysiology. Spherocytosis is characterized by small, sphere-shaped red blood cells that swell from the accumulation of sodium and water. These spheres are rigid, thick, and easily destroyed. Spherocytosis is found in all populations and is inherited as a dominant trait.

Clinical Manifestations. Clinical manifestations include anemia, painful splenomegaly, and jaundice resulting from red cell hemolysis in the spleen and large amounts of bilirubin in the blood. Gallstones are present from the increased level of bilirubin. Infections or chemical exposures may also cause hemolysis.

Medical Diagnosis. The medical diagnosis of spherocytosis is made on the basis of the familial history, the presence of spherocytes in a blood smear, lowered red blood cell count and hemoglobin level, and elevated osmotic fragility.

Medical Management. Medical management involves blood transfusions and a splenectomy. The majority of patients undergoing a splenectomy are free from symptoms but are not completely cured. (Care of the patient with blood transfusions and splenectomy is discussed in Chapter 15.)

Guidelines for Application of the Nursing Process to the Care of the Patient with Hereditary Spherocytosis

Review the medical history and complete a physical assessment of the patient. Observe for jaundice, which will be apparent first in the sclerae and then the mucous membranes, followed by generalized distribution. Check the patient for left upper quadrant fullness and abdominal pain indicating splenomegaly.

Ask the patient about complaints of generalized malaise, weakness, and inability to complete routine daily activities. Look for signs of infection such as fever, cough, dyspnea, fatigue, and chills. Assess the patient's vital signs.

Note the color, consistency, and amount of urine output. Check the skin for dryness, pruritus, and breakdown.

The nursing diagnoses, expected patient outcomes, nursing interventions, and evaluation for patients with hereditary spherocytosis include those described previously under Anemias. The following additional interventions also apply to the care of patients with hereditary spherocytosis. Monitor the patient's vital signs and laboratory studies. Nursing care includes the administration of blood transfusions and pre- and postoperative care if the patient undergoes a splenectomy. Make referrals for genetic counseling if patient is planning to have children.

SICKLE CELL ANEMIA

Etiology and Pathophysiology. Sickle cell anemia is a chronic hereditary hemolytic disorder characterized by an abnormal hemoglobin S. Instead of hemoglobin A in the blood, these abnormal red blood cells become crescent- or sickle-shaped (Fig. 16–1) in the presence of decreased oxygen content in the blood. The elongated, rigid cells become lodged in small vessels, thus slowing or blocking peripheral blood flow or organ perfusion. The accumulation of damaged cells also causes the blood to become more viscous, which further decreases blood flow.

High stress levels, caused by factors including work, exercise, anorexia, and pregnancy, may precipitate a sickle cell crisis. Sickle cell symptoms may also be precipitated by exposure to low oxygen tensions, which occurs in mountain climbing or flying in a nonpressurized aircraft.

Sickle cell anemia primarily affects Africans and black Americans and, to a lesser degree, Mediterra-

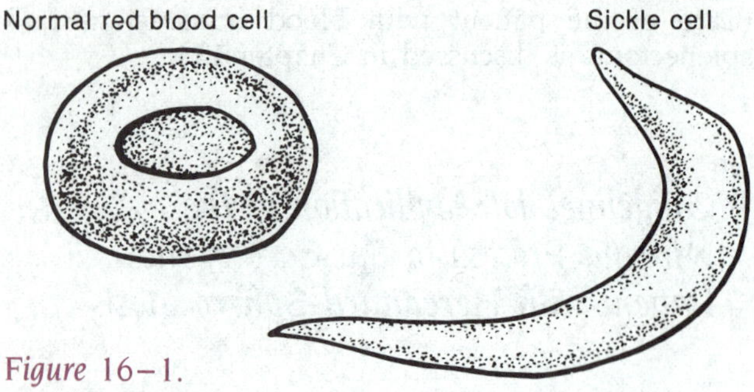

Figure 16–1.

Drawing of normal cell and deoxygenated sickle cell.

neans and Arabs. Sickle cell trait occurs in approximately 8% of blacks in the United States and is present in those who are heterozygous for sickle cell hemoglobin. These individuals usually have no symptoms. Figure 16–2 illustrates the probabilities of children inheriting sickle cell anemia and sickle cell trait from parents heterozygous for hemoglobin S. Individuals with sickle cell trait have approximately 25% to 40% hemoglobin S, whereas individuals who are homozygous for hemoglobin S or those with sickle cell anemia have approximately 80% to 100% hemoglobin S.

Clinical Manifestations. Clinical manifestations include tachycardia, cardiomegaly, fatigue, dyspnea, joint pain, and ischemic leg ulcers. Painful leg ulcers develop from sickled cells blocking blood vessels, resulting in peripheral anoxia. As anoxia increases, thrombosis and infarction develop, resulting in tissue necrosis. Tenderness and enlargement of the liver, spleen, and penis occur from the pooling of sickled red blood cells causing the blood to thicken. It is common for male patients to experience a sudden, painful, persistent penile erection.

The most vulnerable organs are the brain, kidney, heart, lung, skin, bone marrow, and spleen. The gallbladder may also be affected, as demonstrated by tenderness and pain from elevated bilirubin levels and gallstones.

Sickled cells in the pulmonary circulation may result in pulmonary congestion and infection. A decrease in arterial oxygen from sickling cells results in tachycardia and decreased cardiac output. Cardiac dysrhythmias may occur. Joint pain and limited movement are present because of occlusion of the circulatory system. Kidneys have a decreased ability to concentrate urine owing to obstruction of the glomerular capillaries.

Changes in vision or eye pain occur as a result of sickled cells trapped in blood vessels of the eye. Osteoporosis may develop from the rapid growth of bone marrow. The femoral head or vertebra may collapse, leading to compression and deformities.

Medical Diagnosis. The medical diagnosis of sickle cell anemia is made on the basis of the history, physical assessment, and laboratory findings. The laboratory tests include a red blood cell count, stained blood smear, Sickledex test to detect sickle cell hemoglobin, and a hemoglobin electrophoresis test to distinguish sickle cell anemia from sickle cell trait.

Medical Management. Medical management may include surgery to treat gallstones and fractures, antibiotics for infections, transfusions of packed red blood cells to treat anemia, antipyretics to reduce fever, IV fluids to maintain hydration, and localized heat and analgesics to promote joint comfort. Skin grafts may be needed to treat leg ulcers. The primary goal is to prevent complications of cerebral hemorrhage, shock, and uremia leading to renal failure and even death.

Individuals with the disease or trait are offered genetic counseling to help them decide whether or not to have children. All siblings of individuals with sickle cell anemia should be screened for the disorder. Life span is usually approximately 60 years, depending on the frequency of complications.

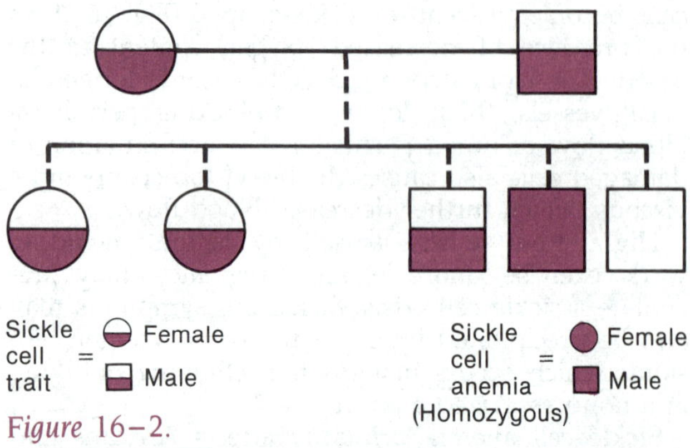

Figure 16–2.

Example of sickle cell anemia heredity from male and female who are heterozygous for hemoglobin S.

Application of the Nursing Process to the Care of the Patient with Sickle Cell Anemia

Assessment

Review the medical history, and complete a physical assessment of the patient. Assess for chest pain, dyspnea, fever, cough, tachypnea, use of accessory muscles, and splinting, which may be indicative of pulmonary congestion and infection. Check for headache, nausea, and confusion.

Observe for jaundice, pallor, and dry skin. Assess for excessive thirst, poor skin turgor, diarrhea, and fatigue, which are indicative of dehydration. Palpate the liver and spleen for tenderness and enlargement.

Assess the level of hydration and urine output to determine renal function. Large amounts of urine may be expected initially owing to interference in renal concentration.

Observe for high stress levels, anorexia, and malaise, which could aggravate a sickling crisis. Assess for changes in vision or eye pain caused from accumulation of sickled cells in the blood vessels of the eye.

Assess for pain in the extremities and reddened, warm or inflamed skin resulting from inadequate circulation and infection. Assess for ulcers in the lower extremities, a common complication caused by impaired circulation. Check all peripheral pulses.

Assess the patient for joint pain, especially in the knees and elbows, due to circulatory occlusion from the sickling. Monitor pain location, duration, and type. Observe the patient's activities. Look for limited movements and inability to move freely or to ambulate without assistance. Pain in weight-bearing bones may be indicative of osteoporosis. Look for signs of guarding or facial grimacing during ambulation.

Nursing Diagnoses and Planning

Nursing diagnoses and related expected patient outcomes most commonly applicable to patients with sickle cell anemia include those previously described under Anemias and the following:

NDx: Pain related to venous stasis and occlusion from sickled cells

Planning: Patient outcomes
1. Patient states there is relief of pain.
2. Patient gradually moves freely without groaning, guarding, or grimacing.
3. Patient completes activities of daily living without interference from severe joint pain.

NDx: Altered tissue perfusion, cardiopulmonary, cerebral, and peripheral, related to decreased arterial oxygen saturation from sickled cells and decreased cardiac output from increased workload

Planning: Patient outcomes
1. Patient's extremities are warm, color is adequate, and pulses are present.
2. Patient's laboratory studies are within normal ranges for the patient.
3. Patient denies headaches, confusion, or nausea.
4. Patient is able to perform activities of daily living without tachypnea, tachycardia, and dyspnea.

NDx: High risk for infection related to increased susceptibility from the systemic effects of the disease

Planning: Patient outcomes
1. Patient's vital signs are within normal ranges for the patient.
2. Patient's laboratory studies are within normal ranges for the patient.
3. Patient denies chills, sore throat, cough, shortness of breath, anorexia, or pain or burning on urination.
4. Patient denies pain in joints and legs (long bones).

Nursing Interventions

NDx: Pain

Help the patient experience minimal joint pain by using pillows to support joints and bony prominences. Reposition the patient frequently. Bed rest may be required to decrease pain, so use passive and active range-of-motion exercises to keep muscles in tone and to retain flexibility. Cleanse and dress leg ulcers carefully. Use a bed cradle to keep the bed linen off the painful area. Give analgesics as prescribed. Remove constricting clothing.

NDx: Altered tissue perfusion, cardiopulmonary, cerebral, and peripheral

Help the patient conserve oxygen needs by encouraging rest and limiting activities. Assist the patient with meals, if needed. Encourage increased intake of fluid to decrease blood viscosity and prevent dehydration. Elevate the head of the bed to aid in chest expansion. Initiate oxygen therapy, if needed.

Keep the patient in a comfortable position and reposition frequently to release pressure. Utilize range-of-motion exercises to stimulate circulation. Monitor vital signs and laboratory studies to assess for changes and improvements in status. Encourage ambulation as tolerated, but provide for frequent rest periods to decrease cardiac workload. Assist the patient when ambulating, because decreased cerebral circulation may cause disorientation and vertigo.

Discourage smoking to avoid vasoconstriction. Remove constricting clothing and keep heavy bed linen from restricting peripheral circulation. Keep the patient's legs in a nondependent position when not ambulating

NDx: High risk for infection

Reposition the patient frequently to stimulate circulation. Tell the patient to cough and take deep breaths, using maximum chest expansion. Monitor the patient's vital signs frequently, observing subtle changes that may indicate early signs of infection. Report any changes noted. Watch for an increasing white blood count on laboratory data.

Culture any wounds on legs. Look for signs of purulent drainage. Use aseptic dressing changes (Chart 16–2).

Promote good nutrition by serving the meals in a relaxed attractive atmosphere. Encourage a high-protein, high-vitamin diet (see Nutrition Box 16–2). Provide oral hygiene frequently to prevent infection and promote better eating habits. Encourage increased fluid intake.

Keep the patient warm, and avoid extreme changes in temperature in the room. Restrict visitors to prevent exposure to infections. Use protective isolation if appropriate.

Chart 16–2.

NURSING GUIDE TO PATIENT EDUCATION FOR SELF-MANAGEMENT: SELF-CARE FOR ULCERS RESULTING FROM SICKLE CELL CRISIS

Instruct the patient with leg ulcers resulting from sickle cell complications to:

Utilize aseptic dressing changes to prevent infection.
Use gloves when handling dressings.
Remove dressings carefully to prevent further trauma.
Apply precribed medications to legs prior to reapplying dressings.
Dispose of dressings in separate plastic bag.
Do not rewrap dressings tight. Check feet for circulation by observing color and temperature.
Do not exercise legs if swollen or if ulcerations are severe.
Rest legs in nondependent position.

Evaluation

Evaluate the effectiveness of nursing care for a patient with sickle cell anemia by comparing the patient's status with the expected patient outcomes. Examples of specific outcomes for patients with sickle cell anemia have been provided in the Planning section.

THALASSEMIA

Etiology and Pathophysiology. Thalassemia is an inherited, chronic hemolytic anemia predominantly affecting individuals with Greek, Italian, and Southern Chinese ancestry. This anemia is characterized by thin, fragile red blood cells known as target cells. Thalassemia minor is a mild anemia and occurs in heterozygotes, whereas thalassemia major or Cooley's anemia is more severe and occurs in homozygotes.

Clinical Manifestations. Clinical manifestations include a mongoloid appearance caused by thickening of the bone marrow activity resulting in thickening of the cranial bones. Cholelithiasis, splenomegaly, and jaundice are present as a result of hemolysis of abnormal cells. Leg ulcers may also be present. Cardiomegaly and fatigue result from increased cardiac workload.

Medical Diagnosis. The medical diagnosis of thalassemia is made on the basis of history, physical assessment, and laboratory studies, including red blood cell count, serum bilirubin, fecal and urinary urobilinogen, and hemoglobin studies.

Medical Management. Medical management involves semimonthly, monthly, or bimonthly blood transfusions of packed red blood cells. Complications may occur from excessive blood transfusions. These include cardiac dysrhythmias and elevated iron levels. They are treated with antiarrhythmics and chelating agents, respectively. A splenectomy may be necessary if the spleen is destroying the transfused cells. Life expectancy is very poor for individuals with thalassemia major. Genetic counseling is encouraged.

Application of the Nursing Process to the Care of the Patient with Thalassemia

The assessment, nursing diagnoses, expected patient outcomes, nursing interventions, and evaluation for patients with thalassemia are similar to those described previously for patients with other anemias. In addition, because patients with thalassemia undergo marked changes in appearance and lifestyle, nursing care includes offering the patient and family support throughout the course of the disease. Help them find coping strategies to deal with the changes in appearance and lifestyle. Make referrals for additional counseling as needed.

GLUCOSE-6-PHOSPHATE DEHYDROGENASE DEFICIENCY

Etiology and Pathophysiology. G6PD deficiency is an inherited sex-linked disorder involving a deficiency of G6PD enzyme, which is important in glucose metabolism by the red blood cells and membrane stability. Hemolysis most frequently occurs when the red cells are affected by certain pharmacologic agents.

The disease affects more than 100 million individuals worldwide. In the United States, approximately 15% of blacks and 2% of whites are affected with this disorder. It is also common among Greeks, Italians, and Arabs.

Like all cells, red blood cells need glucose for energy. When exposed to oxidative food and drugs or following a fever, red blood cells must metabolize an increased amount of glucose. In patients with G6PD deficiency, the red blood cells are unable to metabolize adequate amounts of glucose, resulting in hemolysis. Some of these oxidative agents include sulfonamides, aspirin, thiazide diuretics, oral hypoglycemics, chloramphenicol, antimalarials, and vitamin K derivatives. If individuals are not exposed to these agents, they may remain asymptomatic indefinitely.

Clinical Manifestations. Clinical manifestations include acute intravascular hemolysis lasting for as long as 2 weeks. Generalized anemia, pallor, and jaundice are usually present. Hemoglobin is found in the urine and in higher than normal levels in the blood.

Medical Diagnosis. The medical diagnosis of G6PD deficiency is made on the basis of history and physical assessment, hemoglobinemia, urinalysis for presence of hemoglobin, high serum bilirubin level, reticulocytosis, and the presence of Heinz bodies in red blood cells. High-risk populations should be routinely screened for G6PD deficiency.

Medical Management. Medical management includes removing the food or drug precipitating the disorder. Blood transfusions may be required. Genetic counseling may also be recommended.

Application of the Nursing Process to the Care of the Patient with Glucose-6-Phosphate Dehydrogenase Deficiency

The assessment, nursing diagnoses, expected patient outcomes, nursing interventions, and evaluation for patients with G6PD deficiency are similar to those described previously for patients with other anemias. In the acute phase of the disease, promote frequent rest periods, increased fluid intake, and good nutrition to maximize the patient's health status. Inform the patient and family about the clinical course of the disease and the treatment by reinforcing the physician's instructions and answering any questions they may have. Explain which drugs to avoid to reduce the risk of severe manifestations of the disease.

IMMUNE HEMOLYTIC ANEMIA

Etiology and Pathophysiology. Immune hemolytic anemia is caused by the lysis of red blood cells. This follows the process of red blood cells' combining with antibodies, which then may react with foreign cells, as in a blood transfusion, or with host cells. The red blood cell breakdown that occurs may be severe. The antibodies cover the red blood cells, which are then removed by the spleen. Undestroyed cells are reintroduced into the blood stream as spherocytes, which have a reduced life span.

The disorder may be caused by, or follow, a variety of disorders, such as infections, systemic diseases, transfusion reactions, and snakebites, or fetal-maternal blood exchanges. The resulting anemia may range from mild anemia to severe hemolysis and hyperbilirubinemia.

Clinical Manifestations. Clinical manifestations include fatigue, dyspnea, jaundice, and cardiac arrhythmias. The disorder may be minor enough to produce no apparent symptoms, or extremely severe, resulting in a life-threatening state of shock.

Medical Diagnosis. The diagnosis is made on the basis of the physical findings, history of causative factors, and laboratory studies. The analysis of red blood cells is a definitive study.

Medical Management. The cause of the disorder is determined and removed if possible. Treatment consists of blood transfusions in severe cases, or steroid therapy in mild cases. As the hemolysis decreases, drug treatment is reduced or discontinued. A splenectomy may be necessary if other interventions are not successful in reducing the red blood cell hemolysis.

Application of the Nursing Process to the Care of the Patient with Immune Hemolytic Anemia

The assessment, nursing diagnoses, expected patient outcomes, nursing interventions, and evaluation for patients with immune hemolytic anemia are similar to those described previously for patients with other anemias.

Polycythemias

The polycythemias are a group of disorders characterized by an increase in circulating red blood cells and hemoglobin concentration. Polycythemia vera is the most common disorder in the polycythemia group.

POLYCYTHEMIA VERA

Etiology and Pathophysiology. Polycythemia vera is characterized by overproduction of erythrocytes, leukocytes, and thrombocytes. This results in increased blood viscosity and volume and congestion of all tissues and organs. Polycythemia vera is most common among the middle-aged population and among Jewish men. The cause of the disease is unknown.

Clinical Manifestations. Clinical manifestations include splenomegaly and hepatomegaly as a result of an increase in red blood cells and blood volume. Skin changes such as redness, petechiae, ecchymoses, and hematomas occur from distended blood vessels. Blood pressure, pulse, and respirations are elevated owing to the increased blood volume and viscosity. Headaches and epistaxis may occur because of increased blood pressure and distended vessels. The increased cardiac workload may result in respiratory and circulatory impairment.

Complications include cerebral vascular accident, thrombosis, myocardial infarction, and hemorrhage, resulting from the high blood viscosity and distended blood vessels. Gastrointestinal bleeding and gangrene may occur from impaired circulation. Peptic ulcers are often the result of the high levels of gastric secretions. Increased red blood cell destruction results in high uric acid levels and gout.

Medical Diagnosis. The medical diagnosis of polycythemia vera is based on physical assessment and diagnostic procedures, including complete blood count, especially the red blood cell count and hematocrit, and bone marrow biopsy.

Medical Management. Medical management involves administration of oxygen, radioisotope therapy, or chemotherapeutic agents such as chlorambucil, cyclophosphamide, busulfan, and nitrogen mustard to suppress bone marrow growth. Diet therapy includes foods low in sodium to reduce fluid accumulation. Emergency management includes removing 500 to 2000 ml of blood to decrease the hematocrit level to 45%. Phlebotomies may be repeated every 2 to 3 months, or more often as needed.

Application of the Nursing Process to the Care of the Patient with Polycythemia Vera

Assessment

Check the patient's history and laboratory findings, and complete a thorough physical assessment. Look for changes in skin color and appearance. Ask whether the patient has experienced epistaxis due to congested capillaries and increased blood pressure. Assess for vertigo, headache, tinnitus, blurred vision, shortness of breath, dyspnea, neck vein distention, orthopnea, edema, and fatigue to determine circulatory and respiratory status. Auscultate breath sounds.

Observe for nausea, vomiting, or anorexia. Palpate for enlarged liver and spleen caused by tissue congestion.

Assess for blood in the urine and stools indicative of distended or ruptured vessels. Ask whether the patient has experienced any abdominal pain or heartburn indicative of increased gastric secretions. Check for signs of elevated uric acid levels, as evidenced by edematous and painful joints. Note the big toe, which is frequently the first joint affected. Assess the level of knowledge about the disease, its manifestations, and treatment.

Nursing Diagnoses and Planning

Nursing diagnoses and related expected patient outcomes most commonly applicable to patients with polycythemia vera include the following:

NDx: Fatigue related to increased metabolic requirements and circulatory changes

Planning: Patient outcomes
1. Patient acknowledges increased energy levels.
2. Patient demonstrates interest in surroundings, appears energetic, and is less irritable.
3. Patient completes daily activities without complaints of fatigue.

NDx: Altered tissue perfusion, cardiopulmonary and peripheral, related to increased arterial pressure and interruption of arterial and venous blood flow

Planning: Patient outcomes
1. Patient presents stable vital signs, palpable pulses, and appropriate level of consciousness.
2. Patient's urine output is adequate, with no apparent signs of blood.
3. Patient's skin is warm and dry, with no evidence of pallor.
4. Patient performs moderate activities without dyspnea, tachypnea, or tachycardia.

NDx: Knowledge deficit: nature of the disease, treatment, and potential alteration in lifestyle needed

Planning: Patient outcomes
1. Patient relates accurate information about the cause, effects, and clinical course of the disorder.
2. Patient lists strategies to cope with the disorder and the adjustments in lifestyle that both the patient and family can achieve.
3. Patient chooses a diet low in sodium and avoids gas-producing and highly acidic foods and fluids.

Nursing Interventions

NDx: Fatigue

Instruct the patient to note fatigue levels, when the fatigue is most severe, when the peak energy level occurs, and what activities are performed at those times. Assist the patient in creating a schedule of daily activities that capitalizes on the patient's ability to function well at certain times and allows for rest during times of exhaustion. Review the activities in the patient's daily routine and prioritize them with the patient. Help the patient look for ways to delegate tasks and reduce energy-using activities. Tell the patient to ask for assistance with self-care or other activities of daily living when fatigued.

Identify coping strategies with the patient and family. Explain the effects of stress on energy levels. Teach the patient about the benefits of moderate exercise, and assist with the planning of a realistic program of daily exercise with frequent rest periods. Stress the need for uninterrupted sleep periods.

Provide time for the patient and family to discuss their feelings and concerns about the disease, its effect on the patient, and the potential alterations in lifestyle needed.

NDx: Altered tissue perfusion, cardiopulmonary and peripheral

Help the patient conserve oxygen needs by encouraging rest and limiting activities. Elevate the head of the bed to aid in lung expansion. Initiate oxygen therapy if needed. Assist the patient with activities of daily living, if needed, to conserve energy.

Keep the patient in a comfortable position and reposition frequently to release pressure. Utilize range-of-motion exercises to stimulate circulation. Monitor vital signs and laboratory studies to assess for changes and improvements in status. Encourage ambulation as tolerated, but provide for frequent rest periods to decrease cardiac workload. Discourage smoking to avoid vasoconstriction. Discuss strategies to reduce stress, which could cause increased blood pressure. Remove constricting clothing and keep heavy bed linen from restricting peripheral circulation. Keep the patient's legs in a nondependent position when not ambulating.

Provide a low sodium diet to reduce fluid retention. Instruct the patient to avoid gas-forming and highly acidic foods and fluids. Give prescribed medications to promote increased circulation and diuresis as needed. Monitor laboratory studies to assess pulmonary, circulatory, and renal function.

NDx: Knowledge deficit: nature of the disease, treatment, and potential adjustments in lifestyle needed

Explain the disease to the patient and family in understandable terms. Allow for questions and discussion about concerns, fears, and misunderstandings. Tell the patient that medical care must now continue throughout his or her lifetime. Explain the need for phlebotomies every 2 to 3 months, or more frequently, to reduce the volume of circulating blood. Describe all prescribed medications, noting the dose, time, frequency, side effects, and toxic effects. Write out specific instructions for the patient and family to take with them upon discharge.

Teach the patient about diet modifications appropriate to reduce some of the complications of the disease. Give examples of menu plans incorporating low-sodium, low–gas-producing, and low-acid foods. Ask for consultation from a dietitian.

Teach the patient the signs and symptoms of complications of the disease, such as bleeding, and when to seek medical intervention. Advise the patient to avoid stimulants and to try to stop smoking to reduce vasoconstriction, which may increase blood pressure.

Teach strategies to reduce stress and how to balance rest with exercise. Demonstrate range-of-motion exercises to promote good circulation.

Discuss the lifestyle changes necessary to cope with the complications of the disease, such as fatigue and circulatory problems. Find ways the family can assist the patient. Seek assistance from clergy or counseling if appropriate.

Evaluation

Evaluate the effectiveness of nursing care for a patient with polycythemia vera by comparing the patient's status with the expected patient outcomes. Examples of specific outcomes for patients with polycythemia vera have been provided in the Planning section.

Leukocyte-Related Disorders

Agranulocytosis

Etiology and Pathophysiology. Agranulocytosis is characterized by a reduced number of leukocytes (leukopenia) and neutrophils (neutropenia) in the blood. The cause of agranulocytosis is usually a drug toxicity or hypersensitivity to phenothiazines, antithyroid drugs, sulfonamides, or other drugs. High doses of chemotherapeutic drugs and extended radiation therapy also cause neutropenia. The disorder is more common in women than in men.

Clinical Manifestations. The primary clinical manifestation of agranulocytosis is infection, which produces symptoms of fever, chills, fatigue, and ulcerations of mucous membranes. Because the number of the patient's granulocytes is significantly reduced, the body's defense against infection is impaired. A variety of disorders other than anemias and infections, such as tuberculosis, typhoid fever, malaria, and uremia, are also associated with agranulocytosis.

Medical Diagnosis. The medical diagnosis is made on the basis of history of exposure to a causative agent, physical assessment, and laboratory studies, including white blood cell count; throat, blood, urine, and stool cultures; and a bone marrow examination.

Medical Management. Medical management includes removing the causative agent, treating infections with antibiotics, and reducing fever with antipyretics. Sedatives for sleep may also be necessary.

Agranulocytosis can be fatal without immediate treatment. With treatment, the production of granulocytes resumes.

Application of the Nursing Process to the Care of the Patient with Agranulocytosis

Assessment

Review the history and potential cause of the disorder, and perform a physical examination. Ask the patient what medications, if any, have been or are presently being taken. Observe for toxic signs if the patient is taking drugs known to increase the risk of agranulocytosis.

Check the skin and mucous membranes for redness. Assess for anorexia, severe fatigue, weakness, persistent cough, sore throat, ulcerations of the mouth or throat, and dysphagia. Also check for prostration, fever, dehydration, diaphoresis, weak, rapid pulse, and severe chilling. Any of these may indicate the presence of infection. Palpate for enlarged lymph nodes. Ask about problems with elimination such as constipation.

Nursing Diagnoses and Planning

Nursing diagnoses and related expected patient outcomes applicable to patients with agranulocytosis may vary with the cause (such as specific drug). Those most commonly applicable in all cases of agranulocytosis include the following:

NDx: High risk for infection related to decreased body defenses against microorganisms

Planning: Patient outcomes
1. Patient's vital signs are within normal limits for the patient.
2. Patient's laboratory studies are within normal limits for the patient.
3. Patient denies cough, chills, fever, ulcerations, or other signs of infection.

NDx: Knowledge deficit: nature of the disorder and prevention of complications

Planning: Patient outcomes
1. Patient states the cause and effects of the disorder.
2. Patient recognizes early signs of infection.
3. Patient verbalizes strategies to prevent infection.
4. Patient states the importance of avoiding self-medicating without a physician's approval.
5. Patient recognizes when to seek medical intervention.

Nursing Interventions

NDx: High risk for infection

Assist the patient in remaining infection-free by utilizing protective isolation. Restrict visitors, and prevent personnel with colds from caring for the patient.

Encourage increased fluid intake to prevent dehydration. Offer six to eight small meals per day that are high in protein and vitamins to promote energy and increase the patient's nutritional status. Soft, bland foods may be ordered if the patient is experiencing a sore mouth or throat. Give meticulous mouth care. Encourage warm, saline irrigations of the throat every hour to prevent bacterial accumulation.

Assist the patient in bowel elimination by diet and fluid therapy and the addition of stool softeners if necessary. Tell the patient not to strain with defecation because tearing of the rectal mucosa could lead to infection. Enemas may be harsh and should also be avoided.

Encourage active and passive range-of-motion exercises every hour as tolerated. Turn the patient and encourage him or her to cough and breathe deeply to prevent hypostatic pneumonia. Encourage adequate rest periods and even bed rest, if necessary, to minimize oxygen requirements to conserve energy. Relieve fever with tepid baths, but prevent chilling.

NDx: Knowledge deficit: nature of the disorder and prevention of complications

Teach the patient and family about the nature of the disease, possible causes, and preventive measures. Allow time for questions and verbalization of concerns. Give the patient literature about agranulocytosis, as appropriate, to refer to in the future. Speak in terms the patient and family can understand.

Inform the patient about the importance of avoiding infections. List signs and symptoms of infections for the patient, and explain the need for early medical intervention if any symptoms appear. Tell the patient not to take any medications without the approval of the physician.

Explain the importance of good nutrition, moderate exercise, and frequent rest periods to prevent infections. Tell the patient to avoid drafts, extreme changes in temperature, and chilling.

Evaluation

Evaluate the effectiveness of nursing care for a patient with agranulocytosis by comparing the patient's status with the expected patient outcomes. Examples of specific outcomes for patients with agranulocytosis have been provided in the Planning section.

Neoplasias

LEUKEMIAS

Etiology and Pathophysiology. Leukemia is the term used to categorize a group of disorders in which a neoplastic growth of white blood cells occurs in the bone marrow. The leukemic cells multiply while suppressing bone marrow functions, resulting in a decreased production of red blood cells, platelets, and other types of granulocytes. The spleen and lymph nodes are also involved. The etiology of leukemia remains unknown; however, studies indicate some genetic predispositions and viral implications. Leukemia has a high incidence in individuals previously exposed to excessive radiation and chemical agents.

Leukemia occurs in approximately eight to nine individuals per 100,000 per year. It is a common cause of death among children.

Leukemias are classified according to their onset, cell maturity, and prognosis. Each type affects a different age group. Acute leukemia has a rapid onset and involves blood-forming organs. The leukocytes produced are immature cells. It is usually fatal within days to months if untreated. Acute leukemia occurs most frequently in children and young adults. Chronic leukemia has an insidious onset. The cells produced are more mature and differentiated white cells. Most patients affected by chronic leukemia are between 25 and 60 years of age at onset and survive 5 years or more.

Leukemias are also classified according to white cell type and tissue involved, such as lymphocytes, myelocytes, or monocytes. They are then further delineated as acute or chronic.

There are six primary categories of leukemias. Four of the most common types are discussed here.

1. Acute lymphocytic leukemia (ALL)
2. Acute myelocytic (granulocytic) leukemia (AML)
3. Acute monocytic leukemia (rare)
4. Chronic lymphocytic leukemia (CLL)
5. Chronic myelocytic (granulocytic) leukemia (CML)
6. Chronic monocytic leukemia (rare)

Approximately 60% of all leukemias are acute, 25% are chronic lymphocytic leukemias, and 15% are chronic myelocytic leukemias.

Acute Lymphocytic Leukemia. ALL is characterized by malignant growth of lymphoblasts in the marrow and peripheral tissues that spread to surrounding organs. Hepatosplenomegaly and lymphadenopathy are present in 70% to 80% of patients with ALL. Bone or joint pain occurs in approximately 25% of these patients.

Eighty percent of individuals affected by ALL are children. The peak incidence of ALL in children is between 2 and 4 years old, with a significant decrease at age 10. ALL rarely occurs after age 15.

ALL is usually treated with a variety of drugs, including vincristine, L-asparaginase, prednisone, daunorubicin, and doxorubicin. These and other chemotherapeutics may be used individually or in combination.

ALL has the best prognosis of all the leukemias. With chemotherapy, the median survival time is approximately 5 years, and if untreated, the survival time is 4 to 6 months. When treated, approximately 50% of children with ALL are considered cured. In adults, only 10% to 15% are considered cured following treatment. In children, a complete remission rate of 80% to 95% can be expected, whereas in adults the rate is 50% to 70%. In cases of ALL, the older the patient, the lower the remission rate.

Acute Myelocytic Leukemia. AML is characterized by immature myeloblasts in bone marrow that infiltrate various organs. It most commonly occurs in adolescence and after age 55. If untreated, the median survival rate is approximately 2 to 4 months.

Chemotherapies frequently used include vincristine, prednisone, and other drugs given singularly or concurrently. With chemotherapy, complete remission occurs in 50% to 75% of all patients. The median survival rate is approximately 2 to 3 years. Approximately 20% of treated patients are in complete remission after 5 years.

Chronic Lymphocytic Leukemia. CLL is characterized by a slow growth of lymphoid cells within the lymph nodes, bone marrow, liver, and spleen. It can occur at any age but is most common between the ages of 50 to 70, and it is three times more common in men. CLL occurs in approximately three individuals per 100,000 annually. The average survival time for an individual with CLL without treatment is 4 to 6 years, and with treatment is 7 years. Chemotherapeutic agents used for patients with CLL include chlorambucil, COP (Cytoxan, Oncovin, prednisone), or other similar drugs.

Chronic Myelocytic Leukemia. CML is characterized by a slow, abnormal growth of granulocytic cells. Primary symptoms include long bone pain due to bone marrow engorgement, anemia, and massive splenomegaly. CML occurs in approximately one individual per 100,000 annually. It occurs at any age but is most common in individuals between 40 and 60 years of age, and it is more common in men. The average survival time for individuals with CML is 3 to 4 years. Chemotherapy does not increase the life span but does produce prolonged asymptomatic periods. Drugs used to arrest CML include busulfan, hydroxyurea, DAT (daunorubicin, ara-C, thioguanine), and others in combination with these.

Clinical Manifestations. Clinical manifestations of the leukemias include respiratory complications caused by an increased metabolic rate from the overproduction of leukocytes and increased susceptibility to infections, anemia, and bleeding tendencies from decreased red blood cells, low hemoglobin levels, and thrombocytopenia. Malnutrition may be evident with anorexia, nausea, and vomiting. Mouth soreness also contributes to the anorexia. Infiltration into the central nervous system, meninges, and cranial nerves may cause headaches, visual problems, nausea, vomiting, tinnitus, and vertigo. Fatigue and weakness are present from hypoxia.

Systemic or local infections with fever develop as a result of an increased susceptibility to invading microorganisms. Pus is usually absent because of the low white blood cell count. Infections may also cause mouth and throat ulcerations to appear. These ulcers, along with some of the effects of the therapies, contribute to anorexia.

Splenomegaly, hepatomegaly, enlarged lymph nodes, and engorged bone marrow occur as a result of tissue distention from an increase in white blood cells. Abdominal pain and distention are also complications of tissue distention. Gradually leukemic cells invade all tissues and organs in the body.

Joint, sternum, bone, and nerve pain occur from deposits of blast cells in chronic myelogenous leukemia and from the pressure of enlarged lymph nodes, usually more common in chronic lymphocytic leukemia.

Uric acid levels are increased because of purine metabolism and chemotherapy destroying the white blood cells. When abnormal white blood cells invade the kidneys, uremia and renal failure result. Neurologic changes occur as well.

Medical Diagnosis. The medical diagnosis of leukemia is made on the basis of history, physical assessment, and laboratory studies of a white blood cell count, differential leukocyte count, presence of blast cells in the blood, and a bone marrow examination for the presence of abnormal leukocytes. Blood, wound, throat, urine, and stool cultures are obtained to determine which organisms are present.

Medical Management. Chemotherapy is the primary treatment for patients with acute leukemias. (See Chapter 11 for discussion on care of the patient receiving chemotherapy.) Refer to Table 16–1 for specific chemotherapeutic agents. Radiotherapy may be used in patients who are drug resistant, especially in CML.

Table 16–1. COMMON CHEMOTHERAPEUTIC AGENTS FOR LEUKEMIAS

ACUTE LYMPHOBLASTIC LEUKEMIA (ALL)	
	Vincristine (Oncovin)
	Prednisone (Deltasone, Merticorten, et al.)
	Daunorubicin (Daunomycin)
	Doxorubicin (Adriamycin)
	L-Asparaginase (L-ASP, Elspar)
	Methotrexate (MTX, amethopterin)
	6-Mercaptopurine (Purinethol)
CHRONIC LYMPHOCYTIC LEUKEMIA (CLL)	
COP	Chlorambucil (Leukeran)
COP	Cyclophosphamide (Cytoxan)
COP	Vincristine (Oncovin)
COP	Prednisone (Deltasone, Merticorten, et al.)
	COP + doxorubicin (Adriamycin)
	COP + carmustine, melphalan
ACUTE MYELOBLASTIC LEUKEMIA (AML)	
	Vincristine (Oncovin)
	Prednisone (Deltasone, Merticorten, et al.)
	Cytarabine (Cytosar, Ara-C)
	Daunorubicin (Daunomycin)
	Doxorubicin (Adriamycin)
CHRONIC MYELOCYTIC LEUKEMIA (CML)	
	Busulfan (Myleran)
	Hydroxyurea (Hydrea)
DAT	Doxorubicin (Adriamycin)
DAT	Daunorubicin (Daunomycin)
DAT	Cytarabine (Cytosar, Ara-C)
DAT	6-Thioguanine
	6-Mercaptopurine (Purinethol)

A splenectomy may be indicated. (See Splenectomy, Chapter 15.) Autografting and bone marrow transplantation may be conducted in patients with CML. (See Bone Marrow Transplant, Chapter 9.)

Medical management includes analgesics for mild pain. Narcotics and tranquilizers may be ordered for severe pain and to enhance other drug actions. Nonaspirin antipyretics are used to control fever. Aspirin should be avoided because it interferes with platelet function.

Stool softeners are ordered to promote bowel elimination. Allopurinol, potassium acetate or citrate, and sodium bicarbonate are ordered to alkalinize the urine and to prevent gout. The patient is hydrated with 3 to 4 L of intravenous fluids per day if uric acid levels are elevated.

Antibiotics may be ordered to treat infections. Studies are being conducted on the development of specific antibiotics to treat leukemic cells. Chest x-ray films may be used to diagnose pneumonia and determine the degree of disease involvement.

Granulocytes are administered to patients with severe neutropenia. Red blood cells and platelets are transfused, when necessary, to treat severe anemia or to prevent or treat acute hemorrhage. The use of leukapheresis (lymphocyte removal from the blood) is under investigation.

Application of the Nursing Process to the Care of the Patient with Leukemia

Assessment

Review the patient's history and laboratory findings, and perform a physical examination. Ask whether the patient has had recent exposure to chemicals, chemotherapy, or radiation. Look for signs of infection, bleeding of the gums, ecchymoses, or pain.

Observe for fatigue, weakness, malaise, cyanosis, dyspnea, tachycardia, and weight loss from increased metabolic rate. Assess for petechiae, purpura, bruising, pallor, shortness of breath, headache, weakness, and tachycardia indicative of anemia.

Note any tender, reddened areas on mucous membranes. Assess for fever, ulcerations, and bleeding gums, indicating a localized mouth infection. Also assess for systemic infections that may be manifested by changes in vital signs.

Ask about burning, pain, and frequency of urination, which may indicate an infection. Assess the color and consistency. Observe for elimination patterns. Check the stool for blood. Note any constipation or diarrhea episodes.

Check for anorexia, nausea, vomiting, and sore throat and mouth, which may interfere with nutritional intake. Ask whether the patient has been experiencing gastric irritation.

Assess for tenderness, pain, or enlargement of the liver, spleen, and lymph nodes. Note changes in degree and site of pain. Observe for muscle weakness and edema, which can further aggravate pain levels. Assess for joint, bone, or nerve pain. Subcutaneous lumps due to proliferating deposits of blast cells may be present in advanced stages of CML. Pain may be caused by pressure from enlarged lymph nodes. In CLL, lymph nodes are smooth, mobile, discrete, and nontender and vary in size (Nursing Care Guide 16–2).

Observe for presence of gout as manifested by heat, redness, or tenderness in one or more peripheral joints, especially the great toe. Assess for blood levels of uric acid. Check the diet for a high level of purine foods.

Assess for headaches, confusion, restlessness, changes in vision, retinal hemorrhages, and papilledema, indicating abnormal white blood cell infiltration into the central nervous system.

Observe for crying episodes, withdrawal, inability to concentrate, loss of appetite, insomnia, irritability, depression, and threats of suicide, indicating a high stress level. Assess the patient's and family's coping mechanisms. See which strategies seem to be most functional. Note any support systems.

Assess the patient's level of knowledge about leukemia. Find out whether the patient and family understand the effects of the disease and the treatments used to arrest the course of the disease.

Nursing Diagnoses and Planning

Nursing diagnoses and related expected patient outcomes most commonly applicable to patients with leukemia include the following:

NDx: High risk for infection related to the compromised immune response

Planning: Patient outcomes
1. Patient's vital signs and results of laboratory studies are within normal limits for the patient.
2. Patient exhibits no signs of infection, such as cough, chills, fever, sore throat, ulcerations of the mouth, or burning on urination.
3. Patient identifies signs of infections and measures to prevent them.
4. Patient is in protective isolation.

NDx: Altered nutrition, less than body requirements related to anorexia, secondary to sore mouth, chemotherapy, or radiation sickness

Planning: Patient outcomes
1. Patient eats well-balanced meals, choosing high-protein and high-vitamin foods as listed in Nutrition Box 16–2.
2. Patient chooses nonirritating foods.
3. Patient eats six to eight small meals per day to conserve energy and avoid distention.
4. Patient increases fluid intake to keep well hydrated.

NDx: Sensory/perceptual alterations; visual, auditory, and kinesthetic related to malignant infiltration into the central nervous system

Planning: Patient outcomes
1. Patient reports decrease or absence of headache, visual impairment, vertigo, nausea, and vomiting.
2. Patient requests assistance as needed when ambulatory to prevent injury.
3. Patient is alert and oriented to time, place, and person.

NDx: Pain related to enlarged nodes, chemical treatments, and bone infiltration

Planning: Patient outcomes
1. Patient reports that pain is controlled with analgesics.
2. Patient states comfort measures to help relieve pain.
3. Patient states coping measures to help relieve or tolerate pain.

Text continued on page 660

Nursing Care Guide 16–2.

PATIENTS WITH CHRONIC LYMPHOCYTIC LEUKEMIA

Assessment Findings: Patient complains of fatigue, weakness, hypoxia, dyspnea, tachycardia, malaise; exhibits decreased levels of Hgb and RBCs and thrombocytopenia.

Nursing Diagnosis: Activity intolerance related to overall weakness and an increased metabolic rate from the overproduction of leukocytes

Patient Outcomes	Nursing Interventions	Rationale
Patient completes activities of daily living without complaints of fatigue or weakness.	Allow for frequent rest periods. Provide a quiet environment and encourage energy-saving techniques.	Adequate rest periods throughout the day prevent extreme fatigue, save energy stores, and decrease oxygen demands.
Patient states that he or she is free of insomnia and sleeps well at night.	Offer sedatives as indicated. Encourage at least 8 hours of sleep every night. Provide quiet without interruptions.	Increasing sleep periods restores energy and reduces fatigue.
Patient is free from labored respirations; vital signs are within normal ranges.	Elevate head of bed, and monitor vital signs. Auscultate lungs every shift. Encourage patient to fully expand chest with respirations.	Changes in vital signs may indicate increasing problems of oxygen deficiency or other complications.

Evaluation: Compare the patient's status with the expected patient outcomes. If the outcomes are achieved, evaluate nursing care as successful. If not, reassess the patient, formulate new nursing diagnoses, and revise expected patient outcomes and nursing interventions as appropriate.

Assessment Findings: Patient complains of fever; mouth ulceration; respiratory distress; bleeding gums; hypertrophy of mouth, throat, and gums; vital sign changes; tender, reddened areas; elevated WBC count; burning or pain with urination, frequency of urination, odor or dark amber coloration of urine; perirectal abscess; blood in urine and stool; diarrhea; constipation; signs of septicemia; and pneumonia.

Nursing Diagnosis: High risk for infection related to increased susceptibility from inadeqaute primary and secondary defenses

Patient Outcomes	Nursing Interventions	Rationale
Patient's temperature and vital signs are within normal limits.	Monitor temperature. Apply ice packs; use hypothermia units or cool body sponging and nonaspirin antipyretics.	Keeping the patient's temperature within normal limits is important to prevent complications of hyperthermia.
Patient identifies actions taken to prevent infections and reduce risk of contamination.	Encourage 3000 to 4000 ml of fluid daily to prevent dehydration. Tell the patient to refrain from association with others when they have respiratory infections.	The patient with insufficient defenses against secondary infections needs increased awareness of methods to prevent infections.

(continued)

Nursing Care Guide 16–2. *(continued)*

PATIENTS WITH CHRONIC LYMPHOCYTIC LEUKEMIA

Patient Outcomes	Nursing Interventions	Rationale
	Instruct patient to avoid venipunctures and injections when possible to prevent organisms from entering the blood stream.	Multiple venipunctures may increase the patient's risk of septicemia or a localized infection.
	Place patient in reverse isolation (i.e., laminar air flow). Obtain blood, throat, urine, stool, and / or wound culture to determine type of organism present.	Reverse isolation protects the patient from external contaminants. This may be necessary, particularly during acute exacerbations of the disease.
Patient denies pain or burning with urination, frequency of urination, and odor and dark coloration of urine. Patient experiences adequate bladder and bowel elimination.	Provide and encourage increased fluids. Offer the urinal or bedpan frequently, or assist the patient to the restroom. Provide stool softeners to reduce irritation. Inspect skin for reddened areas, lesions, and so on.	Continual flushing of the urinary tract decreases risk of an infection. Eliminating straining with bowel movements may prevent breakdown and abscesses around the anal area.
Patient maintains skin integrity.	Promote good hygiene. Offer sitz baths to promote circulation and healing. Turn the patient frequently, and massage reddened areas	The patient with decreased immune function is at increased risk for skin breakdown and infection when on bed rest. Stimulating circulation to the skin surfaces helps alleviate some of the potential problems.

Evaluation: Compare the patient's status with the expected patient outcomes. If the outcomes are achieved, evaluate nursing care as successful. If not, reassess the patient, formulate new nursing diagnoses, and revise expected patient outcomes and nursing interventions as appropriate.

Assessment Findings: Patient experiences nausea, vomiting, anorexia, diarrhea, constipation, abdominal distention, flatus, and sore mouth from ulcers.

Nursing Diagnosis: Altered nutrition, less than body requirements related to anorexia, secondary to a sore mouth and radiation sickness

Patient Outcomes	Nursing Interventions	Rationale
Patient's appetite improves. Patient consumes foods high in calories, protein, and vitamins.	Promote good oral hygiene. Offer six to eight small meals. Encourage diet high in calories, protein, and vitamins. Encourage high fluid intake. Monitor fluid intake and output.	Appropriate nutrition is essential for healing, maintenance of normal body functions, and prevention of infections.

(continued)

Nursing Care Guide 16–2. *(continued)*

PATIENTS WITH CHRONIC LYMPHOCYTIC LEUKEMIA

Patient Outcomes	Nursing Interventions	Rationale
Patient maintains appropriate weight level.	Weigh patient daily on same scale with similar clothing. Commend the patient for achieving the appropriate weight as recommended.	Positive reinforcement encourages the patient to continue to progress.
Patient relates adequate knowledge regarding proper food intake.	Teach patient about appropriate diet and hygiene habits. Allow time for questions and concerns about the nutritional needs.	An understanding of the type of nutrition intake necessary may prevent future problems for the patient. Having the patient restate the information reinforces the learning and allows for corrections if there are misunderstandings.
	Have the patient reiterate the directions provided by the physician and nurse. Note bowel elimination pattern.	With inadequate nutrition, the patient may experience altered elimination patterns.
Patient's elimination patterns are adequate.	Offer stool softeners as needed. Encourage increased fluid intake.	

Evaluation: Compare the patient's status with the expected patient outcomes. If the outcomes are achieved, evaluate nursing care as successful. If not, reassess the patient, formulate new nursing diagnoses, and revise expected patient outcomes and nursing interventions as appropriate.

Assessment Findings: Patient complains of red, sore tongue; mouth ulcers; sore throat; bleeding gums; anorexia; thirst; and dry mouth.

Nursing Diagnosis: Altered oral mucous membrane related to disease or treatment

Patient Outcomes	Nursing Interventions	Rationale
Patient states food intake does not irritate mouth.	Offer six to eight small meals of soft, bland food to reduce irritation to the mouth. Encourage 3000 to 4000 ml of fluids per day.	Small amounts of bland food at frequent intervals are less irritating to the oral mucosa.
Patient states mouth discomfort has subsided.	Instruct patient that mouth lesions will subside when remission is achieved.	Exacerbations of the disorder and the treatments initiated increase the susceptibility to oral mucosal breakdown.
	Encourage oral hygiene every 2 hours using a soft cotton-tipped applicator. Keep lips well lubricated.	Frequent oral hygiene helps reduce infections and breakdown within the oral cavity.

(continued)

Nursing Care Guide 16–2. *(continued)*

PATIENTS WITH CHRONIC LYMPHOCYTIC LEUKEMIA

Patient Outcomes	Nursing Interventions	Rationale
Patient's oral cavity is free from ulcers, bleeding, and lesions.	Have patient rinse mouth with hydrogen peroxide and water and gargle before eating.	Hygiene prior to meals makes foods more palatable.
	Offer cold foods high in protein (e.g., ice cream), chilled fruit, vegetable juices. Avoid hot or spicy foods and acidic juices. Inspect mouth three times daily. Ensure that oral hygiene regimen is being completed every 2 to 3 hours throughout the day and every 6 hours during the night.	Cold foods are more soothing to the oral mucosa. Spicy foods may feel as if they are burning the mucosa if lesions are present. Continued proper oral hygiene prevents further mouth problems.

Evaluation: Compare the patient's status with the expected patient outcomes. If the outcomes are achieved, evaluate nursing care as successful. If not, reassess the patient, formulate new nursing diagnoses, and revise expected patient outcomes and nursing interventions as appropriate.

Assessment Findings: Patient experiences joint, bone, or nerve pain; muscle weakness; edema; and heat, redness, or tenderness in joints, especially toes, ankles, knees, hands, and elbows, demonstrating gout. Enlarged, smooth, mobile, discrete, nontender subcutaneous nodes causing pain.

Nursing Diagnosis: Pain related to tissue distention, muscle wasting, edema, or chemotherapy

Patient Outcomes	Nursing Interventions	Rationale
Patient moves without signs of severe pain, such as grimacing, moaning, or guarding.	Investigate complaints of discomfort. Encourage relaxation exercises and deep diaphragmatic breathing. Position patient for comfort. Support joints and extremities with pillows.	Relaxation exercises may help reduce pain. Keeping bony prominences padded eliminates pressure to the area and increased discomfort.
Patient reports that pain is relieved or controlled.	Offer analgesics for mild pain, and narcotics for severe pain. Offer tranquilizers to enhance drug actions. Encourage patient's coping mechanisms. Massage areas of pain.	

Evaluation: Compare the patient's status with the expected patient outcomes. If the outcomes are achieved, evaluate nursing care as successful. If not, reassess the patient, formulate new nursing diagnoses, and revise expected patient outcomes and nursing interventions as appropriate.

(continued)

Nursing Care Guide 16–2. *(continued)*

PATIENTS WITH CHRONIC LYMPHOCYTIC LEUKEMIA

Assessment Findings: Patient exhibits behaviors of crying, withdrawal, inability to concentrate, loss of appetite, insomnia, irritability, depression, and threats of suicide.

Nursing Diagnosis: Anxiety related to diagnosis and concerns of death or dying

Patient Outcomes	Nursing Interventions	Rationale
Patient verbalizes fears and concerns.	Allow patient to ventilate feelings regarding disease and treatment process in a nonjudgmental environment.	Free verbalization of anxiety helps relieve some of the fear and concerns.
Patient and family demonstrate reduced anxiety and fear.	Encourage family to participate. Reassure patient and family that feelings of fear, anxiety, and depression are very common. Allow for friends and clergy to visit. Maintain eye contact with patient.	Encouraging family or other significant others to participate helps provide support systems for the patient.
Patient exhibits coping mechanisms to deal effectively with problems.	Offer professional counseling referrals. Assist patient and family in identifying coping strategies.	Appropriate coping with the trauma of disease is important to the healing process.

Evaluation: Compare the patient's status with the expected patient outcomes. If the outcomes are achieved, evaluate nursing care as successful. If not, reassess the patient, formulate new nursing diagnoses, and revise expected patient outcomes and nursing interventions as appropriate.

Assessment Findings: Patient asks questions when in doubt; states that he or she does not understand disease process, prevention techniques, and treatment.

Nursing Diagnosis: Knowledge deficit: nature of disease, treatment, and prevention of complications

Patient Outcomes	Nursing Interventions	Rationale
Patient verbalizes accurate information about disease, treatment, and self-care.	Explain disease process to patient. Provide literature. Provide information about nutritional requirements, fatigue prevention, and comfort measures. Instruct patient to avoid contact sports, razors, and alcohol intake to prevent or minimize bleeding.	Explanation of the disorder and typical treatment plan reinforces the physician's information and helps the patient understand the disease and health care needs.

(continued)

Nursing Care Guide 16–2. *(continued)*

PATIENTS WITH CHRONIC LYMPHOCYTIC LEUKEMIA

Patient Outcomes	Nursing Interventions	Rationale
	Explain to patient that aspirin should be avoided because it interferes with platelet functions and may enhance bleeding.	
Patient relates the importance of reporting signs and symptoms of infection to the health care team. Patient exhibits health promotion behaviors such as choosing proper foods, inspecting mouth and gums, and so on.	Encourage patient and family to observe and report signs of developing infection. Provide a list of signs and symptoms of infections for the patient. Explain that early detection and treatment may limit the severity of infection. Discuss the importance of preventing constipation and rectal pain and bleeding. Teach the patient good oral hygiene techniques.	Having the patient relate information for preventions given provides opportunity to assess the patient's understanding of the disorder and to correct any misunderstandings. Having the family involved gives additional support to the patient. Compliance is more likely if the patient and family understand the importance of prevention of complications.
Patient relates the side effects of therapy and coping strategies to minimize them.	Inform patient of common side effects of antileukemic therapy (e.g., gastrointestinal disturbances, diarrhea).	Information about the side effects alerts the patient to be prepared for them and to attempt to prevent their occurrence.
Patient states names, dosage, action, and side effects of medication.	Explain treatment of chemotherapy or radiotherapy if applicable. Explain importance of taking antibiotics on schedule. Explain that platelet and white blood cell transfusions are routine in treatment. Red blood cells may be transfused in patients with anemia, and platelets may be used to treat hemorrhage. Teach patient some strategies for coping with or alleviating the side effects of therapy.	Knowledge of the medications and therapy used is important to prevent additional problems and to promote patient participation in the treatment regimen.

Evaluation: Compare the patient's status with the expected patient outcomes. If the outcomes are achieved, evaluate nursing care as successful. If not, reassess the patient, formulate new nursing diagnoses, and revise expected patient outcomes and nursing interventions as appropriate.

NDx: Activity intolerance related to weakness, poor nutrition, and depressed energy stores from anemia, complications of treatment, and stress

Planning: Patient outcomes

1. Patient reports increased ability to perform activities of daily living.
2. Patient demonstrates no shortness of breath upon mild exertion.
3. Patient reports less weakness with increased tolerance for activity.
4. Patient sleeps 6 to 10 hours per night without difficulty.

NDx: Anxiety related to health status, fear of death or treatment outcomes, and complications of the disease

Planning: Patient outcomes

1. Patient's anxiety is lessened as evidenced by stable vital signs, relaxed appearance, and calm, positive attitude.
2. Patient states strategies to cope with the disease manifestations.
3. Patient verbalizes fears and concerns.

NDx: Knowledge deficit: nature of illness and complication of bleeding related to thrombocytopenia

Planning: Patient outcomes

1. Patient reports accurate information about the nature of the disease.
2. Patient states accurately the signs of bleeding and when to notify the physician.
3. Patient presents no signs or symptoms of bleeding such as petechiae, ecchymoses, epistaxis, dark stools, and so on.
4. Patient verbalizes the preventive measures necessary to prevent bleeding as listed in Chart 16–1.

Nursing Interventions

NDx: High risk for infection

Keep the patient warm, and avoid extreme changes in temperature in the room. Restrict visitors to prevent exposure to infections. Use protective isolation if appropriate.

Monitor the patient's vital signs frequently, observing subtle changes that may indicate early signs of infection. Report any changes noted.

Promote good nutrition by serving the meals in a relaxed, attractive atmosphere. Encourage a high-protein and high-vitamin diet. Provide oral hygiene frequently to prevent infection and promote better eating habits.

Encourage mouth cleansing every 2 hours with a nonirritating substance. Keep the patient's lips well lubricated to prevent skin breakdown. Have the patient use a mixture of hydrogen peroxide and water, especially when bleeding is present, to help prevent the growth of organisms.

Explain the importance of preventing constipation, because it can cause irritation, bleeding, and infection of the rectal mucosa. Use stool softeners when indicated. Diarrhea caused by chemotherapy is treated by careful cleaning of the rectal area after each episode. Give antidiarrheal medications as prescribed.

Since early identification and treatment may limit the severity of the infection, teach patients and their families to continually observe for signs of developing infection upon discharge and to notify the physician if such signs appear.

NDx: Altered nutrition, less than body requirements

Encourage the patient to eat a diet high in calories, protein, and vitamins (see Nutrition Box 16–2). Offer six to eight small meals per day of soft, bland foods to reduce irritation and trauma to the mouth and gastrointestinal tract.

Serve the meals in an attractive manner. Allow the patient time to eat, and assist with eating if necessary. Provide rest periods prior to eating so that the patient will not be too fatigued to eat.

NDx: Sensory/perceptual alterations; visual, auditory, and kinesthetic

Teach the patient to use safety measures at all times. Explain to the family the need for their assistance to the patient to prevent injury. Have the patient request assistance when getting out of bed and ambulating. Keep the bed rails up, and place frequently used articles within the patient's reach.

Check the patient frequently for orientation to time, place, and person. Speak loudly if auditory problems are evident. Decrease the external stimuli, and provide periods of rest. Give analgesics as prescribed to control headaches.

NDx: Pain

Place the patient in comfortable positions, and reposition frequently. Use pillows to support bony prominences. Assess when the pain is most severe, and allow the patient to rest during those periods. Give pain medications as ordered prior to activity periods so that the patient can better tolerate the movement.

Help the patient find alternate methods to alleviate or to be able to tolerate the pain. Show the patient and family relaxation techniques and how to perform massage. Teach the patient the use of patient-controlled analgesia (PCA) if ordered.

NDx: Activity intolerance

Instruct the patient to develop a regimen of activity with frequent rest periods throughout the day. Encourage the patient to do range-of-motion exercises frequently while lying in bed to maintain muscle tone and strength. Tell the patient to avoid sudden movements, such as getting out of bed quickly, because this decreases the blood supply to the brain, aggravating vertigo and disorientation. Have the patient practice deep breathing exercises to increase oxygen and blood to the brain.

Teach the patient to practice energy-saving techniques to reduce fatigue and shortness of breath. Place frequently used articles within the patient's reach.

Provide and encourage frequent rest periods while delivering patient care. Prevent interruptions during rest periods and at night, whenever possible. Reduce any disturbing noises and limit visitors as necessary.

Provide warm clothes and blankets to prevent chilling. Avoid unnecessary exposure to drafts and extreme changes in temperature.

Encourage good nutrition to increase the patient's energy level. Offer four to six meals per day. This is less tiring for the patient and prevents gastric overdistention.

NDx: Anxiety

Allow the patient to verbalize concerns about the disease, its effects on the patient and family, and fears about death. Help the patient and family find coping strategies that are effective to deal with their anxiety level. Allow time for questions from the patient and the family.

Teach the patient relaxation techniques to help reduce the anxiety. Explain how stress can aggravate the complications of the disease. Tell the patient to rest frequently during the day. Provide comfort measures, both physical and emotional, to the patient and family.

Explain the disease process, the treatments, and potential results so that the patient has a better understanding of the disease and its progression. Allow time for the patient and family to be alone when needed. Seek assistance from clergy or other professional counselors when appropriate. Make referrals as needed to social service agencies.

NDx: Knowledge deficit: nature of disease and complication of hemorrhage

Instruct the patient about the clinical course of leukemia and the complication of hemorrhage. Teach the patient signs of bleeding to observe for and when to seek medical assistance. Explain the need for avoiding sharp objects, straight razors, contact sports, and injections and venipuncture whenever possible. Tell the patient to watch for discoloration of urine or stools.

Explain proper oral hygiene methods necessary to prevent further irritation and ulceration of mucous membranes. Instruct the patient to use a soft toothbrush and to use mouthrinse frequently. Show how to inspect the oral cavity, checking the tongue and gums for early signs of irritation. Teach the patient to avoid extremely hot, spicy foods and acidic drinks to lessen oral and gastrointestinal irritation (Chart 16–3).

Evaluation

Evaluate the effectiveness of nursing care for a patient with leukemia by comparing the patient's status with the expected patient outcomes. Examples of specific outcomes for patients with leukemia have been provided in the Planning section.

HODGKIN'S DISEASE

Etiology and Pathophysiology. About half of all lymphomas are Hodgkin's disease, a chronic, malignant disorder of unknown etiology that originates in the lymphatic system and spreads to other organs and structures in the later stages. Hodgkin's disease is characterized by large atypical tumor cells or abnormal histiocytes called Reed-Sternberg cells. These cells invade the lymph nodes, spleen, and liver. As they multiply, they replace normal cells and cause necrosis and fibrosis. Hodgkin's disease is classified by stages according to lymph node involvement, appearance, severity, and prognosis. Hodgkin's disease usually occurs in individuals between 20 and 50 years of age and is twice as likely to occur in men as in women.

Prognosis varies by stage at the time of diagnosis. Ninety-five percent of patients with localized Hodgkin's disease can be cured or have a 10-year survival without recurrence when treated early. Patients in Stages I and II are usually cured with radiation treatment if the disease has not spread to the lymph node chains, spleen, and nasopharynx. Patients in Stages III and IV cannot be cured but usually experience symptomatic relief when treated with both radiotherapy and chemotherapy or combination chemotherapy. Eighty percent of patients undergoing combination chemotherapy experience complete remissions. If clients are not treated, they have a 5-year life expectancy.

Clinical Manifestations. Early clinical manifestations include pruritus, weakness, and intermittent fever. Respiratory changes, edema, and cyanosis result from enlarged lymph nodes pressing on the superior vena cava. Pressure on the nerves and esophagus may result in laryngeal paralysis and dysphagia.

Infection occurs from immunodeficiency, the result of chemotherapy, and the invasion of the malignancy into the viscera. High- and low-grade fevers are common. Pneumonia, septicemia, and urinary infections are the most frequently acquired infections.

Chart 16–3.

NURSING GUIDE TO PATIENT EDUCATION FOR SELF-MANAGEMENT: SELF-CARE FOR PREVENTION OF COMPLICATIONS OF LEUKEMIA

To prevent complications associated with leukemia, instruct the patient to:

Prevent infections by:

- Avoiding contact with persons with coughs, colds, and fevers.
- Developing good hygiene practices such as frequent hand washing, careful wound or abrasion cleaning, and good oral care.
- Recognizing early signs of infections and seeking treatment immediately.
- Avoiding sharp instruments, razors, injections, and venipunctures to prevent breaks in the skin that could provide entry for microorganisms.
- Getting adequate rest and eating properly to maintain general resistance levels.

Prevent bleeding by:

- Avoiding shaving with razors, using sharp instruments, having injections or venipunctures, and participating in contact sports.

Promote good nutrition and prevent irritation by:

- Eating a diet high in calories, protein, and vitamins.
- Eating six to eight small feedings of soft, bland foods.
- Rinsing mouth every 2 hours with a mixture of hydrogen peroxide and water.
- Avoiding hot spicy foods.
- Drinking up to 4000 ml of fluids daily.
- Avoiding high purine foods such as liver, kidneys, sweetbreads, brains, sardines, and anchovies.

Prevent pain by:

- Explaining the usage, dosages, and side effects of medication prescribed for pain by the physician.
- Teaching relaxation methods.
- Providing strategies for developing comfort measures to be used at home.

Renal impairment is present as a result of invasion of the kidneys by abnormal leukocytes. Gout may be present because of the increased production of uric acid in the blood as a result of increased cell production.

The central nervous system may be affected as a result of infiltrating abnormal white blood cells. Dehydration may result from fever and diaphoresis.

Anemia is present as a result of red blood cell destruction. Prolonged lymphatic obstruction results in accumulation of fluid in the lungs and abdomen, usually present in later stages of the disorder.

Low blood counts indicate that the bone marrow and spleen are affected. Lymph nodes are painless and enlarged from the massive growth of abnormal cells. Splenomegaly and hepatomegaly are present, indicating organ involvement. Jaundice is present with liver damage and bile duct obstruction. Bilirubin is present in the blood.

Bone or mediastinal pain lasting as long as 1 hour occurs when alcohol is ingested. The cause of this symptom is unknown. Nerve pain resulting from nerve root compression may be present. If the spinal cord is compressed, paralysis occurs. Fractures or vertebral compression may occur if the disorder has spread to the bone.

Medical Diagnosis. The medical diagnosis of Hodgkin's disease is made on the basis of history, physical assessment, and laboratory findings. Lymph node biopsy with the presence of Reed-Sternberg cells and a chest x-ray film or computed tomography (CT) scan to determine mediastinal involvement are the primary diagnostic tests. Blood tests are done to determine the presence of anemia.

A staging laparoscopy may be used to determine visceral involvement.

Medical Management. Medical management for Stages I and II includes high-dose radiation therapy for 4 to 6 weeks. Stages III and IV are treated with radiation or chemotherapy, or both. The most common chemotherapy combination is the MOPP regimen, which includes mechlorethamine (Mustargen), vincristine (Oncovin), procarbazine, and prednisone (Table 16–2). Other chemotherapy combinations may be used if MOPP is not effective or if the treatment is for a recurrence following initial remission. Disease management may involve surgical removal of a large pressure-causing tumor. Antipyretics are ordered to reduce fever, and transfusions are given when anemia is present. (See Chapter 11 for care of the patient receiving chemotherapy.)

Complications of treatment include mouth and throat ulcers, anemia, and immunodeficiency that may occur as a result of chemotherapy. Thrombocytopenia leading to hemorrhage may result from decreased levels of red blood cells and hemoglobin. Radiation sickness may result from the high-dose radiation therapy.

Application of the Nursing Process to the Care of the Patient with Hodgkin's Disease

Assessment

Review the history, and conduct a physical examination. Question the patient about a recent history of pruritus, fever, and weakness. Assess for dyspnea, cough, stridor, chest pain, cyanosis, and pleural effusion, indicating pulmonary involvement. Check the results of the laboratory studies.

Observe for facial and neck edema and cyanosis resulting from enlarged lymph nodes. Assess the patient's speech and swallowing for changes caused by pressure.

Observe for high fever alternating with prolonged low-grade fever, indicative of infection. Assess for night sweats, extreme fatigue, weight loss, and malaise, indicative of anemia. Assess for changes in urine output, indicating spread of the disease to the urinary system.

Assess for complications from radiation or chemotherapy as manifested by dysphagia, dry mouth, nausea, vomiting, skin rashes, and hair loss. Palpate for painless enlargement of lymph nodes, especially on sides of the neck, axillae, and groin.

Check the patient's dietary pattern. Observe for signs of inadequate intake, such as poor skin turgor and weight loss. Monitor fluid intake and output. Observe for signs of fatigue from malnutrition.

Look for edema of extremities from pressure on veins. Palpate for an enlarged spleen and liver, indicating possible spread of the disease to those organs.

Assess for vertebral compression and fractures, indicating spread of the disease to bone. Observe for paralysis, indicative of spinal cord compression.

Assess for anxiety, as evidenced by crying, withdrawal, lack of concentration, loss of appetite, insomnia, irritability, depression, and threats of suicide.

Nursing Diagnoses and Planning

Nursing diagnoses and related expected patient outcomes most commonly applicable to the patient with Hodgkin's disease include the following:

NDx: Ineffective breathing pattern related to tracheobronchial obstruction from enlarged lymph nodes and pleural effusion

Planning: Patient outcomes

1. Patient's vital signs are within normal ranges for the patient, with no signs of cyanosis, dyspnea, tachypnea, or tachycardia.
2. Patient uses good lung expansion techniques.
3. Patient is able to perform activities of daily living without respiratory distress.
4. Patient's blood gas levels are within normal ranges for the patient.

NDx: High risk for infection related to immunodeficiency, effects of chemotherapy, and the invasion of malignant cells into viscera

Table 16–2. MOPP COMBINATION CHEMOTHERAPY REGIMEN FOR HODGKIN'S DISEASE*

CHEMOTHERAPY	DOSAGE	ROUTE	TIME
Nitrogen Mustard (Mustargen)	6 mg/m^2 of body surface area	IV	Day 1 and day 8
Vincristine (Oncovin)	1.4 mg/m^2	IV	Day 1 and day 8 (not to exceed 2 mg/dose)
Procarbazine	100 mg/m^2	p.o.	Day 1 through day 14
Prednisone	40 mg/m^2	p.o.	Day 1 through day 14 in 1st and 4th cycle only

*Minimum of six 2-week cycles with 2-week rest between cycles. Doses of Mustargen, Oncovin, and procarbazine are reduced as WBC falls below 4000 cu mm and platelets fall below 100,000/cu mm, or if neurotoxicity develops.

Dose is stopped if WBC reaches 1000/cu mm and platelets reach 50,000/cu mm. Hemorrhage is possible at counts below 20,000/cu mm.

Modified from Le Blanc DH. People with Hodgkin disease: The nursing challenge. *Nurs Clin North Am* 1978; 13(2):282.

Planning: Patient outcomes
1. Patient presents no evidence of cough, dyspnea, sore throat, or mouth ulcers.
2. Patient denies pain or burning with urination.
3. Patient identifies actions needed to prevent infections.
4. Patient's vital signs are within normal ranges for the patient.

NDx: Altered nutrition, less than body requirements related to anorexia from treatments, fatigue, and complications of disease

Planning: Patient outcomes
1. Patient chooses foods appropriate to replace dietary deficiencies.
2. Patient avoids irritating foods and fluids.

NDx: Activity intolerance related to reduced energy stores, decreased oxygen from ineffective breathing pattern, and inadequate nutrition

Planning: Patient outcomes
1. Patient follows a regimen of planned activities and rest periods each day.
2. Patient verbalizes feeling less fatigued and demonstrates signs of increased activity.
3. Patient is able to perform activities of daily living.
4. Patient's vitals signs are within normal ranges for the patient.
5. Patient denies shortness of breath on mild exertion.

NDx: Anxiety related to inability to cope with the manifestations of the disease, fear of treatments, and threat of death

Planning: Patient Outcomes
1. Patient relates concerns about illness to the nurse or other appropriate member of the health care team.
2. Patient and family verbalize accurate information about the disorder, complications, and therapy.
3. Patient expresses feelings of reduced anxiety and fear.
4. Patient displays physical signs of decreased anxiety; vital signs are within normal ranges, patient is resting well, appears calm, and eats well.

Nursing Interventions

NDx: Ineffective breathing pattern
Have the patient turn, cough, and breathe deeply hourly while awake to prevent respiratory infection and increase oxygen intake. Teach the patient to use full chest expansion. Elevate the head of the bed to assist with chest expansion and free movement of the diaphragm.

Encourage good nutrition with increased fluid intake for maintenance of health and hydration. Provide a diet high in protein and vitamins (see Nutrition Box 16–2). Allow time for meals and provide rest periods prior to eating to prevent poor eating habits due to fatigue and respiratory difficulty. Assist the patient with eating if necessary.

Remove tight clothing to maximize respiratory efforts and promote circulation. Administer oxygen as needed. Have emergency equipment by the bedside for airway and respiratory support.

NDx: High risk for infection
Keep the patient warm, and avoid extreme changes in temperature in the room. Restrict visitors to prevent exposure to infections. Use protective isolation if appropriate.

Monitor the patient's vital signs frequently, observing subtle changes that may indicate early signs of infection. Report any changes noted. Ask the patient to report any signs of infection such as cough, dyspnea, sore throat, or pain or burning with urination.

NDx: Altered nutrition, less than body requirements
Help the patient maintain adequate nutrition by providing an attractive meal in a pleasant atmosphere. Encourage patient to eat foods high in protein and vitamins. Provide six to eight small meals to prevent distention and reduce fatigue. Provide oral hygiene frequently to prevent infection and promote better eating habits. Ask for consultation with the dietitian.

Instruct patient to avoid foods that are gas-forming, because they cause abdominal distention that may decrease the appetite and also interfere with respiratory efforts. Avoid hot, spicy foods and acidic fluids to decrease gastrointestinal irritation when present. Encourage increased fluid intake to prevent constipation and promote adequate hydration. Monitor the patient's fluid intake and output.

NDx: Activity intolerance
Instruct the patient to develop a regimen of activity with frequent rest periods throughout the day. Encourage the patient to do range-of-motion exercises frequently while lying in bed to maintain muscle tone and strength. Tell the patient to avoid sudden movements, such as getting out of bed quickly, because this decreases the blood supply to the brain, aggravating vertigo and disorientation. Have the patient practice deep breathing exercises to increase oxygen and blood to the brain.

Teach the patient to practice energy-saving techniques to reduce fatigue and shortness of breath. Place frequently used articles within the patient's reach.

Provide and encourage frequent rest periods while delivering patient care. Prevent interruptions during rest periods and at night whenever possible.

Table 16–3. CATEGORIES OF NON-HODGKIN'S LYMPHOMAS

FAVORABLE HISTOLOGY	UNFAVORABLE HISTOLOGY
Nodular poorly differentiated lymphocytic lymphoma (NPDL)	Nodular histiocytic lymphoma (NHL)
Nodular mixed lymphocytic and histiocytic lymphoma (NML)	Diffuse poorly differentiated lymphocytic lymphoma (DPDL)
Well-differentiated lymphocytic lymphomas of the nodular (NWDL) or diffuse (DWDL) type	Diffuse histiocytic lymphoma (DHL)
	Diffuse mixed lymphoma (DML)
	Diffuse undifferentiated lymphoma (DUL)

Reproduced by permission from Xistris DM. In Phipps, WJ, Long, BC, Woods NF (eds). *Medical-surgical nursing*. 3rd ed. St. Louis: CV Mosby, 1987.

Reduce any disturbing noises and limit visitors when necessary.

Provide warm clothes and blankets to prevent chilling. Avoid unnecessary exposure to drafts or extreme changes in temperature.

Encourage good nutrition to increase the patient's energy level. Offer four to six meals per day. This is less tiring for the patient and prevents gastric overdistention.

NDx: Anxiety

Allow patient to verbalize concerns about the disease, its effects on the patient and family, and fears about death. Help the patient and family find coping strategies that are effective to deal with their anxiety level. Allow time for questions from the patient and the family.

Seek assistance from clergy or other professional counselors when appropriate. Make referrals as needed to social service agencies.

Evaluation

Evaluate the effectiveness of nursing care for a patient with Hodgkin's disease by comparing the patient's status with the expected patient outcomes. Examples of specific outcomes for patients with Hodgkin's disease have been provided in the Planning section.

NON-HODGKIN'S LYMPHOMAS

Etiology and Pathophysiology. Non-Hodgkin's lymphomas usually occur in individuals between 50 and 60 years of age. Non-Hodgkin's lymphomas consist of several lymphoid malignancies with varying histopathologies, clinical disease courses, and treatment responses. The cause of the lymphomas is unknown.

Non-Hodgkin's lymphomas are categorized into lymphocytic, histiocytic, and mixed cell types, each being nodular or diffuse on a microscopic examination. These are further categorized as favorable or nonfavorable histology, depending on their response to treatment (Table 16–3). Generally, a nodular cell structure has a more favorable prognosis than a diffuse cell structure, and a lymphocytic cytology is more favorable than a histiocytic cytology.

Clinical Manifestations. Clinical manifestations are similar to those of Hodgkin's disease with some exceptions. Individuals with non-Hodgkin's lymphomas have involvement of several sites early in the course of the disease rather than involvement of only one site, as is typical in Hodgkin's disease.

Initial painless lymphadenopathy occurs usually on one side of the body only. Abnormal cells spread to the bone marrow and eventually to the liver and spleen, causing hepatomegaly and splenomegaly. Gastrointestinal disturbances and nervous system changes are evident. Pressure on these areas creates pain and numbness, leading to paralysis. Anemia, fever, weight loss, weakness, and anorexia result from red blood cell destruction and infections.

Medical Diagnosis. The medical diagnosis of non-Hodgkin's lymphoma is made on the basis of history, physical assessment, and laboratory findings. Lymph node biopsies; bone, chest, and abdominal x-ray films and scans; and blood studies are the commonly used tests.

Medical Management. Medical management involves a lower dose of radiotherapy for localized non-Hodgkin's lymphoma than for Hodgkin's disease because the bone marrow is involved and it is more sensitive. Chemotherapy is given for nonlocalized non-Hodgkin's lymphoma. (Refer to Table 16–4 for common chemotherapeutic regimens used to treat non-Hodgkin's lymphomas.)

The prognosis varies for the non-Hodgkin's lymphomas. The chemotherapy combination COP (Cytoxan, Oncovin, and prednisone) produces some response in 90% of patients and complete response in

Table 16–4. CHEMOTHERAPY FOR NON-HODGKIN'S LYMPHOMAS

COP	CHOP	CHOP-BLEO	COPP	BACOP
Cyclophosphamide (Cytoxan)	Cytoxan	Cytoxan	Cytoxan	Bleomycin
Vincristine (Oncovin)	Doxorubicin Hydrochloride (Adriamycin)	Doxorubicin Hydrochloride	Oncovin	Doxorubicin Hydrochloride (Adriamycin)
Prednisone	Oncovin	Oncovin	Procarbazine	Cytoxan
	Prednisone	Prednisone	Prednisone	Oncovin
		Bleomycin		Prednisone

Nursing Care Guide 16–3.

PATIENTS WITH LYMPHOMAS

Assessment Findings: Patient complains of dyspnea, chest pain, hoarseness, cyanosis, and nonproductive cough.

Nursing Diagnosis: Ineffective airway clearance related to tracheobronchial obstruction, enlarged nodes, airway edema, or superior vena cava syndrome

Patient Outcomes	Nursing Interventions	Rationale
Patient exhibits a decrease in labored respirations without signs of pallor or cyanosis.	Assess respiratory status, rate, and rhythm. Observe for dyspnea, cyanosis, pallor, and cough. Auscultate chest.	Changes in respiratory pattern may indicate an airway problem.
Patient's chest is fully expanded, with respiratory rate maintained within normal range.	Teach patient how to maximize chest expansion. Administer oxygen as needed.	Maximizing chest expansion increases effectiveness of inspiratory pattern.
Patient completes activities of daily living without signs of respiratory difficulty or complaints of fatigue.	Promote rest and relaxation. Identify energy-saving techniques. Provide a quiet environment. Assist patient with activities of daily living. Administer cough suppressants as indicated.	Increased rest periods decrease fatigue and respiratory efforts.

Evaluation: Compare the patient's status with the expected patient outcomes. If the outcomes are achieved, evaluate nursing care as successful. If not, reassess the patient, formulate new nursing diagnoses, and revise expected patient outcomes and nursing interventions as appropriate.

Assessment Findings: Patient experiences anorexia, dysphagia, unexplained weight loss, and edema.

Nursing Diagnosis: Altered nutrition, less than body requirements, related to enlarged nodes, pressure on esophagus, or anorexia

Patient Outcomes	Nursing Interventions	Rationale
Patient's appetite improves.	Encourage frequent small meals. Serve attractive meals of patient's choice of foods.	Frequent small meals served attractively help promote a better nutritional intake.
Patient verbalizes information regarding proper food intake.	Tell the patient to eat a diet high in calories, protein, and vitamins. Use soft or puréed foods if dysphagia persists.	Proper nutrition is necessary for general health maintenance and promotion of healing.

(continued)

Nursing Care Guide 16–3. *(continued)*

PATIENTS WITH LYMPHOMAS

Patient Outcomes	Nursing Interventions	Rationale
Patient maintains appropriate weight level.	Weigh patient daily. Keep accurate intake and output. Commend the patient for following the plan and maintaining a proper weight level. Offer frequent snacks between meals.	Monitoring the patient's progress with encouragement to continue to follow diet plan increases patient's self-esteem and promotes compliance with the treatment.

Evaluation: Compare the patient's status with the expected patient outcomes. If the outcomes are achieved, evaluate nursing care as successful. If not, reassess the patient, formulate new nursing diagnoses, and revise expected patient outcomes and nursing interventions as appropriate.

Assessment Findings: Patient exhibits behavior of crying, irritability, withdrawal, anger, and fear; threatens harm to self.

Nursing Diagnosis: Anxiety related to diagnosis and fear of dying

Patient Outcomes	Nursing Interventions	Rationale
Patient verbalizes fears and concerns.	Encourage patient to verbalize concerns, fears, and questions regarding disease process and prognosis. Refrain from making judgments about the patient's fears.	Verbalization in a nonthreatening environment alleviates some of the distress and allows for free expression.
Patient and family demonstrate reduced anxiety and fear.	Encourage the family to participate.	Including the family gives support to the patient and allows them to freely express their concerns.
Patient exhibits coping mechanisms to deal effectively with problems.	Reassure patient that the fears are common and are experienced by most patients. Seek professional counseling assistance. Invite friends and clergy to visit. Identify coping strategies in patient and family.	Finding effective coping strategies is important to alleviate the anxiety. At times, professional assistance is necessary.

Evaluation: Compare the patient's status with the expected patient outcomes. If the outcomes are achieved, evaluate nursing care as successful. If not, reassess the patient, formulate new nursing diagnoses, and revise expected patient outcomes and nursing interventions as appropriate.

(continued)

Nursing Care Guide 16–3. *(continued)*

PATIENTS WITH LYMPHOMAS

Assessment Findings: Patient asks questions about disease process and treatment; expresses concerns about self-care.

Nursing Diagnosis: Knowledge deficit: nature of disease, treatment, and health care needed

Patient Outcomes	Nursing Interventions	Rationale
Patient verbalizes accurate information about disease, treatment, and self-care.	Explain the disease process, treatments, and health care needs the patient will experience. Give patient written information when possible.	An understanding of the disease and its treatment and prognosis is important to increase the patient's compliance and prevent complications.
Patient relates the importance of health maintenance and complication prevention.	Have the patient reiterate the information provided by the physician and the nurse. Include family or significant others in the education sessions. Teach patient self-care health behaviors. Describe complications of the disease and prevention methods.	Reinforcement of information helps ensure understanding and allows for corrections to be made if misinformation is present. Including the family adds additional reinforcement and provides support for the patient.
Patient states names and dosages of the medications and the side effects of each.	Inform patient of the medications used, side effects, and dosages.	Knowledge of the medications may decrease medication problems such as misuse or incorrect dosage once the patient is at home.
Patient relates the treatment strategies, coping mechanisms to assist in reducing side effects, and self-care necessary.	Discuss the importance of preventing infections, maintaining adequate nutrition, and getting maximum rest. Teach patient how to utilize coping mechanisms to reduce stress, pain, and other side effects.	Increased knowledge of self-care and prevention of complications decreases patient's risk of problems.

Evaluation: Compare the patient's status with the expected patient outcomes. If the outcomes are achieved, evaluate nursing care as successful. If not, reassess the patient, formulate new nursing diagnoses, and revise expected patient outcomes and nursing interventions as appropriate.

60% to 70% of patients. Cytoxan taken orally results in complete remissions in 55% of patients, with a median survival time of more than 5 years.

In patients with diffuse histiocytic lymphoma (DHL), combination chemotherapy is also preferred over single agents. COP, COPP (COP and Procarbazine), MOPP, CHOP (COP and Adriamycin), and others result in complete responses in 40% to 50% of patients, whose median survival time is more than 3 years. Patients with nodular lymphocytic and histiocytic lymphoma have had complete responses with single agents, and 50% to 70% of patients treated with COP, COPP, MOPP, and other regimens have experienced a median survival time of 4.5 years for those who attained a complete response and 13 months for those with a partial response.

Application of the Nursing Process to the Care of the Patient with Non-Hodgkin's Lymphoma

The assessment, nursing diagnoses, expected patient outcomes, nursing interventions, and evaluation for patients with non-Hodgkin's lymphomas are similar to those described previously for patients with Hodgkin's disease (Nursing Care Guide 16–3).

MULTIPLE MYELOMA

Etiology and Pathophysiology. Multiple myeloma is a malignant disease characterized by the growth of plasma cells, invading bone marrow, lymph nodes, liver, spleen, and kidneys. The cause of the disease is unknown. Multiple myeloma develops slowly over a period of time and occurs in clients older than 40 years of age. It is twice as common in men as in women. Usually, bone marrow is 5% plasma cells, but in multiple myeloma, bone marrow is 30% to 95% plasma cells, most of which are immature and malignant.

Clinical Manifestations. Clinical manifestations include the development of pneumonia, anemia, thrombocytopenia, and vascular insufficiency. Anemia, hemorrhage, and infection may occur as a result of impaired production of red blood cells, white blood cells, and platelets, resulting from replacement of bone marrow with plasma cells.

Neurologic complications result from the tumor pressing on the spinal cord, causing paraplegia. Skeletal changes may occur from osteoporosis, pathologic fractures, and bone deformities.

Increased bilirubin and sedimentation rates and low sodium and chloride levels occur because of an increased susceptibility to infection as a result of impaired antibody formation. This is caused by plasma cell abnormalities in the bone marrow. Folate deficiency is present when the tumor absorbs the folate or the individual consumes a low amount of dietary folate.

Hypercalcemia, uremia, and renal stones may be present owing to inactivity and calcium and phosphorus lost in damaged bones. Bence Jones protein may be present in urine. These particles of protein are produced by malignant plasma cells in the bone tumors and may block convoluted tubules, resulting in renal disorders or failure. Osteolysis occurs if the tumor cells cause the marrow cavity to expand. Osteoporosis, backache, or bone pain results from skeletal involvement. Skeletal deformities occur in the sternum and ribs. The spine may be shortened. Multiple osteolytic lesions in the skull may be present.

Amyloidosis occurs in approximately 10% of all patients. Symptoms depend on the organ involved.

Medical Diagnosis. The medical diagnosis of multiple myeloma is made on the basis of history, physical assessment, and laboratory studies, including serum electrophoresis and Bence Jones protein in urine. Skull x-ray films are ordered to detect the presence of lesions. Bone marrow aspiration and biopsy are repeated every 6 to 12 months. Serum electrophoresis and urine protein electrophoresis are completed with each course of therapy and every 2 to 3 months during remission to determine the progress of the disorder.

Medical Management. Medical management involves chemotherapy to reduce pain and bone tumor size and growth. Melphalan (Alkeran) and cyclophosphamide (Cytoxan) are two common alkylating agents used to treat individuals with multiple myeloma. Alkeran, the most successful drug, has side effects of bone marrow depression and pancytopenia. Cytoxan has side effects of leukopenia, nausea, alopecia, and hemorrhagic cystitis. Blood counts are monitored weekly to determine occurrence of myelosuppression.

Radiotherapy is used to treat spinal cord compression and pain unrelieved by chemotherapy. However, its use is limited because it may suppress marrow, which would limit the use of chemotherapy. Research studies also demonstrate that interferon has antitumor activity against multiple myeloma.

Anemia is treated with transfusions of packed red blood cells, and infections are treated with broad-spectrum antibiotics. Hypercalcemia, nausea, vomiting, and bone pain are treated with diuresis, prednisone, and mithramycin to help increase the secretion and catabolism. Allopurinol is used to treat and prevent hyperuricemia. Pain is also treated with a variety of analgesics.

The median survival time for untreated patients is less than 1 year; and for treated patients, it is 20 to 30 months. Fewer than 10% of patients survive more than 5 years.

Application of the Nursing Process to the Care of the Patient with Multiple Myeloma

Assessment

Review the history, and complete a physical assessment. Assess for diminished or absent breath sounds over the involved areas. Listen for inspiratory rales and decreased resonance over areas of infiltration. Check for pallor, dry skin with poor turgor, nostril-flaring cyanosis, use of accessory muscles, elevated temperature, rapid pulse, and tachypnea.

Observe for symptoms related to the presence of renal stones and changes in urinary output. Monitor the laboratory data for the presence of Bence Jones protein in the urine. Check for signs of dehydration resulting from poor intake and vomiting caused by chemotherapy.

Observe for somnolence, polydipsia, anorexia, peripheral neuropathy, and constipation, which are indicative of hypercalcemia or uremia. Assess for dilated and tortuous retinal veins, papilledema, retinal hemorrhages, and epistaxis. Check the laboratory studies for the presence of calcium in blood or urine.

Observe for changes in activity and ambulation. Assess the patient for pathologic fractures of the ribs and weight-bearing bones and compression fractures of the spine due to osteoporosis. These may be evidenced by sudden, severe pain usually related to lifting or bending. Other clinical signs include kyphosis and loss of height. Check for changes in the pelvis, spine, and ribs that worsen with movement.

Dysrhythmias, ecchymoses, peripheral nerve involvement, and gastrointestinal disturbances are common symptoms of amyloidosis, a complication of the disease.

Assess the patient's level of anxiety regarding the disease and prognosis. Check for an understanding of the treatment necessary and the complications.

Nursing Diagnoses and Planning

Nursing diagnoses and related expected patient outcomes most commonly applicable to patients with multiple myeloma include those previously described under Hodgkin's disease and the following:

NDx: Pain related to malignant infiltration into bone

Planning: Patient outcomes

1. Patient reports pain is controlled with analgesics.
2. Patient states comfort measures to help relieve pain.
3. Patient states coping measures to help relieve or tolerate pain.

Nursing Interventions

NDx: Pain
Place the patient in comfortable positions and reposition frequently. Use pillows to support bony prominences. Assess when the pain is most severe, and allow the patient to rest during those periods. Give pain medications as ordered prior to activity periods so that the patient can better tolerate the movement.

Help the patient find alternate methods to alleviate or to be able to tolerate the pain. Show the patient and family relaxation techniques and how to perform massage. Teach the patient the use of patient-controlled analgesia (PCA) if ordered.

Additional Interventions
Assist the patient in counteracting calcium overload by promoting increased fluid intake to as much as 4000 ml/day. Record intake and output, and note the color and consistency of the urine.

Prevent the complications of hypercalcemia and osteoporosis. Encourage ambulation and range-of-motion exercises as tolerated, as well as the use of canes, crutches, or a brace if necessary. Assist the patient with ambulation.

Promote good safety measures. Keep the side rails up. Use a trapeze for easier patient movement. Place personal items within reach of the patient.

Provide comfort by repositioning frequently and using pillows for support. Give good skin care without using harsh soap or rough towels. Use lotion on dry skin. Massage easily but frequently.

Evaluation

Evaluate the effectiveness of nursing care for a patient with multiple myeloma by comparing the patient's status with the expected patient outcomes. Examples of specific outcomes for patients with multiple myeloma have been provided in the Planning section.

Infections

Infectious Mononucleosis

Etiology and Pathophysiology. Infectious mononucleosis is a benign, self-limiting disease with mild, widespread effects throughout the body. It is caused by a herpes-like virus called the Epstein-Barr virus. Incubation period can be as long as several weeks. Mononucleosis commonly occurs in individuals with impaired body defenses and low resistance. It is estimated that 50% to 80% of the world's population

is infected with the Epstein-Barr virus, but only individuals with antibodies to the virus develop infectious mononucleosis.

Infectious mononucleosis is most common in children between 3 and 5 years of age and young persons between 15 and 30 years of age. The exact mode of transmission is unknown.

Clinical Manifestations. Symptoms include the presence of lymphocytosis, headache, sore throat, fever, chills, malaise, and generalized weakness and fatigue. Painful enlargement of the cervical, axillary, and groin lymph nodes is common. The acute phase may last as long as a month, followed by an extended recovery period.

Splenomegaly may cause pain in the left upper quadrant. Hepatomegaly may indicate rare liver involvement. The nervous system may be affected by the increase in mononuclear leukocytes and pressure of enlarged organs or nerves.

Medical Diagnosis. The medical diagnosis of infectious mononucleosis is made on the basis of history, physical assessment, and laboratory studies such as white blood cell count, positive heterophile agglutination test results, and an increase in mononuclear leukocytes.

Medical Management. The primary management of mononucleosis is symptomatic. Bed rest is recommended. Salicylates are prescribed to reduce the fever, and antibiotics are used to suppress infections. The prognosis is excellent, and recovery usually occurs in 2 to 4 weeks. Rarely, a splenic rupture may occur from increased lymphocytes in the spleen. This may be evidenced by abdominal pain and shock. Emergency surgery is required to treat a splenic rupture.

Guidelines for Application of the Nursing Process to the Care of the Patient with Infectious Mononucleosis

Check the history, and complete a physical examination of the patient. Observe for a sore throat, increased nasal secretions, generalized aches, and symptoms typical of influenza. Palpate for an enlarged liver and lymph nodes predominantly in the posterior cervical, axillary, and groin regions. Assess for left upper quadrant pain, indicating splenic enlargement. Look for the presence of a macular rash. Check the nutritional status of the patient. Assess for headaches and vertigo, indicating nervous system involvement. Observe for activity level changes such as weakness and inability to perform activities of daily living owing to extreme fatigue.

The nursing diagnoses, expected patient outcomes, nursing interventions, and evaluation for patients with infectious mononucleosis are similar to those described previously for patients with anemia. The patient with infectious mononucleosis is rarely hospitalized for treatment unless there are complicating factors present such as other infections or debilitation and extreme fatigue from long-term poor nutrition. If this is the case, also focus on the specific manifestations of the complications.

Bleeding Disorders

Bleeding disorders are classified as either purpuras, an extravasation of a small amount of blood into the tissues and mucous membranes, or coagulation disorders. Purpuras are further divided into vascular purpuras or purpuras due to platelet disorders. Coagulation disorders include disseminated intravascular coagulation (DIC), acquired hypoprothrombinemia, and hemophilia. Major deficiencies underlying bleeding disorders include weak, damaged vessels prone to rupture, platelet deficiency or thrombocytopenia, impairment or lack of one of the clotting factors, and impaired fibrinolysis.

Purpuras

Etiology and Pathophysiology. Purpuras are either vascular, resulting from vessel damage or rupture; or thrombocytopenic, resulting from platelet deficiency. In vascular purpuras, bleeding into the tissues occurs when pressure on the small blood vessels causes tearing. This can result from exposure to chemicals and drugs, allergies, uremia, infections, injuries, and malnutrition.

Spontaneous bleeding into surrounding tissues may occur when the platelets are less than 100,000/mm^3. This low platelet count is referred to as thrombocytopenic purpura. There are two types of thrombocytopenic purpura: idiopathic thrombocytopenic purpura (ITP) and secondary thrombocytopenic purpura.

In ITP, the platelets are destroyed prematurely by antiplatelet antibodies. The cause is unknown, but the disorder frequently follows viral infections. Children tend to acquire acute ITP, whereas adults acquire chronic ITP. Unlike ITP, secondary thrombocytopenic purpuras result from drug sensitivity or from a primary disorder.

Clinical Manifestations. Clinical manifestations of purpuras include small amounts of bleeding into the tissues and mucous membranes, resulting in petechiae and ecchymoses. Epistaxis and prolonged oozing from small wounds are common. Hepatomegaly, splenomegaly, and hematuria may be present as a result of increased blood loss and the body's compensatory mechanisms.

Medical Diagnosis. The medical diagnosis is made on the basis of history, physical assessment, and laboratory studies, including platelet count, bleeding time, capillary fragility, partial thromboplastin time (PTT), prothrombin time (pro time), and fibrinogen level.

Medical Management. Medical management for purpuras in general includes removing the causative agent and administering platelet transfusions. Steroid therapy, such as prednisone, is used to reduce bleeding tendencies and to elevate the platelet count. Bleeding usually ceases within 2 days with steroid therapy, and platelet counts rise within a week.

A splenectomy may be required, which results in remission in 60% to 80% of patients (see Splenectomy, Chapter 15). Immunosuppressive drugs may be used if the splenectomy does not correct the problem.

Complications include hemorrhaging of the gastrointestinal tract and cerebral vessels. Nerve pain is evident by numbness and tingling of extremities. Paralysis may occur if a hematoma presses on a nerve or on brain tissue. Acute renal failure may be due to a severe complication. Prognosis for recovery without medical management is 10% to 20% for adults. With treatment, the prognosis is excellent.

Application of the Nursing Process to the Care of the Patient with Purpura

Assessment

Check the patient's history for the cause of the disorder, and complete a physical assessment. Assess for bleeding into the joints by checking for pain or edema. Look for other signs of bleeding such as ecchymoses, petechiae, hematomas, or epistaxis. Check the urine and stools for blood. Note the duration and severity of the bleeding. Check the laboratory studies for abnormal bleeding times and platelet counts.

Observe for faintness, tachycardia, hypotension, confusion, and air hunger indicative of hemorrhage. Check cardiopulmonary status. Monitor vital signs. Check peripheral pulses. Assess the level of consciousness and orientation to person, time, and environment.

Ask whether the patient has recently taken anticoagulants, aspirin, or drugs that suppress bone marrow function such as chloramphenicol or antineoplastic drugs. Assess for jaundice, and palpate the liver and spleen for enlargement.

Ask for the patient's history of any bleeding episodes or familial bleeding tendencies. Check the patient's level of understanding about bleeding disorders and prevention of hemorrhaging.

Nursing Diagnoses and Planning

Nursing diagnoses and related expected patient outcomes most commonly applicable to patients with purpuras include the following:

NDx: Altered tissue perfusion, cardiopulmonary, peripheral, and cerebral, related to destruction of platelets causing excessive bleeding

Planning: Patient outcomes
1. Patient's extremities are warm, color is adequate, and pulses are present.
2. Patient's laboratory studies are within normal ranges for the patient.
3. Patient denies headaches, confusion, or nausea.
4. Patient is able to perform activities of daily living without tachypnea, tachycardia, and dyspnea.

NDx: Knowledge deficit: nature of disease and prevention of complication of hemorrhage

Planning: Patient outcomes
1. Patient relates accurate information about the bleeding disorder, its clinical course, and the complication of hemorrhage.
2. Patient accurately states the signs of bleeding and when to notify the physician.
3. Patient presents no signs or symptoms of bleeding such as petechiae, ecchymoses, epistaxis, dark stools, and so on.
4. Patient verbalizes the measures necessary to prevent bleeding as listed in Chart 16–1.

Nursing Interventions

NDx: Altered tissue perfusion, cardiopulmonary, peripheral, and cerebral

Help the patient conserve oxygen needs by encouraging rest and limiting activities. Assist the patient with meals, if needed. Administer oxygen as needed. Elevate the head of the bed to aid in chest expansion.

Keep the patient in a comfortable position, and reposition frequently to release pressure. Utilize range-of-motion exercises to stimulate circulation. Monitor vital signs and laboratory studies to assess for changes and improvements in status. Encourage ambulation as tolerated, but provide for frequent rest periods to decrease cardiac workload. Assist the patient when ambulating, because decreased cerebral circulation may cause disorientation and vertigo.

Discourage smoking to avoid vasoconstriction. Remove constricting clothing, and keep heavy bed linen from restricting peripheral circulation. Keep the patient's legs in a nondependent position when not ambulating. Prevent any bleeding episodes if possible.

NDx: Knowledge deficit: nature of disease and complication of hemorrhage
Instruct the patient about the clinical course of the disease and the complication of hemorrhage. Teach the patient signs of bleeding to observe for and when to seek medical assistance. Explain the need for avoiding sharp objects, straight razors, contact sports, and injections and venipuncture whenever possible. Tell the patient to watch for discoloration of urine or stools (see Chart 16–1).

Explain proper oral hygiene methods necessary to prevent further irritation and ulceration of mucous membranes. Instruct the patient to use a soft toothbrush and to use mouthrinse frequently. Show how to inspect the oral cavity, checking the tongue and gums for early signs of irritation. Teach the patient to avoid extremely hot, spicy foods and acidic drinks to lessen oral and gastrointestinal irritation.

Tell the patient to carry an identification card listing the blood disorder, patient's name and address, name of physician, blood type, and a family member to call in an emergency.

Check the laboratory data for the bleeding times and platelet count. Be prepared for an emergency episode of bleeding. Tell the patient not to take aspirin because it may increase the bleeding time.

Evaluation

Evaluate the effectiveness of nursing care for a patient with purpura by comparing the patient's status with the expected patient outcomes. Examples of specific outcomes for patients with purpura have been provided in the Planning section.

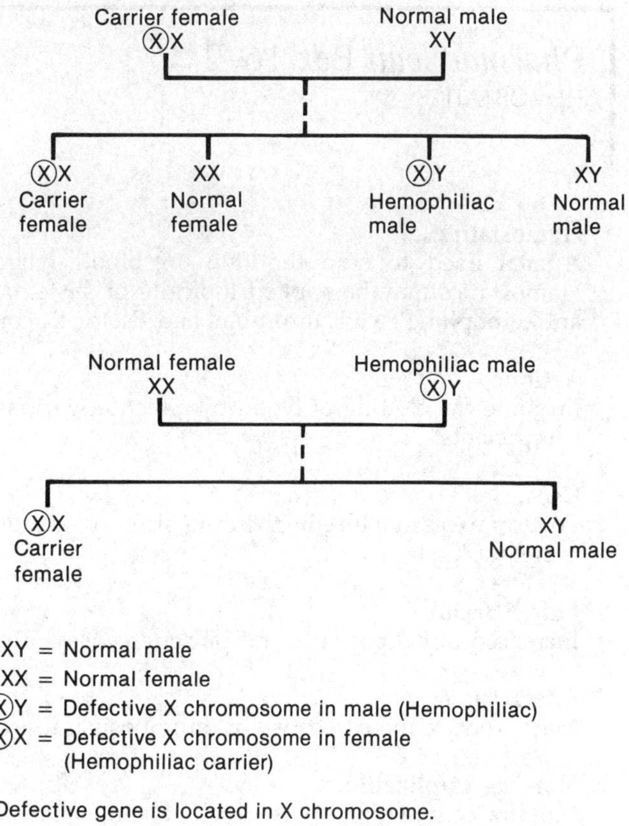

Figure 16–3.

Hemophilia heredity pattern.

Coagulation Disorders

Coagulation disorders may be hereditary or acquired and occur as a result of a decrease or absence of one or more clotting factors. The hereditary disorders are labeled as hemophilia A, B, or C and von Willebrand's disease. The most common acquired disorders are hypoprothrombinemia and disseminated intravascular coagulation (DIC).

HEMOPHILIAS

Etiology and Pathophysiology. The hemophilias, hereditary coagulation disorders, consist of four major types: hemophilia A (classic hemophilia), hemophilia B (Christmas disease), hemophilia C (Rosenthal's disease), and von Willebrand's disease. Hemophilia A is caused by an inherited deficiency of factor VIII, whereas hemophilia B is caused by an inherited deficiency of factor IX. Both are sex-linked recessive disorders transmitted by females, usually occurring in males and rarely in homozygous females. An example of the hereditary pattern of hemophilia is demonstrated in Figure 16–3. Hemophilia A occurs predominantly in children. Almost 80% of all hemophilias are hemophilia A.

Hemophilia C, an extremely rare type of hemophilia, is transmitted as an autosomal dominant trait. It is a deficiency of clotting factor XI. Only 2% of the hemophilias are hemophilia C.

Von Willebrand's disease is a bleeding disorder occurring in both males and females equally. It is caused by an inherited deficiency of factor VIII and impaired platelet function. It is transmitted as an autosomal dominant trait in both sexes.

Clinical Manifestations. Clinical manifestations of hemophilia include severe bleeding episodes from minor injuries. Coagulation time in hemophilia A and B is prolonged, whereas the bleeding time is normal. In von Willebrand's disease, both coagulation and bleeding times are prolonged with decreased platelet adhesiveness.

The nose, gums, and mouth may bleed with the slightest irritation because the clotting factor is absent. Minor trauma may result in slow, prolonged bleeding. On the other hand, the patient may expe-

Pharmacology Box 16–2.
HEMOSTATICS

Hemostatics:
Agents used to stop the flow of blood whenever excessive bleeding is or has been occurring. Hemostatics may be applied topically or systemically. Common hemostatics include aminocaproic acid, antihemophilic factor, thrombin, and Factor IX complex.

Action:
Promote the clotting of blood by affecting various components in the clotting cycle or replacing missing components.

Uses:
To stop excessive bleeding during surgery or after trauma, or to replace clotting factors in various types of hemophilia.

Side Effects:
Increased blood pressure and pulse rate. May also cause tingling, fever, chills, or headache.

Interactions:
May produce increased risk of thrombosis if used with aminocaproic acid.

Nursing Implications:
Monitor coagulation times; check patient's vital signs frequently. Report any significant changes.

rience a cut that does not bleed initially but begins to bleed days later. Bleeding into the joints (hemarthrosis) impedes movement of the extremities, while causing severe pain. Hematuria, gastrointestinal bleeding, or bleeding into the central nervous system may result from spontaneous bleeding or from increased intraabdominal or intracranial pressure. It is important to note that even the slightest injury may result in massive hemorrhaging because there is no mechanism for clotting present.

Medical Diagnosis. The medical diagnosis of hemophilia is made on the basis of history, physical assessment, and laboratory studies of coagulation and bleeding times, presence of factor VIII, IX, or XI, and platelet adhesiveness.

Medical Management. Medical management includes administering the deficient clotting factors, parenteral administration of plasma, cryoprecipitate, whole blood, or commercially prepared antihemophilic factor (AHF) (Pharmacology Box 16–2).

Joint pain and edema are controlled with analgesics and corticosteroids. Blood may be aspirated from the joint to alleviate pain. If bleeding into the joints is untreated, permanent damage is likely.

Complications include permanent joint deformity from hemarthrosis, and permanent nerve damage with paralysis from hematomas that compress the nerves.

Guidelines for Application of the Nursing Process to the Care of the Patient with Hemophilia

Check the patient's history for the type of hemophilia, treatment instituted, and frequency of bleeding episodes. Complete a physical assessment. Note any signs of bleeding, joint pain, hematomas, and limited movement. Assess the patient's level of understanding of the clinical course of the disease and prevention of complications.

The nursing diagnoses, expected patient outcomes, nursing interventions, and evaluation for patients with hemophilia are similar to those described previously for patients with purpuras. Focus nursing interventions on preventing further bleeding, promoting comfort, and teaching the patient and family about the disease, the necessary lifelong treatment, signs and symptoms of complications, and preventive measures (see Chart 16–1).

Stop any bleeding immediately by direct pressure. In hemarthrosis, pack the joints in ice to control the bleeding and edema. Assist the patient in preventing injury by promoting safety measures and avoiding the use of sharp objects around the patient. Teach the patient how to prevent bleeding. Promote a diet high in iron to replace losses from hemorrhage (see Nutrition Box 16–1).

The National Hemophilia Foundation serves as a resource for individuals with hemophilia and their families. Refer the patient to this organization for further assistance and information about the disease. Have the patient carry an identification card, noting the disease, physician, and blood type, at all times.

ACQUIRED HYPOPROTHROMBINEMIA

Etiology and Pathophysiology. In this disorder, there is a deficiency of prothrombin in the blood caused by either lack of vitamin K or excessive coumarin anticoagulants.

Clinical Manifestations. Clinical manifestations include ecchymosis and epistaxis resulting from minor trauma. Hematuria, gastrointestinal bleeding, postoperative hemorrhage from an incision, and prolonged bleeding from a venipuncture site may also be present.

Medical Diagnosis. The medical diagnosis of acquired hypoprothrombinemia is based on history, physical assessment, and prothrombin time.

Medical Management. Medical management involves the oral or parenteral administration of vitamin K and the discontinuation of the anticoagulant. Vitamin K may be administered intravenously for acute hemorrhage.

Application of the Nursing Process to the Care of the Patient with Acquired Hypoprothrombinemia

The assessment, nursing diagnoses, expected patient outcomes, nursing interventions, and evaluation for patients with acquired hypoprothrombinemia are similar to those described previously for patients with other bleeding disorders.

DISSEMINATED INTRAVASCULAR COAGULATION

Etiology and Pathophysiology. DIC is characterized by widespread coagulation in the arterioles and capillaries throughout the body. This coagulation results in disseminated fibrin deposits and microthrombi formation in the microcirculation, with subsequent depletion of clotting factors. Circulatory impairment results in infarcts and necrosis of tissues and organs. Renal failure associated with obstruction of the renal capillaries is especially common.

With the depletion of clotting factors, prolonged bleeding may occur spontaneously from mucous membranes or internal tissues or organs, or result from minor trauma or venipunctures. Bleeding episodes may vary from minimal oozing to massive hemorrhage.

Although the exact cause of DIC is unknown, it is usually associated with serious illness. Among the conditions that may predispose to DIC are metastatic cancer, acute leukemias, hemolytic transfusion reactions, massive tissue trauma, septicemia, abruptio placentae, septic abortion, surgery, and shock. Any individual with a predisposing condition who develops purpura, bleeding tendencies, or signs of renal failure should be evaluated for DIC.

Clinical Manifestations. Clinical manifestations include petechiae and ecchymoses, hematuria, and bleeding from any body orifice or venipuncture site. Gastrointestinal bleeding, oliguria, acute renal failure, convulsions, coma, and death may result from internal hemorrhage.

Medical Diagnosis. The medical diagnosis is based on history, physical assessment, and laboratory studies of prothrombin time, partial thromboplastin time, thrombin time, platelet count, and fibrinogen levels.

Medical Management. Medical management involves correcting the underlying condition, controlling the bleeding, and slowing the widespread coagulation. Administration of heparin slows the clotting process and allows restoration of clotting factors to normal levels. Severe hemorrhage is treated by transfusions of packed red blood cells and, possibly, clotting factors.

Guidelines for Application of the Nursing Process to the Care of the Patient with Disseminated Intravascular Coagulation

Assess the patient at risk for bleeding tendencies, internal bleeding, pain caused by pressure from hematomas, oliguria, and altered level of consciousness. Look for changes in vital signs indicating shock from hemorrhage. Watch laboratory data for changes in bleeding times and platelet counts. Prepare to deal with an acute hemorrhage.

The nursing diagnoses, expected patient outcomes, nursing interventions, and evaluation for patients with DIC are similar to those described previously for patients with other bleeding disorders.

The Elderly: Special Considerations

The older adult with disorders of the blood or blood-forming organs is usually at a higher risk of developing complications of the disease or the treatments than the younger adult. The decreased gastric motility, altered mucous membranes, diminished respiratory capacity, decreased circulation, and renal function in the aged all contribute to this high-risk status.

Of the hematologic disorders, anemia is the most common one found in the older adult. Generally, the cause of the anemia is poor dietary intake or inability to absorb dietary nutrients. Typically, the elderly patient presents a poor nutritional history. This may be due to financial status, lack of knowledge, or physical limitations affecting the ability to prepare food. Symptoms of anemia in the older adult may be attributed to other than a disease state. Fatigue is frequently attributed to the normal aging process rather than to an anemic condition. In most anemias, the oxygen-carrying capacity of the blood is decreased. Disorientation, headaches, weakness, dyspnea, and tachycardia caused by inability of the blood to carry enough oxygen to tissues may also be attributed to the normal aging process or to senility rather than to the disease.

Some of the types of leukemias are commonly found in the older adult. The older the individual, the more severe the symptoms and the progression of the disease. Chemotherapy or radiation therapy is often the choice for medical intervention in leukocyte disorders. The geriatric patient does not tolerate drug therapy well if the drugs have high toxicity levels, as do most chemotherapeutic agents. Reduced gastric motility, as well as other gastrointestinal changes, causes a significant increase in drug absorption. This enhances the chance of problems with the side effects of the therapy. The older adult is also more susceptible to other complications of drug and radiation therapy than the younger adult.

Anorexia is a major side effect of several therapeutic interventions for leukocyte disorders. In the older adult, anorexia may already be present prior to the therapy, and the therapy only aggravates it. It becomes a nursing challenge to improve the nutritional status of the aged patient receiving treatment for hematologic disorders. Mouth problems due to the disease process, the treatments, and to ill-fitting teeth are common. Nutritional supplements and soft, bland foods may be necessary if the patient has mouth problems that contribute to a malnourished state.

Disorders of the blood-forming organs in the elderly are usually due to other than hematologic problems. Cancer of the gastrointestional system that metastasizes to the spleen, lymph, bone, or liver is common. Cancer of the liver as the primary site is also frequently found in the aged. Males with prostatic cancer are often found to have metastasis to the bone. Interference with these organs can be manifested in symptoms of reduced oxygen-carrying capacity due to decreased numbers of red blood cells and bleeding problems caused by interference with production of the clotting factors.

It is extremely important to listen to the elderly patient, make astute observations, and review the patient's history to accurately diagnose and care for problems associated with the hematologic system. The older adult affected by disorders of the blood or blood-forming organs may be in a life-threatening state. Nursing interventions must be specific to the patient's needs and the disorder.

Bibliography

Alavi J. Sickle cell anemia: Pathophysiology and treatment. Med Clin North Am 1984; 68(3):545.

Ali N. Teaching osteoporosis prevention. Adv Clin Care 1991; 6(2):32.

Andres R, Bierman EL, Hazard W. Principles of geriatric medicine. New York: McGraw-Hill, 1985.

Baquie M. What matters most in chronic pain management. RN 1989; 52(3):46.

Baserga S, Benz E. Hematologic abnormalities: Approach to blood disorders in elderly patients. Consultant 1984; 24:309.

Bates B. A guide to physical examination. Philadelphia: JB Lippincott, 1989.

Block M. Text-atlas of hematology. Philadelphia: Lea & Febiger, 1976.

Brocklehurt JC. Textbook of geriatric medicine and gerontology. 3rd ed. New York: Churchill Livingstone, 1985.

Brown B. Hematology: Principles and procedures. 3rd ed. Philadelphia: Lea & Febiger, 1980.

Brown M, Kiss M. Standards of clinical nursing practice for leukemia: Anorexia, nausea and vomiting and fluid volume deficit. Cancer Nurs 1984; 7(1):62.

Brown M, Kiss M. Standards of clinical nursing practice for leukemia: Neutropenia and thrombocytopenia. Cancer Nurs 1983; 6(6):487.

Bulechek GM, McCloskey JC. Nursing interventions: Treatments for nursing diagnoses. Philadelphia: WB Saunders, 1985.

Bullock BL, Rossendahl PP. Pathophysiology adaption and alterations in function. Philadelphia: JB Lippincott, 1992.

Burggraf W, Donlon B. Assessing the elderly: System by system. Part one. Am J Nurs 1985; 85(9):974.

Carpenito LJ. Nursing diagnosis: Application to clinical practice. 3rd ed. Philadelphia: JB Lippincott, 1989–1990.

Cartlidge J. Haemophilia. Nurs Mirror 1984; 158(7):i.

Cassileth BR, Cassileth PA. Clinical care of the terminal cancer patient. Philadelphia: Lea & Febiger, 1982.

Cline M. Haskell C. Cancer chemotherapy. 3rd ed. Philadelphia: WB Saunders, 1980.

Dickinson R. Our way, VI ulcers heal. RN 1990; 90:32.

Doenges M, Jeffries MF, Moorhouse MF. Nursing care plans, nursing diagnoses in planning patient care. Philadelphia: FA Davis, 1984.

Fischer D, Marsh J. Cancer therapy. Boston: GK Hall Medical Publishers, 1982.

Fontana JA. Amyloidosis: A pathologic and clinical review. Crit Care Nurse 1989; 9(9):38.

Froberg J. The anemias: Causes and course of action. Part 1. RN 1989; 52(1):24.

Froberg J. The anemias: Causes and courses of action. Part 2. RN 1989; 52(3):52.

Froberg J. The anemias: Causes and courses of action. Part 3. RN 1989; 52(5):42.

Gill F. Congenital bleeding disorders: Hemophilia and Von Willebrand's disease. Med Clin North Am 1984; 68(3):601.

Greenspan E. Clinical interpretation and practice of cancer chemotherapy. New York: Raven Press, 1982
Greifu S, Radjeski D, Winnick B. Oral care is part of cancer care. RN 1990; 53(6):43.
Gunz F. (ed). Leukemia. 4th ed. New York: Grune & Stratton, 1983.
Hagan SJ. Bring help and hope to the patient with Hodgkin's disease. Nursing 83. 1983; 14:58.
Hagemeister FB, Fuller LM. Lymphoma and Hodgkin's disease: New imaging techniques help guide diagnosis and referral. Consultant 1984; 24:129.
Haller D. Non-Hodgkin's lymphomas. Med Clin North Am 1984; 68(3):741.
Henderson ML. Assessing the elderly: Altered presentations. Part 2. Am J Nurs 1985; 85(10):1103.
Ho MT, Saunders CE. Current emergency diagnosis and treatment. 3rd ed. Norwalk, CT: Appleton & Lange, 1990.
Illustrated manual of nursing practice. Springhouse, PA: Springhouse, 1991.
Iyer P, Taptich B, Bernocci-Losey D. Nursing process and nursing diagnosis. Philadelphia: WB Saunders, 1986.
Kellermeyer RW. General principles of the evaluation and therapy of anemias. Med Clin North Am 1984; 68(3):533.
Koch P. Thrombocytopenia: Don't let it make a big problem out of nothing. Nursing 84 1984; 84:55.
Krupp M, Schroeder S, Tierney L. Current medical diagnoses and treatment 1987. Norwalk, CT: Appleton & Lange, 1987.
Lankford TR, Steward PMJ. Foundations of normal and therapeutic nutrition. New York: John Wiley & Sons, 1986.
Leavell BS, Thorup OA. Fundamentals of clinical hematology. 4th ed. Philadelphia: WB Saunders, 1976.
Louria DB. Introduction and epidemiology: Infectious complications of neoplastic disease. Am J Med 1984; 76:414.
Marino LB. Cancer nursing. St. Louis: CV Mosby, 1981.
McGillick K. DIC: The deadly paradox. RN 1982; 45(8):41.
Miale J. Laboratory medicine: Hematology. 5th ed. St Louis: CV Mosby, 1977.
Moosa AR, Robson MC, Schimpff SC. Comprehensive textbook of oncology. Baltimore: Williams & Wilkins, 1986.
Newman K. The leukemias. Nurs Clin North Am 1985; 20(1):227.
Oken MM. Multiple myeloma. Med Clin North Am 1984; 68(3):757.
Pilot H. Fundamentals of oncology. 3rd ed. New York: Marcel Dekker, 1986.
Porth C. Pathophysiology, concepts of altered states. 3rd ed. Philadelphia: JB Lippincott, 1990.
Portlock D. Hodgkin's disease. Med Clin North Am 1984; 68(3):729.
Reiss BS, Melick ME. Pharmacological aspects of nursing care. 2nd ed. Albany, NY: Delmar Publishers, 1987.
Rivers R, Williamson N. Sickle cell anemia: Complex disease, nursing challenge. RN. 1990; 90(6):24.
Steffl BM. Handbook of gerontological nursing. New York: Van Nostrand Reinhold, 1984.
Taber's cyclopedic medical dictionary. 16th ed. Philadelphia: FA Davis, 1989.
Terry B. Hodgkin's disease and non-Hodgkin's lymphomas. Nurs Clin North Am 1985; 20(1):207.
Ulrich S, Canale SW, Wendell S. Nursing care planning guides: A Nursing diagnosis approach. Philadelphia: WB Saunders, 1986.
Williams W. Hematology. 3rd ed. New York: McGraw-Hill, 1983.
Wintrobe M. Clinical Hematology. 8th ed. Philadelphia: Lea & Febiger, 1981.
Wyngaarden J, Smith L. Cecil Textbook of Medicine. 17th ed. Vol 1. Philadelphia: WB Saunders, 1985.
Yurick AG, Spier BE, Robb SS, Ebert NJ. The aged person and the nursing process. 2nd ed. Norwalk, CT: Appleton-Century-Crofts, 1984.

Unit Six

ADULTS WITH CIRCULATORY DYSFUNCTION

Learning Objectives

AFTER COMPLETING THIS UNIT, THE LEARNER WILL BE ABLE TO:

Chapter Seventeen

1. Explain the normal anatomy and physiology of the heart.
2. Describe common clinical manifestations of cardiac dysfunction.
3. Compare and contrast the common cardiac rhythms found in specific cardiac disorders.
4. Identify the risk factors associated with coronary disease and the information and physical examination data essential to the assessment of cardiac status.
5. Identify the most common laboratory and radiologic studies used to diagnose cardiac disorders.
6. Describe medical management and surgical procedures commonly used in the treatment of patients with cardiac disorders.
7. Identify data essential to the assessment of patients undergoing treatment of cardiac disorders.
8. State nursing diagnoses and related expected patient outcomes commonly applicable to patients undergoing treatment of cardiac disorders.
9. Describe nursing interventions, with their rationales, commonly applicable to patients undergoing treatment of cardiac disorders.
10. Explain the basis for evaluation of nursing care provided to patients undergoing treatment of cardiac disorders.
11. Identify special considerations for the elderly patient with altered cardiac function.

Chapter Eighteen

1. Describe common cardiac disorders in terms of etiology, pathophysiology, clinical manifestations, diagnostic procedures, and medical management.
2. Identify common pharmacologic agents used to treat cardiac disorders.
3. Describe the health teaching appropriate for the patient who is at high risk for coronary artery disease.
4. Identify information and physical examination data essential to the assessment of patients with common cardiac disorders.
5. State nursing diagnoses and related expected patient outcomes commonly applicable to patients with cardiac disorders.
6. Describe nursing interventions, with their rationales, commonly applicable to patients with cardiac disorders.
7. Explain the basis for evaluation of nursing care provided to patients with common cardiac disorders.
8. Identify special considerations for the elderly patient with a cardiac disorder.

Chapter Nineteen

1. Explain the normal anatomy and physiology of the vascular system.
2. Identify the important risk factors for vascular disorders.
3. Describe common clinical manifestations of vascular dysfunction.
4. Identify information and physical examination data essential to the assessment of vascular status.
5. Compare and contrast the diagnostic studies used to identify vascular problems.
6. Describe medical management and surgical procedures commonly used in the treatment of patients with vascular disorders.
7. Describe the healing stages of leg ulcers.
8. Identify data essential to the assessment of patients undergoing treatment of vascular disorders.
9. State nursing diagnoses and related expected patient outcomes commonly applicable to patients undergoing treatment of vascular disorders.
10. Describe nursing interventions, with their rationales, commonly applicable to patients undergoing treatment of vascular disorders.
11. Explain the basis for evaluation of nursing care provided to patients undergoing treatment of vascular disorders.
12. Identify special considerations for the elderly patient with altered vascular function.

Chapter Twenty

1. Describe common vascular disorders in terms of etiology, pathophysiology, clinical manifestations, diagnostic procedures, and medical management.
2. Compare the common pharmacotherapeutic agents used to treat vascular disorders.
3. Identify information and physical examination data essential to the assessment of patients with common vascular disorders.
4. State nursing diagnoses and related expected patient outcomes commonly applicable to patients with vascular disorders.
5. Describe nursing interventions, with their rationales, commonly applicable to patients with vascular disorders.
6. Explain the basis for evaluation of nursing care provided to patients with common vascular disorders.
7. Identify special considerations for the elderly patient with a vascular disorder.

Chapter Seventeen

KNOWLEDGE BASIC TO THE NURSING CARE *of Adults with Cardiac Dysfunction*

Human life cannot exist without a functioning heart. The heart is unique in many ways when compared with other organs of the body. The heart's function is purely mechanical. It does not secrete, excrete, or produce any substances: It only pumps blood. The heart does not filter blood or exchange oxygen or any other products. It propels blood through a vast network of vessels to all body tissues. The heart's delivery system requires it to beat approximately 60 times per minute, 3600 times per hour, and 86,400 times per day for the lifetime of the individual. It is a very durable organ, able to accomplish this task without tiring or stopping to rest for many years in the healthy individual. The heart compensates quickly with a variety of insults to its own tissues and fails only in later stages of disease processes.

Anatomy and Physiology

The heart is a hollow, muscular pump that lies in the middle portion of the chest slightly to the left side. It is surrounded by the lungs on both the right and left sides. It sits between the sterum and ribs anteriorly and the vertebral column and attached ribs posteriorly.

Surrounding the heart is the pericardium, a fibrous sac filled with a small amount of fluid, which allows free motion of the pumping heart. The pericardium forms a barrier that protects the heart from infections of the lung and mediastinum and from external trauma to the chest wall.

Heart

The heart is composed of three layers: epicardium, myocardium, and endocardium. The epicardium is the outermost layer and covers the surface of the heart and the great vessels (pulmonary artery and aorta) and becomes continuous with the inner lining of the pericardium. The myocardium is the muscular portion of the heart and is the part responsible for pumping blood. The endocardium is the innermost layer, which is a thin, delicate sheath of tissue lining the inside of the cardiac chambers and covering the surface of the cardiac valves.

Cardiac Chambers and Great Vessels

The heart contains four chambers: two on the left side and two on the right. The right atrium lies laterally on the right side, whereas the right ventricle, the most anterior chamber of the heart, lies just beneath the sterum. The left atrium is the most posterior chamber of the heart. The left ventricle lies laterally on the left side (Fig. 17–1).

The chambers of the heart and the great vessels are separated by the heart valves and the septum. The valves keep the blood in a forward flow through all chambers of the heart. The septum separates the right and left sides of the heart. The right atrium receives blood from the head, arms, chest, legs, and abdomen, collectively called the systemic circulation (Fig. 17–2). The blood from the systemic circulation is venous blood, which is unoxygenated.

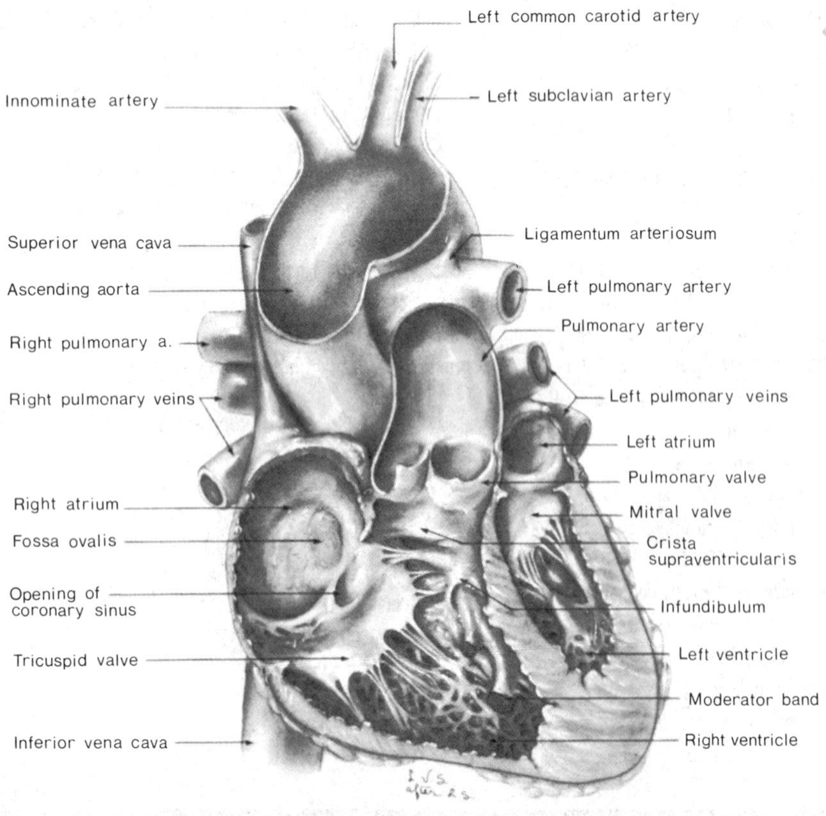

Figure 17–1.

Structures of the heart and their anatomic positions. (From Sanderson RG, Kurth CL. The cardiac patient. 2nd ed. Philadelphia: WB Saunders, 1983, p 5.)

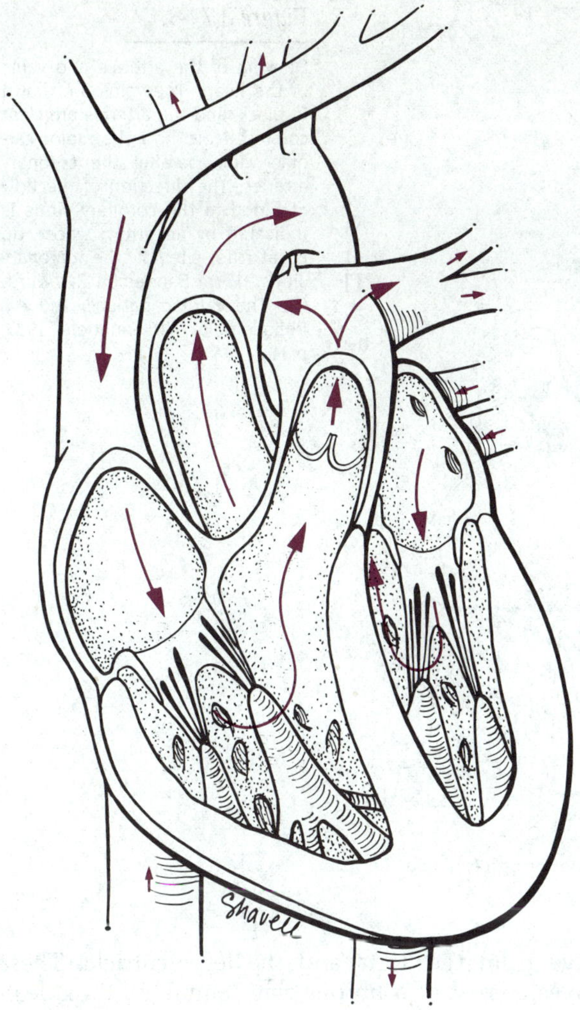

Figure 17–2.

Blood flows in a forward motion through the chambers of the heart, with the valves opening and closing in a coordinated manner.

The blood flows into the right atrium with greater force during inspiration because the right atrial pressure is lower than vena cava pressure during inspiration (chest expands, diaphragm descends, and pressure inside the chest cavity decreases). Because pressure in the venous system outside the chest cavity is higher than vena cava pressure, blood flows from the area of higher pressure to the area of lower pressure. The veins that lead directly into the right atrium are the superior vena cava (draining the upper part of the body), the inferior vena cava (draining the lower part of the body), the coronary sinus (draining blood from the circulation of the heart), and the multiple thebesian veins (draining blood directly from the atrial wall itself) (Fig. 17–3).

The right atrium is separated from the left atrium by the interatrial septum. During fetal life there is an opening in the interatrial septum to allow shunting of blood from the right atrium to the left atrium. The opening normally closes soon after birth, and there is no further shunting of blood across the interatrial septum.

The right atrium is separated from the right ventricle by the tricuspid valve (see Fig. 17–2). When the tricuspid valve opens, blood flows from the blood-filled right atrium to the right ventricle. The right atrium then contracts and empties its total contents of blood into the right ventricle, and the tricuspid valve closes. The outflow tract from the right ventricle is the pulmonary artery; the pulmonic valve allows blood to flow from the right ventricle to the main pulmonary artery. The pulmonic valve opens as the right ventricle contracts and propels blood through the pulmonary artery to the lungs. The main pulmonary artery branches into the right and left pulmonary arteries so blood is carried to both lung fields.

In the lungs, the blood exchanges carbon dioxide for oxygen and then returns to the left atrium via the network of pulmonary veins. The left atrium is separated from the left ventricle by the mitral valve. When the left atrium is filled with blood, the mitral valve opens and blood flows into the left ventricle. Again, the left atrial contraction occurs in conjunction with right atrial contraction, and blood is forced into the left ventricle for filling. The two ventricles are separated by the interventricular septum. The outflow tract from the left ventricle is the aorta; the aortic valve allows blood to flow into the aorta. When the aortic valve opens, blood is propelled by left ventricular contraction into the aorta. Aortic (arterial) blood is oxygenated and distributed to all body tissues.

The left atrium and ventricle are more muscular than the right atrium and ventricle. The left ventricle is the most muscular of all the heart chambers. The left ventricle generates pressures of 120 mm Hg or more to pump blood into arterial circulation. In comparison, the right ventricle generates pressures of about 20 mm Hg to pump blood into the pulmonary system. Left atrial pressure is approximately 5 to 10 mm Hg, and right atrial pressure is approximately 2 to 7 mm Hg normally.

Cardiac Valves

The tricuspid and mitral valves are called atrioventricular (AV) valves because they are situated between the atrium and ventricle on each side of the heart. The tricuspid valve is on the right side, and the mitral valve is on the left. The AV valves are composed of a fibrous supporting ring called the annulus, leaflets, supporting strands called chordae tendineae, and papillary muscles, which connect the chordae tendineae to the ventricular wall (Fig. 17–4).

The mitral valve has two leaflets or cusps, which is why it is also called the bicuspid valve. The cusps descend into the left ventricle during diastole, allowing a wide opening through which blood can flow. The two leaflets rise out of the ventricle and abut each other during systole to form a blood-tight seal against regurgitation of blood. The leaflets come

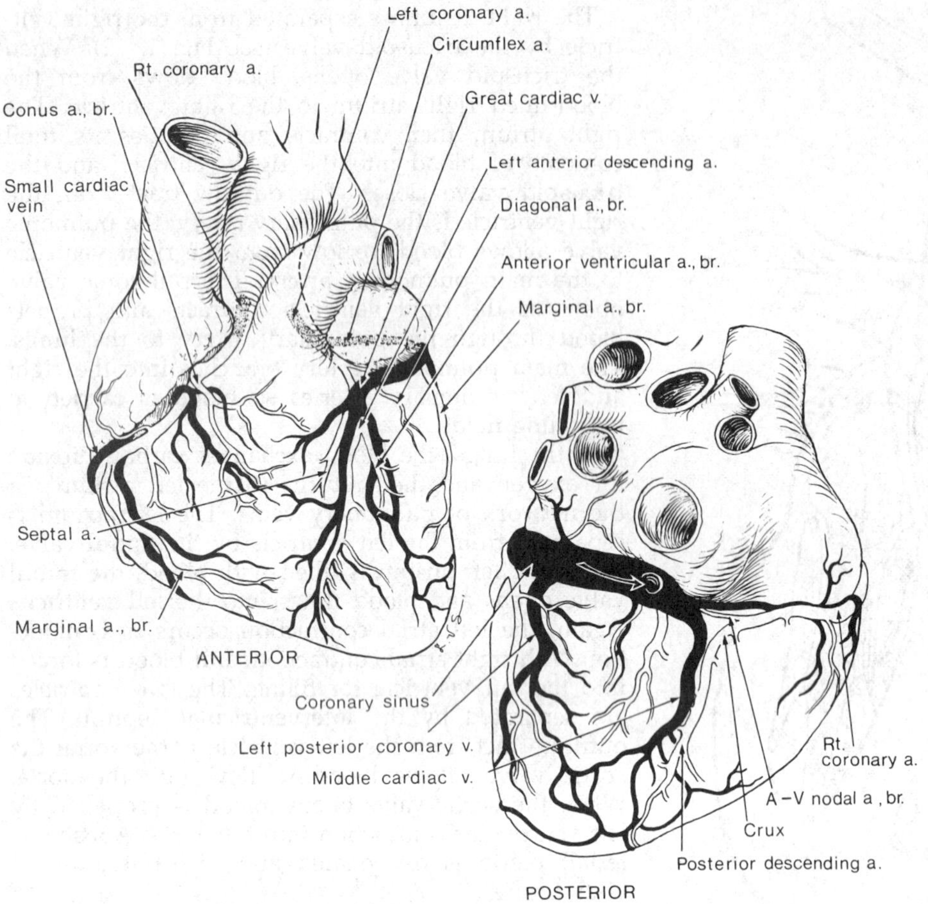

Figure 17–3.

Drawing of the arteries and veins of the heart. The veins are drawn in black, and the arteries are clear colored. Note how the major cardiac veins parallel the coronary arteries. The direction of the flow of blood in the coronary sinus is indicated by an arrow, whose tip is at the site of the coronary sinus. (From Sanderson RG, Kurth CL. The cardiac patient. 2nd ed. Philadelphia: WB Saunders, 1983, p 12.)

together and join with the annulus in junctional areas called commissures (Fig. 17–5).

The tricuspid valve has three leaflets or cusps, thus the name tricuspid valve (Fig. 17–6). The three leaflets abut each other during systole to form a seal so blood does not regurgitate into the right atrium.

The pulmonic and aortic valves are semilunar valves that separate the ventricular cavities from the arterial vessels: the pulmonic valve from the pulmonary artery and the right ventricle, and the aortic valve from the aorta and the left ventricle. These valves consist of a fibrous ring (annulus), three leaflets (cusps), and a small recess or outpocketing above each leaflet called the sinus of Valsalva in the aortic valve.

The three leaflets of the aortic valve float upward and toward the side walls of the aorta during ventricular systole, making a wide opening and allowing blood to be ejected into the aorta. During ventricular diastole, the leaflets descend and the edges

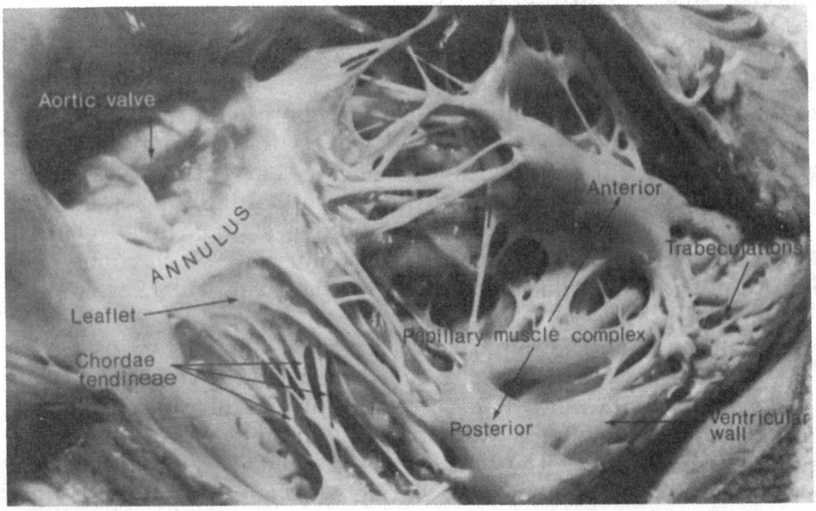

Figure 17–4.

Photograph of a mitral valve and its supporting structures—chordae tendineae, papillary muscles, and ventricular wall. (From Sanderson RG, Kurth CL. The cardiac patient. 2nd ed. Philadelphia: WB Saunders, 1983, p 7.)

meet, preventing regurgitation of blood through the valve.

The pulmonic valve lies between the right ventricle and the main pulmonary artery. It is composed of the same parts as the aortic valve, the annulus, and the three cusps, but its sinuses are not as well defined as those of the aortic valve.

Coronary Arteries

The coronary arteries supply the cardiac muscle with blood, oxygen, and nutrients for its continued function. Each coronary artery originates from a small opening in the wall of the aorta called an orifice or ostium. The left coronary artery (LCA) arises from above the left coronary cusp of the aortic valve, and the right coronary artery (RCA) arises from the right coronary cusp of the aortic valve. The third cusp of the aortic valve is the noncoronary cusp and is not associated with a coronary artery. The coronary arteries traverse the epicardial surface of the heart and are embedded in the fat that surrounds them. Branches of arteries grow off the sides of each artery and penetrate through to the myocardium to supply it with blood. The terminal portions of the arteries end in a collection or plexus of small vessels just inside the inner lining of the cardiac chambers, and they supply blood to the papillary muscles.

The RCA exits from the anterior surface of the aorta, passes diagonally toward the right side of the heart, and descends in the groove between the right atrium and right ventricle (see Fig. 17–3). It gives off a marginal branch that descends along the lateral margin of the heart to the apex and supplies blood to both the anterior and posterior surfaces of the right ventricle. The RCA continues right to left high across the posterior surface of the right ventricle. At the site of the sharp angulation or the crux, the RCA gives off a small branch to the AV node. The RCA

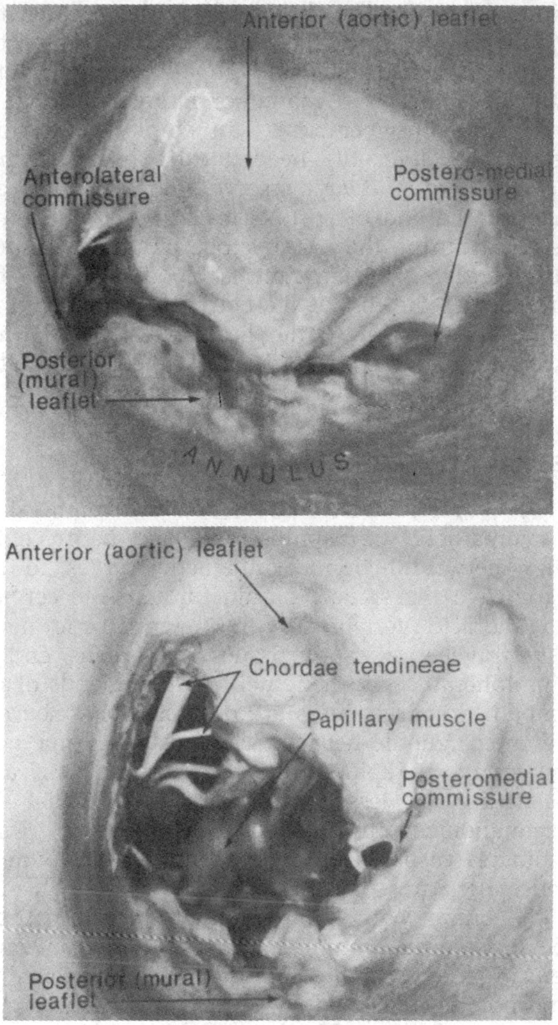

Figure 17–5.

Photograph of the mitral valve in the open (diastole, *bottom*) and closed (systole, *top*) positions. The joining of the leaflets into their commissures can be seen. (From Sanderson RG, Kurth CL. The cardiac patient. 2nd ed. Philadelphia: WB Saunders, 1983, p 8.)

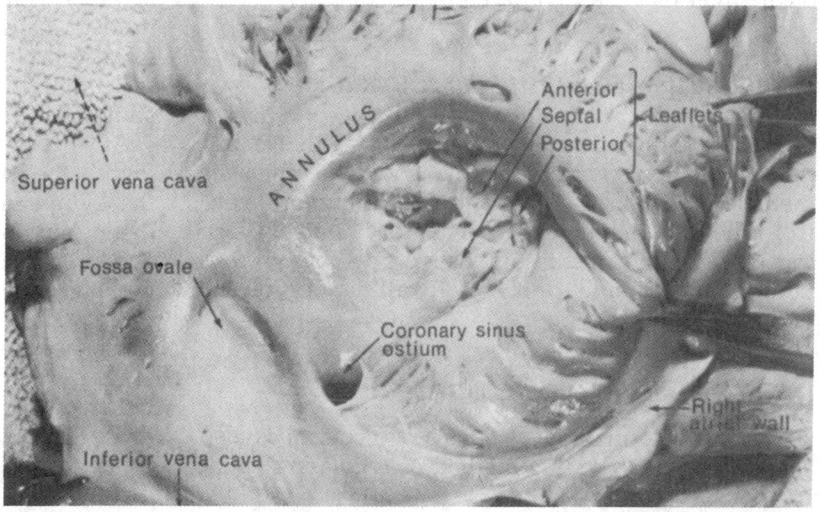

Figure 17–6.

Photograph of the interior of the right atrium, showing the three leaflets of the tricuspid valve, the opening of the coronary sinus, and the fossa ovale. (From Sanderson RG, Kurth CL. The cardiac patient. 2nd ed. Philadelphia: WB Saunders, 1983, p 9.)

ends in the posterior descending branch of the artery as it descends in the posterior interventricular groove. The RCA supplies blood to anterior portions of the right and left ventricles, the posterior portion of the right ventricle, the AV node, and the posterior portion of the interventricular septum. When the RCA provides the descending branch, as it does in about 80% of the cases, the RCA is said to be "predominant." In the remaining 20% of the cases, the LCA provides the posterior descending branch. In these cases, a left coronary system is said to be "predominant."

The LCA exits from the posterior surface of the aorta (see Fig. 17–3). It passes behind the pulmonary artery, gives off small arteries to the left atrium, and then separates into its two major divisions: the left anterior descending (LAD) artery and the circumflex (CF) artery. The LAD artery descends on the anterior surface of the heart in the groove between the right and left ventricles. It gives off septal branches that supply the anterior portion of the interventricular septum and anterior ventricular branches that supply the anterior surface of the left ventricle. A large diagonal branch supplies the lateral margin of the left ventricle. The circumflex artery passes around the left atrium and flows from the right to left high across the posterior surface of the heart in the AV groove in close association with the coronary sinus. Its major branch is the obtuse marginal branch, which supplies much of the posterior surface of the left ventricle.

Coronary Veins

The venous drainage system of the heart closely parallels the arterial inflow (see Fig. 17–3). Coronary veins accompany each of the major coronary arteries. All of the coronary veins flow into the coronary sinus, which is the large vein that passes from left to right high across the posterior cardiac surface and ends in the right atrium at the coronary sinus ostium between the tricuspid valve and the opening of the inferior vena cava (see Fig. 17–3).

Regulatory Mechanisms for Circulation

There are three regulatory mechanisms that maintain circulation of blood in the body: the intrinsic method of control, neural control, and humoral control. The three methods of circulatory control work together to give maximum delivery of blood containing oxygen and nutrients to all tissues of the body.

INTRINSIC METHOD OF CONTROL

The intrinsic method of circulatory control is also called the Frank-Starling method of regulating circulation. According to this method, the greater the amount of blood in the ventricles, the greater the amount of blood that is pumped during systole. Thus, if there is a demand for more blood at any given time, the ventricles can empty more completely to deliver the needed extra blood supply. Because there is always reserve volume in the ventricles at the end of systole, it can be emptied into the aorta during the next systolic pumping episode, thus increasing the amount of blood flow into the aorta and to the rest of the body. In a circular fashion, venous return to the heart is increased, thus increasing the amount of blood pumped through the heart and into the arterial system to tissues.

NEURAL CONTROL

The neural control of circulation is a combination of sympathetic, parasympathetic, and baroreceptor reflex nerve function. Sympathetic nerves to the heart leave the spinal column through the cervical and thoracic vertebrae. Other sympathetic nerve fibers travel to all body tissues and organs, ending in peripheral sympathetic nerves. At the ends of the sympathetic nerve fibers are postganglionic neurons and preganglionic neurons. The postganglionic neurons secrete norepinephrine, which stimulates vasoconstriction of vessels in tissues and organs. The preganglionic neurons secrete acetylcholine, which stimulates vasodilation of the same vessels. Sympathetic fibers are controlled by the vasomotor center in the brain. With stimulation of the sympathetic fibers, powerful vasodilation occurs in skeletal muscle, cardiac muscle and the brain. The fight or flight syndrome is explained by these sympathetic effects because to fight or flee the individual needs an increased amount of blood circulated to the brain and the skeletal muscles for quick thinking and quick action. To obtain an increased blood flow, vasoconstriction shunts blood from the kidneys (which reduces urine output), from the gut (which decreases digestion), from the spleen, and from the skin (which causes chills), to the core of the body (which is the heart and brain) and to the skeletal muscles as needed. During any stressful event, these changes usually occur. This requires a concomitant increase in heart rate and blood pressure. The heart is also stimulated by an increase in circulating epinephrine.

At the end of the stressful situation (fight or flight), the parasympathetic nervous system buffers the sympathetic nervous system. The parasympathetic nervous system contains both postganglionic and preganglionic neurons as does the sympathetic nervous system, but at both its preganglionic and postganglionic endings acetylcholine is secreted. Because acetylcholine stimulates vasodilation, this is the only effect the parasympathetic nervous system exerts on the vessels. Thus, blood flow is increased to the kidneys, gut, spleen, and skin, while the increased flow, needed during stress, is diverted away from skeletal muscle, cardiac muscle, and the brain. These areas are not vasoconstricted because they need high blood flow to maintain normal functions. With parasympathetic stimulation, there is a resultant decrease in heart rate and blood pressure.

The baroreceptors reside in the walls of large systemic arteries such as the internal carotid arteries and aortic arch. They have a spraylike nerve ending and are stimulated when they are stretched by an increase in pressure caused by increased blood flow through the internal carotid arteries and the aorta. Stimulation of the baroreceptors causes inhibition of the vasomotor center in the brain (decreased sympathetic stimulation) and excitation of the vagal center (increased parasympathetic stimulation). The result is decreased blood pressure and heart rate. Stimulation of the baroreceptors usually does not occur with an increase of 0 to 50 mm Hg; an increase of 50 to 200 mm Hg stimulates a maximum response; and an increase of more than 200 mm Hg stretches the receptors to a point at which they can no longer respond. A rising pressure stimulates more of a response than a stationary or falling pressure.

HUMORAL CONTROL

Humoral control of circulation is accomplished by release of epinephrine and norepinephrine from the adrenal medulla. Epinephrine and norepinephrine both are vasoconstricting substances and can divert blood from peripheral areas of the body to the core when needed. Secretion of aldosterone by the adrenal cortex aids in fluid control by providing retention of sodium and water in the vascular system when the body needs to conserve its fluid. Circulating epinephrine and norepinephrine cause an increase in blood pressure and heart rate.

Conduction System

Cardiac muscle is contractile tissue. The muscle cells of the heart are capable of initiating their own rhythmic action potentials without any nervous intervention or other stimulation. Rhythmic waves of contraction occur repeatedly to activate the pumping mechanism of the heart. The contractile characteristics of cardiac muscle reside in biochemical properties of the substances found in the tissue itself. Changes in the chemicals induce changes in cardiac rhythm and rate.

The electrolyte primarily responsible for the electrical charge at the cardiac cell membrane is potassium. In the sinoatrial (SA) node, there is continuous movement of potassium and sodium across the cellular membrane. As sodium moves into the cell, potassium moves out, causing the cell to fire. This impulse moves from cell to cell until all cardiac cells have fired. This total involvement of all cardiac cells is called depolarization. At the end of depolarization, sodium moves out of the cell and potassium moves back into the cell, causing repolarization. The electrochemical changes occurring as sodium and potassium move across the cellular membrane can be detected on the surface of the body and recorded. The resultant recording is the electrocardiogram (ECG or EKG).

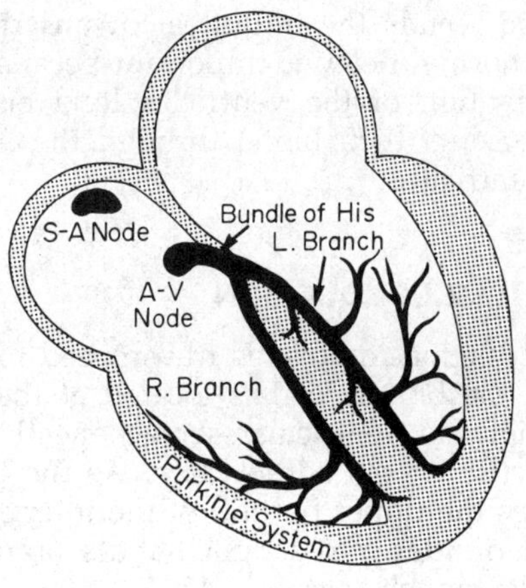

Figure 17–7.

Diagrammatic illustration of the conducting tissues. (From Sanderson RG, Kurth CL. The cardiac patient. 2nd ed. Philadelphia: WB Saunders, 1983, p 13.)

SINOATRIAL NODE

Normal cardiac conduction begins at the SA node, which is termed the pacemaker of the heart (Fig. 17–7). Its innate rate is about 60 to 100 beats per minute. Thus, in an adult, a heart rate of 60 to 100 beats per minute is considered to be normal. The SA node lies at the medial aspect of the junction between the superior vena cava and the right atrium. It is supplied with blood by a small atrial branch of the RCA.

ATRIOVENTRICULAR NODE

Transmission of the impulse occurs from the SA node to the AV node (see Fig. 17–7) through internodal tracts in the atrial muscle. The AV node is also called the AV junction or junctional pacemaker of the heart. Its innate rate is about 40 to 60 beats per minute and is the secondary pacemaker that takes over if the SA node is damaged or diseased and can no longer maintain its pacemaking responsibility. Because the AV node fires at a slower rate than the SA node, slower heart rates will be found if the AV node is setting the heart rate. The AV node lies at the base of the atrial septum just beneath the right atrial endocardium and rests very close to the coronary sinus ostium and to the septal leaflet of the tricuspid valve. The AV node receives its signals from the atrium and, after a delay of approximately

0.04 second, sends the impulses toward the ventricles. This normal delay is important because it postpones activation of the ventricles long enough for the atria to eject their blood through the AV valves into the ventricles.

VENTRICULAR CONDUCTION

The conduction impulse is transmitted to the ventricles via the bundle of His located at the junction of the atrial and ventricular septa beneath the noncoronary cusp of the aortic valve. As the bundle of His reaches the upper portion of the interventricular septum, it divides into a right bundle branch and a left bundle branch (see Fig. 17–7). These branches then descend in the interventricular septum and terminate in the Purkinje fibers, which carry the impulse to the ventricular musculature. The left bundle branch divides into parts as it exits the septum: the left anterior bundle branch and the left posterior bundle branch, which supply electrical conduction to the large left ventricle. The ventricles are capable of initiating their own action potentials and may do so if both the SA and AV nodes are incapable of providing pacemaking for the heart. The innate rate of the ventricles is approximately 20 to 40 beats per minute, a heart rate that is not very compatible with an active life. Therefore, an artificial pacemaker is implanted in cases in which the ventricles pace the heart.

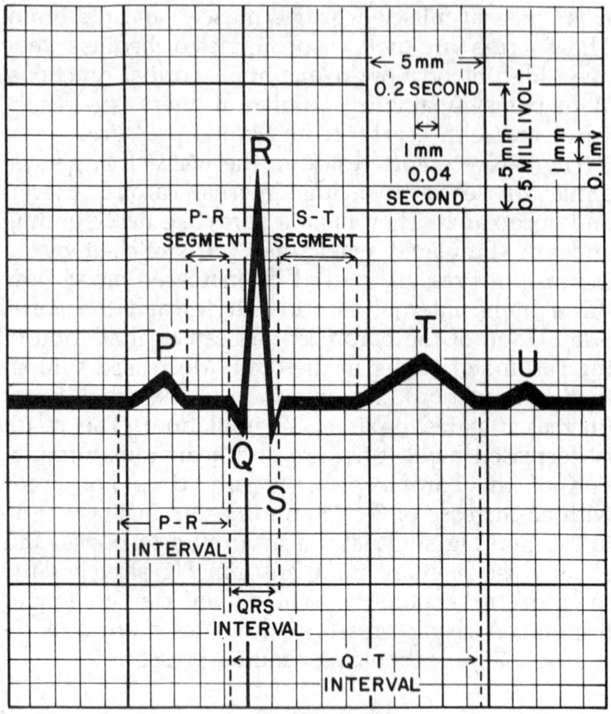

Figure 17–8.

Normal electrocardiogram (ECG) complex. The complex is superimposed on the standard electrocardiographic paper at customary amplitude (1 mm = 0.1 mv) and paper speed (25 mm per second). (From Sanderson RG, Kurth CL. The cardiac patient. 2nd ed. Philadelphia: WB Saunders, 1983, p 129.)

ELECTROCARDIOGRAM

Wave patterns are generated by the electrical impulses as they travel through the different parts of the cardiac conduction system. As the wave patterns are recorded on the ECG, they are labeled P, Q, R, S, T, and U.

As atrial excitation begins in the SA node and spreads through the right and left atria, atrial depolarization is initiated. Atrial depolarization is represented on the ECG as a P wave (Fig. 17–8). In normal rhythm, the P wave should be the first wave seen in the cardiac cycle. The upstroke of the P wave represents the beginning of atrial depolarization, and the return of the P wave to baseline marks the completion of atrial depolarization. Thus, the width of the P wave represents the time necessary for the atrial activation process.

After atrial depolarization, an absence of electrical activity is noted on the ECG for a brief period, representing passage of the impulse from the atria through the AV node and the bundle of His to the ventricular myocardium. This flat, or isoelectric, line represents the early phase of atrial repolarization. The passage of time is labeled as the PR interval and is measured from the beginning of the P wave to the beginning of the QRS complex (see Fig. 17–8).

Ventricular depolarization is represented on the ECG by the waveform labeled QRS (see Fig. 17–8). The Q wave is always the first downward or negative deflection, and the R wave is always the first upward or positive deflection. If there is a second negative deflection after the R wave, it is labeled an S wave. In certain leads of the ECG, a Q wave may not be obvious. Even if a Q wave is not obvious, the ventricular depolarization wave is still called the QRS complex. The QRS waveform represents ventricular depolarization, and it is during this period of time that actual atrial repolarization occurs. It is important to remember that electrical depolarization occurs before cardiac muscle contraction and that electrical repolarization follows cardiac muscle contraction.

After ventricular activation, ventricular repolarization begins. The ST segment is a flat (isoelectric) line between the S wave and the T wave, and it represents the early phases of ventricular muscle recovery (see Fig. 17–8). The T wave represents the actual recovery, or repolarization, of the ventricular muscle. Occasionally, an additional waveform, a U wave, can be observed after the T wave. The origin of the U wave is not well understood, but it is considered a significant finding in hypokalemic states. Figure 17–8 represents one cardiac cycle and the various electrical events that occur in the cycle.

The ECG recording paper is run at a uniform

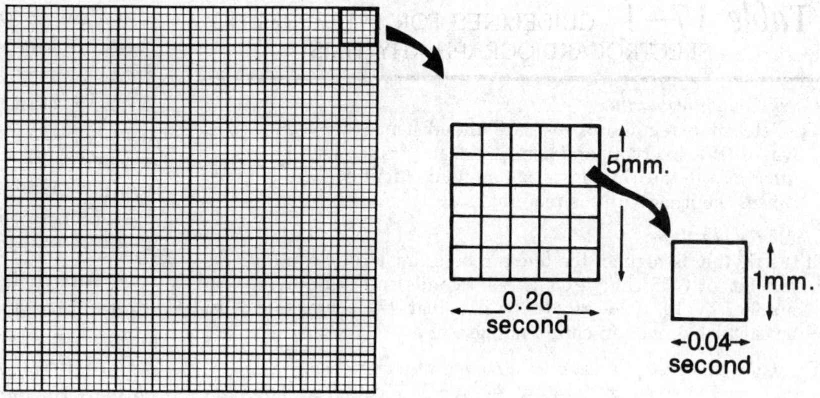

Figure 17–9.

One large ECG square is equivalent to 0.20 second. One small ECG square is equivalent to 0.04 second. (From Sanderson RG, Kurth CL. The cardiac patient. 2nd ed. Philadelphia: WB Saunders, 1983, p 129.)

speed of 25 mm/second to facilitate time measurement of the various electrical events. ECG paper is subdivided horizontally and vertically with 1-mm and 5-mm boldfaced, spaced lines (Fig. 17–9). The vertical lines represent time intervals, and the space between two 1-mm lines, or the space in one small square, represents 0.04 second. Thus, two small squares represent 0.08 second, three small squares represent 0.12 second, and so forth. The space across five small squares or one large square represents 0.20 second (Fig. 17–9).

For convenience, ECG recording paper displays a marker every 3 seconds (Fig. 17–10). There are 15 large (5 mm) squares per 3-second marker. Fifteen large squares, the distance between two markers, represent 3.0 seconds. Two of these distances is equal to 6.0 seconds; thus, the number of QRS complexes in a 6.0-second period can be counted. This is multiplied by 10 to obtain an approximate heart rate per minute.

Normal conduction time from the atria, through the AV node, and to the ventricular myocardium is between 0.12 and 0.20 second and is represented by the PR interval. The PR interval is measured from the beginning of the P wave to the beginning of the QRS complex, not including the Q wave (see Fig. 17–8). A deviation from this "normal" PR interval represents pathology that either accelerates or delays conduction of the impulse.

Normal ventricular depolarization time should occur in less than 0.12 second and is represented by the QRS interval. The QRS interval is measured from the beginning of the Q wave to the point at which the S wave ends or reaches baseline (ST segment) (see Fig. 17–8).

The physiologic pacemaker of the heart is the SA node because of its high rate of automaticity. The rhythm that is generated by the SA node is known as a sinus rhythm and is characteristically regular. To determine regularity, the distance between two R waves is measured and that distance is then compared with other R-R intervals. Normal sinus P waves have smooth contours and appear uniform across the monitor tracing. A P wave precedes each QRS complex. The QRS complexes are uniform in appearance and follow each P wave by the same distance. Each rhythm that is interpreted is done so in comparison with its deviation from a sinus rhythm; therefore, the normal sinus rhythm characteristics should be known by all practitioners responsible for interpreting ECG rhythms. Guidelines for interpreting ECG rhythms are helpful and can be used to interpret all types of rhythms. Basic guidelines are provided in Table 17–1.

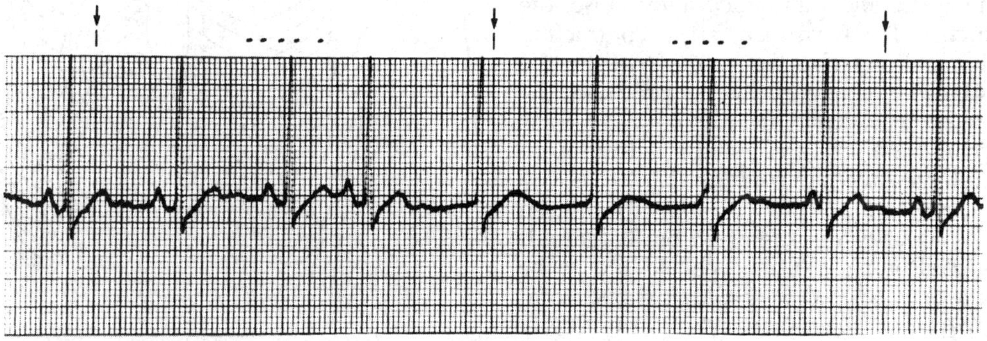

Figure 17–10.

The arrows at the top of the ECG strip note the 3-second markings displayed on standard ECG recording paper. An approximate heart rate can be calculated by counting the number of QRS complexes between two sets of markings (6.0 seconds) and multiplying by 10. (From Sanderson RG, Kurth CL. The cardiac patient. 2nd ed. Philadelphia: WB Saunders, 1983, p 130.)

Table 17–1. GUIDELINES FOR INTERPRETING ELECTROCARDIOGRAPH RHYTHMS

Check rhythm regularity.
To determine regularity, measure the distance between two R waves (R-R interval), and compare that distance with other R-R intervals. If the rhythm is not regular, identification of what causes the irregularity is required.

Check the heart rate.
If the rhythm is regular, the rate can be estimated by counting the number of QRS complexes in 6.0 seconds and multiplying that number by 10. If the rhythm is irregular, the actual rate must be calculated over an entire minute.

Check the relationship between the atria and the ventricles.
Look for P waves in front of every QRS complex. Look for uniform P waves. Determine whether the P waves are of equal distance from every QRS complex. If P waves are absent, are not uniform, or have a varying PR interval, the abnormalities must be explained.

Check the QRS complexes for normalcy.
They should all look the same. The QRS interval should be normal. Variation in the QRS complexes in the tracing must be explained. The reason for the extra complexes or missing complexes should be determined. Assessing and describing abnormalities will help the practitioner determine possible pathology, its location, and the possibilities for treatment.

Heart Sounds

Heart sounds are produced by the closing of the heart valves. They are best heard with a stethoscope in the cardiac auscultatory sites, as illustrated in Figure 17–11.

Normal heart sounds are labeled S_1 and S_2. The first heart sound, S_1, is produced by the simultaneous closure of the mitral and tricuspid valves. As the mitral and tricuspid valves close, the aortic and pulmonic valves open, ventricular contraction occurs, and blood flows out of the ventricles during systole. The mitral valve produces most of the first heart sound, so S_1 is best heard in the mitral area. This is on the left side, fifth intercostal space, midclavicular line (see Fig. 17–11).

The second heart sound, S_2, is produced by the simultaneous closure of the aortic and pulmonic valves. As the aortic and pulmonic valves close, the mitral and tricuspid valves open, atrial contraction occurs, and blood flows into the ventricles from the atria during diastole. The aortic valve produces the major portion of the second heart sound, so S_2 is heard loudest in the aortic area. This is on the right side, second intercostal space (see Fig. 17–11).

The third heart sound, S_3, is normal in children and may be heard until the age of 25 or 30 years. If the S_3 is heard after age 30, it is considered to be pathologic and is produced by rapid, passive atrial filling of a partially filled ventricle during early diastole when the mitral and tricuspid valves are open. In right or left ventricular failure, the ventricle is unable to initiate a contraction adequate to eject the blood it receives, resulting in a partially filled chamber during diastole. As blood flows into the partially filled ventricle during early diastole, turbulent flow is produced and is heard as a low-pitched thud. A left ventricular S_3 is best heard in the apical area. This is on the left side at the apex of the heart. A right ventricular S_3 is best heard in the right ventricular area near the left sternal border. The timing sequence of S_1, S_2, and S_3 can be compared with the timing of the syllables in the word *Kentucky*. S_3 closely follows S_2 with a normal separation of S_1 and S_2 (Fig. 17–12).

A fourth heart sound, S_4, is produced by high-velocity blood flow during atrial contraction as the blood enters a noncompliant ventricle, causing turbulent flow. An S_4 is always pathologic and may be caused by cardiomyopathy, aortic and pulmonic stenosis, pulmonary hypertension, systemic hypertension, myocardial infarction, heart block, or coronary artery disease. A left atrial S_4 is best heard in the apical (mitral) area, whereas a right atrial S_4 is best heard in the right ventricular area close to the left sternal border. The timing of S_1, S_2, and S_4 can be compared with the timing of the syllables in the word *Tennessee*. The S_4 closely precedes S_1 with a normal separation of S_1 and S_2 (Fig. 17–13).

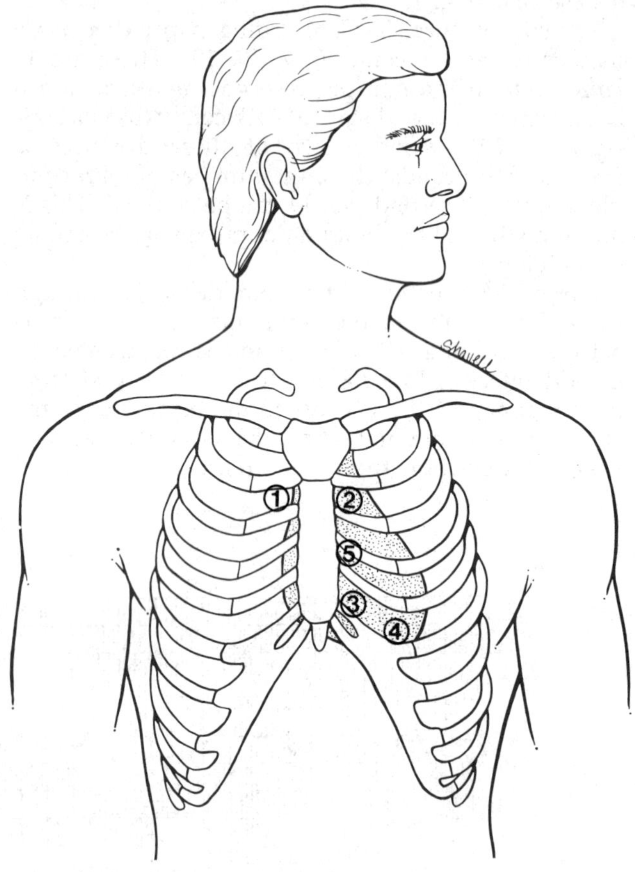

Figure 17–11.

Listen with a stethoscope to these auscultatory sites: *1*, aortic (second right intercostal space; *2*, pulmonic (second left intercostal space); *3*, tricuspid (lower left sternal border); *4*, mitral (fifth intercostal space, midclavicular line); and *5*, right ventricular (near left sternal border and over sternum).

Figure 17–12.

Heart sounds as they occur in the cardiac cycle. Use of the word *Kentucky* exemplifies the first, second, and third heart sounds. (Modified from Sanderson RG, Kurth CL. The cardiac patient. 2nd ed. Philadelphia: WB Saunders, 1983, p 79.)

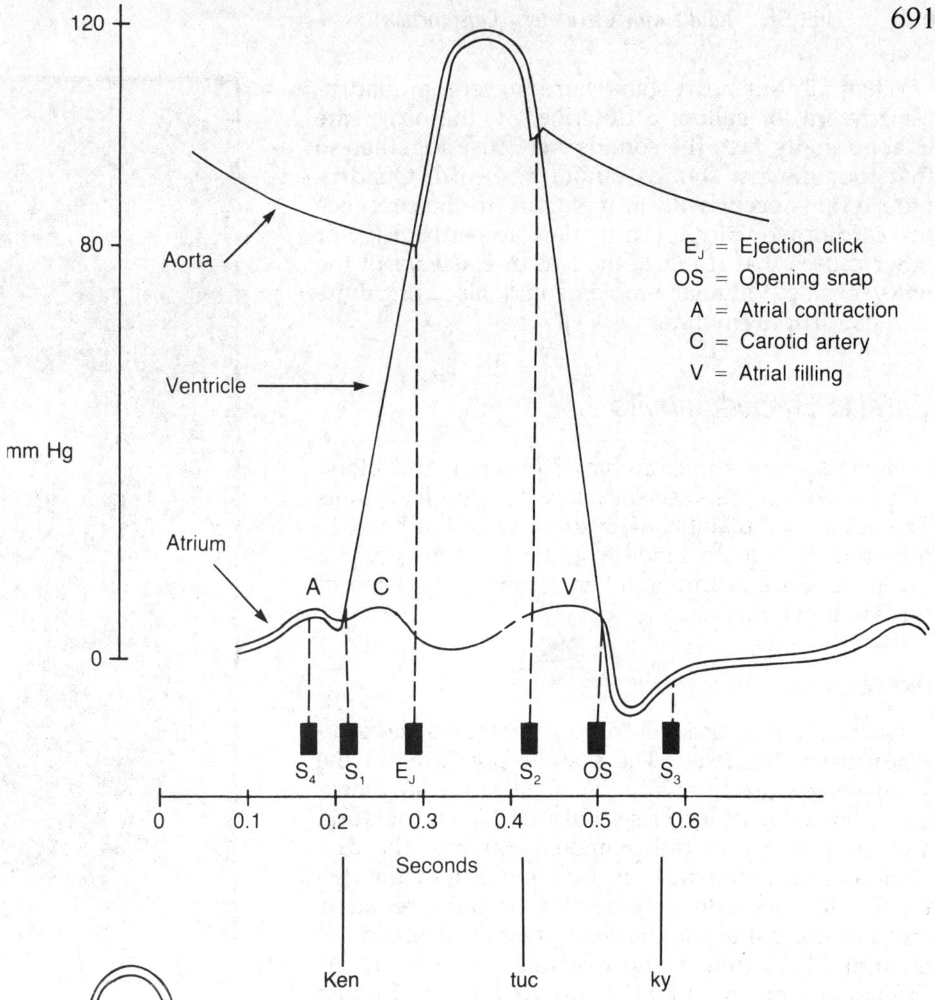

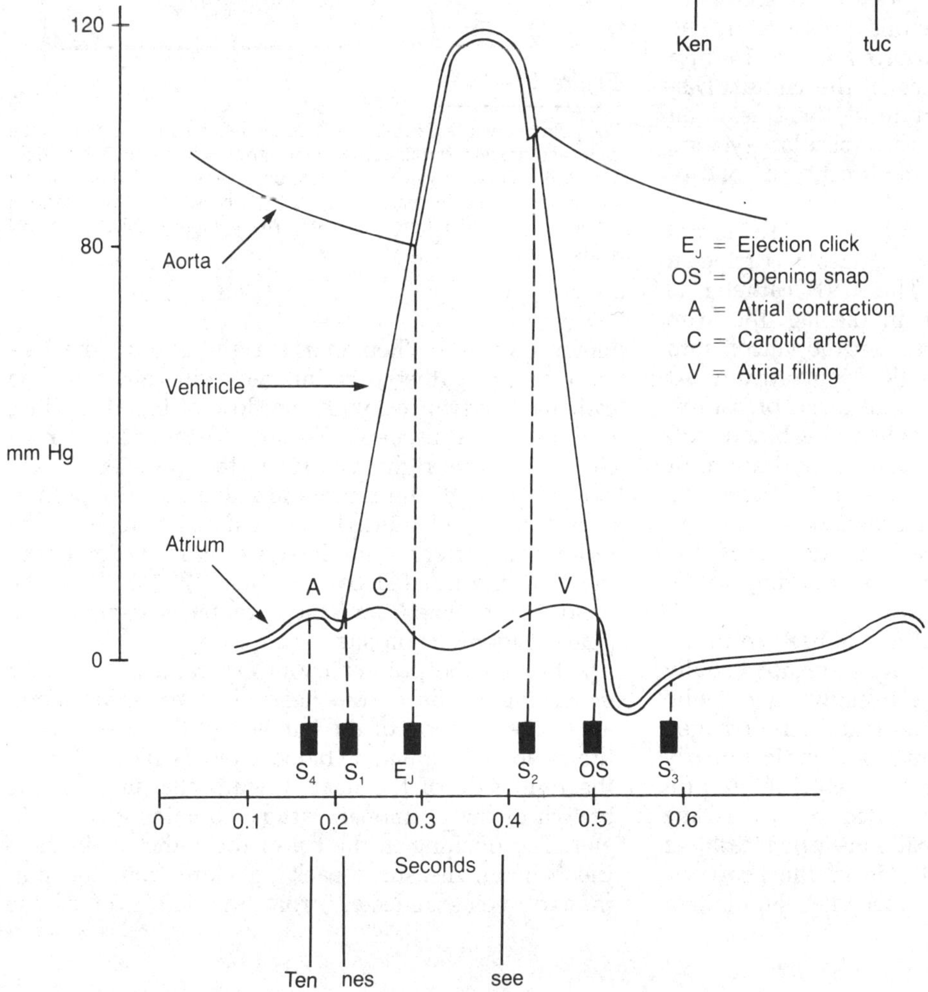

Figure 17–13.

Heart sounds as they occur in the cardiac cycle. Use of the word *Tennessee* exemplifies the fourth, first, and second heart sounds. (Modified from Sanderson RG, Kurth CL. The cardiac patient. 2nd ed. Philadelphia: WB Saunders, 1983, p 79.)

When all four heart sounds are present, a quadruple rhythm, or gallop, is described. If the heart rate is abnormally fast, the sounds may fuse together so that four distinct sounds cannot be heard. Quadruple rhythms occur with heart failure in the presence of cardiomyopathy, ventricular hypertrophy, or other causes that result in the loss of elasticity of the left ventricle. Valvular problems may also contribute to a quadruple rhythm.

Cardiac Hemodynamics

Hemodynamics refer to blood pressure and blood volume within the vascular space at any given time. The ability (or inability with disease) of the heart to distribute adequate blood volume by generating a given pressure is important in treating problems of cardiac function.

PRESSURES

Normal atrial and ventricular pressures have already been discussed. The systolic pressures in the great vessels are normally the same as in the ventricles from which they arise: 120 mm Hg in the aorta and 25 mm Hg in the pulmonary artery. The diastolic pressure depends on the resistance of the distal circuit. The systemic arterioles are quite resistive, and the normal aortic diastolic pressure descends to 80 mm Hg, whereas the diastolic pressure in the pulmonary artery drops to approximately 10 mm Hg, reflecting the low resistance in the circuit. Disease processes, plus drug and fluid therapies, can change pressures throughout the vascular system. Balancing pressures for optimum function is one of the goals of medical treatment.

Central venous pressure (CVP), or right atrial pressure, is useful for detecting changes occurring in the right side of the heart. The CVP catheter is threaded through a large vein in the leg, the arm, the neck, or the subclavian area and advanced into the vena cava until it reaches the right atrium. At this point, the catheter reflects right atrial pressures. Right atrial pressure changes when the blood volume changes, as occurs in bleeding, dehydration, or vigorous diuresis. As blood returns to the heart via the large veins, the pressure it exerts is the CVP. If blood volume returning to the heart decreases, the CVP decreases, and if blood volume returning to the heart increases, the CVP increases.

Pulmonary artery pressure (PAP) is used to monitor a failing heart. Volume changes are not usually sudden in cardiac patients, especially those who have myocardial infarctions (no acute hemorrhage). Consequently, CVP readings may not indicate early hemodynamic changes of the left ventricle. A pulmonary artery catheter (also called a Swan-Ganz catheter) is a flow-directed, balloon-tipped catheter that is inserted into the right side of the heart via the venous system (brachial, subclavian, jugular, or

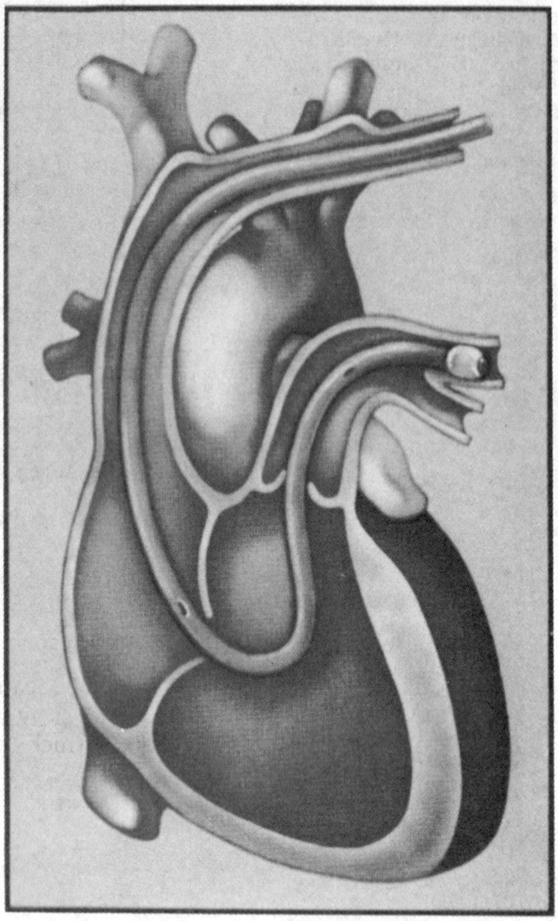

Figure 17–14.

The pulmonary artery catheter enters the heart via the superior vena cava and travels through the right atrium, tricuspid valve, right ventricle, pulmonic valve, and pulmonary artery and into a distal branch of the pulmonary artery, where it wedges (with balloon inflated). (Modified from Lalli SM. The complete Swan-Ganz. RN 1978; 41:66.)

femoral veins). When in the right atrium, the balloon of the catheter is inflated with air, and the catheter is advanced with the flow of blood, pulling it through the tricuspid valve into the right ventricle. From the right ventricle, the catheter is advanced through the pulmonic valve into the pulmonary artery and guided into a distal branch of the pulmonary artery until it stops or is wedged into place by the inflated balloon (Fig. 17–14). Then the balloon is deflated, and the catheter is secured into place at its insertion site.

Although the pulmonary artery catheter is placed in the right side of the heart, it gives information about the function of the left side of the heart. When the balloon is inflated, blood flow is blocked from the right side of the heart toward the lungs in the branch of the pulmonary artery containing the catheter. The opening in the tip of the catheter, distal to the balloon, measures back pressure from the pulmonary veins reflected from the left side of the heart. During ventricular diastole, when the mitral valve is open, the pressure in the left ventricle is reflected in the left atrium, which is turn is reflected in the pulmonary veins and against the tip of the pulmonary artery catheter with the balloon inflated. This is called the pulmonary wedge pressure (PWP). Thus, PWP (balloon inflated) is a good indication of left ventricular end-diastolic pressure (LVEDP). Further, PWP correlates very closely with pulmonary artery diastolic pressure.

Normal PAP is 25/10 mm Hg, with a mean pressure of 10 to 20 mm Hg. Normal PWP is 5 to 12 mm Hg and is also called pulmonary capillary wedge pressure (PCWP), or pulmonary artery occluded (PAO) pressure. PAP is monitored continuously on an oscilloscope, and PWPs are obtained as needed. The balloon is inflated with the amount of air needed to change the PAP curve into a PWP curve (Fig. 17–15). Usually 0.6 to 0.8 ml of air is sufficient to inflate the balloon to a wedge position. Air is never forced into the balloon, because it may break and cause injury to the pulmonary artery tissue. When the PWP has been obtained, the balloon is deflated. The balloon is not left inflated because, during inflation, no blood is able to pass by the balloon to the pulmonary artery branch, which contains the pulmonary artery catheter. Patients who require PAP monitoring are critically ill and should be cared for in an intensive care setting.

CARDIAC OUTPUT

Cardiac output is the amount of blood propelled forward by the heart. Cardiac output can be determined at the bedside and in the cardiac catheterization laboratory by several different methods. It is measured in liters of blood per minute. In an average-size adult at rest, cardiac output is approximately 6 L/minute. In disease states the cardiac output is usually less than normal and may be so low that an adequate blood supply to the body's tissues, especially in times of stress, cannot be delivered.

Cardiac output measurements can be obtained at the bedside when a four-lumen pulmonary artery catheter (thermodilution catheter) is inserted into the patient. The four-lumen catheter contains lumens for measurement of CVP, PAP, and PWP plus a lumen containing a thermistor for measurement of blood temperature in the heart. A bolus of 10 ml of cold or room-temperature (cooler than body temperature) intravenous fluid is injected into the external port of the CVP portion of the catheter. As the fluid exits into the right atrium, it cools the blood that is in the right atrium. This volume of cooled blood moves into the right ventricle and then into the pulmonary artery. In the pulmonary artery, the thermistor senses the temperature change as the cooled blood passes over it. The pulmonary artery temperature monitoring port (containing the thermistor) will record a decrease in temperature followed by a gradual return to the patient's body temperature as the cold solution is "washed out." The resulting temperature-time curve is analyzed by a computer and cardiac output is thereby calculated.

Clinical Manifestations of Cardiac Dysfunction

All body systems are affected by cardiac changes because the systems are dependent on the heart to supply oxygenated blood and nutrients to the tissues. Clinical manifestations of cardiac disorders will be found throughout the body during assessment for cardiac changes.

Activity Alterations

Exercise places a demand for increased blood flow on arterial circulation. Diseased arteries cannot dilate to supply oxygen to the heart muscle, which demands increased oxygen for metabolic processes. The result of a decreased oxygen supply to the myocardium is ischemic muscle tissue and the onset of chest pain (angina pectoris).

A decreased cardiac output may be sufficient to

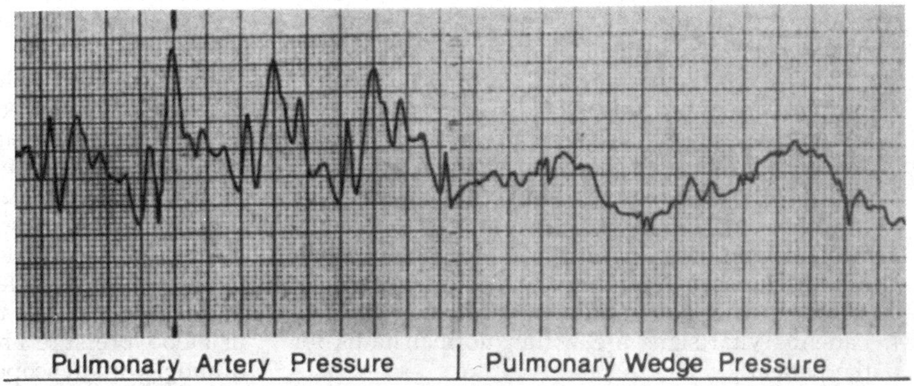

Figure 17–15.

When the balloon of the pulmonary artery catheter is inflated, the wedge pressure waveform changes from pulmonary artery pressure to pulmonary wedge pressure. (Modified from Bolognini V. The Swan-Ganz pulmonary artery catheter: Implications for nursing. Heart Lung 1974; 3:980.)

supply the body's muscles at rest, but, with activity and the inability to increase cardiac output, fatigue results. Patients with chronic decreased cardiac outputs do not feel like participating in activities of daily living that involve the use of large muscles such as walking, bathing, dressing, feeding oneself, cooking, or household work. Even if individuals feel like performing the activities of daily living, they may be limited by fatigue, weakness, and respiratory difficulty.

Application of the Nursing Process to the Care of the Patient with Activity Alterations

Assessment

Assess for tachypnea, shortness of breath on exertion, tachycardia, and fatigue as a result of the lack of oxygen to the heart, causing a decreased cardiac output. Observe the skin for pallor and cyanosis, especially around the mouth and distally in the fingers and toes. Check all pulses. Review the laboratory data, noting the hemoglobin levels and blood gas levels.

Ask the patient about the ability to complete activities of daily living. Check the patient's sleep and rest patterns. Find out whether the symptoms are intermittent or persistent. Check the extremities for weakness, tingling, numbness, and paresthesia.

Assess for chest pain. Ask about the frequency, duration, and intensity. Check whether a particular activity precipitates the episode of angina and what is used to relieve the pain.

Nursing Diagnoses and Planning

The nursing diagnosis and related expected patient outcomes most commonly applicable to patients with decreased cardiac output resulting in fatigue and activity alterations are as follows:

NDx: Activity intolerance related to decreased oxygenation secondary to decreased cardiac output or coronary artery disease

Planning: Patient outcomes

1. Patient verbalizes decreased feelings of fatigue and demonstrates an increased activity level.
2. Patient follows a regimen of planned activity and rest each day.
3. Patient completes activities of daily living with minimal assistance and without signs of fatigue, dyspnea, chest pain, and tachycardia.
4. Patient's vital signs are within normal limits for the patient.

Nursing Interventions

NDx: Activity intolerance

Instruct the patient to practice energy-saving techniques to reduce the demand on the heart for increased output. Place frequently used articles within the patient's reach. Allow for rest periods during the delivery of nursing care. Prevent interruptions during the patient's rest time and at night. Reduce any disturbing noise, and limit visitors if necessary.

Encourage good nutrition to increase the patient's energy level. Offer frequent small meals to avoid fatigue while eating. Feed the patient if necessary to prevent cardiac strain and to keep the nutritional status from becoming deficient.

Help the patient develop a regimen of activity with frequent rest and relaxation times throughout the day. Encourage the patient to slowly build up a tolerance for increased activity. Referral to an exercise therapist may be beneficial.

Evaluation

Evaluate the effectiveness of nursing care for a patient with decreased cardiac output resulting in fatigue and activity intolerance by comparing the patient's status with the expected patient outcomes. Examples of specific outcomes for patients with fatigue and activity intolerance have been provided in the Planning section.

Circulatory Alterations

The heart rate and strength of peripheral pulses vary depending on the type of cardiac disease present. With stress, excitement, or anxiety, the heart rate elevates above normal levels. Rhythm changes may also occur. If the rhythm is irregular, an ECG is obtained to diagnose the irregularity. The heart rate is monitored apically as well as peripherally. There may be a pulse deficit between the apical and peripheral pulses, which needs further examination. Pulses are detected and recorded for arteries in the temporal, carotid, brachial, radial, femoral, popliteal, posterior tibial, and dorsalis pedis areas.

Normally venous pulses cannot be palpated. In right-sided heart failure, however, the jugular veins may be distended (JVD) and thus palpable. JVD varies with the elevation of the patient's head. If the distention is present with the head elevated 90 degrees, it is significant.

Blood pressure is measured and compared with the patient's normal blood pressure if it is known. Blood pressure is elevated in chronic hypertension, in stress, and when the patient is in pain. Decreases in blood pressure are noted in patients with dehydration, with syncope, or in shock.

Patients with low cardiac output may experience orthostatic hypotension. This is assessed by measuring the blood pressure and pulse in a supine position and in a standing position. A decrease in systolic pressure of 10 to 20 mm Hg and a decrease in diastolic pressure of 10 mm Hg, together with an increase in pulse rate, are indicative of orthostatic hypotension.

Right-sided heart failure leads to peripheral edema of the feet, ankles, fingers, and hands. Patients seeking medical assistance often report tightness when wearing shoes. Patients with chronic heart failure may exhibit peripheral edema and oliguria during the day, whereas at night the excess peripheral fluids escape from the extremities while the patient is in s supine position. The fluid returns to the kidneys, resulting in nocturnal urinary frequency (nocturia). Patients on bed rest exhibit edema in dependent areas such as the sacral area, particularly if the head of the bed is elevated. Edema is found in the feet if the knees are elevated while in bed or in the legs if they are in a dependent position.

A common symptom of cardiac disease is chest pain or angina pectoris. Many patients do not describe their angina as distinct pain so evaluation of the "feeling" of the patient is crucial. The patient may describe it as a "heavy" feeling on the chest. It should be evaluated as to severity, intensity, duration, exact location, and radiation. An episode of angina may occur at rest or with activity. Its duration is usually less than 15 minutes without interruption. Within a given patient, the pain does not usually vary except in severity, radiation, and duration. The character, or quality, of the pain is identical each time it occurs; only the magnitude changes. Varying forms of angina pectoris are expressed by adding terms to the word *angina* (Table 17–2).

Chest pain is usually the result of ischemic myocardial tissue. It may also be due to pericarditis, dissection of the aorta, pulmonary emboli, or reflex esophagitis associated with hiatal hernia. A complete history of the chest pain differentiates its cause.

Table 17–2. TYPES OF ANGINA PECTORIS EXPLAINED BY DIFFERENT TERMS ADDED TO THE WORD ANGINA

Types of Angina	Characteristics
Stable angina	Frequency and severity unchanged for several months
Unstable angina	Increasing frequency, severity, or duration occurring with lessened activity or at rest; recent-onset angina also considered unstable
Crescendo angina or preinfarction angina	A form of unstable angina in which there is high likelihood that myocardial infarction will occur within next few days
Angina de cubitus	Angina while lying down
Atypical angina, variant angina, or Prinzmetal's angina	Represents an unusual form in which the pain generally occurs at rest or long after activity, is prolonged, and is accompanied by ST elevation rather than ST depression on the electrocardiogram during pain
Intractable angina	Angina that is continued, frequent, and limiting despite treatment

Data from Sanderson RG, Kurth CL. The cardiac patient. 2nd ed. Philadelphia: WB Saunders, 1983, p. 393.

Application of the Nursing Process to the Care of the Patient with Circulatory Alterations

Assessment

Observe for tachycardia, bradycardia, tachypnea, cyanosis, orthopnea, palpitations and dyspnea. Check all peripheral pulses. Examine skin color, especially distally. Check the nail beds for discoloration and capillary refill. Review the laboratory data such as the complete blood count (CBC) and blood gas levels. Check the vital signs. Examine the ECG if available.

Ask the patient about episodes of chest pain. Determine the frequency, type, precipating factors, duration, and relief methods. Ask specific questions about the patient's pain. Be sure the patient understands that the questions relate to pain or any other chest discomfort that is experienced.

Observe for edema in the extremities and lungs. Check for JVD. Auscultate the chest thoroughly, checking for adventitious sounds and abnormal cardiac rhythms.

Check for signs of orthostatic hypotension. Ask the patient about episodes of syncope, dizziness, confusion, restlessness, and weakness. Feel the patient's skin for moisture or coolness. Check the patient's orientation and level of alertness. Assess for confusion caused by decreased oxygen to cerebral tissue.

Nursing Diagnoses and Planning

Nursing diagnoses and related expected patient outcomes most commonly applicable to patients with circulatory alterations include the following:

NDx: Decreased cardiac output related to mechanical failure and damaged or weakened myocardial tissue; primary or secondary to other disease states

Planning: Patient outcomes

1. Patient's vital signs are within normal ranges for the patient.
2. Patient has a balanced intake and output and is free of peripheral and central edema.

3. Patient's skin is warm, color is appropriate, no cyanosis is present, and peripheral pulses are palpable.
4. Patient maintains an adequate cardiac output as seen by the hemodynamic monitoring.

NDx: High risk for injury related to orthostatic hypotension secondary to circulatory changes with cerebral hypoxia

Planning: Patient outcomes
1. Patient states need for assistance when out of bed and ambulating to prevent injury.
2. Patient states preventive measures such as resting in upright position for a few minutes before getting out of bed and requesting support when needed.
3. Patient conforms to the safety measures.
4. Patient remains free from injury.

NDx: Altered tissue perfusion, cardiopulmonary, related to inadequate cardiac output caused by weakened myocardial muscle

Planning: Patient outcomes
1. Patient demonstrates increased perfusion as noted by warm, dry skin, strong pulses, absence of edema, and cyanosis.
2. Patient's vital signs are within normal ranges for the patient.
3. Patient demonstrates changes in behaviors that promote improved circulation such as mild exercise, cessation of smoking, and relaxation techniques.

NDx: Pain related to inadequate oxygenation of cardiac tissue

Planning: Patient outcomes
1. Patient states chest pain is absent or diminished.
2. Patient relates methods to relieve chest pain.

Nursing Interventions

NDx: Decreased cardiac output
Monitor the patient's vital signs both at rest and during activity. Encourage the patient to take frequent rest periods throughout the day to prevent fatigue and strain on the myocardium. Instruct the patient to stop activity if it initiates episodes of chest pain or aggravates chest discomfort.

Use telemetry monitoring whenever possible, especially if the patient experiences dysrhythmias or if the patient is taking antidysrhythmic drugs. Review the results of laboratory studies and hemodynamic monitoring.

Check the patient's fluid intake and output, observing for adequacy and balance. Keep the patient's legs in a nondependent position while sitting. Provide support for the extremities while the patient is sitting or lying in bed. Pad bony prominences to prevent breakdown from pressure and poor circulation.

Teach the patient relaxation techniques and range-of-motion procedures to increase circulation while lying in bed. Keep the patient warm and comfortable. Prevent constriction of circulation as a result of tight clothing or bed linen.

NDx: High risk for injury
Teach the patient to ask for assistance when getting out of bed or ambulating. Keep the bed rails in the upright position and the patient's call light within reach. Explain the effects of orthostatic hypotension, its origin and safety measures to prevent injury. Teach the patient to sit for a few moments before rising after being in a supine position. Be sure the patient is mentally alert and physically stable before being allowed the freedom to get out of bed or walk without assistance.

NDx: Altered tissue perfusion, cardiopulmonary
Help the patient conserve oxygen needs by encouraging rest and limiting activities. Elevate the head of the bed to aid in lung expansion. Initiate oxygen therapy if needed. Assist patient with activities of daily living, if needed, to conserve energy.

Keep the patient in a comfortable position, and reposition frequently to release pressure. Use range-of-motion exercises to stimulate circulation. Monitor vital signs and laboratory studies to assess for changes and improvements in status. Encourage ambulation as tolerated, but provide for frequent rest periods to decrease cardiac workload. Discourage smoking to avoid vasoconstriction. Discuss strategies to reduce stress, which could cause increased blood pressure. Remove constricting clothing, and keep heavy bed linen from restricting peripheral circulation. Keep the patient's legs in a nondependent position when not ambulating.

Provide a low-sodium diet to reduce fluid retention. Give prescribed medications to promote increased circulation and diuresis as needed. Monitor laboratory studies to assess pulmonary, circulatory, and renal function.

NDx: Pain
Give prescribed antianginal drugs as needed. Document all episodes of chest pain. Have the patient describe the pain. Look for nonverbal signs of pain such as restlessness, gasping, clenched fists, stiffness, grimacing, and facial flushing. Obtain a 12-lead ECG during an acute episode of chest pain for diagnostic purposes. If no relief is obtained from repeated medication, notify the physician. Administer oxygen if needed.

Teach the patient about the medications prescribed for chest pain. Have the patient keep a log of the time and date the medication is taken, the results, and whether repeated doses had to taken.

Teach the patient some relaxation techniques for pain relief. Have the patient relate potential coping strategies that have worked previously for relaxation during periods of stress or pain. Allow the patient to rest after acute episodes of chest pain.

Evaluation

Evaluate the effectiveness of nursing care for a patient with circulatory alterations from cardiac dysfunction by comparing the patient's status with the expected patient outcomes. Examples of specific outcomes for patients with circulatory alterations have been provided in the Planning section.

Integumentary Alterations

A patient with suspected cardiac disease may have skin pallor from increased systemic vascular resistance or anemia. With a slow peripheral flow rate, which occurs in heart failure, capillary refill time is prolonged. Normally, capillary refill time is less than 5 seconds. When the arterial blood contains a larger than normal portion of unoxygenated hemoglobin (blue to purple in appearance), the skin color becomes pale and dusky blue, or cyanotic. Peripheral cyanosis is a result of decreased circulation. Such cyanosis is usually first noted in the fingers and toes around the nail beds.

Chronic hemoglobin desaturation, which occurs in congenital heart disease and chronic lung disease, leads to clubbing of the fingers and toes along with peripheral cyanosis. Central cyanosis is indicative of a decreased blood flow rate or ineffective exchange of oxygen and carbon dioxide. Central cyanosis is noted when the skin around the mouth, the mucous membranes, the lips, and ear lobes becomes a dusky blue. Cyanosis should not be used to gauge hypoxia because it can be a late sign of hypoxia, and cardiac arrest may be imminent when central cyanosis is noted.

Temperature changes of the skin are also found when there are autonomic nervous system changes. With normal function, the hands and feet feel warm to the touch. In stressful situations, or with moderate sympathetic stimulation, the hands and feet feel cool and may also be moist. With severe sympathetic stimulation, as in shock, the extremities become cold and clammy because of the severe vasoconstriction that occurs.

Application of the Nursing Process to the Care of the Patient with Integumentary Alterations

Assessment

Assess the patient's temperature frequently. Feel the extremities, and observe for discoloration. Check all peripheral pulses. Observe for signs of cardiogenic shock, which may cause the temperature alteration. Look for signs of stress and anxiety in the patient, which may cause increased vasoconstriction, aggravating the symptoms.

Nursing Diagnoses and Planning

Nursing diagnoses and related expected patient outcomes most commonly applicable to patients with integumentary alterations from cardiac problems include those discussed under circulatory alterations and the following:

NDx: High risk for altered body temperature, less than normal, related to cardiac disease causing severe vasoconstriction, decreased circulation, or decreased oxygenation to tissues*

Planning: Patient outcomes

1. Patient remains warm and comfortable without chills and signs of decreased circulation to extremities such as weak pulses, cool skin, and cyanosis.
2. Patient's temperature is within normal range for the patient.
3. Patient reports feeling relaxed and nonstressed.

Nursing Interventions

NDx: High risk for altered body temperature, less than normal

Instruct the patient to report any early signs of temperature changes such as chilling or cold feet. Check and document the patient's temperature every 4 hours or more frequently as needed. Apply extra blankets to keep the patient warm and comfortable. Eliminate drafts in the patient's room if possible. Avoid providing cold foods and fluids. Observe for and report early signs of circulatory or pump failure problems.

Assist the patient to relax by providing a calm,

* This diagnosis could also have been listed under Circulatory Alterations.

quiet atmosphere. Allow for uninterrupted rest periods. Teach the patient some relaxation techniques. Limit interruptions and visitors.

Evaluation

Evaluate the effectiveness of nursing care for a patient with integumentary alterations from cardiac dysfunction by comparing the patient's status with the expected patient outcomes. Examples of specific outcomes for patients with integumentary alterations have been provided in the Planning section.

Renal Alterations

A decreased cardiac output results in decreased perfusion of the kidneys via the renal arteries, causing oliguria. Further decreases in renal perfusion may lead to anuria and acute tubular necrosis (ATN) (see Chapter 26 for a discussion of ATN). Activation of the renin-angiotensin-aldosterone system is a response to decreased renal blood flow. The result is an increased blood pressure with retention of sodium and water in the vascular system.

With prolonged renal vasoconstriction, the kidneys lose their ability to filter, excrete, and reabsorb necessary particles. Urinary output falls to 20 to 30 ml/hour or less. A disproportionate rise in blood urea nitrogen (BUN) and serum creatinine is noted. Urinary sodium concentration is high because the kidneys are unable to reabsorb sodium. As the kidneys lose the ability to concentrate urine, the urine osmolarity drops, and the urine specific gravity decreases. Metabolic wastes plus metabolic by-products of drugs given to the patient are recirculated when the kidneys are unable to filter them from the blood. Thus, drug toxicity symptoms may be seen in patients with renal alterations from cardiac malfunction.

Application of the Nursing Process to the Care of the Patient with Renal Alterations

Assessment

Assess the patient's intake and output. Examine the color, consistency, and amount of urine. Observe for signs of urine retention such as oliguria, edema, rales, wheezing, and increased blood pressure. Check for disorientation, confusion, memory loss, and other such cerebral signs indicating high levels of circulating toxic wastes. Assess for signs of drug toxicity (specific to the drugs the patient is taking) because decreased renal function may exacerbate toxicity. Review the laboratory data related to renal function.

Nursing Diagnoses and Planning

Nursing diagnoses and related expected patient outcomes most commonly applicable to patients with renal alterations from cardiac dysfunction include those discussed under cardiac alterations and the following:

NDx: Altered urinary elimination, decreased, related to decreased renal perfusion secondary to decreased cardiac output

Planning: Patient outcomes
1. Patient's output is at least 30 ml/hour.
2. Patient's laboratory data are within normal ranges for the patient.
3. Patient remains well hydrated without edema.
4. Patient's circulation is adequate.

Nursing Interventions

NDx: Altered urinary elimination, decreased
Record fluid intake and output hourly. Continue to hydrate the patient unless otherwise indicated. Check edematous areas, and document the severity. Keep edematous areas elevated when possible. Note the color, consistency, and amount of urine. Notify the physician if the output falls below 30 ml/hour. Change the patient's position frequently to increase circulation and prevent skin breakdown. Assist the patient in getting out of bed and in ambulating if confusion or disorientation is present. Note the patient's medications, and document any exaggerated side effects. Promote activities that increase tissue perfusion, which will then increase renal perfusion, such as exercise and relaxation. Also help the patient to decrease anxiety, which causes vasoconstriction. Counsel the patient to cease smoking. Provide warmth and avoid chilling. (See Chapters 25 and 26 for the care of patients with renal dysfunction.)

Evaluation

Evaluate the effectiveness of nursing care for a patient with renal alterations from cardiac dysfunction by comparing the patient's status with the expected patient outcomes. Examples of specific outcomes for patients with renal alterations have been provided in the Planning section.

Respiratory Alterations

Cardiac patients frequently exhibit tachypnea, wheezing, cyanosis, and extreme shortness of breath if they are having pain, are anxious, or are in a state of congestive failure. Left-sided heart failure leads to crackles heard only in the lung bases in early failure but throughout the lung fields as the failure progresses. A dry, hacking cough may be indicative of pulmonary congestion or a history of cigarette smoking. Acute pulmonary edema is evidenced by pink, frothy sputum (hemoptysis), along with tachypnea and wheezing as the small airways are filled with fluid.

Dyspnea is a common complaint of patients with cardiac disease. With left ventricular failure and mitral and aortic valve disease, left ventricular pressure is increased. As a result, left arterial, pulmonary venous, and pulmonary capillary pressures also increase. When hydrostatic pressure in the pulmonary capillary bed exceeds the oncotic pressure of plasma proteins, fluid escapes into the surrounding lung tissue. The process of breathing becomes more difficult as oxygen and carbon dioxide exchange occurs in the remaining alveoli that are not fluid filled. Dyspnea is usually related to exertion when it is of cardiac origin. Dyspnea associated with pulmonary disease occurs at rest as well as with exertion. The increased effort of inspiration leads to fatigue of the respiratory muscles and may result in pulmonary arrest.

Orthopnea is the term used to describe the inability to breathe easily while lying flat. This is a common manifestation of respiratory and cardiac dysfunction. The patient may use several pillows to obtain a position comfortable for easy breathing while sleeping. The patient may report inability to sleep uninterrupted if the pillows are not used.

If the patient awakens from a sound sleep with acute shortness of breath and must stand or sit to breathe easily and feel comfortable, it is called paroxysmal nocturnal dyspnea (PND). This condition usually lasts only a few minutes, but it is extremely frightening to the patient. PND may occur only one or several times per night.

Application of the Nursing Process to the Care of the Patient with Respiratory Alterations

Assessment

Assess the respiratory status by observing for tachypnea, cyanosis, dyspnea, orthopnea, wheezing, and tachycardia. Check for increased dyspnea on exertion. Auscultate the chest, listening for rales and wheezes. Review the blood gas levels.

Nursing Diagnoses and Planning

The nursing diagnosis and related expected patient outcomes most commonly applicable to patients with respiratory alterations from cardiac dysfunction are as follows:

NDx: Ineffective breathing pattern related to increased anxiety, chest pain, or inadequate oxygenation secondary to cardiac disease state, resulting in pulmonary edema

Planning: Patient outcomes

1. Patient breathes easier and effectively as evidenced by lack of dyspnea, cyanosis, tachypnea, or orthopnea.
2. Patient's blood gas levels are within normal ranges for the patient.
3. Patient denies shortness of breath on exertion.

Nursing Interventions

NDx: Ineffective breathing pattern

Promote maximum respirations by repositioning the patient. Have the patient stay in a semi-Fowler's position while in bed for better chest expansion. Allow frequent rest periods while administering care so the patient does not become fatigued and dyspneic. Teach the patient deep-breathing techniques. Tell the patient to seek assistance if activities cause more difficult breathing or extreme fatigue. Administer oxygen as needed.

Observe for signs of respiratory distress, and administer treatments and medications as ordered. Watch for changes in the blood gas levels, indicating early respiratory difficulty. (See Chapters 12 to 14 for care of the patient with respiratory dysfunction.)

Evaluation

Evaluate the effectiveness of nursing care for a patient with respiratory alterations from cardiac dysfunction by comparing the patient's status with the expected patient outcomes. Examples of specific outcomes for patients with respiratory alterations have been provided in the Planning section.

Gastrointestinal Alterations

Patients with right-sided heart failure may complain of abdominal discomfort, nausea, or vomiting. Liver engorgement occurs with decreased venous return to the heart secondary to right-sided heart failure, causing pressure and pain in the abdominal cavity.

Severe vasoconstriction causes detrimental changes in the pancreas. As the pancreatic cells become ischemic and necrotic, they release amylase and lipase into the circulating blood. Measuring serum amylase and lipase gives an indication of the severity of the pancreatic injury. Pancreatic injury leads to pancreatitis, pancreatic hemorrhage, and peritonitis, which may be life threatening.

Application of the Nursing Process to the Care of the Patient with Gastrointestinal Alterations

Assessment

Assess the patient for gastric discomfort and abdominal distention. Ask the patient about nutritional habits and ability to eat. Check the intake, noting the foods and fluids consumed, and whether any particular food stimulates the distress. Determine whether the patient is too fatigued to eat or whether eating causes respiratory distress, making it more difficult for the patient to consume the entire meal. Note any diarrhea or vomiting. Ask about episodes of nausea and anorexia. Check the amount usually served at the meal and the type of foods the patients likes. Ask about weight loss. Look for signs of hypovolemia and malnutrition such as poor skin turgor, dry skin, weakness, brittle nails and hair, mucous membrane ulcerations, and depression.

Nursing Diagnoses and Planning

The nursing diagnosis and related expected patient outcomes most commonly applicable to patients with gastrointestinal alterations from cardiac dysfunction are as follows:

NDx: Altered nutrition, less than body requirements, related to gastrointestinal distress secondary to decreased perfusion, cardiac disease state, or congestive heart failure

Planning: Patient outcomes

1. Patient eats well-balanced meals as prescribed.
2. Patient tolerates small, frequent meals without fatigue and gastric distress.
3. Patient is well hydrated and well nourished and maintains an appropriate weight.
4. Patient is free from anorexia, nausea, or vomiting.

Nursing Interventions

NDx: Altered nutrition, less than body requirements

Help the patient maintain adequate nutrition by providing an attractive meal in a pleasant atmosphere. Serve food the patients likes when possible. Encourage the patient to eat foods high in potassium and fiber, low in sodium, and low in saturated fat (Nutrition Boxes 17–1, 17–2, and 17–3). Provide six to eight small meals to prevent distention and to reduce fatigue.

Instruct the patient to avoid foods that are gas-

Nutrition Box 17–1.
POTASSIUM-RICH FOODS

Meats
- Beef
- Ham
- Pork
- Veal
- Liver
- Chicken
- Goose
- (Note: Meats in general are not as high in potassium as fruits or vegetables.)

Seafood
- Scallops
- Clams
- Sardines
- Tuna

Fruit
- Bananas
- Cantaloupe
- Honeydew
- Nectarine
- Oranges
- Peaches
- Plums
- Raisins
- Avocado
- Rhubarb

Vegetables
- Beans, dried
- Green beans
- Artichokes
- Asparagus
- Greens
- Carrots
- Cabbage
- Cauliflower
- Chard
- Cucumber
- Potatoes
- Peas
- Pumpkin
- Spinach
- Squash

Dairy
- Powdered milk
- Whole milk
- Skim milk
- Ice cream

Other
- Peanuts

Nutrition Box 17–2.

FOODS HIGH IN SATURATED FAT AND FOODS HIGHER IN UNSATURATED FAT THAN SATURATED FAT

Saturated Fat	Unsaturated Fat
Bacon	Chicken breast
Butter	Corn oil
Cheese	Dressings (made with the oils on this list)
Coconut oil	Fish (freshwater)
Gravies	Imitation foods (bacon, cheese)
Lard	Plant foods
Most meats	Polyunsaturated margarine
Nondairy creamer	Safflower oil
Palm oil	Soybean oil
Poultry skin	Sunflower oil
Salad dressings	
Sauces	
Whipped dairy dessert toppings	

forming because they cause abdominal distention, which may decrease the appetite, and also interfere with respiratory efforts. Avoid hot, spicy foods and acidic fluids to decrease gastrointestinal irritation when present. Encourage increased fluid intake, unless contraindicated, to prevent constipation and to promote adequate hydration. Monitor the patient's intake and output.

Review the cause, symptoms, and nutritional implications of the gastrointestinal problems with the client and family. Allow time for questions and verbalization of concerns and misunderstandings. (See Chapters 21 to 24 for the care of the patient with gastrointestinal dysfunction.)

Evaluation

Evaluate the effectiveness of nursing care for a patient with gastrointestinal alterations from cardiac dysfunction by comparing the patient's status with the expected patient outcomes. Examples of specific

Nutrition Box 17–3.

HIGH- AND LOW-SODIUM FOODS

High Sodium	Low Sodium
Bacon	Canned low-sodium meat or fish
Canned meat or fish	Fresh fish
Canned fruit drinks	Fresh fruit
Canned vegetables	Fresh vegetables
Cheese	Popcorn (unsalted)
Cold cuts	Poultry
Glazed fruit/candied fruit	Puffed rice and wheat
Ice cream	Shredded wheat
Kidney	Skim milk
Peanut butter	Unsalted breads and cereals
Seafood	Unsalted butter or margarine
Sauces	Unsalted dressings

outcomes for patients with gastrointestinal alterations have been provided in the Planning section.

Neurologic Alterations

The level of consciousness is assessed frequently in patients with cardiac dysfunction because it may change quickly. With cardiac failure and its concomitant decrease in circulating oxygen, the brain may not receive the necessary amount of oxygen for normal functioning. This oxygen deficit alters the level of consciousness. Restlessness is usually the first sign of decreased circulation of oxygen to the brain.

Syncope may be associated with periods of severe bradycardia or transient asystole. Aortic stenosis and aortic insufficiency may lead to decreased blood flow to the brain and result in syncopal episodes. Syncope also has many noncardiac causes, but patients who experience syncope should be evaluated for possible cardiac dysfunction.

Periods of disorientation and confusion are common. This can lead to safety problems for the patient.

Application of the Nursing Process to the Care of the Patient with Neurologic Alterations

The assessment, nursing diagnoses, expected patient outcomes, nursing interventions, and evaluation for patients experiencing neurologic alterations as a result of cardiac dysfunction are similar to those described previously for patients experiencing circulatory alterations caused by cardiac dysfunction. (See also Chapters 37 and 38 for the care of the patient with neurologic dysfunction.)

Application of the Nursing Process to the Care of the Patient with Clinical Manifestations of Cardiac Dysfunction

The nursing diagnoses, expected patient outcomes, and nursing interventions already discussed relate to specific clinical manifestations of cardiac dysfunction. The typical patient with a cardiac disorder, however, also presents with signs and symptoms of anxiety and a lack of understanding of the cardiac disease state.

Assessment

Assess for nervousness, clenching of hands, episodes of crying, depression, and irritability, which may indicate anxiety. Look for changes in vital signs such as increased heart rate, respiratory rate, and blood pressure. Ask the patient about palpitations, inability to sleep, and frequent gastric upset.

Question the patient about the disease state, the potential effects, diagnostic tests, and treatments to determine the level of understanding. Allow the patient to ask questions in return to assess the knowledge base better. Determine what the physician has explained and what misunderstandings the patient may have about that information.

Nursing Diagnoses and Planning

Nursing diagnoses and related expected patient outcomes most commonly applicable to patients with various clinical manifestations of cardiac dysfunction include those already discussed and the following:

NDx: Anxiety related to fear of the disease, possible complications and treatments, disability, or death

Planning: Patient outcomes
1. Patient states a relief of anxiety and fear.
2. Patient is relaxed and sleeps without interruption.
3. Patient's vital signs are within normal ranges for the patient.
4. Patient denies palpitations, inability to rest and sleep, or apprehension about condition.

NDx: Knowledge deficit: nature of disease and self-management

Planning: Patient outcomes
1. Patient identifies preventive health measures for cardiac disease.
2. Patient lists personal risks factors and how to modify them.
3. Patient verbalizes accurate information about the disease process, possible treatments, and expected outcomes.
4. Patient initiates lifestyle changes necessary to maintain and improve health and cardiac function.

Nursing Interventions

NDx: Anxiety

Allow the patient to verbalize concerns about the disease, its effects on the patient and family, and fears about disability or death. Help the patient and family find coping strategies that are effective to deal with their anxiety level. Allow time for questions from the patient and the family.

Teach the patient relaxation techniques to help reduce the anxiety. Explain how stress can aggravate the complications of the disease. Tell the patient to rest frequently during the day. Provide comfort measures, both physical and emotional to the patient and family.

Orient the patient to the environment, and explain actions and therapies as they are instituted. Emphasize signs of progress to give the patient hope and to encourage continued progress. Promote diversional activities and exercise, as tolerated, to reduce stress. Administer drugs, as prescribed, to lessen anxiety and to promote rest.

Explain the disease process, treatments, and potential results so the patient will have a better understanding of the disease and its progression. Allow time for the patient and family to be alone when needed. Seek assistance from clergy or other professional counselors when appropriate. Make referrals as needed to social service agencies.

NDx: Knowledge deficit: nature of disease and self-management

Describe the basic anatomy and physiology of the heart to the patient in understandable terms. Explain the cause and effect of the specific disease process and the clinical manifestations. Explain the origin of chest pain, its relief, and the effects of the prescribed medications.

Help the patient identify cardiac risk factors and how they are affecting the patient's life. Discuss possible lifestyle changes and how to implement them. Review diet modifications, the need to stop smoking, appropriate exercises, and stress-reduction techniques.

Provide appropriate printed material about the risk factors, the disease process, and the medications ordered. Allow the patient and family to review the literature and to voice questions and concerns. Assist the patient and family in locating community resources to help them cope with the effects of the cardiac dysfunction and the lifestyle changes needed.

Evaluation

Evaluate the effectiveness of nursing care for a patient with clinical manifestations of cardiac dysfunction by comparing the patient's status with the expected patient outcomes. Examples of specific outcomes for patients with clinical manifestations of cardiac dysfunction have been provided in the Planning section.

Assessment of Cardiac Status

The cardiac health history and the identification of risk factors for heart disease are the most important parts of diagnosing a cardiac problem. A cardiac physical assessment follows the history so that specific problems can be identified and a plan for care established.

Patient History

The cardiac health history is an organized method of eliciting comprehensive, pertinent information from a patient regarding past and present state of health to formulate a data base for problem identification. The health history serves as a basis for directing attention toward specific body systems during the physical examination and allows observation of how the patient's personality structure interrelates with activities of daily living. Time must be allowed during the health history to establish a relationship of trust with the patient by listening attentively, and with concern and by allowing the patient to assume an active, integral, participatory role in health care.

Patients must be allowed to describe their complaints in their own words, such as "I have chest pressure with exercise." The assessment determines when the problem began and if the problem occurs at rest or only with exercise, after meals, and so forth. The duration of the complaint, what brings it on, and how it subsides (with medication or rest) are important. Some patients have associated symptoms such as pain that radiates to a shoulder, arm, or jaw, nausea, diaphoresis, or lightheadedness, and these must be elicited from the patient as the history is obtained.

Questions eliciting information about the ability to perform activities (even activities of daily living) will give an indication of the patient's level of fatigue or other limiting factors such as orthostatic hypotension, edema, and the occurrence of chest pain. As the patient answers questions and tells the cardiac history, notations are to be made about the onset of dyspnea, coughing, or inability to "catch one's breath." Asking the patient about appetite, usual eating patterns, and elimination patterns are important to determine changes that have occurred acutely or over a period of time. The patient may have noted edema of the hands or feet along with weight gain. A loss of weight may be associated with anorexia or abdominal discomfort. Asking about rest patterns will give information about the ability to sleep, the use of multiple pillows for sleep, and PND.

Risk Factors

One part of the cardiac health history is designed to elicit the possible risk factors for heart disease from the patient. Some risk factors can be modified and some cannot. It is important to distinguish the different types of risk factors and help the patient plan care that will modify risk factors. The family history will reveal whether there are any familial diseases that affect the heart or other systems.

NONMODIFIABLE RISK FACTORS

Coronary artery disease is the most common acquired cardiac disease. It is preceded by atherosclerosis. (Risk factors for developing atherosclerosis are identified in Chapter 18.) Nonmodifiable risk factors for coronary artery disease include the following:

Positive Family History. A patient whose father, mother, uncle, brother, or other close blood relative who has had chest pain diagnosed as angina or who suffered a myocardial infarction gives host susceptibility for atherosclerosis. The magnitude of familial risk depends on the sex of the relative (males give a higher risk) and the age of onset of coronary artery disease in the person at risk.

Increasing Age. As a result of the aging process, there is an increase in the arterial deposition of cholesterol, an accumulation of calcium deposits in the coronary arteries, reduced elasticity of the vessels, and an increase in blood pressure. Together these changes increase the risk of coronary artery disease in the older patient.

Male Sex. Males acquire coronary artery disease more frequently and at an earlier age than females. Men are at the highest risk between the ages of 40 and 55 years. There is a decreased incidence of coronary artery disease in females before menopause. After menopause the risk increases. Coronary artery disease is the leading cause of death in females after the age of 65 years.

MODIFIABLE RISK FACTORS

The modifiable risk factors play a very important role in planning long-term care for the patient with identified heart disease. Modifiable risk factors include the following:

Hyperlipidemia. Circulating lipids in the blood are cholesterol lipoproteins: high-density lipoproteins (HDL), low-density lipoproteins (LDL), and very-low-density lipoproteins (VLDL). When the lipids are elevated in the serum, there is a higher risk that they will collect in the coronary arteries (as well as other arteries of the body) and over a period of time clog the arterial opening, leading to decreased blood flow to myocardial tissue, ischemia, and angina. A diet low in animal fats (saturated fats), high in fiber, and calorically balanced to maintain appropriate body weight can decrease the risk of coronary artery disease.

High Blood Pressure. Fluctuations of blood pressure are normal in all persons, but a sustained high blood pressure over a period of years leads to atherosclerosis. The mechanism of atherosclerosis secondary to high blood pressure is thought to be the mechanical damage of arterial linings that accompanies elevated pressure.

Diabetes Mellitus and Glucose Intolerance. High insulin levels induced by the insulin therapy for insulin-dependent diabetics have been implicated in the development of coronary artery disease. Arterial wall exposure to abnormally high levels of circulating insulin causes proliferation of smooth muscle cells, inhibition of glycolysis, and synthesis of cholesterol, triglycerides, and phospholipids. Diabetes mellitus and glucose intolerance are associated with hyperlipidemia, high blood pressure, and obesity, thus increasing the risk of atherosclerosis.

Obesity. The obese patient has an increase in cholesterol synthesis and usually a decrease in HDL, possibly caused by inactivity. Obesity appears to be a major determinant of glucose intolerance and of adult-onset diabetes mellitus. Obesity probably contributes to the development of coronary artery disease through its association with the other risk factors of hypertension, hyperlipidemia, and diabetes mellitus.

Cigarette Smoking. Cigarette smoking independently increases the risk of coronary artery disease 2½ times in persons who smoke two or more packs per day. Because the effect of cigarette smoking on the incidence of coronary artery disease is reversible, it is reasonable to suspect that smoking triggers cardiovascular events rather than being primarily atherogenic in nature or that atherogenesis may depend on the continuation of smoking. Mechanisms that have been suggested to explain the increased risk in smokers are as follows:

1. Vasoconstriction secondary to nicotine inhalation;
2. Neutralization of heparin, which promotes thrombus formation;
3. Platelet aggregation and the release of products during aggregation that may lead to vasospasm;
4. Increases in catecholamines, which lead to increases in heart rate and blood pressure;
5. Dysrhythmias, which diminish cardiac output and may precipitate fatal rhythms in vulnerable persons; and
6. Decreases in vital capacity of the lungs. Also, carbon monoxide reduces the oxygen-carrying capacity of the blood, thus reducing the duration of smokers' exercise tolerance.

Use of Oral Contraceptives. It is not known how oral contraceptives contribute to coronary artery disease. Serum lipids, specifically triglyceride, cholesterol, LDL, and VLDL levels, are elevated by oral contraceptives. Abnormalities of clotting factors and platelet functions have also been noted with the use of oral contraceptives. Users of oral contraceptives have elevated mean blood pressures with systolic increases rather than diastolic increases. The risk from cigarette smoking acts synergistically with the risk from oral contraceptives to increase the risk of coronary artery disease in women at least fivefold.

Sedentary Lifestyle. Physical exercise raises HDL cholesterol, which is protective against development of coronary artery disease. Exercise has also been shown to reduce resting heart rates, control obesity, and increase vital capacity of the lungs, thus promoting oxygenation. Physical activity also helps dispel some of the effects of emotional stress on the cardiovascular system.

Type A Personality. The Type A behavior pattern is characterized by an increased sense of time urgency, a profound eagerness to compete, and a persistence for recognition. These behaviors lead to profound stress, a higher serum cholesterol level, increased amounts of circulating norepinephrine and adrenocorticotropic hormone (ACTH), elevated serum triglyceride levels, and increased sludging of red blood cells, particularly during episodes of hypertriglyceridemia—all risk factors for developing coronary artery disease.

Emotional Stress. Stress is present in daily life, and what is stressful for one individual may not be stressful for another. The stress components of our lifestyle include sociocultural mobility (major changes in residence, occupation, and cultural situations), socioeconomic status, educational level (the higher the level of education, the lower the incidence of coronary artery disease mortality), anxiety, depression, sleep disturbances, life dissatisfaction, and life changes (marriage, divorce, major illnesses, and death). Reducing stress and learning to deal with life's changes are necessary components of good cardiac health.

Physical Examination

Physical assessment follows the attainment of the cardiac health history. The four components of physical assessment—inspection, palpation, percussion, and auscultation—are used to gather data about cardiac functioning. The physical assessment is completed in a systematic, structured method.

INSPECTION

Observation of the patient will give immediate, useful information about the current cardiac status. The patient who is fatigued may look unkempt, pale, and haggard. Dyspnea may be noted, with an increased respiratory rate and difficulty answering questions during the assessment. Pallor of the skin may be noted if increased systemic vascular resistance or anemia is present. Peripheral cyanosis, the result of decreased circulation, may be noted in the fingernail or toenail beds.

PALPATION

As the peripheral pulses are palpated, temperature and moistness or dryness of the skin are noted. Edema of extremities is also assessed and evaluated. Normally, the liver cannot be palpated, but with right-sided failure and back-up of venous fluid, the liver may be palpable at the lower edge of the right rib cage. An engorged liver may also be painful when palpated.

PERCUSSION

Percussion of the chest may reveal areas of lung consolidation from fluid-filled spaces. Left-sided heart failure causes excess fluid to back up into alveoli that are normally filled with air. Air-filled alveoli give a hollow sound when percussed, whereas fluid-filled airways give a dull sound.

Percussion of the abdomen should produce a tympanic sound over the stomach and the liver and spleen. A fluid-filled bladder also produces a dull sound, whereas an empty bladder produces a tympanic sound.

AUSCULTATION

Using a stethoscope, auscultate the heart sounds by placing the diaphragm on the chest wall in the apical (mitral) area of the heart. After listening for the normal heart sounds, S_1 or S_2, listen for extra heart sounds, S_3 or S_4, that may be present. Then move the stethoscope to the aortic, pulmonic, tricuspid, and right ventricular areas (see Fig. 17–1) while listening to the heart sounds. For sounds that are difficult to hear, use the bell of the stethoscope placed lightly on the chest wall. The apical pulse rate is determined using auscultation and counting the beats that occur in 1 minute.

Lung sounds are auscultated by moving the diaphragm of the stethoscope across all lobes of the lungs anteriorly and posteriorly. As air passes through alveoli containing fluid, crackles (rales) are heard. If airways are narrowed by inflammation or disease, wheezes are heard during inspiration or expiration.

Diagnostic Procedures

A variety of diagnostic procedures are used to confirm suspected cardiac diagnoses. Explanations and expectations of the tests are given to the patient and family for each procedure. Some of the diagnostic procedures for determining cardiac dysfunction are noninvasive, and others are invasive. Most invasive studies require informed consent forms to be signed before the study.

X-Ray Studies

The most common x-ray examination ordered for cardiac patients is the routine chest x-ray film. Anatomic abnormalities can be clearly identified, and physiologic alterations can be inferred from the chest x-ray film. The silhouette of the heart, its chambers, the great vessels, and the placement of these structures in the chest cavity can be seen on the chest x-ray film. Radiographic density of the heart made up of muscle and blood is different from the surrounding structures such as the air-filled lungs, pericardial fat, and the esophagus when filled with barium for the purposes of x-ray definition. Chest x-ray films should be taken with the patient in an erect position during deep inspiration. A posteroanterior (PA) film is taken with the x-ray plate in front of the patient's chest. For an anteroposterior (AP) chest x-ray film, the x-ray plate is placed in back of the patient's chest, but there are significant changes in the contour of the cardiac silhouette if the AP film is used. The same considerations must be kept in mind if a supine chest x-ray film is taken.

Normally the lungs are filled with air, but with disease processes, fluid may accumulate in the lungs or pleural cavities. Fluid is detected as a dense area on the chest x-ray film. Pulmonary edema causes fluffy densities around the root of the lung, and pleural effusions obscure the sharp costophrenic angles.

A chest x-ray film may be taken in the x-ray department, which gives the best contrast films for diagnostic purposes, or in the patient's room with a portable x-ray machine when the patient cannot be moved. Many intensive care unit patients who must be continually monitored have a portable chest x-ray film ordered. In portable chest films, the heart and great vessels assume a different size and configuration because of the placement of the chest plate at a shorter distance from the machine (about 4 feet versus 6 feet in the x-ray department). A portable chest film should not be compared with an x-ray department film because of these changes.

Fluoroscopy

Heart, lung, and vessel movements are viewed on a luminescent x-ray film screen (or monitor) in a darkened room during fluoroscopy. Fluoroscopy allows analysis of the motion of the intrathoracic structures, such as the heart beating, the lungs expanding, and intravenous or intra-arterial catheters and pacemakers. Cardiac catheterization, which uses fluoroscopy extensively, is discussed later.

Stress Test

The stress test is the recording of the ECG during exercise. A resting ECG may be normal, but with exercise (or stress) changes occur that are significant and that need therapy for control. The purposes of exercise testing are to detect latent coronary artery disease, evaluate sequentially the exercise response in patients who have known coronary artery disease, evaluate the effects of medical or surgical treatment, and monitor the effects of cardiac rehabilitation programs.

The graded exercise stress test (GEST) is carried out in stages. Each stage is 3 minutes in duration. An increase in workload is accomplished by increasing the speed or the incline of the treadmill used to exercise the patient. Before the test, a baseline resting ECG is taken, and resting blood pressure is determined. During the entire test, the electrical pattern of the heart is constantly monitored, and blood pressure readings are obtained as each workload comes to an end. The test is continued until the patient reaches his or her maximal heart rate, previously determined by age (Table 17–3) or until there is an indication to stop the test. Absolute indications to stop the exercise include hypotension, three consecutive premature ventricular contractions, ST depression of 1 mm or more, physical exhaustion, severe angina, and a staggering gait.

Table 17–3. AGE-RELATED HEART RATES

Age	Maximal Heart Rate	90%	60%
35	185	166	111
45	180	158	108
50	170	153	102
55	165	149	99
60	160	144	96
65	155	140	93
70	150	135	90

From Sanderson RG, Kurth CL. The cardiac patient. 2nd ed. Philadelphia: WB Saunders, 1983, p. 512.

ECG monitoring is continued for 5 to 10 minutes after the exercise while the patient's heart rate and blood pressure responses return to normal. A high correlation is found between significant obstructive coronary artery disease and a positive stress test.

Complications of stress testing are cardiac dysrhythmias, which may lead to cardiac arrest and myocardial infarction. Monitoring the cardiac rhythm for several hours after stress testing may be indicated for this reason.

Ambulatory Electrocardiogram Monitoring

A Holter monitor provides ambulatory monitoring of the ECG for a 24-hour period or more while the patient is at home or at work. The patient is connected to the recording box (like a cassette tape recorder) via electrodes on the chest and wears the electrodes and recorder for the duration of the recording time. A common fear of many patients is that electricity will be transmitted from the leads to their bodies. The patient should be assured that this will not occur.

The ECG monitor records the electricity being generated by the action potential of the patient's heart. The patient is instructed to keep a diary of daily activities and to note the time of those activities. Most Holter monitors have a recording clock so variations in the ECG can be compared with activities in the diary by using the times recorded. The patient can mark events by pushing a button on the recorder when symptoms such as chest pain, dizziness, or palpitations are experienced. If the symptoms are caused by a change in the cardiac rhythm, this type of ambulatory ECG recording will help diagnose the problems and provide answers in planning care for the patient.

At the end of the recording period, the patient returns the Holter monitor to the physician, clinic, or hospital, and the tape is scanned by special equipment that can evaluate a 24-hour period in just a few minutes. ECG abnormalities are identified by the scanner and recorded at normal ECG paper speed for careful consideration and diagnosis by the physician.

Ambulatory monitoring is also done in hospitals via telemetry units. Patients who have had an acute cardiac event or dysrhythmias or who have been started on cardiac medications that may affect heart rhythm wear electrodes connected to a battery-powered unit. The ECG is viewed on a monitor at a nurse's station in a critical care or telemetry unit. The patient's cardiac rhythm is monitored as activities of daily living are completed. If dysrhythmias occur during eating, bathing, walking, or other activities, they can be treated before the patient is discharged.

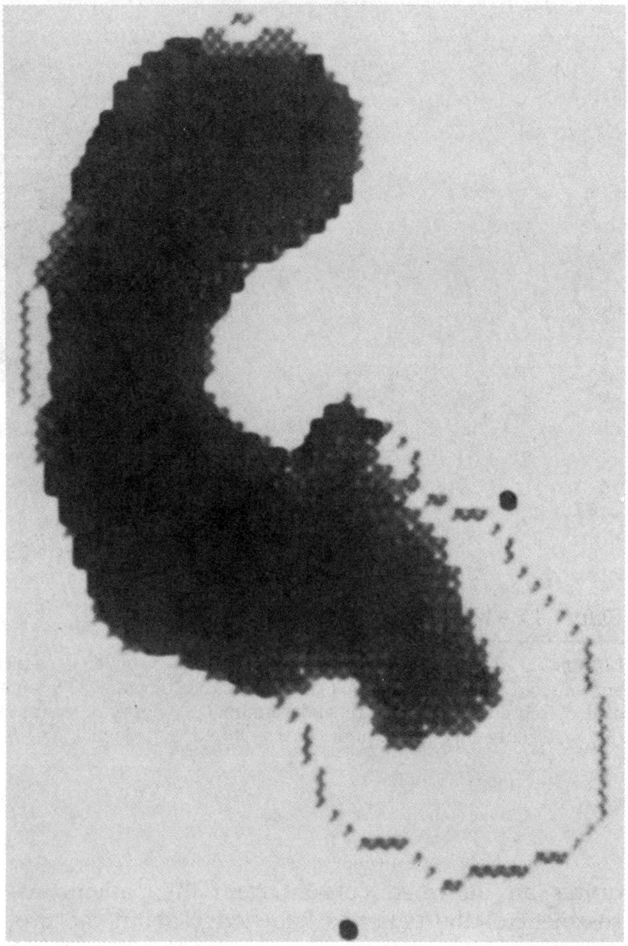

Figure 17–16.

First-pass angiocardiography (technetium). In this computer-processed image, the outlines of the left ventricle are easily seen in end-diastole (outer, single-line image) and in end-systole (inner, darkly shaded image). The ascending aorta also can be seen (in upper left portion) as the radioactive technetium is visualized by the gamma camera in its passage out of the heart. (From Sanderson RG, Kurth CL. The cardiac patient. 2nd ed. Philadelphia: WB Saunders, 1983, p 102.)

Radioactive Imaging

The technique of radioactive imaging uses radioactive isotopes that have an affinity for specific types of tissue. Radioactive thallium 201 is used to evaluate myocardial ischemia because it is selectively diminished in areas of myocardial ischemia. Technetium stannous pyrophosphate has a particular affinity for areas of acute myocardial necrosis and is used to confirm a diagnosis of acute myocardial infarction.

The radioactive agent is injected into a peripheral vein. The patient is placed beneath a scintillation gamma camera, a device that detects gamma radiation. The images that are recorded on magnetic disc or tape exemplify the areas where the radioactive agent was absorbed or not absorbed by the tissue (Fig. 17–16). Complications of radioactive imaging are rare.

Echocardiography

High-frequency sound waves are emitted from a transducer that is placed on the anterior chest wall of the patient. Because the frequencies of the sound waves that are used are above the audible range, they are called ultrasound waves. As the ultrasound waves pass through the chest wall, they encounter the cardiac wall or other tissue and bounce, or echo, back to the transducer. The echoes are then recorded. The recording depicts the depth of a cardiac structure (wall, chamber, septum, valve) by converting to distance the time taken by the echo to travel to the reflecting surface and return to the transducer (Fig. 17–17). The echocardiogram is a noninvasive procedure that gives information about the thickness and function of the cardiac valves, size of cardiac chambers, thickness of ventricular and atrial walls, and size of intracardiac shunts.

Cardiac Catheterization

The technique of cardiac catheterization has been improved over the past 20 years so that a variety of intracardiac abnormalities—anatomic, hemodynamic, and functional—can be detected. Cardiac catheterization is an invasive procedure that re-

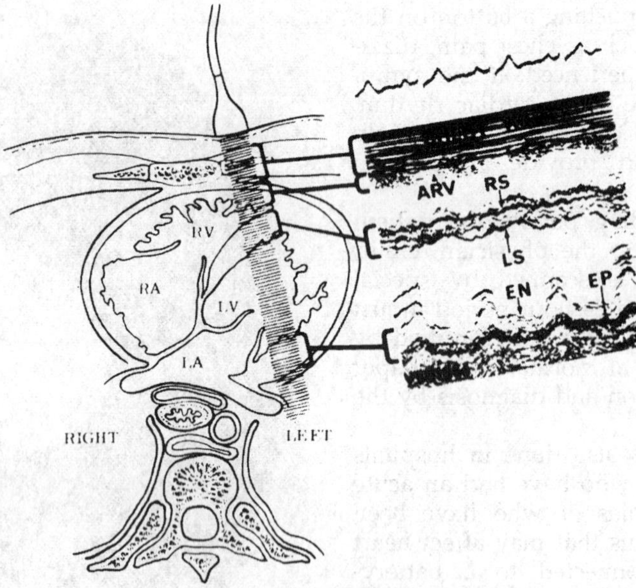

Figure 17–17.

Diagram of the chest wall and heart transversed by an "ice-pick" beam of echoes and an echocardiogram depicting the structures encountered along with a simultaneous electrocardiogram. ARV, anterior wall right ventricle; RS, right side of interventricular septum; LS, left side of septum; EN, posterior endocardium; EP, posterior epicardium. Lung tissue produces the echoes below the posterior epicardium. (From Feigenbaum H. Echocardiography. 3rd ed. Philadelphia: Lea & Febiger, 1981. Reprinted with permission.)

quires an informed consent from the patient. Assessment of the patient's knowledge about the procedure is important. The physician and nurse provide information to relieve anxiety about the planned procedures (Nursing Care Guide 17–1).

Before catheterization, the patient is given a mild sedative to aid in relaxation during the procedure. The patient is to remain awake while the cardiac catheterization procedure is progressing, because the patient is frequently instructed by the physician to cough or change breathing patterns. Such actions change the pressures in the chest cavity and aid circulation as it is viewed on the oscilloscope in the catheterization laboratory. Before catheterization, the patient should be told that participation is expected during the procedure.

During cardiac catheterization and angiography, a radiopaque contrast dye is injected into cardiac chambers and coronary arteries to view blood flow through these areas. The patient is assessed for known allergy to the substance to be used. Allergy to iodine and seafood is a contraindication for using most radiopaque dyes without prior preparation to combat the potential allergic reaction. The patient is told to expect a warm, tingling sensation when the dye is injected. If the patient experiences chest pain, appropriate analgesics are administered.

After catheterization, the patient is assessed for pain, stability of vital signs, bleeding, edema, and temperature change. Pulses distal to the catheter insertion site are palpated and compared with the opposite side. Changes in peripheral pulses, which indicate compromised circulation, such as a weakened thready pulse are reported immediately.

Arterial puncture sites are bandaged with pressure dressings. The dressings are monitored for blood saturation and tightness by palpating pulses distal to the site every 15 minutes to 1 hour as ordered. The patient is on bed rest for 8 to 10 hours after the procedure to ensure stability of vital signs and absence of bleeding. Before discharge, the patient is given instructions for self-management at home (Chart 17–1).

RIGHT-SIDED HEART CATHETERIZATION

A small plastic catheter is inserted into a peripheral vein (femoral or anticubital) and advanced through the venous system into the right atrium. The catheter can be manipulated under fluoroscopic control through the tricuspid valve into the right ventricle, through the pulmonic valve, and into the main pulmonary artery. From there, the catheter can be advanced into the smaller branches of the pulmonary vessels until it becomes wedged in a very small peripheral branch. As the catheter passes through the various chambers of the right side of the heart, pressures can be recorded and blood samples can be drawn for analyses. The oxygen and carbon dioxide content are the most important measurements.

Nursing Care Guide 17–1.

PATIENTS UNDERGOING CARDIAC CATHETERIZATION

Precatheterization

Assessment Findings: Patient presents with signs of restlessness, nervousness, and increased respiratory and heart rate, asks questions about procedures, clenches hands, and cries.

Nursing Diagnosis: Anxiety related to fear of procedure, diagnosis, and future medical/surgical management

Patient Outcomes	Nursing Interventions	Rationale
Patient is less anxious, as evidenced by patient smiling and lack of restlessness, crying, or nervousness.	Explain the procedure to the patient and family. Allow time for questions and concerns.	An understanding of the procedure may alleviate the stress induced from the unknown or misunderstandings.
Patient's vital signs are within normal limits for the patient.	Teach relaxation techniques. Allow time for rest; provide a quiet, comfortable atmosphere.	Practicing relaxation techniques alleviates tension, as indicated by normal vital signs.
Patient states relief of anxiety.	Help the patient find coping strategies that help alleviate the stress and anxiety.	Appropriate coping strategies may reduce levels of anxiety.

Evaluation: Compare the patient's status with the expected patient outcomes. If the outcomes are achieved, evaluate nursing care as successful. If not, reassess the patient, formulate new nursing diagnoses, and revise expected patient outcomes and nursing interventions as appropriate.

Assessment Findings: Patient asks questions about procedure, seems uninformed about pre- and postprocedure care and treatments; patient and family voice concerns about risks and necessity for the procedure.

Nursing Diagnosis: Knowledge deficit: nature of procedure and postprocedure care

Patient Outcomes	Nursing Interventions	Rationale
Patient reports accurate information about the procedure, the necessity for it, and the expectations after procedure.	Be certain the physician has discussed the procedure, risks, complications, and expectations with the patient. Allow the patient to ask questions, and try to expand on the understanding about the procedure for the patient and family. Have the patient state the information received from the physician so any misconceptions can be eliminated.	Checking the information the patient has received reinforces the understanding. Allowing time for questions gives the patient a chance to be fully knowledgeable about the procedure. Asking the patient to repeat the information allows for correction of misinformation.

(continued)

Nursing Care Guide 17–1. *(continued)*

PATIENTS UNDERGOING CARDIAC CATHETERIZATION

Patient Outcomes	Nursing Interventions	Rationale
Patient and family state they have an understanding of the procedure, the risks, and the postprocedure care needed.	Explain the postprocedure care needed to both the patient and the family, and tell the patient it will be repeated before discharge (see Chart 17–1).	Giving information to both patient and family provides support and reinforcement for the patient, especially after discharge. It also alleviates some of the anxiety for the family.

Evaluation: Compare the patient's status with the expected patient outcomes. If the outcomes are achieved, evaluate nursing care as successful. If not, reassess the patient, formulate new nursing diagnoses, and revise expected patient outcomes and nursing interventions as appropriate.

Postcatheterization

Assessment Findings: Patient is diaphoretic, and weak and exhibits pallor, tachycardia, tachypnea, and wheezing.

Nursing Diagnosis: Fluid volume deficit related to extreme diuresis from effect of contrast dye

Patient Outcomes	Nursing Interventions	Rationale
Patient remains well hydrated. Vital signs are within normal limits for the patient.	Encourage increased fluid intake to match the output. Observe for signs of hypovolemia such as poor skin turgor, dry, cracked lips, and vital sign changes.	Increased intake of fluids replaces losses. Vital sign changes and dry skin and mucous membranes may reflect dehydration.
Patient's output is adequate without excess.	Check the patient's output frequently. Compare fluid intake and output amounts.	Increased output is a side effect that should be noted.

Evaluation: Compare the patient's status with the expected patient outcomes. If the outcomes are achieved, evaluate nursing care as successful. If not, reassess the patient, formulate new nursing diagnoses, and revise expected patient outcomes and nursing interventions as appropriate.

(continued)

Nursing Care Guide 17–1. *(continued)*

PATIENTS UNDERGOING CARDIAC CATHETERIZATION

Assessment Findings: Patient complains of confusion, disorientation, paresthesia, weakness, or syncope.

Nursing Diagnosis: Altered tissue perfusion, cerebral, related to potential complication of blood clot or plaque being dislodged during procedure and traveling to the brain

Patient Outcomes	Nursing Interventions	Rationale
Patient remains alert and oriented.	Watch for signs of confusion, dizziness, altered level of consciousness, and lethargy. Notify the physician if these signs are evident.	Although a clot or plaque embolus may not be preventable, observe for early signs of decreased cerebral tissue perfusion so early intervention can occur.
Patient experiences no further complications from the results of the procedure.	Assist the patient in getting out of bed when able if dizzy or confused or if blood pressure is low.	Because the patient may have some weakness and orthostatic hypotension, assistance is needed to prevent injury.

Evaluation: Compare the patient's status with the expected patient outcomes. If the outcomes are achieved, evaluate nursing care as successful. If not, reassess the patient, formulate new nursing diagnoses, and revise expected patient outcomes and nursing interventions as appropriate.

Assessment Findings: Patient asks questions about necessary home care and other discharge instructions.

Nursing Diagnosis: Knowledge deficit: self-management after discharge

Patient Outcomes	Nursing Interventions	Rationale
Patient states accurate information about discharge care. Patient states when to report to the physician for follow-up.	Give the patient written instruction for self-care after discharge as listed on Chart 17–1. Have patient repeat information. Allow time for questions and concerns, and correct misunderstandings. Explain in terminology the patient can understand, and ask for the patient's perception of what was said.	Written instructions reinforce verbal information and allow for review after discharge. Having patient repeat information and providing time for questions allow further patient education and correction of misunderstandings.
Patient and family report an understanding of the instructions given.	Include the family in the discharge instruction session. Allow time for questions.	Including the family gives additional support to the patient, especially if the patient cannot provide the self-care necessary on discharge.

Evaluation: Compare the patient's status with the expected patient outcomes. If the outcomes are achieved, evaluate nursing care as successful. If not, reassess the patient, formulate new nursing diagnoses, and revise expected patient outcomes and nursing interventions as appropriate.

Chart 17–1.

NURSING GUIDE TO PATIENT EDUCATION FOR SELF-MANAGEMENT: DISCHARGE INSTRUCTIONS AFTER CARDIAC CATHETERIZATION

On discharge, instruct the patient who has had a cardiac catheterization to:

Watch for bleeding or swelling at dressing sites (puncture sites).
If bleeding occurs, apply direct pressure over dressing and notify physician.
Observe for signs of circulatory impairment of extremities such as discoloration, numbness, tingling, or lack of warmth.
Report any of the above untoward symptoms to physician.
Expect some pain at puncture sites. Take analgesic as ordered.
Increase fluid intake for 24 hours, unless contraindicated, to assist in the removal of the contrast medium.

When the catheter is wedged in a peripheral pulmonary artery branch, the pressure reflected is the PWP, or PCWP. The wedged catheter obstructs pulmonary artery blood flow in that small vessel and senses the pressure transmitted by the pulmonary veins and the left atrium, thus reflecting indirectly the pulmonary venous or left atrial pressures.

LEFT-SIDED HEART CATHETERIZATION

A catheter is placed into the left side of the heart by inserting it into a peripheral artery (femoral or brachial) and advancing it through the aorta and the aortic valve into the left ventricle, through the mitral valve, and into the left atrium. At times the catheter cannot be advanced into the left atrium because of the action and pressures of blood flowing through the mitral valve. Therefore, access to the left atrium is gained by transseptal puncture. The right-sided heart catheter, with a catheter-sheathed needle on its end, is advanced through the interatrial septum from the right atrium to the left atrium.

Patients who have had an aortic valve replacement or who have a stenotic aortic valve may require percutaneous puncture through the chest wall for access to the left ventricle. As in right-sided heart catheterization, pressure measurements can be made and blood samples withdrawn anywhere along the catheterization route. Cardiac output is usually determined as a measure of hemodynamic function.

ANGIOGRAPHY

During cardiac catheterization, the chambers and great vessels are visualized along with the coronary arteries and the flow of blood through the heart. A contrast agent (iodinated water-soluble compound) that is opaque to the x-ray beam is injected into the circulation at different sites. Rapidly changing films record the dynamics of the passage of the contrast agent through the vascular tree starting at the injection site. The film recording of these angiographic studies is known as cineangiography. The recordings can be studied at various speeds for detailed diagnosis of coronary artery and cardiac chamber problems.

Complications of the procedure include allergic reactions to the contrast agent, bleeding at the catheter site, and puncture of vessels during the procedure. Rarely does angiography produce more severe symptoms.

Blood Studies

The usual diagnostic studies for cardiac disorders include CBC, electrolytes, cholesterol, lipids, and enzymes. If specific enzymes are elevated in the blood, further delineation is accomplished by determining isoenzymes. Additional blood studies may be ordered for patients with complicating problems such as diabetes. If a patient has a family history of other diseases, further blood studies may also be ordered.

COMPLETE BLOOD COUNT AND DIFFERENTIAL COUNT

The CBC and differential count are a series of peripheral blood tests that provide information about the hematologic system and other organs. This information also provides clues to cardiac problems, especially those related to oxygenation. A complete discussion of the tests and possible abnormalities is found in Chapter 15.

ELECTROLYTES

Routine determination of serum electrolytes includes sodium (Na), potassium (K), chloride (Cl), and carbon dioxide (CO_2). Sodium and potassium are the necessary electrolytes for cardiac electrical conduction. Normal conduction demands appropriate electrolyte balance in the blood. As sodium and potassium vary from the normal level, dysrhythmias may be seen on the ECG. The normal levels for sodium and potassium are 136 to 145 mEq/L and 3.5 to 5.0 mEq/L, respectively. Chloride maintains electrical neutrality as a salt with sodium and serves as a buffer in acid-base balance. The normal level for chloride is 98 to 106 mEq/L. Carbon dioxide content of the blood plays a major role in acid-base balance, which also affects the normal conduction system of the heart. The normal level for carbon dioxide is 22 to 30 mEq/L. Acid-base imbalances may produce cardiac dysrhythmias that will be noted on the ECG.

GLUCOSE

Hyperglycemia is present in diabetes mellitus and is an acute stress response to surgery, myocardial infarction, or other traumatic cardiac events. Other metabolic diseases may also be diagnosed by evaluating the serum glucose level. A complete discussion of glucose levels is found in Chapter 30.

BLOOD UREA NITROGEN/SERUM CREATININE

Kidney function is assessed by evaluating the BUN and serum creatinine. Urea is formed in the liver as an end product of protein catabolism and is excreted entirely by the kidney. Therefore, the BUN is directly related to the excretory function of the kidney. In primary renal diseases, there is inadequate excretion of urea, and the blood concentration rises above normal. Cardiac patients with changing hemodynamics will have varying BUN levels from day to day because of decreased renal perfusion. The normal BUN is 8 to 20 mg/dl.

Creatinine is excreted entirely by the kidneys and is directly proportional to renal excretory function. Creatinine is a catabolic product of creatine, which is used in skeletal muscle contraction. The daily production of creatine, and subsequently creatinine, depends on muscle mass, which fluctuates very little. The normal serum creatinine level is 0.6 to 1.3 mg/dl.

The BUN is affected by dehydration, malnutrition, and hepatic function, whereas the creatinine is not. When the BUN rises out of proportion to the creatinine level, dehydration, gastrointestinal bleeding, and malnutrition are suspected. When both the BUN and creatinine levels rise, the patient is assessed for kidney disease or failure. Low protein intake, overhydration, or severe liver failure will reduce the BUN level but not the creatinine level.

ERYTHROCYTE SEDIMENTATION RATE

The erythrocyte sedimentation rate (ESR, or sed rate) is a nonspecific test used to detect inflammatory response, infection, or necrotic processes. The ESR is not diagnostic for any specific disorder or disease, but it is useful to detect inflammatory disease that is not otherwise suspected or to confirm a disease that is suspected such as endocarditis, rheumatic fever, or pericarditis.

PROTHROMBIN TIME AND PARTIAL THROMBOPLASTIN TIME

The prothrombin time (pro time or PT) is used to evaluate the adequacy of the extrinsic clotting system. The partial thromboplastin time (PTT) is used to assess the intrinsic clotting system. Both of these tests are discussed in detail in Chapter 15. They are useful for monitoring the patient on anticoagulant therapy. Heparin, an anticoagulant, is frequently given during cardiac and vascular surgery and is also used for thromboembolic episodes such as pulmonary embolism, arterial embolism, and thrombophlebitis.

SERUM LIPIDS

A serum lipid study usually includes total blood lipids, cholesterol, triglycerides, phospholipids, and cholesterol lipoproteins. Lipids, such as cholesterol, triglycerides, and phospholipids, are transported in the blood by combining with proteins and, therefore, are called lipoproteins. The lipoproteins can be separated by electrophoresis and fractionated into HDL, LDL, and VLDL. LDL and VLDL have a strong association with coronary artery disease, whereas HDL is protective against coronary artery disease and is associated with a decreased risk of myocardial infarction.

ENZYMES

Enzymes are proteins formed by the protoplasm of all cells. When cell membranes are damaged or broken, as occurs when cardiac cells are damaged by a myocardial infarction, enzymes inside the cells are released through the damaged membranes into the circulating blood. Three enzymes are specific to cardiac tissue: lactic dehydrogenase (LDH), serum aspartate aminotransferase (AST), formerly measured as serum glutamic oxaloacetic transaminase (SGOT), and creatine kinase (CK) or creatine phosphokinase (CPK).

CK is the first enzyme that elevates after any cardiac damage. It elevates within 3 to 6 hours of the onset of ischemia, peaks in 18 hours, and returns to normal within 3 days (Fig. 17–18). In addition to being found in cardiac muscle, CK is also found in skeletal muscle and brain tissue. Patients who are suspected of having an acute cardiac disease should not be given any intramuscular injections because the needle damage to skeletal muscle may elevate the CK and mask an increase that is actually due to cardiac damage.

The AST elevates within 6 hours after cardiac

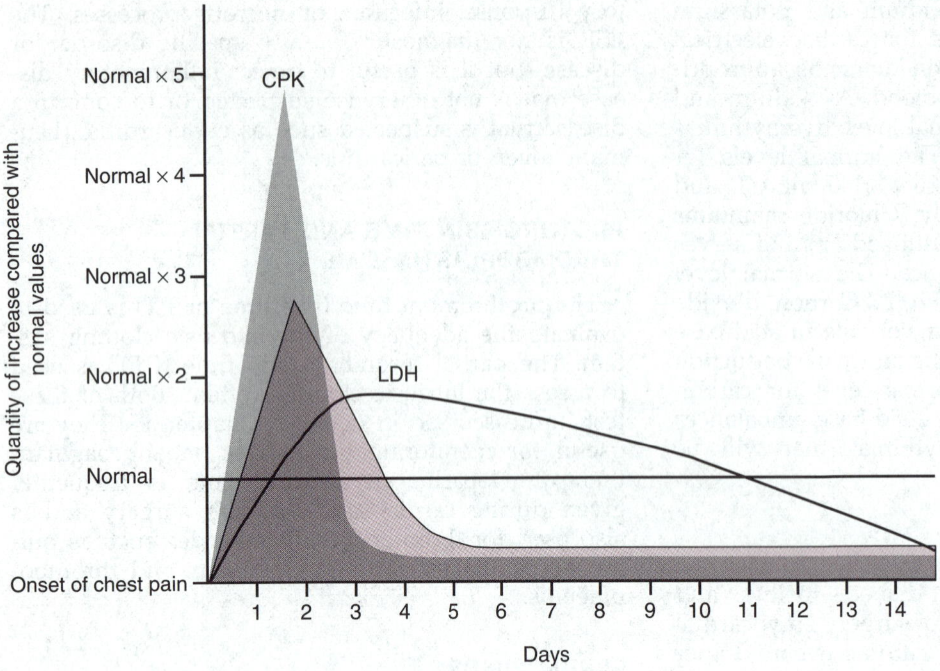

Figure 17–18.

Serum enzyme level elevation and return to normal following an acute myocardial infarction.

Pharmacology Box 17–1.

CARDIAC GLYCOSIDES

Cardiac Glycosides:
Class of drugs derived from natural sources containing a glycoside, a steroid, and a lactone.

Action:
Exert a positive inotropic action on the heart and may exert a negative chronotropic action and a negative dromotropic action.

Uses:
Treatment of congestive heart failure.

Side Effects:
Anorexia, nausea, vomiting, headache, weakness, restlessness, confusion, and cardiac arrhythmias.

Interactions:
May interact with drugs such as antacids and antidiarrheal agents.

Nursing Implications:
Check heart rate before administering; if less than 60 beats per minute, check with physician.
If administering intravenously, give deep in large muscle.
Some glycosides are best absorbed in liquid form.
Give tablets with food to decrease gastric irritation.
Protect intravenous solution from light.
Observe for side effects and toxicity.
Monitor cardiac status, checking for bigeminy or other dysrhythmias.
Check laboratory data for potassium level.
Encourage patient to eat potassium-rich foods.
Instruct patient about medication, side effects, and to check heart rate.

damage, peaks in 12 to 14 hours, and returns to normal in 4 days (see Fig. 17–18). It is found in cardiac muscle, skeletal muscle, liver, pancreas, and kidney tissue.

The LDH elevates within 24 hours after cardiac damage, peaks within 72 hours, and returns to normal within 14 days (see Fig. 17–18). Besides being found in cardiac muscle, LDH is found in red blood cells, skeletal muscle, brain, liver, kidney, lung, and skin tissue.

ISOENZYMES

The CK can be fractionated into three isoenzymes: MM, BB, and MB. These isoenzymes may show whether the CK came from the heart muscle (MB) or from skeletal muscle (MM). The isoenzyme MB provides a unique marker for damaged myocardial cells. The CK-MB level does not rise after angina without myocardial infarction present. For this reason, it is a more valuable test for evidence of myocardial infarction than the total CK. The CK-BB isoenzyme is found primarily in the brain and lungs, whereas the CK-MM isoenzyme is found primarily in skeletal muscle.

There are five LDH isoenzymes, LDH-1 to LDH-5, which may be separated by electrophoresis. LDH-1 is primarily found in the heart and red blood cells. Normally LDH-2 is greater than LDH-1, but in cardiac cellular damage LDH-1 becomes greater than LDH-2. This is called an LDH flip. An LDH flip is diagnostic of an acute myocardial infarction.

Medical Management

Nonsurgical Management

Once the risk factors for cardiac dysfunction have been identified, the goal of nonsurgical management is reduction of risk for myocardial disease. Some risk factors, such as heredity, cannot be altered, but many others can be modified or eliminated, thus changing the risk for future cardiac problems.

REDUCTION OF RISK FACTORS

Hyperlipidemia is reduced by adhering to a diet low in animal fats and other saturated fats and high in fiber. Calories are balanced to maintain an appropriate body weight. For some individuals, this may mean a reduction in caloric intake to achieve weight loss. Caloric intake is regulated to achieve the target body weight, with a normal glucose level and without excessive strain on the heart. Because obesity is also a risk factor for cardiac disease, weight reduction is a goal to be achieved.

Associated disease processes need to be controlled. High blood pressure is treated with a combination of diet changes, exercise, and antihypertensive drug therapy. Diabetes mellitus is controlled by drug therapy and diet, with the goal of keeping the glucose level stable and within normal limits.

Cessation of smoking is the only method to combat the risk smoking plays in cardiac disease. Medical management in smoking cessation may include referral to education and support classes for smokers or nicotine-replacement drug therapy.

Physical exercise is recommended as a component of every individual's daily life. The specific exercise prescription is modified for each patient on the basis of history, ability, and other interfering disorders or limitations.

Individuals with Type A personality patterns are confronted with their behaviors that aggravate stress levels such as time urgency, competitiveness, compulsive work schedules, and interrupted sleep patterns. A frank explanation of the risk of cardiac disease from these continued behaviors is usually necessary. Referral to stress-management seminars or relaxation sessions may be indicated. Professional assistance from a psychiatrist, psychologist, or counselor may also be beneficial.

Women taking oral contraceptives are periodically tested for serum lipid, triglyceride, and cholesterol levels. Baseline levels are determined before initiating contraceptive therapy. Any significant elevation in the values after introduction of oral contraceptives is evaluated. Other birth-control measures may be recommended if the values indicate an increased risk of cardiac disease. Blood pressure measurements are taken along with the serum testing because an elevation in blood pressure may accompany oral contraceptive use. Cigarette smoking is highly discouraged because smoking and oral contraceptive use together increase the risk of coronary artery disease at least five times.

PHARMACOLOGIC THERAPY

There are a multitude of pharmacologic agents available for the treatment of cardiovascular disease. Most of the drugs can be categorized into five groups that are used to treat cardiac failure, angina pectoris, blood pressure variations, and dysrhythmias. The five groups are cardiac glycosides, vasodilators, catecholamines, antiarrhythmics, and diuretics. The drugs in each category have many similar characteristics, but individual drugs in each group also have some unique properties, side effects, routes of administration, and nursing implications.

CARDIAC GLYCOSIDES

Cardiac glycosides are used to treat patients with congestive heart failure. They strengthen cardiac muscle contractions, which results in more efficient pumping of blood by the heart. Thus, more blood flows to the kidneys and is filtered to remove fluid and properties that are not needed by the body. Intravascular volume decreases as urine output increases, thus reducing venous congestion and easing the workload of the heart (Pharmacology Box 17–1).

Pharmacology Box 17–2.
ANTIANGINAL DRUGS

Antianginal Drugs:
Group of drugs used for symptomatic relief of chest pain.

Action:
Reduce oxygen consumption by coronary vessels, relieving ischemia; relax coronary smooth muscle, producing vasodilation; and increase coronary blood flow.

Uses:
Treatment of angina pectoris; they provide relief of cardiac ischemia, thus relieving angina.

Side Effects:
Headache, flushing of face, nausea, vomiting, dizziness, hypotension, and confusion.

Interactions:
May enhance effects of alcohol, and alcohol in turn may aggravate side effects of the antianginal agents.

Nursing Implications:
Instruct patient to take oral tablets on empty stomach and not drink alcohol while taking medication.
Watch for signs of hypotension; check blood pressure.
Store tablets in a tightly closed container.
Give at first symptom of anginal attack.
Teach patient when to take tablets, and place at the bedside or tell patient to notify nurse immediately when pain occurs.
Instruct patient about medication, how and when to repeat dose, side effects, and how to apply medication if using nitroglycerin patches.

Cardiac glycosides also slow the transmission of electrical impulses from atrial to ventricular tissue in the heart. Thus, patients who have supraventricular dysrhythmias (coming from above ventricular tissue) may benefit from drug therapy that slows their heart rate, thus increasing cardiac filling time and resulting in an increase in cardiac output.

The most commonly used cardiac glycoside is digoxin. Other drugs in the cardiac glycoside category are deslanoside, digitoxin, and ouabain. The side effects of the drugs in this group are similar for the different preparations. They include nausea, vomiting, weakness, heart block, and visual disturbances such as seeing halos around lights and greenish-yellow hues. Serum digoxin levels should be monitored when patients begin digoxin therapy, when dosages are changed, if they exhibit toxicity signs or if signs of ineffectiveness occur. Serum digoxin levels should be drawn 4 to 6 hours after an intravenous administration and 6 to 8 hours after an oral dose.

Hypokalemia and hypercalcemia make a patient hypersensitive to digoxin; thus, toxicity may result with low serum levels of digoxin. Patients taking nifedipine, verapamil, or quinidine may have high serum digoxin levels, thus indicating that their doses of digoxin need to be lowered while concurrently taking these drugs.

Symptoms of toxicity are the more severe side effects of digoxin. Toxicity is usually treated by discontinuing the drug or giving a lower dose. The physician is notified of toxicity symptoms so orders to treat the problem may be obtained. If dysrhythmias are severe, they are treated with the appropriate antiarrhythmic drug therapy or a pacemaker if indicated.

VASODILATORS

Vasodilators act on the smooth muscle walls of blood vessels to widen the vascular lumen, thus decreasing resistance to blood flow and increasing flow through the vessels. Some vasodilators act primarily on the walls of veins, some on the walls of arteries and some on both. Those that act primarily on veins are called venodilators and are used to prevent angina and to treat acute anginal attacks (Pharmacology Box 17–2). Common venodilators are nitroglycerin, isosorbide dinitrate, and other nitrates. They dilate veins and venules so that more blood collects in these capacitance vessels rather than returning to the heart. Blood is said to "pool" in these peripheral vessels. Pooling of blood away from the heart reduces the "preload" to the heart, allowing the heart to expend less oxygen to empty its chambers. A myocardial oxygen deficit that causes angina is less likely to occur when preload is reduced. Venodilators may also dilate coronary arteries, thus improving collateral circulation to the heart tissues. Myocardial ischemia is further reduced when this occurs. Venodilators may also alleviate congestive heart failure because of a reduction of preload.

Vasodilating medication is easiest to administer in sublingual form. A nitroglycerin tablet is placed under the patient's tongue just before engaging in activities that are known to provoke angina (exercising, going out into cold weather, eating a heavy meal, sexual intercourse, or dealing with an emotionally stressful situation). When angina occurs, the patient is taught to place a nitroglycerin tablet under the tongue every 3 to 5 minutes until three tablets have been used. If relief is not obtained with three sublingual nitroglycerin tablets, the patient needs to seek immediate medical assistance because a heart attack may be occurring and further use of nitroglycerin tablets will not relieve the angina.

Oral and transdermal nitrates give continuous protection against angina. They take effect more slowly than sublingual nitrates, but they last longer. Some transdermal patches last up to 24 hours; thus, the patient has to apply a new patch only once each day.

Arterial dilators relax the walls of arteries and make it easier for the heart to expel blood from the left ventricle into the arterial circulation. Cardiac output increases when the heart does not have to pump against a highly resistant system. The most common arterial dilators are diazoxide, hydralazine, and minoxidil. Patients who have arterial hypertension will achieve a lowered blood pressure with the use of arterial dilators.

Balanced vasodilators control blood pressure by widening the lumens of arteries and veins. Drugs that contain both arterial and venous dilating properties are nitroprusside and prazosin. Both of these drugs directly relax vascular smooth muscle, and prazosin also blocks sympathetic $alpha_1$-adrenoceptors, interfering with nerve impulses that cause vascular smooth muscles to contract.

Blocking the conversion of angiotensin I to angiotensin II, the most powerful vasoconstrictor produced by the body, is achieved with the use of captopril, enalapril, lisinopril, and other enzyme inhibitors. By inhibiting angiotensin II production, captopril also indirectly reduces production of aldosterone. As a result, the body excretes more sodium and water, thus reducing blood volume and causing a decrease in blood pressure. Refer to Chart 17–2 for patient education information.

CATECHOLAMINES

Catecholamines are most often used in cardiac emergencies because of their positive inotropic and vasopressor action. They increase cardiac output, blood pressure, and systemic vascular resistance.

Dopamine is a naturally occurring catecholamine, a precursor of norepinephrine. It stimulates sympathetic $alpha_1$-receptors in the smooth-muscle walls of arterioles. The arterioles contract and increase arterial blood pressure. Dopamine also acts on cardiac $beta_1$-receptors to increase the strength and rate of

Chart 17–2.

NURSING GUIDE TO PATIENT EDUCATION FOR SELF-MANAGEMENT: SELF-MEDICATION WITH CORONARY VASODILATORS

Instruct the patient taking coronary vasodilators at home to:

Place sublingual tablets under the tongue.
Swallow tablet whole if it is not noted to be sublingual.
Lie down or sit in a chair when taking medication. Stay in that position for 5 to 10 minutes because of potential weakness or dizziness.
Repeat dose of sublingual medication (if pain is not relieved immediately) every 5 minutes for up to three doses.
Notify the physician if pain persists.
Avoid alcohol when taking medication.
Watch for side effects such as headache, weakness, confusion, dizziness, nausea, and vomiting.
Document episodes of pain and number of doses of medication taken. Report this to the physician.
Store medication in a tightly closed, dark container.

cardiac contraction. This combination of effects may prevent a patient from going into shock. Before dopamine therapy, any pre-existing hypovolemia should be corrected so there is enough vascular volume to contribute to an increase in cardiac output.

Dobutamine is a synthetic catecholamine that is primarily a myocardial $beta_1$ stimulator. Its peripheral vascular effects are minimal even in high doses. It increases stroke volume and cardiac output without as much increase in cardiac rate as produced by dopamine. Thus, it uses less cardiac energy and tends to produce fewer dysrhythmias.

Dobutamine may be used with the balanced vasodilator nitroprusside to sharply decrease preload and circulating blood volume in patients with severe refractory heart failure. It can also be used with dopamine because dopamine will improve renal blood flow while dobutamine is increasing cardiac output.

Patients receiving catecholamine therapy should be in a critical care area with continuous ECG monitoring and invasive hemodynamic monitoring. Small dosage changes in catecholamines may mean life-threatening changes in blood pressure and cardiac rate. Such patients need close nursing observation and intervention as indicated by changes in their status.

ANTIARRHYTHMICS

Antiarrhythmic drugs suppress the cardiac automaticity, thus altering the rate of conduction, the refractory period, or the shift in impulse. There are several drugs in the antiarrhythmic category. The drug used is chosen on the basis of the patient's history, concomitant problems, specific drug effect, and tolerability (Pharmacology Box 17–3).

Lidocaine decreases the irritability of the ventricles and is used to control ventricular tachycardia, ventricular fibrillation, and premature ventricular contractions (PVCs). It is given by an intravenous bolus, followed by an intravenous drip titrated to control the undesired arrhythmia. Procainamide hydrochloride is given to patients who do not respond to lidocaine, and it can be given orally for long-term

Pharmacology Box 17–3.
ANTIARRHYTHMIC AGENTS

Antiarrhythmic Agents:
Class of drugs that suppress cardiac automaticity. They may be subdivided into four categories on the basis of other electrophysiologic effects of the drugs.

Action:
Alter rate of conduction and refractory period or correct shift in impulse origin or automaticity of cardiac tissue.

Uses:
Treatment of rhythm disturbances.

Side Effects:
Anorexia, nausea, vomiting, dry mouth, blurred vision, cardiac arrhythmias, systemic lupus erythematosus, urinary retension, drowsiness, tremors, and paresthesia.

Interactions:
Some antiarrhythmic agents may elongate bleeding times, potentiate actions of other drugs such as antihypertensives and diuretics, react with other drugs to cause dysrhythmias, and enhance the action of curariform drugs and antibiotics.

Nursing Implications:
Give with meals to prevent gastrointestinal distress.
Observe for liver distress because many of the drugs are metabolized in the liver.
Check laboratory studies for liver function and bleeding times.
Observe for side effects (as listed above).
Monitor electrocardiographic reading and blood pressure.
Check output; watch for signs of renal insufficiency.
Observe for signs of bleeding.
Instruct patient about medications and side effects.

Pharmacology Box 17–4.

DIURETICS (ANTIHYPERTENSIVES)

Diuretics:
Class of drugs affecting sodium and water excretion. Some cause potassium depletion; others are potassium sparing.

Action:
Varies with type of diuretic; generally, they inhibit sodium and chloride absorption, thus promoting their excretion along with excess fluid.

Uses:
Treatment of high blood pressure and hypervolemia; as well as pulmonary edema, peripheral edema, and congestive heart failure.

Side Effects:
Hypokalemia, cardiac dysrhythmias, postural hypotension, weakness, dizziness, dehydration, nausea, vomiting, headache, and confusion.

Interactions:
May cause digitalis toxicity because of hypokalemic state; may potentiate effects of alcohol; may react with probenecid; and may enhance effects of other antihypertensive drugs.

Nursing Implications:
Give early in day to prevent nocturia.
Monitor intake and output.
Check laboratory data and electrolytes, especially potassium level.
Observe for signs of hypokalemia. (If patient is taking a potassium supplement, also observe for hyperkalemia.)
Monitor weight and blood pressure.
Check for symptoms of digitalis toxicity.
Provide potassium-rich foods. (If patient is taking a non-potassium sparing diuretic). Instruct patient about medication, side effects, and possible hypotensive episodes.

management of ventricular arrhythmias. Quinidine sulfate is similar in action to lidocaine and procainamide. It is used for the treatment of chronic ventricular tachycardia and paroxysmal atrial tachycardia.

Verapamil is useful in supraventricular tachycardia because it slows conduction in the AV node. It also slows the ventricular response to atrial flutter and fibrillation because of the slowing of conduction in the AV node. Thus, patients who have fast heart rates because of atrial flutter or fibrillation with a resultant decrease in cardiac output can improve with the administration of intravenous or oral verapamil.

Adenosine given by intravenous bolus is used to convert supraventricular tachycardia without the side effect of hypotension, which may occur with verapamil. Adenosine's half-life is 10 to 15 seconds; thus, possible side effects of chest pain, dyspnea, or transient arrhythmias disappear very rapidly.

Atropine sulfate increases sinus node automaticity and AV node conduction. It is used for the treatment of sinus bradycardia because of its ability to speed conduction and cause an increase in heart rate. Atropine is given as an intravenous bolus.

DIURETICS

Diuretics are used frequently in the treatment of cardiac disease because cardiac failure causes retention of fluid (Pharmacology Box 17–4). Excess fluid may collect in the pulmonary system and lead to pulmonary edema. Peripheral edema may also result from cardiac failure. Furosemide is a potent, rapidly acting diuretic used to decrease total body fluid. It inhibits reabsorption of sodium and chloride in the ascending loop of Henle in the kidneys. The onset of diuresis after an intravenous dose of furosemide is about 10 minutes, with a total diuretic effect that lasts approximately 6 hours. Furosemide may also be given orally. Less potent diuretics, such as hydrochlorothiazide, spironolactone, as well as a variety of others, may be used for the treatment of

Chart 17–3.

NURSING GUIDE TO PATIENT EDUCATION FOR SELF-MANAGEMENT: SPECIAL INSTRUCTIONS FOR PATIENTS TAKING DIURETICS

Instruct the patient taking diuretic medications to:

Expect the amount of urine and the frequency of voiding to increase.
Avoid restricting normal fluid intake, unless specifically ordered, because of the increased output.
Take medication early in the morning to prevent nocturia. If ordered twice a day, take early in the morning and early in the evening.
Eat meals that include potassium-rich foods.
Observe for signs of hypokalemia such as fatigue, anorexia, vomiting, paresthesia, and palpitations.
Observe for signs of hyperkalemia (if also taking a potassium supplement) such as muscle weakness, nausea, respiratory distress, and diarrhea.
Observe for signs of hypovolemia such as dry skin, hypotension, weakness, dizziness, and excessive thirst.
Report any of the above untoward signs to the physician.
Be safety conscious; hypotension may occur, causing weakness, dizziness, and syncope.

Pharmacology Box 17–5.

ANTIHYPERTENSIVES (NONDIURETICS)

Antihypertensives:
Group of drugs used to reduce hypertension by means other than sodium and water excretion (as diuretics act).

Action:
Varies with specific drug.

Uses:
Treatment of high blood pressure.

Side Effects:
Drowsiness, weakness, headache, constipation, postural hypotension, confusion, convulsions, and nephropathy.

Interactions:
Vary with specific drug.

Nursing Implications:
Monitor blood pressure.
Instruct patient to avoid postural hypotension by rising from bed slowly, sitting for a few moments before rising.
Check for oversedation, drowsiness, confusion, dizziness, and headache.
Keep side rails up.
Monitor laboratory data.
Check intake and output; watch for signs of renal complications.
Observe for fluid retention.

chronic cardiac failure and are usually given orally. Refer to Chart 17–3 for patient education information.

Diuretics also have an antihypertensive effect from the reduction in circulating volume. Many other cardiac drugs have an antihypertensive effect but are not in the diuretic group (Pharmacology Box 17–5).

THROMBOLYTIC THERAPY

The lysing or dissolving of clots within the coronary arteries may prevent myocardial damage from prolonged ischemia. If a clot can be lysed and blood flow restored through the coronary artery to the myocardium, ischemia will be reversed.

Streptokinase is a nonenzymatic enzyme excreted by group C beta-hemolytic streptococci. It generates the proteolytic enzyme plasmin, which lyses clots (Fig. 17–19). Activase is a form of tissue plasminogen activator (t-PA), a naturally occurring protein that plays a major role in dissolving clots (Fig. 17–20). Eminase is a thrombolytic agent that can be given as a single dose because its duration is much longer than that of streptokinase or activase.

Thrombolytic therapy is contraindicated in patients with active internal bleeding; history of cerebral vascular accident (CVA); recent surgery or trauma (usually within the last 2 months); intracranial neoplasm; arteriovenous malformation or aneurysm; severe, uncontrolled hypertension; or any bleeding disorder. Patients with any other condition in which bleeding would constitute significant risk or a management problem are not candidates for thrombolytic therapy.

MECHANISM OF ACTION

Streptokinase (SK)

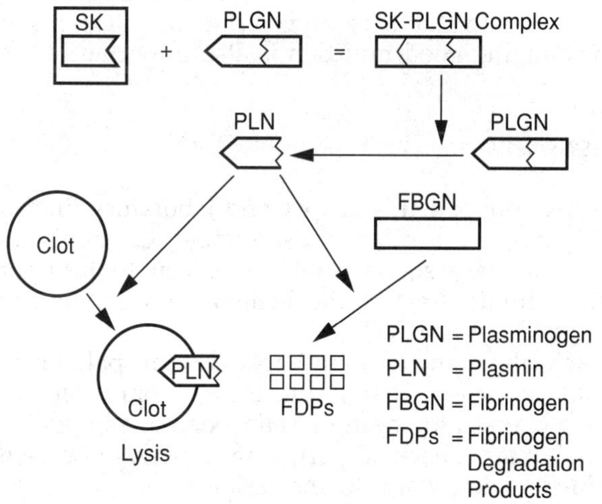

Figure 17–19.

Diagram showing the mechanism of action of streptokinase. The ultimate goal is lysis of clots as shown at the bottom of the diagram. (From Davis P. Pathophysiology of acute MI: Comparison of agents. In Thrombolytic therapy in acute MI: Nursing implications. AACN International Conference 88, September 1988, p 2. Genentech, Inc., 460 Point San Bruno Blvd., South San Francisco, CA 94080.)

MECHANISM OF ACTION

Tissue Plasminogen Activator (t-PA)

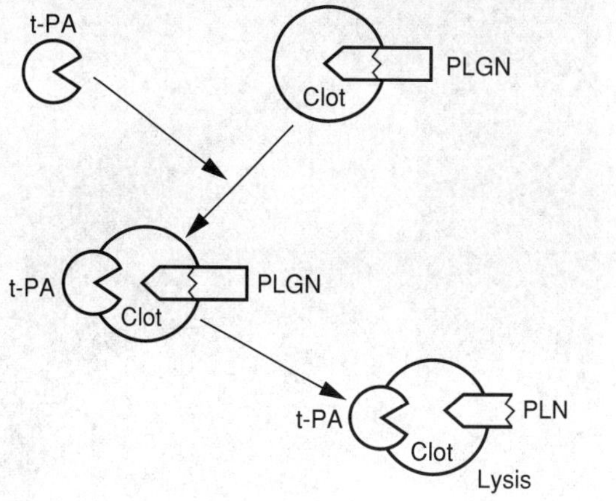

Figure 17–20.

Diagram showing the mechanism of action of tissue plasminogen activator (t-PA). Lysis of clots is the goal of therapy. (From Davis P. Pathophysiology of acute MI: Comparison of agents. In Thrombolytic therapy in acute MI: Nursing implications. AACN International Conference 88, September 1988, p 2. Genentech, Inc., 460 Point San Bruno Blvd., South San Francisco, CA 94080.)

Surgical Management

Cardiac surgical procedures are classified as open or closed. Open-heart procedures involve the use of the heart-lung machine for oxygenation and circulation support during surgery. Closed-heart procedures do not involve the use of the heart-lung machine because the oxygenation and circulation of blood to the brain is not impaired, or is impaired for a very short period of time but not long enough to cause death of cells.

CORONARY ARTERY BYPASS GRAFTING

Coronary artery bypass grafting (CABG) is the most common cardiac surgical procedure. It is used for revascularization of the myocardium in atherosclerotic coronary artery disease. The goal of the procedure is to bring an improved blood supply to the ischemic myocardium. A conduit of the patient's own tissue, such as the saphenous vein, cephalic vein, or internal mammary artery, is used to bring blood from the aorta to the coronary artery distal to or downstream from the obstruction (Fig. 17–21). Thus, blood flow to the myocardium is replenished. The coronary arteries are on the surface of the heart and are easily accessible for the bypass procedure. Multiple arteries are usually involved, and patients may receive one to five bypasses during the surgery to improve blood supply to the myocardium.

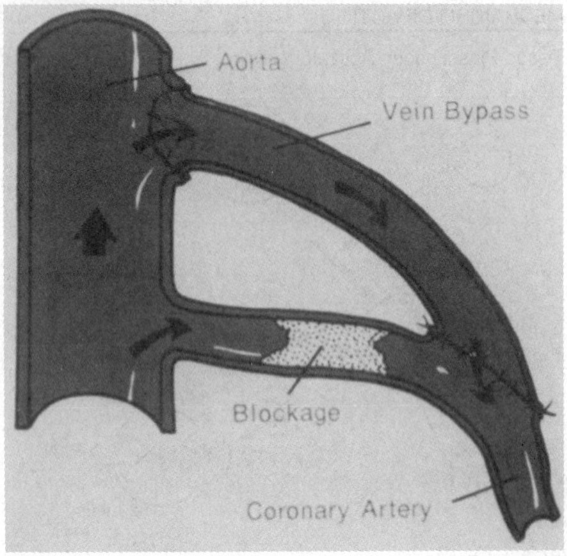

Figure 17–21.

Diagram of aortocoronary bypass graft. Blood flows out of the heart, into the aorta, down the vein graft, and into the coronary artery distal to the obstruction. In this course, the graft bypasses the obstruction in the patient's native circulation. (Reprinted with permission of the Arizona Heart Institute.)

CABG is begun with opening of the chest using a midline incision and cannulation of arteries and veins with connection to the heart-lung machine, which drains blood from the heart, oxygenates it, and then pumps it back into the body (Fig. 17–22). Large cannulas are inserted through the right atrium into the superior and inferior venae cavae for the drainage of blood from the heart. After oxygenation, the blood is returned to the body via cannulas in the ascending aorta or one of the femoral arteries.

The heart-lung machine also cools the blood as it is drained from the body. Metabolic processes are slowed as body temperature is reduced, and hypoxia is tolerated better by body organs at a reduced temperature. At the conclusion of the operative procedure, the blood is rewarmed before being pumped into the body, thus rewarming the patient before removal from the heart-lung machine. The degree of hypothermia is determined by the surgeon but is usually between 35°C and 28°C (95°F and 82.4°F).

To prevent blood from clotting in the extracorporeal circuit, the patient is anticoagulated with relatively high doses of heparin: a loading dose of 300 to 400 units of heparin per kilogram of body weight and supplemented by additional heparin every hour. At the completion of the bypass, protamine sulfate is administered to reverse the heparin anticoagulation. Because of the different rates of metabolism of heparin and protamine, this reversal is often imperfect, and activated clotting times may remain prolonged for several hours. Additional protamine sulfate may be required postoperatively.

Other components of blood-clotting mechanisms may also be depressed with use of the heart-lung machine. Platelets usually are depleted, and patients with low preoperative platelet counts may need platelet administration. Red blood cells are hemolyzed because of the mechanical trauma of the pump and suction systems of the heart-lung machine. The products of red blood cell breakdown impose a burden on the liver and kidneys, which metabolize and excrete them. Red blood cell replacement is usually needed in the postoperative period.

Embolus is a complication that may be encountered whenever the heart-lung machine is used. Embolization of calcium, air, or thrombi from the operative field into the patient's arterial system may occur, and precautions are taken to avoid such emboli. Calcifications of valves or arteries are removed from the operative field using a separate suction system (not the suction of the heart-lung machine). Before closing the heart in any open-heart surgical procedure, all air is evacuated and replaced by blood. If embolization results, central nervous system damage may occur regardless of whether the emboli are calcium, air, or blood clots.

Application of the Nursing Process to the Care of the Patient Having a Coronary Artery Bypass Graft

PREOPERATIVE NURSING CARE

Preparation of the patient undergoing CABG focuses on assessment and education. Enhancing the patient's health status by preventing complications and encouraging good nutrition is also important.

Assessment

Review the patient's history and laboratory findings, and complete a physical assessment. Check the cardiopulmonary status carefully. Listen to heart and lung sounds. Review the hemodynamic monitoring results. Look for JVD.

Ask the patient about episodes of palpitations, dyspnea, chest pain, dizziness, confusion, and edema. Look for cyanosis and edema, especially in distal areas. Check all peripheral pulses. Observe the skin for color, warmth, and lesions.

Check the intake and output. Note the color, consistency, and amount of urine. Ask about episodes of gastrointestinal distress. Look for abdominal distention.

Assess the patient's and family's understanding of the cardiac disease and surgical treatment required. Observe for signs of anxiety such as nervous twitch-

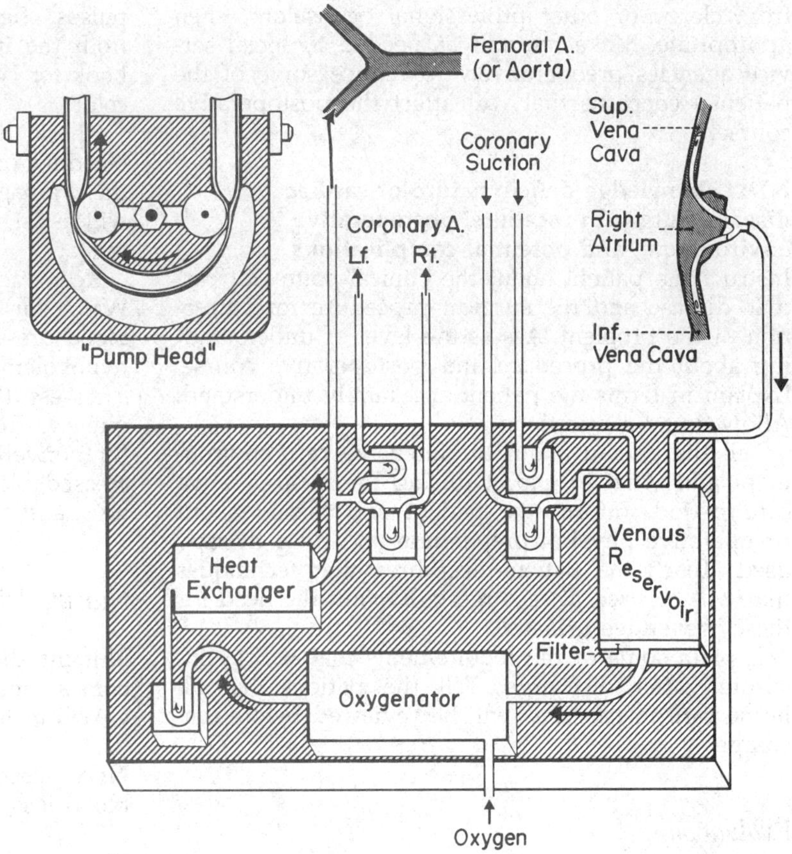

Figure 17–22.

Schematic diagram of the heart-lung machine. Unoxygenated blood is drained from the heart and is emptied into the venous reservoir along with the blood retrieved by the coronary suction system. It then passes to the oxygenator, which adds oxygen to the blood until it is fully saturated. In the heat exchanger, the temperature of the blood is raised or lowered. The blood is then pumped back into the body; separate circuits (like the coronary artery system) also may be perfused. The insert depicts the roller "pump head," which propels the blood forward. (From Sanderson RG, Kurth CL. The cardiac patient. 2nd ed. Philadelphia: WB Saunders, 1983, p 416.)

ing, crying, respiratory distress, or inability to communicate.

Nursing Diagnoses and Planning

Nursing diagnoses and related expected patient outcomes most commonly applicable to patients undergoing CABG include the following:

NDx: Anxiety related to fear of death, potential complications of surgery, and potential lifestyle changes

Planning: Patient outcomes

1. Patient's anxiety is lessened as evidenced by stable vital signs, relaxed appearance, and calm, positive attitude.
2. Patient states strategies to cope with the stressors.
3. Patient and family verbalize fears and concerns.

NDx: Knowledge deficit: nature of cardiac disease, surgical procedure, postoperative environment, and potential complications

Planning: Patient outcomes

1. Patient reports accurate information about the nature of the disease and surgery for correction of problems.
2. Patient relates information about the intensive care environment, the support equipment used, and the probable postoperative treatment course.
3. Patient explains the need for the preoperative preparation instituted.

Nursing Interventions

NDx: Anxiety

Allow the patient to verbalize concerns about the disease and impending surgery, its effect on the patient and family, and fears about death. Help the patient and family find coping strategies that are effective to deal with their anxiety level. Allow time for questions from the patient and the family. Provide comfort measures, both physical and emotional, for the patient and family.

Teach the patient relaxation techniques to help reduce the anxiety. Explain how stress can aggravate the complications of the disease and the usual postoperative events. Tell the patient about the intensive care environment and the support equipment that will be present.

Explain the disease process, the surgery, and expected results so the patient will have a better understanding of the surgical intervention and the postoperative course. Allow time for the patient and family to be alone when needed. Seek assistance from clergy or other professional counselors when appropriate. Make referrals as needed to social service agencies preoperatively to reduce some of the patient's concerns that will affect the postoperative course.

NDx: Knowledge deficit: nature of cardiac disease, surgical procedure, postoperative environment, and potential complications
Instruct the patient about the clinical course of cardiac disease and the surgical procedure for correction of the problem. Assess the level of understanding about the procedure and postoperative course. Explain in terms the patient and family understand. Allow time for questions.

Tell the patient about the intensive care environment and what to expect during the postoperative care period. Inform the patient and family about preoperative physical preparation and drug therapy used. Teach the patient deep-breathing techniques that will be used after surgery. Explain the need for these preventive measures.

Explain some of the requirements that will be instituted after discharge. Tell the patient that all home care instructions will be reviewed before discharge.

Evaluation

Evaluate the effectiveness of nursing care for a patient having CABG by comparing the patient's status with the expected patient outcomes. Examples of specific outcomes for patients undergoing CABG have been provided in the Planning section.

POSTOPERATIVE NURSING CARE

The postoperative course for the patient having CABG begins in the intensive care unit. In this highly specialized area, the patient is stabilized, carefully monitored, and prepared for transfer to a surgical unit or department. The patient is usually in the intensive care unit for 12 to 48 hours or longer depending on the prior disease state and complications of the surgery. Once the patient is stable, extubated, and presumed free from acute surgical complications such as hemorrhage or respiratory failure, transfer to another care unit is instituted for the rest of the patient's in-hospital recuperative period.

Assessment

Assess the patient's cardiopulmonary status. Observe for dyspnea, cyanosis, rales or rhonchi, tachypnea, and chest expansion. Check blood gas results. Check blood pressure, heart rate, and all peripheral pulses. Review hemodynamic monitoring results from the intensive care unit and the present ECG. Look for JVD. Observe the skin for temperature and color.

Check the chest and leg dressings. Note any bleeding or other drainage on the dressings. Circle the drainage periphery and document the time. This will assist in determining further episodes of bleeding.

Keep accurate records of intake and output. Watch for signs of fluid overload such as increased blood pressure and edema. Also observe for signs of hypovolemia because of blood loss.

Assess the patient for pain. Ask about the frequency, duration, intensity, and location. Observe for nonverbal signs of pain such as grimacing, increased blood pressure, clenching of teeth, restlessness, and anxiety.

Nursing Diagnoses and Planning

Nursing diagnoses and related expected patient outcomes most commonly applicable to patients after CABG include the following:

NDx: Decreased cardiac output related to surgical blood loss and myocardial inadequacy

Planning: Patient outcomes
1. Patient's vital signs are within normal ranges for the patient.
2. Patient shows signs of adequate cardiac output such as good peripheral pulses, appropriate color and warmth of extremities, and adequate urine output.

NDx: Pain related to surgical intervention and manipulation

Planning: Patient outcomes
1. Patient states pain is relieved or reduced to a tolerable level.
2. Patient relates relaxation techniques for pain relief.
3. Patient does not display nonverbal signs of pain.

NDx: Knowledge deficit: signs and symptoms of complications, preventive measures, when to seek medical assistance, and restrictions and self-care necessary on discharge

Planning: Patient outcomes
1. Patient relates accurate information about the signs and symptoms of complications and when to seek medical assistance.
2. Patient lists restrictions on activities as ordered by the physician.
3. Patient states self-care measures necessary on discharge.

Chart 17–4.

NURSING GUIDE TO PATIENT EDUCATION FOR SELF-MANAGEMENT: DISCHARGE INSTRUCTIONS AFTER CORONARY ARTERY BYPASS GRAFTING (CABG)

On discharge, instruct the patient who has undergone a CABG to:

Adhere to a designated regimen of rest and excercise, as prescribed. Sleep 6 to 10 hours per night and intermittently throughout the day. Begin a moderate excercise program starting with light housekeeping, and walking, as prescribed. Do not lift heavy objects, and avoid pushing/pulling activities that may stress the chest area.

Observe for signs of infection such as elevated temperature, chest pain, cough, dyspnea, redness, or drainage from the surgical sites. Notify the physician if any of these symptoms or other unusual signs appear.

Eat a well-balanced diet, as prescribed, avoiding saturated fats and salty foods. Eat frequent small meals to avoid gastric distress and fatigue.

Prevent straining with bowel movements by using a stool softener, drinking fluids, and including some fiber in the diet unless otherwise contraindicated.

Nursing Interventions

NDx: Decreased cardiac output

Monitor the patient's vital signs both at rest and during activity when he or she is able to get out of bed. Encourage the patient to take frequent rest periods to prevent fatigue and strain on the myocardium. Instruct the patient to stop activity if it initiates episodes of chest pain or aggravates chest discomfort.

Use telemetry monitoring whenever possible, especially if the patient experiences dysrhythmias or if the patient is taking antidysrhythmic drugs. Review the results of postoperative laboratory studies and hemodynamic monitoring.

Check the patient's fluid intake and output, observing for adequacy and balance. Keep the patient's legs in a nondependent position while sitting. Provide support for the extremities while sitting or lying in bed. Pad bony prominences to prevent breakdown from pressure and poor circulation.

Teach the patient relaxation techniques and range-of-motion procedures to increase circulation while lying in bed. Keep the patient warm and comfortable. Prevent constriction of circulation from tight clothing or bed linen.

NDx: Pain

Have the patient describe the pain. Give prescribed analgesic drugs as needed. Check for relief after administration of analgesics. If no relief is obtained from repeated medication, notify the physician. Reposition the patient for comfort. Document all episodes of pain. Look for nonverbal signs of pain such as restlessness, gasping, clenched fists, stiffness, grimacing, and facial flushing. Obtain a 12-lead ECG during an acute episode of pain for diagnostic purposes because it may be difficult to determine whether the pain is anginal or surgical.

Teach the patient some relaxation techniques for pain relief. Have the patient relate potential coping strategies that have worked previously for relaxation during acute episodes of stress or pain. Administer oxygen if pain causes respiratory distress.

NDx: Knowledge deficit: signs and symptoms of complications, preventive measures, when to seek medical assistance, and restrictions and self-care necessary on discharge

Describe potential complications of the surgery such as bleeding, cardiac arrhythmias, respiratory distress, and infection. Teach the patient and family signs and symptoms of these complications to watch for. Tell the patient to seek medical assistance if any unusual symptoms appear (Chart 17–4).

Prepare the patient for discharge by explaining the home-care restrictions as ordered by the physician. Tell the patient to begin a regimen of planned mild exercise with frequent rest periods, gradually increasing the activities as tolerated and prescribed. Explain that lifting heavy objects or pushing and pulling heavy objects may cause chest trauma and should be avoided.

Explain the need for good nutrition. Encourage the patient to follow a diet low in saturated fat and sodium (see Nutrition Boxes 17–2 and 17–3). Give the patient lists of food and fluids to avoid and some sample meal plans to follow. Explain the need to prevent straining with bowel movements. Tell the patient to drink fluids frequently and to eat high-fiber foods if not contraindicated.

Additional Interventions

Postoperatively, the patient is vulnerable to several complications. Assess frequently for bleeding. Some bloody drainage is expected, but excessive bleeding early in the postoperative period should be reported. Check the vital signs and look for signs of hypervolemia. In particular, observe for increasing outlines of drainage on the dressing indicating continued bleeding.

The patient may have gas-exchange problems and thus inadequate oxygenation to tissues. After extubation, observe the patient's respiratory status frequently. Look for increasing restlessness, cyanosis, dyspnea, tachypnea, and tachycardia. Administer oxygen and order blood gas studies if indicated. Position the patient for maximum chest expansion. Encourage deep breathing and repositioning. Control the patient's pain, because intense pain may restrict the patient's ability to deep breathe and move freely.

Prevent fluid volume deficits or overloads by carefully monitoring the intake and output. Encourage good nutrition when the patient is allowed to resume food and fluids.

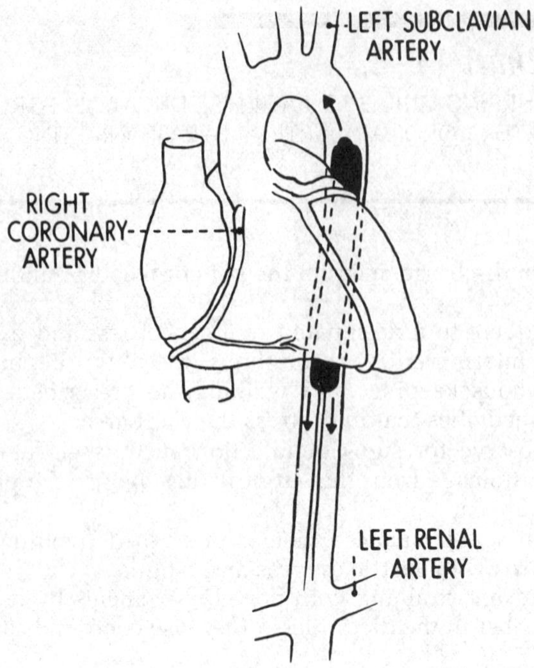

Figure 17–23.

The intra-aortic balloon in place, distal to the left subclavian artery and proximal to renal arteries. (From Frazee S, Nail L. New challenge in cardiac nursing: The intra-aortic balloon. Heart Lung 1973; 2:527.)

Evaluation

Evaluate the effectiveness of nursing care for a patient after CABG by comparing the patient's status with the expected patient outcomes. Examples of specific outcomes for patients after CABG have been provided in the Planning section.

INTRA-AORTIC BALLOON PUMP SUPPORT

Some patients who experience myocardial infarction or who undergo surgery for treatment of cardiac disease may demonstrate the signs and symptoms of cardiogenic shock. Cardiogenic shock has a high mortality rate of 80% to 90% and therefore should be prevented. Cardiogenic shock patients have left ventricular function that cannot maintain the cardiac output necessary for perfusion of vital organs, and they may need intra-aortic balloon pump (IABP) support. The two main goals of IABP are afterload reduction and diastolic augmentation. Preload occurs with a high pulmonary venous pressure produced by excess fluid in the lungs. Afterload occurs with a high systemic vascular resistance. Preload reduction is accomplished by administration of intravenous diuretics, nitroglycerin, rotating tourniquets, or phlebotomy. Afterload reduction is accomplished by arteriolar dilating drugs given intravenously such as nitroprusside, prazosin, or hydralazine and use of IABP. IABP increases perfusion of the body's organs and tissues during diastole by increasing the time interval for diastolic filling of the heart. The result is diastolic augmentation. Peripheral vascular resistance and the workload of the heart are decreased, and afterload reduction is thereby achieved.

The balloon is positioned in the thoracic aorta after it is passed through the femoral artery via a cutdown or a percutaneous insertion. The balloon will be positioned below (distal to) the left subclavian artery as it branches off of the aortic arch and above (proximal to) the renal arteries as they branch off of the descending aorta (Fig. 17–23).

The balloon is inflated during diastole when the aortic valve is closed. Blood is forced from the aorta in two directions: upward into the coronary arteries and the arteries going to the head and upper extremities, and downward into the renal arteries and the arteries going to the lower extremities. Perfusion of blood and oxygen to the myocardium, brain, and kidneys increases. Myocardial function, cardiac output, and renal function improve.

Deflation of the balloon occurs just before and during the beginning of systole. Because most of the blood has been pushed out of the aorta by the inflated balloon during diastole, the heart is pumping against low peripheral vascular resistance, which reduces the workload of the left ventricle. Patients requiring balloon catheter treatments are critically ill, so nursing care is focused on life-sustaining interventions. These patients are monitored and cared for in intensive care units.

VENTRICULAR ASSISTANCE

Ventricular assistance is frequently required for the patient with a failing heart. A ventricular assist device (VAD) is a mechanical pump that is used to maintain life until another procedure can be implemented or until the heart can recover and support itself. It is most frequently used in patients with severe cardiomyopathy, myocarditis, endocarditis, myocardial infarction, or a rejected transplanted heart. The VAD can support the right, left, or both ventricles. However, it is the left ventricle that usually needs the assistance.

When the VAD is attached to the heart surgically, blood can be shunted from the inadequate ventricle to a battery-run pump, which does not replace the work of the ventricle but only assists it in its function. The pump and battery may be implanted in the patient's chest, or they may be attached externally with internal tubes to the heart.

Complications are common in patients with VADs. The most common complication is the formation of thrombi. This leads to pulmonary emboli, cerebral clots, and peripheral thrombophlebitis. Even with heparin therapy, clots tend to develop.

A VAD is generally considered to be only a temporary therapy to sustain life for a patient with a serious cardiac dysfunction. Many patients receiving ventricular assistance are awaiting a heart transplant. However, patients with severe cardiac disease who are not candidates for transplantation may have a permanent VAD implanted in the chest. This is still considered a palliative treatment.

PERCUTANEOUS TRANSLUMINAL CORONARY ANGIOPLASTY

The patient who experiences angina without evidence of cardiac damage may be a candidate for percutaneous transluminal coronary angioplasty (PTCA) (Fig. 17–24). In the cardiac catheterization laboratory, a coronary arteriogram is performed to confirm stenosis of a coronary artery. A coronary artery guide wire is passed into the aorta (as in cardiac catheterization) and positioned in the orifice of the stenosed coronary artery to be dilated. A special double-lumen catheter with a nonelastic dilating balloon and a soft wire tip is advanced through the guide wire into the coronary artery and positioned so the catheter tip is beyond the atherosclerotic obstruction and the dilating balloon is within the stenotic area (see Fig. 17–24). The dilating balloon is inflated for 3 to 4 seconds and then deflated. The coronary arteriogram is repeated to document the effect of the forceful dilation on the obstructing lesion. It is thought that the balloon causes compression of the soft atheromatous material of the stenotic lesion, a "flattening out" of the obstruction, which opens the lumen to permit increased blood flow. Careful selection of patients for PTCA is important. Some qualifying conditions include the following:

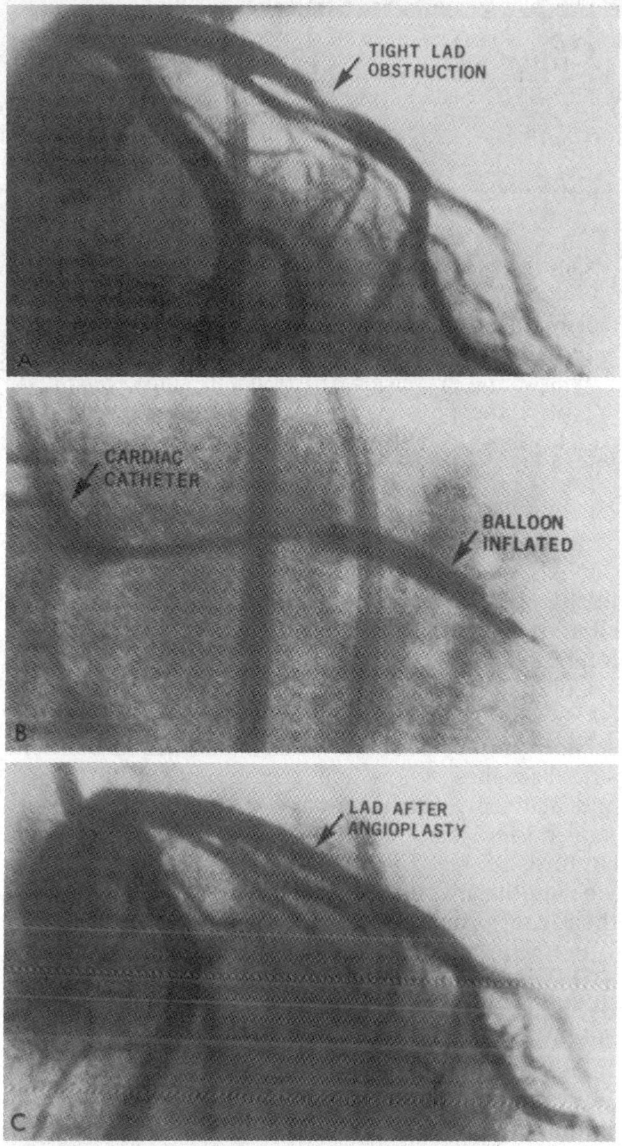

Figure 17–24.

Percutaneous transluminal coronary angioplasty. A, Preliminary coronary arteriogram demonstrates high-grade obstruction in the left anterior descending (LAD) coronary artery. B, Dilating balloon is shown distended (in the obstructed artery). C, Postdilatation coronary arteriogram, showing reduction of coronary obstruction from approximately 80% to less than 20%. (From Sanderson RG, Kurth CL. The cardiac patient. 2nd ed. Philadelphia: WB Saunders, 1983, p 120.)

1. The atherosclerotic disease should be restricted to a single vessel.
2. The lesion should be short (less than 1 cm long).
3. It should be noncalcified.

A short history of anginal pain, less than 1 year, usually indicates a soft, distensible atheroma that is

Chart 17–5.

NURSING GUIDE TO PATIENT EDUCATION FOR SELF-MANAGEMENT: DISCHARGE INSTRUCTIONS AFTER A PERCUTANEOUS TRANSLUMINAL CORONARY ANGIOPLASTY (PTCA)

On discharge, instruct the patient who has had a PTCA to:

Schedule a postprocedure follow-up appointment with the physician.
Observe for signs of latent bleeding at the puncture sites.
Follow the exercise restrictions, as stated by the physician, until the next office visit.
Notify the physician if any other untoward symptoms appear such as weakness, confusion, dizziness, tingling, and so on.

likely to be dilated successfully. Resting ECGs should rule out previous (or present) myocardial infarction.

Complications of PTCA include the complications of routine cardiac catheterization plus possible dissection of the coronary artery, blocking one of the side branches where the atheroma is compressed, and acute myocardial infarction. Immediate surgery may be indicated when complications of dissection, rupture, or bleeding of coronary arteries occur, as well as the inability to open the lesion, which may then lead to myocardial infarction.

Both during and after the procedure, the patient is assessed for complications and monitored for hemodynamic status. The patient is observed for signs of rhythm changes, bleeding, or respiratory distress. Intake and output are monitored while intravenous fluid therapy is progressing. Vital signs are checked frequently.

Before discharge, instructions for home care are given to the patient and family (if present). The patient is taught to observe for signs of bleeding at the puncture site and to report any unusual symptoms to the physician. Usually, activity as tolerated is resumed on discharge unless otherwise contraindicated (Chart 17–5).

VALVE REPLACEMENT

Heart valves that become stenotic or inadequate because of disease states or congenital anomalies cause regurgitation of blood into the ventricles, increasing the workload on the myocardium. Diseased valves may require replacement with prosthetic devices. The aortic and mitral valves are more frequently affected than the tricuspid or pulmonic valves.

Mechanical and biologic valves are available for implantation. Each type has positive and negative features. The choice of valve is made on the basis of the patient's history, preceding factors, complications, potential for compliance with the therapy needed, and ease of implantation.

The patient receiving a mechanical valve requires extensive postoperative anticoagulant therapy to prevent clot formation. Cerebral and pulmonary emboli are common complications of the mechanical valve replacement. A biologic valve replacement also presents risks to the patient. The biologic valve is less sturdy than the mechanical valve so it tends to malfunction. It also causes some clot formation, so the patient is on heparin therapy for a short time postoperatively. Other complications of valve-replacement surgery include infections and valve failure.

HEART TRANSPLANTATION

This procedure, although seemingly common in today's medical field, is still a highly complicated, high-risk procedure that is performed only in limited health care institutions. It may be the last hope for the patient with a dying heart or for the newborn with severe cardiac anomalies. Many patients selected for a heart transplant have had a history of coronary artery disease or ventricular fibrosis.

Postoperative complications include tissue rejection and infection. The complications are treated with antibiotics, immunosuppressive drugs, and antibiotics. The treatment of immunosuppression often increases the patient's risk for development of even more infectious processes.

The patient undergoing a heart transplant is carefully assessed and counseled before the surgery. Both the patient and family are actively involved in the process from the onset. Extensive teaching and counseling are imperative. Discussions are held with the entire support team of health care personnel.

Tissue typing and crossmatching are required, as is an available matched donor organ. Patients and families suffer a great deal emotionally waiting for the donor heart to become available.

Postoperatively, the patient is in a special intensive care unit in protective isolation. The heart transplant patient is carefully monitored for signs of infection, hemodynamic problems, respiratory complications, early signs of failure or rejection, other complications of therapy, and the overall response to the new organ. Support equipment includes chest tubes, monitor leads, trachea tube and ventilator, chest dressings, catheters, and arterial and venous catheters. This support equipment is continually monitored and adjusted to maintain the patient's status within acceptable ranges as predetermined by the physician. The nursing role in the care of the heart transplant patient is highly specialized.

The Elderly: Special Considerations

Physiologic changes in the cardiovascular system present in a variety of ways in the older person. Throughout the adult years, the heart muscle loses its efficiency and contractile strength, resulting in reduced cardiac output. Adjustment to this change is made by pacing activities: for example, driving rather than walking long distances, taking an elevator rather than walking up several flights of stairs. Elevated pulse rates in the elderly may not be as high as in younger persons, but tachycardia experienced with activity or stress in the elderly will last for longer periods of time. Stroke volume may increase as the heart tries to increase cardiac output in stressful situations, resulting in an elevated blood pressure and a bounding pulse.

The increased rigidity of vessel walls and narrowing of lumens that occur with aging necessitate increased force from the heart to pump blood through the vessels. Thus, systolic and diastolic blood pressures rise. Heart valves become thick and rigid as a result of sclerosis and fibrosis, compounding the need for increased force to deliver adequate blood and oxygen to all of the body's tissue. There is controversy among physicians about treating elevated blood pressures in the elderly because some elevation is necessary to compensate for changes associated with the aging process.

The elderly may be spared the lethal complications associated with myocardial infarction because over the years they have developed collateral circulation of the myocardium. They may instead have compromised tissue perfusion because of increased peripheral vascular resistance resulting from the arteriosclerosis of the peripheral vessels. Just as the heart ages, so do the other organ systems of the body. With acute cardiac disease, the elderly often acquire problems such as renal failure because of a decreased cardiac output in congestive heart failure, respiratory failure from fluid accumulation in congestive heart failure, and disorientation, syncope, or coma resulting from inadequate circulation to the brain.

Medication therapy deserves specific mention in the elderly. The older adult takes medications frequently, both prescription and over the counter. Some of their health problems may result from adverse reactions to medications. Many elderly take more than one medication, so possible drug interactions must be monitored. Decreased blood flow to the liver diminishes hepatic drug metabolism, whereas decreased blood flow to the kidneys decreases drug elimination. Thus, the common adult dosages of many cardiac medications must be reduced for the elderly. Their responses to medications are monitored and dosages altered according to each individual's response. Laboratory tests that measure drug levels in the blood may be needed to adjust specific medications. Signs of toxicity for any medication must be assessed, documented, and reported when caring for elderly patients.

Anginal pain in the elderly is more diffuse and less severe than in younger patients. It may be regarded as not bothersome and therefore not reported until cardiac damage has resulted. Dyspnea, rather than pain, may be the most prominent symptom of acute myocardial infarction in an older adult.

Peripheral edema may be due to nutritional deficiencies rather than ventricular dysfunction. A low serum albumin level associated with edema in all soft tissue areas is indicative of inadequate nutrition in the elderly.

There are age-related changes in all systems of the body. These changes mandate that nursing assessment, planning, implementation, and evaluation be examined in relationship to the aging process. Cardiac problems in the elderly should be evaluated for each individual and a plan of care developed accordingly. The goal of nursing care is to help the aging patient remain a functioning, contributing member of society.

Bibliography

Abrams J. Update on nitroglycerin and nitrates. Drug Ther 1992; 22(4):67.

Andreoli KG, Zipes DP, Wallace AG, Kinney MR, Fowkes VK. Comprehensive cardiac care. 6th ed. St. Louis: CV Mosby, 1987.

Appel-Hardin S, Dente-Casidy AM. How to use a noninvasive temporary pacemaker. Nursing 1991; 21(5):58.

Braddy PK. Cardiac assessment tool. Crit Care Nurse, 1989; 9(9):71.

Brenner ZR. Nursing elderly cardiac clients. Crit Care Nurse 1987; 7(2):78.

Carbajal E, Deedwania PC. Silent myocardial ischemia: Mechanisms, diagnosis, prevalence. Prim Cardiol 1991; 17(10):30.

Carpenito LJ. Handbook of nursing diagnosis. 2nd ed. Philadelphia: JB Lippincott, 1987.

Castello R, Alegria E. Exercise testing for evaluating the patient with coronary artery spasm. Prim Cardiol 1991; 17(10):20.

Cerrato P. Hypertension: The role of diet and lifestyle. RN 1990; 90:46.

Contrades S. Altered cardiac output: An assessment tool. Dimens Crit Care Nurs 1987; 6(5):274.

Crouse LJ, Kramer AH. Exercise cardiography—A creditable cor-

onary artery disease screening test. Cardiol Board Rev 1992; 9(4):101.
Culliford AT, Galloway AC, Colvin SB, et al. Octogenarians are not too old for aortic valve replacement. Cardiol Board Rev 1992; 9(4):84.
Dalal JN, Jain AC. Chronic stable angina pectoris: Risk stratification and treatment. Postgrad Med 1992; 91(4):165.
Das BN, Banka VS. Coronary artery disease in women: How it is and isn't unique. Postgrad Med 1992; 91(4):197.
Eliopoulos C. Gerontological nursing. 2nd ed. Philadelphia: JB Lippincott, 1987.
Feury D, Nash D. Hypertension: The nurse's role. RN 1990; 53(11):54.
Guzzetta CE, Dossey BM. Cardiovascular nursing: Bodymind tapestry. St. Louis, MO: CV Mosby, 1984.
Holloway NM. Medical-surgical care plans. Springhouse, PA: Springhouse Corporation, 1988.
Johnson LJ. Nuclear cardiology: New techniques and tracers. Cardiovasc Rev Rep 1992; 13(4):26.
Kaplan RM. Health-related quality of life in cardiovascular disease. J Consult Clin Psychol 1988; 56:382.
Kee JL. Laboratory and diagnostic test with nursing implications. 2nd ed. Norwalk, CT: Appleton & Lange, 1987.
Kunkel DB. Cardiac glycosides: Part 1. Updating Foxglove's toxic heritage. Emerg Med Clin North Am 1987; 19(13):154.
Kunkel DB. Cardiac glycosides: Part II. Nature's storehouses. Emerg Med Clin North Am 1987; 19(14):185.
McGinty MK, Chase SL, Mercer ME. Pharmacy-nursing discharge counseling program for cardiac patients. Am J Hosp Pharm 1988; 45(7):1545.
McHale DJ, Riggs KL, Thurman L. Epicardial pacing after cardiac surgery. Crit Care Nurse 1991; 11(8):62.
Morrissey JJ. Exercise and chronic heart disease. Geriatr Nurs 1987; 8(3):138.
Mutnick AH, Fecitt S, Rogers B. Cardiac drugs: Inotropic and chronotropic agents. Nursing 1987; 17(1):58.
Pagana KD, Pagana TJ. Diagnostic testing & nursing implications: A case study approach. 2nd ed. St. Louis: CV Mosby, 1986.
Reger MJ, Hermann F, Ried LD. Effectiveness of a printed leaflet for enabling patients to use digoxin side-effect information. Drug Intell Clin Pharm 1987; 21(2):200.
Sanderson RG, Kurth CL. The cardiac patient: A comprehensive approach. 2nd ed. Philadelphia: WB Saunders, 1983.
Stanley M. Cardiovascular physiology in the elderly. Crit Care Nurse 1985; 5(6):69.
Thompson V. Chest pain: Your response to a classic warning. RN 1989; 52(4):32.
Todd B. Update: Cardiac emergency drugs. Geriat Nurs 1986; 7(5):263.
Tresch DD, Troup PJ, Thakur RK, Wetherbee JN. Benefits of cardioverter/defibrillator implantation for elderly patients. Cardiol Board Rev, 1992; 9(4):63.
Underhill SL, Woods SL, Sivarajan ES, Halpenny CJ. Cardiac nursing. Philadelphia: JB Lippincott, 1982.
Vaska PL. Biventricular assist devises. Crit Care Nurse 1991; 11(8):52.
Weeks LD. Advanced cardiovascular nursing. Boston: Blackwell Scientific Publications, 1986.
Yacone L. The nurse's guide to cardiovascular drugs. RN 1988; 51(8):36.

Chapter Eighteen

NURSING CARE of Adults with Cardiac Disorders

The basic treatments for the variety of cardiac disorders are similar regardless of cause. The primary goal of medical and surgical treatment of cardiac disease processes is to restore the person to optimum cardiac function with minimal restrictions in daily activities. Many of the cardiac disorders present similar signs, symptoms, and complications. The impact of cardiac disorders on the other organs must always be considered, because the heart is responsible for delivering oxygen and nutrients via the blood to all parts of the body.

Infections and Inflammations

Cardiac Infections

ETIOLOGY AND PATHOPHYSIOLOGY

The cardiac tissues can become infected just as other tissues of the body. Cardiac infections may be acquired from procedures that introduce bacteria into the blood stream, such as cardiac catheterization, insertion of pulmonary artery catheters, or surgical processes. Infections may also be acquired from general viral or bacterial infections that invade cardiac tissue, such as those caused by staphylococcus, beta-hemolytic streptococcus, or pneumococcus.

ENDOCARDITIS

Endocarditis is an inflammatory process involving the endocardial surface of the heart, which includes the valves. Inflammatory endocarditis may be the result of collagen-vascular disease and rheumatic fever. Infective endocarditis can be an acute or subacute process from direct bacterial, fungal, or rickettsial invasion. Most episodes of bacterial endocarditis occur on previously abnormal valves (rheumatic, congenital, or insufficient valves of any cause), but acute bacterial endocarditis (ABE) may occur on normal valves. This is commonly found in drug addicts who inject a large bacterial inoculum intravenously along with the drug when they use unsterile needles or drugs. Patients with ABE experience sudden fevers and exhibit symptoms of septicemia, valvular insufficiency, and congestive failure. Patients with subacute bacterial endocarditis (SBE) have low-grade fevers, weight loss, anemia, splenomegaly, and heart murmurs that continue over a period of time, and they may not be diagnosed as having SBE for months.

MYOCARDITIS

Myocarditis is an inflammation of the heart muscle itself, which can be caused by a variety of agents such as bacteria, viruses, fungi, or parasites. The cardiac problems encountered are similar regardless of the infecting organism. Cardiac dilation and hypertrophy result from weakening of the muscle as it is infected. Thrombi form on the valves and within the chambers and can be dislodged into both the pulmonary and systemic circulations. Lymphocytes and leukocytes infiltrate the circulating blood cells around the small coronary vessels and between the muscle fibers. This leads to degeneration of the cardiac muscle fibers, which results in further dilation, hypertrophy, and eventually heart failure.

Inflammation of the myocardium sometimes accompanies other systemic diseases such as the collagen-vascular diseases. Examples are lupus erythematosus, periarteritis, scleroderma, and rheumatoid arthritis. In sarcoidosis, portions of the myocardial wall are replaced with sarcoid granulomas.

CLINICAL MANIFESTATIONS

Changes that occur in the endocardium and valves produce permanent and disabling effects. The mitral and aortic valves are most often affected, although the tricuspid and pulmonic valves can also be damaged. With acute inflammation, the valves become reddened and edematous. Small vegetative lesions develop on the valve leaflets and proceed to turn into fibrous scar tissue. With these changes, the valve leaflets contract and become deformed in relation to their original shape. The edges of the leaflets may not approximate each other, leading to valvular insufficiency, or the edges of the leaflets may fuse together, leading to valvular stenosis. Valvular changes result in murmurs heard during auscultation. There may also be cardiomegaly noted on the chest x-ray film, signs of pericarditis, a friction rub, and congestive heart failure (CHF).

The inflammatory process of the rheumatic fever affects the synovial membrane of joints and causes edema, heat, pain, and redness of the joint. The combination of these symptoms is called polyarthritis and limits joint motion. The polyarthritis may be so severe that the patient becomes completely immobile. The larger joints are most often affected and include the hips, knees, ankles, shoulders, elbows, and wrists.

MEDICAL DIAGNOSIS

The diagnosis is made on the basis of clinical and laboratory findings. A history of positive throat cultures for streptococcus with fever and an elevated erythrocyte sedimentation rate (ESR) are usually found in a patient with rheumatic fever. The clinical symptoms of carditis and polyarthritis, along with positive laboratory data, lead to the diagnosis.

Bacterial endocarditis is diagnosed with positive blood cultures. A series of blood cultures are usually needed for diagnosis. They are obtained during a 3- to 4-day period to ensure adequate sampling of the blood containing the bacteria causing the inflammatory response.

Pharmacology Box 18–1.

BROAD-SPECTRUM ANTIBIOTICS FOR CARDIAC INFECTIONS

Broad-Spectrum Antibiotics:
Group of anti-infective agents that is effective against both gram-negative and gram-positive bacteria and other microorganisms.

Action:
Inhibit growth of microorganisms by interrupting cell membrane function, protein synthesis, or cell metabolism.

Uses:
Inflammations and infections.

Side Effects:
Vary considerably with the particular drug. They may include drug sensitivity resulting in anaphylaxis, development of secondary infections, and drug toxicity as well as diarrhea, gastrointestinal distress, and impaired kidney function.

Interactions:
Vary with the specific drug.

Nursing Implications:
Check for allergic reactions.
Observe for signs of secondary infections such as abnormal discharge from the vagina, a coated tongue, and so on.
Check vital signs.
Instruct the patient to note any signs of secondary infections and to report them to the attending physician.
Note that some antibiotics should be taken with food.

MEDICAL MANAGEMENT

Treatment of rheumatic fever is aimed at controlling the acute inflammatory process and preventing cardiac damage, complications, and recurrence of the disease. Broad-spectrum antibiotics such as high-dose intravenous penicillin or a semisynthetic penicillin plus streptomycin, vancomycin, or gentamicin are used to treat cardiac infections (Pharmacology Box 18–1). Antibiotic therapy must be continued for 4 to 6 weeks, preferably intravenously.

Anti-inflammatory agents such as salicylates and corticosteroids are given to reduce the edema, pain, and general inflammation of the joints. Restriction of physical activities until joint edema and pain are relieved decreases future joint problems.

If bacterial destruction of the valve is widespread, valvular replacement may be needed within 1 year of the acute illness. Valve-replacement surgery cannot be done until all traces of bacterial infection are eliminated, because sutures into bacteria-invaded tissue will not hold and the prosthetic valve will ultimately disengage.

To prevent recurrences of the disease, prophylactic use of penicillin or another antibiotic may be given for a period of 3 to 5 years. After this period of prophylaxis, the patient will still need to take antibiotics before any procedure that may result in bacteria entering the blood stream, such as dental procedures or urinary tract manipulations.

Application of the Nursing Process to the Care of the Patient with a Cardiac Infection

Assessment

Review the patient's history, present symptoms, and diagnostic test results. Assess the patient's vital signs. Obtain a thorough history of strep throat, rheumatic fever, congenital heart disease, and cardiac surgery. Assess for fatigue, weakness, dyspnea, palpitations, and fainting spells. Auscultate the heart sounds to determine whether any abnormal sounds are present such as an S_3 or S_4, rubs, or murmurs. Examine the patient for evidence of painful or swollen joints to determine whether there are systemic symptoms as well as cardiac symptoms.

Nursing Diagnoses and Planning

Nursing diagnoses and related expected patient outcomes most commonly applicable to patients with cardiac infections include the following:

NDx: Pain related to inflammation of the myocardium and pericardium and local or systemic infection

Planning: Patient outcomes

1. Patient verbalizes relief or controlled pain levels.
2. Patient demonstrates use of relaxation skills and diversional activities that decrease the sense of pain.
3. Patient's vital signs are within normal ranges for the patient.

NDx: Activity intolerance related to inflammation and degeneration of myocardial muscle cells, reduced cardiac output, and painful, inflamed joints

Planning: Patient outcomes

1. Patient demonstrates a decrease in physiologic signs of activity intolerance.
2. Patient demonstrates an increase in physiologic signs of activity tolerance such as stable blood pressure, normal pulse rate, and absence of dyspnea with increased activity levels.

NDx: Knowledge deficit: nature of inflammatory cardiac diseases, the need for long-term therapy and follow-up, and ways to prevent recurrence or complications

Planning: Patient Outcomes

1. Patient verbalizes understanding of inflammatory process, treatment program, possible complications, and prevention plan.
2. Patient displays behavior changes in lifestyle that will prevent recurrence and complications of inflammatory cardiac processes.

Nursing Interventions

NDx: Pain
Investigate all complaints of chest pain and joint pain. Document onset of pain and factors that aggravate and relieve the pain. Provide a quiet environment for the patient with comfort measures that may include medications, positioning, back rubs, and emotional support. Teach relaxation exercise to assist in the relief of pain. Give prescribed medications for pain as necessary.

NDx: Activity intolerance
Assess the patient's response to activity and the types of activity that may not be possible. Severe joint pain may not allow the patient to be ambulatory. Note accompanying symptoms of dyspnea, weakness, and fatigue. Maintain bed rest during febrile periods and until painful, edematous joints can tolerate increased movement. When the patient is out of bed, note the response of blood pressure, heart rate, and respiratory rate to increased activity.

Allow uninterrupted sleep periods to reduce the fatigue. Limit interruptions and restrict visitors as needed so the patient can have lengthy periods of rest. Have the patient perform range-of-motion exercises frequently during the day to maintain and increase strength and endurance. Assist the patient with activities as necessary. Provide six small meals during the day to conserve strength and energy.

NDx: Knowledge deficit: nature of inflammatory cardiac diseases, the need for long-term therapy and follow-up, and ways to prevent recurrence or complications
Explain the effects of inflammation on the heart and other affected tissues. Educate the patient about signs and symptoms of recurrence, symptoms to report, and actions to take that will reduce the possibility of future recurrence (Chart 18–1). Discuss the use of prophylactic antibiotics, the time period of their use, and procedures that require prophylaxis throughout the lifetime (i.e., dental procedures).

Evaluation

Evaluate the effectiveness of nursing care for a patient with cardiac inflammation by comparing the patient's status with the expected patient outcomes. Examples of specific outcomes for patients with a cardiac infection have been provided in the Planning section.

Pericardial Disease

ETIOLOGY AND PATHOPHYSIOLOGY

The pericardium protects the heart from trauma and infection, although it is not essential for life. A few milliliters, 30 to 50, of pericardial fluid are present within the pericardial sac to help lubricate the pumping action of the heart. When the amount of fluid within the pericardium increases, the result is a pericardial effusion. Pericardial effusions may develop rapidly or slowly over a period of days or weeks. Rapidly developing pericardial effusions of a few milliliters can cause cardiac tamponade, with

Chart 18–1.

NURSING GUIDE TO PATIENT EDUCATION FOR SELF-MANAGEMENT: DISCHARGE INSTRUCTIONS FOR THE PATIENT RECOVERING FROM A CARDIAC INFECTION

On discharge instruct the patient recovering from a cardiac infection to:

Take the prescribed antibiotics exactly as ordered for the full length of time specified. Even though it may be for several weeks, it is imperative that they be taken as ordered to clear the infection completely and to prevent other infections from developing while the patient is recuperating.
Restrict physical activities until joint pain and edema are relieved to prevent future joint problems.
Avoid close contact with individuals with infections, colds, or influenza.
Return to the physician's office, as designated, for follow-up assessment.
Report any untoward symptoms of the medications, intolerable joint pain, or symptoms of a recurring infection to the attending physician immediately.
Notify the attending physician if planning to undergo any procedure that has risk of bacteria entering blood stream, such as dental procedures or invasive diagnostic procedures. Prophylactic antibiotics may be given prior to the procedure.

resultant deteriorating hemodynamics. Slowly developing pericardial effusions may be as large as 1000 to 2000 milliliters of fluid as the pericardium slowly stretches to accommodate the fluid.

Inflammation of the sac surrounding the heart, the pericardium, is called pericarditis. It can be caused by a wide variety of disease processes. The most common infectious causes are viral, bacterial, fungal, and parasitic. Inflammatory causes of pericarditis include rheumatic and collagen-vascular diseases. Metabolic causes include uremia, myxedema, and amyloidosis. Autoimmune pericarditis is a response to nonspecific pericardial trauma such as myocardial infarction (MI). The most common type of pericarditis is acute idiopathic pericarditis, which has no apparent predisposing or causative factors.

All types of pericarditis develop an exudate between the heart and the pericardium as a result of the inflammation. There may be bleeding into the pericardial space, with fibrous tissue invading the space and forming scar tissue. Scar tissue and adhesions may constrict the movement of the heart, leading to cardiac failure.

CLINICAL MANIFESTATIONS

A pericardial effusion that occurs suddenly may increase pressure within the pericardial cavity to a level that hinders myocardial movement, leading to a condition called cardiac tamponade. Chest pain, a pericardial friction rub, and electrocardiogram (ECG) changes are manifestations of pericarditis. The inflammatory response also causes a leukocytosis and an elevated ESR.

The chest pain is described as a sharp pain that begins in the precordial area and may radiate to the neck, back, or abdomen. It is usually worse with deep breathing, coughing, or lying on the left side.

The pericardial friction rub is heard when the stethoscope is placed on the left chest in the apical area or along the left sternal border. The rub results from the movement between the inflamed pericardial surfaces. The sound of a friction rub is like that of two pieces of leather being rubbed together or the sound of a "squeaky" shoe. The rub may come and go throughout the inflammatory period of 7 to 10 days.

ECG changes associated with pericarditis are specific to the ST segment. In the early stages of pericarditis, the ST segment elevates. It then becomes inverted and, with resolution of the inflammation, the ST segment returns to normal.

MEDICAL DIAGNOSIS

The diagnosis is made on the basis of history, symptoms, x-ray film, and other diagnostic studies. An important diagnostic sign of cardiac tamponade is the appearance of pulsus paradoxus. It is measured by auscultating the Korotkoff sounds as the blood pressure cuff is lowered by 4 mm Hg per respiratory cycle. The inspiratory drop in systolic pressure is the pulsus paradoxus. Normally the pulsus paradoxus should not exceed 8 mm Hg. In acute cardiac tamponade, it always exceeds this amount.

MEDICAL MANAGEMENT

Tamponade, an increase in the pericardial fluid to the point that ventricular movement is restricted, is a medical emergency. If not relieved, cardiac arrest will follow. Excess pericardial fluid is immediately removed (pericardiocentesis) by needle aspiration of the fluid through needle puncture of the chest wall into the pericardium.

Antipyretics are used to treat fever associated with pericarditis as well as the inflammatory process. Dyspnea may be associated with pericarditis because of the pain of breathing, or it may be a result of pericardial effusion (i.e., tamponade). Antibiotics specific for the causative agent of pericarditis are prescribed.

Application of the Nursing Process to the Care of the Patient with Pericardial Disease

The assessment, nursing diagnoses, expected patient outcomes, nursing interventions, and evaluation for patients with pericardial disease are similar to those described previously for patients with cardiac infection.

Functional Disorders

Congestive Heart Failure

ETIOLOGY AND PATHOPHYSIOLOGY

CHF is present when the cardiac output is not sufficient to meet the metabolic demands of the body. The hemodynamics of heart failure are inadequate renal blood flow and increased ventricular filling pressures.

When the left ventricle cannot pump its volume of blood out into the systemic circulation, it fails, and the term left-sided heart failure is given to the process. Likewise, when the right ventricle cannot pump its blood volume into the pulmonary artery, it fails. This process is termed right-sided heart failure. Congestive failure can be strictly from one side of the heart, but more frequently there is a combination of both left-sided and right-sided heart failure. CHF may begin on the left side, and as the lungs become saturated with excess fluid, the process backs up into the right ventricle, leading to right-sided heart failure.

CLINICAL MANIFESTATIONS

Many heart diseases, as well as other systemic pathologies, result in CHF. When the left ventricle cannot empty its blood volume, the blood backs up into the pulmonary veins and ultimately into the lungs. The patient with left-sided heart failure is dyspneic, coughs from the increased fluid in the lungs, and, if severe failure is present, may produce frothy, pink sputum. The dyspneic patient will prefer to sit upright to enhance breathing and to increase the intake of oxygen. Loud crackling (rales) and, in some patients with narrowed airways, wheezing can be heard in the lung fields during auscultation. With right-sided heart failure, edema occurs in the periphery. It can be seen in the ankles and pretibial, genital, and sacral areas in addition to the jugular veins. Fluid collects in any dependent part of the body. The liver and abdominal areas become engorged with fluid, leading to anorexia, nausea, and vomiting.

MEDICAL DIAGNOSIS

The diagnosis is made on the basis of symptoms presented, history, and diagnostic studies. Clinical assessment of the patient reveals either pulmonary or peripheral congestion or both. Vital signs may be abnormal with either increased or decreased values depending on the severity of the failure. A chest x-ray film reveals cardiac enlargement with pulmonary congestion. The ECG is not diagnostic for CHF, but its abnormalities may reflect the underlying heart disease causing the failure, such as a recent MI.

MEDICAL MANAGEMENT

Treatment is aimed at relieving the symptoms of failure, discovering the underlying cause, and correcting the problems if possible. Oxygen administration to improve oxygenation of the myocardium and other body organs is essential. The pharmacologic therapy instituted may include a variety of cardiac drugs, depending on the patient and the response to treatment.

VASODILATOR DRUGS

Morphine sulfate dilates the coronary arteries and the peripheral vasculature. Dilating the periphery diverts some of the excess fluid from the core of the body to the periphery, allowing increased expansion of the lungs and thus improving oxygenation. Intravenous morphine sulfate will also help sedate the patient and decrease the workload, because anxiety and panic cause increased respiratory effort. Venous pooling, decreased cardiac return, and reduction in pulmonary capillary pressure (preload reduction) is achieved by the administration of nitroglycerin.

AFTERLOAD REDUCING AGENTS

Afterload reducing agents, which reduce systemic vascular resistance and blood pressure, make it easier for the heart to empty, thus increasing cardiac output. Common afterload reducing agents include sodium nitroprusside (Nipride), prazosin (Minipress), and hydralazine (Apresoline).

DIURETICS

Intravenous furosemide (Lasix) is used to venodilate systemic and pulmonary beds with ultimate diuresis as excess fluid is filtered through the kidneys (see Pharmacology Box 17–4). For control of chronic CHF, the reduction of sodium in the diet may be advocated along with drug therapy.

DIGITALIS

Digitalis glycosides improve myocardial contractility, improve stroke volume, reduce ventricular filling pressures, and increase cardiac output (see Pharmacology Box 17–1). The results of digitalis therapy are not apparent for several hours after administration, which is why these preparations are not the first choice for pharmacologic therapy in acute CHF episodes. Adjunctive administration plus chronic administration of digitalis may decrease or eliminate the need for further diuretic administration.

Application of the Nursing Process to the Care of the Patient with Congestive Heart Failure

Assessment

Review the history and laboratory data, and complete a physical assessment. Assess the patient's physical abilities, because the patient with CHF reports feeling fatigued to the point of exhaustion. Ask the patient whether the fatigue is intermittent or continuous during the day. Ask about sleep and rest patterns, strength and endurance, and ability to complete activities of daily living.

Assess the vital signs. Note whether the patient is dyspneic during activity or during rest. Ask whether the patient has experienced any chest pain. If so, obtain a description of the frequency, severity, duration, relief methods, and radiation. Auscultate the chest for rales or wheezing, because left-sided heart failure results in adventitious lung sounds throughout the lung fields and is accompanied by a productive or nonproductive cough. Check for tachycardia with the presence of dysrhythmias such as atrial fibrillation, premature ventricular contractions, (PVCs) and heart blocks. Peripheral pulses may be diminished, with central pulses that are bounding with visible jugular, carotid, or abdominal pulsations. Check the blood pressure, which may be low, normal, or high depending on the degree of failure.

Observe for edema of the ankles, sacrum, and liver or abdominal enlargement, because right-sided heart failure results in peripheral edema. Also look for jugular vein distention. Check for tenderness in the abdomen. Assess capillary refill in the nail beds, which is usually slow in congestive failure. Note the skin color, looking for paleness, cyanosis, duskiness, or an ashen appearance.

The fluid retention may cause the patient to complain of recent weight gain, loss of appetite, nausea and vomiting, and diarrhea or constipation. Assess the patient for gastrointestinal system problems resulting from the CHF. Ask whether clothes or shoes seem tight in recent days or weeks. Weigh the patient, and record the data for baseline information. If the patient is being diuresed, the baseline weight is an important measuring point for later comparisons of the effect of the diuretic. Observe for signs of cerebral edema such as behavior changes, confusion, and disorientation.

Nursing Diagnoses and Planning

Nursing diagnoses and related expected patient outcomes most commonly applicable to patients with CHF include the following:

NDx: Decreased cardiac output related to altered myocardial contractility and alterations in rate, rhythm, or electrical conduction

Planning: Patient outcomes
1. Patient's vital signs are within acceptable ranges for the patient.
2. Patient demonstrates absence or control of dysrhythmias.
3. Patient participates in activities consistent with abilities.
4. Patient is free of dyspnea.

NDx: Activity intolerance related to generalized weakness or an imbalance between the oxygen supply and the oxygen demand

Planning: Patient outcomes
1. Patient increasingly participates in activities without intolerable dyspnea or fatigue.
2. Patient demonstrates energy-saving activities and seeks assistance as needed.
3. Patient sets a daily schedule that allows for intermittent periods of rest as needed.
4. Patient verbalizes understanding of the need for oxygen, medications, and supportive equipment that may increase tolerance for activity.

NDx: Fluid volume excess, related to reduced glomerular filtration rate (GFR) secondary to reduced cardiac output, increased antidiuretic hormone (ADH) production, and sodium and water retention

Planning: Patient outcomes
1. Patient maintains a balanced intake and output.
2. Patient's breath sounds are clear to auscultation.
3. Patient's daily weights are as expected for the patient, and edema is absent.
4. Patient verbalizes dietary and fluid restrictions.

NDx: High risk for impaired skin integrity related to decreased tissue perfusion and edema

Planning: Patient outcomes
1. Patient's skin remains intact without edema, redness, or lesions.
2. Patient demonstrates behaviors used to prevent skin breakdown such as turning, keeping feet and legs out of dependent positions, and keeping skin clean, dry, and supple.

NDx: Ineffective breathing pattern related to extensive pulmonary edema secondary to CHF

Planning: Patient outcomes
1. Patient's vital signs are within normal ranges for the patient.
2. Patient denies dyspnea, tachypnea, or productive cough.
3. Patient is able to complete activities of daily living without breathing difficulties.

Nursing Interventions

NDx: Decreased cardiac output
Monitor the patient's vital signs both at rest and during activity. Encourage the patient to have frequent rest periods throughout the day to prevent fatigue and strain on the myocardium. Note any dyspneic episodes and precipitating factors. Ask whether the patient is getting enough rest and sleep. Prevent disturbances in the room, especially at night.

Use telemetry monitoring whenever possible, especially if the patient experiences dysrhythmias or is taking antidysrhythmic drugs. Auscultate the apical pulse, noting the rate and rhythm. Review the results of laboratory studies and hemodynamic monitoring.

Check the patient's intake and output, observing for adequacy and balance. Keep the patient's legs in a nondependent position while sitting. Provide support for the extremities while sitting or lying in bed. Pad bony prominences to prevent breakdown from pressure and poor circulation.

Teach the patient relaxation techniques and range-of-motion procedures to increase circulation while lying in bed. Keep the patient warm and comfortable. Prevent constriction of circulation from tight-fitting clothing or bed linen.

NDx: Activity intolerance
Instruct the patient to develop a regimen of activity with frequent rest periods as needed. Encourage the patient to do range-of-motion exercises frequently while lying in bed to maintain muscle tone and strength. Provide supplemental oxygen as needed. Have the patient practice deep-breathing exercises to increase oxygen and blood flow to the brain.

Teach the patient to practice energy-saving techniques to reduce fatigue and shortness of breath. Place frequently used articles within the patient's reach. Have the patient seek assistance when needed.

Provide and encourage frequent rest periods while delivering patient care. Prevent interruptions during rest periods and at night whenever possible. Reduce any disturbing noises and limit visitors as necessary. Encourage acceleration of activity, and monitor progress as the patient moves through the rehabilitation process.

Encourage good nutrition to increase the patient's energy level. Offer four to six meals per day. This is less tiring for the patient and will prevent gastric overdistention and prevent dyspneic episodes during meals.

NDx: Fluid volume excess
Help the patient exercise, when able, to assist in the dissemination of fluid. Give prescribed diuretics, and provide a bedside commode for the patient if he or she is unable to ambulate to the bathroom. Teach the patient about the effects of the medications, the necessity for fluid-intake restrictions, and the dietary changes needed such as a low-sodium meal plan (Nutrition Box 18–1). Monitor the patient's intake and output carefully, and document the results. Weigh the patient daily, and record the weight.

Inspect the skin for edematous areas and potential sites of skin breakdown. Keep the patient's legs elevated and supported when sitting to prevent dependent edema. Have the patient maintain a semi-Fowler's or high Fowler's position to maximize the respiratory effort. Check frequently for noisy respirations.

NDx: High risk for impaired skin integrity
Inspect the skin frequently, noting skeletal prominences, presence of edema, or areas of redness that may be prone to breakdown. Reposition the patient hourly if necessary to prevent pressure areas and to stimulate circulation. Massage the skin to enhance circulation to prevent ischemic sites. Keep the skin clean, dry, and supple. Use lotions to prevent dry, cracked skin.

NDx: Ineffective breathing pattern
Promote maximum respirations by repositioning the patient. Have the patient stay in a semi-Fowler's or high Fowler's position while in bed for better chest expansion. Allow frequent rest periods while administering care so the patient does not become fatigued and dyspneic. Teach the patient deep-breathing techniques. Tell the patient to seek assistance if activities cause more difficult breathing or extreme fatigue. Administer oxygen as needed.

Observe for signs of respiratory distress, and administer treatments and medications as ordered. Watch for changes in the blood gas values, indicating early respiratory difficulty. Auscultate the chest

Nutrition Box 18–1.

NUTRITIONAL TIPS FOR THE PATIENT WITH CONGESTIVE HEART FAILURE

Instruct the patient with congestive heart failure to follow these diet therapy tips:

Follow a sodium restricted diet: This may vary from only eating foods that contain no sodium to very low sodium to just avoiding salty foods and avoiding salting foods before eating. The amount of sodium ingested daily should be based on the severity of the disease and the amount of edema present. The exact amount of sodium allowed may be prescribed by the physician.
Learn to use other seasonings that enhance food flavor but contribute no sodium to the diet.
Read food labels for the sodium content, and avoid foods high in sodium, presalted, or preserved with salt.
Limit caloric intake to maintain weight or reduce weight if obese.
Eat frequent small meals to prevent gastric distention, fatigue, and cardiac or respiratory distress from increased workload on the myocardium.
Eat low-fat, easily digested foods.

for changes in the adventitious sounds. (See Chapters 12 to 14 for care of the patient with respiratory dysfunction.)

Evaluation

Evaluate the effectiveness of nursing care for a patient with CHF by comparing the patient's status with the expected patient outcomes. Examples of specific outcomes for patients with CHF have been provided in the Planning section.

Dysrhythmias

ETIOLOGY AND PATHOPHYSIOLOGY

With disease and other metabolic disturbances of the body, the conduction system of the heart may be disrupted. Causes of the disruption of normal conduction in the heart are varied. Because normal conduction is dependent on the movement of potassium and sodium ions across the cardiac cellular membrane, a loss or gain of these ions, especially potassium, can cause disruption in the conduction tissue of the heart. A change in the acid-base balance of the body, and thus in the circulating blood through the cardiac circulatory system, may also cause dysrhythmias. Surgery with resultant cardiac edema or incision of conduction pathways may result in dysrhythmias. Ischemia or infarct of the myocardial tissue and conduction tissue results in abnormal conduction patterns.

BRADYCARDIA

A heart rate of lower than 60 beats per minute is termed bradycardia. It may be the result of vagal stimulation, hypothermia, increased intracranial pressure, MI, drug actions of digitalis and propranolol, obstructive disease, or myxedema (Fig. 18–1).

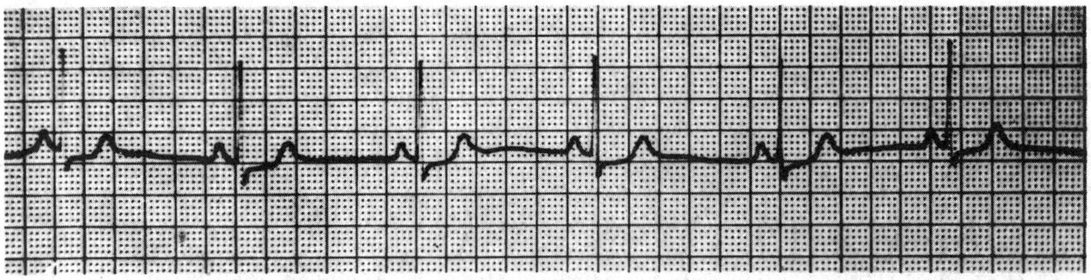

Figure 18–1.

Sinus bradycardia at a rate of fewer than 60 beats per minute. (From Sanderson RG, Kurth CL. The cardiac patient. 2nd ed. Philadelphia: WB Saunders, 1983, p 140.)

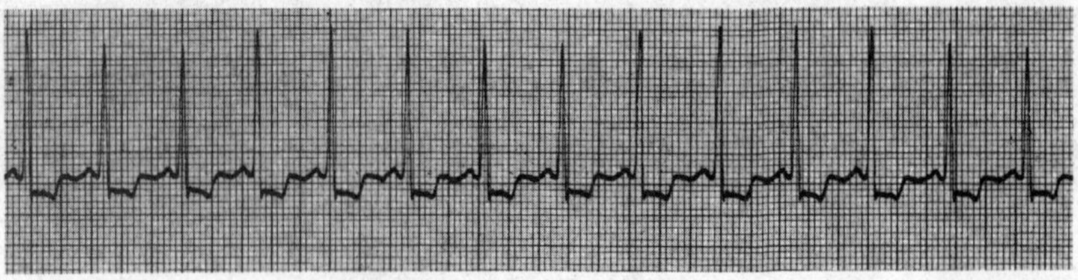

Figure 18–2.

Sinus tachycardia at a rate of 115 beats per minute. (From Sanderson RG, Kurth CL. The cardiac patient. 2nd ed. Philadelphia: WB Saunders, 1983, p 140.)

Increased vagal stimulation may result from pain, ischemia, and fear. Unless the bradycardia is symptomatic (mental confusion, disorientation, lethargy), it is usually observed rather than treated. Atropine administered intravenously is the treatment of choice when bradycardia must be chemically treated.

TACHYCARDIA

A heart rate of more than 100 beats per minute is termed tachycardia. If tachycardia arises from the sinoatrial node (SA), it is termed sinus tachycardia (Fig. 18–2). Tachycardia may be caused by increased sympathetic tone, fever, exercise, emotion, and MI. A variety of disorders such as pulmonary embolism, heart failure, anemia, thyrotoxicosis, and pericarditis may result in sinus tachycardia. The treatment for sinus tachycardia is directed at correcting the underlying disorder.

Ventricular tachycardia arises from disruptions in ventricular conduction tissue and is a life-threatening event (Fig. 18–3). It is almost always associated with organic heart disease and requires prompt treatment to prevent death. Ventricular tachycardia may be interrupted by rapid administration of intravenous lidocaine. If lidocaine therapy is unsuccessful in converting the ventricular tachycardia to a more physiologic rhythm, electrical cardioversion synchronized to the R wave of the ECG tracing is the treatment of choice, especially if the patient is showing signs of severe hemodynamic impairment.

If ventricular tachycardia is not promptly converted, it may deteriorate into ventricular fibrillation. Ventricular fibrillation represents uncoordinated, chaotic depolarization of the ventricles (Fig. 18–4). The ventricular tissues are electrically fragmented so there is no coordinated ventricular activity. The ECG tracing is erratic with no PQRST waveforms evident. Because there is no effective pumping action present, cardiac output is insufficient to sustain life. The patient loses consciousness and may also go into a seizure secondary to anoxia. Ventricular fibrillation is a medical emergency. The treatment of choice is electrical defibrillation. Cardiopulmonary resuscitation (CPR) is instituted on recognition of the dysrhythmia and should be continued until an effective cardiac rhythm is established. Lidocaine may be administered concurrently with resuscitation efforts to prevent return of ventricular fibrillation after successful defibrillation.

CLINICAL MANIFESTATIONS

The symptoms accompanying dysrhythmias vary depending on the specific dysrhythmia that is occurring. The symptoms are discussed with each of the dysrhythmias just outlined.

MEDICAL DIAGNOSIS

The diagnosis is based on assessment of symptoms and diagnostic testing.

MONITORING METHODS

Electrocardiac monitors are used to detect changes in cardiac rate and rhythm. Monitors may be hard cable units that connect leads on the patient's chest to a bedside oscilloscope. The ECG pattern is usu-

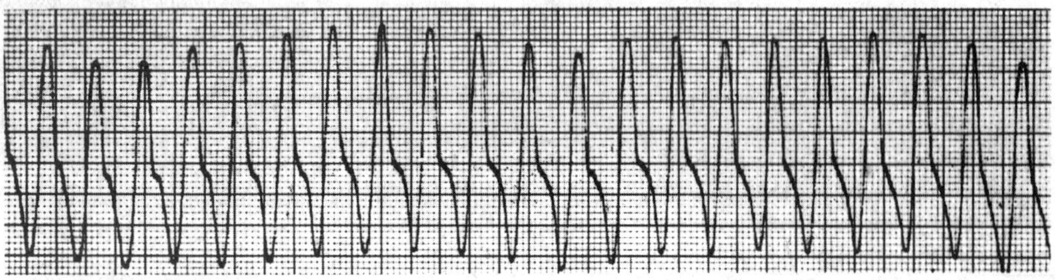

Figure 18–3.

Sustained ventricular tachycardia. (From Sanderson RG, Kurth CL. The cardiac patient. 2nd ed. Philadelphia: WB Saunders, 1983, p 156.)

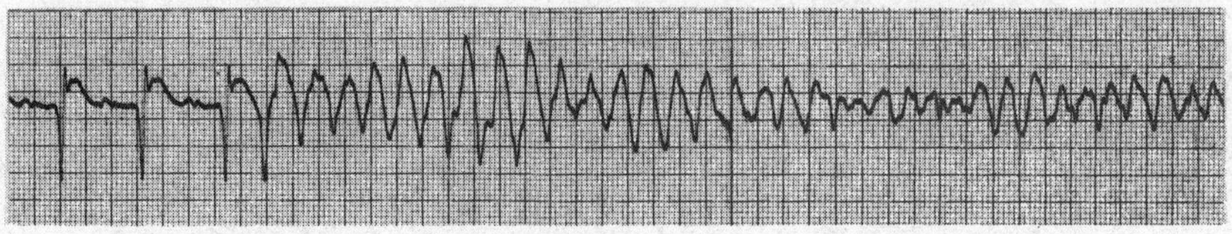

Figure 18–4.

Ventricular tachycardia and fibrillation after a premature ventricular contraction that occurs during the T wave of the preceding beat. (From Sanderson RG, Kurth CL. The cardiac patient. 2nd ed. Philadelphia: WB Saunders, 1983, p 159.)

ally also seen on an oscilloscope at the nurse's station for continuous monitoring. Such monitors limit the patients' movements, because they can ambulate only as far as the cable to the monitor reaches.

Patients who have increased ambulation expectations may wear telemetry units powered by batteries, which allow them to walk greater distances from their assigned rooms. Telemetry units also allow continuous ECG monitoring at the nurse's station.

Individuals who need to have their ECG pattern documented while performing usual activities at home or work can be connected to a Holter monitor. A Holter monitor is battery powered and contains a tape that records the electrical pattern continuously for 24 hours or more. The tape is then transcribed to paper by a machine in the ECG laboratory and interpreted by a physician. (See Chapter 17 for a thorough discussion of the diagnostic use of cardiac monitors.)

MEDICAL MANAGEMENT

The treatment of choice for most dysrhythmias is usually drug therapy. The most common drugs used for the treatment of each dysrhythmia are discussed with the description of the dysrhythmia. Other treatments may include implantation of a pacemaker for either permanent or temporary support.

PACEMAKERS

Patients may require implantation of an artificial pacemaker if a cardiac conduction block, which is incompatible with life, develops. In a diseased heart, a conduction impulse that arises from the SA node and travels through the conduction pathways may be blocked by disease, ischemia, edema, scar tissue, surgical incision of conduction tissue, or other cardiac abnormalities. If the conduction impulse cannot proceed through the atrioventricular node or into the ventricles, depolarization of the heart will not occur, the heart will not contract, and there will be no cardiac output for the impulse. When this situation occurs, life may be threatened, and the immediate installation of a temporary pacemaker may be required. If the conduction defect does not resolve spontaneously, with resolution of edema, ischemia, and so on, a permanent pacemaker is implanted.

Most pacemakers are powered by safe, reliable, and long-lasting lithium batteries. The battery is placed subcutaneously in the patient's chest or abdominal area and is connected to the pacemaker leads (Fig. 18–5). The type of pacemaker used depends on the conduction problem that must be corrected and physician reference. Leads are surgically placed into the heart. Atrial and ventricular leads are placed via a vein (usually the right or left cephalic) under local anesthesia in the operating room or cardiac catheterization laboratory. Postoperatively, the patient is monitored for 12 to 36 hours to ensure that the pacemaker is functioning properly. Adjustments can be made if necessary. Many of the pacemakers used today are programmable, and numerous functions can be changed noninvasively once the pacemaker is implanted (Nursing Care Guide 18–1).

Text continued on page 746

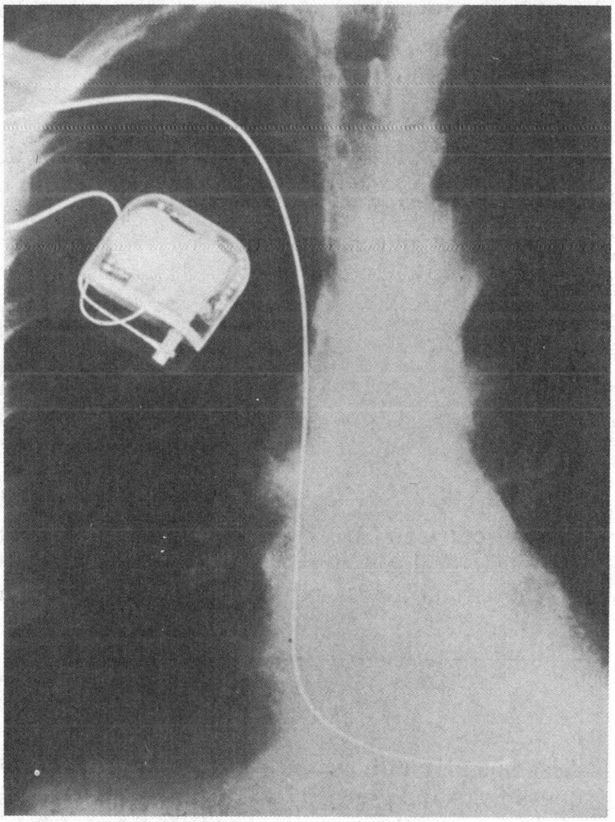

Figure 18–5.

Chest x-ray film showing right ventricular lead placement attached to an implanted pacemaker. (From Sanderson RG, Kurth CL. The cardiac patient. 2nd ed. Philadelphia: WB Saunders, 1983, p 229.)

Nursing Care Guide 18–1.

PATIENTS UNDERGOING INSERTION OF A PACEMAKER

Preoperative Care

Assessment Findings: Patient appears nervous, withdraws from conversation, clenches hands; blood pressure, pulse, and respirations are slightly elevated for the patient; patient makes statements indicating concern about the procedure and results of medical intervention.

Nursing Diagnosis: Anxiety related to uncertainty about procedure, potential risk factors and outcome

Patient Outcomes	Nursing Interventions	Rationale
Patient states methods to relax and release tension, and practices the techniques.	Teach the patient relaxation techniques. Reassure the patient about the necessity of the pacemaker. Teach deep-breathing techniques.	Relaxation exercises help reduce stress and tension.
	Explain the procedure to the patient, and allow time for questions and expression of concerns. Explain each step of the preoperative preparation.	An understanding of the procedure may help reassure the patient and reduce anxiety.
	Have the patient repeat the instructions.	Having the patient reiterate the instructions allows for correction of misunderstandings and reinforces the information.
Patient reports feeling less nervous, appears relaxed, and is able to rest well, and vital signs are within normal ranges for the patient.	Provide a quiet, calm environment with periods of rest during the delivery of nursing care. Ask for supportive assistance from clergy or the patient's significant others.	Frequent rest periods may assist in reducing the patient's anxiety about the procedure.
	Tell the patient it is normal to be worried about the procedure and its outcome.	Reassurance of the normality of feelings of anxiety helps alleviate some of the fear.
	Check vital signs after the patient is rested and more relaxed, and note any changes.	Changes in vital signs may reflect the patient's state of anxiety.

Evaluation: Compare the patient's status with the expected patient outcomes. If the outcomes are achieved, evaluate nursing care as successful. If not, reassess the patient, formulate new nursing diagnoses, and revise expected patient outcomes and nursing interventions as appropriate.

Assessment Findings: Patient and family seem very concerned about the procedure; they ask several questions about the surgical procedure, the preparation before surgery, the pacemaker, the expectations of the intervention, possible complications, and expected outcome.

(continued)

Nursing Care Guide 18–1. *(continued)*

PATIENTS UNDERGOING INSERTION OF A PACEMAKER

Nursing Diagnosis: Knowledge deficit: nature of surgery, expected outcome, and possible complications

Patient Outcomes	Nursing Interventions	Rationale
Patient accurately describes the purpose and function of the pacemaker and the necessity for its insertion and relates information about the procedure, complications, and expected results as presented to the patient by the physician.	Explain to the patient the procedure, the preoperative preparation, and the expected outcomes. Have the patient relate what the physician has explained, and clear up any misunderstandings. Allow time for questions from the patient or the family. Give the patient literature explaining the pacemaker and its function.	An understanding of the procedure enhances cooperation and compliance with instructions. Having the patient reiterate the information reinforces the instructions and allows for correction of misunderstandings.
Patient reports an understanding of the preoperative preparation necessary.	Explain all preoperative nursing interventions as they are delivered.	An explanation of the preoperative procedures enhances cooperation from the patient.

Evaluation: Compare the patient's status with the expected patient outcomes. If the outcomes are achieved, evaluate nursing care as successful. If not, reassess the patient, formulate new nursing diagnoses, and revise expected patient outcomes and nursing interventions as appropriate.

Postoperative Care

Assessment Findings: Patient grimaces, moans, and complains of discomfort at insertion site; patient's blood pressure, pulse, and respiratory rate are elevated.

Nursing Diagnosis: Pain related to invasive surgical procedure

Patient Outcomes	Nursing Interventions	Rationale
Patient reports relief of pain, appears relaxed and comfortable, and is able to rest well.	Give prescribed analgesics for control of postoperative pain. Make patient comfortable, and provide a quiet atmosphere for rest after surgery.	Early intervention for pain relief reduces potential for complications and allows for restful periods for the patient.
	Check insertion site for signs of infection, which may increase pain at site.	
	Tell the patient to practice relaxation techniques taught before surgery.	Practicing relaxation exercises may help relieve discomfort and promote rest.

(continued)

Nursing Care Guide 18–1. *(continued)*

PATIENTS UNDERGOING INSERTION OF A PACEMAKER

Patient Outcomes	Nursing Interventions	Rationale
Patient's vital signs are within normal ranges.	Monitor vital signs, and document the results.	Changes in vital signs may indicate changes in pain levels or the presence of complications.

Evaluation: Compare the patient's status with the expected patient outcomes. If the outcomes are achieved, evaluate nursing care as successful. If not, reassess the patient, formulate new nursing diagnoses, and revise expected patient outcomes and nursing interventions as appropriate.

Assessment Findings: Patient seems overly anxious, withdraws from conversations, seems reluctant to listen to home care instructions, and states concerns about complications.

Nursing Diagnosis: Fear related to potential complications such as pacemaker failure or disengagement and possible cardiac arrest

Patient Outcomes	Nursing Interventions	Rationale
Patient states an understanding of the methods necessary to manage the potential complications of the procedure and having the pacemaker.	Explain the complications to the patient in understandable terms. Include the patient's family in the education sessions. Tell the patient it is quite normal to have fears about the future. Allow time for questions and expression of concerns.	An understanding of the procedure and the self-care management necessary enhances cooperation and reduces fear and anxiety.
Patient and family relate signs of problems and when to seek medical intervention.	Give the patient written instructions for home care. Tell the patient and family to seek medical intervention if any untoward signs occur, such as fainting, dizziness, chest pain, dyspnea, tachycardia, bradycardia, or any other symptom that the patient senses as unusual.	Written and verbal instructions reinforce the information provided. Including the family allows for further reinforcement and assistance for the patient if needed after discharge.
	Teach both the patient and the family how to monitor the heart rate.	

Evaluation: Compare the patient's status with the expected patient outcomes. If the outcomes are achieved, evaluate nursing care as successful. If not, reassess the patient, formulate new nursing diagnoses, and revise expected patient outcomes and nursing interventions as appropriate.

(continued)

Nursing Care Guide 18–1. *(continued)*

PATIENTS UNDERGOING INSERTION OF A PACEMAKER

Assessment Findings: Patient relates concern about discharge plans, changes in lifestyle needed, when to seek medical assistance, and how to manage self-care; patient and family ask many questions about the postoperative course and home needs; both patient and family seem nervous and extremely concerned about the patient's status.

Nursing Diagnosis: High risk for impaired home maintenance management related to fear and concerns about care after discharge

Patient Outcomes	Nursing Interventions	Rationale
Patient relates accurate information about the home care required and the need for follow-up care with the physician.	Describe the signs requiring immediate medical intervention such as pain or discomfort at insertion point, fever, chills, dizziness, fainting, excessive fatigue, shortness of breath, and pulse rate below the preset rate or double the preset rate.	An understanding of the self-care needed and the potential complications after discharge may enhance compliance and promote early intervention if complications occur.
Patient describes lifestyle changes needed, such as the preventive care for invasive procedures, the need to refrain from lifting arms for several weeks, the need for monitoring of pulse rates, and the need for carrying an identification card.	Teach the patient and family how to monitor the pulse rate accurately, and tell them to keep a record of it. Tell the patient to carry an identification card stating name and address, type of pacemaker, manufacturer, preset rate, and physician's name and telephone number. Because pacemakers can set off security alarms (such as in an airport), tell the patient to report this before entering a security area.	Preparing the patient for the lifestyle changes that may be necessary will prevent complications.

Evaluation: Compare the patient's status with the expected patient outcomes. If the outcomes are achieved, evaluate nursing care as successful. If not, reassess the patient, formulate new nursing diagnoses, and revise expected patient outcomes and nursing interventions as appropriate.

Application of the Nursing Process to the Care of the Patient with Dysrhythmias

Assessment

Review the patient's medical history and diagnostic results for the type of dysrhythmia present. Assess for fatigue and generalized weakness, which is usually present in patients with dysrhythmias that cannot be attributed to any specific change in living pattern. Ask about a history of cardiac dysrhythmias or disease processes. Check vital signs and note changes with activity. Examine the ECG results. Ask about anorexia, nausea, vomiting, and resultant weight loss. Auscultate the lungs for rales indicating some degree of left-sided heart failure. Assess for signs of right-sided heart failure such as edema, jugular vein distention, and an engorged, painful liver.

Check for signs of mental status changes that occur with decreased cardiac output. Look for disorientation, confusion, memory loss, or changes in level of consciousness. Decreased perfusion of the brain also leads to behavior changes such as combativeness, lethargy, and hallucinations.

Nursing Diagnoses and Planning

Nursing diagnoses and related expected patient outcomes most commonly applicable to patients with dysrhythmias include the following:

NDx: Decreased cardiac output related to altered electrical conduction

Planning: Patient outcomes
1. Patient achieves adequate cardiac output as evidenced by normal vital signs.
2. Patient participates in activities that reduce the myocardial workload.
3. Patient demonstrates a reduced frequency of dysrhythmias causing decreased cardiac output.

NDx: Anxiety related to fear of the potential life-threatening dysrhythmia, treatment regimen necessary, and fear of death

Planning: Patient outcomes
1. Patient reports reduced anxiety and fear of disorder.
2. Patient appears relaxed and is able to rest and sleep well.
3. Patient's vital signs are within normal ranges for the patient.
4. Patient does not present outward signs of anxiety such as nervousness, clenching of hands, withdrawal, hyperventilation, or twitching.

NDx: Knowledge deficit: electrical conduction of the heart, nature of dysrhythmias (specify the particular dysrhythmia), and the drug intervention or other therapies required

Planning: Patient outcomes
1. Patient verbalizes accurate information about the electrical conduction of the heart and the nature of the dysrhythmia present.
2. Patient reports an understanding of the medications prescribed, the dose, side effects, and expected therapeutic results.
3. Patient accurately checks heart rate and records it.

Nursing Interventions

NDx: Decreased cardiac output
Monitor the patient's vital signs both at rest and during activity, and document the data. Encourage the patient to take frequent rest periods throughout the day to prevent fatigue and strain on the myocardium. Note any dyspneic episodes and precipitating factors. Ask whether the patient is getting enough rest and sleep, and prevent disturbances.

Use telemetry monitoring whenever possible, especially if the patient experiences dysrhythmias or is taking antidysrhythmic drugs. Auscultate the apical pulse, noting the rate and rhythm. Review the results of laboratory studies and hemodynamic monitoring.

Check the patient's intake and output, observing for adequacy and balance. Keep the patient's legs in a nondependent position while sitting. Provide support for the extremities while sitting or lying in bed. Pad bony prominences to prevent breakdown from pressure and poor circulation.

Teach the patient relaxation techniques and range-of-motion exercises to increase circulation while lying in bed. Keep the patient warm and comfortable. Prevent constriction of circulation from tight-fitting clothing or bed linen.

NDx: Anxiety
Help the patient find effective relaxation methods. Teach relaxation techniques that the patient can practice throughout the day. Allow the patient and family time to be alone. Provide for plenty of rest periods. Give explanations that the patient can understand, and allow for patient input in the daily care plan. Teach the patient about the disease and medications used to control the effects of the disorder.

Answer the patient's questions in a professional, informative manner. Help the patient find coping strategies that relieve stress and anxiety. Ask for assistance from clergy or counseling staff if necessary.

NDx: Knowledge deficit: electrical conduction of the heart, nature of dysrhythmias (specify the particular dysrhythmia), and the drug intervention of other therapies required
Plan for education sessions with the patient when rested and relaxed. Provide time for questions and concerns to be voiced. Include the family in the teaching. Review the normal cardiac function and electrical conduction with the patient using terminology the patient can understand. Explain the specific changes in rhythm in relation to the normal patterns. Identify symptoms of the dysrhythmia such as fatigue, edema, anorexia, and changes in mentation.

Instruct the patient about the prescribed medications, the side effects, dosages, frequency, and when to seek medical intervention if untoward symptoms are present. Provide written instructions about the medications. Tell the patient to keep a record of pulse rates, untoward symptoms, and medication administration for physician perusal at the next visit.

Evaluation

Evaluate the effectiveness of nursing care for a patient with a dysrhythmia by comparing the patient's status with the expected patient outcomes. Examples of specific outcomes for patients with dysrhythmias have been provided in the Planning section.

Myocardial Infarction

ETIOLOGY AND PATHOPHYSIOLOGY

Myocardial infarction (MI) results when a coronary artery becomes completely obstructed. An obstructed artery cannot carry blood to the heart muscle it supplies. If that portion of the heart muscle is supplied by other nearby vessels, called collateral vessels, they can take over when there is insufficient blood supply to the myocardium. If there are no collateral vessels available to bring blood to the heart muscle, the muscle becomes ischemic for an extended period. In angina pectoris alone, the ischemia usually lasts only for a short period of time before it is relieved. Prolonged ischemia leads to death of the cells in the affected area, a process called infarction. Because the infarcted area is in the myocardium, the result is an MI. The infarction can involve almost any area of the heart but usually affects the left ventricle. It may involve the inferior wall (an inferior MI), the anterior and lateral walls (an anterolateral MI), or the septum along with an adjoining wall (anteroseptal or posteroseptal MI).

CLINICAL MANIFESTATIONS

The most significant symptom of infarction is acute pain. The pain is usually described as crushing, heavy, or constricting the chest. Substernal pain may radiate to the neck, jaw, or left arm. The pain differs from angina by being prolonged and unrelieved by rest or nitroglycerin tablets. Vagal stimulation results in epigastric distress, leading to nausea and vomiting in addition to pain. Patients may view the epigastric distress as indigestion and try to relieve it with antacids. This treatment usually delays seeking medical intervention, which may increase the myocardial damage as the infarction proceeds. The decreased circulation to the myocardium may lead to hypotension and cardiogenic shock.

MEDICAL DIAGNOSIS

The diagnosis is made on the basis of symptoms, history, and clinical and laboratory tests. The patient usually has a history of risk factors for coronary disease such as obesity, smoking, and familial history of cardiac disease. An ECG is obtained, although it may be negative for cardiac damage if it is taken early in the course of the infarction. Only after tissue damage has been done will the ECG be positive for an infarction. Ischemic changes and early dysrhythmias can be noted on the ECG. Serial serum enzymes are evaluated. Release of cellular enzymes occurs with cell damage and death. The most common enzymes evaluated for diagnosis of cardiac damage are creatine kinase (CK), lactate dehydrogenase (LDH), aspartate aminotransferase (AST) (formerly serum glutamic oxaloacetic transaminase [SGOT]). (Refer to cardiac diagnostic tests in Chapter 17.)

MEDICAL MANAGEMENT

The treatment of MI initially includes rest, analgesia, oxygen, and early detection and treatment of dysrhythmias. Bed rest is ordered for the first 48 to 72 hours to allow the myocardium to rest and attempt to recuperate and to prevent further damage. The patient is allowed out of bed only to use the bedside commode. Once the patient has been on bed rest for several days and the chest pain is relieved, the patient is allowed to sit in a chair for short periods of time. Indications for prolonged bed rest are the development of unstable vital signs, dysrhythmias, pericarditis, or shock.

Sufficient analgesia should be administered to control the severe chest pain, as evidenced by the patient's ability to sleep. Morphine sulfate is the analgesic of choice because of its peripheral vasodilating properties, leading to a decrease in cardiac workload, plus its ability to give the patient a feeling of euphoria, thus decreasing anxiety. Small intravenous doses of 2 to 5 mg are titrated to bring the patient to a state of pain relief or to somnolence or both. The concomitant use of intravenous or intramuscular promethazine (Phenergan) or hydroxyzine (Vistaril) is strongly advised, because they accomplish the same effect with much lower doses of narcotics and produce fewer side effects of nausea, vomiting, vagotonia, and urinary retention.

Oxygen is usually administered at a flow rate of 2 to 4 L/minute by nasal prongs. If the patient also has evidence of chronic obstructive pulmonary disease with carbon dioxide retention, the oxygen flow rate or method of administration may be altered. Oxygen helps to relieve ischemia of the myocardium by raising the blood oxygen level.

Electrical conduction of the heart is constantly monitored. Ischemia and death of cardiac muscle cells cause alteration of electrical conduction through the muscle. Necrotic or dead tissue is electrically inert and unable to be depolarized. This disruption in tissue conductivity leads to irritable cells as they die or are salvaged. Such irritability produces extraventricular beats noted, or PVCs on the ECG (Fig. 18–6). In the presence of MI, PVCs predispose the patient to ventricular tachycardia and ventricular fibrillation, which may lead to death.

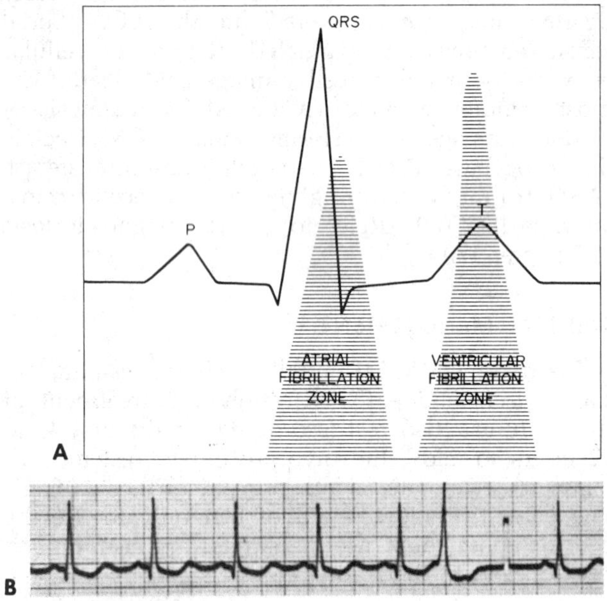

Figure 18–6.

A, The vulnerability zones related to the ECG are shown. The shaded areas indicate the times when an induced electrical current can produce atrial or ventricular fibrillation. The peak of the T wave is the most critical time for producing ventricular fibrillation. A premature ventricular contraction occurring during the vulnerable T wave period may induce ventricular fibrillation. *B*, The "R on T" phenomenon is shown. The R wave of the PVC (beat 6) occurs near the peak of the T wave of the preceding beat. (From Sanderson RG, Kurth CL. The cardiac patient. 2nd ed. Philadelphia: WB Saunders 1983, p 153.)

Intravenous lidocaine is used to suppress ventricular dysrhythmias such as PVCs. The initial dose is given as a bolus of 50 to 100 mg over 1 to 2 minutes (25 to 50 mg/minute). Then a lidocaine drip of 2 g in 500 ml of 5% dextrose in water is begun at 1 to 4 mg/minute. The total hourly dose, bolus plus drip, should not exceed 250 mg/hour. Other antiarrhythmic drugs may be used if lidocaine does not suppress the ventricular arrhythmias or if the patient needs long-term control. Some of the common ventricular antiarrhythmic drugs are procainamide (Pronestyl, Procan), quinidine (Quinidex), propranolol (Inderal), phenytoin (Dilantin), or bretylium (Bretylol).

Patients who present at a treatment facility within fewer than 6 hours from onset of symptoms and with more than 30 minutes of continuous chest pain (angina) unrelieved by nitroglycerin or nifedipine may be candidates for thrombolytic therapy. Streptokinase (Streptase, Kabikinase), alteplase (Activase), and anistreplase (Eminase) are some of the agents commonly used for thrombolytic therapy (Pharmacology Box 18–2).

Patients are maintained on a nothing by mouth order with intravenous therapy for 24 to 72 hours depending on their condition and response to treatment. Clear liquids, advancing to solid, bland food, are given as the patient is recuperating. Meals are given in small, frequent portions to prevent increasing the workload on the myocardium and to prevent anginal episodes (Nutrition Box 18–2).

Application of the Nursing Process to the Care of the Patient with a Myocardial Infarction

Assessment

Assess the patient for pain immediately, determining the duration, severity, and radiation. Check the patient's respiratory status, cardiac rhythm, and vital signs. Seek medical assistance as soon as possible.

Nursing Diagnoses and Planning

Nursing diagnoses and related expected patient outcomes most commonly applicable to patients with MI include the following:

NDx: Pain related to tissue ischemia secondary to coronary artery occlusion

Planning: Patient outcomes

1. Patient verbalizes relief or control of chest pain.
2. Patient demonstrates a relaxed manner and release of tension and is able to rest quietly.
3. Patient's vital signs are within normal ranges for the patient.

Pharmacology Box 18–2.
THROMBOLYTIC AGENTS

Thrombolytic Agents:
Enzymes such as alteplase, streptokinase, and urokinase.

Action:
Convert plasminogen to plasmin, which breaks up fibrin clots.

Uses:
Lysis of thrombi after an acute myocardial infarction or for pulmonary emboli.

Side Effects:
Excessive bleeding and bruising, bleeding at puncture site, internal hemorrhage, and fever or headache.

Interactions:
Risk of bleeding is increased if used in combination with anticoagulants.

Nursing Implications:
Check vital signs.
Monitor the electrocardiogram.
Watch for bleeding every 15 minutes for 8 hours and then every hour for 8 hours, especially at the puncture site.
Hold pressure on any needle stick sites for 5 minutes.
Protect the patient from bruising and bleeding.
Avoid overmanipulation of the patient.
Teach the patient signs of bleeding to observe for and how to prevent bleeding episodes.
Explain to the patient to report any signs of bleeding that occur.

Nutrition Box 18–2.
DIET RECOMMENDATIONS FOR THE PATIENT RECOVERING FROM A MYOCARDIAL INFARCTION

After the patient has recovered from the critical stage of a myocardial infarction, the following diet plan may be followed:

For the first few days of allowed solid food after intravenous or clear liquids, provide only soft, bland, easily tolerated foods.
Avoid spicy foods, gas-producing foods, and extremely hot or cold foods.
Provide frequent, small meals (six to eight per day) to prevent gastric distention, fatigue, respiratory distress, or increased workload on the myocardium.
Provide a low-calorie diet of low-sodium, low-fat, high-protein foods.
After rehabilitation begins and the diet can be advanced, provide four to five meals per day, if the patient begins to tolerate more food at a time and has the endurance to eat a slightly larger meal at a sitting. The continued plan of providing small, frequent meals prevents the problems mentioned above.
Increase the caloric content of the diet as needed by the patient to maintain weight and provide energy. If the patient is obese, a reduction diet is ordered.
Continue to provide foods low in fat and sodium.
Provide foods according to the patient's food preferences as much as possible.
Provide a quiet, pleasant atmosphere for the mealtime, and allow the patient to rest after eating.

Chart 18–2.

NURSING GUIDE TO PATIENT EDUCATION FOR SELF-MANAGEMENT: DISCHARGE INSTRUCTIONS FOR THE PATIENT RECOVERING FROM A MYOCARDIAL INFARCTION

Instruct the patient being discharged after recovery from an MI to:

Modify activities of daily living. Avoid overexertion, tiring activities, or any activity that induces fatigue or chest pain. Add a few new activities daily as tolerated without dyspnea, fatigue, or other untoward signs.

Begin an exercise regimen that is designed specifically for the patient's ability and limitations. Build strength and endurance slowly but steadily. If symptoms reappear with the exercise, modify it to a previous level, and repeat the gradual increase in activities.

Avoid extreme temperature changes, associating with individuals who are ill, and other exposures that put the patient at high risk for acquiring an infection.

Follow the prescribed diet therapy plan, reducing caloric intake if overweight, and eat low-fat, well-balanced, frequent, small meals.

Rest and relax frequently throughout the day to decrease stress and decrease the workload on the myocardium during the healing period.

Cease smoking, and avoid gatherings at which people are smoking.

Adhere to the prescribed medication regimen carefully.

Follow the physician's instructions for follow-up care. If any untoward symptoms such as chest pain, palpitations, extreme dyspnea, dizziness, or peripheral edema appear, notify the physician immediately.

NDx: Anxiety related to change in health status, possible death, or loss of socioeconomic status

Planning: Patient outcomes
1. Patient states feelings about health status and identifies causes for the feelings.
2. Patient verbalizes a reduction in anxiety.
3. Patient demonstrates positive problem-solving skills.
4. Patient appears relaxed and less anxious and is resting well.

NDx: Decreased cardiac output related to changes in cardiac rate, rhythm, or electrical conduction

Planning: Patient outcomes
1. Patient demonstrates a decrease in dysrhythmias as seen by hemodynamic monitoring.
2. Patient demonstrates an increase in activity tolerance.
3. Patient experiences decreased episodes of dyspnea.
4. Patient's vital signs are within normal ranges for the patient.

NDx: Knowledge deficit: nature of MI and coronary artery disease, treatment, expected outcomes, and potential lifestyle change

Planning: Patient outcomes
1. Patient verbalizes understanding of heart disease, present condition, and symptoms that require immediate attention.
2. Patient verbalizes understanding of lifestyle changes such as diet, exercise, or cessation of smoking, as listed in Chart 18–2.
3. Patient states the purposes of prescribed medications, the dose, time, frequency, and side effects.

Nursing Interventions

NDx: Pain

Monitor and document the characteristics of the chest pain as described by the patient. Note nonverbal signs of pain as well as hemodynamic changes such as heart rate, respiratory rate, and blood pressure as the pain changes. Instruct the patient to report any chest pain immediately. Explain the medications and procedures that are used to relieve the pain (Nursing Care Guide 18–2). Provide a calm, quiet environment and comfort measures to ensure effectiveness of the pain medications. Teach the patient to use relaxation techniques to reduce pain reduction and to relieve anxiety. Approach the patient in a calm, confident manner. Check vital signs before administering medication for pain. Administer oxygen by nasal cannula as indicated to promote oxygen perfusion of the myocardium.

Nursing Care Guide 18–2.
PATIENTS TAKING ANTIANGINAL DRUGS

Assessment Findings: Patient complains of pressure in the chest area, a heavy feeling across the chest, or unrelieved chest pain episodes.

Nursing Diagnosis: Pain related to ischemia of the myocardium secondary to coronary artery disease

Patient Outcomes	Nursing Interventions	Rationale
Patient reports relief of chest pain or a decrease in chest pain to a tolerable level.	Give prescribed antianginal medications at the onset of chest pain. Repeat doses as necessary to obtain pain relief.	Early intervention when pain episodes occur may reduce the intensity and duration of the episode.
	Document episodes of angina, noting the intensity, radiation, and duration, along with the number of doses needed to obtain relief.	Accurate documentation is useful for comparisons with future episodes of angina to follow the progression of the attacks.
	Allow patient to rest after episode of intense pain. Provide a calm quiet environment.	Rest and relaxation time after the anginal episode reduce the cardiac workload.
	Teach methods to deal with the pain, such as relaxation techniques.	Relaxation exercises can be helpful for pain tolerance.
	Assist the patient with activities of daily living as needed.	Decreasing the workload on the heart may reduce the number of anginal attacks experienced.
Patient's vital signs are within normal ranges for the patient.	Check vital signs, and note elevations, which may indicate increased pain episodes.	Changes in vital signs such as elevations in pulse, respirations, or blood pressure often indicate increases in pain.

Evaluation: Compare the patient's status with the expected patient outcomes. If the outcomes are achieved, evaluate nursing care as successful. If not, reassess the patient, formulate new nursing diagnoses, and revise expected patient outcomes and nursing interventions as appropriate.

(continued)

Nursing Care Guide 18–2. *(continued)*

PATIENTS TAKING ANTIANGINAL DRUGS

Assessment Findings: Patient complains of weakness and dizziness when getting out of bed; patient is unsteady when ambulating; blood pressure drops when patient is in upright position.

Nursing Diagnosis: High risk for injury related to orthostatic hypotension as side effect of pharmacologic therapy

Patient Outcomes	Nursing Interventions	Rationale
Patient relates safety measures to prevent injury and implements safe behaviors as instructed.	Instruct the patient about the effects of the medication. Ask the patient to repeat the information.	Explaining the side effects of the medications warns the patient of potential harm. Having the patient reiterate the information allows for correction of any misunderstandings.
	Tell the patient to seek assistance when getting out of bed and ambulating. Keep the bed rails in the up position. Put the call light within reach, and instruct the patient about its use. Place frequently used articles close to the patient. Have the patient sit on the side of the bed for a few minutes before getting out of bed. Instruct the family about the effects of the medication and the need for assistance for the patient when ambulating.	Practicing safety measures may prevent injury.
Patient's vital signs are within normal ranges; patient denies weakness or dizziness and remains free from injury.	Check vital signs frequently, noting changes, especially in blood pressure. Check blood pressure while the patient is lying and sitting.	A decreasing blood pressure may represent the hypotensive effect of the medication.

Evaluation: Compare the patient's status with the expected patient outcomes. If the outcomes are achieved, evaluate nursing care as successful. If not, reassess the patient, formulate new nursing diagnoses, and revise expected patient outcomes and nursing interventions as appropriate.

(continued)

Nursing Care Guide 18–2. *(continued)*

PATIENTS TAKING ANTIANGINAL DRUGS

Assessment Findings: Patient asks questions about medication regimen; patient seems to have misunderstandings about the drugs, the dosages, and frequency; patient does not understand the side effects of the medications.

Nursing Diagnosis: Knowledge deficit: nature of medications, time, dosage, frequency, side effects, and expected therapeutic effects

Patient Outcomes	Nursing Interventions	Rationale
Patient relates accurate information about the medications, side effects, dosages, and therapeutic expectations. Patient demonstrates appropriate use of the medications.	Explain to the patient about the specific antianginal medications prescribed, the dosage, number of times to repeat it (if allowed), frequency, side effects, and expected therapeutic effects. Have the patient repeat the information. Tell the patient to rest or lie down after taking the medication in case dizziness occurs. Have the patient keep a record of the anginal episodes and the medication taken, including the dose and number. Tell the patient to avoid alcoholic beverages while taking medication because more intense side effects might occur. Encourage the patient to avoid activities that might precipitate anginal attacks, such as stress, smoking, or extreme exercise.	Providing information to the patient about the medications, appropriate dosage, and side effects may prevent misuse or other pharmacologic problems after the patient is discharged. Having the patient reiterate the information allows for correction of misunderstandings.
Patient states when to seek medical intervention.	Tell the patient to observe for side effects and to notify the physician if any are apparent.	Follow-up care by the attending physician is important for proper monitoring of the patient's progress.

Evaluation: Compare the patient's status with the expected patient outcomes. If the outcomes are achieved, evaluate nursing care as successful. If not, reassess the patient, formulate new nursing diagnoses, and revise expected patient outcomes and nursing interventions as appropriate.

NDx: Anxiety
Acknowledge the patient's anxiety and the perception of the threat of the situation. Encourage expression of feelings of anger, fear, and grief. Orient the patient to routine procedures, and explain all activities that occur in the patient's room. Allow the family to express feelings and ask questions. Keep both the patient and the family apprised of changes in the patient's status or treatment plans. Seek assistance from clergy or significant others if necessary to help allay the patient's anxiety. Answer all questions factually, and provide consistent reinforcement, because the ability to understand and remember may be temporarily impaired. Accept but do not reinforce the use of denial. Support grieving behavior, and let the patient know it is a normal response. Encourage independence, self-care, and decision-making.

NDx: Decreased cardiac output
Promptly treat life-threatening dysrhythmias. Provide a bedside commode to decrease expenditure of energy that is required when using a bedpan or ambulating to the bathroom. Administer supplemental oxygen as indicated. Elevate the head of the bed to allow for maximum lung expansion to increase oxygen intake. Place needed utensils near the patient to save energy from excessive movement. Feed the patient if necessary, when allowed to eat, to conserve energy. Allow the patient time to rest between treatments, and limit visitors and extra activity in the room.

NDx: Knowledge deficit: nature of myocardial infarction and coronary artery disease, treatment, expected outcomes, and potential lifestyle changes
Explain the cause, effects, and clinical course of coronary artery disease and the resulting MI to the patient. Allow time for questions from the patient. Allow the patient to verbalize concerns and fears. Evaluate discharge needs of the patient and family (see Chart 18–2).

Alert the patient to signs and symptoms of MI for the future and the complications. Teach the patient to use safety measures or to ask for assistance when out of bed or when ambulating until strength and endurance inproves.

Instruct the patient about dietary modifications needed to reduce risk or to prevent complications of the disorder (see Nutrition Box 18–2). If the patient is obese, explain the need for a weight-reduction diet. Give the patient meal plans based on the predetermined caloric limitation. Explain the need for decreases in dietary fats and cholesterol to prevent the effects of the disease and increases in protein and vitamins to promote good health and healing. Initiate counseling with a dietitian to assist with meal planning if needed.

Teach the patient about the effects of smoking and the importance of quitting. Refer the patient to a smoking cessation program. Plan a post-discharge exercise regimen that gradually increases the intensity and endurance of the exercise, as prescribed by the physician.

Teach the patient dosage, route, time, frequency, side effects, and toxic effects of any medication prescribed (see Nursing Care Guide 18–2). Explain the diagnostic studies completed and the need for any follow-up studies after discharge. Include the family in any of the teaching sessions when applicable.

Evaluation

Evaluate the effectiveness of nursing care for a patient with MI by comparing the patient's status with the expected patient outcomes. Examples of specific outcomes for patients with MI have been provided in the Planning section.

Cardiomyopathy (Myocardiopathy)

ETIOLOGY AND PATHOPHYSIOLOGY

Cardiomyopathy is disease of the heart muscle. It is considered to be a vague pathologic entity because the causes of cardiomyopathy are not well understood. Acute injury such as a vitamin deficiency (thiamine or beriberi), myocarditis, an antigen-antibody reaction, chronic alcohol intake, or pregnancy, especially in the postpartum period, may lead to cardiomyopathy. Varying degrees of ventricular hypertrophy occur depending on the severity of the heart disease. Thrombi may develop in both ventricles. Thickening of the endocardium has been noted, with diffuse infiltration of fibrous tissue into the myocardium.

Primary cardiomyopathies are those heart diseases of unknown cause. The onset is often covert, and extensive cardiac damage is done.

CLINICAL MANIFESTATIONS

Cardiomyopathy produces a diseased heart that is extremely dilated, has varying degrees of ventricular hypertrophy, and functions poorly. Thickening of the endocardium is seen as well as mural thrombi of one or both ventricles. Patients present with heart failure, dysrhythmias, or thromboembolic episodes that may be pulmonary or systemic.

MEDICAL DIAGNOSIS

The diagnosis is made on the basis of symptoms and diagnostic studies. The patient's chest x-ray film shows a large heart as a result of dilation and hypertrophy. The ECG may show bundle branch block, atrial fibrillation, and ventricular ectopia. Auscultation of the heart sounds may reveal the presence of S_3 or S_4, or both, plus mitral or tricuspid regurgitation, or both.

MEDICAL MANAGEMENT

Treatment of cardiomyopathy varies according to the underlying cause. Primary therapy usually consists of digitalis and diuretics for CHF, and antiarrhythmics for the dysrhythmias, especially ventricular ectopia. Long-term anticoagulation may be used in an effort to reduce pulmonary and systemic emboli. Bed rest is used in the initial treatment of CHF. Specific infections are treated with appropriate antibiotics, and anti-inflammatory agents may be used to decrease the symptoms of an inflammatory process.

In patients with debilitating and life-threatening cardiomyopathy, the only hope of survival may be a heart transplant (see Chapter 17 for discussion of heart transplantation).

Application of the Nursing Process to the Care of the Patient with Cardiomyopathy

Assessment

Review the patient's history and diagnostic testing, and complete an assessment. Because CHF is the usual presenting problem in cardiomyopathy, assess for symptoms that are common to congestive failure. Ask the patient about episodes of fatigue and general exhaustion. Find out when the periods of fatigue are most profound, what precipates them, and whether rest for a short time relieves the symptoms. Check for inability to rest or sleep well. Assess for chest pain, dyspnea, and tachycardia. Check the patient's vital signs at rest and after activity.

Auscultate the heart sounds and lung sounds for abnormalities. Look for edema, both central and in the periphery. Assess for neck vein distention, noisy respirations, and severe dyspnea. Weigh the patient, and compare it with the patient's usual weight. Check all pulses. Note any dysrhythmias on the ECG.

Examine the patient's skin, observing for areas of breakdown. Check for pressure sites, lesions, or constriction. Assess the skin for color, circulation, and temperature.

Nursing Diagnoses and Planning

Nursing diagnoses and related expected patient outcomes most commonly applicable to patients with cardiomyopathy include the following:

NDx: Decreased cardiac output related to altered myocardial contractility and alterations in rate, rhythm, or electrical conduction

Planning: Patient outcomes
1. Patient's vital signs are within acceptable ranges for the patient.
2. Patient demonstrates absence or control of dysrhythmias.
3. Patient participates in activities consistent with abilities.
4. Patient is free of dyspnea.

NDx: Activity intolerance related to generalized weakness or an imbalance between the oxygen supply and the oxygen demand

Planning: Patient outcomes
1. Patient increases participation in activities without intolerable dyspnea or fatigue.
2. Patient demonstrates energy-saving activities and seeks assistance as needed.
3. Patient sets a daily schedule that allows for intermittent periods of rest as needed.
4. Patient verbalizes understanding of the need for oxygen, medications, and supportive equipment that may increase tolerance for activity.

NDx: Fluid volume excess related to reduced glomerular filtration rate secondary to reduced cardiac output, increased ADH production, and sodium and water retention

Planning: Patient outcomes
1. Patient maintains a balanced intake and output.
2. Patient's breath sounds are clear to auscultation.
3. Patient's daily weights are as expected for the patient, and edema is absent.

NDx: High risk for impaired skin integrity related to decreased tissue perfusion and edema

Planning: Patient outcomes
1. Patient's skin remains intact without edema, redness, or lesions.
2. Patient demonstrates behaviors used to prevent skin breakdown such as turning, keeping feet and legs out of dependent positions, and keeping skin clean, dry, and supple.

NDx: Ineffective breathing pattern related to extensive pulmonary edema secondary to CHF

Planning: Patient outcomes
1. Patient's vital signs are within normal ranges for the patient.
2. Patient denies dyspnea, tachypnea, or productive cough.
3. Patient is able to complete activities of daily living without breathing difficulties.

Nursing Interventions

NDx: Decreased cardiac output
Monitor the patient's vital signs both at rest and during activity, and document the data. Encourage the patient to have frequent rest periods throughout the day to prevent fatigue and strain on the myocardium. Note any dyspneic episodes and precipitating factors. Ask whether the patient is getting enough rest and sleep, and prevent disturbances whenever possible.

Use telemetry monitoring, especially if the patient experiences dysrhythmias or is taking antidysrhythmic drugs. Auscultate the apical pulse, noting the rate and rhythm. Review the results of laboratory studies and hemodynamic monitoring.

Check the patient's intake and output, observing for adequacy and balance. Keep the patient's legs in a nondependent position while sitting. Provide support for the extremities while sitting or lying in bed. Pad bony prominences to prevent breakdown from pressure and poor circulation.

Teach the patient relaxation techniques and range-of-motion exercises to increase circulation while lying in bed. Keep the patient warm and comfortable. Prevent constriction of circulation from tight-fitting clothing or bed linen.

NDx: Activity intolerance
Instruct the patient to develop a regimen of activity with frequent rest periods as soon as possible. Encourage the patient to do range-of-motion exercises frequently while lying in bed to maintain muscle tone and strength. Provide supplemental oxygen as needed. Have the patient practice deep-breathing exercises to increase oxygen and blood to the brain.

Teach the patient to practice energy-saving techniques to reduce fatigue and shortness of breath. Place frequently used articles within the patient's reach. Have the patient seek assistance when needed.

Provide and encourage frequent rest periods while delivering patient care. Prevent interruptions during rest periods and at night, whenever possible. Reduce any disturbing noises, and limit visitors as necessary. Encourage acceleration of activity, and monitor progress as the patient moves through the rehabilitation process.

Encourage good nutrition to increase the patient's energy level. Offer four to six meals per day. This is less tiring for the patient and will prevent gastric overdistention and prevent dyspneic episodes during meals.

NDx: Fluid volume excess
Help the patient exercise, when able, to assist in the dissemination of fluid. Give prescribed diuretics, and provide a bedside commode for the patient if he or she is unable to ambulate to the bathroom. Teach the patient about the effects of the medications, the necessity for fluid-intake restrictions, and the dietary changes needed such as a low-sodium meal plan. Monitor the patient's intake and output carefully, and document the results. Weigh the patient daily, and record the weight.

Inspect the skin for edematous areas and potential sites of skin breakdown. Keep the patient's legs elevated and supported when sitting to prevent dependent edema. Have the patient maintain a semi-Fowler's or high Fowler's position to maximize the respiratory effort. Check frequently for noisy respirations.

NDx: High risk for impaired skin integrity
Inspect the skin frequently, noting skeletal prominences, presence of edema, or areas of redness that may be prone to breakdown. Reposition the patient hourly if necessary to prevent pressure areas and to stimulate circulation. Massage the skin to enhance circulation to prevent ischemic sites. Keep the skin clean, dry, and supple. Use lotions to prevent dry, cracked skin.

NDx: Ineffective breathing pattern
Promote maximum respiration by repositioning the patient. Have the patient stay in a semi-Fowler's or high Fowler's position while in bed for better chest expansion. Allow frequent rest periods while administering care so the patient does not become fatigued and dyspneic. Teach the patient deep-breathing techniques. Tell the patient to seek assistance if activities cause more difficult breathing or extreme fatigue. Administer oxygen as needed.

Observe for signs of respiratory distress, and administer treatments and medications as ordered. Watch for changes in the blood gas values, indicating early respiratory difficulty. Auscultate the chest for changes in the adventitious sounds.

Evaluation

Evaluate the effectiveness of nursing care for a patient with cardiomyopathy by comparing the patient's status with the expected patient outcomes. Examples of specific outcomes for patients with cardiomyopathy have been provided in the Planning section.

Cardiac Arrest

ETIOLOGY AND PATHOPHYSIOLOGY

Cardiac arrest is defined as the cessation of effective cardiac output. It is evident by the absence of a pulse in a major artery such as the carotid or femoral artery. The common dysrhythmias that are noted at the time of arrest include ventricular fibrillation, ventricular tachycardia, or asystole (complete cessation of ventricular electrical activity). A cardiac arrest may immediately precede or follow a respiratory arrest. When one system ceases to function effectively, the other system also fails rapidly. A cardiac arrest may follow hemorrhage, shock, MI, severe congestive failure, systemic infections, anaphylactic reaction, or several other medical conditions and emergencies.

CLINICAL MANIFESTATIONS

Hypoxemia, followed by acidemia, occurs rapidly when circulation slows or stops. Cardiac output ceases, the skin becomes cool and cyanotic, and death ensues unless there is immediate reversal of the situation.

MEDICAL DIAGNOSIS

The first indication of cardiac arrest for the hospitalized patient on a cardiac monitor is the appearance of a life-threatening dysrhythmia such as asystole, ventricular tachycardia, or ventricular fibrillation. Unresponsiveness and the inability to arouse the patient may be the first indication of a cardiac arrest in the unmonitored patient.

MEDICAL MANAGEMENT

CPR is an organized method of aiding the victim of a cardiac or respiratory arrest by supporting the cardiac and respiratory systems. Using the basic life-support guidelines, an airway must be established first. Opening the airway may be as simple as tilting the head back and lifting the chin, or it may require intubation and artificial respiration. A cardiac monitor is applied for direct observation of the cardiac rhythm. Cardiac output is reestablished by resuscitation. Hypoxemia is treated with supplemental oxygen. Acidemia is monitored using arterial blood gas reports and is reduced via drug intervention. Pharmacologic agents to improve cardiac output and to restore myocardial contractility are given. Hypotension is reversed with drugs such as dopamine hydrochloride (Intropin), dobutamine hydrochloride (Dobutrex), levarterenol (norepinephrine, Levophed), or metaraminol (Aramine). Other drugs, as discussed earlier under specific dysrhythmias, may be used to control the dysrhythmias occurring during the resuscitation process.

Guidelines for Application of the Nursing Process to the Care of the Patient in Cardiac Arrest

Nursing care of the patient in cardiac arrest is directed toward saving the patient's life and preserving maximum function. Immediate reaction is required to treat changes that occur in the patient who survives a cardiac arrest. The patient is admitted to an intensive care unit and is carefully monitored for hemodynamic and physical response. Continued nursing care is provided on the basis of the symptomatology, reaction to treatment, and ensuing complications (Nursing Care Guide 18–3).

Structural Disorders

Coronary Artery Disease

The most common form of heart disease is coronary artery disease (CAD). It is responsible for nearly half a million deaths in the United States each year. Although a few unusual diseases result in coronary artery obstruction (collagen-vascular disease, coronary spasm, embolic events), esssentially all coronary artery disease is the result of atherosclerosis.

Just as the heart is composed of three layers, so are the coronary arteries. The outer supporting wall of the artery is called the adventitia. The middle layer, the media, is composed of smooth-muscle cells separated on either side by sheets of elastic tissue. The internal wall of the artery is the intima, and is composed of a thin, fibrous lining and a very thin sheet of cells, the endothelium, which lines the lumen of the vessel.

ATHEROSCLEROSIS OF THE CORONARY ARTERIES

ETIOLOGY AND PATHOPHYSIOLOGY

Coronary artery disease is the result of atherosclerosis. The atherosclerotic process develops slowly over many years. Usually the diagnosis is made when the obstructive process reaches such proportion that blood flow to the myocardium is impaired sufficiently to result in clinical symptoms such as angina pectoris, MI, dysrhythmias, CHF, or even sudden death. The exact cause of atherosclerosis leading to coronary artery disease is not known. A number of risk factors have been identified as contributing to the disease process. (See Chapter 17 for a discussion of risk factors.)

Atherosclerosis is characterized by the accumulation of lipids and fibrous tissue in the wall of the coronary artery, causing obstructions to variable degrees. The earliest lesion is usually an *atheroma*. An atheroma is formed when fatty material, composed of crystals of cholesterol, accumulates beneath the intima, causing that layer to be raised and to project into the blood stream (into the lumen of the vessel).

Text continued on page 762

Nursing Care Guide 18–3.
PATIENTS SURVIVING A CARDIAC ARREST

Assessment Findings: Patient is nervous, restless, and tense; withdraws from others; expresses feeling of fear, helplessness, and concern about the future.

Nursing Diagnosis: Anxiety related to fear of cardiac disease, uncertainties about the future, and the possibility of death

Patient Outcomes	Nursing Interventions	Rationale
Patient appears relaxed with no visible signs of anxiety such as nervousness, restlessness, or clenching of the hands; vital signs are within normal ranges.	Allow time for discussion of the patient's concerns and fears without expressing opinions about the patient's status. Invite questions about the patient's condition, and share the information with the family. Provide rest periods and time for privacy.	Accepting but not encouraging denial of the patient's condition or seriousness of the illness leaves the atmosphere open for free expressions of feelings.
	Assess vital signs.	Vital signs within normal ranges may indicate decreased anxiety.
Patient reports feeling less anxious, verbalizes methods for coping with illness, joins in conversations, and participates in care regimen.	Help the patient find effective coping strategies to manage the lifestyle changes that may be necessary. Teach relaxation techniques. Acknowledge that feelings of fear are normal and expected after such a traumatic event. Encourage participation in the daily care regimen.	Using proven coping techniques may help alleviate the patient's stress. Relaxation techniques assist in anxiety reduction and allow for rest. Encouraging patient participation in the care acknowledges the patient's worth.

Evaluation: Compare the patient's status with the expected patient outcomes. If the outcomes are achieved, evaluate nursing care as successful. If not, reassess the patient, formulate new nursing diagnoses, and revise expected patient outcomes and nursing interventions as appropriate.

(continued)

Nursing Care Guide 18–3. *(continued)*

PATIENTS SURVIVING A CARDIAC ARREST

Assessment Findings: Patient presents altered hemodynamics, decreased output, poor peripheral circulation, and cyanosis.

Nursing Diagnosis: Decreased cardiac output related to electrical and mechanical malfunction

Patient Outcomes	Nursing Interventions	Rationale
Patient preserves a cardiac rhythm that is stable enough to support an adequate cardiac output and demonstrates a decrease in dysrhythmias as seen by the hemodynamic monitoring.	Promptly treat life-threatening dysrhythmias. Assist the patient in turning and performing other self-care activities. Perform passive range-of-motion exercises as tolerated. Administer oxygen, and raise the head of the bed for maximum chest expansion. Allow the patient frequent rest periods during delivery of nursing care. Use a bedside commode to conserve patient energy.	Immediate intervention may prevent arrest. Assisting the patient and performing passive range-of-motion exercises stimulate circulation but conserve the patient's energy and reduce the workload on the myocardium.
	Limit visitors, and reduce disturbances. Plan care to reduce interruptions.	Reducing external stimuli allows for rest and reduces cardiac strain.
	Monitor the heart rate and rhythm continuously. Assess for dysrhythmias.	Careful monitoring provides for early interventions if problems arise.
Patient's vital signs are within normal ranges for the patient.	Assess vital signs frequently, noting any changes. Notify physician according to protocol.	Vital signs within normal ranges may indicate patient stability.

Evaluation: Compare the patient's status with the expected patient outcomes. If the outcomes are achieved, evaluate nursing care as successful. If not, reassess the patient, formulate new nursing diagnoses, and revise expected patient outcomes and nursing interventions as appropriate.

(continued)

Nursing Care Guide 18–3. *(continued)*
PATIENTS SURVIVING A CARDIAC ARREST

Assessment Findings: Patient complains of pressure, heaviness, or pain in the chest and states pain is radiating into the neck and arm.

Nursing Diagnosis: Pain related to tissue ischemia secondary to coronary artery occlusion

Patient Outcomes	Nursing Interventions	Rationale
Patient verbalizes relief or control of chest pain and is able to rest comfortably and sleep well.	Give prescribed pharmacologic agents for anginal pain, and repeat as ordered. Teach relaxation techniques. Position the patient for comfort.	Antianginal agents given appropriately may quickly reduce the anginal episode or prevent another attack. Relaxation and comfort measures may help reduce the pain or make it more tolerable for the patient.
Patient states relaxation methods and coping strategies to assist in the control or prevention of anginal episodes.	Support the patient in the use of coping methods that help patient to relax and relieve or prevent episodes of pain. Feed the patient if necessary, and place articles within reach. Help prevent anginal episodes by teaching the patient to use energy-saving activities.	Relaxation techniques assist the patient to rest and reduce anxiety, which increases the effort of the myocardium. Energing-saving practices reduce the workload of the myocardium.

Evaluation: Compare the patient's status with the expected patient outcomes. If the outcomes are achieved, evaluate nursing care as successful. If not, reassess the patient, formulate new nursing diagnoses, and revise expected patient outcomes and nursing interventions as appropriate.

(continued)

Nursing Care Guide 18–3. *(continued)*
PATIENTS SURVIVING A CARDIAC ARREST

Assessment Findings: Patient is dyspneic, tachypneic, and cyanotic; blood pressure is elevated, and tachycardia is present; some confusion, dizziness, and a headache are present; urine output is decreased; gastric distress and distention are evident; peripheral pulses are diminished; toes are pale and cool.

Nursing Diagnosis: Altered tissue perfusion, cardiopulmonary, cerebral, renal, peripheral, and gastrointestinal, related to decreased cardiac output secondary to cardiac malfunction

Patient Outcomes	Nursing Interventions	Rationale
Patient demonstrates appropriate functioning of all body systems as seen on hemodynamic monitoring, and by appropriate orientation to time, place, and person; lack of gastrointestinal or neurologic symptom complaints; and adequate output.	Monitor and assess the adequacy of cardiac function, respiratory status, urine output, mentation, gastrointestinal functioning, and peripheral circulation. Provide frequent, small, nonirritating meals as described in Nutrition Box 18–1. Complete range-of-motion exercises, and reposition the patient frequently to stimulate circulation. Have the patient take frequent deep breaths with good chest expansion to increase oxygen intake. Keep the patient in a high Fowler's position, and administer oxygen by nasal cannula.	Decreased cardiac output may affect all body systems. Careful monitoring for changes and the promotion of activities that improve circulation are important to the patient's progress. Early intervention may reduce the effects of the disorder.
Patient is warm, presents good skin color, has palpable pulses in the periphery, and shows no signs of tissue ischemia.	Check for skin breakdown caused by decreased circulation to the extremities. Keep the patient warm, and remove constricting clothing. Note vital signs frequently. Give prescribed medications to increase circulation. Do not allow patient to smoke, which causes vasoconstriction. Teach the patient to use relaxation methods to reduce stress and thus reduce vasoconstriction and high blood pressure, and help prevent ischemic attacks, which cause angina.	Maintenance of skin integrity is important. Decreased circulatory status predisposes the patient to skin breakdown and infections.

Evaluation: Compare the patient's status with the expected patient outcomes. If the outcomes are achieved, evaluate nursing care as successful. If not, reassess the patient, formulate new nursing diagnoses, and revise expected patient outcomes and nursing interventions as appropriate.

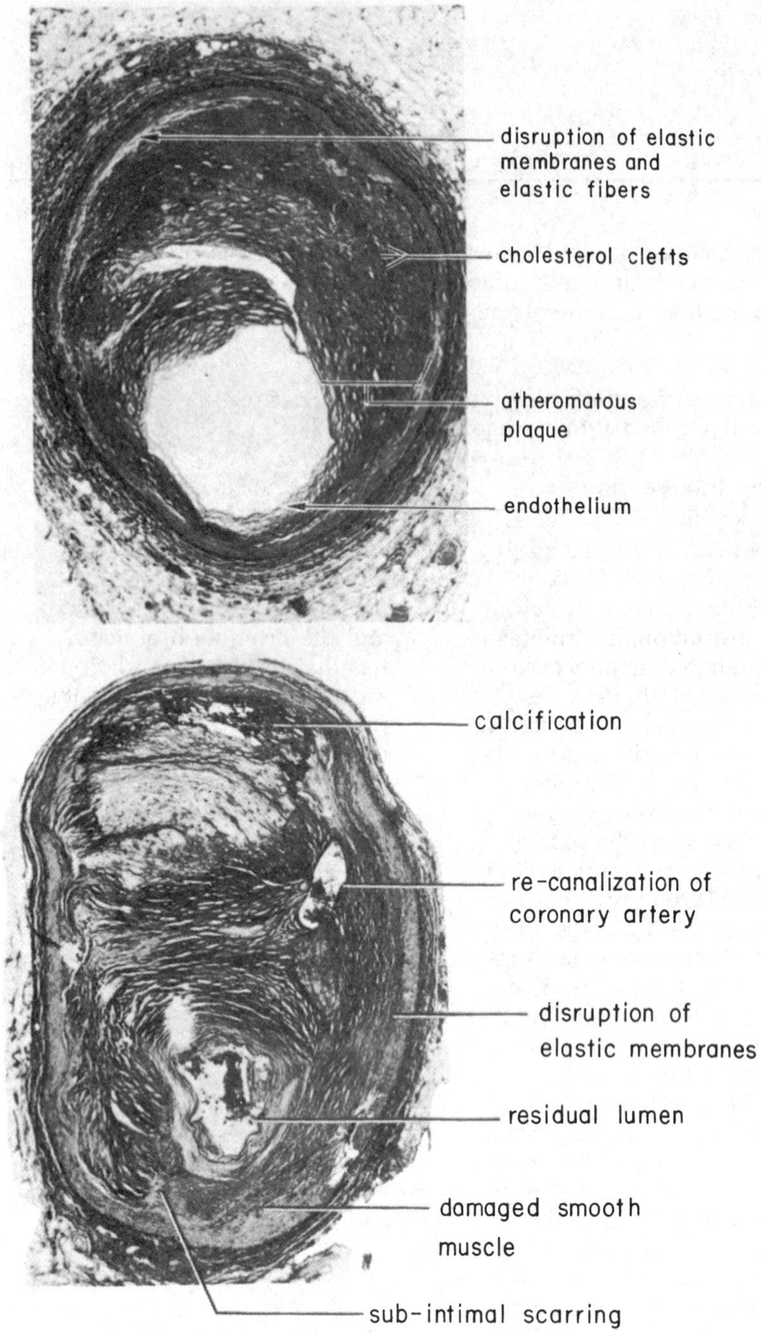

Figure 18–7.

Different stages of coronary artery narrowing are shown in microscopic sections. The section at the top shows early atheroma, whereas the bottom section shows an almost completely obstructed vessel caused by the atheromatomous process. (From Sanderson RG, Kurth CL. The cardiac patient. 2nd ed. Philadelphia: WB Saunders, 1983, p 39.)

Fibrous tissue response to this lipid accumulation results in scarring of the vessel wall, which later becomes calcified. The atheroma, may occupy only a small segment of the vessel or may involve its total circumference (Fig. 18–7). As the atheroma projects into the lumen of the vessel, it causes roughening of the intima. Fibrin and platelets accumulate at the site, resulting in a small blood clot. In addition, hemorrhage into the atheroma, either through the central blood stream or via the tiny blood vessels that supply the wall of the coronary artery itself, causes the atheroma to increase in size. The elastic membranes of the media are damaged by the hemorrhage, a fibrous tissue response occurs, and the artery loses its ability to stretch and contract.

As these processes of lipid accumulation and subintimal hemorrhage are repeated, the vessel becomes more and more narrow, limiting the amount of blood that can pass through it. Finally, the lumen becomes so narrow that a blood clot (thrombus) forms and the arterial obstruction is complete. Sometimes, as the thrombus becomes organized with fibrous tissue, new blood vessels grow into it, allowing very small amounts of blood to flow once again. This process is called recanalization.

The rate of development of coronary narrowing is

variable from patient to patient. Some patients have lesions that remain stable for many years, whereas others have obstructions that progress from a minor to a critical problem in less than a year. In order for the heart muscle to function effectively, it must receive an adequate amount of blood through the coronary arteries. When the atherosclerotic disease process exceeds approximately 65% to 70% obstruction of the vessel lumen, a significant reduction in blood flow through the vessel results. Obviously, multiple obstructing lesions in the same artery reduce the blood flow even more severely. When the blood supply fails to meet the heart's demand, angina pectoris or MI may result.

CLINICAL MANIFESTATIONS

The most common symptom experienced by patients with coronary artery disease is chest discomfort called angina pectoris. Many patients do not describe the symptom as "pain," so practitioners must carefully assess the symptoms of the patient. It is better to use the term *discomfort* and allow the patient to describe the feeling. It is frequently described as a heavy feeling, pressure, or weight on the chest. It may also be described as severe or mild, oppressive or sharp, and located in the chest, neck jaws, back, or inner aspect of the arm. It may occur at rest or with exercise. The duration of the pain is always more than a few seconds—generally several minutes, rarely hours, and never days—and without interruption. In a given patient, the pain usually does not vary except in severity, radiation, and duration. The character, or quality, of the pain is identical each time it occurs; only the magnitude changes.

Angina pectoris occurs when the myocardium does not receive enough oxygen through narrowed coronary arteries to maintain its usual pumping action. Cells of the myocardium thus become ischemic, and nerve endings around the cells send pain messages to the brain. The sensation of chest pain usually causes the patient to stop any activity, lie down, or seek medical assistance to obtain relief from the pain.

Angina may slowly increase over a period of months as the coronary arteries become more obstructed. Any activity that causes the heart to increase its output may bring on an attack of angina such as eating a large meal, walking in cold weather, or emotional stress.

MEDICAL DIAGNOSIS

The diagnosis of atherosclerosis of the coronary arteries is made on the basis of history, present symptoms, lifestyle assessment, and diagnostic testing (see Chapter 17). Laboratory studies of cholesterol levels—low-density lipoprotein (LDL) and high-density lipoprotein (HDL)—may add support to the diagnosis. High cholesterol levels, with a high LDL and low HDL, are common in atherosclerosis.

The diagnosis of angina may be made on the basis of the history, findings from the assessment for the diagnosis of atherosclerosis, the response to nitroglycerin tablets, and exercise stress testing. Because exercise stress testing forces the heart to pump faster, thus increasing its output, angina appears if an increased blood flow is unable to pass through the coronary arteries.

MEDICAL MANAGEMENT

The treatment of atherosclerosis of the coronary arteries is based on reducing risk factors and managing the effects of the disease process (see Chart 18–3 and discussion of atherosclerosis in Chapter 20). The patient is educated about lifestyle changes needed such as diet modifications, cessation of smoking, and initiation of a mild exercise regimen. A low-cholesterol, low-fat diet is encouraged. The patient may be referred to a smoking cessation program. Surgical intervention may be necessary to either clear the arteries or bypass them. (Refer to Chapter 17 for the discussion of surgical management of cardiac disorders.)

The treatment of angina pectoris consists of reducing the demand for oxygen by the myocardium and increasing the delivery of oxygen to the myocardium. Rest, nitrates (which dilate coronary arteries and increase blood flow), and β-adrenergic blocking agents (which decrease sympathetic activity to the cardiac muscle, smooth muscle of the bronchi, and smooth muscle of the blood vessels) are prescribed. Heart rate decreases with the use of β-adrenergic blocking agents so that myocardial oxygen consumption is decreased. Calcium channel blocking agents cause coronary and peripheral artery dilation as well as decreased myocardial contractility (Pharmacology Box 18–3). A decreased amount of oxygen is required by the myocardium when these drugs are used (Table 18–1). Because rest decreases the amount of oxygen needed by all tissues of the body, it is usually the first step used to gain relief from angina.

Application of the Nursing Process to the Care of the Patient with Atherosclerosis of the Coronary Arteries

Assessment

Assess for pain, noting the onset, intensity, duration, radiation, and location. Determine whether the pain is present only during exercise or at rest. Look for signs of pain such as grimacing, clenching of hands,

Chart 18–3.

NURSING GUIDE TO PATIENT EDUCATION FOR SELF-MANAGEMENT: RISK REDUCTION FOR PREVENTION OF ATHEROSCLEROSIS

Instruct the patient with coronary artery disease from atherosclerosis to modify lifestyle and to lower risk by:

Reducing serum lipid levels. The blood cholesterol level directly relates to the development of atherosclerosis. Increased cholesterol levels can be modified by following a low-fat, low-cholesterol diet and exercising daily.

Reducing high blood pressure or preventing high blood pressure. The risk for atherosclerosis may double with high blood pressure. It can be lowered by reducing weight, reducing stress levels, and participating in a regular exercise program.

Ceasing smoking. Because nicotine is a vasoconstrictor, blood flow through arteries is decreased in smokers.

Keeping diabetes mellitus under control. If the patient is diabetic, risk for atherosclerosis is increased because of the high levels of blood lipids, but it may be less severe if the diabetes is well controlled.

Reducing weight. The patient who is obese is at high risk for atherosclerosis. This can be corrected by following a weight-reduction plan and an exercise plan.

Changing from a high-fat diet to a low-fat diet. A diet that is high in fat contributes to elevated blood lipid levels, which is a major risk factor for atherosclerosis. Following a low-fat (low saturated fat) diet helps prevent atherosclerosis, contributes to weight loss, and decreases the workload on the myocardium.

moaning, or guarding when the patient is moving in bed or ambulating or after ambulation when the patient is at rest. Ask the patient to explain the feeling in the chest. Look at the patient's history of risk factors.

Assess for any skin changes. Ask the patient about numbness, tingling, or paresthesia of the extremities, indicating decreased cardiac output. Check the vital signs. Auscultate for bruits over occluded arteries. Monitor serum cholesterol levels and other laboratory data.

Check the patient's physical mobility. Ask about assistance needed to perform activities of daily living. Determine the patient's flexibility, range of motion, and strength in the extremities.

Assess the patient's level of knowledge about the disorder and treatment. Ask about the patient's lifestyle and associated risk factors. Assess the level of adaptation to the disorder and ability to manage the disease process and its manifestations.

Nursing Diagnoses and Planning

Nursing diagnoses and related expected patient outcomes most commonly applicable to patients with atherosclerosis of the coronary arteries include the following:

NDx: Pain related to ischemia of the myocardium secondary to the disease process causing occlusion of the arteries

Planning: Patient outcomes

1. Patient verbalizes relief of pain.
2. Patient states methods to prevent anginal episodes and to cope with them.
3. Patient reports a decrease in the frequency, duration, and severity of the anginal episodes.

NDx: Activity intolerance related to fatigue and weakness from inadequate cardiac functioning or chest pain with exertion

Planning: Patient outcomes

1. Patient verbalizes activities that aggravate pain and fatigue.
2. Patient demonstrates energy-saving activities and seeks assistance as needed.
3. Patient sets a daily schedule that allows for intermittent periods of rest as needed.

Pharmacology Box 18–3.

CALCIUM CHANNEL BLOCKING AGENTS

Calcium Channel Blockers:
Group of drugs such as nifedipine, verapamil, and nicardipine that cause arterial dilation.

Action:
Inhibit movement of extracellular calcium into cardiac muscle, thus slowing conduction and reducing cardiac workload; they dilate coronary arteries and prevent coronary spasms.

Uses:
Management of anginal episodes; control of ventricular rate in atrial fibrillation and flutter and supraventricular arrhythmias; and control of hypertension.

Side Effects:
Headache, dizziness, weakness, confusion, edema, and constipation.

Interactions:
May be less effective if taken with calcium tablets; may be enhanced by cimetidine (Tagamet); may be enhanced by the additions of beta blockers; may cause increased serum digoxin levels; and may cause decreased blood pressure if taken with beta blockers.

Nursing Implications:
Monitor blood pressure for hypotension.
Monitor the electrocardiogram for bradycardia and dysrhythmias.
Observe for side effects.
Assess for symptoms of congestive heart failure such as edema, cough, changes in vital signs, and decreased circulation.
Check laboratory data, especially liver function studies, because some enzymes may be increased.

Table 18–1. COMMOMLY USED CARDIAC DRUGS

NITRATES
Nitroglycerin (NTG)
Erythrityl tetranitrate (Cardilate)
Isosorbide dinitrate (Isordil)

β-ADRENERGIC BLOCKING AGENTS
Atenolol (Tenormin)
Metoprolol (Lopressor)
Propranolol (Inderal)
Nadolol (Corgard)
Timolol (Timoptic)
Penbutolol (Levatol)

CALCIUM CHANNEL BLOCKING AGENTS
Verapamil (Isoptin)
Nicardipine (Cardene)
Nifedipine (Procardia)
Diltiazem (Cardizem)

ANTIARRHYTHMICS
Lidocaine (Xylocaine)
Procainamide (Pronestyl)
Quinidine (Quinate)
Propranolol (Inderal)
Phenytoin (Dilantin)
Bretylium tosylate (Bretylol)

AFTER-LOAD REDUCING AGENTS
Nitroprusside (Nipride)
Prazosin (Minipress)
Hydralazine (Apresoline)

CARDIAC GLYCOSIDES
Digitalis (Digitoxin)
Digitoxin (Crystodigin)
Deslanoside (Cedilanid)

DIURETICS
Ethacrynic acid (Edecrin)
Furosemide (Lasix)
Bumetanide (Bumex)
Mannitol (Osmitrol)
Spironolactone (Aldactone)
Hydrochlorothiazide (HydroDIURIL)
Chlorothiazide (Diuril)
Metolazone (Zaroxolyn)

4. Patient verbalizes understanding of the need for oxygen, medications, and supportive equipment that may increase tolerance for activity.
5. Patient is able to perform activities of daily living without fatigue.

NDx: Altered health maintenance related to a knowledge deficit about the disease state, reduction of risk, and management of manifestations of disease

Planning: Patient outcomes
1. Patient reports accurate information about the disease process, the risk factors, and the possible manifestations of the disease.
2. Patient states lifestyle changes needed to prevent recurrence of disease (see Chart 18–3).
3. Patient states information about the medications, including the time, route, dosage, and potential side effects.

Nursing Interventions

NDx: Pain
Instruct the patient to notify the nurse when anginal pain occurs. Administer prescribed medication, and assess and document the pain episode, noting the duration, severity, and patient's response to the medication. Observe for associated signs and symptoms such as dyspnea, nausea and vomiting, dizziness, or palpitations. Evaluate complaints of pain in the jaw, neck, shoulder, arm, or hand (typically on the left side). Place the patient at complete rest during the anginal episode, elevate the head, and administer oxygen if dyspnea is present. Monitor the vital signs every 5 minutes during the anginal episode and stay with the patient (see Nursing Care Guide 18–2).

NDx: Activity intolerance
Instruct the patient to develop a regimen of activity with frequent rest periods throughout the day. Encourage the patient to do range-of-motion exercises frequently while lying in bed to maintain muscle tone and strength. Provide supplemental oxygen as needed. Have the patient practice deep-breathing exercises to increase oxygen and blood flow to the brain.

Teach the patient to practice energy-saving techniques to reduce fatigue and shortness of breath. Place frequently used articles within the patient's reach. Have the patient seek assistance when needed.

Provide and encourage frequent rest periods while delivering patient care. Prevent interruptions during rest periods and at night whenever possible. Reduce any disturbing noises, and limit visitors as necessary.

Encourage good nutrition to increase the patient's energy level. Offer four to six meals per day. This is less tiring for the patient and will prevent gastric overdistention.

NDx: Altered health maintenance
Explain the cause, effects, and clinical course of coronary artery atherosclerosis to the patient. Allow time for discussion with the patient whenever questions arise. Provide appropriate literature about atherosclerosis for the patient and family to review. Allow the patient to verbalize concerns and fears. Evaluate discharge needs of the patient and family.

Alert the patient to signs and symptoms of coronary artery atherosclerosis and the complications such as acute chest pain and activity intolerance. Teach the patient to use safety measures or to ask for assistance when out of bed or when ambulating. Refer the patient to an exercise therapist to plan a program of exercise to reduce the risk of disease.

Instruct the patient about dietary modifications needed to reduce risk or prevent complications of the disorder (see Chart 18–3). If the patient is obese, explain the need for a reduction diet. Give the patient meal plans based on the predetermined caloric limitation. Explain the need for decreases in dietary fats and cholesterol to prevent the effects of the disease and for increases in protein and vitamins to promote good health and healing. Initiate counseling with a dietitian to assist with meal planning if needed.

Teach the patient about the effects of smoking and the importance of quitting. Refer the patient to a smoking cessation program.

Teach the patient the dosage, route, time, frequency, side effects, and toxic effects of any medication prescribed. Explain the diagnostic studies completed and the need for any follow-up studies after discharge. Include the family in any of the teaching sessions when applicable.

Evaluation

Evaluate the effectiveness of nursing care for a patient with coronary artery disease from atherosclerosis by comparing the patient's status with the expected patient outcomes. Examples of specific outcomes for patients with coronary artery disease from atherosclerosis have been provided in the Planning section.

Cardiac Valvular Disease

ETIOLOGY AND PATHOPHYSIOLOGY

Cardiac valvular abnormalities are classified as pure stenosis, pure insufficiency, or mixed with both stenosis and insufficiency. *Stenosis* is the term used to describe the condition in which the valve opening is narrowed, causing an obstruction of blood flow. *Insufficiency* is the term used to describe the condition when the valve is incapable of preventing retrograde blood flow, thus allowing blood to regurgitate through the valve's orifice. When both stenosis and insufficiency are present, it is termed a mixed lesion. The pathology is usually advanced in the mixed lesion. Cardiac valve disease may be the result of illnesses such as rheumatic fever or cardiac inflammatory processes. It may also result from congenital defects, trauma, MI, and degenerative changes.

CLINICAL MANIFESTATIONS

AORTIC VALVE STENOSIS

Aortic valve stenosis results in left ventricular failure with the associated symptoms of fatigue, dyspnea, and possibly syncope. Angina pectoris may be present if the cardiac output is decreased to the point of not being able to adequately perfuse the coronary arteries. Exertion usually increases the symptoms of left ventricular failure. Auscultation of heart sounds reveals a systolic murmur.

AORTIC VALVE REGURGITATION

Aortic valve regurgitation also results in left ventricular failure. Dyspnea, fatigue, syncope, and angina pectoris are common symptoms. Diastolic and systolic murmurs may be heard on auscultation.

MITRAL VALVE STENOSIS

Mitral valve stenosis results in right ventricular failure. Symptoms include fatigue, weakness, ascites, hepatomegaly, chest pain, dyspnea, on exertion, and palpitations. A diastolic murmur is heard on auscultation of the heart sounds.

MITRAL VALVE REGURGITATION

Mitral valve regurgitation results in left-sided heart failure. Common manifestations are fatigue, weakness, dyspnea, and palpitations. A systolic murmur is heard on auscultation.

MITRAL VALVE PROLAPSE

Many cases of mitral valve prolapse can be asymptomatic. If symptoms appear, they are like those of mitral valve regurgitation: fatigue, weakness, dyspnea, and palpitations. Anxiety with hyperventilation, lightheadedness, and panic attacks may accompany the symptoms of left-sided heart failure. Atypical chest pain may be present. For most patients with mitral valve prolapse, the psychological effects of the diagnosis are more disabling than the disease itself.

MEDICAL DIAGNOSIS

The diagnosis is made on the basis of physical assessment and other diagnostic studies. Cardiac valvular disease may be noted by auscultation of the heart sounds. As blood is forced through a stenotic valve or regurgitates through an insufficient valve, it is heard as a murmur. Diagnosis may be confirmed by an echocardiogram, a phonocardiogram, or cardiac catheterization.

MEDICAL MANAGEMENT

Medical treatment for cardiac valvular disease may include pharmacologic therapy as well as surgical intervention. Because CHF on either the right or left side, or both, may be present, depending on which valve is involved, control of failure is initiated early in the treatment regimen. This is accomplished through the use of diuretics, digoxin, and activity limitations. Dysrhythmias that occur with valvular disease are treated with appropriate antiarrhythmics.

Several surgical procedures can relieve the problems associated with cardiac valvular disease. Valvotomy is the procedure in which a stenotic valve is exposed and the stenotic areas are incised to relieve the obstruction. In some cases, tissue surrounding the valve, such as muscle around the aortic valve, must be resected or incised to prevent the muscle from constricting the outflow tract. Valvotomy is usually an open-heart procedure, requiring the use of the heart-lung machine as heart tissue is explored and incised as needed.

Commissurotomy is a procedure in which either the surgeon's finger or an expandable dilator is inserted through a stenosed valve to "crack open" or "split" the fused commissures of the valve. Commissurotomy is usually a closed-heart surgery but may be performed with the heart-lung machine as an open-heart procedure in some cases.

Valve replacement is used when a valve cannot be repaired, such as when the leaflets have lost their flexibility, when calcification is present to a marked degree, or when papillary muscles are infarcted to the degree that they cannot support the valve in its correct position. Prosthetic valves may be made of plastic, metal, or a combination of materials surrounded by grafting materials such as Dacron or nylon that can be sutured to viable tissue. Biologic valves from porcine or bovine tissue are commonly used. Valves have an expected longevity of 8 to 10 years and may involve long-term anticoagulation to prevent clots from forming on the "foreign" tissue implanted in the patient's body. Cardiac valve replacements are open-heart surgical procedures. (Refer to Chapter 17 for the discussion of valvular surgery.)

Application of the Nursing Process to the Care of the Patient with Cardiac Valvular Disease

Assessment

Review the patient's history, present problems, and diagnostic study results to determine the specific disorder and thus the assessment needed. Because many patients with valvular disease present with symptoms of CHF, assess the patient for dyspnea, weakness, fatigue, syncopal episodes, cough, and tachycardia. Look for edema in the periphery. Take vital signs, and compare with normal ranges. Look for a history of rheumatic fever, streptococcal infection, or congenital heart problems that involve the valves. Auscultate the heart sounds. Check the ECG for abnormal patterns in rate or rhythm. Assess the skin for paleness or cyanosis. Ask about any numbness and tingling in the extremities.

Nursing Diagnoses and Planning

Nursing diagnoses and related expected patient outcomes most commonly applicable to patients with cardiac valvular disease include the following:

NDx: Altered tissue perfusion, peripheral, related to the imbalance between oxygen supply and oxygen demand secondary to cardiac valvular disease (specify valve[s])

Planning: Patient outcomes
1. Patient demonstrates a decrease in peripheral edema.
2. Patient reports a decrease in numbness and tingling in the extremities.
3. Patient's skin color remains appropriate without paleness or cyanosis.

NDx: Knowledge deficit: nature of cardiac valvular disease and misconceptions about the disease process and treatments

Planning: Patient outcomes
1. Patient verbalizes understanding about the disease process.
2. Patient reports accurate information about the treatments, including drug therapy and lifestyle changes.
3. Patient demonstrates cooperation with the treatment plan and follow-up care.

Nursing Interventions

NDx: Altered tissue perfusion, peripheral
Help the patient conserve oxygen needs by encouraging rest and limiting activities. Assist with ambulation. Elevate the head of the bed to aid in lung expansion. Initiate oxygen therapy if necessary. Assist patient with activities of daily living such as feeding, if needed, to conserve energy. Have the patient move in bed frequently to stimulate circulation.

Keep the patient in a comfortable position, and reposition him or her frequently to release pressure. Use range-of-motion exercises to stimulate circulation. Monitor vital signs and laboratory studies to assess for changes and improvements in status. Encourage ambulation as tolerated, but provide for frequent rest periods to decrease cardiac workload. Discourage smoking to avoid vasoconstriction. Remove constricting clothing, and keep heavy bed linen from restricting peripheral circulation. Keep the patient's legs in a nondependent position when not ambulating. Massage the legs to stimulate circulation.

Provide a low-sodium diet to reduce fluid retention. Give prescribed medications to promote increased circulation and diuresis as needed. Monitor laboratory studies to assess pulmonary, circulatory, and renal function.

NDx: Knowledge deficit: nature of cardiac valvular disease and misconceptions about the disease process and treatments
Explain the cause, effects, and clinical course of cardiac valvular disease and the resulting complications to the patient. Allow time for questions from the patient at any time. Allow the patient to verbalize concerns and fears. Evaluate discharge needs of the patient and family. If the patient is to have surgery, explain the preoperative and postoperative courses to the patient (refer to Chapter 17 for a discussion of the surgical intervention and care).

Instruct the patient about dietary modifications needed to reduce risk or prevent complications of the disorder. If the patient is obese, explain the need for a weight-reduction diet. Give the patient meal plans based on the predetermined caloric limitation. Explain the need for decreases in dietary sodium to prevent fluid accumulation and for increases in protein and vitamins to promote good health and healing. Initiate counseling with a dietitian to assist with meal planning if needed.

Teach the patient the dosage, route, time, frequency, side effects, and toxic effects of any medication prescribed. Explain the diagnostic studies completed and the need for any follow-up studies after discharge. Include the family in any of the teaching sessions when applicable.

Teach the patient how to participate in a moderate exercise program to increase circulation and to maintain strength and endurance. Modify the program to meets the patient's needs and abilities.

Evaluation

Evaluate the effectiveness of nursing care for a patient with cardiac valvular disease by comparing the patient's status with the expected patient outcomes. Examples of specific outcomes for patients with cardiac valvular disease have been provided in the Planning section.

Trauma

Cardiac Trauma

ETIOLOGY AND PATHOPHYSIOLOGY

Cardiac trauma is usually divided into two categories: penetrating trauma and blunt trauma. Only approximately one half of the patients receiving stab wounds to the heart survive long enough to obtain medical treatment. If the patient is transported to a trauma center with the capability of immediate open-heart surgery, the survival potential increases significantly. Gunshot wounds to the heart are even more severe. The survival rate is only 10% to 15%. The chambers of the heart that are damaged and the amount of blood lost determine the survival of most cardiac trauma patients. Crushing injuries to the heart from automobile accidents or other blunt truma incidents usually cause damage to multiple chambers of the heart, valves, and great vessels. The damage inflicted may not be compatible with life.

CLINICAL MANIFESTATIONS

Massive blood loss is common in traumatic injuries to the myocardium. Trauma to the chest injures not only the heart but also the large vessels, the lungs, and possibly the liver. These multiple-organ injuries compound the blood loss from the injury. Hypotension and shock result from massive hemorrhage. The trauma may also cause cardiac tamponade.

MEDICAL DIAGNOSIS

The diagnosis is made on the basis of assessment of the trauma site, symptoms, and diagnosic tests. Immediate assessment is made to determine life-threatening symptoms. Vital signs and the overall clinical condition are used to determine the amount of damage present. X-ray films, cardiac catheterization, or immediate open-heart surgery is necessary to reveal the specific damage and to repair the injuries.

MEDICAL MANAGEMENT

Patients with cardiac trauma who survive long enough to reach a major trauma center usually must undergo corrective surgery. The initial surgery may be only the life-saving intervention, and several other reconstructive surgeries will have to follow. The prognosis for such injuries is usually grave.

Application of the Nursing Process to the Care of the Patient with Cardiac Trauma

Nursing management of the patient with cardiac trauma may vary with the type of trauma the patient experienced and the medical intervention necessary to correct the effects of the cardiac trauma. Because of the typical effects of most cardiac trauma, the assessment, nursing diagnoses, expected patient outcomes, nursing interventions, and evaluation for patients with cardiac trauma are similar to those described previously for patients with cardiac valvular disease. If the patient undergoes surgery for correction of the damage from the trauma, the nursing care may change. (See Chapter 17 for care of the patient undergoing cardiac surgery.)

Neoplasia

Cardiac Tumors

ETIOLOGY AND PATHOPHYSIOLOGY

Although tumors within the heart are rare, those diagnosed may be either primary site tumors or metastatic tumors. The metastatic tumors implanting on the heart are usually from primary cancers of the breast, bronchus, or lymph nodes or from malignant melanoma.

CLINICAL MANIFESTATIONS

All cardiac tumors can cause pericardial effusion and constriction and may even grow into the heart muscle, impairing contractility or obstructing blood flow. By the time symptoms of a cardiac tumor occur, the tumor is usually large and has thoroughly invaded the surrounding tissue. Some tumors arise from the endocardial tissue of the valve leaflets and grow to obstruct blood flow through the involved valve.

MEDICAL DIAGNOSIS

The diagnosis is made on the basis of symptoms, x-ray films, and other diagnostic tests. The patient usually presents with symptoms of fatigue, dyspnea,

CHF, or pain. Pericardial effusion may be present. Chest x-ray films and cardiac catheterization are done to reveal the presence of a tumor and the involved structures.

MEDICAL MANAGEMENT

Surgical intervention may be indicated for cardiac tumors that obstruct major vessels or valves. Cardiopulmonary bypass is necessary for cardiac tumor excision, except when the tumor is only in the epicardial area. If the tumor is not causing a major obstruction, treatment focuses on the presenting symptoms. Fluid accumulation is reduced with diuretic therapy. Other cardiac drugs specific to the dysrhythmias present are ordered.

Application of the Nursing Process to the Care of the Patient with Cardiac Tumors

Assessment

Before the physical assessment of the patient, review the medical notes and the diagnostic studies completed to determine the structures involved. Assess for interferences with all systems, because impaired blood flow through the cardiac chambers or valves affects the lungs, kidneys, digestive tract, and neurologic function. Look for signs of respiratory difficulty such as dyspnea, tachypnea, wheezes, or cyanosis. Observe for changes in intake and output, edema, digestive problems, and either constipation or diarrhea. Ask the patient whether there have been episodes indicating neurologic dysfunction such as confusion, dizziness, or memory lapses. The symptoms are usually progressive, and the patient may not have sought medical treatment until the symptoms were no longer tolerable.

Nursing Diagnoses and Planning

Nursing diagnoses and related expected patient outcomes most commonly applicable to patients with cardiac tumors vary with the type and the location of the tumor. The nursing diagnoses, patient outcomes, and nursing interventions previously discussed under cardiomyopathy are applicable to the patient with a cardiac tumor. In addition, the following nursing diagnosis, patient outcomes, and nursing interventions apply:

NDx: Fear related to the negative diagnosis of cardiac tumor and perceived threat of death

Planning: Patient outcomes

1. Patient appears relaxed and reports reduced anxiety and fear to a manageable level.
2. Patient acknowledges and discusses fears and concerns.
3. Patient demonstrates appropriate behavior to cope with the diagnosis and possible outcomes of the condition.

Nursing Interventions

NDx: Fear

Acknowledge the reality of the patient's fears and concerns, and encourage expression of feelings. Accept but do not reinforce the patient's behaviors of denial. Involve the patient and family in discussions, planning, and education sessions for short-term and long-term therapy. Provide information in a professional, empathetic manner, and allow time for questions and concerns. Use the services of professional counseling or clergy if appropriate. Help the patient to identify coping strategies and to use them effectively.

Evaluation

Evaluate the effectiveness of nursing care for a patient with a cardiac tumor by comparing the patient's status with the expected patient outcomes. Examples of specific patient outcomes for patients with a cardiac tumor have been provided in the Planning section.

The Elderly: Special Considerations

Because of the aging of the cardiovascular system, complications can occur in the older adult. There is less elasticity of the aorta and arteries; the valves become thick and rigid as a result of fibrosis and sclerosis; and the heart muscle contains increased collagen and scar tissue. Cardiac output is reduced about 1% each year beginning at approximately 25 years of age. Maximum coronary blood flow at age 60 is estimated to be 35% less than that of younger persons. Systolic blood pressure rises to compensate for the inelasticity and increased resistance of peripheral vessels.

Pain described by the elderly person may be atypical for cardiac disease as a result of altered pain sensation in the aged. Because of other organ dysfunction associated with aging, cardiac pain may be interpreted by the individual as respiratory, gastric, or musculoskeletal.

Edema associated with CHF or other cardiac problems may lead to skin breakdown in older individuals who have fragile skin. Protective padding for pressure points and gentle changes of position are important nursing measures to prevent problems. Intravenous fluids are monitored carefully in the elderly because excessive fluid infusion results in hypervolemia and may lead to CHF in the older adult.

Temperature elevations increase metabolism, thereby increasing the body's requirements for oxygen as the heart muscle works harder. For every degree of temperature elevation, the heart rate increases approximately 10 beats per minute. Older hearts cannot tolerate this type of stress very well. Therefore, temperature elevations need to be treated promptly to decrease the stress on the heart muscle.

Anorexia that accompanies some forms of cardiac disease may lead to decreased nutritional status in the older adult. Several small meals throughout the day help to compensate for a poor appetite and reduce the workload on the heart as it supplies blood to the digestive system.

A healthy cardiac lifestyle that begins in childhood can prevent many of the cardiac problems that occur in later life. Individuals who do not begin the habit of cigarette smoking, who develop lifelong exercise programs, who eat low-fat, low-cholesterol foods, and who learn to manage life's stressors in a healthy manner are less likely to experience the common cardiac disorders in their elderly years. Prevention is the best treatment for potential cardiac disorders, even with the older adult. Education programs for the elderly focusing on exercise (designed for their age and ability), appropriate nutrition and meal planning, and information about other lifestyle changes can contribute to decreasing severe cardiac disease in the older adult or assist them in managing the effects of the disorder.

Bibliography

Andreoli KG, Zipes DP, Wallace AG, et al. Comprehensive cardiac care. 6th ed. St. Louis: CV Mosby, 1987.

Barbash GI, Keren G, Motro M. Thrombolytic therapy reduces postinfarction left ventricular thrombus risk. Cardiol Board Rev 1992; 9(4):52.

Braddy PK. Cardiac assessment tool. Crit Care Nurs 1989; 9(9):71.

Brenner ZR. Nursing elderly cardiac clients. Crit Care Nurse 1987; 7(2):78.

Carbajal E, Deedwania PC. Silent myocardial ischemia: Mechanisms, diagnosis, prevalence. Prim Cardiol 1991; 17(10):30.

Carpenito LJ. Handbook of nursing diagnosis. 2nd ed. Philadelphia: JB Lippincott, 1987.

Carpenito LJ. Nursing diagnosis. 2nd ed. Philadelphia: JB Lippincott, 1990–1991.

Castello R, Alegria E. Exercise testing for evaluating the patient with coronary artery spasm. Prim Cardiol 1991; 17(10):20.

Cerrato P. Hypertension: The role of diet and lifestyle. RN 1990; 53(12):46.

Dudek SG. Nutrition handbook for nursing practice. New York: JB Lippincott, 1987.

Eliopoulos C. Gerontological nursing. 2nd ed. Philadelphia: JB Lippincott, 1987.

Feury D, Nash D. Hypertension: The nurse's role. RN 1990; 53(11):54.

Gawlinski A. Saving the cardiogenic shock patient. Nursing 1989; 19(12):34.

Gleeson B. After myocardial infarction: How to teach a patient in denial. Nursing 1991; 21(5):48.

Gollub CO. An up-to-date guide to acute myocardial infarction. Mod Med 1992; 60(5):52.

Guzzetta CE, Dossey BM. Cardiovascular nursing: Bodymind tapestry. St. Louis: CV Mosby, 1984.

Holloway NM. Medical-surgical care plans. Springhouse, PA: Springhouse Corporation, 1988.

Hussar DA. Update 91: New drugs. Nursing 1991; 21(5):41.

Kaplan RM. Health-related quality of life in cardiovascular disease. J Consult Clin Psychol 1988; 56(3):382.

Kee JL. Laboratory and diagnostic test with nursing implications. 2nd ed. Norwalk, CT: Appleton & Lange, 1987.

Kloner RA, Pfeffer MA. The guide to cardiology: Aortic and peripheral artery disease. Cardiovasc Rev Rep 1992; 13(4):18.

Kunkel DB. Cardiac glycosides: Part 1. Updating foxglove's toxic heritage. Emerg Med 1987; 19(13):153.

Kunkel DB. Cardiac glycosides: Part II. Nature's storehouses. Emerg Med 1987; 19(14):185.

Lankford TR, Jacobs-Steward PM. Foundations of normal and therapeutic nutrition. New York: John Wiley & Sons, 1986.

Levy W, Cannom DS, Cohen LS. The nontransmural myocardial infarction in perspective. Cardiovasc Rev Rep 1992; 13(4):8.

McCance KL, Huether SE. Pathophysiology: The basis for disease in adults and children. St. Louis: CV Mosby, 1990.

McGinty MK, Chase SL, Mercer ME. Pharmacy-nursing discharge counseling program for cardiac patients. Am J Hosp Pharm, 1988; 45(7):1545.

McHale DJ, Riggs KL, Thurman L. Epicardial pacing after cardiac surgery. Crit Care Nurse 1991; 11(8):62.

Mohandas MS, Khanna A, Ansari M. Hypertrophic myopathy: Why is it so often overlooked in elderly patients? Postgrad Med 1991; 90(5):187.

Morrissey JJ. Exercise and chronic heart disease. Geriatr Nurs 1987; 8(3):138.

Mutnick AH, Fecitt S, Rogers B. Cardiac drugs: Inotropic and chronotropic agents. Nursing 1987; 17(1):58.

Pagana KD, Pagana TJ. Diagnostic testing & nursing implications: A case study approach. 2nd ed. St. Louis: CV Mosby, 1986.

Phillips P. Women's angina risk probed. Chronic Care, 1991; 32(10):10.

Reger MJ, Hermann F, Ried LD. Effectiveness of a printed leaflet for enabling patients to use digoxin side-effect information. Drug Intell Clin Pharm 1987; 21(2):200.

Reiss BS, Melick ME. Pharmacological aspects of nursing care. New York: Delmar Publishing, 1987.

Sanderson RG, Kurth CL. The cardiac patient: A comprehensive approach. 2nd ed. Philadelphia: WB Saunders, 1983.

Shaw M (ed). Illustrated manual of nursing practice. Springhouse, PA: Springhouse Publishing, 1991.

Stanley M. Cardiovascular physiology in the elderly. Crit Care Nurse 1985; 5(6):69.

Thompson V. Chest pain: Your response to a classic warning. RN 1989: 52(4):32.

Todd B. Update: Cardiac emergency drugs. Geriatr Nurs 1986; 7(5):263.

Underhill SL, Woods SL, Sivarajan ES, Halpenny CJ. Cardiac nursing. Philadelphia: JB Lippincott, 1982.

Vasek JL. Diagnosing syncope: With an emphasis on cardiac causes. Postgrad Med 1991; 90(5):175.

Vaska PL. Biventricular assist devices. Crit Care Nurse 1991; 11(8):52.

Weeks LD. Advanced cardiovascular nursing. Boston: Blackwell Scientific, 1986.

Yacone L. The nurse's guide to cardiovascular drugs. RN 1988; 51(8):36.

Chapter Nineteen

KNOWLEDGE BASIC TO THE NURSING CARE *of Adults with Vascular Dysfunction*

The peripheral vascular system consists of the vascular structures that transport the blood leaving the left side of the heart to the tissues of the body. These transportation vessels are termed the systemic circulatory system. The major components of the systemic vasculature are arteries, capillaries, and veins (Fig. 19–1). The lymphatic system is integrally related to circulatory function and is also discussed in this chapter.

Anatomy and Physiology

Vascular Structure

The vascular structures found in the transport loop of the systemic circulation have many structural similarities. With the exception of capillaries, the blood vessels are composed of three distinct layers (Fig. 19–2). The tunica adventitia, or externa, is the outermost layer. It is composed of fibrous and connective tissue that provides support to the vascular structure. The tunica media, or middle layer, is predominantly smooth muscle. This smooth muscle layer is important in that it is most responsive to neural and chemical input that regulates the diameter of blood vessels. The tunica intima, the innermost layer, is composed of connective tissue and a smooth endothelial inner surface for blood to transit the system. This slippery surface prevents blood from clotting. Blood vessels vary in density and size relative to their function and anatomic position in the vascular system (Fig. 19–3).

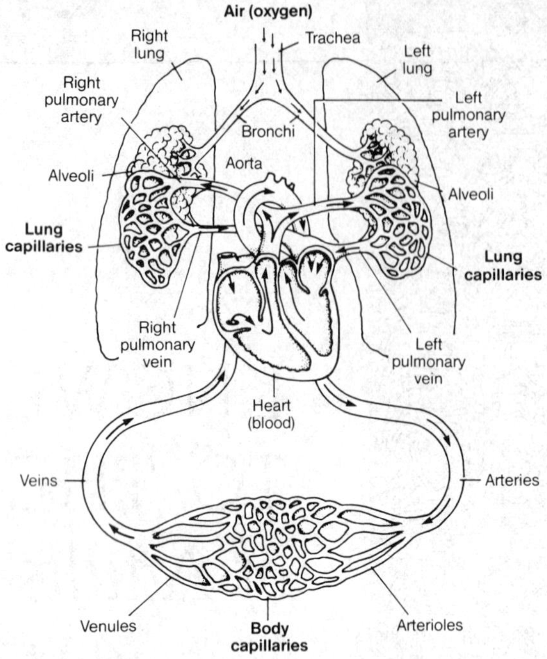

Figure 19–1.

Schematic drawing of systemic circulation (start at bottom of figure). Loaded with carbon dioxide, blood from the body capillaries goes through venules and veins into the right atrium of the heart. The blood is pumped into the lungs. Here it drops carbon dioxide and picks up oxygen and returns to the left atrium of the heart. Blood is pumped through the aorta into the systemic circulation (arteries and arterioles) until it reaches the capillaries, where it gives up oxygen and picks up carbon dioxide and cellular metabolic waste products. (Courtesy of the American Lung Association.)

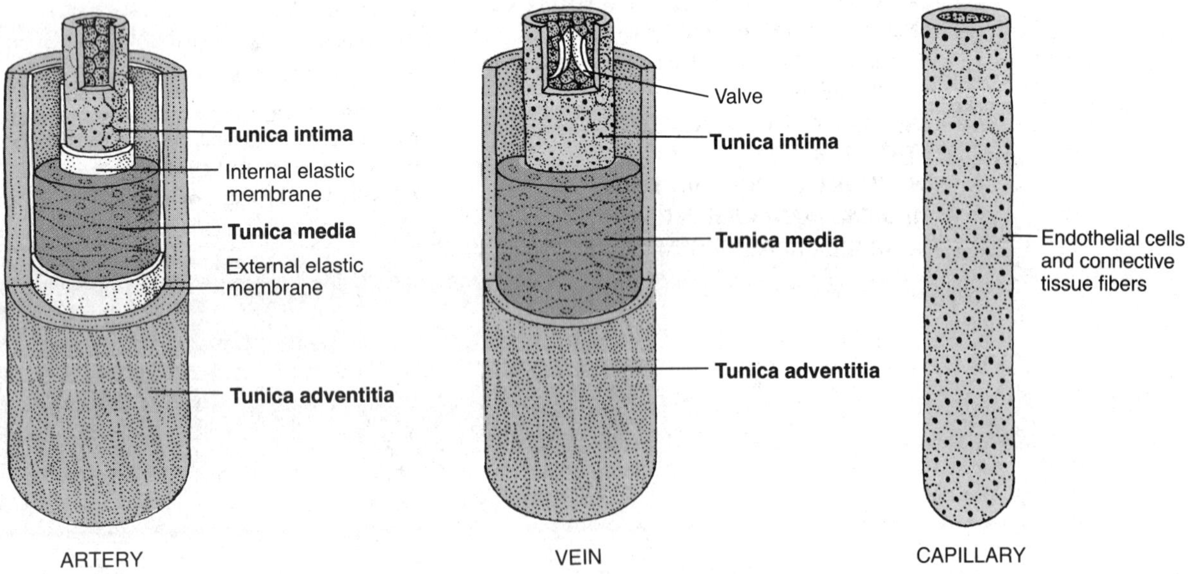

Figure 19–2.

Microscopic anatomy of an artery, a vein, and a capillary. (From Ignatavicius DD, Bayne MV. Medical-surgical nursing: A nursing process approach. Philadelphia: WB Saunders, 1991, p 2083.)

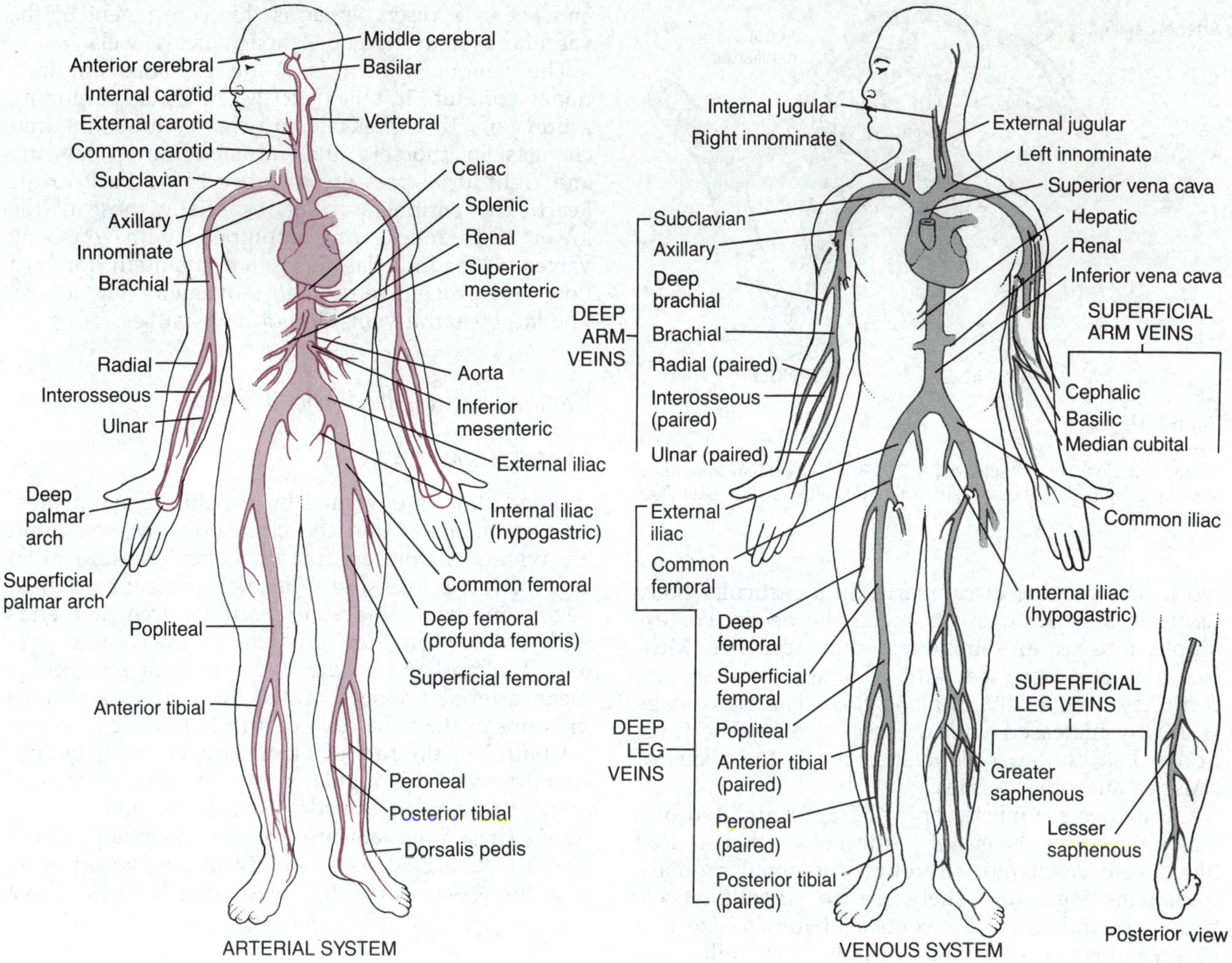

Figure 19–3.

Left, Anatomy of the arterial system. *Right*, Anatomy of the venous system. (From Ignatavicius DD, Bayne MV. Medical-surgical nursing: A nursing process approach. Philadelphia: WB Saunders, 1991, p 2082.)

ARTERIES AND ARTERIOLES

The arterial tree of vessels begins the transport of oxygenated blood in the aorta and culminates its high-pressure conduits in the arterioles. The large arteries are thick walled and quite elastic. They stretch in response to cardiac systole and recoil during diastole. This structural characteristic propels blood forward rapidly.

The arterioles are just a few millimicrons in length, have diameters of 8 to 50 μ and are composed predominantly of smooth muscle. They branch many times to supply as many as 100 capillaries. The contraction or relaxation of this smooth muscle changes the diameter of the vessel, thus influencing resistance in the peripheral vascular system. Arterioles are high-resistance vessels innervated by the sympathetic fibers of the autonomic nervous system. Sympathetic stimulation results in vasoconstriction. Decreased sympathetic activity results in vasodilation; thus, arterioles have a major influence on blood pressure and blood distribution to the capillaries. Precapillary sphincters located at the termination of some arterioles act as control valves through which blood is released into the capillaries.

Arterioles may also connect directly with capillaries or first connect with precapillaries (metarterioles). These structures serve as either thoroughfare channels or pipelines to supply the capillary network. Blood transits through the arterial system rapidly. Approximately 20% of the total circulating volume is contained within the high-pressure arterial component at any one time.

CAPILLARIES

Blood flow through the capillary system accomplishes the nutritional delivery and waste-product removal of the circulation. There are approximately 10 billion capillaries in the peripheral vascular net-

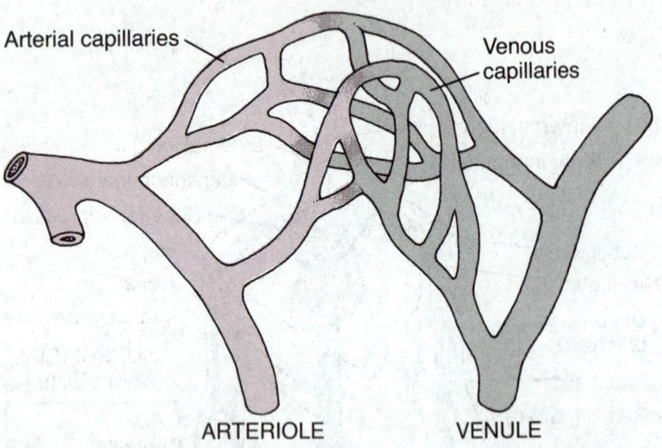

Figure 19–4.

Microcirculation. (From Ignatavicius DD, Bayne MV. Medical-surgical nursing: A nursing process approach. Philadelphia: WB Saunders, 1991, p 2083.)

work. The number of capillaries in a particular body tissue is dependent on its metabolic needs. For example, muscles are abundant with capillaries. Muscles comprise more than 40% of total body tissue. At rest, they receive 20% of blood flow. This percentage is greatly increased with exercise to 85%. The functional distribution of capillaries meets the needs of muscles and other tissues.

Capillaries are microscopic and are composed of a single-thickness layer of endothelial tissue. Red blood cells must move through the small capillary lumen in single file. There are no smooth muscle fibers in capillaries. The control of lumen size is a passive effect of alterations in either precapillary or postcapillary resistance. They contain small pores, which make the capillary bed extremely permeable to the exchange between blood and tissue cells or gases, nutrients, and metabolic wastes. Fluid volume transfer between plasma and interstitial fluid occurs in the capillary system. The capillaries contain 5% of the total circulating blood volume. Arterioles, capillaries, and venules as a unit are referred to as the microcirculation (Fig. 19–4).

Arteriovenous anastomoses are found in some capillary beds. Blood passes directly from arteriole to venule in these structures. They are believed to be local thermoregulation centers between the body and the external environment.

VEINS AND VENULES

The venules connect with capillaries and veins and begin the conduit of vessels for blood returning to the right atrium of the heart. Venules are thin-walled transit tubules. White blood cells can enter or exit the circulatory system through the venule.

Veins have a thinner tunica media, so the walls are extremely distensible or collapsible. They are capable of holding large volumes of blood: up to 75% of total volume. This characteristic ability to stretch and act as a reservoir earns this component of the vascular system the name capacitance vessels.

The venous system is a low-pressure unidirectional conduit. It relies on the muscular pumping action of the skeletal muscle contraction and changes in thoracic and intraabdominal pressure and right atrial pressure to move blood back to the heart. The peripheral veins, especially those of the lower extremities, are equipped with one-way valves or endothelial flaps that maintain forward flow and prevent retrograde movement (Fig. 19–5). The large central veins do not have valves.

Factors That Affect Blood Flow

STRUCTURAL FACTORS

Blood flow is governed by the difference in pressure gradients within the circulatory system. Fluid always flows from an area of higher pressure to an area of lower pressure. The high-pressure gradient begins in the high-pressure arterial tree and ends with the low-pressure gradient in the venous system. The pressure gradient ranges from an average mean arterial pressure of 100 mm Hg to a venous pressure in the vena cava of 4 to 0 mm Hg.

Control of the rate of blood flow through the circulatory system is regulated by a number of factors. Some mechanisms impede or cause resistance to the flow. These mechanisms are the diameter of the vessel, the elastic recoil ability of the vessel wall, and the viscosity of the blood itself. These three

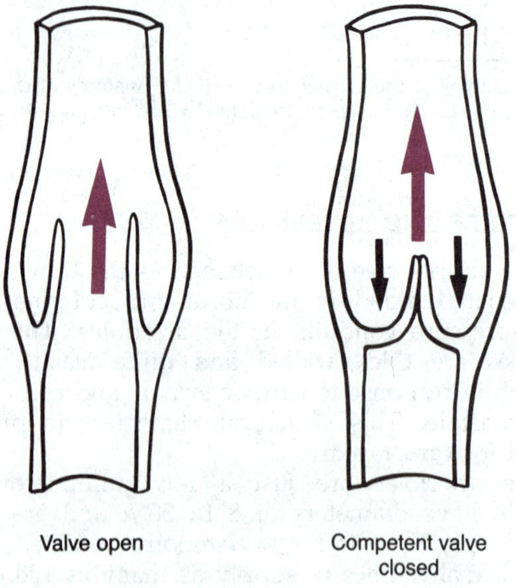

Figure 19–5.

The normal venous valve in the open and the closed positions. The colored arrows in both valves signify the forward flow of blood (toward the heart). A competent venous valve in the closed position prevents retrograde flow of blood, signified by the black arrows. Thus, the valves help maintain the movement of blood back to the heart.

contribute to the hemodynamic or peripheral vascular resistance.

DIAMETER OF THE VESSEL

The velocity of the flow of any liquid is inversely proportional to the cross-sectional areas of the lumen or opening through which the fluid must flow. In the vascular system, the differences in the lumens of the arteries, capillaries, and veins exert an influence on the rate of flow. Arterioles, the smallest and most distant branches of the arterial tree, alter their diameter in response to the metabolic needs of the tissues and various chemical and hormonal stimulation. These vessels are often called resistance vessels because of the effect of their changing lumen size on blood flow to the capillaries and blood pressure.

ELASTIC RECOIL

Arteries have thick muscular walls and thus have a considerable amount of recoil ability that facilitates the movement of blood under high pressure quickly to the capillary networks. Capillaries alter diameter negligibly and have little recoil ability with their single-cell-layer thickness. Veins with less muscular walls and the great capacity for distensibility and collapsibility provide no impedance to blood flow if valves are competent.

Blood moves through healthy vessels smoothly because of streamlined or laminar flow. In this type of flow, the blood components are layered. Plasma is in closest proximity to the vessel wall, and erythrocytes, platelets, and cellular components move through the center of the vessel. Narrowing of the lumen of the vessel at anatomic bifurcations, or by atherosclerosis or other structural changes in vessel integrity, can lead to turbulence or eddy currents of blood flow. These areas of turbulent flow may produce a murmur, or bruit, that can be auscultated with a stethoscope.

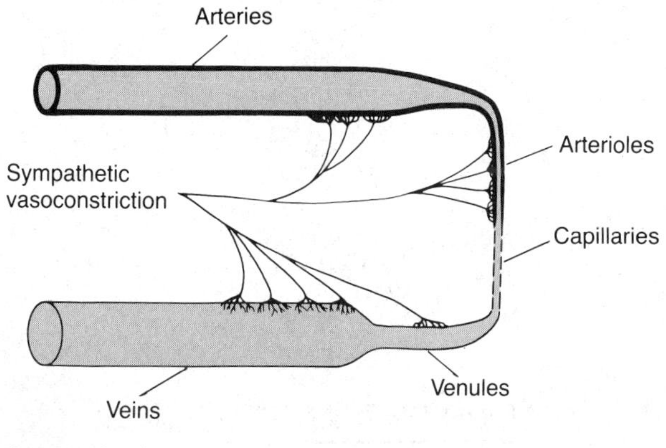

Figure 19–6.

Sympathetic innervation of circulation. (From Guyton, AC. Textbook of medical physiology. 8th ed. Philadelphia: WB Saunders, 1991, p 195.)

VISCOSITY OF BLOOD

The last basic controller of the rate of blood flow is the viscosity of blood itself. This factor is usually of little consequence with normal red blood cell concentrations, but if the hematocrit increases to an adult level of 55%, the "thicker" blood flows more slowly. This viscous blood will have a greater tendency to clot and contribute to impeded flow.

DIRECT CONTROL OF BLOOD FLOW

There are three mechanisms that influence blood flow by direct effects on the vessels:

1. Local control.
2. Neural control.
3. Humoral control.

LOCAL CONTROL

Local control of blood flow in all body tissues is governed by each particular tissue's need for nutrition and perfusion. The tissues regulate flow independently of the autonomic nervous system through a mechanism of metabolic autoregulation. Although the mechanism of autoregulation is not fully understood, it appears to be regulated by a lack of oxygen or accumulation of tissue metabolites. When oxygen and the level of other cellular nutrients decrease or metabolites increase, arterioles and metarterioles dilate to increase blood flow. During exercise, muscles demand an increased flow and vasodilation of arterioles occurs. At rest, the arterioles constrict and blood flow is directed to other parts of the body. Local autoregulation is a major controller of vasoconstriction or vasodilation and thus of blood flow by variation in lumen size.

NEURAL CONTROL

Neural control of blood flow is mediated by the sympathetic branch of the autonomic nervous system. The sympathetic pathway begins in the vasomotor center located in the lower pons and medulla. The vasomotor center also receives input from the hypothalamus. All blood vessels except capillaries are supplied with sympathetic nerve fibers (Fig. 19–6). Sympathetic input impacts the blood vessels, producing selective vasoconstriction rapidly, within 1 to 30 seconds. The sympathetic nerve fibers secrete norepinephrine, a potent vasoconstricting neurotransmitter. The effect of this vasoconstriction in the arterioles is a rise in arterial blood pressure. The effect of norepinephrine on veins is venoconstriction, which will cause an increase in venous return to the heart.

HUMORAL CONTROL

Various substances released into or circulating in the blood can influence blood flow. Hormones are released from the adrenal medulla in response to acute stress as part of the "fight or flight" response. The hormones epinephrine and norepinephrine (catecholamines) act directly on the smooth muscle of blood vessels to cause vasoconstriction and some selective vasodilation. Other substances found in circulation that influence the diameter of the lumen of vessels, and thus blood flow, are listed in Table 19–1.

Lymphatic Vascular System

The lymphatic system is integrally related to the systemic vascular system. It consists of lymph capillaries, vessels, ducts, nodes and the lymph that flows through its channels to return to the venous system. Figure 19–7 illustrates the lymphatic network. Lymphatic vessels serve as an accessory route for the transport of fluid, proteins, and large particulate matter away from the interstitial spaces. They remove excess interstitial fluid or plasma that the venous capillaries are unable to reabsorb (Fig. 19–8). The lymphatic system plays an important role in immunity and in the prevention of edema in body tissues.

The lymphatic capillaries are thin-walled, endothelially lined, and slightly larger than systemic circulatory capillaries. They have varying diameters. These capillaries have wider spaces between endothelial cells than venous capillaries, so they are more permeable to large molecules of protein and colloids. With the exception of the central nervous system and in nonvascular structures such as cartilage,

Table 19–1. SUBSTANCES AFFECTING BLOOD FLOW

VASOCONSTRICTORS	
Angiotensin	Released in response to a decreased arterial pressure or a decrease in sodium. It is formed after activation of the renin-angiotensin system of the kidney. (It is the most potent vasoconstrictor known.)
Cold	Direct application causes local vasoconstriction.
Serotonin	Particularly potent in cutaneous arterioles. It is found in platelets, gastrointestinal mucosa, and cancerous tumors.
Trauma	Arterial injury causes local reaction.
VASODILATORS	
Bradykinin	Vasoactive polypeptide found in plasma that also increases capillary permeability.
Heat	Direct application causes local reaction.
Histamine	Released from injured body cells and affects arterioles. It also increases the porosity of capillaries, causing them to leak fluid and plasma proteins into tissues.
Muscle metabolites	The most common muscle metabolite is lactic acid.

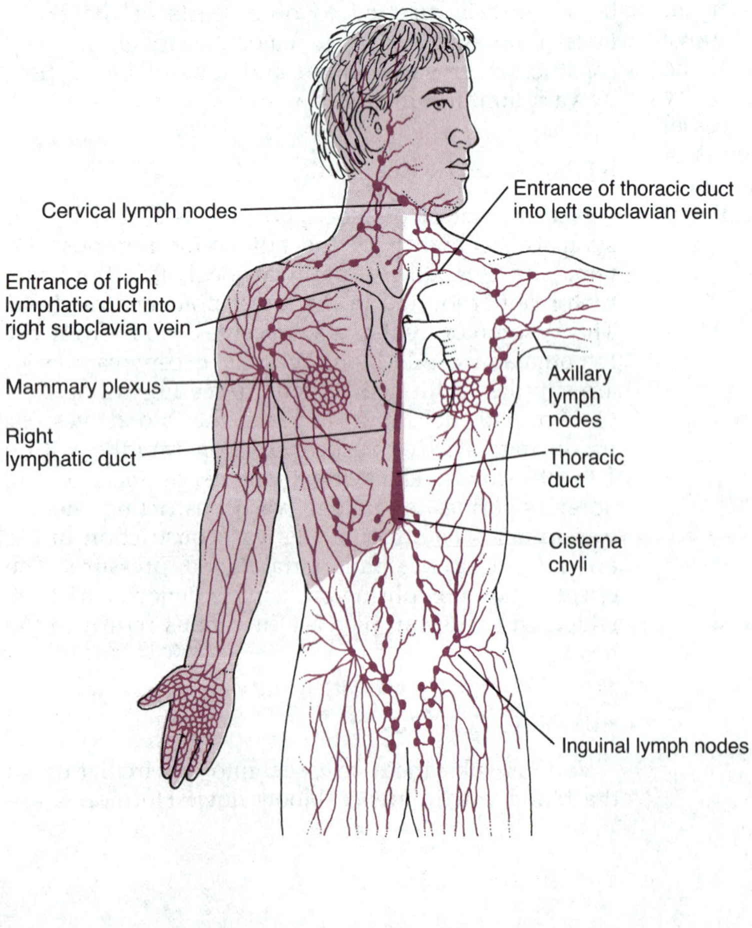

Figure 19–7.

The lymphatic system. Lymph in the shaded area returns to the right lymphatic duct. Lymph in the rest of the body returns through the thoracic duct. (From Ignatavicius DD, Bayne MV. Medical-surgical nursing: A nursing process approach. Philadelphia: WB Saunders, 1991, p 2085.)

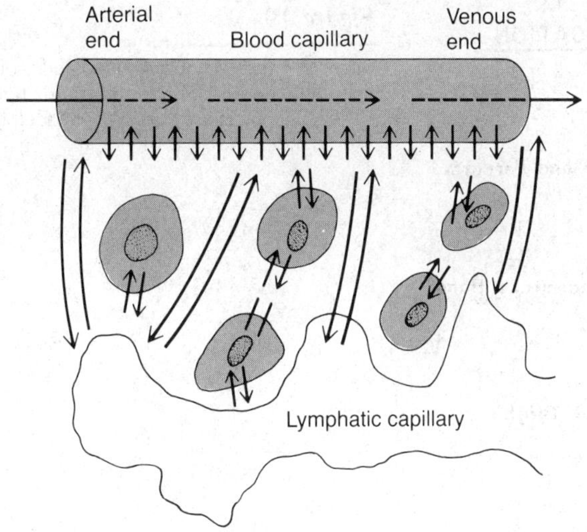

Figure 19–8.

Diffusion of fluid between capillary and interstitial fluid spaces and the lymphatics. (From Guyton, AC. Human physiology and mechanisms of disease. 5th ed. Philadelphia: WB Saunders, 1992, p 125.)

lymphatic capillaries are found at the venous end of most body tissues.

The lymphatic capillaries and vessels have one-way valves, as does the venous system, but they are more numerous. At the capillary level, the valvular structure originates between the spaces of the endothelial cell wall. These valve flaps are attached to filaments that pull inward, allowing excess interstitial fluid to enter the capillary but preventing backflow.

Lymphatic capillaries increase in diameter to form lymphatic vessels. The lymphatic network propels lymph forward to enter the venous circulation. Lymph empties into two major ducts: the thoracic duct and the right lymphatic duct. The thoracic duct receives lymph from most of the body. The right lymphatic duct empties the right side of the head, neck, arm, and thorax. These ducts empty directly into the venous system at the junction of the subclavian and internal jugular veins.

Lymph nodes are small, ovoid masses of lymphatic tissue located along the circuit of lymphatic channels. The internal structure of the node is spongy, enabling it to serve as a filter for bacteria. Granulocytes, macrophages, and lymphocytes are able to pass into the lymph nodes and return to systemic circulation via the lymphatic network.

Lymph has many similarities to plasma. It is pale yellow to milky white in color, depending on the concentration of molecules of digested fats. The fluid also contains lymphocytes, granulocytes, enzymes, hormones, antibodies, and excess interstitial fluid. Because it is deficient in fibrinogen, erythrocytes, and platelets, it coagulates very slowly. Lymph movement is generated by the contraction of the lymphatic walls and is additionally propelled by the compression of tissues through skeletal muscle activity.

Clinical Manifestations of Vascular Dysfunction

The clinical manifestations of vascular dysfunction are due to impaired blood flow that deprives tissues of adequate perfusion of oxygen and nutrients or of the removal of waste products of metabolism. Complete obstruction of blood flow results in rapid tissue death. The progression of symptomatology depends on several variables:

1. Origin: arterial or venous.
2. Duration and onset: acute or chronic.
3. Obstruction: partial or complete.
4. Presence of collateral or alternate vessels to perfuse an area.

The chief clinical manifestations are pain and changes in tissue integrity and characteristics in areas of poor perfusion.

Pain

Pain is often an omnipresent clinical manifestation of vascular dysfunction. It is related to tissue hypoxia or ischemia from obstructed blood flow that causes a decrease in tissue oxygenation or the accumulation of the waste products of metabolism. Although the exact mechanism is unknown, pain is believed to be the result of a metabolic factor that is released from the ischemic tissues. This factor irritates peripheral sensory nerve endings. The intensity of pain will vary with acuity of the particular disease process.

Pain is often chronic and unrelenting, affecting the quality of life. The duration and intensity may push an individual to the limit of endurance. Pain may interfere with sleep-rest cycles, appetite, physical activity, concentration, and interpersonal relationships. Emotional stress brought on by constant pain manifests in irritability, anger, crying, withdrawal, depression, and even suicide. The pain may be resolved only by nerve block or amputation of the ischemic area.

INTERMITTENT CLAUDICATION

Intermittent claudication is a severe aching or cramplike pain most frequently experienced in the calf muscles. It is precipitated by walking or muscular contractions of the lower extremities and is relieved by rest. The pain is usually bilateral and can be replicated in a given individual at the previous claudication walking distance. Claudication pain is associated with arterial insufficiency caused by atheromatous plaque, creating obstruction of blood flow to the extremities. The femoral artery is usually the occlusive site for calf claudication. Occlusions of the aortic and iliac arteries cause claudication pain

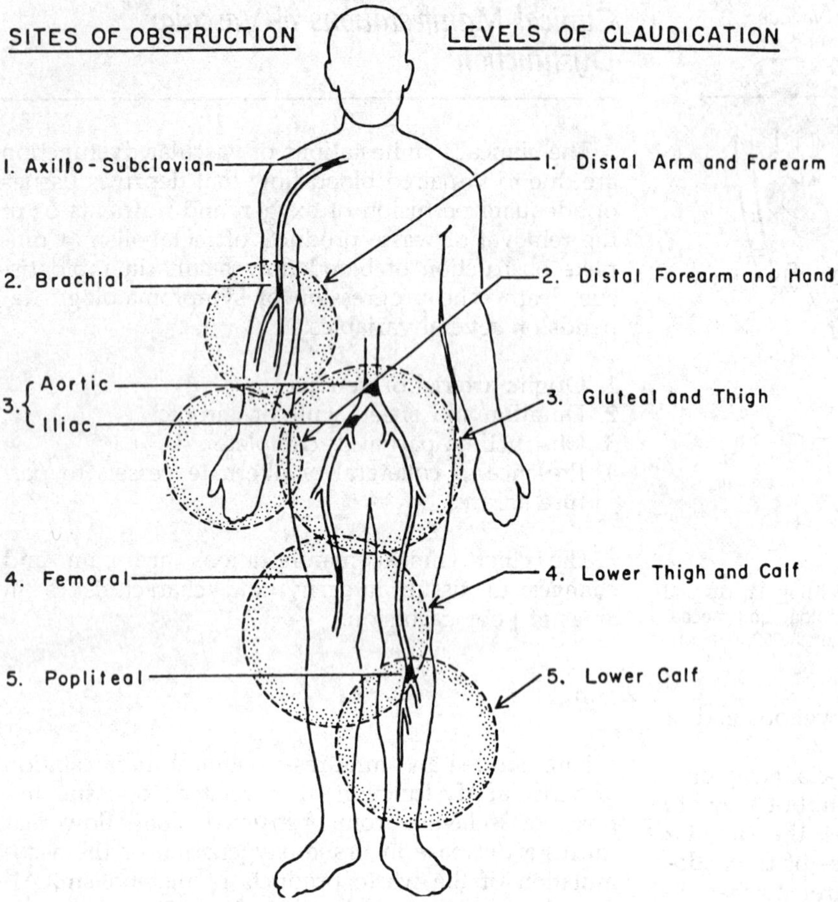

Figure 19–9.

Sites of arterial obstruction and corresponding levels of claudication. (From Fahey VA. Vascular nursing. Philadelphia: WB Saunders, 1988, p 61.)

in the hip or thigh. Figure 19–9 illustrates sites of obstruction and corresponding levels of claudication.

The circulatory needs of muscles for oxygen and metabolite removal are increased with exercise. The mechanically impaired arteries are not able to dilate to increase blood flow through the obstruction. The pain of intermittent claudication appears to be related in order of occurrence:

1. Tissue ischemia.
2. Metabolite accumulation in tissue.
3. Painful muscle spasm.

REST PAIN

Rest pain is a sign of acute arterial insufficiency and is associated with severe ischemia. It is often the precursor to gangrene. It is described as a severe ache, throbbing, gnawing, or burning pain. The discomfort is often more severe at night and may last for interminable hours. The pain of arterial insufficiency is aggravated by elevation of the affected part. It may be relieved by placing the part dependent to the level of the heart.

Many patients may be able to rest only by sitting in a chair or by dangling the affected extremity from the bed. The individual often rubs and cradles the ischemic leg in their lap in an effort to alleviate the pain.

PAIN OF VENOUS INSUFFICIENCY

Venous dilation, congestion, edema, and stasis from incompetent valves produce a heaviness or dull, aching pain in the affected extremity. Some individuals experience leg cramps, especially at rest. Elevation of the congested extremity facilitates venous return of excess blood volume and often relieves the pain.

Stasis of deoxygenated blood that is additionally unable to remove the toxic by-products of cellular metabolism causes tissue deterioration. Stasis ulceration develops. These ulcerations produce localized pain in the area of deterioration.

PAIN OF ISCHEMIC NEUROPATHY

This type of pain manifests late in the course of acute arterial insufficiency and is described as a shocklike sensation occurring in both the leg and the foot. Paresthesias often accompany progressive ischemia. The pain is believed to be associated with irritation of the peripheral sensory nerves by the effects of chronic ischemia.

PAIN OF ULCERATION OR GANGRENE

The pain of arterial ulcerations or gangrene is described as aching, sharp, stabbing, and unrelenting. It is so intense that rest and sleep are greatly impaired. This type of severe rest pain is the result of acute or progressively chronic ischemia and is frequently the precursor to amputation. Venous stasis ulcerations are less painful than ischemic arterial ulcers.

Application of the Nursing Process to the Care of the Patient with Pain

Assessment

Obtain a patient history and description of the pain. Include identification of the location, intensity, and quality. Have the patient rate the intensity of pain on a scale of 0 to 10. Include their present pain level, the most severe level, and the least severe level experienced on this scale. Use the patient's own words to describe the quality of the pain. Ask about the onset, duration, and any variations or rhythms to the occurrence of pain. Determine precipitating factors such as exercise or exposure to cold. Evaluate activity and exercise tolerance, such as distances walked when pain occurs, to establish a baseline.

Claudication pain is usually elicited at approximately the same walking distance in a particular individual. By obtaining this history or activity baseline, planning for slow progressive exercise is begun. Inquire about measures that have helped alleviate the pain, such as rest or position changes.

Inquire about the effects of pain on sleep-rest patterns, appetite, physical activity, and relationships with others. Evaluate the patient's ability to cope with the pain and the effects on emotional stability.

Assess the patient's level of knowledge of what is causing the pain, and instruct accordingly. Evaluate the effectiveness of pain-management measures.

Nursing Diagnoses and Planning

The nursing diagnosis and related expected patient outcomes most commonly applicable to patients with peripheral vascular pain are as follows:

NDx: Pain related to impaired peripheral circulation

Planning: Patient outcomes
1. Patient verbalizes a decrease in the level of pain.
2. Patient follows a regimen of exercise and rest.
3. Patient participates in relaxation techniques to help manage pain.

Nursing Interventions

NDx: Pain
Because the cause of the pain is impaired circulation, measures that improve blood flow help alleviate or lessen the discomfort. Tell the patient to begin a slow, progressive, moderate exercise program of walking short distances several times a day followed by rest periods. This is helpful for many patients with intermittent claudication. Note the distance or amount of muscular activity the patient can tolerate before pain occurs. Exercise promotes not only blood flow and removal of metabolites that cause muscle spasm but also the development of collateral circulation channels that bypass areas of blockage. Walking assists the venous pump by causing muscular contractions to return blood to the heart. It is helpful in individuals with venous insufficiency if followed by a period of elevation.

Position the patient for pain relief. Place the extremities in a dependent position to the torso with arterial insufficiency. This works with the force of gravity, helping circulatory perfusion. Do not elevate the extremities for any extended period because it usually increases pain and further compromises circulation. Elevation of the extremity is *contraindicated* with arterial insufficiency.

Elevate the extremities in venous disorders. This assists in relieving venous engorgement, edema, and pain. Instruct the patient to elevate the extremities several times throughout the day. Tell the patient to avoid standing for prolonged times in one position but to shift the weight from side to side. Encourage flexion and dorsiflexion of the ankles when at rest. These muscular contractions assist the venous muscular pumping action.

Administer prescribed analgesics, tranquilizers, vasodilators, and sleep medications, and evaluate their effectiveness. These medications may relieve or lessen the severity of pain and make it possible for the patient to participate more actively in exercise that improves circulation. Encourage adequate rest and sleep to maintain psychological integrity.

Teach relaxation exercises such as deep abdominal breathing with a focal point, guided imagery, and autogenic training. These produce a sense of control over pain and decrease feelings of powerlessness. Physiologic production of the relaxation response decreases sympathetic vasoconstriction in peripheral vessels. Peripheral vessels dilate and increase cutaneous temperature during the relaxation response.

Sit down at the bedside, and practice relaxation exercises with the patient. These exercises are most successful when the nurse is actively involved rather than just providing a relaxation tape or written instructions. Once the patient has learned the technique, reinforce it with alternate material. Provide back and neck massage. This promotes relaxation and circulation. Massage of the calves of the legs, however, is *contraindicated* in any patient on bed rest or with limitations in mobility or after surgery because it could release a thrombus, causing embolization.

Evaluation

Evaluate the effectiveness of nursing care for a patient experiencing peripheral vascular pain by comparing the patient's status with the expected patient outcomes. Examples of specific outcomes for patients experiencing peripheral vascular pain have been provided in the Planning section.

Changes in Skin Color, Temperature, and Integrity

The clinical manifestations vary with arterial or venous dysfunction. Table 19–2 compares and summarizes changes in skin, color, temperature, and integrity.

TROPHIC CHANGES

Trophic changes are the result of prolonged lack of cellular nutrition and ischemia. The growth of nails, hair, and skin are affected.

COLOR CHANGES

Cyanosis, or bluish discoloration, develops in tissues that contain blood deficient in oxygenated hemoglobin. Many individuals with venous insufficiency acquire positional cyanosis when the legs are in a dependent plane. Mottling, or cyanotic discoloration, of the toes or foot is present in end-stage arterial obstruction and is a precursor to ischemic gangrene. The extremity assumes a normal coloration when elevated.

Pallor is caused by deficient blood supply. Normal blood flow through a tissue manifests in a pink or rosy hue. Extremities with advanced arterial disease become extremely pale when elevated above the level of the heart.

Rubor (redness) in chronic arterial insufficiency is the result of a permanent dilation of the arterioles caused by damage of the vascular smooth muscle layer. Arterioles lose their basic vasomotor tone and responsiveness. They become dilated with blood. Muscle metabolite accumulation of lactic acid also has a vasodilating effect that produces rubor.

Rubor is produced as a rebound response to placing the arterially affected extremity in an elevated position (becomes pale) and then lowering it dependent to the heart (becomes ruddy). Pallor followed by rubor is a sign of severe arterial disease.

Rubor localized in the hands and feet is characteristic of arterial spasms or occlusions. Exposure to cold temperatures often precipitates spasms in individuals with arterial vessel dysfunction.

Brownish pigmentation is often present on the anterior surface of the lower leg in venous insufficiency. This coloration is due to chronic stasis and poor cellular nutrition and waste removal.

Table 19–2. CLINICAL MANIFESTATIONS OF CHANGES IN SKIN TEMPERATURE, COLOR, AND INTEGRITY WITH ARTERIAL AND VENOUS INSUFFICIENCY

ASSESSMENT	ARTERIAL	VENOUS
Extremity characteristics	Extremities often exhibit muscular atrophy and decreased hair growth; skin is dry, smooth, shiny in appearance; toenails are thickened, discolored	Brownish pigmentation on anterior surface of lower leg and ankle; skin thickened, rough; dermatitis
Skin color	Ghostly white pallor when elevated; rebound rubor when placed in dependent position; blotchy cyanosis as severe ischemia progresses	Feet and lower leg become cyanotic with prolonged dependent position; normal coloration to rosy when elevated
Skin temperature	Poikilothermy (decreased temperature); cool feet; extremity becomes cold below the level of occlusion with acute blockage	Warm; cooler with presence of tissue edema
Edema	Not characteristically present	Persistent chronic swelling, especially in prolonged dependent position; elevation will decrease venous dilation and swelling
Pathologic ulcerations	Caused by prolonged small artery and arteriole constriction; acutely painful; pale grayish base; located on heel, lateral malleolus of ankle, toes, top of the foot.	Caused by venous stasis or pooling of blood; chronic slow healing moderately painful; pink base; found on medial malleolus of ankle
Gangrene	Dry gangrene starting with the toes. Dry, hard, black, shriveled appearance; toes may autoamputate; pregangrenous areas appear dark purple and do not change color with pressure	Not present
Paresthesia	Tingling, numb, or prickly sensation with progressive ischemia	Not present

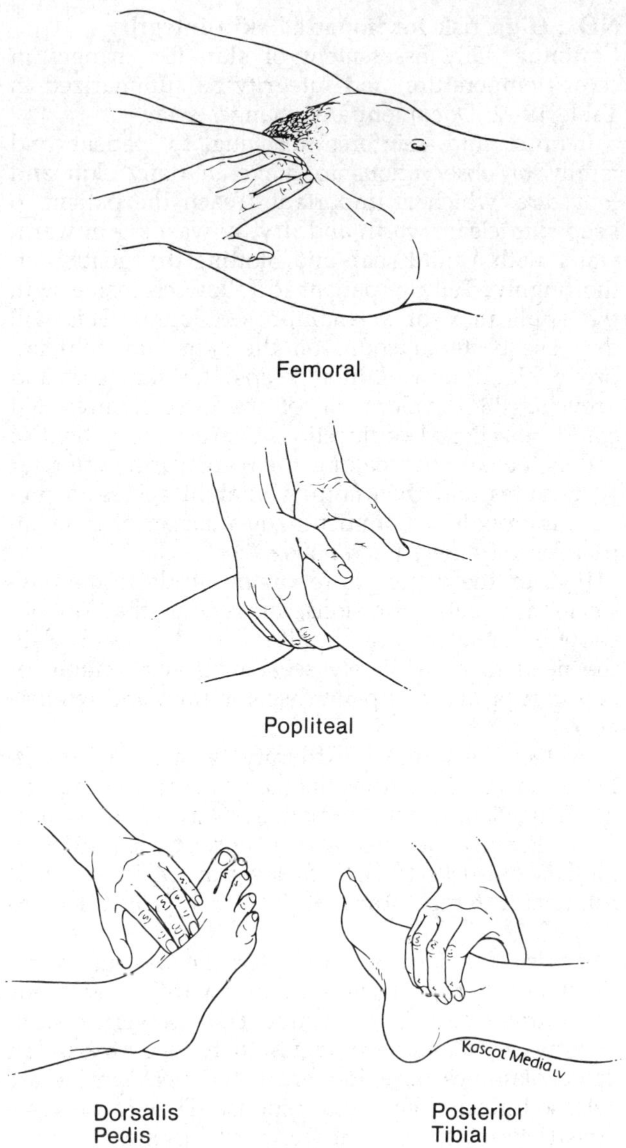

Figure 19–10.

Palpation of pulses. (From Fahey VA. Vascular nursing. Philadelphia: WB Saunders, 1988, p 64.)

TEMPERATURE CHANGES

Skin temperature is a reflection of the adequacy of the blood circulation. Coolness of an extremity denotes deficient blood supply. A rapid change to coldness signifies an acute occlusion. Emergency measures must be taken to salvage the limb.

ULCERATION

In arterial disorders, ulcerations are caused by chronic occlusion of arterioles and small arteries. In venous insufficiency, the precipitating factor is venous stasis and the accumulation of deoxygenated blood. The nutrition of tissues is impeded, making them vulnerable to bacterial growth and tissue breakdown or ulceration.

GANGRENE

Gangrene is characterized by black devitalized tissue. It is the net result of tissue death from severe ischemia. Gangrene most often is confined to one extremity.

Application of the Nursing Process to the Care of the Patient with Changes in Skin Color, Temperature, and Integrity

Assessment

Review the medical history to determine how long symptoms have been present. Perform a physical examination of the affected extremity for evidence of the manifestations of peripheral vascular dysfunction. Table 19–2 summarizes assessment parameters of skin integrity in vascular disorders. Thoroughly examine all extremities for changes in skin color, temperature, or presence of ulcerations or gangrene.

Palpate the distal pulses bilaterally, and note their presence, absence, and quality. Move up the extremity if the distal pulses are absent. Use Doppler ultrasonography if pulses are not palpable (Figs. 19–10 and 19–11). Assessment of pulses gives an estimation of the degree of vascular dysfunction. Pulses are present with venous disorders but are characteristically diminished or absent in arterial insufficiency. Check capillary refill in extremities. It should be less than 3 seconds if perfusion is adequate.

Observe skin color or temperature changes while the extremity is positionally elevated or dependent to the heart. Ask the patient about skin-color changes with exposure to cold temperatures. Ask whether the patient perceives coolness or warmth in the part. Examine toenails and skin for changes in thickness, pigmentation, or coloration. Check for the

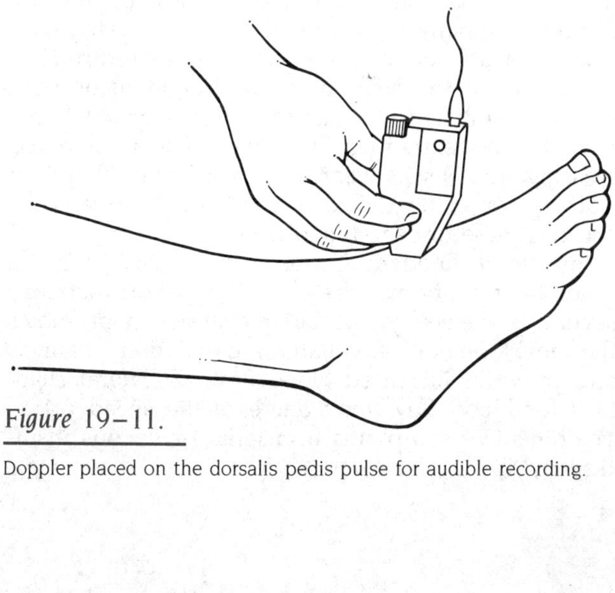

Figure 19–11.

Doppler placed on the dorsalis pedis pulse for audible recording.

presence of edema, ulceration, gangrene, or paresthesia.

If ulceration or gangrene is present, carefully document the location, color, shape, and presence of qualities of healing or granulation. Measure the area precisely for baseline data for future comparison. Ask how ulcerations are presently being cared for. Assess learning needs for wound care. Gangrene is end-stage ischemia, and amputation is most likely a reality. Provide support in the grieving process for limb loss.

Nursing Diagnoses and Planning

Nursing diagnoses and related expected patient outcomes most commonly applicable to patients with changes in skin color, temperature, and integrity include the following:

NDx: Altered tissue perfusion, peripheral, related to compromised blood flow

Planning: Patient outcomes
1. Patient exhibits improved blood supply to the affected extremity as evidenced by improvement in color, temperature, and integrity.
2. Patient participates in exercises and positioning that facilitate blood flow.

NDx: High risk for impaired skin integrity related to impaired circulation

Planning: Patient outcomes
1. Patient maintains or reestablishes skin integrity with no signs of tissue damage.
2. Patient demonstrates daily protective measures in skin care and activities.

Nursing Interventions

NDx: Altered tissue perfusion, peripheral

Determine whether the altered tissue perfusion is the result of arterial or venous insufficiency or both. Position the patient appropriately: feet elevated with venous insufficiency to promote venous return; feet dependent to the heart or on a straight plane with arterial insufficiency to assist with the gravitational flow to the extremity. Tell the patient to avoid crossing the legs, wearing constrictive shoes or clothing, or using the knee gatch on hospital beds because these impede blood flow.

Encourage moderate muscular activity such as graded extremity exercise or walking short distances several times a day. Muscular contraction promotes the development of collateral circulation channels and provides increased blood flow. Collateral channels for blood flow may decrease the speed of development of symptoms in arterial or venous insufficiency.

NDx: High risk for impaired skin integrity

Continue daily assessment of skin for changes in color, temperature, and integrity as summarized in Table 19–2. Document any changes seen.

Instruct and reinforce teaching to patient and family of observations to make in daily skin and foot care, which is important. Teach the patient to keep skin clean, warm and dry by washing in warm water with a mild soap and blotting dry gently and thoroughly. Tell the patient to follow cleansing with the application of a lanolin-based lotion. This will decrease bacterial count on the skin and help improve blood flow. Lotion keeps the skin soft and prevents the development of cracks or fissures that could be a portal of infection. Instruct the patient to soften toenails by soaking them in warm water for 10 minutes and then cutting straight across to prevent ingrowth. Recommend consultation of a podiatrist for extremely thick nails.

Instruct the patient to report promptly to the physician any cuts, abrasions, or lesions that do not show evidence of healing after 2 or 3 days. Explain the need to immediately seek medical attention for any abrupt onset of pain, discoloration, and temperature.

Protect the affected extremity from injury resulting from pressure from linens by placing a bed cradle if needed. Teach the patient to avoid direct heat from heating devices and to use nonconstricting footlets or socks to keep feet warm. Maintain environmental temperature at 70°F to 74°F (21°C to 23.5°C).

Assess risk factors, and assist the patient in understanding the importance of control over them. Discourage smoking; nicotine is a powerful vasoconstrictor. Discuss strategies to reduce stress. The catecholamines norepinephrine and epinephrine are released during the stress response. They cause vasoconstriction, especially in peripheral tissues.

Manage ulcerations per physician's protocol. Carefully document progression of wound healing.

Evaluation

Evaluate the effectiveness of nursing care for a patient experiencing changes in skin color, temperature, and integrity by comparing the patient's status with the expected patient outcomes. Examples of specific outcomes for patients experiencing changes in skin color, temperature, and integrity have been provided in the Planning section.

Assessment of Vascular Status

The health history, along with identification of risk factors for vascular disease, is the most important part of diagnosing a peripheral vascular problem. A physical assessment follows the history so that specific problems can be identified and a plan for care established.

Patient History

The health history is an organized method of eliciting comprehensive, pertinent information from a patient regarding past and present state of health in relation to the peripheral vascular status to formulate a data base for problem identification. The health history serves as a basis for directing attention toward specific body systems during the physical examination and allows observation of the patient during the responses to the questions. Time must be allowed during the health history to establish a relationship of trust with the patient by listening attentively and with concern and by allowing the patient to assume an active, integral role in his or her health care.

Collect the appropriate data using understandable terminology, and allow the patient to respond fully and voice concerns. Ask the patient about the history of the present illness or disorder. Inquire as to the patient's chief complaint. Obtain a detailed description of the complaint. If pain is the most significant problem, ask for the location, intensity, duration, precipitating factors, and relief methods. For example, the patient may indicate that pain occurs in the calves but only after walking short distances and it stops after resting for a few moments. Ask whether this happens every time the patient walks or just at specific times. Find out how severe the pain becomes and if it is always relieved by rest.

Ask the patient about past medical problems, medications, and surgeries. Also ask about the family history of illness. Determine the patient's usual activities of daily living and whether the present condition interferes with the normal daily routine. Complete a brief review of the systems, determining whether dysfunctions in any other system are affecting the peripheral vascular status. Carefully document the information obtained.

Risk Factors

The risk factors for peripheral vascular disease (PVD) are essentially the same as those for coronary artery disease (see Chapter 18). Review these with the patient to assess risk for peripheral vascular dysfunction. Determine the patient's understanding of the risk factors and the importance of reducing risk for vascular disease when possible. Age and sex are nonmodifiable risk factors. Men older than 50 years of age have a higher incidence of peripheral vascular dysfunction than women of the same age. Elderly male diabetic smokers have the highest incidence of PVD.

Elevated cholesterol levels are associated with atherosclerosis and resultant peripheral vascular problems. Current recommended blood cholesterol levels are as follows:

Less than 200 mg/dl: desirable
200 to 239 mg/dl: borderline to high
240 mg/dl or greater: high risk

Most cholesterol is contained in low-density lipoproteins (LDL). High-density lipoproteins (HDL) remove cholesterol from the blood and return it to the liver. Table 19–3 summarizes modifiable risk factors for peripheral dysfunction.

Table 19–3. MODIFIABLE RISK FACTORS

Elevated lipid levels	Directly associated with atheromatous plaque buildup Diet and exercise can lower levels of LDLs.
Obesity	Raises blood lipid levels, increasing deposition of atheromatous plaque Greater tissue needs for circulation Associated with decreased physical mobility and activity, which raises the level of LDL
Sedentary lifestyle	Increased LDL; exercise promotes utilization of lipids and raises level of beneficial HDL
Stress	Blood coagulates more easily Vasoconstriction of peripheral vessels Related to an increase in LDLs Decreases immune response
Cigarette smoking	Direct stimulation of the sympathetic nervous system; peripheral vasoconstriction immediate, lasting as long as 1 hour; after one cigarette, effects platelets, making them more "sticky," and increases platelet aggregation Carbon monoxide damages red blood cells' ability to carry oxygen to nourish tissues Increased chance of blood clot formation
Hypertension	Arterial walls damaged from elevated blood pressure; become thickened and demand more oxygenation.
Diabetes	Associated with high incidence and accelerated rate of peripheral vascular disease, especially in distal vessels. Damage to microcirculation Poor wound healing as a result of tissue malnourishment

Abbreviations: LDL, low-density lipoproteins ("bad cholesterol"); HDL, high-density lipoproteins ("good cholesterol").

Physical Examination

Complete a general inspection of the patient, focusing on the overall appearance of the patient and the extremities. In particular, note the skin color, temperature, and integrity. Note obvious venous insufficiency, which may be evident by torturous veins and peripheral edema. Poor color, a cool skin temperature, or the presence of edema or lesions indicate potential peripheral vascular dysfunction. Check the nail beds for color and clubbing. The hair

Table 19–4. COMMON ARTERIAL DIAGNOSTIC STUDIES

STUDY	PURPOSE	PROCEDURE
NONINVASIVE		
Doppler ultrasonography	Detection of flow disruption in arteries or veins caused by stenosis, occlusion, thrombus; used when pulses not palpable; sound frequencies heard related to blow flood and velocity	Conductive jelly applied to skin; Doppler flowmeter detects flow through vessels and magnifies sound; differences in pitch noted. Doppler ultrasonogram can be attached to blood pressure cuff to obtain thigh, calf, ankle pressures
Doppler treadmill	Measurement of ankle pressures with exercise to test for intermittent claudication	Patient walks on treadmill after Doppler study until claudication pain develops; Doppler ultrasonogram again records extremity pressures
Cold stimulation test	Determination of temperature changes in fingers; used to diagnose Raynaud's phenomenon	Thermistors are attached to fingers and baseline temperature obtained; fingers submerged in ice water 20 sec; temperature measured every 5 min until pretest temperature established
INVASIVE		
Arterial angiography or arteriography	Visualize arteries and assess blood flow; detect obstruction, narrowing, or aneurysm, collateral circulation	Iodine-based contrast medium injected into artery; x-ray films taken; test takes 1–2 hr
Digital subtraction angiography (DSA)	Visualize arteries and assess blood flow; detect obstruction, narrowing, or aneurysm, collateral circulation	Injection of contrast media into venous system via vena cava; fluoroscopic image intensifier displays vessel; data fed to computer; images not required are subtracted to provide detailed image of desired area of study
Lumbar sympathetic block	Determination of the feasibility of sympathectomy to provide increased flow in extremity by blocking vasoconstriction input from sympathetic nervous system	Procaine hydrochloride, a local anesthetic, is injected to block sympathetic nerves at the level of 2nd–3rd lumbar vertebra; patient observed for warming of the extremity or decrease in pain

Table 19–5. COMMON VENOUS DIAGNOSTIC STUDIES

STUDY	PURPOSE	PROCEDURE
NONINVASIVE		
Impedance plethysmography	To evaluate presence of iliac or femoral veins; gives information on changes in venous volume after impedance; measures electrical resistance in veins as related to blood volume	Electrodes wrapped around calf; pressure cuff on thigh inflated to impede venous flow; cuff deflated rapidly and measurement of venous flow taken; normally impedance would increase venous volume; if volume remains the same, test is positive for blockage caused by clot along with the presence of Homans' sign or other symptoms of DVT
Perthes' test	To evaluate the competence of valves in saphenous vein or varicose veins or DVT.	Tourniquet applied around thigh or knee; patient asked to walk; previously distended veins collapse if valves are competent; veins remain distended if obstruction or incompetency of valves is present.
Doppler ultrasonogram	To detect auditory signs of blood flow; sound waves bounced off RBCs in vein or artery can detect incompetent valves; sounds of retrograde flow can be discriminated	Conductive jelly applied to skin; Doppler flowmeter detects flow through vessels and magnifies sound; differences in pitch noted; Doppler monitor can be attached to BP cuff to obtain thigh, calf, ankle pressures
INVASIVE		
Venogram or venography	To visually examine veins and valves; has been definitive examination for visualization of clots	Injection of 50 ml of contrast media into veins; procedure is dangerous; contraindicated in patients with suspected or acute phlebitis; exam can precipitate thrombophlebitis
Radionuclide venography	To detect early thrombi in leg veins; useful in patients too ill for venogram; not useful for thrombus in pelvis or femoral area	Radioactive fibrinogen 125 is injected; if thrombi present, iodine isotope will combine with existing clot; clot then can be detected with scintillator scan counter; scan done 12 and 24 hr after injection

Abbreviations: DVT, deep venous thrombosis; BP, blood pressure; RBCs, red blood cells.

on the extremity may be thick, fragile, and shiny, which is indicative of poor circulation to the area. Note any areas of localized redness or cyanosis.

Assessment of the pulses is a first-line diagnostic test. This assessment is ongoing after many invasive diagnostic procedures, vascular surgery, and daily nursing care of the patient with PVD. Evaluation of the pulses is an essential and reliable indicator of the progression or severity of peripheral arterial insufficiency or arterial occlusive disease.

Compare both extremities at one time, and evaluate pulses for their presence or absence. Note the intensity, amplitude, equality, rate, and rhythm of the pulse. Pulses are rated on a scale of 0 (not present) to 4 (full, bounding pulse).

Begin with the most distal pulses and proceed upward. If an abnormality exists, the pulses below the level of the occlusion are affected. Begin assessment of pulses in this order: dorsalis pedis, posterior tibial, popliteal, and femoral. Congenital absence of either the dorsalis pedis or posterior tibial can occur, but this defect does not affect both of these distal pulses in any one individual. Use Doppler ultrasonography on sites of absent pulses because it often establishes the presence of blood flow that was not palpable. Auscultate with a stethoscope for bruits, especially over the popliteal, femoral, and abdominal areas.

Assess the arterial flow by having the patient lie flat with the arms (or legs) raised above the level of the heart. Have the patient wave the extremities for a few moments. Then have the patient sit upright. The extremity appears slightly pale at first, but color should return within 10 seconds. Delayed pallor or mottling indicates an arterial insufficiency problem. Compare the extremities bilaterally, and document all findings.

Table 19–6. NURSING ACTIONS FOR INVASIVE CONTRAST MEDIA STUDIES: ARTERIOGRAPHY AND VENOGRAPHY

ACTION	RATIONALE
BEFORE PROCEDURE	
1. Obtain baseline data: Check extremities: Pulse Color, sensation Temperature, movement Vital signs	Baseline data are used for post-procedure comparison; changes in neurovascular parameters after procedure indicate increased occlusion and limb-threatening ischemia.
2. Assess patient for allergy to iodine or seafood.	Iodine is used in contrast media injected during the procedure. Allergic reaction and anaphylactic shock could occur.
3. Clarify purpose and patient involvement during procedure, and explain that contrast medium causes feeling of warmth or burning during injection.	Clarification will alleviate anxiety and ensure patient cooperation.
4. Obtain permit.	These are invasive procedures; legal documentation of patient informed consent is required.
DURING AND AFTER PROCEDURE	
1. Observe for allergic reaction signs and symptoms: Dyspnea Flushing or hives Nausea or vomiting Tachycardia or hypotension Numbness in extremity	Allergic reactions may occur during or even a few hours after procedure.
2. Monitor and compare baseline vital signs, extremity pulses, and neurovascular integrity, per recovery protocol, beginning with every 15 min and then hourly for up to 4 hr.	Changes in vital signs may indicate complications.
3. Check extremity for the following: Pulses Pallor Cyanosis Decrease in temperature Numbness or paralysis	Bleeding and neurovascular compromise can be life- or limb-threatening.
4. Maintain patient on bed rest with extremity extended 4–6 hr after procedure.	Rest promotes reduction in bleeding.
5. Check injection site dressing for bleeding or hematoma formation with each vital sign and neurovascular assessment.	Bleeding may indicate serious complications.
6. Encourage oral fluids.	Consumption of oral fluids enhances excretion of contrast media.

Diagnostic Procedures

There are numerous diagnostic studies used in a workup for peripheral vascular dysfunction. These are classified as noninvasive or invasive. Tables 19–4 and 19–5 summarize arterial and venous diagnostic testing, respectively.

The purpose and procedure involved in the diagnostic examination is explained to the patient to alleviate anxiety and elicit cooperation. Time is provided for the patient to ask questions (Nursing Care Guide 19–1). All invasive diagnostic procedures require a signed informed consent. Table 19–6 summarizes nursing actions for patients undergoing invasive venography or arteriography.

Medical Management

The overall objective of medical management of patients with peripheral vascular dysfunction is to increase blood flow to the ischemic tissues. The approaches taken depend on the acuity of the disease process. Specific management is discussed with each disorder in Chapter 20. Some general approaches to management are addressed in this chapter.

Nursing Care Guide 19–1.

PATIENTS UNDERGOING DIAGNOSTIC TESTING FOR PERIPHERAL VASCULAR DYSFUNCTION

Assessment Findings: Patient presents with signs of restlessness, nervousness, increased respiratory, and heart rate; asks questions about procedures; and clenches hands and cries.

Nursing Diagnosis: Anxiety related to fear of procedure, diagnosis, and future medical/surgical management

Patient Outcomes	Nursing Interventions	Rationale
Patient practices relaxation techniques for relief of tension and anxiety.	Teach relaxation techniques. Help the patient find coping strategies that help alleviate the stress and anxiety.	Implementation of relaxation exercises reduces stress and anxiety.
Patient appears less anxious, as evidenced by smiling; lack of restlessness, crying, or nervousness; and vital signs within normal limits.	Explain the diagnostic procedure to the patient and family. Allow time for questions and concerns. Check vital signs.	An understanding of the procedure may alleviate some of the fear and anxiety. Vital signs within normal limits may indicate relief of anxiety.

Evaluation: Compare the patient's status with the expected patient outcomes. If the outcomes are achieved, evaluate nursing care as successful. If not, reassess the patient, formulate new nursing diagnoses, and revise expected patient outcomes and nursing interventions as appropriate.

(continued)

Nursing Care Guide 19–1. *(continued)*

PATIENTS UNDERGOING DIAGNOSTIC TESTING FOR PERIPHERAL VASCULAR DYSFUNCTION

Assessment Findings: Patient and family ask questions about the diagnostic procedure and seem uninformed about preprocedure and postprocedure care, if necessary. Patient and family voice concerns about risks and necessity for the procedure, especially if an invasive test is to be done.

Nursing Diagnosis: Knowledge deficit: nature of the diagnostic procedure and postprocedure care

Patient Outcomes	Nursing Interventions	Rationale
Patient and family state they have an understanding of the diagnostic procedure, the risks, and the postprocedure care needed, if applicable.	Be certain the physician has discussed the procedure, risks, complications, and expectations to the patient.	An understanding of the procedure is important to increase patient compliance and reduce fears about the diagnostic testing.
	Give the patient and family literature about the procedure if available. Allow the patient to ask questions, and try to expand on the understanding about the procedure for the patient and family.	Including the family in the sessions reinforces the information provided. Misinformation can be corrected during the question session.
Patient reports accurate information about the diagnostic procedure, the potential risks, and the necessity for it.	Have the patient restate the information received.	Reiteration of the information allows for an assessment of the patient's understanding.
	Explain the postprocedure care needed.	
	Tell the patient to notify the physician if any untoward symptoms occur after discharge.	Follow-up care is necessary to prevent complications.

Evaluation: Compare the patient's status with the expected patient outcomes. If the outcomes are achieved, evaluate nursing care as successful. If not, reassess the patient, formulate new nursing diagnoses, and revise expected patient outcomes and nursing interventions as appropriate.

Pharmacology Box 19–1.

LIPID-LOWERING DRUGS (HYPOLIPEMICS)

Hypolipemics:
Lipid-lowering drugs used in patients with levels of hyperlipoproteinemia that are associated with an increased risk of atherosclerosis and its complications.

Action:
The prototype drug, cholestyramine (Questran), lowers cholesterol level by binding with bile acids in the intestine, changing cholesterol into an insoluble complex that is eliminated in feces. Lovastatin (Mevacor) blocks the enzyme nesessary for the synthesis of cholesterol in the liver.

Use:
As adjunct therapy when diet, exercise, weight reduction, and other nonpharmacologic methods of risk-factor control have failed to reduce blood lipid levels.

Side Effects:
May interfere with or enhance the oral absorption of anticoagulants; the bile-sequestering resins may interfere with absorption of vitamin K and thus reduce prothrombin; they can produce flatulence, constipation, liver function abnormalities, diarrhea, abdominal pain, or heartburn; they interfere with absorption of digitalis, folic acid, and corticosteroids.

Interactions:
Bile acid sequestrants and vitamins A, D, E, and K (may bind with the vitamins).

Nursing Implications:
Establish baseline lipid levels before therapy is begun and periodically during therapy. Administer routine medications before meals or 4 hr after. Monitor for bleeding tendencies. Assess for constipation, especially in the elderly. Report gastrointestinal symptoms that persist. Lipid-lowering drugs are contraindicated in pregnancy.

Nonsurgical Management

Conservative approaches to management include reduction of risk factors, exercise, and medication. Nonsurgical procedures such as angioplasty and laser thermal angioplasty are common noninvasive techniques used for some patients to improve peripheral circulation.

REDUCTION OF RISK FACTORS

A reduction in modifiable risk factors is accomplished through diet, exercise, and other lifestyle adjustments. For patients with high cholesterol levels, drug therapy may be instituted. Cigarette smoking is discouraged. Routine medical evaluation with laboratory assessments is prescribed.

EXERCISE

A slow, progressive exercise program can be effective for patients with intermittent claudication if there is no contraindication or performance deficit such as severe respiratory, cardiac, or musculoskeletal dysfunction. Exercise is also beneficial for reducing some of the modifiable risk factors (see Table 19–3). The patient may be referred to an exercise therapist for a prescribed regimen of physical activity.

MEDICATIONS

A combination of drugs may be used in arterial PVD, but their efficacy in improving circulation is questionable because the basic problem of atherosclerosis is irreversible. At best, they may provide some relief of symptoms or prevent further arterial plaque accumulation. These medications include vasodilators, hypolipemics, anticoagulants, defibrination agents, and antiplatelet therapy (Pharmacology Boxes 19–1 and 19–2). Drug therapy may improve blood flow at rest but has negligible effect on the increased tissue oxygenation needs with activity. Table 19–7 summarizes some representative drugs used.

Pharmacology Box 19–2.
ANTICOAGULANTS

Anticoagulants:
Drugs that affect the ability of the blood to form fibrin clots; includes heparin, warfarin sodium, and dicumarol.

Action:
Inhibit various stages of the blood-clotting cycle depending on the specific anticoagulant.

Uses:
Treatment of deep venous thrombosis, pulmonary emboli, myocardial infarction, rheumatic heart disease, and prevention of clot formation.

Side Effects:
Excessive anticoagulation, causing petechiae, bruising, hematomas, ecchymoses, and hemorrhage.

Interactions:
May interact with other protein-bound drugs such as salicylates. Metabolism of anticoagulants may also be enhanced by drugs that increase liver enzyme production.

Nursing Implications:
Check coagulation studies before giving each dose of anticoagulant and intermittently throughout the patient's hospital stay. Check frequently for signs of bleeding such as petechiae and ecchymoses. Teach the patient to practice safety measures to prevent cuts and scratches, which may bleed excessively.

Geriatric Considerations:
Bruising, especially on the hands, arms, and legs, and bleeding of mucous membranes may be more prominent. Special safety and care measures are needed to prevent injury and bleeding episodes because capillaries are more fragile in the older adult.

ANALGESICS

Pain management is a challenge. Pain relief may not be fully accomplished until measures are taken to remove the source of pain: the obstructed blood flow. Both narcotic and nonnarcotic analgesics are used to control the pain of advanced ischemia. The patient often requires increasing doses as the disease progresses. It is important to keep the analgesic level even. Instruct the patient to ask for medication before the pain becomes intolerable. Patient-controlled analgesia (PCA) is often used. It has the

Table 19–7. MEDICATIONS USED IN PERIPHERAL VASCULAR DISEASE

CLASSIFICATION	DRUG	EFFECTS
Vasodilator	Isoxuprine hydrochloride (Vasodilan)	Acts directly on vascular smooth muscles. High doses also inhibit platelet aggregation and decrease blood viscosity.
Antiplatelet or defibrination agent	Pentoxifylline (Trental)	Makes RBCs more flexible, thereby facilitating movement through the capillary. It decreases platelet and RBC aggregation and decreases blood viscosity.
Antiplatelet	Aspirin	Powerfully inhibits platelet aggregation. Effects may persist 3–8 days.
Antiplatelet and vasodilator	Dipyridamole (Persantine)	Vasodilation effects are only slight in peripheral arteries. Drug inhibits platelet aggregation. It is usually prescribed with aspirin.
Anticoagulant	Heparin	Prevention of clot (thrombosis) formation by blocking several factors essential to normal blood clotting. It is used prophylactically or in acute disease states.

added benefit of increasing the patient's sense of control and decreasing powerlessness in coping with the pain.

Sustained-action morphine sulfate (MS Contin) is a 12-hour sustained-release tablet that may provide relief. Sympathetic nerve blocks are occasionally used when other analgesia has failed.

ANGIOPLASTY

Peripheral angioplasty is a nonsurgical but invasive procedure. Percutaneous transluminal angioplasty (PTA) involves the insertion of an inflatable balloon-tipped catheter into an identified area of arterial blockage. The balloon is inflated, compressing atherosclerotic plaque and thereby enlarging and smoothing the lumen of the affected vessel and increasing blood flow. Blockages in the iliac and femoral arteries have had the greatest success with PTA. The procedure can be repeated if the vessel reoccludes. Reocclusion of the artery may be immediate. Thirty percent of vessels reocclude during the first 6 months. Many arteries remain patent from 1 to 5 years. The procedure is of benefit for patients who are poor surgical risks, because local anesthesia is used. Successful angioplasty restores pulses, improves extremity tissue integrity, and abates or lessens claudication pain.

Complications of angioplasty include stenosis, thrombi formation, embolism, or bleeding. Heparin is often given for 3 days after the procedure. The patient is prescribed home-maintenance antiplatelet therapy with aspirin and dipyridamole.

LASER THERMAL ANGIOPLASTY

Laser thermal angioplasty can be performed in conjunction with PTA. The laser-tipped fiberoptic catheter heats to approximately 400°C, vaporizes the atherosclerotic plaque, and opens a channel for blood flow. Laser probe angioplasty is believed to produce a smoother vessel lumen and a decreased frequency of reocclusion.

Guidelines for Application of the Nursing Process to the Care of the Patient Undergoing Angioplasty

Nursing care for the patient undergoing angioplasty is essentially the same as with an arteriography (see Table 19–6). Preoperatively, the patient is allowed *nothing by mouth* (NPO). The groin area is prepared with a surgical scrub. The physician may order the area shaved before the scrub.

After the procedure, the patient is on bed rest, with the affected extremity maintained in straight alignment for 6 to 8 hours. Monitor laboratory values for prolonged clotting times because the patient is often heparinized during and after the procedure. Blood coagulation studies include prothrombin time (PT), partial thromboplastin time (PTT), and activated clotting time (ACT). ACT can be done at the bedside. Desirable levels for these laboratory tests to maintain vessel patency is two times the control.

Assess for bleeding or hematoma formation at the angioplasty insertion site. Palpate the tissues around the site for distention from hematoma. Measure abdominal girth every 4 hours for patients with iliac artery angioplasty. They are more likely to manifest retroperitoneal bleeding. Monitor for signs of shock from retroperitoneal hemorrhage. (See Chart 19–1 for discharge instructions.)

Surgical Management

Management by surgical intervention is necessary when ischemic pain interferes with activity and threatens tissue loss. Thre are many surgical procedures that can restore circulation and thus decrease pain and improve tissue integrity. These procedures enable an individual to improve the quality of life.

SYMPATHECTOMY

Sympathectomy is a palliative surgery. It consists of excision of the second and third lumbar sympathetic ganglia. It blocks vasoconstricting input, thus reducing pain and improving peripheral blood flow, especially to the skin of the lower extremities. It may be of benefit to patients with chronic arterial occlusive disease. A diagnostic lumbar sympathetic block is performed before the surgical procedure. A sympathectomy is considered if the extremities warmed in response to the block. Warming of the extremity establishes the presence of adequate collateral blood flow, which is recommended for a sympathectomy to be successful. This procedure permanently dilates blood vessels, thus improving collateral circulation.

Arteries and arterioles made "stiff" from atherosclerosis are unable to dilate. These patients are poor candidates for sympathectomy. The procedure permanently dilates blood vessels, thus improving collateral circulation. It is seldom done with the advent of angioplasty and other surgical procedures that directly improve blood flow.

GRAFTS

A patch graft removes the diseased part of the artery and replaces it with a "patch" from the pa-

Chart 19–1.

NURSING GUIDE TO PATIENT EDUCATION FOR SELF-MANAGEMENT: GENERAL DISCHARGE INSTRUCTIONS AFTER ANGIOPLASTY

Instruct the patient who has undergone peripheral angioplasty to:

Observe for active bleeding or bruising at the puncture sites.
Observe the extremities for pallor, coldness, discoloration, numbness, or tingling.
Drink an increased amount of fluid, unless otherwise contraindicated, to assist the excretion of the contrast media.
Check temperature for elevation, which may be indicative of an infection.
Check the puncture sites for drainage (other than bleeding) or swelling, which may indicate localized infection.
Notify the physician if any of the above untoward symptoms occur.

tient's vein, usually the saphenous vein. This method is preferred over a synthetic graft made of Dacron or Teflon because thrombosis is less likely to occur. A vein patch may also be used to widen an artery.

A bypass graft leaves the diseased area intact but bypasses it with a graft, either the patient's saphenous vein or a synthetic material. The saphenous vein is the preferred grafting material, but many patients have concomitant coronary artery disease and may need the saphenous vein for a future coronary artery bypass graft. Before grafting, an arteriography is done to determine the presence of blood flow in vessels below the obstruction and the best location for the graft. Bypass grafting is preferred over excision and replacement grafting because collateral circulation is maintained. The success rate of grafting is better in larger vessels. The successful reestablishment of blood flow is evidenced by return of pulses, warming of the extremity, and decreased ischemic pain.

PHYSICAL PREPARATION OF THE PATIENT

Inform the patient about the procedure, its risks, and the postoperative course. Begin physical preparation after the operative permit is signed. Prepare the surgical site per protocol. Administer prophylactic antibiotics if they are ordered.

POSTOPERATIVE COURSE

If the surgically revascularized vessel remains patent, the postoperative course is usually uneventful, and the patient is ambulating the first postoperative day. Anticoagulation therapy is frequently instituted with heparin or low-molecular-weight dextran to prevent thrombus formation. Postoperative noninvasive arterial studies give baseline information for future management.

COMPLICATIONS

The most common postoperative complication is graft occlusion, usually occurring in the first 24 hours. Other complications include bleeding, infection, and delayed wound healing resulting from the effects of prolonged tissue ischemia.

EMBOLECTOMY

An embolectomy is the surgical removal of a clot (thrombus) in the vessel. This procedure is performed when a major vessel is acutely occluded, thus impeding the flow of blood to a large area of tissue. Ischemia is severe. Distal extremities become cyanotic and mottled. The surgery is often an emergency and is most successful when performed within 8 to 10 hours after the clot has formed. Anticoagulant therapy is used postoperatively to prevent further thrombus formation (see Pharmacology Box 19–2).

ENDARTERECTOMY

Endarterectomy is the surgical removal or "reaming out" of fatty plaques from the inner (tunica intima) and middle (tunica media) layers of vessel walls. The artery is incised, cleaned out, and then sutured closed. An endarterectomy is most successful if the atheromatous plaque accumulation is localized. This procedure is contraindicated in patients with aneurysmal (vessel wall weakening and dilation) changes, total occlusion of the aortic branch to renal arteries, or a major aortic occlusion that extends into the iliac and femoral arteries.

AMPUTATION

Amputation—surgical removal of part or all of an extremity—is often the only therapeutic option when areas are hopelessly ischemic, painful, and gangrenous. It is often the culmination of months of ischemic rest pain and progressive tissue degeneration. Individuals with PVD have the highest amputation incidence, 85%, compared with traumatic or infectious causes.

The elderly with PVD constitute the largest amputation population group. Of this group, diabetic elderly male smokers have the highest amputation rate. Even though the surgical procedure provides relief to the ischemic pain, it represents a major assault to the independence and coping ability of an elderly individual.

The level of amputation is dictated by peripheral vascular diagnostic studies. Arterial obstructive gangrene requires identification of circulation adequacy proximal to the amputation level for optimal tissue healing after the procedure.

A long rehabilitation course to functional upright ambulation is dependent on stump healing, adequacy of circulation in the remaining leg, the patient's overall health, and motivation. Ambulation with a prosthesis requires a tremendous expenditure of energy and coordination. It may not be a viable option for the individual with a PVD-induced amputation. Wheelchair independence and acceptance may be the optimal goal.

Loss of an extremity is always a devastating event. The grieving process may have been underway through the period preceding the amputation. Support of the patient throughout care hastens the acceptance phase of a changed body image.

Many PVD-induced amputations could be prevented by meticulous foot care and prevention of cuts and abrasions of the extremities. The foot is quite vulnerable, being the most distal to the area of ischemic flow. Wound healing is impaired because of a lack of normal tissue nutrition.

Dry, gangrenous toe tips with no evidence of infection or cellulitis may be allowed to autoamputate. This is a nonsurgical spontaneous separation of the devitalized tissue. Chapter 35 presents a detailed description of amputation and rehabilitation aspects.

Application of the Nursing Process to the Care of the Patient Undergoing Peripheral Vascular Surgery

PREOPERATIVE NURSING CARE

Assessment

Obtain a history, and perform a complete physical assessment to evaluate the health status of all body systems. Determine risk factors presented by nutritional deficits, lifestyle, and involvement of cardiac, respiratory, or endocrine systems that could complicate surgery.

Nursing Diagnoses and Planning

The nursing diagnosis and related expected patient outcomes most commonly applicable to patients scheduled for peripheral vascular surgery are as follows:

NDx: Knowledge deficit: surgical procedure and postoperative course

Planning: Patient outcomes

1. Patient states accurate information about the surgical procedure and expected results.
2. Patient describes the typical postoperative course.

Nursing Interventions

NDx: Knowledge deficit: surgical procedure and postoperative course

Assess the patient's understanding about the surgical procedure, its risks, the usual postoperative course, and self-care responsibilities after discharge. Explain all facets of the procedure, the recovery period, and the postoperative care required. Tell the patient about medications, activity progression, and routine postoperative deep-breathing exercises. Provide time for the patient and family to ask questions and verbalize concerns.

Evaluation

Evaluate the effectiveness of nursing care for a patient who is scheduled for peripheral vascular surgery by comparing the patient's status with the expected patient outcomes. Examples of specific outcomes for patients scheduled for peripheral vascular surgery have been provided in the Planning section.

POSTOPERATIVE NURSING CARE

Assessment

Assess the patient's dressing for bleeding and the patient's vital signs, level of consciousness, respiratory pattern, skin temperature, and color. Check the integrity of the intravenous site. Evaluate the patient's level of pain.

Complete a critical assessment of pulses and other parameters of neurovascular compromise that indicate thrombosis or reocclusion. Monitor blood coagulation; study results for abnormal bleeding times.

Nursing Diagnoses and Planning

Nursing diagnoses and related expected patient outcomes most commonly applicable to patients undergoing peripheral vascular surgery include the following:

NDx: Altered tissue perfusion, peripheral, related to thrombus formation or reocclusion induced by the previous existing vascular dysfunction or excessive bleeding

Planning: Patient outcomes

1. Patient exhibits palpable pulses, adequate temperature, sensation, and color in extremities.
2. No excessive bleeding develops.
3. Patient experiences no ischemic pain.
4. Patient's laboratory coagulation studies are within safe range.

NDx: High risk for infection related to surgical incision, location, length, and presurgical tissue integrity

Planning: Patient outcomes

1. Patient demonstrates a dry, nondraining wound with no evidence of erythema or swelling.
2. Patient is free of signs of infection (afebrile, normal white blood cell count).

NDx: Pain related to incision or acute postsurgical thrombus occlusion

Planning: Patient outcomes

1. Patient states pain is relieved.
2. Patient is able to mobilize freely without extreme discomfort.
3. Patient is able to participate in self-care.

NDx: Altered health maintenance related to lack of knowledge of self-care after discharge

Planning: Patient outcomes

1. Patient relates accurate information on wound care, medications, potential complications, and the need to seek medical attention if these occur.
2. Patient palpates pulses and inspects incision and skin daily for changes in color, temperature, and integrity.
3. Patient is able to increase activity as prescribed.
4. Patient states the need for follow-up care.

Nursing Interventions

NDx: Altered tissue perfusion, peripheral

Monitor neurocirculatory status for signs of reocclusion. Ask the patient to report changes in color or sensation. Assess pulses, mark location of distal pulses, and use Doppler ultrasonography for nonpalpable pulses. Check color, sensation, temperature, and motor ability in the affected extremities, and document the changes. Notify the physician of abnormalities, because sudden changes indicate acute occlusion, requiring emergency medical intervention.

Ask the patient to wiggle the toes and to perform dorsiflexion and flexion of the plantar area of the foot. Note any complaints of pain in the extremity at rest or excessive pain with movement, and check for paresthesia. Measure the girth of the extremity, and check for swelling. Document findings for a postoperative baseline. Some swelling is expected as the result of surgical tissue trauma and as a rebound effect of tissues becoming revascularized after a period of ischemic flow. Edema can also be caused from hemorrhage into the tissues from a leaking graft. Excessive accumulation of fluid in the muscle compartment can compromise tissue perfusion and cause nerve compression and result in compartment syndrome. The classic signs of compartment syndrome are excessive pain at rest that is increased with movement and paresthesias. Notify the physician immediately; an emergency fasciotomy may be required.

Keep the extremity in straight alignment per physician's protocol, usually 24 hours after major grafting. Position the patient off of the graft site or drains. Avoid extreme flexion of the extremity. These interventions prevent trauma to the graft, and promote optimal circulation.

Monitor vital signs for evidence of shock. Maintain blood pressure at the prescribed level. An elevated blood pressure can place too much stress on the graft and cause rupture and hemorrhage.

NDx: High risk for infection

Use strict aseptic techniques when changing dressings or handling intravenous equipment. Monitor temperature and white blood cell count reports. Inspect the incision for warmth, erythema, swelling, unusual drainage, and wound approximation.

Observe and prevent skin breakdown by position changes and early mobilization of the patient. Have the patient cough and deep breath every 2 hours to prevent respiratory infection.

NDx: Pain

Manage operative pain with prescribed analgesics, and note patient responses. Encourage verbalization of discomfort before pain becomes intolerable; PCA is often used. Incisional pain is usually the greatest during first 4 postoperative days. Revascularization pain is sometimes experienced as a throbbing sensation. The return of ischemic pain indicates reocclusion; notify the physician immediately.

NDx: Altered health maintenance

Teach the patient about the care of the surgical incision and how to complete an aseptic dressing change. Explain the signs and symptoms of complications and when to seek medical intervention. Inform the patient of activity restriction such as avoiding long periods of sitting, leg crossing, extreme flexion, and heavy lifting. Reinforce teaching of the prescribed progression of ambulation. Teach how to perform pulse checks and assess extremities. Reinforce teaching on the importance of daily foot care and the reduction of risk factors for peripheral vascular dysfunction.

Evaluation

Evaluate the effectiveness of nursing care for a patient undergoing peripheral vascular surgery by comparing the patient's status with the expected patient outcomes. Examples of specific outcomes for patients undergoing peripheral vascular surgery have been provided in the Planning section.

The Elderly: Special Considerations

PVD is essentially an age-related dysfunction. The elderly comprise the largest PVD population group. Elderly male smokers have the highest incidence of disorders of the vascular system.

Changes in the integrity of the blood vessels occur as the result of progressive atherosclerosis. The aorta becomes thicker and less elastic; thus, additional strain is placed on the left ventricle of the heart to pump blood into the systemic circulation.

All the arterial vessel layers can be affected by the aging process. The outer layer develops increased connective tissue. The smooth muscle fibers in the middle layer become less responsive to hormonal influence and vasoconstrictor input from the sympathetic nervous system. Calcium deposition in the medial layer makes the vessel stiffer and less distensible. The intimal layer of the vessel is affected by the buildup of atherosclerotic plaque.

Veins also lose elasticity with age. The vessel walls become weakened. Varicosities or abnormal dilation of the veins can result from overdistention of these weakened veins. Decreased muscular activity as a result of chronic multisystem effects of aging impede venous return. Venous stasis from bed rest, surgery, and immobility in the elderly is associated with a high incidence of venous thrombus formation, embolization, and death.

Capillaries are also altered in the aging process. The single-layer endothelial cells rest on a collagen-like material called the basement membrane. This membrane also thickens with age, hampering cellular nutrition and waste-product removal. Persistent lack of cellular nutrition makes the elderly person a greater risk for infection and poor wound healing. The healing abilities of the elderly are already compromised by a decreased immunologic response and changes in other body systems.

Chronic PVD in the elderly is an assault to physiologic and psychological integrity. Pain, limitations of mobility, and disruptions in skin integrity can produce a feeling of powerlessness in the elderly individual with PVD. All nursing measures that assist the person to have knowledge of the disease process, preventive factors, participation in care, and decision making lessen this response.

Bibliography

Alspach J (ed). American Association of Critical Care Nurses. Core curriculum for critical care nursing. 4th ed. Philadelphia: WB Saunders, 1991.

Appleton DL, Ouaglia JD. Vascular disease and postoperative nursing management. Crit Care Nurse 1985; 4:34.

Baquie M. What matters most in chronic pain management. RN 1989; 52(3):46.

Baum PL. Heed the early warning signs of peripheral vascular disease. Nursing 1985; 15(3):50.

Beasley-Dixon M, Nunnelee J. Arterial reconstruction for atherosclerotic occlusive disease. J Cardiovasc Nurs 1987; 1(2):36.

Benson JL, Allastair KM. In situ artery bypass. AORN J 1987; 45:40.

Blank C, Irwin G. Peripheral vascular disorders: Assessment and intervention. Nurs Clin North Am 1990; 25(4):777.

Blankenship D, Clegg L, Powell D. Post arteriographic pressure dressings: Two types. Crit Care Nurse 1991; 11(5):92.

Borkowski-Weller D. Urokinase: Restoring circulation without surgery. RN 1990; 53(10):44.

Brooks G, Fahey T. Exercise physiology: Human bioenergetics and its applications. New York: Macmillan, 1985.

Carpenito L. Nursing care plans and documentation: Nursing diagnoses and collaborative problems. New York: JB Lippincott, 1991.

Dickinson R. Our way, VI ulcers heal. RN 1990; 53(7):32.

Dixon MB, Nunnelee J. Arterial reconstruction for atherosclerotic occlusive disease. J Cardiovasc Nurs 1987; 1(2):36.

Ernest C, Stanley J (eds). Current therapy in vascular surgery. 2nd ed. Philadelphia: BC Decker, 1991.

Fahey VA. Vascular nursing. Philadelphia: WB Saunders, 1988.

Fellows E, Jocz AM. Getting the upper hand on lower extremity arterial disease. Nursing 1991; 21(8):34.

Govoni L, Hayes J. Drugs and nursing implications. 6th ed. Norwalk, CT: Appleton & Lange, 1988.

Guyton AC. Human physiology and the mechanisms of disease. 5th ed. Philadelphia: WB Saunders, 1992.

Guyton AC. Textbook of medical physiology. 8th ed. Philadelphia: WB Saunders, 1991.

Haimovci H. Vascular surgery: Principles and techniques. 2nd ed. New York: Appleton-Century-Crofts, 1984.

Helden ER. The cholesterol enigma. J Soc Peripheral Vasc Nurs 1987; 4:5.

Herman J. Nursing assessment and nursing diagnosis in patients with peripheral vascular disease. Nurs Clin North Am 1986; 21:219.

Hill S. Interventions for the elderly amputee. Rehabil Nurs 1985; 10(3):23.

Howard P. Elevated cholesterol: A nurse's guide to drug therapy. RN 1991; 54(8):26.

Hubner C. Exercise therapy and smoking cessation for intermittent claudication. J Cardiovasc Nurs 1987; 1(2):50.

Huisman MV, Buller HR, Ten Cate JW, Vreeken J. Serial impedance plethysmography for suspected deep venous thrombosis in out-patients. N Engl J Med 1986; 314:823.

Ignatavicius D, Bayne M. Medical-surgical nursing: A nursing process approach. Philadelphia: WB Saunders, 1991.

Kannel WB, McGee DL. Update on some epidemiologic features of intermittent claudication: The Framingham study. J Am Geriatr Soc 1985; 33(1):13.

Matteson M, McConnell E. Gerontological nursing: Concepts and practice. Philadelphia: WB Saunders, 1988.

Merry J. Take your assessment all the way down to the toes. RN 1988; 51(1):60.

Miller R, Evans W. Nurse and patient: Allies preventing amputation. RN 1988; 51(7):38.

National Cholesterol Education Program. Report of the Expert Panel on Population Strategies for Blood Cholesterol Reduction (NIH publication no. 90-3046). Washington, DC: U.S. Department of Health and Human Services.

Paul M, Halfman-Franey M. Laser angioplasty in peripheral vascular disease. Crit Care Nurse 1990; 10(5):65.

Porth C. Pathophysiology: Concepts of altered health states. 2nd ed. Philadelphia: JB Lippincott, 1986.

Sakallaris BR. Laser therapy for cardiovascular disease. Heart Lung 1987; 16(5):465.

Sanborn TA, Haudenschild CC, Garber GR, et al. Angiographic and histologic consequences of laser thermal angioplasty: Comparison with balloon angioplasty. Circulation 1987; 75(6):1281.

Tretbar LL. Chronic venous insufficiency of the legs: Pathogenesis of venous ulcers. J Enterostomal Ther 1987; 14:105.

Turner JA. Nursing interventions in patients with peripheral vascular disease. Nurs Clin North Am 1986; 21:233.

Witztum JL, Simmons D, Steinberg D, et al. Intensive combination drug therapy of familiar hypercholesterolemia with lovastatin, probucol, and colestipol. Circulation 1989; 79(1):16.

Zacca NM, Raizner AE, Noon GD, et al. Treatment of symptomatic peripheral atherosclerotic disease with a rotational atherectomy device. Am J Cardiol 1989; 62:77.

Chapter Twenty

NURSING CARE *of Adults with Vascular Disorders*

Vascular disorders encompass all diseases of the blood vessels, arteries and veins, and lymphatic vessels. The most common disorders of the vessels are the obstructive disorders such as atherosclerosis and arteriosclerosis. Many of the changes in the vessels occur with the aging process, but lifestyle has been found to be a significant contributing factor to the incidence of vessel occlusive diseases. Disorders of the vascular system may cause pain, decrease mobility, interefere with peripheral circulation, and exacerbate other disease processes.

Many of the diseases of the vascular system are chronic and debilitating. This presents specific implications for nursing care. Because the elderly, in particular, are prone to vascular disorders, long-term care planning, home care instructions, and follow-up care are all important facets of nursing interventions. Referrals to other agencies outside the hospital for continued care may be necessary for the patient with a vascular disorder because of the chronicity of the disease.

Common Arterial Vascular Disorders

The collective group of common arterial vascular disorders includes inflammatory conditions such as Buerger's disease and inflammations of the aorta; functional and structural problems that are obstructive in nature, such as Raynaud's disease or atherosclerosis and arteriosclerosis; and other structural abnormalities, such as aneurysms.

Thromboangiitis Obliterans (Buerger's Disease)

ETIOLOGY

Thromboangiitis obliterans is a chronic imflammatory process involving the medium-size arteries and veins, leading to arterial vessel occlusion. Early stages are characterized by acute inflammation followed by remission lasting weeks to years. The disease most often affects male smokers between 20 and 45 years of age. The greatest incidence occurs among Jewish and Asian individuals. Although the exact cause is unknown, it is thought to be due to a reaction to the excessive use of nicotine over a long period of time. The incidence of the disease has decreased in recent years.

PATHOPHYSIOLOGY

The arteries of the lower extremities are most often involved. Large arteries and veins are rarely involved unless it is late in the disease process. Lesions consisting of abscesses develop in specific areas. The arteries contract in the region of the destruction, and occlusion occurs. Cellular proliferation of the intima predisposes to thrombi development in the vessels, contributing to the occlusion and causing intense pain.

Although the disease affects both arteries and veins, arteries are more commonly and more severely affected. Spasms may also occur in the vessels, further decreasing the blood flow and causing increased ischemia.

CLINICAL MANIFESTATIONS

Peripheral vascular ischemia results in cold extremities. The distal portions of the hands and feet are extremely pale. In the later stages of the disease, rubor may be present when the extremity is in a dependent position. Pain is one of the most common and most severe manifestations of thromboangiitis obliterans. In the early stages, it may affect only the palm of the hand and the arch of the foot. As the disease progresses, the pain may be excruciating. Rest pain, numbness, burning, and impaired sensation result from ischemic neuropathy.

Pulses of the dorsalis pedis, posterior tibial, ulnar, and radial arteries are weak or absent from the decreased blood supply to the periphery. The extremities may become edematous in advanced stages. Nail ulcers and gangrene may result from infections and tissue necrosis.

MEDICAL DIAGNOSIS

The diagnosis is made on the basis of the history, physical assessment, and laboratory studies. Arteriography of the extremities, oscillometry, skin temperature studies, and x-ray films may also be used to determine the diagnosis. The peripheral pulses are checked with a Doppler ultrasonogram.

MEDICAL MANAGEMENT

Smoking is prohibited because nicotine produces vasoconstriction and exacerbates the disease. Pharmacologic intervention includes analgesics for pain control and vasodilators to increase blood flow to the extremities. A sympathectomy may be done to promote vasodilation, enhance circulation to the skin, and relieve rest pain. Buerger-Allen exercises are prescribed to promote vasodilation (Chart 20–1 and Fig. 20–1). Amputation of the fingers and toes or a below-the-knee amputation may be necessary if gangrene is present or if pain cannot be controlled.

Application of the Nursing Process to the Care of the Patient with Thromboangiitis Obliterans

Assessment

Review the patient's history and diagnostic findings. Perform a physical assessment, focusing on the cir-

Chart 20–1.

NURSING GUIDE TO PATIENT EDUCATION FOR SELF-MANAGEMENT: DISCHARGE INSTRUCTIONS FOR THE PATIENT WITH BUERGER'S DISEASE; BUERGER-ALLEN EXERCISES

Teach the patient with Buerger's disease to perform Buerger-Allen exercises to improve the circulation to the legs and feet (see Fig. 20–1). Instruct the patient to:

Elevate the feet and legs to a 45-degree to 90-degree angle or until the color of the skin of the legs blanches, and support them in this position for 2 to 3 minutes.
Lower the legs and feet to a position beneath the rest of the body or until the color of the skin of the legs turns red, and support them in this position for 5 to 10 minutes.
Raise the legs and feet to a flat position, even with the body in a supine position, and rest them on the bed in this position for 10 minutes.
Repeat the routine to the patient's level of tolerance.

culation of the extremities. Palpate distal pulses bilaterally. Note the presence, rate, regularity, and intensity of each. Assess the extremities for color, temperature, and sensation. Assess for the presence of pain, noting the location, intensity, precipitating factors, duration, frequency, radiation, and relief methods. Check for edema, lesions, or gangrene of the extremities. Note whether the patient is taking any medications or smokes cigarettes.

Nursing Diagnoses and Planning

Nursing diagnoses and related expected patient outcomes most commonly applicable to patients with thromboangiitis obliterans include the following:

NDx: Pain related to the inflammation and ischemia secondary to the disease state

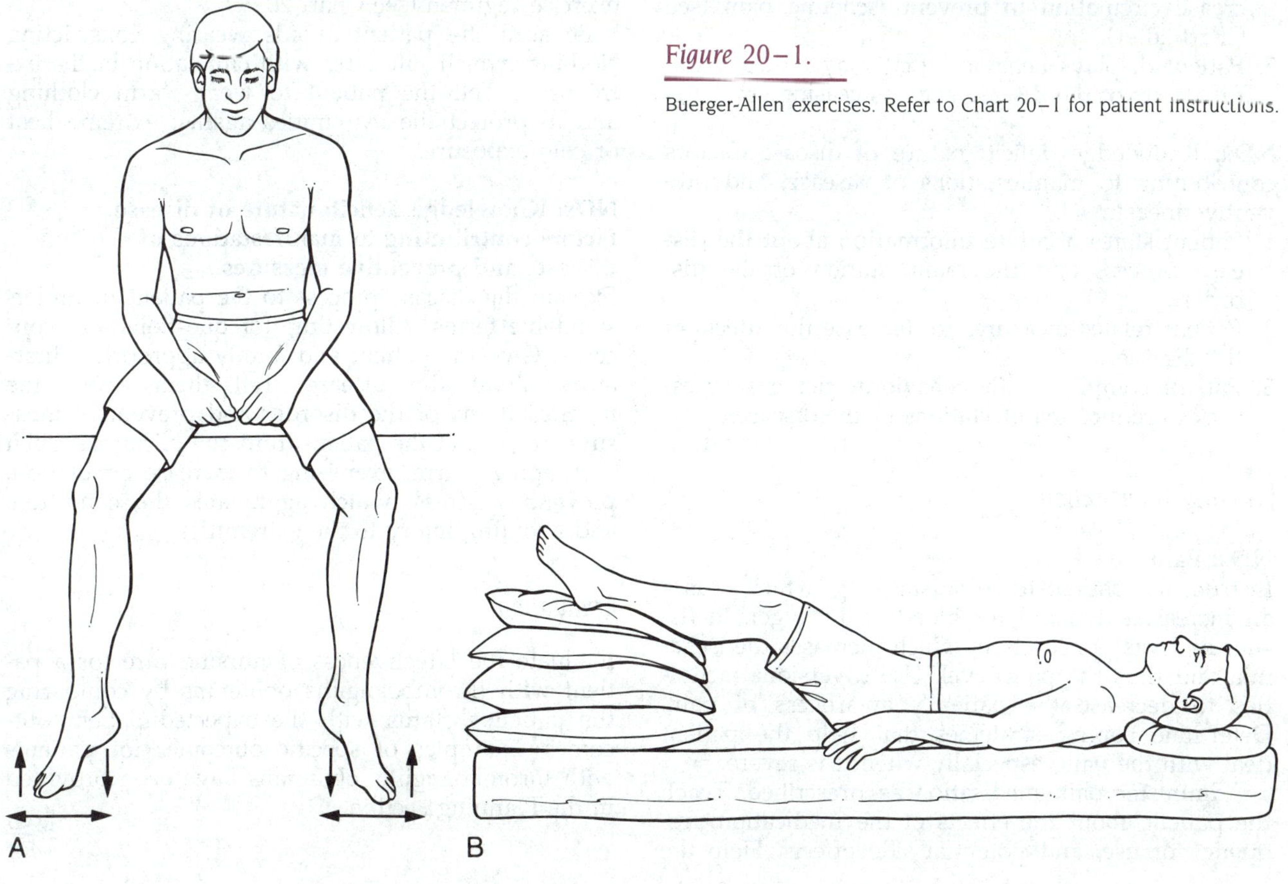

Figure 20–1.

Buerger-Allen exercises. Refer to Chart 20–1 for patient instructions.

Chart 20–2.

NURSING GUIDE TO PATIENT EDUCATION FOR SELF-MANAGEMENT: RELAXATION EXERCISES FOR THE PATIENT WITH VASCULAR DISORDERS

Instruct the patient to:

Sit or lie in a comfortable position with loose clothing in a quiet, dark room.
Close the eyes, and breathe slowly and naturally.
Starting at the head, tighten and relax each muscle, ending with the feet.
Continue to breathe slowly and deeply.
Repeat the words *relax, peace,* and so on each time exhalation occurs.
Disregard all outside thoughts and concerns.
Focus on each muscle being relaxed more and more with each exhalation.

Tell the patient this exercise should take only about 10 minutes or so to complete. Visualizing a favorite quiet place (the beach, woods, mountain, and so on) may be helpful to relax the mind and muscles.

Planning: Patient outcomes

1. Patient reports an absence or reduction in pain.
2. Patient does not display signs of pain such as grimacing, clenching hands, or guarding.
3. Patient states methods of relaxation to reduce pain and coping strategies to deal with the pain.
4. Patient describes and practices exercises to increase circulation to prevent ischemic pain (see Chart 20–1).
5. Patient displays behaviors that may reduce painful effects of the disease such as ceasing smoking.

NDx: Knowledge deficit: nature of disease, factors contributing to manifestations of disease, and preventive measures

1. Patient states accurate information about the disease process and the manifestation of the disorder.
2. Patient relates measures to decrease the effects of the disease.
3. Patient complies with behavioral changes necessary to reduce manifestations of the disease.

Nursing Interventions

NDx: Pain

Instruct the patient to cease smoking, which causes an increased demand for blood and oxygen to tissues and vasoconstriction, which increases the ischemia and thus the pain level. Use diversional activities to decrease the patient's awareness of pain. Determine coping strategies that help the patient deal with the pain, especially when it is severe.

Administer pain medication as prescribed. Teach the patient about the effects of the medication, frequency of use, and potential side effects. Help the patient decrease stress and tension through the use of relaxation methods to relieve the pain caused by increased vasoconstriction (Chart 20–2). Allow for periods of rest during episodes of intense pain.

Teach the patient Buerger-Allen exercises to increase circulation to the extremities to reduce the ischemia. Encourage continued participation in the exercise regimen (see Chart 20–1).

Be sure the patient avoids wearing constricting clothing, which interferes with circulation in the extremities. Tell the patient to wear warm clothing and to protect the extremities against extreme heat or cold exposure.

NDx: Knowledge deficit: nature of disease, factors contributing to manifestations of disease, and preventive measures

Explain the disease process to the patient in understandable terms. Allow time for questions and concerns. Give the patient and family appropriate literature about the disease. Tell them about the manifestations of the disorder and preventive measures to protect the patient from complications, such as keeping warm, exercising to increase circulation, preventing stress, which aggravates the condition, and avoiding injury to the extremities.

Evaluation

Evaluate the effectiveness of nursing care for a patient with thromboangiitis obliterans by comparing the patient's status with the expected patient outcomes. Examples of specific outcomes for patients with thromboangiitis obliterans have been provided in the Planning section.

Inflammations of the Aorta

Inflammation of the aorta (aortitis) occurs primarily in the aortic arch. Blood flow to the vessels branching from the the aortic arch may be impaired because of the inflammation, which leads to tissue and organ ischemia. Arteriosclerosis, dissecting aneurysms, tuberculosis, septicemia, and rheumatoid disease may cause inflammation of the aorta.

TAKAYASU'S ARTERITIS

ETIOLOGY AND PATHOPHYSIOLOGY

The cause of the disorder, which is also called the pulseless disease, is unknown. In Takayasu's arteritis, the aortic arch becomes inflamed, causing the arterial walls to become thick and rigid. Stenosis of the aorta and occlusion of the lumen by thrombosis occur, which decrease the blood flow to branches supplied by the aorta and result in an absent pulse in the affected sites. The disorder affects women more frequently than men. It is also more common in the Japanese population.

CLINICAL MANIFESTATIONS

Blood vessels leading from the aortic arch to the brain, arms, and legs become inflamed and occluded, causing ischemia of the tissues. The aortic arch syndrome may be present. It is manifested by cerebral ischemia, vertigo, visual disturbances, claudication of the arms with exercise, intermittent claudication of the muscles in the jaw while chewing, and impaired pulses in the arms.

Dyspnea, cough, and edema may be present from impaired oxygen exchange. If the coronary arteries are involved, angina pectoris may occur. Fever, arthralgia, and an elevated sedimentation rate may be present as a result of the inflammation.

MEDICAL DIAGNOSIS

The diagnosis is made on the basis of the history, present symptoms, and aortography, which depicts dilation, stenosis occlusion, and wall thickness of the aortic arch.

MEDICAL MANAGEMENT

Inflammation is managed with adrenal corticosteroids. A good response usually occurs if treated early. Surgical excision with grafting may be necessary.

SYPHILITIC AORTITIS

ETIOLOGY AND PATHOPHYSIOLOGY

Syphilitic aortitis occurs as a lesion in the late stages of acquired syphilis. This usually appears 10 to 30 years after contact with the infectious agent. It is more common in men than in women. The smooth muscle and elastic tissues are necrosed, and the medial layers of the aorta are damaged. The ascending aorta may be dilated and calcified. Coronary arteries become narrowed and stenosed. This leads to aortic insufficiency in some cases and aortic aneurysms in others.

CLINICAL MANIFESTATIONS

Clinical manifestations are not usually apparent until the patient is 30 to 50 years of age. If aneurysms develop, substernal chest pain, spreading to the sternum and vertebrae, is present from the ischemia and necrosis. Rupture of the aneurysm is possible. Distended jugular veins may indicate occlusion of the superior vena cava as a result of pressure from the aneurysm.

Atelectasis of the left lung and compression of the left bronchus may result from an aortic arch aneurysm. Pressure may also cause ulceration of the trachea or bronchi, causing hemoptysis or rupture of the esophagus.

MEDICAL DIAGNOSIS

The diagnosis is made on the basis of the history, physical assessment, aortography, and computed tomographic (CT) scans. A positive VDRL (Venereal Disease Research Laboratory) test result is common, but in patients older than 65 years the test is not a reliable indicator of previous infection.

MEDICAL MANAGEMENT

Benzathine penicillin or procaine penicillin given intramuscularly for several weeks is the treatment of choice for syphilitic aortitis. The aortic wall damage may be irreversible, and complications may continue even with treatment because of the nature of the primary disease process. Surgical resection with grafting may be used to treat a syphilitic aortic aneurysm if the patient is a candidate for surgery.

Application of the Nursing Process to the Care of the Patient with Inflammation of the Aorta

The assessment, nursing diagnoses, expected patient outcomes, nursing interventions, and evaluation for patients with inflammation of the aorta are similar to those described subsequently for patients with obstructive arterial vascular disorders and arterial aneurysms. Also refer to Chapter 19 for application of the nursing process to the patient undergoing peripheral vascular surgery.

Obstructive Disorders

The obstructive vascular disorders are more commonly found in the older adult. Several of the diseases, such as atherosclerosis, are insidious in the development and are influenced by lifestyle. Because many of the disorders have similar characteristics and effects on the patient, there are several commonalities of nursing care applicable to patients with an obstructive arterial vascular disorder.

Application of the Nursing Process to the Care of the Patient with Obstructive Arterial Vascular Disorders

Assessment

Review the history and diagnostic studies results for the patient. Complete a physical assessment. Check the patient for circulatory impairment, especially in the periphery. Palpate all distal pulses, and compare them bilaterally. Auscultate for bruits in the major arteries. Note the temperature, color, and sensation in the extremities. Look for signs of poor capillary refill, indicating decreased circulation.

Ask the patient about pain in the extremities. Obtain a description of the pain, including onset, duration, precipitating factors, and relief measures.

Check for signs of injury caused by falls, burns, or cuts. Ask the patient about the amount of sensation in the extremities. Check for numbness, tingling, and equal feeling bilaterally.

Observe for breaks in the skin. Look for tears, ulcerations, necrotic spots, or gangrene. Note any drainage from lesions.

Nursing Diagnoses and Planning

Nursing diagnoses and related expected patient outcomes most commonly applicable to patients with obstructive arterial vascular disorders include the following:

NDx: Altered tissue perfusion, peripheral, related to the disease state, causing arterial vessel occlusion and decreased circulation to the extremities

Planning: Patient outcomes

1. Patient demonstrates increased perfusion as noted by warm, dry skin; strong pulses; absence of edema; and cyanosis in the extremities.
2. Patient's vital signs are within normal ranges for the patient.
3. Patient demonstrates changes in behaviors that promote improved circulation such as mild exercise, cessation of smoking, and relaxation techniques.

NDx: High risk for injury related to decreased sensation in the extremities secondary to arterial occlusion, causing hypoxia

Planning: Patient outcomes

1. Patient states need for assistance when out of bed and ambulating to prevent injury.
2. Patient states preventive measures such as requesting assistance when needed and following foot-care guidelines as described in Chart 20–3.

Chart 20–3.

NURSING GUIDE TO PATIENT EDUCATION FOR SELF-MANAGEMENT: SELF-CARE FOR PREVENTION OF FOOT PROBLEMS IN VASCULAR DISORDERS

Instruct the patient with vascular problems to institute the following foot-care measures to prevent complications:

Wear soft, comfortable shoes that are not too tight and that do not have any pressure areas.
Cleanse feet frequently. Be sure to dry them well, especially between the toes.
Apply skin moisturizer if feet are excessively dry or cracked.
Put on clean antiembolic stockings or socks daily.
Massage the feet frequently to promote circulation.
Keep toenails trimmed short. When trimming, be extremely careful not to cut the skin and not to cut the nails too short, causing bleeding.
Check the feet daily for discoloration, edema, bleeding, blisters, or any other lesions.
Consult a physician if any of these symptoms become apparent.

3. Patient conforms to the safety measures.
4. Patient remains free from injury.

NDx: Impaired skin integrity in the extremities related to inadequate oxygen and nutrients secondary to decreased circulation

Planning: Patient outcomes
1. Patient's skin remains intact without evidence of shearing, infection, ulcerations, or gangrene.
2. Patient states appropriate skin-care measures to prevent impairment of skin integrity.

Nursing Interventions

NDx: Altered tissue perfusion, peripheral
Help the patient conserve oxygen needs by encouraging rest and limiting activities. Elevate the head of the bed to aid in lung expansion. Initiate oxygen therapy if needed. Assist patient with activities of daily living, if needed, to conserve energy.

Keep the patient in a comfortable position, and reposition frequently to release pressure. Use range-of-motion exercises to stimulate circulation. Monitor vital signs and laboratory studies to assess for changes and improvements in status. Encourage ambulation as tolerated, but provide for frequent rest periods to decrease cardiac workload. Discourage smoking to avoid vasoconstriction. Discuss strategies to reduce stress, which could cause increased blood pressure. Remove constricting clothing, and keep heavy bed linen from constricting peripheral circulation.

Give prescribed medications to promote increased circulation. Discuss risk factors and preventive health care measures with the patient. Explain lifestyle changes that will promote good circulation and decrease risk of further arterial occlusion.

NDx: High risk for injury
Teach the patient to ask for assistance when getting out of bed or ambulating. Keep the bed rails in the upright position and the patient's call light within reach. Explain the effects of decreased circulation to the extremities and safety measures to prevent injury.

Instruct the patient to use care when bathing the extremities. With decreased sensation, it is easy to burn the feet or legs by using water that is too hot. Give the patient and family a list of foot-care measures (see Chart 20–3). Teach the patient to use special care when trimming toenails.

NDx: Impaired skin integrity
Handle the patient's legs and feet with care, especially if the skin is not intact. Use aseptic technique when bathing or dressing areas where the skin is broken to prevent infection. Keep linen off the extremities with the use of a bed cradle. Have the patient avoid wearing constricting clothing. Keep the extremities warm and dry at all times.

Check peripheral circulation frequently. Observe for early signs of problems developing as a result of decreased circulation such as pressure spots, absent pulses, coldness, and discoloration. Report any untoward signs. Have the patient change position frequently to stimulate circulation and prevent pressure sores. Use heel pads to prevent skin breakdown if the patient is in bed for long periods of time.

To promote healing and minimize tissue damage, teach the patient to eat a diet high in protein and vitamins. Encourage the consumption of food low in cholesterol and triglycerides to decrease the formation of atherosclerotic plaques.

Evaluation

Evaluate the effectiveness of nursing care for a patient with an obstructive arterial vascular disorder by comparing the patient's status with the expected patient outcomes. Examples of specific outcomes for patients with an obstructive arterial vascular disorder have been provided in the Planning section.

VASOSPASTIC DISORDER (RAYNAUD'S DISEASE)

ETIOLOGY

Vasospastic disorder, also called Raynaud's disease, has an unknown cause. The incidence of this disorder is higher in individuals with immunologic disorders. The disease is more common in women and usually begins between 20 and 30 years of age. It is often associated with other diseases but is not precipitated by any one condition. The onset is insidious, with initial episodes occurring in the winter months. The characteristic vasospastic episodes usually affect the fingers, last from just a few minutes to hours, and may occur several times per day or may not occur for weeks at a time. They are frequently precipitated by a chilly or damp environment.

PATHOPHYSIOLOGY

Raynaud's disease is characterized by paroxysmal, bilateral digital ischemia induced by cold or emotional stress. The vasospastic episodes may end spontaneously or be relieved by a warm environment or by placing the fingers in warm water. The ischemia is due to constriction of the digital and plantar arteries, which overreact to vasospastic stimuli. As the disease progresses, the intima of the arteries becomes thick and the muscular layers hypertrophy. Thrombosis of small arteries and gangrene of the digit tips may result.

Raynaud's phenomenon is a condition with the same symptoms of Raynaud's disease that may occur in conjunction with other diseases or conditions. It may result from collagen disorders such as scleroderma, arterial disorders causing occlusion such as Buerger's disease, drug or chemical exposures, or neuropathy such as carpal tunnel syndrome. Raynaud's phenomenon is a temporary disorder without the pathology of Raynaud's disease.

CLINICAL MANIFESTATIONS

Vasospastic disease or Raynaud's disease, is characterized by intermittent episodes of vasospasms in the fingers, causing pallor and cyanosis. It rarely occurs in the thumbs or toes and may be confined to two or three digits of the hand. Although it is usually bilateral and symmetric, more digits of one hand may be affected than of the other hand. Initially, one or two digits may by symptomatic, but eventually all fingers extending to the distal palm area become affected.

During a vasospastic episode, the digits become pale, cold, and cyanotic from vasoconstriction of the small cutaneous vessels. Pulses are usually still palpable. As the vasospasm ends, the fingers become bright red (rubor) starting at the base from the increased blood flow and blood volume. Throbbing pain and a burning sensation accompany the return of circulation.

Numbness, edema, and decreased sensations may develop as the disease progresses through repeated ischemic episodes. Trophic changes occur such as atrophy of the fingers; smooth, shiny, stretched skin; slow-growing, ridged nails; infections; blisters; and small painful gangrenous areas on the tips of the digits. These changes may occur 1 to 4 years after onset of the disorder because of obstruction of the digital blood vessels.

MEDICAL DIAGNOSIS

The diagnosis is made on the basis of the history, physical assessment, patient description of vasospastic episodes, arteriography, and plethysmography. Nerve conduction tests may be done to rule out carpal tunnel syndrome when the symptoms are unilateral. The Doppler ultrasonogram is used to determine the presence of digital pulses. Although Raynaud's disease is not a fatal disorder, it may cause deformity or disability in severe cases.

MEDICAL MANAGEMENT

Medical care includes avoiding precipitating factors, especially by protecting the hands from exposure to a cold and damp environment. Sedatives or tranquilizers may be prescribed to help relieve symptoms by relaxing the patient. Large doses of vasodilators are prescribed in some cases to increase blood flow to the distal areas, but they are frequently of limited value. Reserpine may be injected directly into veins in the hands to promote vasodilation and to produce symptomatic relief for up to 2 weeks. Because this is a very temporary treatment, it is not commonly used. A sympathectomy can be performed to help alleviate the symptoms. In most cases, the disease is treated conservatively through prevention methods. Chart 20–4 provides discharge instructions for the patient with Raynaud's disease.

Application of the Nursing Process to the Care of the Patient with Vasospastic Disorder (Raynaud's Disease)

The assessment, nursing diagnoses, expected patient outcomes, nursing interventions, and evaluation for patients with vasospastic disorder (Raynaud's disease) are similar to those described previously for patients with thromboangiitis obliterans and ob-

Chart 20–4.

NURSING GUIDE TO PATIENT EDUCATION FOR SELF-MANAGEMENT: DISCHARGE INSTRUCTIONS FOR THE PATIENT WITH RAYNAUD'S DISEASE

On discharge, instruct the patient with Raynaud's disease to observe the following preventive and safety measures:

Avoid exposure to chilly, damp, or cold temperatures.
Wear protective clothing such as gloves and heavy socks when out in cold or damp weather.
Use relaxation exercises to decrease stress levels.
Try to get plenty of rest and sleep every day.
Cease smoking.
Stop activity during an episode of vasospasm to protect the area until sensations return.

Nursing Care Guide 20–1.

PATIENTS WITH VASOSPASTIC DISORDER (RAYNAUD'S DISEASE)

Assessment Findings: Patient experiences numbness in digits of hands progressing to pain; fingers are blanched; radial pulses are present.

Nursing Diagnosis: Altered tissue perfusion, peripheral, related to obstructed circulation secondary to vasospasms

Patient Outcomes	Nursing Interventions	Rationale
Patient exhibits improved blood supply to ischemic areas as seen by warm, pink digits.	Provide warmth, especially for the extremities, and prevent drafts. Assess pulses. Assess the skin temperature, color, and texture frequently. Document any changes.	Providing warmth to the extremities may prevent some problems resulting from the circulatory deficiency. Observation for problems leads to early intervention and prevention of complications.
Patient identifies activities to improve circulation and prevent vasospasmic episodes.	Teach the patient to wear warm clothing, protect the digits from exposure, and avoid damp, chilly environments. Instruct about the effects of smoking, and encourage the patient in the cessation of smoking. Have the patient reiterate the information provided.	Some vasospasmic episodes may be prevented by removing the precipitating factors such as sudden chilling or smoking. Having the patient repeat the information allows for correction of misunderstandings and reinforcement of the information.
Patient ceases smoking.	Talk to the attending physician about smoking cessation programs. Make a referral to a smoking cessation program.	There are a variety of programs for assisting patients in quitting smoking such as nicotine patch programs and behavioral modification programs.

Evaluation: Compare the patient's status with the expected patient outcomes. If the outcomes are achieved, evaluate nursing care as successful. If not, reassess the patient, formulate new nursing diagnoses, and revise expected patient outcomes and nursing interventions as appropriate.

(continued)

structive arterial vascular disorders (Nursing Care Guide 20–1.)

ARTERIAL EMBOLUS AND THROMBUS

ETIOLOGY

An arterial embolism is characterized by fragments of atheromatous material or thrombi (the embolus) that enter the arterial system and obstruct a vessel. The embolus is carried by the blood flow to the site where it lodges.

A thrombus may also block an artery at the site where it develops rather than traveling to another site of lodgment. It usually develops in an artery damaged by atherosclerosis or inflammation. Thrombus formation may be due to rheumatic heart disease, accounting for about one quarter of cases, and arteriosclerotic heart disease, accounting for about two thirds of cases. Other cardiac and vascular disorders such as fibrillation and aneurysms are also associated with the development of thrombi. Symptoms do not usually appear until the vessel is occluded.

PATHOPHYSIOLOGY

A thrombus may develop at the point where blood flow is restricted in the vessel from a lesion,

Nursing Care Guide 20–1. *(continued)*

PATIENTS WITH VASOSPASTIC DISORDER (RAYNAUD'S DISEASE)

Assessment Findings: Patient reports pain in digits after vasospasmic episode; at times, the pain is extreme.

Nursing Diagnosis: Pain related to aftereffects of vasospasms in digits

Patient Outcomes	Nursing Interventions	Rationale
Patient reports absence of pain or that pain is reduced to tolerable level.	Give analgesics as prescribed. Allow patient to rest and relax frequently. Keep the patient free from chilling.	Analgesics reduce the pain sensations. Prevention of vasospasms reduces the number of pain episodes the patient experiences.
Patient states methods to deal with pain and measures to prevent vasospasms from occurring.	Teach relaxation exercises, as described in Chart 20–2. Help the patient find coping methods to deal with the pain after the vasospasms.	Relaxation techniques may reduce some of the pain or help the patient tolerate it better.
	Instruct the patient on how to avoid the vasospasms as described in Chart 20–4.	Prevention of the vasospasms or a reduction in the occurrence reduces the painful episodes after spasm.

Evaluation: Compare the patient's status with the expected patient outcomes. If the outcomes are achieved, evaluate nursing care as successful. If not, reassess the patient, formulate new nursing diagnoses, and revise expected patient outcomes and nursing interventions as appropriate.

Assessment Findings: Patient presents cold, numb, and pale digits; there is potential for lesions or gangrene.

Nursing Diagnosis: Impaired skin integrity related to decreased circulation to the digits secondary to disease process

Patient Outcomes	Nursing Interventions	Rationale
Patient's skin on digits remains intact, warm, pink, and smooth without signs of breakdown or gangrene.	Instruct the patient to observe for early signs of breakdown and seek medical assistance if symptoms appear.	Early recognition and intervention may prevent severe complications.

(continued)

Nursing Care Guide 20–1. *(continued)*

PATIENTS WITH VASOSPASTIC DISORDER (RAYNAUD'S DISEASE)

Patient Outcomes	Nursing Interventions	Rationale
	Tell the patient how to protect the digits from the vasospasmic episodes.	Prevention of vasospasmic episodes reduces the risk of complications.
	Explain the necessity of keeping the hands warm and covered in cold weather. Instruct on skin care if any breakdown is apparent such as keeping skin clean, using aseptic dressing, if needed, and moisturizing the dry areas to prevent cracks.	Patient education is important because the patient needs to observe for signs of skin problems and to properly care for the skin after discharge.

Evaluation: Compare the patient's status with the expected patient outcomes. If the outcomes are achieved, evaluate nursing care as successful. If not, reassess the patient, formulate new nursing diagnoses, and revise expected patient outcomes and nursing interventions as appropriate.

Assessment Findings: Patient asks questions about care of hands and prevention of vasospasms; seems anxious about managing effects of disease; is unsure about future effects of disease.

Nursing Diagnosis: Knowledge deficit: nature of disease and preventive care

Patient Outcomes	Nursing Interventions	Rationale
Patient states accurate information about the disease process and the preventive measures, as listed in Chart 20–4.	Explain the disease process to the patient in understandable terms. Give the patient appropriate literature about the disease. Explain the preventive measures, as listed in Chart 20–4.	An understanding of the disease process and the preventive behaviors may increase patient compliance with the medical regimen and prevent complications of the disease process.
	Allow time for questions, concerns, and repeated explanations. Have the patient repeat the information provided.	Planning time for questions and having the patient repeat the information allow for correction of any misunderstandings.

Evaluation: Compare the patient's status with the expected patient outcomes. If the outcomes are achieved, evaluate nursing care as successful. If not, reassess the patient, formulate new nursing diagnoses, and revise expected patient outcomes and nursing interventions as appropriate.

fatty plaques, inflammation, or any other obstruction. The term *thrombosis* refers to the process of the development of a thrombus. Any disease, drug, or process that slows circulation in the system, especially in the peripheral circulatory system, may place the patient at risk for thrombus formation. If a piece of a fatty plaque or a thrombus breaks loose and travels to another location in the circulatory system and obstructs a vessel, the blockage is an embolus and the state of having a blockage is an embolism.

CLINICAL MANIFESTATIONS

When an embolism lodges in a vessel or when a thrombus develops in a vessel in the extremities, pain occurs distal to the site of occlusion. The pain may be either gradual or sudden depending on the blockage. Numbness, tingling, and a cold sensation may precede the pain. The pain is described as a burning or aching type of discomfort in most patients. Exercise aggravates the discomfort in the extremity. Tenderness directly over the site of the blockage may be present. Muscle weakness or paralysis of the affected part can also occur.

Mottling, rigidity, collapsed veins, and impaired reflexes are present. The extremity may display pale to blotchy discoloration. Arterial pulses are absent distal to the occlusion if the blockage is in a large artery.

MEDICAL DIAGNOSIS

The diagnosis is made on the basis of physical assessment with the confirmation from diagnostic studies. An angiogram is used to determine the presence of ulcerative atherosclerotic lesions or abnormalities of blood flow caused by the arterial obstruction. A Doppler ultrasonogram may be used to locate the obstruction.

MEDICAL MANAGEMENT

The goal of medical care is to improve blood flow through the affected vessel. Heparin is administered to prevent further clot formation. The patient is placed on long-term anticoagulant therapy once the acute phase has passed and is monitored for effects of the therapy. Thrombolytic therapy may be used to dissolve the clot and restore circulation. Procaine or lidocaine (Xylocaine) may be injected into the subarachnoid space of the spinal column as a lumbar sympathetic block to relieve constriction and spasms of the affected vessel. Vasodilators may be prescribed as adjunct therapy. Analgesics are given for pain relief.

If the embolus or thrombus is completely occluding a major vessel so that circulation is severely compromised or interrupted in the extremity, surgical intervention is required. A thromboendarterectomy or an arterial graft may be done. (Refer to Chapter 19 for a discussion of endarterectomy and grafts.)

The prognosis depends on the location and extent of the blockage, age of the patient, and other complicating conditions. Early treatment is essential for a good prognosis. Removing or treating the underlying cause is important. The recurrence of thrombi and emboli is common, particularly if the cause is atherosclerotic disease.

Application of the Nursing Process to the Care of the Patient with an Arterial Embolus or Thrombus

Assessment

Review the patient's history and diagnostic studies. Assess the patient for changes in sensation, color, temperature, strength, and endurance. Palpate for the presence of pulses in the affected area. Note any pain and determine its onset, duration, intensity, radiation, and location.

Check the patient's understanding of the disorder, the treatment, and expected outcomes of the treatment, especially if surgery is indicated. Observe for signs of anxiety such as increased blood pressure and heart rate, nervousness, withdrawal, twitching, and continual questions related to the medical intervention. If the condition is highly acute—complete occlusion of a major vessel—the patient may fear surgery, the risk of death, or loss of a limb.

Nursing Diagnoses and Planning

Nursing diagnoses and related expected patient outcomes most commonly applicable to patients with an arterial embolus or thrombus include those discussed under obstructive arterial vascular disorders and the following (also refer to Chapter 19 for application of the nursing process to the patient undergoing peripheral vascular surgery):

NDx: Anxiety related to the disease state, treatment, and possible surgical intervention

Planning: Patient outcomes
1. Patient states accurate information about the disease, its effect on the extremities, potential treatment, and expected outcomes.
2. Patient exhibits signs of decreased anxiety such as normal vital signs; a cheerful, relaxed posture; and lack of nervousness or twitching.
3. Patient reports feeling less anxious.

Nursing Interventions

NDx: Anxiety
Explain the disease process, the typical interventions, and expected outcomes to the patient. If the situation requires surgery, explain the necessity of the surgery and all preoperative preparations as they are instituted. Allow the patient time to adjust to the information and to voice concerns. Encourage questions, and give explanations in terms the patient can understand. Include the family in the discussions when appropriate.

Encourage rest, and teach relaxation techniques to reduce the anxiety (see Chart 20–2). Provide uninterrupted rest periods throughout the day. Seek assistance from clergy or other professionals as needed.

Evaluation

Evaluate the effectiveness of nursing care for the patient with an arterial embolus or thrombus by comparing the patient's status with the expected patient outcomes. Examples of specific outcomes for patients with an arterial embolus or thrombus have been provided in the Planning section.

ATHEROSCLEROSIS

ETIOLOGY

The most common occlusive disorder of the arteries is atherosclerosis. The exact cause of atherosclerosis is unknown; however, the fatty tissue found in the disease may be the continuation of a fatty streak that is present at birth in the vessels. The fatty plaques occur most frequently in the peripheral arteries, particularly of the lower extremities. In the aorta, the abdominal section is affected with atherosclerosis more often than the ascending section.

Atherosclerosis is primarily recognized in adults 20 years of age or older and is most commonly found in the older adult. It is the major cause of death in the individual older than 65 years. Risk factors associated with atherosclerosis include increased cholesterol, particularly low-density lipoproteins (LDL), cigarette smoking, hypertension, diabetes and a familial history of heart disease.

PATHOPHYSIOLOGY

In atherosclerosis the wall of the artery becomes calcified from fatty plaques. The plaques are white fibrous tissue and yellowish fatty deposits of cells, lipids, carbohydrates and calcium in the intima of the vessel. Thrombosis develops, causing obstruction of the vessel.

Calcium deposits in the wall of the vessel prevent dilation and contraction. The lumen of the artery becomes narrowed and weak and loses its flexibility. As the intima thickens with age, vessels become more rigid, resulting in a rise in peripheral resistance and increased cardiac workload. An aneurysm may develop, causing obstruction or occlusion of the vessel and leading to fibrosis of tissues and organs from lack of blood supply. Calcification, necrosis, and rupture of the vessel may also occur. Any arterial vessel may be involved, but the aorta, iliac arteries, carotid arteries, and coronary arteries are the most commonly affected.

CLINICAL MANIFESTATIONS

Clinical manifestations of atherosclerosis depend on the location and the extent of arterial occlusion. Ischemia in the lower extremities is seen if the atherosclerotic area is in the abdominal aorta or iliac or femoral arteries. Manifestations of the ischemia include decreased or absent pulses, cold feet, gangrene of the toes or feet, intermittent claudication, and aneurysms.

If the blockage is in the carotid arteries, manifestations include dizziness, confusion, transient ischemic attacks, and cerebrovascular accidents. Atherosclerotic plaques in the coronary arteries usually cause angina pectoris and myocardial infarction. Hypertension may be caused by occlusion in the renal arteries.

MEDICAL DIAGNOSIS

The diagnosis of atherosclerosis is determined by history, physical assessment, and diagnostic studies. Present symptoms, palpation of peripheral pulses, and skin temperature studies are also used for determining the diagnosis. A treadmill exercise test and Doppler ultrasonogram demonstrate the quality of peripheral blood flow and the presence of intermittent claudication. Angiography, tomography, and magnetic resonance imaging evaluate blood flow and the severity of the obstruction or narrowing of the arteries. Laboratory studies of cholesterol levels, LDL and high-density lipoproteins (HDL), may add support to the diagnosis. High cholesterol levels, with a high LDL and low HDL, are common in atherosclerosis.

MEDICAL MANAGEMENT

The medical management of atherosclerosis depends on the location and severity of the disorder. It may consist of palliative treatment, supportive care, or pharmacologic intervention. The patient is educated about lifestyle changes needed such as diet modifications, cessation of smoking, and initiation of a mild exercise regimen. A low-cholesterol, low-fat diet is encouraged. The patient may be referred to a smoking cessation program. Exercise increases the circulation to the periphery, so a regular exercise program is prescribed on the basis of the patient's ability and other influencing factors. Antiplatelet therapy may be prescribed for carotid arterial occlusion.

Surgical intervention may be necessary to enhance blood flow to the affected areas. Sympathectomy, angioplasty, and grafts are the most common surgeries performed for atherosclerotic disorders. Refer to Chapter 19 for a discussion of the surgeries for vascular disorders.

Application of the Nursing Process to the Care of the Patient with Atherosclerosis

Assessment

Assess for pain, noting the onset, intensity, duration, radiation, and location. Determine whether the pain is present only during exercise or at rest. Look for signs of pain such as grimacing, clenching of hands, moaning, or guarding when the patient is moving in bed or ambulating or after ambulation when the patient is at rest.

Assess for any skin changes. Ask the patient about numbness, tingling, or paresthesia of the extremities. Check the temperature and color of the extremities when the patient is elevated and when he or she is in a dependent position. Observe the condition of the feet. Palpate for pulses and compare bilaterally. Look for signs of skin breakdown. Auscultate for bruits over occluded arteries. Monitor serum cholesterol levels and other laboratory data.

Check the patient's physical mobility. Ask about assistance needed to perform activities of daily living. Determine the patient's flexibility, range of motion, and strength in the extremities.

Assess the patient's level of knowledge about the disorder and treatment. Ask about the patient's lifestyle and associated risk factors. Assess the level of adaptation to the disorder and ability to manage the disease process and its manifestations.

Nursing Diagnoses and Planning

Nursing diagnoses and related expected patient outcomes most commonly applicable to patients with atherosclerosis include those discussed under obstructive arterial vascular disorders and the following:

NDx: Pain related to ischemic tissues secondary to decreased circulation from disease process

Planning: Patient outcomes
1. Patient reports an absence or reduction in pain when ambulating or at rest.
2. Patient does not present nonverbal signs of pain such as grimacing, clenching hands, or guarding.
3. Patient states methods of relaxation to reduce pain and coping strategies to deal with the pain.

NDx: Impaired physical mobility related to pain and decreased strength and sensation secondary to disease state

Planning: Patient outcomes
1. Patient reports increased mobility, strength, and endurance.
2. Patient is able to perform activities of daily living.

NDx: Knowledge deficit: nature of the disease, nutritional needs, treatments, and measures to reduce risk

Planning: Patient outcomes
1. Patient describes cause, effects, and risk factors associated with atherosclerosis.
2. Patient lists symptoms and treatments for the complications of the disorder.
3. Patient relates the nutritional therapy for lowering cholesterol levels.
4. Patient states the self-care needed to prevent risk or complications of atherosclerosis.

NDx: Self-esteem disturbance related to chronic illness, changes in lifestyle to manage disease and reduce risk factors, and inability to perform activities of daily living

Planning: Patient outcomes
1. Patient states methods to cope with illness.
2. Patient denies feelings of inadequacy, helplessness, or dependency.
3. Patient appears positive, friendly, and cheerful and actively participates in plans for discharge and patient education sessions.
4. Patient takes responsibility for self-care.

Nursing Interventions

NDx: Pain

Instruct the patient to cease smoking, which causes an increased demand for blood and oxygen to tissues and vasoconstriction, which increases the ischemia and thus the pain level. Use diversional activities to decrease the patient's awareness of pain. Determine coping strategies that help the patient deal with the pain, especially when it is severe. Be sure the patient avoids wearing constricting clothing, which interferes with circulation in the extremities.

Administer pain medication as prescribed. Teach the patient about the effects of the medication, fre-

Nutrition Box 20–1.

DIET GUIDELINES FOR PREVENTION OF ATHEROSCLEROSIS

- Eat only the number of calories to maintain an ideal weight or reduce calories to achieve target weight.
- Decrease fat intake to 30% to 35% of total calories.
- Decrease intake of saturated fat.
- Decrease intake of cholesterol to 300 mg/day.
- Decrease sodium to 130 mg/day.
- Maintain protein intake at 12% to 15% of total calories.
- Increase carbohydrate intake to 50% to 55% of total calories.
- Eat no more than three egg yolks per week.
- Use more poultry meats (white meat, skinless).
- Use skim milk dairy products.
- Remove visible fat from meat, use more polyunsaturated fats, and add no salt to cooking.
- Eat more fresh fruits and vegetables.

Data from American Heart Association. The American Heart Association diet: An eating plan for healthy Americans. Dallas, TX: American Heart Association, 1991.

quency of use, and potential side effects. Help the patient decrease stress and tension through the use of relaxation methods to relieve the pain caused by increased vasoconstriction. Allow for periods of rest during episodes of intermittent claudication.

NDx: Impaired physical mobility

Assist the patient when getting out of bed and ambulating. Use durable medical equipment accessories, when appropriate, to assist the patient in maintaining mobility. Teach the patient to perform range-of-motion exercises to increase circulation and to maintain or improve strength and endurance.

Prepare a daily exercise schedule for the patient, increasing the level as tolerable. Tell the patient to walk slowly and avoid stairs or inclines at first, if necessary, and to stop for a few minutes when pain occurs.

Encourage the patient to persist in the exercise regimen, even if it must be moderated at times of pain or lack of endurance. Praise the patient on progress made.

NDx: Knowledge deficit: nature of the disease, nutritional needs, treatments, and measures to reduce risk

Explain the cause, effects, and clinical course of atherosclerosis to the patient. Allow opportunities for the patient to ask questions at any time. Provide appropriate literature about atherosclerosis for the patient and family to review. Allow the patient to verbalize concerns and fears. Evaluate the discharge needs of the patient and family.

Alert the patient to signs and symptoms of atherosclerosis and complications, such as impaired mobility, skin breakdown, and infection or gangrene of the extremities. Teach the patient to use safety measures or to ask for assistance when out of bed or when ambulating.

Instruct the patient about dietary modifications needed to reduce risk or prevent complications of the disorder. Explain the need for decreases in dietary fats and cholesterol to prevent the effects of the disease and increases in protein and vitamins to promote good health and healing (Nutrition Box 20–1). Initiate counseling with a dietitian to assist with meal planning if needed.

Teach the patient how to achieve comfort by frequent repositioning and padding bony prominences. Show family members how to massage the patient with lotion to promote circulation and to prevent skin breakdown. Tell the patient to avoid using heating pads because thermoreceptors in the tissue may be dulled from oxygen deprivation. Explain the use of a bed cradle to prevent pressure on joints and sensitive areas.

Teach the patient dosage, route, time, frequency, side effects, and toxic effects of any medication prescribed. Explain the diagnostic studies completed and the need for any follow-up studies after discharge. Include the family in any of the teaching sessions when applicable.

NDx: Self-esteem disturbance

Teach the patient self-care measures, encouraging participation and decision making by the patient.

Explain how changes in lifestyle can benefit the patient and significant others. Allow time for expression of concerns, questions, and clarification of misunderstandings. Praise the patient for knowledge gained about the disorder, for attempts at lifestyle change, and for participation in self-care.

Seek assistance from clergy, family members, or other professionals when appropriate. Make referrals for the patient on discharge as needed.

Evaluation

Evaluate the effectiveness of nursing care for a patient with atherosclerosis by comparing the patient's status with the expected patient outcomes. Examples of specific outcomes for patients with atherosclerosis have been provided in the Planning section.

CHRONIC ARTERIAL OCCLUSIVE DISEASE (ARTERIOSCLEROSIS OBLITERANS)

ETIOLOGY

The cause of chronic arterial occlusive disease is usually atherosclerosis, resulting in gradual blockage of the large vessels. It may also be caused by thrombosis or chronic inflammation. Chronic arterial occlusive disease is most common in men older than 50 years and primarily affects the vessels of the lower extremities. Diabetes mellitus is frequently a precursor of the disorder because of the prevalence of hyperlipedemia in the disease. Chronic arterial occlusive disease affects the distal part of the aorta and the iliac, femoral, and popliteal arteries.

Arteriosclerosis of smaller arterial vessels is considered to be part of the aging process. This may cause a hypertensive state in the patient if it is severe in the renal arterioles.

PATHOPHYSIOLOGY

Fatty plaques or atheromas gradually occlude the arterial vessel, causing the symptoms of the disease. Occlusions of the aorta and iliac arteries usually occur proximal to the bifurcation of the common iliac arteries or distal to the aortic bifurcation. Complete occlusion may also be present. Occlusion of the femoral and popliteal arteries usually begins distal to the femoral artery and spreads into the popliteal artery. The superficial femoral artery is the most commonly affected area.

CLINICAL MANIFESTATIONS

The clinical manifestations of chronic arterial occlusive disease result from ischemia distal to the occluded blood flow. Occlusion of the aorta and iliac artery produces intermittent claudication in the calf muscles, thighs, buttocks, and lower back. Occlusion in the femoral and popliteal arteries produces intermittent claudication in the calf muscles and the feet. The pain increases with exercise.

Rest pain usually results from ischemia of the distal tissues and nerves. It is worse at night when cardiac output is decreased. Elevation of the affected extremity aggravates the condition.

Dependent rubor results from the inadequate blood supply, causing anoxia and paralysis of the capillaries. The presence of dependent rubor indicates moderate to severe arterial occlusive disease. When the extremity is in a dependent position, the amount of color change is directly related to the severity of the disease. Pallor occurs when the extremity is elevated.

As a result of the decreased arterial blood flow, the lower leg and foot display hair loss; thin, dry, shiny skin; and decreased musculature. If the foot is elevated, immediate blanching is present. When the foot is lowered, venous filling is delayed. The foot is usually cold and often numb. The toenails may be hypertrophied. Ulcerative lesions appear on the extremities because of a lack of oxygen and nutrients from the diminished circulation. Gangrene develops from bruising, shearing, and trauma to the tissue.

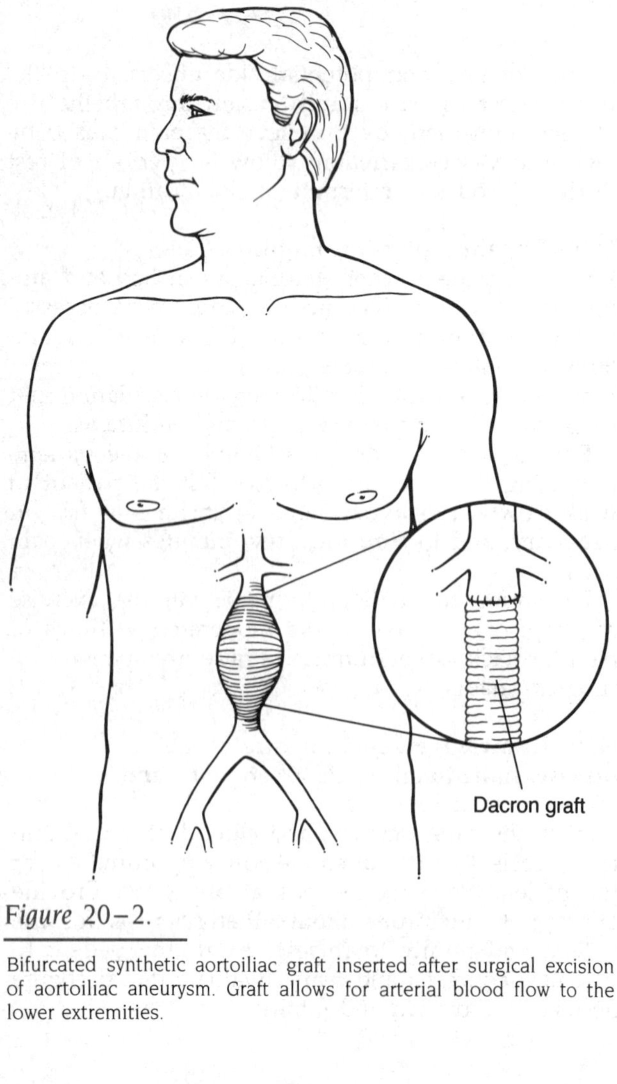

Figure 20–2.

Bifurcated synthetic aortoiliac graft inserted after surgical excision of aortoiliac aneurysm. Graft allows for arterial blood flow to the lower extremities.

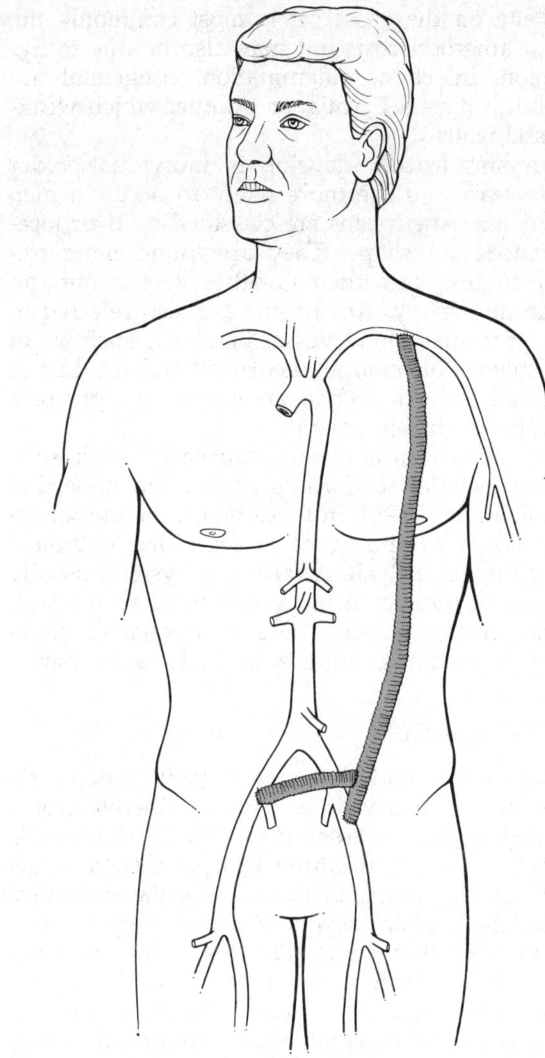

Figure 20–3.

The axillobifemoral bypass graft. The ancillary artery is connected to the femoral artery, with a branch graft connecting to the other femoral artery.

The extremities usually become very painful from the lesions. The development of secondary infection, which aggravates and spreads the ulcerations, is common.

Edematous extremities may be evident, especially if the patient keeps them in a dependent position for long periods of time. Edema may range from mild to the severe, pitting type. The edema is the result of position and obstruction in the vessel.

Popliteal or pedal pulses are usually absent. Pulsation in the abdominal aorta may be present. Bruits are audible with a stethoscope over the occluded arteries. If pulses are palpable, they tend to be obscure with exercise if an obstruction of the artery is present.

MEDICAL DIAGNOSIS

The diagnosis of chronic arterial occlusive disease is made on the basis of history, present symptoms, physical assessment, and diagnostic studies. Arteriography may be conducted if heart disease is also present. Ultrasonography, oscillometry, plethysmography, and a Doppler ultrasonogram may be used to determine the degree of occlusion.

MEDICAL MANAGEMENT

The goal of treatment is to restore blood flow through the narrow or occluded artery and to relieve the patient's symptoms. Conservative treatment includes reduction of risk factors to slow the progression of the disease and to improve blood flow. Medical management also includes pharmacologic therapy such as vasodilators and anticoagulants to enhance circulation.

Surgical intervention may be required to bypass the occluded artery. An aortofemoral graft or an aortoiliac graft may be necessary to bypass the blockage. An aortoiliac graft is illustrated in Figure 20–2. A graft from the axillary artery to the femoral artery may also be required (Fig. 20–3). A femoropopliteal bypass graft or a longer graft extending to the tibioperoneal trunk or ankle may be performed (Fig. 20–4). The patient's saphenous vein is used as the bypass graft to prevent complications of throm-

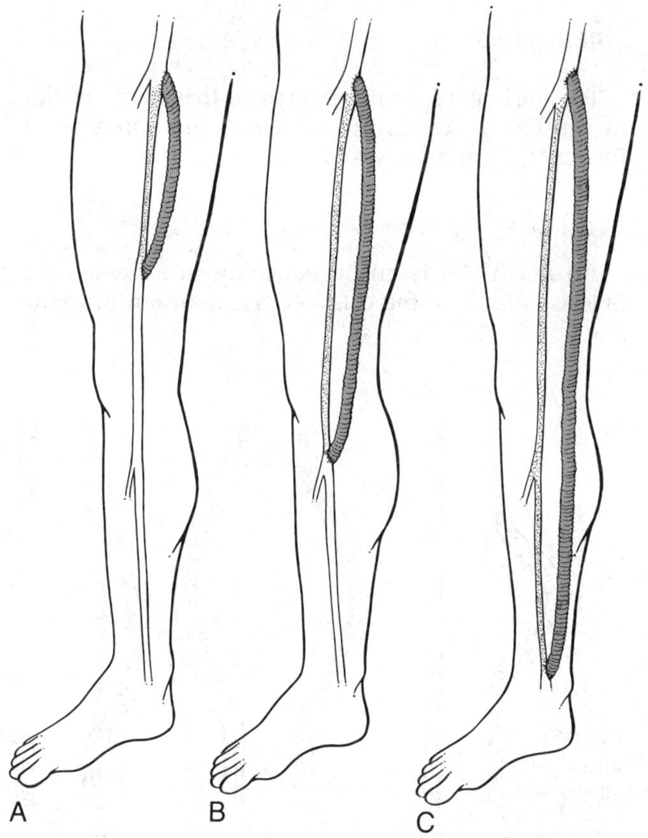

Figure 20–4.

A, A femoropopliteal bypass graft. *B*, A graft extending to the tibioperoneal trunk. *C*, A long graft extending to the ankle.

bosis and sepsis. (Refer to Chapter 19 for a discussion of bypass grafts.)

A thromboendarterectomy may be done for occlusions in the common iliac and femoral arteries. A sympathectomy may be performed to dilate the arteries permanently, causing increased blood supply to the lower legs and feet. Amputation may be necessary if the artery is completely occluded, especially if gangrene is present. (Refer to Chapter 19 for a discussion of endarterectomy, sympathectomy, and amputation.)

Application of the Nursing Process to the Care of the Patient with Chronic Arterial Occlusive Disease

The assessment, nursing diagnoses, expected patient outcomes, nursing interventions, and evaluation for patients with chronic arterial occlusive disease are similar to those described previously for patients with atherosclerosis and obstructive arterial vascular disorders.

Aneurysms

The various types of aneurysms that may develop in the blood vessels are structural abnormalities of the arterial vascular system.

ETIOLOGY

An aneurysm is an outpouching of a vessel wall or sac caused by the dilation or expansion of a particular site on the vessel. It is most commonly the result of atherosclerosis but may also be due to hypertension, infection, inflammation, congenital abnormalities of vessel walls, or trauma, which weakens vessel walls.

Aneurysms usually develop in individuals older than 60 years and are more likely to occur in men than women. Aneurysms are classified by their location, cause, and shape. They are found more frequently in the aorta than in other vessels but can occur in any artery. Aneurysms are also referred to by the particular blood vessel involved, such as an aortic, splenic, or femoral aneurysm, and the part of the vessel involved, such as an ascending aortic or a descending aortic aneurysm.

A true aneurysm is usually caused by atherosclerosis and includes fusiform, saccular, and dissecting aneurysms (Fig. 20–5). In these types, the outpouching or sac is composed of at least one unbroken layer of the vessel wall. A false aneurysm is usually the result of trauma to the vessel wall, so the wall does not remain intact. There is leakage of blood into the surrounding tissue from a false aneurysm.

PATHOPHYSIOLOGY

Although the underlying pathologic process resulting in an aneurysm is usually atherosclerosis, other pathologic processes may also be responsible for arterial changes resulting in a weakened vessel wall. Over the years, increased vascular pressures and stretching of the layers of the damaged vessel result in the outpouching. The aneurysm gradually increases in size and may rupture. This is a critical situation that requires immediate medical intervention. A ruptured cerebral aneurysm produces one type of cerebrovascular accident.

A small aneurysm may be present for years before diagnosis because a very small one will present few, if any, symptoms. Most large aneurysms are palpa-

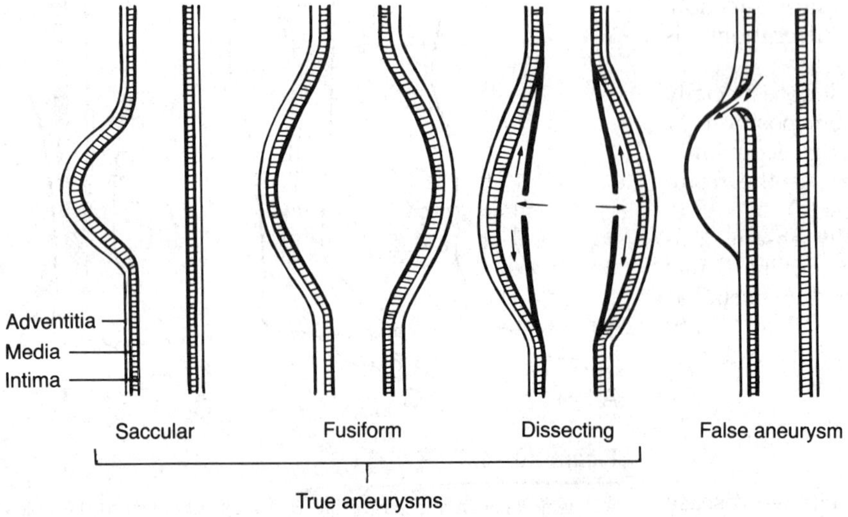

Figure 20–5.

Classification of aneurysms. True aneurysms include the saccular, fusiform, and dissecting types. A false aneurysm occurs from a rupture in the vessel wall with leakage of blood in an outpouching of the tissue.

ble and are found during a routine physical examination.

FUSIFORM ANEURYSM

A fusiform or spindle-shaped aneurysm is the most common type of aneurysm diagnosed. The entire circumference of the vessel is dilated by the aneurysm. A fusiform aneurysm occurs most commonly in the abdominal aorta and iliac arteries and is usually caused by atherosclerosis.

SACCULAR ANEURYSM

A saccular aneurysm is an outpouching or saclike aneurysm of the artery that involves only a part of the vessel wall. The primary cause of a saccular aneurysm is trauma to the site and thinning and stretching of the medial layer of the vessel. Saccular aneurysms occur most commonly in the abdominal aorta and popliteal and femoral arteries. Aneurysms occurring in the transverse and descending thoracic aorta are also frequently saccular. A saccular aneurysm in the circle of Willis in the brain (berry aneurysm) is due to a congenital anomaly.

DISSECTING ANEURYSM

A dissecting aneurysm occurs when blood penetrates the intimal layer of the aortic wall and separates the layers of the arterial wall, forming a hematoma. The intima and medial layers are torn in most cases, and the hematoma extends to the adventitia layer. The separation may extend in either direction. The separation may obstruct an artery branching from the aorta, or the hematoma may rupture, causing a life-threatening situation.

If the dissecting aneurysm is in the ascending aorta, it is a type A dissecting aneurysm; if the aneurysm is in the descending aorta, it is a type B dissecting aneurysm. Predisposing factors to a dissecting aneurysm include hypertension and left ventricular hypertrophy. They occur more frequently in men than in women and are usually located in the thoracic arch of the aorta. Surgical intervention is the usual treatment for a dissecting aneurysm.

ABDOMINAL AORTIC ANEURYSM

ETIOLOGY AND PATHOPHYSIOLOGY

Most abdominal aortic aneurysms develop in the abdominal aorta below the renal arteries. They may also extend to the iliac arteries. Atherosclerosis is the most common predisposing factor for developing an abdominal aortic aneurysm. Other causes include infection, trauma, or congenital abnormalities. The medial layer of the vessel wall is weakened, affecting the elastin and collagen, and the adventitia layer becomes inflamed.

An abdominal aortic aneurysm is usually of the fusiform type and contains ulcerated plaques, thrombi, and necrotic material. It may vary in size from 10 to 15 cm. The incidence of abdominal aortic aneurysms has increased in recent years, primarily because of longevity with an increase in atherosclerotic problems. It is more common in individuals older than 60 years who have a history of cardiovascular disease, including myocardial infarction, hypertension, angina pectoris, and congestive heart failure.

CLINICAL MANIFESTATIONS

Typically, individuals with an abdominal aortic aneurysm are asymptomatic. Complications are just as likely to occur in an asymptomatic patient as a symptomatic patient. Abdominal pain from pressure on the somatic sensory nerve is a common manifestation. The pain ranges from mild to severe and may be localized in the lumbar, midabdominal, or pelvic area. It may also radiate to the lower extremities. Low back pain may indicate impending rupture.

The patient may feel a throb or pulsation in the abdomen, especially when supine. This pulsation may also be auscultated as a bruit over the abdomen. Large aneurysms can easily be palpated and may cause some abdominal distention. Tenderness with palpation may be present directly over the aneurysm. Extremities may be pale, cold, or mottled and pulses absent if the aneurysm dissects, enlarges, or ruptures, interrupting blood flow to the periphery.

Because approximately half of the patients with an abdominal aortic aneurysm have hypertension, systolic readings in the thigh, which are normally higher than in the arm, may be decreased as a result of arterial occlusion of the femoral artery. Occlusion of arteries related to abdominal aneurysms is illustrated in Figure 20–6.

MEDICAL DIAGNOSIS

The diagnosis is made on the basis of physical assessment and diagnostic test results. Approximately one third of the asymptomatic abdominal aortic aneurysms are discovered by palpation; the others are too small to palpate. In extremely obese patients, palpation may be of limited use. The aneurysms are diagnosed by the presence of a systolic bruit or pulsation over the abdominal mass. Ultrasonography and CT scans are used to detect the size and location of the aneurysm and to determine the condition of the renal, carotid, and coronary arteries.

MEDICAL MANAGEMENT

Surgical resection is the treatment of choice for most abdominal aortic aneurysms. If the patient is a poor surgical risk or in extremely poor health or has a history of cardiac dysfunction, the surgery may be

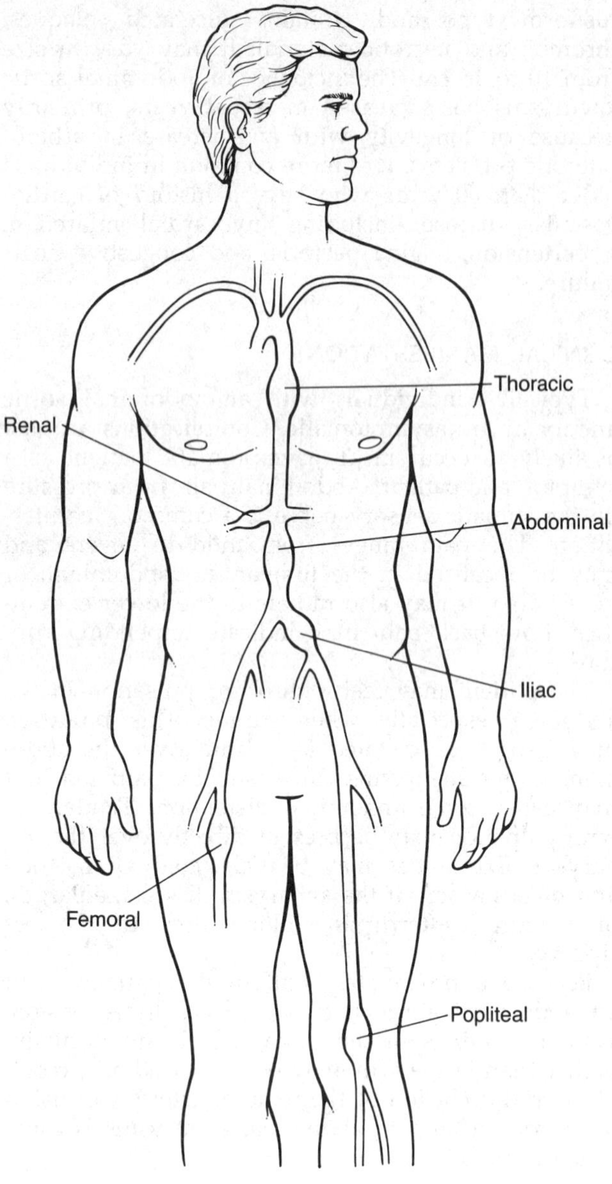

Figure 20–6.

The relative location of arterial occlusion and arterial aneurysms.

delayed. If the aneurysm is very small, the prognosis may still be good without surgery.

Patients having elective surgery for resection of an abdominal aortic aneurysm have a good prognosis. Mortality is usually associated with myocardial infarction. If untreated, rupture of the aneurysm with hemorrhage is the most common cause of death.

The larger the aneurysm, the more likely it is to rupture. The presence or absence of symptoms has no effect on the likelihood of rupture or development of other complications. Less than 30% of abdominal aortic aneurysms rupture.

Symptoms of a ruptured aneurysm include sudden back or abdominal pain, a decrease in blood pressure, increased pulse rate, and ecchymoses in the lower back area. Laboratory findings show a decreased red blood cell count and hemoglobin related to the hemorrhage. Even with surgery, the prognosis can be poor after rupture, especially if the patient is older than 65 years or has a history of other disorders.

Other complications may develop from compression of a large aneurysm on adjacent structures. Pressure on the duodenum can result in blockage of the intestine or bleeding from ulcerations caused by inadequate blood flow to the organ.

THORACIC AORTIC ANEURYSM

ETIOLOGY AND PATHOPHYSIOLOGY

Atherosclerosis is the primary cause of thoracic aortic aneurysms. They occur most often in men between 40 and 70 years of age. Thoracic aneurysms are frequently dissecting aneurysms, but they may also be fusiform or another type.

CLINICAL MANIFESTATIONS

Thoracic aortic aneurysms are usually asymptomatic. Patients with symptoms may experience constant pain in the chest or upper back, neck, and shoulders. The pain may be more prominent when the patient is supine. Dyspnea may result from pressure of the aneurysm against the trachea, bronchi, or lungs. A brassy cough, stridor, hoarseness, and weak voice are caused by pressure on the trachea and laryngeal nerve. Dysphagia occurs from pressure on the esophagus. Pressure on the cervical sympathetic nerve chain causes unequal dilation of the pupils. The aneurysm may compress large veins in the chest, causing edema, cyanosis, and dilated superficial veins of the neck, chest, and upper extremities. Neck vein distention occurs from pressure on the superior vena cava.

MEDICAL DIAGNOSIS

A thoracic aortic aneurysm is diagnosed by physical assessment and history, if symptomatic, chest x-ray film, aortography, and CT scan, which help determine the exact location of the aneurysm and the surrounding vessels that are involved.

MEDICAL MANAGEMENT

Surgical resection of the aneurysm with a vascular graft is the treatment of choice (see Chapter 19 for a discussion of grafts). Antihypertensive medications are given to keep the systolic pressure below 120 mm Hg, thus reducing the pressure in the aorta. Other medications such as propranolol may be prescribed to reduce cardiac contractions and to decrease the pulsating flow of blood.

With treatment, most patients survive several

years. The prognosis worsens if the patient is older than 50 years or has a history of hypertension or if the aneurysm is extremely large. Death from rupture of the aneurysm occurs in approximately one third of patients. A small asymptomatic aneurysm may not be treated unless it enlarges.

PERIPHERAL ARTERIAL ANEURYSMS

ETIOLOGY AND PATHOPHYSIOLOGY

Peripheral aneurysms occur more often in the lower extremities than in the upper extremities. Two thirds of all peripheral arterial aneurysms occur in the popliteal artery, and about one third occur in the femoral artery. Flexion of the knee may predispose the popliteal artery to dilation.

Aneurysms of the peripheral vessels are usually a result of atherosclerosis. Other causes include infection and trauma. Most peripheral aneurysms occur in men. They are often bilateral and multiple.

Popliteal aneurysms are located in the popliteal fossa and appear as a pulsating mass. The aneurysm is usually elongated and fusiform (Fig. 20–7). Symptoms are absent in approximately half the patients. Almost all popliteal aneurysms occur in men between 50 and 80 years of age. Femoral aneurysms also appear as a pulsating mass located along the femoral artery.

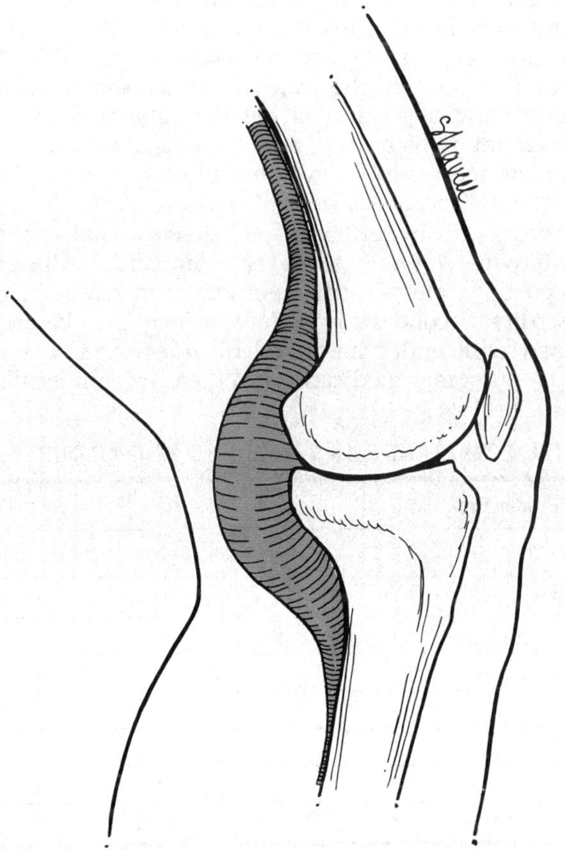

Figure 20–7.

Fusiform aneurysm of the popliteal artery.

CLINICAL MANIFESTATIONS

Clinical manifestations of peripheral arterial aneurysms include intermittent claudication from arterial insufficiency in the lower legs and feet. Rest pain or gangrene may occur from thrombosis or embolism. Tenderness, pain, edema, coldness, and numbness in the lower extremities are caused by pressure on the nerves, veins, and arteries.

MEDICAL DIAGNOSIS

The diagnosis is made on the basis of the symptoms present, physical assessment, and diagnostic studies such as angiography and ultrasonography.

MEDICAL MANAGEMENT

Surgical resection of the aneurysm with a prosthetic or saphenous graft is the treatement of choice. Prognosis is excellent after surgery if the patient takes steps to reduce the risk factors associated with atherosclerosis. The most common postoperative complication is bleeding. (Refer to Chapter 19 for a discussion of grafts.)

Without surgery, complications develop within 8 years in most patients. Thrombosis may result in ischemia and possible loss of the extremity. The aneurysm may cause pressure on surrounding veins and nerves, causing occlusion and pain. Other complications include rupture, which is rare, infection, and gangrene from interruption of the circulation.

Application of the Nursing Process to the Care of the Patient with an Aneurysm

The assessment, nursing diagnoses, expected patient outcomes, nursing interventions, and evaluation for patients with an aneurysm are similar to those described previously for patients with arterial embolus or thrombus and obstructive arterial vascular disorders. Refer to Chapter 19 for application of the nursing process to the patient undergoing peripheral vascular surgery.

The following additional assessments apply to the care of patients with aneurysm. Assess the cardiopulmonary and renal statuses by observing hemodynamic monitoring, laboratory tests, and output. Check for tenderness and distention of the abdomen. Auscultate arteries for bruits. Do not use deep palpation if a dissecting aneurysm is suspected. Assess all pulses to determine occlusion of arteries. Observe the color and temperature of the extremities. Look for venous distention and edema. Check for pain in the back, neck, shoulders, or extremities. Observe for ecchymoses on the lower back.

Assess changes in respiratory status. Observe for fever and leukocytosis, indicating pulmonary complications. Auscultate for wheezes and crackles, indicating pulmonary congestion from increased hydrostatic pressure in the pulmonary vascular system. Respiratory distress may indicate impending shock from hemorrhage after rupture of the aneurysm. Observe for other changes in the patient indicating a ruptured aneurysm such as sudden, intense pain and vital sign changes.

The following additional interventions apply to the care of patients with aneurysm. If the patient is high risk, surgery may be delayed or not recommended. Explain the effects of the disorder to the patient and family. Teach the signs of rupture, and tell the patient to seek immediate medical assistance if any of the signs become apparent. Explain the lifestyle restrictions prescribed by the physician. Allow the patient and family time to ask questions and to voice fears and concerns about the patient's future. Make appropriate referrals for home-care assistance as needed.

Hypertensive Vascular Disease

Hypertensive vascular disease is defined as a persistent systolic blood pressure greater than 140 mm Hg and a persistent diastolic blood pressure greater than 90 mm Hg. A persistent systolic blood pressure greater than 140 mm Hg with a diastolic pressure less than 90 mm Hg is termed *systolic hypertension.* In 1992 federal health officials released a new system for classifying blood pressure, dividing levels of hypertension into four stages (Table 20–1).

Hypertensive vascular disease is the most common cardiovascular disorder in the United States. It is estimated that at least 20% of the adult population may be affected. In the elderly, the numbers are significantly higher. Approximately 65% of the black elderly and 40% to 50% of the white elderly are hypertensive. Because individuals with hypertension are often free of symptoms until complications develop, only approximately 50% of the individuals with hypertension are diagnosed. Of those diagnosed, only roughly 50% comply with their prescribed treatment plan.

The incidence of hypertension in the United States is higher among men than women and is highest in the black population. In addition to a higher incidence of hypertension, these individuals also tend to have a more severe disease state and a higher incidence of mortality associated with the disease.

Classification of Hypertension

Hypertension is classified as either primary (essential) hypertension or secondary hypertension. Approximately 90% of all individuals who have hypertension have primary hypertension. The onset is usually between 25 and 55 years of age. Primary hypertension is further categorized as benign, which has a slow onset and is initially asymptomatic, or malignant, which is a rare form characterized by sudden onset, rapid development of symptoms, and accelerated progression of the disease.

Secondary hypertension is characterized by an underlying known cause that impairs peripheral blood flow, alters cardiac output, or increases blood viscosity. Secondary hypertension may also be associated with endocrine gland disorders and side effects of some medications. When the underlying

Table 20–1. CLASSIFICATION OF BLOOD PRESSURE FOR ADULTS 18 YEARS OLD AND OLDER

AVERAGE DIASTOLIC BLOOD PRESSURE (mm Hg)	AVERAGE SYSTOLIC BLOOD PRESSURE (mm Hg)						
	LESS THAN 120	120–129	130–139	140–159	160–179	180–209	210 OR OVER
Less than 80	Optimal*	Normal	High Normal	1	2	3	4
80–84	Normal	Normal	High Normal	1	2	3	4
85–89	High Normal	High Normal	High Normal	1	2	3	4
90–99	1	1	1	1	2	3	4
100–109	2	2	2	2	2	3	4
110–119	3	3	3	3	3	3	4
120 or over	4	4	4	4	4	4	4

Note: White areas denote normal pressure. Shaded areas denote hypertension (Stages 1–4)

*Unusually low readings should be evaluated for clinical significance.

From National Heart, Lung, and Blood Institute, National Institutes of Health. National High Blood Pressure Education Program. Washington, DC: U.S. Government Printing Office, 1992.

Table 20–2. RISK FACTORS ASSOCIATED WITH HYPERTENSION

RISK FACTORS	RATIONALE
Age	Loss of arterial elasticity
Sex	Higher blood pressure in males younger than 40 years
Race	Blood pressure higher in blacks; cause unknown, possibly a result of high-fat dietary intake, genetics
Obesity	Extra weight increases cardiac workload and adds strain on vessels
Smoking	Nicotine constricts vessels
Caffeine	Vasoconstriction
Sodium	Water retention causes volume expansion
Stress	Vasoconstriction

cause is treated, the hypertension resolves. Secondary hypertension occurs in 10% of all individuals with hypertension.

ETIOLOGY

Primary hypertension has no known cause; however, a variety of factors contribute to its occurrence. These factors, which are identified in Table 20–2, include heredity, age, and lifestyle patterns. A diet high in fat and sodium also increases the risk of hypertension. There is a direct relationship between the incidence of hypertension and atherosclerosis. Hypertension is a risk factor in the development of atherosclerosis, and atherosclerosis, with its associated impairment of arterial blood flow, contributes to the development of hypertension.

PATHOPHYSIOLOGY

Peripheral vascular resistance and cardiac output directly affect blood pressure. Resistance is determined by the diameter of the blood vessels and blood viscosity. Primary benign hypertension is characterized by narrowed arteries, which cause an increase in peripheral resistance. In many instances, it is unclear whether increased peripheral resistance precedes or is the result of increased blood pressure.

In some individuals with primary hypertension, pathologic response to stress causes excessive stimulation of the sympathetic nervous system. Increased sympathetic nervous system stimulation produces peripheral vasoconstriction and increased heart rate, which results in increased blood pressure.

In some cases of hypertension, excess quantities of renin are secreted by the kidneys. Excess renin may be secreted in response to sympathetic nervous system stimulation or in the absence of any stimulating factors. Renin converts angiotensinogen into angiotensin I, which is subsequently converted by an enzyme to angiotensin II. Angiotensin II causes arteriole constriction and stimulates the adrenal cortex to increase the secretion of aldosterone. Aldosterone promotes sodium and water retention, which increases extracellular fluid volume. The combination of excess peripheral vasoconstriction and an increase in the blood volume results in pathologic elevation in blood pressure (Fig. 20–8).

In the early stages of primary benign hypertension, changes in the blood vessels and organs are not apparent. However, as the disorder progresses, changes can be detected in blood vessels and the major target organs such as the heart, kidneys, brain, and eyes.

Under constant stress of abnormally high pressure, the intima of the arteries is damaged, resulting in edema, fibrin accumulation, and clot formation. Arterial walls weaken, and the vessels become sclerosed and tortuous. As the lumens narrow, the blood flow to the major target organs and peripheral tissues decreases. Because the blood supply to organs and peripheral tissues is impaired, ischemia, atrophy, fibrosis, and loss of function occur. Damaged vessels may eventually become occluded or may hemorrhage as a result of weakened vascular walls.

Cardiovascular disorders associated with hypertension are the result of the heart's attempt to overcome increased peripheral resistance. When the blood vessels constrict, the heart pumps harder, resulting in cardiac hypertrophy, especially of the left ventricle. This, in turn, may lead to left ventricular failure, progressing to right ventricular failure and congestive heart failure. Venous congestion occurs throughout the entire vascular system. Figure 20–9 illustrates the events in hypertensive vascular disease that lead to target organ destruction.

Decreased arterial blood flow to the kidneys may cause ischemia and necrosis of renal nephrons and may lead to renal failure. Weakened arteriosclerotic vessels under prolonged above-normal pressure may

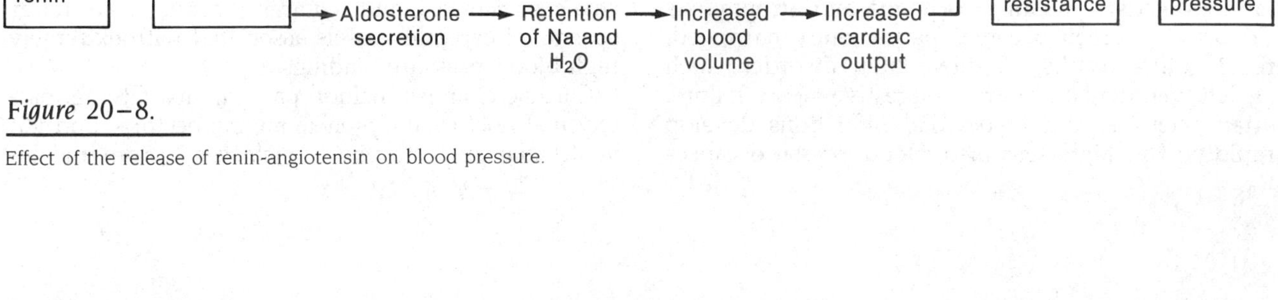

Figure 20–8.

Effect of the release of renin-angiotensin on blood pressure.

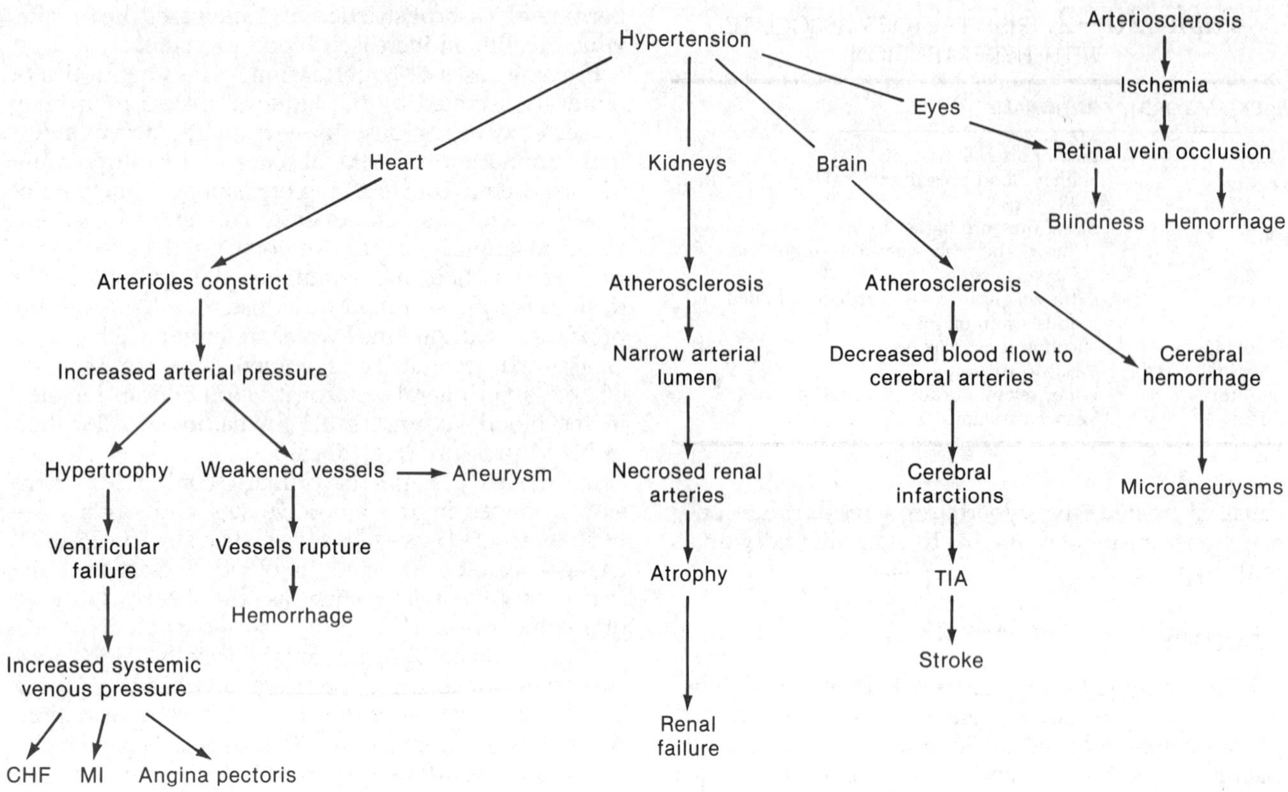

Figure 20–9.

Major target organs affected by hypertension. CHF, congestive heart failure; MI, myocardial infarction; TIA, transient ischemic attack.

rupture or develop aneurysms. Cerebral aneurysms may result in cerebral hemorrhage, transient ischemic attacks, cerebral infarctions, or cerebrovascular accidents. Arteriosclerosis, ischemia, and hemorrhage of retinal vessels may result in visual disturbances and blindness. Arterial atherosclerosis with reduced blood flow to the lower extremities results in arterial peripheral vascular disease, ischemia, and intermittent claudication. The incidence of these long-term degenerative changes associated with hypertension is greatly reduced if the condition is adequately controlled.

The pathologic deterioration associated with malignant hypertension is more severe and may progress more rapidly than in benign hypertension. In malignant hypertension, the blood pressure rises suddenly, possibly as high as 200/140 mm Hg. It occurs most commonly in individuals 40 to 50 years of age. More than 50% of the individuals experiencing malignant hypertension have an underlying chronic kidney disease.

Hyperplasia of the intima of the arteries in the kidneys leads to nephron ischemia and atrophy. As the arterial lumen becomes permanently narrowed, renal failure results. Cardiovascular disorders such as left ventricular failure, congestive heart failure, arteriosclerosis, and myocardial infarctions develop rapidly. The high sustained blood pressure causes papilledema, hemorrhage, and exudates in the retinas. Without treatment, the mortality rate is approximately 100% within 2 years and roughly 80% within 1 year.

CLINICAL MANIFESTATIONS

An absence of symptoms in the initial stages is typical of benign hypertension. This is one reason why rates of early diagnosis and compliance to treatment regimens are so low. Initially the patient feels well even without treatment.

Ophthalmoscopic examination of the retina shows hemorrhages, crossing over, narrowing, and nicking of the retinal arteries, tortuous vessels, patchy white areas with indefinite edges (cotton wool exudates), and papilledema with blurring of the disk margins.

Cerebrovascular manifestations include epistaxis, vertigo, lightheadedness, tinnitus, occipital headaches in the early morning, and blurred vision. Decreased sensations and hemiplegia may indicate a transient ischemic attack or stroke. Personality changes, nausea, and vomiting result from reflex spasms of cerebral vessels associated with extremely high blood pressure readings.

Cardiac changes include palpitations, fatigue, paroxysmal nocturnal dyspnea, angina pectoris, and left ventricular hypertrophy, which result from the increased workload on the heart, and tissue ischemia from impaired blood supply.

Renal involvement results in nocturia, hematuria, and increased blood urea nitrogen and creatinine levels. Skin changes such as discoloration and edema may indicate vessel inflammation.

MEDICAL DIAGNOSIS

The medical diagnosis is made on the basis of the findings from the history, physical assessment, and blood pressure measurements. The blood pressure measurements over a period of a few days to several weeks are obtained. The recorded blood pressure at each measurement is the average of three readings taken at least 2 minutes apart. On the first measurement, the patient's pressure is obtained in both arms while he or she is lying, sitting, and standing.

A chest x-ray film and an electrocardiogram are done to determine cardiac changes, and a urinalysis is completed to detect protein. Complete blood count, fasting blood sugar, blood urea nitrogen, serum creatinine, and urinary specific gravity help determine the extent of renal damage.

Renal function studies, renal angiography, intravenous urograms, and tomography are used to detect secondary causes. Urine is tested for excessive serum catecholamines. Studies are conducted to evaluate plasma renin, angiotensin, and aldosterone. A serum potassium level is determined because hypokalemia may be indicative of primary aldosteronism. Thyroid studies are conducted because hyperthyroidism can cause excessively high blood pressure and heart rate, leading to vasoconstriction and hypertension. High serum cholesterol and triglyceride levels may predispose to the development of atheromatous plaques.

MEDICAL MANAGEMENT

The medical management goal for primary hypertension is to reduce the blood pressure. Minimizing risk factors by low-cholesterol, low-salt diet, weight loss, relaxation exercises, and a regular regimen of moderate exercise may be the treatment of choice in patients whose diastolic blood pressure is less than 100 mm Hg. If the diastolic blood pressure is consistently greater than 105 mm Hg, drug therapy may be indicated. Table 20–3 outlines detection and treatment guidelines recommended by the National Institutes of Health. The goal in drug therapy is to use the least amount of medication with the most effectiveness and the least significant side effects.

The drugs of choice for hypertension vary with physician preference, patient history, concurrent medications, and tolerability. Commonly prescribed antihypertensive drugs are listed in Table 20–4. Diuretics may be used to suppress renal tubular reabsorption of sodium. Sympathetic blocking agents or beta blockers and vasodilators may be added. The medications are given to relax smooth-muscle walls, decrease cardiac output, block or interfere with sympathetic impulses, decrease release of renin, and decrease peripheral resistance and arterial constriction (Pharmacology Box 20–1).

NONCOMPLIANCE TO TREATMENT

Noncompliance to treatment regimens for hypertension is extremely common. It is estimated that only approximately one ninth of all patients with hypertension are being treated adequately. Of the newly diagnosed patients, approximately one half discontinue the therapy within 1 year of treatment, and almost three fourths discontinue therapy within 5 years.

Many theories have been proposed to explain why noncompliance is so high among patients with hypertension. The disorder is usually asymptomatic in its early stages, and treatment requires lifestyle changes and, in some cases, medications. The patient may feel well without treatment and may even feel ill when taking medication because of the side effects. It is difficult to motivate patients to adhere to a treatment regimen when benefits are not easily apparent. Other factors associated with noncompliance include long waiting times at clinics or physician's offices, treatment and medication costs, and poor follow-up care.

With asymptomatic diseases such as hypertension, patients have a 50% appointment failure and more than 60% noncompliance rate with medications. It is estimated that one third of patients almost always

Table 20–3. RECOMMENDED ACTION FOR PERSONS WITH HIGH SYSTOLIC OR HIGH DIASTOLIC READINGS

RECOMMENDED ACTION FOR PERSONS WITH HIGH SYSTOLIC READINGS

SYSTOLIC READINGS WITH DIASTOLIC ≤90 mmHg	RECOMMENDED ACTION
≥200	Immediate evaluation and treatment no later than 2 weeks
140–199	Reevaluate within 1–2 months
<140	Reevaluate in 2 years

RECOMMENDED ACTION FOR PERSONS WITH HIGH DIASTOLIC READINGS

DIASTOLIC READINGS	RECOMMENDED ACTION
≥115	Immediate evaluation and treatment
105–114	Evaluation/treatment no later than 2 weeks
90–104	Reevaluate within 1–2 months
<90	Reevaluate in 1 year

From The Joint National Committee on Detection, Evaluation and Treatment of High Blood Pressure. The Fourth Report of the Joint National Committee on Detection, Evaluation and Treatment of High Blood Pressure (JNC IV). Bethesda, MD: National Institutes of Health, 1988.

Table 20–4. ORAL ANTIHYPERTENSIVE MEDICATIONS

MEDICATION	ACTION	CONTRAINDICATIONS	SIDE EFFECTS
THIAZIDE DIURETICS			
Bendroflumethiazide (Naturetin) Benzthiazide (Exna, Aquatag) Chlorothiazide (Diuril) Chlorthalidone (Hygroton) Cyclothiazide (Anhydron) Hydrochlorothiazide (Esidrix, HydroDIURIL, Oretic) Hydroflumethiazide (Saluron) Indapamide (Lozol) Metolazone (Zaroxolyn, Diulo) Methyclothiazide (Ethon, Enduron) Polythiazide (Renese) Trichlormethiazide (Metahydrin, Naqua) Quinethazone (Hydromox)	Renal excretion of Na^+, H_2O, K^+; initial decrease in blood volume and cardiac output	Renal failure Hepatic disease Lactation/pregnancy Hypokalemia Gout Diabetes Peripheral vascular disease	↑ BUN ↑ Uric acid ↑ Blood glucose ↑ Calcium ↓ Potassium Restlessness Lethargy, weakness, vertigo, thirst, dry mouth GI disturbances Muscle cramps Hypotension, tachycardia Polyuria Leukopenia Agranulocytosis
LOOP DIURETICS			
Furosemide (Lasix) Ethacrynic acid (Edecrin) Bumetanide (Bumex)	Same as thiazides	Same as thiazides	Similar to thiazides Hypocalcemia Hypovolemia Dehydration Gynecomastia Photosensitivity
POTASSIUM SPARING (NONTHIAZIDES)			
Spironolactone (Aldactone)	Renal excretion of Na^+ and H_2O; retention of K^+	Renal failure Hyperkalemia Diabetes Calcium channel blocking agents	↑ BUN Hyperkalemia Hyponatremia Gynecomastia Hirsutism Irregular menses Rash Lethargy, ataxia Confusion
Triamterene (Dyrenium) Amiloride (Midamor)			Hyperkalemia, hyperchloremic acidosis, diarrhea, nausea, vomiting, rash, photosensitivity, blood dyscrasias
Spironolactone with HCTZ (Aldactazide, Dyazide)	Blocks reabsorption of Na^+		Vertigo, headache, dry mouth, GI disturbances
ADRENERGIC INHIBITORS			
Beta Blockers			
Acebutolol (Sectral) Atenolol (Tenormin) Metoprolol (Lopressor) Nadolol (Corgard) Pindolol (Visken) Propranolol (Inderal) Timolol (Blocadren)	Decreases cardiac output, sympathetic stimulation, and renin secretion	Bronchial asthma Rhinitis Cardiomegaly CHF Peripheral vascular disease Bradycardia Diabetes, hypoglycemia MAO inhibitors Bronchodilators Liver disease Pheochromocytoma Pregnancy, lactation	Lethargy, fatigue, depression, vertigo, insomnia, headache Bronchospasm Dyspnea Bradycardia, palpitations, orthostatic hypotension Raynaud's phenomenon GI disturbances, nausea, vomiting, diarrhea, fluid retention Hypoglycemia Thrombocytopenia Rash, fever, nasal stuffiness Impotence

(continued)

Table 20–4. (continued) ORAL ANTIHYPERTENSIVE MEDICATIONS

MEDICATION	ACTION	CONTRAINDICATIONS	SIDE EFFECTS
ADRENERGIC INHIBITORS (*continued*)			
Alpha Inhibitors			
Prazosin (Minipress)	Decreases peripheral vascular resistance, vasodilation		
Beta/Alpha Combined			
Labetalol (Normodyne, Trandate)	Same as prazosin		
Central Inhibitors			
Clonidine (Catapres)	Initially decreases cardiac output; decreases peripheral vascular resistance and heart rate	Hepatic disease Pregnancy Tricyclic antidepressants Mental depression	Orthostatic hypotension, vertigo, sedation, rash, constipation, dry mouth, headache, fatigue, anorexia, bradycardia, fluid retention, insomnia, nightmares
Guanabenz (Wytensin)			Drowsiness, dry mouth, fluid retention, rash, postural hypotension, loss of libido, dark or blue urine
Methyldopa (Aldomet)			Same as clonidine Fever, anemia, impotence
Peripheral Inhibitors			
Guanadrel (Hylorel) Guanethidine (Ismelin) Reserpine (Serpasil, Serpalan, Serpate)	Relaxes smooth muscle, decreases peripheral vascular resistance, heart rate, and blood pressure when upright	CHF, pheochromocytoma, peptic ulcer, surgery, ulcerative colitis, bronchial asthma, tricyclic antidepressants, MAO inhibitors, orthostatic hypotension, severe coronary artery or cerebrovascular disease, mental depression	Orthostatic hypotension, bradycardia, diarrhea, edema, impotence, decreased libido, depression, nasal congestion, increased appetite, weight gain, gastric hyperacidity, salt and H_2O retention, drowsiness, bizarre dreams
VASODILATORS			
Diazoxide (Hyperstat) Hydralazine (Apresoline) Minoxidil (Loniten) Sodium nitroprusside (Nipride)	Relaxation of arteriolar smooth muscle resulting in vasodilation; initial increase in cardiac output; decreased peripheral vascular resistance	Coronary artery disease CHF Lupus erythematosus Cerebrovascular disease Migraine	Headache, vertigo, fever, flushing, tachycardia, palpitations, nausea, anorexia, diarrhea, dyspnea, rash, angina, fluid retention, muscle aches, tremors, cramps, lupus-like syndrome with long-term usage
CALCIUM CHANNEL BLOCKING AGENTS			
Diltiazem (Cardizem) Nifedipine (Procardia) Verapamil (Calan, Isoptin)	Inhibits calcium into smooth muscle cells; arteriolar vasodilation, decreases peripheral vascular resistance; increases cardiac output, with the exception of verapamil.	CHF Heart block Beta blocking agents	Headache, vertigo, weakness, palpitations, tachycardia, arrhythmia, flushing, rash, hypotension, peripheral edema, nausea, constipation, diarrhea, fluid retention, bradycardia, muscle aches, tremors, cramps
ANGIOTENSIN-CONVERTING ENZYME INHIBITORS			
Captopril (Capoten) Enalapril (Vasotec)	Decreases peripheral vascular resistance	Renal insufficiency Renal artery stenosis	Hypotension Hyperkalemia Granulocytopenia, hemolytic anemia, proteinuria, stomatitis, loss of taste, tongue ulcers, fever, rash

Abbreviations: Na^+, sodium ion; H_2O, water; K^+, potassium ion; BUN, blood urea nitrogen; GI, gastrointestinal; HCTZ, hydrochlorothiazide; CHF, congestive heart failure; MAO, monoamine oxidase.

Pharmacology Box 20–1.
β-ADRENERGIC BLOCKING AGENTS

Beta Blockers:
Drugs that block receptor sites affected by catecholamines.

Action:
Exhibit effective blocking at specific receptor sites, resulting in decreased heart rate, slowed conduction, decreased plasma renin, and decreased force of myocardial contraction.

Uses:
To reduce hypertension, arrhythmias, aortic stenosis, and other noncardiovascular effects.

Side Effects:
May be selective depending on the particular drug; they include drowsiness, malaise, nausea, tingling, paresthesia, dizziness, and decreased heart rate.

Interactions:
May interact with cardiac depressants, may be inactive when used in conjunction with sympathomimetic drugs, may antagonize the bronchodilating effect of theophylline, may increase problems with orthostatic hypotension, and may enhance neuromuscular blocking agents.

Nursing Implications:
Watch for signs of drug interactions as listed above.
Monitor vital signs while patient is on medications; especially observe for bradycardia and measure the blood pressure frequently to monitor the effect of the drug if given for hypertension.
Tell the patient being discharged on medication to return, as ordered, for follow-up laboratory studies to check kidney, liver, cardiac, and respiratory function.
Give the medication before meals except when otherwise indicated, because most beta blockers should be taken before meals.

Geriatric Considerations:
Caution the elderly patient to change positions slowly because the drug may cause orthostatic hypotension. This could be a safety concern for older adults, especially those with physical mobility impairment. Tell the patient the drug may cause increased sensitivity to cold, which is a common problem in the elderly.

take the prescribed medications, one third take the prescribed medication sometimes, and one third never take the prescribed medication. It is difficult to predict which patients will be noncompliant with the prescribed treatment regimen. Evidence suggests that increased patient education regarding the disease and treatment modalities may enhance compliance.

COMPLICATIONS

HYPERTENSIVE CRISIS

Excessively high blood pressure requiring immediate treatment is termed *hypertensive crisis*. Less than 5% of patients with primary hypertension progress to a hypertensive crisis. During a crisis the diastolic pressure may be as high as 130 mm Hg. Retinal hemorrhages, exudates, and papilledema are usually present. The patient may be restless and confused and experience blurred vision, headache, nausea, and vomiting. A cerebrovascular accident, renal failure, or cardiac failure may occur within days. A hypertensive crisis is a medical emergency. The patient is admitted to an intensive care unit for close monitoring of the blood pressure and target organ damage. Quick-acting parenteral medications such as the vasodilators, sympathetic inhibitors, and diuretics identified in Table 20–5 are administered to lower the blood pressure rapidly.

Application of the Nursing Process to the Care of the Patient with Hypertension

Assessment

Review the patient's history and diagnostic studies, and complete a physical assessment. Assess the blood pressure while the patient is lying, sitting, and standing. Take the measurements in both arms and legs to determine the baseline data and note any differences bilaterally. Before taking the blood pressure, have the patient rest quietly for at least 5 minutes. Compare the readings with previous data. Measurements may be affected by the time of day taken, the patient's emotional status, pain, smoking, eating, talking, coldness, bladder distention, or drugs. Blood pressure readings are often higher at midmorning and noon.

Palpate the apical pulse at the midclavicular line in the fifth intercostal space and the peripheral pulses to determine the rate, rhythm, and amplitude. Palpate extremities for edema. Auscultate for dysrhythmias, tachycardia, or abnormal breath sounds, which may indicate cardiac involvement.

Ask about episodes of angina, and obtain a description of the pain as to intensity, precipitating factors, duration, radiation, and relief methods. Examine the neck for enlarged thyroid or vein distention. Observe for decreased urinary output or increased output if the patient is on diuretic therapy.

Table 20–5. PARENTERAL MEDICATIONS USED IN TREATING HYPERTENSIVE CRISIS

MEDICATION	ACTION	INDICATIONS	NURSING CONSIDERATIONS
DIURETICS			
Furosemide (Lasix)	Inhibits reabsorption of Na^+ and chl by the renal tubule; large amounts of Na^+ and chl are excreted; smaller amounts of K^+ and bicarbonate ion are excreted	Malignant hypertension Hypertensive encephalopathy CHF Intracranial hemorrhage Pulmonary edema Lymphedema	Never use with ethacrynic acid; assess for electrolyte losses (i.e., chest pain, calf and pelvic pain); do not give with whole blood or its derivatives; assess for vestibular disturbance with renal impairment; assess for vascular thrombosis and embolism, especially in elderly
Ethacrynic acid (Edecrin, Edecril)	Same as for Lasix	Same as for Lasix	Same as for Lasix; pain and irritation at injection site when given IM and SC
VASODILATORS			
Sodium nitroprusside (Nipride)	Vasodilation of peripheral arterioles	Hypertensive encephalopathy Malignant hypertension CHF, pheochromocytoma Intracranial hemorrhage	Monitor BP closely; check for excessive hypotensive effect
Diazoxide (Hyperstat)	Vasodilation of peripheral arterioles	Hypertensive encephalopathy Intracranial hemorrhage Malignant hypertension	Potent diuretic; assess BP before each bolus dose; inject rapidly within 30 sec into peripheral vein; keep patient flat 30 min after injecting
Hydralazine (Apresoline)	Vasodilating effect on vascular smooth muscle and CNS effects (reflex action)	Malignant hypertension Eclampsia	Assess BP within 5 min after injecting; may cause headaches, palpitations, arrhythmias; weigh daily; observe for edema, I & O
SYMPATHETIC INHIBITORS			
Methyldopa (Aldomet)	Depresses sympathetic nervous system, relaxes smooth muscle	Malignant hypertension Intracranial hemorrhage	Weigh daily; observe for edema, I & O; usually used with other antihypertensive drugs
Reserpine (Serpasil)	Same as Aldomet	Malignant hypertension	Same as above
GANGLIONIC BLOCKER			
Trimethaphan (Arfonad)	Dilates blood vessels, increases heart rate and cardiac output	Malignant hypertension Hypertensive encephalopathy Pulmonary edema Dissecting aortic aneurysm Ischemic heart disease	Instruct patient with history of angina that it may precipitate an attack; monitor BP closely; assess for peripheral vascular collapse (i.e., hypotension; rapid pulse; cold, clammy skin; cyanosis)

Abbreviations: Na^+, sodium ion; chl, chloride; K^+, potassium ion; CHF, congestive heart failure; IM, intramuscular; SC, subcutaneous; BP, blood pressure; CNS, central nervous system; I & O, intake and output.

Palpate the abdomen for masses and bruits indicative of aneurysms or stenosis of the abdominal aorta or renal arteries.

Assess the neurologic status to detect changes associated with altered cerebral perfusion, cerebrovascular accident, or hemorrhage. Assess for pallor, diaphoresis, and vertigo when the patient rises from a supine position, which may indicate orthostatic hypotension.

Assess for skin and retinal changes indicative of progressive hypertension. Obtain height and weight measurements to determine obesity. Review the patient's dietary pattern; check caloric levels and the amount of fat, cholesterol, and sodium regularly consumed. Determine food preferences and financial influences on food choices.

Assess the patient's level of knowledge, stressors, and risk factors such as smoking, obesity, and lack of exercise. Determine whether the patient is taking birth-control pills, diet pills, cold medications, amphetamines, or alcohol, which may be associated with hypertension. Check the family history for hypertension, other cardiovascular diseases, or diabetes.

Nursing Diagnoses and Planning

Nursing diagnoses and related expected patient outcomes most commonly applicable to patients with hypertension include the following:

NDx: Decreased cardiac output related to increased workload of the heart and vasoconstriction

Planning: Patient outcomes
1. Patient's vital signs are within normal ranges for the patient.
2. Patient has a balanced intake and output and is free of peripheral and central edema.
3. Patient's skin is warm, color is appropriate, no cyanosis is present, and peripheral pulses are palpable.
4. Patient maintains an adequate cardiac output as seen by the hemodynamic monitoring.

NDx: Altered nutrition, more than body requirements, related to lifestyle, resulting in obesity, atherosclerosis, and hypertension

Planning: Patient outcomes
1. Patient states accurate information about an appropriate diet plan for weight loss, including low-fat, low-cholesterol, and low-sodium foods.
2. Patient chooses food as allowed on the diet plan.
3. Patient's weight decreases.

NDx: Self-esteem disturbance related to hypertensive disease state, changes in lifestyle to manage disease and reduce risk factors, or inability to comply with the treatment plan

Planning: Patient outcomes
1. Patient states methods to cope with illness.
2. Patient denies feelings of inadequacy, helplessness, or dependency.
3. Patient appears positive, friendly, and cheerful and actively participates in plans for discharge and patient education sessions.
4. Patient takes responsibility for self-care and complies with treatment plan.

NDx: Knowledge deficit: nature of the disease, nutritional needs, treatments, and measures to reduce risk

Planning: Patient outcomes
1. Patient describes cause, effects, and risk factors associated with hypertension.
2. Patient lists symptoms and treatments for the complications of the disorder.
3. Patient relates the nutritional therapy for lowering cholesterol levels and consumes low-fat, low-sodium meals.
4. Patient states the self-care needed to prevent risk or complications of hypertension.

NDx: Noncompliance to treatment regimen related to asymptomatic disorder, side effects of medications, financial problems, inability to make lifestyle adjustments, or lack of education about disease state

Planning: Patient outcomes
1. Patient relates accurate information about the disease and the importance of following the prescribed treatment plan.
2. Patient states the potential consequences or risks of not following the prescribed treatment plan.
3. Patient demonstrates compliance with the plan.
4. Patient's vital signs stay within normal ranges for the patient.

Nursing Interventions

NDx: Decreased cardiac output

Monitor the patient's vital signs while he or she is lying, sitting, and standing. Encourage the patient to have frequent rest throughout the day to prevent fatigue and strain on the myocardium. Instruct the patient to stop activity if it initiates episodes of chest pain, aggravates chest discomfort, or causes headache, confusion, or dizziness, indicating possible neurologic problems.

Use telemetry monitoring whenever possible, especially if the patient experiences dysrhythmias or if the patient is taking antidysrhythmic drugs. Review the results of laboratory studies and hemodynamic monitoring.

Check the patient's intake and output, observing for adequacy and balance. Keep the patient's legs in a nondependent position while sitting to prevent edema. Provide support for the extremities while sitting or lying in bed.

Teach the patient relaxation techniques and range-of-motion procedures to increase circulation while lying in bed. Keep the patient warm and comfortable. Prevent constriction of circulation from tight-fitting clothing or bed linen.

NDx: Altered nutrition, more than body requirements

Teach the patient about dietary modifications needed to reduce weight. Give the patient literature explaining the caloric content of foods and the fat, cholesterol, and sodium content. Plan a dietary regimen for the patient including foods of choice when able, and give sample menus to the patient and family to follow at home. Seek dietary counseling with the dietitian as needed.

Devise an exercise regimen for the patient that will help burn calories and increase circulation as well as make the heart more efficient and lower the blood pressure. Encourage the family to participate with the patient in the exercise program.

NDx: Self-esteem disturbance

Teach the patient self-care measures, encouraging participation and decision-making by the patient. Explain how changes in lifestyle can benefit the patient by reducing blood pressure and risk of other disorders. Allow time for expression of concerns, questions, and clarification of misunderstandings. Praise the patient for knowledge gained about the disorder, for attempts at lifestyle change, and for participation in self-care.

Seek assistance from clergy, family members, or other professionals when appropriate. Make referrals for the patient on discharge as needed.

NDx: Knowledge deficit: nature of the disease, nutritional needs, treatments, and measures to reduce risk

Explain the cause, effects, and clinical course of hypertension to the patient. Provide opportunities for the patient to ask questions at any time. Provide appropriate literature about hypertension for the patient and family to review. Allow the patient to verbalize concerns and fears. Evaluate discharge needs of the patient and family (Chart 20–5). Teach the patient or family how to take a blood pressure reading.

Alert the patient to signs and symptoms of uncontrolled hypertension and the complications such as impaired renal function, hemorrhage, and neurologic disturbances.

Instruct the patient about dietary modifications needed to reduce risk, reduce weight, or prevent complications of the disorder. Explain the need for decreases in dietary fats and cholesterol to prevent the effects of the disease and increases in protein and vitamins to promote good health and healing (see Nutrition Box 20–1). Also instruct the patient to follow a reduced-sodium diet (Nutrition Boxes 20–2 and 20–3). Devise a diet plan for weight reduction as needed and appropriate for the patient. Initiate counseling with a dietitian to assist with meal planning if needed.

Teach the patient dosage, route, time, frequency, side effects, and toxic effects of any medication prescribed. Explain the diagnostic studies completed and the need for any follow-up studies after discharge. Include the family in any of the teaching sessions when applicable.

Chart 20–5.

NURSING GUIDE TO PATIENT EDUCATION FOR SELF-MANAGEMENT: STEPPED-CARE GUIDELINES FOR THE PATIENT WITH HYPERTENSION

The Joint National Committee on Detection, Evaluation, and Treatment of High Blood Pressure recommends the following guidelines for hypertensive patients:

Upon discharge, instruct the patient to:

Set a plan for lifestyle changes to reduce weight.
Cease smoking.
Reduce the dietary intake of salt.
Consume no more than 2 oz of hard liquor, 8 oz of wine, or 24 oz of beer per day.

Adapted from the National Committee on Detection, Evaluation, and Treatment of High Blood Pressure. 1988 report. Bethesda, MD: National Institutes of Health, 1988.

Nutrition Box 20–2.

SOME COMMON FOODS TO AVOID ON A LOW-SODIUM DIET

- Any presalted canned foods, meats, or snacks
- Foods preserved by sodium addition
- Soups, bouillon, and gravies
- Condiments and sauces
- Cheese, butter, and cheese spreads
- Seasonings prepared with salt such as garlic salt or onion salt
- Frozen fish, pizza, or sausage products

Nutrition Box 20–3.

HERBS AND SPICES TO SUBSTITUTE FOR SALT

Allspice	Ground meats, stews, tomatoes, peaches
Almond extract	Pudding, fruits
Basil	Fish, lamb, ground meats, stews, salads, soups, sauces
Bay leaves	Meats, stews, poultry, soups, tomatoes
Caraway seeds	Meats, stews, soups, salads, breads, cabbage, noodles
Chives	Salads, sauces, soups, meat dishes, vegetables
Cinnamon	Fruits, breads, pie crust, desserts
Curry powder, cumin	Lamb, chicken, fish, tomatoes, soup
Dill	Fish, soups, salads
Garlic powder	Meats, soups, salads, vegetables
Lemon juice	Meats, fish, poultry, salads, vegetables
Dry mustard	Meats, eggs, salads
Nutmeg	Fruits, cottage cheese, pie crust, potatoes
Onion powder	Meats, vegetables, salads
Paprika, parsley	Meats, eggs, fish, soups, salads, vegetables, potatoes
Peppermint	Puddings, fruits, desserts
Rosemary	Chicken, veal, beef, pork, sauces, potatoes, peas
Sage	Meats, stews, biscuits, beans
Savory	Salads, ground meats, soups, beans, squash, peas
Thyme	Veal, pork, sauces, onions, peas, tomatoes
Turmeric	Meats, fish, rice

I, ____________________, will ______________________________

Patient Name) *(Behavior to be changed)*

by ____________________ for ______________________________

(Deadline) *(Reward)*

____

Patient's Signature

____

Nurse's Signature

Figure 20–10.

Example of a contract to change behavior. (See also Chart 20–6.)

NDx: Noncompliance to treatment regimen

Encourage the patient to comply with the prescribed treatment plan by explaining the consequences and risks of noncompliance and the benefits of compliance. Refer the patient to a support group if applicable. Seek assistance of social services for financial counseling and support. Encourage the family to become involved with the treatment regimen, especially the lifestyle changes. Have a family member check the patient's blood pressure and weight, if needed, weekly. Praise the patient for compliance to the regimen. Institute a behavior-modification program using a contract signed by the patient and the nurse to improve compliance (Fig. 20–10 and Chart 20–6).

Evaluation

Evaluate the effectiveness of nursing care for a patient with hypertension by comparing the patient's status with the expected patient outcomes. Examples of specific outcomes for patients with hypertension have been provided in the Planning section.

Chart 20–6.

NURSING GUIDE TO PATIENT EDUCATION FOR SELF-MANAGEMENT: A BEHAVIOR MODIFICATION PROGRAM FOR IMPROVING COMPLIANCE WITH A TREATMENT PLAN

Using a behavior modification program can assist with improving the patient's compliance with a treatment program. Set up the program with the patient as follows:

Identify the behavior to be changed with the patient's approval.
Write the behavior that is to be changed in the form of a goal-oriented contract (see Fig. 20–10.)
Identify a reward for the patient if the behavior is achieved.
Be sure the contract is realistic, measurable, positively stated, dated, and timed with a deadline.
Have both the nurse and the patient sign the contract, and give each party a copy.
Be sure that follow-up occurs on the stated date. Renegotiation may be done if necessary.

Common Venous Vascular Disorders

The collective group of venous vascular disorders includes those that are inflammatory in nature such as thrombophlebitis and those, such as varicose veins, that are the result of other vascular problems.

Thrombophlebitis

ETIOLOGY

Thrombophlebitis, or venous thrombosis, is the development of a clot in the vein with inflammation of the vessel walls. If inflammation is not present but a clot is, the condition is referred to as phlebothrombosis. The clot, or thrombus, causes partial or complete occlusion of the vein. The primary cause of venous thrombosis is venous stasis. Immobilization and surgical procedures predispose patients to venous stasis. Bed rest reduces blood flow in the legs by 50%. Injury to the vessel wall and increased blood coagulation when anticoagulants are suddenly withdrawn may also cause a thrombus to form. The estrogen oral contraceptives affect the clotting mechanism of the blood by increasing platelet adhesiveness, increasing the risk of clot formation. Some blood dyscrasias and dehydration may increase the risk by increasing the platelets and the blood viscosity (Table 20–6).

It is estimated that approximately one third of all patients older than 40 years having major surgery acquire small thrombi in the deep calf veins within 24 hours postoperatively. Patients with cerebrovascular accidents or hip fractures have a 50% or greater chance of acquiring thrombi as a result of immobilization from prescribed extended bed rest.

Phlebitis is the inflammation of a vein without thrombosis, most commonly occurring in the lower extremities. Phlebitis of deep veins is more common than of superficial veins. It is found in women more often than men, and the occurrence increases with age.

Table 20–6. RISK FACTORS ASSOCIATED WITH THROMBOPHLEBITIS

Obesity
Pregnancy (10 days after delivery)
Oral contraceptives
Intravenous therapy
Smoking
Bed rest, immobilization
Prolonged sitting or standing
Hypercoagulability of blood (malignant neoplasms)
Blood dyscrasias
Infections (pneumonia)
Trauma (accidents, fractures)
Surgery (postoperative venous stasis)
Dehydration

PATHOPHYSIOLOGY

The thrombus or clot formation process (thrombosis) begins with an aggregation of platelets on the vein wall. Platelets may be released in the blood in the presence of viruses, bacteria, endotoxins, some diseases, and trauma to the vein wall. The platelets adhere to the vessel wall within 7 to 10 days, forming deposits of fibrin, white blood cells, and red blood cells. As the thrombus develops, it causes further scarring and damage to the vessel. A free-floating tail is present on the thrombus and may break off, particularly if from a deep vein thrombus, and travel to other parts of the body, such as the lungs, causing an embolus. Thrombi from superficial veins rarely become dislodged.

The thrombi tend to develop from the outer edges toward the center. They may occlude the vessel completely or only partially. If the thrombi develop in superficial veins, collateral circulation usually compensates for the blockage. If the thrombus develops in larger veins, collateral circulation may not be sufficient to carry the amount of blood flow necessary to the affected extremity, and symptoms will appear.

CLINICAL MANIFESTATIONS

Many patients with thrombophlebitis present no symptoms, especially if the inflammation is in superficial veins. When symptoms do develop, they tend to appear suddenly and last 1 to 2 weeks after the onset of the inflammation. The clinical manifestations vary with the amount of involvement and vein affected.

Deep venous thrombophlebitis causes severe pain, fever, chills, edema, and cyanosis along the affected vein. It frequently produces complications of venous insufficiency and varicosities. Homans' sign, calf pain with dorsiflexion of the foot, may be present in deep venous thrombophlebitis, but it is not diagnostic of the condition.

Superficial thrombophlebitis may cause minor pain, edema, rubor, warmth, and topical tenderness along the affected vein. Needle trauma to superficial veins may cause septic phlebitis, resulting in red, warm, tender inflamed areas. The veins feel hard and thready when palpated. Fever and leukocytosis may also occur.

MEDICAL DIAGNOSIS

The diagnosis is made on the basis of history, physical assessment, and diagnostic studies. Phlebography is used to detect the location and degree of attachment of the thrombus and to confirm the diagnosis of thrombophlebitis. Plethysmography measures changes in blood volume and shows decreased circulation distal to the thrombus. A radioactive fibrinogen uptake test determines the presence of small thrombi in the calf. Angiogram,

Table 20–7. ANTICOAGULANTS

MEDICATION	ACTION	CONTRAINDICATIONS	SIDE EFFECTS
Heparin sodium (parenteral)	Delays clotting time, prevents thrombus formation; does not resolve clot; used first 7–14 days of thrombus development Administration: IV bolus 100 units/kg initially, then 1500 units in D_5 infused per hour; SC 15–20,000 units every 12 hr if veins cannot be used Dosage: determined by hematocrit and coagulation tests	Hypertension CHF Uremia Duodenal ulcer GI bleeding Recent trauma or surgery Blood dyscrasias Aneurysms Alcoholism Renal and liver diseases Pregnancy Women older than 60 years	Alopecia, flushing, bleeding, hematuria, ecchymosis, bleeding gums, thrombocytopenia, GI bleeding, osteoporosis, epistaxis, rashes Caution: If heparin is given SC, do not stretch skin or rub injection site to prevent hematomas. Use smaller doses in elderly.
Coumarin (oral) Dicumarol (bishydroxycoumarin) Warfarin sodium (Coumadin)	Inhibits synthesis of clotting factors II, VII, IX, X Administration: On 5th day of heparin, start coumarin 10–15 mg/day in first 48 hr, then 2.5–7.5 mg/day as maintenance up to 6 months Dosage: determined by prothrombin time	Same as heparin	Avoid drugs that may enhance or inhibit effects (see Table 20–8).

Abbreviations: IV, intravenous; D_5, dextrose 5%; SC, subcutaneous; CHF, congestive heart failure; GI, gastrointestinal.

venogram, and Doppler venous flow studies may detect further damage to the vessels.

MEDICAL MANAGEMENT

The goal of therapy is to control thrombosis, relieve symptoms, prevent complications, and prevent recurrence of the disorder. The primary treatment is bed rest with elevation of the affected extremity, application of warm compresses, analgesics for pain, and anticoagulant therapy. The dosage, action, side effects, and contraindications for anticoagulant therapy are presented in Table 20–7.

Heparin is the drug of choice for initial anticoagulation and short-term therapy, although it can be used for long-term therapy as well. Heparin is administered by intravenous or subcutaneous routes. The injection site is monitored to ensure that the locations are rotated. While the patient is on heparin therapy, minor trauma, injections, use of razor blades, and aspirin use are avoided to prevent bleeding.

Baseline coagulation studies such as clotting time, prothrombin time, partial thromboplastin time, and platelets are evaluated before the initiation of the therapy and throughout the administration of the anticoagulants. Heparin doses are determined by maintaining the coagulation time within a preset therapeutic range, usually one and one-half to two and one-half times the control. (Refer to Chapter 15 for a discussion of coagulation times.)

Oral anticoagulants are used for long-term therapy. Coumarin derivatives prevent synthesis of clotting factors and may be administered for several months after discharge to prevent recurrence of the thrombosis. The coagulation studies may be monitored at 1-week to 4-week intervals on an outpatient basis depending on the case.

Bleeding complications can occur from the anticoagulant therapy. Bleeding usually develops after the first 3 days of therapy. If the venous occlusion is severe enough to cause total obstruction of the blood flow, ischemia of the extremity and gangrene may result. Approximately one half of the patients with deep venous thrombosis acquire chronic venous insufficiency or stasis dermatitis within 5 years. Venous stasis ulcers develop in about 20% of the patients with chronic venous insufficiency. Varicose veins may develop secondary to deep thrombophlebitis as a result of incompetent valves.

Pulmonary embolism may result if parts of the thrombus break loose and travel through the right side of the heart into the pulmonary artery. The pulmonary blood flow is obstructed, resulting in pulmonary infarction from ischemia and necrosis. Venous pressure in the pulmonary artery is increased. A pulmonary embolism is characterized by an abrupt onset, dyspnea, chest pain, cough, hemoptysis, fever, restlessness, petechiae, and shock.

Thrombolytic agents such as streptokinase and urokinase may be used to dissolve fresh clots, but they are more frequently used for major arterial blockages rather than venous blockages. Complications of thrombolytic therapy include bleeding and anaphylaxis.

A femoral vein thrombectomy may be performed in the presence of massive venous occlusion. Vein ligation or interruption of the inferior vena cava may be performed to prevent pulmonary embolism. This is accomplished by implanting a filter in the inferior vena cava to preserve blood flow while preventing clots from moving to the lungs. Prognosis improves after 2 to 3 weeks if the patient remains free from pulmonary embolism. (Refer to Chapter 19 for the discussion on peripheral vascular surgery.)

Application of the Nursing Process to the Care of the Patient with Thrombophlebitis

Assessment

Review the patient's history and diagnostic study results. Palpate and compare the lower extremities for edema, discoloration, and tenderness. Measure the circumference of the limbs. Ask about pain in the extremities, noting the intensity, location, and duration. Assess skin temperature of both limbs. Check for the presence of Homans' sign.

Review the laboratory studies, especially the hematocrit and coagulation time results, if the patient is on heparin therapy. Ask whether the patient is taking any drugs that may potentiate or inhibit the anticoagulant (Table 20–8). Check the urine for presence of blood, and assess the stools for occult blood. Observe for ecchymoses, petechiae, epistaxis, or bleeding from the gums.

Check the patient's activity level. If the patient is on bed rest, observe for complications of immobility such as skin breakdown, infection, and pressure areas. Observe for signs of pulmonary embolism, including sudden chest pain, dyspnea, restlessness, diaphoresis, and cyanosis. Auscultate breath sounds to check for wheezes or crackles indicative of respiratory distress from infection or embolus.

Assess the patient's level of understanding about the disorder and the complications. Note the patient's history and risk assessment.

Nursing Diagnoses and Planning

Nursing diagnoses and related expected patient outcomes most commonly applicable to patients with thrombophlebitis include the following:

NDx: Pain in extremities related to venous inflammation

Planning: Patient outcomes
1. Patient reports absence of pain or decrease in pain to a tolerable level.
2. Patient states comfort measures to help relieve pain such as positioning and relaxation techniques.
3. Patient does not present nonverbal signs of pain such as grimacing, withdrawal, nervousness, and clenching of hands.

Table 20–8. DRUGS AFFECTING ANTICOAGULANTS

DRUGS THAT POTENTIATE ORAL ANTICOAGULANTS	DRUGS THAT INHIBIT ORAL ANTICOAGULANTS
Anabolic steroids	Griseofulvin
Aspirin	Barbiturates
Phenylbutazone (Butazolidin)	Cholestyramine
Chloral hydrate	Corticosteroids
Chloramphenicol	Glutethimide (Doriden)
Neomycin	Oral contraceptives
Glucagon	Ethchlorvynol (Placidyl)
Quinidine	Tranquilizers

NDx: Altered tissue perfusion, peripheral, related to impaired venous flow from thrombus formation

Planning: Patient outcomes
1. Patient demonstrates increased perfusion as noted by warm, dry skin; absence of edema; and cyanosis in the extremities.
2. Patient's vital signs are within normal ranges for the patient.

NDx: Impaired physical mobility related to extended bed rest and pain secondary to disease state

Planning: Patient outcomes
1. Patient reports increased mobility, strength, and endurance.
2. Patient is able to perform activities of daily living.

NDx: Impaired skin integrity in the extremities related to immobility

Planning: Patient outcomes
1. Patient's skin remains intact without evidence of shearing, infection, ulcerations, or gangrene.
2. Patient states appropriate skin-care measures to prevent impairment of skin integrity.

NDx: Knowledge deficit: nature of the disease, complications of bed rest, treatments, and measures to reduce risk

Planning: Patient outcomes
1. Patient describes cause, effects, and risk factors associated with thrombophlebitis.
2. Patient lists symptoms and treatments for the complications of the disorder.
3. Patient states the self-care needed to prevent risk or complications of thrombophlebitis.

Nursing Interventions

NDx: Pain
Instruct the patient to cease smoking, which causes an increased demand for blood and oxygen to tis-

sues, and vasoconstriction, which increases the ischemia and thus the pain level. Use diversional activities to decrease the patient's awareness of pain. Determine coping strategies that help the patient deal with the pain, especially when it is severe.

Administer pain medication as prescribed. Teach the patient about the effects of the medication, frequency of use, and potential side effects. Help the patient decrease stress and tension through the use of relaxation methods to relieve the pain caused by inflammation (see Chart 20–3). Allow for periods of rest during episodes of intense pain. Apply warm, moist compresses to the extremities to decrease edema, relieve spasms, and promote comfort.

Be sure the patient avoids constricting clothing, which interferes with circulation in the extremities and may exacerbate the complications of the disorder. Avoid placing a pillow behind the knees, which can be constricting. Tell the patient to wear warm clothing and to protect the extremities from extreme heat or cold exposure.

NDx: Altered tissue perfusion, peripheral

Help the patient conserve oxygen needs by encouraging rest and limiting activities. Elevate the head of the bed to aid in lung expansion. Initiate oxygen therapy if needed. Assist the patient with activities of daily living, if needed, to conserve energy.

Keep the patient in a comfortable position, and reposition frequently to release pressure. Use range-of-motion exercises, when allowed, to stimulate circulation. Monitor vital signs and laboratory studies to assess for changes and improvements in status. Encourage ambulation when the patient is off bed rest, as tolerated, but provide for frequent rest periods to decrease cardiac workload. Discourage smoking to avoid vasoconstriction. Remove constricting clothing, and keep heavy bed linen from restricting peripheral circulation. Keep the patient's legs in an elevated position when not ambulating.

Give prescribed medications to reduce inflammation, prevent further thrombosis, and thus increase circulation. Discuss risk factors and preventive health-care measures with the patient. Explain lifestyle changes that will promote good circulation and decrease risk of futher venous disorders (Chart 20–7).

NDx: Impaired physical mobility

Assist the patient when he or she is allowed out of bed. The patient may be very weak after being on extended bed rest. Use durable medical equipment accessories, when appropriate, to assist the patient in maintaining mobility. Teach the patient to perform range-of-motion exercises to increase circulation and to maintain or improve strength and endurance.

Prepare a daily exercise schedule for the patient as soon as he or she is allowed to be mobile again, increasing the level as tolerable. Tell the patient to walk slowly and avoid stairs or inclines at first, if necessary, and to stop for a few minutes of rest when tired. Encourage the patient to persist in the exercise regimen, even if it must be moderated at times for lack of endurance. Praise the patient on achievements accomplished.

NDx: Impaired skin integrity

Handle the patient's legs and feet with care, especially if the skin is not intact. Use aseptic technique when bathing or dressing areas where the skin is broken to prevent infection. Keep linen off the extremities with the use of a bed cradle. Instruct the patient to avoid wearing constricting clothing. Keep the extremities warm and dry at all times.

Check peripheral circulation frequently. Observe for early signs of problems developing because of decreased circulation such as pressure spots, absent pulses, coldness, and discoloration. Report any untoward signs. Have the patient change position frequently to stimulate circulation and prevent pressure sores. Use heel pads to prevent skin breakdown if the patient is in bed for long periods of time. Apply antiembolic stockings during the acute phase to decrease venous stasis and promote circulation, thus preventing further skin problems. To promote healing and minimize tissue damage, promote a diet high in protein and vitamins.

NDx: Knowledge deficit: nature of the disease, complications of bed rest, treatments, and measures to reduce risk

Explain the cause, effects, and clinical course of thrombophlebitis to the patient. Allow opportunities for the patient to ask questions at any time. Provide appropriate literature about the disorder for the patient and family to review. Allow the patient to verbalize concerns and fears. Evaluate the discharge needs of the patient and family (see Chart 20–7).

Alert the patient to signs and symptoms of thrombophlebitis and complications such as impaired mobility, pain, skin breakdown, and infection of the extremities. Teach the patient to use safety measures or to ask for assistance when out of bed or when ambulating. Instruct the patient on exercises that can be performed after bed rest restrictions are removed to increase strength and endurance.

Teach the patient how to achieve comfort by frequent repositioning and padding bony prominences. Explain the use of a bed cradle to prevent pressure on joints and sensitive areas. Teach the patient how to apply the elastic hose, which compresses superficial veins to enhance circulation to deep veins and decreases the chance of recurrence of the disorder (Chart 20–8).

Teach the patient the dosage, route, time, frequency, side effects, and toxic effects of any medication prescribed. If the patient is on heparin and is being discharged with orders for coumadin therapy, explain the signs of bleeding to the patient and pro-

Chart 20–7.

NURSING GUIDE TO PATIENT EDUCATION FOR SELF-MANAGEMENT: DISCHARGE INSTRUCTIONS FOR THE PATIENT WITH THROMBOPHLEBITIS

Upon discharge, instruct the patient with thrombophlebitis to do the following:

Prevent recurrence of the disorder by:

Avoiding crossing the legs when sitting or lying in bed.
Exercising the toes and feet frequently by dorsiflexion while sitting or lying in bed.
Participating in a walking exercise program to strengthen leg muscles and assist venous return.
Avoiding sitting with the legs in a dependent position.
Avoiding standing in place for long periods of time.
Ceasing smoking to prevent vasoconstriction.
Avoiding wearing tight, constricting clothing on the extremities.

Prevent complications of anticoagulant therapy by:

Understanding the dosage, actions, and side effects of the medication prescribed.
Avoiding over-the-counter medications without checking with the physician to prevent the potentiating or inhibiting effects of other medications.
Taking the anticoagulant medication at the same time each day to maintain the appropriate blood level.
Taking the medication until discontinued by a physician's order.
Returning to the physician's office as needed for medical and laboratory follow-up studies.
Notifying dentist and other medical personnel that an anticoagulant is being taken and bleeding precautions are necessary.
Carrying or wearing an identification card stating name and address, which anticoagulant is being taken, blood type, and physician's name and telephone number.
Being especially careful around sharp instruments or while shaving with a razor blade.
Avoiding contact sports or other rough physical activities.

Assess for signs and symptoms of excessive anticoagulation by:

Observing for petechiae, ecchymoses, bleeding gums when brushing teeth, and prolonged bleeding when cut or nicked while shaving.
Checking for blood in the urine or dark stools, indicating occult blood.
(Notify the physician if any of these complications are apparent.)

vide instructions on when to seek medical attention. Include the family in any of the teaching sessions when applicable.

Evaluation

Evaluate the effectiveness of nursing care for a patient with thrombophlebitis by comparing the patient's status with the expected patient outcomes. Examples of specific outcomes for patients with thrombophlebitis have been provided in the Planning section.

Chronic Venous Insufficiency

Chronic venous insufficiency results from valve destruction, which occurs in chronic venous inflammation and venous stasis. Most patients in whom chronic venous insufficiency develops have a history of deep venous thrombosis with repeated episodes of phlebitis.

The valves of the veins in the legs are unable to close completely because of thrombus formation, scarring, or fibrosis. Incompetency of the veins occurs from the prolonged high venous pressure in the extremities. As illustrated in Figure 20–11, the veins become weak, overstretched, and distended from the extensive pressure. The valve no longer

Chart 20–8.

NURSING GUIDE TO PATIENT EDUCATION FOR SELF-MANAGEMENT: APPLICATION OF ELASTIC ANTIEMBOLIC STOCKINGS TO PREVENT VENOUS STASIS

Instruct the patient with elastic antiembolic stockings prescribed to:

Apply the elastic stockings to both legs, even if only one is affected, to give support to the extremities and to increase circulation.
Pull stockings up until they are smooth and free of wrinkles.
Be sure stockings feel tight but not constrictive to the extremities. If they feel too constrictive or if there is numbness in the feet or toes, they should not be worn, but instead returned for a better fitting pair.
Put the stockings on before getting out of bed in the morning. They may be removed for 30 minutes every 6 hours or as prescribed.
Observe the skin after removal for irritation, dryness, lesions, pressure areas, or discoloration.
Wash the stockings in a mild detergent without bleach to prevent skin irritation when reapplied. Have a second pair available for use when one pair is being washed.

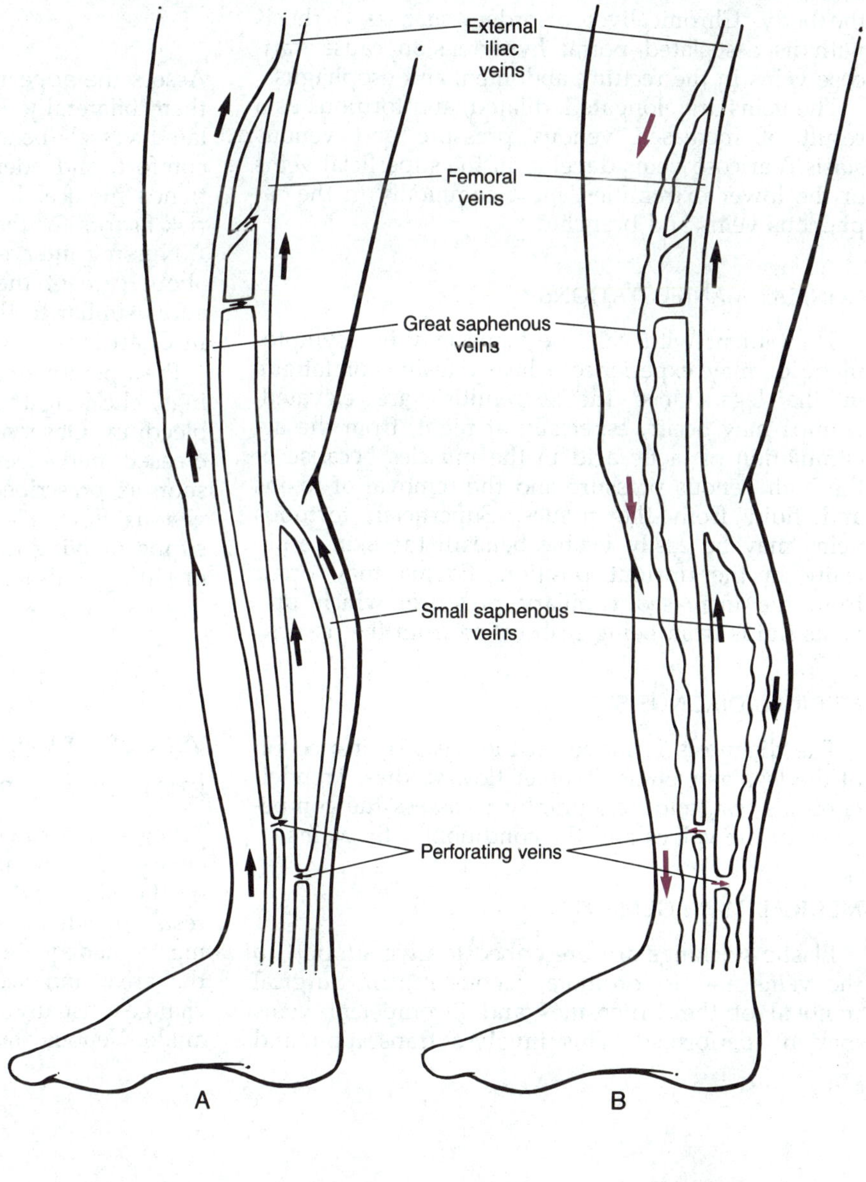

Figure 20–11.

A, Drawing of normal (superficial and deep) venous flow. *B,* Venous flow in varicosities caused by incompetent valves.

closes completely, thus allowing the blood to flow back into the dilated veins. Venous stasis and increased venous pressure result in varicosities and venous ulcers.

VARICOSE VEINS

ETIOLOGY AND PATHOPHYSIOLOGY

Abnormal dilation of the veins as a result of venous insufficiency with valvular malfunction results in varicose veins. This may be the result of congenital malformations of the vein walls and valves, repeated episodes of thrombophlebitis, or conditions that cause venous stasis such as pregnancies or prolonged standing and sitting. A genetic predisposition to varicose veins is common in many individuals. Heavy lifting and obesity may also cause high venous pressure, resulting in varicosities. Deep venous thrombosis, obstruction, or inflammation may cause varicose veins through valvular destruction.

Some disease processes may also predispose the individual to varicosities of veins in other parts of the body. Chronic liver disorders such as cirrhosis with its associated portal hypertension cause varicose veins in the rectum, abdomen, and esophagus.

The veins are elongated, dilated, and tortuous as a result of increased venous pressure and venous stasis. Varicose veins develop in the superficial veins of the lower extremities, most commonly in the saphenous veins and branches.

CLINICAL MANIFESTATIONS

The patient with varicose veins may be asymptomatic or may experience a heavy feeling or fatigue in the legs. Once the extremities are elevated, cramps may occur, especially at night, from the accumulation of lactic acid in the muscles because of the high venous pressure and the removal of toxins and fluid from the tissues. Superficial, tortuous veins may be easily visible beneath the skin, especially in the upright position. Edema may occur from the increased capillary pressure, which prevents fluids from being reabsorbed from the tissues.

MEDICAL DIAGNOSIS

The diagnosis is made on the basis of inspection of the legs as well as Doppler flow studies, Trendelenburg's test, and venography to assess the competency of the valves and the condition of the veins.

MEDICAL MANAGEMENT

Elastic stockings are prescribed to give support to the veins and to promote venous return. Surgical removal of the varicosities and incompetent veins may be performed. This involves transection and ligation of the saphenous vein and its stripping or removal. The vein is ligated in the groin area while a wire is passed through the vein to the ankle. The vein is stripped as the wire is removed. The legs are elevated during surgery to minimize bleeding. Complications of the surgery include infection, thrombosis, and nerve damage. (Refer to Chapter 19 for discussion of peripheral vascular surgery.)

Small varicosities may be treated with sclerotherapy by aspirating the blood in the vein and injecting a sclerosing solution. This produces fibrosis and blocks the opening to the vein. Complications of sclerotherapy include phlebitis, tissue necrosis, and, rarely, infection. Treatment of any type will not prevent the recurrence of varicosities. Reducing risk factors, however, may help prevent further development of additional varicose veins.

Guidelines for Application of the Nursing Process to the Care of the Patient with Varicose Veins

Assess the appearance of the extremities, comparing them bilaterally. Palpate for superficial, tortuous, dilated vessels beneath the skin. Assess for pain, discomfort, and edema in the legs. Determine the patient's medical history of thrombophlebitis or other risk factors for the development of varicosities.

Nursing interventions include teaching the patient about care of the extremities and preventive measures similar to those for thrombophlebitis, as listed in Chart 20–7. (Also see Nursing Care Guide 20–2.)

Postoperative care includes applying elastic stockings, checking the dressings sites, and assessing for bleeding. Observe for edema, discoloration, or decreased nerve sensation. Encourage ambulation as soon as prescribed to decrease edema and promote venous flow. Elevate the legs when the patient is sitting or lying in bed. Discourage standing in place or sitting with legs crossed.

VENOUS STASIS ULCERS

ETIOLOGY AND PATHOPHYSIOLOGY

Leg ulcers associated with chronic venous insufficiency occur from extensive damage to the integrity of the skin and subcutaneous tissues. This is the result of edema, decreased venous circulation leading to inadequate supply of oxygen and nutrients to the area, and accumulation of toxic wastes. These changes usually occur in the lower leg near the ankle. Venous stasis ulcers are more common in the elderly with compromised circulation and limited mobility.

CLINICAL MANIFESTATIONS

The clinical manifestations of venous stasis ulcers include brownish skin pigmentation from small vein rupture; dry, cracked skin from inadequate oxygen and nutrients to the area; and infections from exposed skin breaks. Edema from vein dilation and backup of venous flow from incompetent valves may also occur.

MEDICAL DIAGNOSIS

The diagnosis is made on the basis of history and physical findings. Doppler ultrasound studies and venography are used to confirm the cause of the ulcerations.

MEDICAL MANAGEMENT

Venous stasis ulcers are treated with compresses of isotonic saline solution or Burow's solution. Daily whirlpool therapy promotes circulation, comfort, and healing. A local corticosteriod and systemic antibiotics may be necessary to treat the infectious organisms. Systemic rather than local antibiotics are preferred to prevent the development of skin sensitivity, which impedes the healing process. Skin grafts may be necessary to promote the healing process for large ulcers. Debridement may be done to promote granulation. Dextranomer (Debrisan) beads may be applied to the affected area to absorb secretions and necrotic tissue. A semirigid boot may be applied to the leg after the swelling has subsided to promote venous return while compressing the superficial veins. The boot is changed every 1 to 2 weeks depending on the presence of edema and drainage from the ulcer.

Application of the Nursing Process to the Care of the Patient with Venous Stasis Ulcers

Assessment

Assess the affected area for discoloration, warmth, drainage, and edema. Ask the patient about pain, tenderness, or sensation in the affected limb. Note the color and amount of drainage.

Assess the patient's knowledge level regarding the disorder, the medications prescribed, and measures to prevent recurrence of the ulcerations. Observe the patient's activity level, and note whether mobility is impaired as a result of the leg ulcerations. Review the patient's typical meal plan, and check for vitamin and protein content of the food choices.

Nursing Diagnoses and Planning

Nursing diagnoses and related expected patient outcomes most commonly applicable to patients with venous stasis ulcers include the following:

NDx: Impaired skin integrity in the extremities related to immobility

Planning: Patient outcomes
1. Patient reports increased mobility, strength, and endurance.
2. Patient is able to perform activities of daily living.

NDx: Impairment of skin integrity in the extremities related to immobility

Planning: Patient outcomes
1. Patient's skin remains intact without evidence of infection, ulcerations, or gangrene.
2. Patient states appropriate skin-care measures to prevent impairment of skin integrity.

NDx: Knowledge deficit: nature of the disease, its complications, treatments, and measures to reduce risk

Planning: Patient outcomes
1. Patient describes cause, effects, and risk factors associated with venous stasis ulcers.
2. Patient lists symptoms and treatments for the complications of the disorder, including how and when to apply elastic hose (as described in Chart 20–8) and care of the ulcerations at home.
3. Patient states the self-care needed to prevent risk or complications of venous stasis ulcers.
4. Patient chooses foods that promote health and healing.

Nursing Interventions

NDx: Impaired physical mobility
Assist the patient when he or she is allowed out of bed. The patient may be very weak after being on bed rest. Use durable medical equipment accessories, when appropriate, to assist the patient in maintaining mobility. Teach the patient to perform range-of-motion exercises to increase circulation and to maintain or improve strength and endurance.

Prepare a daily exercise schedule for the patient as soon as he or she is allowed to be mobile again, increasing the level as tolerable.

Nursing Care Guide 20–2.

PATIENTS WITH VARICOSE VEINS

Assessment Findings: Patient complains of dull, aching pain in legs, especially after long periods of standing or sitting with legs in a dependent position; vein distention and dilation are visible; some edema of ankles and feet is present.

Nursing Diagnosis: Pain related to effects of valvular insufficiency, venous stasis causing vein distention and blood pooling in the extremities

Patient Outcomes	Nursing Interventions	Rationale
Patient reports decrease in discomfort or absence of pain in legs and feet.	Give analgesics for leg aches as prescribed. Keep heavy linens elevated with a bed cradle.	Keeping pressure off the legs and administering pain medications as occasion requires help relieve painful episodes.
Patient states methods to reduce or prevent pain in the legs and feet.	Teach the patient how to prevent effects of the valvular disorder by preventing venous stasis by avoiding standing or sitting in one position for lengthy periods of time, elevating legs when sitting, wearing shoes that are comfortable and not too tight, massaging legs to promote venous return, unless contraindicated, and wearing elastic support stockings.	An understanding of preventive methods may reduce the number of painful episodes the patient experiences.

Evaluation: Compare the patient's status with the expected patient outcomes. If the outcomes are achieved, evaluate nursing care as successful. If not, reassess the patient, formulate new nursing diagnoses, and revise expected patient outcomes and nursing interventions as appropriate.

Assessment Findings: Patient asks questions about care of legs and feet, especially why there is so much edema and discomfort; seems anxious about managing effects of the disorder; is unsure about potential surgery for correction of the disorder; wants to know if self-care measures can prevent further effects of the disorder.

Nursing Diagnosis: Knowledge deficit: nature of disease and preventive care

Patient Outcomes	Nursing Interventions	Rationale
Patient states accurate information about the development of varicosities and the preventive measures.	Explain the disease process to the patient in understandable terms. Give the patient appropriate literature about the disease to review. Explain the preventive measures. Tell the patient about the medications, dose, side effects, time and route, and expected results.	An understanding of the disorder and the events that exacerbate the condition may improve patient compliance to the management regimen.

(continued)

Nursing Care Guide 20–2. *(continued)*

PATIENTS WITH VARICOSE VEINS

Patient Outcomes	Nursing Interventions	Rationale
	Teach the patient how to apply the support stockings. Allow time for questions and concerns to be voiced. Allow the patient's family to participate in the education sessions.	
Patient explains the surgical procedure and the risks and long-term implications of having surgery for varicose veins.	Find out whether the physician has explained to the patient about the surgical procedure for varicosities, the potential risks, and future implications. Assist the patient in clearing up any misconceptions about the procedure.	An understanding of the procedure may reduce the patient's fear and anxiety.

Evaluation: Compare the patient's status with the expected patient outcomes. If the outcomes are achieved, evaluate nursing care as successful. If not, reassess the patient, formulate new nursing diagnoses, and revise expected patient outcomes and nursing interventions as appropriate.

Assessment Findings: Patient is unable to walk without assistance; legs are extremely edematous; patient complains of pain in extremities; physician orders bed rest.

Nursing Diagnosis: Impaired physical mobility related to exacerbation of effects of disorder and physician's response to patient's symptoms

Patient Outcomes	Nursing Interventions	Rationale
Patient reports decrease in pain when ambulating and is able to ambulate without aggravating effects of disorder.	Encourage range-of-motion exercises while on bed rest. Keep legs elevated above the patient's heart. Give diuretics and analgesics, as prescribed.	Exercises help venous return to reduce edema while maintaining muscle strength and endurance. Elevating the legs reduces edema and aids in venous return.
Patient practices preventive measures when able to ambulate again, such as not standing or sitting for long periods of time and wearing elastic support stockings.	Explain preventive measures that can prevent further episodes of acute exacerbation requiring bed rest.	An understanding of preventive measures may reduce the risk of complications.

Evaluation: Compare the patient's status with the expected patient outcomes. If the outcomes are achieved, evaluate nursing care as successful. If not, reassess the patient, formulate new nursing diagnoses, and revise expected patient outcomes and nursing interventions as appropriate.

NDx: Impaired skin integrity
Maintain the patient on bed rest during the acute phase. Elevate the legs to decrease venous pressure. Culture any drainage from the ulcerations. Teach the patient to perform dorsiflexion while on bed rest to promote blood flow.

Cleanse the ulcerations daily with the prescribed solution. Use an aseptic technique to prevent infection. Wet saline or Burow's solution compresses may be used to promote the healing process. Apply lotion to the surrounding skin to prevent dryness.

Reposition the patient frequently to prevent pressure areas. Use pads for heels, and keep bed linen off the limbs by using a bed cradle.

Teach the patient measures to prevent recurrence of the ulcers such as wearing elastic hose and elevating the legs periodically to promote venous flow. Discourage standing in place or sitting with the legs in a dependent position for long periods of time. Encourage leg exercises such as walking to increase circulation to the distal limbs. Instruct the patient to avoid wearing constrictive clothing and extreme hot or cold temperatures.

Encourage the patient to eat a diet high in vitamin C, protein, and minerals to enhance healing and maintain tissue integrity. Seek dietary counseling if necessary.

NDx: Knowledge deficit: nature of the disease, its complications, treatments, and measures to reduce risk
Explain to the patient the cause, effects, and treatments for venous stasis ulcers. Allow opportunities for the patient to ask questions at any time. Allow the patient to verbalize concerns and fears. Evaluate discharge needs of the patient and family.

Alert the patient to the complications of ulcerations such as impaired mobility, pain, and infection of the extremities. Teach the patient to use safety measures or ask for assistance when out of bed or when ambulating. Instruct the patient on exercises to increase strength and endurance that can be performed after bed rest restrictions are removed.

Teach the patient how to achieve comfort by frequent repositioning and the padding of bony prominences. Explain the use of a bed cradle to prevent pressure on joints and sensitive areas. Teach the patient how to apply the elastic hose, which compresses superficial veins to enhance circulation to deep veins and decreases the chance of recurrence of the disorder (see Chart 20–7). Explain how to apply the compresses if the patient is to continue the dressings at home.

Teach the patient the dosage, route, time, frequency, side effects, and toxic effects of any medication prescribed. Explain the benefit of a diet high in vitamins and protein, and give the patient lists of appropriate foods. Have a dietitian assist with the meal planning if needed. Include the family in any of the teaching sessions when applicable.

Evaluation

Evaluate the effectiveness of nursing care for a patient with venous stasis ulcers by comparing the patient's status with the expected patient outcomes. Examples of specific outcomes for patients with venous stasis ulcers have been provided in the Planning section.

Common Lymphatic Disorders

The lymph system drains excess fluids and proteins from the interstitial spaces. It is important in maintaining control of tissue fluid volume. In lymphatic disorders, obstruction of the lymph vessels interrupts the normal tissue fluid volume control, resulting in edema. Several factors may contribute to this process.

Lymphangitis and Lymphadenitis

ETIOLOGY AND PATHOPHYSIOLOGY

Lymphangitis and lymphadenitis are both inflammations of the lymph system. Lymphangitis refers to an inflammation of the vessels, usually caused by a bacterial infection. Lymphadenitis refers to inflammation of the lymph nodes. Both disorders may contribute to lymphedema. The bacteria invades the skin and spreads to the lymph nodes through the lymphatic vessels.

CLINICAL MANIFESTATIONS

The inflamed area may be only superficial, or an abscess may form. Red streaks appear along the pathway of the lymphatic vessels. Lymph nodes enlarge and become very tender. Local inflammation, pitting edema, and red discoloration in the extremity may occur as a response to the bacterial invasion. Cellulitis often occurs, causing throbbing pain in the affected part. The heart rate may be elevated to compensate for increased blood supply to the inflamed area. Fever, chills, malaise, anorexia, headache, nausea, and vomiting may result as a systemic reaction to the infection.

MEDICAL DIAGNOSIS

The diagnosis is made on the basis of history, present symptoms, and laboratory studies such as white blood cell count. Culture of the wound exudate determines the type of organism present.

MEDICAL MANAGEMENT

Systemic antimicrobial agents are administered on the basis of blood culture results. Penicillin is the usual drug prescribed for a streptococcal infection.

Erythromycin or a cephalosporin may be ordered if the patient is allergic to penicillin.

If an abscess is present, fluid may be drained from the wound. Incision and drainage are avoided in the presence of cellulitis to prevent spread of the infection. Early detection and treatment are important because the infection may progress rapidly and lead to septicemia or even death in rare cases. With treatment, the prognosis is excellent.

Guidelines for Application of the Nursing Process to the Care of the Patient with Lymphangitis or Lymphadenitis

Observe the extremities for skin changes such as discoloration, extreme warmth, or edema. Check for pain in the affected extremity. Palpate for pulses and tenderness. Assess vital signs for increased heart rate, fever, or respiratory difficulty, indicating systemic infection.

Promote healing of the affected extremity by preventing further trauma. Keep the extremity elevated to reduce edema. Apply warm compresses frequently to the site. Use aseptic technique when changing dressings. Provide for frequent rest periods to conserve energy. Keep the patient warm, and prevent drafts. After the inflammation has subsided, elastic support bandages or hose may be used to prevent further edema.

Give prescribed antibiotics and analgesics or antipyretics as needed. Teach the patient about the medications, frequency, amount, dosage, and side effects before discharge.

Lymphedema

ETIOLOGY AND PATHOPHYSIOLOGY

Lymphedema is defined as edema of the extremities from inadequate control of fluid volume in the tissues or interstitial spaces. Primary lymphedema (congenital lymphedema [Milroy's disease] or lymphedema praecox) is due to obstructed lymph vessels. It may be visible at birth but is usually diagnosed later. Primary lymphedema is more common in females, ages 10 to 25 years, than in males.

Secondary lymphedema is caused by inflammation of the lymphatic vessels or obstruction of the lymph flow as a result of pressure on the lymph nodes or vessels from neoplasms or other structures. Secondary lymphedema may result from a disruption of the lymphatic system that occurs postmastectomy or from varicose veins, phlebitis, or irradiation. Secondary lymphedema usually occurs after 40 years of age and may be found in either men or women. It is usually unilateral but may be bilateral depending on the cause.

Lymph accumulates distally because of the blockage of the lymph vessels or nodes. The lymphatic pressure rises in the periphery, causing incompetent valves and dilation of the vessel walls. The edema is the result of accumulation of lymph in the interstitial spaces.

CLINICAL MANIFESTATIONS

Clinical manifestations of lymphedema include fluid accumulation beginning in the distal limb. In the lower extremities, edema begins in the foot and extends proximally. Prolonged standing, extremely warm weather, obesity, and pregnancy may aggravate lower limb lymphedema.

Primary lymphedema is insidious in onset, usually with bilateral, soft, pitting edema initially followed by firm, nonpitting edema. The skin is thick, and hair follicles are prominent. Pain is usually absent, but the patient may complain of a dull, heavy sensation in the affected extremities.

Secondary lymphedema is characterized by painless edema of the affected extremities. Pain appears if infection is present or if the edema is so severe as to cause extreme stretching of the skin and pressure in the affected limb. If the condition becomes chronic, the affected area is usually severely edematous, with thick, hard skin resulting in deformity. The condition is then termed *elephantiasis*.

MEDICAL DIAGNOSIS

The diagnosis is made on the basis of physical assessment, lymphangiography, and redioactive isotope studies.

MEDICAL MANAGEMENT

Treatment of lymphedema includes a low-sodium diet, oral diuretics such as the thiazides, and the use of an external pneumatic compressor to decrease edema. The extremity is kept elevated to prevent further edema. The underlying cause of secondary edema may also need to be treated. Antibiotics are prescribed if infection is present. The prognosis depends on the cause of the lymphedema, but it is usually very good. In most cases, the disorder can be controlled with treatment.

Guidelines for Application of the Nursing Process to the Care of the Patient with Lymphedema

Review the patient's history, and assess present physical symptoms. Observe the extremities for color changes, pitting edema, and circulation states. Palpate for pulses in the extremities, checking presence, intensity, and regularity. Assess for pain or tenderness in the affected limb. Measure the circumference of the extremity daily to determine changes.

Nursing interventions include measures to relieve the edema, promote lymph drainage, and prevent infection. Elevate the extremity, and wrap it with elastic bandages or hose for support. Assist the patient in ambulation if necessary. Massage the affected extremity manually or mechanically to force the lymph drainage toward the trunk of the body. Instruct the patient on the use of the mechanical device to promote lymph drainage after discharge if needed.

Explain the dosage, frequency, time, and side effects of prescribed medications. Encourage the patient to express feelings and concerns about the disorder, especially if it is chronic. The patient's self-image may suffer because of the appearance of the edematous extremity. Refer the patient to counseling if necessary.

The Elderly: Special Considerations

Physiologic changes of the aging process must be considered when delivering care to the elderly patient with vascular disorders. The blood vessel walls become thickened with age, leading to a decrease in elasticity of the smaller arteries. Vessels become dilated, elongated, and tortuous, and plaques collect in the inner vessel walls, resulting in vessel weakness. Inefficient valve function causes a decreased blood supply to the lower extremities. The blood tends to pool in the distal limbs. Most older adults experience some degree of atherosclerosis, which can be accentuated by changes in the cardiovascular system as a result of the aging process.

The elderly patient may think pain and discomfort experienced in the lower limbs are a normal part of the aging process and may thus delay seeking treatment for a vascular disorder. Pain sensation may be diminished from other disease processes interfering with neurotransmission. The older adult may not recognize early trauma to the skin integrity because of decreased sensation.

Cardiac output is decreased as a result of fibrosis and sclerosis in the endocardium and thickening of the left ventricular wall, which results in myocardial hypertrophy and decreased blood flow to the extremities. Dependent edema may be present in the elderly patient because of thickening and dilation of vessels. Decreased renal flow causes impaired renal function, leading to increased sodium and water retention.

Medication for the relief of pain resulting from vascular disorders in the elderly must be administered with extreme caution because drug toxicity can result from the reduced blood flow to the liver and decreased gastric motility with increased drug absorption. A decreased cardiac output reduces renal blood flow, thereby diminishing glomerular filtration rate and tubular reabsorption of the medication.

When teaching exercises to the elderly patient to promote circulation, use slow, rhythmic motions because bone brittleness and joint stiffness from degenerative changes may be present. There is a decrease in the speed and power of muscle contractions and a decrease in muscle strength, endurance, and agility resulting from calcification of ligaments and a reduction in muscle fibers after 50 years of age. If the exercise program is too rigid, the patient may become frustrated and not comply with the plan.

The elderly patient experiences a variety of problems from arterial vascular occlusion. Skin changes resulting from decreased arterial blood flow may already be apparent in the elderly from fragile capillaries, loss of collagen fibers, and decreased blood flow to the skin. This makes identification of trophic changes caused by arterial vascular disorders difficult to differentiate. Thinning of hair or hair loss is usually due to the aging process and is not a reliable symptom of arterial vascular disorders. The older adult experiences a decreased sensation to extreme hot and cold temperatures and is more prone to burns or frostbite injuries. These injuries are aggravated by the decreased circulation to the skin for healing.

A diet low in fat and cholesterol may not be palatable to the older adult who has eaten foods high in fat content for years. Dietary planning should include the patient's choices within the list of appropriate foods. Food preparation habits should be assessed because the individual may eliminate some fats in the food choices but may still prepare the food by deep frying in fat.

Special considerations are taken into account when caring for the elderly patient with hypertension. Increasing age is associated with a gradual increase in both systolic and diastolic blood pressure. Increased peripheral vascular resistance is the major cause of the increases in blood pressure. This occurs because of structural changes in the vessels, collagen deposition and calcium deposition in the vessel walls, and changes in connective tissues. These changes and target organ damage may be the result of the aging process and not be associated with a disease state. Rigid arteries develop in the older adult because of decreased elasticity and thickening of vessel walls. This increases peripheral vascular resistance, resulting in hypertension.

The autonomic nervous system response in the aged is slowed, resulting in systolic hypertension or orthostatic hypertension. The patient is instructed to move slowly when changing position to avoid dizziness and falling. Assistance may be needed for ambulation.

Hypertension in the older adult is aggravated by declines in renin levels as a result of the aging process. This may interfere with the therapeutic effects of antihypertensive agents. Some elderly patients with hypertension are less responsive to beta blocker pharmacologic therapy than younger patients. Many elderly patients cannot tolerate an exercise regimen to assist in lowering blood pressure, so they are dependent on pharmacologic interventions. The goal of the therapy in the elderly is to lower the blood pressure without reducing the blood flow to the extremities or causing increased problems from side effects.

Noncompliance with the hypertension treatment regimen is often higher in the elderly because of lack of understanding, misconceptions, forgetfulness, financial problems, and reduced motivation. Depression, confusion, and weakness may be related to the aging process but may also be caused by the antihypertensive medications. These side effects may contribute to the patient's noncompliance.

The older adult with hypertension is frequently on a low-sodium, calorie-restricted diet. Special care must be give to menu planning to assist the patient to comply with the diet therapy. Aged individuals experience a decreased sense of smell from diminished olfactory fibers and a decreased taste discrimination from reduced numbers of taste buds and saliva production. This may contribute to the poor dietary habits of the elderly and noncompliance to the prescribed plan.

Venous vascular disorders in elderly patients are extremely common. In the older adult, the veins become thick, dilated, and fibrosed. These changes lead to varicosities, edema, and stasis ulcers. Skin changes commonly seen in venous vascular disorders may be the result of the aging process and not of a vascular disease.

If bed rest is required for treatment of venous vascular disorders in the elderly, complications can develop rapidly. Decreased respiratory function potentiates the likelihood of respiratory complications such as pneumonia in the elderly patient on bed rest. Increased fragility of the skin enhances the likelihood of skin breakdown while the patient is on bed rest. Healing is slower in the older adult because of poor nutrition, decreased circulation, and other complicating disorders. Venous vascular disorders often result in necrotic areas and gangrene of the affected limb.

When ambulation is resumed, the elderly patient may experience increased muscle weakness because glucose mobilizes more slowly in response to exercise, and protein synthesis in muscle cells is decreased in the older adult.

Guidelines for home care should be given to the patient verbally and in writing to help reinforce compliance and to promote understanding. Family or friends need to be included to assist the patient and to offer reassurance in coping with the vascular disorder. Referrals to other health care agencies may be necessary because many elderly patients with vascular disorders are discharged from the hospital with specific self-care treatments to be continued in the home.

Bibliography

Abernathy DR. Clinical pharmacology in older hypertensive patients. Hypertension: New Approaches Drug Ther 1991; 3(1):9.

Andres R, Bierman EL, Hazard W. Principles of geriatric medicine. New York: McGraw-Hill, 1985.

Badger C. The swollen limb. Nurs Times 1986; 82(31):40.

Ballenger MJ. Dissecting aneurysms. *Emergency* 1985; 40(11):42.

Bang NU. Thrombosis and atherosclerosis. New York: Year Book Medical Publishers, 1982.

Baum PL. Taking the P.V.D. patient's history . . . peripheral vascular disease. Nursing 1986; 16(5):30.

Bergan JJ, Yao J. Aneurysms: Diagnosis and treatment. New York: Grune & Stratton, 1982.

Bergan JJ, Yao J. Evaluation and treatment of upper and lower extremity circulatory disorders. New York: Grune & Stratton, 1984.

Bernhard VM, Towne JB (eds). Complications in surgery. 2nd ed. New York: Grune & Stratton, 1985.

Blakenhorn DH. Preventive treatment of atherosclerosis. New York: Addison-Wesley, 1984.

Bullock BL, Ronndahl PP. Pathophysiology: Adaptations & alterations in function. Boston: Little, Brown, 1984.

Burggraf V, Donlon B. Assessing the elderly: Part 1, System by system. Am J Nurs 1985; 85(9):974.

Carpenito LJ. Nursing diagnosis: Application to clinical practice, 3rd ed. Philadelphia: JB Lippincott, 1989.

Cerrato P, Hypertension: The role of diet and lifestyle. RN 1990; 53(12):46.

Cooley DA. Surgical treatment of aortic aneurysms. Philadelphia: WB Saunders, 1986.

Cox HC, Hinz MD, Lubuno MA, et al. Clinical applications of nursing diagnosis, Philadelphia: FA Davis, 1989.

Dale WA. Management of vascular surgical problems. New York: McGraw-Hill, 1985.

Dardik H. Arterial reconstruction in the lower extremity. New York: McGraw-Hill, 1986.

DeBakey ME. Atherosclerosis: Patterns and rates of progression. In Gotto AM, Smith LC, Allen B (eds). Atherosclerosis. New York: Springer-Verlag, 1980.

D'Epiro P. Hypertension: Tips for better compliance. Patient Care 1986; 19(4):54, 63.

Doenges M, Jeffries MF, Moorhouse MF. Nursing care plans: nursing diagnoses in planning patient care. Philadelphia: FA Davis, 1984.

Eliopoulos C. Gerontological nursing. 2nd ed. Philadelphia: JB Lippincott, 1987.

Epstein M, & Oster JR. Hypertension: A practical approach. Philadelphia: WB Saunders, 1984.

Fellows E, Jocz AM. Getting the upper hand on lower arterial extremity disease. Nursing '91 1991; 21(8):34.

Feury D, Nash D. Hypertension: The nurse's role. RN 1990; 53(11):54.

Fregly MJ, Kare MR. The role of salt in cardiovascular hypertension. New York: Academic Press, 1982.

Gaspar MR, Barker WF. Peripheral arterial disease. 3rd ed. Philadelphia: WB Saunders, 1981.

Gavras H, Gavras I. Hypertension in the elderly. New York: John Wright, PSG, 1983.

Glassock RJ. Current therapy in nephrology and hypertension. St. Louis: CV Mosby, 1987.

Goldhaber SZ. Pulmonary embolism and deep venous thrombosis. Philadelphia: WB Saunders 1985.
Goodfriend TL. Hypertension essentials: Current concepts of cause and control. New York: Grune & Stratton, 1983.
Goodman RP. Mild hypertension: Pros and cons of drug and non-drug therapies. Consultant 1986; 26(4):141.
Guzzetta CE, Dossey BM. Cardiovascular nursing: Bodymind tapestry. St. Louis: CV Mosby, 1984.
Haimovici H (ed). Vascular surgery: principles and techniques. 2nd ed. New York: Appleton-Century-Crofts, 1984.
Hall WD, Saunders E, Shulman NB. Hypertension in blacks: Epidemiology, pathophysiology and treatment. New York: Year Book Medical Publishers, 1985.
Hirsh J, Genton E, Hull R. Venous thromboembolism. New York: Grune & Stratton, 1981.
Holloway NM. Medical-surgical care plans. Springhouse, PA: Springhouse, 1988.
Horowitz O, McCombs P, Roberts B. Diseases of blood vessels. New York: Lea & Febiger,1985.
Iyer P, Taptich B, Bernocci-Losey D. Nursing process and nursing diagnosis. Philadelphia: WB Saunders, 1991.
Jarrett F, Hirsch S. Vascular surgery of the lower extremity. St. Louis: CV Mosby, 1985.
Kaplan RM. Health-related quality of life in cardiovascular disease. J Consult Clin Psychol, 1988; 56(3):382.
Kee JL. Laboratory and diagnostic tests with nursing implications. 2nd ed. Norwalk, CT: Appleton & Lange, 1987.
Kempczinski RF. The ischemic leg. New York: Year Book Medical Publishers, 1985.
Kerstein MD, Moulder PV, McLane AM. Pocket guide to nursing diagnoses. St. Louis: CV Mosby, 1984.
Krupp MA, Chatton MJ. Current medical diagnosis and treatment. New York: Lange Medical Publications, 1987.
Krupp M, Schroeder S, Tierney L. Current medical diagnoses and treatment 1987. Norwalk, CT: Appleton & Lange, 1987.
Kwaan HC, Bowir EJ. Thrombosis. Philadelphia: WB Saunders, 1982.
Lankford TR, Steward PMJ. Foundations of normal and therapeutic nutrition. New York: John Wiley & Sons, 1986.
Lotchen JM, McKean HE, Kotcher TA. Blood pressure trends with aging. Hypertension (Suppl III), 1982; 4:128.
Mayes JR. Peripheral vascular disease: Laboratory tests and treatment, Part 2. Physician Assist, 1986; 10(7):97.
Melmon KL. Getting the most out of antihypertensives. Emerg Medicine Clin North Am 1986; 18(2):80.
Messerli FH. The age factor in hypertension. Hosp Pract 1986; 21(1):103.
Morrison LM, Schjeide OE. Arteriosclerosis: prevention, treatment and regression. Springfield, IL: Charles C Thomas, 1984.
Moser M. Stepped-care approach to hypertension: Is it still useful? Physician Assis 1986; 10(2):63.
Narjarian JS, Delaney JP. Advances in vascular surgery. New York: Year Book Medical Publishers, 1983.
National Heart, Lung, and Blood Institute, National Institutes of Health. National High Blood Pressure Education Program. Washington, DC: U.S. Government Printing Office, 1992.
Phillips HP. Blood pressure control and quality of life in the elderly patient. Hypertension: New Approaches to Drug Ther 1991; 3(1):21.
Pilliam B. Encouraging compliance with antihypertensive treatment. Nurs Life 1986; 6(3):31.
Reidenberg MM. Drugs in the elderly. Med Clin North Am 1982; 66:1073.
Reiss BS, Melick ME. Pharmacological aspects of nursing care. 2nd ed. Albany, NY: Delmar Publishers, 1987.
Rodman MJ. Hypertension: First-line drug therapy. RN 1991; 91(1):32.
Rutherford RB, Johnson G. Nonoperative management of chronic venous insufficiency. In Rutherford RB, (ed). Vascular surgery. 2nd ed. Philadelphia: WB Saunders, 1984.
Schulze C. Aortic dissection—An ICU crisis. RN 1990; 53(8):36.
Shaw M (ed). Illustrated manual of nursing practice. Springhouse, PA: Springhouse, 1991.
Sowers JR. Physiology of hypertension in the elderly. Hypertension: New Approaches Drug Ther 1991; 3(1):4.
Spittell JA (ed). Clinical vascular disease. Philadelphia: FA Davis, 1983.
Stanley M. Cardiovascular physiology in the elderly. Crit Care Nurse 1985; 5(6):69.
Steffl BM. Handbook of gerontological nursing. New York: Van Nostrand Reinhold, 1984.
Taber's cyclopedic medical dictionary. 16th ed. Philadelphia: FA Davis, 1989.
Wagner MM, Beaver BM. Peripheral vascular dysfunction. Nurs Clin North Am 1986; 21(2):195.
Wolfe JHN, Kinmonth JB. The prognosis of primary lymphedema of the lower limbs. Arch Surg 1981; 116:1157.
Wyngaarden JB, Smith LH. Cecil textbook of medicine. 17th ed. Philadelphia: WB Saunders, 1987.
Yacone L. The nurse's guide to cardiovascular drugs. RN, 1988; 51(8):36.
Zoler ML. BP drug acts selectively in brain. Chronic Care 1991; 31(10):8.

Unit Seven

ADULTS WITH GASTROINTESTINAL DYSFUNCTION

Learning Objectives

AFTER COMPLETING THIS UNIT, THE LEARNER WILL BE ABLE TO:

Chapter Twenty-one

1. Explain the normal anatomy and physiology of the digestive system and its accessory organs.
2. Describe common clinical manifestations of gastrointestinal (GI) dysfunction.
3. Identify information and physical examination data essential to the assessment of gastrointestinal status.
4. Describe basic diagnostic tests and modalities of medical management (GI intubation, enteral and parenteral nutrition) used in the treatment of patients with GI disorders.
5. Describe basic surgical procedures (gastrectomy, intestinal resection, colostomy, ileostomy, ileoanal endorectal pull-through) used in the treatment of patients with GI disorders.
6. Identify data essential to the assessment of patients undergoing treatment of GI disorders.
7. State nursing diagnoses and related expected patient outcomes commonly applicable to patients undergoing treatment of GI disorders.
8. Describe nursing interventions, with their rationales, commonly applicable to patients undergoing treatment of GI disorders.
9. Explain the basis for evaluation of nursing care provided to patients undergoing treatment of GI disorders.
10. Identify special considerations for the elderly patient with altered GI function.

Chapter Twenty-two

1. Describe common upper GI disorders in terms of etiology, pathophysiology, clinical manifestations, diagnostic procedures, and medical management.
2. Identify information and physical examination data essential to the assessment of patients with common upper GI disorders.
3. State nursing diagnoses and related expected patient outcomes commonly applicable to patients with upper GI disorders.
4. Describe nursing interventions, with their rationales, commonly applicable to patients with upper GI disorders.
5. Explain the basis for evaluation of nursing care provided to patients with common upper GI disorders.
6. Identify special considerations for the elderly patient with an upper GI tract disorder.

Chapter Twenty-three

1. Describe common lower GI disorders in terms of etiology, pathophysiology, clinical manifestations, diagnostic procedures, and medical management.
2. Identify information and physical examination data essential to the assessment of patients with common lower GI disorders.
3. State nursing diagnoses and related expected patient outcomes commonly applicable to patients with lower GI disorders.
4. Describe nursing interventions, with their rationales, commonly applicable to patients with upper GI disorders.
5. Explain the basis for evaluation of nursing care provided to patients with common lower GI disorders.
6. Identify special considerations for the elderly patient with a lower GI tract disorder.

Chapter Twenty-four

1. Describe common disorders of the accessory organs of digestion in terms of etiology, pathophysiology, clinical manifestations, diagnostic procedures, and medical management.
2. Identify information and physical examination data essential to the assessment of patients with common disorders of the accessory organs of digestion.
3. State nursing diagnoses and related expected patient outcomes commonly applicable to patients with disorders of the accessory organs of digestion.
4. Describe nursing interventions, with their rationales, commonly applicable to patients with disorders of the accessory organs of digestion.
5. Explain the basis for evaluation of nursing care provided to patients with common disorders of the accessory organs of digestion.
6. Identify special considerations for the elderly patient with a disorder of the accessory organs of digestion.

Chapter Twenty-one

KNOWLEDGE BASIC TO THE NURSING CARE *of Adults with Gastrointestinal Dysfunction*

Ingestion, digestion, and absorption of nutrients essential for life and growth are functions of the gastrointestinal tract, as is the excretion of solid waste from the body. Patterns of gastrointestinal function vary both within and among individuals. Different people vary in patterns of intake, ability to tolerate various types of foods, and patterns of elimination. Likewise, an individual's intake, tolerance of various foods, and pattern of elimination vary from time to time such that transient episodes of anorexia, distention, flatulence, or stool that is dryer or looser than normal are considered normal variations in function. This fact presents a challenge to the health care provider because these same variations can represent disease. Thus, a clear understanding of the anatomy and physiology of the gastrointestinal tract and the pathophysiology underlying the major clinical manifestations of gastrointestinal disease is essential to accurate assessment and effective intervention.

Anatomy and Physiology

The gastrointestinal (GI) tract is a continuous tube of varying diameter approximately 9 m (30 feet) long. It begins with the mouth and extends through the pharynx, esophagus, stomach, small intestine, and large intestine to the anus. The accessory organs of digestion are the teeth, tongue, salivary glands, gallbladder, pancreas, and liver.

The primary function of the GI tract is to convert complex food substances into simpler compounds that can be absorbed into the blood stream and utilized by the cells of the body. It also excretes solid waste from the body.

Basic Structure of the Gastrointestinal Tract

From the lower third of the esophagus to the anus, the GI tract is composed of four layers of tissue: the inner layer, or mucosa; the submucosa; the muscularis; and an outer layer, the serosa.

The mucosa is composed of a surface layer of epithelium, a layer of loose connective tissue rich in blood and lymphatic vessels called the lamina propria, and a thin layer of smooth muscle. Mucus and digestive juices are secreted by the cells of the mucosa.

The submucosa is composed of loose connective tissue. It connects the mucosa to the underlying muscularis and allows for movement and change in size of the tract.

The muscularis is composed of smooth muscle arranged in two layers. An inner circular layer of fibers surrounds the tube, and an outer layer of longitudinal fibers runs parallel with its long axis. Each of these layers provides a specific type of motility necessary for maximal efficiency of digestion and absorption. Contraction of the longitudinal muscles causes a motion called peristalsis to occur. Peristalsis primarily causes the propulsion of nutrients down the tube. Contraction of the circular muscle causes segmentation. This enhances the mixing of food with the various digestive juices and also forces food close to the mucosal lining of the tract, thus facilitating absorption.

The outer layer or serosa consists of epithelial and connective tissue. The serosa is also called the visceral peritoneum.

Peritoneum

The organs of the GI tract below the esophagus are located in the abdominal cavity and are covered with the peritoneum, the largest serous membrane of the body. The peritoneum is composed of two layers: the parietal layer, which lines the walls of the abdominal cavity, and the visceral layer, which covers some of the organs within the cavity. Between the parietal and visceral portions of the peritoneum is a potential space called the peritoneal cavity, which contains serous fluid. The peritoneum contains several large folds that pass between the viscera of the abdomen and pelvis. These folds connect the organs to one another and to the walls of the cavity. They also contain blood and lymph vessels along with nerves that supply the organs in the abdomen.

Mouth

The mouth is the structure through which food enters the GI tract. Within the mouth are the tongue with its taste receptors, the teeth, and the salivary glands.

The mouth is bounded laterally by the cheeks and anteriorly by the lips. The hard palate forms the anterior portion of the roof of the mouth, and the soft palate forms the posterior portion. The tongue, along with its associated muscles, forms the floor of the mouth.

Mucous membrane lines the oral cavity. It contains many small glands, called buccal glands, which secrete small amounts of saliva. The salivary glands, however, secrete the major amount of saliva. The three pairs of salivary glands are the parotid, submandibular, and sublingual. Each of these pairs supplies different proportions of ingredients to saliva. The parotid gland secretes serous fluid that contains the enzyme salivary amylase. The sublingual gland secretes mucus, which is a thicker fluid and contains a small amount of enzyme. The submandibular gland secretes both mucus and serous fluid.

The process of digestion begins in the mouth with chewing or mastication. Chewing mechanically breaks up large food particles and mixes food and saliva. This not only facilitates swallowing but initiates the first phase of chemical digestion, which is the breakdown of starches by salivary amylase (ptyalin) contained in the saliva.

Swallowing, or the act of deglutition, is the process by which chewed food, now called a bolus, moves from the mouth to the stomach. This process has three distinct stages: the oral, the pharyngeal, and the esophageal. In the oral phase, which is under voluntary control, the bolus is moved by the tongue into the oropharynx. Upon entering the oropharynx, the process becomes involuntary. Impulses are sent to the swallowing center in the medulla oblongata. Returning impulses cause the epiglottis to move and cover the tracheal opening to prevent aspiration of food into the lung, and the bolus passes through the pharynx and into the esophagus. During the third or esophageal phase, the bolus is forced through the esophagus by involuntary peristaltic waves.

Pharynx

The pharynx, or throat, is a musculomembranous tube that is approximately 13 cm (5 inches) long. It extends from the base of the skull to the esophagus and lies in front of the cervical vertebrae. The pharynx has openings that communicate to the ears, nose, mouth, larynx, and esophagus. It is divided into three parts: the nasopharynx, the oropharynx, and the laryngopharynx. The nasopharynx is situated behind the posterior nares and above the soft palate. It connects with the posterior nares, thus allowing the passage of air during breathing. It also contains the openings of the auditory tubes through which air enters the middle ear. The oropharynx extends from the soft palate to the hyoid bone, and the laryngopharynx extends from the hyoid bone to the esophagus. The oropharynx and the laryngopharynx serve as a passageway for both the digestive and the respiratory tracts.

Esophagus

The esophagus is a muscular tube approximately 24 cm (9 inches) long that lies behind the trachea. It extends from the distal portion of the pharynx, passes through the mediastinum in front of the vertebral column, penetrates the diaphragm through an aperture called the esophageal hiatus, and terminates in the upper portion of the stomach.

Peristaltic waves down the esophagus transport food and fluids from the oral cavity to the stomach. To facilitate this process, esophageal glands secrete mucus, which lubricates the food bolus and helps prevent damage to the esophageal wall.

Just above the diaphragm and 2 to 5 cm above the esophageal gastric junction, nutrients pass through the lower esophageal sphincter (LES). The LES (see Fig. 21–1) is an area of the esophageal smooth muscle that remains tonically constricted except when it relaxes as part of the swallowing reflex to permit the passage of the bolus into the stomach. Its primary purpose is to prevent reflux of gastric contents, which are highly acidic and contain protein-digesting enzymes, into the upper esophagus during contractions of the stomach.

Also preventing reflux of gastric contents is a physiologic valvelike mechanism at the end of the esophagus just under the diaphragm. This is a pressure-controlled closure, whose action is due to the fact that three quarters of the esophagus is in the thoracic cavity under negative pressure, whereas the one quarter distal to the diaphragm is in the abdominal cavity under positive pressure. This pressure difference forces the lower end of the esophagus closed, thus preventing the high pressure in the stomach from forcing gastric contents back into the esophagus. This is less efficient than a true valve would be, and any compromise of the diaphragmatic opening can result in incompetence and development of related pathology. The passage of liquids and very soft foods from the mouth to the stomach takes approximately 1 second. Semisolid or solid foods pass through in approximately 4 to 8 seconds.

Stomach

The stomach is the dilated portion of the alimentary canal. It is situated in the left upper part of the abdomen and lies directly under the diaphragm. The upper part of the stomach communicates with the distal portion of the esophagus, and the lower part communicates with the duodenum. The size and shape of the stomach vary according to the amount of stomach contents, the stage of digestion, the condition of the muscular wall, and the status of the adjacent intestines.

The parts of the stomach are the cardia, the fundus, the body, the antrum, and the pylorus (Fig.

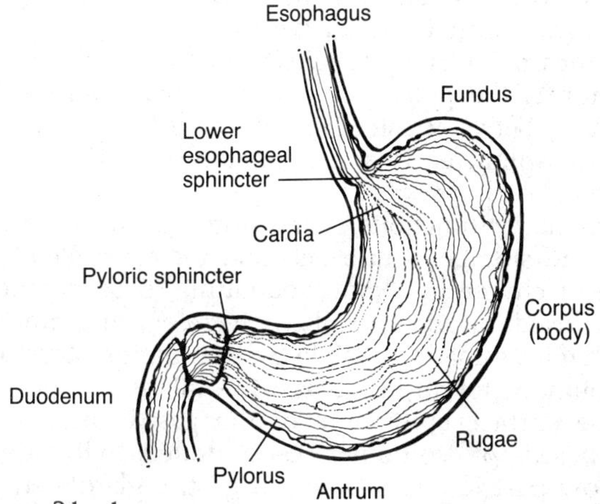

Figure 21–1.

Physiologic anatomy of the lower esophagus and the stomach. Note the location of the lower esophageal sphincter (LES). Note also the regions of the stomach: cardia, fundus, body, antrum, and pylorus.

Table 21–1. HORMONE AND HORMONE-LIKE SUBSTANCES INVOLVED IN THE REGULATION OF GASTRIC SECRETION, MOTILITY, AND EMPTYING

HORMONE	SOURCE	STIMULUS	FUNCTION
Gastrin	Enteroendocrine cells in gastric mucosa	Partially digested proteins, caffeine, and other chemicals in food present in stomach	Increases secretion of hydrochloric acid, pepsinogen by gastric glands Relaxes ileocecal valve
Serotonin	Enteroendocrine cells in gastric mucosa	Presence of food in the stomach	Contracts gastric muscles
Histamine	Enteroendocrine cells in gastric mucosa	Presence of food in the stomach	Stimulates secretion of hydrochloric acid by parietal cells
Somatostatin	Enteroendocrine cells in gastric mucosa	Presence of food in the stomach	Inhibits gastric secretion, motility, and emptying Inhibits pancreatic secretion Inhibits absorption in the small intestine by decreasing blood flow
Intestinal gastrin	Duodenal mucosa	Presence of acidic, partially digested food in duodenum	Stimulates secretion by gastric glands
Secretin	Duodenal mucosa	Acid chyme, irritants, or partially digested protein in chyme, hypertonic, or hypotonic fluids	Inhibits gastric secretion during gastric phase Increases production of bicarbonate ion–rich pancreatic juice Stimulates increased production of bile
Cholecystokinin (CCK)	Jejunal mucosa	Presence of fats in the intestinal contents	Stimulates gallbladder to contract and eject bile. Simultaneously relaxes sphincter of Oddi and stimulates release of pancreatic juice
Gastric inhibitory peptide (GIP)	Duodenal mucosa	Presence of fats in the duodenum and, to a lesser degree, presence of carbohydrates	Decreases motor activity of the stomach and slows emptying of gastric contents into the duodenum

21–1). The cardia is the upper area of the stomach that surrounds the lower esophageal sphincter. The fundus is the rounded portion above and to the left of the cardia. The body, or corpus, is below the fundus and is the central portion of the stomach. The pylorus is the narrow, inferior portion of the stomach, the first part of which is sometimes called the antrum. A ringlike muscle in the pyloric opening forms the pyloric sphincter, which controls the opening between the stomach and duodenum. The pyloric sphincter is a true anatomic valve and remains closed at rest.

The major functions of the stomach are the direction and storage of nutrients and the controlled passage of chyme into the duodenum. These functions are carried out via specialized secretory and motility mechanisms made possible by the unique structural adaptations found in the gastric wall.

The surface epithelium of the gastric mucosa is composed of columnar cells dotted with deep, narrow gastric pits into which gastric glands empty their secretions. Gastric glands in different regions of the stomach contain different types of secretory cells and hence produce different secretions.

The four main types of secretory cells are chief (zymogenic or peptic) cells, parietal cells, mucous cells, and enteroendocrine cells. Chief cells secrete pepsinogen, the precursor of the protein-digesting enzyme pepsin. Parietal cells secrete hydrochloric acid, which creates the acidic environment necessary for the conversion of pepsinogen into pepsin. They also secrete intrinsic factor, which is essential for the absorption of vitamin B_{12} in the terminal ileum. Mucous cells secrete a sticky, alkaline mucus that adheres to the epithelial surface and helps protect the gastric wall against damage from acid gastric secretions. Enteroendocrine cells secrete a variety of hormone and hormone-like substances that are involved in the regulation of gastric secretion, motility, and emptying (Table 21–1). These include gastrin, histamine, and serotonin. The secretions of the chief, parietal, and mucous cells are collectively referred to as gastric juice and total approximately 3000 ml per day.

The glands in the cardiac area of the stomach primarily secrete mucus, whereas those in the fundus and the body of the stomach secrete almost all the hydrochloric acid, pepsinogen, and intrinsic factor. The pyloric glands secrete mucus and the hormone gastrin.

Secretion of gastric glands is under both nervous and hormonal control and occurs in three phases: cephalic, gastric, and intestinal.

In the cephalic phase, gastric secretion is stimulated by the sight, smell, taste, or thought of food. This is a reflex response mediated by the vagus nerve. It serves to prepare the stomach for the arrival of foodstuffs requiring digestion.

In the gastric phase, gastric distention initiates secretion of gastric juice, but the major source of stimulation is the hormone gastrin. Gastrin-secreting (enteroendocrine) cells are directly activated by foodstuffs such as partially digested proteins and caffeine. The gastrin secreted then directly stimulates other gastric secretory cells to increase the production of gastric juice, with its greatest effect being on the hydrochloric acid–producing parietal cells.

Gastrin secretion is controlled by a negative feedback mechanism based on the pH of the stomach contents. When protein, which acts as a buffer, enters the stomach, the pH rises and gastrin and hydrochloric acid are secreted. As protein digestion occurs and the pH falls to 2, secretion is inhibited.

The intestinal phase of gastric secretion begins when partially digested food enters the duodenum. This stimulates release of a hormone called intestinal gastrin, which stimulates continued gastric secretion.

Gastric juice is also secreted in response to histamine that is produced by enteroendocrine cells in the gastric mucosa.

Another way in which the stomach wall differs from the wall in the rest of the gastrointestinal tract is that the muscularis contains an innermost oblique layer of smooth muscle in addition to the longitudinal and circular layers. This allows gastric contents not only to be propelled through the stomach but to be churned and pummeled to effectively mix and liquefy the bolus of food. It also contributes to the great distensibility of the stomach.

As a bolus of food enters the stomach, peristaltic movements pass over the stomach every 15 to 25 seconds. These movements macerate the bolus and mix it with the gastric secretions to form a thinner substance called chyme. As digestion continues, more forceful movements begin in the body of the stomach and increase as they reach the pylorus. When the chyme reaches the pylorus, a small amount is forced through the pyloric splinter into the duodenum with each peristaltic movement. The remaining chyme is forced back into the stomach, where further mixing occurs (Fig. 21–2). Another wave pushes the chyme forward again, and a little more is forced or "squirted" into the duodenum. This forward and backward movement of stomach contents accounts for most of the mixing in the stomach.

Like gastric secretion, gastric motility is under both hormonal (see Table 21–1) and nervous control. Parasympathetic stimulation via the vagus and its branches results in increased secretion and mobility, whereas sympathetic stimulation has an inhibiting effect on gastrointestinal function.

Chemical digestion in the stomach consists of the breakdown of proteins into smaller molecules called peptides through the action of pepsin. Digestion of starches, which began in the mouth, ceases as the salivary amylase is inactivated by the highly acid gastric environment. There is no absorption of basic nutrients in the stomach. Substances that are absorbed are water, alcohol, and aspirin.

Small Intestine

The small intestine, approximately 7 m (23 feet) long and 2.5 cm (1 inch) in diameter, is divided into three segments: the duodenum, the jejunum, and the ileum. The duodenum, the shortest of the three, begins at the pyloric valve of the stomach and continues approximately 25 cm (10 inches) until it unites with the jejunum. The pancreatic and bile ducts, joined as the common bile duct, empty into the duodenum through the sphincter of Oddi. The jejunum, the middle segment, is approximately 2.5 m (8 feet) long and merges with the ileum, which is approximately 3.5 m (12 feet) in length. The ileum connects with the large intestine at the ileocecal valve, which guards the entrance to the cecum. The valve, which is usually closed to increase absorption time and to prevent movement of bacteria from the large intestine into the small intestine, opens to allow passage of chyme into the cecum.

The small intestine is the principal organ of digestion and absorption, and structural adaptations in the form of plicae circulares, villi, and microvilli have developed to support these functions (Fig. 21–3).

The plicae circulares are deep, permanent circular folds in the mucosa and submucosa, which force chyme to move in a spiral direction. This enhances mixing with digestive juices and slows forward movement of the chyme, prolonging contact time with both intestinal enzymes and the absorptive surface of the mucosa. Villi, finger-like projections clustered over the entire mucosa, and microvilli, which are minute projections of the plasma membrane of the mucosal absorptive cells, serve to increase the absorptive surface. Microvilli, which form the so-called brush border on the absorptive cells, also contain digestive enzymes. Each of the villi, which project approximately 1 mm and give the small intestine the texture of velvet, contains a dense capillary bed and a modified lymphatic vessel called a lacteal. They absorb digested nutrients and transport them via the capillary bed or the lacteal into the blood stream.

Between the villi, the mucosa is dotted with pits, which lead into the crypts of Lieberkühn (intestinal crypts). These glands secrete both intestinal juice

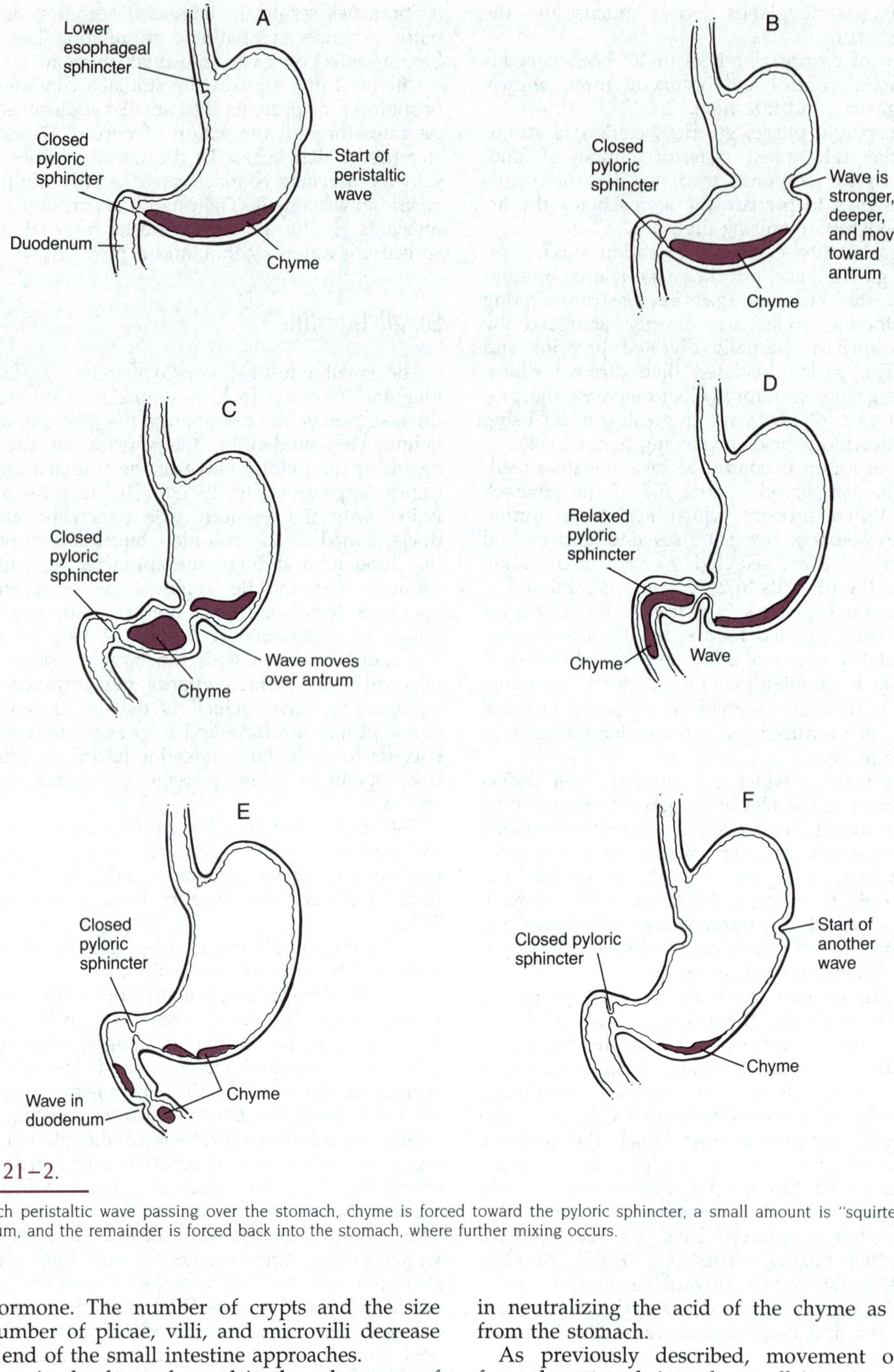

Figure 21–2.

With each peristaltic wave passing over the stomach, chyme is forced toward the pyloric sphincter, a small amount is "squirted" into the duodenum, and the remainder is forced back into the stomach, where further mixing occurs.

and hormone. The number of crypts and the size and number of plicae, villi, and microvilli decrease as the end of the small intestine approaches.

Brunner's glands are located in the submucosa of the duodenum. These glands secrete an alkaline mucus that protects the wall of the small intestine from the action of the digestive enzymes and assists in neutralizing the acid of the chyme as it enters from the stomach.

As previously described, movement of chyme from the stomach into the small intestine is a slow process carefully controlled by the pyloric valve. It is essential for two reasons that only small amounts of chyme enter the duodenum at one time. First, chyme is usually hypertonic, and large amounts would pull water by osmosis into the intestine and could seriously decrease blood volume. Second, chyme from the stomach is highly acidic, and the pH must be raised for the digestive enzymes in the small intestine to function.

Once in the small intestine, chyme is subjected to two types of movement: segmentation and peristalsis. Segmentation, which consists of alternate contractions of the circular muscle fibers, mixes the chyme with the digestive juices and brings it into contact with the villi. Peristaltic waves then move the chyme forward in the small intestine. Both these movements are initiated by the distention of the intestine and are under the control of the autonomic nervous system.

The chyme that enters the small intestine contains partially digested carbohydrates, partially digested proteins, and for the most part, undigested lipids. The completion of the digestion of these nutrients is a combined effort of bile, pancreatic juice, and intestinal juice.

Starches entering the small intestine are hydrolized by pancreatic amylase into disaccharides, which in turn are broken down into absorbable monosaccharides by disaccharases in the intestinal juices. Similarly, proteoses (protein fragments) that enter the duodenum are split into peptides by trypsin, chemotrypsin, and other proteases found in the pancreatic juice. The peptides in turn are split into amino acids by peptidases in the intestinal juice.

Fats entering the small intestine are emulsified by bile to prepare them to be acted on by pancreatic lipase, which breaks them down into fatty acids and glycerides. Bile then renders the fatty acids water-soluble so they can be absorbed across the intestinal mucosa.

Large Intestine

The large intestine is approximately 1.5 m (5 feet) in length and 6.5 cm ($2\frac{5}{8}$ inches) in diameter. It extends from the ileum to the anus and is divided into four parts: the cecum, colon, rectum, and anal canal. The cecum is a blind pouch approximately 6 cm ($2\frac{3}{8}$ inches) long. Attached to the lower portion of the cecum is a narrow coiled tube called the vermiform appendix. The opening from the ileum into the cecum is protected by a large fold of mucous membrane called the ileocecal valve, which allows the digestive by-products from the small intestine to pass into the large intestine.

The colon extends from the cecum to the rectum and is divided into the ascending, transverse, descending, and sigmoid colon. The ascending colon passes upward on the lower right side of the abdomen to become the transverse colon at the hepatic flexure. The transverse colon crosses the mid abdomen, bends downward at the splenic flexure on the left side, and becomes the descending colon. At the level of the iliac crest, the colon curves like the letter S and is called the sigmoid colon, which terminates at the rectum. The rectum continues from the sigmoid colon and ends at the anal canal. The terminal portion of the large intestine, or the anal canal, is

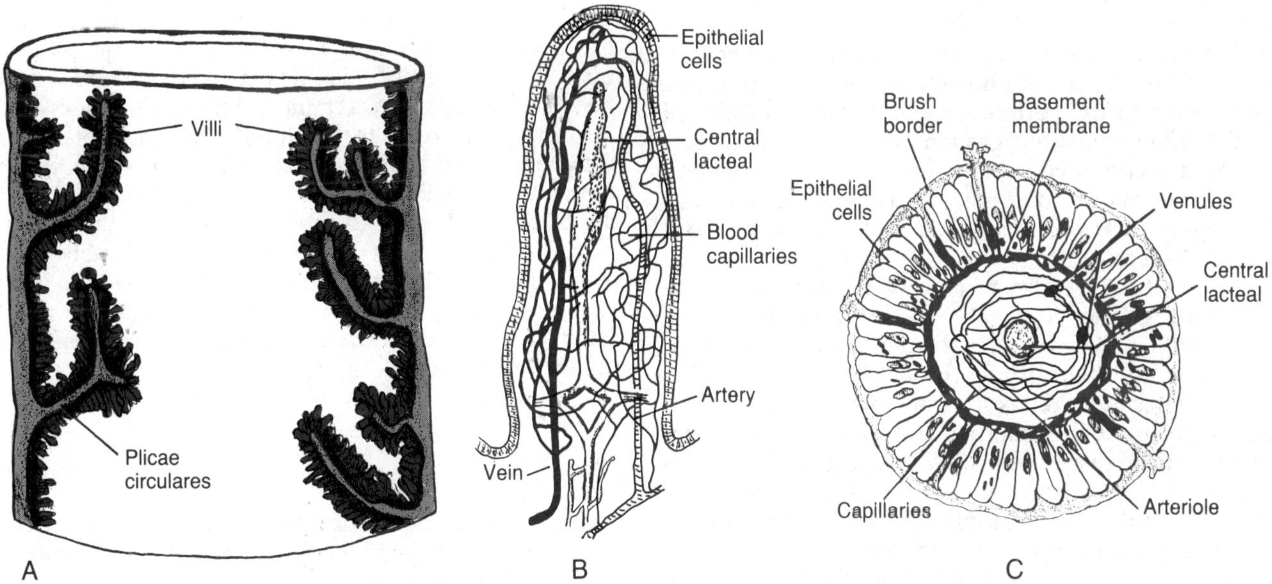

Figure 21–3.

Structural adaptations found in the wall of the small intestine that facilitate its digestive and absorptive functions are the plicae circulares, villi, and microvilli. *A*, Longitudinal section of the small intestine showing the plicae circulares covered with villi. *B*, Longitudinal section of a villus. *C*, Cross section of a villus showing the brush border of microvilli. (From Guyton AC. Textbook of medical physiology. 8th ed. Philadelphia: WB Saunders, 1991, p 730.)

approximately 2 to 3 cm (1 inch) long. The opening of the anal canal to the exterior, called the anus, is guarded by an internal and an external sphincter. These sphincters remain closed except during the act of defecation, when the residue of digestion is expelled.

The mucosa of the large intestine differs from that of the small intestine in that it does not have villi or circular folds. It does, however, contain simple columnar epithelium with numerous goblet cells, which absorb water and secrete mucus that lubricates the residue as it passes through the colon.

The muscularis of the colon is also unique in that it does not completely surround the colon but rather forms three bands called the taeniae coli. These bands, when contracted, gather the colon into a series of pouches called haustra, giving it a puckered appearance.

Movement in the large intestine consists of peristalsis, which is mild and slow, haustral churning, and mass movements. Haustral churning refers to the action of smooth muscle in individual haustra. As chyme passes through the ileocecal valve, it fills and distends the first haustrum in the cecum. This distention causes the smooth muscle in the haustrum to contract and thus mixes and propels the chyme to the next haustrum.

Mass movements are long, slow, strong waves of muscular contraction that start in the transverse colon and propel colonic contents into the rectum. They occur three or four times daily, usually during or just after eating, as a result of the gastrocolic and gastroduodenal reflexes (presence of food in the stomach or duodenum reflexly stimulates mass peristalsis in the colon). These mass movements become stronger as the amount of bulk in the diet is increased.

The large intestine reabsorbs water and electrolytes, particularly sodium and chloride, and stores feces prior to defecation. No enzymes are produced in the colon, and no digestion occurs. However, any remaining carbohydrates or amino acids are metabolized by colonic bacteria, releasing gases such as hydrogen, carbon dioxide, and methane, which contribute to fecal odor.

Colonic bacteria also produce vitamin K and some B vitamins, and these are absorbed by the colon along with water and electrolytes. Finally, they provide bulk and help propel the stool into the rectum.

The defecation reflex is stimulated by distention of the rectum. The internal and external sphincters involuntarily relax when this happens, but there is an overriding central nervous system control by which an individual voluntarily suppresses the urge to defecate by contraction of the external sphincter.

Nearly 10,000 ml of fluid pass through the GI tract of the average adult every 24 hours. This includes 1 to 2 L of saliva, 3000 ml of gastric fluid, 500 ml of bile, 1000 ml of pancreatic juice, and 2000 ml of intestinal secretions in addition to the average 1 to 2 L per day that is ingested. Feces that are evacuated contain approximately 150 ml of water.

Liver

The liver is the largest organ of the body. It has multiple functions that affect many different body systems (see Chapter 27). These functions include the storage and metabolism of nutrients that have been digested and absorbed, the detoxification of noxious substances, and the production of bile.

Bile, which is continuously produced by the liver, prepares lipids to be broken down by the enzyme lipase. This is done by the bile salts, mainly cholic acid and chenodeoxycholic acid, which emulsify fats (i.e., break them into small droplets and distribute them throughout the watery chyme). The result is a large surface area on which lipase can act. Bile salts also facilitate fat and cholesterol absorption and, with lecithin, make cholesterol soluble.

The pigment chiefly responsible for the greenish-yellow color of bile is bilirubin. Bilirubin is metabolized by bacteria in the small intestine, and a breakdown product, urobilinogen, gives feces their characteristic brown color. Without urobilinogen, feces are pale gray to white.

Gallbladder

The gallbladder is a pear-shaped muscular sac located below the liver. It is approximately 8 cm (3 inches) long and 2.5 cm (1 inch) wide. Its major function is to store and concentrate bile secreted by the liver. The liver secretes bile continuously, but the sphincter of Oddi, through which bile passes into the duodenum, is closed when bile is not needed for digestion. At these times, bile backs up into the gallbladder to be stored until fats enter the duodenum and stimulate the release of cholecystokinin (CCK). This intestinal hormone stimulates the gallbladder to contract and eject bile into the cystic duct, from which it flows into the common bile duct, through the sphincter of Oddi, and into the duodenum (Fig. 21–4). CCK simultaneously stimulates release of pancreatic juice and relaxes the sphincter of Oddi.

Pancreas

The pancreas is the primary producer of digestive enzymes. It is a large gland approximately 12.5 cm (6 inches) long and 2.5 cm (1 inch) wide and is divided into the head, the body, and the tail. The pancreas lies behind the stomach, with its head lying in the curve of the duodenum and the tail reaching to the spleen.

The pancreas is both an endocrine and an exo-

Figure 21–4.

Anatomic relationships of the liver, gallbladder, pancreas, and duodenum. Color indicates path of bile flow.

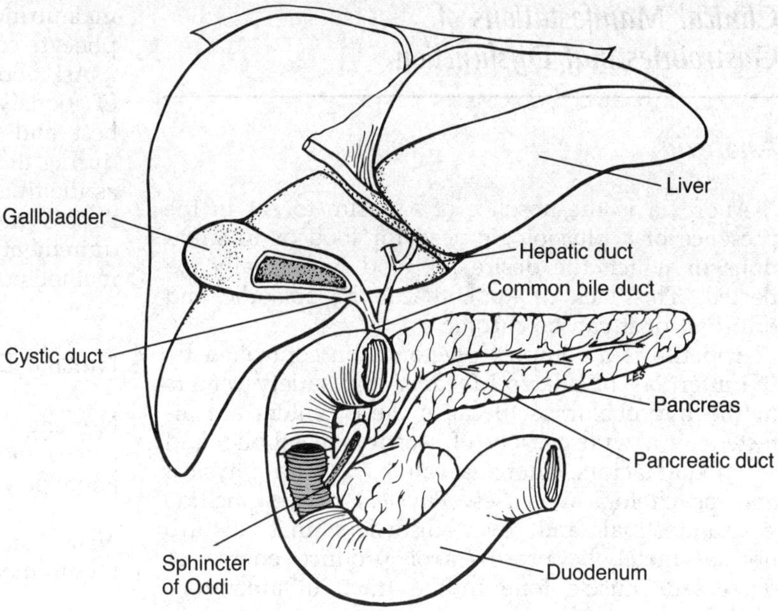

crine gland. Its endocrine cells secrete insulin and glucagon (see Chapter 29), and the exocrine, or acinar, cells secrete a high bicarbonate solution and enzymes specific to the digestion of each of the three basic nutrients.

The watery, very alkaline solution with a high content of sodium bicarbonate is produced by specialized cells in the head of the pancreas. This solution neutralizes acid chyme and raises the pH to the level needed for effective action of pancreatic and intestinal enzymes. It is secreted in response to stimulation by the hormone secretin, which is released when hydrochloric acid enters the small intestine.

The secretion of enzyme-rich pancreatic fluid is stimulated by CCK, the same hormone that stimulates the gallbladder to contract. Intestinal CCK is released when proteoses, peptones, or fats are present in the upper small intestine. Pancreatic fluid contains the following enzymes: pancreatic amylase, which hydrolyzes starch into maltose and chains of glucose molecules; pancreatic lipase, which breaks emulsified fats into fatty acids and monoglycerides; and trypsin, chemotrypsin, and other proteases, which split proteoses into peptides. The last three all are secreted in inactive form to prevent digestion of the pancreatic cells themselves.

Pancreatic juice leaves the pancreas through the pancreatic duct, which enters the duodenum near the common bile duct.

A summary of the digestive secretions including their source, pH, daily volume, component enzymes, and role in chemical digestion is presented in Table 21–2.

Table 21–2. SUMMARY OF DIGESTIVE SECRETIONS AND ENZYMES

SECRETION	VOLUME PER DAY	pH	ENZYME	SOURCE	ACTION AND PRODUCTS
Saliva	1–1.5 L	6.8	Salivary amylase	Salivary glands	Hydrolyzes starch to maltose
Gastric juice	1.5–2.5 L	2–4	Pepsin	Gastric mucosa	Breaks down protein into proteoses, peptones, and polypeptides
Pancreatic juice	600–800 ml	8–8.4	Trypsin	Pancreas	Splits proteins into amino acids and polypeptides
			Chymotrypsin	Pancreas	Splits proteins
			Pancreatic amylase	Pancreas	Splits starch into maltose
			Pancreatic lipase	Pancreas	Hydrolyzes fats into fatty acids and monoglycerides
Intestinal juice	2–3 L	7–9	Intestinal lipase	Intestinal glands	Splits fats into fatty acids and glycerol
			Peptidase	Intestinal glands	Splits polypeptides into amino acids
			Enterokinase	Duodenal mucosa	Activates trypsin
			Maltase, Sucrase, Lactase	Intestinal glands	Split disaccharides into monosaccharides

Clinical Manifestations of Gastrointestinal Dysfunction

Anorexia

Anorexia is the absence of a desire to eat in the presence of a physiologic need for food or in situations in which the desire for food is normally expected. This lack of appetite can be episodic and transient or it can be chronic.

Appetite is a complex phenomenon controlled by the interplay of bilateral feeding and satiety centers in the hypothalamus. Because these centers are affected by a wide variety of sensory, metabolic, and hormonal factors, anorexia can have both physical and psychological causes. Physical causes include gastrointestinal and liver disorders that disturb normal metabolic processes or produce edema or decreased muscle tone in the tract, inflammatory disorders, severe pulmonary disease, uremia, congestive heart failure, and cancer. Anorexia is also associated with poor oral hygiene, abdominal distention, and drugs such as amphetamines. Psychological causes of anorexia include fear, anxiety, depression, and offensive sights, odors, and conversations, as well as association of eating or of particular foods with unpleasant past experiences.

Prolonged anorexia can lead to malnutrition and ultimately to life-threatening fluid and electrolyte imbalance. Medical management is focused on treatment of the underlying condition and correction of nutritional deficiencies. The latter may include supplemental feedings or total parenteral nutrition, or both.

Application of the Nursing Process to the Care of the Patient with Anorexia

Assessment

Begin assessment of the anorexic patient with a dietary history. Determine the types and amounts of foods usually eaten. Compare this with the patient's report of current dietary intake. Determine when the anorexia began, and explore its relationship to any other symptoms, environmental factors, or life events.

Assess the patient's general nutritional status. Check current weight, and determine whether loss has occurred and over what period of time. Observe for signs of malnutrition such as dull, thin, brittle hair, tired apathetic facial expression, dry skin and nails, and muscle wasting. Review laboratory values such as albumin levels, lymphocyte counts, and serum electrolyte levels for changes indicative of malnutrition (albumin level less than 3.5 g/dl, lymphocyte count below 1500 cu mm).

Ask about the patient's likes and dislikes in terms of foods and fluids, and determine which are the best and least well tolerated. Find out the times during the day when the patient usually eats as well as the time when the patient is usually most hungry. Assess the patient's understanding of dietary requirements, the nutritional value of foods, and methods of food preparation.

Nursing Diagnoses and Planning

Nursing diagnoses and related expected patient outcomes most commonly applicable to patients with anorexia include the following:

NDx: High risk for altered nutrition: less than body requirements related to lack of appetite

Planning: Patient outcomes
1. Patient eats a *(specify for individual)* calorie diet per day.
2. Patient consumes *(specify for individual)* grams of protein per day.
3. Patient maintains current weight.

NDx: High risk for altered health maintenance related to insufficient knowledge of dietary requirements, nutritional value of specific foods, or methods of adjusting food preparation or service to make the food more appetizing

Planning: Patient outcomes
1. Patient describes his or her daily dietary requirements.
2. Patient identifies nutritional value of specific foods relative to his or her dietary needs.
3. Patient describes ways to make foods more appetizing.

Nursing Interventions

NDx: High risk for altered nutrition: less than body requirements

Offer the patient foods that are well liked and that meet the patient's nutritional needs. Avoid offering foods that will fill the patient up but are of little nutritional value. Urge the family to provide favorite foods if not otherwise available.

Encourage the patient to eat at the time of day when he or she is most hungry. Before serving food, be certain that the patient does not need to go to the bathroom; that hands, face, and mouth are clean; and that he or she is positioned appropriately and is as comfortable as possible. Provide small portions attractively served. Make sure that utensils are spotlessly clean and that cold foods are cold and hot foods hot. Keep the environment calm, neat, and free of odors or offensive sights and sounds. Explore the possibility of communal dining or guest trays for visitors to enhance the social quality of dining.

NDx: High risk for altered health maintenance

Explain the patient's individual dietary needs so they are clearly understood by the patient and any significant other who has a key role in food selection and preparation. Describe the nutrient value of various foods, and identify those best suited to the patient's needs. Discuss methods of preparation that maximize nutritional value and also tend to be appetizing. Explain the importance of personal comfort, a clean, stress-free environment, and attractively served food in promoting appetite. Arrange for teaching by a dietitian whenever necessary.

Evaluation

Evaluate the effectiveness of nursing care for a patient with anorexia by comparing the patient's status with the expected patient outcomes. Examples of specific outcomes for patients with anorexia have been provided in the Planning section.

Nausea and Vomiting

Nausea is a disagreeable feeling of revulsion toward food usually accompanied by symptoms of altered autonomic nervous system activity such as diaphoresis, increased salivation, pallor, tachycardia, dizziness, and faintness.

Nausea usually precedes the act of vomiting, which is the expulsion of upper gastrointestinal contents through the mouth as a result of reverse peristalsis and relaxation of the lower esophageal sphincter.

There are two centers in the medulla involved with vomiting: the vomiting center and the chemoreceptor trigger zone (CTZ). The vomiting center is stimulated directly by the autonomic nervous system. Such stimulants as gastrointestinal distention, irritants and toxins, injury to the viscera, pain, and even emotional upheaval can cause nausea and vomiting in this direct way. The vomiting center can also be directly stimulated by the local pressure that occurs when there is increased intracranial pressure.

Indirect stimulation of the vomiting center occurs when an emetic agent stimulates the CTZ, which in turn causes the vomiting center to respond. Emetic agents include such drugs as morphine, meperidine (Demerol), ergot derivatives, and digitalis preparations, as well as metabolic substances resulting from uremia, infection, and radiation. Motion in the semicircular canals of the ears is also believed to cause nausea and vomiting through the indirect trigger zone route.

A specific type of vomiting is projectile vomiting, which is associated with increased intracranial pressure and pyloric obstruction. It occurs without warning and is so forceful that the emesis is projected a distance from the mouth. Retching is contraction of the stomach as in vomiting but without emesis because the stomach is empty.

The medical management of nausea and vomiting focuses both on the treatment of the underlying disorder and on removal of the immediate precipitating cause of the reflex. For example, gastric lavage or suction may be used to remove irritating substances from the stomach, a nasogastric tube may be inserted to reduce gastric distention, drugs known to stimulate the CTZ are discontinued, metabolic disorders that result in circulating "toxins" that stimulate the CTZ are corrected, and antiemetic drugs may be ordered to depress the sensitivity of the CTZ.

The major complication of vomiting is fluid and electrolyte imbalance. Gastric acid contains large amounts of potassium and chloride as well as hydrogen ions. Excessive losses of these substances can result in metabolic alkalosis and hypokalemia as well as dehydration.

A second serious complication of vomiting is aspiration of vomitus into the lungs, which can cause asphyxia, atelectasis, or pneumonitis.

Application of the Nursing Process to the Care of the Patient with Nausea and Vomiting

Assessment

Question the patient about the occurrence of nausea and vomiting. Ask about time(s) of onset, duration, precipitating factors, associated symptoms, and types of remedies tried as well as their effectiveness in providing relief. Also ask about the appearance, amount, and odor of vomitus. When possible, inspect vomitus for presence of undigested food, which can indicate gastric irritation so acute that food is immediately vomited; mucus, which can indicate chronic gastritis or rhinopharyngitis; parasites; or foreign bodies. Note also the color of the vomitus, which can be black or have a coffee-ground appearance owing to the presence of old blood; red, owing to blood from recent bleeding; green, owing to bile if vomitus has come from the duodenum beyond the entrance of the bile duct; or brown, owing to feces, indicating that the vomitus has come from the large intestine.

Nursing Diagnoses and Planning

The nursing diagnosis and related expected patient outcomes most commonly applicable to patients with nausea and vomiting are as follows:

NDx: High risk for fluid volume deficit related to loss of fluids from the gastrointestinal tract secondary to vomiting

Planning: Patient outcomes
1. Skin turgor is firm.
2. Oral mucous membranes are moist and shiny.
3. Serum electrolyte levels remain in normal range.

Nursing Interventions

NDx: High risk for fluid volume deficit
Avoid exposing the patient to stimuli likely to produce or worsen nausea, which in turn can precipitate vomiting and concomitant fluid loss. Maintain a calm, quiet environment, limiting visitors if necessary. Avoid moving the patient suddenly or unnecessarily. Encourage the patient to take deep breaths when feeling nauseated, and apply cold compresses to the forehead if comforting to the patient.

Keep the room well ventilated and free of strong or disagreeable odors. Discard vomitus and remove soiled clothing or linens immediately. Assist the patient in rinsing and cleansing the mouth after each episode of vomiting.

Administer antiemetics and intravenous fluids as ordered. Measure all vomitus, and maintain a careful record of all fluid intake and output.

When oral intake is resumed, give clear fluids such as water or ginger ale in small amounts (i.e., 20 ml every 30 minutes). If this is tolerated, gradually increase amounts, adding foods like gelatin, tea, and consommé. Progress to small, frequent meals of toast, cereal, chicken, and other easily digested bland foods. Encourage the patient to take fluids an hour before or after a meal but not with it, because fluids with meals can precipitate vomiting.

Avoid giving foods high in fat and those like orange juice that are known to stimulate peristalsis.

If foods high in potassium are needed for replacement, include tea, bananas, dry whole milk, and cheese in the diet as tolerated.

Additional Interventions
Position the patient in a side-lying or semi-Fowler's position to prevent aspiration. Remove dentures. If necessary, remove vomitus from the mouth of comatose, anesthetized, or otherwise impaired patients.

Evaluation

Evaluate the effectiveness of nursing care for a patient with nausea and vomiting by comparing the patient's status with the expected patient outcomes. Examples of specific outcomes for patients with nausea and vomiting have been provided in the Planning section.

Intestinal Gas

Symptoms caused by intestinal gas are eructation, abdominal distention, and excessive flatus.

Eructation is belching (i.e., escape of gas from the GI tract through the mouth).

This can be due to disease such as gastric dilatation or outlet obstruction but most often is the result of air swallowing by anxious individuals.

Abdominal distention or bloating is caused by abnormal motility of the intestine. It is not due to excessive amounts of gas. In some areas of the intestine, motility is increased, while other areas are in spasm. When gas being propelled through the intestine more rapidly than normal encounters areas of resistance due to spasm, the proximal bowel dilates, stretching the smooth muscle, and distention and cramping result.

Flatus is gas passed through the rectum. Seven to 10 L of gas ordinarily enter the large intestine daily. Part of this gas comes from swallowed air and part is the result of bacterial action in the large intestine. Of this, only 0.6 L is normally expelled, with the remainder being absorbed.

Increased flatus can result either from excessive production of gas or from impaired absorption of gas. Excessive gas production occurs as a result of the ingestion of the so-called gas-forming foods such as beans, cabbage, onions, cauliflower, and corn, many of which contain nonabsorbable carbohydrates that serve as a medium for bacterial growth. Impaired absorption occurs when intestinal motility is increased and gases are passed through the large intestine so quickly that there is insufficient time for absorption. This may be caused by the ingestion of irritating foods.

Constipation

Constipation is the infrequent (in relationship to the individual's normal pattern) passage of hard, dry stool. Stool becomes hard and dry because of an abnormally long time spent in the large intestine, where water is constantly being removed from it. This prolonged transit time in the intestine can be due to disorders such as a stricture or partial obstruction of the intestinal lumen by a tumor but in most cases relates to personal habits. Specific factors that contribute to constipation include lack of adequate amounts of dietary fiber or roughage, inadequate fluid intake, lack of exercise, and irregular bowel habits (e.g., suppressing the urge to defecate because of inopportune time of the urge or fear of discomfort, as with hemorrhoids). Constipation can also be due to compromised ability to increase intraabdominal pressure, as with emphysema or poor abdominal muscle tone. It can occur as a side effect to medications such as anticholinergics, tranquilizers, morphine derivatives, and antacids with aluminum. It can also be due to progressive weakening of the reflexes involved in defecation secondary to the prolonged use of laxatives.

Symptoms that often accompany constipation are a feeling of pressure or fullness in the rectum, back pain, headache, anorexia, and malaise. Streaks of blood may appear in the stool as a result of irritation of the rectal and anal mucosa from the hard stool as it passes. If an incomplete obstruction of the bowel is causing the constipation, loose portions of the stool seep around it, and the patient passes a colored watery mucus. Occasionally, constipation may become so severe that a fecal impaction forms. This is a condition in which exceedingly hard feces block the rectum. When this occurs, the impaction may need to be mechanically removed with a gloved finger. Prolonged constipation may result in a true obstruction of the colon, a pathologic state that is discussed in Chapter 23.

Medical treatment of constipation is directed at eliminating or alleviating the cause. Laxatives (Pharmacology Box 21-1) and enemas are prescribed only when all natural efforts have failed, because these agents decrease muscle tone and mucus production and do not resolve the underlying problem. Stool softeners may be utilized for patients who have potential for becoming constipated, such as the bedridden or those taking narcotics on a long-term basis.

Application of the Nursing Process to the Care of the Patient with Constipation

Assessment

Obtain a bowel history to serve as a basis of assessment. Ask the patient how often bowel movements normally occur and obtain a description of the stool in terms of color, amount, and consistency (formed, mushy, frothy, or liquid). Determine the time of day that defecation usually occurs and any associated events such as drinking hot coffee, eating, or smoking. Keep in mind that bowel pattern varies from person to person such that two bowel movements per day may be normal for one patient, whereas one bowel movement every three days may be normal for another. Ask about any symptoms related to defecation, such as abdominal distention, cramping, straining, or bleeding. Determine current bowel status, noting time of last bowel movement, type of stool, and any accompanying distress. Explore personal habits and lifestyle characteristics with a potential impact on bowel function. Obtain information about diet, exercise, and use of medications including laxatives. Auscultate bowel sounds, noting frequency and pitch. Gently palpate and percuss for abdominal distention. Inspect the anal area for hemorrhoids, fissures, or irritation. Inspect stool specimens when available.

Nursing Diagnoses and Planning

The nursing diagnosis and related expected patient outcomes most commonly applicable to patients with constipation are as follows:

NDx: Constipation related to lifestyle factors and/or lack of knowledge of normal bowel function

Planning: Patient outcomes
1. Patient passes soft, formed stool at regular intervals.
2. Patient reports absence of uncomfortable straining at stool.

Nursing Interventions

NDx: Constipation
Explain to the patient the relationship of fluids and dietary fiber to normal bowel function. Stress the need for 8 to 10 glasses of fluid per day, and teach about good sources of dietary fiber such as fruits, vegetables, grain products, and nuts. Suggest adding bran to cereal to meet the need for fiber. Instruct the patient to begin with a small amount of added bran and to gradually increase the amount as tolerated until 2 g are added.

Explain the importance of exercise, and encourage walking and abdominal muscle exercises such as leg lifts and sit-ups when possible. Encourage bedridden patients to move frequently, do range-of-motion exercises, leg raising, or bicycle exercises as their condition allows.

To facilitate defecation, provide privacy and assist the patient to the most normal position possible. Take the time to help the patient to the bathroom or to a commode rather than onto a bed pan, which should be used only as a last resource. Support the patient's usual schedule of evacuation, and encourage defecation at the time the gastrocolic reflex is most active (i.e., following a meal, particularly breakfast).

Evaluation

Evaluate the effectiveness of nursing care for a patient with constipation by comparing the patient's

Pharmacology Box 21–1.
LAXATIVES

Laxatives:
Drugs used to facilitate or stimulate passage of feces.
Classified by action into bulk formers, surfactants, contact laxatives, saline laxatives, and miscellaneous.
Classified by effect into the following categories:
Group I—act in 2–6 hours and produce watery stool
Group II—act in 6–12 hours and produce semifluid stool
Group III—act in 1–3 days and produce soft, formed stool

Action:
Bulk Formers—These nondigestible, nonabsorbable substances swell with water to form a gel that softens and enlarges the fecal mass, thus stretching the intestinal wall and stimulating reflex peristalsis (e.g., psyllium [Metamucil]).
Surfactants—Soften stool by lowering its surface tension, allowing absorption of water. Also inhibit fluid absorption by intestinal wall and stimulate secretion of water and electrolytes into lumen (e.g., docusate sodium [Colace]).
Contact Laxatives—Promote secretion of water and electrolytes into the intestine, and decrease their absorption, softening feces and stimulating peristalsis (e.g., bisacodyl [Dulcolax], castor oil).
Saline Laxatives—Pull water into intestine by osmotic action, swelling and softening feces and stimulating peristalsis (e.g., magnesium hydroxide [milk of magnesia]).
Miscellaneous—Mineral oil lubricates feces and inhibits water absorption.

Uses:
Bulk Formers—Temporary treatment of constipation; symptomatic relief of diarrhea in patients with a colostomy or ileostomy. Also used in irritable bowel syndrome and diverticulosis.
Surfactants—Used to prevent straining at stool in postoperative cardiac patients and those with anal or rectal diseases.
Contact Laxatives—Few therapeutic uses other than preparing the bowel for diagnostic tests.
Saline Laxatives—High-dose therapy used for bowel preparation, to eliminate ingested poisons, or to remove dead parasites after treatment with antihelmintic agents.

Side Effects:
Repeated laxative use depresses the reflexes involved in defecation, leading to further dependence on laxatives. It can also cause dehydration, electrolyte imbalance, and colitis.

Interactions:
None with stimulant, bulk-forming, or hyperosmolar agents. Mineral oil can interfere with absorption of fat-soluble vitamins, oral contraceptives, and anticoagulants. Also interferes with the anti-infective action of nonabsorbable sulfonamides.

Nursing Implications:
Administer bulk-forming laxatives with a full glass of water or juice to prevent esophageal obstruction. Also give a full glass of water with surfactant and saline laxatives.
Make castor oil more palatable by chilling and giving with juice.
Instruct patients in regard to bowel function:
- Individuals have different elimination patterns.
- Quality of stool is more important than quantity or frequency.
- The urge to defecate should not be ignored.
- Dietary fiber, as found in fruits, vegetables, and bran, is needed for proper bowel function.
- Daily exercise promotes good bowel function.
- Laxatives should be taken only when absolutely necessary and in the smallest effective dose.

status with the expected patient outcomes. Examples of specific outcomes for patients with constipation have been provided in the Planning section.

Diarrhea

Diarrhea is the increased frequency of passage of abnormally liquid stool. It results from the presence of an excessive amount of water in the intestinal contents, from changes in intestinal motility, or as is often the case, a combination of the two. Abnormally large amounts of water in the intestinal contents can occur as a result of impaired absorption or increased secretion of electrolytes and water by the cells of the intestinal wall owing to the actions of toxins such as the salmonella enterotoxin or hormones such as serotonin, as seen in malignant carcinoid syndrome. It may also be due to the presence of substances that pull water into the intestine by osmosis. Such substances may be poorly absorbable solutes, such as bran, that have been ingested, products of maldigestion, or a dietary nonelectrolyte, such as glucose, that has failed to be transported into the cells.

Changes in intestinal motility most often contribute to diarrhea by increasing peristalsis and therefore the speed with which intestinal contents pass through the tract. This decreases the time that intestinal contents are in contact with the cells of the intestinal wall, and thus decreases the absorption of water. Increased peristalsis may be due to abnormal bowel contents, intrinsic irritability of the bowel, or inflammation of the bowel. Examples of specific disorders that are characterized by diarrhea due to one or more of these mechanisms are irritable bowel syndrome, enteritis, ulcerative colitis, and Crohn's disease.

Symptoms that often accompany diarrhea are abdominal cramping; appearance of mucus, blood, or fat in unformed stool; urgency such that involuntary expulsion of stool may occur if there is any delay in reaching the toilet; tenesmus (painful straining to empty the bowel without evacuation of feces); and perianal discomfort. Often there is also a feeling that the rectum has not been completely emptied.

Uncorrected diarrhea can lead to severe fluid and electrolyte imbalance. Water loss as high as 10,000 ml in 24 hours accompanied by loss of sodium, potassium, and bicarbonate can lead to dehydration, electrolyte imbalances, metabolic acidosis, and malnutrition. Irritation and breakdown of the anal area can also occur as a result of contact with the diarrheal stool.

In addition to identifying and treating the cause of the diarrhea, a major concern of medical management is the prevention or treatment of fluid and electrolyte imbalances and acidosis. In cases of moderate to severe diarrhea, fluids are administered intravenously and potassium is added once adequate renal function is established.

Application of the Nursing Process to the Care of the Patient with Diarrhea

Assessment

Assess the patient as described under constipation. Be certain to question the patient about urgency and anal discomfort. Assess for signs and symptoms of dehydration and electrolyte imbalance, and review related laboratory values. If the diarrhea is possibly infectious in origin, question the patient about exposure to persons with similar symptoms, ask about foods eaten in the last 24 to 48 hours, and determine whether the patient has traveled recently.

Nursing Diagnoses and Planning

Nursing diagnoses and related expected patient outcomes most commonly applicable to patients with diarrhea include the following:

NDx: Diarrhea related to *(specify)*

Planning: Patient outcomes
1. Patient passes formed stool at regular intervals.
2. Patient reports decrease in frequency and liquidity of stools.

NDx: High risk for fluid volume deficit related to excessive water loss in the stool

Planning: Patient outcomes
1. Skin turgor is firm.
2. Mucous membranes are moist.
3. Urinary output is at least 50 ml/hour.
4. Urinary specific gravity is within normal range.
5. Serum electrolyte levels are within normal range.

NDx: High risk for impaired tissue integrity related to irritation of the anal area by diarrheal stool

Planning: Patient outcomes
1. Anal skin and mucous membrane are free of erythema.
2. Anal skin and mucous membrane are intact.
3. Patient denies tenderness or burning in the anal area.

Nursing Interventions

NDx: Diarrhea
Recognize that diarrhea, particularly when accompanied by urgency and loss of control, is a source of embarrassment to most people. Be sensitive to the

Pharmacology Box 21–2.

NONSPECIFIC ANTIDIARRHEAL AGENTS

Antidiarrheal Agents:
Drugs used in the treatment of diarrhea. Specific antidiarrheal drugs are used to treat the underlying cause of the diarrhea. Nonspecific antidiarrheals act on or within the bowel to relieve diarrhea without regard to its cause.

Action:
Opioids, the most effective nonspecific antidiarrheal agents, stimulate receptors in the GI tract that suppress peristalsis and promote absorption of water and electrolytes (e.g., diphenoxylate [Lomotil], loperamide [Imodium]).

Uses:
Decrease the fluidity of feces and the frequency of defecation.

Side Effects:
When used in cases of infectious diarrhea, lengthen the time the infecting organisms remain in the GI tract and can prolong the infection. No other side effects at dose used to treat diarrhea.

Interactions:
Can decrease absorption of digoxin if given at the same time. Kaolin and pectin mixtures decrease the absorption of lincomycin if given 2 hours before or 3 to 4 hours after it.

Nursing Implications:
Monitor frequency, amount, and appearance of stool. Monitor for related systemic manifestations: fever, pain, dehydration, and electrolyte imbalance. Caution against excessive use because morphine-like side effects can occur.

patient's need for privacy, and ensure that the room is well ventilated and odor free. Maintain easy access to the bed pan or toilet, and if the patient needs assistance, respond as quickly as possible. Maintain a quiet, stress-free environment, and encourage bed rest, because activity stimulates peristalsis.

Administer prescribed antidiarrheal medications (Pharmacology Box 21–2), and limit oral intake in accord with physician's orders, because ingestion of food or fluids stimulates peristalsis. In cases of mild diarrhea, the patient is generally allowed nothing by mouth (NPO status) for at least 4 hours. When oral intake is resumed, offer small amounts of liquids such as weak tea, bouillon, Jell-O, and then thin-cooked cereal, which will replace lost electrolytes but not stimulate the intestine. Progress as tolerated to a low-residue diet that includes foods such as tender beef, veal, chicken, boiled or steamed rice, and hard-boiled eggs. Avoid cold liquids, caffeine, and concentrated sweets.

NDx: High risk for fluid volume deficit
Administer intravenous fluids as ordered. Maintain a record of fluid intake and output, being certain to measure liquid stool and count it as output. Check urine specific gravity and weigh the patient daily. Monitor laboratory values for indications of fluid and electrolyte balance, such as increased serum osmolality, increased hematocrit, and hypokalemia.

NDx: High risk for impaired tissue integrity
Wipe the anal area with soft toilet tissue, then wash gently with warm water and gentle soap, rinse thoroughly, and pat dry after every bowel movement. Follow with the application of a protective salve such as petroleum jelly. If irritation develops or persists despite this routine, try washing and drying with warm water and absorbent cotton. Also eliminate the use of ointments, because they restrict perspiration and may contribute to irritation in some cases.

Give sitz baths for 10 minutes two or three times per day to promote healing and comfort. Apply witch hazel–soaked soft pads, such as Tucks, as an additional comfort measure if needed.

If leaking of fecal matter is a problem, place a piece of absorbent cotton over the anus and hold in place with snug underwear. This allows good air circulation to the area and is easily replaced as frequently as required.

Evaluation

Evaluate the effectiveness of nursing care for a patient with diarrhea by comparing the patient's status with the expected patient outcomes. Examples of specific outcomes for patients with constipation have been provided in the Planning section.

Pain

Pain from the viscera and the peritoneum is mediated by the sympathetic nervous system. It is usually due to anoxia, inflammation, or stretching of smooth muscle or organ capsules.

Pain from hollow viscera is called visceral pain. It begins in the midline and is perceived as dull regardless of the specific organ involved. Subsequently as inflammation or ischemia progresses, it localizes at a site specific to the affected organ (Table 21–3). For example, the pain of appendicitis starts in the periumbilical region and over a period of hours localizes to the lower right quadrant.

Quality of pain also differs according to tissues affected. Pain related to stretching of the smooth muscle of the intestinal tract or the common bile duct is colicky and unaffected by movement. Pain from peritoneal irritation, in contrast, is described as sharp and severe and is exacerbated by jarring or moving.

Gastrointestinal Bleeding

Bleeding can occur in any part of the GI tract. It is referred to as upper GI bleeding if it originates in the esophagus, stomach, duodenum, and lower GI bleeding if it occurs in the jejunum, ileum, colon, or rectum. It is called multifocal GI bleeding when lesions are present throughout the tract.

GI bleeding may be acute or chronic. Acute bleeding occurs in minutes to hours and may be massive (more than 1000 ml blood loss) or discrete (less than 100 ml blood loss). Chronic bleeding occurs over a period of weeks or months and may be recurrent, intermittent, or persistent. Recurrent bleeding is bleeding that recurs after completely stopping; intermittent bleeding occurs at regular or irregular intervals; and persistent bleeding is continuous or ongoing.

ETIOLOGY

GI bleeding results when the GI mucosa is irritated and its blood vessels disrupted. This can be due to inflammation as seen secondary to ingestion of alcohol or irritating medications; mechanical trauma as seen in Mallory-Weiss syndrome, in which an esophageal tear occurs from forceful vomiting and retching; erosion by an expanding neoplasm; or corrosion by gastric acid or pepsin as in peptic ulcer disease. It may also be related to a vascular defect such as esophageal varices, systemic disease such as nonthrombocytopenic purpura, or toxic reaction such as antibiotic-induced colitis.

CLINICAL CHARACTERISTICS

Clinical characteristics vary with the magnitude and location of the bleeding. Bleeding may be occult or may present as melena, hematochezia, rectorrhagia, or hematemesis.

Occult bleeding is not visible to the naked eye but is detected by chemical test (e.g., guaiac test or Hematest). It indicates chronic GI bleeding and can originate anywhere from the mouth to the anus. It is often identified as part of a routine examination or as a result of diagnostic studies on a patient with iron deficiency anemia. Occult blood can be found

Table 21–3. LOCATION OF PAIN FROM VARIOUS ORGANS OF THE GASTROINTESTINAL TRACT

SOURCE OF PAIN	PERCEIVED LOCATION OF PAIN
Esophagus	Over the site of the lesion Occasionally, lower esophageal pain felt at suprasternal notch or neck or, if severe, in the back
Stomach and duodenum	Right epigastric or midepigastric
Jejunum and ileum	Periumbilical
Distal ileum	Periumbilical or lower right quadrant
Colon	Lower abdomen, often poorly localized
Rectum	Posterior over the sacrum
Gallbladder and common bile duct	Right upper quadrant or epigastrium. If pain is severe, referred to back, between the shoulder blades
Pancreas	Midepigastric or left epigastric, radiating to midline of upper back Pain in tail of pancreas may be referred to shoulder
Diaphragmatic pleura	Trapezius ridge of the shoulder

in the stool for as long as 3 weeks after bleeding has occurred.

Melena is the passage of black, tarry, sticky, foul-smelling stool that contains a large amount of digested blood. It occurs with bleeding from the upper GI tract or from lesions in the jejunum or ileum.

Hematochezia, or the passage of obviously bloody stools, usually indicates lower GI bleeding. Blood mixed with stool is characteristic of inflammatory bowel disease, whereas blood on the surface of the stool suggests the presence of polyps or a malignant tumor. Blood that appears after the passage of formed stool is characteristic of hemorrhoids. Hematochezia may also be seen with upper GI bleeding if it is massive and rapid, because such bleeding can increase intestinal motility.

Rectorrhagia is the passage of red blood from the rectum in the absence of feces. It generally indicates anorectal disease.

Hematemesis, or the vomiting of blood, is ordinarily due to upper GI bleeding. The vomitus may contain frank red blood or appear dark red, brown, mahogany, or black. Since color darkens as a result of exposure to gastric secretions, the longer the blood has been in the stomach, the darker it tends to be in color. If blood has clotted in the stomach and the clots have begun to be digested, vomitus will have a "coffee grounds" appearance.

In cases of acute, massive bleeding of more than 500 ml, nausea, thirst, diaphoresis, orthostatic hypotension, and syncope develop. If the blood loss continues, hypovolemic shock manifested by pallor, cold, clammy skin, hypotension, and tachycardia ensues.

MEDICAL MANAGEMENT

The first priority in the management of the patient with GI bleeding is to assess blood loss and return the patient to hemodynamic stability. Focus then turns to identification of the bleeding source and the diagnosis and treatment of the underlying disorder.

Blood loss is estimated on the basis of vital signs, physical assessment data, and laboratory data. As a general principle, blood loss in a person with normal blood pressure is considered severe if the systolic pressure is lower than 100 mm Hg or if the pulse rate is higher than 100 and is accompanied by pallor and postural hypotension (Meeroff, 1986, p. 154). More specifically, a systolic pressure of 70 to 90 mm Hg with a pulse of 110 to 130 is consistent with loss of 25% to 40% of total blood volume (1500 ml). A systolic blood pressure of lower than 70 mm Hg with a pulse rate of more than 130 is consistent with loss of 40% of the total blood volume (2000 ml) and severe shock (Patras et al, 1988, p. 72). In uncertain cases, the tilt test is used to assist in estimating blood loss. For this test, the pulse and blood pressure are measured with the patient in a supine position and again after sitting up for 60 seconds. An increase in pulse rate of 20 to 25 beats per minute is considered indicative of a blood loss of less than 500 ml, and a greater increase in pulse rate accompanied by a drop in blood pressure is indicative of blood loss in excess of 500 ml. A tilt test is not done if the patient is already hypotensive when supine or if cardiac or cerebrovascular disease is present.

Hemoglobin and hematocrit values are also analyzed, although blood loss is not reflected in these values for 12 to 24 hours after the onset of bleeding. A persistent decrease in these values indicates a continuous loss of blood.

To stabilize a patient with acute bleeding, normal saline or Ringer's lactate is given until blood pressure rises, signs of peripheral vasospasm disappear, and urinary output returns to 30 ml/hour. When shock is severe, plasma expanders are given until typed and crossmatched blood is available for transfusion. A central venous pressure (CVP) line (or, for patients with cardiac compromise or in need of massive fluid replacement, a Swan-Ganz line) is inserted to monitor circulatory volume. The patient is placed in a head-down left lateral position to increase cerebral blood flow and prevent aspiration. Volume of urinary output and urine specific gravity are monitored via an indwelling catheter. Oxygen may be administered.

Measures to locate the site of bleeding begin with insertion of a nasogastric tube to check for blood or clots in the stomach. Other diagnostic tests are then used as indicated. These may include upper and lower flexible endoscopy to attempt to directly visualize the lesion, air contrast studies, arteriography to demonstrate extravasation of blood into the GI lumen or alterations in the vasculature, and radioisotopic scintigraphy.

Treatment of bleeding varies with the cause and the location. Immediate treatment of gastric bleeding is gastric lavage, because upper GI bleeding regardless of cause generally stops when the acid-blood contents are removed from the stomach and are replaced by a neutral solution. Cool saline is the solution of choice for this procedure, although iced tap water is sometimes used. Water breaks up large clots more readily than saline but is also more likely to contribute to electrolyte imbalance. The cool solution is instilled 50 to 100 ml at a time, left for a short interval, and then aspirated. This volume is small enough to prevent distention but sufficient to cause vasoconstriction owing to its cold.

Pharmacologic agents such as antacids (Pharmacology Box 21–3) and H_2-receptor antagonists (see Pharmacology Box 22–2) that reduce gastric acidity are given to treat bleeding from inflammatory, erosive, or ulcerative upper GI lesions. Other drugs used regardless of the source of bleeding are vasoconstrictors and antifibrinolytic agents. If the bleeding is from esophageal varices, a Sengstaken-Blakemore tube (see Fig. 21–8) may be used to directly compress the varices and promote hemostasis. Embolization therapy (injection of a natural or synthetic

Pharmacology Box 21–3.
ANTACIDS

Antacids:
Over-the-counter alkaline compounds that neutralize gastric acid.

Action:
React with gastric acid to produce neutral or low acidity salts, thereby raising pH and inactivating pepsin at pH of 5 or higher.

Uses:
Decrease destruction of gut wall in peptic ulcer disease, provide prophylaxis against stress ulcers, and provide symptomatic relief of heartburn due to reflux esophagitis.

Side Effects:
Altered bowel function: constipation or diarrhea. Antacids causing constipation include aluminum hydroxide and calcium carbonate; those causing diarrhea include magnesium hydroxide and magnesium carbonate.

Antacids with high sodium content may induce fluid retention and exacerbate hypertension and congestive heart failure.

Hypermagnesemia, which can lead to respiratory or mental depression and coma, can develop in patients with renal failure taking magnesium compounds; similarly, hyperaluminemia and hypophosphatemia may occur.

Interactions:
Affect dissolution and absorption of many drugs as a result of raising the gastric pH. Also interfere with the action of the local anti-ulcer drug sucralfate.

Nursing Implications:
- Teach patients to combine use of constipating and diarrhea-producing antacids to counteract effect of each and maintain normal bowel function.
- Shake liquid preparations well before administering.
- Instruct patient to chew antacid tablets thoroughly and follow with a full glass of water.
- Allow 1 hour between the administration of antacids and other medications to minimize drug interactions.
- Explain that stools may appear white or speckled as a result of antacid therapy.
- Instruct patients with a sodium or potassium restriction to check label on antacids for amounts of these ions.

clot into the bleeding vessel), endoscopy with electrocoagulation or laser photocoagulation, and surgery for uncontrolled hemorrhage are other treatment options.

Guidelines for Application of the Nursing Process to the Care of the Patient with Gastrointestinal Bleeding

Nursing care of the patient with GI bleeding varies according to the severity and location of the bleeding and the method of treatment. Thus, it may include measures discussed under the care of the patient in shock, the care of the patient with ruptured esophageal varices, the care of the patient with a gastrectomy, or the care of the patient with an intestinal resection. Regardless of cause or treatment, basic assessment data for any patient presenting with an acute bleeding episode include level of consciousness, vital signs, color, appearance of neck veins, capillary refill, and condition of the abdomen (i.e., presence or absence of bowel sounds, distention, and guarding).

Assessment of Gastrointestinal Status

Patient History

Obtain a diet history. Ask the patient to describe his or her usual diet in terms of amount and type of foods eaten and daily pattern of intake, for example, three meals per day, snacks throughout the day, or no breakfast, lunch, dinner, and bedtime snack. Ascertain what if any foods or food groups are not eaten. Ask whether vitamin, mineral, or other supplements are taken and, if so, the amount and frequency. Inquire about the general condition of the teeth, and note the date of the last dental examination. Ascertain whether the patient has dentures and whether they are comfortable and worn regularly. Ask about usual pattern of bowel elimination, noting frequency, color, and consistency of stool. Be certain to also note measures such as daily bran or laxatives routinely used to promote bowel function. Obtain specific data regarding GI symptoms experienced. Ask about difficulty chewing, difficulty swallowing, soreness of the mouth, anorexia, nausea, vomiting, belching, indigestion, abdominal distention, abdominal pain, diarrhea, flatulence, constipation, pencil-shaped stools, straining at stool, painful defecation, and blood in the stool or from the rectum. If symptoms are reported, determine onset, duration, and severity. Explore the relationship of symptoms to specific foods, use of alcohol, or specific activities or events. Also determine what measures or over-the-counter drugs have been used to treat symptoms, the frequency of use, and their effectiveness.

Review the patient's past medical history. Ask specifically about previous GI disorders and abdominal surgery, noting date of occurrence, treatment, and results.

Inquire about previous diagnostic tests, including the most recent rectal examination and examination of stool for occult blood. Note the patient's general health status, other current medical problems, and all medications being taken. Keep in mind that the last factor is particularly important because so many medications have side effects related to GI function.

Physical Examination

Examine the mouth and pharynx using a flashlight and tongue blade to ensure good visibility of all areas. Begin by asking the patient to remove any dental appliances. Proceed by noting the condition of the lips: color, moistness, suppleness, symmetry, and the presence of any lesions such as cracks, cold sores caused by the herpes simplex virus, or areas of leukoplakia. Using a tongue blade to move the tongue out of the way and a flashlight for good visibility, inspect the teeth and gums. Note absence of teeth; presence of loose teeth; caries, and plaque; color of the gums; gum recession or hypertrophy; any evidence of bleeding gums; ulcerated areas; and other signs of malfitting dentures. Keep in mind that normally the mucosa of the gums is light pink and may be shiny and thin in older individuals. Also remember that gum recession is a normal occurrence with advancing age. Observe the mucous membranes in the mouth, including that under the tongue. Look for areas of redness or swelling, as well as for lesions such as ulcerations, white patches of thrush or leukoplakia, and nodules. Observe the color and condition of the tongue. Keep in mind that a smooth, red tongue can be indicative of nutritional deficiency, and a thickly coated tongue can indicate inadequate oral hygiene. Using the tongue blade to depress the tongue, inspect the pharynx and tonsils for redness, swelling, and exudate. Finally, note the odor of the patient's breath, which can be indicative of substances such as alcohol or garlic recently ingested, poor oral hygiene, local infection (foul odor), or systemic disease such as diabetic acidosis (acetone odor) or liver disease (ammonia odor).

Next examine the abdomen. Assist the patient into a supine position with arms at sides, and uncover the abdomen from the xiphoid process to the symphysis pubis. In good light, inspect the abdomen. Note color and texture of the skin, contour (flat, hollow, rounded, or protuberant), and whether or not it is symmetric. Note presence and location of scars, striae, dilated veins, or other abnormality. Examine the umbilicus for signs of inflammation or hernia. Observe for peristaltic waves, keeping in mind that except for slow waves in very thin people, peristalsis is not normally visible. Auscultate all four quadrants for bowel sounds and note their frequency and character. Normal bowel sounds, clicking, and gurgling noises, which occur from 5 to 34 times per minute, are generally loudest in the right lower quadrant of the abdomen. Remember always to auscultate first and then proceed to percussion and palpation.

Percuss all four quadrants of the abdomen to determine areas of tympany and dullness. Tympany is normal over most of the abdomen owing to the presence of a small amount of air in the bowel. Dullness is heard over bowel filled with stool, over areas of ascites, over organs such as the liver, and over solid or fluid-filled masses. Dullness in the suprapubic area may be due to a full bladder or an enlarged uterus. After percussion, proceed to palpate the abdomen. Perform light palpation using the pads of the finger tips to check for muscle tenderness and resistance, as well as for superficial masses. Palpate gently with the fingers together in each quadrant. If the patient has localized abdominal pain, palpate the painful area last. If the abdomen is involuntarily rigid or "boardlike" (rigid on expiration despite the patient's breathing through the mouth with the jaw dropped open [Bates, 1991, p. 350]), stop the examination and notify the physician, because this may indicate acute peritonitis. Follow light palpation with deep palpation to check for other than superficial masses and areas of tenderness. Perform deep palpation only if trained in the technique, because it is not a routine part of basic nursing care.

The lower edge of the normal liver is usually palpable under the costal margin at the midclavicular line. It is normally felt as soft, clearly defined, regular, and smooth. To palpate for it, place your dominant hand on the right side of the abdomen at the midclavicular line below the level of percussed liver dullness. Press the fingers gently inward and upward as you instruct the patient to take a deep breath. Feel for the edge of the liver, striking your finger as it is moved downward by the flattening of the diaphragm on inspiration. When it is felt, raise your fingers slightly to let the liver slip beneath them and thus allow palpation of its anterior surface.

Finish assessment of the GI tract with examination of the anal region. Inspect the perianal area for the presence of hemorrhoids, fissures, ulcerations, or other lesions. Note any drainage, abnormal odor, or change in skin color. If a rectal examination is to be done, insert a gloved and lubricated finger gently through the anal sphincter. Palpate for nodules and note presence of stool. Upon withdrawing the gloved finger, observe for presence of blood or mucus and note color of any stool.

Diagnostic Procedures

Gastric Analysis

A gastric analysis is a procedure in which the contents of the stomach are examined. It is usually done to determine whether hydrochloric acid is present and in what amount, although it can also demonstrate the presence of occult blood, malignant cells, bacteria, and parasites. It is useful in the diagnosis of ulcer disease, which is characterized by high gastric acidity, and pernicious anemia in which gastric acid is absent. It also aids in evaluating the effects of a vagotomy (cutting of the vagus nerve to decrease production of gastric acid) and in the diagnosis of malignant tumors of the stomach.

Physical Preparation of the Patient. The evening before a gastric analysis, the patient receives a light meal or clear fluids. After midnight, the patient is placed on NPO status. Smoking is not allowed on the morning of the test because it can stimulate the production of gastric acid and affect test results.

Procedure. A nasogastric tube is inserted through the mouth or nose into the stomach and is taped in place. Gastric contents are withdrawn using a syringe and gentle suction. When hydrochloric acid production is being measured, this initial aspiration provides a baseline level, and subsequent aspirations of secretions are then obtained at 15- to 20-minute intervals for 1 to 2 hours. A stimulus in the form of a carbohydrate meal of dry toast and tea, 50 ml of alcohol or caffeine, or an injection of histamine is usually given to stimulate gastric secretion.

Complications. Nausea and vomiting may occur during ingestion of the stimulus or following the procedure. If histamine is used as a stimulus, an allergic reaction may occur.

Guidelines for Application of the Nursing Process to the Care of the Patient Having a Gastric Aspiration

Make certain the preparation for the procedure including limitations on smoking and diet is understood. Just prior to the procedure, explain to the patient that a tube will be passed into the stomach to obtain gastric secretions and that she or he will be asked to swallow while the tube is being inserted. Explain about any stimulus to be given, and in the case of histamine, tell the patient that he or she should be prepared for a hot, flushing sensation and for frequent measurements of pulse and blood pressure.

Assess each patient for a history of allergies because this may contraindicate the use of histamine.

Monitor the patient immediately after the procedure for any discomfort, nausea, or vomiting. Give mouth care using a toothbrush or mouthwash to remove any dried secretions from the oral mucosa. Instruct the patient to resume diet as tolerated.

Upper GI Series

An upper GI series is an x-ray examination of the esophagus, stomach, and duodenum. Barium sulfate, a white, chalky, radiopaque substance, is used to allow x-ray visualization of the structures. This procedure is used to detect esophageal tumors, esophageal varices (dilated veins prone to rupture and hemorrhage), gastric ulcers, and gastric tumors. It also allows visualization of any esophageal strictures or swallowing disorders. As the barium progresses through the small intestine, obstructions, inflammations, or diverticula can be identified (Fig. 21–5).

If only the esophagus is examined, the procedure is called a barium swallow. If the jejunum and ileum are also visualized, it is an upper GI series with a small bowel examination.

Physical Preparation of the Patient. Basic preparation for an upper GI series consists of having the patient remain on NPO status after midnight before the examination. In some instances, a low-residue diet is followed for 2 to 3 days, and narcotic and anticholinergic drugs are avoided for 24 hours so that motility of the bowel will be normal.

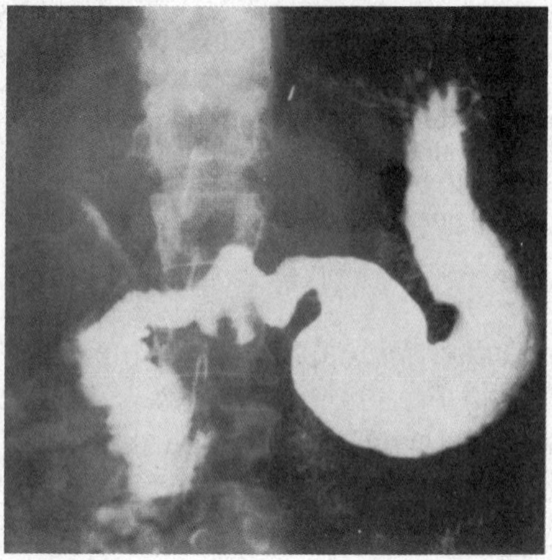

Figure 21–5.

Upper GI series showing barium in the lower end of the esophagus, stomach, and small intestine. (From Sleisinger MH, Fordtran JS. Gastrointestinal disease: Pathophysiology, diagnosis, management. 4th ed. Philadelphia: WB Saunders, 1989, p. 956.)

Procedure. The patient, in an upright position behind a fluoroscopic screen, swallows the contrast medium. X-ray films are taken with the patient tilted in various positions on a tilt table as the barium progresses through the upper GI tract. For visualization of the jejunum and ileum, additional barium is swallowed and films are taken at half-hour intervals.

Postprocedure Course. Because barium sulfate is a constipating substance that can cause obstruction of the GI tract if not eliminated, cathartics are given following the procedure. A common order is for 30 ml of milk of magnesia or half a bottle of magnesium citrate.

Complications. A major complication of an upper GI series is perforation of the stomach or intestine. If this occurs, barium can escape into the peritoneum and peritonitis can result.

If cathartics are not taken as ordered after the test, severe constipation, impaction, or intestinal obstruction may occur in 1 to 2 days.

Occasionally, nausea occurs from swallowing the barium.

Guidelines for Application of the Nursing Process to the Care of the Patient Having an Upper GI Series

Assess the patient's understanding of the procedure, making certain that the restrictions on diet and medications to be observed prior to the test are clearly understood. The patient should also know that she or he will be asked to drink a thick, chalky substance at the beginning of the test, that she or he will be tilted on a table into various positions so that all areas of the upper GI tract can be seen and x-rayed, and that the procedure can take 1 to 2 hours or longer. If a knowledge deficit is identified, provide information as needed.

Following a barium swallow, assess the patient's tolerance of the procedure and note any nausea. Encourage the patient to rest, and allow resumption of food and fluids as ordered and tolerated. Because there is a potential for constipation caused by the barium, instruct the patient regarding the use of cathartics and basic measures to promote good bowel function, such as intake of adequate amounts of fiber and water in the diet. Tell the patient to expect white stools for 48 to 72 hours and, if an out-patient, to report if bowel movements do not occur. If an in-patient, check for the passage of barium and chart it in the patient record.

Barium Enema

A barium enema is a radiologic examination of the rectum and colon. It is used to diagnose problems in the large intestine such as tumors, polyps, and diverticula. It can also identify filling defects that could be ulcerative in nature, such as seen in Crohn's disease and ulcerative colitis.

A barium enema should precede an oral barium study because it takes several days for swallowed barium to pass completely out of the GI tract and any residual barium can distort the results of a barium enema.

Physical Preparation of the Patient. A bowel preparation is done prior to the procedure in order to adequately cleanse the bowel of any feces, which would interfere with the test and produce inaccurate results. For a basic bowel preparation, oral intake the day before the examination is limited to clear fluids. That evening four tap water enemas are given, and an oral cathartic such as magnesium sulfate is administered. On the morning of the examination, a suppository and an enema are given.

Alternative bowel preparation better suited to the out-patient consists of Fleet enemas or the use of an osmotic solution such as GoLYTELY that induces diarrhea. With the GoLYTELY, a clear liquid dinner is eaten the night before the examination. Then 8 ounces of GoLYTELY is drunk every 10 to 15 minutes until a clear diarrhea develops. This takes approximately 2 to 3 hours. No food or fluids are taken after midnight, and on the morning of the examination, Fleet enemas are administered. If a patient is on daily medication, it may be taken with a small amount of fluid on the morning of the examination provided the physician gives permission. Patients may also be instructed to avoid taking aspirin for 10 days prior to the examination to decrease the risk of bleeding.

Procedure. Barium is instilled into the large intestine through the rectum. If needed, a rectal tube with an inflatable balloon is used to help the patient retain the barium during the examination. The progress of the barium is followed on a fluoroscopy screen, and x-ray films are taken with the patient in different positions. When this is completed, the patient is allowed to expel the barium, and additional films are taken of the entire lower GI tract.

Postprocedure Course. After a barium enema, an oral cathartic such as magnesium sulfate or an oil retention enema is ordered to aid the elimination of the barium and prevent impaction of it in the bowel.

Complications and Contraindications. The major complications of a barium enema are severe constipation and impaction of barium in the bowel. The test is usually contraindicated in patients with toxic megacolon or perforation or obstruction of the GI tract.

Guidelines for Application of the Nursing Process to the Care of the Patient Having a Barium Enema

Assess the patient's ability to tolerate the extensive bowel preparation necessary for this examination. This includes checking hydration and electrolyte status, sphincter control, and ability to get to the bathroom. Assess the patient's understanding of the procedure, and provide information as needed to enable the patient to describe the test and its preparation accurately in general terms.

Ensure that the preparation is completed as ordered, and evaluate its effectiveness by checking that the returns of the enema given on the morning of the test are clear.

Following the test, encourage oral fluids and give cathartics or enemas as ordered to prevent constipation or impaction due to the barium. Tell the patient that stools will be white for 24 to 72 hours, and document passage of barium in the patient's record.

Oral Cholecystogram

An oral cholecystogram is an x-ray visualization of the gallbladder. It is used to evaluate gallbladder function and aids in the diagnosis of gallstones or other gallbladder disease.

Physical Preparation of the Patient. Normal dietary intake of fat should be maintained during the days preceding the test in order to empty the bile from the gallbladder. The evening before the test, the patient has a fat-free supper. This prevents contraction of the gallbladder and allows accumulation of the contrast substance needed for x-ray visualization. After midnight, the patient is placed on NPO status.

Procedure. An oral cholecystogram is dependent on the absorption of orally ingested radiopaque dye tablets from the small intestine, removal of the dye from the blood by the liver, excretion of the dye with the bile from the liver, concentration of the bile and the dye in the gallbladder, and excretion of the bile and the dye through the common bile duct in response to a fatty meal.

The dye tablets are taken early (about 7 P.M.) on the evening prior to the test. The most commonly used are Telepaque, which come in 500 mg tablets. Because the dose is calculated on body weight, six or more tablets may be needed. To minimize nausea, tablets are given 5 minutes apart with small sips of water.

On the following day, initial films are taken to determine the position of the gallbladder and to ensure that it has opacified. After the gallbladder is visualized, a fatty meal is given to stimulate contraction and emptying of the gallbladder. This takes 15 to 20 minutes, after which additional x-ray films are taken. If gallstones are seen on the first x-ray film, no fatty meal is given and no additional films are taken. If the gallbladder cannot be visualized, it is indicative of biliary obstruction or inappropriate preparation, and the test may be repeated the next day.

Complications. Severe diarrhea and vomiting with subsequent dehydration can be caused by the Telepaque tablets. A severe anaphylactic reaction can occur if the patient is allergic to iodine, which is present in the dye. Liver and kidney damage can occur if the dye is not properly excreted.

Guidelines for Application of the Nursing Process to the Care of the Patient Having an Oral Cholecystogram

Assess the patient's understanding of the oral cholecystogram. The patient should be able to say why it is being done, state the dietary restrictions involved, and describe the procedure in general. The patient should know that the procedure will be done in the x-ray department and will take approximately 1 hour.

Assess the patient for an allergy to iodine. Explore the patient's history to determine whether other tests using an iodine-based dye have been done and, if so, whether any untoward reactions occurred. Also determine whether the patient ever had an untoward reaction after eating shellfish.

Administer the dye tablets, taking care to give them as scheduled to ensure that the dye has adequate time to be absorbed prior to the test. Then assess for nausea, vomiting, abdominal cramps, and dysuria, which may occur as side effects of the Telepaque. If vomiting or diarrhea occurs, inspect the vomitus or stool for Telepaque tablets. Whether tablets can be identified or not, notify the x-ray department and the physician, because expulsion would affect the uptake of the dye and result in an inaccurate test.

When planning care for a patient who is to have an oral cholecystogram, check to see whether the patient is to have any other tests done that involve the use of iodine. If so, schedule them prior to the oral cholecystogram. Schedule any tests using barium after the cholecystogram, or the gallbladder will not be accurately visualized.

After the test, assess the patient's hydration status. Monitor urinary output and check skin turgor. Also assess for nausea and vomiting, and instruct the patient to resume the prescribed diet when GI function appears stable.

Cholangiogram

A cholangiogram is an x-ray examination in which a contrast medium is used to outline the hepatic, cystic, and common bile ducts. In intravenous cholangiography, dye is given slowly into a vein, and x-ray films are taken as the dye is excreted by the liver. In some cases, a fatty meal is then ingested and additional x-ray films are taken to show the contraction of the gallbladder. In operative and postoperative cholangiography, dye is injected into the common bile duct via a drainage tube; and in percutaneous transhepatic cholangiography, injection of dye is through the skin of the abdomen into the liver. In endoscopic retrograde cholangiography, the contrast medium is instilled via a cannula inserted through the ampulla of Vater by means of a flexible fiberoptic duodenoscope.

Cholangiography takes approximately 4 hours and is contraindicated by severe liver disease or jaundice. For an intravenous cholangiogram, the patient is assessed for allergy to shellfish or contrast media, is placed on NPO status after midnight, and has a laxative or enema to cleanse the bowel. The patient is also told to expect a brief burning sensation when the dye is injected. After the procedure, rest is promoted, fluids are encouraged, and diet is resumed as tolerated.

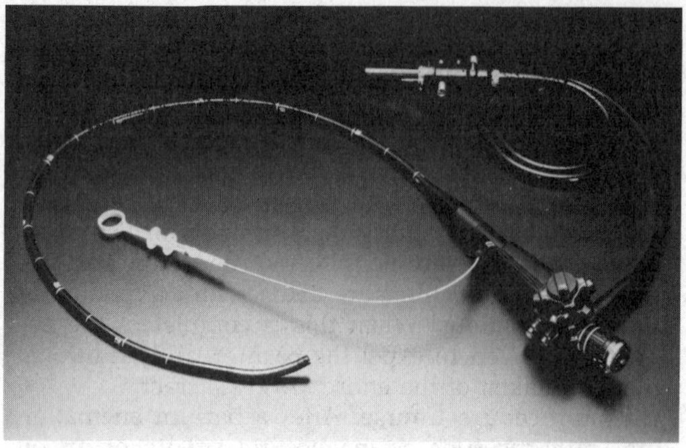

Figure 21–6.

Upper GI flexible endoscope. (From Zuidema GD. Shackelford's surgery of the alimentary tract. 3rd ed, Vol 1. Philadelphia: WB Saunders, 1991, p 80.)

Endoscopy

Endoscopy is the visualization of the inside of a body cavity by means of a lighted tube. Most endoscopic examinations of the upper and lower GI tract are done with a flexible fiberoptic scope, which can provide an undistorted image of the body cavity even when completely bent. Illumination is provided by an external light source, and the scope is designed to allow passage of instruments so that pictures can be taken, biopsies obtained, polyps and foreign objects removed, and bleeding areas cauterized. The scope varies in length depending on the area in which it will be used (Fig. 21–6).

ESOPHAGOGASTRODUODENOSCOPY

Esophagogastroduodenoscopy is the direct visualization of the esophagus, stomach, and the beginning of the duodenum by means of an endoscope passed through the patient's mouth (Fig. 21–7).

This upper GI endoscopy is performed primarily as an adjunct to x-ray evaluation or as an emergency procedure in patients with acute upper GI bleeding. It is used in the diagnosis of hiatus hernia, esophageal varices, esophagitis, ulcer disease, polyps, and malignant tumors. It is also used to identify areas of bleeding in the upper GI tract, to obtain biopsy specimens, and to detect small or surface lesions that do not show up on x-ray film.

Physical Preparation of Patient. Unless the procedure is performed on an emergency basis, all food and fluids as well as antacids are withheld for 8 hours prior to the examination to ensure optimum visualization and to prevent aspiration. If the procedure is done on an emergency basis, stomach contents are aspirated beforehand through a nasogastric tube.

Usually a sedative such as Valium is given intravenously with or without Demerol at the onset of the procedure to decrease anxiety. The dose is titrated to achieve the degree of sedation required. Occasionally, atropine is also given to decrease salivary and gastric secretions.

Procedure. The throat is anesthetized either by swabbing it or by having the patient gargle with a local anesthetic. When the gag reflex has disappeared, the patient is placed in a lateral recumbent position and the endoscope is guided through the mouth to the hypopharynx. The patient is instructed to swallow, and the scope is further advanced to the anatomic area to be examined. Because it is essential that the patient lie perfectly still during the procedure, a general anesthetic may be necessary for patients who are unable to cooperate. Optimal visualization is achieved by the insufflation of air through the scope to distend the area being examined. Photographs of lesions, biopsy specimens and brushings for cytologic examination are taken when indicated.

Postprocedure Course. The patient rests until the sedation has worn off and then may return to usual activity. Foods and fluids are resumed when the gag reflex returns, which is usually in 1 to 2 hours.

Complications. The major complication is perforation of the GI tract, with the possibility of excessive bleeding and subsequent infection. Aspiration is a risk if food and fluids have not been withheld prior to the procedure.

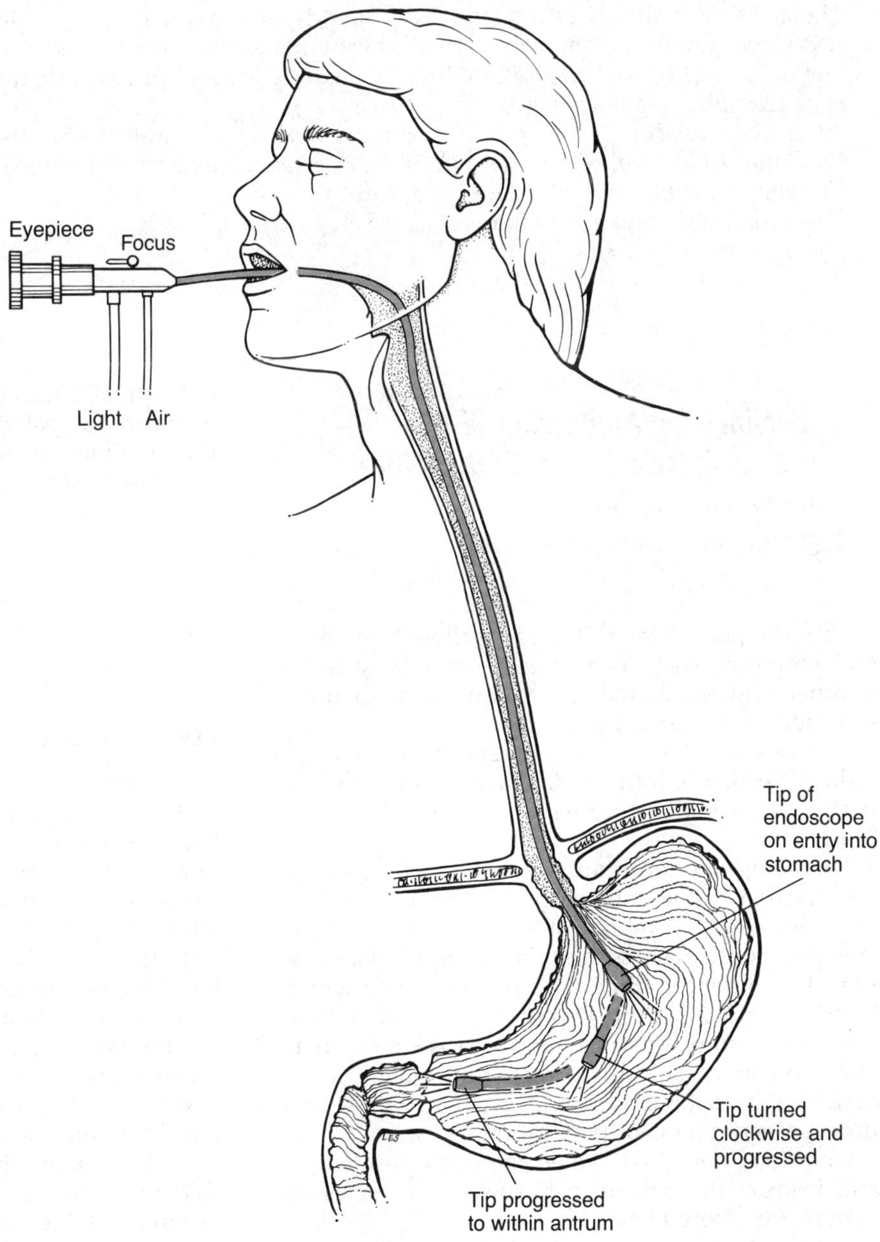

Figure 21–7.

Flexible endoscope shown passed through the mouth and the esophagus to the stomach. Dotted lines show how the endoscope is moved to allow visualization of all areas of the stomach.

Chart 21–1.

NURSING GUIDE TO PATIENT EDUCATION FOR SELF-MANAGEMENT: INFORMATION FOR THE PATIENT HAVING AN ESOPHAGOGASTRODUODENOSCOPY

Explain to the patient that:

The procedure is uncomfortable and very tiring but not painful.
Food and fluids must not be taken for at least 8 hours prior to the procedure.
Dentures, eyeglasses, and jewelry will be removed prior to the procedure.
A sedative will be given to promote relaxation (but not sleep) before the procedure is begun.
The procedure will be done in the ________. (endoscopy suite, treatment room on the unit, or out-patient department)
The throat will be anesthetized, and this can make the tongue and throat feel swollen.
The gag sensation will be lost, but swallowing is unimpaired.
It is important to remain perfectly still during the examination.
She or he will be told to swallow to help pass the tube. If air is insufflated, a feeling of fullness, bloating, or cramping may occur.
After the procedure, vital signs will be taken and activity limited until the sedation has worn off.
Food and fluids will be withheld until the gag reflex has returned, which is usually 1 to 2 hours.
The throat may be sore after the procedure.
The procedure takes 15 to 60 minutes.

Guidelines for Application of the Nursing Process to the Care of the Patient Having an Esophagogastroduodenoscopy

Assess the patient for ability to swallow; presence of GI symptoms such as nausea, vomiting, pain, abdominal distention, and GI bleeding; and for understanding of the procedure.

In assessing the patient's understanding and providing needed information, make certain that the patient knows the information presented in Chart 21–1.

Following the procedure, assess the physiologic stabilization of the patient by monitoring vital signs and checking for return of the gag reflex. Assess level of consciousness and keep side rails raised until the patient is fully alert. Assess the patient for bleeding and for pain. Report and record immediately any complaints of sharp, intense pain in the abdomen or chest. Also report immediately a sudden rise in temperature and tachycardia, because these are symptoms of perforation.

Give food and fluids when the gag reflex returns, and instruct the patient in the use of lozenges and gargles for a sore throat.

If the upper GI endoscopy is being done on an out-patient basis, make certain someone is available to escort the patient home after it is completed and the sedation has worn off. Provide instruction about the resumption of food and fluids and about symptoms that should be reported to the health care professional.

COLONOSCOPY

A colonoscopy is a procedure in which the lining of the large intestine all the way to the ileocecal valve is directly visualized through a fiberoptic colonoscope. A colonoscopy can help distinguish inflammatory from neoplastic diseases. It is indicated when the patient has a history of undiagnosed constipation and diarrhea, anorexia, persistent rectal bleeding, or lower abdominal pain. It is also used to check for recurring polyps or malignant tumors.

Physical Preparation of the Patient. A bowel preparation as described previously under Barium Enema is done to allow proper inspection of the colon. In some cases, the patient may also be kept on NPO status for 8 hours. Medication such as Demerol, Versed and Valium may be given intravenously at the onset of the procedure to promote comfort and relaxation.

Procedure. With the patient in left Sims' position, a digital rectal examination is done to dilate the rectum and rule out an obstruction. The colonoscope is inserted into the rectum, and a small amount of air is insufflated to distend the bowel lumen. The scope is then advanced through the rectum and into the sigmoid colon, past the splenic flexure, and on through the transverse colon and the cecum to the ileocecal valve. The scope is then slowly withdrawn for detailed visualization. If needed, suction is used to remove blood or secretions obstructing the view. Biopsy and cytology specimens may be obtained, polyps excised, and photographs taken if required.

Complications. Infrequent but possible complications of a colonoscopy are bleeding and perforation of the bowel wall. If either of these occurs, surgical intervention may be necessary.

Guidelines for Application of the Nursing Process to the Care of the Patient Having a Colonoscopy

Assess the patient's understanding of the colonoscopy as a procedure and as a diagnostic test. If a knowledge deficit is identified, provide information to ensure that the patient understands the prescribed preparation and knows that the test permits examination of the large intestine, that a flexible instrument is passed through the anus and may cause a feeling of needing to have a bowel movement or a cramping sensation, and that the test takes from 30 to 60 minutes. Careful assessment of the patient's understanding of the bowel preparation is particularly important when the test is done on an out-patient basis and the patient is responsible for following the instructions accurately.

Following the procedure, assess the patient for signs of perforation—sudden temperature elevation, tachycardia, or abdominal pain. Observe stools for red blood and take vital signs every 2 hours until stable. Instruct the patient to expel all air from the rectum. Encourage rest for 30 to 60 minutes. Give food and fluids once the patient has passed flatus.

When the test is done on an out-patient basis, be certain the patient has arranged to be driven home, because sedatives used during the procedure may temporarily impair the ability to drive. Also provide instructions for self-care as presented in Chart 21–2.

Ultrasonography

Ultrasonography is a noninvasive procedure that uses high frequency, inaudible sound waves to form images of internal structures. Sound waves are directed at the area to be studied by a transducer that is rubbed slowly on the lubricated skin surface. As the sound waves hit internal organs, they are reflected back and converted to an image on a screen. Photographs of these images can be taken as desired.

Ultrasonic examination of the gallbladder and biliary system helps diagnose cholelithiasis (gallstones) and cholecystitis when results of the cholecystogram are inconclusive.

Liver ultrasonography can detect metastasis, abscesses, and hematomas. Pancreatic ultrasound studies aid in the diagnosis of pancreatitis, pseudocysts,

Chart 21–2.

NURSING GUIDE TO PATIENT EDUCATION FOR SELF-MANAGEMENT: SELF-CARE AFTER COLONOSCOPY

Instruct the patient to:

Avoid driving or operating any power-related machinery if you received medication before or during the procedure.
Avoid making important decisions for 24 hours if you received medication before or during the procedure.
Resume oral intake gradually, starting with a light meal and progressing to a regular diet.
Remember that feelings of gassiness or bloatedness are caused by the air that is instilled in the bowel during the procedure.
Remember that abdominal tenderness may occur as a result of stretching of the abdominal muscles during the procedure.

and pancreatic cancer. Abdominal sonograms can detect tumor masses in the abdominal cavity.

Ascites and extreme obesity interfere with ultrasonic studies. So too can barium. For this reason, ultrasonography should be scheduled before tests using barium.

Minimal preparation is required for ultrasonic studies of the GI tract. The patient is instructed to avoid carbonated beverages and large amounts of carbohydrates for 48 hours before the test to help decrease intestinal gas.

The test is painless, and all that is required of the patient is to lie still and hold his or her breath for 20- to 30-second intervals as directed.

Computed Tomography

Computed tomography (CT) of the abdomen produces three-dimensional images of abdominal tissues. It is used to identify tumors and other diseases of the abdominal organs including the gallbladder, biliary ductal system, pancreas, and peritoneum. A contrast medium may be used to visualize the biliary tract or to highlight differences in pancreatic tissue density.

The patient is placed on NPO status for 8 to 12 hours before an abdominal CT scan and is assessed for allergies to shellfish and contrast media. During the scan, which takes 45 minutes to 1 hour, a supine position must be maintained.

Since barium can interfere with the CT scan, barium studies should be scheduled after the scan or at least 4 days prior to it.

Magnetic Resonance Imaging

Magnetic resonance imaging (MRI) produces cross-sectional images of tissue. It can be used to study blood flow in the abdomen as well as to identify areas of infection or malignancy. The procedure takes 1 to 1½ hours and requires that the patient lie still. Contraindications to MRI include pregnancy and the presence of a pacemaker, a metallic implant, or an infusion pump.

Medical Management

Gastrointestinal Intubation

GI intubation refers to the insertion of a tube into the stomach or intestine. This may be for the purpose of removing toxic substances by suction, removing fluids and gas by suction or gravity drainage, instilling irrigating solutions (lavage) or medications, controlling bleeding, or administering enteral feeding. Different types of tubes are used for different purposes (Fig. 21–8). Tubes may be inserted through the nose or via a surgical stab wound into the abdomen.

INTUBATION FOR DECOMPRESSION AND DRAINAGE

Intubation is done to remove contents of the stomach or intestines when the GI tract is unable to properly propel and absorb its secretions such as when an obstruction is present or peristalsis is greatly reduced as a result of the effects of anesthesia and surgery. Patients are also intubated after surgery on the stomach or intestines to remove gas and secretions from the area of the suture line until healing takes place, after a drug overdose, and as a diagnostic procedure.

TYPES OF TUBES USED FOR DECOMPRESSION AND DRAINAGE

Nasogastric or short tubes are used to intubate the stomach. Examples of short tubes used for decompression and drainage are the Levin and Salem sump tubes (Fig. 21–8). The Levin tube is a single-lumen tube approximately 3 feet long with a solid tip and holes along the sides. The Salem sump is a double-lumen tube (a tube within a tube). In the Salem sump, the small vent tube within the larger tube prevents suction damage to the gastric mucosa by preventing greater than 25 mm Hg of pressure at the openings in the distal end of the tube.

Intestinal tubes (see Fig. 21–8) are designed to enter the small intestine through the pyloric

Figure 21–8.

Comparison of design and function of selected gastrointestinal tubes. *A*, Lavacuator tube. An orogastric tube with a large suction lumen and a smaller lavage/vent lumen that provides continuous suction because irrigating solution enters the lavage lumen while stomach contents are removed through the suction lumen. Used to remove toxic substances from the stomach. *B*, Levin tube. A plastic or rubber single-lumen tube with a solid tip that may be inserted into the stomach via the nose or the mouth. Used to drain fluid and gas from the stomach. Single lumen must be used for irrigation and drainage, so continuous irrigation is not possible. *C*, Salem sump tube. A short double-lumen tube. The small vent tube within the large suction tube prevents mucosal suction damage by maintaining the pressure in open eyes at the distal end of the tube at less than 25 mm Hg. *D*, Miller-Abbott tube. A long double-lumen tube used to drain and decompress the small intestine. One lumen leads to a balloon that is filled with mercury once it is in the stomach; the second is for irrigation and drainage. *E*, Cantor tube. A single-lumen long tube with a small inflatable bag at the distal end. Five to ten ml of mercury are injected with a needle (gauge 21 or smaller or balloon may leak) and syringe into the bag prior to insertion of the tube. *F*, Sengstaken-Blakemore tube. A stiff rubber tube with an esophageal and a gastric balloon used for tamponade. The Sengstaken-Blakemore tube does not provide esophageal suction, but a gastric tube (e.g., Levin tube) may be inserted in the opposite naris or via the mouth and allowed to rest on top of the esophageal balloon. Esophageal suction is then possible, and the risk of aspiration is reduced. *G*, Weighted flexible feeding tube with stylet. Access port with irrigation adaptor allows maintenance of the tube without disconnecting the feeding set.

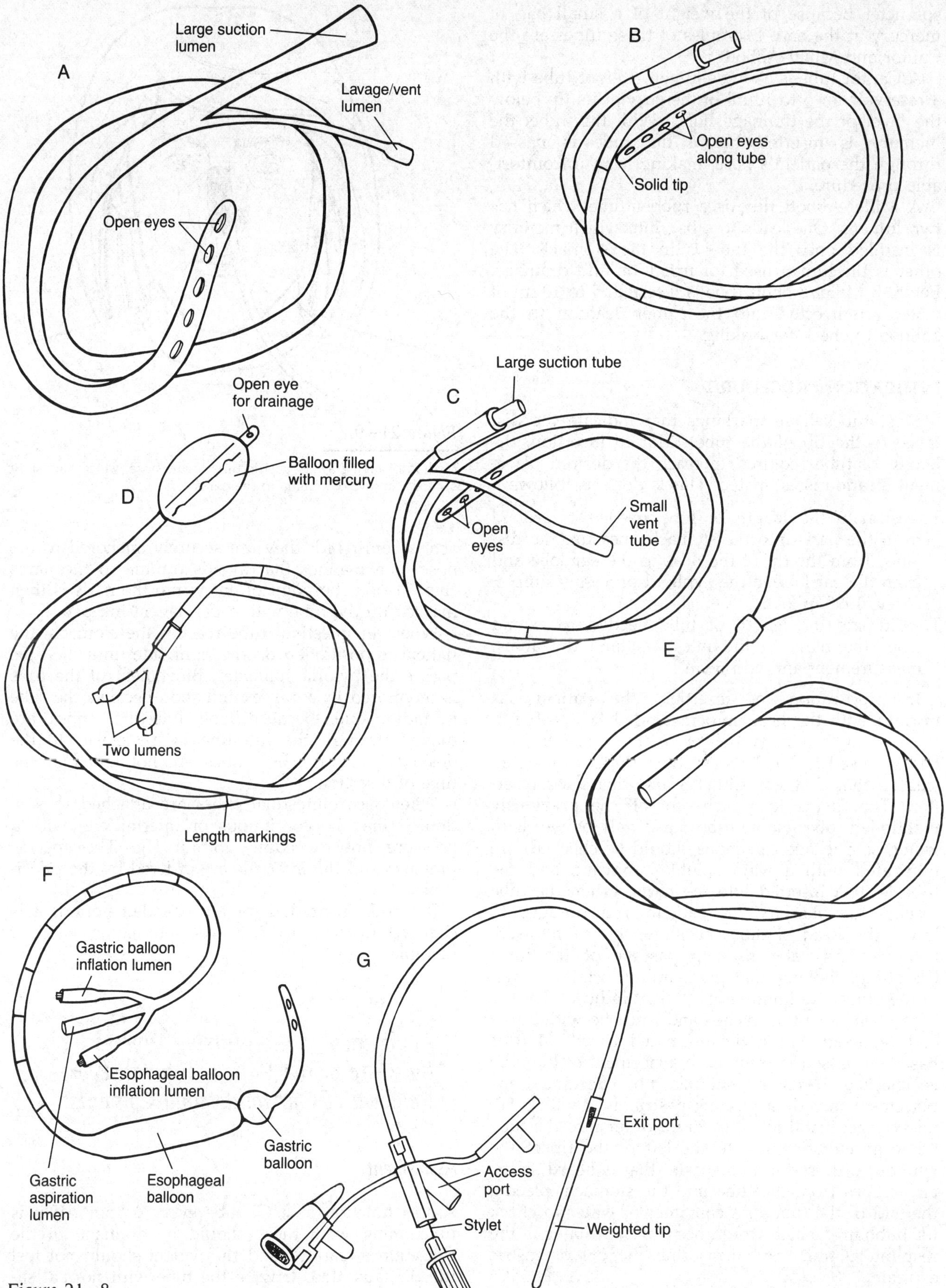

Figure 21–8.

See legend on facing page

sphincter because of the weight of a small bag of mercury at the end. Examples of these tubes are the Cantor and Miller-Abbott.

A Cantor tube is a single-lumen, 10-foot tube with a reservoir for 5 to 10 ml of mercury at its tip below the level of the drainage holes. With this tube, the mercury is inserted before the tube is passed through the patient's nose, making it an uncomfortable procedure.

A Miller-Abbott tube is a rubber tube which has two lumens. One leads to a bag into which mercury is instilled once the tube is in the stomach. The other is the lumen used for irrigation and drainage. Before a Miller-Abbott tube is inserted, 5 to 10 ml of water are injected into the lumen leading to the balloon to check for leaking.

INTUBATION PROCEDURE

Most tubes have markings that indicate the distance to the tip of the tube. Prior to insertion, the length of tube required to reach the desired placement location is estimated. This is done as follows:

To estimate the length of tube needed to extend from the naris into the stomach, measure the distance from the tip of the nose to the ear lobe and from the ear lobe to the xyphoid process (Camp & Otten, 1990, p. 61).

To estimate the length of tube needed to extend from the naris to the intestine, take the above measurement and add 5 cm.

In preparation for insertion, the patient sits upright with the head hyperextended if possible. If the patient is unconscious or unable to sit up, the bed is raised to Fowler's position. Rubber tubes are iced so that they are stiff, because this eases insertion. The first 1 to 4 inches of all the previously mentioned tubes (some tubes need only be wet with water, so package directions should be checked) are lubricated with a water-soluble lubricant, and the tube is then inserted into the naris. When the tube reaches the pharynx, the patient is encouraged to lower the head slightly, swallow, and if allowed, take sips of water to help passage of the tube. Coughing, choking, and the inability to talk or hum in the otherwise unimpaired patient indicate that the tube is entering the trachea and must be withdrawn and repassed. When the estimated length of tube has been passed into the nose, placement of the tube is checked. Bedside methods for checking tube placement include aspirating gastric juice with a 50-ml syringe; instilling 10 to 20 ml of air into the tube while auscultating just to the left of the tip of the xyphoid process for a "swoosh" that is heard as the air escapes from the tube into the stomach; placing the end of the tube in a container of water to check for bubbling, which would occur if the tube is in the respiratory tract; and measuring the pH of gastric aspirate.

When placement of nasogastric tubes in the stomach is confirmed, they are securely anchored to the nose in a manner that avoids trauma to the nares (Fig. 21–9). The point of entry into the naris is then marked on the tube with a permanent-ink pen.

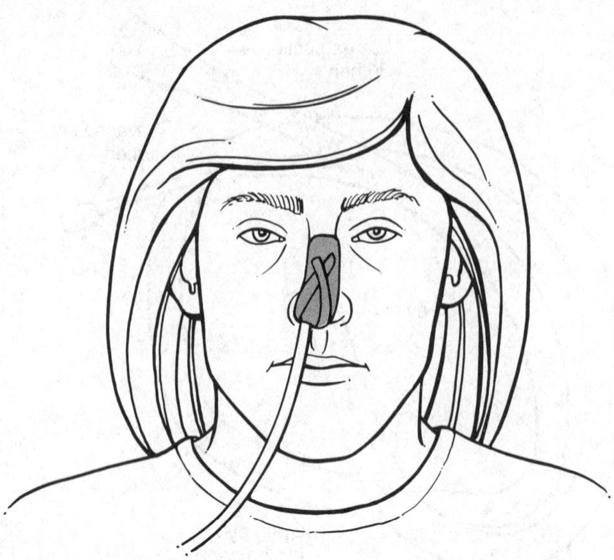

Figure 21–9.

Method of taping a nasogastric tube to the nose, which anchors it securely but avoids trauma to the nares.

When an intestinal tube reaches the stomach, the patient is positioned on the right side until the tube passes the pyloric sphincter. Movement of the tube is monitored by x-ray examination because the tube is radiopaque. Because long intestinal tubes are moved through the intestine by peristalsis to the desired location, these tubes are not taped at the time of insertion.

When gastrointestinal tubes are attached to suction, it may be continuous or intermittent, with a pressure not exceeding 25 mm Hg. The specific pressure and the intervals are ordered by the physician.

If a tube is needed for an extended period, it is changed every 2 to 3 weeks, alternating nares if possible.

Application of the Nursing Process to the Care of the Patient Intubated for Removal of Gastrointestinal Contents

Assessment

Assess function of a GI tube every 4 hours. If it is functioning well, there should be drainage in the collection apparatus and the patient should not feel full or nauseated. Irrigate the tube with normal saline to determine patency if needed.

Note amount, color, and consistency of drainage as well as any changes occurring in these parameters. Normal gastric secretions are yellow-green. If blood is present from previous bleeding, drainage is dark brown and has a "coffee grounds" appearance as a result of the action of hydrochloric acid on the hemoglobin. Immediately report the presence of bright red blood because it indicates frank, current bleeding. Be alert for the passage of flatus or bowel movement, and if either occurs, report it to the physician, because this may indicate that there is no longer a need for the tube.

Assess the patient for signs of fluid, electrolyte, and acid-base imbalance, which can occur because of excessive losses from the gastrointestinal tube. Record fluid intake and output, including amounts of irrigating solutions instilled and returned. Measure body weight, check skin turgor, and monitor serum electrolytes.

Also assess the patient for redness, bleeding, and discomfort of the nares, where the tube may exert pressure, and for a sore throat because the pharynx is irritated by the tube.

Nursing Diagnoses and Planning

Nursing diagnoses and related expected patient outcomes most commonly applicable to intubated patients include the following:

NDx: High risk for altered oral mucous membrane related to mouth breathing and limitation on oral intake

Planning: Patient outcomes

1. Oral mucous membrane is pink and moist.
2. Lips are supple, moist, and free of cracks.
3. Patient denies soreness or dryness of mouth and lips.

NDx: High risk for fluid volume deficit related to drainage rather than reabsorption of gastrointestinal secretions

Planning: Patient outcomes

1. Skin turgor is firm.
2. Mucous membranes are moist.
3. Urinary output is at least 50 ml/hour.
4. Urinary specific gravity is between 1.003 and 1.035.
5. Serum electrolyte levels and acid-base parameters are within normal range.

NDx: High risk for impaired tissue integrity related to mechanical irritation from the nasogastric or nasointestinal tube

Planning: Patient outcomes

1. Skin and mucous membranes of the nares are free of erythema.
2. Skin and mucous membranes of the nares are intact.
3. Bleeding from the nares is absent.

Nursing Interventions

NDx: High risk for altered oral mucous membrane

Because most intubated patients breathe through the mouth, meticulous mouth care is essential for comfort and protection of the mucous membrane. Assist the patient in brushing the teeth and rinsing the mouth every 4 hours while awake. Use a soft toothbrush to avoid accidental trauma. Avoid lemon and glycerin swabs as well as commercial mouthwashes containing alcohol because these further dry the mucous membrane. If the patient is unconscious, clean the mouth with saline- or hydrogen peroxide–moistened swabs four to six times each day. Apply a water-soluble lubricant to the lips to keep them supple and prevent cracking.

When permitted, allow the patient to "mist" the mouth with a spray bottle of water or offer gum, small amounts of Gatorade, warm saline gargles, or anesthetic throat lozenges to help wet mucous membranes of the mouth and soothe an irritated pharynx. Do not allow the patient to swallow sips of water or suck on ice chips unless specifically ordered because these small amounts of hypotonic fluid can add up rapidly and contribute to significant fluid and electrolyte imbalance.

NDx: High risk for fluid volume deficit

Monitor laboratory data, skin turgor, and condition of mucous membranes for signs of dehydration. Remember that oral mucous membrane reflects changes caused by mouth breathing and restricted oral intake as well as by dehydration. Administer replacement fluids and electrolytes as ordered. Maintain an accurate and complete fluid intake and output record, always being certain to subtract any fluids given by mouth or tube from the total amount of gastrointestinal drainage. Obtain daily weights and monitor central venous pressure or other hemodynamic parameters to ensure adequate but not overreplacement of fluid.

NDx: High risk for impaired tissue integrity

Cleanse the area around the nares gently using warm water or saline. Gently remove any crusts that have formed as a result of increased nasal secretions secondary to irritation from the tube. Apply a protective water-soluble lubricant.

Question the patient about discomfort from the tube and adjust accordingly. To prevent pull on the tube, loop an elastic band around it, then loop the tube above the elastic around the patient's ear, and use a safety pin inserted through the elastic band to pin the tube to the patient's gown or pajamas. Inspect both the naris and the skin behind the ear frequently for signs of irritation, and if present, reinsert the tube through the opposite naris or change the position of the tube over the ear.

Because the skin beneath the anchoring tape becomes oily, loosening the tape and creating the risk of the tube's being pulled out, remove the tape anchoring the tube in place daily, being careful to avoid stripping the epidermis. Wash the area thoroughly, wipe with an alcohol swab, shave male patients, and apply new tape. If skin irritation is a problem, use a transparent, moisture- and vapor-permeable dressing such as Op-Site, which can remain in place for as long as 7 days.

Additional Interventions
Explain the purpose of intubation and describe what to expect during insertion to help allay the patient's anxiety. Provide ongoing explanations about intubation and related treatments as needed. This is especially important for the patient with a long intestinal tube who is constantly being x-rayed and repositioned.

Mark the tube at the end of the naris right after insertion so it is possible to tell later whether the tube's position has changed.

Irrigate GI tubes as ordered to maintain patency. Use the type and amount of solution specified by the physician. If the tube is in place to protect a suture line in the GI tract, follow strict sterile technique during the procedure. Instill irrigating fluid manually, and then reattach the tube to suction. Monitor returns and be certain to record the irrigating fluid as intake. Keep in mind that a clogged tube can result in gastric distention, which can lead to shock if unrelieved.

If a mercury-weighted tube is inserted, record the amount of mercury instilled in the patient's record. When the tube is removed, follow institutional procedure for collection and disposal of the mercury, which is a toxic substance. Remember that in the event that the mercury escapes into the GI tract, it is allowed to pass normally because it is not absorbed and is therefore not toxic to the patient.

Evaluation

Evaluate the effectiveness of nursing care for an intubated patient by comparing the patient's status with the expected patient outcomes. Examples of specific outcomes for intubated patients have been provided in the Planning section.

REMOVAL OF GASTROINTESTINAL TUBES

Before removal of a GI tube that has been inserted for decompression and drainage, gastrointestinal function is assessed. Bowel sounds are auscultated, the abdomen is observed for distention, the patient is asked whether flatus has been passed, and the patient's tolerance of ice chips or clamping of the tube, or both, is noted. Also noted is the volume of drainage, which should have decreased prior to removal of the tube.

For removal of the tube, the patient is raised to a semi-Fowler's position and a towel is placed across the chest. The patient is told that some gagging, sneezing, or nasal discomfort may occur, and tissues are provided. With the health care professional wearing gloves, the tube is flushed with 10 ml of normal saline to cleanse it of debris and move it away from the mucosa. Next the tube is clamped by being folded in the hand, and the patient is told to take a deep breath and exhale slowly. The tube is withdrawn during exhalation (Short, 1989). When the tube is removed, it is placed in the towel and removed from the immediate environment. Long intestinal tubes are withdrawn slowly a few inches at a time because rapid withdrawal can cause vomiting. Mouth care is given, and the procedure is documented in the patient's record. Subsequently the patient is assessed for nausea, vomiting, and abdominal distention.

Enteral and Parenteral Nutrition

Adults ordinarily need 1500 to 2000 calories and 0.5 g/kg of protein per day for normal activity. When the patient is acutely ill, as with serious infection or major surgery, requirements can increase to as much as 10,000 calories and 4 g/kg of protein. This increased need is complicated by the fact that the patient is often unable to maintain minimal nutrition because of lack of appetite or physical impediments to eating. Enteral feedings and hyperalimentation are two methods that provide supplemental nutrition to patients unable to meet their needs through oral feedings.

ENTERAL NUTRITION

Enteral nutrition is another term for tube feeding. It is used to maintain weight in patients with severe anorexia or increased metabolic needs and in patients who cannot eat by mouth because of dysphagia obstruction of the upper GI tract, decreased level of consciousness, surgery of the GI tract or the head and neck region, malabsorptive syndromes such as Crohn's disease, or anorexia nervosa.

Enteral therapy requires a functional GI tract. It is contraindicated when conditions such as persistent vomiting, upper GI bleeding, obstruction, or inflammatory bowel disease are present.

TYPES OF TUBE FEEDINGS

Feedings are primarily absorbed in the upper small intestine with minimal digestion needed. Most enteral feedings provide one calorie per ml of feed-

Table 21–4. FEEDING TUBES: TYPES, PLACEMENT, AND ADVANTAGES

TYPE OF TUBE	PLACEMENT	ADVANTAGES
Nasogastric tube	Passed via nose into stomach	No surgical wound
Nasointestinal tube	Passed via nose into intestine	Placement beyond pyloric sphincter is thought to reduce backflow No surgical wound
Esophagostomy tube	Passed directly into the esophagus through a surgically created opening in the cervical area	Decreased risk of aspiration Bypasses operative area in patients who have had head and neck surgery, while allowing maximal normal function of the GI tract
Gastrostomy tube	Passed directly into the stomach through an opening created in the abdominal wall	Good for long-term use Prevents pharyngeal irritation Decreased risk of aspiration Is not immediately visible
Jejunostomy tube	Passed into the jejunum through an opening created in the abdominal wall	Good for long-term use Bypasses pathology of the upper GI tract Decreases risk of aspiration

ing; and 2000 to 3000 ml can be given during a 24-hour period. An important factor to consider in enteral therapy is osmolarity. Feedings should be as close to the normal body osmolarity of 340 mOsm/L as possible to avoid the shifting of fluid from one body space to another.

Tube feedings can be made by blenderizing various foods until they are thin enough to pass through the tube. Although this type of feeding is nutritious and less expensive, the convenience and standardization of commercial products far outweigh the possible economic savings for most people. Commercial products are consistently smooth and easy to administer, there is minimal chance of contamination, and the contents are clearly stated on the label. They also have the advantage of not requiring refrigeration until opened, and they can be stored for long periods of time.

Commercial products may be divided into three categories. First are chemically defined (polymeric) formulas. These do not provide complete nutritional requirements but are used in conjunction with oral or hyperalimentation therapy. Defined formulas are hyperosmolar and therefore must be diluted before being given. If they are not diluted, the body will shift intracellular fluid to achieve isosmolarity, possibly causing diarrhea. Most of the calories in defined formulas (50% to 90%) are carbohydrates, with about 8% protein content. Examples of defined formulas are Vivonex and Vital, powdered products that must be dissolved before administration.

Meal replacement feedings constitute a second category of commercial preparation. These are isosmolar and are nutritionally complete. Approximately 50% of the calories are carbohydrates, 15% are proteins, and 15% are fats. Ensure, Isocal, and Osmolite are examples of meal replacement feedings.

A third category of tube feedings is called supplemental. These are dominant in one nutrient and are given along with other nourishment. Amin-Aid and Polycose are examples of these.

METHODS OF DELIVERY

Tube feedings may be given by bolus or by intermittent or continuous drip.

In bolus feedings, 300 to 400 ml of formula is infused for several minutes every 4 to 6 hours, usually through an Asepto syringe or a funnel. This type of feeding is generally not well tolerated and therefore the least often used.

Intermittent feedings can be given either by gravity drip or pump infusion. They are generally given five to eight times per day over a period of a few hours.

Continuous feedings are given by pump at a slow, constant rate in amounts of 75 to 150 ml/hour. They are given when large amounts of formula cannot be tolerated at one time. They are used for patients with nasointestinal or jejunostomy tubes as well as for selected patients with nasogastric or gastrostomy tubes.

The type of delivery method selected is based on the needs of the individual patient. Factors considered in selecting a method include the patient's physical and nutritional status, tolerance of the feedings, mobility, comfort, and psychological well-being.

ROUTES OF DELIVERY

Feedings may be given directly into the stomach by nasogastric or gastrostomy tube, into the esophagus by esophagostomy tube, or into the small intestine by nasointestinal tube. Types of feeding tubes and their placement and advantages are outlined in Table 21–4.

Nasogastric Feeding

Nasogastric tubes are inserted through the nose and esophagus into the stomach. Nasogastric feeding requires intact gag and swallow reflexes, a competent lower esophageal sphincter, and the capacity to handle a high-osmotic load. An intermittent feeding schedule is preferred whenever possible because the stomach normally functions as a reservoir for food injected at intervals.

Nasointestinal Feeding

Nasointestinal tubes are inserted through the nose, esophagus, and stomach into the duodenum (nasoduodenal) or the jejunum (nasojejunal). Nasointestinal feeding is used when the potential for aspiration is high, when there is dysfunction of the gastric outlet, or when digestive processes are impaired so that a simple nutrient formula is required.

Feedings are administered on a continuous schedule via a nasointestinal tube because the intestine normally receives nutrients from the stomach in slow peristaltic waves.

Gastrostomy

In a gastrostomy, a tube is passed directly into the stomach through the abdominal wall. It provides a permanent access and hence is excellent for long-term enteral nutrition. The two major types of gastrostomy are the traditional surgical gastrostomy and the newer percutaneous gastrostomy.

Surgical Gastrostomy. A surgical gastrostomy is performed with the patient under general anesthesia and involves a laparotomy. A permanent stoma is created by suturing the stomach wall to the abdominal wall, and a large diameter tube is inserted. Postoperative ileus is usually present for 24 to 48 hours following the procedure, and enteral feeding cannot be started until peristalsis has resumed.

Percutaneous Endoscopic Gastrostomy. A percutaneous endoscopic gastrostomy (PEG) is a procedure in which an endoscope is inserted into the stomach, the light from which shines against the abdominal wall and allows visualization of the tube placement site. A large-gauge needle and suture are passed through the abdominal and stomach walls, and a snare or biopsy forceps is used to bring the inner end of the suture up through the endoscope into the patient's mouth. The PEG tube is tied to the suture and is then pulled through the mouth down into the stomach and out through the abdominal wall. The tube is held in place by an anchor system such as an internal and external rubber bumper, or an internal retention balloon and outer disk (Fig. 21–10). In several weeks a fibrous track forms between the gastric wall and the exit site.

A percutaneous gastrostomy has several advantages over a surgical gastrostomy. There is less risk because it is performed while the patient is under intravenous sedation rather than general anesthesia.

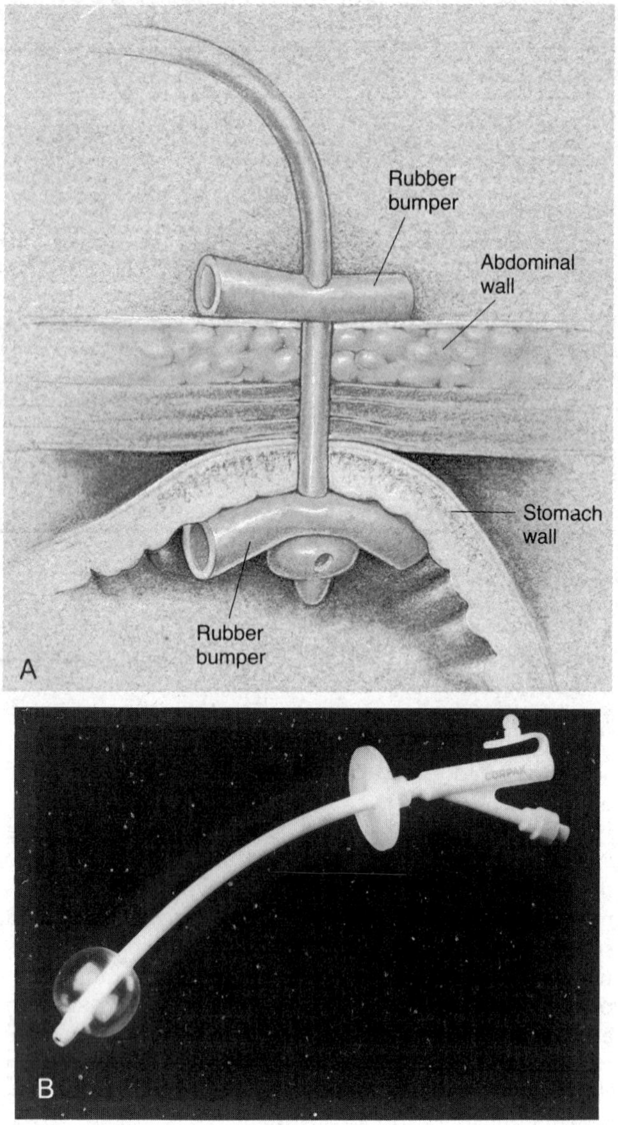

Figure 21–10.

A, PEG tube in place anchored with rubber bumpers. (Modified from Starkey JF, Jefferson PA, Kirby DF. Taking care of percutaneous endoscopic gastrostomy. Am J Nurs 1988; 88(1):43. Copyright Bob L. Shepherd.) *B*, Gastrostomy tube designed for initial placement during a surgical gastrostomy as well as for replacement of a PEG tube. (Courtesy of Corpak, Wheeling, IL.)

Recovery is faster and there is less discomfort because there is no laparotomy. Feeding can be started within 24 hours (as soon as bowel sounds return). Finally, the procedure can be done in the endoscopy suite or at the bedside, so it is less costly.

In preparation for PEG, the patient is kept on NPO status for 24 hours to empty the stomach and decrease the risk of aspiration. If the patient was receiving tube feedings prior to the procedure, feedings are withheld for 8 hours. During the procedure, vital signs, color, and level of consciousness are monitored. Suctioning is used as necessary because secretions can accumulate in the mouth.

Complications of gastrostomy are aspiration, peritonitis, accidental tube removal, and wound cellulitis.

Jejunostomy

In a jejunostomy, a tube is passed into the jejunum through an opening in the abdominal wall. As with a gastrostomy, a surgical or a percutaneous approach may be used.

Percutaneous endoscopic jejunostomy (PEJ) is an extension of a PEG; that is, a small tube is passed through a PEG and guided via an endoscope into the duodenum. The tube is then propelled by peristalsis into the jejunum.

Jejunostomy tubes must be of very small diameter, given the small size of the jejunum. Therefore they can easily become clogged. They can also be moved back into the stomach by vomiting, in which case the tube must be repositioned under endoscopy.

Feedings are given on a continuous basis, given the small size of the tube and the fact that the jejunum is not normally a reservoir for nutrients. Since no residual feeding is present in the jejunum, placement can be confirmed by x-ray film only after injection of a contrast medium.

DELIVERY SYSTEMS

Feeding Tubes

Nasoenteric tubes in use today for enteric feedings are predominantly small bore, made of Silastic, and very flexible. The majority are weighted usually with tungsten or silicone, and many are inserted and removed with a stylet. The stylet is designed to assist in passage of the newer, soft flexible tubes. Wire stylets or guide wires are stiff and straight and provide easy insertion but are associated with the risk of perforation. Plastic stylets do not have this risk but coil easily and may be difficult to insert into the feeding tube. Stylets are removed once the tube is inserted. They are stored in a plastic bag or other container labeled with patient identification information in case tube reinsertion is required.

Most feeding tubes are coated with a lubricant that is activated by water, therefore they are wet rather than lubricated prior to insertion. These tubes are generally comfortable, are unaffected by contact with digestive juices, help prevent reflux esophagitis, and allow oral intake while in place. Disadvantages of these tubes include a tendency to clog if not routinely irrigated and the need for very slow administration and the use of a feeding pump owing to the small lumen.

Feeding Administration Sets

Administration sets consist of a container to hold the formula and tubing to connect to the feeding tube itself. The basic type of container is an open system: a plastic bag with attached tubing, which can be filled with feeding and when empty may be washed and refilled for a 24-hour period. Some of these bags, such as the Kangaroo (Fig. 21–11*A*), have an outside pocket designed to hold a Polar pack of ice to keep the formula cool and discourage bacterial growth. A second type is a closed administration set featuring a disposable prefilled bottle that is used with a spike set, that is, tubing attached to a cap with a spike that perforates the seal on the formula container when put in place (Fig. 21–11*B*). Bottles are replaced when empty, and spike sets are replaced every 24 hours.

Feeding Pumps

Infusion pumps are used to provide constant slow administration of formula, which helps prevent symptoms such as feelings of excessive fullness, abdominal cramping, and diarrhea. Use of a pump also permits administration of thicker consistency feedings than would pass through a small-bore tube by gravity alone.

There are a variety of pumps available. All feature a mechanism to set the drop rate in milliliters per hour and an alarm that signals an empty feeding bag or an occlusion of the tube. Many also have an alarm that signals a change in flow rate. Most can be operated by battery for some time interval and indicate when battery charge is low. All are small and easy to use, simply requiring that the drip rate be set, the tubing primed and threaded around the drive, and a button pushed to start (Fig. 21–12).

Application of the Nursing Process to the Care of the Patient Receiving Enteral Feedings

Assessment

Assess the patient's nutritional status in response to therapy. Observe for physical signs of improved nutrition such as weight gain and better condition of hair, nails, and skin, as well as for increased energy and subjective statements of feeling stronger.

Auscultate for bowel sounds, and check placement of feeding tube before each intermittent feeding and every 4 hours during continuous feeding to ensure delivery to the intended area and to prevent aspiration. Remember that the small intestine is not a reservoir, and therefore no residual formula can be aspirated. The only way placement in the duodenum or jejunum can be checked is by x-ray film after injection of a contrast medium.

Assess for tolerance of feedings. Be alert to complaints of nausea or cramping, and observe for abdominal distention, vomiting, or diarrhea. Check respirations and airway clearance to assess for

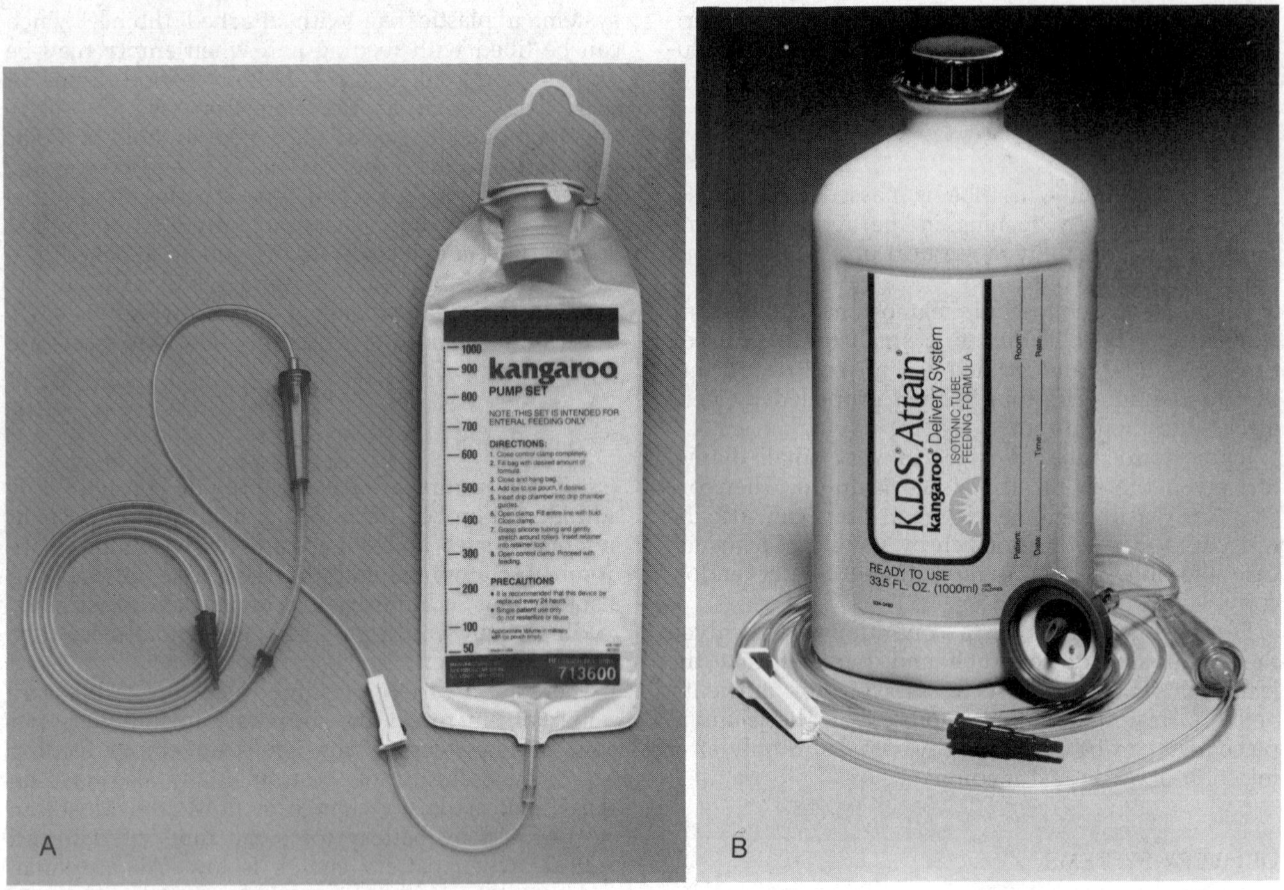

Figure 21–11.

Open and closed feeding administration sets. *A*, Kangaroo refillable pump set. *B*, Prefilled bottle with spike set. (Courtesy of Sherwood Medical, St. Louis, MO.)

aspiration. Assess for hyperglycemia: observe for thirst, polyuria, and confusion; test urine for glucose and acetone; and check blood glucose levels daily. Observe for signs of dehydration, which can result from inadequate fluid intake or excess fluid loss. Check for "tenting" of the skin due to loss of turgor, thirst, changes in mentation, rapid weight loss, and urinary specific gravity greater than 1.018. Inspect the condition of the area around the tube insertion site. Look for signs of infection or irritation such as redness, excoriation, bleeding, or purulent drainage. If the patient has a PEG or PEJ, expect a small amount of drainage for about a week owing to the tissue reaction to the tube, which is a foreign body. When assessing the wound, slide the outer bumper approximately 1 cm away from the skin to check for redness and breakdown. Gently press around the tube to check for drainage. Also inspect the tube for signs of wear.

Assess the patient's psychological reaction to the feeding system. If the patient is to be discharged home with it, assess both the patient's and significant other's understanding of and ability to manage and cope with this therapy. Also assess the need for follow-up visits by a home health nurse.

Nursing Diagnoses and Planning

Nursing diagnoses and related expected patient outcomes most commonly applicable to patients on enteral feedings include high risk for impaired tissue integrity and altered oral mucous membrane previously described under Intubation as well as the following:

NDx: Altered nutrition: less than body requirements related to inadequate intake or absorption of nutrients

Planning: Patient outcomes

1. Patient maintains weight or shows slow, steady weight gain.
2. Patient is in positive nitrogen balance.
3. Serum electrolyte and protein levels are within normal range.

NDx: High risk for aspiration related to enteral feeding

Planning: Patient outcomes
1. Abrupt coughing and gagging are absent.
2. Respirations are silent and easy.
3. Lungs are clear on auscultation.

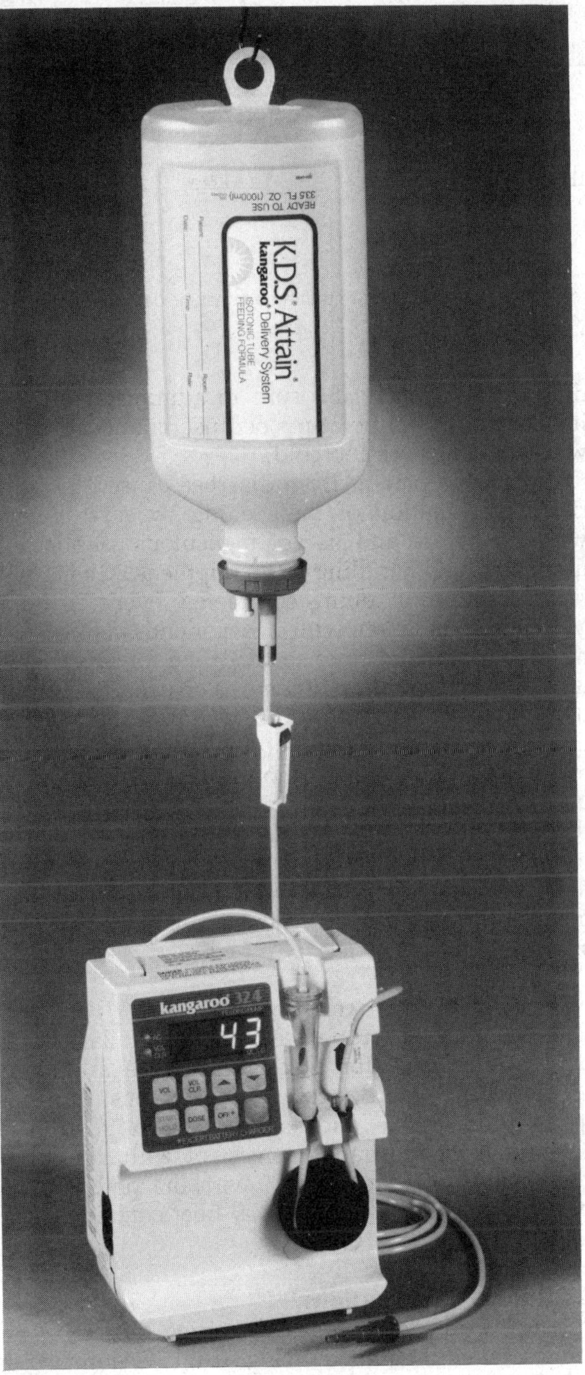

Figure 21–12.

Kangaroo 324 pump. (Courtesy of Sherwood Medical, St. Louis, MO.)

NDx: High risk for diarrhea related to intolerance of formula administered

Planning: Patient outcomes
1. Patient passes formed stool at regular intervals.
2. Patient denies abdominal cramping.

NDx: High risk for constipation related to enteral feeding formula

Planning: Patient outcomes
1. Patient passes soft, formed stool at regular intervals.
2. Patient denies uncomfortable straining at stool.

Nursing Interventions

NDx: Altered nutrition: less than body requirements

Administer enteral feedings as per physician's order. Record fluid intake and output, and weigh the patient daily at the same time of day and on the same scale. Report any rapid weight gain or loss to the physician. This is important because rapid weight gain may indicate the patient is retaining fluid and is overhydrated, whereas rapid loss may indicate dehydration.

Give additional water throughout the day. Give the amount needed to have daily intake exceed output by 500 ml.

If it is necessary to decrease the administration rate because of lack of tolerance, calculate the patient's daily caloric intake at the new rate (calories per ml of formula × number of ml given per hour × number of hours of administration per day). Compare this with the caloric intake ordered. Record change on chart, and if the patient is receiving significantly fewer calories per day because of the decrease in administration rate, notify the physician.

NDx: High risk for aspiration

The patients at greatest risk for aspiration of tube feedings are the unconscious, the confused, the seriously debilitated, the elderly, those with tracheostomies or large-bore feeding tubes, and those whose gag reflexes are impaired or who cannot sit upright. Protect the patient from aspiration by keeping the head elevated at least 30 degrees during feeding and for 1 hour thereafter. If this is not possible, position the patient on the right side. Check placement of the feeding tube before every intermittent or bolus feeding and every 4 hours during continuous feeding. If you question the placement of the tube, delay feeding until correct placement is confirmed. Also check for gastric residual, because overloading the stomach predisposes to reflux and regurgitation. Check before each intermittent or bolus feeding and every 2 to 4 hours during continuous feeding. If the residual is more than 30 ml, discontinue the feeding for

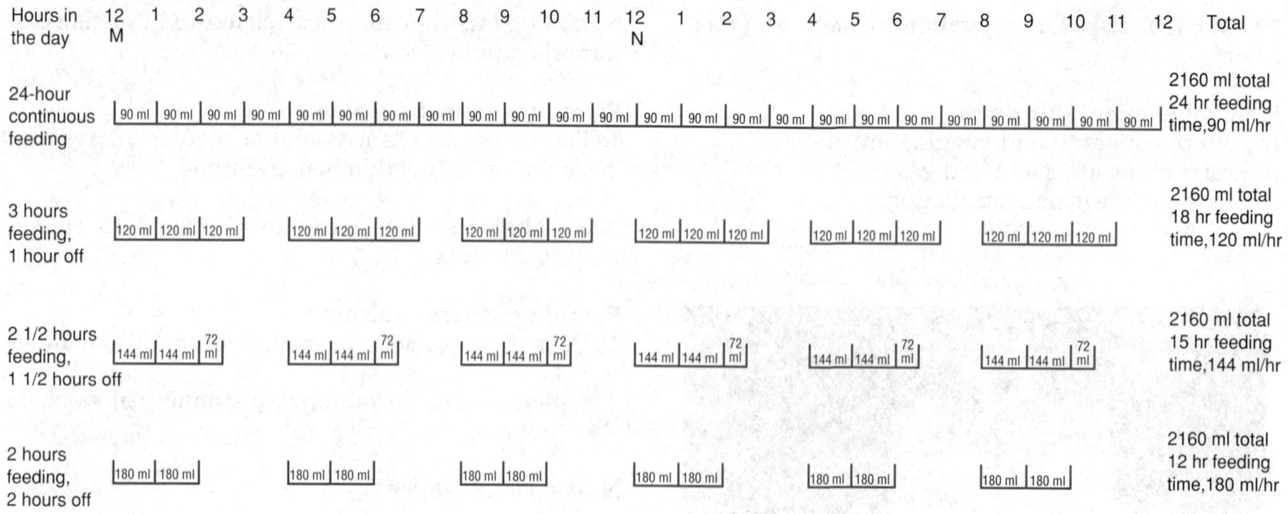

Figure 21–13.

Graphic representation of gradually increasing the rate and time between enteral feedings while maintaining a constant daily caloric intake.

30 to 60 minutes and then recheck. If a residual of more than 30 ml still persists, notify the physician. Remember that difficulty in checking for residual can occur as a result of malposition of the tube in the GI tract. For example, if the plunger on the syringe cannot be withdrawn, the end of the tube may be lodged against the stomach wall. If only air can be aspirated, the tube may be curled up in the esophagus or in the stomach above the level of the gastric contents. Attempt to reposition the tube by rotating it, advancing it a few inches, pulling it back slightly, changing the patient's position, or injecting a little air to push the tube away from the stomach wall if this is the problem. Try again to obtain a residual. If nausea or vomiting occurs, discontinue the feeding and notify the physician.

NDx: High risk for diarrhea

Diarrhea is usually the result of feedings that are too rapidly administered, too high in lactose, or incompatible in osmolality. It may also be due to bacterial contamination of the feeding.

Build the patient's tolerance to feedings by initially administering slowly over long periods of time and then gradually increasing the rate and the time between feedings (Fig. 21–13).

Dilute formulas with water if needed for tolerance. This is often necessary at the start of enteral therapy. Hypertonic formulas generally need to be diluted half with water, but even full-strength isotonic feeding may not be tolerated initially by patients who have been ill for a period of time and have become malnourished. Increase diluted formulas to full strength gradually. Do not attempt to increase rate and strength of feeding at the same time. Focus first on developing the patient's tolerance to full-strength formula, because diluted formula is providing fewer calories per ml and therefore the patient is at risk for not receiving adequate daily caloric intake. Be sure to administer all feedings at room temperature because cramping occurs when feedings are too cold.

Protect the patient from diarrhea caused by bacterial contamination of the feeding by careful handwashing before and use of meticulous aseptic technique during handling of equipment. Change the feeding bag and tubing completely every 24 hours. Mark each new set with the patient's name, room number, date, and time so that time for replacement is easily and accurately known. Never let formula hang longer than the time recommended by the manufacturer, and never store formula in the refrigerator for longer than 24 hours. If refillable bags are used, never add new formula to that remaining in the bag; rather, rinse the bag and tubing with warm water, then fill with new formula. Remember that diarrhea can be due to viral disease or change in medication as with any other patient. Report persistent diarrhea.

NDx: High risk for constipation

Patients receiving tube feedings, particularly those on tube feedings for a long time, are at risk for constipation. Guard against this by ensuring adequate fluid intake and exercise when possible. If changes in bowel habits consistent with developing constipation appear, explore with the physician the possibility of switching to a fiber-containing formula.

Additional Interventions

Attempt to unclog a blocked feeding tube by aspirating formula behind the clog. If this is not successful, flush the tube with warm water. Use at least a 30-ml syringe, because anything smaller could build up pressure and rupture the tube.

Prevent clogging of the feeding tube by flushing with 30 ml of water every 3 to 4 hours during continuous feedings and both before and after intermittent or bolus feedings. Do not flush with fruit juice because this merely curdles the formula. Cola is sometimes used to discourage clogging. If this is done, immediately flush with water to remove the stickiness. If formula is thick, squeeze or shake the container at intervals. When administering medications via a feeding tube, request the liquid form when possible. If pills or tablets must be given, crush thoroughly (remember that some medications cannot be safely crushed) and mix with a small amount of water. Pull the mixture up in a syringe and feed it into the tube. Flush the feeding tube with 5 ml of water between each medication and with 25 ml of water when the last medication is given.

When giving medications directly into the jejunum, dilute with 50 to 100 ml of water to prevent mucosal damage. Never give bulk-forming agents via the tube.

Protect against damage to the naris and the oral mucous membranes caused by nasogastric or nasointestinal tube as described previously. If the patient has a gastrostomy or jejunostomy tube, cleanse it daily with hydrogen peroxide, being certain to move outer bumper on PEG or PEJ away from the skin surface. Dry thoroughly, replace bumper if present, and leave exposed to the air. Cover the area with a dressing only immediately following the creation of the ostomy because dressings tend to hold moisture to the skin and thus support maceration and bacterial growth. Change any dressing in use at least once a day and immediately if wet, noting date and time on tape. Never place a dressing under a PEG or PEJ bumper.

If the patient is to go home while still receiving enteral feedings, begin teaching well in advance of discharge. Along with teaching administration of feedings, be certain that the patient and significant others know when to purchase needed supplies and have an identified resource to contact in the event of a problem. Make home health care referrals and referrals to community resources as needed.

Evaluation

Evaluate the effectiveness of nursing care for patients on enteral feedings by comparing the patient's status with the expected patient outcomes. Examples of specific outcomes for patients on enteral feedings have been provided in the Planning section.

TOTAL PARENTERAL NUTRITION (HYPERALIMENTATION)

Total parenteral nutrition (TPN), also called intravenous hyperalimentation (IVH) or simply hyperalimentation, is the intravenous administration of nutrients in amounts needed to produce a state of anabolism. It is used when the individual's nutritional needs cannot be met satisfactorily through the gastrointestinal tract. Thus, it is used in a wide variety of clinical conditions such as inflammatory bowel disease, pancreatitis, trauma, large burns, or acute renal failure and following extensive bowel surgery.

SOLUTIONS

Basic components of solutions are synthetic, highly usable essential and nonessential amino acids, large amounts of dextrose to provide protein-sparing calories, electrolytes, vitamins, minerals, and trace elements. To some degree, these components can be modified to meet the needs of individual patients. For example, additional sodium or potassium may be added; insulin may be added; or in the case of patients with renal failure, all protein may be in the form of essential amino acids.

ADMINISTRATION

Because solutions are highly concentrated and hypertonic, they must be administered into a wide-diameter vessel with a rapid blood flow so that they are diluted quickly before they can cause sclerosis of the vessel. Thus, the only veins into which the catheter tip can be safely placed are the innominate, the intrathoracic subclavian, and the superior vena cava, with the middle of the superior vena cava being the most ideal site.

The insertion of the catheter for TPN is most often through the subclavian or internal jugular vein. It is done at the bedside but involves strict surgical asepsis. During insertion of the inside-the-needle catheter, when the needle is open to the air and while the catheter is being threaded into position, the patient is instructed to take a deep breath, hold it, and bear down slightly. This Valsalva maneuver increases central venous pressure and thus protects against air emoblism. Once the catheter is in place, the needle is withdrawn and covered with a plastic guard to prevent inadvertent puncture of the catheter. A single suture anchors the catheter at the insertion site to prevent accidental dislodgement or back-and-forth movement, which could contaminate the wound with microorganisms from the skin. A dressing is applied, and a chest x-ray film is taken immediately at the bedside to confirm accurate placement of the catheter. An isotonic intravenous solution is run at a rate sufficient to keep the catheter open until placement is verified, and then the infusion is begun.

COMPLICATIONS

Complications of TPN fall into two categories: those associated with catheter insertion and those related to ongoing infusion.

Major complications of insertion include pneumothorax due to accidental pleural puncture, hemothorax due to damage to the subclavian or nearby vessels, and hydrothorax due to the catheter's passing through the vein, resulting in the infusion of solution into the chest. Symptoms of these complications are sharp chest pain and decreased breath sounds. Treatment varies with the severity of the condition, and in some cases insertion of a chest tube may be necessary.

Inadvertent arterial puncture can also occur during catheter insertion. If not noted at the time of occurrence, symptoms that develop include a rapidly expanding hematoma, signs and symptoms of tracheal compression, and respiratory distress. Treatment consists of direct pressure on the artery for a minimum of 5 minutes.

Major complications of ongoing TPN are infection, hyperglycemia, and hypoglycemia. Infection, the most dreaded complication because it can lead to sepsis, can occur because of in-line contamination or can be caused by the migration of organisms along the catheter from the insertion site. Infection typically presents as a low-grade fever of several days' duration, which then becomes a high fever. In some cases, however, glycosuria or a dramatic spike in temperature may be the first symptom to develop. Whenever fever occurs, a history and physical examination are done, and cultures not only of the invasive line site but of urine, sputum, feces, and any wound drainage are obtained. When the temperature has spiked suddenly, the intravenous lines are changed, new solution hung, and the discontinued materials sent for culture. Removal of the catheter itself may be necessary to prevent sepsis.

Glucose imbalance is the most common metabolic complication of TPN. Hyperglycemia occurs when the glucose load in the TPN solution exceeds the body's ability to metabolize it. Symptoms include nausea, weakness, excessive thirst, excessive urination, and headache. This may be a transient state at the beginning of TPN because of the fact that the beta cells of the pancreas are not yet producing the increased amount of insulin demanded by the glucose load. When this is the case, treatment simply consists of slowing the rate of infusion to give the pancreas time to adjust. At other times, hyperglycemia may be due to actual compromised glucose tolerance caused by factors such as old age, diabetes, stress, shock, sepsis, hepatic or renal failure, starvation, and medication such as particular diuretics and tranquilizers. In these cases, exogenous insulin is added to the TPN solution. It is administered in this way to achieve a more constant serum level than is possible with intermittent, subcutaneous injections.

Progressive hyperglycemia can result in osmotic diuresis with dehydration and electrolyte imbalance, which can lead to coma and death.

Hypoglycemia can result from the body's overproduction of insulin in response to the increased glucose load or from sudden interruption of therapy. It occurs because serum insulin levels stay high for a period of time after serum glucose drops. The infusion can be interrupted accidentally because of the tubing's becoming kinked or bent as the patient changes position. The symptoms of hypoglycemia are weakness, headache, chills, tingling in the mouth or extremities, thirst, hunger, diaphoresis, and apprehension.

Air embolism is a potential complication of TPN therapy because it can occur whenever the central venous system is open to air. Thus, there is a risk of air embolism during insertion, during tubing changes, during infusion if an accidental disconnection of the line occurs, and through the track left after removal of the catheter. To protect against air embolism, the patient is positioned in a Trendelenburg or flat position and asked to perform the Valsalva maneuver whenever the catheter is to be open to the air. In addition, all junctures in the line are taped, and when the catheter is removed, an airtight dressing is immediately put in place and left for 48 hours to allow full closure of the track.

If an embolism does occur, symptoms, which vary with its severity, include dyspnea, apnea, hypoxia, disorientation, tachycardia, hypotension, and precordial murmur. The immediate treatment is to place the patient on the left side, with the feet higher than the head. This is done to trap air in the right atrium, from where it can be removed by direct intracardiac aspiration if necessary.

Application of the Nursing Process to the Care of the Patient Receiving Total Parenteral Nutrition

Assessment

Assess the patient's baseline condition prior to the start of TPN. Review the patient's medical history and determine current status in relationship to symptoms and treatment of the problem underlying the need for TPN. Note patient's weight and observe for signs of nutritional deficiency and fluid and electrolyte imbalance.

Assess the patient's understanding of TPN therapy and level of anxiety regarding it.

Once TPN is begun, assess for signs of complications. Immediately following catheter insertion, assess for sharp chest pain and decreased breath sounds, which can indicate pneumothorax, hemothorax, or hydrothorax. Observe also for signs of a rapidly expanding hematoma, tracheal compression, and respiratory distress, which may indicate accidental arterial puncture.

Assess for infection. Check temperature every 4 hours and observe for malaise. When changing the dressing, assess the insertion site for erythema, edema, skin ulceration, and drainage. Make ongoing assessments of fluid and electrolyte status and acid-base balance. Be alert to signs of vitamin and trace element deficiency or toxicity.

Assess carefully for signs of glucose imbalance because this is the most common metabolic complication. Check serum glucose daily.

Observe for diuresis, dry skin, and thirst, which may indicate hyperglycemia. Also observe for weakness, diaphoresis, and pallor, which may indicate hypoglycemia.

Assess for therapeutic responses to TPN therapy. Weigh the patient daily. Review laboratory data, and watch for signs of improved healing.

Nursing Diagnoses and Planning

Nursing diagnoses and related expected patient outcomes most commonly applicable to patients receiving TPN include the following:

NDx: Anxiety related to the TPN procedure

Planning: Patient outcomes
1. Patient describes the procedures involved with TPN.
2. Patient attends to instructions.
3. Patient states anxiety is under control.
4. Overt signs of excessive anxiety are absent.

NDx: Altered nutrition: less than body requirements related to inability to take in needed amounts of nutrients via the GI tract

Planning: Patient outcomes
1. Patient is in positive nitrogen balance.
2. Patient gains *(specify amount)* of weight per week.

NDx: High risk for infection related to in-line contamination or migration of organisms along the catheter from the insertion site

Planning: Patient outcomes
1. Patient is afebrile.
2. Insertion site is free of erythema, edema, and drainage.
3. Skin around insertion site is intact.

Nursing Interventions

NDx: Anxiety

Prepare the patient for what to expect during the insertion of the catheter. Tell the patient that the physician will wear a mask, gown, and gloves and that other persons at the head of the bed will wear masks to guard against infection. Explain that the Trendelenburg position is used to distend the vein and facilitate positioning of the catheter. Tell the patient that a small towel roll will be placed under the back to hyperextend the neck and raise the collar bone and that the face will be turned to the side and loosely covered but that there will be no difficulty breathing or seeing. Describe the preparation that is done with acetone, iodine, and alcohol to cleanse the skin of microorganisms. Explain that a local anesthetic will be given to numb the shoulder and that it can feel like a bee sting until it starts to work. Tell the patient to expect a strange feeling of pressure or even pain within the chest as the catheter is introduced, and stress that this is a normal occurrence. Show the patient the tubing and point out how thin it is. Reassure the patient that removal of the catheter is a quick, simple, painless procedure, not anything like the insertion procedure.

If the patient is highly anxious despite explanation and reassurance, indicate this to the physician and suggest an order for an antianxiety agent.

Following insertion of the catheter, keep the patient informed about his or her care and progress. For example, explain that the chest x-ray film taken after insertion is standard procedure to check catheter placement and not an indication that a problem has occurred. Similarly explain the dressing and tubing change procedures and inform the patient of positive responses to therapy such as weight gain or signs of improved healing.

NDx: Altered nutrition: less than body requirements

Administer TPN solutions according to physician's orders. Check labels on all solution containers carefully for accuracy. Maintain a constant rate of infusion around the clock, keeping in mind that initially solution is infused slowly at a rate of 60 to 80 ml/hour for the average adult. The rate is then increased by 25 ml/hour/day to allow time for the pancreatic beta cells to increase the production of insulin to meet the need created by the TPN solution. Use a mechanical controller or pump. Check the rate every 30 minutes and reset as necessary. Remember that too rapid administration can cause a hyperglycemic reaction or even hyperosmotic, nonketotic coma. Never adjust rate to compensate for past increases or decreases. Mark the container in hourly amounts to aid in assessing the accuracy of the flow rate.

Maintain accurate fluid intake and output records, and weigh the patient daily at the same time, on the same scale, and in the same clothing.

NDx: High risk for infection

Infection as a complication of TPN may be caused by in-line contamination or by migration of organisms along the catheter from the site of insertion. Guard against in-line contamination by keeping all prepared TPN solutions refrigerated until used. When hanging a new container, examine it carefully for cracks or small punctures. Also inspect the solution against a bright light to check for turbidity or particulate matter, which can indicate bacterial contamination. Change IV tubing and filters every 24 hours using strict aseptic technique. Do this at the same time the solution container is changed because each time the line is disconnected there is a risk of contamination. Do not use the TPN line for central venous pressure monitoring, drawing blood, or administering medications.

Decrease the risk of infection originating at the site of insertion by meticulous cleansing and dressing of the area while maintaining strict aseptic technique. This is so important in the prevention of sepsis that some agencies have a special team responsible for maintaining catheter dressings and others require staff nurses to be "certified" before assuming this responsibility. Such certification typically consists of an in-service program, assigned readings, demonstration, and satisfactory performance of a supervised dressing change. Although precise protocols for dressing changes vary somewhat in different agencies, most are based on the technique developed by Grant and Dudrick, outlined here.

Change the dressing over the catheter insertion site every 48 hours or three times per week and whenever wet or contaminated. If the airtight seal of the dressing is broken, do not reinforce the dressing —change it.

Using sterile gloves and a sterile clamp to hold the swabs, scrub the catheter site with acetone to defat the skin. Scrub until the sponges come away clean. Follow with tincture of iodine, which has an antifungal and antibacterial effect. Apply a full 2 minutes, allow to air dry, and then use alcohol to remove the iodine because it can cause irritation or burning if left on the skin. Again air dry—do not fan or blow. Throughout this procedure, be certain to work in concentric circles going from clean to dirty areas (i.e., from the site of insertion outward). Also be certain to clean the catheter and all its parts. After cleansing, apply a topical antimicrobial ointment to the insertion site and cover with two small gauze sponges. Spray tincture of benzoin on exposed skin to protect against breakdown and cover with an occlusive dressing, being certain not to touch the side of the dressing being placed against the patient's skin. Place a slit piece of tape under the catheter for occlusion while allowing easy access for tubing changes. Seal all edges of the dressing with tape. Also tape all tubing junctions to protect against accidental separation. Anchor the filter to the dressing to eliminate pull on the insertion site (Fig. 21–14). If keeping the dressing dry is a problem, cover with a plastic drape or use a dressing such as Op-Site, a thin transparent waterproof dressing that allows vapor to escape while maintaining sterility.

Monitor condition of the insertion site with each dressing change. Notify the physician if drainage or skin irritation is noted, and obtain cultures as ordered.

Take the patient's temperature every 6 hours and report an increase to the physician. Keep in mind that certain drugs and disease states inhibit the fever response, so although a temperature of higher than 37.7°C (100°F) orally should always be reported, judge each patient individually. If a sudden high temperature elevation occurs, culture and change the IV tubing and hang new solution immediately. If new solution is unavailable, hang 20% dextrose with insulin if ordered.

Additional Interventions

Keep the patient lying flat when changing the tubing. Also instruct him or her to perform a Valsalva maneuver when the catheter is open to the air to further protect against an air embolism.

Evaluation

Evaluate the effectiveness of nursing care for a patient receiving TPN by comparing the patient's status with the expected patient outcomes. Examples of specific outcomes for patients receiving TPN have been provided in the Planning section.

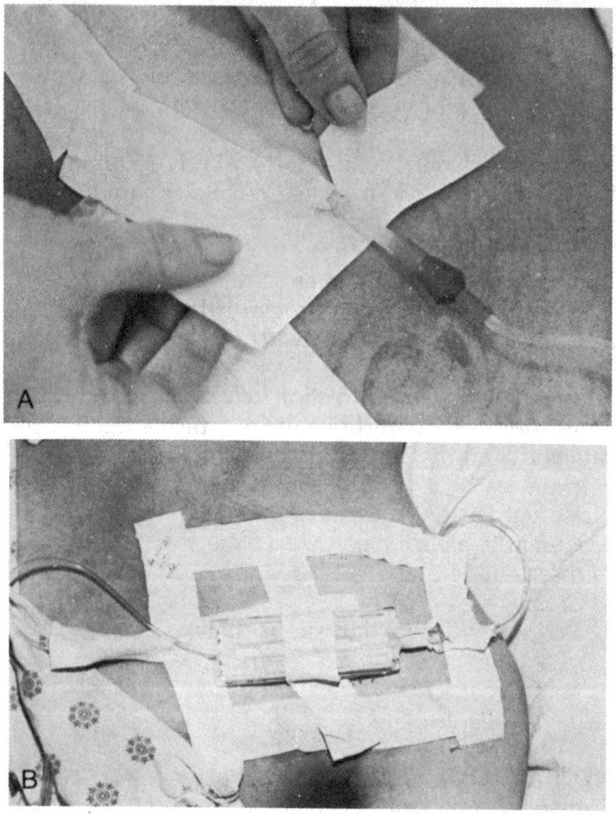

Figure 21–14.

Method of dressing the exit site of a TPN catheter. *A*, A slit piece of tape is placed under the catheter and along all edges of the dressing to ensure air occlusion. *B*, All tubing junctions are sealed with tape, and the filter is anchored to the dressing to prevent pull. (Reprinted with permission from Plumer AL. Principles and practice of intravenous therapy. 4th ed. New York: Little, Brown, 1987, pp 401, 402.)

INTRAVENOUS LIPIDS

Fats are needed to prevent or treat essential fatty acid deficiency (EFAD), which is characterized by poor wound healing; dry, scaling skin; thin hair; thrombocytopenia; and liver function changes. Fat is also a major source of calories, generating 9 kcal/g, as opposed to the 4 kcal/g from carbohydrates.

Fats may be given alone or simultaneously with the basic TPN solution through a Y-connector just proximal to the catheter hub.

If fat is used as a major source of calories, the amount of glucose in the TPN solution is decreased, and administration through a peripheral vein is possible, although a pump must be used if the solution is still hypertonic. Ten percent fat emulsions are isotonic and can also be administered via a peripheral vein.

When administering lipids, do not keep the solution refrigerated; but before hanging the bag, do examine the emulsion carefully for signs of separation or an oily appearance. Check recommendations for type of tubing to be used, because conventional tubing contains a plasticizer that can be extracted by fat-containing fluids unless specifically stated to the contrary on the package insert. Add nothing to fat solutions because the stability of the emulsion may be disturbed.

Do not use a filter, because it clogs or disturbs the emulsion. Never store or reuse a partially used container, and never leave a container hanging for longer than 12 hours.

Maintain flow rate strictly within the manufacturer's guidelines, remembering that initial rate is very slow and the patient must be observed for adverse reactions. These include nausea and vomiting, headache, flushing, perspiration, insomnia, vertigo, chills, and fever. Never exceed the maximum daily dose.

Necessary fats may also be provided through use of a total nutrient admixture that contains carbohydrates, proteins, and fats in a single solution.

HOME TOTAL PARENTERAL NUTRITION

Many patients who require TPN over long periods are now taught to administer the solution at home. Some are even able to tolerate cyclic rather than continuous feedings. When this is the case, the solution is generally run at night, leaving the patient free during the day to carry on with usual lifestyle activities. Home total parenteral nutrition (HTPN) is administered either through a long catheter tunneled subcutaneously to an exit point easily accessible to the patient (Fig. 21–15) or through an implantable infusion device.

The two basic catheters used for home TPN are the Broviac catheter, which has a narrow lumen, and the Hickman, which has a larger bore size through which blood can be withdrawn or medications administered. Newer catheters, double- and triple-lumen, represent the fusion of the two and have the advantage of allowing one port and line to be maintained for administration of TPN solution only. These long catheters are generally inserted with the patient under general anesthesia. Then either continuous or cyclic infusion via volumetric pump is immediately begun. Volumetric pumps must be used to maintain flow because of the long length and small diameter of these catheters. The pump used must be a low-pressure one to guard against rupture of the catheter and resultant embolism and contamination.

Gastrointestinal Surgery

Abdominal Incisions. Laparotomy is a term used to refer to the surgical opening of the abdomen. Of the many types of incisions that can be used to open the abdomen, the specific one used depends on the organ or area to be operated on, the type of procedure to be done, the ease of entry, ease of making the incision larger if the need occurs, ease of closure, and postoperative wound strength. Table 21–5 describes and illustrates common abdominal incisions.

Complications. Patients having surgery of the GI tract are at risk for a number of complications. These include infection, wound dehiscence, paralytic ileus, atelectasis, and urinary retention.

Infection. For some unknown reason, the abdominal wall is particularly susceptible to infection. In addition, the GI tract is not sterile, so when the lumen is opened, organisms can spill into the abdomen. Infection is a greater risk with intestinal surgery than with gastric surgery because fewer microorganisms are found in the acid environment of the stomach.

Wound Dehiscence. Abdominal suture lines are subjected to stress from breathing, coughing, and straining during movement or at the time of defecation. This stress predisposes to dehiscence. To help prevent dehiscence as well as to protect against impaired blood clotting and impaired liver tolerance to anesthesia, the patient's fluid, electrolyte, and nutritional status is carefully assessed preoperatively, and measures are instituted to correct any imbalances or deficiencies. Adequate protein and vitamin C are particularly important to support wound healing. A nasogastric tube is used postoperatively to prevent distention, which also creates stress on the suture line and can contribute to dehiscence.

Ileus. Handling of the GI tract along with the effects of preoperative medications and anesthesia results in some degree of paralytic ileus (impaired movement of intestinal contents through the intestine owing to reduced or absent peristalsis) in almost all patients. For this reason, all patients are placed on NPO status until peristalsis returns, as indicated by the presence of normal bowel sounds and the passage of flatus.

Atelectasis. Because breathing is difficult and painful, particularly with an upper abdominal incision, shallow respirations and chest splinting may occur. Secretions may pool in the lungs, bronchi can

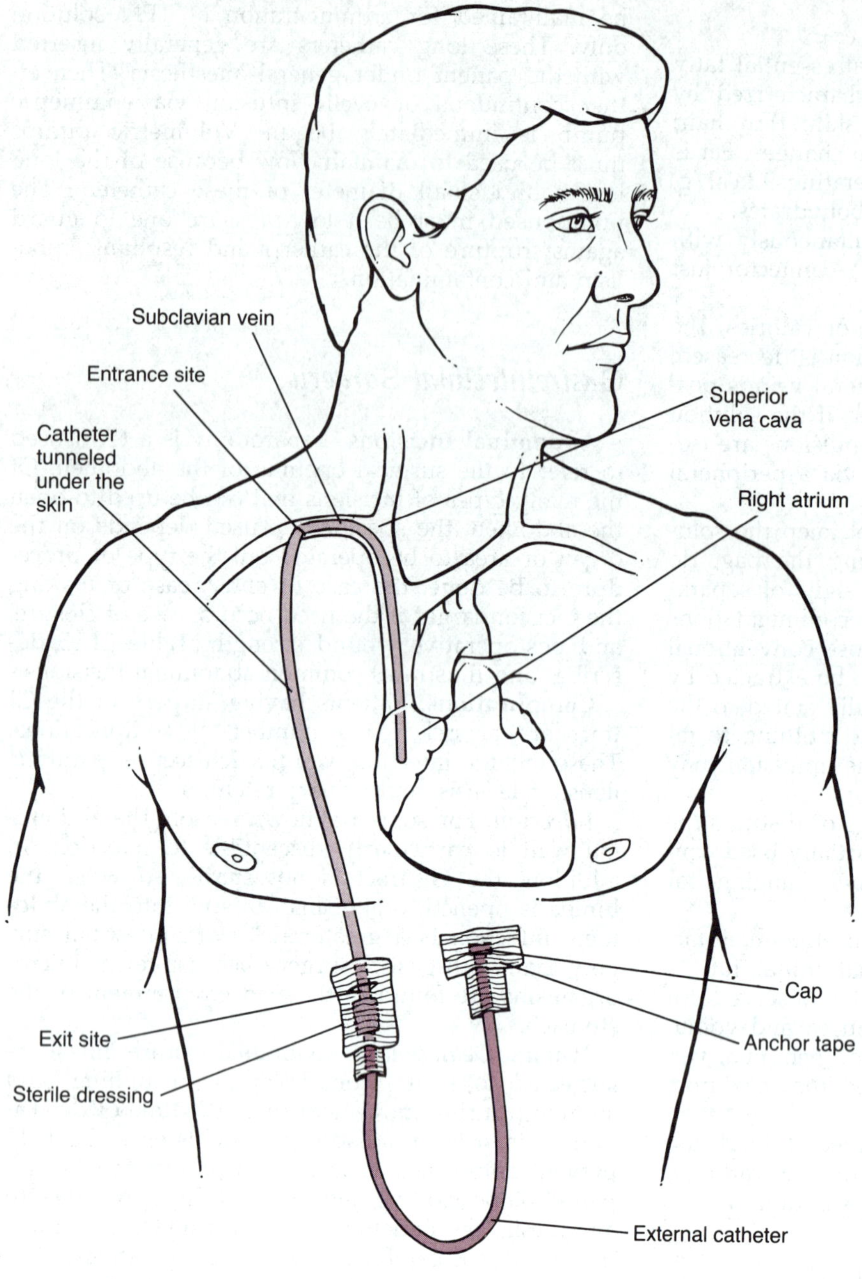

Figure 21–15.

Placement of a long tunneled tube for TPN therapy.

be clogged with mucus, and atelectasis and pneumonia can result.

Urinary Retention. The pain of an abdominal incision along with the effects of medications and anesthesia can result in the inability to empty the urinary bladder.

GASTRECTOMY

Gastrectomy refers to the surgical excision of the stomach. In a total gastrectomy, the entire stomach is removed, and the esophagus is sutured to either the duodenum or the jejunum (Fig. 21–16). In a subtotal gastrectomy, a part of the stomach is removed.

Uses. Total or subtotal gastrectomy is done to remove benign or malignant tumors of the stomach or to remove a chronic peptic ulcer. It may also be performed to stop hemorrhage from a perforating ulcer.

Procedure. Two procedures involving a subtotal gastrectomy are the Billroth I and the Billroth II (Fig. 21–17). In the Billroth I procedure, the pyloric portion of the stomach is removed and the remaining stomach is anastomosed to the duodenum (gastroduodenostomy) (Fig. 21–17*B*). In a Billroth II procedure, the pylorus is removed, the proximal end of the duodenum is sutured closed, and the remaining portion of the stomach is anastomosed to the jejunum (gastrojejunostomy) (Fig. 21–17*C*). The Billroth II is preferable in the treatment of duodenal ulcers because it reduces the chances of reulceration.

Text continued on page 897

Table 21–5. COMMON ABDOMINAL INCISIONS

INCISION	DIAGRAM	PRIMARY USES	COMMENTS
Upper midline	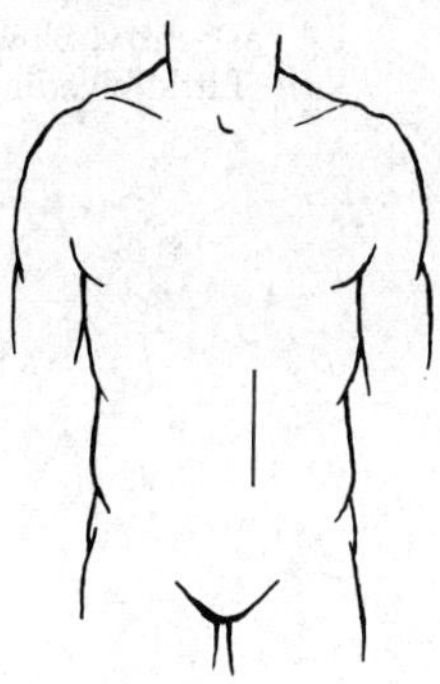	Gastrectomy	Simple, fast, good exposure of upper abdomen. Wound weak. High incidence of dehiscence.
Lower midline	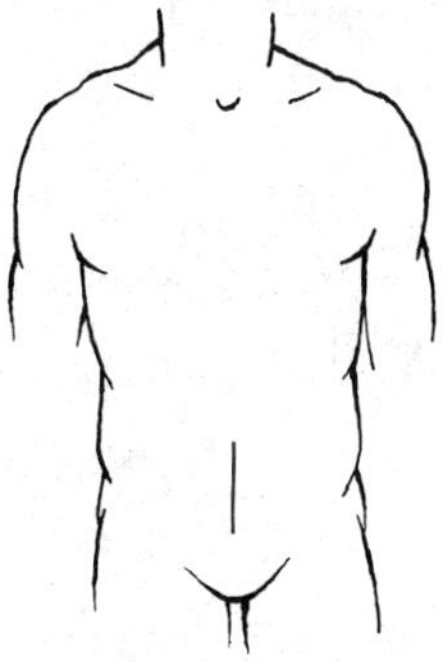	Genitourologic procedures	Simple, fast, good exposure of sigmoid colon and other pelvic organs. High incidence of dehiscence.
Upper paramedian (upper rectus) Right	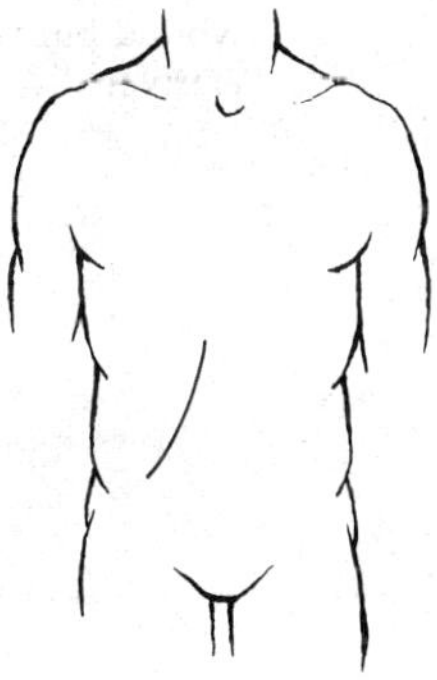	Biliary surgery	Fast entry, slow but strong closure. Little bleeding. No nerve injury.
Left	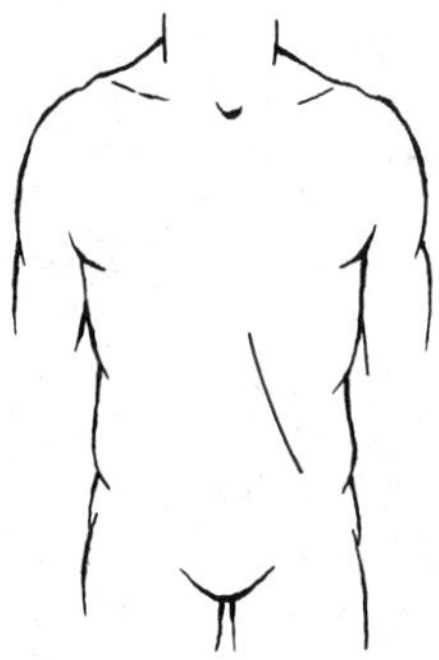	Gastrectomy Vagectomy Repair of hiatus hernia	

(continued)

Table 21–5. (continued) COMMON ABDOMINAL INCISIONS

INCISION	DIAGRAM	PRIMARY USES	COMMENTS
Lower paramedian (lower rectus) Right	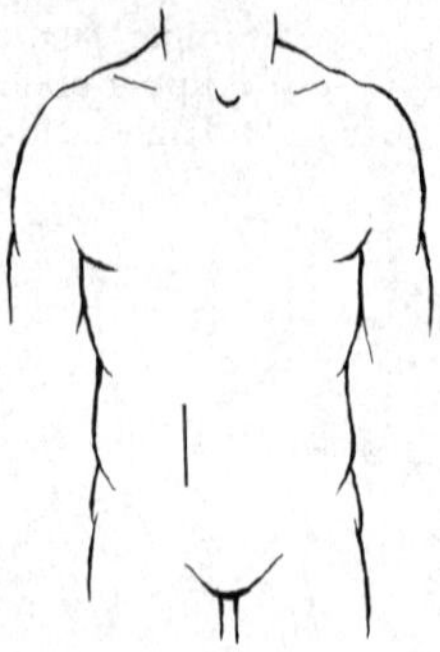	Appendectomy Small bowel resection	Fast entry. Slow but strong closure. Little bleeding. No nerve injury.
Left	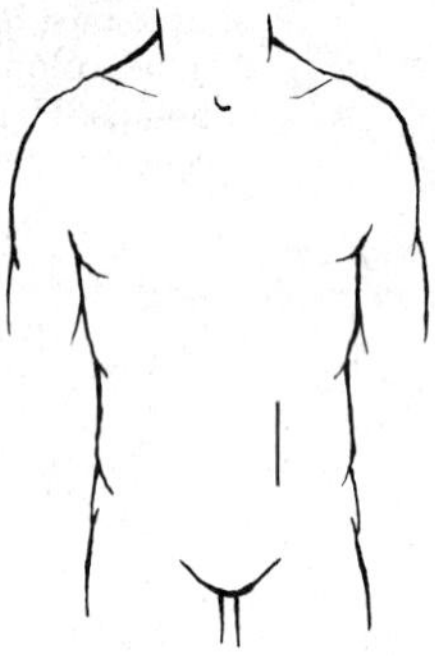	Sigmoid colon surgery	
Subcostal			Oblique incision. Very strong wound but very painful postoperatively.
Right	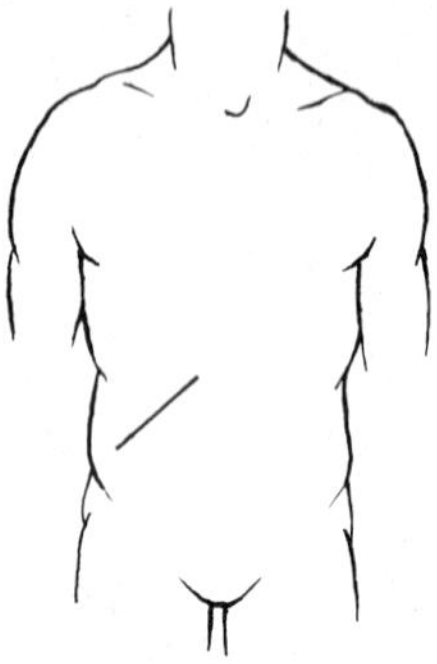	Biliary surgery	
Left	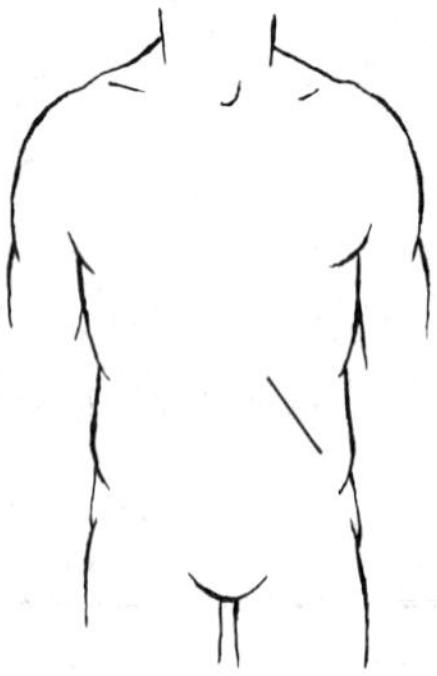	Operations on spleen and pancreas	

(continued)

Table 21–5. *(continued)* COMMON ABDOMINAL INCISIONS

INCISION	DIAGRAM	PRIMARY USES	COMMENTS
Gridiron (McBurney)	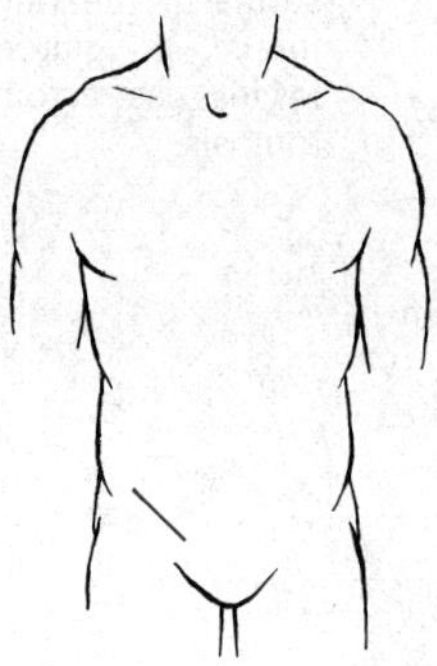	Appendectomy	
Upper transverse	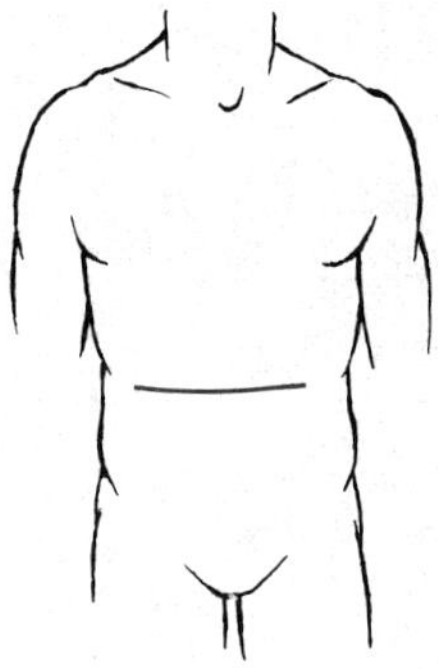	Transverse colostomy or colon resection pancreatic procedures	
Pfannenstiel	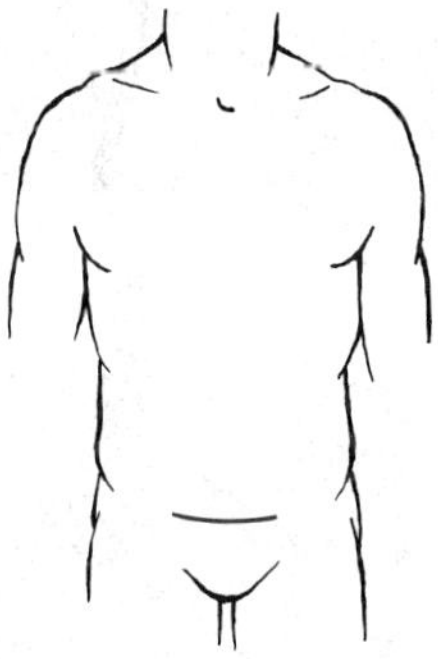	Gynecologic procedures	

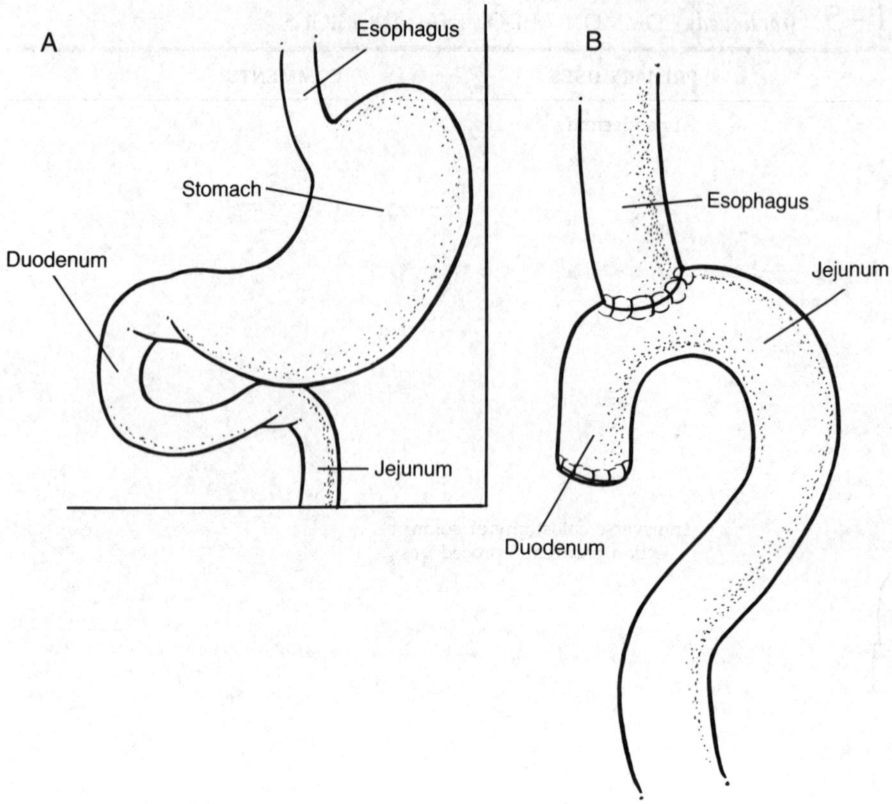

Figure 21–16.

Total gastrectomy. *A*, Normal anatomic relationship of the esophagus, the stomach, the duodenum, and the jejunum. *B*, Anatomic relationships following gastrectomy with jejunal anastomosis.

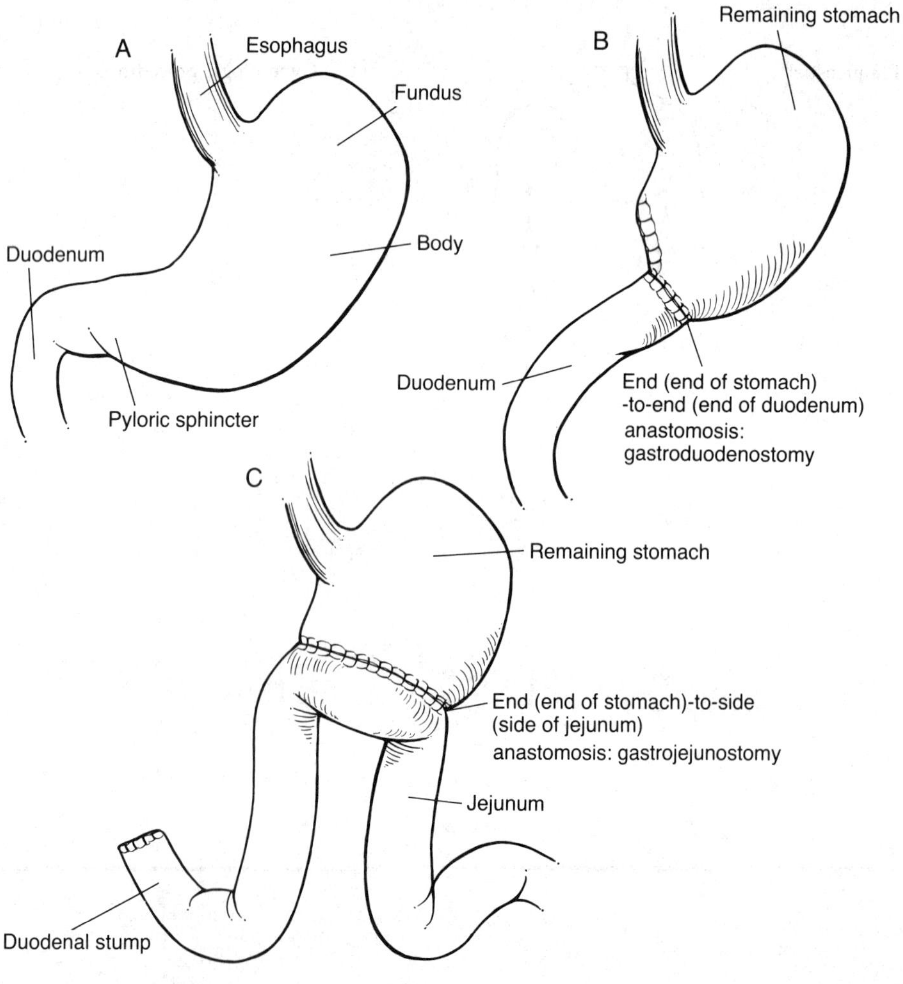

Figure 21–17.

Subtotal gastrectomy procedures. *A*, Normal stomach and small intestine. *B*, Billroth I procedure. *C*, Billroth II procedure.

Table 21–6. COMPLICATIONS OF GASTRECTOMY

COMPLICATION	CAUSE	SYMPTOMS	TREATMENT
Hemorrhage			
Early	Splenic injury Slipped ligature	Persistent bloody drainage from nasogastric tube	Saline gastric lavage Blood replacement Reoperation
7th to 10th day	Sloughing at anastomosis	Recurrence of bloody gastric drainage	Cool saline lavage
Acute gastric dilation	Swallowed air distends stomach, stimulating gastric secretions, which can lead to dehydration and a fall in plasma volume	Epigastric pain, feeling of fullness, hiccoughs, gagging, tachycardia, and hypertension	Nasogastric suction Fluid replacement to restore plasma volume
Alkaline reflux gastritis	Reflux of intestinal contents including bile salts injures gastric mucosal barrier	Persistent pain and epigastric "burning" that is worse after meals; nausea and vomiting	Semi-Fowler's position Antacid or histamine blocker therapy
Dumping syndrome	Rapid entry of large amounts of hypertonic chyme into the small intestine causes fluid to move into bowel lumen, decreasing plasma volume and causing vasomotor symptoms. Resultant distention of intestine causes GI symptoms.	Tachycardia, palpitations, fainting, hypertension, flushing, diaphoresis, bloating, cramping, diarrhea, and nausea occurring with eating 1–3 weeks postoperatively Disappears in 1 hour Usually resolves in 3–6 months postoperatively	Avoid drinking fluid with meals. Eat six small meals per day of dry foods. Avoid concentrated carbohydrates. Lie down for 30 to 60 minutes after eating. Avoid very hot and very cold food. Anticholinergic drugs taken 30 minutes before eating.
Postprandial hypoglycemia	Increased insulin release following carbohydrate ingestion	Weakness, faintness, perspiration, hunger, nausea, anxiety, tremors, and palpitations occurring 2 to 3 hours after eating	Ingestion of sugar or hard candy relieves symptoms. More frequent meals low in sugar prevent attacks
Impaired absorption of iron	Deficiency of gastric acid, which is needed to increase solubility of iron for absorption to occur	Anemia	Iron taken orally, with recumbent position after ingestion to promote absorption
Impaired vitamin B_{12} absorption	Lack of intrinsic factor caused by atrophy of gastric mucosa	Pernicious anemia	Parenteral administration of vitamin B_{12}
Impaired calcium absorption	Deficiency of gastric acid, which is needed to increase solubility of calcium for absorption to occur	Osteoporosis	
General nutritional deficiency	Reduced capacity of stomach causes a feeling of satiation after ingesting small amounts of food Malabsorption from decreased gastric acid or pancreatic enzymes	Failure to gain or maintain weight	Small meals 6 times per day

Physical Preparation of the Patient. Fluid and electrolytes are given as needed to make up for deficiencies caused by the underlying disease and losses from preoperative tests. In some cases, TPN is used for protein replacement and vitamins K and C are administered to promote clotting and wound healing. The patient is usually on a fluid diet for 24 hours and then is placed on NPO status after midnight prior to surgery. The abdomen is prepared from nipple line to symphysis pubis.

Postoperative Course. The patient remains on NPO status and is maintained on intravenous fluids until bowel sounds return and the nasogastric tube, which is inserted to remove secretions and prevent distention and vomiting, is removed. Oral intake is then begun, usually with sips of warm tea because cold liquids tend to cause distress. Intake is very gradually increased until the patient is eating six small, bland meals per day and drinking 120 ml of fluid in between.

On the evening of surgery, the patient is gotten out of bed and is progressively ambulated.

See Table 21–6 for potential complications of gastrectomy, as well as their causes, symptoms, and treatment.

Application of the Nursing Process to the Care of the Patient Having a Gastrectomy

PREOPERATIVE NURSING CARE

Assessment

Question the patient about symptoms related to the underlying disease process (e.g., nausea, vomiting, heartburn, anorexia, bleeding), and determine whether they affect immediate care needs. Assess nutritional status. Review the patient's usual dietary patterns, and ask about any weight loss. Examine for signs of dehydration, and review laboratory data such as serum electrolyte and serum albumin levels, which are indicative of nutritional status.

Explore the patient's understanding of the disease and the planned surgery. Be alert to signs of excessive anxiety or ineffective coping.

Nursing Diagnoses and Planning

Nursing diagnoses and related expected patient outcomes most commonly applicable to patients scheduled for a gastrectomy include the following:

NDx: Anxiety related to anesthesia and surgery

Planning: Patient outcomes
1. Patient practices relaxation as instructed.
2. Patient reports feeling more relaxed.
3. Patient expresses an optimistic view about the surgical outcome.
4. Patient rests quietly.

NDx: Knowledge deficit: preoperative preparation, postoperative course

Planning: Patient outcomes
1. Patient describes preoperative preparation.
2. Patient describes usual postoperative procedures and course.
3. Patient describes importance of coughing, deep breathing, and leg exercises in the prevention of complications.
4. Patient demonstrates coughing and deep breathing.
5. Patient demonstrates postoperative leg exercises.

Nursing Interventions

NDx: Anxiety
Reassure the patient that some anxiety prior to surgery is normal and in fact helps prepare the body for the stress and promotes recovery. Offer reassurance about the success of surgery, as appropriate. Depending on the individual situation, you might reassure the patient about his or her general state of health and therefore fitness for surgery, mention the frequency of the procedure and its success rate, or describe the professionals who participate in surgery, noting their roles in protecting the patient and their competency. Keep in mind that many times the patient's concerns stem from misconceptions about normal anatomy and physiology, so the patient may be unable or too embarrassed to ask questions.

Review relaxation techniques with the patient, or provide the patient with a relaxation tape and orient the patient to its use. Maintain a quiet, calm environment and administer sedatives as ordered.

NDx: Knowledge deficit: preoperative preparation, postoperative course
Review preoperative events with the patient. Explain that many tests, including a physical examination, x-ray examinations, and blood tests, will be done to determine general state of health and identify any problems that need special consideration. Reassure the patient that the specific nature and purpose of each test will be explained before it is done.

Describe the preoperative preparation. Explain that it is important that the GI tract be empty when the operation is done, so only liquids will be allowed for 24 hours before surgery and a bowel preparation will be given the day before surgery to clean out the large bowel. Explain that the abdomen will be shaved and scrubbed from nipple line to symphysis pubis to remove as many bacteria as possible but that the incision will be much smaller than the area prepared. (If the patient is to receive IV fluids or hyperalimentation therapy to make up nutritional deficiencies before surgery, describe these to the patient. Also explain if a nasogastric tube is to be inserted prior to surgery to empty the stomach, as in cases of pyloric obstruction.)

Prepare the patient for postoperative events. Inform the patient of the following:

There will be a tube going from the stomach out through the nose to drain stomach secretions into a bottle on the wall and that the drainage may be red initially. Explain that because the purpose of the tube is to keep the stomach empty to promote healing of the suture line, no foods or fluids will be given by mouth for the several days that the tube is in place. Assure that the tube does not cause pain, although the nostrils may feel a bit sore and the mouth dry, symptoms which will be eased by salves and mouth rinses.

Intravenous fluids will be given until peristalsis returns, the nasogastric tube is removed, and oral intake is reestablished.

Oral intake will begin with clear fluids once bowel function has returned, as indicated by the presence of bowel sounds and passage of flatus. Full fluids and then bland foods will be added as tolerated. Eating patterns will be altered and return to former eating habits will be slow if in fact they can be completely resumed.

Evaluation

Evaluate the effectiveness of nursing care for a patient scheduled for a gastrectomy by comparing the patient's status with the expected patient outcomes. Examples of specific outcomes for patients scheduled for a gastrectomy have been provided in the Planning section.

POSTOPERATIVE NURSING CARE

Assessment

Monitor and record vital signs every 4 hours or more frequently if necessitated by the patient's condition, and assess for pain. Check the dressing for drainage, and inspect the suture line for signs of infection and dehiscence.

Check the patency of the nasogastric tube, and observe and record the amount and character of the drainage from it. Normally, drainage is bloody for 24 hours postoperatively and then changes to brown-tinged and then to yellow or clear. Remember that if a total gastrectomy has been done, gastric drainage is less than that with a subtotal gastrectomy because the stomach is no longer present to produce secretions or to hold them and that the amount of secretions decreases as peristalsis returns.

Note odor of gastric aspirate, because a fecal smell can indicate regurgitation of large intestine contents into the operative area.

Auscultate for bowel sounds and question the patient about passage of flatus to determine when peristalsis has resumed and oral intake may be begun. Measure abdominal girth to detect development of distention.

Once bowel function has returned and oral intake is resumed, assess tolerance of food and fluids. Note nausea, vomiting, diarrhea, and other signs of dumping syndrome. Record all intake and output and assess overall nutritional status, because the reduced size and functional capacity of the stomach can cause decreased appetite and difficulty gaining weight.

Nursing Diagnoses and Planning

Nursing diagnoses and related expected patient outcomes most commonly applicable to patients who have had a gastrectomy include the following:

NDx: Pain related to trauma from surgery and irritation of the nostril by the nasogastric tube

Planning: Patient outcomes
1. Patient moves without loud moans, complaints of severe pain, or signs of severe pain such as pallor and tachycardia.
2. Patient states abdominal pain is relieved.
3. Patient appears relaxed (e.g., lips are not pressed together, face does not appear drawn).
4. Patient denies nostril discomfort.

NDx: High risk for ineffective airway clearance related to shallow breathing secondary to diaphragmatic splinting accompanying upper abdominal surgery

Planning: Patient outcomes
1. Patient moves, coughs, and breathes deeply as directed.
2. Lung sounds are clear on auscultation.

NDx: High risk for trauma (internal suture line) related to gastric distention, vomiting, or movement of the nasogastric tube

Planning: Patient outcomes
1. Patient is afebrile.
2. Abdomen is soft.
3. Patient states pain is decreasing.

NDx: High risk for altered oral mucous membrane related to mouth breathing and NPO status

Planning: Patient outcomes
1. Oral mucous membrane is pink and moist.
2. Lips are free of cracks.
3. Patient reports mouth and lips feel soft and supple.

NDx: High risk for infection related to contamination of the abdominal wound

Planning: Patient outcomes
1. Wound is odorless and free of purulent drainage.
2. Wound edges are approximated.

NDx: Altered nutrition: less than body requirements related to postoperative dietary restrictions, early satiety, or dumping syndrome

Planning: Patient outcomes
1. Patient ingests a nutritionally balanced diet.
2. Patient achieves and maintains recommended weight.

NDx: High risk for altered health maintenance related to insufficient knowledge of need for follow-up care

Planning: Patient outcomes
1. Patient lists symptoms to be reported to the physician.
2. Patient states when to return for follow-up.

Nursing Interventions

NDx: Pain

Administer pain medication as ordered. Keep the head of the bed elevated to decrease pull on the incision. Splint the incision with a pillow when the patient is turning, coughing, or deep breathing. Apply a binder as ordered to support incision when the patient is moving.

Encourage the patient to relax. Play soft music, and prompt the patient to concentrate on slow, even breathing or contemplate a calm, pleasant scene permeated by a relaxing color.

Clean the nostril through which the nasogastric tube passes with applicators dipped in water and apply water-soluble lubricant.

NDx: High risk for ineffective airway clearance

Have the patient turn, cough, and breathe deeply every 2 hours while on bed rest. Splint incision to decrease pain when the patient is turning, coughing, and deep breathing. Ambulate patient as ordered.

NDx: High risk for trauma (internal suture line)

Keep the nasogastric tube connected to suction as ordered to drain secretions and prevent gastric distention and vomiting. Irrigate the tube gently with normal saline as ordered to keep it patent. Reinforce or replace the tape holding the tube in place as needed. Be careful not to move the tube when adding or changing tape. Notify the physician if abdominal girth increases.

NDx: High risk for altered oral mucous membrane

Assist the patient in brushing and flossing the teeth after eating. Assist the patient in rinsing the mouth frequently. Offer throat lozenges or gum if allowed. Apply water-soluble lubricant to lips to prevent drying and cracking.

NDx: High risk for infection

Caution patient against touching the abdominal dressing or the surrounding area. Use strict aseptic technique when caring for the wound. Reinforce dressing as needed unless dressing is wet with predominantly bloody drainage, in which case it should be changed.

NDx: Altered nutrition: less than body requirements

Administer intravenous fluids and electrolytes as ordered (usually for approximately 4 days). When bowel motility has returned, give clear fluids, preferably beginning with sips of warm tea, because cold liquids tend to cause distress. Gradually introduce full fluids and progress to a bland diet as tolerated. Give iron and vitamin supplements as ordered. Give six small feedings per day. Give liquids before or after but not with feedings to combat early satiety.

To combat dumping syndrome, instruct the patient to avoid hypertonic liquids and high-carbohydrate foods; assume low Fowler's position during meals; lie down for a half-hour after eating to delay gastric emptying; avoid fluids with meals; and take antispasmodics as ordered to aid in delay of gastric emptying.

NDx: High risk for altered health maintenance

Instruct the patient to report continuous epigastric distress that increases after eating because it may indicate alkaline reflux gastritis. Also stress the need to report persistent fatigue because it may be related to iron or vitamin B_{12} deficiency.

Evaluation

Evaluate the effectiveness of nursing care for a patient who has had a gastrectomy by comparing the patient's status with the expected patient outcomes. Examples of specific outcomes for patients who have had a gastrectomy have been provided in the Planning section.

INTESTINAL RESECTION

An intestinal resection is a procedure in which a part of the small intestine or large intestine is excised.

Uses. Intestinal resection is used in the treatment of problems such as intestinal malignancy, obstruction, inflammatory bowel disease, perforated diverticulum, and ischemic or traumatic injury.

Physical Preparation of the Patient. To ensure that the bowel is clean and empty of stool, an extensive bowel preparation is done. The patient is placed first on a low-residue diet and then, for the 24 hours immediately preceding the operation, on a liquid diet so that stool does not accumulate in the bowel. To empty the bowel of any stool already present, an oral preparation such as GoLYTELY or Colyte and a series of enemas are given. To decrease the bacteria in the bowel and thus help prevent postoperative infection, oral anti-infectives are given. The anti-infective must be nonabsorbable so that it passes through the entire intestinal tract, where its action is needed. Anti-infectives that can be used for this purpose include neomycin, erythromycin, kanamycin sulfate (Kantrex), and succinylsulfathiazole (Sulfasuxidine).

Fluids and electrolytes are ordinarily given preoperatively to make up losses from dietary restrictions, preparation for preoperative diagnostic tests, and the operation itself, as well as for deficiencies that may have resulted from the disease process and its symptoms. Often, it is necessary to give vitamins C and K parenterally to ensure amounts adequate for blood clotting and wound healing.

For some patients, TPN may be needed for protein replacement.

On the day of, or during, surgery a nasogastric tube is inserted. This removes gastric secretions and prevents vomiting until gastrointestinal function returns. If a long tube is used in place of a nasogastric tube, it may be inserted 24 to 48 hours before the operation, to allow time for it to pass into the intestine. A long tube in addition to removing secretions from the operative area also causes the intestine to "gather up on it," resulting in more operative space.

An indwelling catheter is also inserted because urinary retention is common after surgery on the intestines, particularly the distal colon or rectum. The catheter keeps the bladder empty during surgery, thereby giving more space in the surgical field and decreasing the chances of accidental injury to it.

Procedure. The preferred type of resection is one in which the diseased part of the bowel is removed and the two remaining ends are anastomosed (surgically joined together). This restores the continuity of the bowel and preserves normal defecation. In a second type of resection, the diseased part of the bowel is removed and the functioning end of the remaining intestine is brought out onto the surface of the abdomen, forming an ostomy. Subsequently, it is through this artificial opening that fecal matter exits from the GI tract. The opening is called an ileostomy when it is the ileum that is brought out onto the abdominal surface, and a colostomy when it is the colon.

Postoperative Course. The nasogastric or nasointestinal tube remains in place attached to low suction until bowel sounds return and the suture lines have begun to heal. During this time, which is usually approximately 5 days, the patient is maintained on intravenous fluid and electrolytes and in some cases on TPN. After the tube is removed, oral intake is resumed, beginning with clear fluids and progressing to full fluids and a regular diet as tolerated.

Ambulation is begun 24 to 48 hours postoperatively because thrombophlebitis and pulmonary embolism are potential complications, particularly between the seventh and tenth postoperative days.

Various difficulties can accompany the resumption of oral intake, depending on the location and extent of the resection. For example, resection of the jejunum results in malabsorption of fluids, electrolytes, fat, and the fat-soluble vitamins (A, D, E, K). Resection of the ileum results in malabsorption of fat and vitamin B_{12}, and resection involving the ileocecal valve often results in diarrhea.

Postoperative weight loss occurs following almost all bowel resections, and weight and strength are slowly regained over a period of months.

Application of the Nursing Process to the Care of the Patient Having an Anastomosed Intestinal Resection

PREOPERATIVE NURSING CARE

The assessment, nursing diagnoses, expected patient outcomes, nursing interventions, and evaluation for patients scheduled for an anastomosed intestinal resection are similar to those described previously for patients scheduled for a gastrectomy, with the following consideration. Review the patient's normal bowel habits to provide a baseline for postoperative assessment of bowel function.

POSTOPERATIVE NURSING CARE

Assessment

Postoperatively, assess physiologic stabilization by monitoring vital signs and observing the wound for bleeding. Assess the patient for pain and note location, type, and intensity. Check the nasogastric or intestinal tube every 4 hours for patency. Note the amount of drainage, which should decrease during the first 24 to 48 hours. Also note the color and consistency of the drainage and observe it for the presence of blood. Question the patient about nausea and check for abdominal distention, both of which indicate a malfunction in the gastrointestinal suction that if not corrected can cause injury to the suture line.

Assess fluid and electrolyte status. Measure fluid intake and output. Observe for signs and symptoms of dehydration or overhydration, and review serum electrolyte values.

Carefully assess respiratory status because hypoxia secondary to ineffective ventilation is a potential complication of an intestinal resection. Observe for normal chest excursion, note color, and auscultate the lungs every 4 hours for the first 72 hours postoperatively. Also assess for signs of thrombophlebitis. Observe for redness and swelling and check for heat and pain in the calf. Check for a positive Homans' sign. Be alert to signs of urinary tract infection. Note color and clarity of urine, and question the patient regarding pain.

Check temperature throughout the postoperative period. Keep in mind that an elevation in the evening with a return to normal by morning is a characteristic of infection. When this occurs early in the postoperative period, aspiration pneumonia or urinary tract infection is likely. Fever that occurs 4 to 7 days after surgery suggests a leak at the anastomosis or a wound abscess. As the postoperative period progresses, assess the patient for return of bowel function. Listen for bowel sounds every 4 hours and question the patient about the passage of flatus and then the passage of feces.

Obtain daily weights. When oral intake is resumed, monitor food intake and assess the patient's tolerance of it. Check for singultus, nausea, vomiting, abdominal distention, diarrhea, or other gastrointestinal distress.

Nursing Diagnoses and Planning

Nursing diagnoses and related expected patient outcomes most commonly applicable to patients who have had an intestinal resection with anastomosis include the following:

NDx: Pain related to surgical trauma to the abdomen

Planning: Patient outcomes
1. Patient moves without signs of severe pain such as moaning, pallor, and tachycardia.
2. Patient rests quietly without signs of discomfort such as clenched hands, groaning, and crying.
3. Patient states pain is relieved.

NDx: High risk for ineffective breathing pattern related to shallow breathing secondary to incisional pain on deep breathing

Planning: Patient outcomes
1. Patient coughs and breathes deeply as directed.
2. Cyanosis is absent.
3. Arterial blood gas levels are within normal range.

NDx: High risk for altered oral mucous membrane related to NPO status and presence of a nasogastric or nasointestinal tube

Planning: Patient outcomes
1. Oral mucous membrane is moist and free of cracks.
2. Lips are supple, moist, and free of cracks.
3. Patient denies dryness of the mouth.

NDx: High risk for altered nutrition: less than body requirements related to inadequate intake or malabsorption

Planning: Patient outcomes
1. Patient maintains expected weight.
2. Patient resumes oral intake of a nutritionally balanced diet.
3. Patient takes nutritional supplements as directed.

NDx: High risk for infection related to surgical incision of the skin and opening of the peritoneal cavity and bowel

Planning: Patient outcomes
1. Wound is approximated and free of erythema and drainage.
2. Abdomen is soft and nondistended.
3. Patient is afebrile.

NDx: High risk for altered peripheral tissue perfusion related to thrombophlebitis secondary to venous stasis

Planning: Patient outcomes
1. Patient does foot and leg exercises as directed.
2. Calves and upper thighs are free of redness, swelling, heat, and pain.
3. Homans' sign is negative.

NDx: High risk for altered health maintenance related to insufficient knowledge of discharge instructions

Planning: Patient outcomes
1. Patient explains instructions for self-care at home.
2. Patient lists symptoms to be reported to the physician.
3. Patient states time of follow-up appointment.

Nursing Interventions

NDx: Pain
Give prescribed analgesics every 3 to 4 hours for 72 hours. Assist the patient into semi-Fowler's position to relieve stress on the suture line. To relieve gas pains associated with the return of peristalsis, encourage ambulation and use a rectal tube to remove flatus as needed.

NDx: High risk for ineffective breathing pattern
Teach the patient to splint the abdomen with pillows, and assist in turning, coughing, and deep breathing every 2 hours for 72 hours after surgery. Instruct in the use of an incentive spirometer. Reassure the patient that coughing and deep breathing, despite the fact that they may hurt, do not damage the incision. When the patient is able, ambulate him or her at least three times per day.

NDx: High risk for altered oral mucous membrane
Assist the patient in brushing the teeth at least three times per day. Encourage frequent mouth rinses, but avoid the use of solutions with a drying effect on mucous membranes. Apply a water-soluble lubricant to the lips to keep them supple and prevent cracking.

NDx: High risk for altered nutrition: less than body requirements
Administer TPN if ordered. When oral intake is resumed, give small amounts of clear fluids of the patient's choice. If these are tolerated without singultus, nausea, vomiting, or other discomfort, gradually progress to full fluids and then to a regular

diet. Give nutritional supplements as ordered, and alert the physician to any weight loss promptly.

NDx: High risk for infection

Monitor for signs of peritoneal irritation caused by leaking of the suture line.

Use strict aseptic technique when doing wound care. Reinforce or change the dressing when wet to prevent the transfer of microorganisms from the environment by capillary action.

NDx: High risk for altered peripheral tissue perfusion

Guide the patient in foot and leg exercises ten times each every 2 hours while on bed rest. Apply antiembolic stockings or Ace bandages to further support venous return. Avoid gatching the bed to elevate the knees, pillows under the knees, or any other form of pressure in the popliteal space. Assist the patient out of bed, and begin ambulation as ordered in 24 to 48 hours after surgery. Instruct the patient to avoid crossing the legs or sitting for long periods.

NDx: High risk for altered health maintenance

Review the physician's instructions in regard to care of the incision, diet, and limitations on activities after discharge. Be certain the patient understands that although stool softeners may be used to prevent constipation and straining, laxatives must be avoided because of their irritating effects on the bowel. Instruct the patient to report bleeding, abdominal distention, abdominal rigidity, or fever and to return for a follow-up appointment at the designated time.

Evaluation

Evaluate the effectiveness of nursing care for a patient who has had an anastomosed intestinal resection by comparing the patient's status with the expected patient outcomes. Examples of specific outcomes for patients who have had an anastomosed intestinal resection have been provided in the Planning section.

COLOSTOMY

A colostomy is a surgically created opening between the colon and the abdominal wall through which fecal matter is expelled.

Depending on its location in the colon, it is referred to as an ascending, transverse, descending, or sigmoid colostomy. The fecal output from an ascending colostomy is predominantly liquid because it passes through only a small area of water-absorbing large bowel prior to exit. From a transverse colostomy, fecal output is mushy; from a descending colostomy, it is semi-formed; and from a sigmoid colostomy, it is almost identical to that which would be evacuated from the rectum.

Uses. Temporary colostomies are done to divert fecal matter from diseased or injured intestine in order to rest the affected area of the bowel and allow healing. Conditions that can require a temporary colostomy include diverticulitis, ischemia of the bowel, volvulus, perforation of the bowel, and gunshot or stab wounds.

Permanent colostomies are constructed when the distal bowel must be removed or is obstructed and inoperable. Colorectal cancer is the most common condition for which a permanent colostomy is done.

Physical Preparation of the Patient. The physical preparation of a patient for colostomy surgery is the same as for an anastomosed intestinal resection but with one addition. The patient scheduled for a colostomy may have the stoma site identified and marked on the abdomen preoperatively by either an enterostomal therapist or the surgeon. When this is done, the abdomen is inspected with the patient lying supine, sitting up, and standing so that all folds, creases, scars, and bony prominences are avoided.

Procedure. Colostomies are surgically constructed as an end colostomy, a double-barrel colostomy, or a loop colostomy.

An end colostomy (Fig. 21–18*A*) is one in which there is a single stoma on the abdomen created from the end of the proximal bowel (that section of bowel that remains connected to the upper GI system and through which intestinal contents will pass). This end is brought out through an opening in the abdominal wall, is folded on itself in a cuff, and is sutured to the skin. Thus, the surface of the stoma is actually the mucosal lining of the bowel. The distal portion of the bowel (that section of bowel connected only to the rectum) may either be removed or be left in place within the abdominal cavity. An end colostomy is usually a permanent procedure that may be necessitated by a malignancy in the large bowel, abdominal trauma, or other pathologic conditions in which the distal colon is nonfunctional.

A double-barrel colostomy (Fig. 21–18*B*) is one in which two separate stomas are created on the abdominal wall. The proximal stoma is the end of the functioning colon that is continuous with the upper GI tract, whereas the distal stoma, also referred to as a mucous fistula, opens into the nonfunctioning section of colon that is continuous with the rectum. Most often, this is a temporary colostomy that is done to rest an area of bowel and will be closed at a future time.

As the name suggests, a loop colostomy is formed by bringing a loop of bowel through an incision in the abdominal wall. A glass rod or rubber tube is slipped under the loop to hold it in place outside the abdomen until sufficient healing has occurred to maintain it in this position. An incision is made in

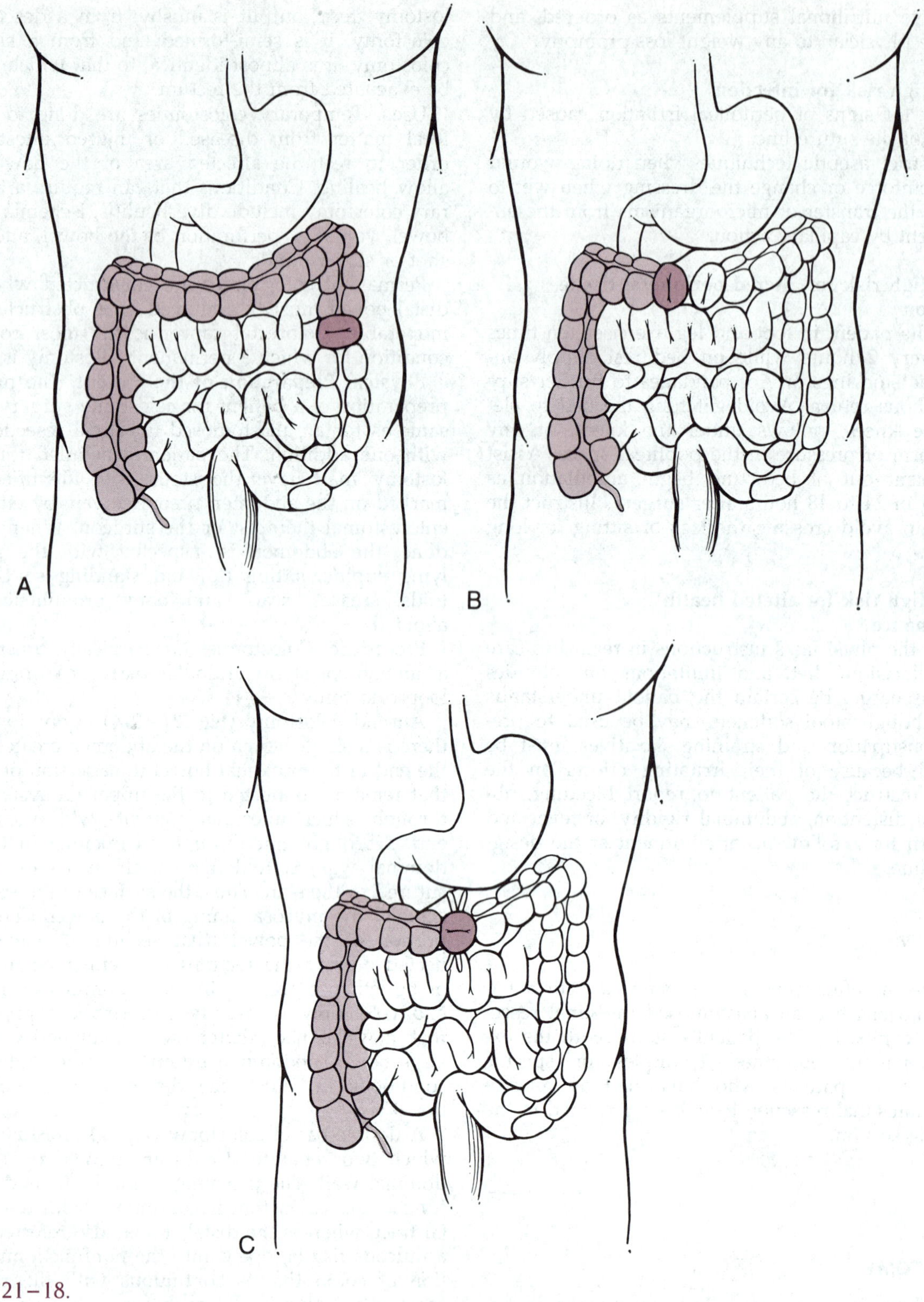

Figure 21–18.

Types of colostomy. *A*, End colostomy. *B*, Double-barrel colostomy. *C*, Loop colostomy.

its anterior wall, which results in an opening leading to the proximal bowel and an opening leading to the distal bowel within the single stoma (Fig. 21–18C). This opening of the bowel may be done in the operating room but is often done several days later in the patient's room. This delay decreases the chance of infection by allowing the wound to seal off before the contaminated bowel is opened. There is minimal bleeding with this procedure because an electrocautery is used, and it is pain-free because there is no sensory innervation in the bowel wall. There is, however, an odor of burning tissue, and good ventilation should be provided during and after the procedure. Within 7 to 10 days, adhesions form that prevent retraction of the stoma into the abdomen, and at this time the supporting glass rod or rubber tube is removed. A loop colostomy is often done as a temporary emergency procedure to divert the fecal stream from an area of bowel that is obstructed or perforated.

Postoperative Course. For 24 to 48 hours after surgery, there is mucus and serosanguineous drainage from the stoma. As peristalsis returns, large amounts of malodorous flatus are passed, followed by fecal drainage usually within 72 hours. Initially the feces are liquid, but their consistency changes when the patient starts to ingest solid foods. Fecal output from a sigmoid colostomy generally resumes the form and consistency of normal stool within a few weeks, whereas feces from a transverse colostomy eventually have the consistency of toothpaste but continue to drain several times per day.

The nasogastric or nasointestinal tube is removed and the patient started on clear fluids when bowel function has completely returned. Intravenous fluids are discontinued when oral intake is tolerated well, and the diet is gradually progressed to a full low-residue diet. After 4 to 6 weeks, a high-carbohydrate, high-protein general diet is taken as tolerated. The patient is ambulated in 24 to 48 hours and is discharged in 5 to 10 days.

Complications. Potential complications of colostomy surgery include infection, hemorrhage, obstruction, and stomal problems such as necrosis, retraction, stenosis, prolapse, and mucocutaneous separation.

Stomal necrosis can develop as a result of impaired circulation. It begins as a dusky, dark discoloration of the stoma usually appearing between 24 and 72 hours postoperatively. If the necrosis extends below the level of the facia, the stoma is surgically revised to prevent perforation and peritonitis, otherwise the affected area of the stoma is debrided and subsequently evaluated.

Stomal retraction (Fig. 21–19) is a condition in which the stoma does not protrude from the abdomen. This can develop at any time as a result of either poor surgical technique or significant weight gain. Stomal retraction makes pouching and hence maintenance of the peristomal skin difficult, and in some cases, surgical revision may be required.

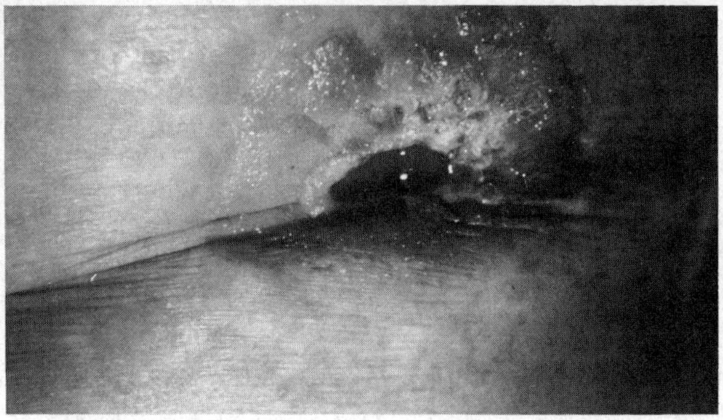

Figure 21–19.

Stomal retraction. (Courtesy of Convatec, Princeton, NJ.)

Stenosis of the stoma is a narrowing of the opening at either the level of the skin or the fascia. Typically the patient complains of constipation and a sense of pressure when stool is passed, and although the stoma may appear normal, a tight band is felt on digital examination. Treatment of stomal stenosis varies with its severity and the condition of the patient. Temporary relief measures consist of stool softeners, irrigations, and stomal dilation. The only long-term corrective measure is surgical revision.

Prolapse of the stoma is a condition in which all layers of the bowel protrude through the stoma (Fig. 21–20), which appears swollen and elongated. Protrusion occurs after discharge and is painless. It occurs most frequently following a loop colostomy and when the bowel was distended at the time of surgery. If circulation to the stoma is unimpaired, the patient may be taught to manually reduce the protrusion and to wear a binder or abdominal support belt. In other cases surgical correction is done.

Mucocutaneous separation is a disruption of the suture line at the base of the stoma with a resultant open wound. This occurs early in the postoperative period and is often preceded by redness of the skin

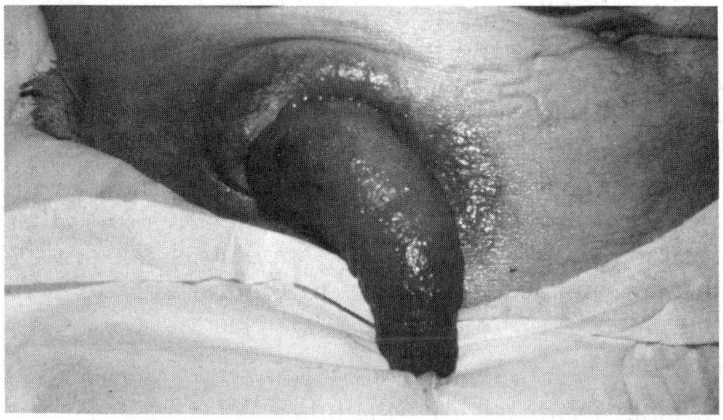

Figure 21–20.

Stomal prolapse. (Courtesy of Convatec, Princeton, NJ.)

around the base of the stoma. Once the separation has occurred, the patient complains of pain or burning when the effluent (drainage) from the ostomy comes in contact with the wound. Treatment varies with the extent of the wound. Shallow wounds are filled with paste or solid skin barrier, whereas deep, draining wounds are irrigated and packed. All wounds are left to heal by secondary intention.

Application of the Nursing Process to the Care of the Patient with a Colostomy

PREOPERATIVE NURSING CARE

Assessment

When assessing a patient scheduled for a colostomy, include those assessments that apply to any surgical patient and those for the patient having an intestinal resection with an anastomosis. In addition, thoroughly assess the patient's ability to accept and deal with the ostomy.

Assess the patient's emotional reaction to the scheduled surgery. Keep in mind that the alteration in body function and structure that occurs with this surgery can precipitate an intense emotional response. Observe for signs of anxiety and manifestations of grieving such as denial, anger, depression, and withdrawal.

Question the patient about any previous experience with an ostomy. Determine whether the patient has ever seen a colostomy, knows what it is and how it works, or knows anyone with an colostomy. If so, what are the patient's perceptions about the colostomy based on this experience? Are there any misconceptions due to type of ostomy, changes in surgical procedures, available appliances, or methods of care?

Assess the patient's perception of the effects of the colostomy on his or her lifestyle. Is the patient aware that the colostomy will require certain adjustments in the pattern of daily living, that supplies will be needed, and that time will be required for its care? Does the patient perceive colostomy care as able to be incorporated into the daily routine and expect that life will resume a usual pattern?

Assess sources of support available to the patient. Keep in mind that the closest relative or other seemingly obvious source of support is not always the person most acceptable to or best able to help the patient.

Nursing Diagnoses and Planning

Nursing diagnoses and related expected patient outcomes most commonly appliable to patients scheduled for colostomy surgery include the following:

NDx: Anxiety related to the outcome of the surgery and ability to live with and manage the colostomy

Planning: Patient outcomes
1. Patient expresses confidence in the decision to have the surgery.
2. Patient cooperates with preoperative preparation.
3. Signs of excessive anxiety such as trembling, inability to direct attention, tachycardia, and dry mouth are absent.

NDx: Knowledge deficit: appearance and function of the colostomy, need for an appliance, and need for learning self-care measures

Planning: Patient outcomes
1. Patient describes what the stoma will look like, where it will be located, how the colostomy will function, and what kind of appliance will be in place after surgery.
2. Patient asks questions about care of the colostomy or states that care procedures will have to be learned.

Other nursing diagnoses that may apply to the patient depending on the underlying intestinal disorder include the following: fluid volume deficit related to disease symptoms such as diarrhea, vomiting, and anorexia or dietary restrictions for diagnostic tests and surgery; and altered nutrition: less than body requirements related to effects of the disease process or dietary restrictions for diagnostic tests and surgery.

Nursing Interventions

NDx: Anxiety
Provide time, privacy, and encouragement for discussion of the patient's concerns. Acknowledge that feelings of anxiety are normal and expected when facing colostomy surgery. Do not give false reassurance, but do stress the expected beneficial effects of the surgery and the competence of the persons responsible for patient care. Assure the patient that having a colostomy does not dramatically change the quality of life and that most activities—work, personal and recreational—can be resumed, and offer to arrange a visit from an ostomate (i.e., a person who has had a colostomy, adjusted well to it, and acts as a volunteer in helping others adjust both before and after surgery). Guide the patient in the use of relaxation exercises, and provide diversion such as radio, television, or reading materials as appropriate to the patient's condition.

Remember too that the need for a colostomy can be as upsetting to significant others as to the patient. Be certain therefore to provide significant others with the opportunity to ventilate their feelings and concerns so that they are able to support the patient in coping.

NDx: Knowledge deficit: appearance and function of a colostomy, need for an appliance, and need for learning self-care measures
Provide the patient with basic information about the planned colostomy and its function. Include a simple description of the normal structure and function of the GI tract illustrated by an uncomplicated drawing; an explanation of how a colostomy is formed and its effect on bowel function; a definition of terms such as stoma, appliance, and pouch; and a description of the location and appearance of the stoma as well as the characteristics of the drainage. If there is a doll set up for teaching ostomies, let the patient see and handle the equipment to reduce fear of the unknown. Explain that daily routines of self-care for the colostomy will be necessary, that they will be taught, and that with time they become part of everyday living, like taking a bath or shaving. Show the patient the type of collection pouch that will be in place after surgery, and let him or her examine it if desired.

Adjust the information given to the needs of the individual patient. Add more depth and detail when desired by the patient, but avoid providing unnecessary, unwanted material that will only serve to increase the patient's anxiety. If reading materials are given to the patient, make sure they contain only information pertinent to the patient, to avoid confusion and anxiety. Also be certain to arrange a follow-up discussion so that any questions or concerns can be addressed.

Additional Interventions
When possible, check for sensitivity to colostomy care products such as skin barriers and sealants to be used postoperatively by doing a patch test. Apply small amounts of these products to the skin of the upper back, and cover with an airtight dressing. Remove this dressing in 48 hours, leave the area exposed to the air for a half-hour, and then inspect for signs of a skin reaction.

Evaluation

Evaluate the effectiveness of nursing care for a patient scheduled for colostomy surgery by comparing the patient's status with the expected patient outcomes. Examples of specific outcomes for patients scheduled for colostomy surgery have been provided in the Planning section.

POSTOPERATIVE NURSING CARE

Assessment

Make postoperative assessments as described for the patient following an anastomosed intestinal resection. In addition, make assessments related to ostomy structure, function, and care and patient acceptance.

Assess the condition of the stoma. Observe its shape, which may be perfectly round or somewhat irregular, depending on its surgical construction. Note its color and consistency. Keep in mind that it should feel soft or slightly firm to the touch and be deep pink to red, shiny, and moist, like the mucous membrane inside the mouth. A dark red to purple color to the stoma indicates poor circulation, and light pink indicates either poor circulation or anemia.

Inspect for signs of bleeding, and note the amount of edema present. In the immediate postoperative period, expect to see small amounts of pinpoint bleeding on the stoma as a result of the high vascularity of the intestine. Also expect significant edema, which should disappear gradually over 4 to 6 weeks.

Examine the collection pouch to determine the amount and characteristics of the drainage from the stoma. Remember that mucus and serosanguineous drainage are expected for the first 24 to 72 hours after surgery.

Assess for the return of bowel function. Listen for bowel sounds, and check for the passage of flatus. When the colostomy begins to function note the color, consistency, and amount of fecal drainage. Inspect the peristomal skin for signs of impaired circulation, irritation, and excoriation. Also check that the skin surrounds the stoma closely about its entire circumference.

Continue to assess the response of the patient and significant others to the colostomy as well as the patient's readiness for teaching related to colostomy care. Remember that a person who is in a state of shock and disbelief and who has not looked at the stoma is not ready for teaching. Remember also that teaching will not be effective when the patient is angry or depressed. Be alert to questions from the patient about the colostomy or related care, because these are generally good indicators of readiness for learning.

Nursing Diagnoses and Planning

Nursing diagnoses and related expected patient outcomes most commonly applicable to patients following colostomy surgery include those previously described under the care of the patient with an anastomosed intestinal resection and the following:

NDx: Bowel incontinence related to the formation of a colostomy and loss of rectal function

Planning: Patient outcomes
1. Patient uses the selected pouching system effectively to collect fecal drainage.
2. Patient identifies factors such as change in diet and times of eating that affect pattern of colostomy function.

NDx: High risk for impaired skin integrity related to irritation of the peristomal skin from contact with ostomy output, from removal of adherent appliances, or from sensitivity to adhesives and other materials

Planning: Patient outcomes
1. Peristomal skin is free of erythema and blisters.
2. Peristomal skin is intact.

NDx: High risk for altered nutrition: less than body requirements related to omission of foods with essential nutrients from the diet because of flatulence, odor, or diarrhea

Planning: Patient outcomes
1. Patient describes components of a nutritionally balanced diet.
2. Patient is able to select a nutritionally balanced diet from foods that are tolerated well.
3. Patient identifies specific foods that are likely causes of flatulence, odor, or diarrhea.

NDx: High risk for body image disturbance related to loss of bowel control, presence of the stoma, release of fecal material onto abdomen, passage of flatus, odor, and need for an appliance

Planning: Patient outcomes
1. Patient verbalizes acceptance of self with the colostomy.
2. Patient identifies own strengths.
3. Patient expresses pleasure at visits from relatives and friends.
4. Patient discusses resumption of work, household, and social activities from a positive perspective.

NDx: High risk for altered sexuality patterns related to fear of rejection because of the presence of a stoma or an appliance

Planning: Patient outcomes
1. Patient discusses concerns about the effects of the colostomy on sexual function.
2. Patient verbalizes confidence in ability to participate in a satisfying sexual relationship.

NDx: High risk for altered health maintenance related to insufficient knowledge of care of the colostomy, effect on lifestyle, and support services

Planning: Patient outcomes
1. Patient demonstrates correct appliance application.
2. Patient identifies symptoms that should be reported to the health care professional.
3. Patient correctly demonstrates cleaning and deodorizing of the appliance.
4. Patient identifies potential effects of the colostomy on individual lifestyle without exaggeration or denial.
5. Patient describes available support services, including how to contact the United Ostomy Association.

Nursing Interventions

Carry out basic postoperative interventions as for the patient with an intestinal resection with an anastomosis.

Encourage the patient to cough and breathe deeply every 2 hours to enhance lung expansion and decrease the risk of pulmonary congestion and pneumonia. Guide the patient in foot and leg exercises every hour while the patient is awake and on bed rest to foster venous return and help prevent thrombus formation and pulmonary embolism. Begin ambulation 24 to 48 hours after surgery.

NDx: Bowel incontinence
Use a colostomy appliance to collect the feces expelled involuntarily from the colostomy. In most cases a collection pouch, usually translucent plastic, is placed over the colostomy at the completion of the operation. Monitor this pouch for the accumulation of flatus and drainage, and empty or change it as necessary. Do not allow the pouch to get too full, because back pressure can damage the suture lines and disrupt the pouch seal. Subsequently assist the patient in the selection of a collection system for daily use that is best suited to his or her needs. If the patient is unable to perform self-care and will be dependent on a spouse or significant other for assistance, include that person in the selection process.

There are various types of colostomy equipment available, and selection of the appliance system appropriate to the individual patient is essential if problems with leaking and skin irritation are to be prevented (Fig. 21–21). Factors that influence the appropriateness of specific systems include the location of the colostomy, abdominal size and shape, physical and mental capabilities, and personal preference of the patient.

Appliances are either disposable or reusable and come as one- or two-part systems. (A two-part system includes both a collection pouch and a skin barrier.) Collection pouches come in both clear and opaque plastic and can be odorproof. Pouch covers of soft material that make the pouch more comfortable to wear can be purchased or made.

Appliances must be sized to fit the stoma. Because of the progressive decrease in postoperative edema, check the size after 3 weeks and determine final stoma size at 3 to 4 months after surgery.

Once a system is selected, use it consistently to eliminate confusion for patients and make learning the required care skills easier. Similarly, if caring for a patient with a preexisting colostomy, follow the patient's usual method of care. Make suggestions if appropriate, but do not try to force change if the existing system is effective.

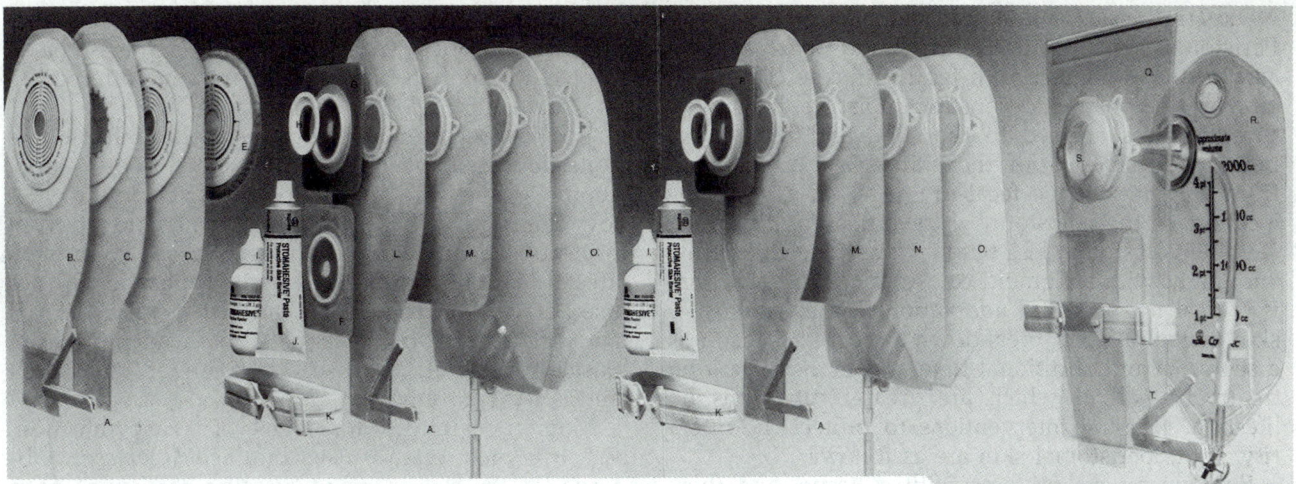

Figure 21–21.

Examples of the various types of colostomy equipment patients may use: *A*, Active Life/Sur-Fit Tail Closure; *B*, Active Life One-Piece Drainable Custom Pouch; *C*, Active Life One-Piece Drainable Pouch with pre-cut openings; *D*, Active Life One-Piece Closed-End Pouch; *E*, Active Life One-Piece Stoma Cap; *F*, Sur-Fit Flexible; *G*, Stomahesive Wafer with Sur-Fit Flange; *H*, Sur-Fit Disposable Convex Insert; *I*, Stomahesive Protective Powder; *J*, Stomahesive Paste; *K*, Adjustable Belt; *L*, Sur-Fit Drainable Pouch; *M*, Sur-Fit Closed-End Pouch; *N*, Sur-Fit Urostomy Pouch; *O*, Sur-Fit Urostomy Pouch with Accuseal Tap; *P*, Durahesive Wafer with Flange; *Q*, Sur-Fit Irrigation Sleeve; *R*, Visi-Flow Irrigation System; *S*, Sur-Fit Adapter Faceplate; *T*, Sur-Fit Irrigation Sleeve Tail Closure. (Courtesy of Convatec, Princeton, NJ.)

Inform patients with a sigmoid or descending colostomy that control over fecal expulsion may be gained in time by means of a regular diet or periodic colostomy irrigation, although this latter method is seldom used today. Explain that if control is achieved, a collection pouch will not be necessary all of the time because something as simple as a gauze pad covered with Saran Wrap over the stoma is sufficient, although some persons choose to continue with a small, lightweight collection appliance for security. In assisting patients to establish control, instruct in basic dietary considerations as presented in Nutrition Box 21–1 and in the importance of maintaining a regular pattern of eating and exercise.

Nutrition Box 21–1.

NUTRITION: SPECIAL CONSIDERATIONS FOR PATIENTS WITH A COLOSTOMY

Instruct patients with a colostomy to:

Eat a low-residue diet for 4 to 6 weeks after surgery.
Progress to a high-carbohydrate, high-protein general diet after this 4- to 6-week period.
Add new foods one at a time to determine their effect.
Try each food at least three times before eliminating from the diet.
Consider the effects of specific foods on the gastrointestinal system when selecting the diet:
Constipating foods: cheese, nuts, chocolate, corn, raisins
Laxative foods: prunes, fresh fruits, broccoli, spinach, green beans, liver, highly spiced foods, beer
Gas-forming foods: nuts, cabbage, sauerkraut, corn, cauliflower, broccoli, spinach, peas, beans, apples, avocados, watermelon, cucumbers, carbonated beverages
Odor-causing foods: alcohol (particularly beers), onions, beans, cabbage, turnips, asparagus, mushrooms, radishes, cucumbers, eggs, fish, highly spiced foods
Deodorizing foods: parsley, beet greens, spinach, buttermilk, yogurt
Remember that milk and milk products are often not tolerated well and should be limited.

NDx: High risk for impaired skin integrity
Peristomal skin irritation and breakdown can occur as a result of contact with fecal drainage containing enzymes, exposure to constant moisture, sensitivity to substances applied to the skin, and removal of pouch adhesives from the skin. Risk of irritation from enzymes in the fecal drainage varies with the location of the colostomy. It is highest with an ascending colostomy, less with a transverse colostomy, and slight with a sigmoid colostomy. Good skin care is critical to successful adaptation to a colostomy. If skin irritation and breakdown occur, the result is discomfort and additional time and money spent on treatment—all of which are greater intrusions on lifestyle. Nursing interventions to protect the integrity of the peristomal skin are as follows.

Remove mucus or feces with a tissue, and thoroughly wash the peristomal skin to remove all traces of intestinal discharge. Rinse carefully to remove all soap residue, and dry gently and completely. If the patient is an elderly person whose skin tends to be dry, omit the soap and wash with warm water only. Do not use oily soaps or emollients, because they interfere with the adherence of the collection pouch.

Use a skin barrier to protect the eighth of an inch of exposed skin between the stoma and the pouch opening from exposure to fecal drainage. The usual type of skin barrier used today is a pectin-based wafer that is cut to fit closely around the base of the stoma. It can be used with a variety of pouches and is warmed by placing it under the patient's upper back or between the hands to increase its adhesiveness to the skin.

Skin barriers also come in the form of powders and pastes. Use pastes in conjunction with wafers to fill in creases and folds to obtain a better and longer-lasting pouch seal for patients whose colostomy is in a difficult location.

Apply a skin sealant to the peristomal skin area where adhesive will be applied to hold the collection pouch in place. Skin sealants are sprays, liquids, gels, or wipes that coat the skin with a clear film so that when the adhesive substance is removed, the protective film rather than the epidermis is torn off.

Apply the pouch snugly and monitor routinely for leaking. Change the pouch immediately if leaking occurs. When removing the pouch, follow the directions accompanying it carefully to ensure the least traumatic removal.

If needed, remove hair from the peristomal skin regularly to decrease the risk of folliculitis caused by trauma of the hair follicles. Use an electric or straight razor according to personal preference, but avoid depilatories because of the risk of sensitivity to them.

If skin irritation does occur, institute immediate treatment. When the skin around the stoma is reddened, change the appliance every 1 to 2 days. Wash the area with warm water, pat dry, and then expose to a heat lamp with a 60-watt bulb positioned 12 to 16 inches from the stoma for 20 minutes. Place gauze wet with saline over the stoma to protect it. Apply a skin barrier carefully patterned to the stoma and a collection appliance.

If the skin around the stoma is broken, change the collection appliance daily. Wash the skin and apply compresses of Burow's solution for 30 minutes. Follow this with a heat lamp treatment, and apply a protective preparation such as Orabase to broken areas. Reapply a skin barrier and appliance. Do not use antacids on the skin because they raise the pH and predispose to infection. Also avoid aluminum paste because it decreases adhesion of the pouch and is hard to remove.

Monitor carefully for signs of yeast infection, which is most often caused by *Candida albicans*. Observe for the characteristic irregular patches of deep erythema with papular lesions and the appearance of dry, scaling areas of skin as the process progresses.

NDx: High risk for altered nutrition: less than body requirements
Review basic principles of nutrition with the patient. Discuss the components of a nutritionally balanced diet, the use of the basic food groups in planning a balanced diet, and the need for at least 2500 ml of fluid per day. Explain to the patient that there are no specific dietary restrictions following a colostomy: some patients are able to eat anything, whereas other patients find that specific foods cause constipation, diarrhea, odor, or excessive flatus. Teach the patient which foods are most likely to cause these effects, as listed in Nutrition Box 21–1. Stress, however, that food tolerance is an individual thing and that desired foods should be tried one at a time and at least three times before being eliminated from the diet.

NDx: High risk for body image disturbance
Acknowledge to the patient that negative feelings about the colostomy are normal and that it takes time to accept and adjust to this body change. Recognize that patients often experience fear of rejection, disgust, or shame. Be certain, therefore, that facial expressions and other nonverbal behaviors convey acceptance, not revulsion, distaste, or pity, which would reinforce the patient's distress. Recognize too that denial is common after ostomy surgery, and allow the patient to experience denial, while gently fostering acceptance of the reality. Do this by not forcing the patient to look at the stoma or participate in care but by using the terms colostomy and stoma and by describing their appearance and giving brief, matter-of-fact explanations of the colostomy care being given. Touch the stoma to show that it does not hurt, is not easily damaged, and is not revolting. Provide an opportunity for the patient to look at or touch the stoma, as by leaving it uncovered while supplies are obtained. Be alert to

patient's comments and questions that indicate that the stoma has been looked at, and encourage discussion of related feelings and concerns.

Protect the patient from unnecessary embarrassment related to the colostomy by ensuring privacy for discussion, teaching, and colostomy care and by controlling odor. Empty the collection pouch of malodorous flatus or fecal drainage prior to meals and visiting hours. Provide good ventilation, and deodorize the room immediately. Do not put pin holes in the disposable plastic pouch used in the early postoperative period to allow flatus to escape as it is being produced, because this results in unpredictable, uncontrolled odor. In helping the patient to select an appliance for long-term use, recommend one that is odor free, that is, no odor except when emptying or if the outlet is not cleaned. Such an appliance may cost somewhat more initially but the subsequent need to purchase deodorizers is eliminated.

Encourage the patient to be well groomed. Stress that with some attention to the style of clothing purchased, the ostomy and the pouch cannot be noticed. Suggest a visit from an ostomate as one way of demonstrating this fact. Throughout the recovery period, foster the patient's sense of control. Involve the patient in decision-making, and help the patient identify personal strengths. Encourage the family to treat the patient normally and to engage in a frank discussion of feelings.

NDx: High risk for altered sexuality patterns

Encourage the patient to discuss resumption of sexual activity, and provide basic information in this regard.

Affirm that sexual intercourse, conception, and pregnancy are all possible following a colostomy. If a collection appliance is worn, suggest that it be emptied prior to intercourse, and recommend different positions if needed to accommodate the appliance.

Acknowledge that concerns about sexual activity are normal, and encourage the patient to discuss them openly with spouse or significant other. Provide privacy and time for such discussion. Provide access to written material such as "Sex and the Male Ostomate," published by the United Ostomy Association. Refer to an enterostomal therapist or sex therapist if needed.

NDx: High risk for altered health maintenance

Begin teaching the patient to care for the colostomy as soon as possible postoperatively. It is true that learning occurs best when teaching coincides with the time the patient is most ready to learn, but this is not always possible today when patients may be discharged in as few as 5 or 6 days because of changes in reimbursement. As a result, teaching must sometimes be done while the patient is still struggling to accept to reality of the ostomy and to express feelings regarding it. Keep in mind, however, that although this increases the challenge of effective teaching, that learning self-care can lead to a sense of control and a confidence in the ability to cope that can help overcome negative feelings about the ostomy.

Teach the patient first to care for the colostomy: to identify needed supplies, to empty the pouch, to change the pouch, to control odor, to clean the appliance, and to care for the peristomal skin. Adapt the teaching to the patient's needs within the confines of the situation. For example, consider initially teaching the patient to use the clamp on the pouch and to empty the pouch and allowing the patient to simply observe a pouch change and skin care. Subsequently, when teaching the patient to change the pouch, recognize that the pouch may have to be changed every day regardless of need to ensure that the patient will have sufficient opportunity to learn the procedure before discharge. When teaching colostomy care, also be certain to have the patient do it in the manner in which it is best done after discharge—for example, sit on the toilet to empty the bag—because the way it is first learned tends to remain the way it is done.

Be certain to instruct the patient to empty the pouch when it is one-third full and at bedtime. Suggest that for a few days after discharge an alarm clock be set to ensure that the patient is awakened in time to empty the pouch. Stress the importance of always using one hand to support the skin while lifting adhesive with the other when changing the pouch. For maximum convenience and ease, suggest changing the pouch first thing in the morning before eating or drinking because the colostomy is usually not functioning at this time. Instruct the patient to dispose of pouches in plastic bags, first wrapping them in aluminum foil if it is desired to disguise what is being disposed of.

Explain that odor is best controlled by the use of an odorproof pouch but that if necessary deodorant substances such as Nilodor or baking soda may be put in the bag. Instruct the patient to wash reusable appliances with soap and water and expose to fresh air to not only clean them and prolong their use but to keep them odor free. If odor persists, instruct the patient to soak the appliances in a commercially available deodorizer.

Inform the patient that any type of clothing can be worn, including girdles and panty hose.

Also inform the patient that physical activities are unrestricted: showers and tub baths may be taken, and swimming, tennis, and exercise programs may be resumed, usually within 8 weeks after surgery. Explain that there is no restriction on travel; it is simply necessary to carry supplies for colostomy care so they are easily accessible. Remind the patient to wear seat belts above or below the stoma.

Describe to the patient ostomy clubs and support groups available in the community, and give information as to how to contact them. Explain that the

United Ostomy Association has meetings in every city to provide ostomy patients with assistance and psychological support.

Provide the patient with written instructions regarding care upon discharge. This is important because information given in stressful situations is often forgotten or confused and review is necessary. In addition, when making referrals for follow-up care in the home, be certain to specify the type of appliance system being used and carefully describe the teaching that has been done with the patient.

Evaluation

Evaluate the effectiveness of nursing care for a patient who has had colostomy surgery by comparing the patient's status with the expected patient outcomes. Examples of specific outcomes for patients who have had colostomy surgery have been provided in the Planning section.

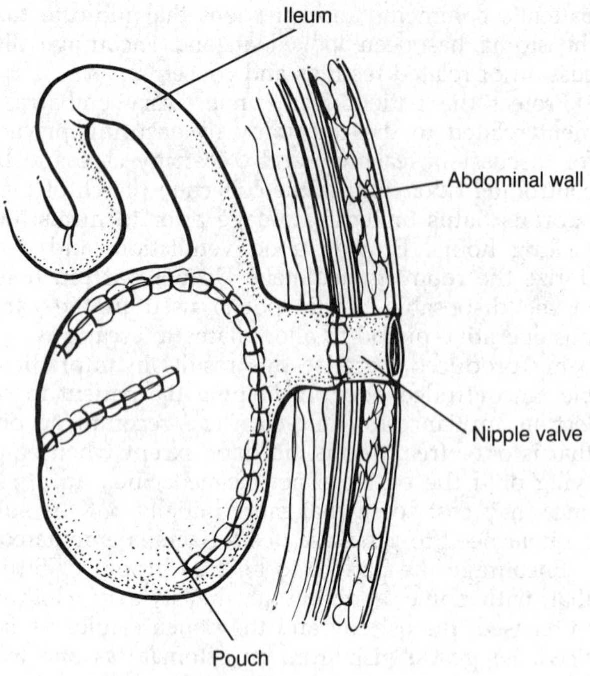

Figure 21–22.

Continent ileostomy or Kock pouch. Pouch to hold fecal matter is created surgically from a loop of ileum folded back on itself.

ILEOSTOMY

An ileostomy is a surgically created opening between the ileum and the abdominal wall through which fecal matter is expelled. The major difference between an ileostomy and a colostomy is the type of fecal output. The output from an ileostomy is a malodorous, enzyme-rich, caustic yellow, green, or brown liquid. Exactly how liquid, and therefore what the volume of output is, depends on where in the ileum the ostomy is located. Because the terminal ileum begins to take over the water-absorbing function of the colon, the closer the ileostomy is to the junction of the large bowel, the less liquid is the output.

Uses. Ileostomies are most often used in the treatment of ulcerative colitis, an inflammatory disease of the colon, and for cancer of the colon.

Physical Preparation of the Patient. The preparation of the patient is the same as for a colostomy.

Procedure. The three types of ileostomy are conventional (end or Brooke ileostomy), loop ileostomy, and continent ileostomy or Kock pouch.

A conventional ileostomy is formed in a manner similar to an end colostomy. The proximal end of the ileum is pulled through the right abdominal wall. It is then cuffed to form a stoma that protrudes approximately an inch beyond the skin surface to decrease the risk of effluent coming in contact with the skin and causing irritation. The distal ileum may either be removed or be left in place with the end sutured closed.

When a loop ileostomy is formed, the intact ileum is pulled through the right abdominal wall and a rod is inserted through the loop to support the ileum in this position. The top portion of the loop is then incised to allow drainage. This is a temporary procedure used to divert fecal matter from an unhealed anastomosis between the distal ileum and the anus.

In a continent ileostomy, an internal pouch to hold stool is created by suturing two loops of ileum together. A nipple valve is then constructed by intussuscepting the ileum (Fig. 21–22). This controls the passage of feces and gas, because as the pouch fills, pressure forces the valve to close. The pouch initially holds 100 to 600 ml but gradually stretches with use up to a capacity of 1000 ml in about 6 months. This procedure is designed to eliminate the need for an external collection appliance. It cannot be used for patients with short bowel syndrome or Crohn's disease, nor can it be used when patients are obese, on high doses of steroids, or unable to perform the required self-care.

Postoperative Course. Ileostomies begin expelling flatus and then dark green odorless liquid in 12 to 72 hours, with those just proximal to the ascending colon taking the longest. Initially the amount of effluent is between 1000 and 2000 ml daily. With the resumption of oral intake, volume decreases noticeably and the effluent turns dark green to yellow to brown. It also develops a distinctive odor. In 3 to 6 months, as the ileum begins to absorb more water, the effluent becomes like a fluid paste.

With a conventional or loop ileostomy, the greatest amount of fecal discharge generally occurs 4 to 6 hours after meals, but discharge does occur in smaller amounts at unpredictable intervals. As a result, it is necessary for the patient to wear an appliance (pouch) at all times to collect the fecal output.

One type of appliance is an open-ended bag that can be emptied every 4 to 6 hours or whenever the patient urinates. This type of bag is changed if leakage around the stoma occurs or after 3 to 4 days.

With a continent ileostomy (Kock pouch), a catheter is inserted into the internal pouch at the time of surgery. It is attached to suction to keep the pouch empty until the suture lines have healed.

During this time, the catheter is irrigated with 10 to 20 ml of normal saline every 3 hours to keep it patent. The saline is generally instilled with a syringe, and return is by gravity drainage. The catheter is removed in 10 to 14 days. Subsequently, a catheter is reinserted to drain the pouch every 3 to 4 hours. The interval is gradually increased until this is done not more than three times per day. Eventually the patient becomes aware of pressure in the pouch and begins to drain it as needed.

Because mucus is expelled from the ileostomy, an absorbent dressing is needed, although an external pouch is not.

Other aspects of the postoperative course parallel those following a colostomy.

Complications. A major problem after any ileostomy is the potential for fluid and electrolyte imbalance.

Because the output is high in fluid and electrolyte content, the patient with an ileostomy is at risk for dehydration, potassium and sodium deficiencies, and acidosis as a result of the loss of bicarbonate. These problems can occur quickly, particularly if diarrhea develops, whether from illness, dietary changes, or in response to medications such as antibiotics that alter the flora that develops in the ileum. Laxatives are never given to these patients, nor is the ileostomy irrigated. If a bowel preparation is required, the patient simply adheres to a liquid diet for 24 hours.

Malabsorption of fat, iron, folate, and vitamin B_{12} may occur, and there is the risk of infection, hemorrhage, or obstruction.

Other complications that can occur with a conventional ileostomy include skin excoriation from contact with the caustic effluent and stomal problems as described under Colostomy.

Complications of a continent ileostomy include incontinence caused by valve malfunction, difficult intubation, perforation, and pouchitis due to bacterial overgrowth.

Application of the Nursing Process to the Care of the Patient with an Ileostomy

PREOPERATIVE NURSING CARE

Preoperative assessment, nursing diagnoses, expected patient outcomes, nursing interventions, and evaluation for patients having ileostomy surgery are similar to those described previously for patients having colostomy surgery.

Because many ileostomies are done for uncontrollable inflammatory bowel disease, however, there is a greater likelihood that patients having an ileostomy will need longer, more intensive fluid, blood, and protein therapy preoperatively to make up for existing deficiencies. Be certain, therefore, to assess for signs of fluid and electrolyte imbalance, particularly hypokalemia, hyponatremia, and fluid deficit. Maintain accurate fluid input and output records at all times.

POSTOPERATIVE NURSING CARE

Postoperative assessment, nursing diagnoses, expected patient outcomes, nursing interventions, and evaluation for patients who have had ileostomy surgery are similar to those described previously for patients who have had colostomy surgery. Nutritional considerations and patient teaching information specific to the patient with an ileostomy are presented in Nutrition Box 21–2 and Chart 21–3.

ILEOANAL ENDORECTAL PULL-THROUGH

An ileoanal endorectal pull-through is a procedure in which the entire colon and proximal two thirds of the rectum are removed, the mucosa of the remaining rectum is stripped away, and a pouch is created from two or three loops of ileum (ileoanal reservoir), which is then stapled to the anus.

Uses. An ileoanal endorectal pull-through is used in the treatment of ulcerative colitis and familial polyposis. It is designed to preserve the anal sphincter and retain sensation and control over elimination from the large bowel.

Physical Preparation of the Patient. A medical workup is performed up to one month prior to the scheduled surgery in order to ascertain the status of the rectal mucosa (Becker & Parodi, 1989, p. 271). This examination includes a flexible sigmoidoscopy and anorectal manometry. Anorectal manometry is done to assess anal function, including tone and contraction of the sphincter, and is also indicative of rectal capacity (Becker & Parodi, 1989, p. 272).

To ensure that the bowel is clean and empty of stool at the time of surgery, a mechanical preparation is done. The patient is given a clear liquid diet to decrease the formation of feces, and a laxative such as Fleet Phospho-Soda (30–45 ml only) for its gentle purgative action. A soapsuds enema is administered the day prior to surgery and may be repeated on the morning of surgery. Oral antibiotics such as neomycin or erythromycin are given prophylactically to decrease bacterial flora and help prevent postoperative infection. The usual dosage of

Nutrition Box 21–2.

NUTRITION: SPECIAL CONSIDERATIONS FOR PATIENTS WITH AN ILEOSTOMY

Instruct patients with an ileostomy to:

Eat foods such as clear soups, cottage cheese, dry cheese, liver, lean meat, rice, tea, and coffee during the initial period of adjustment to the ileostomy.
Resume ingestion of high-fiber foods one at a time after ileostomy function has stabilized to allow tolerance of them to be evaluated.
Try each new food three times before deciding that it cannot be tolerated.
Record problem foods in a food diary for future reference.
Chew all foods well.
Avoid foods such as corn, popcorn, celery, Chinese food, peanuts, coconut, and skins of raw fruits, which could block the stoma.
Drink six to eight glasses of water per day to guard against dehydration because the water-absorbing surface if the intestine is decreased.
Ingest electrolyte replacement solutions such as Gatorade in the summer or at other times when heavy perspiration occurs.
Decrease the amount of dietary fiber if the ileostomy output is too liquid.
Eat pasta, boiled rice, or low-fat cheese to thicken stool.
Add salt to the diet if the ileostomy output is too dry.

Chart 21–3.

NURSING GUIDE TO PATIENT EDUCATION FOR SELF-MANAGEMENT: SELF-CARE AFTER ILEOSTOMY

Instruct the patient to:

Expect the ileostomy to be noisy initially as a result of tissue edema but be assured that this will decrease with time.
Expect undigested foods such as seeds and kernels to pass through the stoma.
Give meticulous care to the skin surrounding the stoma because this is more critical with an ileostomy than with a colostomy owing to the increased danger of skin excoriation from enzymes in the effluent.
Make ongoing assessments of self for signs of dehydration, hypokalemia, and hyponatremia.
Ingest a mixture of 1 tsp of table salt, 1 tsp of baking soda, and 1 quart of water as ordered by the physician if diarrhea occurs to correct acidosis secondary to the loss of bicarbonate.
Avoid laxatives.
Treat blockage of the ostomy lumen by a mass of undigested high-fiber foods as follows:
- Assume knee-chest position.
- Gently massage area below the stoma.
- Call physician if lumen remains blocked, because a lavage by bulb syringe with 30 to 50 ml of normal saline may be required.
- Adjust pouch, because stoma swells with blockage.
- Increase fluid intake after removal to compensate for the resultant diarrhea.
- Expect abdominal pain around the stoma for 3 to 5 days.

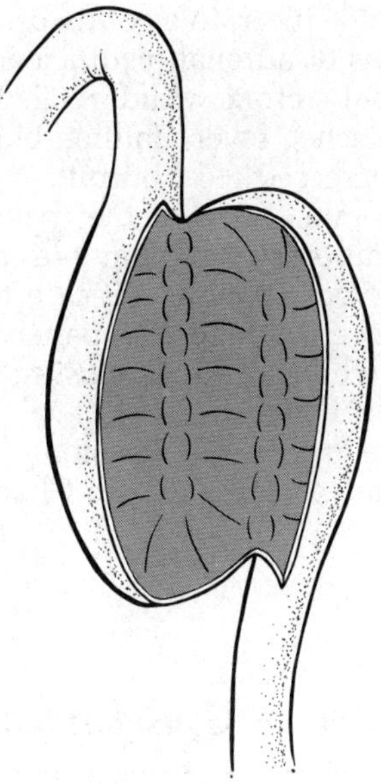

Figure 21–23.

Creation of an S pouch for ileoanal endorectal pull-through.

these antibiotics is 0.5 g every hour for 4 hours, then 0.5 g every 4 hours. Steroids or sulfasalazine may also be given preoperatively for the anti-inflammatory effect.

The patient is kept on NPO status after midnight before the day of surgery. If the surgery is scheduled late in the afternoon, an intravenous line may be inserted to maintain fluid and electrolyte balance.

Procedure. The anus is dilated, and the mucosa is stripped and removed from the lower rectum through an anoscope. The abdomen is then opened through a midline incision, and the colon and rectum down to the level of the mucosectomy are removed. Next a J or S pouch (Fig. 21–23) is created using loops of terminal ileum. The end of the pouch (or in the case of the S pouch, the distal end of the ileum) is pulled through the rectal stump and anastomosed to the anus.

Gowns and gloves are then changed, and a loop ileostomy is created through a predetermined site in the abdominal wall (Fig. 21–24*A*). The abdominal wound is closed, and an ileostomy appliance is put in place.

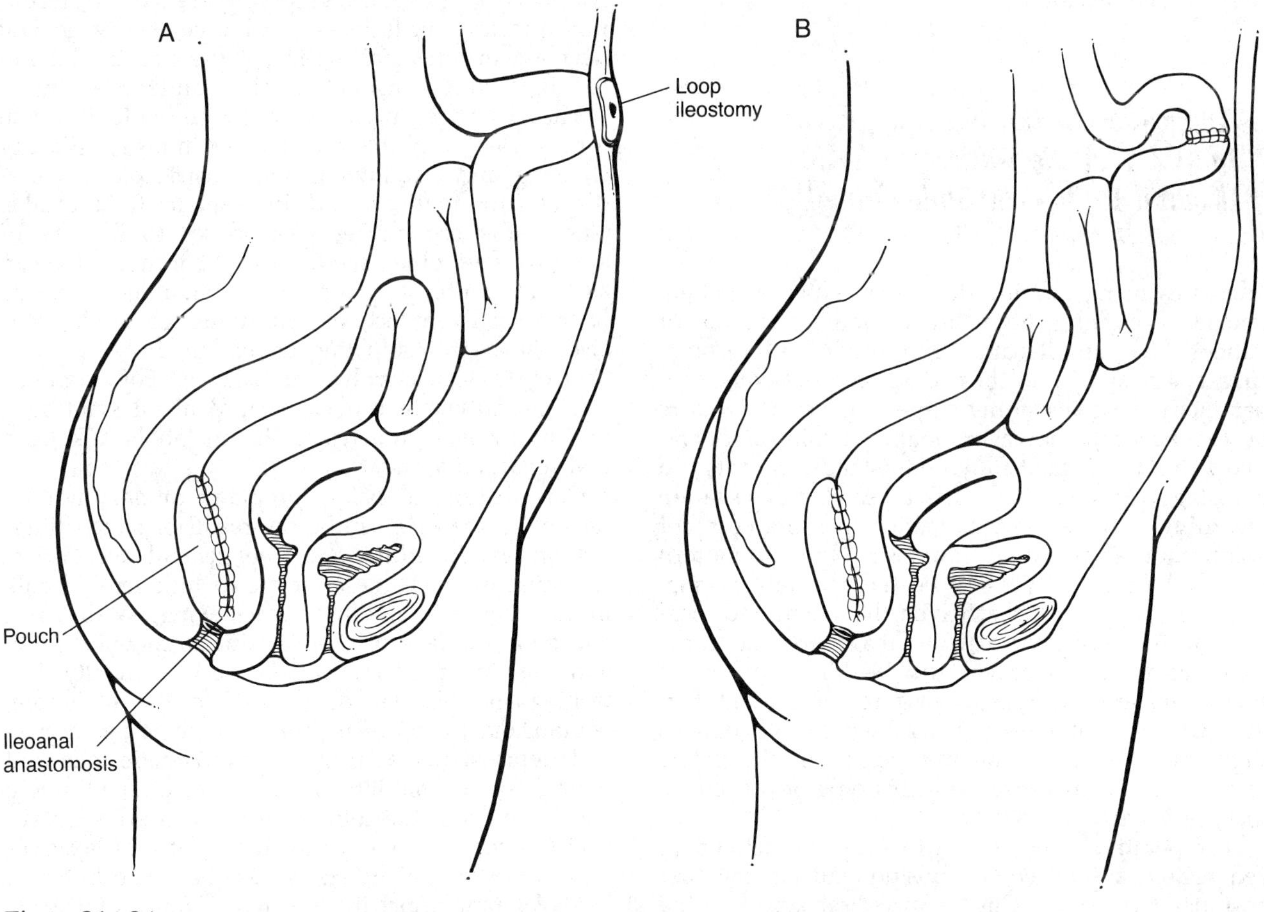

Figure 21–24.

Ileoanal endorectal pull-through. *A*, Anatomic relationships of the lower gastrointestinal organs following initial surgery. *B*, Anatomic relationships of the lower gastrointestinal organs following closure of the ileostomy.

Postoperative Course. The loop colostomy is maintained for approximately 3 months to allow complete healing of the internal suture lines. A second operation to close the ileostomy and restore bowel continuity is done (Fig. 21–24*B*). After this second operation, stool is once again passed via the rectum and no collection appliance is needed. Bowel elimination does not return to normal, however; for although the ileoanal reservoir slows stool down, patients may have as many as 20 loose bowel movements per day during the first week after closure, and three to eight bowel movements per day and one at night thereafter. In some cases, it is necessary to intubate the anus to drain it for 6 to 16 months. In others, medications or bulk formers are needed to provide acceptable control.

After the procedure, patients are examined at regular intervals with sigmoidoscopy and biopsy to check for recurrence or malignancy.

Complications. Potential complications of ileoanal endorectal pull-through include incapacitating diarrhea, irritation of the perianal skin from leaking stool, leak or stricture at the anastomosis, pouchitis, incontinence especially at night, and urgency. In addition, there is the risk of recurrence of the primary disorder in the rectal stump, creating the need for a conventional ileostomy.

Application of the Nursing Process to the Care of the Patient with an Ileoanal Endorectal Pull-through

The assessment, nursing diagnoses, expected patient outcomes, nursing interventions, and evaluation for patients having ileoanal endorectal pull-through surgery are similar to those described previously for patients having ileostomy surgery. Given the nature of the surgery, however, make certain preoperatively that the patient fully understands that this is a two-stage procedure and has a realistic expectation regarding ultimate bowel function (i.e., the need for a collection appliance is eliminated, but the pattern of bowel function will not be the typically normal one). Also recognize that, given the extent and location of the surgery, patients may have concerns about its effect on sexual and bladder function. If such fears are expressed, reassure the patient that the risk of impotence or bladder dysfunction is slight because the autonomic nerves in the pelvic region are not disturbed with this type of procedure (Becker & Parodi, 1989).

Postoperatively, be certain to keep the patient on bed rest in a semi-Fowler position during the first postoperative day. This reduces tension on the ileoanal anastomosis and is critical to the success of the surgery. If the patient has been on long-term steroid therapy for ulcerative colitis prior to surgery, monitor for signs of adrenal insufficiency during the period of gradual steroid withdrawal. These include weakness, headache, fever, falling blood pressure, diarrhea, and increased fecal output.

To boost morale, remind the patient that the ileostomy is temporary and that the anal sphincter has been preserved. Provide self-care teaching on a daily basis and encourage the patient to function independently while awaiting closure of the ileostomy.

Following closure of the ileostomy, instruct the patient in self-care as presented in Chart 21–4.

The Elderly: Special Considerations

Age-related changes occur throughout the gastrointestinal tract. In the mouth, taste sensation is diminished, gingival tissue is resorbed, and teeth are often lost. Production of saliva decreases, and dryness of the mouth and difficulty swallowing ensue. Esophageal and gastric emptying are slowed, resulting in feelings of fullness and indigestion. A general decrease in intestinal motility gives rise to abdominal discomfort, constipation, and flatulence.

These changes place the older individual at risk for a variety of problems. Changes in taste, difficulty chewing and swallowing, and gastric distress predispose to anorexia and inadequate fluid intake. Gastric distress further predisposes to the use of antacids and other medications that not only can alter GI motility (magnesium-containing antacids have a laxative effect, and aluminum-containing antacids have a constipating effect) but in some cases contribute to electrolyte imbalance. For example, calcium carbonate can cause milk-alkali syndrome, which involves hypercalcemia, metabolic alkalosis, and renal impairment.

Constipation, a major complaint among individuals older than 60, can be the result of many different factors. In addition to the general decrease in intestinal motility, these factors include lack of bulk in the diet due to difficulty chewing, swallowing, and anorexia; lack of exercise due to mobility problems; limited fluid intake because of difficulty controlling the bladder or getting to the bathroom; hemorrhoids; emotional problems including sadness and depression that increase sympathetic tone and inhibit colonic motility; side effects of medication; and ischemia of the colon caused by arteriosclerosis. Constipation predisposes to the overuse of laxatives or, in cases in which laxative use has contributed to its development, predisposes to continued abuse.

When caring for a geriatric patient, carefully assess for these age-related changes in the GI system

Chart 21–4.

NURSING GUIDE TO PATIENT EDUCATION FOR SELF-MANAGEMENT: SELF-CARE AFTER COMPLETION OF AN ILEOANAL ENDORECTAL PULL-THROUGH

Instruct the patient to:

Use a mirror daily to inspect the perianal area for redness or excoriation.
Cleanse the perianal area with warm water after each bowel movement. Avoid use of soap, which can be irritating. Pat dry gently and thoroughly with cotton balls or unscented white tissue. If preferred, blow dry with a hand-held hair dryer set on its lowest setting.
Apply a protective skin barrier such as Vitamins A & D or Desitin ointment to the perianal area after each cleansing.
Avoid use of products containing alcohol or fragrance on the perianal area.
Wear loose underpants to promote air circulation and prevention of moisture in the perianal area.
Report perianal redness, excoriation, itching, or burning to the physician.
Use a thin sanitary shield to protect clothing from fecal leaking.
Perform perianal exercises four times per day to promote sphincter control: Tighten the anus as though trying to prevent a bowel movement, count to 10, relax, and repeat five or six times.
Avoid evening snacks to discourage nighttime incontinence.
Report anorexia, abdominal discomfort, or bloody diarrhea, all of which are signs of pouchitis, to the physician.

Adapted from Dalton-Loehner D, Conner P. Beyond ileostomy: Surgery for a normal life. RN 1989; 52(7):31–32.

as well as for contributing factors and resultant patient problems. To assist the individual in coping with these age-related changes, encourage use of mouthwash for dry mouth, daily brushing and flossing to promote healthy gums and teeth, and regular dental care. To combat anorexia, feelings of fullness, and gastric distress, suggest small, frequent meals and use of selected spices to compensate for decreased taste and make food appealing. Also suggest that the patient remain in an upright position after eating to facilitate passage of food through the upper GI tract. To promote bowel elimination, encourage a fluid intake of at least 2500 ml/day (unless contraindicated by the presence of another disease), inclusion of fiber in the diet, and exercise compatible with overall physical status. Be certain to teach about the proper use of laxatives, antacids, and other over-the-counter products and their effects on GI function.

Just as age-related changes in the digestive system have implications for the care of all older individuals, changes in other areas of body function affect the care of the geriatric patient with a GI disorder.

Perception of abdominal pain appears to be diminished in the elderly, and abdominal muscles are frequently weak, flabby, and unable to display the true rigidity characteristic of peritoneal irritation. This make assessment of the abdomen difficult, and even more so if because of mental changes the individual has difficulty being specific about the chronology and character of the pain. In these cases, use questions that are specific, unhurried, and related to other activities (e.g., "What happens to the pain when you turn on your side?").

The functional reserve of the elderly is decreased. As a result, increased demand on the body systems may exceed the reserve capacity and homeostasis may not be maintained. Thus, GI diagnostic procedures that involve extensive bowel preparation and GI surgery, particularly procedures of the upper GI tract that are complex, lengthy, and have a direct effect on respiratory function, present major risks to the geriatric patient. Physiologic status must be closely monitored, and actions to support homeostasis aggressively pursued. In the case of diagnostic tests, preparation may be adjusted to the patient's tolerance or alternative tests selected. Expected progress following surgery may also be different for the geriatric patient. For example, start of drainage from a colostomy is not as rapid as in a younger person because of decreased peristalsis and mucus production.

Age-related changes also affect the geriatric patient's capacity for self-care and thus determine type and content of patient teaching. For instance, impaired motor skills and decreased vision can make use of an appliance and related skin care difficult for the patient with an ostomy.

Bibliography

Alltop SA. Teaching for discharge: Gastrostomy tubes. RN 1988; 51(11):42.

Alterescu KB. The ostomy: What about special procedures? Am J Nurs 1985; 85(12):1363.

Alterescu KB. Colostomy. Nurs Clin North Am 1987; 22(2):281.

Alterescu V. The ostomy: What do you teach the patient? Am J Nurs 1985; 85(11):1250.

Anderson BJ. Tube feeding: Is diarrhea inevitable? Am J Nurs 1986; 86(6):704.

Andres R, et al (eds). Principles of geriatric medicine. New York: McGraw-Hill, 1985.

Andresen G. A fresh look at assessing the elderly. RN 1989; 52(8):28.

Bates, B. A guide to physical examination and history taking. 5th ed. Philadelphia: JB Lippincott, 1991.

Becker JM, Parodi JE. Total colectomy with preservation of the anal sphincter. Surg Annu 1989; 21:263.

Berk JE, Haubrich WS, Kalser MH, et al (eds). Bockus gastroenterology. 4th ed. Vols 1–7. Philadelphia: WB Saunders, 1985.

Boarini J. The ostomy: What can go wrong. Am J Nurs 1985; 85(12):1358.

Bope ET. Lower gastrointestinal bleeding. Prim Care 1988; 15(1):93.

Brandt LJ. Gastrointestinal disorders of the elderly. New York: Raven Press, 1984.

Brewer C. Jejunostomy: Highlights of care. J Enterostom Ther 1987; 14(4):163.

Broadwell D, Jackson BS. Principles and practices of ostomy care. St. Louis: CV Mosby, 1982.

Brozenec S, Patras A. Gastrointestinal surgery. In Shekleton M, Litwack K (eds). Critical care nursing of the surgical patient. Philadelphia: WB Saunders, 1991, pp 436–463.

Bruckstein DC. Percutaneous endoscopic gastrostomy. Geriatr Nurs 1988; 9(2):92.

Bryant R, Boarini J. Gastrointestinal surgical procedures. J Enterostom Ther 1986; 13(1):34.

Burnside IM. Nursing and aged: A self approach. 3rd ed. New York. McGraw-Hill, 1988.

Caird FI, Grimley-Evans J. Advanced geriatric medicine. Vol 6. Stoneham, MA: Butterworth, 1987.

Calkins E, Ford AB, Katz PR. The practice of geriatric medicine. 2nd ed. Philadelphia: WB Saunders, 1992.

Camp D, Otten N. How to insert and remove nasogastric tubes quickly and easily. Nursing 1990; 20(9):59.

Carnevali D. Nursing management for the elderly. 2nd ed. Philadelphia: JB Lippincott, 1988.

Carroll M, Brue LJ. A nurse's guide to caring for elders. New York: Springer Publishing, 1988.

Carroll PF. Aspirated feeding solution. Nursing 1986; 16(1):33.

Chwals WJ, Blackburn GL. Perioperative nutritional support in the cancer patient. Surg Clin North Am 1986; 66(6):1137.

Colley R, Fischer JE. Understanding hyperalimentation: A patient's guide. Cincinnati, OH: Bermon Printing, 1981.

Curtas S, Chapman G, Meguid MM. Evaluation of nutritional status. Nurs Clin North Am 1989; 24(2):301.

Dalton-Loehner D, Connor P. Beyond ileostomy: Surgery for a normal life. RN 1989; 52(7):29.

Decker S. The life-threatening consequences of a GI bleed. RN 1985; 48(10):18.

Drossman DA (ed). Manual of gastroenterologic procedures. 2nd ed. New York: Raven Press, 1987.

Eisenberg P. Enteral nutrition: Indications, formulas, and delivery techniques. Nurs Clin North Am 1989; 24(2):315.

Esberger KK. Nursing care of the aged. Norwalk, CT: Appleton & Lange, 1989.

Feickert D. Gastric surgery: Your crucial pre- and postop role. RN 1987; 50(1):24.

Flynn KT, Norton LC, Fisher RL. Enteral tube feeding: Indications, practices and outcomes. Image J Nurs Sch 1987; 19(1):16.

Freedman J. Speaking out on nasogastric feeding. Geriatr Nurs 1987; 8(1):7.

Gauderer MWL, Stellato TA. Gastrostomies: Evolution, techniques, indications, and complications. Curr Probl Surg 1986; 23(9):661.

Given B, Simmons S. Gastroenterology in clinical nursing. St. Louis: CV Mosby, 1984.

Govoni LE, Hayes JE. Drugs and nursing implications. 6th ed. Norwalk, CT: Appleton & Lange, 1988, pp 1181–1183.

Griffin JP. Be prepared for the bleeding patient. Nursing 1986; 16(6):34.

Groth K. Age-related changes in the gastrointestinal tract. Geriatr Nurs 1988; 9(5):278.

Gruendemann BJ, Meeker M. Alexander's care of the patient in surgery. 6th ed. St. Louis: CV Mosby, 1987.

Hakki A, Hakki A, Iskandrian A, et al. A simple formula for monitoring parenteral infusion. Crit Care Nurse 1986; 6(3):57.

Hamilton H. Gastrointestinal disorders. Springhouse, PA: Springhouse, 1985.

Hatchett-Cohen L. Nasoduodenal tube feeding. Geriatr Nurs 1988; 9(2):88.

Heymsfield SB, Erbland M, Casper K, et al. Enteral nutritional support: Metabolic, cardiovascular, and pulmonary interrelations. Clin Chest Med 1986; 7(1):41.

Hill L, Kozarek R, McCallum R, Mercer CD. The esophagus: Medical and surgical management. Philadelphia: WB Saunders, 1988.

Kahn R. Renewing the commitment to oral hygiene. Geriatr Nurs 1986; 7(5):244.

Kaushik SP, Ralphs DNL, Hobsley M. Influences on the occurrence of dumping syndrome. Am J Gastroenterol 1983; 78(3):155.

Kohn CL, Keithley JK. Enteral nutrition: Potential complications and patient monitoring. Nurs Clin North Am 1989; 24(2):339.

Lamy PP. Treating GI upset in older adults. J Gerontol Nurs 1985; 11(7):40.

Lancaster JR. Upper gastrointestinal bleeding. Prim Care 1988; 15(1):31.

Longman AJ, Dewalt EM. A guide for oral assessment. Geriatr Nurs 1986; 7(5):252.

Malloy C, Hartshorn J. Acute care nursing in the home. Philadelphia: JB Lippincott, 1989.

Matteson MA, McConnell ES. Gerontological nursing: Concepts and practice. Philadelphia: WB Saunders, 1988.

McGee L. Feeding gastrostomy. J Enterostom Ther 1987; 14(5):201.

Meeroff JC. Management of massive gastrointestinal bleeding. Hosp Prac 1986; 21(5):93.

Meguid MM, Meguid V. Preoperative identification of the surgical cancer patient in need of postoperative supportive total parenteral nutrition. Cancer 1985; 55(suppl 1):258.

Mertes JE. Action STAT! G.I. bleeding. Nursing 1989; 19(8):37.

Metheny N. Measures to test placement of nasogastric and nasointestinal feeding tubes: A review. Nurs Res 1988; 37(6):324.

Metheny NM. 20 ways to prevent tube feeding complications. Nursing 1985; 15(1):47.

Mettlin C. Dietary factors for cancer of specific sites. Surg Clin North Am 1986; 66(5):917.

Moore, MC. Do you still believe these myths about tube feeding? RN 1987; 50(5):51.

Ofstehage JC, Magilvy K. Oral health and aging. Geriatr Nurs 1986; 7(5):238.

Patras AZ, Paice JA, Lanigan K. Managing GI bleeding. Nursing 1988; 18(4):68.

Plumer AL. Principles and practice of intravenous therapy. 4th ed. Boston, Little, Brown, 1987.

Quigley M. Upper gastrointestinal hemorrhage. In Parrillo J (ed). Current therapy in critical care medicine. Philadelphia: BC Decker, 1991, pp 279–283.

Rajaratnam R. Method for anchoring nasogastric feeding tubes. Laryngoscope 1985; 95(2):219.

Ricci J. Alcohol-induced upper GI hemorrhage. Crit Care Nurse 1987; 7(1):56.

Ricker LE, Williams J, Dunfee C, et al. Colorectal carcinoma. AORN J 1989; 50(5):1046.

Rideout BW. The patient with an ileostomy. Nurs Clin North Am 1987; 22(2):253.

Sabiston DC (ed). Textbook of surgery: The biological basis of modern surgical practice. Philadelphia: WB Saunders, 1991.

Saleh JW. Laparoscopy. Philadelphia: WB Saunders, 1988.

Salmon PR, Jong M. Endoscopic haemostasis of the upper gastrointestinal tract. Clin Gastroenterol 1986; 15(2):321.
Schiller KFR, Cockel R, Hunt RH. A colour atlas of gastrointestinal endoscopy. Philadelphia: WB Saunders, 1987.
Shellito PC, Malt RA. Tube gastrostomy: Techniques and complications. Ann Surg 1985; 201(2):180.
Short NM. Gastrointestinal intubations: Nursing considerations. Gastroenterol Nurs 1989; 12(1):43.
Sleisenger MH, Fordtran JS. Gastrointestinal disease: Pathophysiology, diagnosis, management. 4th ed. Philadelphia: WB Saunders, 1989.
Smith CE. Detecting acute abdominal distension: What to look for, what to do. Nursing 1985; 15(9):39.
Smith CE. Assessing bowel sounds: More than just listening. Nursing 1988; 18(2):42.
Smith DB. The ostomy: How is it managed? Am J Nurs 1985; 85(11):1246.
Smith LH, Thier SO. Pathophysiology: The biological principles of disease. 2nd ed. Philadelphia: WB Saunders, 1985.
Sodeman WA Jr, Saladin TA, Boyd WP Jr. Geriatric gastroenterology. Philadelphia: WB Saunders, 1989.
Starkey JF, Jefferson PA, Kirby DF. Taking care of percutaneous endoscopic gastrostomy. Am J Nurs 1988; 88(1):42.
Stelzner M, Fonkalsrud E. Endorectal ileal pull through procedure for patients with ulcerative colitis and familial polyposis with carcinoma. Surg Gynecol Obstet 1989; 169(3):187.
Surratt S, Ryan A, Hallenbeck P, et al. Troubleshooting a sump tube. Am J Nurs 1993; 93(1):42.
Thurlow PM. Bedside enteral feeding and tube placement into duodenum and jejunum. J Parenter Enteral Nutr 1986; 10(1):104.
Toranes S. Ileal pull-through surgery. Nursing 1987; 17(11):92.
Watt RC. The ostomy: Why is it created? Am J Nurs 1985; 85(11):1242.
Welch JP. Bowel obstruction: Differential diagnosis and clinical management. Philadelphia: WB Saunders, 1990.
Wilhelm L. Helping your patient "settle in" with TPN. Nursing 1985; 15(4):60.
Williams SR. Nutrition and diet therapy. St. Louis: Times Mirror/Mosby, 1989.
Wright B. Enteral feeding tubes as drug delivery systems. Nutr Support Serv 1986; 6(2):33.
Wroblewski B, Young L. Topics in parenteral nutrition for the 1990s. Focus Crit Care 1991; 18(4):276.
Young CK, White S. Preparing patients for tube feeding at home. Am J Nurs 1992; 92(4):46.
Zuidema GD (ed). Shackelford's surgery of the alimentary tract. 3rd ed. Philadelphia: WB Saunders, 1991.

Chapter Twenty-two

NURSING CARE *of Adults with Disorders of the Upper Gastrointestinal System*

Upper gastrointestinal disorders are among the most common health problems of adults and range in severity from simple cold sores to gastric cancer. Regardless of the specific problem, normal ingestion or digestion of nutrients, or both, are affected, and there is potential for nutritional imbalance, pain, and in most cases for life-threatening complications.

The chronic nature of many upper gastrointestinal disorders has specific implications for nursing care. The need for long-term care and follow-up requires that the nurse be able to provide appropriate patient or family teaching; act as a liaison between such resources as the community health nurse, the physician, and the pharmacist; and provide support over an extended period of time.

Infections and Inflammations

Oral Infections

There are many different types of oral infection. Generally they are due to an interaction of factors such as poor oral hygiene, poor nutritional habits, and stress, although in some instances, they may be related to a systemic disorder. For the most part, they simply cause discomfort and are a nuisance. However, if they are not cared for properly, more serious complications can occur.

The etiology, pathophysiology, clinical manifestations, medical diagnosis, and medical management of the most common oral infections are presented in Table 22–1.

Application of the Nursing Process to the Care of the Patient with an Oral Infection

Assessment

When assessing a patient with an oral infection, wear a mask and gloves. Begin with careful inspection of the mouth. Use a penlight and tongue blade to visualize all areas of the mouth, including under the tongue and inside the lips, which are retracted with the tongue blade. Examine the lips for color, hydration, and the presence of lesions, especially in the angles. Check the gums for retraction, inflammation, edema, bleeding, and lesions. Note the odor of the breath, and question the patient about any taste or areas of soreness in the mouth.

Review the patient's usual pattern of oral hygiene, and explore recent activities or stresses that may have predisposed to the development of a specific oral infection.

Assess the patient's general nutritional status. Be certain to inquire about any changes in diet necessitated by the problem with the mouth. If these changes are significant and prolonged, review the current diet for nutritional adequacy and check for weight loss and signs of nutritional deficiency.

Also assess for any misconceptions related to the infection, particularly in terms of its contagion and its cause.

Nursing Diagnoses and Planning

Nursing diagnoses and related expected patient outcomes most commonly applicable to patients with oral infections include the following:

NDx: Pain related to irritation of ulcerated areas in mouth when eating or speaking

Planning: Patient outcomes
1. Patient uses pain medication or topical anesthetic as needed.
2. Patient avoids irritating foods and fluids.
3. Patient states mouth is less sore.
4. Lesions are decreasing in size and number.

NDx: High risk for altered health maintenance related to insufficient knowledge of nature of the infection, treatment, and measures to prevent recurrence

Planning: Patient outcomes
1. Patient describes the infection, stating cause, usual duration, and degree of contagion.
2. Patient explains treatment regimen to be followed at home.
3. Patient describes relationship of oral hygiene, nutrition, and stress to the development of oral infections.
4. Patient demonstrates good oral hygiene.

Nursing Interventions

NDx: Pain

Minimize discomfort and aid healing by administering mild analgesics and topical anesthetic preparations such as viscous Xylocaine as prescribed. Instruct the patient in the use of mouth rinses, which can be medicated solutions or simply one-quarter strength hydrogen peroxide and water solution, used every 1 to 2 hours.

Limit the diet to soothing foods such as Jell-O, pudding, egg nogs, cool drinks, and custards.

NDx: High risk for altered health maintenance

Explain the cause, expected course, usual duration, and contagion of the infection to the patient. Review the treatment regimen, making certain that the pa-

Table 22–1. COMMON INFECTIONS OF THE MOUTH

TYPE OF INFECTION	ETIOLOGY AND PATHOPHYSIOLOGY	CLINICAL MANIFESTATIONS	MEDICAL DIAGNOSIS	MEDICAL MANAGEMENT
Herpes labialis (cold sores)	Caused by herpes simplex virus. Latent virus appears to be activated by an external factor such as cold or fever. Vesicles form scab, and heal in 1 to 3 weeks without scarring. Wide variation in individual susceptibility.	Clear vesicles, most often located at the mucocutaneous junction of the lips and face, which scab.	Based on clinical appearance and history.	No specific treatment available. Symptomatic relief is provided by topical anesthetics.
Aphthous ulcers (canker sore or ulcerative stomatitis)	Cause is unknown, although hereditary predisposition and involvement of Ig-E–bearing lymphocytes appear to be involved. Occur more often in women.	Painful, shallow, pseudomembranous covered ulcers with a ring of erythema, occurring on the oral mucosa.	Based on clinical appearance and history.	Topical anesthetics such as viscous lidocaine or the antihistamine diphenhydramine held in the mouth provide symptomatic relief, as do bland washes and mild analgesics. Antibiotic suspensions such as tetracycline, 250 mg/ml, held on ulcers for 2 minutes four to five times per day, promote healing. Short courses of corticosteroids (e.g., 40 mg prednisone o.d., 2–3 days) control severe symptoms.
Acute gingivitis (acute necrotizing ulcerative gingivitis, trench mouth, or Vincent's disease)	Noncontagious, acute infection of the gums, often associated with fusiform bacilli or a spirochete. No epidemiologic pattern is seen. Malnutrition, stress, fatigue, and poor oral hygiene appear to be predisposing factors.	Foul taste in the mouth. Malaise. Occasional fever and lymphadenopathy.	Based on clinical symptoms and response to treatment.	Good oral hygiene. Hydrogen peroxide mouthwashes. Balanced diet. Penicillin or erythromycin, 250 mg PO q.i.d., if fever or lymphadenopathy is present.
Chronic gingivitis	Related to poor mouth care, irritating fillings, or poorly fitting dentures.	Often asymptomatic, although gums may be reddened and edematous and may be painful and bleed after brushing or flossing.	Based on history and physical findings.	Improved oral and dental care.
Moniliasis (thrush)	Infection with the fungus *Candida albicans,* which is part of the normal flora of the mouth. Often associated with dentures, poor oral hygiene, diabetes mellitus, and the use of antibiotics. Apparently noncontagious.	Creamy white patches of fungus on the mucous membranes that resemble milk curds and are surrounded by erythematous mucosa.	Based on smear or culture showing the fungus.	Nystatin suspension, chewable tablets, or lozenges, 100,000 units three to four times o.d.

tient understands the importance of taking antibiotics on a consistent schedule and of taking all the doses ordered even if symptoms have disappeared.

Instruct the patient and the family on the value and technique of good oral hygiene, the importance of good nutrition, and the control of stress in the prevention of recurrences.

Evaluation

Evaluate the effectiveness of nursing care for a patient with an oral infection by comparing the patient's status with the expected patient outcomes. Examples of specific outcomes for patients with an oral infection have been provided in the Planning section.

Esophagitis

ETIOLOGY

Esophagitis is an inflammation of the esophagus. As with any inflammation, esophagitis may be triggered by a variety of thermal, chemical, physical, and mechanical factors. These include smoking, intake of alcohol or spicy foods, ingestion of caustic agents such as lye or ammonia, reflux of acidic gastric contents into the esophagus, friction from the movement of a sliding hiatus hernia, prolonged gastric intubation, and bacterial or viral invasion of the esophageal wall. Of these, reflux of gastric contents is most often the causative factor.

PATHOPHYSIOLOGY

The effects of the inflammatory process on the esophagus range from a local area of hyperemia to edema, necrosis, and ulceration depending on the nature of the causative agent and the amount and duration of exposure to it. With prolonged or recurrent inflammation, the esophageal wall may become thickened and fibrotic.

CLINICAL MANIFESTATIONS

The onset of symptoms of esophagitis may be sudden or gradual. Classic symptoms are burning, retrosternal discomfort (pyrosis or heartburn); pain on swallowing, which may radiate into the arms, neck, back, or jaw; and eructation or acid regurgitation. If the esophageal lumen is narrowed from edema or fibrosis, dysphagia for solid foods may be present. In severe cases in which mucosal erosion is present, bleeding manifested as hematemesis or melena may occur.

MEDICAL DIAGNOSIS

Diagnosis of esophagitis is made on the basis of symptomatology, history of recent exposure to irritating factors, and if needed, direct examination of the mucosa with an esophagoscope.

MEDICAL MANAGEMENT

Treatment of esophagitis is directed at eliminating the causative factor and promoting an environment within the esophagus that is conducive to healing. For patients with simple esophagitis, a bland diet, elimination or reduction of smoking, and antacids (Pharmacology Box 22–1) to be taken at bedtime and when pain occurs are prescribed.

If reflux of gastric contents is contributing to the esophagitis, drugs such as cimetidine or ranitidine (Zantac) that block the histamine receptors may be ordered to reduce gastric acid (Pharmacology Box 22–2).

Treatment must be continued until the esophagus is completely healed and not merely until symptomatic relief is obtained. Early discontinuation of treatment is a common cause of recurrence.

Surgical resection of the esophagus is indicated if obstruction, perforation, or hemorrhage occurs or severe pain persists. When gastric reflux is a problem, a procedure such as vagotomy with antrectomy or a pyloroplasty may be required.

Application of the Nursing Process to the Care of the Patient with Esophagitis

Assessment

Since pain is the most prominent symptom of any esophageal disorder, determine the type, severity, and location of pain experienced by the patient. Question the patient about odynophagia (painful swallowing), pyrosis, and diffuse epigastric pain as well as the relationship of the onset of pain or its increased severity to factors such as meals, ingestion of specific foods, eating at particular times, smoking, body position, or activity. Also question the patient about related symptoms such as eructation, dysphagia, regurgitation, and hematemesis.

Assess the patient's current nutritional status. Identify the normal daily diet, and explore any changes in eating patterns necessitated by the presence of symptoms. An example of the latter would be the elimination of specific types of foods from the diet that were previously enjoyed. Nonprescription remedies may cause undesirable side effects, such as the acid rebound effect and potential for metabolic

Pharmacology Box 22–1.

ANTACIDS

Antacids:
Over-the-counter medications that neutralize gastric acid. Most in current use are nonabsorbable and are bases of magnesium, aluminum, or calcium.

Action:
Antacids that are weak bases combine with hydrochloric acid in the stomach to form salts and water and thus raise gastric pH and decrease the proteolytic action of pepsin.

Uses:
Treatment of peptic ulcer disease, esophagitis due to reflux, gastritis, and symptomatic relief of pyrosis.

Side Effects:
Increase of gastric pH with predisposition to gastrointestinal infection is a side effect of all antacids. Other side effects are specific to the type of antacid used. Those containing magnesium can cause diarrhea, dehydration, and in patients with renal insufficiency, hypermagnesemia with neurologic, muscular, and cardiovascular changes. Those containing aluminum include constipation, impaction, and with long-term use, hypophosphatemia, which can cause osteomalacia and myopathy. Calcium carbonate can cause acid rebound and milk-alkali syndrome.

Interactions:
Antacids are capable of interacting with virtually all other drugs through effects on their absorption owing to chemical binding, a change in gastric pH, or a change in gastric emptying time. Drugs whose absorption is impaired by antacids include tetracyclines, anticholinergics, cardiac glycosides, phenothiazides, indomethacin, isoniazid, and phenylbutazone. Drugs whose absorption is accelerated include weak bases and enteric-coated preparations.

Nursing Implications:
Shake liquid preparations well, and follow with a small amount of water. If given by nasogastric tube, flush with at least 60 ml of water to prevent caking on the sides of the tube and subsequent blockage.
Instruct patients to chew chewable tablets thoroughly and follow with a full glass of water.
Give other medications 2 to 3 hours before or after antacids.
Instruct patients taking aluminum- or calcium-based antacids to drink at least 2500 ml of fluid per day to prevent constipation. Instruct those taking magnesium preparations to add bananas, rice, applesauce, and tea to the diet to combat diarrhea.
Instruct all patients to report persistent problems with bowel function as well as symptoms of electrolyte imbalance.
Warn patients that antacid therapy may cause stools to be white or speckled in appearance.

Geriatric Considerations:
The elderly are at risk for hypermagnesemia and other fluid and electrolyte imbalances when taking magnesium-containing antacids.

The elderly, especially those with dehydration, decreased bowel motility, or renal disease, are at risk for severe constipation and impaction when taking calcium- or aluminum-containing antacids.

Pharmacology Box 22–2.

HISTAMINE$_2$-RECEPTOR ANTAGONISTS

Histamine$_2$-Receptor Antagonists:
Drugs that block the H_2-histamine receptor sites as opposed to H_1-receptor sites blocked by traditional antihistamines.

Action:
Block the H_2-receptor sites on the gastric parietal cells, inhibiting the secretion of hydrochloric acid (HCl). Also decrease HCl secretion in response to other chemical and nervous stimuli. Have no significant cardiovascular effects at the doses used to treat gastric disease.

Uses:
Treatment of peptic ulcer disease, Zollinger-Ellison syndrome and other hypersecretory disorders, and gastrointestinal reflux. Prevention of stress ulcers.

Side Effects:
Infrequent with cimetidine and ranitidine.
Cimetidine—Occasional mild diarrhea, nausea, dizziness, rash, and muscle aches. May also cause impotence, decreased sperm count, and gynecomastia in males and galactorrhea in females because of antiandrogenic effects.
Ranitidine—Headache, nausea, and constipation.
Famotidine—Headache, diarrhea, dizziness, and constipation.

Interactions:
Antacids decrease the absorption of H_2-receptor antagonists.
Cimetidine mildly inhibits the cytochrome oxidase system of the liver and thereby increases the half-life of drugs such as diazepam, flurazepam, and theophylline; also beta-blockers, phenytoin, salicylates, and quinidine.
Cimetidine plus morphine can cause muscle twitching, confusion, and apnea.
Cimetidine can decrease serum levels of dioxin, decrease absorption of ketoconazole, and increase effects of carbamazepine and procainamide.

Nursing Implications:
Give H_2 blockers at least 1 hour before of after antacids.
Do not dilute with sterile water for injection; use a compatible solution as listed on the label.
Observe elderly patients on cimetidine for confusion.
Monitor fluid intake and output of elderly patients and those with impaired renal function. Instruct patients to: take with meals so that the peak effect coincides with the time of maximum secretion of gastric acid; avoid cigarette smoking because it impairs the effect of H_2 blockers; do not self-dose for pain—take prescribed doses only; and report persistent or worsening side effects.
Explain the need for periodic blood counts and tests of renal and hepatic function when taking H_2 blockers for longer than 4 weeks.

Geriatric Considerations:
Mental confusion, agitation, depression, and hallucinations may occur in the elderly. These effects are most common with cimetidine and are usually associated with decreased renal function.

acidosis associated with the use of bicarbonate of soda as an antacid. Therefore, elicit the frequency of their use and their effects.

When the medical diagnosis has been made and treatment prescribed, assess the patient's level of understanding. Assess for other factors that are likely to promote or prevent compliance with the treatment regimen. These include economic factors, home and family situation, and psychological response to the disorder and the treatment.

Nursing Diagnoses and Planning

Nursing diagnoses and related expected patient outcomes most commonly applicable to patients with esophagitis include the following:

NDx: Pain related to esophageal inflammation

Planning: Patient outcomes

1. Patient explains proper self-administration of antacids as presented in Pharmacology Box 22–1.
2. Patient describes the potential for aggravation of the pain by alcohol and nicotine.
3. Patient states the discomfort has decreased.
4. Patient rubs area over sternum and belches less frequently.
5. Patient reports absence of discomfort when swallowing nonirritating foods and fluids.

NDx: High risk for constipation or diarrhea related to use of antacids (specify)

Planning: Patient outcomes

1. Patient describes effects of antacids on bowel activity.
2. Patient lists measures to promote normal bowel activity.
3. Patient reports regular passage of soft, formed stool.

NDx: High risk for altered health maintenance related to insufficient knowledge of nature of the disorder, dietary modifications, measures to limit gastric reflux, and use of prescribed medications

Planning: Patient outcomes

1. Patient describes the causes, effects, and usual clinical course of esophagitis.
2. Patient lists symptoms to be reported such as hematemesis or melena.
3. Patient lists foods to be avoided.
4. Patient describes benefit of small, frequent feedings.
5. Patient states plan for implementing dietary changes.
6. Patient verbalizes the importance of and a realistic plan for reducing or eliminating smoking.
7. Patient explains relationship of tight clothing and body positions to reflux of gastric contents into the esophagus.
8. Patient identifies name, use, dose, time, route of administration, and side effects of each prescribed drug.

Nursing Interventions

NDx: Pain

Administer or teach the patient to self-administer antacids prescribed for pain as described in Pharmacology Box 22–1. Encourage the use of relaxation techniques to assist the patient in handling the pain. Caution the patient against smoking or drinking alcoholic beverages in an attempt to relax and relieve the pain, because these activities can in fact aggravate the condition.

NDx: High risk for constipation or diarrhea

Explain to the patient that aluminum- or calcium-based antacids have a tendency to cause constipation and magnesium-based antacids can cause diarrhea. If the patient is on an aluminum- or calcium-based antacid, review the importance of plenty of fluids and roughage in the diet as well as the value of regular exercise in preventing constipation. If the patient is taking a magnesium-based antacid, advise that large amounts of fresh fruits and vegetables and other foods such as licorice that stimulate bowel function be avoided. In all cases, instruct the patient to report uncomfortable constipation or diarrhea, because it is possible to use antacids in combination and thus control these side effects.

NDx: High risk for altered health maintenance

Explain the causes, effects, and usual clinical course of esophagitis to the patient at a level he or she can understand. Describe the role of gastric reflux as a causative or exacerbating factor. Alert the patient to symptoms such as hematemesis and melena that should be promptly reported.

Instruct the patient and the family about dietary modifications that facilitate healing and help prevent recurrence. Stress the need to avoid alcohol, caffeine, and any food that causes pain. Because gastric reflux is a factor in the vast majority of cases of esophagitis, recommend small, frequent meals to help reduce the secretion of gastric acid. Initiate a consultation with a dietitian to assist the patient with meal planning if needed. To further aid in preventing gastric reflux, instruct the patient to avoid eating for 2 to 3 hours prior to bedtime, to remain in an upright position for 2 to 3 hours after eating, and to avoid bending and the wearing of tight clothing.

Teach the patient the dose, route, time, frequency, expected side effects, and signs of toxic effects of all prescribed medications.

Evaluation

Evaluate the effectiveness of nursing care for a patient with esophagitis by comparing the patient's status with the expected patient outcomes. Examples of specific outcomes for patients with esophagitis have been provided in the Planning section.

Acute Gastritis

Acute gastritis is a self-limiting inflammation of the stomach mucosa. It may be diffuse or localized. In the diffuse form, all areas of the stomach are affected, whereas in the localized form only a specific area is involved.

ETIOLOGY

Acute gastritis can result from any chemical, thermal, bacterial, or mechanical factor that injures the gastric mucosa. Examples of these factors are drugs such as aspirin, digitalis, and phenylbutazone (Butazolidin); alcohol; excessive amounts of irritating foods such as tea, coffee, pepper, and other spices; foods that are very rough, very hot, or contaminated with *Staphylococcus;* corrosive substances; and exposure to radiation. Acute gastritis is also found to develop in association with severe medical problems such as acute respiratory failure, sepsis, renal failure, advanced carcinomatosis, hypovolemic shock, and extensive trauma.

PATHOPHYSIOLOGY

Regardless of the specific precipitating factor, the involved mucosa exhibits vascular congestion, edema, petechial hemorrhages, and areas of erosion and superficial ulceration. All of these are reversible, although healing time varies with the cause.

CLINICAL MANIFESTATIONS

Acute gastritis is often asymptomatic. When symptoms do occur, they include one or more of the following: epigastric pain, abdominal tenderness, nausea, vomiting, and eructation. If the gastritis is of the hemorrhagic type as caused by aspirin or stress, hematemesis or melena also occurs, accompanied by a decreased hematocrit level and an elevated blood urea nitrogen level.

MEDICAL DIAGNOSIS

The diagnosis of acute gastritis is made on the basis of endoscopy or biopsy.

MEDICAL MANAGEMENT

Acute gastritis is treated only when symptoms are present. Treatment consists of removal of the precipitating factor when possible, antiemetics to control nausea and vomiting, or antacid and H_2-antagonist therapy to decrease gastric secretions that can further irritate inflamed areas.

In cases of acute hemorrhagic gastritis, parenteral fluid and blood replacement as well as nasogastric lavage may also be required.

Application of the Nursing Process to the Care of the Patient with Acute Gastritis

Assessment

History and the subjective description of symptoms are critical to the assessment of the patient with gastritis. Carefully question the patient regarding location, onset, duration of pain and factors that relieve or aggravate pain. Collect information about changes in appetite and eating habits as well as data about eructation, weight changes, and color and character of stool. If emesis is reported, question the patient about its characteristics, such as the presence of red blood, "coffee grounds," or bile, as well as its relationship to nausea. Elicit information related to possible precipitating factors. Ask the patient about use of prescription or over-the-counter medications; ingestion of alcoholic beverages, tea, and coffee; and types of foods included in the usual daily diet.

Assess the patient's understanding of and reaction to the problem and its treatment. Keep in mind that anxiety over prognosis is common, especially in patients with hematemesis.

During physical examination, check for upper abdominal tenderness and signs of dehydration. Also observe for signs of systemic disease that might be related to the gastritis.

Nursing Diagnoses and Planning

Nursing diagnoses and related expected patient outcomes most commonly applicable to patients with acute gastritis include the following:

NDx: Pain related to inflammation of the gastric mucosa

Planning: Patient outcomes
1. Patient states pain is decreased or absent.
2. Behavioral signs of pain such as moaning and holding the upper abdomen are absent.

NDx: High risk for fluid volume deficit related to vomiting and limited fluid intake

Planning: Patient outcomes
1. Skin turgor is firm.
2. Mucous membranes are moist.

3. Urinary output is at least 50 ml/hour or 1500 ml/day.
4. Serum electrolyte levels are within normal range.
5. Symptoms of electrolyte imbalance are absent.

NDx: High risk for altered health maintenance related to insufficient knowledge of causes and prevention of acute gastritis

Planning: Patient outcomes
1. Patient names any identified causative factors.
2. Patient describes how to avoid causative factors in the future.
3. Patient lists irritating substances that can contribute to gastritis.
4. Patient identifies changes in eating habits necessary to avoid irritating food substances.
5. Patient identifies substitute foods or food seasonings for those to be avoided as well as correct methods of food preparation.

Nursing Interventions

NDx: Pain
Administer prescribed antacids to neutralize gastric acid and raise gastric pH and H_2-antagonists to inhibit gastric acid secretion. Encourage the patient to avoid cigarette smoking, because nicotine increases gastric acidity. Provide restful diversion such as soft music, and encourage the use of controlled breathing or other relaxation techniques.

NDx: High risk for fluid volume deficit
Initiate interventions to control vomiting. Keep the patient on NPO status, administer antiemetics as ordered, and maintain a quiet environment. Monitor intravenous fluids, and maintain an accurate record of fluid intake and output. Review electrolyte values daily.

When the acute phase has passed, start the patient on clear fluids and progress to a full bland diet divided into several small feedings, as tolerated.

NDx: High risk for altered health maintenance
Explain the causative factor to the patient if a specific one, such as a drug or contaminated food, is identified. Provide information needed to enable the patient to avoid exposure to it in the future. For example, if aspirin is involved, explain that it is found in many over-the-counter medications such as Alka-Seltzer, and instruct the patient to read labels or consult with the pharmacist prior to using these products. If contaminated food was responsible, review the patient's knowledge of proper food storage and preparation techniques. In all cases, explain the role of irritating foods, and assist the patient in identifying desirable changes in his or her daily diet. When indicated, initiate a consult with a dietitian.

Additional Interventions
Maintain the patient on bed rest during the acute phase, and check all emesis for signs of bleeding.

Evaluation

Evaluate the effectiveness of nursing care for a patient with acute gastritis by comparing the patient's status with the expected patient outcomes. Examples of specific outcomes for patients with acute gastritis have been provided in the Planning section.

Chronic Gastritis

Chronic gastritis is a long-term progressive disease. It affects women more often than men, and its overall frequency increases with advancing age.

ETIOLOGY

The etiology of chronic gastritis is unknown, although many factors have been theorized to contribute to its development. These include radiation exposure, nutritional deficiencies, endocrine disorders, immune disturbances, alcohol or drug abuse, and reflux of duodenal secretions into the stomach.

PATHOPHYSIOLOGY

Chronic gastritis begins as superficial gastritis in which the inflammatory changes are limited to the upper portion of the mucosa. As the process invades the mucosa more deeply, it is referred to as atrophic gastritis. In this stage, the mucosa becomes thin, and parietal and chief cells are absent. The progressive decrease in gastric acid secretion results in altered digestion, and diminished secretion of intrinsic factor results in vitamin B_{12} deficiency and pernicious anemia.

Gastric cancer occurs more often in patients with chronic gastritis than in the general population. No causal relationship has been established, however.

CLINICAL MANIFESTATIONS

Chronic gastritis is often asymptomatic. When symptoms do occur, they are often similar to those of peptic ulcer disease or gastric cancer. Epigastric fullness, burning or pain, nausea, vomiting, and flatulence may occur, especially following large meals. Anorexia, weight loss, and symptoms of anemia also develop.

MEDICAL DIAGNOSIS

Definitive diagnosis of chronic gastritis is based on endoscopy with gastric biopsy. Since the disease process may be localized, several biopsies from different areas of the stomach are required.

MEDICAL MANAGEMENT

There is no specific treatment for chronic gastritis. Symptomatic relief is generally obtained with ant-

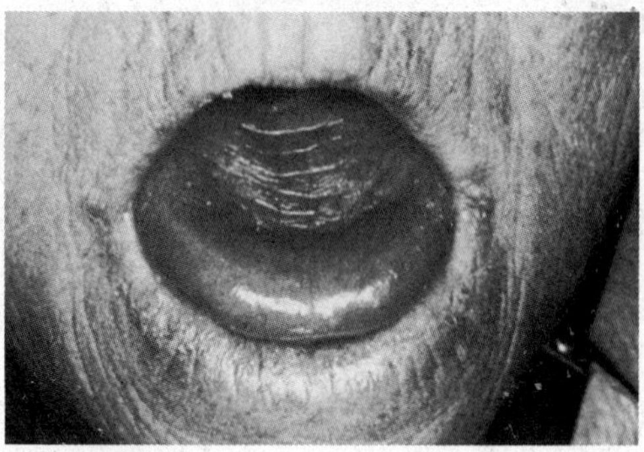

Figure 22–1.

Severe atrophic glossitis. The tongue is painful, smooth, shiny, and bright red as a result of the atrophy of papillae. (From Sleisenger MH, Fordtran JS. Gastrointestinal disease: Pathophysiology, diagnosis, management. 4th ed. Philadelphia: WB Saunders, 1989, p xxxv.)

acid therapy and bland diet taken in small, frequent feedings throughout the day. Patients are followed to monitor for development of pernicious anemia, which requires monthly injections of vitamin B_{12} for life, as well as for the occurrence of gastric cancer.

Application of the Nursing Process to the Care of the Patient with Chronic Gastritis

The assessment, nursing diagnoses, expected patient outcomes, nursing interventions, and evaluation for patients with chronic gastritis are similar to those described previously for patients with acute gastritis, with the following considerations.

Because the nursing diagnosis of high risk for altered health maintenance related to insufficient knowledge of the need for follow-up care commonly applies to patients with chronic gastritis, explain to the patient the relationship of pernicious anemia and gastric cancer to chronic gastritis. Describe what pernicious anemia is and how it is treated. Explain the importance of observing for and reporting symptoms of vitamin B_{12} deficiency such as stomatitis and glossitis (Fig. 22–1).

Structural and Functional Disorders

Peptic Ulcer Disease

Peptic ulcer is a general term that refers to a sharply defined break in the muscularis mucosae in any part of the gastrointestinal tract that is exposed to gastric juice containing acid and pepsin. Thus, a peptic ulcer can occur in the distal esophagus, the stomach, the duodenum, or any part of the intestinal tract that has been surgically connected to the stomach. When referring to an ulcer, it is necessary to identify it by location, for example a gastric ulcer or a duodenal ulcer, because there are differences in incidence and etiology.

Ulcers are a common disorder and are responsible for approximately 10% of all adult hospital admissions. The ratio of duodenal ulcers to gastric ulcers is 3:2, and the male-to-female ratio has recently changed from 3:1 to 1:1. Peak incidence of duodenal ulcers is in the fifth and sixth decades, although diagnosis of the disorder in 20- and 30-year-olds is not uncommon. Gastric ulcers, in contrast, are more common in persons between the ages of 60 and 80 years. Both types of ulcer can occur in the same person, and this in fact occurs twenty times more often than would be expected by chance alone.

A unique form of peptic ulcer is the stress ulcer, which is discussed later.

ETIOLOGY

Ulceration of the gastrointestinal mucosa is believed to result from an imbalance between the resistance of the mucosa to injury and the amount of gastric secretions. Although the precise determinants of these two variables are unknown, many different factors have been implicated. The finding that gastric ulcers are more common in persons with type A blood, whereas duodenal ulcers are more common in those with type O blood suggests that a hereditary or genetic relationship exists. The use of such drugs as salicylates, indomethacin, phenylbutazone, ibuprofen, and the glucocorticoids is highly correlated with the development of gastric ulcers. Also linked to the development of ulcers is infection with the common bacteria *Helicobacter pylori.* Smoking is associated with an increase in incidence of both gastric and duodenal ulcers, a higher incidence of complications, and slower healing of the ulcers.

Personality characteristics such as compulsive, "Type A" behavior as well as life stress are also considered to play a role in the development of ulcers. Although direct evidence may be lacking, the fact that emotional stress increases gastric secretion, blood flow, and motility and constricts blood vessels in the duodenum supports the relationship.

PATHOPHYSIOLOGY

Gastric ulcers apparently result from decreased mucosal resistance to the effects of gastric acid, whereas duodenal ulcers are due to increased exposure of the mucosa to highly acidic materials.

In the person with a gastric ulcer (Fig. 22–2), the amount of gastric secretion is normal or even reduced, and gastric emptying time is unchanged. There is, however, an abnormally high back diffusion of hydrogen ions into the mucosa. This in-

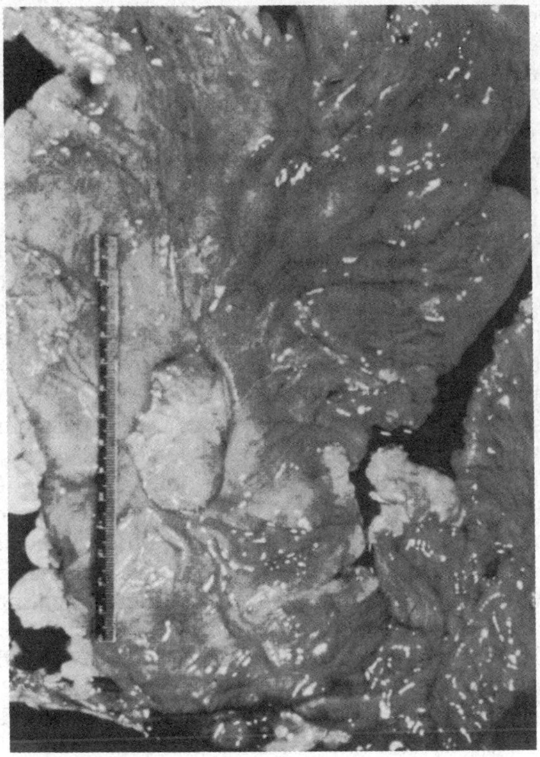

Figure 22–2.

Large, deeply excavated peptic ulcer in the prepyloric region of the stomach along the lesser curvature. (From Cotran RS, Kumar V, Robbins SL. Robbins pathologic basis of disease. 4th ed. Philadelphia: WB Saunders, 1989, p 849.)

creased back diffusion is postulated to result from a break in the "mucosal barrier," which is a hypothetical barrier allowing the passage of hydrogen ions into the gastric lumen without injury to the mucosa. Possible causes of such a break in the mucosal barrier include reflux of bile acids into the stomach and decreased blood flow to the gastric mucosa.

In the person with a duodenal ulcer, the mucosal resistance is normal, but there is an increase in the number of parietal cells in the stomach, a parallel increase in the volume of gastric acid, and a more rapid emptying of stomach contents into the duodenum. The effect of these changes is that the duodenal mucosa is exposed to an abnormally low pH for an extended period of time.

Regardless of type or cause, progressive ulceration can result in massive hemorrhage if the wall of a large blood vessel is eroded, or peritonitis if the wall of the stomach or intestine is perforated. If an ulcer is in the narrow pyloric area, associated edema can result in partial or total obstruction of the gastrointestinal tract.

CLINICAL MANIFESTATIONS

The major symptom of uncomplicated peptic ulcer is pain. Associated symptoms are change in appetite and weight, and very rarely nausea and vomiting.

Ulcer pain may be described as a feeling of pressure, burning, heaviness, or hunger. The pain, which can vary from mild to severe, is sharply localized near the midline of the epigastrium in an area that the patient can usually point to with one finger.

Generally there is a relationship between the onset of pain and gastric activity, with pain occurring a few hours following meals, at bedtime, and in the middle of the night, when gastric activity is high and there is no food to act as a buffer. Because of the increased acidity and emptying time associated with a duodenal ulcer, the pain takes on a pain-food-relief-pain pattern. Because food relieves the pain, these patients have good appetites and often even gain weight.

With gastric ulcer, the pain has no clear pattern and some patients have relatively constant pain. Because of this, patients with gastric ulcer tend to be anorexic and experience weight loss.

Ulcer pain may worsen under conditions of emotional stress, tension, fatigue, or exposure to cold.

MEDICAL DIAGNOSIS

The diagnosis of peptic ulcer disease is suggested by the patient's history of pain and confirmed by endoscopy. Barium studies are of little value because they cannot locate the exact lesion or determine the extent of mucosal damage. Similarly, physical examination yields few significant data.

MEDICAL MANAGEMENT

Medical management is designed to relieve symptoms, promote mucosal healing through the control of gastric acid, prevent or detect the development of complications, and prevent recurrences. Treatment is similar regardless of the location of the ulcer and is based on a program of dietary modification, rest, and medication.

DIET

Dietary therapy for the patient with an ulcer today is much more flexible than in the past. The traditional ulcer diet used to involve elimination of all potentially irritating food from the diet and ingestion of large amounts of milk and cream. Since research failed to support the effectiveness of this regimen, dietary modification is now based on the patient's tolerance of specific foods. If a food causes pain, its intake should be reduced or it should be eliminated from the diet entirely. Substances that are likely to fall into this category are heavily spiced foods, fresh fruits, and alcohol. Caffeine is also restricted because it stimulates gastric acid secretion.

In addition to avoiding pain-producing foods, patients may be encouraged to eat smaller, more frequent meals because this results in a more continual neutralization of gastric acid. All these dietary factors are determined individually for each patient. Absence of pain indicates manageable acid levels and is the best guide to determining diet changes.

DRUG THERAPY

Medications used in the treatment of ulcer disease are predominantly of two types: antacids and histamine H_2-receptor antagonists.

Antacids (see Pharmacology Box 21–1) neutralize acid present in the stomach and thereby relieve pain. Antacids do not heal the ulcer, but they do provide an environment conducive to healing. They are usually taken at bedtime and 1 to 3 hours after meals because the presence of food in the stomach delays gastric emptying and prolongs the time the antacid is in the stomach. Nonetheless, their effect lasts only 30 to 60 minutes, and so they may be required much more frequently by some patients. If the patient is awakened by pain during the night, antacids may be taken routinely approximately 1 hour before the time at which the pain usually occurs.

The histamine H_2-receptor antagonists (see Pharmacology Box 21–2) such as cimetidine and ranitidine decrease the basal secretion of gastric acid to almost zero and the food-induced secretion of acid by 75%. This decrease in gastric acid reduces further irritation to the mucosa and thus facilitates healing. Duration of action is 6 to 7 hours for cimetidine and 10 to 12 hours for ranitidine. However, because studies have failed to show that ulcers heal faster in response to treatment with histamine H_2-receptor antagonists as opposed to antacids, the main reason for their use is convenience. Because they are effective for 6 to 12 hours, it is only necessary for the patient to take one tablet two or four times per day as opposed to four or more 30-ml doses of liquid antacid.

Also used in the treatment of peptic ulcer disease is sucralfate (Carafate). This drug promotes healing by coating the ulcer, thus protecting it against further damage from acid and pepsin. Sucralfate is not absorbed, has minimal side effects, and neither neutralizes acid nor decreases acid secretion.

Proton pump inhibitors constitute a new class of anti-ulcer drugs currently being investigated. These drugs inhibit the enzyme that produces gastric acid and thus can suppress both basal and stimulated gastric acid release. Omeprazole (Prilosec) is the prototype drug of this class. When taken orally once a day, omeprazole has been shown to surpass cimetidine in suppressing gastric acid secretion.

To further control acid in the duodenum, patients with ulcer disease are advised to reduce or quit smoking. This is because nicotine reduces the bicarbonate content of pancreatic secretions and therefore decreases the degree of gastric acid neutralization in the duodenum. Because alcohol and aspirin are directly absorbed across the gastric mucosa, they should be avoided also.

Sedatives or tranquilizers may be prescribed to promote physical and psychological rest.

SURGERY

When a complication (hemorrhage, obstruction, or perforation) occurs or in cases in which conservative treatment is unsatisfactory, surgery is performed.

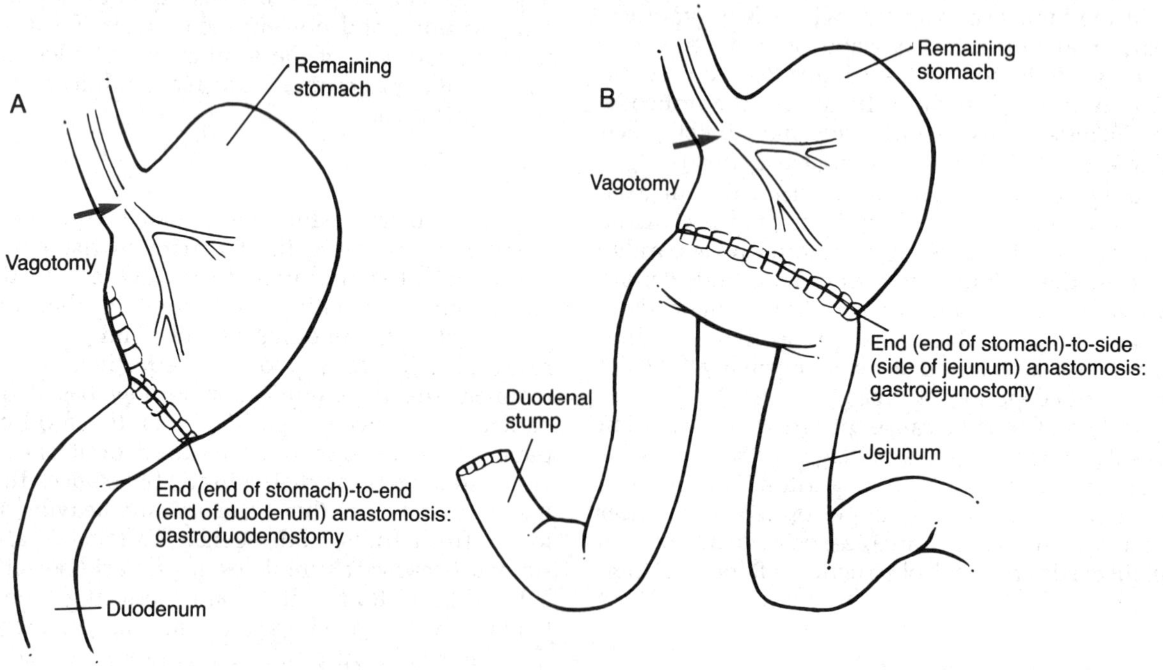

Figure 22–3.

A, Billroth I with vagotomy. *B*, Billroth II with vagotomy.

Among the most common surgical procedures for peptic ulcer disease are gastric resection, vagotomy, and pyloroplasty.

In a gastric resection or subtotal gastrectomy done for peptic ulcer disease, the distal portion of the stomach including the antrum and the pylorus is removed. The remaining stomach is then attached either to the duodenum via an end-to-end anastomosis as in a Billroth I procedure or to the jejunum via an end-to-side anastomosis as in a Billroth II procedure. With this type of surgery not only is the ulcer removed, but also a large portion of the parietal cells, which produce hydrochloric acid, and the antrum, which secretes gastrin, the hormone that stimulates the secretion of both hydrochloric acid and pepsinogen. A Billroth II procedure is generally preferred in the treatment of duodenal ulcers because gastric contents bypass the duodenum and there is less incidence of reulceration.

Vagotomy, or cutting of the vagus nerve, is done to eliminate parasympathetic stimulation of gastric secretion (Fig. 22–3). If the vagus nerves are cut as they enter the stomach (truncal vagotomy), gastric secretion is decreased, but intestinal motility is also decreased and gastric emptying delayed. The latter effects are sometimes avoided by a selective vagotomy in which only those branches of the vagus nerve that innervate the parietal cells are cut. Vagotomy is often done in conjunction with other surgical procedures for ulcers to ensure continued reduction of acid secretion and to reduce the potential for reulceration.

A pyloroplasty is a procedure in which the pylorus is incised and resutured to relax the muscle and enlarge the opening of the stomach into the duodenum to increase the rate of gastric emptying. It is done to relieve or prevent obstruction in the pylorus caused by the effects of vagotomy or the presence of scar tissue.

COMPLICATIONS OF PEPTIC ULCER

The three major complications of peptic ulcer disease are hemorrhage, gastrointestinal obstruction, and perforation.

HEMORRHAGE

Hemorrhage occurs when the wall of a large blood vessel is eroded through. It is manifested by vomiting of frank blood, by the presence of coffee-ground material in emesis or nasogastric drainage, or by melena. The preferred treatment is nonsurgical because the bleeding patient is a poor surgical risk. One approach to treatment consists of continuous gastric lavage with cool saline and administration of vasoconstrictive medications intravenously or directly into the bleeding vessel. A second approach is transendoscopic treatment such as sclerotherapy, topical therapy with tissue adhesives or coagulative agents, electrocoagulation, or laser photocoagulation. Once the bleeding is controlled, the classic ulcer medication and diet regimen are slowly reinstated.

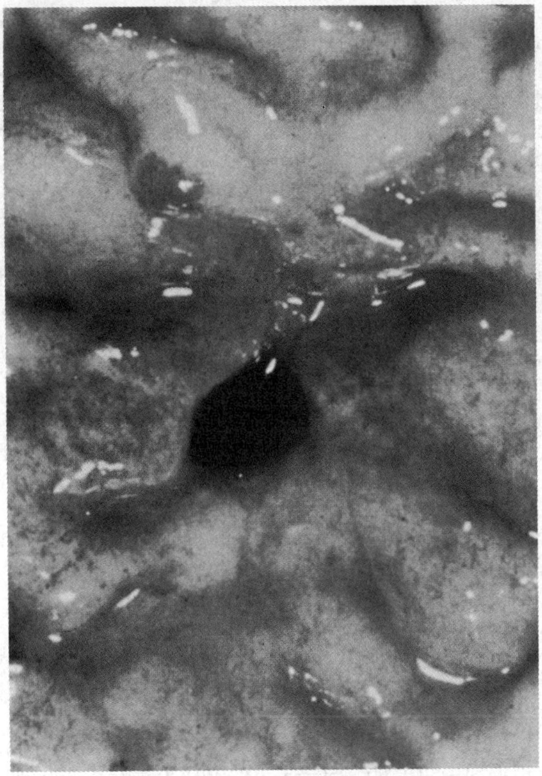

Figure 22–4.

Close-up view of a small, completely penetrating duodenal ulcer. (From Robbins SL, Cotran RS, Kumar V. Pathologic basis of disease. 3rd ed. Philadelphia: WB Saunders, 1984, p 819.)

OBSTRUCTION

Obstruction occurs secondary to edema or scarring, most often in the narrow pyloric region. Its primary symptoms are a sensation of fullness followed by vomiting of partially digested gastric contents and abdominal distention. Conservative treatment comprises maintenance of fluid and electrolyte balance by means of intravenous therapy and nasogastric suction of stomach contents until healing occurs.

PERFORATION

Perforation occurs when the ulcerative process has extended through the entire thickness of the gastric or duodenal wall, creating an opening through which gastrointestinal contents may spill into the peritoneal cavity (Fig. 22–4). The result of such spillage is an immediate chemical peritonitis and subsequent bacterial peritonitis caused in most cases by *Escherichia coli*, staphylococcus, or a streptococcus.

Posterior perforations may self-seal or manifest as an abscess.

Symptoms of perforation depend upon the size and location of the defect. Acute gastric perforation is characterized by sudden, sharp, intolerably severe pain beginning in the midepigastric area and spreading over the abdomen, which becomes rigid and boardlike. Referred pain to the shoulder may also occur via the phrenic nerve as a result of irritation of the diaphragm. Nausea is common and is occasionally accompanied by vomiting. Peristalsis decreases and paralytic ileus develops. Respirations are rapid and shallow, with minimum movement of painful abdominal muscles. Hypovolemic shock occurs, and the patient develops tachycardia, pallor, cold clammy skin, and a decreased blood pressure. Progression of peritonitis is very rapid and may result in death in 72 hours.

With perforation of the duodenum, symptoms generally parallel those just listed, although vital signs may remain within normal range.

In cases of very small perforations that close almost immediately by adhering to adjoining tissues and therefore are accompanied by little or no spillage of gastrointestinal contents, the immediate symptoms are similar to those previously listed but quickly subside. Abscess formation may follow in some cases, however.

Immediate treatment of perforation consists of suction to prevent further spillage of gastrointestinal contents into the peritoneal cavity, fluid and electrolyte replacement, and antibiotic therapy to resolve or prevent peritonitis. With this treatment, small perforations heal completely. Larger defects require emergency surgical closure.

Application of the Nursing Process to the Care of the Patient with Peptic Ulcer Disease

Assessment

Obtain a comprehensive history of the patient's pain. Include type, location, time of onset, precipitating factors, and remedies employed such as taking a particular antacid or eating food and their effectiveness. Question the patient about the presence of other symptoms such as nausea, vomiting, and change in appetite and weight.

Obtain information about any family history of ulcer disease as well as lifestyle factors known to be associated with its development. Question the patient about smoking, use of prescription and nonprescription drugs, and use of alcohol. Explore the patient's dietary patterns and eating habits. Ask the patient to name favorite types of foods and beverages and to describe the number and schedule of meals and snacks per day. Have the patient validate this information by listing the time, amount, and type of foods eaten during the past 48 hours.

Explore sources of stress of the patient and his or her coping mechanisms. Be certain to ascertain the patient's perception of the amount of stress and the effectiveness of coping.

Assess the patient's and the family's knowledge of the disease and its treatment as well as the probability of compliance with treatment.

Assess the patient hospitalized with ulcer disease on an ongoing basis for intolerance to specific foods, response to therapy, and development of complications. Changes in the character of pain, the presence of bloody or coffee-ground emesis or nasogastric drainage, and melena are classic indications that a complication may have occurred.

Nursing Diagnoses and Planning

Nursing diagnoses and related expected patient outcomes most commonly applicable to the patient with uncomplicated peptic ulcer disease include the following:

NDx: Pain related to the irritating effects of gastric acid on injured tissue

Planning: Patient outcomes
1. Patient lists prescribed medications aimed at reducing pain, stating name, dose, route, and frequency of each.
2. Patient describes dietary modifications conducive to pain reduction.
3. Patient selects or plans nutritionally balanced meals that exclude pain-producing foods.
4. Patient reports that pain is relieved.
5. Patient sleeps through the night without pain.

NDx: High risk for altered health maintenance related to insufficient knowledge of disease process, aggravating factors, promotion of physical and psychological rest, and need for follow-up care

Planning: Patient outcomes
1. Patient describes the relationship among gastric acidity, mucosal damage, and symptomatology.
2. Patient lists substances known to aggravate the disease process.
3. Patient describes the relationship of stress to the disease process.
4. Patient describes a plan to reduce stress and promote physical rest.
5. Patient lists symptoms to be reported.

NDx: High risk for noncompliance related to dietary modifications, reduction of smoking, or medication regimen

Text continued on page 939

Nursing Care Guide 22–1.

PATIENTS UNDERGOING SUBTOTAL GASTRECTOMY FOR DUODENAL ULCER DISEASE

Preoperative Care

Assessment Findings: Patient states, "I hope everything goes all right tomorrow. I'll sure be glad to be rid of my ulcer, but it makes me really nervous to think about being put to sleep and opened up." Patient also complains of feeling jittery and not being able to sit still.

Nursing Diagnosis: Anxiety related to experience of anesthesia and surgery

Patient Outcomes	Nursing Interventions	Rationale
Patient practices relaxation as instructed. Patient reports feeling more relaxed. Patient expresses an optimistic view about the surgical outcome. Patient rests quietly.	Reassure patient that some anxiety prior to surgery is normal and in fact helps prepare the body for the stress and promotes recovery.	Encourages patient to share feelings and thus receive support by allaying fears of being negatively perceived because of anxiety.
	Offer reassurance about the success of surgery as appropriate. Possible examples include: reassure patient about his or her general state of health and therefore fitness for surgery; mention the frequency of the procedure and its success rate; describe the professionals that participate in surgery, noting their roles in protecting the patient and their competency.	Provides the patient with positive facts on which to focus and base hope for a successful surgical outcome.
	Review relaxation techniques with the patient and/or provide patient with a relaxation tape and orient patient to its use.	Helps control anxiety; although some anxiety can be beneficial in preparing the body for the stress of surgery, excessive anxiety is detrimental.
	Maintain a quiet, calm environment.	Facilitates relaxation, rest, and action of sedative medications.
	Administer sedatives as ordered.	Promotes rest and relaxation.

Evaluation: Compare the patient's status with the expected patient outcomes. If the outcomes are achieved, evaluate nursing care as successful. If not, reassess the patient, formulate new nursing diagnoses, and revise expected patient outcomes and nursing interventions as appropriate.

(continued)

Nursing Care Guide 22–1. *(continued)*

PATIENTS UNDERGOING SUBTOTAL GASTRECTOMY FOR DUODENAL ULCER DISEASE

Assessment Findings: Patient says, "Tell me what to expect, I've never had surgery before except to have my tonsils out when I was 4, and I really don't remember very much. Am I going to have a lot of pain when I wake up? Will I be able to eat? Will I have a lot of tubes?"

Nursing Diagnosis: Knowledge deficit: preoperative preparation, postoperative course.

Patient Outcomes	Nursing Interventions	Rationale
Patient describes preoperative preparation. Patient describes usual postoperative procedures and course. Patient describes importance of coughing, deep breathing, and leg exercise in the prevention of complications. Patient demonstrates coughing and deep breathing. Patient demonstrates postoperative leg exercises.	Explain to the patient that: ■ Many tests including a physical examination, x-ray examination, and blood tests will be done prior to surgery to determine general state of health and identify any problems that need special consideration. ■ The specific nature and purpose of each test will be explained before it is done. ■ It is important that the gastrointestinal tract be empty when the operation is done, so only liquids will be allowed for 24 hours before surgery, and enemas may be given the day before surgery to clean out the large bowel. ■ The abdomen will be shaved and scrubbed from nipple line to symphysis pubis to remove as many bacteria as possible, but the incision will be much smaller than the area prepared. (If the patient is to receive intravenous fluids or hyperalimentation therapy to make up nutritional deficiencies before surgery, explain this to the patient. Also explain if a nasogastric tube is to be inserted to empty the stomach as in cases of pyloric obstruction.) ■ After surgery, there will be a tube going from the stomach out through the nose to drain stomach secretions into a bottle on the wall. Drainage may be red initially.	Prepares the patient for perioperative events, thus involving the patient in the plan of care, promoting cooperation, and decreasing the risk of anxiety over routine measures.

(continued)

Nursing Care Guide 22–1. *(continued)*

PATIENTS UNDERGOING SUBTOTAL GASTRECTOMY FOR DUODENAL ULCER DISEASE

Patient Outcomes	Nursing Interventions	Rationale
	Because the purpose of the tube is to keep the stomach empty to promote healing of the suture line, no foods or fluids will be given by mouth for the several days that the tube is in place. The tube does not cause pain, although the nostrils may feel a bit sore and the mouth dry—symptoms that will be eased by salves and mouth rinses. ■ Intravenous fluids will be given until peristalsis returns, the nasogastric tube is removed, and oral intake is reestablished. ■ Coughing, turning, and deep breathing will be encouraged every 2 hours while on bed rest in order to promote lung expansion, clear secretions from the airways, and prevent respiratory infection. ■ Leg exercises should be done five times every 1 to 2 hours to promote movement of blood in the veins and discourage the formation of blood clots. ■ Ambulation usually begins on the first postoperative day. ■ Oral intake will begin with clear fluids once bowel function has returned as indicated by the presence of bowel sounds and passage of flatus; full fluids and then bland foods will be added as tolerated. Demonstrate, and have the patient practice, turning, coughing, and deep breathing with a pillow used to splint the abdomen. Demonstrate leg exercises.	

Evaluation: Compare the patient's status with the expected patient outcomes. If the outcomes are achieved, evaluate nursing care as successful. If not, reassess the patient, formulate new nursing diagnoses, and revise expected patient outcomes and nursing interventions as appropriate.

(continued)

Nursing Care Guide 22–1. *(continued)*

PATIENTS UNDERGOING SUBTOTAL GASTRECTOMY FOR DUODENAL ULCER DISEASE

Postoperative Care

Assessment Findings: Patient states, "I have so much pain. It hurts when I lie still, but it's even worse when I move." Patient moans softly on moving. Face appears tense and strained. Patient also complains of nostril discomfort and asks if the nasogastric tube can be removed.

Nursing Diagnosis: Pain related to trauma from abdominal surgery and irritation of the nostril by the nasogastric tube

Patient Outcomes	Nursing Interventions	Rationale
Patient moves without loud moans, complaints of severe pain, or signs of severe pain such as pallor and tachycardia.	Administer pain medication.	Pain relief promotes rest, which facilitates the healing process.
	Keep the head of the bed elevated.	Decreases pull on the incision line.
Patient states abdominal pain is relieved.	Splint the incision with a pillow when turning, coughing, deep breathing.	Decreases discomfort by reducing pull on incised tissues.
Patient appears relaxed (i.e., lips are not pressed together, face does not appear drawn).	Encourage the patient to relax.	Relaxation decreases muscle spasm.
Patient denies nostril discomfort.	Play soft music, and prompt the patient to concentrate on slow, even breathing or to contemplate a calm, pleasant scene permeated by a relaxing color.	
	Clean the nostril through which the tube passes with applicators dipped in water, and apply water-soluble lubricant.	Removes secretions, which can form crusts and irritate the nares. Lubricant protects area from contact with irritating secretions, decreases friction, and keeps tissues moist and supple.

Evaluation: Compare the patient's status with the expected patient outcomes. If the outcomes are achieved, evaluate nursing care as successful. If not, reassess the patient, formulate new nursing diagnoses and revise expected patient outcomes and nursing interventions as appropriate.

Assessment Findings: Patient has had a gastric resection with anastomosis of the remaining stomach to the small intestine.

Nursing Diagnosis: High risk for trauma (internal suture line) related to gastric distention, vomiting, or movement of the nasogastric tube

(continued)

Nursing Care Guide 22–1. *(continued)*

PATIENTS UNDERGOING SUBTOTAL GASTRECTOMY FOR DUODENAL ULCER DISEASE

Patient Outcomes	Nursing Interventions	Rationale
Signs of leakage at the anastomosis are absent: Patient is afebrile. Increased pain is absent. Abdomen is soft.	Keep the nasogastric tube connected to suction as ordered.	Gastric distention and vomiting place stress on the suture line and can lead to disruption of the anastomosis and leakage of gastric contents into the abdominal cavity.
	Irrigate the tube gently with normal saline as ordered to keep it patent.	Maintains drainage, thereby preventing stress on the anastomosis from gastric distention. Gentle irrigation protects the suture line from disruption. Normal saline is isotonic and therefore maintains osmotic pressure and minimizes loss of electrolytes from the stomach.
	Reinforce or replace the tape holding the tube in position as needed. Be careful not to move the tube when adding or changing tape.	Prevents movement of the nasogastric tube, which could lead to trauma to the anastomosis.

Evaluation: Compare the patient's status with the expected patient outcomes. If the outcomes are achieved, evaluate nursing care as successful. If not, reassess the patient, formulate new nursing diagnoses, and revise expected patient outcomes and nursing interventions as appropriate.

(continued)

Planning: Patient outcomes
1. Patient reduces smoking.
2. Patient adheres to dietary and medication regime.
3. Complications are absent.

Nursing Interventions

NDx: Pain

Administer or teach self-administration of antacids, histamine antagonists, or other prescribed medications, adhering strictly to the ordered schedule to promote healing. Encourage the patient to avoid cigarette smoking and foods that commonly cause an exacerbation of ulcer pain. These include highly spiced foods and those that contain caffeine, such as cola, tea, coffee, and chocolate. Explain that foods that cause pain vary from person to person, and instruct the patient to keep a daily record of foods eaten and amount of pain experienced so that specific foods that should be avoided can be identified. If needed, enlist the dietitian to assist the patient in selecting and planning a well-balanced diet based on the foods that are tolerated well.

Instruct the patient to eat small frequent meals to help keep the gastric acid neutralized and to drink six to eight glasses of water per day to dilute it. Also instruct the patient to eat slowly and to chew foods thoroughly because large chunks of food are associated with increased secretion of hydrochloric acid.

Stress the importance of both physical and psychological rest. For the hospitalized patient, provide the physical care needed to keep the patient comfortable and maintain a quiet environment, which may mean limiting visitors and telephone calls. When attempting to create a restful atmosphere, consider not only how much activity the patient can

Nursing Care Guide 22–1. *(continued)*

PATIENTS UNDERGOING SUBTOTAL GASTRECTOMY FOR DUODENAL ULCER DISEASE

Assessment Findings: Patient has had major abdominal surgery and was intubated for general anesthesia. Respirations are shallow and secretions can be heard in the large airways.

Nursing Diagnosis: Ineffective airway clearance related to shallow breathing secondary to diaphragmatic splinting accompanying upper abdominal surgery

Patient Outcomes	Nursing Interventions	Rationale
Patient moves, coughs, and breathes deeply as directed. Lung sounds are clear on auscultation.	Turn, cough, and deep breathe every 2 hours while on bed rest.	Promotes elimination of inhalation anesthetics in the immediate postoperative period. Also promotes aeration of alveoli, and moves secretions into larger respiratory passages for expectoration.
	Splint incision to decrease pain and anxiety when turning, coughing, and deep breathing.	Minimizes discomfort and promotes willingness to turn, cough, and breathe deeply.
	Ambulate patient as ordered.	Promotes maximum lung expansion and movement of secretions.

Evaluation: Compare the patient's status with the expected patient outcomes. If the outcomes are achieved, evaluate nursing care as successful. If not, reassess the patient, formulate new nursing diagnoses, and revise expected patient outcomes and nursing interventions as appropriate.

Assessment Findings: Patient is mouth breathing because of the nasogastric tube in the nose and is on NPO status.

Nursing Diagnosis: High risk for altered oral mucous membrane related to mouth breathing and NPO status

Patient Outcomes	Nursing Interventions	Rationale
Oral mucous membranes are pink and moist. Lips are supple and intact. Patient states mouth and lips feel moist and free of discomfort.	Assist the patient in brushing and flossing the teeth after eating.	Cleanses the mouth and provides feeling of freshness and comfort.
	Assist the patient in rinsing the mouth frequently.	Moistens mucous membranes of the mouth.
	Offer throat lozenges or gum if allowed.	Increases saliva, thereby relieving dryness of the oral mucous membranes.
	Apply water-soluble lubricant to lips.	Helps keep the lips moist, supple, and free of cracks.

Evaluation: Compare the patient's status with the expected patient outcomes. If the outcomes are achieved, evaluate nursing care as successful. If not, reassess the patient, formulate new nursing diagnoses, and revise expected patient outcomes and nursing interventions as appropriate.

(continued)

Nursing Care Guide 22–1. *(continued)*

PATIENTS UNDERGOING SUBTOTAL GASTRECTOMY FOR DUODENAL ULCER DISEASE

Assessment Findings: Patient has an upper abdominal wound.

Nursing Diagnosis: High risk for infection related to contamination of the abdominal wound

Patient Outcomes	Nursing Interventions	Rationale
Wound is odorless and free of purulent drainage. Wound edges are approximated.	Caution patient against touching the abdominal dressing or the surrounding area.	Protects against introduction of pathogens from the patient's hands to the area of the surgical wound.
	Use strict aseptic technique when caring for the wound.	Protects against contamination of the wound with pathogens.
	Reinforce dressing as needed, unless dressing is wet with predominantly bloody drainage, in which case it should be changed.	Environmental pathogens can move by capillary action through wet dressings.

Evaluation: Compare the patient's status with the expected patient outcomes. If the outcomes are achieved, evaluate nursing care as successful. If not, reassess the patient, formulate new nursing diagnoses, and revise expected patient outcomes and nursing interventions as appropriate.

(continued)

tolerate but how much inactivity can be tolerated. It may be less stressful to the patient if some phone calls and some work is allowed than if these are prohibited entirely.

NDx: High risk for altered health maintenance

Teach the patient about the basic pathophysiology of ulcer disease and the relationship among gastric acidity, mucosal damage, and symptoms experienced. Explain the effect of smoking, caffeine, and drugs containing aspirin on the process and hence the need to avoid them. Discuss the importance of psychological and physical rest, and explore with the patient ways to reduce stress and to organize activities so that time for rest periods is available. Instruct the patient in the importance of follow-up care. Stress the need to report promptly severe abdominal pain, nausea, vomiting, abdominal distention, or persistence of original symptoms despite compliance with treatment.

NDx: High risk for noncompliance

Allow the patient to express feelings about limitations on diet, need to avoid smoking, and the need for daily medication. Stress that the patient is taking control of his or her life when the decision is made to adopt lifestyle changes to promote healing as opposed to being controlled by these changes. Identify with the patient factors seen as interfering with compliance and explore ways of dealing with them. Involve the family or significant others in planning for self-care and recommend counseling or support groups as needed.

Evaluation

Evaluate the effectiveness of nursing care for a patient with peptic ulcer disease by comparing the patient's status with the expected patient outcomes. Examples of specific outcomes for patients with uncomplicated peptic ulcer disease have been provided in the Planning section.

See Nursing Care Guide 22–1 for the care of the patient undergoing a subtotal gastrectomy for duodenal ulcer disease.

Nursing Care Guide 22–1. *(continued)*

PATIENTS UNDERGOING SUBTOTAL GASTRECTOMY FOR DUODENAL ULCER DISEASE

Assessment Findings: Patient has had part of the stomach removed, is on NPO status, and is at risk for early satiation and dumping syndrome on resumption of oral intake.

Nursing Diagnosis: Altered nutrition: less than body requirements related to dietary restrictions related to surgery, early satiety, or dumping syndrome

Patient Outcomes	Nursing Interventions	Rationale
Patient ingests a nutritionally balanced diet. Patient achieves and maintains recommended weight.	Administer intravenous fluids and electrolytes as ordered (usually for about 4 days).	Replaces fluids and electrolytes lost through nasogastric drainage, wound drainage, and normal elimination processes, because patient is on NPO status after surgery and only gradually resumes oral intake once bowel motility has resumed.
	Give clear fluids when bowel motility has returned.	Clear fluids are easiest to digest and absorb and least likely to cause nausea and vomiting.
	Gradually introduce full fluids, and progress to a bland diet as tolerated.	Gastric capacity is significantly decreased because of the partial gastrectomy. Nausea and vomiting can occur from oral intake that is "too much, too fast."
	Give iron and vitamin supplements as ordered.	Prevents deficiency due to insufficient oral intake.
	Give six small feedings per day and liquids before or after but not with feedings.	Decreases risk of early satiation.
	To combat dumping syndrome: ■ Avoid hypertonic liquids and high-carbohydrate foods. ■ Position patient in low Fowler's position during meals. ■ Instruct patient to lie down for a half-hour after eating to delay gastric emptying. ■ Avoid fluids with meals. ■ Take antispasmodics as ordered to aid in delay of gastric emptying.	Rapid entry of large amounts of hypertonic chyme into the small intestine precipitates dumping syndrome.

Evaluation: Compare the patient's status with the expected patient outcomes. If the outcomes are achieved, evaluate nursing care as successful. If not, reassess the patient, formulate new nursing diagnoses, and revise expected patient outcomes and nursing interventions as appropriate.

(continued)

Nursing Care Guide 22–1. *(continued)*

PATIENTS UNDERGOING SUBTOTAL GASTRECTOMY FOR DUODENAL ULCER DISEASE

Assessment Findings: Patient has no previous experience with surgery.

Nursing Diagnosis: High risk for altered health maintenance related to lack of knowledge of prevention of recurrence, need for follow-up care

Patient Outcomes	Nursing Interventions	Rationale
Patient describes importance of avoiding aspirin products, alcohol, and cigarette smoking. Patient identifies sources of stress. Patient identifies ways of relieving or coping with stress. Patient lists symptoms to be reported to the physician.	Instruct the patient to avoid aspirin-containing over-the-counter drugs such as Contac and Alka-Seltzer, use of alcohol, and cigarette smoking.	Decreases the risk of ulcer recurrence.
	Help the patient identify sources of lifestyle stress.	Sources of stress must be identified before strategies to reduce stress can be planned.
	Explore with the patient methods of decreasing or lowering stress.	Stress is associated with exacerbation of peptic ulcer disease, although its role as a causative factor remains in question.
	Refer to stress reduction groups or other professonal help as necessary.	In some cases, external support is needed to help the patient plan and carry through with stress-reducing strategies.
	Instruct the patient to report: ■ Continuous epigastric distress that increases after eating. ■ Persistent fatigue.	Continuous epigastric distress may indicate alkaline reflux gastritis. Persistent fatigue may indicate iron or vitamin B_{12} deficiency.

Evaluation: Compare the patient's status with the expected patient outcomes. If the outcomes are achieved, evaluate nursing care as successful. If not, reassess the patient, formulate new nursing diagnoses, and revise expected patient outcomes and nursing interventions as appropriate.

Additional Assessments and Interventions

Monitor and record vital signs every 4 hours or more frequently if necessitated by the patient's condition.

Observe and record the amount and character of the drainage from the nasogastric tube. Normally, drainage is bloody for 24 hours postoperatively, then changes to brown-tinged and then to yellow or clear. Amount of secretions decreases as peristalsis returns.

Note odor of gastric aspirate, because a fecal smell can indicate regurgitation of large intestine contents into the operative area.

Auscultate for bowel sounds, and question the patient about passage of flatus to determine when peristalsis has resumed and oral intake may begin.

Record all intake and output.

Acute Stress Ulcers

Acute stress ulcers are a form of peptic ulcer disease that occur in patients who have suffered a major physiologic insult. They are distinct from chronic peptic ulcer in pathophysiology and in clinical presentation.

ETIOLOGY

Many different kinds of physiologic stress are associated with the development of acute stress ulcers. These include acute respiratory insufficiency, sepsis, renal failure, advanced carcinomatosis, and severe traumatic injuries. Stress ulcers also occur following burn injuries, brain injury, trauma, or a cerebral vascular accident. Stress ulcers following burn injury are sometimes called Curling's ulcers, and those following brain injury are called Cushing's ulcers.

PATHOPHYSIOLOGY

Acute stress ulcers are multiple superficial lesions that occur primarily in the gastric fundus, often in the middle of an area affected by acute gastritis (Fig. 22–5). Although the exact pathophysiology of their development is not known, it is believed that the intensive stress response causes mucosal ischemia, which results in backflow of hydrogen ions and a deficiency of mucus that normally coats the wall of the stomach. Stress ulcers following brain injury or lengthy cranial surgery (Cushing's ulcers) are thought to be caused by hypersecretion of gastric acid. It is known that although not the cause per se, gastric acid must be present for stress ulcers to develop. Reflux of bile salts and pancreatic enzymes from the duodenum into the stomach are also thought to contribute to the process.

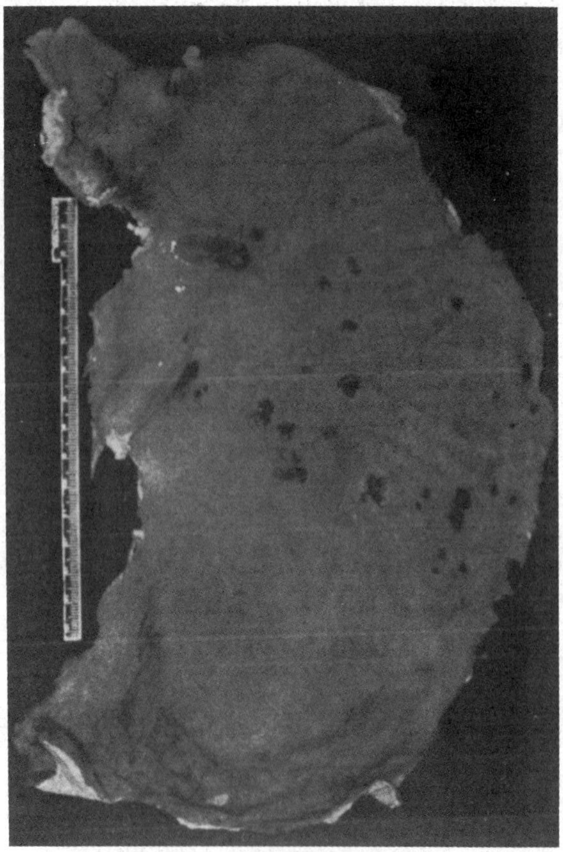

Figure 22–5.

Acute stress ulcers in a patient dying of severe burns. (From Cotran RS, Kumar V, Robbins SL. Robbins pathologic basis of disease. 4th ed. Philadelphia: WB Saunders, 1989, p 848.)

CLINICAL MANIFESTATIONS

The only symptom of stress ulcers is painless hemorrhage, indicated by hematemesis or melena, occurring 2 to 10 days following the physiologic insult.

MEDICAL DIAGNOSIS

Positive diagnosis of acute stress ulcers depends on visualization of the lesions during gastroscopy. This requires that the patient's stomach be lavaged with ice water prior to the procedure to remove clots that could obscure the lesions. Radiologic studies are of no value in the diagnosis of stress ulcers because the ulcers are too superficial to be identified.

MEDICAL MANAGEMENT

The most effective treatment of stress ulcers is prevention. H_2-receptor antagonists are given intravenously around the clock to suppress the secretion of gastric acid. Antacid therapy may also be employed.

Although studies indicate a high incidence of gastric lesions in patients suffering from massive trauma, only a small proportion of them bleed. If bleeding does occur, there is a 50% mortality rate. Hourly titration of antacid therapy to maintain the gastric pH at 4.0 or greater is the most effective method of preventing bleeding from stress ulcers (Shoemaker et al, 1989, p. 1300). It does not, however, control bleeding, which must be treated aggressively as a medical emergency. Treatment of bleeding may involve the standard techniques of gastric lavage and vasoconstrictive medication or may consist of electrocoagulation during endoscopy.

Once the patient is no longer critical and can tolerate medication by mouth, a regimen of oral antacids and H_2 blockers is continued for 4 to 6 more weeks.

Guidelines for Application of the Nursing Process to the Care of the Patient with Stress Ulcers

Identify patients at risk for the development of stress ulcers and observe for hematemesis, blood or coffee-ground material in the gastric drainage, and melena.

Other assessments and interventions relate to the prescribed regimen for prevention of stress ulcers as well as to the patient's primary medical problem.

Hiatus Hernia

A hiatus hernia is a protrusion of part of the stomach into the thoracic cavity through the opening in the diaphragm through which the esophagus passes. It occurs more often in women than in men and is the most common pathologic condition of the upper gastrointestinal tract.

ETIOLOGY

Normally, the opening or hiatus in the diaphragm through which the esophagus passes encircles the esophagus tightly and prevents the stomach from ascending into the thoracic cavity. A congenitally short esophagus, trauma, or weakening of the diaphragmatic muscle around the hiatus can permit movement of the lower esophagus and upper stomach into the chest cavity. Weakening of the diaphragmatic muscle may be congenital, with symptoms occurring later in life, or it may be the result of aging. The major contributing factor in the development of hiatus hernia is increased intraabdominal pressure. This can result from bending, straining, lifting heavy objects, coughing, vomiting, obesity, pregnancy, and the like.

PATHOPHYSIOLOGY

Ninety percent of hiatus hernias are classified as "sliding," that is, the top of the stomach enters the thoracic cavity when the individual is supine but slides back into the abdomen when a vertical position is assumed (Fig. 22–6). The mechanical irritation caused by the friction along with the reflux regurgitation of acidic gastric contents into the lower

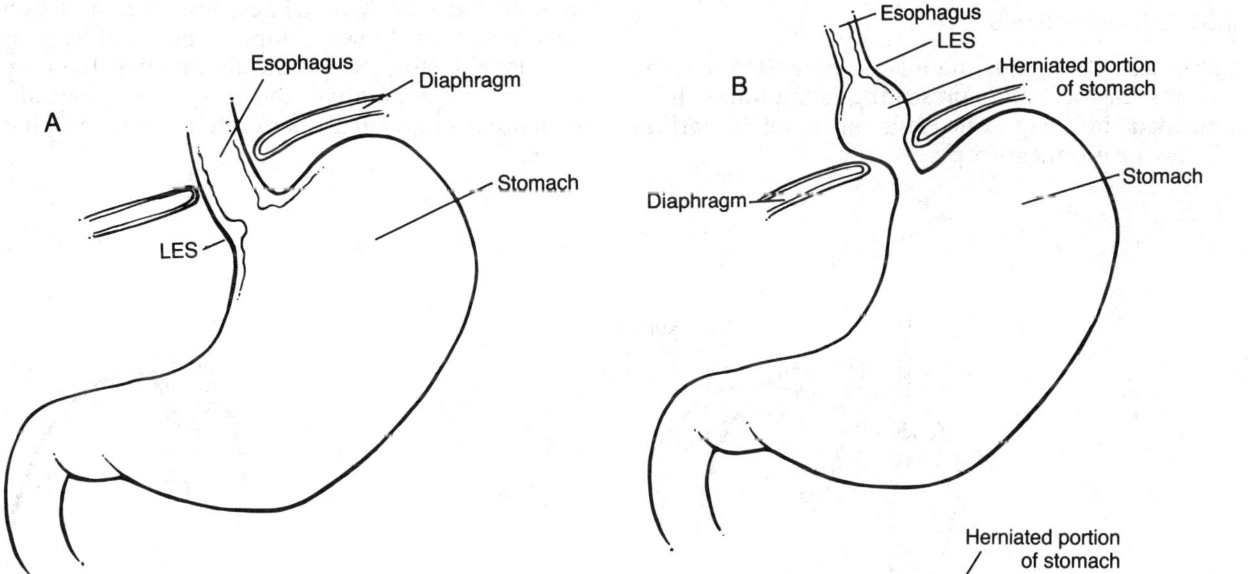

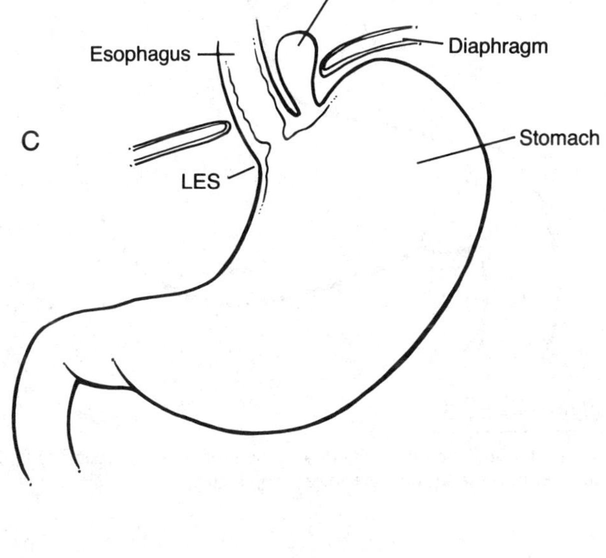

Figure 22–6.

A, Normal relationship of esophagus, diaphragm, and stomach. *B*, Sliding hiatus hernia. Note top of the stomach above the diaphragm in the thoracic cavity. *C*, Rolling (paraesophageal) hiatus hernia. Note part of the stomach other than that adjoining the esophagus in the thoracic cavity. (LES, lower esophageal sphincter.)

esophagus results in esophagitis, the pain and swelling of which can lead to aspiration and malnutrition.

A second type of hiatus hernia is a paraesophageal or "rolling" hernia (see Fig. 22–6). In this type, a portion of the stomach other than that directly adjoining the esophagus moves up through the diaphragmatic opening and protrudes into the thoracic cavity. If this protruding portion of the stomach becomes incarcerated, circulation can be impaired and ulceration or tissue necrosis can result.

CLINICAL MANIFESTATIONS

Hiatus hernia is often asymptomatic and may remain undetected unless discovered by chance. When symptoms do occur, the most frequent is heartburn. With the common sliding hernia, pyrosis (heartburn) and acid regurgitation occur from reflux of acidic gastric contents into the esophagus. If this leads to air swallowing, eructation (belching) and flatulence also occur. Dysphagia (difficulty swallowing) appears if irritation of esophageal tissue leads to scarring and decreased motility. Symptoms are aggravated by any increase in intraabdominal pressure.

MEDICAL DIAGNOSIS

Diagnosis of hiatus hernia is suggested by the patient's history and presenting symptoms. It is confirmed by diagnostic tests such as a barium swallow or esophagoscopy.

MEDICAL MANAGEMENT

Treatment of hiatus hernia is usually conservative, with surgery reserved for severe cases in which symptoms cannot be adequately controlled. Conservative treatment consists of a bland diet taken in small, frequent feedings; positioning in a semi-Fowler's position after eating to promote movement of ingested foods into the stomach and to discourage esophageal reflux; raising the head of the patient's bed at home on 6-inch blocks to reduce reflux during the night; and antacids for symptomatic relief of pyrosis. Often histamine receptor–blocking agents such as cimetidine (Tagamet) or ranitidine (Zantac) are also ordered to reduce the amount of acid in the stomach.

If surgical intervention is required, a procedure such as a Nissen fundoplication is done (Fig. 22–7). In this operation, the fundus of the stomach is wrapped around the lower esophagus, creating a one-way valve to control the flow of upper gastrointestinal contents. Other surgical procedures used to treat hiatus hernia are the Hill and Belsey procedures, which also increase resistance at the gastroesophageal junction and therefore inhibit gastric reflux. As with any major surgery, there is a postoperative risk of hemorrhage, infection, and pulmonary embolus. Other complications that can occur because the surgery specifically involves the esophagus are postoperative dysphagia, esophageal obstruction, esophageal perforation, and esophageal fistula.

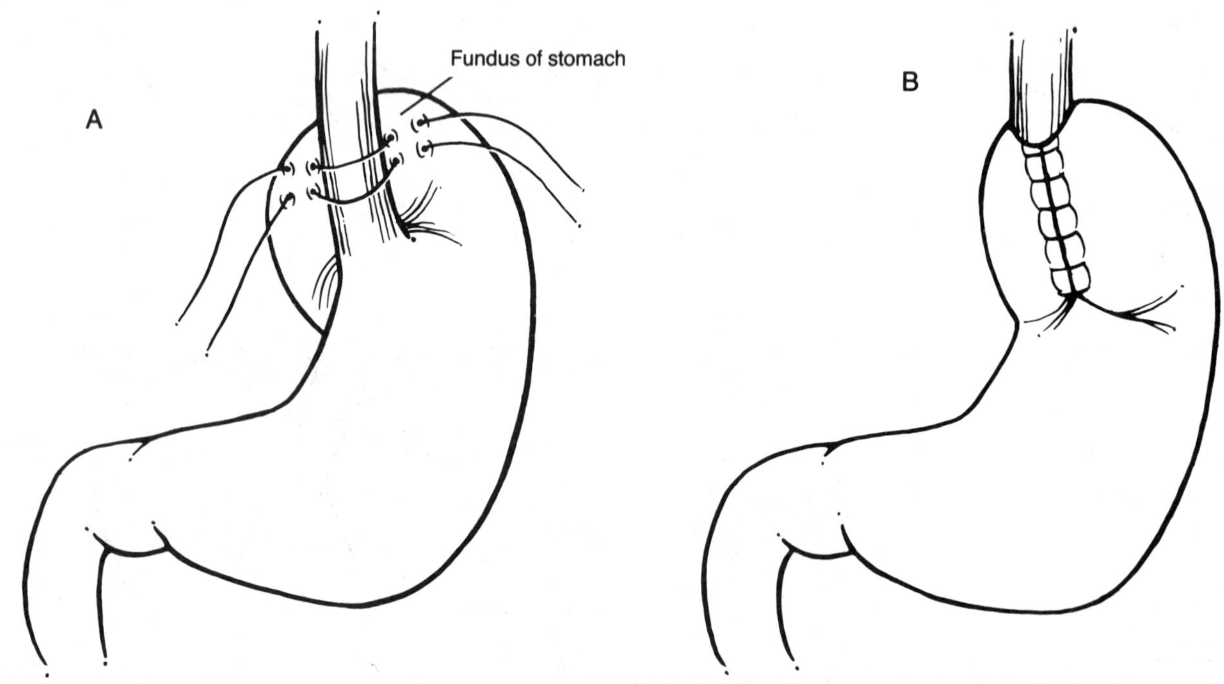

Figure 22–7.

Nissen fundoplication. *A*, Fundus of the stomach has been brought up in preparation for being wrapped around the esophagus. *B*, Fundus is sutured in place around the lower esophagus.

Chart 22–1.

NURSING GUIDE TO PATIENT EDUCATION FOR SELF-MANAGEMENT: USE OF ANTACIDS

To promote safe, effective self-administration of antacids, instruct the patient to:

Shake all liquid antacids well before taking.
Chew chewable tablets thoroughly and take with a full glass of water because antacid must be in liquid form in order to work.
Check the expiration date on the bottle and discard outdated medication because antacids become less effective as they age.
Adhere to the prescribed schedule of doses.
Always measure the antacid dose; do not drink from the bottle.
Consult with the physician or pharmacist before changing antacids because different antacids contain different ingredients, some of which may be contraindicated for particular patients.
Check with the physician or the pharmacist about the scheduling of other medications while taking antacids because antacids alter the gastric pH and can affect the absorption of many medications, including antibiotics, cardiac glycosides, and enteric-coated tablets. As a general rule, medications should be taken 2 to 3 hours before or after an antacid.
Drink at least 2500 ml of fluids per day if taking antacids that contain calcium or aluminum to help prevent constipation and impaction.

Application of the Nursing Process to the Care of the Patient Receiving Nonsurgical Treatment for Hiatus Hernia

Assessment

Assess the type and extent of the patient's discomfort and its relationship to meals, to ingestion of specific foods, or to specific activities. Examples of such relationships are pyrosis occurring after eating spicy food or after eating a large meal and then lying down. Identify remedies that the patient uses for relief of symptoms; determine the frequency of their use as well as their effectiveness. Assess the patient's general nutritional status and identify dietary changes made because of discomfort.

Because medical management is not 100% effective in relieving symptoms, it is also important to identify the patient's understanding of the disease process and expectation of treatment.

Nursing Diagnoses and Planning

Nursing diagnoses and related expected patient outcomes most commonly applicable to patients undergoing nonsurgical treatment for a hiatus hernia include the following:

NDx: Pain related to esophageal irritation secondary to reflux of acidic gastric contents

Planning: Patient outcomes

1. Patient describes the proper use of antacids as presented in Chart 22–1.
2. Patient reports that pain is relieved.

NDx: High risk for altered health maintenance related to insufficient knowledge of nature of the disorder and prevention and control of symptoms

Planning: Patient outcomes

1. Patient describes the basic pathology of hiatus hernia.
2. Patient describes measures to reduce the severity of symptoms.
3. Patient reports that pyrosis occurs no more than twice per day.

Nursing Interventions

NDx: Pain

Instruct the patient in the use of antacids for pain, as described in Chart 22–1. Warn against the use of alcohol for pain relief because this reduces pressure in the lower esophageal sphincter and thus worsens the problem. Instead, encourage the use of relaxation measures and diversion to cope with discomfort.

NDx: High risk for altered health maintenance

Describe what a hiatus hernia is, how it produces symptoms, and how changes in diet, activities, and

Nutrition Box 22–1.

NUTRITION: SPECIAL CONSIDERATIONS FOR PATIENTS WITH HIATUS HERNIA

Patients with a hiatus hernia should:

Eat small, frequent meals to prevent distention of the stomach, which increases acid secretion.

Eat a high-protein diet because protein stimulates gastrin secretion and increases lower esophageal sphincter pressure.

Avoid fat in the diet because fat decreases pressure in the lower esophageal sphincter.

Avoid substances such as tea, coffee, cola, and chocolate that contain caffeine, which stimulates gastric acid secretion.

Avoid irritating foods such as citrus fruits and tomato products.

Drink water after eating to cleanse the esophagus.

Promote the passage of food into the stomach by gravity by not lying down for 2 to 3 hours after eating, eating slowly, and chewing food well.

Lose weight if overweight to improve posture and general body mechanics.

personal habits can aid in preventing or controlling symptoms.

Instruct the patient in the selection of foods and other dietary considerations as outlined in Nutrition Box 22–1. Also instruct the patient to avoid activities that increase intraabdominal pressure such as bending, lifting, wearing clothing that constricts the abdomen, straining at stool, and vigorous coughing. Suggest that the patient sleep on the right side and elevate the head of the bed 6 inches on blocks so that gravity will aid in preventing reflux. Discourage eating close to bedtime as well as smoking, which increases gastric secretion.

Evaluation

Evaluate the effectiveness of nursing care for a patient with a hiatus hernia by comparing the patient's status with the expected patient outcomes. Examples of specific outcomes for patients with a hiatus hernia have been provided in the Planning section.

Guidelines for Application of the Nursing Process to the Care of the Patient Receiving Surgical Treatment for Hiatus Hernia

The nursing care of a patient having surgery for a hiatus hernia involves the general preoperative and postoperative measures required by any major surgery (see Chapter 4), with the following considerations.

Owing to the fact that the operative area is in close proximity to the diaphragm, postoperative coughing and deep breathing are often difficult and painful. This puts the patient at risk for pulmonary complications. Preoperative assessment of respiratory status and patient teaching about the need for and technique of postoperative turning, coughing, and deep breathing are of critical importance. If the patient smokes, stress the importance of decreasing or eliminating cigarettes for at least a few days prior to surgery.

Postoperatively, assessment of respiratory status continues to be critically important, and a nursing diagnosis of high risk for infection related to inadequate airway clearance is applicable to all patients. Assist the patient in turning, coughing, and deep breathing until he or she is ambulatory, to promote good ventilation, move secretions, and prevent respiratory infection. Evaluate these interventions as effective if the lungs are clear to auscultation, no purulent sputum is produced, and body temperature remains within normal range.

Because eructation can also be difficult postoperatively because of the closeness of the operative area to the diaphragm, assess for postoperative distention. Also assess for dysphagia, which may occur temporarily as a result of edema of the distal esophagus. When gastric suction is discontinued, start the patient on a liquid diet and progress to a full diet as tolerated. Encourage the patient to eat slowly to prevent swallowing air. Avoid carbonated beverages and gas-producing foods as the diet is progressed.

Achalasia

ETIOLOGY AND PATHOPHYSIOLOGY

Achalasia is a motor disorder of the lower two thirds of the esophagus in which peristalsis is decreased or absent, the lower esophageal sphincter fails to relax and allow swallowed food to pass into the stomach, and the esophagus above the sphincter dilates (Fig. 22–8). The exact cause of achalasia is unknown, but a disturbance of the intrinsic innervation of the smooth muscle appears to be involved.

CLINICAL MANIFESTATIONS

Symptoms of achalasia are odynophagia and dysphagia. Odynophagia (painful swallowing) typically occurs 5 to 8 seconds after swallowing and can range from mild discomfort to severe pain described as sharp and crushing. It is commonly substernal and often radiates to the back, neck, jaw, and arms.

Dysphagia associated with achalasia may be intermittent or continuous. It may occur with the ingestion of both solids and liquids. Regurgitation, which can lead to aspiration, may also occur.

Symptoms appear to worsen with emotional stress, with rapid eating, and with ingestion of large amounts of very hot or very cold foods.

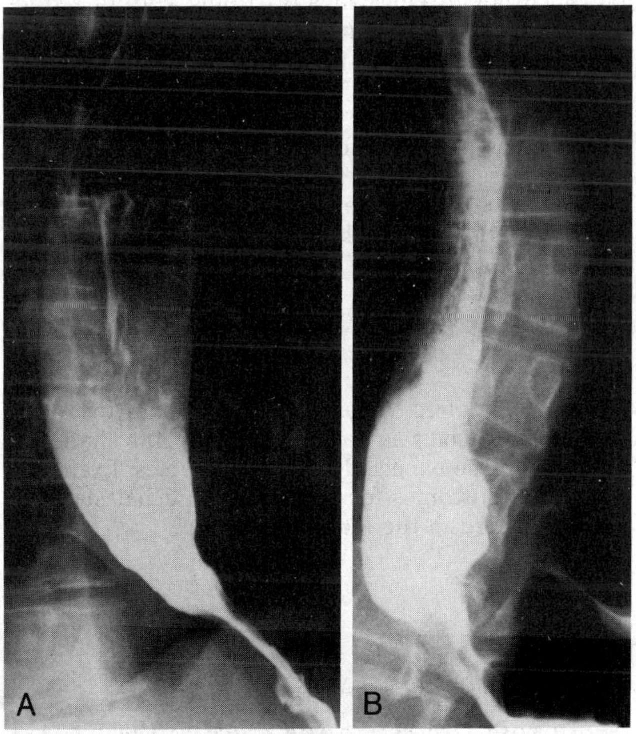

Figure 22–8.

A, Achalasia with a narrowed, elongated esophagogastric junction (rat-tail sign). *B,* Widening of the esophagogastric junction in a patient with achalasia following balloon dilation. (From Zuidema GD [ed]. Shackelford's surgery of the alimentary tract. 3rd ed, Vol 1. Philadelphia: WB Saunders, 1991, p 69.)

MEDICAL DIAGNOSIS

Diagnosis of achalasia is made on the basis of radiologic and manometric studies. Dilation of the esophageal body with a narrowed distal end can be seen during a barium swallow. Manometry directly measures pressure and function of the lower esophageal sphincter as well as motility of the esophagus. With achalasia, there is a high resting pressure at the sphincter, little or no relaxation of the sphincter on swallowing, and absence of peristalsis in the lower two thirds of the esophagus.

MEDICAL MANAGEMENT

Medical management of achalasia is aimed at alleviating the obstruction at the lower end of the esophagus caused by the aperistaltic esophagus and failure of the lower esophageal sphincter to relax.

The three basic management options are esophageal dilatation, drug therapy, and surgery. The most effective nonsurgical intervention is pneumatic dilatation. In this procedure, which takes only a few minutes and requires only a day in the hospital, a balloon-tipped dilator is passed through the mouth and positioned in the lower esophageal sphincter under radiologic guidance. It is then abruptly inflated to partially rip the muscle of the sphincter. After the dilatation, the patient remains on NPO status for approximately 6 hours and is monitored for signs of esophageal perforation, which is the major risk associated with the procedure. Because an emergency thoracotomy is required in the event that perforation occurs, this procedure is not done on elderly patients or on those with significant cardiovascular, renal, or pulmonary disease. If dilatation is unsatisfactory, a myectomy may be done. This is direct cutting of the muscle of the lower esophageal sphincter to enlarge the opening into the stomach so that food can pass through more readily. A myectomy may be done through either an abdominal or a thoracic incision. It is important to remember that neither dilatation nor myectomy corrects the underlying neurologic problem.

Anticholinergic agents and calcium antagonists such as nifedipine are sometimes used to decrease the tone and contraction of the esophageal smooth muscle. Their use is generally limited to patients who are poor surgical risks or who have had esophageal dilatation with less than the desired effect.

Application of the Nursing Process to the Care of the Patient with Achalasia

Assessment

Explore the patient's symptoms, including severity, frequency, and relationship to any specific factor

Chart 22–2.

NURSING GUIDE TO PATIENT EDUCATION FOR SELF-MANAGEMENT: DYSPHAGIA

To facilitate swallowing, instruct the patient to:

Sit up straight when eating. Keep the head upright and tilted slightly forward.
Allow sufficient time for meals and eat slowly.
Take small bites of solid foods and small sips of liquids.
Eat textured foods that need to be chewed.
Avoid sticky foods like bananas, mashed potatoes, and peanut butter.
Avoid very hot or cold foods.
Take fluids to wash down solid food.

such as type of food eaten or a stressful situation. Assess the patient's nutritional status and usual daily diet. Identify changes in diet necessitated by symptoms, including changes in size and timing of meals, consistency of foods, foods avoided, or foods newly included in the diet. Determine the effect of such changes as well as of any other home remedies used.

In preparation for patient teaching, assess the patient's understanding of the disorder, the proposed treatment, and its expected result. Also assess the resources available to the patient that could support compliance with the treatment program.

Nursing Diagnoses and Planning

Nursing diagnoses and related expected patient outcomes most commonly applicable to patients with achalasia include the following:

NDx: Impaired swallowing related to motor dysfunction of the esophagus

Planning: Patient outcomes
1. Patient identifies measures to aid swallowing.
2. Patient describes both the plan and its importance for reducing stress.
3. Patient ingests a nutritionally balanced diet composed of a variety of foodstuffs without stated or other overt signs of discomfort.

NDx: Pain related to swallowing

Planning: Patient outcomes
1. Patient reports that pain on swallowing is decreased.
2. Behavioral signs of discomfort such as posturing and avoidance of increasing numbers of foods are absent.

Nursing Interventions

NDx: Impaired swallowing
Instruct the patient in measures to facilitate swallowing as presented in Chart 22–2. Explain the relationship of stress to exacerbation of symptoms. Discuss sources of stress to the patient, and assist the patient in identifying ways of coping with or reducing it. Particularly emphasize the importance of avoiding stress at meal times.

NDx: Pain
Intervene as described for difficulty swallowing food because ease of swallowing reduces discomfort. Instruct the patient to elevate the head of the bed to help prevent nocturnal regurgitation and tracheal aspiration.

Evaluation

Evaluate the effectiveness of nursing care for a patient with achalasia by comparing the patient's status with the expected patient outcomes. Examples of specific outcomes for patients with achalasia have been provided in the Planning section.

Guidelines for Application of the Nursing Process to the Care of the Patient Undergoing Surgical Treatment for Achalasia

Nursing care of the patient undergoing an esophageal myectomy for the relief of achalasia combines the care required by any patient undergoing major surgery, that necessitated by opening the thoracic or abdominal cavity (depending on the approach used in the specific case), and that necessitated by the effects on the esophagus.

Because gastric reflux may develop subsequent to the surgical procedure, be sure to assess the patient for related symptoms, and if they occur, institute nursing interventions related to diet, position, and avoidance of factors that increase intraabdominal pressure as described in Application of the Nursing Process to the Care of the Patient with a Hiatus Hernia.

Trauma

Many types of traumatic injury can affect the mouth and other organs of the upper gastrointestinal tract (Table 22–2). These include abrasions, lacerations, penetrating injuries, blunt force injuries, and chemical or thermal injuries. They can be minor, requiring little or no treatment, or severe, potentially life-threatening events that require intensive, prolonged therapy.

Fracture of the Mandible

ETIOLOGY AND PATHOPHYSIOLOGY

Most fractures of the mandible or lower jaw result from a blow to the face or chin. They may be simple fractures without bone displacement, or in the case of severe accidents, there may be both marked displacement and loss of tissue. Occasionally the mandible is fractured as part of a planned surgical correction of a deformity.

CLINICAL MANIFESTATIONS

Symptoms of a fractured mandible are pain on movement, abnormal mobility of the lower jaw, malocclusion, and irregularity of the dental arch.

MEDICAL DIAGNOSIS

The diagnosis of mandibular fracture is suggested by palpation and confirmed by x-ray examination.

MEDICAL MANAGEMENT

Simple fractures of the mandible can be managed by intermaxillary fixation. In this procedure, wires are placed around the upper teeth and around the lower teeth on both sides of the fracture. Then,

Table 22–2. SELECTED TYPES OF UPPER GASTROINTESTINAL TRAUMA

TYPE OF TRAUMA	ETIOLOGY	CLINICAL MANIFESTATIONS	TREATMENT
Esophageal damage from medication	Lodging of medications such as tetracycline, doxycycline, quinidine, and ascorbic acid in the esophagus causes localized, shallow mucosal ulcer	Steady burning chest pain and odynophagia 4 to 6 hours after taking medication	Symptomatic with antacids and soft, bland diet. Healing occurs in approximately 1 week. Teach prevention: take capsules in an upright position and with a large glass of water.
Chemical burns	Accidental ingestion of strong acid or base such as lye Suicide attempt	Acute pain, possible respiratory distress secondary to pharyngeal edema or mucus block, fever, shock	Emergency treatment for respiratory distress and shock. If these are not present, sips of water to dilute chemical. Analgesics for pain. Nasogastric tube to keep esophagus patent. Corticosteroids to decrease inflammatory response. Antibiotics to combat infection. Tube feedings, daily dilation with a bougie, starting approximately 1 week after the insult.
Esophageal obstruction by a foreign body	Accidental ingestion of pins, fishbones, tooth, or a large bolus of meat or other food Suicide attempt	Pain, dysphagia, and possible dyspnea	Removed with an esophagoscope. Bolus of meat may be dissolved with proteolytic enzymes.
Esophageal perforation	Stab or bullet wounds, accidental perforation with a surgical instrument, spontaneous rupture with vomiting	Retrosternal pain followed by dysphagia, hyperpnea, cervical tenderness, subcutaneous emphysema, fever, leukocytosis, and sometimes severe hypotension	Semi-Fowler's position and nasogastric tube to limit reflux. Patient is placed on NPO status with hyperalimentation. Broad-spectrum antibiotics to combat mediastinitis. Chest tubes to drain the chest, and if a large perforation, surgical repair.

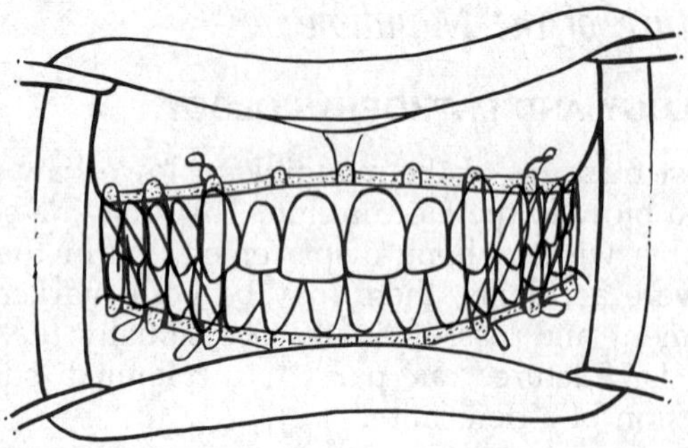

Figure 22–9.

Intermaxillary fixation. Note wires surrounding tops of upper and lower teeth and the bands attached to them, holding the lower jaw firmly in place against the upper jaw.

using these wires as sources of attachment, wires or rubber bands are applied, holding the top teeth to the bottom teeth and thus firmly holding the lower jaw against the upper jaw (Fig. 22–9). In cases in which teeth are lost or bone is displaced, alternative means of immobilization such as metal arch bars in the mouth or pins into the bone are used.

The patient is generally out of bed on the first postoperative day and discharged in 2 to 3 days, but the jaw remains immobilized for 6 to 8 weeks.

Application of the Nursing Process to the Care of the Patient with a Mandibular Fracture

PREOPERATIVE NURSING CARE

Give basic preoperative care as discussed in Chapter 4. Remember that in most cases fixation of the mandible represents emergency rather than elective surgery. Be certain that the patient understands what is to be done and how it will look. Reassure the patient regarding postoperative ability to breathe and swallow. Explain that speech may be difficult at first but within a few days should be understandable. Plan for an alternative means of communication during the first postoperative days.

POSTOPERATIVE NURSING CARE

Assessment

Make assessments as for any postoperative patient. Pay particular attention to respiratory status. Assess amount of secretions and the need for suctioning. Use a tongue blade and flashlight to inspect accessible areas of the mouth for cleanliness and for irritation from the wires. Observe and record the patient's intake and his or her response to the blenderized diet. Question the patient about constipation and passage of excessive flatus.

Nursing Diagnoses and Planning

Nursing diagnoses and related expected patient outcomes most commonly applicable to patients with a fractured mandible include the following:

NDx: High risk for ineffective airway clearance related to inability to open mouth and clear throat effectively

Planning: Patient outcomes
1. Respiratory rate is within normal limits.
2. Respirations are silent and easy.
3. Lungs are clear on auscultation.

NDx: High risk for aspiration related to inability to open mouth and clear throat effectively

Planning: Patient outcomes
1. Signs of regurgitation are absent.
2. Signs of respiratory distress are absent.

NDx: High risk for infection related to break in the oral mucous membrane and limited ability to clean the oral cavity

Planning: Patient outcomes
1. Patient denies areas of irritation from the wires.
2. Gums are pink and smooth.
3. Breath is free of offensive odor.

NDx: Impaired verbal communication related to inability to open mouth

Planning: Patient outcomes
1. Patient uses alternative communication techniques.
2. Patient's needs are understood.

NDx: High risk for altered nutrition: less than body requirements related to inability to eat other than by sucking liquids through a straw or from a spoon

Planning: Patient outcomes
1. Patient maintains body weight.

NDx: High risk for constipation related to a liquid, high-carbohydrate diet

Planning: Patient outcomes
1. Patient describes interventions to combat constipation.
2. Patient has soft, formed bowel movement at least every third day.
3. Patient denies excessive flatus.

NDx: High risk for altered health maintenance related to insufficient knowledge of self-care following discharge

Planning: Patient outcomes

1. Patient describes measures to prevent airway obstruction, including how and when to cut wires or bands.
2. Patient describes the selection and preparation of a high-protein, high-calorie, liquid diet.
3. Patient demonstrates oral hygiene.
4. Patient lists signs and symptoms to report.
5. Patient states date of follow-up visit.

Nursing Interventions

NDx: High risk for ineffective airway clearance

Keep wire cutters (scissors if rubber bands are used) taped to the head of the bed and suction equipment at the bedside. Maintain the patient in a side-lying position with the head elevated until fully awake. Wearing gloves, suction the nose with a small catheter to remove secretions as needed. To suction the mouth, move the cheek away from the teeth with a tongue blade. Gently run the suction catheter in the space created, and insert it into the oral cavity itself either through a space between teeth or around the back of the third molar. If the patient is able, teach him or her to self-suction as needed.

If the patient is in respiratory distress and suctioning is not effective, cut the wires or bands in order to clear the airway.

NDx: High risk for aspiration

Give ordered antiemetics as needed to prevent vomiting. In the event vomiting occurs, tilt the patient's head forward or to the side and use suction to remove the vomitus. If there is a nasogastric tube, keep it patent and attached to low suction.

NDx: High risk for infection

Maintain meticulous oral hygiene. Give warm alkaline mouthwashes or oxygenating rinses every 2 hours and after eating. Cleanse the teeth with a soft toothbrush if permitted, or use an oral syringe to irrigate between the teeth and along the outer gum line.

Lubricate the lips with a water-soluble lubricant to prevent cracking.

NDx: Impaired verbal communication

Provide the patient with pencil and paper, chalkboard, Magic Slate, or other means of communication during the first few postoperative days, when speech is at best difficult to understand. Respond to the patient's call signal in person rather than by intercom during this time.

NDx: High risk for altered nutrition: less than body requirements

Start the patient on clear fluids through a straw. Progress as tolerated to a full blenderized diet. Give foods such as Jell-O or custard that can be sucked in off a spoon as desired. Administer high protein supplements as ordered. Follow each feeding with water.

Before discharge, arrange for the patient to see a dietitian for help in planning a high-calorie, high-protein blenderized diet with variation in taste. This is very important because the patient will be on the diet for 6 to 8 weeks and the risk of less than optimal nutrition is great because it becomes boring and tiresome eating a blenderized diet through a straw. This is attested to by the fact that a weight loss of 10 to 20 lb is not unusual in patients with wired jaws.

NDx: High risk for constipation

Tell the patient about the potential for excessive flatus and constipation owing to a liquid, high-carbohydrate diet and the intake of air when sucking through a straw or from a spoon. Encourage ambulation and exercise to promote good bowel function. If needed, provide prune juice and give a bulk-forming laxative as ordered.

NDx: High risk for altered health maintenance

Instruct the patient in self-care following discharge as specified in Chart 22–3.

Additional Interventions

If an appliance is in place outside the mouth, alert the patient to its presence and caution against turning over onto it.

Evaluation

Evaluate the effectiveness of nursing care for a patient with a fractured mandible by comparing the patient's status with the expected patient outcomes. Examples of specific outcomes for patients with a fractured mandible have been provided in the Planning section.

Neoplasia

Oral Cancer

Cancer of the oral cavity is primarily a disease of the elderly. Its incidence increases between ages 50 and 70, and it is more common in men. It can occur on the lip, on the tongue, or inside the mouth.

ETIOLOGY

Two clearly identified causes of oral cancer are the use of tobacco and the use of alcohol, which are thought to interfere with local defense mechanisms. Tobacco use includes smoking cigarettes, pipes, and

Chart 22–3.

NURSING GUIDE TO PATIENT EDUCATION FOR SELF-MANAGEMENT: DISCHARGE INSTRUCTIONS AFTER INTERMAXILLARY FIXATION

Instruct the patient to:

Protect against airway obstruction.
- Keep a wire cutter (or if rubber bands were used, a scissors) with him or her at all times.
- Avoid carbonated beverages because their foam can be difficult to clear from the throat.
- Avoid alcoholic beverages because they depress the reflexes needed to keep the airway clear.
- Do not swim because it can be difficult to remove water from the throat.

Prevent oral infection.
- Brush teeth regularly if permitted.
- Rinse mouth with water, mouthwash, dilute hydrogen peroxide, or saline after eating and at bedtime.
- Use a Water Pik or oral syringe as desired to cleanse the mouth, but keep the stream of solution gentle.
- Apply paraffin to the ends of the wires to avoid injury to the mouth.

Maintain a balanced nutritional intake.
- Blenderize foods.
- Select foods high in protein and carbohydrate.
- Select a variety of foods.
- Drink at least 2500 ml of fluid per day.

Obtain necessary follow-up care.
- Report any irritation, swelling, or unusual pain.
- Report to the physician immediately if the wires or bands are cut.
- Return for scheduled visits.

cigars and the use of chewing tobacco and snuff. Irritation from prolonged exposure to sun and wind or from a hot pipe stem contributes specifically to the development of cancer of the lip. Other factors believed to contribute to the development of cancer of the mouth but whose roles have not been proved include poor oral hygiene with subsequent bacterial invasion and physical trauma as from jagged teeth or improperly fitting dentures. Malnutrition, syphilis, and cirrhosis have also been found to be present in large numbers of patients with this disease.

PATHOPHYSIOLOGY

The majority of oral malignant lesions are squamous cell carcinomas. Most often these tumors occur on the lips, the lateral aspects of the tongue, or the floor of the mouth, although any part of the oral cavity including the pharynx and sinuses can be affected.

Cancer of the mouth spreads primarily by local extension and via the regional lymph nodes of the head and neck. Cancer of the lip has a good prognosis because it is well localized and is easily detected before extensive tissue involvement occurs.

Cancers of the tongue and the floor of the mouth have a poorer prognosis because the tumors are not as readily noticeable in their early stages. In addition, the extensive vascular and lymphatic supply of the mouth facilitates metastasis.

CLINICAL MANIFESTATIONS

Malignant lesions of the lip tend to arise in areas of leukoplakia, that is, white, nodular, patchy areas on the mucosa that cannot be easily rubbed off (Fig. 22–10). The cancer may appear as a blister, as a nonhealing sore that crusts and bleeds, or as a painless, hard, white, fixed mass. As tumor growth progresses, secondary infection occurs, resulting in ulceration, tenderness, edema, and surrounding erythema.

Malignant lesions of the mouth and tongue usually are white or yellowish ulcerated lesions, although in earliest stages they may appear simply as a red or white surface patch. Initially the lesions are

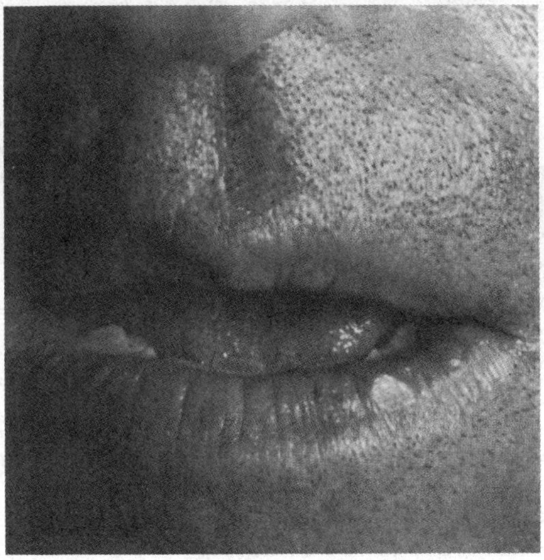

Figure 22–10.

Small patch of leukoplakia on the left lower lip. (From Moschella SL, Hurley HJ. Dermatology. 2nd ed, Vol 2. Philadelphia: WB Saunders, 1985, p 1867.)

asymptomatic, although depending on the location, sometimes the patient is aware of feeling a roughened area with the tongue. As the tumor enlarges, symptoms develop that vary with the location and extent of spread. With cancer of the anterior, mobile portion of the tongue, pain or soreness can occur when eating hot or spicy foods, and as mobility of the tongue becomes impaired, speech can become slurred. Swallowing is painful, and as neighboring structures are affected, pain in the area of the temporomandibular joint and the outer ear along with increased salivation and blood-tinged sputum can occur. With tumors of the base of the tongue, odynophagia, unilateral sore throat, and salivary changes occur.

MEDICAL DIAGNOSIS

Any oral lesion that does not heal in 3 weeks or less should be evaluated as a possible oral malignancy. Oral exfoliative cytology in which the suspicious lesion is scraped and the cells examined microscopically can support the diagnosis of cancer. However, only a biopsy provides a definitive benign diagnosis. Submental, submaxillary, and cervical nodes are palpated to determine metastases. Malignant lesions of the mouth are often found by the patient's dentist during a routine dental examination.

MEDICAL MANAGEMENT

Treatment mode depends on the location, type, size, and lymphatic spread of the tumor.

Nonmetastasized cancers of the lip are effectively treated either by external beam radiation or by simple surgical excision, usually under local anesthesia. If metastasis to the lymph nodes has occurred, surgical resection is combined with postoperative radiation therapy.

Small tumors located on the anterior portion of the tongue may be treated by either radiation or surgical excision, whereas larger tumors require partial glossectomy (removal of part of the tongue) and subsequent radiation. If tumor involves the floor of the mouth near the lower jaw, removal of the mandible (mandibulectomy) and a radical neck dissection may also be required. This surgery is also followed by radiation and then by reconstructive procedures because removal of the mandible results in a noticeable cosmetic deficit.

For tumors on the base of the tongue, surgical treatment involves a total glossectomy and a laryngectomy, with follow-up radiation and chemotherapy. Because this is extremely disfiguring and incapacitating surgery that is accompanied by a large incidence of tumor recurrence, radiation only may be elected in some cases. A radical neck dissection is performed in conjunction with surgical treatment of any of the oral cancers with follow-up radiation and chemotherapy if lymph node metastasis has occurred.

Application of the Nursing Process to the Care of the Patient Having Surgery for Oral Cancer

PREOPERATIVE NURSING CARE

Assess the patient's readiness for surgery as described in Chapter 4. Pay particular attention to the patient's nutritional, fluid, and electrolyte status because oral cancer frequently interferes with eating owing to soreness and difficulty swallowing. Check for weight loss. Review recent patterns of dietary intake, and review laboratory data related to nutrition and fluid and electrolyte balance. Carefully assess respiratory status because the patient is at risk for problems with airway clearance postoperatively.

Assess the patient's understanding of the proposed surgery and his or her psychological response to it. This is critical because oral surgery can result in unconcealable disfiguration and impairment in the basic functions of speaking, swallowing, and eating. If the patient will be unable to speak, discuss alternative forms of communication. Review with the patient expected postoperative procedures such as oral suctioning, nasogastric suction, and wound care.

With extensive surgery such as total glossectomy and removal of the palate and mandible, prostheses of the palate and jaw may be constructed to replace portions of tissues that have been resected. If prostheses are to be made, impressions will be taken preoperatively, so be certain to explain this process to the patient.

Institute nutritional support measures as ordered. These may consist of supplemental feedings, vitamin supplements, or hyperalimentation therapy to maximize the patient's nutritional status for surgery.

Cleanse the patient's mouth, and ensure that other preoperative preparations are carried out as ordered.

POSTOPERATIVE NURSING CARE

Assessment

Make usual postoperative assessments as outlined in Chapter 4. If the parotid gland has been resected, assess the patient's capacity for facial movement by asking him or her to raise eyebrows, frown, smile, show teeth, and pucker lips. Assess for nutritional problems when oral foods and fluids are reinstated. Also assess the psychological response to the surgery. Be alert for signs of reluctance to interact with other people; anxiety about resumption of personal responsibilities, prognosis, or self-care; and any other nonadaptive response. Explore the patient's coping mechanisms and available support systems.

Nursing Diagnoses and Planning

Nursing diagnoses and related expected patient outcomes most commonly applicable to patients who have had surgery for a neoplasm of the oral cavity include the following:

NDx: High risk for ineffective airway clearance related to edema, difficulty swallowing or handling secretions

Planning: Patient outcomes
1. Patient coughs and deep breathes as directed.
2. Respirations are easy, quiet, and symmetric.
3. Lungs are clear on auscultation.

NDx: Pain related to surgical tissue trauma

Planning: Patient outcomes
1. Patient describes self as at least fairly comfortable.
2. Behavioral signs of pain such as grimacing or moaning are absent.
3. Patient reports decreasing pain throughout postoperative course.

NDx: High risk for altered nutrition: less than body requirements related to inability to ingest foods and fluids orally

Planning: Patient outcomes
1. Patient's daily caloric intake meets basic requirements as identified by the dietitian.
2. Serum albumin and albumin-globulin ratio are within normal limits.
3. Patient maintains weight.

NDx: Impaired verbal communication related to removal of oral tissues, postoperative restrictions on mouth movement

Planning: Patient outcomes
1. Patient uses alternative communication techniques.
2. Patient's needs are understood.

NDx: High risk for body image disturbance related to changes in appearance secondary to surgery

Planning: Patient outcomes
1. Patient looks at self in mirror.
2. Patient indicates interest in appearance.
3. Patient welcomes visitors.
4. Patient interacts with other patients.

NDx: High risk for infection related to the location of the surgical incision

Planning: Patient outcomes
1. Purulent drainage from wound is absent.
2. Foul odor from the wound is absent.
3. Patient is afebrile.

NDx: High risk for altered health maintenance related to insufficient knowledge of self-care following discharge

Planning: Patient outcomes
1. Patient demonstrates care of the wound.
2. Patient demonstrates self-examination for facial and oral cancer.

Nursing Interventions

NDx: High risk for ineffective airway clearance

Immediately following surgery, place the patient in a side-lying position to facilitate drainage. When the patient is alert, assist him or her into Fowler's position if desired. Suction the mouth as needed, or allow saliva and other drainage to drain into an emesis basin via a gauze wick. Turn the patient frequently, and assist with coughing and deep breathing every 2 hours. If a tracheostomy was done to facilitate breathing, provide care as described in Chapter 12.

NDx: Pain

Administer prescribed pain medication as needed. This can range from viscous lidocaine to anesthetize a painful area of the mouth after removal of a small, localized malignancy to systemic analgesics like meperidine hydrochloride for severe, more generalized pain after extensive surgery. Provide the patient with a soft, nonirritating diet and avoid any trauma to the mouth during oral hygiene.

NDx: High risk for altered nutrition: less than body requirements

Because a high-protein, high-calorie diet is needed to promote healing, supplemental tube feedings may be given, and, in some cases, hyperalimentation therapy may be ordered. When oral intake is allowed, place small amounts of bland fluids on the back of the tongue with an Asepto syringe or a soft feeding tube. As the patient's tolerance permits, increase the diet to include nonirritating foods such as Jell-O, pudding, custard, and pureed foods. Avoid acidic foods and very hot and very cold foods.

Teach the patient to eat slowly, take small sips or bites of food, eat small amounts frequently, avoid using a fork (which may cause tissue injury), and drink water after eating to clear the mouth of food particles. Provide privacy, sufficient time, and a comfortable upright position so that the patient can be successful in learning how to manage food and fluids.

NDx: Impaired verbal communication

If the patient is unable to speak because of a tracheotomy or restricted movement of the mouth, use an alternative form of communication such as a Magic Slate or flash cards as discussed preoperatively. Keep the patient's call light within reach at all times, and alert all members of the health care team to the fact that the patient cannot speak.

When speech is possible, encourage the patient to speak slowly. Maintain an unhurried, undemanding atmosphere, and provide for privacy as the patient "relearns" to speak. Initiate referral to speech therapy as necessary.

NDx: High risk for body-image disturbance

Provide an accepting, nonthreatening environment. Be sensitive to and acknowledge the patient's feelings. Be straightforward about the patient's appearance, but be certain to avoid comments or actions that could be construed by the patient as indicating distaste or pity. Do not force the patient to look at the wound. When the patient does look at it, remind the patient that it is not yet healed and so there is still swelling and inflammation.

Assist the patient with good grooming. Be certain that hair is combed and male patients are shaved. Encourage makeup for female patients. Get patients up and dressed as soon as allowed.

NDx: High risk for infection

To cleanse the oral cavity and promote wound healing and comfort, irrigate the oral area with sterile water, dilute hydrogen peroxide, or soda bicarbonate solution. Use a cotton-tipped applicator to cleanse the teeth and gums if needed, but do not use any commercial toothbrush because it may cause tissue damage. Avoid commercial mouthwashes and lemon glycerin swabs because of their drying effect on mucous membranes.

Meticulous care of the incision lines is important. Use a cotton-tipped applicator to gently clean the incision with dilute hydrogen peroxide. If an antibiotic ointment such as bacitracin is ordered, apply it lightly to the incision line. If the patient has a wound suctioning device to facilitate drainage, monitor every 4 hours for proper functioning and amount and character of drainage.

NDx: High risk for altered health maintenance

Instruct the patient in self-care following discharge. Keep in mind that each patient who has had surgery for oral cancer has specific needs for teaching depending on the type of surgical procedure done. If needed, provide instructions for wound care as outlined in Chart 22–4. Instruct all patients in self-examination for facial and oral cancer as specified in Chart 22–5 and in the need for medical follow-up, because a patient with one of these cancers is at great risk for developing another.

Additional Interventions

If drooling is a problem, encourage the patient to consciously swallow more often. Keep tissues and a disposal bag readily available to the patient at all times. Administer anticholinergics such as atropine or belladonna compounds as ordered to decrease salivation.

Evaluation

Evaluate the effectiveness of nursing care for a patient having surgery for oral cancer by comparing the patient's status with the expected patient outcomes. Examples of specific outcomes for patients having surgery for oral cancer have been provided in the Planning section.

Guidelines for Application of the Nursing Process to the Care of the Patient Receiving Supportive Treatment for Oral Cancer

If the patient with oral cancer is not having surgery, nursing care is primarily planned to enable the patient to be comfortable, to maintain oral intake for as long as possible, and to cope with a terminal illness. Provide food, fluids, and oral hygiene as described previously. Give medication for pain as needed in accordance with the physician's orders. Provide

Chart 22–4.

NURSING GUIDE TO PATIENT EDUCATION FOR SELF-MANAGEMENT: BASIC WOUND CARE AFTER SURGERY FOR ORAL CANCER

Instruct the patient to:

Mix equal amounts of hydrogen peroxide and sterile saline in a sterile container. Always mix new solution each time wound care is done. Discard remaining solution when finished.

Place several cotton applicator sticks into the container. Do not touch any part of the applicator beyond the end of the stick.

Beginning at the top of the wound, gently cleanse the incision with a damp applicator. Do not go back over any area that has been touched. Use a new applicator as needed.

Go over an area with a dry applicator as needed if the peroxide has caused a lot of bubbling.

Apply a *thin* layer of any prescribed ointment to the incision with a dry applicator. Use the same technique as with cleansing—do not retrace over areas already touched and use a new applicator as needed. When squeezing the ointment onto the applicator, do not let the tip of the applicator touch the tube itself.

Chart 22–5.

NURSING GUIDE TO PATIENT EDUCATION FOR SELF-MANAGEMENT: SELF-EXAMINATION FOR FACIAL AND ORAL CANCER

Instruct the patient to use a mirror and good light and examine himself or herself monthly for signs of facial or oral cancer as described here:

Examination of the face and neck

Inspect your face and neck for any differences in shape between the right side and the left side.

Observe the skin on the face and neck for changes in color, changes in a mole, lumps, or sores. Be certain to remove glasses and inspect the skin around the eyes and on the bridge of the nose.

Press along the sides and front of the neck with your finger tips, feeling for tender areas or lumps.

Examination of the mouth

Remove dentures and partial plates in preparation for examination of the inside of the mouth.

Pull the lower lip down, and inspect for sores or color changes. Palpate for lumps.

Pull the top lip up and back. Inspect for sores or color changes, and palpate for lumps.

Grasp the upper lip on one side of the nouth with one hand and the lower lip on the same side with the other. Pull out and to the side to expose the inside of the cheek.

Observe for discoloration and sores. Repeat with other cheek.

Check for lumps and tenderness in the cheek. Put your thumb on the inside of the cheek and your index finger on the outside. Gently compress the tissue between them. Repeat with other cheek.

Open your mouth and tilt your head back. Inspect the roof of the mouth for discoloration, raised areas; sores, or swelling.

Open your mouth wide and touch the roof of the mouth with the tip of your tongue. Look for discoloration and raised areas or sores on the floor of the mouth and the bottom of the tongue.

Press the floor of the mouth with your fingers to detect lumps or tender areas.

Stick the tongue out and look at its top surface for discoloration or sores.

Grasp the tongue with a piece of gauze or tissue. Pull it forward and to each side in turn. Inspect for discoloration, raised areas, sores, or other lesions.

psychological support in terms of allowing time and opportunity to verbalize feelings and facilitating visits by family, chaplain, or hospice worker.

Cancer of the Esophagus

The incidence of cancer of the esophagus varies greatly throughout the world. In the United States, it occurs most often in males between 60 and 80 years of age, with black, Chinese, and Japanese men affected more frequently than white men.

ETIOLOGY

The wide variation in geographical distribution suggests that environmental factors have a definite role in the development of esophageal carcinoma. Implicated factors are smoking, alcohol abuse, poor oral hygiene, and poor nutritional habits. Esophageal cancer also appears to be related to untreated achalasia and the presence of strictures caused by the ingestion of lye.

PATHOPHYSIOLOGY

There are primarily two types of cancer that affect the esophagus: squamous cell carcinoma and adenocarcinoma. Squamous cell carcinoma, by far the more common of the two, usually involves the upper or middle third of the esophagus. Adenocarcinoma, in contrast, most often arises in the stomach and extends secondarily into the esophagus.

The tumor appears as an ulcerating mass that projects into the lumen. It tends to extend around the total inner circumference as well as up and down the esophagus. As it enlarges, the normal distensibility of the esophagus is overcome, and the passage of ingested food past the tumor is progressively obstructed. Unfortunately, by the time obstruction is sufficient to cause symptoms, spread of the cancer has usually occurred into lymph nodes and adjacent tissues (Fig. 22–11). For this reason, the prognosis is very poor.

The pattern of spread is specific to the location of the original tumor. Tumors of the upper third of the esophagus spread to the cervical nodes, trachea, larynx, and thyroid gland; middle third tumors spread to the lymph nodes of the lungs; and lower tumors spread to the lungs and the liver.

With advanced disease, extensive mediastinal or pericardial involvement can occur as well as tracheoesophageal fistula or aortic erosion with exsanguinating hemorrhage.

CLINICAL MANIFESTATIONS

Esophageal cancers tend to be asymptomatic until relatively far advanced. When symptoms do occur, the most common is dysphagia, which develops

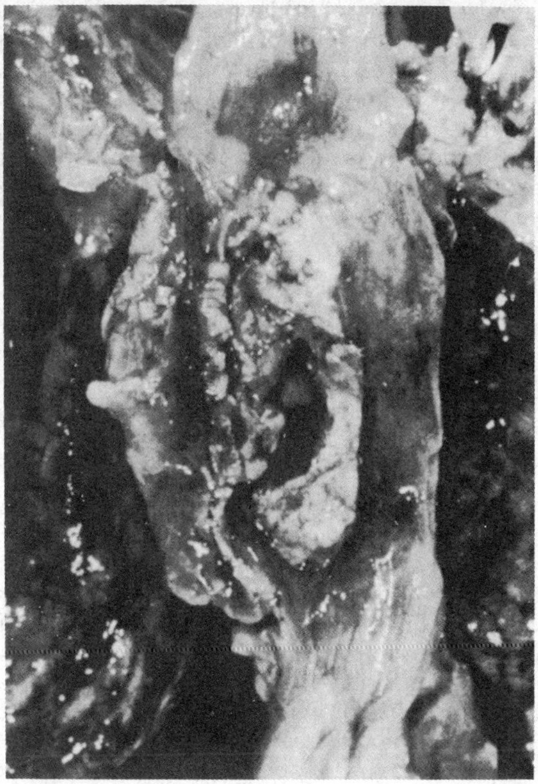

Figure 22–11.

Carcinoma of the esophagus with a large defect in the central necrotic portion. Tumor has directly invaded the trachea to produce an esophagotracheal fistula. (From Cotran RS, Kumar V, Robbins SL. Robbins pathologic basis of disease. 4th ed. Philadelphia: WB Saunders, 1989, p 836.)

when the mass begins to occlude the esophageal lumen. Over a period of 6 to 8 months, the dysphagia progresses from difficulty with solid foods to difficulty with liquids and finally with saliva. The dysphagia is insidious in that the patient eliminates foods that are difficult to swallow one by one over a period of time and often does not realize the extent of the problem until the diet is essentially liquid. Occasionally dysphagia is accompanied by vague substernal discomfort or a feeling of fullness after ingestion of only a small amount of food.

As the disease advances, halitosis, anorexia, weight loss, and emaciation occur. Nausea and vomiting of undigested food occur if obstruction is complete, and cough occurs if a tracheoesophageal fistula or other tracheal involvement is present. A steady, boring pain on swallowing or hoarseness, or both, develop with extensive mediastinal involvement.

MEDICAL DIAGNOSIS

Diagnosis of esophageal carcinoma is based on an x-ray esophagram with barium swallow. This demonstrates the tumor by showing a narrowing of the esophagus in the area of the mass. The pathologic type of the malignancy is determined by means of an esophagoscopy with biopsy and cytologic brushings. Subsequently, the patient is scheduled for a variety of procedures, the results of which are needed to stage the disease and plan therapy. These procedures include bronchoscopy, organ scanning, liver function tests, chest x-ray examination, and computed tomography (CT) scan for mediastinal spread.

MEDICAL MANAGEMENT

Treatment of esophageal cancer varies with the location of the tumor, the overall condition of the patient, and the stage of the disease.

SURGICAL RESECTION OR BYPASS

When possible, surgical resection is the treatment of choice for esophageal cancer because the obstruction is removed and the continuity of the gastrointestinal tract and ability to swallow are restored. Two types of resection are esophagogastrostomy and esophagectomy with interposition of colon. Esophagogastrostomy, which is done for tumors of the distal esophagus, involves bringing the stomach up into the thoracic area for anastomosis to the remaining esophagus. Esophagectomy with interposition of a section of colon is used when such a large segment of the esophagus is removed that a conduit between the remaining esophagus and the stomach is needed. Interposition of colon is usually done as a second-stage procedure following recovery from the esophagectomy.

In esophageal bypass surgery, the stomach or colon is anastomosed to the esophagus above the tumor, thus bypassing the obstruction and restoring the ability to swallow.

Intensive preparation for surgery is necessary because most patients with esophageal cancer are poor surgical risks as a result of malnutrition with resultant decreased blood volume, protein depletion, fluid and electrolyte imbalances, and loss of resistance to infection.

Postoperatively, the patient is kept on NPO status for approximately 5 days. A nasogastric tube is in place to prevent pressure on the suture line for approximately 1 week. If the thoracic cavity is opened, a chest tube is inserted to reexpand the lungs. In some cases, a tracheostomy may also be done to manage airway clearance.

Postoperative complications include respiratory infection and leaking at the anastomosis. The patient is prone to respiratory infection owing to the location of the incision and the related difficulty in coughing and deep breathing to clear the airways of secretions. The patient is also at risk for aspiration pneumonia secondary to the reflux of gastric contents.

Leaking of the anastomosis is a major, frequently fatal development that occurs more often in the esophagus than in any other part of the GI tract. It can be due to tension on the suture line, poor healing, or impaired blood supply. Symptoms include low-grade fever, substernal pain, elevated pulse and respiratory rates, and shock. Occasionally subcutaneous emphysema or symptoms mimicking pulmonary embolism occur. Treatment consists of draining accumulated fluid from the thoracic cavity or, in some cases, repeat surgery for reanastomosis.

RADIATION

For tumors of the upper or middle esophagus, preradiation and postradiation therapy are often combined with surgery. When surgery is not an option because of the size of the tumor and existing metastases, radiation alone may be used to shrink the tumor and provide symptomatic relief.

Side effects of radiation to the upper and middle thirds of the esophagus include retrosternal discomfort, pain on swallowing, increased salivation, and nausea.

LASER PALLIATION

Laser therapy may be used in place of or in conjunction with surgery or radiation to reduce tumor size, maintain a patent esophageal lumen, and reduce dysphagia and discomfort. With the patient under local anesthesia, a laser passed through an endoscope is used to vaporize the obstructing tumor mass. This is a long procedure, and treatments are usually scheduled on alternating days until a patent lumen is established. A temporary increase in dysphagia and discomfort occurs immediately following this therapy, but within a few days after the last treatment an oral diet is gradually resumed.

Major advantages of this treatment are that it can be repeated an unlimited number of times, there are no undesirable systemic effects, and it can be used regardless of where the tumor is located in the esophagus (Ragan, 1990, p. 693). Potential complications of laser palliation include aspiration, bleeding, and perforation of the esophagus.

PROSTHETIC INTUBATION

In cases in which other measures fail, a pliable tube may be inserted into the esophagus to keep the lumen open and allow the patient to eat fairly normally for a period of time. A tube prosthesis may also be inserted to bypass a tracheoesophageal fistula and prevent aspiration of ingested food.

An example of a tube prosthesis is the Celestin tube, which is semirigid and held open by a wire coil. Under fluoroscopy, with the patient heavily sedated, it is pulled into place in the esophagus from below through an opening into the stomach.

A prosthetic tube may also be placed in the esophagus via endoscopy. The difficulty with this procedure is that the prosthesis tends to slip.

The swallowing reflex is unaffected by a tube prosthesis, but swallowing is initially uncomfortable and difficult. Patients start with sips of water and gradually add other fluids and foods as they learn how much of a substance can be swallowed at one time.

A major problem associated with tube prostheses is reflux of gastric contents and subsequent aspiration pneumonia. This is a problem because the tube interferes with normal peristalsis in the esophagus, leaving only the effect of gravity to prevent reflux. Thus, patients with a tube prosthesis can never lie flat but must keep the head elevated even at night.

GASTROSTOMY

As a last recourse, a gastrostomy tube is inserted as a means of maintaining nutrition. In some cases, a surgical gastrostomy is done in which the anterior wall of the stomach is sutured to the abdomen, creating a permanent fistula that allows the tube to be easily inserted and replaced. With increasing frequency, however, the percutaneous endoscopic gastrostomy is the procedure of choice.

Application of the Nursing Process to the Care of the Patient Having Esophageal Surgery for Cancer

Nursing care of patients having surgery for esophageal cancer combines the basic care of any operative patient, the care of the patient who has had chest surgery, and the care of any patient with a diagnosis of cancer.

PREOPERATIVE NURSING CARE

Assessment

Perform a complete assessment of the patient scheduled for surgery for esophageal cancer, as for any patient having major surgery. Pay particular attention to assessment of nutritional status and fluid and electrolyte balance because surgery is often preceded by a long period of dysphagia during which foods and fluids in the diet are progressively eliminated or decreased. Question the patient about changes in appetite and food intake. Check for loss of weight. Review laboratory studies for electrolyte imbalances, decreased serum albumin level, decreased total protein level, and decreased serum transferrin level or iron-binding capacity.

Assess the patient's pulmonary function. Because the surgical procedure involves opening the thoracic cavity and manipulation in the area of the diaphragm, postoperative coughing and breathing will be painful and the patient will have an increased risk of respiratory complications.

Observe the patient for signs of infection because resistance may be low as a result of malnutrition secondary to progressive dysphagia.

Because cancer of the esophagus is generally far advanced at the time of diagnosis, and surgery is therefore palliative rather than curative, carefully assess the emotional response of the patient and family, their usual coping mechanisms, and available support systems.

Nursing Diagnoses and Planning

Nursing diagnoses and related expected patient outcomes most commonly applicable to patients scheduled for esophageal resection for cancer of the esophagus include the following:

NDx: Knowledge deficit: operative procedure and its expected outcome, postoperative course, and treatments

Planning: Patient outcomes
1. Patient describes the operative procedure and its expected effect in general terms.
2. Patient verbalizes understanding of postoperative equipment and treatments.
3. Patient demonstrates coughing and deep breathing.
4. Patient describes how nourishment will be maintained after surgery.

NDx: Anxiety related to the surgical experience, the resultant report on the extent of disease and its prognosis

Planning: Patient outcomes
1. Patient expresses concerns about the surgical experience and its effect on body functions.
2. Patient cooperates with preoperative preparation.
3. Signs of excessive anxiety such as trembling, crying, and pacing are absent.

NDx: Altered nutrition: less than body requirements related to inability to swallow foods or fluids prior to surgery

Planning: Patient outcomes
1. By time of surgery, patient's weight approximates ideal body weight.
2. Nitrogen balance is positive.
3. Serum electrolyte values, albumin level, and albumin-globulin ratio are within normal limits.

Nursing Interventions

NDx: Knowledge deficit: operative procedure and its expected outcome, postoperative course, and treatments
Clarify the patient's understanding of the surgery and its expected outcomes. Explain the usual postoperative procedures. Prepare the patient for the presence of a nasogastric tube and chest tube. Explain that blood transfusions are commonly given and that intravenous fluids can be expected for

about a week. Discuss how and when oral intake will be resumed.

Teach techniques of coughing and deep breathing, and describe the use of incentive spirometers and intermittent positive pressure breathing (IPPB). Explain the importance of these in preventing postoperative respiratory infection and promoting a rapid recovery. Encourage deep abdominal breathing every 2 hours while awake in preparation for surgery. Discourage smoking.

NDx: Anxiety

Acknowledge that anxiety over the surgery and disease prognosis is normal. Encourage the patient and family to verbalize concerns and ask questions about the surgery. Seek to identify specific worries such as ability to eat subsequent to surgery, ability to breathe with the nasogastric tube in place, or risk of acquired immunodeficiency syndrome (AIDS) or hepatitis associated with the blood transfusions. Correct any misconceptions, and provide reassuring information when possible.

Maintain a calm environment. Suggest the use of relaxation techniques. Administer sedatives as ordered.

NDx: Altered nutrition: less than body requirements

Carry out measures to restore nutritional, fluid, and electrolyte balance as ordered. These generally include administration of intravenous solutions; vitamin supplements (particularly vitamins B, C, and K); high-protein, high-caloric feedings; and even hyperalimentation therapy. Record all intake and output.

Additional Interventions

Thoroughly cleanse the mouth. Brush and floss teeth. Clean dentures. Use a swab or gauze to scrub the tongue and other areas in the mouth. Use milk of magnesia and mineral oil or the equivalent to remove crusts.

Evaluation

Evaluate the effectiveness of nursing care for a patient scheduled for surgery for esophageal cancer by comparing the patient's status with the expected patient outcomes. Examples of specific outcomes for patients scheduled for surgery for esophageal cancer have been provided in the Planning section.

POSTOPERATIVE NURSING CARE

Assessment

Assess the patient's return to physiologic stability. Check vital signs, color, skin temperature, responsiveness, wound drainage, and fluid intake and output. Assess the function of both the chest tube and the nasogastric tube. Note the amount and color of drainage from each. In the early postoperative period, when the stomach is still atonic, observe carefully for signs of reflux and aspiration.

Assess the patient for pain, and note the response to pain medication. Make frequent checks of respiratory status. Note rate, depth, and symmetry of respirations, and listen for abnormal breath sounds. Observe for signs of dehydration, and review laboratory data related to fluid and electrolyte balance as it becomes available. If the patient is on IPPB, note pulse rate, color, chest expansion, and amount and character of the expectorate, as well as the patient's general reaction to each treatment.

Assess for signs of leaking at the anastamosis: question the patient about substernal pain; check for fever, increased pulse or respiratory rate, and signs of shock; and be alert for subcutaneous emphysema or symptoms mimicking those of a pulmonary embolism.

When oral intake is started, assess tolerance of various food substances. Note development of nausea, vomiting, or any other distress. Be alert to signs of nutritional deficiency such as negative nitrogen balance and weight loss.

Nursing Diagnoses and Planning

Nursing diagnoses and related expected patient outcomes most commonly applicable to patients after esophageal resection for carcinoma include the following:

NDx: Pain related to thoracic/upper abdominal surgery

Planning: Patient outcomes

1. Patient states that pain is relieved.
2. Patient coughs, breathes deeply, and moves without moaning, crying out, or exhibiting pallor or other sign of distress.

NDx: High risk for ineffective airway clearance related to splinted respirations secondary to thoracic and epigastric pain, presence of chest tube, and poor cough effort

Planning: Patient outcomes

1. Respirations are easy, silent, and symmetrical.
2. Lungs are clear on auscultation.

NDx: Altered nutrition: less than body requirements related to inability to ingest foods or fluids orally

Planning: Patient outcomes

1. Patient's intake is nutritionally adequate.
2. Patient maintains weight.
3. Electrolyte values, albumin level, and albumin-globulin ratio are within normal limits.

NDx: High risk for infection related to the presence of a surgical incision or leaking of the esophageal anastomosis

Planning: Patient outcomes

1. External incision line is clean and approximated.
2. Foul wound drainage is absent.
3. Patient is afebrile.
4. Pulse, respiration, and blood pressure are within normal limits.
5. Patient denies substernal pain.

Nursing Interventions

NDx: Pain
Medicate for pain as ordered. Avoid overmedicating and depressing the cough reflex and respiratory center. Pay careful attention to positioning and other basic comfort measures. Provide a quiet environment, and encourage the use of breathing, visualization, and other relaxation techniques.

NDx: High risk for ineffective airway clearance
Assist the patient to a semi-Fowler's position to encourage lung expansion. Turn, cough, and deep breathe every 2 hours. Encourage the use of an incentive spirometer. If the patient is receiving IPPB treatments, ensure that each treatment is followed by supervised coughing, otherwise its effectiveness is lost.

NDx: Altered nutrition: less than body requirements
When oral intake is initiated, usually on the fifth or sixth day after surgery, give small sips (approximately 5 ml) of water every 15 to 30 minutes. Over the next few days, increase the amount taken at one time to 10 or 15 ml, and give plain tea in addition to water. Subsequently, give other bland fluids, and by the end of 2 weeks, allow the patient a soft diet as tolerated. Teach the patient to swallow only small amounts at a time. To prevent reflux and aspiration, instruct the patient to avoid lying down after eating and to keep the head of the bed elevated at night.

If the patient has had a pliable tube prosthesis inserted into the esophagus, swallowing can be very difficult, although the swallowing reflex is intact. Start oral intake with small sips of water until the patient learns how much can be swallowed at one time without difficulty. Add other fluids and soft foods to the diet as tolerated. Because pneumonia resulting from the reflux and aspiration of gastric secretion is the primary problem associated with the use of pliable tube prostheses, do not allow the patient to lie flat, and monitor for signs of aspiration.

Also monitor the patient for obstruction of the prosthesis, which can be caused by blockage with solid food, pills, or mucosal prolapse.

NDx: High risk for infection
Cleanse the mouth thoroughly and frequently with dilute hydrogen peroxide to decrease oral bacteria. Tape the nasogastric tube securely to the nose. Do not reposition or manipulate it because this could traumatize the anastomosis.

Use meticulous aseptic technique in caring for the patient's wounds.

Additional Interventions
Position the patient in semi-Fowler's position to discourage reflux of gastric secretions. Keep the nasogastric tube patent.

Evaluation

Evaluate the effectiveness of nursing care for a patient who has had surgery for esophageal cancer by comparing the patient's status with the expected patient outcomes. Examples of specific outcomes for patients who have had esophageal surgery for cancer have been provided in the Planning section.

Gastric Cancer

Gastric cancer is seen throughout the world but, like esophageal cancer, exhibits a wide variation in its occurrence. Its incidence is greatest among men in their late sixties who belong to a low socioeconomic group.

The incidence of gastric cancer has been steadily decreasing in the United States, although it still remains one of the leading causes of cancer deaths.

ETIOLOGY

The cause of gastric cancer is unknown, but many different factors have been postulated to influence its development. Among these are dietary factors such as smoked foods, reuse of cooking fats that contain many carcinogens, and foods preserved with nitrites and ingestion of few fresh fruits and vegetables. Other correlations include a history of chronic gastritis or pernicious anemia and infection with the bacteria *Helicobacter pylori.* Heredity is also thought to be a possible factor because gastric cancer occurs significantly more often in individuals with type A blood.

PATHOPHYSIOLOGY

The majority of gastric carcinomas occur in the pyloric region of the stomach in the area adjacent to the antrum. All are adenocarcinomas, and most present as a bulky mass projecting into the gastric lumen and are characterized by a deep central ulcer.

The remaining tumors appear either as an infiltrating lesion that causes narrowing of the lumen, a polypoid mass with or without a stalk, or a diffuse lesion that spreads superficially over the mucosa.

Gastric carcinoma spreads by direct invasion of adjacent tissues such as the lower esophagus, pancreas, transverse colon, and peritoneum and by way of the lymphatics to the pancreas and the liver. Late in the disease, hematogenous spread occurs to the bone, the brain, and the lung.

CLINICAL MANIFESTATIONS

Early gastric cancer is asymptomatic. When symptoms do occur, they consist of anorexia, weight loss, fullness, and vague epigastric discomfort. This discomfort most often occurs after eating and is unrelieved by antacids. As the disease progresses, bloating, dysphagia, boring epigastric pain, and vomiting due to obstruction occur. Since gastric tumors tend to bleed, anemia with its accompanying weakness and fatigue is also a frequent finding. In a few instances, the presence of a palpable abdominal mass and ascites is the first noticeable sign.

MEDICAL DIAGNOSIS

Typically, the diagnosis of gastric cancer is suggested by barium studies and confirmed by gastroscopy, biopsy, and cytologic studies.

MEDICAL MANAGEMENT

The only curative treatment for gastric cancer is surgery. The type of surgery done depends on the location, type, and extent of the tumor mass, and the effectiveness depends on how early the diagnosis is made. Gastrectomy, either partial or complete (see Chapter 21), is the usual procedure, with total gastrectomy the procedure of choice for a large cancer.

If surgery is contraindicated because of advanced disease, chemotherapy may be used to provide relief of symptoms. As indicated, gastric cancers are often not diagnosed until too late for any effective results from surgery.

Guidelines for Application of the Nursing Process to the Care of the Patient with Gastric Cancer

Nursing care of patients with gastric cancer varies with the stage of the disease and the type of treatment prescribed.

Individualize care for patients with gastric cancer regardless of stage or treatment based on careful assessment of the individual's needs. Assess the current physical and psychological status of all patients. Explore current symptoms and carefully assess nutritional status. Question the patient about changes in appetite and food intake; check for weight loss; and review laboratory studies for electrolyte imbalances, decreased serum albumin level, decreased total protein level, and decreased serum transferrin level or iron-binding capacity.

Review the patient's history. Note when the gastric cancer was diagnosed, what treatments were subsequently given, and the patient's subsequent course. Assess the patient's response to the current hospitalization. Determine the patient's expectations, the patient's and family's understanding of the disease and treatment prescribed, and the support systems available to them.

The Elderly: Special Considerations

Gastrointestinal disorders are the most common source of chronic distress among the elderly. Nonetheless, there are no gastrointestinal diseases that are unique to the aged, nor are diseases of the GI tract more prevalent in the aged than in the rest of the population. The incidence of certain diseases of the upper GI system does increase with age. However, many gastrointestinal symptoms in the aged result from changes in the cardiovascular or central nervous system, whose functions affect that of the GI system.

Disorders of the Mouth

Perhaps the most marked oral change in the aged is the loss of teeth. Despite improvements in dental care over the last decades, approximately one half of people in the United States age 65 or older wear dentures. This not only results in a decrease in chewing ability but increases the risk of both gingivitis and oral cancer.

Disorders of the Esophagus

In the esophagus, age changes give rise to a condition called presbyesophagus. This is a condition in which there is an abnormal increase in nonperistaltic contractions and overall weak muscular contraction in the esophagus, accompanied by inadequate relaxation of the lower esophageal sphincter. These motility changes are generally asymptomatic. Thus, complaints of difficulty swallowing or pain on swallowing cannot be attributed to benign age changes without thorough evaluation.

Esophageal diseases whose incidence increases with age include hiatus hernia, esophageal diverticula, and esophageal cancer. The dramatic increase in hiatus hernia is believed to be caused by weakening of the diaphragmatic musculature. The presence of diverticula appears to be associated with weakening of the muscular layer of the esophagus.

Sometimes symptoms of esophageal disorders in the elderly are similar to those seen in other age groups. At other times, typical symptoms are absent and the presence of disease is indicated by either repeated instances of aspiration pneumonia or signs of malnutrition secondary to progressive but unnoticed dysphagia. When pain is present, it must be carefully differentiated from cardiac pain. Findings consistent with esophageal pain include onset with lying down and relief following administration of antacids.

Gastric Disorders

With age, there is marked atrophy of the gastric mucosa accompanied by decreased secretion of hydrochloric acid (hypochlorhydria) or even absence of hydrochloric acid (achlorhydria). These changes are associated with the chronic gastritis and pernicious anemia common in the elderly.

Peptic ulcer disease also affects the elderly. In fact, onset of the disease occurs after age 60 in a significant number of patients. Contributing factors include decreased blood flow to the gastric mucosa because of atherosclerosis and increased use of drugs such as aspirin and steroids for arthritic conditions. Onset in the aged is often insidious. Symptoms can be atypical or even absent, with the first sign of disease being an episode of upper GI bleeding.

Bibliography

Baer CL, Williams BR. Clinical pharmacology and nursing. Springhouse, PA: Springhouse, 1988.
Bennett JR. Practical gastroenterology. New York: Macmillan, 1988.
Berk JE, Haubrich WS, Kalser MH, et al (eds). Bockus gastroenterology. 4th ed. Vols 2 and 7. Philadelphia: WB Saunders, 1985.
Bongiovanni GL. Essentials of clinical gastroenterology. 2nd ed. New York: McGraw-Hill, 1988.
Bouchier I, Allan R, Hodgson J, Keighley M. Textbook of gastroenterology. London: Bailliere Tindall, 1984.
Brandt LJ. Gastrointestinal disorders of the elderly. New York: Raven Press, 1984.
Bruckstein AH. Peptic ulcer disease: New concepts, new and current therapeutics. Consultant 1986; 26(4):157.
Brugere J, Guenel P, Leclerc A, Rodriguez J. Differential effects of tobacco and alcohol in cancer of the larynx, pharynx, and mouth. Cancer 1986; 57(2):391.
Burtis G, Davis J, Martin S. Applied nutrition and diet therapy. Philadelphia: WB Saunders, 1988.
Chwals WJ, Blackburn GL. Perioperative nutritional support in the cancer patient. Surg Clin North Am 1986; 66(6):1137.
Cormack D (ed). Geriatric nursing—A conceptual approach. Oxford: Blackwell Scientific Publications, 1985.
Crawshaw JP. Managing acid reflux: A stepped approach. Patient Care 1986; 20(7):72.
Drossman DA (ed). Manual of gastroenterologic procedures. 2nd ed. New York: Raven Press, 1987.
Eagon J, Miedema B, Kelly K. Postgastrectomy syndromes. Surg Clin North Am 1992; 72(2):445.
Eastwood GL. Core textbook of gastroenterology. Philadelphia: JB Lippincott, 1984.
Eisenberg P. Monitoring gastric pH to prevent stress ulcer syndrome. Focus Crit Care 1990; 17(4):316.
Esberger KK, Hughes ST Jr. Nursing care of the aged. Norwalk, CT: Appleton & Lange, 1989.
Feickert DM, Jillson E, Palazzo T. Gastrectomy for stomach cancer. AORN J 1988; 47(6):1396.
Gambert SR (ed). Handbook of geriatrics. New York: Plenum Press, 1987.
Given B, Simmons S. Gastroenterology in clinical nursing. 4th ed. St. Louis: CV Mosby, 1984.
Greenberger NJ. Gastrointestinal disorders. 4th ed. Chicago: Year Book, 1990.
Groth K. Age-related changes in the gastrointestinal tract. Geriatr Nurs 1988; 9(5):278.
Grundy A, Belli A. Balloon dilatation of upper gastrointestinal tract strictures. Clin Radiol 1988; 39:229.
Ham RJ, Sloane PD. Primary care geriatrics. 2nd ed. St. Louis: Mosby–Year Book, 1991.
Hamilton H. Gastrointestinal disorders. Springhouse, PA: Springhouse, 1985.
Heatley RV, et al (eds). Clinical nutrition in gastroenterology. New York: Churchill Livingstone, 1986.
Hill L, Kozarek R, McCallum R, Mercer CD. The esophagus: Medical and surgical management. Philadelphia: WB Saunders, 1988.
Hocking MP, Vogel SB (eds). Woodward's postgastrectomy syndromes. 2nd ed. Philadelphia: WB Saunders, 1991.
Holt KM, Isenberg JI. Peptic ulcer disease: Physiology and pathophysiology. Hosp Pract 1985; 20(1):89.
Iber FL, Baum RA. Gastroenterology: A concise textbook. (Concise Textbook Series, Vol 21). New York: Elsevier, 1987.
Jamieson GG, Duranceau A. Gastroesophageal reflux. Philadelphia: WB Saunders, 1988.
Jarvis C. Physical examination and health assessment. Philadelphia: WB Saunders, 1992.
Kahn R. Renewing the commitment to oral hygiene. Geriatr Nurs 1986; 7(5):244.
Kaushik SP, Ralphs DNL, Hobsley M. Influences on the occurrence of dumping syndrome. Am J Gastroenterol 1983; 78(3):155.
Klass A. Lasers in diseases of the digestive tract. In Fuller TA (ed). Surgical lasers: A clinical guide. New York: Macmillan, 1987, pp 170–193.
Laskin DM. Oral and maxillofacial surgery. St. Louis: CV Mosby, 1985.
Lawrence W. Gastric cancer. CA 1986; 36(4):216.
Levin LS, Johns ME. Lesions of the oral mucous membranes. Otolaryngol Clin North Am 1986; 19(1):87.
Longman AJ, Dewalt EM. A guide for oral assessment. Geriatr Nurs 1986; 7(5):252.
Luce EA. Carcinoma of the lower lip. Surg Clin North Am 1986; 66(1):3.
Lye M (ed). Acute geriatric medicine. Lancaster, England: MTP Press, 1985.
Malseed RT, Harregan GS. Textbook of pharmacology and nursing care. Philadelphia: JB Lippincott, 1989.
Mathewson M. Pharmacotherapeutics—A nursing process approach. Philadelphia: FA Davis, 1986.
Matteson MA, McConnell ES. Gerontological nursing: Concepts and practice. Philadelphia: WB Saunders, 1988.
McCallum RW. The management of esophageal motility disorders. Hospital Practice 1988; 23(2):239.
Meeker MH. Alexander's care of the patient in surgery. 9th ed. St. Louis: CV Mosby, 1991.
Meguid MM, Meguid V. Preoperative identification of the surgical cancer patient in need of postoperative supportive total parenteral nutrition. Cancer 1985; 55(suppl 1):258.

Mettlin C. Dietary factors for cancer of specific sites. Surg Clin North Am 1986; 66(5):917.
Ofstehage JC, Magilvy K. Oral health and aging. Geriatr Nurs 1986; 7(5):238.
Paunder R (ed). Recent advances in gastroenterology, No. 7. New York: Churchill Livingstone, 1988.
Ragan JA. Lasers in gastroenterology. Nurs Clin North Am 1990; 25(3):685.
Richter JE, Castell DO. Diffuse esophageal spasm: A reappraisal. Ann Intern Med 1984; 100(2):242.
Robinson MG. Management of reflux esophageal disease. Am J Med 1984; 77(5B):106.
Sabiston DC (ed). Textbook of surgery: The biological basis of modern surgical practice. 14th ed. Philadelphia: WB Saunders, 1991.
Schrier RW. Geriatric medicine. Philadelphia: WB Saunders, 1990.
Schroeder S, et al (eds). Current medical diagnosis and treatment. Norwalk, CT: Appleton & Lange, 1988.
Shoemaker WC, Ayres S, Grenvik A, et al. Textbook of critical care. 2nd ed. Philadelphia: WB Saunders, 1989.
Sleisenger MH, Fordtran JS. Gastrointestinal disease: Pathophysiology, diagnosis, management. 4th ed. Philadelphia: WB Saunders, 1989.
Smith CE. Detecting acute abdominal distension: What to look for, what to do. Nursing 1985; 15(9):39.
Smith LH, Thier SO. Pathophysiology: The biological principles of disease. 2nd ed. Philadelphia: WB Saunders, 1985.
Sodeman WA, Saladin TA, Boyd WP Jr. Geriatric gastroenterology. Philadelphia: WB Saunders, 1989.
Sontag SJ. Prostaglandins and acid peptic disease. Am J Gastroenterol 1986; 81(11):1021.
Steffl B. Handbook of gerontological nursing. New York: Van Nostrand Reinhold, 1984.
Sutherland J. Gastroesophageal reflux disease. Postgrad Med 1992; 89(7):45.
Sweny SR. Managing esophagogastric disorders. In EW Jackson (pub). Nursing photobook performing GI procedures. Horsham, PA: Intermed Communications, 1987, pp 33–37.
Swonger AK, Matejski MP. Nursing pharmacology. Boston: Scott, Foresman/Little, Brown, 1988.
Turnberg J. Clinical gastroenterology. Chicago: Mosby–Year Book, 1989.
Williams SR. Nutrition and diet therapy. St. Louis: Times Mirror/Mosby, 1985.
Zuidema GD (ed). Shackelford's surgery of the alimentary tract. 3rd ed. Philadelphia: WB Saunders, 1991.

Chapter Twenty-three

NURSING CARE *of Adults with* Disorders *of the* Lower Gastrointestinal System

The major work of the gastrointestinal (GI) system takes place in the small and large intestines. It is primarily here that the digestion and absorption of nutrients occur; the final excretion of waste products is the principal function of the colon.

Disorders of the lower GI system present a challenge to nurses for several reasons. Many of these diseases are obstructive in nature, and their signs and symptoms are vague and difficult to define. This often results in the delay of diagnosis of a problem until it is too late for effective treatment. Other disorders such as the inflammatory bowel diseases continue to elude efforts to determine their cause, making efforts for prevention and early detection difficult. Finally, some lower GI disorders are uncomplicated in themselves but become difficult to manage when presented in the elderly. For example, appendicitis, a relatively minor problem in a young adult, can be very dangerous in the geriatric patient.

Infections and Inflammations

Peritonitis

Peritonitis is an inflammation of the peritoneum, which is the thin membrane that lines the abdominal cavity and covers the abdominal organs.

ETIOLOGY

Bacterial infection is the most common cause of peritonitis. Specific causative organisms include *Escherichia coli,* alpha-hemolytic and beta-hemolytic streptococci, *Staphylococcus aureus,* enterococci, and gram-negative rods. These organisms enter the peritoneal cavity by escape from the intestinal tract through an opening in its wall or by extension of an infection through the wall of a hollow organ. Thus, conditions that can lead to bacterial peritonitis include appendicitis; perforated peptic ulcer; perforated diverticulum; necrosis of the intestine secondary to obstruction, infection, or malignancy; acute salpingitis; and continuous ambulatory peritoneal dialysis.

Peritonitis may occur also as a result of chemical irritation secondary to the introduction of GI secretions into the peritoneal cavity. This can occur with acute hemorrhagic pancreatitis. It also occurs as a result of leakage of an internal suture line at the liver, pancreas, or stomach.

PATHOPHYSIOLOGY

The classic inflammatory reaction characterized by vascular dilation, increased capillary permeability, and a serous or slightly turbid exudate occurs after bacterial or chemical invasion of the peritoneal cavity. Subsequently, the exudate becomes fibrinous and purulent and may be copious. In some cases, it remains localized as abscesses or pockets of pus, whereas in other cases it becomes generalized and involves the entire peritoneal cavity.

When generalized peritonitis occurs, sympathetic nervous stimulation causes peristaltic activity to decrease, and paralytic ileus results. The loss of large amounts of fluid from both the bowel lumen and the peritoneal cavity results in hypovolemia and hemoconcentration, which can lead to shock and oliguria or even to acute tubular necrosis.

Resolution of peritonitis can take various forms in different individuals. In some, the exudate disappears without residual effects. In others, walled-off abscesses remain that either eventually heal or serve as the source of a new infection. In still others, the exudate forms fibrous adhesive bands called adhesions that bind abdominal tissues together and interfere with normal function.

CLINICAL MANIFESTATIONS

The primary symptom of peritonitis is severe abdominal pain localized to the involved area and intensified by movement. The abdomen is rigid, and nausea, vomiting, a sudden spike in temperature, and leukocytosis occur. Oliguria, tachycardia, hypotension, sweating, and pallor develop in severe cases of generalized peritonitis as shock secondary to hypovolemia and sometimes septicemia ensue.

MEDICAL DIAGNOSIS

The diagnosis of peritonitis is usually made on the basis of the presenting symptoms coupled with a history of a predisposing event. Diagnosis can be difficult, however, in the elderly and in patients taking corticosteroids, because symptoms can be masked or suppressed. In such cases, tachycardia or unexplained hypotension may be the only early symptom, and definitive diagnosis may depend on x-ray demonstration of free air in the peritoneal cavity or paracentesis to confirm the presence of polymorphonuclear leukocytes and bacteria.

MEDICAL MANAGEMENT

Initially, large doses of broad-spectrum intravenous antibiotics are given to combat the infection. If necessary, the antibiotic regimen is adjusted later on the basis of the results of peritoneal fluid cultures.

Fluid, electrolyte, and colloid replacement is begun immediately. Nasogastric suction is instituted to help relieve abdominal distention, and an indwelling urinary catheter is inserted to allow for accurate monitoring of urinary output. If ventilation is impaired because of pressure on the diaphragm from fluid within the abdominal cavity, oxygen is given and, if needed, assisted ventilation with a tracheostomy is instituted.

Eliminating the cause of the problem is also an essential part of management. Thus, a ruptured appendix is excised, a suture line repaired, an abscess drained, a perforation repaired, or an intestine resected. In cases of intestinal pathology, a temporary ostomy is usually the initial procedure of choice. Generally, surgery is done as quickly as possible. In selected cases, such as when the patient is a poor operative risk, medical treatment aimed at supporting localization may be used, with surgical drainage performed at a later date.

Application of the Nursing Process to the Care of the Patient with Peritonitis

Assessment

If peritonitis is a potential problem, monitor the patient's pain. Report severe, well-localized abdominal pain, especially if it is experienced as a sudden change from the previous pain pattern. Palpate the abdomen for tenderness and rigidity, and check for diminished or absent bowel sounds every 2 to 4 hours. Check temperature and other vital signs every hour.

If peritonitis has been diagnosed, assess vital signs and bowel sounds at least every 2 to 4 hours.

Assess the patient's discomfort, and observe for abdominal distention. Assess for fluid and electrolyte imbalance. Review laboratory values. Check skin turgor. Measure intake and output carefully. Be certain to include nasogastric drainage. If a surgical drain is in place, note the color and consistency of the drainage and include the amount on the intake and output record. If a central venous pressure (CVP) catheter is in place to guide fluid replacement, check pressure, keeping in mind that normal CVP is 4 cm to 10 cm of water and that a low CVP is indicative of hypovolemia, whereas a pressure of 15 cm or higher may indicate circulatory overload. Check urine specific gravity, skin turgor, and condition of mucous membranes.

Assess effectiveness of ventilation, and observe for proper function of oxygen, nasogastric tube, or other equipment in use.

Nursing Diagnoses and Planning

Nursing diagnoses and related expected patient outcomes most commonly applicable to patients with peritonitis include the following:

NDx: Pain related to inflammation of the peritoneum

Planning: Patient outcomes
1. Patient states abdominal pain is relieved.
2. Signs of severe pain, such as knees pulled up, are absent.
3. Patient rests quietly.

NDx: High risk for altered oral mucous membrane related to mouth breathing and nothing-by-mouth (NPO) status.

Planning: Patient outcomes
1. Oral mucous membranes are pink and moist.
2. Lips are smooth and free of cracks.

NDx: Fear related to treatment and prognosis

Planning: Patient outcomes
1. Patient acknowledges and discusses fears.
2. Patient verbalizes accurate knowledge of the situation.
3. Patient rests quietly.

Nursing Interventions

NDx: Pain
Position the patient in a semi-Fowler's position to minimize discomfort and to promote localization of the infection in the abdominal area. Give analgesics as ordered. Because of the risk of masking symptoms, these may be given sparingly, so use of nonpharmacologic methods of pain control is critical. Keep the environment quiet and calm. Keep the bedding clean and free from wrinkles. Provide comfort measures frequently such as a back rub, change in position, or a fluffed pillow.

NDx: High risk for altered oral mucous membrane
Assist the patient in brushing teeth and cleaning and rinsing the mouth frequently. Avoid use of lemon and glycerine swabs and commercial mouthwashes that contain alcohol because these further dry the mucous membrane. Apply a water-soluble lubricant to the lips to prevent drying and cracking.

NDx: Fear
Acknowledge the patient's fear, and give permission for feelings to be expressed. Allow sufficient time for the patient to express feelings. Clarify the patient's understanding of the situation so that groundless fears are eliminated. Provide opportunities for questions, and give honest answers. Allow the patient to make decisions on care when possible, and explain procedures at a level the patient can

understand and within the boundaries of what he or she desires to know.

Additional Interventions
Maintain bed rest, and administer intravenous antibiotics as ordered. Monitor the patient for side effects and for the expected therapeutic responses. Indications that the antibiotics are effectively eliminating the infection include softening of the abdomen, return of bowel sounds, passage of flatus, defecation, and return to normal body temperature.

Replace fluids, electrolytes, and plasma expanders as ordered. Administer oxygen as ordered. If a nasogastric tube is in place, keep it taped securely to the nose and maintain its function. Apply water-soluble lubricant to the nares as needed to prevent irritation and discomfort.

When peristalsis returns, start the patient on clear fluids as ordered. Progress as tolerated in accordance with the prescribed diet.

Evaluation

Evaluate the effectiveness of nursing care for a patient with peritonitis by comparing the patient's status with the expected patient outcomes. Examples of specific outcomes for patients with peritonitis have been provided in the Planning section.

Appendicitis

Appendicitis is an acute inflammation of the vermiform appendix. It is a common disorder, with a peak incidence among 20- to 30-year-olds.

ETIOLOGY

Obstruction of the appendix appears to be the precipitating factor in appendicitis. Possible causes of obstruction include calculi (fecaliths) in the appendix, parasites, lymphoid hyperplasia secondary to viral infection, twisting of the appendix by adhesions, and malfunction of a valve system at the appendiceal opening.

PATHOPHYSIOLOGY

Obstruction results in increased intraluminal pressure, which in turn may collapse the blood vessels in the wall of the appendix and predispose to invasion by local bacteria such as *E. coli*, enterococci, and beta-hemolytic streptococci.

In early acute appendicitis, there is scant neutrophilic exudation throughout the wall, the subserosal vessels are congested, and the serosa becomes a dull, granular red. Subsequently, the neutrophilic exudation increases, a suppurative exudate covers the serosa, abscesses form within the wall, and ulcerations and areas of necrosis appear in the mucosa. If unchecked, large areas of hemorrhagic ulceration develop in the mucosa, areas of gangrenous necrosis develop in the wall, and rupture occurs.

Complications of appendicitis are perforation with generalized peritonitis; paralytic ileus; subphrenic, pelvic, or lumbar abscess; pylephlebitis and thrombosis of the portal veins; and septicemia. Table 23–1 provides information concerning how to recognize and manage some of these complications.

CLINICAL MANIFESTATIONS

The principal symptom of appendicitis is persistent pain. In the classic presentation, pain begins as a vague, mild discomfort over the epigastric or periumbilical areas. Over a period of approximately 4 hours, it increases in intensity, becomes colicky, and localizes in the right lower quadrant (Fig. 23–1). This pattern, however, does not occur in all patients. Variations include diffuse pain, pain in the lower abdomen, pain referred to the right thigh or testicle if the appendix is behind the cecum, or even pain in the left lower quadrant.

Table 23–1. RECOGNITION AND MANAGEMENT OF COMPLICATIONS OF APPENDICITIS

COMPLICATION	SYMPTOMS	MANAGEMENT
Perforation with generalized peritonitis	Severe pain Fever of 37.7°C (100°F) or higher Abdominal rigidity Vomiting Tachycardia	IV electrolyte and amino acid solutions Nasogastric suction Antibiotics Surgical drainage when localized
Abscess Subphrenic Lumbar Pelvic	Chills, fever, diaphoresis Tachycardia Anorexia Diarrhea with a pelvic abscess Increased leukocytosis	Parenteral antibiotics to help localize infection Surgical drainage Appendectomy in 6 weeks
Paralytic ileus	Absent bowel sounds	Nasogastric suction Intravenous fluids and electrolytes

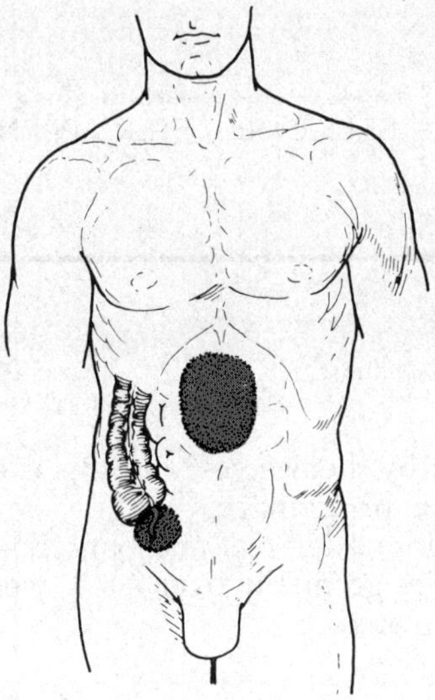

Figure 23–1.

In classic appendicitis, pain begins in the epigastric or periumbilical region and becomes localized over McBurney's point (midpoint on a line between the umbilicus and the right anterosuperior iliac spine) in a period of approximately 4 hours. (From O'Toole M. Miller-Keane encyclopedia and dictionary of medicine, nursing, and allied health. 5th ed. Philadelphia: WB Saunders, 1992, p. 111.)

With rupture of the appendix, pain may be suddenly relieved, only to be followed by pain resulting from localized or generalized peritonitis.

In addition to pain, anorexia and nausea with or without vomiting are the most frequent symptoms of appendicitis. Occasionally, constipation occurs, but diarrhea is rare. Temperature is usually between 38°C and 38.6°C (100.4° and 101.4°F) unless the appendix has ruptured, in which case it is higher. Dysuria is not common.

Physical examination findings vary with the age of the patient and the stage of the inflammation. The most significant finding is tenderness when pressure is applied over McBurney's point, which is located midway between the umbilicus and the right anterior iliac spine. Other frequent findings are rigidity of the right rectus muscle, rebound tenderness (pain when deep pressure on the abdomen is released), exacerbation of pain associated with coughing, right lower quadrant pain triggered by palpation of the left lower quadrant, and leukocytosis (10,000/cu mm or more) with an elevated neutrophil count.

MEDICAL DIAGNOSIS

The diagnosis of acute appendicitis is not easy given the variability of presenting symptoms and the large number of other conditions that can cause an acute abdomen. The diagnosis is especially difficult in the very young and in the elderly. It requires expert clinical judgment based on the patient's history, physical findings, and laboratory and x-ray studies.

MEDICAL MANAGEMENT

The patient who presents with a question of appendicitis is kept on NPO status. No analgesics are given until the decision to operate is made because they may mask symptoms needed for differential diagnosis. No cathartics or enemas are given because the resultant stimulation of peristalsis irritates the already inflamed area and can precipitate perforation. Intravenous antibiotics are begun, and an appendectomy is performed as soon as possible because the longer the duration of symptoms, the greater the likelihood of perforation.

APPENDECTOMY

An appendectomy is the surgical removal of the vermiform appendix. The appendix is removed through a lower right quadrant incision and may be done under either general or local anesthesia.

PHYSICAL PREPARATION OF THE PATIENT

An intravenous infusion is started, and prophylactic antibiotics are given. In some cases, aspirin is also given to reduce fever. A nasogastric tube is inserted if paralytic ileus is suspected; the patient is asked to void; the abdomen is shaved and scrubbed; and preoperative medications are administered.

POSTOPERATIVE COURSE

In an uncomplicated appendectomy, oral fluids may be given as soon as the patient is awake, and the patient is progressed to a regular diet as soon as tolerated. If the temperature is normal and discomfort is not excessive, the patient may return home on the day of operation, although a hospital stay of 3 to 4 days is usual. Sutures are removed at a follow-up visit between the fifth and seventh postoperative days. Physically stressful activities need to be avoided for several weeks until the wound is completely healed.

Application of the Nursing Process to the Care of the Patient Having an Appendectomy

PREOPERATIVE NURSING CARE

Because an appendectomy is usually an emergency procedure, the time for preoperative nursing care is limited. Nonetheless, make certain to assess the pa-

Chart 23–1.

NURSING GUIDE TO PATIENT EDUCATION FOR SELF-MANAGEMENT: SELF-CARE AFTER APPENDECTOMY

Instruct the patient to:

Gently wash the incision with soap and water daily, and pat dry.
Be aware that if Steri-Strips are in place, they will eventually fall off by themselves, and this is expected.
Inspect the incision daily, and report any incisional redness, swelling, or drainage.
Avoid clothing that places pressure on the incision line, such as bikini underwear and pantyhose.
Avoid heavy lifting and strenuous exercises. Resume normal activities gradually over 2 to 3 weeks.
Eat small, frequent, high-calorie meals and gradually increase as tolerated.
Report any chills, fever, or increased pain.
Return for follow-up visit on *(specify date and place).*

tient for coexisting physical problems that have implications for nursing care. For example, observe for signs of respiratory infection, and question the patient or significant other about any chronic disease and routine use of medication.

Make the patient as comfortable as possible through positioning. Keep in mind that bending the right knee on the abdomen often provides relief. Administer analgesics when prescribed. When pain medication is not allowed, be certain to explain to both the patient and significant others that the medication may mask symptoms and thus interfere with correct diagnosis.

Tell the patient what is being done, but do so briefly because the discomfort is generally so severe that the patient cannot attend to and is not desirous of a long explanation.

Anxiety regarding surgery is generally not a major problem for the patient because it is seen as "the way out of the pain."

POSTOPERATIVE NURSING CARE

Assessment

Make usual postoperative assessments: Take vital signs, measure intake and output, and check the dressing for intactness and for drainage. Also assess for pain and for good respiratory excursion and airway clearance. Check bowel sounds, and assess tolerance of oral intake when resumed.

Nursing Diagnoses and Planning

Because of the lack of time for preoperative teaching, the nursing diagnosis and related expected patient outcomes most commonly applicable to patients who have had an appendectomy are as follows:

NDx: High risk for altered health maintenance related to lack of knowledge of operative procedure, postoperative activities, and discharge instructions.

Planning: Patient outcomes

1. Patient coughs, deep breathes, splints the incision, and ambulates as directed.
2. Patient states that questions regarding the surgery have been answered satisfactorily.
3. Patient describes self-care at home, as outlined in Chart 23–1.

Nursing Interventions

NDx: High risk for altered health maintenance

Explain the importance of coughing and deep breathing after general anesthesia, and guide the patient in performing these activities correctly. Show the patient how to splint the incision with the hands or with a pillow to make coughing and moving easier. Explain how oral intake and ambulation will be resumed.

Ask the patient whether these are any questions about the surgery. Provide the requested information, or tell the patient how to acquire it.

Instruct the patient in self-care after discharge as outlined in Chart 23–1.

Additional Interventions

Place the patient in a Fowler's position after recovery from anesthesia. Have the patient cough and deep breathe every 2 hours. Give oral fluids when desired, and progress the patient to a regular diet as tolerated. Medicate for pain every 3 or 4 hours as prescribed. Get the patient out of bed and begin to ambulate when he or she is alert and in stable condition.

Evaluation

Evaluate the effectiveness of nursing care for a patient who has had an appendectomy by comparing the patient's status with the expected patient outcomes. Examples of specific outcomes for patients who have had an appendectomy have been provided in the Planning section.

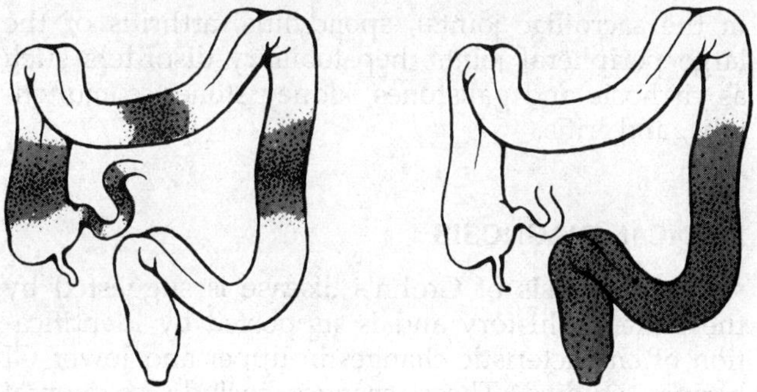

Figure 23–2.

Crohn's disease (*left*) and ulcerative colitis (*right*). Whereas Crohn's disease typically involves the small and large intestine in a segmental manner with intervening "skip" areas, ulcerative colitis is generally a disease of contiguity that starts in the rectum and progresses in a retrograde fashion to involve varying lengths of the colon. (From Cotran RS, Kumar V, Robbins SL. Robbins pathologic basis of disease. 4th ed. Philadelphia: WB Saunders, 1989, p. 887.)

Crohn's Disease

Crohn's disease is a form of inflammatory bowel disease (IBD) that is chronic and is characterized by exacerbations and remissions. Its incidence is highest in adults between 20 and 40 years of age, and it occurs in males and females alike. It is prevalent in the Jewish population and is infrequently seen in blacks.

ETIOLOGY

The cause of Crohn's disease is unknown, although immunologic dysfunction, allergy to foods such as cow's milk or other specific protein, and heredity are all postulated to contribute to its development. Infection is also suggested as a possible etiologic factor or a secondary effect because intestinal bacteria counts are increased in Crohn's disease, fever is a common symptom, and antibiotics as well as parenteral nutrition in place of oral nutrition, both of which decrease intestinal bacteria, can be effective treatment. Psychogenic factors, which for many years were thought to cause the disease, are now seen as merely contributing to exacerbations.

PATHOPHYSIOLOGY

Crohn's disease most often involves the terminal ileum and the adjacent right colon, although any part of the GI tract can be affected.

Inflamed areas occur randomly in the affected areas, producing a patchy distribution of lesions (Fig. 23–2). The affected areas of the bowel are swollen and hyperemic with ulcerations and longitudinal fissures. Adhesions develop between loops of bowel, and the serosal surface has deposits of mesenteric fat. The mesentery itself is thickened with engorged lymphatic vessels and enlarged lymph nodes.

As the disease progresses, deep ulcers and fissures extend into the muscle layers of the wall. These lesions, which surround small islands of mucosa, give rise to the characteristic "cobblestone" appearance of advanced disease. Often fistulas develop from these lesions into adjacent segments of the intestine, into other abdominal organs such as the gallbladder, urinary bladder, and uterus, or through the abdominal wall. Ultimately, the intestinal wall becomes permanently fibrosed, thickened, and narrowed. Absorption is impaired, and small-bowel obstruction may result.

CLINICAL MANIFESTATIONS

Crohn's disease affecting the region of the terminal ileum is characterized by episodes of abdominal pain most often occurring after eating and accompanied by fever and mild (not more than four or five stools per day), usually nonbloody diarrhea. Over time, these episodes increase in frequency, duration, and severity; the pain eventually localizes in the right lower quadrant. Weight loss and a history of recurrent oral aphthous ulcers are common, accompanied in some cases by persistent right lower quadrant tenderness or a palpable mass. Weight loss is more profound and pain more diffuse when the jejunum is affected, whereas diarrhea and crampy abdominal pain predominate when primarily the colon is involved.

Weakness, fatigue, anorexia, anemia, and other symptoms of malabsorption and protein-losing enteropathy occur with advanced disease, and perirectal and perianal fistulas are common.

Complications of Crohn's disease that can occur outside of the GI system include erythema nodosum, which manifests as raised, dull red, painful lesions on the legs, sacroiliitis (painful inflammation in the sacroiliac joints), spondylitis, arthritis of the large peripheral joints, hepatobiliary disorders such as cirrhosis and gallstones, kidney stones, conjunctivitis, and iritis.

MEDICAL DIAGNOSIS

The diagnosis of Crohn's disease is suggested by the patient's history and is supported by identification of characteristic changes in upper and lower GI barium studies. These changes include segmental narrowing of the bowel, absence of the normal mucosal pattern, presence of intestinal fistulas, and the "string sign" (i.e., narrowed terminal ileum seen when the disease is localized to the terminal ileum and adjacent colon). Proctosigmoidoscopy and colonoscopy may be done to determine the extent of involvement; in a few cases, intestinal biopsy may be necessary to confirm the diagnosis.

MEDICAL MANAGEMENT

Treatment is palliative because there is no known cure for Crohn's disease. It is aimed at restoring and maintaining normal nutritional status, suppressing inflammation, preventing complications, and minimizing the discomforts of pain and diarrhea.

Management of nutrition depends on the severity of the patient's condition. During periods of relatively mild disease, a low-fiber, low-fat diet is prescribed to help control cramping and diarrhea. If lactase deficiency exists, high-lactose foods are eliminated.

During acute stages of the disease, enteral feedings with a low-residue defined formula or total parenteral nutrition (TPN) is usually required.

Pharmacologic therapy also varies somewhat with the severity of the disease. Corticosteroids in the form of corticotropin (ACTH), prednisone, or hydrocortisone are used to suppress inflammation in acutely ill patients. These drugs are then tapered off and discontinued when the acute symptoms subside. Parenteral anti-infectives such as metronidazole are also given in acute cases, despite the fact that no causative infective organism has been identified, because their use is sometimes associated with clinical improvement. Similarly, oral antimicrobials may be prescribed in milder cases. Sulfasalazine (Asulfidine), an anti-infective with anti-inflammatory properties, is also often used.

Other drugs that may be used in the treatment of Crohn's disease are immunosuppressant and antidiarrheal agents.

Surgery is not ordinarily a part of the treatment plan for patients with Crohn's disease because the disease almost always recurs in the remaining bowel. It is done only when absolutely essential, such as when obstruction, perforation, or a fistula has developed. It is also done in selected cases of intractable disease in which the patient is so incapacitated by intestinal or systemic symptoms that an acceptable quality of life is not possible. When surgery is essential, the procedure most often done for Crohn's disease is total proctocolectomy (excision of the rectum and the colon) with ileostomy, although a total colectomy with an ileosigmoid, ileorectal, or ileoanal anastomosis may also be done.

Application of the Nursing Process to the Care of the Patient with Crohn's Disease

Assessment

Obtain a history and description of the patient's symptoms. Ask about abdominal pain, and note the type, location, severity, duration, and relationship to eating, stress, or other identifiable factors. Question the patient about diarrhea, determining the number of stools per day, their color, consistency, and odor. Ask specifically about whether any blood has been seen in the stool.

Assess the patient's nutritional status. Check for weight loss, question the patient about anorexia, and explore the patient's usual diet both before and after the onset of symptoms. Assess for signs of fluid and electrolyte imbalance, and gently palpate the abdomen for tenderness or a mass. Take the temperature, and inspect the perineal area for irritation, skin breakdown, and fistula formation.

Assess also for signs of extraintestinal complications of Crohn's disease. Inspect the legs for the dull, red, raised nodules of erythema nodosum. Question the patient about stiffening of the spine and joint pain, and observe for movement limitations.

Inspect the conjunctiva for signs of inflammation, and look for redness in the iris. Question the patient about pain on pupil dilation (pain that is worse in the dark) characteristic of iritis.

Question about a family history of Crohn's disease and about any known allergies, particularly to milk.

Explore sources of stress in the patient's life and the relationship of episodes of stress to exacerbations of the disease. Identify the individual's mode of handling stress as well as sources of support.

Nursing Diagnoses and Planning

Nursing diagnoses and related expected patient outcomes most commonly applicable to patients with Crohn's disease include the following:

NDx: Pain related to inflammation of the intestinal wall

Nutrition Box 23–1.

NUTRITION: SPECIAL CONSIDERATIONS FOR PATIENTS WITH CROHN'S DISEASE

Instruct patients with Crohn's disease to:

Eat foods that are high in protein (eggs, meat, cheese) and calories to promote healing.
Limit fat intake, especially if steatorrhea (fatty stools) is present by avoiding all fried foods and most dairy products except for skim milk.
Eat a low- or minimum-residue diet to reduce fecal output. Avoid raw fruits and vegetables, dried fruit and beans, whole-grain breads and cereals, bran, seeds, and nuts.
Avoid foods that stimulate intestinal peristalsis such as prune juice, coffee, and carbonated beverages.
Take note of which foods cause discomfort or diarrhea because individual food intolerances are common. Eliminate these foods from the diet.
Ensure adequate intake of vitamins and minerals, especially vitamin C (found in citrus fruits and juices), folic acid (found in green, leafy vegetables), and zinc (found in red meat). If foods high in these substances are not tolerated in the diet, take supplements as directed.
Promote a restful environment while eating.
Eat slowly, and chew foods well.

Planning: Patient outcomes
1. Patient reports pain has decreased.
2. Patient ingests prescribed diet without subsequent nonverbal signs of abdominal pain.

NDx: Diarrhea related to impaired absorption of sodium and water secondary to mucosal inflammation

Planning: Patient outcomes
1. Patient passes no more than three stools per day.
2. Stools are formed.

NDx: High risk for impaired skin integrity related to perianal irritation secondary to diarrhea

Planning: Patient outcomes
1. Patient denies perirectal soreness.
2. Perirectal skin is free of redness.
3. Perirectal skin is intact.

NDx: High risk for altered nutrition: less than body requirements, related to limited intake of nutrients as a result of anorexia and fear of exacerbating symptoms and malabsorption

Planning: Patient outcomes
1. Patient describes nutritional guidelines as presented in Nutrition Box 23–1.
2. Patient is in positive nitrogen balance.
3. Patient maintains or regains normal weight.

NDx: Ineffective individual coping related to the unpredictable nature of the disease and the inability to manage the stress of changes, common situational crises, and general life demands

Planning: Patient outcomes
1. Patient identifies own ineffective coping behaviors.
2. Patient identifies own strengths.
3. Patient identifies effective methods of coping.
4. Patient identifies available resources to support coping ability.

Nursing Interventions

NDx: Pain
Encourage the patient to report abdominal pain and accept medication. Administer analgesics and antispasmodics as prescribed, and monitor their effectiveness. Position the patient with the knees flexed, and apply heat to the abdomen if allowed. Encourage deep breathing and the use of other relaxation exercises.

NDx: Diarrhea
Maintain the patient on bed rest during severe exacerbations to decrease peristalsis. Keep a bedpan and toilet tissue readily available for the patient because episodes of diarrhea are sudden. Place a deodorizer in the room, and empty the bedpan immediately to control disagreeable and embarrassing odor. Administer prescribed antidiarrheal agents, and document the frequency, color, and consistency of stools. Keep the patient on NPO status, or give small, frequent meals low in residue.

NDx: High risk for impaired skin integrity
Monitor for perianal skin irritation and fissures. Wash area well after each bowel movement. Use tap

water for irritated areas and mild, soapy water for surrounding areas. Rinse and pat dry thoroughly. Apply an emollient or topical anesthetic for comfort.

NDx: High risk for altered nutrition: less than body requirements
Administer intravenous fluid and electrolytes, TPN, or nutritional supplements as prescribed. Administer prescribed anticholinergics one-half hour before meals to decrease bowel motility.

Encourage the patient to avoid smoking, which increases peristalsis, and record intake, output, and weight daily. Instruct the patient in nutritional guidelines as presented in Nutrition Box 23–1.

NDx: Ineffective individual coping
Encourage the patient to discuss fears and feelings related to the disease. Remember that the attacks are unpredictable and can be exhausting and incapacitating, forcing the patient to be out of work and unable to make plans. Acknowledge understanding of these difficulties, and provide a private, nonrushed environment for discussion of them.

Assist the patient to identify measures to be used at home to limit the disruptive effect of the disease. For example, suggest the purchase of a bedpan or a commode if getting to the bathroom is a problem during acute attacks. If time spent in the bathroom is distressing, help the patient identify activities such as sewing or reading that can be done during this time.

Explore with the patient his or her usual method of coping with stress caused by change, situational crises, or general life demands. Assist the patient in identifying those coping mechanisms that were effective and those that were ineffective. Encourage the patient to identify new effective strategies to reduce stress, and aid in the identification and selection of available resources such as support groups. Support the patient in evaluating lifestyle and in identifying sources of stress. Identify what can be changed and what cannot. Discuss the importance of obtaining adequate rest and avoiding fatigue in relation to coping ability. Refer to a support group or, if indicated, to professional therapy.

Evaluation

Evaluate the effectiveness of nursing care for the patient with Crohn's disease by comparing the patient's status with the expected patient outcomes. Examples of specific outcomes for patients with Crohn's disease have been provided in the Planning section.

Ulcerative Colitis

Ulcerative colitis is a form of inflammatory bowel disease (IBD), characterized by exacerbations and remissions, that involves the mucosa and submucosa of the colon. It is primarily a disease that occurs in young adults, although a significant number of cases develop between the ages of 55 and 60 years. The disease is much more common among whites than blacks. It is also more prevalent among females and those of Jewish descent.

ETIOLOGY

The cause of ulcerative colitis is unknown. However, the same factors that are implicated in the development of Crohn's disease are thought to play a role in the development of ulcerative colitis. These include immunologic dysfunction, allergy to specific proteins, viral or bacterial infection, and heredity.

PATHOPHYSIOLOGY

Ulcerative colitis most often begins in the rectum and spreads proximally (see Fig. 23–2). In the majority of cases, spread is limited to the sigmoid and descending colon, although involvement of the transverse and ascending colon can occur. The disease is characterized by diffuse continuous inflammation of the bowel mucosa, which becomes engorged, red, and friable. Multiple small hemorrhages appear as do scattered yellowish spots, which are microabscesses in the mucous membrane. These abscesses subsequently develop into larger, multiple, irregular, open ulcerations that give the mucous membrane a moth-eaten appearance (Fig. 23–3). As the disease progresses, these ulcers join to form large, denuded areas where the lining of the colon has been destroyed.

As a result of these changes in the mucosa, the absorption of sodium and water is impaired, leading to watery diarrhea. Potassium resorption is also impaired and can lead to significant loss because intestinal juices are high in potassium. In addition, protein is lost through the damaged areas, and hypoalbuminemia results. Iron deficiency anemia eventually develops because of blood loss from the hemorrhagic mucosa.

With repeated attacks of inflammation, the bowel becomes fibrosed, the muscularis mucosae becomes hyperplastic, and the haustrations disappear. This results in a narrowed, shortened bowel with a smooth, tubular appearance. In severe cases, the inflammation also leads to perforation or to dilation and thinning of the bowel wall. Cancer of the colon has been found to occur in direct proportion to the duration of ulcerative colitis and extent of colonic involvement (Greenberger, 1990, p. 223).

CLINICAL MANIFESTATIONS

Symptoms of ulcerative colitis may develop gradually or have a sudden, acute onset, which sometimes follows a stressful event, minor infection, or even antibiotic therapy. The most frequent symptoms are rectal bleeding, diarrhea, abdominal pain,

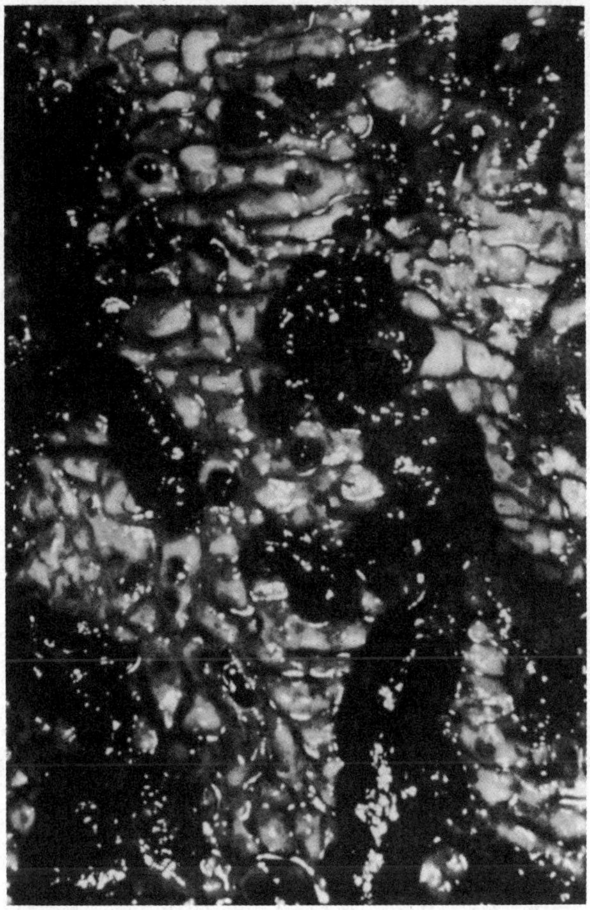

Figure 23–3.

The dark, irregular pattern constitutes ulcerations that have in many instances coalesced, leaving virtual islands of residual, paler mucosa. (From Cotran RS, Kumar V, Robbins SL. Robbins pathologic basis of disease. 4th ed. Philadelphia: WB Saunders, 1989, p 887.)

weight loss, and fever. Other symptoms are those associated with anemia from the chronic blood loss in the stools; dehydration and electrolyte imbalances from the loss of fluid and electrolytes in the diarrhea; and nutritional problems related to the chronic malabsorption of specific nutrients.

Depending on the symptoms, the disease is classified as mild, moderate, or severe (fulminant). In mild ulcerative colitis, the symptoms occur gradually and consist of more frequent bowel movements, rectal bleeding, lower abdominal discomfort, and malaise. With moderate disease, onset is more abrupt with four or five loose, bloody stools per day and abdominal cramps severe enough to awaken the patient from sleep. Low-grade fever, fatigue, and extraintestinal manifestations such as the dull, red, painful lesions of erythema nodosum on the legs, back pain and stiffening, arthritis in the large peripheral joints, inflammations of the eye, and kidney stones may also occur. Severe ulcerative colitis is characterized by profuse diarrhea, rectal bleeding, rectal urgency, high fever, anorexia, and weight loss. Pallor, tachycardia, hypertension, and even shock are not uncommon.

MEDICAL DIAGNOSIS

The diagnosis of ulcerative colitis is made on the basis of the patient's history of symptoms, the visualization of inflammation on proctoscopy or sigmoidoscopy, negative stool cultures, and absence of parasites on stool examination.

Colonoscopy is contraindicated in moderate to severe cases because of the risk of perforation and hemorrhage. Barium enema is also contraindicated because of the bowel preparation involved and its effects on the inflamed mucosa.

MEDICAL MANAGEMENT

Medical management of ulcerative colitis is similar to that of Crohn's disease. Mild to moderate cases are controlled by a low-roughage diet without milk or milk products, anticholinergics to decrease peristalsis and GI secretion, antidiarrheal drugs to reduce the frequency of bowel movements, and anti-infective drugs such as sulfasalazine. In addition, corticosteroids and immunosuppressive drugs may be prescribed.

Anti-infectives and corticosteroids are also used to treat severe disease in conjunction with intravenous fluids and electrolytes, blood transfusions, and a nasogastric tube attached to low-suction.

Surgery is indicated for unremitting disease and for complications such as perforation or hemorrhage. The most common surgical treatment of ulcerative colitis is a total colectomy with ileostomy (Fig. 23–4) (or proctocolectomy with ileostomy if the rectum is severely involved), which is considered to be curative. Two alternatives to this procedure are the continent ileostomy or Kock pouch and an ileoanal anastomosis with or without an ileal reservoir (see Chapter 21).

See Table 23–2 for a summary comparison of Crohn's disease and ulcerative colitis.

Application of the Nursing Process to the Care of the Patient with Ulcerative Colitis

The assessment, nursing diagnoses, expected patient outcomes, nursing interventions, and evaluation for patients with ulcerative colitis are similar to those described previously for patients with Crohn's disease. When a total colectomy with ileostomy is done, provide care as presented in Nursing Care Guide 23–1.

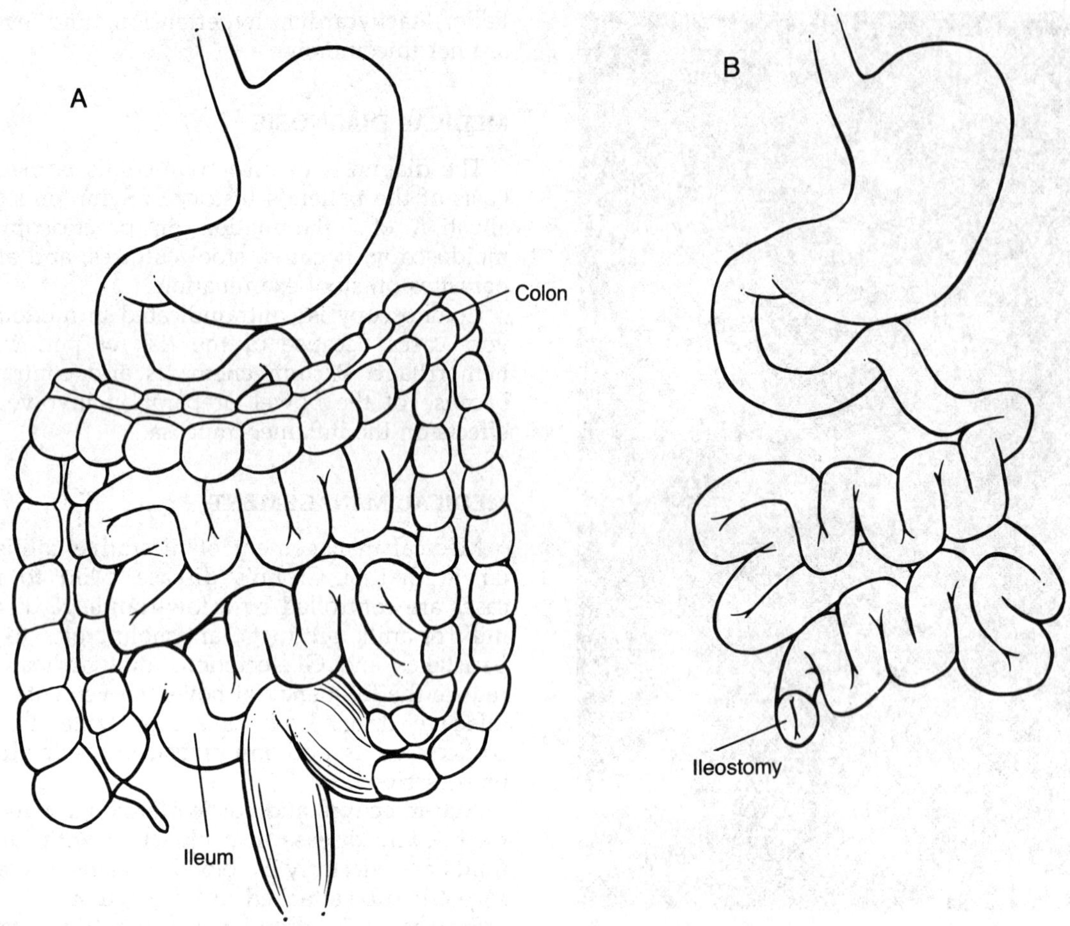

Figure 23–4.

A, Lower gastrointestinal tract prior to total colectomy. *B*, Lower gastrointestinal tract after total colectomy with ileostomy.

Table 23–2. SIMILARITIES AND DIFFERENCES BETWEEN CROHN'S DISEASE AND ULCERATIVE COLITIS

Etiology	Cause is unknown. Similar factors are postulated to contribute to both: heredity, immunologic dysfunction, allergy.
Pathophysiology	Crohn's disease can affect any area of the gastrointestinal tract and is characterized by segmental involvement, linear ulcers, cobblestone appearance, and fistulas. Ulcerative colitis affects primarily the lower colon and is characterized by continuous symmetric inflammation; engorged, friable mucosa, with a moth-eaten appearance because of multiple, large, irregular, open ulcers.
Clinical manifestations	Mild diarrhea accompanied by right lower quadrant abdominal pain but without rectal bleeding and a palpable abdominal mass are characteristic symptoms of Crohn's disease. Diarrhea, often severe, with rectal bleeding is characteristic of ulcerative colitis. Extraintestinal complications that may occur are the same in both diseases. They include erythema nodosum, spondylitis, arthritis in the large joints, cirrhosis, cholelithiasis, kidney stones, conjunctivitis, and iritis.
Medical diagnosis	The diagnosis of both diseases is suggested by the patient's history. The diagnosis of Crohn's disease depends on characteristic findings on upper and lower intestinal contrast studies. The diagnosis of ulcerative colitis depends on visualization of diffuse inflammation during proctosigmoidoscopy in the presence of negative stool cultures and examination for parasites. Occasionally, a biopsy is necessary to confirm either diagnosis.
Medical management	Palliative management of Crohn's disease and ulcerative colitis is similar: low-fiber, low-fat diet also low in lactose if lactase deficiency exists, enteral feedings with a low-residue defined formula or total parenteral nutrition if needed; corticosteroids to suppress inflammation; anti-infectives, sulfasalazine, immunosuppressive or antidiarrheal therapy. In Crohn's disease, surgery is not a treatment of choice because of almost certain disease recurrence in the remaining bowel. In ulcerative colitis, a colectomy is considered curative.

Anorectal Abscess

An anorectal abscess is a localized infection with a collection of pus in the anorectal area.

ETIOLOGY AND PATHOPHYSIOLOGY

Rectal abscesses begin as inflammations of the rectal crypts. Later cysts form that extend into the submucosal layer. Abscess formation occurs secondary to infection with normal rectal flora such as *E. coli, Proteus,* staphylococci, or streptococci.

An anorectal fistula (Table 23–3) may develop as a complication of an anorectal abscess (Fig. 23–5).

Persons with Crohn's disease and immunodeficiency disorders are at risk for anorectal abscess.

CLINICAL MANIFESTATIONS

A classic symptom of anorectal abscess is constant, throbbing pain that is aggravated by sitting and by defecation. Other symptoms are tenderness and swelling in the area of the abscess; foul-smelling, purulent drainage; and fever.

MEDICAL DIAGNOSIS

A diagnosis of anorectal abscess is suggested by the presence of the characteristic rectal pain. It is confirmed by digital palpation of the abscess externally or internally or, in some cases, by visualization during proctoscopy.

MEDICAL MANAGEMENT

Treatment of an anorectal abscess is incision and drainage followed by antibiotic therapy. Often the wound is packed with Vaseline gauze and is allowed to heal by granulation. In some cases, this is done as a day-surgery procedure.

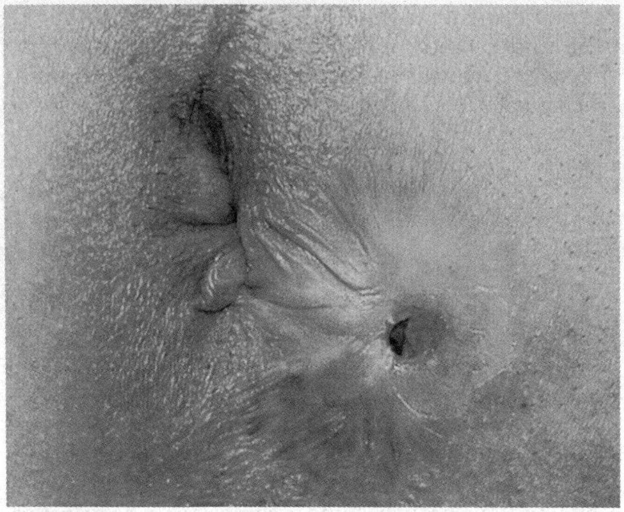

Figure 23–5.

Anal fistula. (From De Los Rios E. Atlas of therapeutic proctology. Philadelphia: WB Saunders, 1984, p 106.)

Application of the Nursing Process to the Care of the Patient Having Incision and Drainage of a Rectal Abscess

PREOPERATIVE NURSING CARE

Preoperative nursing care of a patient scheduled for incision and drainage of an anorectal abscess involves the basic assessments and interventions that apply to any surgical patient. Keep the patient on NPO status, prepare the bowel, and administer pre-

Table 23–3. ANORECTAL FISSURES, FISTULAS, AND CYSTS

	ANAL FISSURE	ANORECTAL FISTULA	PILONIDAL CYST
Description	Ulcer or crack in lining of anal wall	Hollow tract connecting anal canal or rectum with perianal skin	Cyst lined with dermoid tissue and hair found at the base of the spine about 5 cm (2 in.) above anus
Etiology	Anal trauma such as passage of a hard, large stool	Rupture or incision and drainage of anorectal abscess, cancer, radiation therapy, Crohn's disease	Congenital defect
Clinical manifestations	Severe, burning pain on defecation; small amount of bleeding; painful spasms of anal sphincter; constipation from fear of pain on defecation	Constant irritating drainage of blood, pus, mucus, and sometimes stool	Asymptomatic unless infected, in which case pain, swelling, and drainage occur
Medical management	Comfort measures such as local anesthetics, sitz baths, and stool softeners until healed; chronic cases may require surgical excision	Fistulotomy (opening of the tract) or fistulectomy (excision of the tract); wound is packed with gauze and allowed to heal by granulation; treatment of underlying disorder	Incision and drainage; wound either closed or packed and left to heal by granulation; sitz baths
Nursing care	Same as for hemorrhoidectomy	Same as for hemorrhoidectomy	Same as after incision and drainage of anorectal abscess

operative medications as ordered. Be certain the patient understands what is to be done, its expected effect, and the usual postoperative course. Provide additional explanation as needed.

POSTOPERATIVE NURSING CARE

Assessment

Assess the patient's return to physiologic stability after surgery. Make ongoing assessments of the patient's discomfort. Inspect the operative area for bleeding and drainage, being careful not to dislodge any rectal packing inserted during surgery. Note the amount, color, and odor. Measure urinary output, and check the frequency and consistency of bowel movements, because some degree of urinary retention and constipation are likely to occur.

Nursing Diagnoses and Planning

Nursing diagnoses and related expected patient outcomes most commonly applicable to patients who have had an incision and drainage of an anorectal abscess include the following:

NDx: Pain related to surgical trauma in the anorectal area

Planning: Patient outcomes
1. Patient states that he or she is comfortable.
2. Patient tolerates a sitting position 24 hours postoperatively.

NDx: High risk for infection (recurrent) related to contamination and poor healing of the wound

Planning: Patient outcomes
1. Pink granulation tissue is evident in the wound.
2. Wound is free of odor and purulent drainage.
3. Patient is afebrile.

Nursing Interventions

NDx: Pain
Administer prescribed analgesics as needed. This is generally every 4 hours during the immediate postoperative period, and after the immediate postoperative period, before dressing changes and bowel movements. Keep the patient in a side-lying position for the first 24 hours to prevent pressure on the surgical area. Subsequently, allow the patient to sit for short periods of time and provide a flotation pad or foam doughnut cushion for comfort. Give sitz baths, or apply warm, moist compresses as ordered.

Provide a high-fiber diet, and encourage the patient to drink large amounts of fluids daily to promote passage of soft, formed stools. Give bulk-forming stool softeners as ordered to prevent constipation and trauma to the operative area from passage of hard stool.

NDx: High risk for infection (recurrent)
Use a T-binder to anchor a dressing over the wound while drainage persists. If packing is in place, it is ordinarily changed daily. Remove packing gently after soaking loose with saline or half-strength hydrogen peroxide or soaking in a sitz bath.

Use strict sterile technique when caring for the wound. Explain to the patient the importance of careful cleansing of the area after defecation, and instruct the patient to take a sitz bath after each bowel movement.

Before discharge, teach the patient how to care for the wound at home. Stress the need to avoid any potential contamination to the area and to report signs of recurrent infection such as increased pain, purulent drainage, or fever.

Evaluation

Evaluate the effectiveness of nursing care for a patient who has had an incision and drainage of an anorectal abscess by comparing the patient's status with the expected patient outcomes. Examples of specific outcomes for patients who have had an incision and drainage of an anorectal abscess have been provided in the Planning section.

Functional Disorders

Mechanical Ileus

Mechanical ileus is a condition in which movement of intestinal contents through the intestine is impaired because of mechanical obstruction.

ETIOLOGY

Mechanical obstruction can result from problems outside the intestine, within the wall of the intestine, or within the lumen of the intestine. Problems outside the intestine that can cause mechanical obstruction include adhesions and hernias. Problems within the intestinal wall include stricture, hematomas, and intramural tumors. Foreign bodies, intussusception, volvulus (twisting of the bowel), and epithelial tumors are examples of problems within the intestinal lumen (Fig. 23–6).

PATHOPHYSIOLOGY

Movement of air, food, and secretions in the direction of the rectum ceases. The bowel proximal to the obstruction dilates, and the distal bowel tends to collapse. Absorption is diminished, whereas intes-

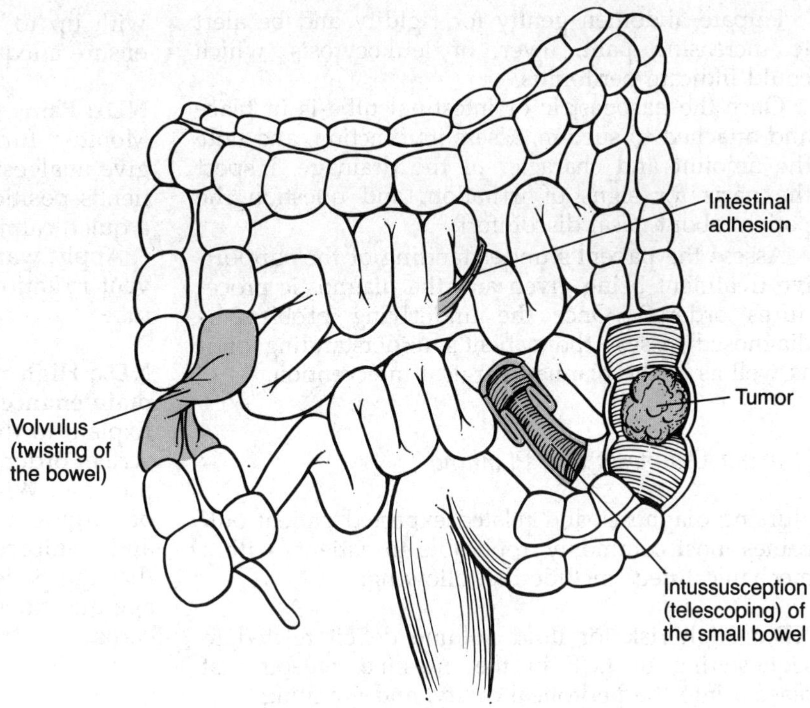

Figure 23–6.

Causes of mechanical intestinal obstruction. Illustrated here are volvulus (twisting of the bowel), adhesion, tumor, and intussusception (telescoping of the bowel).

tinal secretion increases. Intraluminal pressure increases and ultimately results in ischemia and necrosis of the bowel. Bacteria multiply.

Fluid and electrolyte imbalances that occur are hyponatremia and the loss of hydrogen ions and chloride as a result of vomiting gastric contents, metabolic alkalosis, and hypochloremia. In unresolved intestinal obstruction, large amounts of extracellular fluid (ECF) become sequestered in the intestine and plasma weeps into the peritoneal cavity. Hypovolemia and shock can ensue.

CLINICAL MANIFESTATIONS

The predominant symptoms of mechanical ileus are vomiting, cramping, abdominal pain, distention, and inability to pass stools or flatus. When the obstruction is high in the intestine, vomiting is marked and abdominal distention limited. Conversely, when the obstruction is low there is marked distention but little vomiting. Bowel sounds are high pitched, frequent, and rushing (periodic loud bursts). Sometimes they disappear late in the course of the obstruction. With loss of extracellular fluid into the intestine and vomiting, symptoms of dehydration and hypovolemia occur.

MEDICAL DIAGNOSIS

Diagnosis of mechanical bowel obstruction or ileus is made on the basis of the history and physical findings. It can be confirmed by plain x-ray films of the abdomen, which show air-fluid levels in the obstructed bowel. Once obstruction is confirmed, diagnostic measures to determine its cause are begun.

MEDICAL MANAGEMENT

Initial treatment of mechanical bowel obstruction is supportive. The patient is on NPO status, and a nasogastric or intestinal tube is inserted to decompress the intestine and prevent vomiting. Intravenous fluids and electrolytes, and in some cases TPN, are given as needed to maintain homeostasis. Antibiotics are given to combat infection. Analgesics may be given for pain. Once the underlying condition is diagnosed and the patient is stable, surgical correction is performed.

Application of the Nursing Process to the Care of the Patient with a Mechanical Ileus

Assessment

Ascertain symptoms and their time of onset. Assess for abdominal pain. If present, note type, location, and severity. Ask about vomiting, and determine amount, color, odor, and consistency of the vomitus. Listen for bowel sounds, and check for abdominal distention. Determine when the patient last had a bowel movement and passed flatus.

Observe for signs of dehydration and hypovolemia. Inspect oral mucous membranes for dryness, and check skin turgor. Take vital signs to check for increased temperature; rapid, weak pulse; rapid respirations; and hypotension. Check urinary output, and review laboratory values of hematocrit and serum electrolytes.

Palpate abdomen gently for rigidity and be alert to increasing pain, fever, or leukocytosis, which could indicate peritonitis.

Once the nasogastric or intestinal tube is in place and attached to suction, assess its function, and note the amount and character of the drainage. Inspect the naris for signs of irritation, and question the patient about nasal discomfort.

Assess the patient's understanding of the supportive treatment being given and the diagnostic procedures ordered. Once the underlying problem is diagnosed, assess the patient's understanding of it as well as of the planned surgical intervention.

Nursing Diagnoses and Planning

Nursing diagnoses and related expected patient outcomes most commonly applicable to patients with a mechanical ileus include the following:

NDx: High risk for fluid volume deficit related to sequestering of ECF in the intestine, weeping of plasma into the peritoneal cavity, and vomiting

Planning: Patient outcomes
1. Blood pressure, pulse, and respirations are within the patient's normal range.
2. Urinary output is 50 ml or more per hour.
3. Serum electrolytes and osmolarity are within normal limits.

NDx: Pain related to increased intraluminal pressure

Planning: Patient outcomes
1. Patient states pain is relieved.
2. Patient rests without verbal or nonverbal signs of pain.

NDx: High risk for altered health maintenance related to insufficient knowledge of supportive treatment, diagnostic tests, diagnosis, and surgical intervention

Planning: Patient outcomes
1. Patient states reasons for supportive treatment such as NPO status and nasogastric suction.
2. Patient states purpose of ordered diagnostic tests.
3. Patient describes simply but accurately the diagnosis underlying the disorder.
4. Patient describes the surgical procedure and its expected effect.

Nursing Interventions

NDx: High risk for fluid volume deficit
Administer intravenous fluid and electrolytes prescribed to replace lost water, sodium, chloride, and potassium. These might consist of isotonic sodium chloride alternating with 5% dextrose and water with up to 40 mEq of potassium. Monitor CVP to ensure adequate replacement and prevent overload.

NDx: Pain
Monitor function of the nasogastric suction, and give analgesics as ordered for pain. Change the patient's position frequently for comfort, and maintain a quiet, calm environment.

Apply water-soluble lubricant to the naris to prevent irritation from the nasogastric or nasointestinal tube.

NDx: High risk for altered health maintenance
Explain to the patient the reason for treatments. Describe ordered diagnostic tests, and explain their purpose. When the underlying problem and a plan of surgical intervention have been identified, clarify and reinforce the physician's explanation to ensure that the patient and the family understand. Encourage questions, and allow time for expression of concerns.

Evaluation

Evaluate the effectiveness of nursing care for a patient with mechanical ileus by comparing the patient's status with the expected patient outcomes. Examples of specific outcomes for patients with mechanical ileus have been provided in the Planning section.

Paralytic (Adynamic) Ileus

Paralytic, or adynamic, ileus is the impaired movement of intestinal contents through the intestine because of reduced or absent peristalsis.

ETIOLOGY

Paralytic ileus can result from severe physiologic stress such as burns, peritonitis, blunt traumatic injury to the abdomen, intraabdominal vascular accident, or severe electrolyte imbalance. It is most commonly seen, however, after abdominal surgery. In fact, it is said that ileus occurs to some extent in every patient who has had an abdominal operation.

PATHOPHYSIOLOGY

Excessive sympathetic nervous system activity is believed to cause the decrease or absence of peristalsis, which in turn, causes the intestine to become flaccid and functionally obstructed. Fluid accumulates in the bowel lumen because intestinal secretion is normal but absorption and motility are impaired. There is little increase in intraluminal pressure, however, because the fluid is evenly distributed throughout the tract; hence, there is little risk of ischemia of the intestinal wall. There is a risk of dehydration, which can lead to shock and renal failure as a result of loss of accumulated fluid from the intestine by vomiting or suction if fluid and electrolytes are not replaced.

CLINICAL MANIFESTATIONS

The major symptoms of paralytic ileus are decreased to absent bowel sounds, abdominal distention, and vomiting or increased nasogastric drainage. If dehydration results, oliguria, tachycardia, poor skin turgor, and dry mucous membranes may present. Tenderness or pain is minimal or absent unless the ileus is associated with peritonitis.

MEDICAL DIAGNOSIS

Paralytic ileus is diagnosed primarily on the basis of the patient's history and presenting symptoms (i.e., decreased or absent bowel sounds, failure to pass flatus, emesis, or excessive GI tube drainage). A plain abdominal x-ray film showing uniform distention of the intestinal lumen throughout the small and large bowel substantiates the diagnosis.

MEDICAL MANAGEMENT

Paralytic ileus resolves spontaneously in an average of 3 to 5 days. Therefore, symptomatic treatment consisting of nasogastric suction for intestinal decompression, and fluid and electrolyte replacement is provided while waiting for the parasympathetic nervous system to override the sympathetic nervous system and allow return to normal function. Ambulation is encouraged if possible because it promotes bowel function. Rarely, drugs that stimulate the parasympathetic nervous system are given.

Application of the Nursing Process to the Care of the Patient with Paralytic Ileus

Assessment

Assess all postoperative patients, especially those having abdominal procedures, for signs and symptoms of paralytic ileus. Check bowel sounds every 4 to 8 hours, and check the abdomen for distention. Note vomiting because, although some emesis is not unusual after general anesthesia, profuse vomiting is indicative of paralytic ileus. Observe the amount and quality of any GI tube drainage every 4 hours. Question the patient about the presence and passage of flatus, and assess frequency of bowel movements.

Nursing Diagnoses and Planning

Nursing diagnoses and related expected patient outcomes most commonly applicable to patients with paralytic ileus include the following:

NDx: High risk for fluid volume deficit related to vomiting or excessive GI drainage

Planning: Patient outcomes
1. Intake approximates output.
2. Skin turgor is good.
3. Mucous membranes are moist and pink.

NDx: Anxiety related to meaning of vomiting, distention, insertion of a nasogastric tube, and prolonged NPO status

Planning: Patient outcomes
1. Patient describes paralytic ileus as a basically benign response to surgery that disappears with time.
2. Patient states the reason for a nasogastric tube and NPO status.
3. Patient expresses confidence that the ileus will resolve without negative sequelae.

Nursing Interventions

Although there is no specific treatment for paralytic ileus, interventions that diminish existing distress and promote peristalsis are used.

NDx: High risk for fluid volume deficit
Administer intravenous fluids as ordered. Record intake and output, including emesis and nasogastric drainage. Monitor laboratory data, skin turgor, and condition of mucous membranes for signs of dehydration.

NDx: Anxiety
Explain to the patient what paralytic ileus is, and stress that it is a common response to abdominal surgery and that normal intestinal function returns spontaneously usually within a week. Explain the need for nasogastric drainage and being NPO.

Additional Interventions
If allowed, encourage the patient to move about and walk, explaining that these activities promote normal bowel function.

Maintain NPO status until peristalsis returns, then give small amounts of fluid, and progress the diet as tolerated in accordance with the physician's order.

Evaluation

Evaluate the effectiveness of nursing care for a patient with paralytic ileus by comparing the patient's status with the expected patient outcomes. Examples of specific outcomes for patients with paralytic ileus have been provided in the Planning section.

Malabsorption Syndrome

Malabsorption syndrome refers to the signs and symptoms that result from the impaired passage of proteins, carbohydrates, fats, vitamins, and minerals across the intestinal wall and into the circulation. In its full-blown form, absorption of all of these major nutrients is impaired. In less severe cases, the impaired absorption is limited to one or more of the nutrients.

ETIOLOGY AND PATHOPHYSIOLOGY

The causes of malabsorption are many. Any factor that interferes with chemical or mechanical digestion, and thus affects the condition in which nutrients are presented to the intestinal wall for absorption, or that shortens the length of time in which they are in contact with the wall can result in malabsorption. Examples of these conditions are pancreatic insufficiency, deficiency of conjugated bile acids, and gastrectomy. Any conditions that alter the intestinal mucosa or decrease the absorptive surface can also cause malabsorption.

These conditions include gluten-induced enteropathy, Crohn's disease, and intestinal resection. Additional causes of malabsorption are obstruction to the intestinal lymphatic system (as can occur with lymphoma), tuberculosis, infections, disease of the distal ileum, and drugs such as cholestyramine, colchicine, kanamycin, bacitracin, polymyxin, neomycin, and irritant laxatives.

For unknown reasons, malabsorption can also accompany thyroid disorders and diabetes mellitus.

CLINICAL MANIFESTATIONS

The clinical manifestations of malabsorption vary with the nutrients affected and the severity of the problem (Table 23–4). The classic symptoms of full-blown malabsorption syndrome are weight loss, muscle wasting, bloating, borborygmus, and passage of frequent bulky, gray, greasy, foul-smelling stools indicative of steatorrhea.

In cases in which malabsorption is less severe or intermittent, the primary symptoms may be chronic fatigue, lack of drive, and depression.

MEDICAL DIAGNOSIS

The diagnosis of malabsorption and identification of the underlying cause require extensive diagnostic testing. Diagnostic findings compatible with malabsorption syndrome are decreased serum albumin, carotene, calcium, cholesterol, potassium, magnesium, vitamin B_{12} and folic acid, elevated prothrombin time, and an increase in stool fat based on the chemical analysis of a 72-hour stool collection obtained while the patient is ingesting 80 to 100 g of fat per 24 hours.

Other diagnostic tests include tolerance tests for D-xylose, glucose, lactose, sucrose, and vitamin B_{12}; breath tests for fat absorption and bacterial overgrowth; ultrasonography, computed tomographic (CT) scans, and x-ray films to identify abnormalities in the GI tract; and, in some cases, biopsies of the intestinal mucosa.

MEDICAL MANAGEMENT

Medical management depends on the specific underlying cause. Measures to restore fluid, electrolyte,

Table 23–4. MANIFESTATIONS OF NUTRITIONAL DEFICIENCY IN MALABSORPTION SYNDROME

MALABSORBED NUTRIENT	CLINICAL MANIFESTATIONS
Protein	Weight loss, muscle wasting, alopecia, peripheral edema
Carbohydrate	Weight loss, diarrhea, flatulence, abdominal distention
Fat	Weight loss, diarrhea, steatorrhea, dermatitis
Vitamin A	Epithelial keratinization, follicular hyperkeratosis, skin and mucous membrane infections
Thiamin (B_1)	Anorexia, constipation, fatigue, depression, apathy, neuritis in the legs, cardiac failure
Riboflavin (B_2)	Glossitis, cheilosis, dermatitis, photophobia
Folic acid	Macrocytic and megaloblastic anemia, glossitis, cheilosis, dermatitis
Niacin	Dermatitis, weakness, anorexia, diarrhea, apathy, depression, mental confusion
Pyridoxine	Nervous irritability, weakness, hypochromic and microcytic anemia, seborrhea-like skin lesions
Vitamin B_{12}	Pernicious anemia, glossitis, cheilosis, peripheral neuropathy, paresthesias
Vitamin D	Softening of the bones, bone deformity, bone pain, fractures, muscle weakness, tetany
Vitamin K	Bruising, bleeding, hematuria, hypoprothrombinemia, prolonged clotting time
Calcium	Positive Trousseau's and Chvostek's signs, tetany, osteoporosis, osteomalacia, bone pain, fractures, hypertension
Iron	Brittle nails, anemia, glossitis, cheilosis, stomatitis, decreased resistance to infection
Sodium	Muscle cramps, weakness
Zinc	Dermatitis
Potassium	Muscle flaccidity, weakness, decreased tendon reflexes, cardiac dysrhythmias
Magnesium	Neuromuscular dysfunction, muscle spasms, tremors, tetany, anorexia, nausea, decreased tendon reflexes, apathy, personality changes, cardiac dysrhythmias
Phosphate	Osteomalacia
Water	Dehydration

and nutritional balance are an essential part of the management of all patients.

Guidelines for Application of the Nursing Process to the Care of the Patient with Malabsorption Syndrome

The nursing care of patients with malabsorption syndrome varies with the medical management of the underlying cause. In all cases, however, thoroughly assess nutritional status, and administer replacement or supplementary fluids, electrolytes, and nutrients as ordered.

Gluten-Induced Enteropathy

Gluten-induced enteropathy is a disorder of absorption also referred to as nontropical sprue or celiac sprue. It varies in severity and occurs more often in females than in males.

ETIOLOGY

As the name suggests, gluten-induced enteropathy is due to an immunologic sensitivity to the protein gluten. Large amounts of gluten are found in wheat and in rye; smaller amounts are found in oats and barley.

PATHOPHYSIOLOGY

In sensitive persons, gluten causes atrophy of the intestinal mucosa and flattening of the villi (Fig. 23–7). The result is impaired absorption, as a result of decreased uptake and transport, of proteins, fats, and carbohydrates and often the fat-soluble vitamins, vitamin B_6, vitamin B_{12}, iron, folate, and the trace elements.

In some cases, a temporary intolerance to lactose (milk sugar) also occurs. This is due to a deficiency of the enzyme lactase, which develops as a result of the changes in the intestinal mucosa.

CLINICAL MANIFESTATIONS

Gluten-induced enteropathy presents with the classic symptoms of malabsorption, which vary in degree with the severity of the disorder. GI symptoms include the frothy, gray, foul-smelling, bulky stools that float in the toilet bowl because of their gas content, indicative of steatorrhea; abdominal distention; crampy abdominal pain; anorexia; and sometimes diarrhea. Other symptoms are chronic fatigue, weight loss, and anemia. In cases of delayed diagnosis and severe disease, muscle wasting, edema, bleeding, hypotension, and symptoms of hypocalcemia may be present.

MEDICAL DIAGNOSIS

There is no diagnostic text specific for gluten-induced enteropathy. An intestinal biopsy showing atrophy of the villi is considered essential to the diagnosis but does not exclude other possible disorders. Definite diagnosis requires a demonstrated remission of the disease in response to the elimination of dietary gluten.

MEDICAL MANAGEMENT

The management of gluten-induced enteropathy is based on the total elimination of gluten from the diet. Such a gluten-free diet requires avoidance of all cereal grains except for rice and corn. This diet must be followed for life because, even though the intestinal mucosa returns to normal when the diet is followed, reexposure to gluten causes a reactivation of the pathology. A therapeutic response to the gluten-free diet is seen as early as in a week and, in the majority of patients, in no more than 8 weeks.

In the initial period of treatment, a high-calorie, high-protein diet with vitamin and mineral supplements is often given to help the patient regain normal nutritional status. If lactose intolerance is a problem, milk and milk products are limited until improvement occurs.

Corticosteroids may be used temporarily in patients who are critically ill or in long-term patients who are unresponsive to a gluten-free diet.

Application of the Nursing Process to the Care of the Patient with Gluten-Induced Enteropathy

Assessment

Assess the patient for symptoms of malabsorption. Explore the patient's symptoms. Question the patient about bowel elimination patterns. Note the frequency of bowel movements and the characteristics of the stool. Ask specifically about the occurrence of frothy, foul-smelling, bulky stools that float, because these are characteristic of steatorrhea. Also ask the patient about abdominal pain, cramping, and distention. Obtain current weight. Determine whether weight loss has occurred and over what period of time. Question the patient about anorexia. Obtain a

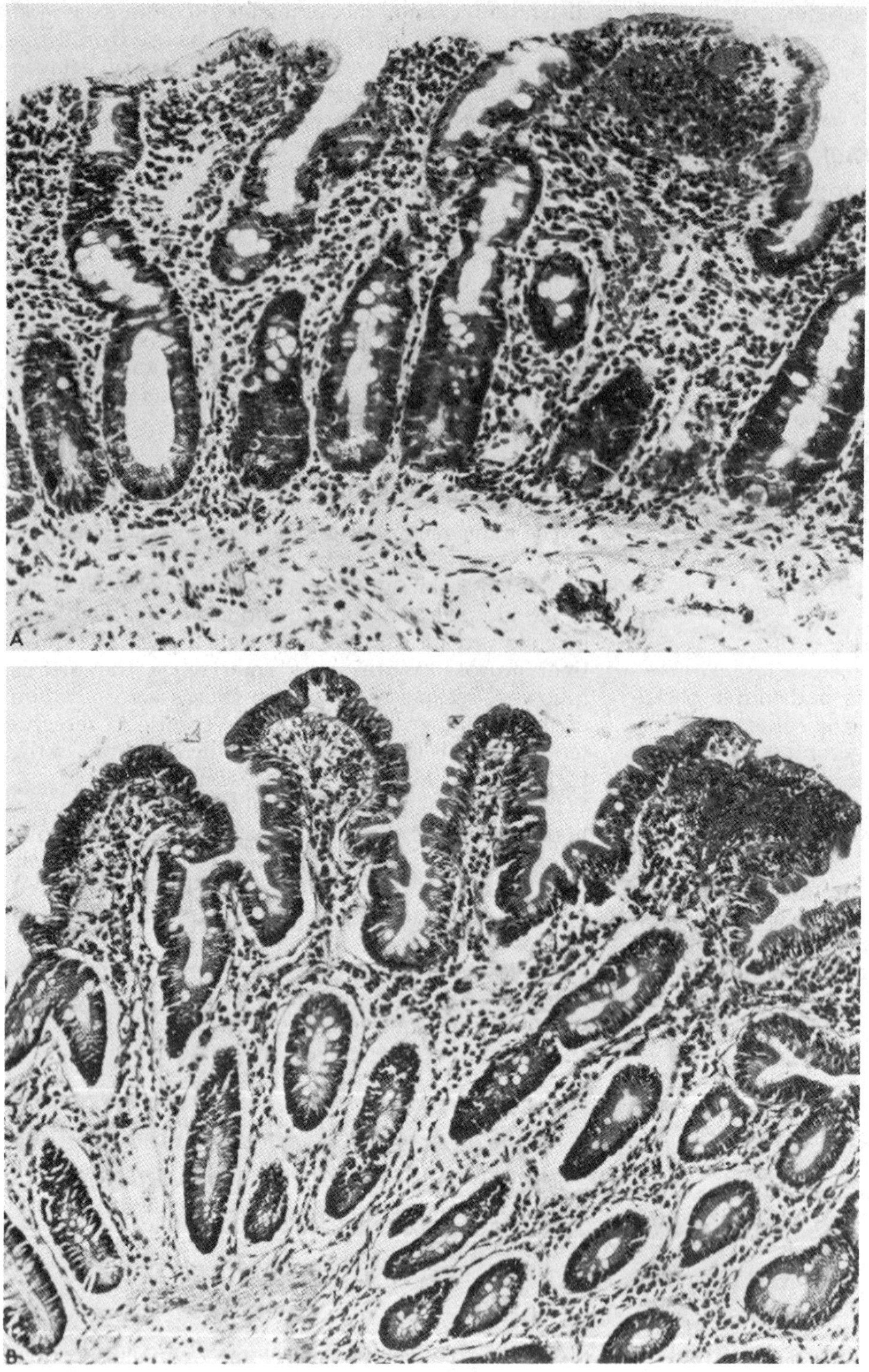

Figure 23–7.

A, Mucosal changes in gluten-induced enteropathy. Note the flattening of the villi and atrophy of the mucosa. *B,* Mucosa after 5 days on a gluten-free diet. (From Cotran RS, Kumar V, Robbins SL. Robbins pathologic basis of disease. 4th ed. Philadelphia: WB Saunders, 1989, p 878.)

diet history that includes types and amounts of foods usually eaten. Compare this with the patient's report of current dietary intake, and explore the relationship of eating to symptoms. Also question about fatigue, and check for signs of anemia. Observe for muscle wasting, and note the condition of the skin, hair, and nails. Assess for signs of vitamin deficiency and fluid and electrolyte imbalance.

Once gluten-induced enteropathy is diagnosed, assess the patient's understanding of the disorder and its treatment. Also assess the patient's motivation and ability to comply with the therapeutic diet.

Nursing Diagnoses and Planning

Nursing diagnoses and related expected patient outcomes most commonly applicable to patients with gluten-induced enteropathy include the following:

NDx: High risk for altered health maintenance related to insufficient knowledge of cause, prognosis, and treatment of the disorder

Planning: Patient outcomes

1. Patient describes the disorder as caused by a sensitivity to the protein gluten.
2. Patient explains that if gluten is eliminated from the diet, symptoms will disappear, but that symptoms will return any time gluten is eaten.
3. Patient lists foodstuffs to be avoided and allowable substitutes.

NDx: High risk for noncompliance related to gluten-free diet

Planning: Patient outcomes

1. Patient verbalizes intent to comply with the diet.
2. Symptoms have regressed by the time of follow-up.

Nursing Interventions

NDx: High risk for altered health maintenance

Clarify and reinforce the patient's understanding of the relation between the ingestion of gluten, the changes in the intestine, and the resultant symptoms. Stress that elimination of gluten results in a rapid improvement in symptoms but that a gluten-free diet must be followed for life or symptoms will return. If needed, use an example familiar to the patient to illustrate this fact. One such example might be the skin reaction to poison ivy that occurs in response to each exposure to the oil of the plant.

Also clarify and reinforce the patient's understanding of the requirements of a gluten-free diet as presented in Nutrition Box 23–2. Explain that, because many of the grains permitted on this diet are refined and unenriched, supplementary multivitamins with minerals are recommended.

NDx: High risk for noncompliance

Explain the importance of maintaining a gluten-free diet not only to the patient but also to the family or significant others to encourage them to support the patient's compliance with the diet rather than to discourage it.

Nutrition Box 23–2.

NUTRITION: SPECIAL CONSIDERATIONS FOR PATIENTS WITH GLUTEN-INDUCED ENTEROPATHY

Instruct patients with gluten-induced enteropathy to:

Eliminate from the diet all foods containing wheat, rye, oats, and barley.

When cooking, substitute soybean flour, corn flour or cornmeal, or potato or rice flour for wheat flour.

Remember that cereal grains are used in many processed foods including:

- creamed soups and vegetables
- ice cream
- cakes, cookies, breads
- pasta
- processed cheese
- commercial salad dressing
- hot dogs and luncheon meats
- beer and ale
- malted milk

Read the list of ingredients on all food labels carefully to check for cereal, starch, flour, thickening agents, emulsifiers, gluten, and stabilizers.

- Avoid foods that list hydrolyzed vegetable protein because this may be soybean, corn, wheat, or a combination of these.
- Avoid foods that list vegetable protein because this can be soybeans, corn, wheat, rye, oats, or barley.
- Do use foods that list starch as long as they are made in the United States, because this refers to cornstarch.

To further facilitate compliance with the diet, make sure the patient is provided with a basic list of foods to be avoided and foods that are allowed as well as recipes for preparing gluten-free meals. Also make certain that the patient is familiar with gluten-free products such as soy flour and rice flour and knows where they can be purchased. Refer the patient to resources for additional recipes, and explain that lists of gluten-free products can be obtained from the major food companies.

Evaluation

Evaluate the effectiveness of nursing care for a patient with gluten-induced enteropathy by comparing the patient's status with the expected patient outcomes. Examples of specific outcomes for patients with gluten-induced enteropathy have been provided in the Planning section.

Lactase Deficiency

Lactase deficiency is a condition marked by low levels or absence of the enzyme lactase in the intestine. It is so prevalent among certain ethnic groups as to be almost considered normal for them. These groups include the Japanese, Filipinos, black Americans, Native Americans, and Greenland Eskimos.

ETIOLOGY

Lactase deficiency occurs as a primary or a secondary disorder. Primary lactase deficiency occurs in rare instances as a congenital disorder but predominantly develops for unknown reasons in late adolescence or early adulthood. Secondary lactase deficiency accompanies disorders such as inflammatory bowel disease (IBD), gastroenteritis, and gluten-induced enteropathy, which damage the intestinal mucosa.

PATHOPHYSIOLOGY

Lactase is the enzyme that breaks down lactose, the predominant disaccharide in milk and milk products, into galactose and glucose as part of the digestive process. Without sufficient lactase, lactose remains undigested and is fermented by bacteria in the intestine into lactic and other organic acids. Water is then pulled into the intestinal tract by the osmotic pressure of these substances.

Lactase deficiency has no known effect on the absorption of protein, fat, calcium, or other nutrients.

CLINICAL MANIFESTATIONS

The symptoms of lactase deficiency are bloating, borborygmus, cramping abdominal pain, flatulence, and diarrhea. These symptoms can develop anytime from one-half to several hours after ingestion of lactose. Anorexia or significant weight loss is rare. The development of symptoms varies with the amount of lactose consumed; only 20% to 30% of lactose-deficient individuals develop symptoms in response to the lactose load found in 240 ml (8 oz) of milk. Development of symptoms also varies with the type of dairy food eaten. Because cottage cheese, ice cream, and yogurt contain less lactose than milk and hard cheese, these foods cause fewer symptoms.

Symptoms are also fewer when dairy foods are eaten in conjunction with other foods that delay emptying of the stomach.

MEDICAL DIAGNOSIS

The diagnosis of lactase deficiency is suggested by a rise in blood sugar of less than 20 mg/dl after the oral administration of lactose and a normal rise in blood sugar after oral administration of an equal amount of glucose and galactose. The diagnosis can be confirmed by low lactase activity in a jejunal biopsy specimen.

The simplest diagnostic test is a hydrogen breath test. This test is based on the fact that hydrogen is a product of the metabolism of unabsorbed carbohydrate by bacteria in the colon. Thus, in the person with lactase deficiency, the ingestion of lactose, which cannot be absorbed, causes an increase in hydrogen in the breath two to eight times the normal level.

MEDICAL MANAGEMENT

Lactase deficiency is managed by decreasing the amount of lactose in the diet to a level that can be tolerated by the patient or by using a commercially available enzyme to predigest lactose or to supplement the body's lactase thereby increasing tolerance.

Enzyme (LactAid) can be purchased over the counter in the form of drops, which are added to milk and allowed to incubate for 24 hours, or caplets, which are taken immediately before meals and are effective for lactose challenge equal to 240 ml (8 oz) of milk. Enzyme-supplemented, low-fat and nonfat ready-to-drink milk is also available in supermarket dairy cases.

Application of the Nursing Process to the Care of the Patient with Lactase Deficiency

Assessment

Obtain a complete description and history of the patient's symptoms. Question carefully about anorexia and weight loss. Review the patient's diet, and

Nutrition Box 23–3.

NUTRITION: SPECIAL CONSIDERATIONS FOR PATIENTS WITH LACTASE DEFICIENCY

Instruct patients with lactase deficiency to do the following:

Eliminate milk and milk products from the diet until symptoms have disappeared and then gradually reintroduce these products as tolerated.

Resume intake of fermented dairy products such as yogurt, cottage cheese, buttermilk, sour cream, and hard cheeses first because they contain bacteria that break down lactose.

Use whole milk rather than skim milk, or substitute soy milk if necessary.

Drink milk only with meals because this is when it is best tolerated.

Limit milk consumption to one glass at a time.

Read labels on drug and food products carefully because lactose can be used as a filler in foods such as breads, pastries, candy, liquid diet aids, instant cocoa mix, french fries, hot dogs, sausages, artificial sweeteners, puddings, gravies, and powdered eggs. Look for words such as "milk fat solids," "nonfat milk solids," and "whey."

Try using LactAid, a commercially available enzyme that breaks down lactose with milk to increase tolerance.

Maintain an adequate supply of calcium for the body despite limited amounts of dairy products in the diet by eating other high-calcium foods such as salmon, sardines, spinach, rhubarb, and Tang beverages or by taking calcium supplements.

explore relationships between diet and the onset of symptoms. Have the patient keep a log of foods eaten and symptoms experienced if needed.

Nursing Diagnoses and Planning

The nursing diagnosis and related expected patient outcomes most commonly applicable to patients with lactase deficiency are as follows:

NDx: High risk for altered health maintenance related to insufficient knowledge of the disorder and its treatment

Planning: Patient outcomes

1. Patient describes relationship between lactose and symptoms.
2. Patient identifies sources of lactose.
3. Patient explains self-care measures as described in Nutrition Box 23–2.

Nursing Interventions

NDx: High risk for altered health maintenance

Reinforce the patient's understanding of the relationship between the ingestion of lactose and the development of symptoms, and identify sources of lactose. Explain that lactose intolerance varies in severity and that dairy products can often be tolerated to some degree depending on type and amount. Instruct the patient in dietary guidelines as presented in Nutrition Box 23–3.

Evaluation

Evaluate the effectiveness of nursing care for a patient with lactase deficiency by comparing the patient's status with the expected outcomes. Examples of specific outcomes for patients with a lactase deficiency have been provided in the Planning section.

Structural Disorders

Diverticular Disease

Diverticula are outpouchings of mucosa through the muscular wall of the intestine (Fig. 23–8). They can occur in any part of the intestine but are most common in the sigmoid colon.

Diverticulosis is one form of diverticular disease. It is characterized by the presence of noninflamed diverticula and in many cases is asymptomatic. Diverticulitis is a form of diverticular disease in which there is inflammation of a diverticulum.

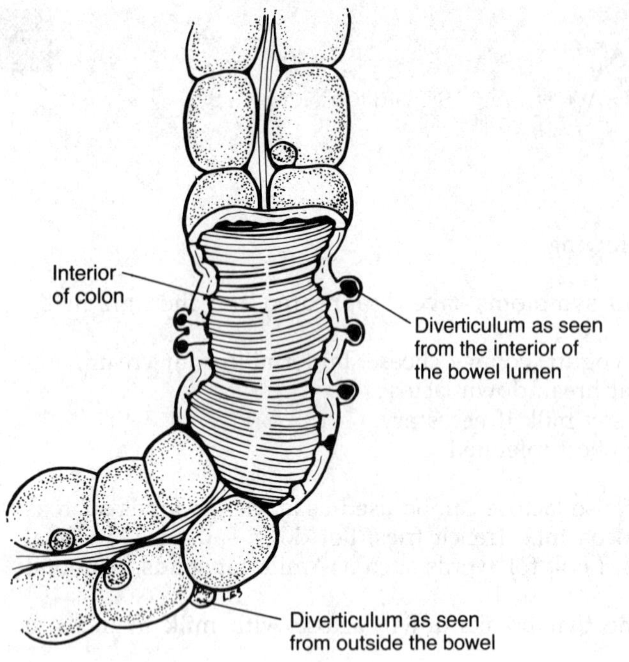

Figure 23–8.

Diverticular disease.

Diverticular disease is the most common pathologic condition of the colon in the United States. Its incidence increases with age, beginning at approximately 35 years. It is estimated that approximately one third of the population is affected by 60 years of age.

ETIOLOGY AND PATHOPHYSIOLOGY

Diverticula appear to be caused by increased pressure within the lumen of the bowel, which forces herniation of the mucosa through weak areas of the muscular wall. Such weak areas occur naturally at points where blood vessels penetrate or may develop as a result of the atrophy of the intestinal muscle, which occurs with aging. Increased intraluminal pressure is believed to result from small, scant stools, which increase the force and alter the mechanical characteristics of the peristaltic waves needed to propel them. This change in peristalsis causes hypertrophy of the muscle such that the muscular ridges thicken and almost touch during contractions, producing temporary obstruction and increased pressure in the affected segment of bowel.

Lack of fiber in the diet, which leads to low-bulk stools and prolonged transit time in the intestine, is considered to be a prime precipitating factor in this sequence of events because diverticular disease is rare in cultures in which high-residue diets are the norm.

Inflammation in a diverticulum is believed to occur when increased pressure results in micro- or macroperforation of the mucosal pouch. The inflammation spreads around the diverticulum into the pericolic fat and can cause fibrosis of the colonic wall. If the perforation is large, pericolic abscesses, fistula formation into the bladder or vagina, or generalized peritonitis may occur.

CLINICAL MANIFESTATIONS

Clinical manifestations of both symptomatic diverticulosis and diverticulitis include left quadrant pain, which typically begins as intermittent crampy pain and in the case of diverticulitis subsequently becomes constant and may radiate to the back; constipation sometimes alternating with diarrhea; abdominal distention; and palpation of a sausage-shaped mass in the lower left quadrant. Symptoms unique to diverticulitis are fever and leukocytosis.

Bleeding may accompany both diverticulosis and diverticulitis. Many times it is occult. However, it can also occur in significant amounts in otherwise asymptomatic patients, especially among the elderly.

MEDICAL DIAGNOSIS

Diverticular disease is generally diagnosed by colonoscopy or barium enema, although the latter is not done during the acute stage of diverticulitis because of the danger of massive perforation. In many asymptomatic or mild cases, diverticula are found by chance during examination for another reason. Cancer of the colon must be ruled out as part of the diagnostic process because the presenting symptoms are so similar.

MEDICAL MANAGEMENT

Management of diverticulosis is aimed at increasing stool bulk and preventing constipation and increased intraluminal pressure in the bowel. Thus, a high-fiber diet and bulk-forming laxatives such as Metamucil are prescribed. Stool softeners such as dioctyl sodium sulfosuccinate or a suppository such as bisacodyl may be used to prevent straining at stool. Spasmolytic anticholinergics such as propantheline bromide are taken before meals and at bedtime, and nonopiate analgesics are given for pain. Narcotic analgesics are avoided because they increase intraluminal pressure.

Patients with uncomplicated diverticulitis are treated with clear fluids to rest the bowel and parenteral antibiotics such as gentamycin, 1.0 to 1.5 mg/kg, and clindamycin, 600 mg every 8 hours. With high fever and signs of abscess formation, the patient is NPO, has nasogastric suction, and is on intravenous fluids.

Surgical intervention such as a bowel resection and sometimes a temporary colostomy is required when complications such as perforation (Fig. 23–9), hemorrhage, obstruction, or abscess formation occur. When a colostomy is formed, the distal bowel stump may be oversewn or exteriorized as a mucous fistula.

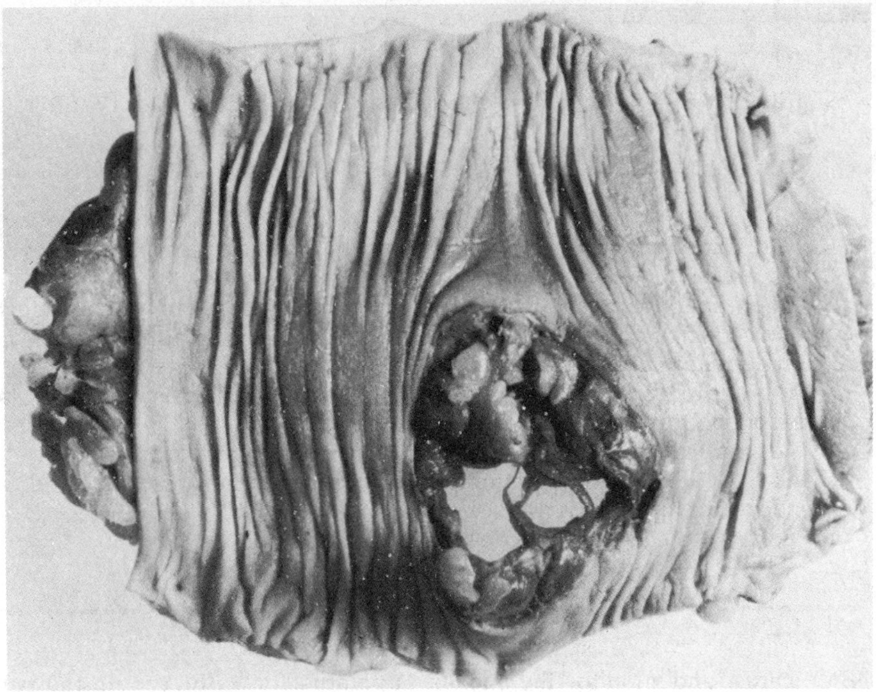

Figure 23–9.

Large perforation of the sigmoid colon secondary to diverticulitis. (From Killingback M. Management of perforative diverticulitis. Surg Clin North Am 1983; 63(1):105.)

Application of the Nursing Process to the Care of the Patient with Diverticular Disease

Assessment

Assess the patient's pain. Ask about its onset, type, location, and intensity. Check for abdominal distention, and question the patient about bowel function. Determine elimination pattern, appearance, size and consistency of stool, occurrence of rectal bleeding, and whether the patient strains at stool. Ask about the use of laxatives or enemas.

Review the patient's usual diet. Ascertain the types and amounts of foods ingested as well the pattern of eating.

Check for fever, and review white blood cell count and sedimentation rate values for indications of infection. Also check for abdominal rigidity and tenderness, tachycardia, and hypotension, which can indicate perforation.

Nursing Diagnoses and Planning

Nursing diagnoses and related expected patient outcomes most commonly applicable to patients with symptomatic diverticulosis include the following:

NDx: Pain related to increased pressure within an area of the intestine

Planning: Patient outcomes
1. Patient reports decrease in pain.
2. Signs of abdominal discomfort, such as pressing on abdomen or flexing legs on abdomen, are absent.

NDx: Constipation related to scant stool with prolonged transit time in the intestine

Planning: Patient outcomes
1. Patient passes soft, formed stool of normal size.
2. Straining at stool is absent.

NDx: High risk for altered health maintenance related to insufficient knowledge of prevention of recurrence

Planning: Patient outcomes
1. Patient describes self-care measures to prevent recurrence of symptoms.
2. Patient states time of any follow-up visit.

Nursing Interventions

NDx: Pain

Administer or teach the patient to self-administer analgesics and spasmolytics as prescribed. Encourage rhythmic deep breathing and use of progressive relaxation exercises to promote pain relief.

For patients with diverticulitis, give clear fluids or a low-residue diet as ordered to rest the bowel. If a nasogastric tube is in place, keep the patient on

Nutrition Box 23–4.

NUTRITION: SPECIAL CONSIDERATIONS FOR PATIENTS WITH DIVERTICULAR DISEASE

Instruct patients with diverticular disease to do the following:

Eat high-fiber foods to add bulk to the stool and speed its passage through the bowel. Examples of foods to include are fresh fruits with skins such as apples, pears, and plums; bananas; dried fruits; whole-wheat bread and crackers; and raw vegetables such as lettuce, carrots, and cauliflower.

Add bran to food on a daily basis. Begin with 1 teaspoon per day and gradually progress to 2 teaspoons three times per day.

Avoid high-roughage foods such as nuts, popcorn, and raw celery.

Drink 8 to 10 glasses of water per day (unless otherwise contraindicated) because fiber retains water and decreases its absorption.

Avoid large meals and the consumption of alcohol.

NPO status, and monitor the suction apparatus for proper function.

NDx: Constipation

Explain the role of diet, fluid intake, exercise, and a schedule for eating and defecation in promoting good bowel function. Teach the patient about a high-fiber diet and fluid intake as described in Nutrition Box 23–4.

Administer or teach the patient to self-administer prescribed bulk-forming laxatives and stool softeners. Caution the patient against the use of other types of laxatives.

NDx: High risk for altered health maintenance

Instruct the patient in self-care measures to prevent recurrence of symptoms as described in Chart 23–2. Be certain the patient knows when to return for any needed follow-up.

Additional Interventions

Administer intravenous fluid and antibiotics as ordered. Maintain function and placement of the nasogastric tube, and keep the patient NPO. Give frequent mouth care, and apply water-soluble lubricant to the naris. When oral intake is resumed, give clear liquids, progressing to a low-residue diet as ordered. Be certain to explain to the patient that these dietary restrictions are designed to rest the bowel and to allow the inflammation to subside. If the patient is on bed rest, encourage frequent turning, as well as foot and leg exercises, to prevent skin breakdown and venous stasis. Encourage periodic coughing and deep breathing if the patient is at risk for respiratory complications.

Chart 23–2.

NURSING GUIDE TO PATIENT EDUCATION FOR SELF-MANAGEMENT: PREVENTION OF RECURRENCE OF SYMPTOMATIC DIVERTICULOSIS OR DIVERTICULITIS

Instruct the patient to:

Follow the dietary guidelines as set forth in Nutrition Box 23–4.

Maintain weight within the accepted range for his or her age and sex.

Avoid activities such as lifting, bending, stooping, coughing, vomiting, and straining at stool that increase intraabdominal pressure.

Avoid strong enemas or purgative products: Use hydrophilic colloid laxatives (Metamucil) and stool softeners such as dioctyl sodium sulfosuccinate if needed to prevent constipation and straining at stool.

Evaluation

Evaluate the effectiveness of nursing care for a patient with diverticular disease by comparing the patient's status with the expected Patient outcomes. Examples of specific outcomes for patients with diverticular disease have been provided in the Planning section.

See Nursing Care Guide 23–1 for the care of the patient who has had a temporary colostomy for diverticular disease.

Intestinal Adhesions

Intestinal adhesions are bands of fibrous tissue that develop as a result of trauma or infection within the peritoneal cavity.

ETIOLOGY

Adhesions develop as part of the healing process. They form when fibrin, which is deposited after injury, becomes organized with an ingrowth of capillaries and fibroblasts rather than being absorbed. Most adhesions result from abdominal surgery, but they can also occur secondary to intraabdominal inflammatory disease.

PATHOPHYSIOLOGY

Adhesions result in intestinal obstruction by causing angulation (folded on itself), torsion (twisting), or constriction of the bowel.

CLINICAL MANIFESTATIONS

The patient with adhesions presents with the signs and symptoms of moderate to severe obstruction, depending on the degree of luminal narrowing. Abdominal distention, decreased or absent bowel sounds, and sometimes vomiting and abdominal cramping occur.

MEDICAL DIAGNOSIS

Diagnosis of adhesions is made on the basis of the presenting signs and symptoms, a history of recent abdominal surgery or infection, and absence of other causes of obstruction. A distended bowel is seen on abdominal x-ray films.

MEDICAL MANAGEMENT

Medical management is aimed at relieving the obstruction. A long intestinal tube such as a Miller-Abbott tube is used to treat small adhesions because the weighted end may be enough to dilate the constricted area and relieve the obstruction. If this is unsuccessful or if the adhesion is large, surgical release (lysis) or excision is performed.

Application of the Nursing Process to the Care of the Patient with Intestinal Adhesions

The assessment, nursing diagnoses, expected patient outcomes, nursing interventions, and evaluation for patients with adhesions that are obstructing the bowel are similar to those described previously for patients with mechanical ileus. Pay particular attention to the patient's anxiety level and need for knowledge. This is important because many of these patients have a history of serious illness and extensive abdominal surgery and attribute the current symptoms to further critical disease with poor prognosis.

Intestinal Hernias

An intestinal hernia is a protrusion of peritoneum, omentum, and intestine out of the abdominal cavity through an abnormal opening in the muscle of the abdominal wall.

On the basis of location, hernias are classified as inguinal, femoral, or ventral (umbilical). (Fig. 23–10). Inguinal hernias are most common and occur in males more often than females.

ETIOLOGY

The basic defect underlying the development of an intestinal hernia is a congenital or acquired weakness of the abdominal wall. Actual herniation occurs as a result of the effect of prolonged increased intraabdominal pressure on the weakened area. Such increased intraabdominal pressure can result from obesity; pregnancy; chronic, strenuous coughing; heavy lifting; straining; or an enlarging tumor.

PATHOPHYSIOLOGY

The peritoneum pouches out through the weakened abdominal wall, forming the hernial sac. In the early stages, tissues such as omentum and intestine enter the sac when the patient stands or strains. They spontaneously reenter the abdominal cavity when the patient sits and intraabdominal pressure is lowered. Once formed, hernias tend to enlarge, and soon tissues remain in the hernial sac at all times. If the herniated tissues can be replaced in the abdominal cavity by manual manipulation, the hernia is referred to as reducible. If they cannot be replaced

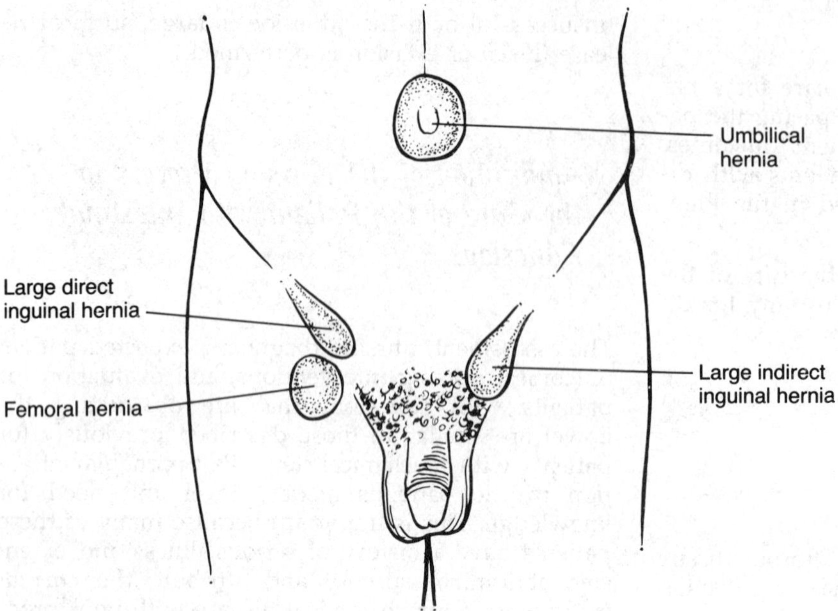

Figure 23–10.

Types of hernias.

in the abdominal cavity, the hernia is irreducible or incarcerated. A hernia is strangulated when twisting or swelling of the tissues in the sac or constriction of the ring of tissue through which the sac protrudes blocks the flow of blood to the intestine and obstructs the passage of materials through it (Fig. 23–11). Such acute obstruction leads to necrosis and gangrene.

CLINICAL MANIFESTATIONS

An uncomplicated hernia presents as a bulge that may only be apparent or that may increase in size on exertion.

The bulge is soft to the touch and often tender. The symptoms of a strangulated hernia are those of an acute intestinal obstruction: severe pain, nausea, vomiting, distention, and fever.

MEDICAL DIAGNOSIS

Diagnosis of hernia is made on the basis of the patient's history and visualization or palpation of the hernia on physical examination. When examining for an inguinal or femoral hernia, the patient is asked to strain downward to increase intraabdominal pressure and cause a reducible hernia to enter the hernial sac where it can be seen or palpated. Similarly, when an incisional or umbilical hernia is suspected but not visible, the patient is asked to raise the head and shoulders off the examining table because this maneuver usually causes the hernia to bulge.

MEDICAL MANAGEMENT

The treatment of choice for incisional, inguinal, and femoral hernias is surgical repair because it

Text continued on page 1005

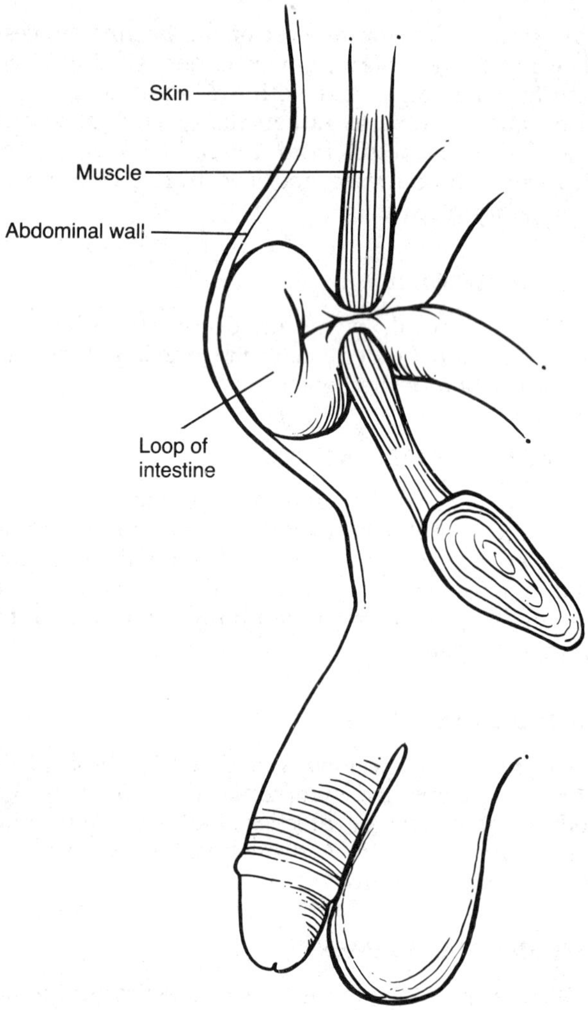

Figure 23–11.

Strangulated hernia. Note compression of the herniated loop of intestine by the ring of tissue through which it passes.

Nursing Care Guide 23–1.

PATIENT CARE AFTER A TEMPORARY COLOSTOMY FOR DIVERTICULAR DISEASE

Assessment Findings: Patient complains of abdominal pain and grimaces and groans on moving.

Nursing Diagnosis: Pain related to surgical trauma to the abdomen

Patient Outcomes	Nursing Interventions	Rationale
Patient moves without signs of severe pain such as moaning, pallor, and tachycardia.	Give prescribed analgesics every 3–4 hours for 72 hours.	Early analgesic administration provides more effective pain relief.
Patient rests quietly without signs of discomfort such as clenched hands, groaning, and crying.	Place the patient in semi-Fowler's position.	Decreases stress on the suture line.
	Encourage ambulation.	Stimulates return of bowel function and relief from gas pains.
Patient states pain is relieved.	Use a rectal tube to remove flatus.	Decreases distention and relieves associated pain.

Evaluation: Compare the patient's status with the expected patient outcomes. If the outcomes are achieved, evaluate nursing care as successful. If not, reassess the patient, formulate new nursing diagnoses, and revise expected patient outcomes and nursing interventions as appropriate.

Assessment Findings: Patient is restless, and face appears tense. Patient states he or she feels apprehensive, inadequate, and helpless.

Nursing Diagnosis: Anxiety related to prognosis and ability to live with and manage the colostomy

Patient Outcomes	Nursing Interventions	Rationale
Physical signs of high anxiety such as trembling, tachycardia, and dry mouth are absent.	Provide time, privacy, and encouragement for discussion of the patient's concerns.	Allows for feedback, provides perspective, and permits a supportive relationship.
Patient attends to directions and information.	Provide desired information about prognosis, reason of surgery, and function and care of the colostomy.	Patient has had limited preoperative preparation because of the emergency nature of the surgery and lack of knowledge predisposes to anxiety.
Patient expresses confidence in ability to cope with the colostomy and its care.		
	Acknowledge that feelings of anxiety are normal and expected after emergency colostomy surgery.	Allays patient concerns about being judged negatively because of anxiety.
	Guide the patient in relaxation techniques if needed.	Reduces tension level and diverts patient's attention.
	Arrange for a visit from an ostomate if desired.	Provides the patient with concrete evidence that a normal lifestyle can be maintained despite the presence of a colostomy. It also allows for sharing of realistic, practical answers to concerns and questions.

(*continued*)

Nursing Care Guide 23–1. *(continued)*

PATIENT CARE AFTER A TEMPORARY COLOSTOMY FOR DIVERTICULAR DISEASE

Evaluation: Compare the patient's status with the expected patient outcomes. If the outcomes are achieved, evaluate nursing care as successful. If not, reassess the patient, formulate new nursing diagnoses, and revise expected patient outcomes and nursing interventions as appropriate.

Assessment Findings: Patient has had a resection of the large bowel and formation of a descending colostomy.

Nursing Diagnosis: Bowel incontinence related to the formation of a colostomy and loss of rectal function

Patient Outcomes	Nursing Interventions	Rationale
Patient uses the selected pouching system effectively to collect fecal drainage. Patient identifies factors such as change in diet and times of eating that affect pattern of colostomy function.	Monitor the collection pouch placed over the colostomy at the time of operation for the accumulation of flatus and drainage.	Indicates functional status of the bowel.
	Empty or change the pouch when it is no more than half full.	Back pressure can damage suture lines and disrupt the pouch seal.
	Assist the patient in the selection of a collection system for daily use that is best suited to his or her needs after discharge. If the patient is unable to care for self, include a significant other in the selection process.	Eliminates unnecessary frustration and thus promotes adaptation and correct self-management.
	Use the selected system consistently.	Assists the patient in mastering self-care and adapting to the demands of the colostomy.
	Explain to the patient that some control over fecal expulsion may be obtained eventually by means of a regular dietary intake and irrigations.	Provides the patient with a positive but realistic fact on which to focus.
	Irrigate the colostomy if ordered.	Promotes bowel emptying.

Evaluation: Compare the patient's status with the expected patient outcomes. If the outcomes are achieved, evaluate nursing care as successful. If not, reassess the patient, formulate new nursing diagnoses, and revise expected patient outcomes and nursing interventions as appropriate.

(continued)

Nursing Care Guide 23–1. *(continued)*

PATIENT CARE AFTER A TEMPORARY COLOSTOMY FOR DIVERTICULAR DISEASE

Assessment Findings: Patient has a descending colostomy and uses a collection system that is applied to the abdomen with adhesive.

Nursing Diagnosis: High risk for impaired skin integrity related to irritation of the peristomal skin from contact with fecal matter, removal of collection systems, or sensitivity to adhesives or other materials

Patient Outcomes	Nursing Interventions	Rationale
Peristomal skin is free of erythema and blisters. Peristomal skin is intact.	Remove mucus and feces from the stoma with a tissue.	Prepares area for washing.
	Wash the peristomal skin to remove all traces of drainage.	Removes substances that can irritate the skin.
	Avoid use of oily soaps and emollients.	Oily substances interfere with adherence of the collection system.
	Omit soap, and wash with water only if the patient is elderly with a tendency for dry skin.	Soap dries the skin.
	Rinse thoroughly and dry gently.	Removes all irritating soap residue and avoids irritation from friction.
	Fit the appliance to the stoma so that there is $\frac{1}{8}$ in. of skin between the pouch opening and the stoma.	Prevents loosening of appliance due to moisture from stoma.
	Use a skin barrier between the pouch opening and the stoma.	Protects the skin from contact with fecal drainage.
	Apply a skin sealant to the area of skin that will be covered with adhesive when collection system is applied.	Prevents damage to the epidermis when the appliance is removed.
	Apply the pouch snugly.	Helps prevent leakage of irritating material onto the skin.
	Monitor the pouch for leaking, and change immediately if it occurs.	Prevents prolonged contact between irritating drainage and the skin.
	Institute a vigorous treatment regimen immediately if peristomal skin irritation does occur.	Irritation can progress rapidly to skin breakdown.

Evaluation: Compare the patient's status with the expected patient outcomes. If the outcomes are achieved, evaluate nursing care as successful. If not, reassess the patient, formulate new nursing diagnoses, and revise expected patient outcomes and nursing interventions as appropriate.

(continued)

Nursing Care Guide 23–1. *(continued)*

PATIENT CARE AFTER A TEMPORARY COLOSTOMY FOR DIVERTICULAR DISEASE

Assessment Findings: Respirations are shallow. Patient states that "it hurts to take a deep breath."

Nursing Diagnosis: High risk for ineffective breathing pattern related to incisional pain on deep breathing

Patient Outcomes	Nursing Interventions	Rationale
Patient coughs and deep breathes as directed. Cyanosis is absent. Arterial blood gases are within normal range.	Teach the patient to splint the abdomen with pillows.	Pain decreases patient's willingness to turn, cough, and deep breathe.
	Assist patient in turning, coughing, and deep breathing every 2 hours for 72 hours postoperatively.	Promotes good ventilation and airway clearance.
	Reassure the patient that coughing and deep breathing, although they may hurt, will not harm the incision.	Promotes cooperation with the therapeutic plan by allaying fear of injury.
	Ambulate the patient at least three times a day (tid) as soon as able.	Promotes good ventilation and airway clearance.

Evaluation: Compare the patient's status with the expected patient outcomes. If the outcomes are achieved, evaluate nursing care as successful. If not, reassess the patient, formulate new nursing diagnoses, and revise expected patient outcomes and nursing interventions as appropriate.

Assessment Findings: Patient is under nothing by mouth orders (NPO), has a nasogastric or nasointestinal tube in place that is connected to low suction, and is mouth breathing.

Nursing Diagnosis: High risk for altered oral mucous membrane related to NPO status and presence of a nasogastric or nasointestinal tube

Patient Outcomes	Nursing Interventions	Rationale
Oral mucous membrane is moist and free of cracks.	Assist patient to brush teeth at least tid.	Cleanses and moistens the mouth.
Lips are supple, moist, and free of cracks.	Encourage frequent mouth rinses.	Moistens oral mucous membranes.
Patient denies dryness of the mouth.	Avoid use of rinses that are drying.	Helps prevent drying and cracking.
	Apply water-soluble lubricant to the lips.	Keeps lips supple and reduces cracking by maintaining tissue moisture.

Evaluation: Compare the patient's status with the expected patient outcomes. If the outcomes are achieved, evaluate nursing care as successful. If not, reassess the patient, formulate new nursing diagnoses, and revise expected patient outcomes and nursing interventions as appropriate.

(continued)

Nursing Care Guide 23–1. *(continued)*

PATIENT CARE AFTER A TEMPORARY COLOSTOMY FOR DIVERTICULAR DISEASE

Assessment Findings: Patient has had abdominal surgery under general anesthesia and is on bed rest.

Nursing Diagnosis: High risk for altered peripheral tissue perfusion related to thrombophlebitis secondary to venous stasis

Patient Outcomes	Nursing Interventions	Rationale
Calves are free of redness, swelling, heat, and pain. Homans' sign is negative.	Guide the patient in foot and leg exercises 10 times every 2 hours while on bed rest.	Muscle contraction promotes venous return by its squeezing action on the veins and thus reduces the risk of thrombus formation.
	Apply antiembolic stockings or Ace bandages.	Supports venous return by enhancing the squeezing action of the muscles on the veins.
	Avoid use of knee gatch or any other source of pressure on the popliteal space.	Eliminates obstruction to venous return as a result of bending or compressing veins and thus decreases stasis, which predisposes to thrombus formation.
	Ambulate the patient as soon as ordered.	Muscle contraction promotes venous return by its squeezing action on the veins and thus reduces the risk of thrombus formation.
	Instruct patient to avoid crossing legs or sitting for long period of time.	Eliminates obstruction to venous return caused by bending or compressing veins and thus decreases stasis, which predisposes to thrombus formation.

Evaluation: Compare the patient's status with the expected patient outcomes. If the outcomes are achieved, evaluate nursing care as successful. If not, reassess the patient, formulate new nursing diagnoses, and revise expected patient outcomes and nursing interventions as appropriate.

(continued)

Nursing Care Guide 23–1. *(continued)*

PATIENT CARE AFTER A TEMPORARY COLOSTOMY FOR DIVERTICULAR DISEASE

Assessment Findings: Patient has had the bowel surgically opened without standard bowel preparation because of the emergency nature of the surgery.

Nursing Diagnosis: High risk for infection related to surgical incision of the peritoneal cavity and bowel

Patient Outcomes	Nursing Interventions	Rationale
Suture line is approximated and free of erythema and purulent drainage. Abdomen is soft and nondistended. Patient is afebrile.	Monitor for signs of peritoneal irritation: muscle rigidity and rebound tenderness.	Muscle rigidity and rebound tenderness are early signs of peritonitis.
	Use strict aseptic technique when doing wound care.	Protects against wound infection as a result of cross-contamination.
	Reinforce or change dressing when wet.	Microorganisms can travel through wet dressings by capillary action.

Evaluation: Compare the patient's status with the expected patient outcomes. If the outcomes are achieved, evaluate nursing care as successful. If not, reassess the patient, formulate new nursing diagnoses, and revise expected patient outcomes and nursing interventions as appropriate.

Assessment Findings: Patient has a new colostomy and verbalizes negative feelings about it and fear of negative reaction from family and friends, stating "This thing is disgusting. No one is going to want to come near me."

Nursing Diagnosis: Body image disturbance related to loss of bowel control, presence of the stoma, release of fecal material onto abdomen, passage of flatus, odor, need for a collection system

Patient Outcomes	Nursing Interventions	Rationale
Patient verbalizes acceptance of self with a colostomy. Patient verbalizes interest in grooming. Patient expresses pleasure at visits from relatives and friends. Patient discusses resumption of work, social activities, and so on in a positive way.	Acknowledge to the patient that negative feelings about the colostomy are normal and that it takes time to accept and adjust to this body change.	Reassures patient that his or her negative feelings are not abnormal and that feelings will ease with time.
	Be certain facial expressions and other nonverbal behaviors convey acceptance, not revulsion, distaste, or pity.	Nonverbal communication can contradict and "speak more loudly" than verbal communication. Negative, nonverbal communication acts to reinforce patient's negative perceptions of self.

(continued)

Nursing Care Guide 23–1. (continued)

PATIENT CARE AFTER A TEMPORARY COLOSTOMY FOR DIVERTICULAR DISEASE

Patient Outcomes	Nursing Interventions	Rationale
	Touch the stoma to show it does not hurt, is not easily damaged, and is not revolting.	Allays patient's fears and connotes acceptance.
	Provide opportunity for the patient to look at the stoma and express feelings about it.	Looking at the stoma and verbalizing feelings about it are essential to accepting and caring for the colostomy.
	Provide privacy for care and teaching.	Protects the patient from embarrassment.
	Empty the pouch of malodorous fecal drainage or flatus before meals, visiting hours, and the like.	Prevents embarrassment, promotes socialization, and prevents anorexia that may result from unpleasant odor.
	Provide good ventilation and deodorize the room as needed.	Prevents embarrassment as a result of odor.
	Do not put pinholes in a plastic pouch to allow release of flatus.	This creates unpredictable, uncontrollable odor.
	Encourage good grooming.	Promotes patient's sense of well-being.
	Stress that, with a little attention to style, the pouch is not visible beneath clothing.	Guides the patient in strategies for minimizing effect of colostomy on appearance and preventing unnecessary embarrassment.
	Help the patient to identify personal strengths.	Helps place feelings about the negative effect of the colostomy on self in perspective.
	Include patient in decision making.	Fosters a sense of control.
	Encourage frank discussion of feelings with significant others.	Allows for validation of feelings and a supportive relationship.

Evaluation: Compare the patient's status with the expected patient outcomes. If the outcomes are achieved, evaluate nursing care as successful. If not, reassess the patient, formulate new nursing diagnoses, and revise expected patient outcomes and nursing interventions as appropriate.

(continued)

Nursing Care Guide 23–1. *(continued)*

PATIENT CARE AFTER A TEMPORARY COLOSTOMY FOR DIVERTICULAR DISEASE

Assessment Findings: Patient states, "I suppose this is the end of good eating. No more fresh fruits and vegetables, gravy, spices, and other good things."

Nursing Diagnosis: High risk for altered nutrition: less than body requirements, related to omission of foods because of flatulence, odor, or diarrhea

Patient Outcomes	Nursing Interventions	Rationale
Patient describes components of a nutritionally balanced diet. Patient is able to select a nutritionally balanced diet from foods that are tolerated well. Patient identifies specific foods that are likely causes of flatulence, odor, or diarrhea.	Review basic principles of nutrition with the patient.	A nutritionally balanced diet is needed to heal the wound and maintain overall state of health. In adjusting to a new colostomy, patients are at risk for inadvertently adopting a nutritionally imbalanced diet.
	Discuss the use of the food pyramid in planning a balanced diet.	The food pyramid is one of the simplest methods available for selecting a generally balanced diet. Because of its simplicity, it is easily complied with and is suitable for virtually all patients.
	Explain the importance of drinking at least 2500 ml per day.	Extra fluid intake is needed because more fluid is lost through a colostomy than is lost with normal stool passing through the rectum.
	Provide the patient with a list of foods likely to cause flatulence, odor, or diarrhea (see Nutrition Box 21–1).	Allows patient to minimize problems by avoiding these foods until colostomy is well established.
	Instruct the patient initially to avoid high-roughage foods such as nuts, popcorn, and raw celery.	High-fiber foods stimulate bowel activity and increase the volume of stool. In some cases, fiber can accumulate and block the stoma.
	Instruct the patient to try new foods one at a time and at least three times before eliminating them from the diet.	Allows the patient to accurately determine effects of individual foodstuffs on the gastrointestinal tract.

Evaluation: Compare the patient's status with the expected patient outcomes. If the outcomes are achieved, evaluate nursing care as successful. If not, reassess the patient, formulate new nursing diagnoses, and revise expected patient outcomes and nursing interventions as appropriate.

(continued)

Nursing Care Guide 23–1. *(continued)*

PATIENT CARE AFTER A TEMPORARY COLOSTOMY FOR DIVERTICULAR DISEASE

Assessment Findings: Patient states, "I may have to learn how to care for this bag but I guess I don't have to worry about birth control while I have this thing."

Nursing Diagnosis: High risk for altered sexuality patterns related to fear of rejection because of the presence of a stoma and a collection system

Patient Outcomes	Nursing Interventions	Rationale
Patient discusses concerns about the effects of the colostomy on sexual function. Patient verbalizes confidence in ability to participate in a satisfying sexual relationship.	Acknowledge that concerns about sexual activity after a colostomy are normal.	Helps put the patient at ease with his or her concerns and thus helps make the patient feel comfortable in discussing them.
	Encourage the patient to discuss sexual concerns openly with spouse or significant other.	Allows for mutual support and problem solving.
	Provide privacy and time for discussion of sexual concerns.	This establishes an environment conducive to open communication.
	Explain that sexual intercourse, conception, and pregnancy are all possible after a colostomy.	Provides factual information to combat misconceptions about functional changes resulting from a colostomy.
	Recommend that the collection pouch be emptied before intercourse.	Protects against spillage as a result of accidental disruption of the seal and contributes to comfort.
	Suggest positions that accommodate the collection pouch.	Protects against spillage as a result of accidental disruption of the seal and contributes to comfort.
	Provide access to written materials about sex and a colostomy such as the pamphlets published by the United Ostomy Association called "Sex and the Male Ostomate" and "Sex and the Female Ostomate."	Allows patient to review information when desired in a private and comfortable environment of choice.
	Refer to a sex therapist if needed.	Provides a source of additional help if other coping strategies prove insufficient.

Evaluation: Compare the patient's status with the expected patient outcomes. If the outcomes are achieved, evaluate nursing care as successful. If not, reassess the patient, formulate new nursing diagnoses, and revise expected patient outcomes and nursing interventions as appropriate.

(continued)

Nursing Care Guide 23–1. *(continued)*

PATIENT CARE AFTER A TEMPORARY COLOSTOMY FOR DIVERTICULAR DISEASE

Assessment Findings: Patient is newly postoperative from colostomy surgery, has no previous knowledge of colostomy function or care, and asks questions regarding it.

Nursing Diagnosis: High risk for altered health maintenance related to insufficient knowledge of care of the colostomy and effects on lifestyle

Patient Outcomes	Nursing Interventions	Rationale
Patient identifies supplies needed for colostomy care and where to obtain them. Patient empties, changes, and cleans the pouch effectively. Patient demonstrates peristomal skin care. Patient states guidelines for performing colostomy care. Patient describes the effect (or lack thereof) of the colostomy on day-to-day activities. Patient identifies services available from the United Ostomy Association.	Teach the patient to care for the colostomy as soon as possible postoperatively. Include information on needed supplies and on emptying and changing the pouch, cleaning the pouch, controlling odor, and caring for the peristomal skin.	Provides a sense of control and allows independence, both of which are essential to adjusting to the colostomy and resuming a normal lifestyle.
	Instruct the patient to empty the pouch when it is one-third full and at bedtime.	Guards against back pressure, which can disrupt the suture line and the pouch seal.
	Suggest that an alarm clock be set the first few nights after discharge to wake the patient to empty the bag.	Ensures that the patient awakes to empty the bag.
	Suggest changing the pouch first thing in the morning before eating or drinking.	Allows maximum convenience and ease because the colostomy usually does not function at this time.
	Explain that physical activities are unrestricted and can be resumed in full usually within 8 weeks after surgery. Be certain to stress that showers and baths may be taken, any type of clothing may be worn, including girdles and pantyhose, and that travel is possible as long as supplies are kept available and seat belts are worn above the stoma.	Provides patient with lifestyle guidelines for self-care after discharge.
	Inform the patient about the services available through the United Ostomy Association.	Makes patient aware of community resources and how to access them.
	Provide the patient with written instructions regarding self-care.	Provides a ready reference for use after discharge because information learned during periods of stress is not generally retained in full.

Evaluation: Compare the patient's status with the expected patient outcomes. If the outcomes are achieved, evaluate nursing care as successful. If not, reassess the patient, formulate new nursing diagnoses, and revise expected patient outcomes and nursing interventions as appropriate.

eliminates the risk of strangulation. In rare cases—for example, when a patient must be stabilized medically before surgery is possible—a truss or girdle may be used to prevent protrusion of the hernia after manual reduction. A truss is a pad placed over the hernia that is held in place with a belt. It should be worn as consistently as possible, and activities that increase intraabdominal pressure should be avoided. Potential complications of a truss are skin irritation and strangulation of the hernia.

HERNIORRHAPHY

Herniorrhaphy is the permanent surgical reduction of a hernia. It is most often an elective procedure but is a surgical emergency in cases of incarceration and strangulation.

The surgical approach varies depending on the location and severity of the problem. Basically, it consists of opening the hernial sac, replacing the protruding organs into the abdominal cavity through the abnormal opening, and removing the sac. If closure is reinforced with synthetic sutures of mesh, the procedure is referred to as a hernioplasty. If the herniated portion of the intestine is necrotic, an intestinal resection may be necessary.

Inguinal herniorrhaphy may be done as an overnight or day surgery procedure with spinal or local anesthesia.

Complications

Complications of herniorrhaphy, although uncommon, can occur. They include infection, hemorrhage, and compromise of the vas deferens or impaired blood supply to the testes in men. Infection is signaled by soreness in the operative area and fever. It is treated with antibiotics, warm compresses, and incision and drainage.

Application of the Nursing Process to the Care of the Patient Having a Herniorrhaphy

PREOPERATIVE NURSING CARE

Assessment

Assess the patient's physical status as before any surgical procedure. Make certain to assess carefully for respiratory infection, chronic cough, or allergies. Because postoperative coughing or sneezing can disrupt the repair, the procedure may be postponed or palliative medications such as antihistamines prescribed.

Assess the patient's understanding of the surgical procedure and the expected postoperative course as well as the psychological response to the scheduled surgery. This is particularly important when the patient is a male with an inguinal hernia because there is the potential for misunderstanding and anxiety about the effect of the surgery on sexual activity.

Nursing Diagnoses and Planning

The nursing diagnosis and related expected patient outcomes most commonly applicable to patients scheduled for herniorrhaphy are as follows:

NDx: Knowledge deficit: surgical procedure, perioperative routines, and usual postoperative course

Planning: Patient outcomes

1. Patient describes perioperative events.
2. Patient describes expected postoperative discomforts.

Nursing Interventions

NDx: Knowledge deficit: surgical procedure, perioperative routines, and usual postoperative course

Describe the surgical procedure and perioperative routines in accord with the type of anesthesia to be used and the expected length of hospitalization. Explain that urination may be difficult right after surgery and that pain and scrotal swelling may last for 24 to 48 hours.

Evaluation

Evaluate the effectiveness of nursing care for a patient scheduled for a herniorrhaphy by comparing the patient's status with the expected patient outcomes. Examples of specific outcomes for patients scheduled for a herniorrhaphy have been provided in the Planning section.

POSTOPERATIVE NURSING CARE

Assessment

Assess return to physiologic stability. Take vital signs, and inspect the dressing for drainage.

Assess ability to empty the bladder, particularly in men who have had an inguinal hernia repaired, because difficulty voiding is not uncommon, especially in the first 8 postoperative hours. Measure intake and output. Observe and palpate the suprapubic area for signs of bladder distention. Also observe for scrotal edema.

Assess patients for pain as well as for coughing, sneezing, or other strenuous movements.

Nursing Diagnoses and Planning

Nursing diagnoses and related expected patient outcomes most commonly applicable to patients who have had a herniorrhaphy include the following:

NDx: Pain related to surgical trauma to the groin

Planning: Patient outcomes
1. Patient states pain is relieved.
2. Patient moves without grimaces or other behavioral signs of pain.
3. Scrotal swelling is decreased or absent.

NDx: High risk for urinary retention related to effects of anesthesia and surgical trauma

Planning: Patient outcomes
1. Patient voids adequate amounts (200–300 ml) within 8 hours.
2. Urinary bladder distention is absent.

NDx: High risk for impaired tissue integrity related to stress on the wound secondary to increased intra-abdominal pressure

Planning: Patient outcomes
1. Patient splints incision if coughing is necessary.
2. Patient sneezes with mouth open.
3. Straining at stool is absent.

NDx: High risk for altered health maintenance related to insufficient knowledge of self-care after discharge

Planning: Patient outcomes
1. Patient describes limitations on activity.
2. Patient explains good body mechanics.
3. Patient identifies measures to prevent constipation.
4. Patient lists symptoms to be expected and those to be reported.

Nursing Interventions

NDx: Pain
Administer prescribed analgesics as needed. Elevate the scrotum, and apply ice packs while in bed to decrease pain and swelling. Apply a scrotal support when out of bed.

NDx: High risk for urinary retention
Assist the patient to a standing position to void. Use inducements such as running water as needed. Report bladder distention to the surgeon because catheterization will generally be required.

NDx: High risk for impaired tissue integrity
Encourage the patient to turn and deep breathe. Do not encourage coughing. Instruct the patient to splint the incision with hands or a pillow if coughing is unavoidable. Instruct the patient to sneeze with the mouth open if sneezing is unavoidable. Explain the importance of not straining at stool, and assist the patient to limit pull on the incision when moving.

NDx: High risk for altered health maintenance
Instruct the patient in self-care after discharge as specified in Chart 23–3. Remember that restrictions on activities vary from surgeon to surgeon, with some imposing no limitations whatsoever.

Evaluation

Evaluate the effectiveness of nursing care for a patient who has had a herniorrhaphy by comparing the patient's status with the expected patient outcomes. Examples of specific outcomes for patients who have had a herniorrhaphy have been provided in the Planning section.

Hemorrhoids

Hemorrhoids are dilated, swollen rectal veins. Internal hemorrhoids protrude within the anal canal and are covered with mucous membrane. External hemorrhoids protrude at the anal opening and are covered with anoderm and perianal skin (Fig. 23–12).

ETIOLOGY AND PATHOPHYSIOLOGY

Stasis in the anal venous system is believed to play a principal role in the development of hemorrhoids. Thus, straining at stool, prolonged sitting on the toilet, heavy lifting, pregnancy, infiltrating cancer, and portal hypertension secondary to liver disease are predisposing factors.

CLINICAL MANIFESTATIONS

Symptoms of internal hemorrhoids are pain and bleeding on defecation. Bleeding is more red than dark and is often slight, appearing as red streaks on the stool or toilet tissue. It is chronic, however, and over time can be sufficient to cause iron deficiency anemia.

External hemorrhoids appear as lumps of pink to red tissue at the anus. If they are thrombosed, they are very tender, tense, and blue. Rectal itching is common with external hemorrhoids.

MEDICAL DIAGNOSIS

External hemorrhoids are diagnosed by visual examination. Internal hemorrhoids are diagnosed

Chart 23–3.

NURSING GUIDE TO PATIENT EDUCATION FOR SELF-MANAGEMENT: SELF-CARE AFTER HERNIORRHAPHY

Instruct the patient to:

Expect pain and scrotal swelling for 24 to 48 hours.

Resume nonstrenuous activities gradually over 5 to 7 days.

Use good body mechanics.

Avoid heavy lifting and sexual activities for 6 to 8 weeks or in accordance with surgeon's instructions.

Avoid straining at stool.
- Eat a high-residue diet.
- Drink at least 2000 ml of fluid per day.
- Take stool softeners as ordered.

Report immediately incisional soreness or drainage, fever, or difficult urination.

through history, rectal examination, and visualization through an anoscope.

MEDICAL MANAGEMENT

Treatment of uncomplicated hemorrhoids is symptomatic. Sitz baths and topical preparations such as dibucaine ointment and witch hazel are used to shrink mucous membranes and relieve pain.

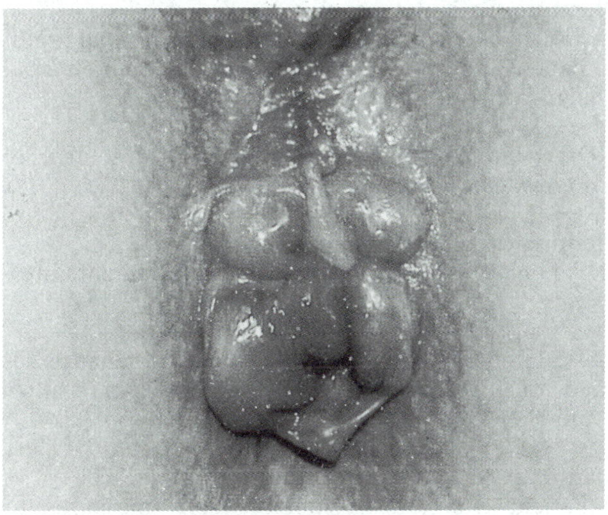

Figure 23–12.

Location and appearance of internal and external hemorrhoids. (From De Los Rios E. Atlas of therapeutic proctology. Philadelphia: WB Saunders, 1984, p 37.)

A high-fiber diet, 2000 ml of fluid per day, and stool softeners or mild laxatives are used to prevent constipation and to keep the stool soft and formed.

Internal hemorrhoids are sometimes treated with a sclerosing agent or rubber band ligation. In the former, a sclerosing agent such as 5% phenol in oil is injected into the subcutaneous tissue between and around the internal hemorrhoids, causing the tissue to fibrose and shrink, resulting in a reduction in the size of the mass. This is done on an out-patient basis but requires one to four injections 5 to 7 days apart.

Rubber band ligation is also done on an outpatient basis and requires multiple visits depending on the number of hemorrhoids present. In this procedure, rubber bands are put around the base of internal hemorrhoids that bleed or are prolapsed. This results in ischemia followed by necrosis and sloughing in about a week. No anesthesia is required for this procedure, and subsequent discomfort is readily controlled with aspirin or the like.

Neither injection of a sclerosing agent nor rubber band ligation is used for external hemorrhoids because of the pain that would occur as a result of the sensory innervation of the area.

For patients with multiple prolapsed or thrombosed hemorrhoids and severe symptoms, hemorrhoidectomy is the treatment of choice. In this procedure, which may be done under regional anesthesia, the anal canal is first dilated and inspected with an anoscope. Each hemorrhoid is then grasped and excised and the base sutured. When all hemorrhoids are removed, petrolatum gauze packing may be placed in the anal canal and a dressing and T-binder applied.

Application of the Nursing Process to the Care of the Patient with Hemorrhoids

Assessment

Question the patient about rectal pain, itching, and bleeding. Note the frequency and severity of each. Determine the type and effectiveness of treatment measures used to relieve symptoms. Assess for lifestyle factors such as prolonged standing on the job, heavy lifting, or frequent pregnancy, which may contribute to the development or worsening of hemorrhoids.

Obtain information about bowel habits, because constipation, with straining at stool and sitting on the toilet for long periods of time, contributes to anal venous stasis. Explore the patient's usual diet and type of exercise, because these factors affect bowel function and can cause straining.

Nursing Diagnoses and Planning

The nursing diagnosis and related expected patient outcomes most commonly applicable to patients with hemorrhoids are as follows:

NDx: High risk for altered health maintenance related to insufficient knowledge of self-management of hemorrhoids

Planning: Patient outcomes
1. Patient describes measures to obtain symptomatic relief of hemorrhoids.
2. Patient explains relationship of constipation and other activities to hemorrhoids.
3. Patient lists symptoms that require medical evaluation.

Nursing Interventions

NDx: High risk for altered health maintenance
Review with the patient measures that are generally effective in providing symptomatic relief of hemorrhoids such as sitz baths, cold witch hazel compresses, and preparations such as dibucaine cream. Discuss constipation, straining at stool, and activities such as heavy lifting and prolonged standing as aggravating factors. Explain the importance of dietary fiber, large amounts of fluid, and daily exercise in preventing constipation.

Instruct the patient to obtain medical care if excessive pain, bleeding, or prolapse of hemorrhoids occurs.

Evaluation

Evaluate the effectiveness of nursing care for a patient with hemorrhoids by comparing the patient's status with the expected patient outcomes. Examples of specific outcomes for patients with hemorrhoids have been provided in the Planning section.

Application of the Nursing Process to the Care of the Patient After Hemorrhoidectomy

Assessment

Check vital signs, and assess the patient's discomfort. Inspect the rectal area for bleeding every 2 to 4 hours during the first 24 hours after surgery.

Measure urinary output, because difficulty voiding is not unusual.

Assess for anxiety over defecation.

Nursing Diagnoses and Planning

Nursing diagnoses and related expected patient outcomes most commonly applicable to patients who have had a hemorrhoidectomy include the following:

NDx: Pain related to surgical trauma to the anal area

Planning: Patient outcomes
1. Patient reports that pain is relieved by analgesics.
2. Patient moves freely without verbal or nonverbal signs of pain.

NDx: High risk for constipation related to fear of pain on defecation

Planning: Patient outcomes
1. Patient passes soft, formed stool at regular intervals.

NDx: High risk for altered health maintenance related to insufficient knowledge of self-care after hemorrhoidectomy

Planning: Patient outcomes
1. Patient describes or demonstrates measures to promote healing.
2. Patient lists measures to decrease the risk of recurrence.

Chart 23–4.

NURSING GUIDE TO PATIENT EDUCATION FOR SELF-MANAGEMENT: SELF-CARE AFTER HEMORRHOIDECTOMY

Instruct the patient to:

Report symptoms of complications such as bleeding, increased pain, purulent drainage, or fever.

Take sitz baths after bowel movements for 1 to 2 weeks for cleanliness and comfort.

Prevent constipation.
- Take stool softener as ordered.
- Eat high-fiber diet.
- Drink at least 2000 ml/day.
- Exercise regularly.

Avoid prolonged sitting or standing.

Lose weight if obese.

Nursing Interventions

NDx: Pain
Do not underestimate the extent of the patient's discomfort because hemorrhoidectomy, although not major surgery, is very painful. Give analgesics as ordered. Provide a flotation pad or soft ring cushion for the patient when lying supine to relieve pressure. Give sitz baths, which promote comfort and healing by helping keep the area clean and reducing edema.

Monitor the patient during the first sitz baths because dilation of the pelvic veins can cause hypotension during the early postoperative period. Limit sitting to short periods of time, and provide a soft ring cushion for the patient to sit on if needed. If ordered, apply ice packs, warm compresses, or analgesic ointments.

NDx: High risk for constipation
Be alert to anxiety over having a bowel movement. Explain that some discomfort will occur but that it is expected. Administer stool softeners as ordered to keep the stool easy to pass. If the patient has not defecated by the second or third postoperative day and oil enemas are ordered, medicate for pain in advance and insert a well-lubricated enema tip gently into the rectum.

NDx: High risk for altered health maintenance
Instruct the patient in self-care measures, as specified in Chart 23–4, to promote uncomplicated healing and to decrease the risk of recurrence.

Additional Interventions
Help the patient out of bed to void. If difficulty voiding persists, give a sitz bath. Use a dressing held in place with a T-binder to absorb drainage if needed.

Evaluation

Evaluate the effectiveness of nursing care for a patient who has had a hemorrhoidectomy by comparing the patient's status with the expected patient outcomes. Examples of specific outcomes for patients who have had a hemorrhoidectomy have been provided in the Planning section.

Neoplasia

Polyps of the Colon

ETIOLOGY AND PATHOPHYSIOLOGY

Polyps are the most common benign tumor of the bowel, although their cause is unknown. Polyps arise from the mucosa of the bowel and project into its lumen. They may be single or multiple and hyperplastic, pedunculated (on a stalk), or flat (sessile) (Fig. 23–13).

Polyps are generally considered to be associated with some risk of cancer. This risk is greatest when

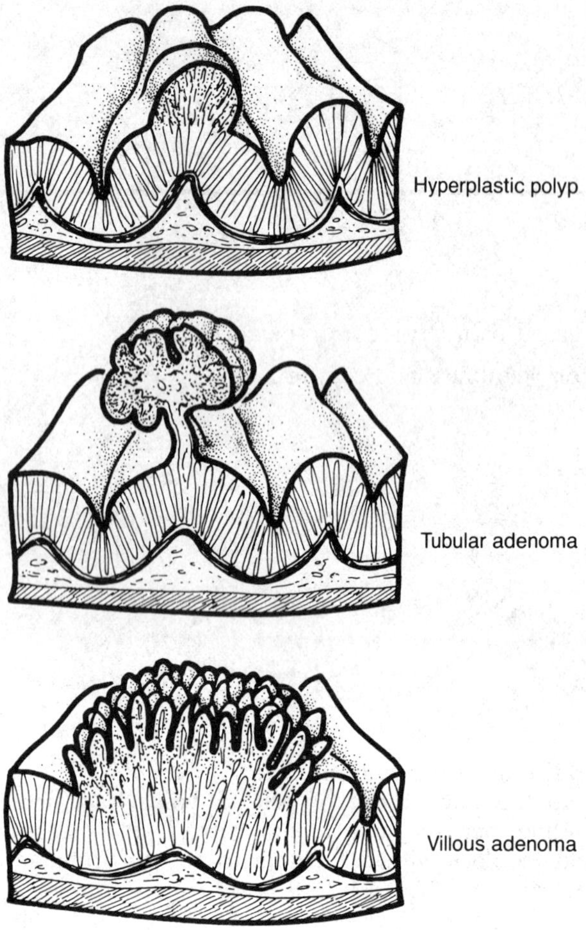

Figure 23–13.

A diagrammatic representation of the three principal forms of colonic polyps. The hyperplastic polyp (*above*) sits as a hemispheric dome on top of the mucosal fold. The tubular (pedunculated) adenoma (*middle*) has a slender stalk and a knobby raspberry-like head. The sessile villous adenoma (*below*) has a broad base and myriad delicate papillae protruding into the lumen. (From Robbins SL, Kumar V. Basic pathophysiology. 4th ed. Philadelphia: WB Saunders, 1987, p 552.)

polyps are multiple, larger than 2 cm in diameter, and histologically of the villous type. The risk is further increased if there is a family history of cancer. In familial polyposis, a rare genetic disorder in which there are multiple polyps along the intestine, there is a 100% association with cancer by age 40 years.

CLINICAL MANIFESTATIONS

Polyps are usually asymptomatic, although rectal bleeding and symptoms of iron deficiency anemia occasionally occur. Very large polyps can partially obstruct the colon and cause abdominal pain.

MEDICAL DIAGNOSIS

Polyps are most often diagnosed by sigmoidoscopy or barium studies of the colon. A biopsy is usually done in conjunction with sigmoidoscopy to rule out cancer. Small polyps in the rectal area can be diagnosed by digital rectal examination.

MEDICAL MANAGEMENT

Removal is the treatment of choice for polyps because of their malignant potential. In most cases, polyps can be removed by cautery snare through a colonoscope. Surgical excision may be used for large, sessile polyps.

After endoscopic polypectomy, a repeat colonoscopy is done 1 year later and then at least every 3 years.

Guidelines for Application of the Nursing Process to the Care of the Patient with a Polyp of the Colon

Nursing care of the patient with polyps of the colon primarily involves patient education. Explain the relationship between polyps and cancer of the colon. Be alert for signs of excessive anxiety in regard to this. Stress the effectiveness of follow-up rectal examinations and colonoscopies in identifying early malignant changes that can be effectively treated.

Cancer of the Colon and Rectum

The majority of cancers originating in the GI tract occur in the colon or the rectum. Of these, two thirds or more arise in the rectosigmoid area, with a significant portion within reach of the finger on rectal examination.

The incidence of cancers of the colon and rectum is equal in men and women and is highest between the ages of 50 and 65 years.

There is a good prognosis for persons with these cancers provided they are diagnosed and treated early. Unfortunately, in many cases the patient does not seek treatment until the cancer is too far advanced for successful treatment.

ETIOLOGY

The cause of colorectal cancer is unknown. However, it occurs most often among populations with diets low in fiber, high in refined carbohydrates, high in fats, and high in meat. Thus, it is suggested that prolonged transit time for stool in the intestine may predispose to carcinogenic changes.

Other risk factors associated with the development of colorectal cancer are a familial history of the disease, familial polyposis, rectal polyps, and active inflammatory bowel disease of at least 10 years' duration.

PATHOPHYSIOLOGY

Colorectal cancers are primarily adenomas and develop from the epithelial lining of the intestine (Fig. 23–14). The tumor may project into the lumen of the bowel or encircle the bowel, causing stenosis, ulceration, or perforation. Spread occurs by invasion through the bowel wall into adjacent organs such as the small intestine and uterus. It also occurs by metastasis via the lymphatic vessels and the portal vein. The liver is the most common metastatic site, although metastases to the lungs, kidneys, and bones also occur. The survival rate is proportional to the depth of the lesion and the number of lymph nodes involved at the time of surgery.

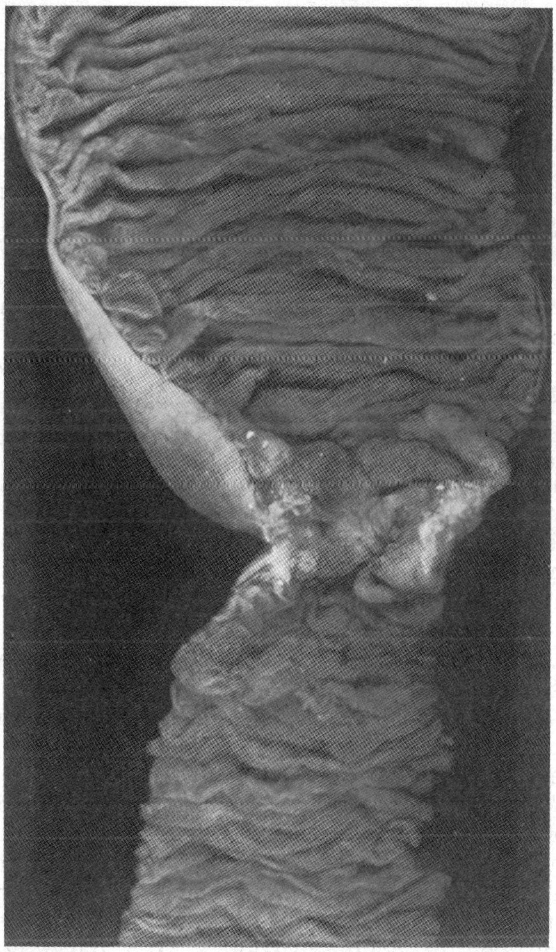

Figure 23–14.

Carcinoma of the rectosigmoid. Narrow annular lesion has caused obstructive dilatation of the proximal bowel above. (From Robbins SL, Kumar V. Basic pathophysiology. 4th ed. Philadelphia: WB Saunders, 1987, p 557.)

CLINICAL MANIFESTATIONS

Colorectal cancer is frequently asymptomatic in its early stages. When symptoms do occur, they vary somewhat according to the location of the tumor.

The first symptoms of left colon tumors are changes in bowel function that often go unnoticed as significant by the patient. These changes consist of constipation or diarrhea along with the gradual development of flat, ribbon-like, or pencil-shaped stools.

Other symptoms of left colon tumors are crampy gas pains, blood in the stool, which is bright red and coats the stool, and ultimately progressive abdominal distention and vomiting as obstruction becomes more complete.

Characteristic symptoms of right colon tumors include vague, dull abdominal pain, which is exacerbated by walking, and blood mixed in the stool, which appears dark red or mahogany. Symptoms of rectal cancer are straining at stool, a feeling of incomplete evacuation, a mucous discharge, bright red bleeding and, with advanced disease, pain.

Late symptoms of any colorectal cancer are weakness, anorexia, weight loss, and anemia. Once metastasis has occurred, signs of liver, respiratory, or renal failure may develop or complaints of back pain because of bone involvement may present.

MEDICAL DIAGNOSIS

The diagnosis of colorectal cancer is suggested when a patient presents with a combination of these symptoms. To establish the diagnosis, a rectal examination, barium studies, and colonscopy are done. Liver function tests, an intravenous pyelogram (IVP), and other studies are done to detect metastases and stage the disease.

MEDICAL MANAGEMENT

Medical management depends on the location of the tumor and the stage of the disease. Surgery is the treatment of choice because it is most effective. When possible, the section of bowel containing the tumor, along with a section of bowel on either side, is excised to eliminate the area of immediate lymphatic spread. The remaining bowel is then rejoined in an end-to-end anastomosis. Thus, for a tumor of the right colon, a right colectomy with an ileotransverse anastomosis is done, whereas for a tumor of the descending colon, a left colectomy is done with the transverse colon anastomosed to the sigmoid colon. For tumors low in the sigmoid or in the rectum where reanastomosis of the bowel is impossible, an abdominal perineal resection is done (see later discussion).

In some cases of widespread disease, palliative surgery is done. For example, when symptoms of obstruction are present, the involved area may be resected or bypassed or, if necessary, a colostomy is created proximal to the obstructed bowel.

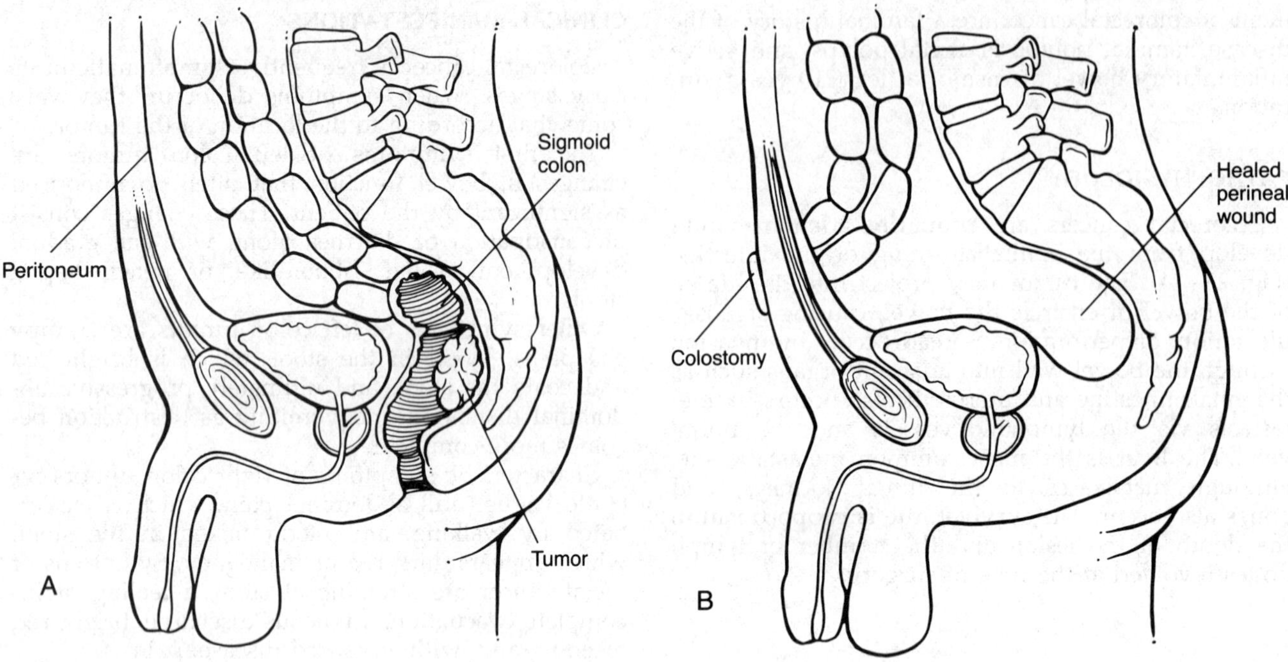

Figure 23–15.

Abdominal perineal resection. *A*, Anatomy prior to surgery. *B*, Anatomy after surgery.

Radiation may be given preoperatively to shrink the size of the tumor, and chemotherapy is occasionally given postoperatively to patients with extensive invasion or metastases. Radiation and chemotherapy are also used for palliation when tumors are inoperable.

Late in the disease, treatment simply consists of comfort measures and nutritional support. This may include continuous analgesic infusion via implantable pump and tube feedings or TPN given in the home, hospital, or hospice.

Abdominal Perineal Resection. An abdominal perineal resection is a procedure in which a colostomy is created and the distal sigmoid colon, rectum, and anus are removed (Fig. 23–15).

Physical Preparation of the Patient. Fluid and electrolyte imbalances are corrected. Nutritional status is improved through a high-calorie diet or even TPN depending on the patient's condition. Iron supplements or blood transfusions are given to correct anemia.

To reduce the risk of contamination at the time of operation, the bowel is emptied and cleansed. The patient is on a low-residue diet and then, for 2 to 3 days immediately before surgery, a liquid diet to prevent accumulation of feces. Laxatives and enemas are given to empty the bowel, and intestinal anti-infectives such as neomycin or kanamycin are administered to decrease the bacteria in the bowel.

A nasogastric tube is inserted for decompression as is an indwelling urinary catheter to keep the bladder empty during surgery.

Because formation of a colostomy is part of the surgical procedure, preparatory sessions with the enterostomal therapist are also an essential part of the patient's preparation.

Procedure. An abdominal perineal resection is a two-step procedure. First the abdomen is opened, the sigmoid colon cut above the level of the tumor, and the proximal end of the sigmoid brought out through a stab wound in the abdominal wall to form a colostomy. After closure of the abdominal incision, a perineal incision is made and the lower sigmoid, rectum, and anus, along with the skin, muscle, fat, and lymphoid tissue in the area, are removed. The perineal wound is then (1) closed completely with a suction drainage tube in place in the wound through incisions made on either side of it, (2) partially closed with a Penrose drain in place in the midline, or (3) left open and packed to heal by granulation. Generally the first method is preferred except in cases of contamination or active infection.

Postoperative Course. Immediately after surgery, profuse serosanguineous drainage is expected. Suction drainage tubes are left in place attached to low, continuous suction or to a portable suction apparatus such as a Hemovac until drainage is less than 50 ml per 24 hours, usually 3 to 5 days. Both Penrose drains and packing are removed gradually over a period of 5 to 7 days. An indwelling catheter is in place for 5 to 7 days to prevent urinary retention and pressure of a full bladder on the perineal wound. It also helps keep the perineal dressing dry.

The patient is on NPO status and receives intravenous fluid and electrolytes until bowel function returns and stool is passed through the colostomy, which is usually in 5 to 7 days.

Parenteral nutrition may also be given during this time if the patient's nutritional status needs improvement.

The patient is ambulatory in 24 to 48 hours and is usually discharged in 10 to 12 days. The perineal wound can heal in 2 to 4 months, although 6 to 8 months is not uncommon.

After hospitalization, the patient is monitored closely for signs of recurrence of the malignancy. This often includes repeated tests for carcinoembryonic antigens (CEA), antigens normally present in the fetus but which, when found in the adult, are thought to be specific for cancerous tumors. A drop in the CEA level after surgery is consistent with complete tumor removal. No decrease or an increase is indicative of residual tumor or spread.

Complications. Complications of abdominal perineal resection are many. They include hemorrhage, infection, impaired wound healing, persistent draining perineal sinus tract, urinary dysfunction, and impotence.

Application of the Nursing Process to the Care of the Patient Having an Abdominal Perineal Resection

PREOPERATIVE NURSING CARE

Preoperative nursing care of a patient scheduled for an abdominal perineal resection involves the basic assessments and interventions that apply to any surgical patient. Pay particular attention to GI and nutritional status in terms of immediate care needs, ability to tolerate the preoperative tests and bowel preparation, and the propensity for a successful surgical outcome.

POSTOPERATIVE NURSING CARE

Assessment

Assess the patient's return to physiologic stability. Check blood pressure, pulse, and respiration at least every 15 minutes and then at increasing intervals. Inspect the stoma for signs of hemorrhage. Remember that a small amount of oozing is expected; frank bleeding is not. Also assess adequacy of blood supply to the stoma by observing its color, which should be a moist, deep pink to red. Note the degree of edema, keeping in mind that significant edema is normal as a result of surgical trauma but that it should decrease progressively over time.

Inspect the abdominal dressing for drainage. Later, when the dressing is changed or removed, observe the wound for approximation of the suture line, redness, edema, and drainage. Also check for abdominal distention, which can lead to dehiscence of the incision.

Inspect the perineal wound. If it is a closed wound, check the amount and color of drainage in the collection container. Observe the wound itself for signs of separation or infection. If it is a semiclosed or packed wound, examine for bleeding, excessive drainage, or unusual odor. Be certain to note any signs of necrosis.

Assess the patient for abdominal and perineal pain. Remember that perineal discomfort is worsened by sitting, so be certain to assess the amount of discomfort at this time. Also question about perineal itching because this is a common problem after perineal resection.

Assess for return of peristalsis. Listen for bowel sounds, and check for the passage of flatus. When the colostomy begins to function (usually within 72 hours after surgery, although it may take up to 5 days), note the color, consistency, and amount of stool. Be certain to also inspect the peristomal skin for signs of irritation or excoriation.

Assess fluid, electrolyte, and nutritional status. Measure intake, output, and daily weight. Review serum electrolyte data, and observe for signs of dehydration.

Assess function of the urinary tract. Observe for signs of infection. Note the color of the urine and its clarity. When the catheter is removed, check for retention and, in men, for incontinence, which can occur as a result of the surgery.

Throughout the postoperative period, assess the patient's emotional reaction to the surgery and coping ability. Note willingness to speak of the surgery and its effects and whether or not the patient looks at the wounds and the stoma or asks questions about them. Note the degree of patient cooperation with and participation in care as well as the patient's outlook toward the future.

Nursing Diagnoses and Planning

Nursing diagnoses and related expected patient outcomes most commonly applicable to patients who have had an abdominal perineal resection include the following:

NDx: Pain related to surgical trauma to the abdomen and perineum

Planning: Patient outcomes

1. Patient moves without signs of severe pain such as moaning, pallor, and tachycardia.
2. Patient rests quietly without signs of discomfort such as clenched hands, groaning, and crying.
3. Patient reports pain is relieved.

NDx: High risk for ineffective breathing pattern related to shallow breathing secondary to incisional pain on deep breathing

Planning: Patient outcomes
1. Patient coughs and deep breathes as directed.
2. Lung sounds remain clear to auscultation.
3. Arterial blood gases are within normal range.

NDx: Impaired tissue integrity related to presence of large perineal wound

Planning: Patient outcomes
1. Drainage is serosanguineous and decreases progressively over 4 to 5 days.
2. Suture line of a closed wound is approximated.
3. Granulation tissue forms in open wounds.

NDx: Bowel incontinence related to the formation of a colostomy and loss of rectal function

Planning: Patient outcomes
1. A selected pouching system is used effectively to collect fecal drainage.
2. Patient identifies factors such as change in diet and times of eating that affect the pattern of colostomy function.

NDx: High risk for altered nutrition: less than body requirements, related to inadequate intake of nutrients and/or impaired absorption

Planning: Patient outcomes
1. Patient maintains expected weight.
2. Patient resumes oral intake of a nutritionally balanced diet.
3. Patient takes nutritional supplements as directed.

NDx: High risk for impaired skin integrity related to irritating effects of colostomy drainage and removal of adhesives on the peristomal skin

Planning: Patient outcomes
1. Peristomal skin is intact.
2. Peristomal skin is free of erythema.
3. Patient denies burning or soreness of the peristomal skin.

NDx: High risk for altered oral mucous membrane related to NPO status and presence of a nasogastric or nasointestinal tube

Planning: Patient outcomes
1. Oral mucous membrane is moist and free of cracks.
2. Lips are moist, supple, and free of cracks.
3. Patient denies dryness of the mouth.

NDx: High risk for altered peripheral tissue perfusion related to thrombophlebitis secondary to venous stasis

Planning: Patient outcomes
1. Patient does foot and leg exercises as directed.
2. Calves and upper thighs are free of redness, swelling, heat, and pain.
3. Homans' sign is negative.

NDx: Body image disturbance related to loss of bowel control, presence of a perineal wound and a stoma, release of fecal material onto the abdomen, passage of flatus, odor, need for an appliance

Planning: Patient outcomes
1. Patient verbalizes acceptance of self with the colostomy and the perineal wound.
2. Patient identifies own strengths.
3. Patient expresses pleasure at visits from relatives or friends.
4. Patient verbalizes interest in grooming and appearance.

NDx: High risk for sexual dysfunction related to the effects of the abdominal and perineal surgery

Planning: Patient outcomes
1. Patient discusses sexual concerns openly.
2. Patient describes potential effects of the surgery on sexual function.
3. Patient verbalizes optimism about resuming a sexual relationship.

NDx: High risk for altered health maintenance related to insufficient knowledge of self-care after discharge

Planning: Patient outcomes
1. Patient demonstrates wound care and colostomy care.
2. Patient describes dietary regimen.
3. Patient lists prescribed medications, giving name purpose, dose, route, time, and side effects.
4. Patient identifies community resources.
5. Patient lists symptoms to be immediately reported.

Nursing Interventions

NDx: Pain
Give prescribed analgesics every 3 to 4 hours for 72 hours. Remember that the patient will have a great deal of pain not only from the abdominal incision but also from the perineal incision. Keep the patient physically comfortable to aid in the effectiveness of the analgesics. Place the patient in a side-lying position with the knees flexed to reduce stress on the incision line. Have the patient change position every 2 hours. Avoid the dorsal recumbent position, which is uncomfortable because of pressure on the perineal wound and may interfere with drainage and healing.

Teach the patient to splint the abdominal incision when turning, coughing, and deep breathing, and time wound care so that it is done when analgesics given are at their peak effectiveness. Give sitz baths, and apply antipruritics for discomfort from perineal itching, which is a common occurrence as the wound begins to heal. When the patient is out of bed, encourage short walks rather than sitting in a chair. When sitting is necessary, provide a soft foam ring to increase comfort.

If "phantom" rectal pain is a problem, explain that it occurs because the sympathetic nerves, which used to control the rectum, are still intact even though the rectum was removed. Reassure the patient that it is not an indication of a complication and should disappear with time.

NDx: High risk for ineffective breathing pattern

Teach the patient to splint the abdomen with pillows, and assist in turning, coughing, and deep breathing every 2 hours for 72 hours after surgery. Instruct the patient in the use of an incentive spirometer. Reassure the patient that coughing and deep breathing, despite the fact that they may hurt, will not damage the incision or the ostomy. When the patient is able, ambulate at least three times per day.

NDx: Impaired tissue integrity

Reinforce and change the perineal dressing as often as needed to keep the area dry. Cleanse the rectal area frequently to prevent odor and skin irritation. Use a T-binder or similar device to hold the dressing in place without the use of adhesive tape.

If the perineal wound is closed with drains attached to suction, monitor the function of the apparatus, and record the amount and color of the drainage. Expect the drains to be removed when drainage has decreased to less than 50 ml per 24 hours, which is usually in 3 to 5 days.

After their removal, give sitz baths three times per day to promote comfort and healing both before and after the drains are removed. If the perineal wound is semiclosed with Penrose drains in place, give sitz baths three times a day after the drains are removed.

Irrigate open wounds as ordered at least four times per day after the packing is removed 3 to 4 days postoperatively. Use a hand-held shower device or an Asepto syringe. Irrigate gently, because too much force can damage granulation tissue and increase the risk of introducing bacteria. Hold the tip several inches from the wound, and irrigate with a normal saline, hydrogen peroxide, or antibiotic solution as per the surgeon's orders. Apply streptokinase or streptodornase if ordered to debride the wound chemically.

NDx: Bowel incontinence

Use a colostomy appliance to collect the feces expelled involuntarily from the colostomy. In most cases, a clear plastic, open-ended collection pouch is placed over the colostomy at the time of surgery. Monitor this pouch for the accumulation of flatus or drainage and empty or change as necessary. Subsequently, assist the patient in the selection of a collection system for daily use that is best suited to his or her needs. If the patient is unable to perform self-care and will be dependent on a spouse or significant other for assistance, include that person in the selection process. Once a system is selected, use it consistently to eliminate confusion and facilitate the patient's learning of self-care.

Explain that control over fecal expulsion may be gained in time by means of a regular diet or periodic irrigation and that a collection pouch may not be needed all the time. To assist the patient in achieving control, instruct the patient in basic dietary considerations as presented in Nutrition Box 21–1 and in the importance of maintaining a regular pattern of eating and exercise.

NDx: High risk for altered nutrition: less than body requirements

If the patient is vomiting, give antiemetics as prescribed. Administer TPN if ordered. When oral intake is resumed, give small amounts of clear fluids of the patient's choice. If these are tolerated without singultus, nausea, vomiting, or other discomfort, gradually progress to full fluids and then to a regular low-residue diet. Give nutritional supplements as ordered, and promptly alert the physician to any weight loss.

NDx: High risk for impaired skin integrity

Remove mucus or feces with a tissue, and thoroughly wash the peristomal skin. Rinse carefully to remove all soap residue, and dry gently and completely. Omit the soap if dry skin is a problem, but do not use oily soaps or emollients because these interfere with the adherence of an appliance. Use a skin barrier to protect the eighth of an inch of exposed skin between the stoma and the pouch opening from exposure to fecal drainage. Apply a skin sealant to the peristomal skin areas where adhesive will be used, and position the collection pouch snugly in place. Monitor for leaking from the pouch, and change immediately should it occur. If skin irritation develops, institute immediate treatment as described in Chapter 21.

NDx: High risk for altered oral mucous membrane

Assist the patient to brush the teeth at least three times per day. Encourage frequent mouth rinses with dilute mouthwash or saline solution. Avoid the use of solutions with a drying effect on mucous membranes. Apply water-soluble lubricant to the lips to keep them supple and prevent cracking.

NDx: High risk for altered peripheral tissue perfusion

Guide the patient in foot and leg exercises 10 times each every 2 hours while on bed rest. Apply antiembolic stockings or Ace bandages to further support venous return. Avoid use of the knee gatch, pillows under the knees, or any other form of pressure in the popliteal space. Assist the patient out of bed, and begin ambulation as ordered in 24 to 48 hours after surgery. Instruct the patient to avoid crossing the legs or sitting for long periods of time.

NDx: Body image disturbance
Acknowledge to the patient that ambivalent feelings about the surgery are normal because on the one hand it is a potentially life-saving procedure, yet on the other hand it involves a change in both body appearance and function. Recognize that patients often experience fear of rejection, disgust, or shame, and be certain that comments, facial expressions, or other nonverbal behaviors convey acceptance and not revulsion, distaste, or pity.

Recognize that denial is a common reaction to this surgery, and permit its use while also promoting acceptance. Describe the appearance of the stoma and the perineal wound, and refer to them by name when giving care. Also offer to provide a mirror for the patient to view the wounds if desired. Do not force the patient to look at the wounds, but be certain to indicate that there is nothing abnormal in wanting to see the effects of the surgery on the body.

Protect the patient from undue embarrassment by providing privacy during care, discussions, and teaching and by taking steps to keep the patient and the environment odor free.

Encourage the patient to be well groomed, and discuss how the ostomy and pouch are not visible under clothing if styles are selected with a bit of care. Foster a sense of control by allowing the patient to make decisions whenever possible and assisting the patient to incorporate colostomy care into the daily routine.

Promote communication of feelings between the patient and significant others, and encourage family and friends to treat the patient normally.

NDx: High risk for sexual dysfunction
Encourage the patient to express feelings and ask questions about sexual function, and whenever possible include the spouse in the discussion. Make certain that the male patient understands that, although sexual dysfunction is a potential complication of this surgery, erection, ejaculation, and orgasm involve different nerve pathways so that sexual dysfunction, if it occurs, is not necessarily complete. Also inform the patient that if impotence should occur and persist for more than 3 months, a penile implant could be considered.

NDx: High risk for altered health maintenance
Instruct the patient in the care of the abdominal wound, the perineal wound, and the colostomy. Begin teaching as soon as the patient's condition allows postoperatively. Provide the information the patient needs and requests, but avoid unnecessary detail, which may create anxiety or confusion. Encourage participation of family members who will be assisting with the patient's care or purchasing supplies and equipment. Repeat information as needed, and provide written care instructions because what is explained under stress tends to be easily forgotten. Teach the patient to change the appliance, do peristomal skin care, take sitz baths, and eat a balanced diet while avoiding foods that cause constipation or diarrhea. Also teach the patient about the action, purpose, side effects, and administration of prescribed drugs. Inform him or her about available community resources such as the United Ostomy Association and the American Cancer Society, which offer information, counseling, and other support services.

Instruct the patient to report stenosis, prolapse, or retraction of the stoma, irritation of the peristomal skin, bleeding, abdominal distention or rigidity, and persistent diarrhea. Also instruct the patient to weigh him or herself weekly and to report the loss of more than 2 pounds.

Evaluation

Evaluate the effectiveness of nursing care for a patient who has had an abdominal perineal resection by comparing the patient's status with the expected patient outcomes. Examples of specific outcomes for patients who have had an abdominal perineal resection have been provided in the Planning section.

The Elderly: Special Considerations

There is no lower GI disorder that is unique to the aged, nor is the overall prevalence of these disorders greater among the elderly than the rest of the population. Nonetheless, lower GI diseases are an important cause of both morbidity and mortality among the aged.

With aging, there is atrophy of the muscle and the mucosa throughout the small and large intestines, but there does not appear to be significant changes in either motor or secretory function. There does appear to be some decrease in absorption, particularly in the absorption of fats and vitamin B_{12}, however, because of the decrease in intestinal epithelial cells. Malabsorption syndromes in the elderly differ from those in the younger adults in the presenting symptoms. Diarrhea is the most common symptom among the younger groups, whereas symptoms caused by the secondary effects of malabsorption such as fatigue from anemia or bone pain from osteomalacia predominate in the elderly.

Diverticular disease occurs with increasing frequency as age advances, affecting approximately 40% of all individuals older than 70 years. It is thought that the increase in duodenal diverticula found in the aged contributes to the development of bacterial overgrowth, which in turn can cause malabsorption.

Ischemia of the small intestine can occur in the elderly because of acute occlusion of the mesenteric vessels, thrombosis of the mesenteric vessels, or a decrease in cardiac output secondary to shock, myocardial infarct, or sepsis. Symptoms of intestinal ischemia resulting from an acute embolism are abdominal pain, distention, and fever. When ischemia is widespread, diarrhea, which may be bloody, leukocytosis, and hemoconcentration also occur. Ischemia caused by thrombosis, on the other hand, develops over a number of hours or days and is characterized by nonspecific abdominal pain. Management of these mesenteric vascular disorders consists of replacement of intravascular volume, correction of acidosis, and surgical resection of the intestine with or without vascular bypass or endarterectomy.

Another form of intestinal ischemia that occurs in the elderly is abdominal angina. This is a chronic disease caused by atherosclerosis of the mesenteric vessels. It is characterized by severe, crampy pain occuring 20 to 30 minutes after eating and is often accompanied by diarrhea, steatorrhea, and marked weight loss. It is diagnosed by angiography and is treated with small, frequent feedings or surgical revascularization.

Inflammatory bowel disease is also a problem in the elderly. A significant number of cases of ulcerative colitis develop after the age of 60 years. In many of these, the initial attack is more severe than when the disease develops at a younger age, and there is a greater incidence of megacolon and peritonitis. It is also true, however, that if this initial attack is severe, the older patient is less likely to experience a relapse.

Another common lower GI problem of the elderly is hemorrhoids. These may develop in old age or may be a recurrence of an earlier problem. The immediate precipitating factor is often chronic constipation, but multiple pregnancies and years of work requiring one to stand on the feet are common predisposing factors.

Appendicitis is an example of a disorder that is usually minor in younger patients but can be very serious in the elderly. Its occurrence is rare in the older population because of the tendency for lymphoid atrophy, which obliterates the lumen of the appendix. When it does occur, however, there are two major problems. First, the reduced lymph tissue, which normally prevents infections, makes systemic infection more likely. Second, the reduced blood flow to this area of the colon means that appendicitis in the elderly is often associated with gangrene. In addition, the initial signs and symptoms of appendicitis may be absent or atypical in the older patient, but a rapid, severe course may follow. Peritonitis readily develops, and mortality rates are 12% in those older than 60 years and 30% in those older than 70 years.

Bibliography

Baer CL, Williams BR. Clinical pharmacology and nursing. Springhouse, PA: Springhouse, 1988.

Bennett JR. Practical gastroenterology. New York: Macmillan, 1988.

Berk JE, Haubrich WS, Kalser MH, et al. (eds). Bockus gastroenterology. 4th ed. Philadelphia: WB Saunders, 1985.

Bongiovanni GL. Essentials of clinical gastroenterology. 2nd ed. New York: McGraw-Hill, 1988.

Bouchier I, Allan R, Hodgson J, & Keighley M. Textbook of gastroenterology. London: Bailliere Tindall, 1984.

Brandt IJ. Gastrointestinal disorders of the elderly. New York: Raven Press, 1984.

Bryant R. Diverticular disease. J Enterostom Ther 1986; 13(3):114.

Burtis G, Davis J, Martin S. Applied nutrition and diet therapy. Philadelphia: WB Saunders, 1988.

Chwals WJ, Blackburn GL. Perioperative nutritional support in the cancer patient. Surg Clin North Am 1986; 66(6):1137.

Cooke D. Inflammatory bowel disease: Primary health care management of ulcerative colitis and Crohn's disease. Nurse Pract 1991; 16(8):27.

Cormack D (ed). Geriatric nursing—Conceptual approach. Oxford, England: Blackwell Scientific Publications, 1985.

De Los Rios E. Atlas of therapeutic proctology. Philadelphia: WB Saunders, 1984.

Deters G. Managing complications after abdominal surgery. RN 1987; 50(3):27.

Eastwood GL. Core textbook of gastroenterology. Philadelphia: JB Lippincott, 1984.

Edwards J, et al. Helping the emergency colostomy patient through reality shocks. Nursing 1987; 17(7):63.

Esberger KK, Hughes ST Jr. Nursing care of the aged. Norwalk, CT: Appleton & Lange, 1989.

Finne CO. Cancer of the colon. J Enterostom Ther 1986; 13(5):196.

Flynn KT, Norton LC, Fisher RL. Enteral tube feeding: Indications, practices and outcomes. Image: J Nurs Scholarship 1987; 19(1):16.

Gambert SR (ed). Handbook of geriatrics. New York: Plenum Press, 1987.

Given B, Simmons S. Gastroenterology in clinical nursing. 4th ed. St. Louis: CV Mosby, 1984.

Greenberger NJ. Gastrointestinal disorders. 4th ed. Chicago: Year Book Medical Publishers, 1990.

Groth K. Age-related changes in the gastrointestinal tract. Geriatr Nurs 1988; 9(5):278.

Ham RJ, Sloane PD. Primary care geriatrics. 2nd ed. St. Louis: Mosby Year Book, 1991.

Hamilton H. Gastrointestinal disorders. Springhouse, PA: Springhouse, 1985.

Hively-Petillo M. Psychologic factors and inflammatory bowel disease. J Enterostom Ther 1985; 12(6):214.

Hoexter B, Labow SB, Moseson M. Common diseases of the anus and rectum. Hosp Med 1985; 21(9):110.

Iber FL, Baum RA. Gastroenterology: A concise textbook (concise textbook series, Vol. 21). New York: Elsevier, 1987.

Jarvis C. Physical examination and health assessment. Philadelphia: WB Saunders, 1992.

Kinash RG. IBD: Implications for patients, challenges for nurses. Rehab Nurs 1987; 12(2):82.

Kirsner J, Shorter RG (eds). Inflammatory bowel disease. 3rd ed. Philadelphia: Lea & Febiger, 1988.

Krause M, Mahan L. Food, nutrition & diet therapy. 7th ed. Philadelphia: WB Saunders, 1984.

Lamy PP. Treating GI upset in older adults. J Gerontol Nurs 1985; 11(7):40.
Maize-Grochowski A. When the Dx is Crohn's disease. RN 1991; 54(2):52.
Malseed RT, Harregan GS. Textbook of pharmacology and nursing care. Philadelphia: JB Lippincott, 1989.
Mathewson M. Pharmacotherapeutics—A nursing process approach. Philadelphia: FA Davis, 1986.
Matteson MA, McConnell ES. Gerontological nursing: Concepts and practice. Philadelphia: WB Saunders, 1988.
McConnell EA. Meeting the challenge of intestinal obstruction. Nursing 1987; 17(7):34.
McCormack A, Itkin J, Cloud C. If your patient develops peritonitis. RN 1987; 50(3):31.
Meeker MH. Alexander's care of the patient in surgery. 9th ed. St. Louis: CV Mosby, 1991.
Meguid MM, Meguid V. Preoperative identification of the surgical cancer patient in need of postoperative supportive total parenteral nutrition. Cancer 1985; 55(Suppl 1):258.
Messner R, Gardner S, Lewis S. Crohn's disease—More than a chronic illness. Occup Health Nurs 1985; 33(12):604.
Messner RL, Gardner SS. Stop a killer with early detection . . . colorectal cancer. J Gerontol Nurs 1985; 11(11):8.
Messner RL, Gardner SS, Webb DD. Early detection: The priority in colorectal cancer. Cancer Nurs 1986; 9(1):8.
Mettlin C. Dietary factors for cancer of specific sites. Surg Clin North Am 1986; 66(5):917.
Nelson RL, Nyhus LM. Surgery of the small intestine. Norwalk, CT: Appleton & Lange, 1987.
Newfildt J. Helping the IBD patient cope with the unpredictable. Nursing 1987; 17(8):47.
Pounder R (ed). Recent advances in gastroenterology, No. 7. New York: Churchill Livingstone, 1988.
Ricker LE, et al. Colorectal carcinoma. AORN J 1989; 50(5): 1046.
Sabiston DC (ed). Textbook of surgery: The biological basis of modern surgical practice. 14th ed. Philadelphia: WB Saunders, 1991.
Savaiano DA, Kotz C. Recent advances in the management of lactose intolerance. Contemp Nutr 1988; 13(9):10.
Schrier RW. Geriatric medicine. Philadelphia: WB Saunders, 1990.
Sleisenger MH, Fordtran JS. Gastrointestinal disease: pathophysiology, diagnoses and management. 4th ed., Philadelphia: WB Saunders, 1988.
Smith CE. Detecting acute abdominal distention: What to look for, what to do. Nursing 1985; 15(9):39.
Smith, LH, Thier SO. Pathophysiology. The biological principles of disease. Philadelphia: WB Saunders, 1985.
Sodeman WA, Saladin TA, Boyd WP Jr. Geriatric gastroenterology. Philadelphia: WB Saunders, 1989.
Spiro H. Clinical gastroenterology. 3rd ed. New York: Macmillan, 1983.
Swonger AK, Matejski MP. Nursing pharmacology. Boston: Scott, Foresman/Little, Brown, 1988.
Turnberg J. Clinical gastroenterology. Chicago: Year Book–Mosby, 1989.
Weinrich SP, Blesch KS, Dickson GW, et al. Timely detection of colorectal cancer in the elderly. Cancer Nurs 1989; 12(3):170.
Welch JP. Bowel obstruction: Differential diagnosis and clinical management. Philadelphia: WB Saunders, 1990.
Williams SR. Nutrition and diet therapy. St. Louis: Times Mirror/Mosby, 1989.
Zadeh, AT, Kirchner B. Outpatient hemorrhoidectomy: Laser treatment and care results. AORN J 1986; 44(6):966.
Zuidema GD (ed). Shackelford's surgery of the alimentary tract. 3rd ed. Philadelphia: WB Saunders, 1991.

Chapter Twenty-four

NURSING CARE *of Adults with Disorders of the Accessory Organs of Digestion*

The exocrine pancreas and the gallbladder are accessory gastrointestinal organs in that each plays a role in the normal digestive process. The exocrine pancreas secretes pancreatic amylase, lipase, and proteases, enzymes that break down carbohydrates, fats, and proteins, respectively. The gallbladder stores bile, which emulsifies fat, stimulates pancreatic secretion, and activates pancreatic lipase.

Because of these functions, common symptoms of pancreatic and gallbladder disease relate to changes in the digestive process. Similarly, management of these disorders generally includes measures to promote return to normal digestion.

Infections and Inflammations

Cholecystitis

ETIOLOGY AND PATHOPHYSIOLOGY

Cholecystitis, or inflammation of the gallbladder, is almost always associated with cholelithiasis. Cholelithiasis refers to the presence of stones in the gallbladder, cystic duct, or common bile duct (Fig. 24–1). The exact cause of stone formation is unknown; however, bile stasis, imbalances in cholesterol metabolism, and infection seem to be precipitating factors. Stones, once formed, may remain in the gallbladder or migrate to the cystic or common bile duct, causing inflammation and obstruction.

In acute cholecystitis, vascular congestion, edema, and distention of the gallbladder develop within 24 to 48 hours after injury. Later, a cellular reaction occurs, which can lead to organ anoxia, necrosis, or gangrene.

Chronic cholecystitis is a persistent inflammation of the gallbladder probably caused by chemical or mechanical irritation from the stones. The chronic irritation results in a thickened, fibrotic mucosa and subsequent disorders of organ function.

CLINICAL MANIFESTATIONS

Early symptoms of cholecystitis include intolerance to fatty foods, nausea with or without vomiting, flatulence, elevated temperature, and right upper quadrant (RUQ) discomfort. In acute episodes, RUQ pain is intense and may radiate to the right scapula and shoulder. If the flow of bile is obstructed, jaundice, clay-colored stools, and dark-colored urine also are present.

MEDICAL DIAGNOSIS

Laboratory data indicative of cholecystitis include an elevated white blood cell count (WBC), alkaline phosphatase, aspartate aminotransferase (AST, formerly serum glutamic oxalo-acetic transaminase [SGOT]), and lactate dehydrogenase (LDH). If biliary obstruction is present, serum bilirubin levels are also elevated.

Diagnosis of cholelithiasis is confirmed by the visualization of gallstones. This may be accomplished through the use of cholecystosonography, cholecystogram, nuclear imaging, intravenous (IV) cholangiogram, or endoscopic retrograde cholangiopancreatography.

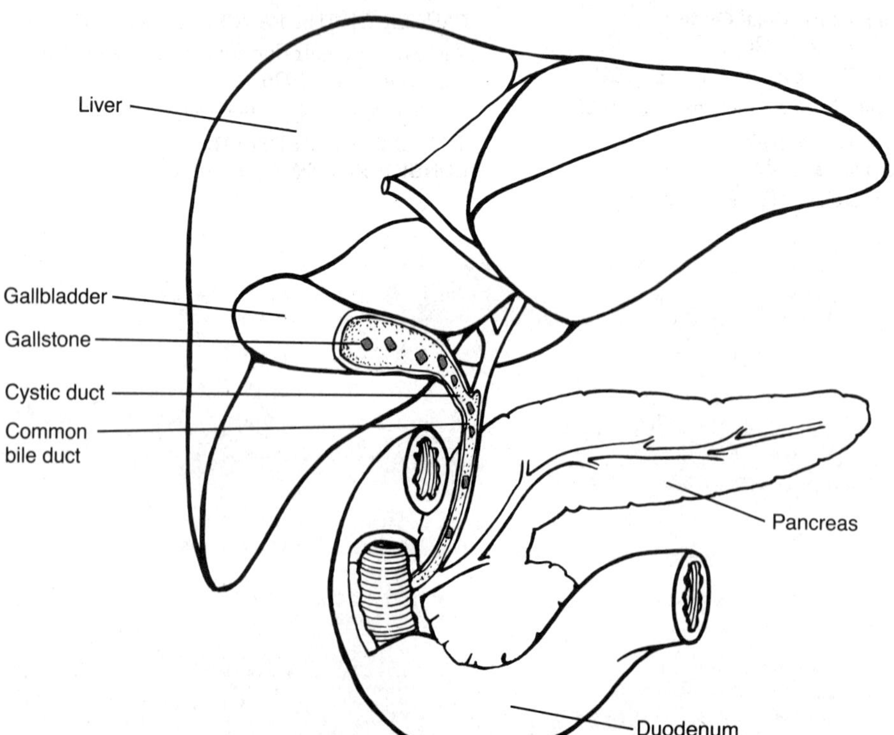

Figure 24–1.

Common locations of stones within the biliary tract.

MEDICAL MANAGEMENT

SUPPORTIVE MEASURES

Supportive treatment for acute cholecystitis includes the control of pain through the use of analgesics and anticholinergic drugs and the control of infection through the use of IV antibiotics. If nausea and vomiting are present, the patient is maintained on a nothing-by-mouth (NPO) order and has a nasogastric tube attached to suction in place. Fluid and electrolyte balance is maintained through replacement therapy. When tolerated, oral intake is begun with a low-fat, clear-liquid diet or minimal-fat, full-liquid diet, which is progressed gradually to a restricted but soft diet.

Supportive treatment of chronic cholecystitis includes a low-fat diet (Nutrition Box 24–1) and in some cases long-term therapy with oral gallstone-dissolving drugs such as chenodeoxycholic acid (CDCA) and ursodeoxycholic acid (see later discussion).

GALLSTONE DISSOLUTION THERAPY

Contact Solvents

Contact solvents are substances that, on contact, chemically react with cholesterol gallstones and cause them to dissolve.

Monooctanoin (Moctanin) is a contact solvent used to treat patients with large residual or newly formed gallstones in the bile duct after cholecystectomy. Monooctanoin is infused through a nasobiliary tube at a rate of 2 to 7 ml per hour for 1 to 3 weeks. During this time, a cholangiogram is done every 3 days to monitor the dissolution of the stones.

Anorexia, nausea, vomiting, and abdominal pain are potential side effects of this therapy. To help prevent them, the infusion is stopped during meals. In addition, the patient may be placed on a bland diet. When gastric upset occurs despite these measures, the infusion rate is slowed and antiemetics or antidiarrheals are given if necessary.

A second contact solvent, whose use in dissolving cholesterol stones present in the gallbladder is being investigated, is methyl tertiary butyl ether (MTBE). MTBE is instilled directly into the gallbladder by transhepatic catheter or by nasobiliary catheter inserted by endoscopic retrograde cannulation of the gallbladder (Foerster et al, 1990). Once the catheter is in place, the bile is aspirated from the gallbladder and the MTBE is instilled. After several minutes when the MTBE is saturated with dissolved cholesterol, it is aspirated and fresh MTBE is instilled. This is continued until fluoroscopy, which is done at 1- to 2-hour intervals, shows dissolution to be complete. The time for dissolution ranges from 45 minutes to 14 hours. It appears that the time is shorter when MTBE is instilled via nasobiliary catheter than by transhepatic catheter (Foerster et al, 1990).

Preparation for the procedure consists of an oral contrast dye given the night before fluoroscopy. Postprocedure care after transhepatic catheter insertion is similar to that after a liver biopsy (see Chapter 27). No specific care is required after nasobiliary catheter insertion.

Oral Bile Acids

CDCA (chenodiol) and ursodeoxycholic acid are bile acids. They facilitate the gradual dissolution of cholesterol gallstones by decreasing the amount of cholesterol in the bile and increasing cholesterol solubility. These drugs are taken daily and have been shown to dissolve small cholesterol stones successfully. This can take 6 months or more, and treatment for up to 2 years is common.

Side effects of bile acid therapy include diarrhea, which in most cases can be controlled by reducing the dose; gastritis, which can lead to gastric ulcers; and liver damage characterized by elevated liver enzymes. Oral bile acids also interfere with the action of oral contraceptives. When therapy is discontinued, gallstones may recur.

Oral bile acid therapy is used primarily for patients who are poor surgical risks or as prophylaxis against formation of new calculi in patients with recurrent cholecystitis. It is also used for patients after contact solvent therapy or lithotripsy (see later discussion) to promote dissolution of remaining stone fragments. Oral bile acid therapy is contraindicated for patients with gastric ulcers, liver disease, and atherosclerosis.

ENDOSCOPIC SPHINCTEROTOMY

Endoscopic sphincterotomy is a procedure in which the sphincter of Oddi, which surrounds the common bile duct where it empties into the duodenum, is incised. Stones may then be removed or allowed to pass spontaneously from the duct.

Physical Preparation of the Patient

For an endoscopic sphincterotomy, the patient is kept on NPO status from midnight before the procedure and in some cases receives prophylactic antibiotics.

Procedure

The patient is sedated with IV diazepam (Valium), and the throat is sprayed with lidocaine to eliminate the gag reflex. An endoscope is advanced through the mouth to the opening of the common bile duct in the duodenum. The opening of the duct is widened by cutting into the sphincter muscle, which surrounds it, with an electrodiathermy knife attached to the endoscope. If stones are to be removed, a tiny collapsed basket or deflated balloon on an accessory tip of the endoscope is maneuvered into the duct and past the stones. The basket is then opened and the stones scooped out or the balloon is inflated and the stones pulled out into the duodenum.

Nutrition Box 24–1.

NUTRITION: SPECIAL CONSIDERATIONS FOR PATIENTS WITH CHOLECYSTITIS

Instruct patients with chronic cholecystitis and those for whom gallbladder surgery is planned in the following:

To achieve a general decrease in dietary fat:

- Avoid fatty meats, sauces, and gravies.
- Avoid cream and rich desserts.
- Avoid fried and other fatty foods.

To limit total fat intake to a specific number of grams while not totally eliminating specific foods from the diet:

- Use a Fat Portion Exchange List (Table 24–1) to select type and amount of foods in the daily diet.
- Remember that the specified amount of each food item on the list provides five grams of dietary fat and is equal to one fat portion.
- Select the number of portions per day equal to the total amount of fat allowed in the daily diet. Example: For a daily diet containing 50 g of fat, select 10 portions.

Postprocedure Course

The patient remains on NPO status until the gag reflex returns, and then oral intake is resumed beginning with liquids as tolerated. IV fluid is discontinued when oral fluid intake is reestablished. Bed rest is maintained for 6 to 8 hours and normal routine is resumed within 4 or 5 days. Abdominal discomfort, which may persist for a couple of weeks, is treated with analgesics such as acetaminophen with codeine. The patient is told to observe for signs of bleeding (e.g., tarry stools, red or coffee-ground vomitus) and to report these or any fever or pain immediately.

Complications

Pancreatitis, perforation of the duodenum, and bleeding are potential complications of endoscopic sphincterotomy.

LITHOTRIPSY

Lithotripsy is a general term referring to the crushing of a stone. Lithotripsy procedures vary in the type of force used to crush the stone as well as the location of the stone in the body.

Mechanical Lithotripsy of Common Duct Stones

Mechanical lithotripsy is a variation on the endoscopic removal of stones from the common bile duct described previously. It is used for stones that are too large to be removed intact by a basket or balloon even with sphincterotomy. In a mechanical lithotripsy, the endoscope attachment inserted into the duct traps the stone in a basket device and then crushes it into small fragments, which can be expelled into the duodenum (Fig. 24–2). Sphincterotomy may or may not be done. In some cases, follow-up oral bile acid therapy may be prescribed.

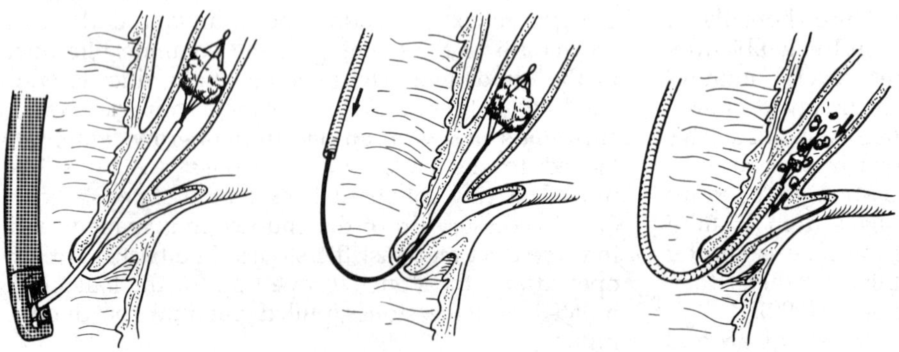

Figure 24–2.

Artist's illustration of a basket contained in a flexible cord spring sheath, with stone entrapped, handle attached, and stone crushed. (From Siegel JH, Ben-Zvi JS, Pullano WE. Mechanical lithotripsy of common duct stones. Gastrointest Endosc 1990; 36(4):353. © by the American Society of Gastrointestinal Endoscopy.)

Table 24–1. FAT PORTION EXCHANGE LIST

FOOD	AMOUNT EQUAL TO ONE FAT PORTION
FATS AND OILS	
Margarine, diet	1 tbsp
Margarine, soft	1 tsp
Mayonnaise, diet	1 tbsp
Mayonnaise, regular	$1\frac{1}{2}$ tsp
Avocado	2 tbsp
Bacon fat, lard	1 tsp
EGGS	
Egg yolk	1
Whole egg	1
DAIRY GROUP	
Evaporated whole milk	$\frac{1}{4}$ cup
1% milk, buttermilk	2 cups
Whole milk, regular, homogenized	$\frac{1}{2}$ cup
Cream cheese	1 tbsp
Heavy cream, fluid	1 tbsp
Egg nog	$\frac{1}{4}$ cup
Ice cream	$\frac{1}{3}$ cup
Ice milk	1 cup
American, blue, brick, colby cheese	$\frac{1}{2}$ oz
MEAT AND POULTRY*	
Beef, lean (choice-grade cooked, boneless, trimmed of all fat)	3 oz, most lean
Beef, rib roast, or steak	1 oz
Canadian bacon	2 oz
Chicken breast without skin	1 breast (5–6 oz)
Chicken breast with skin	$\frac{1}{4}$–$\frac{1}{3}$ breast
Ham, cured, extra lean	3 oz
Ham, cured, regular	$1\frac{1}{2}$ oz
Pepperoni	$\frac{1}{2}$ oz ($\frac{1}{2}$ slice)
Turkey ham	4 oz
Veal (except breast)	3 oz
FISH AND SEAFOOD†	
Cod, flounder, grouper, haddock, scallops, shrimp, lobster, sole	unlimited‡
Pike, pollock, turbot	16 oz
Tuna, canned in oil	2 oz
PROTEIN ALTERNATIVES	
Legumes, cooked; lima beans, split peas	6 cups
Tofu (soybean curd)	2–3 oz
CANNED SOUPS (made with water)	
Chicken noodle	$2\frac{1}{2}$ cups
Cream of celery, chicken, or mushroom	$\frac{3}{4}$ cup
Tomato	$2\frac{1}{2}$ cups
BREAD AND STARCH (high-fat snacks and desserts)	
Baked custard	$\frac{1}{2}$ cup
Cheesecake, pie	$\frac{1}{3}$ average piece
Corn bread	1 piece (2 in. × 3 in.)
Corn chips, potato chips	$\frac{1}{2}$ oz ($\frac{1}{2}$ small bag)
Croissant, danish	$\frac{1}{3}$ of one whole
Pancake, waffle, Pop-Tart, muffin	1
SWEETS	
Caramel, peanut brittle	2 oz (six small caramels)
Cocoa powder, unsweetened	6 tbsp
Fudge	1 oz

* Weight after cooking; no fat added.
† Raw weight.
‡ All fish and seafood for which the amount is unlimited contain so little fat that, if prepared without any added fat, the fat content is negligible.
Data from Boyar AP, Loughridge JR. The fat portion exchange list: A tool for teaching and evaluating low-fat diets. J Am Diet Assoc 1985; 85(5):589. Copyright Boyar/Loughridge AHF 1985. Reprinted by permission.

Extracorporeal Shock Wave Lithotripsy

Extracorporeal shock wave lithotripsy (ESWL) is a noninvasive, outpatient procedure that uses high-pressure or high-energy sound waves to break gallstones into small fragments, which can pass through the common bile duct into the duodenum. The machine that generates the shock waves is called a lithotriptor. All lithotriptors generate the waves in a liquid medium. These waves can then be propagated through living tissue because of its high water content, provided that the body is in contact with the water medium in which the shock wave was generated. "Coupled" refers to this contact of the body with the water medium. With "wet" lithotriptors, coupling is accomplished by placing the patient in a shallow pool of water or via a porthole in the lithotriptor table that opens to the fluid medium. With a dry lithotriptor (Fig. 24–3), the patient is coupled by lying on a flexible membrane, which in turn is in contact with the water medium. An ultrasound gel is placed on the surface of the membrane to couple it with the patient's body.

Physical Preparation of the Patient. Patients use a bisacodyl suppository the evening before lithotripsy and do not eat or drink for 12 hours before. This helps to decrease the risk of vomiting during the procedure as well as to decrease the gas in the intestine. Because intestinal gas interferes with shock waves, 80 mg of simethicone is taken after each meal, at bedtime, and on awakening in the morning beginning 24 hours before the procedure.

Procedure. An IV infusion is started to allow for administration of drugs if necessary. The lower chest and abdomen are exposed, and the patient is coupled to the lithotriptor. Because electrocardiogram (ECG), blood pressure, and oxygen saturation are monitored throughout the procedure, ECG leads, blood pressure cuff, and pulse oximetry monitor are put in place. The gallbladder is then imaged on an ultrasonogram so the stones can be targeted (to visualize stones in the common bile duct, a contrast medium must be introduced) and shock waves are begun. Approximately 1500 shocks are given during a period of 1 to 2 hours. The shock waves are synchronized with the heart rate to avoid triggering a dysrhythmia. As each is generated, a popping sound is heard and as it is propagated the patient may feel fluttering or a mild blow. Basically, lithotripsy is a painless procedure, although toward the end of the procedure some discomfort may result from lying in one position for an extended length of time and from the passage of stone fragments through the common bile duct. Because sudden movements and muscle tension can interfere with the procedure, a short-acting analgesic such as alfentanil is often given IV to maintain the patient's comfort.

Postprocedure Course. Because lithotripsy does not require general anesthesia or sedation, patients may return home and resume full activity as soon as the effects of any analgesic given have worn off. Transient gross hematuria may occur after treat-

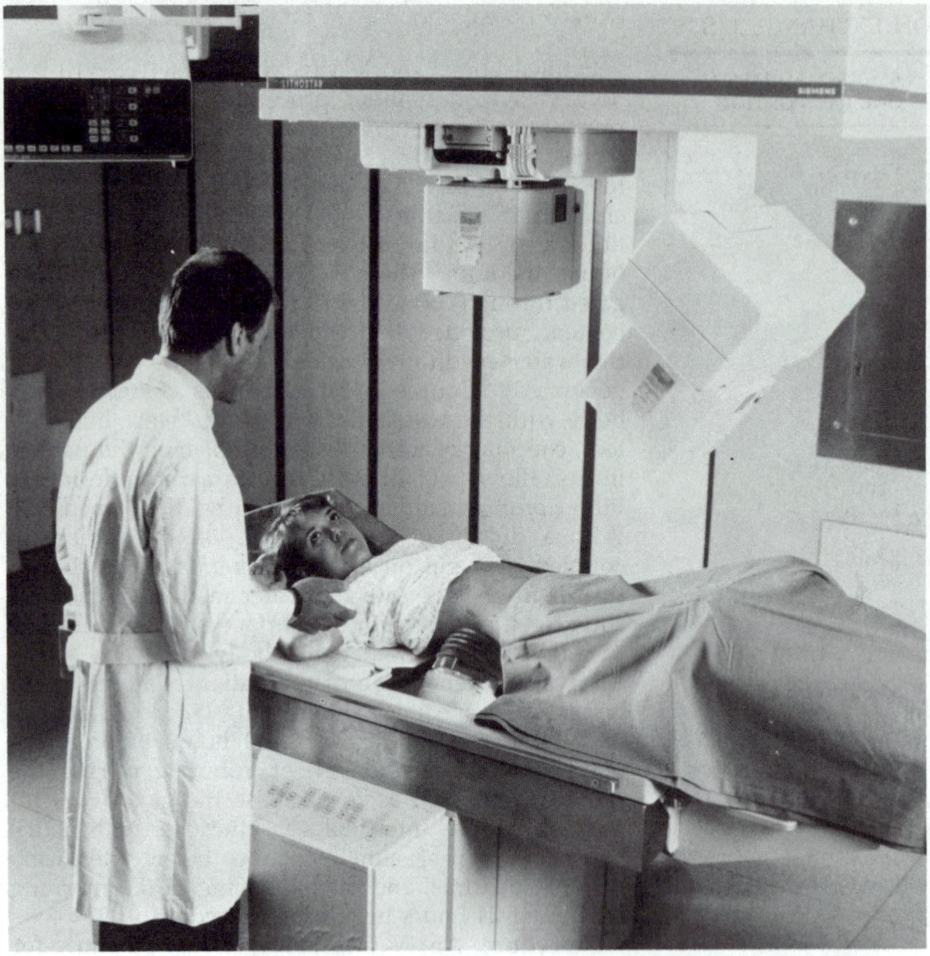

Figure 24–3.

Patient positioned on a dry lithotriptor. Note that the patient is lying on a flexible membrane that is in contact with the liquid medium in which the shock waves are generated. (Courtesy of Siemens Medical Systems, Inc.)

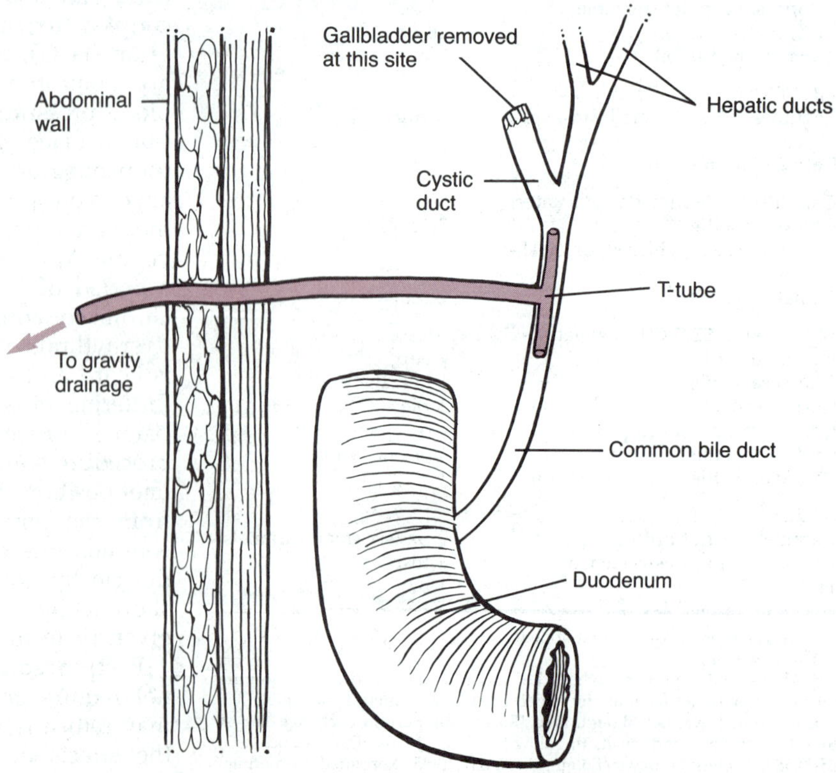

Figure 24–4.

Placement of a T-tube following cholecystectomy.

ment, and the patient may experience episodes of RUQ pain for 2 to 3 months as fragments of stone pass through the common bile duct. Adjuvant oral bile acid therapy is begun immediately, and the patient returns in 6 weeks for follow-up. At this time, an ultrasonogram is done to check the size of remaining stone fragments, and liver function tests are done to check for liver damage secondary to the oral bile acid therapy. Subsequent follow-ups are at 3-month intervals. Oral bile acids are continued until the patient is free of stone fragments on two successive follow-up visits. Patients are instructed to report fever, severe nausea and vomiting, jaundice, abdominal pain, and persistent hematuria.

Complications. Potential complications of ESWL are accidental damage to the gallbladder and surrounding tissues, acute cholecystitis, bile duct obstruction by stone fragments, pancreatitis, and stone recurrence.

SURGICAL INTERVENTION

A variety of surgical procedures are performed in the treatment of cholelithiasis and cholecystitis. These include cholecystectomy, the removal of the gallbladder; cholecystotomy, the opening of the gall bladder for decompression and drainage; choledochostomy, the creation of an opening into the common bile duct; and choledocholithotomy, the removal of a stone from the common bile duct. Of these, cholecystectomy is the procedure most often performed.

Cholecystectomy

Cholecystectomy is the surgical removal of the gallbladder. The two basic types of cholecystectomy are open cholecystectomy and laparoscopic cholecystectomy.

Physical Preparation of the Patient. Preoperative preparation for patients undergoing a cholecystectomy includes restriction of foods and fluids, cleansing enemas, and nipple-to-groin surgical skin preparation. If nausea and vomiting are present, a nasogastric tube attached to suction is used for gastric decompression. Patients with obstructive jaundice have their prothrombin time monitored and, if needed, are given vitamin K before surgery. Before laparoscopic cholecystectomy, a urinary drainage catheter and a nasogastric tube are inserted for decompression to decrease the risk of accidental puncture of the bladder or the stomach when the trocar (sharp-pointed instrument equipped with a cannula) is inserted. The urinary catheter and nasogastric tube are generally inserted in the operating suite and are removed in the recovery area.

Conventional Open Cholecystectomy

Procedure. Through a high right subcostal incision, the cystic duct is ligated and the gallbladder excised. A Penrose drain is inserted in the wound to prevent accumulation of drainage in the operative area. This drain exits through a stab wound on the abdominal wall close to the incision. If the patient is suspected of having stones in the bile duct, a choledocholithotomy, or incision into the common bile duct and removal of stones, is performed. Following this, a T-tube is placed in the duct to ensure its patency until the edema produced by the procedure subsides. The T-tube also prevents narrowing of the tube secondary to healing. Because the T-tube does not completely occlude the duct, some bile flows around the T-tube into the duodenum, and some flows into the drainage collection system (Fig. 24–4).

Postoperative Course. Postoperatively, breathing tends to be shallow because of the effect of anesthesia and the patient's reluctance to breathe deeply as a result of the pain, which is caused by the proximity of the incision to the diaphragm.

A sterile dressing covers the RUQ incision. Serosanguineous drainage with a small amount of bile is expected from the Penrose drain for the first 24 hours. Drainage then decreases and the Penrose drain is removed, usually in 48 hours. If a T-tube was inserted during surgery, the end of the tube leading to the drainage collection system is securely fastened to the dressing (Fig. 24–5). Drainage that is initially bloody and then turns green-brown is measured as output, with the amount ranging from 500 to 1000 ml per day. Excess bile drainage may be returned to the patient via the nasogastric tube to

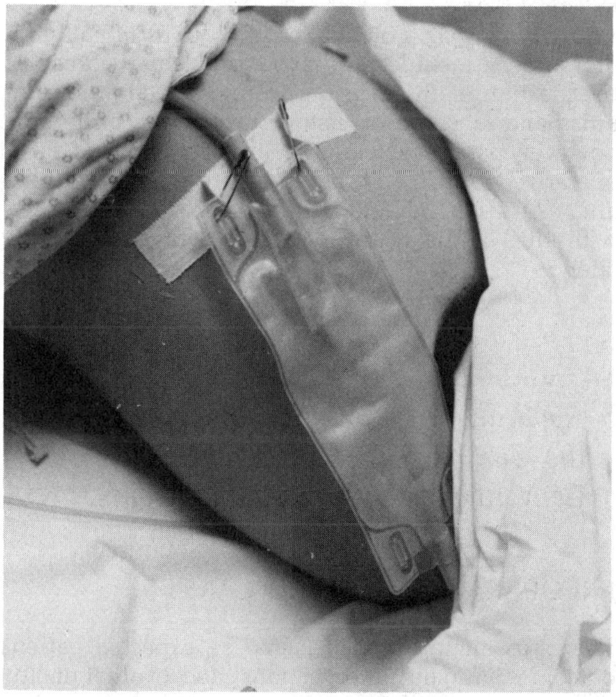

Figure 24–5.

Bile drainage bag in place. Note tape on abdomen, which allows bag to be pinned in such a way that the tube will not be dislodged.

prevent electrolyte imbalance, or replacement with synthetic bile salts such as dehydrocholic acid (Decholin) may be ordered. When drainage diminishes, a cholangiogram is done to confirm patency of the common bile duct, and then the surgeon removes the T-tube. Before this, the T-tube may be clamped for 1 hour before and after meals to allow bile to flow into the duodenum and to determine the patient's tolerance to the elimination of external drainage. If distress develops, the tube is immediately unclamped and the surgeon notified.

Fluids are administered intravenously for 24 to 48 hours. The patient's diet is then progressed as tolerated from clear fluids to soft, regular foods. Because bile flows continuously into the duodenum after removal of the gallbladder rather than periodically in response to fat intake, a few patients may be temporarily unable to tolerate large amounts of fat. For these patients, limited fat intake may be needed for up to a month. Fried food may need to be avoided by all patients despite an otherwise normal diet.

Generally, the patient is progressively ambulated beginning 8 hours after surgery. Return to work is generally in about 4 weeks.

Some ambulatory surgical centers are performing uncomplicated conventional cholecystectomies on selected patients. In these cases, patients can be discharged to the care of family members as few as 4 hours after surgery. They are instructed to remain on bed rest with bathroom privileges and a clear liquid diet for 24 hours, after which both activity and diet can be gradually increased. Follow-up is with a home health nurse and a visit to the surgeon in 1 or 2 days.

Complications. Potential complications of gallbladder surgery include respiratory problems because of the location of the incision, wound infection, peritonitis, and abscess or fistula formation. Generally, however, patients experience an uncomplicated postoperative course and are discharged 3 to 5 days after surgery. Sometimes patients are discharged with the T-tube clamped, which will be removed later.

Application of the Nursing Process to the Care of the Patient Having a Conventional Open Cholecystectomy

PREOPERATIVE NURSING CARE

The assessment, nursing diagnoses, expected patient outcomes, nursing interventions, and evaluation for patients scheduled for a cholecystectomy are similar to those for any other preoperative patient (see Chapter 4), with several considerations. After cholecystectomy, breathing tends to be shallow because deep breathing is painful as a result of the location of the incision. Therefore, assess respiratory status and teach prophylactic measures such as coughing and deep breathing carefully. Keep in mind that respiratory complications occur more frequently among patients who smoke.

In patients with obstructive jaundice, monitor the serum prothrombin, because a decrease in prothrombin increases the usual risk of postoperative bleeding.

POSTOPERATIVE NURSING CARE

Assessment

After a cholecystectomy, assessments are those required by any patient who has had major surgery. Take vital signs, measure intake and output, observe wound drainage for color and amount, monitor fluid intake, and observe IV site for signs of infiltration and irritation.

Assess respiratory excursion every hour for the first 6 hours, then every 2 to 4 hours for the remainder of the first 24 hours postoperatively. Auscultate the lungs every 4 hours for the next 2 to 3 days. Note shallow or guarded breathing, weak cough, and decreased or adventitious breath sounds.

Check for displacement of the T-tube. Every 2 hours, check for patency of the T-tube, and note the amount, color, consistency, and odor of the drainage. Keep in mind that drainage is initially bloody but changes to green-brown, that 500 to 1000 ml of drainage is expected in 24 hours, and that little or no drainage may indicate duct obstruction by a retained stone. Check the T-tube exit site for signs of infection and for bile drainage, which may indicate dislodgement of the tube.

Observe the color and amount of drainage from the Penrose drain. Inspect the suture line for signs of infection and the surrounding skin for signs of irritation caused by drainage from the Penrose drain.

Inspect sclerae for jaundice, and review WBC counts for elevation over 10,000/mm.[3] If a nasogastric tube is in place, check the amount and characteristics of drainage. Auscultate for bowel sounds and palpate for abdominal distention, because return of bowel sounds and a soft, nondistended abdomen indicate that oral intake may be resumed.

Nursing Diagnoses and Planning

Nursing diagnoses and related expected patient outcomes most commonly applicable to patients who have had a cholecystectomy include the following:

NDx: High risk for impaired gas exchange related to shallow breathing secondary to pain on deep breathing

Planning: Patient outcomes
1. Rate and depth of respirations are within patient's normal range.
2. Lungs are clear to auscultation.
3. Arterial blood gas values are within patient's normal limits.

NDx: High risk for impaired skin integrity related to copious drainage from the T-tube site

Planning: Patient outcomes
1. Skin is free from excoriation.
2. Dressing remains dry and intact.

NDx: High risk for altered tissue perfusion; peripheral, related to obstruction in venous return

Planning: Patient outcomes
1. Patient wears elastic stockings as instructed.
2. Patient performs foot and leg exercises as instructed.
3. Patient ambulates with assistance.
4. Calves and thighs are free of redness, tenderness, and heat.

NDx: High risk for altered health maintenance related to insufficient knowledge of self-care after discharge

Planning: Patient outcomes
1. Patient lists signs and symptoms that should be reported to a health care professional.
2. Patient demonstrates care of the wound.
3. Patient states date of follow-up appointment.

Nursing Interventions

NDx: High risk for impaired gas exchange
Medicate the patient every 3 to 4 hours for the first 24 to 48 hours after surgery because respiratory excursion is painful as a result of the location of the incision. Expect to administer an analgesic such as meperidine hydrochloride (Demerol) rather than morphine sulfate because the opiate drugs may increase biliary duct spasm. Thereafter, administer a milder analgesic as ordered to provide relief. Splint the incisional area while encouraging the patient to cough and deep breathe every hour in the early postoperative period. Place the patient in a low Fowler's position while in bed to reduce pressure on the diaphragm. Turn the patient every 2 hours and ambulate as soon as allowed.

NDx: High risk for impaired skin integrity
Change dressings frequently for the first 24 hours if a Penrose drain is in place, because the drainage contains bile that is very irritating to the skin. Use Montgomery straps to minimize skin irritation from frequent removal of tape. Cleanse the suture line and around the T-tube site with a sterile solution of normal saline or an antiseptic at each dressing change.

Avoid altering the position of the T-tube during dressing changes because if it becomes dislodged, surgical replacement may be required.

NDx: High risk for altered tissue perfusion; peripheral
Apply antiembolic stockings to help prevent thrombosis formation. Remind the patient to do foot and leg exercises every hour while awake as taught preoperatively. Encourage ambulation when permitted, and instruct ambulatory patients to avoid sitting or standing in one position for a long time.

NDx: High risk for altered health maintenance
Instruct the patient in self-care after discharge as presented in Chart 24-1. Be certain to explain the principles of asepsis as well as the ordered protocol for care of the wound and of the T-tube if present. Allow the patient to practice with supervision. Correct technique and answer questions as needed. Provide instruction to significant others, and initiate a referral to a home-care agency if needed.

Additional Interventions
Attach the T-tube to the patient's gown to prevent pull on the tube from the weight of the drainage bag. Keep the tubing free of kinks and the bag below the level of the suture line to prevent reflux of bile. Position the patient off the tube to maintain free flow of drainage. Never irrigate, aspirate, or clamp a T-tube: The resultant back pressure could disrupt the suture line.

Report T-tube drainage in excess of 1000 ml per day. If ordered, return excess bile to the patient via the nasogastric tube. Also report purulent or foul-smelling drainage or a sudden increase in amount of drainage after it has diminished; the latter can indicate an obstruction below the T-tube.

Keep the patient on NPO status, and maintain the nasogastric tube to suction as ordered until peristalsis returns. Administer antiemetics as ordered for episodes of postoperative nausea. When peristalsis is reestablished and the nasogastric tube removed, give clear fluids as tolerated. Progress gradually to a full diet.

Evaluation

Evaluate the effectiveness of nursing care for a patient who has had a cholecystectomy by comparing the patient's status with the expected patient outcomes. Examples of specific outcomes for patients who have had a cholecystectomy have been provided in the Planning section.

Chart 24–1.

NURSING GUIDE TO PATIENT EDUCATION FOR SELF-MANAGEMENT: DISCHARGE INSTRUCTIONS AFTER CONVENTIONAL CHOLECYSTECTOMY WITH T-TUBE INSERTION

Instruct the patient to:

Keep the T-tube drainage bag below the level of the T-tube.
Prevent pull on the tube by coiling the drainage tubing and securing to the abdomen with tape or other fastener.
Avoid tight-fitting clothing, which can irritate the wound or put pressure on the T-tube.
Expect possible bile leakage, and select clothing that can be washed in a solution of detergent, bleach, and baking soda if staining occurs.
Open the drain spout and empty the T-tube drainage bag each day at the same time. Be sure to note the amount of drainage in the bag so that changes in the amount of drainage can be identified.
Change the dressing around the T-tube daily. While holding the tube in place, remove the old dressing, wipe skin area around the tube with an antiseptic, apply a clean precut dressing, and tape in place.
Take showers, not tub baths, to help prevent bacteria from entering the wound.
Avoid strenuous activities, which could place strain on the wound.
Report increased, purulent, or foul-smelling drainage; redness, swelling, warmth, or pain at the incision line; oral temperature greater than 100°F (37.7°C); abdominal pain; nausea or vomiting.
Return for a follow-up cholangiogram on *(specify date, time, and place).*

Open Laser Cholecystectomy. Laser cholecystectomy is a variation on the conventional open cholecystectomy. After laser surgery, patients have been found to have less discomfort and to be ready to resume usual activities more quickly. In one study, patients were generally discharged on the second postoperative day, resumed usual at-home activities in 10 to 14 days, and returned to work in 15 to 17 days (Swazuk et al, 1989, p. 1005).

Laparoscopic Cholecystectomy. Laparoscopic cholecystectomy is less invasive than an open cholecystectomy. There is minimal postoperative pain, the procedure is done on an outpatient or overnight basis, and recovery time is shorter. The procedure is contraindicated in cases in which the gallbladder is so severely inflamed it could rupture and when multiple adhesions are present.

Procedure. Laparoscopic cholecystectomy is done under general anesthesia. A long, narrow, cylindrical laparoscope is inserted through a 1-cm incision in the abdomen (usually in the lower aspect of the umbilicus) after insufflation with carbon dioxide. This scope visualizes the internal organs and projects their image onto a video monitor, which the surgeon watches as the procedure is performed. Three smaller incisions are made through which other instruments are inserted for dissection, coagulation, irrigation, and suction. The excised gallbladder is removed through the umbilical incision. When a laser is used for incision and cauterization, the procedure is called a laser laparoscopic cholecystectomy or laser endoscopic cholecystectomy.

Complications. Potential complications of laparoscopic cholecystectomy are accidental bowel or bladder puncture and uncontrolled bleeding.

Guidelines for Application of the Nursing Process to the Care of the Patient Undergoing Laparoscopic Cholecystectomy

Nursing care for patients undergoing laparoscopic cholecystectomy is similar to that for any patient having surgery under general anesthesia. A nursing diagnosis unique to the patient who has had a laparoscopic cholecystectomy is pain (referred right shoulder) related to the pressure of the insufflated carbon dioxide on the diaphragm. To relieve this pain, place the patient in semi-Fowler's position and apply heat to the right shoulder. Also encourage ambulation to increase the body's absorption of the gas. Administer or teach self-administration of oral analgesics as prescribed for 24 to 48 hours. Instruct the patient to gradually resume normal activities over a 3-day period but to avoid heavy lifting for approximately 10 days.

Acute Pancreatitis

Acute pancreatitis is a diffuse inflammation of the pancreas caused by the activation of pancreatic enzymes within the organ itself, which precipitates a process of pancreatic autodigestion. It is a serious disorder with a significant mortality risk.

ETIOLOGY

Acute pancreatitis can be associated with the excessive use of alcohol, thiazide diuretics, steroids, acetaminophen, or oral contraceptives; biliary tract disease; abdominal surgery or other trauma; penetrating duodenal ulcer; metabolic disorders; mumps; or bacterial infection. Nonetheless, the precise reason for pancreatic enzymes being activated in the pancreas rather than in the intestine is unknown. It is hypothesized, however, that obstruction of the pancreatic ducts and reflux of duodenal contents into the pancreas through a dilated sphincter of Oddi may be significant factors.

PATHOPHYSIOLOGY

Regardless of cause, the basic factor in the onset of acute pancreatitis is the presence of activated trypsin within the pancreas. Trypsin is thought to initiate pancreatic digestion and activate elastase, kinins, and phospholipase.

Elastase dissolves the elastic fibers of the blood vessels within the pancreas, resulting in blood loss or hemorrhage. Activated kinins cause systemic vasodilation and increased vascular permeability, thus predisposing the person with acute pancreatitis to hypovolemic shock. The activity of phospholipase A results in pancreatic parenchymal and fat necrosis.

Acute pancreatitis often resolves without residual damage, although in some cases it may progress to the chronic form of the disease.

CLINICAL MANIFESTATIONS

Sudden onset of intense left upper quadrant abdominal pain radiating to the midback or left shoulder is the most outstanding symptom of acute pancreatitis. Onset of pain is often acute and frequently occurs 24 to 48 hours after a heavy meal or heavy use of alcohol. The pain is unrelieved by antacids and is usually accompanied by nausea and vomiting and in some cases by symptoms of circulatory shock. Examination of the abdomen reveals muscle guarding and rigidity with rebound tenderness. If there is seepage of bloody exudate from the pancreas, periumbilical bruising (Cullen's sign) and bruising of the flanks (Grey Turner's sign) may be seen. Respiratory distress may also occur.

MEDICAL DIAGNOSIS

A serum amylase level of more than 500 units/dl (normal is 60 to 160 units/dl), an elevated urinary amylase level, and an elevated serum lipase level are diagnostic of acute pancreatitis. The WBC, serum glucose, blood urea nitrogen (BUN), and LDH levels are also usually elevated.

MEDICAL MANAGEMENT

During the critical stage, pancreatic activity is diminished by keeping the patient on NPO status, administering anticholinergic drugs, and instituting nasogastric suction, which relieves abdominal distention and removes hydrochloric acid before it can enter the duodenum and stimulate the pancreas. Pain is usually controlled by Demerol in combination with the anticholinergics. Morphine is avoided because it can cause spasm in the sphincter of Oddi.

If hypovolemic shock is present, volume replacement is initiated immediately with Ringer's lactate followed by administration of whole blood, packed cells, or plasma expanders. Central venous pressure (CVP) or pulmonary capillary wedge pressure (PCWP) is used to monitor the response to fluid replacement, and urinary output is measured hourly.

Blood gases are monitored and if hypoxemia occurs, oxygen therapy and even intubation and ventilation are used, if necessary.

Antibiotic therapy is usually instituted to defend against secondary infections, and in some cases, exudate is removed from the peritoneal cavity by peritoneal dialysis. Insulin is given if hyperglycemia develops.

When the critical phase is over, oral intake is begun. Clear fluids are given first followed by carbohydrate foodstuffs or elemental protein feedings, which do not stimulate pancreatic secretion. Gradually a bland, low-fat diet with six feedings per day is introduced. If glucose tolerance is impaired, the amount of carbohydrate in the diet is restricted.

Application of the Nursing Process to the Care of the Patient with Acute Pancreatitis

Assessment

Assess the patient's response to prescribed pain medication. Keep in mind that the patient with acute pancreatitis is in persistent, intense pain and often assumes the fetal position in an attempt to minimize it.

Assess vital signs, hemodynamic status, and urinary output every hour because the patient is prone to hypovolemic shock as a result of vomiting, blood loss, systemic vasodilation, and increased vascular permeability. Measure all intake and output including nasogastric drainage. Weigh the patient daily, and observe for the appearance of ascites. Measure abdominal girth daily if ascites is suspected.

Observe for signs of sodium, chloride, and potassium deficits resulting from vomiting, gastric suctioning, and fluid shifts. Observe also for signs of hypocalcemia because serum calcium levels decrease in acute pancreatitis, possibly owing to fat necrosis that results in binding of calcium with free fatty acids. Report signs of muscle twitching, tremors, and irritability immediately. Have intravenous calcium gluconate on hand in case it is needed to prevent tetany.

Inspect the oral and nasal mucosa for dryness and cracking. This is important because the patient is on NPO status, has nasogastric suction, and is receiving anticholinergic drugs, which decrease salivary and respiratory secretions.

Assess for signs of respiratory infection because the patient's breathing is typically shallow and guarded as a result of peritoneal irritation. Auscultate the lungs, and record the patient's temperature every 4 hours.

Auscultate the abdomen for bowel sounds every 4 hours. Remember that they will initially be diminished or absent as a result of peritoneal irritation and gastric suctioning. When oral intake is resumed, monitor the patient's response to foods and fluids. Also ascertain the patient's understanding of dietary restrictions and willingness and ability to comply with them.

Nursing Diagnoses and Planning

Nursing diagnoses and related expected patient outcomes most commonly applicable to patients with acute pancreatitis include the following:

NDx: Pain related to the inflammatory process in the abdomen

Planning: Patient outcomes
1. Patient states pain is diminished.
2. Patient assumes a high Fowler's position without verbal or nonverbal signs of discomfort.

NDx: High risk for fluid volume deficit related to vomiting, gastric suction, and activation of pancreatic enzymes

Planning: Patient outcomes
1. Skin turgor is normal.
2. Mucous membranes are moist.
3. Capillary refill is within normal limits.
4. Vital signs are within patient's baseline ranges.
5. Fluid intake approximates fluid output.

NDx: Altered oral mucous membrane related to drying effects of NPO status and anticholinergic drugs

Planning: Patient outcomes
1. Oral mucous membranes are moist and supple.
2. Oral mucous membranes are free of cracks.

NDx: High risk for ineffective airway clearance related to shallow, guarded respirations

Planning: Patient outcomes
1. Patient coughs and deep breathes as directed.
2. Lungs are clear on auscultation.

NDx: High risk for altered health maintenance related to insufficient knowledge of self-care after discharge

Planning: Patient outcomes
1. Patient describes dietary and other lifestyle adjustments to be followed after discharge.
2. Patient verbalizes intent to comply with lifestyle adjustments.

Nursing Interventions

NDx: Pain
Medicate the patient as ordered for pain before the pain becomes so severe as to render the medication relatively ineffective. Maintain a calm, quiet environment; give back rubs; and assist the patient in changing position to further promote comfort. Guide the patient in relaxation exercises and provide background distraction in the form of soft music if appropriate.

NDx: High risk for fluid volume deficit
Monitor vital signs every hour, or more frequently if necessary, until fluid volume stability is evident. Monitor the amount of nasogastric tube drainage, and check it and the stool for signs of bleeding. Measure urinary output hourly.

Maintain the patency of the IV line, and administer IV solutions as ordered. Monitor laboratory data related to fluid and electrolyte status.

NDx: Altered oral mucous membrane
Encourage the patient to rinse the mouth every 1 to 2 hours while awake. Avoid the use of glycerin as well as commercial mouthwash, which contain drying agents. Apply water-soluble lubricant to the lips as needed to keep them soft and supple.

NDx: High risk for ineffective airway clearance
Maintain the patient in Fowler's position to promote respiratory expansion. Turn the patient frequently, and encourage coughing and deep breathing every 2 hours when awake to decrease the risk of atelectasis and pooling of secretions.

NDx: High risk for altered health maintenance
Explain to the patient and the family that the recovery period from this serious illness is extended. Stress that the patient will need rest and only with time will regain strength and be able to resume usual activities.

Nutrition Box 24–2.

NUTRITION: SPECIAL CONSIDERATIONS FOR PATIENTS WITH PANCREATITIS

Instruct patients with pancreatitis to:

Avoid large meals.
Eat small amounts of food high in carbohydrates (450 g) and proteins (120 g).
Eat only small amounts of fats (30 g) until there is no evidence of steatorrhea.
Limit fiber intake because this may increase steatorrhea.
Eliminate coffee, tea, and spices from the diet because they stimulate pancreatic secretion.
Avoid alcohol completely because it stimulates the pancreas and can precipitate acute attacks of pancreatitis.
Report as directed for vitamin B_{12} injections.
Take prescribed enzyme replacements with or immediately after meals, being certain to swallow them whole and not disrupt their protective coating with hot foods or liquids.

Reinforce to both the patient and significant others the relationship of alcohol to pancreatitis and the necessity of avoiding it completely. If this is likely to be a problem for the patient, provide information on community resources such as Alcoholics Anonymous. If appropriate to the individual patient, also explain the relationship of particular medications to pancreatitis.

In all cases, reinforce the patient's understanding of the therapeutic diet (Nutrition Box 24–2) and its effect in preventing recurrence.

Additional Interventions
Apply water-soluble lubricant to the naris to lessen irritation from the nasogastric tube. When bowel sounds have returned to normal, give small frequent feedings as per order.

Evaluation

Evaluate the effectiveness of nursing care for a patient with acute pancreatitis by comparing the patient's status with the expected patient outcomes. Examples of specific outcomes for patients with acute pancreatitis have been provided in the Planning section.

Chronic Pancreatitis

ETIOLOGY

The cause of chronic pancreatitis is similar to that of acute pancreatitis except it does not occur in association with biliary tract disease. It is estimated that 70% to 80% of the cases of chronic pancreatitis in the United States are associated with chronic alcoholism.

PATHOPHYSIOLOGY

There are three fundamental pathologic changes in the pancreas with chronic pancreatitis. These are the formation of protein plugs in the ducts, some of which are calcified; a decrease in the number of acinar cells, which produce digestive enzymes; and fibrosis of the pancreatic tissue. These changes lead to obstruction of the ducts, a decrease in digestive enzymes, and hence malabsorption and nutritional deficiencies. Eventually, the islet cells are affected and diabetic mellitus results. Chronic pancreatitis is complicated by the development of pseudocysts, abscesses, and external fistulas.

CLINICAL MANIFESTATIONS

Chronic pancreatitis is characterized by acute attacks of upper abdominal and back pain often accompanied by vomiting. These attacks increase in frequency and duration over time. The pain accompanying each attack becomes progressively more severe even to the point at which opiates are ineffective in relieving it.

Another prominent symptom is weight loss. Early in the disease, this may be due to inadequate nutritional intake secondary to anorexia or fear that eating will precipitate an attack. Late in the disease, it results from malabsorption and is accompanied by vitamin deficiencies and the frothy, foul-smelling stools indicative of steatorrhea.

MEDICAL DIAGNOSIS

Patients with chronic pancreatitis generally seek medical help when they are experiencing an acute

Pharmacology Box 24–1.
PANCREATIC ENZYMES

Pancreatic Enzymes:
Classified as digestants, oral pancreatic enzymes are usually derived from pork pancreas.

Action:
Pancreatic enzymes aid in the digestion and absorption of carbohydrates, fats, and proteins.

Uses:
These enzymes replace or supplement exocrine pancreatic secretions in malabsorption syndrome precipitated by acute and chronic pancreatitis, cancer of the pancreas, and cystic fibrosis.

Side Effects:
Holding tablets in the mouth may cause ulceration. Nausea, diarrhea, and hyperuricemia may occur with high dosage.

Interactions:
None are known.

Nursing Implications:
Direct patient to take medication with meals unless otherwise advised. Instruct patient to report loss of appetite or constipation because these may be signs that the dosage is too high. Check for pork allergy and, if present, arrange for a bovine preparation. Do not crush enteric tablets.

exacerbation of the disease and diagnosis is primarily made on the basis of the presenting symptoms and the patient's history. Laboratory tests confirming chronic pancreatitis are increased alkaline phosphatase, increased serum glucose, and a secretion challenging test revealing a decreased secretion of pancreatic juices. A glucose tolerance test is done to evaluate islet cell function.

MEDICAL MANAGEMENT

Treatment of chronic pancreatitis centers around the prevention of severe episodes by minimizing the work of the pancreas. A low-fat, high-carbohydrate, high-protein bland diet with abstention from alcohol and caffeine is instituted. If there is insufficient enzyme production, oral pancreatic enzymes (Pharmacology Box 24–1) to be taken with meals are prescribed. Anticholinergic drugs, antacids, and gastric acid inhibitors are also given to decrease gastric acid, which stimulates pancreatic function. Because the absorption of vitamin B_{12} is impaired in many cases, parenteral administration may be necessary.

Patients with hyperglycemia are treated with insulin or, if the islet cells can be stimulated, with oral hypoglycemic agents.

Pain control is the most difficult part of the medical management of chronic pancreatitis. Because of the chronic nature of the disease and the nature of the pain, the risk of opiate tolerance is high. Thus, nonopiate pain control measures are generally used, although with limited success. Surgery is indicated when pain becomes intractable or complications such as abscesses and fistulas compromise the patient's quality of life. The goal of surgery is to provide drainage of pancreatic secretions into the intestine. To this end, a variety of procedures such as pancreaticojejunostomy, revision of the sphincter of Oddi, and even pancreatectomy are done. However, the results are generally unsuccessful because of a high morbidity and mortality rate associated with the procedures and recurrence of symptoms as a result of progression of the disease.

Application of the Nursing Process to the Care of the Patient with Chronic Pancreatitis

Assessment

Assess location and intensity of pain. Determine the time of onset, and ask for the name and frequency of any pain medication taken at home. Assess the effectiveness of the pain medication, and ask about any other interventions used successfully to reduce pain. Ask the patient about the presence of nausea and vomiting, and obtain a description of stools. Question specifically about frothy, bulky, foul-smelling stools. Ascertain what the patient has had to eat and drink in the 48 hours preceding the attack, because there is usually a correlation between dietary intake and the development of pain and distressing abdominal symptoms.

Obtain the patient's weight, and assess general nutritional status. When the patient is able, obtain a complete history of attacks and their treatment. Assess the patient's understanding of the disease and the dietary restrictions necessary for its control (see Nutrition Box 24–2). Determine whether oral pancreatic enzymes are prescribed and the patient's understanding of their use. Assess the patient's compliance with the treatment regimen, and seek to identify factors that affect it negatively.

Assess blood and urinary glucose levels, because patients with chronic pancreatitis frequently acquire diabetes mellitus. Ascertain the patient's knowledge about diabetic diets and medication if a diagnosis of diabetes mellitus has already been made.

Nursing Diagnoses and Planning

Nursing diagnoses and related expected patient outcomes most commonly applicable to patients with chronic pancreatitis include the following:

NDx: Pain related to the inflammatory process in the abdomen

Planning: Patient outcomes
1. Patient states abdominal pain has diminished.
2. Patient moves without groans, grimaces, or other signs of discomfort.

NDx: High risk for noncompliance related to medication regimen and diet therapy

Planning: Patient outcomes
1. Patient self-administers oral pancreatic enzymes and antacids as prescribed.
2. Patient describes dietary regimen.
3. Patient chooses low-fat, bland foods and decaffeinated coffee from the regular hospital menu.
4. Patient reports intent to avoid alcoholic beverages because alcohol can exacerbate symptoms.

NDx: Altered nutrition: less than body requirements related to decreased intake or malabsorption

Planning: Patient outcomes
1. Patient eats foods served at mealtime.
2. Patient takes vitamin supplements as prescribed.
3. Patient maintains weight or gains a specified amount.

Nursing Interventions

NDx: Pain

Acknowledge the severity of the patient's pain, and give prescribed medications as necessary. Discuss with the patient other methods of relieving pain (i.e., focusing, biofeedback, relaxation techniques, and diversional activities). Explain that the pain is related to digestive activity and that diet and gastric-related medications help limit discomfort.

NDx: High risk for noncompliance

Review with the patient the prescribed medication regimen and diet program, as outlined in Nutrition Box 24–2. Explain the reason for taking the prescribed pancreatic enzymes (see Pharmacology Box 24–1) and antacids. Ask the patient to monitor the response to the regimen. Tell the patient to note whether less abdominal discomfort is experienced and whether stools return to normal, because compliance is enhanced when the patient associates treatment with a lessening of symptoms. Obtain a written order allowing the patient to self-administer oral pancreatic enzymes and antacids as prescribed while hospitalized, because self-care begun in the hospital is more likely followed up on discharge. Be certain to observe that the patient takes the medication as prescribed.

Include the family in discussions about medication and diet therapy. Family support facilitates compliance with the long-term therapeutic regimens that patients with chronic pancreatitis are required to follow.

NDx: Altered nutrition: less than body requirements

Because anorexia is frequently a problem, enhance the patient's feeling for food by ensuring a clean, quiet environment for eating and providing foods of the patient's choice when possible. Acknowledge that some people are fearful of eating lest an acute attack be precipitated, but stress that adequate nutrition is necessary if health is not to deteriorate further and that only foods on the prescribed diet are being offered.

Stress the importance of taking pancreatic enzymes as prescribed and receiving parenteral vitamin B_{12} if needed.

Evaluation

Evaluate the effectiveness of nursing care for a patient with chronic pancreatitis by comparing the patient's status with the expected patient outcomes. Examples of specific outcomes for patients with chronic pancreatitis have been provided in the Planning section.

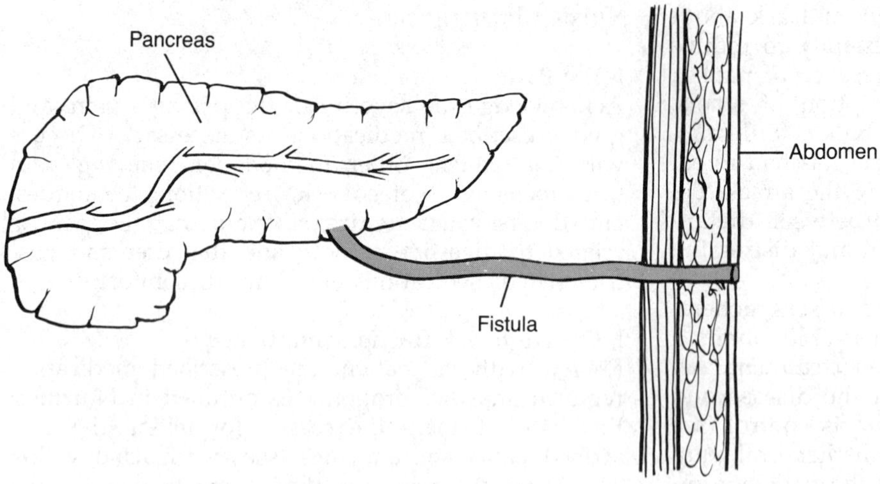

Figure 24–6.

Schematic internal view of a pancreatic fistula.

Structural Disorders

Pancreatic Fistula

ETIOLOGY

Pancreatic fistulas are most commonly the result of pancreatic abscesses, which develop secondary to acute pancreatitis.

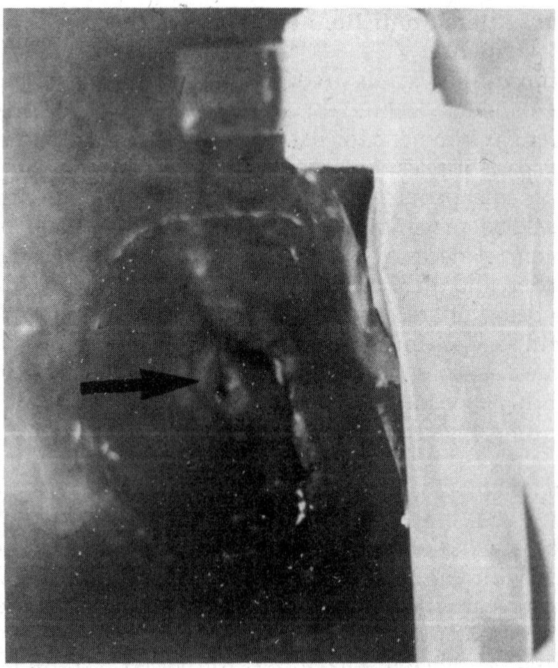

Figure 24–7.

External appearance of a pancreatic fistula.

PATHOPHYSIOLOGY

Once a pancreatic abscess has formed, an abnormal tract or tunnel develops, connecting the internal abscess site with the abdominal wall (Fig. 24–6). The fistula or tunnel ultimately erodes through the abdominal wall and begins to drain. Very quickly, the opening enlarges, and copious amounts of purulent drainage appear (Fig. 24–7).

CLINICAL MANIFESTATIONS

The patient with a pancreatic fistula appears acutely ill and has an elevated temperature. Examination of the abdominal wall discloses a small, reddened area that is warm to the touch if the abdominal wall has not yet been broken through. If it has broken through, the fistula opening as well as purulent, foul-smelling drainage is evident.

MEDICAL DIAGNOSIS

Diagnosis is made on the basis of examination of the wound. Sonography and computed tomographic (CT) scan may be used to define the source of the fistula. The WBC count is elevated.

MEDICAL MANAGEMENT

The offending organism is identified by wound culture, and appropriate IV antibiotic therapy is instituted. The wound may be irrigated with one-half strength normal saline and hydrogen peroxide, several times daily. Because the fistula should heal from the inside out, the wound is sometimes packed with sterile gauze after each wound irrigation. Acetaminophen is given for discomfort as well as for fever.

Application of the Nursing Process to the Care of the Patient with a Pancreatic Fistula

Assessment

Take vital signs every 4 hours because an elevated temperature and pulse rate accompany pancreatic fistulas. Observe the amount and character of the drainage, and obtain a culture of it before administration of antibiotics. Assess the condition of the abdominal skin because it is prone to excoriation from the drainage.

Because a secondary fistula tract sometimes develops either to a hollow organ or to the body surface, gently palpate the abdomen for signs of increased tenderness. Auscultate bowel sounds, and observe for signs of urinary tract infection.

Nursing Diagnoses and Planning

Nursing diagnoses and related expected patient outcomes most commonly applicable to patients with a pancreatic fistula include the following:

NDx: High risk for impaired skin integrity related to irritating wound drainage

Planning: Patient outcomes
1. Skin surrounding fistula opening is intact.
2. Skin surrounding fistula opening is free of erythema.

NDx: High risk for altered health maintenance related to insufficient knowledge of wound care

Planning: Patient outcomes
1. Patient demonstrates wound irrigation.
2. Patient demonstrates care of skin around fistula site.
3. Patient demonstrates proper application of dressing.

Nursing Interventions

NDx: High risk for impaired skin integrity
Irrigate fistula with prescribed irrigant. Note color and odor of drainage. Cleanse area around fistula with normal saline and pat dry. Keep skin surrounding fistula dry and free of drainage because purulent drainage can cause excoriation. If prescribed, pack fistula tunnel with sterile gauze to hasten inside-out healing and to minimize leakage of drainage onto surrounding skin. Use Montgomery straps if drainage is copious and if dressing changes are frequent to prevent irritation of the skin from frequent use of tape. Instruct the patient to notify the nurse when the dressing appears to be damp or wet. An ostomy-type appliance may be used to contain the drainage and protect the skin.

NDx: High risk for altered health maintenance
Because the patient will most likely be discharged before the fistula has completely closed, wound irrigation and dressing must be taught. Explain that irrigating the wound is necessary to facilitate healing, and show the patient how it is done. Have the patient demonstrate irrigating the wound several times before discharge. Similarly, teach proper dressing technique and have the patient demonstrate the procedure.

Evaluation

Evaluate the effectiveness of nursing care for a patient with a pancreatic fistula by comparing the patient's status with the expected patient outcomes. Examples of specific outcomes for patients with a pancreatic fistula have been provided in the Planning section.

Neoplasia

Cancer of the Pancreas

Cancer of the pancreas is increasing in incidence and ranks second to colon cancer as the most common cause of death from cancers of the gastrointestinal tract. It is twice as common in men as in women and has its peak incidence between 50 and 70 years of age.

ETIOLOGY

The cause of cancer of the pancreas is unknown, but possible predisposing factors have been identified. These include alcoholism, diabetes, ingestion of a high-fat diet, and carcinogens in cigarette smoke, food, and the environment.

PATHOPHYSIOLOGY

Pancreatic cancers are usually adenocarcinomas that originate from the epithelial lining of the duct areas of the organ. Sixty percent to 70% of the time they originate in the head of the pancreas. As the tumor mass grows, it causes blockage of the ducts and frequently extends into nearby structures such as the stomach, liver, and intestines as well as into the lymph nodes. The tumor usually grows quickly and rapidly metastasizes to the liver, lungs, or bones and hence is associated with a poor prognosis.

CLINICAL MANIFESTATIONS

Many of the symptoms of pancreatic cancer are nonspecific and late in onset, thus contributing to the fact that the disease is often far advanced at the time of diagnosis. Symptoms include anorexia, vague abdominal discomfort, upper or midabdominal pain, boring pain in the midback, nausea, and vomiting. There is also weight loss and, in 80% to 90% of patients, jaundice, which is indicative of impairment of liver or biliary function. The weight loss is rapid and progressive and in most cases is why medical help is sought. Fluid and electrolyte imbalances, steatorrhea, bleeding tendencies caused by vitamin K deficiency, and ascites also occur. If the islet cells are involved, diabetes may be the first indication of the malignancy with glycosuria, hyperglycemia, and abnormal glucose tolerance presenting.

Because of the location of the pancreas, the tumor is not usually palpable. However, the liver may enlarge during the course of disease as may the gallbladder.

MEDICAL DIAGNOSIS

The diagnosis of cancer of the head of the pancreas is strongly suggested by the appearance of painless jaundice and unexplained weight loss. Ultrasonography and tomography help differentiate between enlargement of the pancreas from inflammation as opposed to tumor. Also useful in diagnosis are cholangiography, endoscopic retrograde cholangiopancreatography (ERCP), and angiographic visualization showing engorgement of the small arteries of the pancreas, which is indicative of cancer.

Percutaneous fine-needle aspiration biopsy may be done to confirm the diagnosis and to guide in selecting the surgical approach to be used for those patients who are scheduled for surgery.

MEDICAL MANAGEMENT

The usual treatment for cancer of the pancreas is surgical. If the head of the pancreas is involved and there is no evidence of distant metastasis, a radical pancreatoduodenectomy (Whipple procedure) is performed.

In patients with cancer of the body or tail of the pancreas, a curative operation cannot be performed because of the location of the tumor and probable extensive metastasis. Thus, the treatment goal is palliation of symptoms through a combination of a simple surgical procedure such as a cholecystojejunostomy (Fig. 24–8), radiation, and chemotherapy. Chemotherapy and radiation therapy have little or no influence on the primary tumor but can relieve the pain of tumor pressure as the disease advances. Other aspects of palliative treatment include pain control, nutritional support, and control of complications.

RADICAL PANCREATODUODENECTOMY (WHIPPLE PROCEDURE)

A radical pancreatoduodenectomy is a very extensive surgical procedure that involves the removal of the proximal pancreas, duodenum, lower half of the stomach, and the gallbladder. The pancreatic duct is implanted into the jejunum, as is the remaining stomach and hepatic duct (see Fig. 24–8). The purpose of this procedure is to allow gastric, hepatic, and pancreatic secretions to empty into the jejunum so that reasonably normal digestion may take place. This procedure offers the possibility of a cure but has a high mortality rate, and a low 5-year survival rate after the operation.

Physical Preparation of the Patient

Preparation of the patient for a Whipple procedure is intensive and often requires an extended period of time because of the extensiveness of the procedure and the fact that most times the patient is malnourished and in poor physical condition. The patient is hydrated and is usually given parenteral nutrition. Blood transfusions are often used to correct anemia, and vitamin K is given to correct prothrombin deficiency. Because postoperative infection is a major risk, antibiotics such as kanamycin or neomycin are often started 3 to 4 days before surgery.

Postoperative Course

After surgery, the patient is usually admitted to a surgical critical care unit. IV fluids and electrolytes are administered, and transfusions may be given to replace blood lost during the operation. An arterial catheter is in place to monitor arterial pressure, and an indwelling urinary catheter is in place to monitor urinary output. To minimize pancreatic secretion and to decompress the stomach and thus prevent stress on internal suture lines, the patient is maintained on NPO status and nasogastric suction is in place.

Parenteral nutrition is continued, with oral intake gradually resumed when bowel function has fully returned. Vasopressor drugs are used to combat hypotension, which can occur during the first 48 hours after pancreatic resection, and prophylactic antibiotics are given.

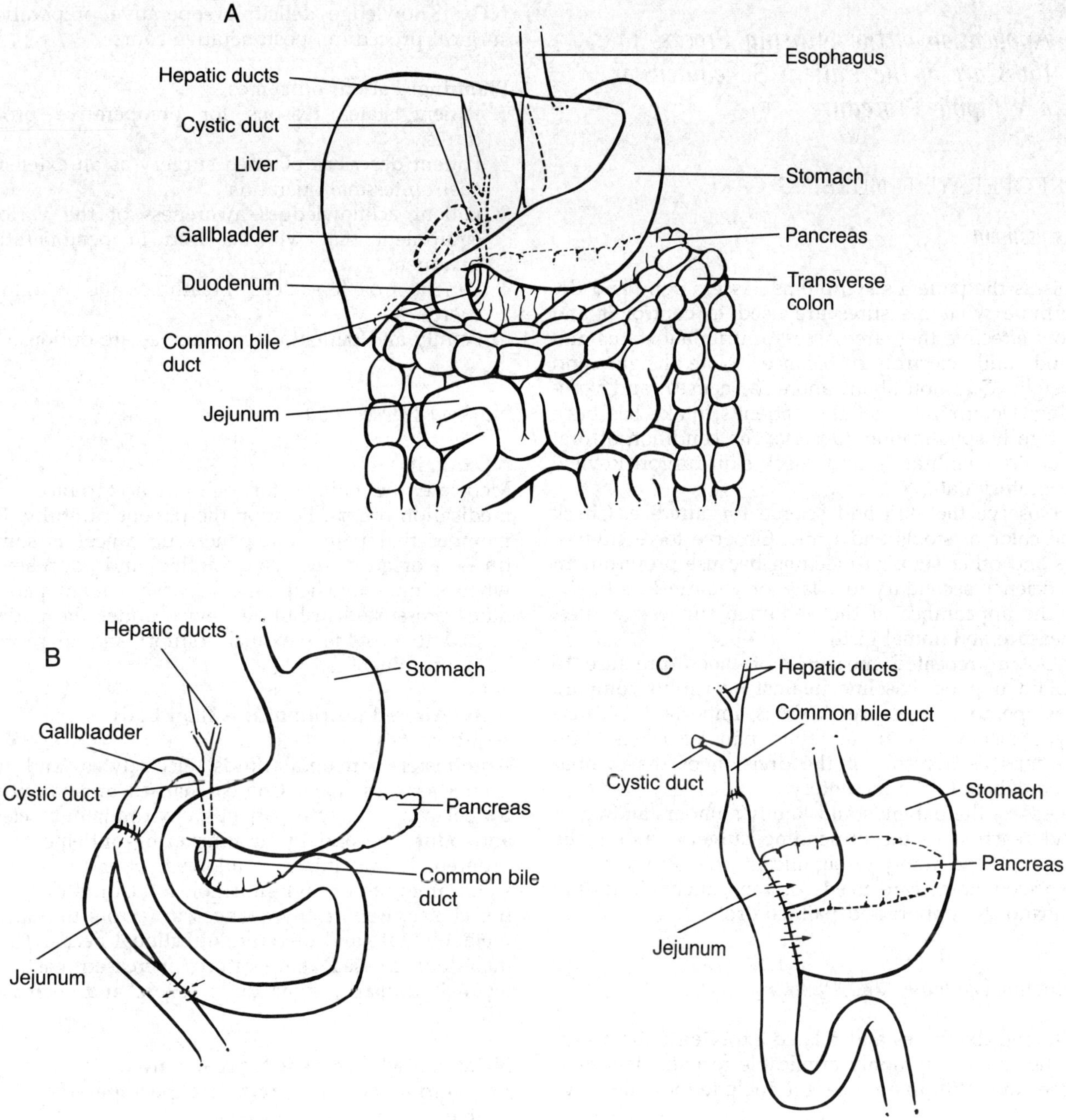

Figure 24–8.

A, Normal relationship of upper abdominal organs. *B,* Cholecystojejunostomy. Note the anastomosis between the gallbladder and the jejunum, which allows bile to flow directly into the intestine, bypassing obstruction caused by an inoperable tumor of the head of the pancreas. *C,* Upper abdominal contents following a Whipple procedure. Note the removal of the proximal pancreas, duodenum, lower half of the stomach, and gallbladder.

Complications

Major complications of a Whipple procedure are hemorrhage, necrosis, and fistula formation (which occur as a result of the action of pancreatic enzymes) and hepatorenal failure and vascular collapse. Pulmonary complications such as pneumonia, atelectasis, and pleural effusion also are prevalent, given the proximity of the operative area to the diaphragm and the chest. The incidence of complications is high not only because of the extent of the surgery but because patients tend to be at increased risk as a result of a history of alcohol or drug abuse, diabetes, and malnutrition.

Application of the Nursing Process to the Care of the Patient Scheduled for a Whipple Procedure

PREOPERATIVE NURSING CARE

Assessment

Assess the patient's symptoms. Assess pain, and determine what measures are used to control it and how effective they are. Assess nutritional status and fluid and electrolyte balance. Note height and weight. Question about anorexia, nausea, and vomiting. Determine what the patient's intake has been before hospitalization. Observe the condition of oral mucous membranes, and check skin turgor. Review laboratory data.

Observe the skin and sclerae for jaundice. Check the color of stools and urine. Observe for ecchymosis and other signs of bleeding because prothrombin deficiency secondary to a lack of vitamin K is likely. If the appearance of the abdomen suggests ascites, measure abdominal girth.

Obtain repeated measures of blood pressure to obtain a good baseline against which to compare postoperative pressure. This is important because hypotension can occur after pancreatic resection perhaps as a result of the division of the sympathetic fibers to the mesentery.

Assess the patient's and family's understanding of and reaction to the impending surgery. Assess the ability of the family or significant others to meet the expected home-care needs of the patient, including nutritional support and pain control.

Nursing Diagnoses and Planning

Nursing diagnoses and related expected patient outcomes most commonly applicable to patients scheduled for a Whipple procedure include the following:

NDx: Pain related to pressure on and destruction of intraabdominal structures from carcinoma

Planning: Patient outcomes
1. Patient states pain is reduced to at least a level that is bearable with use of medication or other pain control strategies.
2. Patient rests quietly without groaning or moaning.

NDx: Altered nutrition: less than body requirements related to anorexia and malabsorption

Planning: Patient outcomes
1. Patient maintains or increases body weight.

NDx: Knowledge deficit: preoperative preparation, surgical procedure, postoperative course

Planning: Patient outcomes
1. Patient states reasons for preoperative procedures.
2. Patient describes planned surgery as an extensive gastrointestinal operation.
3. Patient acknowledges awareness of the various equipment that will be used in postoperative treatment.
4. Patient practices deep breathing and coughing exercises.
5. Family and patient discuss home-care options.

Nursing Interventions

NDx: Pain
Medicate the patient for pain in accordance with medication orders. Position the patient carefully. Remember that pain from pancreatic cancer is sometimes worsened by lying supine and is relieved when sitting hunched forward. Use a foam pad or other pressure-distributing device under the patient in bed to provide maximal comfort and to protect bony prominences.

NDx: Altered nutrition: less than body requirements
Administer parenteral fluids, electrolytes, and nutrients as prescribed. Combat nausea and vomiting by ensuring that the patient's environment is clean and odor free and by administering antiemetics as ordered. If oral intake is allowed, offer the patient small amounts of high-nutrition foodstuffs of his or her choice. Report any changes in factors that affect metabolic rate and therefore nutritional needs. These include increased temperature, increased gastrointestinal drainage, signs of infection, and increased stress.

NDx: Knowledge deficit: preoperative preparation, surgical procedure, postoperative course
Review preoperative procedures, the surgical procedure, and the postoperative course with the patient and family. Be sure to explain that the surgical procedure takes several hours to complete, because frequently a family equates extended time in the operating room with occurrence of serious complications. Also begin discussion of preparation for discharge. This focuses the patient and family on a positive goal and allows the family time to mobilize the resources that will be required on discharge.

Keep in mind that the patient is critically ill and may not have the physical energy or mental concentration to follow lengthy explanations. Remember also that both the patient and family are likely to be very anxious over the outcome of the surgery and may have difficulty attending to and remembering information.

Evaluation

Evaluate the effectiveness of preoperative nursing care for a patient scheduled for a Whipple procedure by comparing the patient's status with the expected patient outcomes. Examples of specific outcomes for patients scheduled for a Whipple procedure have been provided in the Planning section.

POSTOPERATIVE NURSING CARE

Assessment

Take vital signs, check CVP, and measure urinary output every hour. Read the operative report, and check placement of all drainage tubes. Make certain they are free of stress or kinks and that they are in a dependent position. Note the characteristics and amount of drainage from each. Keep in mind that serosanguineous drainage is normal and that clear, bile-tinged, or bloody drainage can indicate disruption of an anastomosis. Carefully assess functioning of the nasogastric suction because removal of gastrointestinal drainage and secretions is necessary to prevent stress on the anastomosis sites. As with the drains, check for pull or binding. Also check suction gauge at regular intervals.

Observe for signs of fluid and electrolyte imbalance because patients lose large amounts of protein and fluid into the peritoneal cavity and the intestinal tract. Measure all intake and output. Monitor serum electrolytes, serum albumin, serum and urine osmolality, hematocrit levels, arterial blood gas levels, and pH. Monitor for signs of the third-spacing phenomenon: increase in weight, fluid in the lungs, pitting edema in the extremities, and dependent edema in the back and over the sacrum. Check blood sugar levels because removal of islet cells may necessitate administration of insulin to prevent hyperglycemia.

Assess the patient's pain, and note the effectiveness of medication and other comfort measures. When analgesics are given that depress the central nervous system, assess for any depressant effect on the respiratory system that would increase the risk of complications in this area.

Observe the wound for signs of hemorrhage, and monitor prothrombin levels because the potential for impaired coagulation exists. Observe both the wound and the entry site of the total parenteral nutrition (TPN) catheter for signs of infection: redness, purulent drainage, and foul odor. Also check for signs of peritonitis by watching for a sudden increase in temperature and palpating the abdomen for rigidity. Observe skin areas in contact with pancreatic drainage for excoriation.

Assess general nutritional status. Obtain daily weights. Listen for the return of bowel sounds, and observe for passage of flatus and stool. When oral intake is resumed, observe for signs of malabsorption such as steatorrhea and diarrhea and assess for dumping syndrome. Inspect the skin for signs of breakdown for which the patient is at risk because of bed rest and impaired nutrition.

Assess the patient's emotional status. Look for signs of depression, anger, and anxiety. Explore coping mechanisms of both the patient and the family.

Nursing Diagnoses and Planning

Nursing diagnoses and related expected patient outcomes most commonly applicable to patients who have had a Whipple procedure include the following:

NDx: High risk for impaired gas exchange related to lengthy anesthesia and location of surgical trauma

Planning: Patient outcomes
1. Rate and depth of respirations are within patient's normal range.
2. Lungs are clear on auscultation.
3. Arterial blood gas values are within baseline limits.

NDx: Pain related to surgical trauma and irritation of the naris by the nasogastric tube

Planning: Patient outcomes
1. Patient reports that pain is relieved to at least a bearable level after medication.
2. Patient performs routine postoperative exercises without complaints or signs of severe pain such as pallor and tachycardia.
3. Patient denies nostril discomfort.

NDx: High risk for fluid volume deficit related to effects of pancreatic surgery, presence of multiple drainage tubes, and limited oral intake

Planning: Patient outcomes
1. Hourly urinary output is 50 ml or more.
2. IV intake approximates urinary and nasogastric tube output.
3. Skin turgor is good.
4. Serum electrolyte levels are within normal limits.

NDx: High risk for altered nutrition: less than body requirements related to inadequate intake of nutrients or malabsorption

Planning: Patient outcomes
1. Patient maintains or gains weight.
2. Patient is in positive nitrogen balance.

NDx: High risk for trauma to the internal suture lines related to gastrointestinal distention

Planning: Patient outcomes
1. Nasogastric suction is functioning.
2. Abdomen is soft.
3. Patient states that pain is decreasing over time.

NDx: High risk for altered oral mucous membrane related to mouth breathing secondary to the nasogastric tube and NPO status

Planning: Patient outcomes
1. Oral mucous membranes are pink and moist.
2. Lips are free of cracks.
3. Patient states that lips are supple and pain free.

NDx: High risk for infection related to contamination of the abdominal wound or catheter site or to contamination or disruption of an internal anastomosis, presence of a parenteral nutrition catheter

Planning: Patient outcomes
1. Patient remains afebrile.
2. Patient's WBC count is within normal limits.
3. Wound drainage is nonpurulent.
4. Abdomen is soft to palpation.
5. TPN catheter site is nonreddened and free of foul odor or purulent drainage.

NDx: High risk for altered health maintenance related to insufficient knowledge of self-care after discharge

Planning: Patient outcomes
1. Patient demonstrates sterile dressing change.
2. Patient describes signs and symptoms to be reported to physician.

Nursing Interventions

NDx: High risk for impaired gas exchange
Place the patient in semi-Fowler's position to promote lung expansion and also to reduce pull on the suture line. Establish and maintain a consistent pulmonary hygiene routine that includes turning, coughing, deep breathing, ambulation, and the use of an incentive spirometer.

NDx: Pain
Medicate the patient for pain as often as prescribed. Assist the patient to splint the incisional area when moving, coughing, or deep breathing. When ambulatory, plan to get the patient out of bed while pain medication is effective. Encourage relaxation, and provide a calm, quiet environment. Use other pain-relieving strategies such as imaging and distraction as appropriate.

Ascertain what pain medication the patient will use after discharge. Instruct the patient and family about the administration and side effects of the drug.

To prevent or ease nasal discomfort from the nasogastric tube, wash the nostril with applicators wet with water and apply a water-soluble lubricant. Make certain that the tube is taped in place in a manner that does not exert pressure on the naris.

NDx: High risk for fluid volume deficit
Administer fluids as ordered. Monitor urinary output. Report an output less than 25 ml hourly to the physician. Record all intake and output.

NDx: High risk for altered nutrition: less than body requirements
Administer parenteral nutrition as prescribed. When oral intake is allowed, advance the patient's diet as tolerated, to a full high-carbohydrate, high-protein, high-vitamin diet as ordered. Administer prescribed vitamin and mineral supplements as well as any prescribed pancreatic enzymes.

NDx: High risk for trauma
Keep the nasogastric tube free of kinks and connected to suction as ordered to drain secretions and to prevent distention. Irrigate the tube gently with normal saline (usually 10 to 20 ml) as ordered to keep it patent. Reinforce or replace the tape holding the tube in place as needed. Avoid moving the tube when adding or moving tape. Keep the patient on NPO status until bowel function has completely returned to avoid distention and vomiting.

NDx: High risk for altered oral mucous membranes
Give mouth care frequently. Encourage the patient to rinse mouth with water often when able.

NDx: High risk for infection
Administer prophylactic antibiotics as ordered. Use strict aseptic technique when doing wound care and handling catheters and related equipment. Reinforce dressing as needed unless wet with predominantly bloody drainage, in which case it should be changed. Institute a skin-care protocol before signs of irritation from drainage are noted. Use paste or salve to prevent contact of drainage with the skin surface.

Change the dressing at the TPN catheter site regularly, using strict technique as described in Chapter 21. Caution the patient against touching the abdominal dressing or the dressing at the TPN catheter site.

NDx: High risk for altered health maintenance
Because the patient will most likely be discharged before the surgical wounds are completely healed,

demonstrate to the patient and the family techniques to be used for wound care and dressing changes. Observe as patient or a family member performs wound care and one or more dressing changes.

Teach the patient and family about signs of wound infection, and instruct them to notify the physician at the first sign of infection.

Additional Interventions

Support the patient's and family's coping mechanisms. Use additional sources of support such as social services and pastoral care as needed. Make referrals as needed to ensure care at home.

Evaluation

Evaluate the effectiveness of nursing care for a patient who has had a Whipple procedure by comparing the patient's status with the expected patient outcomes. Examples of specific outcomes for patients who have had a Whipple procedure have been provided in the Planning section.

The Elderly: Special Considerations

The incidence of biliary stones increases with advancing age. The associated clinical manifestations may be atypical, with symptoms of septic shock being the first sign of disease. When surgery is required, it is ideally performed as an elective procedure. This allows a thorough preparation of the patient and thus decreases the risk of complications from coexisting disease.

Pancreatic disease is also common among the elderly, and pancreatic enzyme replacement is often needed. When such replacement is ordered for an elderly patient who has difficulty swallowing, be sure to request the powdered form. Mix it well with applesauce or other fruit, but do not mix with foods containing protein. Do not let the enzymes stay on the lips or the skin because tissue breakdown can occur. Never crush enteric coated tablets.

Bibliography

Baer DL, Williams BR. Clinical pharmacology and nursing. Springhouse, PA: Springhouse, 1988.

Bagg AM. Whipple's procedure. Crit Care Nurse 1988; 8(5):34.

Bennet JR. Practical gastroenterology. New York: Macmillan, 1988.

Berk JE, Haubrich WS, Kalser MH, et al (eds). Bockus gastroenterology. 4th ed. Philadelphia: WB Saunders, 1985.

Bogiovanni GL. Essentials of clinical gastroenterology. 2nd ed. New York: McGraw-Hill, 1988.

Brandt IJ. Gastrointestinal disorders of the elderly. New York: Raven Press, 1984.

Burtis G, Davis J, Martin S. Applied nutrition and diet therapy. Philadelphia: WB Saunders, 1988.

Drossman DA (ed). Manual of gastroenterologic procedures. 2nd ed. New York: Raven Press, 1987.

Esberger KK. Nursing care of the aged. Norwalk, CT: Appleton & Lange, 1989.

Fischer JM. Cholecystectomy in the ambulatory setting: A case study. J Post Anesthesia Nurs 1988; III(5):342.

Foerster EC, Matek W, Domschke W. Endoscopic retrograde cannulation of the gallbladder: Direct dissolution of gallstones. Gastrointest Endosc 1990; 36(5)444.

Given B, Simmons S. Gastroenterology in clinical nursing. 4th ed. St. Louis: CV Mosby, 1984.

Greenberger NJ. Gastrointestinal disorders. 4th ed. Chicago: Year Book, 1990.

Groth K. Age-related changes in the gastrointestinal tract. Geriatr Nurs 1988; 9(5):278.

Guilbeau AM, Young LS, Kirshenbaum G. Laser laparoscopic cholecystectomy. AORN J 1990; 52(4):780.

Iber FL, Baum RA. Gastroenterology: A concise textbook. Concise textbook series, Vol 21. Amsterdam: Elsevier, 1987.

Jackson DC, Martin T, Evans MM, Rubio PA. Endoscopic laser cholecystectomy. AORN J 1990; 51(6):1546.

Lauschner U. Endoscopic therapy of biliary calculi. Clin Gastroenterol 1986; 15(2):333.

Mack E. Chemical dissolution of biliary stones. Contemp Surg 1986; 28(6):20.

Malseed RT, Harregan GS. Textbook of pharmacology and nursing care. Philadelphia: JB Lippincott, 1989.

Marta MR. Endoscopic retrograde cholangiopancreatography. Focus Crit Care 1987; 14(5):62.

Matthews K. Endoscopic cholecystectomy: A new approach. Todays OR Nurse. 1990; 12(8):17.

Meeker MH, Rothrock, JC. Alexander's care of the patient in surgery. 9th ed. St. Louis: CV Mosby, 1990.

Meguid MM, Meguid V. Preoperative identification of the surgical cancer patient in need of postoperative supportive total parenteral nutrition. Cancer 1985; 55(Suppl. 1):258.

Mettlin C. Dietary factors for cancer of specific sites. Surg Clin North Am 1986; 66(5):917.

Munn NE. When the bile duct is blocked. RN 1989; 52(1):50.

Nahrwold D, et al. Biliary lithotripsy. Curr Probl Surg 1990; 27(11):727.

Ondrusek RS. Cholecystectomy: An update. RN 1993; 56(1):28.

O'Reilly M, Mulry K. Cholelithotripsy. AORN J 1989; 49(6):1520.

Paunder R (ed). Recent advances in gastroenterology. No. 7. New York: Churchill Livingstone, 1988.

Rowland GA, Marks DA, Torres WE. The new gallstone destroyers and dissolvers. Am J Nurs 1989; 89(11):1473.

Sabiston DC Jr (ed). Textbook of surgery: The biological basis of modern surgical practice. 14th ed. Philadelphia: WB Saunders, 1991.

Schmalz MJ, Geenen JE, Hogan WJ, et al. Pain on common bile duct injection during ERCP: Does it indicate sphincter of Oddi dysfunction? Gastrointest Endosc 1990; 36(5):458.

Schrier RW. Geriatric medicine. Philadelphia: WB Saunders, 1990.

Shi W, Papaioannou T, Daykhovsky L, et al. Fragmentation of biliary stones with a 308 nm excimer laser. Lasers Surg Med 1990; 10(3):284.

Siegel JH, Ben-Zvi JS, Pullano WE. Mechanical lithotripsy of common duct stones. Gastrointest Endosc 1990; 36(4):351.

Sleisenger MH, Fordtran JS. Gastrointestinal disease: Pathophysiology, diagnosis and management. 4th ed. Philadelphia: WB Saunders, 1989.

Smith LH, Thier SO. Pathophysiology: The biological principles of disease. 2nd ed. Philadelphia: WB Saunders, 1985.

Sodeman WA Jr, Saladin TA, Boyd WP Jr. Geriatric gastroenterology. Philadelphia: WB Saunders, 1989.

Swazuk K, Mueller BG, Daly CJ. Laser cholecystectomy. AORN J 1989; 50(5):998.

Swonger AK, Matejski MP. Nursing pharmacology. Boston: Scott, Foresman/Little, Brown, 1988.

Urban MH. Endoscopic retrograde cholangiopancreatography. AORN J 1989; 50(3):572.

Williams SR. Nutrition and diet therapy. 6th ed. St. Louis: Times Mirror/Mosby, 1989.

Unit Eight

ADULTS WITH URINARY TRACT DYSFUNCTION

Learning Objectives

AFTER COMPLETING THIS UNIT, THE LEARNER WILL BE ABLE TO:

Chapter Twenty-five

1. Explain the normal anatomy and physiology of the urinary system.
2. Describe common clinical manifestations of urinary tract dysfunction.
3. Identify information and physical examination data essential to the assessment of the urinary system.
4. Identify the most common laboratory and radiologic studies used to diagnose urinary disorders.
5. Describe medical management and surgical procedures commonly used in the treatment of patients with urinary disorders.
6. Identify data essential to the assessment of patients undergoing treatment of urinary disorders.
7. State nursing diagnoses and related expected patient outcomes commonly applicable to patients undergoing treatment of urinary disorders.
8. Describe nursing interventions, with their rationales, commonly applicable to patients undergoing treatment of urinary disorders.
9. Explain the basis for evaluation of nursing care provided to patients undergoing treatment of urinary disorders.
10. Identify special considerations for the elderly patient with altered urinary function.

Chapter Twenty-six

1. Describe common urinary disorders in terms of etiology, pathophysiology, clinical manifestations, diagnostic procedures, and medical management.
2. Identify common pharmacologic agents used to treat urinary disorders.
3. Explain the effects of acute and chronic renal failure.
4. Describe the health teaching appropriate for the patient who is at high risk for urinary infections.
5. Identify information and physical examination data essential to the assessment of patients with common urinary disorders.
6. State nursing diagnoses and related expected patient outcomes commonly applicable to patients with urinary disorders.
7. Describe nursing interventions, with their rationales, commonly applicable to patients with urinary disorders.
8. Explain the basis for evaluation of nursing care provided to patients with common urinary disorders.
9. Identify special considerations for the elderly patient with a urinary disorder.

Chapter Twenty-five

KNOWLEDGE BASIC TO THE NURSING CARE *of Adults with* Urinary Tract Dysfunction

The urinary system is responsible for maintaining a homeostatic state by reabsorbing and retaining materials needed by the body for a variety of activities, and filtering and excreting waste materials. Any dysfunctions in the system may also cause disruption in other systems, such as the cardiovascular system; gastrointestional, liver, and biliary systems; neurologic system; and even the integumentary system.

Anatomy and Physiology

The urinary tract consists of the paired kidneys and ureters, the urinary bladder, and the urethra. These structures are essentially the same in both sexes with the exception of the urethra, which is longer in the male (Fig. 25–1). Dysfunction in the system has a profound effect on almost all other body systems because function of the urinary tract is critical to the maintenance of overall homeostasis.

Kidneys

The kidneys are paired organs that lie lateral to the vertebral column between the twelfth thoracic (T-12) and the third lumbar (L-3) vertebrae. The kidneys lie in an oblique position. They are found retroperitoneally against the posterior abdominal wall in the right and left upper abdominal quadrants. The average size kidney measures approximately 12 to 14 cm in length, 5 to 7 cm in width, and 3 cm in thickness; the adult kidney weighs approximately 150 g (5 oz). The left kidney is usually slightly larger than the right, and the position of the liver causes the right kidney to be somewhat lower in position than the left.

Externally, the hilum is a concave notch on the medial side of the kidney. In addition to the ureter, the renal artery, the renal vein, nerves, and lymphatic vessels enter the kidney through the hilum. The parenchyma is the functional tissue and consists of the cortex and the medulla. The kidneys are enclosed in the thin, fibrous renal capsule. The capsule is supported by layers of perineal fat and Gerota's fascia. The capsule covers all areas of the kidney except the hilum. The muscles of the back, flank, and abdomen also provide support and protection to the kidneys.

On cross section, the kidney is composed of two main parts: the cortex and the medulla (Fig. 25–2). The medulla is below the cortex. The medulla is divided into 10 to 20 triangle-shaped wedges referred to as the renal pyramids. The base of each pyramid faces the cortex, and the apex or renal papilla faces the center of the kidney. The papillae carry formed urine into the collecting system. The pyramids of the medulla have a somewhat striated appearance as contrasted with the smoother texture of the cortical substance. The cortex extends inward between each of two pyramids, forming the renal columns. The apices of the renal pyramids form a "cupping" effect, or the minor calices. Each minor calix joins one or two other minor calices to form a major calix; there are approximately eight minor calices and three major calices. The major calices come together at the center of the medulla to form the renal pelvis.

The renal pelvis is a cone-shaped structure that extends from the center of the medulla. It exits the kidney through the hilum and curves downward to form the ureter. The kidney pelvis normally holds 5 to 7 ml of urine.

The cortex of the kidney, or outer layer, contains the nephrons. The nephron is the functioning unit of the kidney (Fig. 25–3). It contains the glomeruli, which are a tuft of capillaries. Blood enters into the glomerulus via the afferent arterioles and exits via the efferent arterioles. The glomerulus is enclosed in Bowman's capsule. Bowman's capsule is the beginning of the tubular system of the nephron. The tubular system consists of the proximal convoluted tubule (PCT), the loop of Henle, and the distal convoluted tubules (DCT). This structure twists and turns throughout the parenchyma of the kidney. The distal convoluted tubules terminate in one of the many collecting ducts that pass through the papillae and calyces, emptying into the renal pelvis.

The renal artery is the major blood supply of the kidneys. The kidneys receive 25% of the total cardiac output. The renal artery arises from the abdominal aorta, branching into the right and left renal arteries. The renal veins empty into the inferior vena cava.

The kidneys have both sympathetic and parasympathetic innervation. Innervation is through the lesser splanchnic nerves. Blood vessels, lymphatics, and nerves all exit through the hilus.

The renal system's overall function can generally be described as the maintenance of the body's internal homeostasis. It does so by the use of glomerular filtration, tubular reabsorption and secretion, and excretion. A more definitive description of this function is (1) excretion of the body's metabolic waste (primary function), (2) regulation of fluid and electrolyte balance, (3) maintenance of the body's acid-base balance, (4) assistance with calcium metabolism and regulation of blood pressure, and (5) regulation of red blood cell production. Renal function can be affected by the kidney's response to the composition, pressure, and volume of blood flowing through the kidneys.

Approximately 180 L of plasma, approximately 125 ml/minute, are filtered through the kidneys in 25 hours. In that time, 1 L becomes urine and the other 179 L are reabsorbed, as is two thirds of the solute. The kidneys selectively reabsorb those essential substances needed to maintain normal body fluid composition and excrete unneeded substances in the urine (Fig. 25–4).

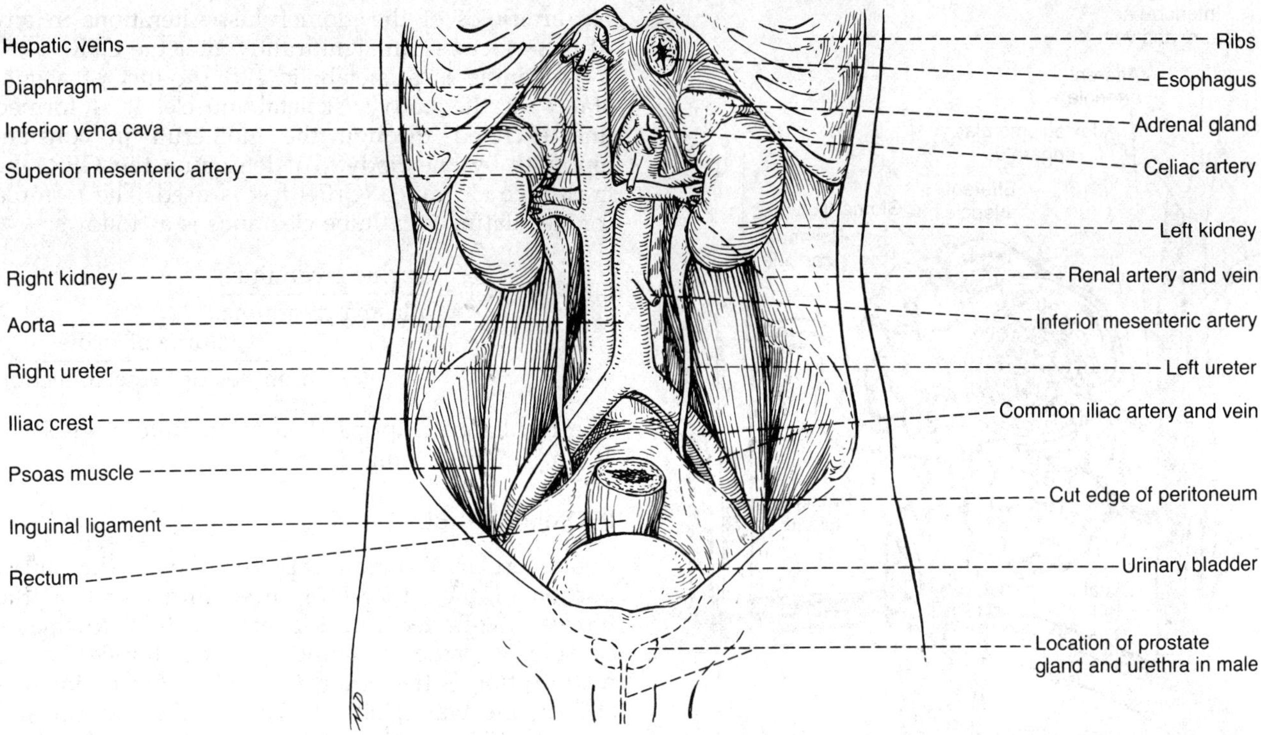

Figure 25–1.

Kidney and related structures. (From Black JM, Matassarin-Jacobs, E. Luckmann and Sorenson's medical-surgical nursing. 4th ed. Philadelphia: WB Saunders, 1993, p 1406.)

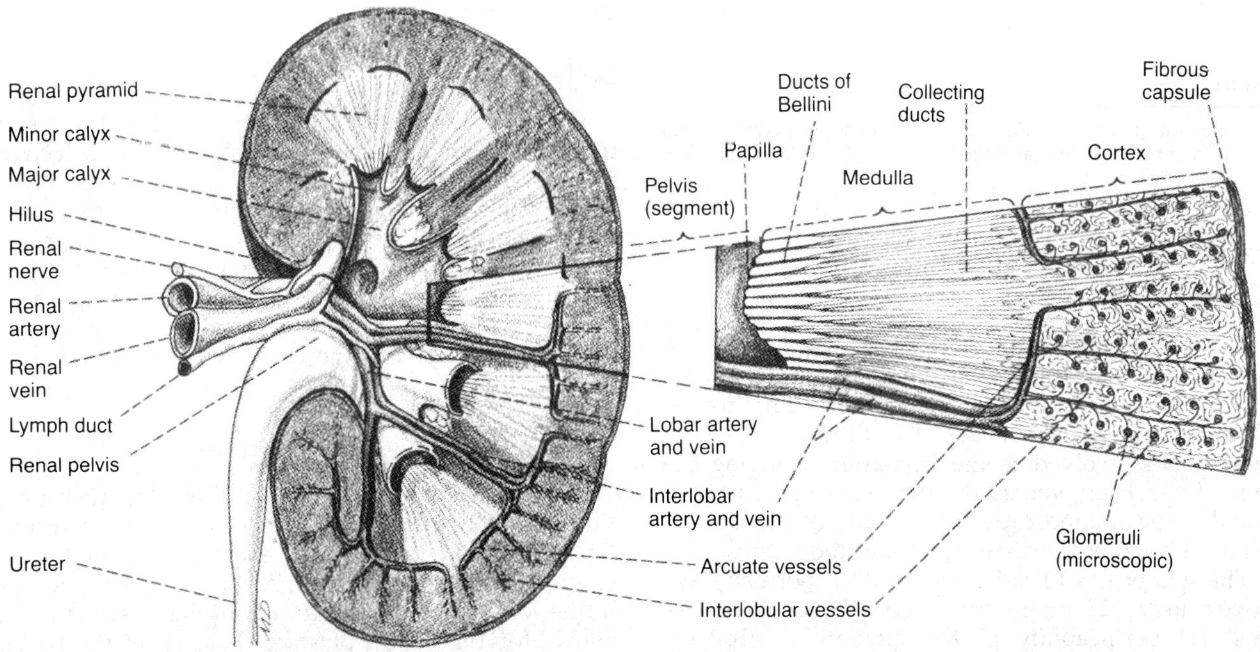

Figure 25–2.

Anatomy of the kidney, and enlargement of a segment of the kidney. (From Black JM, Matassarin-Jacobs, E. Luckmann and Sorenson's medical-surgical nursing. 4th ed. Philadelphia: WB Saunders, 1993, p 1406.)

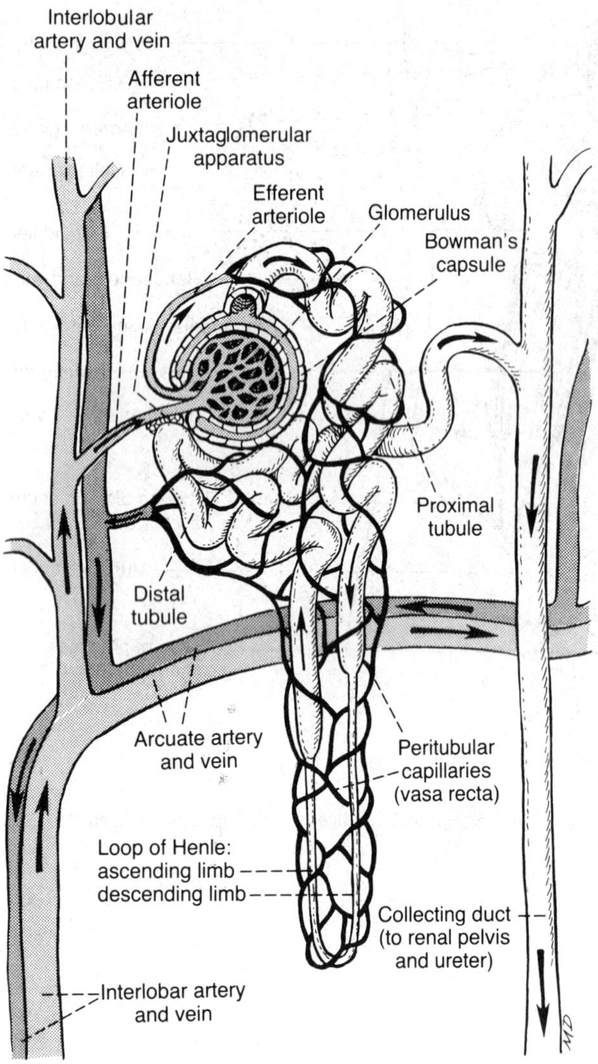

Figure 25–3.

The nephron. (From Black JM, Matassarin-Jacobs, E. Luckmann and Sorenson's medical-surgical nursing. 4th ed. Philadelphia: WB Saunders, 1993, p 1407.)

URINE FORMATION AND EXCRETION

GLOMERULUS

The primary function of the kidneys, that of the excretion of metabolic waste, begins in the glomerulus. In the glomerulus, or capillary tuft, filtration of plasma is the principal task. The filtration pressure mechanism involved is the hydraulic pumping action of the heart versus the opposing osmotic (colloidal) pressure and capsular pressure of the kidney. When these pressures are equal, filtration stops.

The gomerular filtration rate (GFR), normally approximately 125 ml/minute, depends on three factors: (1) permeability of the glomerular capillary walls, (2) blood pressure, and (3) effective filtration process. It is also regulated and kept constant by the contraction and relaxation of the afferent and efferent arterioles of the glomerulus. Alterations in any of these factors can significantly alter the GFR.

Creatinine is a metabolic end product of a substance in the body's skeletal muscle. It is formed and excreted through the glomeruli in constant amounts by the body. To determine the GFR, the creatinine clearance (CrCl) test is used. The formula for calculating creatinine clearance is as follows:

$$\text{GFR} = \text{CrCl} = \frac{\text{urine creatinine}}{\text{plasma creatinine}} \times \frac{\text{volume of urine}}{\text{minutes of urine collection}}$$

The results are expressed in ml/minute, with 90 to 100 ml/minute being normal.

PROXIMAL TUBULE

Glomerular filtration represents only the initial portion of the process of urine formation. As the filtrate is collected into the space within Bowman's capsule, it passes into the proximal tubule, where reabsorption is the primary function. Approximately 80% of the water, 50% to 70% of the sodium and chloride, 85% of all electrolytes, and normally all of the filtered glucose are reabsorbed here.

LOOP OF HENLE

The filtrate continues through the loop of Henle. As the blood supply of the nephron runs parallel to the loop of Henle, the formation and maintenance of the osmotic gradient by the reabsorption of sodium chloride is the primary function of this portion of the nephron.

DISTAL TUBULE

The continued flow of the filtrate is into the distal tubule and on into the collecting duct, as selective reabsorption and secretion of certain substances convert the filtrate into urine. The urine flows into the ducts of the renal papillae, into the minor calices, the major calices, and finally into the renal pelvis. Here the urine flow is promoted by the renal intraluminal pressure and ureteral peristaltic activity. The urine is transported down the ureter into the bladder.

REGULATION OF FLUID AND ELECTROLYTES

By altering the processes of filtration, reabsorption, and secretion, fluids and electrolytes are regulated. If renal blood flow is adequate, the nephrons control fluid volume through concentration and dilution of urine. Dilute urine in the distal tubule allows for regulation of water balance in the body. If the body is dehydrated, antidiuretic hormone (ADH) is released and water is reabsorbed. If the body is hydrated, ADH is not released and water is

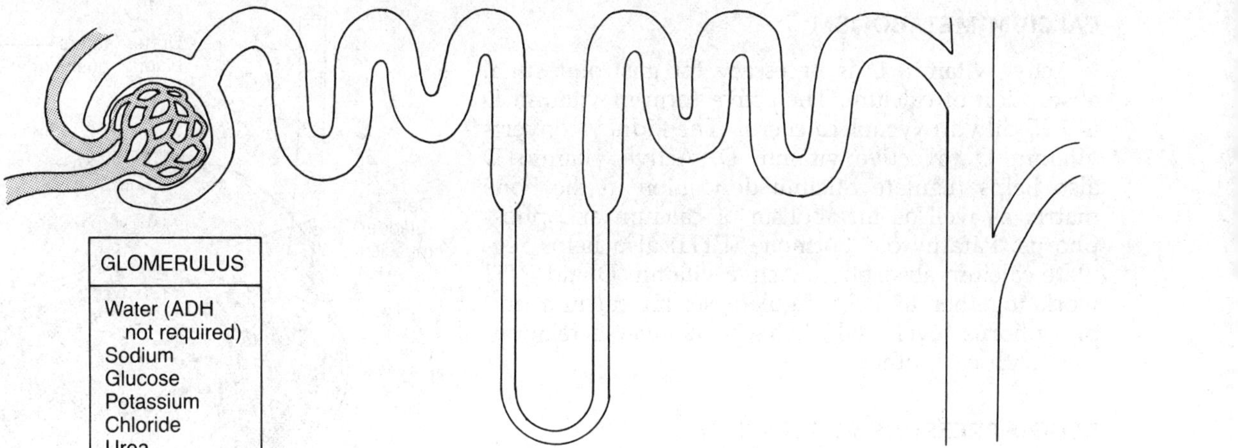

	GLOMERULUS	PROXIMAL TUBULE	LOOP OF HENLE	DISTAL TUBULE	COLLECTING DUCT
FILTRATION (from blood)	Water (ADH not required) Sodium Glucose Potassium Chloride Urea Urate Uric acid Proteins Amino acids Bicarbonate Creatinine Phosphate Inulin PAH	Isotonic filtrate	Hypertonic filtrate	Isotonic or hypotonic filtrate	Hypertonic or hypotonic filtrate
REABSORPTION (into blood)		Water (ADH not required) Sodium Glucose Potassium Chloride Urea Urate Uric acid Proteins Amino acids Carbon dioxide	Water Sodium Chloride Urea Urate Carbon dioxide	Water (ADH required) Sodium Chloride Urea Urate Carbon dioxide	Water (ADH required) Sodium Chloride Urea Urate Carbon dioxide
SECRETION (from blood)		Creatinine Hydrogen PAH		Potassium Uric acid Hydrogen	Potassium Hydrogen

Figure 25–4.

Normal physiologic function of the nephron in urine formation. Although inulin and para-aminohippuric acid (pah) are not normally present, they are important test substances. (From Black JM, Matassarin-Jacobs, E. Luckmann and Sorenson's medical-surgical nursing. 4th ed. Philadelphia: WB Saunders, 1993, p 1411.)

excreted. The distal tubule and collecting ducts need ADH to become permeable to water.

Electrolyte balance is influenced by hydrostatic and osmotic pressures. The majority of electrolytes are reabsorbed in the proximal convoluted tubule. The regulation of electrolytes occurs in the distal tubules. Depending on the concentration of the electrolytes in the urine, the tubular cells secrete or further reabsorb electrolytes in the urine. This takes place through diffusion and active transport.

REGULATION OF ACID-BASE BALANCE

Regulation of acid-base balance is done by both the respiratory and the renal systems. The kidneys are the primary regulator of pH. The renal tubule cells normally secrete equal amounts of hydrogen and bicarbonate. In response to acidosis, excess hydrogen ions are secreted into the proximal and distal tubules and the collecting ducts and excreted in the urine. The kidneys can also regenerate bicarbonate that is reabsorbed. In an alkalotic state, bicarbonate can be excreted in the urine.

STIMULATION OF RED BLOOD CELL PRODUCTION

The renal parenchyma is believed to produce erythropoietin. Erythropoietin is needed to stimulate the bone marrow to produce red blood cells. As a result of deficit of erythropoietin, the client becomes anemic.

CALCIUM METABOLISM

Active vitamin D is necessary for gastrointestinal absorption of calcium. The active form of vitamin D is 1,25-dihydroxycholecalciferol. The kidney converts vitamin D to active vitamin D. Active vitamin D also helps regulate calcium deposition in the bone matrix as well as metabolism of calcium and phosphorus. Parathyroid hormone (PTH) also helps regulate calcium absorption. Active vitamin D and PTH work together to help regulate serum calcium and phosphorus levels, which have an inverse relationship with each other.

BLOOD PRESSURE REGULATION

The kidneys help regulate blood pressure through regulation of plasma volume, the renin-angiotensin-aldosterone system, and prostaglandins. Plasma regulation is done through reabsorption of water and by controlling the composition of extracellular fluid.

The renin-angiotensin-aldosterone system plays an important role in blood pressure regulation. The release of the hormone renin is caused by a decrease in blood flow or volume or a decrease in serum sodium, or both. Renin is released by the juxtaglomerular apparatus of the nephron. Renin stimulates the conversion of angiotensinogen to angiotensin I in the liver. Angiotensin I is a mild vasoconstrictor. Angiotensinase converts angiotensin I to angiotensin II in the lungs. Angiotensin II is a powerful vasoconstrictor and stimulates the release of aldosterone. Aldosterone is a mineralocorticoid that increases the reabsorption of sodium. The increased sodium increases the amount of water reabsorbed. The increase of water absorbed and vasoconstriction increase blood pressure.

Prostaglandins are substances produced in the kidney and other tissues in the body. It is believed they have either vasoconstricting or vasodilating properties that facilitate regulation of glomerular filtration, vascular resistance, and renin production. Research on the role and function of prostaglandins is in progress because their actual mechanism is not completely understood.

Ureters

The ureters are paired, cylindrical, fibromuscular tubes that transport urine by peristalsis from the renal pelvis to the bladder. They are approximately 30 to 33 cm in length and vary in diameter from 2 to 8 cm. Points of narrowing in the ureters occur at (1) the ureteropelvic junction, (2) the point where they enter the bony pelvis as they cross over the iliac vessels, and (3) the ureterovesical junction. There is no true valve or sphincter at the location where the ureters enter the bladder, but their oblique pathway into the bladder creates a type of mucosal fold that, in the normal state, prevents urine from flowing black up the ureters to the kidneys (reflux) during voiding or bladder emptying.

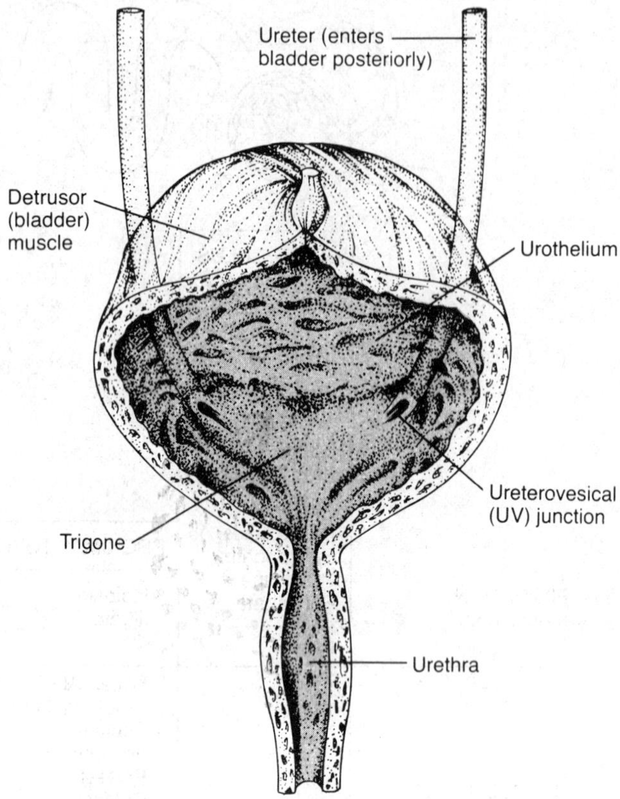

Figure 25–5.

Gross anatomy of the urinary bladder. (From Ignatavicius D, Bayne M. Medical-surgical nursing. Philadelphia: WB Saunders, 1991, p 1806.)

The ureters' function is to propel urine from the renal pelvis to the urinary bladder. This is done through peristaltic contractions of the smooth muscle fibers of the middle layer of the ureters.

Bladder

The bladder is a hollow, muscular organ that serves as a reservoir for urine (Fig. 25–5). The adult bladder normally has a capacity of 350 to 450 ml. When empty, it lies between the rectum and pubis in the male and in front of the vagina and uterus in the female. When distended, it projects well into the abdomen and can be easily palpated or percussed.

There are three openings (orifices) on the floor of the bladder, one anteriorly for the urethra and two posteriorly and laterally for the paired ureters. The triangular area outlined by these three openings is called the trigone.

The inner lining, or mucosal layer, of the bladder is composed of transitional epithelium. Beneath the mucosa is a submucosal layer made up largely of connective and elastic tissue. External to the submucosa is the muscular layer, the detrusor muscle. This muscle is a mixture of smooth muscle fibers arranged in a circular, longitudinal, and spiral manner.

The bladder neck, sometimes called the involuntary internal sphincter, is not a true circular sphincter. Rather, it is a thickening formed by the interlaced fibers of the muscular layer of the bladder as they pass distally to become the smoother urethral musculature.

By the process of micturition (voiding), the bladder is emptied as urine is passed through the urethra and excreted via the urinary meatus. Micturition is a highly coordinated and complicated process. However, the normal micturition cycle can be simply separated into two phases: urine storage and bladder emptying. Both phases are controlled and coordinated through innervation by the sympathetic, parasympathetic, and central nervous systems.

During urine storage (or the filling phase), there is a slow rise in intravesical pressure as a result of the increasing volume of urine in the bladder. As pressure increases, stretch receptors in the bladder wall convey afferent impulses via the pelvic nerve to the spinal cord. This action then stimulates the sympathetic efferent supply, located in spinal cord segments T-11 to L-2, and impulses are conveyed back to the bladder and urethra via the hypogastric nerves. The result is the activation of the internal sphincter to maintain continence, and the inhibition of a vesical contraction to allow for more complete bladder filling.

When intravesical pressure reaches a critical point and the bladder is sufficiently distended, nerve impulses are transmitted from the spinal cord to the brain. Although many areas of the brain may be involved in the voiding process, it is the brain stem that is considered to be the actual organizational center for micturition.

Bladder emptying (or voiding) occurs by parasympathetic facilitation and sympathetic inhibition. Initiation of voiding is achieved when the efferent pelvic nerve, which originates in spinal cord segments S-2 to S-4, stimulates the bladder to contract and permits the bladder neck and urethra to open. At this same time, relaxation of the external urethral sphincter and perineal muscles occurs through inhibition of the pudendal nerve, which also originates in the sacral spinal cord.

Micturition is considered a nerve-mediated event. Thus, any interruption between the sacral spinal cord and the brain stem may result in neurogenic voiding dysfunction.

There are other factors that also contribute to normal micturition. Urine storage requires appropriate bladder sensations during filling, a closed bladder outlet at rest, and the absence of involuntary bladder contractions. Bladder emptying requires a strong and well-maintained bladder contraction, as well as the absence of anatomic obstruction. Conditions that interfere or alter these requirements compromise normal voiding.

Urethra

The urethra is the hollow muscular tube that conveys urine from the bladder to the urinary meatus (opening) for excretion. In the female, the urethra is approximately 4 cm in length and extends from the bladder neck to the meatus. It is slightly curved and lies beneath the pubis symphysis just anterior to the vagina. The epithelial lining of the female urethra is squamous in its distal portion and transitional in the remainder. The submucosal layer consists of both connective and elastic tissue. External to the submucosa is a layer of smooth muscle that is continuous with the inner longitudinal layer of the bladder's muscle wall. Surrounding this is a heavy layer of circular smooth muscle fibers that extends from the external muscular layer of the bladder. These fibers constitute the true involuntary internal urethral sphincter (bladder neck). External to this is the circular, striated, voluntary, external sphincter that surrounds the middle third of the urethra.

The urethra in the male is approximately 15 cm long and is described as being made up of five portions. In descending order they are the prostatic, membranous, bulbous, penile (pendulous), and glandular portions. The prostatic urethra and the membranous urethra are sometimes referred to as the posterior urethra; the bulbous, penile, and glandular portions are referred to as the anterior urethra. The mucosal layer in the male urethra is also made up of squamous epithelium distally; proximally it is transitional in type. The internal sphincter is formed of the same muscle fibers previously described. The external sphincter in the male surrounds the urethra at the narrowest portion, the membranous urethra.

The urethra serves as a conduit for the elimination of urine from the body. When pressure in the urethra falls, it facilitates movement of urine from the bladder into the urethra. The female urethra empties by gravity, while the male urethra empties by several contractions of the bulbocavernous muscle.

Clinical Manifestations of Urinary Tract Dysfunction

The elimination of urine is a normal physiologic process that most people take for granted until changes occur that disrupt what are considered normal and usual bladder habits. Because of fear, some will choose to ignore such changes; however, prompt urologic consultation is always advised. The discussion that follows defines and describes the most common symptoms associated with disorders of the urinary tract.

Dysfunctional Voiding

Despite the many disease processes that alter urination, symptoms of dysfunctional voiding are similar in that they represent a problem at the level of the lower urinary tract. The similarity among these symptoms further extends to possible complications, which include chronic urinary tract infections, hydronephrosis, and a decrease in the overall integrity and function of the bladder and urethra.

FREQUENCY

Frequency is the most common urologic symptom and refers to how often an individual urinates. During the daytime, the normal adult usually voids every 3.5 to 4 hours, and at night, no more than once. The patient who complains of frequency may be voiding as often as every 1 to 2 hours during the day and night. There are many causes of frequent urination, including an increased volume of urine, decreased bladder capacity, inflammation with increased sensitivity of the urinary tract, pressure from abdominal masses, incomplete bladder emptying, and even anxiety.

URGENCY

Urgency is a sudden and very strong desire to urinate that is difficult to suppress. This symptom suggests an irritation of the bladder, which may be caused by an infection, tumor, or neurologic disease. Often, urinary urgency is triggered by everyday events such as the sound of running water, an abrupt change in position (e.g., sitting to standing), and the sensation of warm water on the skin.

DYSURIA

Dysuria is the term that refers to painful or difficult urination. Frequency and urgency are symptoms that usually accompany dysuria; together they suggest an inflammation or irritation of the lower urinary tract. The location of the discomfort may be a clue to the cause of dysuria. For instance, pain at the beginning of urination points to a problem in the urethra, whereas pain during or after urination suggests a problem in the bladder.

NOCTURIA

Nocturia is a nighttime frequency and is generally related to an increase in urine production at night. This symptom may be suggestive of a decrease in the function of the renal parenchyma. However, nocturia often occurs in the absence of any disease process. An individual who drinks large amounts of fluid in the evening is likely to experience nocturia. Similarly, the diuretic effect of coffee and alcohol, if consumed in the evening, produces nocturia. Medication-induced nocturia is common in one who takes diuretics for congestive heart failure, especially if the medication is taken in the evening. Additionally, the elderly person who experiences generalized fluid retention during the day, will have nocturia caused by the movement of fluid with rest. Unexplained nocturia is a disturbance that should be investigated if it occurs two or more times each night.

NOCTURNAL ENURESIS

Nocturnal enuresis is the involuntary release of urine during sleep—in other words, bedwetting. This symptom is sometimes confused with nocturia, but the two are distinctly different. The patient with nocturia awakens with the need to urinate and has sufficient time to get to the bathroom; the patient with nocturnal enuresis is unaware of the need to urinate and awakens only after the bed has been wet with urine. The manifestation of nocturnal enuresis in the adult is highly suggestive of a neurologic disorder.

HESITANCY

Hesitancy is a delay in the start of urination. In men, this symptom may be accompanied by the complaint of a slow or weak urine stream, an intermittent stream, or postvoid dribbling. Together these symptoms suggest a blockage of the lower urinary tract, which is commonly caused by an enlarged prostate or urethral stricture.

URINARY RETENTION

Urinary retention is the inability to effectively empty the bladder. Acute retention occurs postoperatively but may also be medication-induced or the result of injury to the lower back or pelvis. Chronic retention is related to longstanding obstruction of the lower urinary tract, as well as neurologic and psychogenic disorders. Most patients who experience urinary retention are completely unable to urinate; depending upon the cause of retention, the urge to void may or may not be present. It should be noted that one is also considered to have urinary retention if a stream can be produced but there is residual urine in the bladder. Residual urine should be no more than 50 ml.

Application of the Nursing Process to the Care of the Patient with Urinary Retention

Assessment

Assess the patient's usual urinary elimination pattern. Ask the patient how often he or she voids and the amount of urine voided. Ask whether the patient has experienced any frequency, urgency, fullness, or suprapubic discomfort. Assess the patient for distention by palpating the bladder area and above the symphysis pubis. Check the intake and output record for the past 24 hours. Assess for residual urine by catheterizing the patient immediately after voiding. The amount of urine obtained should be measured and recorded.

Nursing Diagnoses and Planning

The nursing diagnosis and related expected patient outcomes most commonly applicable to patients experiencing urinary retention are as follows:

NDx: Urinary retention related to postoperative complications

Planning: Patient outcomes
1. Patient voids adequate amounts within reasonable intervals.
2. Patient denies frequency, urgency, fullness, or suprapubic discomfort.
3. Patient has no visible or palpable bladder distention.
4. Patient has balanced fluid intake and output within 48 hours after surgery.

Nursing Interventions

NDx: Urinary retention
Collect data regarding usual urinary elimination patterns. Assess for sign and symptoms of urinary retention such as complaints of frequency, urgency, fullness, or bladder discomfort; bladder distention; and small frequent voidings.

Monitor fluid intake and output. Fluid input and output should be balanced within 48 hours after surgery. In the initial postoperative period, urinary output is expected to decrease as a result of increased blood loss that increases the secretion of ADH and aldosterone. Notify the physician if there is no urinary output within 6 to 12 hours postoperatively.

Instruct the patient in measures to prevent urinary retention. Teach the patient to void when the urge is felt. Provide privacy; allow the patient to get up to go to the commode unless contraindicated; pour warm water over the perineum, run water, or put the patient's hand in warm water. Encourage the patient to try to void after 2 to 3 hours.

Evaluation

Evaluate the effectiveness of nursing care for a patient with urinary retention by comparing the patient's status with the expected patient outcomes. Examples of specific outcomes for patients with urinary retention have been provided in the Planning section.

INCONTINENCE

Incontinence is a symptom; it is not a disease. It is defined, according to the International Continence Society, as "an involuntary loss of urine sufficient in quantity and/or frequency to be a social or health problem." Urologic and neurologic disorders can cause incontinence. Many factors, including the aging process, can contribute to incontinence. Incontinence is one of the most disruptive disorders of the urinary system. It causes stress for both the patient and the caregiver. It is often a major factor in the decision to seek long-term care. There are five types of urinary incontinence and the pathophysiology is different for each (Table 25–1).

Total Incontinence. Total incontinence is the constant and involuntary dribble of urine. This is pri-

Table 25–1. CLASSIFICATION OF URINARY INCONTINENCE

TYPE	FEATURE	CAUSE
Total incontinence	Continuous and unpredictable passage of urine	Injury to the lower urinary tract, sphincter trauma, surgery, or childbirth
Functional incontinence	Difficulty or inability to reach the toilet in time as a result of environmental barriers, disorientation, and/or physical limitations	Intact lower urinary tract but factors such as immobility, severe cognitive impairment, musculoskeletal impairments, and restricted access to toilets cause the incontinence
Urge incontinence	Strong desire to urinate with an uncontrolled emptying	Bladder irritation or reduced bladder capacity after radiation treatment, urinary tract infection, increased urine concentration, the use of caffeine or alcohol, or an enlarged prostate
Stress incontinence	Immediate involuntary loss of urine as a result of an increase in intraabdominal pressure (coughing, laughing, straining)	Decreased pelvic muscle tone caused by menopause, childbirth, obesity, or surgical procedure interfering with the normal structure
Reflex incontinence	Constant urine loss	Neurologic abnormalities such as spinal cord lesions, also drugs, tumors, benign strictures, and prostatic hypertrophy

marily caused by neurologic disorders, trauma, or anatomic problems.

Reflex Incontinence. Reflex incontinence is associated with urinary retention. It is caused by a grossly distended bladder that leaks as more urine is produced and as intraabdominal pressure is exerted on the full bladder. It is common among those who have sustained a spinal cord injury and is seen in autonomic neuropathies and bladder neck obstruction.

Urge Incontinence. Urge incontinence results when the feeling to urinate is so strong and so severe that uncontrolled bladder emptying occurs. This may be due to bladder inflammation from tumor or infection. However, urge incontinence is more frequently due to uninhibited bladder contractions that are related to neurologic disorders, such as spinal cord injuries.

Stress Incontinence. Stress incontinence is the unexpected loss of small amounts of urine when there is a rapid rise in intraabdominal pressure, either from coughing, laughing, straining, or physical activity. In most instances, the pelvic muscles supporting the bladder have weakened, and the normal anatomic position of the bladder and urethra has changed. This type of incontinence is more common in females. Causes of stress incontinence include childbirth trauma, as well as loss of muscle tone secondary to obesity or aging.

Functional Incontinence. Functional incontinence is an involuntary, unpredictable passage of urine. The patient cannot control micturition owing to environmental barriers, physical limitations, or disorientation. The patient is unable to reach the bathroom in time to void.

Application of the Nursing Process to the Care of the Patient with Incontinence

Nursing diagnoses have been identified by North American Nursing Diagnosis Association (NANDA) for the five types of incontinence. Much of the nursing care is similar. The problem of total incontinence is discussed here.

Assessment

Ask the patient for a detailed voiding history. Questions should relate to time, place, and amount of urine. Ask the patient about awareness of the passage of urine and whether a stimulus can be identified. Ask about past history of urologic or neurologic disease and dementia. Ask about symptoms of hesitancy, urgency, polyuria, dysuria, and nocturia. An accurate history is very important in assessing the incontinent patient. Keep an accurate record of fluid input and output. Assess the characteristic of the urine. Assess the mental status of the patient.

Nursing Diagnoses and Planning

The nursing diagnosis and related expected patient outcomes most commonly applicable to patients with total incontinence are as follows:

NDx: Total incontinence related to independent contraction of detrusor reflex due to trauma or surgery

Planning: Patient outcomes

1. Patient and significant other demonstrate bladder regimen.
2. Patient's voiding occurs on a planned schedule.
3. Patient's skin is intact.
4. Patient has decrease in episodes of incontinence.
5. Patient and significant other manage bladder elimination.
6. Patient verbalizes feelings of self-worth.

Nursing Interventions

NDx: Total incontinence

Establish a bladder training program, and assist the patient and significant other in carrying out this program. Set up a schedule for toileting. Ensure that all staff involved know the schedule and adhere to it. The patient may or may not require the placement of an indwelling catheter. Check frequently for incontinence. To prevent skin breakdown, it is essential that the patient remain dry.

Teach the patient and family the bladder regimen, and give support and encouragement. Praise both patient and family for maintenance of the program and for any decrease in the incontinent episodes. Allow the patient and family time to talk about their feelings related to this problem. Answer all questions in terminology the patient can understand.

Evaluation

Evaluate the effectiveness of nursing care for a patient with total incontinence by comparing the patient's status with the expected patient outcomes. Examples of specific outcomes for patients with total incontinence have been provided in the Planning section.

Pain

The primary reason a patient seeks urologic consultation is because of pain within the urinary tract. Discomfort may be localized to a specific organ or part, or it may refer from one area of the urinary tract to another. Generally, pains within the urinary

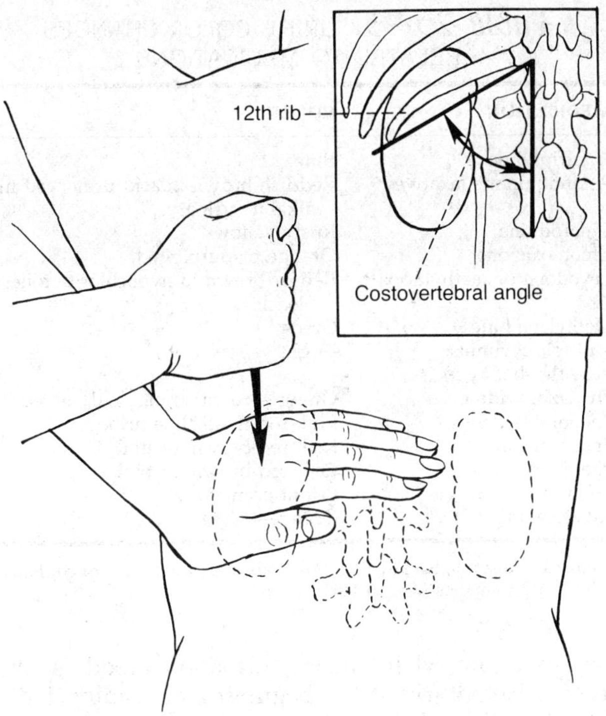

Figure 25–6.

Percussion over the costovertebral angle. (From Black JM, Matassarin-Jacobs, E. Luckmann and Sorensen's medical-surgical nursing. 4th ed. Philadelphia: WB Saunders, 1993, p 1420.)

tract originate from distention or inflammation of the system.

RENAL PAIN

Renal pain manifests as a constant and dull ache in the area of the costovertebral angle below the twelfth rib (Fig. 25–6). This type of pain may also be sharp or paroxysmal and may radiate to the lower abdomen and inguinal area. It is important to note that some disorders of the kidney, such as cancer and tuberculosis, are not painful, owing to the slow development of the disease process.

URETERAL PAIN

Ureteral pain is colicky in nature and among the most severe types of pain known. It is caused by sudden obstruction, usually from a calculus, that produces hyperperistalsis and spasm of the ureter. A stone obstructing the upper ureter produces symptoms similar to those of renal pain, but may also radiate pain to the testis or labia. Pain generated by obstruction of the lower ureter causes suprapubic discomfort, but may also be felt in the bladder, penis, or urethra.

BLADDER PAIN

Bladder pain due to overdistention causes local discomfort in the suprapubic area. Infection and inflammation of the bladder produce a sharp burning pain that radiates to the distal urethra; it intensifies with urination.

Application of the Nursing Process to the Care of the Patient Experiencing Urinary Tract Pain

Assessment

Assess the characteristics of the pain, including type, location, duration, severity, frequency, and any precipitating factors. Assess for tenderness or pain with palpation. Ask about methods of pain relief and what lessens the pain. Observe the patient's reaction to the pain.

Nursing Diagnoses and Planning

The nursing diagnosis and related expected patient outcomes most commonly applicable to patients experiencing urinary tract pain are as follows:

NDx: Pain related to distention or inflammation

Planning: Patient outcomes
1. Patient reports that pain is controlled with analgesics.
2. Patient identifies comfort measures to help relieve pain.
3. Patient states coping measures such as relaxation techniques to help relieve, lessen, or tolerate pain.

Nursing Interventions

NDx: Pain
Place the patient in comfortable positions, and reposition frequently. Assess when pain is most severe, and allow the patient to rest during those periods. Administer pain medications as ordered prior to activity so that patient can tolerate the activity better.

Assist the patient in finding alternate methods to alleviate, lessen, or be able to tolerate the pain. Show the patient and family relaxation techniques that may help. Encourage the patient to practice them frequently.

Evaluation

Evaluate the effectiveness of nursing care for a patient experiencing urinary tract pain by comparing the patient's status with the expected patient outcomes. Examples of specific outcomes for patients experiencing urinary tract pain have been provided in the Planning section.

Change in Urine Characteristics

Urine color normally ranges from pale yellow to deep gold, depending on its concentration. Significant changes in color may be disease-related; however, an alteration in urine color may also be caused by foods or medications (Tables 25–2 and 25–3). Turbidity refers to the clarity of urine. Upon visualization, a normal urine specimen should be clear. A cloudy specimen is noted when a urinary tract infection is present, owing to the large number of white blood cells in the urine. Benign cloudiness occurs at an alkaline pH and is caused by the precipitation of phosphates in the urine but also occurs when a urine specimen has been left standing at room temperature for a long period of time.

Urine has an odor that at most times is nonspecific. In certain instances, though, the scent given off by a freshly voided urine specimen may be a clue to an underlying disease process. For example, a foul-smelling urine is typically associated with a bacterial infection; a strong, pungent odor suggests gram-negative bacteriuria. The presence of ketone bodies gives urine a sweet, fruity smell, whereas urine odor that resembles maple syrup or sweaty feet suggests a metabolic disorder.

Hematuria

The presence of blood in the urine, whether grossly visible or only a microscopic finding, is always a serious situation that requires evaluation. In the young adult, trauma, urinary tract infection, and urinary calculi are among the most common causes of hematuria. In the middle-aged to elderly patient, hematuria is highly suggestive of a tumor within the urinary tract, although infection, calculi, benign prostatic hypertrophy, vascular malformation of the kidney, and medications may also induce bleeding.

To help pinpoint the site of bleeding, it is important to know when during urination blood is observed. Hematuria at the beginning of voiding indicates bleeding of the anterior urethra. Hematuria at the end of the stream suggests posterior urethral, bladder neck, or trigone bleeding. Total hematuria, which is blood throughout the entire urine stream, denotes a site within or above the bladder.

Table 25–2. URINE COLOR CHANGES RELATED TO PATHOLOGIC DISORDERS

COLOR	PATHOLOGIC
Red	Bleeding in the lower urinary tract
Dark red or smoky gray	Bleeding in the upper urinary tract
Tea colored	Release of myoglobin from severely damaged tissue
Dark yellow	Presence of urobilinogen or bilirubin
Green	Presence of *Pseudomonas* organisms

Table 25–3. URINE COLOR CHANGES RELATED TO MEDICATIONS

MEDICATION	COLOR
Amitriptyline	Blue
Anthraquinone laxatives	Reddish-brown in acid urine; red in alkaline urine
Chloroquine	Rusty-yellow
Chlorzoxazone	Orange or purple-red
Levodopa or methyldopa	Red or brown in hypochlorite toilet bleach
Methylene blue	Green
Multiple vitamins (with riboflavin)	Bright yellow
Phenazopyridine	Orange-brown, orange-red, or red
Phenolphthalein	Pink-red in alkaline urine
Phenothiazine	Red, red-brown, or pink
Phenytoin	Red, red-brown, or pink
Rifampin	Bright orange-red
Sulfasalazine	Orange-yellow

From Luckmann J, Sorensen KC. Medical-surgical nursing. 3rd ed. Philadelphia: WB Saunders, 1987, p 1163.

When assessing the patient with hematuria, it is helpful to know whether or not pain is associated with the bleeding. Painful hematuria occurs in association with infections or the passage of a calculus. Painless hematuria is more ominous and is considered to be a symptom of a urinary tract neoplasm, unless studies suggest another etiology. In addition to noting the presence or absence of pain, it is also important to note the color of urine. Depending upon the number of red blood cells in the urine, as well as the source and time of bleeding, urine color varies from a light pink to bright red or dark brown.

Change in Urine Volume

Anuria refers to urine output that is 100 ml or less in a 24-hour period. Oliguria refers to a urine output that is usually between 100 and 400 ml in a 24-hour period. These terms represent varying degrees of decreased urinary output. Both conditions may be the result of acute renal failure, fluid-electrolyte imbalance, bilateral ureteral obstruction, or urethral obstruction.

Polyuria is the excessive secretion of urine, which is generally more than 2500 ml in a 24-hour period. Common causes of polyuria include a decrease in the concentrating ability of the kidneys, an increase in fluid intake (e.g., psychogenic water drinking), diabetes insipidus, diabetes mellitus, and intake of diuretics.

An accurate evaluation of a change in urine volume requires the careful recording of fluid intake and output, as well as astute observations by the nurse. Patient education about the measurement of fluid intake and output is essential to ensure compliance with a procedure that may last for several days.

Assessment of the Urinary System

The health history and detailed descriptions of urinary problems the patient is experiencing are important components in the process of diagnosing urinary system dysfunction. A physical assessment follows the history so that specific problems can be identified and a plan for care established.

Patient History

The health history is an organized method of eliciting comprehensive, pertinent information from a patient regarding past and present state of health in relation to the urinary function to formulate a data base for problem identification. The health history serves as a basis for directing attention toward specific body systems during the physical examination and allows observation of the patient during the responses to the questions. Time must be allowed during the health history to establish a relationship of trust with the patient through attentive, concerned listening and by allowing the patient to assume an active, integral role in participating in health care.

Collect the appropriate data using understandable terminology, and allow the patient to respond fully and voice concerns. Ask the patient about the history of the present illness or disorder. Ask what is the patient's chief complaint. Get a detailed description of the complaint. If incontinence is the most significant problem, ask about the time during the day or night it most frequently occurs, whether there is a precipitating event, and whether fluids were ingested prior to the episode. Ask whether the patient experiences difficulty in urinating, whether burning is present, or whether frequency is a problem. Determine whether the color and consistency of the urine is within normal ranges. Ask whether pain with urination is present. Check whether a discharge is present with urination or is present around the meatus. Ask the patient to describe the discharge by color and odor. Determine the usual amount of fluids that are ingested daily and the approximate amount of output.

Ask the female patient about urine leaks with exercise, coughing, or sneezing. Determine the severity of the problem. Ask the male patient whether he has been circumcised and whether the foreskin retracts easily. Also ask the male patient whether he experiences dribbling or nocturnal frequency or has any known prostate problems.

Ask the patient about past medical problems, medications, and previous surgeries. Also, ask about the family history of illness. Determine the patient's usual activities of daily living and whether the present condition interferes with the normal daily routine. Complete a brief review of the systems, determining whether dysfunctions in any other system are affecting the urinary system status. Carefully document the information obtained.

Physical Examination

Begin the examination with a general inspection of the patient. Note the fluid status of the patient, which may be evidenced by skin turgor, signs of edema, and comparisons of daily fluid intake and output. If edema is present, assess the severity of it. Check the mucous membranes in the mouth. Look for dry, cracked skin and sunken eyes indicative of dehydration. Weigh the patient and compare the results with the patient's stated weight. Check vital signs, noting the blood pressure in particular. Observe the patient's skin color, checking for signs of jaundice.

Check the patient's abdomen for signs of ascites. Note whether the patient seems distended near the symphysis pubis. Wearing gloves, inspect the urethral meatus, looking for redness, deviation, or discharge. Ulcerations in the area may be indicative of a sexually transmitted disease.

Using the stethoscope on the abdomen, auscultate the renal arteries for bruits, which may be indicative of artery stenosis or hypertension. Palpation of the kidneys and bladder is completed to diagnose lumps or masses. Have the patient void in a specimen container prior to palpating the bladder. This prevents discomfort from pressure on a full bladder and the urgency to void during the examination and allows for assessment of the urine. Observe the urine for color, consistency, and amount. Ask the patient whether a feeling of urgency is still present after voiding or whether the bladder does not feel empty. Palpate the kidneys bilaterally, and note any evidence of masses or tenderness. Palpate the bladder, noting the size and the presence of any lumps or tender areas.

Document the findings from the physical examination in detail, using schematics, when appropriate, to describe location. Also note statements from the patient that may explain the findings or present more data about any abnormalities found.

Diagnostic Procedures

To diagnose disorders of the urinary tract, a variety of diagnostic procedures may be used. Examina-

Table 25–4. NORMAL FINDINGS AND SIGNIFICANCE OF ABNORMAL FINDINGS IN URINALYSIS

CHARACTERISTIC	NORMAL FINDINGS	SIGNIFICANCE OF ABNORMAL FINDINGS
Color	Pale yellow	Dark amber indicates concentrated urine. Very pale yellow indicates dilute urine. Dark red or brown indicates blood in the urine; brown also may indicate increased urinary bilirubin level. Other color changes may result from diet or medications.
Odor	Specific aromatic odor, similar to ammonia	Foul smell indicates possible infection or dehydration.
Turbidity	Clear	Cloudy urine indicates infection or sediment.
Specific gravity	Usually 1.015–1.025; possible range 1.010–1.030	Changes reflect a disturbance in the concentrating and diluting function of the tubules. Specific gravity is influenced by many factors. Specific gravity may become fixed in renal insufficiency.
pH	6; possible range 4.6–8.0	Changes are caused by diet, medications, infection, acid-base imbalance, and altered renal function.
Glucose	None or < 15 mg/dl	Presence may indicate decreased tubular reabsorption capacity or hyperglycemia that exceeds this capacity.
Ketones	None	Presence reflects incomplete metabolism of fatty acids, as in diabetes mellitus.
Protein	2–8 mg/100 ml	Increased levels may indicate stress, infection, strenuous exercise, or glomerular disorders.
Red blood cells	1 or 2 per high-power field	Increased levels are normal with indwelling or intermittent catheterization or menses but may reflect tumor, stones, or glomerular disorders.
White blood cells	1–3 per high-power field	Increased levels may indicate infectious or inflammatory processes.
Bilirubin	None	Presence suggests hepatic or biliary disease or obstruction.
Casts	A few or none, composed of red blood cells or white blood cells, protein, or tubular cell casts.	Increased levels indicate presence of bacteria or protein, which is seen in severe renal disease.
Crystals	None	Presence of normal or abnormal crystals may indicate that the specimen has been allowed to stand.
Bacteria	< 1000 colonies/ml	Increased levels indicate need for urine culture to determine the presence of urinary tract infection.

From Ignatavicius D, Bayne M. Medical-surgical nursing. Philadelphia: WB Saunders, 1991, pp 1816–1817.

tion of the urine is important for all patients regardless of the disorder, but it is even more significant in determining dysfunction of the urinary system. Other tests used to evaluate function of the urinary system include hematologic tests, diagnostic imaging, and invasive diagnostic tests such as cystoscopy and biopsy.

Studies on Urine

URINALYSIS

Urinalysis is the simplest and most frequently performed diagnostic procedure; it is an essential component of the urologic evaluation. Macroscopic urinalysis includes assessment of color, turbidity, odor, and specific gravity, in addition to dipstick testing for pH, protein, glucose, ketones, bilirubin, and blood. Microscopic examination of urine sediment is done to detect red and white blood cells, epithelial cells, casts, crystals, bacteria, fungi, and fat globules (Table 25–4). A midstream sample from the first or second urination of the morning is desired for this routine examination.

URINE CULTURE

A urine culture is indicated when symptoms suggest a urinary tract infection. It is done to identify the bacteria infecting the urine so that the proper medication is selected and treatment initiated. A clear, uncontaminated urine sample is necessary when a culture is to be performed. Once the specimen has been obtained, it should be sent to the laboratory immediately to prevent the overgrowth of bacteria, which may alter the actual bacterial count. If a delay of 20 minutes or longer is anticipated between the collection of the urine and the receipt of the specimen in the laboratory, then the sample should be refrigerated; however, refrigeration must not exceed 24 hours.

URINE CYTOLOGY

Urine cytology is the microscopic examination of urine to detect the presence of atypical epithelial cells that have been shed from the surface of the urinary tract. This laboratory examination is used as a screening procedure for individuals considered at risk of developing cancer within the urinary system;

it is used in the follow-up examination of persons with known urinary tract malignancy; and it is used to diagnose inflammatory and infectious disease processes.

To perform a cytologic evaluation, a minimum of 50 ml of urine is needed. At least three specimens should be collected and examined at different times within a 3-month period. Although the first morning specimen is preferred for urine cytology studies, other types of urine samples may also be used, including a random daytime sample or a catheterized urine sample. Urine samples obtained after bladder irrigation or prostatic massage, as well as those obtained from an ileal conduit or suprapubic aspiration, are also acceptable.

24-HOUR URINE COLLECTION

A 24-hour urine collection is considered to be a valid and reliable diagnostic measure for substances excreted in the urine (Table 25–5). With regard to the urinary system, this test is commonly done to measure creatinine and protein excretion in patients with known or suspected renal disease. In stone-forming patients, it is used to measure, among other things, calcium and uric acid, which are primary components of urinary calculi.

To collect a 24-hour urine specimen, the patient should be given a container with a tight-fitting lid that holds up to 2 L. A form or piece of paper on which to make notations is also helpful.

The day and time the collection are to be started is not particularly important. However, for the sake of convenience, the patient should be advised to start the urine collection after rising in the morning and to stay home for the day. If the test is completed while the patient is hospitalized, the nurse tells the patient when to start collecting the urine.

On the morning the collection is to begin, the patient should note the exact time of awakening and then immediately void and *discard* the first-voided urine. Every voiding after this time is collected and saved. The collection period ends the next morning at the same time it was started, after saving that morning's first-voided urine.

Thorough patient instruction is necessary to ensure that the collection of a 24-hour urine specimen is done properly. Accurate results are dependent on the careful documentation of the beginning and end of the collection period as well as the compulsive saving of urine. Patients should be reminded that all urine voided during the collection times must be saved, even urine voided at night. In addition, the container filled with urine should be kept refrigerated, or on ice, while the collection is in progress and until the specimen is delivered to the laboratory. Adherence to this entire procedure is essential because misleading results may be obtained from a specimen improperly collected.

Table 25–5. NORMAL VALUES FOR A 24-HOUR URINE COLLECTION

SUBSTANCE	VALUE
Chloride	110–250 mEq
Creatinine	0–100 mg for men 0–200 mg for women
Glucose	0–0.5 g
Potassium	25–100 mEq
Sodium	30–200 mEq
Urea nitrogen	10–15 g

Hematologic Tests

COMPLETE BLOOD COUNT

With respect to urologic patients, the complete blood count is generally ordered as a screening procedure in patients with problems such as hematuria and urinary tract infections. Of special interest would be values for hematocrit and hemoglobin and white blood cell count.

BLOOD CHEMISTRY STUDIES

Blood chemistry studies are also ordered for screening purposes, especially in individuals with a history of urinary calculi formation. For those with renal failure, oliguria, or suspected fluid-ion imbalance, the frequent measurement of serum electrolytes offers a means of assessing the patient's status, as well as the effectiveness of medical treatments.

SERUM CREATININE AND BLOOD UREA NITROGEN

Serum creatinine and blood urea nitrogen (BUN) are two tests commonly used to measure glomerular filtration. The difference between these measurements relates to the rate of absorption of creatinine and urea by the renal tubules.

Creatinine is secreted in very small amounts by the renal tubules, and reabsorbed very slowly. Thus, when a rise in the creatinine occurs, it reflects an actual decrease in glomerular filtration. For this reason, the serum creatinine is considered a reliable indicator of renal function. The normal adult value for serum creatinine is 0.7 to 1.5 mg/dl. With aging, the glomerular filtration tends to decrease and the serum creatinine levels increase. After age 70, a normal creatinine level may be as high as 1.8 mg/dl.

In contrast, urea is more rapidly reabsorbed by the renal tubules. Because the level of reabsorption is directly related to the rate of urine flow through the kidneys, a mere slowing of this action quickly produces a measurable increase of urea. The BUN is a valid test, but an increase does not always imply

Table 25–6. DRUGS AFFECTING SERUM CREATININE AND BLOOD UREA NITROGEN (BUN) LEVELS

SERUM CREATININE	BUN
Amphotericin B	Bacitracin
Cefazolin	Cephaloridine
Cephalothin	Gentamicin
Gentamicin	Kanamycin
Kanamycin	Chloramphenicol
Methicillin	Methicillin
Ascorbic acid	Neomycin
Barbiturates	Vancomycin
Lithium carbonate	Methyldopa
Mithramycin	Guanethidine
Methyldopa	Sulfonamides
Phenolsulfonphthalein (PSP)	Propranolol
Bromosulfophthalein (BSP)	Morphine
Triamterene	Lithium carbonate
	Salicylates
	Hydrochlorothiazide
	Ethacrynic acid
	Furosemide
	Triamterene

the presence of renal disease. In the adult, the normal BUN level is 6 to 23 mg/dl.

Nursing Implications. Explain that the purpose of the testing is to determine how well the kidneys are excreting wastes. Instruct the patient that there is no food or water restriction before the test. Because these tests are often routinely ordered, medications that can influence the test results may not be withheld prior to the testing, but this is considered when interpreting the test results. If ordered, hold medications that influence test results for 24 hours prior to the test (Table 25–6). On the laboratory slip, list any drugs that cannot be withheld. Recognize the clinical problems associated with high levels and assess the patient accordingly. An elevated BUN level can indicate dehydration, high protein intake, gastrointestinal bleeding, or prerenal failure. An elevated serum creatinine level indicates acute and chronic renal failure or prolonged shock and can be used with other tests and procedures as a diagnostic tool for many other medical disorders. Check both the blood urea nitrogen and the creatinine levels. If both are elevated, the problem is most likely renal in nature.

Radiologic Studies

There are several radiologic studies used routinely to aid in diagnosing or ruling out disorders of the urinary tract in adults. Those studies most commonly performed are outlined in Table 25–7. Also described are several newer studies that are being used with increasing frequency as technologies are improved. Magnetic resonance imaging (MRI) and various nuclear medicine studies are very useful for patients who are allergic to contrast dye. A decade ago, such an allergy would have required extensive invasive testing or steroid preparation. Because these newer technologies are not available in all hospitals, invasive tests and steroid preparations are additionally described because they continue to be used.

The excretory urogram, also called intravenous urogram or intravenous pyelogram (IVP) remains the mainstay of urologic diagnostic tests. Along with cystoscopy, an excretory urogram is usually ordered for virtually every urologic disorder, from microscopic hematuria to renal cancer. Table 25–7 describes in detail nursing care of the patient having an excretory urogram as well as clinical uses, complications, and nursing care of other commonly performed radiologic studies.

Patients who have never had radiologic studies using contrast dye may not know that they are allergic to it. An inability to tolerate iodine-containing foods, most often shellfish, is a strong indicator of a contrast dye allergy. Patients who are allergic may know only that they had a reaction during an x-ray examination done for an entirely different disorder and thus may not relate it to any urologic tests.

The most severe complication in patients who are allergic to contrast dye is an anaphylactic reaction that causes respiratory and cardiac distress or arrest. Identification of patients at risk before the excretory urogram prevents such a disaster. An excretory urogram can be done safely even when an allergy to contrast dye exists by administering corticosteroids for 24 hours before, the day of, and 24 hours after the test, along with an antihistamine (usually diphenhydramine) 1 hour before the test. Frequently the excretory urogram is scheduled with an anesthesiologist present for careful patient monitoring in addition to the steroid preparation.

Patients with chronic diseases known to affect renal function should also receive careful assessment before any diagnostic study using contrast dye. Elevated BUN and creatinine levels should alert the nurse to possible complications, because compromised renal function makes it difficult for the kidneys to clear the dye. Alternative studies are used to evaluate the kidneys of patients with renal disease, such as a retrograde pyelogram, renal ultrasonogram, or a nuclear medicine study.

Application of the Nursing Process to the Care of the Patient Undergoing an Excretory Urogram

Assessment

By far the most important factors that must be assessed in the urology patient about to have any radiologic testing are allergy to contrast dye and

Table 25–7. MOST COMMONLY PERFORMED RADIOLOGIC AND OTHER STUDIES OF THE URINARY TRACT

DEFINITION AND DESCRIPTION	CLINICAL USES	COMPLICATIONS	NURSING CARE
KUB (KIDNEYS, URETERS, AND BLADDER)			
A plain radiographic film of the abdomen that visualizes the major organs of the urinary tract.	To identify radiopaque stones, large masses, or gross abnormalities of the kidneys, ureters, and bladder. Frequently used as an initial diagnostic test for acute flank pain or as follow-up after treatment for stone diseases.	None Contraindicated in pregnancy	Physician may order a mild laxative the night before KUB if not done on an emergency basis. Patients may require reassurance about exposure to x-rays.
EXCRETORY UROGRAM			
A radiographic study using contrast dye. The dye is injected for several minutes intravenously and then observed through a series of films as it passes through the urinary tract. A final film is taken after the patient voids the contrast dye.	Evaluation of the kidneys, ureters, and bladder. An IVP identifies the location of stones or masses and aids in diagnosis congenital anomalies. Renal function can be grossly assessed by the kidney's ability to clear the dye. The postvoid film can identify a signficant residual volume.	An unknown allergy to contrast dye may result in severe anaphylactic reaction. In rare cases, use of contrast dye can lead to acute renal failure. Hypersensitivity to contrast dye may result in pruritus, skin flushing, or difficulty breathing.	Question the patient about an allergy sensitivity to contrast dye, iodine, or iodine-containing foods (shellfish). Patients with renal failure, labile diabetes, or myeloma in those in severely dehydrated states should not undergo the test. It is also contraindicated in pregnancy. Patients with a known allergy to contrast dye can usually tolerate the test safely after a steroid prep. Explain the events that will occur before, during, and after the test. Explain the laxative preparation and dietary restrictions; assist patient in adhering to the preparation, and evaluate results. (The test preparation usually consists of a routine bowel cleansing preparation given to the patient during the evening before the test. Also a clear liquid diet may be given the day before. NPO status is maintained after midnight the night before the test is done.) After the test, provide nourishment and encourage fluid intake. Monitor, intake and output. Observe for symptoms of hypersensitivity reaction. Notify the patient's physician if nausea or vomiting occur; intravenous hydration may be ordered to ensure that the dye is flushed out of the urinary tract completely.

(continued)

renal function. Careful questioning during a nursing history can provide valuable information that can prevent dangerous complications.

Assess the patient's knowledge about the procedure, risk, and potential findings. Ask the patient about fears or anxiety related to the tests. Look for nonverbal signs of anxiety, such as nervousness; increased pulse, respirations, and blood pressure; and withdrawal from participation in conversations. Note whether the patient asks frequent questions or relates inaccurate information about the procedure.

Check the patient's fluid intake and output for several days after the procedure. Assess the color, consistency and amount of urine every 8 hours. Check whether the patient is having difficulty voiding or whether pain or burning on urination is present. Look at the results of the urinalysis and other diagnostic tests completed.

Table 25–7. (continued) MOST COMMONLY PERFORMED RADIOLOGIC AND OTHER STUDIES OF THE URINARY TRACT

DEFINITION AND DESCRIPTION	CLINICAL USES	COMPLICATIONS	NURSING CARE
RETROGRADE/ANTEGRADE PYELOGRAM *Retrograde pyelogram:* This procedure is performed in the cystoscopy suite. With the patient under local or regional anesthesia, a cystoscope is inserted (see Cystogram). A ureteral catheter is passed into the ureter, and contrast dye is injected.	Either of these studies may be ordered when IVP has failed to visualize the kidneys or ureters, or in patients with a known allergy to contrast dye. Retrograde pyelogram is the least invasive of the two procedures and is preferred for that reason. Antegrade pyelogram may be necessary in patients with ureteral abnormalities that prevent passing a ureteral catheter. It is commonly done after percutaneous renal surgery for kidney stones, because a nephrostomy catheter is already in place. Retrograde pyelogram is frequently done before ESWL in patients with radiolucent stones or as part of a follow-up regimen for patients with urologic cancer who are allergic to contrast dye.	Retrograde pyelogram: ■ Ureteral perforation ■ Perforation of the renal pelvis ■ Infection ■ Urinary retention Antegrade pyelogram: ■ Renal puncture or damage ■ Hematuria ■ Infection ■ Urinary retention ■ Perinephric hematoma	Explain the procedure and type of anesthesia to be used. Retrograde pyelogram may be done under local anesthesia only; however, both procedures are done under spinal or general anesthesia. Ensure dietary restrictions before the procedure; administer premedications if ordered. After the procedure, monitor vital signs and intake and output, and observe the patient for symptoms of systemic infection secondary to instrumentation. Urine output should be assessed for quantity and for hematuria. Puncture wounds from antegrade pyelogram should be dressed and observed for urine drainage or infection.
CYSTOGRAM A radiologic study of the bladder only. The patient is catheterized, and contrast dye is instilled through the catheter into the bladder, until the bladder is filled. Several films are taken, then the dye is drained out through the catheter and the catheter is removed. A final film is then taken.	Evaluation of the bladder for gross abnormalities. Commonly done after bladder surgery to check for extravasation. This study can detect large tumors or diverticula and can identify vesicoureteral reflux. Although not the primary diagnostic test for this, a cystogram can also identify causes of urethral obstruction and some voiding disorders. Also used in trauma patients with suspected bladder injury and in patients with enteritis diverticulitis or endometriosis when bladder involvement is suspect.	None The amount of contrast dye that extravasates through a small bladder perforation is harmless. Systemic absorption of contrast dye through the bladder wall is rarely enough to cause a reaction in the patient allergic to contrast dye.	Explain the procedure to the patient. There is usually no need for anesthesia or any preparation for a cystogram. Contraindicated in pregnancy. Patients who are allergic to contrast dye may receive a steroid preparation.
VOIDING CYSTOURETHROGRAM A radiologic study that captures on film the dynamics of voiding: how the bladder fills and how it empties. A urethral catheter is inserted, and dye is instilled into the bladder until the patient feels an urge to void. The catheter is removed and the patient is asked to void. Films are taken during filling, voiding, and after voiding.	Evaluation of the lower urinary tract, the urethra, and in some cases, the distal ureters. Commonly used as a diagnostic aid for patients with voiding disorders or anomalies when significant vesicoureteral reflux is suspected.	Same as for cystogram.	Same as for cystogram.

(continued)

Table 25–7. *(continued)* MOST COMMONLY PERFORMED RADIOLOGIC AND OTHER STUDIES OF THE URINARY TRACT

DEFINITION AND DESCRIPTION	CLINICAL USES	COMPLICATIONS	NURSING CARE
ULTRASONOGRAPHY *Renal ultrasonography:* A transducer is passed over the flank or lateral abdomen, depending on the patient's position. Transmission gel is applied to the skin and transducer. *Bladder ultrasonography:* A transducer is passed over the suprapubic and lower abdominal area.	Renal ultrasonography is used as a diagnostic aid in evaluating the kidneys for congenital anomolies, inflammatory conditions, calcifications, hydronephrosis, renal failure, and masses. Patients with suspicious areas on IVP are sent for ultrasonographic examination to determine whether these areas are cysts or solid masses. Renal ultrasonography is also frequently used to evaluate kidneys after renal transplant. Bladder ultrasonography is sometimes used in the evaluation of voiding dysfunction. Residual urine can be estimated. Any large lesions within the bladder, tumor or diverticula, or outside the bladder can be identified.	None. There is no contraindications to ultrasonography.	Explanation of the procedure helps allay fears. Most ultrasonographic studies are painless. Bladder ultrasonography requires a full bladder. As with the other urologic procedures, several of the ultrasonographic studies require exposure of the genitalia and thus can be embarrassing to the patient.
COMPUTED TOMOGRAPHY (CT) CT scan may be ordered to study all or part of the urinary tract. A CT scan of the pelvis visualizes the lower structures of the urinary tract. The patient is usually given an oral dose of an iodine-containing preparation prior to the testing. During the procedure, the patient lies supine on a table while scans are taken at intervals of 1–2 cm. Some CT scans include intravenous as well as oral injection of contrast medium.	CT scans are clinically useful in evaluating many urologic disorders. A broad categorization would include renal masses, chronic infections, vascular lesions, nephrolithiasis, and other renal diseases, and metastatic evaluations.	CT scan has no post-test complications other than a potential delayed hypersensitivity reaction to the contrast material used. Patients with known allergy to contrast dye receive a steroid preparation before any CT scan in which contrast dye will be used. Oral contrast preparations are not absorbed, so alone they are safe. However, the decision to inject contrast dye is often made during the scan; therefore, a steroid preparation is routine for contrast-allergic patients. Hypersensitivity reactions include pruritus, urticaria, skin flushing, and breathing difficulties.	Assessment for allergy to contrast dye or hypersensitivity to iodine-containing foods should be done on admission. Explain the CT scanner to the patient, including the room and the use of oral and intravenous contrast dye. As with any study, the injection of contrast dye intravenously may cause a flushing or warm feeling. Patients often find it hard to lie still for long periods and find the hard, flat table uncomfortable. After CT scan, monitor intake and output, observe for symptoms of a hypersensitivity reaction, and encourage fluid intake to flush out remaining dye.
MAGNETIC RESONANCE IMAGING (MRI) A study based on the reaction of protons and electrons in living tissues to a magnetic field. Images are obtained by measuring the energy utilized by the protons and electrons during this reaction to the magnetic field.	Useful in urology for imaging of the retroperitoneum, pelvic area, bladder, and prostate. Images can be obtained in three planes: coronal, sagittal, and transverse. Most urologists feel that MRI does not, at this time, replace CT scanning. Continued use of the MRI is necessary. It is quite valuable in patients with an allergy to contrast dye.	Contraindicated in patients with pacemakers. Difficult to obtain clear images with the slightest motion, even cardiac, respiratory, or bowel. Surgical clips, implants, or any metallic devices within the body will cause artifact. There are no known complications from MRI.	There is usually no preparation for an MRI study. The patient must be sure to remove all jewelry and anything metallic, even credit cards, before entering the MRI area. Describe the procedure and the possibility of feeling claustrophobic during the test. Sedation may be ordered for relaxation.

(continued)

Table 25–7. (continued) MOST COMMONLY PERFORMED RADIOLOGIC AND OTHER STUDIES OF THE URINARY TRACT

DEFINITION AND DESCRIPTION	CLINICAL USES	COMPLICATIONS	NURSING CARE
NUCLEAR MEDICINE STUDIES			
Nuclear medicine studies involve the injection of radioactive tracers into the circulatory system, then following their progression through the various organs using a specialized camera. There are several types of radioactive tracers used, some of the more common being DTPA, DMSA, Hippuran I 131.	Nuclear medicine studies are clinically useful in a variety of urologic disorders and in patients in whom the administration of contrast dye is contraindicated. For example: acute or chronic renal failure, evaluation of masses, hydronephrosis and hydroureter, renal transplant evaluation, and trauma. For most urologic disorders, radiography and CT scans are preferred. Bone scans are commonly done as part of a metastic evaluation. Renal scans are often used to evaluate renal blood flow and function in patients with renal disease.	Contraindicated in pregnancy. Hypersensitivity reactions to the radioactive tracers are very rare.	There is no patient preparation for nuclear medicine studies. The radioactive tracer is injected at a specified time before the study, allowing it to concentrate in the desired organ(s). Commercially manufactured kits are available for out-patient use. Intake and output should be monitored after the test, and fluid intake encouraged. In some institutions, patients are placed on radiation precautions for 24 hours. The institution's recommended protocols for disposal of waste products and linen should be followed.

Abbreviations: NP, intravenous pyelogram; ESWL, extracorporeal shock wave lithotripsy; DTPA, diethylene triamine pentaacetic acid; DMSA, dimercaptosuccinic acid.

Nursing Diagnoses and Planning

Nursing diagnoses and related expected patient outcomes most commonly applicable to patients undergoing an excretory urogram include the following:

NDx: Knowledge deficit: nature of the diagnostic test, the purpose, preparation, and procedure

Planning: Patient outcomes
1. Patient verbalizes an understanding of the events that will occur before, during, and after the procedure.
2. Patient identifies allergies or contraindications before the procedure that may predispose to complications.

NDx: Anxiety related to unfamiliar and presumably uncomfortable tests

Planning: Patient outcomes
1. Patient verbalizes a reduction in anxiety.
2. Patient demonstrates positive problem-solving skills.
3. Patient seems relaxed and less anxious and is resting well.

NDx: Altered patterns of urinary elimination related to complications from radiologic procedures

Planning: Patient outcomes
1. Patient maintains adequate urinary output and fluid intake in the postprocedure period.
2. Patient denies pain or burning on urination after the procedure.

Nursing Interventions

NDx: Knowledge deficit: nature of the diagnostic test, the purpose, preparation, and procedure

Identify allergy to contrast dye or compromised renal function before any study in which contrast dye is used. Explain the procedure to the patient, providing information about any injections or invasive procedures, the room where the study will be done, and any unfamiliar machines or equipment. Ask the patient what he or she already understands about the procedure, and reinforce accurate facts and correct any misunderstandings. Explain that the patient will need to drink increased fluids after the test and that the output will be closely monitored.

NDx: Anxiety

Acknowledge the patient's anxiety and the perception of the threat of the situation. Encourage expression of feelings of anger, fear, or grief. Orient the patient to the procedure, and explain all activities that will take place in the diagnostic laboratory and afterwards in the patient's room. Allow the family to express feelings and ask questions.

Seek assistance from clergy or significant others if necessary to help allay the patient's anxiety. Answer all questions factually, and provide consistent reinforcement. Encourage questions, self-care, and decision-making as much as possible.

NDx: Altered patterns of urinary elimination

After the study, encourage fluid intake and monitor intake and output closely. Provide fluids of choice for the patient to increase the fluid intake. Evaluate urine for color, consistency, and quantity.

Observe the patient for hypersensitivity reactions after the use of any dyes or injectable materials; particular attention should be paid to indications of pruritus, rashes, breathing difficulties, generalized edema, or urinary retention.

Evaluation

Evaluate the effectiveness of nursing care for a patient undergoing an excretory urogram by comparing the patient's status with the expected patient outcomes. Examples of specific outcomes for patients undergoing an excretory urogram have been provided in the Planning section.

Cystoscopy

Cystoscopy or cystourethroscopy is an examination of the urinary bladder and urethra by direct visualization. Cystoscopy involves the passage of a metal sheath into the urethra. A bridge is connected to the end of the sheath, and through these two parts are passed telescopes that allow for visual inspection of the bladder and urethra. Any urine in the bladder is emptied through the sheath. An irrigating solution, usually sterile saline, is allowed to flow by gravity into the bladder. A fiberoptic light end, connected to a powerful light source, is attached to the telescope. Telescopes with two standard lenses are used; the 30-degree and 70-degree lenses provide direct and wide-angle viewing. The urethra is visualized by looking through one of the telescopes as the sheath is passed through it (Fig. 25–7).

Several types of specimens can be obtained during cystoscopy. Saline washings may be sent for cytologic examination. Biopsy forceps can be passed through the sheath to allow for biopsies of suspicious areas. Bridges with specialized ports allow for the passing of ureteral catheters during cystoscopy. Other specialized instruments can be used for various purposes.

Routine cystoscopy is performed under local anesthesia. Regional, spinal, or general anesthesia is sometimes used when patient tolerance prohibits local anesthesia, when the physician prefers it, or when multiple biopsies or other painful procedures are anticipated.

Clinical Uses. Along with the excretory urogram, cystoscopy is a mainstay of the urologic diagnostic evaluation. There is no other test that can take the place of directly visualizing the interior of the bladder. Cystoscopy is the primary diagnostic method and follow-up regimen for bladder tumors. It is also an essential part of the diagnostic evaluation for many urologic disorders, including prostatism, voiding disorders, fistulae, diverticula, recurrent urinary tract infections, and some congenital anomalies.

The presence of a urinary tract infection is a contraindication to cystoscopy. Significant bladder outlet obstruction from prostatism is considered by some physicians to be a contraindication to out-patient cystoscopy, because hematuria, urinary retention, and bladder neck edema are common after any urethral instrumentation. In such patients, assessment includes questioning about voiding patterns and a check for a recent negative urine culture result.

Complications. Serious complications after simple cystoscopy are quite uncommon. Minor complications are possible, and the patient should be advised of symptoms of these complications before leaving for home.

Infection is always a possibility after any urethral instrumentation, including cystoscopy. The patient should be advised to report any fever, persistent burning on urination, or frequency. Hematuria occurs more frequently in men than in women, and after any biopsies. A slightly blood-tinged urine should clear up within 24 to 48 hours. Gross hematuria with clots may require hospitalization and continuous bladder irrigation. Urinary retention is also more common in men, especially in those with enlarged prostates. If unable to void after 6 to 8 hours, the patient should return to the physician's office or to the hospital. Pushing oral fluids copiously can help prevent all these complications.

Serious complications include urethral, bladder, or ureteral perforation. Fortunately, these complications are rare. Any sudden and severe pain in the lower

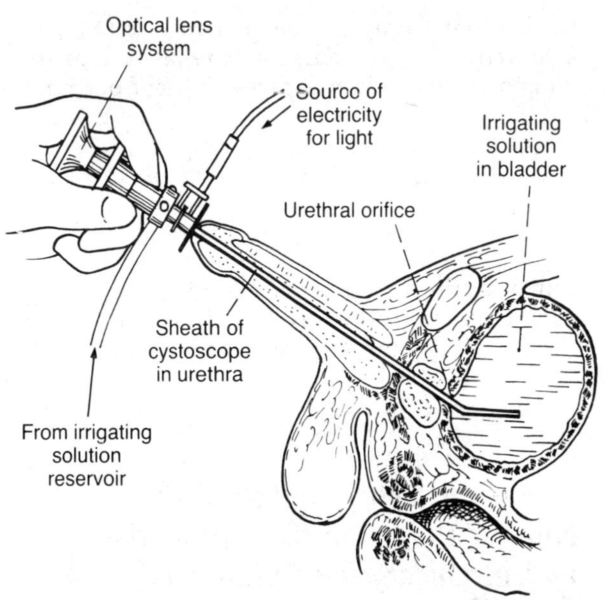

Figure 25–7.

Cystoscope in the male bladder. (From Black JM, Matassarin-Jacobs, E. Luckmann and Sorenson's medical-surgical nursing. 4th ed. Philadelphia: WB Saunders, 1993, p 1437.)

Nursing Care Guide 25–1.
PATIENTS UNDERGOING CYSTOSCOPY

Preoperative Care

Assessment Findings: Patient presents signs of restlessness, nervousness, increased respiratory and heart rates, asks questions about procedures, clenches hands, cries.

Nursing Diagnosis: Anxiety related to fear of procedure, diagnosis, and future treatments or medical management

Patient Outcomes	Nursing Interventions	Rationale
Patient is less anxious as evidenced by smiling; lack of restlessness, crying, or nervousness; and vital signs within normal limits.	Explain the procedure to the patient and family. Describe the preoperative preparation.	An understanding of the procedure may reduce anxiety.
	Allow time for questions and concerns.	Providing time for questions relieves some of the patient's fear of the unknown and allows for correction of misunderstandings.
	Check vital signs, and observe for signs of relaxation in the patient.	Changes in vital signs may indicate reduced anxiety.
Patient verbalizes feeling less anxious.	Teach relaxation techniques. Help the patient find coping strategies that help alleviate the stress and anxiety.	Relaxation exercises promote relief of stress and anxiety.
	Allow time for rest; provide a quiet, comfortable atmosphere.	Rest periods and quiet may promote a reduction in stress and anxiety.

Evaluation: Compare the patient's status with the expected patient outcomes. If the outcomes are achieved, evaluate nursing care as successful. If not, reassess the patient, formulate new nursing diagnoses, and revise expected patient outcomes and nursing interventions as appropriate.

(continued)

abdomen during cystoscopy calls for immediate termination of the procedure. Likewise, any sudden change in vital signs requires termination of cystoscopy.

Guidelines for Application of the Nursing Process to the Care of the Patient Undergoing Cystoscopy

Review the history and other completed diagnostic studies. Assess the patient's anxiety level regarding the cystoscopy. The nature of cystoscopy provokes great anxiety in some patients, requiring repeated reassurances and explanations. Evaluate any physical limitations that would prevent the patient from lying in a lithotomy position. Patients with a history of unstable cardiac, neurologic, or psychiatric conditions are not good candidates for cystoscopy under local anesthesia. Communicate these findings to the physician so that alternative or adjunctive measures can be taken.

The nursing diagnoses, related expected patient outcomes, and nursing interventions most commonly applicable to patients undergoing a cystoscopy include those described previously for patients undergoing an excretory urogram. (Also see Nurs-

Nursing Care Guide 25–1. *(continued)*

PATIENTS UNDERGOING CYSTOSCOPY

Assessment Findings: Patient asks questions about procedure, seems uninformed about pre- and postprocedure care and treatments; patient and family voice concerns about risks and necessity for the procedure.

Nursing Diagnosis: Knowledge deficit: nature of procedure and postprocedure care

Patient Outcomes	Nursing Interventions	Rationale
Patient reports accurate information about the procedure, the necessity for it, and the expectations postprocedure.	Be certain the physician has discussed the procedure, risks, complications, and expectations with the patient.	Having the patient reiterate the information provided allows for an assessment of the patient's understanding of the procedure.
	Allow the patient to ask questions, and try to expand on the understanding about the procedure for the patient and family.	Providing time for questions allows for correction of misunderstandings.
	Explain the postprocedure care needed, and tell the patient that the information will be repeated prior to discharge.	Providing some information about postprocedure expectations helps relieve anxiety about the postprocedure care needed.
Patient and family state that they have an understanding of the procedure, the risks, and the postprocedure care needed.	Include the family in the education sessions. Allow time for questions and concerns. Explain all information in understandable terms.	Inclusion of the family provides reinforcement for the patient, relieves family anxiety, and gives support to the patient.

Evaluation: Compare the patient's status with the expected patient outcomes. If the outcomes are achieved, evaluate nursing care as successful. If not, reassess the patient, formulate new nursing diagnoses, and revise expected patient outcomes and nursing interventions as appropriate.

(continued)

ing Care Guide 25–1.) The following additional interventions also apply to the care of patients undergoing cystoscopy.

The procedure is often embarrassing to many patients because there is manipulation of the genitalia, and patients may develop increased anxiety prior to the cystoscopy. Explain the necessity of the procedure to the patient and the details of what is to be done.

If intravenous sedation or anesthesia (regional, spinal, or general) is to be used during cystoscopy, the patient receives nothing by mouth (NPO) after midnight prior to the surgery. Teach the patient relaxation methods during the preoperative period. Most patients can tolerate the procedure under local anesthesia when they are well-prepared and practice relaxation techniques prior to and during the examination.

After the cystoscopy, monitor fluid intake and output carefully. Encourage increased fluid intake. Notify the physician if the patient does not void within 8 hours or if excessive bleeding or pain is present. Note any hematuria or change in the appearance of the urine. Dysuria and frequency are common for 24 to 48 hours. If an indwelling catheter is present, monitor for patency, and measure the output. Document both the color and amount of urine. Medicate the patient as necessary for discomfort from bladder spasms.

Give the patient written discharge instructions.

Nursing Care Guide 25–1. *(continued)*

PATIENTS UNDERGOING CYSTOSCOPY

Postoperative Care

Assessment Findings: Patient is unable to void even with increased fluid intake; patient has difficulty starting stream; patient complains of discomfort with voiding and is able to produce only some dribbling; or patient complains of frequency of urination with small amounts voided each time.

Nursing Diagnosis: Altered patterns of urinary elimination related to irritation of urethra secondary to instrumentation

Patient Outcomes	Nursing Interventions	Rationale
Patient resumes normal patterns of urinary elimination with adequate output.	After the procedure, encourage increased fluid intake (8–10 glasses of water unless contraindicated).	Increased intake of fluids helps restore normal urinary pattern and flushes the system, helping prevent infection.
	Have the patient attempt to void frequently, and measure amount. Ask the patient whether it seems as though the bladder has been emptied.	Frequent voiding prevents accumulation of urine, which may promote bacterial growth or overdistend the bladder.
Patient denies difficulty with urination.	Have the patient report any difficulty with urination. Ask whether there are feelings of burning or irritation. Check the color, consistency, and amount of the urine.	Early assessment for problems may prevent serious complications.

Evaluation: Compare the patient's status with the expected patient outcomes. If the outcomes are achieved, evaluate nursing care as successful. If not, reassess the patient, formulate new nursing diagnoses, and revise expected patient outcomes and nursing interventions as appropriate.

Assessment Findings: Patient asks questions about home care necessary and other discharge instructions.

Nursing Diagnosis: Impaired home maintenance management related to insufficient knowledge about home care

Patient Outcomes	Nursing Interventions	Rationale
Patient states accurate information about discharge care, including when to report to the physician.	Give the patient written instructions for self-care after discharge, and have the patient repeat the information.	Written instructions reinforce the verbal information provided. A reiteration of the instructions allows for an assessment of the patient's understanding of the information.
	Tell the patient to observe for any change in color or consistency of the urine.	

(continued)

Nursing Care Guide 25–1. *(continued)*

PATIENTS UNDERGOING CYSTOSCOPY

Patient Outcomes	Nursing Interventions	Rationale
	Explain that some discomfort may occur from bladder spasms or irritation of the urethra.	An explanation of the possible complications prepares the patient for them and for early intervention.
	Tell the patient to notify the physician if bleeding, extreme pain, changes in the color or consistency of the urine, or inability to void occurs.	An explanation of follow-up care needed and when to seek medical assistance may prevent problems.
	Encourage the patient to continue to drink copious amounts of fluid at home to wash out urinary tract.	Continued intake of increased amounts of fluids helps flush the urinary system and prevent complications.
Patient and family verbalize an understanding of the instructions given.	Explain all information to the patient's family, and have them repeat the information. Be sure to use terminology that is understandable to them. Allow time for questions.	Including the family reinforces the information and provides support for the patient. Reiteration of the instructions allows for an assessment of the understanding of the information.

Evaluation: Compare the patient's status with the expected patient outcomes. If the outcomes are achieved, evaluate nursing care as successful. If not, reassess the patient, formulate new nursing diagnoses, and revise expected patient outcomes and nursing interventions as appropriate.

Review the information verbally in understandable terms. Also explain the home care needed to the family. Allow time for questions or concerns (see Nursing Care Guide 25–1).

Bladder Biopsy

Bladder biopsies may be performed for a number of reasons. Patients with a history of transitional cell carcinoma of the bladder frequently have biopsies of suspicious areas seen on radiographic studies or during cystoscopy. Patients with symptoms indicative of a carcinoma of the bladder, ureter, or renal pelvis may require biopsies of any of these areas. Lastly, some infectious conditions or diseases, such as interstitial cystitis, must be diagnosed by pathologic or cystologic evaluation of tissue specimens.

Bladder biopsies are easily performed during cystoscopy, using biopsy forceps to obtain a "cold cup" specimen (a snip of tissue) to send to the pathology laboratory. One or two superficial biopsies can be done under local anesthesia. More extensive biopsies, often called superficial and deep or random bladder biopsies, are usually done under regional or general anesthesia.

Specimens of ureteral or renal pelvic tissue can be obtained using several instruments that are passed up the ureter during cystoscopy. Small brushes that collect cells and minute pieces of tissue for cytologic evaluation are used to perform brush biopsies. Careful, methodologic specimens can be collected in this manner to determine the origins of suspicious cells found in urinary cytology when no obvious lesions can be found.

Urethral biopsies can be obtained using the same method as bladder biopsy when urethral malignancy is suspected.

Clinical Uses. Bladder biopsies are indicated for diagnosis of transitional cell carcinoma, squamous cell carcinoma, or adenocarcinoma of the bladder; for various infectious processes within the bladder wall, and for interstitial cystitis. Random biopsies of several areas within the bladder mucosa are indicated for staging of bladder cancer or for identification of a site of origin of suspicious or malignant cells found on urinary cytology. Biopsies of suspicious areas seen on cystoscopy are always indicated.

Brush biopsy of the ureter or renal pelvis is indicated when suspicious areas are seen on radiographic studies or when malignant cells are present in a urinary cytology and no bladder lesions are present. Because transitional cell carcinoma can recur anywhere in the urothelial lining of the urinary tract, such examinations are sometimes necessary as part of a thorough follow-up regimen (although periodic excretory urography, cystoscopy, and urinary cytology may suffice).

Complications. Patients on anticoagulant therapy or those with known bleeding disorders should not undergo bladder biopsy because hemorrhage may result. (Anticoagulants should be discontinued 3 to 5 days before biopsy when possible.) Bladder biopsy should not be performed when an active urinary tract infection is present because sepsis may result.

Complications during bladder biopsy include bladder perforation with urinary extravasation, and prolonged bleeding. Biopsies of the ureter or renal pelvis can be complicated by perforation of either of these areas, again with urinary extravasation. Complications after any of these biopsies include persistent bleeding, urinary tract obstruction from edema, sepsis, stricture, formation, and scar tissue formation.

Application of the Nursing Process to the Care of the Patient Undergoing a Bladder Biopsy

Assessment

Assess for the presence of any bleeding disorders. Check bleeding times preoperatively, and question the patient about excessive bleeding from minor cuts or frequent bruising. Assess current medications. Identify patients on nonsteroidal, anti-inflammatory drugs or those who frequently take aspirin or aspirin-containing compounds, as well as those on anticoagulant therapy. All these drugs should be discontinued 3 to 5 days before any biopsies.

Check the results of the urine studies. A recent urine culture should be free of infection. Note the color, consistency, and amount of urine for baseline data to be used in postbiopsy comparisons.

Assess for any physical limitations that would prohibit the patient from lying in a lithotomy position. Assess the patient's understanding of the procedure before teaching is begun. Look for signs of anxiety.

Nursing Diagnoses and Planning

Nursing diagnoses and related expected patient outcomes most commonly applicable to patients undergoing a bladder biopsy include those described previously for patients undergoing an excretory urogram and the following:

NDx: Pain related to irritation from biopsy site

Planning: Patient outcomes

1. Patient denies pain or discomfort after the procedure.
2. Patient resumes a normal pattern of urinary elimination after the procedure.

Nursing Interventions

NDx: Pain

After completion of the procedure, monitor fluid intake and output; assess urinary output for degree of hematuria. If no Foley catheter is present, the patient should void within 8 hours after the procedure. If a Foley catheter is present, it must remain patent. A continuous or intermittent bladder irrigation may be necessary when significant hematuria is present. Ask the patient about feelings of discomfort, especially when voiding if no catheter is present. Irritation from the biopsies or from the Foley catheter is often uncomfortable enough to warrant medication. Give the prescribed medication as necessary. Belladonna and opium suppositories or anticholinergic drugs may relieve bladder spasms, and a mild pain medication may relieve vague feelings of discomfort.

Evaluation

Evaluate the effectiveness of nursing care for a patient undergoing a bladder biopsy by comparing the patient's status with the expected patient outcomes. Examples of specific outcomes for patients undergoing a bladder biopsy have been provided in the Planning section.

Renal Biopsy

Two techniques of renal biopsy are available. Needle biopsy of the kidney, also called closed renal biopsy, is described here. Open renal biopsy is a surgical procedure, which is not described.

Needle biopsy of the kidney involves a percutaneous puncture made through the flank into the lower pole parenchyma of either kidney. The kidney may be localized using ultrasonography or fluoroscopy or simply by determining its location in relation to the eleventh or twelfth rib on a recent radiologic study. A local anesthetic is used, usually 1% lidocaine, using a spinal needle. The needle's placement in the kidney is determined by its movement during inspiration and expiration (if ultrasonography or fluoroscopy are not used). One of several standard biopsy needles then replaces the spinal needle, and a core of tissue is sent to the pathology laboratory for analysis.

Closed renal biopsy is usually performed in the ultrasound or radiology departments or, in rare cases, at the patient's bedside.

Clinical Uses. Renal biopsy is used to diagnose renal disease, or to evaluate response to treatment or progression of disease in patients with a previously diagnosed renal disorder. It is much more clinically useful in nephrology than in urology. Urologists occasionally use closed renal biopsy to aspirate specimens from suspicious areas seen on ultrasonogram or x-ray film in order to differentiate between simple cysts and malignancies. In these cases, adjunctive ultrasonography, fluoroscopy, and occasionally computed tomography scanning are used.

Complications. The most common complication of closed renal biopsy is bleeding. Prolonged bleeding in the form of gross hematuria or a perinephric hematoma represents a complication. Rarely is bleeding severe enough to cause circulatory collapse. Late hemorrhage occurs in some patients 7 to 10 days after biopsy. Other infrequent complications are arteriovenous aneurysm and inadvertent biopsy of an organ other than the kidney.

Closed renal biopsy is contraindicated in patients with severe hypertension, pyelonephritis, coagulopathies, and renal tuberculosis. It is also not recommended in patients with a solitary kidney or a kidney in an unusual anatomic position.

Application of the Nursing Process to the Care of the Patient Undergoing a Renal Biopsy

Assessment

Assess all medications the patient is currently taking. Assess routine use of aspirin, aspirin-containing compounds, or nonsteroidal anti-inflammatories, and notify the physician of the information. Assess for signs of bleeding postoperatively. Check the urinary output for color, and note any drop in blood pressure.

Check vital signs. Evaluation of the patient's vital signs may indicate an infectious process (fever) or previously undiagnosed hypertension, both of which increase the risk of postbiopsy complications. After the biopsy, vital sign changes may indicate fluid volume deficits caused by bleeding.

Assess the patient's anxiety level and knowledge regarding the procedure. This is essential, because patient cooperation is an important component in the procedure's success. To assess the level of understanding, ask the patient to explain the information the physician has stated.

Nursing Diagnoses and Planning

Nursing diagnoses and related expected patient outcomes most commonly applicable to patients undergoing renal biopsy include the following:

NDx: Knowledge deficit: nature of the procedure, the purpose, and risks for renal biopsy

Planning: Patient outcomes
1. Patient verbalizes an understanding of the procedure and the need for cooperation during the procedure.
2. Patient recovers from the procedure without serious complications.
3. Patient tolerates the procedure and adheres to postbiopsy mobility restrictions.

NDx: High risk for fluid volume deficit related to possible bleeding of biopsy site

Planning: Patient outcomes
1. Patient maintains adequate fluid volume as evidenced by lack of signs of bleeding and adequate output.
2. Patient's vital signs remain within normal ranges for the patient.

Nursing Interventions

NDx: Knowledge deficit: nature of procedure, the purpose, and risks

Explain the events that will occur during renal biopsy. Prebiopsy teaching may require several repetitions for the anxious patient. When it is possible for the nurse to be present during the procedure, descriptions of what is occurring and the use of relaxation techniques are advantageous.

The patient will be asked to take deep breaths, hold their breath, and lie very still during the procedure. After biopsy, patients often must lie prone for 1 hour, then remain on bed rest for a specified time period up to 24 hours. If gross hematuria or bleeding from or around the biopsy site persists, bed rest may be ordered for longer periods. Monitor vital signs for several hours after the procedure, and

Table 25–8. URODYNAMIC PROCEDURES

DEFINITION AND DESCRIPTION	CLINICAL USES	COMPLICATIONS	NURSING CARE
URINARY FLOW RATE			
A measure of the volume of urine expelled from the bladder during a given period of time; it is an assessment of the joint action of the bladder and outlet. Rate is calculated and expressed as ml/sec. It is the easiest, most informative, and only noninvasive urodynamic procedure. Patient is simply required to urinate into a special commode with measuring device attached.	To assess patients with symptoms of outflow obstruction (e.g., BPH, urethral strictures). Before and after any procedure designed to improve urine flow. As a screening procedure for those with dysfunctional voiding prior to initiating other invasive urodynamic tests.	None	Explain that a full bladder is needed in order to obtain a valid and reliable study. Make sure that the patient understands that this is a test to assess voiding, not defecation; stool interferes with the validity of the test. Instruct the patient to force fluids and delay voiding until time for the test.
CYSTOMETROGRAM (CMG)			
A measure of bladder pressure (in cm H_2O) during the filling and storage phases of micturition. Procedure requires that a catheter be inserted and the bladder slowly filled with water or gas (CO_2) until capacity is reached. Notation is made of amount of fluid or gas infused and of patient's sensations to filling.	To evaluate all types of urinary incontinence; in those with enuresis; for sure or suspected neurogenic voiding dysfunction.	A UTI may result from instrumentation of the urethra. Procedure is contraindicated if UTI is present or if patient is experiencing diarrhea.	Fully explain the procedure: Check to see whether the patient is taking any medication that could interfere with results of the tests (cholinergics and anticholinergics have direct effect upon the bladder). Check to see whether patient had a recent negative result on urine culture. After the procedure, an increase in fluid intake helps reduce discomfort felt when voiding and dilutes urine to prevent infection.
ELECTROMYOGRAPHY (EMG)			
The recording of electrical activity generated by the striated muscles of the external urethral sphincter. To establish the recording, two needle, wire, or surface electrodes are strategically placed on the perineum and connected to the urodynamics machine.	To evaluate the coordination of the external urethral sphincter and perineum with detrusor activity during bladder filling and emptying. Aids in diagnosing detrusor-sphincter dyssyneriga. Always done in conjunction with other urodynamic tests.	Some pain may be experienced during the insertion of wire or needle electrodes.	Explain the procedure and assure the patient that it involves only temporary discomfort.
COMBINED MICTURITION STUDY			
The simultaneous recording of urine flow, intravesical pressure, intraabdominal (usually via the rectum) pressure, and sphincter EMG activity during the emptying phase of micturition. Requires that the patient be transferred to commode chair following bladder filling (done during CMG) with monitoring equipment attached.	When used in conjunction with CMG, this study offers the clinician the opportunity to evaluate the entire micturition cycle. Helpful in cases of complicated voiding dysfunction to differentiate between outflow obstruction and weak detrusor.	Dizziness may occur during the procedure as a result of the change in position.	Same as for previous studies.
VIDEOURODYNAMIC STUDY			
The synchronous recording of previously described urodynamic parameters and cystourethrography.	Complicated neurologic disease; complicated incontinence; when clinical impression differs from urodynamic findings; unsuccessful therapeutic results from medications or surgery.	Same as for previous studies.	Same as for previous studies.
URETHRAL PRESSURE PROFILE (UPP)			
A study of the pressures along the length of the urethra. Requires that a special #8 to #10 French catheter be inserted into the bladder and then pulled back through the urethra at a fixed rate as water or gas is infused.	To determine urethral incompetency; to locate areas of increased resistance of obstruction; before and after artificial sphincter implants; in the operating room during surgery for bladder neck reconstruction.	Same as for CMG.	Same as for previous studies.

Abbreviations: BPH, benign prostatic hypertrophy; UTI, urinary tract infection.

report any significant changes to the physician immediately. Dress the biopsy site with a small dressing or adhesive bandage, and observe frequently for bleeding.

NDx: High risk for fluid volume deficit
Monitor vital signs frequently after biopsy to check for impending shock related to decrease in fluid volume from bleeding. Check urine for changes in color. Check the biopsy site for bleeding. Keep a small pressure dressing over the puncture site, and apply digital pressure if any bleeding is noted.

Evaluation

Evaluate the effectiveness of nursing care for a patient undergoing a renal biopsy by comparing the patient's status with the expected patient outcomes. Examples of specific outcomes for patients undergoing a renal biopsy have been provided in the Planning section.

Urodynamics

Urodynamics refers to a series of diagnostic techniques used for the evaluation of voiding disorders. The use of urodynamic procedures to measure urinary tract function is analogous to pulmonary function tests that measure lung function.

There are various components of urodynamic testing, which incorporate measures of flow, volume, pressure, and electrical response. Used individually or in combination with one another, these measurements provide valuable insight and understanding about the process of micturition.

The need for urodynamic testing is based, in part, upon findings from the history, physical examination, radiographic investigation, and endoscopic evaluation. The extent of testing required depends upon the patient's problem, the urologist's preference for various procedures, and the availability of urodynamic testing equipment.

Without question, simple urodynamic assessment is essential in the evaluation of patients with suspected neurogenic voiding dysfunction. For those with unusual disorders or inconclusive findings from previous studies, sophisticated multichannel studies (or videourodynamics) may be necessary.

Until recently, urodynamic testing was used solely for the purpose of assessing lower urinary tract function. However, research and newer measurement techniques have extended the use of these procedures to assessment of the upper urinary tract. Table 25–8 describes the various urodynamic procedures, including clinical uses, complications, and nursing care.

Application of the Nursing Process to the Care of the Patient Undergoing Urodynamic Testing

Assessment

Assess the patient for any signs or symptoms that indicate the presence of a urinary tract infection. Check for elevated temperature. Note the urine culture results. Check the color and consistency of the urine. If there are signs of a urinary infection, notify the physician. The testing should be postponed. Irritation of the urinary tract from infection adversely alters test results, and repeated instrumentation could lead to sepsis.

Evaluate the patient's physical condition, because multiple position changes are usually required during the course of the procedure. Check whether the patient can transfer from a bed to a commode with ease. Note whether the patient is able to walk alone or whether assistance is needed. Check whether the patient has the strength to undergo testing at the time it is scheduled. Although urodynamic testing is often performed in the patient with impaired mobility, a more complete evaluation can be obtained if the patient feels physically able to cooperate with the testing and is able to freely move about.

Evaluate the patient's mental status, because study results are correlated with the individual's description of sensations during the procedures. If the patient is disoriented, confused, or unable to take instructions, then the patient is probably *not* a candidate for urodynamic testing.

Review current medications prescribed for the patient to see whether any are being taken that directly alter bladder function. Make note of cholinergic and anticholinergic agents, musculotropic relaxants, polysynaptic inhibitors, beta-adrenergic stimulants, and tricyclic antidepressants. Although these drugs are helpful in treating voiding symptoms as well as a variety of other medical problems, they also interfere with urodynamic test results and prevent evaluation of true urinary tract function.

Nursing Diagnoses and Planning

Nursing diagnoses and related expected patient outcomes most commonly applicable to patients undergoing urodynamic testing include the following:

NDx: Knowledge deficit: nature of urodynamic testing techniques

Planning: Patient outcomes
1. Patient verbalizes an understanding of the events that will occur before, during, and after the testing.

2. Patient denies lack of understanding about the testing and verbalizes lack of anxiety about it.

NDx: High risk for infection related to instrumentation of the urinary tract

Planning: Patient outcomes
1. Patient denies burning or pain on urination, which may be signs of infection.
2. Patient's vital signs are within normal ranges.
3. Patient presents clear urine with no trace of bacteria on urinalysis.

NDx: Altered urinary elimination related to irritation of urethra caused by catheterization

Planning: Patient outcomes
1. Patient denies having difficulty voiding.
2. Patient increases fluid intake after the test.
3. Patient's fluid intake and output are adequate.

Nursing Interventions

NDx: Knowledge deficit: nature of urodynamic testing techniques
Explain each urodynamic procedure; however, before proceeding with a detailed description of the tests to the patient, it is wise to call the urodynamic facility to inquire about any special testing techniques utilized. Emphasize that these studies are neither passed or failed; rather, they are used to collect information about a person's voiding pattern.

Prior to testing, dress the patient in a hospital gown only. The limited clothing is necessary owing to the amount of equipment attached to the patient during the urodynamic procedures.

Explain to the patient that there will be no premedication given for this test. Although premedicating patients with sedatives or analgesics is common prior to many procedures, it is not done prior to urodynamic testing (unless ordered for a specific reason). These drugs can affect bladder function, but more importantly, they alter a patient's perception and threaten safety during the procedure.

Tell the patient that after urodynamic testing, there may be some perineal discomfort generally caused by repeated instrumentation. Because of irritation, the patient may also be reluctant to void. Encourage the pateint to take an increased fluid volume for 24 to 36 hours after the studies to increase urine output and stimulate voiding and to dilute urine and flush out bacteria.

NDx: High risk for infection
Because a urinary tract infection can also occur after urodynamic testing, instruct the patient to report suggestive signs and symptoms such as burning or pain with urination or discharge. For patients who are prone to developing a urinary tract infection, prophylactic antibiotics may be prescribed. Explain the frequency, dosage, and side effects of the medication to the patient. Encourage increased fluid intake to clear out bacteria.

NDx: Alteration in patterns of urinary elimination
After the study, encourage fluid intake and monitor intake and output closely. Provide fluids of choice for the patient to increase the fluid intake. Evaluate urine for color, consistency, and quantity. Check for burning with urination, bloody urine, or meatal pain. Provide a bedside receptacle if the patient cannot get up to go to the bathroom.

Observe the patient for hypersensitivity reactions after the use of any dyes or injectable materials; particular attention should be paid to indications of pruritus, rashes, breathing difficulties, generalized edema, or urinary retention. Tell the patient to report any difficulty in urination or other side effects of the testing procedure.

Evaluation

Evaluate the effectiveness of nursing care for a patient undergoing urodynamic testing by comparing the patient's status with the expected patient outcomes. Examples of specific outcomes for patients undergoing urodynamic testing have been provided in the Planning section.

Medical Management

Nonsurgical Management

Nonsurgical management of urinary tract dysfunctions involves a combination of treatment modalities. Catheterization, pharmacologic agents, bladder retraining, nutritional therapy, and self-directed measures are some of the interventions used to assist patients with urinary problems.

CATHETER DRAINAGE

The primary purpose of a catheter is to remove urine from the bladder when the patient is incapable of totally emptying the bladder. A catheter may be used in emergency situations or following certain surgical interventions or traumatic injuries. Additionally, a catheter can be used for instilling medication into the bladder, for diagnostic procedures, and for monitoring urinary output more accurately. In severe cases of urinary incontinence, when other medical problems exist, a catheter is sometimes used to temporarily manage the incontinence until a more permanent means of control is established.

Catheters come in a wide variety of shapes and sizes and should be chosen according to the needs of the patient. Pediatric sizes (#10 to #14 French [Fr]) are available for the young adult but are also used in patients with atrophy of the meatal urethra. Large sizes (#25 or greater Fr) are used during bladder irrigation procedures. Coudé-tip catheters are useful in males with enlarged prostates, and the mushroom-shaped or winged catheter may be used for suprapubic or nephrostomy placement. In the most difficult cases, a stylet or filiform catheter may be used by the physician to achieve catheter insertion. Samples of the catheter materials are latex, Silastic, silicone-coated, solid silicone, and variations of the above.

INDWELLING CATHETERS

Indwelling catheters are used for the continuous drainage of urine from the bladder. They may be employed temporarily after a surgical procedure or be required for long-term management of urinary retention. Regardless of use, all indwelling catheters should be maintained as a sterile, closed drainage system and should be inserted using strict aseptic technique by qualified personnel.

Indwelling catheters can lead to many negative side effects, such as inflammation of the urethra, strictures, urinary tract infections, renal and bladder calculi, hydronephrosis, and in males, epididymitis and penoscrotal complications. Table 25–9 provides nursing guidelines for prevention of such side effects.

Table 25–9. NURSING GUIDELINES FOR PREVENTION OF COMPLICATIONS OF INDWELLING CATHETERS

To minimize the complications associated with indwelling urinary catheters, follow these guidelines:

Use aseptic technique in catheter insertion.
Determine appropriate type and size of catheter before insertion.
Employ a closed drainage system. If irrigations are ordered, all efforts must be made to prevent contamination of the system.
Ensure that drainage bag stays below the level of the bladder at all times.
Remove catheter as soon as possible.
Use aseptic technique when taking urine samples from the aspiration port.
Change catheter only when it becomes obstructed or contaminated; catheters should not be changed on a routine basis.
Empty drainage bags every 8 hours or more often if volume is excessive.
Clean the outlet valve each time, and prevent contact contamination by the measuring container.
Ensure that each catheterized patient has an individualized, labeled measuring container.
Ensure that all catheterized patients maintain adequate hydration; 2 to 3 L/day of water is recommended except in the presence of cardiac insufficiency or renal failure.
Anchor the catheter securely to the leg or lower abdomen by use of tape or catheter strap.
Assess the catheterized patient on a routine basis. Assess fluid intake and output levels; patency of the system, color and odor of urine, evidence of sediment, presence/absence of patient discomfort, fever, and hematuria.
Remove catheter by aspirating fluid from the inflation port with a syringe. Because varied amounts of fluid are used to inflate catheter balloons, be sure to check the insertion record before aspiration to determine the amount of fluid used.

The presence of an indwelling catheter increases the hospitalized patient's risk of nosocomial infection by 40% to 50%. Patients especially at risk for infection are pregnant women, the elderly, diabetics, and those who are immunosuppressed.

Nursing measures such as the application of antimicrobial agents at the urethral meatus have proved ineffective in reducing the risk of catheter-related infections and may in fact promote infections by acting as an irritant to meatal tissue. In addition, repeated washing of the meatus with soap and water may increase the risk of infection, owing in part to the manipulation of the catheter and the introduction of exogenous bacteria into the bladder. Instillation of antiseptic solutions such as hydrogen peroxide, or chlorhexidine into the urinary drainage bag has also proved to be ineffective in reducing catheter-induced urinary tract infections. Thus, routine perineal care during the daily bath is generally sufficient to minimize infection from the indwelling catheter.

In any hospitalized patient with an indwelling catheter, bacteriuria will be present after 24 to 72 hours. Therefore, routine urine cultures are indicated only when symptoms of an upper urinary tract or systemic infection are present. Routine catheter changes, once done to impede bacterial growth, are also not necessary unless the closed drainage system has been broken. Although continuous bladder irrigations may be used after transurethral surgery, routine bladder irrigations are contraindicated except on the express orders of a physician when clots or other residue has blocked catheter drainage.

For patients requiring catheter drainage at home, a low-dose prophylactic antibiotic may be prescribed to control bacterial growth. Some of these patients may also require a routine catheter change or catheter irrigation to prevent occlusion of the catheter from crystals that tend to form on the tip. However, if the tube is patent and draining well, there is really no reason to change or irrigate it. In addition, patients should be instructed about the procedure for transferring the catheter from a drain bag to a urinary leg bag. They should also be advised to rinse the drain bags overnight at least two or three times each week in a solution of equal parts white vinegar and water, which helps to clean and deodorize them.

SUPRAPUBIC CATHETERS

A suprapubic catheter may be used in place of a urethral catheter when there is urethral injury, prostatic obstruction, or strictures. It is also used after gynecologic surgery and may be used for long-term catheterization. Insertion of the catheter may be done in the patient's bed as opposed to an operating room or cystoscopy room. The catheter is inserted into the bladder using a trocar-cannula device that is inserted directly above the pubic bone. The catheter is held in place either internally by the design of the catheter or externally by a disk or sutures. Initially, the insertion site is cleaned and redressed every day. After healing has occurred, a permanent suprapubic opening should be cleaned and observed several times per week. A dressing may no longer be necessary. Catheters are changed only if they show evidence of obstruction. Suprapubic catheters should be changed only by qualified personnel. Irrigations may be ordered to maintain patency and should be performed using clean technique.

The catheter must be connected to either a drain bag or a urinary leg bag. Use of the leg bag is beneficial to patients who are ambulatory or wish to sit in a wheelchair without having a cumbersome drain bag present for everyone to see. One advantage of a suprapubic catheter is that it does not interfere with sexual activity as an indwelling catheter does.

INTERMITTENT SELF-CATHETERIZATION

Generally referred to as clean intermittent self-catheterization, the technique was reinstituted in the early 1970s as an alternative to indwelling catheterization. The procedure may be used on a long- or short-term basis, depending on the bladder's ability to return to normal function. Paraplegic or quadriplegic patients seldom are able to discontinue the process, but some patients with mildly neurogenic bladders or who have had gynecologic surgery may use the program for only a few weeks or months.

The theory behind the effectiveness of clean intermittent self-catheterization is the physiologic capacity of the bladder to hold approximately 500 ml. When the amount goes over 500 ml, two problems can occur: (1) The blood flow to the bladder is decreased, lowering the defense mechanism of the bladder wall; and (2) bacteria present in the urine multiplies rapidly. The longer contaminated urine is allowed to stay in the bladder, the higher the bacteria count. Consequently, the natural defense mechanism of the bladder wall is decreased as the fluid volume increases. For this reason, patients should be taught the importance of regular and complete bladder emptying in order to prevent recurrent urinary tract infections.

It is important for the patient to understand the necessity of learning the procedure and that the desired results will not occur without compliance. Self-care and the willingness to overcome certain fears must be within the value system of the individual in order for a self-catheterization program to succeed. Table 25–10 provides nursing guidelines for clean intermittent self-catheterization.

Application of the Nursing Process to the Care of the Patient with an Indwelling Catheter

Assessment

Review the patient's history and diagnostic studies completed. Monitor the patient's fluid intake and output. Note conditions that would prevent increased fluid intake, such as congestive heart failure or renal failure. Assess the patency of the catheter. Check the color, amount, and odor of the urine. Check vital signs routinely, being alert to an elevated temperature. Check the results of the laboratory data to assess the white blood count for indications of infection. Assess patient for chills, back pain or suprapubic pain, and burning with urination.

Nursing Diagnoses and Planning

The nursing diagnosis and related expected patient outcomes most commonly applicable to patients with indwelling catheters are as follows:

NDx: High risk for infection related to catheter, lack of appropriate perineal hygiene

Planning: Patient outcomes

1. Patient has negative results on urine cultures.
2. Patient remains afebrile.
3. Patient denies signs and symptoms of infection, such as burning or pain, cloudy urine, or a discharge.
4. Patient's white blood cell count is within normal limits.

Nursing Interventions

NDx: High risk for infection

Monitor vital signs every 4 hours, and report temperature elevations. Maintain fluid intake of 2500 ml/day unless contraindicated. Observe urine for signs and symptoms of urinary tract infection, such as cloudy or very turbid urine. Wash hands prior to each contact with patient. Use gloves as necessary. Use aseptic technique when cleansing around the catheter. Maintain patency of catheter and tubing. Do not raise catheter above the level of the bladder, because this allows urine to run back into the bladder. Monitor results of complete blood count, and report white blood count abnormalities. Collect cultures as ordered, and note any abnormalities. Teach the patient and family necessary interventions to prevent infection (see Table 25–9).

Table 25–10. NURSING GUIDELINES FOR CLEAN INTERMITTENT SELF-CATHETERIZATION (CISC)

Provide all teaching in a private and comfortable environment.
Review the individual's need for the procedure and history.
Individualize the teaching plan based on the assessment of the individual's needs.
Select the appropriate catheter for the individual based on sex, ability to move, individual requirements, and preference.
Explain the procedure.
Describe the basic location of anatomic structures.
Encourage the visualization of anatomic structures.
Utilize a mirror with female patients.
Be aware that the individuals may not know how to view their genital organs and may have many reservations and concerns about their anatomy.
Describe hand-washing techniques necessary prior to insertion.
Explain the need for some individuals to utilize clean gloves, specifically health care professionals and those persons who are immunosuppressed, have genital lesions, or are in long-term care facilities.
Describe the need for a water-soluble lubricant to increase the ease of insertion. Note that water may be substituted in an emergency situation.
Demonstrate the insertion procedure with a mannequin, or have the patient view a video on the procedure.
Encourage the patient to become familiar with the equipment.
Clarify any misconceptions and questions.
Assess the individual readiness to perform CISC.
Talk the individual through the procedure, assisting him or her as needed.
For women, explain that insertion is in an upward direction toward the umbilicus. If there is a vaginal prolapse, it may be necessary to perform the procedure in a recumbent position or utilize a vaginal pessary.
For the men, instruct them to hold the penis by the sides, perpendicular to the body, in order to facilitate the passage of the catheter. If there is resistance at the level of the prostate, one can utilize deep breathing or relaxation exercises, or it may require the use of a coudé-tip (bent stiff tip that does not bend against an obstacle) catheter to facilitate the catheterization.
Explain how to perform the Credé maneuver to facilitate complete bladder emptying.
Correct errors, while remembering to encourage and praise the patient's progress.
Explain how to clamp or stop the drainage of urine if it exceeds 500 ml in the first few minutes.
Review the individual's catheterization schedule.
Discuss the need to monitor fluid intake and output.
Describe the importance of assessing the urine output, specifically the color, clarity, amount, and odor.
Emphasize the importance of performing CISC on schedule rather than just when convenient.
Explain how CISC can be performed in public facilities.
Explain alternative means to performing CISC when in a public bathroom. For example, women can perform the CISC while standing up with one foot on the toilet seat to maintain balance, utilizing as clean a technique as possible.
Describe cleansing regimens for the daily care of the catheter. Simple cleansing with soap and water after each use is sufficient; soaking the catheter in a solution of half-strength white vinegar and water overnight once per week to clean out exudate and decrease odors.
Discuss the appropriate storage of the catheter in a clean, closed container. Catheters may be stored in any closed container and reused for 4–6 weeks, after which time they are discarded. Catheters with cracks should be discarded.

Evaluation

Evaluate the effectiveness of nursing care for a patient with an indwelling catheter by comparing the patient's status with the expected patient outcomes. Examples of specific outcomes for patients with indwelling catheters have been provided in the Planning section.

MEDICATIONS

Many urologic problems can be treated nonsurgically using a variety of medications, singly or in combinations. The approach to infections of the urinary tract is either to employ broad-spectrum antibiotics or to use genitourinary-specific antibacterials. In some instances, urinary acidifiers are used to lower the pH and control bacterial growth.

Pharmacologic management of dysfunctional voiding is often successful in correcting or improving problems associated with urine storage and bladder emptying. Drugs used to treat these problems act by either blocking, modifying, or mimicking substances that influence lower urinary tract function, such as acetylcholine, norepinephrine, histamine, dopamine, the prostaglandins, 5-hydroxytryptamine, and kinins.

For patients with recurrent ureterolithiasis, medications are prescribed to reduce stone formation. The specific agent used depends upon where in the urinary tract the stone was formed as well as its composition.

The goal of drug therapy in acute and chronic renal failure is to maintain fluid and electrolyte balance and ultimately to minimize complications. However, in some situations, drugs are used to prevent or limit the degree of renal failure.

Bladder irrigants are helpful in treating some urologic problems. Irrigants are especially useful to locally administering medications. Using either intermittent or continuous delivery of irrigant solution permits fluid to flow into and out of the urinary tract without systemic absorption.

Many chemotherapeutic agents used to treat other malignancies are also used to treat urinary carcinomas. One group of chemotherapeutic agents unique to urology is the intravesic drug category. These drugs are used to treat superficial bladder tumors. The preparations are instilled directly into the bladder via a catheter and offer direct treatment of lesions without systemic side effects associated with other medications. Each medication is discussed in detail with the specific disorder in Chapter 26.

SELF-HELP MEASURES

Urology nursing is different from other specialties because many care activities are directed toward teaching patients self-care practices. Self-catheterization, a common self-help technique for urinary tract dysfunctions, was discussed previously in the chapter. Other self-care measures include Credé voiding, Kegel exercises, bladder drill, and trigger voiding.

CREDÉ OR VALSALVA VOIDING

The purpose of the Credé method is to aid in the passage of urine out of the bladder. A gentle massage is applied to the bladder in a downward direction during and after urination, or the patient might rock back and forth while sitting on the toilet. In another technique, called Valsalva voiding, the patient is instructed to bear down as in passing fecal matter. The Valsalva maneuver for voiding is not recommended for cardiac or elderly patients in poor health because of the effect on the vagus nerve.

KEGEL OR PELVIC FLOOR EXERCISES

This method of controlling involuntary loss of urine was first developed in the early 1950s for women with simple stress incontinence. It combines an exercise technique with biofeedback. The technique has proved to be effective for both women with stress incontinence and some men after prostate surgery.

Learning the technique is rather simple and provides positive reinforcement for the compliant individual. (Refer to Chart 25–1 for the patient instructions.) A perineometer is used to measure contractile ability. Another measure of successful muscle contraction is to insert one finger into the vagina and instruct the patient to tighten as if holding urine back. This assists the patient in identifying which muscles to contract when practicing the procedure.

There is some controversy as to whether the patient should practice the technique at various intervals during the day or complete the exercise in one sitting, but it is usually recommended that it be practiced repetitively, several times per day. Kegel exercises are highly successful when performed on a regular basis. The patient should practice them whenever urination occurs and at other times throughout the day. The combination of pelvic floor exercises and local or topical estrogen has been helpful for many postmenopausal women with stress incontinence.

Chart 25–1.

NURSING GUIDE TO PATIENT EDUCATION FOR SELF-MANAGEMENT: KEGEL EXERCISES

Phase I: Instruct the patient to:

Sit or stand with legs apart.
Pull up the rectum, vagina, and urethra.
Hold the muscles in this position for 4–5 sec.
Repeat the exercises 5 or 6 times, gradually increasing the number of times. (As the muscle strengthens, the individual will be able to do 25 or more exercises at one time.)
Repeat the exercise several times a day, increasing the total number to 200 times.
Exercise while driving, sitting at a desk, or watching television.

Phase II: Instruct the patient to:

Sit on the toilet and start to urinate.
Stop the urine flow by pulling up and tightening the rectum, vagina, and urethra.
Hold this position for 4–5 sec.
Release the muscles and start the stream again.
Repeat the exercise 5 or 6 times with each urination.

Chart 25–2.

NURSING GUIDE TO PATIENT EDUCATION FOR SELF-MANAGEMENT: BLADDER DRILL INSTRUCTION

Instruct the patient to:

Increase oral fluid intake. Encourage the patient to drink up to 200–300 ml of fluids per day unless otherwise medically contraindicated. Tell the patient to avoid natural diuretics such as caffeine products and alcohol.

Establish a voiding pattern. Tell the patient to attempt to urinate every 2 hours, and keep a record of the time and amount. Also note whether the patient was incontinent prior to the voiding time.

Begin the voiding schedule. Start when the patient awakens in the morning. Have the patient void at that time and then every 2 hours throughout the day, extending the time to every 3 to 4 hours at night.

Lengthen the schedule. As the patient is able to halt periods of incontinence, lengthen the time between voidings by 30 minutes until the patient is toileting every 3 to 4 hours throughout the day.

Monitor fluid intake and output. Throughout the process, check the patient's fluid intake and measure the output. Note inadequacies in either measurement.

Reward efforts to comply with the schedule. Give positive reinforcement to the patient for compliance with the routine, and ignore periods of incontinence. The plan needs to be individualized and advanced as the patient progresses.

BLADDER DRILL

This technique is also referred to as bladder training and is designed to regain urinary control through routine scheduling. It requires the cooperation of both the care provider and the patient. The patient's intake of oral fluids should be up to 2000 to 3000 ml unless otherwise contraindicated. Natural diuretics such as caffeine products and alcohol are to be avoided. The patient is taught to follow a routine voiding pattern as described in Chart 25–2. High level success is achieved when the plan is individualized, when all participants are motivated in working toward a specific goal, and when the fluid intake and output is considered to be adequate.

TRIGGER VOIDING

A variety of techniques may be employed to achieve voiding on cue. Mothers have often used the simple trigger technique of turning on a water faucet while trying to toilet train a young child. Similar types of trigger mechanisms may also be used for patients experiencing difficulty in starting the process of urination. Among the techniques used are stroking the inner thighs or abdomen, gently pulling on the pubic hair, using the Credé method, suprapubic tapping, putting oil of wintergreen in the bedpan, using an alarm clock or timer (enuresis alarm systems), and running tap water, dipping the hands in warm water, or pouring warm water over the perineum. Individual assessment is made for each patient to determine which trigger mechanism is most effective.

ADDITIONAL TREATMENT OPTIONS

Urinary continence in women may be assisted by the use of a vaginal ring, pessary, or tampon. These are nonsurgical approaches that temporarily reposition the bladder and vaginal walls.

Transurethral Teflon injection for urinary incontinence has been available for more than 20 years, but has only recently come to the attention of the health consumer. The 20- to 30-minute procedure creates a bulge in the urethra, thus blocking the leakage of the urine. Teflon injections are considered experimental at this time and are performed only by specially trained physicians.

DIET THERAPY

Management of the patient with a urinary tract disorder usually includes some dietary modificaions. For the patient with chronic renal failure, diet therapy is directed toward control of edema and malnutrition by monitoring protein, sodium, potassium, and water. The basic objectives of the treatment by diet therapy are described in Nutrition Box 25–1. The objectives are achieved by providing a low-sodium, low-potassium, low-protein, and high-carbohydrate diet.

Nutrition Box 25–1.

DIET THERAPY TREATMENT OBJECTIVES FOR CHRONIC RENAL FAILURE

For the patient with chronic renal failure, diet therapy is directed toward control of edema and malnutrition by monitoring protein, sodium, potassium, and water intake. The overall treatment plan has the following six objectives:

1. Minimize protein catabolism.
2. Avoid overhydration or dehydration.
3. Maintain acid-base balance by correcting or preventing acidosis.
4. Correct electrolyte depletions and avoid excesses.
5. Control fluid and electrolyte losses from vomiting and diarrhea.
6. Maintain nutritional intake and weight appropriate for the patient.

The above objectives are achieved by providing a low-sodium, low-potassium, low-protein, and high-carbohydrate diet. The patient is carefully monitored for problems. Medications are used as adjunct therapy to correct or prevent episodes of vomiting and diarrhea and to maintain acid-base balance.

Patients predisposed to urinary calculus formation also benefit from a change in diet. The most common type of calculus is composed of calcium oxalate. Therefore, a calcium-restricted diet may be recommended for the patient with urinary lithiasis. This diet limits foods that are high in calcium (Nutrition Box 25–2).

In addition to dietary restrictions, encourage patients to practice high-volume fluid flushing, up to 3000 to 4000 ml/per day (except in the presence of cardiac or renal complications). A high oral intake followed by bladder emptying every 2 hours is a practice that should be taught regardless of the stone composition.

For patients requiring catheterization or those with recurrent urinary tract infections, diet modifications to acidify urine are recommended because a lower urinary pH is known to decrease the rate of bacterial multiplication. Advise patients to consume food such as meat, nuts, prunes, plums, cranberries, and wholegrain cereals and breads. Large quantities of milk, fruits, and vegetables are to be avoided because they produce a more alkaline urine. Discourage consuming caffeine products, carbonated

Nutrition Box 25–2.

FOODS TO AVOID ON A CALCIUM-RESTRICTED DIET

Instruct the patient predisposed to calcium oxalate urinary calculus formation to avoid or severely limit the following calcium-containing foods:

- Dairy products
- Green leafy vegetables
- Whole grains

The patient should also limit the intake of the following foods:

- Citrus fruits
- Cranberry juice
- Nuts
- Chocolate

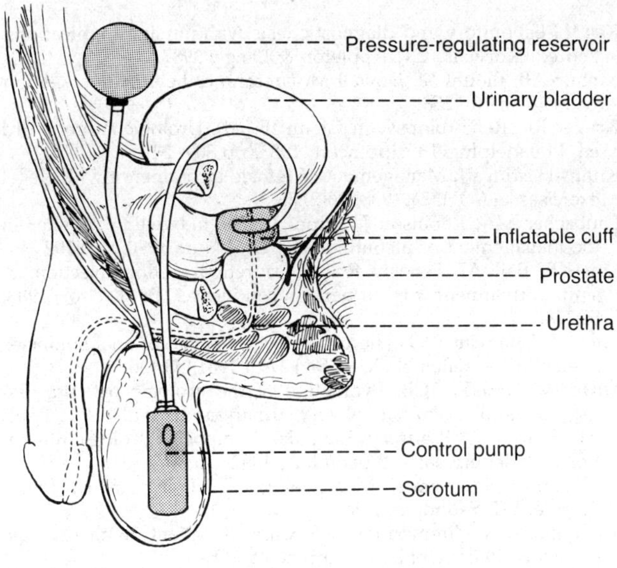

Figure 25–8.

Artificial urinary sphincter. (From Black JM, Matassarin-Jacobs, E. Luckmann and Sorenson's medical-surgical nursing. 4th ed. Philadelphia: WB Saunders, 1993, p 1458.)

beverages, and alcohol together. The exception to these restrictions is for patients taking sulfonamides, which require an alkaline urine for maximum effectiveness.

This brief overview is designed to focus attention on the relationship between urologic problems and a patient's diet. For more specific guidelines, a nutrition book should be consulted.

Surgical Management

One treatment option that is still considered experimental is the implantation of an artificial sphincter. A hydraulic pump mechanism is installed that contains a reservoir, urethral cuff, and pump. Inflation of the urethral cuff prevents leakage of urine until it is deactivated at the time of urination (Fig. 25–8). It enables the patient to urinate by deflating the cuff that encircles the bladder neck. The cuff is deflated by squeezing the control pump in the scrotum. The cuff then automatically reinflates.

Other surgical interventions for urinary tract disorders are specific to each disorder and thus are discussed with the appropriate problem in Chapter 26.

The Elderly: Special Considerations

In many instances, a urinary tract problem in the elderly patient can be attributed to a specific disease or disorder. The illnesses more prevalent in the geriatric population that produce some form of urinary tract dysfunction include cerebrovascular accident (CVA), Alzheimer's disease, diabetes mellitus, Parkinson's disease, alcoholic neuropathy, and vascular disease. Additionally, medications prescribed for the elderly patient, including antidepressants and drugs containing antihistamines, belladonna alkaloids, and phenothiazines, also alter elimination.

The absence of a specific disease or disorder in the geriatric patient suggests that changes in the urinary system are the result of normal aging. In the older adult, there is a decrease in the muscle tone of the bladder and urethra, which causes the bladder to empty less efficiently. Also, there is a decrease in the functional capacity of the bladder and a diminished sensation to fullness. These age-related changes produce problems such as urinary frequency, urgency, and nocturia.

In the older woman, a decrease in the estrogen level causes tissue changes in the urethra and the vagina, as well as relaxation of the pelvic floor muscles. Urethral, vaginal, and uterine prolapse occur, producing restricted urine flow and some retention. However, the most common problem in the older female as a result of these changes is stress incontinence.

The nurse caring for the older adult with a urinary tract problem should complete a thorough health assessment in order to determine the cause of urinary symptoms. This may be time-consuming and difficult because most older adults are reluctant to objectively and openly discuss their bladder habits and problems. The nurse should demonstrate patience, professionalism, and concern for the patients and their problems during this first encounter to lay the groundwork for a successful and therapeutic nurse-patient relationship directed toward practical and simple management of urinary problems. For instance, the elderly patient with nocturia should be advised to maintain an adequate fluid intake during the day but to limit beverages in the evening. The patient should also be advised to leave a nightlight on near the bathroom as a safety precaution to prevent injury from a fall.

For the elderly patient experiencing frequency, urgency, or incontinence, time-voiding may be suggested as a means of establishing a safe and accident-free pattern of urinary elimination. Another alternative is to recommend the use of continence products, such as pants liners and special briefs. These items are widely available and provide an added protection against possible embarrassing events.

Urinary dysfunction as a result of normal aging is considered to be a problem manageable by the nurse. In addition to the interventions previously mentioned, there are a number of other nursing techniques that are effective in reversing or managing urinary problems in the older adult. Most of these are described within the chapter and may be appropriate for all patients with urinary tract dysfunction. Caring for the geriatric patient with a urinary tract dysfunction presents a unique opportunity that allows the independent application of nursing knowledge and skills to aid a specific segment of the population.

Bibliography

Abdellah F. 1988; Incontinence: Implications for health care policy. Nurs Clin North Am 23(1):291.

Baer CL. Assessing flank pain. Nursing 1989; 19(10):75.

Baer CL. Investigating dysuria. Nursing 1989; 19(5):108.

Bluestein D, Archer L. The sensitivity, specificity, and predictive value of diagnostic information: A guide for clinicians. Nurse Pract 1991; 16(7):39.

Brendler CB. Perioperative care. In Walsh PC, Retik AB, Stamey TA, Vaughan ED (eds). Campbell's urology. 6th ed, (Vol 3). Philadelphia: WB Saunders, 1992, pp 2315–2359.

Brinsko V. It's in the bag. J Urol Nurs 1989; 8(1):563.

Britton PM. Nursing care of catheterized patients. Prof Nurse 1990; 5(5):231.

Burggraf V, Donlon B. Assessing the elderly: Part I—System by system. Am J Nurs 1985; 85(9):973.

Burke JP, Garibaldi RA, Britt M, et al. Prevention of catheter-associated urinary tract infections: Efficacy of daily meatal care regimens. 1981; 70(2):655.

Burke JP, Jacobson JA, Garibaldi RA, et al. Evaluation of daily meatal care with poly-antibiotic ointment in prevention of urinary catheter-associated bacteriuria. Urol 1983; 129:331.

Ciaravino YM. Nursing care of the patient receiving urodynamic testing. AUAA 1984; 5(1):12.

Clay E. Habit retraining: A tested method to regain urinary control. Geriatr Nurs 1980; 1(4):252.

Colling J. Educating nurses to care for the incontinent patient. Nurs Clin North Am 1988; 23(1):279.

Corriere JN. Essentials of urology. New York: Churchill Livingstone, 1986.

Cos K, Cos LR. Hematuria revisited. AUAA J 1984; 5(2):4.

Crow R, Mulhall A, Chapman R. Indwelling catheterization and related nursing practice. 1988; 13(4):489.

Demmerle B, Bartal MA. Nursing care for the incontinent person. Geriatr Nurs 1980; 1(4):246.

Devine CJ, Jordan GH, Schlossberg SM. Surgery of the penis and urethra. In Walsh PC, Retik AB, Stamey TA, Vaughan ED (eds). Campbell's urology 6th ed, Vol 3. Philadelphia: WB Saunders, 1992, pp 2957–3032.

Engram BW. Do's and don'ts of urologic nursing. Nursing 1983; 13(10):49.

Friedman FB. Why not use a foley? RN 1982; 45(11):71.

Gittes RS. Hematuria. AUAA J 1980; 2(2):27.

Greengold BA, Ouslander JG. Bladder retraining: A program for elderly patients with post-indwelling catheterization. J Gerontol Nurs 1986; 12(6):31.

Hanno PM, Woin AJ. A clinical manual of urology. Norwalk, CT: Appleton-Century-Crofts, 1986.

Harper WE. An appraisal of 12 solutions used for bladder irrigation or instillation. Br J Urol 1982; 53:433.

Harvey AM, Johns RJ, McKusick VA, et al. Principles and practice of medicine. 21st ed. Norwalk, CT: Appleton-Century-Crofts, 1984.

Hough E. Effective management of urinary drainage systems in critical care areas. Intensive Care Nurs 1989; 5(2):82.

Ignatavicius D, Bayne M. Medical surgical nursing. Philadelphia: WB Saunders, 1991.

Islam AK, Chapman J. Closed catheter drainage and urinary infection—A comparison of two methods of catheter drainage. Br J Urol 1977; 49:215.

Jeter K, Faller N, Norton C. Nursing for continence. Philadelphia: WB Saunders, 1990.

Joyce JM, Croft BY, Teates CD. Nuclide studies. In Gillenwater JY, Grayhack JT, Howards SS, Duckett JW (eds). Adult and pediatric urology. Chicago: Year Book Medical Publishers, 1987, pp 169–190.

Kaschak ND. The treatment of urinary incontinence in adults. Nurse Pract 1989; 14(6):21.

Kaufman JJ Current urologic therapy. 2nd ed. Philadelphia: WB Saunders, 1986.

Kee JL. Laboratory and diagnostic tests with nursing implications. 2nd ed. Norwalk, CT: Appleton & Lange, 1987.

Kinney AB, Blount M, Dowell M. Urethral catheterization. Geriatr Nurs 1980; 1(6):258.

Kruger RP. Renal biopsy. In Glenn JF (ed). Urologic surgery. 3rd ed. Philadelphia: JB Lippincott, 1983, pp 309–315.

Kuhns-Hastings J. Management of female incontinence with Kegel exercises. AAOHN J 1988; 36(2):78.

Laubacher MA, Robinson J, Shipes E, The indwelling catheter in the management of incontinence. J Urol Nurs 1990; 9(1):792.

Lim KB, Ball AJ, Feneley RCL. Periurethral Teflon injection: A simple treatment for urinary incontinence. Br J Urol 1983; 55:208.

Low AI, Donovan WD. The use and mechanism of anal sphincter stretch in the reflex bladder. Br J Urol 1981; 53:430.

Lowe FC, Brendler CB. Evaluation of the urologic patient: History, physical examination, and urinalysis. In Walsh PC, Retik AB, Stamey TA, Vaughan ED (eds). Campbell's urology. 6th ed, Vol 1. Philadelphia: WB Saunders, 1992, pp 307–331.

Luckmann J, Sorensen K. Medical-surgical nursing. 3rd ed. Philadelphia: WB Saunders, 1987.

McConnell EA, Zimmerman MF. Care of patients with urologic problems. Philadelphia: JB Lippincott, 1983.

McCormick K, Scheve A, Leahy E. Nursing management of urinary incontinence in geriatric inpatients. Nurs Clin North Am 1988; 23(1):231.

McGuire EJ. Identifying and managing stress incontinence in the elderly. Geriatrics 1990; 45(6):44.

National Institutes of Health. Summary of the NIH Consensus Development Conference on Urinary Incontinence in Adults. Bethesda, MD: NIH, 1988.

Palmer MH. Urinary incontinence. Thorofare, NJ: MJ Slack, 1985.

Pein FD, Landers JQ. Indwelling urinary catheter infections in small community hospital: Role of urinary drainage bag. Urology 1983; 22:255.

Pieper B, Cleland V, Johnson DW, O'Reilly JL. Inventing urine incontinence devices for women. Image J Nurs Sch 1989; 21(4):205.

Planatemoli LV. When the patient has a foley. RN 1984; 47(3):42.

Pollack HM, Banner MP. Diagnostic uroradiology. In Hanno PM, Woin AJ (eds). A clinical manual of urology. Norwalk, CT: Appleton-Century-Crofts, 1987, pp 79–118.

Race GJ, White MG. Basic urinalysis. Hagerstown, MD: Harper & Row, 1979.

Resnick NM. Urinary incontinence in the elderly. Medical Grand Rounds 1984; 3(3):281.

Resnick NM, Yalla SV. Current concepts: Management of urinary incontinence in the elderly. N Engl J Med 1985; 313(13):800.

Roe B, Brocklehurst J. Study of patients with indwelling catheters. J Ad Nurs 1987; 12(6):713.

Rous SN. Urology: A core textbook. Norwalk, CT: Appleton-Century-Crofts, 1985.

Samples JT, Dougherty MC, Abrams RM, Batich CD. The dynamic characteristics of the circumvaginal muscles. JOGNN 1988; 18(3):194.

Sawyer DL. Potential for infection: A nursing diagnosis for the patient with an indwelling catheter. Focus Crit Care 1989; 16(1):46.

Schumann JL. Urinalysis for the office practice: Part I. Reagent strip testing. AUAA J 1986; 6(4):14.

Schumann JL. Urinalysis for the office practice: Part II. Standardized urine microscopy. AUAA J 1986; 7(1):8.

Schumann JL. Urinalysis for the office practice: Part III. Urine cytology and advanced laboratory techniques. AUAA J 1987; 7(3):6.

Shapiro JI, Schrier RW. Etiology, pathogenesis, and management of renal failure. In Walsh PC, Retik AB, Stamey TA, Vaughan ED (eds). Campbell's urology. 6th ed, Vol 2. Philadelphia: WB Saunders, 1992, pp 2045–2064.

Smith DR. General urology. 11th ed. Los Altos, CA: Lange Medical Publications, 1984.

Taylor K, Henderson J. Effects of biofeedback and urinary stress incontinence in older women. J Gerontol Nurs 1986; 12(9):25.

Chapter Twenty-six

NURSING CARE *of Adults with* Urinary Tract Disorders

Urinary tract disorders are some of the most common health problems individuals experience. Although the disorders are not often life-threatening, morbidity from urinary tract problems is still a threat, especially when damage to the kidney occurs. Because the urinary system assists the body in maintenance of homeostasis through fluid and electrolyte balance, disorders of the system have a profound effect on the entire body's functioning.

Infections and Inflammations

The most common urologic disorders are infections and inflammations of the urinary tract. This type of problem is prevalent in three quarters of the patients seeking urologic consultation and accounts for more than 40% of nosocomial infections.

By definition, an infection exists in the urinary tract when specific microorganisms can be identified through urine culture. To meet the definition of urinary tract infection (UTI), there must be more than 10^5 (100,000) organisms per ml in a clean catch urine specimen. UTIs are described in relation to the anatomic area involved, such as cystitis, urethritis, or pyelonephritis.

Cystitis

ETIOLOGY AND PATHOPHYSIOLOGY

Cystitis is the inflammation of the bladder, which usually results from the invasion of bacteria into the urinary tract. In the female patient, bacteria that enter the urinary tract usually originate from either the rectum or the vagina and ascend upward via the urethra. In the male patient, cystitis is usually the result of an existing problem in the urinary tract, such as prostatitis or benign prostatic hypertrophy.

Cystitis is more common in women, and it is estimated that 10% to 25% of the female population experience the problem at least once in their lifetime. This is due to the length of the urethra (1–1½ inches) and the proximity of the meatus to the vagina and rectum. Cystitis can occur following instrumentation of the urinary tract or be the result of incomplete bladder emptying. The incidence of cystitis is also associated with sexual intercourse and pregnancy. In some instances, cystitis develops when bacteria travel to the bladder via the vascular or lymphatic systems from a site elsewhere in the body.

When bacteria enter the bladder, they adhere to and multiply in the bladder's mucosal surface. As the infection intensifies, the surface of the bladder becomes reddened and edematous; areas of ulceration may also develop. Symptoms of pain and urinary urgency result when urine comes in contact with the irritated surface of the bladder. This irritation is exacerbated when the bladder becomes even slightly distended with urine.

CLINICAL MANIFESTATIONS

The patient with cystitis usually presents with one or more of the following symptoms: dysuria, frequency, urgency, nocturia, nocturnal enuresis, incontinence, urethral pain, low back pain, suprapubic pain, and fever. The patient may also describe episodes of painful straining that are ineffective in producing urine, called tenesmus. Hematuria is not uncommon in the patient with cystitis, and urine often has a strong odor.

Chart 26–1.

NURSING GUIDE TO PATIENT EDUCATION FOR SELF-MANAGEMENT: SELF-CARE FOR PREVENTION OF URINARY TRACT INFECTIONS

Instruct the patient to:

- Drink 2 to 3 L of fluid daily.
- Notify the physician if urgency, frequency, burning, or difficulty in urinating is experienced.
- Empty the bladder as soon as the urge is felt.
- Clean the perineum from front to back (women only).
- Avoid irritating substances such as bubble bath, nylon underwear, and scented toilet paper (women only).
- Wear cotton underwear.
- Take all of medication, even after symptoms subside, to prevent recurring infections.
- Schedule a follow-up visit with the physician to have a repeat urine culture.

MEDICAL DIAGNOSIS

Although information from patients' history and knowledge of their presenting symptoms are helpful in making a diagnosis, it is the urine culture that confirms the presence of an infection in the bladder. A urine culture that grows more than 100,00 colonies of bacteria per ml of urine documents the existence of an infection. A complete blood count with differential shows an elevated white blood count with a "shift to the left." This shift indicates that there is an increase in the number of immature white blood cells, which would be a response to the infection. In instances when the colony count is less than 100,000, additional studies such as intravenous pyelography (IVP) and cystoscopy may need to be done and the findings correlated with other data to make the diagnosis. IVP, computed tomography (CT), and ultrasonography may provide evidence of obstruction.

MEDICAL MANAGEMENT

Patients with uncomplicated, acute cystitis are usually treated with an antimicrobial agent. The specific medication used is determined by sensitivity testing for the bacteria found growing in the urine; those most commonly prescribed include ampicillin, amoxicillin, trimethoprim-sulfamethoxazole, and sulfisoxazole. In most instances of acute cystitis, patients are treated for 7 to 10 days. However, there are studies that suggest that 1-day therapy, or even single-dose therapy, is equally effective in women with acute, uncomplicated cystitis. For patients with chronic recurrent cystitis, antimicrobial therapy may be required for several months. Analgesics, urinary antiseptics, and anticholinergics are also used to treat the pain and bladder spasms that often accompany UTIs. Chart 26–1 describes self-care measures for prevention of urinary tract infections.

Application of the Nursing Process to the Care of the Patient with Cystitis

Assessment

Obtain a health history, including a review of the patient's current status and symptoms. Assess for uropenia, hesitancy, frequency, and dysuria. Ask about voiding patterns. Obtain information about the color and odor of the urine. Ask whether there is any blood or mucus in the urine. Ask the patient to describe any pain or discomfort that has occurred. Since medical treatment most often involves the administration of an antimicrobial agent, the patient should also be asked about any drug allergies or sensitivities.

Inspect the lower abdomen and the meatus to determine whether tissues are inflamed. Palpate the urinary bladder for distention or pain.

Review the patient's daily hygiene and dietary practices, as well as discussing activities that may predispose the patient to cystitis. Ask whether the onset of symptoms associated with cystitis occur after sexual intercourse. Check whether the patient frequently takes bubble baths. Note whether the patient wears tight-fitting blue jeans. Ask whether the patient is able to empty the bladder at regular intervals, or whether voiding is often delayed for several hours. The answers to these questions are extremely important and will be helpful in developing a teaching plan aimed at preventing a recurrence of cystitis.

Assess the patient's level of knowledge about the disorder, treatment, and care needed. Note the patient's questions and concerns. Invite the family to participate when appropriate, and assess their level of knowledge about the condition.

Nursing Diagnoses and Planning

Nursing diagnoses and related expected patient outcomes most commonly applicable to patients with cystitis include the following:

NDx: Altered patterns of urinary elimination related to inflammation and irritation

Planning: Patient outcomes
1. Patient adheres to established voiding schedule.
2. Patient reports relief of irritative voiding symptoms.
3. Patient resumes normal voiding pattern.

NDx: Pain related to inflammation and irritation

Planning: Patient outcomes
1. Patient reports comfort and pain relief.
2. Patient is able to void without pain or burning.

NDx: Knowledge deficit related to factors that may predispose to cystitis and/or treatment regimen

Planning: Patient outcomes
1. Patient lists factors that predispose to cystitis.
2. Patient describes medical and dietary regimen.
3. Patient verbalizes measures to prevent cystitis.

Nursing Interventions

NDx: Altered patterns of urinary elimination
Nursing intervention for the patient with cystitis includes the implementation of measures to alleviate the irritative voiding symptoms. Administer antimicrobial medications as ordered to sterilize the urine, and antispasmodics or analgesics as ordered to relieve the accompanying suprapubic discomfort brought on by bladder spasms. An increased oral

fluid intake of up to 3000 ml/day should be encouraged (unless contraindicated for other medical reasons) because a more dilute urine lessens the irritation to the bladder mucosa.

Quite often, a patient delays voiding because of the pain and discomfort brought on by urination. Encourage voiding at regular intervals. Frequent bladder emptying decreases intravesical irritation and prevents stasis of urine.

NDx: Pain
Administer analgesics and antispasmodics as ordered. Offer a warm sitz bath to relieve perineal or suprapubic discomfort. This may be done 2 or 3 times per day. Encourage the patient to drink 2 to 3 L/day.

NDx: Knowledge deficit
Incorporate information about the dosage and potential side effects of the medication prescribed; a reminder to complete the entire course of therapy even though symptoms have subsided is also necessary. Instruct the patient to drink 2 to 3 L/day and obtain adequate rest and nutrition. Review the practice of proper hygiene. Most importantly, teach the patient activities that may be performed to prevent a recurrence of the cystitis. For example, if the patient's bladder infection occurred following sexual intercourse, then the patient should be taught the practice of voiding immediately after coitus; similarly, if the patient experiences irritative voiding symptoms after taking a tub bath, then showering should be encouraged to prevent the ascent of bacteria into the urinary tract from the bath water. Teach the patient to recognize symptoms of UTI and report them to the physician. Explain the diagnostic studies completed and the need for any follow-up studies after discharge. Include the family in any of the teaching sessions when applicable.

Evaluation

Evaluate the effectiveness of nursing care for a patient with cystitis by comparing the patient's status with the expected patient outcomes. Examples of specific outcomes for patients with cystitis have been provided in the Planning section.

Urethritis

ETIOLOGY AND PATHOPHYSIOLOGY

Urethritis is an inflammation of the urethra. The patient presents with signs and symptoms very similar to those of cystitis. Urethritis can be acute or chronic.

Urethritis is found in both males and females. In males the most common cause is gonorrhea. Urethritis is often associated with venereal disease. Some of the organisms more commonly associated with urethritis are *Ureaplasma*, *Chlamydia*, and *Trichomonas vaginalis*. Urethritis can also be caused by irritants such as soaps, perfumed toilet paper and sanitary napkins, and bubble baths.

CLINICAL MANIFESTATIONS

The patient with urethritis presents with burning, frequency, and nocturia. There may be difficulty with urination. Males usually have a discharge from the urethral meatus, but females do not usually have meatal discharge. Patients often complain of lower abdominal discomfort.

MEDICAL DIAGNOSIS

Urethritis is diagnosed on the basis of the patient's history and current complaints. Examination of the urine may reveal pus or bacteria. If pyuria (pus in the urine) is found without significant bacteria, the patient should be examined for an infection elsewhere in the urinary tract.

MEDICAL MANAGEMENT

If the urethritis is caused by bacterial invasion, the patient is treated with systemic or topical antibiotics, or both. If it is caused by an irritant, the irritant should be removed. The patient is encouraged to avoid factors that can contribute to the problem. A high fluid intake and sitz baths are also encouraged.

Application of the Nursing Process to the Care of the Patient with Urethritis

The assessment, nursing diagnoses, expected patient outcomes, nursing interventions, and evaluation for patients with urethritis are similar to those described previously for patients with cystitis.

Pyelonephritis

ETIOLOGY AND PATHOPHYSIOLOGY

Pyelonephritis is an infection of the upper urinary tract that produces pain and edema in the kidney, renal pelvis, and surrounding structures. Its onset is usually acute, with symptoms that are often mistaken for muscle strain in the lower back. It can become chronic, resulting in hypertension and uremia in some patients. Pyelonephritis is the original diagnosis in one third of patients with renal failure.

The most common cause of pyelonephritis is the reflux of infected urine from the bladder to the upper urinary tract. However, stasis of urine in the system as a result of obstruction can also lead to pyelonephritis.

Patients at risk for developing pyelonephritis are those who have had recent instrumentation of the urinary tract, those with diabetes mellitus, those with a history of analgesic abuse, and those with voiding disorders associated with incomplete bladder emptying. Elderly patients and pregnant women are also susceptible to developing the problem.

The source of bacteria contaminating the urinary tract is usually fecal flora. Once these microorganisms enter the system they adhere to and multiply in uroepithelial tissue. An *Escherichia coli* infection is the most common, although pyelonephritis caused by *Proteus, Pseudomonas, Enterobacter, Klebsiella,* enterococcus, *Serratia, Morganella,* and *Staphylococcus* is not uncommon.

CLINICAL MANIFESTATIONS

The patient with acute pyelonephritis complains of a persistent ache in the flank or back, cystitis-like symptoms, fever with chills, and general malaise accompanied by nausea, vomiting, and diarrhea. Upon examination, there may be tenderness in the area of the costovertebral angle (CVA) and an elevated pulse rate, as well as pus, bacteria, and white cell casts in the urine. Patients with chronic pyelonephritis are usually asymptomatic, except for some vague and intermittent flank pain, an occasional elevated temperature, and evidence of persistent, unresolved bacteriuria.

MEDICAL DIAGNOSIS

The diagnosis of pyelonephritis is made primarily on the basis of the patient's history, physical examination, and findings from urinalysis, urine culture, blood count, and radiographic studies. A positive urine culture result and an elevated white blood cell count along with x-ray results that demonstrate changes in the appearance of the kidney and ureter consistent with a long-standing infection confirm the diagnosis.

MEDICAL MANAGEMENT

Once pyelonephritis has been diagnosed, oral or intravenous antibiotic therapy is immediately instituted and continued for at least 2 weeks; for patients with chronic pyelonephritis, intense antibiotic therapy may be required for as long as 6 months to clear the infection. Relief of symptoms includes aspirin for an elevated temperature, antiemetics to control nausea and vomiting, oral or intravenous fluids to prevent dehydration and increase urine output, pain medications and urinary antiseptics to relieve discomfort, and bed rest.

In some cases, surgery may be done to relieve obstruction or eradicate intractable infection. Stones could be removed by performing extracorporeal shock wave lithotripsy, percutaneous ultrasonic pyelolithotomy, or pyelotomy. A nephrectomy could be done, as a last resort, to eradicate infection. The care of the patient undergoing these procedures is discussed later in this chapter.

Application of the Nursing Process to the Care of the Patient with Pyelonephritis

Assessment

Review the patient's health history and medical management. It is important to note whether this is the first occurrence of pyelonephritis. Assess the patient for pain, malaise, fatigue, chills, and fever. Inspect the area of the CVA for asymmetry or swelling, which would indicate inflammation. Encourage the patient to feel free to talk about the signs and symptoms. Many patients feel embarrassed and anxious about discussing problems of the urinary tract.

Nursing Diagnoses and Planning

Nursing diagnoses and related expected patient outcomes most commonly applicable to patients with pyelonephritis include the following:

NDx: Pain related to inflammation and infection

Planning: Patient outcomes
1. Patient verbalizes relief from pain.
2. Patient is able to resume usual activities of daily living.

NDx: Activity intolerance related to fatigue

Planning: Patient outcomes
1. Patient follows a regimen of planned activities and rest periods each day.
2. Patient verbalizes feeling less fatigued and demonstrates signs of increased activity.
3. Patient is able to resume usual activities of daily living.

NDx: Knowledge deficit related to medical diagnoses and treatment regimen

Planning: Patient outcomes

1. Patient describes cause, effects, and clinical course of pyelonephritis.
2. Patient lists symptoms of pyelonephritis and treatment.
3. Patient states self-care needed to prevent recurrence or complications of pyelonephritis.

NDx: Fear related to the potential development of chronic renal failure

Planning: Patient outcomes

1. Patient verbalizes fear relating to potential complications of diagnoses.
2. Patient states self-care needed to prevent recurrence or complications of pyelonephritis.

Nursing Interventions

NDx: Pain
Administer analgesics and antiseptics as ordered to relieve pain and discomfort. Administer antiemetics as ordered to alleviate nausea and vomiting. Assist patient in achieving comfortable positions while on bed rest.

NDx: Activity intolerance
Encourage bed rest during the acute stages. Encourage the patient to do range-of-motion exercises frequently while lying in bed to maintain muscle tone and strength. As symptoms subside, instruct the patient in developing a regimen of activity with frequent rest periods throughout the day.

NDx: Knowledge deficit
Explain the cause, effects, and clinical course of the disorder to the patient. Allow for questions from the patient at any time. Provide appropriate literature for the patient and family to review.

Alert the patient to signs and symptoms of pyelonephritis that should be attended to when they occur. Teach the patient measures to prevent urinary tract infections. Stress the importance of balancing rest and activity. Instruct the patient to follow a balanced diet with increased fluid intake.

Teach the patient dosage, route, time, frequency, side effects, and toxic effects of any medication prescribed. When the patient suffers from chronic pyelonephritis, stress the importance of compliance with an extended medication regimen. Include the family in any of the teaching sessions when applicable.

NDx: Fear
Encourage the patient to verbalize feelings related to the disease. Discuss the patient's perception of the danger of developing renal failure. Provide information to reduce distortions. Assist the patient in the use of coping skills. Teach the patient measures to prevent the recurrence of pyelonephritis.

Evaluation

Evaluate the effectiveness of nursing care for a patient with pyelonephritis by comparing the patient's status with the expected patient outcomes. Examples of specific outcomes for patients with pyelonephritis have been provided in the Planning section.

Perinephric Abscess

ETIOLOGY AND PATHOPHYSIOLOGY

A perinephric abscess is a fluid-filled mass that forms outside the kidney but within its supportive tissue structures. It is associated with chronic upper urinary tract infections, often causes necrosis to surrounding tissues, and usually occurs because of extravasation of infected urine. *E. coli, Pseudomonas,* and *Staphylococcus* are the most common causative organisms.

CLINICAL MANIFESTATIONS

Signs and symptoms of a perinephric abscess are similar to those for pyelonephritis. A persistent fever despite the administration of antibiotics for a suspected upper urinary tract infection is considered characteristic. Additionally, palpation of a flank mass and observed edema of the skin over the affected area are possible. If the abscess is unusually large, other internal structures such as the diaphragm and the spine are displaced. The eruption of skin lesions over the abscess may also occur if the infecting organism is *Staphylococcus.*

MEDICAL DIAGNOSIS

The diagnosis is confirmed by radiologic examination. Ultrasonography or computer tomographic scans of the affected kidney are the procedures of choice. A kidney, ureter, and bladder (KUB) x-ray examination and an excretory urogram may also be done.

MEDICAL MANAGEMENT

Once the abscess has been detected and located, immediate percutaneous drainage is required. Antibiotic therapy is also necessary to prevent sepsis and further extension of the disease. Failure to intervene quickly once the diagnosis is made can result in the death of the patient because of sepsis. In some instances, surgical removal of the abscess and correction of an underlying urinary tract problem are necessary.

Application of the Nursing Process to the Care of the Patient with a Perinephric Abscess

The assessment, nursing diagnoses, expected patient outcomes, nursing interventions, and evaluation for patients with a perinephric abscess are similar to those described previously for patients with pyelonephritis. The assessment, nursing diagnoses, expected patient outcomes, nursing interventions, and evaluation for patients undergoing percutaneous drainage of the abscess are similar to those described previously for patients undergoing renal biopsy (see Chapter 25).

Glomerulonephritis

ETIOLOGY AND PATHOPHYSIOLOGY

Glomerulonephritis is an inflammation of the kidney that affects the capillary loops in the glomeruli. Its onset is usually secondary to an infection of the upper respiratory tract, most commonly caused by beta-hemolytic streptococci. However, glomerulonephritis can be the result of a primary infection elsewhere in the body and be caused by staphylococcus, pneumococcus, or a virus. Glomerulonephritis can occur at any age; it has a higher incidence in males than females.

Glomerulonephritis is caused by an immunologic reaction (Table 26–1). The antigen that initiates the process may be endogenous or exogenous. Endogenous antigens are believed to be already present in the glomerulus or other tissues of the body. Exogenous antigens are from infections occurring in the body. Because of the antigen-antibody response, glomerular injury occurs.

The antigen-antibody complexes are trapped within the glomerulus. This trapping produces an inflammatory response that damages the glomeruli. The glomeruli are unable to filter out the plasma proteins, and they are instead spilled into the urine. As the inflammation persists, there is destruction of renal tissue, scarring, and hypertrophy, which impinges upon unaffected tubules.

CLINICAL MANIFESTATIONS

Patients with glomerulonephritis often present with a sore throat, an elevated temperature, microscopic hematuria, proteinuria, a decreased urinary output, swelling of the face and lower extremities, costovertebral angle tenderness, and flank pain likened to renal colic. As the disease progresses, the patient experiences shortness of breath, lethargy, and anorexia. Signs and symptoms of uremia may become evident. Hypertension often develops, and the blood urea nitrogen and creatinine levels are elevated.

MEDICAL DIAGNOSIS

The diagnosis of glomerulonephritis is made on the basis of findings from the patient's history, physical examination, and urinalysis. A renal biopsy may be performed to confirm the presence of glomerular inflammation.

MEDICAL MANAGEMENT

Glomerulonephritis is a serious condition that could lead to end-stage renal disease if not treated promptly. The goal of medical intervention is to treat the inflammation and accompanying symptoms in order to restore the kidney to normal function. Because the primary infecting organism is often beta-hemolytic streptococci, patients are generally treated with penicillin for 7 to 10 days. Salt restriction may be required to combat the associated edema and hypertension. Bed rest is essential during the acute phase of the disease process and may be necessary for a longer period of time, until renal function has stabilized and proteinuria and hematuria are no longer evident. The usual course of illness is 14 days. The proteinuria and hematuria may last several months. If symptoms do not subside within 2 years, the patient will more than likely be afflicted with chronic glomerulonephritis.

Table 26–1. CAUSES OF GLOMERULONEPHRITIS

Glomerulonephritis, primary
Acute glomerulonephritis
Postinfectious glomerulonephritis
Infectious glomerulonephritis
Membranoproliferative glomerulonephritis
Rapidly progressive glomerulonephritis
Idiopathic membranous glomerulonephritis
IgA nephropathy
Chronic glomerulonephritis
Lipoid nephrosis
Focal glomerular sclerosis
Glomerulonephritis, secondary to systemic disease
Goodpasture's syndrome
Hemolytic-uremic syndrome
Henoch-Schönlein syndrome
Polyarteritis
Progressive systemic sclerosis
Systemic lupus erythematosus
Wegener's granulomatosis

From Luckmann J, Sorensen K. Medical-surgical nursing. 3rd ed. Philadelphia: WB Saunders, 1987, p 1205.

Application of the Nursing Process to the Care of the Patient with Glomerulonephritis

Assessment

Assess the patient with glomerulonephritis by checking the history and laboratory data. Then inquire about any previous infections that may have occurred. Of special interest would be a recent upper respiratory tract infection, skin infection, pericarditis, or lower urinary tract infection.

Next, evaluate the current status of the patient. This includes an examination of the patient for signs of renal failure, respiratory distress, circulatory congestion, and systemic infection. Also note the patient's nutritional status and current eating habits, the type and location of any pain, the appearance of the urine, and any physical limitations brought on by the associated weakness, lethargy, and fatigue.

Finally, review the laboratory values for quantitative information from the urinalysis, complete blood count, and blood chemistry.

Nursing Diagnoses and Planning

Nursing diagnoses and related expected patient outcomes most commonly applicable to patients with glomerulonephritis include the following:

NDx: Activity intolerance related to fatigue, fluid volume excess, and loss of energy

Planning: Patient outcomes

1. Patient follows a regimen of planned activities and rest period each day.
2. Patient verbalizes feeling less fatigued and demonstrates signs of increased activity.
3. Patient is able to resume usual activities of daily living.

NDx: Fluid volume excess related to decreased glomerular filtration rate

Planning: Patient outcomes

1. Patient exhibits decreased edema.
2. Patient does not experience signs and symptoms of fluid overload.
3. Patient demonstrates knowledge related to therapeutic regimen to decrease fluid.

NDx: Altered nutrition: less than body requirements related to anorexia, nausea, and vomiting

Planning: Patient outcomes

1. Patient increases oral intake as evidenced by eating 75% of meals.
2. Patient describes the rationale and procedure for treatment.
3. Patient maintains desired weight.
4. Patient experiences no nausea and vomiting.

Nursing Interventions

NDx: Activity intolerance
Assist the patient in maintenance of bed rest. This is very important because there is a direct relationship between physical activity and the presence of proteinuria and hematuria. Even ambulation a short distance must be restricted until the kidney has had time to heal and there is little or no protein and blood in the urine. Patient education and the encouragement of a caring nurse ensure compliance with this temporary but difficult alteration in the patient's activity level. As symptoms improve, instruct the patient in developing a regimen of activity with frequent rest periods throughout the day.

NDx: Fluid volume excess
Assess the patient frequently for signs and symptoms of fluid overload. Weigh the patient every morning. Monitor fluid intake and output. Instruct the patient in diet that is low in sodium. Assist patient in coping with any fluid restriction that is ordered. Protect edematous skin from injury. Assess the patient's knowledge of diet and medical regimen. Instruct the patient as needed, including family when necessary.

NDx: Altered nutrition: less than body requirements
Explain to the patient the importance of consuming adequate amounts of nutrients. Monitor intake and output, and weigh patient daily. Instruct in prescribed diet. If there is severe edema, hypertension, or oliguria, a low-protein, low-sodium diet with fluid restriction is ordered. Teach the patient to use spices to help improve the taste of food. Plan care so that unpleasant procedures do not take place before meals. Medicate the patient for pain or nausea 30 to 45 minutes before meals as ordered. Provide a pleasant, relaxed atmosphere for meals. Assist the patient in resting or relaxing before meals. Encourage small, frequent feedings. Provide good oral hygiene. Allow the patient to choose food items as much as possible. Encourage support from family.

Evaluation

Evaluate the effectiveness of nursing care for a patient with glomerulonephritis by comparing the patient's status with the expected patient outcomes. Examples of specific outcomes for patients with glomerulonephritis have been provided in the Planning section.

Renal Failure

Renal failure or renal insufficiency is the condition of partial or total loss of kidney function. Failure does not occur until there is functional loss of 75% of the kidney's nephrons, the functioning unit of the kidney.

Renal failure may be either acute or chronic, depending on the course of onset. Regardless of the type of failure, the body undergoes significant biochemical changes that, without treatment, will result eventually in death. Table 26–2 presents terminology related to renal failure.

Table 26–2. TERMS RELATED TO RENAL FAILURE

Acute renal failure (ARF): Loss of functional ability of the kidney that is rapid in onset and usually reversible. It may be prerenal, renal, or postrenal in nature.
Acute tubular necrosis (ATN): Acute renal failure that is renal in nature. The cause is ischemic or toxic injury.
Anuria: Urinary output of less than 100 ml/day.
Azotemia: Buildup of nitrogenous waste products in the blood, specifically BUN and creatinine.
Chronic renal failure (CRF): Chronic, progressive loss of renal function that is irreversible. Causes of chronic renal failure are numerous.
Metabolic waste products: By-products of protein metabolism that are excreted in the urine.
Oliguria: Urinary output of less than 400 ml/day.
Uremia: The clinical manifestations associated with an accumulation of nitrogenous waste products in the blood, typically associated with renal failure.

Acute Renal Failure

ETIOLOGY AND PATHOPHYSIOLOGY

Acute renal failure occurs suddenly and is often reversible. It generally follows an ischemic or toxic trauma to the kidney. Recovery from acute renal failure is dependent on the cause and underlying disease process. If the renal failure is a result of an extensive disease process, the mortality rate is high. The cause of acute renal failure has three distinct sources: prerenal, renal, and postrenal (Fig. 26–1).

Prerenal failure is caused by interference with renal blood flow. The kidney is dependent on an adequate blood flow to maintain function. A decrease in perfusion results in decreased glomerular filtration. Causes of prerenal failure include decreased volume states caused by diarrhea, vomiting, hemorrhage, excessive use of diuretics, burns, and glycosuria; states that are caused by shifts of volume such as vasodilation and sepsis; states of decreased cardiac output, such as congestive heart failure, pericardial tamponade, and acute pulmonary embolus; states of decreased vascular resistance such as anesthesia and hepatorenal syndrome; and states of vascular obstruction, such as dissecting aneurysm and bilateral renal artery occlusion.

Renal causes are those conditions that cause direct kidney damage or changes. These include nephrotoxic substances such as aminoglycosides and heavy

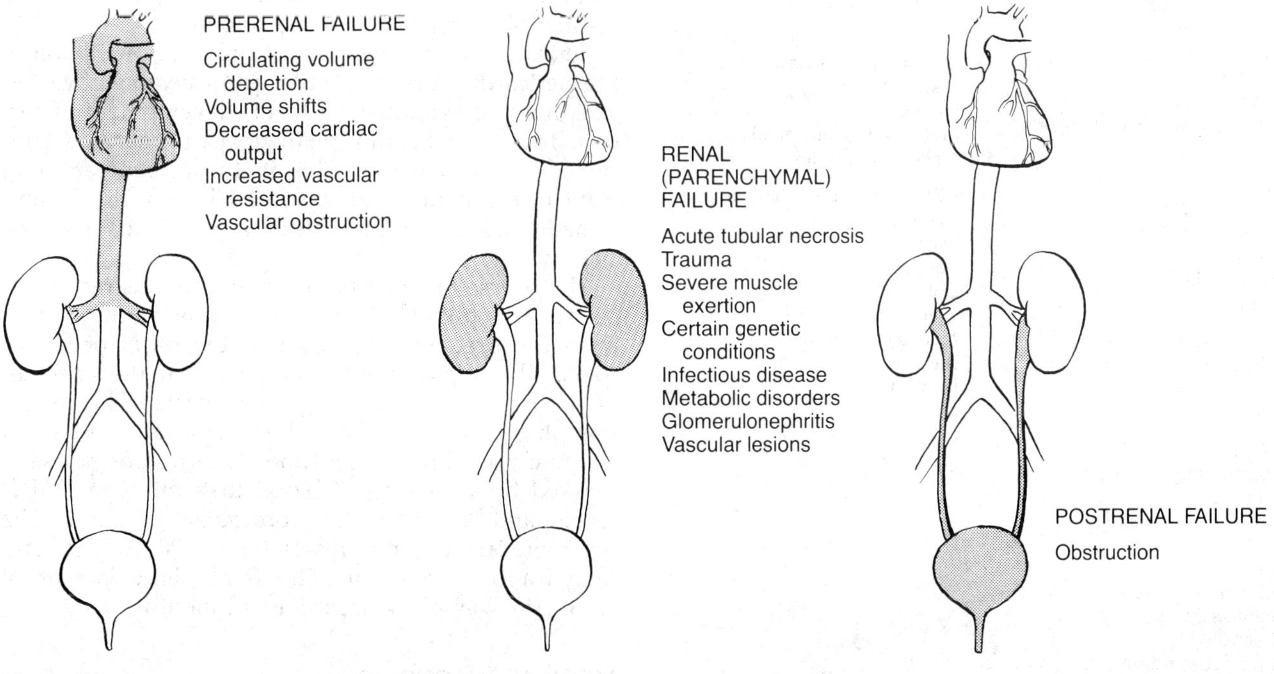

Figure 26–1.

Causes of acute renal failure: prerenal, renal, and postrenal. (From Black JM, Matassarin-Jacobs E. Luckmann and Sorensen's Medical-surgical nursing. 4th ed. Philadelphia: WB Saunders, 1993, p 1500.)

metals and ischemia. Acute tubular necrosis (ATN) is the most common renal cause of acute renal failure. Other renal causes include acute glomerulonephritis, trauma, severe muscle exertion, genetic and metabolic disorders, and renal vascular lesions.

Postrenal causes are related to obstruction in the urinary tract from the renal tubules to the urethral meatus. The obstruction can be caused by urethral or bladder cancer, renal calculi, atony of bladder, prostatic hyperplasia or cancer, cervical cancer, postsurgical or traumatic interruption, or retroperitoneal fibrosis.

Acute renal failure is caused by two major mechanisms: (1) ischemic changes to renal cells or (2) renal cell changes as a result of toxic substances. Ischemia may be a result of decreased perfusion leading to the death of renal cells and compromised renal function. Toxic substances decrease renal function by attacking the renal cell membranes and destroying their ability to maintain hemostasis. Some nephrotoxic substances are listed in Table 26–3.

CLINICAL MANIFESTATIONS

Symptoms of acute renal failure are rapid on appearance and are a result of retention of fluids and metabolic wastes and inability to regulate electrolytes (Table 26–4). In general, the individual is acutely ill. Biochemical changes occur rapidly and give the person little time to adjust to the altered internal environment. The individual may exhibit either oliguria (urine output of less than 400 ml/day) or anuria (urine output of less than 100 ml/day).

Table 26–3. NEPHROTOXIC SUBSTANCES

DRUGS	OTHER SUBSTANCES
ANTIBIOTICS/ANTI-INFECTIVES	ORGANIC SOLVENTS
Amphotericin	Carbon tetrachloride
Colistimethate	Ethylene glycol
Methicillin	NONDRUG CHEMICAL AGENTS
Polymyxin B	Radiographic contrast dye
Rifampin	Pesticides
Sulfonamides	Fungicides
Tetracycline hydrochloride	Myoglobin (from breakdown of skeletal muscle)
Vancomycin	
AMINOGLYCOSIDES	HEAVY METALS AND IONS
Gentamicin	Arsenic
Kanamycin	Bismuth
Neomycin	Copper sulfate
Netilmicin sulfate	Gold salts
Tobramycin	Lead
ANTINEOPLASTICS	Mercuric chloride
Cisplatin	Mercury
Cyclophosphamide	Uranium
Methotrexate	
OTHER DRUGS	
Acetaminophen	
Captopril	
Fluorinated anesthetics	
Indomethacin	
Lithium	
Mercurial diuretics	
Penicillamine	
Phenacetin	
Phenazopyridine hydrochloride	
Quinine	

From Ignatavicius D, Bayne M. Medical-surgical nursing. Philadelphia: WB Saunders, 1991, p 1919.

Table 26–4. EFFECTS OF ACUTE RENAL FAILURE

Fluid and electrolyte imbalances	Gastrointestinal disorders
Fluid excess or deficit	Anorexia
Hyperkalemia	Nausea and vomiting
Hyponatremia	Diarrhea
Hypocalcemia	Constipation
Hypermagnesemia	Uremic encephalopathy
Acidosis	Apathy
Increased susceptibility to secondary infections	Defective recent memory
	Episodic obtundation
Anemia	Tremors
Platelet dysfunction	Convulsions
	Coma

Data from Luckmann J, Sorensen K. Medical-surgical nursing. 3rd ed. Philadelphia: WB Saunders, 1987, p 1221.

Fluid overload is exhibited by edema and hypertension when the intake of fluids exceeds the urinary output and insensible losses. When the overload becomes severe, the signs and symptoms of congestive heart failure and pulmonary edema are present.

Retention of electrolytes and metabolic wastes (such as urea and creatinine) produce a group of symptoms known as uremia. These include nausea, vomiting, drowsiness, fatigue, and shortness of breath. Confusion, convulsions, coma, or gastrointestinal bleeding may also be present.

Pericarditis may develop as a result of irritation of the pericardium by the buildup of metabolic wastes. This may be exhibited by fever, development of cardiac friction rub, and pleuritic pain. Cardiac tamponade may develop. This is the accumulation of fluid in the pericardial sac (see Chapter 18). If tamponade has developed, pulsus paradoxus may be present.

The course of renal failure is usually characterized by several phases. The onset phase is the period from the precipitating event to the onset of symptoms. The oliguric phase occurs from the onset of symptoms, lasting as long as 8 weeks. The longer this phase lasts, the worse the prognosis. The patient is acutely ill during this time. The diuretic phase is marked by a leveling of blood urea nitrogen (BUN) levels and a return to glomerular filtration. The urine output may be greater than 2000 ml/day, and dehydration can occur. The final phase is that of recovery. This phase lasts 3 to 12 months.

MEDICAL DIAGNOSIS

Medical diagnosis is made on the basis of symptoms and findings from blood chemistries. These include decreased or absent urinary output; increased levels of serum BUN, creatinine, sodium, potassium, and chloride; and a decrease in serum calcium, carbon dioxide (bicarbonate), hemoglobin, and hematocrit levels.

MEDICAL MANAGEMENT

Medical interventions during the oliguric phase are designed to prevent hyperkalemia, severe acidosis, severe fluid overload and pulmonary edema, infection, convulsions, and pericarditis, which may become life-threatening. Drugs used to treat renal failure are described in Table 26–5. When administering any drugs, drug metabolism must be considered, because of the altered metabolism seen with renal failure. Fluid replacement must be done carefully because fluid overload can easily occur. The amount of fluid given is usually based upon the previous days' output plus an amount to account for the body's insensible loss (400–500 ml). The physician determines this amount. Central venous pressure (CVP) monitoring or pulmonary artery monitoring is used to evaluate hemodynamic status.

Dialysis is used to control the buildup of electrolytes, metabolic wastes, and fluids. Hemodialysis is often the preferred method of dialysis in acute renal failure.

Dietary restrictions of protein and potassium are enforced to help reduce the accumulation of electrolytes and metabolic wastes. Fluid and sodium are restricted during the oliguric phase to decrease fluid overload (Nutrition Box 26–1).

During the diuretic phase of acute renal failure, interventions are designed to maintain fluid and electrolyte balance. Interventions vary depending on the excretion of metabolic wastes and electrolytes.

Complete recovery of renal function is slow and requires from several days to months. Return of the renal function to normal or near normal levels is evidenced when the kidney can both conserve and dilute urine and when the serum electrolyte and nonprotein nitrogen levels become normal.

Application of the Nursing Process to the Care of the Patient with Acute Renal Failure

Assessment

When acute renal failure has been diagnosed, assess for the following subjective data: voiding patterns, weight gain, nausea, family history of renal disease, recent history of flulike symptoms, and any medications taken recently. Obtain the objective data: amount of urine excreted in 24 hours, blood pressure (including postural changes), daily weights, fluid status, peripheral edema, assessment of breath sounds, skin turgor, changes in mental status, and changes in pulse rate and rhythm.

These patients excrete less urine or no urine. The patients may tell you that they have not voided all day. Weight gain is indicative of fluid retention and is noted especially in the oliguric phase. Assess for nausea, often one of the first signs exhibited with retention of metabolic wastes. Assess the family history and check for flulike symptoms, which may give an indication as to the cause of acute renal failure. Ask about the medication history because it may also be helpful in identifying nephrotoxic substances that have been ingested (see Table 26–3).

During the oliguric phase, the 24-hour urine output is diminished or absent. During the diuretic phase, output may be greatly increased. Daily weights may increase rapidly during the oliguric phase and decrease during the diuretic phase. Edema, decreased or wet breath sounds, and skin turgor all are signs of fluid status. Observe for changes in mentation, which are symptoms of uremia and electrolyte imbalances. Changes in cardiac rate and rhythm may be indicative of hyperkalemia or hypokalemia. Electrolyte values and arterial blood gases (ABGs) must be monitored closely (Table 26–6).

Assess the patient's knowledge level regarding renal failure and the prescribed treatment. Find out whether the patient and family understand the effects of the disease and the treatments used. Assess the patient's and family's coping mechanisms. Identify any support systems.

Nursing Diagnoses and Planning

Nursing diagnoses and related expected patient outcomes most commonly applicable to patients with acute renal failure include the following:

NDx: Fluid volume excess related to malfunctioning kidneys

Planning: Patient outcomes
1. Patient exhibits decreased peripheral, facial, and sacral edema.
2. Patient exhibits systemic signs of fluid overload.
3. Patient relates causative factors and treatments to alleviate overload.
4. Patient has a balanced fluid intake and output.
5. Patient's electrolyte levels are within safe limits.

NDx: Altered nutrition: less than body requirements related to renal failure and dietary restrictions

Planning: Patient outcomes
1. Patient's weight is within accepted range.
2. Patient verbalizes need for dietary changes.
3. Patient follows prescribed diet.
4. Patient eats 75% of meals.

Table 26–5. DRUGS USED IN THE TREATMENT OF RENAL FAILURE

DRUG	INDICATIONS	INTERVENTIONS	RATIONALES
CARDIOTONICS			
Digoxin Digitoxin	Decreased stroke volume Decreased strength of cardiac contractions	1. Monitor for signs of digoxin toxicity and hypokalemia.	1. Digoxin remains in the body longer when renal function is impaired.
		2. Monitor for bradycardia (pulse < 60 beats per minute).	2. This is a symptom of digoxin toxicity.
		3. Give after dialysis.	3. Effective levels of digoxin are reduced during dialysis.
VITAMINS AND MINERALS			
Folic acid	Dietary supplement	1. Usually give after dialysis.	1. Water-soluble vitamins are removed during dialysis.
Ferrous sulfate	Anemia	1. Monitor for constipation.	1. This is a frequent and uncomfortable side effect associated with oral iron supplements.
		2. Note change in stools, which normally become blackish green.	2. Color is caused by the presence of unabsorbed iron and is harmless.
Calcium gluconate	Dietary supplement	1. Give only when serum phosphorus levels are normal.	1. Calcium supplements may cause a *decrease* in the serum phosphorus levels because these two minerals exist in the blood in a balanced *reciprocal* relationship.
PHOSPHATE BINDERS			
Aluminum hydroxide gel (Amphojel, ALternaGEL, Alu-Cap) Aluminum carbonate gel (Basaljel)	Phosphate binder; prevention of renal osteodystrophy	1. Monitor for constipation, which occurs frequently.	1. This is a frequent side effect of many drugs that bind phosphorus.
		2. Monitor for signs of hypophosphatemia.	2. Drugs can prevent intestinal absorption of phosphorus to the extent that the client develops hypophosphatemia.
STOOL SOFTENERS AND LAXATIVES			
Docusate sodium (Colace) Bisacodyl (Dulcolax)	Prevention of constipation caused by limited fluid intake, iron supplements, and phosphate binders	1. Observe for abdominal cramps and diarrhea.	1. These indicate drug overdose.
ANTIHYPERTENSIVES			
Hydralazine hydrochloride (Apresoline) Methyldopa (Aldomet) Metroprolol tartrate (Lopressor) Prazosin (Minipress) Propranolol (Inderal) Clonidine hydrochloride (Catapres)	Hypertension	1. Monitor for hypotension.	1. These drugs decrease peripheral resistance and lower the diastolic and mean arterial blood pressures, which could cause the client to experience hypotension.
		2. Avoid giving before dialysis.	2. Blood pressure drops during and immediately after dialysis. If these agents are given just before dialysis, the client is at greater risk for hypotension.

(*continued*)

NDx: Hopelessness related to discomfort secondary to uremia

Planning: Patient outcomes

1. Patient verbalizes relief of discomforts related to uremia (i.e., pruritus, nausea and vomiting, and paresthesia).
2. Patient exhibits relaxed facial expression and body positioning (see Nursing Care Guide 26–1).

Nursing Interventions

NDx: Fluid volume excess

Assess and report signs and symptoms of fluid volume excess, which include significant weight gain, increased blood pressure and pulse, change in mental status, dyspnea, orthopnea, crackles in the lungs, edema, distended neck veins, and elevated CVP. Monitor chest x-ray results. Monitor fluid intake and

Table 26–5. *(continued)* DRUGS USED IN THE TREATMENT OF RENAL FAILURE

DRUG	INDICATIONS	INTERVENTIONS	RATIONALES
DIURETICS			
Osmotic Diuretics (act on proximal convoluted tubule)			
Mannitol Urea	Causes rapid diuresis (e.g., after contrast medium infusion)	1. Measure fluid intake and output.	1. Severe dehydration is possible.
Thiazide and Thiazide-like Diuretics (act on cortical diluting site of ascending limb of loop of Henle)			
Chlorothiazide (Diuril) Hydrochlorothiazide (HydroDIURIL) Chlorthalidone (Hygroton) Metolazone (Zaroxolyn)	Hypertension Congestive heart failure with edema	1. Observe for signs and symptoms of electrolyte imbalance.	1. Common complications of this therapy include hypokalemia and hypercalcemia.
Loop Diuretics (act on ascending limb of loop of Henle)			
Furosemide (Lasix) Bumetanide (Bumex) Ethacrynic acid (Edecrin)	Hypertension Congestive heart failure Edema (when creatinine clearance is <25–50 ml/min)	1. Observe for orthostatic hypotension. 2. Monitor for possible hyponatremia and hypokalemia.	1. Rapid fluid volume depletion may occur. 2. These agents increase excretion of both sodium and potassium.
Potassium-Sparing Diuretics (act on distal convoluted tubule)			
Spironolactone (Aldactone) Triamterene (Dyazide)	Primary aldosteronism Hypertension (with other drugs to decrease potassium loss)	1. Observe for signs and symptoms of electrolyte imbalance.	1. Hyperkalemia with cardiac manifestations is a common complication of this drug therapy.
ANTIANEMICS			
Epoetin alfa (Epogen)	Reverse anemia of chronic renal failure	1. Observe for limb tenderness or pain after injection. 2. Observe for chills and sweats.	1. Common side effect. 2. Noted side effects.

From Ignatavicius D, Bayne M. Medical-surgical nursing. Philadelphia: WB Saunders, 1991, pp 1899–1900.

Nutrition Box 26–1.

DIETARY RESTRICTIONS FOR PATIENTS WITH RENAL FAILURE

Dietary Component	Chronic Uremia	Renal Failure	Peritoneal Dialysis
Protein	0.55–0.60 g/kg of body weight per day	1.0–1.3 g/kg of body weight per day	0.8–1.5 g/kg of body weight per day
Fluid	1500–3000 ml/day	700 ml/day plus amount of urinary output	Restriction based on fluid weight gain and blood pressure
Potassium	70 mEq/day	70 mEq/day	Usually no restriction
Sodium	1–3 g/day	1–2 g/day	Restriction based on fluid weight and blood pressure
Phosphorus	700 mg/day	700 mg/day	800 mg/day

From Ignatavicius D, Bayne M. Medical-surgical nursing. Philadelphia: WB Saunders, 1991, p 1915.

Table 26–6. ELECTROLYTE AND ACID-BASE IMBALANCES AND TREATMENT IN RENAL FAILURE

MANIFESTATIONS OF ELECTROLYTE IMBALANCE

ELECTROLYTE IMBALANCE	MANIFESTATIONS
Hyponatremia (decreased sodium)	Headache, muscle weakness, fatigue, apathy, confusion, coma, postural hypotension, anorexia, nausea, vomiting, abdominal cramping, weight loss
Hypernatremia (increased sodium)	Dry mucous membranes, decreased urinary output, rubbery skin turgor, excitement, tachycardia
Hypokalemia (decreased potassium)	Anorexia, nausea, vomiting, abdominal distention, lethargy, confusion, mental depression, weakness, decreased standing blood pressure, arrhythmias, electrocardiographic changes, thirst, increased urine output
Hyperkalemia (increased potassium)	Nausea, vomiting, diarrhea, irritability, weakness, oliguria, arrhythmias, electrocardiographic changes, sudden death, numbness, tingling
Hypocalcemia (decreased calcium)	Osteoporosis, fractures, tingling, convulsions, muscle spasms, tetany, calcium deposits in tissue, nausea, vomiting, diarrhea, arrhythmias
Hypercalcemia (increased calcium)	Renal calculi, coma, decreased reflexes, lethargy, arrhythmias, muscle fatigue, bone pain, osteoporosis, fractures
Acidosis (decreased bicarbonate)	Headache, malaise, rapid deep respirations, disorientation, stupor, coma, hyperkalemia

ELECTROLYTE IMBALANCES AND TREATMENT GOALS

ELECTROLYTE	NORMAL VALUE	CHANGE IN RENAL FAILURE	GOAL OF TREATMENT
Sodium (Na)	135–145 mEq/L	Increase or decrease	125–145 mEq/L
Potassium (K)	3.5–5 mEq/L	Increase	3–6 mEq/L
CO_2 (bicarbonate)	22–30 mEq/L	Decrease	>15 mEq/L
Calcium (Ca)	9–11 mg/dl	Decrease	9–11 mg/dl
Phosphate (PO_4)	2.5–4.8 mg/dl	Increase	3–5 mg/dl
Albumin	4–4.5 g/dl	Decrease	>3.5 g/dl
Urea nitrogen (BUN)	10–20 mg/dl	Increase	<100 mg/dl
Creatinine	0.6–1.7 mg/dl	Increase	<15 mg/dl
Uric acid	2.2–8 mg/dl	Increase	<12 mg/dl

output. Maintain fluid restrictions as ordered. Restrict sodium intake as ordered. Monitor and document the therapeutic effect and side effects of prescribed medications. Weigh the patient at the same time each day. Alert the physician if signs and symptoms persist or worsen. Prepare the patient and family for dialysis if needed.

NDx: Altered nutrition: less than body requirements

Weigh the patient daily. Assess nutritional status on a regular basis, and document the patient's food intake. Monitor intake and output. Assess the patient for any problems that could be associated with poor intake. These include anorexia, nausea, vomiting, fatigue, and mouth discomfort.

Administer antiemetics as ordered. Encourage the patient to take slow, deep breaths if nauseated. Provide oral hygiene frequently. Provide small, frequent meals. Ensure that the environment is clean, relaxed, and pleasant. Provide a rest period before meals to minimize fatigue.

Obtain a dietary consultation if needed. Encourage the patient and family to discuss needs with the dietitian. Encourage the family to bring in favorite foods that meet dietary requirements.

NDx: Hopelessness

Assess for nonverbal signs of discomfort. Assess for complaints of nausea, vomiting, pruritus, muscle cramps, or paresthesia. Assist patient with position changes as needed. Teach relaxation techniques. Administer medications as ordered. More specific interventions for relieving discomforts can be found in Nursing Care Guide 26–1.

Patient education is essential in the strict regimen and restrictions that must be employed. Education along with other psychosocial support mechanisms may also help decrease anxiety. Compliance with the medical regimen is essential; therefore, measures must be instituted to aid in compliance.

Evaluation

Evaluate the effectiveness of nursing care for a patient with acute renal failure by comparing the patient's status with the expected patient outcomes. Examples of specific outcomes for patients with acute renal failure have been provided in the Planning section.

Chronic Renal Failure

ETIOLOGY AND PATHOPHYSIOLOGY

Chronic renal failure (CRF) is irreversible. It is characterized by progressive reduction of nephrons until the remaining nephrons can no longer maintain the body's internal environment. Owing to the wide variety of causes of CRF, the early stages of the disease vary. The end result for the person with renal failure is either uremia and death, or treatment by dialysis or transplant.

The causes of CRF are numerous; including chronic glomerulonephritis, acute renal failure, polycystic kidney disease, obstruction, repeated pyelonephritis, and nephrotoxins. Systemic diseases such as diabetes mellitus, hypertension, lupus erythematosus, polyarteritis, sickle cell disease, and amyloid disease may also lead to renal failure.

The specific pathophysiologic mechanisms of renal failure are dependent on the underlying disease process. As nephrons are destroyed, the total glomerular filtration rate falls and clearance is reduced. BUN and creatinine levels rise. It is believed that remaining nephrons hypertrophy as a result of increased workload. The glomerular filtration rate remains effective until 70% to 80% of renal function is lost.

Early in the disease the kidneys can maintain excretion of solutes or waste products by decreasing water reabsorption. The ability to concentrate urine is lost, and urinary output increases. These are early signs of CRF and can cause severe dehydration. As renal failure progresses, serum BUN level rises and urinary output decreases.

The course of CRF begins with the stage of diminished renal reserve. Kidney function decreases, but no wastes are accumulated. The second stage is renal insufficiency. The remaining healthy kidney tissue can no longer compensate. Glomerular filtration rate falls, and metabolic wastes begin to accumulate. The final stage is end-stage renal disease. Serum BUN and creatinine levels rise excessively. Homeostasis cannot be maintained, and without dialysis, death will occur.

CLINICAL MANIFESTATIONS

The course of chronic renal failure is highly individualized; however, there are common features of the disease process (Table 26–7). The manifestations seen are those related to (1) imbalance of fluids and electrolytes, (2) alterations of the body's regulatory mechanisms, and (3) retention of metabolic wastes. Uremia, anemia, and acidosis are always present. Fluid and sodium are either abnormally retained or excreted; thus, urinary volume may be increased, normal, or decreased.

Hypertension is very common in CRF but not always present. The most common cause of a higher blood pressure is an increase in total body water and sodium.

No body system remains unaffected by renal failure. The cardiovascular changes exhibited are fluid overload, hypertension, tachycardia, arrhythmias, congestive heart failure, or pericarditis. These changes are related to the increased fluid volume, buildup of metabolic wastes, changes in the renin-angiotensin mechanism, and chronic hypertension.

Effects on the gastrointestinal system are anorexia, nausea and vomiting, gastrointestinal bleeding, abnormal distention, diarrhea, constipation, or halitosis. These changes are related to buildup of uremic toxins, electrolyte imbalances, changes in platelet activity, and the conversion of urea to ammonia by saliva.

The patient may exhibit lethargy, confusion, convulsions, stupor, coma, sleep and behavioral disturbances, or muscle irritability. Neurologic symptoms are related in part to uremic toxins, electrolyte imbalances, or cerebral swelling caused by fluid shifts.

Osteoporosis, renal rickets, and joint pain are manifestations in the skeletal system of decreased calcium absorption and decreased phosphate excretion. Integumentary changes include pallor, itching, bruising, or uremic frost as a result of anemia, decreased activity of sweat and oil glands, dry skin, and phosphate deposits in the skin.

Genitourinary manifestations are decreased urine output, decreased specific gravity of the urine, protein in the urine, casts and cells in the urine, or decreased sodium in the urine. These are all caused by the damage to the nephron.

Other clinical manifestations are anemia, leukocytosis, and defects in platelet function and number. The manifestations are related to suppression of red blood cell production caused by decreased production of erythropoietin, decreased red cell survival time, loss of blood through bleeding and dialysis, and decreased activity of platelets.

Table 26–7. CLINICAL MANIFESTATIONS OF RENAL FAILURE

Cardiovascular	Hypervolemia, hypertension, tachycardia, arrhythmias, congestive heart failure, pericarditis
Hematologic	Anemia, leukocytosis, decreased platelet function, thrombocytopenia
Gastrointestinal	Anorexia, nausea, vomiting, abdominal distention, diarrhea, constipation, bleeding
Neurologic	Lethargy, confusion, convulsions, stupor, coma, sleep disturbances, behavioral disturbances, muscle irritability
Dermatologic	Pallor, pigmentation, pruritus, ecchymosis, excoriation, uremic frost
Urinary	Decreased urine output, decreased specific gravity, proteinuria, casts and cells in the urine

MEDICAL DIAGNOSIS

Diagnosis of renal failure is made on the basis of the history, symptomatology, and laboratory studies. The most definitive of these are serum creatinine and creatinine clearance. A rise in serum creatinine level and a fall in creatinine clearance are indicative of renal failure.

MEDICAL MANAGEMENT

The focus of conservative management is regulation of fluids, electrolytes, and metabolic wastes through dietary and volume controls along with medication, treatment of concurrent disorders, and patient comfort. Treatment goals are as follows:

1. Stabilization of internal environment
2. Control of fluid and electrolyte imbalances
3. Absence of infection
4. Absence of bleeding
5. Control of blood pressure
6. Control of concurrent illness
7. Absence of toxicity of medications that are inadequately excreted
8. Sufficient nutrient intake to maintain positive nitrogen balance
9. Control of anorexia and nausea
10. Control of itching (pruritus)

Fluid and sodium excretion vary significantly from patient to patient. Most patients have a tendency toward hypervolemia because of the inability to excrete sodium and water. Other patients are unable to conserve sodium and water because of an inability to concentrate the urine and therefore tend to be hypovolemic. The desired effect is to maintain the person in a normotensive, normovolemic state.

Virtually every electrolyte and mineral is affected in renal failure. The goal of treatment here is to maintain electrolyte levels within an acceptable limit (see Table 26–6). Control of electrolytes is accomplished through dietary restriction or medication, or both. Because of the chronic nature of the disease, these patients may be able to tolerate electrolyte imbalance without the symptoms seen in patients without renal disease.

Dietary restrictions can significantly reduce metabolic wastes. Protein restrictions may range from 20 to 80 g/day. The restriction is dependent on the ability of the person to excrete wastes from the body. The quality of protein allowed must be high in order to maintain positive nitrogen balance, thus decreasing urea production from muscle wasting. Calories for energy needs are supplied by carbohydrates and fats (see Nutrition Box 26–1).

Anemia is present in all renal failure patients owing to multiple causes. Anemia may be treated with iron supplements and folic acid supplementation. The drug epoetin alfa (Epogen) has greatly reduced the problem of anemia. Transfusions are used in cases of severe anemia when the patient is symptomatic.

Gastrointestinal symptoms of these patients range from nausea to gastrointestinal bleeding. Treatment of these manifestations includes administration of antacids and antiemetics, dietary control of nitrogenous wastes, and maintenance of fluid and electrolyte balances.

Hypertension is treated vigorously in this population. A stepwise approach to treatment may be instituted as follows: (1) sodium and fluid restriction, (2) diuretic therapy, (3) beta blockers, and (4) vasodilators.

Sources of infection, such as an indwelling catheter, are avoided. When infection occurs, immediate action is taken to treat the infection.

Patient comfort is promoted. These patients are prone to muscle cramping, pruritus, headaches, ocular irritation, insomnia, and fatigue. Muscle cramping is often associated with sodium depletion. Measures instituted to control the cramping include local heat and massage. Primary treatment is control of the electrolyte imbalance. Pruritus is described as a sensation of deep itching that may be related to the uremic frost or associated with phosphate deposits in the skin. Treatment for pruritus is aimed at decreasing the phosphorus with administration of phosphate binders such as Basaljel. Local and systemic agents may be administered to decrease the itching. Ocular irritation is exhibited by burning and watery eyes, thought to be caused by calcium deposits in the conjunctiva. Treatment is aimed at decreasing the plasma phosphate levels; "artificial tears" may be utilized for local comfort. Insomnia and fatigue are related to uremia and possibly psychosocial disturbances. Treatment is designed to decrease metabolic waste buildup and psychosocial support. If necessary, medications are used with caution for sleep. Changes in drug metabolism related to decreased renal function must be considered when administering all medications.

Application of the Nursing Process to the Care of the Patient with Chronic Renal Failure

The assessment, nursing diagnoses expected patient outcomes, nursing interventions, and evaluation for patients with CRF can be found in Nursing Care Guide 26–1.

Text continued on page 1104

Nursing Care Guide 26–1.

PATIENTS WITH CHRONIC RENAL FAILURE

Assessment Findings: Patient experiences weight gain, hypertension, tachycardia, dyspnea, crackles in lungs, increasing central venous pressure (CVP), and decreased mentation.

Nursing Diagnosis: Fluid volume excess related to retention of sodium and water secondary to decreased number of functioning nephrons and decreased glomerular filtration

Patient Outcomes	Nursing Interventions	Rationale
Patient's vital signs are within normal limits, chest is clear, no shortness of breath is apparent, and CVP is appropriate.	Maintain fluid restrictions as ordered. Restrict sodium intake.	Restricting fluids and sodium decreases the workload on the kidneys.
	Monitor vital signs and CVP frequently. Auscultate chest sounds.	Assessment of vital signs allows for early intervention if problems occur.
	Elevate the head of the bed and administer oxygen if needed.	This allows for easier respiratory effort.
Patient presents a decrease in peripheral edema.	Assess signs of edema in extremities. Check for pitting. Look for signs of compromised circulation.	Decreased edema in the periphery indicates a reduction in the fluid volume excess.

Evaluation: Compare the patient's status with the expected patient outcomes. If the outcomes are achieved, evaluate nursing care as successful. If not, reassess the patient, formulate new nursing diagnoses, and revise expected patient outcomes and nursing interventions as appropriate.

Assessment Findings: Patient experiences muscle cramps, numbness, burning, tingling, and restless leg syndrome (crawling, itching sensation).

Nursing Diagnosis: Pain related to peripheral neuropathies associated with electrolyte imbalances and nitrogenous waste accumulation

Patient Outcomes	Nursing Interventions	Rationale
Patient denies muscle cramps and paresthesia.	Observe the patient's reaction to discomfort. Explain the cause of the problems.	Understanding the cause of the discomfort may help the patient accept the problem.
	Provide a footboard, and instruct the patient to push feet against the board. Instruct patient to move legs while lying in bed. Keep linens off extremities.	Exercising while in bed helps relieve some of the symptoms of restless leg syndrome.
	Apply cool packs if ordered for comfort. Administer pharmacologic agents as ordered for discomfort.	Cool packs are soothing.

(continued)

Nursing Care Guide 26–1. *(continued)*
PATIENTS WITH CHRONIC RENAL FAILURE

Patient Outcomes	Nursing Interventions	Rationale
Patient completes activities of daily living without complaints of discomfort.	Assist the patient in completing daily self-care activities as needed. Explain alternative methods for performing tasks, and encourage the patient to do as much as possible.	Helping the patient complete tasks of self-care and encouraging self-participation promotes independence in the patient and prepares the patient for discharge.
	Teach the patient exercises and relaxation techniques.	Exercises and relaxation techniques may help relieve symptoms of the syndrome.

Evaluation: Compare the patient's status with the expected patient outcomes. If the outcomes are achieved, evaluate nursing care as successful. If not, reassess the patient, formulate new nursing diagnoses, and revise expected patient outcomes and nursing interventions as appropriate.

Assessment Findings: Patient scratches and rubs skin continually. Patient complains of severe itching.

Nursing Diagnosis: Impaired skin integrity related to atrophy of sweat glands, accumulation of urate crystals and calcium phosphate crystals on the skin

Patient Outcomes	Nursing Interventions	Rationale
Patient refrains from scratching and rubbing skin.	Assess for pruritus. Tell patient about the effects of continued scratching of the skin.	Assessment of symptoms of pruritus provides for early interventions.
	Apply cool moist packs. Use lotion on the skin as needed.	Cool packs are soothing to the skin. Lotion prevents dryness.
	Discourage frequent bathing. Use mild soaps and tepid water for bathing. Dry skin completely.	Frequent bathing is drying to the skin. Mild soap and water is less irritating.
	Provide diversional activities for the patient.	This takes the patient's mind off the constant feelings of skin irritation.
Patient denies pruritus and presents no evidence of skin irritation.	Monitor the patient for signs of skin breakdown. Look for scratches, signs of infection, reddened areas, and extreme dryness.	Assessing for pruritus and problems associated with it allows for early intervention to prevent skin breakdown.

Evaluation: Compare the patient's status with the expected patient outcomes. If the outcomes are achieved, evaluate nursing care as successful. If not, reassess the patient, formulate new nursing diagnoses, and revise expected patient outcomes and nursing interventions as appropriate.

(continued)

Nursing Care Guide 26–1. *(continued)*

PATIENTS WITH CHRONIC RENAL FAILURE

Assessment Findings: Patient is disoriented, experiences poor judgment and reasoning ability. Patient has short attention span, poor memory, irritability, and confusion.

Nursing Diagnosis: Altered thought processes related to accumulation of nitrogenous wastes and electrolyte imbalances

Patient Outcomes	Nursing Interventions	Rationale
Patient verbalizes orientation to time, place, and person.	Check the patient's orientation frequently. Reorient the patient to time, place, and person as needed. Explain to the patient all procedures and equipment used.	Assessing the patient's orientation provides baseline and continual data on the patient's neurologic status. This assists in orienting the patient to the present.
	Decrease external stimuli to a minimum.	Reducing stimuli prevents more confusion for the patient.
Patient presents improvement in thought processes.	Assess for alterations in thought processes. Allow time for patient to make decisions.	Presenting information slowly allows for comprehension by the patient.
	Explain the physiologic basis for the change in mentation to the patient and family.	An understanding of the basis for the disturbances may help the patient and family accept and adjust to the situation.
	Repeat instructions as needed. Assist the patient in decision-making when appropriate.	Some assistance in decision-making may be needed because of inability to process information appropriately.

Evaluation: Compare the patient's status with the expected patient outcomes. If the outcomes are achieved, evaluate nursing care as successful. If not, reassess the patient, formulate new nursing diagnoses, and revise expected patient outcomes and nursing interventions as appropriate.

(continued)

Nursing Care Guide 26–1. *(continued)*

PATIENTS WITH CHRONIC RENAL FAILURE

Assessment Findings: Patient experiences weakness, fatigue, and decreased endurance. Patient complains of inability to complete activities of daily living.

Nursing Diagnosis: Activity intolerance related to anemia and uremia

Patient Outcomes	Nursing Interventions	Rationale
Patient denies weakness and fatigue.	Assist the patient in identifying activities that result in extreme fatigue.	Restricting activities that cause extreme fatigue preserves the patient's energy.
	Provide uninterrupted rest periods throughout the day.	Frequent rest is necessary to promote increased energy levels.
	Teach the patient energy-saving techniques. Help the patient establish goals for increased endurance.	Using energy-saving techniques reduces the workload on the patient.
	Encourage good nutrition habits. Teach the patient to consume foods that are high in iron.	Good nutrition promotes increased energy.
Patient completes activities of daily living such as self-care practices without complaints of fatigue and weakness.	Assist the patient with self-care as needed. Teach family members how to assist the patient.	Assisting the patient with some activities preserves strength.
	Have the patient organize the day for maximum activity during periods of maximum strength and energy level.	Careful planning for the day may allow for maximun utilization of the patient's abilities.
	Refer the patient to an exercise therapist for assistance in developing a planned routine of daily exercise.	Prescribed exercises may increase strength and endurance.

Evaluation: Compare the patient's status with the expected patient outcomes. If the outcomes are achieved, evaluate nursing care as successful. If not, reassess the patient, formulate new nursing diagnoses, and revise expected patient outcomes and nursing interventions as appropriate.

Assessment Findings: Patient and family ask questions about the disease process and treatment regimen.

Nursing Diagnosis: Knowledge deficit: nature of disease process and the need for follow-up care and treatment

(continued)

Nursing Care Guide 26–1. *(continued)*

PATIENTS WITH CHRONIC RENAL FAILURE

Patient Outcomes	Nursing Interventions	Rationale
Patient verbalizes an understanding of the disease process, the dietary restrictions, and measures to control problems associated with the disease.	Instruct the patient about the disease process, the dietary implications, and the methods for control of complications associated with the disease. Reinforce fluid and dietary restrictions as described in Nutrition Box 26–1.	Understanding the disease may promote compliance with the treatment regimen.
	Provide the patient with written instructions and information. Include the patient's family in the education sessions when appropriate.	Written instructions reinforce the verbal information. Including the family provides additional support for the patient.
	Have the patient repeat the information, and correct any misunderstandings. Allow the patient and family to ask questions.	Reiteration of the information allows for correction of misinformation.
Patient demonstrates an ability to weigh self and to monitor fluid intake and output appropriately.	Teach the patient how to monitor weight and fluid intake and output. Tell the patient to record the results and to present the information to the physician at the follow-up visit.	Recording of the weight and fluid intake and output provides the physician with data about the patient's progress and renal status after discharge.
Patient identifies signs and symptoms that are to be reported to the physician, and verbalizes the need for follow up care and compliance with treatment plan.	Explain to the patient the signs and symptoms of potential problems that should be reported to the physician, such as weight gain greater than 1 lb/day, uncontrolled nausea and vomiting, increased weakness or confusion, abnormal bleeding, unrelieved itching, skin breakdown, shortness of breath, increased muscle crampling, tremors, or seizures.	Understanding the disease process, the complications, and when to seek assistance may prevent problems for the patient after discharge.
	Explain the importance of follow-up care and compliance with the treatment plan.	Continued medical monitoring of the patient and compliance with the treatment plan are essential to the appropriate management of the disease and prevention of complications.

Evaluation: Compare the patient's status with the expected patient outcomes. If the outcomes are achieved, evaluate nursing care as successful. If not, reassess the patient, formulate new nursing diagnoses, and revise expected patient outcomes and nursing interventions as appropriate.

Dialysis

Dialysis was first utilized in 1960 by means of an artificial kidney with chronic intermittent hemodialysis. When the irreversibility of renal damage was established, treatment was then withdrawn. This practice continues in many countries worldwide where resources are limited.

In 1972, the United States government established legislation to provide payment for the health care costs of citizens with end-stage renal disease (ESRD). Payment is provided to persons with documented ESRD through Medicare. At present, more than 80,000 people are being treated with some form of dialysis.

Dialysis occurs with the movement of fluids and particles across a semipermeable membrane. This treatment is used to restore fluid and electrolyte balance and acid-base balance and to remove wastes and toxic materials from the body. This treatment is an augmentation of renal function to sustain life in acute and chronic situations.

Dialysis is based on three principles: diffusion, osmosis, and ultrafiltration. Diffusion is the movement of particles across a semipermeable membrane from areas of a higher concentration to those of a lower concentration. Diffusion is used to clear solutes from the body in both hemodialysis and peritoneal dialysis. Osmosis is the passage of solvent (water) across a semipermeable membrane from an area of lesser solute concentration to an area of greater solute concentration. Osmosis is used to remove extra fluid, especially in peritoneal dialysis. Ultrafiltration is the movement of fluid across a semipermeable membrane as a result of an artificially created pressure gradient. Ultrafiltration is more efficient in removing fluids from the body than is osmosis. Ultrafiltration is used to remove excess fluids in hemodialysis. During dialysis diffusion, osmosis, and ultrafiltration occur simultaneously.

Dialysis of some form is implemented when the following conditions occur:

1. Unmanageable hyperkalemia
2. Intractable acidosis
3. Volume overload
4. Uremia

There are four main goals of dialysis therapy:

1. Removal of metabolic waste products
2. Maintenance of safe concentration of electrolytes
3. Correction of acid-base balance
4. Removal of excess fluids

These goals can be met through the use of hemodialysis or peritoneal dialysis. The two methods of dialysis vary significantly in procedure, benefits, time required to complete, cost, and appropriateness for the patient. Some of the similarities and differences between hemodialysis and peritoneal dialysis are described in Table 26–8.

Table 26–8. COMPARISON OF HEMODIALYSIS AND PERITONEAL DIALYSIS

HEMODIALYSIS	PERITONEAL DIALYSIS
ADVANTAGES	
More efficient clearance	Easy access; fewer hemodynamic complications
Short time needed for treatment	
COMPLICATIONS	
Disequilibrium syndrome	Protein loss
Muscle cramps	Peritonitis
Hemorrhage	Hyperglycemia
Air embolus	Respiratory distress
Hemodynamic changes (hypotension, cardiac arrhythmias, and anemia)	Bowel perforation
CONTRAINDICATIONS	
Hemodynamically unstable	Extensive peritoneal adhesions
	Peritoneal fibrosis
	Recent abdominal surgery
ACCESS	
Vascular access route	Intraabdominal catheter
PROCEDURE	
Complex	Simple
Specially trained registered nurses required	Special training not needed
NURSING IMPLICATIONS	
Vascular access care	Abdominal catheter care
Restricted diet	More flexible diet

From Ignatavicius D, Bayne M. Medical-surgical nursing. Philadelphia: WB Saunders, 1991, p 1901.

Peritoneal Dialysis

Peritoneal dialysis involves the instillation of hypertonic fluid into the peritoneal cavity, where it is allowed to remain for a prescribed period of time before it is drained. Fluids and solutes from the blood stream are transferred through the peritoneum. Solutes, which carry fluids, move from an area of higher concentration in the body to an area of lower concentration in the dialyzing fluid. It is used for both acute and chronic renal failure and can be performed in the hospital or at home (Fig. 26–2).

Peritoneal dialysis offers many advantages to the patient, including the following:

1. Maintenance of steady state of blood chemistry
2. Opportunity for patient independence in dialysis therapy
3. Simplicity of learning procedure
4. Fewer dietary restrictions
5. More control over daily life
6. Safe usage in hemodynamically unstable patients

The contraindications for peritoneal dialysis include the following:

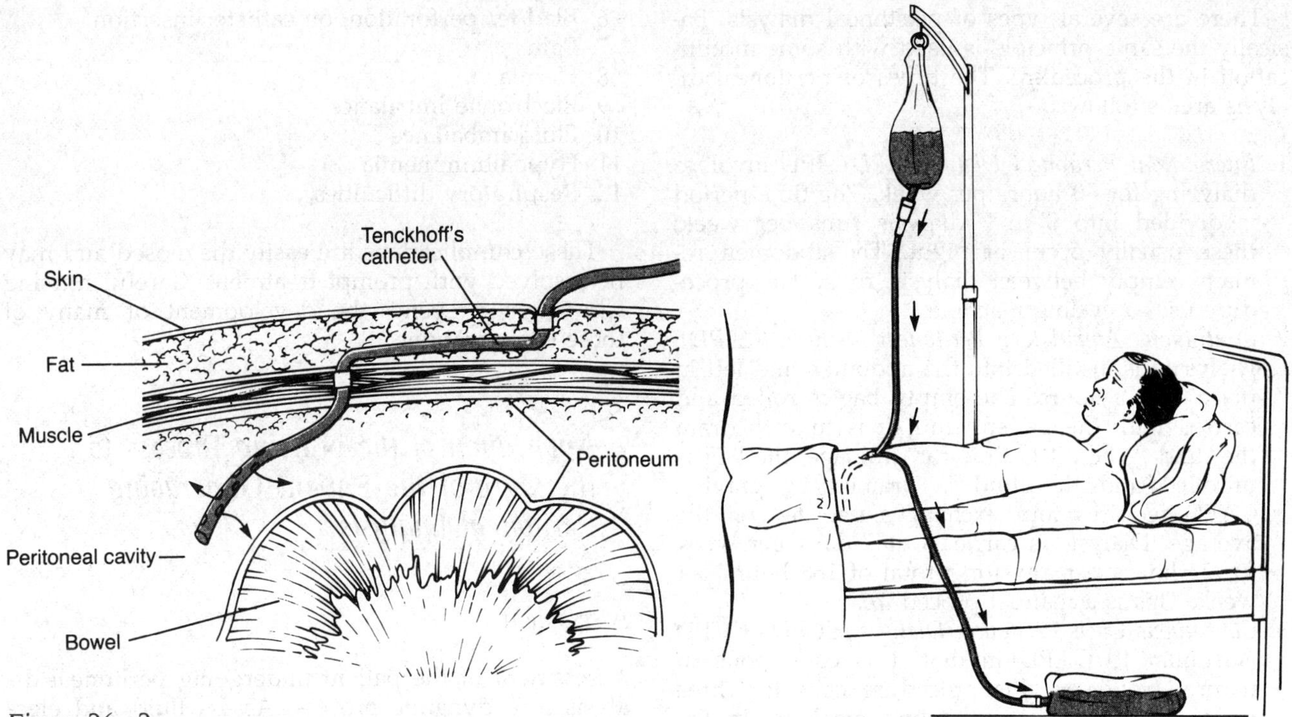

Figure 26–2.

Manual peritoneal dialysis via an implanted abdominal catheter (Tenckhoff's catheter). (From Ignatavicius D, Bayne M. Medical-surgical nursing. Philadelphia: WB Saunders, 1991, p 1909.)

1. Tight abdominal muscles
2. Diaphragmatic tears
3. Abdominal drains
4. Diffuse bowel disease
5. Respiratory insufficiency
6. Intraabdominal cancer
7. Extensive abdominal adhesions
8. Infection in the abdomen

PROCEDURE

Access to the peritoneal cavity is gained through placement of a catheter. If the catheter is to be used for an acutely ill patient, a catheter is placed for each dialysis. The physician will choose the appropriate type catheter (Fig. 26–3). For chronic use, a permanent catheter is placed.

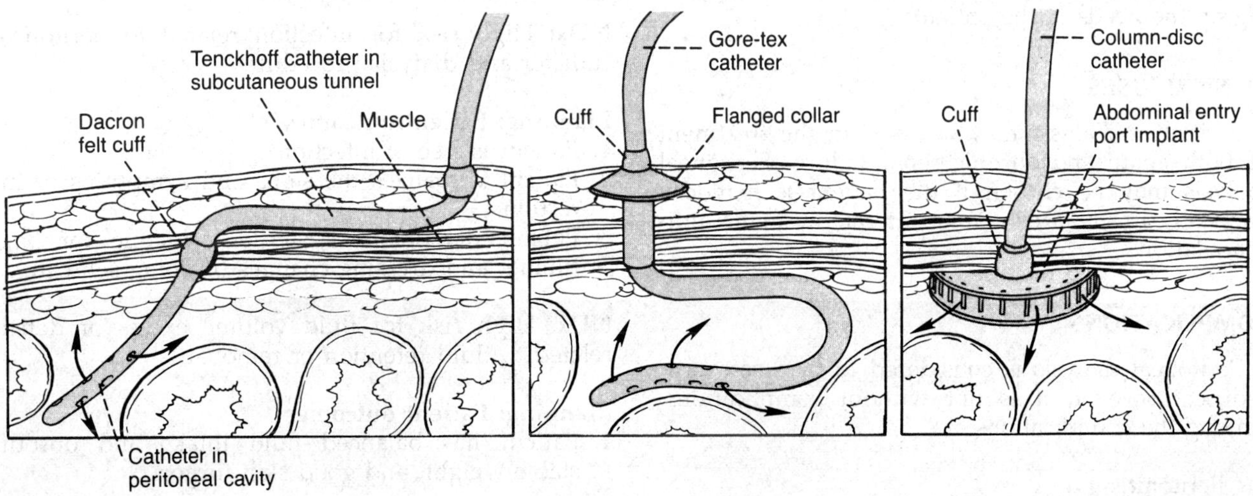

Figure 26–3.

Three types of peritoneal dialysis catheters. Tenckhoff's catheter has two Dacron felt cuffs that hold the catheter in place and prevent dialysate leakage and bacterial invasion. Subcutaneous tunnel also helps prevent infection. The Gore-Tex catheter has a Dacron cuff above a flanged collar. The column-disc catheter has a cuff and large abdominal entry port implant. (From Black JM, Matassarin-Jacobs E. Luckmann and Sorenson's Medical-surgical nursing. 4th ed. Philadelphia: WB Saunders, 1993, p 1511.)

There are several types of peritoneal dialysis. Basically the same principle is used with some modification in the procedure. The types of peritoneal dialysis are as follows:

1. *Intermittent Peritoneal Dialysis (IPD).* IPD involves dialyzing for 40 hours per week. The time period is divided into 3 to 7 dialysis runs per week; these usually occur at night. The abdomen remains empty between dialysis runs. The procedure uses a cycling machine.
2. *Continuous Ambulatory Peritoneal Dialysis (CAPD).* Dialysate is instilled into the abdomen and left in place 4 to 8 hours. The empty bag is rolled and carried with the patient until it is time to drain the fluid. When it is time for drainage, the bag is unrolled and the fluid is drained by gravity. CAPD requires four exchanges per day on the average. Dialysis is carried out 7 days per week for 24 hours per day for a total of 168 hours per week. This is a manual procedure.
3. *Continuous Cycle Peritoneal Dialysis (CCPD).* CCPD is similar to CAPD in that it is continuous in nature. However, this procedure calls for three cycles to be run via a cycling machine. In the morning, fresh dialysate is instilled into the abdomen and allowed to remain until it is drained just prior to initiation of the nightly cycles.

Commercial dialysate comes in both 1.5% and 4.26% dextrose, in 2-L bottles or bags. Usual instillation for adults is 2 L per exchange.

Peritoneal dialysis is carried out under strict sterile technique. Mask should always be worn by nurses performing peritoneal dialysis. Povidone-iodine should be used for cleansing the catheter both for connection and disconnection.

Drugs or other substances may be added to the dialysate under sterile technique. These may include potassium, antibiotics, heparin, and insulin, depending on the needs of the patient.

CLINICAL USES

Peritoneal dialysis may be used in the treatment of both acute and chronic renal failure. Peritoneal dialysis may be chosen if the patient is hemodynamically unstable or cannot tolerate systemic anticoagulation.

COMPLICATIONS

Peritoneal dialysis is considered to be a safe procedure; however, it is not without complications. Among the complications are

1. Peritonitis
2. Catheter plugging or displacement
3. Constipation
4. Fluid leakage
5. Bowel perforation, on catheter insertion
6. Bladder perforation, on catheter insertion
7. Pain
8. Hernia
9. Electrolyte imbalance
10. Fluid imbalance
11. Hypoalbuminemia
12. Respiratory difficulties

These complications are easily diagnosed and may be resolved with prompt treatment. Careful nursing care often prevents the development of many of these complications.

Application of the Nursing Process to the Care of the Patient Undergoing Peritoneal Dialysis

Assessment

Assessment of the patient undergoing peritoneal dialysis is a dynamic process. Assess fluid and electrolyte status on a continual basis. Monitor fluid intake and output. Assess blood pressure and vital signs before, during, and at the completion of dialysis. Monitor and record infusion and drainage of dialysate. Assess for signs of respiratory distress, pain, and discomfort. Assess the patency of the catheter. Assess for any signs of infection. Evaluate the patient's knowledge related to the procedure.

Nursing Diagnoses and Planning

Nursing diagnoses and related expected patient outcomes most commonly applicable to patients undergoing peritoneal dialysis include the following:*

NDx: High risk for infection related to peritoneal catheter and dialysis procedure

Planning: Patient outcomes
1. Patient is free of infection.
2. Patient verbalizes the signs and symptoms of infection.
3. Patient demonstrates sterile technique for bag, tubing, and dressing changes (if doing self-care).

NDx: High risk for fluid volume excess or deficit related to fluid retention or removal

Planning: Patient outcomes
1. Patient has balanced fluid intake and output, stable weight, and good skin turgor.

* Other nursing diagnoses that apply to both peritoneal dialysis and hemodialysis are covered in the section on hemodialysis.

2. Patient's vital signs and CVP are within normal limits.
3. Patient's dialysate outflow is greater than or equal to inflow.

NDx: Altered nutrition: less than body requirements related to protein loss in dialysate

Planning: Patient outcomes
1. Patient has stable weight.
2. Patient has adequate protein intake (1.2–1.5 g/kg body weight/day) and a normal serum albumin level (3.5–5.5 g/dl).

Nursing Interventions

NDx: High risk for infection
Observe for and report signs and symptoms of peritonitis. These include fever, abdominal pain, cloudy outflow, nausea, and malaise. Maintain sterile technique when changing dialysate bags, connecting and disconnecting the catheter, and performing catheter care (Table 26–9). Maintain sterility of dialysate.

Assess the catheter site for redness, drainage, tenderness, or foul odor. If exudate is present, it should be cultured. Observe for leakage at the site. Continuous leakage can lead to peritonitis.

Instruct the patient in the procedure and the needed care to maintain dialysis at home if needed. Allow patient and family to ask questions.

NDx: High risk for fluid volume excess or deficit
Observe for and report signs and symptoms of fluid overload. These include hypertension, tachycardia, dyspnea, crackles in lungs, distended neck veins, and increased CVP. Record accurately the measurement of inflow and outflow.

Observe for and report signs of outflow problems. Outflow problems may include catheter obstruction by omentum, catheter occlusion by fibrin, and a full colon. For a full colon, administer stool softeners and provide a high-fiber diet. Enemas can be used if necessary. If the catheter is occluded by fibrin, obtain an order to irrigate with heparinized saline. If the omentum obstructs the catheter, turn the patient from side to side, elevate the head of the bed, or apply firm pressure to the abdomen. Notify the physician if outflow problems continue.

Monitor intake and output. Weigh the patient daily. Raise the head of the bed, and drain the dialysate; notify the physician if respiratory distress occurs.

Assess for signs and symptoms of fluid deficit. These include hypertension, tachycardia, decreased CVP, and poor skin turgor.

NDx: Altered nutrition: less than body requirements
Monitor intake and output. Weigh the patient daily. Provide adequate dietary protein. Consult with dietitian as necessary. Instruct patient in proper diet. Provide a list of restricted and encouraged food with menus. Assist the patient in developing a plan for meals prior to discharge. Allow the patient and family to ask questions.

Evaluation

Evaluate the effectiveness of nursing care for a patient undergoing peritoneal dialysis by comparing the patient's status with the expected patient out-

Table 26–9. NURSING CARE GUIDELINES FOR PERITONEAL DIALYSIS CATHETER CARE

INTERVENTIONS	RATIONALES
1. Mask yourself and your client. Wash your hands.	1. This decreases the risk of airborne contamination and prevents cross contamination.
2. Put on sterile gloves. Remove the old dressing. Remove the contaminated gloves.	2. The dressings should be changed daily and whenever it becomes soiled to prevent infection. Gloves should be worn while removing contaminated dressings to avoid cross contamination.
3. Assess area for signs of infection, such as swelling, redness, or discharge around the catheter site.	3. Early recognition of infection facilitates treatment by antibiotics and limits systemic involvement.
4. Use aseptic technique.	4. Peritonitis is a constant threat to anyone receiving peritoneal dialysis. The best protection is strict aseptic technique.
a. Open the sterile field on a flat surface and place two precut 4 × 4 inch gauze pads on the field.	a. Movement of microorganisms into insertion site is inhibited.
b. Place three cotton swabs soaked in povidone-iodine on the field. Put on sterile gloves.	b. Povidone-iodine solution provides an antiseptic barrier against bacteria.
5. Use cotton swabs to clean around the catheter site. Use a circular motion starting from the insertion site and moving away toward the abdomen. Repeat with all three swabs.	5. Aseptic technique is maintained by avoiding contamination of the already cleaned area nearest the catheter.
6. Apply precut gauze pads over the catheter site. Tape only the edges of the gauze pads.	6. This method prevents infection while allowing the skin around the catheter to breathe.

From Ignatavicius D, Bayne M. Medical-surgical nursing. Philadelphia: WB Saunders, 1991, p 1910.

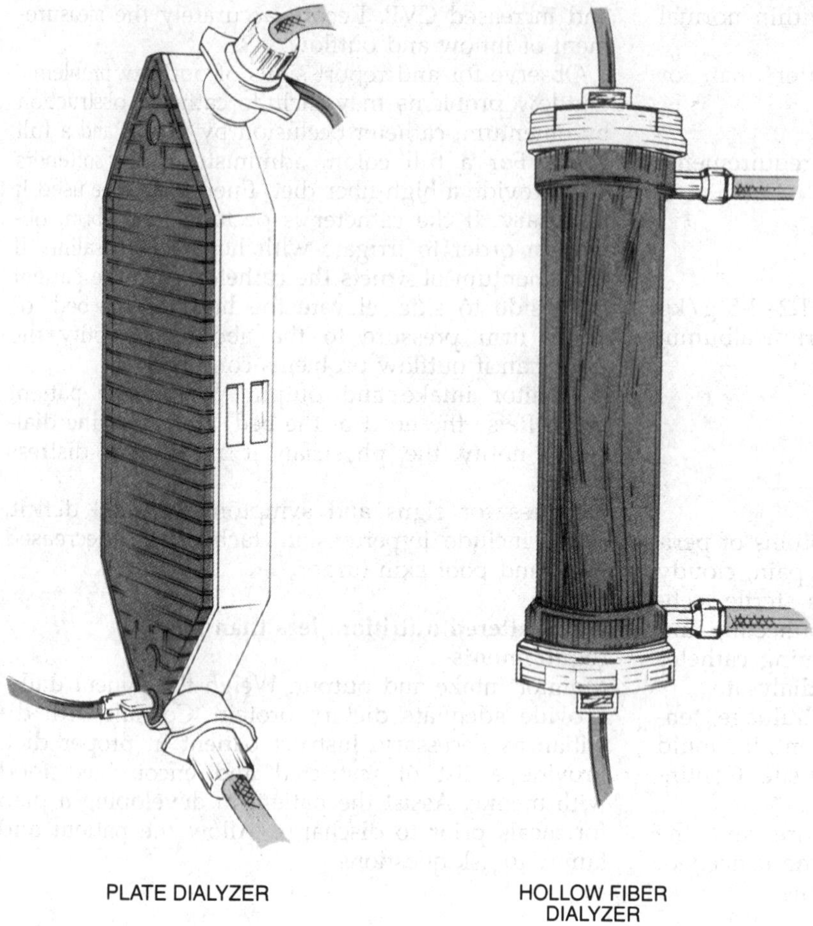

Figure 26–4.

Artificial kidneys (dialyzers) used in hemodialysis. (From Ignatavicius D, Bayne M. Medical-surgical nursing. Philadelphia: WB Saunders, 1991, p 1902.)

comes. Examples of specific outcomes for patients undergoing peritoneal dialysis have been provided in the Planning section.

Hemodialysis

In hemodialysis, blood is removed from a vascular access. The blood is heparinized and pumped through a dialyzer (Fig. 26–4) and then returned to the patient's circulation. Diffusion and ultrafiltration occur, allowing the blood to be filtered.

PROCEDURE

A hemodialysis system includes a dialyzer, dialysate, vascular access routes, and hemodialysis machine. There are several different designs of dialyzers. The dialyzer has a blood compartment and a dialysate compartment. The two compartments are separated by a semipermeable membrane. The dialysate is an electrolyte solution that can be modified to meet the patient's needs. Toxins and wastes diffuse across the semipermeable membrane from the blood to the dialysate.

There are many different models of hemodialysis machines, but their basic function is similar.

Heparin is used for anticoagulation to prevent clots from forming in the dialyzer and tubing. Dosage is based on each patient's individual need. Clotting studies, such as activated partial thromboplastin times (APTT) and partial thromboplastin time (PTT), are done to monitor the drug's effect. The antidote for heparin is protamine sulfate. The hemodialysis circuit is illustrated in Figure 26–5.

Hemodialysis involves shunting the patient's blood from the body through a dialyzer in which diffusion and ultrafiltration occur and then returning filtered blood to the patient's circulation. Vascular access is necessary in order to perform hemodialysis. There are several techniques instituted to establish this access.

1. Arteriovenous fistula
2. Arteriovenous graft
3. External arteriovenous shunt
4. Femoral vein catheterization
5. Subclavian vein catheterization

The first three are permanent access techniques. The last two are temporary access techniques.

Arteriovenous (AV) fistulas are created surgically by joining or anastomosing an artery and a vein.

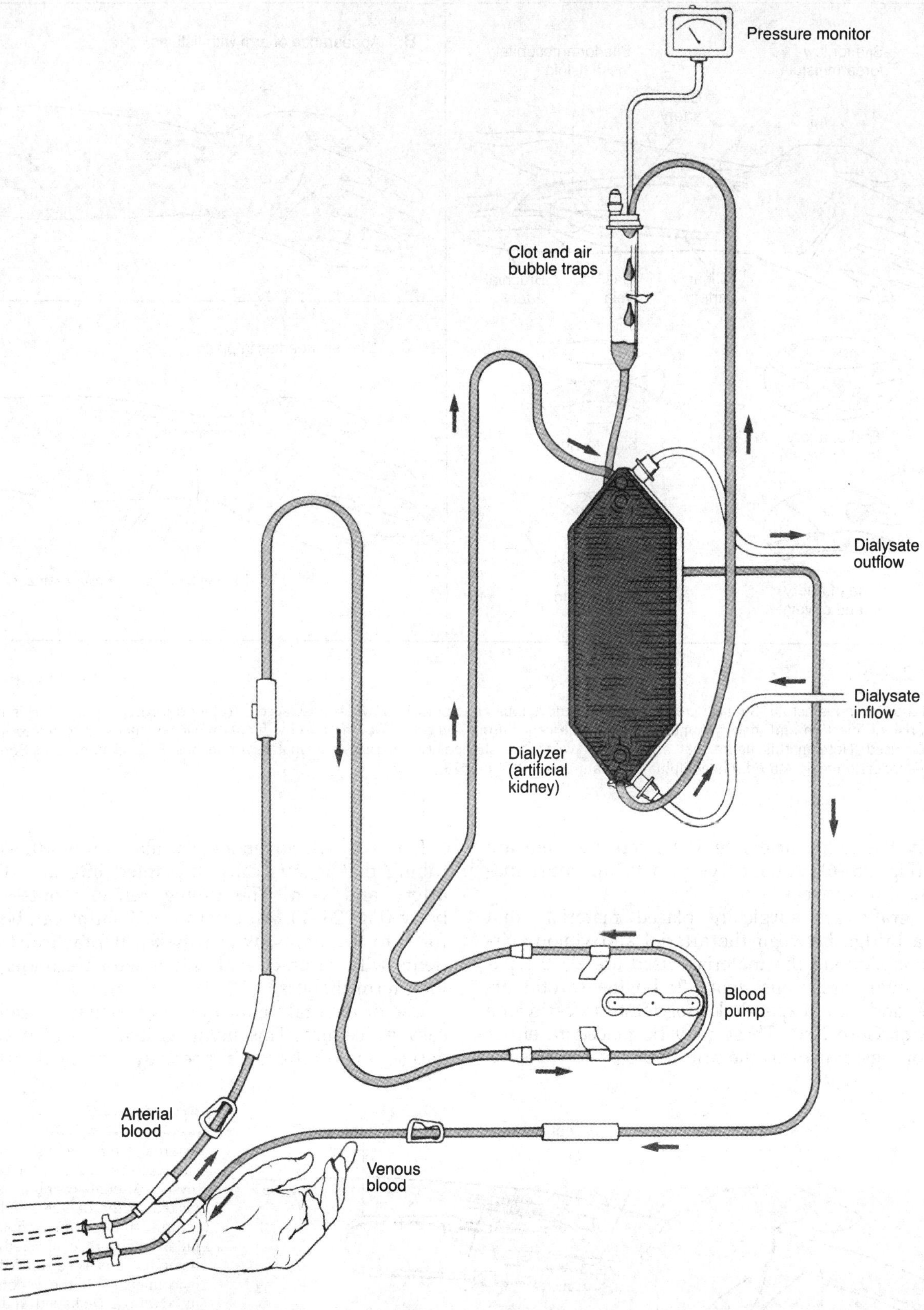

Figure 26–5.

Hemodialysis circuit. (From Ignatavicius D, Bayne M. Medical-surgical nursing. Philadephia: WB Saunders, 1991, p 1903.)

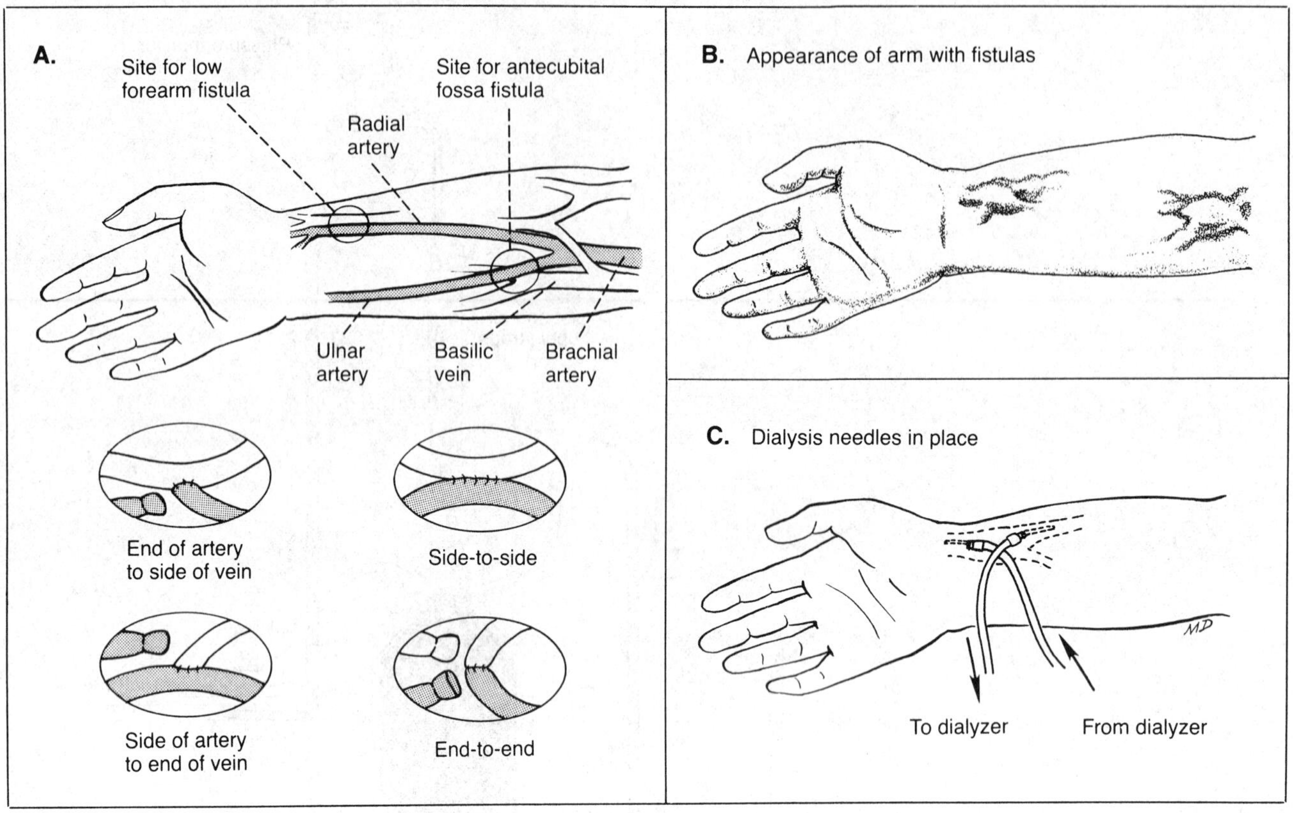

Figure 26–6.

Internal arteriovenous fistula. Surgical creation of an arteriovenous anastomosis provides easy access to blood for hemodialysis. This method reduces risk of infection and makes shunts unnecessary except during hemodialysis. The internal fistula must be created 2 to 6 weeks before it can be used. Note in this figure that arteries, not veins, are shaded. (From Black JM, Matassarin-Jacobs E. Luckmann and Sorensen's Medical-surgical nursing. 4th ed. Philadelphia: WB Saunders, 1993, p 1513.)

Usually the radial artery and the cephalic vein are used (Fig. 26–6). After surgery, a fistula must mature for 6 to 12 weeks.

AV grafts are surgically placed materials that form a bridge between the arterial and venous circulations. Among the materials used are (1) the patient's own saphenous vein, (2) bovine carotid arteries, and (3) expanded polytetrafluoroethylene (PTFE or Gore-Tex). These may be placed in either arms or legs; however, the arm is the preferred site.

External arteriovenous shunts are Silastic-Teflon tubing that is surgically implanted into an adjacent artery and vein. The tubing remains outside the body (Fig. 26–7). An external AV shunt can be used for 6 to 9 months, which makes it practical for patients with chronic renal failure who are undergoing long-term dialysis.

Use of femoral vein catheters is usually a safe and easy procedure. This involves insertion of two #16-gauge angiocaths or a specially designed catheter

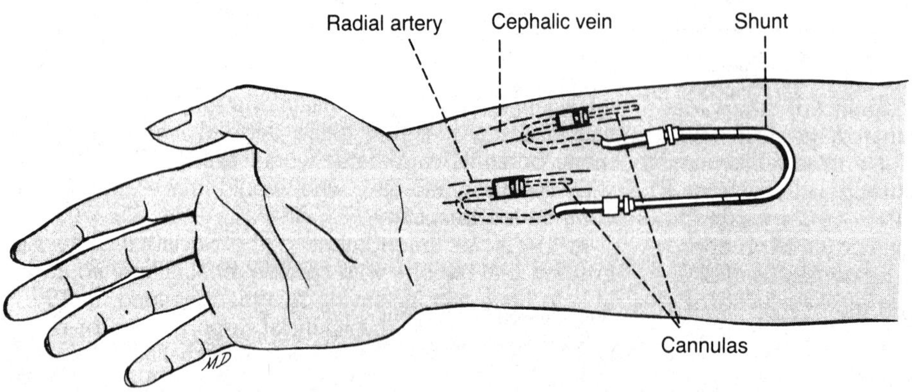

Figure 26–7.

External arteriovenous shunt provides access to blood for hemodialysis. Arterial cannula is connected to the dialyzer, and blood returns through the venous cannula. When not connected to the hemodialyzer, the arterial cannula is connected to the venous cannula with a U-shaped shunt and secured carefully to the skin. (From Black JM, Matassarin-Jacobs E. Luckmann and Sorensen's Medical-surgical nursing. 4th ed. Philadelphia: WB Saunders, 1993, p 1512.)

Table 26–10. COMPLICATIONS OF HEMODIALYSIS

Complications related to vascular access:
- Clot formation in the graft, fistula, or catheter
- Stenosis or narrowing of the anastomosis
- Infection
- Aneurysm formation
- High-output cardiac failure

Complications related to the dialysis procedure:
- Hypovolemia
- Shock
- Blood loss
- Electrolyte imbalance
- Air embolus

into the femoral vein. These catheters must be removed after each dialysis treatment.

Subclavian vein catheterization involves the placement of a specially designed catheter into the subclavian vein under sterile technique. The advantage of the subclavian catheter is that it can be left in place for repeated use. Care of these types of vascular access is discussed within the context of the nursing process.

CLINICAL USE

Hemodialysis is usually performed in a hospital or free-standing dialysis clinic. The procedure is usually carried out three times per week. Home dialysis is available for select patients. Hemodialysis may be used in the treatment of both acute and chronic renal failure.

COMPLICATIONS

The complications of hemodialysis are divided into two categories: (1) those involving the vascular access, and (2) those involving the dialysis process (Table 26–10).

Application of the Nursing Process to the Care of the Patient Undergoing Hemodialysis

Assessment

Assessment of the patient undergoing hemodialysis is related to control of fluid and electrolyte balance, prevention of complications, and maintenance of vascular access. Cardiac status is of utmost importance. Assess postural changes of blood pressure, especially at the completion of dialysis. Check all vital signs. Assess heart and lung sounds. Monitor heart rhythm. Assess CVP, if line is present, and status of neck veins.

Assess fluid status before and after the procedure. Monitor intake and output. Weigh patient before and after dialysis. Assess mental status. Mental status changes may indicate disequilibrium dementia or electrolyte imbalance. Monitor electrolyte values.

Check the patency of the vascular access by auscultating for a bruit and palpating for a thrill. The presence of the bruit and thrill is indicative of an adequate blood flow through the access. Observe and report any numbness, pain, or swelling in the extremity distal to the access. The vascular access is the lifeline of the patient on hemodialysis and must be monitored closely and handled with care. Assessments and care of a vascular access are listed in Table 26–11.

Assess the patient's and family's knowledge con-

Table 26–11. NURSING CARE GUIDELINES FOR CARING FOR THE VASCULAR ACCESS

TYPE	INTERVENTION	RATIONALE
Fistula	Inspect needle puncture sites after dialysis. If bleeding occurs, apply pressure to stop bleeding; release pressure to check site every 5 to 10 minutes.	Prevents hemorrhaging.
	Do not take blood pressure, perform venipuncture, or draw blood from arm with fistula. Avoid tight clothing or restrictive bands or jewelry. Palpate for thrill and auscultate for bruit every shift. Report absence of thrill or bruit.	Prevents clotting and allows for early intervention at signs of clotting.
	Observe for signs and symptoms of infection. Culture and report any drainage.	Prevents infection and allows for early intervention at signs of infection.
Shunt	Wrap shunt securely with gauze. Tape all connections. Do not use scissors to remove dressings. Keep bulldog or rubber-shod clamp at bedside for use if disconnection occurs. Apply firm pressure at site if shunt pulls out, and notify physician immediately.	Prevents hemorrhaging and disruption of shunt.
	Expose a portion of the loop to check for patency every shift. Palpate for thrill and auscultate for bruit above exit site every shift.	Prevents clotting and allows for early intervention at signs of clotting.
	Use aseptic technique with dressing changes. Observe for signs of infection. Culture any drainage.	Prevents infection and allows for early intervention at signs of infection.

cerning dialysis, vascular access, and dietary and medical regimen. Assess support systems and the patient's coping mechanisms.

Nursing Diagnoses and Planning

Nursing diagnoses and related expected patient outcomes most commonly applicable to patients undergoing hemodialysis include the following:

NDx: High risk for fluid volume excess or deficit related to renal failure or fluid removal

Planning: Patient outcomes
1. Patient has balanced intake and output, stable weight, and good skin turgor.
2. Patient's vital signs and CVP are within normal limits.
3. Patient's dialysate outflow is greater than or equal to inflow.

NDx: High risk for injury related to blood loss from access site

Planning: Patient outcomes
1. Patient exhibits normal vital signs, normal skin temperature and color, and brisk capillary refill.
2. Patient's access has audible bruit and palpable thrill.

NDx: High risk for infection related to vascular access

Planning: Patient outcomes
1. Patient is afebrile.
2. Patient's access site is free of erythema, warmth, exudate, swelling, and tenderness.

NDx: Ineffective individual coping related to effects of long-term hemodialysis

Planning: Patient outcomes
1. Patient expresses a realistic view of the situation and coping resources available.
2. Patient discusses changes in self and family as a result of renal failure.
3. Patient verbalizes feelings to health care professional and family.
4. Patient identifies changes in family roles and processes as a result of renal failure.
5. Patient identifies alternative coping behaviors.

Nursing Interventions

NDx: High risk for fluid volume excess or deficit
Observe for and report signs and symptoms of fluid overload. These include hypertension, tachycardia, dyspnea, crackles in lungs, distended neck veins, and increased CVP. Record accurately the measurement of inflow and outflow.

Observe for and report signs of outflow problems. Outflow problems may include catheter obstruction from kinking or catheter occlusion by fibrin. If the catheter is occluded by fibrin, obtain an order to irrigate with heparinized saline. Notify the physician if outflow problems continue.

Monitor intake and output. Weigh the patient daily. Raise the head of the bed, and notify the physician if respiratory distress occurs. Assess for signs and symptoms of fluid deficit. These include hypertension, tachycardia, decreased CVP, and poor skin turgor.

NDx: High risk for injury
Provide adequate site care (see Table 26–11). Monitor for complications. Report severe or unrelieved pain, numbness, tingling, or swelling of the extremity distal to the access. Observe for symptoms of blood loss. Maintain and monitor equipment.

NDx: High risk for infection
Provide adequate site care. Use aseptic technique when doing dressing changes. Monitor vital signs. Observe for redness, swelling, warmth, exudate, and tenderness at site. Culture any drainage. Teach patient and family to recognize signs and symptoms of infection.

NDx: Ineffective individual coping
It often takes several weeks for the full impact and permanency of dialysis to be realized. The most common psychosocial problems seen are (1) change in body image, (2) dependency-independency conflict, and (3) difficulty in facing potential death. Relationships with family, relatives, and friends are likely to change. Many patients have much difficulty coping with these changes and problems.

Instruct the patient and family in all areas of the treatment regimen. Allow for questions and verbalization of fears and concerns. Identify the patient's normal patterns of coping. Provide support for decisions made by the patient and family, and accept the patient's reactions to dialysis. Encourage active participation in the patient's care by the patient and the family.

Evaluation

Evaluate the effectiveness of nursing care for a patient undergoing hemodialysis by comparing the patient's status with the expected outcomes. Examples of specific outcomes for patients undergoing hemodialysis have been provided in the planning section.

Renal Transplantation

Renal transplantation is the surgical transfer of a functioning kidney from one person to another. This is a treatment option for irreversible renal failure. In 1984, there were approximately 7000 renal transplants performed and another 7000 people on the waiting lists for transplantation.

Donors for transplantation come from two sources. The first group consists of living-related donors, and the other group consists of cadaveric donors. The preferred donor is the living-related donor because genetic matching is closer or even identical. There is a third source of donors that is gaining popularity. This is the living-nonrelated donor. At present some centers are utilizing this source of donors.

The major factors in donor and recipient determination are blood type and histocompatibility typing. Kidneys are not transplanted across blood types. Therefore, if the recipient has type A blood, the donor must have type A blood also. In histocompatibility typing, the human leukocyte antigens (HLA) are examined. There are three areas that are examined. They are A, B, and DR loci. In living-related donors, the ideal is to have an identical match; however, a half match is acceptable. In cadaveric transplantation, there may be no match at all except the blood type. The matching of donor and recipient varies from center to center; some using only blood type and others using HLA matching in choosing the recipient. The final determining factor in the recipient is called a final crossmatch. In this test, the donor's and recipient's blood are mixed and examined for a reaction. If there is a reaction, the recipient and donor are not compatible, and, therefore, the transplant will not take place.

Cadaveric kidneys may be maintained for as long as 72 hours before transplant depending on the preservation method. This allows kidneys to be transported long distances for transplantation.

Donors must meet certain criteria for transplantation. These criteria can be found in Table 26–12.

Table 26–12. DONOR CRITERIA FOR RENAL TRANSPLANTATION

1. Heart beating
2. Functioning organs
3. No history of chronic disease
4. No history of cancer outside of the central nervous system
5. Younger than 65 years of age

Procedure

After removal from the donor, the kidney is preserved on ice or on a perfusion pump. When the donor is cadaveric, there may be multiple organs harvested. Due to the preservation of the kidneys, they are the last organs to be harvested. Both kidneys are removed along with the aorta, vena cava, and ureters.

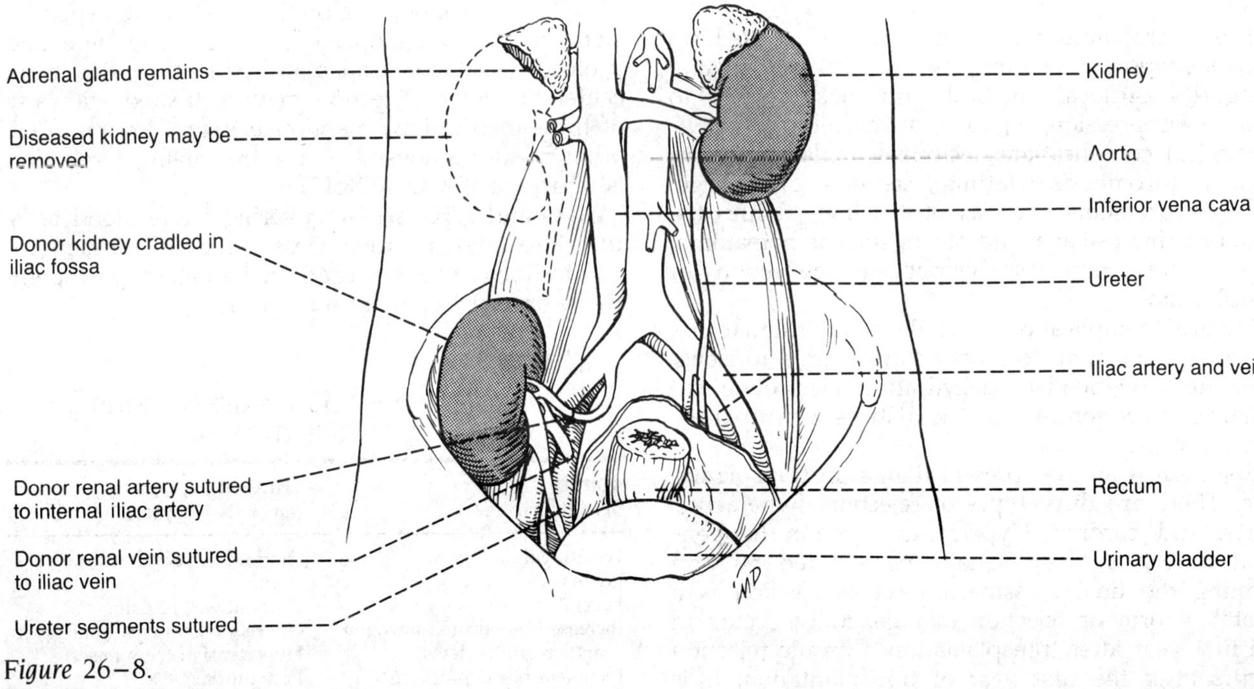

Figure 26–8.

Transplanted kidney placement. (From Black JM, Matassarin-Jacobs E. Luckmann and Sorensen's Medical-surgical nursing. 4th ed. Philadelphia: WB Saunders, 1993, p 1517.)

When the donor is living-related, a single kidney is removed through a flank incision. In this nephrectomy, the kidney, renal vein and artery, and ureter are removed together. The transplanted kidney is placed in the iliac fossa. Either kidney may be used, and that determines the side of transplant (Fig. 26–8).

The recipient has a hockey-stick incision in either the lower lower left or right quadrant of the abdomen, depending on the kidney used. The renal artery and vein are attached to the iliac artery and vein. The surgery is performed without entering the peritoneum; therefore, the patient may eat or drink after recovering from anesthesia.

Depending on the surgeon's preference, the patient returns from the operating room with at least one intravenous line and usually a Foley catheter and some sort of abdominal drain.

In some centers, the patient may go to the intensive care unit for 24 to 48 hours. In other centers, the patient returns to the transplant floor.

Clinical Use

Renal transplantation is a means of restoring renal function to normal in most patients, and thus allowing them to return to a healthy lifestyle. Geriatric patients are not candidates for transplantation, because most centers limit the upper range for receiving a transplant to the age of 55 to 60 years.

Complications

There are numerous complications related to transplantation. These may be grouped into several categories: surgical, medical, and those related to immunosuppression, rejection, or infection.

Surgical complications include vascular problems such as thrombosis (clotting), stenosis, or leakage; urologic problems such as obstruction, reflux, fistula, or urine leakage; and others such as hematoma, abscess formation, or lymphocele (collection of lymph fluid).

Medical complications include acute tubular necrosis (a form of acute renal failure related to ischemia), fluid overload or dehydration, electrolyte imbalances, hypertension, gastric distress, constipation, and diarrhea.

Rejection is an ever-present danger in transplantation. There are three types of rejection: hyperacute, acute, and chronic. Hyperacute rejection happens immediately, but can usually be avoided by performing the final crossmatch. Acute rejection is a treatable form of rejection that generally occurs in the first year after transplantation. Chronic rejection occurs after the first year of transplantation; it is untreatable and generally results in the loss of the graft. See Table 26–13 for signs and symptoms of rejection.

Infection is the plague of all patients taking immunosuppressive medications because these drugs decrease the body's ability to fight off infection. The infections may be bacterial, viral, or fungal in nature. Bacterial infections are the easiest to treat because of the broad spectrum of antibiotics available. The most common fungal infection is caused by yeast and can be treated with amphotericin and, if oral, with Mycelex. Viral infections can be the most troublesome to transplantation. The most common viral infection is caused by cytomegalovirus; if not detected and treated early, it can eventually result in graft loss or even death of the patient. The other menacing viral infection of the transplant patient is the herpes virus, which can show many forms in the immunosuppressed patient. It can range from simple outbreaks of "fever blisters," to herpes zoster or shingles, to a systemic form that is extremely detrimental to the patient's health. Zovirax has become instrumental in the treatment of these patients.

The complications related to immunosuppressive medications are varied and range from a marked decrease in white blood cell counts to an increased risk of cancer. All immunosuppressive medications increase the risk of infection.

Immunosuppression

Immunosuppressive medications are given to prevent rejection of the transplanted organ. There are five medications given as therapy immediately after transplant. These are antilymphocyte globulin (ALG), antithymocyte globulin (ATG), cyclosporine, steroids, and azathioprine (Imuran). The type and protocol used for transplant patients varies from center to center. Rejection may be treated with any of these medications mentioned except Imuran. One other medication used in the treatment of rejection is muromonab-CD3 (OKT3).

ALG and ATG act by covering white blood cells, therefore making them less effective. These two medications may be used immediately postoperatively or as a treatment for rejection.

Table 26–13. MANIFESTATIONS OF REJECTION

ACUTE (less than 1 year)	CHRONIC (more than 1 year)
Weight gain	Gradual decrease in urine output
Edema	Gradual weight gain
Fever	Gradual rise in creatinine level
Increased blood urea nitrogen and creatinine levels	Hypertension (new onset)
Increased blood pressure	Proteinuria
Swelling and tenderness at graft site	
Electrolyte imbalances	

Steroids (prednisone and Solu-Medrol) affect the immune system by decreasing the inflammatory response, sensitivity, and the number of some of the white blood cells. These medications are not without side effects. They include increases in blood sugar level, retention of sodium and water, decreased wound healing, stress ulcer formation, mood swings, muscle wasting, steroid acne, and rarely cataracts and degeneration of the weight-bearing joints. Steroids are used for maintenance therapy and treatment of rejection.

Cyclosporine acts directly on T cells to prevent rejection. This medication is extremely expensive. The side effects include toxicity of the kidney and liver, increased hair growth on the face, hypertension, tremors, and rarely seizures.

Imuran acts by decreasing white cell activity. Side effects include increased risk of infection and malignancy, hair loss, decrease in number of platelets, nausea, and vomiting.

Muromonab-CD3 (OKT3) is a new treatment for rejection. The major side effect of this medication is pulmonary edema, especially with the first dose. This medication should never be given to a fluid-overloaded individual. Other side effects are fever and malaise.

Obviously, immunosuppressive medications have many disturbing side effects. Therefore, the patient must be educated to expect these. Noncompliance with the medication schedule is often associated with the patient's inability to tolerate the side effects from immunosuppressive drugs as well as afford their high cost.

Application of the Nursing Process to the Care of the Patient Who has Undergone Renal Transplantation

Assessment

Assess the patient's vital signs and breath sounds. Record intake and output. Weigh the patient daily. Assess the wound status and graft site. Evaluate the patient's mental and nutritional status. Determine the patient's understanding of the surgery. Check for anxiety or concerns about the procedure. Monitor complete blood count, serum electrolytes, and BUN and serum creatinine levels.

Nursing Diagnoses and Planning

Nursing diagnoses and related expected patient outcomes most commonly applicable to patients who have undergone renal transplantation include the following:

NDx: High risk for infection related to immunosuppressive drug therapy

Planning: Patient outcomes

1. Patient exhibits normal vital signs.
2. Patient is free from redness or purulent drainage at wound site.
3. Patient verbalizes the signs and symptoms of infection.

NDx: Fear related to possibility of rejection

Planning: Patient outcomes

1. Patient verbalizes specific fears related to transplantation.
2. Patient verbalizes realistic expectations related to transplantation.
3. Patient verbalizes decreased fear.

NDx: Altered health maintenance related to lack of knowledge about signs and symptoms of rejection, side effects of immunosuppressive drugs, and the need to protect the vascular access.

Planning: Patient outcomes

1. Patient verbalizes signs and symptoms of rejection
2. Patient verbalizes side effects of immunosuppressive drugs.
3. Patient verbalizes importance of protecting vascular access.

Nursing Interventions

NDx: High risk for infection

Monitor vital signs. Report fever and unexplained tachycardia. Observe for infections in other body systems. Use aseptic technique with all invasive procedures and dressing changes. Instruct patient in measures to avoid infection (Chart 26–2).

NDx: Fear

Encourage the patient to verbalize subjective feelings, perceptions of illness, perception of own coping skills, and need for assistance from the nursing staff. Initiate teaching to decrease knowledge deficit. Teach patient what to expect during hospitalization and after discharge. Monitor level of fear, and encourage patient to verbalize fear.

NDx: Altered health maintenance

Explain and teach the patient and family about signs and symptoms of infection and rejection and the importance of protecting the vascular access (see Chart 26–2). Allow the patient and family to ask questions. Give them written instructions and printed literature explaining the postoperative care needed.

Chart 26–2.

NURSING CARE GUIDE TO PATIENT EDUCATION FOR SELF-MANAGEMENT: SELF-CARE FOR THE RENAL TRANSPLANT PATIENT

Instruct the patient to:

Recognize and report fever and tachycardia.
Be alert to signs and symptoms of common infections:
- Urinary tract infection—cloudy, odorous urine; urinary burning; frequency; and urgency
- Upper respiratory tract infection—productive cough with purulent, colored, copius sputum
- Otitis media—malaise, earache
- Impetigo—inflamed, drainage pustules on skin

Avoid contact with individuals with known infections.
Recognize and report immediately the signs of rejection:
- Oliguria
- Tenderness over kidney (in iliac fossa)
- Sudden weight gain
- Fever
- Malaise
- Increased blood pressure

Protect the vascular access because it may be needed if rejection occurs.
Forbid venipuncture, blood drawing, or blood pressure to be taken in the access extremity.

Evaluation

Evaluate the effectiveness of nursing care for a patient who has undergone renal transplantation by comparing the patient's status with the expected patient outcomes. Examples of specific outcomes for patients who have undergone renal transplantation have been provided in the Planning section.

Obstruction

Urinary tract obstruction can be defined as blockage of the normal glomerular filtrate flow anywhere along the urinary tract. Obstruction of the urinary tract poses serious pathophysiologic consequences for the renal parenchyma in the form of dilation and thinning of the renal tubules with eventual atrophy of the renal substance itself.

Any disorder that interferes with the peristaltic movement of urine is obstructive, and an obstruction can occur at any point in the urinary tract.

Classification systems denoting obstruction vary. One method is to classify obstructions according to congenital or acquired causes. Congenital anomalies in the urinary tract are found more commonly than in any other organ system, and these anomalies are generally obstructive in nature. Acquired causes are many and may be found either within the urinary tract, invading the tract, or compressing the tract. Other means of classifying obstruction include the duration (acute or chronic), the degree (partial or complete), and the level at which it occurs in the urinary tract (upper or lower).

Pathophysiologic changes secondary to obstruction occur only in those segments of the urinary tract proximal to the obstruction. These changes do not occur throughout the urinary tract all at once; each portion of the tract tends to protect those parts more proximal to the obstruction. For example, when there is obstruction of the bladder neck, the bladder undergoes changes, but the ureter is protected until the bladder can no longer compensate.

Initially, obstruction causes back pressure because of stasis of urine in the segment of the urinary tract just above the obstruction. The hydrostatic pressure of the accumulated urine opposes the peristaltic force of the urine flow. In response to the back pressure, the affected segment dilates to accommodate the stagnated urine. In most instances, dilatation stretches the muscle fibers, stimulating hypertrophy. The hypertrophied muscle contracts more strongly in an effort to force urine through the area of obstruction; the affected segment compensates, which means it undergoes changes in order to maintain function.

If obstruction is not relieved, increasing dilatation overstretches the muscle fibers, decreasing muscle tone and the ability to contract. The segment decompensates and is unable to maintain its function of elimination. The area becomes increasingly dilated, and the atonic muscle wall may become thinned and weakened. Increased back pressure is transmitted to the next proximal segment in the urinary tract, and this cycle of compensation-decompensation occurs in succession to all segments up to the renal pelvis and calices.

Any obstruction of the urinary tract can lead to an increased pressure in the renal pelvis and calices, otherwise known as hydronephrosis (Fig. 26–9). Such pressure can damage the renal parenchyma and interfere with renal function; renal blood flow may also be compromised. If infection is present, the damage to the kidney could be more severe.

The long-term effects of hydronephrosis and how much function returns after relief of the obstruction are determined by several factors such as severity (complete or partial obstruction), duration, totality (bilateral or unilateral obstruction), and presence of infection.

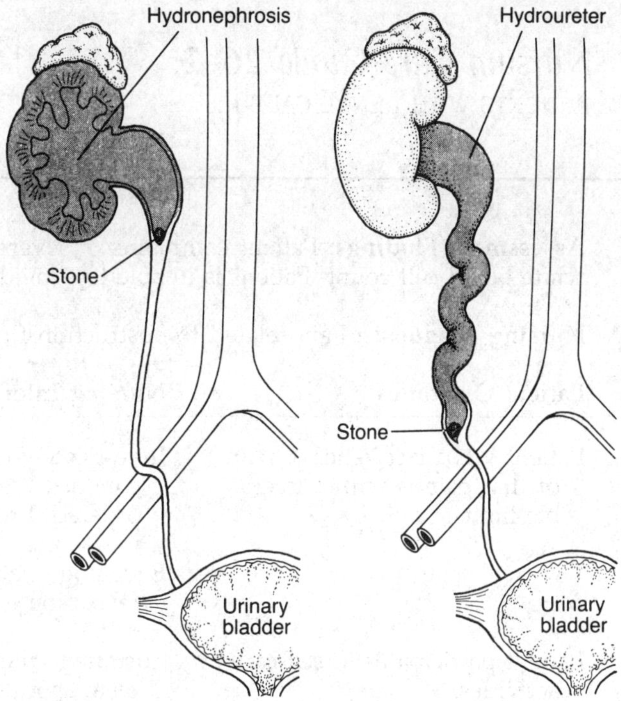

Figure 26–9.

Hydronephrosis is caused by obstruction in the upper part of the ureter; hydroureter is caused by obstruction in the lower part of the ureter. (From Ignatavicius D, Bayne M. Medical-surgical nursing. Philadelphia: WB Saunders, 1991, p 1964.)

Postobstructive Diuresis

Following relief of obstruction, urine output may increase three- to ten-fold. This response, called postobstructive diuresis, is usually mild and self-limiting, but in some cases it can be severe. This state of markedly excessive, dilute urine output is caused by the impaired ability of renal tubules to concentrate and absorb body fluids and electrolytes (primarily sodium) effectively. This impairment of renal function is secondary to renal damage caused by increased pressure on the tubules as a result of urinary tract obstruction.

Diuresis can be defined as a urine output that is more than 2000 ml in an 8-hour period. In a broader sense, any urine output above normal (which in adults can range from 700 to 2000 ml) may be considered to be a postobstructive diuresis, if only because of its life-threatening potential.

Postobstructive diuresis is characterized by an excessive loss of both water and electrolytes. If judicious treatment is not undertaken in a timely manner, this dramatic polyuria and "salt-losing" may result in rapid depletion of extracellular fluid volume, vascular collapse, and death. Fluid and electrolytes must be replaced appropriately until renal function (concentrating ability) improves.

Urinary Calculi

ETIOLOGY AND PATHOPHYSIOLOGY

Urinary calculus, or urolithiasis, is the presence of stones in the urinary tract. It is one of the most common urologic problems for adults. Twelve percent of the population of the United States develops a urinary tract calculus at some time in their lives. For some this may mean a small stone that passes easily and painlessly through the urinary tract. In extreme cases, patients suffer recurrent urinary tract infection or loss of renal function from large, obstructing or infected renal stones.

Passing a urinary calculus can be a very painful experience. Stones that grow too large to pass spontaneously are treated using a variety of medical and surgical techniques. The recent advent of the use of shock waves to disintegrate stones without the need for surgery has drastically reduced the morbidity formerly associated with this disease.

Approximately 80% of persons with urinary calculus disease are found to have a metabolic or dietary cause for stone formation. In the remaining 20%, diet, fluid intake, and geographic location are thought to be major factors. Generally, persons whose diet includes a high intake of calcium and animal proteins, persons whose fluid intake is chronically low, and persons who live in the Southeast, Southwest, and Northwest United States are at greater risk for urinary calculus formation.

Urinary calculi occur most commonly in the 20-50-year-old age group. Stones associated with infection are more common in women. It is believed that stones form when chemicals and other elements

Nursing Care Guide 26–2.

PATIENTS WITH RENAL CALCULI

Assessment Findings: Patient complains of severe pain in back and flank area; has fever and increased white blood cell count. Patient is unable to provide self-care as a result of the extreme pain.

Nursing Diagnosis: Pain related to obstruction from renal calculi

Patient Outcomes	Nursing Interventions	Rationale
Patient verbalizes relief of pain or that pain is within tolerable limits.	Investigate complaints of discomfort. Medicate for pain as ordered. Provide comfort measures.	Assessing the patient's pain provides baseline data for comparisons at a later time.
	Encourage patient to practice relaxation exercises.	Relaxation techniques may provide additional relief for the patient.
Patient participates in self-care activities.	Encourage the patient to complete as much self-care as able. Assist the patient when necessary.	Participating in the care may ease some of the emotional stress associated with the condition.
	Medicate for pain prior to self-care activities.	Medicating the patient prior to activity may promote more participation from the patient.
	Encourage ambulation and increased fluid intake, as tolerated.	Ambulating and drinking increased amounts of fluids may help pass the calculi, thus eliminating the pain.

Evaluation: Compare the patient's status with the expected patient outcomes. If the outcomes are achieved, evaluate nursing care as successful. If not, reassess the patient, formulate new nursing diagnoses, and revise expected patient outcomes and nursing interventions as appropriate.

Assessment Findings: Patient experiences nausea and/or vomiting and is unable to eat or drink fluids.

Nursing Diagnosis: Altered nutrition: less than body requirements related to nausea and vomiting secondary to extreme pain from renal calculi

Patient Outcomes	Nursing Interventions	Rationale
Patient verbalizes relief of nausea and vomiting.	Evaluate the factor causing the nausea. Administer analgesics and antiemetics as ordered. Monitor the patient's fluid intake and output.	Analgesics relieve the pain that may result in relief of the nausea. Antiemetics relieve the nausea and vomiting.

(continued)

Nursing Care Guide 26–2. *(continued)*

PATIENTS WITH RENAL CALCULI

Patient Outcomes	Nursing Interventions	Rationale
	Encourage relaxation techniques such as slow, deep breathing. Position the patient for comfort.	Relaxation exercises may provide stress relief and make the patient more comfortable as well as relieve some of the pain.
	Provide small frequent sips of fluids as tolerated.	Replacing fluids slowly may prevent aggravation of the nausea.
	Provide oral hygiene frequently. Encourage the patient to rinse mouth as necessary.	Providing oral hygiene reduces foul odor and taste and prevents increased bacterial growth in the mouth.

Evaluation: Compare the patient's status with the expected patient outcomes. If the outcomes are achieved, evaluate nursing care as successful. If not, reassess the patient, formulate new nursing diagnoses, and revise expected patient outcomes and nursing interventions as appropriate.

Assessment Findings: Patient complains of urgency, bladder fullness, and suprapubic discomfort. The patient's bladder is distended and easily palpable; intake is greater than output, and pain is increasing.

Nursing Diagnosis: Altered patterns of urinary elimination related to obstructed ureter

Patient Outcomes	Nursing Interventions	Rationale
Patient denies feelings of urgency, fullness, or discomfort.	Assess for increasing pain and bladder fullness.	Assessing for bladder distention, discomfort, and dysuria provides a baseline for comparisons at a later time. It also promotes early intervention for problems found.
	Administer analgesics as ordered.	Analgesics may relieve some of the discomfort.
Patient's voiding pattern returns to normal; fluid intake and output are adequate.	Monitor the fluid intake and output, strain all urine, and insert Foley catheter if necessary to relieve pressure. Note the color and consistency of the urine.	Monitoring the fluid intake and output provides for early intervention if problems arise. Straining urine may reveal passage of the calculi.
	Encourage increased fluid intake.	Increased fluids help wash out system and may promote the passage of the calculi.

Evaluation: Compare the patient's status with the expected patient outcomes. If the outcomes are achieved, evaluate nursing care as successful. If not, reassess the patient, formulate new nursing diagnoses, and revise expected patient outcomes and nursing interventions as appropriate.

commonly found in urine become concentrated and lead to the formation of crystals. The crystals begin to cling together to eventually form a calcification or calculus. The elements that lead to crystal formation may be present in large amounts in the urine as a result of one of many metabolic disorders, diet, or fluid intake.

Most urinary tract stones are formed in the kidney. Ureteral stones are usually renal stones that have moved down the ureter. Bladder stones are common in patients with indwelling urinary drainage tubes or an inability to empty their bladder when voiding.

CLINICAL MANIFESTATIONS

Pain is the most common symptom patients with urinary calculi experience. Renal calculi cause flank pain on the same side as the affected kidney, which may radiate to the groin or the genitalia. Ureteral stones cause pain in the flank and abdominal area, which may also radiate to the genitalia. When the discomfort is dull and aching, the patient may visit the doctor's office. Most patients, however, go to the emergency room during an episode of renal ureteral colic.

Colic occurs when the muscular components of the lining of the urinary tract go into spasm in response to irritation from the calculus. Episodes of colic are excrutiatingly painful, have a sudden onset, and are often accompanied by severe nausea and vomiting. Large doses of pain medication are often required to relieve the pain. Fever and an elevated white blood cell count may be present if the stone has caused an infection.

MEDICAL DIAGNOSIS

Diagnosis of a urinary calculus or calculi is made on the basis of the presenting symptoms and on a series of radiographic tests. A plain abdominal film will identify most calculi, although some are composed of elements that are radiolucent. An excretory urogram further outlines the calculus and allows evaluation of its location in the kidney or ureter and any effect the calculus has had on the surrounding tissue. Retrograde pyelogram may be necessary to diagnose renal or ureteral stones in patients with radiolucent stones or in those with an allergy to contrast dye. The urinalysis may show red blood cells, white blood cells, and bacteria.

MEDICAL MANAGEMENT

The treatment for urinary calculus disease depends on the size, number, location, and content of the stone or stones. Eighty to ninety percent of stones that are smaller than 5 mm in diameter pass spontaneously. Hospitalization may be required to treat the symptoms of colic that may occur as the stone passes. Infected stones, even if smaller than 5 mm, may cause pyelonephritis requiring antibiotic therapy.

Patients with multiple stones, very large impacted stones, or stones that obstruct the urinary tract usually require surgical treatment.

SURGICAL INTERVENTION

Extracorporeal shock wave lithotripsy (ESWL) is now commonly used to treat renal or ureteral calculi. Surgical interventions are reserved for patients in whom ESWL is contraindicated or would be unsuccessful. A variety of surgical approaches are used, ranging from procedures performed through a small flank incision using flexible ultrasonic instruments (used to break up and remove renal stones) to major surgeries such as nephrolithotomy or nephrectomy.

Lower ureteral or bladder stones are usually removed using instruments that are passed through a cystoscope. Bladder stones that are very large require open surgical removal.

Application of the Nursing Process to the Care of the Patient with Urinary Calculi

The assessment, nursing diagnoses, expected patient outcomes, nursing interventions, and evaluation for patients with urinary calculi are provided in Nursing Care Guide 26–2 and Nutrition Box 26–2.

Upper Urinary Tract Obstruction

URETEROPELVIC JUNCTION OBSTRUCTION

ETIOLOGY AND PATHOPHYSIOLOGY

Ureteropelvic junction (UPJ) obstruction is a term that refers to the anatomic site of obstruction. Causes of this type of urinary tract disorder are varied, but can usually be attributed to congenital anomalies such as a ureter that has developed abnormally high in the renal pelvis. Inflammation, ischemia, tumors, and calculi are examples of acquired causes of UPJ obstruction.

In most cases of UPJ obstruction, regardless of the cause, there is hydronephrosis and dilatation of the kidney pelvis and calices. With longstanding obstruction, there is deterioration of renal function. Other pathophysiologic changes can occur but are related to specific causes of the obstruction.

Nutrition Box 26–2.

DIETARY NEEDS RELATED TO TYPE OF CALCULUS

Calculus Type	Dietary Needs
Calcium phosphate	Decrease dairy products to reduce calcium content in urine. Increase meats, eggs, fish, prunes, grapes, and cranberry juice to acidify urine.
Calcium oxalate	Decrease dairy products to reduce calcium content in urine. Decrease colas, coffee, nuts, chocolate, rhubarb, and spinach to decrease oxalate content in urine.
Uric acid	Increase legumes, green vegetables, and fruits (except prunes, grapes, cranberries, and citrus fruits) to increase alkalinity of the urine. Decrease purine sources such as organ meats, gravies, red wines, goose, venison, and seafoods.
Struvite (magnesium ammonium phosphate)	Increase eggs, fish, prunes, and cranberries to increase the acidity of the urine. Decrease nuts, poultry, milk, cheese, peas, and corn to decrease phosphate content in the urine.
Cystine	Increase legumes, green vegetables, and fruits (except grapes, prunes, and cranberries) to increase the alkalinity of the urine.

CLINICAL MANIFESTATIONS

The patient with UPJ obstruction usually describes symptoms of several years' duration. Flank or back pain is the most common symptom. The discomfort felt is usually vague but intensifies with diuresis following an excessive fluid intake. Pyuria, hematuria, and bacteriuria may be present. A flank mass may occasionally be palpable.

MEDICAL DIAGNOSIS

Information from the history and physical examination is correlated with radiographic findings to establish the diagnosis. An excretory urogram is performed. Results usually indicate delayed excretion of urine from the affected kidney, as well as variable dilation of the renal pelvis and calices. Hydronephrosis may also be evident. In some instances, hydration or drug-induced diuresis may accentuate the effects of the obstructive lesion and facilitate diagnosis. Ultrasonography and computed tomography are sometimes done to document the nonfunctional status of the kidney.

MEDICAL MANAGEMENT

Treatment for UPJ obstruction is directed toward restoring renal function, providing relief of symptoms, eliminating infection, and correcting anatomic abnormalities. When renal function has not been compromised, pyeloureteroplasty is the procedure of choice for correcting UPJ obstruction. Various surgical techniques are utilized, but all are focused on restoring normal anatomic structure and function to the kidney. When prolonged and untreated obstruction has resulted in irreversible renal damage, a nephrectomy may be indicated.

URETEROVESICAL JUNCTION OBSTRUCTION

The ureterovesical junction (UVJ) is that part of the urinary system where the ureters enter the bladder. Normally, orifices are located on either side of the proximal border of the trigone area.

ETIOLOGY AND PATHOPHYSIOLOGY

The causes of obstruction at the UVJ are relatively few and are not always clearly defined. Obstruction may occasionally be caused by structure formation following an operative procedure, or it may be the result of an inflammatory process precipitated by ureteral instrumentation. More commonly, the cause is secondary to an infective or neoplastic condition or the presence of a stone at the junction. Certain anatomic pathologies can also cause blockage of the flow of urine through the UVJ. These include ureteroceles, bladder diverticula, and a condition referred to as obstructive megaureter (large or dilated ureter).

Pathophysiologic changes that occur as a result of obstruction at the UVJ are the same as those that occur with UPJ obstruction. Depending upon the degree of obstruction, vesicoureteral reflux may also occur.

CLINICAL MANIFESTATIONS

The presenting symptoms of UVJ obstruction are fever, flank pain, and varying degrees of gastrointestinal disturbances. When the blockage is the result of an obstructed megaureter, adult patients may complain of abdominal pain and hematuria.

MEDICAL DIAGNOSIS

The diagnosis of UVJ obstruction is made on the basis of findings from radiographic studies. Excretory urography, intravenous pyelography (IVP), and retrograde pyelography are the procedures most commonly performed.

MEDICAL MANAGEMENT

Treatment of UVJ obstruction is dependent on the cause of the problem. In general, obstruction that is the result of an infection, tumor, or urinary calculus is first managed medically; surgical intervention for these types of problems is considered on an individual basis. When the obstruction is related to presence of a ureterocele, diverticula, or megaureter, surgical removal is usually indicated.

URETERAL STRICTURE

ETIOLOGY AND PATHOPHYSIOLOGY

A ureteral stricture is an abnormal narrowing of the ureter. Although stricture formation can occur an any point in the ureter, there are three areas that are particularly prone to the development of this abnormality: the UPJ, the midureter, and the distal ureter above the UVJ.

The narrowing of the ureter can sometimes be attributed to congenital malformation or congenital stenosis. More often, this abnormality is acquired as a result of trauma, which can occur with operative procedures or instrumentation of the ureter, the passage or presence of stones within the ureter, or the inadvertent ligation of the ureter. Infections such as renal tuberculosis and retroperitoneal fibrosis can induce ureteral stricture formation. Cancerous tumors and their metastases, radiation therapy, and transplanted kidneys can also be etiologic factors for stricture formation in the ureter. Predisposing factors that have been identified include urinary extravasation, infection, and ischemia to the ureter.

The formation of ureteral strictures is due to a series of fibrotic tissue changes that lead to scar formation and increasing constriction of the ureter. Prolonged constriction decreases the perfusion of the tissues involved, impedes the development of a collateral vascular supply, and interrupts the flow of urine from the kidney to the bladder. As with other types of upper urinary tract obstruction, an untreated ureteral stricture can eventually lead to hydronephrosis and damage of the renal parenchyma.

CLINICAL MANIFESTATIONS

Frequently, patients with ureteral strictures are asymptomatic. The stricture may be found during a radiographic examination being performed for another problem. Symptoms include fever, flank pain, gastrointestinal disturbances, and hematuria. Abdominal pain may simulate the pain of appendicitis if the right ureter is obstructed. If the involved kidney is enlarged, it may be palpated or percussed on physical examination. Tenderness of the kidney may be present if infection exists.

MEDICAL DIAGNOSIS

Together with history and physical examination, the diagnosis of ureteral stricture is generally made by excretory urography and retrograde ureteropyelography. These studies often reveal the obstructive lesion, usually with varying degrees of hydronephrosis.

MEDICAL MANAGEMENT

The treatment of a ureteral stricture depends upon its location. For a stricture at the UPJ, a pyeloplasty may be necessary. Midureteral strictures are often treated by surgical excision of the stenotic area, followed by ureteroureterostomy (end-to-end anastomosis of the remaining portions of the ureter). Lower ureteral strictures and UVJ strictures may be treated by excision of the strictured portion of the ureter, followed by reimplantation of the ureter into the bladder wall. For cases involving extreme hydronephrosis, nephrectomy may be necessary.

Balloon dilation of ureteral strictures, utilizing a

special balloon catheter, has become a popular and successful treatment option for certain situations. The better success rate has been demonstrated with strictures caused by inflammatory processes or those that have been diagnosed on newly operated patients. This technique has not been successful with strictures caused by cancerous tumors or failed pyeloplasties or by radiation-induced strictures.

Application of the Nursing Process to the Care of Patients with Upper Urinary Tract Obstruction

PREOPERATIVE NURSING CARE

Assessment

Assess for signs of fever, flank pain, abdominal pain, and gastrointestinal disturbances. Note changes in the patient's voiding pattern as well as any signs of infection. As with any presurgical candidate, the patient's understanding of the condition, the procedure to be performed, and the postoperative routine is evaluated.

Nursing Diagnoses and Planning

Nursing diagnoses and related expected patient outcomes most commonly applicable to the preoperative patient with upper urinary tract obstruction include the following:

NDx: Knowledge deficit related to proposed treatment plan

Planning: Patient outcomes
1. Patient asks questions that are appropriate and related to presurgical teaching.
2. Patient demonstrates an understanding of the treatment plan.

NDx: Anxiety related to outcome of care and obstruction

Planning: Patient outcomes
1. Patient verbalizes reasons for anxiety.
2. Patient demonstrates decreased levels of anxiety.
3. Patient demonstrates effective coping skills.

Nursing Interventions

NDx: Knowledge deficit
Because most upper urinary tract obstructions are treated surgically, preoperative nursing interventions are directed toward preparing the patient for the upcoming surgical procedure. In addition to those activities, which are a part of the routine preoperative case, develop a teaching plan that describes the series of events that will take place. Provide an illustration of the urinary tract to reinforce the physician's explanation of the surgical procedure; this simple visual aid enhances preoperative teaching, and helps the patient understand the problem and proposed treatment plan. Because the patient will return from surgery with multiple drainage tubes, point out locations for drainage tube placement.

NDx: Anxiety
In addition to explaining the preoperative preparation and the surgical intervention to the patient, teach the patient some relaxation techniques. Allow time for the patient to express fears and concerns, and answer all questions as honestly as possible. Seek support from clergy or significant others when appropriate.

Evaluation

Evaluate the effectiveness of preoperative nursing care for a patient with upper urinary tract obstruction by comparing the patient's status with the expected patient outcomes. Examples of specific outcomes for patients with upper urinary tract obstruction have been provided in the Planning section.

POSTOPERATIVE NURSING CARE

Assessment

Postoperative assessment of the patient who has undergone surgical correction of an upper urinary tract obstruction includes determination of renal function. Check the patency of urinary drainage tubes, such as a nephrostomy tube or ureteral stent. Inspect the skin surrounding the insertion site of urinary drainage tube. Note any leakage of urine. Observe any urine drainage (whether outside the tube or within the tube) for its color and degree of hematuria. Monitor intake and output, and observe the patient for signs of fluid and electrolyte imbalance.

In addition to evaluating the function of the urinary system, check dressings over the surgical site for excessive or unusual drainage, and continually assess the patient for signs of infection, either of the surgical incision or of the urine and the urinary tract. Assess routine postoperative needs.

Nursing Diagnoses and Planning

Nursing diagnoses and related expected patient outcomes most commonly applicable to postoperative patients with upper urinary tract obstruction include the following:

NDx: Altered patterns of urinary elimination related to surgical procedure

Planning: Patient outcomes
1. Patient's urinary drainage tubes are patent.
2. Patient's urinary output is adequate in relation to their intake.

NDx: High risk for infection related to risk of urine stasis within drainage tubes

Planning: Patient outcomes
1. Patient is free of signs and symptoms of urinary tract infection.
2. Patient exhibits normal vital signs and laboratory data.

NDx: Impaired skin integrity related to leakage of urine around drainage tubes

Planning: Patient outcomes
1. Patient's skin around the drainage tube remains clean and dry and without signs of irritation.
2. Patient's skin around the drainage tube remains intact.

Nursing Interventions

NDx: Altered patterns of urinary elimination
Assess urinary drainage for patency. Ensure that urine drains freely. Monitor fluid intake and output. As the patient's mobility increases, ensure that urinary drainage bags are secure and draining freely. Empty bags at regular intervals.

NDx: High risk for infection
Observe for signs and symptoms of a urinary tract infection. Note color, consistency, and amount of urine. Monitor vital signs, reporting fever or unexplained tachycardia. Monitor white blood count, urinalysis, and urine culture for infection.

NDx: Impaired skin integrity
Keep skin around drainage tubes clean and dry. Reinforce or change dressings as needed. Observe the skin around drainage tubes for redness or breakdown.

Evaluation

Evaluate the effectiveness of postoperative nursing care for a patient with upper urinary tract obstruction by comparing the patient's status with the expected patient outcomes. Examples of specific outcomes for patients with upper urinary tract obstruction have been provided in the Planning section.

Lower Urinary Tract Obstruction

URETHRAL STRICTURE

ETIOLOGY AND PATHOPHYSIOLOGY

Urethral stricture is defined as a pathologic narrowing of the urethra. It is a problem that is more common in males because of the anatomic structure and length of the urethra. Females do develop urethral strictures, but it is more often a functional obstruction rather than an anatomic obstruction.

Urethral strictures can be congenital or acquired. Chronic infection, sexually transmitted diseases, and trauma to the lower urinary tract or pelvis all are causes of stricture formation. In females, trauma following intercourse, childbirth, vaginal surgery, or chronic urethritis can lead to the development of a urethral stricture. There are also iatrogenic causes of stricture formation; these include manipulation of the lower urinary tract during diagnostic procedures and transurethral surgery as well as the long-term use of indwelling urethral catheters. In some instances, neoplasms, venereal warts, and urethral polyps are underlying causes of urethral stricture formation.

A stricture develops because of the formation of collagen and fibrous tissue at the area of insult within the urethra. This leads to a narrowing and a loss of elasticity of the passageway. Consequently, urine flow out of the bladder is restricted, and dilation of the system proximal to the strictured area occurs.

CLINICAL MANIFESTATIONS

Patients with a urethral stricture usually have obstructive and irritative voiding symptoms. Obstructive symptoms include (1) decreased force of the urinary stream (one of the most common complaints), (2) hesitancy in initiating the urinary stream, (3) double voiding (patient voids and then is able to void again within 5 to 10 minutes), (4) postvoid dribbling, (5) interrupted urinary stream, (6) urinary retention (generally a slow developing, chronic problem), and (7) overflow incontinence. Irritative voiding symptoms include (1) dysuria, (2) frequency, (3) nocturia, and (4) urgency and urge incontinence.

MEDICAL DIAGNOSIS

A general and urologic history, coupled with selected diagnostic procedures, confirms the diagnosis of a urethral stricture. Diagnostic studies that are usually performed include urine cultures to identify the presence of any urinary tract infection, urine flow studies to measure the amount of decrease in the force of the urinary stream, and radiologic studies, such as a voiding cystourethrogram and urethrogram, to visualize the location and extent of the obstruction.

MEDICAL MANAGEMENT

The goal of treatment is to relieve the obstruction and eradicate any existing infection. The type of treatment selected depends on the location, length, and density of the stricture area.

Mechanical dilation of strictures is among the most common therapy instituted. It is a nonsurgical procedure that involves the use of urethral sounds (curved metal rods) that graduate in size up to #36 French. A local anesthetic is usually instilled into the urethra prior to the procedure. The sounds are then passed (starting with the smaller and working up to the larger sizes) into the urethra and through the strictured area to open it to approximately #22 French.

Another procedure often performed is the internal urethrotomy. This involves an incision of the strictured area under direct visualization through a specially designed endoscope. To prevent recurrence of the stricture after incision, a program of intermittent self-catheterization is sometimes recommended.

Urethroplasty, or surgical repair of the strictured area, is indicated when there is recurrence of a previously treated stricture, when dilation of the area is needed more frequently than every 6 months, when the strictured area is too large for treatment by dilation or urethrotomy, and when the stricture is the result of severe traumatic urethral injury (e.g., severed urethra). Urethroplasty is performed as either a one- or two-stage procedure. In the one-stage operation, the stricture is excised, and anastomosis of remaining urethral ends is carried out; a tissue graft over the anastomosed area may be used. In the two-step procedure, which is thought by some to have the higher success rate, the area of stricture is marsupialized (formation of a pouchlike structure) and allowed to heal. After about a 6-month period, the tissue is reapproximated to form a new urethra.

The newest treatment alternative for urethral strictures is laser photoradiation. Those using this therapy have had mixed results. Consequently, its place in the treatment of urethral strictures is still unknown.

MEATAL STENOSIS

ETIOLOGY AND PATHOPHYSIOLOGY

Stenosis of the external meatus is a problem that is seen in both adults and children. Meatal stenosis (or distal urethral stenosis, as the problem is sometimes referred to in women) can be either congenital or acquired. Congenital meatal stenosis in males is rare but is occasionally associated with hypospadias. In females, congenital distal urethral stenosis is a condition that is problematic in early childhood, but which typically disappears after puberty, possibly because of the production of estrogens.

Acquired meatal stenosis is caused by inflammation secondary to an infectious process. In females, it can also occur as a result of the trauma of a vaginal delivery.

In the male patient, meatal stenosis is seen as a membranous web of tissue running across the external urinary meatus. In females, there is a ring of stenosis that forms just inside the external urinary meatus; it is the result of collagen and inelastic tissue formation, similar to that which occurs during stricture formation. When severe meatal stenosis exists, complete bladder emptying could be compromised. However, the problem primarily affects the quality and control of the urinary stream.

CLINICAL MANIFESTATIONS

The signs and symptoms of meatal stenosis are much the same as those described for urethral stricture. In addition, the male patient may describe difficulty directing his urinary stream, which causes urine to deflect all over the bathroom; he may also find it necessary to hold the penis down during the act of voiding. A fine forceful stream, a prolonged voiding time, and terminal hematuria are other common complaints.

MEDICAL DIAGNOSIS

To confirm the diagnosis of meatal stenosis, a urethral calibration (measurement of the internal diameter of the urethral meatus with special sounds) is usually performed. In some male patients, this procedure may not be necessary because visible evidence of meatal stenosis may be seen upon examination of the penis. Additional diagnostic techniques, such as radiographic studies, are usually not done unless other problems within the urinary system are suspected.

MEDICAL MANAGEMENT

Meatal stenosis can be corrected by dilation with catheters up to #24 to #26 French. This is done at regular intervals over a specified period of time. To prevent infection during the course of the treatment period, antibiotic therapy is usually initiated.

Surgical intervention such as meatotomy may be performed in the male patient under local anesthesia. This procedure quite simply involves making an incision through the web of membranous tissue. If surgical intervention is indicated for the female with distal urethral stenosis, urethroplasty is performed.

Application of the Nursing Process to the Care of the Patient with Lower Urinary Tract Obstruction

PREOPERATIVE NURSING CARE

Assessment

Question the patient with lower urinary tract obstruction about the incidence of any previous urinary tract obstructions, urinary tract infections, injuries to the pelvis, or abdominal surgeries. Identify all symptoms the patient may be experiencing, and distinguish whether these are truly symptoms. Assess the patient for signs and symptoms of a urinary tract infection such as burning with urination or cloudy urine. Ask whether the patient has a discharge from the urethra.

Nursing Diagnoses and Planning

Nursing diagnoses and related expected patient outcomes most commonly applicable to the preoperative patients with lower urinary tract obstruction include the following:

NDx: Altered patterns of urinary elimination related to blockage of the urinary outlet

Planning: Patient outcomes
1. Patient voids at regular intervals.
2. Patient does not strain excessively or use force to empty the bladder.

NDx: Urinary retention related to obstruction of urine flow

Planning: Patient outcomes
1. Patient voids at regular intervals.
2. Patient expresses a sense of complete bladder emptying.

NDx: High risk for infection related to stasis of urine

Planning: Patient outcomes
1. Patient is free of signs and symptoms of a urinary tract infection.
2. Patient exhibits normal vital signs and laboratory data.

Nursing Interventions

NDx: Altered patterns of urinary elimination
Monitor closely the patient's pattern of urinary elimination. If appropriate, instruct the patient to keep a record of the time and amount of each void. Teach the patient to relax throughout urination rather than trying to strain or force the stream.

NDx: Urinary retention
Monitor the patient's fluid intake and output. Provide adequate fluids. Palpate the bladder for fulness. If retention is suspected, obtain an order for catheterization. Catheterize for residual urine.

NDx: High risk for infection
Observe for and document any signs and symptoms of a urinary tract infection. Monitor vital signs, reporting fever or unexplained tachycardia. Monitor white blood count, urinalysis, and urine culture for infection. Note the color, consistency, and amount of urine. Report any abnormalities.

Evaluation

Evaluate the effectiveness of preoperative nursing care for a patient with lower urinary tract obstruction by comparing the patient's status with the expected patient outcomes. Examples of specific outcomes for patients with lower urinary tract obstruction have been provided in the Planning section.

POSTOPERATIVE NURSING CARE

Assessment

The patient who has undergone surgical correction of a lower urinary tract obstruction is likely to have some type of urinary drainage tube, usually an indwelling Foley catheter. Check this tubing to be sure it is draining freely without obstruction. Note the color and quality of the urine passing through the tube.

Bladder spasms are not uncommon when the lower urinary tract has been manipulated. Assess the patient for any pain or discomfort that has resulted from the surgical treatment.

The development of a urinary tract infection can also occur following instrumentation of the urethra. Assess the patient for signs and symptoms of an infectious process.

Nursing Diagnoses and Planning

Nursing diagnoses and related expected patient outcomes most commonly applicable to postoperative patients with lower urinary tract obstruction include the following:

NDx: High risk for infection related to instrumentation of the lower urinary tract

Planning: Patient outcomes
1. Patient is free of signs and symptoms of a urinary tract infection.
2. Patient exhibits normal vital signs and laboratory data.

NDx: Pain related to the occurrence of bladder spasms

Planning: Patient outcomes
1. Patient expresses relief of pain and bladder spasms.
2. Patient gradually increases activity without discomfort.

Nursing Interventions

NDx: High risk for infection
Observe for and document any signs and symptoms of a urinary tract infection. Monitor vital signs, reporting fever or unexplained tachycardia. Monitor white blood count, urinalysis, and urine culture for infection. Note the color, consistency, and amount of urine. Report any abnormalities.

NDx: Pain
Any manipulation or instrumentation of the lower urinary tract causes discomfort. Administer analgesics and antispasmodics as necessary to provide the patient with relief of pain or bladder spasms. Limit the patient's activity because too much physical stress can precipitate bladder spasms as well as hematuria.

Evaluation

Evaluate the effectiveness of postoperative care for a patient with lower urinary tract obstruction by comparing the patient's status with the expected patient outcomes. Examples of specific outcomes for patients with lower urinary tract obstruction have been provided in the Planning section.

Trauma

Renal Trauma

Renal trauma is not uncommon and occurs in various blunt or penetrating injuries. In patients with severe multiple trauma, renal injuries are deferred to the priorities of resuscitation and stabilization of vital signs. Severe renal injuries require immediate surgical intervention at the same time that injuries to other vital organs (if present) are treated.

ETIOLOGY AND PATHOPHYSIOLOGY

The usual cause of renal trauma is blunt or penetrating injury to the kidney. Blunt renal trauma occurs more frequently than penetrating trauma. Approximately 60% to 85% of the renal trauma cases are blunt trauma injuries. Blunt trauma is caused by direct blows, sports injuries, or rapid deceleration injuries such as motor vehicle accidents or falls from heights. Penetrating renal trauma is caused by stabbing or gunshot wounds.

The kidneys are located in the upper retroperitoneal space, in front of the lower thoracic cage and beneath the liver, spleen, and diaphragm. Under normal circumstances, the kidneys are somewhat mobile. They are surrounded by fat, called Gerota's fascia, and are held in place only by their major blood vessels, which are attached to the aorta and vena cava. The renal capsule is a tough membrane that resists rupture.

Blunt renal trauma occurs when the kidney is violently and suddenly jarred out of its normal position. In the presence of bony fractures, such as lower rib or upper lumbar vertebral fractures, Gerota's fascia and the renal capsule may be penetrated, causing damage to the kidney's internal structure. If the trauma is great enough to rupture the major renal blood vessels, shock quickly occurs and represents a life-threatening emergency.

Penetrating renal trauma is frequently associated with other abdominal injuries that require immediate surgical repair. The severity of the trauma to the kidney depends on the location of the entry and exit wounds or the force of the blunt blow to the kidney.

CLINICAL MANIFESTATIONS

If the patient is conscious, blunt renal injuries may cause flank or upper abdominal pain. Other possible symptoms include flank or abdominal bruising, masses, or tenderness in the area of trauma. Lower rib fractures or injuries to nearby organs greatly increase the likelihood of renal injuries. Hematuria, either gross or microscopic, is common after renal trauma. The amount of hematuria is not a good indicator of the severity of the injury.

Penetrating renal injury is suspected when an entrance wound is present in the renal area. Symptoms reported by the conscious patient are not specific enough to diagnose renal injury. Because major blood loss and shock are likely when major blood vessels are involved, the patient must be closely monitored. Patients with gunshot wounds are transferred to the operating room, usually immediately after assessment, and after the diagnostic studies can be performed if time permits.

MEDICAL DIAGNOSIS

Classification of renal injury is necessary before treatment decisions are made. The four categories of renal injury are (1) contusion, (2) minor laceration, (3) major laceration, and (4) multiple laceration or shattered kidney.

Diagnostic studies are done as quickly as possible when renal trauma is evident. Urinalysis involves an evaluation for hematuria as well as the presence of other abnormalities. Hematuria is usually present with renal trauma; however, 10% to 40% of the patients with renal trauma do not have hematuria. The amount of hematuria does not correlate with the severity of the trauma, and the absence of hematuria does not rule out renal trauma.

When the patient is stable, an excretory urogram using high doses of contrast material is done to evaluate the renal injury. Blunt renal injury may be difficult to see on the urogram, and nephrotomograms or a CT scan may be necessary. When a kidney cannot be seen at all on a urogram, an emergency arteriogram or CT scan is done if time permits. The number of preoperative diagnostic studies performed depends upon the patient's condition. In severly injured patients, diagnosis may be made intraoperatively, and excretory urograms are performed with the patient on the operating table.

MEDICAL MANAGEMENT

Conservative treatment is appropriate for most patients with blunt trauma and few patients with penetrating renal trauma. Patients with minor injuries, microhematuria, and a normal urogram are discharged on limited activity for a time period. Patients with contusion or minor laceration are admitted and treated with bed rest. Urine evaluations are done to determine the presence and severity of the hematuria. Antibiotics may be administered. Most patients recover from these minor injuries without complications. Follow-up after discharge is necessary because late complications, including late bleeding and hypertension, may occur.

For patients with severe blunt renal trauma, and for most patients with penetrating renal trauma, surgical intervention is necessary. Approximately 15% of blunt injuries and 85% of penetrating injuries require exploration and repair. A midline abdominal incision is performed so that abdominal exploration can be done at the same time. As much functioning kidney as posssible is salvaged during the surgical repair. When a shattered kidney or multiple lacerations are present, a nephrectomy may be necessary.

The only exception to immediate surgery in severe renal trauma is when the need for a nephrectomy is evident in a clinically stable patient. In this case, the nephrectomy can be performed hours or days later.

Follow-up for up to 1 year after the penetrating renal trauma is important to rule out the potential for latent complications of surgical repair, including calcification, areas of nonfunction, and hypertension.

Application of the Nursing Process to the Care of the Patient with Renal Trauma

Assessment

Initial assessment of the patient with suspected renal trauma involves assessment of other systems in order of priority. Check the patient's respiratory and cardiovascular status first. Next, complete a neurologic assessment, following that with the assessment of any abdominal or pelvic injuries once the patient is stabilized. Specific renal injuries may not be apparent on assessment; thus, complete a general abdominal assessment, noting any bruising or penetrating wounds in the flank area. Ask the patient about areas of pain or tenderness, and observe for hematomas or swelling. Blunt injuries are the most difficult to assess and are not usually found without radiologic studies. If a penetrating wound is present, note the location of entrance and exit wounds and amount of bleeding and determine the type of wound (gunshot, stab). Check the urine for gross hematuria.

Nursing Diagnoses and Planning

Nursing diagnoses and related expected patient outcomes most commonly applicable to patients with renal trauma include the following:

NDX: Altered tissue perfusion, renal, related to hemorrhage from injury

Planning: Patient outcomes
1. Patient's renal function is adequate, without evidence of bleeding.
2. Patient's vital signs are within normal limits for the patient.

NDx: Pain related to trauma and manipulation during treatment

Planning: Patient outcomes
1. Patient reports a decrease in pain or that pain is tolerable.
2. Patient rests without interruptions from pain.

NDx: Anxiety related to traumatic event and fear of damage to the kidney

Planning: Patient outcomes
1. Patient expresses feelings about events that occurred and potential outcomes after treatment.
2. Patient reports decreased anxiety and appears relaxed.

Nursing Interventions

NDx: Altered tissue perfusion, renal
During the initial evaluation of the injury in the trauma suite or emergency room, focus nursing interventions on stabilizing the patient. Closely observe the patient for vital sign changes, which may indicate bleeding and impending shock. Note the amount of urine produced hourly, and document the data. Keep the patient on bed rest to prevent further trauma and to aid in healing of minor blunt trauma injuries.

If the patient required surgical intervention, during the postoperative period monitor the output carefully. Observe for gross hematuria. Check the flank incision for drainage. Take vital signs frequently, watching for changes. Monitor the laboratory data, noting the urinalysis and BUN and creatinine levels to assess for renal function. Report an output of less than 30 ml/hour to the attending physician.

NDx: Pain
Evaluate the patient's pain tolerance. Give analgesics as prescribed. Position the patient for comfort. Medicate the patient prior to engaging in care activities. Encourage the patient to practice relaxation exercises.

NDx: Anxiety
Explain all nursing activities to the patient, and allow the patient to participate in the care decisions. Let the patient verbalize fears and concerns about the injury and outcomes. Keep the patient informed about the renal status. Help the patient find coping strategies that are effective. Provide periods of rest and quiet as needed.

Evaluation

Evaluate the effectiveness of nursing care for the patient with renal trauma by comparing the patient's status with the expected patient outcomes. Examples of specific outcomes for patients with renal trauma have been provided in the Planning section.

Ureteral Trauma

Injuries to the ureter occur far more frequently from penetrating trauma than from blunt trauma. In either case, ureteral trauma is relatively rare, accounting for only a small percentage of injuries seen in trauma. Unfortunately, ureteral injury does not usually manifest itself until several days after the occurrence of the injury.

ETIOLOGY AND PATHOPHYSIOLOGY

The spinal column and large muscles of the back protect the ureters posteriorly. The abdominal wall and contents protect the ureters anteriorly. Because of this protection, only severe blunt trauma (such as falls from extreme heights) can cause ureteral trauma. The type of ureteral injury most frequently sustained during blunt trauma is disruption of the ureter at the UPJ.

Penetrating injuries, especially gunshot wounds, account for 95% of ureteral trauma from external causes. A bullet or stab wound can sever or nick the ureter at any point along its course from the kidney to the bladder. Injury to the ureter during difficult abdominal surgeries is much more common than penetrating or blunt causes of ureteral injury.

CLINICAL MANIFESTATIONS

There are no specific symptoms that lead to suspicion of ureteral injury. In most cases, the symptoms of ureteral trauma appear several days after the injury. Hematuria is present in most cases of ureteral injury from external causes. As with renal trauma, the amount of hematuria is not a good indicator of the severity of the injury. Penetrating ureteral trauma is suspected when entrance or exit wounds are in the ureteral area. Since most wounds are explored surgically, little time exists for symptomatic evaluation of the patient. Symptoms of a ureteral injury that have been present for several days include fever, flank pain, and infection with generalized abdominal symptoms of pain, tenderness, rigidity and nausea, vomiting, and paralytic ileus.

MEDICAL DIAGNOSIS

Diagnosis of ureteral injury is achieved by radiographic examinations or during surgery. Blunt trauma is usually evaluated with an excretory urogram. Extravasation of contrast material from the site of the ureteral disruption demonstrates the injury. Penetrating trauma is evaluated by exploratory surgery in most cases. Ureteral trauma is diagnosed at that time by intraoperative urogram or intravenously injected indigo carmine, which causes a blue discoloration of the tissue surrounding the site of injury.

MEDICAL MANAGEMENT

Ureteral trauma usually requires surgical repair. The type of surgery depends upon which section of the ureter has been injured. Upper ureteral injuries are repaired by pyeloplasty. Lower ureteral injuries are repaired by reimplantation into the bladder. Injuries in the middle of the ureter are corrected by an end-to-end anastomosis. Varying amounts of debridement of surrounding tissue may be necessary after bullet wounds. In most patients, ureteral stents or nephrostomy tubes are used postoperatively to divert urine away from the surgical area. Penrose drains or sumps may also be used.

Application of the Nursing Process to the Care of the Patient with Ureteral Trauma

The assessment, nursing diagnoses, expected patient outcomes, nursing interventions, and evaluation for patient with ureteral trauma are similar to those described previously for patients with renal trauma.

Bladder Trauma

The urinary bladder's anatomic location deep in the pelvis usually protects it from injury. Bladder trauma can occur, however, from blunt or penetrating injuries. Penetrating injuries account for only approximately one fourth of all bladder injuries. The more frequent cause of bladder trauma is blunt injuries that occur in pelvic fractures.

ETIOLOGY AND PATHOPHYSIOLOGY

The type of injury the urinary bladder sustains depends upon the amount of urine in the bladder at the time of injury. The empty bladder is more likely not to be injured or to receive less injury than the full bladder. Penetrating trauma is usually due to gunshot wounds or stab wounds. Blunt trauma is classified into three types of injuries: contusion, extraperitoneal, or intraperitoneal. Contusion is not usually a serious injury and does not require surgery. A contusion is often a partial thickness tear of the bladder wall. Penetration of the bladder wall by a bone fragment during pelvic fracture is an extraperitoneal rupture. Urine leaks out of the bladder into the area directly surrounding the bladder. Intraperitoneal rupture occurs when a severe blow to the lower abdomen causes intolerable strain on a full bladder. In response to the sudden increase in pressure, the full bladder ruptures at its weakest point, the dome, which is located at the top of the bladder. Urine leaks into the peritoneal cavity, around the bowel and nearby organs.

CLINICAL MANIFESTATIONS

Most patients with bladder trauma have gross hematuria. Other symptoms frequently seen are lower suprapubic or lower abdominal pain. There may be evidence of pelvic hematoma on rectal examination. The patient may report having received a direct blow to the abdomen.

Symptoms of shock are uncommon when the bladder injury is the only injury the patient sustained. However, additional injuries are frequently present, causing symptoms other than those noted. The multiple trauma patient may suffer from shock and require evaluation of life-threatening injuries initially.

MEDICAL DIAGNOSIS

A plain radiographic film of the abdomen is done initially to observe for pelvic fracture, calcifications, foreign bodies, or bullets. An intravenous urogram is performed to rule out ureteral or renal injury and to evaluate the shape of the bladder. The bladder injury may be seen on the urogram, but a cystogram is the best diagnostic tool for diagnosing the extent of the bladder injury. Because this requires catheterization, urethral trauma is first ruled out. Once the catheter is in place, small amounts to large amounts of contrast dye are instilled into the bladder. Small amounts of dye will demonstrate injuries at the base of the bladder. Large amounts are instilled to demonstrate injuries to the the top of the bladder. In female patients, a thorough pelvic examination is necessary to detect urethral or vaginal injury in addition to the bladder injury.

MEDICAL MANAGEMENT

Conservative management of minor bladder injuries consists of urinary catheter drainage until the wounds heal. A Foley catheter or suprapubic catheter is used, depending on the location of the injury. The progress of healing is evaluated periodically by cystogram until no extravasation of contrast dye is seen. Small amounts of sterile urine leaking into the area surrounding the bladder are usually not harmful to the patient and are gradually absorbed into the interstitial fluid. Antibiotics may be used during the prolonged catheter therapy to prevent urinary tract infections.

Penetrating wounds are surgically explored and repaired. Surrounding organs and tissue are assessed for damage, and the bladder injury is closed with absorbable sutures. A suprapubic catheter is used to divert drainage of urine away from the healing suture line. A large suprapubic tube is used for men, and a Foley catheter or a suprapubic tube is used for women, depending upon the location of the injury. Penrose drains may be used on either side of the bladder.

Patients with intraperitoneal and extraperitoneal bladder rupture caused by blunt trauma are usually treated with the same type of surgical intervention. Occasionally, in patients with minor ruptures, conservative treatment is used rather than surgery.

Application of the Nursing Process to the Care of the Patient with Bladder Trauma

Assessment

Treat the patient with a pelvic fracture as though a bladder injury exists. Evaluate the urine for hematuria. If the patient cannot void, do not catheterize the patient until a urethral injury is ruled out. If the patient is able to void easily, the injury is probably minor. Serious pelvic fractures with bladder injury involve profound blood loss and shock, thus genitourinary assessment may be delayed until the patient is stabilized.

After assessment of vital signs, assess for symptoms of genitourinary injury. Ask the patient about the nature of the trauma sustained and whether a blow to the abdomen occurred. Patients with severe intraperitoneal ruptures may appear to have an "acute abdomen," especially if several hours have passed since the injury. If the patient reports an inability to void since the injury, bladder rupture is possible.

Nursing Diagnoses and Planning

Nursing diagnoses and related expected patient outcomes most commonly applicable to patients with bladder trauma are similar to those described previously for patients with renal trauma and also include the following:

NDx: Urinary retention related to trauma

Planning: Patient outcomes
1. Patient has an adequate balanced intake and output.
2. Patient resumes normal pattern of voiding after treatment of injury.

NDx: High risk for infection related to disruption of the urinary system

Planning: Patient outcomes
1. Patient's vital signs remain within normal ranges for the patient.
2. Patient presents no signs of infection such as bacteremia, bacteriuria, fever, or dysuria.

Nursing Interventions

NDx: Urinary retention
Check the catheter drainage for patency. Encourage increased fluid intake if not contraindicated. Administer analgesics and antispasmotics as prescribed to relieve spasms and pain and to prevent interference with urinary output. Monitor the patients laboratory data. Note hematuria and document the data. After the catheter is removed, encourage the patient to void frequently and measure each voiding. Note the color, consistency, and amount of urine. Use strategies to assist the patient with voiding if there is difficulty.

NDx: High risk for infection
Monitor the patient for symptoms of peritonitis, such as increased abdominal pain, tenderness, fever, and unstable vital signs. Check the incision for signs of infection, and keep drainage from Penrose drains away from the suture line. Assess the urine for cloudiness, sediment, or foul odor. Report any early signs of infection to the attending physician. Keep catheters patent and the drainage system closed, and use aseptic dressing changes when removing and replacing the surgical dressings. Tell the patient to report any untoward symptoms. Review the urinalysis and urine cultures for indications of infection.

Evaluation

Evaluate the effectiveness of nursing care of the patient with bladder trauma by comparing the patient's status with the expected patient outcomes. Examples of specific outcomes for patients with bladder trauma have been provided in the Planning section.

Urethral Trauma

Injuries to the urethra are far more common in men than in women, and are much more difficult to repair in men. In women, the urethra is entirely internal and somewhat mobile. The male urethra has some nonmobile areas, which are more susceptible to injury than other parts of the urethra. When trauma occurs to these areas, it is difficult to diagnose and correct. Long-term complications are common.

ETIOLOGY AND PATHOPHYSIOLOGY

The urogenital diaphragm is an important anatomic landmark because male urethral injuries are classified as to whether they occur above it or below it. Anterior urethral injuries occur below the urogenital diaphragm. The anterior portion of the urethra is very mobile, and it is injured most frequently from straddle-type injuries such as a fall in which the patient lands sitting, or by a direct blow or penetration along the course of the lower urethra.

Posterior urethral injuries occur between the bladder neck and the urogenital diaphragm. The presence of the prostate gland and the numerous ligaments make this portion of the urethra immobile in the male. The cause of injuries to the posterior urethra is usually severe blunt trauma such as pelvic fracture.

Anterior and posterior urethral injuries may be either complete or partial. Other causes of urethral injury are self-manipulation injury from a variety of objects or injury during medical instrumentation.

CLINICAL MANIFESTATIONS

The presence of blood at the urinary meatus is a sign of urethral injury. The patient may complain of difficulty voiding or may be unable to void at all. Pain is present at the site of injury or throughout the lower abdomen, depending upon the extent of the trauma and cause. Evidence of penile or perineal hematoma is common. Anterior urethral injuries are usually easy to see. The penis may be swollen with blood and urine if the patient has tried to void.

If the urethral injury has been present for several hours or days, symptoms of inflammation and sepsis result. Swelling can involve the penis, scrotum, and perineal area in the male and the entire perineal area in the female. In complete posterior urethral disruption, a rectal examination yields only the presence of a hematoma because the prostate and bladder are displaced superiorly.

MEDICAL DIAGNOSIS

A plain abdominal film is completed initially to check for pelvic fracture. When blood is present at the urethral meatus, a retrograde urethrogram is done. This reveals the site of injury by demonstrating extravasation of contrast dye. If no extravasation is seen, the injury is likely to be either a contusion or a small tear. Urethroscopy may be done to confirm the diagnosis of minor injuries. Excretory urogram and cystogram are done to complete the evaluation when urethral continuity is largely intact.

MEDICAL MANAGEMENT

Urethral contusions with minimal hematuria in a patient who is able to void does not require treatment. Urethral tears without extravasation on urethrogram are treated with a Foley catheter for 7 to 10 days or suprapubic drainage, allowing the injury to heal. Most urethral injuries are treated in this manner.

If surgery is necessary, the type of surgical repair performed depends upon the severity of the injury. When serious multiple injuries exist, urinary diversion by placement of a suprapubic cystostomy is performed, and urethral reconstruction is delayed until other injuries can be treated. When only urethral injury exists, particularly a posterior injury, surgical reconstruction is performed immediately. Anterior tears are repaired by suturing the tear or laceration.

Guidelines for Application of the Nursing Process to the Care of the Patient with Urethral Trauma

Ask the patient to describe the injury sustained and the length of time that has passed since it occurred. When serious multiple injuries exist, assess vital systems initially. Once the patient is stable, assess the genitourinary injuries.

In the male, assess the external genitalia. Assess the location and type of visible external penetrating wounds. Inspect the penis, scrotum, and perineal area for hematomas or swelling. In inflamed areas, palpation may reveal fluid underneath, the result of extravasation of urine during voiding. Assess the patient for symptoms of infection if significant time has passed since the injury.

In the female, check the perineal area for hematomas. Ask whether the patient has difficulty voiding. Note any bloody discharge. Ask about pain or burning during urination.

In all patients, examine the urinary meatus for blood. If blood is present, do not catheterize the patient until further medical examination has occurred. Ask the patient when the last voiding occurred. Send a voided specimen to the laboratory for assessment for hematuria and bacteria.

The nursing diagnoses, related expected patient outcomes, and nursing interventions most commonly applicable to patients with urethral trauma are similar to those described previously for patients with renal or bladder trauma.

Neoplasia

A neoplasia or tumor is a pathologic overgrowth of tissue, which can be either benign or malignant, solid or cystic, superficial or invasive, as well as primary or metastatic. Many types of tumors can be found in the urinary tract, and eventually, all neoplasias will affect its function. This section discusses those tumors that are the most common and that pose the biggest threat to the integrity of the urinary system—primary malignant tumors.

Cancer of the Kidney

ETIOLOGY AND PATHOPHYSIOLOGY

Malignant tumors of the kidney are the second most frequently occurring cancers in the urinary tract; bladder cancers are more common. As many as 18,000 new cases of renal cancer are diagnosed in the United States each year, and approximately 45%

of those with the disease die annually. The incidence of kidney cancer is higher (2:1) in males than in females and increases in frequency with age.

The types of malignant tumors generally found in the kidney are renal cell carcinoma (adenocarcinoma of the kidney), tumors of the renal collecting system (transitional cell epithelioma), Wilms' tumor (nephroblastoma), and sarcoma. Of these, renal cell carcinoma is the most frequently diagnosed tumor and accounts for more than 80% of all cases of kidney cancer. It is a disease that causes great concern, yet is challenging to diagnose and treat. Because of the predominance of renal cell carcinoma over other types of malignant renal tumors, the discussion that follows is specific to this condition.

The cause of renal cell carcinoma is unclear, and research continues in an attempt to identify sources of the disease, as well as groups at risk for developing it. Facts that are known about renal cell carcinoma include the following: (1) it primarily affects men older than age 40; (2) it is more often seen in urban areas than in rural areas; and (3) it is associated with the use of tobacco, especially that used in pipes and cigars.

Renal cell carcinoma usually affects only one kidney, and apparently originates in the proximal convoluted tubule. The tumor typically grows into the renal medulla, but can extend downward to the renal pelvis or out to the renal capsule and perinephric fat. Not uncommon is the extension of the tumor into the renal vein and inferior vena cava. In some instances, a renal cell carcinoma may grow large enough to impinge upon or invade surrounding muscles and abdominal organs. Enlargement of the affected kidney, as well as hemorrhage and necrosis, is the direct result of tumor growth.

Metastasis of a renal cell carcinoma occurs in about one fourth of cases. Common sites for metastasis are the lungs, lymph nodes, adrenal gland, liver, opposite kidney, brain, and bone.

CLINICAL MANIFESTATIONS

Gross or microscopic hematuria, flank pain, and a palpable flank mass are considered classic symptoms of the presence of a renal cell carcinoma. Ironically, this triad of symptoms is probably present in less than half of the patients with the disease. More often, patients with renal cell carcinoma present with symptoms unrelated to the urinary tract; these are usually vague complaints that are common to a number of other conditions. For example, a persistent fever or gastrointestinal disturbances (anorexia, constipation, nausea, or vomiting) may be the first and only symptoms in a patient with renal cell carcinoma.

MEDICAL DIAGNOSIS

The diagnosis of renal cell carcinoma is made on the basis of findings from radiographic evaluation. An excretory urogram is the study most frequently performed, because it allows for visualization of the kidney's collecting system and permits full assessment of renal contour. Other examinations such as nephrotomograms, renal sonography, CT scan, angiography, or magnetic resonance imaging are used to more specifically define the extent of the tumor or when findings from the intravenous urogram are inconclusive.

MEDICAL MANAGEMENT

Treatment for renal cell carcinoma is immediate surgical removal of the tumor. A radical nephrectomy is usually performed. This procedure is done through a transabdominal, thoracoabdominal, or extrapleural interspace incision and involves removal of the affected kidney as well as Gerota's fascia, the upper ureter, and at times, the adrenal gland. In some instances, lymph nodes are also excised. When the tumor has invaded the abdomen or vena cava, it is removed and resected as completely as possible.

Application of the Nursing Process to the Care of the Patient Undergoing a Nephrectomy for Cancer of the Kidney

Assessment

In the preoperative period, assess the overall health of the patient with renal cell carcinoma. Because the tumor can affect a number of different abdominal structures and can metastasize to several different locations in the body, a system-by-system approach should be taken to establish the patient's current condition. Note the patient's nutritional status, including eating habits. Check the urinary status, assessing for signs of infection such as fever, discolored urine, or difficulty with urination.

Assess the patient's understanding of the disease process and the treatment plan. Note any misunderstandings.

In the immediate postoperative period, assess the patient's fluid and electrolyte status, because a significant amount of blood is lost during radical nephrectomy. Find out exactly how much blood was lost during the procedure. If replacement fluid was given during surgery, determine the type and amount administered. Assess vital signs, fluid intake and output, hemoglobin and hematocrit results, and urine specific gravity.

Evaluate the patient's respiratory status, because breathing may be compromised as a result of the location and size of the incision necessary for the radical nephrectomy. Respiratory function may also be limited if the patient is experiencing significant discomfort. Assess for pain and the need for analgesia.

Infection is always a threat when the urinary tract has been manipulated or disrupted. Assess for signs and symptoms of infection, noting any temperature elevation, redness at the surgical site, cloudy urine, or discharge.

Assess the patency of any urinary or wound drainage tubes. Note the color and quantity of drainage fluids. Because excessive drainage (sometimes urine) from the surgical site is not uncommon, inspect the area carefully, and note the need for dressing reinforcement or change of dressing.

Once the immediate postoperative period has passed, assess the patient's incision for evidence of wound healing. Evaluate the pattern of bowel elimination. Check the patient for the presence of paresthesia over the surgical site, because peripheral nerves are cut during surgery.

Nursing Diagnoses and Planning

Nursing diagnoses and related expected patient outcomes most commonly applicable to patients undergoing a nephrectomy for cancer of the kidney include the following:

NDx: Ineffective breathing pattern related to pain from the surgical site

Planning: Patient outcomes
1. Patient maintains an effective breathing pattern.
2. Patient coughs, turns, and breathes deeply every 2 hours.
3. Patient's lungs are clear to auscultation.

NDx Fluid volume deficit related to excessive loss from surgery

Planning: Patient outcomes
1. Patient's vital signs remain stable.
2. Patient has balanced fluid intake and output.
3. Patient's hemoglobin and hematocrit values remain within normal limits.
4. Patient's blood chemistry levels remain within normal limits.

NDx: Anxiety related to the diagnosis of cancer and the uncertain outcome of treatment

Planning: Patient outcomes
1. Patient verbalizes fears and concerns related to diagnosis and treatment.
2. Patient asks questions related to fears and concerns.
3. Patient reports decrease in anxiety and appears relaxed.

NDx: Pain related to manipulation during surgery

Planning: Patient outcomes
1. Patient states that pain is decreased or relieved by analgesia.
2. Patient participates in care without apparent discomfort.
3. Patient is able to rest without interruption from pain.

NDx: Knowledge deficit: nature of surgery and follow-up care

Planning: Patient outcomes
1. Patient verbalizes the procedure as discussed by the physician and the measures necessary to maintain health of the remaining kidney after discharge.
2. Patient asks questions about the follow-up care.
3. Patient reports accurate information about the directions given.

Nursing Interventions

NDx: Ineffective breathing pattern
Auscultate the breath sounds frequently, and note any abnormalities. In the postoperative period, respiratory function may be compromised. Check for dyspnea, shallow breathing, or tachypnea. Position the patient to facilitate maximum respiratory efforts, such as in a semi-Fowler's position. Encourage the patient to cough, deep breathe, and turn frequently, at least every 2 hours. Also encourage the patient to use incentive spirometer, as instructed, every hour while awake.

NDx: Fluid volume deficit
Nursing care postoperatively is centered on preventing complications. Check the fluid intake and output carefully, assessing it every 4 hours or more frequently as needed. The immediate postoperative period is the most critical in terms of fluid volume. The electrolyte and fluid balance is very labile at this time. Watch for vital sign changes indicating a change in volume status. Check the laboratory data such as the urine specific gravity and the hemoglobin and hematocrit values. Note changes and report them. Increase intravenous fluids as ordered to maintain appropriate output and blood pressure. Measure output hourly and document the results.

NDx: Anxiety
Allow time for the patient to express fears and concerns, and answer all questions as honestly as possible. Seek support from clergy or significant others when appropriate. Include the family in counseling sessions. Allow the patient to make choices about care when appropriate. Explain all procedures prior to initiating them. Schedule time for the patient to rest as needed. Encourage relaxation exercises.

NDx: Pain
For severe postoperative pain, administer analgesics as prescribed. In addition to relief of pain, this aids in respiratory function by promoting a more effective breathing pattern because the respiratory mus-

Chart 26–3.

NURSING GUIDE TO PATIENT EDUCATION FOR SELF-MANAGEMENT: SELF-CARE FOR MAINTAINING THE HEALTH OF THE REMAINING KIDNEY

Instruct the patient to:

Drink at least six to eight glasses of liquid per day.
Void when the urge is felt.
Maintain a program of moderate activity.
Maintain acidity of urine by eating meats, eggs, poultry, fish, grapes, whole grains, and cranberry and prune juice; limit intake of milk and carbonated beverages.
Wipe perineum from front to back (women only).
Keep pernineal area clean and dry.
Take prophylactic anti-infectives as prescribed.
Report signs and symptoms of an infection immediately.
Notify physician if a cold or other infection persists for more than 3 days or if unable to maintain fluid intake.
Inform health care workers of nephrectomy so that measures can be taken to protect kidney.
Avoid activities that could cause trauma to remaining kidney (e.g., contact sports, horseback riding).
Consult physician before taking any medications that may be nephrotoxic.
Follow instructions to prevent stone formation if nephrectomy was done for calculi.
Follow instructions for controlling blood pressure if nephrectomy was done because of hypertension.

Data from Ulrich SP, Canale SW, Wendell SA. Nursing care planning guides. 2nd ed. Philadelphia: WB Saunders, 1990, pp 531–532.

cles are not restricted by discomfort. Administer analgesics prior to treatments and prior to sleep. Use relaxation techniques to relieve tension, stress, and pain, and position the patient for comfort. Teach the patient how to use patient-controlled analgesia (PCA), if ordered.

NDx: Knowledge deficit: nature of surgery and follow-up care
Explain the surgical procedure to the patient, including the expectations postoperatively. Describe the equipment the patient will see postoperatively and the necessity for it. Discuss the discharge plans with both the patient and family. Include information about the signs and symptoms of wound infection prior to discharge as well as other complications. Allow time for questions. Caution the patient against lifting heavy objects until allowed by the physician. Encourage the patient to avoid activities that would strain the flank area. Explain interventions to maintain the health of the remaining kidney as described in Chart 26–3.

Evaluation

Evaluate the effectiveness of nursing care for a patient undergoing a nephrectomy for cancer of the kidney by comparing the patient's status with the expected patient outcomes. Examples of specific outcomes for patients undergoing a nephrectomy for cancer of the kidney have been provided in the Planning section.

Cancer of the Renal Pelvis and Ureter

ETIOLOGY AND PATHOPHYSIOLOGY

Primary malignant tumors of the renal pelvis and ureter are extremely rare and account for fewer than 7% of all urinary tract carcinomas. The most common type of tumor found in this part of the urinary tract is transitional cell carcinoma that develops from the uroepithelium. This is also the most frequently occurring tumor in the bladder. Its incidence is three times greater in males than in females. Chemical carcinogens, phenacetin, cigarette smoking, and chronic infection and inflammation of the upper urinary tract are possible causes of tumor growth. The presence of a transitional cell carcinoma in the renal pelvis or ureter increases the likelihood of the same type of tumor developing in the bladder.

CLINICAL MANIFESTATIONS

The most common symptoms in patients with a tumor of the renal pelvis or ureter are hematuria and flank pain. Some patients also present with costovertebral angle tenderness or generalized symptoms such as weight loss and anorexia. The majority of patients, however, are asymptomatic.

MEDICAL DIAGNOSIS

Tumors of the renal pelvis and ureter are difficult to detect; therefore, a number of different diagnostic tests are performed to locate the lesion, define its extent, and confirm the diagnosis. Radiologic examination includes one or more of the following: excretory urogram, retrograde pyelogram, renal ultrasound, CT scan, and renal angiography. A ureteroscopy may also be performed in order to directly visualize the area in question, and voided urine samples or brush biopsy specimens may be obtained for cytologic examination. (Refer to Chapter 25 for an explanation of the diagnostic tests.)

MEDICAL MANAGEMENT

Treatment for cancer of the renal pelvis and ureter is surgical removal of the tumor. The actual procedure performed depends upon the location and extent of the tumor and may be either a partial nephrectomy, nephrectomy, or radical nephrectomy.

Application of the Nursing Process to the Care of the Patient with Cancer of the Renal Pelvis and Ureter

The assessment, nursing diagnoses, expected patient outcomes, nursing interventions, and evaluation for patients with cancer of the renal pelvis and ureter are similar to those described previously for patients with cancer of the kidney. When there is extension of the tumor into the bladder, nursing care activities as described for the patient with cancer of the bladder would apply.

Cancer of the Bladder

ETIOLOGY AND PATHYSIOLOGY

Malignant tumors of the bladder are the most frequently occurring tumors within the urinary system. However, when the entire genitourinary system is considered, prostate tumors are far more prevalent. Over 40,000 new cases of bladder cancer are diagnosed each year. The number of deaths from the disease are more than 10,000 annually. Five-year survival rates are as high as 90% for patients who have received treatment of superficial tumors. When tumor growth is extensive, the 5-year survival rate drops to approximately 10% to 50%.

The cause of bladder cancer has been attributed to a number of environmental and occupational health hazards. Among the most common are chemicals used by industrial workers in dyestuff manufacture, rubber manufacture, coal gas production, sewage work, and textile printing. It has been theorized using cigarettes and artificial sweeteners as well as coffee drinking can increase one's risk of bladder cancer. Patients who have undergone pelvic irradiation, who have a history of chronic infection and inflammation of the urinary tract, who have been treated with cyclophosphamide, or who were born with extrophy of the bladder (a congenital condition in which the bladder develops outside the abdomen) are also at risk for developing cancer of the bladder.

The incidence of bladder cancer is three times greater in men than in women and affects whites twice as often as blacks. It is a condition generally seen in patients older than the age of 40.

There are three types of tumors found in the bladder: transitional cell carcinoma, squamous cell carcinoma, and adenocarcinoma. Of these, transitional cell carcinoma is the most common, accounting for approximately 90% of all bladder cancers.

Transitional cell carcinoma develops in the epithelial lining of the bladder. The tumors can appear in many different forms but are generally identified as being papillary or nonpapillary lesions. Papillary tumors are usually superficial lesions that grow outward from the mucosa. Nonpapillary tumors are solid growths that tend to extend deep into the bladder wall and that are more likely to metastasize. Common sites of metastasis are the lymph nodes, liver, lungs, and bone.

CLINICAL MANIFESTATIONS

The most common symptom in patients with cancer of the bladder is hematuria. The presence of blood in the urine may be a gross or microscopic finding and can occur with each voiding or intermittently. As was previously mentioned, the amount and severity of hematuria do not correlate with the presence or absence of a disease state. However, it is important to note that in the patient with hematuria, cancer is considered as a valid diagnosis until disproven.

In addition to hematuria, the patient may experience irritative voiding symptoms such as frequency, urgency, and dysuria. These symptoms are often associated with cancer in situ.

MEDICAL DIAGNOSIS

The medical diagnosis is made on the basis of symptoms, history, and diagnostic tests. The goal is to determine the extent of the cancerous lesion in order to classify it according to the stage of penetration or invasiveness into the bladder wall. This dif-

Table 26–14. STAGING AND TREATMENT FOR BLADDER CANCER

STAGE	DESCRIPTION	TREATMENT
O	Carcinoma in situ Papillary tumor—no invasion	1. Transurethral resection 2. Intravesical chemotherapy 3. Lasers 4. Interstitial irradiation 5. Intravesical immunotherapy
A	Papillary tumor—lamina propria invasion	
B1	Superficial muscle invasion	
B2	Deep muscle invasion	1. Radical cystectomy and urinary diversion 2. Radiation therapy in inoperable patients
C	Invasion of perivesical fat	
D1	Invasion of contiguous viscera Involvement of pelvic nodes	1. External radiation 2. Systemic chemotherapy
D2	Involvement of juxtaregional nodes Distant metastases	

ferentiation of bladder tumors helps to delineate the appropriate method of treatment (Table 26–14).

To diagnose cancer of the bladder, voided urine samples are collected for cytologic examination. Radiologic studies, which may include an excretory urogram or a CT scan, are then performed. Finally, a cystourethroscopy is performed and a biopsy taken of the suspect lesion. In many instances, random biopsies of apparently normal tissue are also obtained to help determine the extent of disease.

MEDICAL MANAGEMENT

The type of treatment initiated for cancer of the bladder depends upon the form of tumor (papillary versus nonpapillary) and the stages of the disease. A variety of therapies for treatment of bladder cancer exist. These are reviewed here.

TREATMENT OF PAPILLARY OR SUPERFICIAL BLADDER CANCER

1. Transurethral Resection. This surgical procedure is the initial and most common treatment for superficial bladder cancer. It involves endoscopic removal of the tumor(s). Assessment of the urinary tract for the recurrence of cancerous lesions is required every 3 to 6 months following tumor resection.
2. Intravesical Chemotherapy. This therapy allows for high concentrations of chemotherapeutic agents to be instilled directly into the bladder. The advantage to this treatment is that patients avoid toxic side effects that occur with systemic administration of the chemotherapeutic agents. Intravesical chemotherapy is used when superficial bladder cancer is widespread and transurethral resection would not be effective. More frequently though, it is used as an adjunctive treatment after transurethral resection surgery to decrease the number of tumors and the time between recurrences of the tumors.
3. Laser Therapy. The use of lasers to treat superficial bladder tumors is becoming increasingly common. One advantage to this type of treatment is that multiple tumors can be eradicated without administering anesthesia to the patient. Additionally, blood loss is minimized, trauma to the normal tissue surrounding the tumor is avoided, and tumor spread is prevented by vaporization of the cancerous tissue.
4. Interstitial Radiation. Although external radiation of superficial bladder tumors has not been effective, recent studies from other countries suggest that radium implants are successful in preventing extension and recurrence of the disease.

TREATMENT OF NONPAPILLARY OR MUSCLE INVASIVE BLADDER CANCER

1. Segmental or Partial Cystectomy. This procedure may be performed when there is a single, well-defined tumor in the bladder that is not accessible to treatment by transurethral resection. The overall objective is to remove only that portion of the bladder affected by tumor without disrupting or injuring the ureters, bladder neck, or prostate.
2. Intravesical Immunotherapy. Some urologists have had success in managing, or curing, selected patients with nonpapillary disease by intravesical immunotherapy. The treatment involves the instillation of bacille Calmette-Guérin (BCG) into the bladder. A schedule is established in which the instillation of the BCG is repeated as often as every 5 to 7 days for a 6-week course. At a designated time after the treatments are discontinued, the bladder is rebiopsied. If the tumor has recurred, other treatment options are considered. If there is no evidence of tumor, the patient status is monitored by cystoscopy every 3 months initially, then 6 months to 1 year.
3. Radical Cystectomy. This procedure is performed when the bladder cancer is not treatable by conservative measures or when there is recurrence of disease (and the cancer has invaded the muscle wall) following treatment by conservative therapies. In the male patient, radical cystectomy involves removal of the bladder as well as the prostate, seminal vesicles, and proximal urethra. A total urethrectomy is performed if the prostatic urethra is affected by the tumor. In the female patient, the bladder, entire urethra, anterior vaginal wall, uterus, cervix, fallopian tubes, and ovaries are removed. Excision of pelvic lymph nodes is routine in either instance.

Once a radical cystectomy is complete, a means of urinary diversion is created. This procedure is done at the same time as the cystectomy. The

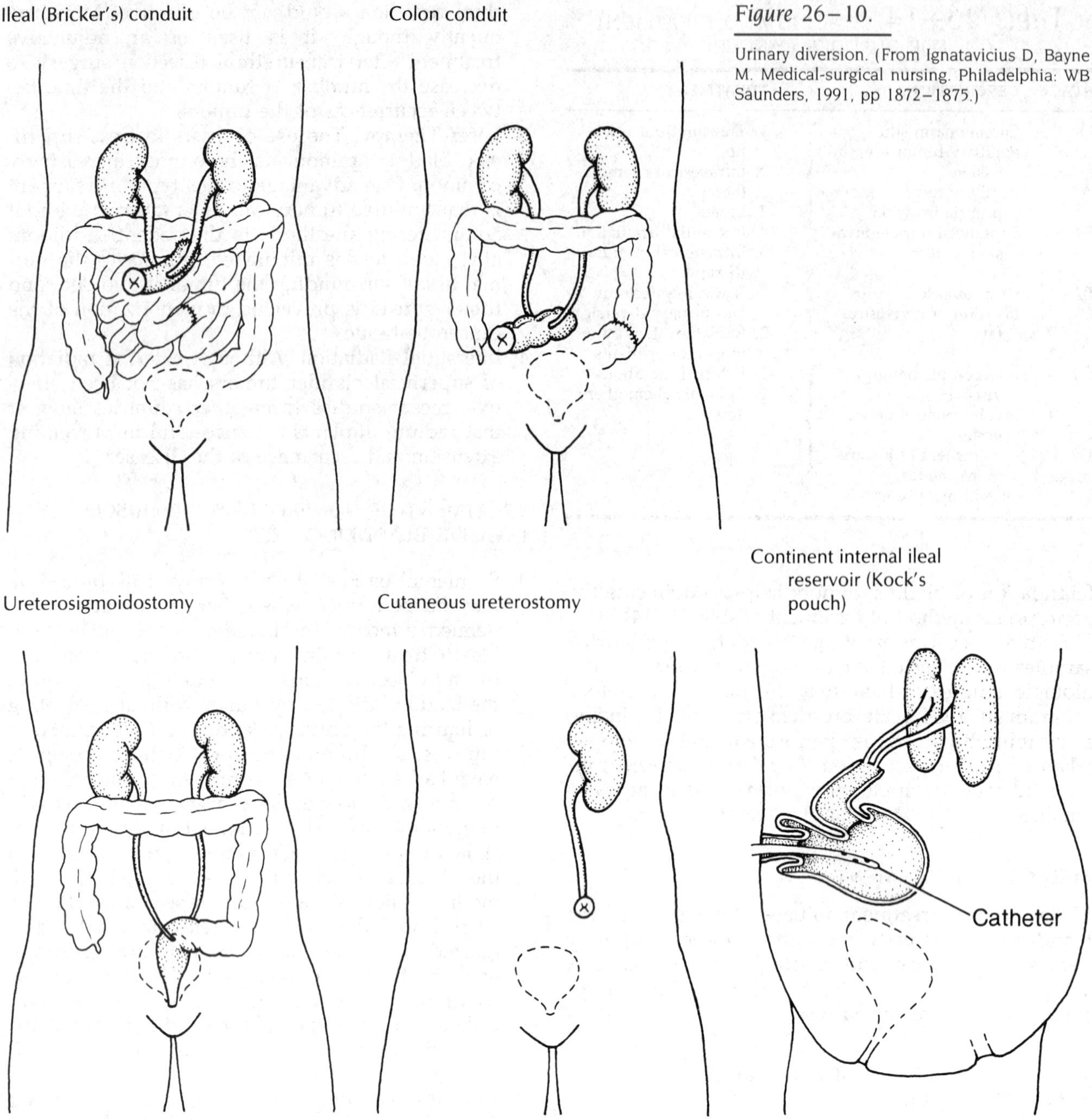

Figure 26–10.

Urinary diversion. (From Ignatavicius D, Bayne M. Medical-surgical nursing. Philadelphia: WB Saunders, 1991, pp 1872–1875.)

types of urinary diversions most frequently constructed are the ileal conduit, the colon conduit, the cutaneous ureterostomy, and the continent internal ileal reservoir (Fig. 26–10). A ureterosigmoidostomy may also be constructed, but it has many disadvantages and thus is not the surgery of choice in most cases.

4. Radiation Therapy. External radiotherapy is used to treat, and sometimes cure, malignant bladder tumors in very elderly patients thought to be poor surgical candidates, or those who have tumors that are considered to be inoperable. Radiation therapy may also be done preoperatively to shrink a bladder tumor prior to a cystectomy. In patients with advanced metastatic cancer, it is used as a palliative treatment. The use of interstitial radiation to treat nonpapillary tumors is also promising. For these types of tumors, irridium needles are inserted through an open bladder directly into the tumor. They are left in place for a period of several days, then removed percutaneously.
5. Systemic Chemotherapy. Chemotherapeutic agents such as cisplatin and doxorubicin (Adriamycin) are administered to patients for palliative treatment of nonpapillary bladder tumors. In some instances, patients experience remission of the disease after treatment.

Application of the Nursing Process to the Care of the Patient with Papillary or Superficial Bladder Tumors

Assessment

Check the patient's history and current findings, focusing on any predisposing or risk factors that may have precipitated the development of a bladder tumor. Evaluate the patient's usual pattern of urinary elimination, and note any irritative or unusual voiding symptoms. Obtain a urine specimen to check for the presence of hematuria. Review laboratory results, noting the urine culture and the presence of bacteria. Explore generalized complaints such as weight loss, fatigue, anorexia, diarrhea, constipation, or fever. Finally, assess the patient's level of understanding about the disease and the proposed treatment plan. This assessment is applicable in the pretreatment and posttreatment phases for the patient with a papillary or superficial bladder tumor.

Nursing Diagnoses and Planning

Nursing diagnoses and related expected outcomes most commonly applicable to patients with papillary or superficial bladder tumors include the following:

NDx: Altered patterns of urinary elimination related to vesical irritation from the presence of bladder tumors

Planning: Patient outcomes
1. Patient expresses relief of voiding symptoms.
2. Patient's urine has a decrease in blood and an absence of bacteria.
3. Patient voids appropriate amounts of urine.

NDx: Knowledge deficit: nature of the disorder and the treatment plan

Planning: Patient outcomes
1. Patient asks questions that are appropriate to health teaching.
2. Patient verbalizes an understanding of the disorder and the proposed treatment plan.

Nursing Interventions

NDx: Altered patterns of urinary elimination
Offer measures to help the patient relieve irritating voiding symptoms. Warm baths, a routine of timed voiding, or the administration of analgesia may lessen the urinary tract discomfort. Since bleeding is a common problem, obtain urine specimens regularly, and perform dipstick checks for hematuria. Encourage fluids unless contraindicated. If an infection is suspected, send a urine specimen for culture to the laboratory.

NDx: Knowledge deficit: nature of the disorder and treatment plan
Because patient education is the most important nursing measure for the patient with cancer of the bladder, explain all nursing and medical interventions to the patient. Provide general information to the patient about the diagnosis, with specific information about the particular type of bladder tumor. Instruct the patient about the events that are to occur in relation to the treatment plan, specifying all information about the pre- and postoperative care and guidelines for the patient to follow.

Stress the importance of complying with the long-term treatment plan and follow-up care. Patients often assume that once treatment has been instituted, the tumor is gone forever. However, as many as 70% of the patients treated for superficial bladder cancers have recurrence of the disease at some time. Depending on the physician's preference and the patient's condition, repeat assessment of the urinary tract is performed every 3 to 6 months initially, then every 6 to 12 months, for the rest of the patient's life. Encourage the patient to follow this reassessment schedule.

Evaluation

Evaluate the effectiveness of nursing care for a patient with papillary or superficial bladder tumors by comparing the patient's status with the expected patient outcomes. Examples of specific outcomes for patients with papillary or superficial bladder tumors have been provided in the Planning section.

Application of the Nursing Process to the Care of the Patient with Nonpapillary or Muscle-Invasive Bladder Cancer

Because a radical cystectomy with urinary diversion is the primary method of treatment for patients with these tumors, the application of the nursing process is specific to this type of intervention.

Assessment

Preoperatively, evaluate the patient's overall physical, nutritional, and respiratory status. Ask the patient about usual eating habits. Note the patient's weight in relation to height, and observe for signs of malnutrition. Check for dyspnea, tachypnea, or abnormal breath sounds. Assess the patient's view of sexuality and pattern of sexual activity. This information is valuable in the postoperative period as the patient adjusts to the presence of an ostomy. Assess the patient's anxiety in relation to the surgery and to the physical changes that will occur as a result of the surgical intervention. Determine the patient's understanding of the disease and the surgical intervention. Determine the patient's ability to cope with the upcoming lifestyle changes. Find out what support systems are available to the patient and who will be at home to assist the patient.

Postoperatively, assess the patient for any respiratory distress such as difficulty breathing, extreme tachypnea, or wheezing. Note the patient's circulatory status. Assess pulses, color of extremities, heart rate, and blood pressure. Evaluate fluid and electrolyte status frequently. Determine the need for pain relief. As in all types of abdominal surgery, assess the wound frequently for excessive drainage or signs of infection. Assess all drains for patency. Evaluate the color and appearance of the stoma as well as the condition of the surrounding skin. Assess the ostomy appliance every shift and as necessary for placement, leaking around the system, and need for replacement or emptying.

In addition to the assessment of the various physical parameters, assess the patient and family for their reaction to the appearance of the stoma and for their readiness to learn about stoma care. Once past the immediate postoperative period, assess the patient for an understanding of the basics of the stoma care as well as the ability to perform the procedure.

Nursing Diagnoses and Planning

Nursing diagnoses and related expected patient outcomes most commonly applicable to patients with nonpapillary or muscle-invasive bladder cancer who are undergoing a cystectomy include the following:

NDx: Fluid volume deficit related to the surgical intervention

Planning: Patient outcomes
1. Patient's fluid intake and output is balanced.
2. Patient's urinary output is 30 ml/hour or more.
3. Patient's vital signs are within normal ranges for the patient.

NDx: Impaired skin integrity related to leakage of urine around the stoma

Planning: Patient outcomes
1. Patient's skin remains intact.
2. Patient's skin remains clean and dry.
3. Patient remains free of infection around stoma.

NDx: Anxiety related to surgical procedure and lifestyle changes

Planning: Patient outcomes
1. Patient communicates fears and concerns about surgery, body image, and coping with stoma care.
2. Patient identifies relaxation techniques and other coping mechanisms.

NDx: Altered patterns of urinary elimination related to the urinary diversion

Planning: Patient outcomes
1. Patient's urinary output is 30 ml/hour or more.
2. Patient's urine is clear, with normal characteristic odor.
3. Patient is able to maintain an appropriate fluid intake and output.

NDx: Body image disturbance related to the urinary stoma

Planning: Patient outcomes
1. Patient expresses feelings related to the stoma.
2. Patient expresses fears and concerns.
3. Patient asks questions about the care of the stoma.
4. Patient looks at the stoma with the appearance of acceptance.

NDx: Altered health maintenance related to lack of knowledge about the surgical intervention and postoperative stoma care

Planning: Patient outcomes
1. Patient relates accurate information about the surgical procedure and postoperative expectations.
2. Patient asks questions about the home care necessary.
3. Patient demonstrates appropriate care of the stoma.

Nursing Interventions

NDx: Fluid volume deficit
Monitor the patient's fluid status frequently. Check the fluid intake and output, and document the data. Note any signs of fluid deficit such as changes in vital signs. Monitor the cardiovascular status, checking the patient's blood pressure and pulse rate as per unit protocol. Observe the wound for excessive drainage or signs of hemorrhage. Check drains, and note the amount of drainage. Report any signs of excessive fluid loss, especially hemorrhage. Measure all drainage bag amounts, and document the results.

NDx: Impaired skin integrity
Check the newly created stoma every 2 to 4 hours during the first 24 hours. Note the color, size, and general appearance. Report any excessive bleeding

around the stoma. Check the pouch covering the stoma for leakage, and change as ordered and needed. Cleanse the skin frequently, as prescribed, to prevent excoriation from the drainage. Place a skin barrier around the peristomal skin for protection. Observe for early signs of skin breakdown, such as redness around the stoma or other discoloration or lesions.

NDx: Anxiety
Permit the patient to verbalize feelings about the diagnosis, stoma, and changes in lifestyle and body image. Allow time for questions and concerns from the patient. Refer the patient to clergy or other counseling groups for assistance with the emotional trauma. Invite a member of an ostomy group to visit the patient. Have the patient practice relaxation techniques as frequently as needed to allay anxiety episodes.

NDx: Altered patterns of urinary elimination
Check the patient's fluid intake and output frequently, especially in the early postoperative period. Note any extreme imbalances, and report them to the attending physician. Once the patient is able to take oral fluids, encourage increased fluid intake unless otherwise contraindicated. Patients with urinary diversions often restrict fluids to prevent continuous drainage of urine. Explain to the patient the necessity for continuing to take increased oral fluids. The patient may subconsciously dehydrate from continued self-restriction of fluids. Increased fluid intake also assists in infection prevention.

NDx: Body image disturbance
Provide opportunities for the patient to verbalize feelings and concerns about the changes experienced. Prior to surgery, show the patient examples of the appliances that may be used. Have a member of an ostomy group visit the patient to assist in providing the needed emotional support. Discuss the family's feelings about the surgery and the changes in the patient's physical appearance. Ask the patient what information the physician has provided about sexual activity. (Male patients will be impotent.) Be accepting of the patient's demonstration of feelings, but do not reinforce denial.

NDx: Altered health maintenance
Extensive preoperative teaching, based on the patient's readiness, is necessary to ensure a successful outcome from the surgery. Verify what the physician has explained to the patient and family about the operation, and review these points with the patient. Use illustrations to explain the procedure and the outcome in terms of changes in body image. Help the patient visualize the anatomic structures and identify the location of the incision area and stoma placement. Describe the appearance of the stoma to the patient.

Familiarize the patient with the postoperative equipment and treatments that are to be completed, such as the stoma care, wound care, and intravenous therapy. Explain the need for not allowing the patient to receive anything by mouth (NPO status) and for the use of analgesics.

Because the patient may be admitted to an intensive care unit for the immediate postoperative period, explain the appearance of the unit to the patient. Also explain the equipment and care that will be given in the unit.

Postoperatively, when the patient is stable, begin discharge planning. Consult with an enterostomal therapist for a teaching plan for the patient and family and for continued follow-up care that may be needed. The enterostomal therapist can assist the patient with the transition from hospital care to home care. Several teaching sessions are usually necessary for the patient to understand the stoma care. Refer the patient to an ostomy support group if one is available in the area. This group is extremely helpful in getting the patient to accept the stoma and change in lifestyle necessary to cope with the diagnosis and future. A representative of the group may visit the patient while still in the hospital to assist the patient in understanding the care needed and to give emotional support. A visiting nurse may also provide assistance with the stoma care when needed.

Prior to discharge, instruct the patient to observe for latent postoperative complications such as wound infection and obstruction of the stoma. Arrange for a follow-up visit with the physician and the enterostomal therapist to answer questions that may arise after discharge and to evaluate the patient's competency with the ostomy care.

Additional Interventions
Additional nursing interventions for the patient undergoing a radical cystectomy with urinary diversion include preparing the patient both physically and emotionally for the surgery. Implement the nursing activities common to all patients undergoing major abdominal surgery, including bowel preparation. Postoperatively, monitor the patient closely for life-threatening problems. Assess all systems continuously until the patient is considered stable.

Evaluation

Evaluate the effectiveness of nursing care for a patient with nonpapillary or muscle-invasive bladder cancer undergoing a cystectomy by comparing the patient's status with the expected patient outcomes. Examples of specific outcomes for patients undergoing a cystectomy for bladder cancer have been provided in the Planning section.

Cancer of the Urethra

ETIOLOGY AND PATHOPHYSIOLOGY

Primary malignant tumors of the urethra are extremely rare, but they are the only urinary tract carcinomas with a higher incidence in the female than in the male. The cause of the tumors is unknown, although urethral irritation, urethral polyps, and urethral diverticulum are suggested as possible causes of the disease.

CLINICAL MANIFESTATIONS

Clinical manifestations of urethral cancer are nonspecific, making the medical diagnosis difficult.

MEDICAL DIAGNOSIS

The diagnosis is ultimately confirmed by biopsy of suspicious areas within the urethra.

MEDICAL MANAGEMENT

Medical treatment is always surgical removal of the lesion in the urethra.

Guidelines for Application of the Nursing Process to the Care of the Patient with Urethral Cancer

Nursing care of the patient with cancer of the urethra depends on the location and extent of the cancer. Because surgery is the treatment of choice, care is directed at preparing the patient for the surgery and postoperative prevention of complications. If the cancer is extensive, the patient may undergo extensive surgery. In that case, the care is similar to that of the patient with cancer of the bladder with a urinary diversion.

The Elderly: Special Considerations

Urinary tract disorders in the elderly are similar to those in adults of any age. Many of the problems that arise are the result of the normal aging process. The most common problem in the geriatric patient is incontinence, which is described in Chapter 25.

The second most frequent disorder of the urinary tract in the older adult is lower tract infection. Frequency of urinary tract infection increases in the aged population equally in males and females. Urinary tract infections are attributed to instrumentation such as catheterization and cystoscopy, bladder outlet changes, diabetes, neurologic disease, and medication use.

Catheterization is one of the leading causes of urinary tract infections. Many infections are associated with multiple and indwelling catheters. When inserting and caring for catheters in the elderly patient, the use of aseptic technique is essential. It is also important for the patient to increase fluid intake unless contraindicated.

Physical changes that occur in females can contribute to the development of urinary tract infections. The urethral orifice can become displaced into the vaginal outlet because of relaxed musculature and atrophy of the periurethral structures. Because of these changes, bacteria from the vagina and rectum may enter the urethra and cause a urinary tract infection. Owing to decreased bladder capacity and problems with incontinence, the older adult may deliberately decrease fluid intake. This contributes to the development of more urinary tract infections.

When caring for the elderly patient, it is important to assess and review the patient's history to identify urinary tract problems and potential causes. Always encourage increased fluid intake unless contraindicated. Other nursing interventions must be specific to each patient's needs, likes and dislikes, and medical management.

Bibliography

Baer CL. Acute renal failure: Recognizing and reversing its deadly course. Nursing 1990; 20(6):34.

Bahnson R. Urosepsis. Urol Clin North Am 1986; 13(4):627.

Bass M. Infection in renal transplantation: The first six months. Crit Care Nurs Clin North Am 1990; 2(1):133.

Beier-Holgersen R, Bruun J. Voiding pattern of men 60 to 70 years old: Population study in an urban population. J Urol 1990; 143(3):531.

Bell D, Rosenthal J. Arteriovenous graft life in chronic hemodialysis. Arch Surg 1988; 123:1169.

Bellinger MF. The history of urinary diversion and undiversion. J Enterostom Ther 1989; 16(1):39.

Benet A, Abarbanel J, Lask D, Kimche D. Surgical management of long urethral strictures. J Urol 1990; 143(5):917.

Birolini D, Steinman E, Utiyama E, Arroyo A. Open pelviperineal trauma. J Trauma 1990; 30(4):492.

Brendler C, Schlegel P, Walsh P. Urethrectomy with preservation of potency. J Urol 1990; 144(8):270.

Brettschneider NR, Orihuela E. Carcinoma of the bladder. Urol Nurs 1990; 10(1):14.

Cardona V, Hurn P, Mason P, et al. Trauma nursing from resuscitation through rehabilitation. Philadelphia: WB Saunders, 1988.

Carroll P, McAninch J. Staging of renal trauma. Urol Clin North Am 1989; 16(2):193.

Coe F, Parks J. Pathophysiology of kidney stones and strategies for treatment. Hosp Pract 1988; 23(3):185.

Coleman EA. When the kidneys fail. RN 1986; 49(7):28.

Erlich L. Use of EPOGEN for treatment of anemia associated with chronic renal failure. Crit Care Nurs Clin North Am 1990; 2(1):101.

Faris MH. When your kidneys fail. Los Angeles: National Kidney Foundation of Southern California, 1984.
Fedric T. Immunosuppressive therapy in renal transplantation. Crit Care Nurs Clin North Am 1990; 2(10):123.
Flanigan R, Rapp R, McRoberts W. Nutritional assessment and therapy in advanced urothelial cancer. Urol Clin North Am 1984; 11(4):671.
Fowler J. Urinary tract infections in women. Urol Clin North Am 1986; 13(4):673.
Gharbieh PA. Renal transplant: Surgical and psychologic hazards. Crit Care Nurse 1980; 8(6):58.
Glassock R, Cohen A, Danovitch G, Parsa K. Human immunodeficiency virus (HIV) infection and the kidney. Ann Intern Med 1980; 112(1):35.
Greig BJ. A new option for cystectomy patients. RN 1990; 53(9):34.
Guerriero W. Ureteral injury. Urol Clin North Am 1989; 16(2):237.
Held J, Volpe H. Bladder preserving combined modality therapy for invasive bladder cancer. Oncol Nurs Forum 1991; 18(1):49.
Innerarity S. Electrolyte emergencies in the critically ill renal patient. Crit Care Nurs Clin North Am 1990; 2(1):89.
Javadpour N (ed). Cancer of the kidney. New York: Thieme-Stratton, 1984.
Kott S, Kaiser J. Emergency nursing: A physiologic and clinical perspective. Philadelphia: WB Saunders, 1990.
Krieger J. Urinary tract infections in women: Causes, classification, and differential diagnoses. Urol 1990; 35(1)(Suppl):4.
LeBouton J. Nursing aspects of bacillus Calmette-Guerin immunotherapy for superficial bladder cancer. Urol Nurs 1990; 10(4):9.
Lingeman JE. Kidney stones: Acute management. Patient Care 1990; 24(13):20.
Marshall B. Laser lithotripsy: A nursing perspective. Urol Nurs 1991; 11(2):25.
Mee S, McAninch J. Indications for radiographic assessment in suspected renal trauma. Urol Clin North Am 1989; 16(2):187.
Morrison A. Advances in the etiology of urothelial cancer. Urol Clin North Am 1984; 11(4):557.
Pearlstein G. Renal system complication in HIV infection. Crit Care Nurs Clin North Am 1990; 2(1):79.
Pryor J, Jenkins AD. Use of double-pigtail stents in extracorporeal shock wave lithotripsy. J Urol 1990; 143(3):475.
Reilly N, Torosian L. The new wave in lithotripsy: Implications for nursing. RN 1988; 51(3):44.
Richard C. Comprehensive nephrology nursing. Boston: Little, Brown, 1986.
Rivers R. Nursing the kidney transplant patient. RN 1987; 50(8):46.
Rober P, Smith J, Pierce J. Gunshot injuries of the ureter. J Trauma 1990; 30(1):83.
Roberto P. Diabetic nephropathy: Causes, complications, and considerations. Crit Care Nurs Clin North Am 1990; 2(1):55.
Roth R, Bechmann C. Complications of extracorporeal shockwave lithotripsy and percutaneous nephrolithotomy. Urol Clin North Am 1988; 15(2):155.
Schneider E, Rowe J (eds). Handbook of the biology of aging. 3rd ed. New York: Academic Press, 1990.
Smith DB. Patient adjustment to an ideal conduit after radical cystectomy. J Enterostom Ther 1989; 16(6):244.
Smith DB. Continent diversions: An overview. Dimens Oncol Nurs 1990; 3(4):18.
Smith M. Renal trauma: Adult and pediatric considerations. Crit Care Nurs Clin North Am 1990; 2(1):67.
Sommers MS. Blunt renal trauma. Crit Care Nurse 1990; 10(3):38.
US Renal Data System. 1990 USRDS Annual Report. Bethesda, MD: USRDS, 1990.
Weiskittel P, Sommers S. The patient with lower urinary tract trauma. Crit Care Nurse 1989; 9(1):53.

Unit Nine

ADULTS WITH HEPATIC DYSFUNCTION

Learning Objectives

AFTER COMPLETING THIS UNIT, THE LEARNER WILL BE ABLE TO:

Chapter Twenty-seven

1. Explain the normal anatomy and physiology of the liver.
2. Describe common clinical manifestations of liver dysfunction.
3. Identify information and physical examination data essential to the assessment of liver function.
4. Describe diagnostic procedures commonly used in the diagnosis of liver disorders.
5. Describe medical management and surgical procedures commonly used in the treatment of patients with liver disorders.
6. Identify data essential to the assessment of patients undergoing treatment of liver disorders.
7. State nursing diagnoses and related expected patient outcomes commonly applicable to patients undergoing treatment of liver disorders.
8. Describe nursing interventions, with their rationales, commonly applicable to patients undergoing treatment of liver disorders.
9. Explain the basis for evaluation of nursing care provided to patients undergoing treatment of liver disorders.
10. Identify special considerations for the elderly patient with altered liver function.

Chapter Twenty-eight

1. Describe common liver disorders in terms of etiology, pathophysiology, clinical manifestations, diagnostic procedures, and medical management.
2. Identify information and physical examination data essential to the assessment of patients with common liver disorders.
3. State nursing diagnoses and related expected patient outcomes commonly applicable to patients with liver disorders.
4. Describe nursing interventions, with their rationales, commonly applicable to patients with liver disorders.
5. Explain the basis for evaluation of nursing care provided to patients with common liver disorders.
6. Identify special considerations for the elderly patient with a liver disorder.

Chapter Twenty-seven

KNOWLEDGE BASIC TO THE NURSING CARE *of Adults with* Hepatic Dysfunction

The liver plays a vital role in the digestion, absorption, metabolism, and storage of nutrients. It is the major "biochemical factory" in the body, performing more than 400 chemical functions. Patients with hepatic disorders have clinical manifestations that result from interference with the liver's normal functions. Major manifestations include jaundice, ascites and portal hypertension, bleeding, hepatic encephalopathy, and nutritional deficiencies. A complete history and physical examination, including blood, urine, stool, and visualization studies, play an important role in the diagnosis and treatment of liver disorders.

Anatomy

The liver, weighing approximately 1500 g or $3\frac{1}{2}$ pounds in the adult, is the largest organ in the body and performs the greatest number of functions. The liver is located in the right upper quadrant of the abdomen and extends across the midline to the left upper quadrant. It extends up under the ribs 6 to 12 cm in the right midclavicular line and 4 to 8 cm in the midsternal line. The liver is composed of two major lobes: a large right lobe and a smaller left lobe. These lobes are separated by the falciform ligament, a fold of visceral peritoneum that fastens the liver to the anterior abdominal wall. Two smaller lobes are present on the posterior surface of the liver: the quadrate lobe near the gallbladder and the caudate lobe near the inferior vena cava. The entire organ is covered by a dense connective tissue called the capsule of Glisson. Figure 27–1 illustrates the anterior surface of the liver.

Each lobe is composed of 50,000 to 100,000 hepatic lobules, the functional unit of the liver. Lobules, as shown in Figure 27–2, are made up of layers of hepatocytes (hepatic cells) only one or two cells thick that radiate outward from a central vein. The portal vein brings about 75% of the blood supply to the liver. This blood is rich in nutrients from the intestine and flows to the hepatic sinusoids, large capillaries that separate the layers of hepatocytes. This venous pathway through the liver is known as the hepatic portal system. The remaining 25% of the blood supply to the liver is delivered via the hepatic artery. This blood is rich in oxygen and mixes with the portal blood in the sinusoids. Approximately 1450 ml of mixed arteriovenous blood flows through the liver per minute. From the hepatic sinusoids, blood flows to the central vein of each lobule and is carried through a series of merging vessels into the hepatic vein. The hepatic vein empties into the inferior vena cava. Although there are two sources for blood flow into the liver—the portal vein and the hepatic artery—all blood leaves the liver via the same route: the hepatic vein to the inferior vena cava.

Each hepatic lobule also has specialized bile ducts called canaliculi, which drain bile that has been produced by the hepatocytes. The canaliculi flow into the larger hepatic ducts, which then empty into the common bile duct. The cystic duct, a branch of the common bile duct, carries bile to the gallbladder, where it can be stored.

Physiology

The functions of the liver are summarized in Table 27–1. In addition to the metabolism of carbohydrates, lipids, and proteins, the liver manufactures and secretes bile; filters blood; detoxifies drugs, toxins, and hormones; and serves as a storage depot.

Carbohydrate Metabolism

The regulation of blood glucose levels involves the secretion of two pancreatic hormones. Insulin, produced by the beta cells of the pancreas, acts on the liver to stimulate the formation of glycogen from glucose, inhibits the conversion of noncarbohydrates into glucose, and aids the diffusion of glucose through the cell wall, thus preventing excessive blood glucose levels. Glucagon, produced by the alpha cells of the pancreas, acts to increase blood glucose levels by stimulating the liver to produce glucose when blood levels fall below normal.

When blood glucose levels are within normal range, glucose is transported from the intestines to the liver via the portal circulation, where it is converted to glycogen. This process, called glycogenesis, prevents large amounts of glucose from entering the blood stream when it is not needed. The glycogen is

Table 27–1. LIVER FUNCTIONS

FUNCTION	DESCRIPTION
METABOLISM	
Carbohydrate	Converts glucose to glycogen for storage (glycogenesis)
	Breaks down glycogen into glucose for energy (glycogenolysis)
	Converts protein and fat to glucose for energy (gluconeogenesis)
Lipid	Oxidizes fatty acids and glycerol for energy
	Reforms triglycerides
	Produces cholesterol and ketones
Protein	Synthesizes new amino acids, albumin, alpha and beta globulins, fibrinogen, prothrombin, and clotting factors V, VII, VIII, and X
	Converts ammonia to urea
SECRETION	Produces and secretes bile needed for fat digestion
FILTRATION	Removes foreign substances from the blood, including bacteria and aged red blood cells
DETOXIFICATION	Chemically modifies drugs, toxins, and hormones and makes them more suitable for excretion
STORAGE	Stores glycogen; vitamins A, D, B_{12}, K_1, and K_2; folic acid; iron; manganese; copper; and zinc

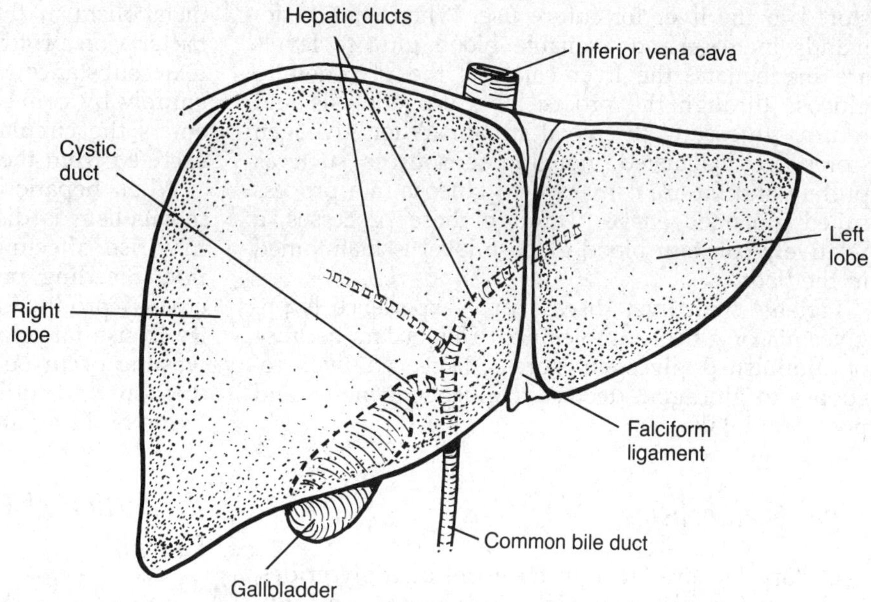

Figure 27–1.

Anterior view of the liver.

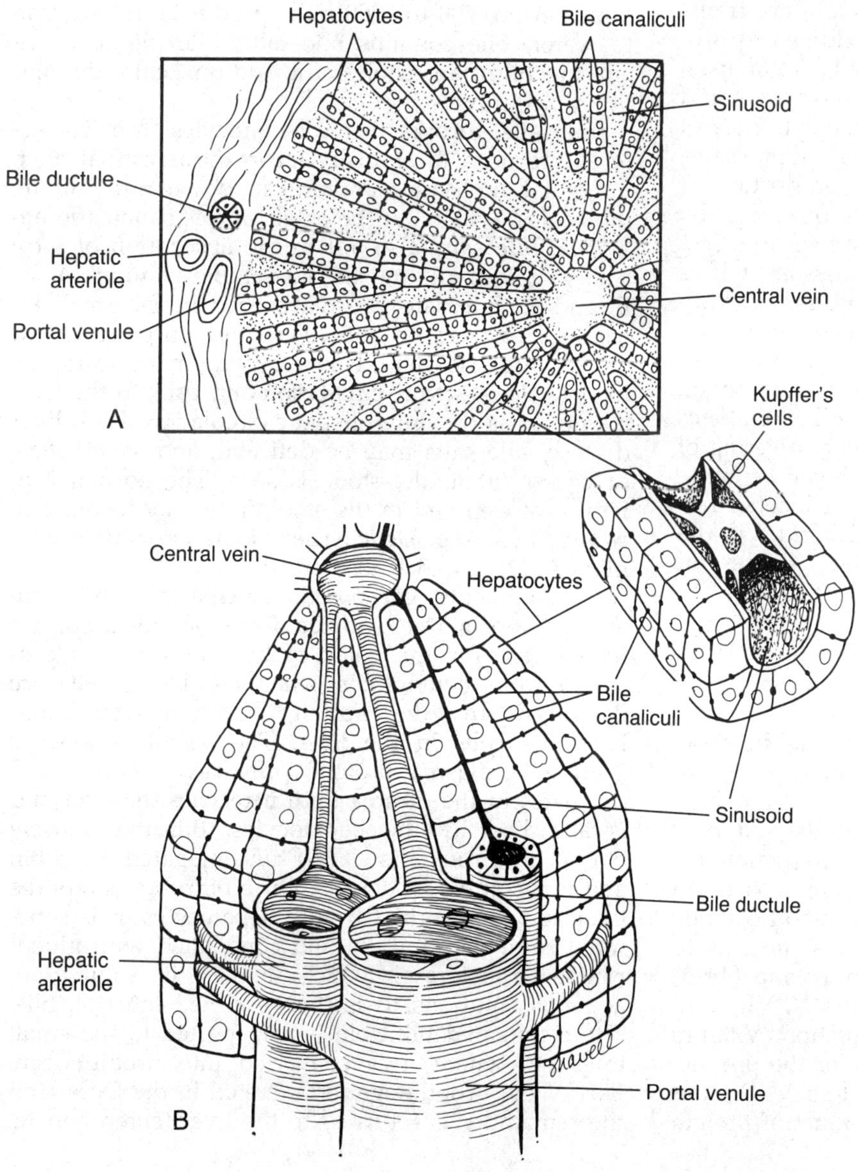

Figure 27–2.

A, Overview of a liver lobule. B, Representation of the relationship of structures within the lobules of the liver.

stored in the liver for future use. When energy demands increase and available blood glucose levels are inadequate, the liver converts the glycogen to glucose through the process of glycogenolysis and returns glucose to the blood stream. When glycogen stores are exhausted, nonglucose sources such as protein and fat are converted to glucose in a process called gluconeogenesis. Through these processes, a relatively constant blood glucose level is maintained in the body.

Patients with liver disease may experience hypoglycemia or glucose intolerance. This occurs because of diminished glycogen stores, decreased liver response to glucagon, decreased gluconeogenesis, and poor oral intake.

Lipid Metabolism

Dietary fat, primarily in the form of triglycerides, is digested in the small intestines under the influence of pancreatic lipase and bile salts. Fatty acids, the end products of dietary fat digestion, are transported to the liver, where they are oxidized to produce energy when glucose is not available, or used to reform triglycerides or to produce cholesterol and ketones. Cholesterol is important in the synthesis of liver cell membranes, for the production of bile salts, which aid fat digestion, and for the production of various sex hormones and hormones produced by the adrenal gland. Ketones, in the form of acetoacetic acid, are transported to peripheral tissues, where they are used for energy. When glucose is not available and fat is used for energy, ketones are formed in large quantities, resulting in the accumulation of ketones in the blood. This occurs with prolonged fasting or starvation and in uncontrolled diabetes mellitus. If not treated, ketosis leads to a lowering of the pH of body fluids (acidosis), which can be fatal.

Persons who ingest large amounts of alcohol frequently have an accumulation of triglycerides in the liver. This condition, called fatty liver, causes an enlarged liver and abnormal liver function.

Protein Metabolism

Amino acids are the end products of the digestion of protein in the small intestine. Amino acids are transported via the portal vein to the liver, where they are used to form new compounds and new amino acids, and into the systemic circulation for use by body tissues. The liver uses amino acids to produce albumin, needed to maintain blood osmotic pressure; the alpha and beta globulins, needed to transport lipids and fat-soluble vitamins; and fibrinogen, prothrombin, and clotting factors V, VII, VIII, and X, major factors in blood coagulation. Vitamin K, a fat-soluble vitamin, is necessary for the production of prothrombin and clotting factors V, IX, and X. Ammonia is formed as an end product of protein metabolism in the liver as well as by the action of bacteria on proteins in the intestine. This potentially toxic substance is removed from the blood almost entirely by conversion to urea in the liver. The urea enters the circulation, travels to the kidney, and is excreted from the body in urine.

When hepatic disorders are present, liver protein metabolism is disrupted and blood ammonia levels may rise, affecting acid-base balance and brain function. Bleeding problems develop as a result of decreased production of clotting factors and the inability to use fat-soluble vitamin K. Fatigue and muscle wasting occur because of decreased amino acid production and utilization, which prevents adequate tissue building and repair.

Production of Bile and Conjugation of Bilirubin

Bile, a yellowish-green fluid, is continually manufactured and secreted by the hepatocytes. In a 24-hour period, 700 to 1200 ml is produced. In addition to water, bile contains bile salts, bile pigments including bilirubin, cholesterol, sodium, chloride, and other electrolytes.

Bile salts, formed in the hepatocytes from cholesterol, are used to emulsify fat in the intestinal tract. Large fat molecules are broken down into minute molecules, which can be acted on by pancreatic enzymes. Bile salts also aid in the absorption of fatty acids, cholesterol, and the fat-soluble vitamins A, D, E, and K. Bile salts are reabsorbed in the small intestine, returned to the liver, and once again excreted into the bile. This recycling path from the liver to the systemic circulation and back to the liver is known as the enterohepatic circulation. With liver disease, bile salts may be deficient, and steatorrhea, or excess fat in the stool, is seen. The normal 2 to 5 g of fat excreted in the stool daily may increase to as much as 60 g. Deficiencies of the fat-soluble vitamins A, D, E, and K also occur.

Bile pigments, composed principally of bilirubin and biliverdin (an oxidized form of bilirubin), are responsible for the color of bile. Bilirubin is produced from hemoglobin when red blood cells are destroyed by the spleen, bone marrow, and Kupffer's cells in the liver. The bilirubin attaches itself to a plasma protein, primarily albumin, and circulates in the plasma until it reaches the liver and is absorbed by the hepatocytes. Bilirubin loosely bound to protein is called unconjugated bilirubin and is insoluble in plasma. Once bilirubin enters the liver and is absorbed by the hepatocytes, it is separated from the albumin and conjugated with glucuronide transferase, which makes it soluble in aqueous solutions. It is then excreted into the bile. The conjugated bilirubin is transported to the small intestine, where it is converted into urobilinogen. Part of the urobilinogen is excreted in the feces, and the remainder is returned to the liver (enterohepatic

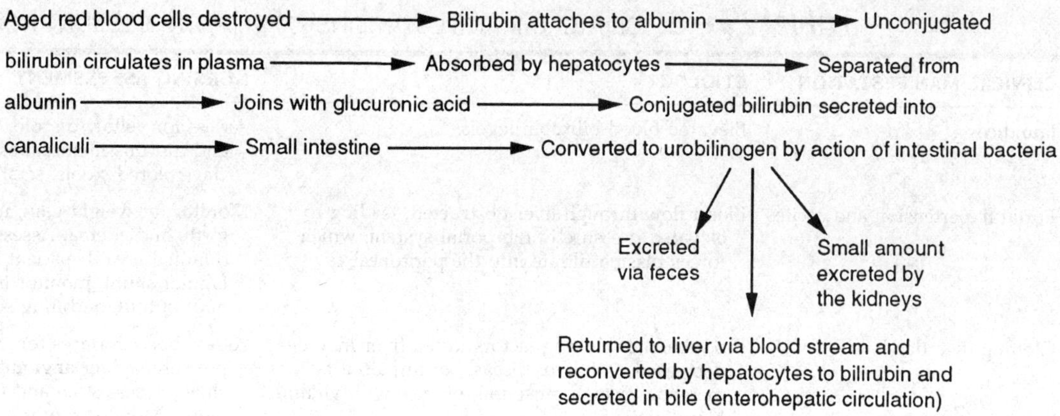

Figure 27–3. Bilirubin metabolism.

circulation), where it is removed from the blood. Traces of urobilinogen that are not removed from the blood by the liver are carried to the kidneys and excreted in the urine. Figure 27–3 summarizes bilirubin metabolism.

An increased level of unconjugated bilirubin is seen with increased destruction of red blood cells or hemolytic disease; an increased level of both unconjugated and conjugated bilirubin is seen with liver disease.

Blood Filtration

As blood flows through the intestinal capillaries, many intestinal bacteria are picked up. Kupffer's cells, large mononuclear phagocytic cells lining the hepatic sinusoids, cleanse the blood as it passes through the liver. Less than 1% of bacteria from the intestine succeed in passing to the systemic circulation. In addition to bacteria, Kupffer's cells also phagocytize aged erythrocytes. Through a series of enzyme reactions, amino acids and iron from the erythrocytes are salvaged and reused, and the heme portion of the erythrocyte is used to produce bilirubin.

Detoxification

The liver chemically modifies a wide variety of drugs, toxins, and hormones. Under normal conditions, the liver inactivates these substances or alters them to make them more suitable for excretion. When hepatic disorders are present, the liver's ability to chemically modify substances may be impaired. As a result, increased sensitivity to certain drugs may occur (e.g., sedatives and hypnotics); the effects of hormones may be enhanced (e.g., increased conversion of androgens to estrogens, resulting in male breast enlargement); or toxins usually metabolized and excreted via the liver may be returned to the circulatory system (e.g., increased ammonia levels, which affect acid-base balance and brain function).

Storage Depot

Approximately 450 ml of blood, or 10% of the total blood volume, is normally circulating through the liver at a given time. During periods of hypotension and shock, the liver is capable of shunting extra blood to the systemic circulation. Because the liver is highly vascular, it has the capability of storing as much as 1 L of blood if the total blood volume rises above normal and the pressure in the vena cava increases.

In addition to glycogen and amino acids, the liver stores vitamins A, D, and B_{12}, folic acid, and iron. Manganese, copper, and zinc, although found in other body tissues, are most concentrated in the liver. Vitamin K_1, found in foods that are ingested, and vitamin K_2, which is produced by bacteria in the intestine, both are stored to a limited degree in the liver. In the presence of liver disease, many of these stored substances may be depleted.

Clinical Manifestations of Hepatic Dysfunction

The major clinical manifestations associated with hepatic dysfunction are jaundice, ascites and portal hypertension, clotting disorders, hepatic encephalopathy, and nutritional deficiencies. Patients experiencing liver failure will exhibit all of these manifestations. Table 27–2 summarizes the major clinical manifestations of hepatic dysfunction. Nursing Care Guide 27–1 summarizes the nursing care of the patient with liver failure who is experiencing the major clinical manifestations of hepatic dysfunction.

Jaundice

Jaundice, also known as icterus, is yellow discoloration of the skin, sclerae, and mucous membranes caused by elevated bilirubin levels in the blood. Jaundice is classified as hemolytic (prehepatic), hep-

Table 27–2. CLINICAL MANIFESTATIONS OF HEPATIC DYSFUNCTION

CLINICAL MANIFESTATION	ETIOLOGY	NURSING ASSESSMENT
Jaundice	Elevated blood bilirubin levels	Assess for yellow discoloration of skin, sclerae, and mucous membranes; dark urine; light or clay-colored stools; scratch marks or scratching.
Portal hypertension and ascites	Blood flow through liver obstructed, leading to elevated pressure in the portal system, which forces plasma filtrate into the peritoneal cavity	Monitor for weight gain, increased abdominal girth, and edema. Assess for taut skin over abdominal area. If patient has had a peritoneojugular shunt, monitor hematocrit levels, urinary output, and lung sounds.
Clotting disorders	Production of clotting factors in the liver may be decreased with liver disease, or impaired fat metabolism may cause interference with vitamin K utilization	Assess body surfaces for evidence of bleeding: purpura, spider angiomas, ecchymoses, petechiae. Assess stool and urine for presence of blood. Monitor prothrombin time.
Hepatic encephalopathy	Liver unable to metabolize toxic substances produced in the intestines; exact pathophysiology unknown	Assess for change in mental status. Monitor blood ammonia levels and precipitating factors, especially diuretic therapy. Assess for fetor hepaticus and asterixis.
Nutritional deficiencies	Liver unable to metabolize, produce, or store essential nutrients	Assess for symptoms shown in Table 27–5.

atocellular (hepatic), or obstructive (intrahepatic or extrahepatic).

PATHOPHYSIOLOGY

Hemolytic jaundice occurs when red blood cells are destroyed at a rate that exceeds the liver's ability to remove bilirubin from the blood. A higher than normal amount of unconjugated bilirubin is present in the blood stream. Hemolytic jaundice is seen in pernicious anemia, in sickle cell anemia, and in transfusion reactions.

In hepatocellular jaundice, liver cells are unable to metabolize bilirubin because of infection, chemical or drug toxicity, or hepatocyte necrosis. The uptake, conjugation, and excretion of bilirubin are usually impaired. When there is damage to the hepatocytes, intracellular enzymes are released into the circula-

Nursing Care Guide 27–1.

PATIENTS WITH LIVER FAILURE

Assessment Findings: Patient with ascites complains of "feeling tired almost all the time." Shortness of breath is noted after walking more than a few steps. Respirations are 26 per minute and shallow.

Nursing Diagnosis: Ineffective breathing pattern related to pressure on the diaphragm from ascites

Patient Outcomes	Nursing Interventions	Rationale
Patient's vital signs remain within normal limits, with respirations between 12 and 20 per minute with full chest expansion.	Elevate the head of the bed 45–90 degrees.	Promotes maximum chest expansion and relieves pressure from ascites.
	Instruct patient to deep breathe every 2 hours.	Encourages maximum chest expansion.
	Monitor vital signs and auscultate lungs every 4 hours.	Facilitates early identification of decreased air exchange and oxygen deficit.

(continued)

Nursing Care Guide 27–1. *(continued)*

PATIENTS WITH LIVER FAILURE

Evaluation: Compare the patient's status with the expected patient outcomes. If the outcomes are achieved, evaluate nursing care as successful. If not, reassess the patient, formulate new nursing diagnoses, and revise expected patient outcomes and nursing interventions as appropriate.

Assessment Findings: Patient indicates pants are tight around the waist and a 10- to 12-lb weight gain has been noticed over the past 2 weeks. Abdomen is distended, shiny, and taut, with striae. Edema of both ankles is present.

Nursing Diagnosis: Fluid volume excess related to accumulation of fluid in the peritoneal cavity and dependent areas of the body

Patient Outcomes	Nursing Interventions	Rationale
Patient's abdominal girth and weight decrease daily.	Monitor intake and output.	Fluid intake that exceeds output over a 3-day period indicates fluid retention.
	Administer prescribed diuretics.	Diuretics increase fluid excretion.
	Restrict fluids to 1500 ml daily, including fluids given with medications. Divide allowance as follows: 750 ml from 8 A.M. to 4 P.M.; 600 ml from 4 P.M. to 11 P.M.; 150 ml from 11 P.M. to 8 A.M.	Restriction limits fluid accumulation. The largest amount of fluid is given during waking hours. The majority of the total allowance will be allocated to meals.
	Provide oral hygiene every 4 hours; *do not* use lemon–glycerin swabs.	Mouth care decreases thirst. Glycerin dries mucous membranes.
	Weigh the patient daily before breakfast but after he or she has voided.	Weight loss or gain may indicate fluid loss or gain.
	Measure abdominal girth daily. Mark point at which girth is measured.	Decreasing girth indicates a decrease in ascitic fluid. Measuring at the same point ensures accuracy.

Evaluation: Compare the patient's status with the expected patient outcomes. If the outcomes are achieved, evaluate nursing care as successful. If not, reassess the patient, formulate new nursing diagnoses, and revise expected patient outcomes and nursing interventions as appropriate.

(continued)

Nursing Care Guide 27–1. *(continued)*

PATIENTS WITH LIVER FAILURE

Assessment Findings: Patient indicates loss of appetite and reports frequent vomiting after eating. Patient has not finished a "full meal" in the past 3 weeks.

Nursing Diagnosis: Altered nutrition: less than body requirements related to anorexia, vomiting, and inadequate dietary intake

Patient Outcomes	Nursing Interventions	Rationale
Patient eats 80–100% of each meal.	Give largest meal in morning.	Appetite is greatest early in the day and decreases later in the day.
	Provide five or six small meals during the day.	Small portions are more appetizing and better tolerated.
Patient demonstrates steady weight gain with no evidence of fluid retention.	Provide oral hygiene before meals.	Refreshes mouth and stimulates appetite.
	Administer antiemetics 30–45 minutes before meals if necessary.	Most antiemetics require 20–30 minutes to reach effective levels.
	Maintain low-sodium diet.	Decreases risk of fluid retention.
	Offer juice of patient's choice between meals.	Juice provides calories and vitamins.

Evaluation: Compare the patient's status with the expected patient outcomes. If the outcomes are achieved, evaluate nursing care as successful. If not, reassess the patient, formulate new nursing diagnoses, and revise expected patient outcomes and nursing interventions as appropriate.

(continued)

tion. Alanine aminotransferase (ALT), previously referred to as serum glutamic-pyruvic transaminase (SGPT), and aspartate aminotransferase (AST), previously referred to as serum glutamic-oxaloacetic transaminase (SGOT), will be elevated when hepatocellular jaundice is present. The level of both these enzymes is determined to differentiate between hemolytic jaundice and jaundice caused by liver disease. Hepatocellular jaundice is seen with hepatitis and cirrhosis.

Obstructive jaundice occurs when the flow of bile is obstructed. The obstruction can be intrahepatic or extrahepatic. Intrahepatic obstruction is obstruction of bile ductules within the liver. It can result from pressure created by inflammatory processes, as is seen in hepatitis. With intrahepatic jaundice, both unconjugated and conjugated levels of serum bilirubin are elevated. Extrahepatic obstructive jaundice results from an obstruction to bile flow through the common bile duct. Elevated conjugated bilirubin levels are seen with this form of jaundice. Elevated serum alkaline phosphatase levels are also present because alkaline phosphatase, an enzyme produced by the liver, is normally excreted with bile. Gallstones, strictures of the bile ducts, and bile duct tumors can cause extrahepatic jaundice.

CLINICAL CHARACTERISTICS

The patient with jaundice has yellow discoloration of the skin and mucous membranes. Usually the first site of yellow discoloration is the sclerae of the eye, an area rich in elastin, which has a special affinity for bilirubin. General skin color may range from a light yellow tint to a deep bronze color. Pruritus occurs when bile salts, which are an irritant, are deposited in the skin.

Because bile is not entering the intestine in normal quantities, the stool is lighter in color, progressing to a clay color in the absence of bile. Urine becomes a deep orange color and foams when shaken because bile is now excreted through the kidney.

Nursing Care Guide 27–1. (continued)

PATIENTS WITH LIVER FAILURE

Assessment Findings: On the third day of hospitalization, the patient's skin, mucous membranes, and sclerae are light yellow. Patient is observed scratching upper arms and abdomen; reports feeling "kind of itchy." Urine is darker than usual and has a strong odor. Spider angiomas are noted on upper torso, and multiple ecchymotic areas are visible on arms and legs.

Nursing Diagnosis: High risk for impaired skin integrity related to pruritus, ascites, edema, and interference with clotting mechanisms

Patient Outcomes	Nursing Interventions	Rationale
Patient's skin is free of scratch marks.	Administer baths with cool water and use lightweight bed clothing.	Warmth increases blood flow and increases bile salt deposits on skin.
	Use a mild soap or soap substitute.	The alkalinizing effects of soap dry the skin.
	Pat skin dry. *Do not* rub.	Rubbing stimulates nerve endings and increases pruritus.
	Gently apply lotion to the skin every 8 hours.	Lotion has a cooling effect and minimizes dryness.
	Trim and file nails.	Prevents injury from scratching.
	Administer bile acid sequestrants as prescribed.	Relieves pruritus by decreasing bile acid deposits on the skin.
	Provide diversional activities: television, books, magazines, and so on.	Activities lessen awareness of pruritus.
Patient experiences no excessive bleeding.	Use a soft toothbrush.	Minimizes risk of bleeding from gums.
	Use electric razor for shaving.	Protects from facial cuts.
	Monitor temperature orally.	Rectal irritation may develop when rectal route is used.
	Group venipunctures, and apply pressure for 5 minutes after venipunctures.	Decreases the number of skin punctures and potential bleeding sites. Direct pressure promotes coagulation.
Patient's skin remains intact during hospitalization.	Inspect skin surfaces daily for lesions or open areas.	Early detection and intervention minimizes skin damage.
	Do not administer injections in edematous sites.	Drugs act as irritants when not absorbed.
	Teach patient to reposition self every 2 hours in bed or chair.	Frequent position changes relieve pressure and increase local blood flow.
	Place trapeze over bed and teach patient to use it to lift the body during position changes.	Lifting the body off the bed prevents injury from shearing force.
	Keep bed linens dry.	Moisture predisposes to skin breakdown.

Evaluation: Compare the patient's status with the expected patient outcomes. If the outcomes are achieved, evaluate nursing care as successful. If not, reassess the patient, formulate new nursing diagnoses, and revise expected patient outcomes and nursing interventions as appropriate.

(continued)

Nursing Care Guide 27–1. *(continued)*

PATIENTS WITH LIVER FAILURE

Assessment Findings: On the fourth day of hospitalization, patient is apathetic and responds slowly to questions. Speech is slurred. Patient answers appropriately when asked name but cannot identify location or month of the year. Handwriting is difficult to read, whereas admission writing sample is clear and distinct. Irregular, jerking movements are noted when arms are extended. Serum potassium level is within normal limits. Blood ammonia level is elevated.

Nursing Diagnosis: High risk for injury related to altered thought processes secondary to impaired liver detoxification

Patient Outcomes	Nursing Interventions	Rationale
Patient remains free of injury.	Monitor level of consciousness, orientation, rate of speech, and response time every 4 hours.	Changes in level of consciousness, orientation, speech, and response time indicate a change in condition.
	Monitor for asterixis every 4 hours.	Most common sign of impending coma due to hepatic encephalopathy.
	Obtain daily writing sample.	Difficulty writing indicates deterioration in condition.
	Restrict protein intake.	Reduces ammonia production.
	Monitor serum potassium level.	Decreased potassium levels can precipitate hepatic coma.
	Administer neomycin and lactulose as prescribed.	Lower blood ammonia levels.
	Keep bed in low position, with side rails up and call bell in reach.	Minimizes risk of injury.

Evaluation: Compare the patient's status with the expected patient outcomes. If the outcomes are achieved, evaluate nursing care as successful. If not, reassess the patient, formulate new nursing diagnoses, and revise expected patient outcomes and nursing interventions as appropriate.

MEDICAL MANAGEMENT

Because jaundice is a symptom of an underlying disorder, no specific medical interventions are used to treat it in the adult. Bile acid sequestrants, described in Pharmacology Box 27–1, may be prescribed to relieve pruritus.

Application of the Nursing Process to the Care of the Patient with Jaundice

Assessment

Monitor skin, urine, and stool color daily. Diminished evidence of jaundice in the skin, a decrease in the color intensity of the urine, and a return of color to the stool indicates an improved clinical status. Note evidence of scratching. Increased scratching indicates an increase of bile salt deposits in the skin, which accompanies an increase in the level of circulating unconjugated bilirubin. Observe the patient for evidence of decreased interpersonal relationships or decreased involvement in self-care activities. Because jaundice changes the physical appearance, the patient may withdraw or verbalize negative feelings.

Nursing Diagnoses and Planning

Nursing diagnoses and related expected patient outcomes most commonly applicable to patients with jaundice include the following:

NDx: High risk for impaired skin integrity related to pruritus secondary to bile salt accumulation

Planning: Patient outcomes

1. Patient's skin remains intact with no evidence of scratch marks.
2. Patient verbalizes a decrease in pruritus.

NDx: Body image disturbance related to altered skin pigmentation

Planning: Patient outcomes

1. Patient verbalizes an acceptance of self in present condition.
2. Patient takes an active part in grooming activities.

Nursing Interventions

NDx: High risk for impaired skin integrity
Administer cool-water baths, 90° to 100°F (32° to 37.8°C). Apply lightweight bedding, and advise the patient to wear lightweight clothing. Warmth increases blood flow to an area and results in increased bile salt deposits, leading to increased pruritus. Use a mild soap or a soap substitute for bathing, and apply lotion gently to the skin every 8 hours. The alkalinizing effects of soap dry the skin, which intensifies pruritus. Lotion minimizes dryness and has a cooling effect. Cornstarch, oatmeal powder, and baking soda baths every 12 hours, if prescribed, have a soothing effect on the skin, which decreases pruritus. However, caution patients that bathing more than once a day may increase pruritus because of the drying effects of water. At all times, pat skin dry rather than rubbing. Rubbing stimulates nerve endings and increases patient discomfort.

Trim and file nails to prevent injury to the skin. Mittens can be worn by confused patients. Administer bile acid sequestrants, if prescribed.

Provide diversional activities. Television, radio, books, board games, or other activities of interest distract the patient and lessen awareness of the pruritus.

Pharmacology Box 27–1.

BILE ACID SEQUESTRANTS

Bile Acid Sequestrants:
Drugs that bind bile acids in the gastrointestinal tract. They are available as cholestyramine resin (Cholybar, Questran) and colestipol hydrochloride (Colestid).

Action:
Bind with bile acids to form an insoluble complex that is excreted in the feces; they also increase cholesterol excretion.

Uses:
Relieve pruritus associated with elevated levels of bile acids and are used to lower the cholesterol level in patients at risk for heart disease who do not respond to dietary treatment.

Side Effects:
Constipation, nausea, and abdominal discomfort.

Interactions:
May bind with oral drugs concurrently administered and prevent their absorption. They decrease absorption of fat-soluble vitamins A, D, E, and K.

Nursing Implications:
Administer other drugs 1 hour before or 4 hours after to prevent drug binding. Must not be taken in dry form; esophageal irritation or blockage may result. Put dose on top of 4–6 oz of water, milk, or juice and let stand for 1–2 minutes. Stir and drink medication while it is suspended in solution; will not dissolve in fluid. Supplemental vitamin therapy may be necessary. Monitor bowel movements. Constipation occurs in 20% of patients. Encourage high-bulk diet and adequate fluid intake (2500–3000 ml/day) if allowed. A stool softener may be required.

Geriatric Considerations:
The elderly are at increased risk for constipation and are more likely to develop a fecal impaction.

NDx: Body image disturbance
Reinforce positive progress. Inform the patient when bilirubin levels are decreasing, urine color is less intense, and stool color is returning. Explain that these are indications that normal bile flow is returning and jaundice will be decreasing. Clarify misconceptions that the patient may have. Explain that jaundice will not remain after the underlying cause is treated. Provide reliable, accurate information to establish a trusting nurse-patient relationship.

Assist the patient with grooming activities to improve personal appearance. Encourage the patient to wear his or her own pajamas rather than a hospital gown. Assist the patient in choosing clothing colors that do not accentuate the jaundice. Assist the patient with grooming activities, such as applying makeup. These interventions allow the patient to maintain control and encourage social interaction.

Evaluation

Evaluate the effectiveness of nursing care for a patient with jaundice by comparing the patient's status with the expected patient outcomes. Examples of specific outcomes for patients with jaundice have been provided in the Planning section.

Portal Hypertension and Ascites

PATHOPHYSIOLOGY

Portal hypertension is elevated pressure within the portal venous blood vessels of the liver. This condition is usually associated with cirrhosis or cancer of the liver, although it can occur in some hematologic and cardiovascular diseases. In liver disease, portal hypertension develops when blood flow through the liver is obstructed because of destruction of hepatocytes, fat deposits, and fibrous tissue formation.

As portal blood flow through the liver becomes obstructed, collateral blood vessels and portal branch vessels enlarge as venous blood seeks an alternate route to the systemic circulation that bypasses the liver. Enlarged collateral channels develop between the portal and systemic veins that supply the esophagus, stomach, spleen, and rectum and in the umbilical veins of the falciform ligament. The collateral vessels dilate because of high intravascular pressure caused by the shunting of blood from the portal vessels. They become tortuous and may rupture, as seen in esophageal varices, a complication of portal hypertension. The management of esophageal varices is discussed in Chapter 28. An enlarged spleen (splenomegaly) results from splenic vein congestion caused by the high pressure in the portal system.

Ascites, the accumulation of fluid in the peritoneal cavity, occurs when the elevated portal vessel pressure in the liver causes increased resistance to blood flow and forces protein-rich plasma filtrate into the hepatic lymphatic vessels. This protein-rich plasma filtrate oozes from the liver surface into the peritoneal cavity because the lymphatic vessels are unable to absorb the large quantity of filtrate.

The amount of ascitic fluid is further increased because the damaged hepatocytes are unable to produce albumin, which is essential for maintaining the oncotic pressure within the circulatory system. Decreased albumin levels (hypoalbuminemia) cause decreased oncotic pressure, which results in a loss of fluid from the circulating blood volume and hemoconcentration. Fluid leaves the plasma and enters the peritoneal cavity as well as the extracellular spaces. The fluid in the extracellular spaces results in tissue edema.

In response to decreased circulating volume, the kidneys release renin, which increases the secretion of aldosterone from the adrenal cortex and antidiuretic hormone from the hypothalamus. As a result, sodium and water are retained. This further increases both ascites and edema. Figure 27–4 illustrates the mechanism of ascites formation in the presence of liver disease.

CLINICAL CHARACTERISTICS

Portal hypertension will not be evident unless the patient has visibly dilated abdominal blood vessels, bleeding from collateral blood vessels, or ascites.

Ascites is suspected when a patient complains of increased abdominal girth, or unexplained weight gain, or both. As the amount of fluid increases in the peritoneal cavity, the abdomen becomes distended and the umbilicus may evert because of the pressure exerted by the fluid. When fluid accumulation approaches 1000 ml, a dull sound is heard when the patient is in the supine position and the abdomen is percussed over the fluid-filled area. If the patient is turned on the side, fluid shifts with gravity and a dull sound is percussed in the dependent area. Distended abdominal veins and striae (stretch marks) may also be present.

The accumulation of fluid in the peritoneal cavity may cause respiratory difficulty because of pressure on the diaphragm. Total lung expansion is prevented and respirations are shallow.

MEDICAL MANAGEMENT

Treatment of portal hypertension requires that the underlying cause be identified. Medical management of ascites includes bed rest with sodium and fluid restriction, pharmacotherapy with diuretic agents, administration of albumin, paracentesis, and surgical intervention.

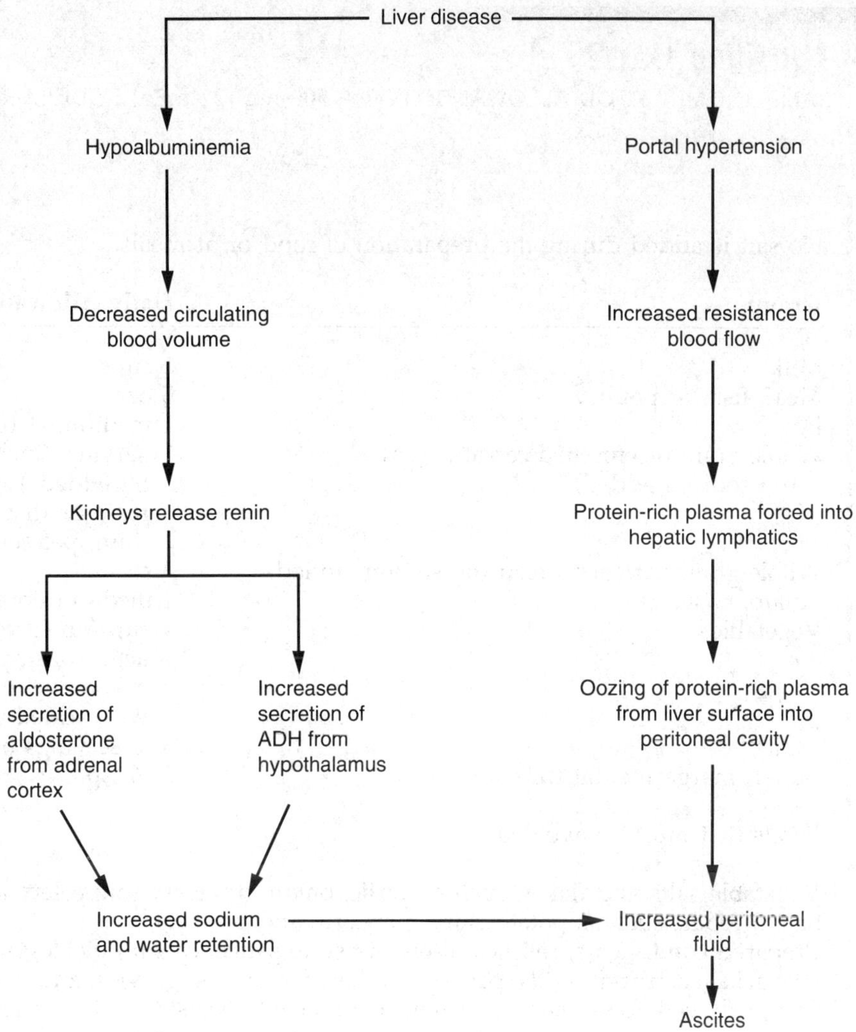

Figure 27–4.

Mechanism of ascites formation in liver disease. (ADH, antidiuretic hormone.)

DIETARY INTERVENTION

Ascitic fluid accumulation occurs when patients are in positive sodium balance as a result of excess aldosterone secretion. Therefore, sodium restriction decreases or stops the accumulation of ascitic fluid. A diet containing 250 to 500 mg of sodium is usually prescribed. Nutrition Box 27–1 describes the daily food allowance for a patient on a 500-mg (22-mEq) sodium-restricted diet. A fluid restriction of 1000 to 1500 ml daily is maintained when patients have decreased blood serum sodium levels (hyponatremia), which usually reflects excess body water rather than decreased sodium levels.

PHARMACOTHERAPY

If there is no decrease in ascitic fluid accumulation with sodium restriction alone, diuretics are added to the treatment plan. Diuretics cause a loss of fluid from the plasma, which is replaced by the reabsorption of ascitic or edema fluid. Spironolactone (Aldactone) is the diuretic of choice for patients with mild to moderate sodium retention. This medication blocks the action of aldosterone and promotes sodium loss and potassium retention. If spironolactone does not produce adequate fluid loss within 1 week, furosemide (Lasix) is prescribed in combination with spironolactone. Chart 27–1 summarizes patient information related to the use of diuretic therapy.

ALBUMIN THERAPY

Salt-poor human albumin is administered to increase the plasma colloid osmotic pressure and to promote reabsorption of ascitic fluid. Because this therapy is very expensive and the results are only temporary, it is not a therapy of choice.

PARACENTESIS

Paracentesis is a procedure that removes fluid from the peritoneal cavity. A trocar is inserted into the peritoneal cavity through an incision below the umbilicus. Tubing is connected to the trocar, and fluid drains from the peritoneal cavity over a period

Nutrition Box 27–1.

SAMPLE DAILY FOOD ALLOWANCE FOR A 500-mg (22-mEq) SODIUM-RESTRICTED DIET

No salt is added during the preparation of food or at meals.

Group	Daily Allowance
Milk	2 cups
Meat, fish, or poultry	5 oz
Egg	1 medium (1 oz meat may replace egg)
Whole-grain or enriched cereal (no sodium added)	1 serving (includes Puffed Wheat, Puffed Rice, Shredded Wheat, farina; no quick-cooking cereals or dry cereals with more than 5 mg sodium per serving)
Whole-grain enriched bread (no sodium added)	3 slices
Potato, pasta, rice	1 medium potato or 1 cup cooked pasta or rice
Vegetables	1 cup (no carrots, kale, beet greens, chard, spinach, frozen peas, frozen lima beans, beets, celery, or white turnips; no vegetables packaged with added sodium)
Fruit	3–5 servings (includes 1 serving citrus fruit)
Butter, margarine, fat (unsalted)	3–6 tsp

Foods that must be avoided:

Vegetable salts and flakes, such as garlic, onion, or celery salt; celery and parsley flakes
Salted foods, such as potato chips, popcorn, and pretzels
Prepared condiments, relishes, Worcestershire sauce, catsup, pickles, soy sauce, mustard, and olives
Prepackaged frozen foods, packaged mixes for sauces, gravies, and casseroles
Salt-preserved foods such as salted or smoked meats (bacon, corned beef, frankfurters, ham, kosher meats, luncheon meats), salted or smoked fish (herring, anchovies, frozen fish fillets), and sauerkraut
Canned soups
Meat extracts, bouillon cubes, and meat sauces
All canned meats and vegetables unless prepared without sodium
Cheese and peanut butter unless prepared without sodium
Packaged baking mixes or flour mixes unless prepared without sodium

of 30 to 60 minutes. When repeated paracentesis is indicated, an 18-gauge angiocatheter or needle may be used in place of a trocar to minimize trauma. The procedure is carried out at the bedside. Table 27–3 describes the nurse's role before, during, and after paracentesis.

The fluid removed from the peritoneal cavity contains large amounts of albumin, sodium, and potassium. Because this fluid rapidly reforms in the peritoneal cavity after removal, paracentesis is not a practical treatment for all patients with ascites. However, large-volume paracentesis (the removal of 1 to 2 L of fluid) remains an effective treatment for patients who are resistant to diuretic therapy and for patients who have respiratory difficulty because of pressure on the diaphragm from the ascitic fluid. Concomitant administration of 50 ml of intravenous (IV) salt-poor albumin for each liter of fluid removed helps to slow the reaccumulation of ascitic fluid. Small-volume paracentesis (50 to 100 ml) is used for diagnostic purposes when the cause of the ascites is unknown. Larger quantities of fluid may be removed when the fluid interferes with diagnostic visualization studies such as x-ray examinations or abdominal ultrasonography.

LeVEEN SHUNT

Patients who have severe and incapacitating ascites that does not respond to diuretic therapy are candidates for a surgical procedure that drains ascitic fluid from the peritoneal cavity into the superior vena cava. The LeVeen peritoneojugular shunt is a silicone catheter inserted and positioned surgically,

Chart 27–1.

NURSING GUIDE TO PATIENT EDUCATION FOR SELF-MANAGEMENT: DIURETIC THERAPY

Diuretics are a class of drugs that increase water and electrolyte elimination via the kidneys. The mechanism of action varies depending on the medication prescribed. With all diuretics, except the potassium-sparing diuretics, potassium is excreted in addition to sodium. When a potassium-sparing diuretic is prescribed with other diuretics, potassium balance is usually maintained.

Instruct the patient to do the following:

Take the medication early in the day to avoid the need to urinate during the night.
Report vomiting, leg cramps, or muscle weakness. These may indicate a potassium level less than 3.5 mEq/L.
Report signs of dehydration: thirst, altered mental status, decreased urine output, and decreased skin turgor.
Notify physician if vomiting or diarrhea occurs that lasts longer than 1 day. This can cause electrolyte imbalances.

If the patient is switched to a potassium-sparing diuretic or is taking a potassium-sparing diuretic in addition to another diuretic, caution the patient to omit all potassium supplements that may have been ordered previously. Hyperkalemia can result.

Table 27–3. PARACENTESIS

NURSING ACTIONS	RATIONALE
BEFORE PROCEDURE	
Obtain written consent.	Invasive procedure
Have patient void immediately before procedure.	Prevents accidental puncture of the bladder
Position patient upright in a chair or on edge of bed with feet and back supported.	With patient in upright position, air inside the intestines allows them to float away from needle insertion site
Assess vital signs.	Baseline data for comparison
Cleanse skin below umbilicus with antiseptic solution.	Removes surface organisms to reduce risk of infection
DURING PROCEDURE	
Remain with patient.	Nurse's presence provides support
Monitor vital signs.	Close observation detects complications early; vascular collapse is evidenced by increased pulse and decreased blood pressure
AFTER PROCEDURE	
Apply sterile pressure dressing to site, and allow patient to assume a comfortable position.	A break in the skin is a potential site for infection; pressure reduces risk of bleeding
Monitor vital signs and check dressing every 15 minutes for 1 hour, every 30 minutes for 2 hours, every hour for 2 hours, and then every 4 hours for 24 hours.	Patient is monitored for evidence of delayed complications; hypovolemic shock can result from shift of fluid from circulatory system to peritoneum to replace aspirated fluid

as illustrated in Figure 27–5. One end of the catheter is implanted in the peritoneal cavity, and the other end is channeled through the subcutaneous tissue to the superior vena cava where the end is implanted. A one-way pressure-sensitive valve regulates the flow of ascitic fluid. When the patient inhales, the diaphragm descends and pressure in the peritoneal cavity increases. This causes the valve to open and fluid is transported to the superior vena cava. During exhalation, the valve closes and prevents backflow. Diuretic therapy is usually prescribed in conjunction with the LeVeen shunt.

The Denver shunt is a modification of the LeVeen shunt and is used when ascites results from malignancy. Malignant ascites contains particulate matter that may block flow through the tubing. The Denver shunt has a subcutaneous pump that can be compressed manually to irrigate the tubing.

The emptying of large amounts of fluid into the superior vena cava may additionally benefit the patient by producing hemodilution, an increase in cardiac output, improved renal blood flow, and a decrease in serum aldosterone level. Complications of the shunting procedure include infection, occlusion of the shunt, leakage of peritoneal fluid, and disseminated intravascular coagulation (DIC). As a result of endotoxins and coagulant precursors in the ascitic fluid, some degree of DIC develops in all patients. Normal clotting factors are depleted, anticoagulants are released, and uncontrolled bleeding may occur. Usually the degree of bleeding is insig-

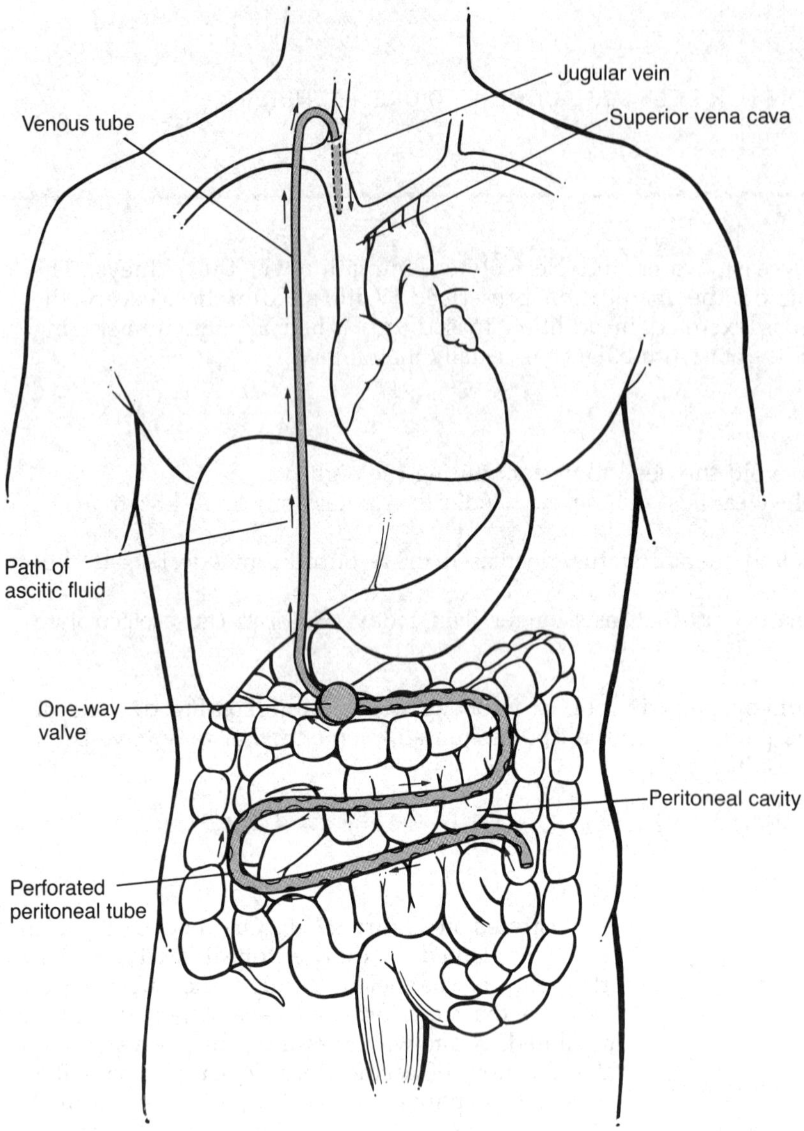

Figure 27–5.

LeVeen shunt. Arrows show direction of flow of ascitic fluid out of the peritoneal cavity, through the shunt, into the superior vena cava.

nificant. However, if excessive bleeding occurs, the shunt is removed.

Although the shunt procedure provides patients with temporary relief from the symptoms of ascites, it does not correct the underlying problem. Usually a shunt remains patent for a few days to 3 years. Approximately half are patent after 1 year.

Application of the Nursing Process to the Care of the Patient with Ascites

Assessment

Assess for changes in weight, abdominal girth, and degree of edema. Increasing weight, abdominal girth, and edema indicate fluid retention. Note the appearance of taut, shiny skin over the abdomen caused when fluid accumulates in the peritoneal cavity and stretches the skin. Observe the patient for difficulty breathing. Ascites causes pressure on the diaphragm and prevents total lung expansion. Examine all skin surfaces for evidence of redness or skin breakdown. Fluid accumulation in the tissues places the patient at risk for skin breakdown. Imposed bed rest increases the risk even further.

Assess the postoperative patient who has had a peritoneojugular shunt to determine shunt function. Assess abdominal girth, body weight, hematocrit level, and urinary output to establish a baseline for comparison with later measurements. A decrease in girth, body weight, and hematocrit level and an increase in urinary output indicate that the shunt is operating effectively.

The patient is also observed for early signs of DIC. These include bleeding of the mucous membranes, hematuria, and oozing of blood from intravenous or puncture sites. Coagulation studies will indicate low levels of fibrinogen and prolonged prothrombin times (PT) and thromboplastin times. These findings are immediately reported to the physician.

Observe the dressing site for evidence of peritoneal fluid leakage, which may predispose the patient to infection.

Nursing Diagnoses and Planning

Nursing diagnoses and related expected patient outcomes most commonly applicable to patients with ascites include the following:

NDx: Ineffective breathing pattern related to pressure on the diaphragm from ascites

Planning: Patient outcomes

1. Patient's respiratory rate remains between 12 and 20 per minute.
2. Patient has full chest expansion with each respiration.
3. Patient verbalizes ability to breathe with less difficulty.

NDx: Fluid volume excess related to the accumulation of fluid in the peritoneal cavity and dependent areas of the body

Planning: Patient outcomes

1. Patient's abdominal girth decreases daily.
2. Patient's body weight decreases daily.

NDx: High risk for impaired skin integrity related to ascites and edema

Planning: Patient outcomes

1. Patient's skin remains intact.

Nursing diagnoses and related expected patient outcomes most commonly applicable to patients who undergo a peritoneojugular shunt procedure include the following:

NDx: High risk for fluid volume deficit related to diuretic therapy and too rapid removal of fluid from the peritoneal cavity to the superior vena cava

Planning: Patient outcomes

1. Patient's electrolyte values remain within normal limits.
2. Patient's respirations remain clear and unlabored.

NDx: High risk for altered health maintenance related to lack of knowledge of signs of shunt failure

Planning: Patient outcomes

1. Patient states intent to weigh self daily.
2. Patient demonstrates ability to weigh self accurately.
3. Patient verbalizes situations that require physician notification.

Nursing Interventions

NDx: Ineffective breathing pattern
Position the patient in a semi-Fowler's or high Fowler's position as tolerated to promote maximum chest expansion by decreasing the pressure of the ascitic fluid and the internal organs on the diaphragm. Instruct the patient to deep breathe every 2 hours to promote maximum lung expansion. Auscultate the lungs for diminished breath sounds every 4 hours. Compare the right upper and lower lobes with the left upper and lower lobes. Diminished breath sounds, especially in the lower lobes, indicate inadequate chest expansion. Monitor vital signs every 4 hours to identify early indications of oxygen deficit. Manifestations of hypoxemia include a rising, bounding pulse; a rising systolic blood pressure; and rapid respirations.

NDx: Fluid volume excess
Monitor fluid intake and output daily. In a healthy person, the fluid intake from all sources equals the fluid output from all sources over a 3-day period. Fluid intake exceeding output indicates fluid retention. Limit fluids to prescribed amount spread out over a 24-hour period and administer prescribed diuretics. Half of the allotted fluids are given between 8 A.M. and 4 P.M. An additional two fifths of the total is given between 4 P.M. and 11 P.M., and the remainder is permitted between 11 P.M. and 8 A.M. Notify the dietary department and determine how much fluid will be served with meals. Subtract this from the total fluid allowance to prevent excess intake. Remember that fluids given with medications are included in the daily fluid intake. Provide the patient with mouthwash for oral hygiene every 4 hours to decrease thirst. Do not use lemon-glycerin swabs to moisten the mouth. Glycerin, an astringent, has a drying effect on mucous membranes.

Weigh the patient daily before breakfast but after he or she has urinated. Have the patient wear similar clothes and use the same scale each day to ensure accuracy. A change of 2 lb is equivalent to 1 L of fluid. As much as 6 to 8 lb can be gained before physical signs of ascites or edema are evident. Measure the abdominal girth daily. Mark the abdomen with a pen to indicate the point at which the measurement is taken to ensure valid comparison with previous measurements. Abdominal girth decreases as ascites decreases.

NDx: High risk for impaired skin integrity
Inspect the patient's skin daily for evidence of redness or skin breakdown, especially in dependent body areas (e.g., sacral area for a patient on bed rest; lower extremities for a patient out of bed). Edema causes pressure on the blood vessels and impedes blood flow to peripheral vessels. Obstructed capillary blood flow leads to tissue ischemia and necrosis. Use pressure-relieving pads on the bed and chair to provide more even weight distribution. Teach the patient the importance of changing position every 2 hours. Provide a bed trapeze if

Chart 27–2.

NURSING GUIDE TO PATIENT EDUCATION FOR SELF-MANAGEMENT: LeVEEN SHUNT

Instruct the patient to do the following:

Use strict aseptic technique when caring for the incision.
Examine wound daily for signs of infection: redness, edema, purulent discharge, increasing tenderness.
Perform deep breathing at frequent intervals during the day to maintain shunt patency.
Measure abdominal girth daily.
Record weight obtained each day before breakfast but after voiding.
Report the following symptoms to the physician immediately: increased weight, increased abdominal girth, decreased urinary output, respiratory distress, edema.
Keep appointments for follow-up evaluations by the physician.

the patient is capable of using it. The trapeze bar allows the patient to lift rather than pull the body when repositioning and therefore decreases shearing force, a major contributor to skin breakdown. A footboard to prevent the patient from sliding down in bed further minimizes shearing force. If the patient is permitted out of bed, limit time in the chair to no more than 2 hours unless the patient can shift his or her weight unassisted.

Avoid injections when possible. If injections must be administered, inspect injection sites carefully. Do not administer injections in sites that are edematous. The absorption of drugs is decreased in these areas because of fluid accumulation and decreased blood supply. Drugs injected into edematous areas can also act as irritants and predispose to skin breakdown.

Keep bed linens and bed clothing dry. Moisture increases the incidence of skin breakdown fivefold. Keep the skin dry, and apply a thin layer of lotion daily. Moisture, as well as excessive dryness, decreases the skin's resistance to infection. Application of lotion massages the skin and increases blood supply to the area.

NDx: High risk for fluid volume deficit (LeVeen shunt)

Monitor electrolytes and hematocrit every 4 hours during the immediate postoperative period to identify early signs of excess hemodilution. Monitor respiratory status, and auscultate the lungs for crackles (rales) every 2 hours. Excess hemodilution, dyspnea, tachycardia, or pulmonary edema indicates that fluid is being removed too quickly from the peritoneal cavity. To slow the rate of fluid flow from the peritoneal cavity, place the patient in a sitting position. This action increases the difference in pressures between the peritoneal and thoracic cavities, thus interrupting the flow of peritoneal fluid into the superior vena cava. Exhaling against a closed glottis also decreases flow. Assist the patient to turn and deep breathe every 2 hours. Monitor intake and output. Examine skin and mucous membranes daily. Decreased skin turgor and dry mucous membranes indicate fluid depletion.

NDx: High risk for altered health maintenance (LeVeen shunt)

Instruct the patient to weigh himself or herself each morning before eating breakfast but after urinating to monitor fluid volume status. Observe the patient carry out the procedure without assistance to determine accuracy and evaluate learning. Teach the patient to notify the physician if clothing becomes tight at the waist, a weight gain of more than 1 lb/day or 3 lb/week is noted, urinary output decreases, or breathing difficulty is experienced. Chart 27–2 provides guidelines for education for self-management for the patient with a LeVeen shunt.

Evaluation

Evaluate the effectiveness of nursing care for a patient with ascites by comparing the patient's status with the expected patient outcomes. Examples of specific outcomes for patients with ascites have been provided in the Planning section.

Clotting Disorders

PATHOPHYSIOLOGY

Bleeding is frequently seen in patients with hepatic dysfunction. Clotting factors V, VII, IX, and X, fibrinogen, and prothrombin are synthesized by the healthy liver. With liver disease, production may decline. Altered fat metabolism also interferes with the utilization of vitamin K, which further decreases the synthesis of clotting factors.

CLINICAL CHARACTERISTICS

Bleeding may be noted from the gums after brushing the teeth, from the nose after forceful blowing, as petechial hemorrhages of the eye, or as skin or mucous membrane lesions that result from the spontaneous rupture of small blood vessels. The most common lesions are petechiae, pinhead-size, purplish hemorrhagic areas; purpura, larger hemorrhagic areas up to 1 cm in diameter; ecchymoses, large irregularly shaped hemorrhagic areas; and spider angiomas, small hemorrhagic areas with numerous dilated vessels radiating outward. Bleeding, although not always visible, may also be present in the urine and stool.

MEDICAL MANAGEMENT

A parenteral aqueous solution of vitamin K is prescribed when prothrombin production is decreased because of obstruction of bile flow. Parenteral vitamin K is absorbed in the absence of bile and can be used for the production of prothrombin. If the liver has ceased to produce clotting factors because of hepatocyte damage, fresh plasma, or whole-blood-replacement therapy may be indicated.

Application of the Nursing Process to the Care of the Patient at Risk for Bleeding

Assessment

Observe all body surfaces and mucous membranes daily to identify bleeding sites, precipitating factors, and amount of bleeding. Monitor PT and other clotting factors. Monitor all body fluids for the presence of blood. Observe for excessive menstrual bleeding.

Nursing Diagnoses and Planning

Nursing diagnoses and related expected patient outcomes most commonly applicable to patients at risk for bleeding include the following:

NDx: High risk for injury related to interference with the clotting mechanism

Planning: Patient outcomes

1. Patient avoids activities that increase the risk of bleeding.

Nursing Interventions

NDx: High risk for injury

Instruct the patient to avoid all substances and activities that may precipitate bleeding. These include alcohol; all nonprescription drugs, including aspirin; coarse foods; and large meals. Gastrointestinal bleeding is precipitated when the gastrointestinal tract is irritated. Forceful coughing, straining at stool, and heavy lifting are also contraindicated. Excessive pressure within the thoracic or abdominal cavities may cause bleeding. Test all urine, stool, and emesis for occult blood because small amounts of bleeding may not be visible to the naked eye. Provide a soft toothbrush to minimize gum bleeding while brushing, and substitute foam toothettes if bleeding continues. Male patients should shave with an electric razor. Take temperatures orally to minimize irritation to the blood vessels in the rectal area. If the patient is confused or agitated, pad side rails to decrease the risk of injury.

Because frequent diagnostic blood studies are required with hepatic disorders, group tests to limit the number of venipunctures and use the smallest gauge needle possible. Apply pressure at all venipuncture sites for 3 to 5 minutes or until bleeding stops. Coagulation may require 5 to 10 minutes with some patients.

Evaluation

Evaluate the effectiveness of nursing care for a patient at risk for bleeding by comparing the patient's status with the expected patient outcomes. An example of a specific outcome for patients at risk for bleeding has been provided in the Planning section.

Hepatic Encephalopathy

The term *hepatic encephalopathy* is used to describe a group of manifestations of impaired neurologic function that are experienced by patients with advanced liver disease. The syndrome is frequently referred to as hepatic coma.

PATHOPHYSIOLOGY

The exact pathophysiology of hepatic encephalopathy is unclear. However, it is known that the inability of the liver to metabolize and cleanse the blood of ammonia and mercaptans, toxic substances produced in the intestines, is a major contributor to the problem. Ammonia is produced by intestinal bacteria as an end product of protein metabolism. Mercaptans are produced when sulfur-containing compounds are metabolized in the intestine. These substances alter metabolism in the central nervous system possibly by interfering directly with brain carbohydrate metabolism or indirectly by causing the formation of other neurotoxic substances. Actual blood ammonia levels do not always correlate directly with the severity of hepatic encephalopathy, but decreasing ammonia levels are associated with successful treatment.

The most common factors that precipitate hepatic encephalopathy in the patient with liver disease are the excessive ingestion of protein and gastrointestinal bleeding. The metabolism of blood protein in the intestine results in ammonia production. Other causes include the overzealous use of chlorothiazide diuretics, which can cause potassium depletion. In this instance, the diuretic causes hypokalemic metabolic alkalosis and increased absorption of ammonia from the renal tubules and gastrointestinal tract and ultimately increases the amount of ammonium hydroxide that enters the brain. When the potassium level is maintained within normal limits, this problem is not encountered.

Factors unrelated to ammonia levels may also be associated with hepatic encephalopathy. These include the use of sedatives, tranquilizers, or narcotics; severe infection; and operative procedures.

CLINICAL CHARACTERISTICS

Hepatic encephalopathy must be suspected in any patient with liver disease who experiences abnormal neurologic signs and symptoms. Initial signs are apathy, restlessness, and a shortened attention span. The patient picks at the bedclothes and has a "far-away look," slowed thought processes, and slurred speech. Simple tasks become difficult. Sometimes, a sweet, musty odor (fetor hepaticus) resulting from the breakdown of mercaptans may be noted from the breath. The most common and reliable sign that hepatic encephalopathy is developing is the presence of asterixis, often referred to as liver flap or hepatic tremor. Asterixis is irregular flapping movements of the fingers and wrists when the hands and arms are outstretched, with the palms down, wrists

Table 27–4. STAGES OF HEPATIC ENCEPHALOPATHY

STAGE	CHARACTERISTICS
1: Prodromal	Shortened attention span, slowed thought processes, apathy, or euphoria present; mild confusion, slight tremor may be noted; picking at bedclothes and yawning common; reversal of usual sleep pattern
2: Impending coma	Disorientation, asterixis, peculiar "musty" odor to breath (fetor hepaticus), sleeping most of time but easily aroused, incontinent
3: Stupor	Deep sleep but can be aroused, incoherent speech
4: Coma	Stage 4A: patient responds to painful stimuli Stage 4B: no response

Nutrition Box 27–2.

SAMPLE DAILY FOOD ALLOWANCE FOR A 30-g PROTEIN-RESTRICTED DIET

1 cup of milk
1 oz of meat or 1 egg
3 slices of bread
$\frac{1}{2}$ cup of cereal
2 small potatoes
1 cup of vegetables
2 servings of salad (fruit or vegetable)
2 servings of fruit
$\frac{1}{2}$ cup of fruit or fruit juice
2 tbsp of cream
Butter
Jelly
Sugar
Nonprotein foods to supply caloric requirements

Protein is reduced to 15 g if the milk and 1 oz of meat or one egg is deleted.

The following protein sources are known to raise the ammonia level to a greater degree than other protein sources and are therefore avoided: American cheese, buttermilk, cheddar cheese, blue cheese, chicken, gelatin, ground beef, ham, potatoes, and salami.

Pharmacology Box 27–2.

NEOMYCIN SULFATE

Neomycin Sulfate:
Aminoglycoside antibiotic; antiinfective.

Action:
Destroys bacteria by inhibiting protein synthesis; broad-spectrum antibacterial activity.

Uses:
Reduces the number of ammonia-producing organisms in the intestine and is used for preoperative intestinal asepsis.

Side Effects:
Ototoxicity and nephrotoxicity. Mild laxative effect; diarrhea, nausea, vomiting; vitamin B_{12} malabsorption–like syndrome.

Interactions:
Increased risk for ototoxicity when neomycin sulfate is administered with loop diuretics (furosemide and ethacrynic acid). May decrease absorption of cyanocobalamin.

Nursing Implications:
Monitor for evidence of ototoxicity: diminished hearing, tinnitus, vertigo, loss of balance, or altered gait in ambulatory patients. Monitor urinary output. Notify physician if output decreases. Provide adequate hydration. Visually inspect urine for evidence of cells or casts in the urine. Compare baseline and periodic audiometric and renal studies for early detection of toxicity.

bent up, and fingers spread. Jerking muscle tremors can also be seen in the feet and the tongue. Progression to deep coma can occur gradually or suddenly. Table 27–4 summarizes the stages of hepatic encephalopathy.

MEDICAL MANAGEMENT

The presence of altered neurologic signs and advanced liver disease and the exclusion of other causes of neurologic impairment are sufficient to arrive at a diagnosis of hepatic encephalopathy. Precipitating factors that can be corrected, such as hypokalemia or gastrointestinal bleeding, are addressed by the physician. When these are corrected and no improvement in neurologic function occurs, treatment includes dietary restriction of protein and bowel cleansing.

DIETARY INTERVENTION

To reduce ammonia production in the early stages of hepatic encephalopathy, protein intake is restricted to 15 to 50 g daily with sufficient carbohydrate to provide 2000 kcal/day. Vitamin and mineral supplements are also prescribed. Protein is eliminated totally if the patient is in an advanced stage of hepatic encephalopathy. As neurologic signs and symptoms resolve, protein intake is increased by 10 to 15 g per week. If neurologic manifestations recur, protein is once again decreased. Nutrition Box 27–2 illustrates the daily intake for a patient on a 30-g protein-restricted diet.

BOWEL CLEANSING

The purpose of bowel cleansing is to decrease enteric organisms which produce ammonia when they break down nitrogenous substances. Bowel cleansing is achieved in a number of ways. Neomycin, a poorly absorbed antibiotic excreted in the stool, is administered orally, 1 to 2 g every 6 hours. Neomycin reduces ammonia-forming bacteria in the intestine. Neomycin enemas containing 4 g of the drug are administered to cleanse the lower bowel. Lactulose, a nonabsorbable disaccharide, is used to decrease bowel ammonia absorption. Lactulose is metabolized by colonic bacteria to organic acids, which prevent the diffusion of ammonia through the intestinal mucosa. Lactulose syrup, 50 ml every 2 hours, is administered until diarrhea develops. The dose is then decreased to the amount necessary to produce two to four soft stools per day. Lactulose and neomycin can be prescribed together. Pharmacology Boxes 27–2 and 27–3 describe neomycin and lactulose.

Pharmacology Box 27–3.

LACTULOSE

Lactulose:
Colonic acidifier; hyperosmotic laxative.

Action:
Acidifies colonic contents, resulting in the retention of ammonia in the colon as ammonium ion. Because the colon is more acidic than the blood, ammonia migrates from the blood to the colon to form ammonium ion. The laxative action of lactulose then expels the trapped ammonium ion from the colon.

Uses:
Reduces blood ammonia level in hepatic encephalopathy by 25% to 50%.

Side Effects:
Cramps, borborygmi, distention, flatulence, and diarrhea; hypernatremia due to water loss.

Interactions:
Nonabsorbable antacids inhibit desired effect of lactulose.

Nursing Implications:
Assess patient's mental status frequently during therapy. Improvement usually occurs within 24–48 hours. Monitor stools for diarrhea, which indicates dose should be decreased until patient has three to four soft stools per day. Lactulose enemas may be used when oral administration is contraindicated because of the danger of aspiration or if the patient is intubated. Three hundred ml of lactulose and 700 ml of water are administered rectally and must be retained for 30–60 minutes.

Geriatric Considerations:
The elderly are at increased risk for hypernatremia because of reduced capacity to adjust to fluid loss.

Application of the Nursing Process to the Care of the Patient with Hepatic Encephalopathy

Assessment

Assess the patient for changes in mental function. Note the presence of apathy, restlessness, slowed thought processes, and slurred speech. Determine orientation to time, person, and place. Assess for changes in psychomotor functions. Request a handwriting sample for comparison with later samples. Assess for presence of asterixis and fetor hepaticus. Note blood ammonia levels and potassium levels. Increasing blood ammonia levels or decreasing potassium levels may indicate the development of hepatic encephalopathy. Assess for the presence of precipitating factors such as diuretic therapy, gastrointestinal bleeding, and surgical procedures that place the patient at increased risk for hepatic encephalopathy. Assess family members' understanding of hepatic encephalopathy. Family members may not be prepared to deal with the rapid deterioration in mental function.

Nursing Diagnoses and Planning

Nursing diagnoses and related expected patient outcomes most commonly applicable to patients with hepatic encephalopathy include the following:

NDx: High risk for injury related to altered thought processes secondary to impaired liver detoxification

Planning: Patient outcomes
1. Patient remains free of injury.

NDx: Altered family processes related to family member with hepatic encephalopathy

Planning: Patient outcomes

1. Family members verbalize their concerns to nursing staff.

Nursing Interventions

NDx: High risk for injury

Monitor level of consciousness, orientation, rate of speech, and response time every 4 hours. Ask the patient to state his or her name, the date, and month and to identify present location. Request a daily sample of handwriting, either a short sentence or the patient's name. A decreasing level of consciousness, disorientation, slurred speech, prolonged response time, and difficulty writing indicate that the patient's condition is deteriorating. Monitor for the irregular, jerking movements of asterixis every 4 hours. This is the most common sign of impending coma. Restrict protein intake, and administer neomycin or lactulose, or both, as prescribed. Decreased ammonia levels correlate with improvement in the patient's condition. Provide increased carbohydrates for energy and to spare protein from being broken down. Monitor daily serum potassium levels. Decreased potassium levels, which may occur with diuretic therapy, can precipitate coma. The use of potassium-sparing diuretics minimizes this risk.

Keep side rails up and the bed in low position at all times. If the patient is disoriented or comatose, continue to identify yourself on entering the room and explain all procedures. Keep a night-light on during sleeping hours.

NDx: Altered family processes

Provide an explanation of hepatic encephalopathy in understandable terms. Keep the family informed of the patient's progress on a daily basis. Allow family members to visit with minimal interruption. Include family in care if they desire to take part. Provide a place away from the patient's room for family to ask questions and discuss progress. Include the family in nursing care conferences when possible. Illness of one family member affects the family unit. Successful coping strategies require that the family, with the support of the professional health care team, acknowledge the problem, accept it, and adjust to its consequences.

Evaluation

Evaluate the effectiveness of nursing care for a patient with hepatic encephalopathy by comparing the patient's status with the expected patient outcomes. Examples of specific outcomes for patients with hepatic encephalopathy have been provided in the Planning section.

Nutritional Deficiencies

Because the liver performs so many varied functions, hepatic disorders can affect digestion, absorption, metabolism, and storage of nutrients.

PATHOPHYSIOLOGY

Anorexia, the absence of hunger, is frequently seen with hepatic disorders. The hypothalamus is responsible for regulating food intake by controlling feeding centers located at separate sites in the hypothalamus. The satiety centers are stimulated by high blood levels of glucose and free fatty acids after a meal and cause a decreased desire for food. Although the exact cause of anorexia is unknown, the slowed metabolism of fatty acids may be a factor that causes a feeling of "fullness" and, therefore, a lack of appetite. Nausea and vomiting, also seen in the patient with hepatic dysfunction, may result from slowed or incomplete metabolism of body wastes by the liver. The presence of anorexia, nausea, and vomiting presents a challenge to health care providers because nutrients are essential for the regeneration of hepatocytes, and stored nutrients are exhausted when intake is inadequate to meet the body's needs.

The most pronounced nutritional deficiencies are seen in patients with alcohol-related liver disease. In the liver, alcohol is converted to acetaldehyde, and excessive amounts of hydrogen result from the reaction. The acetaldehyde is a toxic substance to the liver and causes inflammation and hepatocyte necrosis. The hydrogen replaces fatty acid as a fuel, and fat accumulates in the liver. Because this fat occupies most of the volume of the hepatocytes, normal cell functions are interrupted. When alcohol consumption is stopped, fat deposits disappear within 3 to 6 weeks.

In addition to the problems caused directly by alcohol intake, the chronic alcoholic is usually malnourished because of inadequate nutrient intake. Alcohol replaces food in the diet. When nutrients are ingested, there is malabsorption of thiamine, vitamin B_{12}, folic acid, and ascorbic acid as a result of inflammation of the gastrointestinal tract. Because hepatocytes are inflamed, they cannot activate vitamins D and B_6 and thiamine. To metabolize the alcohol, increased amounts of the B vitamins are needed by the body, and liver stores are depleted.

Regardless of the cause, all patients with liver disease are at risk for nutritional deficiencies when the hepatocytes cannot perform normal functions. Protein synthesis is impaired and stored proteins are exhausted, which results in muscle wasting, inability to repair and regenerate damaged tissues, and decreased levels of the plasma proteins needed to maintain intravascular oncotic pressure and fluid balance. Interference with carbohydrate metabolism causes glycogen stores to be depleted, and proteins are used for energy, further depleting protein stores.

Hypoglycemia results when both glycogenolysis and gluconeogenesis are no longer possible. Inadequate production of bile salts causes malabsorption of fats and fat-soluble vitamins. Fats that cannot be absorbed are excreted in the stool (steatorrhea) and deprive the body of substantial calories, which contributes to weight loss and malnutrition. Because calcium binds to fatty acids, calcium is excreted in the stool and calcium deficits occur.

CLINICAL CHARACTERISTICS

Patients with nutritional deficiencies exhibit a wide variety of signs and symptoms. Table 27–5 summarizes the major clinical characteristics of nutrient deficiencies associated with hepatic disorders.

MEDICAL MANAGEMENT

A high-protein, moderate-fat, high-carbohydrate diet is recommended for patients with liver disease to promote positive nitrogen balance, correct undernutrition, replenish plasma protein, and promote regeneration of functioning liver tissue to minimize the risk of hepatic encephalopathy. Protein is restricted when hepatic encephalopathy is present. Sodium restriction is required if ascites and edema are present.

A vitamin supplement containing vitamin B complex, especially folic acid, is recommended. Water-soluble forms of vitamins A, D, and E are given if steatorrhea is present. Vitamin K is administered if prothrombin time is prolonged. Antiemetic agents may be prescribed to relieve symptoms of nausea and vomiting.

Table 27–5. CLINICAL CHARACTERISTICS OF NUTRITIONAL DEFICIENCIES ASSOCIATED WITH HEPATIC DISORDERS

DEFICIENT NUTRIENT	CLINICAL CHARACTERISTICS
Protein	Muscle wasting Impaired tissue repair Decreased synthesis of plasma proteins
Carbohydrate	Hypoglycemia
Fat	Steatorrhea
Vitamin A	Overgrowth of epidermal cells
Vitamin D	Osteomalacia (bone softening)
Calcium	Osteomalacia
Vitamin K	Clotting disorder
B complex vitamins	Dermatitis, neuritis
Niacin	Muscle weakness, anorexia
Folic acid	Anemia
Vitamin B_{12}	Anemia, neuritis, glossitis
Vitamin C	Anemia, weakness, decreased appetite, inflamed gums, delayed wound healing
Iron	Anemia

Application of the Nursing Process to the Care of the Patient with Nutritional Deficiencies

Assessment

Obtain a complete dietary history to determine dietary patterns. One method to assess nutritional intake is to ask the patient to recall all intake for the previous 3-day period. Include between-meal and bedtime snacks as well as meals. Determine drinking habits, including how long the patient has consumed alcohol, how often consumption occurs, the amount consumed, and the type of alcoholic beverage. Assess for the clinical manifestations of specific nutrient deficiencies, as shown in Table 27–5.

Nursing Diagnoses and Planning

Nursing diagnoses and related expected patient outcomes most commonly applicable to patients with nutritional deficiencies include the following:

NDx: Altered nutrition: less than body requirements related to nausea, vomiting, anorexia, or inadequate dietary intake

Planning: Patient outcomes
1. Patient eats 80% to 100% of all meals.
2. Patient has a steady weight gain with no evidence of fluid retention.
3. Patient outlines a 3-day meal plan.

Nursing Interventions

NDx: Altered nutrition: less than body requirements

If the patient is vomiting, administer prescribed antiemetic agent 30 to 45 minutes before meals. Most antiemetic drugs require at least 20 to 30 minutes to reach effective levels. Provide mouth care before each meal to remove unpleasant tastes and stimulate a desire for food. Offer clear liquids (gelatin, tea, ginger ale, or cola), 60 ml/hour, to the patient who cannot tolerate solid food. Gradually increase the amount as tolerated by the patient.

Provide five or six small meals rather than three large meals when anorexia is present. Large meals are unappealing when anorexia is present and may discourage the patient. Consider patient food preferences in planning meals. Provide the largest amount of food at the first meal of the day. Appetite is usually greatest on awakening and may decrease during the day. Offer fruit juices between meals. Juices provide vitamins and extra calories.

As the patient's condition improves, explain his or her nutritional needs, and assist in choosing meals for the next day. Provide the patient with written information describing the prescribed diet and the basic food groups. Review materials with the patient daily. When the patient can outline the prescribed diet, ask him or her to outline a 1-day meal plan for home use. If successful, ask him or her to outline a 3-day plan.

Evaluation

Evaluate the effectiveness of nursing care for a patient with nutritional deficiencies by comparing the patient's status with the expected patient outcomes. Examples of specific outcomes for patients with nutritional deficiencies have been provided in the Planning section.

Assessment of Hepatic Function

Patient History

When collecting a history, determine whether the patient has any complaints related to the clinical manifestations of liver disease. Areas to focus on are reports of increased fatigue, shortness of breath, changes in skin color, bruising, itching, recent weight gain, and changes in stool or urine color. Ask specifically about tightness of clothing, especially at the waistline, or pain or discomfort in the abdomen. Determine whether there has been any change in eating, sleeping, or elimination patterns. Determine the patient's present and former use of alcohol. Specifically ask the amount of alcohol consumed daily. Ask whether any prescribed medications, over-the-counter medications, or recreational drugs are currently being or have recently been used. Review any past hospitalizations and the reason for admission. Ask whether the patient has received blood or blood products. Blood and blood products can transmit viral hepatitis. Ask the female patient if she has noted menstrual irregularities. Question the male patient about enlargement of breast tissue or change in body hair distribution. Impaired liver function may interfere with hormone metabolism.

Physical Examination

Examine the skin, sclerae, and mucous membranes for jaundice. Inspect the skin for evidence of scratching, petechiae, purpura, ecchymosis, and spider angiomas, seen most often on the shoulders and upper trunk. Note breast enlargment in the male. Measure abdominal girth. Examine the abdomen for prominent veins caused by obstructed portal blood flow and for a glistening, taut appearance caused by stretching of the skin with ascites. Note the presence of striae and abdominal distention.

Percuss the abdomen in the supine position to determine the presence of fluid laterally. The abdomen is normally tympanic on percussion; fluid produces a dull sound. Turn the patient on the left and right sides, and percuss again. Fluid shifts to the dependent side, causing bulging and shifting dullness. As shown in Figure 27–6, percuss the liver starting at an area below the umbilicus at the midclavicular line. Continue percussing upward until dullness over the liver is noted. Then start at the fourth intercostal space, midclavicular line, and percuss downward until dullness is noted. The vertical span of liver dullness should be 6 to 12 cm ($2\frac{1}{2}$ to $4\frac{1}{2}$ in.). If midclavicular percussion indicates liver enlargement, percuss the liver in the midsternal line, where it is normally 4 to 8 cm ($1\frac{1}{2}$ to 3 in.) and note span.

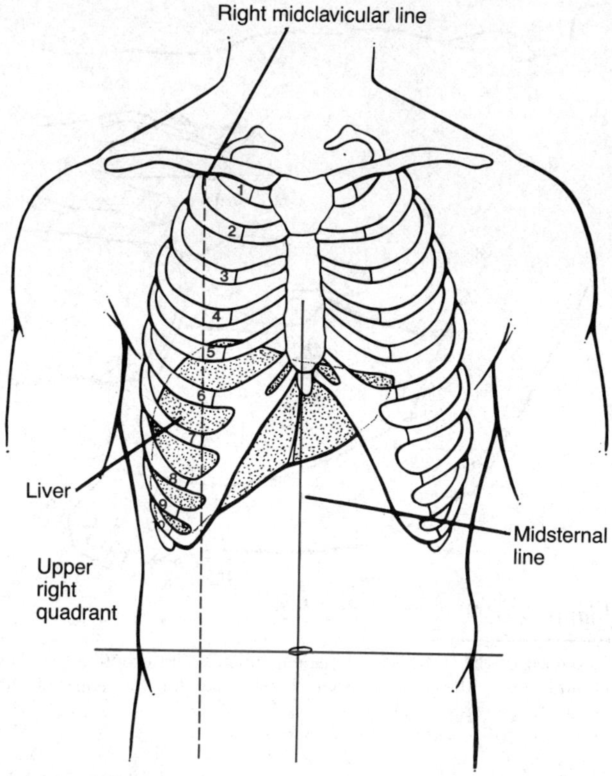

Figure 27–6.

Anatomic landmarks for percussion of the liver.

Palpate the abdomen to determine the size and location of the liver. To palpate, place your left hand under the patient at the eleventh and twelfth ribs and lift upward toward the abdominal wall, as shown in Figure 27–7. Place your right hand on the abdomen so that the tips of the fingers rest on the right midclavicular line below the level of dullness. Fingers may point toward the head or be positioned slightly oblique to the midclavicular line. Press your right hand in and up as you instruct the patient to take a deep breath. Usually the liver is not felt. In some thin individuals and in liver enlargement, it may be felt as a firm, smooth, even, nontender mass that slides under the fingers of the right hand.

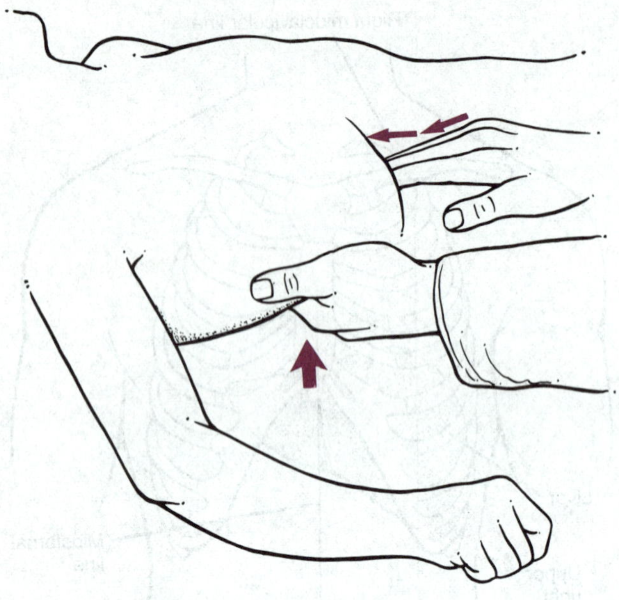

Figure 27–7.

Palpation of the liver. As the patient inhales, the examiner presses in and up at the midclavicular line to feel for the edge of the descending liver.

Observe and palpate for muscle wasting. Muscle tone should be firm, not doughy. Test muscle strength in the upper and lower extremities by asking the patient to flex a limb and then resist you when you apply opposing force against the flexion. Instruct the patient to extend the arms to test for asterixis.

To assess cognitive abilities, ask the patient to describe the similarities between two objects, such as a peach and a pear. Provide a series of four or five numbers, and ask the patient to repeat them to test recent memory. Have the patient write a short sentence or his or her name or draw a picture to test coordination.

Diagnostic Procedures

Hepatic function is evaluated by blood studies to assess metabolic function, urine and fecal examinations, noninvasive procedures such as ultrasonography, computed tomography (CT) scans and magnetic resonance imaging (MRI), and liver biopsy, an invasive procedure. All blood tests and invasive procedures place the patient at risk for bleeding because of altered clotting mechanism. Application of the nursing process to the care of the patient at risk for bleeding was discussed earlier in this chapter under Clotting Disorders. Common diagnostic studies used to assess liver function are summarized in Tables 27–6 and 27–7.

Blood Studies

LIVER ENZYMES

Enzymes, intracellular protein catalysts that enhance chemical reactions, are released when cellular damage occurs. Elevated levels of enzymes known to exist in an organ are useful indicators of cellular damage to that specific organ. Aspartate aminotransferase (AST), formerly known as serum glu-

Table 27–6. COMMON DIAGNOSTIC STUDIES OF LIVER FUNCTION

STUDY	NORMAL VALUE	PROCEDURE/INTERPRETATION
SERUM ENZYMES		
AST	Men: 8–46 U/L Women: 7–34 U/L	5-ml venous sample obtained; elevated with acute hepatitis, active cirrhosis, and hepatic necrosis
ALT	10–30 IU/ml	5-ml venous sample obtained; high concentration of this enzyme normally found in the liver is more specific than AST for liver disease
LDH	70–250 U/L	5-ml venous sample obtained
Isoenzymes		
LDH_4	5–15% of total	Liver contains high concentrations of LDH_4 and LDH_5, isoenzymes of LDH; both levels are elevated with liver disease
LDH_5	2–20% of total	
Alkaline phosphatase	20–130 U/L	3-ml venous sample obtained; elevation associated with elevated AST and bilirubin
Isoenzymes		
5′-Nucleotidase	0–1.6 U	Elevation supports hepatobiliary disorder
Gamma glutamyl transpeptidase	Men: 6–37 U/L Women: 6–37 U/L	Elevated with hepatic carcinoma and hepatobiliary tract obstruction
BILIRUBIN METABOLISM		
Total serum bilirubin	0.3–1.2 mg/dl	5-ml venous sample with 4-hour fast before sample
Direct (conjugated)	0.1–0.4 mg/dl	Elevated unconjugated bilirubin associated with increased destruction of RBCs; elevated conjugated bilirubin seen with most liver disease
Indirect (unconjugated)	0.3–1.1 mg/dl	

(continued)

Table 27–6. COMMON DIAGNOSTIC STUDIES OF LIVER FUNCTION (*continued*)

STUDY	NORMAL VALUE	PROCEDURE/INTERPRETATION
BILIRUBIN METABOLISM (*continued*)		
Urine bilirubin	Negative	Examine urine within 1 hour of sample collection; should be performed on every routine urinalysis; early indicator of liver disease
Urine urobilinogen	1–4 mg/24 hr	Usually a 24-hour urine collection; increased in any condition that causes increased bilirubin and any disease that prevents removal of reabsorbed urobilinogen from the portal circulation
Fecal urobilinogen	40–200 mg/24 hr	Stool specimen obtained; decreased or absent when normal amounts of bilirubin are not excreted into intestinal tract; decreased values seen with severe liver disease
PROTEIN METABOLISM		
Total serum protein	6.6–7.9 g/dl	5-ml venous sample obtained; decreased total protein with insufficient protein intake or decreased formation in the liver
Serum albumin	3.3–4.5 g/dl	Decreased albumin levels occur with hepatocellular disease
Serum globulin	2.0–4.2 g/dl	Elevated levels in advanced cirrhosis and chronic active hepatitis
A/G ratio	1.5:1–2.5:1	When total protein increases and albumin is unchanged or decreased while globulins increase, proportion of albumin falls; occurs in acute liver disease
Serum protein electrophoresis	Total protein: Albumin, 52–68% Globulin, 32–48% $alpha_1$ globulin, 2.4–5.3% $alpha_2$ globulin, 6.6–13.5% beta globulin, 8.5–14.5% gamma globulin, 10.7–21%	5-ml venous blood sample; percentage of $alpha_1$, $alpha_2$, beta, and gamma globulin is determined; total percentage of globulin increases as a result of increased levels of these immunoglobulins when infectious and diffuse inflammatory liver disease is present; occurs with chronic hepatitis and advanced cirrhosis
Blood ammonia	40–100 μg/dl	Fasting 3-ml venous sample obtained; elevated levels occur when liver cannot convert ammonia to urea for excretion from the body; elevated levels seen in liver failure
LIPID METABOLISM		
Total cholesterol	Varies with age and diet Desirable level <200 mg/dl	Fasting venous blood sample; decreased levels associated with liver disease
Cholesterol esters	60%–75% of total cholesterol	Percentage of cholesterol esters decreases with liver diseases as a result of a decrease of lecithin cholesterol acryl transferase, an enzyme needed to esterize cholesterol
CARBOHYDRATE METABOLISM		
Serum glucose	60–110 mg/dl	Fasting 5-ml venous sample; hypoglycemia (40–60 mg/dl) occurs with 50% of patients who have acute viral hepatitis; caused by depleted glycogen stores, decreased gluconeogenesis, and poor intake
COAGULATION STUDIES		
Prothrombin time (PT)	Males: 9.6–11.8 sec Females: 9.5–11.3 sec	7-ml venous sample; PT is prolonged when liver is unable to use vitamin K or form protein; because patient may have a coagulation disorder, apply pressure to the puncture site for 3–5 minutes after needle is withdrawn
TUMOR MARKER		
Alpha-fetoprotein (AFP)	<30 ng/ml	5-ml venous sample; levels of 10,000–100,000 ng/ml are seen with hepatic carcinoma or metastatic lesions involving liver; successful treatment response causes immediate drop in levels; with recurrence of hepatic carcinoma, levels rise 1–6 months before symptoms occur

Normal values and procedures are guidelines. Reported reference ranges may vary depending on the method used for testing as well as the population tested. Contact laboratory performing test for absolute values, interfering substances, specimen preservation, and specific collection procedures.

Abbreviations: AST, aspartate aminotransferase (formerly SGOT, serum glutamic-oxaloacetic transaminase); ALT, alanine aminotransferase (formerly SGPT, serum glutamic-pyruvic transaminase); LDH, lactate dehydrogenase; RBC, red blood cell; A/G, albumin/globulin ratio.

Table 27–7. VISUALIZATION PROCEDURES TO EVALUATE LIVER FUNCTION

STUDY	PURPOSE/DESCRIPTION
Liver scan	Size, shape, position, and function of the liver are determined. A tracer dose of a radioactive material, usually technetium, is given intravenously 30 minutes prior to the scan. The procedure takes approximately 60 minutes and causes no patient discomfort. Pregnancy is a contraindication for the procedure because of fetal exposure to the isotope. Pregnant health care personnel should not care for patients who have had a scan for 48 hours after the procedure. In the normal liver, technetium uptake is uniform. "Cold" spots, areas with decreased uptake of the isotope, indicate lesions. Use of this procedure is decreasing because of improved results with ultrasonography, computed tomography (CT), and magnetic resonance imaging (MRI).
Abdominal ultrasonography	Harmless, high-frequency sound waves are used to differentiate tissues within the abdominal cavity, including the liver. Fluid-filled structures within the liver, such as cysts, transmit ultrasound waves easily, whereas solid tumors transmit poorly. Ascites, even in small quantities, can be identified. A conductive gel is placed on the abdomen, and the patient must lie still for about 30 minutes.
Computed tomography (CT)	Computer processing of x-ray images provides cross-sectional views of the liver. An intravenous iodinated contrast agent may be used to enhance results. Before the procedure, question the patient regarding allergy to shellfish or iodine. CT is useful for identifying tumors, cysts, and abscesses.
Magnetic resonance imaging (MRI)	MRI produces a cross-sectional image of tissues in the body by generating a magnetic field between the machine and hydrogen atoms in the body. MRI is the most sensitive study for detecting lesions. The major disadvantages of MRI are the long time required for scanning (more than an hour in many cases) and the need for the patient to remain absolutely still during the procedure. Patients with cardiac pacemakers, surgical clips, and metallic prostheses cannot have MRI because of the magnetic field.
Endoscopy	
Esophagoscopy	An endoscope is inserted via the oral cavity to visualize the esophagus and identify esophageal varices. Patient is kept on NPO status for 8 hours before procedure. A local anesthetic in the form of a gargle or spray is administered to prevent gagging during tube insertion. The examination takes approximately 20–30 minutes. Assess patient for return of gag reflex before allowing oral food or fluids after the procedure.
Peritoneoscopy	A laparoscope is introduced through an incision in the abdominal wall. Patient usually receives a sedative before the procedure, and local anesthetic is used at the insertion site. Direct visualization of the liver is possible. Procedure is most commonly done to obtain samples of liver tissue. Total examination time is approximately 1 hour. Patient usually has a small dressing over the incision site. Monitor site for bleeding or discharge.

Abbreviation: NPO, nothing by mouth.

tamic-oxaloacetic transaminase (SGOT), is found in the largest quantities in cardiac, liver, and skeletal muscle and in kidney cells. Damage to any one of these organs will result in elevated blood levels. Alanine aminotransferase (ALT), formerly known as serum glutamic-pyruvic transaminase (SGPT), occurs in relatively high levels in liver tissue and low levels in other organs. Therefore, an elevated ALT is a more specific indicator of liver damage, and decreasing levels can be monitored to determine improvement in liver function.

Alkaline phosphatase (ALP) is found in the liver, bone, and intestine. When this enzyme is elevated and no clinical symptoms indicate the source of the elevation, isoenzyme studies are indicated. Isoenzymes are forms of an enzyme that are characteristic of a specific tissue. 5′-Nucleotidase (5′-N) and gamma glutamyl transpeptidase (GGT), isoenzymes of ALP, are found in greatest concentrations in hepatobiliary tissue. Lactate dehydrogenase (LDH), although widely distributed in the body, exists in five isoenzymes. Elevated levels of LDH_4 and LDH_5 are associated with liver damage.

BILIRUBIN LEVELS

Bilirubin, produced by the cells of the reticuloendothelial system, circulates loosely bound to protein (unconjugated or direct bilirubin) and is removed from the body by the liver, where it is conjugated with glucuronide transferase and excreted into the bile. If the total bilirubin level is elevated or if jaundice is present, both conjugated and unconjugated levels of bilirubin are determined. Elevated levels of unconjugated bilirubin are usually associated with increased destruction of red blood cells. Elevated levels of conjugated bilirubin are seen with most liver diseases.

PROTEIN STUDIES

Protein studies are done to determine the liver's ability to carry out protein metabolism. Total serum protein normally consists of approximately 60% albumin and 40% globulin. In some liver diseases, such as chronic active hepatitis, total protein level remains normal despite altered liver function because globulin levels increase as albumin levels decrease. The albumin/globulin (A/G) ratio is determined to identify this shift. With other liver diseases, total protein is decreased.

Ammonia, an end product of protein metabolism, is converted to urea in the liver and excreted by the kidneys. With impaired hepatocellular function, ammonia levels rise. Elevated ammonia levels do not directly correlate with the risk of hepatic encephalopathy, but decreasing levels indicate the condition is improving.

LIPID STUDIES

Cholesterol, a lipid, is synthesized by the liver. Hepatocyte damage causes interference with synthesis and thus a decreased cholesterol blood level.

ALPHA-FETOPROTEIN

Alpha-fetoprotein (AFP) is the major serum protein during fetal life. It is produced in large quantities by the liver until about the 32nd week of gestation. Only small quantities are produced after the first year of life. Rapidly multiplying liver cells resume production of AFP. Elevated levels are seen when patients have hepatocellular carcinoma or metastatic lesions affecting the liver. Although levels may rise to thousands of times the normal level, 30% to 50% of patients with hepatocellular carcinoma do not have elevated AFP. When levels are elevated, successful treatment of hepatic carcinoma results in an immediate drop in AFP levels.

PROTHROMBIN

The prothrombin time (PT) represents the time required for a firm fibrin clot to form after coagulation factor III and calcium are added to a blood sample. Prothrombin, a vitamin K–dependent protein necessary for blood coagulation, is formed by the liver. Any condition that impairs the liver's ability to use vitamin K or to form proteins will prolong the PT and increase the risk of bleeding.

Urine and Fecal Studies

Bilirubin metabolism is also assessed by examining urine and stool samples. Under normal circumstances, no bilirubin is excreted in the urine, and only a small amount of urobilinogen is present. Bilirubin appears in the urine when increased amounts of conjugated bilirubin enter the blood stream.

Urobilinogen, normally secreted into the intestine with bile, appears in feces. When bilirubin metabolism is impaired, urobilinogen levels are decreased in the feces and increased in the urine. Because blood and urine samples are easier to obtain, fecal urobilinogen levels are done infrequently.

Visualization Procedures

Liver scan, ultrasonography, CT scan, MRI, esophagoscopy, and peritoneoscopy are useful diagnostic tools that provide a pictorial image of the liver.

Liver Biopsy

Liver biopsy, usually performed at the bedside, is used to obtain a specimen of liver tissue for examination. It is performed by inserting a special needle through the intercostal space between the sixth and seventh or eighth and ninth ribs and removing a liver tissue sample. It may also be done by direct visualization via laparoscopy. Ultrasonography or CT scan may be used to identify specific sites to undergo biopsy. Direct visualization is the preferred method because tissue samples can be taken from specific areas of the liver. This is important when isolated lesions are present, such as in the early stage of hepatic carcinoma.

Although the procedure is relatively safe, complications can occur. Improper placement of the biopsy needle upward into the chest cavity can result in pneumothorax. Laceration of a bile duct causes leakage of bile into the peritoneal cavity, resulting in peritonitis. Puncture of a blood vessel within or surrounding the liver can cause hemorrhage.

Table 27–8 explains nursing responsibilities before, during, and after a liver biopsy.

Table 27–8. LIVER BIOPSY

NURSING ACTIONS	RATIONALE
BEFORE PROCEDURE	
Obtain written consent.	Invasive procedure
Verify that coagulation studies are within normal limits.	Bleeding tendencies may be present as a result of liver disease
Preferably, patient is maintained on NPO status for 6 hours before procedure.	Complications requiring surgery can occur
Assess vital signs.	Baseline data for comparison
Administer prescribed medications 30–60 minutes before procedure.	Medication to calm an anxious patient requires time to act
Position patient in supine or left lateral position with right arm extended above the head.	Widens the intercostal spaces and fully exposes the hepatic area
DURING PROCEDURE	
Stand on the patient's left side, hold patient's left hand, and place one hand lightly on right arm.	Nurse's presence provides support and distracts patient during procedure; touching right arm allows nurse to quickly restrain it from movement during the procedure
When the physician is ready to insert biopsy needle, instruct patient to inhale deeply, exhale fully, and hold breath on exhalation while specimen is obtained.	On exhalation, the diaphragm ascends and risk of pneumothorax and liver laceration is minimized
AFTER PROCEDURE	
Place sterile dressing over needle insertion site, and position patient on right side with folded towel under costal margin.	This position compresses the liver capsule against the chest wall, minimizing leakage of blood or bile
Monitor vital signs every 15 minutes for 1 hour, every 30 minutes for 2 hours, and then hourly until stable.	Bleeding or bile peritonitis causes change in vital signs
Assess patient for pain.	Some pain in RUQ and right shoulder is common because of leakage of small amounts of bile, blood, or both from biopsy site; if pain is severe, notify physician immediately

Abbreviations: NPO, nothing by mouth; RUQ, right upper quadrant.

Application of the Nursing Process to the Care of the Patient Undergoing Diagnostic Studies of Hepatic Function

Assessment

Before all diagnostic procedures, question the patient to determine familiarity with the procedure. Observe the patient for physiologic and emotional signs and symptoms of anxiety. These include diaphoresis, trembling, restlessness, difficulty sleeping, crying, and inability to concentrate.

Nursing Diagnoses and Planning

Nursing diagnoses and related expected patient outcomes most commonly applicable to patients undergoing diagnostic studies of hepatic function include the following:

NDx: Anxiety related to lack of knowledge of diagnostic procedures

Planning: Patient outcomes
1. Patient describes the procedure.
2. Patient explains the purpose of the procedure.
3. Patient verbalizes concerns related to procedure.
4. Patient verbalizes decreased anxiety after teaching.

Nursing Interventions

NDx: Anxiety
Assist the patient in reducing anxiety level. Explain the procedure using terminology the patient can understand. Provide time for the patient to ask questions and to repeat the information provided. When possible, provide the patient with written material explaining the procedure. Return to the patient after 20 to 30 minutes and answer any questions. Repeated explanations may be necessary because anxiety can interfere with learning. Acknowledge patient's fears and anxiety regarding the procedure. Reassure the patient that some anxiety is normal. Provide a quiet environment. Excess stimulation can increase anxiety. Remain with the patient during liver biopsy to ensure safety and provide reassurance and comfort.

Evaluation

Evaluate the effectiveness of nursing care for a patient undergoing diagnostic studies of hepatic function by comparing the patient's status with the expected patient outcomes. Examples of specific outcomes for patients undergoing diagnostic studies of hepatic function have been provided in the Planning section.

The Elderly: Special Considerations

Both the size and the weight of the liver decrease after 50 years of age. As a result of decreased cardiac output, hepatic blood flow also decreases. However, liver function tests remain normal, with the exception of serum albumin levels, which tend to decline very slightly. This may be due to decreased albumin synthesis or decreased protein intake.

The most consistent finding associated with the aging process is a decrease in liver enzymes needed for drug metabolism and detoxification. Smaller doses of all drugs are recommended for elderly patients. Drug interactions and cumulative drug effects occur with higher frequency in the aged.

A number of factors contribute to a prolonged recovery time for elderly patients with liver disease. Delayed diagnosis is one factor. Gallbladder disease or biliary obstruction, conditions common in the elderly person, are frequently diagnosed when the real problem is liver disease because the symptoms are similar. Days or weeks may be spent treating biliary conditions before an actual diagnosis of liver disease is made. Early signs of hepatic encephalopathy are often overlooked when forgetfulness and confusion are attributed to the normal aging process. In addition, although the precise mechanism is not known, elderly patients have a decreased immunologic response to many infectious and inflammatory disorders; thus, symptom development is delayed. Even with prompt diagnosis and treatment, chronic health problems such as diabetes mellitus, congestive heart failure, hypertension, and malignancy experienced by many elderly can cause a prolonged recovery time for patients having concurrent liver disease.

Normal aging changes in other body systems can also affect the elderly patient with liver disease and intensify symptoms. Thinning of epidermal skin layers, a decrease in subcutaneous fat, and decreased sebum production contribute to dry skin and make the skin more prone to trauma. When jaundice is present, itching is intensified and skin injury from scratching is more likely. Diminished salivary flow and changes in the sense of smell may decrease appetite. Anorexia, experienced by many patients with liver disease, becomes even more problematic to treat in the elderly.

Bibliography

Bosch J, Navasa M, Garcia-Pagán JC, et al. Portal hypertension. Med Clin North Am 1989; 73(4):931.

Boyer TD. Cirrhosis of the liver and its major sequelae. In Wyngaarden JB, Smith LH Jr, Bennett JC (eds). Cecil textbook of medicine. 19th ed, Vol 1. Philadelphia: WB Saunders, 1992, pp 786–796.

Braunwald E, et al. (ed). Harrison's principles of internal medicine. 11th ed. New York: McGraw-Hill, 1987.

Byrne CJ, et al. Laboratory tests: Implications for nursing care. 2nd ed. Reading, MA: Addison-Wesley, 1986.

Carpenito LJ. Nursing diagnoses: Application to clinical practice. 4th ed. Philadelphia: JB Lippincott, 1992.

Cella JH, Watson J. Nurse's manual of laboratory tests. Philadelphia: FA Davis, 1989.

Dudley FJ. Pathophysiology of ascites formation. Gastroenterol Clin North Am 1992; 21(1):215.

Ebersole P, Hess P. Toward healthy aging. St. Louis: CV Mosby, 1990.

Fishbach FT. A manual of laboratory diagnostic tests. 4th ed. Philadelphia: JB Lippincott, 1992.

Gammal SH, Jones A. Hepatic encephalopathy. Med Clin North Am 1989; 73(4):793.

Goiella EC, Bevil CW. Nursing care of the aging client: Promoting healthy adaptation. Norwalk, CT: Appleton-Century-Crofts, 1985.

Groth K. Age-related changes in the gastrointestinal tract. Geriatr Nurs 1987; 9(5):278.

Guyton AC. Human physiology and mechanisms of disease. 4th ed. Philadelphia: WB Saunders, 1987.

Hole JW Jr. Human anatomy and physiology. 5th ed. Dubuque, IA: William C Brown, 1990.

Karb VB, Queener SF, Freeman JB. Handbook of drugs for nursing practice. St. Louis: CV Mosby, 1989.

Kemp BB, Pillitteri A, Brown P. Fundamentals of nursing: A framework for practice. 2nd ed. Glenview, IL: Scott, Foresman, 1990.

Matteson MA, McConnell ES. Gerontological nursing: Concepts and practice. Philadelphia: WB Saunders, 1988.

North American Nursing Diagnosis Association: NANDA nursing diagnoses: Definitions and classifications. St. Louis: North American Nursing Diagnoses Association, 1992.

Ockner RK. Approaches to the diagnosis of jaundice. In Wyngaarden JB, Smith LH Jr (eds). Cecil textbook of medicine. 18th ed. Philadelphia: WB Saunders, 1988, pp 817–818.

Potter PA, Perry AG. Basic nursing: Theory and practice. St. Louis: CV Mosby, 1987.

Reynolds TB. Renaissance of paracentesis in the treatment of ascites. In Stollerman GH (ed). Advances in internal medicine. Vol 35. Chicago: Year Book Medical, 1990, pp 365–391.

Rustgi AK, Saini S, Schapiro RH. Hepatic imaging and advanced endoscopic techniques. Med Clin North Am 1989; 73(4):895.

Schamburek RD, Farrar JT. Disorders of the digestive system in the elderly. N Engl J Med 1990; 322(7): 438.

Scharschmidt BF. Bilirubin metabolism and hyperbilirubinemia. In Wyngaarden JB, Smith LH Jr, Bennett JC (eds). Cecil textbook of medicine. 19th ed, Vol 1. Philadelphia: WB Saunders, 1992, pp 756–760.

Seidel HM, Ball JW, Dains JE, Benedict GW. Mosby's guide to physical examination. 2nd ed. St. Louis: CV Mosby, 1991.

Sherlock S. Diseases of the liver and biliary system. 8th ed. Boston: Blackwell Scientific, 1989.

Weisiger RA. Hepatic metabolism in liver disease. In Wyngaarden JB, Smith LH Jr, Bennett JC (eds). Cecil textbook of medicine. 19th ed, Vol 1. Philadelphia: WB Saunders, 1992, pp 754–756.

Williams SR. Essentials of diet and nutrition and diet therapy. 5th ed. St. Louis: Times Mirror/Mosby College Publishing, 1990.

Chapter Twenty-eight

NURSING CARE *of Adults with Hepatic Disorders*

Patients with hepatic disorders have signs and symptoms that reflect alterations in normal liver functions. The major hepatic disorders include infectious and inflammatory conditions, structural abnormalities, trauma, and neoplasms.

Infections and Inflammations

Viral hepatitis and liver abscess are the most common hepatic infectious processes. Inflammation results when an individual ingests, inhales, or receives parenteral substances that have a poisonous effect on the liver.

Viral Hepatitis

Acute viral hepatitis is characterized by inflammation and necrosis of hepatic cells. Although the major forms of hepatitis differ from each other with regard to incubation period, route of transmission, antigenic properties, and progression to chronicity, they all produce an inflammatory response in the liver. Table 28–1 presents a comparison of the hepatitis viruses.

ETIOLOGY

HEPATITIS A

Hepatitis A virus (HAV) is found worldwide and almost exclusively spread by the fecal-oral route. It occurs sporadically from close person-to-person contact or epidemically from the ingestion of water, milk, or food (especially shellfish) that is contaminated with human waste. HAV infection can be spread from one family member to another, via food handlers in restaurants, and from resident to resident in an institutional setting. Lack of toilet training and hand-to-mouth contact can lead to outbreaks of hepatitis A in preschool settings.

HAV is endemic in underdeveloped countries and is related to poor personal hygiene, overcrowding, and poor sanitation. Sexual transmission of HAV is also seen in individuals who have oral-anal-genital contact.

HEPATITIS B

Hepatitis B virus (HBV) is also distributed worldwide and is increasing in frequency. This is attributed to an increase in intravenous (IV) drug use and sexual activity with multiple partners. The parenteral route is the major route of transmission. Groups at risk for infection via the parenteral route include patients and staff in hemodialysis units, IV drug users, surgeons, dentists, nurses, blood bank employees, and laboratory technicians.

HBV is found in semen and saliva in addition to blood. Two nonparenteral routes for transmission are sexual contact and perinatal transmission. Individuals at risk for infection via the nonparenteral route include spouses and sexual contacts of persons with active hepatitis B, family members of chronically infected patients, and residents and staff of institutions for the mentally retarded. Research studies indicate that up to 30% of persons with Down's syndrome are hepatitis B carriers. This is believed to be due to a genetic predisposition to the disease.

Perinatal transmission, rare in the United States but common in the Far East and in developing countries, occurs in infants born to healthy carrier mothers or mothers with acute hepatitis B during the third trimester of pregnancy. It is unclear whether mother-to-infant infection occurs in utero or at the time of delivery. Hepatitis B infection is not related to breast feeding.

HEPATITIS D

The hepatitis D virus (HDV), or delta agent, is regarded as a complication of hepatitis B. The hepatitis B surface antigen must be present for the HDV to replicate. It is most common among drug users, hemodialysis patients, and recipients of multiple transfusions.

HEPATITIS C

Patients with viral hepatitis who do not show evidence of HAV or HBV or the delta agent in blood tests are diagnosed as having hepatitis C, formerly parenterally transmitted non-A, non-B hepatitis, and commonly referred to as posttransfusion hepatitis. The hepatitis C virus (HCV) is present in 1% of the blood donor population. Approximately 90% of posttransfusion hepatitis is diagnosed as HCV. It is more common when paid donors are used. Hemophiliacs who receive clotting factor concentrates from commercial sources and renal dialysis patients are particularly at risk for HCV. It is believed that the incidence of posttransfusion hepatitis will decline dramatically with the screening of all blood donations for HCV required since May 1990. Although research has not been completed, preliminary reports indicate that hepatitis C may be a common cause of chronic liver disease and linked to the development of hepatocellular carcinoma.

HEPATITIS E

The hepatitis E virus (HEV), formerly enterically transmitted non-A non-B hepatitis, is transmitted via the enteric route and has characteristics similar to those of the HAV. Hepatitis E is a leading cause of acute viral hepatitis in young to middle-aged adults in developing countries. The mortality rate for infected pregnant women is close to 20%. There is no

Table 28–1. COMPARISON OF HEPATITIS VIRUSES

VARIABLE	HEPATITIS A	HEPATITIS B	HEPATITIS D	HEPATITIS C	HEPATITIS E
Causative agent	Hepatitis A virus (HAV)	Hepatitis B virus (HBV)	Hepatitis D virus (HDV)	Hepatitis C virus (HCV)	Hepatitis E virus (HEV)
Other names	Infectious hepatitis	Serum hepatitis	Delta agent hepatitis	Post-transfusion hepatitis; parenterally transmitted non-A, non-B hepatitis	Enterically transmitted non-A, non-B hepatitis
Incubation period	15–50 days; mean, 28–30 days	45–160 days; mean, 60–90 days	Unknown; HBV must be present	15–180 days; mean, 6–9 weeks	15–64 days; mean, 26–42 days
Mode of transmission	Fecal-oral route; may be sexually spread	Infected blood or body fluids; sexually spread	Infected blood or body fluids; sexually spread	Infected blood or body fluids; sexual spread rare	Fecal-oral route
Sources of infection	Direct contact with infected persons; poor sanitation; infected food handlers; contaminated food, especially shellfish, water, milk; persons with subclinical infections	Contaminated needles and syringes; blood products; sexual contact; perinatal transmission; asymptomatic carriers			Direct contact with infected persons; contaminated water (rare in United States)
High-risk groups	Preschoolers, family members, homosexuals	Intravenous drug users, recipients of commercial blood transfusions, health care workers, dialysis patients			Homosexuals; young adults, primarily males
Laboratory confirmation	HAV-Ab/IgM	HB_sAg, HB_cAb	Delta antigen in serum	HCV-Ab	Elimination of other forms of hepatitis
Mortality	<0.6%	1%–2%	Concurrent HDV infection increases risk of fulminant HBV infection	Rare	Unknown; 20% in pregnant women in the third trimester
Prophylaxis	Good sanitation, hygiene; ISG; vaccine under development	HBIG; hepatitis B vaccine	HBIG; hepatitis B vaccine (hepatitis D occurs only if HBV present)	None	Good sanitation, hygiene; ISG not effective
Geriatric considerations	Most fatalities in the aged population	More severe clinical course, greater progression to chronicity, higher mortality rate			Uncommon in elderly
Postrecovery considerations	No carrier or chronic state; lifelong immunity to HAV reinfection	5%–10% develop carrier state or chronic hepatitis; chief cause of cirrhosis and hepatocellular cancer in United States; lifelong immunity to HBV reinfection	Higher incidence of chronic active hepatitis and cirrhosis than with HBV alone	Frequent carrier state and chronic hepatitis; increased risk of cirrhosis and hepatocellular cancer; reinfection possible	No evidence of chronic or carrier state
Special precautions	Blood, tissue, organ, and sperm donations cannot be made by individuals with a history of hepatitis.				

Abbreviations: Ab, antibody; IgM, immunoglobulin M; HB_sAg, hepatitis B surface antigen; HB_cAb, antibody to hepatitis B core antigen; ISG, immune serum globulin; HBIG, hepatitis B immune globulin.

evidence of a chronic form. Diagnosis depends on exclusion of other forms of hepatitis, especially HAV. At present there is no serologic test for HEV.

PATHOPHYSIOLOGY

All forms of viral hepatitis are characterized by liver cell necrosis, inflammation, and cell regeneration. The regular organizational pattern of the hepatocytes is disrupted as a result of the inflammatory process and cellular damage. Bile flow is impaired because of hepatocyte inflammation. Liver cell necrosis occurs in a spotty, piecemeal manner. Hepatocytes adjacent to blood vessels show the first evidence of damage. Even as cell necrosis is occurring, previously destroyed cells are regenerating. During the recovery period, hepatocytes regain their normal appearance and function.

CLINICAL MANIFESTATIONS

The incubation period, the period of time between infection and actual symptoms, and the severity of viral hepatitis depend on the organism responsible for the infection.

Hepatitis A, often referred to as infectious hepatitis, has an incubation period of 15 to 50 days. It is characterized by an acute onset that produces a mild illness lasting approximately 6 weeks. Infection with HAV does not produce a carrier state and does not

Table 28–2. CLINICAL MANIFESTATIONS AND LABORATORY DATA ASSOCIATED WITH THE PREICTERIC, ICTERIC, AND POSTICTERIC PHASES OF HEPATITIS

PHASE	MANIFESTATIONS	LABORATORY FINDINGS
Preicteric (occurs 1 to 3 weeks before onset of jaundice)	Fatigue Anorexia Nausea Vomiting Abdominal discomfort Joint pain Pharyngitis Cough Coryza	Elevated enzyme levels (especially AST and ALT), elevated urine bilirubin levels
Icteric (may last from 2 to 6 weeks)	Jaundice appears Appetite remains poor Right upper quadrant pain Stool color lightens Urine color darkens Pruritus	Same as preicteric phase with addition of elevated serum levels of direct bilirubin
Posticteric (lasts from 2 to 12 weeks)	Jaundice subsides Stools return to normal color Urine returns to normal color Appetite improves Fatigue may continue	All laboratory values return to normal

Abbreviations: AST, aspartate aminotransferase; ALT, alanine aminotransferase.

lead to chronic liver disease. The mortality rate for HAV is less than 0.6%.

Hepatitis B, often referred to as serum hepatitis, has an incubation period of 45 to 160 days. The clinical course is usually more prolonged than that of hepatitis A, and it is more likely to cause serious illness in the elderly and the debilitated. Infection with HBV can cause chronic hepatitis and lead to a carrier state, and may also increase the risk of liver cancer. Simultaneous infection with HBV and the delta agent does not increase the risk that chronic hepatitis will occur. However, when a patient is chronically infected with HBV and has an acute infection with the delta virus, the condition usually results in chronic active hepatitis. Acute delta infection can result in liver failure. The mortality rate for hepatitis B is approximately 2%.

The incubation period for HCV ranges from 2 to 26 weeks, with an average of 6 to 9 weeks. A carrier state can occur, and more than 25% of patients with HCV develop chronic hepatitis, but for most patients this is mild and symptoms disappear after a year. The incubation period for HEV is 15 to 64 days; incubation for HDV in humans has not been established.

From the onset of infection, clinical and biochemical recovery from uncomplicated viral hepatitis takes approximately 6 months. The earliest symptoms are usually nonspecific and are often mistaken for influenza or an upper respiratory tract infection. Although some patients experience no further symptoms, the usual course of hepatitis includes the preicteric, icteric, and posticteric phases. Table 28–2 summarizes the clinical manifestations and laboratory data commonly seen in each phase.

PREICTERIC PHASE

The preicteric phase is characterized by nonspecific complaints: fatigue, anorexia, nausea, pharyngitis, cough, coryza, abdominal discomfort, and joint pain. It begins 1 to 3 weeks before the appearance of jaundice. During the final 1 to 5 days of the preicteric phase, the patient may note that urine is becoming darker and stools are lighter in color. Laboratory results indicate elevated enzyme levels, especially aspartate aminotransferase (AST) and alanine aminotransferase (ALT), and elevated urine bilirubin levels.

ICTERIC PHASE

The icteric phase begins with the appearance of jaundice. Laboratory tests show elevated levels of direct bilirubin. Because of obstructed bile flow, decreased urobilinogen is excreted in the feces, resulting in a lighter stool color, whereas increased excretion of urobilinogen in the urine causes its color to darken. The symptoms seen in the preicteric phase subside, but appetite remains poor. Right upper quadrant pain is common because of the enlarged liver. Pruritus is associated with worsening jaundice and increased bile salt deposits in the skin. Clinical manifestations associated with decreased production of clotting factors are rare, but a few spider angiomas may be seen. The icteric phase usually lasts from 2 to 6 weeks.

POSTICTERIC PHASE

The recovery period is characterized by decreasing jaundice and, in uncomplicated cases, lasts from

2 to 12 weeks. Stool and urine color return to normal and appetite improves. Patients may continue to complain of fatigue.

MEDICAL DIAGNOSIS

The diagnosis of viral hepatitis is made on the basis of information obtained from the patient's history, physical examination, and laboratory findings, including specific serologic tests. If viral hepatitis is suspected, the physician questions the patient regarding possible sources of the virus. This includes contact with jaundiced individuals, recent travel to countries where hepatitis is endemic, injections, IV drug use, tattooing, dental treatments, blood transfusions, and shellfish ingestion. Physical examination confirms a tender, palpable liver with hepatomegaly and splenomegaly.

Laboratory data include elevated liver enzyme levels as a result of hepatocyte necrosis, an elevated erythrocyte sedimentation rate (ESR) caused by hepatic inflammation, and leukopenia associated with viral infections. Serum bilirubin levels, especially conjugated bilirubin, are elevated in the presence of jaundice. In severe cases, the prothrombin time is prolonged because of the liver's inability to produce clotting factors.

Specific serologic tests are available to identify HAV, HBV, HCV, and the delta antigen. A diagnosis of HEV is made by excluding HAV, HBV, and HCV and the patient's history of probable risk factors. Table 28–3 summarizes the significance of the various hepatitis markers commonly used to diagnose and monitor a patient's progress. Serologic identification of the delta antigen is not widely used.

To differentiate hepatitis A and hepatitis B, the first marker tested is the antibody to HAV, which is immunoglobulin M specific (HAV-Ab/IgM). This is present between 4 and 6 weeks after infection and indicates an acute stage of hepatitis A infection. The remaining two markers are the B surface antigen and the B core antibody. The HBV surface antigen (HB_sAg) is detected 2 to 8 weeks before the onset of jaundice. It may appear before liver enzymes rise and clinical symptoms appear and remains detectable during and beyond the icteric phase of acute hepatitis B. Shortly after the appearance of the surface antigen, the hepatitis B core antibody (HB_cAb) appears and is detectable for a period of 6 to 14 weeks.

Tests to identify serologic markers that indicate resolution of the infection may be ordered after symptoms subside. These include the HAV antibody, which is specific to immunoglobulin G (HAV-Ab/IgG) and indicates previous exposure and immunity to hepatitis A, and the hepatitis B surface antibody (HB_sAb), which appears 2 to 10 months after infection and indicates previous exposure and permanent immunity to hepatitis B.

MEDICAL MANAGEMENT

There is no specific treatment for acute viral hepatitis. Hospitalization is reserved for patients with an uncertain diagnosis, the severely ill, or those patients who have a delayed recovery.

Rest is advised, but strict bed rest is not necessary. The amount of activity the patient can tolerate is usually dictated by the patient's level of fatigue. No specific dietary interventions are necessary provided the patient is receiving a well-balanced diet that is tolerated. A low-fat, high-carbohydrate diet is often more tolerable to a patient with anorexia and nausea. If vomiting is present and the patient cannot tolerate oral feedings, IV fluid replacement and small doses of antiemetic agents may be prescribed. Alcoholic beverages are contraindicated during the course of the illness.

Table 28–3. COMMON HEPATITIS MARKERS AND THEIR SIGNIFICANCE

TYPE	APPEARANCE	IMPLICATIONS
HEPATITIS A		
HAV-Ab/IgM	4–6 weeks after infection	Indicates current acute infection with HAV
HAV-Ab/IgG	8–12 weeks after infection	Indicates previous exposure and immunity to HAV
HEPATITIS B		
HB_sAg	4–12 weeks after infection	Present in most cases of acute and chronic infection with HBV
HB_eAg	4–12 weeks after infection	Indicates "highly infectious" state
HB_cAb	6–14 weeks after infection	Indicates past infection with HBV
HB_sAb	2–10 months after infection	Indicates previous exposure and immunity to HBV
HEPATITIS C		
HCV-Ab	5–12 months after infection	Present in up to 90% of patients with chronic post-transfusion hepatitis C. Found in 1% of normal volunteer blood donors as well as patients with hepatocellular carcinoma

Abbreviations: HAV, hepatitis A virus; Ab, antibody; IgM, immunoglobulin M; IgG, immunoglobulin G; Hb_sAg, hepatitis B surface antigen; HBV, hepatitis B virus; HB_eAg, hepatitis B e antigen; HB_cAb, antibody to hepatitis B core antigen; HB_sAb, antibody to hepatitis B surface antigen; HCV, hepatitis C virus.

PROPHYLAXIS

Hepatitis A

The administration of immune serum globulin (ISG) provides temporary passive immunity to hepatitis A for people who are planning travel to the tropics and developing countries where the incidence of hepatitis A is high. Protection is afforded for up to 3 months. Repeat immunization is required for longer stays. ISG can also be given to close contacts of patients diagnosed with hepatitis A. It should be administered within the first few days of exposure. Casual work or school contacts do not require ISG unless there has been mutual handling of food and beverages or if hygiene practices are poor.

Hepatitis B

Hepatitis B immune globulin (HBIG) provides passive immunity to hepatitis B and is indicated in certain circumstances. Because the cost is extremely high—$250 to $300 for the recommended two doses 4 weeks apart—it should be administered only when indicated. HBIG is recommended in the following situations:

1. Inoculation of material known to be contaminated with HBV, such as an accidental cut or puncture with a contaminated needle or instrument from an HB_sAg-positive patient.
2. Splashing of HB_sAg-positive material into the eye or on an open skin wound.
3. Ingestion of HB_sAg material during laboratory procedures using pipettes.

The use of HBIG requires that the source of the virus be known and that the recipient of the HBIG actually be at risk. The usual procedure is to test blood for HB_sAg from both the source and the exposed person. If the exposed person is already positive for HB_sAg or immune, there is no reason to administer HBIG.

Active immunity to hepatitis B is provided by the hepatitis B vaccine. It is recommended for all adults at high risk for hepatitis B and for all infants and children. Those in high-risk categories include travelers to countries where hepatitis B is endemic, clients and staff of institutions for the mentally retarded, health-care workers, hemodialysis patients, homosexually active males, and household and sexual contacts of HBV carriers. The vaccine is administered three times over a period of 6 months. The second dose follows the first by 1 month; the third dose is given 6 months after the first dose.

COMPLICATIONS

Previously healthy individuals in whom hepatitis develops usually recover completely with no complications. However, elderly patients, the chronically malnourished, and those with chronic medical problems (congestive heart failure, diabetes mellitus, malignancy) may have a prolonged recovery. After complete recovery, second episodes of the same type of hepatitis are rare, although the possibility of infection with another hepatitis virus does exist. Drug addicts, because of poor hygiene practices and the use of dirty needles and syringes, experience a higher incidence of repeat occurrences, most frequently HCV. The major complications associated with hepatitis infection are chronic hepatitis and fulminant hepatitis.

CHRONIC HEPATITIS

Chronic hepatitis is possible in patients who have had HBV or HCV hepatitis. There are two types of chronic hepatitis: chronic persistent hepatitis and chronic active hepatitis.

Chronic persistent hepatitis is characterized by inflammation of the portal tracts with no hepatocyte necrosis. In chronic persistent hepatitis, there is a delayed convalescent period marked by fatigue, anorexia, hepatomegaly, and right upper quadrant pain. Moderate increases in serum enzyme levels and bilirubin are seen. Symptoms may persist for 10 years or longer. Usually no specific treatment is indicated; however, recombinant alpha interferon has been approved for the treatment of chronic hepatitis. Prognosis is favorable because no further liver damage occurs.

Chronic active hepatitis is a more serious form of chronic hepatitis because it may progress to cirrhosis and liver failure. Approximately one third of the patients acquire cirrhosis, and one fifth die of liver failure within 4 years. Active hepatocellular necrosis occurs. Diagnosis requires liver biopsy. Although research findings are contradictory, there is some agreement that corticosteroids should be used to treat chronic active hepatitis to suppress the inflammatory response seen on biopsy.

FULMINANT HEPATITIS

Fulminant hepatitis is seen in less than 1% of patients with viral hepatitis. Massive cell necrosis occurs, and the liver is unable to regenerate functional tissue. There is rapid liver decompensation within a few weeks after onset of hepatitis. The patient enters Stage III or IV of hepatic encephalopathy and may die within a week.

Application of the Nursing Process to the Care of the Patient with Hepatitis

Nursing care for the patient with jaundice is discussed in Chapter 27. Nursing Care Guide 28–1 summarizes nursing management of a patient with hepatitis. Strict adherence to Universal Precautions prevents the transmission of hepatitis via blood and body fluids. Universal Precautions include the use of gloves when blood or body fluids are handled, gowns when clothing may be contaminated, and face shields or goggles and masks when splashing of blood or body fluids is possible. If the patient with hepatitis A is incontinent or has poor hygiene practices, enteric isolation precautions are instituted and a private room is required to prevent the spread of the virus to other patients.

Assessment

Question the patient regarding known or possible exposure to contaminated food, water, needles, surgical equipment, blood transfusions, or individuals with the hepatitis. Assess for the clinical manifestations of hepatitis. Palpate and percuss the liver to identify hepatomegaly and tenderness or pain. Question the patient regarding activity level, appetite, and the presence of nausea or vomiting.

Nursing Diagnoses and Planning

Nursing diagnoses and related expected patient outcomes most commonly applicable to patients with hepatitis include the following:

NDx: High risk for altered health maintenance related to insufficient knowledge of viral hepatitis disease process and transmission

Planning: Patient outcomes
1. Patient explains the cause of viral hepatitis.
2. Patient verbalizes precautions to prevent transmission of the disease.

NDx: Activity intolerance related to fatigue

Planning: Patient outcomes
1. Patient participates in activities of daily living without experiencing fatigue.
2. Patient increases ambulation distance daily.

Nursing Interventions

NDx: High risk for altered health maintenance
Explain the mode of transmission to the patient and significant others. For HAV and HEV, explain that the virus is passed in the stool and is spread to others when the organism remains on the hands after toileting and is spread to items touched by the patient, such as food, dishes, and glasses. Explain the purpose of enteric isolation to the patient, family members, or significant others and the importance of hand washing to remove the organism. Teach correct hand washing procedure. For HBV, HCV, and HDV, explain that blood, semen, and saliva can spread the disease, and teach the patient and significant others how to prevent transmission.

Instruct the patient to refrain from kissing and sexual contact until liver enzyme test results return to normal. Caution the patient to refrain from consuming alcohol and using all drugs, unless prescribed by the physician. Explain that because alcohol and drugs are metabolized by the liver, use of these substances can lead to further liver damage.

Explain to the patient that blood, tissue, sperm, and organ donations cannot be made by persons who have a history of hepatitis.

NDx: Activity intolerance
Explain that activity should not exceed what the patient is comfortable doing. Fatigue is a normal response to hepatic cellular damage, and activity tolerance will increase as liver inflammation subsides. Provide rest periods between activities. Allow 60 to 90 minutes for rest between meals and hygiene or other activities. Explain to the patient and family that visitors are important during illness, but they must not interfere with sleep and rest. If bed rest is not prescribed, encourage the patient to ambulate short distances each day. Provide a rest period before ambulation. Increase the distance walked by 10 to 20 feet each succeeding day. Monitor pulse rate before and after ambulation to determine the effect of ambulation on the cardiovascular system.

Evaluation

Evaluate the effectiveness of nursing care for a patient with hepatitis by comparing the patient's status with the expected patient outcomes. Examples of specific outcomes for patients with hepatitis have been provided in the Planning section.

Toxic and Drug-Induced Hepatitis

ETIOLOGY

Toxic hepatitis is an inflammatory condition caused by ingestion, inhalation, or parenteral administration of substances that have a poisonous effect on the liver. Table 28–4 illustrates some common hepatotoxins with their source. These agents produce liver damage with predictable regularity.

Table 28–4. COMMON HEPATOTOXINS AND THEIR SOURCE

TOXIN	SOURCE
Carbon tetrachloride	Dry-cleaning fluid
Trichloroethylene	Cleaning fluid (often sniffed by adolescents)
Toluene	Glue (often sniffed by adolescents)
Chlorophenothane	Insecticide
Vinyl chloride	Use in the production of synthetics
Muscarine	Poisonous mushrooms
Arsenic	Garden and household pesticides, Fowler's solution used in the treatment of psoriasis
Yellow phosphorus	Rat poison, firecrackers

Nursing Care Guide 28–1.

PATIENTS WITH HEPATITIS

Assessment Findings: Patient is admitted to the hospital with a diagnosis of hepatitis. Patient verbalizes no understanding of disease or method of transmission.

Nursing Diagnosis: High risk for altered health maintenance related to insufficient knowledge of hepatitis disease process and transmission

Patient Outcomes	Nursing Interventions	Rationale
Patient verbalizes precautions to prevent spread of disease.	Explain mode of transmission: hepatitis A, fecal-oral; hepatitis B and hepatitis C, blood or body fluids.	Appropriate personal hygiene and good sanitation prevent spread of hepatitis.
	Demonstrate hand washing. Explain Universal Precautions.	Hand washing and Universal Precautions minimize risk of transmission of virus.
	Assist patient in identifying close contacts who may have been exposed to the hepatitis virus.	Immune serum globulin or hepatitis B immune globulin may be indicated to provide contacts with passive immunity.
Patient verbalizes an understanding of treatment plan.	Provide written dietary instructions. Stress need to abstain from alcohol and all drugs unless prescribed by physician. Explain importance of rest and exercise.	A well-balanced diet, avoidance of hepatotoxins, and rest aid hepatocyte regeneration.
	Instruct patient not to donate blood, organs, tissue, or sperm.	Prevents transmission of virus.

Evaluation: Compare the patient's status with the expected patient outcomes. If the outcomes are achieved, evaluate nursing care as successful. If not, reassess the patient, formulate new nursing diagnoses, and revise expected patient outcomes and nursing interventions as appropriate.

Assessment Findings: Patient complains of fatigue and lack of interest in usual activities.

Nursing Diagnosis: Activity intolerance related to fatigue

Patient Outcomes	Nursing Interventions	Rationale
Patient participates in activities of daily living.	Provide rest periods between activities; 60–90 minutes between meals and procedures.	When activities are not spaced, fatigue results and tolerance for activity is reduced.
	Encourage participation in self-care according to ability.	Success in accomplishing self-care activities is an incentive to accomplish further activities.

(continued)

Nursing Care Guide 28–1. *(continued)*

PATIENTS WITH HEPATITIS

Evaluation: Compare the patient's status with the expected patient outcomes. If the outcomes are achieved, evaluate nursing care as successful. If not, reassess the patient, formulate new nursing diagnoses, and revise expected patient outcomes and nursing interventions as appropriate.

Assessment Findings: Jaundice develops on the third day of hospitalization. Patient refuses to see family or friends and requests that lights in room remain off.

Nursing Diagnosis: Body image disturbance related to altered skin pigmentation

Patient Outcomes	Nursing Interventions	Rationale
Patient verbalizes acceptance of self in present condition.	Explain pathophysiologic basis for jaundice. Reinforce positive progress: decreasing bilirubin levels, improved stool and urine color.	Jaundice is temporary and will diminish as condition improves.
	Allow time for patient to express fears or concerns.	Providing reliable, accurate information and active listening establish a trusting nurse-patient relationship.
Patient takes part in grooming activities.	Encourage use of own pajamas or clothing. Choose colors that do not accentuate jaundice.	Encourages social interaction and allows patient to maintain control.
	Assist with grooming activities.	Prevents excess fatigue.

Evaluation: Compare the patient's status with the expected patient outcomes. If the outcomes are achieved, evaluate nursing care as successful. If not, reassess the patient, formulate new nursing diagnoses, and revise expected patient outcomes and nursing interventions as appropriate.

Drug-induced toxic hepatitis is usually an idiosyncratic response. The patient may have a unique susceptibility to the medication or an immunologic response. Drugs are responsible for 2% to 5% of all hospital admissions for jaundice in the United States. Certain drugs account for 20% to 50% of the cases of fulminant hepatic failure. Table 28–5 presents the medications most commonly associated with drug-induced toxic hepatitis and their potential hepatotoxic effect.

PATHOPHYSIOLOGY

The specific liver changes associated with toxic hepatitis depend on the offending agent. Exposure to vinyl chloride over many years leads to sclerosis of the portal venules and subsequent portal hypertension. Ingestion of poisonous mushrooms causes massive cell destruction. Drug-induced liver disease is classified as cytotoxic, cholestatic, or mixed. Cytotoxic injury causes damage to hepatic cells. Cholestatic injury causes arrested bile flow. Mixed injury has simultaneous characteristics associated with both cytotoxic and cholestatic injury. Isoniazid, used as a prophylactic agent in patients with a positive tuberculin test, produces liver necrosis in susceptible individuals. If isoniazid is administered in combination with rifampin for treatment of active tuberculosis, the patient is at even greater risk for liver damage. Chlorpromazine produces cholestasis in 1%

Table 28–5. DRUGS COMMONLY ASSOCIATED WITH HEPATOTOXICITY

DRUG	TOXIC EFFECT
Acetaminophen (Tylenol)	Has a predictable, dose-dependent effect; causes liver cell necrosis; acute liver failure and death in doses >10–15 g at one time; cell necrosis may also occur at therapeutic doses of 3–8 g/day; cellular injury reversed if drug discontinued
Acetylsalicylic acid (Aspirin)	Elevated liver serum enzyme levels and abnormal liver function tests with doses >3 g/day; mechanism of liver injury not known; reversible if drug discontinued
Chlorpromazine (Thorazine)	Impaired secretion of bile with cellular inflammation and cell necrosis
Erythromycin estolate (Ilosone)	Impaired secretion of bile and liver cell necrosis; documented cases of patients who had unnecessary gallbladder surgery on basis of presenting signs and symptoms
Isoniazid (INH)	Symptoms mimic viral hepatitis infection; seen in approximately 1% of patients taking drug as prophylaxis against tuberculosis; of this group, 10% may have fatal reaction; incidence exceeds 2% in those older than 50 years; usually occurs 2–3 months after starting drug but can occur up to 12 months later; elevated enzyme levels seen in 10%–20% of patients taking isoniazid, although no actual symptoms are present
Phenobarbital (Luminal)	Lowers serum bilirubin levels by inducing increased production of glucuronyl transferase; increases excretion and flow of bile salts; altered liver function and jaundice more common with long-term use
Diazepam (Valium)	Long-term use alters liver function by unclear mechanism, manifested by jaundice
Oral contraceptives	May cause interference with bile secretion and bile flow, cause hepatic vein thrombosis and predisposition to cholesterol gallstone formation; symptoms and effects resolve if drug discontinued

to 2% of patients receiving the drug. Phenobarbital and diazepam produce mixed injury.

CLINICAL MANIFESTATIONS

The person with toxic hepatitis experiences signs and symptoms similar to those of viral hepatitis. Initially, gastrointestinal and influenza-like symptoms appear. Depending on the toxic agent, the degree of exposure, and the extent of liver damage, jaundice, hepatomegaly, and other signs of hepatic necrosis may be present.

The onset of symptoms depends on the type of reaction experienced. Drug-induced liver disease may develop within days of exposure to a known hepatotoxic agent. It may take several weeks for symptoms caused by a hypersensitivity or drug allergy to appear. Weeks or months often pass before manifestations of metabolic idiosyncratic reactions to drugs appear.

MEDICAL DIAGNOSIS

If symptoms of chronic active hepatitis are present, but serologic tests for viral hepatitis are negative, a complete history of exposure to hepatotoxins is obtained. Liver biopsy may be performed to identify the extent of liver damage.

MEDICAL MANAGEMENT

Treatment of toxic hepatitis requires removal of the suspected hepatotoxin. In most cases of drug-induced hepatitis, hepatic damage will resolve if the offending agent is discontinued.

Guidelines for Application of the Nursing Process to the Care of the Patient with Toxic Hepatitis

Nursing assessment of the person with toxic hepatitis includes close observation for all of the clinical manifestations of hepatitis previously mentioned. Obtain a complete list of all medications taken currently and within the past 3 months, including over-the-counter medications. Ask specifically about any past exposure to hepatotoxic agents. Nursing diagnoses reflect the patient's response to the clinical manifestations and the need to teach the patient to avoid exposure to the hepatotoxic agent or use of the hepatotoxic drugs.

Liver Abscess

ETIOLOGY

A pyogenic liver abscess is a collection of pus within the liver that results from bacterial infection. The organisms most commonly associated with this condition are the enteric flora, *Escherichia coli* and *Klebsiella*, and *Staphylococcus aureus*. In approximately two thirds of all cases, multiple bacterial species are present. Anaerobic bacteria are present in one half or more of all cases. Since the introduction of antibiotics, the incidence of liver abscess is low.

Organisms reach the liver in a number of ways. The most common source is biliary tract disease, such as acute cholecystitis. Other sources of liver abscess include infections in areas drained by the portal system, such as the appendix and diverticulum; direct extension from an adjacent structure, such as a subphrenic abscess; organisms introduced from outside the body as a result of a gunshot or knife wound; and organisms introduced via the hepatic artery as a result of bacteremia.

In areas of the world where sanitation is poor, liver abscess may be caused by the ameba *Entamoeba histolytica*. This ameba invades the intestinal mucosa, causing a colitis, and may travel via the blood stream to the liver.

The mortality rate for patients with a pyogenic abscess ranges from 10% to 60%. Multiple abscesses that cannot be surgically drained, advanced age, underlying malignancy, and spread of the organism to other locations adversely affect the prognosis. Uncomplicated amebic liver abscess has a mortality rate less than 1%.

PATHOPHYSIOLOGY

Imaging studies, such as ultrasonography and computed tomography (CT), reveal single or multiple collections of pus encased in fibrous tissue. Approximately two thirds of the patients with this condition have multiple abscesses. The right lobe is involved more often than the left, most likely because it is larger and receives more blood.

CLINICAL MANIFESTATIONS

The clinical manifestations of liver abscess are usually those of a systemic infectious process. Fever may precede other symptoms. Abdominal pain, weight loss, and anorexia are the characteristic complaints. Jaundice is present in up to 20% of the cases and usually indicates biliary tract disease. On physical examination, 50% of the patients have hepatomegaly with right upper quadrant pain or tenderness.

MEDICAL DIAGNOSIS

Laboratory data indicate the presence of leukocytosis, but liver function test results may be only slightly altered if the abscess is located to a small area of the liver. Most commonly, alkaline phosphatase levels are elevated. Blood cultures are positive in 40% of cases.

X-ray examination of the chest reveals elevation of the right hemidiaphragm in about one half of patients with liver abscess. Ultrasonography and CT scan are ordered to visualize abscess formation. Ultrasonography is most useful in differentiating liver abscess from neoplasms, hematomas, and cysts. CT has the advantage of being able to reveal abscesses high up in the right lobe that may be missed by ultrasonography. When amebic abscess is suspected, contents of the abscess can be aspirated guided by ultrasonogram or CT scan.

MEDICAL MANAGEMENT

Initial treatment for patients with liver abscess includes combination intravenous antibiotic therapy. An aminoglycoside or third-generation cephalosporin is prescribed to destroy gram-negative organisms, clindamycin is prescribed to destroy anaerobic organisms, and ampicillin is prescribed to destroy gram-positive organisms. Specific antibiotic therapy is instituted when blood and abscess cultures are complete. Antibiotic therapy may need to be continued for up to 16 weeks. Oral preparations are usually prescribed after the third week.

When etiologic factors indicate that amebic liver abscess is present, metronidazole (Flagyl) is prescribed for 5 to 7 days. Metronidazole is described in Pharmacology Box 28–1.

Percutaneous closed drainage may be used for bacterial liver abscess. It is used for amebic liver abscess only if the patient fails to respond to oral medication. A catheter is inserted into the abscess under radiologic guidance and remains in place for drainage from 3 to 20 days. Surgical incision and drainage may be required when additional disease, such as bile duct obstruction, is present.

Guidelines for Application of the Nursing Process to the Care of the Patient with Liver Abscess

Assess the patient for pain, and note changes in severity of pain. Monitor vital signs, especially temperature, to determine the response to antibiotic therapy. Administer antibiotics at prescribed intervals to maintain therapeutic blood levels. Because patients may think they can stop taking medication when their physical condition improves, teach them the rationale of long-term antibiotic therapy and the importance of continuing therapy for the prescribed length of time.

Structural Disorders

Cirrhosis

Cirrhosis of the liver is a chronic, degenerative process that follows hepatocellular necrosis. It is

Pharmacology Box 28–1.
METRONIDAZOLE (FLAGYL)

Metronidazole:
Antiprotozoal agent.

Action:
Metabolized by anaerobic organisms to products that disrupt DNA synthesis.

Uses:
Drug of choice for treating acute intestinal amebiasis and for liver abscess caused by *Entamoeba histolytica*. It is also used for the treatment of anaerobic bacterial infections of the abdomen, bones or joints, lower lung, and central nervous system.

Side Effects:
Previously unrecognized *Candida* infections may present more prominent symptoms and require treatment. Nausea, dry mouth, headache, and dizziness may occur. Toxicity may precipitate seizures, and peripheral neuropathy may occur. The appearance of abnormal neurologic signs requires discontinuation of the drug.

Interactions:
Potentiates the anticoagulant effect of warfarin and other oral anticoagulants, resulting in a prolonged prothrombin time. Simultaneous administration of phenytoin or phenobarbital causes lower plasma levels of metronidazole. Alcohol consumption during therapy and for 1 day after therapy causes abdominal cramps, nausea, vomiting, headache, and flushing. Disulfiram, used for alcohol avoidance, taken concurrently with metronidazole can cause psychotic reactions. Disulfiram should be discontinued 2 weeks before therapy begins.

Nursing Implications:
Instruct the patient to avoid all alcoholic beverages during and immediately after therapy. Caution against the use of hazardous equipment if dizziness occurs. Notify the physician immediately if seizures or abnormal neurologic signs are present. Instruct the patient to report evidence of numbness or paresthesia of an extremity. Patients with edema may not be able to tolerate the 28 mEq of sodium in each gram of metronidazole.

Table 28–6. COMPARISON OF MAJOR TYPES OF CIRRHOSIS

	LAENNEC'S	PRIMARY BILIARY	POSTNECROTIC
Occurrence	Most common type in North America and Western Europe	No specific distribution	Most common form worldwide
Cause	Most commonly alcohol consumption	Unknown	Previous hepatitis, toxic drug or chemical reaction, or autoimmune disease
Sex affected	Males most often, but females seen more frequently as drinking habits change	Women 30–65 years of age	Men and women equally
Other names	Alcoholic cirrhosis Fatty cirrhosis Micronodular cirrhosis		Toxic cirrhosis Cryptogenic cirrhosis Coarsely nodular cirrhosis
Major clinical features	Muscle wasting Jaundice Portal hypertension Ascites	May be asymptomatic for years; eventually portal hypertension, ascites, and jaundice occur	Usually resembles active hepatitis in early stage and Laennec's cirrhosis in late stage

characterized by nodule formation and generalized liver fibrosis. Three forms of cirrhosis are commonly identified: Laennec's, primary biliary, and postnecrotic. Although each type has a different cause, the ultimate outcome is essentially the same. Table 28–6 compares the major types of cirrhosis.

ETIOLOGY

LAENNEC'S CIRRHOSIS

Laennec's cirrhosis, also known as alcoholic, portal, or fatty cirrhosis, is the most common type of cirrhosis in North America and Western Europe. It usually results from excessive alcohol (ethanol) ingestion over a long period of time. However, cirrhosis does not develop in all alcoholics. Several studies have shown that the disorder develops in less than 20% of individuals who consumed an average of 160 g of ethanol per day, equivalent to two six-packs of beer, for more than 10 years. However, females who ingest large quantities of alcohol have disproportionately more significant liver injury than males consuming the same amount of alcohol. This is attributed to a specific gender-linked factor that affects the stomach's ability to metabolize alcohol before it reaches the systemic circulation and ultimately the liver as well as decreased liver enzyme activity affecting alcohol metabolism. Nutrition is also implicated as a possible reason for the development of Laennec's cirrhosis. Frequently, alcoholics do not maintain a balanced diet and consume only the calories supplied by the alcoholic beverage. However, Laennec's cirrhosis develops in many alcoholics even in the presence of a balanced diet. Because conflicting evidence does not support one specific cause for alcoholic cirrhosis, it is believed that genetic, nutritional, and environmental factors may all play a role in its development.

The first indication of liver damage as a result of alcohol use is fatty infiltration of the liver. Large droplets of fat gradually occupy most of the volume of the hepatocyte cells. Patients in this stage rarely have symptoms. These cellular changes usually resolve within 3 to 6 weeks if alcohol is withdrawn and the patient consumes a diet with adequate protein, calories, and vitamins. If alcohol intake continues, alcoholic hepatitis may develop. This condition, an acute liver inflammation, is often a precursor of Laennec's or alcoholic cirrhosis.

PRIMARY BILIARY CIRRHOSIS

Primary biliary cirrhosis, also known as cholangitic or obstructive cirrhosis, is reported in all races and in most geographic areas of the world. More than 90% of the patients are women, and the typical age of onset is between 30 and 65 years. A high rate of breast cancer has also been reported in women who have primary biliary cirrhosis. Because of the high incidence in females, estrogen or progesterone is thought to be a factor in the development of this disease. A genetic factor may also be important because the disease has been reported in mothers and daughters, siblings, and twins.

Primary biliary cirrhosis starts in the bile ducts with obstruction of bile flow (cholestasis). Gradual scarring and destruction of hepatocytes occur, and bands of fibrous tissue extend to adjacent structures in the liver.

POSTNECROTIC CIRRHOSIS

Postnecrotic cirrhosis, also known as cryptogenic, toxic, or macronodular cirrhosis, is any cirrhosis in which the cause is unknown. Liver tissue is replaced with small to large nodules of fibrous tissue. It is believed that most cases represent the end stage of a previously active, chronic, or recurrent hepatitis, or an autoimmune disease. Some cases have been linked to a toxic drug or chemical response. Patients with postnecrotic cirrhosis can remain asymptomatic for a number of years. Cirrhotic changes may be detected during evaluation for an unrelated problem or when symptoms develop.

PATHOPHYSIOLOGY

Regardless of the type of cirrhosis, the end result is extensive destruction of hepatocytes and interference with liver function. Destroyed hepatocytes are replaced with dense, fibrous scar tissue and nodules. The nodules impede portal blood flow, and portal hypertension occurs. This leads to development of ascites, varices, and splenomegaly. The thin-walled varices, especially in the mucosa of the gastric fundus and esophagus, may bleed slowly or rupture and cause massive and possibly fatal hemorrhage. Decreased hepatic synthesis of coagulation factors and decreased platelets as a result of splenomegaly further complicate the control of bleeding. The pathophysiology of portal hypertension is discussed in Chapter 27.

CLINICAL MANIFESTATIONS

Patients with Laennec's cirrhosis usually note symptoms at an average age of 50 years. Most often, they seek medical advice because of ascites or jaundice. Complaints of generalized weakness and nonspecific gastrointestinal symptoms such as anorexia, nausea, indigestion, flatulence, and possibly right upper quadrant pain made worse by sitting up or leaning forward are common. Peripheral edema may be present before ascites, but frequently they appear together. Weight loss is common, but, because of fluid retention, it is not apparent. Some patients do not seek medical attention until massive gastrointestinal hemorrhage from ruptured esophageal or gastric varices occurs.

Table 28–7 presents the major clinical manifestations of cirrhosis and corresponding pathophysiol-

Table 28-7. CLINICAL MANIFESTATIONS OF CIRRHOSIS

CLINICAL MANIFESTATION	PATHOPHYSIOLOGY
Gastrointestinal symptoms	Venous congestion of gastrointestinal tract
Palpable liver	Fatty infiltration of liver cells causes liver enlargement and nodule formation
Fever (low grade)	Hepatic inflammation and necrosis
Weakness, fatigue, and muscle wasting	Interference with synthesis of tissue proteins and utilization of nutrients
Bleeding tendencies	Decreased absorption of vitamin K or decreased production of clotting factors
Ascites and edema	Portal hypertension, decreased serum albumin level, decreased ability of liver to metabolize aldosterone
Striae	Stretching of abdominal skin because of ascites
Jaundice	Failure of liver cells to metabolize bilirubin
Spider angiomas	Arterial lesions formed by dilation of groups of small blood vessels
Gynecomastia; scant hair on chest, pubic area, and axilla	Inability of liver to detoxify estrogen
Palmar erythema (liver palms)	Bright red palms and soles of feet believed to be caused by high estrogen levels
Distended abdominal blood vessels	Obstructed liver blood flow, leading to formation of collateral blood vessels
Impaired neurologic function (hepatic encephalopathy): shortened attention span, slurred speech, asterixis, hyperactive muscle reflexes, grimacing, blinking, appearance of sucking and grasp reflexes, loss of consciousness. Table 27–4 lists additional characteristics of impaired neurologic function.	Formation of toxic products, most notably ammonia and mercaptans, which interfere with brain metabolism

ogy. The severity and number of manifestations are generally proportional to the extent of liver damage. Because of the many and varied functions of the liver, every body system is affected in some way. The clinical manifestations and medical and nursing management of jaundice, ascites, and hepatic encephalopathy are discussed in detail in Chapter 27.

MEDICAL DIAGNOSIS

A diagnosis of cirrhosis is made on the basis of presenting clinical manifestations, patient history, liver function tests, visualization studies, and liver biopsy.

In Laennec's cirrhosis, the patient is usually anemic as a result of the direct toxic effect of alcohol on the bone marrow, a nutritional deficiency of folic acid and pyridoxine, and the possibility of chronic gastrointestinal blood loss. Leukopenia may also be present as a result of the bone marrow depression caused by alcohol. Liver function studies indicate elevated alkaline phosphatase, AST, ALT, and bilirubin levels. Prothrombin time is prolonged, and blood ammonia levels may be increased because of the shunting of blood around the liver. Ultrasonography and CT scan confirm the presence of fibrous tissue and impaired hepatic blood flow. An endoscopy or upper gastrointestinal barium study verifies the presence of varices. A liver biopsy confirms a diagnosis of cirrhosis but may be contraindicated if the patient has a coagulation disorder.

MEDICAL MANAGEMENT

Medical management depends on the stage of the disease and the presenting clinical manifestations. Abstinence from alcohol in all types of cirrhosis is of the utmost importance. Continued alcohol use with Laennec's cirrhosis reduces the 5-year survival rate to approximately 40% versus more than 60% for those who abstain.

No dietary restrictions are imposed unless ascites or hepatic encephalopathy are present. Patients are encouraged to consume a well-balanced diet, with between 2500 and 3000 calories daily. At least 1 g of protein per kilogram of body weight is recommended to promote regeneration of hepatocytes. Vitamin and folic acid supplements are usually prescribed because of malabsorption of the fat-soluble and B-complex vitamins. If symptoms of hepatic encephalopathy occur, protein is restricted. With ascites, sodium restriction is instituted.

COMPLICATIONS

ESOPHAGEAL VARICES

Bleeding from esophageal varices is a major, life-threatening complication of portal hypertension. The varices, usually located in the lower one third of the esophagus, may extend into the stomach. Slow bleeding can occur, but hemorrhage is most common. The exact cause of bleeding from esophageal varices remains controversial. However, the theory that bleeding results from esophageal irritation caused by eating solid foods, which cause trauma to the thin-walled vessels, has been abandoned. It is now believed that a combination of factors, including increased portal hypertension and thinning of the walls of the varices, leads to rupture.

The most common manifestation of ruptured esophageal varices is hematemesis with rapid development of hemorrhagic shock and severely compromised blood flow to vital organs. Hemorrhagic shock is treated with parenteral fluid replacement and blood transfusions as described in Chapter 15. Bleeding from ruptured varices stops spontaneously in 60% of patients, but recurrent episodes are common. There is no way to identify in which patients bleeding will spontaneously stop and those who, without treatment, will continue to bleed.

Initial treatment to control bleeding usually consists of pharmacologic therapy and insertion of a large-bore nasogastric tube to aspirate blood from the stomach. As discussed earlier, digestion of blood in the gastrointestinal tract places the patient at risk for elevated serum ammonia levels and hepatic encephalopathy. The nasogastric tube may also be used for gastric lavage, gentle irrigation of the stomach with normal saline to facilitate complete removal of blood and blood clots. Use of iced saline to promote vasoconstriction of bleeding varices is controversial. The benefits are questionable, especially if the bleeding is esophageal rather than gastric.

Once the gastric aspirate clears with lavage, or at least shows partial clearing of clots, immediate endoscopy is performed to confirm the diagnosis and rule out other sources of bleeding. Patients with cirrhosis frequently bleed from nonvariceal causes, such as hemorrhagic gastritis and peptic ulcers. When bleeding from varices is confirmed, treatment may include injection sclerotherapy and possible balloon tamponade. Long-term control of bleeding may require additional sclerotherapy or surgical intervention.

Pharmacologic Therapy

Pharmacologic therapy is initiated early in a bleeding episode. Drugs can be administered even before the patient reaches the hospital or immediately on admission to the emergency room. Vasopressin (Pitressin), a potent vasoconstrictor, is most often used to decrease portal blood flow and decrease portal pressure. Vasopressin is administered as a bolus via a peripheral vein. Temporary control of bleeding is achieved in approximately 50% of patients; however, rebleeding within 24 to 48 hours after vasopressin therapy is discontinued is as high as 45%. Because of its vasoconstrictive effects, vasopressin must be used with caution in patients who have coronary artery disease.

Nitroglycerin, a potent systemic vasodilator, is often administered via the IV or sublingual route in combination with vasopressin. Nitroglycerin causes vasodilation of the portosystemic collateral blood vessels. It enhances portal pressure reduction and reduces side effects associated with vasopressin alone. Studies indicate that combination therapy is effective in controlling acute bleeding in 64% of patients.

Propranolol and nadolol, beta-blocking agents, are used to prevent initial and recurrent variceal hemorrhage but are not widely used for acute variceal bleeding because of their potential impairment of cardiovascular response to hemorrhage. These drugs reduce portal pressure by reducing portal and collateral blood flow.

Sclerotherapy

Endoscopic sclerotherapy is the procedure of choice for long-term control of actively bleeding esophageal varices. This procedure involves the injection of a sclerosing agent directly into the varices until they are obliterated. It requires a high degree of skill and is effective in stopping bleeding in 75% to 90% of patients.

Follow-up endoscopies are recommended at 6-month intervals to monitor for recurrence of varices. Prophylactic sclerotherapy, performed before any bleeding episodes, remains highly controversial. Some studies indicate that patients may experience an increased risk rather than decreased incidence of bleeding after the procedure.

Balloon Tamponade

The Sengstaken-Blakemore tube, illustrated in Figure 28–1, controls bleeding from esophageal varices by exerting direct pressure on bleeding sites. It is a triple-lumen tube with ports for gastric aspiration, inflation of a gastric balloon, and inflation of an esophageal balloon. The gastric balloon applies pressure at the cardioesophageal junction. This decreases blood flow to the esophageal varices and directly compresses gastric varices. The esophageal balloon directly compresses the esophageal varices. Balloon tamponade is used when sclerotherapy cannot be performed because of excessive bleeding or when pharmacotherapy is ineffective. It stops bleeding in approximately 78% of patients, but up to 50% rebleed after the tube is removed.

The Sengstaken-Blakemore tube is passed via the nares into the stomach. The gastric balloon is inflated with air, clamped, and pulled tightly against the cardiac portion of the stomach to tamponade bleeding sites. Traction is applied to maintain the gastric balloon snugly in place. One method for maintaining traction is to use a pulley system with a 0.5-kg weight (500 ml of saline in a plastic bottle). Another method is fitting the patient with a football helmet and taping the tube to the chin guard under tension. If bleeding does not stop with inflation of the gastric balloon, the esophageal balloon is inflated to 25 to 45 mm Hg. Inflation pressure is constantly monitored by manometer to prevent esophageal necrosis from overinflation. X-ray examination of the upper abdomen and chest using portable equipment confirms balloon placement. Gastric contents and blood are aspirated by gastric lavage or intermittent suction via the gastric aspiration port.

When the esophageal balloon is inflated, the patient cannot swallow. Secretions accumulate above the level of the balloon and place the patient at risk

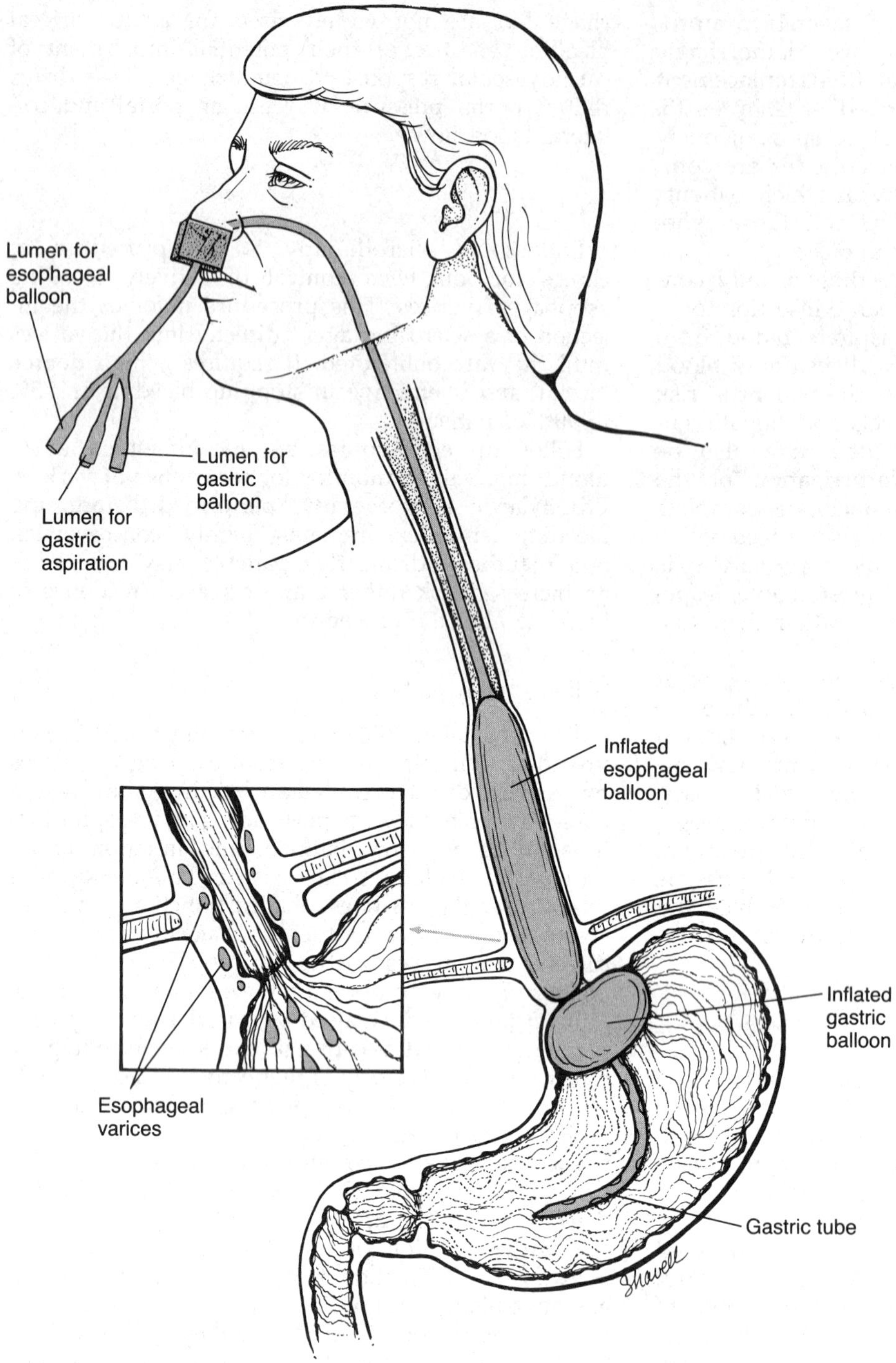

Figure 28–1.

Sengstaken-Blakemore tube.

for pulmonary aspiration. To minimize the risk, a nasogastric tube is inserted in the opposite naris, passed to the level of the esophageal balloon, and connected to intermittent suction to aspirate esophagopharyngeal secretions. If a Salem sump tube is used, it is connected to low, continuous suction. Stuporous or comatose patients may require endotracheal intubation to prevent aspiration.

The Minnesota esophagogastric tamponade tube, a four-lumen balloon tube, is a modification of the Sengstaken-Blakemore tube. The Minnesota tube has an additional lumen for aspirating esophagopharyngeal secretions. When this tube is used, an additional nasogastric tube is unnecessary. The Linton tube has only one balloon for gastric tamponade and esophageal and gastric ports for suctioning. Studies indicate no specific superiority or lower complication rate with the use of any particular tamponade tube.

In addition to pulmonary aspiration, major complications associated with balloon tamponade therapy are mechanical airway obstruction and esopha-

Figure 28–2.

Normal portal system and selected surgical shunts. *A*, Normal portal system. *B*, End-to-side portacaval shunt. Portal hypertension is reduced and gastroesophageal varices are decompressed by improving blood flow through the small gastric vein and coronary vein and anastomosing the portal vein to the inferior vena cava. *C*, Distal splenorenal shunt. The coronary vein is ligated to reduce portal hypertension, and gastroesophageal varices are decompressed by anastomosing the splenic vein to the renal vein.

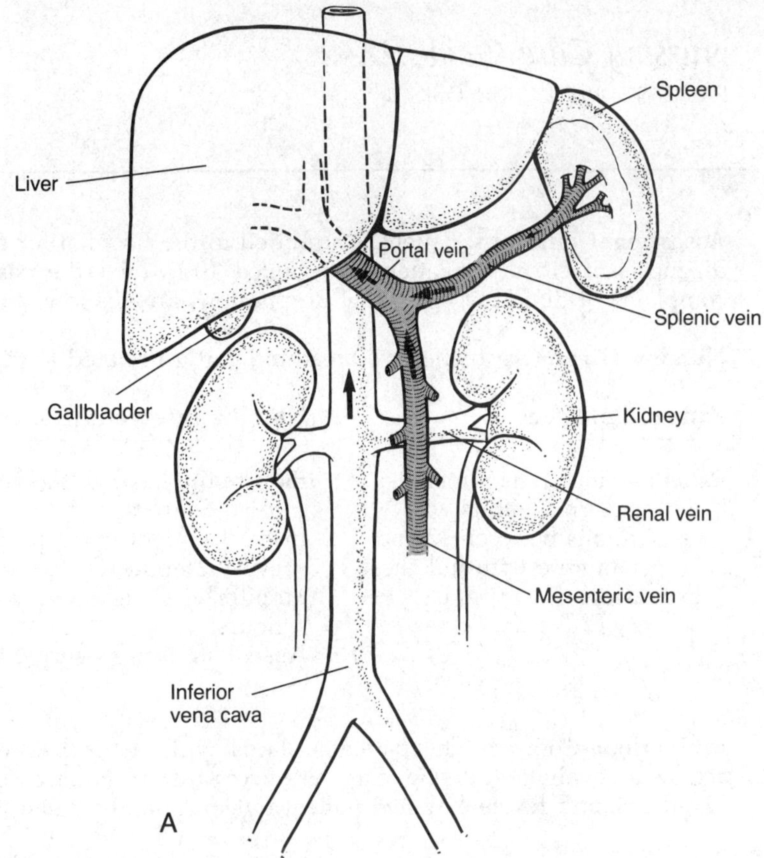

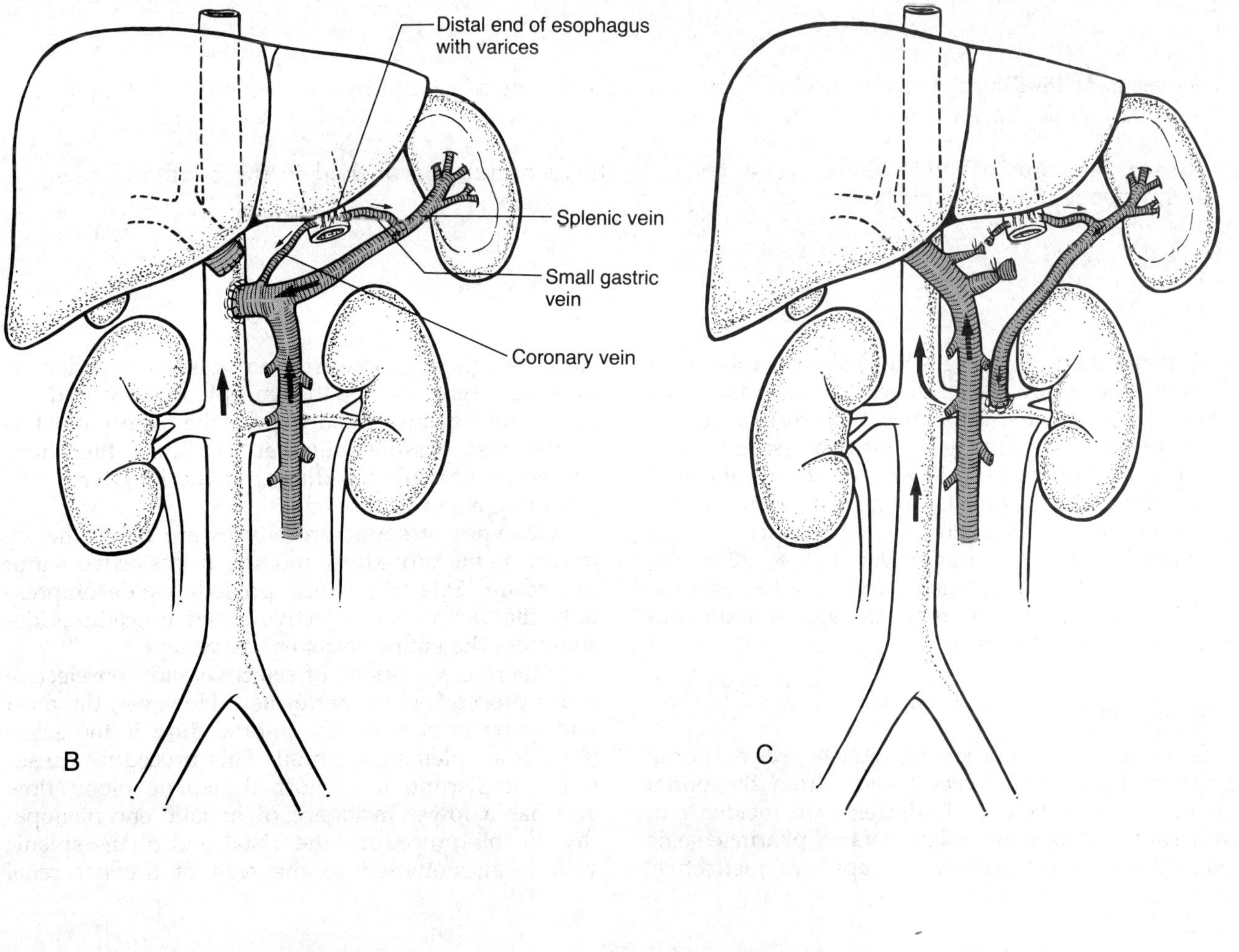

Nursing Care Guide 28–2.
PATIENTS WITH CIRRHOSIS

Assessment Findings: Patient is admitted to the hospital for the third time in the last 18 months with a diagnosis of cirrhosis. Patient has gained 10 lb over the past 3 days. Abdomen is distended. Patient complains of difficulty breathing. Respirations are shallow, and dyspnea is noted.

Nursing Diagnosis: Ineffective breathing pattern related to pressure on the diaphragm from ascites

Patient Outcomes	Nursing Interventions	Rationale
Patient's vital signs remain within normal limits with respirations between 12 and 20 per minute with full chest expansion.	Elevate the head of the bed 45 to 90 degrees.	Promotes maximum chest expansion.
	Instruct patient to deep breathe every 2 hours.	Encourages maximum chest expansion.
	Monitor vital signs every 4 hours.	Identify early indicators of oxygen deficit.
	Auscultate lungs every 4 hours.	Identify respiratory problems in early stage.

Evaluation: Compare the patient's status with the expected patient outcomes. If the outcomes are achieved, evaluate nursing care as successful. If not, reassess the patient, formulate new nursing diagnoses, and revise expected patient outcomes and nursing interventions as appropriate.

Assessment Findings: Abdominal girth increased 4 inches since last admission. Abdomen is shiny and taut with striae. Lower extremities are edematous.

Nursing Diagnosis: Fluid volume excess related to the accumulation of fluid in the peritoneal cavity and dependent areas of the body

(*continued*)

geal perforation. If the gastric balloon ruptures or deflates, the entire tube moves upward and may obstruct the airway. Esophageal necrosis resulting from prolonged esophageal tube pressure causes esophageal perforation. Most experts recommend that esophageal balloon tamponade therapy be discontinued in 24 hours; however, the gastric balloon tamponade may be maintained for 48 to 72 hours. Some authorities recommend deflating the esophageal balloon for 30 to 60 minutes every 8 hours, but this practice is not universal.

Surgical Procedures

Surgical shunt procedures, which reduce portal pressure by diverting blood away from the portal circulation, may be used to decrease the incidence of variceal bleeding when sclerotherapy, pharmacologic interventions, and balloon therapy are ineffective. However, these procedures may place the patient at increased risk for hepatic encephalopathy and remain quite controversial. Even when the patient is in the best possible physical condition, the shunt procedure controls bleeding, but the long-term survival rate is not improved.

Two types of shunt procedures are done: the selective shunt procedure and the nonselective shunt procedure. Selective shunt procedures decompress only the varices; nonselective shunt procedures decompress the entire portovenous system.

Numerous variations of selective and nonselective shunt procedures are performed. However, the most widely recommended shunt procedure is the selective distal splenorenal shunt. This procedure causes minimal disruption of normal hepatic blood flow and has a lower incidence of hepatic encephalopathy. In this procedure, the distal end of the splenic vein is anastomosed to the side of the left renal

Nursing Care Guide 28–2. *(continued)*

PATIENTS WITH CIRRHOSIS

Patient Outcomes	Nursing Interventions	Rationale
Patient's abdominal girth and weight decrease daily.	Monitor intake and output.	Fluid intake that exceeds output over a 3-day period indicates fluid retention.
	Administer prescribed diuretics.	Diuretics promote loss of fluid.
	Consult with dietitian to restrict fluids to 1500 ml daily. Administer: 750 ml from 8 A.M. to 4 P.M.; 600 ml from 4 P.M. to 11 P.M.; 150 ml from 11 P.M. to 8 A.M. Include fluids given with medications.	Limits fluid accumulation. Largest amount of fluid is given during waking hours to minimize thirst.
	Provide mouth care every 4 hours: *Do not* use lemon-glycerin swabs.	Decreases thirst. Glycerin dries mucous membranes.
	Weigh the patient daily before breakfast but after he or she has voided, wearing similar clothes each time.	Weight loss or gain may indicate fluid loss or gain.
	Measure abdominal girth daily. Mark point at which girth is measured.	Decreasing girth indicates a decrease in ascitic fluid. Measuring at the same point ensures accuracy.

Evaluation: Compare the patient's status with the expected patient outcomes. If the outcomes are achieved, evaluate nursing care as successful. If not, reassess the patient, formulate new nursing diagnoses, and revise expected patient outcomes and nursing interventions as appropriate.

(continued)

vein. Blood is diverted from the high-pressure varices to the low-pressure renal vein. The portocaval shunt is the most common nonselective shunt procedure. It creates an anastomosis between the portal vein and the inferior vena cava. This procedure results in total loss of portal blood flow to the liver and is associated with an increased incidence of hepatic encephalopathy. The portocaval shunt is usually used in emergency situations when all other nonsurgical treatment options have failed. Figure 28–2 illustrates the normal portal system, the distal splenorenal shunt, and the portocaval shunt.

The transjugular intrahepatic portosystemic shunt is a new nonsurgical procedure under investigation for the treatment of acute and recurrent variceal hemorrhage. In this procedure a stent is inserted into a new pathway created under radiologic guidance by balloon dilation of the tissue between the hepatic vein and the portal vein in the liver. This artificial shunt creates a new pathway for unobstructed blood flow and results in reduced portal venous pressure and decompression of esophageal varices. Periodic portal venograms confirm patency of the shunt.

Application of the Nursing Process to the Care of the Patient with Esophageal Varices

Esophageal varices are a complication of cirrhosis of the liver. Nursing Care Guide 28–2 summarizes the nursing management of a patient with cirrhosis, which includes monitoring for jaundice, ascites, he-

Nursing Care Guide 28–2. *(continued)*

PATIENTS WITH CIRRHOSIS

Assessment Findings: Sacral edema is present with ascites.

Nursing Diagnosis: High risk for impaired skin integrity related to ascites and edema

Patient Outcomes	Nursing Interventions	Rationale
Patient's skin remains intact during hospitalization.	Inspect skin surfaces daily for lesions or open areas.	Early intervention minimizes skin damage.
	Do not administer injections in edematous sites.	Drugs act as irritants when not absorbed.
	Teach patient to reposition self every 2 hours in bed or chair.	Frequent position changes increase blood flow.
	Place trapeze over bed.	Prevents injury from shearing force.
	Keep bed linens dry.	Moisture predisposes to skin breakdown.

Evaluation: Compare the patient's status with the expected patient outcomes. If the outcomes are achieved, evaluate nursing care as successful. If not, reassess the patient, formulate new nursing diagnoses, and revise expected patient outcomes and nursing interventions as appropriate.

Assessment Findings: Patient vomits large volume of blood. Blood pressure decreases from 136/86 mm Hg to 102/64 mm Hg. Pulse increases from 78 to 106 per minute. Sengstaken-Blakemore tube is inserted.

Nursing Diagnosis: High risk for aspiration related to retained secretions or balloon rupture

Patient Outcomes	Nursing Interventions	Rationale
Patient's respirations remain within normal limits with no evidence of respiratory distress.	Suction esophagus every 15–30 minutes.	When Sengstaken-Blakemore tube is in place, patient cannot swallow and secretions accumulate above the esophageal balloon.
	Monitor respirations, and auscultate lungs every 15–30 minutes.	Aspiration can occur as a result of loss of swallowing ability.
	Monitor patient closely. Keep scissors at bedside.	Airway obstruction is a major danger. All balloon lumens must be cut immediately if respiratory distress occurs.

Evaluation: Compare the patient's status with the expected patient outcomes. If the outcomes are achieved, evaluate nursing care as successful. If not, reassess the patient, formulate new nursing diagnoses, and revise expected patient outcomes and nursing interventions as appropriate.

(continued)

Nursing Care Guide 28–2. *(continued)*
PATIENTS WITH CIRRHOSIS

Assessment Findings: Bleeding is controlled, and the Sengstaken-Blakemore tube is removed. Patient becomes apathetic. Patient responds slowly to questions, and speech is slurred. Patient answers appropriately when asked name but cannot identify location or month of year. Handwriting is difficult to read, but admission sample is legible.

Nursing Diagnosis: High risk for injury related to alteration in thought processes secondary to impaired liver detoxification (hepatic encephalopathy)

Patient Outcomes	Nursing Interventions	Rationale
Patient remains free from injury.	Monitor orientation, rate of speech, and response time every 4 hours.	Changes in level of orientation, speech, and response time indicate a change in patient condition.
	Monitor for asterixis every 4 hours.	Most common sign of impending hepatic coma.
	Obtain daily handwriting sample.	Deterioration indicates deterioration in patient condition.
	Restrict protein intake.	Reduces ammonia production.
	Monitor potassium level.	Decreased potassium levels can precipitate hepatic coma.
	Administer neomycin and lactulose, as prescribed.	Lower blood ammonia levels.
	Keep bed in low position, side rails up, and call bell in reach.	Minimizes risk of injury.

Evaluation: Compare the patient's status with the expected patient outcomes. If the outcomes are achieved, evaluate nursing care as successful. If not, reassess the patient, formulate new nursing diagnoses, and revise expected patient outcomes and nursing interventions as appropriate.

(continued)

patic encephalopathy, and nutritional deficiencies. Nursing care for patients with jaundice, ascites, hepatic encephalopathy, and nutritional deficiencies is described in Chapter 27.

Assessment

Question the patient regarding the use of alcohol, including type, amount, and length of use. Examine the patient to detect the presence of jaundice, ascites, and edema. Assess mental status to determine the presence of hepatic encephalopathy. Question the patent regarding hematemesis or black, tarry stools, indicating blood in the stool.

If pharmacologic therapy with vasopressin is instituted, assess for side effects related to vasoconstriction and cardiotoxicity. These include bradycardia, dysrhythmias, hypertension, and chest pain. Assess fluid and electrolyte balance. Vasopressin may cause dilutional hyponatremia.

With active variceal bleeding, assess vital signs for evidence of hypovolemic shock. The patient in shock is restless and has cool, clammy skin, a decrease in blood pressure, tachycardia, and a decrease in urinary output. Note the frequency and amount of hematemesis and blood in the stool.

If balloon tamponade therapy is instituted, frequent respiratory assessment is indicated to identify accumulation of secretions above the level of the esophageal balloon. Monitor rate and quality of respirations. Auscultate the lungs for evidence of aspiration. Esophageal perforation caused by balloon tamponade is suspected if the patient complains of back pain or upper abdominal pain or if shock is evidenced. Perforation requires immediate surgical intervention.

Assessment after a surgical shunt procedure is

Nursing Care Guide 28–2. *(continued)*

PATIENTS WITH CIRRHOSIS

Assessment Findings: Family members are standing in hall outside patient's room pacing back and forth. Patient's sister is crying intermittently. Patient's brother is heard raising his voice in response to questions or comments by other family members.

Nursing Diagnosis: Altered family processes related to family member with impending hepatic encephalopathy

Patient Outcomes	Nursing Interventions	Rationale
Family members verbalize concerns to nursing staff.	Explain hepatic encephalopathy in terms family can understand.	Family must face the diagnosis and its implications if successful coping is to be achieved.
	Keep family informed of patient's progress, and arrange a specific time for family members to meet with health care team to discuss concerns.	Open communication between family and health care team facilitates adjustment to the illness and prognosis.
	Allow family members to assist with care, if they desire.	Promotes self-esteem of individual family members and continued contact with patient.

Evaluation: Compare the patient's status with the expected patient outcomes. If the outcomes are achieved, evaluate nursing care as successful. If not, reassess the patient, formulate new nursing diagnoses, and revise expected patient outcomes and nursing interventions as appropriate.

similar to that of a patient having abdominal surgery discussed in Unit 7. In addition, the patient is assessed for signs of hepatic encephalopathy and thrombus formation at the anastomosis site. Pain, fever, distention, and nausea indicate thrombus formation.

Nursing Diagnoses and Planning

Nursing diagnoses and related expected patient outcomes most commonly applicable to patients with esophageal varices and who are undergoing balloon tamponade therapy include the following:

NDx: High risk for aspiration related to retained secretions or balloon displacement secondary to balloon tamponade therapy

Planning: Patient outcomes

1. Patient's respirations remain between 12 and 20/minute with no evidence of respiratory distress.
2. Lungs are clear on auscultation.

Nursing Interventions

NDx: High risk for aspiration

Constant nursing observation is necessary when balloon tamponade therapy is in progress. Monitor respirations and auscultate the lungs every 15 to 30 minutes. Maintain intermittent suction to nasogastric tube or esophagopharyngeal port of Minnesota tube, if used. Maintain low, continuous suction if a Salem sump tube is used. Suction esophagopharyngeal secretions every 15 to 30 minutes if the Sengstaken-Blakemore tube is used without an accompanying nasogastric tube. Retained secretions lead to aspiration and occlude the airway. Observe the patient for sudden respiratory distress, which occurs if the gastric balloon ruptures and the entire tube moves upward. Gasping, dyspnea, and cyanosis will be evident. If this occurs, immediately cut all balloon lumens. A scissors must be kept at the patient's bedside at all times. Supply the patient with tissues to expectorate oral secretions.

To provide comfort, remove dried blood from the nares and mouth with a solution of equal parts hydrogen peroxide and normal saline. Apply a water-soluble lubricant to the nares to protect the skin.

Evaluation

Evaluate the effectiveness of nursing care for a patient with esophageal varices who is undergoing balloon tamponade therapy by comparing the patient's status with the expected patient outcomes. Examples of specific outcomes for patients with esophageal varices who are undergoing balloon tamponade therapy have been provided in the Planning section.

Trauma

Blunt and Penetrating Injuries

ETIOLOGY

Liver trauma usually results from an automobile accident, fall, stab wound, or gunshot wound. Blunt or nonpenetrating hepatic injuries result from direct blows, compression between the lower right ribs and spine, or shearing secondary to rapid deceleration. Blunt hepatic injuries are common in victims of motor vehicle accidents. Unrestrained drivers and front-seat passengers involved in frontal collisions are especially at risk. Stab wounds or gunshot wounds below the right nipple or in the right upper abdominal quadrant are most likely to cause penetrating hepatic injuries.

PATHOPHYSIOLOGY

Liver trauma may result in hepatic contusions, simple lacerations, or small intrahepatic hematomas. More serious injuries include hemorrhage resulting from major hepatic lacerations as well as damage to the hepatic veins or retrohepatic vena cava.

CLINICAL MANIFESTATIONS

The diagnosis of liver trauma is difficult to make if physical signs are minimal. After a serious accident, obvious injuries are often treated first, and "hidden" injuries may not be immediately diagnosed.

Fractured lower right ribs, bruising, and pain in the right upper quadrant or posteriorly may indicate liver trauma. Because the liver is highly vascular, severe internal hemorrhage is possible. Restlessness, decreasing blood pressure, and tachycardia indicate hypovolemic shock as a result of blood loss. If blood and bile leak into the peritoneal cavity, peritonitis occurs. This is suspected if the patient has abdominal tenderness, rebound tenderness, and decreased or absent bowel sounds. In some cases, the presence of blood in peritoneal lavage is the only sign of liver trauma.

MEDICAL DIAGNOSIS

When a patient is admitted with known right upper quadrant trauma, abdominal distention, and profound hypotension only temporarily responsive to blood and fluid administration, immediate surgical intervention is indicated. The diagnosis of liver trauma is confirmed in the operating room. In stable asymptomatic or minimally symptomatic patients, diagnosis is based on peritoneal lavage to detect bleeding into the peritoneal cavity and CT scan to detect the presence and magnitude of the injury.

MEDICAL MANAGEMENT

Small lacerations or intrahepatic hematomas with no evidence of active bleeding require nonoperative management. Repeat CT examinations document healing. Hemorrhage caused by minor injury is treated by simple suture and drainage. Deeper lacerations and damage to the intrahepatic vessels require blood vessel ligation and deep sutures. Severe liver trauma may require hepatic segmentectomy (removal of a portion of the liver).

COMPLICATIONS

The most common complications after surgical intervention for hepatic injury are intrahepatic abscess formation, recurrent hemorrhage, sepsis, pneumonia, and renal failure. Injuries to the hepatic veins or retrohepatic inferior vena cava are almost always fatal.

Guidelines for Application of the Nursing Process to the Care of the Patient with Liver Trauma

The patient with liver trauma is admitted to a surgical intensive care unit for close observation and hemodynamic monitoring. Monitor vital signs hourly, maintain strict intake and output, and review laboratory results of hemoglobin, hematocrit, and electrolyte levels to detect changes in hemodynamic status. Assess for abdominal pain, tenderness, and presence of bowel sounds to detect changes in gastrointestinal function. Nursing care of postoperative patients is discussed in detail in Chapter 4, and nursing care after gastrointestinal surgery is discussed in Unit 7.

Neoplasia

Benign Hepatic Tumors

The most common benign hepatic tumor is the hemangioma. This tumor, found most often in females, is usually discovered incidentally during surgery. When manifestations of an abdominal mass are present, surgical resection is performed.

Benign hepatic adenomas, although rare, are also found almost exclusively in females during the childbearing years. Hormonal factors are believed to influence adenoma development. The incidence of this disorder increases with the use of oral contraceptives. If oral contraceptives are discontinued, the lesions usually regress.

Although hepatocellular adenoma is not considered premalignant, hepatocellular carcinoma has developed in a small number of patients. Symptoms of adenoma include abdominal pain, leukocytosis, and fever. Intraabdominal hemorrhage develops in approximately one third of patients, with a mortality rate of approximately 20%. Complete surgical excision is usually performed when the tumor is identified. However, if a patient is taking oral contraceptives and the tumor has not ruptured, a trial period during which the drugs are discontinued may be indicated. Visualization studies, usually a liver scan, are performed to monitor tumor regression.

Malignant Hepatic Tumors

Primary hepatic malignancies are hepatocellular carcinoma (arising in the liver cell), cholangiocellular carcinoma (arising in the bile duct cell), or a combination of both. Primary hepatocellular carcinoma is the most common type, but it remains relatively uncommon in the United States and Western Europe. It is one of the most frequently encountered malignancies in other areas of the world, including sub-Saharan Africa, Southeast Asia, Japan, and Greece.

Although primary hepatocellular carcinoma occurs infrequently, the liver is a major site for metastatic lesions. Only cirrhosis surpasses metastatic carcinoma of the liver as a cause of fatal liver disease.

ETIOLOGY

Primary hepatocellular carcinoma is predominantly a disease affecting males and occurs frequently in a cirrhotic liver. Development of hepatocellular carcinoma is higher in patients with chronic HBV infection. Other factors linked to the development of hepatocellular carcinoma include exposure to carcinogens and the use of androgenic steroids.

The rich blood supply and lymphatic flow in the liver make it a prime site for the growth of cancerous cells originating elsewhere in the body. Liver metastasis is common for tumors originating in the stomach, colon, pancreas, lung, oropharynx, and bladder.

PATHOPHYSIOLOGY

Malignant cells multiply randomly and invade liver tissue. Normal liver functions are compromised. In cases in which cirrhosis is present, the growth of malignant cells further compromises a failing liver. Nodules are usually present in advanced stages of the disease.

CLINICAL MANIFESTATIONS

The most common complaint associated with primary or metastatic hepatic carcinoma is abdominal pain localized in the upper abdomen or right upper quadrant. An abdominal mass may be present. Hepatomegaly is evident in two thirds of patients and weight loss is noted. A friction rub or vascular bruit is heard over the liver.

MEDICAL DIAGNOSIS

Liver function studies commonly reveal elevated alkaline phosphatase and serum enzyme levels, but these tests are not specific for carcinoma. An increased or progressively rising alpha-fetoprotein level is strongly suggestive of hepatocellular carcinoma, but many patients have only a low-level elevation, which is nonspecific.

Scanning techniques, ultrasonography, CT scan, and magnetic resonance imaging (MRI) are used to identify the presence of a liver mass and to localize the area for liver biopsy. A definitive diagnosis is made via biopsy.

MEDICAL MANAGEMENT

The results of treatment for both primary and secondary hepatocellular carcinoma are poor. Most patients die within 6 months of diagnosis.

Treatment for hepatic carcinoma includes hepatic resection, liver transplantation, radiation therapy, and chemotherapy. For many patients, there is no appropriate treatment because the lesion is discovered in an advanced stage of the disease. Supportive care is provided.

If a solitary tumor is located, hepatic resection is possible. Because the liver has excellent regenerative abilities, up to 90% can be removed. Liver transplantation may be performed in some patients. However, the survival rate for both procedures is poor unless the tumor is detected at an early stage.

Radiation therapy is occasionally used, but success rates are extremely poor. Chemotherapy with doxorubicin (Adriamycin) and 5-fluorouracil administered individually, as well as combination therapy with multiple agents, yields similarly poor results. Although chemotherapy produces tumor regression, the survival rate is not improved.

Chemotherapeutic agents may be administered via hepatic artery infusion or an implantable pump. Hepatic artery infusion requires the placement of a catheter into the hepatic artery either percutaneously or via laparotomy. The catheter is brought out of the abdomen via a stab wound and attached to an external pump, which administers the chemotherapeutic agent at a prescribed rate directly into the liver. Complications include sepsis, hemorrhage, and thrombosis. This technique usually requires hospitalization and may limit the patient's activities.

The implantable pump also delivers a continuous flow of cytotoxic drugs to the liver. This device is implanted under the skin on the chest or abdominal wall. An outlet catheter is surgically implanted inside the hepatic artery. Drugs are instilled by injection through the skin into a chamber in the center of the pump. Heparin is used to maintain pump patency when chemotherapy is not being administered. The pump is usually filled every 1 to 2 weeks. Patients have fewer complications and increased independence when an implantable pump is used.

Patients with hepatic neoplasias require the same support and nursing care as patients with other oncologic disorders described in Chapter 11.

Orthotopic Hepatic Transplant

Orthotopic hepatic transplant is removal of the liver and replacement with a donor liver. The first hepatic transplant was performed in 1963, but the procedure remained experimental until 1983. Increased use of the procedure at major medical centers is possible because of better preservation techniques for donor organs, revised criteria for recipients, improved surgical techniques, better control of complications, and the use of improved immunosuppressive therapy to prevent organ rejection by the liver recipient. Although figures vary among transplant centers, the 1-year survival rate is approximately 85%, the 4- to 5-year survival rate is approximately 60%.

Selection Criteria for Hepatic Transplant Recipients

Each transplant center develops specific criteria for choosing liver transplant recipients. These criteria are based on the outcomes of previous transplant surgeries. Although some differences may exist, criteria generally include several common factors. The candidate for liver transplant must be in the final stage of hepatic disease. If the cause of liver failure is alcohol related, the patient must be free from alcohol use for a period determined by the transplant center.

Factors that contraindicate hepatic transplant include bacterial or fungal infections outside the hepatobiliary system, malignancies outside the hepatobiliary system, advanced cardiac disease, psychological instability, and lack of adequate support systems. These factors have been found to increase significantly the risk of death after transplant surgery. For patients with advanced renal disease, combined liver-kidney transplants are performed at many major transplant centers.

Selection Criteria for Hepatic Transplant Donors

Generally, liver donors must be between the ages of 3 months and 50 years with no history of liver disease, drug or alcohol abuse, malignancy, syphilis, tuberculosis, or acquired immunodeficiency syndrome (AIDS). Ideally, the donor's height and weight approximate that of the recipient for a proper "fit." However, the increasing use of "pared-down livers" allows the use of larger donor organs.

Typical donors present with head injuries, or cerebral vascular accidents or are victims of homicide or suicide. Brain death must be diagnosed and documented. The donor is ventilator dependent with no evidence of sepsis.

The donor liver is removed during a surgical procedure that takes 3 to 4 hours. The liver is placed in a potassium-rich preserving solution and must arrive within 8 to 12 hours at the transplant center. Newer preservative solutions may extend this period to 24 hours.

Surgical Procedure

The recipient's liver is removed at a time that coincides with the arrival of the donor liver. With removal of the diseased organ, the splanchnic and vena cava circulations are occluded and a venous bypass system may be used. Heparinized shunts are placed in the femoral vein and the axillary vein to shunt blood back to the heart through the axillary system. The donor liver is flushed with Ringer's lactate solution to remove the preserving potassium solution, which could cause hyperkalemia in the recipient. The portal venous system, hepatic artery, and biliary systems are anastomosed. A removable T-tube for bile drainage is brought out through the abdominal wall. Prompt outflow of bile through the T-tube is an early indicator of proper function of the transplanted liver.

During the surgical procedure, the patient is placed on a heating blanket to prevent hypothermia. Fluids and blood products are administered as needed. An arterial catheter, nasogastric tube, and

Pharmacology Box 28–2.
CYCLOSPORINE

Cyclosporine:
Immune suppressant.

Action:
Inhibits cell-mediated immune reactions, specifically T lymphocytes. Bone marrow function is not affected.

Uses:
Protects transplanted organs from rejection by the host. It is often used in combination with prednisone for liver transplant recipients.

Side Effects:
The major reactions seen with this therapy are tremor, hypertension, hirsutism, gum hyperplasia, and renal dysfunction, which is dose dependent. Gastrointestinal symptoms may include diarrhea, nausea, and vomiting. Natural defenses against bacterial, viral, fungal, and other types of infections are lowered. Patients are at risk for infection from all causes.

Interactions:
Medications causing nephrotoxicity should not be administered concurrently. Rifampin, phenytoin, and phenobarbital increase the metabolism of cyclosporine and decrease its plasma levels. Plasma concentrations are increased with high doses of methylprednisolone, erythromycin, and antifungal agents.

Nursing Implications:
Caution patient to avoid hazardous equipment if tremor develops. Monitor blood pressure, and teach patient or family members to monitor at home. Inspect mouth and gums at frequent intervals. Teach patient importance of oral hygiene, including brushing, flossing, and regular dental checkups. Monitor weight, intake, and output. Assess blood urea nitrogen (BUN) and serum creatine levels for evidence of nephrotoxicity. Instruct patient to report any sign of infection immediately, including fever, sore throat, increased fatigue, urinary frequency or dysuria, coughing or chest congestion, and skin eruptions. Stress the importance of avoiding persons with infections. Review hand-washing technique with patient and family.

indwelling urinary catheter are in place. After surgery, immunosuppressive drug therapy, usually begun in the preoperative period, is continued. Cyclosporine, prednisone, and azathioprine (Imuran) are the pharmacologic agents most often used in combination to prevent organ rejection. Pharmacology Box 28–2 describes cyclosporine, the most commonly used maintenance drug.

Postoperative Complications

After surgery, hepatic transplant recipients require close observation and monitoring by specially trained nurses. Signs of organ rejection must be recognized early. Other possible complications in the postoperative period include hemorrhage; fluid and electrolyte imbalances; pulmonary problems, most often right-sided portal vein thrombosis; infection; and some degree of renal failure caused by the nephrotoxicity of cyclosporine.

Guidelines for Application of the Nursing Process to the Care of the Patient Who Has Had an Orthotopic Hepatic Transplant

Nursing care for patients who have had an orthotopic liver transplant is similar to that described previously in Unit 7 for the patient who has had abdominal surgery. In addition, the nurse monitors for signs of obstruction, rejection, and hepatic or biliary infection.

A T-tube is inserted at the time of surgery. Thick, dark-green bile drainage indicates good liver function. A sudden drop in amount or a change in color to light yellow suggests liver dysfunction. The T-tube usually remains in place for several months, but it is clamped after 2 or 3 weeks. If fever, abdominal pain, or cramping develops within 24 hours after the tube is clamped, the T-tube is reconnected to drainage, and evaluation for biliary infection or obstruction begins.

Because liver transplant patients receive large doses of steroids and immunosuppressants to prevent liver rejection, the patient is at increased risk for infection. Suppression of antibodies prevents rejection of the implanted liver but also makes the patient less responsive to other antigens, such as bacteria or viruses. Symptoms of infection are masked by the immunosuppression therapy and complicated by possible rejection of the organ.

Rejection and infection result in fever, decreased quantity and quality of bile, loss of appetite, vague abdominal pain, and joint pain. To determine the cause of the problem, liver biopsy; CT scan; ultrasonography; blood, sputum, urine, and drainage cultures; and chest x-ray examinations may be performed. If rejection is identified, dosage of immunosuppressive drugs is increased. If infection is the problem, less immunosuppressive drug is given, and antibiotic therapy is instituted. Because immunosuppressive therapy is lifelong, patient education related to drug therapy and recognition of complications is instituted early in the postoperative period.

Patients who undergo liver transplant experience a great deal of stress both before and after the procedure. A long waiting period for a donor liver followed by the realization that rejection of the transplanted organ is an ever-present possibility requires ongoing support by a multidisciplinary team. It is imperative that patients understand the importance of life-long drug therapy and follow-up visits.

The Elderly: Special Considerations

The Elderly Patient with Hepatitis

Elderly persons who have undergone numerous surgical procedures and received a number of blood transfusions are at increased risk for hepatitis B and hepatitis C. In the geriatric patient, both hepatitis B and hepatitis C are associated with a more severe clinical course, a greater progression to chronicity, and a higher mortality rate.

Hepatitis infection in the elderly is often misdiagnosed as gallstones or malignancy because these conditions are frequently seen in older patients. Elderly patients are rarely diagnosed or treated in early stages of hepatitis because there is often a delay in the onset of symptoms, believed to be a result of immunologic factors. In addition, the hospital stay for older patients may be prolonged and complicated because of the existence of other chronic conditions.

The Elderly Patient with Toxic Hepatitis

Older individuals are at greater risk for drug-induced hepatitis because of the numerous medications they take. Many drugs are metabolized in the liver, and because of the decreased production of liver enzymes needed for drug metabolism and the decreased protein synthesis associated with aging, the geriatric patient may experience a prolonged effect from these drugs. The potential for toxicity and cumulative effects increases with aging. Careful monitoring for signs of drug related hepatic impairment is indicated for all geriatric patients.

The Elderly Patient with Cirrhosis

Cirrhosis in elderly patients is frequently of unknown origin. Individuals in whom cirrhosis develops in the middle years, most often related to alcohol abuse, usually do not survive into old age. When cirrhosis does occur in the elderly, the complications are similar to those in the younger population, but hepatic encephalopathy occurs with greater frequency and the prognosis is worse.

A condition known as cardiac cirrhosis is seen in elderly patients; however, many authorities do not consider this a true cirrhosis. Severe, prolonged right-sided heart failure leads to hepatic congestion, which results in cellular necrosis and fibrosis. Often the hepatic damage is overshadowed by the cardiac problem and resulting symptoms. Hepatic damage can be reversed if the heart failure is controlled.

Bibliography

Arroyo V, Gines P, Planas R. Treatment of ascites in cirrhosis. Gastroenterol Clin North Am 1992; 21(1):237.

Beckerman S, Galloway S. Elective resection of the liver: Nursing care. Crit Care Nurse 1989; 9(10):40.

Benenson AS (ed). Control of communicable diseases in man. 15th ed. Washington, DC: American Public Health Association, 1990.

Boyer TD. Cirrhosis of the liver and its major sequelae. In Wyngaarden JB, Smith LH Jr, Bennett JC (eds). Cecil textbook of medicine. 19th ed, Vol 1. Philadelphia: WB Saunders, 1992, pp 786–796.

Burnett DA, Rikkers LF. Nonoperative emergency treatment of variceal hemorrhage. Surg Clin North Am 1990; 70(2):291.

Carpenito LJ. Nursing diagnoses: Application to clinical practice. 4th ed. Philadelphia: JB Lippincott, 1992.
Carruth AK, Boss BJ. More than they bargained for: Adverse drug reactions. J Gerontol Nurs 1990; 16(7):27.
Cuthbert JA. Southwestern Internal Medicine Conference: Hepatitis C. Am J Med Sci 1990; 299(5):346.
Doherty MM, Carver DK. Transjugular intrahepatic portosystemic shunt: New relief for esophageal varices. Am J Nurs 1993; 93(4):58.
Ebersole P, Hess P. Toward healthy aging. St. Louis: CV Mosby, 1990.
Esteban JI, González A, Hernández JM, et al. Evaluation of antibodies to hepatitis C virus in a study of transfusion associated hepatitis. N Engl J Med 1990; 323(16):1107.
Feliciano DV. Surgery for liver trauma. Surg Clin North Am 1989; 69(2):273.
Fishbach FT. A manual of laboratory diagnostic tests. 4th ed. Philadelphia: JB Lippincott, 1992.
Hudak CM, Gallo BM, Benz JJ. Critical care nursing: A holistic approach. 5th ed. Philadelphia: JB Lippincott, 1990.
Karb VB, Queener SF, Freeman JB. Handbook of drugs for nursing practice. St. Louis: CV Mosby, 1989.
Lewis JH, Zimmerman HJ. Drug induced liver disease. Med Clin North Am 1989; 73(4):775.
Lieber CS, Guadagnini KS. The spectrum of alcoholic liver disease. Hosp Prac 1990; 25(2A):51.
Matloff DS. Treatment of acute variceal bleeding. Gastroenterol Clin North Am 1992; 21(1):103.
Matteson MA, McConnell ES. Gerontological nursing: Concepts and practice. Philadelphia: WB Saunders, 1988.
Miller H. Liver transplantation: Postoperative ICU care. Crit Care Nurse 1988; 8(6):19.
Porth CM. Pathophysiology: Concepts of altered health states. 3rd ed. Philadelphia: JB Lippincott, 1990.
Rikkers LF, Sorrell WT, Jin G. Which portosystemic shunt is best? Gastroenterol Clin North Am 1992; 21(1):179.
Robinson CH, et al. Normal and therapeutic nutrition. 17th ed. New York: Macmillan, 1986.
Schamburek RD, Farrar JT. Disorders of the digestive system in the elderly. N Engl J Med 1990; 322(7):438.
Semonin-Holleran R. Critical nursing care for abdominal trauma. Crit Care Nurse 1988; 8(3):48.
Sheets L. Liver transplantation. Nurs Clin North Am 1989; 24(4):881.
Sherlock, S. Diseases of the liver and biliary system. 8th ed. Cambridge, MA: Blackwell Scientific, 1989.
Terblanche J, Burroughs AK, Hobbs KE. Controversies in the management of bleeding esophageal varices—Part 1. N Engl J Med 1989; 320(21):1393.
Terblanche J, Burroughs AK, Hobbs KE. Controversies in the management of bleeding esophageal varices—Part 2. N Engl J Med 1989; 320(22):1469.
Van Dam J, Zeldis JB. Hepatic diseases in the elderly. Gastroenterol Clin North Am 1990; 19(2):459.
Vargo RL, Rudy EB. Infection as a complication of liver transplant. Crit Care Nurse 1989; 9(4):52.
Whiteman K, et al. Liver transplantation. Am J Nurs 1990; 90(6):68.
Williams SR. Essentials of nutrition and diet therapy. 5th ed. St. Louis, MO: Times Mirror/Mosby College, 1990.

Unit Ten

ADULTS WITH ENDOCRINE DYSFUNCTION

Learning Objectives

AFTER COMPLETING THIS UNIT, THE LEARNER WILL BE ABLE TO:

Chapter Twenty-nine

1. Explain the function of the endocrine system and hormone receptors.
2. Describe regulation of hormone secretion.
3. Identify the endocrine glands and the hormones secreted from each.
4. Explain the three common types of endocrine dysfunction.
5. Identify essential information and physiologic and psychological alterations commonly assessed in patients with endocrine dysfunction.
6. Describe guidelines for application of the nursing process to the care of patients with endocrine dysfunction.

Chapter Thirty

1. Explain the normal physiology of insulin and the hormonal regulation of blood glucose levels.
2. Describe diabetes mellitus in terms of its classifications, etiology, pathophysiology, clinical manifestations, diagnostic procedures, and medical management.
3. Identify information and physical examination data essential to the assessment of patients with diabetes mellitus.
4. State nursing diagnoses and related expected patient outcomes commonly applicable to patients with diabetes mellitus.
5. Describe nursing interventions, with their rationales, commonly applicable to patients with diabetes mellitus.
6. Explain the basis for evaluation of nursing care provided to patients with diabetes mellitus.
7. Describe the acute complications and long-term degenerative changes of diabetes mellitus in terms of etiology, pathophysiology, clinical manifestations, diagnostic procedures, medical management, and prevention.
8. Identify special considerations for the elderly patient with diabetes mellitus.

Chapters Thirty-one, Thirty-two, Thirty-three, and Thirty-four

1. Explain the normal anatomy and physiology of the endocrine glands and related structures.
2. Describe the function of the pituitary, adrenal, thyroid, and parathyroid hormones.
3. Describe common endocrine gland disorders in terms of etiology, pathophysiology, clinical manifestations, diagnostic procedures, and medical and surgical management.
4. Identify information and physical examination data essential to the assessment of the thyroid gland.
5. Identify information and physical examination data essential to the assessment of patients with common endocrine gland disorders.
6. State nursing diagnoses and related expected patient outcomes commonly applicable to patients with endocrine gland disorders.
7. Describe nursing interventions, with their rationales, commonly applicable to patients with endocrine gland disorders.
8. Explain the basis for evaluation of nursing care provided to patients with common endocrine gland disorders.
9. Identify special considerations for the elderly patient with altered pituitary, adrenal, thyroid, or parathyroid function.

Chapter Twenty-nine

KNOWLEDGE BASIC TO THE NURSING CARE *of Adults with* Endocrine Dysfunction

In order to survive, the human organism must regulate a multitude of functions and communicate among millions of cells. The endocrine system and the nervous system have evolved to meet this need.

The endocrine system is a group of ductless glands and tissues that produce and secrete chemical substances called hormones, which regulate cell functions. These hormones are discharged directly into the blood or lymph system and then circulated throughout the body. Although the glands of the endocrine system are the primary source of hormone synthesis and secretion, recent research has demonstrated that many hormones are also produced in minute amounts at multiple sites in the body.

Hormone Receptors

Hormones have diverse molecular structures and physiologic properties. Most hormones can be categorized as (1) proteins and polypeptides, (2) steroids, or (3) amines and amino acid derivatives. Each hormone may affect a specific organ or tissue, called a target organ or target tissue, or may have a general effect on the entire body. The cells of the target tissue contain receptors that recognize and bind strongly with specific hormones and reject inappropriate substances. Hormone receptor sites may be on the cell membrane or in the interior of the cell. A cell does not respond to a hormone unless it has receptor sites for that hormone. Cells with fewer receptor sites for a specific hormone bind with less hormone than cells with many receptor sites for that hormone. In addition, abnormalities in, or absence of, specific hormone receptors can result in a pathologic state as a result of complete rejection of that receptor site's hormone by the target cells.

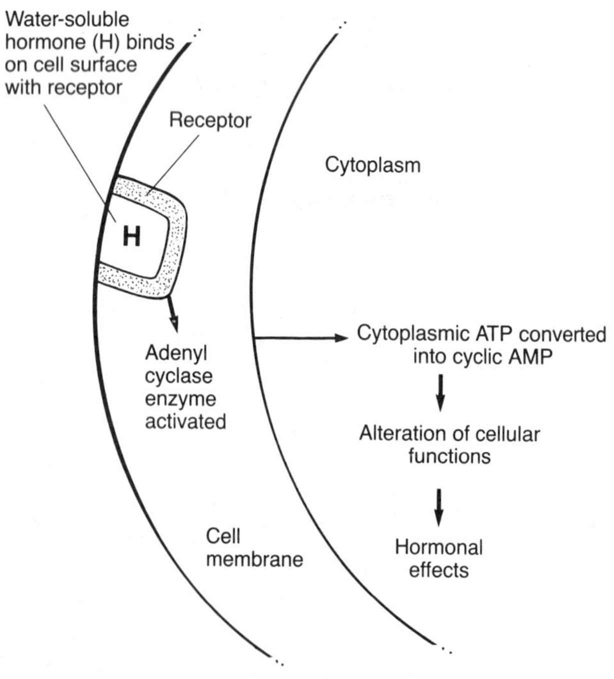

Figure 29–1.

The mechanism by which water-soluble hormones alter the cellular function of target cells to produce short-term hormonal effects. ATP, adenosine triphosphate; AMP, adenosine monophosphate.

Cell Membrane Receptors

Protein and peptide hormones, and most amine and amino acid derivative hormones, are water soluble and cannot readily penetrate the lipid barrier of the cell membrane. As illustrated in Figure 29–1, they interact first with receptors on the surface of the cell, activating the enzyme adenyl cyclase within the cell membrane. The adenyl cyclase enzyme then causes conversion of cytoplasmic adenosine triphosphate (ATP) into short-acting cyclic 3′,5′-adenosine monophosphate, or cyclic AMP, inside the cell. Once formed, cyclic AMP acts as an intracellular hormonal messenger. As a "second messenger," cyclic AMP diffuses throughout the cell and alters cellular functions to produce the hormonal effects inside the cell. This response can occur almost instantly, requiring only a few seconds or minutes to complete.

Intracellular Receptors

Because of their smaller size and chemical composition, the lipid-soluble steroid hormones readily penetrate the cell membrane to bind directly with intracellular protein receptors (Fig. 29–2). These combined hormone-receptor molecules diffuse into the cell nucleus and activate specific genes within the nuclear DNA to produce messenger RNA. The messenger RNA diffuses out of the nucleus into the cytoplasm, where it promotes synthesis of a specific protein within the cell, which, in turn, alters cell function, growth, or differentiation. The effect of steroid hormones takes about 45 minutes to begin, and several hours or days for the full effect to occur.

Regulation of Hormone Secretion

The secretory function of the endocrine glands may be affected by the nervous system, by chemical substances in the blood, or by other hormones. Because hormones are very potent substances, their concentration in the blood must be maintained at a relatively constant level. One way this is accomplished is through negative feedback control, which is illustrated in Figure 29–3. As the concentration in the blood serum of a hormone or of a substance affected by a hormone rises, further secretion of that hormone is inhibited. When the serum levels fall, hormone production is stimulated.

Secretion of hormones by the pineal gland, adre-

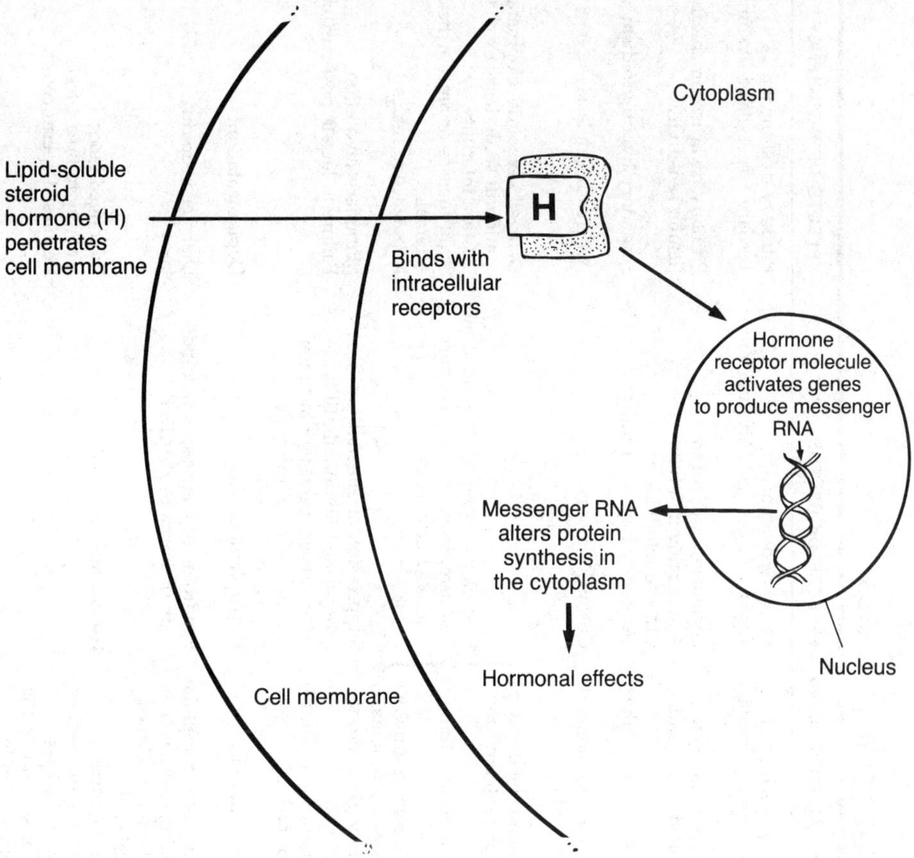

Figure 29–2.

The mechanism by which lipid-soluble steroid hormones alter the cellular function of target cells to produce long-term hormonal effects.

nal medulla, posterior pituitary, and hypothalamus can be affected directly by neurologic stimuli in addition to regulation of secretion by negative feedback control.

Endocrine Glands

As illustrated in Figure 29–4, the endocrine glands are located throughout the body. Although the location and function of each gland vary widely, the system as a whole is interrelated, and the secretion of one gland often affects other glands in the body. Table 29–1 summarizes the endocrine glands, the hormones they secrete, and the effects of these hormones on the body and on each other.

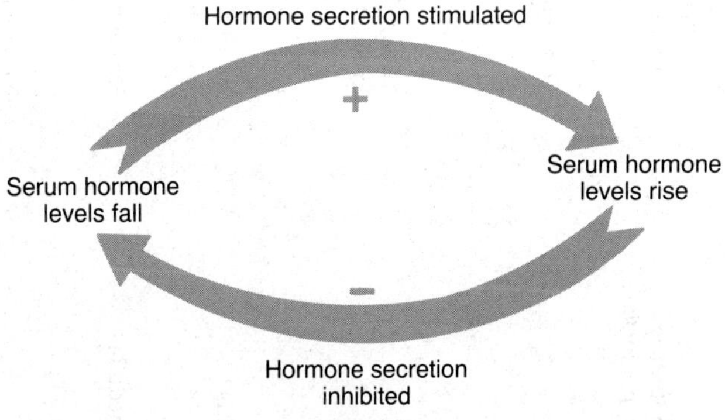

Figure 29–3.

Negative feedback control. As the endocrine gland secretes its hormone, serum levels of the hormone rise and inhibit further secretion from the gland.

Thymus Gland

The thymus gland consists of two flattened lobes of lymphoid tissue located in the mediastinal cavity just below the clavicle. Its principal secretion is thymopoietin, which stimulates the development of mature immunologic lymphocytes called T cells. The thymus gland is important in the development of the immune response in the newborn and the maintenance of immunologic competence in the adult.

Pineal Gland

The pineal gland, sometimes called the pineal body, is a small pine cone–shaped structure located in the cranial cavity behind the midbrain and the third ventricle. It produces and secretes melatonin, and possibly other hormones that interact with the hypothalamic-pituitary system to affect and respond to the circadian release of many of the endocrine hormones. In sighted individuals, activity of the pineal gland responds to cycles of light and dark-

Table 29–1. THE ENDOCRINE GLANDS

GLAND	HORMONES	PRIMARY HORMONAL FUNCTIONS	EFFECTS OF EXCESS	EFFECTS OF DEFICIENCY
Hypothalamic neurosecretory cells	Releasing hormones Inhibiting hormones	Control secretion of specific hormones from the anterior pituitary gland.	Pituitary dysfunction Tertiary target gland dysfunction	Pituitary dysfunction Tertiary target gland dysfunction
Anterior pituitary (adenohypophysis)	Somatotropin (STH) or growth hormone (GH)	Stimulates growth of cells, bones, muscles, and soft tissue. Insulin antagonist.	Gigantism in children Acromegaly in adults Glucose intolerance	Pituitary dwarfism in children Insulin sensitivity
	Thyrotropin or thyroid-stimulating hormone (TSH)	Regulates secretory activity of the thyroid gland.	Secondary hyperthyroidism	Secondary hypothyroidism
	Adrenocorticotropic hormone (ACTH)	Stimulates secretion of hormones from the adrenal cortex.	Cushing's disease	Adrenal hypoplasia
	Gonadotropic hormones Luteinizing hormone (LH)	Induces ovulation and the development of the corpus luteum in females. Stimulates testosterone secretion in males.	Precocious sexual development, hirsutism, alteration in secondary sex characteristics (LH and FSH)	Delayed sexual development, alteration in secondary sex characteristics, infertility Scant menses or amenorrhea in females Impotence in males
	Follicle-stimulating hormone (FSH)	Stimulates graafian follicle growth and estrogen secretion in females.		
	Prolactin	Stimulates mammary gland development and lactation. Suppresses secretion of gonadotropin releasing hormones.	Suppression of gonadal function, depressed libido, infertility Amenorrhea, persistent lactation (galactorrhea) in females Impotence in males	Mammary involution Failure to lactate post partum
	Melanocyte-stimulating hormone (MSH)	Stimulates melanin synthesis.	Hyperpigmentation	Depigmentation
Posterior pituitary (neurohypophysis)	Antidiuretic hormone (ADH)*	Regulates osmolality of extracellular fluids by increasing reabsorption of water from the renal tubules. Also has vasopressive effect.	Syndrome of inappropriate antidiuretic hormone (SIADH)	Diabetes insipidus
	Oxytocin*	Stimulates uterine contraction. Initiation of breast milk expression (let-down reflex) in females. Increases ejection of sperm into the semen during ejaculation in males.	(Under investigation)	Prolonged labor Inability to breast-feed Decreased sperm count
Thyroid	Thyroxine (T_4) Triiodothyronine (T_3)	Regulate metabolism, energy production, and growth and development.	Primary hyperthyroidism Graves' disease	Primary hypothyroidism Myxedema Juvenile hypothyroidism Cretinism in infants
	Calcitonin	Increases the rate at which calcium is deposited into the bones.	Increased bone density Hypocalcemia	Osteoporosis Hypercalcemia
Parathyroids	Parathormone, or parathyroid hormone (PTH)	Regulates serum calcium and phosphate levels. Promotes resorption of calcium from the bones.	Hyperparathyroidism Hypercalcemia, osteoporosis	Hypoparathyroidism Tetany, hypocalcemia
Adrenal medulla	Epinephrine, or Adrenalin	Instantaneous stress reaction. "Fight or flight" response. Raises metabolism, blood glucose levels, cardiac output.	Pheochromocytoma, severe hypertension (epinephrine and norepinephrine)	No known disease or effect
	Norepinephrine	Generalized vasoconstriction.		

Adrenal cortex	Glucocorticoids Cortisol Cortisone Corticosterone	Mediate the stress response. Promote protein and fat catabolism to raise blood glucose levels. Promote sodium and water retention, potassium excretion. Suppress ACTH secretion.	Inhibit the inflammatory response Cushing's syndrome	Addison's disease
	Mineralocorticoids Aldosterone Deoxycorticosterone (DOC)	Promote sodium and water retention, potassium excretion.	Primary aldosteronism	
	Sex hormones Androgens Estrogen	Development and maintenance of secondary sex characteristics and libido. Source of testosterone in females, estrogen in males.	Virilism	
Pancreas				
Beta cells	Insulin	Regulates fat, protein, carbohydrate metabolism. Lowers blood glucose levels by promoting glucose transport into the cells.	Hyperinsulinism Hypoglycemia	Diabetes mellitus
Alpha cells	Glucagon	Raises blood glucose levels by promoting hepatic glycogenolysis. Promotes glyconeogenesis (gluconeogenesis). Insulin antagonist.	Glucose intolerance and hyperglycemia	(Under investigation; probable hypoglycemia)
Delta cells	Somatostatin†	Inhibits diverse endocrine functions. Inhibits the release of insulin, glucagon, and somatotropin (STH).	Hyperglycemia	(Under investigation)
Gonads				
Ovaries (female)	Estrogen Progesterone	Development, maturation, and cyclic function of the reproductive system. Development of breasts and secondary sex characteristics.	Infertility, alteration in menstrual cycle, alteration in secondary sex characteristics	Amenorrhea, infertility, spontaneous abortion, regression of secondary sex characteristics, decreased libido
Testes (male)	Testosterone	Development, maturation, and function of the reproductive system and secondary sex characteristics. Stimulates growth of skeletal muscles, bones, skin, and hair. Stimulates closure of the epiphyseal plates at puberty.	Suppresses gonadotropic activity, thereby causing testicular atrophy, infertility, impotence Precocious sexual development, premature epiphyseal closure in children	Impotence, infertility Cryptorchidism in children
Thymus	Thymopoietin	Development of the immune response in the newborn. Maintenance of immunologic response in the adult.	(Under investigation)	Immunodeficiency disorders
Pineal	Melatonin	Influences and responds to the body's circadian rhythms.	(Under investigation)	(Under investigation)

* Antidiuretic hormone and oxytocin are produced in the hypothalamus, but stored in and secreted from the posterior pituitary.

† Somatostatin is also produced in the hypothalamus, many regions of the central and peripheral nervous system, retina, thymus, adrenal medulla, placenta, and delta cells of the stomach and intestine. It may also function as a neurotransmitter in the central nervous system.

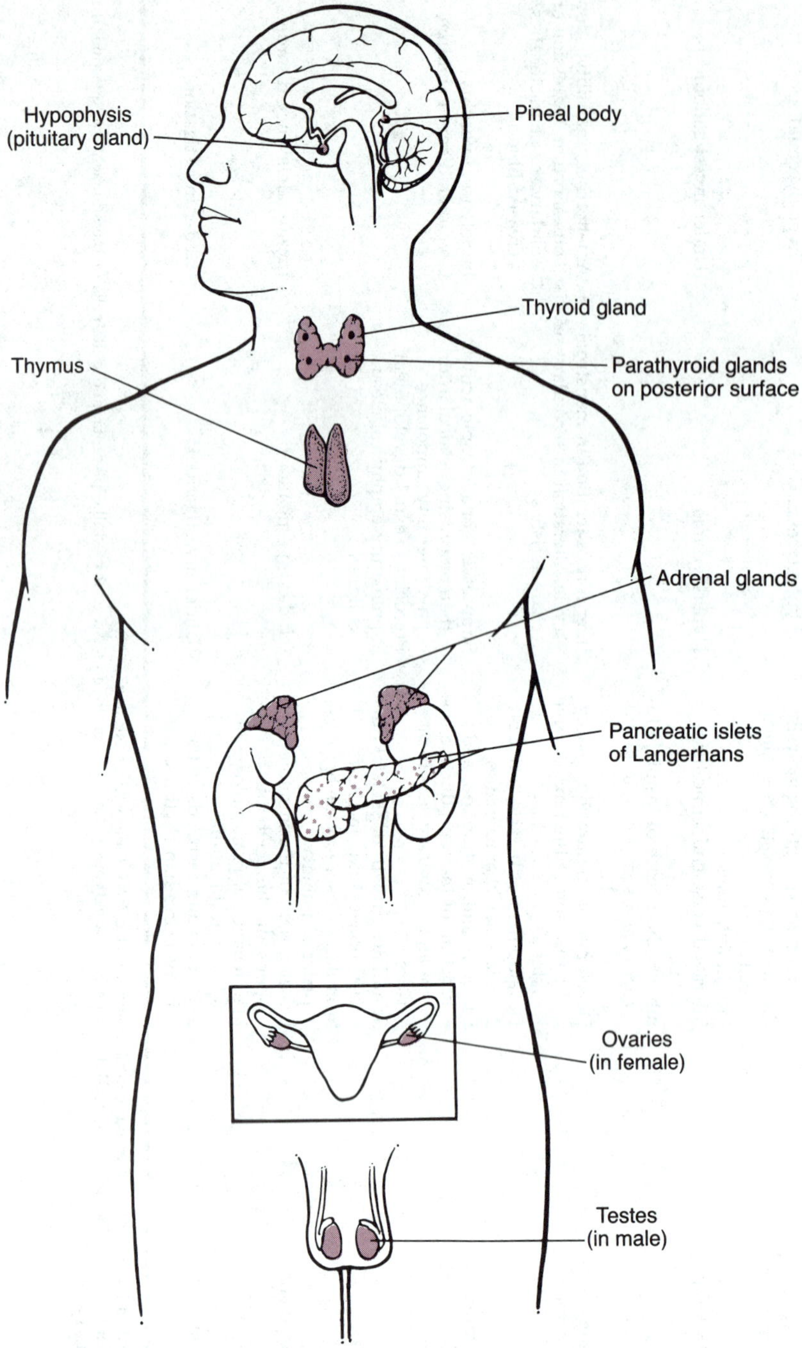

Figure 29–4.

Anatomic location of the glands of the endocrine system.

ness and to the wavelength (color) of light. Melatonin levels are highest during the daily periods of darkness. Some research indicates that melatonin may affect the sleep-wake cycle by inducing drowsiness. In blind humans, melatonin levels fluctuate in a 24.7-hour cycle.

Although the effects, if any, of melatonin on the human reproductive cycle are unclear, the amount of melatonin in the circulation has been shown to vary with the phases of the menstrual cycle. Higher melatonin levels occur in the days immediately preceding menstruation.

Hypothalamus

The hypothalamus region of the brain lies beneath the thalamus and forms the floor and part of the lateral walls of the third ventricle. Special neurosecretory cells in the hypothalamus synthesize and secrete hypothalamic hormones, which regulate the secretory functions of the anterior pituitary gland. The hypothalamic hormones that stimulate pituitary secretions are called releasing hormones. Those that inhibit pituitary secretions are inhibiting hormones. These hormones are transported via the hypotha-

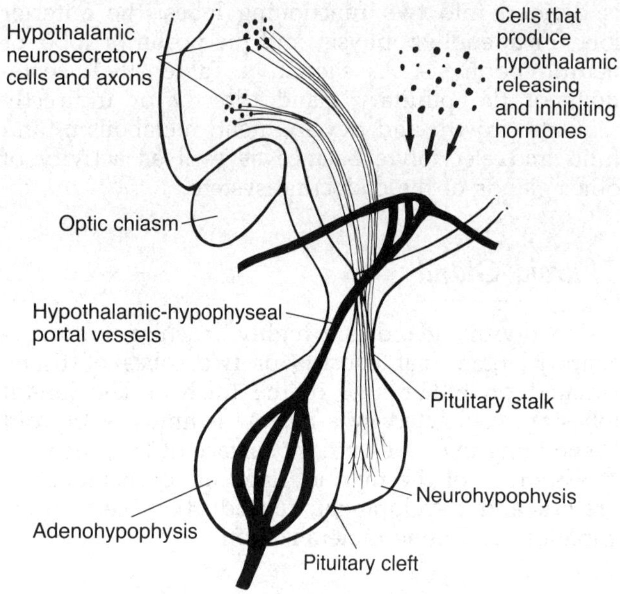

Figure 29–5.

Anatomic relationship of the hypothalamus and the pituitary gland, with vascular and neurologic connections. Hypothalamic releasing and inhibiting hormones enter the hypothalamic-hypophyseal vessels for transport to the adenohypophysis (anterior pituitary). Antidiuretic hormone and oxytocin produced by hypothalamic neurosecretory cells pass down the axons to the neurohypophysis (posterior pituitary).

lamic-hypophyseal portal vessels to the anterior lobe of the pituitary, which is located directly below the hypothalamus and connected to it by the pituitary stalk. Figure 29–5 illustrates the anatomic relationship of the hypothalamus and pituitary gland. A partial list of the hypothalamic secretions and their effects on pituitary function is given in Table 29–2.

Other neurosecretory cells in the hypothalamus produce two hormones, antidiuretic hormone and oxytocin, which pass down the cell axons to the posterior pituitary, where they are stored. These hormones are later released in response to neurostimulation of the posterior pituitary by the hypothalamus. Another example of neuroregulation of hormone secretion by the hypothalamus is the secretion of epinephrine and norepinephrine from the adrenal medulla in response to impulses transmitted via a direct nerve pathway that connects the adrenal medulla to the hypothalamus.

By analysis of input from nerve circuits that connect it to almost all parts of the brain and from information received from the blood passing through it, the hypothalamus constantly monitors the body's homeostasis. Through the dynamic processes of feedback and regulation, almost the entire endocrine system is controlled by either hormonal secretions or nervous signals from the hypothalamus.

Table 29–2. HYPOTHALAMIC SECRETIONS

HYPOTHALAMIC SECRETION	FUNCTION
Somatostatin (SS) or growth hormone inhibiting hormone	Inhibits secretion of somatotropin (STH)
Growth hormone releasing hormone (GH-RH)	Stimulates growth hormone (GH) secretion
Thyrotropin releasing hormone (TRH)	Stimulates thyroid-stimulating hormone (TSH) secretion
Corticotropin releasing hormone (CRH)	Stimulates adrenocorticotropic hormone (ACTH) secretion
Luteinizing hormone releasing hormone (LH-RH)*	Stimulates secretion of luteinizing hormone (LH) and follicle-stimulating hormone (FSH)
Follicle-stimulating hormone releasing hormone (FSH-RH)*	Stimulates FSH secretion
Prolactin releasing hormone (PRH)	Stimulates secretion of prolactin
Prolactin inhibiting hormone (PIH)	Inhibits secretion of prolactin
Melanocyte-stimulating hormone releasing hormone	Stimulates melanocyte-stimulating hormone (MSH) secretion
Melanocyte-stimulating hormone inhibiting hormone	Inhibits secretion of MSH

* These two releasing hormones are sometimes grouped and designated as gonadotropin releasing hormone (Gn-RH).

Pituitary Gland

The pituitary gland, or hypophysis, is an oval pea-sized organ located in the sella turcica of the sphenoid bone of the skull. It is attached to the underside of the hypothalamic portion of the brain by a pituitary stalk, or infundibulum. Within the infundibulum are the hypothalamic-hypophyseal portal vessels, which vascularize the anterior lobe of the pituitary after passing through the hypothalamus, and the specialized neurons that transmit impulses from the hypothalamus to the posterior lobe of the pituitary. These vascular and neural pathways form the primary vital connection between the central nervous system and the endocrine system necessary to maintain homeostasis.

As illustrated in Figure 29–5, the pituitary gland

is divided into two functioning lobes: the anterior lobe, or adenohypophysis, and the posterior lobe, or neurohypophysis. As shown in Table 29–1, secretions of the pituitary gland directly or indirectly regulate growth and development, metabolism, and fluid and electrolyte balance as well as activity of other glands of the endocrine system.

Thyroid Gland

The thyroid gland is a highly vascular, butterfly-shaped organ that consists of two lobes of tissue situated on either side of the trachea. The lateral lobes are connected by a narrow isthmus of thyroid tissue lying over the anterior surface of the trachea.

Secretions of the thyroid gland affect metabolism, growth and development, reproduction, cell differentiation, and bone mineralization.

Parathyroid Glands

The parathyroid glands are usually four in number and are imbedded on the posterior aspect of the thyroid gland. Each gland has a flattened oval shape and is smaller than the pituitary gland. Parathyroid hormone regulates serum calcium and phosphorus levels.

Adrenal Glands

The adrenal glands, or suprarenal glands, are pyramid-shaped organs that sit on the top of each kidney. Each adrenal gland is composed of two distinctly different structures, each one with its own functions. The adrenal medulla is an extension of the sympathetic nervous system and mediates the body's response to stress. The adrenal cortex secretes a group of steroid hormones that regulate metabolism and sodium and potassium balance, mediate the inflammatory response, and affect secondary sex characteristics. The adrenal cortex is essential for life.

Pancreatic Islets

The islets of Langerhans of the pancreas secrete three hormones that regulate the metabolism of carbohydrates, fats, and proteins. The functions of these hormones are discussed at length in Chapter 30.

Gonads

The gonads are the sex glands. The female sex glands, the two ovaries, are located on either side of the uterus. The male sex glands, the two testes, are located in the scrotal sac. The gonads are responsible for regulating the reproductive cycle and the development and maintenance of secondary sex characteristics and maturation.

Endocrine Dysfunction

Endocrine dysfunction arises from the effects of an imbalance in the production of one or more hormones or from the effects of an alteration in the body's ability to use the hormones produced. Endocrine dysfunction can originate at almost any point in the production-secretion-feedback-regulation cycle. Dysfunction of one endocrine gland is likely to affect the function of one or more of the others.

Primary Endocrine Gland Dysfunction

Primary endocrine gland dysfunction implies that an endocrine gland is secreting either too much or too little hormone because of a defect in the gland itself. Secretion of excessive amounts of hormone is called hypersecretion. Secretion of inadequate amounts of hormone is called hyposecretion or hormone deficiency.

Primary hypersecretion from an endocrine gland is usually the result of either a secreting benign or malignant tumor or idiopathic hyperplasia. Idiopathic hyperplasia is an increase in the size of the gland and proliferation of the number of active secreting cells as a result of unknown causes.

Primary hyposecretion by an endocrine gland can result from anything that destroys glandular tissue or interferes with the ability of the gland to function. Common causes of glandular hypofunction are a destructive benign or malignant tumor, an inflammatory or infectious process, a destructive autoimmune response, and mechanical damage to the gland.

Secondary Endocrine Gland Dysfunction

Secondary endocrine gland dysfunction implies that a gland is secreting too much or too little hormone secondary to factors outside of the gland itself. Depending upon the cause of the dysfunction and how long it has been present, secondary glandular dysfunction may be temporary or permanent. If the gland is structurally sound, normal function may return once the causative factor is corrected.

Inability to Use Hormone Produced

Inability of the body to use a hormone secreted may produce clinical manifestations of glandular hyposecretion when the endocrine gland is actually producing normal or even increased amounts of hormone. Two common causes of inability to use a hormone produced are production of a biologically inactive hormone and production of autoantibodies that destroy a specific hormone or hormone receptors.

Assessment of Endocrine Function

Clinical manifestations and nursing care of specific endocrine disorders are discussed in detail in Chapters 30 through 34. Because each hormone affects numerous functions throughout the body, an individual with endocrine dysfunction has many health problems and nursing needs. Accurate assessment, reporting, and documentation of clinical manifestations, changes in condition, and response to treatment are especially important in the care of these patients because they often demonstrate rapid fluctuations in physical and emotional status. As a group, endocrine disorders commonly produce alterations in the function of multiple body systems. Table 29–3 lists alterations commonly assessed in patients with endocrine dysfunction. The focus of the physical examination of a patient with an endocrine disorder varies with the specific gland involved and is discussed in the appropriate chapters.

Patient History

In collecting a history from a patient with an endocrine disorder, it is sometimes helpful to have someone familiar with the patient present because altered cognitive function caused by the disorder may cause the patient to misunderstand questions or give vague or inaccurate answers. Assess alertness, mental processes, and speech patterns while collecting the history.

Determine the individual's reason for seeking medical care and knowledge about the diagnosis and treatment. Obtain a description of the symptoms, when they were first noted, whether the onset was sudden or gradual, the duration of each symptom, and current status. Determine whether the symptoms progressed steadily or had cyclic periods of exacerbation and remission. Ask specifically about unusual fatigue or lethargy, because it is often the earliest manifestation of endocrine dysfunction. Determine the patient's perception of the severity of the symptoms and what impact they have had on daily activities.

Question the patient about recent illness, injury, or physical or emotional stress, because stress is often a precipitating factor in the onset or exacerbation of endocrine disorders. Determine whether the patient is currently, or has recently, been taking any prescription or nonprescription medication or drug, because the side effects of some drugs may mimic or precipitate endocrine dysfunction. Review the family history for endocrine, developmental, or growth disorders, because heredity is a factor in many endocrine diseases.

Table 29–3. ALTERATIONS COMMONLY ASSESSED IN PATIENTS WITH ENDOCRINE DYSFUNCTION

GENERAL ALTERATIONS IN BODY STRUCTURE AND FUNCTION
Fatigue or lethargy
Altered rest and activity patterns
Altered growth and development patterns
Changes in appearance and body characteristics
Atypical skin pigmentation and/or texture
Changes in hair texture and/or distribution
Disturbances in sexual function and reproduction
Changes in secondary sex characteristics
PSYCHOSOCIAL ALTERATIONS
Changes in body image and role performance
Changes in cognitive function
Personality changes
Emotional lability
Disturbances in coping mechanisms and support systems
Anxiety or fear
ALTERATIONS IN NUTRITION AND ELIMINATION
Changes in appetite and fluid intake
Weight loss or gain
Changes in bowel elimination pattern
Changes in urinary pattern and/or quantity
Deficiencies or excesses of nutritional elements
ALTERATIONS IN GASEOUS TRANSFER
Altered cardiac output
Fluid and electrolyte imbalances
Dependent edema or anasarca
Changes in pulse rate and/or blood pressure
Changes in peripheral circulation
Anemia
Altered respiratory rate or pattern
ALTERATIONS IN BODY DEFENSES
Elevated or subnormal body temperature
Decreased resistance to inflammation and infection
Impaired wound healing and recovery from illness
Impaired stress response
ALTERATIONS IN SENSORIMOTOR FUNCTION
Bone and joint abnormalities
Muscle wasting and atrophy
Altered balance and gait
Tetany, paresthesias, and muscle cramps
Visual disturbances
Headaches

Determine whether the patient has noted any changes characteristic of the alterations common in endocrine disorders, as identified in Table 29–3. Collect information on the patient's usual coping patterns and support systems, because endocrine disorders frequently require surgical intervention and usually require lifelong self-management and follow-up care.

Guidelines for Application of the Nursing Process to the Care of the Patient with Endocrine Dysfunction

Diagnostic procedures to evaluate endocrine gland function are initially determined by the patient's

Chart 29–1.

NURSING GUIDE TO PATIENT EDUCATION FOR SELF-MANAGEMENT: ENDOCRINE DYSFUNCTION

Instruct the patient in the following:

The correct medical term for the diagnosis.
Pathophysiology, disease progression, and patient prognosis.
Prescribed therapeutic regimen, its rationale, and expected results.
Self-administration of medications and/or treatments and schedule.
Expected action and side effects of medications.
Dietary alterations.
Alterations in lifestyle and activities.
What to do if unable to follow prescribed regimen because of illness.
Self-monitoring of the effectiveness of treatment.
Symptoms of a recurrent hormone imbalance.
Symptoms that should be reported to the physician.
Need to carry or wear emergency medical information and identification.
Plans for follow-up care.
Information on community and national support groups.
Referral to community agencies.

history and clinical manifestations. Patients are often acutely ill during the diagnostic phase. Nursing care is planned to provide physical and emotional support while facilitating accurate and timely collection of specimens and rapid completion of diagnostic procedures. Specimens must be collected and preserved correctly for results to be accurate. Many diagnostic procedures for endocrine disorders are timed and require special preparation and specimen collection for a period of hours or days. Patient teaching and cooperation are essential.

Emotional support and teaching regarding lifelong adjustments in lifestyle, medications, and indications of impending hormonal imbalance are probably the most important nursing functions in terms of helping the individual live successfully with an endocrine disorder. Important topics to include in the patient teaching plan are identified in Chart 29–1. Ample opportunity must be provided for the patient and family to share concerns and to discuss perceptions of the effects the condition will have on lifestyle and responsibilities. Success is determined by the patient's ability to achieve short-term goals and hormonal balance while in the hospital and ability to continue to maintain hormonal balance after discharge while adapting to required lifestyle changes.

The Elderly: Special Considerations

The normal aging process is accompanied by changes in the function of the endocrine glands. With advancing years, the amount of hormones secreted by many of the endocrine glands changes. One of the most noticeable age-related changes is a decrease in the elderly individual's ability to adapt to stress and respond to environmental changes. These adaptations are mediated by hypothalamic-pituitary-adrenal gland interactions. Pancreatic and thyroid secretions also diminish, altering digestion and metabolism. Normal gonadal secretions diminish, with resultant deterioration of secondary sex characteristics and, in females especially, the onset of osteoporosis. The interaction between pineal gland activity and the endocrine effects of the aging process is under investigation.

The incidence of many endocrine dysfunctions increases with age. Therefore, as the population ages, more and more individuals develop specific endocrine disorders. With replacement therapy and dietary adjustment, most of these disorders are compatible with long life.

The geriatric patient with an endocrine disorder presents many special nursing challenges. Alterations in fluid and electrolyte balance, so prevalent in these conditions, are more difficult to assess in the elderly because of loss of skin tone, muscle tremors, and deteriorating thought processes. Many elderly have chronic cardiovascular problems, which make it difficult to determine the cause of changes in cardiovascular status. These conditions, plus long-standing problems related to mobility, sight, hearing, elimination, and nutritional intake, can interfere with accurate diagnosis as well as evaluation of treatment and the patient's understanding of instructions in self-care.

The liver and kidney also deteriorate with age. This interferes with the metabolic breakdown of replacement hormones and puts the elderly individual at higher risk to develop undesirable side effects. Hormone replacement therapy for the elderly must be initiated cautiously and the dosage increased slowly, with close assessment of the therapeutic effects, to prevent accumulation of the drug and to avoid overloading the cardiovascular system by increasing the workload of the heart.

Bibliography

Abrams AC. Clinical drug therapy: Rationales for nursing practice. 3rd ed. Philadelphia: JB Lippincott, 1991.

Booth D. Hypoparathyroidism: The overlooked disorder. Gerontol Nurs 1990; 16(6):16.

Bullock BL, Rosendahl PP. Pathophysiology: Adaptations and alterations in function. 2nd ed. Boston: Little, Brown, 1988.

Chenevey B. Overview of fluids and electrolytes. Nurs Clin North Am 1987; 22(4):749.

Cooper JAD, Pappas PG. (eds). Cecil review of general internal medicine. 5th ed. Philadelphia: WB Saunders, 1992.

DeGroot LJ (ed). Endocrinology. 2nd ed. Philadelphia: WB Saunders, 1989.

Dudek SG. Nutrition handbook for nursing practice. Philadelphia: JB Lippincott, 1987.

Eliopoulos C. Gerontological nursing. 3rd ed. Philadelphia: JB Lippincott, 1993.

Gambert SR (ed). Handbook of geriatrics. New York: Plenum Press, 1986.

Greenspan FS. Basic and clinical endocrinology. Norwalk, CT: Appleton & Lange, 1991.

Griffin J, Ojeda S (eds). Textbook of endocrine physiology. New York: Oxford University Press, 1988.

Guyton G. Textbook of medical physiology. 8th ed. Philadelphia: WB Saunders, 1991.

Kidd PS, Murakami RY. Common pathologic conditions in elderly persons: Nursing assessment and intervention. J Emerg Med 1987; 13(1):27.

Lloyd RV. Endocrine pathology. New York: Springer-Verlag, 1990.

Malseed RT, Harrigan G. Textbook of pharmacology and nursing care: Using the nursing process. 2nd ed. Philadelphia: JB Lippincott, 1989.

Mathewson MK. Antidiuretic hormone. Crit Care Nurse 1986; 6(5):88.

Mathewson MK. Thyroid disorder. Crit Care Nurse 1987; 7(1):74.

Matteson MA, McConnell ES. Gerontological nursing: Concepts and practice. Philadelphia: WB Saunders, 1988.

Moran S. Innovative geriatric care. Nurs Manage 1987; 18(6):26.

Price AP, Wilson LM. Pathophysiology: Clinical concepts of disease processes. 4th ed. St. Louis: Mosby Year Book, 1992.

Raffensperger EB. Clinical nursing handbook. Philadelphia: JB Lippincott, 1986.

Robbins SL, Kumar V. Basic pathology. 4th ed. Philadelphia: WB Saunders, 1987.

Schultz PN. Hypopituitarism in patients with a history of irradiation to the head and neck area: Diagnosis and implications for nursing. Oncol Nurs Forum 1989; 18(6):823.

Sheeky SB. Metabolic and endocrine emergencies. J Emerg Nurs 1985; 11(1):49.

Sowers J, Felicetta J (eds). Endocrinology of aging. New York: Raven Publishing, 1988.

Wilson JD, Foster DW (eds). Williams textbook of endocrinology. 8th ed. Philadelphia: WB Saunders, 1992.

Chapter Thirty

NURSING CARE *of Adults with Diabetes Mellitus*

Diabetes mellitus is a chronic disorder of altered carbohydrate, fat, and protein metabolism caused by either a relative or absolute lack of insulin or the inability of the tissues to respond to insulin. Diabetes mellitus is characterized by persistent hyperglycemia, impaired leukocyte activity, and long-term vascular and neurologic degeneration. It is one of the oldest diseases known to man and was recorded as early as 1500 B.C. The term *diabetes* is derived from the Greek verb meaning to "run through" and the Latin word *mellitus,* meaning "honey," because of the association noted by physicians that these patients had polyuria and that their urine was sweet.

Hormonal Regulation of Blood Glucose Levels

Insulin

Insulin is a hormone secreted by the beta cells in the islets of Langerhans in the pancreas. It is a small protein composed of two amino acid chains that are connected to each other by disulfide linkages. The primary function of insulin is to transport glucose into muscle and fat cells to be used for energy. Insulin affects carbohydrate, fat, and protein metabolism and lowers blood glucose levels. Box 30–1 presents a glossary of terms frequently used in discussion of insulin and diabetes mellitus.

CARBOHYDRATE METABOLISM

The effects of insulin on carbohydrate metabolism are to increase the rate of glucose metabolism, decrease blood glucose concentration, and increase glycogen stores. Insulin binds with the cell's receptor sites, which causes the rapid uptake, storage, and use of glucose by most cells in the body. Insulin promotes the transport of glucose across the cell wall by a process known as facilitated diffusion, thereby providing the body with energy. Following a meal, insulin promotes storage of excess glucose in the liver by converting glucose into glycogen, a process called glycogenesis. Between meals, when blood glucose levels fall, the liver converts glycogen back into glucose, a process called glycogenolysis.

FAT METABOLISM

Insulin promotes fatty acid synthesis by converting glucose into fatty acids. These fatty acids are subsequently deposited as fat in adipose tissue. Although most of this synthesis occurs in the liver, a small proportion occurs in the fat cells themselves. The conversion of glucose into fatty acid is called lipogenesis.

PROTEIN METABOLISM

Insulin promotes the entry of amino acids into cells and inhibits the catabolism of protein. Insulin also decreases the rate at which amino acids are released from cells, especially muscle cells. Insulin inhibits the rate of gluconeogenesis, which is the formation of glucose from fats and protein, by decreasing the activity of enzymes that promote gluconeogenesis.

Regulation of Insulin Secretion

Insulin is normally secreted at a continuous basal rate, with increased secretion in response to food. At

Box 30–1.

TERMS FREQUENTLY USED IN NURSING CARE OF THE PATIENT WITH DIABETES MELLITUS

- Anabolism – The synthesis of complex molecules from simple molecules.
- Catabolism – The breakdown of complex molecules to simple molecules with the release of energy.
- Diffusion – The means by which molecules or solutes move across a selectively permeable membrane from a higher concentration to a lower concentration.
- Facilitated Diffusion – The means by which glucose crosses a membrane. Glucose combines with a carrier substance, insulin, to cross the cell membrane.
- Glycogen – A polysaccharide formed from glucose and stored in the liver and muscle cells.
- Glycogenesis – The synthesis of glycogen from glucose.
- Glycogenolysis – The breakdown of glycogen to glucose.
- Gluconeogenesis – The conversion of fat or protein to glycogen and then to glucose in the liver.
- Lipogenesis – The conversion of glucose and triglycerides into fat for storage.
- Lipolysis – The breakdown of fat to glucose.

the normal fasting blood glucose level, insulin secretion is minimal. When blood glucose concentration is increased, such as after eating a meal, insulin secretion increases. Insulin secretion in response to glucose stimulation is rapid and occurs within minutes. This rise in insulin allows the transport of glucose into muscle, liver, and other cells, thereby reducing blood glucose concentration. The reduced blood glucose level then causes a decrease in the secretion of insulin. Between meals and during overnight fasting, insulin and glucose levels fall. If the period of fasting is prolonged, stored glucose is released from the liver, protein is released from muscle, and fat is released from adipose tissue to provide energy for the cells.

Counterregulatory Hormones

Blood glucose concentrations are also influenced by counterregulatory hormones, all of which oppose the action of insulin and are therefore also known as insulin antagonists. These counterregulatory hormones are glucagon, epinephrine, cortisol, growth hormone, and somatostatin (growth hormone inhibiting hormone).

Glucagon is secreted by the alpha cells of the islets of Langerhans in the pancreas. It increases blood glucose concentration by causing glycogenolysis (the breakdown of glycogen into glucose) and by increasing gluconeogenesis (formation of glucose from amino acids). Glucagon is essential for recovery from hypoglycemia and is the primary counterregulatory hormone.

The effect of epinephrine on blood glucose concentration is similar to that of glucagon, although not quite as strong.

Cortisol increases the blood glucose concentration by increasing the rate of gluconeogenesis and decreasing glucose utilization by the cells. Further information on the physiologic effects of epinephrine and cortisol is provided in Chapter 32.

Growth hormone (somatotropin) is secreted by the anterior pituitary gland. Long-term growth hormone excess limits glucose transport into cells and results in elevated blood glucose levels.

Somatostatin is a hormone secreted by the hypothalamus. It inhibits the release of both somatotropin from the anterior pituitary gland and certain hormones such as glucagon and insulin.

Absence of Insulin

The absence of insulin results in hyperglycemia (elevated blood glucose) by impairing glucose uptake in the cells, especially in muscle cells and the liver. Cellular starvation occurs despite elevated blood glucose levels because glucose transport into the cells is impaired. Impaired protein synthesis and excessive protein catabolism also occur, causing an increase in glucogenic amino acids. This leads to increased hepatic glucose production and causes further increase in blood glucose levels. The conversion of protein to glucose is called gluconeogenesis.

When severe insulin deficiency exists, lipolysis occurs. Lipolysis is the formation of excessive amounts of glycerol and free fatty acids through the hydrolysis of triglycerides. Glycerol increases hepatic glucose production, causing a higher level of hyperglycemia. At the same time, in an attempt to provide energy, ketone bodies are formed in the liver from the free fatty acids.

Hyperglycemia causes osmotic diuresis, which leads to fluid losses, dehydration, and electrolyte depletion. The presence of ketone bodies causes the development of ketoacidosis, an acute complication of type I (insulin-dependent) diabetes mellitus. Figure 30–1 compares the normal physiologic response to the ingestion of food with the pathophysiologic response in diabetes mellitus.

Diabetes Mellitus

Incidence

According to the American Diabetes Association (ADA), approximately 6% of the United States population, or 11 million people, have diabetes mellitus. Of these, only 6 million have been diagnosed, and the remainder do not know they have diabetes. Eighty percent of the diabetic population have type II diabetes, or non–insulin-dependent diabetes mellitus (NIDDM), and 20% have type I diabetes, or insulin-dependent diabetes mellitus (IDDM). The number of individuals with diabetes increases by 6% annually. By the year 1999, the ADA predicts that there will be 20 million people in the United States with diabetes mellitus.

The effects of diabetes mellitus are both physical and economic. Diabetes is considered to be a major chronic health care problem. It is known to be the third leading cause of death, and the leading cause of new cases of blindness in adults between the ages of 20 and 74. It accounts for 30% of new cases of end-stage renal disease, 50% to 60% of adult deaths due to coronary heart disease, and 40% to 50% of nontraumatic amputations due to foot or ankle ulcers. Total hospital usage for diabetes has amounted to 11.5 million days, with the direct cost of $7.87 billion for in-patient care and $1.73 billion for out-patient care annually.

The impact of diabetes on the health care system can be directly affected by the way the individual with diabetes manages the disease and maintains control of blood glucose levels. Studies have confirmed that optimum control can help delay or prevent the onset of long-term degenerative changes. Modern technology has provided individuals who have diabetes mellitus with the methods necessary

Relationship between insulin secretion and blood glucose levels after food ingestion in the non-diabetic individual

Ingestion of food—carbohydrate, protein, fat

↓

Blood glucose levels rise

↓

Insulin is produced by the pancreas, resulting in the following:

Glucose is stored as glycogen in the liver and muscle

Fat is stored in adipose tissue

Protein is synthesized into amino acids

Blood glucose levels fall

Pathophysiologic response to the ingestion of food in diabetes mellitus

Ingestion of food—carbohydrate, protein, fat

↓

Blood glucose levels rise

↓

Absence of insulin causes the following:

Glucose entering the body from the ingestion of food is not converted into glycogen (decreased glycogenesis)
There is decreased utilization of glucose by the cells, causing cellular starvation

Proteins and fats are mobilized rather than stored

Amino acids convert to glucose (increased gluconeogenesis)
Free fatty acids are released by adipose tissue and converted to ketone bodies (ketoacidosis) by the liver for energy

Blood glucose levels continue to rise

Figure 30–1.

Comparison of the effects of the presence of insulin (normal physiology) with those of the absence of insulin (pathophysiology of diabetes mellitus) after the ingestion of food.

to help achieve and maintain good control. Despite this, studies have shown that three of five diabetic individuals measure insulin dosages incorrectly; two thirds of all diabetic individuals do not know how to follow a prescribed diet and do not know their prescribed caloric intake; one third have not received the formal teaching that is necessary to gain the knowledge to manage the disease; and approximately 40% do not test or monitor diabetic control at home.

Etiology

Progress in the fields of molecular biology and virology, protein chemistry, genetics, and immunology has helped increase knowledge of the etiology of diabetes. Although some controversy exists, most research indicates that type I diabetes, or IDDM, is an autoimmune disease. Studies have shown that more than 90% of patients with IDDM have antibodies directed against their own islet cells. These autoantibodies bind to a substance inside the islet cells, causing destruction of these cells and leading to the inability of the pancreas to produce insulin. Furthermore, these autoantibodies have been found in diabetic patients long before the symptoms of diabetes appear, suggesting that they play a role in causing the disease. However, the mechanism that triggers the immunologic attack is still unknown.

Research has also made progress in searching for the genes that determine susceptibility to diabetes. Individuals at risk for diabetes mellitus are those with a strong family history of diabetes; blacks, Hispanics, and Native Americans; persons who are obese; and those who have a morbid obstetric history and a history of delivering infants weighing more than 9 lb. It has long been known that among identical twins with one twin having type I diabetes (IDDM), there is a 50% chance of the disease developing in the other twin. Twin studies of type II diabetes (NIDDM) show a 90% concordance. This has led to the search to identify which genes determine susceptibility to diabetes. Studies have focused on human leukocyte antigen (HLA) molecules, which are proteins found on the surface of cells in the body. The focus of these studies is to determine exactly how the HLA genes contribute to susceptibility to the disease.

A major breakthrough in research occurred when the 64K protein was identified as the protein involved in the development of diabetes mellitus. The

64K protein is found on the beta cells of the pancreas, which produce insulin. Antibodies to the 64K protein appear in the blood stream up to 7 years before diabetes is diagnosed and can be detected in 80% of the people in whom diabetes develops. Hopefully, identification of the 64K protein will enable researchers to develop a simple, inexpensive assay for the 64K antibody and a test to identify potential diabetics long before symptoms of the disease develop.

The ability to prevent the onset of diabetes mellitus in individuals at high risk is becoming a reality. Clinical trials are being done to test for the presence of islet cell antibodies in these individuals. The immunosuppressant drug azathioprine (Imuran) has been used successfully in preventing diabetes from developing in some patients.

Pathophysiology

Diabetes mellitus is the inability of the body to produce adequate insulin in response to rising blood glucose levels or inability to utilize the insulin produced. As shown in Figure 30–2, when a nondiabetic person eats a meal, the beta cells in the pancreas produce exactly the right amount of insulin to maintain normal blood glucose levels. When blood glucose levels start to fall, such as between meals, the pancreas decreases the amount of insulin it produces. This is an ongoing continuous process to maintain normal blood glucose levels.

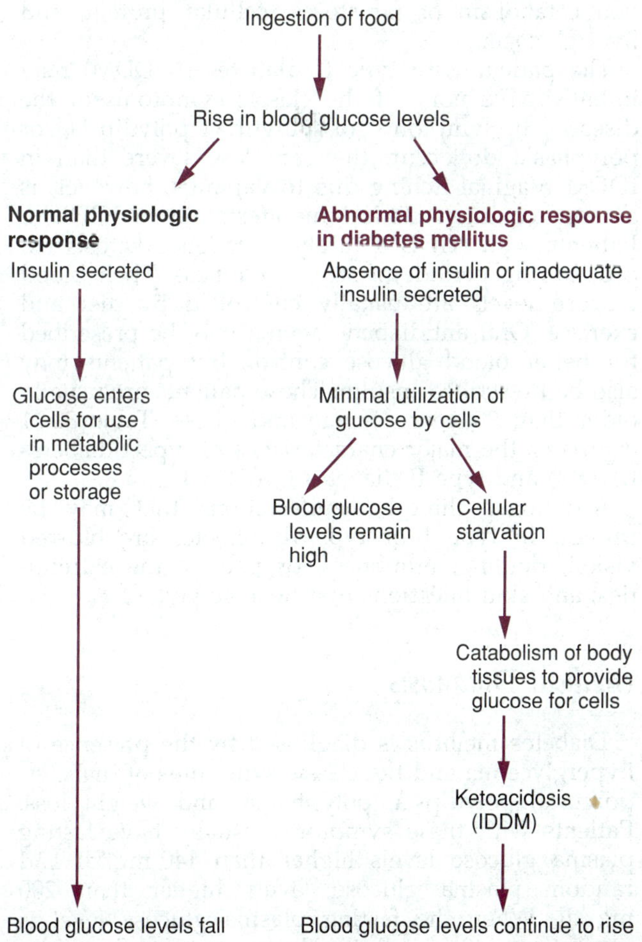

Figure 30–2.

Comparison of the physiologic response to food ingestion in the nondiabetic individual and the diabetic individual.

When a person has diabetes mellitus, there is either a lack of insulin produced by the beta cells of the pancreas, or the insulin it produces is ineffective. As illustrated in Figure 30–2, this in turn causes a decreased utilization of glucose by the cells, resulting in increased blood glucose levels that can range as high as 800 mg/dl; increased mobilization of fats from fat storage areas, resulting in abnormal fat metabolism and deposits of lipids in vascular walls causing atherosclerosis; and loss of protein from tissues in the body.

As the blood glucose levels rise, glucose enters the kidney tubules and spills into the urine. This usually occurs when the blood glucose level reaches 180 mg/dl. This is called the *renal threshold* and can vary somewhat from person to person. The increase in blood glucose levels results in dehydration of tissue cells, because glucose cannot diffuse through the cell wall without insulin, and as the osmotic pressure increases in the extracellular fluid, there is an osmotic transfer of water out of the cells. The loss of glucose in the urine causes diuresis, because the osmotic effect of glucose in the tubules of the kidney prevents tubular reabsorption of fluids. The overall effect is dehydration that is associated with hypovolemia.

As the body shifts from metabolizing carbohydrates to metabolizing fats for energy, there is an increase in the production of ketones, resulting in ketosis. These ketones cause a decrease in sodium concentration, because they combine with sodium derived from extracellular fluid for excretion in the urine. Hydrogen ions replace the sodium, increasing the acidosis. Metabolic acidosis occurs, leading to Kussmaul's respirations, which is deep and rapid breathing with increased expiration of carbon dioxide. There is a marked decrease in the bicarbonate level of extracellular fluid and, as a compensatory mechanism to correct the acidosis, chloride ions are excreted by the kidneys. In diabetic ketoacidosis, coma and death can occur within hours.

CLASSIFICATION OF DIABETES MELLITUS

In 1979, the National Diabetes Data Group of the National Institutes of Health sponsored development of a classification system for diabetes based on etiology and pathogenesis. Diabetes mellitus is currently classified as follows:

1. Type I diabetes, or insulin-dependent diabetes mellitus (IDDM)

2. Type II diabetes, or non–insulin-dependent diabetes mellitus (NIDDM)
3. Other types (secondary to other diseases)

TYPE I DIABETES (INSULIN-DEPENDENT DIABETES MELLITUS)

Type I diabetes, or insulin-dependent diabetes mellitus (IDDM), was formerly known as juvenile diabetes. Type I diabetes occurs mostly in people younger than the age of 40 but can also occur in older adults, thus the change in name from juvenile diabetes to type I diabetes. With type I diabetes, there is a marked decrease in the number of beta cells in the pancreas, leading to a lack of insulin and elevation of blood glucose level. Therefore, the person with type I diabetes (IDDM) must have daily insulin injections to control blood glucose concentration and is dependent upon exogenous insulin.

TYPE II DIABETES (NON–INSULIN-DEPENDENT DIABETES MELLITUS)

Type II diabetes, or non–insulin-dependent diabetes mellitus (NIDDM), is the most prevalent form of diabetes in this country today, usually occurring in adults older than the age of 40. The major characteristic of type II diabetes (NIDDM) is insulin resistance. The amount of endogenous insulin produced by the pancreas may be normal, decreased, or even increased. The problem lies in the fact that the available insulin is unable to bind with cell receptor sites to promote the transport of glucose into the cells for use or storage. This has been attributed to a defect either at the receptor site of the cell, in the number of receptor sites, or at the postreceptor site, which is located inside the cell. Insulin injections usually are not necessary to treat type II diabetes (NIDDM) but at times may be required to control blood glucose levels.

OTHER TYPES OF DIABETES

The third major classification of diabetes is "other types." Included in this grouping are disorders of temporary carbohydrate and glucose intolerance that are associated with, or are secondary to, other physical or mechanical problems. Examples are gestational diabetes; pancreatic disease or pancreatectomy; various endocrine disorders such as acromegaly, Cushing's syndrome, or pheochromocytoma; and the administration of medications or hormones, such as cortisone preparations, that cause hyperglycemia.

IMPAIRED GLUCOSE TOLERANCE

A diagnosis of impaired glucose tolerance is made when plasma glucose levels are higher than normal but not high enough to diagnose as diabetes. The terms *chemical, latent, borderline, subclinical,* and *asymptomatic* diabetes were formerly used to identify this condition, but these terms have been discontinued. Because approximately 25% of patients with impaired glucose tolerance eventually develop diabetes, these patients should frequently be reevaluated.

Clinical Manifestations

The clinical manifestations of type I diabetes (IDDM) and type II diabetes (NIDDM) differ. The patient with type I diabetes (IDDM) usually has a sudden onset of polyuria (frequent urination), polydipsia (extreme thirst), and polyphagia (hunger). In addition, there are symptoms of weight loss despite increased food intake, extreme fatigue, and pruritus and vaginal itching. The patient is usually a thin individual and younger than 40 years of age. Patients with type I diabetes (IDDM) are prone to developing ketosis during episodes of hyperglycemia and must take daily insulin injections. Ketoacidosis results from the excess circulating ketone bodies and is manifested by Kussmaul's respirations; loss of sodium, potassium, chloride, and water; and continued catabolism of fat stores, cellular protein, and liver glycogen.

The patient with type II diabetes (NIDDM) may initially have none of the classic symptoms of the disease. If symptoms of polyuria, polydipsia, or polyphasia do occur, they are less severe than in IDDM. Vaginal itching due to vaginitis, however, is a more common clinical manifestation in NIDDM. Patients with NIDDM rarely experience ketosis except during periods of stress or illness. Their blood glucose levels are usually controlled by diet and exercise. Oral antidiabetic agents may be prescribed for better blood glucose control, but patients may also be prescribed insulin. These patients are usually older than 30 years of age and obese. Table 30–1 compares the major characteristics of type I diabetes (IDDM) and type II diabetes (NIDDM).

Additional clinical manifestations that may be present in type I or type II diabetes are blurred vision; tingling, numbness, or pain in the extremities; and skin infections that heal slowly.

Medical Diagnosis

Diabetes mellitus is diagnosed by the presence of hyperglycemia and the classic symptoms of diabetes: polyuria, polydipsia, polyphagia, and weight loss. Patients with these symptoms usually have fasting plasma glucose levels higher than 140 mg/dl and random plasma glucose levels higher than 200 mg/dl. When the fasting plasma glucose level is lower than 140 mg/dl, the diagnosis is confirmed by an oral glucose tolerance test.

The criteria for diagnosis of diabetes mellitus in nonpregnant adults, gestational diabetes, and im-

Table 30–1. CHARACTERISTICS OF TYPE I DIABETES (IDDM) AND TYPE II DIABETES (NIDDM)

	IDDM	NIDDM
Incidence	20%	80%
Endogenous insulin production	None	Normal, decreased, or increased
Clinical manifestations	Polyuria Polydipsia Polyphagia Pruritus Vaginal itching Weight loss Dehydration Ketosis Fatigue	Classic symptoms of polyuria, polydipsia, and polyphagia are usually absent Vaginal itching Obesity Pruritus
Characteristics	Usually younger than age 40 at onset Ketosis-prone	Usually older than age 40 at onset Not ketosis-prone
Treatment	Insulin Diet Exercise	Oral antidiabetic agents Diet Exercise Insulin if blood glucose levels cannot be controlled with diet, oral antidiabetic agents, and exercise

paired glucose tolerance, established by the National Diabetes Data Group, are summarized in Table 30–2.

FASTING BLOOD SUGAR

The fasting blood sugar (FBS) test measures the amount of glucose in the blood after fasting for 10 hours. It is done both as a diagnostic test and to measure the glucose levels of the already diagnosed diabetic to monitor control. Venous blood is usually used in laboratories and hospitals, and capillary blood is used by individuals testing their own blood for glucose at home with a self-testing glucose meter.

Nursing Implications. The patient is instructed to have nothing to eat or drink for 10 hours prior to the test. If the fasting blood glucose level is higher than 140 mg/dl on more than one occasion, the diagnosis of diabetes mellitus can be made. If the fasting blood glucose level is normal or near normal, an oral glucose tolerance test has to be done to confirm a diagnosis of diabetes. Factors that cause the glucose level to rise in the absence of diabetes include stress, illness, trauma, and some drugs.

Table 30–2. CRITERIA FOR DIAGNOSIS OF DIABETES MELLITUS AS DEVELOPED BY THE NATIONAL DIABETES DATA GROUP

CRITERIA FOR DIAGNOSIS IN NONPREGNANT ADULTS

1. Random plasma glucose level of 200 mg/dl or higher, plus the classic symptoms of polydipsia, polyuria, polyphagia, and weight loss.
2. Fasting plasma glucose level of 140 mg/dl or higher on at least two occasions.
3. Fasting plasma glucose level of less than 140 mg/dl, but sustained elevated plasma glucose levels during at least two oral glucose tolerance tests; the 2-hour sample and at least one other between 0 and 2 hours should be 200 mg/dl or higher after a 75-g glucose load.

CRITERIA FOR DIAGNOSIS OF GESTATIONAL DIABETES

Following an oral glucose load of 100 g of glucose, two venous plasma glucose levels must be equal to or higher than the following values:

Fasting	105 mg/dl
1 hour	190 mg/dl
2 hours	165 mg/dl
3 hours	145 mg/dl

CRITERIA FOR IMPAIRED GLUCOSE TOLERANCE IN NONPREGNANT ADULTS

All of the following have to be present:

1. Fasting blood glucose level of 140 mg/dl or lower
2. Two-hour oral glucose tolerance test result between 140 and 200 mg/dl
3. Intervening oral glucose tolerance test result of 200 mg/dl or higher.

ORAL GLUCOSE TOLERANCE TEST

The oral glucose tolerance test is done to diagnose diabetes when the fasting plasma glucose is at or below 140 mg/dl.

Procedure. A blood sample is drawn to obtain a fasting blood glucose level. Next, the patient drinks a solution of 75 g of glucose for nonpregnant adults, 100 g for pregnant adults, and 1.75 g/kg of ideal body weight (not to exceed 75 g) for children. Blood samples are obtained at 30 minutes, and then every hour for up to 5 hours. The patient should remain quiet for the duration of the test.

Nursing Implications. The oral glucose tolerance test is considered to be a sensitive test for diabetes mellitus, but if the guidelines for the preparation and procedure are not strictly followed, erroneous results could occur. The test is done in the morning prior to any other activities, and the patient is instructed to have nothing to eat or drink for the previous 10 hours. During the test, the patient is

Table 30–3. CRITERIA FOR INTERPRETING THE RESULTS OF THE ORAL GLUCOSE TOLERANCE TEST

Diabetes mellitus in the nonpregnant adult is diagnosed when:
The 2-hour plasma glucose level is 200 mg/dl or higher
and
Either the ½-hour, 1-hour, or 1½-hour glucose level is greater than 200 mg/dl

instructed to sit or lie quietly and not to smoke or drink any liquid except water.

For 3 days before the test, medications should be discontinued when possible, and the diet should contain at least 150 g of carbohydrate daily. Patients who have had gastric surgery should have an intravenous glucose tolerance test rather than an oral glucose tolerance test, because the oral glucose quickly passes into the small intestine and is rapidly absorbed, giving an abnormal result.

Nonhospitalized individuals having this test may need written instructions to ensure adequate preparation.

Table 30–3 summarizes interpretation of the oral glucose tolerance test in non-pregnant adults.

Medical Management

The medical management of diabetes mellitus includes diet, exercise, and the addition of insulin or oral antidiabetic agents as appropriate. To ensure success, the patient must be an active member of the health care team and is instructed in all aspects of diabetes and its treatment. No longer is the diabetic patient a passive recipient of health care. He or she must assume responsibility for self-management of his or her condition. Therefore, it is essential to provide the patient with the knowledge necessary to correlate blood sugars, diet, medications, and exercise so that the ultimate goal of preventing acute complications and minimizing the effects of long-term degenerative changes can be realized.

DIET

The diabetic diet is the cornerstone of treatment for the diabetic patient. However, diet therapy is often ineffective and has been identified as the one area of self-management most responsible for poor control of diabetes because of lack of adherence to the prescribed diet. To ensure success, it is necessary to individualize the diet to the needs of the patient and to provide adequate teaching to the patient and family or care partners. The goals of dietary management of diabetes are to have the patient attain and maintain ideal body weight or at least an improved goal weight, to provide adequate nutrition for growth and development in children and in pregnant women, to achieve blood glucose levels as close to normal as possible, to prevent acute complications such as ketoacidosis and hypoglycemia, and to prevent or delay the development of long-term, degenerative complications associated with diabetes mellitus.

The most widespread and currently accepted approach to diet therapy is the use of the Exchange Lists for Meal Planning by the American Diabetes Association. This diet is based on the principle that foods within the same exchange list contain approximately the same amount of calories, carbohydrates, fats, and proteins and therefore can be eaten interchangeably. It provides flexibility in selecting foods and enhances the ability of patients to adhere to the diet.

The number of exchanges a patient can have at each meal are calculated according to the number of prescribed daily calories. Many combinations can be developed. Nutrition Box 30–1 contains sample meal plans using the exchange lists. The timing of meals and snacks is very important for patients taking insulin and oral antidiabetic agents in order to maintain stable blood glucose levels and prevent episodes of hypo- and hyperglycemia.

The American Diabetes Association recommends that 55% to 60% of the total calories consumed be carbohydrate, preferably complex carbohydrate; 15% to 20% protein; and less than 30% fat. The diet should contain less than 10% polyunsaturated fats, less than 10% saturated fats, and only 10% to 15% monounsaturated fats.

The American Diabetes Association further recommends that individuals with diabetes limit their cholesterol intake to less than 300 mg/day and their sodium intake to less than 3 g/day. The ADA Exchange Lists for Meal Planning highlight foods that exceed these amounts.

Recent evidence has shown that foods with a high soluble fiber content may lower plasma glucose and cholesterol levels. Soluble fibers are found in fruits, legumes, and oats. The ADA Exchange Lists for Meal Planning also highlight foods containing high amounts of fiber.

Although the intake of alcohol is not recommended, moderate amounts of alcohol may be allowed in the diabetic diet. When alcohol is included in the meal plan, the calories are accounted for by reducing the fat intake (pure alcohol is 7 cal/g). Alcohol intake in patients who are malnourished or fasting may cause hypoglycemia.

There are some foods considered free foods; that is, they contain less than 20 calories per serving. Examples of these are sugar-free carbonated drinks, coffee, tea, lettuce, sugar-free gelatin, and 1 tbsp catsup. Seasonings are also free, such as basil, cinnamon, and garlic. Free foods are not restricted and can be eaten in any desired amounts at any time.

Implementation of the diabetic diet requires patient education and often behavior modification as detailed in the Application of the Nursing Process later in this chapter.

Nutrition Box 30–1.

GUIDELINES FOR MEAL PLANNING FOR PATIENTS WITH DIABETES MELLITUS

Exchange List	Samples of Equivalent Meals		
Breakfast			
1 Fruit	4 oz orange juice	½ banana	½ grapefruit
2 Starch/Bread	1 bagel	2 slices toast	1 cup oatmeal
1 Fat	1 tbsp cream cheese	1 slice bacon*	1 tsp butter
1 Milk	8 oz skim milk	8 oz plain nonfat yogurt	8 oz 1% milk
Lunch			
2 Starch/Bread	2 slices bread	1 pita (6 in.)	1 hamburger bun
3 Meat†	½ cup tuna*	3 oz ground turkey	3 oz ground beef
1 Vegetable	1 large tomato	1 cup raw vegetables	4 oz vegetable juice*
1 Fruit	1 apple	4 oz apple cider	12 cherries
1 Fat	1 tsp salad dressing	1 tsp mayonnaise	1 tsp oil
1 Milk	8 oz skim milk	8 oz lowfat buttermilk	⅔ cup nonfat dry milk
Dinner			
2 Starch/Bread	1 cup corn	1 small baked potato	1 cup pasta (cooked)
3 Meat†	3 oz steak	3 oz chicken	3 oz veal cutlet (unbreaded)
2 Vegetable	1 cup raw vegetables *and* ½ cup carrots	1 cup broccoli	½ cup green peppers *and* ½ cup onions
1 Fruit	1¼ cup strawberries	1 peach	1¾ cup blueberries

* 400 mg or more of sodium in two or more exchanges
† Medium fat meat exchange (7 g protein, 5 g fat, 75 calories)
All foods within each exchange list contain approximately the same amount of carbohydrates, proteins, and fats and therefore can be eaten interchangeably. However, foods from one list or exchange cannot be substituted for foods from another list or exchange.

EXERCISE

Exercise is an important component in the treatment of diabetes mellitus. The benefits include improvement in insulin sensitivity, potential improvement in glucose tolerance in some patients, the promotion of weight loss and attainment of goal body weight, improved cardiovascular status, reduction of cholesterol and triglyceride levels, potential reduction in insulin and oral antidiabetic agent requirements, and an improved sense of well-being.

An exercise program should be tailored to meet the individual needs of the patient with diabetes. Factors to be considered are the type of diabetes the patient has, the patient's age and medical condition, and the presence of long-term degenerative changes.

If the patient is taking insulin, it is important to consider the type of insulin, the time it is administered, when the insulin reaches its peak, and the injection site used. Insulin is absorbed faster when injected into a site that is exercised. The abdomen, rather than the leg, should be used for an injection site when the individual will be walking or running.

A blood glucose test done prior to exercising lets the patient know whether a snack should be eaten. Unless a meal has just been completed, a fruit exchange equal to 15 g of carbohydrate is usually eaten before engaging in moderate exercise. This snack is in addition to food allowed in the regular meal plan. The patient taking antidiabetic medication should always carry a simple carbohydrate snack when exercising and should be prepared to treat hypoglycemia if it occurs.

Exercise should not be done if the blood glucose level is higher than 250 mg/dl or when ketones are present in the urine. Exercise at this point will raise blood glucose levels by increasing secretion of glucagon and growth hormone, thereby causing the liver to release more glucose.

Because obesity and inactivity are characteristics of the patient with NIDDM, exercise may have a positive effect on controlling hyperglycemia for these patients. Increased physical activity is an important part of any weight reduction program because it increases energy expenditure, increases muscle mass, and decreases body fat. When combined with diet, exercise is an excellent way to at-

Table 30–4. CATEGORIES OF INSULIN

CATEGORY	ONSET	PEAK ACTION	DURATION
Rapid-acting	½–1 hr	2–4 hr	5–7 hr
Intermediate-acting	2–4 hr	8–12 hr	18–24 hr
Long-acting	4–6 hr	18–24 hr	>36 hr

tain and maintain ideal or goal body weight. The patient with NIDDM who is not taking insulin or oral antidiabetic agents does not have to eat a snack before exercising.

Exercise may be contraindicated in patients with poor metabolic control and those with active proliferative retinopathy, significant cardiovascular disease, or peripheral neuropathy. Patients with these conditions can exercise only following a thorough medical assessment.

INSULIN THERAPY

INSULIN INJECTIONS

The beta cells in the islets of Langerhans in the pancreas stop producing insulin in patients with IDDM. Therefore, these patients must have insulin injections to survive. Insulin can be administered only by injection, because it is a protein and would be destroyed by digestive enzymes if taken orally.

Insulin for injection was originally derived from animal sources by extracting insulin from beef and pork pancreata. Biosynthetic and semisynthetic human insulins are now manufactured and widely prescribed. Human insulin is identical to the insulin produced by the human pancreas and is nearly free of the foreign substances in animal-source insulins. It is, therefore, less likely to stimulate formation of insulin antibodies. Some research has shown that these antibodies may temporarily bind to animal-source insulin and then release it, causing unpredictable blood levels of insulin and, therefore, poor control of blood glucose. Lipoatrophy at the injection site has also been related to animal insulin impurities.

Insulin is categorized as short- or rapid-acting, intermediate-acting, and long-acting. These categories refer to the onset, or when the insulin begins to work; the peak, or when the insulin provides the maximum effect; and the duration, or the length of time the insulin is active in the body. Table 30–4 summarizes the categories of insulin, and Table 30–5 provides a list of insulin preparations and manufacturers.

Table 30–5. PARTIAL LIST OF INSULIN PREPARATIONS

CATEGORY	INSULIN	FORM	MANUFACTURER
Rapid-acting	Humulin R	Human	Lilly
	Novolin R	Human	Novo Nordisk
	Velosulin R	Human	Novo Nordisk
	Velosulin R	Pork	Novo Nordisk
	Iletin II R	Pork	Lilly
	Iletin I R	Beef/Pork	Lilly
	Purified Pork R	Pork	Novo Nordisk
	Purified Pork S	Pork	Novo Nordisk
	Regular	Pork	Novo Nordisk
	Semilente	Beef	Novo Nordisk
Intermediate-acting	Humulin L	Human	Lilly
	Humulin N	Human	Lilly
	Insulatard NPH	Human	Novo Nordisk
	Novolin L	Human	Novo Nordisk
	Novolin N	Human	Novo Nordisk
	Iletin I Lente	Beef/Pork	Lilly
	Iletin I NPH	Beef/Pork	Lilly
	NPH	Beef	Novo Nordisk
	Iletin II Lente	Pork	Lilly
	Iletin II NPH	Pork	Lilly
	Insulatard NPH	Pork	Novo Nordisk
	Purified Pork Lente	Pork	Novo Nordisk
	Purified Pork N	Pork	Novo Nordisk
Long-acting	Humulin U	Human	Lilly
	Iletin II PZI	Beef or Pork	Lilly
	Purified Beef U	Beef	Novo Nordisk
	Iletin I PZI	Beef/Pork	Lilly
	Ultralente	Beef	Novo Nordisk
Mixtures	Mixtard (70% NPH, 30% Regular)	Pork	Novo Nordisk
	Novolin 70/30	Human	Novo Nordisk
	Humulin 70/30	Human	Lilly

Insulin is currently available in two concentrations: U-100 and U-500. The most widely used concentration is U-100. U-500 is used in cases of severe insulin resistance. Insulin is measured in United States Pharmacopeia (USP) units, which does not refer to volume but to a standard of insulin activity. The concentration refers to the number of units in one milliliter (ml). For example, a vial of U-100 insulin has 100 units in 1 ml, and a vial of U-500 insulin has 500 units in 1 ml. Syringes and insulin vials are clearly labelled U-100. Because there is no U-500 syringe, the amount of insulin to administer has to be calculated in milliliters.

The goal of insulin treatment is to mimic the pattern of normal insulin secretion. In the nondiabetic, there is a continuous basal secretion of insulin, with secretion of additional insulin after eating, in response to increased blood glucose levels. Therefore, the type I diabetic patient may receive one to several insulin injections a day. Many patients take one or two injections of a mixture of short-acting and intermediate-acting insulins, but some patients take an injection of short-acting insulin before each meal in addition to one daily long-acting insulin basal dose to control hyperglycemia. Research has shown that three or more insulin injections a day, with dosage based on blood glucose levels, produce better control of blood glucose and delay the onset and reduce the severity of the long-term degenerative changes associated with diabetes mellitus. Figure 30–3 illustrates several patterns of insulin administration. Chart 30–1 contains patient information guidelines for preparing and administering insulin injections.

Occasionally, there may be what is known as a "honeymoon" phase or temporary remission in patients with IDDM; that is, the beta cells begin to produce insulin again. As endogenous insulin secretion begins, the patient experiences hypoglycemic reactions. Exogenous insulin injections need to be reduced or even eliminated during this temporary remission. The honeymoon phase is more common in the late teenage years and in young adults and can last from several months to approximately a year.

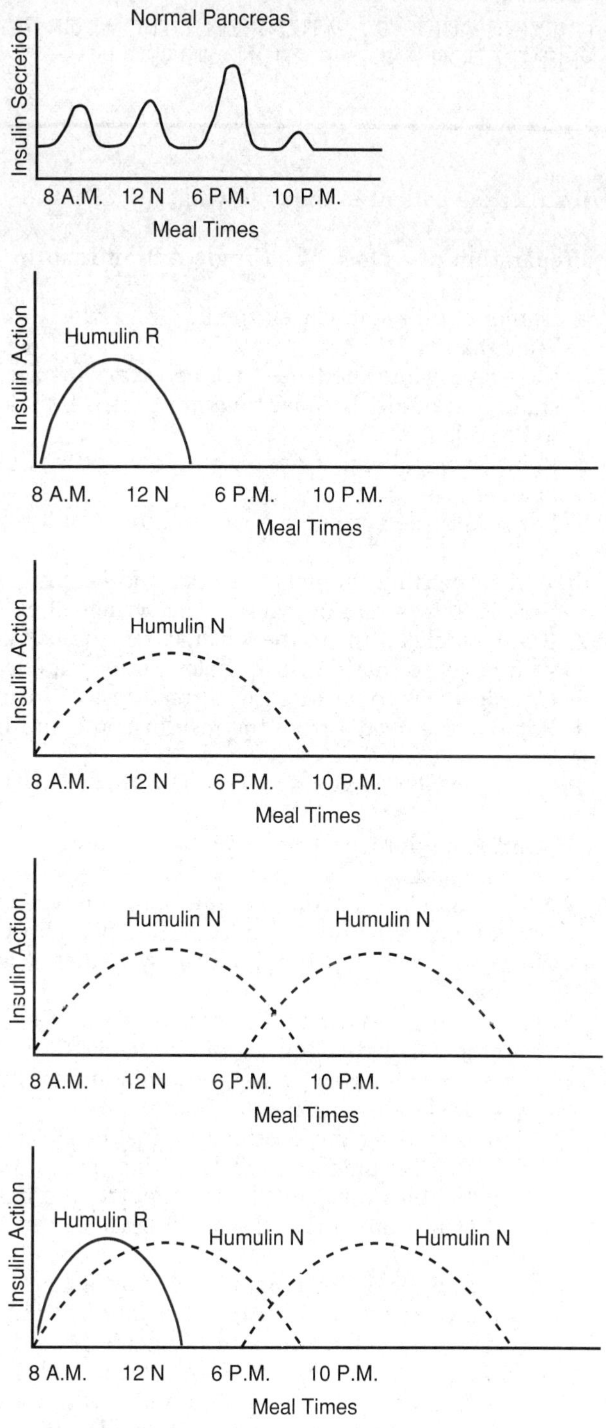

Figure 30–3.

Relationship between food intake and the onset, peak, and duration of different patterns of insulin injections and preparations.

OTHER MODES OF INSULIN ADMINISTRATION

Insulin Pumps

Another method of administering insulin is by use of a device known as an insulin pump or continuous subcutaneous insulin infusion (CSII). This mode of insulin delivery provides a steady basal dose of insulin throughout the day and night, as well as a bolus of insulin when food is eaten. The insulin pump is designed to mimic the action of the normal pancreas and replaces insulin injections. It is usually recommended when multiple injections of insulin are not effective in controlling glucose levels.

CSII is called an open-loop infusion system because it does not contain a glucose sensor that automatically adjusts the insulin infusion rate. It is operated by the patient, who must test blood glucose levels to determine the amount of insulin to take. Approximately 40% of the patient's total daily insulin requirement is administered at the basal rate,

Chart 30–1.

NURSING GUIDE TO PATIENT EDUCATION FOR SELF-MANAGEMENT: GUIDELINES FOR PREPARATION AND INJECTION OF INSULIN

Instruct the patient in the following:

Preparation of a Dose of a Single-Action Insulin

1. Gather equipment. Check medication order.
2. Wash hands.
3. If using an intermediate- or long-acting insulin, roll the bottle between your hands to mix it. Do not shake the bottle, because shaking causes bubbles to form. Regular, short-acting insulin does not have to be rolled.
4. Remove metal cap if opening a new bottle. Clean the rubber top with an alcohol swab if previously opened.
5. Draw into the syringe the same amount of air as insulin prescribed, and inject this air into the insulin bottle.
6. While inverting the insulin bottle and keeping the needle tip below the level of insulin, withdraw the prescribed amount of insulin. The syringe should be held vertically at eye level.
7. If air bubbles form in the syringe, tap the barrel of the syringe and move the needle tip above the insulin level so that the air bubbles can be expelled from the syringe and into the air space in the bottle.
8. Double-check to be sure the correct dose of insulin is in the syringe.
9. Remove the needle from the insulin bottle and inject into selected site.

Preparation of a Mixture of Two Insulins with Different Actions (Insulin Mix)

1. Gather equipment. Check medication order.
2. Wash hands.
3. Roll the delayed-acting insulin bottle between your hands to mix it. Do not shake the bottle, because shaking causes bubbles to form. Regular, short-acting insulin does not have to be rolled.
4. Remove metal cap if opening new bottles. Clean the rubber top with an alcohol swab if previously opened.
5. Draw into the syringe the same amount of air as delayed-acting insulin prescribed, and inject this air into the delayed-acting insulin bottle. Withdraw needle empty.
6. Draw into the syringe the same amount of air as short-acting insulin prescribed, and inject this air into the short-acting insulin bottle.
7. While inverting the short-acting insulin bottle and keeping the needle tip below the level of insulin, withdraw the amount of short-acting insulin prescribed. The syringe should be held at eye level.
8. If air bubbles form in the syringe, tap the barrel of the syringe and move the needle tip above the level of insulin so that the air bubbles can be expelled from the syringe and into the air space in the bottle.
9. Withdraw prescribed amount of short-acting insulin, and remove syringe from bottle.
10. Carefully insert needle into the delayed-acting insulin bottle, and with bottle inverted, pull the plunger down to the total amount of insulin prescribed (short-acting plus delayed-acting = total dose).
11. If an air bubble develops in the syringe while withdrawing the delayed-acting insulin, withdraw the needle, discard the medication and syringe, and start over. This is necessary because in an attempt to expel the air bubble, some of the insulin mixture may inadvertently be expelled also.
12. Withdraw needle and inject into selected site.

Insulin Injection

1. Select the injection site. See Figure 30–4 for sites.
2. Wipe the site with an alcohol swab. Holding the syringe like a pencil, gently pinch a large portion of skin, and insert the needle quickly at a 90-degree angle into subcutaneous tissue. Insert the needle at a 45-degree angle if you have less than an inch of skin when you pinch.
3. Push the plunger down to inject the insulin.
4. Release the skin and withdraw the needle.
5. Press site with alcohol swab but do not massage.

Chart 30–1. *(continued)*

NURSING GUIDE TO PATIENT EDUCATION FOR SELF-MANAGEMENT: GUIDELINES FOR PREPARATION AND INJECTION OF INSULIN

Additional Patient Teaching Instructions

- Store unopened insulin bottles in the refrigerator. Store opened insulin bottles that will be used within 1 month at room temperature of 80°F (26.7°C) or less.
- It is best to bring refrigerated insulin to room temperature before injecting. When cold insulin is injected, absorption rates are delayed because of initial capillary vasoconstriction, and the injection is more painful.
- Do not expose insulin to direct sunlight. Do not freeze insulin.
- Check the expiration date on insulin bottles before purchase. Do not use insulin past the expiration date.
- When traveling, carry insulin and syringes on your person and do not check with baggage.
  When preparing an insulin mix, always inject air into the intermediate- or long-acting insulin bottle first and then into the regular short-acting insulin bottle. Withdraw the regular insulin first. Do this to avoid contamination of the regular insulin by the intermediate-acting insulin.
- Be sure to remove all air bubbles from the syringe before injecting, because air bubbles take the place of insulin. If air bubbles are injected, you recieve less insulin than prescribed.
- When possible, give mixed insulins within 15 minutes after preparation, because after that time, the action of the regular insulin may blunted.
- Do not inject within 1 inch of the previous injection site. Rotate injection sites to avoid lipodystrophy (lumps or indentations) and to maximize absorption of the insulin. Researchers at the University of Minnesota recommend abandoning site rotation plans in favor of injecting insulin in the abdomen only for maximum glucose control.
- Do not inject areas that are going to be exercised that day.
- Give insulin injections at the same time each day to ensure continuity of onset, peak, and duration of action.
- When taking less than 50 units of insulin, use low-dose insulin syringes. These syringes hold ½ cc and measure up to 50 units. Each line on the syringe equals one unit of insulin.
- When taking more than 50 units of insulin, use a 1-cc insulin syringe that measures up to 100 units. Each line on the syringe equals two units of insulin.
- Never reuse disposable insulin syringes. Never wipe the needle tip with alcohol before using.

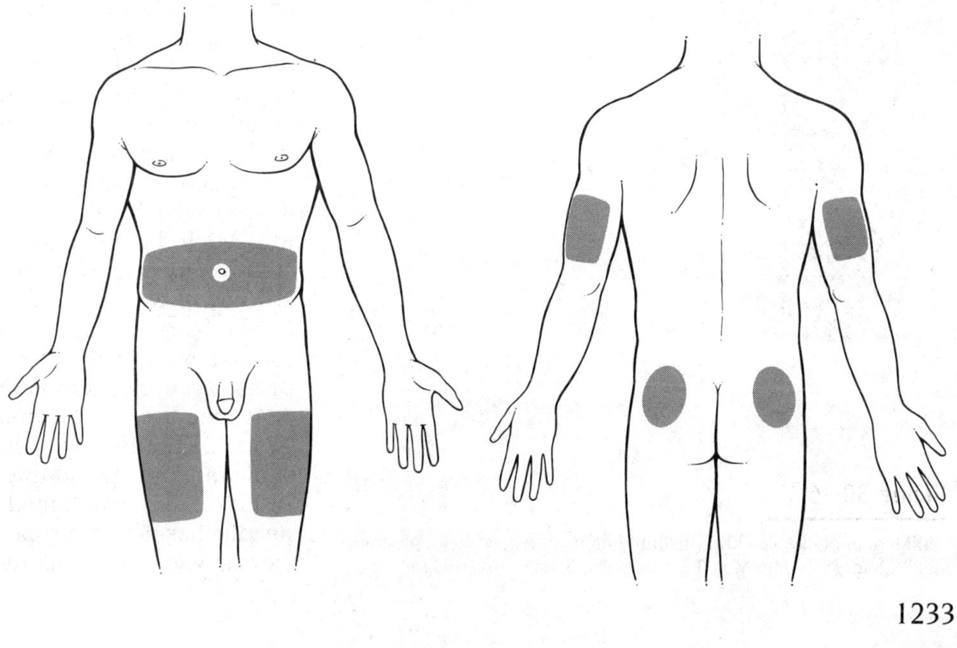

Figure 30–4.

Insulin injection sites.

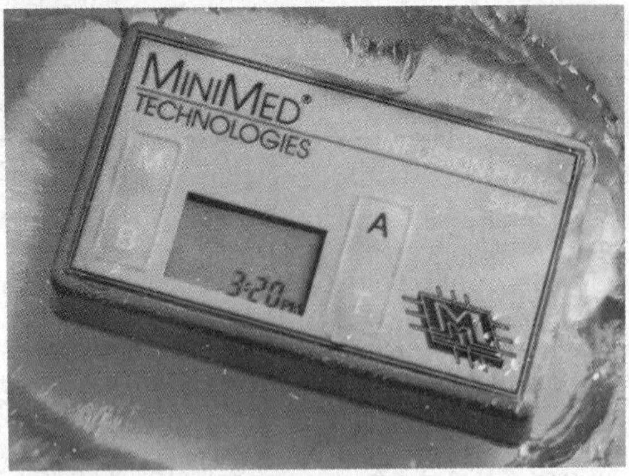

Figure 30–5.

MiniMed Model 504-S Splash Proof Insulin Pump. (Courtesy of MiniMed Technologies, Sylmar, CA 91342.)

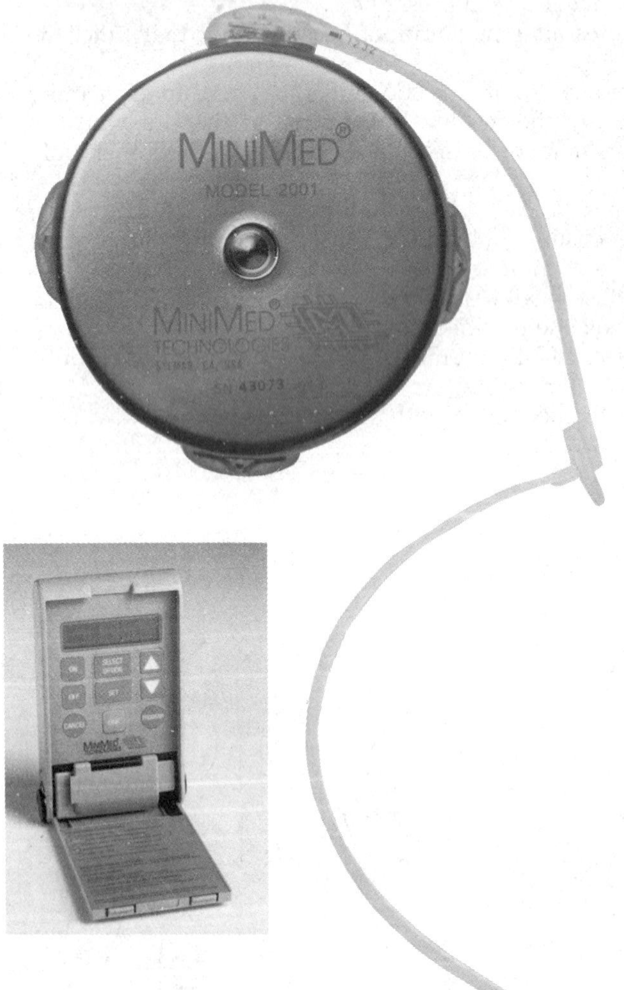

Figure 30–6.

MiniMed Implantable 2001 Insulin Pump and hand-held programmer. (Courtesy of MiniMed Technologies, Sylmar, CA 91342.)

and the remainder is divided among meals and snacks.

A needle or catheter attached to a thin, narrow lumen tube is inserted into the subcutaneous tissue of the abdomen or the thigh, and the tube is connected to a syringe filled with regular insulin in the pump. The infusion site is usually changed every 3 days. The only type of insulin used in a pump is regular insulin. The insulin is slowly pushed automatically from the syringe, thereby providing a basal rate of insulin infusion 24 hours a day. The insulin pump can be programmed to change delivery rates throughout the day. Boluses are given by manual programming before meals. The insulin pump is the size of a beeper and weighs only a few ounces. It is worn on a belt, in a pocket, or under clothes. The cost of an insulin pump is approximately $3800. Figure 30–5 shows the MiniMed Model 504-S Splash Proof Insulin Pump.

Besides providing more effective control of glucose levels, the use of an insulin pump offers greater lifestyle flexibility and convenience. Frequently, patients on multiple insulin injections a day prefer to use the insulin pump. The selection of patients is very important to ensure a successful outcome. The patient should be mature, have some technical ability, and have the financial resources necessary for this therapy.

Complications associated with the use of an insulin pump include the increased risk of rapid onset of ketoacidosis as a result of pump failure and the possibility of infection at the infusion site. Although ketoacidosis among patients using insulin pumps can be fatal, it is avoidable with proper patient education and self–blood glucose monitoring as well as technical improvements and alarm systems in the pump. Infection at the site of the infusion is a more common complication. Some causes of infection are mechanical irritation from motion of the needle or catheter during activity and sensitivity to the needle or catheter. Patients with infections are treated with oral antibiotics and topical therapies.

Another complication of using the insulin pump is the increased risk of hypoglycemic episodes and hypoglycemic coma. Patients should be aware of this possibility and do frequent self–blood glucose monitoring as a precaution.

Implantable insulin pumps may soon be available if approved by the Food and Drug Administration. MiniMed Technologies is currently conducting a clinical investigation to demonstrate the safety and efficacy of the MIP-2001, shown in Figure 30–6. This implantable insulin pump is a 7-oz disk-shaped titanium device that automatically releases a constant, preprogrammed amount of insulin into the peritoneal membrane. The pump is refilled approximately every 3 months by inserting a needle through the skin and into the pump. Because the pump's drug reservoir is maintained at negative pressure, the needle has to be properly seated inside the pump for the vacuum in the reservoir to draw insulin from

Table 30–6. CHARACTERISTICS OF SULFONYLUREAS (ORAL ANTIDIABETIC AGENTS)

BRAND NAME	GENERIC NAME	DAILY DOSAGE	DURATION
FIRST-GENERATION SULFONYLUREAS			
Orinase	Tolbutamide	500–3000 mg	6–12 hr
Diabinese	Chlorpropamide	100–500 mg	up to 60 hr
Dymelor	Acetohexamide	250–1500 mg	12–18 hr
Tolinase	Tolazamide	100–1000 mg	12–24 hr
SECOND-GENERATION SULFONYLUREAS			
Micronase, Diaβeta	Glyburide	1.25–20 mg	16–24 hr
Glucotrol	Glipizide	5–40 mg	12–24 hr
Glynase PresTab	Micronized glyburide	1.5–12 mg	16–24 hr

the syringe. This mechanism prevents the risk of accidentally injecting insulin directly into the patient. Insulin delivery is controlled by a hand-held external programmer and is customized for each patient by the physician. Patients using an implantable pump must continue to monitor their blood glucose levels as often as four to six times a day. The pump costs between $9000 and $12,000, not including the physician's charges or the hospital expenses for surgery. The major problem in some patients is blockage of the catheter that delivers insulin. One goal of current research is to develop a pump that not only infuses insulin but also monitors blood glucose levels, which would be comparable to an artificial pancreas.

Insulin Nasal Spray

Research is being conducted in the use of an insulin nasal spray as an alternate insulin delivery route. Insulin nasal spray acts within 10 minutes and lasts for just 1 hour. It would be used at mealtimes to lower blood glucose levels following a meal. The advantage of using insulin nasal spray rather than an injection of short-acting insulin before meals is the lower risk of hypoglycemia developing 3 or 4 hours later.

ORAL ANTIDIABETIC AGENTS

SULFONYLUREA COMPOUNDS

The sulfonylurea oral antidiabetic agents are effective for stable, non–insulin-dependent, nonketotic type II diabetics who cannot be treated by diet alone or who are unwilling or unable to take insulin. They should not be used in children, insulin-dependent type I diabetics, during pregnancy or lactation (because the effects on the fetus and newborn are unknown), or for patients with allergies to sulfonylurea compounds.

Sulfonylureas are effective only in people who have some functioning beta cells and who continue to secrete some endogenous insulin. They stimulate the beta cells to produce more insulin, reduce the accelerated rates of hepatic glucose production in type II diabetes, partially reduce the postreceptor defect in cells, and increase the number of cellular insulin receptors. See Table 30–6 for the complete list of sulfonylureas, or oral antidiabetic agents. Chart 30–2 contains patient education guidelines for administration of sulfonylureas and includes their side effects and drug interactions.

CURRENT RESEARCH IN THE MANAGEMENT OF DIABETES

PANCREATIC TRANSPLANTS

The first pancreatic transplant was done in 1966 at the University of Minnesota. Currently, 400 to 500 transplants worldwide are performed each year. The largest number of these have been done at the University of Minnesota, where patient survival following pancreas transplant alone is 98% and pancreas transplant function remains consistently at 60%. Patients who have had a pancreas-kidney transplant have a success rate of 71%.

Most transplants are whole organs from cadavers. The donor must be free of pancreatic trauma, pancreatitis, and diabetes and have no history of hepatitis, syphilis, or acquired immune deficiency syndrome (AIDS). After blood and tissue samples are matched to the recipient, the organ is usually transplanted within 30 hours of harvesting. The only transplant center currently using living related donors is the University of Minnesota Hospital. An HLA-identical sibling is considered the ideal living donor because the recipient may not need immunosuppression. The related donor is given a glucose tolerance test and C peptide measurement and must be 10 years older than the age at which the recipient developed diabetes. The donor must also be free of islet cell autoantibodies. The success rate for patients with a living related donor is higher than with a cadaver. However, the use of living donors appears to be limited, because although only the distal half of the pancreas is removed, which alone does not cause diabetes in the donor, abnormal glucose tolerance has developed postoperatively in most HLA-identical donors.

Patients selected as the best candidates for pancreatic transplant are those who are most likely to die within a few years from long-term degenerative

Chart 30–2.

NURSING GUIDE TO PATIENT EDUCATION FOR SELF-MANAGEMENT: GUIDELINES FOR TAKING SULFONYLUREAS

Instruct the patient in the following:

Sulfonylureas or oral antidiabetic agents are not insulin. Insulin is a protein that, if swallowed, would be destroyed by digestion.

Side effects can occur when taking sulfonylureas: Skin rashes in 2% of patients; gastrointestinal disturbances in 5% of patients; and when chlorpropamide is taken with alcohol, 35% of patients have a disulfiram-like effect.

Hypoglycemic reactions can occur when taking sulfonylureas, especially in the elderly, in malnourished patients, in alcoholics, and in patients with impaired renal or hepatic function. Teach the signs, symptoms, and treatment of these reactions (Table 30–7).

Hypoglycemic reactions can be prolonged and difficult to reverse because of the long duration of action of some of the agents.

Sulfonylureas should be used cautiously in patients with a history of allergy to sulfonamides.

The hypoglycemic action of sulfonylureas is enhanced by sulfonamides, phenylbutazone, anticoagulants, and salicylates. Propanolol can mask the symptoms of hypoglycemia.

Thyroid preparations, corticosteroids, and thiazide diuretics oppose the action of sulfonylureas.

Alcohol may produce a disulfiram-like reaction with any sulfonylurea.

changes. Therefore, the severity of the complications of diabetes overshadows the risks of the procedure and immunosuppressive therapy. Candidates for the procedure are usually insulin-dependent diabetics and between the ages of 18 and 50. In addition, one of the following conditions must be present: renal disease, with proteinuria higher than 150 mg/24 hours; autonomic neuropathy, identified as severe orthostatic hypotension, gastroparesis, or abnormal cardiovascular autonomic reflexes; or poor blood glucose control despite an appropriate insulin regimen, namely, patients who have had six or more hypoglycemic insulin reactions in a 1-month period that required emergency treatment, or four or more unexplained episodes of ketoacidosis. Also, patients who have been hospitalized for more than 90 days in a 1-year period for poor control may qualify for a transplant.

Patients who do not qualify for a transplant are those with a severe psychiatric disorder, severe coronary artery disease, active infection, or peptic ulcers and patients with a creatinine clearance of less than 60 ml/minute. Major problems associated with pancreatic transplants continue to be rejection of the transplant by the body's immune system and the development of insulitis, which is an autoimmune reaction that destroys the beta cells of the transplanted organ.

Immediately after surgery, patients are given intravenous antilymphocyte globulin and cyclosporine to prevent rejection of the new organ. They are subsequently changed to an oral regimen of either cyclosporine and prednisone, or azathioprine, prednisone, and low doses of cyclosporine. This becomes a lifelong treatment. Patients on immunosuppressive therapy have a lifelong increased risk of infection.

An early symptom of tissue rejection is hyperglycemia. Therefore, the patient should test blood glucose levels four times a day initially after discharge from the hospital, gradually reducing this to once a week. Other symptoms of rejection are tenderness over the graft area, malaise, and fever. Rejection can occur months or years after surgery.

A pancreatic transplant (without complications) including evaluation, the surgical procedure, and 1 year of follow-up costs a minimum of $125,000. Half the transplant candidates are denied insurance coverage and must use personal resources or seek research funding to cover the cost. The potential benefits of a successful transplant are the freedom from insulin injections and the elimination of glucose control issues. In addition, evidence is now suggesting that some of the long-term effects of diabetes may be stabilized.

Management During Illness

Stress and short-term illness such as fever, influenza, vomiting, and diarrhea can rapidly lead to hyperglycemia in the patient with diabetes mellitus. These conditions cause an increased need for insu-

Table 30–7. CHARACTERISTICS OF HYPOGLYCEMIA AND HYPERGLYCEMIA

HYPOGLYCEMIA (INSULIN SHOCK, INSULIN REACTION)	HYPERGLYCEMIA (DIABETIC KETOACIDOSIS)
CAUSES	
Too much insulin	Not enough insulin
Excess dose of oral antidiabetic agent	Insufficient dose of oral antidiabetic agent
Too little food	Eating too much or eating sweets
Unusual physical activity	Illness or infection
	Stress
SYMPTOMS	
Shaking	Polyuria
Sweating	Polydipsia
Dizziness	Fatigue
Anxiety	Abdominal pain
Palpitations	Headache
Tachycardia	Blurred vision
Headache	Nausea
Behavioral changes	Vomiting
Mental confusion	Kussmaul's respiration
Slurred speech	Fruity odor on the breath
Loss of coordination	Coma
Drowsiness	
Coma	
TREATMENT	
Glucose or glycogen	Insulin
Food	Fluids
	Electrolytes

lin, and the pancreas may be unable to produce sufficient insulin to meet this demand. Stress and illness also cause an increased secretion of the counterregulatory hormones glucagon, epinephrine, and cortisol, thereby raising blood glucose levels. The hyperglycemia leads to osmotic diuresis in which glucose, fluids, and electrolytes are lost. This results in dehydration, electrolyte depletion, and loss of nutrients. Patients with type I diabetes (IDDM) rapidly develop ketoacidosis. However, patients with type II diabetes (NIDDM) are more at risk of developing hyperglycemic hyperosmolar nonketotic syndrome (HHNKS), a life-threatening condition.

During illness, it is important for any patient with diabetes to monitor blood glucose levels every 4 to 6 hours until symptoms of the illness subside and to check urine ketone levels when the blood glucose level is higher than 250 mg/dl. Fluid intake is increased to minimize the risk of dehydration. Patients who are nauseated or vomiting are advised to take fluids containing glucose and electrolytes, such as regular soda and diluted fruit juices, gelatin, and chicken bouillon. The physician is notified when a blood glucose level higher than 250 mg/dl and ketonuria last more than 6 hours, when signs of dehydration occur (dry mucous membranes, lightheadedness, lethargy, decreased urine output), when symptoms of ketoacidosis occur (fruity odor on the breath, abdominal pain, air hunger), when the patient is unable to retain fluids or food for 4 hours, or when the illness becomes unmanageable. Patients are instructed never to stop taking insulin when sick. Insulin doses may need to be increased, and at times supplemental injections of insulin are necessary in the patient with IDDM. Patients with NIDDM may require insulin injections when acutely ill or if unable to tolerate oral antidiabetic agents.

MANAGEMENT DURING SURGERY

The goal of management during surgery is to prevent both hyperglycemia and hypoglycemia. Hyperglycemia, which results from stress and the physiologic effects of surgery, can lead to ketoacidosis, especially in the patient with type I insulin-dependent diabetes. Hypoglycemia, if unrecognized and untreated, can be life-threatening.

Preoperative care includes a complete history and physical examination and laboratory evaluation to determine the degree of diabetes control. Factors to consider preoperatively are the type of diabetes the patient has, blood glucose levels, and whether there are long-term degenerative changes present. For example, the presence of renal disease can affect the amount of fluids and medications tolerated. Also, if the patient is in poor metabolic control and is losing glucose in the urine, the body uses protein and fat stores for energy. This could prevent a surgical wound from healing properly.

One of three methods is usually used to administer insulin perioperatively: omitting the short-acting insulin and administering one-third to one-half the usual intermediate-acting insulin before surgery; adding 10 to 20 units of regular insulin to an intravenous infusion of 1 L of 5% dextrose in 0.45% sodium chloride; or adding 100 units of regular insulin to 500 ml of sodium chloride and piggybacking this to an infusion of 5% dextrose in 0.45% sodium chloride. The rate of infusion is adjusted according to the blood glucose level, which is monitored every 1 to 2 hours in the perioperative period. In addition to testing blood glucose levels, the urine is tested for ketones if the blood glucose level is higher than 250 mg/dl.

Patients with NIDDM who are taking oral antidiabetic agents may require insulin during surgery and postoperatively. Therefore, most oral agents are discontinued approximately 24 hours before surgery, with the exception of chlorpropamide, which is discontinued 2 to 3 days before surgery. Patients who are controlled by diet alone need to be monitored for hyperglycemia because the physiologic stress of the surgery may raise blood glucose levels and alter glucose tolerance.

Postoperative care includes maintaining blood glucose levels between 150 and 250 mg/dl to prevent acute complications of hypoglycemia and hyperglycemia. Blood glucose levels are usually measured every 4 to 6 hours. Hypoglycemia can be difficult to identify in the patient recovering from anesthesia, because the usual symptoms may be masked. The patient is also observed for signs of infection such as inflammatory wound changes or drainage and elevated temperature. Pain management is important because pain causes the release of counterregulatory hormones that increase the blood glucose level. Patients with diabetic neuropathy are susceptible to developing footdrop and foot ulcerations, so pressure areas are monitored and preventive measures implemented.

Evaluation of Therapy

SELF-BLOOD GLUCOSE MONITORING

Self-blood glucose monitoring (SBGM) is standard practice in managing diabetes and is the key to obtaining and maintaining optimum control of blood glucose levels. Its development has had a great impact on the treatment of diabetes. The importance of accuracy in obtaining blood glucose results has led to the development of meters, such as the one shown in Figure 30-7, that are simple to use, small in size, and easy to learn how to operate. A meter that measures blood glucose by infrared light so that patients will no longer have to prick their finger is in development.

Before selecting a specific meter, the patient is assessed for the cognitive and psychomotor skills necessary to perform the procedure correctly. Patients with learning difficulties or with poor dexterity need a meter that is simple to operate. It is also possible to test blood glucose levels by using a reagent strip without a meter. This provides a visual reading based on color changes and gives an approximate blood glucose value. This method cannot be used by patients who are color blind. Chart 30-3 presents patient education guidelines for self-blood glucose monitoring and factors that can affect test results.

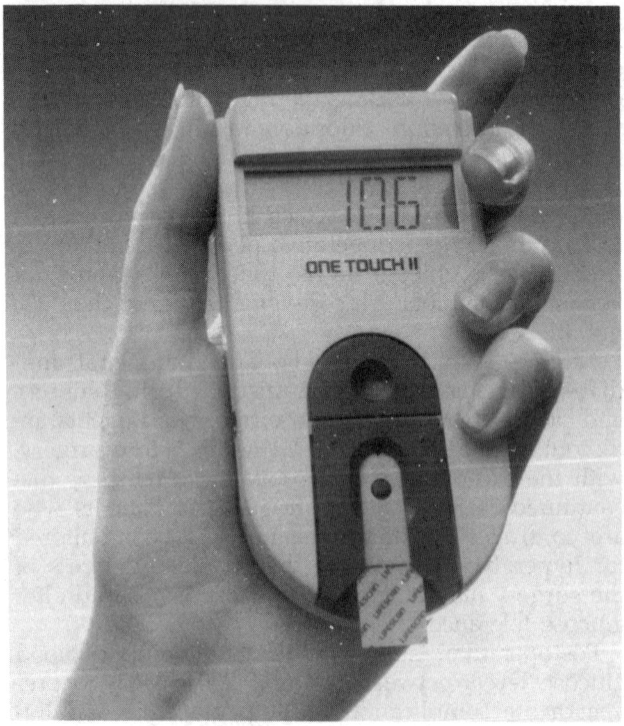

Figure 30-7.

Lifescan One Touch II blood glucose meter for home use. (Courtesy of Lifescan, Inc., Milpitas, CA 95035.)

The frequency of testing depends upon the patient's state of health and the type of diabetes the patient has. The insulin-dependent diabetic patient with fluctuating glucose levels may have to test four to six times a day, whereas the controlled non-insulin-dependent patient can test several times a week. All patients are advised to keep accurate records of the results and to report them to the physician on a regular basis.

The major advantage of using self-blood glucose monitoring is immediate feedback of results for the patient, which is important in diagnosing hypoglycemia and hyperglycemia and in regulating insulin doses. Diabetics who monitor their blood glucose levels are taught to adjust food intake and insulin dose in response to blood glucose levels or to compensate for anticipated changes in physical activity. Self-blood glucose monitoring allows the person with diabetes to be an integral member of the health care team and an active participant in his or her own health care.

Disadvantages of self-blood glucose monitoring include the cost of the meter, testing strips, and lancets if they are not covered by insurance; discomfort caused by piercing the finger; and the potential for infection if good handwashing technique is not followed.

URINE TESTING FOR GLUCOSE

Testing the urine for glucose is no longer considered an accurate measurement of diabetic control because of several disadvantages. First, a patient's blood glucose level has to be at least 180 mg/dl, the minimum renal threshold, before the result of the urine test for glucose is positive. Furthermore, urine testing cannot detect hypoglycemia, because a negative urine test result shows only that the blood glucose is below the renal threshold of 180 mg/dl. Other disadvantages related to urine glucose testing include the lag time between the time the glucose is elevated in the blood and when it spills into the urine, the variances in individual renal thresholds, the false-positive and false-negative results that can occur when certain medications are taken, and the social stigma attached to handling urine.

Despite the disadvantages, urine testing is less expensive than blood testing, and for those patients who choose to test their urine, there are several agents available. They all contain instructions and have a color chart for reading results. All tests re-

Chart 30–3.

NURSING GUIDE TO PATIENT EDUCATION FOR SELF-MANAGEMENT: GUIDELINES FOR SELF–BLOOD GLUCOSE MONITORING

Instruct the patient in the following:

1. Obtain a large drop of blood from the finger tip or earlobe with a lancet device. Blood flow is enhanced by sticking the side of the finger tip, holding the finger under warm water before sticking, and lowering the hand. To use a reagent strip, place the drop of blood on a fresh reagent strip for the time period specified by the manufacturer. Blot the blood off the strip, and either read the reagent strip visually or insert it into a glucometer. To perform the visual reading, compare the color on the strip to a color chart that comes with the strips. To use a direct-read glucometer, place the drop of blood directly on the meter window.
2. The following factors affect test results:
   - The drop of blood must cover the designated part of the reagent strip or meter window and must be applied as directed by the manufacturer.
   - The timing must be exact according to manufacturer's directions. If the elapsed time is too short, the test results will be lower than they actually are; and if the elapsed time is too long, the test results will be higher than they actually are.
   - The window of the meter must be clean for accurate results.
   - The meter and strips must not be exposed to temperatures higher than 85°F (95.4°C).
   - Reagent strips must not be used after the expiration date.
3. The nurse wears gloves when testing a patient's blood glucose level, but patients do not wear gloves when self-testing.
4. When testing different patients with the same lancet holder device, the nurse changes the lancet and platform between patients. Patients using their own lancet holder device need only change the lancet for each test.
5. Although most meters are calibrated internally when they are manufactured, they can be checked for accuracy with control solutions provided by the manufacturer according to directions.

quire specific timing for valid results. Each agent has an expiration date; outdated agents may give inaccurate results and should be discarded.

URINE TESTING FOR KETONES

Urine is frequently tested for ketones in patients with type I insulin-dependent diabetes because these individuals are prone to developing ketosis. Patients who are testing their urine for glucose also test for ketones if the urine glucose level is 1% or higher. Patients who are testing their blood for glucose are instructed to test their urine for ketones if the blood glucose level is more than 250 mg/dl. In addition, all pregnant women with diabetes are advised to test their urine for ketones on a daily basis, because the presence of ketones without an elevated blood glucose level in a pregnant woman indicates starvation ketosis. Starvation ketosis can be caused by inadequate carbohydrate intake by the mother or can result from nocturnal hypoglycemia. If ketones are present, the patient should notify the physician for a change in diet or insulin. The presence of ketones and elevated blood glucose levels during pregnancy significantly increase the risk of fetal morbidity and mortality. Therefore, it is important for the pregnant diabetic patient to test for ketones and glucose, especially in the morning after fasting for the night.

There are several agents available for testing urine for ketones or acetone, one type of ketone. Manufacturers' directions should be followed when using these agents. Each agent has an expiration date; outdated agents may give inaccurate results and should be discarded.

GLYCOSYLATED HEMOGLOBIN

Measurement of glycosylated hemoglobin, also called hemoglobin A_{1c} (HbA_{1c}), can provide an overview of a person's blood glucose levels over the previous 3 months. The red blood cell, of which hemoglobin is a part, has a life span of approximately 120 days. As glucose enters the blood stream, some attaches or glycosylates to hemoglobin molecules in an irreversible bond. The higher the amount of glucose in the blood stream, the more hemoglobin is glycosylated.

HbA_{1c} levels are not affected by recent food intake, exercise, or stress. The results reveal blood glucose levels during the previous 3- to 4-month timespan, so patients can no longer be especially careful about complying with the diet and taking medication for a few days before visiting the physician. The HbA_{1c} replaces the isolated blood glucose level formerly obtained at office visits to monitor control.

The normal HbA_{1c} level ranges from 4% to 7%. However, depending on the method used to measure the components of the glycosylated hemoglobin, actual test results vary from laboratory to laboratory. Good diabetic control is indicated by a HbA_{1c} level of less than 9%.

Recent studies have identified several factors that can affect the results of the HbA_{1c} test. The results can be lower if the patient has hemolytic anemia, chronic blood loss, or abnormal hemoglobins (S, C, or D). The results can be elevated if the patient has hyperglycemia, thalassemia, or chronic renal failure; is on dialysis; had a splenectomy; or has elevated triglyceride or hemoglobin F levels.

Acute Complications of Diabetes Mellitus

DIABETIC KETOACIDOSIS

Diabetic ketoacidosis (DKA) is a major, life-threatening complication of diabetes that results from insulin deficiency. It is considered a medical emergency.

ETIOLOGY AND PATHOPHYSIOLOGY

The causes of diabetic ketoacidosis are summarized in Table 30–7. The condition is characterized by severe disturbances in protein, fat, and carbohydrate metabolism resulting from a profound insulin deficiency. The levels of the counterregulatory hormones glucagon, epinephrine, cortisol, and growth hormone are markedly elevated and antagonize the effects of insulin. The patient develops severe hyperglycemia, osmotic diuresis and dehydration, hyperlipidemia, and metabolic acidosis. Electrolyte depletion occurs as ketones are lost in the urine.

CLINICAL MANIFESTATIONS

The clinical manifestations of DKA usually include hyperglycemia, polyuria, polydipsia, weakness, lethargy, anorexia, nausea, vomiting, blurred vision, headache, muscle aches, and abdominal pain. As hyperglycemia persists, cellular dehydration occurs, which causes sodium and potassium depletion. Dehydration also causes thirst, dry mucous membranes, loss of skin turgor, sunken eyeballs, renal failure, and hypovolemic shock.

The patient in metabolic acidosis has Kussmaul's respirations (deep, rapid breathing), a fruity odor on the breath from the ketones, and nausea and vomiting. Hyperkalemia occurs as potassium moves out of the cell with water in exchange for hydrogen ions. Depression of the central nervous system, and eventually coma, may result from acidosis. The arterial pH is less than 7.35, plasma bicarbonate is less than 15 mEq/L, blood glucose level is higher than 250 mg/dl, and ketones are present in the blood and urine.

MEDICAL MANAGEMENT

The major goals for the treatment of DKA are to correct the hyperglycemia, fluid volume depletion, hyperosmolarity, acidosis, and potassium deficiency. Hyperglycemia is treated with an intravenous infusion of regular insulin in 0.45% normal saline. When the blood glucose level falls to 300 mg/dl, the infusion rate is reduced, and 5% dextrose is added to maintain a blood glucose level of approximately 250 mg/dl or until the patient recovers from ketosis.

To correct fluid volume depletion, 1 to 2 L of 0.45% sodium chloride are infused within the first 2 to 3 hours. Intravenous fluids are then administered more slowly, with the rate depending on the state of dehydration. Adequate volume replacement is determined by a systolic blood pressure between 90 and 140 mm Hg, a pulse rate between 60 and 100 beats per minute, and a urine output of at least 30 ml/hour.

Patients in ketoacidosis have a serum osmolarity of more than 330 mOsm/L. The normal range for serum osmolarity is 280 to 300 mOsm/L. Treatment consists of hypotonic fluid, usually 0.45% saline. Serum osmolarity is corrected as saline is given to correct hypovolemia. Acidosis is corrected by the administration of insulin and fluids. The use of sodium bicarbonate to correct this acidosis is avoided because it can precipitate a further drop in serum potassium levels.

Electrolyte imbalance is restored through the administration of intravenous potassium. Initially, the potassium level may be normal or high because potassium leaves the cell and enters the plasma as the cells dehydrate. However, as insulin is administered, potassium moves back into the cells and the serum potassium level falls. Twenty to 40 mEq potassium chloride per liter of intravenous fluid is given even if initial serum potassium levels are normal. As DKA is resolved, the rate of the potassium infusion is decreased. Potassium level is determined every 2 hours during the first 8 hours of treatment.

HYPERGLYCEMIC HYPEROSMOLAR NONKETOTIC SYNDROME

Hyperglycemic hyperosmolar nonketotic syndrome (HHNKS) is a life-threatening, emergency situation more commonly seen in the elderly type II non–insulin-dependent diabetic patient or undiagnosed diabetic patient. Because the initial symptoms of HHNKS can go unnoticed for several weeks and they are often confused with other medical conditions, the mortality rate is high. Type II diabetics who are most likely to develop HHNKS are elderly patients whose fluid intake is poor and hospitalized patients who are not receiving adequate fluid intake.

ETIOLOGY AND PATHOPHYSIOLOGY

HHNKS is usually precipitated by an acute illness or infection, fluid loss from osmotic diuresis secondary to hyperglycemia, severe burns, severe diarrhea, hemodialysis, peritoneal dialysis, myocardial infarction, uremia, arterial thrombosis, hypertonic enteral feedings, or pharmacologic agents such as thiazides, propranolol, phenytoin, and steroids.

HHNKS is similar to DKA, but because it occurs primarily in type II non–insulin-dependent diabetics, the lack of insulin is not absolute and lipolysis or fat breakdown does not occur. Therefore, ketones are not produced. However, as a result of the precipitating event, insulin needs increase, but the pancreas cannot compensate to produce enough insulin for normal metabolism to take place. This results in severe hyperglycemia, with a blood glucose level often higher than 800 mg/dl, and hyperosmolality.

CLINICAL MANIFESTATIONS

HHNKS is evidenced by profound hyperglycemia and dehydration, absence of ketosis, and the presence of neurologic changes ranging from depressed sensorium to coma.

The onset of HHNKS is gradual, with a history of increasing polyuria and polydipsia. These early symptoms are frequently missed, especially in the elderly, which is one reason dehydration is more severe than in DKA. The dehydration or loss of fluids also causes electrolyte depletion, hyperosmolality, and hypovolemia.

Patients can also have neurologic signs similar to those of a cerebrovascular accident, which are reversible when the condition subsides. Despite severe hyperglycemia, there are no ketones in the blood or urine, and there are fewer complaints of gastrointestinal symptoms than in DKA. Table 30–8 compares the characteristics of DKA and HHNKS.

MEDICAL MANAGEMENT

The primary goals of treatment are to rehydrate the patient to restore fluid volume and to correct electrolyte deficiency. The amount of fluid replacement depends on the level of dehydration and the patient's cardiovascular status. Intravenous fluid replacement is similar to that administered in DKA. Blood glucose levels and osmolality decrease as the patient is rehydrated. Elderly patients and those

Table 30–8. CHARACTERISTICS OF DIABETIC KETOACIDOSIS (DKA) AND HYPERGLYCEMIC, HYPEROSMOLAR, NONKETOTIC SYNDROME (HHNKS)

DKA	HHNKS
Usually occurs in insulin-dependent diabetes mellitus (IDDM)	Usually occurs in diagnosed or undiagnosed non–insulin-dependent diabetes mellitus (NIDDM)
Blood glucose level between 300 and 800 mg/dl	Blood glucose level between 600 and 1200 mg/dl or higher
Ketones produced	No ketones produced
Blood pH below 7.35	Blood pH normal
Serum osmolality less than 350 mOsm/kg	Serum osmolality more than 350 mOsm/kg

with a previous history of cardiovascular disease are monitored by central venous pressure or Swan-Ganz catheter. Potassium replacement is guided by continuous cardiac monitoring and frequent serum potassium determinations.

Insulin is another important component in the treatment of HHNKS and is given according to the same guidelines as in DKA. Blood glucose and electrolyte levels are monitored every 1 to 2 hours until stable.

HYPOGLYCEMIA

Acute hypoglycemia occurs when blood glucose levels fall below 50 mg/dl. Hypoglycemia is dangerous because the brain relies solely on glucose for energy and it cannot metabolize fats for energy as the rest of the body can when glucose is not available.

ETIOLOGY AND PATHOPHYSIOLOGY

Hypoglycemia is an acute complication that can occur in patients taking medication for diabetes. The most common causes are too much insulin, inadequate food intake, excessive or prolonged physical activity, and ingestion of alcohol, especially when not eating.

The diabetic patient can have a hypoglycemic insulin reaction from too much insulin if an error is made in preparing the medication, if the insulin is absorbed more rapidly than normal as a result of injection into an extremity that is being exercised, or if the type of insulin is changed from animal-source insulin to human insulin or other highly purified preparation. Hypoglycemia may also develop in patients when their blood glucose levels approach normal and insulin requirements decrease.

Hypoglycemia can occur if snacks or meals are late or omitted. All prescribed exchanges of the meal plan have to be eaten on schedule. Hypoglycemia may also occur when there is delayed or impaired absorption of carbohydrates as a result of gastrointestinal neuropathy.

Physical activity can lower blood glucose levels for as long as 24 hours following the exercise. The presence of insulin normally inhibits the production of glucose by the liver, so in the nondiabetic person, endogenous insulin production decreases during exercise, thereby allowing for increased hepatic glucose production. However, the diabetic patient who receives a set amount of exogenous insulin may have a relative excess of insulin, which would inhibit the production of glucose by the liver during exercise. Exercise also increases sensitivity of muscle tissue to insulin and promotes increased glucose uptake by muscle to replenish stores of glycogen depleted by exercise. The combination of decreased glucose production by the liver and increased glucose utilization by muscle can lead to hypoglycemia both during and after exercise.

Ingestion of alcohol or ethanol causes hypoglycemia by inhibiting glucose production by the liver (gluconeogenesis). This can occur with as little as 2 or 3 oz of alcohol on an empty stomach.

Hypoglycemia can also occur when taking propranolol, which can mask the early symptoms of a hypoglycemic reaction; at the onset of menses, when there is a decrease in progesterone levels, which decreases insulin requirements; and during the immediate postpartum period, when there is a reduction in placental hormones that are antagonistic to insulin.

CLINICAL MANIFESTATIONS

Hypoglycemia can be classified as mild, moderate, or severe, depending upon the symptoms the patient has. Although the severity of the hypoglycemic reaction is poorly correlated with blood glucose levels because the exact blood glucose level at which symptoms begin varies from patient to patient, most patients develop symptoms when blood glucose is between 50 and 60 mg/dl.

The patient who has mild hypoglycemia exhibits sudden tremors, palpitations, diaphoresis, and hunger, which are symptoms associated with stimulation of the autonomic nervous system. The patient remains alert and capable of self-treatment, such as ingesting 10 to 15 g of simple carbohydrate (4 to 6 oz of juice or six to ten Life Savers). Following treatment, the symptoms subside quickly.

Moderate hypoglycemia causes impaired function of the central nervous system. In addition to manifestations of stimulation of the autonomic nervous system, the patient may experience headache, mood changes, irritability, inability to concentrate, confusion, slurred speech, irrational behavior, blurred vision, impaired judgment, and drowsiness. The patient is able to request assistance and may require a second dose of simple carbohydrate to correct the hypoglycemia.

A severe hypoglycemic reaction is one in which the patient needs the assistance of another person for treatment because of severely impaired neurologic function. The patient is unresponsive and may have convulsions. Treatment consists of parenteral glucagon or intravenous glucose.

MEDICAL MANAGEMENT

The major goal of the treatment of hypoglycemia is rapid reversal of the condition by administration of glucose to prevent injury or residual central nervous system damage. It is also important to review principles of self-management with the patient to prevent further hypoglycemic episodes. The production of counterregulatory hormones assists in the recovery from hypoglycemia if glycogen stores are not depleted. An elevated circulating insulin level delays recovery.

Treatment depends on the patient's history, resources, and severity of the hypoglycemic episode. All levels of hypoglycemia in both type I and type II diabetic individuals are treated immediately. Review Table 30–7 for a comparison of the causes, symptoms, and treatment of hypoglycemia and hyperglycemia.

SOMOGYI PHENOMENON

The Somogyi phenomenon is characterized by periods of hypoglycemia followed by rebound hyperglycemia. Typically, the Somogyi phenomenon occurs during the night, but it can occur any time a hypoglycemic episode occurs. The phenomenon begins with hypoglycemia, followed by oversecretion of counterregulatory hormones. The counterregulatory hormones stimulate the liver to produce glucose, causing hyperglycemia.

Diagnosing the Somogyi phenomenon may be difficult because the pattern of hypoglycemia followed by rebound hyperglycemia may also be caused by developing insulin resistance. Somogyi phenomenon is suspected in patients whose blood glucose levels fluctuate between hypoglycemia and severe hyperglycemia, those whose blood glucose levels increase despite increasing doses of insulin, and patients who awaken with headaches, complain of restless sleep, nightmares, or enuresis or who have unexplained nausea and vomiting.

Diagnosis of the Somogyi phenomenon requires measuring blood glucose levels between 2:00 A.M. and 4:00 A.M. and again at 7:00 A.M. If the blood glucose levels between 2:00 A.M. and 4:00 A.M. are below 50 to 60 mg/dl and the 7:00 A.M. blood glucose level is more than 180 to 200 mg/dl, the Somogyi phenomenon probably occurred.

Treatment for the Somogyi phenomenon is to decrease the evening insulin dose to a level that no longer causes nocturnal hypoglycemia. A bedtime snack is also recommended to counter the duration of the effects of intermediate- and long-acting insulins during the night.

DAWN PHENOMENON

The dawn phenomenon is a condition that can occur in some insulin-dependent patients and is characterized by an increase in fasting blood glucose levels between 5:00 A.M. and 9:00 A.M. It is not preceded by an episode of hypoglycemia. A possible cause is the release of growth hormone or cortisol during rapid-eye-movement (REM) sleep in the early morning hours, which increases glucose levels.

Diagnosis requires measuring blood glucose levels at 3:00 A.M. If this blood glucose level is normal and the level at 6:00 A.M. or 7:00 A.M. is elevated, the dawn phenomenon is suspected.

Treatment consists of delaying the intermediate-acting evening insulin dose until 10:00 P.M. and eating a bedtime snack. The intermediate-acting insulin would prevent a rise in blood glucose after 3:00 A.M.

Long-Term Degenerative Changes of Diabetes Mellitus

The discovery of insulin and oral antidiabetic agents, along with improved technology and methods of managing diabetes, has enabled people with diabetes to live longer. As they live longer, diabetic patients are at an increased risk of developing the long-term, chronic degenerative changes associated with the disease. Although degenerative changes can develop in all patients with diabetes mellitus, research has confirmed that good control of blood glucose levels may delay, or possibly prevent, their onset and can reduce their severity.

DEGENERATIVE VASCULAR CHANGES

MACROVASCULAR DISEASE

Macrovascular disease, or macroangiopathy, is an atherosclerotic process of large and moderate-size blood vessels that can occur in any individual whether or not diabetes mellitus is present. However, over the past 2 decades, research has shown that people with diabetes are at greater risk of developing these changes at an earlier age. It is now recognized that macrovascular disease is responsible for most of the morbidity and mortality seen in patients with diabetes. Macrovascular disease at least doubles the risk of coronary artery, cerebral vascular, and peripheral vascular disease in the diabetic patient. In addition to the usual risk factors of cigarette smoking, hypertension, and elevated cholesterol and triglyceride levels, hyperglycemia is an independent risk factor in the diabetic patient. Research to determine why atherosclerosis occurs more frequently in people with diabetes continues, but there is no conclusive evidence as yet.

People with diabetes are advised of the increased risk of macrovascular disease and to take steps to reduce the risk factors associated with its development.

MICROVASCULAR DISEASE

Microvascular disease, or microangiopathy, refers to small vessel disease that affects the arterioles, venules, and capillaries. It is characterized by thickening of the capillary basement membrane that surrounds the endothelial cells of the capillary, increased capillary permeability, and capillary occlusion. It primarily affects the eyes, kidneys, nervous system, and peripheral circulation. Microangiopathy results in diabetic retinopathy, peripheral nephropathy, and diabetic neuropathy. Guidelines for patient teaching to monitor and minimize the risks associated with microvascular degenerative changes are presented in Chart 30–4.

Diabetic Retinopathy

Diabetic retinopathy is characterized by progressive deterioration of the small blood vessels in the retina. It is the leading cause of blindness in the United States and is related to the length of time the patient has had diabetes. After 10 years of having diabetes, 50% of all diabetic patients and 90% of those with poorly controlled blood glucose levels have some form of retinopathy.

There are three stages of diabetic retinopathy. The first and earliest stage is nonproliferative background retinopathy characterized by microaneurysms, which are seen as tiny red dots in the retina. Other changes associated with background retinopathy are the appearance of yellow lipid deposits commonly called hard exudates, small intraretinal hemorrhages that appear as red smudges on the retina, and the presence of macular edema. Blurred central vision caused by the macular edema develops in 10% of diabetic patients and may be the only subjective symptom. Macular edema may progress to loss of central vision in later stages.

The second stage of diabetic retinopathy is preproliferative retinopathy characterized by progression of background retinopathy and further destruction and occlusion of retinal capillaries. The retinal veins become tortuous and bulging, and multiple clustered blot hemorrhages appear, indicating weakened capillary walls. Poor retinal perfusion may stimulate initial growth of abnormal new blood vessels. Areas of retinal ischemia produce soft exudates or cotton-wool spots, which are white, fluffy-looking lesions.

In patients with severe preproliferative retinopathy, there is a 50% chance that the third stage, proliferative retinopathy, will develop within 1 year. This stage is characterized by the growth of networks of new abnormal blood vessels on the surface of the retina and extending into the vitreous. This growth of new blood vessels is called neovascularization and occurs in response to ischemia in the diseased retina. Light transmission through these areas is diminished.

These new blood vessels are very brittle and can easily hemorrhage, sometimes filling the vitreous

Chart 30–4.

NURSING GUIDE TO PATIENT EDUCATION FOR SELF-MANAGEMENT: GUIDELINES FOR SELF-CARE AND MONITORING LONG-TERM DEGENERATIVE CHANGES OF DIABETES MELLITUS

Instruct the patient in the following for diabetic retinopathy:

Have an eye examination annually by an ophthalmologist.

Make an appointment with the ophthalmologist immediately if blurred vision occurs or if there is a change or decrease in vision.

Instruct the patient in the following for diabetic peripheral neuropathy:

Foot-Care Instructions:

Follow a foot-care routine daily to prevent long-term complications.

Inspect the feet daily for sores, blisters, swelling, redness, and tenderness. Report skin infections or nonhealing sores immediately to the physician. Loss of sensation caused by diabetic neuropathy can lead to infection, gangrene, and possible amputation if not detected and treated early.

Wash the feet daily using a mild soap. Pat the feet dry and apply lotion (do not apply lotion between the toes). Use lotion containing lanolin, not petroleum jelly. Test the temperature of the water before submerging the feet to prevent burns. Do not soak the feet.

Wear properly fitting shoes with smooth linings.

Do not walk in bare feet either in the house or outside.

Avoid using a heating pad or hot water bottle on the feet.

Cut the toenails straight and even with the toe itself. If the toenails are thick and hard to cut or if vision is poor, have a physician or podiatrist cut them.

Make an appointment with a podiatrist for treatment of corns, calluses, warts, thickened or rough skin, splinters, or injuries. Do not attempt to treat corns, calluses, or warts with nonprescription preparations or instruments.

Do not cross the legs at the knees or ankles when sitting.

Instruct the patient in the following for diabetic nephropathy:

Renal function is monitored by checking the urine for the presence of protein during physician visits. If overt proteinuria is present, renal function tests are done.

For advanced uremia:

- Follow a protein-restricted diet.
- Monitor blood glucose levels closely, because insulin requirements decrease with uremia and there is an increased likelihood of having a hypoglycemic reaction.

with blood. As the damaged vessels heal and blood is resorbed from the vitreous, fibrous scar tissue forms. The growth of fibrous scar tissue is called fibrous proliferation. As the fibrous tissue contracts, it can place traction on the retina, resulting in retinal detachment. Loss of vision caused by vitreous hemorrhage or retinal detachment can be the patient's first symptom of proliferative retinopathy. Any diabetic patient complaining of spots floating in the field of vision, rapid visual changes, or fogged vision should be referred to an ophthalmologist immediately.

The primary treatment for diabetic retinopathy is argon laser photocoagulation. In patients with high-risk characteristics of proliferative retinopathy, panretinal photocoagulation is most beneficial. This is a procedure in which 1200 to 1600 laser burns, each measuring 500 μm, are placed throughout the midperipheral retina but not in the macular region. Macular edema is treated by focal argon laser photocoagulation. The Early Treatment Diabetic Retinopathy Study has shown during a 3-year period that patients receiving this treatment have had the rate of visual loss reduced by 50%.

Laser photocoagulation is a relatively painless procedure performed on an outpatient basis with anesthetic eye drops. The patient can usually resume activities of daily living the following day, with possible restrictions on heavy lifting. However, multiple treatments may result in night blindness, decreased visual acuity, or loss of peripheral vision.

The treatment for vitreous hemorrhage is a vitrectomy. In this procedure, both the hemorrhagic area of the vitreous and the fibrous proliferation are removed and replaced with sterile saline.

All diabetic patients are advised to have an eye examination by an ophthalmologist annually, including an intraocular pressure measurement and a dilated pupil fundus examination. Fluorescein angiography is done to assess retinal vessels and macular edema.

Diabetic Neuropathy

Diabetic neuropathy is the most common complication of diabetes. It occurs in 70% of diabetic patients and is already present in 12% of patients at the time of diagnosis. The incidence and prevalence of neuropathy increase with the age of the patient and the severity of hyperglycemia.

Diabetic neuropathy is a group of neurologic complications related to the abnormal metabolism of diabetes that affects the peripheral and autonomic nervous systems. The pathology can be metabolic or vascular and results in a loss of large and small myelin nerve fibers (demyelination), connective tissue proliferation, and thickening of the capillary basement membrane.

A common theory for the pathology of diabetic neuropathy is a disturbance of the polyol pathway of glucose metabolism in nerve tissue during periods of hyperglycemia.

Diabetic neuropathies are classified according to the anatomic distribution of the lesions, type of nerve involvement, degree of vascular involvement, and extent of nerve damage. Diabetic mononeuropathies include nerves chronically exposed to external pressure, such as those affected in carpal tunnel syndrome, extraocular motor paralysis, and footdrop. The symptoms are numbness, tingling, burning, and sudden pain. Medical management includes correction of the nerve entrapment. Pain is treated by splinting, local injections of glucocorticoids, or nerve block. Recovery usually occurs within 3 months. Without treatment, muscle weakness and wasting could result.

Distal symmetric polyneuropathy, also referred to as peripheral neuropathy, is the most common form of diabetic neuropathy. The symptoms include numbness, tingling, burning, dull ache, and cramping that begins in the digits and progresses to the foot and hand. The symptoms are usually worse during the night. Eventually, the pain increases, and the skin may become so sensitive that the patient is unable to tolerate pressure from bed sheets. As the neuropathy progresses, the patient develops muscle weakness, sensory loss, an unbalanced gait, foot ulcers, and loss of fine motor skills. Sensory neuropathy leads to loss of pain and pressure sensation and increases the risk of undetected injury, tissue ischemia, or infection. Medical management includes control of hyperglycemia and medication to relieve pain and allow the patient to sleep at night.

Autonomic neuropathy involves nerves of the small blood vessels, the sweat glands of the skin, the gastrointestinal tract, the genitourinary tract, the cardiovascular system, and the adrenergic system. This type of neuropathy usually occurs in combination with peripheral neuropathy. The symptoms depend on the system involved. Orthostatic hypotension and mild, persistent tachycardia are common manifestations of cardiovascular autonomic neuropathy. When the nerves of the sweat glands are involved, there can be frequent attacks of profuse sweating when eating, and drying and cracking of the skin of the feet. Involvement of the gastrointestinal tract, known as gastroparesis, can cause delayed emptying of the gastric contents, retention and decreased ability to expel gastric contents, and nausea and vomiting of undigested food. Involvement of the small intestine causes watery diarrhea, often at night without warning, followed by constipation. Involvement of the genitourinary tract causes urinary retention, overflow incontinence, and frequent urinary tract infections.

Sexual dysfunction occurs in 50% of male diabetic patients and 35% of the females after 20 years of having diabetes. The symptoms in males are impotence, retrograde ejaculation, and inability to maintain an erection. Females have a reduction in the ability to have an orgasm and changes in vaginal lubrication.

Diabetic Nephropathy

Diabetic nephropathy is characterized by proteinuria, hypertension, edema, and renal insufficiency. It occurs in patients who have had diabetes for more than 10 years and is the third most commonly listed diagnosis of patients being treated for end-stage renal disease (ESRD). ESRD requiring dialysis eventually develops in 30% to 40% of patients with diabetes mellitus. In addition, 97% of patients with ESRD have diabetic retinopathy, and 50% are either blind or have significant loss of vision. This is known as renal-retinal syndrome.

Pathology and early renal changes develop without clinical signs, and deterioration of renal function is often ongoing for many years before detection. During this time, glomerular changes are taking place—basement membrane thickening, mesangial expansion, and arteriosclerosis of the afferent and efferent blood vessels. The effectiveness of glomerular filtration decreases. Urinary creatinine clearance decreases as the glomerular filtration rate deteriorates. Next, there is formation of nodular and diffuse lesions throughout the glomerulus, which is called Kimmelstiel-Wilson syndrome. These changes occur in both IDDM and NIDDM patients, often earlier in patients with NIDDM.

The first clinical sign that kidney damage has occurred is the presence of protein in the urine as a result of increased glomerular capillary permeability caused by thickening of the basement membrane. Proteinuria usually develops within 15 to 20 years after the onset of clinical symptoms of diabetes. Protein can be detected by the dipstick method of testing a single specimen of urine or by testing a 24-hour urine collection. Nephrotic syndrome is diagnosed when the amount of protein excreted exceeds 3.5 g/day. As protein is excreted, plasma albumin concentration falls, leading to protein tissue wasting, sodium and water retention, weight gain, and edema.

Diabetic patients are tested regularly for proteinuria. When proteinuria is present, serum creatinine and urea nitrogen concentrations are also measured, and a 24-hour urine test to quantitate the total protein excreted and creatinine clearance may be done.

Hypertension is the most important factor in the progression of diabetic nephropathy. Controlling and treating hypertension has been shown to slow the progression of established renal disease. Normal blood pressure, maintained through the use of diuretics and antihypertensive drugs, decreases the rate at which the glomerular filtration rate declines, reduces proteinuria, and helps prevent cerebrovascular and coronary artery disease.

Renal insufficiency is characterized by proteinuria, hypertension, a glomerular filtration rate below 25 to 30 ml/minute (normal is approximately 125 ml/minute), and elevated serum creatinine and blood urea nitrogen levels.

The patient has uremia when the glomerular filtration rate is below 15 ml/minute and the serum creatinine level is greater than 4 to 5 mg/dl. The clinical signs at this stage include nausea, vomiting, lethargy, anemia, hypertension, and acidosis. In addition, blood glucose levels fluctuate greatly, and insulin needs decrease as uremia advances because about 25% of insulin is catabolized by the kidneys.

Medical management includes placing the patient on a protein-restricted diet. Patients with ESRD require either a kidney transplant or dialysis, or death will occur. Patients with diabetic nephropathy are at increased risk for acute renal failure after a radiocontrast procedure such as intravenous pyelography and computed tomography scan. Therefore, a minimum amount of dye is given and the patient is well hydrated before the procedure. In addition, intravenous mannitol is often administered before the procedure and continued for 24 hours following the procedure. Serum creatinine concentration is measured daily for 2 to 3 days afterward.

Application of the Nursing Process to the Care of the Patient with Diabetes Mellitus

Assessment

Nursing assessment of the patient with diabetes mellitus is based on the type of diabetes the patient has, the duration of the disease, the frequency of acute complications, and the presence of long-term degenerative changes. Assessment includes a complete history and physical assessment, as presented in Box 30–2. The history identifies factors that affect glucose levels, such as dietary and exercise habits, whether the patient takes insulin or oral antidiabetic agents, and the patient's level of knowledge and compliance in managing the disease. The physical assessment confirms physical changes in the multiple body systems affected by diabetes mellitus.

Because diabetes requires self-management, it is important to assess the patient's readiness, willingness, and ability to learn the self-care regimen. Patients who are newly diagnosed may not be ready to learn as a result of feelings of loss associated with loss of freedom and loss of control over their lives. These feelings are indicative of a grieving process. The patient may demonstrate anxiety, fear, denial, anger, and depression before accepting the disease. Some patients never accept the disease and may fluctuate back and forth between these stages throughout life.

Patients who are not newly diagnosed are assessed for assimilation of diabetes management practices into their lifestyle. Interview the patient, and explore aspects of the diabetic treatment plan that have been easy for the patient to assimilate versus those that have been more difficult. For example, the patient who is able to work through the stages of grief and who accepts responsibility for self-care by making lifestyle changes to adhere to the treatment regimen, who keeps abreast of new information, and who uses self–blood glucose monitoring to manage the disease has coped well. The patient who has not progressed through the grief process and does not take responsibility for self-care needs assistance in exploring what has not been accomplished and in developing ways to make these accomplishments a reality.

Assessment also includes determination of the patient's desire and ability to learn. Ask about prior health care experiences the patient has had with diabetes, what the patient wants to learn and the most immediate concern for learning, the patient's level of formal education and reading ability, and the patient's goals. In order for patient teaching to be successful, the teaching plan has to be centered around the needs of the patient. For example, if the

Box 30–2.

NURSING GUIDELINES FOR ASSESSMENT OF A PATIENT WITH DIABETES MELLITUS

History

Obtain information concerning the following:

- *Duration of diabetes.*
- *Reason for admission or appointment.*
- *Diet patient follows.* Ask patient to write down from memory everything eaten for the previous 2 days to determine whether patient understands and complies with a previously taught diet.
- *Insulin therapy.* If patient has been administering insulin at home, observe patient prepare and administer insulin in the hospital. Ask patient to state the name and dose of the insulin and time taken and to describe its action according to onset, peak, and duration.
- *Sulfonylureas.* If patient takes oral antidiabetic agents, ask patient to state the name of the agent. Ask patient whether he or she knows the difference between insulin and oral antidiabetic agents.
- *Self–blood glucose monitoring.* If the patient has been doing this procedure at home, observe while it is done. Ask patient to describe how he or she interprets the results.
- *Knowledge of acute complications.* Ask patient to state the causes, symptoms, and treatment of hypoglycemia and hyperglycemia and ketoacidosis.
- *Knowledge of sick-day management.* Ask patient to describe how he or she manages sick days regarding diet and medication. Determine whether patient understands implications of illness, especially infection, nausea and vomiting, and diarrhea.
- *Foot-care routine.* Ask patient to describe how he or she takes care of the feet. Determine whether patient understands implications of foot-care problems.
- *Exercise.* Determine whether the patient leads a sedentary or active lifestyle and whether he or she understands the effects of exercise on blood glucose levels.
- *Basic physiology of diabetes.* Ask patient to explain what diabetes is and how it affects the body.
- *Long-term degenerative changes.* Ask patient to list the long-term changes that can occur with diabetes and how to delay their onset.
- *Personal history.* Find out whether patient lives alone or with others; lifestyle, including occupation, hobbies, and weekend activities; whether patient receives social assistance; and whether there is a family history of diabetes.
- *Diabetic identification.* Ask to see the diabetic identification the patient wears or carries.

Physical Assessment

Physical assessment includes the following:

- Assess for the presence or history of *Candida albicans* in the groin, the axillae, and under the breasts, and vaginal yeast infections in females.
- Examine the tibial area for the presence of "shin spots," known as diabetic dermopathy, and for necrobiosis, which is characterized by raised reddened lesions with sharply defined borders.
- Examine the elbows and knees for xanthomas, which are yellow fat deposits.
- Examine insulin injection sites for the presence of lipodystrophy.
- Examine the feet and legs for sores, blisters, reddened areas, or ulcers.
- Examine the toenails to see whether they are thick and hard to cut.
- Palpate the dorsalis pedis and posterior tibial pulse.
- Examine the dorsal part of the foot for hair loss.
- Assess weight, blood pressure, and pulse.
- Assess for symptoms of cardiovascular disease—dyspnea, irregular apical or brachial pulse, dependent edema, orthostatic hypotension.
- Palpate ankles for edema.
- Examine hands for sores, burns, or muscle atropy.
- Assess for gastrointestinal disturbances such as diarrhea, especially at night.
- Assess for urinary tract infections.
- Assess for impotence or other reproductive problems.
- Assess for loss of sensation in extremities.

patient shows a desire to learn how to prepare and administer insulin, the nurse should begin teaching this first. If the patient is unable to read, teaching methods must include the use of audio-visuals and discussion rather than printed material.

Assessment of the diabetic patient also includes identifying available support systems, such as the family and significant others. It is advisable to include these individuals in the patient teaching process because personal relationships are sometimes affected by the disease.

The nursing assessment of the diabetic patient also includes a physical assessment. Diabetes affects every system in the body. Therefore, the skin, mouth, eyes, and cardiovascular, peripheral vascular, renal, and neurologic systems are assessed. Box 30–2 outlines physical assessment guidelines for the diabetic patient.

Nursing Diagnoses and Planning

Nursing diagnoses and related patient outcomes most commonly applicable to patients with diabetes mellitus include the following:

NDx: Anticipatory and/or dysfunctional grieving related to loss of freedom and required changes in lifestyle

Planning: Patient outcomes

1. Patient verbalizes negative feelings about diabetes, such as anger, fear, and depression.
2. Patient verbalizes questions and concerns.
3. Patient states desire to participate in self-care activities.

NDx: Ineffective individual coping related to realization that diabetes is a chronic condition requiring lifelong self-management, medical supervision, and lifestyle changes to prevent long-term degenerative changes

Planning: Patient outcomes

1. Patient verbalizes perception of disease, benefits of care, and barriers to care.
2. Patient identifies coping patterns and personal strengths to promote effective coping.
3. Patient demonstrates a desire to participate in learning and self-care activities.
4. Patient identifies individual stressors.
5. Patient participates in developing a realistic plan for incorporating changes into lifestyle using appropriate problem-solving techniques.
6. Patient recognizes and uses available support systems.

NDx: Fluid volume deficit related to loss of fluids associated with diarrhea, vomiting, and osmotic diuresis from hyperglycemia

Planning: Patient outcomes

1. Patient maintains adequate intake of fluids and electrolytes as evidenced by:
   a. Normal skin turgor
   b. Moist mucous membranes
   c. Blood pressure and pulse within normal range for patient
   d. Balanced intake and output
   e. Urine specific gravity between 1.010 and 1.030
   f. Normal serum sodium, chloride, magnesium, phosphorus, and potassium levels
   g. Absence of nausea, vomiting, and diarrhea

NDx: Altered tissue perfusion related to degenerative vascular changes of diabetes

Planning: Patient outcomes

1. Patient maintains adequate systemic tissue perfusion as evidenced by:
   a. Blood pressure and pulse within normal range for patient
   b. Palpable peripheral pulses
   c. Skin warm and of normal color
   d. Capillary refill time of less than 3 seconds
   e. Urine output greater than 30 ml/hour
   f. Verbalization of increased sensation and decreased tingling and numbness in extremities
   g. Decreased edema in extremities
   h. Verbalization of increased comfort
   i. Maintenance of skin integrity

NDx: High risk for trauma related to muscle weakness and atrophy, sensory and motor loss secondary to peripheral neuropathy, and symptoms of hypoglycemic insulin reactions

Planning: Patient outcomes

1. Patient identifies factors that increase the potential for trauma.
2. Patient verbalizes desire to practice measures that prevent trauma.
3. Patient maintains glucose levels below 140 mg/dl, or within target range set by physician, to prevent or delay the onset of degenerative changes.
4. Patient utilizes measures to prevent the onset of hypoglycemic insulin reactions.

NDx: High risk for altered health maintenance related to lack of knowledge of self-care activities

Planning: Patient outcomes

1. Patient verbalizes a basic understanding of the pathophysiology of diabetes.
2. Patient verbalizes an understanding of prescribed medication, including action, dose, side effects, and schedule of administration.
3. Patient demonstrates the ability to prepare and administer insulin correctly.
4. Patient verbalizes an understanding of the prescribed diet and use of exchange lists.

5. Patient demonstrates the ability to perform blood glucose and urine tests correctly and interpret results.
6. Patient verbalizes the causes, symptoms, and treatment for hypoglycemia and hyperglycemia.
7. Patient verbalizes an understanding of proper foot care routine.
8. Patient describes how he or she will incorporate the treatment plan into lifestyle.
9. Patient identifies available support systems.

Nursing Interventions

Nursing care of the patient with diabetes mellitus includes maintaining near normal blood glucose levels, preventing acute complications and long-term degenerative changes, and teaching the patient how to manage the disease at home. Nursing interventions depend on the acuity of the patient's condition, the duration of the disease, the type of diabetes, the reason for admission to the hospital, the presence of long-term degenerative changes, and the patient's level of knowledge of the disease.

NDx: Anticipatory and/or dysfunctional grieving

An analogy to the stages of the grieving process can be made to the stages the diabetic patient goes through before accepting the disease. First determine the patient's perception of the disease and its impact on the future. The patient may have prior knowledge about diabetes that may not be valid, or may have preconceived myths that need to be corrected. Give the patient time to work through the stages of grief by promoting trust, providing a supportive atmosphere of care and concern, and using therapeutic communication to encourage the patient to express feelings. The stage of denial can be prolonged, especially because there are often no manifestations of illness immediately apparent upon diagnosis. It is possible for a patient to have diabetes for years and have no physical symptoms, and it is difficult for these patients to understand why they need to follow a diabetic regimen.

NDx: Ineffective individual coping

Patients who are unable to cope effectively with diabetes may fear the onset of long-term degenerative changes as well as the changes in lifestyle needed to manage a chronic disease. Signs of poor coping ability are sleep disturbances, fatigue, inability to concentrate, inability to solve problems, and verbalization of inability to cope.

The patient may be anxious about learning new information needed to provide self-care, as well as the ability to incorporate a new routine into his or her daily lifestyle. Nursing interventions to assist the patient in coping effectively include identifying the patient's strengths and limitations and encouraging the patient to participate in self-care learning activities. Assist the patient in identifying stressors and in using problem-solving techniques.

Patient teaching and allowing the patient to set goals for self-care give the patient a sense of control and help avoid the development of crisis situations. Individualize teaching at the patient's level of understanding, and provide ample opportunities for the patient to verbalize and demonstrate the acquired knowledge and skills. Review strategies for dealing with anxiety-provoking situations by role-playing and visualizing anticipated events.

Arrange a meeting with other diabetic patients who have coped successfully, and encourage the patient to use available support systems to promote successful coping. Provide information on the American Diabetes Association and local community support groups for diabetics. Initiate a social service referral if appropriate.

NDx: Fluid volume deficit

Determine the causative factors leading to hyperglycemia and fluid volume deficit, and the degree of the deficit. Monitor for the clinical manifestations of dehydration, which include decreased or poor skin turgor, dry mucous membranes, thirst, low blood pressure, weak and rapid pulse, and urine output less than intake with a specific gravity higher than 1.030 (not useful if the patient has diabetic nephropathy).

If nausea and vomiting related to ketoacidosis are the causative factors, the metabolic acidosis is treated. Monitor blood glucose levels, administer insulin, maintain a fluid intake of at least 2500 ml/day as tolerated, and administer intravenous fluids and electrolyte replacement as prescribed. Encourage the patient to take slow, deep breaths, and provide oral hygiene after each emesis to reduce nausea and vomiting.

Observe the patient for electrolyte depletion, and report abnormal laboratory results to the physician. When the patient first has a fluid volume deficit, serum potassium levels are normal as potassium leaves the cell. However, potassium levels can fall when insulin is administered and blood glucose levels start to return to normal, because insulin enhances the movement of potassium back into the cells. Hypokalemia can cause cardiac dysrhythmias and death; therefore, it is extremely important to begin potassium replacement within 1 to 2 hours after starting insulin. In addition, if the patient is receiving sodium bicarbonate, additional potassium should be given, because bicarbonate can aggravate hypokalemia by promoting the movement of potassium back into the cells.

Once the patient is stabilized, discuss the events that led to hyperglycemia and fluid volume deficit to identify actions the patient could take to avoid a recurrence.

NDx: Altered tissue perfusion

Monitor for the manifestations of altered tissue perfusion on a daily basis. These include a significant decrease in blood pressure, a resting pulse of more than 100 beats per minute, a decrease in systolic blood pressure of at least 15 mm Hg with a simultaneous increase in pulse when the patient changes from a lying to a sitting or standing position, rapid or labored respirations, delayed return of color to feet and lower legs when legs are returned to a dependent position after being elevated for 1 minute, dusky red color of lower legs and feet when in a dependent position, diminished or absent peripheral pulses, capillary refill time of more than 3 seconds, urine output of less than 30 ml/hour, and elevated blood urea nitrogen and serum creatinine levels. Consult with the physician to determine the severity of perfusion impairment indicated by these manifestations, or if they become more severe.

Nursing interventions also include actions to maintain adequate tissue perfusion. Promote improved circulation in the lower extremities by having the patient perform active foot and leg exercises for 10 minutes every 2 hours and by alternating short periods of slow walking with periods of rest. Instruct the patient to avoid crossing the legs, wearing constricting hose, elevating the knees by the use of a knee gatch or pillows, or standing or sitting for long periods. Because exposure to cold causes vasoconstriction, provide a warm room temperature and adequate clothing and blankets. Advise the patient to avoid foods high in fat and cholesterol to slow the progression of atherosclerosis. Discourage cigarette smoking, which causes vasoconstriction. Teach the patient the principles of self-care—prevention and monitoring of the long-term degenerative changes associated with diabetes mellitus (see Chart 30–4)—and which signs and symptoms to report to the physician after discharge.

NDx: High risk for trauma
The diabetic patient with peripheral neuropathy may be unable to perceive movement or position of the extremities and may also have diminished reflexes, muscle weakness, and atrophy. These patients could injure their extremities and not feel the injury, which can ultimately lead to ulcerations, infection, and amputation. Patient instructions in a daily foot care routine that includes inspection of the feet for sores or reddened areas are summarized in Chart 30–4.

Nursing interventions also include teaching the patient how to avoid hypoglycemic insulin reactions and how to treat them if they occur. Insulin reactions usually occur suddenly, and the symptoms progress rapidly from tremors, shaking, sweating, and dizziness to more severe symptoms of irritability, confusion, impaired judgment, unresponsiveness, unconsciousness, and convulsions. Instruct the diabetic patient to have a simple carbohydrate snack always available to ingest if symptoms occur. Delaying the initial treatment of an insulin reaction increases the risk for severe symptoms and the potential for injury to the patient.

NDx: High risk for altered health maintenance
Because diabetes requires lifelong self-care, patient teaching is an integral nursing intervention. After an initial assessment to determine the patient's level of knowledge, develop a teaching plan based on the patient's individual needs. Nursing Care Guide 30–1 provides the details of areas of teaching to promote successful patient self-management.

Evaluation

Evaluate the effectiveness of nursing care for a patient with diabetes mellitus by comparing the patient's status with the expected patient outcomes. Examples of specific outcomes for patients with diabetes mellitus have been provided in the Planning section.

The Elderly: Special Considerations

At the present time, 6.9% of men and 8.9% of women older than 65 years of age have diabetes mellitus, and this number is increasing as the elderly population grows. The incidence of diabetes increases to 10% of men and 20% of women in those older than 80 years of age. Almost 50% of the elderly diabetic patients can be managed by diet alone; 30% require insulin at some time; and 20% to 25% can be treated with a combination of diet and oral antidiabetic agents.

Glucose tolerance declines with increasing age as blood glucose levels tend to increase. The mean blood glucose level 1 hour after ingesting 50 g of oral glucose in a 75-year-old patient is 166 mg/dl, as opposed to 100 mg/dl for a person in the late teens or early twenties. Both the criteria for diagnosing diabetes mellitus and the medical management of the disease in the elderly differ from those of younger and middle-aged adult patients. In addition, signs and symptoms of diabetes are often altered or absent in the elderly. It is important to take these age-related changes into account during screening for diabetes.

Diabetes mellitus in the elderly is diagnosed when the fasting plasma glucose level is equal to or higher than 140 mg/dl on more than one occasion, or if 2 hours following ingestion of up to 75 g of glucose, the plasma glucose level is higher than 200 mg/dl and one other glucose level during the 2-hour oral glucose tolerance test is higher than 200 mg/dl.

The goals of therapy are focused on avoiding hypoglycemia and symptomatic hyperglycemia, and management is individualized to meet the needs of

Text continued on page 1257

Nursing Care Guide 30–1.

PATIENTS WITH DIABETES MELLITUS

Assessment Findings: Patient is a 39-year-old male who was admitted to the hospital 2 days ago for uncontrolled diabetes mellitus and diabetic ketoacidosis (DKA). He is married, has two young children, and works as a salesman, traveling frequently. The patient states that he has had IDDM for 10 years, takes one injection of 25 units U-100 Humulin N and 5 units Humulin R insulin every morning, does not bother to perform self–blood glucose monitoring, does not follow a diabetic diet, and consults with a physician approximately every 6 months if he is not traveling. At the time of admission, the patient was ill with influenza and his blood glucose level was 800 mg/dl.

Nursing Diagnosis: Ineffective management of therapeutic regimen related to lack of understanding of the implications of not following diabetic regimen and difficulty incorporating treatments into personal lifestyle

Patient Outcomes	Nursing Interventions	Rationale
Patient acknowledges insufficient knowledge of diabetic regimen.	Ask the patient how he thinks he developed DKA.	Determines patient's level of knowledge and understanding.
	Observe verbal and nonverbal cues to identify patient's readiness to learn. Use feedback and reflection to confirm observations.	Teaching is not effective unless patient is ready to learn.
	Review the cause and effect relationship between patient behaviors and control of blood glucose levels.	Accurate information corrects misunderstandings and increases patient's knowledge.
Patient acknowledges noncompliant behavior.	Determine reason for noncompliance: ■ Assess cultural and health values of patient and family. ■ Discuss with patient and family their understanding of the implications of noncompliance.	Compliance involves behavioral changes that are influenced by family, cultural, and individual beliefs about health, susceptibility to disease, and seriousness of disease. Cultural practices may affect the learning process.
	Involve patient in identifying desired changes in behavior.	Verbalization of compliant behaviors ensures that the patient understands what he must do to facilitate change.

(continued)

Nursing Care Guide 30–1. *(continued)*

PATIENTS WITH DIABETES MELLITUS

Patient Outcomes	Nursing Interventions	Rationale
Patient demonstrates willingness to learn about disease and to participate in self-care activities.	Implement measures to improve compliance: ▪ Explain diabetes at the patient's level of understanding. ▪ Stress that diabetes is a lifelong chronic condition and that compliance to the treatment plan is necessary to prevent acute complications and to prevent or delay the onset of long-term degenerative changes ▪ Provide complete diabetic teaching to patient and family. Refer to diabetic educator if available.	An assessment of the patient's learning abilities enables the nurse to develop an individual teaching plan and to facilitate effective teaching and learning. The patient needs to be informed about the disease process and its implications in order to make informed decisions on self-care regimen.
	Encourage patient to participate in self-care activities such as insulin injections, self–blood glucose monitoring, and selection of foods using diabetic meal plan from the hospital menu.	Participation in self-care activities provides reinforcement of teaching, enhances learning and retention, and increases self-confidence.
Patient verbalizes intent to modify behavior and incorporate diabetic self-management regimen into lifestyle.	Assist patient in identifying ways to incorporate self-management into lifestyle. Provide positive feedback.	Verbalization of intent and commitment facilitates change in behavior. Positive feedback reinforces learning and motivation.
	Provide written and verbal information on diet plan, medications, activity pattern, symptoms of hyper- and hypoglycemia, what actions to take if they occur, and what to do during periods of illness. Include telephone number of a resource person to answer questions after discharge.	Written information reinforces learning, clarifies verbal instructions, and minimizes the risk of errors. Availability of resource person reduces anxiety.
	Provide information on community resources, diabetic support groups, and diabetic publications. Encourage patient to attend follow-up diabetes education classes. Include patient's wife in teaching, and encourage her support.	Community resources, support groups, publications, and the involvement of family or significant other provide additional support and information that may reduce anxiety and enhance motivation and compliance.

(continued)

Nursing Care Guide 30–1. *(continued)*

PATIENTS WITH DIABETES MELLITUS

Patient Outcomes	Nursing Interventions	Rationale
	Reinforce the benefits of adhering to the prescribed self-management regimen.	Maintenance of blood glucose values below 140 mg/dl slows the progression of the long-term degenerative changes of diabetes.
Patient verbalizes understanding of implications of noncompliance.	Provide information on the pathophysiology of diabetes: ■ Explain effects of hypo- and hyperglycemia on body systems. ■ Explain benefits of latest technology to help maintain normal blood glucose levels. ■ Teach patient that he can control diabetes by accepting responsibility for managing his disease.	The basis of self-management is a sound diabetes education program. A patient who is in control of his or her own disease and able to recognize symptoms is more likely to accept and adhere to the treatment plan.

Evaluation: Compare the patient's status with the expected patient outcomes. If the outcomes are achieved, evaluate nursing care as successful. If not, reassess the patient, formulate new nursing diagnoses, and revise expected patient outcomes and nursing interventions as appropriate.

Assessment Findings: The patient is a 36-year-old single female admitted to the hospital with a diagnosis of newly developed insulin-dependent diabetes mellitus (IDDM). The patient has had symptoms of polyuria, polydipsia, and polyphagia with a 10-lb weight loss over the previous month. Blood glucose level on admission is 400 mg/dl. The patient is a schoolteacher with little knowledge of diabetes or its management.

Nursing Diagnosis: High risk for altered health maintenance related to insufficient knowledge of diabetic self-management

Patient Outcomes	Nursing Interventions	Rationale
Patient verbalizes a basic understanding of the pathophysiology of diabetes mellitus.	Explain the basic pathophysiology of diabetes at patient's level of understanding. Ask the patient to restate information to validate understanding.	In order to manage diabetes, the patient must have some understanding of its pathophysiology.

(continued)

Nursing Care Guide 30–1. (continued)

PATIENTS WITH DIABETES MELLITUS

Patient Outcomes	Nursing Interventions	Rationale
Patient demonstrates ability to plan meals using the American Diabetes Association (ADA) Exchange Lists and stays within prescribed calorie level.	Reinforce diet teaching of ADA Exchange Lists as described in Nutrition Box 30–1. Have patient plan sample menus of preferred foods for breakfast, lunch, dinner, and snack within dietary guidelines. Demonstrate how to adjust diet for changes in activity level and illness.	Diet is a primary component in the successful self-management of diabetes.
	Provide a copy of the ADA Exchange Lists.	Written information reinforces learning, clarifies verbal instructions, minimizes the risk of errors, and allows maximum patient control and flexibility.
Patient verbalizes knowledge of prescribed insulin, dosage, and action.	Explain the pharmacokinetics of prescribed insulin preparation and administration schedule as presented in Tables 30–4 and 30–5.	Insulin is the only antidiabetic agent used to treat IDDM. The patient must have this information to safely self-administer insulin and minimize the risk of complications.
Patient demonstrates ability to prepare and administer insulin correctly.	Teach the procedure according to instructions in Chart 30–1. Observe the patient performing the procedure daily.	Provides opportunity for repeated feedback to reinforce proper technique and correct errors.
Patient demonstrates ability to test blood glucose and correctly interpret results.	Teach patient to test blood glucose according to manufacturer's instructions. Observe patient perform procedure to assess technique, ability to follow instructions, and accuracy of results.	Frequent self–blood glucose monitoring is the best way to evaluate the diabetic treatment plan. Patient must understand and adhere to the manufacturer's instructions to obtain accurate results. Proper technique in obtaining specimen minimizes the risk of infection.
	Provide written information on normal blood glucose values, actions to take when results are abnormal (adjust insulin, modify diet, call physician), and how to adjust for changes in physical activity or illness.	Good diabetic control requires a dynamic balance between diet, insulin, and activity. Adjustment must be made to compensate for changes in any component.

(continued)

Nursing Care Guide 30–1. *(continued)*

PATIENTS WITH DIABETES MELLITUS

Patient Outcomes	Nursing Interventions	Rationale
Patient demonstrates ability to prepare and administer insulin correctly.	Teach patient to test urine for ketones according to manufacturer's directions. Observe patient perform procedure to evaluate technique and accuracy.	Patient must understand and adhere to the manufacturer's instructions to obtain accurate results.
	Instruct patient to test urine for ketones if blood glucose level is higher than 250 mg/dl or if she is ill or pregnant.	Patient is at risk for diabetic ketoacidosis in these situations.
	Provide written instructions on actions to take if ketones are present in the urine. Reinforce the need to notify physician promptly if ketones are present.	Ketonuria indicates incomplete metabolism of body fats. Early detection and treatment minimize the risk of a potentially life-threatening complication. Adjustment in diet or insulin reduces risk of future episodes.
Patient states causes, signs, symptoms, and treatment of hypoglycemia.	Teach patient that: ■ Hypoglycemia is caused by too much insulin, too little food, or a sudden increase in exercise. ■ Signs and symptoms are shaking, sweating, weakness, hunger, dizziness, drowsiness, and confusion. ■ If symptoms occur, take a simple carbohydrate, such as 4 oz fruit juice or regular soda, 2 tsp honey, two lumps of sugar, five or six Life Savers, glucose tablets, or ½ oz of sugar gel icing. Repeat in 10 to 15 minutes if symptoms do not resolve. ■ Follow with a complex carbohydrate and protein snack, such as cheese and crackers and skim milk if the next meal is more than 2 hours away.	Hypoglycemia places the patient at risk for physical injury and irreversible brain damage. It is easily reversed if detected and treated early.
	Teach significant other how to prepare and administer parenteral glucagon if the patient is unconscious.	Glucagon raises blood glucose level by promoting conversion of hepatic glycogen to glucose.

(continued)

Nursing Care Guide 30–1. *(continued)*

PATIENTS WITH DIABETES MELLITUS

Patient Outcomes	Nursing Interventions	Rationale
Patient states causes, signs, symptoms, and treatment of hyperglycemia and ketoacidosis.	Teach patient that: ■ Hyperglycemia and ketoacidosis are caused by insufficient insulin, too much food, not enough exercise, infection, or stress. ■ Signs and symptoms are unusual thirst, frequent urination, weakness, blurred vision, abdominal pain, nausea and vomiting, and blood glucose level higher than goal range of 70 to 140 mg/dl. ■ If symptoms occur, test blood glucose, take insulin if previously instructed in amount to take, drink fluids, and call physician.	Hyperglycemia and ketoacidosis are acute complications of IDDM. Early detection and treatment minimize the risk of a life-threatening situation. Maintenance of blood glucose levels below 140 mg/dl slows the progression of long-term degenerative changes of diabetes.
Patient verbalizes understanding of foot-care routine and other hygiene practices to incorporate into lifestyle.	Teach patient daily foot care as presented in Chart 30–4. Other health care practices include meticulous oral hygiene, dental appointment every 6 months, annual influenza vaccinations, not smoking, and complete physical examination with evaluation of renal function annually or as recommended by physician.	Patients with diabetes are at risk for infection due to impaired leukocyte activity. These health care practices minimize the risk of infection and promote early detection of health problems.
	Instruct patient to have an annual eye examination by an ophthalmologist.	Diabetic retinopathy is usually the earliest degenerative change of diabetes to develop. Early detection and treatment can minimize impairment of vision.

Evaluation: Compare the patient's status with the expected patient outcomes. If the outcomes are achieved, evaluate nursing care as successful. If not, reassess the patient, formulate new nursing diagnoses, and revise expected patient outcomes and nursing interventions as appropriate.

each patient. The patient's lifestyle and other health care needs have to be considered. In planning care for the elderly diabetic patient, carefully assess for special needs associated with altered function that usually occurs with aging, such as poor vision and decreased dexterity, memory impairment or loss, and hearing loss. All these factors can affect the patient's ability for self-care.

Because of advanced age, and because decreased secretion of counterregulatory hormones places the elderly diabetic patient at high risk for hypoglycemia, the advantage of "tight control" to delay the onset of long-term degenerative changes in the elderly patient is questionable. However, most clinicians agree that the problems associated with cataracts, neuropathy, and infection can be decreased by maintaining blood glucose levels below 200 mg/dl in the elderly.

Initially, diet therapy may be the only treatment tried for the newly diagnosed elderly patient, providing blood glucose levels are not higher than 300 mg/dl and the patient is not hyperosmolar. The diabetic regimen is aimed at imposing minimal restrictions and changes in the patient's lifestyle, especially for the newly diagnosed patient. It is important to emphasize the importance of eating nutritious meals on a regular basis. Of course, patients who have been previously diagnosed and who are accustomed to managing diabetes may continue to do so unless failing health requires simplification of the routine.

Although diet therapy may be aimed at reducing calories, a concern when treating the elderly diabetic patient is that of consuming too few calories rather than too many because of financial constraints and because of reduced food intake resulting from decreased taste sensation and limited mobility. Therefore, it is important that a family member or friend supervise the patient's meals to ensure adequate food intake. The elderly diabetic patient can also be referred to Meals On Wheels, a subsidized government agency that can deliver diabetic meals to the home. The diet consists of 60% to 70% carbohydrate, 15% to 20% protein, and 20% fat. The patient taking antidiabetic medication is advised not to fast for religious reasons because of the risk of hypoglycemia.

Although age is not a contraindication for insulin administration, consideration must be given to the patient's ability to prepare the insulin accurately, to monitor control, and to comply with the diet. One or two injections of intermediate-acting insulin or a premixed combination of short-acting and intermediate-acting insulin may be prescribed to be taken before breakfast and supper. In prescribing insulin, the goal is to keep the patient asymptomatic and the blood glucose levels below 200 mg/dl. only. Because there is a decrease in subcutaneous fat in the elderly, it is most important to rotate injection sites. A syringe magnifier can be obtained for the elderly patient with poor vision to ensure accuracy in preparing insulin injections.

Oral antidiabetic agents or sulfonylureas are usually effective in patients who have a blood glucose level below 200 mg/dl. Before prescribing, the individual characteristics of these drugs have to be considered, with special attention paid to the needs of the individual patient. For example, tolazamide has a short half-life, which decreases the risk of hypoglycemia. However, it also has a mild diuretic effect, which may or may not be desirable depending on other medications the patient is taking. Tolbutamide requires two or three daily doses, making compliance a potential problem. The possibility of drug interactions is great because the elderly tend to take many medications such as salicylates, furosemide, thiazide diuretics, and anticoagulants, which are known to have negative interactions with oral antidiabetic agents.

Second-generation sulfonylureas have advantages over first-generation sulfonylureas. Because glipizide is metabolized mostly by the liver, complications resulting from impaired renal function are decreased. Also, hypoglycemia and drug interactions are rare. These drugs are usually taken once a day on an empty stomach, and they are inexpensive.

New technology has made blood glucose testing at home easier. However, if the patient has limited range of motion and dexterity, urine testing may be preferred. Medicare covers the cost of a blood glucose testing device and testing strips. Because short-term memory loss may increase with age, the elderly patient is encouraged to keep a written record of test results. Measurement of glycosylated hemoglobin (HbA_{1c}) several times a year gives an approximation of glucose control. A result of 10% is acceptable for an elderly diabetic patient.

Because the elderly are more prone to upper respiratory infections and pneumonia, the elderly diabetic patient is advised to obtain pneumonia and influenza vaccines. Older people are also more prone to foot problems as a result of the normal physiologic changes of aging, yet they may have difficulty adhering to a regimen of daily foot care as outlined in Chart 30–4. Foot care by a podiatrist every 6 months is recommended. The elderly diabetic patient should always wear diabetic identification.

Because proper management of diabetes depends on the ability of the patient to learn the self-care routine, patient teaching is an important component of the treatment plan. The educational assessment may take longer in the elderly patient, but it is essential in developing teaching strategies. The patient is taught whatever content is necessary to live safely with diabetes and maintain optimum wellness. All verbal instructions are reinforced with clearly printed or large-type, written instruction.

Bibliography

American Diabetes Association. Diabetes facts and figures. Alexandria, VA: National Service Center, 1988.

American Diabetes Association. Physician's guide to insulin-dependent (type I) diabetes, diagnosis and treatment. Alexandria, VA: National Service Center, 1988.

American Diabetes Association. Physician's guide to non-insulin dependent (type II) diabetes, diagnosis and treatment. 2nd ed. Alexandria, VA: National Service Center, 1988.

American Diabetes Association. Goals for diabetes education. Alexandria, VA: National Service Center, 1989.

American Diabetes Association. Managing diabetes in the 1990s. Alexandria, VA: National Service Center, 1989.

American Diabetes Association. Standards of medical care for patients with diabetes mellitus. Alexandria, VA: National Service Center, 1989.

American Diabetes Association and American Dietetic Association. Exchange lists for meal planning. Alexandria, VA: National Service Center, 1989.

Bantle J. Injection site rotation. Practical Diabetology 1990; 9(5):1.

Bartlett EE. The stepped approach to patient education. Diabetes Educ 1988; 14(2):130.

Baum N, et al. Evaluation and treatment of organic impotence in the male with diabetes mellitus. Diabetes Educ 1988; 14(2):123.

Becker S. The risks and rewards of pancreatic transplant. RN 1989; 52(7):54.

Carpenito LJ. Nursing diagnosis: Application to clinical practice. 4th ed. Philadelphia: JB Lippincott, 1992.

Christman C, Bennett J. Diabetes new names, new tests, new diet. Nursing 1987; 17(1):34.

Cooper NA. Nutrition and diabetes: A review of current recommendations. Diabetes Educ 1988; 14(5):428.

Davis ED, Chesnaky P. Site rotation. Diabetes Forecast 1992; 45(3):54.

Davis M. End-stage renal disease. Practical Diabetology 1990; 9(3):5.

De Lawter DE. Beating the odds against peripheral vascular disease. Diabetes Self-Management. 1990; 7(1):34.

Dellasega C. Self-care for the elderly diabetic. Gerontol Nurs 1990; 16(1):16.

DePonti F, Malagelada JR. Diabetes mellitus and the gut. Practical Diabetology 1990; 9(2):8.

Dinsmoor RS. Insulin: A user's guide. Diabetes Self-Management 1991; 8(2):42.

Dinsmoor RS. Should you refrigerate your insulin? Diabetes Self-Management 1991; 8(2):21.

Doenges ME, Moorhouse MF. Nurse's pocket guide: Nursing diagnoses with interventions. 4th ed. Philadelphia: FA Davis, 1993.

Drass J. What you need to know about insulin injections. Nursing 1992; 22(11):40.

Dworetzky T. A bold step in preventing diabetes. Countdown 1991; 12(1):31.

Edson L. Treatment update. Countdown 1990; 11(1):14.

Eliopoulos C. Gerontological nursing. 3rd ed. Philadelphia: JB Lippincott, 1993.

Everetti A, Ferris F. The early treatment of diabetic retinopathy. Diabetes Educ 1988; 14(5):421.

Farkas-Hirsch R, Levandoske LA. Implementation of continuous subcutaneous insulin infusion therapy: An overview. Diabetes Educ 1988; 14(5):401.

Fleckman A. Diabetic ketoacidosis. Practical Diabetology 1991; 10(3): 1.

Franz MJ. Do alcohol and diabetes mix? Diabetes Self-Management 1990; 7(3):25.

Gettrust KV, Brabec PD. Nursing diagnosis in clinical practice. Albany, NY: Delmar Publishers, 1992.

Guthrie D (ed). Diabetes education: A core curriculum for health professionals. Chicago: American Association of Diabetes Educators, 1988.

Guyton AG. Textbook of medical physiology. 8th ed. Philadelphia: WB Saunders, 1991.

Havlin CE, Cryer PE. Hypoglycemia: The limiting factor in the management of insulin-dependent diabetes mellitus. Diabetes Educ 1988; 14(5):407.

Hurxthal K. Quick! Teach this patient about insulin. Am J Nurs 1988; 88(8):1097.

Jackson R. The search for a way to prevent diabetes. Diabetes in the News 1992; 11(2): 6.

Jinks MJ, Evenson LM. Looking at diabetes through older eyes problems and solutions. Diabetes Self-Management 1990; 7(1):38.

Joshu DH, Flavin K, Clutter W. Contrasting type I and type II diabetes. Am J Nurs 1986; 86(11):1240.

Kee JL. Fluids and electrolytes with clinical applications. 4th ed. New York: John Wiley & Sons, 1986.

Kestel F. Using blood glucose meters: What you and your patient need to know. Part I. Nursing 1993; 23(3):34.

Kestel F. Using blood glucose meters: What you and your patient need to know. Part II. Nursing 1993; 23(4):50.

Kestel F. Using blood glucose meters: What you and your patient need to know. Part III. Nursing 1993; 23(5):51.

Lorber DL. Commentary definitions and diagnoses. Practical Diabetology 1990; 9(3):16.

Macheca MKK. Diabetic hypoglycemia: Keeping the threat at bay. Am J Nurs 1993; 93(4):26.

Matheson D, Efantis J. Diabetes and pregnancy: Need and use of intensive therapy. Diabetes Educ 1989; 15(3):242.

Mecklenburg R. Acute complications associated with the use of insulin infusion pumps. Diabetes Educ 1989; 15(1):40.

Mecklenburg RS. Treating ketoacidosis. Practical Diabetology 1990; 9(2):13.

Messana I, Beizer J. Diabetes in the elderly. Practical Diabetology 1991; 10(1):1.

Morley JE. Diabetes in elderly patients. Practical Diabetology 1988; 7(5):6.

Mulkeen H. Diabetes teaching the teaching of self-care. Nurs Times 1989; 85(3):63.

Nelson RL. The OGTT, its practical use. Diabetes Spectrum 1989; 2(4):219.

Nettles AT. Pancreas transplantation: A University of Minnesota perspective. Diabetes Educ 1992; 18(3):232.

North American Nursing Diagnosis Association. NANDA Nursing diagnoses: Definitions and classifications. St. Louis, MO: North American Nursing Diagnosis Association, 1992.

Peragallo-Dittko V. All about insulin. Diabetes Self-Management 1988; 5(4):21.

Petrucci K. Diagnostic reasoning strategies for the elderly person with diabetes. Diabetes Management Issues for the Educator 1988; 5.

Saltiel-Berzin R. Managing a surgical patient who has diabetes. Nursing 1992; 22(4):34.

Saudek CD, et al. Implanted insulin pumps. Practical Diabetology 1990; 9(2):18.

Schuman C. Controlling diabetes during surgery. Diabetes Spectrum 1989; 2(4):263.

Singer A. Peripheral vascular disease and the diabetic foot. Practical Diabetology 1987; 6(4):12.

Steil CF, Deakins DA. Today's insulins: What you and your patient need to know. Nursing 1990; 20(8):34.

Steil CF, Deakins DA. Oral hypoglycemics: What you and your patient need to know. Nursing 1992; 22(11):34.

Taylor DL. Hypoglycemia physiology, signs, and symptoms. Nursing Life 1987; 7(1):36.

Tietyen J. Dietary fiber in foods: Options for diabetes education. Diabetes Educ 1989; 115(6):523.

Timby BK. Clinical nursing procedures. Philadelphia: JB Lippincott, 1989.

Ulrich SP, Canale SW, Wendell SA. Nursing care planning guides: A nursing diagnosis approach. 2nd ed. Philadelphia: WB Saunders, 1990.

Vinicor F. Atherosclerosis and diabetes mellitus. Diabetes Spectrum 1988; 1(5):319.

Wechsler R. What causes diabetes? Countdown 1990; 11(1):10.

Wechsler R. High blood sugar: The root of complications. Countdown 1990; 11(1):20.

Zehrer C, Hansen R, Bantle J. Reducing blood glucose variability by use of abdominal insulin injection sites. Diabetes Educ 1990; 16(6):474.

Chapter Thirty-one

NURSING CARE *of Adults with* Pituitary Disorders

The pituitary gland is a vital link in the hypothalamus-pituitary-endocrine gland axis that maintains homeostasis. Pituitary disorders involve a deficiency or excess of one or more pituitary hormones and are manifested by altered function in target organs and tissues throughout the body. Normal pituitary function and common disorders of the pituitary gland are presented in this chapter. Nurses must integrate understanding of normal gland function with the pathophysiology, etiology, and medical management of pituitary disorders to develop a comprehensive plan of care that meets the needs of these patients.

Anatomy and Physiology

The pituitary gland or hypophysis is a complex structure composed of many independently functioning units, each of which is regulated by the hypothalamus. As discussed in Chapter 29, the pituitary gland is anatomically and physiologically divided into two functioning lobes (see Fig. 29–5, p. 369): the adenohypophysis (anterior lobe) and the neurohypophysis (posterior lobe).

The posterior lobe of the pituitary gland is neural in origin. Its functioning unit is composed mainly of axons, which originate in the hypothalamus and then pass down the hypothalamic-hypophyseal tract in the pituitary stalk or infundibulum to terminate in the neurohypophysis. The posterior pituitary stores and secretes antidiuretic hormone (ADH) and oxytocin, which are produced in the hypothalamus.

The anterior lobe, which accounts for approximately 80% of the entire pituitary, is glandular in structure. It is composed of several different cell types, each of which functions as an almost independent unit in response to hypothalamic stimulation to secrete its own hormone or hormones. Table 31–1 identifies the cell types and the hormones secreted from each.

A review of Table 29–1 (p. 366) identifies the primary functions of each of the hormones secreted by the anterior pituitary gland and the target organ or tissue that each affects. A pituitary hormone may produce its effect either by altering the physiologic function of its target cells or tissue or by altering the secretory function of other endocrine glands. Table 31–2 identifies the target glands and tissues of each of the anterior pituitary hormones.

Table 31–1. ANTERIOR PITUITARY GLAND CELL TYPE AND HORMONE SECRETED

CELL TYPE	HORMONE SECRETED
Somatotrope	Somatotropin (STH, growth hormone)
Thyrotrope	Thyrotropin (TSH)
Corticotrope	Adrenocorticotropic hormone (ACTH)
	Melanocyte-stimulating hormone (MSH)
Gonadotrope	Luteinizing hormone (LH)
	Follicle-stimulating hormone (FSH)
Lactotrope	Prolactin (PRL)

Table 31–2. ANTERIOR PITUITARY HORMONES AND THEIR TARGET GLANDS OR TISSUES

HORMONE	TARGET
Somatotropin (STH)	Body cells
Thyrotropin (TSH)	Thyroid gland
Adrenocorticotropic hormone (ACTH)	Adrenal cortex
Luteinizing hormone (LH)	Ovaries
Follicle-stimulating hormone (FSH)	Ovaries
Prolactin (PRL)	Mammary glands
Melanocyte-stimulating hormone (MSH)	Melanocytes

The pituitary hormones that directly affect the secretory functions of other endocrine glands are referred to as tropic hormones. The presence of a tropic hormone stimulates the target gland to secrete its hormone or hormones. When the tropic hormone is no longer present, secretion from the target gland stops. If pituitary dysfunction causes hyposecretion or hypersecretion of a tropic hormone, the individual shows clinical signs of a corresponding alteration in secretion from the dependent target gland.

Secretion of all anterior pituitary hormones is monitored by the hypothalamus and regulated through negative feedback control. As illustrated in Figure 31–1, a stimulus monitored by the hypothalamus indicates an alteration in the homeostasis of the body. The hypothalamus responds by secreting a releasing hormone. The releasing hormone stimulates one of the secretory cell types in the anterior pituitary to secrete its tropic hormone. The tropic hormone is released into the systemic circulation and stimulates secretion by its target gland. As the target gland secretes its hormone, physiologic changes occur that are monitored by the hypothalamus. These changes may be the rising serum level of the hormone secreted by the target gland, which is monitored directly by the hypothalamus, or other physiologic alterations initiated by the effect of the target gland hormone. The physiologic effects are then monitored by the hypothalamus through impulses transmitted to it by the central nervous system. When the desired physiologic changes have occurred, the hypothalamus stops secretion of the releasing hormone or secretes an inhibiting hormone, and secretion of the tropic hormone from the anterior pituitary ceases.

Because of its role as a regulator of pituitary secretion, dysfunction of the hypothalamus, although rare, can result in pituitary dysfunction.

A number of other disorders can alter pituitary function. Most common among these are secreting and nonsecreting tumors of the gland itself, pressure from tumors in adjacent tissues, genetic disorders,

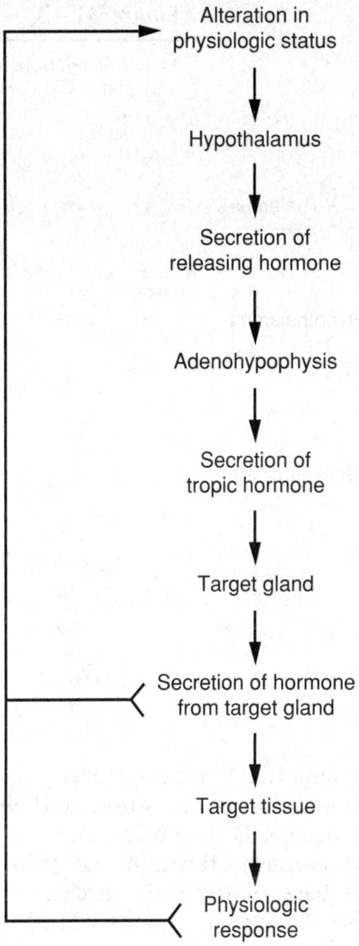

Figure 31–1.

Negative feedback regulation of endocrine secretion.

iatrogenic disorders, and trauma. At the same time, because of its influence on other endocrine glands, pituitary disorders can have wide-ranging and serious effects on the body.

Pituitary disorders are grouped according to the pituitary lobe involved, the dysfunction that results, and the specific hormone affected. They are further classified as primary, caused by a dysfunction within the gland itself, or as secondary, caused by either a dysfunction of the hypothalamus or some other factor outside of the gland itself.

Anterior Pituitary Disorders

Disorders of the anterior lobe of the pituitary can cause an alteration in the function of any one or all of the secretory cell types. Altered function of the secretory cells can result in hyposecretion or hypersecretion of one or more anterior pituitary hormones.

Neoplasia

ETIOLOGY

Pituitary tumors are the most common cause of primary anterior pituitary disorders. Although a pituitary tumor can develop at any age, they are most common in adults, with equal distribution between men and women. The etiologic factors related to their development are unclear.

PATHOPHYSIOLOGY

Pituitary tumors are usually benign secreting adenomas that arise from one cell type and produce clinical manifestations of hypersecretion of one or two pituitary hormones. The individual with a pituitary tumor may also have neurologic manifestations that are caused by pressure exerted on adjacent tissues and structures by the expanding pituitary mass. Pituitary adenomas account for 6% to 18% of all intracranial tumors and are rarely malignant.

CLINICAL MANIFESTATIONS

The majority of individuals with a pituitary adenoma seek medical attention because of the neurologic manifestations of the tumor.

NEUROLOGIC MANIFESTATIONS

Frequently recurring headache unrelated to stress or other apparent physiologic or psychological factors is the most common neurologic manifestation of pituitary adenomas. The headaches are caused by pressure from the expanding mass on the surrounding tissues and vascular structures.

Visual disturbances are the second most common neurologic manifestation. Because of anatomic proximity, as illustrated in Figure 31–2, expansion of the pituitary mass may press on or displace the optic chiasm and optic nerve. Loss of vision in the lateral portions of both visual fields (bitemporal hemianopia) with no change in visual acuity is the most common visual disturbance.

Other neurologic manifestations are rare but may include vascular disturbances and involvement of the cranial nerves.

ENDOCRINE MANIFESTATIONS

The most common pituitary adenomas arise from the lactotrope and somatotrope cells and are discussed later in this chapter. Adenomas of the corticotrope cells are less common, and those of the thyrotrope and gonadotrope cells are rare.

Because of its tropic effect, hypersecretion of a pituitary hormone caused by a secreting adenoma results in increased secretion from the hormone's target gland. For this reason, any individual with

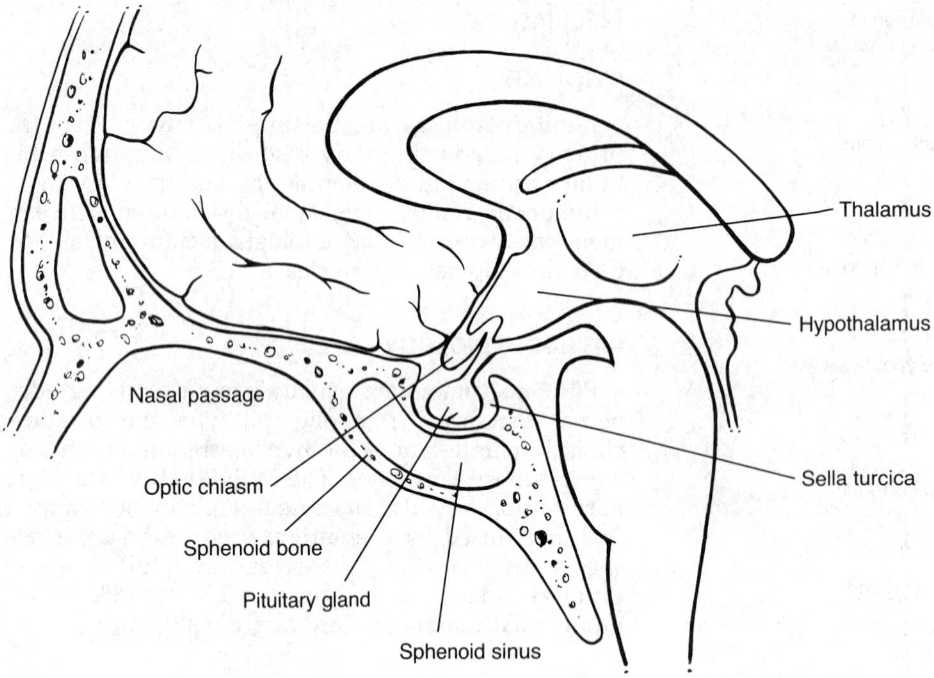

Figure 31–2.

Anatomic relationship of the pituitary gland and the optic chiasm.

clinical manifestations of hypersecretion from an endocrine gland that is under the control of the anterior pituitary must be evaluated for the presence of a pituitary adenoma.

MEDICAL DIAGNOSIS

Medical diagnosis of a pituitary tumor is made on the basis of the patient's history, clinical manifestations, radiologic studies, and serum hormone level determinations. Pituitary hormone levels are elevated in the presence of a secreting pituitary adenoma. Other possible causes of endocrine dysfunction, such as stress or side effects of pharmacotherapy, must be ruled out before confirming a diagnosis of pituitary tumor.

MEDICAL MANAGEMENT

The primary modalities of treatment for a pituitary tumor are surgical excision and irradiation. Tumors of the lactotrope and somatotrope cells have also been found to respond well to pharmacotherapy with bromocriptine (Parlodel).

TRANSSPHENOIDAL MICROSURGERY

Excision of a pituitary adenoma by transsphenoidal microsurgery is the surgical procedure of choice to remove a pituitary tumor while preserving as much normal pituitary tissue as possible. If the entire pituitary gland is removed by the transsphenoidal approach, the surgery is referred to as a total transsphenoidal hypophysectomy.

In transsphenoidal microsurgery, an incision is made at the junction of the gums and upper lip. A surgical microscope is then advanced along the floor of the nasal passage, through the sphenoid sinus, and into the base of the sella turcica, as illustrated in Figure 31–3. Special microsurgical instruments are used to incise the dura mater and to identify and remove the abnormal tissue. Destruction of the abnormal tissue by laser is under investigation. To prevent leakage of cerebrospinal fluid (CSF) after surgery, the dura mater may be patched with a piece of fascia or muscle taken from the leg. The nose is packed, and a gauze dressing or sling is worn under the nose to absorb drainage and to keep the packing in place.

Excision of pituitary adenomas by transsphenoidal microsurgery has a success rate between 70% and 90%. The most common complication is temporary diabetes insipidus (discussed later in this chapter) caused by surgical trauma to the posterior pituitary. Because prophylactic antibiotics are used, meningitis is rare. If a total hypophysectomy is performed, or if normal pituitary tissue is damaged, panhypopituitarism will develop, and the patient will require lifelong hormone-replacement therapy because of the absence of adrenocorticotropic hormone, thyrotropin, and the gonadotropins.

TRANSFRONTAL CRANIOTOMY

If the pituitary adenoma has spread beyond the sella turcica, a total hypophysectomy is performed using a transfrontal craniotomy approach. The preoperative and postoperative care of a patient undergoing a craniotomy procedure is similar to that for transsphenoidal surgery with specific modifications because of the more invasive procedure used. Nursing care after a transfrontal craniotomy is discussed in Chapter 37.

IRRADIATION

Treatment of a pituitary adenoma by external radiation is an alternative to surgery in some cases. Successful reduction of tumor size and neurologic manifestations is similar to that achieved through microsurgery. However, reduction in hormone levels is not as rapid, and it may take up to 2 years for the hormone levels to return to normal.

Stereotaxic radiosurgery is a new method of treating cranial tumors. It uses high-energy, pencil-thin beams of external radiation from a linear accelerator to destroy tumor tissue. Its application to the treatment of pituitary tumors is under investigation.

Nursing care of a patient undergoing conventional and stereotaxic irradiation to the brain is discussed in Chapter 37.

Implantation of radioactive isotopes is seldom performed because of advances in treatment by microsurgery and external radiation and because of the possibility of meningitis and chronic rhinorrhea after the implantation procedure.

Application of the Nursing Process to the Care of the Patient with a Pituitary Neoplasm

Assessment

When obtaining a nursing history from an individual with a pituitary tumor, first determine what clinical manifestations are present. If headaches are present, ask the patient to describe them and to point to the areas of the head involved. Determine when the headaches first began, how often they occur, what precipitates them, and what relieves them.

If visual disturbances are reported by the patient, ask when visual changes were first noticed. Assess visual acuity and visual fields (see Chapter 39) even if a visual disturbance is not reported by the patient. Because visual changes associated with a pituitary tumor develop very gradually, many individuals may not be aware that visual loss has occurred.

Assess the patient's knowledge or interpretation of the cause of neurologic symptoms present. Neurologic disturbances are very frightening to most individuals and are often misinterpreted.

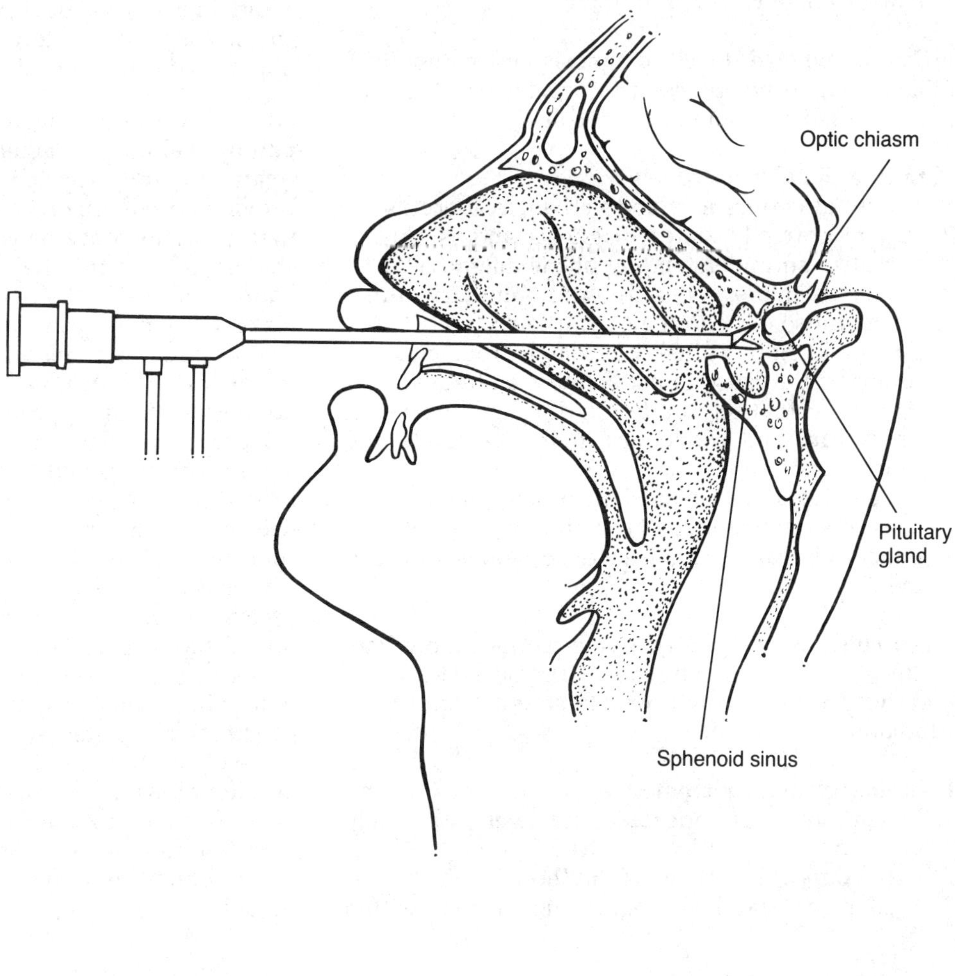

Figure 31–3.

Illustration of the placement of a surgical microscope for transsphenoidal microsurgery.

A complete nursing assessment of a patient with a suspected pituitary adenoma includes assessment for the alterations common to endocrine dysfunctions identified in Chapter 29. The clinical manifestations present will vary according to the specific hormone or hormones affected. Document findings accurately to facilitate diagnosis. Nursing assessments related to altered secretion of specific anterior pituitary hormones are discussed later in this chapter.

Allay preoperative and postoperative anxiety. Determine what the patient knows about the surgery as well as expectations of the postoperative recovery period to identify teaching needs.

Nursing Diagnoses and Planning

Nursing diagnoses and related expected patient outcomes most commonly applicable to patients with a pituitary tumor include the following:

NDx: High risk for trauma related to loss of peripheral vision

Planning: Patient outcomes
1. Patient accurately states degree of loss of peripheral vision.
2. Patient identifies safety measures to avoid trauma.
3. Patient remains free from injury.

NDx: Knowledge deficit: diagnosis and pathophysiology, diagnostic procedures, planned treatment, and expected outcome of treatment

Planning: Patient outcomes
1. Patient asks questions and verbalizes concerns.
2. Patient correctly states diagnosis and is able to verbalize an understanding of the diagnosis.
3. Patient identifies pressure from pituitary tumor as the cause of neurologic symptoms.
4. Patient identifies altered secretion from pituitary tumor as the cause of endocrine manifestations.
5. Patient verbalizes understanding of diagnostic procedures and cooperates in their accurate and timely completion.
6. Patient identifies planned treatment and the reasons this treatment has been chosen.
7. Patient verbalizes realistic expectations of treatment.

NDx: High risk for altered tissue perfusion: cerebral, related to increased intracranial pressure (ICP) secondary to tumor growth or edema after surgery or irradiation

Planning: Patient outcomes
1. Patient remains oriented and alert or easily aroused.
2. Urine output less than 100 ml/hour.
3. Vital signs and neurologic signs remain within normal limits (see discussion of increased ICP in Chapter 37).
4. Patient avoids activities that increase ICP.

NDx: High risk for infection related to surgical incision of the dura mater, oral and nasal mucous membranes, and possibly the leg

Planning: Patient outcomes
1. Patient remains afebrile and free of headaches and nuchal rigidity.
2. Oral and nasal mucous membranes and leg remain free of inflammation, swelling, and purulent drainage.

Nursing Interventions

Nursing care of a patient with a pituitary tumor includes maintaining the patient's safety, monitoring neurologic status, assessing changes in physiologic manifestations of endocrine function, and providing appropriate information and teaching. Changes in vital signs, neurologic signs, and visual fields may indicate growth or regression of the tumor and are reported to the physician promptly.

NDx: High risk for trauma
Assess visual fields and acuity to determine extent of loss. Orient the visually impaired patient to the surroundings, and maintain a safe environment to avoid injury. Explain operation of call bell system, and instruct patient to request assistance before getting out of bed if visual impairment is severe.

NDx: Knowledge deficit: diagnosis and pathophysiology, diagnostic procedures, planned treatment, and expected outcome of treatment
Provide ample opportunity for the patient to express thoughts and concerns about physical changes he or she is experiencing. Reinforce the physician's explanations of the pathology causing the symptoms in terms the patient can understand. Answer questions and correct any misconceptions about symptoms, diagnosis, and treatment. Refer questions you cannot answer to an appropriate resource.

During the diagnostic phase, assess the patient's ability to understand and cooperate with diagnostic procedures. Provide appropriate instruction and necessary assistance to ensure timely and accurate collection of required specimens.

Discuss the planned procedure with the patient preoperatively, and correct any misconceptions or unrealistic expectations about the surgery or expected results. Even though excess hormone secretion will cease after surgery and the patient will feel progressively better, some alterations caused by increased hormone levels, such as excess bone growth or alterations in cardiac function, may be permanent. Be sure to inform the patient if a piece of fascia or muscle is to be removed from the leg so the presence of a second surgical dressing is expected.

Nursing Care Guide 31–1.

POSTOPERATIVE CARE OF PATIENTS UNDERGOING TRANSSPHENOIDAL MICROSURGERY FOR EXCISION OF A PITUITARY ADENOMA

Assessment Findings: Six hours after transsphenoidal microsurgery, a patient who was previously alert and oriented is now becoming restless and vague in responses to questions. Patient complains of blurred vision but denies headache. Pupils react equally but sluggishly to light. Vital signs are stable.

Nursing Diagnosis: Altered tissue perfusion: cerebral related to increased intracranial pressure (ICP) secondary to cerebral edema from surgical trauma

Patient Outcomes	Nursing Interventions	Rationale
Patient remains alert and oriented as evidenced by: 1. is alert or is easily aroused when asleep. 2. correctly identifies person, place, and a realistic time frame. 3. responds appropriately to questions.	Elevate head of bed 30 to 45 degrees. Patient may turn side to side.	Elevation promotes venous drainage and reduces cerebral edema.
	Provide rest periods.	Reduction in external stimuli promotes reduction in cerebral edema.
	Administer prescribed humidified oxygen.	Increases cerebral oxygenation.
	Talk with patient while assessing vital signs and neurologic signs.	Deterioration in mental status is a manifestation of increasing cerebral edema.
Patient avoids activities that increase ICP.	Instruct the patient preoperatively and remind him or her postoperatively not to cough, sneeze, bend from the waist, pull or push with arms, hyperflex the neck, or brush hair vigorously.	These activities increase ICP.
	Before discharge, teach the patient to avoid activities that will increase ICP for up to 2 months.	Avoid activities that increase ICP until the sphenoid sinus and sella turcica heal completely.

(continued)

NDx: High risk for altered tissue perfusion: cerebral

Teach the patient preoperatively to avoid sneezing, coughing, bending, vigorous hair brushing, or any activity that will increase ICP and may cause a CSF leak after surgery. Teach and have the patient practice deep-breathing exercises, which will be used postoperatively to ventilate the lungs and mobilize secretions, because postoperative coughing is prohibited.

Postoperatively, the patient usually feels relatively well, with discomfort similar to a headache. Low doses of narcotic analgesics are prescribed, if needed, for relief. Begin oral fluids as soon as the effects of anesthesia are worn off and progress the diet as tolerated.

Elevate the head of the bed 30 degrees at all times to reduce cerebral edema. The patient may be positioned side to side. Assess vital signs and neurologic signs to detect an increase in ICP from cerebral edema.

Frequently remind the patient to adhere to preoperative instructions to avoid any activity that may increase ICP. Have the patient take five deep breaths every half-hour to prevent pulmonary complications, which could cause increased ICP associated with fever, restlessness, or hypoxia. Assess for the onset of nausea and vomiting, and administer antiemetics promptly because vomiting will cause a rise in ICP.

Monitor intake and output to detect onset of diabetes insipidus. Report an output of more than 100 ml/hour to the physician promptly. Nursing care of the patient who has undergone transsphenoidal microsurgery for excision of a pituitary adenoma is summarized in Nursing Care Guide 31–1.

Nursing Care Guide 31–1. *(continued)*

POSTOPERATIVE CARE OF PATIENTS UNDERGOING TRANSSPHENOIDAL MICROSURGERY FOR EXCISION OF A PITUITARY ADENOMA

Patient Outcomes	Nursing Interventions	Rationale
Patient is free of nausea and vomiting.	Instruct patient to advise nurse at first sign of nausea. Administer prescribed antiemetic promptly.	Vomiting increases ICP.
Patient is alert and oriented, pulse is 60–100 bpm, systolic blood pressure is within 10% of preoperative baseline, respirations are 16–20/minute, urine output is less than 100 ml/hour, strength in bilateral extremities is equal, and pupils react equally to light.	Monitor vital signs, urine output, and neurologic signs hourly for early signs of increased ICP: restlessness, lethargy, confusion, bradycardia, widening pulse pressure, vague headache, dilated pupils, diplopia, blurred vision, progressive muscle weakness, polyuria.	These manifestations indicate impaired cerebral blood flow, decreased tissue oxygenation, and increased pressure on vital brain centers. Early detection of increased ICP prevents cerebral anoxia and irreversible brain damage.
	Administer osmotic diuretics, steroids, or anticonvulsants if prescribed.	Osmotic diuretics reduce cerebral edema. Steroids reduce inflammation of cerebral tissue. Anticonvulsants prevent seizure activity, which can increase cerebral edema and impair tissue oxygenation.

Evaluation: Compare the patient's status with the expected patient outcomes. If the outcomes are achieved, evaluate nursing care as successful. If not, reassess the patient, formulate new nursing diagnoses, and revise expected patient outcomes and nursing interventions as appropriate.

Assessment Findings: Patient has a moderate amount of clear drainage from nasal packing and gauze dressing under the nose.

Nursing Diagnosis: High risk for infection related to surgical incision of the sella turcica and dura mater

Patient Outcomes	Nursing Interventions	Rationale
Patient is free of signs of cerebral spinal fluid (CSF) leak within 72 hours.	Assess for and ask patient about signs of CSF leak: frequent swallowing, sensation of postnasal drip, rapid saturation of gauze pad under nose with clear drainage.	These manifestations indicate leakage of CSF from the sella turcica through the surgical access tract into the posterior nasopharynx. This tract is a possible route for invasion of pathogenic organisms until the dura mater seals. The dura mater should seal within 72 hours.

(continued)

Nursing Care Guide 31–1. *(continued)*

POSTOPERATIVE CARE OF PATIENTS UNDERGOING TRANSSPHENOIDAL MICROSURGERY FOR EXCISION OF A PITUITARY ADENOMA

Patient Outcomes	Nursing Interventions	Rationale
	Test nasal drainage for glucose with a glucose reagent strip. Alternative assessment for CSF is to examine a drop of nasal drainage on a clean cloth or gauze for a pale yellow halo around the pink serosanguineous drainage.	Differentiates between CSF and serous drainage. Glucose is normally present in CSF but not in serous exudate.
Patient remains afebrile and free of nuchal rigidity.	Change dressing under the nose as it becomes moist or soiled.	Moist dressing provides medium for growth of pathogens.
	Assess for fever, nuchal rigidity, headache every 2–4 hours.	Manifestations of meningitis.
	Administer prescribed prophylactic antibiotics.	Prevents meningitis.

Evaluation: Compare the patient's status with the expected patient outcomes. If the outcomes are achieved, evaluate nursing care as successful. If not, reassess the patient, formulate new nursing diagnoses, and revise expected patient outcomes and nursing interventions as appropriate.

Assessment Findings: Patient has a surgical suture line at the junction of the gums and upper lip. Area is slightly edematous, tender, free from inflammation.

Nursing Diagnosis: Altered oral mucous membrane related to surgical incision and sutures

Patient Outcomes	Nursing Interventions	Rationale
Patient avoids mechanical trauma to suture line.	Instruct patient to use foam toothette and dental floss to remove debris from teeth until suture line heals.	Toothbrush with bristles may irritate suture line and delay healing.
Patient rinses oral cavity every 2 hours while awake and after meals until suture line heals in 7–10 days.	Instruct patient to rinse mouth with a solution of equal amounts of hydrogen peroxide and warm water or saline every 2 hours while awake and after meals until suture line heals.	Aids in removal of wound exudate and food particles that can provide a medium for the growth of pathogens and also freshens the mouth.
Patient is free of signs of suture line infection.	Examine suture line and surrounding oral mucous membrane for increasing edema, tenderness, inflammation, purulent drainage twice a day. Advise physician promptly if signs of infection are present.	Early detection and treatment of localized wound infection minimize the risk of delayed healing and meningitis.

(continued)

Nursing Care Guide 31–1. (continued)

POSTOPERATIVE CARE OF PATIENTS UNDERGOING TRANSSPHENOIDAL MICROSURGERY FOR EXCISION OF A PITUITARY ADENOMA

Patient Outcomes	Nursing Interventions	Rationale
Patient demonstrates ability to use a mirror to examine suture line for signs of infection.	If patient is discharged before suture line heals, teach patient to use a mirror to examine area for symptoms of infection just described.	Promotes independence and safety in management of therapeutic regimen. Demonstration provides opportunity to evaluate learning.
Patient states intent to notify physician if increasing edema, tenderness, inflammation, or purulent drainage occurs.	Instruct patient to notify physician promptly if signs of infection are present.	Ensures early detection and treatment of infection.

Evaluation: Compare the patient's status with the expected patient outcomes. If the outcomes are achieved, evaluate nursing care as successful. If not, reassess the patient, formulate new nursing diagnoses, and revise expected patient outcomes and nursing interventions as appropriate.

NDx: High risk for infection
Change the gauze sling or pad under the nose as it becomes soiled to remove a potential site for bacterial growth. Nasal packing is removed after 24 hours by the surgeon. The dura mater usually seals within 72 hours. During this time, assess for CSF leak manifested by frequent swallowing or complaints of a postnasal drip. Test nasal drainage for glucose, which is present in CSF but not in normal nasal secretions. Assess for nuchal rigidity and persistent or severe headache, which are signs of meningitis. Administer prophylactic antibiotics as prescribed.

Provide cool mist humidification if prescribed to prevent dryness of the oral and nasal mucous membranes. Assist the patient with frequent oral hygiene with mouthwash, a solution of hydrogen peroxide and saline, or foam toothette to maintain cleanliness of the incision site. Do not use a bristle toothbrush, which may injure the tissues. Assess mouth and leg incisions each shift for redness, edema, or inflammation.

Evaluation

Evaluate the effectiveness of nursing care for a patient with a pituitary tumor by comparing the patient's status with the expected patient outcomes. Examples of specific outcomes for patients with a pituitary tumor have been provided in the Planning section.

Common Neoplastic Disorders

HYPERSECRETION OF PROLACTIN

ETIOLOGY

Benign secreting adenomas of the lactotrope cells, commonly called prolactinomas, are the most common pituitary tumor. They are more common in women than in men. Although the specific cause is unclear, recent research has indicated that elevated estrogen levels during pregnancy and from contraceptive drugs may be a causative factor in the increasing frequency of this tumor in women.

PATHOPHYSIOLOGY

The primary effect of hyperprolactinemia is suppression of the secretion of gonadotropin releasing hormones from the hypothalamus. This results in decreased secretion of the gonadotropic hormones from the anterior pituitary, which, in turn, causes reproductive disorders, decreased libido, and infertility in both sexes. Excess prolactin levels may also stimulate the mammary glands and cause galactorrhea (lactation not associated with childbirth).

CLINICAL MANIFESTATIONS

Women with prolactinomas usually seek medical attention for persistent amenorrhea or infertility. The individual often gives a history of increasing menstrual irregularity for months or even years before the onset of amenorrhea. Approximately 30% of women of childbearing age with amenorrhea of more than 6 months' duration have hyperprolactinemia. Although galactorrhea is present in fewer than half of the women with prolactin excess, it is considered a characteristic symptom of prolactinomas. Galactorrhea is usually mild but may be profuse. Loss of libido is another common manifestation of prolactinomas.

Men with prolactinomas usually seek medical attention because of the neurologic manifestations of a pituitary tumor: persistent visual disturbances and headaches. A careful history will reveal a progressive loss of libido and impotence in two thirds of these individuals. Gynecomastia is common, but galactorrhea in males is very rare.

MEDICAL DIAGNOSIS

Medical diagnosis of a prolactinoma is made on the basis of the patient history and persistent elevation of plasma prolactin levels in the absence of other causative factors such as stress, hypothalamic dysfunction, and the use of dopamine antagonists. Dopamine antagonists may decrease the secretion of prolactin inhibiting hormone, causing a rise in plasma prolactin levels. Radiologic examinations of the skull, computed tomography (CT) scans, and magnetic resonance imaging (MRI) are also used as diagnostic tools, although many prolactinomas cannot be visualized by these methods.

Plasma Prolactin Levels. The most accurate method of measuring plasma prolactin levels is radioimmunoassay. A fasting blood specimen is colected first thing in the morning, when prolactin levels are the lowest and most stable. The nurse notes on the laboratory requisition whether the patient is receiving a dopamine antagonist, which may increase prolactin secretion, or a dopamine agonist, which may inhibit prolactin secretion.

Normal plasma prolactin levels are 0 to 20 ng/ml. Individuals with prolactinomas have levels exceeding 100 ng/ml. Plasma prolactin levels between 20 and 100 ng/ml are usually caused by secondary factors other than prolactinomas.

MEDICAL MANAGEMENT

Medical treatment depends on the severity of the symptoms and the desires of the individual. If the symptoms are mild—amenorrhea with mild or no galactorrhea—in a woman who does not wish to have children, regular reevaluation but no treatment may be recommended.

If conception is desired or if galactorrhea is profuse, bromocriptine (Parlodel) therapy with periodic diagnostic reevaluation is implemented. Bromocriptine is a dopamine agonist that inhibits prolactin secretion by stimulating release of prolactin inhibiting hormone. Ovulation and ovarian function resume, and conception is possible.

In the presence of neurologic symptoms, the treatment of choice is transsphenoidal microsurgical resection of the tumor with preservation of normal pituitary tissue. External irradiation or stereotaxic radiosurgery may also be an alternative therapy for some individuals.

Guidelines for Application of the Nursing Process to the Care of the Patient with a Prolactinoma

Nursing care of a patient with a prolactinoma incorporates all previously discussed aspects of the care of a patient with a pituitary neoplasm. In addition, assess the patient with a suspected prolactinoma for both the neurologic manifestations of a pituitary tumor and the endocrine manifestations of hypersecretion of prolactin.

Because the clinical manifestations of prolactin excess involve alterations in reproductive function and sex drive, some patients may be embarrassed and will not volunteer important information. Maintain eye contact while asking questions about clinical manifestations to help put the patient at ease and to facilitate collection of a complete history.

Ask both men and women whether any change in sexual desire or function has been noticed during the previous months. Also ask about the presence of any discharge from the nipples. If a discharge has been noted, ask the patient to describe the discharge, its frequency, and amount. The presence of gynecomastia or galactorrhea may be especially embarrassing to men.

Obtain a menstrual history for at least the past year from the female patient. Ask whether she has missed any menstrual periods completely. If medical attention was sought because of infertility, ask how long the patient has been attempting to conceive. Question the patient specifically about past use of oral contraceptives or other estrogen preparations prescribed either for birth control or for treatment of the developing menstrual disorders.

Observe the patient's behavior while obtaining the history, and ask how clinical manifestations have affected relationships with intimates to assess the individual's emotional response to physiologic alterations. Failure to maintain eye contact, lowered voice, or signs of increasing anxiety may indicate the patient is having difficulty coping with the disorder. Confirm this inference, and provide an opportunity for the patient to verbalize by indicating these observations with a statement such as, "You seem uncomfortable. Dealing with these changes in your life must be difficult."

Once the diagnosis is confirmed and the medical treatment planned, assess the patient's understanding of the treatment of choice.

The nursing diagnoses and nursing care plan of a patient with a prolactinoma integrate the patient's clinical manifestations, knowledge of the treatment planned, and teaching needs with the previously discussed nursing care of a patient with a pituitary neoplasm plus aspects of the care of a patient with reproductive or sexual dysfunction. Nursing diagnoses and nursing care related to reproductive disorders are discussed in detail in Chapters 43 to 46. Two such diagnoses that might be appropriate for this patient are sexual dysfunction related to impotence, infertility, or hormonal imbalance and body image disturbance related to clinical manifestations or reproductive dysfunction.

Patient outcomes for the individual with a prolactinoma include criteria previously identified in the care of a patient with a pituitary neoplasm plus patient outcomes for the patient with reproductive or sexual dysfunction. Two such criteria that might be appropriate are as follows:

Patient engages in satisfying sexual relationships and activity.

Patient reports return of desired reproductive function and fertility.

HYPERSECRETION OF SOMATOTROPIN

ETIOLOGY

Excess secretion of somatotropin or growth hormone is a rare condition that can occur at any age but is most commonly diagnosed between the second and fourth decades of life. There is no clear sex, race, or familial predisposition. A secreting benign adenoma of the somatotrope cells is the most common cause of excess somatotropin secretion. Recent studies have identified excess secretion of growth hormone releasing hormone from the hypothalamus as a possible cause of somatotrope hyperplasia. In rare instances, idiopathic hyperplasia of the somatotrope cells may be the cause.

PATHOPHYSIOLOGY

Excess secretion of somatotropin affects all actively growing cells in the body. If it occurs before closure of the epiphyses, gigantism develops with excess growth of the entire skeleton and soft tissues. If it occurs after closure of the epiphyses, acromegaly develops, which is characterized by an increase in connective tissue, cartilage, and soft tissue mass and by growth and an increase in thickness of the bones of the hands and feet and of the flat bones of the face.

Excess somatotropin also alters glucose metabolism by impeding glucose uptake into the cells, resulting in elevated blood glucose levels. Somatotropin is, therefore, referred to as an insulin antagonist, and secondary diabetes mellitus may develop as a result of excess somatotropin secretion. Fat and protein metabolism is also altered, producing elevations in serum lipid levels. Urinary excretion of sodium, potassium, phosphorus, and chloride decreases in the presence of excess somatotropin, thereby increasing serum levels of these electrolytes and promoting fluid retention.

CLINICAL MANIFESTATIONS

The onset of the clinical manifestations of a somatotrope adenoma is insidious. Clinical manifestations include the neurologic manifestations of a pituitary tumor, persistent visual disturbances and headaches, and the endocrine manifestations of excess somatotropin secretion.

In acromegaly, changes in appearance occur so slowly that the disease often goes undetected for years. In retrospect, the individual may remember a progressive increase in ring, shoe, hat, and glove sizes. A review of old photographs, such as those shown in Figure 31–4, will demonstrate a coarsening of the features, with thickening and enlargement of the lips as a result of increased growth of subcutaneous connective tissue. Proliferation of cartilage causes enlargement of the ears and nose, increased circumference of the chest, and arthritic changes in the joints of the long bones and spine. Kyphosis is common. Muscle weakness, osteoporosis, and bowing of the long bones develop as a result of altered protein metabolism and hypertrophy of the periosteum. Overgrowth of the maxilla results in prominent zygomatic arches. Mandibular growth produces prognathism (projection of the lower jaw) with wide spaces between the teeth. A forward slanting forehead results from growth of the supraorbital ridges. The hands and feet become wide and spadelike because of the increase in cartilage and radial growth of the bones. Soft tissue growth is manifested by a deepening or hoarseness of the voice, thickened skin, increased sebum secretion, and enlargement of the tongue and abdominal viscera. Paresthesias may develop as a result of entrapment of nerves by bony or soft tissue overgrowth. Diminished gonad function results in hirsutism, amenorrhea, and infertility in females and in impotence and sterility in males. Cardiomegaly develops as a result of soft tissue changes within the myocardium and the increased cardiac workload produced by the large body mass. These cardiac changes, compounded by the pathologic effects of elevated blood glucose, lipid, and electrolyte levels, contribute to the development of hypertension, coronary atherosclerosis, and congestive heart failure, leading to progressive heart failure and premature death.

In gigantism, linear growth of the child or adolescent progresses steadily until the individual becomes more than three standard deviations above the mean height for his or her age. Growth is symmetric and proportional. The individual may exceed 8 or 9 feet in height and 350 lb in weight. Clinical manifesta-

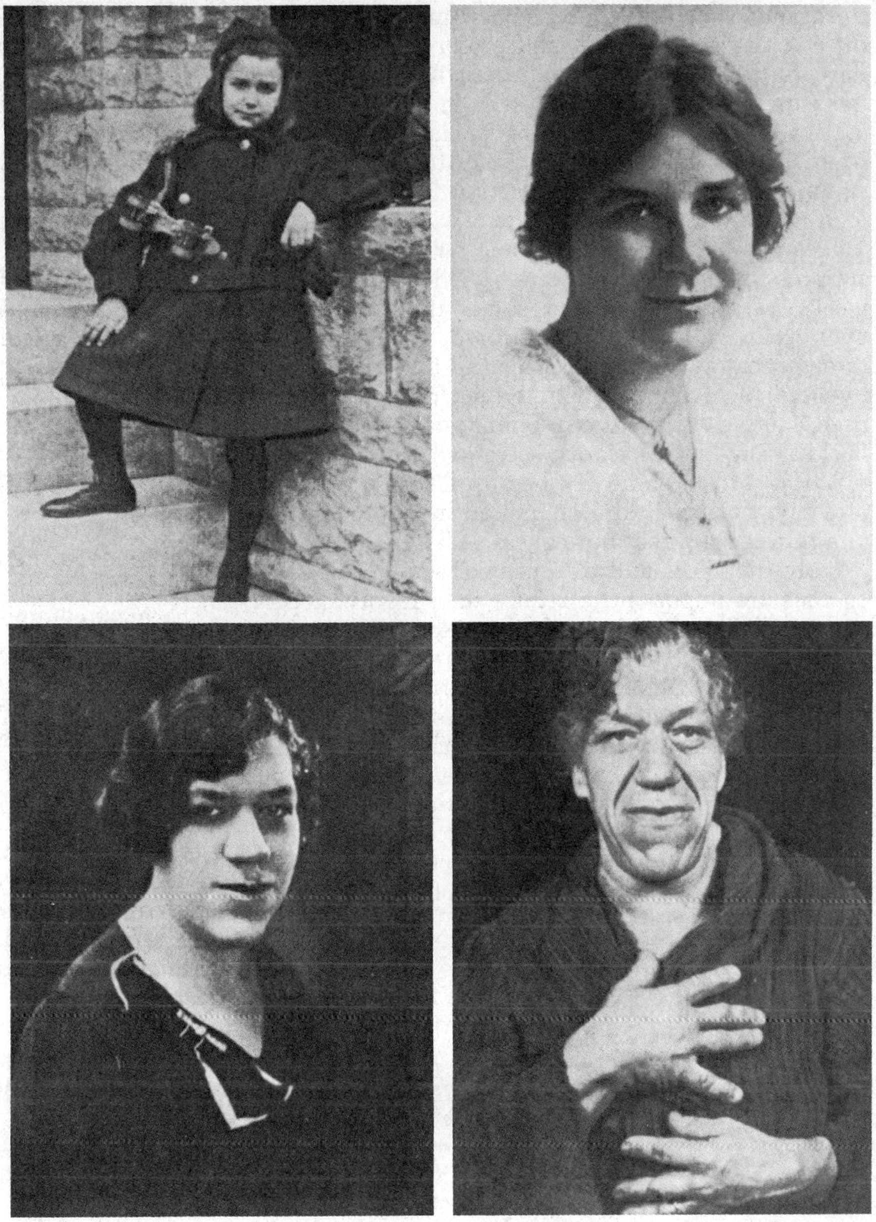

Figure 31–4.

A series of photographs that illustrate the progression of acromegaly in a woman from age 9 to 52. (From Mendeloff AI, Smith DE [eds]. Acromegaly, diabetes, hypermetabolism, proteinuria and heart failure. Clinical Pathological Conference. Am J Med 1956; 20:133.)

tions related to alterations in metabolism are similar to those found in acromegaly. Muscle weakness, osteoporosis, and arthritic changes are common. Cardiac hypertrophy develops at an early age and leads to cardiac failure and premature death.

MEDICAL DIAGNOSIS

Medical diagnosis of excess somatotropin secretion is made on the basis of history, clinical manifestations, old photographs if available, and elevated serum or plasma growth hormone levels. Blood glucose levels remain elevated above normal for more than 2 hours during an oral glucose tolerance test in the presence of altered glucose metabolism. Radiologic examination of the skull, CT scans, and MRI may also be used to visualize the tumor.

Serum or Plasma Growth Hormone Levels. The most accurate measurement of excess serum or plasma growth hormone levels is by radioimmunoassay. To ensure accurate results, the patient fasts from food for 8 to 10 hours and should be free of stress and at complete rest for 30 minutes before specimen collection.

Normal serum or plasma growth hormone levels for adults is less than 10 ng/ml. Levels in children and adolescents may be slightly higher. Individuals with somatotrope adenomas may have levels as high as 400 ng/ml.

MEDICAL MANAGEMENT

Medical treatment depends on the severity of the symptoms. Transsphenoidal microsurgery is the treatment of choice to excise the tumor, rapidly reduce somatotropin levels, and preserve normal pituitary function. A transfrontal craniotomy is used if the tumor has extended to surrounding structures and caused optic or cranial nerve damage. External irradiation is effective, but it may take 2 years for significant hormone level reduction to occur, with 5 to 10 years required for full effect.

Treatment with bromocriptine (Parlodel) produces suppression of somatotropin secretion in about 2 weeks in acromegaly, and some tumor shrinkage may occur. However, serum growth hormone levels rarely decrease to normal, and the long-term effectiveness of treatment with bromocriptine has not been completely evaluated. Somatostatin is effective in lowering somatotropin secretion, but it is not practical for long-term use because it has a duration of action of only 5 to 6 hours and inhibits secretion of a number of other hormones.

Early diagnosis and treatment of somatotrope adenomas are important to reduce the severity of permanent alterations that result from excess somatotropin secretion. Although treatment stops the bone and tissue growth, and features normalize to a degree because of a decrease in soft tissue bulk, there is no reversal of the bone growth that has occurred. Vascular injury from atherosclerosis, cardiovascular damage, and microvascular changes associated with diabetes are irreversible. Blood glucose levels may return to normal, or secondary diabetes may persist. Prognosis depends on the severity of the alterations that remain after treatment.

Guidelines for Application of the Nursing Process to the Care of the Patient with Acromegaly

The nursing care of a patient with acromegaly incorporates all previously discussed aspects of the care of a patient with a pituitary neoplasm with the nursing care of a patient with somatotropin excess. Assess the patient for both the neurologic manifestations of a pituitary tumor and the endocrine manifestations of hypersecretion of somatotropin. Once medical treatment is planned, assess the patient's understanding of the treatment of choice and develop a nursing care plan to meet the patient's needs.

The nursing diagnoses and nursing care plan reflect the patient's clinical manifestations, knowledge of the treatment planned, and teaching needs. Nursing diagnoses specific to the endocrine manifestations of this patient may include high risk for trauma related to osteoporosis and arthritic joint changes, and body image disturbance related to changes in appearance and body characteristics. Nursing diagnoses related to the cardiovascular alterations associated with this condition are discussed in Chapter 18. Patient outcomes will include criteria to maintain patient safety and promote realistic expectations of treatment.

Nursing care includes using side rails for safety and helping the patient to ambulate to promote recalcification of the bones. Position the patient in good body alignment when in bed to prevent deformities and pathologic fractures. Encourage the patient to ask questions about the outcome of treatment, and clarify any misconceptions. Encourage realistic expectations of treatment, and allow the individual to ventilate feelings of anger and grief.

HYPOPITUITARISM

Hyposecretion of any one or of all of the pituitary hormones in the adult may be caused by any lesion or destructive process in or near the pituitary gland. The most common cause is compression or destruction of pituitary cells by a secreting or nonsecreting adenoma. Other causes of hypopituitarism include iatrogenic factors, postpartum necrosis (Sheehan's syndrome), metastatic lesions, and inflammation secondary to infections of the central nervous system.

Clinical manifestations usually develop slowly and depend on which of the pituitary hormones is deficient. Absence of all pituitary hormones is referred to as panhypopituitarism and results in hyposecretion of all of the target glands. Clinical manifestations include lethargy, fatigue, apathy, intolerance to cold, generalized weakness, skin pallor and wrinkling, alterations in secondary sex characteristics, loss of libido, infertility and amenorrhea in women, impotence in men, and a history of poor health.

Medical diagnosis is made on the basis of the clinical manifestations and decreased serum or plasma hormone levels of the pituitary hormones or target gland hormones. Treatment consists of lifelong replacement therapy with adrenocortical and thyroid hormones. Sex hormones and growth hormone may also be prescribed. Nursing care is similar to that of individuals with adrenal cortex and thyroid hypofunction, as discussed in Chapters 32 and 33, respectively.

Posterior Pituitary Disorders

As discussed earlier, the posterior pituitary, or neurohypophysis, stores and secretes antidiuretic hormone (ADH) and oxytocin, which are produced in the hypothalamus. Regulation of ADH secretion is controlled by osmoreceptors in the hypothalamus, which respond to changes in the osmolality of extracellular fluids. When extracellular fluids become highly concentrated, ADH is released and more water is reabsorbed from the renal tubules while electrolytes are excreted. As the extracellular fluid becomes more dilute, ADH secretion stops. ADH also has a vasopressive effect; its secretion may be stimulated by severe blood loss or a decrease in blood pressure.

Disorders of the posterior pituitary are rare and are usually secondary to other primary disorders such as nonendocrine tumors, trauma, and severe infections and inflammatory processes.

Diabetes Insipidus

ETIOLOGY

Diabetes insipidus is a disorder caused by a deficiency in ADH secretion. Primary diabetes insipidus (central or neurogenic diabetes insipidus) is rare and usually occurs as a result of a tumor of the hypothalamus or pituitary gland that destroys the portions of the hypothalamus that manufacture or regulate secretion of ADH. Nephrogenic diabetes insipidus is a rare, inherited genetic defect in which the renal tubules do not respond to ADH and water is not resorbed by the kidney.

Secondary diabetes insipidus is a more common disorder. It develops secondary to head trauma, surgical or irradiation injury, neoplastic or inflammatory processes that exert pressure on the hypothalamus or hypophysis, or idiopathic causes. Secondary diabetes insipidus may be temporary or permanent. Secondary permanent diabetes insipidus will not develop in an individual who has undergone a total hypophysectomy if the pituitary stalk is intact, because the cut axons from the hypothalamus continue to secrete ADH.

PATHOPHYSIOLOGY

In the absence of ADH or failure of the kidneys to respond to ADH, large amounts of fluid and electrolytes are excreted in the urine because the renal tubules do not reabsorb water. As much as 20 L of dilute urine may be excreted daily.

CLINICAL MANIFESTATIONS

Polydipsia and polyuria are the classic symptoms of diabetes insipidus. The urine is pale in color, and the specific gravity is less than 1.006. Anorexia and weight loss occur. If the individual is unable to drink fluids, severe dehydration, with sodium depletion and vascular collapse, rapidly develops.

MEDICAL DIAGNOSIS

Diagnosis is made on the basis of clinical manifestations, dehydration tests, and response to vasopressin.

WATER-DEPRIVATION TEST

The water-deprivation test evaluates the ability of the renal tubules to concentrate urine in the presence of dehydration. All fluids are withheld for 8 to 12 hours or until 3% to 5% of the body weight is lost. Plasma and urine osmolality tests may be done at the beginning and end of the test. The test is positive for diabetes insipidus if the patient continues to excrete large amounts of dilute urine with a low specific gravity despite dehydration.

Nursing implications during the test include frequent assessment of vital signs and monitoring the patient for the clinical manifestations of dehydration and impending hypovolemic shock. The individual needs emotional support because of the insatiable thirst that occurs. Hourly weights are a good indicator of fluid loss. The physician is notified immediately and the test terminated if tachycardia, weight loss of more than 5%, or hypotension develop.

VASOPRESSIN STIMULATION TEST

The vasopressin stimulation test may be done after a positive water-deprivation test to determine whether failure of the renal tubules to concentrate urine is due to renal dysfunction or to pituitary diabetes insipidus. A urine specimen is collected for osmolality before and 1 hour after subcutaneous administration of aqueous vasopressin. The vasopressin stimulation test is positive for diabetes insipidus if there is more than a 5% rise in urine osmolality after vasopressin administration.

MEDICAL MANAGEMENT

Short-term treatment of diabetes insipidus involves parenteral administration of vasopressin, the pharmacologic form of ADH. This is the treatment of choice for patients with temporary diabetes insipidus resulting from cerebral edema. The pharmacokinetics of antidiuretic hormones are described in Pharmacology Box 31–1. Aqueous vasopressin injection (Pitressin) has a short duration of antidiuretic activity and is administered every 6 to 8 hours. Vasopressin tannate (Pitressin Tannate in oil) has a longer half-life and is administered every 36 to 72 hours.

Desmopressin acetate (DDAVP), a synthetic ADH, is the drug of choice for long-term therapy. DDAVP solution is administered intranasally through a straw once or twice daily. Lypressin (Diapid) nasal spray, another synthetic ADH, must be administered three to four times daily.

Nephrogenic diabetes insipidus is usually controlled with a low-sodium, low-protein diet and thiazide diuretics. This combination promotes water and sodium resorption in the proximal renal tubule and reduces water loss in the distal renal tubule, where ADH is necessary. Protein restriction further reduces water loss by reducing the need for solute excretion.

Guidelines for Application of the Nursing Process to the Care of the Patient with Diabetes Insipidus

Assess for the clinical manifestations of diabetes insipidus in all patients who sustained head trauma, cranial surgery, or irradiation; those with metastatic lesions to the brain; and those with a diagnosed pituitary tumor. Monitor vital signs, level of consciousness, urine output, and specific gravity, especially in the unconscious patient who cannot complain of thirst. If urine output exceeds 100 ml/hour for 3 hours with no apparent physiologic cause, notify the physician promptly.

Once diabetes insipidus is diagnosed and therapy is implemented, assess and document the patient's response to treatment. Pharmacology Box 31–1 summarizes pharmacologic information and nursing implications of ADH administration. If Pitressin Tannate is prescribed, warm the vial and shake vigorously to disperse the medication in the oil and to facilitate intramuscular administration. Inject immediately after preparation. If long-term DDAVP or lypressin therapy is required, teach the patient to check the expiration date on the medication, weigh him or herself daily, and report a 3% weight loss to the physician. Weigh the patient the morning of discharge, calculate 3%, and give this number and the total body weight to the patient to avoid confusion. Include the topics identified in Chart 31–1 in the teaching plan of a patient with diabetes insipidus who is taking DDAVP. Observe the patient's technique of self-administration of the prescribed medication to evaluate teaching.

Pharmacology Box 31–1.

ANTIDIURETIC HORMONES

Antidiuretic Hormones:
Class of drugs that promote water conservation by increasing reabsorption of water by the distal portion of the renal tubules.

Action:
Reduce urine volume and increase urine concentration and osmolality by increasing renal tubular reabsorption of water. In doses higher than those required for antidieuretic effect, ADH also has vasopressor effects.

Uses:
To control the symptoms of neurogenic diabetes insipidus.

Side Effects:
Dose related. Water intoxication: changes in mental status, confusion, lethargy, headache, weight gain, convulsions, coma. Shortness of breath, heartburn, nausea, abdominal cramps, vulvar pain, rise in blood pressure, angina.

Interactions:
Alcohol, cyclophosphamide, demeclocycline, epinephrine, heparin, and lithium may decrease antidiuretic response. Oral antidiabetic agents, carbamazepine, and clofibrate may increase antidiuretic response.

Nursing Implications:
Daily weights; monitor fluid intake and output and vital signs; monitor for side effects; notify physician and withhold dose in the presence of chest pain, dyspnea, decreased level of consciousness, sudden weight gain.

Geriatric Considerations:
Risk of water intoxication is especially high in the elderly. Monitor cardiovascular status closely.

Chart 31–1.

NURSING GUIDE TO PATIENT EDUCATION FOR SELF-MANAGEMENT: DESMOPRESSIN ACETATE ADMINISTRATION FOR DIABETES INSIPIDUS

Instruct the patient to:

Expect desmopressin acetate (DDAVP) to reduce frequency and volume of urination and to relieve excessive thirst.
Check expiration date on label. Outdated medication loses its potency rapidly and should be discarded.
Store DDAVP in the refrigerator unless otherwise specified by the manufacturer.
Discard medication and do not use if solution is discolored or if particles are present.
Administer in the evening to control nocturia if a single dose is prescribed.
Monitor pattern of urination. If nocturia or frequent urination during waking hours develops, notify physician. A second morning dose may be prescribed.
Monitor pattern of fluid intake. If frequent thirst develops, notify physician.
Measure dose carefully in calibrated straw.
Inhale high into nasal cavity, not down back of throat.
Weigh daily. Report weight gain of 2 pounds in 1 week to physician.
Report to the physician promptly any of the following: feelings of drowsiness, listlessness, headache, shortness of breath, heartburn, nausea, abdominal cramps, vulvar pain, or severe nasal congestion or irritation.

Syndrome of Inappropriate Antidiuretic Hormone

Excess secretion of ADH is a syndrome that develops in critically ill individuals. The most common cause of the syndrome of inappropriate antidiuretic hormone (SIADH) is secretion of ADH by nonendocrine tumors, especially oat cell carcinoma of the lungs. Other conditions that are associated with SIADH include severe stress, trauma, cerebral hemorrhage, cranial surgery, central nervous system infections, myxedema, and large doses of irradiation and chemotherapy.

In SIADH, the secretion of ADH is not controlled by hypothalamic osmoreceptors and is unrelated to plasma osmolality or extracellular fluid volume. The result is excessive reabsorption of water in the distal renal tubules, leading to expansion of extracellular fluid volume with hemodilution and dilutional hyponatremia.

Assess the patient for clinical manifestations of decreasing urine output with specific gravity of more than 1.030, hyponatremia, weight gain, lethargy, weakness, decreased gastrointestinal motility because of hyponatremia, and decreasing level of consciousness progressing to seizures and coma.

SIADH is best treated by correcting the underlying cause. Fluid restrictions and administration of diuretics, serum albumin, and demeclocycline (Declomycin), a tetracycline that increases free water clearance in the renal tubules, may also be prescribed.

The Elderly: Special Considerations

There is no evidence that the incidence of pituitary disorders is higher in the elderly than in the general population. Indeed, almost all chronic pituitary disorders develop well before senescence. However, in reviewing the normal physiologic changes related to the aging process discussed in Chapter 2 and the complexities of the relationship among the hypothalamus, the pituitary gland, and the target glands and tissues, it is easy to see how the normal aging process could alter the body's response to pituitary function.

Because of the chronicity of physiologic complaints in many elderly individuals, it is often too easy to attribute manifestations of possible pituitary-related disorders to old age rather than to investigate them fully. For example, impotence, a common problem of elderly men readily attributed to the aging process, has been found in some cases to be due to a prolactinoma. Hypofunction of the thyroid gland and adrenal cortex may be due to hypopituitarism caused by altered cerebrovascular blood flow.

Deteriorating neurologic function can alter the transmission of, and response to, stimuli to and from the hypothalamus and pituitary. In addition, chronic undernutrition, common in the elderly, has been found to reduce the secretion of hypothalamic and anterior pituitary hormones.

Several studies have noted that the aged individual is able to maintain urine concentration under normal circumstances but cannot alter urine concentration to adjust for fluid excess or deficit caused by decreased renal response to ADH secretion. To compensate for the decreased renal efficiency, the hypothalamic osmoreceptors become more sensitive in the elderly and ADH secretion increases. This compensatory hypersecretion of ADH is one of the factors in the high incidence of transient SIADH in the elderly after administration of anesthesia. Impaired renal response also places the elderly at higher risk for the untoward effects of drugs that may alter ADH activity. SIADH associated with administration of sulfonylurea compounds, although rare, occurs exclusively in the aged.

Assess all geriatric patients for clinical manifestations of pituitary dysfunction. Evaluate any changes in behavior patterns to rule out the possibility of pituitary neoplasms. Consider any geriatric patient at risk for altered posterior pituitary function caused by fluctuations in extracellular fluid levels, anesthesia, or the response to medications.

Bibliography

Abrams AC. Clinical drug therapy: Rationales for nursing practice. 3rd ed. Philadelphia: JB Lippincott, 1991.

Alfaro-LeFevre R, et al. Drug handbook: A nursing process approach. New York: Addison-Wesley, 1992.

Baer CL. Why does this patient have polyuria? Nursing 1988; 18(10):94.

Brenner ZR. Diagnostic tests and procedures: Applying the nursing process. Norwalk, CT: Appleton & Lange, 1987.

Bullock BL, Rosendahl PP. Pathophysiology: Adaptations and alterations in function. 2nd ed. Boston: Little, Brown, 1988.

Carpenito LJ. Nursing diagnosis: Application to clinical practice. 4th ed. Philadelphia: JB Lippincott, 1992.

Cassel CK, et al. Geriatric medicine. New York: Springer-Verlag, 1989.

Cella JH, Watson J. Nurse's manual of laboratory tests. Philadelphia: FA Davis, 1989.

Chenevey B. Overview of fluid and electrolytes. Nurs Clin North Am 1987; 22(4):749.

Cocchi D. Age related alterations in gonadotropin, adrenocorticotropin and growth hormone secretion. Aging: Clin Exp Res 1992; 4(2):103.

Cooper JAD, Pappas PG. (eds). Cecil review of general internal medicine. 5th ed. Philadelphia: WB Saunders, 1992.

DeGroot LJ (ed). Endocrinology. 2nd ed. Philadelphia: WB Saunders, 1989.

Doenges ME, Moorhouse MF. Nursing diagnoses with interventions. 4th ed. Philadelphia: FA Davis, 1993.

Dudek SG. Nutrition handbook for nursing practice. Philadelphia: JB Lippincott, 1987.

Eliopoulos C. Gerontological nursing. 3rd ed. Philadelphia: JB Lippincott, 1993.

Fischbach F. A manual of laboratory diagnostic tests. 4th ed. Philadelphia: JB Lippincott, 1992.

Germon K. Fluid and electrolyte problems associated with diabetes insipidus and syndrome of inappropriate antidiuretic hormone. Nurs Clin North Am 1987; 22(4):785.

Gordon M. Nursing diagnosis: Process and application. St. Louis: CV Mosby, 1991.

Greenspan FS. Basic and clinical endocrinology. Norwalk, CT: Appleton & Lange, 1991.

Griffin J, Ojeda S (eds). Textbook of endocrine physiology. New York: Oxford University Press, 1988.

Guyton AC. Textbook of medical physiology. 8th ed. Philadelphia: WB Saunders, 1990.

Haverstick LP, et al. Growth hormone: its effect on protein metabolism and clinical implications. Top Clin Nutr 1991; 7(1):52.

Hill MN. Drug compliance: Going beyond the facts. Nursing 1986; 16(10):50.

Jess LW. Assessing your patient for increased ICP. Nursing 1987; 17(6):34.

Kidd PS. Common pathologic conditions in elderly persons. J Emerg Nurs 1987; 13(1):27.

Kositske J. A question of balance: Dehydration in the elderly. J Gerontol Nurs 1990; 16(5):4.

Kumar V, Cotran RS, Robbins SL. Basic pathology. 5th ed. Philadelphia: WB Saunders, 1992.

Lancaster LE. Renal and endocrine regulation of water and electrolyte balance. Nurs Clin North Am 1987; 22(4):761.

Lehne RA. Pharmacology for nursing care. Philadelphia: WB Saunders, 1990.

Lind JM. Ectopic hormone production: Nursing implications. Semin Oncol Nurs 1985; 1(4):251.

Lindaman C. SIADH: Is your patient at risk? Nursing 1992; 22(6):60.

Lloyd RV. Endocrine pathology. New York: Springer-Verlag, 1990.

Malseed RT, Harrigan G. Textbook of pharmacology and nursing care: The nursing process. 2nd ed. Philadelphia: JB Lippincott, 1989.

Mathewson MK. Antidiuretic hormone. Crit Care Nurse 1986; 6(5):88.

Matteson MA, McConnell ES. Gerontological nursing: Concepts and practice. Philadelphia: WB Saunders, 1988.

Moran S. Innovative geriatric care. Nurs Management 1987; 18(6):26.

Patterson LM, Noroian EL. Diabetes insipidus versus syndrome of inappropriate antidiuretic hormone. Dimens Crit Care Nurs 1989; 8(4):226.

Poyss AS. Assessment and nursing diagnosis in fluid and electrolyte disorders. Nurs Clin North Am 1987; 22(4):773.

Price SA, Wilson LM. Pathophysiology: Clinical concepts of disease processes. 4th ed. St. Louis: Mosby–Year Book, 1992.

Reasner CA. Anterior pituitary disease. Crit Care Nurs Q 1990; 13(3):62.

Schultz PN. Hypopituitarism in patients with a history of irradiation to the head and neck area: Diagnoses and implications for nursing. Oncol Nurs Forum 1989; 16(6):823.

Shannon MT, Wilson BA. Govoni & Hayes drugs and nursing implications. 7th ed. Norwalk: Appleton & Lange, 1992.

Sowers J, Felicetta J (eds). Endocrinology of aging. New York: Raven, 1988.

Stachura ME. Human growth hormone: Use and potential abuse. Hosp Formulary 1987; 22(1):48.

Tucker SM, et al. Patient care standards: Nursing process, diagnosis, and outcome. 5th ed. St. Louis, MO: CV Mosby, 1992.

Ulrich SP, Canale SW, Wendell SA. Nursing care planning guides: A nursing diagnosis approach. 2nd ed. Philadelphia: WB Saunders, 1990.

Wilson JD, Foster DW (ed). Williams textbook of endocrinology. 8th ed. Philadelphia: WB Saunders, 1992.

Wyngaarden JB, Smith LH, Bennett JC (eds). Cecil textbook of medicine. 19th ed. Philadelphia: WB Saunders, 1992.

Yucha C. David could have died of thirst yet he never felt thirsty. Nursing 1991; 21(7):42.

Chapter Thirty-two

NURSING CARE *of Adults with Adrenal Disorders*

The two pyramid-shaped adrenal glands lie embedded in fat on the upper pole of each kidney. Each gland measures approximately 5 × 2 × 1 cm and weighs an average of 4 g. Each of the adrenal glands actually consists of two distinct endocrine glands: the adrenal cortex and the adrenal medulla. As illustrated in Figure 32–1, the adrenal cortex is the larger outer structure that surrounds the central adrenal medulla. Each of these structures differs in cellular composition, function, and regulatory mechanism.

Adrenal Cortex

Anatomy and Physiology

The adrenal cortex secretes a group of steroid hormones called corticosteroids. Corticosteroids mediate the body's response to stress and affect metabolism, fluid and electrolyte balance, and secondary sex characteristics.

The adrenal cortex is composed of three distinct layers. The zona glomerulosa, which secretes mineralocorticoids, functions independently of the zona fasciculata and zona reticularis, which secrete glucocorticoids and sex steroid hormones. Figure 32–1 illustrates the three layers of the adrenal cortex and the steroid hormones secreted from each.

The adrenal cortex is the only source of mineralocorticoids and glucocorticoids in the body. They are essential for life. Death will occur within 2 weeks after total loss of these adrenocorticoid hormones.

MINERALOCORTICOIDS

The mineralocorticoids promote sodium retention and potassium excretion in the distal renal tubules. Therefore, they are primary factors in maintaining extracellular fluid volume and electrolyte balance in the body.

Aldosterone is the principal mineralocorticoid secreted by the adrenal cortex. Desoxycorticosterone, an aldosterone precursor, is also secreted in smaller amounts. Aldosterone is secreted in response to increased serum potassium levels, decreased serum sodium levels, and the release of renin-angiotensin into the circulation in the presence of hypovolemia or hypotension. Pituitary adrenocorticotropic hormone (ACTH) also has a weak stimulatory effect on the secretion of aldosterone. Figure 32–2 illustrates the secretion of aldosterone in response to renin-angiotensin release, an important mechanism in homeostatic fluid and electrolyte balance.

GLUCOCORTICOIDS

The glucocorticoids are important in the regulation of carbohydrate, protein, and fat metabolism. Glucocorticoids stimulate gluconeogenesis by the liver and mobilize amino acids from the tissues for

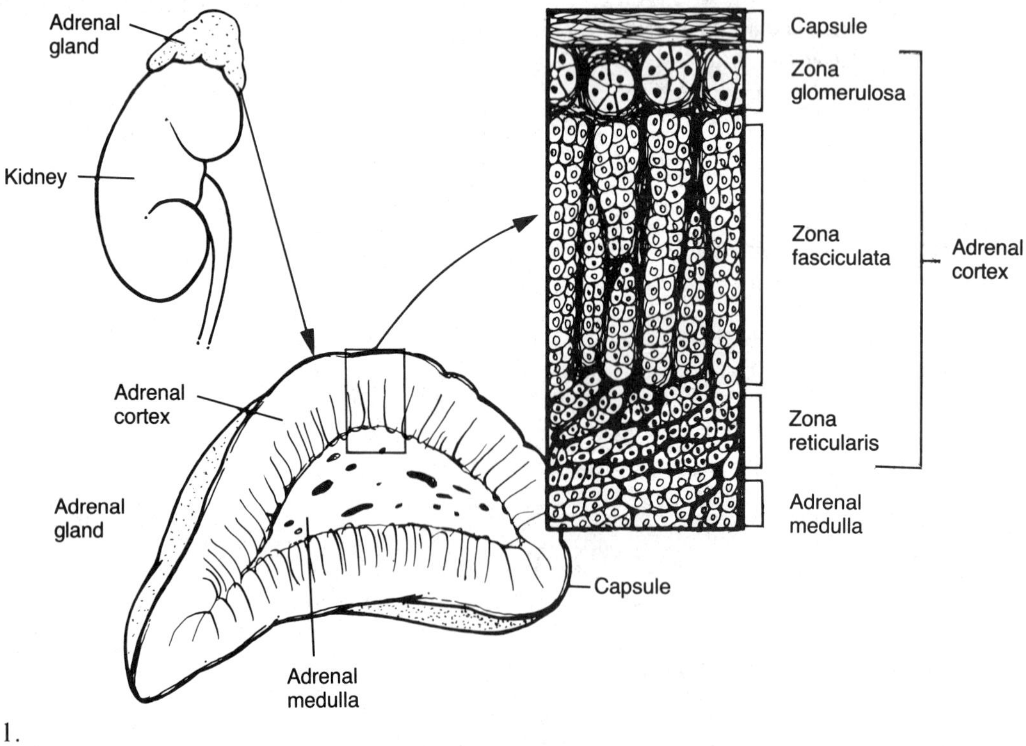

Figure 32–1.

Structures of the adrenal gland. The central adrenal medulla constitutes approximately 20% of the glandular structure and secretes epinephrine and norepinephrine. Insert represents the cellular structure of the adrenal gland with the three zones of the adrenal cortex. The zona glomerulosa secretes mineralocorticoids; the zona fasciculata and zona reticularis secrete glucocorticoids and sex steroid hormones.

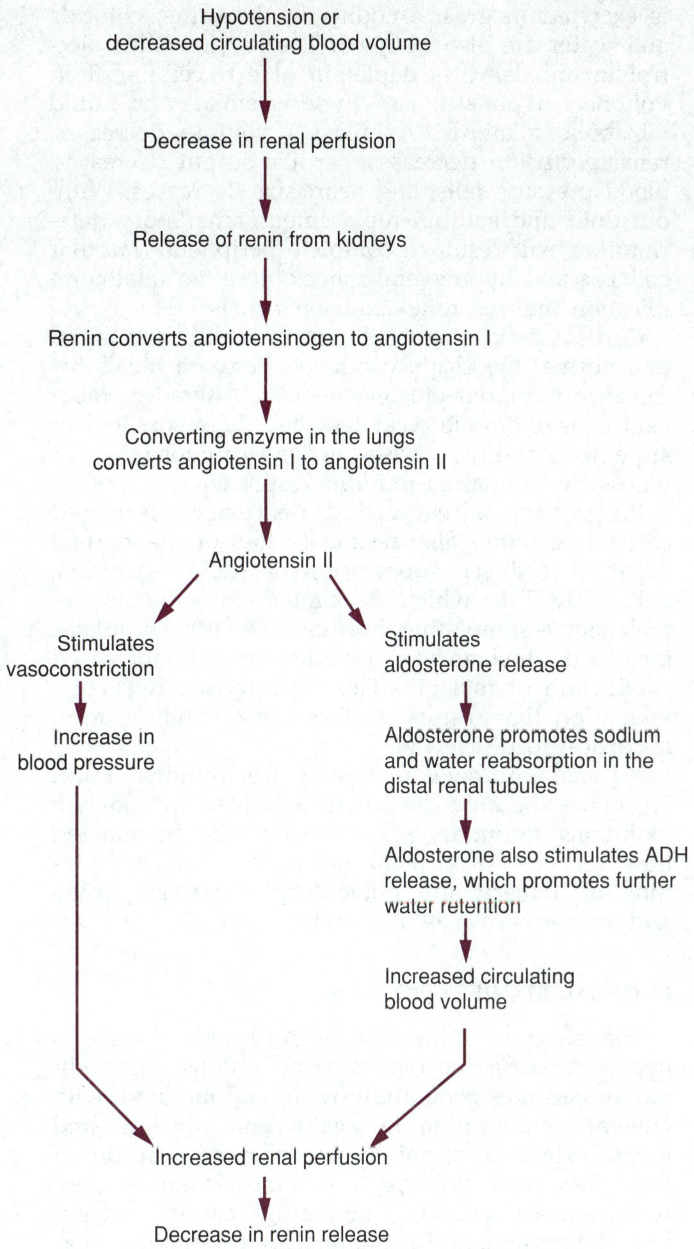

***Figure* 32–2.**

Secretion of aldosterone from the adrenal cortex in response to renin-angiotensin release. Restoration of blood pressure and circulating blood volume inhibits further renin release, completing the negative feedback cycle. (ADH, antidiuretic hormone.)

conversion into glucose. They also decrease glucose and amino acid transport into the cells and glucose utilization by the cells. These effects raise blood glucose levels and reduce protein stores in all body tissues except the liver. The mobilization of amino acids out of the cells results in decreased protein synthesis and increased protein catabolism. In the presence of decreased glucose transport into the cells, fatty acids are mobilized from adipose tissue for energy production, raising serum fatty acid levels. These metabolic effects help maintain blood glucose levels and supply energy for vital tissues between meals and during periods of starvation and fasting. The glucocorticoids also influence cognitive functions and help maintain emotional stability and the individual's ability to respond to stress. In supraphysiologic amounts, the glucocorticoids exert a strong antiinflammatory effect, suppress the immune system, and decrease the number of eosinophils and lymphocytes in the blood.

Secretion of the glucocorticoids is controlled almost entirely by ACTH secretion from the anterior pituitary gland. Secretion of ACTH is initiated by secretion of corticotropin releasing hormone (CRH) from the hypothalamus. CRH is secreted in response to circadian rhythms, physiologic need, and the increased energy demands of acute stress. CRH secretion is inhibited by elevated serum cortisol levels and relief of stress. Regulation of glucocorticoid secretion by this negative feedback cycle is illustrated in Figure 32–3.

Although glucocorticoid secretion varies constantly in response to circadian rhythms, serum levels are usually lowest during sleep, peak near awakening, rise again about 4 to 6 hours later, and then gradually drop through the rest of the day. Because this secretion pattern is characterized by periods of increased production during the daytime, it is referred to as a diurnal secretion pattern. It takes about 48 hours for the cyclic secretion of the glucocorticoids to adjust to changes in daily sleeping habits, one of the reasons for jet lag and excess fatigue in individuals who work different shifts on successive days.

Cortisol, also known as hydrocortisone, is the primary glucocorticoid secreted by the adrenal cortex. Corticosterone and cortisone are also secreted in very small amounts. In addition to their primary metabolic effects, the glucocorticoids also exert a slight mineralocorticoid activity.

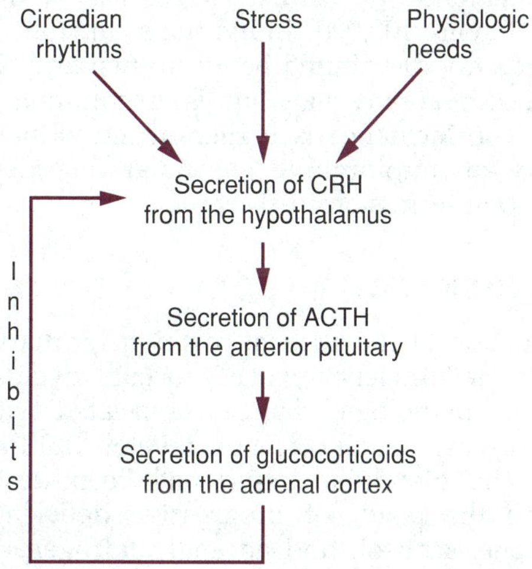

***Figure* 32–3.**

Regulation of glucocorticoid secretion by the corticotropin releasing hormone–adrenocorticotropic hormone (CRH-ACTH) negative feedback cycle.

ADRENAL SEX HORMONES

The adrenal cortex secretes small amounts of both male and female sex hormones. Androgen, the male steroid hormone, is secreted in larger amounts than estrogen and progesterone, the female steroid hormones. The androgenic sex hormones influence the development of secondary sex characteristics.

Adrenocortical Insufficiency: Addison's Disease

Adrenocortical insufficiency is a functional disorder characterized by failure of the adrenal cortex to produce and secrete adrenocortical hormones.

ETIOLOGY

Chronic primary adrenocortical insufficiency, or Addison's disease, most commonly results from idiopathic atrophy or destruction of the adrenal cortex caused by an autoimmune process. It may occur alone or in association with autoimmune-related thyroid disease, insulin-dependent diabetes mellitus, premature gonad failure, and pernicious anemia. Primary adrenocortical insufficiency much less commonly results from destruction of the adrenal cortex by tuberculosis or histoplasmosis organisms, metastatic lesions, or surgical removal of both adrenal glands.

Secondary adrenocortical insufficiency is caused by inadequate secretion of ACTH resulting from either a pituitary or hypothalamic disorder or suppression of adrenal cortex function by administration of exogenous steroid preparations. It may take as long as 9 months after long-term steroid therapy has been discontinued for the hypothalamic-pituitary-adrenal axis to recover sufficiently to respond to acute stress or illness.

The incidence of Addison's disease is approximately 1 per 100,000 individuals in the United States, equally distributed between men and women. It can occur at any age but is uncommon in the elderly. The incidence is higher in individuals with a history of autoimmune glandular disorders and chronic long-term steroid therapy.

PATHOPHYSIOLOGY

Destruction of the adrenal cortex in primary adrenocortical insufficiency usually occurs over several years. The pathologic changes associated with Addison's disease usually do not develop until at least 90% of the glandular tissue has been destroyed. They are the result of progressive deficiencies of aldosterone, cortisol, and adrenal androgen and increased secretion of ACTH.

Aldosterone deficiency results in decreased sodium reabsorption in the distal tubules of the kidneys and increased potassium retention. As sodium is excreted in great amounts in the urine, chloride and water are also excreted. The result of this electrolyte imbalance is depletion of extracellular fluid volume, hyponatremia, hyperkalemia, and mild metabolic alkalosis. As plasma volume decreases, renal perfusion decreases, cardiac output decreases, blood pressure falls, and heart size decreases. Without fluid and sodium replacement, circulatory deterioration will result in complete peripheral vascular collapse and hypovolemic shock, an often fatal complication referred to as Addison's crisis.

Cortisol deficiency results in the inability to maintain normal blood glucose levels between meals because of impaired gluconeogenesis. Altered metabolism causes muscle weakness, loss of vigor, loss of appetite, inability to withstand even minor stress or illness, and impaired immune response.

In primary adrenocortical deficiency, decreased cortisol secretion also results in loss of the normal negative feedback suppression of ACTH secretion. Excess ACTH, which is similar in structure to melanocyte-stimulating hormone (MSH), stimulates increased melanocyte formation and increased production of melanin. The characteristic hyperpigmentation that results is absent in secondary adrenocortical insufficiency.

Adrenal androgen deficiency has minimal effect on males because testicular androgen production maintains secondary sex characteristics. In females, however, loss of adrenal androgen results in thinning of axillary and pubic hair. Decreased libido and amenorrhea may also occur.

CLINICAL MANIFESTATIONS

The onset of symptoms of Addison's disease is insidious, occurring over several months. The individual becomes profoundly weak and fatigued, with general deterioration in health and physical and mental vigor. Postural hypotension as a result of fluid loss, and syncope, muscular weakness, anorexia, nausea, vomiting, abdominal cramps, weight loss, depression, and irritability are common. Generalized bronzing of the skin or patches of hyperpigmentation, especially of the gums and mucous membranes, skin creases, pressure areas, areolae, and genitalia, occur in primary adrenocortical insufficiency. Some patients develop vitiligo, patchy areas of decreased pigmentation surrounded by areas of increased pigmentation, as shown in Figure 32–4.

In Addison's crisis, severe hypotension, hypoglycemia, hyponatremia, hyperkalemia, and dehydration lead to profound shock, cardiac dysrhythmias, and death. Hyperpyrexia and severe abdominal and back pain may also be present. Addison's crisis is usually precipitated by stress, infection, surgery, salt or fluid loss in hot weather or during exercise, or inadequate replacement or sudden withdrawal of exogenous steroids. It may also be precipitated by illness or stress in individuals with previously undiagnosed borderline adrenocortical insufficiency.

MEDICAL DIAGNOSIS

Diagnosis of adrenocortical insufficiency is made on the basis of identification of low levels of circulating plasma cortisol and low 24-hour urinary 17-hydroxycorticosteroids (17-OHCS) and 17-ketosteroids (17-KS). Plasma ACTH levels are elevated in primary adrenocortical deficiency. In secondary adrenocortical deficiency caused by hyposecretion of ACTH from the pituitary, serum ACTH levels are low, and the ACTH stimulation test causes plasma cortisol values to rise. Table 32–1 identifies common diagnostic studies of adrenal cortex function and their nursing implications. The abnormal responses to these studies that are typical in a patient with Addison's disease are summarized in Table 32–2.

Additional laboratory studies demonstrate hyperkalemia, hyponatremia, hypoglycemia, hypochloremia, mild metabolic alkalosis, elevated blood urea nitrogen and serum creatinine, eosinophilia, and lymphocytosis.

MEDICAL MANAGEMENT

Treatment of adrenocortical insufficiency is lifelong hormone replacement. Oral cortisone acetate (Cortone) and hydrocortisone (cortisol, Cortef) are the drugs of choice to replace glucocorticoid activity. The glucocorticoid is administered in divided doses to simulate the body's normal diurnal secretion pattern; two thirds of the total dose on arising and one third in the afternoon. To prevent Addison's crisis, glucocorticoid dosage may be increased two to three times during periods of stress or illness. For some individuals, a diet high in protein and complex carbohydrates is prescribed.

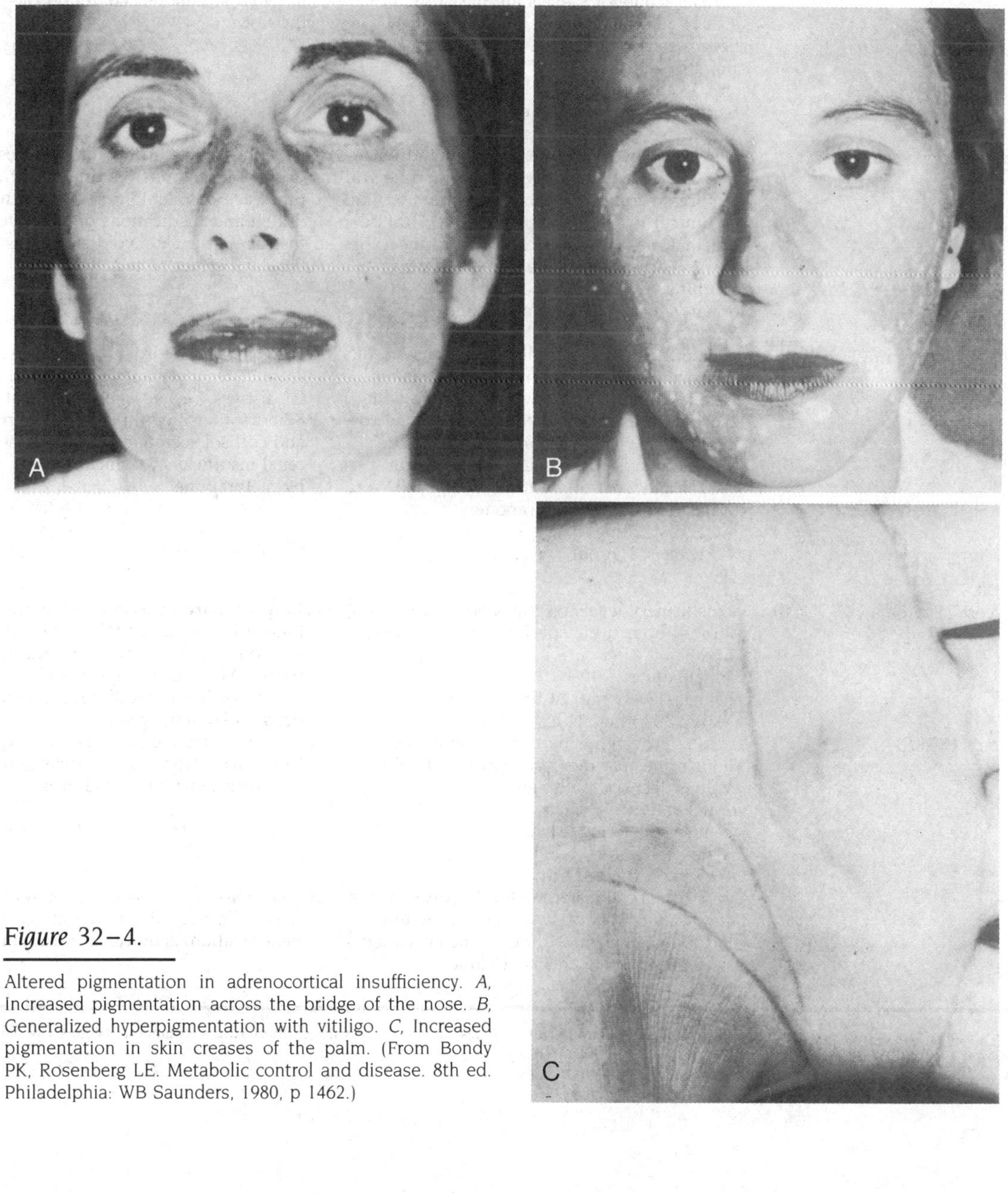

Figure 32–4.

Altered pigmentation in adrenocortical insufficiency. *A*, Increased pigmentation across the bridge of the nose. *B*, Generalized hyperpigmentation with vitiligo. *C*, Increased pigmentation in skin creases of the palm. (From Bondy PK, Rosenberg LE. Metabolic control and disease. 8th ed. Philadelphia: WB Saunders, 1980, p 1462.)

Table 32–1. COMMON DIAGNOSTIC STUDIES OF ADRENAL CORTEX FUNCTION

STUDY	PURPOSE AND PROCEDURE	NURSING IMPLICATIONS
SERUM STUDIES		
Aldosterone	Assess mineralocorticoid production. Measured in conjunction with 24-hour urine to detect aldosteronism. Normal values (upright): Females: 5–30 ng/dl Males: 6–22 ng/dl	Follow physician's dietary and medication instructions. Unrestricted salt intake is preferred. Record diet and medications on laboratory slip.
Cortisol	Assess cortisol production. Levels normally vary with circadian rhythms, with peak level in early morning. Normal values: Morning: 5–25 μg/dl Afternoon: 3–13 μg/dl ($\frac{1}{2}$ of peak level) Evening: $<\frac{1}{2}$ of peak level	Specimen may be collected twice on the same day to evaluate circadian effects on cortisol secretion. Minimize stress to avoid artificially elevated levels. Note time collected on laboratory slip.
ACTH	Assess ACTH production. Levels normally vary with circadian rhythms, with peak level in early morning. Immediately place specimen in ice water. Normal values: Morning: 20–100 pg/ml Afternoon: 10–40 pg/ml ($<\frac{1}{2}$ of peak value)	Implications are the same as for plasma cortisol levels. Single specimen is best collected in early morning. Prepare ice bath before venipuncture.
ACTH stimulation test	Assess response to ACTH in adrenocortical insufficiency. Normally ACTH stimulates increased cortisol production. Baseline serum cortisol laboratory levels are measured. ACTH administered via IV or IM bolus. Serum cortisol levels are drawn 30 and 60 minutes later. Normal values after ACTH: Serum cortisol >20 μg/dl and two to three times baseline	Note on laboratory slip exact time ACTH was administered and specimens were drawn. Check for food restrictions. Instruct patient to avoid strenuous activity on the day before the test.
Dexamethasone suppression test	Assess response to dexamethasone in adrenocortical excess. Normally dexamethasone will suppress cortisol secretion. Baseline morning serum cortisol levels are measured. Oral dexamethasone is administered at bedtime. Serum cortisol levels measured the next morning. Normal values after dexamethasone: Serum cortisol <5 μg/dl.	Check physician's orders for drug restrictions. Cortisol levels must be drawn at the same time each day. Note time specimens were drawn and medications on laboratory slip. Instruct patient to avoid strenuous activity the day before the test.
Metyrapone suppression test	Evaluate the pituitary feedback response to differentiate between adrenal hyperplasia and adrenal tumor. Normally metyrapone will block adrenal cortisol synthesis. Baseline cortisol and ACTH levels are measured. Oral metyrapone is administered at midnight. ACTH and cortisol are measured at 8:00 A.M. Normal values after metyrapone: ACTH: >250 pg/dl Cortisol: <8 μg/dl	Check physician's orders for drug restrictions. Administer metyrapone with food to prevent GI distress. Second specimen must be drawn 8 hours after metyrapone during peak ACTH and cortisol secretion periods. Assess for adrenal insufficiency, which may be induced by metyrapone.
URINE STUDIES		
17-Hydroxycorticosteroids (17-OHCS)	Assess urinary levels of glucocorticoid metabolites. 24-hour urine specimen with preservative. Normal values: Females: 3–13 mg/24 hr Males: 3–15 mg/24 hr	Follow standard collection procedures for 24-hour urine specimen. Note start and end time on collection container and patient record. Many drugs affect results; check physician's orders for restrictions. Note medications on laboratory slip.
17-Ketosteroids (17-KS)	Assess androgen metabolites in the urine. 24-hour urine specimen with preservative. Values decrease with age. Normal values: Females: 5–15 mg/24 hr Males: 8–25 mg/24 hr >65 yr: 4–8 mg/24 hr	Implications are the same as for 17-OHCS. Check with laboratory to determine whether specimen must be kept chilled.
Aldosterone	Assess urinary aldosterone levels. Measured in conjunction with plasma aldosterone to detect aldosteronism. 24-hour urine specimen with preservative and kept chilled. Normal values: 35–80 μg/24 hr	Implications are the same as for serum aldosterone. Test results are not affected by patient position, activity, or circadian rhythms.

Normal values and procedures are guidelines. Contact laboratory performing test for absolute values, interfering substances, specimen preservation, and specific collection procedures.

Abbreviations: IV, intravenous; IM, intramuscular; GI, gastrointestinal.

Table 32–2. TYPICAL RESULTS OF COMMON DIAGNOSTIC STUDIES OF ADRENAL CORTEX FUNCTION IN ADDISON'S DISEASE AND CUSHING'S SYNDROME

	ADDISON'S DISEASE		CUSHING'S SYNDROME		
STUDY	PRIMARY ADDISON'S DISEASE	PITUITARY ACTH-DEPENDENT ADDISON'S DISEASE	CORTISOL-SECRETING ADRENAL TUMOR	PITUITARY ACTH-DEPENDENT CUSHING'S SYNDROME	ECTOPIC ACTH-SECRETING TUMOR
Plasma cortisol	Low	Low	High	High	High
Plasma ACTH	High	Low	High	High	High
17-OHCS	Low	Low	High	High	High
Cortisol response to ACTH stimulation test	None	Normal rise	Marked rise	None	None
Cortisol response to high-dose dexamethasone suppression test			None	Marked drop	None
Cortisol response to metyrapone suppression test			None	Marked rise	Varies

Data represent typical response, but exceptions are possible on rare occasions.
Abbreviation: 17-OHCS, 17-hydroxycorticosteroids.

Fludrocortisone acetate (Florinef) is the drug of choice to replace mineralocorticoid activity. It may be prescribed daily to three times a week. To help prevent sodium depletion, the patient is placed on a diet of unrestricted salt intake. During periods of fluid loss or profuse perspiration, intake of fluid and salt is increased.

Management of acute adrenocortical insufficiency, or Addison's crisis, is a medical emergency. Fluid replacement to reverse hypovolemic shock and steroid replacement are priorities. Hypoglycemia is reversed with parenteral dextrose. Intravenous hydrocortisone every 6 hours and a rapid infusion of isotonic dextrose and saline are administered. Vital signs and serum electrolyte and blood glucose levels are monitored frequently to evaluate fluid, electrolyte, and blood glucose status. Hyperpyrexia is usually corrected with reversal of dehydration. If the patient is admitted to an intensive care unit, sophisticated hemodynamic and cardiac monitoring is implemented.

With properly managed hormone-replacement therapy and patient education to minimize the risk of Addison's crisis, the individual with chronic adrenocortical insufficiency can expect a normal, active life.

Application of the Nursing Process to the Care of the Patient with Adrenocortical Insufficiency: Addison's Disease

Assessment

Obtain a complete nursing history from the patient with diagnosed or suspected chronic adrenocortical insufficiency. Ask specifically about the onset of early symptoms of unusual fatigue, weakness, and lingering minor illnesses. Nonspecific early symptoms are often overlooked by the patient as insignificant or unrelated. Ask about recent or past use of topical, oral, and parenteral adrenocorticosteroid preparations. Obtain baseline weight and vital sign measurements. Assess blood pressure and pulse while the patient is lying and standing to identify the presence of orthostatic hypotension, which is frequently present in fluid volume deficit. Determine presymptomatic weight and blood pressure, if documented or known by patient, and compare with current assessments. Assess mucous membranes and skin turgor for signs of dehydration. Assess for the presence of clinical manifestations associated with Addison's disease. Identify the patient's interpretation of clinical manifestations and knowledge of planned diagnostic procedures and treatment to determine teaching needs.

Assessment of the patient with acute adrenocortical insufficiency is limited to a brief history of the current illness, identification of allergies, and determination of hemodynamic status until intravenous fluids and steroids are initiated. Once the patient is stabilized, obtain a complete history and identification of the events that precipitated the episode of Addison's crisis.

Nursing Diagnoses and Planning

Nursing diagnoses and related expected patient outcomes most commonly applicable to patients with adrenocortical insufficiency (Addison's disease) include the following:

NDx: High risk for fluid volume deficit related to loss of extracellular sodium and water secondary to mineralocorticoid insufficiency

Chart 32–1.

NURSING GUIDE TO PATIENT EDUCATION FOR SELF-MANAGEMENT: CHRONIC ADRENOCORTICAL INSUFFICIENCY—ADDISON'S DISEASE

Instruct the patient to:

Understand the disease process and the need for lifelong replacement therapy.
Take the prescribed replacement therapy; know the names, doses, routes and times of administration, expected effects, side effects of each medication.
Recognize the risk of Addison's crisis, conditions that may precipitate crisis, signs and symptoms of impending crisis, course of action to take.
Notify the physician if unable to ingest or retain food or fluids or if symptoms of crisis develop.
Adjust dosage of prescribed glucocorticoids during illness or increased stress as instructed by the physician.
Carry an emergency syringe of parenteral hydrocortisone at all times and learn how to inject it intramuscularly.
Wear medical alert identification at all times.
Follow a high-complex-carbohydrate, high-protein diet if prescribed.
Maintain high daily sodium intake (up to 8 g), more in hot weather and when diaphoresis is profuse.
Minimize stress and avoid infections and people with infections.
Identify sources of stress, and use relaxation or other techniques to reduce stress.
Avoid fatigue by alternating activity with rest periods.
See physician at least two times a year for follow-up examination and evaluation of treatment regimen.

Planning: Patient outcomes
1. Patient demonstrates adequate extracellular fluid volume as evidenced by the following:
   a. Stable vital signs within normal limits
   b. Moist mucous membranes
   c. Good skin turgor
2. Patient verbalizes understanding of the need for, and intent to take, mineralocorticoid replacement as prescribed.
3. Patient identifies foods and fluids that promote fluid and electrolyte balance.

NDx: High risk for infection related to impaired glucose-regulating mechanisms, impaired immune response, and inability to tolerate stress secondary to glucocorticoid insufficiency

Planning: Patient outcomes
1. Patient verbalizes understanding of the need for, and intent to take, glucocorticoid replacement as prescribed.
2. Patient identifies foods that promote maintenance of blood glucose levels and protein synthesis.
3. Patient remains free of infection.

NDx: Altered tissue perfusion: systemic, related to massive fluid and sodium loss secondary to Addison's crisis

Planning: Patient outcomes
1. Patient maintains adequate tissue perfusion as evidenced by the following:
   a. Stable vital signs within normal limits
   b. Normal neurologic responses
   c. Urine output greater than 30 ml/hour
2. Patient identifies factors that may precipitate Addison's crisis and ways to avoid them.
3. Patient verbalizes understanding of the need for lifelong steroid-replacement therapy and follow-up care.

Nursing Interventions

Nursing care of the individual with adrenocortical insufficiency requires frequent assessment and supportive intervention because of potentially rapid fluctuations in fluid and electrolyte balance and cardiovascular status in addition to adrenocortical hormone replacement. Patient education for self-management of adrenocortical insufficiency and lifelong steroid-replacement therapy to avoid episodes of Addison's crisis is a primary focus. Nursing guidelines for patient education are summarized in Chart 32–1. In developing a teaching plan, it is important to remember that a patient receiving steroid-replacement therapy to correct a deficiency is much less likely to exhibit side effects than a patient receiving supraphysiologic doses to suppress an immune or inflammatory response. Pharmacology Box 32–1 identifies the pharmacokinetics of adrenocorticosteroid preparations.

NDx: High risk for fluid volume deficit

Administer mineralocorticoid replacement as prescribed. Teach the patient dosage and schedule, expected action, and side effects of prescribed mineralocorticoid. Monitor vital signs every 4 hours, and assess skin turgor, mucous membranes, and mental status to detect signs of dehydration. Measure intake and output and weigh the patient daily to identify excess fluid loss. Instruct the patient to report increased thirst or lightheadedness on standing, which may indicate developing fluid loss. Encourage fluid intake to 3000 ml/day with physician approval. Administer intravenous fluids, sodium replacement,

Pharmacology Box 32–1.

ADRENOCORTICOSTEROIDS

Adrenocorticosteroids:
Class of drugs with properties similar to the corticosteroids secreted by the adrenal cortex.

Action:
Mineralocorticoids promote sodium and water retention and potassium excretion by increasing transport through the renal tubular walls. Glucocorticoids promote hepatic gluconeogenesis, alter fat and protein metabolism, and suppress the antiinflammatory and immune response. In supraphysiologic dosages, both groups of corticosteroids exhibit similar properties.

Uses:
Replacement therapy in adrenocortical insufficiency and for suppression of undesirable inflammatory, immune, or allergic responses.

Side Effects:
Side effects rarely develop with replacement therapy or short-term, high-dose therapy. Among side effects are peptic ulcer, steroid diabetes, delayed wound healing and tissue repair, increased susceptibility to infections, osteoporosis, edema, hypertension, amenorrhea, acne, ecchymoses, hirsutism, cataracts, glaucoma, optic nerve damage, atrophy of the adrenal cortex, a Cushing-like syndrome (fat deposits on the face, trunk, neck, shoulders, wasting of arms and legs), mood changes. Adrenocorticosteroids are contraindicated in infectious processes because they mask infections.

Interactions:
Antacids decrease absorption. Hyperglycemic effect may necessitate increased doses of antidiabetic agents. Adrenocorticosteroids increase ulcerogenic effects of salicylates. Their use with antibiotics may result in emergence of resistant strains of microorganisms. Amphotericin B and diuretics increase potassium excretion. Barbiturates, phenytoin, and rifampin decrease effect.

Nursing Implications:
Administer oral preparations with food or milk to decrease ulcerogenic effect. Administer parenteral solutions intravenously or by deep intramuscular injection to avoid tissue atrophy. Avoid the deltoid muscle. Do not alter from prescribed dosage or times of administration. Abrupt withdrawal or dosage reduction may precipitate Addison's crisis. Monitor vital signs, intake and output, daily weight, and urine or blood glucose levels. Assess for dependent edema, mood changes, hypernatremia, hypokalemia, altered vision, and infections. Teach the patient the importance of medical supervision, to consult physician before taking any over-the-counter preparations, and to wear medical alert identification.

Geriatric Considerations:
The elderly are more susceptible to the side effects of this class of drugs and often have preexisting conditions that can be exacerbated by these drugs (e.g., cardiovascular disorders, diabetes mellitus). Treatment is usually initiated with lower doses. Monitor closely for fluid retention, electrolyte imbalance, and hyperglycemia.

Nursing Care Guide 32–1.

PATIENTS WITH ACUTE ADRENOCORTICAL INSUFFICIENCY: ADDISON'S CRISIS

Assessment Findings: Patient with history of chronic adrenocortical insufficiency (Addison's disease) admitted after 24 hours of vomiting and diarrhea. Patient is responsive but lethargic, skin is hot and dry, mucous membranes are dry, temperature is 103.3°F (39.6°C), blood pressure is 90/60 mm Hg, pulse is 110 bpm and thready.

Nursing Diagnosis: Fluid volume deficit related to extracellular sodium and water loss secondary to vomiting, diarrhea, and adrenocortical insufficiency

Patient Outcomes	Nursing Interventions	Rationale
Patient demonstrates adequate extracellular fluid volume by moist mucous membranes, good skin turgor, blood pressure within 10% of normal baseline, pulse 60–100 bpm, urine output >30 ml/hr, and is alert and responds appropriately.	Administer intravenous hydrocortisone and isotonic dextrose and saline as prescribed.	Provides adrenocorticosteroid hormone, fluid, glucose, and sodium replacement.
	Monitor vital signs, neurologic status, urine output, capillary refill hourly. Monitor pulmonary wedge pressure as appropriate, and electrocardiogram if in intensive care unit. Assess for hyperkalemia, and monitor results of serum electrolyte studies.	Evaluates effectiveness of treatment. Hemodynamic parameters indicate perfusion of vital organs. Hyperkalemia may cause cardiac dysrhythmias.
	Administer antiemetic and antidiarrheal if prescribed.	Prevents further fluid loss.
	Provide oral fluids and high-sodium diet as prescribed when patient is alert.	Maintains adequate fluid and sodium replacement.

Evaluation: Compare the patient's status with the expected patient outcomes. If the outcomes are achieved, evaluate nursing care as successful. If not, reassess the patient, formulate new nursing diagnoses, and revise expected patient outcomes and nursing interventions as appropriate.

(continued)

and antiemetics if prescribed. Consult with the dietitian to provide unrestricted salt diet. Assist the patient in selecting high-sodium foods from daily menu. Teach the patient to prevent excess fluid and sodium loss by maintaining adequate salt intake, up to 8 g of sodium daily, and increasing salt intake during hot weather, before strenuous exercise, and if fever, vomiting, or diarrhea occur. Teach the patient and provide in writing the early signs of dehydration, with instructions to notify the physician promptly if they occur to prevent the onset of Addison's crisis.

NDx: High risk for infection

Administer glucocorticoid replacement as prescribed. Teach the patient dosage and schedule, expected action, and side effects of prescribed glucocorticoid. Place the patient in a quiet room, and ensure that roommates are not infectious. Explain all procedures, answer questions, keep environment as free from stress as possible, and encourage communication with the physician and significant others to reduce anxiety. Avoid unnecessary invasive procedures, and protect from chills, drafts, and exposure to staff and visitors with upper respiratory tract infections to minimize chance of infection. Use sterile technique when caring for all skin lesions, venipuncture sites, drains, and wounds to prevent contamination. Monitor vital signs, examine all open areas, and culture suspicious drainage and wounds for prompt identification and treatment of infections. Encourage rest periods to prevent fatigue. In consultation with the dietitian and the physician, teach the patient to select a diet high in complex carbohy-

Nursing Care Guide 32–1. *(continued)*

PATIENTS WITH ACUTE ADRENOCORTICAL INSUFFICIENCY: ADDISON'S CRISIS

Assessment Findings: Patient with chronic adrenocortical insufficiency (Addison's disease) is to be discharged after treatment for an episode of Addison's crisis precipitated by gastrointestinal illness.

Nursing Diagnosis: High risk for altered health maintenance related to insufficient knowledge of self-management of chronic adrenocortical insufficiency and lifelong replacement therapy.

Patient Outcomes	Nursing Interventions	Rationale
Patient identifies recent gastrointestinal illness as precipitating event of this episode of Addison's crisis.	Review disease process and effect of excess fluid and sodium loss and illness on control of Addison's disease. Discuss probability of recent gastrointestinal illness as precipitating event.	Accurate information corrects misunderstandings and increases patient's knowledge.
Patient identifies factors that may precipitate Addison's crisis.	Discuss situations that may precipitate Addison's crisis: hot weather, prolonged excessive perspiration, infection, illness, increased stress, injury. Confer with the patient to identify ways to minimize risks.	Knowledge of possible precipitating factors helps prevent or minimize risk of future crises.
Patient states correct actions to take to minimize risk of Addison's crisis or if signs of dehydration develop.	Teach patient and provide in writing the signs of fluid loss. Teach patient to carry prescribed parenteral hydrocortisone and medical alert identification at all times.	Early detection promotes rapid treatment. Written instructions reinforce learning.
	Teach patient, and a caregiver, and observe return demonstration of correct administration of parenteral hydrocortisone.	Return demonstration provides opportunity to evaluate learning and correct administration technique.
	Instruct patient to notify physician during periods of high risk or if signs of fluid loss develop. Teach patient to increase fluid intake, salt intake, and glucocorticoid preparation as prescribed during periods of high risk.	Increased fluid, sodium, and glucocorticoid intake reduces risk of dehydration and crisis episodes.
Patient states intent to keep twice yearly follow-up appointments.	Reinforce importance of twice yearly follow-up by physician.	Evaluates effectiveness of therapeutic regimen.

Evaluation: Compare the patient's status with the expected patient outcomes. If the outcomes are achieved, evaluate nursing care as successful. If not, reassess the patient, formulate new nursing diagnoses, and revise expected patient outcomes and nursing interventions as appropriate.

drates and protein to promote maintenance of blood glucose levels and protein synthesis. Help the patient identify sources of emotional stress and methods of dealing effectively with them. Discuss situations in daily activities that increase risk of exposure to infectious diseases, and help the patient plan ways to avoid them.

NDx: Altered tissue perfusion: systemic
Monitor vital signs, neurologic status, and urine output hourly during acute adrenocortical insufficiency (Addison's crisis) to assess changes in condition. Monitor results of serum electrolyte studies to evaluate status. If the patient is in an intensive care setting, monitor pulmonary wedge pressures and electrocardiogram as ordered to assess cardiovascular status and to detect dysrhythmias. Administer prescribed intravenous hydrocortisone and isotonic dextrose and saline to re-establish fluid and electrolyte balance. Monitor cardiovascular status and infusion rate hourly to prevent fluid overload because of the risk of heart failure in the presence of cardiac atrophy. Assess infusion sites hourly for early detection of infiltration or inflammation. Nursing Care Guide 32–1 summarizes the nursing care of a patient during Addison's crisis.

Once the patient is stabilized, review events preceding the episode to identify probable precipitating factors. Explain the relationship between the disease process and the need for lifelong steroid-replacement therapy to promote compliance with prescribed therapeutic regimen. Be sure the patient understands the need for increased doses of glucocorticoids during periods of stress and increased salt and fluids during periods of increased perspiration to prevent Addison's crisis. Instruct the patient to carry a kit containing syringes of parenteral hydrocortisone to be administered in an emergency. Teach and have the patient and a caregiver demonstrate intramuscular injection technique. Encourage the patient to wear medical alert identification at all times.

Evaluation

Evaluate the effectiveness of nursing care for a patient with adrenocortical insufficiency (Addison's disease) by comparing the patient's status with the expected patient outcomes. Examples of specific outcomes for patients with adrenocortical insufficiency have been provided in the Planning section.

Adrenocortical Excess: Cushing's Syndrome

ETIOLOGY

Adrenocortical excess, or Cushing's syndrome, is a functional disorder characterized by oversecretion of glucocorticoid hormones, primarily cortisol and, to some degree, adrenal androgen. Hyperplasia of the adrenal cortices, especially the zona fasciculata, is the most common cause of adrenocortical excess. This cortical hyperplasia is usually in response to overproduction of ACTH by a benign secreting adenoma of the anterior pituitary or by an ectopic ACTH-secreting tumor. Bronchogenic and small cell carcinomas of the lung and carcinomas of the pancreas or gastrointestinal tract frequently secrete ACTH. Pituitary-dependent Cushing's syndrome, sometimes referred to as Cushing's disease, may occasionally be caused by oversecretion of CRH by the hypothalamus. Another cause of Cushing's syndrome is a cortisol-secreting tumor of the adrenal cortex. A Cushing-like syndrome can also be induced by prolonged administration of high doses of exogenous glucocorticoids.

Cushing's syndrome is rare in the United States, with approximately 10 cases per million population annually. It most commonly develops in the third and fourth decades of life. Cushing's syndrome resulting from an adrenal tumor or pituitary hypersecretion is more common in women. Ectopic ACTH-secreting tumors are more common in men.

PATHOPHYSIOLOGY

Most pathologic changes associated with Cushing's syndrome are caused by physiologic response to abnormally high levels of cortisol. Increased androgen levels and the mineralocorticoid actions of cortisol also cause pathologic alterations.

Unregulated secretion of cortisol causes increased gluconeogenesis and inhibits the ability of insulin to transport glucose into the cells. Elevated cortisol levels accelerate protein catabolism, impair protein synthesis, and increase mobilization of fat from the extremities. Fat deposits increase on the trunk, supraclavicular areas, between the shoulders, and, to a lesser degree, on the face. Elevated cortisol levels also impair antibody production and inhibit proliferation of lymphocytes. Susceptibility to peptic ulcers increases because cortisol inhibits gastric mucous production while stimulating gastric acid and pepsin production.

The mineralocorticoid actions of supraphysiologic levels of cortisone promote potassium excretion and sodium and water retention. Increased androgen secretion causes virilization in women.

CLINICAL MANIFESTATIONS

Cushing's syndrome may develop gradually or rapidly. Early clinical manifestations are muscular weakness and fatigue. In women, alteration in the menstrual cycle is an early symptom. Truncal obesity, "buffalo hump" between the shoulders, and thin extremities are characteristic. The chest and abdomen may become pendulous. Fat deposits and edema combine to give the face a round, moon-shaped appearance. Hyperglycemia produces "steroid diabetes." Protein catabolism leads to weakness, loss of muscle mass, osteoporosis, bone tenderness, and atrophy of the skin. Osteoporosis may result in pathologic fractures and compression fractures of the vertebrae. The skin becomes thin, fragile, and paper-like, with wide purplish striae caused by deterioration of collagen fibers. Hyperpigmentation, similar to that seen in Addison's disease, may develop in individuals with secondary Cushing's syndrome caused by excess ACTH secretion. Capillary fragility causes large ecchymotic areas to develop either spontaneously or from minor trauma. The face and neck often have a ruddy appearance. Decreased protein synthesis impairs healing and response to injury and infection. Early signs of infection are often suppressed or absent. Rapid mood swings, depression, irritability, euphoria, insomnia, and occasionally psychosis may develop because of the effect of excess cortisol on mental and cognitive functions.

Fluid overload from sodium and water retention may lead to hypertension, edema, cardiac overload, and heart failure. Increased androgen secretion may cause acne, thinning of scalp hair, and decreased libido. In women, oligomenorrhea, amenorrhea, hirsutism, and mild masculinization are common. Figures 32–5 and 32–6 illustrate common clinical manifestations of Cushing's syndrome.

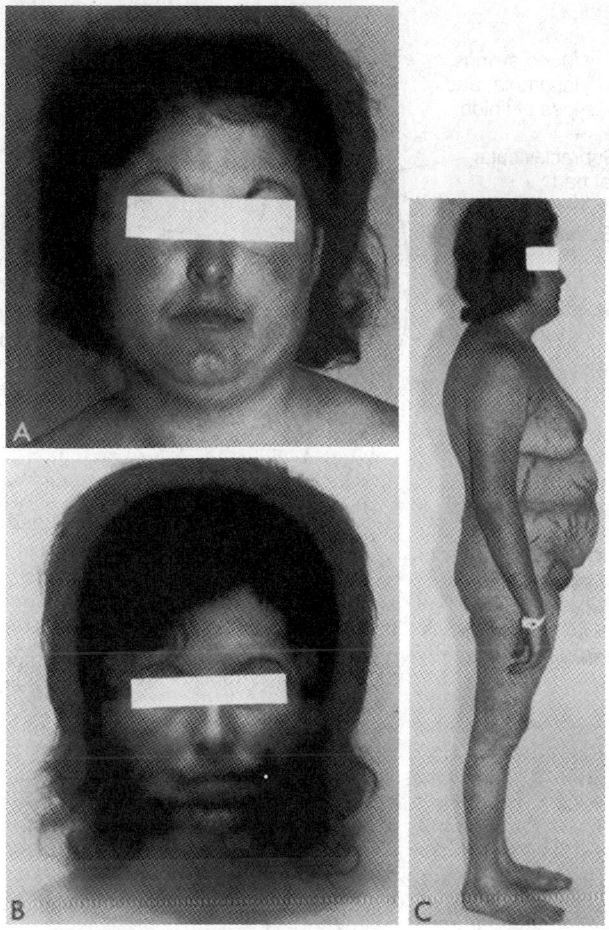

Figure 32–5.

The appearance of a woman with Cushing's syndrome due to adrenal adenoma. Facial features (*A*) before and (*B*) 1 year after treatment. *C*, Profile before treatment. (From Wyngaarden JB, Smith LH, Bennett JC (eds). Cecil textbook of medicine. 19th ed. Philadelphia: WB Saunders, 1992, p 1285.)

MEDICAL DIAGNOSIS

Diagnosis of Cushing's syndrome is made on the basis of the clinical picture and laboratory studies. Circulating plasma cortisol levels are several times higher than normal, and the normal diurnal secretion pattern is absent. In 24-hour urine specimens, 17-OHCS and 17-KS levels are elevated. Plasma ACTH level is elevated in pituitary-dependent Cushing's syndrome and in nonpituitary ACTH-secreting tumors but is decreased if a cortisol-secreting adrenal tumor is present. Cortisol response to the dexamethasone and metyrapone suppression tests varies with the cause. Results of common studies of adrenal function in Cushing's syndrome are presented in Table 32–2.

Additional laboratory studies demonstrate hyperglycemia and impaired glucose tolerance, hypokalemia, hypernatremia, hypercalcemia, and leukocytosis. Erythrocytosis, granulocytosis, lymphopenia, and eosinopenia may also be present. Radiologic studies may show osteoporosis, pathologic fractures, collapsed vertebrae, and cardiac hypertrophy.

Radiologic studies, computed tomography (CT) scans, nuclear magnetic resonance imaging (MRI), angiography, and studies to diagnose neoplastic disorders help to locate adrenal tumors and identify extra-adrenal sources of ACTH.

MEDICAL MANAGEMENT

The primary goal of the medical management of Cushing's syndrome is to return cortisol levels to normal. Without treatment, one half of the individuals with Cushing's syndrome die within 5 years. Prognosis with treatment depends on the severity and duration of the disease at the time of diagnosis plus the severity of residual cardiovascular effects. The earlier the disorder is diagnosed and treated, the better the prognosis.

Treatment of Cushing's syndrome is determined by the cause. The treatment of choice for pituitary-dependent Cushing's syndrome (Cushing's disease) is transsphenoidal microsurgery to remove the ACTH-secreting tumor while preserving normal pituitary function. Pituitary and adrenal function returns to normal in approximately 80% of these patients. In some women, menses returns and pregnancy is possible. If the pituitary tumor is larger than 1 cm in diameter or has extended beyond the sella turcica, a total transsphenoidal hypophysectomy may be performed. After a total hypophysectomy, the patient requires lifelong replace-

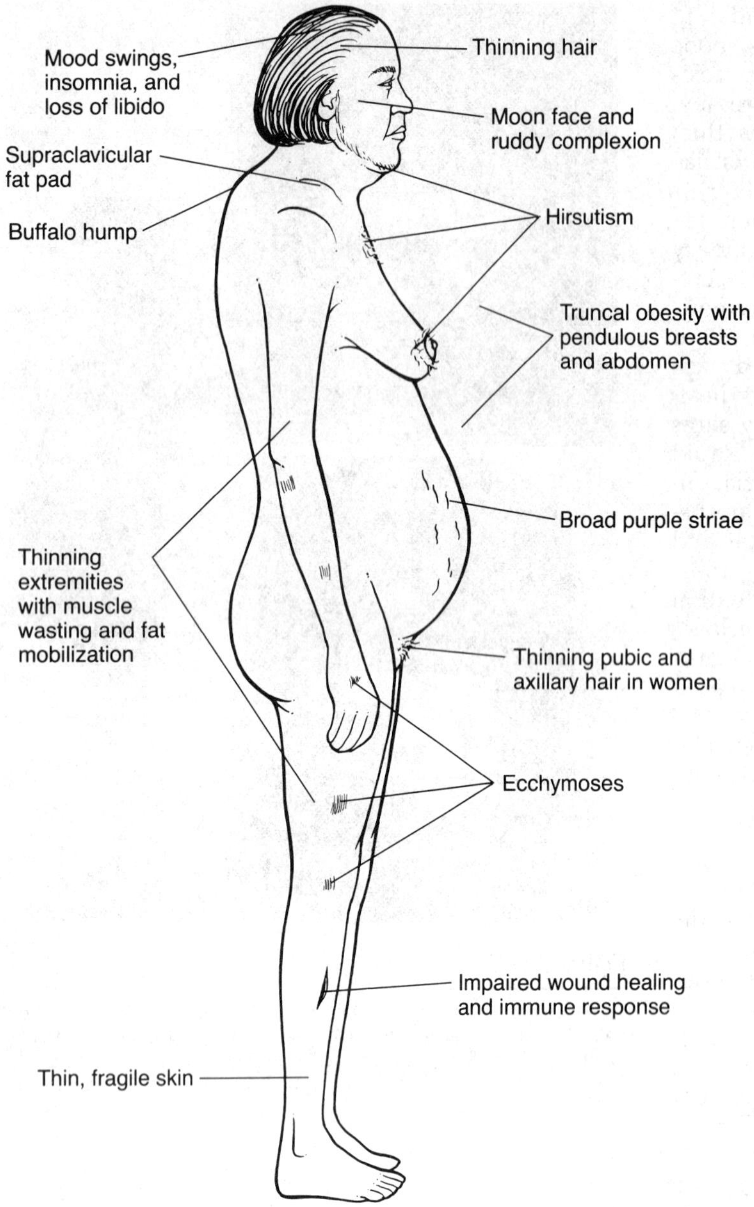

Figure 32–6.

Common clinical manifestations of Cushing's syndrome.

ment of corticosteroids, thyroid hormones, and, in some cases, gonad hormones. Bilateral adrenalectomy, irradiation of the pituitary gland, and administration of adrenal suppressant drugs are alternative treatments if transsphenoidal surgery is contraindicated.

Bilateral or unilateral adrenalectomy is indicated if an adrenal tumor or idiopathic hyperplasia is diagnosed. If a bilateral adrenalectomy is performed, lifelong corticosteroid replacement is required. Ectopic ACTH-secreting tumors respond best by treating the primary neoplasm. If the neoplasm is inoperable, adrenal suppressant drugs are given. The most commonly used adrenal suppressant drugs are mitotane (Lysodren), aminoglutethimide (Cytadren), and metyrapone (Metopirone). Mitotane, the most powerful of these drugs, destroys the adrenal zona fasciculata and zona reticularis. Because it has relatively little effect on the zona glomerulosa, patients treated with mitotane become cortisol deficient but maintain adequate aldosterone secretion. Aminoglutethimide and metyrapone block cortisol synthesis. Nausea and vomiting, central nervous system (CNS) depression, and skin rashes are the most common side effects of adrenal suppressants. Patients are monitored closely for signs of adrenocortical insufficiency during and after treatment of Cushing's syndrome.

If exogenous administration of corticosteroids has resulted in a Cushing-like syndrome, the drug is slowly tapered to the minimal therapeutic level. Corticosteroids required for treatment of long-term chronic conditions can sometimes be administered on an alternate-day schedule that maintains their therapeutic effectiveness while maintaining normal ACTH secretion and adrenal responsiveness to reduce the risk of Cushing-like side effects.

Mineralocorticoid effects of Cushing's syndrome

are treated with spironolactone (Aldactone), a mineralocorticoid antagonist.

Application of the Nursing Process to the Care of the Patient with Adrenocortical Excess: Cushing's Syndrome

Assessment

Obtain a complete nursing history from the patient with diagnosed or suspected adrenocortical excess. Ask specifically about the use of adrenocortical steroid compounds. Obtain weight and vital sign measurements, and compare with presymptomatic assessments if documented or known by the patient. Assess for dependent edema, altered skin integrity, and the presence of clinical manifestations associated with Cushing's syndrome. Determine the patient's activity level and ability to carry out activities of daily living (ADL). Identify the patient's interpretation of clinical manifestations, knowledge of planned diagnostic procedures and treatment, and expectations of the outcome of treatment to determine teaching needs.

Nursing Diagnoses and Planning

Nursing diagnoses and related expected patient outcomes most commonly applicable to patients with adrenocortical excess (Cushing's syndrome) include the following:

NDx: High risk for infection related to impaired immune response and tissue repair

Planning: Patient outcomes
1. Patient identifies activities that increase the risk of infection.
2. Patient participates in activities that reduce the risk of infection.
3. Patient remains afebrile and damaged tissue remains free of localized inflammation, edema, and purulent drainage.

NDx: High risk for altered health maintenance related to insufficient knowledge of how disease process alters carbohydrate, protein, and fat metabolism and increases risk of injury as evidenced by hyperglycemia, skin and capillary fragility, muscle weakness, altered center of gravity, osteoporosis, and increased gastric acid and pepsin secretion

Planning: Patient outcomes
1. Patient verbalizes understanding of the effects of excess cortisol secretion on the body.
2. Patient identifies activities that increase the risk of injury.
3. Patient participates in activities that reduce the risk of injury.
4. Patient remains free of injury.

NDx: Decreased cardiac output related to fluid and electrolyte imbalance

Planning: Patient outcomes
1. Patient demonstrates adequate cardiac output as evidenced by the following:
   a. Stable vital signs within normal limits
   b. Ability to complete self-care activities
   c. Absence of dependent edema, dyspnea, or orthopnea
   d. Lungs clear to auscultation
2. Patient identifies and selects low-sodium foods from daily menu choices.
3. Patient demonstrates stable or decreasing weight.

NDx: Body image disturbance related to physical and behavioral changes characteristic of adrenocortical excess

Planning: Patient outcomes
1. Patient identifies adrenocortical excess as cause of physical and behavioral changes.
2. Patient verbalizes realistic expectations of treatment.
3. Patient verbalizes positive statements about self and future plans.

Nursing Interventions

The focus of nursing care of the individual with adrenocortical excess is to prevent potentially life-threatening infection and injury. Throughout diagnosis and treatment, provide emotional support and information to help the patient and family understand and cope with the physical and mental manifestations of Cushing's disease while developing realistic expectations of treatment.

NDx: High risk for infection
Place the patient in a private room or a room with a noninfectious roommate and protect from visitors and staff with infectious diseases to minimize exposure to pathogens. Discuss the effect of excess cortisol secretion on the body's immune response and tissue repair with the patient. Stress proper hand washing by all personnel, the patient, and visitors. Avoid unnecessary invasive procedures, and use sterile technique when caring for all open lesions, venipuncture sites, and drains to prevent contamination. Monitor temperature every 4 hours, and assess all open areas for signs of infection or inflammation. Culture all suspicious drainage and slow-healing wounds, and monitor results of white blood cell counts to ensure prompt identification of infection, because signs of inflammation may be masked by excess cortisol. Administer prescribed antibiotics on time to ensure therapeutic blood levels. Encourage the patient to deep breathe and

Nursing Care Guide 32–2.

POSTOPERATIVE CARE OF PATIENTS UNDERGOING ADRENALECTOMY FOR CUSHING'S SYNDROME

Assessment Findings: Patient admitted to surgical intensive care unit from postanesthesia care unit after unilateral adrenalectomy for Cushing's syndrome.

Nursing Diagnosis: High risk for altered tissue perfusion: systemic, related to fluid loss and electrolyte imbalance secondary to rapid depletion of adrenocortical hormones and risk of postoperative hemorrhage

Patient Outcomes	Nursing Interventions	Rationale
Patient demonstrates adequate extracellular fluid volume by moist mucous membranes, good skin turgor, blood pressure within 10% of normal baseline, pulse 60–100 bpm, urine output >30 ml/hour, and is alert and responds appropriately.	Administer intravenous hydrocortisone and isotonic dextrose and saline for 24 to 48 hours postoperatively. Administer mineralocorticoid, if prescribed, on the second postoperative day.	Adrenocorticosteroid replacement is necessary to stabilize serum steroid levels during rapid drop in endogenous adrenocortical hormone secretion after surgery. Fluid, glucose, and electrolyte replacement minimizes the risk of Addison's crisis and hypovolemic shock and maintains electrolyte balance.
	Monitor vital signs, neurologic status, urine output, capillary refill hourly. Monitor blood glucose four times daily. Monitor electrocardiogram and pulmonary wedge pressure.	Hemodynamic parameters indicate perfusion of vital organs. Drop in endogenous glucocorticoid secretion places patient at risk for hypoglycemia.
	Examine flank incision and surgical dressings and check under patient frequently for active bleeding. Examine abdomen for hematoma or distension caused by internal bleeding.	Risk of postoperative bleeding is high because adrenal glands and kidneys are highly vascular.
	Provide a noninfectious environment, maintain strict aseptic technique, encourage coughing and deep breathing, and assist with early ambulation to decrease risk of infection.	Risk of infection is high as a result of suppressed immune response, impaired protein synthesis, and delayed wound healing.
	Administer prescribed analgesics.	Promotes patient comfort, reduces stress, and increases patient participation in postoperative activities that decrease the risk of infection and promote healing.
	After 48 hours, administer prescribed decreasing doses of adrenocortical hormones.	Allows the remaining adrenal gland to gradually resume hormone secretion.

(continued)

Nursing Care Guide 32–2. *(continued)*

POSTOPERATIVE CARE OF PATIENTS UNDERGOING ADRENALECTOMY FOR CUSHING'S SYNDROME

Patient Outcomes	Nursing Interventions	Rationale
	Monitor for manifestations of adrenocortical deficiency as exogenous hormones are slowly tapered, and notify the physician immediately if they develop.	Early detection and treatment prevent or minimize the risk of crisis.
	Provide oral fluids, food, and medications 48 to 72 hours postoperatively as tolerated, and discontinue intravenous infusion.	Intravenous access is a potential route of infection.

Evaluation: Compare the patient's status with the expected patient outcomes. If the outcomes are achieved, evaluate nursing care as successful. If not, reassess the patient, formulate new nursing diagnoses, and revise expected patient outcomes and nursing interventions as appropriate.

cough every hour while awake, and assist him or her to turn every 2 hours while in bed to mobilize respiratory secretions and reduce risk of pulmonary infection. Teach the patient to select prescribed high protein diet to promote tissue repair.

NDx: High risk for altered health maintenance

Explain to the patient the effects of excess cortisol secretion on body systems. Confer with the patient to identify potential sources of trauma, activities that increase the risk of injury, and ways to minimize risk during daily activities. Encourage the patient to take several rest periods during the day to conserve energy. Assist with daily activities as needed, but encourage independence as tolerated to promote self-esteem. Provide a safe, obstacle-free environment, and encourage the patient to wear nonskid shoes to prevent falls. Encourage ambulation and assist as necessary to promote muscle tone and calcium deposition in the bones. Use side rails as appropriate for safety or for self-positioning in bed. Assess skin for redness, breakdown, and ecchymosis; gently massage bony prominences; and apply skin lubricants at least twice a day to prevent breakdown. Provide a pressure distribution mattress and elbow and heel protectors. Assist the patient with position changes every 2 hours while he or she is in bed. Monitor blood glucose levels, and administer insulin as prescribed. Unless contraindicated, provide prescribed calorie-restricted, high-protein diet in six small meals a day, and administer prescribed antacid or H_2 receptor antagonist to decrease gastric acidity and prevent peptic ulcers. Report gastrointestinal distress, heartburn, and epigastric pain to the physician promptly.

NDx: Decreased cardiac output

Monitor vital signs and apical heart rate and auscultate breath sounds every 4 hours to detect change in hemodynamic status. Administer prescribed diuretics and antihypertensives. Measure blood pressure daily while patient is lying and sitting or standing to detect orthostatic hypotension. Weigh the patient daily, assess for edema, and monitor intake and output to evaluate fluid balance. Assess for signs of hypokalemia, and administer potassium supplement if prescribed. Assist patient in selection of low-sodium and high-potassium foods from daily menu. Encourage independence in self-care, but provide assistance as needed to prevent overexertion. Discontinue all activity in the presence of tachycardia, dyspnea, fatigue, lightheadedness, or change in blood pressure, which signal activity intolerance, and report symptoms to the physician.

Once a method of treatment is selected, reinforce the physician's explanations, provide opportunity for questions, and correct any misconceptions the patient may have. After surgical excision of an adrenal tumor, a pituitary adenoma, or an ACTH-secreting ectopic neoplasm, the patient is usually in an intensive care setting for 48 to 72 hours to facilitate constant monitoring for rapid changes in cardiac function, electrolyte balance, and hemodynamic status caused by the sudden cessation of excess cortisol secretion. Nursing Care Guide 32–2 presents nursing interventions in the care of a patient after adrenal surgery. To prevent Addison's crisis, the physician prescribes parenteral administration of dexamethasone or other glucocorticoid preoperatively, intraoperatively, and postoperatively, with progressively smaller doses gradually tapered off in the days after surgery. A patient who has had a bilateral adrenalectomy will require adrenocortical hormone replacement for life, as discussed for Addison's disease. Because these patients are at extremely high risk for postoperative infection and delayed wound healing, aggressive pulmonary hygiene, aseptic technique, and meticulous wound care are imperative.

If administration of adrenal suppressant drugs is the selected treatment, teach the patient the name, dose, route of administration, expected effects, and side effects. Be sure the patient understands that the desired effects of these drugs may not become apparent for several weeks. Teach and provide in writing the early signs of adrenocortical insufficiency, and instruct the patient to notify the physician immediately if they develop. If hormone-replacement therapy is necessary after treatment because of adrenocortical insufficiency, follow the nursing guidelines for patient education for self-management identified in Chart 32–1.

NDx: Body image disturbance
Provide factual information regarding the effect of increased levels of circulating cortisol on the body and mental status to help the patient and family understand the changes that have occurred. Encourage the patient to identify and describe feelings about physical changes. Reassure the patient that most physical changes and emotional disturbances resolve with treatment. Assist the patient in identifying relaxation techniques that help control emotions. Maintain a calm, unhurried manner, and explain procedures clearly to promote relaxation and trust. Observe the patient closely during episodes of emotional instability and depression. Some patients may become dangerous to themselves or others. Request a mental health consultation if appropriate. Once the method of treatment is selected, reinforce the physician's explanations of the treatment and expected outcome. Provide opportunity for discussion and questions to correct any misconceptions the patient may have. Be sure the patient understands what pathologic changes, if any, the physician expects to be residual. Reinforce the need for lifelong follow-up for early detection of recurring or developing adrenocortical insufficiency.

Evaluation

Evaluate the effectiveness of nursing care for a patient with adrenocortical excess (Cushing's syndrome) by comparing the patient's status with the expected patient outcomes. Examples of specific outcomes for patients with adrenocortical excess have been provided in the Planning section.

Primary Aldosteronism

ETIOLOGY

Primary aldosteronism is characterized by increased aldosterone secretion. It is most commonly caused by a benign aldosterone-secreting adenoma of the zona glomerulosa. Bilateral adrenal cortex hyperplasia is the cause in less than 30% of individuals with primary aldosteronism. Adrenal carcinoma very rarely causes increased aldosterone secretion.

Primary aldosteronism is diagnosed in approximately 1% of the hypertensive population. It occurs more than twice as frequently in women as in men and usually develops between 30 and 50 years of age.

PATHOPHYSIOLOGY

Unregulated hypersecretion of aldosterone results in increased sodium retention in the distal renal tubules with excess potassium and hydrogen ion excretion and suppression of renin production. As a result of this electrolyte imbalance, increased extracellular fluid volume, hypertension, and hypokalemia develop. Metabolic alkalosis occurs as hydrogen ions are excreted with the potassium. Peripheral edema is either minimal or absent in primary aldosteronism because the proximal renal tubules attempt to compensate for the fluid excess by decreasing sodium reabsorption.

Left ventricular hypertrophy, congestive heart failure, cerebrovascular accidents, and progressive deterioration of renal function and vision result from the pathologic effects of prolonged hypertension.

CLINICAL MANIFESTATIONS

Hypertension and hypokalemia are the most significant clinical manifestations of primary aldosteronism. Edema develops only in the presence of congestive heart failure. Hypertension may be mild to severe. Headaches are common and may be accompanied by visual disturbances and orthostatic hypotension. Hypokalemia results in lethargy, fatigue, muscle weakness, cramps, paresthesias, cardiac dysrhythmias, and decreased ability of the kidneys to concentrate urine. Increased urine volume leads to polyuria, nocturia, and polydipsia. Metabolic alkalosis resulting from hydrogen ion loss correlates to the degree of potassium loss and may result in tetany. Positive Chvostek's and Trousseau's signs indicate the increased neuromuscular irritability that precedes tetany.

MEDICAL DIAGNOSIS

Diagnosis of primary aldosteronism is made on the basis of the presence of hypertension with hypokalemia, low plasma renin levels, and elevated serum and urinary aldosterone levels. Urinary potassium levels exceed 30 mEq/day. Additional laboratory studies demonstrate metabolic alkalosis, hypernatremia, and low urine specific gravity. Impaired glucose tolerance is present in some patients. Mild proteinuria may be present. Renal function studies detect the presence of renal damage.

Radiologic studies, CT scans, MRI, and angiography help to locate adrenal tumors and identify bilateral hyperplasia of the adrenal cortex. Electrocardiograms identify altered electrical conductivity of the myocardium.

MEDICAL MANAGEMENT

The treatment of choice for an aldosterone-secreting adrenal adenoma is unilateral adrenalectomy. Before surgery, hypertension and hypokalemia are corrected by a low-sodium diet, potassium supplements, and administration of spironolactone (Aldactone), an aldosterone antagonist.

Patients with bilateral adrenal hyperplasia are treated medically with spironolactone and a low-sodium, high-potassium diet. Potassium supplements may also be prescribed. If the blood pressure remains elevated, other antihypertensive agents and potassium-sparing diuretics may be added to the regimen.

Guidelines for Application of the Nursing Process to the Care of the Patient with Primary Aldosteronism

Assess for the clinical manifestations of primary aldosteronism in all patients who have hypertension and hypokalemia with no apparent reason for excess potassium loss. Ask specifically about the presence of unusual fatigue, muscle weakness, cramps, palpitations, paresthesias, and frequent urination associated with hypokalemia. Monitor vital signs with apical heart rate every 4 hours to assess blood pressure and cardiac rhythm. Take blood pressure daily while the patient is lying and sitting or standing to detect orthostatic hypotension. Weigh the patient daily, assess for edema, and monitor intake and output to evaluate fluid balance. Monitor results of serum electrolyte and arterial blood gas studies. Administer potassium supplements and spironolactone as prescribed. Assess and document response to therapy. Assist the patient in the timely completion of diagnostic tests. Explain the rationale for the prescribed low-sodium, high-potassium diet, and assist the patient in making appropriate choices from daily menu selections.

Once the diagnosis is confirmed and a method of treatment is selected, reinforce the physician's explanations, provide opportunity for questions, and correct any misconceptions the patient may have. Nursing care after an adrenalectomy was discussed earlier in this chapter. Nursing care after a unilateral adrenalectomy for primary aldosteronism is similar. Because the patient still has one functioning adrenal gland, lifelong steroid-replacement therapy is not necessary.

If surgery is contraindicated and lifelong medical treatment is prescribed, teach the patient the name, dose, route and time of administration, expected effects, and side effects of prescribed medications. Consult with a dietitian to teach and to provide in writing a low-sodium, high-potassium diet. Instruct the patient to report to the physician unusual weight gain, dependent edema, increasing fatigue, dyspnea, or palpitations. Reinforce the need for lifelong follow-up care for early detection of altered response to therapy.

Adrenal Medulla

Anatomy and Physiology

The adrenal medulla and the sympathetic nervous system both develop from the ectodermal tissue of the fetal neural crest. Cells from the ectodermal tissue differentiate to form chromaffin cells and sympathetic ganglion cells. The adrenal medulla is a specialized glandular structure composed of chromaffin cells within the sympathetic nervous system. Any stimulus that activates the sympathetic nervous system can stimulate the adrenal medulla and elicit secretion of medullary hormones. The adrenal medulla functions in conjunction with the sympathetic nervous system to support and prolong the effects of sympathetic stimulation in the body. Because the adrenal medulla is an extension of the sympathetic nervous system, it is not essential for life.

The chromaffin cells of the adrenal medulla secrete two catecholamines: epinephrine and norepinephrine. The adrenal medulla is the primary source of epinephrine in the body. In normal individuals, epinephrine constitutes about 80% of the medullary secretions. Norepinephrine is the principal catecholamine secreted by sympathetic neurons outside the adrenal medulla.

The major effects of epinephrine and norepinephrine secretion are cardiovascular and metabolic. They affect not only the sympathetic nervous system but every cell in the body. Epinephrine primarily stimulates the beta receptors of the sympathetic nervous system. It causes constriction of the peripheral, renal, and gastrointestinal vascular beds. Epinephrine also increases the rate and force of heart contractions, which increases cardiac output and raises systolic blood pressure. These cardiovascular effects shunt blood to the vessels of the heart, brain, and active skeletal muscles, the vital organs necessary for the fight or flight response in an emergency situation. Stimulation of the sympathetic nervous system by epinephrine also dilates the pupils, inhibits peristalsis, increases sphincter tone, stimulates the sweat and apocrine glands, and increases the rate and depth of respirations while dilating the bronchi.

The metabolic effects of epinephrine can raise the body's metabolic rate to 100% above normal. Oxygen consumption and body temperature increase as the metabolic rate rises. Insulin secretion is inhibited, whereas glycogenolysis (the conversion of stored glycogen to glucose) in the liver and muscles increases. These activities result in elevation of blood glucose levels. The increased metabolic activity and rise in blood glucose levels contribute to the increased mental alertness and muscle strength associated with secretion of epinephrine.

Norepinephrine stimulates both the alpha and beta receptors of the sympathetic nervous system but predominantly affects the alpha-adrenergic receptors. It causes generalized vasoconstriction and increases both the systolic and diastolic blood pressures by greatly increasing peripheral resistance. The metabolic and cardiac effects of norepinephrine are not as pronounced as those of epinephrine.

The effects of epinephrine and norepinephrine on the body are summarized in Table 32–3. It is the effects of mass release of the adrenal catecholamines that cause the cold sweat, pounding heart, rapid, deep respirations, tremulousness, and feeling of wide-eyed alertness we all experience in extremely stressful situations.

Table 32–3. PHYSIOLOGIC EFFECTS OF EPINEPHRINE AND NOREPINEPHRINE

EPINEPHRINE
Heart rate increases
Force of heart contractions increases
Cardiac output increases
Peripheral vascular bed constricts
Renal blood vessels constrict
Gastrointestinal vascular bed constricts
Systolic blood pressure rises
Metabolic rate increases to 100% above normal
Oxygen utilization increases
Body temperature rises
Liver and muscle glycogenolysis increases
Insulin secretion inhibited
Blood glucose levels rise
Peristalsis slows
Sphincter tone increases
Sweat and apocrine gland activity increases
Respirations increase in rate and depth
Bronchi dilate
Pupils dilate
Mental alertness increases
Muscle strength increases
NOREPINEPHRINE
Generalized vasoconstriction
Greatly increased peripheral vascular resistance
Moderate cardiac stimulation
Greatly increased systolic and diastolic blood pressures
Mild metabolic effects

Pheochromocytoma

Pheochromocytoma is a rare catecholamine-producing tumor arising from the chromaffin cells of the sympathetic nervous system. It is characterized by unregulated hypersecretion of catecholamines. Pheochromocytoma is the most common pathologic condition associated with the adrenal medulla. There are no known common disorders caused by adrenal medulla insufficiency.

ETIOLOGY

Although the cause of pheochromocytoma is unknown, it is diagnosed most frequently, and at an earlier age, in individuals with a family history of pheochromocytoma or with a history of other endocrine gland neoplasias. It is often associated with hyperparathyroidism, thyroid medullary carcinoma, and multiple endocrine neoplasia (MEN) syndrome.

Pheochromocytomas have been reported to occur throughout the life span, from infancy to the eighth decade of life, but are most common in the 40-year to 60-year age group. Pheochromocytoma is diagnosed in slightly more women than men.

PATHOPHYSIOLOGY

Pheochromocytomas are individual or multiple tumors that can develop from chromaffin cells anywhere along the sympathetic nerve chain. The incidence of multiple tumors increases with a positive family history of pheochromocytoma. More than 90% of these neoplasms occur in the adrenal medulla. The rest develop in extra-adrenal sites along the sympathetic nerve chain in the head or trunk. Extra-adrenal pheochromocytomas are sometimes called paragangliomas.

Most pheochromocytomas are benign. They are well-encapsulated, highly vascular tumors that synthesize, store, and secrete catecholamines. Less than 5% are malignant. Malignant tumors metastasize to the bones, liver, lymph nodes, and lungs. Malignant tumors are resistant to radiation and chemotherapy, and survival after diagnosis rarely exceeds 3 years.

The pathologic changes associated with pheochromocytomas are due to heightened physiologic responses to increased levels of circulating catecholamines. Excess secretion of catecholamines may be continuous or paroxysmal and produces cardiovascular and metabolic disturbances that can be fatal if untreated. Overstimulation of the alpha and beta receptors of the sympathetic nervous system produces increased peripheral vasoconstriction, increased heart rate, increased myocardial contractility and irritability, increased metabolism and oxygen utilization, increased respiratory rate, increased glycogenolysis, decreased peristalsis, stimulation of the sweat and apocrine glands, and pupillary dilation.

CLINICAL MANIFESTATIONS

Hypertension is the most significant clinical feature of pheochromocytoma. Most individuals experience sustained mild to severe hypertension, and many have superimposed paroxysmal episodes of malignant hypertension as high as 300/180 mm Hg or higher. Malignant hypertensive episodes are caused by intermittent release of large amounts of catecholamines from the pheochromocytoma. These episodes may be spontaneous or may be precipitated by stress, a change in position, physical activity, or the Valsalva maneuver. They may last from a few minutes to a few hours. Most episodes subside within 40 minutes. As the disease progresses, paroxysmal hypertensive episodes become more frequent.

Hypertension may be accompanied by a pounding headache, tachycardia, palpitations, hyperventilation, dizziness, visual disturbances, nausea, vomiting, and profuse diaphoresis associated with blanching or flushing of the skin. Patients often experience a feeling of impending doom during a hypertensive episode. Other clinical manifestations include episodes of postural hypotension, abdominal pain, constipation, weakness, fine muscle tremors, hyperreflexia, anxiety, nervousness, insomnia, and increased metabolism and blood glucose levels.

Cardiovascular, pulmonary, and renal problems may develop as a result of sustained hypertension. Congestive heart failure, cerebrovascular accidents, and renal failure are common complications. Death may result from cardiac dysrhythmias, pulmonary edema, or cerebral hemorrhage.

MEDICAL DIAGNOSIS

A diagnosis of pheochromocytoma may be suspected on the basis of physical manifestations and a history of periodic or sustained hypertension with no known cause, but a definitive diagnosis cannot be made without laboratory tests.

Catecholamines are almost completely metabolized into inactive waste products, which are excreted and can be measured in the urine. These metabolites are metanephrine, normetanephrine, and vanillylmandelic acid (VMA). One, and usually all, of these substances are increased in pheochromocytoma. Assay of urinary catecholamines and their metabolites can be performed on a single first-voided morning urine specimen as a screening test or on a 24-hour specimen for definitive diagnosis. Proper patient preparation and collection and preservation of the specimen for urinary catecholamines are necessary to ensure an accurate and timely diagnosis. Timed specimens are difficult to collect, so the procedure must be a high priority in the patient's care. Table 32–4 presents guidelines for collection of a 24-hour urine specimen for catecholamines. The normal values for urinary catecholamines and their metabolites are presented in Table 32–5.

Table 32-4. NURSING GUIDE TO 24-HOUR URINE COLLECTION FOR URINARY CATECHOLAMINES

1. Assess the patient's ability to collect the specimen correctly.
2. Advise the patient of the purpose of the test, the length of time required for the test, how to collect the urine, and where to save it.
3. Instruct the patient to void and discard the urine. The specimen collection begins at the time of this voiding.
4. Record the exact start time and date and end time and date of the collection on the specimen container and patient record.
5. Post a notice in the patient's bathroom and on the patient's record to remind the patient and staff that a 24-hour urine collection is in progress.
6. If any urine is inadvertently discarded, stop the collection and begin a new specimen collection in a new container.
7. At the end of the 24-hour period, instruct the patient to void and add this urine to the specimen container.
8. Many foods and drugs affect urinary catecholamine levels. Restriction of specific substances depends on the evaluation method used. Consult the laboratory to determine which food and drugs must be restricted. Changes in dietary and drug therapies must be ordered by the physician.
9. Explain diet and drug restrictions to the patient.
10. Note any medications administered during the specimen collection on the laboratory requisition.
11. Catecholamines and their metabolites are unstable in urine. A preservative, usually hydrochloric acid, may be added to the specimen container, and the container may be kept on ice or refrigerated during collection. Method of specimen preservation depends on the evaluation method used and is determined by the laboratory.

Because of the effects of excessive catecholamine secretion, the patient also exhibits an increased basal metabolic rate and elevated blood glucose levels. Glycosuria and albuminuria may be present. Radiologic studies, CT scans, MRI, and angiography help locate the tumor and identify extra-adrenal sites.

MEDICAL MANAGEMENT

Although less than 0.5% of the individuals who have hypertension have pheochromocytoma, it is an important disorder because it is curable with treatment in 90% of cases. The treatment of choice is

Table 32–5. URINARY CATECHOLAMINES AND THEIR METABOLITES

LABORATORY TEST	NORMAL VALUES*
Vanillylmandelic acid	<7 mg/24 hr
Epinephrine	0–15 μg/24 hr
Norepinephrine	0–100 μg/24 hr
Metanephrine	0.25–0.8 mg/24 hr

* Normal values are guidelines. Contact laboratory performing test for absolute values.

surgical excision of the tumor or tumors. If the tumors are within the adrenal medullae, a unilateral or bilateral adrenalectomy is performed. With removal of both adrenal glands, the sympathetic nervous system takes over the functions of the missing adrenal medullae. Lifelong corticosteroid therapy, however, is required to replace adrenal cortex functions.

Preoperatively, a stimulant-free diet and bed rest with the head of the bed elevated to 45 degrees are prescribed to help reduce blood pressure and prevent hypertensive episodes. Episodes of hypertensive crisis are controlled by intravenous administration of phentolamine (Regitine), a rapid-acting alpha-adrenergic blocking agent, followed by oral administration of longer acting phenoxybenzamine (Dibenzyline) or prazosin (Minipress). Catecholamine-induced cardiac dysrhythmias are treated with propranolol (Inderal) once alpha-adrenergic blockade has been established. These drugs are also administered for 10 days to 2 weeks before surgery to lessen the chance of intraoperative and postoperative complications. Hypovolemic shock caused by the rapid relaxation of constricted blood vessels is the most common postoperative complication. Transient hypertensive episodes are common.

In the 10% of individuals who are not surgical candidates because of additional medical problems or because of metastasized malignant pheochromocytomas, symptomatic relief can be obtained by administration of phenoxybenzamine or alpha-methyl-para-tyrosine, a catecholamine biosynthesis inhibitor. Five-year survival in this group of individuals is less than 50%.

Application of the Nursing Process to the Care of the Patient with Pheochromocytoma

Assessment

Obtain a complete nursing history. Ask specifically about factors that precipitate hypertensive episodes and the manifestations that accompany an episode. Obtain baseline weight, vital signs, and neurologic signs. Assess for the presence of clinical manifestations common to pheochromocytoma. Identify the patient's interpretation of clinical manifestations, and assess knowledge of planned diagnostic tests and treatment to determine teaching needs.

Postoperatively, the patient is usually in an intensive care setting for constant nursing observation and monitoring of cardiovascular status.

Nursing Diagnoses and Planning

Nursing diagnoses and related expected patient outcomes most commonly applicable to patients with pheochromocytoma include the following:

NDx: High risk for altered tissue perfusion: systemic, related to rapid fluctuations in cardiovascular status

Planning: Patient outcomes
1. Patient avoids activities that precipitate hypertensive episodes.
2. Patient notifies nurse immediately of onset of hypertensive episode.
3. Patient maintains adequate tissue perfusion preoperatively and postoperatively as evidenced by the following:
   a. Stable vital signs within normal limits
   b. Normal neurologic responses
   c. Urine output more than 30 ml/hour
   d. Lungs clear to auscultation

NDx: Anxiety related to overstimulation of the nervous system by increased levels of circulating catecholamines

Planning: Patient outcomes
1. Patient identifies disease process as cause of feelings of anxiety.
2. Patient uses relaxation exercises to reduce anxiety levels.

NDx: Altered nutrition: high risk for less than body requirements related to increased metabolism, abdominal pain, nausea, vomiting, and/or constipation secondary to prolonged catecholamine hypersecretion

Planning: Patient outcomes
1. Patient maintains stable weight within recommended norms.
2. Patient defecates soft, formed stool at least every third day.

NDx: High risk for altered health maintenance related to insufficient knowledge of follow-up care

Planning: Patient outcomes
1. Patient verbalizes understanding of the need for lifelong follow-up care.
2. Patient states intent to advise family members to have screening test for pheochromocytoma.

Nursing Interventions

Nursing care of the individual with pheochromocytoma requires frequent assessment and supportive intervention because of potentially rapid fluctuations in cardiovascular status.

NDx: High risk for altered tissue perfusion: systemic

Monitor vital signs and neurologic signs at least every 4 hours but every 15 minutes during a hypertensive episode. Administer catecholamine-blocking agents as prescribed. Weigh the patient daily, and monitor urine output to identify changes in renal status. Auscultate heart sounds to detect cardiac dysrhythmias and lung sounds to detect congestion and crackles, which may indicate developing pulmonary edema. Maintain head of bed at 30 to 45 degrees to promote orthostatic reduction of blood pressure and to minimize intracranial pressure. Elevate side rails to prevent injury as a result of neurologic manifestations or visual disturbances. Prevent chills and provide frequent skin care during profuse diaphoresis. Minimize patient activity as prescribed, and provide a restful environment free of unnecessary stimuli.

Tell the patient to notify a nurse immediately if symptoms of a hypertensive episode develop. Notify the physician at the onset of a hypertensive episode and have phentolamine and emergency cardiac drugs readily available.

Teach the patient to change position slowly and to avoid rapid movements, bearing down, stress, and any activities that precipitated hypertensive episodes in the past. Do not palpate the patient's abdomen because palpation may stimulate catecholamine release in some individuals. A reminder notice to this effect is posted on the patient's nursing care plan and above the bed. Instruct patient not to smoke and to avoid ingestion of caffeine because nicotine and caffeine stimulate catecholamine secretion.

Postoperatively, the patient will have a midline or transverse abdominal incision. The first 48 hours after surgery are critical because of unstable blood pressure and the risk of postoperative hemorrhage. The patient is usually in an intensive care setting and requires constant nursing observation and monitoring of cardiovascular status. Administer prescribed intravenous fluids to stabilize the blood pressure until the effects of the excess catecholamines and preoperative alpha-adrenergic blockers wear off. This takes about 36 hours.

Examine surgical dressings frequently for bleeding, and assess the abdomen for hematoma, which could indicate internal hemorrhage. Large abdominal incisions are very painful. Administer prescribed analgesics to promote patient comfort, mobility, and participation in performing breathing exercises. However, monitor blood pressure before each dose because many narcotics produce hypotension as a side effect. Monitor urine output hourly for 48 hours after surgery to detect possible kidney damage resulting from surgery or renal failure resulting from profound postoperative shock.

After the immediate postoperative phase, recovery is usually uneventful. The patient is discharged from the hospital once blood pressure readings stabilize and results of a 24-hour urine test for catecholamines and their metabolites are within normal limits. If a bilateral adrenalectomy was performed, the patient will require lifetime replacement with corticosteroids.

NDx: Anxiety

Provide factual information regarding the effect of increased levels of circulating catecholamines on the nervous system. Encourage the patient to identify and describe feelings. Assist the patient in identifying and practicing relaxation techniques that help control anxiety levels. Stay with the patient, and provide emotional support during frightening hypertensive episodes. Many patients believe they are going to die. Speak in a calm, reassuring voice, and maintain a calm, unhurried manner to promote relaxation and trust.

NDx: Altered nutrition: high risk for less than body requirements

Weigh the patient and compare with normal weight range for individuals of same sex, height, and body build. Monitor weight at least three times a week. Monitor blood glucose levels to detect elevation. Provide several small, fiber-rich meals, incorporating the patient's food preferences when nausea is absent. Omit stimulating foods and beverages from the diet. If weight loss is severe, a high-calorie, high-vitamin diet may be prescribed once blood glucose levels are controlled. Administer prescribed stool softeners, laxatives, or enemas to relieve constipation.

NDx: High risk for altered health maintenance

In preparing the patient for discharge, the need for lifelong follow-up is stressed. The recurrence rate of pheochromocytoma after surgery is about 10%. Teach the patient the symptoms of pheochromocytoma, and instruct him or her to report the appearance of symptoms to the physician promptly. Periodic 24-hour urine specimens may be collected for catecholamines. Provide the patient with clearly written instructions on the collection procedure as discussed in the guidelines in Table 32–4.

Because there is a familial tendency to develop pheochromocytomas, an important nursing intervention in the care of these individuals is to advise family members to have a single, first-voided morning urine specimen tested for metanephrines. This test is easier to collect and less expensive than a 24-hour specimen and is an accurate screening test. If results are abnormal, further evaluation for pheochromocytoma is necessary.

Evaluation

Evaluate the effectiveness of nursing care for a patient with pheochromocytoma by comparing the patient's status with the expected patient outcomes. Examples of specific outcomes for patients with pheochromocytoma have been provided in the Planning section.

The Elderly: Special Considerations

Secretion of ACTH and adrenal hormones diminishes with age. Reduced levels of glucocorticoids place the elderly at higher risk for hypoglycemia when food intake is decreased or when the patient must fast for diagnostic procedures or surgery. Although not under the influence of ACTH, less aldosterone is also secreted in the elderly. Lower levels of circulating aldosterone place the elderly at higher risk of excess fluid loss if fluid intake is reduced or if the environment is dry or very warm. It is unclear whether reduced secretion of adrenal sex steroid hormones influences the changes in secondary sex characteristics commonly associated with the aging process.

There is no evidence that the incidence of adrenal disorders is higher in the elderly than in the general population. Tuberculosis-related Addison's disease has been diagnosed in some elderly individuals. By reviewing the normal physiologic changes associated with the aging process discussed in Chapter 2, it is apparent that an elderly individual with an adrenal disorder is at higher risk for complications of fluid and electrolyte imbalance than a younger individual. Orthostatic hypotension develops more rapidly in an elderly person who experiences a change in blood pressure or fluid balance. Elderly individuals receiving glucocorticoid preparations are at higher risk for osteoporosis.

Bibliography

Abrams AC. Clinical drug therapy: Rationales for nursing practice. 3rd ed. Philadelphia: JB Lippincott, 1991.
Alfaro-LeFevre R, et al. Drug handbook: A nursing process approach. New York: Addison-Wesley, 1992.
Benowitz NL. Diagnosis and management of pheochromocytoma. Hosp Pract 1990; 25(6):163.
Besser G, Cudworth A. Clinical endocrinology: An illustrated text. Philadelphia: WB Saunders, 1987.
Brenner ZR. Diagnostic tests and procedures: Applying the nursing process. Norwalk, CT: Appleton & Lange, 1987.
Bullock BL, Rosendahl PP. Pathophysiology: Adaptations and alterations in function. 2nd ed. Boston: Little, Brown, 1988.
Carpenito LJ. Nursing diagnosis: Application to clinical practice. 4th ed. Philadelphia: JB Lippincott, 1992.
Cassel CK, Walsh JR (eds). Geriatric medicine. New York: Springer-Verlag, 1989.
Cella JH, Watson J. Nurse's manual of laboratory tests. Philadelphia: FA Davis, 1989.
Chenevy B. Overview of fluids and electrolytes. Nurs Clin North Am 1987; 22(4):749.
Cocchi D. Age related alterations in gonadotropin, adrenotropin and growth hormone secretion. Aging: Clin Exp Res 1992; 4(2):103.
Cooper JAD, Pappas PG (eds). Cecil review of general internal medicine. 5th ed. Philadelphia: WB Saunders, 1992.
Dedrick CG. Adrenal arteriography and venography. Urol Clin North Am 1989; 16(3):515.
DeGroot LJ (ed). Endocrinology. 2nd ed. Philadelphia: WB Saunders, 1989.
Doenges M, Moorhouse M. Nurse's pocket guide: Nursing diagnosis with interventions. 4th ed. Philadelphia: FA Davis, 1993.
Dudek SG. Nutrition handbook for nursing practice. Philadelphia: JB Lippincott, 1987.
Eliopoulos C. Gerontological nursing. 3rd ed. Philadelphia: JB Lippincott, 1993.
Featherson WE, Ram CVS. Secondary causes of hypertension: Health and cost benefits of making these diagnoses . . . pheochromocytoma and primary aldosteronism. Consultant 1987; 27(8):109.
Feldman JM. Diagnosis and management of pheochromocytoma. Hosp Pract 1989; 24(1):175.
Fischbach F. A manual of laboratory diagnostic tests. 4th ed. Philadelphia: JB Lippincott, 1992.
Gordon M. Nursing diagnosis: Process and application. St. Louis: CV Mosby, 1991.
Green LB, Johns SB. Can you solve this assessment puzzle? RN 1990; 53(11):64.
Greenspan FS. Basic and clinical endocrinology. Norwalk, CT: Appleton & Lange, 1991.
Griffin J, Ojeda S (eds). Textbook of endocrine physiology. New York: Oxford University Press, 1988.
Guyton AG. Textbook of medical physiology. 8th ed. Philadelphia: WB Saunders, 1990.
Guz BV, Straffon RA, Novick AC. Operative approaches to the adrenal gland. Urol Clin North Am 1989; 16(3):527.
Hill MN. Drug compliance: Going beyond the facts. Nursing 1986; 16(10):50.
Ihde DC. Paraneoplastic syndromes. Hosp Pract 1987; 22(8):105.
Kee JL. Laboratory and diagnostic tests with nursing implications. Norwalk, CT: Appleton & Lange, 1987.
Kositske J. A question of balance: Dehydration in the elderly. J Gerontol Nurs 1990; 16(5):4.
Kumar V, Cotran RS, Robbins SL. Basic pathology. 5th ed. Philadelphia: WB Saunders, 1992.
Lancaster LE. Renal and endocrine regulation of water and electrolyte balance. Nurs Clin North Am 1987; 22(4):761.
Lehne RA. Pharmacology for nursing care. Philadelphia: WB Saunders, 1990.
Lind JM. Ectopic hormone production: Nursing implications. Semin Oncol Nurs 1985; 1(4):251.
Lloyd RV. Endocrine pathology. New York: Springer-Verlag, 1990.
Loebl S, et al. The nurse's drug handbook. 5th ed. New York: John Wiley & Sons, 1989.
Malseed RT, Harrigan G. Textbook of pharmacology and nursing care: The nursing process. 2nd ed. Philadelphia: JB Lippincott, 1989.
Matteson MA, McConnell ES. Gerontological nursing: Concepts and practice. Philadelphia: WB Saunders, 1988.
North American Nursing Diagnosis Association. NANDA nursing diagnoses: Definitions and classifications. St. Louis: North American Nursing Diagnosis Association, 1992.
Poyss AS. Assessment and nursing diagnosis in fluid and electrolyte disorders. Nursing Clin North Am 1987; 22(4):773.
Reasner CA. Adrenal disorders. Crit Care Nurs 1990; 13(3):67.
Schwartz MW. Potassium imbalance. Am J Nurs 1987; 87(10):1292.
Segarnick DJ. Steroids. Am Assoc Occup Health Nurses 1987; 35(6):286.
Shannon MT, Wilson BA. Govoni & Hayes drugs and nursing implications. 7th ed. Norwalk, CT: Appleton & Lange, 1992.
Shira MG. Steroid-dependent states and adrenal insufficiency. Nurs Clin North Am 1987; 22(4):837.
Sowers J, Felicetta J (eds). Endocrinology of aging. New York; Raven, 1988.
Staren ED, Conkey C, Morreale B, et al. Surgical intervention for pheochromocytoma. AORN J 1986; 44(5):758.
Toto KH. When the patient has hyperkalemia. RN 1987; 50(4):34.
Toto KH. When the patient has hypokalemia. RN 1987; 50(3):38.
Tucker SM, et al. Patient care standards: Nursing process, diagnosis, and outcomes. 5th ed. St. Louis: CV Mosby, 1992.
Ulrich SP, Canale SW, Wendell SA. Nursing care planning guides: A nursing diagnosis approach. 2nd ed. Philadelphia: WB Saunders, 1990.
Weiner N. Pheochromocytoma. Crit Care Nurs Q 1990; 13(3):14.
Wilson JD, Foster DW (eds). Williams textbook of endocrinology. 8th ed. Philadelphia: WB Saunders, 1992.
Wyngaarden JB, Smith LH, Bennett JC (eds). Cecil textbook of medicine. 19th ed. Philadelphia: WB Saunders, 1992.

Chapter Thirty-three

NURSING CARE *of Adults with Thyroid Disorders*

Disruptions of thyroid function are among the most commonly diagnosed endocrine disorders. Many are autoimmune disorders. Although the pathophysiology and clinical manifestations of each disorder differ, most result in either increased or decreased hormone production and alter metabolism and cellular function throughout the body. The effect may vary from a subtle change in homeostasis to a life-threatening emergency.

Normal thyroid function and common thyroid disorders are presented in this chapter. Some potentially significant disorders that have been recently identified as specific thyroid disorders by improved diagnostic techniques are also included.

Anatomy and Physiology

The thyroid gland is a butterfly-shaped organ situated in the anterior aspect of the neck, posterior to the sternocleidomastoid muscle. It is encapsulated by connective tissue that is continuous with the pretracheal fascia. As illustrated in Figure 33–1, the two lateral lobes of the thyroid lie on either side of the trachea. They are connected by an isthmus that crosses the anterior surface of the trachea just below the cricoid cartilage. A pyramid-shaped extension of the isthmus, usually near the left lobe, exists in approximately 30% of the population. In the adult, the thyroid gland weighs approximately 20 to 30 g, but enlarged thyroid goiters weighing several hundred grams have been reported.

The thyroid gland is a highly vascular organ. The superior thyroid arteries, which branch from the external carotid arteries, and the inferior thyroid arteries, which branch from the subclavian arteries, are the primary arterial vessels. Four to 5 L of blood flow through the gland each hour. In an enlarged gland, the blood flow is even greater and may produce a palpable thrill, or vibration, over the gland. A bruit may be auscultated in an enlarged gland.

The lobes of the thyroid gland are composed of two types of cells: follicular cells and parafollicular cells. Three hormones—thyroxine, triiodothyronine, and calcitonin—are produced and secreted by these cells.

Thyroxine and Triiodothyronine

The follicular cells form tiny, closely packed sacs called follicles or acini. Inside the follicles is a gelatinous iodine-containing colloid and large molecules of thyroglobulin. Thyroxine (T_4) and triiodothyronine (T_3), the primary thyroid hormones, are produced within the thyroglobulin molecules by a process of iodine metabolism and biosynthesis. The hormones are then stored in the follicles, bound to thyroglobulin, until they are released into the circulation. This large reservoir of stored hormone is unique among the endocrine glands and can provide up to 100 days of normal thyroid hormone secretion if thyroid synthesis is interrupted.

In the blood, thyroxine and triiodothyronine are almost entirely bound to circulating plasma proteins. Most of the hormone is bound to thyroxine-binding globulin (TBG). Small amounts are bound to albumin and prealbumin. Only the free unbound hormone in the plasma is biologically active and available for use by body tissues.

Approximately 15% to 20% of the triiodothyronine used by the body is released from the thyroid gland. The rest is produced by a process of monodeiodination of thyroxine (removal of one iodine molecule from thyroxine) that converts thyroxine (T_4) to triiodothyronine (T_3) after thyroxine binds with cell receptor sites in peripheral tissues.

Adequate dietary intake of iodine and protein is necessary for the synthesis of thyroxine and triiodothyronine. The recommended daily intake of iodine is 0.15 mg/day, or approximately 1 mg a week. In the United States, the use of iodized salt and commercial bread products made with dough condi-

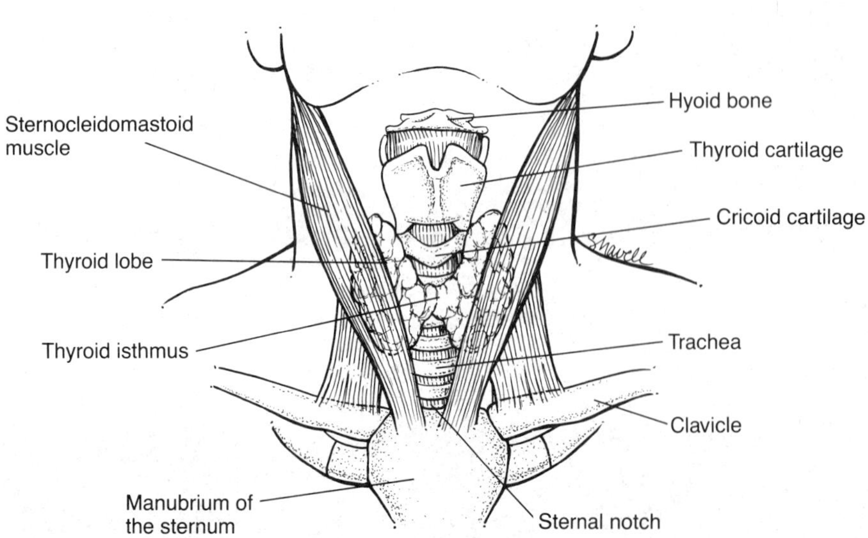

Figure 33–1.

Anterior view of the anatomy of the thyroid gland and surrounding structures.

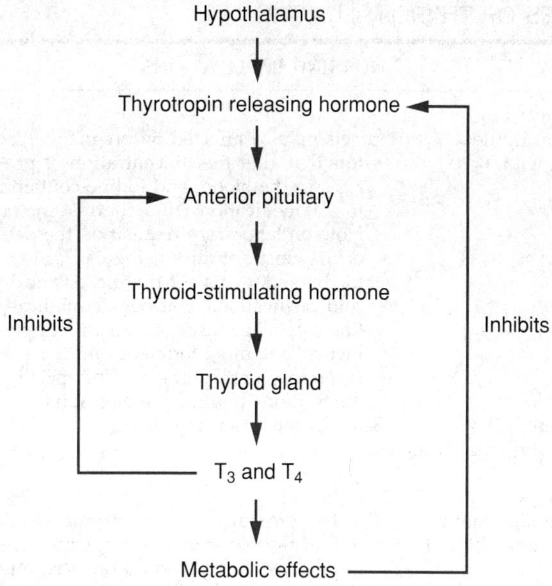

Figure 33–2.

Regulation of thyroid hormone secretion by negative feedback control.

tioners that contain iodine has greatly reduced the risk of inadequate iodine intake.

REGULATION OF SECRETION

The production and secretion of thyroxine and triiodothyronine by the thyroid gland are controlled by secretion of thyroid-stimulating hormone (TSH), also called thyrotropin, from the anterior pituitary gland. Secretion of TSH is initiated by low circulating levels of thyroid hormone and by secretion of thyrotropin releasing hormone (TRH) from the hypothalamus. TRH is secreted in response to the metabolic needs of the body and emotional reactions. TSH secretion is primarily inhibited by increased thyroxine and triiodothyronine levels in the circulation. This feedback mechanism, illustrated in Figure 33–2, maintains an almost constant level of free thyroxine and triiodothyronine in the circulation. TSH secretion may also be inhibited by increased levels of somatostatin, dopamine, corticotropin (ACTH), and glucocorticoid hormones and stimulated by growth hormone and estrogen.

FUNCTIONS OF THYROXINE AND TRIIODOTHYRONINE

The primary function of thyroxine and triiodothyronine is to regulate cell metabolism and energy production. They also influence growth and development and affect cell differentiation in the fetus. The functions of thyroxine and triiodothyronine are detailed in Table 33–1.

In the healthy individual, serum thyroxine (T_4) is present in much larger amounts than triiodothyronine (T_3). The T_4-to-T_3 ratio is approximately 7:1 to 10:1. Triiodothyronine is more potent and more biologically active than thyroxine, but its effects last a shorter time. Triiodothyronine is secreted in increased amounts during severe stress and times of high energy need. Because thyroxine and triiodothyronine have similar functions, they are frequently referred to collectively as thyroid hormone.

Calcitonin

The parafollicular cells (C cells) are interspersed in clusters between the follicles. They produce and secrete calcitonin. Calcitonin lowers serum calcium levels by increasing calcium deposition in the bones. It is an antagonist to parathyroid hormone. Secretion of calcitonin is controlled by serum calcium levels. Increased serum calcium levels stimulate calcitonin secretion, whereas decreased levels inhibit its secretion.

Assessment of the Thyroid Gland

Assessment of the thyroid gland involves inspection, palpation, and auscultation. As illustrated in Figure 33–1, identify the thyroid cartilage with its notched upper edge in the midline of the neck, the cricoid cartilage just below the thyroid cartilage, and the trachea descending below the cricoid cartilage. The thyroid isthmus, if visible, crosses the trachea below the cricoid cartilage. Inspect the trachea for deviation from the midline. Inspect the contour and symmetry of the lower anterior region of the neck.

Table 33–1. PHYSIOLOGIC EFFECTS OF THYROXINE (T_4) AND TRIIODOTHYRONINE (T_3)

Increase basal metabolic rate
Increase metabolic activity of most body tissues (exceptions: brain, retina, spleen, testes, and lungs)
Increase oxygen utilization
Increase rate and depth of respiration
Increase heart rate, contractility, and cardiac output
Increase pulse pressure
Increase cardiac sensitivity to catecholamine secretion (epinephrine and norepinephrine)
Increase utilization of food for energy
Increase protein synthesis and catabolism
Stimulate all aspects of carbohydrate metabolism
Stimulate all aspects of fat metabolism
Increase vitamin metabolism
Stimulate conversion of carotene to vitamin A in the liver
Stimulate mental processes
Stimulate neuromuscular responses
Increase muscle tone
Stimulate red blood cell production
Stimulate activity of other endocrine glands
Promote growth and development in fetuses and children
Promote growth and development of the central nervous system in the fetus and during the first few years of life
Maintain normal reproductive function

Table 33–2. COMMON DIAGNOSTIC STUDIES OF THYROID FUNCTION

STUDY	PURPOSE AND PROCEDURE	NURSING IMPLICATIONS
SERUM STUDIES		
Serum T_4 (total thyroxine)	Assess thyroxine concentration in the blood. Used in conjunction with T_3 to evaluate thyroid function. Normal value: 4.5–13 μg/dl	Levels may be affected by pregnancy, factors that alter the concentration of proteins in the blood, and iodine-containing foods, medications, and contrast media. Note on laboratory requisition the date of diagnostic studies using contrast media and/or use of thyroid or antithyroid medications, goitrogenic medications, or megadoses of mineral supplements containing iodine. Contact laboratory performing test for specific medications that may alter results.
Serum T_3 (total triiodothyronine)	Assess triiodothyronine concentration in the blood. Used in conjunction with T_4 to evaluate thyroid function. Normal value: 70–200 ng/dl	Same as for serum thyroxine.
Free thyroxine (FT_4)	Measurement of the free thyroxine that is unbound to protein in the blood. Not affected by iodine-containing contrast media or medications. Normal value: 0.8–2.4 ng/dl	This test provides a more accurate evaluation of thyroid status in pregnancy and in persons taking medications that alter total thyroxine levels.
Thyroxine-binding globulin (TBG)	Measurement of serum levels of TBG provides an assessment of the thyroxine-binding capacity of the blood. Combined with T_4 to evaluate thyroid function. Normal value: 12–18 μg/dl	Same as for serum thyroxine.
T_3 resin uptake (T_3RU)	Used to indirectly measure the binding of thyroid hormone to TBG in the blood. Radioactive T_3 is added to blood sample to bind with unoccupied sites on TBG. Normal value: 25–35% uptake	Not affected by iodine-containing medications, foods, or contrast media. Other drugs same as for thyroxine.
Thyroid-stimulating hormone (TSH)	Assess circulating levels of TSH secreted by the anterior pituitary gland. Used to differentiate between pituitary dysfunction and primary thyroid dysfunction. Normal value: < 10 μIU/ml	Same as for serum thyroxine. This test is also used to diagnose primary hypothyroidism in neonates.
Thyrotropin releasing hormone (TRH) stimulation test	Assess response of TSH, and sometimes T_3 and T_4, to TRH. Normally TRH stimulates increased TSH production. Baseline TSH level is drawn. TRH bolus is administered intravenously. TSH levels are measured 30 and 60 minutes after TRH is administered. Used to differentiate between hypothyroidism due to hypothalamic, pituitary, or thyroid dysfunction. T_3 and T_4 levels are measured before and 2 hours after TRH administration. Normal values after TRH: TSH increases two times baseline with peak at 30 minutes. T_3 and T_4 rise after TRH administration.	Advise patient of the need for multiple blood samples and of the possibility of transient flushing, nausea, dizziness, and urge to urinate. Monitor for transient effects, and maintain patient safety. Note exact time TRH was administered and specimens drawn on laboratory slip. Same interfering factors as for thyroxine. This test is generally replacing the thyroid-stimulating hormone (TSH) stimulation test.
Antithyroid antibody titer	Detect the presence of thyroid antibodies. Used to differentiate between autoimmune thyroid disorders and toxic thyroid adenoma. Normal value: Titer < 1:100	Antibodies are present in approximately 10% of healthy persons. Results altered by administration of radioactive iodine within 24 hours of test.
Calcitonin	Assess calcitonin concentration in the blood. Used in the differential diagnosis of cancer of the thyroid gland. Normal values: Men: < 19 pg/ml Women: < 14 pg/ml	If basal calcitonin is nondiagnostic, additional blood samples are drawn 1½ and 5 minutes after a pentagastrin injection.

(continued)

Table 33–2. (continued) COMMON DIAGNOSTIC STUDIES OF THYROID FUNCTION

STUDY	PURPOSE AND PROCEDURE	NURSING IMPLICATIONS
NUCLEAR MEDICINE STUDIES		
Radioactive iodine uptake (RAIU) (^{131}I uptake) (^{123}I uptake)	Measure the rate of iodine uptake by the thyroid gland. A trace dose of RAI is administered orally. The amount of RAI absorbed by the gland is measured at intervals by a gamma counter or scintillation counter placed over the gland. Concurrent 24-hour urine specimen may be collected to assess iodine excretion. Often done in conjunction with thyroid scan. Normal values: Absorption by gland: <6% uptake in 2 hr 2–25% uptake in 6 hr 15–45% uptake in 24 hr 24-hour urine: 40–80% RAI excreted in 24 hr	Determine date of last menstrual period in female patients; RAIU is never done during pregnancy or lactation. Same interfering factors as for thyroxine. Ask about seafood and iodized salt intake within the previous 2 weeks. Assure the patient that the amount of radioactive iodine used is very small; it is not harmful to the patient and the patient will not be "radioactive." Explain the need for several uptake measurement sessions and the times they are scheduled. Follow standard procedures for patient education and specimen collection if a concurrent 24-hour urine specimen is needed.
Thyroid scan	Similar to a RAIU, except that a scintillation detector moves back and forth across the gland to produce a scintigraphic image of iodine concentration and distribution throughout the thyroid gland at specified intervals after administration of radioactive iodine. Determines location, size, shape, and functional activity of the gland. Detects hyperactive "hot spots" and hypoactive "cold spots" within the gland, as well as thyroid tissue outside the gland. Results may be plotted by computed tomography scanner to provide a three-dimensional image. Often done in conjunction with RAIU. Normal value: Diffuse tracing with symmetric lobes.	Same as for RAIU. Emphasize the need to lie perfectly still without swallowing during the scanning procedure. Each scan usually takes 20 minutes. Be sure that the patient returns to nuclear medicine department at scheduled intervals, usually 6 and 24 hours after RAI intake. Advise physician and/or nuclear medicine department if patient will not be able to cooperate during scanning procedure.

Normal values and procedures are guidelines. Contact facility performing test for absolute values, interfering substances, patient preparation, and specific procedures.

Normally the neck is symmetric and free from bulges. Tracheal deviation, swelling, or asymmetry may be caused by thyroid enlargement or a neck mass. Ask the patient to extend the neck slightly and swallow or take a sip of water. Observe the normal rise of the thyroid cartilage, cricoid cartilage, and the isthmus of the thyroid gland as the patient swallows.

Next, palpate the thyroid for size, shape, symmetry, consistency, tenderness, and the presence of any nodules. The lobes should be symmetric, feel rubbery, and be free of nodules or tenderness.

The thyroid gland is most frequently palpated from behind the patient. It is easier to palpate in long slender necks than in short stocky ones. Ask the patient to slightly flex the neck. With the finger tips, locate the thyroid and cricoid cartilages. Palpate the thyroid isthmus with the palmar surface of the fingers of one hand while the patient swallows or takes a sip of water. If palpable, it should slide smoothly under the fingers and feel firm and rubbery. The pyramidal lobe, if present, is felt as a pyramid-shaped extension arising from the upper margin of the isthmus.

With the pads of the fingers, palpate downward and laterally between the trachea and each sternocleidomastoid muscle for the lateral lobes of the thyroid gland. Palpation may be facilitated by asking the patient to slightly flex the neck and turn the head toward the side to be examined. The examiner palpates each lateral lobe while using the fingers of the opposite hand to displace the trachea and thyroid toward the side to be examined. Placing the thumb of the palpating hand deep behind the sternocleidomastoid muscle may also aid palpation by displacing the thyroid anteriorly.

If enlargement of the thyroid gland is identified, auscultate over the gland with the bell of the stethoscope for a bruit, a soft rushing sound or vibration caused by increased blood flow.

Any abnormal findings upon assessment of the thyroid gland are documented and reported to the physician. Physical findings are correlated with the patient's history, clinical manifestations, and the results of diagnostic studies of thyroid function to diagnose specific thyroid disorders. Common diagnostic studies used to assess thyroid gland function are identified in Table 33–2.

Infections and Inflammations

Thyroiditis

Thyroiditis is an inflammation of the thyroid gland characterized by enlargement and, often, altered thyroid function. Thyroiditis may be acute, subacute, or chronic. The two most common forms are subacute and chronic.

ACUTE THYROIDITIS

Acute thyroiditis is a rare condition caused by bacterial infection of all or part of the thyroid gland. The patient presents with fever, tenderness on palpation of the thyroid gland, neck pain, swelling, and elevated leukocyte count. Thyroid function is usually normal. Recovery is usually rapid and complete following identification of the causative pathogen and administration of appropriate antibiotic agents.

SUBACUTE GRANULOMATOUS THYROIDITIS

The most common form of subacute thyroiditis is granulomatous thyroiditis, also called de Quervain's thyroiditis and giant cell thyroiditis. It is a self-limiting viral infection of the thyroid gland. Although the incidence is not precisely known, it is not considered a rare disease. Subacute thyroiditis is most commonly diagnosed in women between 30 and 60 years of age several weeks following the mumps or an upper respiratory viral infection. Mild cases may be mistakenly diagnosed as pharyngitis.

Subacute granulomatous thyroiditis is characterized by painful enlargement of the thyroid gland with fever, malaise, dysphagia, hoarseness, leukocytosis, and elevated erythrocyte sedimentation rate (ESR). Pain often radiates to the ear, jaw, or occiput and intensifies with movement of the head or swallowing. The skin overlying the thyroid gland may be warm and red. Signs of hyperthyroidism, such as nervousness, tachycardia, and palpitations, caused by release of stored thyroid hormone from damaged thyroid follicles, are common early in the disease. A subnormal radioactive iodine uptake (RAIU) despite normal or elevated serum thyroxine level is diagnostic of subacute granulomatous thyroiditis.

Treatment is symptomatic. Aspirin or acetaminophen is prescribed for fever and discomfort. In severe cases, an anti-inflammatory glucocorticoid may be administered. Two to 4 weeks after the onset of an episode of subacute granulomatous thyroiditis, many patients experience a transient period of hypothyroidism. The benefit of the use of replacement therapy with thyroid hormone during this period is inconclusive. Several months are required for complete recovery. Close medical evaluation during the recovery period is important to identify the 5% to 10% of patients who develop permanent hypothyroidism as a result of destruction of thyroid follicular epithelial tissue.

SILENT (PAINLESS) THYROIDITIS

Silent, or painless, thyroiditis is a recently identified syndrome thought to have an autoimmune etiology. It is characterized by symptoms of hyperthyroidism associated with subnormal radioactive iodine uptake and normal erythrocyte sedimentation rate. There may be slight enlargement, but no tenderness, of the thyroid gland. The hyperthyroid state may last 2 months and be followed by a transient hypothyroid period. Remission is spontaneous, but the syndrome may recur. Propranolol is prescribed if hyperthyroid manifestations are severe.

CHRONIC THYROIDITIS (HASHIMOTO'S THYROIDITIS)

The most common form of chronic thyroiditis, Hashimoto's thyroiditis, also called chronic lymphocytic thyroiditis, is an autoimmune thyroiditis. It occurs at least ten times more frequently in women than in men and is diagnosed primarily between the ages of 30 and 50. There is often a family history of thyroid disease and other autoimmune disorders. The frequency in individuals with Down's syndrome or Turner's syndrome is very high. The incidence of Hashimoto's thyroiditis is increasing.

Hashimoto's thyroiditis is characterized by destructive lymphocytic infiltration and fibrosis of the thyroid tissue. The earliest clinical manifestation is usually a small to moderate enlargement of the thyroid gland called a goiter. The goiter usually develops slowly, is nontender and free of nodules, has a firm to hard, rubbery consistency on palpation, and moves freely when the patient swallows. The surface may feel smooth or scalloped. Although a goiter caused by Hashimoto's thyroiditis is usually diffuse and symmetric, some asymmetry of the lobes is not unusual. Rarely, a large goiter compresses adjacent structures such as the trachea or esophagus and causes hoarseness or dysphagia. Lymph node enlargement is uncommon. Initially, the patient is euthyroid. If untreated, the goiter gradually increases in size as lymphocytic infiltration and fibrosis of the thyroid tissue progresses, and the individual develops hypothyroidism as a result of loss of functioning thyroid tissue.

The diagnosis of Hashimoto's thyroiditis is confirmed by demonstration of high titers of circulating antithyroid antibodies in the serum. Clinical and diagnostic manifestations of hypothyroidism help confirm the diagnosis, although thyroid function studies may be within normal range if the disease is diagnosed early.

Medical management depends on the size of the goiter and the clinical manifestations present. If the goiter is small and the patient is asymptomatic, no treatment is required. Thyroid hormone therapy is used to treat those with hypothyroidism and to reduce the size of the goiter. Surgery is rare but may be required if thyroid hormone therapy fails to reduce the size of a large unsightly goiter or to relieve pressure symptoms. After surgery, the individual is hypothyroid and requires lifetime maintenance with thyroid hormone replacement. Medical and nursing management of a patient with hypothyroidism and after thyroid surgery is discussed later in this chapter.

Functional Disorders

Functional disorders of the thyroid gland are characterized by altered production of thyroid hormone and are often associated with enlargement of the thyroid gland. They are second only to diabetes mellitus among naturally occurring endocrine disorders.

Table 33–3. CAUSES OF HYPOTHYROIDISM

Chronic thyroiditis	Excess ingestion of food goitrogens:
Pituitary hypofunction	Plant and animal seafood
Hypothalamus hypofunction	Cabbage and related vegetables
Iodine deficiency	Turnips
Idiopathic hypofunction	Rutabaga
Neoplasias	Asparagus
Iatrogenic causes:	Spinach
Thyroidectomy	Soybeans
Hypophysectomy	Peanuts
Irradiation	Peas
Drug goitrogens:	Peaches
Antithyroid agents	Strawberries
Propylthiouracil	
Methimazole	
Iodine in large doses	
Lithium carbonate	
Sulfonamides	
Salicylates	

Hypothyroidism

Hypothyroidism is a metabolic disorder that is usually characterized by a deficiency of the circulating thyroid hormones, thyroxine and triiodothyronine. In rare instances, manifestations of hypothyroidism may be caused by an inability of the target tissues to bind with or use available thyroid hormone. Although it can develop in any age group, hypothyroidism is most common after middle age. Hypothyroidism is five times more prevalent in women than in men.

Hypothyroidism that develops during fetal development or infancy and that results in defective physical development and mental retardation is termed cretinism. Juvenile hypothyroidism develops during childhood after the brain is fully developed but may still result in defective physical development. Early detection and treatment of hypothyroidism in infants and children will prevent mental retardation and promote normal physical development. The reader is referred to a pediatric text for further discussion of hypothyroidism in children.

ETIOLOGY

Primary hypothyroidism is a defect in the thyroid gland itself. The gland is unable to produce or release adequate amounts of thyroid hormone. In the adult, primary hypothyroidism most commonly develops in an individual with a history of chronic thyroiditis (Hashimoto's thyroiditis), an autoimmune disease in which thyroid tissue is gradually destroyed by thyroid antibodies. Hypothyroidism that is characterized by atrophy of the thyroid gland may be caused by failure of the pituitary gland to secrete thyroid-stimulating hormone, referred to as secondary hypothyroidism, or by failure of the hypothalamus to secrete thyroid releasing hormone, referred to as tertiary hypothyroidism.

Iatrogenic causes of hypothyroidism include surgical removal or irradiation of the thyroid gland or pituitary gland and overtreatment of hyperthyroidism with antithyroid agents. Rarely, hypothyroidism may be caused by dietary deficiency of iodine or excess or prolonged ingestion of goitrogens. Goitrogens are drugs and foods that contain thyroid-inhibiting substances that decrease thyroxine production. Although dietary deficiency of iodine is rare in the United States, it is still common in landlocked areas of developing countries. Table 33–3 lists common causes of hypothyroidism.

PATHOPHYSIOLOGY

Pathologic changes associated with hypothyroidism vary with the age of onset of the disorder, its duration before diagnosis, and the severity of the hormone deficiency. The longer its duration and the more severe the hormone deficiency, the more profound the changes in physiologic function. In most cases of hypothyroidism, the physiologic activities identified in Table 33–1 slow as the amounts of circulating thyroid hormone decrease. All body processes are affected as basal metabolism and oxygen consumption by the tissues decrease. Personality changes occur as mental processes and responses to stimuli deteriorate. Individuals with severe hypothyroidism develop a generalized accumulation of hydrophilic mucopolysaccharides in interstitial tissues, which causes a thickened, puffy appearance. This mucinous, nonpitting edema is referred to as myxedema, a term often used synonymously with hypothyroidism.

CLINICAL MANIFESTATIONS

The clinical manifestations of primary hypothyroidism develop insidiously over a period of months or years as the hormone deficiency worsens. All body systems are affected.

Fatigue, lethargy, and increased somnolence are early symptoms. Decreased metabolism and oxygen consumption are manifested by slowed heart rate, decreased cardiac output, decreased blood volume, decreased pulse pressure, decreased respiratory rate, anemia, subnormal basal temperature, and sensitivity to cold. Impaired wound healing, easy bruising as a result of capillary fragility, and hypercholesterolemia, which increases the risk for coronary atherosclerosis, develop.

Anemia combined with decreased cutaneous circulation causes coolness and pallor of the skin. It becomes dry, coarse, and inelastic because of decreased secretions from the sweat and sebaceous glands. Hyperkeratosis may develop. Decreased metabolism of carotene results in hypercarotenemia and a yellow tint in the skin. The hair becomes dull, sparse, and brittle. Loss of hair from the temporal third of the eyebrows is a characteristic feature of hypothyroidism. The nails become brittle and grow slowly.

Severe constipation and decreased appetite result from decreased peristalsis. Generalized myxedema results in weight gain and a puffy appearance. Myxedema is also manifested in bagginess around the eyes, puffiness of the face, and swelling of the subclavicular fossae and dorsa of the hands and feet. The typical facial appearance of a person with myxedema is illustrated in Figure 33–3. Numbness and tingling of the hands or feet due to pressure around peripheral nerve fibers are common. Thick slurred speech and hoarseness are caused by myxedema of the tongue and larynx. Aching and stiffness of muscles and joints are common. Muscle movement and reflexes slow. Women of childbearing age may experience menorrhagia, inability to conceive due to failure to ovulate, and loss of libido. Men may develop loss of libido and impotence.

Decreased cerebral blood flow results in headaches, general slowing of mental processes, slowed speech, apathy, and forgetfulness. Syncope, paranoia, or depressive psychoses may develop. Cerebral hypoxia and decreased metabolism may progress to stupor or myxedema coma.

Although myxedema coma is rare, it has a high mortality rate. It is seen most commonly in the elderly and during winter months and is often preceded by exposure to cold, infection, trauma, or use of central nervous system depressants. Myxedema coma may result in death from cerebral hypoxia, bradycardia with severely decreased cardiac output with congestive heart failure, hypothermia, and hypoventilation progressing to respiratory acidosis or failure. Seizures, intestinal ileus, and fecal impaction may also be present in myxedema coma. Deep tendon reflexes are often absent.

MEDICAL DIAGNOSIS

Medical diagnosis of hypothyroidism is made on the basis of the history, clinical manifestations, and identification of low levels of serum T_4, serum T_3, free thyroxine (FT_4), and T_3 resin uptake. In primary hypothyroidism, serum levels of TSH are elevated. In hypothyroidism caused by pituitary or hypothalamic dysfunction, TSH levels are lower than normal. Table 33–2 identifies common diagnostic studies to evaluate thyroid function and their nursing implications. The abnormal responses to these studies typical in a patient with hypothyroidism are summarized in Table 33–4.

MEDICAL MANAGEMENT

Treatment of primary hypothyroidism requires lifelong thyroid hormone replacement therapy. Levothyroxine (Synthroid, T_4), a synthetic thyroxine, is the drug of choice. Liothyronine (Cytomel, T_3), liotrix (Euthroid, Thyrolar, T_3/T_4), and desiccated thyroid are alternative thyroid preparations. The dosage of thyroid hormone is individualized to achieve a euthyroid, or normal, hormonal state. The dose is gradually increased from initial to maintenance levels at 1- to 2-week intervals while thyroid function is closely monitored.

Treatment of hypothyroidism secondary to a pituitary or hypothalamic dysfunction depends on the

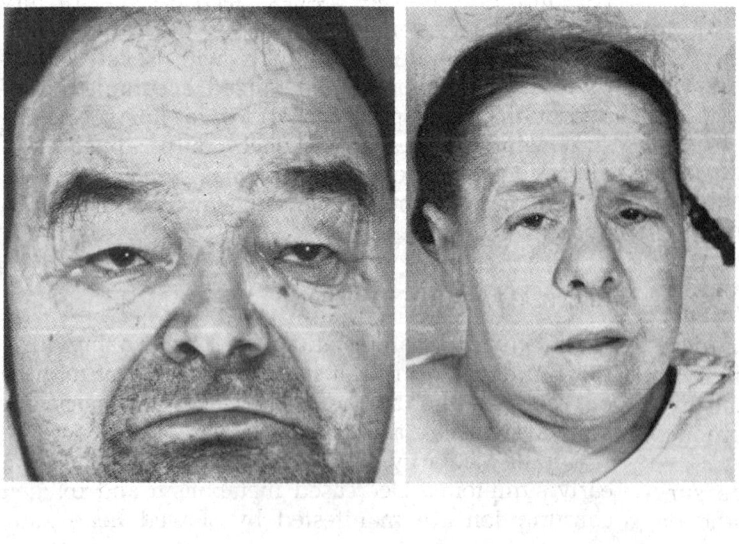

Figure 33–3.

Typical facial puffiness and dull expression of patients with myxedema. (From Larsen PR, Ingbar SH. The thyroid gland. In Wilson JD, Foster DW (eds). Williams textbook of endocrinology. 8th ed. Philadelphia: WB Saunders, 1992, p 451.)

Table 33–4. TYPICAL RESULTS OF COMMON DIAGNOSTIC STUDIES OF THYROID FUNCTION IN HYPOTHYROIDISM AND HYPERTHYROIDISM

	HYPOTHYROID DISORDERS			
	PRIMARY THYROID GLAND DYSFUNCTION	SECONDARY DYSFUNCTION (PITUITARY DYSFUNCTION)	TERTIARY DYSFUNCTION (HYPOTHALAMIC DYSFUNCTION)	HYPERTHYROID DISORDERS
T_4	Low	Low	Low	High
T_3	Low	Low	Low	High
FT_4	Low	Low	Low	High
T_3RU	Low	Low	Low	High
TSH	High	Low	Low	Normal or low
RAIU	Low	Low	Low	High
Change in $T_4:T_3$ ratio	None	None	None	Increase in T_3 proportionately greater than increase in T_4
TSH response to TRH stimulation test	Normal rise	None	Delayed rise	—
T_3/T_4 response to TRH stimulation test	None	None	Rise	—

Table represents typical responses, but exceptions are possible in individual cases.
Abbreviations: T_4, thyroxine; T_3, triiodothyronine; FT_4, free thyroxine; T_3RU, T_3 resin uptake; TSH, thyroid-stimulating hormone; RAIU, radioactive iodine uptake; TRH, thyrotropin releasing hormone.

nature of the dysfunction. The patient may receive temporary thyroid hormone replacement while the underlying disorder is treated, or lifelong replacement if the underlying disorder cannot be corrected.

Hypothyroidism due to inadequate iodine intake is corrected by daily iodine supplements. Hypothyroidism caused by excessive ingestion of goitrogens is corrected, if possible, by decreasing or discontinuing the drug or food involved.

Myxedema coma is reversed by intravenous administration of levothyroxine while the patient is treated for shock with intravenous fluids and hydrocortisone. The underlying precipitating factor is identified and treated. Laboratory studies determine the need for intravenous glucose and electrolytes. Oxygen is administered, and mechanical ventilation may be necessary to correct hypoventilation and respiratory acidosis. The patient is rewarmed passively to prevent rapid increase in oxygen requirements and shunting of blood from the vital organs to the peripheral circulation. If the patient is unconscious, a nasogastric tube may be inserted to prevent aspiration and gastric distention. Once the patient is stabilized, lifelong thyroid hormone replacement therapy is initiated.

Early diagnosis and treatment of hypothyroidism are important to reduce the severity of permanent effects of physiologic changes associated with prolonged thyroid hormone deficiency. Although treatment reverses most clinical manifestations, cardiovascular changes caused by atherosclerosis and some interstitial myxedema may remain.

With early diagnosis and properly managed hormone replacement therapy, the individual with hypothyroidism has an excellent prognosis.

Application of the Nursing Process to the Care of the Patient with Hypothyroidism

Assessment

Obtain a complete nursing history from the patient with diagnosed or suspected hypothyroidism. Ask specifically about the onset of early symptoms of unusual fatigue, lethargy, or somnolence. Nonspecific early symptoms are often overlooked by the patient as insignificant or unrelated to the current illness. Allow extra time for the patient to process and respond to questions because mental functions may be slowed.

Obtain baseline vital signs and apical heart rate to determine cardiovascular status. Weigh the patient, and compare current weight with presymptomatic weight if documented or known by the patient. Note the absence of presence of nonpitting, interstitial myxedema and its distribution. Auscultate for hypoactive bowel sounds. Question the patient and close associates about changes in appearance, behavior, or mental processes. Assess for the presence of clinical manifestations associated with hypothyroidism. As each manifestation is identified, ask the patient how long it has been present. Identify the patient's interpretation of clinical manifestations and knowledge of planned diagnostic studies and treatment to determine teaching needs.

Assessment of the patient in myxedema stupor or coma is limited to determination of hemodynamic

Nursing Care Guide 33–1.

PATIENTS LEARNING SELF-MANAGEMENT OF HYPOTHYROIDISM

Assessment Findings: A 53-year-old woman with a history of progressive slowing of mental processes and lack of energy is diagnosed as having hypothyroidism. Levothyroxine (Synthroid, T_4) has been prescribed.

Nursing Diagnosis: High risk for altered health maintenance related to insufficient knowledge of self-management of hypothyroidism and lifelong thyroid hormone replacement

Patient Outcomes	Nursing Interventions	Rationale
Patient verbalizes understanding of the physiologic effects of thyroid hormones, the pathologic changes that result from their deficiency, and the rationale for the prescribed treatment.	Reinforce in clear, easily understood terms the physician's explanation of hypothyroidism and its treatment.	Understanding of the disease process and treatment increases patient compliance.
	Allow extra time for patient to understand teaching and to ask questions. Provide repetition and reinforcement as necessary. Provide written instructions. Reassure patient that slowed thought processes and lack of energy are manifestations of hypothyroidism that will reverse with treatment.	Hypothyroidism slows mental processes. Repetition reinforces learning. Written instructions reinforce learning and minimize the risk of errors.
Patient states intent to take levothyroxine daily as prescribed.	Teach patient name, dose, administration schedule, expected action, and side effects of levothyroxine. Stress that thyroid replacement is lifelong and that the patient is not to alter dosage without physician instructions. Advise patient to expect diuresis and increased pulse rate as early responses to treatment.	Legally, all persons must have this information to correctly and safely self-administer medication.
	Instruct patient to take as a single dose, before breakfast.	Food interferes with absorption.
	Teach patient to monitor and record the radial pulse before each dose during the adjustment period, and weekly thereafter. Drug is not taken and the physician is notified promptly if the pulse is higher than 100 bpm or is irregular.	Tachycardia is the earliest sign of overdose of thyroid hormone.
	Instruct patient to advise all physicians treating her that she is taking levothyroxine and to wear Medic-Alert identification at all times.	To prevent drug interactions.

(continued)

Nursing Care Guide 33–1. *(continued)*

PATIENTS LEARNING SELF-MANAGEMENT OF HYPOTHYROIDISM

Patient Outcomes	Nursing Interventions	Rationale
	Consult with physician before taking over-the-counter preparations.	
	Consult with physician to determine whether patient is to be instructed to limit ingestion of goitrogens or foods high in iodine.	High iodine intake may alter effectiveness of drug.
	Store in light-resistant container in dry location.	Light and moisture cause deterioration of drug.
Patient states intent to keep monthly appointments for evaluation during dosage adjustment and annual appointments thereafter.	Teach patient that effects of levothyroxine are cumulative and require frequent reevaluation during dosage adjustment. Once a euthyroid state is achieved, annual reevaluation is necessary to monitor response to therapy and to adjust dosage to meet changing metabolic needs associated with aging.	Evaluates effectiveness of treatment and prevents over- or underdosage.
Patient uses energy conservation to complete daily activities.	Teach patient to plan daily activities to allow for frequent rest periods and energy conservation. Example: Plan and complete tasks in one location, rest, begin tasks in another. Remind patient to allow extra time to complete tasks because of slowed mental processes and decreased energy levels. Reassure patient that activity tolerance will increase with treatment.	Euthyroid state will not be attained until several weeks of therapy are completed. Patient will fatigue easily until that time.
	Instruct patient to stop activity and notify the physician if chest pain, palpitations, or tachycardia occurs.	Indicate activity intolerance or possible overdose of levothyroxine.
Patient eats six small meals daily.	Advise patient that six small meals high in protein, carbohydrates, B and C vitamins, and iron will promote optimal nutritional status.	Frequent small meals are better tolerated by individuals with poor appetites than three large meals daily.
	Teach patient to take a few sips of warm liquid 10–15 minutes before eating.	Stimulates peristalsis and improves appetite and digestion.
	Reassure patient that weight loss and increased appetite will occur with treatment.	Indicate increased metabolism.

(continued)

Nursing Care Guide 33–1. *(continued)*

PATIENTS LEARNING SELF-MANAGEMENT OF HYPOTHYROIDISM

Patient Outcomes	Nursing Interventions	Rationale
Patient evacuates soft, formed stool at least once every 3 days.	Determine patient's normal bowel pattern. Discuss the effect hypothyroidism may have on bowel function.	Decreased peristalsis is a manifestation of hypothyroidism and may cause severe constipation.
	Encourage walking or other exercise. Teach patient the importance of fiber and fluids in maintaining normal bowel function throughout life. Provide patient with a list of high-fiber foods.	Exercise stimulates peristalsis and increases abdominal muscle tone. Increased fluids and dietary fiber stimulate peristalsis and soften and provide bulk to the stool to promote bowel evacuation.
Patient uses skin care products that do not dry or irritate the skin.	Instruct the patient to avoid hot water and soap and to apply moisturizers and creams after bathing.	Soap and hot water dry the skin. Emollients restore moisture and counteract dryness.

Evaluation: Compare the patient's status with the expected patient outcomes. If the outcomes are achieved, evaluate nursing care as successful. If not, reassess the patient, formulate new nursing diagnoses, and revise expected patient outcomes and nursing interventions as appropriate.

status until treatment for shock and intravenous thyroid hormone are initiated. Determine baseline vital signs, neurologic status, and renal function for comparison with later assessments. Obtain a brief history and identification of allergies from an individual familiar with the patient if the patient is unable to provide information. Complete the history once the patient is stabilized.

Nursing Diagnoses and Planning

Nursing diagnoses and related expected patient outcomes most commonly applicable to patients with hypothyroidism include the following:

NDx: High risk for altered tissue perfusion: systemic related to anemia, decreased cardiac output, decreased respirations, and hypothermia secondary to decreased basal metabolism

Planning: Patient outcomes
1. Patient maintains adequate tissue perfusion as evidenced by:
   a. Stable vital signs
   b. Basal temperature higher than 96°F (35.5°C)
   c. Pulse higher than 60 bpm and less than 100 bpm and regular
   d. Respirations 8 to 16/minute
   e. Blood pressure higher than 90/60
   f. Capillary refill less than 3 seconds
   g. Alert, oriented to person, place, time
   h. Urine output more than 30 ml/hour

NDx: Activity intolerance related to fatigue, lethargy, altered sensory perception and muscular responses, slowed mental processes

Planning: Patient outcomes
1. Patient displays interest in environment.
2. Patient completes daily activities as independently as possible.
3. Patient safety is maintained.

NDx: Colonic constipation related to decreased mobility, decreased gastrointestinal motility, and anorexia

Planning: Patient outcomes
1. Patient evacuates soft stool at least every 3 days.

NDx: High risk for impaired skin integrity related to loss of elasticity, dryness, and generalized myxedema

Planning: Patient outcomes
1. Patient's skin remains smooth, supple, and free from breakdown.

NDx: High risk for altered health maintenance related to insufficient knowledge of self-administration of thyroid hormone replacement therapy

Planning: Patient outcomes

1. Patient verbalizes understanding of the need for, and intent to take, thyroid hormone replacement as prescribed.
2. Patient states name, dose, administration schedule, timetable for expected effects, and adverse and toxic effects of prescribed thyroid hormone.
3. Patient demonstrates ability to monitor radial pulse.
4. Patient states intent to keep follow-up appointments with physician and to notify physician promptly if pulse is less than 60 bpm, higher than 100 bpm, or irregular.

Nursing Interventions

The majority of patients who have hypothyroidism are diagnosed and treated on an out-patient basis. Therefore, nursing care primarily focuses on patient teaching. Patient teaching for self-management is summarized in Nursing Care Guide 33–1. However, because the manifestations of hypothyroidism develop slowly, some patients remain undiagnosed and untreated for several years. These patients require hospitalization to treat severe hypothyroidism or myxedema coma.

NDx: High risk for altered tissue perfusion: systemic

Evaluate vital functions and neurologic signs of the hospitalized patient with severe hypothyroidism at least twice daily to identify changes in status and response to treatment. Monitor vital signs, capillary refill, and skin color and temperature to determine changes in cardiovascular status. Auscultate rate, depth, and character of respirations to detect respiratory depression and hypoventilation. Monitor fluid intake and output and daily weights to evaluate fluid balance and renal function. Monitor level of consciousness and orientation to person, place, and time to identify cerebral hypoxia. Observe the patient's gait, muscle strength, and reflexes to identify slowed neuromuscular responses and impaired coordination. Maintain a warm environment and provide warm blankets, robe, and socks to conserve body temperature and prevent hypothermia. Administer prescribed thyroid hormone replacement, and monitor the patient's response as basal metabolism increases. Pharmacology Box 33–1 summarizes the pharmacologic actions, side effects, and nursing implications of thyroid hormone replacement preparations.

If the patient is in myxedema coma as a result of severe cerebral hypoxia and decreased perfusion, monitor vital signs, pulse pressure, capillary refill, neurologic status, and renal output hourly. Administer oxygen, parenteral fluids and electrolytes, thyroid hormone, and medications to support cardiovascular function as prescribed. Position the patient on either side to prevent aspiration of oral secretions. The patient may require mechanical ventilation to reverse respiratory depression and acidosis. Provide multiple layers of covers and a warm environment to rewarm the patient passively and slowly while preventing surface burns and increased metabolic requirements.

NDx: Activity intolerance

Orient patient to surroundings, explain call system, and ask the patient to demonstrate how to use it. Monitor level of orientation frequently, and reorient as necessary. Explain procedures and requests clearly and slowly, and reinforce as necessary to promote patient understanding and participation. Provide conversation and nonstressful diversional activities to stimulate interest in activities and surroundings. Reassure the patient and family that current behavior patterns and slowed thought processes are manifestations of hypothyroidism and will reverse with treatment.

Plan care to provide frequent rest periods to conserve energy. Allow patient sufficient time to accomplish activities as independently as possible to promote self-esteem. Place supplies and personal belongings within easy reach to avoid unnecessary exertion. Provide assistance when patient begins to tire to avoid overexertion while promoting patient participation to the extent possible.

Reassess muscle strength and mobility daily. Encourage ambulation and active range-of-motion exercises to promote muscle strength and flexibility. Instruct patient to call for assistance when getting out of bed, remove potential hazards from environment, and provide assistance with ambulation to prevent falls. Keep side rails up if necessary for patient safety. Check the temperature of bath water prior to use to prevent burns. Carefully evaluate need for, and response to, sedatives, narcotics, and barbiturates because of hypersensitivity to these drugs in hypothyroidism.

NDx: Colonic constipation

Determine patient's normal bowel pattern. Monitor for changes in bowel sounds daily. If not contraindicated, provide diet high in fiber and increase fluid intake by offering fluids hourly to soften stool and increase bulk. Six small meals daily are better tolerated by individuals with poor appetites and slow digestion. Administer prescribed stool softeners and peristalsis stimulants, such as docusate sodium and casanthranol (Peri-Colace), to promote defecation. Encourage ambulation and activity as tolerated to increase intestinal motility.

NDx: High risk for impaired skin integrity

Assess skin for redness or breakdown daily. Avoid soap; use oil or lotion in bath water to prevent dryness. Blot skin dry, do not rub, to prevent friction. Massage and lubricate pressure points at least four

Pharmacology Box 33–1.

THYROID HORMONE PREPARATIONS

Thyroid Hormone Preparations:
Class of drugs that increase protein synthesis and stimulate metabolic activity of the cells.

Action:
Exact mechanism of action unknown. By increasing the metabolic activity of the cells, thyroid hormone preparations increase oxygen consumption and energy production; alter carbohydrate, fat, and protein metabolism; and promote growth and maturation of tissues.

Uses:
Replacement therapy in hypothyroid disorders.

Side Effects:
Hypersensitivity reactions (rash, anaphylaxsis) are rare. Side effects appear gradually, primarily result from overdose, and are similar to the manifestations of hyperthyroidism: palpitations, tachycardia, dysrhythmias, elevated pulse pressure, angina pectoris, cardiac failure, headache, tremors, nervousness, insomnia, leg cramps, nausea, diarrhea, anorexia, abdominal cramps, weight loss, heat intolerance, increased basal temperature, sweating, menstrual irregularities.

Interactions:
Cholestyramine and colestipol decrease absorption. Estrogens antagonize action. Thyroid hormone preparations potentiate the effects of anticoagulants, sympathomimetics, and tricyclic antidepressants, and decrease effectiveness of antidiabetic agents and digitalis glycosides.

Nursing Implications:
Administer as a single morning dose before eating. Effects are cumulative. Monitor changes in pulse, blood pressure, appetite, weight, and activity tolerance. Withhold dose and notify physician if pulse is higher than 100 beats per minute or if the rhythm is irregular. Advise patient to expect diuresis and weight loss as the earliest response to therapy. Stress that replacement therapy is lifelong. Emphasize need for monthly evaluations during dosage adjustment and annual evaluations once a euthyroid state is achieved. Store in light-resistant container in dry location. Consult physician for dietary restrictions; ingestion of iodine and goitrogens may be limited.

Geriatric Considerations:
The elderly are especially susceptible to the metabolic effects of thyroid preparations. Dosage must be increased gradually to avoid cardiovascular and cerebral side effects. Assess for angina due to cardiac overload from increased metabolic demands, and for signs of agitation or confusion due to rapid increase in metabolic rate and cerebral perfusion.

times a day, and use elbow and heel protectors to prevent breakdown. Assist and encourage patient to ambulate and change position frequently to promote capillary circulation. Provide diet high in protein, carbohydrates, B and C vitamins, and iron to promote optimal nutritional status and provide elements needed for skin maintenance and repair.

NDx: High risk for altered health maintenance related to insufficient knowledge of self-administration of thyroid hormone replacement therapy
Teach the patient the dosage and schedule, expected action, and side effects of prescribed thyroid hormone replacement preparation. Pharmacology Box 33–1 identifies the pharmacokinetics of thyroid hormone preparations. Advise the patient that diuresis, weight loss, decreasing puffiness, increased pulse rate, increased appetite, and increased activity tolerance are expected early responses to thyroid hormone replacement. Teach the patient that chest pain, shortness of breath, insomnia, and nervousness are early signs of excess thyroid hormone replacement that must be reported to the physician promptly so dosage can be reduced.

Teach the patient how to monitor the radial pulse for one full minute and record the results. Have the patient count the pulse in one wrist while you count it in the other to ensure correct technique. The pulse rate is an important indicator of the body's response to thyroid replacement. It is monitored before each dose during the period of adjustment, and weekly once the patient is euthyroid. The physician is notified promptly if the pulse rate is less than 60 bpm or higher than 100 bpm, or if the rhythm is irregular.

Response to therapy is usually monitored by the physician on a monthly basis until a euthyroid state is achieved, then once yearly. Emphasize that replacement therapy for hypothyroidism is lifelong and that periodic examination to evaluate thyroid function is important. No over-the-counter medications or mineral supplements should be taken without physician approval. Consult with the physician to determine whether the patient is to be instructed to limit intake of foods high in iodine, which may alter response to thyroid replacement therapy.

Evaluation

Evaluate the effectiveness of nursing care for a patient with hypothyroidism by comparing the patient's status with the expected patient outcomes. Examples of specific outcomes for patients with hypothyroidism have been provided in the Planning section.

Hyperthyroidism

Hyperthyroidism is a disorder of hypermetabolism resulting from exposure of the body tissues to excessive quantities of circulating free thyroxine or triiodothyronine, or both. It is second only to diabetes mellitus among naturally occurring endocrine disorders. Heredity is a factor in the incidence of hyperthyroidism, and severe emotional or physical stress often precipitates the onset of overt symptoms. Hyperthyroidism is seven to ten times more common in women and is diagnosed most frequently at puberty, during pregnancy, or in the 30- to 50-year age group. In men, it tends to develop after 50 and is more severe.

The most common form of primary hyperthyroidism is Graves' disease. Toxic nodular goiter, secreting adenoma of the thyroid gland, subacute thyroiditis, a pituitary adenoma that secretes excess thyroid-stimulating hormone, overtreatment of hypothyroidism, and thyroid-stimulating medications may also cause symptoms of hyperthyroidism.

ETIOLOGY

Primary hyperthyroidism, or Graves' disease, is an autoimmune disorder in which immunoglobulins of the IgG class produce thyroid antibodies that are similar in action to thyroid-stimulating hormone (TSH) but exert a stronger and longer-acting effect. These autoantibodies bind at the TSH receptor sites and stimulate thyroid growth, increased vascularity, and hypersecretion of thyroid hormone. The multiple IgG autoantibodies that have been identified in individuals with Graves' disease are referred to collectively as thyroid-stimulating immunoglobulins (TSI).

PATHOPHYSIOLOGY

Graves' disease is a multisystem disorder characterized by hyperthyroidism with diffuse thyroid enlargement and increased vascularity. This enlargement of the thyroid gland in Graves' disease is referred to as a diffuse toxic goiter because it is associated with increased thyroid function. Increased secretion of thyroid hormones produces a sustained hypermetabolic state with increased oxygen consumption and increased sensitivity and stimulation of the sympathetic nervous system. The physiologic activities identified in Table 33–1 increase as the amount of circulating thyroid hormones increases.

Approximately 50% of individuals with Graves' disease also develop infiltrative ophthalmopathy, or exophthalmos, and 5% to 10% develop infiltrative dermopathy. Infiltrative ophthalmopathy results from accumulation of fluid in the fat pads behind the eyeball and inflammatory edema of the extraocular muscles. The increased volume of the orbital contents causes the eyeballs to protrude, as illustrated in Figure 33–4. Inflammation and fibrosis of extraocular muscles may result. Infiltrative dermopathy is a raised, hyperpigmented, nonpitting edema of the pretibial area, ankles, and dorsa of the feet that has an orange-peel appearance. It is sometimes called pretibial myxedema. An example of severe pretibial myxedema is illustrated in Figure 33–5.

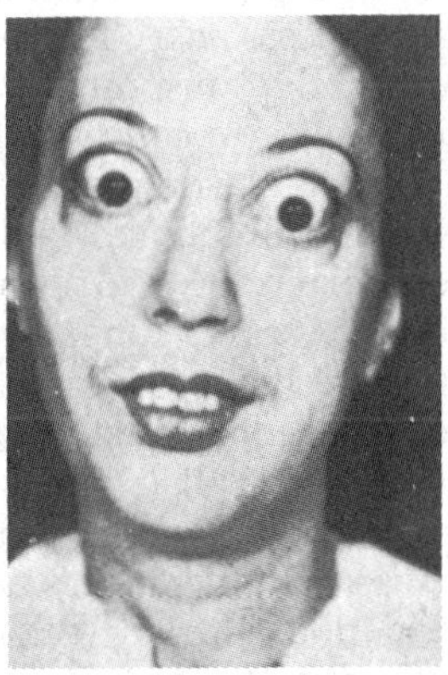

Figure 33–4.

Infiltrative ophthalmopathy, or exophthalmos, in a woman with hyperthyroidism. (From Larsen PR, Ingbar SH. The thyroid gland. In Wilson JD, Foster DW (eds). Williams textbook of endocrinology. 8th ed. Philadelphia: WB Saunders, 1992, p 426.)

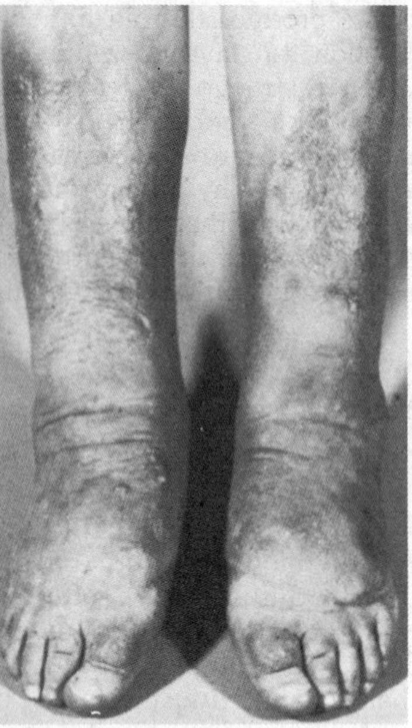

Figure 33–5.

Severe pretibial myxedema sometimes present in hyperthyroidism. (From DeGroot LJ Endocrinology. 2nd ed. Philadelphia: WB Saunders, 1989, p 669.)

The cause of these infiltrative manifestations of Graves' disease is unknown.

CLINICAL MANIFESTATIONS

The severity of the clinical manifestations of primary hyperthyroidism, or Graves' disease, depends on the degree of hormone excess, its duration, how rapidly it developed, and the age of the individual. The disease usually develops gradually over a period of months, or even years. In general, the longer the duration of the disease and the more rapid its onset, the more severe the manifestations.

Exaggerated alertness, nervousness, tremulousness, agitation, irritability, insomnia, a feeling of apprehension, and inability to concentrate are common early symptoms of excess stimulation of the sympathetic nervous system. Emotional lability with inappropriate episodes of crying and euphoria may develop. Increased oxygen consumption due to hypermetabolism and the need to dissipate the excess heat produced are manifested by tachycardia, palpitations, increased cardiac output, a bounding pulse, increased pulse pressure, systolic hypertension, tachypnea, heat intolerance, diaphoresis, and cutaneous vasodilation. Atrial dysrhythmias may develop. Fatigue, muscle weakness, and muscle wasting result from the production of heat rather than energy during metabolism. Weight loss occurs despite an increase in appetite.

Sympathetic nervous system stimulation causes fine muscle and tongue tremors, impaired coordination, hyperreflexia, jerky movement of the eyelids, spasmodic retraction of the eyelids, and a fine tremor of the closed lids. Periorbital edema, as illustrated in Figure 33–6, is common. Photosensitivity, diplopia, and increased lacrimation may develop in conjunction with exophthalmos. The presence of exophthalmos may be masked by the puffiness of periorbital edema.

The skin is warm, moist, smooth, and sometimes flushed. Pruritus may develop. Hard, nonpitting pretibial or ankle edema may be present. The hair is fine, smooth, breaks easily, and does not hold a wave. Hair loss may occur. The nails are soft, easily torn, and the distal nail may separate from the nail bed (onycholysis). Hyperactive bowel sounds with an increase in the frequency of bowel movements and softening of the stools are common. Hypercalcemia and osteoporosis due to bone demineralization may occur. Women experience decreased libido, changes in the menstrual pattern, and reduced fertility. If conception occurs, spontaneous abortion may result. Men experience decreased libido, impotence, and sometimes gynecomastia.

The thyroid gland may be normal in size, or may present as a moderate to massively enlarged diffuse toxic goiter. On palpation, the consistency of the goiter varies from soft to firm and rubbery. It is generally smooth, but may feel lobular. A thrill may be felt over a large goiter, and a bruit can often be auscultated. Figure 33–7 illustrates the physical appearance of an individual with a goiter.

Thyrotoxicosis in Graves' disease is a hypermetabolic state characterized by the presence of all the metabolic and neurologic manifestations of hyperthyroidism. Heart failure due to prolonged tachycardia and atrial dysrhythmias may develop. The difference between hyperthyroidism and thyrotoxicosis is a matter of degree and of the severity of the symptoms present. The terms are sometimes used interchangeably.

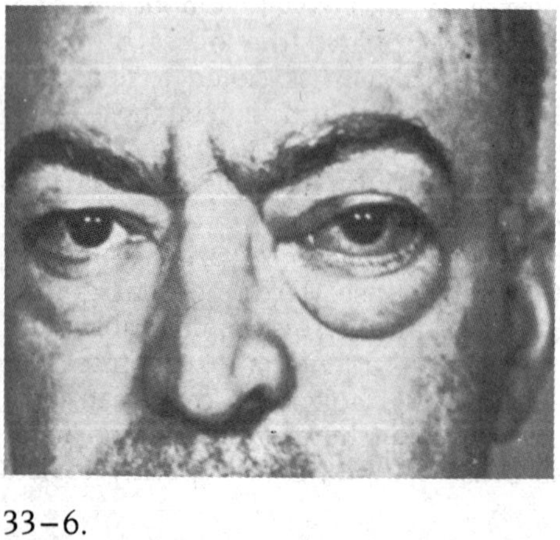

Figure 33–6.

Exophthalmos masked by the periorbital edema common in hyperthyroidism. (From Larsen PR, Ingbar SH. The thyroid gland. In Wilson JD, Foster DW (eds). Williams textbook of endocrinology. 8th ed. Philadelphia: WB Saunders, 1992, p 426.)

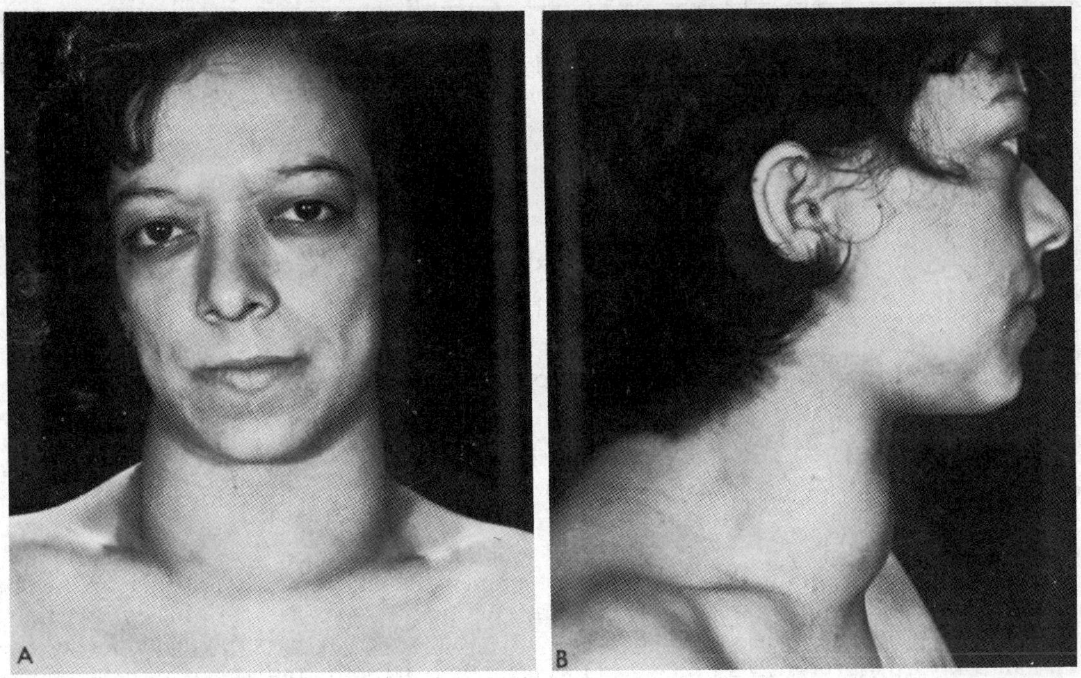

Figure 33–7.

Thyroid enlargement due to goiter. Note enlargement at the base of the neck. (From Larsen PR, Ingbar SH. The thyroid gland. In Wilson JD, Foster DW (eds). Williams textbook of endocrinology. 8th ed. Philadelphia: WB Saunders, 1992, p 425.)

Thyroid storm, or thyroid crisis, is a rare but potentially fatal severe hypermetabolic state characterized by exaggerated clinical manifestations of hyperthyroidism. It may be precipitated by severe stress, infection, surgery, trauma, radioactive iodine therapy, aggressive manipulation of a goiter, and abrupt withdrawal of antithyroid drugs. The clinical manifestations of thyroid storm include fever as high as 106°F (41.1°C), severe tachycardia, profuse diaphoresis, extreme vasodilation, hypotension, atrial fibrillation, hyperreflexia, abdominal pain, delirium, psychosis, nausea, vomiting, diarrhea, and dehydration rapidly progressing to coma and cardiovascular collapse. Hypokalemia may result from the vomiting and diarrhea.

MEDICAL DIAGNOSIS

Medical diagnosis of hyperthyroidism is made on the basis of history, clinical manifestations, and identification of elevated levels of serum T_4, serum T_3, free thyroxine (FT_4), and T_3 resin uptake. In addition, the increase in T_3 is proportionately larger than the increase in T_4 owing, in part, to the increased conversion of free circulating T_4 to T_3. Table 33–2 identifies common diagnostic studies to evaluate thyroid function and their nursing implications. The abnormal responses to these studies typical in a patient with hyperthyroidism are summarized in Table 33–4. Identification of elevated antithyroid antibody titers is useful in differentiating between Graves' disease and toxic thyroid adenoma.

MEDICAL MANAGEMENT

Early diagnosis and treatment is important in the successful management of hyperthyroidism. The primary goal is to suppress secretion of thyroid hormones. This is done either by administration of antithyroid preparations or by destruction or removal of a portion of the thyroid gland. Choice of treatment is determined jointly by the physician and patient, based on consideration of the patient's age, childbearing status, severity of clinical manifestations, and patient preference. Propranolol, a beta-adrenergic blocking agent, is frequently prescribed during treatment for hyperthyroidism to alleviate the cardiovascular effects of thyroid hormone excess. Dexamethasone may be used as an adjunct in the treatment of thyrotoxicosis. When administered in conjunction with antithyroid drugs, it inhibits both the secretion of thyroid hormone and the peripheral conversion of T_4 to T_3, rapidly alleviating symptoms.

Mild exophthalmos is primarily treated symptomatically with lubricating methylcellulose eye drops to prevent corneal dryness and ulcerations until the patient achieves a euthyroid state and spontaneous regression occurs. Treatment of severe cases is controversial. Oral glucocorticoid therapy is commonly prescribed for severe or progressing exophthalmos with extraocular muscle damage or pressure on the optic nerve manifested by changes in visual acuity. Plasmapheresis has been successful in reversing exophthalmos in some patients. Surgical decompression with removal of part of the bony orbit may be necessary to relieve intraorbital pressure and pre-

Pharmacology Box 33–2.
THIOAMIDE ANTITHYROID DRUGS

Thioamide Antithyroid Drugs:
Class of thioamides that inhibit the synthesis of thyroid hormone but do not inhibit the release of stored hormone.

Action:
Interfere with the binding of iodine with the thyroglobulin molecule, which is necessary for the synthesis of thyroid hormone.

Uses:
Used to treat hyperthyroidism and to reduce thyroid gland activity before thyroid surgery or irradiation.

Side Effects:
Bone marrow depression, agranulocytosis, thrombocytopenia, leukopenia, lymphadenopathy, drowsiness, headache, neuritis, vertigo, paresthesias, nausea, vomiting, dyspepsia, loss of taste, swelling of the salivary glands, jaundice, hepatitis, vasculitis, rash, urticaria, pruritus, hyperpigmentation of the skin, abnormal hair loss, drug fever, lupus-like syndrome, arthralgia, hypothyroidism.

Interactions:
Do not give with other drugs that may cause agranulocytosis. Propylthiouracil potentiates anticoagulants.

Nursing Implications:
Administer in equally divided doses at 8-hour intervals. May be taken with food to lessen gastric distress. Monitor for signs of response to therapy after 2 to 3 weeks: weight gain, reduced pulse. Therapy may continue for 6 months to several years. Monitor for side effects. Instruct patient to notify physician immediately if sore throat, chills, fever, skin rash, swelling of the lymph nodes, bruising, or bleeding develops. Stress importance of evaluation of therapy and blood studies every 2 to 3 months. Urge patient not to alter drug regimen or take over-the-counter preparations without consulting physician. Store in light-resistant container in dry environment. Avoid use by pregnant women because these drugs cross the placenta. Avoid use by nursing mothers because these drugs are secreted in breast milk.

Geriatric Considerations:
Agranulocytosis is more likely to develop in the elderly and can develop at any point during therapy.

serve vision. Unfortunately, treatment of hyperthyroidism does not ensure reversal of exophthalmos or complete resolution of its effects.

ANTITHYROID DRUGS

Thioamides are a class of antithyroid drugs that inhibit thyroid hormone synthesis but do not block the release of stored hormone. They are used to treat hyperthyroidism in patients who are not candidates for irradiation and as an initial treatment to reduce thyroid gland activity prior to thyroid surgery or irradiation. Propylthiouracil (PTU) is the drug of choice because it also blocks the conversion of circulating T_4 to T_3. Methimazole (Tapazole) is another commonly used thioamide. They are administered in equally divided doses at 8-hour intervals. Objective manifestations of decreased thyroid function develop in 2 to 3 weeks. Therapy is continued for 6 months to several years, with a higher remission rate in patients who are treated for at least 1 year. Long-term remission is achieved in 25% to 30% of patients. Response to therapy is evaluated every 2 to 3 months. The incidence of adverse reactions to thioamides is low. Agranulocytosis is the most serious side effect. Pharmacology Box 33–2 summarizes the pharmacokinetics of thioamide antithyroid drugs.

IODINE PREPARATIONS

In hyperthyroidism, excess iodine temporarily blocks the release of thyroid hormone and reduces the vascularity and size of an enlarged thyroid gland. Iodine is used in conjunction with antithyroid drugs to rapidly reduce circulating thyroid hormone levels and metabolic activity in hyperthyroid states and before thyroid surgery. The course of therapy is limited to 10 to 14 days because of iodine's temporary effect on hormone release.

Saturated solutions of potassium iodide (SSKI) may be administered to protect the thyroid gland from absorbing radioactivity from the environment after a nuclear power plant accident.

RADIOACTIVE IODINE THERAPY

Radioactive iodine (^{131}I) is an economical, easily administered method of treating hyperthyroidism in nonpregnant individuals older than the age of 30. It is usually administered as a single 4 to 10 mCi dose of oral liquid on an out-patient basis. The patient is instructed to sleep alone for two nights, avoid contact with children, and because body fluids and wastes will be slightly radioactive for 24 to 48 hours, to flush the toilet two or three times after use. Patients receiving doses larger than 30 mCi (common in treatment of secreting thyroid adenomas) require hospitalization with appropriate radiation precautions. The radioactive iodine is absorbed and retained by the thyroid gland, where it irradiates and destroys glandular tissue. It produces the ablative effects of surgical removal of thyroid tissue without the potential risks of surgical complications.

Improvement of symptoms begins 2 to 4 weeks after treatment, with maximum effect in approximately 3 months. Temporary thyroid tenderness immediately after treatment is common. Hypothyroidism develops in approximately 10% of patients the first year after treatment, and in 30% of patients within 5 years. These individuals are maintained on thyroid replacement therapy for life.

SUBTOTAL THYROIDECTOMY

Surgical removal of up to 90% of the thyroid gland is an alternative method of treatment of hyperthyroidism in young adults with severe disease or very large goiters, individuals of childbearing age who are pregnant or who wish to become pregnant soon, and those who either do not respond to pharmacologic therapy or have recurrence after pharmacologic treatment. Subtotal thyroidectomy may also be performed as an elected or recommended procedure in individuals with simple goiter or thyroid nodules.

Complications of thyroid surgery are rare but can be life-threatening. These include hemorrhage; respiratory obstruction caused by edema of the trachea, larynx, glottis, or surrounding soft tissues; and laryngeal nerve damage with vocal cord paralysis. Parathyroid injury or accidental removal during the procedure can result in hypocalcemic tetany with respiratory obstruction caused by vocal cord spasm. Postoperative thyroid storm or crisis is very rare. The risk of hemorrhage and thyroid storm is reduced by administration of antithyroid drugs and iodine before surgery to reduce circulating thyroid hormone levels and the size and vascularity of the thyroid gland.

Use of laser beams guided through fiberoptic operative scopes to vaporize hypertrophic thyroid tissue is a new innovation in thyroid surgery. Laser surgery requires smaller surgical incisions, causes less trauma to surrounding tissues and the residual thyroid tissue, and reduces the risk of hemorrhage and postoperative complications.

Application of the Nursing Process to the Care of the Patient with Hyperthyroidism

Assessment

Obtain a complete nursing history from the patient with diagnosed or suspected hyperthyroidism. Ask specifically about the onset of early symptoms of insomnia, increased alertness and activity despite fatigue, apprehension, agitation, and inability to concentrate. Prompt the patient to think back over at least the past year, because nonspecific early symptoms are often overlooked by the patient as insignificant or unrelated to the current illness.

Obtain baseline vital signs and apical heart rate to identify cardiovascular status. Weigh the patient and compare current weight with presymptomatic weight if documented or known by the patient. Note the absence or presence of exophthalmos and hard, nonpitting pretibial edema. Question the patient and close associates about changes in appearance, behavior, or muscle coordination. Auscultate for hyperactive bowel sounds, and test deep tendon reflexes for hyperreflexia. Assess for fine muscle and eyelid tremors and the presence of other clinical manifestations associated with hyperthyroidism. If possible, compare current handwriting with a sample 6 months to a year old. A change in handwriting smoothness and clumsiness in manipulating buttons are signs of fine muscle tremor of the hands. Examine the thyroid gland to identify size, shape, texture, consistency, tenderness, nodularity, and vascular thrill or bruit. As each manifestation is identified, ask the patient how long it has been present. Identify the patient's interpretation of clinical manifestations and knowledge of planned diagnostic studies and treatment to determine teaching needs.

Assessment of the patient in severe thyrotoxicosis or thyroid crisis is limited to determination of hemodynamic status until treatment for dehydration, hyperthermia, hypermetabolism, and potential cardiovascular collapse is initiated. Obtain a brief history and identification of allergies from an individual familiar with the patient if the patient is unable to provide information. Determine baseline vital signs, neurologic status, and renal function. Obtain a complete history once the patient is stabilized.

Nursing Diagnoses and Planning

Nursing diagnoses and related expected patient outcomes most commonly applicable to patients with hyperthyroidism or Graves' disease include the following:

NDx: Anxiety related to heat intolerance and changes in appearance, behavior, and activity secondary to thyroid hormone excess

Planning: Patient outcomes
1. Patient verbalizes reduction in anxiety.
2. Patient states effect of excess thyroid hormone production on the body.
3. Patient states understanding of thyroid hormone excess as cause of physical and behavioral changes.

NDx: High risk for altered health maintenance related to insufficient knowledge of self-management of pharmacologic therapy during and after treatment with antithyroid drugs, iodine, or radioactive iodine

Planning: Patient outcomes
1. Patient states name, dose, administration schedule, timetable for expected effects, and adverse and toxic effects of prescribed medications.
2. Patient demonstrates ability to monitor radial pulse.
3. Patient states realistic expectations of treatment.
4. Patient states intent to keep follow-up appointments with physician.

NDx: Altered nutrition: less than body requirements related to hypermetabolism, hyperactivity, and increased gastrointestinal motility as evidenced by weight loss

Planning: Patient outcomes
1. Patient states intent to consume high-calorie, high-protein, high-carbohydrate diet until ideal weight and euthyroid state are attained.
2. Patient states intent to drink up to 4000 ml of fluid daily until euthyroid state is achieved.
3. Patient verbalizes understanding of the need to gradually decrease food and fluid consumption to maintain ideal weight as metabolic rate decreases.

NDx: High risk for trauma related to fatigue, fine muscle tremors, ophthalmic changes, and osteoporosis

Planning: Patient outcomes
1. Patient verbalizes understanding of the need for frequent rest periods to conserve energy.
2. Patient requests or accepts assistance with activities that require fine motor coordination.
3. Patient demonstrates ability to self-administer prescribed lubricating eye drops.
4. Patient remains free of injury.

NDx: High risk for altered tissue perfusion: systemic, related to dehydration, hyperthermia, and decreased cardiac output secondary to hypermetabolism and severe thyrotoxicosis or thyroid storm

Planning: Patient outcomes
1. Patient demonstrates adequate tissue perfusion as evidenced by:
   a. Basal temperature within normal limits
   b. Stable vital signs within normal limits
   c. Normal neurologic responses
   d. Urine output of more than 30 ml/hour

NDx: High risk for ineffective airway clearance related to tracheolaryngeal obstruction secondary to possible complications of subtotal thyroidectomy: hemorrhage, edema, laryngeal nerve damage, parathyroid gland damage

Planning: Patient outcomes
1. Patient maintains clear airway as evidenced by:
   a. Stable vital signs within normal limits
   b. Respirations regular and unlabored
   c. Ability to speak and swallow without difficulty

Nursing Interventions

The majority of patients who have hyperthyroidism are diagnosed and treated on an out-patient basis. Therefore, nursing care primarily focuses on patient teaching for self-management. However, because the manifestations of hyperthyroidism develop slowly, some patients remain undiagnosed and untreated for months or years. They may require hospitalization for surgery or to treat severe thyrotoxicosis or thyroid storm.

NDx: Anxiety
Provide factual information to the patient and significant others related to the effect of increased levels of circulating thyroid hormones on heat intolerance, appearance, behavior, and activity. Encourage the patient to identify and describe feelings. Assist the patient in identifying relaxation techniques and diversionary activities that help control anxiety while conserving energy. Establish a schedule of activity and rest periods to provide reassuring routine. Explain procedures in a calm, reassuring voice, and maintain an unhurried manner to promote relaxation and trust. Carefully select roommates, and restrict visitors if necessary to decrease external stimuli. Some patients may require sedation.

The patient with heat intolerance is most comfortable in a cool room with good circulation but free from drafts. Provide lightweight bedding and sleepwear. Frequent hygiene, skin care, and linen changes prevent discomfort and skin breakdown from profuse diaphoresis.

NDx: High risk for altered health maintenance related to insufficient knowledge of self-management of pharmacologic therapy during and after treatment with antithyroid drugs, iodine, or radioactive iodine

Teach the patient the name, dose, administration schedule, time table for expected effects, and side effects of prescribed antithyroid drug, iodine preparation, or radioactive iodine. Pharmacology Box 33–2 summarizes the pharmacologic actions, side effects, and nursing implications of the thioamide antithyroid drugs. Advise patients taking an iodine preparation to take it after meals and to dilute the solution in a full glass of water or juice to prevent gastric irritation, and to drink it through a straw to avoid discoloration of the teeth. Instruct the patient to notify the physician promptly of signs of iodine toxicity: metallic taste, stomatitis, coryza, tenderness of the salivary glands, vomiting, bloody diarrhea, and abdominal pain or distention. Thioamides and iodine preparations are discontinued 3 to 4 days before radioactive iodine therapy to avoid interference with ^{131}I uptake. Instruct the patient to consult the physician before taking any over-the-counter preparations during pharmacologic treatment for hyperthyroidism.

Teach the patient how to monitor the radial pulse for 1 full minute 2 to 3 times weekly and record the results. The pulse rate is an important indicator of the body's response to treatment. The pulse rate should gradually decrease to between 60 and 100 beats per minute. Instruct the patient to notify the physician promptly if the pulse becomes irregular or drops below 60.

Reinforce and clarify the physician's explanations of the expected outcomes of treatment. Encourage the patient to ask questions and verbalize expectations. Inform the physician if the patient expresses unrealistic expectations of treatment so that further discussion and explanation can correct misunderstandings.

The physician monitors response to therapy on a monthly basis until a euthyroid state is achieved, then once or twice yearly. Stress the importance of follow-up thyroid function studies and physical examinations as scheduled. Teach the patient signs of hypothyroidism (which may develop following treatment) and hyperthyroidism (which may signal a recurrence) that should be reported to the physician.

NDx: Altered nutrition: less than body requirements

Weigh the patient, or instruct the patient to weigh himself or herself two to three times a week to determine weight gain or loss. Document food intake. Small frequent high-calorie, high-protein, high-carbohydrate snacks and supplements may be better tolerated, especially if hyperactivity prevents the patient from sitting down for a meal. The patient may require an intake of 4000 to 5000 calories daily to meet metabolic demands. Instruct the patient to avoid caffeine, spicy seasonings, and foods high in bulk or fiber, which may further stimulate intestinal motility and decrease absorption of nutrients. Unless contraindicated by cardiac status, encourage fluid intake up to 4000 ml daily to replace excess fluid lost through profuse diaphoresis and frequent stools. Increased production of metabolic wastes also requires large amounts of fluid to promote their dilution and excretion by the kidneys.

As treatment of hyperthyroidism becomes effective and the patient achieves ideal body weight, the patient must decrease food intake to prevent excess weight gain.

NDx: High risk for trauma

Plan care or help the patient plan activities to allow for frequent rest periods and conservation of energy. Monitor physiologic response to activity. Increased pulse, systolic blood pressure, or respirations, or palpitations indicate overexertion and the need for reduced activity. Provide a nonstimulating environment that is free of hazards. Reassure the patient that fine muscle tremors and difficulty manipulating objects are manifestations of hyperthyroidism, which will improve with treatment. Provide assistance as needed with activities that are difficult for the patient in order to prevent stress, increased anxiety, and injury. Maintain adequate lighting, keep call bell in reach, provide nonskid slippers or shoes, and assist with ambulation as necessary to prevent falls. Administer, or teach the patient with exophthalmos proper administration of, lubricating eye drops to prevent corneal dryness, abrasion, and ulceration.

NDx: High risk for altered tissue perfusion: systemic

Monitor vital signs, pulse pressure, capillary refill, neurologic status, and renal output hourly to identify changes in hemodynamic status in a patient with thyrotoxicosis or in thyroid storm. Institute safety measures if the patient is irrational, delirious, or comatose. Apply a hypothermia blanket or ice packs to reduce hyperthermia. Proplythiouracil and potassium iodide are administered by mouth or nasogastric tube to rapidly reduce circulating thyroid hormone levels. Propranolol is administered to treat cardiac dysrhythmias and reduce sympathetic stimulation. Digoxin, instead of propranolol, is prescribed with cardiac failure. Glucocorticoids and intravenous glucose solutions are administered to treat shock and dehydration and to provide glucose for metabolic requirements. Humidified oxygen is administered to improve tissue oxygenation and meet the high metabolic demands.

NDx: High risk for ineffective airway clearance

The risk of postoperative complications after thyroid surgery is greatly reduced by preoperative preparation of the patient. Antithyroid drugs and iodine preparations are administered to reduce the levels of circulating thyroid hormone and the size and vascularity of the gland. Teach the patient to support the head while moving to prevent tension on the suture line postoperatively. Discuss the planned procedure with the patient, reinforce and clarify the physician's explanations, and provide opportunity for the patient to ask questions and verbalize feelings about the surgery and expected outcome.

Postoperatively, apply an ice collar and place the patient in semi-Fowler's position to reduce edema. Administer humidified oxygen and intravenous fluids to meet metabolic requirements and improve tissue perfusion. Examine dressing and monitor vital signs every 1 to 2 hours for 24 hours, then every 4 hours. Encourage early ambulation to promote optimum respiratory function and mobilization of secretions.

Monitor for and immediately report signs of hemorrhage: a drop in blood pressure; rapid, thready pulse; increased tightness of neck dressing; fullness or pressure at incision site; a choking sensation or difficulty breathing; and excessive bloody drainage on the dressing, pillow, or behind the neck. Hemorrhage and edema can cause respiratory obstruction by compression of the trachea or larynx. Signs of respiratory obstruction are restlessness, respiratory stridor, crowing on respiration, difficulty swallowing, dyspnea, and cyanosis. If hemorrhage or respiratory distress is suspected, release the edges of the dressing to relieve pressure on internal structures and implement measures for hypovolemic shock. Assist with emergency tracheostomy if necessary to maintain airway.

Laryngeal nerve damage may result in temporary or permanent loss of voice or paralysis of the vocal cords, or both. Aphonia immediately after surgery, hoarseness, or high-pitched voice indicates laryngeal nerve damage. Ask the patient to speak every 2 hours to determine voice quality. If the voice is initially clear and then becomes hoarse, edema may be causing temporary pressure on the nerve. Paralysis of the vocal cords can result in respiratory obstruction and may require a tracheostomy. A tracheostomy tray and suction equipment must be available at the bedside for emergency use.

Acute hypocalcemic tetany is discussed in detail in Chapter 34. Hypocalcemic tetany can result from damage to, or accidental removal of, the parathyroid glands during thyroid surgery. The physician is notified immediately if the patient is increasingly irritable or has numbness or tingling of the nose, earlobes, toes, fingers, or circumoral areas; muscle twitching; or painful spasms. Assess muscle irritability by eliciting a positive Chvostek's or Trousseau's sign. If signs of hypocalcemia are present, initiate rebreathing to raise calcium ion levels, institute seizure precautions, and prepare for administration of intravenous calcium chloride or calcium gluconate. Intravenous calcium chloride or calcium gluconate must be available on the unit for emergency use. Tetany can cause respiratory distress as a result of seizures and laryngospasm. A tracheostomy may be required to maintain the airway.

Evaluation

Evaluate the effectiveness of nursing care for a patient with hyperthyroidism by comparing the patient's status with the expected patient outcomes. Examples of specific outcomes for patients with hyperthyroidism have been provided in the Planning section.

Thyroid Hormone Resistance

Thyroid hormone resistance is a recently recognized syndrome characterized by an inability of the target tissues to bind with or use available thyroid hormone. It has a genetic predisposition. The patient presents with manifestations of mild hypothyroidism despite elevated levels of circulating thyroid hormone and normal or elevated levels of thyroid-stimulating hormone (TSH). Thyroid enlargement may be present and lead to misdiagnosis. Thyroid hormone resistance is treated by cautious administration of T_3 to overcome hormone resistance. Liothyronine sodium (Cytomel) is commonly prescribed. Some patients respond well to administration of dopamine, a neurotransmitter that also lowers the serum levels of TSH in both euthyroid and hypothyroid individuals. Antithyroid drugs and thyroidectomy are contraindicated and will worsen the condition.

Structural Disorders

A goiter is an enlargement of the thyroid gland not related to inflammation or neoplasia. A diffuse toxic goiter is common in hyperthyroidism, which was discussed earlier in this chapter. Individuals with nontoxic goiters are usually euthyroid. Goiters are more common in women than men.

Simple Nontoxic Goiter

A simple nontoxic goiter is hyperplasia of the thyroid gland that develops in response to the gland's inability to secrete enough thyroid hormone to meet metabolic needs. The enlarged gland compensates for inadequate hormone production and is able to secrete sufficient amounts of thyroid hormone to maintain a euthyroid state.

Simple goiters are more common in young women. They may develop during periods of increased metabolic demands, such as adolescence or pregnancy. Deficiency of dietary iodine is another cause of simple goiter. Because simple nontoxic goiters caused by iodine deficiency are more common in specific geographic regions far from the seacoast, these goiters are often referred to as endemic goiters.

Clinical manifestations of a simple nontoxic goiter depend on the size of the gland. A large, palpable mass at the base of the neck, as illustrated in Figure 33–7, is the primary manifestation. Displacement or compression of the esophagus or trachea may cause dysphagia, a choking sensation or respiratory difficulty. A very large goiter may impair venous return from the head, neck, and even the upper limbs. Venous engorgement may lead to dizziness and syncope.

Diagnosis is made on the basis of history, clinical manifestations, and the results of thyroid function studies. Once other causes of thyroid enlargement are ruled out, a simple nontoxic goiter is treated by correcting its cause. Temporary thyroid hormone replacement meets metabolic demands while allowing the gland to rest and shrink in size. Iodine supplements or increased dietary iodine is prescribed for individuals with iodine deficiency. Foods high in iodine include seafood, seaplants, and iodized salt. Iodine is also used as a dough conditioner in many commercial bread products. Surgery is not recommended but may be necessary if the goiter does not shrink sufficiently to relieve obstructive symptoms.

Nodular Goiter

A nodular goiter is similar to a simple goiter, except that the glandular enlargement develops as multiple nodules in women older than 40. These multinodular goiters are usually asymptomatic unless very large. Occasionally, a nodule may be hyperfunctioning glandular tissue that shows up as a "hot spot" on the thyroid scan and may be associated with symptoms of hyperthyroidism. Treatment varies according to the age of the individual and clinical manifestations present.

Neoplasia

Thyroid Neoplasms

Benign thyroid cysts and adenomas are firm, well-encapsulated, noninvasive, slow-growing neoplasms of unknown etiology. The incidence is higher in individuals who have received radiation to the head, neck, or chest. Benign neoplasms are usually nonfunctioning and rarely symptomatic. They present as "cold spots" on thyroid scan. Secreting benign adenomas are very rare and are not dependent on TSH to maintain function. Diagnosis of benign neoplasms is confirmed by needle biopsy. Treatment is conservative with annual reevaluation. Functioning adenomas are treated with radioactive iodine or surgery.

Malignant thyroid neoplasms are rare, destructive, non-secreting adenocarcinomas that usually develop as a single, firm nodule. Metastasis to the lungs and bones is common. Thyroid cancer occurs with greater frequency in middle-aged women who have a history of radiation of the head, neck, or chest. There is a familial tendency. Vocal cord paralysis and hoarseness are common with thyroid carcinoma. Thyroid scan, computed tomography or magnetic resonance imaging, and needle biopsy are used to identify probable malignant lesions. Subtotal or total thyroidectomy, sometimes followed by radioactive iodine therapy, is the primary treatment for thyroid cancer. Postoperatively lifelong thyroid hormone replacement is prescribed to suppress thyroid function and minimize the risk of recurrence. Nursing care in relation to these treatments is discussed earlier in this chapter.

Papillary carcinoma is the most common form of thyroid cancer. It usually develops as a firm, solitary nodule identified as a "cold spot" on the thyroid scan. It grows slowly and remains confined to the thyroid gland for many years. Prognosis is excellent if the carcinoma is diagnosed and treated before it spreads outside of the gland.

Follicular carcinoma is slightly more aggressive than papillary carcinoma, and metastasis is more common. These tumors sometimes retain their ability to synthesize and secrete thyroid hormone. Secreting tumors present as a "hot spot" on the thyroid scan. Secreting follicular tumors respond well to treatment with radioactive iodine.

Medullary carcinoma is a cancer of the parafollicular cells. It is more aggressive than follicular cancer and frequently extends into local lymph nodes and surrounding tissues. Medullary tumors secrete calcitonin. Measurement of serum calcitonin levels is used to diagnose the tumor and evaluate the success of treatment. Total thyroidectomy with lymph node dissection is the treatment of choice. Radioactive iodine is not effective. Prognosis is poorer in patients with lymph node involvement.

Undifferentiated carcinoma, also called anaplastic carcinoma, or giant cell or small cell carcinoma, depending on cell structure, is very rare. It rapidly grows into surrounding structures and metastasizes early. Undifferentiated carcinoma is very resistant to treatment, although surgery may be performed to relieve pressure symptoms. Death usually occurs within 6 to 12 months of diagnosis.

The Elderly: Special Considerations

The major significance of functional thyroid disorders in the elderly is not in the differences in incidence, manifestations, or complexity of treatment, but in the potential for inaccurate, delayed, or missed diagnosis because the early signs are incorrectly attributed to manifestations of the aging process. As the individual ages, decreasing thyroid gland function is usually compensated for by decreasing metabolic demands and an increase in the proportion of T_3 to T_4. The ratio of $T_4:T_3$ is closer to 5:1, as compared with 7:1 to 10:1 in younger individuals. The half-life of circulating thyroxine doubles to 9 days.

In patient teaching, always provide the elderly person with large-type or clearly written instructions to reinforce verbal instructions on prescribed medications, pharmacokinetics specific to the elderly, and self-management. Specifically indicate which side effects necessitate immediate notification of the physician.

Hypothyroidism

The incidence of hypothyroidism increases with age. Prevalence in the elderly is estimated to be approximately 10%. Its early manifestations are easy to overlook because of the gradual slowing of metabolism that accompanies the normal aging process. In addition, the slowed mentation, decreased cardiac output, and sensitivity to cold of hypothyroidism may be misidentified as normal manifestations of advanced age. Many elderly persons with hypothyroidism have no symptoms except debilitation and apathy. Diagnosis is made on the basis of clinical manifestations and elevated serum TSH levels.

Thyroid hormone replacement is given with caution in the elderly. Not only are they more susceptible to the metabolic effects of thyroid preparations, but age increases the half-life of thyroxine. Hormone replacement is initiated at a low dose, and increments are made gradually at 4- to 6-week intervals to avoid cardiovascular overload from increased metabolic demands and mental confusion and agitation from the rapid increase in cerebral perfusion. Most elderly individuals achieve a euthyroid state at lower than normal dosages.

Hyperthyroidism

The most common cause of hyperthyroidism in the elderly is toxic nodular goiter. Unlike its higher incidence in women younger than age 60, hyperthyroidism occurs equally in elderly men and women. Alterations in cardiac function are a predominant clinical manifestation. Cardiac disorders, especially atrial fibrillation or congestive heart failure that do not respond to treatment, may be a manifestation of hyperthyroidism in the elderly. Ophthalmic manifestations are uncommon. Anorexia with profound weight loss and muscle wasting, lethargy, depression, and apathy are atypical manifestations that are often seen in the elderly hyperthyroid individual. Diagnosis should rely primarily on thyroid function tests rather than clinical manifestations.

Initial treatment with antithyroid drugs and propranolol followed by radioactive iodine therapy is the treatment of choice in the elderly. A euthyroid state is usually achieved within 6 weeks. Agranulocytosis is the major adverse reaction seen in the elderly. It can develop at any time during therapy with antithyroid drugs. Instruct the patient to notify the physician immediately if manifestations develop.

Bibliography

Abrams AC. Clinical drug therapy: Rationales for nursing practice. 3rd ed. Philadelphia: JB Lippincott, 1991.

Alfaro-LeFevre R, et al. Drug handbook: A nursing process approach. New York: Addison-Wesley Nursing, 1992.

Bates, B. A guide to physical examination and history taking. 5th ed. Philadelphia: JB Lippincott, 1991.

Brenner ZR. Diagnostic tests and procedures: Applying the nursing process. Norwalk, CT: Appleton & Lange, 1987.

Brown SL. Practical points in the postanesthesia assessment and care of the patient having a thyroidectomy. J Post Anesth Nurs 1986; 1(3):191.

Bullock BL, Rosendahl PP. Pathophysiology: Adaptations and alterations in function. 2nd ed. Boston: Little, Brown, 1988.

Bybee DE. Saving lives in thyroid crises. Emerg Med 1987; 19(16):21.

Carpenito LJ. Nursing diagnosis: Application to clinical practice. 4th ed. Philadelphia: JB Lippincott, 1992.

Cassel CK, Walsh JR (eds). Geriatric medicine. New York: Springer-Verlag, 1989.

Cella JH, Watson J. Nurse's manual of laboratory tests. Philadelphia: FA Davis, 1989.

Chambers JK. Metabolic bone disorders: Imbalances of calcium and phosphorus. Nurs Clin North Am 1987; 22(4):861.

Chenevey B. Overview of fluids and electrolytes. Nurs Clin North Am 1987; 22(4):749.

Cooper JAD Jr, Pappas PG. Cecil review of general internal medicine. 5th ed. Philadelphia: WB Saunders, 1992.

DeGroot LJ (ed). Endocrinology. Vol 1, 2nd ed. Philadelphia: WB Saunders, 1989.

Doenges M, Moorhouse M. Nurse's pocket guide: Nursing diagnosis with interventions. 4th ed. Philadelphia: FA Davis, 1993.

Dudek, SG. Nutrition handbook for nursing practice. Philadelphia: JB Lippincott, 1987.

Dunn JT. Teaching hypothyroidism: What are our therapeutic choices? Hospital Formulary 1986; 21(4):456.

Eliopoulos C. Gerontological Nursing. 3rd ed. Philadelphia: JB Lippincott, 1993.

Federman DD. Thyroid. In Rubenstein E, Federman DD (eds). Scientific American medicine. New York: Scientific American, 1992.

Fischbach F. A manual of laboratory diagnostic tests. 4th ed. Philadelphia: JB Lippincott, 1992.

Gallagher MT, Kahn C. Lasers: Scalpels of light. RN 1990; 53(5):46.

Gambert SR (ed). Handbook of geriatrics. New York: Plenum Press, 1986.

Gordon M. Nursing diagnosis: Process and application. St. Louis: CV Mosby, 1991.

Greenspan FS, Rappaport B. Thyroid gland. In Greenspan FS (ed). Basic and clinical endocrinology. Norwalk, CT: Appleton & Lange, 1991.

Griffin J, Ojeda S (eds). Textbook of endocrine physiology. New York: Oxford University Press, 1988.

Guyton AC. Textbook of medical physiology. 8th ed. Philadelphia: WB Saunders, 1991.

Hill MN. Drug compliance: Going beyond the facts. Nursing 1986; 16(10):50.

Ihde DC. Paraneoplastic syndromes. Hosp Pract 1987; 22(8):105.
Isley WL. Thyroid disorders. Crit Care Nurs Q, 1990; 13(3):39.
Kee JL. Laboratory and diagnostic tests with nursing implications. Norwalk, CT: Appleton & Lange, 1987.
Kidd PS, Murakami RY. Common pathologic conditions in elderly persons: Nursing assessment and intervention. J Emerg Med 1987; 13(1):27.
Kraiem Z, Glaser B, Yigla M. et al. Toxic multinodular goiter: A variant of autoimmune hyperthyroidism. J Clin Endocrinol Metab 1987; 65(4):659.
Kumar V, Cotran RS, Robbins SL. Basic pathology. 5th ed. Philadelphia: WB Saunders, 1992.
Lammon CA, Hart G. Recognizing thyroid crisis. Nursing 1993; 23(4):33.
Larsen PR, Ingbar SH. The thyroid gland. In Wilson JD, Foster DW (eds). Williams textbook of endocrinology. 8th ed. Philadelphia: WB Saunders, 1992, pp 357–487.
Lehne RA. Pharmacology for nursing care. Philadelphia: WB Saunders, 1990.
Lloyd RV. Endocrine pathology. New York: Springer-Verlag, 1990.
Lockhart JS, Griffin CW. Postthyroidectomy respiratory distress. Nursing 1987; 17(7):33.
Lockhart JS, Griffin CW. Tetany. Nursing 1988; 18(8):33.
Loebl S, et al. The nurse's drug handbook. 5th ed. New York: John Wiley & Sons, 1989.
Malseed RT, Harrigan G. Textbook of pharmacology and nursing care: The nursing process. 2nd ed. Philadelphia: JB Lippincott, 1989.
Martinelli AM, Fontana JL. Thyroid storm: Potential perioperative crisis. AORN J 1990; 52(2):305.
Mathewson MK. Thyroid disorder. Crit Care Nurse 1987; 7(1):74.
Matteson MA, McConnell ES. Gerontological nursing: Concepts and practice. Philadelphia: WB Saunders, 1988.
Moran S. Innovative geriatric care. Nurs Manage 1987; 18(6):26.
Nordyke RA, Gilbert FI Jr, Harada AS. Graves' disease: Influence of age on clinical findings. Arch Intern Med 1988; 148(3):626.
North American Nursing Diagnosis Association. NANDA Nursing diagnosis: Definitions and classifications. St. Louis: North American Nursing Diagnosis Association, 1992.
Payne NR. Emergency care of the patient with myxedema coma. J Emerg Nurs 1986; 12(6):343.
Shannon MT, Wilson BA. Govoni & Hayes drugs and nursing implications. 7th ed. Norwalk, CT: Appleton & Lange, 1992.
Sowers J, Felicetta J (eds). Endocrinology of aging. New York: Raven Publishing, 1988.
Tucker SM et al. Patient care standards: Nursing process, diagnosis, and outcome. 5th ed. St. Louis: CV Mosby, 1992.
Ulrich SP, Canale SW, Wendell SA. Nursing care planning guides: A nursing diagnosis approach. 2nd ed. Philadelphia: WB Saunders, 1990.
Walpert N. Calcium metabolism disorders. Nursing 1990; 20(7):60.
Wyngaarden JB, Smith LH, Bennett JC (eds). Cecil textbook of medicine. 19th ed. Philadelphia: WB Saunders, 1992.
Yeatts RP, Clontz DM. Graves' ophthalmopathy. J Ophthalmic Nurs Technol 1990; 9(1):16.
Yeomans AC. Assessment and management of hypothyroidism. Nurse Pract 1990; 15(11):8.

Chapter Thirty-four

NURSING CARE *of Adults with Parathyroid Disorders*

Disruptions of parathyroid function are uncommon but potentially life-threatening endocrine disorders. Together with vitamin D and calcitonin secreted from the thyroid gland, parathyroid hormone regulates calcium, phosphate, and magnesium balance in the body. Normal parathyroid function and common parathyroid disorders are presented in this chapter.

Anatomy and Physiology

The parathyroid glands secrete parathyroid hormone (PTH). Most individuals have four ovoid parathyroid glands imbedded on the posterior surface of the thyroid gland, as illustrated in Figure 34–1. Some persons, however, may have as few as two or as many as eight parathyroid glands. Ectopic glands have been found in the mediastinum and in the neck above the thyroid gland. Each gland is approximately 6 × 5 × 2 mm, about the size of a match head. The average weight of each gland is 30 to 40 mg.

The primary function of parathyroid hormone is to regulate serum calcium and phosphate levels by maintaining extracellular ionic calcium concentrations. Parathyroid hormone has a half-life of only a few minutes. Therefore, it must be secreted constantly to maintain serum calcium levels within a very narrow margin of homeostasis. A serum calcium fluctuation as small as 0.5 mg/dl outside a person's normal range may alter body functions. Serum calcium levels rise as parathyroid hormone is secreted. Because there is an inverse relationship between serum calcium and serum phosphorus concentrations, as serum calcium level increases, serum phosphorus level decreases.

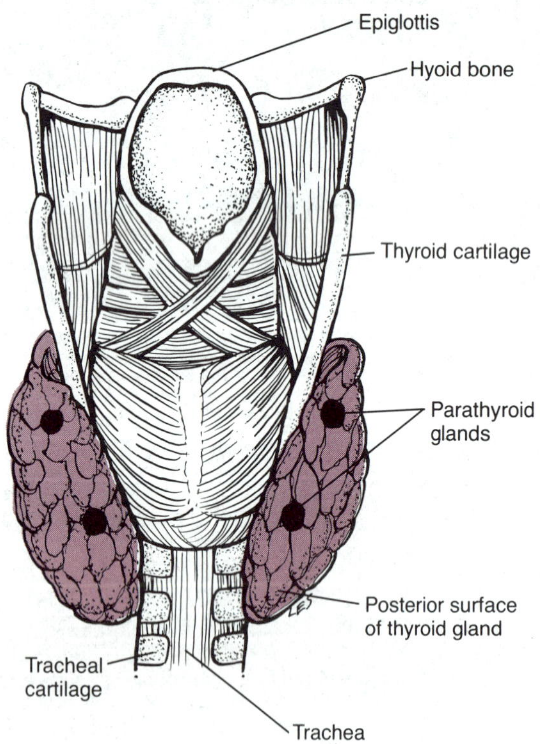

Figure 34–1.

Anatomy of the parathyroid glands, showing their position on the posterior surface of the thyroid gland. Although the parathyroids may be located anyplace on the posterior surface of the thyroid gland, one parathyroid gland is usually located in the upper and one in the lower half of each lobe of the thyroid.

Parathyroid hormone raises serum calcium levels by acting on three target sites in the body: the bones, the kidneys, and the gastrointestinal tract. In the bones, parathyroid hormone stimulates osteoclast activity, causing breakdown of the bone and increased resorption of calcium from the bones. The action of parathyroid hormone on the bones is counterbalanced by the effect of calcitonin, discussed in Chapter 33.

In the kidneys, parathyroid hormone acts directly on the renal tubules to increase reabsorption of calcium and promote excretion of phosphate. In the intestines, parathyroid hormone activates vitamin D, which acts directly on the intestinal mucosa to increase absorption of dietary calcium. Adequate intake of vitamin D is necessary for intestinal absorption of dietary calcium and its utilization by the body. Although there are few natural food sources of vitamin D, it is synthesized in the skin during exposure to ultraviolet light, and in many countries, it is added to pasteurized milk.

The secretion of parathyroid hormone is regulated by negative feedback control in response to the serum concentration of free calcium ions. Free calcium ions, or serum ionized calcium, is the physiologically active form of calcium in the body. As illustrated in Figure 34–2, a fall in the serum ionized calcium level stimulates the parathyroid glands to rapidly secrete parathyroid hormone. Secretion of parathyroid hormone decreases within seconds once serum calcium rises to normal physiologic levels.

Functional Disorders

Functional disorders of the parathyroid glands are characterized by inadequate or excess secretion of parathyroid hormone.

Hypoparathyroidism

Hypoparathyroidism is an acute or chronic disorder of calcium metabolism. It is caused by inadequate secretion of parathyroid hormone or failure of the target cells to respond to it. The latter condition is called pseudohypoparathyroidism and is an extremely rare genetic disorder.

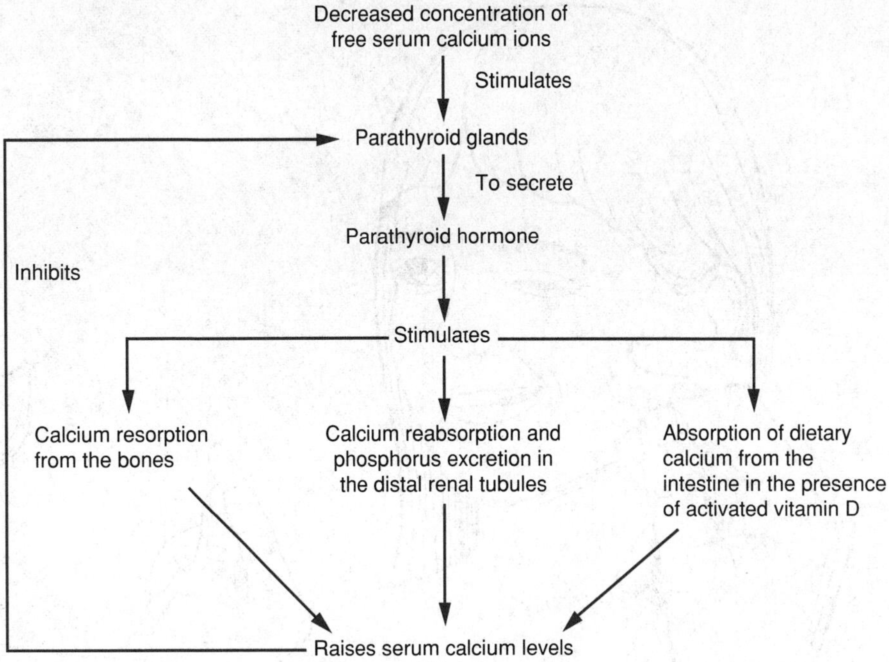

Figure 34–2.

Regulation of parathyroid hormone secretion by negative feedback control.

ETIOLOGY

The most common causes of hypoparathyroidism are iatrogenic. These include damage to, or accidental removal of, the parathyroids during thyroid gland surgery, irradiation of the neck, and surgical removal of the parathyroids to treat neoplasias or hyperparathyroidism. Rarely, hypoparathyroidism develops after destruction of the thyroid gland with radioactive iodine. Autografting of transplanted parathyroid tissue to a muscle of the forearm before procedures with high risk for damage to the parathyroid glands has been successful in preventing iatrogenic hypoparathyroidism.

Idiopathic hypoparathyroidism is less common and is thought to be a familial autoimmune disorder. Chronic hypomagnesemia, frequently associated with alcoholism, malabsorption syndromes, prolonged parenteral nutrition, and the administration of cisplatin and aminoglycoside antibiotics, impairs parathyroid hormone release and impairs the response of body tissues to it. The result is hypocalcemia in the presence of normally functioning parathyroid glands.

PATHOPHYSIOLOGY

Decreased parathyroid hormone activity causes decreased calcium resorption from the bones, decreased intestinal absorption, and decreased reabsorption of calcium in the renal tubules with increased phosphate retention. Hypocalcemia and hyperphosphatemia result. Decreased concentrations of serum ionized calcium increase neuromuscular excitability. Transmission of neuromuscular impulses speeds up, and repetitive responses to a single stimulus may occur. Spontaneous discharge of neuromuscular fibers occurs in severe hypocalcemia. Calcifications in the optic lens and in the basal ganglia develop in chronic hypocalcemic states.

CLINICAL MANIFESTATIONS

The clinical manifestations of hypoparathyroidism are directly related to the decreased serum ionized calcium concentration, its severity, rate of fall, and duration. The more rapid the decrease in serum calcium levels, the more severe the symptoms. Neuromuscular manifestations are most severe in the rapid onset of acute hypocalcemia caused by iatrogenic destruction of, or damage to, the parathyroids.

Early manifestations of acute hypocalcemia include irritability, apprehension, muscle cramps in the extremities and abdomen, and photophobia. Stiffness of the hands and feet and paresthesias characterized by numbness and tingling around the mouth (perioral area), of the nose or earlobes, and in the fingers and toes are common. Tapping the facial nerve in front of the earlobe may elicit spasms of the facial muscle, known as a positive Chvostek's sign. A positive Trousseau's sign is elicited when inflating a blood pressure cuff slightly above the patient's systolic pressure for 1 to 5 minutes causes severe carpopedal spasm. Chvostek's and Trousseau's signs are illustrated in Figure 34–3.

If the serum calcium level continues to fall, general muscle hypertonia and cramping may progress to hypocalcemic tetany characterized by tonic spasms and sustained contraction of individual muscle groups. Respiratory stridor, a crowing on inspiration caused by glottic and laryngeal spasms, bronchospasms, and respiratory arrest may occur as tetany progresses and serum calcium level drops

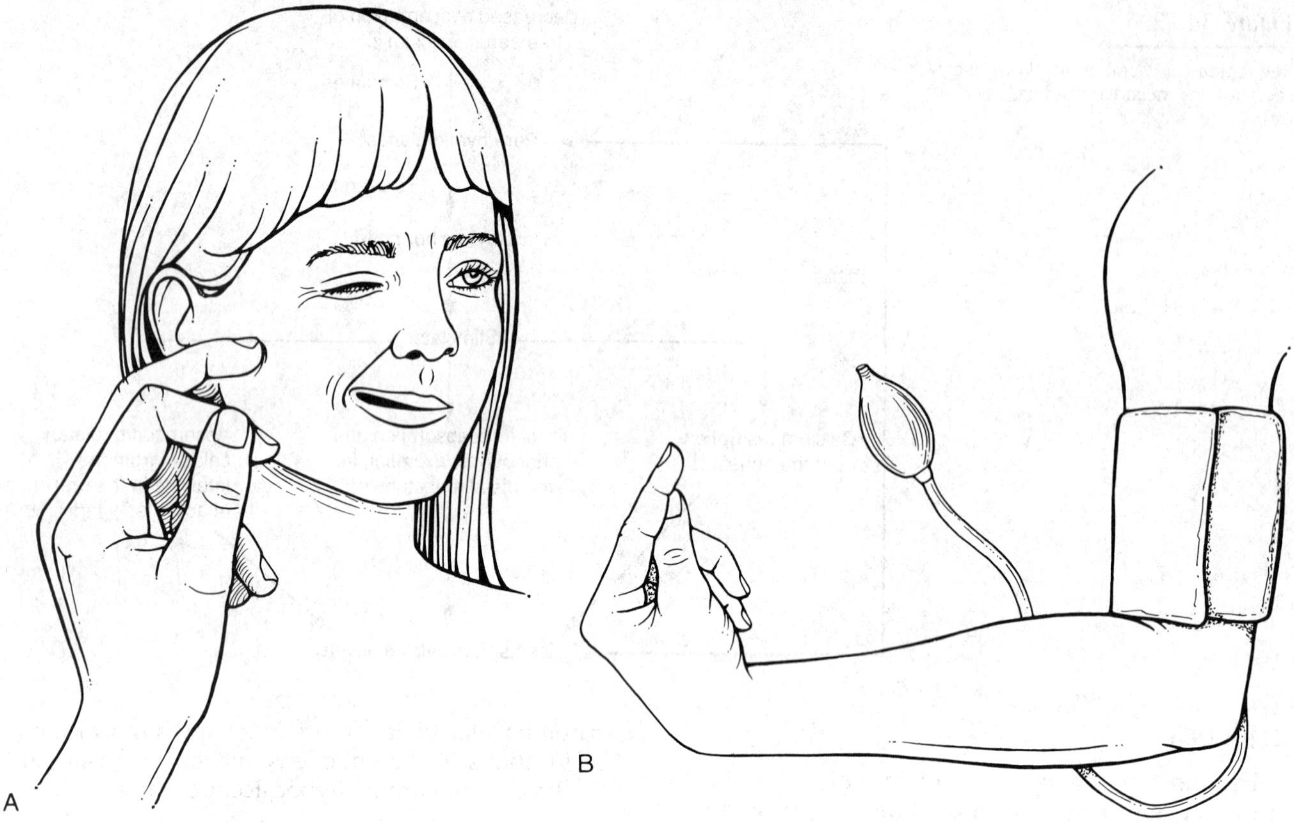

Figure 34–3.

Indications of hypocalcemia: a positive Chvostek's sign (*A*) and a positive Trousseau's sign (*B*).

below 7 mg/dl. Cardiac dysrhythmias can result from decreased myocardial contractility and atony. Generalized tonic-clonic convulsions usually develop if serum calcium level drops below 6 mg/dl. Loss of consciousness and incontinence are rarely associated with hypocalcemic convulsions.

Clinical manifestations in chronic hypocalcemia include irritability, lethargy, and personality changes. The skin becomes dry and scaly, with brittle nails and thin, patchy, prematurely gray hair. Premature cataracts develop as a result of lens calcifications. Calcification in the basal ganglia may result in brain damage, a Parkinson-like syndrome, psychosis, and convulsions. Cardiac dysrhythmias may progress to congestive heart failure.

MEDICAL DIAGNOSIS

Parathyroid hormone levels are determined by radioimmunoassay on an early morning or late evening blood specimen, when PTH secretion is highest. Serum ionized calcium is drawn concurrently. In hypoparathyroidism, the parathyroid hormone level and serum calcium level are low. Serum phosphorus level is elevated. Ectopic calcifications are identified by computed tomography (CT) scans of the brain and ophthalmic examination. Cardiac dysrhythmias and a prolonged QT interval are identified by electrocardiogram.

MEDICAL MANAGEMENT

Treatment of hypoparathyroidism depends on its severity. Acute hypocalcemic tetany is a medical emergency. It is treated by administration of intravenous calcium gluconate or calcium chloride until the serum calcium level is higher than 7.0 mg/dl. Oral calcium and vitamin D therapy is then initiated. Muscle relaxants may also be prescribed if raising the serum calcium level does not control neuromuscular irritability.

Chronic hypoparathyroidism is treated with oral calcium supplements taken concurrently with oral vitamin D supplements. Dihydrotachysterol (Hytakerol) and ergocalciferol (calciferol) are two commonly prescribed vitamin D supplements. A diet high in calcium but low in phosphorus is recommended. Dietary and calcium supplement intake combined should be approximately 2 g daily. Aluminum carbonate gel (Basaljel) or aluminum hydroxide gel (Amphojel) may be prescribed to promote phosphorus excretion. In some cases, thiazide diuretics may be effective in promoting calcium reabsorption from the renal tubules.

The goal in treating chronic hypoparathyroidism is to maintain a serum calcium level between 8.5 and 9.5 mg/dl. It requires lifelong treatment and frequent serum calcium determinations to prevent hypercalcemia from excess calcium and vitamin D intake.

Application of the Nursing Process to the Care of the Patient with Hypoparathyroidism

Assessment

Obtain a complete nursing history from patients with diagnosed or suspected hypoparathyroidism and from patients at risk for acute hypocalcemia. Patients at risk are those with diagnosed chronic hypoparathyroidism or low serum calcium or magnesium concentrations; a history of chronic renal failure, malnutrition, or alcoholism; or a family history of autoimmune endocrine disorders; and those who have undergone thyroid surgery or radioactive iodine therapy. Assess for the presence of clinical manifestations associated with acute and chronic hypoparathyroidism. Obtain baseline vital signs and apical pulse to determine cardiac rhythm. Review laboratory results of serum calcium, ionized calcium, phosphorus, and magnesium values to determine baseline levels. If paresthesias are reported, test for a positive Chvostek's sign or positive Trousseau's sign. Notify the physician immediately if manifestations of impending acute hypocalcemia are present.

Identify the patient's interpretation of the clinical manifestations and knowledge of planned diagnostic studies and treatment to determine teaching needs.

Nursing Diagnoses and Planning

Nursing diagnoses and related expected patient outcomes most commonly applicable to patients with hypoparathyroidism include the following:

NDx: High risk for suffocation, trauma related to increased neuromuscular irritability and tetany secondary to acute hypocalcemia

Planning: Patient outcomes

1. Patient maintains normal neuromuscular activity and respiratory function as evidenced by
   a. Usual mental status
   b. Regular apical pulse, 60 to 100 bpm
   c. Negative Chvostek's and Trousseau's signs
   d. Absence of paresthesias, muscle cramps, tetany, respiratory stridor, convulsions
2. Patient remains free of injury.
3. Patient identifies foods that are high in phosphorus as foods to avoid in diet.

NDx: High risk for altered health maintenance related to insufficient knowledge of chronic hypoparathyroidism, treatment regimen, self-management, and follow-up care

Planning: Patient outcomes

1. Patient verbalizes understanding of the need for, and intent to take, calcium and vitamin D supplements as prescribed.
2. Patient identifies foods that are high in calcium as desirable to include in diet daily.
3. Patient identifies foods that are high in phosphorus as foods to avoid in diet daily.
4. Patient maintains serum calcium level higher than 8.5 mg/dl.
5. Patient states intent to keep follow-up appointments as scheduled.
6. Patient states intent to notify physician promptly if signs of hypocalcemia or hypercalcemia develop.

Nursing Interventions

The nursing priority for the patient with acute or chronic hypoparathyroidism is to prevent the onset of the manifestations of increased neuromuscular irritability and hypocalcemic tetany by maintaining serum calcium level above 8.5 mg/dl. If tetany or convulsions occur, airway maintenance is the first concern.

NDx: High risk for suffocation, trauma

Monitor serum calcium levels, vital signs, and apical pulse of patients at risk for acute hypocalcemia. Place a tracheostomy tray and intravenous calcium gluconate at the bedside of postoperative patients after a thyroidectomy, parathyroidectomy, or radical neck surgery. Provide a nonstimulating environment to minimize neuromuscular stimulation.

Monitor neuromuscular irritability and mental status to identify early signs of acute hypocalcemia. Initiate rebreathing in a paper bag or rebreathing mask, notify the physician immediately, and prepare to administer intravenous calcium gluconate if early signs of hypocalcemic tetany develop. Rebreathing decreases exhaled carbon dioxide, raises serum carbonic acid levels, and lowers serum pH. The resulting mild respiratory acidosis temporarily increases serum ionized calcium levels. Monitor for respiratory stridor caused by glottic and laryngeal spasms. A tracheostomy may be necessary to maintain a patent airway if bronchospasms or convulsions occur. Maintain patient safety if convulsions develop. Nursing care of the patient with acute hypocalcemia is summarized in Nursing Care Guide 34–1.

Nursing Care Guide 34–1.
PATIENTS WITH ACUTE HYPOPARATHYROIDISM: HYPOCALCEMIC TETANY

Assessment Findings: Patient, 12 hours after a total thyroidectomy, is complaining of muscle cramps and numbness and tingling of the nose, fingers, and around the mouth. Patient appears anxious. Positive Chvostek's and Trousseau's signs are elicited.

Nursing Diagnosis: High risk for trauma, suffocation related to increased neuromuscular irritability associated with acute hypocalcemia secondary to damage to the parathyroid glands during thyroid surgery

Patient Outcomes	Nursing Interventions	Rationale
Patient notifies nurse immediately if paresthesia develops.	Teach all patients at risk for acute hypocalcemia to notify the nurse immediately of muscle or abdominal cramps, or tingling of the nose, earlobes, fingers, toes, or perioral area.	Detection and treatment of early manifestations of hypocalcemia can prevent acute hypocalcemic crisis.
Patient remains free of injury.	Place tracheostomy tray and intravenous calcium gluconate at the bedside of patients at risk for acute hypocalcemic tetany.	Emergency supplies and medication should be immediately available if needed.
	Monitor apical heart rate and rhythm, or use a cardiac monitor, to identify dysrhythmias caused by low serum calcium levels. Monitor changes in peripheral sensations, mental status, behavior, response to Chvostek's and Trousseau's tests, and neuromuscular irritability at least every 2 hours for 48 hours.	Cardiac dysrhythmias, altered neurologic status, and neuromuscular irritability are manifestations of hypocalcemia.
	Initiate rebreathing, notify the physician, and prepare to administer intravenous calcium gluconate if signs of increased neuromuscular irritability develop.	Rebreathing produces mild respiratory acidosis and temporarily increases serum calcium levels. Intravenous calcium gluconate rapidly restores serum calcium levels.
Patient's respirations remain clear and unlabored.	Assess for respiratory stridor or obstruction caused by hypocalcemic tetany. Be prepared to assist with emergency tracheostomy if they occur. Maintain patent airway and patient safety if seizures develop.	Acute hypocalcemic tetany may cause laryngospasms, bronchospasms, or seizures.

(continued)

Nursing Care Guide 34–1. (continued)

PATIENTS WITH ACUTE HYPOPARATHYROIDISM: HYPOCALCEMIC TETANY

Patient Outcomes	Nursing Interventions	Rationale
	Monitor parenteral calcium infusion to avoid infiltration. Stop the infusion immediately and notify the physician if infiltration occurs.	Infiltration of calcium may cause tissue necrosis.
	Monitor serum calcium values, vital signs, cardiac rhythm, and patient response during calcium administration.	Evaluates effectiveness of treatment of hypocalcemia and prevents hypercalcemia caused by overtreatment.

Evaluation: Compare the patient's status with the expected patient outcomes. If the outcomes are achieved, evaluate nursing care as successful. If not, reassess the patient, formulate new nursing diagnoses, and revise expected patient outcomes and nursing interventions as appropriate.

NDx: High risk for altered health maintenance related to insufficient knowledge of chronic hypoparathyroidism, treatment regimen, self-management, and follow-up care

Explain the basic concepts of chronic hypoparathyroidism, the function of parathyroid hormone in the body, and reasons for physical and emotional changes the patient has experienced. Provide opportunity for the patient to ask questions and verbalize feelings. Reinforce the physician's explanation of the prescribed therapy, and clarify any misunderstandings.

Teach the patient the dosage, administration schedule, expected action, and side effects of prescribed calcium and vitamin D supplements. Reinforce the benefit of taking these supplements concurrently, preferably with meals, to enhance calcium absorption. Vitamin D toxicity is a potentially serious complication. Instruct the patient to notify the physician promptly if dry mouth, nausea, vomiting, metallic taste, or constipation develops. Constipation is also a side effect of aluminum carbonate gel and aluminum hydroxide gel. Monitor number and consistency of stools. Teach the patient to report the early signs of hypocalcemia to the physician promptly. Teach that frequent urination, thirst, slowed mental processes, muscle weakness, and fatigue are early signs of hypercalcemia that must be reported to the physician promptly.

Reinforce the dietitian's explanation of a high-calcium, low-phosphorus diet. Provide a list of foods high in calcium to include in the diet, and a list of foods high in phosphorus to avoid. Although dairy products and canned fish with bones are high in calcium, they are also high in phosphorus and may be restricted. Consult with the physician and dietitian to determine the precise amount of these foods allowed. High phosphorus levels are found in foods rich in protein (meat, poultry, fish, eggs, legumes, nuts). If aluminum carbonate gel (Basaljel) or aluminum hydroxide gel (Amphojel) is prescribed, stress that it is to be taken with a full glass of water or juice immediately after meals to promote excretion of phosphorus. (When used as antacids, they are taken 1 hour after meals.)

Emphasize that treatment of chronic hypoparathyroidism is lifelong and that periodic examination to evaluate response to treatment and monitor serum ionized calcium levels is necessary to prevent episodes of hypocalcemia or hypercalcemia.

Evaluation

Evaluate the effectiveness of nursing care for a patient with hypoparathyroidism by comparing the patient's status with the expected patient outcomes. Examples of specific outcomes for patients with hypoparathyroidism have been provided in the Planning section.

Hyperparathyroidism

Hyperparathyroidism is a disorder of calcium metabolism caused by excess secretion of parathyroid hormone. It primarily affects individuals older than 50, and females twice as frequently as males. Incidence increases with advancing age. Hyperparathyroidism is being diagnosed more frequently with widespread use of multichannel autoanalyzers that include serum calcium evaluation. Some studies done on individuals older than the age of 50 have found hyperparathyroidism present to some degree in as many as one male in 1000 and two females in 200.

ETIOLOGY

There are several classifications of hyperparathyroidism, each with a different etiology. Of these, primary and secondary hyperparathyroidism are the most common.

Primary hyperparathyroidism is characterized by enlargement of one or more parathyroid glands and increased secretion of parathyroid hormone. Specific etiology is unknown. Single benign adenomas are diagnosed in approximately 85% to 90% of individuals with primary hyperparathyroidism. Other causes include multiple adenomas and single or multiple gland hyperplasia. Parathyroid cancer, which is characterized by serum calcium levels higher than 15 mg/dl, is very rare. The incidence of primary hyperparathyroidism is higher in individuals with a family history of parathyroid disorders or multiple endocrine neoplasias. Irradiation of the neck or thyroid gland also increases risk.

Secondary hyperparathyroidism is a compensatory response by normal glands to chronic mild hypocalcemia. Sustained increase in parathyroid hormone production and secretion results in glandular hyperplasia. Conditions that may precipitate secondary hyperparathyroidism include vitamin D or calcium deficiency, hyperphosphatemia, chronic renal failure, intestinal malabsorption syndromes, rickets, acromegaly, and pseudohypoparathyroidism. Pregnant and lactating women may also experience temporary parathyroid hyperplasia. Secondary hyperparathyroidism usually does not result in hypercalcemia because normal feedback control mechanisms are intact. It is treated by correcting the cause.

PATHOPHYSIOLOGY

Increased parathyroid hormone activity causes increased resorption of calcium from the bones, increased intestinal absorption, and increased reabsorption of calcium in the renal tubules with excess excretion of phosphorus. Hypercalcemia and hypophosphatemia result. Increased concentrations of serum ionized calcium decrease neuromuscular excitability. Transmission of neuromuscular impulses is slowed because of the sedative effect of calcium on nerve fibers. Calcium is deposited in tissues throughout the body, and polyuria and excessive thirst may develop as the body attempts unsuccessfully to excrete excess calcium.

CLINICAL MANIFESTATIONS

The clinical manifestations of primary hyperparathyroidism are directly related to the increased levels of serum ionized calcium. In its mildest form, and often in secondary hyperparathyroidism, the patient may be asymptomatic or have nonspecific clinical manifestations.

Early symptoms include fatigue, general malaise, lethargy, apathy, and drowsiness. Muscle weakness and atrophy, lack of coordination, activity intolerance, memory lapses, poor concentration, and depression result from slowed impulse transmission. Abdominal pain, anorexia, nausea, vomiting, and constipation develop because of decreased gastrointestinal motility. Gastric secretions increase in response to hypercalcemia. This, plus decreased gastrointestinal motility, increases the risk for peptic ulcers. Acute pancreatitis may develop secondary to sustained hypercalcemia.

Renal calculi, formed by precipitation of calcium in the kidneys, are found in the majority of individuals with hyperparathyroidism. Renal colic, urinary tract infections, hematuria, and polyuria occur in conjunction with the renal calculi. Metabolic acidosis due to impaired renal reabsorption of sodium bicarbonate may develop. Cardiovascular manifestations include bradycardia, dysrhythmias, and calcification of arterial walls. Atrioventricular block may lead to cardiac arrest. Hypertension secondary to renal and cardiovascular involvement is common.

Bone demineralization, caused by increased subperiosteal calcium resorption characteristic in hyperparathyroidism of long duration, is most severe in cortical bone. It causes generalized osteoporosis and weakens the bones. Low back pain, bone pain and tenderness, arthralgia, pathologic fractures, and deformity result. Demineralization around the teeth can also occur. Pseudogout, caused by deposition of calcium crystals in articular cartilage, is a complication of hyperparathyroidism. Anemia, calcifications in the cornea of the eye (band keratopathy), and occipital headache are less common manifestations.

Acute hypercalcemic crisis is a rare, life-threatening complication of hyperparathyroidism. It can also occur with some cancers and after chemotherapy or irradiation because of massive cell destruction. In addition to the clinical manifestations already listed, the patient in hypercalcemic crisis is at high risk for severe dehydration, coma, and cardiac dysrhythmias with cardiac arrest in asystole.

MEDICAL DIAGNOSIS

Diagnosis of primary hyperparathyroidism, especially in mild or asymptomatic individuals, is made primarily on the basis of elevated serum parathyroid hormone level after discovery of elevated ionized serum calcium level with decreased phosphorus level, or of elevated 24-hour urinary calcium excretion. An elevated alkaline phosphatase level indicates increased osteoblastic activity of the bones. Radiographic studies may reveal subperiosteal bone resorption, osteoporosis of the skull and other bones, soft tissue calcification, and renal calculi. Bone densitometry identifies loss of bone mass. Cardiac dysrhythmias, atrioventricular block, widened T wave, and shortened QT intervals are confirmed on electrocardiogram.

MEDICAL MANAGEMENT

Early diagnosis and treatment is important in the successful management of primary hyperparathyroidism. The primary goal is to lower serum calcium levels and prevent complications. Because of the risk of progression of the disease, surgery is the treatment of choice in most cases. However, for asymptomatic patients with serum calcium levels lower than 12 mg/dl who have no renal or skeletal manifestations, some physicians favor conservative management with oral phosphate supplements and 4 to 5 L of fluids per day to promote calcium excretion. These patients require frequent follow-up to evaluate treatment and detect hypercalcemia-related complications.

Computed tomography, ultrasonography, magnetic resonance imaging, and arteriography are commonly used to confirm the number and location of the parathyroid glands before surgery. In single gland adenoma, the involved gland is removed. A subtotal parathyroidectomy with removal of $3\frac{1}{2}$ glands is done for multiple gland hyperplasia. Adequate parathyroid hormone will be secreted by the remaining tissue. Some surgeons remove all identified parathyroid glands and graft a portion of one into a muscle of the forearm. This facilitates later removal if hypercalcemia persists.

Serum ionized calcium levels decrease to near normal levels within 24 to 48 hours after surgery. The patient may experience mild symptoms of transient tetany during postoperative adjustment because of the rapid drop in calcium concentration and the rapid absorption of serum calcium by demineralized bone—the "hungry bone syndrome." Once serum calcium level and 24-hour urinary calcium excretion have returned to normal, a high-calcium diet and calcium and vitamin D supplements may be prescribed for several months until bone recalcification is stabilized. Prognosis after surgery is good. However, renal damage may be irreversible, and bone deformities, if present, will persist.

Hypercalcemic crisis is a medical emergency that can occur any time the serum calcium concentration is higher than 12 mg/dl. Intravenous normal saline is rapidly infused to rehydrate the patient and lower serum calcium concentration by expanding fluid volume. Furosemide (Lasix), a loop diuretic, plicamycin (Mithracin), an antibiotic, and calcitonin, a parathyroid hormone antagonist, may also be administered to inhibit bone resorption and promote calcium excretion. The use of intravenous phosphates is limited because of the danger of causing extraskeletal calcification in severely hypercalcemic states. Bisphosphonates have been somewhat effective in inhibiting osteoclastic bone resorption in severe hypercalcemia caused by metastatic bone cancer.

Application of the Nursing Process to the Care of the Patient with Hyperparathyroidism

Assessment

Obtain a complete nursing history from the patient with hyperparathyroidism. Assess for the presence of clinical manifestations associated with hyperparathyroidism. Ask specifically about the onset of early symptoms of hypercalcemia because nonspecific early symptoms are often overlooked by the patient as insignificant or unrelated to the current illness. Obtain baseline vital signs and apical pulse to determine cardiac rhythm. Identify the patient's interpretation of clinical manifestations and knowledge of the planned diagnostic studies and surgery to determine teaching needs. Assess for changes in neuromuscular and mental status and increased urine output, which may indicate deterioration of condition and impending hypercalcemic crisis. Notify physician immediately if condition deteriorates.

Nursing Diagnoses and Planning

Nursing diagnoses and related expected patient outcomes most commonly applicable to patients with hyperparathyroidism include the following:

NDx: High risk for fluid volume deficit related to excess urine output secondary to hypercalcemia

Planning: Patient outcomes
1. Patient consumes 3000 ml of fluid daily.
2. Patient maintains hemodynamic fluid balance as evidenced by
   a. Stable weight
   b. Vital signs within patient's normal range
   c. Stable neurologic status
   d. Moist mucous membranes
   e. Good skin turgor

NDx: High risk for trauma related to impaired neuromuscular function, activity intolerance, and osteoporosis secondary to hypercalcemia

Planning: Patient outcomes
1. Patient remains free of injury.
2. Patient walks for 15 minutes at least three times daily.
3. Patient verbalizes understanding of the need for, and intent to consume, high-calcium diet after surgery.

Nursing Interventions

The priorities of care for the patient with hyperparathyroidism are to lower serum calcium level and prevent renal complications. Postoperative care following a subtotal parathyroidectomy is similar to postthyroidectomy care discussed in Chapter 33. Anticipate and assess for signs of mild hypocalcemic tetany caused by the rapid drop in serum calcium concentration. Monitor closely for the onset of early signs of acute hypocalcemic tetany, a rare early postoperative complication. Notify the physician if they develop.

NDx: High risk for fluid volume deficit
Monitor vital signs, apical pulse, neurologic status, and urine output to identify changes in neuromuscular and cardiac function. Monitor changes in serum calcium determinations. Encourage fluids to 3000 ml daily, unless contraindicated by cardiac status, to maintain hydration, replace fluids lost through excess urine output, and promote excretion of calcium. Record fluid intake and output, and weigh patient daily to assess fluid loss or gain. Adjust intake accordingly. Closely monitor the patient receiving cardiotonics to detect early signs of toxicity. Hypercalcemia potentiates the effects of cardiotonics. Monitor changes in sensorium to detect decreasing alertness, an early sign of dehydration. Examine mucous membranes and test skin turgor to identify signs of dehydration.

Assess for manifestations of renal colic and renal calculi caused by calcium precipitation in the kidneys. Teach patient to consume low-calcium, acid-ash foods and fluids, such as cranberry, tomato, and prune juice, to increase urine acidity and promote calcium excretion. Initiate consultation with dietitian to facilitate patient education. Strain all urine, and send excreted calculi for analysis. Test urine daily with reagent strip to identify hematuria. Encourage mobility to inhibit calcium resorption from the bones. Administer stimulant stool softeners and antiulcer medications to counteract the gastrointestinal effects of hypercalcemia.

A patient in hypercalcemic crisis is placed on a cardiac monitor to facilitate early identification of potentially life-threatening cardiac dysrhythmias. Monitor vital signs, central venous pressure, and urine output hourly during high-volume intravenous infusion with normal saline to prevent fluid overload and assess renal function. Administer prescribed medications to lower serum calcium concentrations. Assess for early signs of hypocalcemic tetany to prevent overtreatment of hypercalcemia.

NDx: High risk for trauma
Explain the pathology of hyperparathyroidism and hypercalcemia as the cause for physical and mental alterations. Provide opportunity for patient to verbalize feelings and ask questions. Support patient in realistic expectations of surgery. Renal damage may not be reversible.

Implement safety measures if mental functions are impaired. Encourage ambulation pre- and postoperatively to diminish muscle atrophy and promote bone recalcification. Maintain an obstacle-free environment to prevent falls. Keep bed in low position with at least one side rail up. Instruct patient to call for assistance before getting out of bed, and place call bell within reach. Supervise or assist with amublation as appropriate. Plan nursing care to allow frequent rest periods to conserve energy.

Teach the patient that a high-calcium diet is important for several months after surgery to maintain adequate serum calcium levels for bone recalcification. Provide a list of foods high in calcium. Review dosage, administration schedule, expected action, and side effects of prescribed calcium supplements. Stress that calcium and vitamin D supplements should be taken together and with meals to enhance absorption. Teach the patient that fatigue, general malaise, lethargy, apathy, and drowsiness are early signs of hypercalcemia, whereas paresthesias, muscle cramps, and irritability are early signs of hypocalcemia. Provide a written list of the signs of calcium imbalance with instructions to notify the physician promptly if they develop. Stress the importance of periodic assessment of serum calcium concentrations to evaluate effectiveness of surgery.

Evaluation

Evaluate the effectiveness of nursing care for a patient with hyperparathyroidism by comparing the patient's status with the expected patient outcomes. Examples of specific outcomes for patients with hyperparathyroidism have been provided in the Planning section.

The Elderly: Special Considerations

As discussed earlier in this chapter, the incidence of hyperparathyroidism increases with age. There is no evidence that the incidence of other parathyroid disorders is higher in the elderly than in the general population. However, poor nutrition in the aged individual increases the risk of altered parathyroid function, and the chance of misdiagnosis or completely missed diagnosis is high. The vague, nonspecific early symptoms of parathyroid disorders may be overlooked as normal changes associated with the aging process. Patients displaying the neurologic alterations of hypocalcemia and hypercalcemia have been misdiagnosed as having Alzheimer's disease or other psychiatric disorders. Parathyroid disorders should be considered as a possibility in all older patients who have altered behavioral or mental status in conjunction with nonspecific neuromuscular or gastrointestinal complaints.

Bibliography

Abrams AC. Clinical drug therapy: Rationales for nursing practice. 3rd ed. Philadelphia: JB Lippincott, 1991.

Alfaro-LeFevre R, et al. Drug handbook: A nursing process approach. New York: Addison-Wesley Nursing, 1992.

Arnaud CD, Kolb FO. The calciotropic hormones & metabolic bone disease. In Greenspan FS (ed). Basic and clinical endocrinology. 3rd ed. Norwalk, CT: Appleton & Lange, 1991.

Avioli LV. Primary hyperparathyroidism: Recognition and management. Hosp Pract 1987; 22 (9):69.

Booth D. Hyperparathyroidism: The overlooked disorder. J Gerontol Nurs 1990; 16(6):16.

Brenner ZR. Diagnostic tests and procedures: Applying the nursing process. Norwalk, CT: Appleton & Lange, 1987.

Brown SL. Practical points in the postanesthesia assessment and care of the patient having a thyroidectomy. J Post Anesth Nurs 1986; 1(3):191.

Bullock BL, Rosendahl PP. Pathophysiology: Adaptations and alterations in function. 2nd ed. Boston: Little, Brown, 1988.

Bybee DE. Saving lives in parathyroid crises. Emerg Med 1987; 19(15):62.

Calloway C. When the problem involves magnesium, calcium, or phosphate. RN 1987; 50(5):30.

Carpenito LJ. Nursing diagnosis: Application to clinical practice. 4nd ed. Philadelphia: JB Lippincott, 1992.

Cassel CK, Walsh JR (eds). Geriatric medicine. New York: Springer-Verlag, 1989.

Cella JH, Watson J. Nurse's manual of laboratory tests. Philadelphia: FA Davis, 1989.

Chambers JK. Metabolic bone disorders: Imbalances of calcium and phosphorus. Nurs Clin North Am 1987; 22(4):861.

Chenevey B. Overview of fluids and electrolytes. Nurs Clin North Am 1987; 22(4):749.

DeGrott LJ (ed). Endocrinology. Vol 2, 2nd ed. Philadelphia: WB Saunders, 1989.

Doenges M, Moorhouse M. Nurse's pocket guide: Nursing diagnoses with interventions. 4th ed. Philadelphia: FA Davis, 1993.

Dudek SG. Nutrition handbook for nursing practice. Philadelphia: JB Lippincott, 1987.

Eliopoulos C. Gerontological nursing. 3rd ed. Philadelphia: JB Lippincott, 1993.

Federman DD. Parathyroid. In Rubenstein E, Federman DD (eds). Scientific American medicine. New York: Scientific American, 1992.

Fischbach F. A manual of laboratory diagnostic tests. 4th ed. Philadelphia: JB Lippincott, 1992.

Gambert SR (ed). Handbook of geriatrics. New York: Plenum Publishing, 1986.

Gordon M. Nursing diagnosis: process and applications. St. Louis; CV Mosby, 1991.

Graves L. Disorders of calcium, phosphorus, and magnesium. Crit Care Nurs Q 1990; 13(3):3.

Griffin J, Ojeda S (eds). Textbook of endocrine physiology. New York: Oxford University Press, 1988.

Guyton AC. Textbook of medical physiology. 8th ed. Philadelphia: WB Saunders, 1990.

Kee JL. Laboratory and diagnostic tests with nursing implications. Norwalk, CT: Appleton & Lange, 1987.

Kidd PS, Murakami RY. Common pathologic conditions in elderly persons: Nursing assessment and intervention. J Emerg Med 1987; 13(1):27.

Kositzke J. A question of balance: Dehydration in the elderly. J Gerontol Nurs 1990; 16(5):4.

Lancaster LE. Renal and endocrine regulation of water and electrolyte balance. Nurs Clin North Am 1987; 22(4):761.

Lehne RA. Pharmacology for nursing care. Philadelphia: WB Saunders, 1990.

Lloyd RV. Endocrine pathology. New York: Springer-Verlag, 1990.

Lockhart JS, Griffin CW. Postthyroidectomy respiratory distress. Nursing 1987; 17(7):33.

Lockhart JS, Griffin CW. Tetany. Nursing 1988; 18(8):33.

Malseed RT, Harrigan G. Textbook of pharmacology and nursing care: The nursing process. 2nd ed. Philadelphia: JB Lippincott, 1989.

Mathewson MK. Thyroid disorder. Crit Care Nurse 1987; 7(1):74.

Matteson MA, McConnell ES. Gerontological nursing: Concepts and practice. Philadelphia: WB Saunders, 1988.

Moran S. Innovative geriatric care. Nurs Manage 1987; 18(6):26.

Poyss AS. Assessment and nursing diagnosis in fluid and electrolyte disorders. Nurs Clin North Am 1987; 22(4):773.

Reiss E. Hyperparathyroidism: Diagnostic strategy. Hosp Med 1986; 22(1):152.

Robbins SL, Kumar V. Basic pathology. 4th ed. Philadelphia: WB Saunders, 1987.

Saxe A, Noell W Jr, Schneider S. Parathyroid autotransplantation: Indications and techniques. AORN J 1986; 44(3):396.

Shannon MT, Wilson BA. Govoni & Hayes drugs and nursing implications. 7th ed. Norwalk, CT: Appleton-Century-Crofts, 1992.

Sherwood LM. Diagnosis and management of primary hyperparathyroidism. Hosp Pract 1988; 12(3):9.

Sowers J, Felicetta J (eds). Endocrinology of aging. New York: Raven Publishing, 1988.

Tucker SM, et al. Patient care standards: Nursing process, diagnosis and outcome. 5th ed. St. Louis: CV Mosby, 1992.

Ulrich SP, Canale SW, Wendell SA. Nursing care planning guides: A nursing diagnosis approach. 2nd ed. Philadelphia: WB Saunders, 1990.

Urrows ST, Freston MS, Pryor DL. Profiles in osteoporosis. Am J Nurs 1991; 91(12):32.

Walpert N. Calcium metabolism disorders. Nursing 1990; 20(7):60.

Wilson JD, Foster DW (eds). Williams textbook of endocrinology. 8th ed. Philadelphia: WB Saunders, 1992.

Wyngaarden JB, Smith LH, Bennett JC (eds). Cecil textbook of medicine. 19th ed. Philadelphia: WB Saunders, 1992.

Yarnell RP, Craig MP. Detecting hypomagnesemia: The most overlooked electrolyte imbalance. Nursing 1991; 21(7):55.

Unit Eleven

ADULTS WITH MUSCULOSKELETAL DYSFUNCTION

Learning Objectives

AFTER COMPLETING THIS UNIT, THE LEARNER WILL BE ABLE TO:

Chapter Thirty-five

1. Explain the normal anatomy and physiology of the musculoskeletal system.
2. Describe common clinical manifestations of musculoskeletal dysfunction.
3. Identify information and physical examination data essential to the assessment of the musculoskeletal system.
4. Identify the most common laboratory and radiologic studies used to diagnose musculoskeletal disorders.
5. Describe medical management and surgical procedures commonly used in the treatment of patients with musculoskeletal disorders.
6. Identify data essential to the assessment of patients undergoing treatment of musculoskeletal disorders.
7. State nursing diagnoses and related expected patient outcomes commonly applicable to patients undergoing treatment of musculoskeletal disorders.
8. Describe nursing interventions, with their rationales, commonly applicable to patients undergoing treatment of musculoskeletal disorders.
9. Explain the basis for evaluation of nursing care provided to patients undergoing treatment of musculoskeletal disorders.
10. Identify special considerations for the elderly patient with altered function of the musculoskeletal system.

Chapter Thirty-six

1. Describe common musculoskeletal disorders in terms of etiology, pathophysiology, clinical manifestations, diagnostic procedures, and medical management.
2. Compare and contrast the various types of fractures in terms of cause, risk factors, treatment, and nursing interventions.
3. Identify common pharmacologic agents used to treat musculoskeletal disorders.
4. Explain the effects of osteoporosis, osteoarthritis, and rheumatoid arthritis.
5. Describe the health teaching appropriate for the patient who is at high risk for musculoskeletal disorders.
6. Identify information and physical examination data essential to the assessment of patients with common musculoskeletal disorders.
7. State nursing diagnoses and related expected patient outcomes commonly applicable to patients with musculoskeletal disorders.
8. Describe nursing interventions, with their rationales, commonly applicable to patients with musculoskeletal disorders.
9. Explain the basis for evaluation of nursing care provided to patients with common musculoskeletal disorders.
10. Identify special considerations for the elderly patient with a musculoskeletal disorder.

Chapter Thirty-five

KNOWLEDGE BASIC TO THE NURSING CARE *of Adults with Musculoskeletal Dysfunction*

The musculoskeletal system is the supporting framework of the body. It is made up of bones, joints, ligaments, muscles, and tendons. These components interact and connect to produce locomotion and to support and protect body structures. Disease or damage to any part of the system can cause pain, immobility, and disability. The musculoskeletal system is intricately related to the individual's overall sense of independence and well-being.

Anatomy and Physiology

Skeletal System

Consisting of 206 bones, the axial and appendicular skeletons form a rigid supporting framework for the human body. The axial or central skeleton is made up of the skull, sternum, ribs, and vertebral column. The appendicular skeleton consists of the shoulder girdle, pelvic girdle, and limbs. In addition to support, the skeletal system has the four other functions of body movement, protection, blood cell formation, and storage of minerals.

Bones and their joints, powered by contracting skeletal muscles, create body motion. Flat bones, such as the skull, ribs, and ileum, provide protection for vital organs. Bones also play a role in homeostasis by producing new blood cells (hematopoiesis) and by serving as a storage space for body minerals such as calcium, phosphorus, magnesium, and sodium. Approximately 99% of the total body calcium and 90% of total body phosphorus are stored in the bones.

Calcium is constantly being deposited in and resorbed (absorbed and removed) from the bones. This constant process is regulated by a number of factors, including local stress to the bone such as weight-bearing, adequate intake and absorption of vitamin D, and circulating blood levels of parathyroid hormone and calcitonin.

MICROSCOPIC ANATOMY

Bone is a dynamic structure composed of 35% organic and 65% inorganic matter. It is continually being produced and absorbed. The organic substance, which consists of cells, blood vessels, and cartilaginous material, gives the bone elasticity. The inorganic substance, which provides hardness, is primarily composed of calcium, with some phosphorus, magnesium, and sodium chloride.

There are three different types of bone cells: osteoblasts, osteoclasts, and osteocytes. Osteoblasts are active bone-building cells that synthesize organic bone matrix or collagen. Osteoclasts are large multinucleated cells that resorb bone. Osteocytes are mature bone cells in a resting state and are positioned in small spaces called lacunae. Osteocytes become active osteoblasts during periods of bone growth or repair.

CLASSIFICATION OF BONE BY CELLULAR STRUCTURE

Bone is classified as cortical or cancellous depending on how the lacunae are organized. As illustrated in Figure 35–1, the hard outer layer of all bones is composed of compact cortical bone. The lacunae, tiny cavities in these bones, are organized in concentric rings or lamellae around haversian canals. The haversian canals contain blood and lymphatic vessels. The lacunae are densely packed and are connected to one another and to the haversian canals by tiny canaliculi, which together form a haversian system or osteon. The osteon is the microscopic functioning unit of mature bone. Haversian canals run parallel to the length of the bone and are connected horizontally by Volkmann's canals (see Fig. 35–1). It is through the Volkmann's canals that bone cells communicate with the inside and outside lining of the bone. This network of canals provides compact bone with a system of blood and lymphatic vessels.

In cancellous or spongy bone, the lacunae are laid out in loosely arranged sheets connected by canaliculi. The sheets of lacunae are arranged in irregular patterns that form open spaces between thin networks of bone and resemble the inside of a sponge. This pattern is organized to withstand compressive and tensile stresses applied to the bone. Cancellous bone is more porous than compact bone and has a rich blood supply. It forms the inside of flat bones and the ends of long bones.

OSSIFICATION

The process of bone formation is called ossification. Ossification is either intramembranous or endochondral. In intramembranous ossification, bone forms from within a membrane. During this process, a fibrous union occurs in which dense connective membrane is directly replaced by deposits of inorganic calcium salts. Flat bones such as the skull, sternum, and ribs are formed by this process.

In endochondral ossification, a cartilage framework exists first and is then resorbed and replaced by bone. Most bones in the body are formed, and fractured bones heal, by the process of endochondral ossification. When bone forms by endochondral ossification, the fibrous union is not created until the cartilage framework is replaced by bone.

By the end of puberty, axial skeletal growth, or growth in the length of the bones, is complete. Although the size of the skeleton in height and build is genetically determined, bone cell content and strength are determined by a counterbalance of resorption and deposit of bone tissue. Throughout life, the osteoblasts deposit newly formed bone while the osteoclasts resorb or thin the bone. Osteoblasts deposit bone on the outer surface while osteoclasts remove bone from the medullary side, so that bone grows in diameter but not in thickness. A balance of these two processes is essential for a strong, healthy skeleton.

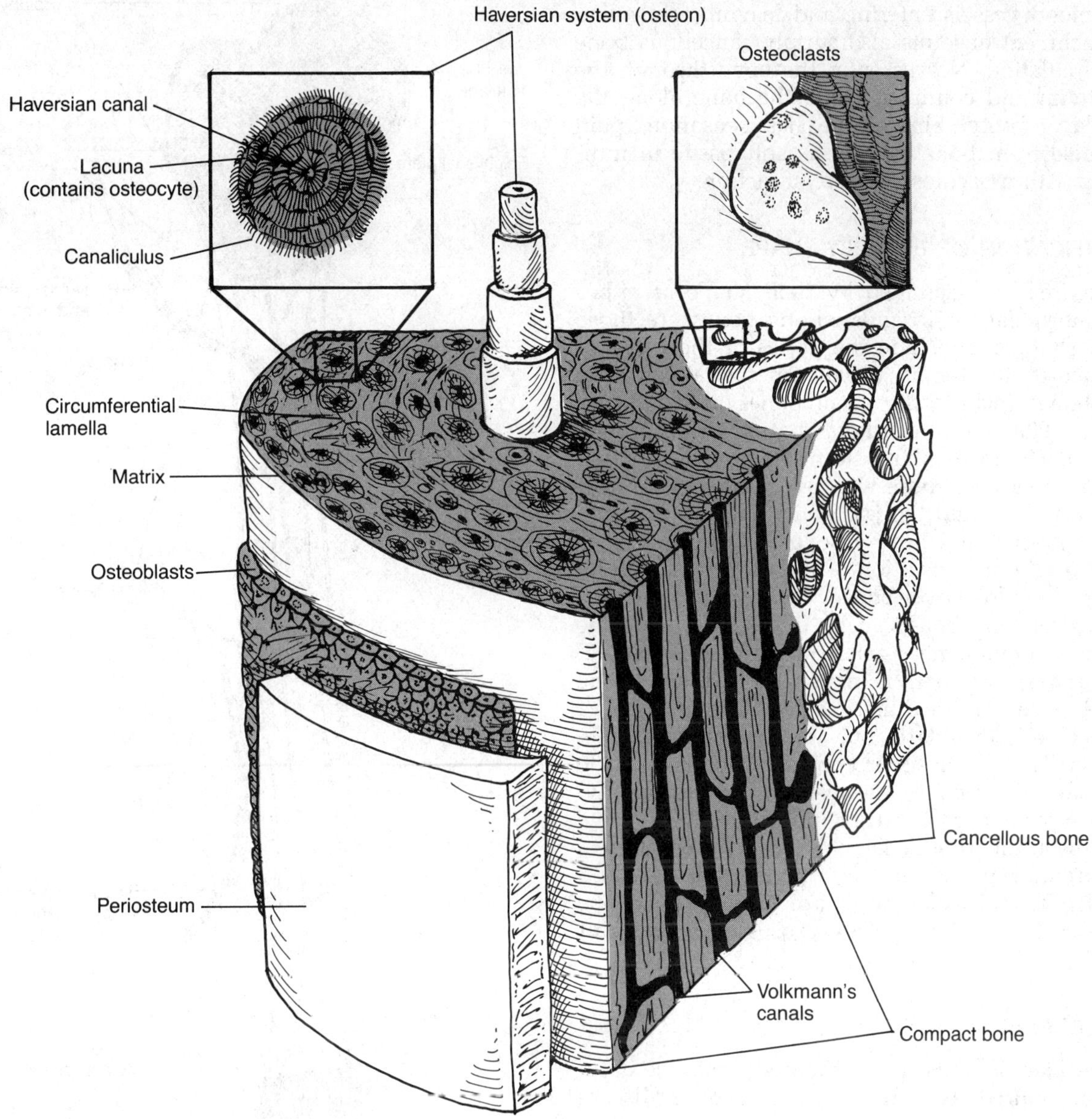

Figure 35–1.

Microscopic anatomy of bone. The section has been enlarged to show periosteum, osteoblasts, haversian system, lacunae, and osteoclasts.

GROSS ANATOMY

All bones, except the joint surfaces, which are covered by articular cartilage, are enclosed in a tough fibrous connective tissue called periosteum. The periosteum provides a supportive structure for blood vessels and nerve tissue and serves as the point of attachment to the bones for muscles, tendons, and ligaments. The periosteum is essential for nourishment, growth, repair, and resorption of bone. The endosteum is a thin membrane that lines the medullary cavity of long bones and the spaces in cancellous bones.

Within the bones there are two types of marrow: yellow and red. Yellow marrow consists mainly of fat cells and is found in the medullary canals of long bones in adults. Red marrow, which is actively involved in hematopoiesis, is found in the cancellous portion of flat bones and in the medullary cavity of growing children.

BLOOD AND NERVE SUPPLY

With its intricate internal microscopic network of vessels, bone is very vascular. Blood circulates to bone by several pathways. One third of compact bone receives its blood from vessels in the periosteum. The medullary or nutrient artery penetrating the long bones supplies blood to the other two thirds of the compact bone and to the cancellous bone; blood vessels entering and leaving the capsular attachment at joints also supply cancellous bone with circulation. Nerves enter the bone through the periosteum and continue inside the bone along the medullary cavity. Since bone has sensation, pain may arise from bone as well as soft tissue in individuals with musculoskeletal dysfunction.

CLASSIFICATION OF BONE BY SHAPE

Bones may be classified by their shape as either long, short, flat, or irregular. Long bones are those with a shaft and include the bones of the extremities, such as the femur, tibia, humerus, and radius. Short bones include the small bones in the hands and feet. Flat bones are those that cover or protect organs, such as the skull, sternum, ribs, and ileum. Irregular bones are those with irregular shapes, such as the vertebrae and the jaw bone. The external surfaces of most bones have grooves and prominences for the origin and insertion of muscles, which allow gliding of tendons over bone.

A typical long bone can be divided into specific structural components as illustrated in Figure 35–2. The diaphysis, or shaft, is made up of compact bone around a central medullary canal. The portion of compact bone that flares out at the ends is the metaphysis. The epiphysis or end of the bone is made up of cancellous bone. The metaphysis and epiphysis are separated by a cartilaginous epiphyseal plate until full adult growth is achieved. The epiphyseal plate provides growth in length of the diaphysis and metaphysis. Its cartilage cells are converted to bone at the end of puberty. This process extends over several years.

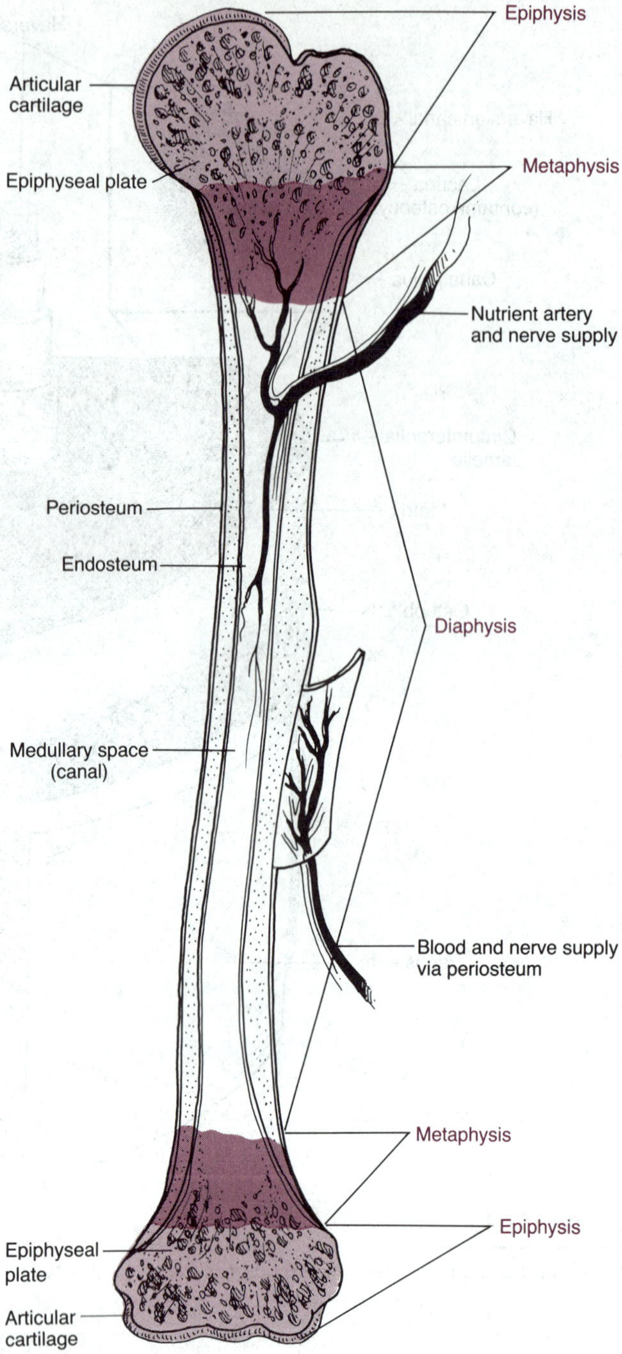

Figure 35–2.

Structure of a long bone. Diagram of the gross anatomy of a long bone, showing the sections of epiphysis, diaphysis, and metaphysis.

BONE REPAIR

Bone, like other tissues in the body, may be damaged or injured as a result of trauma or disease process. The damage or injury may or may not involve tissue surrounding the bone and displacement of bone fragments, or pieces, from their anatomic location. After injury or damage, the process of bone healing or repair occurs in five stages. These stages are listed as they would occur after a fracture or break in the bone.

First, at the time of injury, there is bleeding from within the bone and from surrounding tissue. A clot or hematoma begins to form around the fracture site within 24 hours. Fibroblasts and capillaries invade the clot to form granulation tissue.

During the second stage of bone repair, there is a proliferation of cell formation where the periosteum is torn. Fibroblasts develop from the periosteal region as osteogenic cells from the periosteum and endosteum migrate to and proliferate at the site. The proliferating cells begin to form a callus or bridge across the damaged bone or fracture.

Once callus formation is complete, the third stage begins. During the third stage, the cells differentiate into bone or cartilage, depending on where they are located. Cells nearest the bone surface transform directly into osteoblasts. Less well vascularized cells form cartilage.

The fourth stage is the ossification stage. Inorganic salts are deposited in the new bone matrix to calcify the bone.

During the fifth and final stage of bone repair, consolidation and remodeling of the new bone gradually occurs. Cancellous trabeculae (bony spikes that form a meshwork of spaces for the bone marrow) are absorbed, new lamellae are formed, new haversian systems are developed, and the medullary canal is reestablished. Remodeling continues according to Wolff's law, which states that the structure, function, and shape of a bone are determined by the forces or stress applied to it. Thus, the new bone continues to be remodeled by the stresses placed upon it until it assumes the most efficient shape for its function.

A number of factors can affect how damaged bone heals. These factors include the following:

1. Age.
2. General physical condition of the individual.
3. Type of injury.
4. Degree of displacement of bone fragments.
5. Presence of infection.
6. Adequate immobilization after injury.
7. Vascular sufficiency.
8. Functional periosteum.

Skeletal Muscular System

SKELETAL MUSCLE

Skeletal muscle is sometimes called striated muscle because of its microscopic banded appearance. It is also termed voluntary muscle because its movement can be controlled by conscious effort. Individual muscles are covered and separated by a fibrous membrane called fascia. The fascia is similar to a compartment or envelope. In addition to providing support, the fascia allows skeletal muscle to move smoothly across bones, joints, and muscles and enhances contractility of skeletal muscle.

Skeletal muscle is made up of bundles of cell fibers that are covered and held together by connective tissue. Each muscle fiber contains several myofibrils. Each myofibril is composed of sliding protein filaments called sarcomeres. The sarcomeres are the contractile or working unit of the myofibrils. As the sarcomere filaments slide across one another, they shorten or contract the muscle and lengthen or relax the muscle. This sliding action produces the elastic character of muscle tissue.

Skeletal muscle contracts in response to impulses from the central nervous system. These impulses produce the release of acetylcholine from the motor end plate of the motor neuron, or nerve cell, innervating the muscle. In response to the presence of acetylcholine, calcium ions are released within the muscle cell fibers, and the sarcomeres contract.

The partially contracted quality of muscle fibers at rest produces muscle tone. Abnormal muscle tone is referred to as either flaccid (less than normal tone) or spastic (greater than normal tone). Groups of muscles in a continuous partially contracted state maintain skeletal posture.

Locomotion, or movement, is made possible by muscles working together with the bones and joints. To produce movement, muscles contract over bones. Through the contraction of a variety of muscles, the body is able to produce specific, deliberate movements.

The primary energy source for muscle activity and movement is the breakdown of adenosine triphosphate (ATP) within the cell. Creatine phosphate is a secondary energy source that can be converted to ATP when needed. Since ATP is synthesized by glycolysis (anaerobic process) and the Krebs cycle (aerobic process), during heavy exercise when increased amounts of oxygen are unavailable for efficient functioning of the aerobic process, increased amounts of glucose are necessary. This is provided by glycogen stored in the cells.

LIGAMENTS AND TENDONS

Ligaments are composed of fibrous connective tissue bands that bind bones to other bones. They may either limit or facilitate movement of the joint. Ligaments pass over bone joints, where they remain taut to provide joint stability. Tendons are strong, nonelastic fibrous connective tissue cords. They are an extension of the muscle sheath and attach muscle to the periosteum of the bone.

Where ligaments, tendons, muscle, bone, and skin move across one another there may be friction. Bursae are small sacs of connective tissue that are found where musculoskeletal structures move across one another under pressure. They are lined with a synovial membrane and filled with synovial fluid. Bursae act as cushions to decrease friction between body structures.

JOINTS AND ARTICULATIONS

A joint is the point where two or more bones meet. Joints are classified according to the amount of movement they allow. Joints that allow no movement are classified as synarthrodial joints. Amphiarthrodial joints allow slight movement. Joints that allow free movement are diarthrodial joints. Examples of the different joints in the body are illustrated in Figure 35–3 and listed in Table 35–1. Terms describing movement that diarthrodial joints make possible are defined in Table 35–2.

Most body joints are diarthrodial. The articular surfaces of diarthrodial joints are covered by hyaline cartilage. This cartilage decreases friction as the bones move against one another but does not regenerate. Between the two articulating surfaces is a small space or joint cavity. The entire diarthrodial joint is enclosed by a fibrous capsule of connective tissue that is lined with synovial membrane. This membrane produces synovial fluid which provides

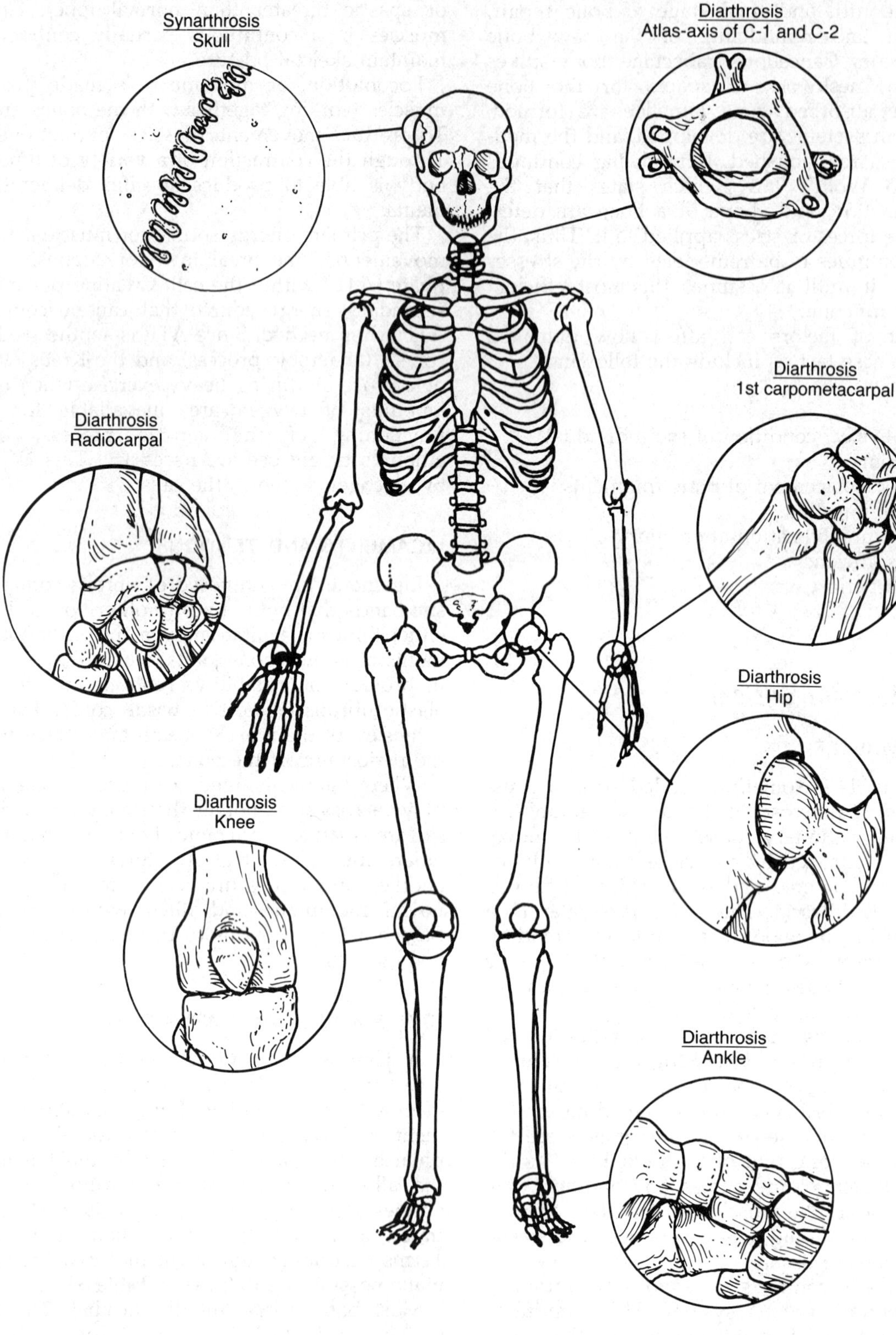

Figure 35–3.

Classification of joints, with examples. Joints are classified as synarthrosis, amphiarthrosis or diarthrosis. Most joints in the body are diarthrodial joints. Diarthrodial joints allow free movement.

Table 35–1. TYPES OF JOINTS

CLASSIFICATION	DESCRIPTION	EXAMPLE
Synarthrosis (allowing no movement)	Suture	Skull
	Synchondrosis	Femur
Amphiarthrosis (allowing slight movement)	Symphysis	Pelvis
	Syndemosis	Tibiofibular
Diarthrosis (allowing free movement)	Ball and socket	Hip and shoulder
	Hinge	Elbow and knee
	Pivot	Top of spine
	Gliding	Vertebrae
	Condyloid	Wrist
	Saddle	Thumb

lubrication for smooth joint motion. The synovial fluid, also provides some nutrients to joint surfaces.

The synarthrodial joints have no cavity. The articulating bone surfaces are connected by fibrous tissue or cartilage, which prevents movement.

CARTILAGE

Cartilage is a smooth, resilient supporting tissue composed of collagen. It provides a smooth, low-friction surface for articulating bones. Because of its elasticity, it also provides a cushion that absorbs shock and reduces stress and strain on joint surfaces. The three types of cartilage in the body are hyaline, elastic, and fibrocartilage. Hyaline cartilage is the most prevalent. It covers the articular surfaces of bone. Hyaline cartilage has no blood vessels. It receives nutrients from synovial fluid, adjacent tissues, or an occasional blood vessel passing through to other tissues. Elastic cartilage contains more elastic fibers and is more flexible than hyaline cartilage. It is found in the outer ear, epiglottis, and larynx. Fibrocartilage contains more collagen fibers and is very resilient. It forms the transitional tissue between hyaline cartilage and the connective tissue of capsules or ligaments and forms the attachment of tendons to bone. Fibrocartilage is also found in the symphysis pubis, the knee meniscus, and the intervertebral discs, where it functions as a shock absorber for the skeleton.

Table 35–2. TERMS DESCRIBING RANGE OF MOVEMENT OF A DIARTHRODIAL JOINT

TERM	DEFINITION
Abduction	Movement away from and out to the side of the body.
Adduction	Movement toward the body or across the midline of the body.
Circumduction	Movement of the limb in a circular fashion from its pivotal point.
Extension	Unfolding or movement from a flexed or bent position to a straight or neutral position.
Flexion	Bending or folding movements going toward the center of the body.
Hyperextension	Extension beyond a straight or neutral position in a direction away from the center of the body.
Pronation	Movement of the palm so that the hand is turned downward or toward the posterior surface of the body.
Rotation	Movement of a bone upon its own axis or pivoting.
Supination	Movement of the palm so the the hand is turned outward with the palm facing the anterior surface of the body.

Clinical Manifestations of Musculoskeletal Dysfunction

The individual with an injury or a disease of the bones, muscles, ligaments, tendons, joints, or cartilage can be expected to present with alteration in movement of individual body parts or a limitation in locomotion, either with or without pain. These symptoms could vary from a change in the normal gait pattern to inability to ambulate. The presence of pain also aggravates the ability for free joint movement and locomotion and may actually be the primary problem causing the musculoskeletal dysfunction. Fractures, multiple trauma, and major diseases affecting the musculoskeletal system produce specific clinical manifestations, which are covered in detail under each disorder in Chapter 36. The extent of musculoskeletal involvement determines how much limitation occurs in ability to perform self-care and other activities of daily living.

Mobility Impairment

Symptoms the individual may experience include limitation in strength, function, or range of motion of the involved musculoskeletal structures. A deformity or change in shape and size of the involved area may be evident as well as local soft tissue inflammation, pain, and edema.

Immobility and disuse resulting from injury or disease affect the entire musculoskeletal system. Muscles develop weakness and atrophy in a short time from lack of use. This is evident in a casted or splinted extremity that has not been exercised. Joints develop stiffness and lose range of motion or develop contractures from immobility and improper positioning. The patient may be unable to perform activities of daily living as a result of weakness and fatigue. Without mobility and normal stresses of use and weight-bearing on the skeleton, bone destruction (osteoclastic activity) and bone resorption occur at a greater rate than bone production and repair. The calcium released from bone destruction results in an alkaline urine, which is likely to result in development of kidney stones and urinary tract infections.

Application of the Nursing Process to the Care of the Patient with Mobility Impairment

Assessment

Complete a thorough movement assessment on the patient. Review history and present mobility problems. Ask the patient to demonstrate mobility of all major joints to evaluate strengths and limitations of movement. Check the patient's ability to perform activities of daily living. Note grip strength, weight-bearing ability, and ability to move freely about the room, with or without assistance. Assess the patient's respiration system, noting shortness of breath after movement. Look for signs of impaired circulation to extremities. Check all distal pulses. Check muscle tone and the patient's ability to repeat a strength exercise without tiring, such as standing on one foot or gripping an object. Ask the patient about symptoms of fatigue after mild exercise. Assess the relation of the symptoms to the patient's disorder or need for assistive devices for movement or locomotion. Observe the type of device used by the patient and its effectiveness. Ask the patient about interferences with movement caused by pain in joints.

Assess the patient frequently for signs of respiratory infection. Look for increased respiratory rate, cough, dyspnea, fever, chills, and shortness of breath. Auscultate lungs for adventitious sounds. Check laboratory results, especially the white blood cell count and urinalysis.

Assess the patient's understanding about the effects of immobility and how to prevent the complications that may occur. Ask the patient about present signs of problems related to immobility. Talk to the patient's family to determine their understanding of the symptoms associated with the hazards of immobility.

See whether the patient experiences any pain or burning on urination or low back pain indicative of a urinary tract infection. Note the color and consistency of the urine.

Assess the patient's extremities, looking for signs of infection from lesions or any areas of breakdown. Note any skin lesions, and report them immediately. Look for purulent drainage from the areas of breakdown or around pin sites. Check distal pulses and the color and temperature of the skin.

Note the patient's ability to perform self-care. Observe the patient's appearance, assessing for poor hygiene, improper dress, or lack of general grooming. Check whether the patient is able to eat without assistance. Ask whether toileting is a problem for the patient or whether assistance is necessary.

Nursing Diagnoses and Planning

Nursing diagnoses and related expected patient outcomes most commonly applicable to patients experiencing immobility problems include the following:*

NDx: Activity intolerance related to fatigue and dyspnea secondary to decreased muscle tone and cardiovascular fitness from lack of exercise or interference with mobility from appliances, deformity, or pain

Planning: Patient outcomes
1. Patient follows regimen of planned activities and rest periods each day.
2. Patient verbalizes decreased feelings of fatigue and demonstrates increased activity level.
3. Patient completes activities of daily living without signs of fatigue and dyspnea such as tachycardia, tachypnea, shortness of breath, and cyanosis.
4. Patient is able to complete some activity, as prescribed, without pain or interference from appliance or in spite of deformity.

NDx: Knowledge deficit: nature of immobility problems and prevention of complications

Planning: Patient outcomes
1. Patient states accurate information about the nature of the potential problems related to immobility.
2. Patient states the signs of complications of immobility and when to seek medical intervention.
3. Patient relates the measures necessary to lessen the risk of complications.
4. Patient shows no evidence of complications, such as extreme fatigue, inability to complete activities of daily living, deformities, skin breakdown, infection, or elimination problems.

NDx: Altered tissue perfusion, peripheral, related to complications of immobility; constriction from casts, traction, or other devices; or bed rest

Planning: Patient outcomes
1. Patient's extremities are warm, color is adequate, and pulses are present.
2. Patient presents no evidence of implications from compromised circulation.

NDx: Impaired skin integrity, related to insufficient peripheral circulation from bed rest or restrictive devices, or related to direct injury from immobilizing devices

* High risk for disuse syndrome may be used instead of the diagnoses listed here, because it incorporates many of the problems associated with immobility. In addition, some patients with musculoskeletal dysfunction have limited periods of immobility, so at any given time it is possible that only one or two of the diagnoses listed here are appropriate.

Planning: Patient outcomes

1. Patient states causes of skin lesions and measures to prevent their occurrence or recurrence.
2. Patient relates appropriate knowledge about skin care.
3. Patient is free of skin complications.

NDx: High risk for infection related to increased susceptibility secondary to bed rest, placement of internal fixation devices, pressure from restrictive devices, or compromised circulation

Planning: Patient outcomes

1. Patient's vital signs are within normal ranges for the patient.
2. Patient displays no signs of infection, such as fever, chills, tachycardia, tachypnea, or pain or burning on urination, or drainage from lesions or at pin sites.
3. Patient identifies early signs of infection and measures to prevent infections.

NDx: Self-care deficit in areas of feeding, hygiene, toileting, or other activities of daily living related to impaired mobility

Planning: Patient outcomes

1. Patient performs activities of daily living, using assistive devices if necessary.
2. Patient states alternative methods to complete tasks that are restricted by musculoskeletal dysfunction or immobilization.

Nursing Interventions

NDx: Activity intolerance

Instruct the patient to develop a regimen of activity with frequent rest periods throughout the day. Encourage the patient to do range-of-motion exercises frequently while lying in bed to maintain muscle tone and strength, or complete passive range-of-motion exercises if necessary. Teach the patient to practice energy-saving techniques to reduce fatigue and shortness of breath. Place frequently used articles within the patient's reach for safety and to prevent overtiring.

Provide and encourage frequent rest periods while delivering patient care. Alternate the rest periods with a planned regimen of appropriate exercises to enable the patient to improve locomotion ability.

NDx: Knowledge deficit: nature of immobility problems and prevention of complications

Instruct the patient about the effects of immobility and the signs of complications, such as elimination difficulty, discoloration of the skin, skin breakdown, diminished pulses, numbness, and the symptoms of infections. Teach the patient when to seek medical assistance. Explain the need for safety measures if locomotion is a problem. Consult with physical and occupational therapists for guidance.

Teach the patient to drink an increased amount of fluids daily to prevent urinary stasis. Provide fiber foods to prevent constipation, especially if the patient is on extended bed rest.

Explain proper methods necessary to prevent further irritation and ulceration of skin where pressure has occurred from bed rest, the appliance, or cast, if present. Allow the patient to ask questions as needed. Include the family in the education sessions when appropriate.

NDx: Altered tissue perfusion, peripheral

Help the patient conserve oxygen needs by encouraging rest and limiting activities. Assist the patient with meals if needed. Administer oxygen if appropriate. Elevate the head of the bed to aid in chest expansion.

Keep the patient in a comfortable position and reposition frequently to release pressure. Use range-of-motion exercises to stimulate circulation. Monitor vital signs and laboratory studies to assess for changes and improvements in status.

Discourage smoking to avoid vasoconstriction. Remove constricting clothing, and keep heavy bed linen from restricting peripheral circulation. Tell the patient to notify the nurse if signs of compromised circulation from constrictive bandages, casts, or other devices seem apparent, such as discoloration, pain, swelling, or numbness of an extremity. Keep the patient's legs in a nondependent position when not ambulating.

NDx: Impaired skin integrity

Teach the patient measures to prevent skin injury from developing. Avoid irritating sheets or garments. Protect the skin from rough edges of immobilizing devices. Have the patient inspect the skin frequently and seek medical assistance if any breakdown or soreness is noted.

Teach the patient to exercise, as tolerated, to promote good circulation. Range-of-motion exercises should be done while on bed rest. Turn the patient frequently, and inspect pressure areas for early signs of breakdown. Keep heavy linen from constricting the peripheral circulation by using a bed cradle. Elevate the patient's legs when sitting in a chair. Inspect the areas distal to constrictive devices for signs of compromised circulation. If lesions are present, use aseptic technique to cleanse them. Wear gloves during the dressing changes. Teach the patient and family members the proper technique for dressing areas of breakdown.

NDx: High risk for infection

Keep the patient warm, and avoid extreme changes in temperature in the room. Turn the patient as needed to stimulate circulation to prevent skin breakdown and skin infections. Have the patient deep breathe and cough frequently to prevent respiratory infections, especially if the patient is on bed rest. Use incentive spirometry if appropriate. Monitor the patient's vital signs frequently, observing for subtle changes that may indicate early signs of infection. Report any changes noted.

Monitor intake and output, and note the color and consistency of the urine. Encourage an increased fluid intake to prevent urinary infections, especially if the patient is on bed rest.

Promote good nutrition for proper healing by serving meals the patient will eat, in a relaxed attractive atmosphere. Encourage a high-protein and high-vitamin diet, and high fiber content to prevent constipation. Provide skin care frequently, especially if areas of breakdown are present. Use aseptic technique to cleanse around pin sites as ordered. Because early identification and treatment may limit the severity of the infection, teach the patient and family to continually observe for signs of developing infection and to notify the physician if such signs appear.

NDx: Self-care deficit
Assist the patient with activities of daily living as needed. Seek alternative methods for the patient to be able to complete the activities when restricted by a disorder or immobilizing device. Teach the patient how to maneuver with the assistance of supportive aids. Explain how to use other extremities to complete a task, or how to move appropriately with the restrictive device in place, such as how to use crutches when the patient's leg is in an immobilizer or fixation device. Seek the assistance of physical therapists or occupational therapists when necessary for consultation or teaching sessions for the patient and family.

Evaluation

Evaluate the effectiveness of nursing care for a patient with immobility problems by comparing the patient's status with the expected patient outcomes. Examples of specific outcomes for patients with immobility problems have been provided in the Planning section.

Pain

A common manifestation of musculoskeletal dysfunction is pain in muscles and joints. The location and type of pain vary with each particular dysfunction. Typically, bone pain is a throbbing, nonlocalized, aching feeling. It may, however, be localized with a fracture or tumor. Pain in the joints may be associated with inflammation and is frequently more severe at the end of the day. Pain associated with inflammation of tendons may be intolerable to the patient during sleeping hours. Rest and anti-inflammatory agents usually relieve the pain of inflammation. Muscle pain ranges from mild tenderness to severe pain with movement or pressure to the affected part. Quick movements may aggravate the sensation of pain in the muscle. Muscle spasms may also accompany the episodes of pain. Pain is treated with a variety of analgesics and skeletal muscle relaxants (Pharmacology Box 35–1).

Application of the Nursing Process to the Care of the Patient with Musculoskeletal Pain

Assessment

Assess the patient for the extent, location, duration, severity, and frequency of the pain and for joint deformities. Look for swelling, redness, and warmth at the site of the pain. Assess for tenderness or pain with pressure applied to the area over the bone or joint. (Palpation should not be done if a fracture is suspected until cleared by x-ray examination.) Check the range of motion of the involved joint and the amount of flexibility or stiffness present. Notice the activity level of the patient and whether the pain restricts the patient's movements, or ability to do self-care or ambulate. Note the area distal to and around devices that may cause constriction of extremities and thus cause pain.

Nursing Diagnoses and Planning

The nursing diagnosis and related expected patient outcomes most commonly applicable to patients with musculoskeletal pain are as follows:

NDx: Pain related to effects of the musculoskeletal disorder

Planning: Patient outcomes
1. Patient reports that pain is controlled with analgesics or relaxants (see Pharmacology Box 35–1).
2. Patient states comfort measures to help relieve pain.
3. Patient states coping measures to help relieve or tolerate pain.

Nursing Interventions

NDx: Pain
Place the patient in comfortable positions, and reposition frequently. Check traction to ensure proper alignment and appropriate weight of pull. Look for signs of pressure causing pain if the patient has a restrictive device applied, such as a cast or splint. Use pillows to support bony prominences.

Pharmacology Box 35–1.
SKELETAL MUSCLE RELAXANTS

Skeletal Muscle Relaxants:
Drugs that promote relaxation of muscles and some sedation.

Action:
These drugs depress the central nervous system in the brain stem, basal ganglia, and spinal cord without altering nerve conduction or muscle excitability.

Uses:
They are used for relief of pain, spasticity, and stiffness in musculoskeletal disorders.

Side Effects:
Drowsiness, gastrointestinal distress, photosensitivity, weakness, sensitivity reactions, ataxia, visual or speech difficulties, and dry mucous membranes.

Interactions:
The drugs interact with alcohol products, antidepressants, and other depressants.

Nursing Implications:
Give the drugs with milk or food to decrease gastric irritation.
Observe for signs of sensitivity reactions such as fever, rashes, or dyspnea.
Tell the patient not to drive or perform tasks requiring alertness.
Teach the patient about the side effects, and caution about taking the drugs with alcohol.

Geriatric Considerations:
Drowsiness may be more severe in the elderly. Gastric irritation may also be more severe. Explain the need to take the medication with food and to refrain from participating in activities that require mental alertness while under the influence of the drug.

Assess when the pain is most severe, and allow the patient to rest during those periods. Give pain medications as ordered before activity periods so that the patient can better tolerate the movement.

Help the patient find alternate methods to alleviate or to be able to tolerate the pain. Show the patient and family relaxation techniques and how to perform massage. Postoperatively, teach the patient the use of patient-controlled analgesia (PCA) if ordered.

Inspect the skin and palpate pulses in distal areas for signs of compromised circulation or skin breakdown caused by constrictive devices that may be the cause of the pain. Tell the patient to report any signs of pain or numbness immediately.

Evaluation

Evaluate the effectiveness of nursing care for a patient with musculoskeletal pain by comparing the patient's status with the expected patient outcomes. Examples of specific outcomes for patients with musculoskeletal pain have been provided in the Planning section.

Assessment of the Musculoskeletal System

The assessment of the musculoskeletal system includes a review of the history of illness or problems with movement and an examination that includes inspection, palpation, measuring the range of motion of joints, grading muscle strength, observing gait, checking neurovascular status, and observing for alterations in activities of daily living.

Patient History

Ask the patient about symptoms of pain, joint stiffness, immobility, swelling, deformity, and any other obvious changes. Get detailed descriptions of the pain experienced by the patient. Note the location, duration, precipitating factors, and effective relief methods. Ask the patient whether any falls or other injuries have occurred recently. Check whether the patient has noticed a recent change in gait, ability to handle utensils, grip strength, posture, joint function, or overall movement ability.

Assess the patient for short- and long-term effects of the musculoskeletal dysfunction on lifestyle, activities of daily living, and potential rehabilitation. This information is elicited through open-ended questions to the patient. Determine the patient's level of independence.

During the patient interview, ask questions that elicit a detailed past history and description of present symptoms. The client's age, sex, and occupation are also important data to document. Muscle strength varies among individuals, but it is expected that a laborer would have greater strength than an office worker. Question the patient about recreational physical activity and activity at the workplace.

Physical Examination

During the assessment, note any abnormalities, and ask questions of the patient about the findings to determine the extent of the problem, its onset, and the potential interferences with activities of daily living. Document each of the responses.

Note the patient's ability to sit, change position, stand, bend over, grasp objects, or walk with ease. These activities are important to manage personal hygiene and grooming needs.

Inspect the patient all over for symmetry, size contour, and random movements on either side of the body. Be sure to compare one side with the other. Note any areas of swelling, discoloration, or obvious malalignment or deformity. Observe the patient in both a standing and a sitting position from the front, sides, and back. The normal spine is straight from the posterior view. Scoliosis is identified by a lateral curvature of the spinal column. From the lateral view, look for a normal forward concave curvature of the cervical spine, a convex curvature of the thoracic spine, and a concave curvature of the lumbar spine. Collapse of one or more vertebral bodies can cause an increased curvature of the involved spine and an overall shortening in height. Excessive convex curvature of the thoracic spine, common in the older adult, is known as kyphosis. Excessive concave curvature of the lumbar vertebral column is termed lordosis. Lordosis may be seen in pregnancy, obesity, and hip deformities.

Observe the appearance of major muscles of the upper extremities and the lower extremities and compare bilaterally. Major muscles may be measured to confirm symmetry.

Palpate all major muscles and joints bilaterally. Note areas of swelling, unusual hardness, localized heat spots, muscle tone, and involuntary movement when palpated. The patient may not complain of pain and tenderness in an affected joint. Observe for nonverbal signs of discomfort such as wincing, contracting, or gasping. Note decreased sensation in any area assessed.

Check the range of motion for the neck, waist, shoulder, elbows, wrists, fingers, hips, knees, ankles, and toes. Note the appropriate range of movement and direction for each. Table 35–3 lists the degrees of movement for each area of assessment. A goniometer is used to acurately measure the range of motion. Place the goniometer against the joint with the arms of the instrument parallel with the axis of each of the bones that connect to form the joint. The angle formed is calibrated on the instrument and represents the amount of flexion or extension of the joint being measured.

Test the patient's muscle strength by applying force to the extremity while the patient tries to hold it in position. Check ocular, facial, neck, arm, wrist, finger, hip, leg, ankle, and foot muscle strength. Compare the findings bilaterally. Note whether the patient exhibited no strength, slight strength, strength without force, or strength with force applied. Document any differences from one side to the other.

Table 35–3. DEGREES OF RANGE OF MOTION OF JOINTS FOR ASSESSMENT

JOINT	MOTION	DEGREES
Neck	Flexion	45
	Extension	55
	Lateral bending (R and L)	40
	Rotation (R and L)	70
Spine/Waist/Hip	Flexion	75+
	Extension	30
	Lateral bending (R and L)	35
	Rotation (R and L)	30
Arms (from shoulder)	Flexion	180
	Extension	50
	Abduction	180
	Adduction	50
	Internal rotation	90
Elbows	Flexion	160
	Extension	0
	Supination	90
	Pronation	90
Wrists	Flexion	90
	Extension (dorsiflexion)	70
	Radial deviation	20
	Ulnar deviation	55
Hip		
Straight knee	Flexion	90
	Hyperextension	15
	Abduction	45
	Adduction	30
	Internal rotation	40
	External rotation	45
Bent knee	Flexion	120
	Extension	0
Ankles/Feet	Plantar flexion	45
	Dorsiflexion	20
	Inversion	30
	Eversion	20

Have the patient walk across the room, turn, and return. If possible, have the patient walk without assistive devices. Note the patient's balance and gait during this procedure. Look for irregular movements, unsteadiness, limping, or abnormal stride. Observe the position of the shoulders and pelvis in relation to the legs, knee joints, and feet.

Normal gait can be divided into two phases: the stance phase, when the leg bears weight, and the swing phase, when the non–weight-bearing leg is in motion. In the normal adult gait pattern, the distance between the heels is 2 to 4 inches and the length of stride is approximately 15 inches. Pain, muscle weakness, instability of joints, and structural deformity are common causes of abnormal gait patterns. Changes in supporting structures, such as decreased elasticity of ligaments and physical changes in weight-bearing joints, can affect gait. The elderly tend to walk with a wide heel base and shorter strides because of structural changes of aging. Also have the patient stand on one foot, then the other foot. Note balance, change in posture, and any involuntary movements. Stand near the patient during this part of the assessment for support and to prevent a fall if the patient wavers or loses balance.

If the patient has a musculoskeletal dysfunction, assess the circulatory status and nerve and muscle function proximal and distal to the defect. This is done to establish a baseline for comparison; then it is monitored frequently to detect changes that may indicate potential complications. Assess the position, color, proximal and distal pulses, capillary refill, motor function, sensation, and temperature of the body part. Evaluation of the motor function indicates that the nerves controlling those muscles are also functioning. Evaluate and compare symmetric sides of the body.

Be aware of the differences in expectations for the elderly patient in all areas of the assessment as compared with the average adult. Normal changes of aging may affect the posture, gait, range of motion, and strength in the older adult.

Diagnostic Procedures

There are numerous diagnostic studies utilized in a workup for musculoskeletal dysfunction. These may be classified as radiologic studies, laboratory studies, or endoscopic studies. The procedures with appropriate nursing interventions are described in Table 35–4.

Medical Management

Medical intervention to treat joint injury, immobilize a fracture, correct a deformity, or provide support for weak joints or muscles may include nonsurgical interventions, such as application of heat or cold, application of casts, and traction, or surgical interventions, such as application of fixation devices or amputation. In some instances more than one therapy may be used concurrently. The type of medical management selected is determined by a number of factors, including the location of the injury, the type and severity of the injury (or defect), and the age and the general health of the patient.

Nonsurgical Management

APPLICATION OF HEAT AND COLD

Heat is applied to sore muscles and joints to promote circulation and provide comfort by relaxing muscles. Heat may be applied by Hydrocollator packs or commercial heating pads with exact temperature settings. The temperature of the heat application should not exceed 37.8°C.(100°F). Heat may be applied intermittently as ordered, as in 15 to 30 minute time periods.

The local application of cold immediately after an injury causes local vasoconstriction, prevents swelling, and aids in pain relief. After the first 48 hours, heat may be applied to increase circulation and promote comfort. Ice bags or commercial cold packs can be used to apply cold to a specific area. Cold is applied intermittently to prevent reflex dilation of blood vessels and frost injury. Cold is applied for 30 minutes or less, then removed for 10 to 15 minutes to allow capillary circulation to return to the affected area.

Application of the Nursing Process to the Care of the Patient Undergoing Heat or Cold Application Therapy

Assessment

Before the prescribed application of heat or cold, assess the patient's skin for lesions or sensitive areas. Caution is necessary in patients with decreased peripheral circulation or decreased sensation because these patients may not feel an extremely hot or cold sensation until trauma to the tissue has occurred. During the treatment, question the patient about subjective sensations of extreme heat or cold, numbness, tingling, or increased pain. Assess for effects of the application such as comfort, relief of pain, or absence of swelling.

Nursing Diagnoses and Planning

The nursing diagnosis and related expected patient outcomes most commonly applicable to patients un-

Table 35–4. COMMON DIAGNOSTIC TESTS FOR MUSCULOSKELETAL FUNCTION

STUDY	DESCRIPTION	NURSING IMPLICATIONS
RADIOLOGIC		
Arthrogram	X-ray film of a joint after a radiopaque dye or air has been injected into the joint cavity. It is used in the diagnosis of intrajoint and cartilaginous disorders.	Assess for allergies to the dye substance or iodine. Determine the patient's understanding of the test, and provide necessary information. Obtain a signed consent if required. After the procedure, assess the site for pain or edema. Also observe for signs of latent allergic reactions.
X-ray examination	General roentgenographic studies of any bone or joint for diagnosis of suspected problems.	Determine the patient's understanding of the test ordered. Explain what is to be done. If the patient is in pain from an injury, give prescribed medication for pain because the affected area may be manipulated during the x-ray examination, causing more pain.
Bone scan	An x-ray examination of skeletal bone using a gamma camera scanner after an injection of a radioactive substance. The dye is picked up in areas of increased metabolism. It is used to diagnose cancer, osteomyelitis, fractures, and osteoporosis.	Assess whether the patient is pregnant or allergic to iodine, because it is contraindicated in these situations. Provide information about the test to the patient. Obtain a signed consent. Give the patient increased fluids prior to the test to aid in the excretion of the medium after the test. If pelvic bones are to be scanned, have the patient void prior to the test, because a full bladder may obscure pelvic bones. After the scan, observe for signs of an allergic reaction, and encourage increased fluid intake.
Computed tomography (CT)	The CT scan combines x-rays with computer technology to produce pictures of internal musculoskeletal structures. A contrast medium may be used. The CT is used to identify tissue tumors, injuries to ligaments or tendons, or fractures.	Assess the patient's knowledge about the procedure, and provide information. Because the machine used is often frightening to the patient, provide reassurance and allow the patient to ask questions and voice concerns. Explain that the patient will be lying flat while passing very slowly through a cylinder-type apparatus. Tell the patient about the importance of lying still and that the scan may take several minutes (20 minutes or more is common).
Arteriography	This is a series of x-ray films taken of the arterial system after injection of a dye. The test is used to diagnose occlusion of blood vessels. Bones do not heal properly and osteomyelitis is more likely if the blood supply to an injured limb is compromised.	Assess the patient's knowledge about the procedure, and provide information needed. Determine whether the patient has allergies to contrast dye. After the procedure, monitor the injection site for signs of hematoma, inflammation, or drainage.
LABORATORY		
Blood analysis	The complete blood count is used to determine possible infection and low hemoglobin level (due to hemorrhage). Blood chemistry is used to determine osteomalacia, some bone tumors, and muscle damage.	Explain the tests to the patient. Reinforce the physician's report of the findings to the patient and family.
Urinalysis	Calcium levels in the urine may increase in some musculoskeletal conditions such as cancer of the bone. The urine may also be tested for bacteria because bladder infections may result from long-term immobility.	Explain why a urine sample is needed. Collect and send the sample to the laboratory according to the set procedure of the institution. Reinforce the results of the tests as reported to the patient by the physician.
Arthrocentesis	A needle puncture into the space of a joint to aspirate fluid. For diagnostic purposes, the fluid is sent to the laboratory for analysis. It is used to determine infection, hemorrhage, or other problems of the joint such as arthritis.	Explain the procedure to the patient. Obtain a signed consent. Assist the physician with the procedure if needed. Observe the puncture site after the test for inflammation, drainage, or swelling, indicative of an infection. An ice bag may be applied.
ENDOSCOPIC		
Arthroscopy	An endoscopic examination of a joint for diagnostic (or corrective) purposes. It is most commonly used for knee disorders. It is performed under aseptic technique in an examining room, or operating room (if corrective), under local or general anesthetic.	Explain the procedure to the patient and obtain a signed consent. If arthroscopy is done for diagnostic reasons only, local anesthesia is usually used, so the patient's preoperative preparation is limited. After the procedure, observe for pain, bleeding, drainage, or swelling at the site. Reinforce the home care instructions from the physician. Check dressings or wrap before the patient's discharge.
OTHER		
Magnetic resonance imaging (MRI)	The MRI uses magnetic force to provide clear three-plane pictures of internal structures. No radiation or contrast medium is used. It is used for diagnosis of any musculoskeletal dysfunction that is not readily diagnosable by other means but is particularly valuable for viewing soft tissues.	Explain the procedure to the patient. Because the equipment is frightening to the patient, mild sedation may be used. Some patients become claustrophobic during the test. Have the patient remove all metal objects. Identify any patient who has internal metal objects such as a fixation device or prosthesis because MRI may cause it to migrate. The MRI is contraindicated for any patient with internal metal objects.

(continued)

Table 35–4. *(continued)* COMMON DIAGNOSTIC TESTS FOR MUSCULOSKELETAL FUNCTION

OTHER *(continued)*		
Electromyography (EMG)	This test determines the electrical activity of skeletal muscle and its ability to respond to a stimulus. An oscilloscope records the activity of the muscle through needle electrodes inserted through the skin. EMG is used to differentiate between neurologic and muscular disorders.	Before the EMG, assess the patient's functional capacity involving specific muscles, such as gait, ability to do range-of-motion exercises, and sensory motor deficits. This is helpful in interpreting the results. Explain the test to the patient. Tell the patient that the test may be lengthy (sometimes up to 2 hours). Obtain a signed consent.
Thermography	An infrared camera is used to determine the amount of heat radiating from soft tissue. The photograph shows variations from cold (blue) to hot (red). It is used to evaluate inflammation of joints, damage to supporting structures, and muscle trauma.	Explain the test to the patient. Tell the patient it is non-invasive and painless. Expose the body part to be tested to room air for 15 minutes prior to the test. The room temperature should be between 20° and 20.9°C (68° and 70°F).

dergoing heat or cold application therapy are as follows:

NDx: High risk for injury: trauma to tissue related to the treatment regimen

Planning: Patient outcomes

1. Patient denies sensation of extreme heat or cold at site of application.
2. Patient's skin remains intact without a burn or frost injury.

Nursing Interventions

NDx: High risk for injury: trauma to tissue
Apply all heat and cold therapy with caution, especially in the patient with decreased peripheral circulation or sensation, as in the elderly or a patient with peripheral vascular disease. Protect the skin from direct contact with the heat or cold source by placing a towel next to the patient's skin. To ensure maximum effectiveness, secure the heat or cold application loosely in the desired position. Leave the application on no longer than 30 minutes at a time, checking the skin frequently for irritation. Tell the patient to report any increased pain, numbness, or burning sensations. Observe for signs of the effectiveness of the therapy, such as absence of edema or decreased edema and tenderness.

Evaluation

Evaluate the effectiveness of nursing care for a patient undergoing heat or cold application therapy by comparing the patient's status with the expected patient outcomes. Examples of specific outcomes for patients undergoing heat or cold application therapy have been provided in the Planning section.

CAST THERAPY

A cast provides circumferential support and protection of an involved body part without prohibiting movement of the entire body. It may be applied to part of an extremity, an entire extremity, the entire body trunk, or part of the trunk. Usually the cast encompasses the joint above and below the bone to be immobilized. If a joint is to be immobilized, then the cast encompasses the bone above and below the joint.

While in a cast, the body part is supported and fixed in one position. The cast is applied while the body part is maintained in a functional position with proper alignment of bone fragments. The cast must fit the specific body part correctly.

The body part to be immobilized, corrected, or rested determines the type of cast applied. Some of the common types of casts are described in Table 35–5 and illustrated in Figure 35–4.

CAST APPLICATION

A cast is applied after abrasions have been cleaned and wounds dressed. The skin should be clean and dry and thoroughly inspected. The body part is maintained in the position in which the cast will harden. If the patient cannot assist, the nurse maintains the position of the body part during cast application. The patient's clothing and bed linen are protected from water and cast residue by a drape during application of the cast.

A layer of tubular stockinet is applied next to the patient's skin. The stockinet may be made of cotton or polyester. Next, a layer of thin padding is applied in a circular fashion. Extra padding may be applied over bony prominences for added protection. The padding is made of cotton or a synthetic material. The cast is then applied over the stockinet and padding.

Most casts are made of polyester, fiberglass, or thermoplastic material, but plaster of Paris casting

Table 35–5. TYPES OF CASTS

CAST	DESCRIPTION	POTENTIAL PRESSURE POINTS
Short arm cast	It extends from the palmar crease of the hand to the elbow. It allows movement of the fingers and thumb and is used for stable fractures or conditions of the metacarpals, carpals, or distal radius. If the thumb is incorporated, the cast is called a gauntlet or thumb spica cast.	Radial and ulnar styloids, also the base of the thumb
Long arm cast	It extends from the palmar crease to the proximal humerus. The elbow is encompassed, and the cast is applied with the elbow flexed in a 90-degree functional position. It is used for unstable fractures of the carpals, stable fractures or conditions of the distal humerus, and fractures and conditions of the radius or ulna.	Radial styloid, olecranon, and lateral epicondyle
Hanging arm cast	It is a heavy, long arm cast used to apply pull or light traction on the humerus. It is suspended by a bandage encircling the neck and attached at the wrist. The patient is maintained in an upright position.	Radial and ulnar styloid, lateral and medial epicondyles, olecranon, and the cervical vertebrae
Short leg cast	It extends from the toes to just below the knee joint. It is used for stable fractures or conditions, such as fusions of the metatarsals, calcaneus, talus, and tarsal bones. It may be fitted with a wedge attached to the foot portion to allow walking and weight-bearing. The attachment may be applied with the initial cast or after complete drying.	Lateral and medial malleolus and fibular head. Pressure to the peroneal nerve may result in footdrop.
Patellar tendon weight-bearing cast	It extends from the toes to the knee. It is molded over the patellar tendon, femoral condyles, and popliteal space. The molded contour controls rotation of the knee. It is used to treat unstable fractures of the tibia and fibula.	Lateral and medial malleous and fibular head
Long leg cast	It extends from the toes to the groin and includes the knee joint. It immobilizes the tibia, fibula, knee, and ankle joint and is used to treat stable injuries of the knee and distal femur. It is applied with the knee slightly flexed to relax the ligaments.	Lateral and medial malleous and the fibular head
Cylinder cast	It extends from just above the malleoli to the upper thigh. It is used to treat stable injuries of the proximal tibia, knee, or distal femur.	Fibular head and malleoli and heel
Spica cast	It encompasses one or more extremities and the body trunk.	Malleoli, fibular heads, and iliac crests for the hip spica casts. Care must taken to prevent pressure on the mesenteric artery from the lower trunk portion of the cast.
One-half hip spica	It encompasses one leg and the lower trunk. It restricts pelvis rotation and limits hip movement.	
One and one-half hip spica	It encompasses one whole leg, the lower trunk, and half of the other leg. It also restricts pelvic rotation and hip movement.	
Double hip spica	It encompasses both legs and the lower trunk. It immobilizes both hip joints. Hip spica casts are used to immobilize the pelvis, hip joints, femur, and knee after injuries or surgery. An abduction bar may be incorporated into the cast for support.	
Shoulder spica	It encompasses one arm and its shoulder and the upper trunk. It is used in unstable fractures of the shoulder girdle, humerus, and elbow joint, or conditions of the shoulder such as a fusion.	Iliac crest, ulnar styloid, lateral and medial epicondyle, and olecranon for the shoulder spica casts
Cast brace	It is used for mid to distal shaft fractures of the femur and utilizes the compression of soft tissue of thigh and upper leg to splint and support a fracture. It is often used after 2 to 6 weeks of skeletal traction or in conjunction with an internal fixation device. It has three sections: a short leg cast, a thigh lacer or contoured thigh cast, and metal or plastic knee hinges. It allows earlier mobilization of the patient with a fractured femur and permits some weight-bearing and movement of the knee joint. An elastic support stocking is worn over the leg, under the cast brace.	Lateral and medial malleoli and the fibular head
Body cast	It encircles the trunk to immobilize the spine. The cervical, thoracic, or lumbar spine may be immobilized for repair of injuries or following operative procedures.	Superior mesenteric artery

material may be used in some instances. Each of the different casting materials requires an agent such as water or heat to prepare the substance for use. Plaster of Paris and polyester casting material are moistened with water. Fiberglass is moistened with water or a special agent. The thermoplastic materials are prepared by hot water or hot air. The various materials differ in characteristics and cost.

Casts made of synthetic materials are ready for weight-bearing within minutes after application. Plaster of Paris casts require several hours for drying of the material. A long leg cast of plaster can take 24 to 48 hours to dry completely and allow weight-bearing.

Synthetic casts weigh less and are more durable than plaster of Paris casts and are immersible in

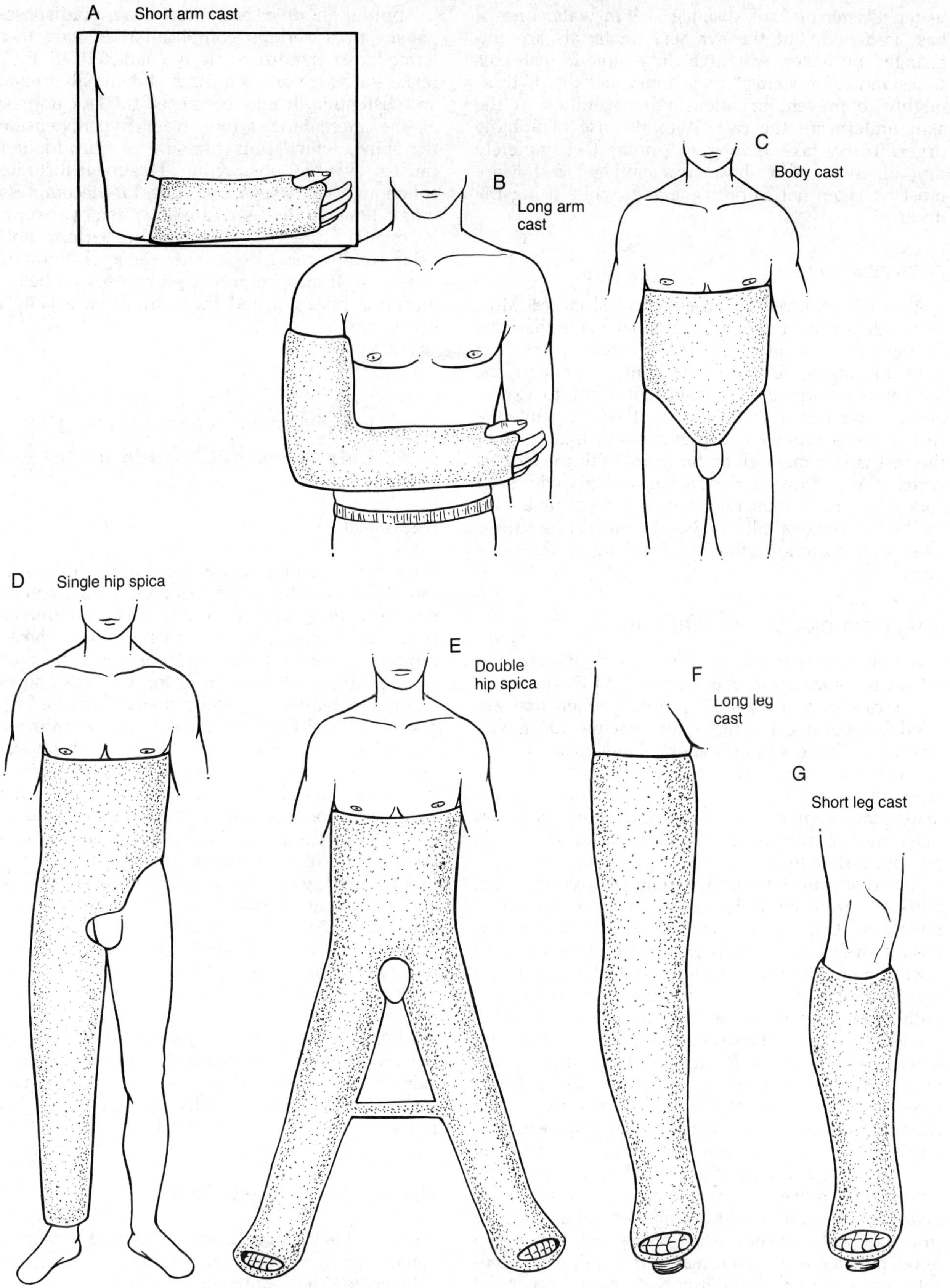

Figure 35–4.

Various types of casts used for musculoskeletal disorders.

water. Plaster of Paris disintegrates in water once it has hardened, but the synthetic materials are unchanged by water. Although the synthetic materials withstand dampening, they must be dried thoroughly to prevent irritation and maceration of the skin underneath the cast. With the use of a blow dryer, it may take as long as 3 hours to completely dry all layers of a short arm synthetic cast. Care must be taken not to burn the skin while using the dryer.

CAST REMOVAL

A cast is removed by an electric cast cutter. Most cast cutters use an oscillating circular blade that cuts through the cast material. These cutters produce a loud buzzing noise that may frighten a patient. The patient is informed in advance of what to expect and is cautioned to avoid moving the limb while the cast is being removed to prevent skin injury. Once the cast is separated along the sides with the electric cutter, the padding and stockinet are cut with scissors. The cast is then removed, top piece first. This method of removal allows the bottom cast half to be used as a posterior splint for handling of the body part.

COMPLICATIONS OF CAST THERAPY

A cast that is too tight constricts circulation and causes pressure areas, skin lesions, and tissue necrosis. A cast may seem to fit properly when first applied but become too tight from edema that develops after the cast application. Conversely, a cast applied to an edematous body part may become too loose when the edema subsides and may provide inadequate support for the affected part. In either case, the cast must be altered or replaced to provide an appropriate fit.

The cast cutter is used to cut through the cast without removing it to release the pressure of a tight cast. Cutting the cast allows edematous soft tissues under the cast to expand without compromising neurovascular function. Once the edema has subsided, the cast is usually sealed and reinforced with an elastic wrap or additional casting material.

Casts, except preformed ones, are applied by layering the materials. Because of the multiple layers of material, any drainage from beneath the cast surfaces to the outside of the cast very slowly. This characteristic of casting material causes difficulty in determining the exact extent of drainage produced at a given time. It may take several days for a small amount of drainage to completely ooze to the outer layer of the cast. Circling and recording time of drainage noted on the surface of the cast, although a good practice in general, may not provide an accurate estimate of the current drainage occurring under the cast or the time it occurred. The patient's subjective sensations of wetness and an assessment of vital signs are the best indicators of hemorrhage under a cast.

Application of a body cast may predispose the patient to a serious complication of cast therapy termed cast syndrome. It is characterized by anorexia, nausea, vomiting, and abdominal discomfort and distention. It may be caused by the compression of the mesenteric artery from hyperextension of the spine, which puts pressure on the duodenum, causing eventual obstruction. Treatment includes instillation of a nasogastric tube for decompression, intravenous fluids, and possibly, removal or readjustment of the cast. This syndrome may not develop until several weeks after the application of the body cast. It may be prevented by use of a belly pad during application and the addition of a belly hole in the cast.

Application of the Nursing Process to the Care of the Patient with a Cast

Assessment

Prior to the casting, assess the skin for lesions, areas of redness, swelling, and irritation. Check and document proximal and distal neurovascular function to establish a baseline. After the casting, check for proper cast fit by assessing neurovascular status of the area involved every hour for 48 hours and every 8 hours thereafter. If distal pulses are covered by the cast, check capillary refill, color, and warmth of the extending part. Observe for skin irritation under and around the cast edge and on bony prominences. Assess for any drainage or foul odors, which may indicate lesions or infection of lesions under the cast. Assess the patient's knowledge about self-care and the care of the cast prior to discharge.

If the patient is in a body cast, observe for signs and symptoms of cast syndrome or restricted chest expansion. Auscultate breath sounds in exposed areas of the chest, if applicable, for early signs of respiratory problems. Observe the perineal area, noting any problems with fecal matter or urine on the cast.

After cast removal, observe the skin for dryness, irritation, or the presence of breakdown. Expect the skin to be somewhat dry, pale, and slightly irritated. Inspect the limb for atrophy, weakness, and loss of range of motion.

Nursing Diagnoses and Planning

Nursing diagnoses and related expected patient outcomes most commonly applicable to patients with a cast include the following:

NDx: Altered tissue perfusion, peripheral, related to constriction of circulation and possible nerve or vascular damage from the cast

Planning: Patient outcomes
1. Patient's extremities are warm, color is adequate, and pulses are present.
2. Patient presents no evidence of complications from compromised circulation.
3. Patient denies pain or decreased sensation in extremities distal to the cast.

NDx: Impaired skin integrity related to insufficient peripheral circulation and/or irritation from the cast over the skin and bony prominences

Planning: Patient outcomes
1. Patient verbalizes factors associated with irritation and skin lesions and measures to prevent the occurrence or recurrence.
2. Patient relates appropriate knowledge about skin care.
3. Patient is free of skin complications.

NDx: Self-care deficit in areas of feeding, hygiene, toileting, or other activities of daily living related to impaired mobility

Planning: Patient outcomes
1. Patient performs activities of daily living, using assistive devices as necessary.
2. Patient states alternative methods to complete tasks that are restricted by musculoskeletal dysfunction and cast therapy.

NDx: Pain related to pressure of the cast, itching, or inability to move freely

Planning: Patient outcomes
1. Patient denies feelings of discomfort, itching, or other irritation from the cast.
2. Patient rests and sleeps well and appears relaxed and able to cope with wearing the cast.

NDx: Impaired home maintenance management related to self-care needed and care of the cast

Planning: Patient outcomes
1. Patient states accurate information about self-care and cast care after discharge (see Chart 35–1).
2. Patient states the signs of complications of cast therapy and when to seek medical intervention.
3. Patient relates the measures necessary to lessen the risk of complications.
4. Patient shows no evidence of complications of cast therapy, such as inability to complete activities of daily living, deformities, skin breakdown, or infection.

Nursing Interventions

NDx: Altered tissue perfusion, peripheral
Keep the patient in a comfortable position, and reposition frequently to release pressure. Use range-of-motion exercises to stimulate circulation. Monitor vital signs and laboratory studies to assess for changes and improvements in status. Encourage ambulation as allowed, but provide for frequent rest periods to decrease cardiac workload and prevent further compromised peripheral circulation.

Discourage smoking to avoid vasoconstriction. Remove constricting clothing, and keep heavy bed linen from restricting peripheral circulation. Tell the patient to notify the nurse if signs of compromised circulation from the cast seem apparent, such as discoloration, pain, swelling, or numbness of an extremity. Keep the patient's legs in a nondependent position when not ambulating.

NDx: Impaired skin integrity
Teach the patient measures to prevent skin lesions from developing. Have the patient inspect the skin frequently around the edges of the cast, and instruct the patient to seek medical assistance if any breakdown or soreness is noted.

Teach the patient to exercise, as tolerated, to promote good circulation to the skin. Range-of-motion exercises should be done while on bed rest. Turn the patient frequently, and inspect pressure areas for early signs of breakdown. Inspect the areas distal to the cast for signs of compromised circulation. If lesions are present, use aseptic technique to cleanse them. Teach the patient and family members the proper technique for dressing areas of breakdown.

Keep the cast and skin around the cast clean and dry. If the cast extends to the perineal area, clean the patient thoroughly after urination or bowel movements. Teach the patient or family to do the same at home to prevent breakdown of the skin in the perineal area.

NDx: Self-care deficit
Assist the patient with activities of daily living as needed. Seek alternative methods for the patient to be able to complete these activities when restricted by the cast. Assist the patient as needed in cleaning the perineal area. Position the patient for maximum comfort for urination.

Teach the patient how to maneuver with the assistance of supportive aids. Explain how to utilize other extremities to complete a task or how to move appropriately with the restrictive device in place, such as how to use crutches when the patient's leg is in a cast. Seek the assistance of physical therapists or occupational therapists when necessary for consultation or teaching sessions for the patient and family.

NDx: Pain
Instruct the patient how to move in bed using assistive devices such as an overhead trapeze or the side rails. Once the patient is able to be out of bed, assist with the changes in balance or weight-bearing, if applicable, when mobile. Help the patient change positions frequently to relieve pressure areas. Give pain medications as prescribed to reduce discomfort. Relieve pressure areas from the cast by cutting windows if ordered.

NDx: Impaired home maintenance management

Instruct the patient about the effects of immobility if the patient is in a full body cast and the effects of disuse of the affected extremity in the case of an arm or leg cast. (See Mobility Impairment in the section on Clinical Manifestations.) Teach the patient and family the signs of complications, such as elimination difficulty, discoloration of the skin, skin breakdown, diminished pulses, numbness, and the symptoms of infections. Tell the patient when to seek medical assistance if symptoms appear. Explain the need for safety measures if locomotion is a problem.

Teach the patient about cast care management as described in Chart 35–1. Explain proper methods necessary to prevent further irritation and ulceration of skin where pressure has occurred from the cast. Allow the patient to ask questions as needed. Include the family in the education sessions when appropriate.

Additional Interventions

Once the cast has been applied and until it is dry, provide firm support for the entire cast. Cleanse any excess casting material from the skin. Have a cast cutter available in case the cast needs to be removed quickly as a result of extreme swelling or just bivalved to release minor pressure from edema. Reposition the patient frequently, maintaining body and cast alignment. Initiate measures to promote comfort and combat itching, such as massaging the skin around the edges of the cast, directing cool air under the cast, or encouraging isometric exercises of the casted body part to increase blood flow and decrease itching, unless contraindicated.

Prepare the patient with a cast for the appearance of dry, scaly skin and lack of muscle strength and tone in the affected part upon the removal of the cast. Also, provide proper care of the body part after removal of the cast by washing the skin gently with a mild soap and water. Gently cleanse the area to remove dead skin. Apply lotion with lanolin as a protective emollient to the dry areas.

If the patient is in a spica or body cast, assess for abdominal distention, nausea, and vomiting, which are symptoms of pressure on the mesenteric artery or abdomen. Place the patient in a prone or side-lying position if any abdominal symptoms occur, and notify the attending physician. Encourage good nutrition to promote healing and to help maintain proper elimination patterns.

Evaluation

Evaluate the effectiveness of nursing care for a patient with a cast by comparing the patient's status with the expected patient outcomes. Examples of specific outcomes for patients with a cast have been provided in the Planning section.

TRACTION THERAPY

Traction is a pulling force applied to a body part while countertraction pulls in the opposite direction. The pulling force is usually generated by a system of weights and pulleys attached to the patient's body. Countertraction is generated by the body's own weight, although it may also be applied by weights and pulleys. The traction or force applied to the body is classified by the direction of the pulling force and the way the force is applied. The direction is either straight or vectored. Straight traction pulls only in one direction, usually in line with the longitudinal axis of the involved bone. Vectored traction is the pulling force that results when traction is applied in two different directions.

Traction is used as a therapeutic intervention for a variety of musculoskeletal problems. Traction may be used to do the following:

1. Reduce a fracture or return the pieces of bone to the original position and proper anatomic alignment.
2. Lessen muscle spasm and prevent muscle contractions that displace fractured bone fragments and create pain.
3. Maintain a reduction while the bone heals.
4. Prevent or correct a deformity by decreasing skin and muscle contractures around a joint or injured part. Traction may be used alone or in conjunction with surgery for this purpose.
5. Lessen the chance of necrosis due to pressure on the articular surfaces of an injured joint and to rest the joint after a fracture within the joint capsule or joint dislocation.

PRINCIPLES OF TRACTION

For any type of traction, to achieve the desired effect of rapid healing with optimum function, the basic principles of traction must be followed. The pull of the traction as well as the use of weights and counterweights, as ordered, must be set up and maintained in an appropriate manner. The principles of traction are detailed in Table 35–6 .

TYPES OF TRACTION

Traction can be applied to the body by manual traction, skin traction, or skeletal traction. Manual traction is applied to a body part when someone, such as the physician, pulls on it. Manual traction is used to reduce a fracture or a dislocated joint. It is effective only as long as the pull is maintained by the individual applying the manual traction. For long-term application of traction, the pulling force is maintained by a system of weights, ropes, and pulleys attached to the patient's skin or skeleton.

Skin traction applies indirect pulling force to the skeleton. It is accomplished by attaching wide strips of adhesive or nonadhesive strapping to the skin from which weights are suspended by ropes and

Chart 35–1.

NURSING GUIDE TO PATIENT EDUCATION FOR SELF-MANAGEMENT: DISCHARGE INSTRUCTIONS AFTER CAST APPLICATION

Instruct the patient to:

Allow air to circulate around the cast until thoroughly dried from the inside out. (For plaster casts only.)
Refrain from using external heat sources to hasten the drying process, as this may result in burns under the cast. (For plaster casts only.)
Refrain from placing plastic or rubber materials around or under a fresh cast because the heat produced by the cast will be directed toward the skin and cause irritation or burns. (For plaster casts only.)
Use the palms of the hands, not the finger tips, when handling the wet cast, to prevent distortion of the cast. (For plaster casts only.)
Protect the wet cast from resting on hard surfaces that might cause distortion of the cast. (For plaster casts only.)
Keep the cast clean and dry. The cast may be wiped clean with a damp cloth. Extra care is needed if the cast extends to the perineal area.
Refrain from inserting sharp objects under the cast, or injury to the skin may result.
Cover rough edges of the cast with tape "petals" to prevent skin irritation and crumbling of the cast edges once it has dried completely.
Observe the cast for areas of softening or indentation, and report observations to the attending physician.
Exercise the joints proximal and distal to the cast if not contraindicated, to prevent muscle atrophy, weakness, and loss of joint motion.
Keep casted extremities elevated above the heart level (whenever possible) to reduce swelling, unless compartment syndrome is suspected.
Report fever or foul odors and drainage from under the cast.
Report swelling, burning, numbness, coldness, discoloration of the skin, decreased sensation, persistent pain, or tingling to the attending physician immediately.
Refrain from using emollient lotions on the skin around the cast because they may run down into the cast, causing dampness and becoming a potential site for bacterial growth.
Refrain from putting talcum powder down the cast because it tends to build up on the skin. Corn starch may be used for perspiration control.
If the cast requires the use of an assistive device for locomotion, such as crutches or a walker, be sure to follow safety instructions for the use of the device. Rearrange the home environment to accommodate the ambulatory aid to prevent falls or other injuries.

Table 35–6. PRINCIPLES OF TRACTION

PRINCIPLE	NURSING IMPLICATION
The pull of traction must be continuous, unless specified otherwise by the attending physician.	Remove or add weights only by a physician's order. Discontinue or release the traction only on the physician's order.
The ropes and weights must be free of friction.	Keep the ropes from becoming entangled in the linen. Be certain the weights hang free at all times. Keep the ropes over the center of the pulley.
There must be sufficient countertraction maintained at all times.	Keep the patient from sliding to the foot of the bed. Keep the patient in side-arm traction in the center of the bed.

pulleys (Figs. 35–5 and 35–6). Belts and halters may be used when a pull is desired on the spine.

Skin traction is used only for temporary management of fractures in adults because the skin cannot tolerate the weight for the long length of time required for healing. Normal skin can tolerate 5 to 7 lb of weight pulling for approximately 3 to 4 weeks without damage.

Skin traction is contraindicated in the presence of skin abrasions or wounds, dermatitis, impaired circulation, varicose ulcers, and peripheral neuropathies. It is used with extra caution on individuals with diabetes mellitus because of the high risk of skin and circulatory disorders in these patients. Skin traction does not control rotation of a body part.

Complications associated with skin traction include allergic reaction to the adhesive; irritation of skin from belts, straps, or halters; peroneal nerve

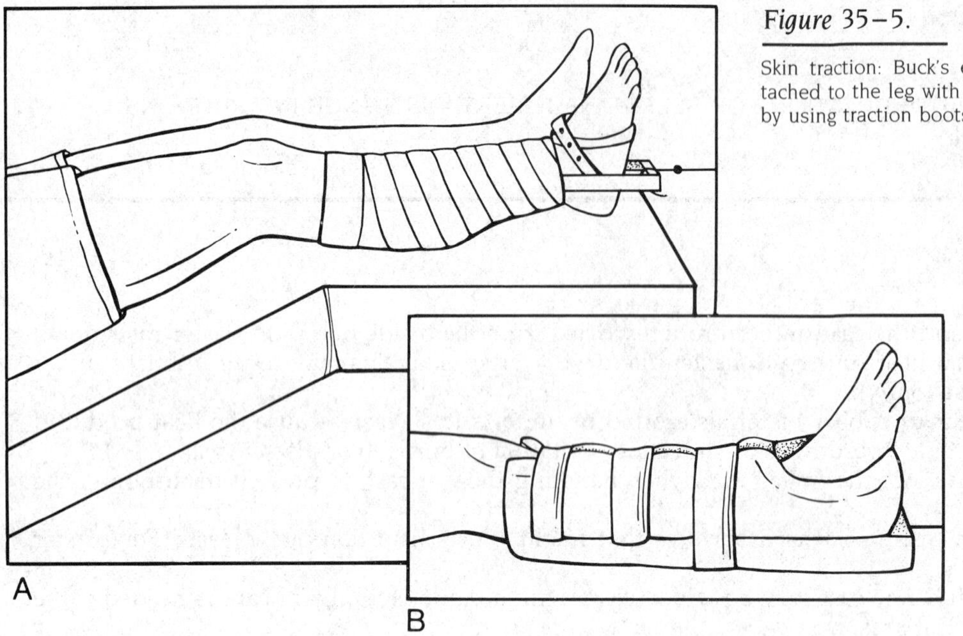

Figure 35–5.

Skin traction: Buck's extension. The traction may be attached to the leg with wraps or skin adhesive strips (A) or by using traction boots (B).

palsy from pressure over the lateral fibular head; and pressure sores around malleoli and radial and ulnar styloids.

Adhesive skin traction is applied to clean, dry skin that has had the hair removed for better adhesion. Hair is best removed by an electric shaver, clipping with scissors, or use of a commercial skin depilatory because shaving with a razor blade can cut the skin. A nonirritating protective adhesive agent may be applied to the skin first. Adhesive strips or material with a hypoallergenic gummed surface that allows air to reach the skin is then applied. A spreader helps keep the pressure off the bony prominences and provides a connection for the rope. The adhesive strips are then wrapped with an elastic bandage. The bandage is wrapped diagonally or in a modified figure eight. It should be snug but not tight or constricting. The adhesive is never applied to bony prominences or over superficial nerves. These areas can be protected with cast padding to prevent adhesion of the tape.

Some conditions may be treated by intermittent skin traction applied by belts or nonadhesive straps. Intermittent skin traction allows removal of the weights for bathing and inspecting the skin, toileting, and some limited activity.

Skeletal traction applies a pulling force directly to a body part by metal pins, screws, or tongs inserted into bone. The metal is made of nonferrous material and is generally placed into cancellous bone distal to the fracture or affected body part. The pins, screws, or tongs for skeletal traction are inserted in the operating room using surgical asepsis.

A small incision is made in the skin, and the metal piece is drilled by hand into the bone. The metal pins, screws, or tongs are then attached to a U-shaped bow or similar device as illustrated in Figure 35–7. The bow is connected by rope to weights via a free-hanging pulley system. Areas away from nerves and blood vessels are selected for insertion sites. The body can tolerate skeletal traction of 20 to 30 lb for as long as 3 or 4 months. The amount of weight applied varies with the condition and part of the body being treated.

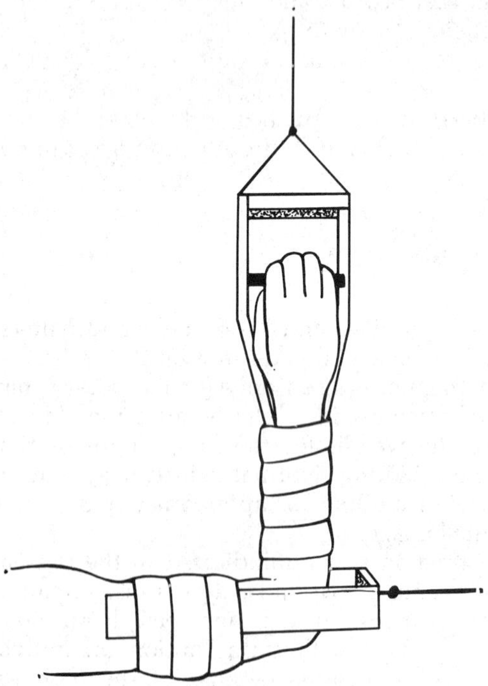

Figure 35–6.

Skin traction: side arm.

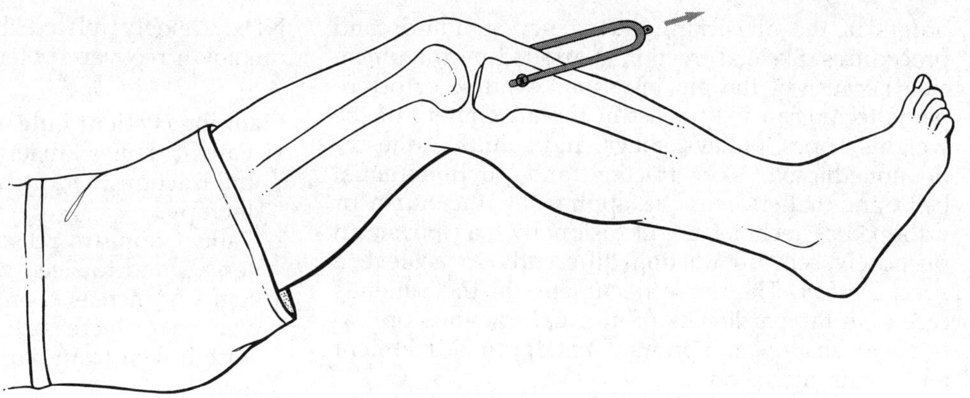

Figure 35–7.

Skeletal traction: Steinmann pin. The pin is inserted through the bone and attached to the bow. Traction is maintained with ropes, pulleys, and weights attached to the top of the bow. This immobilizes and maintains alignment of the body part for extended lengths of time.

Skeletal traction is effective in reducing and maintaining alignment of fracture fragments because it provides control of rotation as well as longitudinal pull. Skeletal traction, applied by use of Steinmann pins or a Kirschner wire, is used primarily for fractures or disorders of the pelvis, acetabulum, and femur. Skeletal traction is seldom used for upper extremity fractures except in the case of complicated distal humerus and elbow injuries or disorders.

Skeletal traction to an arm or leg may be combined with a splint to create a balanced suspension apparatus. The splint maintains suspension and alignment of the limb while other body parts move about freely. A Thomas (or Hodgen) splint is frequently used for balanced suspension to the lower extremity. A Pearson attachment may be clamped to the splint at the level of the knee to permit flexion of the knee and movement of the lower leg. When the leg is suspended in this apparatus, the foot also needs support to prevent footdrop. Remove foot supports regularly for ankle exercise amd to inspect the skin. Elastic or rubber bands attached to a foot splint allow exercise without removing the splint.

Traction to the cervical spine is applied by inserting metal tongs into the parietal prominences of the skull as illustrated in Figure 35–8. Some common types of tongs are Crutchfield, Vinke, Gardner-Wells, and Barton. Screws and a ring or halo may also be used to immobilize the cervical spine. To prevent rotation of the spine, the halo apparatus is connected to a body jacket, vest, or cast (Fig. 35–9).

APPLICATION OF TRACTION

The physician prescribes the type and amount of traction to be applied. Who applies the traction varies according to the type of traction, specific

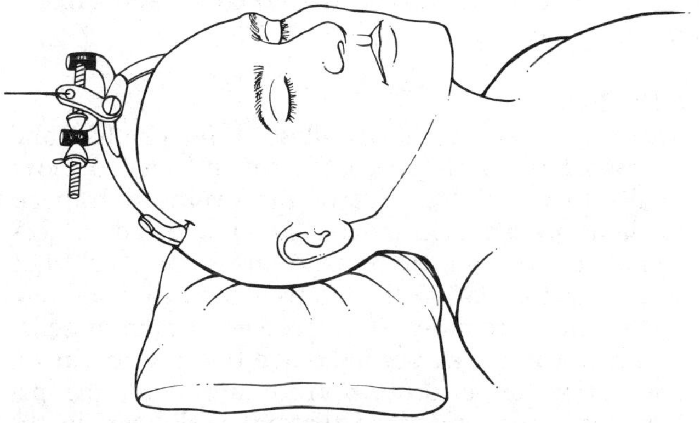

Figure 35–8.

Crutchfield skull tongs. The cervical traction apparatus is attached directly to the skull.

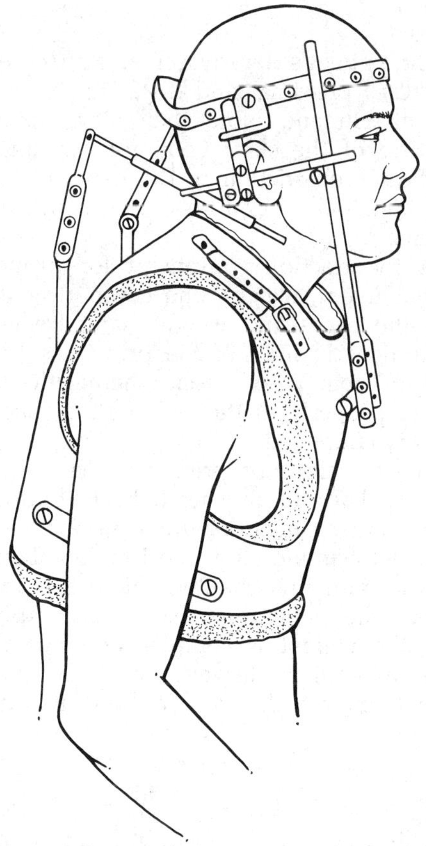

Figure 35–9.

Halo traction apparatus with body brace.

orders of the physician, and agency standards and procedures. Skeletal traction is applied by the physician because of the pin insertion. A nurse or orthopedic technician may assist in the attachment of the weights, ropes, pulleys, slings, and splints. Adhesive or nonadhesive skin traction and circumferential belts and halters may be applied by the nurse or orthopedic technician. Occasionally, a physician purposely sets up traction differently to achieve a special effect. The nurse documents in the patient's care plan the particulars of unusual traction applications to ensure an optimum result from treatment and continuity of care.

The patient in traction is placed in a bed with a firm mattress that allows connection of an overbed frame. This frame is primarily used to attach parts of the traction apparatus but may also be used to attach a trapeze. The trapeze enables the patient to move independently in bed within the limits of the traction apparatus.

Application of the Nursing Process to the Care of the Patient in Traction

Assessment

Assess the patient's neurovascular status frequently. Check pulses proximal and distal to the site of the traction attachment. Note the color, texture, and temperature of the skin. Look for swelling, which may indicate constriction of the extremity. Ask the patient about pain, numbness, or tingling in the affected part.

Assess the traction equipment for proper alignment, attachment, weight, and countertraction. Note whether the ropes and weight hang freely. Assess the equipment in light of the principles of traction as listed in Table 35–6. Check whether the patient is positioned properly in the bed for the type of traction being maintained.

Observe for signs of pressure areas, such as on the elbows, back of the head, back, buttocks, and heels and under slings or wraps. Assess for signs of the hazards of immobility (see Mobility Impairment secton earlier in this chapter). Note the amount of movement the patient is able to accomplish. Ask whether the patient is completing range-of-motion exercises at regular intervals. Check the positioning of the foot, and watch for evidence of footdrop.

Nursing Diagnoses and Planning

Nursing diagnoses and related expected patient outcomes most commonly applicable to patients in traction include those described previously for patients with impaired mobility and the following:

NDx: Anxiety related to fear of the equipment and unknown recovery potential, and discomfort

Planning: Patient outcomes

1. Patient denies anxiety, fear, or nervousness about the traction therapy and potential outcome of the therapy.
2. Patient appears relaxed and is able to rest at intervals and to sleep well.
3. Signs of increased anxiety, such as twitching, nervousness, increased respirations and pulse, or withdrawal from participation in care, are absent.

NDx: Pain related to inability to move well or change positions easily in bed as a result of the traction therapy, pressure from the pulling force or method of attachment of the apparatus, and/or irritation, at site of injury

Planning: Patient outcomes

1. Patient denies pressure, pain, or discomfort.
2. Patient is able to exercise and move somewhat, within the confines of the traction equipment.

Nursing Interventions

NDx: Anxiety

Explain the purpose of all the traction equipment to the patient. Teach the patient how to use the trapeze for readjustment of position in the bed. Explain the necessity of maintenance of body and traction alignment. Prior to performing any procedure on the patient, explain the steps of the procedure and the reason for it. Allow the patient time to ask questions and relay concerns. Check vital signs, and watch for changes indicating increased anxiety. Teach the patient relaxation methods and strategies to cope with the fears of hospitalization. Have the patient practice range-of-motion exercises to help relieve discomfort from the static position and to maintain muscle tone and joint motion. Also, provide diversional activity for the patient to relieve the boredom and anxiety from bed rest.

NDx: Pain

Reposition the patient, as allowed, for comfort and release of pressure. Teach the patient how to move in the bed with the use of the overhead trapeze. Explain how much movement is allowed. Check complaints of pain or pressure areas for cause. Leg wrapping that is too tight causes increased discomfort in the extremities. Give prescribed pain or sedation medications as needed. Give the medication for pain prior to performing procedures with the patient that cause increased discomfort. Be certain the traction equipment is in proper alignment, with the appropriate weight. Incorrect use of the equipment may aggravate the patient's discomfort as well as cause harm to the patient.

Table 35–7. PIN SITE CARE

Regardless of the type of pin, screw, or tong used to maintain traction or immobility of a body part, the care of the pin site is an important nursing responsibility. The nurse provides the following care every shift (or as otherwise prescribed in terms of the care routine and frequency):

1. Assess around the pin site for redness, swelling, increase in tenderness, and the presence of drainage.
2. Examine the pin for breakage, bending, or shifting.
3. Use a prescribed cleansing agent.
4. With gloved hands, clean from the pin site outward using sterile cotton-tipped applicators and the prescribed cleansing agent. Use a separate applicator for each site to eliminate possible cross contamination.
5. Refrain from applying ointments to the site, unless specifically ordered, because they tend to occlude drainage and keep the site moist, which increases the potential for bacterial growth.
6. If drainage is evident, notify the physician, who will determine whether a culture of the drainage should be obtained and if sites are to be covered.

Additional Interventions
To prevent infection at the site of the insertion of pins, wires, or tongs, perform pin site care as described in Table 35–7.

Evaluation

Evaluate the effectiveness of nursing care for a patient in traction by comparing the patient's status with the expected patient outcomes. Examples of specific outcomes for patients in traction have been provided in the Planning section.

Surgical Management

EXTERNAL FIXATION DEVICES

Treatment of musculoskeletal disorders by simple casting or prolonged immobility in traction is not appropriate for all patients or all disorders. In some situations, an external fixation device may be used to stabilize the involved bone or joint.

An external fixation device consists of a metal frame with attached metal percutaneous pins that are held rigidly in place by the frame. The percutaneous pins are inserted into or through the bone above and below a fracture or defect in the bone or joint. An external fixation device is used to compress bone fragments and to maintain alignment for bone, joint, or soft tissue healing. An external fixation device is illustrated in Figure 35–10.

Indications for external fixation therapy include open fractures with nerve and vascular damage, open contaminated fractures with soft tissue damage and infection, severe comminuted fractures, leg lengthening, joints to be removed temporarily, and joint fusions. Access to wounds for assesment of healing and neurovascular function, debridement, dressing changes, irrigations, skin grafting, and burn injury treatment are possible while stabilization of the bone is maintained. An external fixation device can also be used after skeletal traction to maintain alignment until there is complete bone or joint healing. This allows earlier ambulation and discharge, which decreases the risk of complications of immobility.

External fixation may be used for almost any bone. Fractures of long bones of the extremities; elbow, wrist, knee, and ankle disorder; and unstable fractures of the pelvic ring are situations for which external fixation therapy is frequently applied. There are a number of different external fixation systems made by various manufacturers, but the principle of each system is similar.

In some situations, external fixation is used to stabilize a severely injured limb during treatment in an effort to avoid amputation. Despite these efforts, the patient may still lose the limb.

Application of the Nursing Process to the Care of the Patient with an External Fixation Device

Assessment

Assess the pin sites and the neurovascular status of the involved limb. Check the stability of the frame and security of the pins at least once every 4 hours until discharge. Assess any wounds and soft tissue injuries for odor, drainage, inflammation, or necrotic areas. Assess the patient's knowledge about self-care after discharge and about care of the pin site and fixation device.

Nursing Diagnoses and Planning

Nursing diagnoses and related expected patient outcomes most commonly applicable to patients with an external fixation device include the following:

NDx: Anxiety related to the appearance of the device and ability to manage self-care and maintain independence with the device in place

Planning: Patient outcomes
1. Patient denies anxiety, fear, or nervousness about self-care and management with the device in place.
2. Patient looks at the device with acceptance.
3. Patient verbalizes feeling relaxed, resting at intervals, and sleeping well.

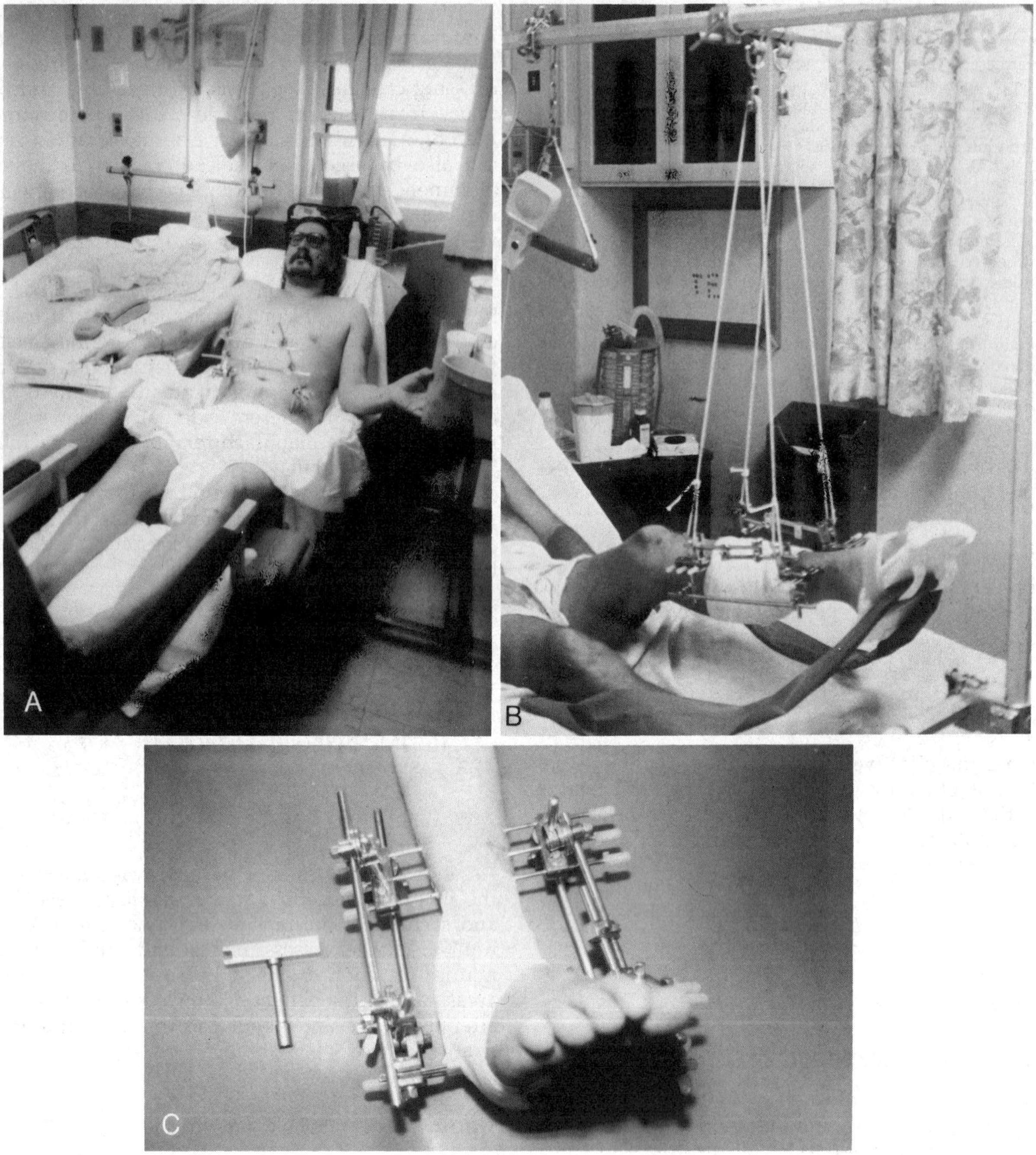

Figure 35–10.

External fixation devices. A, An external fixator applied to the pelvis. Pins are inserted directly into the bone and attached to an external frame. Note that the patient is able to be moved from the bed. B, Suspension of a lower leg in an external fixator. Note that the ropes are used with pulleys to allow movement up and down in bed. The foot splint has been released for better visualization. The foot splint may be worn for 4 to 6 hours and released for 2-hour intervals. C, An external fixator applied to the ankle. Half of the pins are exposed and half are within a wound, covered by dressings. All adjustments for the external scaffolding can be made with the T-handle wrench shown at the side.

4. Signs of increased anxiety, such as twitching, nervousness, and increased respirations and pulse, are absent.

NDx: Impaired home maintenance management related to the external fixation device, pin site care, and mobility management

Planning: Patient outcomes

1. Patient states appropriate information about care and management of the device and when to notify the physician if problems become evident.
2. Patient demonstrates correct pin site care.
3. Patient moves safely with the fixation device intact, using assistive devices if needed.

NDx: High risk for infection related to the pin sites and other soft tissue injuries

Planning: Patient outcomes
1. Patient remains free from infection.
2. Patient's skin shows signs of healing such as new granulation tissue and closure of wounds.
3. Patient verbalizes correct pin site care.

Nursing Interventions

NDx: Anxiety
Reinforce the physician's explanation about the need for the external fixation device and how it will help the patient to become mobile. Prior to the application of the device, show a picture of it to the patient to reduce surprise, fear, and anxiety afterward. Allow time for questions or verbalization of concerns from the patient or family. Assist the patient in finding strategies that enhance effective coping. Refer the patient to social services, physical therapy, or occupational therapy if needed for assistance with adjustment of lifestyle and maintenance of independence. Seek assistance of clergy or a professional counselor if appropriate.

NDx: Impaired home maintenance management
Teach the patient how to care for the fixation device and when to notify the physician if problems arise. Demonstrate pin site care, as detailed in Table 35–7, to the patient, and allow time for the patient to practice it with supervision. Reinforce the physician's instructions about weight-bearing and manipulation of the device. Discuss limitations, if any, and the use of the affected limb. Encourage the patient to continue with the prescribed exercises to maintain muscle strength and range of motion of joints adjacent to the affected part.

Teach the patient the appropriate use of the assistive device, if applicable, or refer the patient to physical therapy or occupational therapy. Provide for the patient's safety by assisting with movement until the patient can securely manage alone or with the assistive device. Discuss any obstacles that may interfere with the patient's safe mobility in the home setting. Help the patient plan modifications of the home environment if needed.

Provide the patient with suggestions on how to modify clothing to fit over the apparatus. Assist with preparations for self-care after discharge. Allow the patient to practice with self-help aids that may be needed to assist with daily hygiene and grooming tasks or other activities of daily living. Teach the patient about dosage, frequency of administration, and side effects of any analgesics or other medications prescribed.

NDx: High risk for infection
Teach the patient to watch for signs of localized infection, such as redness, swelling, increased pain or drainage at the pin sites, and signs of systemic infection, such as fever, increased pulse and respiratory rate, and general malaise. Be certain the patient understands aseptic pin site care. Tell the patient to report any signs of infection to the attending physician.

Evaluation

Evaluate the effectiveness of nursing care for a patient with an external fixation device by comparing the patient's status with the expected patient outcomes. Examples of specific outcomes for patients with an external fixation device have been provided in the Planning section.

INTERNAL FIXATION DEVICES

Internal fixation devices are surgically inserted directly into or attached onto bone to provide support, to fill in a defect, or to achieve and maintain reduction of fracture fragments (Fig. 35–11). Internal fixation allows early ambulation by patients with musculoskeletal disorders.

Internal fixation devices are made of rigid, strong, biologically inert substances, such as polyethylene and nonferrous metal alloys, that can withstand considerable amounts of stress. Although most internal fixation devices are implanted completely under the skin and muscle, some may protrude through the skin and be attached to casts, traction, or external fixation devices.

Internal fixation devices include both temporary

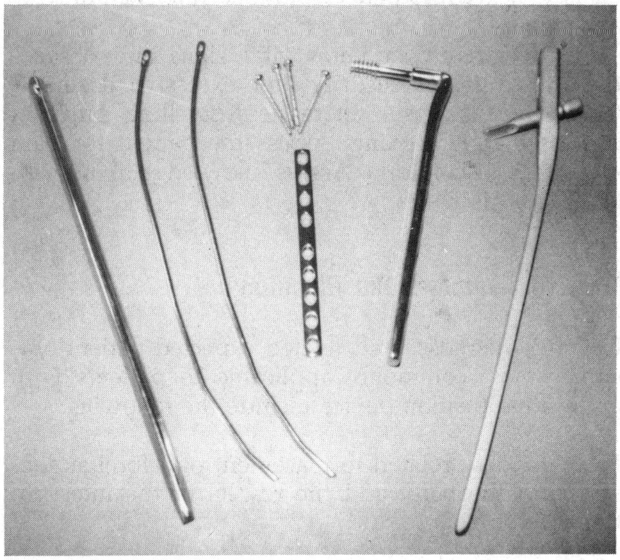

Figure 35–11.

Internal fixation devices. Left to right: K-nail, flexible intermedullary pins, plate and screws, hip compression screw, and a Zickel nail.

and permanent pins, rods, nails, screws, plates, and wires. The type of device selected depends upon the condition to be treated and the physician preference. Intraoperative fluoroscopy and postoperative radiographic studies are used to ensure proper placement of the device and correct bone alignment.

Although internal fixation devices can be of great benefit to the patient, there are complications associated with their use. These include tissue reaction to a foreign substance in the body and breakage or migration of the device. Patients with an internal fixation device may also develop an infection around the device long after surgery. Circulating bacteria from another source such as a decayed tooth or urinary tract infection can lodge on the surface of the device and multiply. Intravenous antibiotic therapy and the removal of the device may be required. To prevent the complication of infection, prophylactic antibiotics are administered before and after surgery.

Application of the Nursing Process to the Care of the Patient with an Internal Fixation Device

Assessment

Preoperatively, assess the neurovascular status of the affected body part as a baseline to detect changes in the postoperative period. Determine the patient's understanding about the surgery and the postoperative course. Ask the patient about feelings of anxiety or other concerns about the surgery. Observe for signs of anxiety, such as twitching, increased heart rate and respiratory rate, withdrawal, and crying.

Postoperatively, monitor vital signs and observe the dressings for security and excessive drainage. Check the suture site for redness, swelling, purulent drainage, and bleeding. Assess the patient for pain and other discomforts. Assess knowledge about self-care after discharge.

Nursing Diagnoses and Planning

Nursing diagnoses and related expected patient outcomes most commonly applicable to patients with an internal fixation device include the following:

NDx: Anxiety related to placement of a foreign substance in the body and the results of the intervention

Planning: Patient outcomes

1. Patient denies anxiety, fear, or nervousness about the surgery and its potential outcome.
2. Patient verbalizes being relaxed, resting at intervals, and sleeping well.
3. Signs of increased anxiety, such as twitching, nervousness, and increased respirations and pulse, are absent.

NDx: Altered health maintenance related to the lack of information about self-care, potential complications, and ability to complete activities of daily living

Planning: Patient outcomes

1. Patient states appropriate information about self-care, avoiding complications, and when to notify the physician if problems become evident.
2. Patient demonstrates correct exercise, as taught, to maintain strength and range of motion.
3. Patient moves the involved part safely, using assistive devices if needed.

NDx: High risk for infection related to the wound, surgical intervention, and foreign device

Planning: Patient outcomes

1. Patient remains free from infection.
2. Patient's suture line shows signs of healing, such as new granulation tissue, and absence of drainage, swelling, or redness.
3. Patient states an understanding for the need to take prophylactic antibiotics prior to some invasive procedures and dental work.

NDx: High risk for injury related to premature weight-bearing and/or failure of the internal fixation device

Planning: Patient outcomes

1. Patient denies problems with mobility or use of the affected part.
2. Patient remains free from injury.

NDx: Pain related to surgical intervention and muscle spasms from manipulation during placement of the device

Planning: Patient outcomes

1. Patient denies discomfort or pain.
2. Patient's affected body part returns to an acceptable level of mobility.

Nursing Interventions

NDx: Anxiety

Reinforce the physician's explanation about the need for the internal fixation device and how it will help the patient to maintain mobility. Allow time for questions or verbalization of concerns from the patient or family. Assist the patient in finding strategies that enhance effective coping. Refer the patient to social services, physical therapy, or occupational

Chart 35–2.

NURSING GUIDE TO PATIENT EDUCATION FOR SELF-MANAGEMENT: DISCHARGE INSTRUCTIONS FOLLOWING APPLICATION OF AN INTERNAL FIXATION DEVICE

Instruct the patient to:

Follow the physician's instructions regarding weight-bearing, limitations on range of motion and use of the involved extremity, and the use of ambulatory aids to prevent problems with the device.
Maintain the physical therapy routine as prescribed.
Observe for signs of infection or reaction to the internal fixation device, such as pain, redness, swelling, or fever.
Observe for signs of migration of the device, such as sudden or continuous pain, protrusion at the site of insertion, and limitation of motion of the joint.
Report any signs of infection or problems immediately to the attending physician.
Wear a MedicAlert tag to inform health care personnel of the internal fixation device, because of the risk for long-term or latent infection of the device and because magnetic resonance imaging may loosen the placement of the device.

therapy, if needed, for assistance prior to discharge. Seek assistance of clergy or a professional counselor if appropriate.

NDx: Altered health maintenance
Teach the patient how to care for the fixation device and when to notify the physician if problems arise. Reinforce the physician's instructions about weight-bearing and manipulation of the involved part. Discuss limitations, if any, and the use of the affected limb. Encourage the patient to continue with the prescribed exercises to maintain muscle strength and range of motion of joints adjacent to the affected part.

Teach the patient the appropriate use of the assistive device if applicable, or refer the patient to physical therapy or occupational therapy. Provide for the patient's safety by assisting with movement until the patient can securely manage alone or with the assistive device. Discuss any obstacles that may interfere with the patient's safe mobility in the home setting. Help the patient plan modifications of the home environment if needed.

Assist with preparations for self-care after discharge, as described in Chart 35–2. Teach the patient about dosage, frequency of administration, and side effects of any analgesics or other medications prescribed.

NDx: High risk for infection
Teach the patient to watch for signs of localized infection, such as redness, swelling, increased pain, or drainage at the suture line (see Chart 35–2). Be certain the patient understands wound care if it is still necessary after discharge. Tell the patient to report any signs of infection to the attending physician. Explain about the need to take prophylactic antibiotics prior to undergoing an invasive procedure or dental work.

NDx: High risk for injury
Reinforce the information that the physician presented to the patient about the surgery and the typical postoperative course. Explain when weight-bearing is appropriate and how to manipulate the limb until that point in time. If an assistive device is needed, teach the patient how to use it safely. Ask a physical therapist or occupational therapist to work with the patient. Teach the patient how to readjust in the home environment to maintain safety.

Tell the patient to report any untoward sign to the physician, such as sudden severe pain at the site, inability to bear weight at the appropriate time, or falls or other blows to the affected area that may occur. Demonstrate exercises that will help develop strength in preparation for weight-bearing.

NDx: Pain
Offer analgesics as prescribed, especially prior to physical therapy and other painful procedures. Position the patient for comfort, and reposition frequently unless otherwise contraindicated. Support the affected part and maintain proper alignment with pillows or blankets until the patient is able to move independently. Avoid extreme adduction or abduction of the involved body part. Elevate the extremity for 48 hours postoperatively to reduce swelling and pressure, unless otherwise ordered.

Evaluation

Evaluate the effectiveness of nursing care for a patient with an internal fixation device by comparing the patient's status with the expected patient outcomes. Examples of specific outcomes for patients with an internal fixation device have been provided in the Planning section.

TOTAL JOINT REPLACEMENT

Total joint replacement involves the surgical removal of deformed or diseased joint surfaces with replacement by smooth artificial surfaces made of metal and plastic. The implant pieces are held in place by a special bone cement called methyl methacrylate, or a special coating on the prosthesis pieces that allows bone growth into the surface of the implant. These biologic ingrowth joint prostheses have a special finish created by a sprayed- or baked-on metal surface that produces a porous finish that eliminates the need for cement. This porous surface allows new bone to grow into the artificial joint pieces and provides a strong bond between the implant and the bone.

Joint prostheses exist for most joints, but replacements for the knee, hip, shoulder, ankle, and wrist and Silastic implants for the phalanges of the fingers and toes are the most common. Numerous manufacturers produce a variety of replacement parts. Joint parts can also be custom made to fit the individual patient. One type of hip joint replacement is illustrated in Figure 35–12.

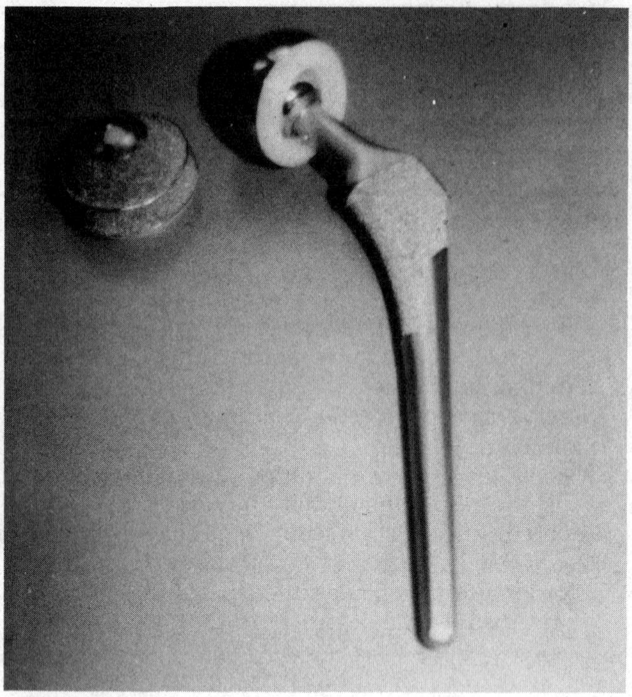

Figure 35–12.

Total hip replacement prosthesis. *Left*, A porous coated acetabular cup; *right*, a femoral stem prosthesis with a porous coating along portions of the stem with a clamp-on acetabular cup.

The purpose of joint replacement is to relieve pain and provide increased range of motion and function of the involved joint. The length of wear for an artificial joint is limited by cracking and loosening of the methyl methacrylate. An active person can expect the standard metal, plastic, and methyl methacrylate joints to last approximately 10 years. The coated or biologic ingrowth implants may provide longer wear.

All patients having a joint replacement should be aware of the potential complications and participation required for successful postoperative rehabilitation. Adverse effects of artificial joints include injury to nerves, producing pain or numbness; infection of the incision or the new joint; thromboembolism; loosening of metal or plastic parts; limb length difference; and dislocation of the new joint.

Loosening and infection within the joint can lead to loss of the implant, and additional surgery, pain, and expense to the patient. Infection may require as much as 6 weeks of intravenous antibiotic therapy. If the joint cannot be corrected, or if another replacement is not an option because of either the patient's choice or physical condition, the joint may be removed or fused.

Application of the Nursing Process to the Care of the Patient with a Total Joint Replacement

The assessment, nursing diagnoses, expected patient outcomes, nursing interventions, and evaluation for patients with a total joint replacement are similar to those described previously for patients with an internal fixation device. (Also see Nursing Care Guide 35–1.)

AMPUTATIONS

An amputation is the removal of an extremity or part of an extremity. Indications for a surgical amputation include circulatory disorders, traumatic injuries including severe thermal or crushing injuries, malignant tumors, uncontrolled infection, gangrene,

Text continued on page 1375

Nursing Care Guide 35–1.

PATIENTS UNDERGOING TOTAL HIP REPLACEMENT

Preoperative Care

Assessment Findings: Patient appears nervous, withdraws from conversation, clenches hands; blood pressure, pulse, and respirations are slightly elevated for the patient; patient makes statements indicating concern about the procedure and results of the surgical intervention, and potential problems with immobility and discomfort.

Nursing Diagnosis: Anxiety related to uncertainty about surgery, potential risk factors, discomfort, and fear of loss of mobility

Patient Outcomes	Nursing Interventions	Rationale
Patient reports feeling less nervous, seems relaxed, and is able to rest well.	Teach the patient relaxation techniques. Provide a quiet, calm environment with periods of rest during the delivery of nursing care. Ask for assistance from clergy or the patient's significant others.	Having an understanding of the procedure lessens fears and reduces anxiety. Telling the patient what to expect prior to initiating procedures for preoperative preparation reduces fear of the unknown.
Patient's vital signs are within normal ranges for the patient.	Check vital signs after the patient is rested and more relaxed, and note any changes.	Changes in vital signs may reflect increasing or decreasing anxiety levels.
Patient states methods to relax and reduce tension.	Teach deep breathing techniques and other relaxation strategies.	Practicing relaxation exercises may decrease anxiety and promote rest.

Evaluation: Compare the patient's status with the expected patient outcomes. If the outcomes are achieved, evaluate nursing care as successful. If not, reassess the patient, formulate new nursing diagnoses, and revise expected patient outcomes and nursing interventions as appropriate.

Assessment Findings: Patient and family seem very concerned about the procedure; they ask several questions about the surgery, the preparation before surgery, the joint replacement device, the expectations of the intervention, and possible complications.

Nursing Diagnosis: Knowledge deficit: nature of prosthetic surgery, preoperative preparations, expected outcome, and possible complications

Patient Outcomes	Nursing Interventions	Rationale
Patient accurately describes the purpose of the surgery and the necessity for the prosthesis.	Explain the procedure to the patient and the expected outcomes. Give the patient literature explaining the procedure and showing what the prosthesis looks like.	Explanations of all the appropriate information about the surgery to the patient and family decreases the knowledge deficit.

(continued)

Nursing Care Guide 35–1. *(continued)*

PATIENTS UNDERGOING TOTAL HIP REPLACEMENT

Patient Outcomes	Nursing Interventions	Rationale
Patient relates information about the procedure, complications, and expected results as presented to the patient by the physician.	Reinforce the information the physician presented to the patient. Have the patient relate what the physician has explained, and clear up any misunderstandings.	Having the patient repeat the information gives opportunity to correct any misinformation.
Patient reports an understanding of the preoperative preparation necessary.	Explain the preoperative preparation and allow time for questions from the patient or the family.	Giving the patient and the family the opportunity to ask questions about the procedure reduces anxiety and may enhance compliance with the preparation.

Evaluation: Compare the patient's status with the expected patient outcomes. If the outcomes are achieved, evaluate nursing care as successful. If not, reassess the patient, formulate new nursing diagnoses, and revise expected patient outcomes and nursing interventions as appropriate.

Assessment Findings: Patient complains of discomfort because of positioning for the traction and inability to move in bed; patient complains of pain in affected hip; patient grimaces frequently, seems apprehensive, and twitches in the bed.

Nursing Diagnosis: Pain related to injury to hip requiring joint replacement surgery, temporary traction, and/or immobility

Patient Outcomes	Nursing Interventions	Rationale
Patient states relief of pain and discomfort.	Administer analgesics as prescribed. Reposition the patient as allowed in the bed. Teach the patient how to move by using the overhead trapeze. Watch for nonverbal signs of pain or discomfort. Check the traction equipment and patient for alignment.	Pain medication administered at regular intervals helps keep pain levels low and vital signs in normal limits. Slight movement in bed releases pressure from bony prominences. Keeping the traction and patient in proper alignment prevents unnecessary extra pulling forces.
Patient displays no nonverbal signs of pain, such as grimacing or twitching in bed.	Observe the patient's nonverbal responses. Check the patient frequently for pressure areas.	Patient may deny pain verbally, but other signs may indicate discomfort.
Patient's vital signs are within normal limits for the patient.	Check vital signs frequently and note changes.	Changes in vital signs may indicate increasing or decreasing discomfort.

Evaluation: Compare the patient's status with the expected patient outcomes. If the outcomes are achieved, evaluate nursing care as successful. If not, reassess the patient, formulate new nursing diagnoses, and revise expected patient outcomes and nursing interventions as appropriate.

(continued)

Nursing Care Guide 35–1. *(continued)*

PATIENTS UNDERGOING TOTAL HIP REPLACEMENT

Postoperative Care

Assessment Findings: Patient has incision site with dressings, an intravenous line, and a urinary catheter and is on bed rest.

Nursing Diagnosis: High risk for infection related to wound site, intravenous line, urinary catheter, and bed rest

Patient Outcomes	Nursing Interventions	Rationale
Patient's wound site remains free from symptoms of infection such as redness, purulent drainage, or excessive swelling.	Check the wound site and suture line for evidence of healing. Watch for signs of infection. Use aseptic technique for dressing changes.	Early diagnosis of complications increases potential for successful treatment. Aseptic technique decreases risk of infection.
Patient denies cough or respiratory distress.	Assess vital signs frequently. Have the patient cough and deep breathe at regular intervals.	Coughing and deep breathing help clear the respiratory system.
Patient's intravenous site remains free from infection.	Check the intravenous site at least each shift, looking for infiltration, redness, or swelling.	Continually assessing for problems allows for early intervention.
Patient remains free from a urine infection as noted by the urinalysis.	Observe the color, consistency, and amount of urine. Encourage increased fluid intake. Use aseptic cleansing around catheter area.	Increased fluid intake and aseptic care of the catheter decrease risk of a urinary infection.
Patient's vital signs are within normal limits for the patient.	Assess vital signs frequently; especially note an increasing respiratory and pulse rate. Also report and document a temperature increase.	Vital sign changes may indicate infection, such as in the respiratory system if patient begins to present an increased respiratory rate and pulse rate and some respiratory distress.

Evaluation: Compare the patient's status with the expected patient outcomes. If the outcomes are achieved, evaluate nursing care as successful. If not, reassess the patient, formulate new nursing diagnoses, and revise expected patient outcomes and nursing interventions as appropriate.

Assessment Findings: Patient grimaces, moans, and complains of discomfort at surgery site; patient's blood pressure, pulse, and respiratory rate are elevated.

Nursing Diagnosis: Pain related to invasive surgical procedure with manipulation, muscle spasms, and previous injury

(continued)

Nursing Care Guide 35–1. *(continued)*

PATIENTS UNDERGOING TOTAL HIP REPLACEMENT

Patient Outcomes	Nursing Interventions	Rationale
Patient reports relief of pain and appears relaxed and comfortable as evidenced by a calm, relaxed manner and willingness to participate in the care.	Give prescribed analgesics for control of postoperative pain. Monitor effects of analgesics given. Make patient comfortable, and provide a quiet atmosphere for rest after surgery.	Relief of postoperative pain allows patient to rest as needed and promotes healing.
	Check insertion site for signs of infection, which may increase pain at site.	Infection inflammation increases pain at the site.
	Tell the patient to practice relaxation techniques taught before surgery.	Practicing relaxation techniques may decrease some of the discomfort.
Patient's vital signs are within normal ranges.	Monitor vital signs, and document the results.	Changes in vital signs may be due to increased pain.

Evaluation: Compare the patient's status with the expected patient outcomes. If the outcomes are achieved, evaluate nursing care as successful. If not, reassess the patient, formulate new nursing diagnoses, and revise expected patient outcomes and nursing interventions as appropriate.

Assessment Findings: Patient seems overly anxious and reluctant to listen to home care instructions; patient is reluctant to work with ambulatory aid and to practice physical therapy; patient states concerns about providing self-care, hygiene, grooming, and activities of daily living when home.

Nursing Diagnosis: Impaired home maintenance management related to inability to manage mobility problems, use of ambulatory aid, fear for safety, and suture line care (if needed)

Patient Outcomes	Nursing Interventions	Rationale
Patient relates accurate information about the home care required, signs of potential problems, and plans for follow-up care with the attending physician.	Describe the signs requiring immediate medical intervention, such as pain or discomfort at surgical site, fever, chills, dizziness, fainting, excessive fatigue, or shortness of breath.	Early diagnosis of potential problems by the patient at home and early medical intervention increase the chance for successful treatment.
Patient demonstrates appropriate use of ambulatory aid.	Assist the patient in practicing using the ambulatory aid. Seek assistance from a physical therapist.	Having the patient practice before discharge reinforces the instructions for use and enhances safety for the patient.
Patient states safety measures for the home environment to prevent falls or other injuries.	Help the patient find ways to increase safety measures in the home environment. Have the patient reiterate the information provided.	Having the patient relate information presented reinforces the information and allows for correction of misconceptions.

Evaluation: Compare the patient's status with the expected patient outcomes. If the outcomes are achieved, evaluate nursing care as successful. If not, reassess the patient, formulate new nursing diagnoses, and revise expected patient outcomes and nursing interventions as appropriate.

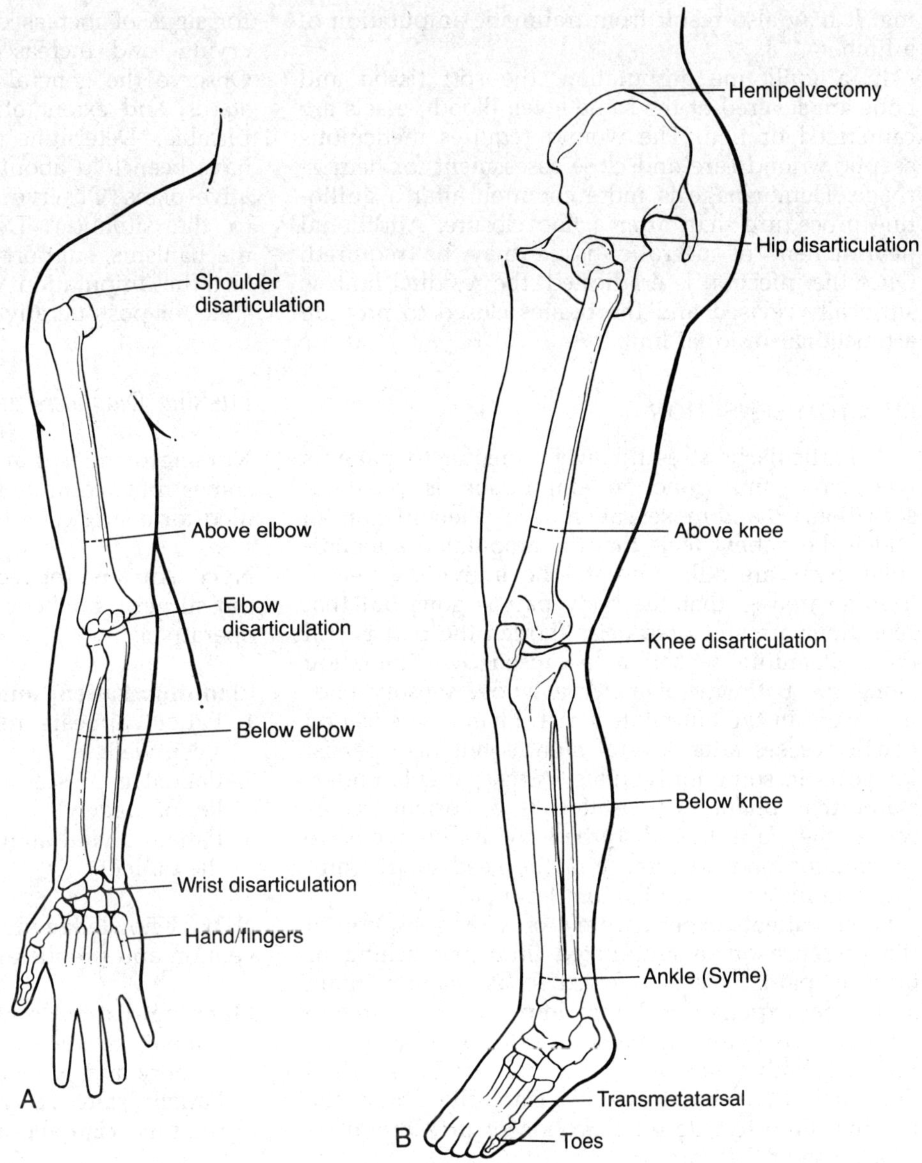

Figure 35–13.
Levels of amputations for the upper extremity (A) and lower extremity (B).

and congenital deformities that result in nonfunctional disfigured limbs.

LEVELS OF AMPUTATIONS

A limb may be amputated at any point along its length (Fig. 35–13). The level of amputation depends on the extent of the disease process, circulation to the area, and optimum function of the residual limb or stump. The terminology used to describe common amputation procedures refers to the level of amputation and is listed in Table 35–8.

TYPES OF AMPUTATIONS

After removal of the body part, the residual limb is either closed with flaps of muscle and tissue or left open. The open type, called a guillotine amputation, is used when infection is present and free drainage of infected material is necessary for heal-

Table 35–8. TERMINOLOGY USED FOR COMMON AMPUTATION PROCEDURES

AMPUTATIONS INVOLVING THE UPPER EXTREMITIES
Finger(s)
Transmetacarpal resection—removal of a portion of the hand
Wrist—removal of the entire hand
Below the elbow
Elbow disarticulation—removal of the forearm at the elbow
Above the elbow
Shoulder disarticulation—removal of the entire arm
AMPUTATIONS INVOLVING THE LOWER EXTREMITIES
Toe(s)
Transmetatarsal resection—removal of a portion of the foot
Total foot removal below the ankle joint
Ankle (Syme)—removal at the ankle joint
Below the knee (BK)
Knee disarticulation—removal of the lower leg at the knee
Above the knee (AK)
Hip disarticulation—removal of the entire leg at the hip
Hemipelvectomy—removal of the entire leg and half of the pelvis

ing. It may also result from traumatic amputation of a limb.

In a guillotine amputation, the soft tissue and bone are severed at the same level. Blood vessels are cauterized or tied. The wound requires meticulous aseptic wound care and close assessment for hemorrhage. Hemorrhage is more common after a guillotine procedure than after a flap closure. Additional debridement of necrotic tissue may be required. Once the infection is eradicated, the residual limb is surgically revised and the tissues closed to provide a functional residual limb.

PHANTOM SENSATION

A particularly stressful event unique to patients who have undergone an amputation is phantom sensation. Phantom sensation is a phenomenon in which the patient feels that the amputated appendicular parts are still present. The individual verbalizes awareness that the body part is gone but that sensations are still present as though the part is still there. Phantom sensation is caused by stimulation along the pathway of a nerve whose sensory endings were in the amputated part. Phantom sensation usually ceases after several months but may persist for years in some individuals. When patients understand that phantom sensation is a normal occurrence, they are less disturbed by it. Preoperative preparation and acceptance of the need for the amputation may reduce phantom limb pain.

Some patients experience not only the sensation of the presence of an amputated limb, but aching or burning pain. This is referred to as phantom pain and is not experienced by all amputees. Measures to help relieve phantom pain include exercise of the residual limb, massaging the end of the residual limb, and diversional activity. Carefully assess the residual limb to rule out infection or pressure areas as a cause of the pain.

In some instances after an amputation, severed nerve endings attempt to regenerate and form a neuroma. The neuroma produces a localized area of numbness and tingling. If discomfort becomes problematic for the patient, the neuroma is surgically removed.

Application of the Nursing Process to the Care of the Patient Undergoing a Surgical Amputation

PREOPERATIVE NURSING CARE

Assessment

Assess the patient's physical and emotional reaction to the planned amputation. Check vital signs. Look for signs of increased anxiety, such as nervousness, crying, and increased pulse and respiratory rate. Observe the general physical condition, nutritional status, and extent of other injuries sustained if applicable. Determine what the patient and family have been told about the surgery and the postoperative plans. Observe their anxiety level and reaction to the situation. Determine the patient's coping mechanisms, support systems, resources, and the effect the amputation will have on the patient's lifestyle for postoperative planning.

Nursing Diagnoses and Planning

Nursing diagnoses and related expected patient outcomes most commonly applicable to patients scheduled for a surgical amputation include the following:

NDx: Anxiety related to the preexisting condition, the surgery, and coping with the amputation postoperatively

Planning: Patient outcomes
1. Patient appears relaxed and is able to rest and sleep well.
2. Patient expresses concerns and acknowledges relief of anxiety.
3. Patient's vital signs are within normal limits for the patient.

NDx: Knowledge deficit: nature of surgical intervention and preoperative preparation

Planning: Patient outcomes
1. Patient relates accurate information about the surgery and preoperative preparation.
2. Patient states correct information presented by the physician about the perioperative course.

Nursing Interventions

NDx: Anxiety
Allow the patient to freely express concerns and ask questions about the surgery and preoperative preparation. Help the patient find relaxation methods that are effective to relieve anxiety. Use the assistance of the patient's support systems, such as family, friends, or clergy. Explain all procedures to the patient prior to performing them. Allow the patient time to rest and sleep as needed.

NDx: Knowledge deficit: nature of surgical intervention and preoperative preparation
Reinforce the information provided to the patient by the physician. Ask the patient to reiterate the information, and correct any misunderstandings. Tell the patient about preoperative plans, such as what treatments and diagnostic tests are to be performed. Allow time for questions and concerns from the patient. Include the family whenever possible.

Evaluation

Evaluate the effectiveness of nursing care for a patient who is scheduled for a surgical amputation by comparing the patient's status with the expected patient outcomes. Examples of specific outcomes for patients scheduled for a surgical amputation have been provided in the Planning section.

POSTOPERATIVE NURSING CARE

Assessment

In addition to the usual postoperative care, observe for hemorrhage or signs of infection in the affected limb. Note drainage through the bandages. Assess the patient for psychological problems related to the absence of the limb. Ask the patient about pain in the residual limb, and determine its intensity and duration and the effect of pain medication. As the residual limb heals, assess the patient's understanding of the instruction for skin care, care of the bandages or prosthesis, if applicable, and home care.

Nursing Diagnoses and Planning

Nursing diagnoses and related expected patient outcomes most commonly applicable to patients after a surgical amputation include the following:

NDx: Self-esteem disturbance related to the absence of a body part

Planning: Patient outcomes
1. Patient relates feelings of self-worth.
2. Patient maintains social activity.
3. Patient is able to look at self with understanding and acceptance.

NDx: Dysfunctional grieving related to loss of a body part

Planning: Patient outcomes
1. Patient freely expresses feelings of grief.
2. Patient verbalizes feelings of improved emotional status.
3. Patient begins to progress through the grief process and returns to daily activities as able.

NDx: Pain related to surgical intervention and postoperative phantom pain

Planning: Patient outcomes
1. Patient denies pain in surgical area.
2. Patient states methods to decrease pain, such as use of relaxation strategies.
3. Patient states an understanding of the cause of phantom pain.
4. Patient reports effectiveness of the prescribed analgesics.

NDx: Impaired mobility (if lower limb) related to inability to manipulate ambulatory aid or prosthesis

Planning: Patient outcomes
1. Patient demonstrates ability to be mobile with some assistance.
2. Patient uses safety tips as presented by the therapist.
3. Patient uses the prescribed ambulatory aid correctly.
4. Patient demonstrates proper locomotion with the prosthesis in place.

NDx: High risk for impaired skin integrity related to improper healing or fit of the prosthesis or improper care of the residual limb

Planning: Patient outcomes
1. Patient relates appropriate skin care as instructed.
2. Patient states signs of infection or improper prosthesis fit and when to seek medical intervention.

NDx: Impaired home maintenance management related to inability to move freely, safety problems, lack of an extremity, and/or unsuitable home environment

Planning: Patient outcomes
1. Patient relates accurate information about alterations in the home environment that are needed for the patient to move freely.
2. Patient verbalizes necessary safety measures.
3. Patient completes activities of daily living with the assistance of the ambulatory aid or prosthesis (upper or lower body).
4. Patient uses resources available to provide assistance with home care.

Nursing Interventions

NDx: Self-esteem disturbance
Allow the patient to vent feelings about the loss of a limb. Provide information about self-help groups. Seek assistance from clergy or professional counseling. Provide diversional activities for the patient until allowed to ambulate. Involve support from the family and other friends. Seek effective coping strategies for the patient. Assist the patient in finding the positive aspects of life to focus on during periods of depression. Have the prosthetist assist the patient with finding artificial parts that are cosmetically appealing

NDx: Dysfunctional grieving
Allow the patient to vent feelings about the surgery and limb loss. Have a professional counselor visit with the patient. Seek assistance from other amputees. Give the patient time to grieve because this process is much the same as losing a loved one. Offer support without making false claims to the patient about how well everything will be. Allow the patient and family to have time alone as needed.

Chart 35–3.

NURSING GUIDE TO PATIENT EDUCATION FOR SELF-MANAGEMENT: CARE OF THE SKIN AND PROSTHESIS AFTER AN AMPUTATION

Instruct the patient to:

Wash the stump daily with warm water and a mild soap to prevent irritation.
Rinse the skin and dry thoroughly to prevent macerated skin.
Wash the stump at night so it can air dry over night before being rewrapped.
Inspect the entire residual stump daily for reddened or open areas, dry skin, or other sign of irritation.
Use a hand mirror to visualize the back of the stump.
Contact the physician for treatment if lesions are present.
Avoid using topical antiseptics, because they may cause further irritation of the skin.
Avoid using lotions unless otherwise instructed by the physician, because they soften the skin and may predispose it to breakdown.
Keep the prosthesis, elastic bandages, and prosthetic socks clean and in good condition.
Follow the prosthetist's instructions for the care of the prosthesis, socks, and straps.
Contact the prosthetist if loosening or pressure from the prosthesis occurs.
Refrain from padding, taping, or altering the prosthesis without consultation with the prosthetist, because this may interfere with the proper fit or use of the device.

NDx: Pain
Help the patient deal with the pain by using alternatives to pain medication such as relaxation exercises. Teach deep breathing techniques and other full-body relaxation strategies. Discuss the cause of phantom pain with the patient. Teach the patient about the use of patient-controlled analgesia if prescribed postoperatively.

When pain is acute, give prescribed analgesics and explain the dosage, frequency, side effects, and expected therapeutic effects of the medications. Caution the patient not to perform tasks that require mental alertness while under the effects of the pain medication. Handle the patient carefully when moving in bed. Caution the patient about weight-bearing on the prosthesis until advised, because that might increase the pain significantly.

Place the patient with a leg amputation in the prone position for 30 minutes four to six times per day as ordered, to prevent flexion contractures of the hip, which also increase the pain.

NDx: Impaired mobility
Teach the patient use of the overhead trapeze while still on bed rest to increase movement in bed, as allowed, to prevent complications of immobility. Reposition the patient frequently to stimulate circulation and prevent skin breakdown. Assist the patient in locomotion, once able, to promote safe use of the ambulatory aid. Use the assistance of the physical therapist and prosthetist to instruct the patient and family about the device or prosthesis. Encourage the patient to perform exercises as described by the therapist. Give analgesics as needed to decrease pain levels that may interfere with the patient's ability to be mobile.

NDx: High risk for impaired skin integrity
Teach the patient to check the residual limb carefully daily as described in Chart 35–3. Have the patient relate potential signs of infection, such as redness, unusual warmth, purulent exudate, or sudden extreme pain. Teach the patient to wrap the residual limb, being careful not to pull the elastic bandages too tight. Have the patient move frequently in bed in the early postoperative course to prevent skin breakdown. Tell the patient to keep the residual limb clean and dry.

Encourage and provide a good, well-balanced meal plan to promote healing and prevent skin problems. Have the patient drink plenty of fluids to maintain good skin integrity and prevent dry, cracked skin.

NDx: Impaired home maintenance management
Provide information to the patient and family about the postoperative course and self-care interventions. Encourage the patient to ask questions and to express fears and concerns. Answer questions honestly, while reinforcing the positive aspects of the patient's life. Encourage and reinforce instructions in the use of medications, prosthesis, and ambulatory aids. Discuss modification of the home environment that will help the patient maintain independence.

Teach the patient about wrapping the residual limb, as described in Table 35–9, and care of the

Table 35–9. WRAPPING A LOWER RESIDUAL LIMB

The steps for wrapping a lower residual limb are illustrated in Figure 35–14 and outlined below.

For a below-the-knee residual limb:

1. Have the patient sit in a semi-Fowler's position.
2. Hold the end of the wrap just above the knee as it is stretched and unrolled diagonally down the back of the limb and over the end of the stump.
3. Pull the wrap up diagonally across the front of the limb and the end of the elastic bandage to secure or anchor it in place.
4. Repeat this figure-eight pattern with one or more elastic bandages until the stump and knee are completely covered.
5. Note that the elastic pull of the bandage is always applied from back to front to avoid causing flexion contractures of the knee.

For an above-the-knee residual limb:

1. Have the patient lie or stand so that the involved hip is hyperextended.
2. Begin the wrap at the top anterior medial aspect of the leg (groin).
3. Pull the wrap diagonally down behind the limb, over the end of the stump, then diagonally up toward the groin and over the end of the bandage to secure it.
4. The wrap may also be brought over the opposite iliac crest, behind the body, diagonally down across the limb, and over the stump and up again.
5. Repeat either pattern until the stump and residual limb are completely covered.
6. The number of wraps around the opposite hip will vary, but one or two layers are sufficient to secure an above-the-knee residual limb wrap.

skin and prosthesis, as described in Chart 35–3. Have the patient demonstrate the technique, and correct any misunderstandings about the care regimen.

Teach the patient about good nutrition to maintain health status and to continue to promote healing. Encourage a diet high in protein, vitamins, and minerals.

Initiate social service referral to help the patient use all resources available to provide financial assistance and to maintain independence. Inform the patient of any local support groups for amputees.

Additional Interventions

Residual limb care is an important part of the nursing care for a patient after an amputation. For the first 48 hours postoperatively, elevate the limb to decrease swelling and promote comfort. Elevation of the lower extremities is done at intervals because elevation for longer periods of time may cause contractures of the hip. To prevent hip contractures, position the patient on the abdomen for 30-minute periods every 4 to 6 hours. Maintain a lower extremity residual limb in alignment while the patient is in the bed or in a chair with rolled towels or sand bags to prevent external rotation and abduction contractures.

The prescribed exercises for the residual limb and proximal joint help maintain the range of motion, prevent contractures, and assist in early conditioning

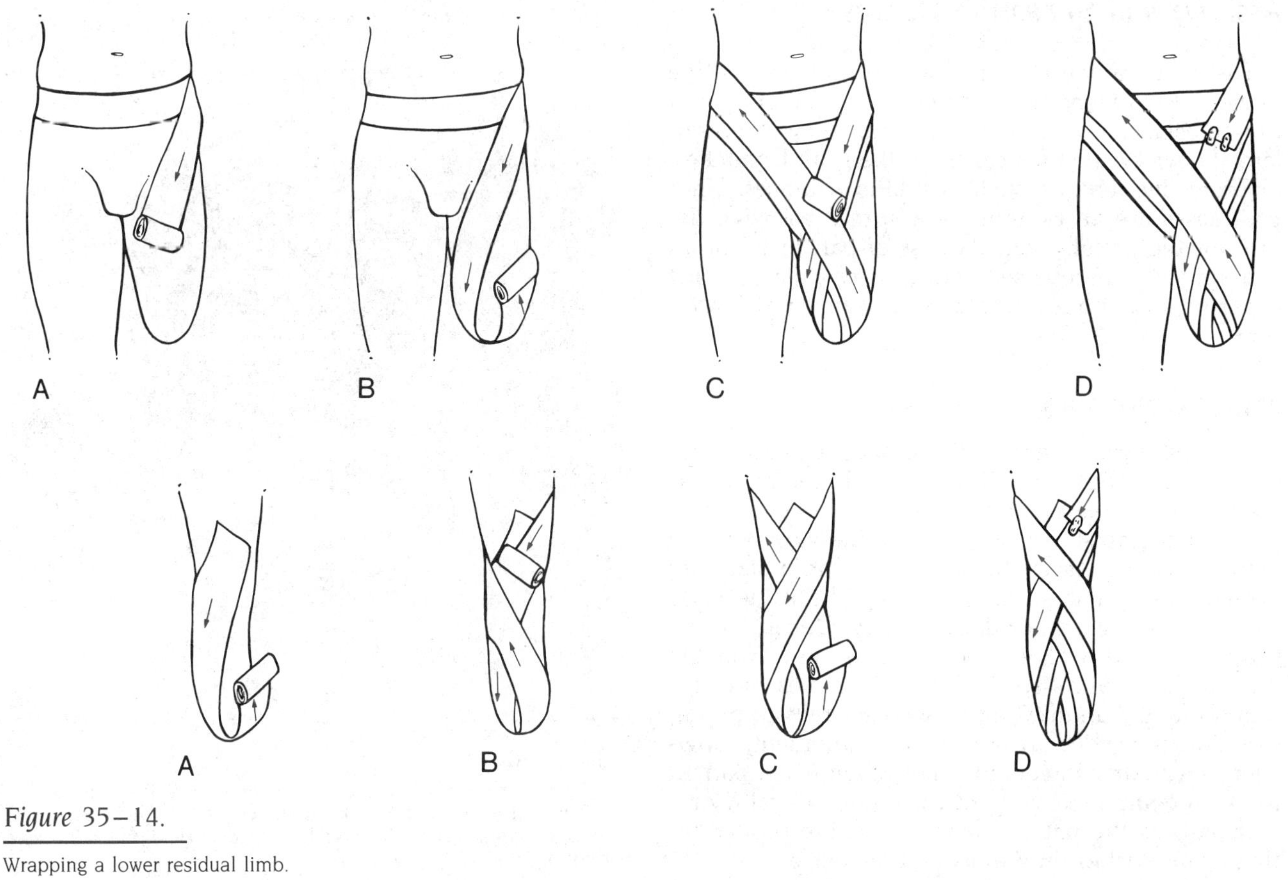

Figure 35–14.

Wrapping a lower residual limb.

of prosthesis fitting. Encourage the patient to practice the exercises as ordered.

Wrapping the residual limb with an elastic bandage helps prevent postoperative edema and, as healing progresses, helps shrink and shape the residual limb to ensure good fit of the prosthesis. Wrap the limb so that all the skin is covered. Tell the patient to leave the wrap on unless a rigid dressing or prosthesis is applied. Reapply the wrap every 8 hours unless otherwise advised, or whenever loosening occurs. Inspect the skin every time the residual limb is rewrapped. Refer to Table 35–9 and Figure 35–14 for a description of the wrapping process.

If the patient experiences throbbing or uncomfortable pressure, rewrap the residual limb. Check the finished wrap for smoothness and secure fastening.

Evaluation

Evaluate the effectiveness of nursing care for a patient after a surgical amputation by comparing the patient's status with the expected patient outcomes. Examples of specific outcomes for patients after a surgical amputation have been provided in the Planning section.

Assistive and Supportive Devices

There are a variety of assistive and supportive devices that can be used in the care of patients with musculoskeletal disorders. These aids may be ambulatory devices, such as canes, walkers, and crutches, or protective devices, such as splints or braces. Limb prostheses are an example of a special assistive device for the patient with the loss of part or all of an extremity. Numerous self-help devices exist to assist a person in adapting to almost any physical limitation.

AMBULATORY AIDS

In most health care settings, the physician prescribes the ambulatory aid to be used. The patient is measured for, and taught to use the device, by a physical therapist. To be correctly measured for an ambulatory aid, the patient should be in a standing position on a flat surface, wearing the same style shoes that are worn for daily activity. Outside of the hospital, canes, walkers, and crutches are available for purchase from surgical supply stores and for rent from community agencies. Generally, no prescription is needed to obtain this equipment. However, third party payers may not reimburse a patient for such equipment without consulting a health professional, or the patient may not receive proper fitting or instruction in the use of the device.

A cane is an ambulatory aid used for balance and to promote a feeling of security. Canes provide only limited support and cannot be used unless the person can tolerate some weight on both lower extremities. The tip of the cane should have a thick, nonskid subber surface for safety. The top curve or handgrip of the cane should be in line with the hip joint. The patient's elbow is slightly flexed when holding the cane correctly positioned at hip height.

Usually a cane is held on the uninvolved side. Thus, if the patient becomes weak or loses control of the involved extremity, the cane provides support on the uninvolved side to which the person will instinctively shift the weight to remain standing. With the cane held on the unaffected side, the typical gait pattern is to move the affected leg and cane forward together, then the unaffected leg.

Walkers provide four points of support, one on each of the four corners surrounding the ambulating patient (Fig. 35–15). They have a wide base, give the most security of all the ambulatory aids, and require less strength for use. The top of the walker should be level with the proximal thumb joints, with the elbow flexed at 25 to 30 degrees. The sides of the walker should be 6 inches from the side of the foot.

Walkers are difficult to maneuver in small places and must have a special attachment to be used on stairs. Most walkers are made of aluminum. Some have unique features such as anterior wheels for ease in moving and modified underarm extensions to accommodate persons with upper extremity limi-

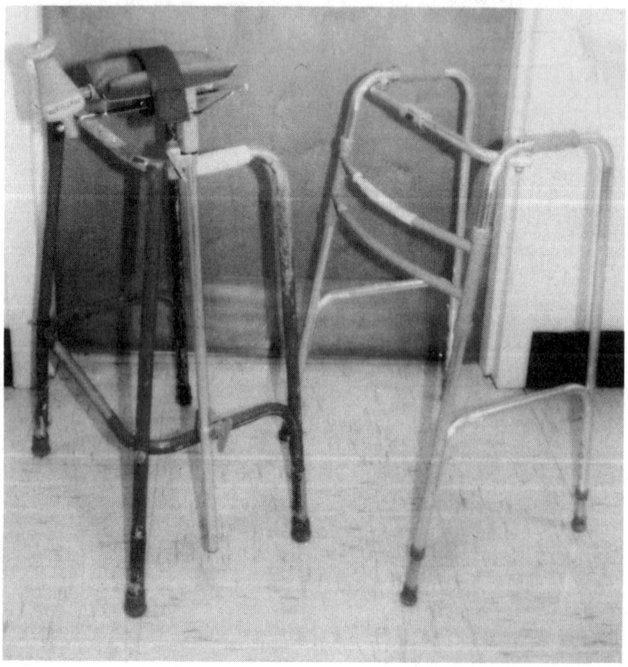

Figure 35–15.

Walkers. *Left*, A platform extension walker for individuals with weak hands or arms. *Right*, The standard model. Note the adjustable height legs.

tations such as weak wrists or fingers or a broken bone.

Walkers create a slow gait pattern. The patient places the walker in front then steps forward. Walkers are primarily used by the elderly or by postoperative patients when they first begin ambulating.

To rise from a sitting position, the individual should not pull on the walker, but rise by using the arms of a chair or some other assistance. Once the patient is in a standing position, the weight of the upper extremities can be placed on the walker for balance and support.

Crutches can be used when no weight-bearing is allowed on one lower extremity or when weight-bearing is allowed on one or both lower extremities (Fig. 35–16). The patient must have upper body strength and arm control to use crutches. The patient's weight is supported on the wrists, hands and shoulders, not on the axillae. Pressure on the axillae can result in nerve damage. Crutches should be measured and fitted by a trained professional. The foam rubber underarm and handgrip pads provide patient comfort, and the thick nonskid tips promote safety.

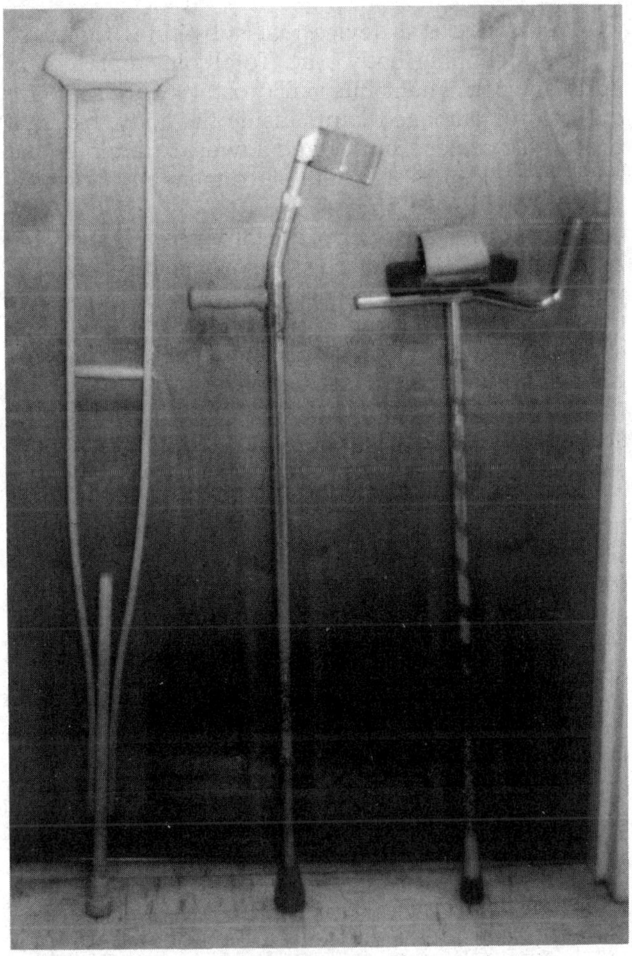

Figure 35–16.

Crutches. Left to right: Standard underarm, wooden, adjustable crutch; metal forearm, Kelly crutch; and forearm gutter crutch for the individual with weak forearms, wrists, or hands.

Before ambulation, the patient is instructed in the proper gait. When ambulating with crutches, the body is kept in good alignment, with the head held high, shoulders back, and stomach and buttocks in. The gait pattern is determined by the physician or therapist. Certain gait patterns are used for specific circumstances. The two-point gait is used if the patient has good coordination and strength. It resembles normal walking and involves moving one leg and the opposite crutch forward, following with the other leg and the other crutch. The three-point gait is used when weight-bearing is not allowed on one extremity. It is slower than the two-point gait and requires the use of both arms, the trunk, and one leg. There are three points of contact with the floor at any point in time. Both crutches are placed in front of the patient, and the patient bears weight on the crutches for half of the gait as the weight-bearing leg is advanced. The four-point gait is used for the weak patient with poor balance who can bear weight on both legs. It requires four points touching the floor as the patient moves forward. One crutch is moved forward, the opposite crutch is then placed forward, then one leg is brought forward, followed by the other leg.

Careful instruction and practice with supervision are necessary to ensure safety for the patient. If the patient has to climb stairs or manipulate in other difficult areas, special instruction sessions are planned with the therapist.

SPLINTS AND BRACES

Splints immobilize or protect a specific body part while allowing motion of nonsplinted areas. They are not circumferential like casts and are usually removable. Splints such as the polyethylene foot-drop splint are also used to treat or prevent the formation of flexion contractures.

Braces serve as functional substitutes to provide support and allow movement of body structures. Lower extremity spring braces provide stability for weight-bearing while allowing mobility for ambulation. Some braces provide anatomic correction as well as support and protection.

Application of the Nursing Process to the Care of the Patient Using an Assistive or Supportive Device for Musculoskeletal Dysfunction

Assessment

If the patient already uses an assistive or supportive device, identify which type the patient uses, why it is needed, and how well the patient maneuvers with the device. Note the patient's gait, balance, and ease of motion. Check whether the patient uses the device correctly. Determine the wearing schedule, fit, and effectiveness. If the patient does not already have an assistive or supportive device but has had one prescribed, determine the patient's knowledge about the device and ability to manipulate it correctly.

Nursing Diagnoses and Planning

Nursing diagnoses and related expected patient outcomes most commonly applicable to patients using assistive or supportive devices for musculoskeletal dysfunction include the following:

NDx: High risk for injury related to improper fit or misuse of the device

Planning: Patient outcomes
1. Patient demonstrates safe use of the prescribed device.
2. Patient denies improper fit or problems with the device.
3. Patient relates safety measures to follow when using the device to prevent injury.

NDx: Impaired home maintenance management related to use of the device, ability to manipulate the device properly in the home, and how to perform activities of daily living while using the device

Planning: Patient outcomes
1. Patient demonstrates proper use of the device.
2. Patient relates strategies for manipulating the device while performing necessary tasks in the home.

Nursing Interventions

NDx: High risk for injury
Teach the patient how to manipulate the device, and have the patient demonstrate its use. Refer the patient to physical therapy for assistance with learning the safe use of the aid. Supervise the patient in the early stages of practice. Be certain the device is properly fitted. Discuss areas of the home that may be potentially hazardous for the patient using an assistive device. Involve the family in the sessions when possible.

NDx: Impaired home maintenance management
Explain the use of the assistive or supportive device prescribed to the patient. Ask the physical therapist to assist in the instruction. Determine the patient's ability to maneuver with the device in an environment with furniture similar to the home setting. If the patient has difficulty, plan instruction to assist the patient in learning how to cope with this problem prior to discharge. Have the patient walk and stand with the equipment to assess proper gait and fit. Encourage the patient to do range-of-motion and strength exercises to build upper body strength, which will be beneficial if the patient is using a walker or crutches. Promote increased independence and encourage progression toward that goal. Also teach the patient proper maintenance of the device.

Evaluation

Evaluate the effectiveness of nursing care for a patient with an assistive or supportive device by comparing the patient's status with the expected patient outcomes. Examples of specific outcomes for patients with an assistive or supportive device have been provided in the Planning section.

External Prostheses

A prosthesis is a device that substitutes for a lost or nonfunctioning body part. Total joint replacement parts are permanent internal prostheses that replace diseased or damaged joints inside the body. External prostheses replace upper and lower extremities that have been lost as a result of congenital deformity, trauma, or disease process.

External prostheses or artificial limbs are available in a variety of designs. They are made of wood, plastic, or lightweight synthetics such as polyurethane. The devices are attached to the body by straps, belts, or suction and may be functional or cosmetic. Functional prostheses may be powered by the individual's own muscles or by the use of levers, springs, cables, locks, gears, and, in some instances such as the knee, a hydraulic mechanism.

Proper selection and fit of an artificial limb requires close collaboration of health team members. The physician prescribes the prosthesis; a prosthetist (one knowledgeable and skilled in the construction and fit of the prosthesis) manufactures and fits the prosthesis. The physical therapist, occupational therapist, and nurse instruct the patient in its use and care. Each has a different but important role in the patient education process. A rehabilitation counselor is also a valuable team member in assisting with establishment of long-range goals for the patient receiving a prosthesis. Because limb prostheses are custom made, expensive, and require extensive teaching and follow-up, a social service referral is important and often necessary.

Factors considered in the selection of an appropriate prosthesis include the following:

1. The general health of the individual and the presence of disorders that might prevent maximum use of the device.

2. The weight, strength, and coordination of the individual. Excessive weight, lack of strength, or poor coordination could prevent the individual from safely using the prosthesis.
3. The lifestyle and activity level of the individual determine the choice between a cosmetic and functional prosthesis.
4. The ability to learn. The individual must be able to understand and follow instructions on the use and care of the prosthesis.
5. The potential for rehabilitation. The individual must be motivated to cooperate in the prescribed exercises and therapy, to care for the residual limb, and to maintain the prosthesis. The individual must also be willing to spend many hours practicing in order to obtain maximum use of a functional prosthesis.

TYPES OF PROSTHESES

There are a variety of prosthetic parts available to match a particular patient's needs. There are artificial parts for the hand, forearm, upper arm, shoulder, foot, ankle, and legs. Temporary artificial parts may be used until a permanent one can be properly fitted or made for the patient.

UPPER EXTREMITY PROSTHESES

The forearm prosthesis is held in place by a strap or harness. There are various hands or terminal devices available, depending on the desired use of the prosthesis or the occupation of the individual. The simplest terminal devices consist of a hook-type mechanism. The hook may be concealed within a cosmetic hand or be undisguised. Some forearm prostheses have several different terminal devices, each with its own function, which may be screwed into the prosthesis according to the individual's need at a given time (Fig. 35–17).

The hand or terminal device is controlled by a cable attached to the patient's muscles in the upper arm or opposite shoulder. Specific muscle movements made by the wearer can elicit motion in the terminal device.

The upper arm prosthesis has an artificial elbow joint and a cable attached to the shoulder or opposite extremity that controls movement of the elbow. Flexion and extension of the elbow maneuver the terminal device for functions such as eating, brushing teeth, and grooming.

With a shoulder prosthesis, there is no elbow or upper arm muscle to trigger movement. Control for the terminal device, the elbow, or for elevation of the prosthetic arm is achieved by cables attached to the muscle of the opposite extremity.

LOWER EXTREMITY PROSTHESES

There are a variety of foot and ankle prostheses available (Fig. 35–18). Foot and ankle prostheses include the Syme prosthesis, which is an artificial foot for an amputation at the ankle joint; the two-way foot or articulating ankle; a solid ankle cushioned heel, or SACH, foot; a flexfoot that allows flexibility for a more normal gait; and the Seattle foot, which has a specially designed heel with a plastic spring and mesh pad that provide a natural lift and forward thrust of the artificial limb. This allows for a more normal gait and running by the amputee. The outer covering of the Seattle foot is made to resemble the individual's other foot, including a sole and toes.

Below-the-knee prostheses replace the lower leg

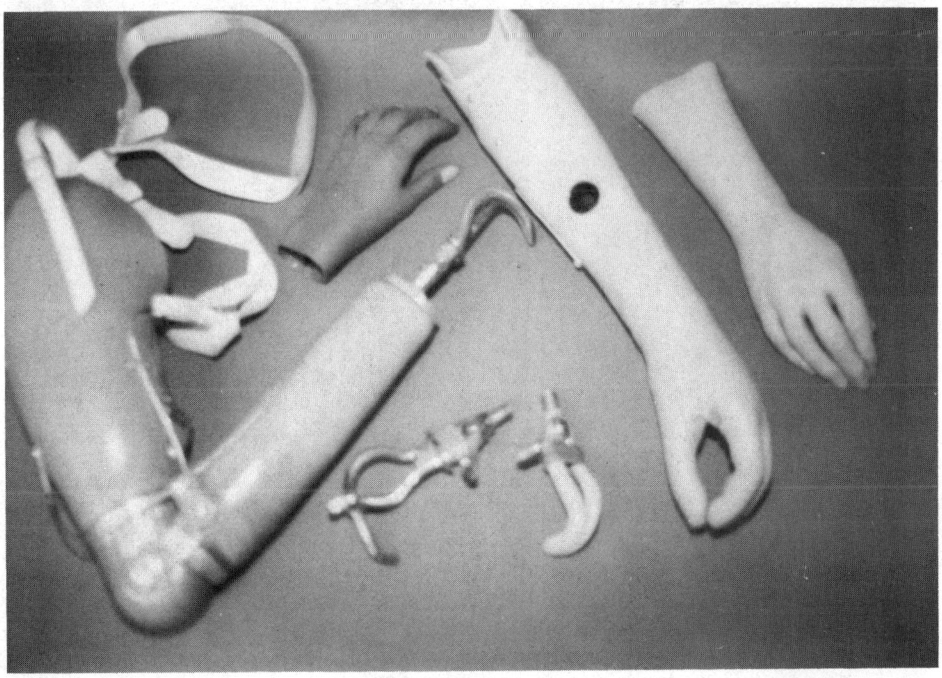

Figure 35–17.

Upper extremity prostheses. Left to right: Upper arm prosthesis with strap, cable, and hook-type terminal device; a dark, short polyethylene cosmetic hand; two different hook terminal devices; a suction-held forearm prosthesis with a polyethylene cosmetic hand; a long polyethylene cosmetic hand.

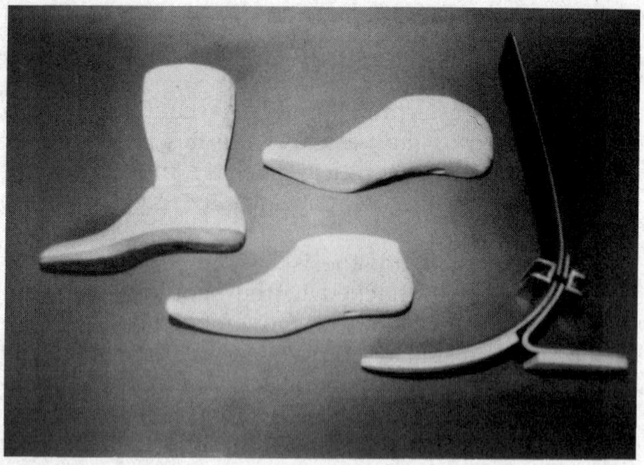

Figure 35–18.

Foot prostheses. Left to right: Two-way or articulating ankle; two SACH feet with different height arches (the top foot can be worn with a higher heel); and the inside support of a flexfoot. (Courtesy of Thomas G. Powell's, Richmond, VA.)

and foot following a below-the-knee amputation (Fig. 35–19). The individual must have an intact knee joint to use a below-the-knee prosthesis. A patellar tendon-bearing (PTB) prosthesis is one type of artificial lower leg. It provides a smooth gait for the wearer and requires less energy to use than some of the other below-the-knee prostheses.

Above-the-knee artificial limbs have different types of knee joints (Fig. 35–19). One type, a Bock safety knee, automatically locks whenever weight is applied to prevent the leg from buckling. This prosthesis is frequently used by elderly or weak persons with poor coordination. An above-the-knee prosthesis with a hydraulic knee provides a smooth gait but requires strength and coordination to use.

TEMPORARY PROSTHESES

Artificial limbs are custom designed for each patient. Final fitting and adjustment of the prosthesis is not possible until all soft tissue has healed, the

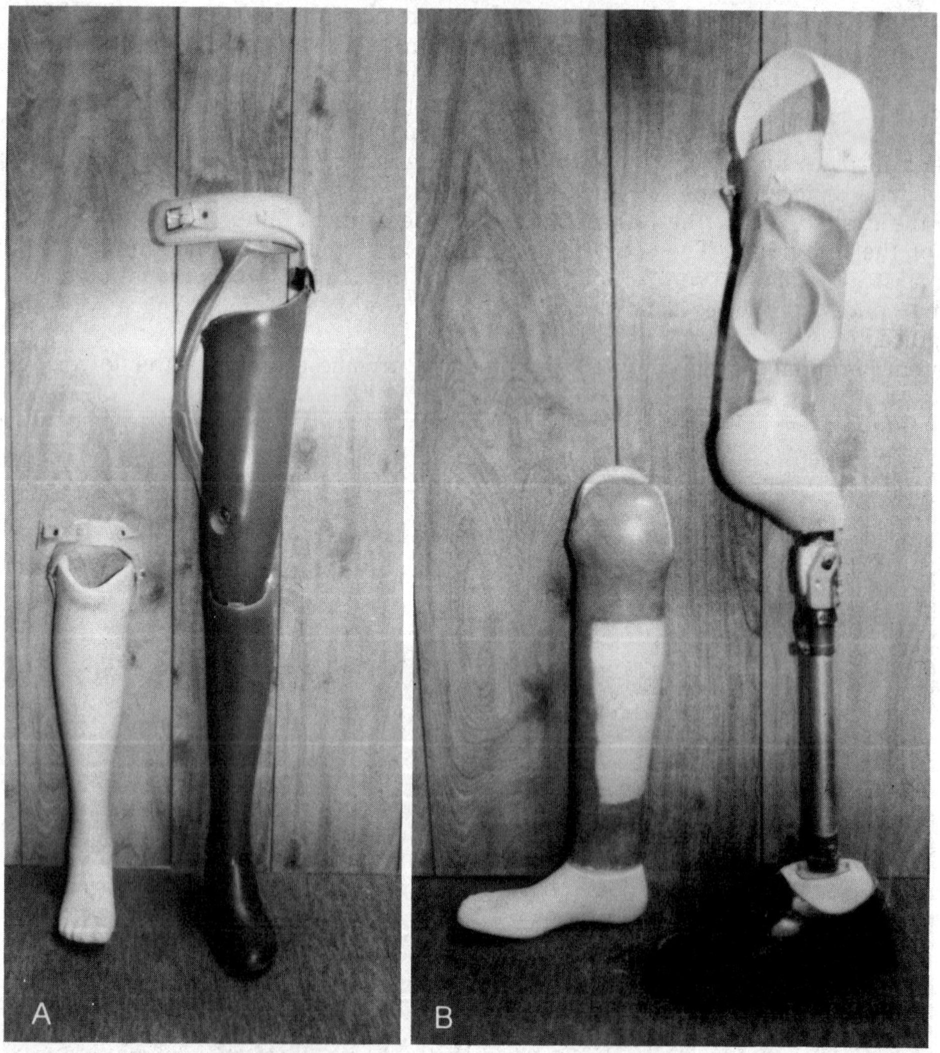

Figure 35–19.

Lower extremity prostheses. A, *Left*, the standard patellar tendon-bearing (PTB) below-the-knee prosthesis; *right*, the standard above-the-knee prosthesis with a pelvic band. B, *Left*, an unfinished PTB below-the-knee prosthesis; *right*, a flexible above-the-knee socket prosthesis with a waist band. The pylon will be covered with polyurethane. Note the safety lock knee. (Courtesy of Thomas G. Powell's, Richmond, VA.)

residual limb is free of edema, and the residual limb size is stable. From amputation to final application of the prosthesis can take 3 to 6 months. Often, a temporary prosthesis is used to prevent postoperative edema, provide support for early ambulation, prevent postoperative contractures of the residual limb, and encourage early rehabilitation and independence. One type of immediate prosthesis consists of a plaster base connected to a metal pylon that is attached to a shoe. An air splint is another device used to decrease edema and assist in early ambulation after amputation. There are a number of commercial brands of air splints, and the instructions for use vary with each type. All types of air splints require frequent inspection of the skin and close monitoring of air pressure.

Self-Help Devices

There are a number of devices available that assist individuals in safely completing self-care activities that they are no longer able to perform independently. The list is too extensive to discuss in detail here; however, the nurse should be aware that such equipment is available and recognize the value of these devices to the patient with musculoskeletal limitations.

Elevated toilet seats, bath benches, and grab bars around toilets, tubs, and showers enable individuals with limited hip and knee range of motion to manage personal hygiene and toileting needs independently. Brushes, combs, and toothbrushes with long-handled extensions permit individuals with limited shoulder and arm strength and range of motion to function more independently in their own grooming. Reachers and dressing appliances such as hooks for zippers and Velcro fasteners assist the individuals with limited movement of multiple joints to dress themselves (Fig. 35–20).

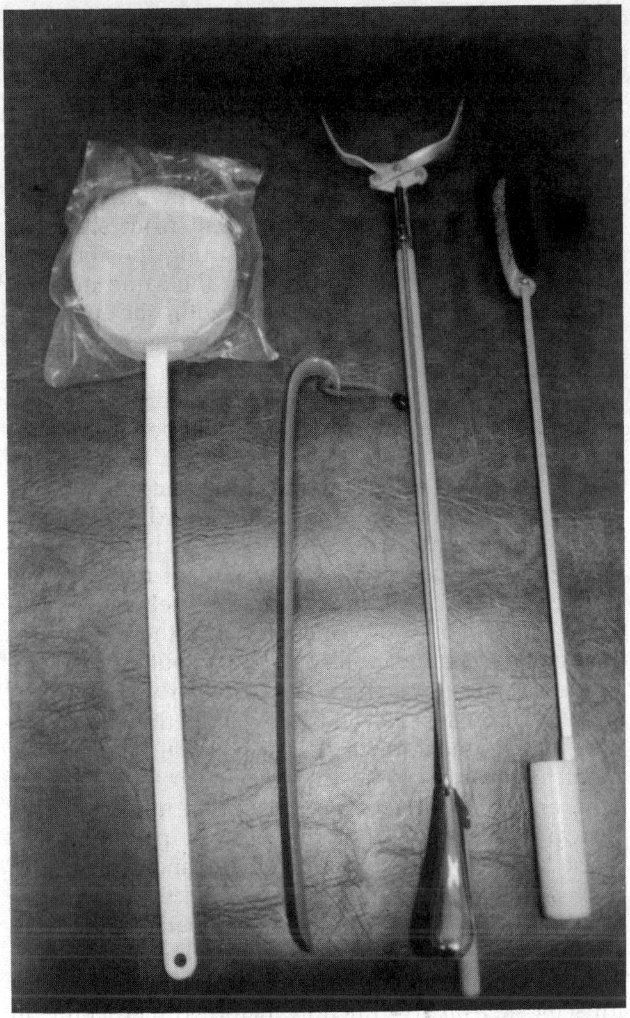

Figure 35–20.

Self-help devices. Left to right: Long-handled sponge, shoehorn, reacher, and long-handled brush.

In most hospitals, the occupational therapist provides information on types of equipment available and how to obtain it and instructs the patient in use of the equipment. During the initial history and assessment, or while observing the patient perform self-care, identify the patient who could benefit from an occupational therapy referral. Also request a social service referral if the patient needs assistive equipment but cannot afford to buy it. Connect the patients with the resources necessary to maximize their potential for independent self-care.

The Elderly: Special Considerations

The normal changes in the musculoskeletal system as a result of the aging process frequently cause the geriatric patient to experience increased discomfort, disability, and deformity. As described in Chapter 2, normal changes occur in muscles and bones or joints resulting in a variety of symptoms. Painful joints, swelling, stiffness, decreased flexibility, muscle cramping and increased susceptibility to injury, especially fractures, are commonalities of the musculoskeletal problems in the older adult.

When assessing the geriatric patient for strength, sensation, motor function, and range of motion, assist the patient as needed to support joints being evaluated. This prevents pressure from interconnecting joints from affecting the findings. The assessment often takes more time with the older adult than a middle-aged or young adult because the older patient may be slower in moving through the steps of range of motion and gait evaluation. Allow time for the patient to rest at intervals during the examination.

Expect some weakness due to normal aging changes. Although the lower extremities may be weaker, there should be equal strength in both lower extremities. It is more important to relate function to strength and range of motion then to compare it with a norm. If extremities are of equal strength and joints bilaterally possess the same range of motion, determine the patient's ability to carry out normal activities of daily living. Limited hip flexion may prevent the patient from sitting in certain chairs, rising from a sitting position, or dressing the lower extremities. In the same manner, limited strength may interfere with the patient's ability to lift items used in feeding, grooming, or household tasks.

The physical musculoskeletal changes of decreased skeletal height, stooped appearance, and muscle atrophy must be incorporated into a new body image. Decreased muscle strength, limited joint range of motion, poor body coordination, and gait changes may demand lifestyle changes and decrease independence. The older patient may become depressed and withdrawn and lose self-esteem because of the loss of function with these physical changes. Decreased ability to carry out normal activities of daily living can be particularly stressful.

Adaptation to change is slower in the elderly. A new environment, such as the hospital, and adjustment to treatments and therapies such as casts, traction, or orthopedic surgery constitute major psychological adjustments for the elderly patient. Time must be allowed for reinforcement and learning of new skills. The use of assistive devices or walking with a prosthesis require extended patience and encouragement from the nurse.

A teaching plan for the geriatric patient with musculoskeletal dysfunction includes instruction on a nutritious well-balanced diet to preserve strength and well-being and to promote healing. Make the patient aware of the increased susceptibility to fractures and the need for a safe environment. Safety from injury, especially falls, is a constant focal point of care planning for all elderly patients.

Extended use of traction therapy is usually not the treatment of choice for the older adult because of the effects of immobility. However, short-term traction is commonly used. When skin traction is applied, proper alignment of the body or affected part may be challenged by the elderly patient's tendency to curl up in a fetal position in the bed. Frequently monitor and correct the improper alignment as needed. The patient may use this posturing because of fear, confusion, or sensations of cold. Offer reassurance to the patient, explain the necessity of maintaining alignment, and be sure the patient is warm. The elderly are more sensitive to changes in room temperature than are other patients. Assess skin temperature, observe the color of the nail beds, and tell the patient to notify the nurse if feeling cold or chilled. Provide extra covers if needed, using a bed cradle to keep the blankets from restricting the traction device.

Short-term traction for a fractured hip, and side-arm or overhead traction for fractures of the humerus, require a supine position with the head of the bed flat. This position may have a harmful effect on the respiratory status of geriatric patients by predisposing them to hypostatic pneumonia. Maintain adequate ventilatory capacity by frequent coughing and deep breathing exercises and use of incentive spirometry. The potential for skin breakdown associated with bed rest for traction therapy is also aggravated by the patient's age. Use special care to prevent skin irritation and breakdown when the elderly patient's freedom of movement is restricted by traction.

Older patients are more prone to the complications of immobility. Plan strategies to prevent these complications and maintain maximum musculoskeletal function. Aging should not be synonymous with dependency. Encourage the geriatric patient to participate in self-care and to remain as mobile and independent as possible.

Bibliography

Andres R, Bierman EL, Hazard W. Principles of geriatric medicine. New York: McGraw-Hill, 1985.

Baquie M. What matters most in chronic pain management. RN 1989; 52(3):46.

Bernhard VM, Towne, JB (eds). Complications in surgery. 2nd ed. New York: Grune & Stratton, 1985.

Bullock BL, Rosenthal PP. Pathophysiology adaption and alterations in function. Philadelphia: JB Lippincott, 1992.

Burggraf V, and Donlon B. Assessing the elderly: Part one; System by system. Am J Nurs 1985; 85(9):974.

Calkins E, Davis P, Ford A. The practice of geriatrics. Philadelphia: WB Saunders, 1986.

Callahan J. Compartment syndrome. Orthop Nurs 1985; 4(4):11.

Carpenito LJ. Nursing diagnosis: Application to clinical practice. 3rd ed. Philadelphia: JB Lippincott, 1989–1990.

Ceccio C, Horosz J. Teaching the elderly amputee to meet the world. RN 1988; 51(9):70.

Ceccio CM. Understanding therapeutic beds. Orthop Nurs 1990; 9(3):57.

Corwin D, Miller C. Get your patient off on the right foot. RN 1990; 53(10):44.

D'Angio G, Evans A. Bone tumors and tissue sarcomas. Baltimore: Edward Arnold, 1985.

Doenges M, Jeffries MF, Moorhouse MF. Nursing care plans: Nursing diagnoses in planning patient care. Philadelphia: FA Davis, 1984.

Edelstein JE. Preprosthetic management of patients with lower or upper limb amputation. Phys Med Rehabil Clin North Am 1991; 2(2);285.

Eliopoulos C. Gerontological nursing. 2nd ed. Philadelphia: JB Lippincott, 1987.

Esquenazi A, Torres MM. Prosthetic feet and ankle mechanisms. Phys Med Rehabil Clin North Am 1991; 2(2):299.

Farrell N. Cast syndrome. Orthop Nurs 1985; 4(4):61.

Geier K, Hesser K. Electrical bone stimulation for treatment of nonunion. Orthop Nurs 1985; 4(2):41.

Holloway NM. Medical-surgical care plans. Springhouse, PA: Springhouse, 1988.

Ignatavicius D, Bayne M. Medical-surgical nursing: A nursing process approach. Philadelphia: WB Saunders, 1991.

Illustrated manual of nursing practice. Springhouse, PA: Springhouse, 1991.

Iyer P, Taptich B, Bernocci Losey D. Nursing process and nursing diagnosis. Philadelphia: WB Saunders, 1988.

Jackson J, Neighbors M. Home care client assessment handbook. Rockville, MD: Aspen Publishers, 1990.
Kee JL. Laboratory and diagnostic test with nursing implications. 2nd ed. Norwalk, CT: Appleton & Lange, 1987.
Krupp MA, Schroeder S, Tierney L. Current medical diagnoses and treatment 1987. Los Angeles: Appleton & Lange, 1987.
Lewis C. Aging: The health care challenge. Philadelphia: FA Davis, 1985.
Malasanos L, Barkauskas V, Moss M, Stoltenberg-Allen K. Health assessment. St. Louis: CV Mosby, 1986.
Malkiewicz J. A pragmatic approach to musculoskeletal assessment. RN 1982; 45(11):57.
Morris L, Kraft S, Tessem S, Reinisch S. Special care for skeletal traction. RN 1988; 51(2):24.
Morris L, Kraft S, Tessem S, Reinisch S. Nursing the patient in traction. RN 1988; 51(1):26.
Olson B, Ustanko L, Warner S. The patient in a halo brace: Striving for normalcy in body image and self-concept. Orthop Nurs 1991; 10(1):44.
Reiss BS, Melick ME. Pharmacological aspects of nursing care. 2nd ed. Albany, NY: Delmar Publishers, 1987.
Resnick D, Niwayama G (eds). Diagnosis of bone and joint disorders. Vol I, II, and III. Philadelphia: WB Saunders, 1981.
Reyburn TV. The "Z" strap: Harnessing modification for patients with upper extremity amputations. Arch Phys Med Rehabil 1991; 72(3):250.
Sabolich J. Prosthetic advances in lower extremity amputation. Phys Med Rehabil Clin North Am 1991; 2(2):415.
Schoen D. The nursing process in orthopaedics. New York: Appleton-Century-Crofts, 1986.
Sculco T. Orthopaedic care of the geriatric patient. St. Louis: CV Mosby, 1986.
Sears, HH. Approaches to prescription of body-powered and myoelectric prostheses. Phys Med Rehabil Clin North Am 1991; 2(2):361.
Sidor ML, Zuckerman JD. Painful hip: Differential diagnosis. Hosp Med 1991; 27(1):55.
Southwick J, Callahan D. A study of blood drainage patterns on synthetic cast materials. Orthop Nurs 1985; 4(2):72.
Taber's cyclopedic medical dictionary. 16th ed. Philadelphia: FA Davis, 1989.
Ulrich SP, Canale SW, Wendell SA. Nursing care planning guides: A nursing diagnosis approach. 2nd ed. Philadelphia: WB Saunders, 1990.
Webb J. Notes on orthopaedic nursing. 2nd ed. New York: Churchill Livingstone, 1985.
Wertz EM. Immobilized. Emergency 1991; 23(8):32.
Wienke VK. Pressure sores: Prevention is the challenge. Orthop Nurs 1987; 6(4):26.
Willey T. High-tech beds and mattress overlays: A decision guide. Am J Nurs 1989; 89(9):1142.
Wyngaarden JB, Smith LH. Cecil textbook of medicine. 17th ed. Philadelphia: WB Saunders, 1987.
Yurick AG, et al. The aged person and the nursing process. 2nd ed. Norwalk, CT: Appleton-Century-Crofts, 1984.

Chapter Thirty-six

NURSING CARE *of Adults with Musculoskeletal Disorders*

The musculoskeletal system provides support and protection for the body. Disorders of the system are often multifaceted and have a variety of underlying causes. The disorders may affect all age groups in the adult population and are particularly common in the older adult. Musculoskeletal disorders affect bones, joints, muscles, tendons, ligaments, and bursae. Major manifestations of musculoskeletal problems include the hazards of immobility, which, in turn, affect many other body systems.

Many of the disorders of the musculoskeletal system are debilitating. This presents specific implications for nursing care. Because the elderly, in particular, are prone to musculoskeletal disorders, many due to the natural aging process, long-term care planning, home care instructions, and follow-up care all are important facets of nursing interventions. Referrals to other agencies outside the hospital for continued care may be necessary for the patient as a result of the problems with immobility and safety associated with musculoskeletal disorders.

Infections and Inflammations

Osteomyelitis

Etiology. Osteomyelitis is an infection of the bone with necrosis of bone and marrow tissue. It weakens the bone and places it at high risk for spontaneous pathologic fractures or fractures with minimum trauma. Osteomyelitis may be caused by bacteria, tubercle bacilli, *Treponema pallidum,* fungi, or the presence of contaminated foreign material such as a bullet or a joint prosthesis. *Staphylococcus aureus* and *Streptococcus pyogenes* are the organisms most frequently associated with osteomyelitis. The pathogens may enter the bone by direct contamination from an open fracture, spread to the bone from another infected body part, or lodge in the bone or marrow from pathogens present in the blood stream. Osteomyelitis may be acute or chronic. Both forms have the same pathologic process occurring but may vary in causative agent, progression, and symptoms.

Pathophysiology. Osteomyelitis involves infection of the haversian canals, bone marrow, and subperiosteal spaces. Initially, bone tissue and blood vessels are destroyed by proteolytic enzymes released by the pathogens. Because of diminished blood flow, removal of debris from the infected area is impaired. As the infection spreads through the bone and subperiosteal spaces, the necrotic debris accumulates. It separates from the rest of the bone and forms a substance known as sequestrum. The sequestrum becomes a reservoir for more bacterial growth.

Damage to the bone and periosteum stimulates osteoblastic activity, and new bone tissue, called involucrum, forms around the sequestrum. Formation of the involucrum and separation of the sequestrum further impair circulation to the diseased bone.

ACUTE OSTEOMYELITIS

Acute osteomyelitis is a condition seen more in children than in adults. It occurs four times more often in males than in females. The prime causative organism is *S. aureus.*

Clinical Manifestations. Clinical manifestations depend upon the extent of the infection and route of contamination. When acute osteomyelitis develops directly from bacteremia, the patient experiences sudden onset of fever and rapid pulse with limited movement and severe pain in the involved body part caused by spasms of surrounding muscles. Osteomyelitis contracted by direct contamination of the bone or by spread from another body part presents fewer systemic effects, but muscle spasms and tenderness over the bone are present.

Medical Diagnosis. Laboratory data include elevated leukocyte count and sedimentation rate. Radiographic changes may not be seen for 1 week to 10 days after the onset of infection. X-ray films then reveal a localized area of destruction surrounded by a zone of decalcified bone. The sequestrum appears as dense areas on x-ray films. Identification of the causative organism is made by blood cultures and aspiration of subperiosteal pus for culture and sensitivity.

Medical Management. The goal of medical management is to rid the body of the infectious organism and prevent spread of the infection to surrounding tissues. Treatment includes debridement of necrotic tissue and large doses of parenteral, then oral, antibiotics until the organism is eradicated. Combinations of antibiotics to prevent growth of resistant organisms may be administered for up to 1 year.

Because the sequestrum and involucrum impair circulation to the infected bone, they must be removed before antibiotic therapy can be effective. Surgical debridement or a closed irrigation system to low suction with normal saline or antibiotic solution may be used to flush away necrotic tissue.

Complications of acute osteomyelitis include septicemia, meningitis, tendosynovitis, and thrombophlebitis. Acute osteomyelitis may also become a chronic infection if inadequately treated.

CHRONIC OSTEOMYELITIS

Chronic osteomyelitis is characterized by gradual progressive development of multiple bone cavities with sequestrum and involucrum throughout the bone.

Clinical Manifestations. The patient with chronic osteomyelitis experiences episodes of pain, caused by the inflammatory activity, and symptom-free periods when the inflammatory activity is decreased. Pain is usually more intense at night. Involved areas are swollen, reddened, warm, and tender to touch. Other symptoms may include deformed bone, dusky skin, atrophied muscles of the involved area, and development of draining sinuses.

Medical Diagnosis. X-ray films show multiple dense areas of sequestrum. Drainage from sinus tracts and aspirated fluid is cultured to identify the causative organism. Sensitivity studies determine antibiotic therapy.

Medical Management. Treatment involves surgical removal of involved tissue, continuous closed suction wound drainage, and combination antibiotic therapy. A windowed cast that allows access for wound care may be applied to support the weakened bone. For particularly resistant or difficult to eradicate cases, a muscle flap transfer that increases blood supply to the involved bone may be done. Hyperbaric oxygen has also been effective in treating some cases. When all conservative measures to control osteomyelitis are unsuccessful, amputation may be required.

Complications of chronic osteomyelitis include muscle contractures, decreased rate of bone growth, nonunion of fractures, and pathologic fracture through the involved bone.

TUBERCULOUS OSTEOMYELITIS

Infection of bone tissue and joints by the tubercle bacillus *Myobacterium tuberculosis* occurs secondary to tubercle lesions elsewhere in the body. Like active tuberculosis, it is more likely to occur in malnourished and physically compromised individuals. Although tuberculous osteomyelitis is uncommon in the United States today, with the current rise in the incidence of active tuberculosis, it may be seen more often in the near future.

Tuberculosis of the bone precipitates the same response in bone tissue as in the lung. The tubercle bacillus invades the bone, and the body's natural immune response encases the organisms within a bone cavitation. The bacillus becomes reactivated when the patient's immune system is weakened.

Clinical Manifestations. The onset of bone tuberculosis is slow and secondary to other organ lesions. The involved areas are warm and tender to the touch. The patient may report pain and muscle spasm, muscle atrophy, and stiff joints. The spine and lower extremities are most often affected. The involved vertebrae may collapse, giving the patient a hunchback appearance. Abscesses and draining sinuses may develop. Neurologic dysfunction from spinal cord compression or inflammation may result in muscular weakness and paralysis. Systemic symptoms include a low-grade fever that is higher at night or in the late afernoon, anorexia, malaise, and weight loss.

Medical Diagnosis. Diagnostic x-ray films show altered bone structure, collapsed vertebrae and compression deformities. Tuberculin skin test results are positive. Acid-fast tubercle bacilli are identified in sputum cultures, joint fluid, or tissue biopsy. Laboratory studies reveal elevated leukocyte count and increased sedimentation rate.

Medical Management. Treatment includes administration of combinations of antitubercular agents to control the infection. Isoniazid, para-aminosalicylic acid, ethambutol, streptomycin, and rifampin are drugs of choice.

OTHER FORMS OF OSTEOMYELITIS

Other causative organisms of osteomyelitis include *T. pallidum*, fungi, and *Salmonella*. Syphilis osteomyelitis affects the bone in the tertiary stage of the disease. It is characterized by a "moth-eaten" appearance of the bone on x-ray film. The patient may complain of bone pain and experience pathologic fractures. Penicillin is used to treat the infection.

Fungal or mycotic osteomyelitis is caused by blastomycosis and coccidioidomycosis. Bone involvement usually begins after respiratory infection. The fungus invades cancellous bone and produces well-defined areas on x-ray film. Amphotericin B is administered to treat the infection.

Salmonella osteomyelitis produces an acute form of osteomyelitis. Individuals with sickle-cell disease are at high risk for this condition. Treatment consists of administration of chloramphenicol or high doses of penicillin or ampicillin.

Application of the Nursing Process to the Care of the Patient with Osteomyelitis

Assessment

Review the patient's history, presenting symptoms, and diagnostic studies. Complete an assessment, observing for outward signs of infection in the affected area. Look for redness, warmth, swelling, and pain. Ask the patient about the severity and duration of the pain and what relief methods have been successful. Check vital signs. Look for additional signs of fever such as flushing, night sweats, and chilling. Determine the patient's understanding of the disease and the treatment regimen.

Nursing Diagnoses and Planning

Nursing diagnoses and related expected patient outcomes most commonly applicable to patients with osteomyelitis include the following:

NDx: Pain related to infection and inflammation

Planning: Patient outcomes
1. Patient denies pain in affected part.
2. Patient states methods to decrease pain, such as using relaxation strategies and reducing swelling and trauma to the affected part.

NDx: Knowledge deficit: nature of disease, treatment, and prognosis

Planning: Patient outcomes
1. Patient states accurate information about the cause of the disease and methods to reduce complications.
2. Patient discusses concerns about the disease and states an understanding of the prognosis and treatment regimen.

Nursing Interventions

NDx: Pain
Give prescribed analgesics and explain the dosage, frequency, side effects, and expected therapeutic effects of the medications. Caution the patient not to perform tasks that require mental alertness while under the effects of the pain medication. Tell the patient to elevate the part to reduce swelling and thus reduce pain. Caution the patient about weight-bearing if contraindicated, because that might increase the pain significantly.

NDx: Knowledge deficit: nature of disease, treatment, and prognosis
Teach the patient about the disease, the cause, methods of prevention of injury to the affected part, and appropriate treatment. Explain that increased swelling, redness, discoloration, or decreased sensation in the affected part may be signs of complications and that the physician should be notified. Reinforce the physician's instruction about weight-lifting (if shoulder, arm, or hand is affected) or weight-bearing (if knee, leg, ankle, or foot is affected). Discuss the antibiotics prescribed, explaining the side effects, expected therapeutic effects, dosage, and frequency.

Evaluation

Evaluate the effectiveness of nursing care for a patient with osteomyelitis by comparing the patient's status with the expected patient outcomes. Examples of specific outcomes for patients with osteomyelitis have been provided in the Planning section.

Arthritis

The general term *arthritis* is defined as inflammation of a joint. It is associated with swelling and pain and can include changes in the structure of involved musculoskeletal tissue. There are more than 100 types of arthritis, each differing somewhat in etiology, pathophysiology and method of treatment. More than 23 million people in the United States are affected by some form of arthritis that is severe enough to require medical attention.

Arthritis is a leading cause of mobility limitation. It can make activities such as dressing, opening a jar, climbing stairs, or getting out of chairs difficult and painful tasks. Persons suffering from arthritis may need more time to perform everyday activities and may also be more dependent on other people. The most prevalent forms of arthritis are rheumatoid arthritis and osteoarthritis.

RHEUMATOID ARTHRITIS

Rheumatoid arthritis is the most serious form of arthritis. It should not be confused with rheumatism, which is a popular lay term used to describe any musculoskeletal symptom of pain or stiffness. Rheumatoid arthritis is a chronic systemic disease characterized by inflammation of the joints and extra-articular manifestations. When it occurs in persons older than 60, it tends to be severe and rapidly progressive.

Etiology. The cause of rheumatoid arthritis is unknown, but it is believed to be an autoimmune disorder. It affects more than 6 million people in the United States.

Pathophysiology. Antibodies produced by the immune system, which usually protect the body, become destructive agents that attack and destroy joint structures. The antibodies first attack the synovium of the joint, causing the joint to become inflamed and swollen with excess synovial fluid. Gradually the articular cartilage and surrounding tendons and ligaments are involved. Chronic congestion and thickening of the synovium produce granulation tissue called pannus, which is Latin for cloth. The pannus causes further erosion of the articular cartilage and invades the joint capsule. As the disease progresses, underlying bone and adjacent connective tissues are damaged. Tough fibrous connective tissue replaces the pannus and fills the joint space. As the fibrous tissue calcifies, the joint becomes ankylosed, or fused. The patient is left with a joint that is painful and often deformed and has very limited or no range of motion.

Clinical Manifestations. Rheumatoid arthritis is more prevalent among females than males and is more likely to develop in persons between 20 and 40 years of age. Rheumatoid arthritis is characterized by remissions, or improvement of symptoms, and exacerbations, or an increase in the severity of symptoms. Exacerbations may be aggravated by emotional or physical stress and illness. Patients usually appear anemic, are anorectic, look and feel ill, have a low-grade fever, and are likely to be underweight.

Joint involvement is symmetric. The joints are

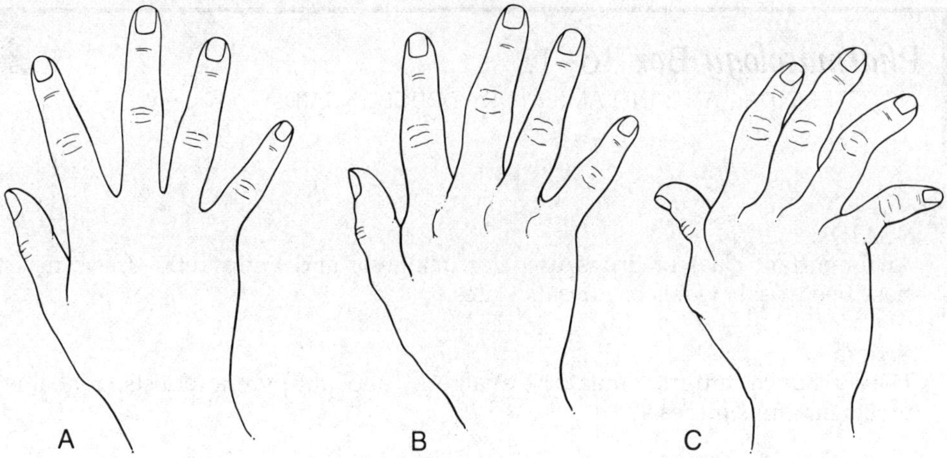

Figure 36–1.

Structure changes in the hand from rheumatoid arthritis. *A*, Early involvement stage; *B*, moderate involvement stage; *C*, advanced involvement stage.

swollen, shiny, reddened, and painful. Joints of the hands and wrists, with the exception of the distal interphalangeal joints, are commonly affected first (Fig. 36–1). Diarthrodial joints are more frequently affected, but any joint of the body may be involved. Pathologic changes in the hand joints commonly result in subluxation of the fingers, hand, and wrist. Classic deformities such as a swan-neck deformity (hyperextension of the proximal interphalangeal joint with fixed flexion of the distal interphalangeal joint), a boutonnière deformity (persistent flexion of the proximal interphalangeal joint with hyperextension of the distal interphalangeal joint), and ulnar deviation of the fingers occur, leaving the hands painful and nonfunctioning. Chronic joint pain of varying intensity, which is more severe upon arising, is experienced by most patients.

Systemic manifestations include muscle atrophy; vasculitis of the smaller peripheral vessels, which can lead to cutaneous ulceration; inflammation of tissue overlying the sclera of the eye; a decrease in salivary and lacrimal secretions (Sjögren's syndrome); carpal tunnel syndrome; and pulmonary nodules and fibrosis. Rheumatoid nodules, which are subcutaneous moveable skin nodules near bony prominences, may occur anywhere on the body.

Medical Diagnosis. Diagnosis is made on the basis of history and radiologic studies. X-ray films reveal clouding of fluid spaces, fraying of inner joint margins, and gradual lessening of joint space.

Although specific blood values are usually abnormal in rheumatoid arthritis, none are considered diagnostic. Laboratory studies show a normal red blood count (RBC) in the early stages, then a decreasing RBC as the disease progresses. An increased white blood count (WBC); elevated erythrocyte sedimentation rate (ESR), which rises with the severity of the disease; and an elevated platelet count are present. The rheumatoid factor (RF), an immunoglobulin that reacts with antibodies produced by lymphocytes in the synovial fluid, is present in 40% to 50% of patients with rheumatoid arthritis in the early stages of the disease, and 80% to 90% of patients with advanced disease. Because the rheumatoid factor may be present in other inflammatory diseases, it is not considered diagnostic for rheumatoid arthritis. Levels of antinuclear antibodies (ANA) and C-reactive proteins may also be elevated. A genetic marker, HLA-Dw4, is present in 50% of patients. Synovial fluid has a high WBC and poor viscosity.

Medical Management. Since there is no cure for rheumatoid arthritis, efforts are directed at improving general health, reducing the inflammatory process, relieving pain, and maintaining mobility of the affected joints. This requires lifelong treatment by numerous health care specialists. Patient understanding and participation and family support are essential factors affecting the course of the disease.

Early management involves educating the patient about the disease process, providing adequate nutrition, having the patient maintain good general health while avoiding physical stress, giving instruction in stress control techniques, and administering drug therapy to decrease the inflammatory reaction. Medications used to decrease the inflammatory process include enteric-coated aspirin in large doses, nonsteroidal anti-inflammatory agents (Pharmacology Box 36–1), and systemic steroids. Other drugs such as parenteral gold preparations, immunosuppressive agents, and penicillamine have been used with success in some patients.

Long-term care includes referrals to different health care personnel and a variety of modes of therapy. A social service referral is usually initiated early in the course of the disease because of its progressively debilitating nature.

Occupational therapists teach the patient how to conserve energy and maintain joint alignment. They also provide splints to protect and support involved joints. Resting splints may be used for night wear and functional splints for protection and support while working.

Physical therapists play an important role in the care of the patient with rheumatoid arthritis. They provide assistive devices to protect weight-bearing joints and assist with ambulation. Physical therapy includes exercises to prevent stiffness and slow loss of joint motion and to maintain muscle size and strength. Passive, active, and stretching exercises

Pharmacology Box 36–1.

NONSTEROIDAL ANTI-INFLAMMATORY DRUGS (NSAIDs)

NSAIDs:
An important class of drugs used for analgesic and antipyretic effects in arthritis treatment. They are classified as salicylates or nonsalicylates.

Action:
They produce anti-inflammatory, analgesic, and antipyretic effects, probably through the inhibition of prostaglandin synthesis.

Uses:
They are used primarily for osteoarthritis and rheumatoid arthritis but may also be prescribed for ankylosing spondylitis, bursitis, or tendinitis.

Side Effects:
Drowsiness, irritability, headache, tinnitus, indigestion, nausea, gastrointestinal bleeding, colitis, pruritus, rashes, and hepatotoxicity.

Interactions:
The interactions may vary with the specific drug. Many of the NSAIDs interact with anticoagulants, alcohol, certain diuretics, aspirin, and other salicylates.

Nursing Implications:
Watch for gastric distress and signs of gastrointestinal bleeding such as dark stools.
Observe for bruising, petechiae, or excessive bleeding from mucous membranes or small skin lesions.
Give the drug with milk or meals to decrease irritation.
Watch for and document side effects or apparent interactions.
Tell the patient to be wary of taking the drug with aspirin.
Teach the patient the correct dose, frequency, side effects, and therapeutic effects of the drug.
Tell the patient to report any untoward effects to the attending physician.
Check liver studies for abnormalities.

Geriatric Considerations:
The older adult should be closely monitored for liver impairment. Renal function should also be checked. Dosages may need to be reduced if nephrotoxicity or hepatotoxicity seems apparent.

may be recommended. During acute exacerbations, joints may remain at rest with only limited passive exercising.

Local heat and cold applications may be used to relieve pain. The patient is instructed in their proper use at home. Although thermal applications do not decrease synovial proliferation and swelling, they provide temporary comfort by decreasing muscle spasms and altering the pain threshold. Generally, cold is used for acute joint pain, and heat is used for chronic joint pain. Cold may be applied by massage with an ice cube until numbness is achieved. Heat may be applied by moist heat packs or paraffin baths.

Another method for controlling chronic pain is the use of transcutaneous electrical nerve stimulation (TENS) to a body part by electrodes attached to the skin. The system is portable and patient controlled. A TENS unit relieves pain and reduces the need for analgesics. Theories to explain how it works suggest that TENS promotes release of endorphins or blocks the passage of pain impulses from the local area to the central nervous system.

When conservative treatment is not adequate, surgery is sometimes used to relieve pain and correct deformities. Types of surgery for rheumatoid arthritis, are synovectomy, osteotomy, arthrodesis, and arthroplasty or total joint replacement.

A synovectomy is the removal of hypertrophied synovium. It is done to delay the destructive process within the joint. Synovectomies are most commonly performed on the elbow, wrist, fingers, and knees.

An osteotomy is the cutting and removal of bone to change joint alignment. This procedure reduces stress on the involved joint, and improved function often results. Arthrodesis is fusion of a joint. Although it causes permanent immobilization of the joint, the joint is more stable and less painful. The joints that are most frequently surgically fused are the wrist and ankle. Arthroplasty with total joint replacement is discussed in Chapter 35.

Application of the Nursing Process to the Care of the Patient with Rheumatoid Arthritis

Assessment

Review the patient's history and current physical problems. Because pain is one of the most significant and chronic problems in arthritis, assess the patient's pain tolerance and its debilitating effects. Check which joints are most severely affected. Determine the patient's perception of the pain experienced, what time of day it is most severe, and what precipitates it. Emotional stress has been associated with exacerbations of rheumatoid arthritis. Ask the patient which, if any, medications have been beneficial in relieving pain, stiffness, or inflammatory reactions.

Examine the affected joints, observing for redness, edema, crepitation, deformity, subluxation, dislocation, ankylosis, and muscle contractions. Look at the affected limbs, noting atrophy, decreased subcutaneous fat, and the presence of subcutaneous nodules. Note mobility problems and difficulties with hand motions.

Determine the patient's and family's understanding of the disease and its progression. Ask the patient about effective coping mechanisms used in the past and what personal support systems are available.

Nursing Diagnoses and Planning

Nursing diagnoses and related expected patient outcomes most commonly applicable to patients with rheumatoid arthritis include the following:

NDx: Pain related to joint or muscle deformity and inflammation

Planning: Patient outcomes
1. Patient denies pain in affected part.
2. Patient states methods to decrease pain such as rest and relaxation therapies.
3. Patient states appropriate use of analgesics or anti-inflammatory agents, and the TENS unit if prescribed.

NDx: Impaired physical mobility related to the rheumatoid disease process and pain

Planning: Patient outcomes
1. Patient moves in bed with the assistance of nursing intervention and an overhead trapeze.
2. Patient performs passive range-of-motion exercises to maintain strength and joint movement during periods of immobility.
3. Patient maintains mobility with the assistance of an ambulatory aid.

NDx: Self-esteem disturbance related to change in appearance from deformities and inability to move freely

Planning: Patient outcomes
1. Patient relates feelings of self-worth.
2. Patient maintains social activity.
3. Patient is able to look at self with understanding and acceptance.

NDx: Self-care deficit: bathing, dressing, or grooming related to decrease in strength and deformities of joints with restricted movement

Planning: Patient outcomes
1. Patient cares for self with little assistance from others.
2. Patient uses assistive devices to provide support for self-care.
3. Patient practices exercises to maintain joint mobility to allow continued independence.

NDx: High risk for injury; falls, related to mobility problems secondary to joint deformity and pain, and improper use of ambulatory aids

Planning: Patient outcomes
1. Patient remains free from injury.
2. Patient demonstrates safe use of ambulatory aid device.
3. Patient states accurate information about the causes of injuries and methods to prevent injury.

NDx: Knowledge deficit: nature of disorder, its progression, and self-care interventions

Planning: Patient outcomes
1. Patient relates accurate information about the disorder.
2. Patient repeats instructions as issued by the physician for home care.
3. Patient has list of referral services and support networks available.

Nursing Interventions

NDx: Pain
Help the patient deal with the chronic pain by using alternatives to pain medication such as relaxation

exercises. Teach deep-breathing techniques and other full body relaxation strategies.

When pain is acute, give prescribed analgesics and anti-inflammatory agents, and explain the dosage, frequency, side effects, and expected therapeutic effects of the medications. Caution the patient not to perform tasks that require mental alertness while under the effects of the pain medication. Handle the patient carefully when moving in bed. Caution the patient about weight-bearing on affected joints without assistance when the disease is in a stage of exacerbation because that might increase the pain significantly.

Apply prescribed heat or cold packs to decrease muscle spasms and promote pain relief. Advise the patient that a warm shower may be helpful in relieving morning pain and stiffness. Reinforce instructions from the therapist in the use of the TENS unit, as ordered. Maintain rest and support of affected inflamed joints.

NDx: Impaired physical mobility

Teach the patient use of the overhead trapeze while still on bed rest to increase movement in bed, as allowed, to prevent complications of immobility. Reposition the patient frequently to stimulate circulation and prevent skin breakdown. Assist the patient in locomotion, once able, to promote safe use of the ambulatory aid. Use the assistance of the physical therapist to instruct the patient and family about the device and to reinforce its safe use. Give analgesics as needed to decrease pain levels that may interfere with the patient's ability to be mobile.

NDx: Self-esteem disturbance

Allow the patient to vent feelings about the disorder. Provide information about self-help groups. Seek assistance from clergy or professional counseling. Provide diversional activities for the patient when on bed rest as a result of exacerbations from the disease. Involve support from the family and other friends. Seek effective coping strategies for the patient. Assist the patient in finding the positive aspects of life to focus on during periods of depression.

NDx: Self-care deficit: bathing, dressing, or grooming

Provide assistance for the patient during bathing and grooming, as needed. Teach the patient methods to complete hygiene tasks that utilize alternative methods. Explain to the family that clothing with Velcro attachments may be easier for the patient to use. Tell the patient to rest frequently while performing the self-care activities to avoid pain and overtiring.

NDx: High risk for injury; falls

Provide assistance during locomotion, as necessary, until the patient becomes skillful with the ambulatory aid. Reinforce the information on the use of the device that was presented by the therapist. Teach the family about safe use of the ambulatory aid. Be sure the patient wears well-fitting shoes with gripper soles while ambulating. Explain how to make the home environment safer for the patient while using the ambulatory aid.

NDx: Knowledge deficit: nature of disorder, its progression, and self-care interventions

Provide information to the patient and family about the disease, its progression, the planned treatment, and self-care interventions. Encourage the patient to ask questions and to express fears and concerns. Answer questions honestly while reinforcing the positive aspects of the patient's life. Encourage and reinforce instructions in the use of medications, splints or braces, and ambulatory aids. Discuss modification of the home environment, which will help the patient maintain independence.

Teach the patient about good nutrition to maintain health status. Encourage a diet high in protein, vitamins, and minerals, with increased fiber to prevent constipation during periods of inactivity.

Initiate social service referral to help the patient use all resources available to provide financial assistance and to maintain role performance and independence. Inform the patient of the local and national support groups for arthritics. The Arthritis Foundation is a voluntary national organization that provides a number of services, including research support, training of specialists, and public and patient information services. The local address is usually found in the yellow pages of the telephone directory. The national organization can be contacted at the Arthritis Foundation, 475 Riverside Drive, New York, NY 10027.

Evaluation

Evaluate the effectiveness of nursing care for a patient with rheumatoid arthritis by comparing the patient's status with the expected patient outcomes. Examples of specific outcomes for patients with rheumatoid arthritis have been provided in the Planning section.

OSTEOARTHRITIS

Also called degenerative joint disease, osteoarthritis is the most common form of arthritis. It is a less destructive, nonsystemic disorder confined to the joint. Osteoarthritis causes degenerative changes in the joint surfaces of weight-bearing joints such as the spine, hips, and knees and in the frequently used joints of the hands. A patient may have both rheumatoid arthritis and osteoarthritis. The prognosis for osteoarthritis is much more positive than that of rheumatoid arthritis because treatment can slow joint destruction and not all joints are involved.

Etiology. There are two types of osteoarthritis: primary and secondary. Primary osteoarthritis is attributed to a genetic predisposition to deterioration of articular cartilage. Primary osteoarthritis is more prevalent in women, and onset may occur as young as 40 years of age. Theories suggest the predisposition may be the result of either an abnormal chemical structure of the articular cartilage or the presence of joints that do not fit together properly and thus develop early wear.

Secondary osteoarthritis, the result of excessive "wear and tear" or trauma of affected joints, is more common after the age of 50. Obesity with continuous excessive stress on joints from excess weight and repeated joint injuries from contact sports are two factors identified as predispositions to secondary osteoarthritis. The accumulated effects of daily stress and wear can also result in secondary arthritis as age advances. X-ray films of most persons older than age 65 reveal some joint deterioration.

Pathophysiology. In both forms of osteoarthritis, as the articular cartilage deteriorates, the surface becomes rough, and soft spots, or malacia, develop. As the softened cartilage is worn away, the joint space narrows and bone surfaces begin to rub against each other. New subchondral bone forms to heal the damaged joint surfaces. As new bone repeatedly forms and is rubbed off, bone spurs, bone cysts, and extended joint margins called osteophytes develop. These abnormal bone growths create joint deformity and pain on motion. Fusion of the joint does not occur.

Clinical Manifestations. Osteoarthritis is characterized by the presence of a dull aching pain in the affected joints. Unlike with rheumatoid arthritis, systemic manifestations are absent and joint involvement is not symmetric. Crepitus, or a grating sound, may be heard and felt on joint movement. Enlargement of the joint and limitation of motion progress over time. The involved fingers often develop painless bony nodules on the dorsolateral surface of the interphalangeal joints. Nodules on the distal interphalangeal joints are Heberden's nodes. Those on the proximal interphalangeal joints are Bouchard's nodes.

Stiffness and joint pain increase as joint deterioration progresses. Stiffness also increases with lack of activity. Pain is usually more severe early in the morning and may be aggravated by cold damp weather. The presence of constant pain and stiff joints leads to fatigue and loss of coordination.

Medical Diagnosis. X-ray film may show lessening of joint space and extension of joint margin as early as 6 months after the onset of the disease. However, radiologic changes are not always consistent with the pain and limitation of motion a patient is experiencing.

No specific laboratory findings are useful in diagnosing osteoarthritis. The patient may have a normal or slightly elevated sedimentation rate.

Medical Management. The management of osteoarthritis is planned to meet the individual patient's needs as determined by the patient's lifestyle and general health. Enteric-coated aspirin or nonsteroidal anti-inflammatory agents are prescribed to relieve pain (see Pharmacology Box 36–1). Parenteral steroids are injected into an acutely inflamed joint. If the patient is overweight, a weight reduction diet may be recommended.

Exercises to preserve joint strength and range of motion, as well as heat or cold applications to relieve pain and relax muscles, are implemented as needed. Joint protection to prevent further joint damage may include avoidance of strenuous activities that create excessive stress on affected joints and the use of assistive devices such as canes, walker, and crutches to reduce weight-bearing.

In situations in which extensive damage of involved joints is present, arthroplasty or total joint replacement may be done to decrease pain and improve function.

Application of the Nursing Process to the Care of the Patient with Osteoarthritis

The assessment, nursing diagnoses, expected patient outcomes, nursing interventions, and evaluation for patients with osteoarthritis are similar to those described previously for patients with rheumatoid arthritis. In addition, see Chart 36–1, which provides discharge instructions for patients with osteoarthritis.

ANKYLOSING SPONDYLITIS

Also called Marie-Strümpell disease, ankylosing spondylitis is a chronic, progressive inflammatory arthritis of the spine and sacroiliac joint. It is characterized by ankylosing and fusion of the spondylus, or vertebra. Once thought to be a form of rheumatoid arthritis, it is actually a distinct type of systemic arthritis.

Etiology. Ankylosing spondylitis has a strong familial tendency, but the exact cause is unknown. It occurs more frequently in families with a history of the disorder and is usually diagnosed in adolescence or early adulthood. It is rare in blacks in the United States.

Pathophysiology. Ankylosing spondylitis begins in the sacroiliac joints and spreads up the spine. As it spreads, succeeding joints become inflamed and fibrotic. As the costovertebral joints and disk spaces deteriorate, they are replaced by bony growth. The spine becomes rigid and ankylosed. Thoracic kyphosis develops with compensating hip flexure, and the ribs, shoulder, neck, and temporomandibular joint

Chart 36–1.

NURSING GUIDE TO PATIENT EDUCATION FOR SELF-MANAGEMENT: DISCHARGE INSTRUCTIONS FOR PATIENTS WITH OSTEOARTHRITIS

Instruct the patient to:

Take prescribed analgesics and/or anti-inflammatory agents as scheduled and before activities that may precipitate episodes of pain.

Maintain the affected joints in a non-flexed, well-aligned position to prevent flexion contractures.

Apply heat or cold packs, as preferred, to decrease muscle spasms and promote pain relief.

Take a warm bath or shower to help relieve morning stiffness.

Perform relaxation techniques, as demonstrated, to help reduce muscle spasms and relieve pain.

Follow prescribed exercise program to maintain range of motion of involved joints.

Refrain from exercising joints beyond the point of pain or fatigue because further injury can occur.

Follow dietary recommendations for weight loss (if overweight) to decrease stress on weight-bearing joints.

Use ambulatory aids, as prescribed, to decrease weight-bearing.

Follow safety instructions while using the ambulatory aid.

Avoid activities that increase stress on involved joints or that may cause additional trauma to the joints.

become involved. Ocular and cardiac involvement can also occur.

Clinical Manifestations. The disease follows an insidious pattern of exacerbations and remissions. Some patients have experienced complete spontaneous remission. The patient usually has a long history of low back pain that is worse at night and upon arising. The pain radiates from the buttocks to the thigh. Although the pain pattern resembles that of sciatica, it does not extend below the knee as does sciatic pain. Involvement is asymmetric and slow in onset. The patient may also experience fever, malaise, and back muscle spasms. Physical examination may reveal a decrease in chest expansion due to costovertebral involvement.

Untreated patients can develop a rigid kyphosis that results in the complication of thoracic organ compression. Patients who develop iritis or other ocular complications are referred to an ophthalmologist. Cardiac dysrhythmias, valve disease, and pulmonary fibrosis may also occur.

Medical Diagnosis. A genetic marker, the human leukocyte-associated antigen with a B27 gene (HLA-B27), is present in 90% of the patients with ankylosing spondylitis. Rheumatoid factor and rheumatoid nodules are absent. The erythrocyte sedimentation rate and levels of alkaline phosphatase and creatine phosphokinase are usually elevated.

X-ray films show fusion of intervertebral bodies with possible calcification on the anterior and posterior longitudinal ligaments of the spinal column. This appearance of the spinal column is referred to as "bamboo spine."

Medical Management. Medical management focuses on providing relief from pain, decreasing the inflammatory process, and preventing and correcting deformity. Pain and inflammation are treated with heat applications, salicylates, and nonsteroidal anti-inflammatory agents. Indomethacin and phenylbutazone have been particularly successful in relieving the symptoms of ankylosing spondylitis. Steroids are sometimes successful in inducing remission.

Rest may be prescribed for acute episodes of inflammation. Spinal extensor strengthening exercises and breathing exercises to maintain chest expansion are recommended. Instruct the patient to maintain an erect posture when sitting or standing to prevent flexion contractures. Wearing special orthotic back braces, sleeping on a firm mattress without a pillow, and sitting in chairs with a high back and firm support help prevent further deformity. Surgical intervention to correct flexion deformities or total hip replacement of ankylosed hip joints may be indicated.

Application of the Nursing Process to the Care of the Patient with Ankylosing Spondylitis

The assessment, nursing diagnoses, expected patient outcomes, nursing interventions, and evaluation for patients with ankylosing spondylitis are similar to those described previously for patients with rheumatoid arthritis.

GOUT

Etiology and Pathophysiology. Gout is a painful metabolic bone disorder in which an inflammatory joint reaction is caused by accumulation of uric acid crystals in the involved joint and soft tissues (Fig. 36–2). The base of the large toe (the first metatarsal phalangeal joint) is primarily affected, but the instep, ankle, knees, elbows, and hands may also be affected.

Gout is caused by a buildup of uric acid in the blood. Primary gout results from a genetic error in purine metabolism, which leads to overproduction or retention of uric acid. Although purines are present in high concentrations in protein and alcohol, high dietary intake of these substances alone does not cause hyperuricemia. However, their ingestion may precipitate an acute episode of gout in a person who already has the disorder. More than 90% of the individuals who have primary gout are men older than age 30. Few women suffer from primary gout. Those who do are usually postmenopausal or older than age 50. Prolonged fasting or excessive drinking increases uric acid in the blood by decreasing excretion through the kidney and can cause secondary gout.

Clinical Manifestations. Initial episodes of acute gout usually involve one joint. The joint becomes red, warm, shiny, swollen, and extremely sensitive to the slightest touch. The patient may have an elevated temperature of 100° to 103°F (38° to 39.5°C). Blood pressure is sometimes elevated, possibly because of the pain response. Nodular deposits of uric acid crystals, called tophi, may be present around the fingers or ear lobes in individuals with chronic severe hyperuricemia. Episodes of acute inflammation usually last less than 10 days. Repeated inflammation may result in joint deformity. Patients are forced by extreme pain to rest the joint and most seek medical attention early in an acute episode.

Medical Diagnosis. Diagnosis of gout is made on the basis of the clinical manifestations, hyperuricemia, and the presence of uric acid crystals in the synovial fluid of the inflamed joint. Blood studies show an increased serum uric acid level of more than 7 mg/100 ml. The erythrocyte sedimentation rate and white blood cell count may be elevated during an acute episode. Twenty-four-hour urine uric acid levels are elevated. X-ray films may show urate deposits in the joints or tophi.

Medical Management. The goals of medical management are to relieve pain, prevent permanent joint damage, and eliminate further acute episodes. Medications and diet are very effective in alleviating symptoms and preventing recurrent episodes of gout.

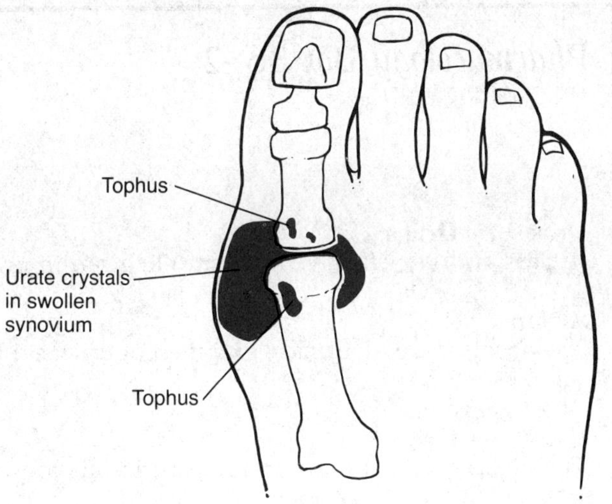

Figure 36–2.

Gouty joint. A tophaceous mass is apparent at the base of the great toe, with urate crystal deposits in the synovium.

Nonsteroidal anti-inflammatory agents such as phenylbutazone (Butazolidin), indomethacin (Indocin), and ibuprofen are used to treat acute episodes. Colchicine, 0.6 mg/hour for up to 10 hours, can bring such rapid relief from an acute episode of gout that many physicians use it as a diagnostic aid. The uricosuric drug allopurinol, 200 to 300 mg daily, is administered to decrease serum uric acid levels in patients with chronic gout. Sulfinpyrazone and probenecid, also uricosuric drugs, may be used prophylactically to prevent reabsorption of uric acid by the kidneys (Pharmacology Box 36–2). Aspirin inactivates uricosurics and therefore should be avoided by persons with a history of gout. Weight reduction is recommended for overweight individuals.

Application of the Nursing Process to the Care of the Patient with Gout

Assessment

Review the patient's history and presenting symptoms. Examine the affected joint for the classic manifestations of an acute episode of gout. Determine the extent of pain and interference with mobility. Question the patient about precipitating events such as trauma, changes in diet, or the use of medications that inhibit the excretion of uric acid.

Pharmacology Box 36–2.
URICOSURIC DRUGS

Uricosuric Drugs:
A class of drugs effective for controlling serum urate levels.

Action:
The agents increase urinary excretion of uric acid by preventing the reabsorption of uric acid in the renal tubules.

Uses:
The drugs are used to control hyperuricemia to prevent attacks of gouty arthritis.

Side Effects:
Headache, dizziness, hypotension, anorexia, nausea, gastric distress, urinary frequency, renal colic, fever, and flushing.

Interactions:
The drugs may interact with salicylates. They can also enhance the effects of hypoglycemic agents and decrease indomethacin excretion.

Nursing Implications:
Tell the patient to avoid alcohol because it increases the urate level.
Inform the patient to avoid all medications that contain aspirin.
Encourage increased fluid intake to maintain an output of 2 to 3 L. This helps prevent hematuria, renal colic, and stone development.
Give the drug with milk or meals to prevent gastric distress.
Teach the patient to avoid high-purine foods as listed in Nutrition Box 36–1.

Geriatric Considerations:
Increased gastric irritation may be present as a result of decreased gastrointestinal motility in the older adult. Give the drug with food and fluids.

Nursing Diagnoses and Planning

Nursing diagnoses and related expected patient outcomes most commonly applicable to patients with gout include the following:

NDx: Pain related to joint inflammation

Planning: Patient outcomes
1. Patient denies acute pain in affected joint.
2. Patient is able to tolerate some discomfort without decreasing mobility.

NDx: Ineffective management of therapeutic regimen related to lack of knowledge about the disease, its cause, prognosis, and information regarding medications and diet therapy

Planning: Patient outcomes
1. Patient relates accurate information about the disease, its cause, and prognosis.
2. Patient states correct information about the drug and diet therapy.
3. Patient chooses food low in purine as listed in Nutrition Box 36–1.

Nursing Interventions

NDx: Pain
Focus on supportive care for the affected joint and effective pain management. Teach the patient about the pain medications prescribed. Tell the patient about the side effects, interactions, and expected therapeutic effects. (see Pharmacology Box 36–2). Give prescribed analgesics and anti-inflammatory agents. Instruct the patient to avoid use of the affected joint until the acute episode subsides.

NDx: Ineffective management of therapeutic regimen
Inform the patient about the disorder, its clinical manifestations, and treatment regimens. Allow the patient to ask questions and voice concerns. Instruct

the patient about prescribed diet therapy to reduce weight and reduce amount of ingested purines (Nutrition Box 36–1). Teach the patient about drug therapy to continue at home (see Pharmacology Box 36–2). Explain side effects of the agents, and inform the patient to notify the physician if untoward effects are present.

Evaluation

Evaluate the effectiveness of nursing care for a patient with gout by comparing the patient's status with the expected patient outcomes. Examples of specific outcomes for patients with gout have been provided in the Planning section.

OTHER MUSCULOSKELETAL INFLAMMATORY DISORDERS

LYME DISEASE

Etiology and Pathophysiology. Lyme disease is a chronic inflammatory disease that is transmitted by the bite of a tick. The causative agent is the tick-borne spirochetal bacterium *Borrelia burgdorferi.* The disease was first identified in the 1970s, although similar disorders were recognized in Europe in the early 1900s. The ticks primarily responsible for transmission are the bear and deer ticks *Ixodes dammini.* However, other ticks of the same family may also transmit the disease.

Lyme disease is most prevalent during the warm weather when the ticks are most numerous. It was named after Lyme, Connecticut, where the first epidemic occurred. The incidence has been reported in 40 states but is more common in the northeast, northern midwest, and far west regions of the United States. The disease usually progresses in stages. In the first stage, the disease appears localized, usually in an extremity. In the second stage, the disease progresses to invade the cardiac and neurologic systems. Neurologic complications also occur in the third stage, but the musculoskeletal involvement is the predominant problem at this level.

Clinical Manifestations. The clinical manifestations include the development of a macule at the site of the tick bite within 20 to 30 days. The macule then forms a larger lesion. This fades over a period of weeks, and the individual may not realize it was present. Some patients have several lesions or a rash, which may be primary or secondary. The primary lesions are usually asymptomatic; the secondary lesions often present symptoms of pruritus, malaise, headache, fever, and chills. Nausea, vomiting, and sore throat may also accompany the influenza-like symptoms.

The second stage of the disease occurs as the organism spreads through the body. Cardiac and neurologic manifestations occur at this time. The problems range from cardiac dysrhythmias to complete heart block. Neurologic complications include meningitis, encephalitis, and neuritis. The seventh cranial nerve is most frequently involved. Other nerves are also commonly involved, so the symptoms may vary from some weakness to pain and dysesthesia.

Nutrition Box 36–1.
HIGH-PURINE AND LOW-PURINE FOODS

High Purine Content	Low Purine Content
Anchovies	Bread (white)
Bouillon	Butter
Broth	Cookies
Gravies	Cereals
Heart	Custard
Kidney	Eggs
Liver	Fruits
Mincemeat	Ice cream
Mussels	Most vegetables (except peas, spinach, asparagus, and beans)
Sardines	Milk
Scallops	Nuts
Sweetbreads	Oils
Yeast (brewer's and baker's)	Popcorn
	Pudding
	Rice

Chart 36–2.

NURSING GUIDE TO PATIENT EDUCATION FOR SELF-MANAGEMENT: PREVENTION OF LYME DISEASE

Instruct individuals in endemic areas to:

Avoid areas of dense foliage and high grasses.
Wear clothing that covers the extremities completely.
Tuck pants legs into socks or boots.
Inspect the skin and clothing for ticks after being outside.
Inspect pets frequently for ticks.
Remove any ticks found on the individual or pets immediately. Be sure to remove the entire tick and dispose of it.
Use repellants such as diethyltoluamide (deet) or permethrin, which are effective against the ticks and safe to use on the skin. Be sure to reapply after bathing or swimming.

Pharmacology Box 36–3.

ORAL CALCIUM SUPPLEMENTS

Oral Calcium Supplements:
This group of drugs includes a variety of over-the-counter and prescription calcium products such as Alka-Mints, Chooz, Tums, Rolaids, Calcium Rich, Cal-600, and others.

Action:
Calcium supplements are prescribed to replace or maintain serum calcium levels at therapeutic ranges.

Uses:
The supplements are indicated for prevention of hypocalcemia, osteomalacia, and osteoporosis, and for other disorders of the bone caused by lack of calcium.

Side Effects:
Side effects include constipation, gastric irritation, chalky taste, nausea, and gastric bleeding.

Interactions:
The supplements may interact with oxalic acid, phytic acid, and phosphorus, causing decreased absorption of the calcium.

Nursing Implications:
Give the drug with food unless otherwise specified to reduce gastric irritation.
Tell the patient to refrain from taking the supplements with milk and other dairy products, bran, or spinach. The acids or phosphorus in these foods may cause decreased absorption of the calcium.
Tell the patient to take only the dosage prescribed because overdosing could precipitate calcium stone formation.

In the third stage, neurologic complications persist but the major manifestation is musculoskeletal involvement, typically arthritis. This begins approximately 4 weeks after the skin lesions appear. The joints, especially the knees, become swollen, warm, and painful. Destruction of the joint may occur from erosion of cartilage and bone.

Medical Diagnosis. The diagnosis is made by assessment, history, and serologic testing. Immunoglobulin antibodies can be detected after approximately 6 weeks. The patient has an elevated erythrocyte sedimentation rate, but this is not specific to the disease. Skin biopsies may isolate the spirochete. A detailed history with an analysis of the presenting symptoms and the exclusion of other disorders are the most common diagnostic tools.

Medical Management. Lyme disease is treated by a variety of regimens, depending on the extent and severity of symptoms and the stage of the disease. Oral antibiotics are used early in the disease process. Cardiac rhythm problems are treated with medication specified for the conduction disorder. Patients are hospitalized and monitored until stable. Steroids may be prescribed, especially if the patient has severe cardiac involvement. The musculoskeletal problems are treated symptomatically. Exacerbations of the disease are common. Intravenous antibiotics are used in later stages of the disease. Ceftriaxone therapy is beneficial in treating Lyme arthritis.

Prognosis is good for patients treated in the early stages. Patient and family education about prevention is an important health issue in areas where the disease is prevalent (Chart 36–2).

BURSITIS

Bursitis is an inflammation of a bursa, such as those located between muscles or tendons and bones. It most commonly occurs in the elbow (tennis elbow), the knee (housemaid's knee), or the shoulder. Bursitis is diagnosed by assessment, history, and x-ray examination to eliminate other musculoskeletal conditions. It is treated by rest, immobilization, heat therapy, and medication. Oral medications used include aspirin or nonaspirin analgesics and nonsteroidal anti-inflammatory agents. The affected joint may also be injected with cortisone or a local anesthetic agent to relieve symptoms and pain.

TENDOSYNOVITIS

Tendosynovitis is the inflammation of a tendon or its sheath. It is a common cause of acute shoulder pain. Calcific tendinitis, a form in which calcium deposits occur in the tendon, causes pain when the arm is abducted 50 to 130 degrees. Treatment of tendosynovitis is directed at decreasing the pain and inflammation. Immobility may be used to relieve the pain.

Structural Disorders

Musculoskeletal structural disorders include metabolic conditions in which bone structure is altered, causing pain, deformity, or fracture. The cause of the disorder may be unknown or may result from dietary or a combination of factors. In any case, potential for injury is significant, and safety becomes an important factor in the care and education of the patient.

Osteomalacia

Etiology and Pathophysiology. Osteomalacia is a metabolic bone disorder characterized by a decrease in calcium and phosphorus deposits in new bone matrix. This results in structurally weak bone mass. Osteomalacia is a condition of adults. In children, whose epiphyseal plates have not closed, the same disorder is known as rickets. The condition in children results in deformed bones, characterized by bowing, and a decrease in skeletal height. Osteomalacia is caused by lack of vitamin D, which is essential for the mineralization of bones.

A number of factors can cause a decrease in vitamin D and result in osteomalacia. A lack of dietary intake of vitamin D is one cause, but this is extremely rare in the United States. Most cases in this country are the result of malabsorption of vitamin D secondary to hepatobiliary disease. A lack of sunlight, chronic pancreatitis, and nontropical sprue are conditions that can lead to osteomalacia.

Clinical Manifestations. The patient with osteomalacia presents with complaints of weakness and vague aches and pains. The bones may be tender to palpation. Vertebral collapse results in kyphosis. The curvature or bowing of the long bones frequently seen in children with rickets may also be found in prolonged adult cases.

Medical Diagnosis. Diagnosis is made on the basis of x-ray films, which show diffuse erosion of the subperiosteal bone. There may be areas resembling fractures that appear as zig-zagging bands of decalcification with callus formation on each side of the bone. These false fractures are known as Looser's zones and occur in areas where fractures are not commonly seen. The serum calcium and phosphorus levels are low, and the alkaline phosphatase level is elevated.

Medical Management. Medical management focuses on treating the underlying cause. Supplements of vitamin D, calcium (Pharmacology Box 36–3), and phosphorus may be prescribed. The disorder responds dramatically to administration of vitamin D. Exercises are helpful in stimulating bone reformation. The patient is counseled to consume a diet of foods high in vitamin D, calcium, and phosphorus and to follow a prescribed program of progressive exercises and weight-bearing to promote recalcification of the bones.

Application of the Nursing Process to the Care of the Patient with Osteomalacia

Assessment

Review the patient's history and presenting symptoms. Complete a physical assessment, noting deformities and areas of weakness. Ask the patient about pain, its onset, intensity, and duration. Look for abnormal curvature of the spine and bowing of the long bones. Assess the patient's nutritional pattern. Determine the intake of vitamin D, calcium, and phosphorus. Ask whether the patient takes supplemental minerals and vitamins. Determine the patient's understanding of the disorder and the treatment program.

Nursing Diagnoses and Planning

Nursing diagnoses and related expected patient outcomes most commonly applicable to patients with osteomalacia include the following:

NDx: Pain related to structural changes in bones and deformities in limbs

Planning: Patient outcomes

1. Patient denies discomfort or extreme pain in limbs.
2. Patient relates accurate information about analgesics prescribed.

NDx: Knowledge deficit: nature of the disorder, its treatment and prevention

Planning: Patient outcomes

1. Patient states accurate information about the disorder, its prognosis, and treatment measures.
2. Patient demonstrates exercises that promote increased bone growth and performs them as prescribed.
3. Patient states accurate information on the appropriate diet and medication therapy.

Nursing Interventions

NDx: Pain
Give prescribed analgesics, and teach the patient about their frequency, dose, side effects, and therapeutic effects. Talk with the patient about relaxation strategies to reduce pain. Tell the patient to refrain from weight-bearing during painful episodes. Pad bony prominences when the patient is in bed. Assist with ambulation to reduce weight-bearing.

NDx: Knowledge deficit: nature of the disorder, its treatment and prevention
Teach the patient about the disorder, explaining its cause, symptoms, and treatment regimens. Tell the patient about the proper use of prescribed medications. Be sure the patient understands the need to take the supplements continually to help reverse the effects of the disorder and to prevent further damage (see Pharmacology Box 36–3). Demonstrate the prescribed exercises, and encourage the patient to practice them frequently because they promote increased bone recalcification and formation.

Review a diet plan with the patient that contains food high in vitamins, calcium (Nutrition Box 36–2), and phosphorus. Teach the patient how to read labels for food content. Note which food the patient chooses from the daily hospital menu, and reinforce good choices.

Evaluation

Evaluate the effectiveness of nursing care for a patient with osteomalacia by comparing the patient's status with the expected patient outcomes. Examples of specific outcomes for patients with osteomalacia have been provided in the Planning section.

Osteoporosis

Etiology and Pathophysiology. Osteoporosis is a metabolic bone disorder characterized by thinning, less dense, or porous bone mass. The chemical composition of the bone tissue remains the same, but there is less bone matter present within the bone, resulting in fragile, easy-to-fracture bones.

Bone production is a dynamic process of constant bone formation and bone resorption. Individuals achieve peak bone mass by approximately 35 years of age. After this time, there is normally a gradual decline in bone mass. It is not known whether the decreased bone mass is due to less new bone being produced, an increase in bone breakdown, or both.

Normal bone loss with aging is referred to as osteopenia. More severe bone loss that is age-related is called primary or senile osteoporosis. Osteoporosis affects more than 15 million people in the United States. Many individuals with osteoporosis develop spontaneous pathologic fractures or experience fractures associated with minimal trauma. Factors putting individuals at high risk of developing osteoporosis include increasing age in white females, low

Nutrition Box 36–2.
CALCIUM CONTENT OF SOME COMMON FOODS

Food	Calcium (mg)
Dairy Products:	
1 cup whole milk	288
½ cup canned evaporated milk	318
⅓ cup dry nonfat milk	293
1 cup skimmed milk	296
1 cup yogurt, low-fat	294
1 cup custard	297
1 oz Swiss cheese	251
1 oz cheddar cheese	213
1 oz American cheese	198
½ cup ice cream	96
8 oz cream cheese	141
1 cup cottage cheese	230
Vegetables:	
1 cup beet greens	144
½ cup collard greens	179
½ cup turnip greens	134
½ cup spinach	84
½ cup rhubarb	106
1 cup asparagus	30
1 cup cooked cabbage	64
1 cup chopped broccoli	136

dietary intake of calcium, immobility, and history of an oophorectomy.

Secondary osteoporosis is loss of bone caused by drugs or disease. Medications that can cause osteoporosis include tetracyclines, corticosteroids, aluminum-containing antacids, and some anticonvulsants, diuretics, and thyroid medications. Diseases involving catabolic hormone excess, such as hyperthyroidism and Cushing's disease, can also produce osteoporosis.

Osteoporosis tends to run in families. In the United States, whites and Asians are affected more often than blacks. Males are seldom affected. It is theorized that the low incidence in men may be because they have more bone mass to begin with and do not normally experience a sudden loss of hormones, as do females.

Idiopathic postmenopausal osteoporosis is the term used to describe the bone loss in women that can be directly related to a decrease in exercise and a decrease in estrogen level. Bones most affected by idiopathic postmenopausal osteoporosis are the femoral neck, wrists, vertebrae, and humeral neck.

Clinical Manifestations. Clinical manifestations of osteoporosis are localized low-back or mid-thoracic pain from vertebral involvement and collapse. The pain increases on sitting and standing. Pain may also be found in other affected parts of the body but seems to be more common in the low back. The patient may develop kyphosis, referred to as dowager's hump, and lumbar lordosis. With collapse of vertebrae, there is also a decrease in height (Fig. 36–3). Involvement of the jaw can result in a loss of teeth. Pathologic fracture of the femoral neck, wrist, or humeral neck is common.

Medical Diagnosis. Early diagnosis of osteoporosis has been difficult in the past because patients are asymptomatic until significant bone loss has occurred. X-ray films show bone loss only after 25% loss has occurred. X-ray films of the hand, wrist bones, and radius at this time reveal diffusely reduced bone density with cortical thinning.

Bone densitometry is a noninvasive diagnostic test with minimal radiation exposure, which can detect bone loss of less than 3%. Some physicians recommend routine bone densitometry for patients older than age 35 who are at high risk in order to identify and treat early osteoporosis and decrease the risk of pathologic fractures. Laboratory values for serum calcium, phosphorus, and vitamin D are normal

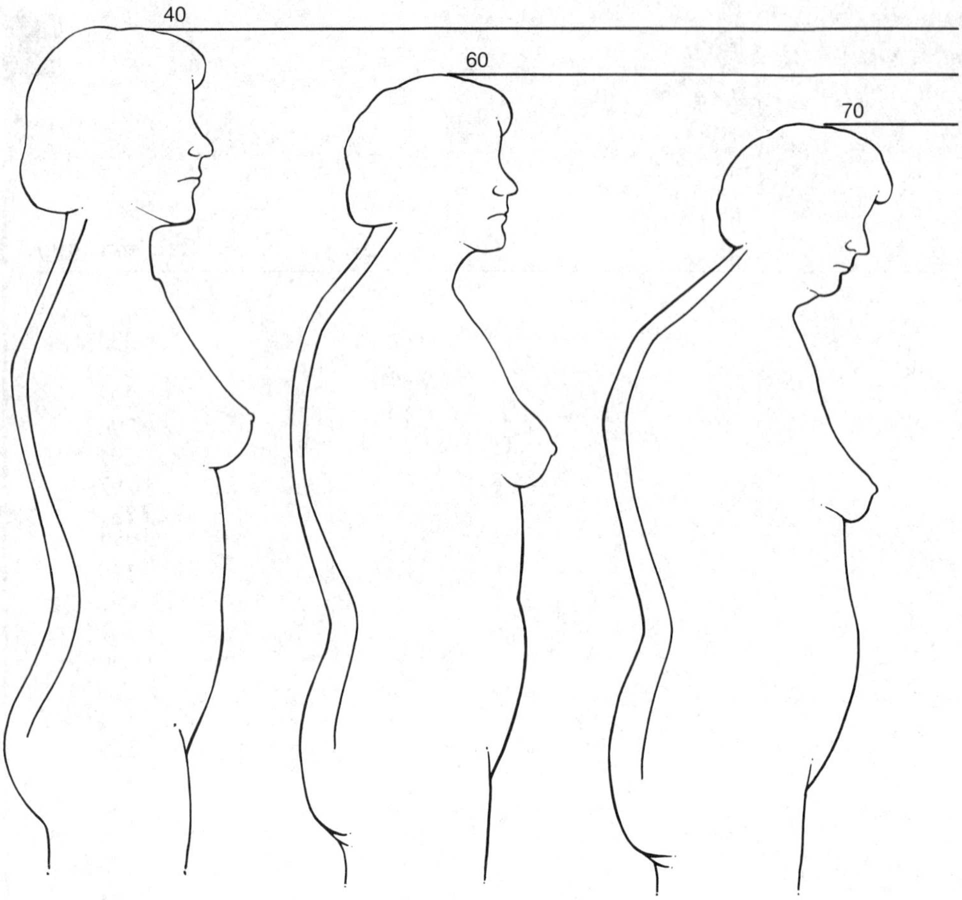

Figure 36–3.

Height and posture changes associated with the process of aging and osteoporosis.

with osteoporosis, but their evaluation may help rule out other conditions.

Medical Management. The goals of medical management are protection from pathologic fracture and prevention of further bone loss. Good body mechanics decreases the risk of pathologic fractures. The patient is taught to avoid lifting heavy objects, straining to open windows, and bouncing in a car over bumps or potholes and to practice safety in the home to prevent slips and falls. A back brace or corset may protect the vertebrae and help relieve back pain.

Calcium and vitamin D supplements and estrogen replacement may be prescribed to maintain bone mass. The recommended dietary allowance (RDA) of calcium for adults is 800 mg. Some research studies recommend that women older than age 35 receive 1000 mg/day. The RDA of vitamin D is 400 IU/day. Most physicians agree that estrogen replacement is necessary in osteoporosis, but controversy exists over how long to continue it and what dosage is optimum. Estrogen administration for 5 years after menopause is generally accepted. Some physicians recommend 10 to 15 years of estrogen therapy with calcium and vitamin D supplements.

Because immobility predisposes a person to bone resorption, planned regular physical activity is important in the prevention of bone loss. A diet that includes the RDA in all food groups to supply adequate vitamins and minerals is important for normal bone growth and development throughout the life span and for the prevention of osteoporosis. Alcohol and caffeine consumption and cigarette smoking have been linked to excess bone loss. The elimination of these substances is recommended in the prevention of osteoporosis.

Application of the Nursing Process to the Care of the Patient with Osteoporosis

Assessment

Review the patient's history, physical findings, and diagnostic studies. Assess the patient's pain, noting the intensity, location, duration, precipitating factors, and relief methods. Ask the patient about any structural changes noticed, such as diminishing height. Complete a musculoskeletal system assessment, noting deformities, strength, and range of motion. Observe the patient's ability to move freely. Assess the patient's knowledge about the disorder, its manifestations, treatment, and prevention methods. Ask the patient whether falls have been a problem. Determine the safety of the patient's environment.

Nursing Diagnoses and Planning

Nursing diagnoses and related expected patient outcomes most commonly applicable to patients with osteoporosis include those previously discussed for the patient with osteomalacia and the following:

NDx: High risk for injury; falls, related to lack of bone integrity, causing weakness and fractures

Planning: Patient outcomes
1. Patient states methods to promote safe mobility.
2. Patient uses ambulatory aids properly.
3. Patient requests assistance when needed to prevent falls.

NDx: Impaired physical mobility related to pain, fractures, and limited range of motion

Planning: Patient outcomes
1. Patient is able to perform activities of daily living.
2. Patient maintains maximum mobility of extremities.
3. Patient states methods to compensate for limited mobility.

Nursing Interventions

NDx: High risk for injury; falls
Teach the patient and family about injury prevention. Help them plan strategies to make the home environment safer for the patient. To prevent a fall, tell the patient to ask for assistance if needed when ambulating. Teach the patient how to use ambulatory aid devices. Observe the patient while using the device, checking for proper handling. Refer the patient to a physical therapist for assistance.

NDx: Impaired physical mobility
Assist the patient in locomotion as needed. Encourage ambulation to prevent the problems of disuse. Use the assistance of a physical therapist to instruct the patient and family about the prescribed ambulatory aid and to reinforce its safe use. Give analgesics as needed to decrease pain levels that may interfere with the patient's ability to be mobile. Encourage participation in a daily exercise program to maintain strength and joint mobility.

Evaluation

Evaluate the effectiveness of nursing care for a patient with osteoporosis by comparing the patient's status with the expected patient outcomes. Examples of specific outcomes for patients with osteoporosis have been provided in the Planning section.

Paget's Disease

Etiology and Pathophysiology. Also called osteitis deformans because of the bone deformity resulting from the disease, Paget's disease is a chronic, progressive metabolic bone disease of unknown cause. It is characterized by excessive bone resorption with replacement by structurally abnormal bone. The bones most frequently involved are the pelvis, spine, sacrum, skull, femur, and humerus.

Osteoclastic resorption in the initial lesion is followed by increased osteoblastic activity. This results in the formation of bone that is normal in mineral content but is structurally thickened and of poor quality. The new bone has a mosaic pattern, which causes it to be weaker and more prone to fracture. Pagetic bone is also more vascular.

Paget's disease occurs in 3% of the population older than age 40 and is more common among males. It mainly affects individuals of Anglo-Saxon descent.

Clinical Manifestations. Clinical manifestations are few and vague in the early stages of the disease. The patient usually seeks medical attention for fractures or bone deformities in later stages of the disease process. Paget's disease may also be detected by laboratory results or radiologic examinations done during a routine physical examination or treatment for another disorder.

In later stages, bone deformity can cause pain and create pressure on nerves. Bones with increased vascularity also feel warm, and pressure on the periosteal lining stimulates pain. The pain experienced is generally a dull aching discomfort. Involvement of spinal vertebrae causes kyphosis and loss of the lumbar curve. Compression fractures of the vertebrae result in a decrease in height and pain from pressure on the spinal nerve roots.

Skull deformity may be identified early and confirmed by x-ray examination. The patient may have noticed an increase in hat size. Skull involvement results in headaches, osteosclerotic hearing loss, tinnitus, and vertigo as a result of an increase in perfusion of blood and pressure on the cranial nerves in the skull. Maxillary and mandibular involvement can cause a change in facial features and loss of teeth. Long bone deformity and bowing are common with progression of the disease. The increased vascularity of pagetic bone can cause stress on the heart by increasing the demand on cardiac output.

The development of sarcoma in pagetic bone is 40 times greater than in normal bone; however, only 1% of patients with Paget's disease develop sarcoma. Some patients develop secondary osteoarthritis as a result of bone deformity adjacent to the joint. Gout is also more common among individuals with Paget's disease.

Medical Diagnosis. Diagnosis is made on the basis of radiologic examination and blood and urine studies. Affected bones have a "cotton wool" appearance in thickened areas such as the skull. X-ray films also reveal a punched-out or mosaic appearance in the bone structure. The bones are more dense than normal, with cortical thickening. New bone is not laid down along lines of stress. A bone scan can reveal the extent of Paget's disease and eliminate the need for numerous skeletal x-ray films.

The serum alkaline phosphatase level is elevated indicating increased osteoblastic activity. Increased osteoclastic activity is indicated by elevated levels of urinary hydroxyproline, as measured in a 24-hour urine specimen.

Medical Management. The goals of medical management are relief of symptoms, protection from pathologic fracture, and prevention of further bone deformity. Nonsteroidal anti-inflammatory agents are generally effective in pain relief. Aspirin, ibuprofen, and indomethacin may also be used as analgesics. Structural changes, especially in the hip, may require surgical correction by a total hip replacement. Spinal changes can be diminished by a supporting corset or brace. Changes in posture require patient education on good body mechanics and safe ambulating techniques. Assistive devices may be necessary for locomotion. Hearing loss may be improved by a hearing aid or referral to a hearing therapist to learn communication skills such as lip reading.

Administration of antipagetic medications can retard the progress of the disease and bring about temporary remission. Calcitonin is used to inhibit osteoclastic bone resorption and produce pain relief. Because calcitonin must be administered subcutaneously for several doses to be effective, the patient or another reliable person is taught to administer the injection. Diphosphonates such as etidronate disodium may be administered to slow the rate of bone resorption and the formation of new bone and to reduce bone vascularity. Teach the patients the administration schedule, expected actions, and side effects of these medications. Lifetime medical follow-up is necessary.

Application of the Nursing Process to the Care of the Patient with Paget's Disease

The assessment, nursing diagnoses, expected patient outcomes, nursing interventions, and evaluation for patients with Paget's disease are similar to those described previously for patients with osteoporosis.

Disorders of the Wrist and Hand

CARPAL TUNNEL SYNDROME

Carpal tunnel syndrome results from compression of the median nerve at the wrist within the carpal tunnel (Fig. 36–4). It is the most common nerve entrapment syndrome. Compression causes sensory motor changes in the hand in sites affected by the median nerve, which includes the thumb, index finger, middle finger, and radial side of the ring

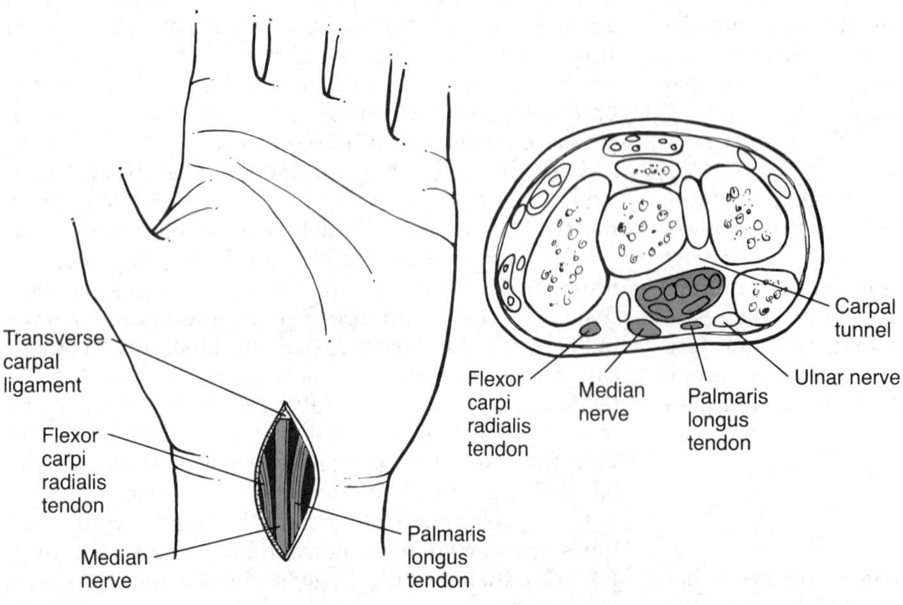

Figure 36–4.

The carpal tunnel in the wrist.

finger. The syndrome occurs most frequently in the summer in individuals between 30 and 60 years of age. It occurs in conditions that cause swelling in the carpal tunnel, which in turn presses the median nerve against the transverse carpal ligament. Rheumatic disorders, tendosynovitis, tumors, tuberculosis, myxedema, and wrist sprain may be causative factors. Carpal tunnel syndrome is aggravated by repeated wrist and hand motions.

Clinical manifestations include pain, numbness, and tingling. The paresthesia affects the thumb, forefinger, and middle fingers. An inability to grasp objects or clench the fist may also be present. Carpal tunnel syndrome is diagnosed on the basis of assessment, history, a compression test, and electromyography, which detects a median nerve conduction delay. Treatment includes rest of the affected wrist and hand, immobilization with a splint to provide neutral extension, and correction of the underlying cause. Because occupation is a contributing factor either to the cause or to increasing the distress of the disorder, the patient is often counseled to seek other employment. If the condition persists or is unrelieved by conservative treatment, surgical decompression may be necessary.

DUPUYTREN'S CONTRACTURE

Dupuytren's contracture is a deformity of the hand in which the ring finger and little finger contract, bending into the palm. Because of the shortening of the palmar fascia, the affected fingers cannot extend. It occurs more frequently in older men who are of Scandinavian origin. Treatment consists of a surgical fasciectomy.

GANGLION

A ganglion is a cystic tumor that develops on a tendon, commonly on the back of the wrist. It develops through a defect in the tendon sheath or capsule. Ganglions are more common in young women than in men. Pain is the chief symptom of a ganglion. Surgically excision may be necessary if the pain is intolerable.

Application of the Nursing Process to the Care of the Patient with a Wrist or Hand Disorder

Assessment

Review the patient's history and presenting symptoms. Determine the patient's ability to use the affected hand. Ask about the effect of the problem on the patient's employment. Check whether the patient's occupation may be a contributing factor to the problem. Determine the patient's ability to perform self-care with the affected extremity.

Nursing Diagnoses and Planning

The nursing diagnosis and related expected patient outcomes most commonly applicable to patients with a disorder of the wrist or hand are as follows:

NDx: Self-care deficit: grooming, bathing, personal hygiene, and activities of daily living related to the deformity or pain

Planning: Patient outcomes
1. Patient maintains maximum use of the affected extremity.
2. Patient adapts to the deformity by using assistive devices or the other extremity.
3. Patient performs activities of daily living and personal self-care tasks.

Nursing Interventions

NDx: Self-care deficit
Assist the patient, as needed, to perform self-care tasks. Teach the patient how to use assistive devices to perform activities that were previously too difficult to perform as a result of pain or the deformities. Have the patient practice using the opposite hand to perform self-care tasks. Give analgesics as prescribed to relieve pain that may be inhibiting the patient's ability to use the affected extremity. Seek assistance from family members when the patient cannot complete activities.

Evaluation

Evaluate the effectiveness of nursing care for a patient with a wrist or hand disorder by comparing the patient's status with the expected patient outcomes. Examples of specific outcomes for patients with a wrist or hand disorder have been provided in the Planning section.

Disorders of the Feet

HALLUX VALGUS (BUNION)

Hallux valgus, commonly known as a bunion, is a progressive disorder in which the great toe deviates laterally (Fig. 36–5). There is also an osseous enlargement of the first metatarsal head (medial aspect), upon which a bursa enlarges from the pressure and inflammation. The cause of a bunion may

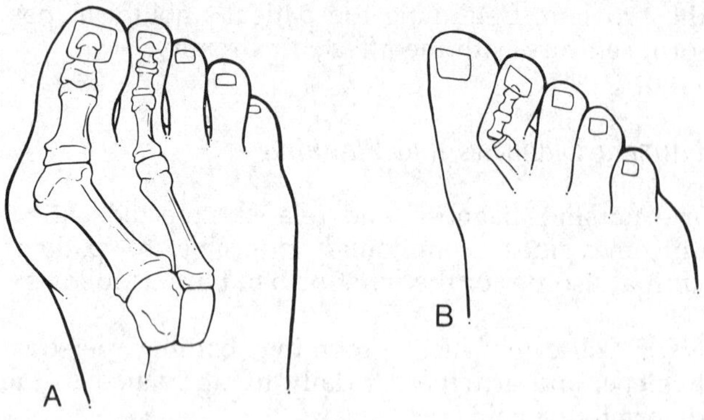

Figure 36–5.

Disorders of the foot. Hallux valgus (bunion) (*A*) and hammer toe (*B*).

be arthritis, improperly fitting shoes, or heredity. Pain, redness, and edema are the typical symptoms presented. The treatment depends upon the severity of the discomfort and deformity. A correctly fitting shoe may be all that is necessary, or surgical excision may be required.

PLANTAR DIGITAL NEUROMA

A plantar digital neuroma (Morton's neuroma) is a swelling of the third lateral branch of the median plantar nerve. It is caused by ischemia of the nerve resulting from digital artery changes. Loss of the transmetatarsal arch may also cause swelling. The most common symptom is a throbbing pain in the foot, which may subside with rest. The pain usually occurs between the third and fourth digits. It is treated with local cortisone or anesthetic injections or, if necessary, by surgical excision or reconstruction of the arch.

HAMMER TOE

Hammer toe is a flexion deformity of the interphalangeal joint (see Fig. 36–5). The condition is usually an acquired disorder from prolonged wearing of ill-fitting shoes. The toe or toes are pulled up, with the ball of the foot pushed downward. Corns usually form on the top of the toes. Treatment consists of exercises, wearing open-toed or well-fitting shoes, and protecting the joints with pads.

PES PLANUS

Pes planus, commonly called flatfoot, is an abnormal lowering and flatness of the metatarsal arch. The condition causes pain in the foot or leg and may interfere with normal foot functioning. It may be an acute or chronic problem. Treatment consists of arch supports, or in severe cases, surgical intervention.

Application of the Nursing Process to the Care of the Patient with a Foot Disorder

Assessment

Assess the severity of the patient's disorder. Determine the effect on mobility and the ability to provide self-care. Ask the patient about pain in the affected area. Determine the onset, duration, intensity, and precipating factors of the pain, and successful relief methods. Watch the patient walk, noting the effect of the disorder on basic movement. Check whether an ambulatory device is necessary for locomotion. Assess the patient's footwear, observing for too-tight fit and nonskid soles. Determine the patient's knowledge about the condition, progression, and potential treatment modalities.

Nursing Diagnoses and Planning

Nursing diagnoses and related expected patient outcomes most commonly applicable to patients with a foot disorder include the following:

NDx: Pain related to structural changes in bones and deformities in feet

Planning: Patient outcomes
1. Patient denies discomfort or extreme pain in feet.
2. Patient relates accurate information about analgesics prescribed.
3. Patient wears well-fitting shoes.

NDx: Altered health maintenance related to lack of knowledge about the disorder, its progression and treatment

Planning: Patient outcomes
1. Patient states accurate information about the disorder, its progression, and treatment measures.
2. Patient wears shoes with appropriate fit for the deformity.

NDx: High risk for injury; falls, related to deformities and/or improper use of ambulatory aids

Planning: Patient outcomes
1. Patient states methods to promote safe mobility.
2. Patient uses ambulatory aids properly.
3. Patient requests assistance when needed to prevent falls.
4. Patient wears shoes with nonskid soles.

NDx: Impaired physical mobility related to pain, deformities, and limited range of motion

Planning: Patient outcomes

1. Patient is able to perform activities of daily living.
2. Patient maintains maximum mobility of extremities.
3. Patient states methods to compensate for inability to move freely.

Nursing Interventions

NDx: Pain

Give prescribed analgesics, and teach the patient about the frequency, dose, side effects, and therapeutic effects. Talk with the patient about relaxation strategies to reduce pain. Tell the patient to refrain from weight-bearing during painful episodes. Assist with ambulation to reduce weight-bearing. Teach the patient about wearing properly fitted shoes to reduce constriction causing pain.

NDx: Altered health maintenance

Teach the patient about the disorder, explaining its cause, symptoms, progression, and treatment regimens. Tell the patient about the proper use of prescribed medications. Reinforce the physician's and physical therapist's instructions. Assist the patient in determining the type of shoes for best fit and mobility.

NDx: High risk for injury; falls

Teach the patient and family about injury prevention. Help them plan strategies to make the home environment safer for the patient. To prevent a fall, tell the patient to ask for assistance if needed when ambulating. Teach the patient how to use the prescribed ambulatory aid. Observe the patient while using the device, checking for proper handling. Refer the patient to a physical therapist for assistance. Be sure the patient wears nonskid shoes when ambulating.

NDx: Impaired physical mobility

Assist the patient in locomotion as needed. Encourage ambulation to prevent the problems of disuse. Use the assistance of the physical therapist to instruct the patient and family about the prescribed ambulatory aid and to reinforce its safe use. Give analgesics as needed to decrease pain levels that may interfere with the patient's ability to be mobile. Encourage participation in a daily exercise program to maintain strength and joint mobility.

Evaluation

Evaluate the effectiveness of nursing care for a patient with a foot disorder by comparing the patient's status with the expected patient outcomes. Examples of specific outcomes for patients with a foot disorder have been provided in the Planning section.

Trauma

Musculoskeletal trauma can involve any of the body's bones, articular cartilage, muscles, ligaments, or tendons. The degree of soft tissue damage and associated nerve, vascular, or organ damage varies with each injury. It is estimated that three fourths of all musculoskeletal trauma involves the appendicular skeleton. Falls, accidents involving motor vehicles, and sports injuries account for most musculoskeletal trauma.

Minor Musculoskeletal Injuries

Minor musculoskeletal injuries are those that do not usually require medical intervention for readjustment or repair of the injured part. Although there may be considerable pain present, the affected part usually heals in time, especially if care is taken not to reinjure it until the healing has occurred.

CONTUSIONS AND STRAINS

Soft tissue trauma with no damage to musculoskeletal structures is a contusion. It is usually the result of a blow or blunt force. Clinical manifestations include swelling and tenderness and localized hemorrhage, with discoloration and ecchymosis from damage to superficial blood vessels in the skin and subcutaneous tissue. Contusions can cause restriction in joint range of motion because of localized tenderness and swelling, but there is no loss of joint stability.

A strain is injury of a muscle that has been stretched beyond its capacity. Small blood vessels in the affected muscle rupture, causing inflammation of surrounding soft tissue structures. The area becomes swollen, tender, and ecchymotic. Painful muscle spasms may occur.

Diagnosis of contusions and strains is made on the basis of examination, history of incident, and ruling out a fracture, dislocation, or ligament injury. Treatment involves prevention of further trauma, bleeding, or swelling. The involved body part is elevated, and ice is applied to prevent or reduce swelling as well as to reduce discomfort. An elastic wrap may be applied to protect it from further damage, relieve pain, and promote comfort. Teach the patient how to apply and remove the wrap. If numbness, tingling, or swelling occurs distal to the elastic wrap, it is too tight. Have the patient demonstrate application of the wrap. Instruct the patient that an elastic wrap provides protection but little support of an affected joint.

SPRAINS

A sprain refers to an injury of a joint. The joint is stretched beyond its normal range of motion, and tearing of the ligaments, capsule, or synovium of the joint results. The most common joints affected are the ankle, knee and wrist. Diagnosis is made on the basis of assessment, history of incident, and x-ray examinations.

The clinical manifestations and treatment of a sprain are dependent on the severity of damage to joint structures. Minor sprains, those with minimal ligament injury, are treated by application of cold, elevation, and an elastic wrap to provide protection and decrease swelling. Use of the joint is restricted for a prescribed period of time to prevent further damage and to allow healing.

Joint weakness and abnormal motion are present when the ligament is torn halfway through. These sprains require restricted use of the joint or immobilization for up to 4 weeks, in addition to the ice, elevation, and wrap.

Major sprain injuries involve complete tearing of the ligament. They are treated by surgical repair of the torn ligament, followed by rigid immobilization in a splint or cast. A tear of the cruciate ligament of the knee is a common sports injury. It is repaired by arthroscopic surgery, usually on an out-patient basis. A full leg immobilizer is worn for up to 4 weeks after the repair (Fig. 36–6). Specific leg exercises are prescribed to restrengthen the affected part.

The individual with a sprained knee or ankle needs crutches for ambulation to maintain non–weight-bearing or limited weight-bearing on the involved joint. In some instances when surgical intervention is not necessary, controlled, passive movement of the involved joint is prescribed to decrease loss of joint function, prevent muscle atrophy, and maintain the strength of other supporting structures during healing. Prescribed passive exercises can be provided by the nurse, a physical therapist, or a joint exercise machine.

There are many types of passive joint exercise machines available today. The most popular machines are used to flex and extend the knee following an injury or surgical repair of a joint. Passive joint movement exercise devices may also be used after total joint replacements. With each type of machine, the physician prescribes the degree of flexion and extension, speed (movements per minute), and length of time for therapy. The extent of movement is usually increased gradually.

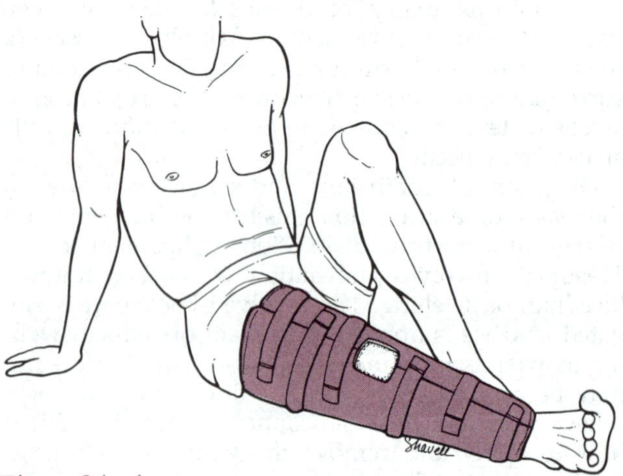

Figure 36–6.

Knee immobilizer used after knee injuries and postoperative knee repair.

MENISCAL TEARS

The meniscus is a fibrocartilaginous semicircular structure within the knee joint. There are two menisci in each knee, one each on the lateral and medial aspects of the joint. They act as a cushion between adjacent articular cartilage and provide stability from rotational forces. One or both of these structures may be injured by knee trauma. Meniscal tears are often associated with moderate or severe knee sprains.

Diagnosis of a torn meniscus is made on the basis of history of injury, physical examination of the knee, loss of knee stability, radiographic studies to rule out fracture, and arthroscopic examination. Treatment is a partial or total meniscectomy by arthroscopy or arthrotomy. This is usually performed on an out-patient basis at the physician's office, in a free-standing surgical clinic, or in the out-patient surgical department of the hospital. Postoperative nursing interventions include assessment of proximal and distal neurovascular function, cold applications, and elevation of the leg for 48 hours. Teach the patient prescribed weight-bearing restrictions, and reinforce instructions in the use of crutches or an immobilization device as needed.

Major Musculoskeletal Injuries

Major musculoskeletal injuries are those that include severe injury to the bone, joint, tendon, or ligament. These injuries require medical intervention for adequate repair or readjustment of the injury.

SUBLUXATIONS AND DISLOCATIONS

Etiology and Pathophysiology. A subluxation is the partial separation of adjacent joint surfaces. A dislocation occurs when normally adjacent joint surfaces become completely separated from one another. Dislocations often occur in combination with fractures of the bone within or near the joint. A subluxation or dislocation may also cause damage to the surrounding ligaments, joint capsule, synovial lining, and the articular cartilage, as well as soft tissue.

Clinical Manifestations. Clinical manifestations include minimal deformity of the joint in a subluxation and marked deformity of the joint with a dislocation. The actual degree of deformity may be masked by the presence of swelling of the injured joint. The joint may be painful, or if major nerves are injured, it may become numb. Loss of joint function varies from slight to complete loss of range of motion. Ecchymosis may result from tearing of adjacent blood vessels. Neurovascular function distal to the injury may be impaired as a result of pressure from displaced joint structures or edema.

Medical Diagnosis. Diagnosis of a subluxation or dislocation is made on the basis of history of an injury or pathologic condition, physical examination, and radiographic studies of the involved area. If distal circulation is impaired, an arteriogram may be performed. However, the dislocation is reduced immediately to restore circulation. During diagnostic procedures, the affected body part is supported and handled carefully to protect it from further injury.

Medical Management. Cold applications and protective elastic wraps or a sling may be prescribed before x-ray examination. Once diagnosis is established by x-ray examination, the joint is reduced or returned to anatomic alignment. In a closed reduction, the physician is able to return the joint structures to anatomic alignment by manipulation and manual traction The patient is usually sedated during closed reduction if the injury is recent. Untreated dislocation of a longer time period may require general anesthesia for reduction.

An open reduction requires hospitalization for surgery under general anesthesia. Following reduction, the joint is immobilized by application of a splint or cast for approximately 3 to 6 weeks. Weight-bearing is avoided for this period of time.

Application of the Nursing Process to the Care of the Patient with a Musculoskeletal Injury

Assessment

Assess the patient's affected part for pain, swelling, discoloration, or malalignment. Check the neurovascular status proximal and distal to the injury by palpating for pulses, feeling for warmth of the part, and assessing for decreased sensation. Ask the patient about numbness or tingling in the extremity. Review how the the injury occurred, and note what treatment was instituted, if any, at the time of the occurrence. Determine the patient's understanding of the injury and treatment necessary.

Nursing Diagnoses and Planning

Nursing diagnoses and related expected patient outcomes most commonly applicable to patients with musculoskeletal injuries include the following:

NDx: Pain related to joint trauma, pressure from edema, and immobilization

Planning: Patient outcomes

1. Patient denies pain in affected part.
2. Patient states methods to decrease pain by reduction of swelling and keeping immobilizer properly applied.

NDx: Altered health maintenance related to lack of knowledge about the injury, management of immobilization device, exercises to perform, and prevention of reinjury

Planning: Patient outcomes

1. Patient states accurate information about the cause of the injury and methods to prevent reinjury.
2. Patient demonstrates proper application of the immobilizer device and states when it is to be in place, how much weight-lifting or weight-bearing is allowed, and when the device may be removed.
3. Patient demonstrates exercises, as taught, to maintain strength and range of motion of joint.

Nursing Interventions

NDx: Pain

Give prescribed analgesics and explain the dosage, frequency, side effects, and expected therapeutic effects of the medications. Caution the patient not to perform tasks that require mental alertness while under the effects of the pain medication. Teach the patient to check for tightness of the immobilizer, looking for signs of swelling or diminished sensation in the distal part of the affected extremity. Tell the patient to elevate the part to reduce swelling and thus reduce pain. Caution the patient about weight-bearing if contraindicated, because that might increase the pain significantly.

NDx: Altered health maintenance

Teach the patient about the injury, the cause, methods of prevention of reinjury, and appropriate treatment. Explain how to apply the immobilizer or wrap to the affected part, and have the patient redemonstrate the process. Check to see that it is not too tight, and tell the patient how to check for improper fit. Explain that increased swelling, discoloration, and decreased sensation in the affected part may be signs of improper fit of the device and that prolonged pressure could cause severe problems if not relieved. Reinforce the physician's instruction about weight-lifting (if shoulder, arm, or hand is affected) or weight-bearing (if knee, leg, ankle, or foot is affected). Demonstrate prescribed exercises to the patient, and encourage participation in the exercise regimen to prevent loss of strength and joint motion.

Evaluation

Evaluate the effectiveness of nursing care for a patient with musculoskeletal injuries by comparing the patient's status with the expected patient outcomes. Examples of specific outcomes for patients with musculoskeletal injuries have been provided in the Planning section.

FRACTURES

A fracture is a crack or break in the continuity of a bone. A fracture may or may not involve damage to tissues or organs surrounding the bone.

Etiology. Fractures may be caused by a direct blow or trauma to the bone, a sudden strong muscle contraction that bends the bone to the breaking point, continuous extreme stress on the bone, or pathologic conditions that cause demineralization of the bone. Demineralization of bones that occurs with prolonged bed rest, decreased weight-bearing, and the aging process increases the risk of bone fracture with minimal stress or trauma.

Pathophysiology. There are many types of fractures. Some of the more common types are illustrated in Figure 36–7. Fractures may be further described by the part of the bone involved and the transverse, linear, or oblique direction of the fracture line.

A closed fracture is one in which the bone is broken but there is no external injury. A closed fracture is not considered a life-threatening injury unless it is an unstable fracture that may damage vital organs or major blood vessels or unless it is associated with internal hemorrhage, shock, or both.

A compound or open fracture is one in which the bone fragments have broken through or penetrated the skin. Because this type of fracture is usually associated with severe tissue damage and blood loss, as well as a high risk of infection, a compound fracture is considered a life-threatening injury.

Clinical Manifestations. A fracture in which the fragments are displaced, or are no longer in their normal alignment, either lies in an abnormal position with angulation where no joint exists, or may present as a shortened or abnormally rotated extremity. In a nondisplaced fracture, the bone remains in normal alignment. Nondisplaced fractures are more difficult to diagnose without radiologic examination.

The degree of pain can vary from tenderness over the fracture site to extreme pain and muscle spasms of the involved body part. Pain may limit motion and use of a fractured bone or adjacent joints, but in some closed nondisplaced fractures, the patient may still have use of the affected body part. Crepitus, a grating sound created by bone fragments scraping against one another, may be heard or felt on movement.

Swelling and ecchymosis of the soft tissue surrounding the injury always occur. This is due to bleeding (which may be considerable) at the fracture site from damage to soft tissue. However, discoloration may not be seen on the skin surface for several days. A decrease in hematocrit and hemoglobin levels indicates the degree of blood loss but may not do so for up to 72 hours after injury. A break in the skin over the fracture site indicates an open or compound fracture. Bone may or may not be visible in the wound.

Injury to nerves and blood vessels near the fracture site is caused by direct trauma from a dislocated joint or fracture fragments at the time of injury. Stretching, tearing, or compression of a nerve or blood vessel is common. Localized swelling, discoloration, and hemorrhage may occur. The danger of further soft tissue damage continues until the injured part is immobilized.

Organ damage can result from direct trauma at the time of injury or from a laceration or puncture caused by the displaced bone fragments. Common organ injuries include cardiac contusions; lung punctures; liver, kidney, and spleen lacerations from fractured ribs; lower abdominal organ injuries from a fractured pelvis; and brain injuries from skull fractures.

Medical Diagnosis. Diagnosis of a fracture is made on the basis of history of an injury or pathologic condition, physical examination, and radiographic studies of the involved area. Computed tomography (CT) scans may be used to identify the exact location and extent of skull, spinal, pelvic, and acetabular fractures. If distal circulation is impaired, an arteriogram may be performed, but the fracture is reduced first to restore circulation. During diagnostic procedures, protect the affected body part from further injury by splinting and careful handling. Explain the diagnostic procedure to the patient, and administer prescribed analgesics as needed for patient comfort.

IMMEDIATE CARE OF THE PATIENT WITH A FRACTURE

Protect known or suspected fractures from further injury until medical intervention is possible. Cover open wounds with sterile or clean white or light-colored lint-free material to prevent further contamination.

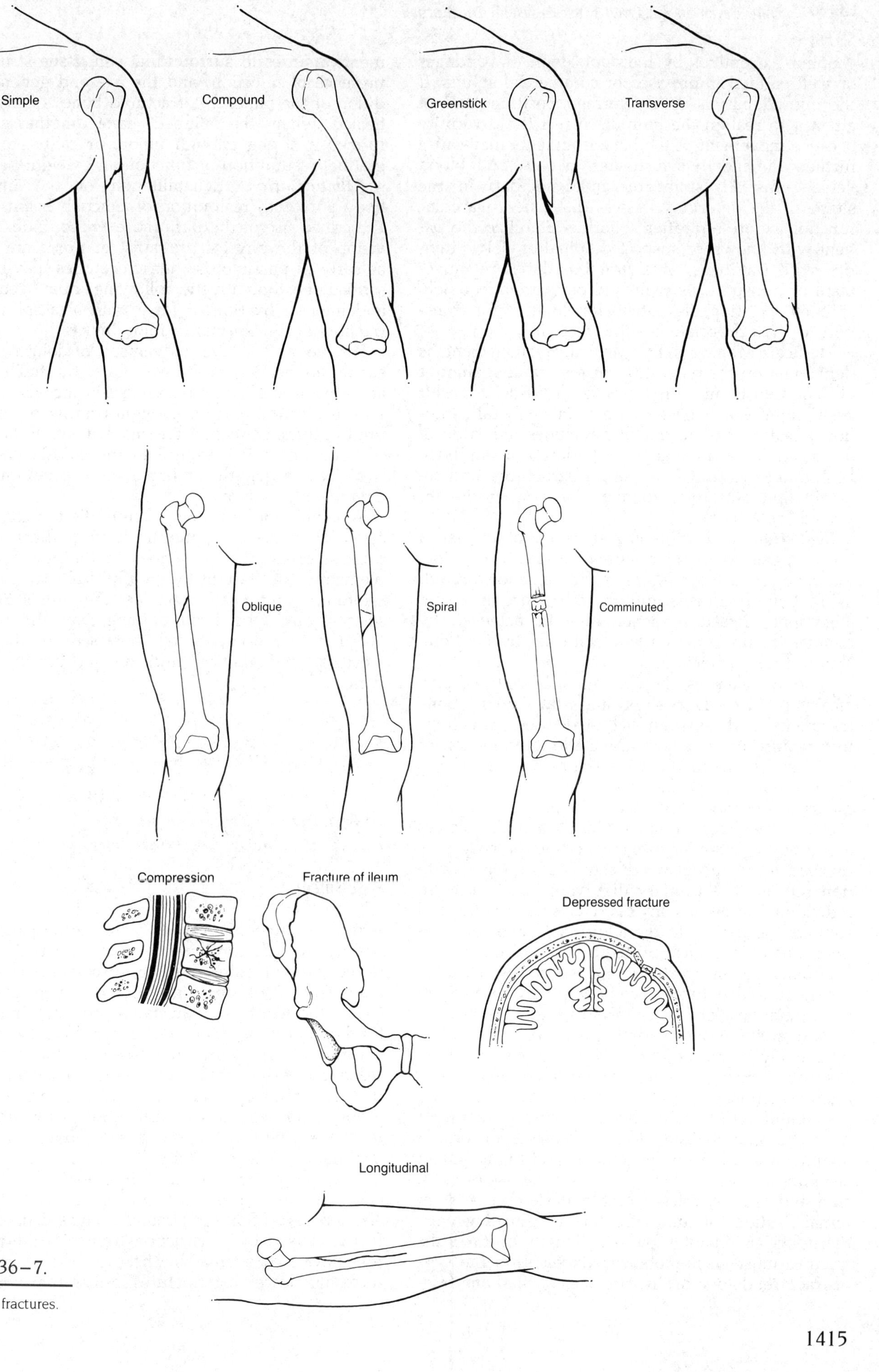

Figure 36–7.

Types of fractures.

Splint extremities by the application of bandages or well-padded improvised or commercial splints. If the injured part is in a deformed position, do not attempt to realign the limb or correct the deformity because movement of the bone fragments may cause further damage to soft tissues, nerves, and blood vessels. Instead, splint the involved part in the shape of the deformity. Assess distal neurovascular function before and after splinting. Stabilize the patient with known or suspected spinal or pelvic injuries with sandbags on a firm board before movement or transport. After injured parts are adequately splinted, position the patient for comfort for transport to an appropriate health care facility.

Medical Management. Medical management is dependent on the type of fracture sustained, amount of blood lost, and the severity of associated soft tissue injuries as well as the patient's general condition. Treatment of all fractures includes reduction of displaced bone fragments, immobilization for bone healing and repair of supporting structures, and rehabilitation and restoration of function of the involved body part.

Reduction. Reduction is restoration of displaced bone fragments to their normal anatomic position. Reduction is achieved by applying traction or pull to the bone fragments until the pieces are in proper alignment. Closed reduction may be achieved by manual traction or gradually achieved by applying skin or skeletal traction.

In some instances, the bone must be reduced surgically to properly position and stabilize the bone fragments and surrounding structures. Situations that require open reduction include interposition of soft tissue between the bone fragments and strong muscle pull or spasms that cause the bone fragments to override each other and prevent stabilization by closed reduction. If internal fixation devices are used to maintain alignment, the procedure is referred to as an open reduction with internal fixation (ORIF). The primary disadvantage of an open reduction is that it converts a closed fracture and subjects the patient to the additional potential complications of a surgical procedure and infection.

Usually, open fractures are surgically cleaned, debrided, and reduced. The patient may receive tetanus immune globulin or toxoid on admission. Parenteral antibiotics are administered pre- and postoperatively to prevent wound and bone infection. Prescribed analgesics are administered before and after reduction.

Immobilization. Dislocated fracture fragments must be immobilized and maintained in proper alignment to allow complete healing of the bone and surrounding tissue. Bone repair and the use of casts, skin and skeletal traction, external fixation, and internal fixation for immobilization and healing were discussed in Chapter 35. The length of time the fracture must be immobilized depends on the type of fracture, degree of displacement of the bone fragments, injuries to surrounding soft tissue structures, presence of infection, and the age and general condition of the patient. A fractured bone is considered healed when the aligned bone fragments have formed a strong enough union, or callus, to allow gradual resumption of function and weight-bearing.

Rehabilitation. Rehabilitation of the involved body part with restoration of function begins early. Prescribed use of the part and exercise under supervision of the physical therapist or nurse are begun as early as possible. Isometric exercises may be prescribed postoperatively following open reduction and internal fixation or for a limb in a splint, cast, traction, or an external fixation device.

Passive and active movement of joints is prescribed as healing progresses. Once the fracture has achieved a solid union, exercise is increased along with use of the part and weight-bearing on the part until optimum function returns. Patients with multiple fractures and complicated musculoskeletal injuries require lengthy rehabilitation programs that continue after discharge.

Rehabilitation requires a multidisciplinary team approach to restore optimum level of function. The exercise program is prescribed by the physician, implemented and taught by the physical therapist, and reinforced and encouraged by the nurse. Support services and specialized training may also be provided by an occupational therapist, social service workers, and dietary and mental health practitioners.

Application of the Nursing Process to the Care of the Patient with a Fracture

Assessment

After the immediate care to stabilize the patient has been provided, continue to assess the patient's affected part for pain, swelling, discoloration, or malalignment. Look for signs of continued bleeding. Check the neurovascular status proximal and distal to the injury by palpating for pulses, feeling for warmth of the part, and assessing for decreased sensation. Assess vital signs, noting changes reflective of ensuing shock, such as decreasing blood pressure and rapid weak pulse rate with increased respiratory effort. Ask the patient about numbness or tingling in the extremity.

After the patient's fracture has been treated medically, continue to assess neurovascular status of the affected part. Look for signs of decreased tissue perfusion caused by constriction from the immobilization device or edema. In the case of forearm fractures and lower leg fractures, assess for symptoms

Nursing Care Guide 36–1.

PATIENTS UNDERGOING SURGERY FOR A FRACTURED FEMUR

Preoperative Care

Assessment Findings: Patient appears nervous, withdraws from conversation, clenches hands; patient states fear about the impending surgery; blood pressure, pulse, and respirations are slightly elevated for the patient; patient makes statements about potential problems with immobility and pain; patient seems concerned about preoperative traction therapy.

Nursing Diagnosis: Anxiety related to fears about surgery, preoperative traction equipment, potential risk factors, pain, and fear of loss of mobility

Patient Outcomes	Nursing Interventions	Rationale
Patient reports feeling less fearful, seems relaxed, and is able to rest well.	Explain all preoperative procedures to the patient. Provide a quiet, calm environment with periods of rest during the delivery of nursing care. Ask for assistance from clergy or the patient's significant others.	Having an understanding of the procedure lessens fears and reduces anxiety. Telling the patient what to expect prior to initiating procedures for preoperative preparation reduces fear of the unknown.
Patient's vital signs are within normal ranges for the patient.	Check vital signs after the patient is rested and more relaxed, and note any changes.	Changes in vital signs may reflect an increase or decrease in anxiety.
Patient states methods to relax and reduce tension.	Teach deep breathing techniques and other relaxation strategies.	Relaxation exercises may decrease anxiety and promote rest.
Patient uses coping mechanisms that are effective.	Explore previous successful coping mechanisms and encourage the patient to use them.	Using previously tried, effective coping methods may help the patient relieve the anxiety and stress present at this time.

Evaluation: Compare the patient's status with the expected patient outcomes. If the outcomes are achieved, evaluate nursing care as successful. If not, reassess the patient, formulate new nursing diagnoses, and revise expected patient outcomes and nursing interventions as appropriate.

(continued)

of compartment syndrome, a limb-threatening complication.

Determine the patient's understanding of the injury and treatment necessary. Assess the patient's ability to perform self-care and to be mobile if a lower extremity is affected.

Nursing Diagnoses and Planning

Nursing diagnoses and related expected patient outcomes most commonly applicable to patients with a fracture include those previously discussed under musculoskeletal injuries and the following (also refer to Nursing Care Guide 36–1 and care of patients with a cast, patients in traction, and patients with fixation devices in Chapter 35):

NDx: Altered tissue perfusion; peripheral, related to the interruption of blood flow secondary to the trauma, edema, thrombus formation, or pressure from the attached device (wrap, cast, traction, or immobilizer)

Nursing Care Guide 36–1. (continued)

PATIENTS UNDERGOING SURGERY FOR A FRACTURED FEMUR

Assessment Findings: Patient seems very concerned about the surgery; patient asks questions about the surgery, the preparation for surgery, the fixation device or cast to be used, the expectations of the intervention, and possible complications.

Nursing Diagnosis: Knowledge deficit: nature of surgery for reduction of the fracture, preoperative preparations, and possible complications

Patient Outcomes	Nursing Interventions	Rationale
Patient accurately describes the purpose of the surgery and the necessity for the traction preoperatively and the immobilizing device postoperatively.	Explain the procedure to the patient, the usual preoperative preparation, and the expected outcomes.	Giving explanations of all the appropriate information about the surgery helps decrease the "unknowns" for the patient.
Patient relates information about the procedure, complications, and expected results as presented to the patient by the physician.	Have the patient relate what the physician has explained, and clear up any misunderstandings. Discuss potential complications with the patient.	Reinforcing the previous information from the physician decreases the knowledge deficit and confirms what the physician stated.
Patient reports an understanding of the preoperative procedures necessary.	Allow time for questions from the patient or the family. Give the patient literature explaining the procedure and showing what the prosthesis looks like.	Having the patient repeat the information gives opportunity to correct any misinformation.

Evaluation: Compare the patient's status with the expected patient outcomes. If the outcomes are achieved, evaluate nursing care as successful. If not, reassess the patient, formulate new nursing diagnoses, and revise expected patient outcomes and nursing interventions as appropriate.

(continued)

Planning: Patient outcomes

1. Patient's affected part has good color, and sensation and pulses are present, with no signs of compromised circulation.
2. Patient denies numbness, tingling, or decreased sensation in the affected part.

NDx: Impaired skin integrity related to bed rest, constriction of device for immobilization, edema, and internal altered circulation

Planning: Patient outcomes

1. Patient states causes of skin breakdown and measures to prevent the occurrence or recurrence.
2. Patient relates appropriate knowledge about skin care.
3. Patient is free of skin complications.

NDx: High risk for infection related to increased susceptibility secondary to bed rest, placement of internal or external fixation devices, pressure from restrictive devices, or compromised circulation

Planning: Patient outcomes

1. Patient's vital signs are within normal ranges for the patient.
2. Patient displays no signs of infection, such as fever, chills, tachycardia, tachypnea, or pain or burning on urination, or drainage from lesions or at pin sites or under the cast.
3. Patient identifies early signs of infection and measures to prevent infections.

NDx: Self-care deficit in areas of feeding, hygiene, toileting, or other activities of daily living requiring

Nursing Care Guide 36–1. *(continued)*

PATIENTS UNDERGOING SURGERY FOR A FRACTURED FEMUR

Assessment Findings: Patient reports discomfort because of positioning and force of the traction and inability to move freely in bed; patient complains of pain in affected leg; patient grimaces frequently, seems apprehensive, and has an increased pulse and respiratory rate.

Nursing Diagnosis: Pain related to fracture of leg, temporary traction, and/or immobility

Patient Outcomes	Nursing Interventions	Rationale
Patient reports relief of pain and discomfort.	Administer analgesics as prescribed. Reposition the patient as allowed in the bed. Teach the patient how to move by using the overhead trapeze. Check the traction equipment and patient for alignment.	Pain medication administered at regular intervals helps keep pain levels low and vital signs in normal limits. Slight movement in bed releases pressure from bony prominences. Keeping the traction and patient in proper alignment prevents unnecessary extrapulling forces.
Patient's vital signs are within normal limits for the patient, and no nonverbal signs of pain such as grimacing, guarding, restlessness in bed are present.	Watch for nonverbal signs of pain or discomfort. Assess vital signs. Check the patient frequently for pressure areas.	Changes in vital signs may reflect increasing pain levels.

Evaluation: Compare the patient's status with the expected patient outcomes. If the outcomes are achieved, evaluate nursing care as successful. If not, reassess the patient, formulate new nursing diagnoses, and revise expected patient outcomes and nursing interventions as appropriate.

Postoperative Care

Assessment Findings: Patient has incision site with dressings and a cast or external fixation device attached to the affected leg.

Nursing Diagnosis: High risk for impaired skin integrity related to wound site, pin sites, or irritation and pressure from cast

Patient Outcomes	Nursing Interventions	Rationale
Patient's wound site and/or pin sites remain free from symptoms of infection such as redness, purulent drainage, or excessive swelling.	Check the wound site and suture line for evidence of healing. Watch for signs of infection. Use aseptic technique during dressing changes. Perform pin care as ordered.	Early diagnosis of complications increases potential for successful treatment. Aseptic technique decreases risk of infection.

(continued)

Nursing Care Guide 36–1. *(continued)*

PATIENTS UNDERGOING SURGERY FOR A FRACTURED FEMUR

Patient Outcomes	Nursing Interventions	Rationale
Patient's skin around and within cast (if applicable) remains intact and free from breakdown.	Tell patient not to put anything into the cast. Check the cast for proper fit.	Putting objects into the cast may cause skin breakdown.
Patient's neurovascular signs are adequate in the affected leg, and vital signs are normal.	Check the neurovascular status proximal and distal to the cast or fixation device.	Pressure from a cast that is too tight may cause tissue breakdown.
	Assess vital signs frequently.	Vital sign changes may indicate infection, especially a systemic one, or compromised circulation in the extremity.

Evaluation: Compare the patient's status with the expected patient outcomes. If the outcomes are achieved, evaluate nursing care as successful. If not, reassess the patient, formulate new nursing diagnoses, and revise expected patient outcomes and nursing interventions as appropriate.

Assessment Findings: Patient grimaces, moans, and complains of discomfort at surgery site; patient's blood pressure, pulse, and respiratory rate are elevated.

Nursing Diagnosis: Pain related to invasive surgical procedure with manipulation, application of external fixation device or cast

Patient Outcomes	Nursing Interventions	Rationale
Patient reports relief of pain; patient appears relaxed and comfortable without signs of distress.	Give prescribed analgesics for control of postoperative pain. Make patient comfortable, and provide a quiet atmosphere for rest after surgery.	Relief of postoperative pain allows patient to rest as needed and assists in keeping vital signs within normal limits.
	Check insertion site for signs of infection, which may increase pain at site.	Infection with inflammation increases pain at the site.
	Tell the patient to practice relaxation techniques taught prior to surgery, such as deep breathing and muscle group relaxation exercises.	Relaxation may reduce anxiety and pain.
Patient's vital signs are within normal ranges.	Monitor the vital signs, and document the results.	Changes in vital signs may indicate changes in pain levels.

Evaluation: Compare the patient's status with the expected patient outcomes. If the outcomes are achieved, evaluate nursing care as successful. If not, reassess the patient, formulate new nursing diagnoses, and revise expected patient outcomes and nursing interventions as appropriate.

(continued)

Nursing Care Guide 36–1. *(continued)*

PATIENTS UNDERGOING SURGERY FOR A FRACTURED FEMUR

Assessment Findings: Patient seems worried about discharge to the home with crutches and self-care instructions for management of the cast or fixation device; patient is reluctant to work with the physical therapist and to practice exercises and locomotion on crutches; patient states concerns about providing self-care, hygiene, grooming, and activities of daily living when home.

Nursing Diagnosis: Altered health maintenance related to inability to manage mobility on crutches, fear for safety, and self-care, skin care, cast care, or external fixation device care

Patient Outcomes	Nursing Interventions	Rationale
Patient relates accurate information about the home care required and signs of potential problems. Patient demonstrates correct care of skin and pin sites or cast, as described in Chapter 35. Patient states plans for follow-up care with the attending physician.	Describe the signs requiring immediate medical intervention, such as severe pain or discomfort at surgical site, fever, chills, dizziness, fainting, excessive fatigue, or shortness of breath. Teach the patient the proper care of the skin and pin sites and/or the cast.	Early diagnosis of potential problems by the patient at home and early medical intervention increase the chance for successful treatment. Having the patient relate information presented reinforces the information and allows for correction of misconceptions.
Patient demonstrates appropriate use of crutches and states safety measures for the home environment to prevent falls or other injuries.	Assist the patient in practicing using the crutches. Help the patient find ways to increase safety measures in the home environment. Make appropriate referrals for assistance in the home if necessary.	Having the patient practice under supervision allows for a check on the patient's progress and safety practices before discharge.

Evaluation: Compare the patient's status with the expected patient outcomes. If the outcomes are achieved, evaluate nursing care as successful. If not, reassess the patient, formulate new nursing diagnoses, and revise expected patient outcomes and nursing interventions as appropriate.

mobility due to interference from immobilization of affected part

Planning: Patient outcomes

1. Patient performs activities of daily living, using assistive devices if necessary.
2. Patient states alternative methods to complete tasks that are restricted by musculoskeletal dysfunction.

Nursing Interventions

NDx: Altered tissue perfusion; peripheral

Help the patient conserve oxygen needs by encouraging rest and limiting activities. Administer oxygen if appropriate. Elevate the head of the bed to aid in chest expansion. Look for signs of compromised circulation. Relieve pressure to the affected part by cutting a window in the cast and padding bony areas. Prevent edema by raising the part.

Keep the patient in a comfortable position and reposition frequently to release pressure. Use range-of-motion exercises to stimulate circulation. Monitor vital signs and laboratory studies to assess for changes and improvement in status.

Discourage smoking to avoid vasoconstriction. Remove constricting clothing, and keep heavy bed linen from restricting peripheral circulation. Tell the patient to notify the nurse if signs of compromised circulation seem apparent, such as discoloration, pain, swelling, or numbness of an extremity. Keep the patient's legs in a nondependent position when not ambulating.

NDx: Impaired skin integrity
Teach the patient measures to prevent skin lesions from developing. Avoid irritating sheets or garments. Have the patient inspect the skin frequently and to seek medical assistance if any breakdown or soreness is noted.

Teach the patient to exercise, as tolerated, to promote good circulation. Range-of-motion exercises should be done while on bed rest. Turn the patient frequently, and inspect pressure areas for early signs of breakdown. Keep heavy linen from constricting the peripheral circulation by using a bed cradle. Elevate the patient's legs when sitting in a chair. Inspect the areas distal to constrictive devices for signs of compromised circulation. If lesions are present, use aseptic technique to cleanse them. Wear gloves during the dressing changes. Teach the patient and family members the proper technique for dressing areas of breakdown.

NDx: High risk for infection
Keep the patient warm, and avoid extreme changes in temperature in the room. Turn the patient as needed to stimulate circulation to prevent skin breakdown and skin infections. Have the patient deep breathe and cough frequently to prevent respiratory infections, especially if the patient is on bed rest. Monitor the patient's vital signs frequently, observing subtle changes that may indicate early signs of infection. Report any changes noted.

Promote good nutrition for proper healing. Encourage a high-protein and high-vitamin diet, and high fiber to prevent constipation. Provide skin care frequently, especially if areas of breakdown are present. Use aseptic technique to cleanse around pin sites as ordered. Because early identification and treatment may limit the severity of the infection, teach the patient and family to continually observe for signs of developing infection and to notify the physician if such signs appear.

NDx: Self-care deficit
Assist the patient with activities of daily living as needed. Seek alternative methods for the patient to be able to complete the activities when restricted by a cast or immobilization device. Teach the patient how to maneuver with the assistance of supportive aids. Explain how to use other extremities to complete a task, or how to move appropriately with the restrictive device in place, such as how to use crutches when the patient's leg is in a cast, immobilizer, or fixation device. Seek the assistance of physical therapists or occupational therapists when necessary for consultation or teaching sessions for the patient and family.

Evaluation

Evaluate the effectiveness of nursing care for a patient with a fracture by comparing the patient's status with the expected patient outcomes. Examples of specific outcomes for patients with a fracture have been provided in the Planning section.

FRACTURES COMMON IN THE GERIATRIC PATIENT

Physical changes accompanying aging, such as changes in posture, a broader-based shuffling gait, poor vision, slower reflexes, weaker muscles, and faulty judgment, make the elderly individual more prone to falls. In addition, the bone structure of the geriatric patient is osteoporotic, or more porous and brittle than the bone structure of younger adults. Osteoporotic bone is more likely to fracture with minimal trauma. Slowing the osteoporotic changes in aging bone with diet, vitamins, and exercise and preventing the number of injuries by identifying individuals at increased risk for falls are measures that could help lower the number of fractures in this population. Some fractures are more common in the elderly patient than in other age groups. The most frequent fractures are those of the hip and the wrist.

Hip Fractures

Etiology. Fractures of the hip with complications compete with heart disease, cancer, and stroke as a leading cause of mortality in the elderly. Most hip fractures occur from falls that involve only slight trauma and would cause little injury in a young adult.

Pathophysiology. A hip fracture refers to a fracture of the proximal end of the femur. The three types of hip fractures are fractures of the femoral neck, intertrochanteric fractures, and subtrochanteric fractures.

Femoral neck fractures occur within the hip joint capsule. They have a high incidence of improper healing and avascular necrosis because the medullary vessels in the femoral neck are torn as the bone fragments shift when the neck is fractured.

Intertrochanteric fractures are extracapsular or outside of the hip joint capsule. Occasionally the fracture line extends into the capsule, and circulatory problems can develop.

Subtrochanteric fractures are extracapsular. These are rarely associated with circulatory impairment or healing problems.

Clinical Manifestations. With nondisplaced intracapsular fractures, the individual may still be able to walk. The involved limb may be of normal length and position, or lateral rotation and shortening of the extremity may be present. Pain is usually felt in the groin and may extend to the knee. It is exacerbated by movement of the hip.

Limbs with intertrochanteric fractures appear shortened and externally rotated. These fractures produce more pain than intracapsular fractures. The history of injury usually includes a direct blow to the trochanter.

Subtrochanteric fractures result from a significant force and create an externally rotated, shortened extremity. Because subtrochanteric fractures can involve blood loss of as much as 1500 ml, the risk of hypovolemic shock is high.

Medical Diagnosis. The diagnosis of a hip fracture is made on the basis of history, physical assessment, and x-ray or CT studies.

Medical Management. Most hip fractures are treated by surgical insertion of an internal fixation device. An ORIF is the most common procedure for displaced fractures. The surgery is usually performed under general or spinal anesthesia. It is important to remember that elderly patients are at increased risk for complications of anesthesia such as paralytic ileus, disorientation, cardiac dysrhythmias, fluid and electrolyte imbalance, and thromboembolism.

The selection of internal fixation device and postoperative care depends upon whether the fracture is intracapsular or extracapsular, and whether the fracture is a stable nondisplaced fracture or an unstable displaced fracture.

Extracapsular fractures may be treated with nails, a nail and plate, multiple pins, or a compression screw device. Intracapsular fractures of the neck are usually treated with a femoral head replacement such as an Austin Moore or Thompson prosthesis or, in complicated fractures, a total hip replacement. Some nondisplaced intracapsular fractures with good circulation may be treated with pins. (Refer to internal fixation devices in Chapter 35.)

Rarely are elderly patients treated by traction for an extended time because of their increased risk of possible complications from prolonged immobility. Intracapsular fractures can take 24 weeks to heal, and extracapsular fractures at least 12 weeks. Buck's skin traction may be used on a short-term basis for preoperative comfort and immobilization. Skeletal traction may replace the Buck's traction if surgery is delayed because of existing medical conditions or other circumstances that prohibit surgery.

Application of the Nursing Process to the Care of the Geriatric Patient with a Hip Fracture

Assessment

Assess for signs and symptoms of complications as discussed under care of the patient with a fracture in the previous nursing process section. This includes looking for signs of compromised circulation, impaired skin integrity, or infection. All these problems may be more common in the older adult. Also assess the patient's extent of immobility and ability to perform self-care activities. Investigate the patient's knowledge about the treatment, self-care needs, care of the surgical site, use of ambulatory aids, and prevention of further injury.

Nursing Diagnoses and Planning

Nursing diagnoses and related expected patient outcomes most commonly applicable to geriatric patients with a hip fracture include those already discussed under fractures and the following:

NDx: Impaired physical mobility related to pain, inability to bear weight, and immobilization device

Planning: Patient outcomes
1. Patient moves in bed with the assistance of nursing intervention and an overhead trapeze.
2. Patient denies pain or discomfort in affected part.
3. Patient is able to be mobile with the assistance of an ambulatory aid.

NDx: High risk for injury; falls related to weakness from immobility and improper use of ambulatory aids

Planning: Patient outcomes
1. Patient demonstrates proper use of a prescribed ambulatory aid.
2. Patient states measures to provide for safe locomotion in the home and elsewhere outside of the hospital.
3. Patient performs prescribed exercises to maintain strength and joint motion.

Nursing Interventions

NDx: Impaired physical mobility
Teach the patient use of the overhead trapeze while still on bed rest to increase movement in bed, as allowed, to prevent complications of immobility. Reposition the patient frequently to stimulate circulation and prevent skin breakdown. Assist the patient in locomotion, once able, to provide safe use of the ambulatory aid. Use the assistance of physical therapy to instruct the patient and family about the device and to reinforce its safe use. Give analgesics as needed to decrease pain levels that may interfere with the patient's ability to be mobile.

NDx: High risk for injury; falls
Provide assistance during locomotion, as necessary, until the patient becomes skillful with the ambulatory aid. Reinforce the information on the use of the device that was presented by the therapist. Teach the family about safe use of the ambulatory aid. Be sure the patient has well-fitting shoes with gripper soles while ambulating. Explain how to make the home environment safer for the patient while using

the ambulatory aid. (Also see Nursing Care Guide 35–1.)

Evaluation

Evaluate the effectiveness of nursing care for a geriatric patient with a hip fracture by comparing the patient's status with the expected patient outcomes. Examples of specific outcomes for geriatric patients with a hip fracture have been provided in the Planning section.

Wrist Fractures

Etiology. The distal radius and ulnar styloid are common sites for osteoporotic fractures in the elderly. A fractured wrist, or Colles' fracture, usually occurs as the individual attempts to break a fall with extended arms and dorsiflexed hands. This type of fracture is extremely common in the elderly and occurs most frequently when the older adult slips and falls on an ice-coated walkway or wet floor.

Pathophysiology. The injury produces an obvious deformity, described as a dinner-fork deformity, with a proximal depression and a fullness in the distal aspect of the wrist. If the median nerve and flexor tendons are involved, sensation and function of all the fingers in the limb may be affected. The elbow and clavicle are also to be inspected for possible injury because force is often transferred along the skeleton.

Clinical Manifestations. Patients with a Colles' fracture present with pain, swelling, tenderness at the point of fracture, and the dinner-fork deformity.

Medical Diagnosis. The diagnosis is made on the basis of physical examination, history, and radiographic studies.

Medical Management. Medical management usually consists of reduction by closed manipulation and immobilization in a short arm cast. If there is comminution of the fracture and extensive swelling or soft tissue involvement, percutaneous pinning, ORIF, or an external fixation device may be used for immobilization.

Application of the Nursing Process to the Care of the Geriatric Patient with a Wrist Fracture

Assessment

Assess the patient's affected wrist for pain, swelling, discoloration, or malalignment. Check the neurovascular status proximal and distal to the injury by palpating for pulses, feeling for warmth of the part, and assessing for decreased sensation. Ask the patient about numbness or tingling in the wrist, hand, or even in the entire arm. Review how the the injury occurred, and note what treatment was instituted, if any, at the time of the occurrence. Be sure to assess the entire patient, because other injuries could have easily occurred in the older patient during the fall. Determine the patient's understanding of the injury and treatment necessary.

Nursing Diagnoses and Planning

Nursing diagnoses and related expected patient outcomes most commonly applicable to geriatric patients with a wrist fracture include the following:

NDx: Pain related to joint trauma, pressure from edema, and immobilization

Planning: Patient outcomes
1. Patient denies pain in affected part.
2. Patient states methods to decrease pain by reduction of swelling and keeping immobilizer properly applied.

NDx: Ineffective management of therapeutic regimen related to lack of knowledge about the injury, management of cast or immobilization device, exercises to perform, and prevention of reinjury

Planning: Patient outcomes
1. Patient states accurate information about the cause of the injury and methods to prevent reinjury.
2. Patient demonstrates proper application of the immobilizer device or care of the cast, how much weight-lifting or weight-bearing is allowed, and when the device may be removed, if applicable.
3. Patient demonstrates proper care of pin sites, if applicable, and signs of infection.
4. Patient demonstrates exercises, as taught, to maintain strength and range of motion of joints.

NDx: Self-care deficit: grooming and basic hygiene related to inability to use wrist or hand of the affected arm

Planning: Patient outcomes
1. Patient demonstrates use of assistive devices if necessary to aid in self-care activities.
2. Patient is able to use opposite arm, wrist, or hand to perform self-care.

Nursing Intervention

NDx: Pain
Give prescribed analgesics and explain the dosage, frequency, side effects, and expected therapeutic ef-

fects of the medications. Caution the patient not to perform tasks that require mental alertness while under the effects of the pain medication. Teach the patient to check for tightness of the cast or immobilizer, looking for signs of swelling or diminished sensation in the distal part of the affected extremity. Tell the patient to elevate the arm to reduce swelling and thus reduce pain.

NDx: Ineffective management of therapeutic regimen
Teach the patient about the injury, how to prevent falls, methods of prevention of further injury to the wrist, and appropriate treatment. Explain how to apply the immobilizer or wrap to the affected part (if not casted) and have the patient redemonstrate the process. Check to see that it is not too tight, and tell the patient how to check for improper fit. Explain that increased swelling, discoloration, and decreased sensation in the affected part may be signs of improper fit of the device or a cast that is too tight, and that prolonged pressure could cause severe problems if not relieved. Reinforce the physician's instruction about weight-lifting with the hand. Teach the patient proper pin care, if applicable, and signs of infection to observe for at the pin site. Demonstrate prescribed exercises to the patient, and encourage participation in the exercise regimen to prevent loss of strength and joint motion.

NDx: Self-care deficit
Assist the patient in performing activities of self-care. Explain how assistive devices may aid the patient in performing self-care. Help the patient learn to use the other hand to complete tasks. Teach the family what they need to do to assist the patient during the healing process.

Evaluation

Evaluate the effectiveness of nursing care for a geriatric patient with a wrist fracture by comparing the patient's status with the expected patient outcomes. Examples of specific outcomes for geriatric patients with wrist fractures have been provided in the Planning section.

TRAUMATIC AMPUTATIONS

A traumatic amputation refers to any injury that cuts off an appendage or body projection. The body part, if it can be recovered, is saved for possible reattachment. It is placed in a plastic bag, which is then put in a container of crushed ice. The amputated part is transported with the patient to the emergency room for continued care. Fingers, toes, arms, hands, and other body parts have been successfully reattached. The patient is stabilized as quickly as possible with intravenous fluids, treatment to other affected areas, and medications. Once this has occurred, the patient is taken to surgery for the microvascular anastomosis of the amputated body part. If reimplantation is not possible, debridement and closure of the residual body part occur. Prognosis varies, depending upon the time since the injury, access to an institution performing microsurgery, degree of damage to the amputated part, and the patient's stability, age, and health status prior to the incident.

Application of the Nursing Process to the Care of the Patient with a Traumatic Amputation Undergoing Reattachment Surgery

Assessment

After the patient has been stabilized, assess the patient's awareness of the situation and knowledge of the impending surgery. Continue to check vital signs. Assess the patient's pain, noting the intensity, whether analgesics have been given, and the patient's response. Determine whether the patient has significant others available for assistance and emotional support. Because the time between the presentation of the patient to the hospital and the initiation of surgical intervention is extremely limited, most nursing interventions, other than the emergency care, occur in the postoperative period.

In addition to the usual postoperative care, as described in Chapter 4, assess the patient's neurovascular status proximal and distal to the surgical site. Palpate pulses and check color, sensation, and edema of the part. If the entire limb is bandaged, assess the bandages for tightness and ask the patient about sensation in the part. It is expected that there may be no sensation for some time. Check for drainage on the bandages.

Assess the patient's anxiety level, coping ability, and understanding of the incident and the treatment regimen. Note the availability of support systems for the patient.

Assess pain and general discomfort. Check whether the patient is able to rest and sleep at intervals.

Nursing Diagnoses and Planning

Nursing diagnoses and related expected patient outcomes most commonly applicable to patients with a traumatic amputation undergoing reattachment surgery include the following:

NDx: Anxiety related to traumatic injury, potential permanent loss of limb, and pain

Planning: Patient outcomes
1. Patient denies anxiety, fear, or nervousness about the surgery and potential outcome of the surgery.
2. Patient appears relaxed and is able to rest at intervals and to sleep well.
3. Patient does not display signs of increased anxiety, such as twitching, nervousness, and increased respirations and pulse.

NDx: Pain related to trauma, manipulation during surgery, and usual postoperative physiologic events

Planning: Patient outcomes
1. Patient denies pressure, pain, discomfort, or alteration in sensation.
2. Patient is able to exercise and tolerate mobility (of unaffected body parts) without interferences from acute pain episodes.

NDx: High risk for infection related to original injury and surgical intervention

Planning: Patient outcomes
1. Patient's vital signs are within normal ranges for the patient.
2. Patient displays no signs of infection, such as fever, chills, tachycardia, tachypnea, pain or burning on urination, or drainage from suture lines or at intravenous site.
3. Patient identifies early signs of infection and measures to prevent infections.

NDx: Impaired home maintenance management related to lack of knowledge about postoperative expectations, potential for rehabilitation and ability to manage self-care, and resources available for assistance

Planning: Patient outcomes
1. Patient states accurate information about the surgical intervention and expected postoperative course as explained by the physician.
2. Patient demonstrates adapted methods for providing self-care.
3. Patient demonstrates exercises for maintenance of mobility of nonaffected extremities and any prescribed for the affected area.
4. Patient recalls resources available for assistance if necessary.

Nursing Interventions

NDx: Anxiety

Explain the purpose of all treatments to the patient. Teach the patient how to reposition in the bed. Prior to performing any procedure on the patient, explain the steps of the procedure and the reason for it. Allow the patient time to ask questions and relay concerns. Reinforce information from the physician to the patient. Give support without offering unrealistic reassurances.

Check vital signs, and watch for changes indicating increased anxiety. Teach the patient relaxation methods and strategies to cope with the fears of hospitalization and medical interventions necessary. Have the patient practice range-of-motion exercises to help relieve discomfort from the static position and to maintain muscle tone and joint motion of unaffected extremities, as allowed. Also, provide diversional activity for the patient to relieve the boredom and anxiety from bed rest.

NDx: Pain

Place the patient in comfortable positions, and reposition frequently. Check the affected extremity to ensure proper alignment and positioning. Look for signs of pressure causing pain, such as from the bandages or positioning of the extremity. Use pillows to support bony prominences.

Give analgesics as prescribed. Assess when the pain is most severe, and allow the patient to rest during those periods. Give pain medications prior to activity periods so that the patient can better tolerate the movement.

Help the patient find alternate methods to alleviate or to be able to tolerate the pain. Show the patient relaxation techniques. Teach the patient the use of patient-controlled analgesia (PCA) if ordered.

Inspect the skin and palpate pulses in distal areas for signs of compromised circulation or skin breakdown caused by constrictive bandages, which may be the cause of the pain. Tell the patient to report any signs of pain, numbness, or change in temperature immediately.

NDx: High risk for infection

Keep the patient warm, and avoid extreme changes in temperature in the room. Turn the patient as needed to stimulate circulation to prevent skin breakdown and skin infections. Massage bony prominences. Have the patient deep breathe and cough frequently to prevent respiratory infections, especially while the patient is on bed rest. Monitor the patient's vital signs frequently, observing subtle changes that may indicate early signs of infection. Report any changes noted.

Promote good nutrition for proper healing by serving meals the patient will eat, in a relaxed attractive atmosphere. Encourage a high-protein, high-vitamin diet. Use aseptic technique when changing bandages and cleansing suture line, as ordered. Check the intravenous site for signs of infection and use aseptic technique when cleansing around insertion site. Because early identification and treatment may limit the severity of the infection, teach the patient and family to continually observe for signs of developing infection and to notify the physician if such signs appear. Stress the importance of taking antibiotics as prescribed.

NDx: Impaired home maintenance management
Explain all interventions to the patient. Tell the patient about the expectations postoperatively. Reinforce the physician's information about recovery and rehabilitation.

Teach the patient about the prescribed medications. Explain the correct dosage, frequency, side effects, and therapeutic effects. Tell the patient when to notify the physician if any problems become evident. Teach the patient signs of complications such as extreme pain, discoloration, intense swelling, temperature change, and decreased sensation after the normal sensation has returned to the affected part.

Assist the patient with activities of daily living as needed. Seek alternative methods for the patient to be able to complete the activities when restricted by the affected extremity. Teach the patient how to maneuver with the assistance of supportive aids if the affected part was a lower extremity. Explain how to use other extremities to complete a task, or how to move appropriately, such as how to use crutches when weight-bearing is not allowed on the reattached extremity. Seek the assistance of physical therapists or occupational therapists when necessary for consultation or teaching sessions for the patient and family.

Provide a list to the patient and family of possible resources for assistance in the community. Make appropriate referrals prior to the patient's discharge.

Evaluation

Evaluate the effectiveness of nursing care for a patient with a traumatic amputation having reattachment surgery by comparing the patient's status with the expected patient outcomes. Examples of specific outcomes for patients with a traumatic amputation having reattachment surgery have been provided in the Planning section.

Complications of Musculoskeletal Injuries

There are a number of complications that can result from major trauma to the musculoskeletal system. Immediate complications may occur following the trauma or up to 3 days thereafter. Delayed complications arise secondary to the initial injury and can develop as long as 6 months to 1 year after the injury. Although all complications are not preventable, early detection and treatment lessen their severity and long-term effects. Thrombophlebitis, deep vein thrombosis, and pulmonary embolism are complications of musculoskeletal injuries that usually occur early in the postinjury course. Refer to Chapters 14 and 20 for discussion of these conditions.

IMMEDIATE COMPLICATIONS

SHOCK

Loss of blood, either internally from a fracture of the pelvis, femur, ribs, or vertebrae or from an open compound fracture, can result in hypovolemic shock. Hypovolemic shock usually develops immediately or within the first 48 hours after injury. The patient becomes restless, agitated, and confused, followed by a decrease in the level of consciousness. The pulse becomes weak and thready as the blood pressure falls. Respirations are rapid, and the patient's skin becomes cool and clammy.

Immediate splinting of suspected fractures prior to transport helps prevent excess blood loss. If profuse external bleeding is apparent, pressure is maintained on the site. If paramedic aid is available, parenteral fluids are started at the scene of the injury. Otherwise, intravenous fluid replacement is initiated immediately upon arrival at the health care facility. Shock and internal bleeding must be treated before the fracture can be reduced and immobilized.

COMPARTMENT SYNDROME

Etiology and Pathophysiology. Compartment syndrome is an increase in the pressure within a fascial muscle compartment. A rise in intracompartmental pressure may occur after a closed fracture injury, crushing injuries, burns, application of a dressing or cast that is too tight, or when a muscle swells after exercise. The forearm and lower leg are most commonly affected by this syndrome. As the pressure within the muscle compartment exceeds diastolic blood pressure, circulation to the muscle is impaired or interrupted completely and necrosis results. Tissue damage can occur within 30 minutes. Elevated pressures for more than 4 hours can result in irreversible damage and limb loss.

Clinical Manifestations. A major clinical manifestation is severe pain in the affected area that is not relieved by narcotics. The pain increases on passive stretching of the muscle. The muscle feels tense and swollen on palpation. The patient may experience numbness and tingling in and distal to an involved muscle as a result of nerve compression. Decrease in sensation, then paralysis, may follow. Loss of the distal pulse is a late sign of compartment syndrome.

Medical Diagnosis. Diagnosis is made on the basis of physical symptoms and measurement of the muscle compartment pressure. Intracompartment pressure is measured by inserting a needle into the muscle compartment. The needle is connected to a saline-filled tube, which is, in turn, connected to a manometer. The specialized monitoring device can provide a constant read-out of compartment pressure.

Medical Management. Abnormal pressure within the muscle compartment is released by fasciotomy, a surgical incision of the fascia, when signs of compromised neurovascular supply develop that cannot be relieved by repositioning, elevation, or ice. A monitored intracompartment pressure of 30 mm Hg or higher is considered sufficient to impair blood flow. A fasciotomy may be done at lower compartment pressures in hypotensive patients. Early diagnosis is the most important step in treating compartment syndrome to prevent limb loss.

FAT EMBOLISM

Etiology and Pathophysiology. Fat embolism is a potentially fatal complication of long-bone fractures and multiple trauma. Theories differ on where the fat globules that form the emboli originate. The mechanical theory hypothesizes that the fracture of the bone releases fat globules from the marrow cavity into the blood stream. The physiochemical theory identifies the stress response of the body and the release of catecholamines by the sympathetic nervous system at the time of injury as the cause. The catecholamines alter the metabolism of fatty acids, which leads to accumulation of fat globules in the blood. Once the fat globules enter the circulation, they cause platelets to clump and form fat emboli. Pulmonary fat emboli damage the alveolar capillary membranes and obstruct capillary blood flow similar to the effects of a pulmonary embolus of vascular origin. Disruption of the exchange of oxygen and carbon dioxide across the capillary membrane results in pulmonary insufficiency, pulmonary infarct, and alveolar collapse. Fat emboli can also lodge in vessels in the heart, brain, kidneys, and other tissues and organs of the body, causing circulatory insufficiency, tissue infarcts, and sudden death.

Clinical Manifestations. The symptoms of fat embolism occur within the first 72 hours after injury. Headache, drowsiness, irritability, memory loss, confusion, rapid pulse, and fever may occur. Pulmonary symptoms include tachypnea, dyspnea, use of accessory muscles, and wheezing caused by blockage of air passages. Inspiratory stridor is caused by obstruction of the upper airways from copious thick white sputum. Petechiae may appear on the neck, upper chest, shoulder, axillae, buccal membranes, and conjunctiva in a small percentage of patients. The petechiae, which result from intravascular thromboses secondary to decreased oxygenation, are characteristic of fat emboli and help differentiate fat embolism from a blood clot embolism and adult respiratory distress syndrome.

Medical Diagnosis. Medical diagnosis is made on the basis of history of a long-bone fracture, diagnostic data, and presenting symptoms. Blood gas values usually indicate a decrease in PaO_2 to lower than 60 mm Hg, a $PaCO_2$ higher than 50 mm Hg, and acidosis. Blood lipase and sedimentation rate are elevated.

Medical Management. The goals of medical management are to improve oxygenation and prevent further deterioration. Oxygen in high concentrations is administered. Coughing and deep breathing or positive end-expiratory pressure (PEEP) mechanical breathing, or both, improve ventilation. Low-molecular-weight dextran intravenous fluids are carefully titrated to prevent both shock and an increase in pulmonary congestion. Steroids are administered to decrease lung inflammation and the cerebral edema associated with hypoxemia. Heparin may be administered to prevent new emboli from forming. Some physicians believe that steroids and heparin should be used prophylactically in high-risk patients, whereas others advocate the use of aspirin. Patients are placed on bed rest to prevent the chance of movement of the bone fragments and release of additional fat globules.

DELAYED COMPLICATIONS

JOINT STIFFNESS AND CONTRACTURES

Joint stiffness is a common sequela of musculoskeletal injuries that involve a diseased or older joint. A loss of range of motion with contracture formation is more likely to occur as a result of a fracture near or into a joint or a fracture associated with joint dislocation. Careful positioning, early passive exercises, and progressive active and resistive exercises are the key to prevention of joint stiffness and contractures. Once intraarticular adhesions occur, manipulation under anesthesia and aggressive physiotherapy may be required to reverse them. Intraarticular structures that have been fractured are also at high risk for development of early osteoarthritis.

INFECTION

A bone infection is called osteomyelitis. Direct contamination of a bone by bacteria may occur as a result of an open fracture, during open reduction of a fracture, or from infection of a superficial wound or surgical incision. Infection of the bone interferes with the process of fracture healing and can result in permanent disability.

Gas gangrene, from gram-positive *Clostridium perfringens,* or tetanus may also develop in grossly contaminated open fractures. Callus formation and union of the fracture fragments may be prevented by the presence of bacteria. Wound infections may aggravate overall healing even though the bone may continue to heal and allow weight-bearing. Wound infections also increase the risk for development of bone infections.

Symptoms of osteomyelitis include pain in the affected area, local erythema, a draining tract, and fever. Local symptoms of gas gangrene include cellulitis engorged with gas bubbles and a foul-smelling watery exudate. The patient may also appear anemic, have a decreased pulse rate, and if untreated, develop septic shock. Symptoms of a wound infection include redness, swelling, and warmth at the site; purulent drainage; and low-grade temperature elevation.

HEALING PROBLEMS

Malunion

A fracture that heals in a position of deformity is referred to as a malunion. This complication leaves a limb at a mechanical disadvantage and may be a severe problem in lower extremities. A malunion is identified on x-ray examination, usually during routine follow-up.

If complete union has not yet occurred, the deformity may be treated by manipulation and recasting. If fracture repair is complete, refracture and alignment or an osteotomy may be necessary.

Delayed Union

A delayed union is identified when the expected average time for a fracture to heal has passed without fracture union. The age, nutritional status, and general health of the individual are considered in the expected time for bone healing. A delayed union is evident on x-ray film. If a cause can be determined, treatment is focused on correcting the cause of the delayed union. A delayed union may progress to a nonunion.

Nonunion

Nonunion is diagnosed when a fracture has failed to heal within the expected time and x-ray films show sclerosed fracture ends, a fluid gap between fragments, or a fibrocartilaginous union. Causes of nonunion include infection, excessive movement of the bone fragments, interposed soft tissue, inadequate blood supply, failed internal fixation, and concurrent pathologic disorders such as metastatic cancer and osteoporosis. As many as 10% of all fractures become delayed unions or nonunions. The distal one third of the tibia is the most common site for delayed union and nonunion healing problems.

Symptoms of nonunion include local pain and instability of the fracture. A nonunion is diagnosed on the basis of assessment, history, and x-ray examination. The goals of medical management are identification and correction of causative factors and promotion of bone healing. Treatments instituted to promote formation of a healthy fibrous union may include bone grafts and use of an electrical bone stimulator. Bone grafts may be autogenous (using the patient's own bone), homogeneous (using bone from another person), or heterogeneous (using a synthetic calcium substance). Autografts are frequently taken from the iliac crest, greater trochanter, or fibula. Surgical incisions at both the donor and graft sites require meticulous wound care to prevent further complications such as osteomyelitis.

An electrical bone stimulator may be used to promote bone healing instead of, or in addition to, bone grafts. Healthy bone possesses a positive electrical potential, which increases with mechanical stress. Fractured bone develops a negative charge. Although scientists are uncertain how it works, electrical stimulation produces an electromagnetic field around the fracture site that promotes new bone growth.

The bone stimulator's electrical current is 1000 times weaker than that of a cardiac pacemaker. Three types of electrical bone stimulators are available: an implanted device similar to a battery in appearance, which requires surgery for insertion and an incision for removal; a semi-invasive device that has percutaneous pins inserted into the fracture site under fluoroscopy and an external battery pack; and a noninvasive apparatus that the patient wears around the fracture site. The external noninvasive device consists of electrical coils within a pack that is wrapped externally around the fracture site. It is worn for 10 to 12 hours a day until healing is complete.

The success rate for all types of electrical bone stimulators is 75% to 85%. The average time for healing is 16 weeks. The decision on the type of device to use is determined by physician preference and patient compliance.

REFLEX SYMPATHETIC DYSTROPHY

Reflex sympathetic dystrophy is a complication of unknown etiology that occurs in severe sprains and fractures of the wrist and ankle. The hand or foot becomes swollen and painful, and range of motion is impaired. X-ray films reveal patchy osteoporosis. The skin over the area appears glossy, reddened, and swollen. Medical management involves aggressive physical therapy and pain management.

PATHOLOGIC OSSIFICATION

Pathologic ossification (also called myositis ossificans) develops in fractures in which the periosteum is stripped from the bone during injury. Ossification extends into the hematoma, soft tissue, and muscle around the fracture site. Fractures of the elbow frequently develop this complication. The symptoms are painful and limited motion of the involved area. Medical management consists of controlled exercise of the involved area and sometimes surgical removal of abnormal bone growth.

AVASCULAR NECROSIS

Necrosis of bone and intraarticular structures can occur from a lack of circulation to the tissue following injury as a result of malalignment, thrombus, or constriction from an immobilizing device or wrap. The ischemic bone becomes necrotic and collapses. Frequent sites of avascular necrosis are the femoral head, the body of the talus bone in the ankle, and the carpal scaphoid bone and lunate bone in the wrist. This complication is most prevalent in the femoral head because the circulatory supply to the intracapsular tissue is disrupted in fractures of the neck of the femur and in hip dislocations posteriorly.

The patient with avascular necrosis experiences increasing pain, limb instability, and decreasing function of the involved area. Diagnosis is confirmed by x-ray films, bone scan, and CT scan that show a collapsing, necrotic bone structure.

Initial medical management attempts to prevent further osteonecrosis. Treatment differs depending on the stage or extent of the necrosis. Protective non–weight-bearing and removal of a core of the cancellous bone through a drill hole in the metaphysis to decrease pressure may halt the degenerative process. When conservative efforts fail to prevent progression of necrosis, a bone graft, bone prosthesis, joint fusion, joint replacement, or amputation may be necessary.

Neoplasia

A neoplasm is any abnormal cell growth that serves no useful purpose and derives its nutrition from, and often destroys, healthy surrounding tissues. Bone tumors are neoplasms that may be either osteoblastic, bone-forming, or osteolytic, bone-destroying. The exact cause of the formation and growth of bone tumors is not known. Bone tumors may be classified by the type of tissue they arise from. Osteogenic tumors arise from osseous or bone tissue. Chondrogenic tumors arise from cartilage. Collagenic tumors arise from connective tissue such as tendons or ligaments. Myelogenic tumors arise from the bone marrow (Table 36–1).

Bone tumors can cause pain, deformity, weakening of the bone structure, and pathologic fractures. Bone necrosis may develop secondary to disruption of vascular supply by pressure from the growing tumor mass or actual destruction of blood vessels. Bone tumors may be further classified by their destructive capacity and cellular activity as either benign or malignant.

Benign Bone Tumors

Etiology and Pathophysiology. Most benign bone tumors occur in children and young adults. They grow slowly and do not metastasize or spread through the blood or lymphatic system to other body parts. Some benign bone tumors are described in Table 36–1.

Clinical Manifestations. Clinical manifestation of benign bone tumors include deformity, swelling over the involved area, and restricted motion. Pain is persistent and may increase with weight-bearing. If the bone structure is weakened or necrosis has developed as a result of impaired circulation, pathologic fractures following minimal or no trauma may occur.

Medical Diagnosis. Preliminary diagnosis of a benign bone tumor is made on the basis of history and physical examination. X-ray films, bone scans, arteriography, and surgical biopsy are used for differential diagnosis. Blood values are usually normal with benign tumors.

Medical Management. The goals of medical management are pain relief and prevention of complications such as pathologic fracture. Surgery is not necessary if tumor growth has stopped, if there is little or no deformity, and if the patient is free of pain.

When surgery is indicated, curettage or resection of the lesion is performed. If the defect from a resected tumor is large, bone grafts may be required. The involved area is protected by splints or casts until the bone heals. Ambulatory aids are used if a lower extremity is involved. To relieve pain, analgesics are prescribed, and the affected area is handled and positioned carefully. Prophylactic antibiotics and aseptic wound care are routine to prevent osteomyelitis. Periodic reevaluation after treatment for a benign bone tumor is important because recurrence of benign lesions is common and malignant tumors may develop.

Application of the Nursing Process to the Care of the Patient with a Benign Bone Tumor

Assessment

Review the patient's history, results of diagnostic studies, and presenting symptoms. Determine the patient's and family's understanding of the diagnosis. Evaluate the site for symptoms of pain, swelling, deformity, or restricted motion. Ask the patient about problems with mobility of the affected part. Note the patient's anxiety level and what coping mechanisms are in place.

Nursing Diagnoses and Planning

Nursing diagnoses and related expected patient outcomes most commonly applicable to patients with a benign bone tumor include the following:

NDx: Anxiety related to diagnosis, potential permanent loss of limb, and pain

Table 36–1. COMMON TYPES OF BONE TUMORS

TYPE	DESCRIPTION
BENIGN TUMORS	
Osteochondroma	A common tumor that appears on x-ray film as a bone spur or projection with a cartilage cap. It usually develops near an epiphyseal growth plate during adolescence. The tumor may stop growing with skeletal maturation. Symptoms include a palpable nodule and mild pain.
Osteoma	An osseofibrous tumor usually found in membranous bones of the face and skull. It may be painful and cause deformity.
Cysts	A unicameral (single-chamber) cyst arises from bone tissue. It contains blood or amber or clear fluid. An aneurysmal bone cyst arises from vascular tissue. It consists of large spaces filled with blood and looks like a "bubble" on x-ray film.
Giant cell tumor	A tumor characterized by large "giant cells" with many nuclei. The tumor looks like soap bubbles on x-ray film. Although it is a benign tumor, it is aggressive, destroys some surrounding tissue, and has the potential to become malignant. It is usually painful. The tumor occurs most frequently in the distal femur, proximal tibia, and distal radius. Females are affected more often than males.
Enchondroma	It is an oval tumor of hyaline cartilage. It usually develops on the small tubular bones of the hands and feet. The inside of the tumor is pale and bluish.
Hemangioma	It is a highly vascular cavernous tumor filled with red bloods cells. It may appear anywhere on the body but is frequently found on the face, skull, or neck.
MALIGNANT TUMORS	
Osteosarcoma	This is the most common malignant bone tumor, characterized by extreme pain, rapid growth, and metastasis. It is more common in young males than other populations. Treatment usually involves resection and chemotherapy.
Chondrosarcoma	The tumor arises from chondroblasts (cartilage tissue). The incidence is highest among middle-aged males. It primarily affects the bones in the trunk, pelvis, and proximal femur. It is slow growing and produces persistent dull pain. The lesions show osseous destruction with the presence of scattered areas of ringlet calcification on x-ray film. This tumor tends to be radioresistant and thus is treated with surgery and chemotherapy.
Fibrosarcoma	The tumor arises from fibrous connective tissue. These tumors are slow growing and can occur at any age. They are found more frequently in males than females. Treatment includes surgical excision with radiotherapy.
Malignant fibrous histiocytoma (MFH)	The MFH tumor arises from fibrous connective tissue. It grows rapidly and is destructive to adjacent bone. MFH lesions can occur at any site but are primarily seen in the long bones. The overlying skin is usually fixed to the tumor. There is no predilection for age or sex. Treatment is similar to that for osteosarcoma.
Ewing's sarcoma	This is a rare highly malignant tumor that originates in the marrow and metastasizes early in its course. It occurs mainly in long bones or the flat bones of the pelvis and ribs. It is more common in young males. Pain is frequently extreme. It is treated with chemotherapy and/or radiation and surgery.
Multiple myeloma	This a primary tumor arising from plasma cells in the bone marrow. It is most common in middle age to old age, with a higher incidence in males. It is rarely diagnosed before bone destruction and metastasis have occurred. Pain is the most common symptom. (See Chapter 16.)

Planning: Patient outcomes

1. Patient denies anxiety, fear, or nervousness about the diagnosis, therapy, and potential outcome of the therapy.
2. Patient appears relaxed and is able to rest at intervals and to sleep well.
3. Patient does not display signs of increased anxiety such as twitching, nervousness, increased respirations and pulse, or withdrawal from self-care activities.

NDx: Pain related to effects of the tumor, swelling, and deformity

Planning: Patient outcomes

1. Patient denies pain in affected part.
2. Patient states methods to decrease pain by reduction of swelling, relaxation strategies, and appropriate use of analgesics.

NDx: Knowledge deficit: nature of disorder, prognosis, management, and prevention of injury of weakened part

Planning: Patient outcomes

1. Patient states accurate information about the cause of the tumor, prognosis, treatment, and methods to prevent injury.
2. Patient reports an understanding of the disorder and the information presented by the physician for management of the condition.

Nursing Interventions

NDx: Anxiety

Explain the purpose of all treatments to the patient. Before performing any procedure on the patient, explain the steps of the procedure and the reason for it. Allow the patient time to ask questions and relay concerns. Reinforce information from the physician to the patient. Give support without offering unrealistic reassurances.

Check vital signs and watch for changes indicating increased anxiety. Teach the patient relaxation methods and strategies to cope with the fears of hospitalization and medical interventions necessary. Also, provide diversional activity for the patient to relieve the boredom and anxiety from bed rest.

NDx: Pain

Give prescribed analgesics, and explain the dosage, frequency, side effects, and expected therapeutic effects of the medications. Caution the patient not to perform tasks that require mental alertness while under the effects of the pain medication. Tell the patient to elevate the part to reduce swelling and thus reduce pain. Caution the patient about weight-bearing, if contraindicated, because that might increase the pain significantly.

NDx: Knowledge deficit: nature of disorder, prognosis and management, and prevention of injury of weakened part

Teach the patient about the tumor, the prognosis, methods of prevention of injury, and appropriate treatment. Explain that increased swelling, discoloration, and decreased sensation in the affected part may be signs of complications or increased tumor growth and that the physician should be notified.

Reinforce the physician's instruction about weight-bearing because the bone structure may be weakened or necrosis may have developed. Weight-bearing on the weak structure may cause increased pain or fracture. Demonstrate prescribed exercises to the patient, and encourage participation in the exercise regimen to prevent loss of strength and joint motion.

Evaluation

Evaluate the effectiveness of nursing care for a patient with a benign bone tumor by comparing the patient's status with the expected patient outcomes. Examples of specific outcomes for patients with a benign bone tumor have been provided in the Planning section.

Malignant Bone Tumors

Etiology and Pathophysiology. Malignant bone tumors grow rapidly, metastasize to other parts of the body by the blood or lymphatic system, and destroy surrounding tissue. Malignant tumors are further described as primary tumors, which arise directly from musculoskeletal tissue, or secondary metastatic tumors, which spread to the bone from a malignancy in some other part of the body. Primary bone tumors include osteosarcomas, Ewing's sarcomas, chondrosarcomas, fibrosarcomas, and malignant fibrous histiocytomas.

Malignant primary bone tumors account for less than 1% of all malignancies. They affect predominantly the young, aged 10 to 30 years old. The prognosis and treatment is dependent on the type and size of the tumor and a staging system based on site and metastatic activity of the tumor.

Clinical Manifestations. Clinical manifestations of malignant tumors include deformity, pathologic fractures, swelling, pain, malaise, fever, and unexplained weight loss. Pain is persistent and usually increases with activity of weight-bearing. Numbness or paresthesias may be present in the distal portion of an involved extremity if the tumor presses on nerves or blood vessels. A palpable soft tissue mass may be present.

Medical Diagnosis. X-ray films, CT scans, or magnetic resonance imaging (MRI) are used to find bone lesions. The bone may have a "moth-eaten" appearance, with many areas of destruction. In multiple myeloma, the formation of an abnormal globulin, called a Bence Jones protein, occurs in the urine.

Medical Management. Once the prognosis for patients with bone malignancies was only 10% to 20% survival even with radical surgery. Technologic advances in nuclear detecting methods, chemotherapy, radiation, and newer surgical procedures such as limb salvage account for improved statistics.

Patients with malignant bone tumors may experience changes in blood coagulation as a result of interference with cell production in the marrow. Thus, they are at high risk for hematologic complications with surgery. Treatment at a comprehensive cancer center with coordination of pathology, radiology, and medical and surgical oncology services is generally considered to be the ideal situation for the treatment of malignant bone tumors.

OSTEOSARCOMA

Etiology and Pathophysiology. Osteosarcoma, or osteogenic sarcoma, is the most common of the malignant bone tumors. It is characterized by rapid growth and metastases. The highest incidence is in adolescent males, but osteosarcoma can also occur in older persons with Paget's disease or individuals who have had bone irradiation. The epiphyseal plate and metaphysis of the long bones are the common sites of osteosarcoma. Today the survival rate for osteogenic sarcoma is 80% to 85% after 5 years after diagnosis. Early metastasis to the lung is common and increases the risk for a poor prognosis.

Clinical Manifestations. The main symptom of osteosarcoma is debilitating pain that is unrelieved by analgesics. This frequently is so severe that it

Nursing Care Guide 36–2.

PATIENTS UNDERGOING SURGERY FOR OSTEOSARCOMA

Preoperative Care

Assessment Findings: Patient appears nervous, withdraws from conversation, clenches hands; blood pressure, pulse, and respirations are slightly elevated for the patient; patient makes statements indicating concern about the procedure and results of the surgical intervention, and potential problems with mobility and discomfort following the surgery and the loss of the limb.

Nursing Diagnosis: Anxiety related to uncertainty about surgery, potential risk factors, discomfort, and fear of loss of mobility

Patient Outcomes	Nursing Interventions	Rationale
Patient reports feeling less nervous, feeling relaxed, and resting well.	Teach the patient relaxation techniques. Provide a quiet, calm environment with periods of rest during the delivery of nursing care. Ask for assistance from clergy or the patient's significant others.	Having an understanding of the procedure lessens fears and reduces anxiety. Telling the patient what to expect prior to initiating procedures for preoperative preparation reduces fear of the unknown.
Patient's vital signs are within normal ranges for the patient.	Check vital signs after the patient is rested and more relaxed, and note any changes.	Changes in vital signs may indicate changes in level of anxiety.
Patient states methods to relax and reduce tension.	Teach deep breathing techniques and other relaxation strategies. Allow the patient to voice concerns about the loss of the extremity.	Relaxation exercises may decrease anxiety and promote rest.

Evaluation: Compare the patient's status with the expected patient outcomes. If the outcomes are achieved, evaluate nursing care as successful. If not, reassess the patient, formulate new nursing diagnoses, and revise expected patient outcomes and nursing interventions as appropriate.

(continued)

causes the patient to awaken at night. Because of the rapid growth of the tumor, the involved area is noticeably larger than normal. Joint motion may also be restricted. The patient has a history of fatigue, lethargy, and weight loss.

Medical Diagnosis. Diagnosis requires radiologic and pathologic examination. X-ray films show the tumor as destructive lesions that extend through the medullary cortex. Soft tissue involvement creates a "sunburst" appearance around the lesions. For suspected lesions, a biopsy is performed in such a way as to allow for complete removal of the biopsy scar and its track if surgery is indicated. Once a diagnosis is confirmed, full lung tomograms, to detect early metastasis to the lung, and bone scans are performed to stage the disease and plan treatment. Blood studies will show an increase in serum alkaline phosphatase level.

Medical Management. Surgical intervention (amputation) in conjunction with radiation and chemotherapy is the treatment of choice. Surgery usually includes wide resection from 7 to 10 cm beyond any involved tissue. Postoperative care depends on the extent of surgery and the need for additional chemotherapy or radiation. Chemotherapy may be administered preoperatively to reduce the size of the tumor and postoperatively to prevent micrometastases.

Because of the risk of tumor recurrence, long-term medical follow-up with repeated x-ray examinations, bone scans, and physical assessment is necessary (Nursing Care Guide 36–2).

Nursing Care Guide 36–2. *(continued)*

PATIENTS UNDERGOING SURGERY FOR OSTEOSARCOMA

Assessment Findings: Patient and family seem very concerned about the procedure; they ask several questions about the surgery, the preparation prior to surgery, the expectations of the intervention, and possible complications.

Nursing Diagnosis: Knowledge deficit: nature of amputation surgery, preoperative preparations, expected outcome, and possible complications

Patient Outcomes	Nursing Interventions	Rationale
Patient accurately describes the purpose of the surgery and the necessity for the amputation and relates information about the procedure, complications, and expected results as presented to the patient by the physician.	Explain the procedure to the patient, the usual preoperative preparation, and the expected outcomes. Have the patient relate what the physician has explained, and clear up any misunderstandings.	Explanations of all the appropriate information about the surgery to the patient and family and reinforcement of the information the physician has provided decrease the knowledge deficit and better prepare the patient for the postoperative period.
Patient reports an understanding of the preoperative preparation necessary.	Allow time for questions from the patient or the family. Give the patient literature explaining the procedure and showing which prosthesis may be used to provide mobility.	Having the patient repeat the information gives opportunity to correct any misinformation.

Evaluation: Compare the patient's status with the expected patient outcomes. If the outcomes are achieved, evaluate nursing care as successful. If not, reassess the patient, formulate new nursing diagnoses, and revise expected patient outcomes and nursing interventions as appropriate.

Postoperative Care

Assessment Findings: Patient has incision site with dressings, an intravenous line, and is on bed rest.

Nursing Diagnosis: High risk for infection related to wound site, intravenous line, and bed rest

Patient Outcomes	Nursing Interventions	Rationale
Patient's wound site remains free from symptoms of infection, such as redness, purulent drainage, or excessive swelling.	Check the wound site and suture line for evidence of healing. Watch for signs of infection. Use aseptic technique during dressing changes.	Early diagnosis of complications increases potential for successful treatment. Aseptic technique decreases risk of infection.

(continued)

Nursing Care Guide 36–2. *(continued)*

PATIENTS UNDERGOING SURGERY FOR OSTEOSARCOMA

Patient Outcomes	Nursing Interventions	Rationale
Patient's vital signs are within normal limits for the patient, and the patient denies cough or respiratory distress.	Assess vital signs frequently. Have the patient cough and deep breathe at regular intervals.	Vital sign changes may indicate infection, such as in the respiratory system if patient begins to present an increased respiratory rate and pulse rate and some respiratory distress.
Patient's intravenous site remains free from infection.	Check the intravenous site at least each shift, looking for infiltration, redness, or swelling.	Checking the intravenous site frequently may prevent complications or allow for early intervention if a problem is evident.

Evaluation: Compare the patient's status with the expected patient outcomes. If the outcomes are achieved, evaluate nursing care as successful. If not, reassess the patient, formulate new nursing diagnoses, and revise expected patient outcomes and nursing interventions as appropriate.

Assessment Findings: Patient grimaces, moans, and complains of discomfort at surgical site and in the absent extremity (phantom pain); patient's blood pressure, pulse, and respiratory rate are elevated.

Nursing Diagnosis: Pain related to invasive surgical procedure with manipulation, muscle spasms, and/or contractures

Patient Outcomes	Nursing Interventions	Rationale
Patient reports relief of pain and reports feeling relaxed and comfortable.	Give prescribed analgesics for control of postoperative pain. Make patient comfortable, and provide a quiet atmosphere for rest after surgery.	Relief of postoperative pain allows patient to rest as needed and assists in keeping vital signs within normal limits.
	Check insertion site for signs of infection, which may increase pain at site.	Infection with inflammation increases pain at the site.
	Explain to the patient about the phenomenon of phantom pain.	
Patient's vital signs are within normal ranges.	Monitor vital signs and document the results. Tell the patient to practice relaxation techniques taught prior to surgery.	Changes in vital signs may be caused by increased pain.

Evaluation: Compare the patient's status with the expected patient outcomes. If the outcomes are achieved, evaluate nursing care as successful. If not, reassess the patient, formulate new nursing diagnoses, and revise expected patient outcomes and nursing interventions as appropriate.

(continued)

Nursing Care Guide 36–2. *(continued)*

PATIENTS UNDERGOING SURGERY FOR OSTEOSARCOMA

Assessment Findings: Patient cries frequently and withdraws from conversations; patient states fear of returning to social life; patient is concerned about the future without the limb and potential mobility problems; patient seems very depressed and refuses to participate in care.

Nursing Diagnosis: Dysfunctional grieving related to loss of lower extremity

Patient Outcomes	Nursing Interventions	Rationale
Patient voices concerns about loss of limb, looks at surgical area, and states feelings about the care necessary.	Allow patient to voice concerns. Be supportive without making false reassurances about the prognosis.	Free expression of grief is therapeutic. Having the patient look at self is important so that the patient will be able to perform self-care and to help the patient get over problems with body image.
Patient returns to social activities and participates in self-care.	Encourage participation in activities with others. Teach the patient to care for the residual limb.	Getting involved in social activities assists the patient in returning to a healthy lifestyle.
Patient talks freely to others about the diagnosis and surgical intervention.	Have the patient visit with other amputees for support.	Talking with other amputees gives the patient strategies to cope with the loss.

Evaluation: Compare the patient's status with the expected patient outcomes. If the outcomes are achieved, evaluate nursing care as successful. If not, reassess the patient, formulate new nursing diagnoses, and revise expected patient outcomes and nursing interventions as appropriate.

(continued)

EWING'S SARCOMA

Etiology and Pathophysiology. A rare but highly malignant bone tumor, Ewing's sarcoma originates in the marrow and metastasizes early. It can occur in major long bones or the flat bones of the pelvis and ribs. Pulmonary involvement is common. Ewing's sarcoma is more prevalent in young males in their early teens to early twenties.

Clinical Manifestations. The clinical manifestations of Ewing's sarcoma are similar to those of osteosarcoma, with the pain more incapacitating, and the malaise, lethargy, and weight loss more pronounced. Pathologic fracture through the lesion is common.

Medical Diagnosis. The diagnosis is made on the basis of history, physical examination, and radiographic studies.

Medical Management. Treatment of Ewing's sarcoma has been most successful with systemic chemotherapy, which includes combinations of two or more drugs, followed by radiation or surgery. The most effective neoplastic agents and the duration of therapy vary among patients. Surgery usually follows chemotherapy or radiation, or both. Because Ewing's sarcoma has a high incidence of recurrence, surgery alone is of little value. Some pelvic masses, inaccessible to radiation and surgery, are treated by chemotherapy alone.

Application of the Nursing Process to the Care of the Patient with a Malignant Bone Tumor

Assessment

Review the patient's history, diagnostic studies, and presenting problems. Assess the affected area, not-

Nursing Care Guide 36–2. *(continued)*

PATIENTS UNDERGOING SURGERY FOR OSTEOSARCOMA

Assessment Findings: Patient seems overly anxious and reluctant to listen to home care instructions; patient is reluctant to work with ambulatory aid and to practice physical therapy; patient states concerns about providing self-care, hygiene, grooming, and activities of daily living when home.

Nursing Diagnosis: Impaired home maintenance management related to inability to manage mobility problems, use of ambulatory aid, fear for safety, and suture line care (if needed)

Patient Outcomes	Nursing Interventions	Rationale
Patient relates accurate information about the home care required and signs of potential problems. Patient states plans for follow-up care with the attending physician.	Describe the signs requiring immediate medical intervention, such as pain or discomfort at surgical site, fever, chills, dizziness, fainting, excessive fatigue, or shortness of breath.	Early diagnosis of potential problems by the patient at home and early medical intervention increase the chance for successful treatment. Having the patient relate information presented reinforces the information and allows for correction of misconceptions.
Patient demonstrates appropriate use of ambulatory aid and states safety measures for the home environment to prevent falls or other injuries.	Assist the patient in practicing using the ambulatory aid. Help the patient find ways to increase safety measures in the home environment.	Having the patient practice under supervision allows for evaluation of patient's ability to practice safe use of ambulatory aids.

Evaluation: Compare the patient's status with the expected patient outcomes. If the outcomes are achieved, evaluate nursing care as successful. If not, reassess the patient, formulate new nursing diagnoses, and revise expected patient outcomes and nursing interventions as appropriate.

ing any swelling, deformity, or pain. Ask the patient about range of motion and mobility problems. Determine whether there is pain and when it is most significant. Note problems with weight-bearing.

Determine the patient's and family's understanding about the diagnosis and possible treatment alternatives. The patient's reaction to the diagnosis of malignancy is important to the care planning. Assess the patient's coping strategies and their effectiveness. Ask about support systems that are available to the patient, such as relatives and friends.

Nursing Diagnoses and Planning

Nursing diagnoses and related expected patient outcomes most commonly applicable to patients with a malignant bone tumor include those discussed previously for patients with a benign bone tumor and the following (also see Chapter 11 for care of the patient with cancer):

NDx: Self-esteem disturbance related to deformity, effects of chemotherapy, or amputation

Planning: Patient outcomes
1. Patient relates feelings of self-worth.
2. Patient maintains social activity.
3. Patient is able to look at self with understanding and acceptance.

NDx: Fear related to forthcoming treatments, prognosis, and uncertain future

Planning: Patient outcomes
1. Patient appears relaxed and is able to rest and sleep at intervals.
2. Patient denies extreme fear about the diagnosis or prognosis and the future.
3. Patient freely expresses concerns about the diagnosis and prognosis.
4. Patient states acceptable coping mechanisms to deal with the fear.

Nursing Interventions

NDx: Self-esteem disturbance

Allow the patient to vent feelings about the diagnosis. Provide information about cancer support groups. Seek assistance from clergy or professional counseling. Provide diversional activities for the patient when bedfast as a result of exacerbations from the disease or the treatment regimen. Involve support from the family and other friends. Seek effective coping strategies for the patient. Assist the patient in finding the positive aspects of life to focus on during periods of depression. Help the patient deal with the altered appearance by suggesting methods of concealment such as the use of appropriate clothing, makeup, or natural looking prosthetic devices.

NDx: Fear

Help the patient cope with the diagnosis and uncertain future. Provide referral to professional counseling services. Assist the patient in the identification of support systems. Talk with clergy and significant others about support for the patient. Explain and reinforce all information provided by the physician regarding the diagnosis and treatment modalities. Allow time for questions and concerns from the patient and family. If appropriate, provide opportunity for the patient and family to talk with others who have successfully faced similar circumstances. Inform the patient about organizations such as the American Cancer Society that provide psychological support, educational services, and other assistance for patients and families.

Evaluation

Evaluate the effectiveness of nursing care for a patient with a malignant bone tumor by comparing the patient's status with the expected patient outcomes. Examples of specific outcomes for patients with a malignant bone tumor have been provided in the Planning section.

Metastatic Bone Tumors

A metastatic bone tumor is cancer of the bone that arises from a primary tumor in another part of the body and metastasizes to bone. The tumor cells metastasize through the circulatory system or lymphatic system. Metastatic bone tumors commonly originate from primary lesions of the breast, kidney, lung, prostate, and thyroid. These tumors can be osteolytic or osteoblastic.

Diagnosis of a metastatic bone tumor is made on the basis of x-ray examination, bone scan, CT, biopsy, and elevated blood levels of alkaline phosphatase and serum calcium. The most common clinical manifestations are pain in the involved bone and pathologic fracture.

Treatment is palliative rather than curative. The goals of medical management and nursing care are pain relief and prevention of complications such as pathologic fractures. The secondary bone tumor may be treated in conjunction with the primary lesion using chemotherapy or radiation, or both. Treatment of pathologic fractures with braces, splints, or internal fixation is often necessary.

The Elderly: Special Considerations

During the aging process, alterations in stature and posture occur, especially among women. This is caused by compression of the spinal column. The older adult also faces many other changes in bone mass, metabolism, and musculature. Loss of agility, flexibility, and mobility are common changes. These alterations may affect the intensity and duration of many musculoskeletal disorders. The changes also put the elderly at high risk for some musculoskeletal problems such as hip fractures, osteoporosis, and arthritis. These conditions have been discussed earlier in the chapter.

Degenerative joint diseases are particularly debilitating for the older adult. Painful or immobile joints may interfere with self-care activities and the ability to maintain locomotion and thus cause the older adult to lose an independent living style.

Pain management with many of the musculoskeletal disorders is a primary problem in the elderly. Appropriate use of medications is imperative to prevent side effects while maintaining adequate control of the pain.

Nursing interventions for the older adult with musculoskeletal disorders are focused on maintenance of mobility, safety, and independence. Continuous activity promotes greater functioning in the geriatric patient. Exercise programs are beneficial to maintain or increase flexibility and strength. Swimming, walking, stretching, and moderate weight-lifting regimens are the most helpful exercise programs and the most attractive to the older adults.

Safety becomes a major problem for the elderly with musculoskeletal disorders because of the loss of mobility, the general physical changes aggravated by the disorder, and the use of ambulatory aids. Patients are taught safe manipulation of the assistive devices, and this is continually reinforced as the older adult patient readies for discharge. Many elderly hospitalized patients are being treated for injuries caused by inability to maneuver an ambulatory aid properly, resulting in a fall and further injuries. The older adult also needs information on making the home environment safe, especially when using an ambulatory aid. Most homes are not designed to allow free movement while using a walker or crutches. The patient may need in-home assistance to modify the environment appropriately.

Dietary evaluation and education may be needed to provide an appropriate meal plan, as prescribed, for healing and health maintenance or to prevent other musculoskeletal disorders. The need for increased vitamins, calcium, and other minerals is stressed.

Medication administration education is also necessary. The geriatric patient reacts to drug therapy differently than the middle aged or young adult. Teach the patient the dosage, frequency, therapeutic effects, and side effects of all prescribed medications and when to notify the physician if problems are apparent. Because gastrointestinal irritation is common, tell the patient to take the medications with milk or meals unless otherwise advised.

The care of the older adult with musculoskeletal disorders is a challenge to nursing staff because these disorders aggravate the changes from the aging process already occurring. The goal is to keep the individual free from injury and as mobile and independent as possible.

Bibliography

Backman C, Mackie H, Harris J. Arthritis hand function test development of a standardized assessment tool. Occup Ther J Res 1991; 11(4):245.

Bullock BL, Rosenthal PP. Pathophysiology adaption and alterations in function. Philadelphia: JB Lippincott, 1992.

Burggraf V, Donlon B. Assessing the elderly: Part one: System by system. Am J Nurs 1985; 85(9):974.

Callahan J. Compartment syndrome. Orthop Nurs 1985; 4(4):11.

Carpenito LJ. Nursing diagnosis: Application to clinical practice. 3rd ed. Philadelphia: JB Lippincott, 1989–1990.

Cassady L, Scaduto J. Thumb reimplantation: A case study. Orthop Nurs 1991; 10(3):24.

Ceccio C, Horoz J. Teaching the elderly amputee to meet the world. RN 1988; 51(9):70.

Ceccio CM. Understanding therapeutic beds. Orthop Nurs 1990; 9(3):57.

Chase JA. Spinal stenosis: When arthritis is more than arthritis. Nurs Clin North Am 1991; 26(1):53.

Corwin D, Miller C. Get your patient off on the right foot. RN 1990; 53(11):44.

D'Angio G, Evans A. Bone tumors and tissue sarcomas. Baltimore: Edward Arnold, 1985.

Dorr LD. Arthritis and athletics. Clin Sports Med 1991; (10(2):343.

Dudek SG. Nutrition for nursing practice. Philadelphia: JB Lippincott, 1987.

Duffy J, Schoen RT, Sigal LH. 1991 update on lyme disease. Patient Care 1991; 25(11):24.

Edelstein JE. Preprosthetic management of patients with lower or upper limb amputation. Phys Med Rehabil Clin North Am 1991; 2(2):285.

Edwards NL. Drugs to lower uric acid levels: How to avoid misuse in gouty arthritis. Postgrad Med 1991; 89(2):111.

Eliopoulos C. Gerontological nursing. 2nd ed. Philadelphia: JB Lippincott, 1987.

Esquenazi A, Torres MM. Prosthetic feet and ankle mechanisms. Phys Med Rehabil Clin North Am 1991; 2(2):299.

Farrara T. Triage decisions. J Emerg Nurs 1991; 17(3):180.

Geier K, Hesser K. Electrical bone stimulation for treatment of nonunion. Orthop Nurs 1985; 4(2):41.

Higgins RM. Reimplantation of digits. Orthop Nurs 1991; 10(3):11.

Holloway NM. Medical-surgical care plans. Springhouse, PA: Springhouse, 1988.

Ignatavicius D, Bayne M. Medical-surgical nursing: A nursing process approach. Philadelphia: WB Saunders, 1991.

Illustrated manual of nursing practice. Springhouse, PA: Springhouse, 1991.

Iyer P, Taptich B, Bernocchi-Losey D. Nursing process and nursing diagnosis. Philadelphia: WB Saunders, 1988.

Jackson J, Neighbors M. Home care client assessment handbook. Rockville, MD: Aspen Publishers, 1990.

Kamper C. Treatment of Lyme disease. J Ped Health Care 1991; 5(2):99.

Kee JL. Laboratory and diagnostic tests with nursing implications. 2nd ed. Norwalk, CT: Appleton & Lange, 1987.

Kleinert HE, Kleinert JM, McCabe SJ, Berger AC. Reimplantation. Clin Symp 1991; 43(2):2.

Krupp MA, Schroeder S, Tierney L. Current medical diagnoses and treatment 1987. Los Angeles: Appleton & Lange, 1987.

Lankford TR, Steward PMK. Foundations of normal and therapeutic nutrition. New York: John Wiley & Sons, 1986.

Lumpkin TH. A great imitator: Lyme disease. J Am Acad Physician Assist 1991; 4(4):284.

Malkiewicz J. A pragmatic approach to musculoskeletal assessment. RN 1982; 45(11):57.

Morris L, Kraft S, Tessem S, Reinisch S. Nursing the patient in traction. RN 1988; 51(1):26.

Morris L, Kraft S, Tessem S, Reinisch S. Special care for skeletal traction. RN 1988; 51(2):24.

Mosher CM. The Papineau bone graft: A limb salvage technique. Orthop Nurs 1991; 10(3):27.

Olson B, Ustanko L, Warner S. The patient in a halo brace: Striving for normalcy in body image and self-concept. Orthop Nurs 1991; 10(1):44.

Piasecki PA. The nursing role in limb salvage surgery. Nurs Clin North Am 1991; 26(1):33.

Reiss BS, Melick ME. Pharmacological aspects of nursing care. 2nd ed. Albany, NY: Delmar Publishers, 1987.

Resnick D, Niwayama G (eds). Diagnosis of bone and joint disorders. Vol I, II, and III. Philadelphia: WB Saunders, 1981.

Reyburn TV. The "Z" strap: Harnessing modification for patients with upper extremity amputations. Arch Phys Med Rehabil 1991; 72(3):250.

Sabolich J. Prosthetic advances in lower extremity amputation. Phys Med Rehabil Clin North Am 1991; 2(2):415.

Schoen D. The nursing process in orthopaedics. New York: Appleton-Century-Crofts, 1986.

Sculco T. Orthopaedic care of the geriatric patient. St. Louis: CV Mosby, 1986.

Sears HH. Approaches to prescription of body-powered and myoelectric prostheses. Phys Med Rehabil Clin North Am 1991; 2(2):361.

Sidor ML, Zuckerman JD. Painful hip: Differential diagnosis. Hosp Med 1991; 27(4):109.

Smarcina CM. Stress fractures in athletes. Nurs Clin North Am 1991; 26(1):159.

Thomas CL (ed). Taber's cyclopedic medical dictionary. 16th ed. Philadelphia: FA Davis, 1989.

Thomas P. Lyme disease tick terror. Harvard Health Letter 1991; 16(9):1.

Ulrich SP, Canale SW, Wendell SA. Nursing care planning guides: A nursing diagnosis approach. Philadelphia: WB Saunders, 1986.

Webb J. Notes on orthopaedic nursing. 2nd ed. New York: Churchill Livingstone, 1985.

Wertz EM. Immobilized. Emergency 1991; 23(8):32.

Willey T. High-tech beds and mattress overlays: A decision guide. Am J Nurs 1989; 89(9):1142.

Willis D. Lyme disease. J Neurosci Nurs 1991; 23(4):211.

Wyngaarden JB, Smith LH. Cecil textbook of medicine. 17th ed. Philadelphia: WB Saunders, 1987.

Unit Twelve

ADULTS WITH NEUROLOGIC DYSFUNCTION

Learning Objectives

AFTER COMPLETING THIS UNIT, THE LEARNER WILL BE ABLE TO:

Chapter Thirty-seven

1. Explain the normal anatomy and physiology of the nervous system.
2. Describe common clinical manifestations of neurologic dysfunction.
3. Identify information and physical examination data essential to the assessment of the nervous system.
4. Describe basic diagnostic tests and modalities of medical management used in the treatment of patients with neurologic disorders.
5. Describe basic intracranial and spinal surgery as used in the treatment of patients with neurologic disorders.
6. Identify data essential to the assessment of patients undergoing treatment of neurologic disorders.
7. State nursing diagnoses and related expected patient outcomes commonly applicable to patients undergoing treatment of neurologic disorders.
8. Describe nursing interventions, with their rationales, commonly applicable to patients undergoing treatment of neurologic disorders.
9. Explain the basis for evaluation of nursing care provided to patients undergoing treatment of neurologic disorders.
10. Identify special considerations for the elderly patient with altered neurologic function.

Chapter Thirty-eight

1. Describe common nervous system disorders in terms of etiology, pathophysiology, clinical manifestations, diagnostic procedures, and medical management.
2. Identify information and physical examination data essential to the assessment of patients with common nervous system disorders.
3. State nursing diagnoses and related expected patient outcomes commonly applicable to patients with nervous system disorders.
4. Describe nursing interventions, with their rationales, commonly applicable to patients with nervous system disorders.
5. Explain the basis for evaluation of nursing care provided to patients with common nervous system disorders.
6. Identify special considerations for the elderly patient with a nervous system disorder.

Chapter Thirty-seven

KNOWLEDGE BASIC TO THE NURSING CARE *of Adults with* Neurologic Dysfunction

The nervous system is a communication network that provides for a constant relay of information to and from the environment. The ability of the central nervous system (CNS) to interpret incoming messages from the environment and then formulate and transmit a response via the peripheral nervous system enables ongoing and evolving interaction between individual and environment.

The CNS underlies the ability to reason, to entertain abstract concepts such as past and future, and to experience emotion. In other words, it is the basis of function as a human being.

In preparation for the study of the nursing care of patients with disorders of this complex system, this chapter begins with a review of the anatomy and physiology of the system. Next, clinical manifestations common to many types of nervous system dysfunction, basic assessment of nervous system function, and frequently used diagnostic tests are discussed. The chapter then proceeds to a discussion of the general care required of patients having cranial or spinal surgery and ends with a section on special considerations relative to the care of the elderly.

Anatomy and Physiology

The nervous system is composed of the CNS and the peripheral nervous system (PNS). The CNS includes the brain and spinal cord. The PNS includes the 12 cranial nerves, 31 pairs of spinal nerves, and the autonomic nervous system (ANS). It is the PNS that connects the CNS with organ systems, skin, and muscles.

Cellular Structure

There are two main types of cells found within the nervous system: neurons and neuroglia. Neurons are the basic functioning units, whereas neuroglial cells are viewed as providing assistance and support to the neurons.

NEURONS

The basic function of neurons is to conduct impulses toward (afferent) or away from (efferent) the CNS. The structure of a neuron (Fig. 37–1) consists of a cell body, in which metabolic activities are carried out, dendrites, which conduct impulses to the cell body, and axons, which conduct impulses away from the cell body.

Nerve cell bodies primarily form the gray matter of the CNS. Nerve cell bodies grouped outside the CNS are known as ganglia.

The white matter of the CNS is made up of the myelinated axons of the neurons. Myelin is a white substance made up of lipids and proteins that encases many axons. Most long axons are myelinated, whereas shorter axons tend not to be.

In the event of neuron trauma or injury, only peripheral nerves possess the ability to recover. Peripheral nerves regenerate at the rate of 1.5 mm/day. The degree of recovery is based on severity of the injury and proximity to the cell body and distal and proximal ends.

NEUROGLIA

The neuroglial cells provide assistance—support, nutrition, and protection—to neurons in the CNS. There are four types of neuroglial cells: oligodendroglia, which form myelin and surround axons and dendrites; astrocytes, which have a star-shaped appearance and provide nutrition and a protective barrier for neurons; microglia, which are known as phagocytic cells; and ependymal cells, which line the cerebral ventricular system and aid in the production of cerebrospinal fluid (CSF) (Fig. 37–2).

Nerve Impulse Transmission

Neurons transmit impulses through the propagation of action potentials along conductive fibers. Action potentials are rapid changes in the membrane potential and consist of three stages: resting, depolarization, and repolarization.

In the resting stage, the neuron has a negative membrane potential (i.e., inside the nerve fiber is more negative than the potential of the intercellular fluid outside the fiber). Because of this large negative difference, the membrane is said to be polarized. In the depolarization stage, the membrane becomes very permeable to sodium. The resultant flow of sodium across the membrane causes the negative potential to be lost and a positive potential to occur. This is followed almost instantly by the repolarization stage, in which the sodium channels close and the potassium channels open wider, leading to an influx of potassium and restoration of the negative resting potential (Fig. 37–3).

Membrane depolarization, which can be initiated by chemical, mechanical, electrical, or thermal means, extends from one neuron to another, resulting in impulse transmission.

The synapse is where nerve impulses are transmitted from neuron to neuron. Nerve transmission at the synapse involves a chemical process. Each axon contains presynaptic neurotransmitters. As the impulse travels down the axon, away from the cell body, neurotransmitters are released at the terminal end and are taken up by the dendrites of the postsynaptic neuron. Neurotransmitters can be excitatory (i.e., dopamine, serotonin, acetylcholine) or inhibitory (i.e., gamma-aminobutyric acid [GABA]) in nature. Neurotransmitters that are excitatory cause the postsynaptic neuron to depolarize, allowing nerve impulse transmission to occur, whereas neurotransmitters that are inhibitory in nature tend not to

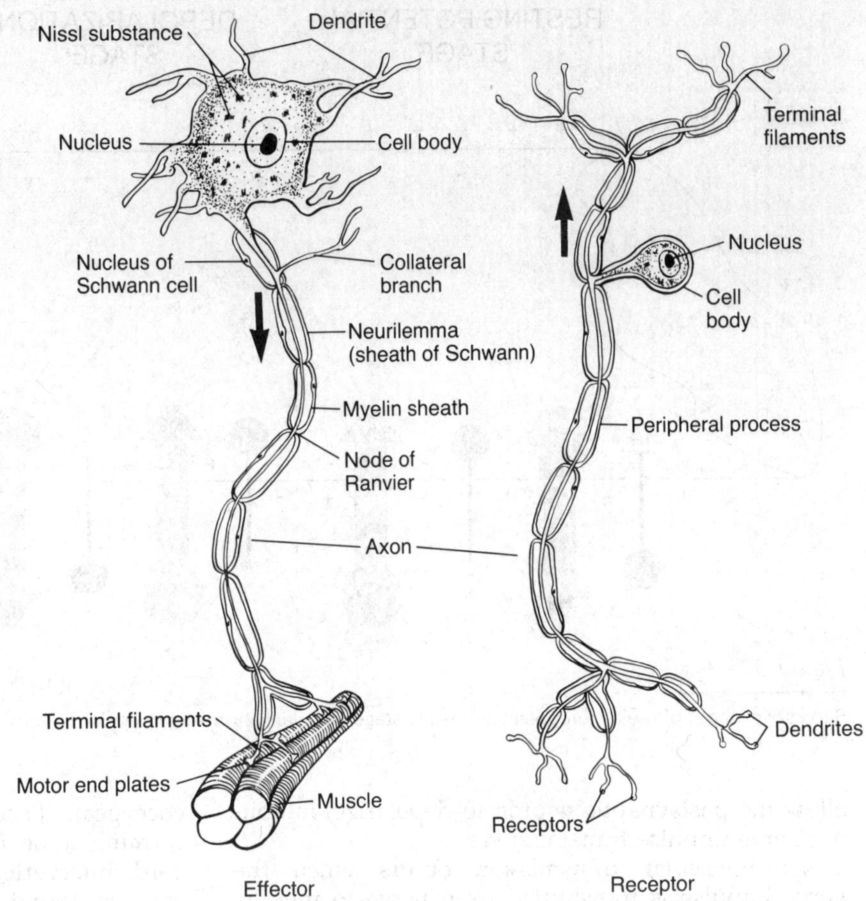

Figure 37–1.

Diagram of a motor (effector) neuron and a sensory (receptor) neuron. Arrows indicate the direction of impulse conduction.

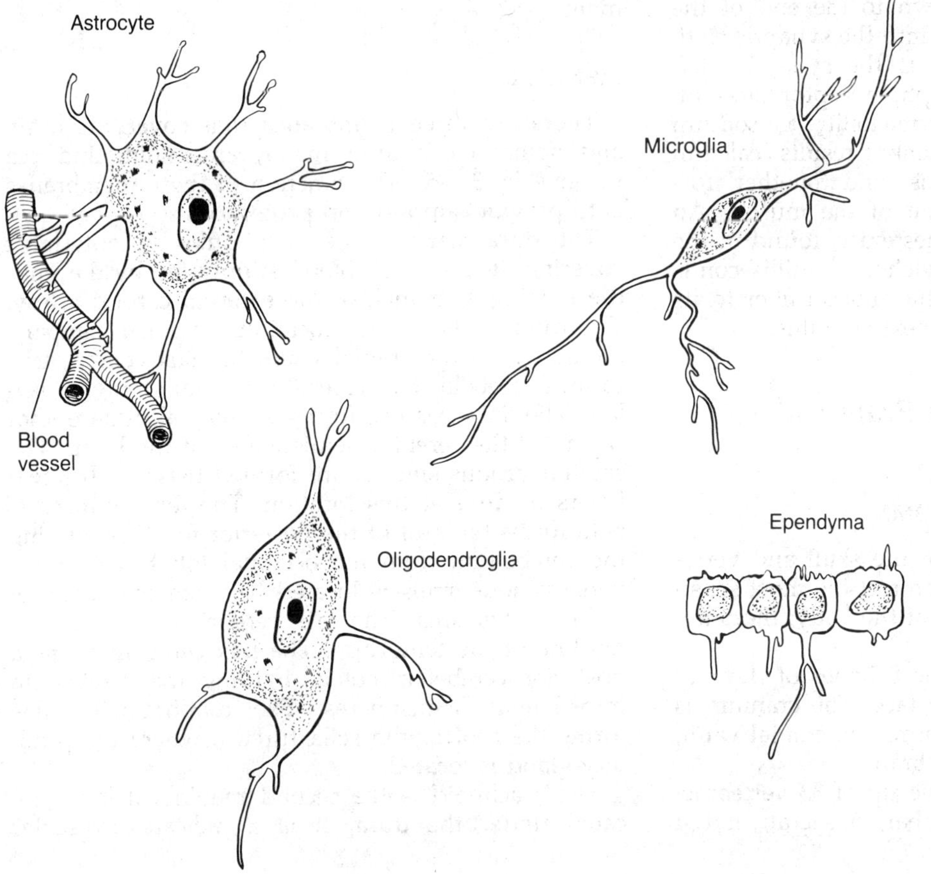

Figure 37–2.

Four types of neuroglial cells, which provide support, nutrition, and protection to neurons in the central nervous system.

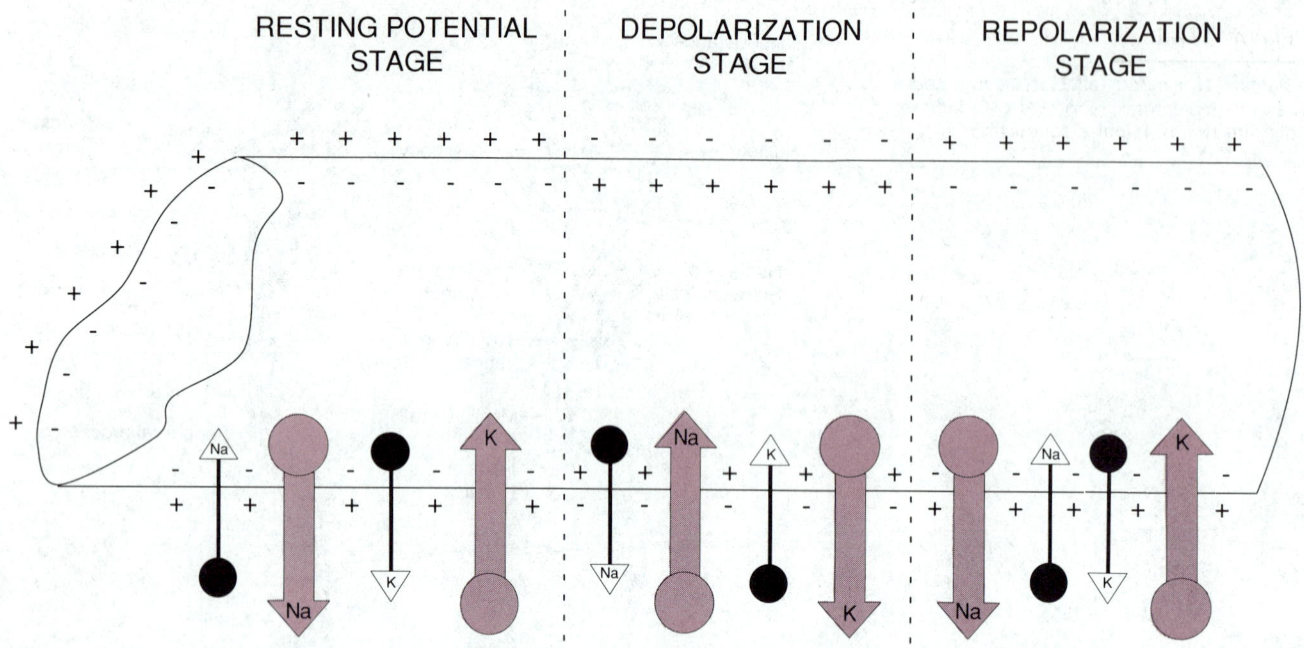

Figure 37–3.

Successive stages of the action potential: resting stage, depolarization stage, repolarization stage.

allow the postsynaptic neuron to depolarize, inhibiting nerve impulse transmission.

Neuromuscular transmission occurs when the nerve impulse is transmitted from nerve to muscle. This takes place at the neuromuscular junction. As the nerve impulse travels down to the end of the axon, acetylcholine is released into the synaptic cleft. The acetylcholine travels across the synaptic cleft and binds with the postsynaptic receptor sites on the muscle, increasing its permeability to sodium and potassium. An action potential results, calcium ions are released, and proteins bind together, formulating the contractile motion of the muscle. An enzyme known as acetylcholinesterase, found in the synapse, inactivates the acetylcholine milliseconds after its release. This returns the muscle fiber to its resting position, ready for the next stimulus.

Protective Coverings of the Brain and Spinal Cord

SKULL AND VERTEBRAL COLUMN

The purpose of the bones of the skull and vertebral column (Fig. 37–4) is to protect the most sensitive and vulnerable structures of the body: the brain and the spinal cord.

The skull is composed of the 8 bones of the cranium and the 14 bones of the face. The cranium is the portion of the skull that forms the cranial vault, the protective covering for the brain.

The vertebral column is made up of 33 vertebrae: 7 cervical, 12 thoracic, 5 lumbar, 5 sacral, and 4 coccygeal. Each vertebra is stacked on another, forming a flexible column that protects the spinal cord. Intervertebral disks of varying shape and size can be found between the individual vertebrae. They act as a cushion for vertebral column movement.

MENINGES

There are three membranes that cover the brain and spinal cord: dura mater, arachnoid, and pia mater (Fig. 37–5). The function of these membranes is to provide support and protection.

The dura mater is the dense, fibrous, outermost covering. It has a rich blood supply fed by the middle meningeal branch of the external carotid artery. The dura folds in four locations to form compartments within the cranial vault: the falx cerebri, tentorium cerebelli, falx cerebelli, and diaphragma sellae. The falx cerebri forms a vertical fissure that separates the cerebral hemispheres of the brain. The sagittal venous sinuses are formed between the two layers of dura at this location. The tentorium cerebelli forms the roof of the posterior fossa, separating the cerebellum from the occipital lobes. The transverse venous sinus is located between the layers of dura in this area. The falx cerebri attaches to the midline of the tentorium. The falx cerebelli forms a posterior cerebellar notch dividing the cerebellum into lateral hemispheres. The diaphragma sellae forms the roof of the sella turcica, where the pituitary gland is located.

The arachnoid is the second meningeal layer, located under the dura. It is a delicate, avascular

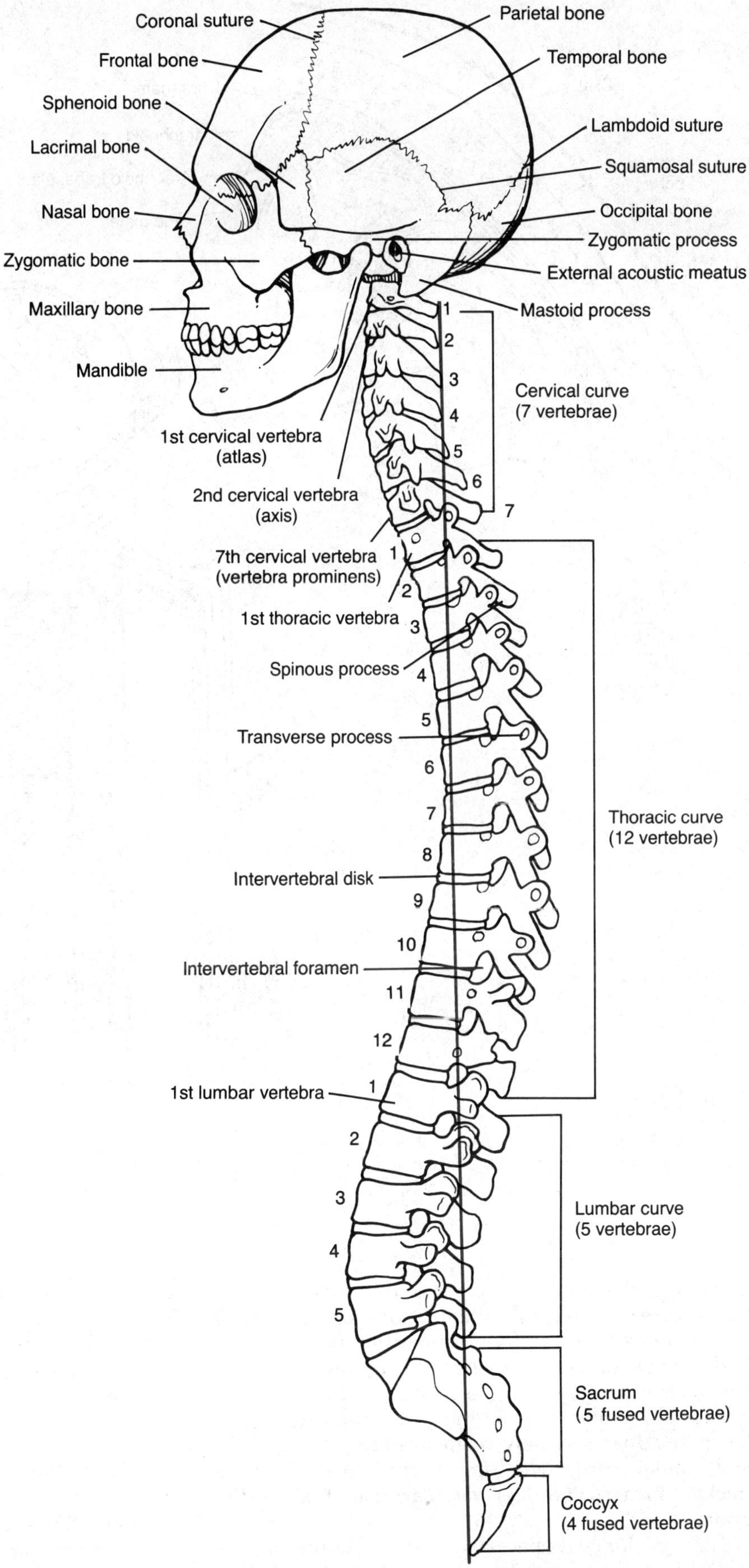

Figure 37–4.

Bony structure of the skull and vertebral column.

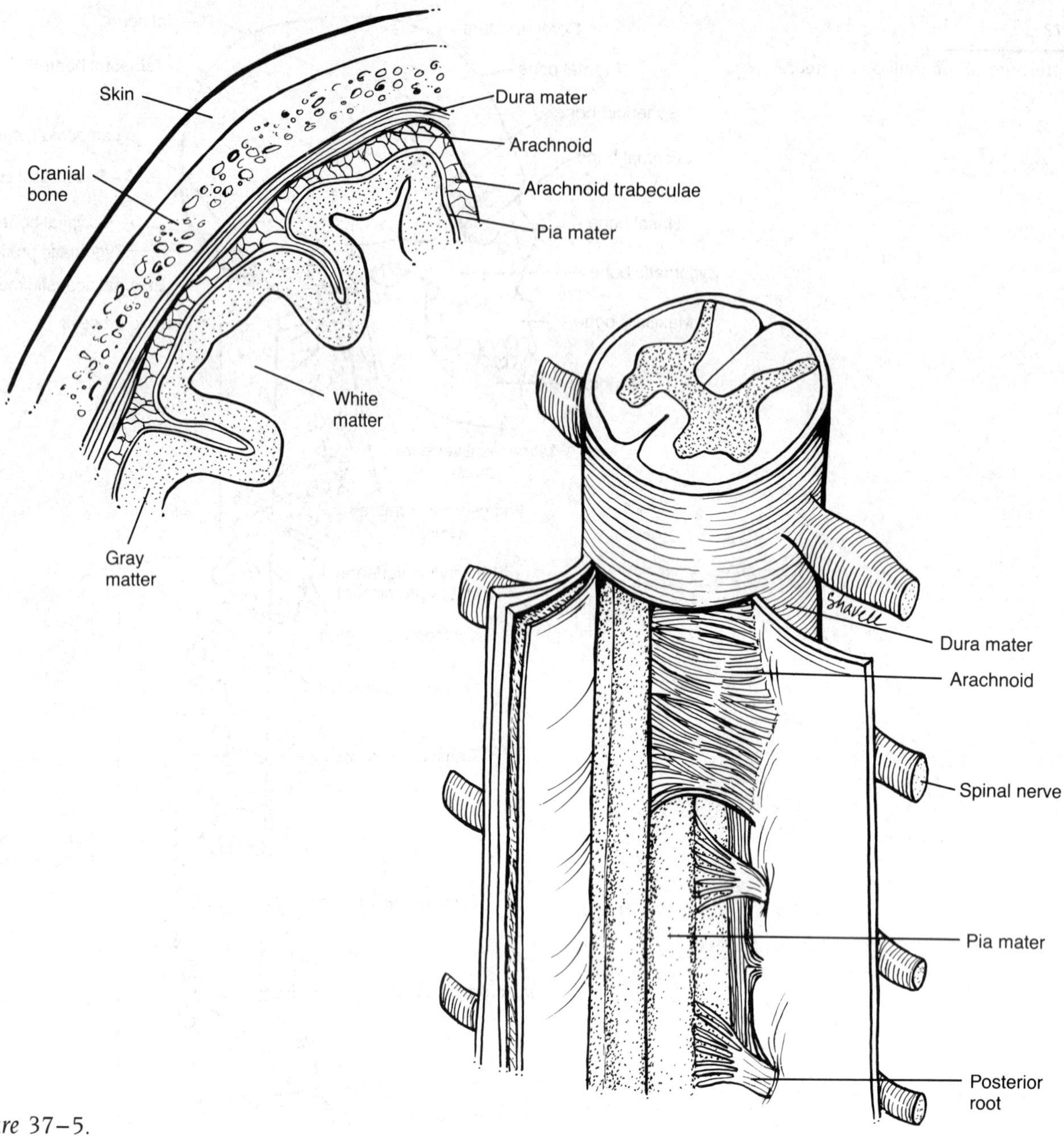

Figure 37–5.

Meninges. The dura mater is of leathery consistency and is the outermost of the three membranes; the arachnoid, which is loose, avascular, and like a spider web, is the middle membrane; and the pia mater is thin, delicate, and closely adherent to the brain and spinal cord.

membrane that loosely surrounds the brain and spinal cord. Arachnoid villi granulations are clusters of arachnoid and can be found projecting into the sagittal venous sinuses, allowing CSF to pass from the subarachnoid space into the venous sinus.

The pia mater is the most delicate meningeal layer. It adheres closely to the surface of the brain and spinal cord. The spinal cord pia mater is thicker, firmer, and less vascular than that of the brain.

Three meningeal spaces are formed by the meninges: the epidural, subdural, and subarachnoid. The epidural space is located between the outer layer of dura and the skull. The subdural space is located below the inner layer of dura and the arachnoid. The subarachnoid space is located between the arachnoid and the pia mater.

Blood Supply and Circulation

Blood flows at a rate of 750 ml/minute in the adult brain, carrying vital supplies of oxygen and glucose. The brain consumes 20% of the body's oxygen supply to oxidize glucose for energy. Without this supply, the brain suffers irreversible damage literally within minutes.

CEREBRAL CIRCULATION

ARTERIAL BLOOD SUPPLY

Arterial blood is supplied to the brain through the internal carotid arteries and the basilar artery. The internal carotid artery originates as the common carotid, which branches from the aorta and subdivides into the internal and external carotid arteries. The basilar artery originates as two vertebral arteries that branch from the subclavian artery and then merge at the level of the pons to form the basilar artery (Fig. 37–6*A*).

The internal carotid arteries and the basilar artery join the circle of Willis, which is located at the base of the skull. There are three major pairs of arterial branches from the circle of Willis that deliver blood to the brain: the anterior, middle, and posterior cerebral arteries (Fig. 37–6*B*).

The anterior cerebral artery (ACA) supplies the medial surface of the frontal and parietal lobes and adjacent cortex. The middle cerebral artery (MCA) supplies the lateral surface of the cerebral hemispheres and comprises 60% of the cerebral circulation. The posterior cerebral artery (PCA) supplies the inferior and medial surface of the temporal and occipital lobes and choroid plexus.

VENOUS DRAINAGE

The cerebral venous drainage is composed of dural venous sinuses. Venous sinuses are located and formed by vascular canals between the two layers of the dura mater. There are no valves, and blood is drained from these sinuses into the internal jugular veins. Three major venous sinuses are the sagittal sinus at the convexity of the brain, the cavernous sinus at the inferior surface, and the transverse sinus at the lateral surface.

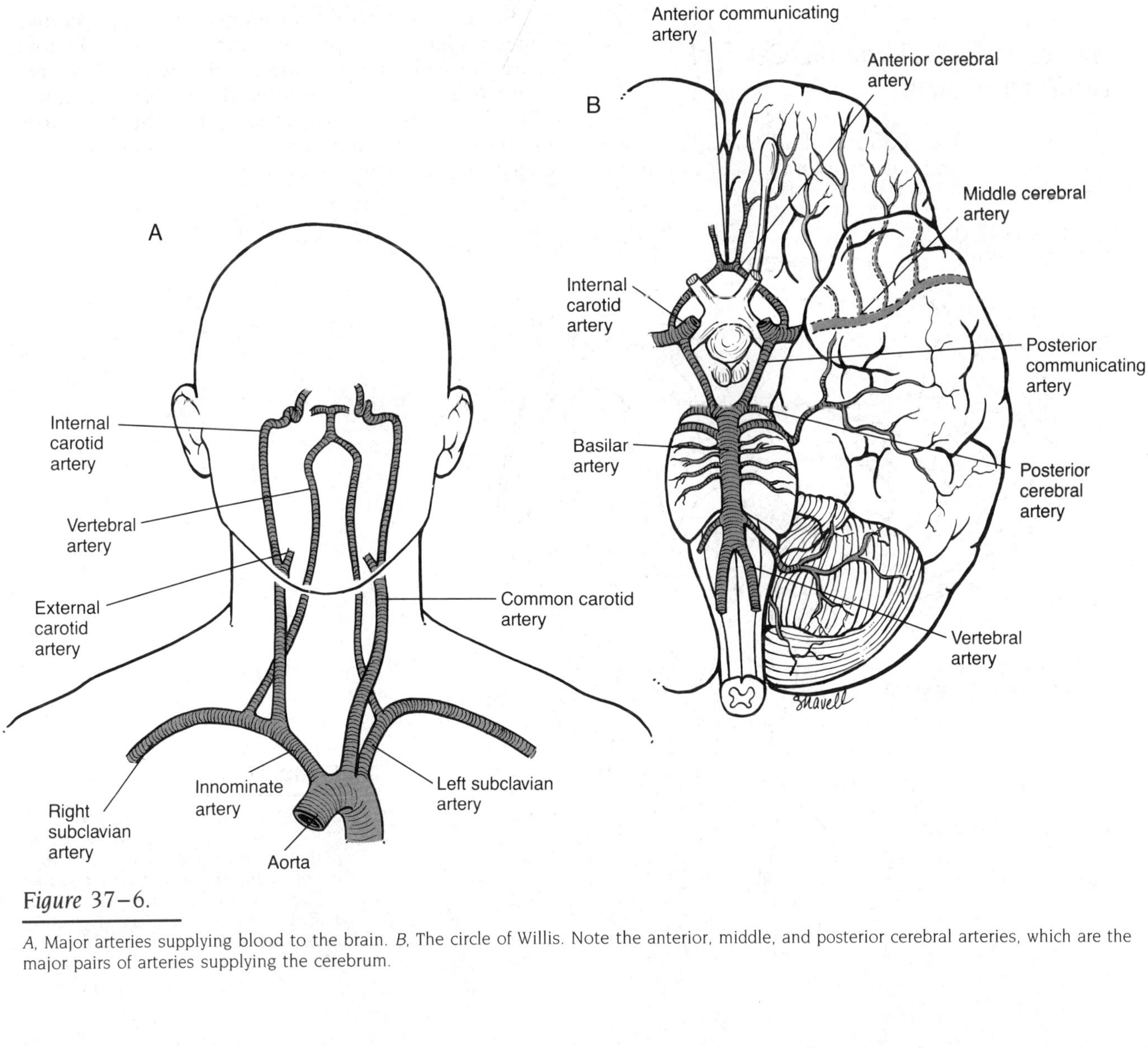

Figure 37–6.

A, Major arteries supplying blood to the brain. *B*, The circle of Willis. Note the anterior, middle, and posterior cerebral arteries, which are the major pairs of arteries supplying the cerebrum.

SPINAL CIRCULATION

The spinal cord primarily receives its arterial blood supply from the spinal arteries, which originate from the vertebral arteries. One anterior spinal artery supplies two thirds of the spinal cord with arterial blood as it runs anteriorly the full length of the cord. Two posterior spinal arteries, each of which runs the full length of the cord, supply the posterior one third of the cord with arterial blood. In addition, there are feeder vessels that support blood supply to the cord.

Blood-Brain Barrier

The blood-brain barrier is composed of capillary epithelium and an astrocyte membrane located in close proximity to the neuron. Because of the tight junction formed at this site, a barrier is formed. This barrier selectively permits substances to pass from the blood into the neuron. Many medications are prohibited from penetrating this barrier, preventing them from affecting the CNS.

Cerebrospinal Fluid and the Cerebral Ventricular System

CSF is a colorless, odorless fluid that fills the cerebral ventricles and subarachnoid spaces to provide a "cushion" for the CNS. This helps to prevent undue injury from sudden or abrupt movements. There is approximately 145 ml of CSF in the adult: 25 ml in the cerebral ventricles, 30 ml in the subarachnoid space, and 90 ml in the lumbar subarachnoid cistern. The CSF pressure, while the individual is in a recumbent position, is normally less than 200 mm water (H_2O) pressure.

CSF is formed primarily in the choroid plexus, a structure found in the lateral ventricles. CSF is excreted constantly at a rate of 25 to 30 ml/hour.

CSF flows in a closed, one-way system (Fig. 37–7). As the CSF is formed in the lateral ventricles, it passes through the foramen of Monro into the third ventricle. It then passes through the aqueduct of Sylvius into the fourth ventricle, exiting through the foramina of Luschka and Magendie into the subarachnoid spaces of the brain and spinal cord.

Enlarged areas of the subarachnoid space that contain a quantity of CSF are known as cisterns. The cisterna magna is located between the medulla and cerebellum, and the lumbar cistern is located at the base of the spinal cord at the L-2 to S-1 vertebral levels.

CSF is reabsorbed constantly into the body's venous system. It passes from the subarachnoid space through the arachnoid villi, which are one-way valve projections into the dural venous sinuses. This allows for a direct pathway for CSF and waste products to enter the venous system and to be excreted by the body.

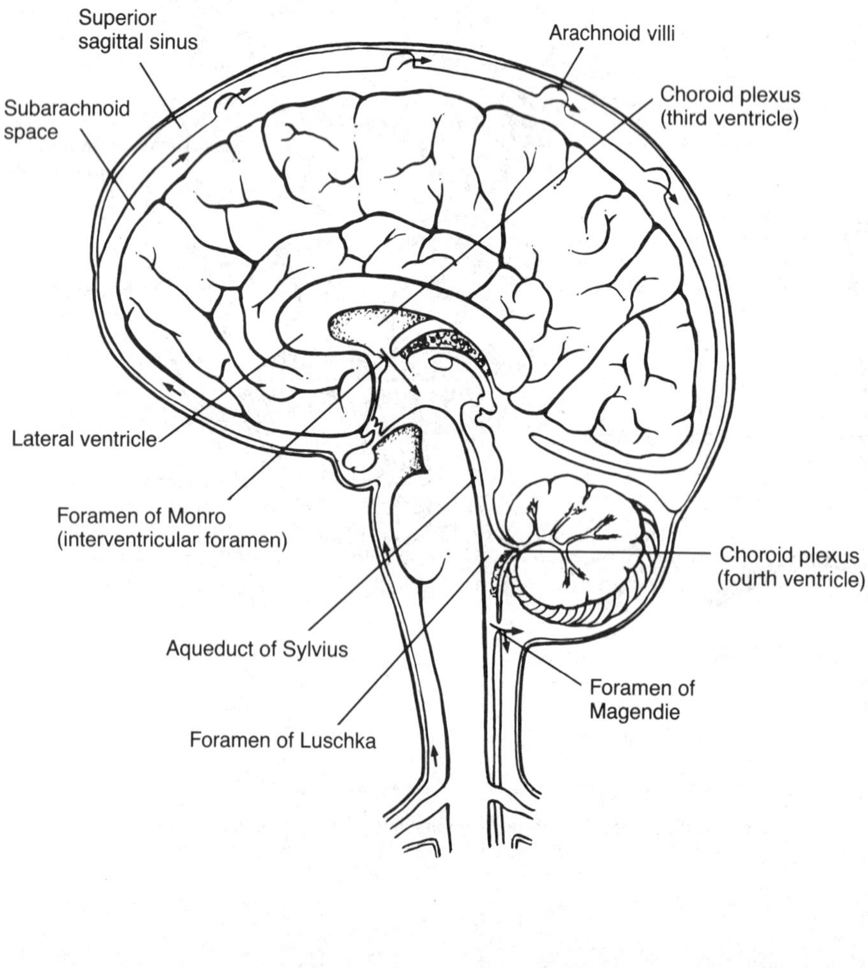

Figure 37–7.

Cerebral spinal fluid (CSF) circulation. CSF is produced by the choroid plexus in the lateral ventricles and flows around the brain and spinal cord until it reaches the arachnoid villi, from which it is absorbed into the venous circulation. Arrows indicate the major pathway of CSF flow.

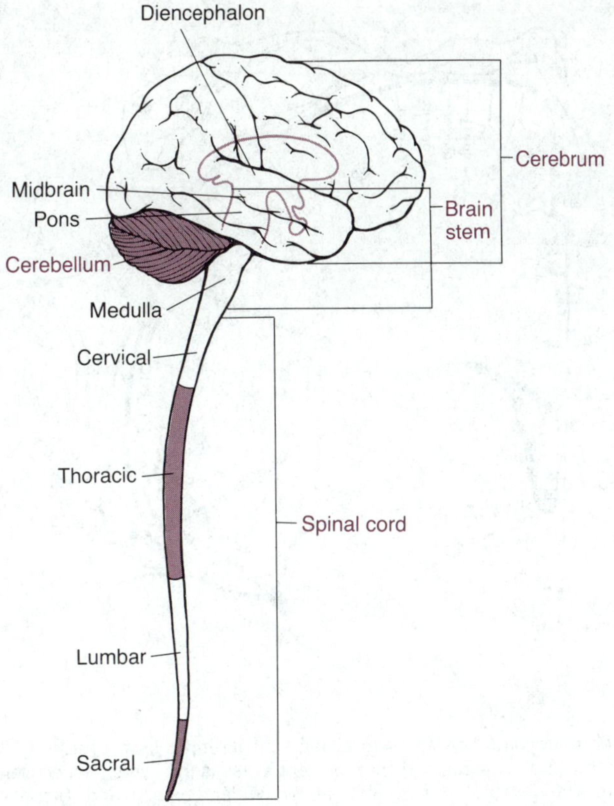

Figure 37–8.

Lateral view of the central nervous system showing its main divisions.

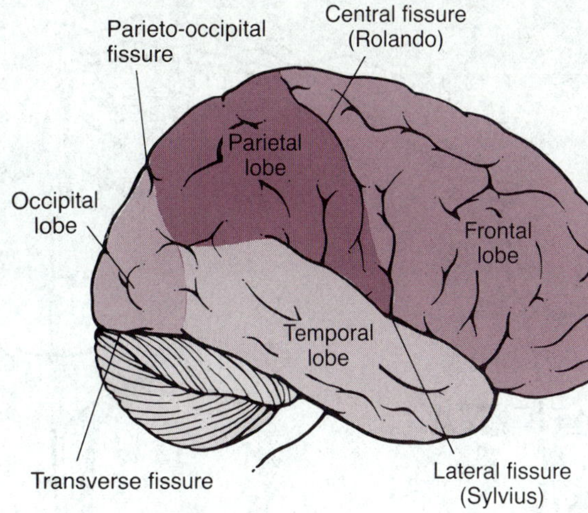

Figure 37–9.

Lobes of the cerebral hemispheres.

Central Nervous System

The CNS, composed of the brain and spinal cord, accounts for approximately 2% of overall body weight (Fig. 37–8). This equates to a volume of approximately 1400 to 1500 ml.

BRAIN

The brain is a highly developed structure and is capable of performing the most complicated activities. It is composed of the cerebrum, brain stem, and cerebellum. The brain not only interprets impulses from and responds to the environment but also stores that information for future use. The brain, its function, and its relation to behavior have been studied as far back as 3000 B.C. Today, it is possible to identify specific localization of function and begin to understand the brain-behavior relationship.

The cerebrum can be further divided into the cerebral hemispheres, diencephalon, and basal ganglia.

CEREBRAL HEMISPHERES

The cerebral hemispheres have a convoluted surface with many peaks, known as gyri (singular, gyrus), and valleys or indentations, known as sulci (sulcus). The hemispheres are connected by a structure known as the corpus callosum. This a thick structure of nerve fibers that directly connects corresponding areas of each hemisphere to one another.

The cerebral hemispheres are subdivided into the lobes of the brain: frontal, temporal, parietal, and occipital (Fig. 37–9). There are corresponding lobes on each cerebral hemisphere. Each lobe has identified areas of specialized function (Fig. 37–10).

The frontal lobes make up approximately one third of the mass of the cerebral hemispheres and are thought to be the seat of the highest cognitive functions (abstract thinking, judgment, emotion). Motor function is also localized in front of the central sulcus on the cerebral motor cortex. The specific areas for motor control can be configured in a topographic scheme (Fig. 37–11). Motor speech (Broca's area) is also located in the frontal lobe of the dominant hemisphere.

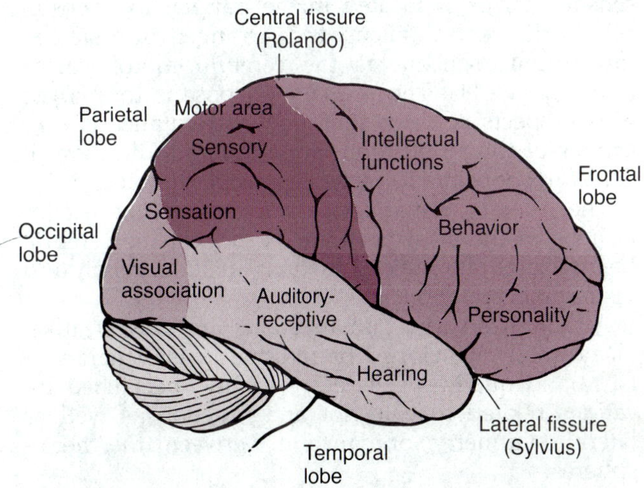

Figure 37–10.

Specialized functions of the lobes of the cerebrum.

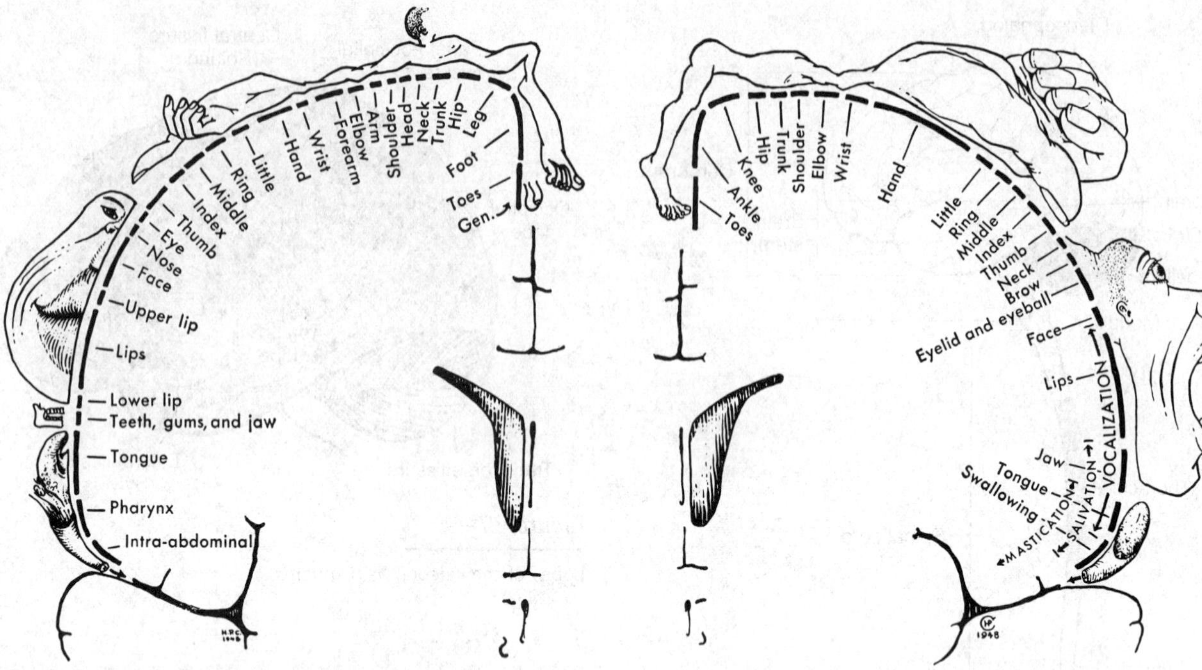

Figure 37–11.

Areas in the cerebral cortex controlling voluntary motor activity of specific body parts and areas receiving sensory input from specific body parts. Diagram is of a frontal section of the cerebrum through the precentral (motor) gyrus and the postcentral (sensory) gyrus, respectively. (Reprinted with the permission of Macmillan Publishing Company from The Cerebral Cortex of Man by Wilder Penfield and Theodore Rasmussen. Copyright 1950 Macmillan Publishing Company; copyright renewed © 1978 Theodore Rasmussen.)

The temporal lobes are located on the lateral aspects of the cerebral hemispheres. Much of the temporal lobes is concerned with perception of verbal material (Wernicke's area, dominant hemisphere), memory, behavior, and emotions.

The parietal lobes are strategically located between the frontal, occipital, and temporal lobes. The anterior border is formed by the central sulcus, whereas the posterior border is formed by the parietooccipital sulcus. The parietal lobe is considered the sensory associative area of the brain. The primary sensory cortex is located in the parietal lobe posterior to the central sulcus. It is arranged in a similar topographic scheme as the cerebral motor cortex (see Fig. 37–11). The primary purpose is to analyze gross aspects of deep sensation and cutaneous sensations of touch, position, pressure, and vibration. It is also responsible for spatial-perceptual abilities.

The primary visual cortex is located in the occipital lobe in the most posterior portion of the cerebral hemispheres. Its major functions include vision and visual interpretation.

Although no two human brains are exactly alike, all normally developed brains share basic characteristics and qualities. There are highly specialized locations related to behavior and function as well as lateral symmetry of function between the hemispheres.

The most obvious functional difference between the hemispheres is that the left hemisphere, in approximately 93% of individuals, is responsible for language (i.e., provides the ability to speak and understand the spoken word). For this reason, the left hemisphere is considered to be dominant. The left hemisphere is the primary mediator of verbal function. Wernicke's area, responsible for the reception of verbal input, and Broca's area, responsible for motor phonation, are located in the left hemisphere.

The right hemisphere, however, does not lie dormant. It is responsible for the processing of information that does not readily lend itself to verbalization. The primary function involved here is the perception of spatial orientation and perspective.

BASAL GANGLIA

The basal ganglia structure is located deep in the cerebral hemispheres. It is composed of gray matter. Its function has been linked with the cerebellum in the coordination and control of fine motor activity.

DIENCEPHALON

The diencephalon, also located deep within the cerebral hemispheres, houses two important structures: the thalamus and the hypothalamus. The thalamus plays a role in one's sleep-wakefulness state, conscious awareness of pain, and relay of ascending impulses to the sensory cerebral cortex. The hypothalamus lies at the base of the diencephalon and is responsible for global actions of body systems (i.e., heart rate, body temperature, water-electrolyte balance, appetite). The hypothalamus works with the ANS and influences the pituitary gland in its release of hormones.

BRAIN STEM

The brain stem is an elongated structure that connects superiorly to the cerebral hemispheres, inferiorly to the spinal cord, and posteriorly to the cerebellum. It houses nerve fibers that form the reticular formation. Motor and sensory neurons gather information regarding muscle activity, and the reticular formation relays motor impulses from the hypothalamus to the ANS and from the extrapyramidal system to voluntary muscles. In addition, sensory impulses ascend through the reticular formation to the

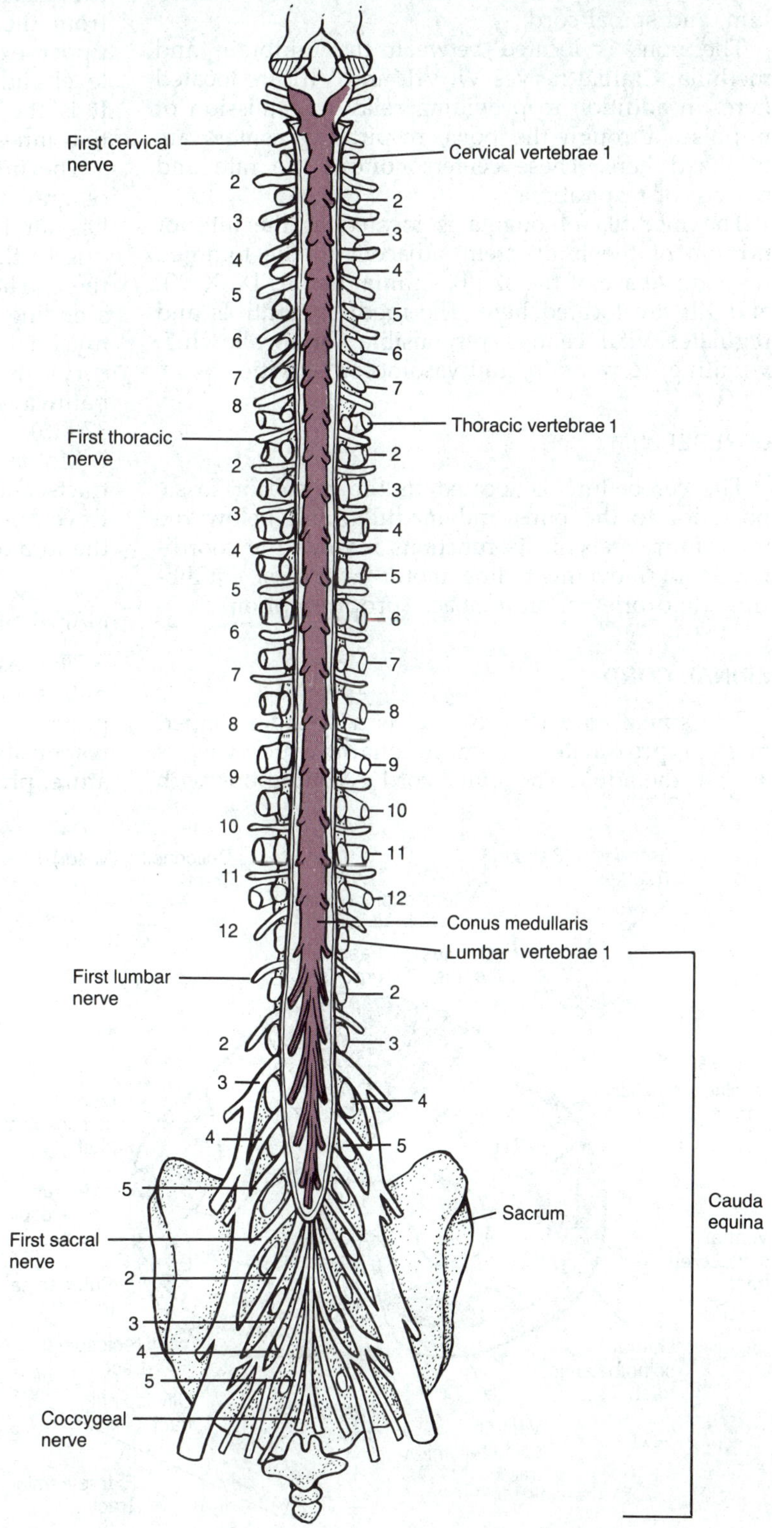

Figure 37–12.

Spinal cord and spinal nerves in relationship to the vertebral column.

cerebral sensory cortex to activate it. This is referred to as the reticular activating system and is responsible for an individual's state of wakefulness.

The brain stem has become known as the "life center" of an individual. It is divided into the midbrain, pons, and medulla oblongata.

The midbrain is the uppermost portion of the brain stem. Cranial nerves III and IV are located here. The midbrain functions as a relay station for impulses among the cerebral hemispheres, cerebellum, and spinal cord.

The pons is located between the midbrain and medulla. Cranial nerves VI, VII, and VIII are located here. In addition to providing relay transmission of impulses through the pons, respiratory centers are localized here. These centers control the rate and pattern of respirations.

The medulla oblongata is located at the inferior portion of the brain stem, adjacent to the foramen magnum (base of the skull). Cranial nerves IX, X, XI, and XII are located here. The medulla controls and regulates vital centers responsible for swallowing, vomiting, respiration, and vasomotor activities.

CEREBELLUM

The cerebellum is located in the posterior fossa, posterior to the pons and medulla, and below the tentorium cerebelli. Its functions involve the coordination of movement, fine motor activities, equilibrium, and orientation in space (proprioception).

SPINAL CORD

The spinal cord (Fig. 37–12) is a cylinder-shaped mass, approximately 43 cm in length, which weighs 35 g in the adult. The spinal cord is continuous with the medulla oblongata, so that a specific line of demarcation between structures is not evident. The spinal cord lies within the vertebral canal with the conus medullaris (caudal end of the spinal cord) extending to the L-1 to L-2 vertebral column level. The three meningeal layers surround the spinal cord to provide protection.

Two enlargements are found in the spinal cord. The first is at the C-5 to T-1 level and is known as the cervical, or brachial, enlargement. It is formed from the volume of motor cells that innervate the upper extremities. The second is at the L-3 to S-2 level and is known as the lumbosacral enlargement. It is the result of the large number of motor cells that innervate the lower extremities.

The internal structures of the spinal cord consist of gray matter and white matter. The gray matter has an H-shaped configuration. The gray color is due to the neuronal cell bodies and synapses found there. The white matter contains ascending and descending pathways, which are mostly made up of myelinated axons. Ascending pathways carry sensory impulses to the brain, whereas descending pathways carry motor impulses from the brain (Fig. 37–13).

Motor and sensory pathways are configured in tracts and are named after the tract in which they travel, the location of the origin of the impulse, and the location of impulse termination.

MAJOR SENSORY (ASCENDING) PATHWAYS

The ascending pathways transmit sensory impulses from the spinal cord to the brain for interpretation. There are three major sensory pathways responsible for the transmission of pain and temperature, proprioception, and light touch.

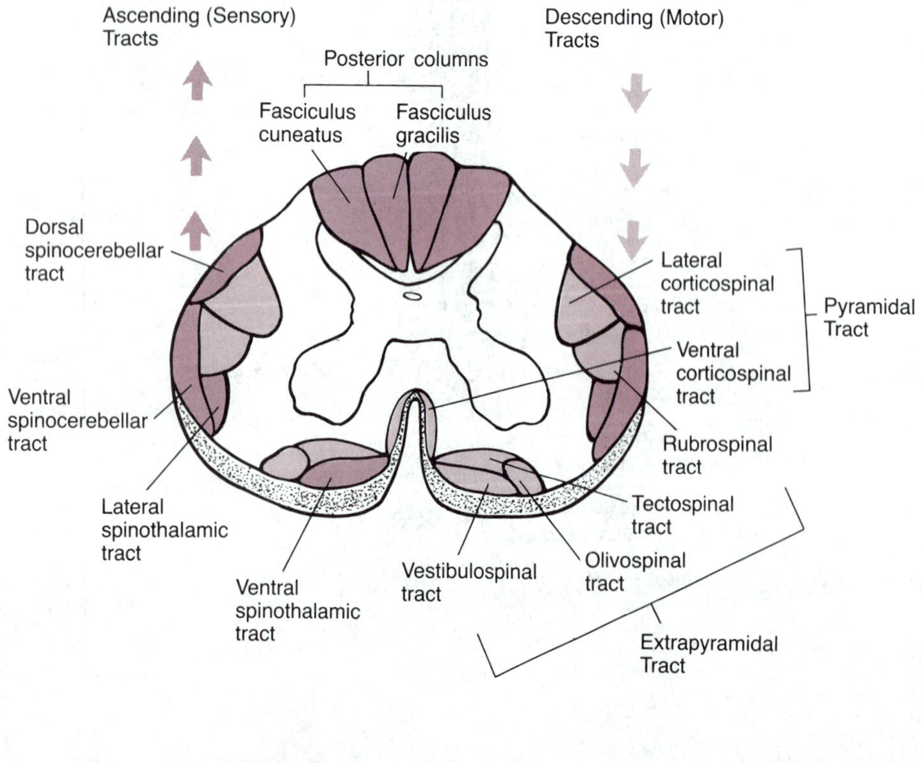

Figure 37–13.

Cross section of the spinal cord showing the major ascending (sensory) pathways and the major descending (motor) pathways.

Table 37–1. CRANIAL NERVES: FUNCTION AND ASSESSMENT

NUMBER	NAME	FUNCTION	ASSESSMENT
I	Olfactory	Olfactory sense (sense of smell)	Patient's eyes are closed. Test one nostril at a time to differentiate odors (spices, peppermint, cloves).
II	Optic	Vision	Assess visual acuity with an eye chart. Using a small object (finger, penlight), test visual field by moving object in from periphery to central vision. Examiner uses own vision to compare results.
III	Oculomotor	Movements of the eyeball and upper eyelid; size of the iris (i.e., constriction and dilation of pupil to regulate amount of light admitted); control of ciliary muscle to regulate degree of refraction by lens	Assess pupil size and shape. Check for ptosis of eyelid. Using a small object (penlight), assess ability for eye movement in all quadrants.
IV	Trochlear	Movement of eyeball by superior oblique muscles	Assessment is the same as for oculomotor nerve.
V	Trigeminal (largest cranial nerve; has three sensory divisions: ophthalmic, maxillary, and mandibular)	Motor function: movement of muscles of mastication Sensory function: pain, touch, temperature of face, nose, teeth, mouth	Ask patient to clench jaw. Touch face with fingertips or cotton swab; have patient close eyes.
VI	Abducens	Movement of eyeball by lateral rectus muscle	Test ability for lateral movement of each eye.
VII	Facial	Motor function: contraction of facial and scalp muscles (facial expression); secretion of saliva by submaxillary and sublingual glands Sensory function: taste (from anterior two thirds of tongue)	Ask patient to frown, smile, raise eyebrows. Note symmetry of facial expressions.
VIII	Auditory (acoustic; has two divisions: vestibular, cochlear)	Sensory function, vestibular branch: equilibrium (position balance) Sensory function, cochlear division: sense of hearing	Ask patient to take a few steps. Note equilibrium. Assess ability for hearing: whisper a phrase, and ask patient to repeat it. Check one ear at a time.
IX	Glossopharyngeal	Motor function: swallowing; reflex control of blood pressure through connection with carotid pressoreceptors; salivary secretion by parotid glands Sensory function: taste and oral and pharyngeal sensations	Test gag reflex by placing applicator against pharynx. Assess ability to swallow.
X	Vagus (has very wide distribution)	Motor function: muscles of pharynx, larynx, thoracic, and abdominal viscera (e.g., regulates gastrointestinal motility or peristalsis, influences cardiac rate); secretion by gastric, intestinal, and pancreatic glands Sensory function: sensations in pharynx, larynx, and thoracic and abdominal viscera	Test gag reflex by placing applicator against pharynx.
XI	Accessory	Movement of shoulder and head by trapezius and sternocleidomastoid muscles	Assess muscle strength by asking patient to shrug shoulders and turn head from one side to the other against resistance.
XII	Hypoglossal	Movements of the tongue	Ask patient to stick out tongue. Note deviation from midline or abnormal movements.

Most motor nerves are considered to also contain some sensory fibers by which information as to the existing conditions in the muscles concerned (proprioceptive data) is transmitted into the central nervous system. The proprioceptive impulses result in appropriate motor responses to facilitate the required pattern of movement.

The lateral spinothalamic tract is the sensory pathway for pain and temperature. Sensory impulses enter the spinal cord and cross almost immediately to the lateral spinothalamic tract, where the impulse is carried upward to the thalamus.

The posterior columns are the pathways for proprioception, deep touch, pressure, and vibration. As impulses enter the spinal cord, they ascend the posterior columns of the spinal cord and cross over at the area between the spinal cord and brain stem.

The ventral (anterior) spinothalamic tract is the pathway for light touch. When the sensory impulse enters the spinal cord, a combination of events occur. The impulse ascends the ipsilateral anterior tract and crosses over to the contralateral anterior tract and also ascends this tract.

Each of these sensory tracts crosses over (decussates) the spinal cord and ends in the thalamus. The thalamus then interprets the impulse and sends it to the corresponding area of the sensory cerebral cortex.

MAJOR MOTOR (DESCENDING) PATHWAYS

The major motor descending pathways transmit motor impulses from the brain to the spinal cord. The impulse is generated in the motor cerebral cortex, descends via the internal capsule (a band of motor fibers from the motor cortex, which synapses with motor pathways in the spinal cord), crosses over at approximately the junction of the brain stem and spinal cord, and travels to the desired spinal level. Thus, motor activities are contralateral from where the specific impulse is generated.

The corticospinal (pyramidal) tract is responsible for voluntary motor movement. The corticospinal tract synapses in the anterior horn of the gray matter before exiting the spinal cord to the PNS. Motor neurons located between the cerebral motor cortex and the anterior horn are known as upper motor neurons (UMNs), whereas motor neurons located below the level of the anterior horn to the PNS are known as lower motor neurons (LMNs).

The extrapyramidal tract, composed of the descending motor pathways excluding the pyramidal tract, functions in conjunction with the basal ganglia and cerebellum to ensure coordination, accuracy, and smoothness of muscle movement.

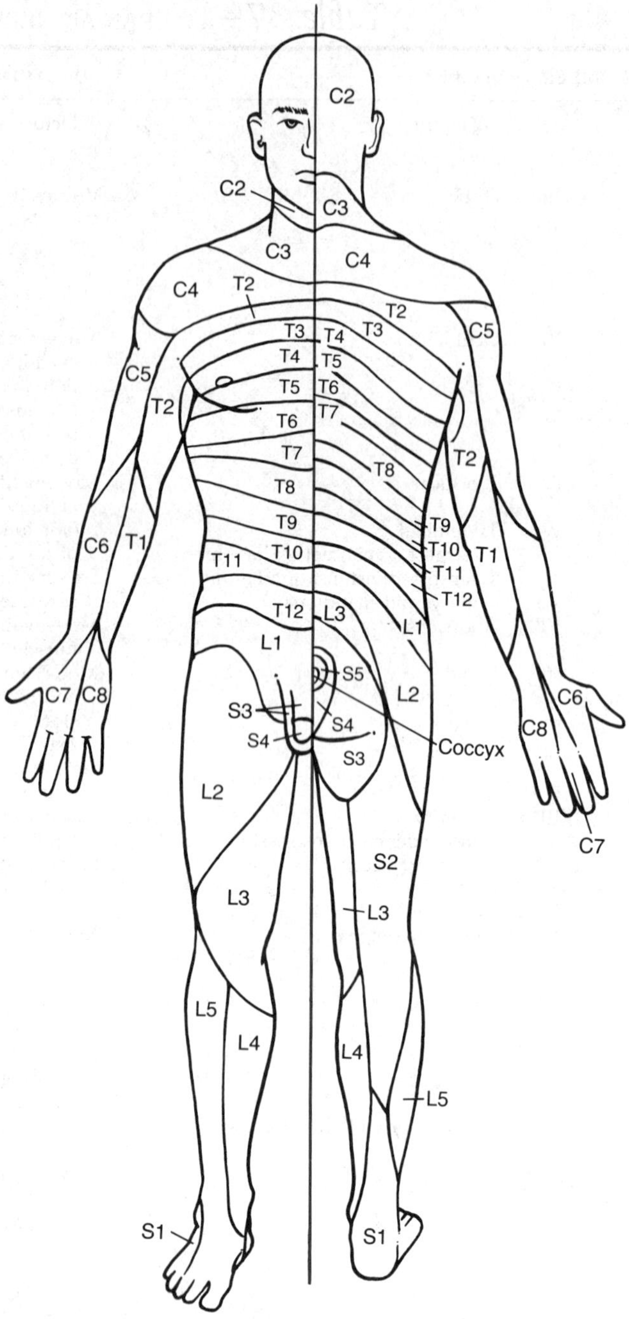

Figure 37–14.

Skin areas innervated by spinal nerves (dermatomes).

Peripheral Nervous System

CRANIAL NERVES

There are 12 pairs of cranial nerves that are part of the PNS. The specific name and function of each are presented in Table 37–1.

SPINAL NERVES

There are 31 pairs of spinal nerves (see Fig. 37–12) that are a part of the PNS. They are symmetrically arranged and exit adjacent to the corresponding level of the vertebral column: 8 cervical, 12 thoracic, 5 lumbar, 5 sacral, and 1 coccygeal. As mentioned previously, the conus medullaris (caudal end of the spinal cord) ends at the L-1 to L-2 level of the vertebral column. Subsequently, the lumbar and sacral spinal nerves develop long roots and are often referred to as the cauda equina or "horse's tail."

Each pair of spinal nerves has a dorsal and a ventral root. The dorsal root carries sensory input (afferent impulses) from the skin and organs of the body to the spinal cord. The ventral root carries motor input (efferent impulses) from the spinal cord to voluntary striated muscles and smooth and cardiac muscles.

Superficial receptors of pain, temperature, and light touch are located throughout the skin in specific regions identified as dermatomes. Dermatome areas correspond to the level of the spinal cord at which the spinal nerves innervating that region enter and exit (Fig. 37–14).

Autonomic Nervous System

The ANS innervates and regulates the activities of the viscera: cardiac muscle, smooth muscle, and glands (Table 37–2). Its function is to maintain the internal homeostasis of the body. This is accomplished by the two antagonistic divisions that comprise the ANS: the sympathetic and parasympathetic nervous systems.

The sympathetic system is associated with the fight or flight response and is activated at the time of stress. It increases heart rate, blood pressure, and blood supply to the body. Noradrenalin is the neurotransmitter associated with this system. This chemical reaction promotes the energy expenditure associated with the sympathetic response.

The parasympathetic system is associated with the conservation of energy, relaxation, and restoration of level of functioning (i.e., decreased heart rate, blood pressure). Acetylcholine is the neurotransmitter associated with this system, which induces a cholinergic effect on the system.

Table 37–2. FUNCTIONS OF THE AUTONOMIC NERVOUS SYSTEM

STRUCTURE OR ACTIVITY	PARASYMPATHETIC EFFECTS	SYMPATHETIC EFFECTS
EYE		
Pupil	Constricted	Dilated
Ciliary muscle	Constricted	Slightly relaxed
Lacrimal glands	Increased secretion	None
CIRCULATORY SYSTEM		
Rate and force of heartbeat	Decreased	Increased
Blood vessels		
In heart muscle	Constricted (α)	Dilated (β_2)
In skeletal muscle	None	Dilated cholinergic, adrenergic (β_2) Constricted adrenergic (α)
In abdominal viscera and the skin	None	Constricted
Blood pressure	Decreased	Increased
RESPIRATORY SYSTEM		
Nasal glands	Copious secretion	Vasoconstriction and slight secretion
Bronchioles	Constricted	Dilated
Rate of breathing	Decreased	Increased
DIGESTIVE SYSTEM		
Tone and peristaltic movements of digestive tube	Increased	Decreased
Muscular sphincters of digestive tube	Relaxed	Contracted (most often)
Secretion of salivary glands	Thin, watery saliva	Thick, viscid saliva
Secretions of stomach, intestine, and pancreas	Increased	Vasoconstriction and slight secretion
Conversion of liver glycogen to glucose	None	Increased
Gallbladder and bile ducts	Contracted	Relaxed
GENITOURINARY SYSTEM		
Urinary bladder		
Muscular walls	Contracted	Relaxed
Sphincters	Relaxed	Contracted
Muscles of the uterus	Relaxed: variable	Contracted under some conditions; varies with menstrual cycle and pregnancy
Blood vessels of external genitalia	Dilated	No direct effect
Penile function	Erection	Ejaculation
INTEGUMENT		
Secretion of sweat	Sweating on palms	Copious secretion
Pilomotor muscles	None	Contracted (gooseflesh)
Secretion of apocrine glands	None	Thick, odoriferous secretion
MEDULLAE OF ADRENAL GLANDS	None	Secretion of epinephrine and norepinephrine
BLOOD		
Coagulation	None	Increased
Glucose	None	Increased
Lipids	None	Increased
BASAL METABOLISM	None	Increased up to 100%

Clinical Manifestations of Neurologic Dysfunction

Altered Levels of Consciousness

Consciousness is defined as awareness of self and the environment. Physiologically, it is divided into two components: content and arousal. The content of consciousness encompasses the ability to think, communicate, and feel, which are functions of the cerebral hemispheres. Arousal refers to the state of wakefulness. Content and arousal are independent components of consciousness, and both can be affected by a variety of neurologic as well as systemic disorders.

ETIOLOGY AND PATHOPHYSIOLOGY

The ascending reticular activating system (ARAS) is responsible for the state of wakefulness. The ARAS is a complex system of neurons with connections to many parts of the brain. The pathways originate in the lower brain stem (medulla), travel upward through the pons and midbrain to the thalamus, and are then dispersed throughout the cerebral cortex. Sensory information is relayed through the ARAS to the cerebral cortex. Arousal and stimulation of cortical neurons occur, inducing a state of alertness. The excited cerebral cortex transmits impulses back through the ARAS to the brain stem, thus establishing a feedback mechanism that maintains wakefulness and cerebral alertness. Impairment of consciousness occurs when there is a disruption in this circuit system. The degree of impairment can vary from slight to complete. Alterations in consciousness can occur secondary to (1) dysfunction in one or both cerebral hemispheres, (2) a localized abnormality in the brain stem affecting the ARAS, or (3) global CNS dysfunction involving the brain stem and the cerebral hemispheres. Specific causes of alterations in consciousness are varied and can include metabolic disorders, systemic failure, toxins, infectious processes, fluid and electrolyte imbalance, structural lesions, and psychiatric disorders.

CLINICAL CHARACTERISTICS

Table 37–3 presents the terms and their defining clinical characteristics commonly used to describe altered states of consciousness.

In describing alterations in consciousness, the focus is on the behavior exhibited by the patient in response to a specific stimulus rather than on labeling the response with a term, because terms alone are subject to individual interpretation. The fully conscious person is awake, alert, appropriate in conversation, and oriented to person, place, and time.

The unconscious person is one who is unable to open the eyes, to obey commands, or to utter recognizable words. The individual experiencing unconsciousness has lost the ability to interact effectively with his or her environment.

MEDICAL DIAGNOSIS

A person is diagnosed as having an altered level of consciousness on the basis of the presence of the clinical manifestations previously described here.

MEDICAL MANAGEMENT

Medical management consists of sustaining vital functions while the underlying problem is identified and treated. In the unconscious patient, the mechanisms essential for awareness and response to comfort, protection, and self-preservation are diminished or absent. The more severe and more prolonged the dysfunction causing the unconscious state, the less likely the recovery. The unconscious individual's survival is directly dependent on the standard of care provided and on the measures taken to prevent complications that could interfere with rehabilitative potential as well as the quality of survival.

Table 37–3. DESCRIPTIONS OF ALTERED LEVELS OF CONSCIOUSNESS

LEVEL OF CONSCIOUSNESS	CLINICAL CHARACTERISTICS
Full consciousness	Patient is awake and alert, appropriate in conversation. Patient is oriented to person, place, and time.
Confusion	Patient has short attention span and poor memory and demonstrates difficulty following commands. Patient experiences increased agitation at night and is disoriented first to time, then place, and possibly self.
Delirium	Patient is restless, agitated, and possibly combative. Patient is disoriented to time and place and is possibly hallucinating.
Obtundation	Patient rouses easily when stimulated and engages in simple but limited conversation and will sleep when undisturbed; lethargy, somnolence, and drowsiness are synonymous terms.
Stupor	Patient is very drowsy and appears unresponsive. When repeatedly and vigorously stimulated, patient will withdraw extremities in a purposeful manner and possibly speak incoherently.
Semicomatose	Patient is unresponsive to stimuli, although painful stimuli to the skin may result in moaning or stirring. Corneal, pupillary, and gag and tendon reflexes (called brain-stem reflexes) are intact.
Comatose	Patient is unarousable and does not stir or moan in response to painful stimuli. Most brain-stem reflexes are intact. Patient may exhibit decorticate or decerebrate posturing.
Deeply comatose	Patient is completely unarousable and unresponsive to all stimuli, including pain. Brain-stem reflexes are absent.

Table 37–4. GLASGOW COMA SCALE

VARIABLE	RESPONSE	SCALE NO.
Eyes	Open spontaneously	4
	Open to verbal commands	3
	Open to pain	2
	No response	1
Best motor response	Obeys verbal command	6
	To painful stimulus	
	Localizes pain	5
	Flexion withdrawal	4
	Flexion abnormal	3
	Extension	2
	No response	1
Best verbal response	Oriented and converses	5
	Disoriented and converses	4
	Inappropriate words	3
	Incomprehensible sounds	2
	No response	1
Total		3–15

Application of the Nursing Process to the Care of the Unconscious Patient

Assessment

Assess neurologic status using the Glasgow Coma Scale (GCS). The GCS (Table 37–4) is a tool that allows for consistency in assessment and documentation. It is based on the assessment of three main components of behavioral response: eye-opening response, motor response, and verbal response. A numerical score is assigned to each response. The minimum score attainable is 3; the maximum is 15. A total score of 7 or less is commonly accepted as a definition of coma.

Check pupils for size, shape, and reaction to light. Assess the corneal reflex, and note and report any decrease in response. Assess for patency of the airway. Note rate, rhythm, and depth of respirations. Auscultate the lung fields for the presence of adventitious breath sounds. Assess adequacy of circulatory function by checking pulse and blood pressure and noting any changes in rate, rhythm, and pattern. Measure temperature rectally to detect hyperpyrexia secondary to urinary tract or respiratory tract infections, wounds, or drug reactions. Inspect the skin carefully whenever the patient is turned and positioned. Observe for redness, indicating possible tissue damage secondary to pressure. Note color, texture, and turgor of the skin. Check muscle tone, muscle size, and joint flexibility. Assess for bowel and bladder function by recording urinary output and bowel movement characteristics and frequency. Palpate the abdomen to detect distention. Auscultate bowel sounds to determine gastrointestinal mobility. Review laboratory values, particularly serum electrolytes, to assess the patient's fluid and electrolyte status. Record all nutritional intake to determine the patient's daily caloric intake.

Nursing Diagnoses and Planning

Nursing diagnoses and related expected patient outcomes most commonly applicable to unconscious patients include the following:

NDx: Ineffective airway clearance related to inability to expectorate and unconscious state

Planning: Patient outcomes
1. Airway remains patent.
2. Patient is free of respiratory distress.

NDx: High risk for impaired skin integrity related to immobility

Planning: Patient outcomes
1. Skin remains intact.
2. Redness or excoriation at pressure points is absent.

NDx: Self-care deficit: total, related to unconscious state

Planning: Patient outcomes
1. Basic needs are met.
2. Patient's dignity is maintained.

NDx: Impaired physical mobility related to inability to participate in movement

Planing: Patient outcomes
1. Joints remain freely mobile.
2. Extremities remain in correct alignment.

NDx: Total incontinence: urinary, related to unconscious state

Planning: Patient outcomes
1. Patient maintains urinary output of 30 ml/hour.
2. Patient is free of urinary tract infection.

NDx: Constipation related to immobility

Planning: Patient outcomes
1. Patient has bowel movement at least every other day.
2. Stool is soft and formed.

Nursing Interventions

NDx: Ineffective airway clearance

Because the unconscious patient cannot take deep breaths in response to instruction, initiate vigorous pulmonary toilet including percussion and postural drainage. Turn the patient from side to side after pulmonary toilet every 2 hours to prevent pooling of secretions in the dependent lung base. Avoid positioning the unconscious patient on his or her back to prevent the tongue from falling back and obstructing the airway. Suction the patient's nasopharynx and oropharynx to remove pooled secretions. If the patient has a tracheostomy, suction after pulmonary toilet. Be certain to preoxygenate before suctioning, and limit suctioning to no more than 15 seconds to prevent hypercapnia. Monitor and document color, consistency, and amount of sputum.

NDx: High risk for impaired skin integrity

The unconscious patient is at high risk for skin breakdown. Turn and position the patient every 2 hours to ensure proper circulation. Blood flow becomes restricted to any body part in which a bone is close to the skin surface if prolonged pressure is maintained. The greater the pressure, the less time that is needed to cause tissue compression and compromised blood flow. If the patient is extremely thin, with more noticeable bony prominences, turn and position him or her more often. Give special attention to ears, shoulders, hips, knees, and ankles. Remember that these areas are direct pressure points when the patient is in a side-lying position, and take care to equitably distribute weight. Place a pillow between the knees to maintain alignment and prevent pressure. Keep the heels from direct contact with the bed. Use lotion to prevent cracking and breakdown of dry skin, and gently massage pressure points to improve circulation. Place an air mattress or other pressure-relieving device on the bed. Avoid many layers of bed protectors and linen because excess bedding can inhibit airflow, limit the pressure-reducing property of the mattress, and trap moisture next to the skin. Keep bed linen free from wrinkles or ridges because wrinkled linen causes excess pressure on bony areas. If the patient is incontinent of urine or feces, gently cleanse the area and dry thoroughly. Constant moisture against the skin renders the tissues more fragile and increases the risk of skin breakdown.

NDx: Self-care deficit: total

Because the unconscious patient is unable to perform his or her own activities of daily living, provide basic hygienic care to maintain cleanliness. Bathe the patient daily and more often if incontinence exists. Provide mouth care to the tongue and gums every 3 to 4 hours using a cotton swab moistened with a nondrying mouthwash. Lubricate the lips with Vaseline or cold cream to prevent drying and encrustation. Brush the teeth with a toothbrush and use a suction catheter to remove excess fluid from the mouth. Wash hair regularly at the bedside according to agency procedure. Inspect fingernails and toenails daily. File and clip nails as necessary to protect the patient from injury. Shave the male patient daily as a part of routine basic care. If the patient is receiving anticoagulant therapy, use an electric razor. Protect the patient at all times from unnecessary body exposure. Provide measures of comfort such as blankets in accordance with the patient's temperature and warmth of the skin. Involve the family whenever possible in the patient's care. The family may wish to provide personal care items for the patient and participate in some activities of daily living (e.g., washing the hair). Ascertain the family's coping strategies while observing their involvement with the patient.

NDx: Impaired physical mobility

The unconscious patient is unable to move spontaneously and thus is at risk for contractures, ankylosis, and muscle atrophy. The patient on bed rest who is unable to weight bear can lose calcium from the bones, predisposing to conditions such as osteoporosis and urinary tract calculi.

Perform passive range-of-motion (ROM) exercises for all joints every 4 hours to prevent joint stiffness and contractures. Position the patient properly in a side-lying position. Position the head in alignment with the spine; place the uppermost hip joint slightly forward and support with a pillow so that it is slightly adducted; flex the upper arm at the elbow and shoulder; flex the upper leg slightly at the hip and knee. Support both the upper arm and upper leg by pillows. Reposition the patient every 2 hours, maintaining correct body alignment. Remember that the unconscious patient is unable to express discomfort if position is misaligned. Support limbs with pillows or hands with a towel roll to prevent dependent edema. Collaborate with the physical therapist if special splints or devices are being used for paralyzed extremities to ensure correct use and to establish a regular on-off use schedule. Teach family members to perform passive ROM exercises. This allows them to actively participate in the patient's therapeutic regimen and allows for sensory stimulation of the patient through touch.

NDx: Total incontinence: urinary

Urinary incontinence may be a result of the unconscious patient being unable to communicate elimination needs or of overall nervous system dysfunction. An indwelling Foley catheter is inserted to prevent skin breakdown secondary to incontinence. For the male patient, a condom-type catheter applied over the penis may be used. For the female patient, incontinence devices are available, but their use usually requires shaving the vulvar area and may predispose the patient to skin breakdown and infection.

Record urinary output every 8 hours; notify physician of output less than 30 ml per hour. Monitor odor and appearance of urine. Obtain urinalysis, and culture and sensitivity specimens as necessary. Monitor temperature every 8 hours because fever may indicate a developing urinary tract infection. Secure the catheter to the inside of patient's thigh with nonirritating tape to prevent traction on the urethra and meatus. Removal of the catheter as soon as possible is strongly recommended.

NDx: Constipation

Because of immobility, the unconscious patient's peristaltic activity is diminished. Constipation and fecal impaction are complications of this decrease and of the lack of a normal diet that would stimulate peristalsis.

Administer stool softeners and mild laxatives daily to facilitate elimination. Provide a fluid intake of at least 2000 ml daily, if not contraindicated, to provide hydration, facilitate digestion, and aid in the softening of stool.

Evaluation

Evaluate the effectiveness of nursing care for an unconscious patient by comparing the patient's status with the expected patient outcomes. Examples of specific outcomes for unconscious patients have been provided in the Planning section.

Increased Intracranial Pressure

Intracranial pressure (ICP) is the pressure exerted within the cranial cavity by its contents, which normally consist of brain tissue, blood, and CSF. The ICP is not a constant: that is, it is a continuously fluctuating phenomenon within a normal range of 80 to 180 mm H_2O or 0 to 15 mm Hg. Activities that increase intrathoracic or intraabdominal pressure, such as coughing, sneezing, or straining at stool (the Valsalva maneuver), cause a momentary increase in ICP. Activities such as sitting or standing up result in a momentary decrease in ICP. Whereas transient increases in pressure are benign, sustained increases in ICP can be life threatening.

ETIOLOGY

Increased ICP can be caused by anything that takes up space within the intracranial compartment and changes the normal ratio of blood, brain, and CSF. Thus, edema of the brain, blood clots, tumors, cysts, abscesses, and hydrocephalus can all cause increased ICP (Table 37–5).

PATHOPHYSIOLOGY

With increased pressure, brain tissue is compressed and lacks blood and oxygen. The end result is brain damage if treatment is not available. Increased blood pressure and decreased pulse are physiologic changes that occur in response to brain tissue being deprived of oxygen. Decreased level of consciousness is a clinical change that results from damage to brain tissue because of lack of nutrition or oxygen. Pupillary reactions change when brain tissue is forced through the uncus, resulting in pressure on the oculomotor nerve. This occurs because of the anatomic relationships of involved structures.

The tentorium is a fold of dura that serves as a shelf on which the cerebral cortex rests. A small space exists between the end of the tentorium and brain stem. This space is called the uncus. With increased ICP, brain tissue is forced through this small opening. This is called uncal herniation. As tissue is forced through the opening, it exerts pressure on the brain stem. It is exactly at this anatomic point that the third cranial nerve (oculomotor) exits from the brain stem. This causes unilateral changes in pupillary response because of compression of the oculomotor nerve. A fixed, dilated pupil is considered to be a late sign of increased ICP.

CLINICAL CHARACTERISTICS

The classic symptoms of increased ICP are decreasing level of consciousness, which is the most sensitive indicator of increased ICP, increasing blood pressure, decreasing pulse, and pupillary changes. Respiratory and motor changes may be present depending on the cause of the increased pressure.

As ICP begins to increase, headache, nausea, restlessness, and drowsiness as well as increasing blood pressure and decreasing pulse may occur. Unilateral motor weakness of the upper and lower extremities may or may not be present depending on the location and extent of the damage.

Late signs of increased ICP are coma, apnea, unilateral pupil changes, high blood pressure, and slow pulse. If untreated, increased ICP causes death.

MEDICAL DIAGNOSIS

ICP may be monitored by three different devices: a ventricular catheter, a subarachnoid screw, and an

Table 37–5. CAUSES OF INCREASED INTRACRANIAL PRESSURE

GENERAL CAUSES	EXAMPLES OF SPECIFIC PATHOLOGY
Increase in brain volume	Tumor
	Cerebral edema, secondary to trauma, surgical manipulation, tumor, tissue hypoxia, infarction
	Brain abscess, encephalitis
Increase in CSF volume	Decreased CSF absorption as a result of meningitis or SAH
	Obstruction of CSF flow because of hydrocephalus
	Tumors compressing the ventricles
	Trauma
Increase in blood volume	Aneurysm or arteriovenous malformations
	Intracranial hemorrhage secondary to hypertension or trauma
	Dilation of cerebral arteries as a result of hypoxemia or hypercapnia
	Obstruction of venous drainage as a result of compression of internal jugular vein, increased CVP
	Hematomas

Abbreviations: CSF, cerebrospinal fluid; SAH, subarachnoid hemorrhage; CVP, central venous pressure.

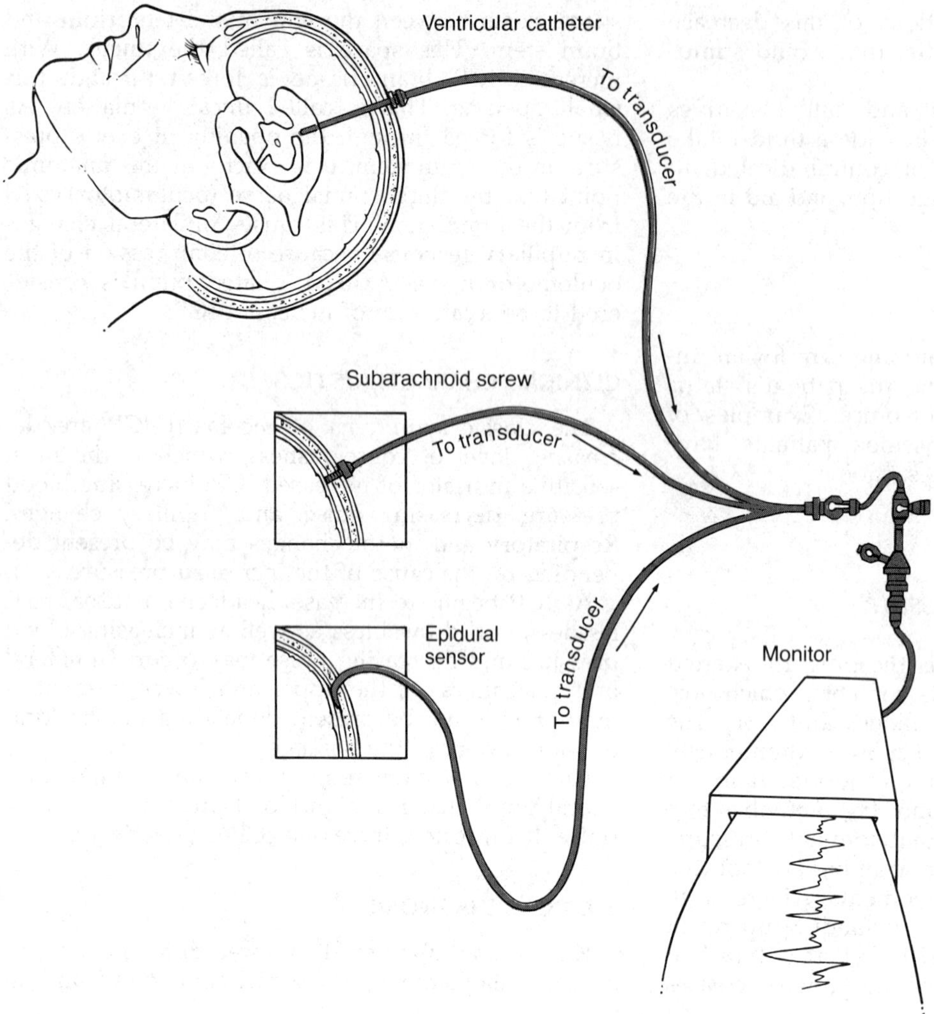

Figure 37–15.

Devices used for monitoring intracranial pressure: a ventricular catheter, a subarachnoid screw, and an epidural sensor.

epidural sensor (Fig. 37–15). No one of these devices is ideal; rather each has specific advantages and disadvantages.

The ventricular catheter allows accurate, direct measurement of ICP and also allows for drainage of CSF, but because it is placed via a burr hole through the cerebrum into a lateral ventricle, there is a risk of both infection and brain damage.

The subarachnoid screw, like the venous catheter, allows direct measurement of pressure and removal of CSF. There is still a risk of infection, although it is not as severe because the screw does not enter the brain tissue but remains in the subarachnoid space. There is also risk that the screw may become obstructed if the brain should swell.

The least invasive and therefore the safest device is the epidural sensor. Unfortunately, it is also the most unreliable because the pressure of the CSF is not measured directly but is measured via a fiberoptic sensor placed in the epidural space. Recent advances in fiberoptic technology have improved the accuracy of epidural sensors, and their use is rapidly becoming widespread. CSF drainage is not possible with this device.

Apart from these devices, medical diagnosis is usually made on the basis of clinical assessment and a computed tomographic (CT) scan. The CT scan will show an area of increased density if a space-occupying lesion is present. A lumbar puncture is generally contraindicated because, by removing spinal fluid, the pressure differential is dramatically changed. This increases the chance of uncal herniation, brain damage, and even death.

MEDICAL MANAGEMENT

Medical management of increased ICP focuses on diagnosing the cause and intervening with appropriate pharmacologic, medical, and surgical therapies.

DRUG THERAPY

There are three general classes of medications used for patients with increased ICP: osmotic diuretics, corticosteroids, and anticonvulsants.

Osmotic diuretics are drugs that are hyperosmolar in nature. The high osmotic concentration of the drug causes water to be drawn from the edematous brain tissue into the vascular system, thus reducing ICP. The most commonly used osmotic diuretic is mannitol (Osmitrol). It is administered intravenously. It acts quickly, and its effect is short term. Mannitol is particularly useful during surgical procedures or as an emergency measure when patients need to be transferred from one location to another for appropriate treatment. The dosage and rate of administration of mannitol (Osmitrol) vary, but the usual dosage is 1.5 to 2 g/kg of body weight. Serum osmolarity levels must be monitored during its use.

Glucocorticoids are effective in reducing focal cerebral edema, particularly if caused by tumors or abscess. Intravenous dexamethasone (Decadron) is the most commonly used glucocorticoid. Large doses are given initially, followed by maintenance doses on a regular basis, usually every 4 to 6 hours. Steroid therapy can potentiate gastrointestinal bleeding, infection, and hyperglycemia. Barbiturate therapy may be used in instances of severe, uncontrolled ICP unresponsive to the usual treatment modalities. Sodium pentobarbital (Nembutal) or thiopental sodium (Pentothal) is administered by continuous intravenous infusion to induce a barbiturate coma. Although the actual mechanism of action is unclear, it is theorized that inducement of barbiturate coma decreases overall cerebral metabolism, glucose utilization, and oxygen demand, allowing brain tissue to better tolerate hypoxia and diminished cerebral perfusion. Barbiturate coma necessitates mechanical ventilation, arterial pressure monitoring, electrocardiogram (ECG) monitoring, and use of an ICP monitoring device in the intensive care setting.

Although anticonvulsants do not specifically treat cerebral edema, they control convulsive or seizure activity of the brain. This is particularly important because, during a seizure, ICP is dramatically increased. If the patient already has increased ICP, the additional pressure produced by the seizure may be incompatible with life.

The most commonly used anticonvulsant medication is phenytoin sodium (Dilantin). The usual dosage is 300 to 400 g/day. The method of administration may be intravenous or oral. Dilantin is poorly absorbed when given intramuscularly.

SUPPORTIVE THERAPY

Maintaining the head of the bed continuously at a 30- to 40-degree angle promotes venous return and decreases cerebral blood volume. Hyperventilation reduces partial pressure of arterial carbon dioxide ($Paco_2$) levels and stimulates cerebral vasoconstriction, thus reducing cerebral blood flow and lowering ICP. $Paco_2$ levels are maintained between 25 and 30 mm Hg. Intubation and mechanical ventilation are usually required.

Hypothermia decreases the metabolic demands of the brain and decreases cerebral blood flow and volume. Therapeutic hypothermia to 90°F induced by a hypothermia blanket cools the body's surface and decreases cerebral metabolism by 35% to 40%. Shivering, which can increase the metabolic rate, is controlled with chlorpromazine (Thorazine).

SURGERY

As an emergency intervention, a small burr hole can be made in the skull for insertion of a ventricular drain. This allows for drainage of CSF and immediately reduces increased ICP. Surgical decompression of the skull (removal of a small segment of bone) may be necessary to relieve pressure. In cases of a space-occupying lesion documented by CT scan, such as an epidural hematoma compressing brain tissue, surgical removal is warranted.

Application of the Nursing Process to the Care of the Patient with Increased Intracranial Pressure

Assessment

Establish a baseline neurologic assessment on all patients with a neurologic problem. Perform frequent assessments on patients at risk for increased ICP. Be sure to document observations in measurable terms. For example, when documenting level of consciousness, state "Rouses easily to verbal stimuli and responds to questions appropriately."

Question the patient about headache, which can be a signal of gradually increasing ICP. Assess quality and type. Remember that headaches that occur with greater intensity on rising from sleep should be reported immediately because the recumbent position decreases venous outflow and can precipitate an increase in ICP.

Because alteration in level of consciousness is an early sign of acutely increasing ICP, assess the patient for subtle behavioral changes, such as restlessness, irritability, drowsiness, confusion, or apathy. Check orientation to person, place, and time. Observe for any difficulties or hesitation in following simple commands or in verbalizing appropriately.

Assess proximal muscle strength by testing for arm drifts. A downward drifting of the extended arm or a pronation of the hand that was not present on baseline examination could indicate a developing hemiparesis. Check handgrips and plantar flexion and dorsiflexion. Note strength and equality. Use a pin or dull needle to test for impaired sensory discrimination in the extremities.

When the patient's baseline level of responsiveness is minimal (i.e., he or she does not follow commands), test motor response by applying a painful

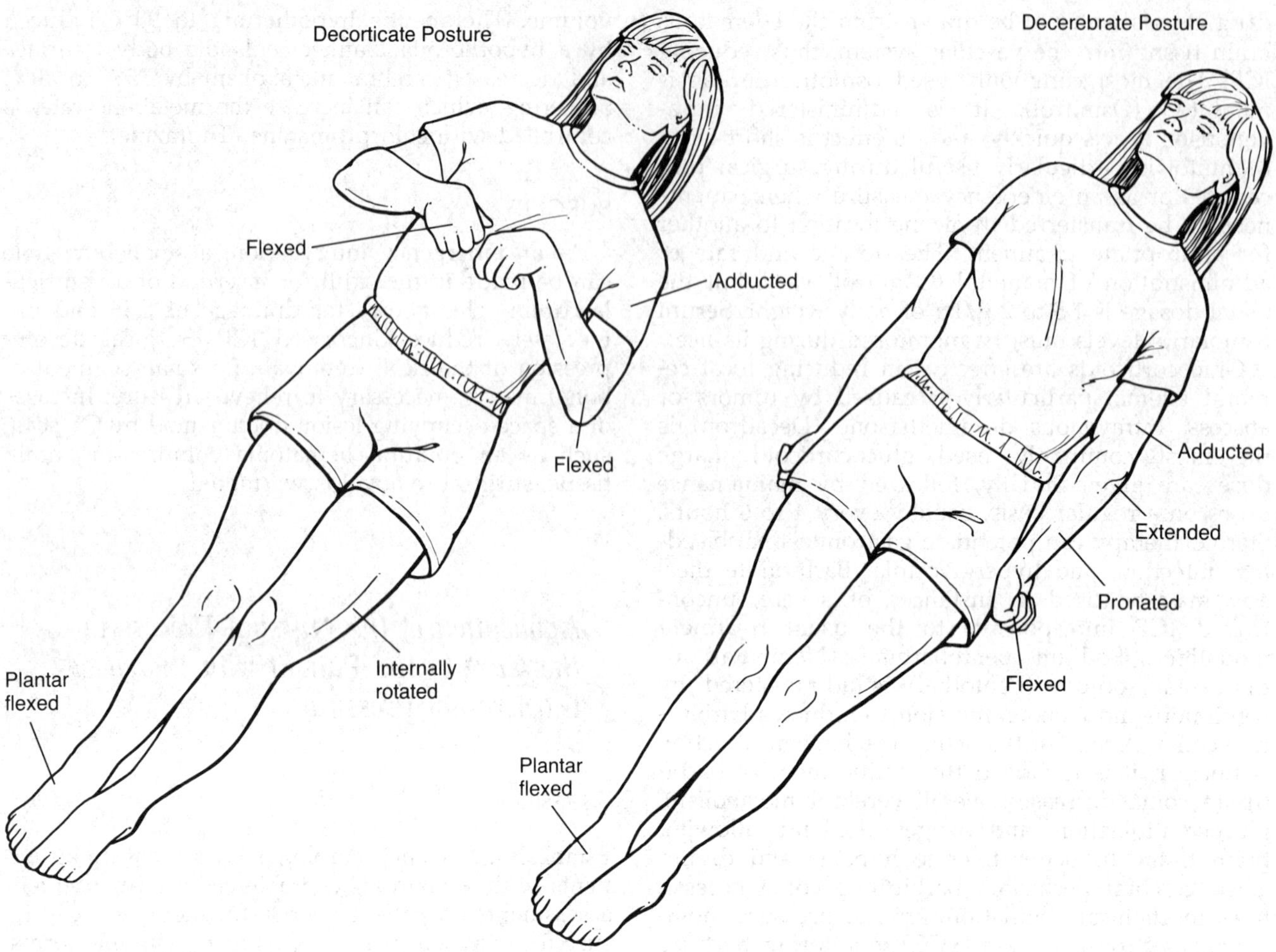

Figure 37–16.

Posturing: decorticate and decerebrate.

stimulus. Press your thumbnail against the patient's nail bed. The unconscious patient usually withdraws the stimulated extremity. Note the symmetry of the withdrawal response from one side of body to the other. An inappropriate response would be posturing. Posturing is a nonpurposeful motor reflex exhibited in one of two ways (Fig. 37–16):

Decorticate posturing (abnormal flexion response): a rigid spine, flexed and adducted arms, extended legs and plantar flexion; indicates dysfunction in the cerebral hemisphere

Decerebrate posturing (abnormal extension response): a rigid and possibly arched spine, rigidly extended arms with palms turned inward, extended legs and plantar flexion; indicates brainstem dysfunction is present

Assess the size and shape of both pupils, noting any deviation from the patient's baseline. Using a penlight, observe the response of each pupil to the light stimulus. Remember that a change in the reaction from brisk to sluggish can indicate increasing ICP and impending herniation. Also keep in mind that pupillary changes generally occur first ipsilaterally (on the same side as the cerebral hemisphere being compressed). Then, as further swelling occurs, both pupils become fixed and dilated (nonresponsive and large in size), an indication that severe and probably nonreversible brain damage has occurred.

Take blood pressure, pulse, and respirations because increasing systolic blood pressure, widening pulse pressure, or bradycardia indicates that the brain is beginning to decompensate. Observe for alterations in respiratory function, such as Cheyne-Stokes respiration, which can lead to respiratory arrest.

Nursing Diagnoses and Planning

Nursing diagnoses and related expected patient outcomes most commonly applicable to patients with increased ICP include the following:

NDx: Altered tissue perfusion: cerebral, related to an increase in brain tissue, intracranial volume, or CSF volume

Planning: Patient outcomes
1. Patient maintains baseline neurologic status.
2. ICP returns to normal range.

NDx: High risk for fluid volume deficit related to osmotic diuretic therapy or fluid restriction

Planning: Patient outcomes
1. Serum electrolytes are within normal range.
2. Serum osmolarity is within normal range.
3. Urine specific gravity is within normal range.

NDx: Ineffective breathing pattern related to alteration in level of consciousness, increased ICP

Planning: Patient outcomes
1. Respiratory rate is regular, between 12 and 24 breaths per minute.
2. Arterial blood gas levels are within normal range.

NDx: High risk for impaired skin integrity related to immobility, hypothermia therapy

Planning: Patient outcomes
1. Skin is free of redness.
2. Skin is intact.

NDx: Altered family processes related to actual or perceived loss of well-being of patient

Planning: Patient outcomes
1. Family verbalizes feelings related to fears.
2. Family verbalizes acceptance of actual or potential altered abilities of patient.
3. Family verbalizes a plan for coping with the actual or potential altered abilities of patient.

Nursing Interventions

NDx: Altered tissue perfusion: cerebral
Document accurate patient behavioral assessments every 1 to 2 hours, and report any deviation from baseline immediately. Maintain adequate venous drainage by elevating the head of the bed 30 to 40 degrees as ordered. This promotes a decrease in cerebral blood volume, thereby preventing a further increase in ICP. Instruct the patient to refrain from activities that increase intrathoracic or intraabdominal pressure such as straining at bowel movement, isometric exercises, coughing, and blowing the nose. A rise in intrathoracic or intraabdominal pressure causes momentary compression of the internal jugular vein and increases cerebral blood volume. Administer medications such as stool softeners and analgesics as necessary, and monitor effectiveness. Minimize the number and length of noxious or invasive nursing procedures such as suctioning or venipuncture whenever possible. Organize nursing care to allow the patient optimal rest periods. Use restraints only when absolutely necessary because agitation increases ICP.

NDx: High risk for fluid volume deficit
Monitor and record intake and output and urinary specific gravity. Monitor pertinent laboratory data such as serum electrolytes, osmolality, and creatine because administration of osmotic diuretics such as mannitol promotes diuresis and can deplete electrolytes. Serum osmolality should not be allowed to exceed 320 mOsm to prevent oversaturation. Monitor vital signs every 1 to 2 hours for tachycardia and hypotension secondary to hypovolemia. Monitor skin turgor for signs of dehydration every 4 hours.

NDx: Ineffective breathing pattern
Maintain a patent airway to prevent hypoxia and hypercarbia. Use airway adjuncts as needed. Auscultate lung fields every 4 hours, and document findings. Administer oxygen therapy as ordered, and document effectiveness. Monitor trends in arterial blood gas values. Use hyperventilation techniques via manual resuscitation bag or via a mechanical ventilator to maintain $Paco_2$ levels between 25 and 30 mm. Monitor for Cheyne-Stokes respiratory pattern, characterized by waxing and waning of respiration with periodic apnea, indicative of increasing ICP affecting the respiratory center in the brain stem.

NDx: High risk for impaired skin integrity
Patients with increased ICP may exhibit a decrease in the level of consciousness, placing them at risk for skin breakdown while bed rest is maintained. Massage bony prominences every 2 hours to promote circulation. Use an air mattress to decrease pressure to total body area. If hypothermia is used to decrease ICP, monitor peripheral circulation, color, and temperature of the skin every 2 to 3 hours.

NDx: Altered family processes
Increased ICP results in a deterioration in the patient's neurologic status. This may be a temporary condition and may have necessitated the patient's transfer to the intensive care unit. Recognize that the uncertainty of the patient's prognosis and the stress of the event can interfere with the family's coping abilities. Explain all procedures to the family. Answer questions, and encourage verbalization of concerns. Provide privacy if needed, and make referrals to other personnel, such as clergy and physician, to assist family in coping with the patient's condition.

Evaluation

Evaluate the effectiveness of nursing care for a patient with increased ICP by comparing the patient's status with the expected patient outcomes. Examples of specific outcomes for patients with increased ICP have been provided in the Planning section.

Speech and Language Dysfunction

Aphasia is defined as a loss or impairment of language function. It can be used to refer to a variety of disturbances including dysfunction of spoken language, writing (agraphia), reading (alexia), or auditory comprehension. The specific dysfunction depends on the area where brain injury has occurred, and so it is rare that a person loses all abilities to communicate. Aphasia is often the result of cerebrovascular accident, tumor mass, hemorrhage, penetrating wounds, or trauma.

The three major types of aphasia syndromes are expressive or motor aphasia, known as Broca's aphasia; receptive or sensory aphasia, known as Wernicke's aphasia; and global aphasia, which is a combination of expressive and receptive aphasia.

EXPRESSIVE APHASIA (BROCA'S APHASIA)

Expressive aphasia is the result of injury to Broca's area, located in the frontal lobe of the dominant hemisphere (Fig. 37–17).

The patient demonstrates difficulty in expressing self through the spoken or written word. Speech is slow, nonfluent, and effortful. Object naming is poor. Comprehension of written or verbal communication is intact.

Patients with Broca's aphasia are aware of their deficits. Often they become frustrated and at times depressed because they are not responding appropriately to their environment and have difficulty communicating their needs.

RECEPTIVE APHASIA (WERNICKE'S APHASIA)

Receptive aphasia is the result of injury to Wernicke's area, located in the temporal lobe of the dominant hemisphere (Fig. 37–17).

The patient experiencing receptive aphasia is unable to comprehend written or verbal communication. Even though sounds are heard, the brain is unable to interpret or give meaning to the sound. The patient has fluent speech with normal rhythm and articulation. The patient conveys information poorly because of the use of empty or incorrect words. Repetition and object naming are poor.

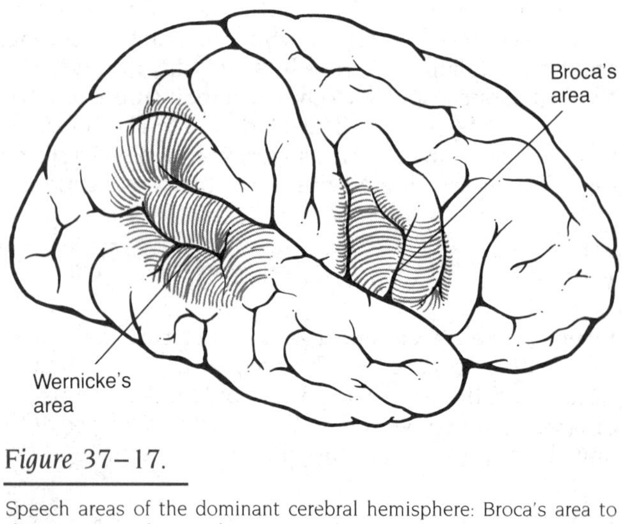

Figure 37–17.

Speech areas of the dominant cerebral hemisphere: Broca's area to the anterior and Wernicke's area to the posterior.

Patients with receptive aphasia may not realize the nature of their deficit. These patients usually have a pleasant disposition and are not depressed.

GLOBAL APHASIA

Global aphasia is a combination of expressive and receptive aphasia. Little of the communication system is intact. These patients experience difficulty in interpreting the verbal or written word as well as expressing their own thoughts or needs by speaking or writing.

Global aphasia is the result of an extensive injury, encompassing both Broca's and Wernicke's areas. Prognosis for these patients is poor.

Application of the Nursing Process to the Care of the Patient with Speech and Language Dysfunction

Assessment

When a patient has sustained a brain insult, assessment of the speech and language system is a basic component of the neurologic baseline assessment. Specifically, assess for the presence of aphasia syndromes. Assess both expressive and receptive language centers through the testing of general behavior and mental status, auditory comprehension, verbal expression, reading, writing, motor speech skills, and verbal fluency. Note any alterations or disturbances in speech and language ability.

When establishing the patient's baseline functional level, be certain to identify and note factors that influence or affect the accuracy of the assessment. Factors to be identified include decreased level of consciousness that would decrease the ability for the patient to respond, visual or hearing deficits or loss, use of prosthetic devices such as dentures and eyeglasses, swallowing difficulties causing garbled speech, and language barriers.

Nursing Diagnoses and Planning

Nursing diagnoses and related expected patient outcomes most commonly applicable to patients with speech and language dysfunction include the following:

NDx: Sensory-perceptual alterations (auditory) related to receptive aphasia

Planning: Patient outcomes

1. Patient communicates needs.
2. Patient demonstrates successful method of communication.
3. Patient uses alternative methods to understand and comprehend interaction with the environment.

NDx: Impaired verbal communication related to expressive aphasia

Planning: Patient outcomes

1. Patient communicates needs.
2. Patient shares frustration when communicating with others.
3. Patient demonstrates alternative methods of communication.

Nursing Interventions

NDx: Sensory-perceptual alterations (auditory)

The patient with receptive aphasia possesses the ability to communicate through means other than comprehension of the spoken word. Therefore, promote communication through the use of alternative devices or techniques such as pad and pencil, touch, pointing, flash cards, pictures, and object communication boards. Face the patient, and establish eye contact to focus communication. Reduce external stimuli, speak slowly, and use simple commands and gestures when addressing the patient. Increase the patient's ability to comprehend by having only one person try to communicate at a time. Provide an accepting environment in which the patient can practice communicating effectively.

NDx: Impaired verbal communication

The patient with expressive aphasia cannot accurately express needs. Encourage the patient to express thoughts and needs through the use of alternative communication devices and techniques such as pantomime, cuing, gestures, pointing, communication boards, or flash cards. Provide the patient with choices by asking questions in a "yes or no" format or by supplying two options. This alleviates the patient's frustration at trying to communicate with phrases that are often unintelligible. Engage the patient in conversation. Allow time for the patient to search for words, and disregard incorrect use of words. Allow the patient to express frustration, and provide accepting atmosphere for him or her to learn and test communication skills.

Evaluation

Evaluate the effectiveness of nursing care for a patient with speech and language dysfunction by comparing the patient's status with the expected patient outcomes. Examples of specific outcomes for patients with speech and language dysfunction have been provided in the Planning section.

Motor System Dysfunction

Dysfunction of the motor system probably is the most marked of all clinical neurologic manifestations. Two major classes of motor system dysfunction are motor neuron disease and movement disorders.

MOTOR NEURON DISEASE

The motor system allows for voluntary motor movements by way of the pyramidal tract of the descending motor pathway, which transmits impulses from the cerebral cortex to the spinal cord and PNS. An alteration in this pathway, whether caused by trauma, infection, degenerative disease, vascular insult or hemorrhage, congenital disorder, or neoplasm, results in a disturbance of motor function and level of mobility. Such alterations are classified as either an upper motor neuron (UMN) lesion or a lower motor neuron (LMN) lesion (Table 37–6).

UMN lesions can be located in the cerebral cortex, internal capsule, brain stem, or spinal cord. Characteristics of UMN lesions include loss of voluntary motor movement, muscle spasticity, hyperreflexia, and atrophy of affected muscle groups related to disuse.

LMN lesions are located in the anterior horn cells of the spinal cord or their axons. Characteristics of LMN lesions include muscle flaccidity, hyporeflexia or areflexia, atrophy of involved muscles related to denervation, and fasciculations.

Lack of voluntary motion in affected muscles is known as paralysis or plegia. Weakness of muscle strength is known as paresis. Hemiplegia or hemiparesis involves extremities on the same side of the body; paraplegia or paraparesis involves both lower extremities; quadriplegia or quadriparesis involves all four extremities. Paresis or paralysis is classified as either spastic or flaccid depending on whether there is UMN or LMN involvement.

MOVEMENT DISORDERS

Coordination, smoothness, and accuracy of motor movement is influenced by the intactness of the extrapyramidal tract of the descending motor pathway in conjunction with the basal ganglia and cerebellum. Neoplasms, degenerative disease, and infection commonly cause interference of motor impulse transmission within the extrapyramidal tract. As a result, the patient experiences movement disorders: bradykinesia (slowness of movement) and involuntary motor movements.

Patients with bradykinesia demonstrate extreme slowness in voluntary motor movement. This condi-

Table 37–6. COMPARISON OF PARALYSIS OF UPPER AND LOWER MOTOR NEURON ORIGIN

VARIABLE	UPPER MOTOR NEURON LESION	LOWER MOTOR NEURON LESION
Involvement	Muscle groups affected	Individual muscles may be involved
Tonus	Increased; muscles spastic; resist passive movement	Absent; muscles flaccid; no resistance offered
Reflexes		
Normal	Normal tendon reflexes exaggerated (hyperactive); abdominal reflex absent or diminished on affected side	Tendon reflexes absent; abdominal reflexes diminished if lesion is at thoracic level
Pathologic	Babinski's sign present (i.e., dorsiflexion of toes, especially the great toe, in response to scratching sole of the foot)	Babinski's sign absent; normal response (plantar flexion of toes) present
	Hoffmann's sign present in hand (flexion of thumb and index finger after sudden release of terminal phalanx of middle finger after it has been flexed)	Hoffmann's sign absent
Muscle atrophy	Only slight atrophy	Marked muscle wasting
Fasciculations (involuntary contractions of small groups of muscle fibers in a muscle)	Absent	May be present

tion is typically seen in patients who have a basal ganglia disorder, such as Parkinson's disease.

Common involuntary motor movements include tremor, dystonia, chorea, and dyskinesia.

Tremor is a rhythmic, quivering, purposeless movement of the extremities or head. A tremor observed when the body part, usually the hand, is at rest is known as a resting tremor. Tremor observed when the patient initiates a movement is known as an intention tremor.

Dystonia is a condition in which there are involuntary twisting movements of the body and trunk. Torticollis is a form of dystonia characterized by the head being pulled to one side of the body as a result of neck muscle spasms. Dystonic movements often involve large muscle groups and produce bizarre movements and appearance.

Choreiform movements are irregular and variable and involve the extremities and facial muscles. Movements may occur at rest and increase when there is purposeful initiation of motor movement.

Dyskinesia is associated with adverse effects of psychotropic medications, such as phenothiazines. It is characterized by involuntary movements of the face, tongue, trunk, and extremities.

Application of the Nursing Process to the Care of the Patient with Motor System Dysfunction

Assessment

The assessment of the patient includes a history and physical examination. Ask the patient whether there is any family history of motor system dysfunction (movement disorders or motor neuron disease). Allow the patient to describe progression of motor dysfunction and how it impacts on ability to function.

Focus physical assessment on the cranial nerves influencing motor function. Assess extraocular movements, chewing, swallowing, facial movement; ability to clear oral secretions; motor speech function; muscle strength of extremities and trunk; and respiratory muscle strength. Observe gait and ability to perform activities of daily living as well as coordination of movements.

Differentiate whether the motor system dysfunction involves the voluntary or involuntary motor movements of the patient. Determine the extent of dysfunction by asking questions such as "Is it limited to a specific area or muscle group?"

Determine whether the motor system dysfunction has had a psychosocial or emotional impact. Ask probing questions, such as "Has this condition changed your lifestyle?", "Have you had to change what you do at home, at work, or with your friends?", "Do you get upset or depressed about your condition?"

Nursing Diagnoses and Planning

Nursing diagnoses and related expected patient outcomes most commonly applicable to patients with motor system dysfunction include the following:

NDx: Impaired physical mobility related to muscle weakness

Planning: Patient outcomes
1. Patient moves, transfers, and ambulates self with or without assistance.
2. Patient remains free of complications of immobility.
3. Patient remains free of self-injury.

NDx: Self-care deficit related to muscle weakness or uncontrolled motor movements

Planning: Patient outcomes

1. Patient hygiene, nutrition, and elimination needs are met.
2. Patient participates in self-care within limitations.

NDx: Impaired gas exchange related to respiratory muscle weakness or uncontrolled motor movements

Planning: Patient outcomes

1. Breath sounds are normal bilaterally.
2. Cyanosis is absent.
3. Patient remains free of aspiration and atelectasis.

NDx: Self-esteem disturbance related to loss of motor function control

Planning: Patient outcomes

1. Patient acknowledges motor dysfunction.
2. Patient willingly expresses feelings.
3. Patient performs activities of daily living within limitations of motor dysfunction.
4. Patient maintains personal and social relationships.

Nursing Interventions

NDx: Impaired physical mobility

To reduce complications related to immobility or subluxation of joints, provide active and passive ROM exercises at least every 6 hours. Allow the patient to do as much for self (moving, transferring, bathing, eating, dressing) as possible.

Arrange for a trapeze to be placed on the bed to allow the patient to aid in positioning self. Maintain good body alignment. Eliminate undue pressure or rotation of joints. Consult with physical and occupational therapists to obtain supportive and assistive devices to be used by the patient for activities of daily living, such as a cane, wheelchair, eating utensils, splints, and slings.

Maintain a turning and positioning schedule every 2 hours. Provide good skin care, and use an air mattress or special bed as necessary. Ensure that clothing and bed sheets are dry and clean.

Plan daily activities so there are rest periods between strenuous activities. Instruct the patient on recognizing signs of fatigue and organizing daily routine to provide optimal rest periods.

NDx: Self-care deficit

Establish patient's ability to meet own self-care needs of hygiene, dressing, eating, ambulating, and toileting.

Encourage the patient to provide self-care within limitations. Provide assistance as necessary in the form of additional support and assistive devices to meet needs.

Because uncontrolled movements may inhibit the patient from feeding self and increase the risk of aspiration, feed the patient if necessary. Consult with the nutritionist and physician to initiate alternative methods to provide nutrition to patient, such as a gastrostomy tube if needed.

Intervene and assist the patient to prevent fatigue or frustration. Ensure that safety measures are followed to avoid injury. For example, instruct the patient to ambulate or transfer with assistance as necessary, and caution him or her not to perform beyond limitations.

Consult with physical and occupational therapists to promote self-care. Consult with social services to assist in discharge planning, and identify available community resources (e.g., home health aide, family involvement).

NDx: Impaired gas exchange

Monitor respiratory status by auscultating lung fields and checking respiratory rate, rhythm, and breath sounds. Position the patient to facilitate drainage of secretions.

Instruct the patient on deep breathing, coughing, and incentive spirometry exercises. Perform suctioning, postural drainage, and chest percussion as necessary.

Instruct the patient to eat in the upright position to avoid aspiration unless contraindicated. Provide foods of appropriate consistency for patient to chew and swallow. Allow adequate time for meals.

NDx: Self-esteem disturbance

Provide an accepting atmosphere in which the patient feels comfortable to discuss feelings and needs by planning time to spend together in a quiet, private area. Encourage the patient to discuss feelings of inadequacies or embarrassment, changes that need to be made in professional, family, and social activities, and the value placed on self-worth.

Identify resources that are available for support and therapeutic intervention, such as self-help groups, church and community resources, and support groups specific to the type of dysfunction or disease process that the patient is experiencing (e.g., multiple sclerosis patient group).

Encourage maintenance of professional, family, and social roles and interactions. Recognize the patient's need to be active and successful in endeavors to increase feelings of self-worth. Assist the patient in identifying effective coping mechanisms. Plan opportunities for the patient to role-play various responses to situations to increase ability to use effective coping mechanisms in unpredictable situations.

Evaluation

Evaluate the effectiveness of nursing care for a patient with motor system dysfunction by comparing the patient's status with the expected patient outcomes. Examples of specific outcomes for patients with motor system dysfunction have been provided in the Planning section.

Sensory System Dysfunction

Sensory system dysfunctions are not easily discernible. However, they have a dramatic impact on the functional level of a patient. Dysfunction of the sensory system manifests as a disturbance in vision, hearing, taste, smell, pain perception, touch sensation, temperature discrimination, or proprioception (awareness of position of body part in space).

VISION

Visual disturbances vary depending on the cause and disease process involved. The visual structures and visual sensory pathway are affected by neurologic conditions including degenerative disease, neoplasms, infection, vascular disease, and hemorrhage. Nystagmus is a condition in which there is tremor-like, oscillating movement of the eyes. This is often seen in patients with cerebellar dysfunction, such as those with multiple sclerosis. Diplopia, also known as double vision, is caused by weakness of the ocular muscles. Scotomata are blind or absent gaps in the visual field. Patients may report alterations of visual acuity, such as blurred vision, clouded vision, or visual loss.

Visual field deficits occur when there is an interruption or lesion of the visual sensory pathway (Fig. 37–18). Patients with pituitary tumors in particular exhibit visual field deficits. As the tumor enlarges, it compresses the optic chiasm, which lies superior to the pituitary gland. Patients complain of hemianopia or loss of vision in one half of their visual field.

HEARING

Hearing disturbances range from diminished to total loss of hearing. Neoplasms, ototoxic medications, head injury, and meningitis are common causes of hearing disturbances. Acoustic neuromas

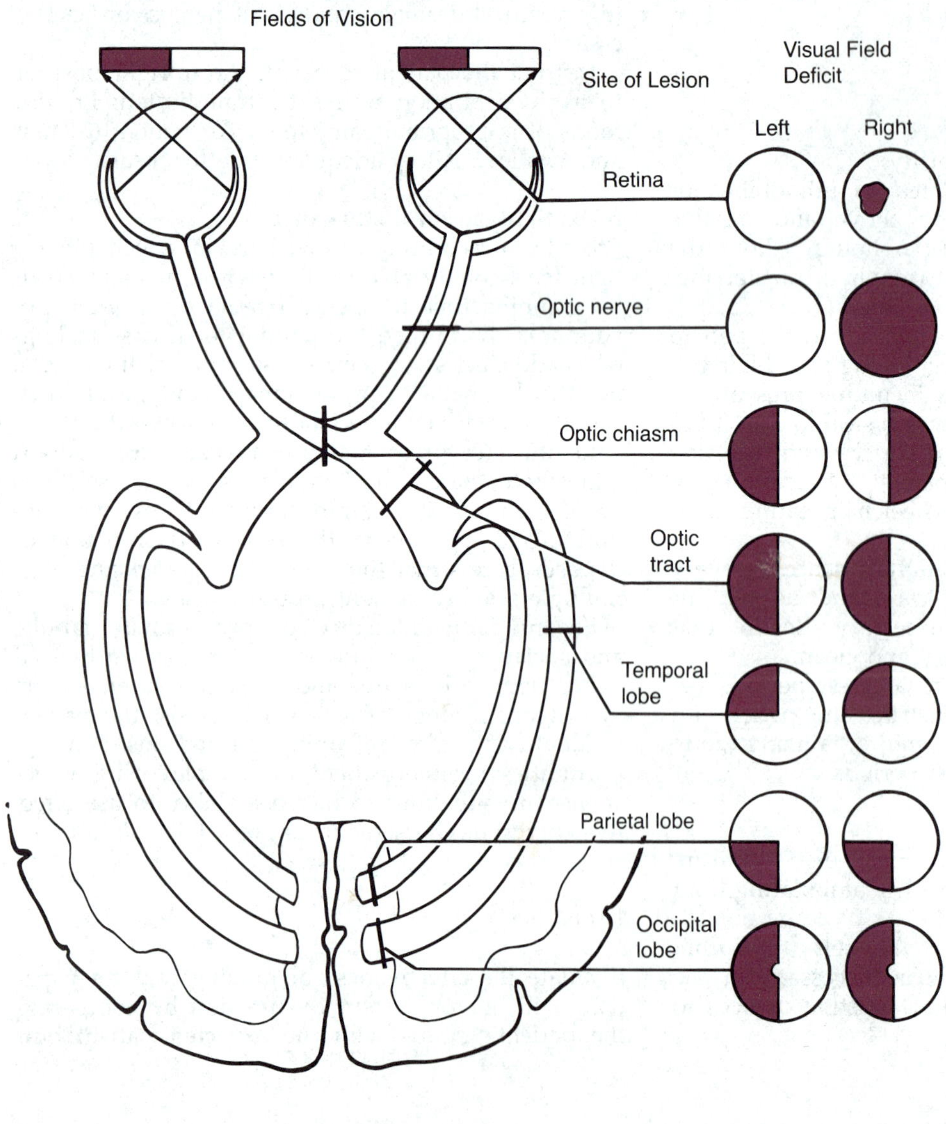

Figure 37–18.

Visual field deficits resulting from interruptions of the visual pathways at various locations.

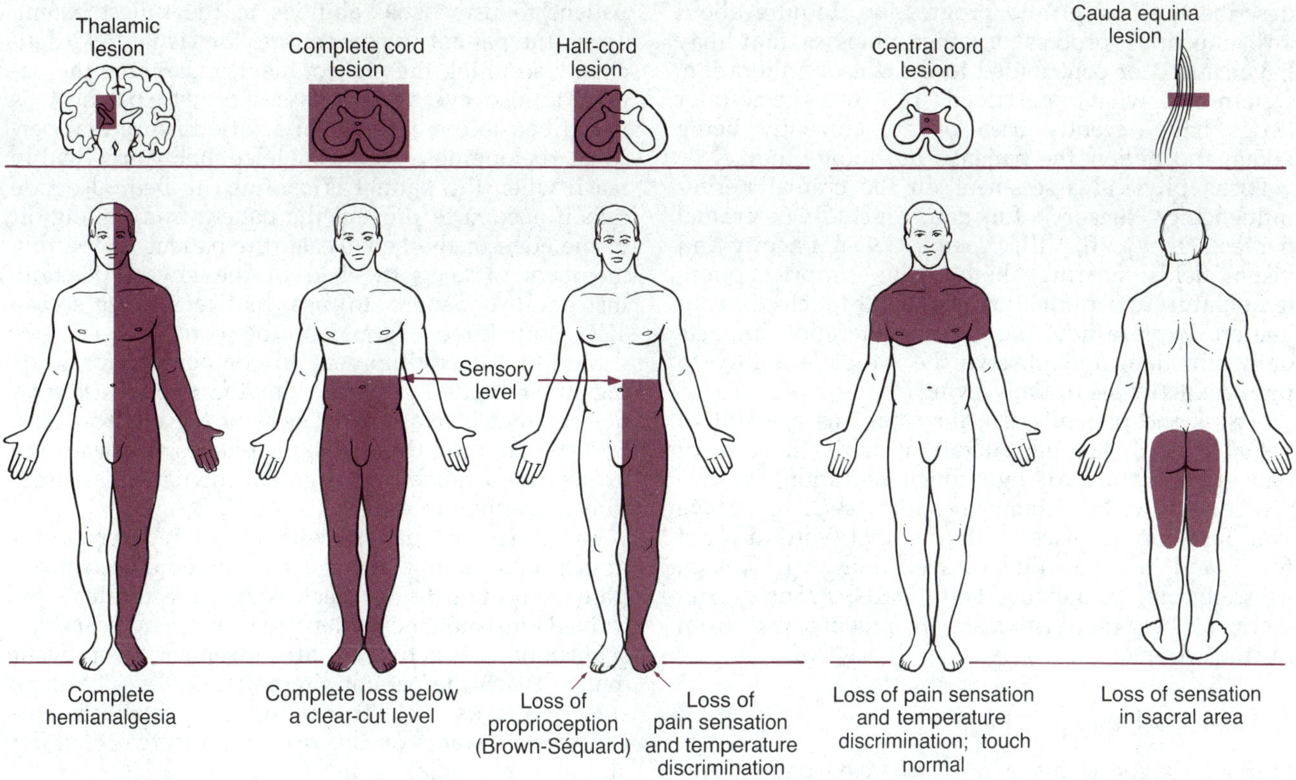

Figure 37–19.

Patterns of altered sensation resulting from various spinal cord lesions.

are tumors that affect cranial nerve VIII, resulting in a hearing impairment or loss.

Tinnitus, conduction deafness, and nerve deafness are three common types of hearing disturbances. Tinnitus is a condition in which the patient complains of a ringing or buzzing in the ear when there is no external source for the sound. Conduction deafness is a hearing loss attributed to lack of sound transmission because of a structural problem in the cochlea or inner ear. Nerve deafness is a hearing loss resulting from a disturbance in the auditory pathway related to a neurologic disease or condition affecting cranial nerve VIII.

PAIN, TEMPERATURE, TOUCH, PROPRIOCEPTION

Disturbances of pain perception, temperature discrimination, proprioception, and touch sensation are caused by impulse transmission interference in the ascending sensory pathways of the spinal cord or the sensory cortex located in the parietal lobe. This interference can be related to varied pathology, such as trauma, neoplasms, hemorrhage, or degenerative changes affecting any portion of the sensory system.

When a complete spinal cord injury occurs, the patient loses all motor and sensory function below the level of injury. There is no recovery of this loss.

When a hemitransection of the spinal cord occurs, the patient manifests what is known as the Brown-Séquard syndrome (Fig. 37–19). This is characterized by ipsilateral (same side) loss of proprioception, ipsilateral paresis or paralysis, and contralateral (opposite side) loss of pain sensation and temperature discrimination.

Complete hemianalgesia results from a thalamic lesion, loss of sensation in the sacral area from a cauda equina lesion, and loss of pain and temperature sense across the upper chest from a central cord lesion (see Fig. 37–19).

The degree and extent of pain, temperature, proprioception, and touch dysfunction are dependent on the extent of injury sustained by the patient. The clinical manifestations may range from paresthesia (abnormal or diminished sensations) to anesthesia (total loss of sensation).

Application of the Nursing Process to the Care of the Patient with Sensory System Dysfunction

Assessment

Obtain a patient history. Ask the patient to identify specific sensory alterations being experienced and to describe their onset and progression. Inquire about any infectious process or other illnesses that may have caused or contributed to the sensory alteration. Determine what prescribed or over-the-counter drugs have recently been or are currently being taken, and review the patient's nutritional intake.

Focus physical assessment on the cranial nerves influencing sensory function, including cranial nerves I, II, V, VII, VIII, IX, and X; visual acuity and visual fields; hearing ability; pain, proprioception, temperature discrimination, and light-touch discrimination. Explore how the sensory alteration impacts daily function, and observe the patient's ability to perform activities of daily living.

Assess the patient's risk for injury as a result of visual deficits; hearing alteration; or dysfunction of pain, temperature, or light-touch sensation, or proprioception. Ask probing questions, such as "Have you had any bruises or burns that you did not feel?" and "Do you find yourself doing tricks, such as squinting, visualizing body parts, or using devices, to help perform tasks or prevent you from hurting yourself?"

Nursing Diagnoses and Planning

Nursing diagnoses and related expected patient outcomes most commonly applicable to patients with sensory system dysfunction include the following:

NDx: High risk for injury related to sensory system dysfunction

Planning: Patient outcomes

1. Patient remains free of injuries such as burns, falls, lacerations, and pressure injuries.
2. Patient uses assistive devices and techniques to compensate for sensory dysfunction.
3. Patient and family demonstrate safety precautions.

NDx: Self-care deficit related to sensory system dysfunction (vision, touch, proprioception, temperature discrimination)

Planning: Patient outcomes

1. Patient performs self-care using compensatory techniques and devices with or without assistance.
2. Patient's hygiene, nutrition, and elimination needs are met.

Nursing Interventions

NDx: High risk for injury

Sensory system deficits compromise a patient's ability to perform activities or tasks safely. The patient has to be protected through his or her own or others' efforts and taught how to meet needs safely.

Maintain a consistent environment for the patient with a visual alteration. Place furniture out of the way so it does not present obstacles. Encourage the patient to use visual abilities to the fullest extent. Teach the patient to compensate for visual field deficits by scanning the environment. Encourage the patient to use eye wear (glasses or eye patches) as prescribed to increase visual acuity. Ensure that personal belongings (tissues, telephone) are within reach when the patient is confined to bed. Use side rails if needed to prevent the patient from falling off of the edge of the bed. Teach the patient and family members to keep the bed in the lowest position. Instruct the patient to use footwear with secure soles; soft slippers should not be worn.

Modify the environment to compensate for hearing impairments. Explore with the patient assistive devices that increase awareness of the environment. Special sounding doorbells, telephones, and warning devices are available to augment the patient's ability to hear various tones.

Encourage the patient with an altered sensorium (touch, pain, temperature discrimination) to concentrate continuously on each step of activities performed. Instruct the patient that awareness and visualization of activities are essential to prevent injury. Teach the patient alternative safety measures, such as the use of a thermometer to establish temperature of water or the use of protective clothing and gloves to shield skin.

When a patient is unaware of position sense (proprioception), instruct him or her to visualize the legs and extremities when walking, sitting, or lying down. Teach the patient to ensure that extremities are in proper body alignment to avoid subluxation of joints or undue pressure.

NDx: Self-care deficit

Establish the patient's ability to meet own self-care needs of hygiene, dressing, eating, ambulating, and toileting. Determine level of additional support and assistive devices needed. Encourage the patient to provide self-care within limitations. Provide assistance to meet needs as necessary.

Encourage the patient to focus on performance of individual steps of self-care when alterations in proprioception, temperature discrimination, pain, or touch sensations are present. This helps to ensure that each step is carried out throughly to avoid inadequate self-care. Teach the patient to visualize steps of psychomotor activities to heighten self-awareness of actions and to avoid injury. Encourage use of a thermometer to determine bath water temperature. Role-play everyday situations, such as using sharp objects (knives), oven, and iron to allow the patient to practice and predict steps he or she needs to perform to accomplish the task without harm.

Evaluation

Evaluate the effectiveness of nursing care for a patient with sensory system dysfunction by comparing the patient's status with the expected patient outcomes. Examples of specific outcomes for patients with sensory system dysfunction have been provided in the Planning section.

Brain Death

Brain death is defined as an irreversible condition in which cerebral function is absent and the brain stem is incapable of maintaining cardiovascular and respiratory vital functions. The heart fails to function within hours or weeks once a person is brain dead and supported on mechanical ventilation. Determination of brain death, as death of an individual, has been the source of moral, social, religious, medical, and legal controversy.

The Harvard University Ad Hoc Committee to Examine the Definition of Brain Death published its criteria for brain death determination in 1968. These criteria included unresponsivity, total lack of reflexes, apnea, and lack of spontaneous movement of the person.

Confirmatory tests for brain death determination include pupils unreactive to light; apnea; and absence of corneal, oculocephalic (doll's eyes), oculovestibular (caloric testing), and gag reflexes. Electroencephalography (EEG), CT scans, and cerebral blood flow studies have been used to document absence of brain function and to support the determination of death.

Confirmatory tests for diagnosis of brain death are repeated in 24 hours to document that no change in the patient's status has occurred. This is critical to rule out the possibility that the patient may be in coma from a reversible event such as drug or metabolic-induced CNS depression, hypothermia, or shock.

The physical care of the patient focuses on maintaining and supporting body functioning while the determination of brain death is in process. The patient does require mechanical ventilation to support respiratory function. The potential of the patient to be an anatomic gift donor needs to be assessed once the determination of death has been confirmed. The option of donation is then presented to the family for their consideration and decision.

Assessment of the Nervous System

Assessment of the nervous system is actually a three-part evaluative process that progresses from the history and description of the patient's complaints and symptoms (subjective data) to a physical examination of nervous system structures and their functions (objective data) to needed diagnostic testing.

Important information that provides a baseline of the patient's functional status is elicited during the data-collection and examination phases of the assessment. In addition, the patient's self-care needs can be identified and can serve as a basis for planning and evaluating progress toward maximizing capabilities.

Patient History

Obtain a careful history before the physical examination of the nervous system. Allow the patient to describe in his or her own words the exact nature of the problem that has prompted a neurologic evaluation. Give special attention to eliciting a chronologic account of the presenting symptoms, noting in particular the nature of onset—sudden or insidious—as well as any circumstances surrounding the initial event. Explore specific details of the present illness in terms of intensity, improvements, or exacerbations. Directly question the patient regarding such symptomatology as numbness or tingling sensations, headaches, seizures, or syncopal episodes as necessary.

Obtain a summary of the patient's medical and surgical history, inclusive of prescription and over-the-counter medications currently and previously used. Ask questions regarding family history of illness because many neurologic diseases are hereditary. Gather psychosociocultural data needed to provide key insights into the patient's and family's coping mechanisms and to serve as the basis for discharge planning. Include the patient's marital status, number and ages of children, past and present occupational status, ethnic background, type of housing, recreational interests, and any financial concerns or constraints. If the patient is unable to provide accurate or complete information, obtain the data from a family member.

Physical Examination

Examination of the nervous system in the conscious adult generally follows a standardized approach, organized into the following components: mental status, speech and language, cranial nerves, motor system, sensory system, and reflexes. Equipment needed for a neurologic examination includes the following:

Cotton
Flashlight
Newspaper (or other printed material)
Ophthalmoscope
Otoscope
Reflex hammer
Safety pins
Snellen's chart
Tape measure
Tongue depressor
Tuning fork
Various objects of different shapes (key, marble, coin)

Vials (stoppered) containing the following:
Peppermint, coffee (smell)
Salt, vinegar (taste)
Hot and cold water (temperature)

MENTAL STATUS

Although the mental status examination is delineated as a separate component of assessment, much of the evaluation of the patient's mental status is integrated throughout the whole interactive process of the neurologic examination. Valuable data are gathered during the interview phase. During this somewhat relaxed conversation, observe the patient's appearance and behavior. Note the overall state of awareness, ability to relax, manner of dress and personal hygiene, facial expressions, quality of speech patterns, and overall mood and thought processes.

Because assessment of a person's mental status is actually an evaluation of cerebral function, ask specific questions that test orientation, judgment, attention span and concentration, memory, intellectual ability, and abstract reasoning.

To assess orientation, ask the patient to correctly state his or her full name, the name of the hospital or facility, and the correct date, including day of week, month, and year. To assess judgment, note whether the patient is able to draw logical conclusions and express thoughts clearly in response to the question "What would you do if there was a fire in the wastebasket?" To assess attention and concentration abilities, ask the patient to repeat a series of five or six digits forward and then backward. Serial 7 testing can also be used. Instruct the patient to start at 100 and subtract 7, then subtract 7 again, and so on. Note the effort required and the speed and accuracy of the answers.

Test both recent and remote memory. Assess remote memory by asking straightforward questions about events in the past that can be validated, such as anniversaries or year of graduation from school. To test recent memory, ask the patient to recall a mutually known event that occurred earlier in the day. Assess immediate recall by giving the patient two or three common objects to remember. Ask the patient to list them after 5 or 10 minutes. Test underlying intelligence by asking general knowledge questions such as "Who is the president of the United States?", "What is the capital city of France?", "What are the four seasons of the year?", or other questions consistent with the patient's cultural and educational background. To assess the capacity to reason abstractly, ask the patient to explain a proverb, such as "A stitch in time saves nine" and to discuss why similar items are alike (e.g., an orange and an apple, or a child and a dwarf).

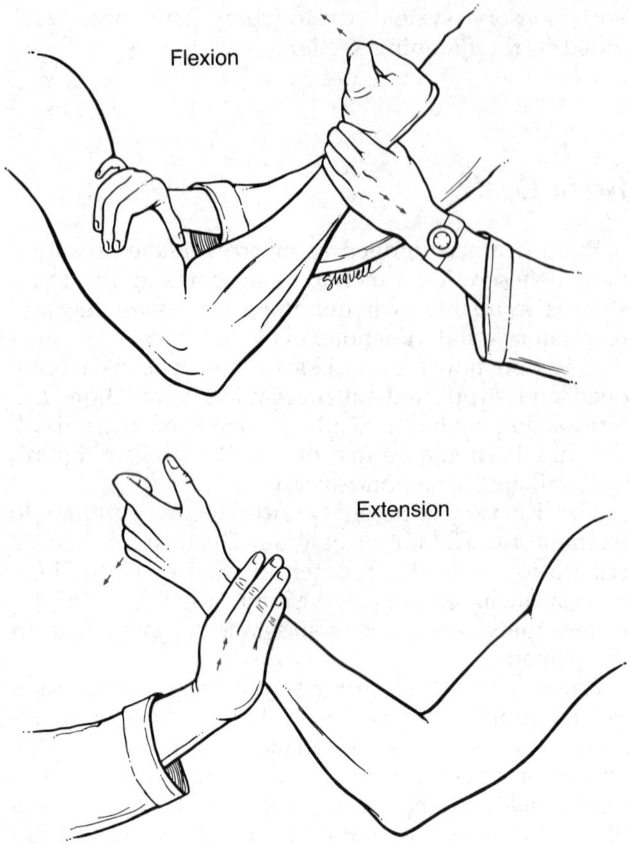

Figure 37–20.

Testing flexion and extension of the upper extremity.

SPEECH AND LANGUAGE FUNCTION

Language is a system in which symbols are used to convey meaning. It can be expressed as the spoken word or in writing. Speech is a mode of communication that uses sounds to represent that symbolic meaning. Speech and language function is a highly complex cerebral process involving coordination between parts of the temporal and frontal lobes of the dominant (usually the left) hemisphere and the occipital lobes. In addition, the muscles of the tongue, palate, pharynx, and lips are necessary for the articulation of speech. Any interference or disruption in the intricate interrelationship of any of these areas results in impairment of communication.

Assessment of speech and language function requires the patient to produce spontaneous speech, repeat phrases, and identify objects. Assess the expressive component of speech by asking the patient to repeat one or two phrases. Note the clarity and fluency of speech as well as the ability to repeat the words without hesitancy or substitution. Show the patient at least five objects, and ask him or her to identify each by name. Note the patient's responses. Keep in mind that the object should not be described by its functional use. For example, a person with a language impairment might be unable to say "hairbrush" but could state that it is "something to use for my hair."

To assess the receptive component of speech, ask the patient to follow a simple one-step command such as "stick out your tongue." If the patient exhibits the ability to follow simple instructions, give more complex commands involving two or three steps. Do not give the patient any visual cues. If the ability to perform complex commands without demonstration is unimpaired, the receptive portion of communication is intact.

To further assess language comprehension as well as the ability to express self in writing, give the patient a paper and pencil. Ask him or her to write his or her name, to draw a picture of a simple object, to write a dictated sentence, and to write a response to an open-ended question.

CRANIAL NERVE FUNCTION

Test the function of the cranial nerves as described in Table 37–1.

MOTOR FUNCTION

The motor system is composed of many intertwining pathways that allow movement to be synchronous, smooth, and coordinated. Assessment of the motor system therefore involves evaluation of gait and posture as well as muscle mass, size, tone, and strength.

Observe the patient's gait, if possible, while the patient is unaware of the observance. Note body posture, rhythm, symmetry of gait, and coordination of movement. For example, if a hemiparesis (i.e., weakness of one side of the body) is present, the normal rhythmic swinging of the arms is reduced on that side (when walking, the right arm should swing with the left leg). Request the patient to lie down in a relaxed manner to assess muscle mass, size, and tone. Inspect and palpate each muscle group, comparing the muscles on the left side of the body with the same ones on the right side. Investigate any suspicion of differences in muscle size by verifying size with a tape measure. Palpate muscle groups to help detect the presence of atrophy or wasting of the muscles.

Tone refers to the resistance detected when a joint is moved through its ROM without any active or voluntary muscle contractions. Passively move each extremity through a full ROM (flexion and extension) to detect hypotonia or hypertonia.

Assess muscle strength by asking the patient to move each of the muscle groups against your active resistance. Compare one side of the body with the same muscle group on the other side. Note symmetry and equality of strength. Test the flexors and extensors of the upper and lower arms and then the flexors and extensors of the upper and lower legs. To test the biceps, hold the patient's wrist and ask him or her to flex the arm as you pull on the wrist. To test the triceps, instruct the patient to extend the arm as you push against the wrist (Fig. 37–20). Test other muscle groups in a similar manner, as illustrated in Figure 37–21. Grade motor strength

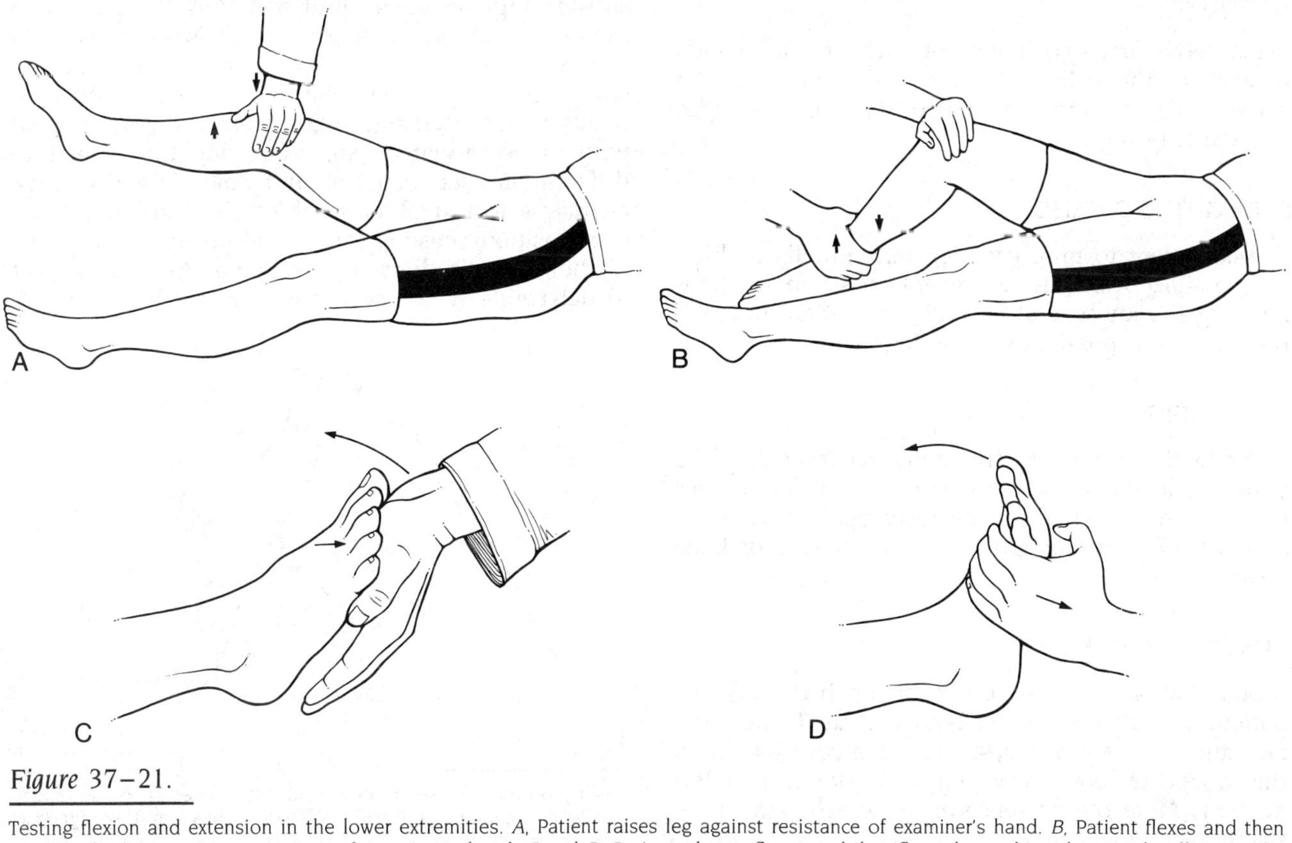

Figure 37–21.

Testing flexion and extension in the lower extremities. *A*, Patient raises leg against resistance of examiner's hand. *B*, Patient flexes and then extends the knee against resistance of examiner's hand. *C* and *D*, Patient plantar flexes and dorsiflexes by pushing down and pulling up the foot against resistance of examiner's hand.

Table 37–7. GRADING SCALE FOR MOTOR STRENGTH

GRADE	DESCRIPTION
5/5	Normal muscle strength (i.e., full range of motion against examiner resistance)
4/5	Full range of motion of muscle but can be overcome with increased examiner resistance
3/5	Full range of motion of muscle against gravity only; is overcome with slight examiner resistance
2/5	Weak movement of muscle but insufficient to overcome gravity
1/5	Slight visible or palpable contraction of muscle noted but no movement results
0/5	Complete paralysis

against gravity and resistance on a scale of 0 to 5 (Table 37–7).

Use the formal testing methods previously described to establish a baseline of the patient's motor function. Make subsequent assessments quickly by using the techniques listed next.

ARM DRIFT

Have patient extend both arms forward, palms up. Ask him or her to close the eyes and hold this position for 10 to 15 seconds. Observe for any downward drift of arms or pronation of hands.

HANDGRIP

Place the first two fingers of each of your hands in each of the patient's hands. Ask him or her to squeeze tightly and simultaneously. Note strength and equality of grips.

STRAIGHT LEG RAISE

Ask patient to raise each leg individually as high as possible from a recumbent position without bending the knees. Note inability of patient to reach the maximum possibility of 90 degrees.

KNEE LIFTS

While the patient is still lying recumbent, place your hands above each kneecap and ask him or her to bend the knees simultaneously against your resistance. Observe for strength and equality of knee bends.

ANKLE DORSIFLEXION

Stand at the foot of the patient's bed. Ask the patient to pull the toes of both feet up toward the face and maintain this position. Place your hands on the dorsa of both feet and pull down simultaneously. Note the presence of decreased patient resistance.

ANKLE PLANTAR FLEXION

Ask the patient to pull the toes up toward the face again. Place the palms of your hands on the soles of the patient's feet and instruct him or her to push down simultaneously. Note the presence of weakness or inability to perform plantar flexion.

SENSORY FUNCTION

Assessment of the sensory system involves evaluation of light-touch, pain, and temperature discrimination, position sense, and vibration. Because these sensory modalities travel on distinct pathways in the nervous system, test each separately. Ask the patient to keep the eyes closed during this portion of the examination to avoid distraction of visual cues from the environment.

To assess light touch, use a wisp of cotton and touch a section of the patient's skin in a stroking manner. Ask the patient to identify the area touched and to describe what is felt. Repeat the procedure in the same area on the opposite side of the body, and compare results. Continue to test light-touch perception in a systematic manner (e.g., begin with the upper arm and progress to the forearm, hand, torso, thigh, lower leg, and foot, remembering to stop and compare right side with left side as each area is tested).

Assess superficial pain sensation by gently touching the point of a pin against the skin in the same systematic manner used for light touch, occasionally substituting the pin's blunt end. Ask the patient to indicate whether the sensation felt is sharp or dull. Determine temperature sensitivity by touching a stoppered vial or test tube of hot water to the patient's abdomen for approximately 1 second. Repeat with the cold-water vial, requesting the patient to differentiate between hot and cold. Use the same technique to test other areas on the extremities. Assess position sense (proprioception) by moving one of the patient's digits up or down. Ask the patient to determine which way the digit has been moved.

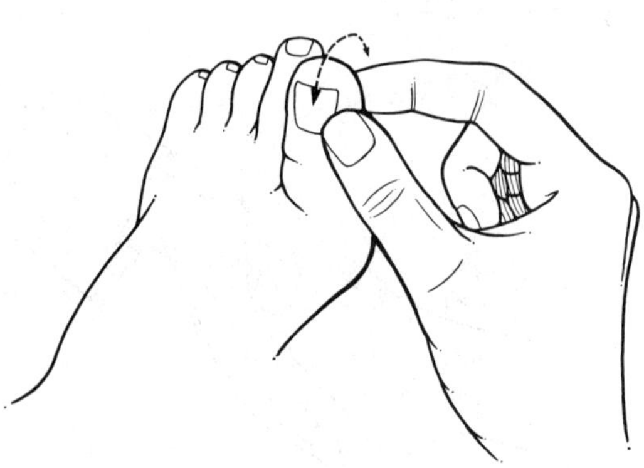

Figure 37–22.

Testing position sense by moving a digit either up or down and asking the patient to identify in which direction the digit was moved.

Check at least three to four digits on each extremity (Fig. 37–22). Assess vibration sense by tapping a tuning fork on the heel of your hand to cause vibration and then placing the base of the fork firmly on the interphalangeal joint of the great toe (Fig. 37–23). Ask the patient to describe what is felt. Repeat this procedure on the bony prominences of the wrists, shoulders, hips, ankles, shins, knees, and elbows. Assess stereognostic function by placing a small common object such as a key in the patient's right hand. Ask him or her to manipulate it in the hand and identify it. Repeat this procedure with a marble and a coin, and then test the left hand with the same objects.

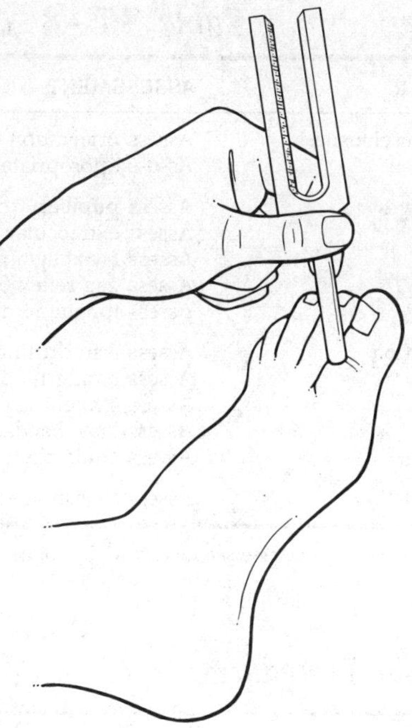

Figure **37–23.**

Testing vibration sense in the great toe.

REFLEX FUNCTION

Assess the deep tendon reflexes with a reflex hammer, as illustrated in Figure 37–24.

Table 37–8 presents a guide to a quick neurologic assessment, which is useful in determining changes in neurologic baseline.

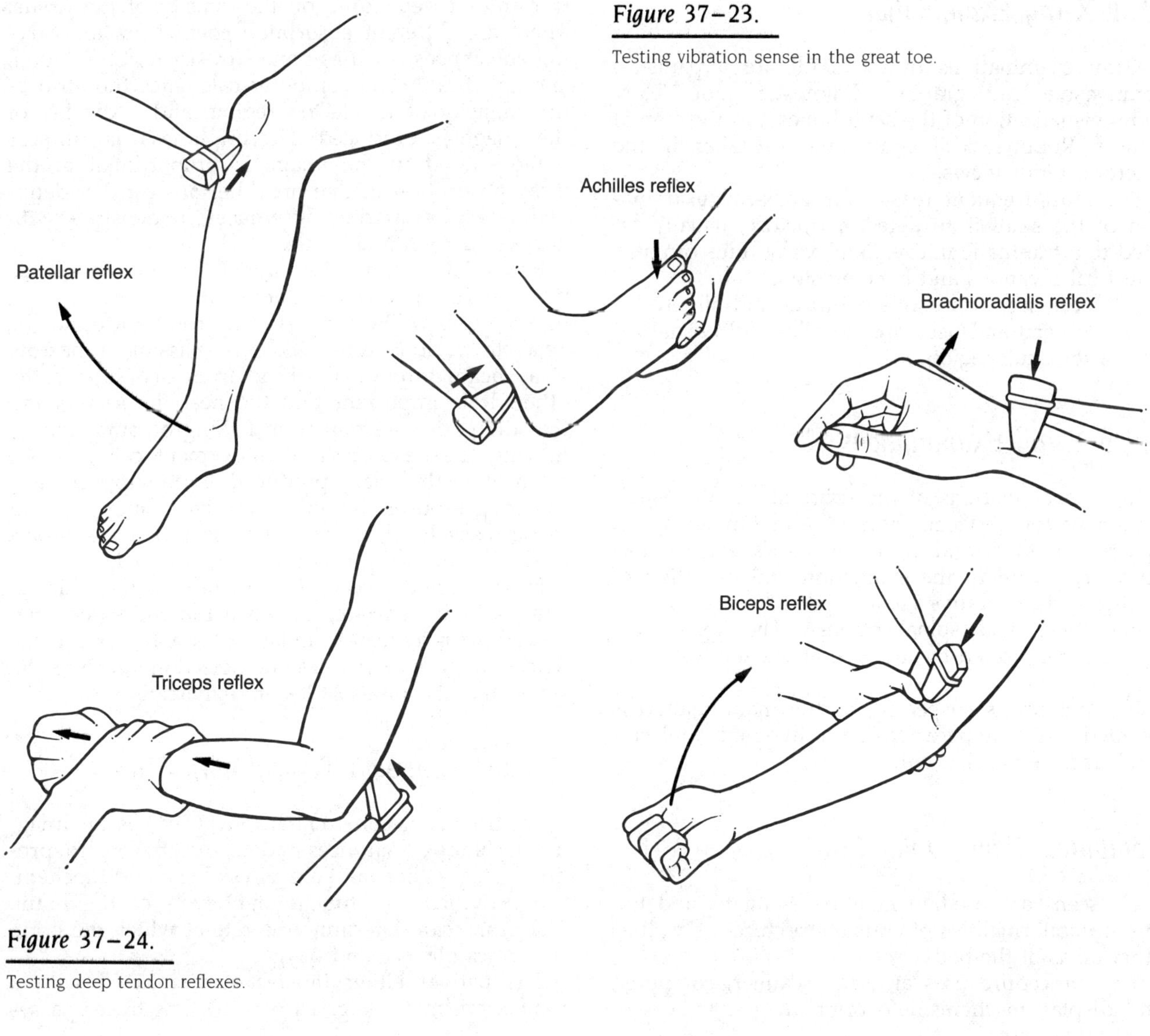

Figure **37–24.**

Testing deep tendon reflexes.

Table 37–8. GUIDE TO A RAPID NEUROLOGIC ASSESSMENT

PARAMETER	ASSESSMENT
Level of consciousness	Assess orientation to person, place, time. Assess appropriateness of speech; note clarity and fluency.
Cranial nerves	Assess pupillary response to light bilaterally (oculomotor nerve). Assess extraocular movements: oculomotor, trochlear, and abducens nerves Assess facial symmetry (facial nerve) Assess gag reflex (glossopharyngeal nerve) Assess tongue in midline when extended (hypoglossal nerve)
Motor function	Assess arm drifting Assess handgrip Assess straight leg raise Assess knee bends Assess ankle plantar flexion and dorsiflexion
Sensory function	Assess sensation to light touch and pinprick in extremities and on trunk, comparing right with left sides

These parameters can be assessed quickly to determine changes in neurologic baseline.

Diagnostic Procedures

Skull X-ray Examinations

X-ray examinations of the skull are a painless, noninvasive radiographic diagnostic tool. They allow visualization of the skull bones and the cranial sinuses. Routine skull x-ray films are taken in the anteroposterior views.

The most frequent reason for an x-ray examination of the skull is to detect a fracture, usually related to a traumatic injury. Skull x-ray films can also detect calcifications and bone erosion.

It is necessary to remove dentures and all jewelry from the head and neck area to allow full visualization of the skull region.

Spine X-ray Examinations

X-ray examinations of the spine allow for visualization of the cervical, thoracic, and lumbar spine. Lateral, anterior, and posterior views are routine. They are useful in the evaluation and detection of fractures, degenerative changes, displacement of the spinal cord, and spinal tumors. The spine area x-rayed is indicated by the type and extent of injury suspected.

If a fracture is suspected, undue manipulation is avoided. Head hyperextension is avoided until cervical fracture is ruled out.

Computed Tomographic Scan

CT scans are used to identify, evaluate, and follow up abnormalities of cranial structures as well as other areas of the body.

This procedure uses an x-ray scanner, computer, and display mechanism to print images. Images of the brain are produced as narrow x-ray beams scan successive layers of the head. As x-ray beams are projected on various planes, they are absorbed or transmitted depending on the density of the tissue. There are different absorption coefficients for varying substances, such as bone, air, tissue, CSF, blood, and calcification. A computer calculates the absorption density of a selected region, and a display of the image is produced. The brightness or dullness demonstrated in the image is proportional to the x-ray absorption in that area. Lesions can be identified when comparing differences in densities with normal surrounding tissue.

For a basic scan, the patient lies in the supine position on an adjustable table with the head resting in a snug cap. The x-ray scanner rotates around the head in various cross sections, passing a narrow x-ray beam through the head from one side to the other. It is important that the head be secure and that the patient refrain from talking or purposefully moving the head, because movement can produce artifacts on the image produced. Extra support, such as sponges on either side of the head, may be used to decrease head movement. It is a painless procedure with no postprocedure care indicated.

In an enhanced scan, the patient receives an intravenous iodinated dye, and then the entire scanning procedure is repeated. Enhanced scans increase the detection of vascular lesion, detection of small lesions, and sharpness of lesion demarcations.

Positron Emission Tomography Scan

Positron emission tomography (PET) is an imaging technique that uses radioactive tracers to produce images that measure physiologic and biochemical activities and functioning levels of the brain. PET scans can determine the rate at which the brain consumes glucose and oxygen.

The patient either inhales or is injected with a radioactive tracer (e.g., carbon 11). The tracer passes through the blood-brain barrier. The positively charged tracer combines with electrons in the brain, thereby creating gamma rays. The scanning equipment, arranged in a circular array of detectors, records the presence of gamma rays. A computer measures the rays and produces an image that corresponds to specific regions of the brain and their cellular functioning.

PET scanning has been useful in diagnostic assessment of patients with neurologic dysfunction. Specific indications include locating brain lesions that alter brain function, identifying metabolic changes such as in patients with Alzheimer's disease, measuring cerebral perfusion, and determining biochemical processes in patients experiencing behavioral disturbances (i.e., depression, schizophrenia).

Magnetic Resonance Imaging

Magnetic resonance imaging (MRI) is one of the newest advances in imaging techniques. MRI can reveal variations in cerebral structures that are subtle and often not seen with other diagnostic modalities. Unlike the CT scan, the MRI does not use x-ray beams. The MRI uses a powerful magnet and radio frequency signals to scan the head and body, and then a computer transforms these signals into images or pictures (Fig. 37–25).

The patient is placed inside a giant, cylinder-shaped electromagnet, which aligns the hydrogen proton atoms found in the water of the cell bodies. Temporary radio-frequency pulsations knock the protons out of alignment. Once the pulsation ends, excess energy is released as the protons return to their resting state (known as relaxation time). This excess energy can be decoded by a computer to give specific information in the form of an image.

MRI is used in the evaluation of patients with cerebral dysfunction as well as other bodily abnormalities. MRI is useful in its ability to demonstrate changes in tissue water content associated with tumor mass; detect necrotic tissue and degenerative changes of the CNS; and visualize the brain stem and structures in the posterior fossa.

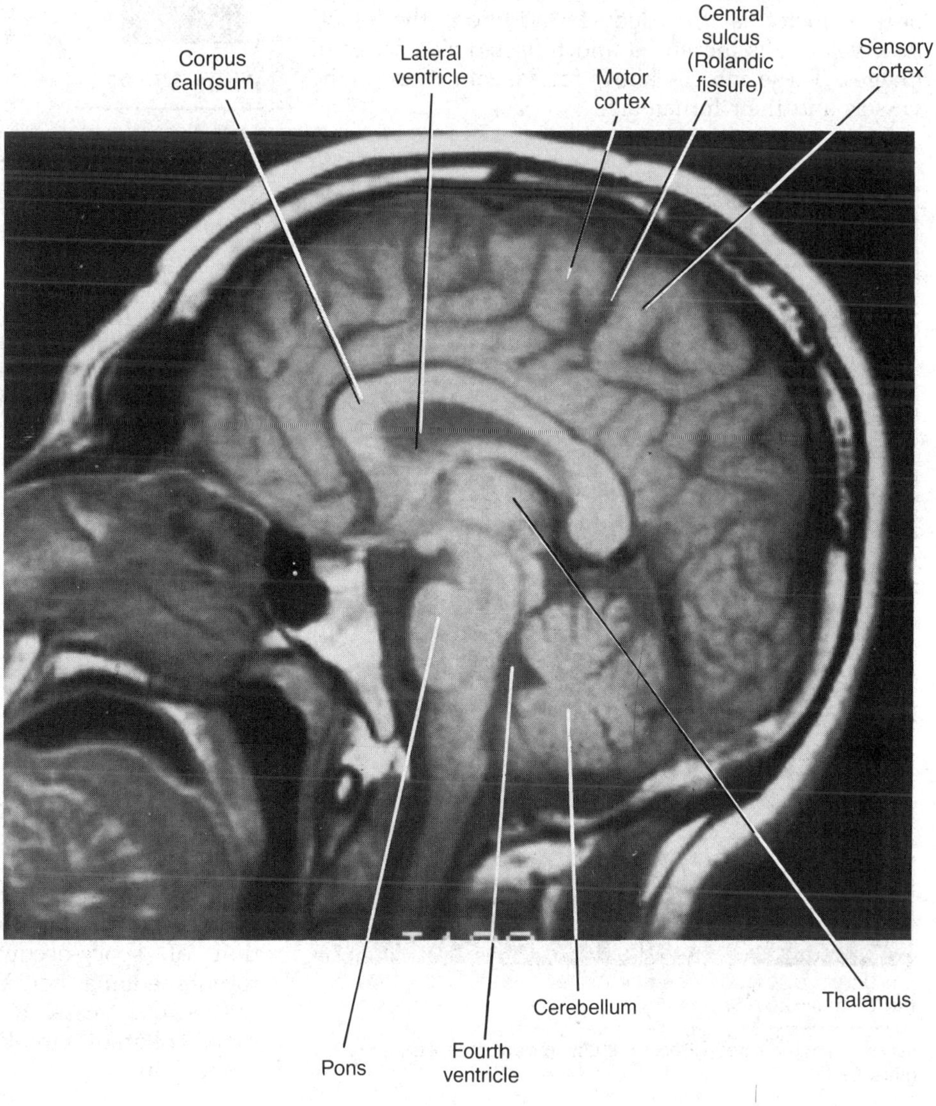

Figure 37–25.

A sagittal midline magnetic resonance (MR) image demonstrating the exquisite detail of discrete anatomic structures possible. (From Marshall SB, Marshall LF, Vos HR, Chesnut RM. Neuroscience critical care: Pathophysiology and patient management. Philadelphia: WB Saunders, 1990, p 128.)

Before the procedure, the patient must remove all metals that would be attracted by the magnet. This procedure is contraindicated for patients with metal implants that cannot be removed such as a pacemaker or internal metallic plate or clip.

Carotid Doppler Studies

Carotid Doppler studies use a Doppler instrument, which emits ultrasound waves to evaluate carotid arterial blood flow.

Ultrasound waves are reflected off moving red blood cells back to the Doppler instrument. The velocity of the blood flow influences reflection of the ultrasound waves. This is evidenced by a change in frequency in sound as recorded by the Doppler instrument.

The patient lies in the supine position, and the Doppler instrument is placed over the neck in the area of the carotid artery (Fig. 37–26). It is moved over the common carotid artery to the bifurcation of the internal and external carotid arteries. As the Doppler instrument receives reflected ultrasound waves, an audible sound is heard and the blood flow velocity is recorded. In addition, the blood flow velocity is measured and reflected as a series of images. These images allow for visualization of the vessels and their lumen size.

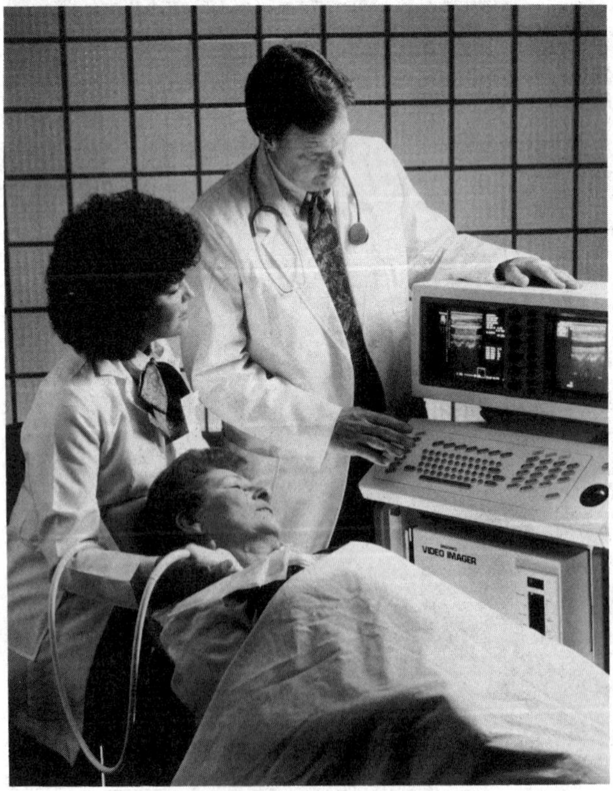

Figure 37–26.

Patient having a carotid Doppler study. (Courtesy of Diasonics, Milpitas, CA.)

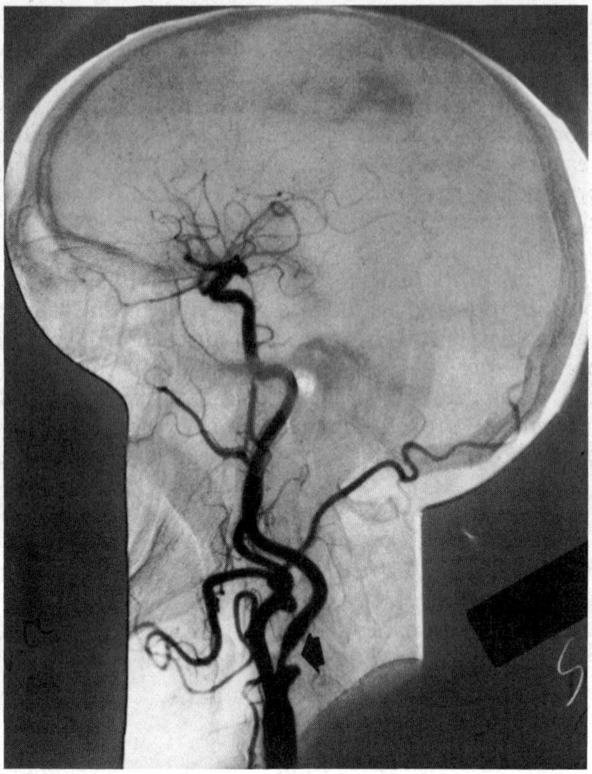

Figure 37–27.

Cerebral angiogram showing internal carotid artery stenosis and ulcerated plaque (*arrow*) in a patient with multiple transient ischemic attacks. (From Marshall SB, Marshall LF, Vos HR, Chesnut RM. Neuroscience critical care: Pathophysiology and patient management. Philadelphia: WB Saunders, 1990, p 135.)

Carotid Doppler studies aid in the detection of turbulent arterial blood flow and anatomic changes in the carotid vasculature, such as stenosis or occlusion. It is a noninvasive, painless, accurate, safe procedure requiring no preprocedure preparation or postprocedure management.

Cerebral Angiography

Cerebral angiography is an invasive procedure that involves the injection of a contrast material into the cerebrovascular circulation (Fig. 37–27).

USES

Cerebral angiography is used to visualize the lumen of vessels and allows the identification of thrombus formation, stenosis, ulceration, and occlusion. It is also used to detect structural abnormalities such as a vascular tumor, aneurysm, or arteriovenous malformation (AVM). It aids in the identification of space-occupying lesions such as cysts, tumors, edema, herniation, or hydrocephalus, which may cause vessel displacement. Angiography also maps collateral circulation, shunting, or variances in blood flow.

PHYSICAL PREPARATION OF THE PATIENT

Patients are asked about allergies to the dye and are given nothing by mouth (NPO status) for 8 hours before angiography. The skin of the puncture site is usually shaved and prepared the night before or at the time of the procedure. Before the start of the procedure, a baseline neurologic assessment is done, and routine measures such as having the patient void and remove dentures and valuables are carried out. If an extremity is to be used for the puncture site, pulses distal to the site are assessed and documented. Sedation is given if ordered, provided the consent form for the procedure has been signed.

PROCEDURE

Angiography is performed by a direct approach, with the contrast material injected into the carotid or vertebral artery, or by an indirect approach, with the contrast material injected into the femoral, brachial, axillary, or subclavian artery with selective catheterization of the cerebral vessels. As the radiopaque dye is injected and passes through the cerebral circulation, films are taken at timed intervals. Angiography is done under local anesthesia or general anesthesia when it is a part of a surgical procedure.

POSTPROCEDURE COURSE

Vital signs and neurologic assessments are monitored frequently for the first 24 hours, as are color, temperature, and pulse distal to the puncture site when it is in an extremity. The puncture site is covered with a pressure dressing and is immobilized for approximately 8 hours to avoid excessive bleeding. Ice is applied to decrease bleeding and edema.

COMPLICATIONS

Potential complications from a cerebral angiography include allergic reaction to the radiopaque dye, vasospasm, thrombosis, hemorrhage, hematoma, embolism, or stroke. These complications may manifest as behavioral, motor, sensory, or language dysfunctions.

Guidelines for Application of the Nursing Process to the Care of the Patient Undergoing Cerebral Angiography

Before the procedure, identify any allergies that contraindicate the use of contrast dye by asking the patient about allergic or sensitive reactions to iodine or shellfish. Perform a neurologic assessment to establish baseline status, with particular attention to the motor and sensory function of the extremities. Assess peripheral circulation. Palpate peripheral pulses, and mark their location with a pen to guide postprocedure assessment. Note strength and presence of the pulses and the warmth and color of skin. Obtain baseline vital signs.

After the procedure, instruct the patient to lie supine for 8 hours and to refrain from bending joints in the extremity with the puncture site. Check vital signs, peripheral pulses, and color and temperature of the extremity distal to the puncture site every 15 minutes for 1 hour, then every half-hour for 1 hour, then every hour until stable. Notify the physician if diminished peripheral pulses or changes in vital signs occur. Monitor the puncture site for bleeding. Should bleeding occur, apply a pressure dressing and notify the physician.

Encourage the patient to drink fluids to decrease the concentration level of the dye in circulation. Notify the physician immediately if difficulty breathing, itching, rash, or other sign of an allergic reaction occurs to allow immediate intervention.

Myelography

Myelography is the introduction of a contrast medium into the subarachnoid space to diagnose alterations of the spinal cord structures by fluoroscopic and x-ray techniques. A myelogram can show one or all segments of the spinal cord.

USES

Myelography is used in the diagnosis of herniated disk, bony changes, congenital lesions, spinal cord tumors, and compression (Fig. 37–28).

PHYSICAL PREPARATION OF THE PATIENT

Monoamine oxidase (MAO) inhibitors, major tranquilizers, and phenothiazine medications are discontinued days before the procedure. Anticonvulsant medications may be continued in some instances.

The patient is checked for allergy and is on NPO status for a minimum of 2 to 4 hours before the procedure. A baseline neurologic assessment is done, and routine measures such as having the patient void are carried out. Preprocedure sedation is given as ordered provided the consent form has been signed.

PROCEDURE

The patient is placed in the prone position on an x-ray table that can be tilted. A spinal needle is inserted in the lumbar subarachnoid cistern (a puncture of the cisterna magna may be indicated if there is suspicion of a cerebellopontine angle tumor). Approximately 10 ml of CSF is removed for laboratory studies, and then the contrast medium is injected. The x-ray table tilts up and down to move the con-

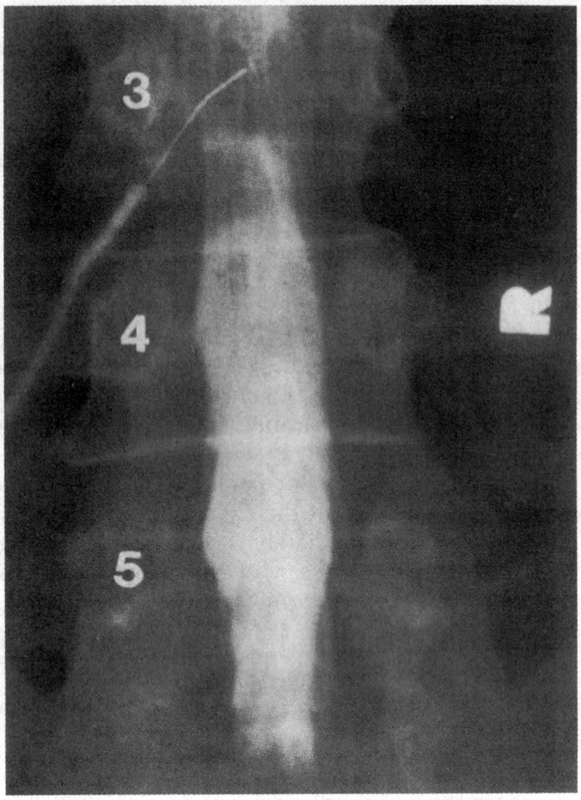

Figure 37–28.

Myelogram. (From Frymoyer JW. The adult spine: Principles and practices. Vol I. New York: Raven Press, 1991, p 314.)

trast material throughout the subarachnoid space, and x-ray films that define the spinal cord, nerve entry roots, and bony structures are periodically taken.

Advances in myelography techniques have focused on the type of contrast medium used. Omnipaque (iohexol), a water-based medium currently used, is absorbed by the body and excreted in the urine. It does not need to be removed manually from the patient after the procedure.

POSTPROCEDURE COURSE

The patient is maintained in Fowler's position with the head elevated 30 to 60 degrees for the first 6 to 8 hours and then in the horizontal position for the next 16 hours after the procedure. This prevents the contrast medium from entering and irritating the cranial structures. The patient is also encouraged to drink fluids to aid in the dilution and excretion of the contrast material. Adverse reactions include headache, nausea, vomiting, and seizures. Phenothiazine antiemetics (e.g., chlorpromazine [Thorazine]) are avoided because of a drug-dye interaction that potentiates seizure activity and other untoward reactions.

If nausea and dehydration occur, intravenous fluid hydration may be indicated. Frequent assessments are made of neurologic status, vital signs, and puncture site and for adverse reactions.

Guidelines for Application of the Nursing Process to the Care of the Patient Undergoing Myelography

Before the myelography, ask the patient about any known allergies or sensitivities. Review the patient's current medical status, and identify any medications such as phenothiazines that would be contraindicated when used with contrast dye. Perform a neurologic assessment to establish baseline status. Also assess the condition of the skin, noting any infections or the presence of a spinal anomaly that would prevent completion of the procedure. Assess the hydration status of the patient. Explain the importance of adequate hydration in reducing the concentration of contrast dye in the circulation, and instruct the patient to drink approximately 2 L of fluid the day before the procedure and every day for several days afterward unless contraindicated by a coexisting medical problem.

After the procedure, instruct the patient to lie with the head elevated 30 degrees for 8 hours when water-based dye is used. Check vital signs every 15 minutes for 1 hour, then every half-hour for an hour, and then hourly until signs are stable. Assess neurologic function for any changes from baseline status. Administer analgesics as ordered for headache, but do not administer phenothiazine medications. Instruct the patient to remain quiet and lie down if headache persists. Notify the physician of complaints of persistent or increased headache. Report any changes in vital signs or untoward reactions, such as seizure activity, nausea, vomiting, or nuchal rigidity, to the physician immediately to allow for immediate intervention and treatment.

Lumbar Puncture

Lumbar puncture is a procedure in which a sterile needle is inserted into the subarachnoid space at the L-4 to L-5 level. This landmark serves to protect the integrity of the spinal cord because in the adult, the spinal cord usually ends at the T-12 level but can extend to the L-1 or L-2 level.

USES

A lumbar puncture is performed to determine CSF pressure and to obtain samples of CSF for laboratory analysis. Routine tests performed on CSF include cell count, protein, glucose, serology, and culture (Table 37–9). Test findings aid in the diagnosis of bacterial meningitis, subarachnoid hemorrhage, pseudotumor cerebri, neurosyphilis, multiple sclerosis, brain tumors, and normal pressure hydrocephalus.

Therapeutic uses of lumbar puncture include serial removal of CSF to reduce ICP and the introduction of spinal anesthetics and intrathecal medications. Medications are given by the intrathecal route when local rather than systemic administration is needed in order for them to exert the desired effect. Medications given by this route include some antibiotics and chemotherapeutic agents.

PROCEDURE

Lumbar puncture is a sterile procedure performed in an outpatient setting or at the bedside. There are no specific preparations or dietary restrictions for this procedure. The patient is placed in either a sitting or a lateral recumbent position and instructed to flex the neck and rest the chin on flexed knees. The puncture site is prepared with an antiseptic agent, the patient draped, and a local anesthetic administered. The physician then introduces the spinal needle through the fourth and fifth lumbar interspace and enters the subarachnoid space while maintaining sterility of the equipment and field (Fig. 37–29). An opening pressure can be obtained by connecting a manometer and a three-way stopcock to the lumbar puncture needle. Spinal fluid for specific laboratory analysis is then collected in sterile tubes. Before the spinal needle is removed, a closing pressure can be obtained by connecting a manometer and a three-way stopcock.

A bandage is placed over the puncture site. A record is maintained of the patient's tolerance of the procedure, opening and closing pressure, and color and characteristics of the CSF.

Table 37–9. CEREBROSPINAL FLUID ANALYSIS

VARIABLE	NORMAL	ABNORMAL
Color	Clear	Cloudy (infection) Initially bloody (traumatic tap) Uniformly bloody (hemorrhage) Xanthochromic (RBC decomposition)
RBC	None	Presence (subarachnoid hemorrhage)
Culture	No organism	Positive (infection)
Pressure	Less than 200 mm H_2O	Above 200 mm H_2O (tumor, hemorrhage edema, obstruction)
Protein	15–45 mg/dl	Elevated values (tumor, infection)
Glucose	50–75 mg/dl	Lower values (tumor, infection)
Serology	Negative	Positive (venereal disease)

Abbreviation: RBC, red blood cells.

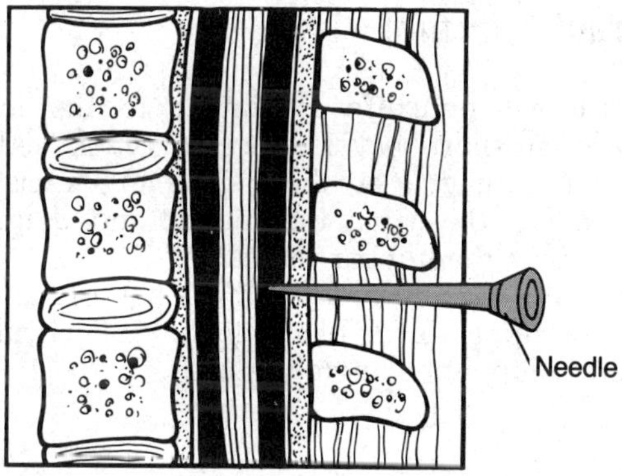

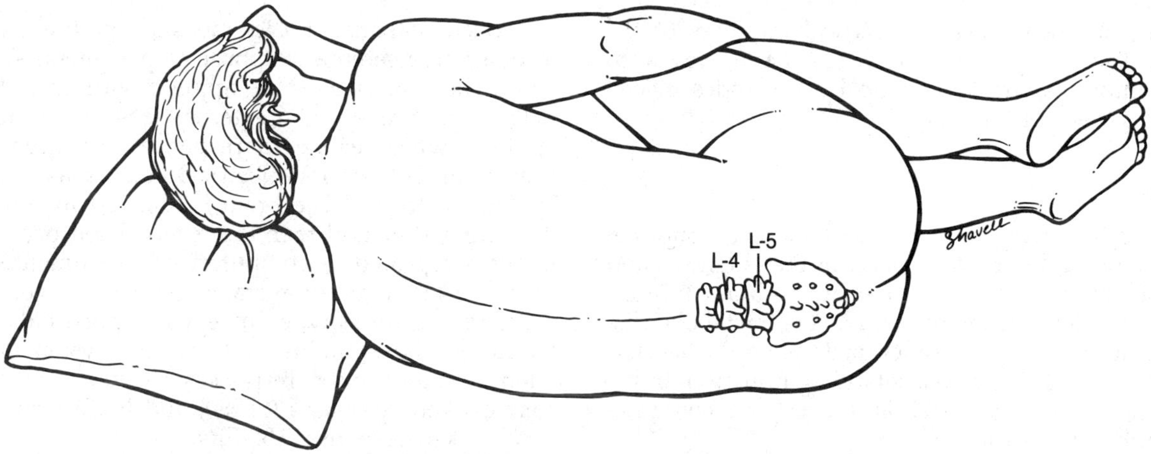

Figure 37–29.

Lumbar puncture. With the patient in a flexed position to maximize the space between vertebrae, the lumbar puncture needle is inserted between L-4 and L-5 to gain entry to the subarachnoid space.

CONTRAINDICATIONS

Lumbar puncture is not performed if there is evidence of high ICP that could result in a herniation syndrome. Other contraindications for lumbar puncture include presence of CSF pathway blockage above the puncture site, spinal anomalies that make puncture difficult or impossible, and skin infection at the puncture site.

POSTPROCEDURE COURSE

The patient is instructed to lie flat for 6 hours after the procedure. Vital signs and neurologic signs are monitored. A mild analgesic such as propoxyphene (Darvon) or codeine may be ordered for discomfort, and the patient is hydrated by forcing oral fluids or by intravenous fluid replacement.

A postlumbar puncture headache occurs in 10% of patients and is caused by leakage of CSF at the puncture site and traction on the meninges. It may occur a few hours to a few days after the lumbar puncture and may be mild or severe. It is typically described as a throbbing in the frontal or occipital area that is aggravated by sitting up or standing. It is not serious but can be disturbing to the patient.

Cisternal Puncture

A cisternal puncture is similar to the lumbar puncture. A short, beveled needle is inserted into the cisterna magna at the C-2 level. A cisternal puncture has the same therapeutic and diagnostic indications as the lumbar puncture.

Cisternal puncture aids in the diagnosis and detection of upper level blockage of CSF circulation and cerebellopontine angle tumors.

Electroencephalography

The EEG measures the electrical impulses of the brain. These impulses, known as brain waves or brain impulses, are picked up by electrodes placed on the surface of the scalp.

USES

An EEG is used to detect and localize abnormal activity of the brain. It is useful in the diagnosis and assessment of patients with seizures, brain tumors, infections, neurobehavioral disorders, metabolic disorders, and other syndromes such as headaches and head injury. EEG is also a vital diagnostic tool in the assessment of electrocerebral silence and confirmation of brain death.

PHYSICAL PREPARATION OF THE PATIENT

Medications and stimulants that influence brain impulses are restricted before an EEG. Patients may also have anticonvulsants discontinued because they can mask electrical impulses in the brain. Stimulants, such as tea and coffee, are restricted to decrease artificial influences on impulse tracings.

PROCEDURE

Surface electrodes are applied with paste to various areas of the patient's scalp to detect electrical impulses, or brain waves. The patient is positioned in a chair or lies supine on a table. The electrodes are connected to the electroencephalograph, which measures the impulses and produces a continuous paper recording.

Brain waves are routinely recorded in four states. First, the patient is asked to lie quietly with eyes closed to establish a baseline recording at rest. The patient is then asked to hyperventilate by breathing through the mouth for 3 to 5 minutes. Recordings continue throughout this period and are maintained to determine the length of time required for the recording to return to baseline. Photic stimulation is the third state. The patient is asked to keep eyes closed and then open them as a light is flickered in front of him or her. Seizure activity may be noted at this time.

Finally, the brain waves are recorded while the patient is asleep. If the patient cannot fall asleep, a hypnotic may be administered. However, the EEG is more accurate if no medications are administered.

POSTPROCEDURE COURSE

This is a safe, painless procedure, and no postprocedure management is required. The EEG paste can be removed with acetone or witch hazel and then by shampooing. The patient resumes routine activities and usual medication regimen immediately.

Evoked Potential Studies

Evoked potential studies measure the brain waves to determine cerebral response to peripheral sensory stimulation. Electrodes are applied with paste to the scalp of the patient. An external sensory stimulus is applied, which evokes a response evidenced by a change in the cerebral electrical activity as detected by the electrodes. The brain is allowed to return to its resting state and then the external sensory stimulation is repeated. A computerized instrument stores data and tabulates an average response curve.

There are three types of evoked potentials, each based on the stimulus and sensory system stimulated: visual evoked responses (VERs), somatosensory evoked responses (SERs), and brain stem auditory evoked responses (BAERs).

In VERs, a strobe light, checkerboard pattern, or unpatterned light is used as stimulation. Electrodes are applied to the posterior portion of the patient's head. With repetition of stimuli, pathways to the occipital cerebral cortex are identified and evaluated.

VERs aid in the diagnosis of multiple sclerosis and lesions of the optic nerve, optic tract, and visual center.

In SERs, an electrical stimulus is applied to peripheral nerves at the wrist or knee. Electrodes are applied to the scalp over the cerebral cortex, contralateral to the stimulus.

SERs are useful in the evaluation of spinal cord function. They aid in the diagnosis of peripheral neuropathies, spinal cord and spinal root injuries, degenerative disease, and tumors.

In BAERs, clicking noises or tone segments are used as stimuli. The stimulus is delivered by an earphone placed over the patient's ears. Electrodes are placed on the top of the scalp and ear lobes.

BAERs allow evaluation of auditory pathways. They aid in the diagnosis of degenerative disease, acoustic neuroma, cerebellopontine angle tumors, and conductive hearing loss.

There is no specific patient preparation or postprocedure management indicated. Evoked potentials may be tested in the hospital setting or in a physician's office. Patients are encouraged to relax and avoid purposeful movements that produce artifacts on the brain wave recordings.

Electromyography

An electromyography (EMG) is the recording of electrical impulses of the muscle fibers and peripheral nerves. Teflon-coated needle electrodes are inserted into skeletal muscles. These electrodes detect electrical activity of skeletal muscle and send the impulse to an oscilloscope, which forms wave tracings. Recordings are made when the muscle groups are at rest and in contraction. When at rest, muscle fibers are silent; when active, muscle fibers have electrical activity.

EMGs aid in differentiating neural from muscular causes of muscular weakness. Therefore, neuromuscular diseases such as myasthenia gravis can be differentiated from disorders of the nerves supplying the muscle, such as amyotrophic lateral sclerosis.

There is no specific patient preparation or postprocedure management indicated. The patient is told there may be some discomfort as the needle electrodes are placed. Mild analgesics may be ordered to relieve discomfort after the procedure.

Nerve Conduction Times

Nerve conduction times study the velocity of conduction of motor and sensory peripheral nerves.

The specific peripheral nerve area to be studied is identified. The nerve is stimulated. The time from nerve stimulation to muscular contraction is recorded by electrodes placed on the skin surface.

Nerve conduction times evaluate the integrity of the myelin and axon of peripheral nerves. They are indicated in the diagnosis of peripheral neuropathies and neuromuscular disorders, such as Guillain-Barré syndrome.

Medical Management

Surgical Management

INTRACRANIAL SURGERY

Conventional intracranial surgery involves opening the skull to perform a surgical intervention on or near any of the intracranial structures. Surgery performed on the cerebral hemispheres is referred to as supratentorial; surgery performed in the brain stem or cerebellar region below the cerebral cortex is referred to as infratentorial.

USES

Intracranial surgery is done to remove a neoplasm, hematoma, or scar tissue causing seizures; clip or ligate an aneurysm; ligate an arteriovenous malformation (AVM) or other vascular abnormality; drain an abscess; repair a skull fracture; remove a foreign object; obtain tissue samples for biopsy; redirect CSF via a shunt; or relieve increased ICP.

PHYSICAL PREPARATION OF THE PATIENT

A written consent for the procedure is obtained. Routine preoperative laboratory tests include a complete blood count, serum electrolytes, coagulation profile, blood typing and crossmatching, an ECG, and chest x-ray examination. As a prophylactic measure, anticonvulsants such as phenytoin (Dilantin) and a glucocorticoid such as dexamethasone (Decadron) may be ordered preoperatively as a treatment for anticipated cortical irritation and cerebral edema. The area of the scalp to be incised is shaved and the area cleansed with antiseptic.

PROCEDURE

Craniotomy is the most common intracranial procedure. A craniotomy is an opening in the skull configured to form a bone flap. This is done by making several burr holes in the skull in the configuration required for exposure. A special saw with a guide wire is inserted into one burr hole under the bone and is brought up through the second burr hole. The surgeon is able to cut through the skull by alternately pulling on each end of the saw, allowing the bone to be cut from the inside of the skull out, avoiding injury to brain tissue. This process is repeated through each burr hole until a bone flap is made (Fig. 37–30). The bone flap is replaced at the conclusion of the surgery. A craniectomy is removal of part of the skull. This may vary from a small burr hole to an area of several centimeters. This approach is used for surgery in the posterior fossa (brain-stem

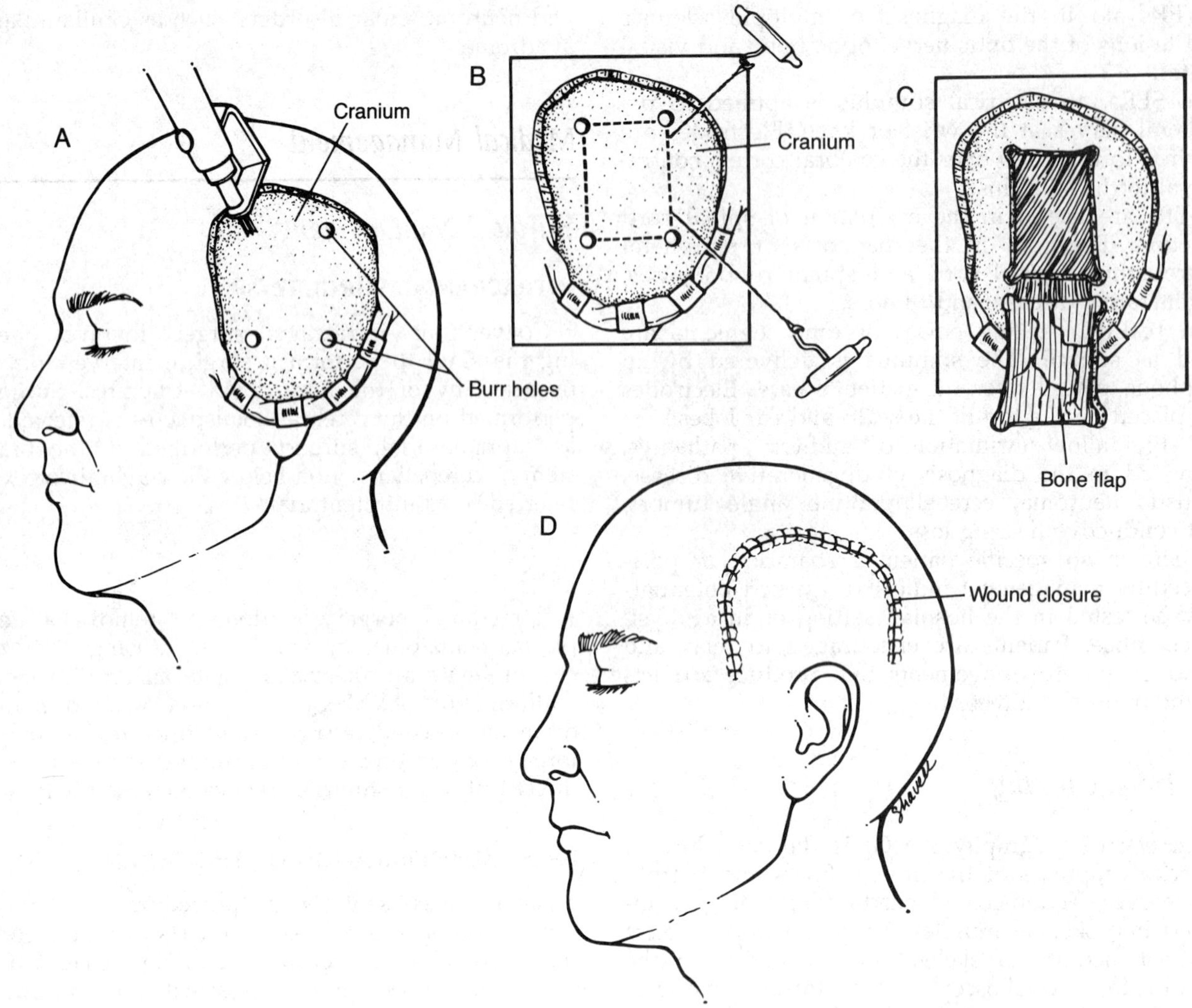

Figure 37–30.

Craniotomy procedure. *A*, Burr holes drilled in skull; *B*, skull cut between burr holes with a surgical saw; *C*, bone flap turned back to expose cranial contents; *D*, bone flap replaced and wound closed.

region). A cranioplasty is the placement of a synthetic plate or bone graft onto an area that is defective or opened. The incision for supratentorial surgery is made behind the hairline. The incision for infratentorial surgery is made just above the nape of the neck.

POSTPROCEDURE COURSE

The prognosis for recovery for a patient who has had a craniotomy is dependent on the nature and location of the brain lesion.

Occasionally patients may have permanent physical and mental handicaps such as paralysis, aphasia, skull defects, personality changes, or severe depression. Residual disorders such as diplopia may be temporary.

A patient who has surgery for the removal of a brain tumor may have received a dye (fluorescein sodium) intravenously to aid in locating the lesion during surgery. The dye causes the skin and sclera of the patient to appear jaundiced for several days after surgery.

If supratentorial surgery was performed, the patient may have generalized facial edema and may be unable to open one or both eyes. Discoloration (ecchymosis) of the skin around the eyes may also be present. These conditions usually improve within 3 to 4 days postoperatively.

Sometimes a catheter is left in place in the lateral ventricle to drain excessive amounts of CSF and to prevent increased ICP. This is usually removed by the neurosurgeon 24 to 48 hours after surgery.

After infratentorial surgery, the head dressing may extend down to the shoulders to prevent movement of the head and neck. Sutures are usually removed by the surgeon on the fifth day after supratentorial surgery and on the seventh day after infratentorial surgery. When the final dressings are removed, the healed wound may be covered by a stockinet cap or scarf or left open to the air.

After infratentorial surgery, the gag and swallowing reflexes may be impaired; therefore, the patient is kept NPO for 24 hours and intravenous fluids are administered. These are given slowly to prevent increased ICP. If difficulty in swallowing persists, tube feedings may be necessary and are usually begun 48 hours after surgery. On the second day after supratentorial surgery, a regular diet is generally ordered as tolerated. Any patient who has had brain surgery is usually fed for 48 hours to prevent overexertion.

Patients are generally not allowed out of bed until the third to fifth postoperative day after infratentorial surgery, but those who have had supratentorial surgery may be allowed to sit in a chair in 24 to 48 hours. See Table 37–10 for a summary comparison of supratentorial and infratentorial surgery.

COMPLICATIONS

Increased ICP may result from brain edema or intracranial bleeding after a craniotomy. A progressive impairment of responsiveness, such as diminishing responses to stimuli, significant changes in vital signs, increased restlessness, paralysis of the extremities, changes in vision, dilated pupils, and increasing headaches, may be indicative of increased ICP.

Respiratory complications and hyperthermia or hypothermia may develop, especially after infratentorial surgery, because the incision is made adjacent to the medulla and vital centers.

Convulsions are not uncommon after any intracranial surgery, but there is an even greater risk after supratentorial surgery. The physician usually orders Dilantin or phenobarbital, or both, to prevent their occurrence.

Other complications that may develop after a craniotomy are meningitis and wound infection.

Application of the Nursing Process to the Care of the Patient Undergoing Intracranial Surgery

PREOPERATIVE NURSING CARE

Assess and document the patient's neurologic status, including level of consciousness, motor and sensory function, pupils, and cranial nerve function. Record vital signs and respiratory status to provide a baseline for intraoperative and postoperative comparisons.

Assess the patient's and family's understanding of the medical problem and the procedure to be performed. Be sure to ascertain whether expectations in regard to the patient's prognosis are realistic.

Recognize that anxiety and apprehension are expected in any patient facing surgery but are greatly intensified in the patient scheduled for brain surgery. The patient and family may be concerned about permanent disability, loss of cognitive abilities, and death. Encourage the patient and family to express their feelings by providing time and privacy and acknowledging a willingness to listen.

Explain in simple terms the preoperative routines, and provide information about the postoperative phase, including routine monitoring equipment used and anticipated tubes such as intravenous catheters and an indwelling urinary catheter. Instruct the patient in effective deep breathing if able.

***Table* 37–10.** COMPARISON OF SUPRATENTORIAL SURGERY AND INFRATENTORIAL SURGERY

VARIABLE	SUPRATENTORIAL	INFRATENTORIAL
Location of surgery	Cerebral hemispheres	Brain-stem or cerebellar region
Postoperative effects	Generalized facial edema Inability to open one or both eyes Ecchymosis around the eyes	Impaired gag and swallow reflexes
Common complications	Convulsions	Respiratory center impairment Hyperthermia Hypothermia
Dressing	Encircles head like a bathing cap	Encircles head and supports neck to prevent flexion
Activity	OOB in 24–48 hours	OOB after 3–5 days
Diet	Fluids when alert Regular diet as tolerated on second postoperative day	NPO status for at least 24 hours If dysphagia persists, tube feedings started after 48 hours
Suture removal	Fifth postoperative day	Seventh postoperative day

Abbreviations: OOB, out of bed; NPO, nothing by mouth.

POSTOPERATIVE NURSING CARE

Assessment

The postoperative care of a patient after a craniotomy is complex and requires keen assessment skills. This care is generally provided in a critical care unit until the patient's condition stabilizes.

Begin assessment of the patient after a craniotomy with the measurement of vital and neurologic signs: temperature, pulse, respirations, blood pressure, pupillary and other reflexes, level of consciousness, arm lifts, handgrips, leg lifts, and ankle plantar flexion and dorsiflexion.

Frequency of these assessments depends on the neurosurgeon's orders and the nurse's judgment of the patient's condition and may range from every 5 to every 30 minutes for the first 6 postoperative hours. As the patient's condition stabilizes, decrease the frequency of these assessments to every 2 to 4 hours. At all times, interpret these findings in view of the baseline data obtained preoperatively, and report any significant changes to the neurosurgeon immediately.

Carefully assess respiratory status. Because surgical trauma may impair the function of the respiratory center, observe depth and pattern of respiration and check blood gas values. Because surgical trauma may also impair the function of the vagus and glossopharyngeal nerves and thus cause paralysis of the muscles involved with swallowing, carefully observe the unconscious patient for the accumulation of secretions, which can be aspirated. Remember that patients who have had infratentorial surgery are at the greatest risk for these effects.

Inspect the patient's head dressing for signs of abnormal bleeding and for clear or yellowish drainage, which may indicate leakage of CSF. Because severe headache may occur during the first 2 postoperative days, assess for signs of restlessness and discomfort. Observe for seizures, which are most common after supratentorial surgery, although they can also follow infratentorial surgery. Also observe for signs of gastrointestinal or urinary tract involvement. When the head dressing is removed, inspect the incision for bulging, redness, drainage, or suture disruption.

Nursing Diagnoses and Planning

Nursing diagnoses and related expected patient outcomes most commonly applicable to patients who have had intracranial surgery include the following:

NDx: Pain related to surgical trauma of the scalp and cranial tissues

Planning: Patient outcomes
1. Patient rests quietly.
2. Patient reports pain is relieved or manageable.

NDx: High risk for impaired gas exchange related to postanesthetic state

Planning: Patient outcomes
1. Patent airway is maintained.
2. Patient maintains regular respiratory pattern of 12 to 24 breaths per minute.

NDx: High risk for altered tissue perfusion: cerebral, related to postoperative cerebral edema

Planning: Patient outcomes
1. Patient maintains or improves neurologic status.

NDx: High risk for infection related to break in skin integrity

Planning: Patient outcomes
1. Patient is afebrile.
2. Incision is clean and approximated.
3. Purulent drainage is absent.

Nursing Interventions

NDx: Pain
Medicate the patient as ordered for head pain, keeping in mind that narcotics and most barbiturates are contraindicated after brain surgery because they can cause respiratory depression and mask signs of increasing ICP. To further promote comfort, keep the patient's environment dim and free of loud noise. Avoid sudden or jarring movement of the patient. Apply ice packs to the head if ordered. Report increasingly severe prolonged or newly occurring headache to the physician because it may indicate increasing ICP.

NDx: High risk for impaired gas exchange
Suction the patient as needed to clear the airway of secretions. Keep in mind that general anesthetic agents may depress the cough reflex as well as cause residual relaxation of muscles in the immediate postoperative phase. Maintaining a patent airway provides adequate air exchange, preventing hypercarbia, which could potentiate an increase in ICP. Administer oxygen therapy as ordered. If the patient is conscious, coach him or her in deep breathing but make certain to instruct the patient not to cough vigorously because this can increase ICP. Turn the patient frequently to further promote adequate ventilation of all lung areas.

NDx: High risk for altered tissue perfusion: cerebral
The patient who has intracranial surgery is at risk for increased ICP secondary to cerebral edema. Position the patient who has had a craniotomy with the head elevated 30 to 45 degrees to promote venous and CSF drainage from the head. Position the patient on the back or on the side opposite the

incision. If the patient is unconscious, make certain the neck is not twisted or flexed because this also inhibits venous return and flow of CSF. Never position the patient with the head lowered, because the increased blood flow to the brain can cause an increase in ICP.

If the patient has had infratentorial surgery, support the head with a small pillow and align carefully because the infratentorial incision disrupts the neck muscles, which support the head.

Administer hypertonic urea, mannitol, or steroids as ordered to decrease postoperative edema. Monitor for both therapeutic and adverse effects. Also restrict fluids as ordered. Because metabolic disturbances, which cause a decrease in urinary output, may occur after intracranial surgery, record fluid intake and output. Also record bowel elimination, keeping in mind that cathartics and enemas are usually contraindicated after intracranial surgery because straining at stool and absorption of fluid can cause an increase in ICP. Alert the neurosurgeon to signs of fecal impaction.

NDx: High risk for infection

The surgical incision site presents an open break in the protective skin barrier and a potential site for normal flora to proliferate and enter the body, producing infection. Record temperature, and report elevations of 2°F or more. Administer prophylactic antibiotics as ordered. Wash hands thoroughly before and after patient contact. Use strict aseptic technique when handling drains at the operative site. Monitor the head dressing for unexpected drainage of blood or CSF. Report drainage to the physician immediately because moisture at the incision provides a medium for bacterial growth. When the dressing is removed, cleanse the operative site as directed by the neurosurgeon.

Additional Interventions

Apply lightweight ice packs to the eyes to decrease periorbital edema after coating the tissues lightly with petrolatum.

After supratentorial surgery, give fluids as desired as soon as the patient is alert provided there is no dysphagia or nausea. Progress to a regular diet as tolerated. Keep in mind that it is critical for the patient to avoid vomiting because it increases ICP. After infratentorial surgery, keep the patient on NPO status for at least 24 hours. Begin giving small amounts of fluid when swallow and gag reflexes return and bowel sounds are heard. Gradually progress diet as tolerated. Provide assistance as needed with feeding because the patient may have problems with actions such as controlling the tongue and raising the arms as a result of the effects of surgery on the cranial nerves.

For the first 48 hours after surgery, provide total nursing care. Thereafter, provide care as required by the type of surgery and the patient's functional ability. Whenever possible, encourage the patient to participate in care, whether it be physical participation or making judgments in terms of timing and sequence of care, what to wear, or what to drink.

Evaluation

Evaluate the effectiveness of nursing care for a patient who has had intracranial surgery by comparing the patient's status with the expected patient outcomes. Examples of specific outcomes for patients who have had intracranial surgery have been provided in the Planning section.

SPINAL SURGERY

USES

Spinal surgery is performed to remove spinal cord tumors, to correct fractures of the vertebrae secondary to trauma, to remove spinal cord AVMs, and, most commonly, to remove a herniated or ruptured intervertebral disk.

PROCEDURE

Laminectomy is the removal of all or part of the vertebral lamina to gain access to the spinal cord and nerve roots. In the case of a herniated or ruptured disk, this procedure allows protruding disk material pressing on the spinal nerve to be removed. Laminectomy is also performed to remove neoplasms of the spine. In this case, the amount of bony lamina removed is larger to allow for a wider exposure for tumor removal. Cervical laminectomy may be done through either an anterior or a posterior approach. A spinal fusion is the union of two or three vertebrae, generally performed after a laminectomy, when indicated, to provide stability to the vertebral column. A microdiskectomy is the excision of displaced intervertebral material using a microscope. The incision is smaller than that required for a laminectomy, resulting in less postoperative discomfort and a shorter hospital stay.

COMPLICATIONS

Complications of spinal surgery include respiratory failure as a result of cord compression and urinary retention caused by irritation of autonomic fibers. There is also the risk of hemorrhage and infection.

POSTPROCEDURE COURSE

The postprocedure course varies with the specific surgical procedure performed and with the underlying medical problem. Whenever laminectomy is done, maintenance of alignment of the spine is critical. Position is restricted, pain is usually significant, and movement is gradually resumed.

With microdiskectomy, there is little limitation on movement and little postoperative pain. The patient is out of bed on the evening of surgery and goes home on about the third postoperative day.

Application of the Nursing Process to the Care of the Patient Undergoing Spinal Surgery

PREOPERATIVE NURSING CARE

Nursing care for patients scheduled for spinal surgery is similar to that for any preoperative patient, with several considerations. Be sure to obtain data regarding initial onset of symptoms, precipitating event (if any), and the degree of pain or discomfort the patient is experiencing. Determine whether the patient is taking medication for pain relief. Assess neurologic status, particularly motor and sensory function. Assess the presence of bowel or bladder involvement, particularly if the cause is related to neoplasm or trauma.

POSTOPERATIVE NURSING CARE

Assessment

Postoperatively, assess neurologic status, and note deviations from baseline. Keep in mind that upper or lower extremity weakness can be the first sign of cord compression and impending paralysis. If the patient has had cervical surgery, assess for sensation in the arms, upper back, shoulder, and neck. If the patient had anterior cervical surgery, also assess for dysphagia resulting from esophageal edema secondary to esophageal trauma during surgery as well as hoarseness and inability to cough because of laryngeal nerve trauma. Assess also for signs of respiratory difficulty as a result of airway compression from bleeding and aspiration. Inspect the neck for swelling, which can be indicative of hemorrhage. Observe the dressing for serosanguineous drainage, which can indicate a dural leak and pose the threat of meningitis. Monitor vital signs for indications of hypovolemia or hyperpyrexia. If the patient has had lumbosacral surgery, check dorsalis pedis and posterior tibial pulses. Note the color and temperature of the legs, and check for sensation in the lower back, buttocks, legs, and toes. Determine the patient's level of comfort, and check the dressing for bleeding or CSF at frequent intervals. Assess for urinary retention. Assess the patient's ability to progress in ambulation. If bone was taken from the iliac crest or fibula for a fusion, monitor the donor site for hematoma formation. Assess the patient's pain at both the site of the spinal surgery and the donor site. Remember that the sudden reappearance of radicular pain can indicate extrusion of the graft.

Nursing Diagnoses and Planning

Nursing diagnoses and related expected patient outcomes most commonly applicable to patients who have had spinal surgery include the following:

NDx: Pain related to edema secondary to tissue trauma and muscle spasms secondary to irritation of nerves intraoperatively

Planning: Patient outcomes
1. Patient rests quietly.
2. Patient states that pain is relieved or manageable.

NDx: High risk for tissue trauma related to displacement of the bone graft after spinal fusion

Planning: Patient outcomes
1. Patient complies with positioning and activity instructions designed to protect the bone graft from extrusion.
2. Sudden reappearance of radicular pain indicative of graft extrusion is absent.

NDx: High risk for injury related to lightheadedness secondary to postural hypotension

Planning: Patient outcomes
1. Patient resumes activities gradually.
2. Patient remains free of injury.

NDx: High risk for urinary retention related to effects of anesthesia or trauma to nerves innervating the bladder

Planning: Patient outcomes
1. Palpable bladder distention is absent.
2. Patient voids sufficient quantity of urine at 3- to 4-hour intervals.

NDx: High risk for altered health maintenance related to insufficient knowledge of self-care after spinal surgery

Planning: Patient outcomes
1. Patient describes self-care requirements after discharge.
2. Patient expresses willingness and ability to comply with self-care requirements.

Nursing Interventions

NDx: Pain

Surgical manipulation causes irritation to the nerves and local edema, which contribute to pain. Administer prescribed analgesics for pain and discomfort caused by the incision and muscle spasm as necessary and at least a half-hour before position changes. After a lumbar laminectomy, pain and spasms occur in the lower body, abdomen, or thighs. After a cervical laminectomy, pain and spasms occur in the upper back, shoulder, neck, or arms. If more than one analgesic is prescribed, determine the severity of the patient's pain, and select the analgesic to be administered accordingly. Monitor for untoward side effects of analgesics, such as respiratory depression, nausea, or constipation. Discuss the pain-management regimen with the patient, and encourage the use of alternate pain-relieving techniques such as the use of imagery and relaxation. For patients with a sore throat, hoarseness, or dysphagia, provide a full liquid to soft diet and anesthetic lozenges as ordered. Also humidify the room, and encourage the patient to rest the voice.

NDx: High risk for tissue trauma

After spinal surgery, maintain correct spinal alignment at all times. For the first 48 hours after surgery, use a turn sheet to logroll the patient for position changes with the help of another nurse or assistant; do not let the patient assist. After this initial period, the patient may be logrolled by one person or may begin to logroll himself or herself.

After cervical surgery, keep the cervical collar on the patient at all times to support the head in a neutral position, thus preventing flexion or extension, which could displace the graft. Place a small pad under the patient's head when in a side-lying position to maintain neck alignment and to protect the ears from pressure. Do not use pillows, which, because of their thickness, alter alignment of the spine. Never position patients who have had posterior-approach surgery on their back. Use a side-lying position only to prevent pressure on the incision. Elevate the head of the bed to a comfortable position per the surgeon's direction. Encourage deep breathing, but do not encourage coughing, because it can lead to extrusion of the cervical bone graft.

After lumbosacral spinal surgery, position the patient off the operative site and keep the bed flat or elevated 5 to 10 degrees. Place a small pillow under the patient's head and at intervals under the knees to relax the muscles of the back. Use a pull sheet to move the patient up in bed.

NDx: High risk for injury

The patient who has undergone spinal surgery is required to remain on bed rest and in some cases has also been on bed rest before surgery. If the patient has been supine for an extended length of time, orthostatic changes may occur when he or she first attempts to sit up. Have the patient sit on the edge of the bed, dangle his or her feet, and breathe deeply for 5 minutes before standing. Check blood pressure while sitting, and compare it with the blood pressure obtained in the supine position. If the systolic pressure has fallen 10 mm Hg or more, consider the patient at risk for postural hypotension when standing. Have two persons provide support for the patient who is getting out of bed for the first time after spinal surgery.

If diminished sensation is present, protect the involved area from injury. For example, instruct the patient to visually check the position and location of the affected extremity.

NDx: High risk for urinary retention

Retention of urine after spinal surgery may be due to the depressant effects of perioperative drugs or to sympathetic fiber stimulation during lumbar laminectomy. An indwelling urinary catheter may be used but is usually removed as soon as possible to minimize the risk of infection. Palpate the bladder for distention. Provide privacy for urination. Use a fracture pan for female patients after lumbar laminectomy. Allow male patients to stand to urinate if allowed. Monitor intake and output accurately. Obtain an order to catheterize the patient if he or she is unable to void within 6 hours of removal of the catheter. If urinary retention is more than a temporary effect, teach the patient to palpate his or her own bladder and to catheterize self intermittently if this is part of the overall plan of care.

NDx: High risk for altered health maintenance

Instruct patients who have had cervical surgery to wear the cervical collar as directed by the surgeon, usually for about 6 weeks.

Instruct patients who have had lumbosacral surgery that activity must be increased only gradually because it takes 6 weeks for the ligaments to heal. Suggest the use of heat to soothe muscle spasms and to promote healing. Caution the patient to avoid activities such as driving that produce strain on the spine. Perform exercises as prescribed by the surgeon, and avoid heavy work for 2 to 3 months.

Additional Interventions

Provide good skin care to prevent the development of pressure sores. Change dressing immediately if contaminated with urine or feces to decrease the risk of infection. Report any bloody or CSF drainage on the dressing.

Encourage the patient to ingest a high-fiber diet and increase fluid intake, because constipation is a risk as a result of decreased activity and perioperative medications that decrease peristalsis.

If a donor site is present, check regularly for bleeding or drainage. Keep the site covered with a dry, sterile dressing, and position the patient to prevent excessive pressure on the area.

Evaluation

Evaluate the effectiveness of nursing care for a patient who has had spinal surgery by comparing the patient's status with the expected patient outcomes. Examples of specific outcomes for patients who have had spinal surgery have been provided in the Planning section.

The Elderly: Special Considerations

Age-Related Changes in the Nervous System

STRUCTURAL CHANGES

Secondary to the aging process, there is a steady loss of neurons in the brain and spinal cord. Neuronal loss is a gradual and variable process, occurring throughout the life span, but is dramatically associated with later life, after age 70, and is most pronounced in the frontal lobes of the cortex. Neuronal losses influence brain weight, contributing to a 10% to 12% brain weight loss by very old age. It has long been postulated that excessive neuronal loss can be linked with Alzheimer's disease. However, research has indicated that the number of cells in the brain of a person with Alzheimer's disease at autopsy is no different from those present in normal individuals of the same age. Neurofibrillar tangles and neuritic plaque formation in the brain occur in small amounts in the normal older adult. However, a large increase in plaques and tangles is found in individuals with senile dementia and Alzheimer's disease.

FUNCTIONAL CHANGES

Reaction time (i.e., the lag between stimulation and the initiation of a response) increases with age. Although the older person may be slower to react to situations and integrate information, the ability to learn is not impaired. Recent memory, also called short-term memory, is affected by the aging process; long-term memory is not. Sleep patterns may be altered in the older adult. The total amount of time of deep sleep decreases, and the aged person tends to wake more during sleep time as well as stay awake more during the night. This is usually compensated for by taking a nap during the day.

CHANGES IN THE SPECIAL SENSES

Normal age-related changes in vision include a decrease in visual acuity, intolerance of glare, inability to adapt to dark and light, and a decrease in peripheral vision. Hearing loss for high-frequency sound is an age-related change. Older persons have difficulty in distinguishing words spoken too fast. Age-related changes occur in taste buds responsible for perception of sweet and salty flavors. Tactile sensation decreases with age, making it difficult to discriminate temperature and perform fine motor tasks.

It is important to remember that age-related changes may occur in varying degrees among individuals. These changes are normal to the aging process. Diseases that tend to occur in later life are not necessarily the expected outcome of aging but rather the result of a pathologic process. Although changes do occur in the nervous system, it cannot be assumed that senility or impairment of cognition is synonymous with aging.

Bibliography

Ad Hoc Committee of the Harvard Medical School to Examine the Definition of Brain Death. A definition of irreversible coma. JAMA 1968; 205:337.

Adams RD, Victor M. Principles of neurology. 4th ed. New York: McGraw-Hill, 1989.

Adams RD, Victor M. Principles of neurology companion handbook. New York: McGraw-Hill, 1991.

Asbury AK, McKhann GM, McDonald WI. Diseases of the nervous system: Clinical neurobiology. 2nd ed. Philadelphia: WB Saunders, 1992.

Burgess KE. "Inside" increased I.C.P. Nurs Life 1985; 5(2):35.

Cammermeyer M, Appeldorn C (eds). Core curriculum for neuroscience nursing. 3rd ed. Chicago: American Association Neuroscience Nurses, 1990.

Carpenito L. Handbook of nursing diagnosis. 4th ed. New York: JB Lippincott, 1991.

Carpenito LJ. Nursing diagnosis: Application to clinical practice. 4th ed. Philadelphia: JB Lippincott, 1992.

Chadwick D, Cartlidge NEF, Bates D. Medical neurology. New York: Churchill Livingstone, 1989.

Dolan JT. Critical care nursing: Clinical management through the nursing process. Philadelphia: FA Davis, 1990.

Esberger KK, Hughes ST. Nursing care of the aged. Norwalk, CT: Appleton & Lange, 1989.

Gilroy J. Basic neurology. 2nd ed. New York: McGraw-Hill, 1990.

Goldberg S. Clinical neuroanatomy made ridiculously simple. North Miami Beach, FL: MedMaster, Inc, 1986.

Grossman RG, Hamilton WJ (eds). Principles of neurosurgery. New York: Raven Press, 1991.

Gunderson CH. Essentials of clinical neurology. New York: Raven Press, 1990.

Guyton AC. Basic neuroscience: Anatomy and physiology. 2nd ed. Philadelphia: WB Saunders, 1992.

Henry GL. Neurologic emergencies: 1. The basic assessment. Emerg Med 1988; 20(30):29.

Hickey J. The clinical practice of neurological and neurosurgical nursing. 3rd ed. New York: JB Lippincott, 1992.

Jacobson AL, Donlon WC. Headache and facial pain: Diagnosis and management. New York: Raven Press, 1990.

Johnson LK. If your patient has increased intracranial pressure, your goal should be: No surprises. Nursing 83 1983; 13(6):58.

Lee BY, Ostrander L, Cochran G, Shaw W (eds). The spinal cord injured patient: Comprehensive management. Philadelphia: WB Saunders, 1991.

Lindsay KW, Bone I, Callander R. Neurology and neurosurgery illustrated. New York: Churchill Livingstone, 1991.

Lower J. Rapid neuro assessment. Am J Nurs 1992; 92(6):38.

Lundgren J. Acute neuroscience nursing: Concepts and care. Boston: Jones and Bartlett, 1986.

Marsden CD, Fowler TJ (eds). Clinical neurology. New York: Raven Press, 1989.

Marshall SB, Marshall LF, Vos HR, Chesnut RM. Neuroscience critical care: Pathophysiology and patient management. Philadelphia: WB Saunders, 1990.

Matteson MA, McDonnell ES. Gerontological nursing concepts and practice. Philadelphia: WB Saunders, 1989.

Mitchell PH, Cammermeyer M, Ozuna J, Woods NF. Neurological assessment for nursing practice. Reston, VA: Reston Publishing, 1984.

Mitchell PH, Hodges LC, Muwaswes M, Walleck CA (eds). AANN's neuroscience nursing. Norwalk, CT: Appleton & Lange, 1988.

Shekleton M, Litwack K. Critical care nursing of the surgical patient. Philadelphia: WB Saunders, 1991.

St. Clair KM, Bove LA. What you can do to prevent increased ICP. Nurs Life 1987; 7(2):50.

Stevens SA, Becker KL. Neurologic assessment: Part 1. Nursing 88 1988; 18(9):54.

Stevens SA, Becker KL. Neurologic assessment: Part 2. Nursing 88 1988; 18(10):51.

Taylor J, Raimond J. Neurological emergencies: Effective nursing care. Rockville, MD: Aspen Systems, 1986.

Chapter Thirty-eight

NURSING CARE *of Adults with* Nervous System Disorders

Disorders of the nervous system can be insidious in onset, with symptoms presenting that are characteristic of many systemic diseases. Neurologic disorders also directly affect function as a human being, that is, the ability to think, to feel, to communicate, and to move. Many neurologic disorders, whether acute or gradual in onset, are chronic in nature and often characterized by progressive deterioration of function. Because the brain cannot regenerate and suffers irreversible damage in a matter of minutes if its supply of oxygen and nutrients is impaired, many neurologic disorders also carry the threat of sudden death. Thus, accurate assessment and rapid intervention paired with sensitivity to the needs of both the patient and significant others are essential to nursing care.

Infections and Inflammations

Meningitis

Meningitis is defined as an inflammation of the meninges of the brain. Two types of meningitis exist: bacterial and viral. The most frequently occurring type of meningitis is bacterial.

BACTERIAL MENINGITIS

ETIOLOGY

The causative organisms responsible for bacterial meningitis are many. The most common ones include *Staphylococcus, Streptococcus,* and *Diplococcus pneumoniae* (gram-positive cocci); *Escherichia coli, Klebsiella* species and *Pseudomonas* (gram-negative rods); *Haemophilus influenzae* (gram-negative cocci); and *Neisseria meningitidis* (gram-negative diplococci).

Staphylococcus, Streptococcus, Diplococcus, N. meningitidis, and *H. influenzae* are normal inhabitants of the oral and nasal cavities. Because of the close proximity to the sinuses, conditions such as sinusitis, otitis media, upper respiratory tract infection or pneumonia, and direct trauma to the ears, nose, or sinuses predispose to entry of these organisms into the central nervous system. *E. coli, Klebsiella, Pseudomonas,* and others can be inadvertently introduced into the central nervous system during neurosurgical procedures, lumbar puncture, and spinal anesthesia or can be introduced secondary to trauma.

PATHOPHYSIOLOGY

Entry of organisms into the central nervous system occurs predominately via the blood stream. The pia mater and arachnoid layers of the meninges as well as the subarachnoid space containing cerebrospinal fluid are affected. The purulent exudate spreads quickly via the free-flowing cerebrospinal fluid. Inflammatory lesions caused by the accumulation of exudate can form, particularly around the base of the brain. The blood vessels of the meninges can become engorged secondary to the inflammatory changes, and thrombosis or rupture may occur. Early treatment of the infectious process is critical to prevent adhesions and scarring, resulting in hydrocephalus.

CLINICAL MANIFESTATIONS

The signs and symptoms manifested by the patient with bacterial meningitis occur in response to the bacterial invasion and are not particular to any one organism. The exception to this is meningococcal meningitis, caused by *N. meningitidis,* in which 50% of patients acquire a petechial rash, purpuric lesions, or ecchymosis.

The patient with bacterial meningitis usually presents with headache and fever. The headache is generally severe and is usually the initial symptom. Variations in level of consciousness may be present in the early stage. These include poor attention span, irritability and restlessness, disorientation, and hallucinations. The patient's level of responsiveness may fluctuate and may decrease with progression of the illness.

Signs of meningeal irritation are also present. These include nuchal rigidity and Kernig's and Brudzinski's signs (Fig. 38–1). Nuchal rigidity or stiff neck is manifested by the patient's tendency to keep the neck extended and immobile. Attempts to flex the neck forward cause pain. Kernig's sign is the inability to extend the leg from a position of 90% flexion at the hip. If attempts to extend the leg cause pain and spasms in the hamstrings, it is considered positive. A positive Brudzinski's sign occurs when passive flexion of the head and neck onto the chest results in a flexion response of the thighs and legs.

Other signs and symptoms that can occur include photophobia, cranial nerve dysfunctions, and generalized convulsions secondary to the irritation of the cerebral cortex.

MEDICAL DIAGNOSIS

A careful history and physical examination are necessary to obtain pertinent information to aid in the diagnosis of meningitis. A history of any preceding infections, particularly involving the ears, sinuses, or respiratory tract, as well as any evidence of recent exposure to individuals known or suspected to have meningitis, provides additional support to the diagnosis. The presence of headache, fever, and meningeal irritation on physical examination is also suggestive of meningitis.

The definitive diagnostic measure is the lumbar puncture. Data that indicate bacterial meningitis include turbid, cloudy fluid, a markedly increased white blood cell count and protein content, and a decreased glucose content. The opening pressure on lumbar puncture is also elevated (greater than

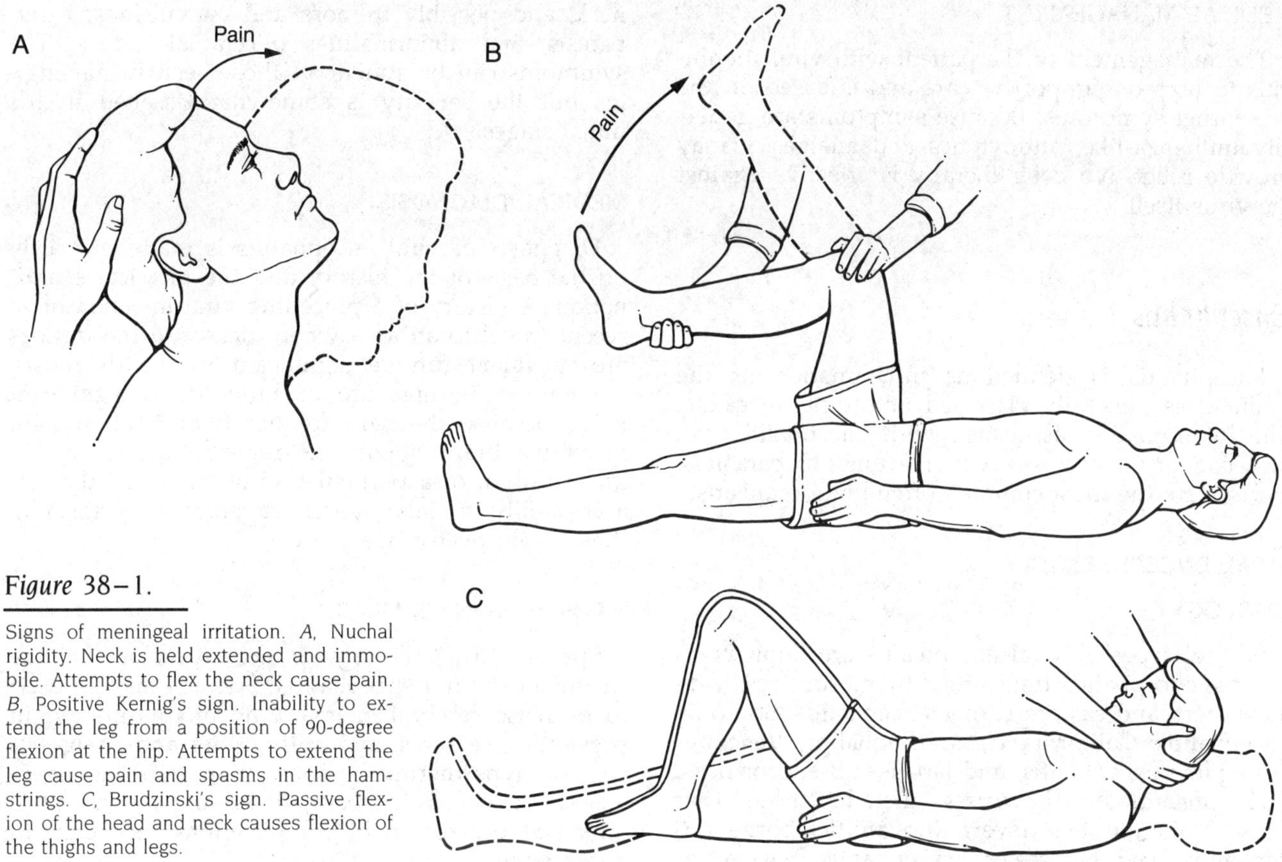

Figure 38–1.

Signs of meningeal irritation. *A*, Nuchal rigidity. Neck is held extended and immobile. Attempts to flex the neck cause pain. *B*, Positive Kernig's sign. Inability to extend the leg from a position of 90-degree flexion at the hip. Attempts to extend the leg cause pain and spasms in the hamstrings. *C*, Brudzinski's sign. Passive flexion of the head and neck causes flexion of the thighs and legs.

180 mm water). Gram's stain and culture reports indicate the causative organism.

Other laboratory findings that may be of significance include skull and sinus x-ray films as well as cultures of the nose, throat, blood, and any other infected sites.

MEDICAL MANAGEMENT

The focus of medical management of the patient with bacterial meningitis is prompt initiation of antibiotic treatment with broad-spectrum antimicrobials before obtaining the culture reports. Once the causative organism is known, drug therapy is continued for at least 10 days, using the most effective drug or drugs specific to that bacteria.

Isolation procedures are not routinely required for the patient with bacterial meningitis. However, respiratory isolation until the patient has received antibiotic therapy for 24 hours is generally adhered to. The individual institution's policies on infection control should be followed.

VIRAL MENINGITIS

ETIOLOGY AND PATHOPHYSIOLOGY

Viral meningitis, also referred to as aseptic meningitis, almost uniformly occurs as a complication of a primary viral infection outside the central nervous system. The most common viruses are the enteroviruses, mumps virus, herpes virus, and arboviruses. The most frequent portals of entry of these viruses are the oral, fecal-oral, or respiratory pathways. Once the virus enters the body, it replicates and spreads to the brain via the blood stream.

CLINICAL MANIFESTATIONS

Viral meningitis usually begins with abrupt onset of fever, headache, stiff neck, and occasional vomiting. Mental status changes such as irritability or slight lethargy may be present. Confusion and severe lethargy are rare. It is often difficult to distinguish between bacterial and viral meningitis on the basis of symptomatology alone.

MEDICAL DIAGNOSIS

The diagnosis of viral meningitis is made on the basis of history and physical examination as well as laboratory data from a lumbar puncture and cerebrospinal fluid analysis. In viral meningitis, the protein content of the cerebrospinal fluid is normal or slightly increased, and the glucose content is normal. No bacteria are reported on Gram's stain or cultures.

MEDICAL MANAGEMENT

The management of the patient with viral meningitis focuses on supportive care and is based on the presenting symptoms. Because symptoms are generally influenza-like, antipyretics and analgesics may provide relief. No drug therapy is effective against the virus itself.

Encephalitis

Encephalitis is defined as inflammation of the brain. It is generally classified according to cause. The inflammation associated with encephalitis can be secondary to viruses, bacteria, fungi, or parasites. Viruses are the most common offending organisms.

VIRAL ENCEPHALITIS

ETIOLOGY

Several types of viral encephalitis are known: arbovirus encephalitis transmitted by mosquitoes, such as western and eastern equine encephalitis; St. Louis encephalitis; California virus encephalitis; Venezuelan equine encephalitis, and Japanese B encephalitis. Tick-transmitted arboviruses include those that cause Colorado tick fever, Russian tick-borne encephalitis, and far eastern encephalitis. Several of these viruses are endemic to certain geographic regions as well as to seasons of the year. Less frequent causes of viral encephalitis include vaccines for smallpox, measles, mumps, and rabies; viral infections such as measles, mumps, infectious mononucleosis, and rubella; and toxins from ingested substances such as lead and arsenic.

PATHOPHYSIOLOGY

Viruses require the assistance of a living host to reproduce. Viruses gain access to the central nervous system through the systemic circulation or through the cranial and peripheral nerves. The virus "takes over" the normal activities of brain cells to reproduce and maintain itself. This process causes inflammation without exudate in the cells of the cortex, resulting in degenerative changes. Widespread edema, compression of blood vessels, hemorrhage, cavitation, and necrosis can occur in a scattered pattern throughout the brain.

CLINICAL MANIFESTATIONS

The onset of symptoms is usually gradual, initially manifested by fever, malaise, headache, listlessness, joint pain, nausea, and vomiting. Within a few days, neurologic symptoms appear. These may include alterations in level of consciousness such as confusion and stupor, ataxia, photophobia, stiff neck, and possibly tremors and convulsions, hemiparesis, and abnormalities of cranial nerves. The symptoms can be similar to those seen in meningitis, but the severity is somewhat lessened in the initial stages.

MEDICAL DIAGNOSIS

Diagnosis of viral encephalitis is made primarily on the basis of the history and the physical examination. A history of a preceding viral infection or of recent travel to an area where ticks and mosquitoes are prevalent can be significant to the diagnosis. Laboratory findings are of little to no significant value because they are frequently normal in viral infections. Brain biopsy and tissue culture can aid in identification of a particular virus provided there is accessibility to laboratories capable of performing these sophisticated analyses.

MEDICAL MANAGEMENT

Specific drug therapy is not available for the treatment of viral encephalitis. Steroids may be used to decrease cerebral edema. Anticonvulsants aid in preventing seizures, and antipyretics and analgesics combat hyperthermia and assist in relieving headaches. The focus of treatment is supportive and is aimed at prevention of complications secondary to encephalitis.

HERPES SIMPLEX ENCEPHALITIS

ETIOLOGY

Herpes simplex encephalitis is the most common nonepidemic form of encephalitis in the United States. It can affect all age groups. It is caused by herpes simplex virus 1 or 2.

Herpes simplex virus 1 is associated with the common cold sore and is present in a dormant state in most people. It is capable of producing acute encephalitis in the adult through reactivation of the latent virus. Although the mechanisms for this reactivation are unclear, fever, emotional stress, and infectious diseases may play a role.

Herpes simplex virus 2 is associated with the sexually transmitted genital disease. It can cause encephalitis only in neonates who acquire it during passage through the birth canal of an infected mother. In adults, herpes simplex virus 2 causes aseptic (viral) meningitis in association with recent genital herpes simplex infections.

PATHOPHYSIOLOGY

The herpes simplex virus attacks the brain, particularly the temporal lobes, and causes destruction and necrosis of neurons. Pronounced cerebral edema occurs, resulting in increased intracranial pressure and possibly a herniation syndrome. It is unclear how the virus enters the central nervous system, but it is postulated that the probable routes of entry are the blood stream and the peripheral nerves. Herpes simplex encephalitis is associated with a 70% mortality if untreated.

CLINICAL MANIFESTATIONS

Generalized symptoms of headache, fever, vomiting, and altered mentation may appear several weeks after a primary infection. Focal neurologic deficits such as hemiparesis, seizures, bizarre behavioral manifestations, and aphasia may develop secondary to involvement of the temporal lobes. Stupor progressing to coma may occur secondary to increased intracranial pressure and diffuse cerebral edema. The mortality rate dramatically increases if progression to a comatose state occurs.

MEDICAL DIAGNOSIS

Diagnosis of herpes simplex encephalitis begins with the history and physical examination. The physical examination reveals an acutely ill patient demonstrating signs and symptoms discussed under Clinical Manifestations. Lumbar puncture may be performed to obtain cerebrospinal fluid for laboratory analysis. Protein content and white blood cell count are elevated. The glucose content is normal to low. Initially, the computed tomographic (CT) scan is normal but focal swelling, particularly in the frontal and temporal lobes, is seen on CT scan a few days after the onset of symptoms. Electroencephalograms (EEGs) show slowing of brain activity in the temporal areas and may indicate seizure activity. For a definitive diagnosis, a brain biopsy is necessary to obtain tissue samples for viral studies to isolate the herpes simplex virus.

MEDICAL MANAGEMENT

Emphasis is placed on the initiation of the limited measures available to treat herpes simplex encephalitis before the development of a comatose state. At present, two controversial methods of treatment with drug therapy exist: vidarabine (ara-A, Vira-A) and acyclovir (Zovirax). Both drugs are antiviral agents that interfere with deoxyribonucleic acid (DNA) synthesis. They are given intravenously, and their efficacy is questionable if not initiated promptly in the early stages of the inflammatory process. Controversy exists because the definitive diagnosis by brain biopsy takes time, and the potency and side effects of the drug therapies pose risks to the patient. Other treatment modalities include glucosteroids, such as dexamethasone (Decadron), to reduce edema and anticonvulsants to treat seizure activity. Intracranial pressure monitoring may be instituted.

Brain Abscess

ETIOLOGY AND PATHOPHYSIOLOGY

A brain abscess is the result of an infectious process either outside or within the central nervous system. Organisms from the infectious process migrate directly to brain tissue, forming a lesion, usually in the white matter of the brain. This lesion is filled with suppurative material and has the ability to enlarge and, therefore, behave as a space-occupying lesion within the cranium. This predisposes not only to the systemic effects of the inflammatory process but to the serious consequences of increased intracranial pressure.

The precipitating factors leading to the formation of a brain abscess are the presence of organisms and the ability of these organisms to gain entry into the brain tissue. Approximately 40% of all brain abscesses extend into the brain directly from middle-ear and mastoid infections. Sinus infections and direct trauma to the brain, allowing for immediate access, are responsible for another approximate 10%. The remaining 50% are the result of infections in other sites within the body that cause septic emboli to travel via the blood stream to the brain. Common sources of septic emboli include the lungs (lung abscesses); the heart (bacterial endocarditis or congenital heart disease); the pelvis (pelvic abscesses); and skin infections.

CLINICAL MANIFESTATIONS

The signs and symptoms exhibited depend on the location of the lesion. Initially, the patient exhibits the general symptomatology associated with an acute infectious process, such as chills, fever, malaise, anorexia, and myalgias. Because brain abscess formation generally occurs secondary to a previously existent infection, these signs may be considered by the patient to be an exacerbation of that illness. As the abscess enlarges, focal neurologic signs may develop, such as headache, nuchal rigidity, and vomiting. The patient continues to experience these symptoms but with increasing severity and persistence. Confusion, drowsiness, seizures, and signs of increased intracranial pressure or cranial nerve palsies may develop as the abscess continues to enlarge and compress surrounding structures.

MEDICAL DIAGNOSIS

Diagnosis of a brain abscess can present some difficulties because of the lack of definitive symptoms and the somewhat confusing clinical picture. A careful history specifically geared to the presence of a previous infection is helpful in suggesting the presence of a brain abscess. X-ray films of the chest, skull, and sinuses may help identify a primary source of infection. Lumbar puncture reveals a markedly elevated pressure (200 to 300 mm water), with protein content and white blood cell count dramatically elevated. Glucose content is normal and the culture and sensitivity are negative because the bacteria are contained within the abscess and have not invaded the cerebrospinal fluid. CT scan, brain scan, or arteriography assist in localizing the lesion and determining its size as well as ascertaining the presence of multiple abscesses.

MEDICAL MANAGEMENT

Prompt initiation of antibiotic therapy is the primary focus of the medical management of the patient with a brain abscess. Anaerobic streptococci and bacteroids are the most common bacteria causing brain abscess formation. Penicillin G and chloramphenicol administered intravenously in divided doses are the usual choices to treat these organisms. In addition, steroid therapy with Decadron is given to combat cerebral edema.

Surgical intervention may be necessary. If the abscess is well encapsulated, it may be removed in its entirety. Aspiration and drainage of the abscess is another option. Antibiotics may be directly injected into the sac once aspiration is completed.

Application of the Nursing Process to the Care of the Patient with Meningitis, Encephalitis, or Brain Abscess

Assessment

The first priority when assessing the patient with meningitis, encephalitis, or brain abscess is to establish a baseline of the patient's neurologic function. Assess level of consciousness, pupils and cranial nerves, movement, and sensation. Note the presence and severity of meningeal signs. Assess the vital signs as part of the neurologic assessment. Observe the patient's sleep-wake cycle, noting any patterns or trends of increased or decreased restlessness in relation to environmental stimuli. Assess skin integrity, color, and turgor. Note whether diaphoresis, dryness, or pallor is present. Test the patient's ability to swallow, and assess the gag reflex. Obtain the patient's weight. Determine the patient's level of comfort on the basis of either subjective complaints of headache, stiff neck, or joint pain or observation of increased irritability in relation to stimulation. Discuss the illness with the patient and the family to assess their level of comprehension of the disease process and anticipated outcome.

Nursing Diagnoses and Planning

Nursing diagnoses and related expected patient outcomes most commonly applicable to patients with meningitis or brain abscess include the following:

NDx: Pain: headache and neck pain related to meningeal irritation

Planning: Patient outcomes
1. Patient exhibits ability to rest.
2. Patient states that pain is decreased.

NDx: High risk for injury related to restlessness, disorientation, seizure activity

Planning: Patient outcomes
1. Patient remains free from injury.

NDx: High risk for altered nutrition: less than body requirements related to anorexia, fatigue, nausea, and vomiting, inability to swallow

Planning: Patient outcomes
1. Weight is maintained within 1 to 2 lb of baseline.
2. Patient is free of symptoms of dehydration.
3. Nausea and vomiting episodes are reduced or eliminated.

NDx: High risk for impaired skin integrity related to immobility, dehydration, and diaphoresis

Planning: Patient outcomes
1. Skin remains intact.
2. Irritation and redness are absent.

NDx: Altered family processes related to critical nature of situation and uncertain prognosis

Planning: Patient outcomes
1. Family members acknowledge difficulty in accepting the illness.
2. Family members identify coping patterns.

Nursing Interventions

NDx: Pain
The patient with meningeal irritation often experiences hyperalgesia and hyperirritability. Minimize unnecessary stimulation by consolidating nursing care activities when feasible. Maintain a quiet environment: Keep the room darkened, and keep environmental noise at a low level. Speak in a quiet voice to avoid startling the patient. Administer analgesics as ordered and monitor for effectiveness. Provide cool compresses to the head. Offer gradual position changes and back massages as needed.

NDx: High risk for injury
A fluctuating level of consciousness may be exhibited by the patient with meningitis or encephalitis as a result of the diffuse inflammation throughout the central nervous system. Seizures are not uncommon. Institute measures to protect the patient from injury during restless or disoriented episodes or during seizure activity. Maintain the bed in the lowest position when the patient is not under observation. Keep side rails up. Place pads or bumpers along the side rails to prevent the patient from striking the extremities against the sides of the bed. Protect intravenous catheters and other tubes such as nasogastric tubes or indwelling urinary catheters from dislodgement. Use restraints when necessary. Institute seizure precautions, and administer anticonvulsant medications as ordered. Monitor laboratory data for therapeutic serum levels of the drug prescribed. Administer sedation if ordered. Remember that sedation may not be prescribed despite restless or agitated behavior because of the potential for an altered level of consciousness to occur secondary to the medication. This may interfere with determination of true changes in mentation versus effects of sedation.

NDx: High risk for altered nutrition: less than body requirements
The patient's nutritional status is at risk secondary to fluctuating levels of consciousness and inability to tolerate oral intake. The infectious process and associated fever increase the body's metabolic and nutritional needs. If the patient is unable to take fluids by mouth because of nausea and vomiting or because of a reduced level of alertness, which poses a risk of aspiration, intravenous fluids will be necessary. Confer with the dietitian to determine the patient's daily caloric requirements. Supplemental feedings by nasogastric tube or total parenteral nutrition (TPN) may be indicated to ensure that an adequate calorie intake is maintained. Monitor intake and output every 8 hours. Weigh the patient every 3 days. If the patient has persistent vomiting, daily weights are necessary. Monitor laboratory values such as blood urea nitrogen (BUN), creatine, and albumin levels. Administer antiemetics as needed.

NDx: High risk for impaired skin integrity
Bed rest and immobility imposed by the acuteness of the infectious process predispose the patient to skin breakdown. In addition, diaphoresis causes the skin to be moist and prone to irritation and ischemic changes, particularly over pressure-sensitive areas. Change the linen frequently to avoid wetness against the skin. Minimize covers and blankets to avoid excess moisture. Turn and position the patient every 2 hours if he or she is unable to shift position without assistance. Inspect the bony prominences for signs of redness or pressure. Protect the heels and elbows. Remember that irritation of these areas occurs quickly, particularly if the patient is restless.

NDx: Altered family processes
In the acute phase of meningitis, encephalitis, or brain abscess, the patient exhibits changes in mentation and level of consciousness. The patient may be restless, irritable, and possibly unable to recognize family members. Realize that this is a frightening experience for the family and that helplessness and anxiety regarding the prognosis may interfere with coping abilities. Encourage the family to express their feelings of fear, anger, and concern. Offer explanations of the disease process and relate patient behaviors and symptoms to the course of the illness. Help the family to identify their supportive strengths as well as behaviors that may be interfering with their abilities to be supportive. Facilitate interaction with the social worker and spiritual counselor if needed.

Evaluation

Evaluate the effectiveness of nursing care for a patient with meningitis, encephalitis, or brain abscess by comparing the patient's status with the expected patient outcomes. Examples of specific outcomes for patients with meningitis, encephalitis, or brain abscess have been provided in the Planning section.

Guillain-Barré Syndrome

Guillain-Barré syndrome is an acute, rapidly progressive inflammation and demyelination of nerve endings of the peripheral nervous system that predominately affects motor function. It is also known as acute idiopathic polyneuritis or postinfectious polyneuritis.

ETIOLOGY

The cause of Guillain-Barré syndrome is unknown. The most widely accepted theory is that it is an autoimmune response. Sixty to 70% of patients with Guillain-Barré syndrome report a mild febrile illness, usually respiratory or gastrointestinal, 1 to 3 weeks before the onset of symptoms. This precipitating illness is believed to be the stimulus for an immune reaction to occur in the body against the body's own peripheral nerves. Guillain-Barré syndrome is nonseasonal and nonepidemic, occurring in the adult population and more frequently between 30 and 50 years of age. There is an equal distribution among both sexes. Viral illnesses and vaccines have also been suggested as causative factors.

PATHOPHYSIOLOGY

The insulatory covering of the axons of nerve fibers, called myelin, is broken down and in some instances destroyed by the inflammatory process associated with Guillain-Barré syndrome. This demyelination process results in slowed or blocked nerve impulse conduction, generally affecting the cranial nerves, the ventral and dorsal roots of the spinal nerves, and the entire length of peripheral nerves. Progressive paralysis of the muscles innervated by these nerves occurs. Remyelination and regeneration of axons occurs spontaneously and completely in approximately 80% of cases.

CLINICAL MANIFESTATIONS

Approximately 1 to 3 weeks after an influenza-like illness, paresthesias, that is, numbness, tingling, or burning sensations, occur in the hands and feet and may progress upward to involve the arms, legs, and trunk. This is quickly followed by weakness of the muscles, again affecting the distal areas of the hands and feet and ascending upward. The weakness may rapidly progress to total paralysis, including the respiratory muscles, necessitating mechanical ventilatory support. Bilateral facial paralysis and difficulty swallowing occur secondary to involvement of the cranial nerves. The severity of the symptoms varies from patient to patient.

In all instances, there is an initial progressive phase, lasting anywhere from a few days to 2 weeks, in which the sensory and motor symptoms occur in a progressive and ascending manner. This is followed by a plateau phase, during which maximum symptomatology exists. This phase generally lasts several days to 2 weeks. The final phase is the recovery, in which there is a progressive return of motor and sensory function. This phase can last from several months to 2 years. Approximately 20% of patients with Guillain-Barré syndrome are left with residual deficits, such as mild motor weakness or diminished reflexes in the lower extremities.

MEDICAL DIAGNOSIS

The diagnosis of Guillain-Barré syndrome is made primarily on the basis of the physical examination and history. An acute onset, rapid progression of weakness and paralysis, lack of reflexes, absence of muscle atrophy in the limbs, and a precipitating febrile illness of either respiratory or gastrointestinal origin are significant. Lumbar puncture for cerebrospinal fluid analysis indicates an increase in the protein count without a significant increase in the cell count. Nerve conduction studies show slowing initially, and abnormalities are seen several weeks after the onset of symptoms.

MEDICAL MANAGEMENT

There is no known cure for Guillain-Barré syndrome. Treatment focuses on supportive therapy and the prevention of complications such as pneumonia secondary to respiratory paralysis and cardiovascular complications resulting from paralysis and immobility. Glucocorticoids such as prednisone and Decadron are often used because of their anti-inflammatory properties, but their efficacy is not clearly documented.

Plasmapheresis may be used. This plasma-exchange treatment is thought to remove antibodies in the blood stream that are destructive to peripheral nervous system tissue. Treatment should be initiated within the first 2 weeks after the onset of symptoms to be effective.

Application of the Nursing Process to the Care of the Patient with Guillain-Barré Syndrome

Assessment

During the acute, initial phase of Guillain-Barré syndrome, obtain a baseline neurologic assessment. Assess motor strength of the extremities, and check for absence of sensation. Compare subsequent evaluations to the baseline assessment to determine ascending progression of sensory loss and weakness. Assess for cranial nerve involvement. Check the patient's ability to swallow; observe for symmetric facial grimacing and frowning and the ability to close the eyes; observe for slurred speech; and test the gag and cough reflexes. Assess respiratory function. Observe for dyspnea and confusion. Note nail bed color. Obtain arterial blood gas levels and vital capacity measurements. Assess cardiovascular status through measurement of blood pressure, heart rate, and peripheral pulses. Check baseline temperature, and obtain the patient's weight.

Assess the patient's anxiety level. Note any expressed verbalizations of fear or anger as the weakness and paralysis progress. Observe the patient and family interaction to determine coping abilities.

Nursing Diagnoses and Planning

Nursing diagnoses and related expected patient outcomes most commonly applicable to patients with Guillain-Barré syndrome include the following:

NDx: Impaired physical mobility related to muscle dysfunction and weakness

Planning: Patient outcomes
1. Patient actively or passively participates in physical activity.
2. Joint mobility is maintained.

NDx: High risk for impaired skin integrity related to immobility

Planning: Patient outcomes
1. Skin remains intact.
2. Pressure areas are free of prolonged erythema.

NDx: Self-care deficit: feeding, bathing/hygiene, dressing/grooming, toileting related to paralysis

Planning: Patient outcomes
1. Patient acknowledges need for assistance with care.
2. Patient performs self-care activities to the extent possible.
3. Patient accepts assistance with self-care.

NDx: High risk for ineffective breathing pattern related to respiratory muscle paralysis

Planning: Patient outcomes
1. Gas exchange with assistance of mechanical ventilator is maintained.
2. Patient is free of cyanosis and other signs of hypoxia.
3. Arterial blood gas levels are within normal limits for the patient.

NDx: Impaired verbal communication, related to cranial nerve paralysis or tracheostomy

Planning: Patient outcomes
1. Effective means of communication are established.
2. Patient expresses needs nonverbally with minimal frustration.

NDx: Powerlessness related to inability to control progression of weakness and paralysis

Planning: Patient outcomes
1. Patient identifies factors contributing to a sense of powerlessness.
2. Patient participates in decision making regarding the plan of care.

Nursing Interventions

NDx: Impaired physical mobility
The weakness associated with Guillain-Barré syndrome often progresses to a flaccid paralysis, which may lead to atrophy and the development of contractures. Reposition the patient or encourage position change every 2 hours. Maintain therapeutic body alignment of shoulders, hips, and extremities. Perform passive range-of-motion exercises every 2 to 4 hours. Support the extremities in functional anatomic positions: Use hand rolls and a footboard to prevent foot drop. Consult with the physical therapist for structured bedside exercises and for the use of splints or other protective devices, if necessary.

NDx: High risk for impaired skin integrity
The paralysis and paresthesias associated with Guillain-Barré syndrome place the patient at risk for skin breakdown. Monitor the patient's skin for intactness, presence of redness, temperature, and turgor every 2 hours. Massage the skin and bony prominences to promote circulation after position changes every 2 hours. Maintain wrinkle-free bed linen. Institute the use of a pressure prevention aid such as an air or egg-crate mattress. Use lotion or cream if the skin appears dry.

NDx: Self-care deficit: feeding, bathing/hygiene, dressing/grooming, toileting
The patient in the acute and plateau phases of Guillain-Barré syndrome lacks the motor ability to perform activities of daily living (ADL) at an optimally functional level. If paralysis is present, the patient is completely dependent on others for feeding, bathing, and toileting. Provide basic hygienic care for the patient daily. Involve the patient in planning a schedule for such activities as hair washing and nail trimming. Feeding needs vary with the patient's ability to swallow. Remember that even if the patient is able to swallow without the risk of aspiration, there will most likely be some degree of weakness in the upper extremities, so provide assistance as needed. Bowel and bladder sphincter control remains surprisingly intact despite diffuse involvement of other sympathetic nerve fibers throughout the nervous system. However, the patient is generally unable to toilet himself or herself because of the motor weakness and paralysis, so assist with toileting as needed.

NDx: High risk for ineffective breathing pattern
Monitor the patient's respiratory rate, rhythm, and depth of respirations every 4 hours in the acute phase. The patient may require emergency intubation or tracheostomy if weakness and paralysis interfere with effective gas exchange. Mechanical ventilation may be required to ensure adequate oxygenation and lung expansion. If the patient requires an artificial airway, such as a tracheostomy, keep the head of the bed elevated to reduce pressure on the diaphragm and to promote chest expansion. Suction the airway, maintaining sterile technique, every 2 hours and as needed to prevent respiratory tract infections. Note the color, amount,

and consistency of secretions. Provide pulmonary toilet and position changes every 2 hours to prevent atelectasis. Monitor arterial blood gas levels for acid-base abnormalities and decreased oxygen saturation.

NDx: Impaired verbal communication
Paralysis of the facial muscles alters the patient's ability to communicate. If a tracheostomy is required to maintain the airway, an additional barrier to verbal communication exists. Explain to the patient why he or she is unable to speak. Ask questions that can be answered by a "yes" or "no" response. Establish an individual pattern of simple communication, if necessary, such as eye blinks. Use flash cards or an alphabet board to facilitate two-way communication. Try to anticipate the patient's needs. Acknowledge the patient's frustration, and provide positive reinforcement when barriers to communication are overcome.

NDx: Powerlessness
Recognize that the immobility imposed by the weakness and paralysis associated with Guillain-Barré syndrome as well as the barriers to communication can contribute to feelings of lack of control and influence over the immediate environment. Encourage the patient to express his or her feelings of powerlessness over the disease progression itself as well as the limitations imposed by the symptoms. Include the patient in decision-making as it pertains to the care routine. Provide explanations and rationales for all care provided and for any treatments or procedures. Establish a trusting relationship with the patient through consistency of care providers if possible.

Evaluation

Evaluate the effectiveness of nursing care for a patient with Guillain-Barré syndrome by comparing the patient's status with the expected patient outcomes. Examples of specific outcomes for patients with Guillain-Barré syndrome have been provided in the Planning section.

Degenerative Disorders

Amyotrophic Lateral Sclerosis

Amyotrophic lateral sclerosis (ALS) is a progressive degeneration and loss of both upper and lower motor neurons. This is the most common motor neuron disease in adults and is often referred to as Lou Gehrig's disease, after the baseball player with this condition. The incidence of ALS is 1.5 per 100,000 individuals in the United States. If affects males three times more often than females.

ETIOLOGY AND PATHOPHYSIOLOGY

The cause of ALS remains unclear. Premature aging, autoimmune response, and genetic or familial factors are suggested causes currently under investigation. Whatever the cause, motor neurons in the brain stem and spinal cord atrophy and die, resulting in progressive motor dysfunction. Estimated survival time after the onset of symptoms is 3 to 4 years.

CLINICAL MANIFESTATIONS

The symptoms experienced by a patient with ALS include muscle weakness, muscle atrophy, hyperreflexia, fasciculations, spasticity, and cramping. No sensory dysfunction is noted.

Weakness usually begins in the upper or lower extremities. There is progressive atrophy and wasting of muscle groups, with absent reflexes in the affected muscle groups and hyperreflexia noted distal to affected areas. As the brain stem is affected, patients present with bulbar signs, which include slurred speech, difficulty swallowing, and inability to clear oral secretions. The respiratory muscles are eventually compromised. Aspiration and respiratory arrest are often the immediate cause of death in these patients.

MEDICAL DIAGNOSIS

A complete history and neurologic examination are performed to identify patterns of motor system involvement with the absence of sensory system dysfunction. CT scan, magnetic resonance imaging (MRI), and cerebrospinal fluid analysis are performed to rule out other disorders or causative factors. Serum creatine kinase (CK) levels are checked because findings of slightly elevated levels correlate with muscle atrophy. An electromyogram is performed to document diminished muscle contraction and fibrillations.

MEDICAL MANAGEMENT

Medical management focuses on supportive and palliative interventions to maintain the patient's highest functional level. Medication is used to control symptomatology. Muscle relaxants (such as diazepam [Valium], baclofen [Lioresal], and dantrolene [Dantrium]) are used to control muscle spasticity. Anticholinergics are used to eliminate or reduce oral secretions and sialorrhea (excessive salivation). Quinine is beneficial in relieving muscle cramps.

Use of supportive measures is discussed and decided with the patient. Supportive measures include enteral feedings and mechanical ventilation. The goal of the decision-making is to retain meaning and value in the patient's life.

Application of the Nursing Process to the Care of the Patient with Amyotrophic Lateral Sclerosis

Assessment

The assessment of the patient includes a history and neurologic examination. Explore any family history of muscle weakness or dysfunction, and ask the patient to review in detail the onset of the current problem. Allow the patient to describe the progression of muscle weakness and how it impacts ability to function. Focus physical assessment on the cranial nerves, determining ability to swallow, speak, chew, and maintain a clear airway, and on motor system function, determining the presence of muscle weakness and atrophy, cramps, and the possibility of joint subluxation.

Explore the psychosocial and emotional impact of the condition. Assess the patient's level of anxiety, and be alert to feelings of hopelessness, anger, and poor self-esteem. Assess the effect of the illness on family functioning.

Nursing Diagnoses and Planning

Nursing diagnoses and related expected patient outcomes most commonly applicable to patients with ALS include the following:

NDx: Impaired physical mobility related to muscle weakness and atrophy

Planning: Patient outcomes
1. Patient participates in ADL.
2. Patient ambulates, transfers, or moves self with or without assistance.
3. Patient avoids complications of immobility: deep venous thrombosis, pulmonary embolism, decubitus formation.

NDx: Altered nutrition: less than body requirements, related to dysphagia and inability to chew

Planning: Patient outcomes
1. Patient remains free of aspiration.
2. Patient ingests adequate volume of food and fluids to meet nutritional needs.
3. Patient maintains optimal body weight.

NDx: Impaired gas exchange related to bulbar and respiratory muscle weakness and inability to clear secretions

Planning: Patient outcomes
1. Arterial blood gas levels are within normal range.
2. Breath sounds are normal bilaterally.
3. Cyanosis is absent.
4. Complications of respiratory insufficiency—atelectasis, pneumonia, aspiration, respiratory arrest—are absent.

NDx: Hopelessness related to irreversible terminal condition

Planning: Patient outcomes
1. Patient acknowledges and shares feelings of hopelessness.
2. Patient and family use resources and support systems available.
3. Patient effectively moves through anticipatory grieving process.

Nursing Interventions

NDx: Impaired physical mobility
To reduce complications related to immobility or subluxation of joints, provide range-of-motion (passive and active) exercises at least every 6 hours. Allow the patient to do as much for self (moving, bathing, dressing, and so on) as possible. Maintain good body alignment, and eliminate undue pressure or rotation of joints. Consult with the physical and occupational therapist to obtain supportive and assistive devices to be used by the patient for ADL, such as a cane, wheelchair, eating utensils, splints, and slings. Maintain a turning and positioning schedule every 2 hours. Provide good skin care, use sheepskin pads, and an air mattress or special bed as necessary.

Plan daily activities so there are rest periods between strenuous activities. Instruct the patient how to recognize signs of fatigue and organize daily routine to provide optimal rest periods.

NDx: Altered nutrition: less than body requirements
Initially weigh patient, and determine optimal body weight; then weigh the patient at least weekly. Determine dietary requirements for the patient, and encourage foods high in protein, carbohydrate, and calories. Select foods that are soft and easy to chew. Consult the dietitian as necessary. Provide patient with approximately 3000 ml of fluids daily. Plan for smaller, frequent meals to allow the patient rest periods and to prevent undue fatigue. Place the patient in a 45-degree to upright position when eating to prevent aspiration. Provide suctioning to prevent aspiration when the patient is unable to swallow, chew, or handle secretions or fluids. Supplemental and enteral feedings may be necessary when the patient cannot ingest optimal calories to maintain body weight.

NDx: Impaired gas exchange
Monitor respiratory status of patient by auscultating the lung fields and checking respiratory rate, rhythm, and breath sounds. Instruct the patient on deep breathing, coughing, and incentive spirometry exercises. Provide chest physiotherapy and postural drainage as necessary. Instruct the patient to suction self to clear secretions that pool in the mouth area.

Have intubation and suction equipment available to support ventilatory efforts if respiratory compromise occurs. If the patient experiences respiratory insufficiency and requires long-term mechanical ventilatory support, provide suctioning to maintain a clear airway. Check ventilator equipment frequently to ensure that it is in proper working order.

NDx: Hopelessness
Provide the patient and family with support to develop effective coping mechanisms. Provide an accepting atmosphere to allow for expression of anxiety, hopelessness, and other emotions. Identify support groups and resources available, such as other persons with ALS, the National Amyotrophic Lateral Sclerosis Foundation, and clergy. Allow the patient and family to express feelings about the terminal condition, and assist and support in preparation for and acceptance of impending death.

Evaluation

Evaluate the effectiveness of nursing care for a patient with ALS by comparing the patient's status with the expected patient outcomes. Examples of specific outcomes for patients with ALS have been provided in the Planning section.

Multiple Sclerosis

Multiple sclerosis (MS) is a progressive neurologic condition characterized by the demyelination and scarring of sites along the central nervous system. Patients with MS experience a variety of alterations of sensory, motor, visual, and emotional functions. Onset most frequently occurs between 15 and 30 years of age. MS is seen more frequently in females, and the average life expectancy is 30 to 40 years after onset of symptoms.

ETIOLOGY

The cause of MS is uncertain. Suggested causes include an autoimmune reaction, an infection by a virus with a long incubation period (known as a slow virus), and a genetic predisposition. Current research has focused on genetic control and the function of the immune system, which supports the theory of an autoimmune-associated dysfunction. MS is not believed to be an infectious or inherited condition; however, familial traits have been identified.

PATHOPHYSIOLOGY

Demyelination and plaque formation occur throughout the central nervous system, predominately affecting the white matter. An inflammatory process occurs and results in edema of the axons. The clinical course of this condition is random and can be silent. Patients experience exacerbations of symptoms that are unpredictable and vary in duration and severity (Fig. 38–2).

CLINICAL MANIFESTATIONS

Because demyelination and plaque formation occur throughout the brain and spinal cord, a wide variety of symptoms can be manifested by patients with MS. Symptoms may initially present alone or in combination with other symptoms. As repeated exacerbations occur, severity of symptoms and residual deficits may increase.

Patients with MS may present clinically with any of the following alterations:

Visual: Diplopia, scotomata, nystagmus, blindness
Sensory: Paresthesia, numbness, tingling, altered position and temperature sense
Motor: Incoordination, ataxia, falling, intention tremor, fatigability, muscle spasms, contractures, paraplegia, dysphagia, impaired speech, bladder/bowel retention/incontinence
Emotional: Euphoria, depression, inappropriate affect, mental deterioration, impaired judgment

MEDICAL DIAGNOSIS

A history is obtained to identify previous episodes of neurologic dysfunction and evidence of more than one lesion. An extensive physical and neurologic examination is conducted to detect visual, motor, sensory, and emotional alterations. Cerebrospinal fluid analysis is performed to establish presence of oligoclonal (immunoglobulin G [IgG]) bands, which is diagnostic of MS. Evoked potential studies (visual, somatosensory, and auditory) and electromyograms are performed to evaluate peripheral nervous system functioning and help to identify clinically silent lesions. CT scans and MRI are done to visualize plaques and identify other pathology.

MEDICAL MANAGEMENT

There is no known cure for patients with MS. Medical management is symptomatic and supportive. High doses of corticosteroids and corticotropin are used to reduce the inflammatory process caused by demyelination of the axons. Antiviral agents such as interferon and immunosuppressive agents such as cyclophosphamide (Cytoxan), cyclosporine, and

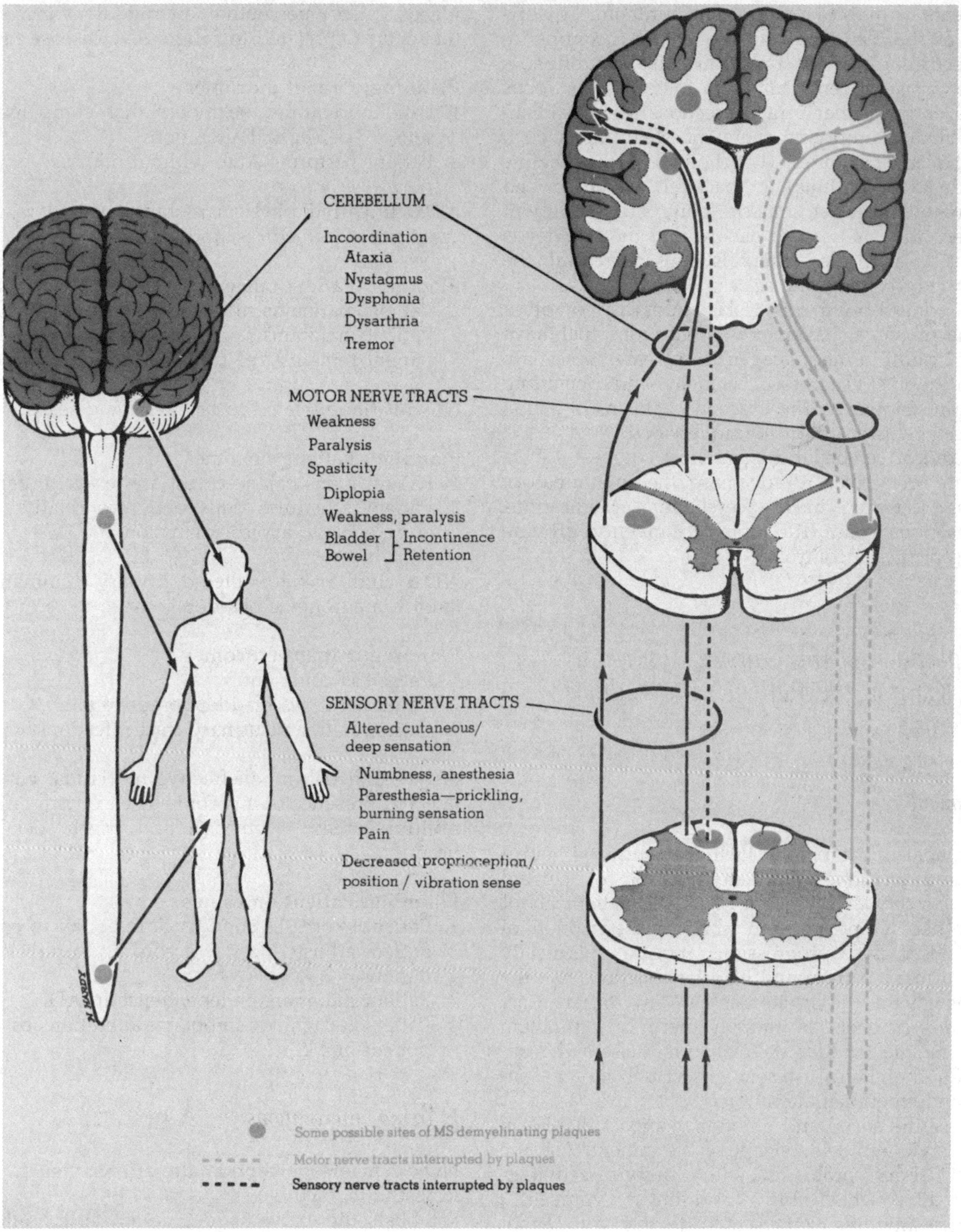

Figure 38–2.

Sites and effects of lesions in multiple sclerosis. (Copyright 1980, The American Journal of Nursing Company. Reprinted from Slater R, Yearwood A. MS: The disease process. Am J Nurs 1980; 80(2):276. Used with permission. All rights reserved.)

methylprednisolone are also used on an experimental basis. Medical intervention focuses on managing the four common symptoms presented by these patients: muscle spasticity, neurogenic bladder, paresthesias, and cerebellar ataxia.

Muscle spasticity impedes the patient's ability to perform routine tasks and ADL. Physical therapy focused on performance of self-grooming, ambulation, gait training, and feeding is prescribed to promote optimal muscle function. In addition, muscle relaxants such as Valium or Lioresal are prescribed to control level of spasticity.

Patients with MS manifest an autonomic disturbance of the bladder characterized by incontinence and recurrent urinary retention. This condition is known as neurogenic bladder. Interventions focus on preventing urinary tract infections and establishing a bladder-emptying regimen. Medications such as bethanechol chloride (Urecholine), propantheline bromide (Pro-Banthine), or baclofen are prescribed to promote bladder muscle control. Intermittent catheterization is used to ensure that the bladder is emptied at scheduled intervals, thus decreasing the incidence of urinary stasis.

The control of paresthesias primarily involves pharmacologic management. Medications that have proven useful in the management of paresthesias are carbamazepine (Tegretol), baclofen, and phenytoin (Dilantin). However, the exact mechanisms of action of these agents are not fully understood.

To control cerebellar ataxia, short courses of steroids are prescribed to decrease the inflammatory process occurring in the cerebellum. Medications such as clonazepam (Klonopin) are given to provide increased muscle control.

Application of the Nursing Process to the Care of the Patient with Multiple Sclerosis

Assessment

Assessment of the patient includes a history, neurologic examination, and determination of current level of safety and function. Ask the patient about his or her symptoms, and obtain a description of their onset and progression. Inquire specifically about urinary pattern and bladder function. Ask the patient whether he or she has had any urinary tract infections or feels as though there is a problem emptying the bladder on urination. Assess the patient for the clinical presence of visual, motor, sensory, and emotional alterations.

Assess the social and emotional impact of MS on the lifestyle and self-concept of the patient. Ask the patient about problems with lifestyle activities: "What do you have difficulty doing for yourself?"; "Is there anything you used to do that you cannot do any more?"; or "Are you injuring or hurting yourself (for example, burns, bruises)?" Question about any sexual alteration, and explore the impact on self-image. Determine strengths and weaknesses as well as effective coping and defense mechanisms.

Nursing Diagnoses and Planning

Nursing diagnoses and related expected patient outcomes most commonly applicable to patients with MS include the following:

NDx: Sensory-perceptual alterations: visual, kinesthetic, tactile; related to progressive disease process

Planning: Patient outcomes
1. Patient identifies behaviors that compensate for sensory-perceptual alterations.
2. Patient performs ADL without injury.

NDx: Impaired physical mobility related to muscle spasticity, contractures, and ataxia

Planning: Patient outcomes
1. Patient maintains motor function.
2. Patient maintains range of motion of joints.
3. Patient remains free from injury.

NDx: Fatigue related to progressive disease process

Planning: Patient outcomes
1. Patient plans balanced rest and exercise periods.
2. Patient schedules daily activities relative to energy levels to avoid exhaustion.

NDx: High risk for altered urinary elimination related to neurogenic bladder

Planning: Patient outcomes
1. Patient is continent.
2. Patient empties bladder completely.
3. Patient is free of urinary tract infections.

NDx: High risk for ineffective individual coping related to presence of a chronic disease with effects on multiple areas of physical and psychosocial functioning

Planning: Patient outcomes
1. Patient expresses confidence in ability to cope.
2. Patient adjusts lifestyle according to physical limitations.
3. Patient maintains independence in ADL.
4. Patient recognizes emotional alterations as a component of MS.

Nursing Interventions

NDx: Sensory-perceptual alterations: visual, kinesthetic, tactile

Establish the patient's degree of visual alteration (i.e., diplopia, blurred vision, field cuts). Encourage patient to wear eyeglasses if prescribed. Instruct the patient on the use of an eye patch to diminish diplopia when present.

Establish the level of impairment in touch sensation, temperature perception, and position sense, and protect the patient from injury associated with these deficits. Because skin impairment is a risk resulting from impaired sensation and immobilization, provide good skin care and encourage the patient to move and ambulate as much as possible. Instruct the patient to use sheepskin, air mattress, paddings, and so on to decrease pressure on joint and bony prominences. Keep the patient off reddened areas and, if needed, establish a turning and positioning schedule every 2 hours.

Instruct the patient to visualize extremities to ensure proper alignment and freedom from injury. Tell the patient to "look where your arms and legs are to make sure you are not injuring them or placing undue pressure on them." Have the patient regulate bath water using a thermometer; use caution with cooling and heating devices; and avoid restrictive clothing. Teach the patient to use visual cues to overcome alteration in position and sense of touch.

NDx: Impaired physical mobility
Encourage the patient to be as physically independent as possible in ADL. Provide active and passive range-of-motion exercises at least every 6 hours. Maintain proper body alignment. Consult with the physical therapist to establish an exercise program and to evaluate the need for supportive and assistive devices (i.e., brace, walker, devices for reaching, eating utensils). Administer ordered muscle relaxants and antispasmodics as necessary.

NDx: Fatigue
Identify high- and low-energy periods of the day. Assist the patient in developing a realistic schedule of activities with rest periods. Perform daily tasks during high-energy times. Divide complicated tasks into steps, allowing for rest between steps. Assist the patient in identifying physical limits; do not push to exhaustion. Instruct the patient on the signs of fatigue (i.e., weakness, tired feeling).

NDx: High risk for altered urinary elimination
Maintain schedule for bladder training. Monitor intake and output. Check for a postvoid residual to determine whether the patient has urinary retention. Establish an appropriate bladder regimen, such as intermittent catheterization, Credé's maneuver, and opportunity to void five times daily.

Instruct the patient on the importance of emptying the bladder and on signs and symptoms of urinary tract infection (i.e., frequency, burning sensation, odor, cloudy urine, and urgency). Administer ascorbic acid (vitamin C) to decrease bacterial growth, and instruct the patient to eat acid ash diet. Administer medications (such as Pro-Banthine and Urecholine, which promote bladder muscle control) as ordered to establish bladder regimen. Teach patient self-straight-catheterization technique for long-term management.

NDx: High risk for ineffective individual coping
Monitor the social and emotional impact of MS on the lifestyle and self-concept of the patient. Encourage expression of feelings and fears. Maintain a supportive and accepting environment. Explore resources available to the patient and family. Facilitate contact with another person with MS, a local support group, or the Multiple Sclerosis Society. Encourage self-care and physical and social activity within physical limitations.

Evaluation

Evaluate the effectiveness of nursing care for a patient with MS by comparing the patient's status with the expected patient outcomes. Examples of specific outcomes for patients with MS have been provided in the Planning section.

Myasthenia Gravis

Myasthenia gravis (MG) is a progressive neuromuscular condition characterized by generalized weakness and fatigue of the skeletal muscles of the body. The term myasthenia gravis comes from Greek and Latin words meaning serious muscle weakness.

MG is not believed to be an inherited condition, although familial tendencies do exist. Females appear to be afflicted three times more frequently than males. The peak onset in women is between 20 and 40 years of age. In men, peak onset is at 40 years of age or older.

ETIOLOGY AND PATHOPHYSIOLOGY

In patients with MG, the acetylcholine (ACH) released at the neuromuscular junction does not appear to be effective in producing an action potential in the muscle group. The exact cause is unclear; however, several theories are under consideration. The most prominent theory at this time suggests an autoimmune mechanism, because antibodies to ACH receptors have been found in 60% to 90% of patients with MG. Other theories suggest decreased release of ACH, excessive cholinesterase in the synapse, abnormally configured receptor sites, and a decreased number of receptor sites (Fig. 38–3). The end result of each of these theorized mechanisms is the same: weakness and inability to perform activity because of lack of action potential in the muscle group.

CLINICAL MANIFESTATIONS

Patients with MG present with weakness that is abnormally increased by continued or repeated use of the muscles at any one time. Weakness is partially relieved by a short period of rest or inactivity of the muscle group. Specific signs and symptoms include ocular muscle weakness (such as ptosis, diplopia), skeletal muscle weakness (facial weakness, dysphagia, difficulty supporting the head in the upright position, generalized muscle weakness), and

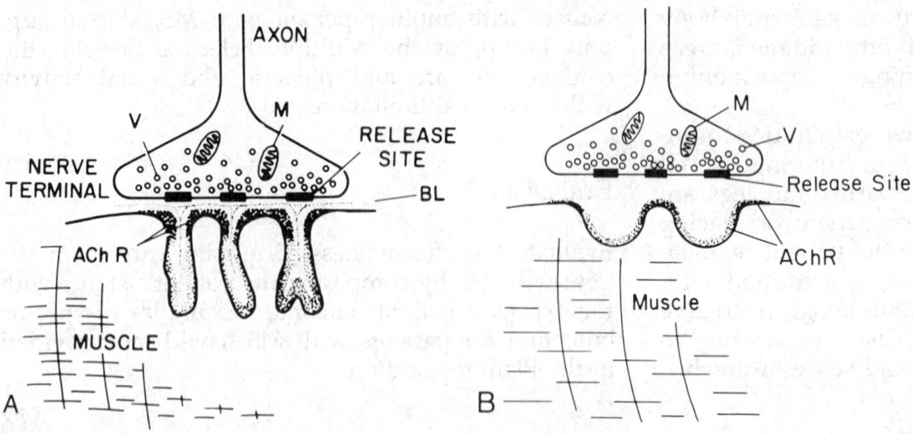

Figure 38–3.

A, Normal neuromuscular junction. *B,* Neuromuscular junction in a patient with myasthenia gravis. Note the reduced numbers of acetylcholine receptors (*stippling*); sparse, shallow postsynaptic folds; widened synaptic space; and normal nerve terminal. V, synaptic vesicle; M, mitochondrion; AChR, acetylcholine receptors; BL, basal lamina. (From Asbury AK, McKhann GM, McDonald WI [eds]. Diseases of the nervous system: Clinical neurobiology. 2nd ed. Philadelphia, WB Saunders, 1992, pp 198, 202.)

respiratory muscle weakness (inability to maintain adequate gas exchange, shallow respirations). The classic symptom is fatigue with continued or repeated use of the muscle group.

Progression of symptomatology is varied and unpredictable. Periods of remission and exacerbations occur. The severity of the condition ranges from:

Mild ocular: Involves one or more ocular muscle group; no mortality

Mild to severe: May involve ocular, bulbar, and skeletal muscle groups, sparing respiratory muscles; low mortality

Acute, severe: Involves ocular, bulbar, skeletal, and respiratory muscles; high mortality rate

Chronic, late severe: Severe symptoms with marked bulbar involvement; high mortality rate

MYASTHENIC/CHOLINERGIC CRISIS

Crisis in a myasthenic patient occurs when there is an inability to maintain respirations that allow for gas exchange. In some cases there may even be a total respiratory arrest. A myasthenic crisis occurs when there is too little ACH available at the neuromuscular junction and, therefore, no action potential is generated for respiratory muscles to maintain adequate respirations. This is often the result of too little anticholinesterase medication, infection, stress, or trauma. A cholinergic crisis occurs when there is too much ACH available at the neuromuscular junction. In cholinergic crisis, the patient experiences total fatigue of respiratory muscles from the constant action potential generated. This results from the administration of an excessive amount of anticholinesterase medication. Each crisis, although having opposing physiology, manifests with the identical outcome ranging from respiratory compromise to respiratory arrest.

MEDICAL DIAGNOSIS

A history and complete physical and neurologic examination are performed to determine symptoms of muscle weakness and the extent of progression. Serum laboratory studies include ACH receptor antibody, lupus erythematosus (LE) cells, electrophoresis of serum proteins, and thyroid function tests to determine level of or alteration in autoimmune function. Chest x-ray examination and CT scans are done to identify the presence of thymoma (tumor of thymus gland). Electromyogram and nerve conduction studies are performed to document abnormal muscle action potential; findings include rapid reduction in amplitude with repetitive stimulation. In addition, drug challenge studies diagnostic of MG are performed, such as edrophonium (Tensilon) test or neostigmine (Prostigmin) test. Two to 10 mg of Tensilon is injected intravenously, or Prostigmin, 1 to 2 mg, is injected intramuscularly. In the myasthenic patient, an increase in muscle strength is noted. This is the result of increasing the amount of available ACH at the neuromuscular junction. If the patient does not have MG, or a decreased level of ACH at the neuromuscular junction, increased weakness occurs, with the potential for respiratory arrest.

MEDICAL MANAGEMENT

Medical management of patients with MG focuses on maintaining optimal respiratory function and muscle strength. Use of anticholinesterase medications (pyridostigmine [Mestinon], Prostigmin) is the most common treatment modality. Anticholinesterase medications maintain an effective chemical balance of ACH and cholinesterase at the neuromuscular junction, allowing for optimal respiratory function and muscle strength. Therefore, timing of anticholinesterase medication is critical. Patients and health care workers need to be instructed to administer this medication on time, not before or after due time, to maintain an effective chemical balance at the neuromuscular junction (Pharmacology Box 38–1).

Other treatment modalities include the use of steroids, plasmapheresis, and thymectomy. Steroids (corticotropin and corticosteroids) have proved effective in preventing the progression and severity of symptoms. Plasmapheresis cleanses the blood stream of the anti-ACH receptor antibodies. Plasmapheresis is a temporary method to control symptomatology; however, it is useful in predicting the patient's response to thymectomy (surgical removal of the thymus gland). The thymus produces antibodies, including the anti-ACH receptor antibody. Thus, thymectomy decreases levels of these antibodies.

Application of the Nursing Process to the Care of the Patient with Myasthenia Gravis

Assessment

Assess for ocular, bulbar, skeletal, and respiratory muscle group involvement and generalized weakness, level of deterioration, and degree of fatigability. Identify functional limitations affecting mobility, self-care, respiratory ability, and activity intolerance.

Assess the extent of ocular muscle weakness. Ask whether the patient has double vision. Observe for facial symmetry and ptosis of the eyelid.

Assess the patient for dysphagia. Explore particular patterns associated with the ability to swallow (i.e., types and consistencies of foods). Ask the patient, "Do you find yourself drooling because you are unable to swallow oral secretions?"

In assessing motor function, determine the level of physical mobility. Ask the patient if he or she tires or fatigues easily, and ask for a description of how he or she feels at that time. Ask to what extent he or she can perform ADL: "Do you need someone to assist in performing personal hygiene, feeding, toileting, moving, and ambulating?"; "Do you find you can perform tasks most easily with the use of assistive devices, such as special eating utensils?"; and "Are there periods of the day when you feel more energetic than others?" Note whether the patient is able to support the head in an upright position with or without assistance. Assess for skin integrity, and note alterations related to undue pressure points.

Assess respiratory status. Ask the patient whether breathing is effortful. Assess the rate and rhythm of respirations. Auscultate the lung fields to assess breath sounds on inspiration and expiration. Determine the effectiveness of respiratory function by ob-

Pharmacology Box 38–1.
CHOLINESTERASE INHIBITORS

Cholinesterase Inhibitors (Anticholinesterase Agents):
These drugs prevent the breakdown of acetylcholine by cholinesterase at the neuromuscular junction. Two widely used drugs in this class are neostigmine (Prostigmin) and pyridostigmine (Mestinon).

Action:
Inhibit destruction of acetylcholine by cholinesterase, thereby enhancing transmission of impulses across the neuromuscular junction.

Uses:
Maintain chemical neurotransmitter balance to optimize muscle strength, respiratory function, and adequate and effective gas exchange in patients with myasthenia gravis.

Side Effects:
Side effects are dose related and include respiratory distress and myasthenic crisis (blurred or double vision, shortness of breath, increased weakness, rapid heartbeat, twitching, dizziness). Other side effects include abdominal cramps, diarrhea, nausea, vomiting, salivation, and sweating.

Interactions:
Atropine inhibits the effect of cholinesterase inhibitors.

Nursing Implications:
Assess patient's ability to swallow before administering oral preparations. Monitor patient for improvement of symptoms within 30 minutes after drug is administered. Monitor patient for side effects. Notify physician if signs of respiratory deterioration (vital capacity below 1 L) or distress occur.

taining a vital capacity (measurement of exhaled volume on a spirometer). Ask the patient, "Are there any activities or times of the day that you feel it is more difficult for you to breathe than other times?"; and "Do you feel stronger and better able to breathe after you take your anticholinesterase medication?"

Nursing Diagnoses and Planning

Nursing diagnoses and related expected patient outcomes most commonly applicable to patients with MG include the following:

NDx: Impaired physical mobility related to weakness of voluntary muscle groups

Planning: Patient outcomes
1. Patient performs ADL.
2. Patient ambulates and transfers with or without assistive devices.
3. Patient maintains muscle strength.

NDx: Fatigue related to repetition of muscle stimulation

Planning: Patient outcomes
1. Patient plans daily schedule with periods of activity and rest.
2. Patient recognizes the signs of fatigue.
3. Patient reports success in controlling or preventing fatigue with scheduling of activities.

NDx: Ineffective breathing pattern related to disease process, myasthenic or cholinergic crisis

Planning: Patient outcomes
1. Respiratory rate and rhythm are within normal limits.
2. Patient maintains optimal tidal volume with or without the support of mechanical ventilation.
3. Breath sounds are normal bilaterally.

NDx: High risk for aspiration related to dysphagia

Planning: Patient outcomes
1. Patient avoids aspiration.
2. Patient clears oral secretions effectively.
3. Breath sounds are normal bilaterally.
4. Patient is afebrile.

Nursing Interventions

NDx: Impaired physical mobility
Monitor and record patient's motor strength and high- and low-energy periods throughout the day. Schedule activities during high-energy periods. Administer anticholinergic medications as prescribed; monitor for effectiveness of medication regimen. Consult physical and occupational therapists as necessary to develop exercise program and to obtain supportive and assistive devices. Encourage the patient to be as independent as possible in activities, ranging from ambulation to turning and repositioning self.

NDx: Fatigue
Encourage the patient to perform activities during high-energy periods. Assist in identifying limits of physical activity. Instruct the patient on signs of fatigue (tired, increasing weakness). Do not push beyond physical limits. Allow rest between daily activities.

NDx: Ineffective breathing pattern
Establish baseline vital capacity and monitor periodically by measuring exhaled volume on a spirometer. Call the physician immediately if vital capacity falls below baseline or 1.0 L. This indicates that the patient is in crisis and needs immediate intervention.

Monitor effectiveness of anticholinesterase medications in maintaining strength of respiratory muscles (i.e., Is the patient able to take a deep breath? Are respiratory rate and rhythm within normal limits?). Instruct the patient to perform coughing and deep-breathing exercises. Provide chest physiotherapy and postural drainage if the lung fields are congested to decrease risk of infection. Provide suction when necessary to clear oral and tracheal secretions.

Notify the physician immediately if vital capacity falls or if the patient exhibits signs of increased secretions or respiratory distress. Ensure that intubation, oxygen, suction, and mechanical ventilation equipment are readily available if the patient experiences a respiratory crisis or arrest.

NDx: High risk for aspiration
Monitor the patient's ability to clear secretions and swallow. Suction as occasion requires to maintain clear airway. Encourage the patient to eat small bites of food at a time. Teach the patient to eat with his or her head at a 30-degree angle or greater to assist in swallowing food. Supervise during meal periods. Provide and instruct the patient on the use of suction and oral catheters to decrease the risk of aspirating by removing pooled oral secretions and food that cannot be swallowed, which is gagging or choking the patient.

Evaluation

Evaluate the effectiveness of nursing care for a patient with MG by comparing the patient's status with the expected patient outcomes. Examples of specific outcomes for patients with MG have been provided in the Planning section.

Muscular Dystrophy: Limb-Girdle

Muscular dystrophy (MD) is a broad classification of specific hereditary neurologic conditions characterized by progressive degeneration and weakness of the voluntary muscles. Although the majority of persons afflicted with MD are children, clinical presentation may occur at any point throughout the life span. Limb-girdle muscular dystrophy is the condition that presents clinically in young adulthood. The earlier the clinical symptoms appear, the more rapid the progression and severity of the disease process.

ETIOLOGY AND PATHOPHYSIOLOGY

Limb-girdle muscular dystrophy has a clinical onset anywhere from the first to the third decade of life. This is an autosomal recessive disease; therefore, both parents need to carry the defective gene for their child to inherit this condition. When both parents carry the defective gene, their children have a 25% chance of being afflicted with the disease, a 50% chance of passing along the defective gene to their offspring, and a 25% chance of being free of the disease. Males and females are affected equally.

CLINICAL MANIFESTATIONS

Clinical onset initially involves the proximal muscles of the pelvic and shoulder girdle. The patient appears to have a forward-stooped appearance. Progression of muscular weakness is variable. When progression is slow, the patient may live a normal life span.

MEDICAL DIAGNOSIS

A complete history and physical and neurologic examination are performed to substantiate muscle weakness. The history focuses on family history, incidence of muscular dystrophies, patient perception of onset of symptoms, and severity of weakness. The physical and neurologic examination focuses on differentiation of the muscle group involvement. A muscle biopsy is performed to demonstrate abnormal characteristics. In addition, an electromyogram, CK, and serum enzyme tests are performed to substantiate the diagnosis and to rule out any underlying pathology.

MEDICAL MANAGEMENT

There is no known cure for limb-girdle muscular dystrophy. Medical management focuses on supportive and palliative interventions to maintain the patient's highest level of functioning. Physical, occupational, and respiratory therapies are prescribed to keep unaffected muscles functioning and to delay development of contractures and skeletal deformities.

Application of the Nursing Process to the Care of the Patient with Limb-Girdle Muscular Dystrophy

Assessment

Patient assessment includes a history and neurologic examination. Inquire about any family history of muscle weakness or dysfunction. Ask the patient to describe the onset of his or her muscle weakness, including how and when it was first noticed, and how it impacts on the ability to carry out tasks and activities. Focus the neurologic assessment on the motor system function. Identify muscle groups involved. Observe the patient for gait disturbances and a forward-stooped appearance. Assess severity of motor system dysfunction, and establish whether the patient is at risk for injury. Determine whether the patient uses any assistive devices such as a wheelchair or cane for mobility. Ask whether falling occurs because of any increase in muscle weakness. Assess the patient for presence of contractures or skeletal deformities. Inspect the extremities and have the patient go through a range of motion.

Assess the psychosocial and emotional impact of this progressive degenerating condition on the patient. Ask questions such as "How does having this condition make you feel?"; "Do you find there is any disruption in your relationships at work, with your family, or with your friends?"; and "Do you feel as though you are the same person you were before the diagnosis of muscular dystrophy?"

Nursing Diagnoses and Planning

Nursing diagnoses and related expected patient outcomes most commonly applicable to patients with limb-girdle muscular dystrophy include the following:

NDx: Impaired physical mobility related to progressive muscular weakness, contractures, skeletal deformities

Planning: Patient outcomes
1. Patient performs ADL within limitations.
2. Patient maintains range of joint motion.

NDx: Powerlessness related to progressive muscular deterioration

Planning: Patient outcomes
1. Patient expresses feelings of powerlessness.
2. Patient identifies areas over which he or she does have control.
3. Patient makes choices in areas over which he or she has control.

4. Patient and family acknowledge and use resources and support systems available.

Nursing Interventions

NDx: Impaired physical mobility
Perform range-of-motion exercises every 6 hours to maintain joint motion and to prevent development of contractures. Allow the patient to do as much for him- or herself as possible (ambulation, feeding, toileting, grooming). Encourage the patient to perform activities using varied muscle groups so that muscles that are still functioning remain healthy. Consult with physical and occupational therapists to obtain supportive devices to be used by the patient for ADL, such as a wheelchair, bathroom lifts, walkers, and braces or supports.

Monitor the patient for any change in motor system function and increased risk of falling. Instruct the patient on signs of weakness and the importance of not pushing beyond limits to prevent self-injury. Encourage the patient to use assistive devices for ambulation when gait is unsteady.

Consult with the social worker for discharge planning. Encourage the patient and family members to actively participate in this process. Because the home environment needs to be prepared to support the optimal functioning level of the patient, the purchase of equipment such as a bed, bathroom equipment, and ramps may be required.

NDx: Powerlessness
Encourage the patient to express fears and feelings of powerlessness. Provide for an accepting atmosphere to allow for expressions of anxiety, powerlessness, and other emotions. Acknowledge to the patient and family that their feelings are legitimate and that it is difficult not to have control over what is happening physically. Reassure that feelings of loss and grieving are normal. Identify and facilitate contact with support groups and resources, such as other persons with muscular dystrophies, clergy, social workers, therapists, and the Muscular Dystrophy Association.

Additional Interventions
Allow the patient and family to express feelings about the irreversible condition and assist and support in preparation and acceptance of impending death when imminent.

Evaluation

Evaluate the effectiveness of nursing care for a patient with limb-girdle muscular dystrophy by comparing the patient's status with the expected patient outcomes. Examples of specific outcomes for patients with limb-girdle muscular dystrophy have been provided in the Planning section

Parkinson's Disease

Parkinson's disease is a neurologic condition characterized by degenerative changes in the basal ganglia, primarily in the area known as the substantia nigra. Parkinson's disease affects men and women equally, with symptoms presenting between the ages of 40 to 70 years. Approximately 1% of the population older than 50 years has Parkinson's disease.

ETIOLOGY

The cause of Parkinson's disease is unknown for the majority of patients afflicted with this condition. Possible causes include viral agents, genetic disposition, and premature aging.

PATHOPHYSIOLOGY

Dopamine, a major neurotransmitter, is manufactured and stored in the area of the brain known as the basal ganglia. Dopamine acts to provide a homeostatic balance of inhibitory and excitatory actions. The degenerative changes associated with Parkinson's disease interfere with the production and storage of dopamine. The symptoms classic of Parkinson's disease (tremors, muscle rigidity, and bradykinesia) are reflective of the imbalance of inhibitory and excitatory actions. This can be directly related to the reduction of available dopamine in these patients.

CLINICAL MANIFESTATIONS

The symptoms experienced by a patient with Parkinson's disease include resting tremors (a pill-rolling motion of the hands when at rest), slowness and rigidity of movement, flexion posture, "stooped" appearance, shuffling gait, inability to stop movement such as walking, fatigue, expressionless, masklike face, drooling, oily skin, dysphagia, urinary hesitancy, and depression (Fig. 38–4). Onset is gradual, usually with unilateral involvement, and progression is slow. Symptoms increase in severity with disease progression.

MEDICAL DIAGNOSIS

Overall history and clinical findings substantiate the diagnosis of Parkinson's disease. Because the progression of symptoms is slow, the diagnosis of Parkinson's disease may not be made initially. Electromyography, EEG, CT scan, and MRI may be ordered to rule out other pathology. The patient's urine and cerebrospinal fluid are tested to document decreased levels of homovanillic acid (HVA), a metabolite of dopamine.

The Unified Parkinson Disease Rating Scale (UPDRS), developed by an international group of neurologists, is used to classify patients with Parkinson's disease. This scale is as follows:

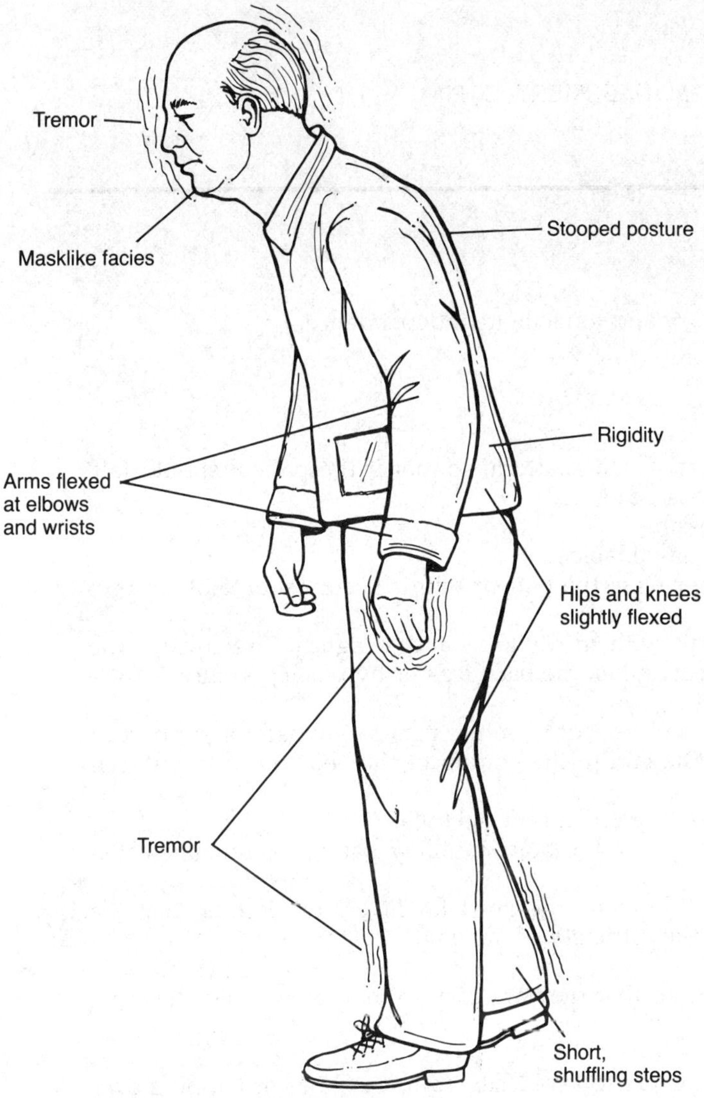

Figure 38–4.

Clinical manifestations of Parkinson's disease.

0 = no sign of disease
1 = unilateral disease
2 = bilateral disease without impairment of balance
3 = mild to moderate bilateral disease with postural instability, still physically independent
4 = severe disability, still able to stand and walk
5 = wheelchair dependent or bedridden

MEDICAL MANAGEMENT

Medical management focuses on the use of drug therapy to control a patient's symptomatology. It is established that decreased levels of dopamine cause the symptoms exhibited by the patient with Parkinson's disease (tremors, muscle rigidity, and bradykinesia). Amantadine (Symmetrel), bromocriptine, levodopa, and carbidopa (Sinemet) are drugs that, once metabolized, break down to the precursor: dopamine. When these drugs are used in various combinations, therefore, the amount of available dopamine at the neuromuscular junction increases and the patient displays decreased or controlled symptoms. Anticholinergics (trihexyphenidyl [Artane], ethopropazine [Parsidol], benztropine [Cogentin]) are used in conjunction with levodopa to increase available dopamine as well as to reduce drooling.

Application of the Nursing Process to the Care of the Patient with Parkinson's Disease

Assessment

Obtain a complete history of the current problem, including symptoms, time of onset, and progression. Proceed to assess current status beginning with motor system functioning. Observe posture and gait. Note muscle rigidity. Check strength, and look for characteristic tremors. Note the ability to swallow and to clear secretions. Assess mental status. Question about depression and altered thought processes, and observe for signs of depression. Determine the patient's ability to communicate. Observe for masklike face, dysarthria, and monotone, whispering voice. Assess for alterations in autonomic system function, such as oily skin and urinary hesitancy.

Explore any medication regimen the patient has been on. Note the name and dose of all medications, and question the patient about their effectiveness in controlling symptoms. Ask the patient whether any specific practices are used to ensure that medications are taken at the right time or intervals.

Assess ability for self-care and the ability to perform ADL. Note the extent and type of assistance required by the patient.

Ask the patient how he or she feels: "How has this condition affected the way you live?" Assess the social and emotional impact of Parkinson's disease on the lifestyle and self-concept of the patient. Allow the patient to describe how Parkinson's disease has impacted on the ability to meet work and family obligations.

Nursing Diagnoses and Planning

Nursing diagnoses and related expected patient outcomes most commonly applicable to patients with Parkinson's disease include the following:

NDx: Impaired physical mobility related to muscular rigidity, bradykinesia, muscle tremors, and loss of postural reflexes

Planning: Patient outcomes
1. Patient performs ADL.
2. Patient maintains current level of mobility with or without assistance.
3. Patient remains free from accidental injury.

Chart 38–1.

NURSING GUIDE TO PATIENT EDUCATION FOR SELF-MANAGEMENT: COPING WITH PARKINSON'S DISEASE

Instruct the patient and/or family to:

Adapt home environment to minimize the risk of injury and to facilitate independence.

- Provide good lighting in all living areas.
- Remove all loose or scatter rugs.
- Remove doorsills that are easily stumbled over.
- Place sharp pointed tables or other objects out of the traffic pattern, so that if the patient should fall, the likelihood of injury from striking a sharp object is decreased.
- Arrange patient's living quarters on one floor if possible.
- Install sturdy stair rails on both sides if stairs are unavoidable.
- Install handles on walls adjacent to doorknobs to provide the patient with a secure source of support while he or she opens doors.
- Facilitate getting in and out of a chair by using chair with sturdy arms and a slightly forward tip. The forward tip can be arranged by having a carpenter lengthen the back legs or by placing secure 2- to 4-inch blocks under them.
- Facilitate getting in and out of bed by placing a heavy piece of furniture next to the bed for support or by tying a loop of rope or a sheet with a knot in the end to the bottom of the bed to use to pull self into a sitting position.
- Install bars on either side of the toilet to facilitate getting on and off the toilet.
- Buy or make a toilet seat that is elevated 2 inches above the bowl to allow patient to remain seated while wiping self.
- Keep home temperature slightly above normal to eliminate the need for layers of clothing that are difficult for the patient to put on and that increase the difficulty of moving.

Select or adapt clothing and other personal use items so that they are easy to manipulate and therefore conserve energy and allow maximum independence.

- Use elastic shoelaces or wear shoes with Velcro fasteners to avoid having to tie shoes or tripping over untied laces.
- Use Velcro patches to fasten clothing; maintain proper appearance by sewing buttons on the top surface.
- Leave neckties knotted; slip over the head and tighten to wear.
- Choose raglan rather than set-in sleeves.
- Contact a rehabilitation center or support group for information about companies in your area that carry especially designed "easy to get in and out of" clothes.

Keep active to prevent physical disability due to disuse and to promote a positive outlook.

- Perform daily home exercises as taught.
- Participate in a formal exercise program once or twice a week; this may be an individual session or a group session offered through a Parkinson patient self-help group.
- Remember that overdoing exercises can be counterproductive, so follow physician's guidelines carefully.
- Remain involved in family and social activities.
- Drive if able, but consider staying in low-traffic areas and having another driver with you to allow breaks if needed.
- Be aware that there is no need to restrict travel, although having a companion along is desirable.

(continued)

Chart 38–1. *(continued)*

NURSING GUIDE TO PATIENT EDUCATION FOR SELF-MANAGEMENT: COPING WITH PARKINSON'S DISEASE

Eat a balanced diet sufficient to prevent weight loss.

- Eat 1500 to 2000 calories per day.
- Eat small, frequent meals because problems with chewing, swallowing, and handling food items make eating a slow, difficult process.
- Reduce dietary protein moderately because proteins reduce the absorption of levodopa; do not drastically reduce protein unless specified by your physician.
- Use an electric warming tray if needed to keep foods warm and palatable during the time it takes to eat.
- Select foods that are easy to handle, chew, and swallow, such as mashed potatoes and other vegetables, meat loaf, and stew.
- Remember that semisolid foods are easier to swallow than liquids or solids and that a commercial product (Thick-It) is available that can be used to thicken fruit juice and carbonated beverages.

Institute measures to cope with sleep pattern disturbances (early to sleep, with awakening in about 3 hours followed by several hours of wakefulness before returning to sleep) that predispose to episodes of nocturnal confusion due to sensory deprivation.

- Keep a light on at night.
- Keep a radio playing softly.
- Consult with the physician if serious sleep pattern disturbance effects persist, because a change in medication may be helpful.

Recognize that caregivers need intervals of relief from responsibilities and plan for respite care accordingly.

NDx: Self-esteem disturbance related to physical limitations and changes in appearance

Planning: Patient outcomes
1. Patient verbalizes positive feelings about self.
2. Patient adjusts lifestyle according to physical limitations.
3. Patient maintains social interactions with family and friends.
4. Patient participates in ADL.

NDx: Impaired verbal communication related to dysarthria and monotone, whispering speech

Planning: Patient outcomes
1. Patient communicates without frustration.
2. Patient uses alternate methods of communication as necessary.

NDx: High risk for altered health maintenance related to insufficient knowledge of self-care

Planning: Patient outcomes
1. Patient and family describe self-care measures presented in Chart 38–1.
2. Patient and family verbalize willingness and ability to follow guidelines presented in Chart 38–1.

Nursing Interventions

NDx: Impaired physical mobility
Encourage the patient to be as physically independent as possible in ADL. Provide active and passive range-of-motion exercises at least every 6 hours. Allow sufficient time to perform ADL by establishing a schedule or routine. Provide for periods of activity and rest.

Administer medications as prescribed to reduce and control muscle rigidity, tremors, and bradykinesia. Evaluate the patient for tolerance of medication. Determine the degree of symptom control and side effects experienced by the patient, such as nausea,

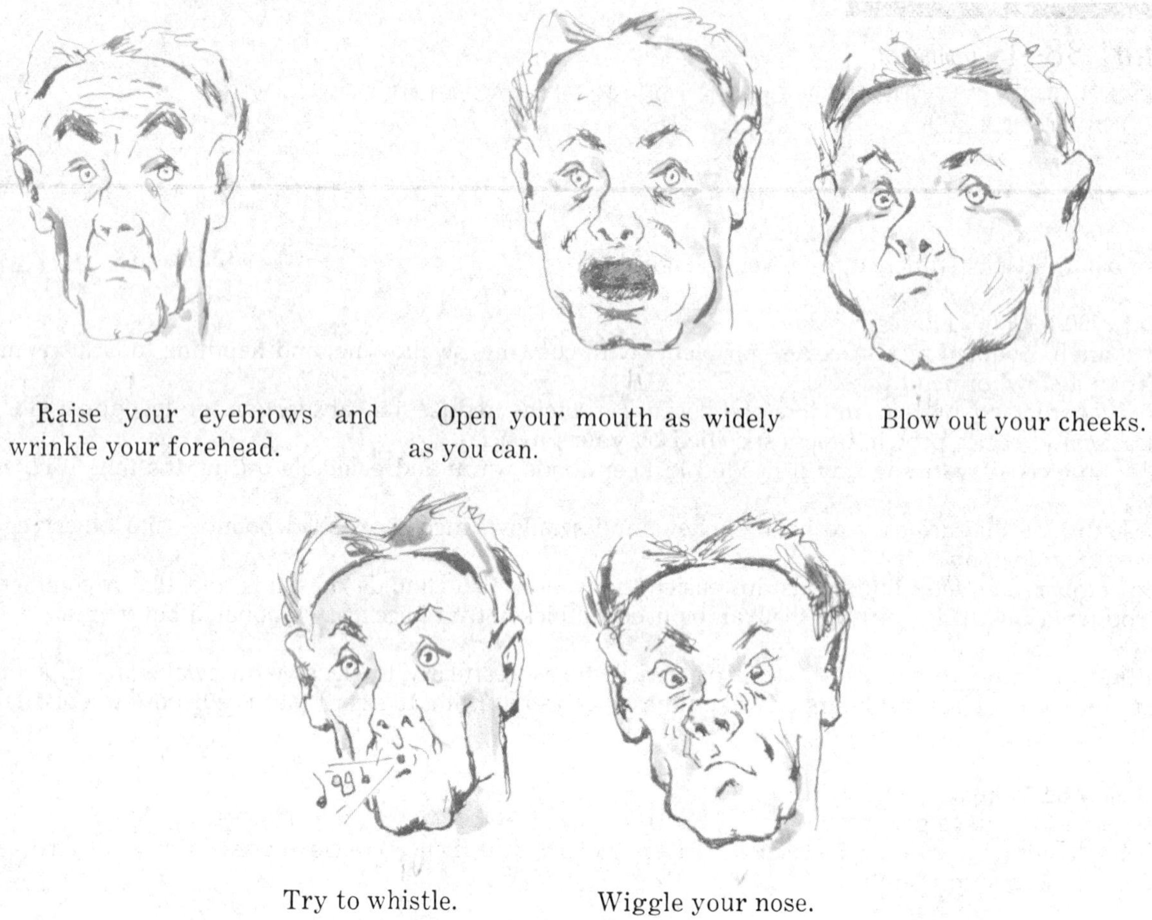

Figure 38–5.

Face and tongue exercises used to promote and maintain muscle strength and hence verbal communication ability in patients with Parkinson's disease. (From Exercises for the Parkinson patient with hints for daily living. Compiled for the Parkinson's Disease Foundation, New York, by L. Côté and G. Riedel. Illustrated by John D. E. Orr.)

vomiting, orthostatic hypotension, dry mouth, dizziness, and "on-off" phenomenon, in which there is periodic loss of symptom control. Instruct the patient to decrease intake of vitamin B_6 and high-protein foods (i.e., multivitamins, milk, eggs, meat) because they facilitate the destruction of dopamine in the liver, thereby decreasing levels of available dopamine.

Consult with the physical and occupational therapists to assist the patient in mobility and to provide assistive devices (i.e., cane, walker). Instruct the patient about safety hazards and how to maintain a safe environment. Explain the importance of removing scatter rugs, maintaining good lighting, avoiding rushing, and allowing time for movements.

NDx: Self-esteem disturbance
Allow the patient to verbalize fears and feelings about loss of function. Inform the patient regarding the resources available such as support groups and the Parkinson's Disease Foundation. Explore strengths and weaknesses as well as effective coping and defense mechanisms. Discuss patient symptoms (e.g., drooling, tremors) and their impact on self-image. Support self-care and physical and social activities within physical limitations.

NDx: Impaired verbal communication
Provide an accepting environment for the patient to communicate, whether attempts are successful or not. This can be accomplished by providing a private, unrushed atmosphere. Decrease external distraction such as noise from television or radio, and move in close proximity when communicating with the patient. This allows for whispers to be heard. Ask questions simply by supplying two options or in a "yes or no" format. Recognize the patient's frustrations when efforts to communicate are unsuccessful. Instruct the patient to perform face and tongue exercises (Fig. 38–5) to maintain optimal

muscle strength. Consult with a speech therapist to evaluate the patient, and develop an individualized program or provide or suggest alternate methods of communication when necessary.

NDx: High risk for altered health maintenance
Instruct the patient and family in self-care measures, as presented in Chart 38-1.

Evaluation

Evaluate the effectiveness of nursing care for a patient with Parkinson's disease by comparing the patient's status with the expected patient outcomes. Examples of specific outcomes for patients with Parkinson's disease have been provided in the Planning section.

Table 38–1. STAGES* OF ALZHEIMER'S DISEASE

EARLY STAGE (2 TO 4 YEARS)
Forgetfulness (may be very subtle and patient may try to cover up using lists and notes)
Declining interest in environment, people, and present affairs
Vague uncertainty and hesitancy in initiating actions
Poor performance at work by end of this stage; may be dismissed from job
MIDDLE STAGE (2 TO 12 YEARS)†
Progressive memory loss
Hesitates in response to questions; shows signs of aphasia
Has difficulty following simple instructions or doing simple calculations
Has episodic bouts of irritability
Becomes evasive, anxious, and physically active
Wanders, particularly at night
Becomes apraxic for many basic activities
Loses important papers
Loses way home in familiar surroundings or loses way in own home
Forgets to pay bills; lets household chores slip and newspapers pile up; does not dispose of garbage; does not take medications
Loses possessions and then claims they were stolen
Neglects personal hygiene (bathing, shaving, dressing)
Loses social graces; behavior can be a major embarrassment to family and friends; usually ends in social isolation of the family and patient
FINAL STAGE (UP TO A YEAR)
Marked loss of weight because of lack of eating; becomes emaciated
Unable to communicate verbally or in writing
Does not recognize family
Incontinent of urine and feces
Possibility of major seizures
Grasping, snout, and sucking reflexes are readily elicited
Finally loses the ability to stand and walk and becomes bedridden
Death is usually caused by aspiration pneumonia

*Stages of Alzheimer's disease vary from patient to patient, but a few time approximations as well as characteristic behaviors can be identified.
†Diagnosis is frequently made in this stage.

Alzheimer's Disease

Alzheimer's disease is a chronic progressive neurodegenerative condition characterized by marked cognitive dysfunction. Its peak onset is between 45 and 65 years of age. Alzheimer's disease is a prominent dementing illness.

ETIOLOGY

The exact cause of Alzheimer's disease is unknown. Theories of cause include genetic tendency, autoimmune reaction, slow virus, and dysfunction of neurotransmitters. Alzheimer's disease is not considered a hereditary disease; however, familial tendencies have been noted.

PATHOPHYSIOLOGY

Cerebral atrophy is noted primarily in the frontal and temporal lobes. Degenerative neuronal changes occur involving the development of neurofibrillary tangles, formation of senile plaques, and loss of neurons. Symptoms manifested by these degenerative changes progress from confusion and memory loss to dementia.

CLINICAL MANIFESTATIONS

Alzheimer's disease has been classified into three stages (Table 38-1). Each stage is characterized by progressive mental and physical dysfunction. Initially, the patient may be forgetful; however, this progresses to memory loss, wandering behavior, and an eventual lack of awareness of the environment, with custodial care required. Death usually occurs in the last stage as a result of aspiration pneumonia.

MEDICAL DIAGNOSIS

A history and neurologic examination are performed to ascertain the level of deterioration of mental and physical functioning. Neurodiagnostic studies include CT scan to demonstrate cerebral atrophy and enlarged ventricles, positron emission tomography (PET) to identify glucose utilization of the brain, and EEG to identify slowing patterns of brain impulses. In some cases, a brain biopsy may be performed.

MEDICAL MANAGEMENT

Medical management of patients with Alzheimer's disease is symptomatic and supportive. There is no known treatment plan that alters progression of the condition or functioning level of the patient. Medications such as vasodilators (papaverine [Pavabid] or ergoloid mesylates [Hydergine]) or psychostimulants (methylphenidate [Ritalin]) are prescribed in an attempt to improve mental status.

Application of the Nursing Process to the Care of the Patient with Alzheimer's Disease

Assessment

Patient assessment includes a history and neurologic examination. Assess for progressive deterioration in mental and physical abilities. Determine the limitations of cognitive function and self-care, and assess risk of injury or self-harm. Also assess the impact of the disease on family members.

Begin with assessment of level of cognitive function, determining orientation to time, place, and person and presence of delusions. Check for loss of recent and remote memory and the ability to retain new information. Assess for errors in judgment, abstract thinking, and loss of insight. Also assess for the presence of aphasia syndromes and difficulty in comprehension.

Assess for behavioral and affective disturbances. Observe for signs of hyperactivity, restlessness, wandering, antisocial behavior, emotional outbursts, paranoia, diminished motivation, and depression.

Determine the level of motor function. Note gait disturbances, seizure activity, and muscle twitching. Assess the ability to carry out purposeful tasks or movements. Identify the ability to perform self-care and ADL. Determine the level of supervision and assistance required to complete tasks.

Explore the impact on family functioning. Ask family members, "How have your lives changed?"; "Are you able to socialize with friends and meet your work responsibilities?"; "Do you feel as though you have enough time for yourself?"; and "Do you find yourself getting frustrated, edgy, or irritable?"

Nursing Diagnoses and Planning

Nursing diagnoses and related expected patient outcomes most commonly applicable to patients with Alzheimer's disease include the following:

NDx: Altered thought processes related to cognitive decline

Planning: Patient outcomes
1. Displays of behavioral dysfunction are minimal.

NDx: Self-care deficit: feeding, hygiene, grooming related to cognitive decline

Planning: Patient outcomes
1. Patient performs self-care within limits of ability.
2. Patient wears clean, neat clothes during daytime.
3. Patient maintains acceptable personal hygiene.
4. Family or significant other identifies personal and community resources that can provide support and assistance.

NDx: High risk for injury related to cognitive decline

Planning: Patient outcomes
1. Patient remains free from injury.

NDx: Ineffective family coping related to constant, total care of family member with Alzheimer's disease

Planning: Patient outcomes
1. Family describes strategies to manage behavioral alterations of the patient.
2. Family identifies personal and community sources of support.

Nursing Interventions

NDx: Altered thought processes
Provide a consistent, structured environment for the patient. Allow the patient to have familiar objects around (e.g., pictures, furniture). Establish daily routines, avoid any variations in day-to-day activities. Do not expect the patient to function or respond beyond capabilities. Anticipate the patient's needs, and eliminate any stress associated with meeting those needs. Eliminate undue noise or disruption of physical surroundings.

NDx: Self-care deficit: feeding, hygiene, grooming
Monitor patient's level and ability to perform ADL. Ensure that the patient attends to daily personal hygiene, wears clean clothing, and eats adequate diet. Allow the patient to maintain self-care activities as long as possible. Encourage the patient to complete self-care. Supervise patient, when necessary, to ensure completion of steps involved in each task. Provide direct care when the patient cannot adequately perform self-care. Consult with nutritionist as necessary to determine nutritional needs. Ensure that the patient is fed and groomed and that hygiene is attended to on a daily basis.

NDx: High risk for injury
Monitor the patient's cognitive function. Identify changes that increase the risk for patient injury, such as wandering, behavioral outbursts, and inattention to what is going on in the environment.

Provide a consistent, familiar environment with good lighting for the patient. Remove obstacles and hazards from the environment (i.e., scatter rugs, candles). Supervise the patient if he or she has a tendency to wander or has potential to inflict self-harm.

NDx: Ineffective family coping
Support the family in developing effective coping mechanisms. Provide for an accepting environment

to allow for expression of anxiety, fear, hopelessness, and other emotions. Allow family members or significant others to express feelings without placing value or judgment on what they say. Ensure that a private area is available to meet with family members or significant others.

Identify support groups and resources available, such as the Alzheimer's Disease and Related Disorders Association. Teach the family strategies that are effective in managing the patient's behavioral alterations (i.e., consistent environment, reduction of stress in environment, consistent manner to handle outbursts and other behaviors). Monitor the family's reaction to caring for the patient. Identify increased periods of stress or difficulty coping with situations. Reinforce with the family their need for respite and support. Encourage family members to meet their own personal needs and not to extend beyond their physical or emotional limitations. Refer to day-care centers and respite centers.

Evaluation

Evaluate the effectiveness of nursing care for a patient with Alzheimer's disease by comparing the patient's status with the expected patient outcomes. Examples of specific outcomes for patients with Alzheimer's disease have been provided in the Planning section.

Herniated Disk Disease

ETIOLOGY

The intervertebral disk lies between two adjacent vertebrae. Its function is to absorb shock and permit motion. Traumatic incidents, such as lifting heavy objects without proper body mechanics or falling, can precipitate a herniation or rupturing of disk material into the spinal canal, where it can impinge on a spinal nerve root (Fig. 38–6). Degenerative changes in the supporting ligaments predispose to

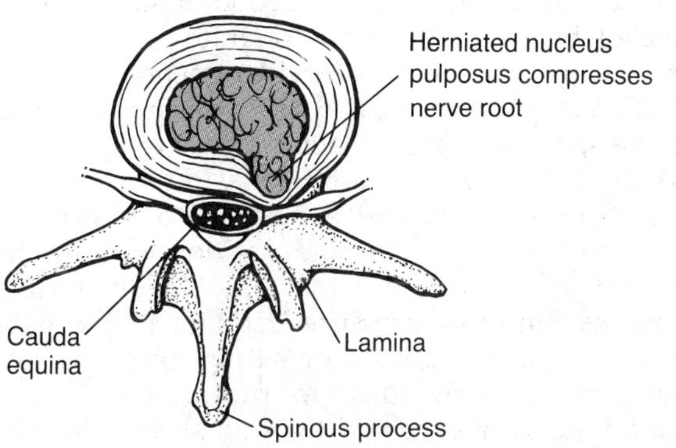

Figure 38–6.

Herniated intervertebral disk.

Table 38–2. CLINICAL MANIFESTATIONS OF NERVE ROOT COMPRESSION SECONDARY TO DISK HERNIATION

COMPRESSED NERVE ROOT*	CLINICAL MANIFESTATIONS
Sixth cervical	Paresthesia and sensory loss in the dorsum of the head Weakness of the biceps Decreased biceps reflex
Seventh cervical	Paresthesias and sensory loss in third and fourth fingers Slight weakness of the triceps Decreased triceps reflex
Fifth lumbar	Pain and paresthesias in the hip, groin, posterolateral thigh, lateral calf, top of the foot to the great and second toes
First sacral	Pain and paresthesias in the midgluteal area, posterior thigh, calf, heel, bottom of the foot to the fourth and fifth toes
Fourth lumbar	Pain in the lower back extending down the anterior surface of the leg to the great toe

*Compressed nerve roots are listed in order of frequency of occurrence.

herniation, and in many cases no specific precipitating event can be identified.

PATHOPHYSIOLOGY

The cervical and lumbar spines are the most flexible and therefore the most susceptible to stress and injury. Herniation of an intervertebral disk in the cervical spine usually takes place between the fifth and sixth or sixth and seventh cervical vertebrae. Herniation of a lumbosacral disk most often occurs between the fourth and fifth lumbar vertebra and results in irritation and compression of the fifth lumbar root. Herniated disks in the thoracic area are rare.

CLINICAL MANIFESTATIONS

The clinical manifestations of a herniated disk vary with the location of the affected disk and the degree of herniation. A small protrusion of a cervical disk causes a stiff neck accompanied by shoulder pain, which radiates down the arm.

Clinical manifestations associated with herniation of lumbar disks include backache, change in posture, and limited motion of the spine. The back pain associated with herniation of a lumbar disk is generally relieved by lying supine on a firm surface with the head slightly elevated and the hips and knees slightly flexed or by lying on the unaffected side with the affected leg flexed at the hip and knee. The pain is aggravated by sitting, standing, bending, coughing, sneezing, and straining.

Larger herniations, whether cervical or lumbar, can compress the nerve root and cause more extensive pain and paresthesias, as described in Table 38–2.

MEDICAL DIAGNOSIS

The diagnosis of herniated disk disease is suggested by the symptoms elicited through the history and physical examination. It is confirmed by CT scan and myelogram. Electromyelography may be done to localize affected nerve roots. The use of MRI, a noninvasive test that provides clear images of spinal cord anatomy, is also being increasingly used. Spinal x-ray films can indicate narrowing of an intervertebral disk but may not show a herniated disk or spinal cord lesion.

MEDICAL MANAGEMENT

Medical management of a herniated disk can consist of conservative or surgical treatment. Conservative treatment consists of enforced bed rest; use of a firm mattress; avoidance of any activity involving flexion of the spine; use of supportive devices such as a corset, brace, or cervical collar; use of pelvic traction (lumbar disk) or halter traction (cervical disk); physiotherapy treatments; and medications to relieve pain and decrease muscle spasm. Surgery is indicated for those patients who do not respond to conservative treatment or whose symptoms warrant immediate surgical intervention.

Application of the Nursing Process to the Care of the Patient with a Herniated Disk

Assessment

Assess the patient's discomfort. Ask the patient to describe the type of pain experienced (aching, burning, tearing, and so on), its severity, its location, any identifiable precipitating factors, such as sitting for a long period of time or writing at a desk, and any pattern to the pain such as an exacerbation in the morning. Ask also about associated symptoms, including limitation of movement, and paresthesias. Explore when the current problem began as well as any history of a similar problem. Determine what treatment measures, if any, have been used and their effectiveness. Observe for changes in posture that suggest the patient is trying to prevent pain or to protect a painful area. Check range of motion, muscle strength, and reflexes in the affected areas.

If this is a recurrent problem, assess the patient's understanding of the cause of the pain and of measures that limit stress on the spine. Also assess the psychosocial effects of the problem on the patient. Explore the patient's ability to work and to participate in household, social, and recreational activities. Assess the patient's feelings about self in relationship to the disorder and the patient's ability to cope and style of doing so.

Nursing Diagnoses and Planning

Nursing diagnoses and related expected patient outcomes most commonly applicable to patients with a herniated disk include the following:

NDx: Pain related to nerve irritation and muscle spasm

Planning: Patient outcomes
1. Patient restricts movement as directed.
2. Patient reports that pain is manageable and decreasing.
3. Patient performs allowed activities without exacerbated pain.

NDx: High risk for altered tissue perfusion related to impaired venous blood flow secondary to thrombophlebitis or pulmonary embolism

Planning: Patient outcomes
1. Patient performs foot and leg exercises as directed.
2. Calves are free of heat, redness, and swelling.
3. Homans' sign (pain in calf on strong, passive dorsiflexion of foot) is negative.

NDx: High risk for altered health maintenance related to insufficient knowledge of measures to reduce stress on the cervical or lumbar spine

Planning: Patient outcomes
1. Patient explains measures to reduce stress on the lumbar spine, as presented in Chart 38–2.
2. Patient expresses willingness to comply with measures to reduce stress on the lumbar spine.
3. Patient expresses confidence in the ability to comply with measures to reduce stress on the lumbar spine.

Nursing Interventions

NDx: Pain
Maintain the patient with herniation of a cervical disk on bed rest with continuous traction while pain is acute. Subsequently, keep the neck immobilized with a collar, and apply traction intermittently as directed by the physician. (Refer to Chapter 35 for the care of the patient in cervical traction.)

Maintain patients on bed rest to control pain and muscle spasm during the acute phase of lumbosacral disk herniation. Make certain that the mattress provides firm support; use a bed board if necessary. Place the patient in a supine position with the head elevated 30 degrees and the hips slightly flexed to minimize intradisk pressure. Explain to the patient that attempting to get up or sitting for even a short time can cause the disk to protrude further and result in another attack. Use a pull sheet, which goes from under the shoulder to midthigh, and a pillow between the legs to move the patient while maintaining correct alignment. Instruct the patient not to

Chart 38–2.

NURSING GUIDE TO PATIENT EDUCATION FOR SELF-MANAGEMENT: MEASURES TO REDUCE STRESS ON THE LUMBAR SPINE

Instruct the patient to:

Maintain good posture: back straight, shoulders back, abdomen and neck tucked in.
Exercise regularly during asymptomatic periods to strengthen the muscles of the back and abdomen. Perform flexion or isometric exercise routine prescribed by the physician.
Sit in a straight-back chair with feet on footstool so knees are flexed above level of hips.
Avoid extended periods of sitting or driving.
Sleep on the back or side, never on the stomach.
Sleep on a mattress with firm support. Use bed board if necessary, but avoid placing the mattress on the floor, because getting up and down may further injure the spine.
Avoid rotating or extending the spine.
Carry objects close to the chest.
Bend at the hips and knees, not at the waist.
Face objects to be lifted directly.
Avoid lifting while bending.
Avoid lifting anything heavier than 10 pounds.
Wear a lumbar corset to protect the back during strenuous activities.
Reduce activity at the first sign of pain.
Use a firm backrest in the car.
Stop and walk at least every 2 hours while riding.
Maintain or regain recommended body weight.

move without assistance. Caution the patient not to raise self by pulling on the side rails, not to stretch to reach for anything, and not to write, do handwork, or hold a book or magazine to read while lying flat because all these activities place further stress on the spine. Also instruct the patient to avoid coughing and sneezing when possible. To facilitate compliance with these instructions, keep the call bell and personal items within easy reach, and provide a reading rack and prism glasses to allow the patient to read or watch television. Give cough suppressants and allergy medications as ordered to control coughing or sneezing.

Administer analgesics every 3 to 4 hours for the first 48 to 72 hours, and have the patient wear a lumbar corset if ordered to immobilize the spine and provide proper alignment. Apply hot, moist packs as ordered every 1 to 2 hours for up to 30 minutes.

Change the patient's position to a side-lying one with knees flexed and the upper knee resting on a pillow when permitted. Recognize that this is often the position of comfort for the patient with leg pain.

Use a fracture pan to meet patient's elimination needs. Place a small pillow on the bed just above the upper edge of the pan to support the spine. Logroll the patient on and off the pan. Caution the patient not to use toilet paper or get off the pan without assistance. Encourage the patient to increase water and roughage in the diet to prevent straining at stool. Administer stool softeners as ordered.

Guide the patient in the progressive exercise program prescribed by the physician. When allowed, provide instruction on how to get out of bed with the least amount of strain on the back. Instruct the patient to turn on the side with the knees flexed and slide (or be moved on a pull sheet) to the edge of the bed. Have the patient next push him- or herself up with the hands while keeping the spine straight and easing the feet and legs over the side of the bed. Instruct the patient to select a straight chair with arm rests and to sit with the back flat against the chair and the knees flexed higher than the hips. Remind the patient to resume activities slowly according to the physician's directions and to sit a maximum of 30 minutes at one time.

NDx: High risk for altered tissue perfusion

Begin foot and leg exercises to promote venous circulation as soon as the acute pain subsides. Instruct the patient to flex the hip and the knee and to slide the heel of the foot along the mattress to the top of the incline created by the knee gatch and then down. Have the patient perform this exercise five times with each leg every 2 to 3 hours while awake. Apply antiembolic stockings if prescribed.

NDx: High risk for altered health maintenance

Instruct the patient in self-care measures to reduce stress on the lumbar spine, as presented in Chart 38–2.

Evaluation

Evaluate the effectiveness of nursing care for a patient with a herniated disk by comparing the patient's status with the expected patient outcomes. Examples of specific outcomes for patients with a herniated disk have been provided in the Planning section.

Functional Disorders

Seizure Disorders

Seizure disorders are chronic conditions characterized by a change in a person's motor or sensory system functioning and behavior. The specific symptoms manifested and their magnitude are dependent on the area of cerebral tissue involved. This change in functioning and behavior results from an uncontrolled excessive discharge of neurons in the cerebral tissue. The period between seizure episodes varies and can range from minutes to days to months to years.

ETIOLOGY

Seizure disorders are caused by factors affecting the cortex of the brain. These factors include genetic disorders, metabolic or electrolyte imbalances, infection, trauma, vascular disease, congenital malformations, encephalopathies, neoplasms, and degenerative diseases.

PATHOPHYSIOLOGY

During a seizure episode, there is an uncontrolled excessive discharge of neurons in the brain. This is accompanied by an increase in the oxygen consumption of the brain and body, an increase in the blood pressure and pulse, and a decrease in the blood oxygen tension (Po_2) level. During the recovery phase between seizure episodes, the body regains homeostasis and no residual brain damage occurs.

Status epilepticus is a state of recurrent seizure activity without interictal recovery between seizures. Without a recovery period, hypoxia results and brain damage is imminent. Status epilepticus is a neurologic emergency and requires *immediate* intervention. Adults often present in status epilepticus as a result of their noncompliance to a prescribed anticonvulsant medication regimen. It may also be a symptom of an underlying structural abnormality (i.e., lesion, tumor mass).

CLINICAL MANIFESTATIONS

The clinical manifestations of the patient during a seizure episode depend on the part of the brain from which the neuron discharge originates, the number of neurons excited, and the extent to which there is spread of activity.

Seizures are often classified into two categories: focal or partial (involving a particular area of the brain) and generalized (involving the entire brain, no focus identified). See Table 38–3 for the characteristics of partial and generalized seizures.

MEDICAL DIAGNOSIS

A complete history and neurologic examination are performed to establish the focal or general characteristics of the seizure disorder. Laboratory serum tests are performed to establish baseline parameters and to identify any metabolic or electrolyte imbalance that could induce seizure activity (glucose, sodium, BUN, calcium). An EEG is performed to document abnormal electrical discharge of the brain. In cases in which temporal lobe involvement may be suspected, a sleep EEG may be performed. CT scans, MRI, and lumbar puncture with cerebrospinal fluid studies may also be done to rule out other underlying pathology.

MEDICAL MANAGEMENT

The first step in planning appropriate medical management for persons with a seizure disorder is to determine the cause. If the seizure disorder is related to a space-occupying lesion, metabolic imbalance, or infectious process, the underlying cause is the focus of treatment.

Anticonvulsant drug therapy (Pharmacology Box 38–2) is the most common treatment mode for patients with seizure disorders. Anticonvulsant therapy is a symptomatic treatment, not a cure for seizure disorders. Certain drugs are more effective for specific types of seizure activity than others. For example, phenytoin (Dilantin), primidone (Mysoline), carbamazepine (Tegretol), divalproex (Depakote), and phenobarbital tend to be more effective for partial and generalized tonic-clonic seizures; ethosuximide (Zarontin), Depakote, and clonazepam (Klonopin) for absence and generalized (non–tonic-clonic) seizures; and diazepam (Valium), phenobarbital, Dilantin, and paraldehyde for status epilepticus.

Anticonvulsants are introduced gradually while serum blood levels are monitored to establish the therapeutic dose for seizure control. Monotherapy is

Table 38–3. SEIZURE CLASSIFICATION

TYPE	DURATION	SEIZURE SYMPTOMS	POSTICTAL SYMPTOMS
PARTIAL SEIZURES			
Simple partial	30 sec	Symptoms vary: sudden jerking, sensory phenomena	No loss of consciousness
Complex partial	1–2 min	May have aura Staring Automatism (e.g., lip smacking, picking at clothes, fumbling) Unaware of environment May wander	Amnesia for seizure events Mild to moderate confusion
GENERALIZED SEIZURES			
Absence (petit mal)	2–15 sec	Stare Eyes fluttering	Amnesia for seizure events No confusion Able to resume activity
Generalized tonic-clonic (grand mal)	1–2 min	A cry Fall Tonicity (rigidity) Clonicity (jerking) May have cyanosis	Amnesia for seizure events Confusion Deep sleep

the goal of most anticonvulsant treatment regimens, but occasionally drugs are used in combination to decrease the potential for toxic effects associated with single-drug therapy.

Just as anticonvulsant drugs are introduced on a gradual basis, withdrawal of therapy is also gradual, using tapered dosages. Sudden withdrawal of anticonvulsants precipitates seizure activity or even status epilepticus.

In certain instances, surgical intervention may be indicated to control seizure activity. These include situations in which medications cannot control seizure activity or surgical procedure would not risk neurologic deficit (language center not involved). The corpus callosum has been surgically divided in patients with severe generalized seizures.

Application of the Nursing Process to the Care of the Patient with a Seizure Disorder

Assessment

Assessment of the patient includes a history and neurologic examination. Ask the patient to describe how the seizure started. "Were there any physical symptoms, such as head or eyes turning to one side, arm or leg rigidity or shaking movements, incontinence?"; "Were there any warning signs or auras?"; "How did the seizure progress?"; "How long did the seizure last?"; "Did you sleep after the seizure was over?"; and "Do you remember anything that was said during the seizure?" In cases in which the patient cannot give complete information, ask a family member or significant other to provide the history and other information.

Ascertain whether anyone else in the family has similar complaints, symptoms, or known seizure disorders. Identify medical or social conditions that would influence or precipitate seizure activity, such as alcohol or drug ingestion, adherence to medication regimen, trauma at birth, cerebrovascular accident, neoplasm, and surgical procedure involving the brain.

Allow the patient to discuss the emotional and psychosocial impact of this condition on self and family functioning. Ask the patient, "Have you changed how you act or what you do when you are at home or at work?"; and "Is there anything you refuse to do because you feel you may get hurt or that it may put you into an embarrassing situation if you were to experience a seizure episode?" Assess the patient's level of safety, compliance with therapeutic plan, alteration of lifestyle, and emotional status.

Nursing Diagnoses and Planning

Nursing diagnoses and related expected patient outcomes most commonly applicable to patients with seizure disorders include the following:

NDx: High risk for injury related to uncontrolled movements during seizure episode

Planning: Patient outcomes
1. Patient remains free from injury.
2. Patient avoids activities or jobs that could cause injury to self or others (powerful machinery, mountain climbing, driving).
3. Patient adheres to prescribed anticonvulsant medication regimen.

Pharmacology Box 38–2.
ANTICONVULSANTS

Anticonvulsants:
These drugs prevent or decrease seizure activity. Major classes of anticonvulsants are barbiturates (e.g., phenobarbital), benzodiazepines (e.g., clonazepam), hydantoins (e.g., phenytoin), oxazolidinedione derivatives (e.g., trimethadione), and succinimides (e.g., ethosuximide).

Action:
Anticonvulsants act on the central nervous system (CNS) in a variety of ways to reduce seizure activity. For example, barbiturates depress impulse transmission across synapses, whereas hydantoins alter the passage of sodium ions across membranes and thus affect impulse generation.

Uses:
Barbiturates are generally effective against generalized tonic-clonic and absence seizures, hydantoins against generalized tonic-clonic and complex partial seizures, and oxazolidinediones and succinimides against absence seizures. However, each anticonvulsant is used for specific types of seizures, so indications for individual drugs should be checked.

Side Effects:
Side effects vary with the individual drug. Common side effects for a drug from each of the major classes of anticonvulsants are as follows:

Barbiturates (phenobarbital): drowsiness, lethargy, nausea, vomiting, rashes, nerve, muscle or joint pain, inflammation
Benzodiazepines (clonazepam): drowsiness, ataxia, behavioral disturbances, increased salivation
Hydantoins (phenytoin): ataxia, slurred speech, confusion, nausea, vomiting, hyperplasia of the gums, dermatitis, nystagmus, double vision, agranulocytosis
Oxazolidinediones (trimethadione): drowsiness, malaise, exfoliative dermatitis, agranulocytosis, aplastic and hypoplastic anemia
Succinimides (ethosuximide): drowsiness, fatigue, dizziness, euphoria, nausea, vomiting, epigastric and abdominal pain, agranulocytosis, aplastic anemia

Interactions:
Interactions vary with the individual drug. Common examples of interactions are as follows:

Phenobarbital: taken with alcohol, narcotic analgesics, other CNS depressants, or monoamine oxidase inhibitors can result in excessive CNS depression; taken with primidone or valproic acid may result in excessive blood levels of phenobarbital; taken with rifampin may have a decreased effect
Clonazepam: None of significance
Phenytoin: taken with alcohol, folic acid, or loxapine results in a decreased effect; taken with oral anticoagulants, antihistamines, chloramphenicol, diazepam, cimetidine, diazoxide, isoniazid, phenylbutazone, salicylates, and sulfamethoxazole results in an increased and potentially toxic effect
Trimethadione: None of significance
Ethosuximide: None of significance

Nursing Implications:
For all anticonvulsants, instruct the patient to do the following:

Avoid activities that demand mental alertness and coordination until the response to the drug is determined.
Call physician immediately if side effects occur.
Never stop taking the drug without consulting the physician because such action can precipitate increased seizure activity.

(continued)

Pharmacology Box 38–2. *(continued)*

ANTICONVULSANTS

Additional nursing implications are as follows:

Phenobarbital: Observe for signs of toxicity: wheezing, cyanosis, clammy skin, hypotension, coma.
- Instruct patient to avoid use of alcohol.
- Explain that full therapeutic effect may not occur for 2 to 3 weeks.
- If ordered intravenously, give drug slowly and monitor respiratory status closely.

Clonazepam: Observe for oversedation.
- Explain need for complete blood count (CBC) and liver function tests.

Phenytoin: Instruct the patient to do the following:
- Carry an identification card indicating that phenytoin is taken and the dose.
- Avoid heavy use of alcohol because it may interfere with effectiveness of the drug.
- Do not change drug brands once stabilized on a drug because untoward effects may occur.
- Explain (1) that drug may color urine pink, red, or reddish brown; (2) the importance of good oral hygiene and regular dental checkups; (3) need for CBC and serum calcium levels every 6 months.
- If ordered intravenously, do not mix with dextrose 5% in water; do not use cloudy solution; administer over 30–60 minutes when possible; begin infusion within 1 hour of mixing and discard after 4 hours.

Trimethadione: Explain the need for CBC, liver function tests, and urinalysis before starting drug and monthly thereafter.
- Instruct the patient to (1) report immediately skin rash, alopecia, sore throat, fever, bruises or nosebleeds; (2) wear sunglasses if vision blurs in bright light and report to physician.

Ethosuximide: Explain the need for a CBC every 3 months.

Chart 38–3.

NURSING GUIDE TO PATIENT EDUCATION FOR SELF-MANAGEMENT: CARE RELATED TO SEIZURES

Instruct the patient and/or family to:

- Maintain a diary/journal of all seizure activity.
- Note time of onset, duration, and description of seizures.
- Take all antiseizure medications on time.
- Report any side effects of medication (i.e., dizziness, unsteady gait, cognitive impairment, visual changes, nausea, or vomiting).
- Practice good oral hygiene.
- Wear medical alert identification.
- Protect the patient from harming self during a seizure.
- Refrain from restraining patient, and never place objects in the patient's mouth.
- Call emergency services if seizure lasts longer than 5 minutes.
- Avoid driving and operating heavy equipment.
- Wear a helmet while bike riding.
- Swim only under close supervision.
- Avoid cigarette smoking.
- Keep regularly scheduled health care appointments.

NDx: High risk for altered oral mucous membrane related to effects of drug therapy on oral tissue

Planning: Patient outcomes
1. Patient performs mouth care daily.
2. Gum hyperplasia is absent.

NDx: Self-esteem disturbance related to unpredictable nature of seizures and embarrassment

Planning: Patient outcomes
1. Patient actively engages in social and job-related activities.
2. Patient expresses feelings of anxiety and concerns.
3. Patient expresses confidence in ability to cope with necessary alteration of lifestyle and family functioning.

NDx: High risk for aspiration related to status epilepticus

Planning: Patient outcomes
1. Patient maintains clear airway.
2. Arterial blood gas values are within normal range.
3. Patient remains afebrile.
4. Patient remains free from aspiration of secretions during seizure episode.

NDx: Impaired gas exchange related to status epilepticus

Planning: Patient outcomes
1. Patient avoids irreversible cerebral damage or hypoxia.
2. Arterial blood gas values remain within normal range.

NDx: High risk for altered health maintenance

Planning: Patient outcomes
1. Patient and family describe self-care measures, as presented in Chart 38–3.
2. Patient and family verbalize willingness and ability to comply with self-care measures presented in Chart 38–3.

Nursing Interventions

NDx: High risk for injury
Provide a safe environment for the patient. Ensure that bed side rails are in working order, and pad side rails for patients with known motor seizures. Do not restrain a patient during seizure activity. Protect the patient's head from hitting a hard surface, such as the floor, by placing a pillow or blanket under the head or by holding it. Call for help. *Do not* leave the patient. Place an oral airway in the mouth when the patient is in a relaxation phase to maintain airway and allow for suctioning as necessary.

Instruct the patient to promote own safety by lying down when an aura is experienced. Encourage normal daily activities. Discuss with the patient those activities that could result in injury or harm and that should be avoided (e.g., operating hazardous machinery, mountain climbing). Conduct an environmental safety review of the home (e.g., hard floors that could be carpeted) and suggest improvements or changes. Explain that a driver's license is granted only with evidence of seizure-free activity between 1 and 3 years, depending on individual state laws.

Instruct the patient on the importance of adherence to anticonvulsant medication regimen. Caution the patient *not* to stop medications if no seizure activity is noted or if he or she feels better.

NDx: High risk for altered oral mucous membrane
Instruct the patient on the importance of good oral hygiene. Allow the patient to redemonstrate steps of oral hygiene to ensure understanding and performance. Explain to the patient that gum hyperplasia is a side effect of some anticonvulsant medications such as Dilantin. If soreness or bleeding of the gums is noticed, inform the physician.

NDx: Self-esteem disturbance
Ask the patient how this condition has affected the ability to carry out daily activities. Support the patient, and encourage sharing of fears, feelings, and anxieties. Assist the patient in identifying strengths and weaknesses, and encourage the use of effective coping mechanisms to manage alterations in lifestyle. Set expectations for social, family, and work interactions. Provide the patient with resources for support, such as the Epilepsy Foundation, other persons with seizure disorders, and support groups.

NDx: High risk for aspiration
Place an oral airway at the patient's bedside, and ensure proper working order of suction equipment for emergency use.

When a patient is in status epilepticus, place an oral airway in the mouth during initiation or relaxation phase of seizure activity. *Do not force* airway in the mouth when the teeth are clenched. Turn the patient on his or her side to allow for drainage of secretions. Administer oxygen and suction patient as necessary to maintain a clear airway.

NDx: Impaired gas exchange
Ensure that properly working oxygen and suction are maintained at the patient's bedside for emergency use. Obtain access to emergency medications used to treat patients in status epilepticus: dextrose 50%, Valium, Dilantin, and phenobarbital injectables.

When a patient is in status epilepticus, maintain patent airway (position head, insert oral airway, suction as needed), administer or give oxygen via nasal cannula, call for physician, prepare intravenous catheter and medications to be administered to interrupt status, assist physician, and maintain safety of patient.

NDx: High risk for altered health maintenance
Instruct the patient and the family in self-care measures, as presented in Chart 38–3.

Evaluation

Evaluate the effectiveness of nursing care for a patient with a seizure disorder by comparing the patient's status with the expected patient outcomes. Examples of specific outcomes for patients with seizure disorders have been provided in the Planning section.

Headache

Headache is probably the most prevalent of complaints and varies in intensity, duration, and frequency.

ETIOLOGY AND PATHOPHYSIOLOGY

The symptom of headache may be caused by an organic factor (intracranial, extracranial lesions, mass, or hemorrhage), stress or muscle tension, vasodilation, or a combination of these. The majority of patients presenting with headache as a chief complaint do not have an underlying neurologic cause for the headache.

CLINICAL MANIFESTATIONS

Clinical manifestations of a patient experiencing a headache are dependent on the type of headache. The most common types of headache include vascular (cluster and migraine) and tension.

Cluster Headaches. Cluster headaches are a type of vascular headache. Alcohol ingestion is the primary precipitating factor that is identified. The headaches occur in clusters: They could occur 8 times a day and even more than 30 times each week. The attacks may be seasonal and even may awaken the patient from sleep. The duration of cluster headaches varies from 30 minutes to hours. Males seem to experience cluster headaches more frequently than females. Patients may also complain of nasal congestion, drooping eyelid (ptosis), tearing of the eyes (lacrimation), and feeling flushed.

Migraine Headaches. Migraine headaches are also a type of vascular headache. They are considered a hereditary condition and are precipitated by vasodilation and increased cerebral blood flow. Females seem to experience migraine headaches more frequently than males. Patients complain of a throbbing sensation, unilateral head pain, nausea, vomiting, photophobia, blurred vision, and nasal congestion.

Tension Headaches (Muscle Contraction Headaches). Tension headaches are also known as muscle contraction headaches. Anxiety and tension are usually the precipitating factors for this type of headache. Common complaints from patients with tension headaches include tightness around the forehead area, dizziness, tenderness in the neck and scalp, and bilateral involvement.

MEDICAL DIAGNOSIS

A history and physical and neurologic examination are performed to determine the type of headache and the underlying cause. The history focuses on familial patterns and the patient's own history of headaches. The physical and neurologic examination focuses on assessment of the body systems to rule out or identify underlying pathology. In addition, neurodiagnostic tests, such as CT scan, MRI, and EEG, are performed to rule out a neurologic cause.

MEDICAL MANAGEMENT

Medical management of the patient with a headache focuses on the symptomatic relief of pain.

The management of vascular headaches (migraine, cluster) includes a combination of drug therapy and awareness and control of precipitating factors. Drug therapy includes the prescription of isometheptene mucate (Midrin), ergotamine tartrate (Gynergen), ergotamine with caffeine (Cafergot), or dihydroergotamine for immediate relief of vascular headache. Midrin and ergotamine have a vasoconstrictive action and are used primarily for treatment of headaches. Other drugs that are useful as a means of prophylactic treatment of vascular headaches include methysergide (Sansert), propranolol (Inderal), and clonidine (Catapres), which inhibit vasodilation of blood vessels.

The management of tension and muscle contraction headaches includes a combination of anxiety and tension relief and drug therapy. Drug therapy includes analgesics and sedatives to relieve anxiety and tension. Analgesics—such as butalbit, aspirin, and caffeine (Fiorinal); oxycodone hydrochloride, oxycodone terephthalate, and aspirin (Percodan); and propoxyphane, aspirin, and caffeine (Darvon) — and sedatives, such as diazepam, phenobarbital, and meprobamate, have proven to be effective. Biofeedback techniques are used to promote reduction of anxiety and tension.

Application of the Nursing Process to the Care of the Patient with Headache

Assessment

Assessment of the patient with headache includes a history and a physical and neurologic examination. The history is extensive and includes a general history, familial history, and a history of headaches. Ask the patient probing questions such as "Have you had any significant injuries, medical conditions, or diseases, such as sinusitis, surgery, infections, or trauma?"; "Does anyone else in your family complain of headaches?"; and "Are there any members of your family with long-standing medical problems such as seizure disorders, a neurologic condition, allergies, or psychiatric illness?" Allow the patient to describe the onset of the headaches, their extent, and duration. Ask the patient questions such as "Is there anything you can do to decrease or eliminate your headache, such as lying down in a dark, quiet room or even trying to calm yourself down from feeling anxious or stressed?" Elicit any patterns that seem to coincide with headaches, such as menstruation in women, argument with a family member or significant other, or stress in the work setting. Focus the physical and neurologic examination on identifying abnormal findings that may be attributed to underlying pathology. Assess for the presence of motor or sensory dysfunction, such as ptosis and photophobia.

Identify any psychosocial or work stress that could precipitate headache. Allow the patient to describe work, family, and social settings. Ask the patient what he or she does for relaxation (i.e., hobbies, sports, activities). Determine whether the people whom the patient is around complain of headaches at the same time to identify an environmental factor as a potential causative agent.

Nursing Diagnoses and Planning

Nursing diagnoses and related expected patient outcomes most commonly applicable to patients with headache include the following:

NDx: Pain related to headache

Planning: Patient outcomes
1. Patient identifies factors that precipitate headaches.
2. Patient performs daily activities without limitations.
3. Headache pain is absent.

NDx: Anxiety related to incidence of headache

Planning: Patient outcomes
1. Patient verbalizes anxiety and concerns.
2. Patient states anxiety is manageable.

NDx: Ineffective individual coping related to recurrent headache

Planning: Patient outcomes
1. Patient uses effective coping strategies.
2. Patient describes knowledge of available resources and supports.

Nursing Interventions

NDx: Pain
Monitor the level of discomfort the patient is experiencing by using a visual analogue scale (scale from 1 to 10, with 10 being the worst pain ever experienced). Encourage the patient to discuss the pain. Monitor and observe for a trend as to how the patient reacts to pain and his or her tolerance to pain. Administer prescribed analgesics and other medications promptly. Observe the patient for relief of headache pain.

NDx: Anxiety
Monitor the patient for signs of anxiety and stress. Explore with the patient feelings of anxiety and circumstances that precipitate an anxious feeling. Encourage the patient to verbalize fears, past experiences, and perceptions of pain. Explain to the patient that anxiety and stress are causative factors of headaches. Explain the relationship of stress and its effect on physiologic functioning (irritability, tension, stomach upset, and headache). Explore with the patient typical work, family, and social situations that elicit anxiety, and identify strategies to control or decrease anxiety. Role-play difficult or confrontational situations to allow the patient to practice responding. Encourage the patient to remove him- or herself from a situation in which he or she has no control over reducing the anxiety level.

NDx: Ineffective individual coping
Establish a trusting relationship with the patient. Provide an accepting environment that allows the patient to express him- or herself freely. Accomplish this by maintaining privacy and a nonjudgmental approach to the patient. Encourage the patient to describe various personal situations and how he or she felt and responded. Explore with the patient alternate responses to the same situation that may have produced a more positive outcome or that allowed him or her to maintain, or even increase, control over personal feelings and actions. This enables the patient to gain insight into circumstances in which he or she may not have coped effectively and to increase awareness of effective coping mechanisms. Role-play to provide the patient with an opportunity to practice responding effectively in difficult and conflicting situations.

Evaluation

Evaluate the effectiveness of nursing care for a patient with headache by comparing the patient's status with the expected patient outcomes. Examples of specific outcomes for patients with headache have been provided in the Planning section.

Structural Disorders

Hydrocephalus

Hydrocephalus is a clinical syndrome in which there is an increase in the volume of cerebrospinal fluid in the cerebroventricular system.

ETIOLOGY AND PATHOPHYSIOLOGY

Hydrocephalus is related to a dysfunction in the production, circulation, or reabsorption of cerebrospinal fluid. There are three types of hydrocephalus: communicating, noncommunicating, and normal pressure.

In communicating hydrocephalus, there is interference in the reabsorption process of cerebrospinal fluid through the subarachnoid villi into the venous blood circulation. This often occurs in patients who have had a subarachnoid hemorrhage (SAH) or meningitis, in which the subarachnoid villi become blocked or occluded from blood, exudate, or other particles. This may be a transient or permanent blockage.

Noncommunicating hydrocephalus, also known as obstructive hydrocephalus, occurs when a blockage exists within the cerebroventricular system. The most significant causes of this obstruction are tumors of the third and fourth ventricles (pinealomas, medulloblastomas). These tumors create a blockage within the ventricles and also impinge on the aqueducts and incisural edge of the tentorium, restricting cerebrospinal fluid circulation and flow to the subarachnoid villi for reabsorption.

Normal pressure hydrocephalus frequently occurs in adults older than 60 years. There is no known cause. There is an increase in the volume of cerebrospinal fluids, causing enlargement of the cerebral ventricles; however, no increased cerebrospinal fluid pressure or signs of increased intracranial pressure are noted.

CLINICAL MANIFESTATIONS

The clinical manifestations of patients with communicating and noncommunicating hydrocephalus are related to increased intracranial pressure. Initial headache, restlessness, and irritability progress to severe headache, projectile vomiting, decreased level of consciousness, blurred vision, diplopia, papilledema, and eventually neurologic deterioration resulting in death if the individual is not treated.

Patients experiencing normal pressure hydrocephalus manifest a classic triad of symptoms: gait disturbance, dementia, and urinary incontinence. Gait disturbance is often the presenting symptom. The patient may be forgetful and have impaired memory function. With treatment, mental functioning can be improved.

MEDICAL DIAGNOSIS

A complete history and neurologic examination are performed to identify onset and progression of symptoms and underlying pathology. A CT scan is used to demonstrate enlarged ventricles, and a lumbar puncture is done to document increased or normal cerebrospinal fluid pressure. MRI and myelogram may be indicated to demonstrate cerebrospinal fluid pathways as well as identify underlying pathology.

MEDICAL MANAGEMENT

The most common method of treatment for hydrocephalus is ventricular shunting, which reestablishes normal routes of cerebrospinal fluid circulation and thus alleviates hydrocephalus. The two types of ventricular shunts are internalized shunts and externalized shunts.

INTERNALIZED VENTRICULAR SHUNTS

Ventriculoperitoneal internal shunts are used to treat adults with hydrocephalus (Fig. 38–7). Insertion of the shunt is a major surgical procedure that takes 1 to 2 hours.

Physical Preparation of the Patient

There is no physical preparation before the patient enters the operating room. Once in the operating room, general anesthesia is administered. To decrease the risk of infection, the head area where the shunt will be inserted is shaved, and the scalp and abdomen are scrubbed with an antiseptic solution.

Procedure

Two incisions are made: one in the head and one in the abdomen. The shunt tube is passed beneath the skin in the fatty tissue. A burr hole is made in the skull. The ventricular shunt catheter tip is passed through the brain into the frontal horn of the lateral ventricle. This is a direct, uncomplicated approach, ensuring accuracy of shunt catheter tip placement. The distal end of the catheter is placed in the peritoneal cavity. The shunt has a standardized, one-way flow valve unit that allows for the outward flow of cerebrospinal fluid from the cerebral ventricles into the peritoneal cavity, where it can be reabsorbed.

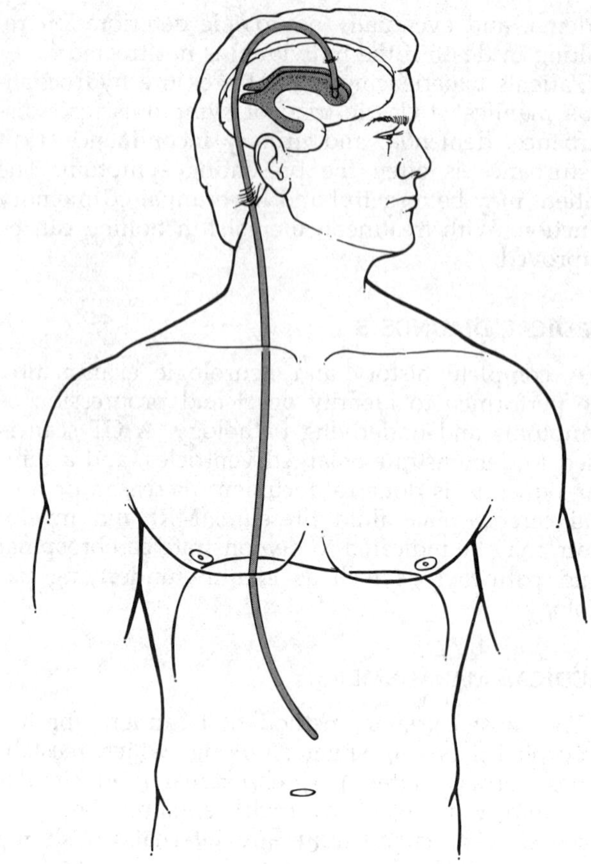

Figure 38–7.

Ventriculoperitoneal internal shunt.

Postoperative Course

The physician determines the progress in activity level after the procedure. The patient initially is on bed rest with no or only minimal head gatch; he or she then slowly increases activity over the following days. This allows the patient's body to adjust to the changes in pressure and return of normal cerebrospinal fluid circulation and reabsorption. Patients are generally up in about 1 to 2 days.

Complications

Common complications of an internal shunt include infection and shunt failure (blockage of the system by debris, blood, or cells; misplacement of catheter tip end; or a break in integrity of shunt components). Shunt failure requires surgical revision of the shunt, whereas infection may necessitate externalization (an exit site incision is made in the neck area through which the distal portion of the shunt is removed and attached to an external cerebrospinal fluid collection device to maintain outflow of cerebrospinal fluid from ventricles to collection device) of the shunt temporarily and initiation of antibiotic treatment regimen. Contamination during the operative placement of the ventricular shunt or infection at the insertion incisional sites increases the risk of tract infections, meningitis, and peritonitis.

EXTERNALIZED VENTRICULAR SHUNTS

Externalized ventricular shunts allow for temporary regulation of intracranial pressure and control of cerebrospinal fluid flow. The external shunt is used during operative procedures and during treatment for an infected internalized shunt that had to be removed. Complications and risks of externalized shunts include infection, overdrainage of cerebrospinal fluid resulting in cortical decompression, and underdrainage of cerebrospinal fluid resulting in increased intracranial pressure. Externalized systems are maintained for up to 5 days, and then they are internalized to reduce the risk of infection.

Application of the Nursing Process to the Care of the Patient After a Ventricular Shunting Procedure

Assessment

Patient assessment includes a history and neurologic examination. Check for signs of increased intracranial pressure to establish a baseline, and assess frequently thereafter for subtle changes, informing the physician immediately of progression of symptoms or complaints. Assess respiratory function by auscultating the lung fields, breath sounds, and respiratory pattern. Observe chest movements, and monitor respiratory pattern and rate. Observe for subtle changes in level of consciousness that may precipitate alteration of respiratory function.

Assess the patient frequently for signs of potential complications: increasing intracranial pressure resulting from underdrainage of cerebrospinal fluid and signs of shock resulting from overdrainage of cerebrospinal fluid.

Assess the incisional sites used for shunt placement for signs of infection. Observe for redness, swelling, and purulent drainage. Note pain or tenderness at the incisional sites and in the peritoneal area. Check the patient's temperature daily. Ask the patient about the presence of chills or other discomfort.

If the patient has an externalized ventricular shunt, assess the character and color of the cerebrospinal fluid in the drainage system. Cerebrospinal fluid is normally colorless and clear. Inspect the drainage system to ensure that the system is closed and intact. Inform the physician immediately of any complications.

Nursing Diagnoses and Planning

Nursing diagnoses and related expected patient outcomes most commonly applicable to patients after a ventricular shunting procedure include the following:

NDx: High risk for ineffective breathing pattern related to increased intracranial pressure secondary to shunt malfunction

Planning: Patient outcomes
1. Respirations are regular and of normal rate and depth.
2. Cyanosis and other signs of hypoxia are absent.

NDx: High risk for infection related to surgical placement of cerebroventricular shunt

Planning: Patient outcomes
1. Patient is afebrile.
2. Redness, swelling, and purulent drainage of shunt placement incisional sites are absent.
3. Signs and symptoms associated with meningitis and peritonitis are absent.

Nursing Interventions

NDx: High risk for ineffective breathing pattern

Externalized Ventricular Shunt
The regulation of cerebrospinal fluid flow is critical to prevent increased intracranial pressure or herniation syndrome. The externalized ventricular shunt has a pressure valve that helps regulate flow. However, both patient activity and changes in the patency of the drainage system can result in inappropriate outflow of cerebrospinal fluid.

Check the physician's orders for activity level, head gatch, and placement level of drainage system collection chamber. Instruct the patient regarding activity level (i.e., bed rest) and limitations. Unplug electric beds to eliminate the risk of altering head gatch and placement level of the collection chamber.

Monitor the system at least once per hour for intactness and patency. Ensure that the system allows for downward flow from the externalization site to the collection chamber. Check the drainage valve every 1 to 2 hours. Inform the physician immediately if drainage is not within ordered parameters (e.g., 15 ml per hour).

Be aware that activities such as suctioning, turning, defecating, and chest physiotherapy increase intrathoracic pressure and therefore inadvertently increase intracranial pressure, which can lead to increased cerebrospinal fluid drainage. To control the volume to be drained, plan patient care to minimize the potential of increasing intracranial pressure, and temporarily clamp tubing to prevent overdrainage of cerebrospinal fluid when indicated. Educate both the patient and visitors about the need for limitations on activities to promote compliance. Monitor respiratory status, and notify the physician immediately of any change.

Ensure that oxygen and suction equipment are at the patient's bedside and in working order. Make intubation and mechanical ventilation support equipment accessible in case a crisis arises (e.g., the patient herniates and respiratory function is compromised).

NDx: High risk for infection

Internalized and Externalized Ventricular Shunt
Inspect integument at incisional sites (neck, chest abdominal regions) every 8 hours. Monitor for signs of infection: redness, swelling, and purulent drainage. Take the patient's temperature daily and when patient complains of being uncomfortable and shivering. Keep incisional sites dry and clean, and protect them with a sterile dressing. Palpate for abdominal tenderness and check for nuchal rigidity.

Externalized Ventricular Shunt
Infection is the major complication of externalized ventricular shunts. Remember that it is critical that the system remain closed and sterile because it is an extension of the patient's cerebrospinal fluid circulatory system. Maintain the integrity of the system by keeping all connections secure and intact, not introducing any fluids into the system, and covering the externalization site with a sterile dressing. Monitor color and character of cerebrospinal fluid, keeping in mind that cloudy fluid with sediment indicates an infectious process.

Inform the physician of any signs of infection. Administer prophylactic antibiotics as ordered.

Evaluation

Evaluate the effectiveness of nursing care for a patient after a ventricular shunting procedure by comparing the patient's status with the expected patient outcomes. Examples of specific outcomes for patients after a ventricular shunting procedure have been provided in the Planning section.

Cerebrovascular Accident

Cerebrovascular accident is a broad term used to describe a condition in which there is an interruption of blood flow to the brain. As a result, there is temporary or permanent dysfunction of a patient's motor, sensory, perceptual, emotional, or cognitive abilities. Symptoms vary depending on the part of the brain affected.

Hippocrates was the first to describe this condition, naming it apoplexy, a Greek term meaning "to strike down." Today this condition is referred to as cerebrovascular accident, apoplexy, or stroke.

Cerebrovascular accident is the third leading cause of death. It afflicts 500,000 persons in the United States each year. There is no gender preference. Incidence increases sharply with age; however, it may be preventable in some cases.

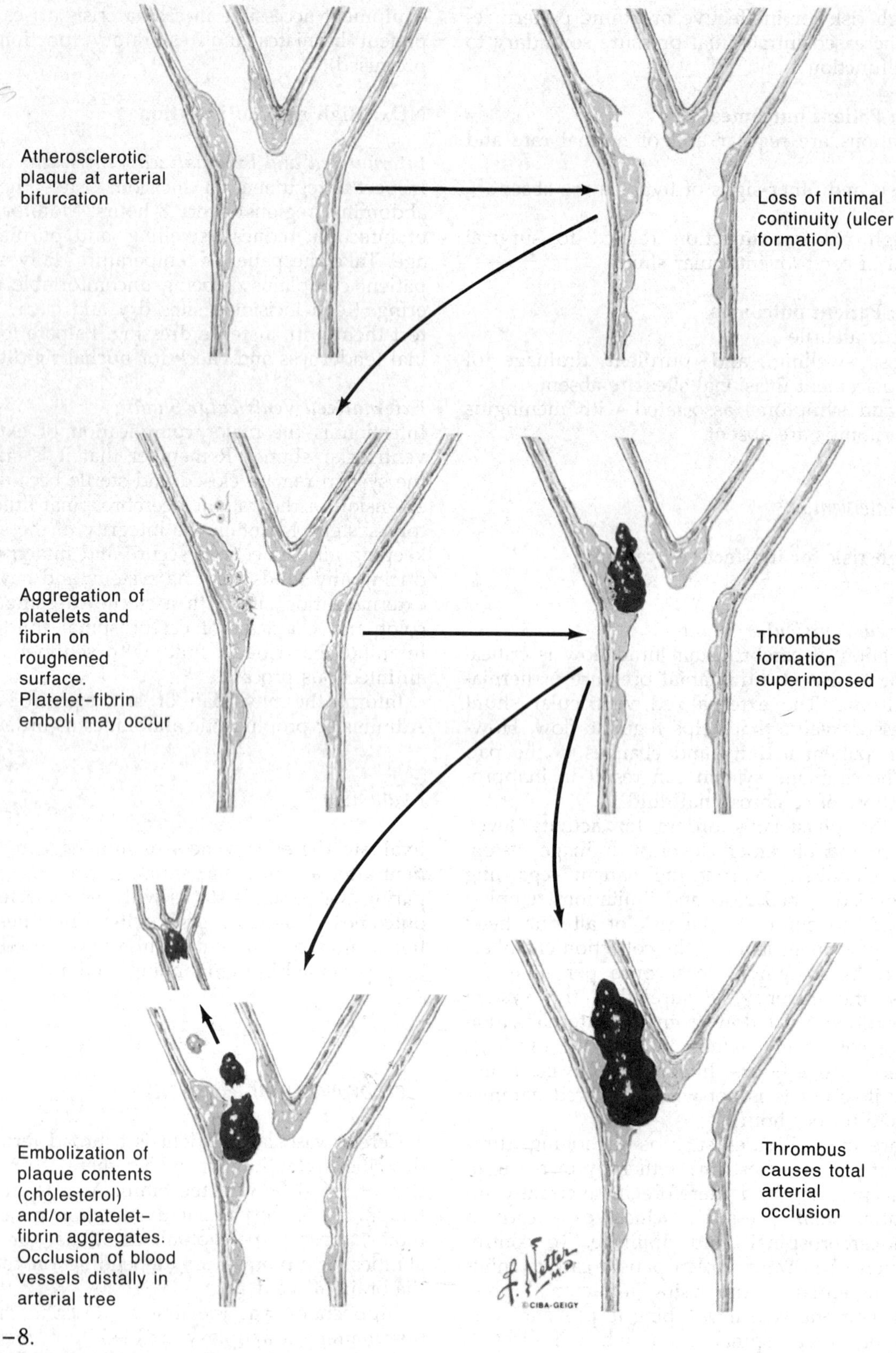

Figure 38–8.

Atherosclerosis, thrombosis, and embolism, which can interrupt blood flow to the brain and cause a cerebrovascular accident or stroke. (©Ciba-Geigy, 1988, Clinical Symposia—Stroke, Vol. 40, Number 4. Illustrated by Frank H. Netter, M.D.)

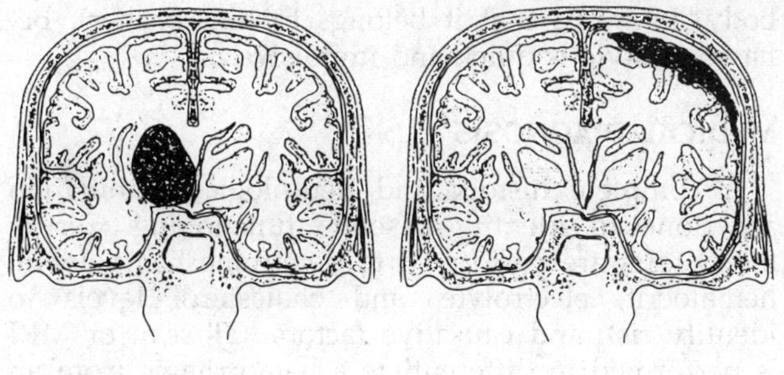

***Figure* 38–9.**

Hemorrhage either within the brain itself (intracerebral) or in the space surrounding the brain (subarachnoid) is a cause of cerebrovascular accident or stroke. (From Stroke—Hope through research [NIH Publication No. 83-2222]. Bethesda, MD: National Institutes of Health, August 1983.)

ETIOLOGY

Cerebrovascular accident is an interruption of blood flow to the brain as a result of occlusive disease (embolic and thrombotic) of the cerebral arteries and vessels (Fig. 38–8) or hemorrhage, either intracerebral or subarachnoid (Fig. 38–9).

The risk factors that predispose one to sustaining a cerebrovascular accident include history of hypertension, heart disease, atherosclerosis, stress, smoking, hypercholesterolemia, hypercoagulopathies, polycythemia, and diabetes mellitus.

PATHOPHYSIOLOGY

Regardless of specific cause, the interruption in blood flow results in decreased oxygen available to an area of cerebral tissue. This leads to anaerobic glycolysis and loss of function. Cerebral ischemia, infarction, and edema may then follow.

There are four major classes of cerebrovascular accidents. They are transient ischemic attack (TIA), reversible ischemic neurologic deficit (RIND), progressive stroke (PS), and complete stroke (CS). The defining characteristics, duration, and type of deficit associated with each of these major classes of cerebrovascular accident are presented in Table 38–4.

CLINICAL MANIFESTATIONS

Neurologic symptomatology is related to the severity of blood interruption and cerebral artery involved. Table 38–5 lists the clinical manifestations associated with interruption of blood flow in each of the main arteries of the brain.

The right and left hemispheres of the brain are not mirror images. Therefore, the clinical presentation of the patient with a cerebrovascular accident is also related to hemispheric involvement (Fig. 38–10). Left hemispheric involvement is characterized by dysfunction of language and speech in 95% of individuals; a slow and cautious behavioral style; and motor plegia of the right side. In right hemispheric involvement, speech and language are usually unaffected. Plegia occurs on the left side, and there is left-sided neglect (patient ignores left side of

***Table* 38–4.** CLASSIFICATION OF CEREBROVASCULAR ACCIDENT

TYPE	DEFINING CHARACTERISTICS	DURATION	DEFICIT
Transient ischemic attack	Onset and disappearance of neurologic deficit within 24 hours caused by temporary disturbance of blood supply to brain	Brief episode of focal neurologic deficit; attacks sometimes occur with considerable frequency, 5–20 times daily; these should be considered as warnings to impending neurologic catastrophe; last several minutes to 2–3 hours; can last up to 24 hours	No residual deficit noted
Reversible ischemic neurologic deficit	Onset and disappearance of focal neurologic deficit within 12 hours, up to days; associated with cerebral emboli	Neurologic deficit persisting longer than 12–24 hours	Minimal to no residual deficits
Progressive stroke	Usually severe, caused by cerebrovascular disease; results from hemorrhagic infarction with edema or progressive thrombosis of a major cerebral vessel; progresses for 12–24 hours	Symptoms persist beyond 24 hours with an associated progressive deterioration of neurologic status	Residual neurologic deficits, most likely related to failure of collateral brain circulation
Complete stroke	Severe, related to cerebrovascular disease	Condition stabilizes and neurologic deficit remains	Optimal recovery has ensued; however, static deficit persists; deficit assumed to be permanent

Table 38–5. CLINICAL MANIFESTATIONS OF INTERRUPTED BLOOD FLOW IN MAJOR CEREBRAL ARTERIES

ARTERY	CLINICAL MANIFESTATIONS
Middle cerebral artery	Contralateral hemiplegia; paralysis of the face alone or limb alone; numbness; hemianopia; dysphasia; agnosia
Anterior cerebral artery	Numbness in opposite lower limb; cognitive decline; impaired judgment and insight; bowel and bladder incontinence
Posterior cerebral artery	Alexia; mental change with memory impairment; hemianopia; cranial nerve III palsy
Internal carotid artery	Monocular blindness, fleeting or permanent
Vertebral basilar artery	Dizziness, syncope, vertigo; loss of muscle coordination; drop attacks; weakness; diplopia; vomiting; impairment of touch sense on face

body, unaware that it belongs to him or her). Behavioral style is quick and impulsive.

MEDICAL DIAGNOSIS

A complete history and neurologic examination are done to identify baseline functioning. Serum blood tests are performed to determine hemoglobin, hematocrit, electrolyte, and cholesterol levels to identify risk and causative factors. CT scan or MRI is performed to differentiate a hemorrhagic from an occlusive cerebrovascular event. Doppler studies may be performed to establish patency of blood flow. An electrocardiogram (ECG) may be indicated to establish any cardiac origin of cerebrovascular accident.

MEDICAL MANAGEMENT

Medical management for a patient experiencing a cerebrovascular accident involves treatment of pre-

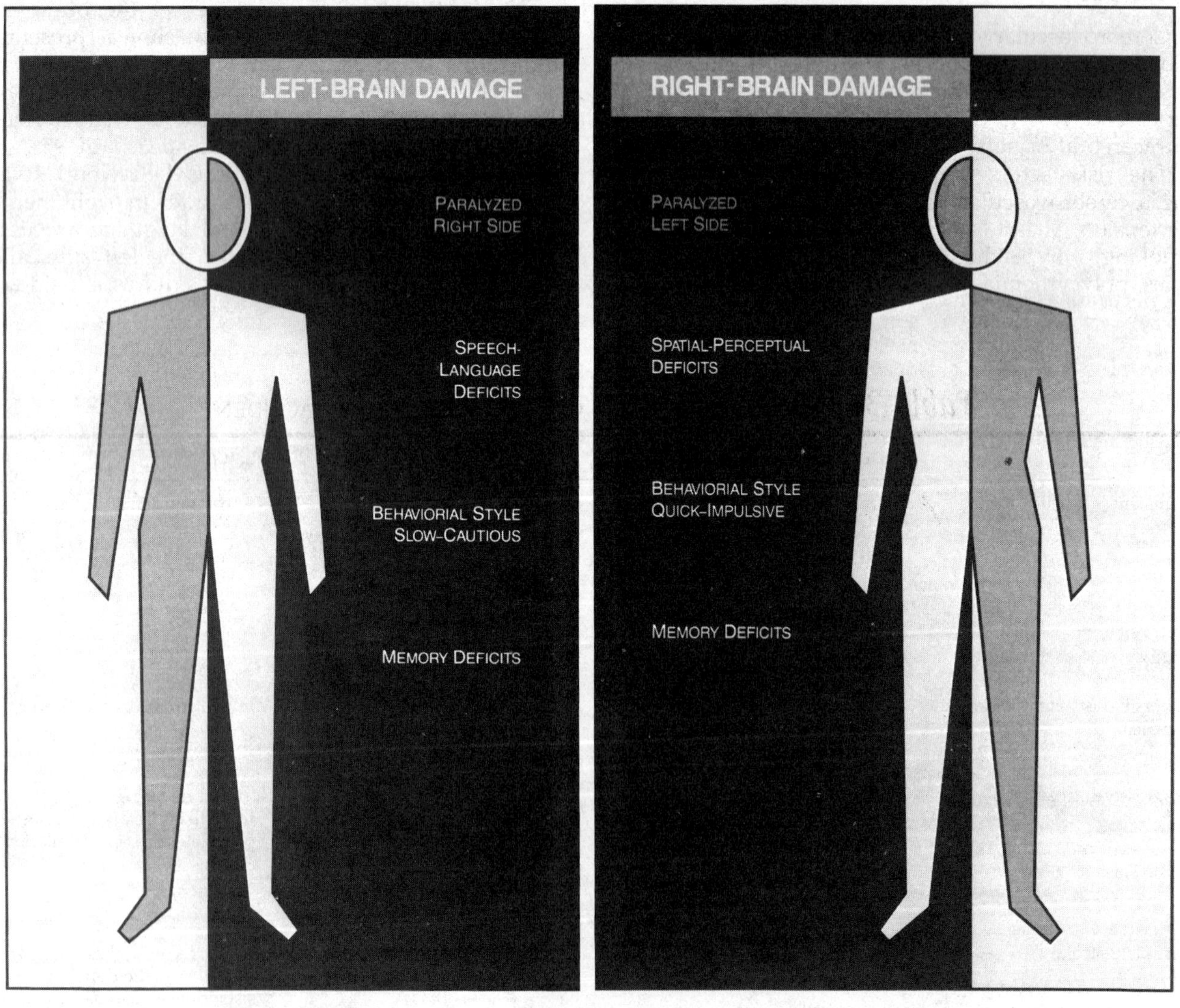

Figure 38–10.

Clinical manifestations of cerebrovascular accidents (stroke). (Reproduced with permission. How Stroke Affects Behavior. 1991. Copyright American Heart Association.)

disposing conditions such as heart disease and diabetes mellitus, control of hypertension, anticoagulant or antiaggregation therapy in nonhemorrhagic events, and possibly surgical intervention.

Control of hypertension is maintained through the use of antihypertensive agents. This decreases the risk for extension of hemorrhagic stroke and promotes adequate cerebral perfusion to the brain.

Anticoagulant therapy is the treatment of choice for patients with an embolic or thrombotic cerebral ischemic event. Heparin is quick acting and of short duration and prolongs blood clotting time by interfering with the conversion of thrombin to fibrinogen and of prothrombin to thrombin. Heparin is initiated immediately and administered intravenously with a goal therapeutic activated partial thromboplastin time (APTT) value 2 to $2\frac{1}{2}$ times the control. Warfarin (Coumadin) is long-term therapy after heparin. Coumadin produces a deficiency of prothrombin and interferes with the conversion of prothrombin to thrombin. The goal therapeutic prothrombin time (PT) value is $1\frac{1}{2}$ times the control. Patients are usually on Coumadin for 3 months and then maintained on aspirin.

Platelet antiaggregation therapy inhibits the initial step of thrombus formation. The two common medications that are effective agents are aspirin and dipyridamole (Persantine).

Surgical intervention may be indicated in certain cases. A carotid endarterectomy is performed to remove a thrombus that totally or partially obstructs the carotid artery. A microvascular bypass procedure may be performed to supply blood, oxygen, and nutrients to an infarcted area.

Application of the Nursing Process to the Care of the Patient with a Cerebrovascular Accident

Assessment

Obtain a history of the onset of the present problem from the patient or significant others. Determine what the initial symptoms were, when they began, and how they progressed. Inquire about any history of similar problems. Question about the presence of risk factors such as hypertension, heart disease, smoking, and history of TIA. Perform a complete physical assessment. Check for the following impairments:

Language: Aphasia syndromes, agnosia, alexia
Motor: Paresis, atáxia, bowel or bladder dysfunction, dysphagia, syncope, vertigo, spasticity
Sensory: Numbness, paresthesia, spatial-perceptual dysfunctions, one-sided neglect
Behavior: Impaired judgment, memory impairment, emotional instability

Assess the impact of neurologic dysfunction on other body system functioning, particularly respiratory. Note any difficulty in clearing secretions, intactness of the gag reflex, breath sounds, and respiratory rate and pattern.

Assess the patient's ability to perform ADL, to be free from injury, to communicate wants and needs, and to maintain appropriate social interaction. Observe the patient, and note any lack of completeness of tasks or unawareness of missed steps. Determine whether the patient is interpreting communication from others and responding appropriately. Assess the extent of supervision or assistance needed. Assess the need for assistive devices to facilitate self-care.

Nursing Diagnoses and Planning

Nursing diagnoses and related expected patient outcomes most commonly applicable to patients with cerebrovascular accidents include the following:

NDx: High risk for ineffective breathing pattern related to muscle weakness and immobility

Planning: Patient outcomes
1. Cyanosis is absent.
2. Arterial blood gas values are within patient's normal range.
3. Bilateral breath sounds are clear.

NDx: High risk for aspiration related to dysphagia

Planning: Patient outcomes
1. Patient avoids aspiration.
2. Mouth and airway are free of secretions.
3. Cyanosis and fever are absent.
4. Breath sounds are normal bilaterally.

NDx: Impaired physical mobility related to plegia

Planning: Patient outcomes
1. Patient participates in ADL.
2. Patient ambulates, transfers, or moves self with or without assistance.
3. Complications of immobility—deep venous thrombosis, pulmonary embolism, decubitus formation, subluxation of joints—are absent.

NDx: Self-care deficit: feeding, bathing and hygiene, dressing and grooming, toileting, related to plegia

Planning: Patient outcomes
1. Patient meets self-care needs with or without assistance.
2. Patient is well groomed.

NDx: High risk for altered nutrition: less than body requirements, related to dysphagia

Planning: Patient outcomes
1. Patient ingests *(specify amount)* calories per day.
2. Patient maintains optimal body weight.
3. Skin turgor is good.

NDx: Unilateral neglect related to behavioral alteration caused by interruption in blood supply to right hemisphere of brain

Planning: Patient outcomes
1. Patient acknowledges the existence of the sensory perceptual impairment.
2. Patient describes protective measures for the affected side.
3. Patient demonstrates behaviors consistent with concern for the affected side.

NDx: High risk for injury related to perceptual loss secondary to interruption of blood flow to left hemisphere

Planning: Patient outcomes
1. Patient uses alternate strategies to compensate for sensory-perceptual loss.
2. Patient performs tasks in appropriate sequence of steps.
3. Patient remains free from injury.

NDx: High risk for constipation related to immobility

Planning: Patient outcomes
1. Stools are soft and formed.
2. Patient passes stool regularly.
3. Patient defecates without straining.

NDx: Altered urinary elimination related to motor system dysfunction

Planning: Patient outcomes
1. Patient is continent.
2. Patient empties bladder completely.
3. Patient is free from urinary tract infections.

NDx: Impaired verbal communication related to aphasia syndromes

Planning: Patient outcomes
1. Patient uses effective alternate communication strategies.
2. Patient successfully communicates needs.

Nursing Interventions

NDx: High risk for ineffective breathing pattern
Monitor respiratory function by auscultating lung fields for breath sounds and noting respiratory pattern. Observe chest movements, and obtain vital signs. Position the patient at a 30-degree head elevation to facilitate respiratory effort. Suction the airway as necessary. Perform chest physiotherapy as needed. Encourage and teach the patient to perform cough and deep-breathing exercises every 2 hours. Provide the patient with an incentive spirometer and instruct in its use. Review the patient's arterial blood gas values.

Monitor the patient for respiratory distress and decreased level of consciousness. Administer oxygen as ordered or when patient is in respiratory crisis (shortness of breath, cyanosis). Have emergency intubation and mechanical ventilation readily available to be used in a respiratory arrest.

NDx: High risk for aspiration
Monitor patient's ability to clear secretions from airway and intactness of gag reflex. Maintain working suction equipment at bedside. Position the patient at a 30-degree (angle) elevation to facilitate drainage of secretions. Suction patient as needed to maintain a clear airway.

Monitor patient during feeding, and suction the airway as needed to prevent aspiration. Encourage the patient to eat semisolid, soft foods such as boneless chicken, custard, and mashed potatoes. Avoid solid and liquid foods that are difficult for the patient with dysphagia to swallow and that increase the risk for aspiration.

NDx: Impaired physical mobility
To decrease the risk of hazards of immobility, perform range-of-motion (passive and active) exercises at least every 6 hours. Allow the patient to do as much for self (moving, bathing, dressing, and so on) as possible. Place a trapeze on the bed to allow the patient to move and turn self. Maintain good body alignment, and eliminate undue pressure or rotation of joints. Consult with occupational and physical therapists to obtain supportive and assistive devices to be used by the patient for ADL, such as a cane, a wheelchair, eating utensils, splints, and slings. Maintain a turning and positioning schedule every 2 hours.

Provide good skin care, and use sheepskin pads, air mattress, or special beds as necessary to prevent injury from immobility. Apply thigh-length antiembolic stockings to prevent venous pooling in extremities and to decrease the risk of deep venous thrombosis. Inspect the lower extremities daily for an increase in calf circumference or redness, and check for Homans' sign. Notify the physician of any change in the patient's condition.

NDx: Self-care deficit: feeding, bathing and hygiene, dressing and grooming, toileting
Encourage the patient to participate actively in self-care (bathing, dressing, grooming, and eating). Allow the patient to perform activities to the limit before actively intervening to complete the task. Explore alternate strategies for the patient to meet self-care needs, and determine the level of additional

support and assistance that is needed. Obtain devices to assist in the completion of self-care (e.g., eating utensils, devices to assist with getting in and out of the bathtub, reaching devices).

Consult with social services to assist in discharge planning and identifying available resources. This allows for preparation of the home environment to promote optimal patient functioning. Special equipment (such as commode, wheelchair, ramp, bed) may need to be purchased. In addition, the family will have the support and knowledge they require to assist the patient in caring for him- or herself at home.

NDx: High risk for altered nutrition: less than body requirements
Obtain a calorie count to establish relationship of intake to nutritional requirements. Monitor and record intake and output. Weigh the patient initially to obtain baseline weight, and then weigh the patient weekly and note variations. Monitor the ability to tolerate feedings and intactness of gag reflex. Place food tray on nonaffected side of patient, and teach the patient to chew on the nonaffected side of the mouth. Ensure that the patient is positioned at a 30-degree angle or higher during feeding. Educate the patient regarding the importance of a low-salt, low-cholesterol diet.

Consult with the nutritionist regarding patient diet, needs, and ability to ingest required calories. Identify the need for supplemental feedings (i.e., high-calorie milkshakes, enteral feedings) when the patient cannot tolerate oral feedings. Monitor the patient's tolerance of oral and enteral feedings. Notify the physician regarding intolerance and the need for parenteral or peripheral nutrition.

NDx: Unilateral neglect
Draw attention to the patient's neglected side. Encourage the patient to turn his or her head to view the full visual field. Place furniture, bed table, eating tray, and personal items on the non-neglected side of the patient. Sit, stand, and talk to the patient on his or her non-neglected side. Reorient the patient to the affected side. Give feedback to the patient about the neglected limb and environment. Use verbal cues, pictures, and repetitive learning opportunities. Teach the patient sitting and balancing exercises. Encourage activities that cause the patient to pass his or her midline, such as placing an object on the patient's affected side and having the patient pick it up using the unaffected hand.

NDx: High risk for injury
Monitor the impact of perceptual loss on the patient's ability to perform tasks. For example, consider whether the patient misjudges distance and hence is at risk for falling, spilling hot liquids, and the like. Encourage the patient to think through steps before initiating tasks and activities. This allows the patient to focus attention on each step of the task to decrease the risk of injury from performing the task incorrectly or impulsively. Establish the extent to which the patient can verbalize and perform ADL without risk of injury or harm. If the patient is unable to verbalize or perform steps of activities, recognize that direct supervision of the patient is required. Eliminate obstructing hazards from the environment such as scatter rugs, electrical cords, and furniture.

Teach the patient alternate strategies such as visual cues and assistive devices for ambulation to compensate for sensory-perceptual alterations. Give one direction at a time, and break tasks into simple, one-step commands. Keep objects on the unaffected side, and approach the patient from the unaffected side. Encourage the patient to scan the entire visual field completely. Teach the patient sitting and balancing exercises.

NDx: High risk for constipation
Establish a bowel regimen acceptable to the patient that is based on the patient's usual pattern of elimination. Administer stool softeners, suppositories, and laxatives as per regimen. Educate the patient regarding necessary daily roughage and fluid intake in diet.

NDx: Altered urinary elimination
Monitor and record intake and output. Ensure a fluid intake of 2500 ml daily. Limit fluid intake after 8:00 P.M. Establish bladder training regimen. Offer opportunity for bladder elimination five times daily. Administer medications such as Urecholine and Pro-Banthine as prescribed to increase bladder muscle control. Check the volume of postvoid residual. Implement straight catheterization protocol if needed.

NDx: Impaired verbal communication
Monitor type and extent of communication deficit present. Identify alternate strategies that can be used to foster patient understanding or expression of patient's needs (pen and paper, picture board). Anticipate the patient's needs. Decrease environmental distractions when communicating with the patient. Give one direction at a time. Limit communication to one person at a time. Allow time for the patient to interpret the message and express needs. Encourage the patient to communicate despite impairment. Consult with speech therapist as needed.

Evaluation

Evaluate the effectiveness of nursing care for a patient with a cerebrovascular accident by comparing the patient's status with the expected patient outcomes. Examples of specific outcomes for patients with cerebrovascular accidents have been provided in the Planning section.

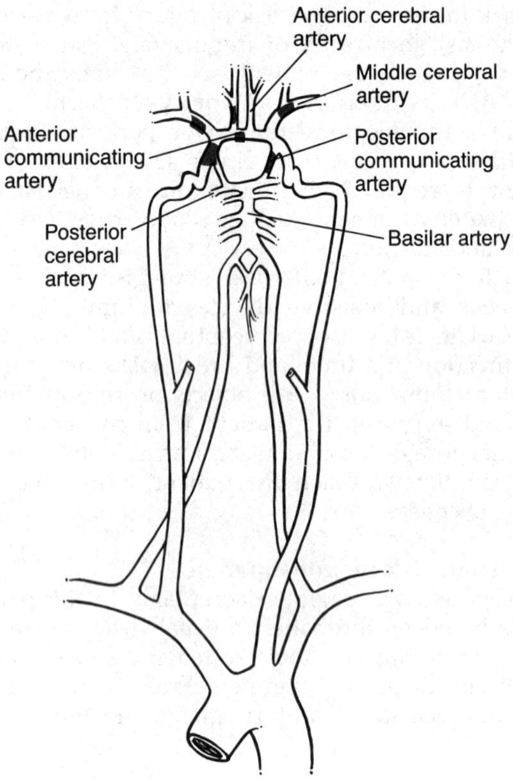

Figure 38–11.

Common sites of cerebral aneurysms.

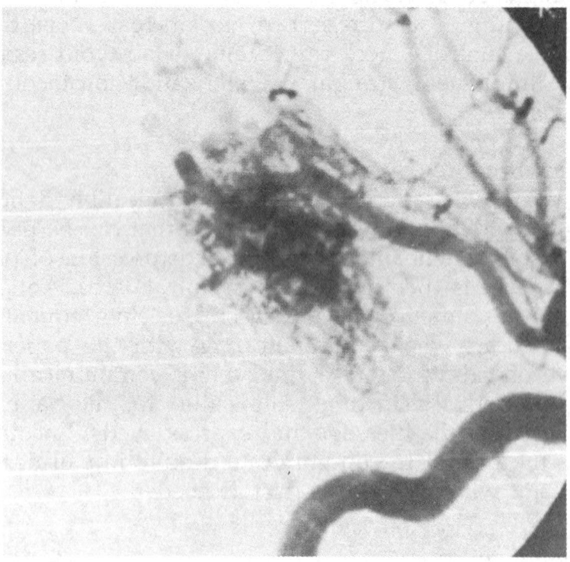

Figure 38–12.

Right internal carotid arteriogram, lateral view, showing an arteriovenous malformation (AVM) supplied by a temporal branch of the right posterior cerebral artery. AVMs are characterized by dilated, tortuous veins and arteries that extend wedge-shaped into the brain tissue. Blood is shunted rapidly and under high pressure through the AVM, leaving ischemic and necrotic areas on the adjoining cortex. (Courtesy of Grant Hieshima, M.D., Radiology Department, University of California, San Francisco.)

Subarachnoid Hemorrhage

SAH accounts for 10% of deaths from cerebral hemorrhage. Peak incidence is between the ages of 35 and 65 years.

There is a high mortality rate associated with SAH. Approximately 30% of patients die from the initial bleed, and 30% of patients rebleed within the first 2 weeks. Of the latter, only about 50% survive.

ETIOLOGY AND PATHOPHYSIOLOGY

The subarachnoid space lies between the pia mater and the arachnoid, two of the protective membranes of the brain. Cerebrospinal fluid fills the subarachnoid space to provide the protective cushion for the brain and spinal cord.

An SAH occurs when blood escapes from a cerebral artery into the subarachnoid space.

Causes of SAH include head trauma, ruptured cerebral aneurysm, and arteriovenous malformations (AVMs).

ANEURYSM

A cerebral aneurysm is an outpouching of an arterial vessel usually found at one of the major bifurcations of the circle of Willis (Fig. 38–11).

Several types of aneurysms have been classified:

Berry, saccular: Most common; congenital anomaly; has a neck to aneurysm
Fusiform: Occurs in conjunction with atherosclerosis; rarely ruptures
Mycotic: Embolus originates from bacterial endocarditis; as embolus lodges in cerebral vessel, inflammatory process develops and vessel wall weakens and dilates
Giant: Large in diameter (greater than 3 mm); mimics a space-occupying lesion; usually has ill-defined neck

An aneurysm is often a congenital weakness in the wall of the artery. Cerebral aneurysms are usually asymptomatic until they rupture. Twenty percent of persons with a ruptured aneurysm are found to have other aneurysms.

ARTERIOVENOUS MALFORMATION

AVMs are a congenital anomaly in which there is an entangled, ill-defined network of arterial, venous, and capillary vessels. The feeding and draining vessels of the AVM become tortuous and distended (Fig. 38–12).

AVMs are often seen in the parietal and occipital regions of the brain, but they can be found elsewhere also. They often present with symptoms of a space-occupying lesion and seizure. Seventy-two percent of AVMs rupture by the time the afflicted person is 40 years of age.

CLINICAL MANIFESTATIONS

The clinical manifestations seen in a patient experiencing an SAH range from minor to severe neurologic deficits. The severity and extent of the deficit are dependent on the type of pathology, area and extent of bleeding, and the presence and degree of vasospasm and hydrocephalus.

The "classic" complaint of patients with an SAH is "All of a sudden I had the worst headache of my life." Other signs and symptoms associated with SAH are altered levels of consciousness (alert to drowsy), restlessness, irritability, photophobia, nuchal rigidity, nausea and vomiting, and focal neurologic deficits (such as weakness, speech and language dysfunction, seizures, sensory alterations, diplopia).

A grading system of the patient's condition has been established by Hunt and Hess. It is used to direct and determine appropriateness of medical treatment and intervention:

Grade I: Asymptomatic, minimal headache, slight nuchal rigidity
Grade II: Moderate to severe headache, nuchal rigidity, cranial nerve III dysfunction
Grade III: Drowsy to confused, nuchal rigidity, minimal focal deficits
Grade IV: Stupor, mild to severe hemiparesis, possibly early decerebrate posturing
Grade V: Deep coma, decerebrate posturing, moribund appearance

MEDICAL DIAGNOSIS

A complete history is taken and a neurologic examination performed to establish baseline function. A CT scan is done to demonstrate presence of an SAH versus an intracerebral hemorrhage or infarction. A lumbar puncture is performed to confirm the diagnosis of SAH by verifying increased opening pressure, presence of blood on a non-traumatic tap, presence of erythrocytes in cerebrospinal fluid, or xanthochromic appearance of cerebrospinal fluid.

Angiographic studies may be done to differentiate the cause of aneurysm or AVM. The angiogram defines location, size, extent, and feeding vessels to the pathology. An angiogram is performed before surgical intervention to fully investigate the cause and to determine an appropriate treatment plan.

MEDICAL MANAGEMENT

In recent years there has been a more aggressive approach to the management of patients with SAH. It is believed that, because the mortality rate is high, prompt intervention and treatment are needed to prevent cerebral ischemia from vasospasm and death from rebleed.

Modes of medical management include the use of volume expanders, blood pressure control, antifibrinolytic therapy, and calcium channel blocking agents. Surgical interventions involve clipping or wrapping aneurysms, carotid ligation to reduce the size of or obliterate an aneurysm, and removal or induced thrombosis of AVMs. Surgery is usually done when the patient is graded in the Hunt and Hess system as I, II, or possibly III.

Environmental precautions for the patient with SAH have been modified during the past decade. Precautions currently involve administration of stool softeners to prevent straining, avoidance of rectal treatments, and limitation of activities to prevent stress or elevated blood pressure.

Guidelines for Application of the Nursing Process to the Care of the Patient with a Subarachnoid Hemorrhage

Focus assessment on onset, duration, and progression of symptoms, including headache, nuchal rigidity, decreased level of consciousness, motor and sensory alterations, nausea and vomiting, and pupillary responses and changes. Obtain a baseline assessment of cardiac and respiratory function, and monitor for ensuing changes. Also monitor for subtle changes in level of consciousness or an increase in headache that may indicate rebleed, increasing intracranial pressure, or herniation syndrome. Notify the physician of any such changes. Ensure that oxygen and suction equipment is at the patient's bedside and in working order. Make intubation equipment and mechanical ventilation equipment accessible in case the patient herniates and sustains respiratory crisis.

Trauma

Head Injury

Trauma is the leading cause of death in persons younger than 40 years. Head trauma accounts for a significant number of these fatalities. Statistical evidence indicates that most head injuries occur in the 16- to 25-year age group, with twice as many occurrences among males as females. Vehicular accidents are the most common cause of head injury. Next most common are head traumas associated with alcohol and drug ingestion; violent acts such as gunshot wounds, stab wounds, and other blunt trauma secondary to assaults; and sports-related injuries and falls.

Recovery from head trauma is directly correlated to the type and severity of the injury sustained and the age and premorbid health of the injured person. Severe head injuries can result in a wide spectrum of disabilities for the patient, ranging from mild cognitive effects to severe functional deficits. The psychological and financial impact for the patient and family can be devastating.

CLASSIFICATION OF HEAD INJURY

Head injury refers to an injury to the scalp, the cranium, or the brain. Frequently, the injury involves all three. The major concern in head injury is the extent of injury to the brain itself. Such injury can occur directly or secondary to other injuries.

SCALP INJURIES

Etiology, Pathophysiology, and Clinical Manifestations

Injuries to the scalp usually occur as abrasions, contusions, or lacerations. An abrasion of the scalp results in a scraping away of the top layer of the scalp. It is generally considered a minor injury, with minimal bleeding noted. A contusion of the scalp is a bruise to the scalp. The integrity of the skin remains intact. Effusion of blood into the subcutaneous layer may occur. A scalp laceration is an actual tear in the tissue of the scalp. Scalp lacerations tend to bleed profusely because of the scalp's extensive vascularity.

Medical Diagnosis

Injuries to the scalp are diagnosed by direct visual inspection. If underlying cerebral damage such as a skull fracture is suspected, x-ray films of the skull are obtained.

Medical Management

No intervention is necessary for scalp abrasions. For a scalp contusion, ice applied soon after injury aids in the prevention of hematoma formation. Profuse bleeding from a scalp laceration can usually be controlled by direct pressure, but suturing of the wound may be necessary in more serious injuries. When suturing is required, the surrounding hair is shaved and the wound cleansed thoroughly with copious amounts of saline to ensure removal of any dirt or foreign material. The wound is debrided if necessary. Prophylactic antibiotic therapy is often ordered.

SKULL FRACTURES

Etiology, Pathophysiology, and Clinical Manifestations

Skull fractures occur in approximately 7% of head injuries. Skull fractures are classified into one of four major categories: linear, comminuted, depressed, or basilar (Fig. 38–13).

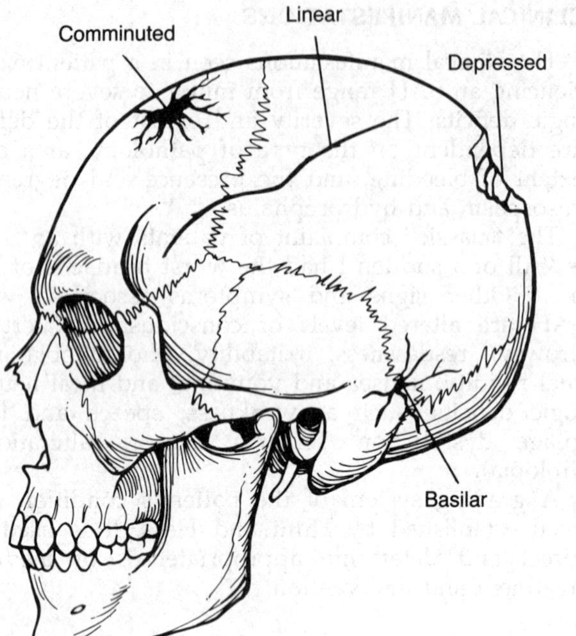

***Figure* 38–13.**

Types of skull fractures.

Linear skull fractures account for 70% to 80% of all skull fractures. Sometimes called a simple fracture, a linear fracture resembles a single line or crack in the skull. There is no displacement of bone.

A comminuted fracture is one in which the bone is broken or crushed into small pieces; a depressed skull fracture is an inward depression of bone fragments, resulting in an indentation in the contour of the skull. Depressed skull fractures are classified as open or closed depending on the presence or absence of scalp lacerations.

A basilar skull fracture occurs at the base of the skull. The dura can be torn in this type of fracture, resulting in the leakage of cerebrospinal fluid from the nose, called rhinorrhea, or from the ear, called otorrhea. Bilateral periorbital ecchymosis, called raccoon's eyes, occurs if the fracture is in the anterior portion of the base of the brain. Ecchymosis over the mastoid bone, called Battle's sign, is another clinical indication of a basilar skull fracture.

Medical Diagnosis

Skull x-ray film is the diagnostic tool used most frequently to diagnose skull fractures. Linear fractures are easily seen on x-ray film. Depressed skull fractures can generally be visualized and palpated. Skull x-ray films are done in addition to inspection of the associated wound to visualize underlying damage to other areas, such as the sinuses.

Basilar skull fractures are extremely difficult to visualize by radiography. The diagnosis is generally made on the basis of the clinical picture. The presence of rhinorrhea or otorrhea is highly suspicious of a basilar skull fracture. Skull x-ray films may disclose the presence of air in the frontal sinuses, indicating the presence of a tear in the dura, which allows air to enter the sinus. Otoscopic examination may reveal the presence of blood or fluid behind the tympanic membrane.

Medical Management

The treatment of a skull fracture depends on the type of fracture and the location. Skull fracture may be only one of several head injuries.

A simple linear fracture generally requires no treatment other than bed rest and observation for underlying brain tissue injury. Depressed skull fractures require surgical intervention, usually within 24 hours of the injury, to debride the wound completely and remove any bone fragments, which may become imbedded in brain tissue or cerebral blood vessels. Elevation of the depressed bone is carried out if possible. A cranioplasty with insertion of acrylic bone may be done at this time or postponed for 3 to 6 months if cerebral edema is present or if concern exists regarding infection. Decadron is administered to reduce cerebral edema. Prophylactic antibiotic therapy is used for 24 to 48 hours postoperatively.

The focus in managing basilar skull fracture centers on preventing both further tears in the dura and infection. Because activities that cause transient increases in intracranial pressure such as the Valsalva maneuver, coughing, sneezing, and blowing the nose may cause further tears in the dura, the patient is instructed to refrain from these activities. In addition, any procedure that requires invasion of the nasal cavity or ear canal is contraindicated. Antibiotic therapy is prescribed to prevent infection. Most cerebrospinal fluid leaks from dural tears resolve spontaneously in 7 to 10 days. If leakage of fluid persists, a craniotomy may be necessary to surgically repair the tear.

BRAIN INJURY

Brain injury can result from a closed head injury or from direct penetration of the cranium and brain such as by a missile.

Closed Brain Injury

Etiology. A closed head injury is a nonpenetrating injury to the head, usually the result of blunt trauma. There is no break between the integrity of the intracranial cavity and the outside environment. Examples of blunt trauma include the head striking a windshield, a fall resulting in hitting or bumping the head, and a blow to the head such as seen in assaults.

Pathophysiology. Concussion and contusion can be the result of closed head trauma. Concussion refers to a transient, temporary neurologic dysfunction secondary to head injury. The word *concussion* is derived from the Latin and means "to shake violently."

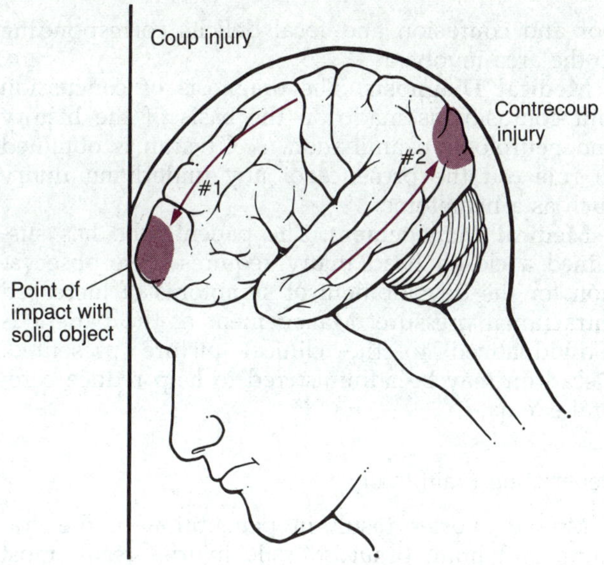

Figure 38–14.

Coup and contrecoup injuries. Forehead impacts on solid surface; brain moves forward, and frontal lobes hit the inside of the skull and are bruised (coup injury). The brain then bounces backward, causing the occipital area to hit the inner skull and become bruised (contrecoup injury).

Contusion refers to an area of brain tissue into which bleeding has occurred. It differs from intracerebral hemorrhage in that the blood is dispersed rather than concentrated in one area of tissue. Contusion is the result of trauma that causes the brain to strike the internal surface of the skull. Areas of bruising or contusion directly beneath the site of trauma are described as coup injuries. Contrecoup injuries are those that occur in an area of the brain opposite the site of impact (Fig. 38–14). Contrecoup injuries are always accompanied by a coup injury but may be significantly greater. Coup and contrecoup injuries frequently follow acceleration-deceleration trauma such as occurs in automobile accidents.

Clinical Manifestations. Concussion can be classified as mild or severe. In mild concussion, there is a temporary neurologic dysfunction without loss of consciousness. Confusion and disorientation occur but clear within seconds to minutes.

Severe concussion, also referred to as classic cerebral concussion, is characterized by temporary neurologic deficit associated with a brief loss of consciousness usually lasting less than 24 hours. Recovery of consciousness is usually associated with a period of confusion and disorientation. A retrograde amnesia occurs, rendering the patient unable to recall the injury as well as the events immediately preceding the injury.

The clinical presentation of the patient with a cerebral contusion depends on the area of the brain that is involved and the extent of the bruising or damage. There is a loss of consciousness, with stupor and confusion and focal deficits corresponding to the area involved.

Medical Diagnosis. The diagnosis of concussion and contusion is made on the basis of the history and neurologic examination. A CT scan is obtained to rule out the presence of any underlying injury such as a hematoma.

Medical Management. The patient who has sustained a closed head injury requires close observation for the development of symptoms of increased intracranial pressure. Management of the patient is individualized to the clinical picture presented. Decadron may be administered to help reduce cerebral edema.

Penetrating Brain Injury

Missile injuries result in penetration of the cranium and brain tissue. Missile injuries result most often from gunshot wounds to the head. The extent of injury depends on the caliber and velocity of the bullet and the direction and action of the bullet within the cranial space.

The damage caused by a bullet includes contusion and laceration of brain tissue, hemorrhage, and cerebral edema. These effects can be localized or can occur diffusely within the brain; the consequences can be fatal. Immediate surgical intervention is necessary on arrival at the emergency room if the patient has survived the initial insult.

COMPLICATIONS OF HEAD INJURY: HEMATOMAS

Head injury may be complicated by the development of intracranial hematomas. These hematomas may develop at initial injury or at a later time. Epidural, subdural, and intracerebral hematomas are three types of intracranial hemorrhages.

Epidural Hematoma

Etiology and Pathophysiology. An epidural hematoma refers to bleeding between the skull and the dura in the epidural space (Fig. 38–15). Epidural hematomas are usually arterial in origin and are most frequently associated with fractures in the temporoparietal bones.

Clinical Manifestations. The patient with an epidural hematoma may be unconscious at the time of the initial injury, become lucid and alert for a few hours or even 1 to 2 days, and then quickly deteriorate in level of consciousness. Headache and vomiting followed by ipsilateral (same side) pupil dilation and contralateral (opposite side) motor paralysis develop, indicative of a herniation syndrome (refer to discussion of increased intracranial pressure).

Medical Diagnosis. Emergency CT scan establishes the location of the hematoma. It further indicates the presence and amount of associated cerebral edema.

Medical Management. Immediate surgical evacuation is necessary. Burr holes are made, and the clot is evacuated. Prognosis is considered to be better with early detection and intervention.

Subdural Hematoma

Etiology and Pathophysiology. A subdural hematoma refers to bleeding between the dura and the arachnoid in the subdural space (see Fig. 38–15). Subdural hematomas are categorized as (1) acute, with symptoms occurring within 48 hours of initial injury; (2) subacute, with symptoms occurring from 2 days to 2 weeks after initial injury; and (3) chronic, more than 2 weeks from initial injury.

Clinical Manifestations. The most common symptoms of acute and subacute subdural hematoma include headache, drowsiness, and confusion, which insidiously worsen. Ipsilateral pupil dilation occurs. Chronic subdural hematomas develop more slowly. Headache, variable levels of consciousness, personality changes, and motor weakness are noted.

Medical Diagnosis. The CT scan is the definitive diagnostic tool to localize the lesion. The slower progression of symptoms helps distinguish between acute and chronic subdural hematomas.

Medical Management. If a subdural hematoma is small, it is generally absorbed. Large acute subdural hematomas require surgical intervention via burr holes to drain the hematoma. Chronic subdural hematomas require surgical removal via craniotomy because the hematoma develops a gelatinous consistency over time and cannot be drained via a burr hole.

Application of the Nursing Process to the Care of the Patient with a Head Injury

Assessment

Initial assessment of the head-injured patient occurs in the emergency room. The first priority involves assessment of the patient's airway. Note the rate

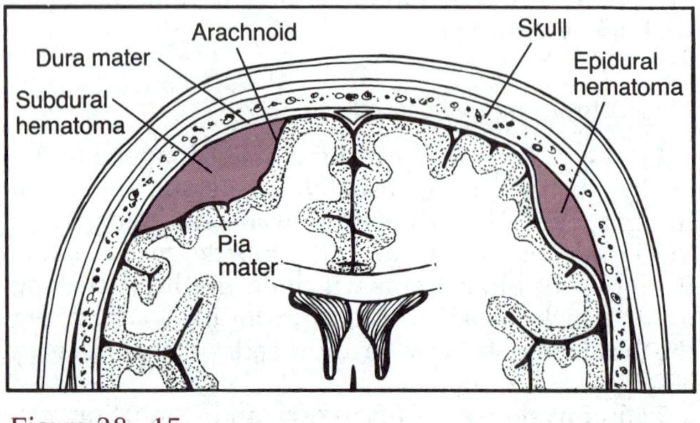

Figure 38–15.

Epidural hematoma and subdural hematoma.

and depth of respirations. Ascertain the patient's level of consciousness. Compare these data to the information available from the scene of the injury. Obtain a description of the cause of injury, and inquire about the patient's use of alcohol or drugs. Perform a baseline neurologic assessment by checking pupils for size and reaction to light and checking motor function of all four extremities. Thoroughly inspect the nose and ears for the presence of blood or cerebrospinal fluid. Note the presence of bruises, lacerations, or abrasions on the scalp, skull, and face. Determine whether the patient lost consciousness at the scene of the injury. Perform a careful examination of the entire patient to determine the presence of other injuries. Assess the patient's and family's emotional reaction to the injury. Because deviations from the patient's baseline neurologic status can indicate the development of hematomas or cerebral edema, reevaluate neurologic function every 2 hours using the Glasgow Coma Scale.

Nursing Diagnoses and Planning

Nursing diagnoses* and related expected patient outcomes most commonly applicable to patients with a head injury include the following:

NDx: High risk for ineffective breathing pattern related to altered level of consciousness and inadequate respiratory function

Planning: Patient outcomes

1. Respiratory rate and depth are within normal limits.
2. Cyanosis is absent.
3. Arterial blood gas levels remain within normal limits for the patient.

NDx: High risk for infection related to impaired integrity of the cranium

Planning: Patient outcomes

1. Patient is afebrile.
2. Local signs of wound infection are absent.

NDx: Ineffective individual coping related to physical disabilities, memory loss, dependence

Planning: Patient outcomes

1. Patient and family verbalize feelings related to loss and grief.
2. Patient and family demonstrate effective coping patterns.

NDx: High risk for altered health maintenance related to insufficient knowledge of treatment and prognosis

Planning: Patient outcomes

1. Patient and family demonstrate knowledge of patient's condition.
2. Patient and family verbalize realistic expectations of patient's rehabilitation potential.

Nursing Interventions

Monitor the patient's neurologic status, and report any changes from baseline immediately. Record vital signs every 2 hours. Administer medications as ordered to control cerebral edema.

NDx: High risk for ineffective breathing pattern
Hypoxia and hypercarbia increase carbon dioxide levels and potentiate an increase in intracranial pressure. Maintain the patient's position on his or her side to maintain a patent airway. Suction the patient as necessary. Obtain arterial blood gas values. Change the patient's position every 2 hours to prevent pooling of secretions.

NDx: High risk for infection
Injuries such as scalp lacerations, depressed skull fractures, and basilar skull fractures increase the risk of introduction of organisms. If the dura mater has been torn or if the sinuses have been involved, bacteria can enter the cerebrospinal fluid and cause meningitis or brain abscess. Monitor the patient's temperature every 4 hours. Monitor wounds for signs and symptoms of infection, such as redness or exudate. Maintain strict aseptic technique. Do not place gauze or packing into the nose or ears if leakage of cerebrospinal fluid occurs. Provide a sterile field to collect drainage and notify physician. Administer antibiotics as ordered and evaluate effectiveness. Monitor white blood cell count.

NDx: Ineffective individual coping
The head-injured patient may have residual cognitive deficits, memory loss, or functional impairments. In the postacute phase, the patient may express frustration and alarm as he or she becomes aware of these deficits. Encourage the patient and family to express feelings of grief and loss and to openly discuss concerns. Assist the patient in relearning necessary aspects of ADL. Encourage the patient to function to maximum capability. Avoid fostering an unnecessary level of dependence. Discourage family members from performing tasks for the patient that he or she can do or can learn to do. Refer the patient and family to social service counseling as needed.

NDx: High risk for altered health maintenance
The unanticipated traumatic event that resulted in the patient's injury may interfere with the family's ability to focus on the reality of the patient's condition. Inform the family of the patient's daily progress, focusing on realistic expectations. Encourage

* Refer to the sections on Increased Intracranial Pressure and Altered Levels of Consciousness for additional nursing diagnoses that might pertain to head-injured patients.

verbalization and questions by the family. Provide support and assistance in the family's decision making regarding discharge and long-term care needs. Suggest utilization of community resources and support groups for the family.

Evaluation

Evaluate the effectiveness of nursing care for a patient with a head injury by comparing the patient's status with the expected patient outcomes. Examples of specific outcomes for patients with a head injury have been provided in the Planning section.

Spinal Injury

Traumatic spinal cord injury affects 12,000 individuals yearly. Statistics indicate that 62% of spinal cord injury victims are between the ages of 15 and 30 years. The causative factors include vehicular accidents, falls, sports injuries, and gunshot wounds. Advances in technology have increased the average expected life span after spinal cord injury to 30 to 40 years. There is a major economic impact associated with spinal cord injuries.

ETIOLOGY

Trauma to the spinal cord is classified as closed or direct (open) trauma. Automobile accidents, falls, and sports such as diving, skiing, football, and lacrosse result in closed injuries; gunshot wounds or stab wounds are examples of direct trauma.

CLOSED INJURIES

Injuries to the spinal cord are usually the result of a force exerted on the vertebral column, which in turn affects the spinal cord. The areas of the vertebral column most vulnerable to injury are the cervical and lumbar areas. These injuries may or may not cause fractures of the vertebrae.

Hyperflexion Injuries

Hyperflexion injuries are the result of extreme flexion of the spine beyond its normal range of motion (Fig. 38–16). Two common illustrations of this type of injury are (1) sudden deceleration in a head-on vehicular collision and (2) diving into shallow water. In flexion injuries, a wedge or compression fracture of the vertebral body is common. The fracture may be dislocated forward onto the lower vertebrae. The degree of damage to the spinal cord is determined by the extent of compression caused by the dislocated or fractured vertebrae. Hyperflexion injuries occur most often in the cervical and lumbar areas.

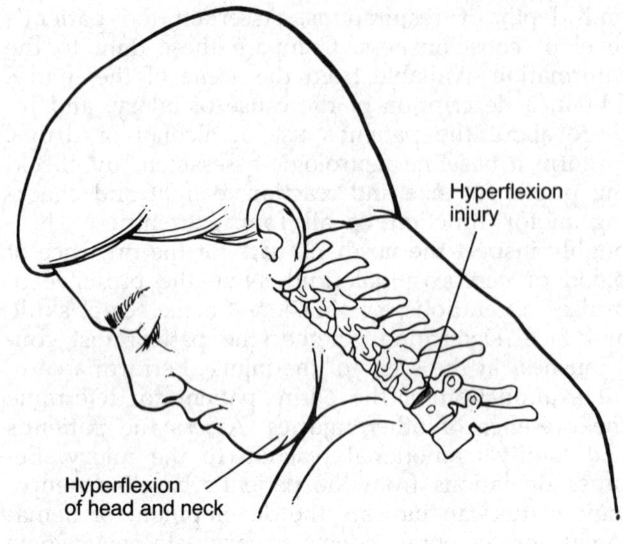

Figure 38–16.

Hyperflexion spinal injury.

Hyperextension Injuries

Hyperextension injuries are caused by extension of the head and neck, which stretches the spinal cord and causes contusion and ischemia (Fig. 38–17). As a general rule, no fractures or dislocations occur, but the contusion and ischemia may produce severe damage to the spinal cord. Examples of this type of injury include falls that involve striking the chin and rear-end vehicular collisions. A less severe form of hyperextension injury is called a whiplash or acceleration injury in which there is stress and

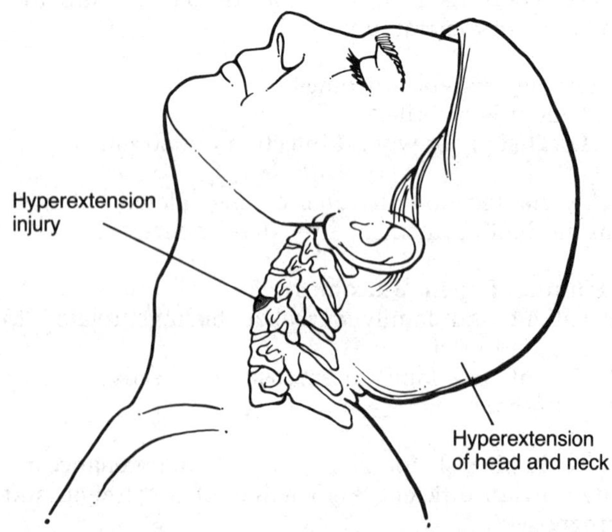

Figure 38–17.

Hyperextension spinal injury.

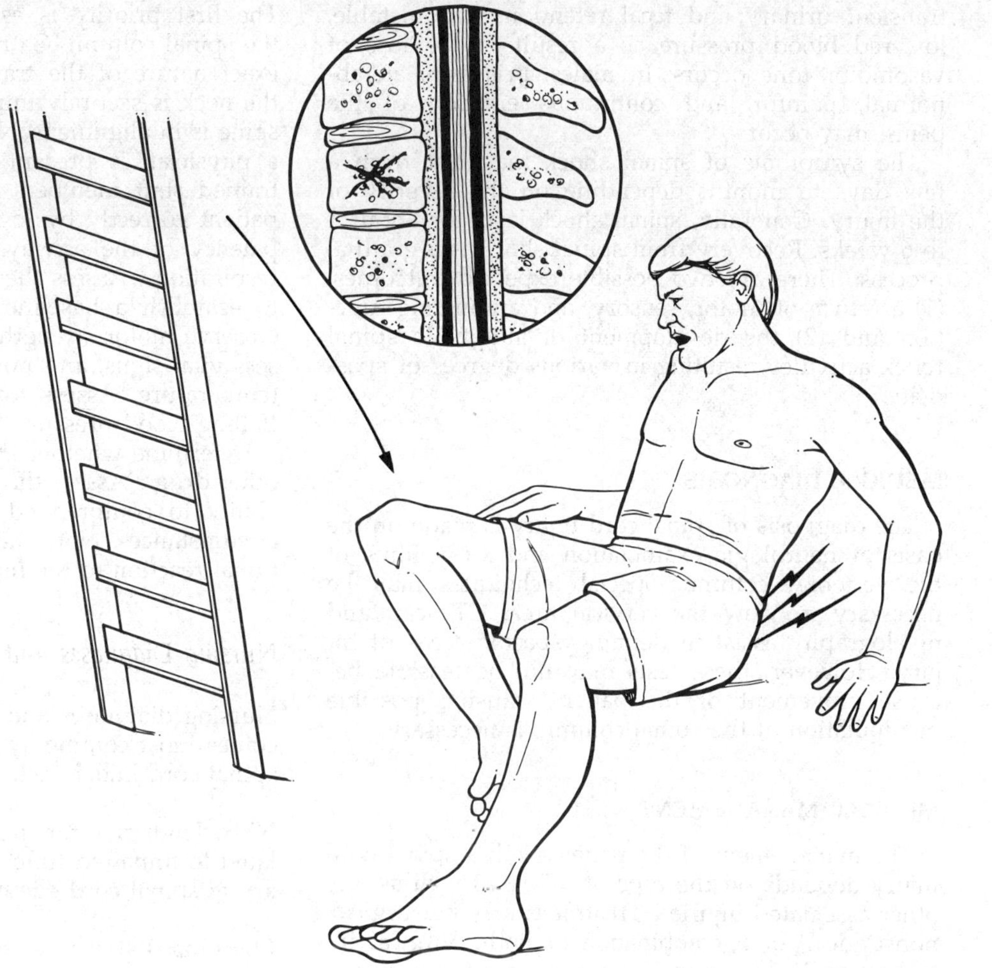

Figure 38–18.
Compression spinal injury.

strain to the soft tissue but no vertebral or cord injury. Hyperextension injuries occur most frequently in the cervical area.

Subluxation Injury

A subluxation deformity is a partial or incomplete dislocation of one vertebra over another. Injury to the spinal cord may or may not occur.

Compression Injury

Compression injuries may occur secondary to falling from a height and landing on the feet or buttocks (Fig. 38–18). There is compression of lower thoracic and lumbar vertebrae severe enough to produce a burst-type fracture.

OPEN INJURIES

Open or direct injuries to the spinal column may be caused by missile wounds (gunshot wounds) or stab wounds. Both these injuries may result in lacerations and transection or severing, of the spinal cord. Direct injury to the spinal cord causes a loss of function below the level of the area injured.

PATHOPHYSIOLOGY

The close anatomic relationship among the vertebrae, ligaments, intervertebral disks, and spinal cord predisposes injury in one of these structures to directly affect one or all of the other structures. Whenever injury has occurred, edema of the spinal cord occurs, similar to the response of injured tissue in other parts of the body. The functional ability of the spinal cord may be temporarily inhibited until the edema has resolved, at which time spinal cord function may return as long as irreversible damage has not occurred.

CLINICAL MANIFESTATIONS

The symptoms exhibited by the patient with spinal cord injury depend on the type of injury sustained and, most importantly, the amount of compression or injury to the spinal cord. Transection of the spinal cord results in spinal shock, which is an immediate response to acute spinal cord injury. Spinal shock is a state of temporary reflex suppression below the level of the injury. There is flaccid paralysis of skeletal musculature and absence of sensation and proprioception below the level of the lesion and transient urinary and fecal retention. An unstable, lowered blood pressure as a result of the loss of vasomotor tone occurs. In males, priapism, an abnormal, painful, and continuous erection of the penis, may occur.

The symptoms of spinal shock may last from a few days to months depending on the severity of the injury. Generally, spinal shock lasts for about 1 to 6 weeks. Recovery from spinal shock is a gradual process. There are two possible expected outcomes: (1) a return of motor, sensory, and autonomic function and (2) the development of automatic spinal reflex activities resulting in various degrees of spasticity.

MEDICAL DIAGNOSIS

The diagnosis of spinal cord injury is made on the basis of neurologic examination and x-ray films of the vertebral column. Special techniques may be necessary to view the cervical area. CT scan and myelography assist in defining specific areas of injury. However, these tests may not be feasible because movement of the patient, causing possible manipulation of the spinal column, is necessary.

MEDICAL MANAGEMENT

The management of the patient with a spinal cord injury depends on the type of injury as well as any other associated injuries. Treatment may be surgical, nonsurgical, or a combination of both. Surgical intervention is indicated if bone fragments secondary to fractures need to be removed from the area of injury, if cord compression is evident, or if a penetrating wound to the spinal cord exists.

Nonsurgical treatment includes the use of immobilization and traction. Cervical fractures are treated by skeletal traction. Cervical tongs (Gardner-Wells, Vinke, Cone, Crutchfield) are used (see Fig. 35–8) with a prescribed amount of weight to provide traction and to re-establish alignment of the vertebrae. The halo device is used to provide skeletal fixation to the cervical area (see Fig. 35–9). The halo device may be used as skeletal traction, similar to cervical tongs, or it may be used with a body vest or jacket, which decreases the length of hospitalization because it allows the patient to be ambulatory.

Application of the Nursing Process to the Care of the Patient with a Spinal Cord Injury

Assessment

Initial assessment of the patient who has sustained a spinal cord injury occurs in the emergency room. The first priority is establishing immobilization of the spinal column. Gather information related to the exact nature of the traumatic incident. Ensure that the neck is securely immobilized and that the lower spine is in alignment. Never move the patient unless a physician is present and a sufficient number of trained staff members are available to transfer the patient correctly by logrolling or lifting. Assess the patency of the airway and the rate and depth of respirations. Assess the patient's neurologic function to establish a baseline for subsequent evaluations. Observe motor strength, sensation, and reflexes. Assess vital signs, and note blood pressure, pulse, and temperature. Assess for symptoms of spinal shock (falling blood pressure, loss of reflexes).

Determine whether the patient ingested alcohol or other drugs. Assess the patient's level of anxiety and ability to comprehend the severity of the present circumstances. Note the patient's and family's emotional reaction to the injury.

Nursing Diagnoses and Planning

Nursing diagnoses and related expected patient outcomes most commonly applicable to patients with a spinal cord injury include the following:

NDx: High risk for ineffective breathing pattern related to impaired function of the diaphragm secondary to spinal cord edema

Planning: Patient outcomes
1. Patient has clear bilateral breath sounds.
2. Arterial blood gas values remain within normal limits for the patient.
3. Patient remains free from pulmonary complications.

NDx: High risk for injury related to unstable vertebral column

Planning: Patient outcomes
1. Baseline neurologic function is maintained.
2. Immobilization device is correctly maintained.

NDx: Impaired physical mobility related to motor and sensory deficits, spine instability

Planning: Patient outcomes
1. Joint flexibility is maintained.
2. Patient demonstrates ability to cope with limitations.

NDx: High risk for infection related to skeletal traction

Planning: Patient outcomes
1. Signs of infection at pin sites are absent.

NDx: Reflex incontinence/urinary retention related to bladder atony secondary to sensory motor deficits

Planning: Patient outcomes
1. Patient empties bladder without residual and retention.
2. Patient remains free from urinary tract infection.

NDx: Constipation related to decreased peristalsis and decreased ability to defecate voluntarily

Planning: Patient outcomes
1. Patient evacuates soft, formed stool at regular intervals.
2. Patient is free from impaction.

NDx: Grieving related to anticipated losses secondary to sensory-motor deficits

Planning: Patient outcomes
1. Patient verbalizes anger.
2. Patient verbalizes perceptions of loss as it relates to self.

Nursing Interventions

NDx: High risk for ineffective breathing pattern
Maintain a patent airway with proper positioning and suctioning as needed. Auscultate breath sounds every 2 to 4 hours. Encourage coughing and deep-breathing exercises every 2 hours to mobilize secretions. Instruct patient in the use of incentive spirometry. Obtain vital capacity measurements every 6 to 8 hours. Use air mister/vaporizer to provide humidity and to assist in breaking up secretions. Administer oxygen as ordered. Obtain arterial blood gas values.

Patients who have sustained a cervical injury are at risk for development of pulmonary complications. Injuries at C4 and above result in loss of innervation of the diaphragm, abdominal, and intercostal muscles. Injury below C-4 leaves the diaphragm intact but impairs the abdominal and intercostal muscles.

NDx: High risk for injury
Injury to the vertebral column can cause compression of the spinal cord if stabilization of the vertebral column is not adequate. Spinal cord compression will result in worsening of any neurologic deficits. Cervical traction provides stability to the cervical spine. Maintain the traction weights at the ordered level. Ensure that they are free-hanging and not resting on the floor or the headboard. Logroll the patient when positioning on his or her side, and use adequate help to maintain proper alignment of the head and neck. Report any deterioration in motor or sensory function immediately.

NDx: Impaired physical mobility
Immobilization of an unstable spinal column places the patient at risk for contracture deformities if motor function is severely impaired. The mobile patient whose activity is restricted is at risk for venous stasis. Maintain the patient in proper alignment at all times. Use supports such as hand rolls or trochanter rolls. Initiate passive range-of-motion exercises every 4 hours. Instruct the patient who is able to move extremities independently in active range-of-motion exercises. Apply antiembolic hose. Remove hose every 8 hours to assess skin integrity and circulatory status.

NDx: High risk for infection
Inspect the skin around the pins of the cervical traction device or halo vest every 8 hours for redness or drainage. Cleanse the area daily according to the specified order for pin care. Maintain aseptic technique. Inspect the pins sites to ensure they are secure.

NDx: Reflex incontinence/urinary retention
Loss of bladder tone occurs as a result of spinal shock, necessitating an indwelling Foley catheter. Once spinal shock has subsided, bladder function may become spastic, predisposing the patient to urinary tract infection.

Maintain accurate intake and output records. Force fluids to ensure an intake of 3000 ml in 24 hours to prevent the formation of urinary tract calculi. Obtain urinalysis, culture, and sensitivity samples as necessary. Provide catheter care twice a day. Tape the catheter to prevent traction on the meatus. If an intermittent catheter regimen is begun, maintain strict aseptic technique. Monitor the patient's temperature every 8 hours. Administer medications such as prophylactic sulfa drugs (sulfisoxazole [Gantrisin]) or internal acidifiers (vitamin C) if ordered.

NDx: Constipation
Encourage fluids and foods high in fiber and roughage to stimulate peristalsis. Consult with the dietitian and the patient to determine what food the patient likes and dislikes. Administer stool softeners, bulk producers, and lubricants as ordered. A bowel-training regimen may be instituted once the patient is considered stable.

NDx: Grieving
Encourage the patient to verbalize fears regarding loss of independence. Allow the patient to express anger. Decrease environmental stress by providing for continuity of care, privacy, and adequate rest periods. Allow the patient to grieve in his or her own way. Provide simple, concrete explanations. Encourage the patient to make choices and become involved in decision-making in care whenever feasible. Provide support and understanding when angry feelings are expressed.

Evaluation

Evaluate the effectiveness of nursing care for a patient with a spinal cord injury by comparing the patient's status with the expected patient outcomes. Examples of specific outcomes for patients with a spinal cord injury have been provided in the Planning section.

Peripheral Nerve Injury

ETIOLOGY

Peripheral nerve trauma can be the result of partial or complete severance; contusion; stretching; compression; ischemia; electrical, thermal, and radiation injuries; and drug injection. A partially or completely severed nerve is usually the result of a sharp cutting instrument. Regeneration is possible in certain circumstances. Contusion to a nerve is the result of direct blows to the nerve, gunshot wounds, or fractures near the nerve. The nerve remains structurally intact, but complete functional ability is impaired. A stretch trauma to a nerve occurs secondary to extreme movement and excessive application of weight such as in orthopedic traction. Compression injury to a nerve is caused by extreme or prolonged pressure on a nerve. Examples include tumors, a herniated intervertebral disk, and narrowed, bony foramina, causing nerve entrapment. Ischemia deprives a nerve of an adequate blood supply. Electrical, thermal, and radiation trauma injuries occur if an electrical wire comes in contact with a peripheral nerve, causing burning and necrosis. An injection of a drug into or near a peripheral nerve causes necrosis and scarring. The sciatic and radial nerves are most commonly affected secondary to improper intramuscular injection techniques.

The most common traumatic syndromes affecting peripheral nerves include (1) brachial plexus injury, (2) upper extremity injuries to the ulnar, radial, or medial nerves (carpal tunnel syndrome), and (3) lower extremity injuries to the femoral, sciatic, and common perineal nerve.

PATHOPHYSIOLOGY

When a nerve in the central nervous system is transected, the entire neuron degenerates because the cell nucleus has been injured. Scar tissue forms secondary to degeneration of the axon. However, if a peripheral nerve has been severed, there is a possibility for self-repair. In the proximal axon, tiny unmyelinated sprouts begin to form, enlarge, and join together. These joined sprouts grow at the rate of 1 mm to 4 mm/day to cross the gap to the distal axon (Fig. 38–19). If realignment is successful, remyelination occurs, growth of the severed axon continues, and eventually 80% of the nerve's former capacity may return.

CLINICAL MANIFESTATIONS

The signs and symptoms of a peripheral nerve injury include a flaccid paralysis or paresis of the muscles supplied by the nerve, loss of reflexes in the affected area, loss of muscle tone, and diminished or complete loss of sensation.

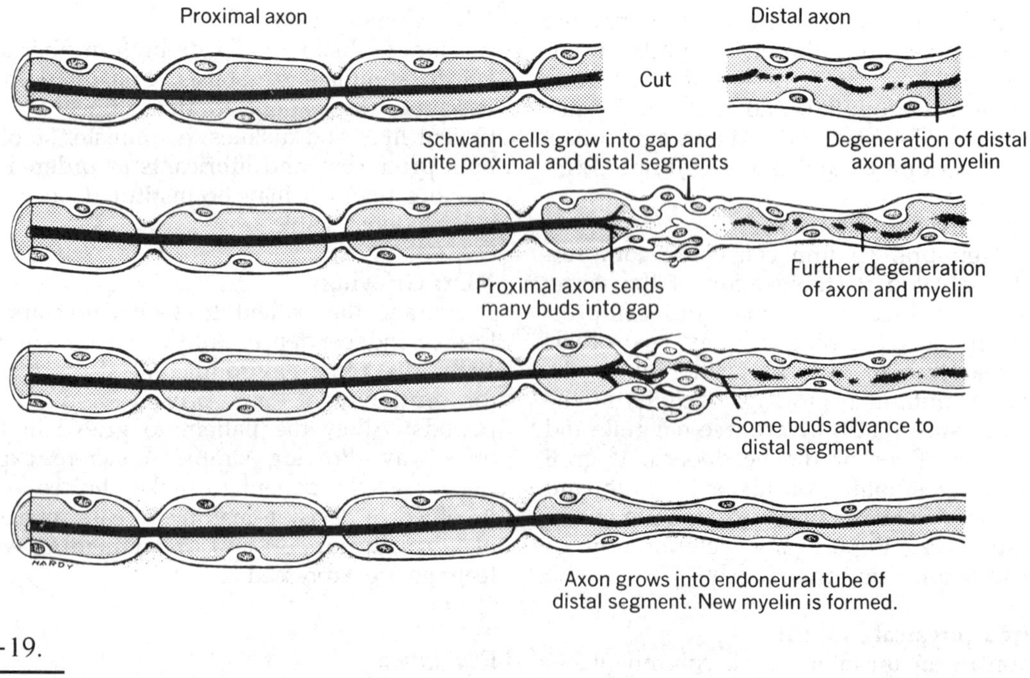

Figure 38–19.

Diagram of changes that occur in a nerve fiber that has been cut and then regenerates. (From Hickey JV. The clinical practice of neurological and neurosurgical nursing. 3rd ed. Philadelphia: JB Lippincott, 1992, p 469.)

MEDICAL DIAGNOSIS

Diagnosis of peripheral nerve injuries is made on the basis of the history and neurologic examination. Electromyography and nerve conduction studies aid in determining the intactness of the nerve. Tinel's sign also indicates nerve function. When percussion is applied over the site of a divided nerve, a tingling or painful sensation is perceived at the distal end of the limb involved. This may indicate the beginning of regeneration of the nerve.

MEDICAL MANAGEMENT

Primary nerve repair is usually scheduled to take place 3 weeks after the injury. Anastomosis of a severed nerve requires the two nerve segments to be dissected to remove scar tissue and aligned so that the slow regeneration process can occur. This may require the patient to have the extremity positioned in exaggerated flexion by a cast or splint. Cable grafting with autologous nerve tissue is a newer surgical technique that may eliminate the need for the exaggerated flexion.

The recovery process is often long and tedious for the patient. The primary concern is joint stiffness and muscle atrophy, which begin to occur almost immediately after injury. A vigorous physiotherapy program is necessary. Daily use of electrical stimulation to the affected muscles, instituted as soon as possible after injury, may facilitate the rehabilitation process.

Guidelines for Application of the Nursing Process to the Care of the Patient with a Peripheral Nerve Injury

Nursing care of the patient with a peripheral nerve injury varies with the specific nerve involved and the method of treatment. In most cases, movement of the affected limb will be limited, and some deficit in mobility or self-care will result.

Neoplasia

Brain Tumors

Intracranial tumors occur as either primary tumors or secondary or metastatic tumors. Primary brain tumors arise or grow from brain tissue. Primary brain tumors occur in people of all ages but are statistically more prevalent in children and middle-aged adults.

Secondary or metastatic brain tumors arise from tissue elsewhere in the body and seed or spread to the brain. The most frequent sites of the primary malignancy are the lungs, breast, skin, gastrointestinal tract, and kidneys. Metastatic brain tumors are much more commonly found in the adult population.

ETIOLOGY

The cause of primary brain tumors is unknown. Environmental agents, familial tendencies, viral implications, and others may be related.

PATHOPHYSIOLOGY

A brain tumor, similar to any other tumor or neoplasm, is an abnormal mass resulting from the excessive multiplication of cells. Brain tumors can grow either as a spherical mass or in a diffusely infiltrating manner, invading surrounding brain tissue without any mass formation. Tumor growth results in compression and invasion of surrounding structures, causing pathophysiologic changes in the brain. Edema develops in the vicinity of the tumor, and signs of increased intracranial pressure are evident as the tumor expands.

Table 38–6 classifies brain tumors according to name, origin, and most frequent site of development.

CLINICAL MANIFESTATIONS

The symptoms exhibited by the patient with a brain tumor can be either focal or generalized. Focal symptoms result from direct compression of surrounding structures, and the signs and symptoms seen are directly correlated to the location. Headache, vomiting, and papilledema are general symptoms associated with most intracranial tumors.

Headache is the only presenting symptom in approximately 20% of patients with brain tumor. The headache is usually intermittent and presents with greater intensity in the morning. Vomiting without a precipitating cause is the initial symptom in about 10% of patients with a brain tumor. Vomiting is indicative of increased intracranial pressure. Papilledema, noted only by visualizing the optic disc with an ophthalmoscope, is present in about 70% to 75% of patients with brain tumors. The optic disk is blurred rather than sharply defined, indicative of an early rise in intracranial pressure.

Other signs and symptoms that may occur include personality changes, decrease in intellectual abilities, and seizures, which are indicative of irritation of the cerebral cortex.

MEDICAL DIAGNOSIS

History and physical examination are the initial steps taken in diagnosing brain tumors. Important

Table 38–6. CLASSIFICATION OF BRAIN TUMORS

NEOPLASM	ORIGIN	MOST FREQUENT SITES	COMMENTS
Gliomas	Neuroglial tissue		Most common type of intracranial neoplasm; rate of growth varies with type of glioma
Astrocytoma	Astrocytes	Adults: cerebrum Children: cerebellum	Most common glioma; grows very slowly; infiltrates surrounding tissue
Glioblastoma	Undifferentiated glial cells	Frontal, parietal, and temporal lobes	Highly malignant
Medulloblastoma	Undifferentiated glial cells	Cerebellum	Rapid extension; highly malignant
Ependymoma	Ependymal cells of lining of ventricle and aqueducts	Fourth ventricle	Rare; frequently papillomatous; may obstruct flow of cerebrospinal fluid
Oligodendroglioma	Oligodendrocytes	Cerebral hemispheres	Rare; grows very slowly; tends to calcify
Meningioma	Meninges	Along the course of the intracranial venous sinuses	Extracerebral, causing compression of brain tissue; usually encapsulated; grows slowly
Hemangiomas			
Angioma	Blood vessel wall	Middle cerebral artery	Not a true neoplasm; congenital mass of tortuous, enlarged vessels; benign but may interfere with adjacent tissues
Angioblastoma	Blood vessel wall	Cerebellum	Tendency to form cysts
Pituitary adenomas			
Chromophobe adenoma	Adenohypophyseal glandular tissue	Anterior pituitary lobe (adenohypophysis)	Encapsulated; compresses pituitary gland tissue and optic nerves, leading to hypopituitarism and impaired vision
Chromophilic adenoma (acidophilic adenoma)	Adenohypophyseal glandular tissue	Anterior pituitary lobe (adenohypophysis)	Seen less often than chromophobe adenoma; causes hypopituitarism (gigantism or acromegaly)
Craniopharyngioma	Embryologic defect in craniopharyngeal duct	Anterior to the pituitary stalk	Produces pressure on surrounding structures, interfering with function
Acoustic neuroma	Eighth cranial (acoustic) nerve		Encapsulated

data are gathered that assist in ruling out diseases that present with similar symptoms. Skull x-ray film, CT scan, and MRI provide information regarding the size and location of the tumor as well as the presence of any bone erosion. Cerebral angiography indicates any displacement of cerebral blood vessels by the invading tumor. Chest films rule out carcinoma of the lung as a primary site. Specific diagnostic procedures are used if the presenting symptomatology suggests localized areas of tumor growth. Examples include audiometric testing if an acoustic neuroma is suspected or endocrinologic studies if a pituitary tumor is suspected.

All patients should have a funduscopic examination to assess for the presence of papilledema. Lumbar puncture should be avoided and may be contraindicated if increased intracranial pressure is present.

MEDICAL MANAGEMENT

Once the diagnosis of brain tumor has been established, the medical management of the patient most often involves surgery, radiotherapy, or chemotherapy alone or in combination. Surgical intervention via a craniotomy approach is the recommended treatment for benign primary tumors. Craniotomy is also performed on the patient with an encapsulated malignant brain tumor that is likely to be easily removed. Radiotherapy or chemotherapy is given postoperatively.

Stereotaxic surgery is rapidly gaining popularity as a method of treating grossly infiltrative tumors that present difficulty for conventional surgical removal. The procedure is usually performed under local anesthesia in the radiology department. The stereotaxic frame is attached to the patient. The CT scanner is used to obtain precise landmarks of the lesion. A burr hole is made and a biopsy obtained for pathology. This allows for prompt initiation of either chemotherapy or radiotherapy once the pathology of the tumor has been determined. The risks to the patient are markedly decreased compared with those of a craniotomy procedure.

Radiotherapy is a treatment modality often used after craniotomy or stereotaxic biopsy. Astrocytomas, glioblastomas, oligodendrogliomas, sarcomas, and craniopharyngiomas are tumors that are often treated with a course of radiotherapy. The total tumor dose is usually from 4000 rad to 7000 rad administered over 4 to 8 weeks.

Chemotherapy is also used in the management of malignant brain tumors. Medulloblastomas and glioblastomas generally respond well to chemotherapy. The drugs used and the dosages depend on the tumor size, location, and general health of the patient.

Guidelines for Application of the Nursing Process to the Care of the Patient with a Brain Tumor

Nursing care for a patient with a brain tumor varies with the stage of the disease and the mode of treatment selected. For patients with terminal disease, the nursing care discussed in Chapter 5 applies; for patients receiving radiation therapy or chemotherapy the care discussed in Chapter 11 applies; and for patients having surgery for a brain tumor the care discussed in Chapter 37 applies.

In all cases, periodic neurologic assessment and observation for worsening headache or vomiting, which can indicate increasing intracranial pressure, are essential.

The Elderly: Special Considerations

Some neurologic disorders are seen more predominately in the elderly population and, in this age group, may differ in clinical presentation, clinical course, and method of treatment. Examples include organic brain syndromes, cerebrovascular accidents, normal pressure hydrocephalus, and subdural hematomas.

Organic Brain Syndrome

Organic brain syndrome (OBS) is a deterioration in brain functioning that may occur in either an acute or a chronic form. Acute OBS, also referred to as delirium or an acute confusional state, is a temporary and usually reversible condition caused by a disturbance of cerebral function and metabolism. Hypoxia, metabolic disorders, trauma, infectious processes, fluid and electrolyte imbalances, and medication reactions can be precipitating factors. Acute OBS often has a sudden onset and is manifested by disorientation, memory loss, and impairment in level of consciousness. Treatment of the underlying condition may reverse the confusional state.

Chronic OBS, also known as dementia, is an irreversible condition. Unlike acute OBS, the onset is usually insidious. Impairment of memory, judgment, affect, and intelligence occurs. Diseases associated with chronic OBS include Alzheimer's disease, Pick's disease, and multi-infarct dementia.

In both acute and chronic organic brain syndromes, nursing management focuses on individualizing a plan of care. Provide orientation on a regular basis, use familiar objects in the environment whenever possible, and ensure that safety is maintained. Involve family members in care, allow time for discussion of anxieties and fears, and suggest support groups or community resources when planning for discharge.

Cerebrovascular Accident

Neurologic deficits suffered as a consequence of a cerebrovascular accident, or stroke, are directly related to the type, location, and extent of damage to cerebral tissue. Aging is not a factor in this physiologic response. However, age may be a factor in the ultimate level of functioning that can be attained after a stroke. The elderly stroke victim is more likely than a younger person to have multiple chronic illnesses. This may prolong the rehabilitation phase secondary to potential complications of those chronic illnesses.

Normal Pressure Hydrocephalus

This disorder is characterized by enlarged ventricles, which compress surrounding cerebral tissue, causing symptomatology. A normal cerebrospinal fluid pressure is noted, as opposed to the elevated cerebrospinal fluid pressure seen in acute hydrocephalus. A distinct triad of symptoms aids in the diagnosis: (1) unsteadiness of gait (ataxia); (2) mild dementia characterized by an insidious onset with impaired memory, apathy, and inattention; and (3) urinary incontinence. Once the disorder is diagnosed, treatment involves surgical placement of a shunt, which often results in alleviation of symptoms.

Subdural Hematoma

A normal consequence of aging is some mild atrophy of brain tissue. This cerebral atrophy allows the bleeding that occurs into the subdural space after mild trauma to accumulate at a slower rate and therefore delay the presentation of symptoms. In the elderly, subdural hematomas often are chronic in nature, and the symptoms of confusion, drowsiness, and cognitive impairment may be unjustly attributed to the aging process.

Resources

American Association of Neuroscience Nurses
224 North Des Plaines
Suite 601
Chicago, IL 60661

American Brain Tumor Association
3725 North Talman Avenue
Chicago, IL 60618

American Cancer Society
1599 Clifton Road NE
Atlanta, GA 30329

American Heart Association National Center
7272 Greenville Avenue
Dallas, TX 75231

American Parkinson Disease Association
116 John Street
New York, NY 10038

American Speech/Language/Hearing Association
10801 Rockville Pike
Rockville, MD 20852

Epilepsy Foundation of America
4351 Garden City Drive
Landover, MD 20785

Guillain-Barré International Foundation
P.O. Box 262
Wynnewood, PA 19096

Hereditary Disease Foundation
1427 7th Street
Suite 2
Santa Monica, CA 90401

Huntington's Disease Foundation of America
140 West 22nd Street
6th Floor
New York, NY 10011

Muscular Dystrophy Association
3561 East Sunrise Drive
Tucson, AZ 85718

Myasthenia Gravis Foundation
53 West Jackson Boulevard
Suite 909
Chicago, IL 60604

National Amyotrophic Lateral Sclerosis Foundation
185 Madison Avenue
New York, New York 10019

National Head Injury Foundation
1140 Connecticut Avenue NW
Suite 812
Washington, DC 20036

National Institute of Neurological and Communicative Disorders and Stroke
National Institutes of Health
Bethesda, MD 20892

National Multiple Sclerosis Society
733 3rd Avenue
6th floor
New York, NY 10017

National Parkinson Foundation
1501 NW Ninth Avenue
Miami, FL 33136

National Spasmodic Torticollis Association, Inc.
P.O. Box 873
Royal Oak, MI 48068

National Spinal Cord Injury Association
600 West Cummings Park
Suite 2000
Woburn, MA 01801

Parkinson's Disease Foundation
William Black Medical Research Building
Columbia University Medical Center
640 West 168th Street
New York, NY 10032

The Stroke Foundation
898 Park Avenue
New York, NY 10021

Tourette Syndrome Association
42–40 Bell Boulevard
Bayside, NY 11361

Bibliography

Adams RD, Victor M. Principles of neurology. 4th ed. New York: McGraw-Hill, 1989.

Asbury AK, McKhann GM, McDonald WI (eds). Diseases of the nervous system: Clinical neurobiology. 2nd ed. Philadelphia, WB Saunders, 1992.

Blount M, Kinney AB, Stackhouse J. Myasthenia gravis: A manual for the nurse. New York: Myasthenia Gravis Foundation, Inc, 1991.

Cammermeyer M, Appeldorn C (eds). Core curriculum for neuroscience nursing. 3rd ed. Chicago, IL: American Association of Neuroscience Nurses, 1990.

Carpenito LJ. Handbook of nursing diagnosis. 4th ed. New York: JB Lippincott, 1991.

Carpenito LJ. Nursing diagnosis: Application to clinical practice. 4th ed. Philadelphia: JB Lippincott, 1992.

Chadwick AT, Oesting HH. Not for specialists only: Caring for patients with spinal cord injuries. Nursing 89 1989; 19(11):52.

Chadwick D, Cartlidge NEF, Bates D. Medical neurology. New York: Churchill-Livingstone, 1989.

Chusid J. Correlative neuroanatomy and functional neurology. 19th ed. Los Altos, CA: Lange Medical Publications, 1985.

Clendaniel B, Fleishell A. An Alzheimer day-care center for nursing home patients. Am J Nurs 1989; 89(7):944.

Cote L, Riedel G. Exercises for the Parkinson patient with hints for daily living. New York: Parkinson's Disease Foundation.

Cote L, Sprinzeles L. The Parkinson patient at home. New York: Parkinson's Disease Foundation.

Diamond S. Headaches that herald intracranial emergencies. Emerg Med 1988; 20(20):20, 27, 31.

Duvoisin RC. Parkinson's disease—A guide for patient and family. 3rd ed. New York: Raven Press, 1991.

Epilepsy Foundation of America. Seizure recognition and observation: A guide for allied health professionals. Landover, MD: Epilepsy Foundation of America, 1981.

Esberger KK, Hughes ST. Nursing care of the aged. Norwalk, CT: Appleton & Lange, 1989.

Fowler RS, Fordyce WE. Stroke: Why do they behave that way? Dallas, TX: American Heart Association, 1983.

Friedman D. Taking the scare out of caring for seizure patients. Nursing 88 1988; 18(2):52.

Gilroy J. Basic neurology. 2nd ed. New York: McGraw-Hill, 1990.

Goldberg S. Clinical neuroanatomy made ridiculously simple. North Miami Beach, FL: MedMaster, Inc, 1986.

Grove TP. A man alone . . . and afraid: Caring for a patient with Guillain-Barré syndrome. Nursing 87 1987; 17(12):44.

Gunderson CH. Essentials of clinical neurology. New York: Raven Press, 1990.

Guyton AC. Basic neuroscience: Anatomy and physiology. 2nd ed. Philadelphia: WB Saunders, 1992.

Hickey J. The clinical practice of neurological and neurosurgical nursing. 3rd ed. New York: JB Lippincott, 1992.

Jacobson AL, Donlon WC. Headache and facial pain: Diagnosis and management. New York: Raven Press, 1990.

Lee BY, Ostrander L, Cochran G, Shaw W (eds). The spinal cord injured patient: Comprehensive management. Philadelphia: WB Saunders, 1991.

Liebman M. Neuroanatomy made easy and understandable. 4th ed. Rockville, MD: Aspen Systems, 1991.

Lindsay KW, Bone I, Callander R. Neurology and neurosurgery illustrated. New York: Churchill Livingstone, 1991.

Lundgren J. Acute neuroscience nursing: Concepts and care. Boston: Jones and Bartlett Publishers, 1986.

Marsden CD, Fowler TJ (eds). Clinical neurology. New York: Raven Press, 1989.

Matteson MA, McConnell ES. Gerontological nursing: Concepts and practice. Philadelphia: WB Saunders, 1989.

Matthews WB, Compston A, Allen IV, Martyn CN. McAlpine's multiple sclerosis. 2nd ed. New York: Churchill Livingstone, 1991.

Mitchell PH, Cammermeyer M, Ozuna J, Woods NF. Neurological assessment for nursing practice. Reston, VA: Reston Publishing, 1984.

Mitchell PH, Hodges LC, Muwaswes M, Walleck CA (eds). AANN's neuroscience nursing. Norwalk, CT: Appleton & Lange, 1988.

Morgante L, Madonna M, Pokoluk R. Research and treatment in multiple sclerosis: Implications for nursing practice. J Neurosci Nurs 1989; 21(5):285.

Nikas DL. Critical aspects of head trauma. Crit Care Q 1987; 10(1):1940.

Olson E. The hazards of immobility. Am J Nurs 1967; 67:788.

Parkinson's Disease Foundation. Parkinson's disease: Progress, promise and hope! (revised). New York: Parkinson's Disease Foundation, 1992.

Plank C. ALS, MS, MD—what's the difference? Am J Nurs 1980; 80(2):282.

Prendergast VP. Bacterial meningitis update. J Neurosci Nurs 1987; 19(2):95.

Price G. MS: The challenge to the family. Am J Nurs 1980; 80(2):284.

Rhynsburger J. How to fight MG fatigue. Am J Nurs 1989; 89(3):337.

Scheinberg LC, Holland NJ. Multiple sclerosis: A guide for patients and their families. 2nd ed. New York: Raven Press, 1987.

Sherman DW. Managing an acute head injury. Nursing 90 1990; 20(4):46.

Slater R, Yearwood A. MS: The disease process. Am J Nurs 1980; 80(2):276.

Smith DB. Epilepsy: Current approaches to diagnosis and treatment. New York: Raven Press, 1990.

Taylor J, Raimond J. Neurological emergencies effective nursing care. Rockville, MD: Aspen Systems, 1986.

U.S. Department of Health and Human Services Task Force on Alzheimer's Disease. Alzheimer's disease: A scientific guide for health professionals. NIH Publication No. 84-2251. Washington, DC: U.S. Government Printing Office, 1984.

Yearwood A. MS: Being disabled doesn't mean being handicapped. Am J Nurs 1980; 80(2):300.

Unit Thirteen

ADULTS WITH SENSORY DYSFUNCTION

Learning Objectives

AFTER COMPLETING THIS UNIT, THE LEARNER WILL BE ABLE TO:

Chapter Thirty-nine

1. Explain the normal anatomy and physiology of the eye.
2. Describe common clinical manifestations of eye dysfunction.
3. Identify information and physical examination data essential to the assessment of the eye.
4. Describe basic diagnostic tests and modalities of medical management used in the treatment of patients with eye disorders.
5. Describe basic ocular surgery.
6. Identify data essential to the assessment of patients undergoing treatment of eye disorders.
7. State nursing diagnoses and related expected patient outcomes commonly applicable to patients undergoing treatment of eye disorders.
8. Describe nursing interventions, with their rationales, commonly applicable to patients undergoing treatment of eye disorders.
9. Explain the basis for evaluation of nursing care provided to patients undergoing treatment of eye disorders.
10. Identify special considerations for the elderly patient with altered ocular function.

Chapter Forty

1. Describe common eye disorders in terms of etiology, pathophysiology, clinical manifestations, diagnostic procedures, and medical management.
2. Identify information and physical examination data essential to the assessment of patients with common eye disorders.
3. State nursing diagnoses and related expected patient outcomes commonly applicable to patients with eye disorders.
4. Describe nursing interventions, with their rationales, commonly applicable to patients with eye disorders.
5. Explain the basis for evaluation of nursing care provided to patients with common eye disorders.
6. Identify special considerations for the elderly patient with an eye disorder.

Chapter Forty-one

1. Explain the normal anatomy and physiology of the ear.
2. Describe common clinical manifestations of ear dysfunction.
3. Identify information and physical examination data essential to the assessment of the ear.
4. Describe basic diagnostic tests and modalities of medical management used in the treatment of patients with ear disorders.
5. Describe basic surgical procedures (tympanoplasty, myringotomy, mastoidectomy) used in the treatment of patients with ear disorders.
6. Identify data essential to the assessment of patients undergoing treatment of ear disorders.
7. State nursing diagnoses and related expected patient outcomes commonly applicable to patients undergoing treatment of ear disorders.
8. Describe nursing interventions, with their rationales, commonly applicable to patients undergoing treatment of ear disorders.
9. Explain the basis for evaluation of nursing care provided to patients undergoing treatment of ear disorders.
10. Identify special considerations for the elderly patient with altered auditory function.

Chapter Forty-two

1. Describe common ear disorders in terms of etiology, pathophysiology, clinical manifestations, diagnostic procedures, and medical management.
2. Identify information and physical examination data essential to the assessment of patients with common ear disorders.
3. State nursing diagnoses and related expected patient outcomes commonly applicable to patients with ear disorders.
4. Describe nursing interventions, with their rationales, commonly applicable to patients with ear disorders.
5. Explain the basis for evaluation of nursing care provided to patients with common ear disorders.
6. Identify special considerations for the elderly patient with an ear disorder.

Chapter Thirty-nine

KNOWLEDGE BASIC TO THE NURSING CARE *of Adults with Dysfunction of the Eye*

Before a nurse can assist in the diagnosis and treatment of patients with ocular disorders, a thorough understanding of anatomy, physiology, and pathophysiology as well as the patient's response to these phenomena is required. It is said that the eye is the window to the body because many diseases and disorders have an ocular component. Therefore, a thorough history and assessment are required.

This chapter reviews normal ocular anatomy and physiology, describes clinical manifestations, outlines the ocular history and assessment processes, and provides basic information on commonly performed diagnostic tests. It features an overview of medical, surgical, and laser therapies as well as the application of the nursing process to the corneal transplant patient.

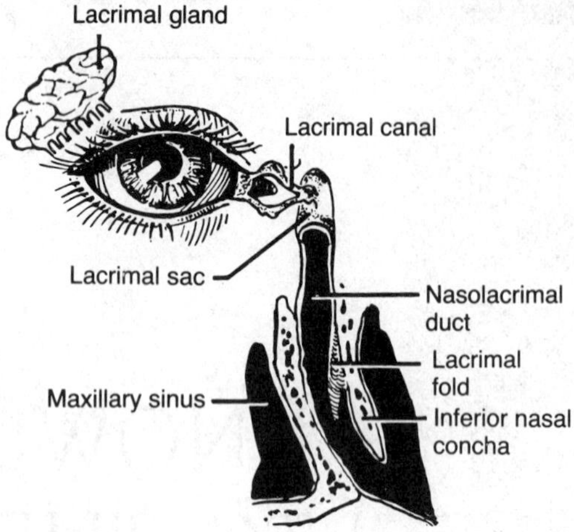

Figure 39–1.

The lacrimal apparatus. (Modified from O'Rahilly R. Basic human anatomy. Philadelphia: WB Saunders, 1983, p. 408.)

Anatomy and Physiology

Protective Structures of the Eye

The bony orbit, lying anteriorly in the skull, protects the globe, or eyeball. The walls of the orbit form the floor of the cerebrum, the roof of the maxillary sinus, and the lateral walls of the nose. The optic foramen, at the posterior portion of the orbit, provides the bony opening through which the optic nerve, central retinal artery, and ophthalmic vein pass on their way to or from the eye.

The accessory structures of the eye, which also help to protect it, are the eyebrows, eyelids, eyelashes, and the lacrimal apparatus.

The eyebrows are arches over the eyes formed by the frontal bone, which are covered by skin rich in sebaceous glands and a ridge of coarse, laterally directed hairs. They help to protect the eye from direct rays of light as well as from perspiration or other foreign material that may come off the brow or forehead.

The upper and lower eyelids, or palpebrae, cover the eyeball from the medial canthus to the lateral canthus. They spread lubricating solutions over the globe and protect the eyes from excessive light and from foreign objects. They also cover the eyes during sleep and prevent drying due to the evaporation of secretions.

The band of connective tissue that gives form to the eyelids is the tarsal plate. Embedded in it are the meibomian glands, whose ducts open onto the margin of each eyelid. These modified sebaceous glands secrete an oily substance that helps prevent the lids from adhering to each other. The eyelids are lined with a mucous membrane called the palpebral conjunctiva. A continuation of this membrane is the bulbar conjunctiva, which covers the sclera, the visible "white of the eye."

The eyelashes are a row of short thick hairs that project from the edge of each eyelid. They help screen the eye from dust and other foreign particles. At the base of these hair follicles are the glands of Zeis, which supply a lubricating substance to the follicle.

The lacrimal apparatus consists of the structures involved in the production and drainage of tears (Fig. 39–1). Tears are produced by the lacrimal gland, which is located in the upper, outer aspect of each orbit. The tears empty through the excretory lacrimal ducts onto the conjunctiva of the upper lid and are spread across the eyeball by blinking. They then enter the lacrimal puncta, which are two small openings located in the inner canthus of each upper and lower eyelid. Tears then pass into the lacrimal canals, the lacrimal sac, the nasolacrimal duct, and finally into the inferior meatus of the turbinate bone of the nose.

Tears contain water, salts, mucus, a bactericidal enzyme called lysozyme as well as other chemical substances. The tear film is also made up of mucins secreted by the conjunctival cells and the oily substance secreted by the meibomian glands. Tears function to clean, lubricate, and moisten the eyeball. Tears wash the surface of the eye at a constant rate but increase dramatically when the eye is exposed to an irritating substance or the emotional stimulus of the parasympathetic nervous system.

Muscles Controlling the Eye

The muscles that control the eye are of two types: those external to the eyeball and those that are internal. The six external muscles are attached to the outside of the eyeball and to the bones of the orbit. They are voluntary, skeletal muscles that function to move the eyeball under the control of cranial nerves III, IV, and VI (Fig. 39–2). Cranial nerve III (oculomotor) innervates the superior rectus, medial rectus, inferior rectus, and inferior oblique muscles. Cranial nerve IV (trochlear) innervates the superior oblique muscle. Cranial nerve VI (abducens) innervates the lateral rectus muscle. Eye movement is coordinated as a result of the joining of cranial nerves III, IV, and VI within the midbrain.

The upper eyelid is raised by the levator palpebrae superioris muscle, which is under the control of cranial nerve III and the sympathetic nervous system. The lid is closed by the orbicularis oculi muscle, which is controlled by cranial nerve VII.

The internal eye muscles include the iris and ciliary muscle, which are controlled through the complex neural network involving the optic nerve (cranial nerve II) and oculomotor nerve (cranial nerve III). The iris and ciliary muscle are smooth, involuntary muscles and function to regulate the size of the pupil and control the shape of the lens in the process of accommodation.

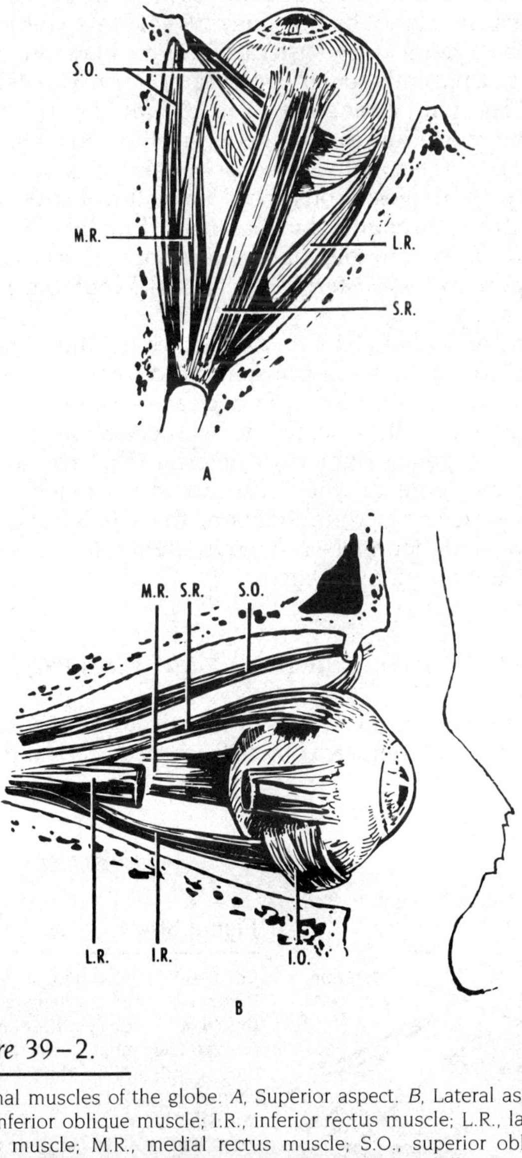

Figure 39–2.

External muscles of the globe. *A*, Superior aspect. *B*, Lateral aspect. I.O., inferior oblique muscle; I.R., inferior rectus muscle; L.R., lateral rectus muscle; M.R., medial rectus muscle; S.O., superior oblique muscle; S.R., superior rectus muscle. (From O'Rahilly R. Basic human anatomy. Philadelphia: WB Saunders, 1983, p. 405.)

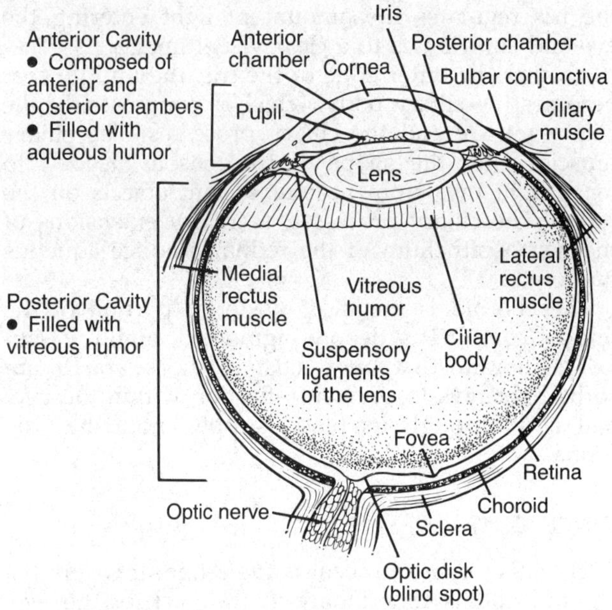

Figure 39–3.

Structure of the eyeball.

Eyeball Structure

The eyeball is spherical and is composed of three distinct layers, or coats, that surround two fluid-filled cavities (Fig. 39–3). The three layers are the external fibrous coat, the middle vascular coat, and the internal nervous coat.

EXTERNAL COAT

The external fibrous coat, which gives the eyeball its shape, has two distinct parts: the cornea and the sclera. The cornea, which covers the iris, is the most anterior portion of the external coat. It is transparent and avascular. The remainder of the external coat is the opaque sclera, part of which is seen as the white of the eye. This visible portion of the sclera is covered with the bulbar conjunctiva whose epithelium is continuous with the layer of epithelium which covers the outer surface of the cornea.

MIDDLE COAT

The middle vascular coat is composed of three parts that together are referred to as the uveal tract. They are the iris, the ciliary body, and the choroid.

The most anterior portion of the middle coat is the iris, or colored area of the eye. The iris muscles constrict and dilate, changing the size of the opening in the center, which is the pupil. By this action the iris regulates the amount of light entering the eye and contributes to a clear visual image.

Around the outer edge of the iris, the middle coat becomes the ciliary body, which is composed of the ciliary muscle and the ciliary processes. The ciliary muscles alter the shape of the lens as needed to focus light rays from near or distant objects on the retina. The ciliary processes, secretory extensions of the neuroepithelium of the retina, produce aqueous humor.

The choroid is the most posterior portion of the middle coat. It is a deeply pigmented, highly vascular membrane that lines most of the sclera. It absorbs light rays to prevent reflection within the eyeball and, through its blood supply, nourishes the retina.

INNER COAT

The inner or neural coat is the retina. It covers the choroid and is found only in the back of the eye. The retina, which forms the visual image, consists of an outer pigmented layer, which stores vitamin A needed for the production of the photopigment rhodopsin, and an inner neural layer. The rods and cones, which are the photoreceptors, are found in the neural layer and are the visual receptors that develop generator potentials. Cones, stimulated only by bright light, are responsible for color vision and visual acuity. Rods allow for vision in dim light and are responsible for perception of different shades of dark and light, shapes, and movement. Rods are located in the peripheral retina, and cones are concentrated in the fovea, the center of a small avascular area called the macula lutea or yellow spot, which is responsible for sharpest vision.

From the photoreceptor cells containing the rods and cones, sensory information is relayed to the bipolar neurons and then to the ganglion cells of the retina. The axons of the ganglion cells exit the retina as the optic nerve in the area known as the optic disk or "blind spot" because of the absence of any photoreceptors.

The optic disk consists of very distensible tissue and can expand well beyond its normal 1.5 mm diameter if capillary pressure is increased. The optic disk is lighter in color than the other parts of the retina and has a characteristic "physiologic cup" at its center, which occupies nearly one third of the disk.

Inner Structure of the Globe

There are two main cavities within the eyeball: the anterior which is further subdivided into an anterior and posterior chamber by the iris, and the posterior cavity. The anterior is filled with aqueous humor, the fluid responsible for maintaining intraocular pressure. Aqueous humor is secreted by the choroid plexuses of the ciliary processes into the posterior chamber at the rate of 2 to 5 mm^3/minute. It then flows through the pupil into the anterior chamber through the trabecular meshwork and ultimately to the canal of Schlemm, a venous sinus found at the junction of the sclera and the cornea, from which it drains into the blood (Fig. 39–4). An automatic feedback regulatory system works to maintain average normal intraocular pressure at approximately 16 mm Hg, with a range of 12 to 20 mm Hg.

The posterior cavity, between the lens and the retina, is filled with vitreous humor. This is a relatively stable gelatinous mass that allows substances to diffuse through it but has little flow of fluid. The mass of the vitreous-filled posterior chamber gives support to the posterior cavity and keeps the retina in place.

The crystalline lens that separates the anterior and posterior cavities is a transparent, colorless, biconvex structure. It is enclosed in a clear capsule and held in place by the suspensory ligaments. The lens refracts or bends light rays entering the eye so that they converge on the retina to form images. In a process called accommodation, the lens changes its shape and hence its refractive ability to adjust for vision at varying distances.

Normal Vision and the Visual Pathways

Light rays from objects in the visual field entering the eye are refracted by the cornea, the aqueous

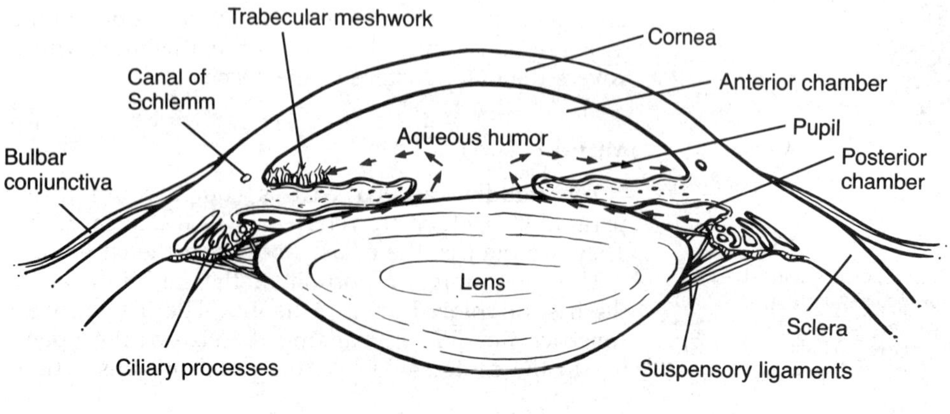

Figure 39–4.

Circulation of aqueous humor. Produced by the epithelial cells of the ciliary processes, it enters the posterior chamber, flows through the pupil, fills the anterior chamber, and flows peripherally through the trabecular meshwork into the canal of Schlemm and ultimately into the venous system.

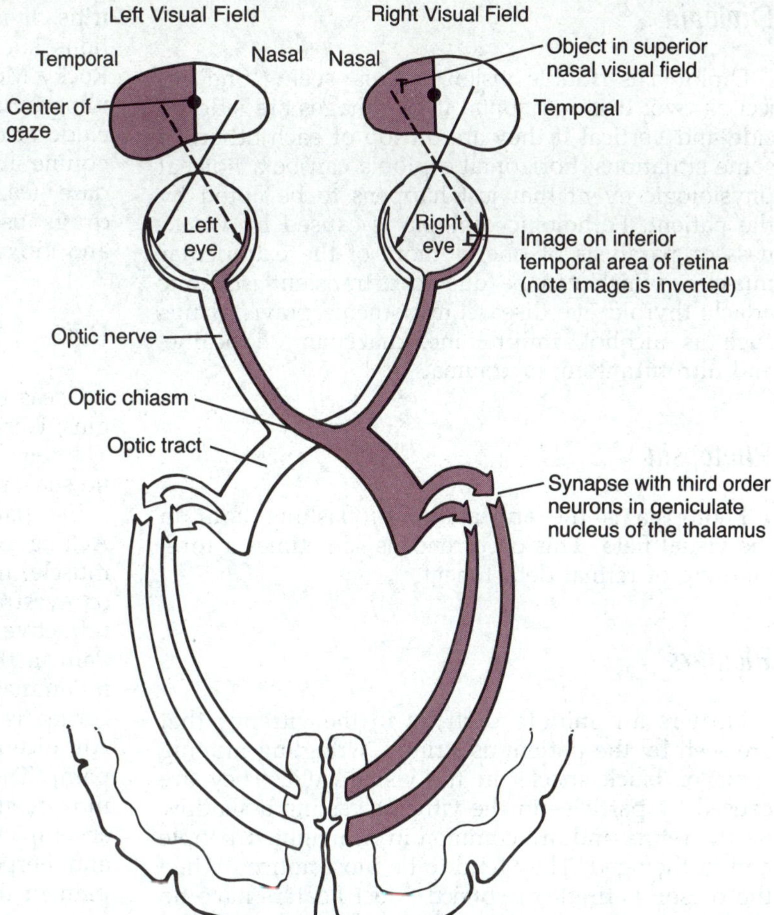

Figure 39–5. Visual pathways.

humor, the lens, and the vitreous humor so that they fall directly on the retina and produce a clear image. Light rays from objects in the nasal half of the visual field of each eye fall on the temporal half of the retina and vice versa. Similarly, light rays from objects in the superior portion of the visual field fall on the inferior portion of the retina. The result is a retinal image that is upside down and reversed right to left.

Stimulation of the retina by light rays initiates the breakdown of photopigments in the photoreceptor neurons and leads to the development of generator potentials and ultimately nervous impulses. These nervous impulses travel along the axons of the ganglion cells while maintaining their spatial relationships to one another and come together to exit the eye as the optic nerve. At the optic chiasm, nerve fibers from the nasal or medial portion of the retina cross to the opposite side. The fibers then continue with the uncrossed temporal fibers as the right or left optic tract to the geniculate nucleus of the thalamus. Here they synapse with third order neurons, which conduct the impulses to the visual area of the right and left occipital lobe, respectively (Fig. 39–5). Thus, the left optic tract receives impulses only from the left side of the retina, and the right optic tract, fibers from the right side of the retina. As a result, visual stimuli from the left side of the visual fields are interpreted in the right occipital lobe, and stimuli from the right side of the visual fields by the left occipital lobe.

Clinical Manifestations of Eye Dysfunction

Blurred Vision

Vision is blurred or misty when there is a lack of sharpness or detail in the visual image. The most common cause of gradual blurring is a refractive error that prevents light rays from objects in the visual field from converging directly on the retina. Other problems originating in the eye that can cause blurred vision are tear film abnormalities, foreign bodies, inflammation of ocular structures, cataract (opacity of the lens), and glaucoma (disease characterized by increased intraocular pressure that results in optic nerve atrophy and blindness). Systemic diseases that can cause blurred vision include diabetes mellitus, hypertension, and kidney diseases. It can also be caused by tobacco and drugs such as alphablockers, phenothiazines, and sulfonamides.

Diplopia

Diplopia is double vision, that is, seeing one object as two. It is horizontal if the images are side by side and vertical if they are on top of each other. In some situations, horizontal diplopia can be a normal physiologic event that just happens to be noted by the patient. Pathologic diplopia is caused by weakness or paralysis of one or more of the extraocular muscles, which can be due to a transient ischemic attack, thyroid eye disease, myasthenia gravis, drugs such as alcohol, imipramine, diazepam, lidocaine, and nitrofurantoin, or trauma.

Photopsia

Photopsia is the appearance of flashing light in the visual field. This occurrence is sometimes a forewarning of retinal detachment.

Floaters

Floaters are minute particles in the vitreous that are seen by the patient as stringy, wriggling moving spots or black specks in the visual field. They are caused by particles in the vitreous casting a shadow on the retina and are common in nearsighted people and in the aged. They tend to be most noticed when the person is tired or worried. Most floaters have no clinical significance, although the presence of many floaters can be a symptom of retinal detachment.

Scotomata

Scotomata are absolute or fixed, nonmoving blind spots in the visual field. They are suggestive of retinal or neurologic lesions. They may also occur as dose-dependent reactions to drugs such as isoniazid, streptomycin, and sulfonamides.

Photophobia

Photophobia is an unusual intolerance to light, which may or may not reflect a pathologic state. It is different from photosensitivity, which is an increased reactivity of the skin and other tissues to ultraviolet light.

The causes of photophobia are varied. It occurs in albino individuals because the choroid is not sufficiently protected from light as a result of a lack of pigment and in individuals whose occupations involve exposure to constant bright sunlight, snow dazzle, constant darkness, furnace heat, or fine, close work. It also occurs with disorders of the anterior segment structures such as acute conjunctivitis, presence of foreign bodies (including contact lenses) on the cornea, keratitis, corneal abrasion, and acute iritis. It is a primary symptom of nonocular conditions such as migraine headaches, meningitis, and Rocky Mountain spotted fever and also occurs as an idiosyncratic effect of some drugs. These drugs include atropine and other cholinergic blockers, chloroquine and other antimalarial drugs, monamine oxidase (MAO) inhibitors, rabies vaccines, and the drugs used in ocular herpes simplex—vidarabine and idoxuridine.

Pain

Areas of the eye sensitive to pain are the lid margins, lacrimal apparatus, cornea, and the uveal tract. The lens and retina are pain-free because they have no sensory innervation.

Eye pain takes many forms and has many causes. Aching of the eyes is associated with fatigue and muscle imbalance. A specific example is asthenopia, or eyestrain, which is pain due to an uncorrected refractive error after long, intensive use of the eyes. Pain in the lid margins is caused by stretching and inflammation and is usually mild to moderate. The cornea is richly supplied with sensory nerve fibers. An ulceration causes stabbing moderate to severe pain. The pain is localized and aggravated by movement of the eye. Moderate to severe pain also accompanies contact with chemical irritants, uveitis, and herpes zoster infections. Severe, deep pressure pain in the eye or eyebrow area is characteristic of increased intraocular pressure.

Loss of Vision

Loss of the ability to see may be gradual or sudden in onset, permanent or temporary, and may involve all or part of the visual field (Table 39–1). Loss of vision may result directly from ocular or orbit dysfunction, from neurologic or systemic disorders, from trauma, or from drugs.

Sudden vision loss is associated with retinal detachment, vitreous hemorrhage, and occlusion of the central retinal artery or vein. Slow central loss is associated with nuclear cataract and macular degeneration; slow peripheral loss is characteristic of open-angle glaucoma.

Assessment of the Eye

Patient History

Begin the history by asking the patient for general information about eye status. Ask questions such as the following:

How is your vision?
When were your eyes last examined?

Table 39–1. VISUAL FIELD DEFECTS

Terminology:
Anopia (anopsia)—Absence of vision
Hemianopia—Blindness in half the visual field in one or both eyes
Homonymous—Referring to the same sides (right or left) of the visual field
Quadrantic—Referring to one quadrant of the visual field

VISUAL DEFECT	DESCRIPTION OF THE DEFECT	ILLUSTRATION
Left anopia	Total blindness on the left side	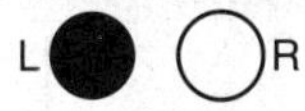
Binasal hemianopia	Blindness on the nasal side of both visual fields	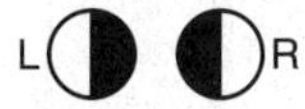
Bitemporal hemianopia	Blindness on the temporal side of both visual fields	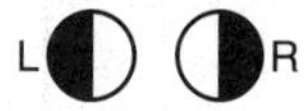
Right homonymous hemianopia	Blindness in the right side of each visual field	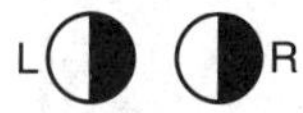
Altitudinal hemianopia	Blindness in the upper or lower half of each visual field	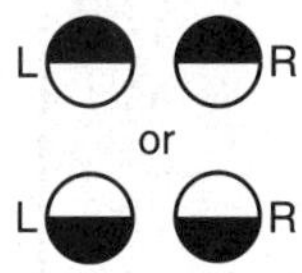
Homonymous left lower quadrantic hemianopia	Blindness in the lower left quadrant of each visual field	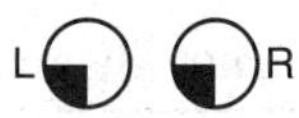

Do you wear eyeglasses or contact lenses? If yes, for what reason—nearsightedness, farsightedness, other? For how long have you worn glasses? When was your lens prescription last changed?
Have you noted any changes in vision—double vision, blurriness, spots before the eyes?
Have you noted any other eye symptoms such as redness, soreness, burning, swelling of the lids or around the eye, itching, excessive tearing, excessive dryness, or discharge or "sleep" from the eye?

Obtain additional clarifying information about any reported changes in vision or other symptoms. Determine time and speed of onset, whether both eyes were affected equally, relationship of the problem to close work or to distance vision, any identifiable precipitating circumstances, any associated systemic symptoms, any treatment instituted, and the response to treatment. If the patient reports spots before the eyes, ask whether they are fixed or moving. If blurred vision or loss of vision is reported, determine whether the entire visual field is involved or whether a particular central or peripheral area is involved.

Ask the patient about any previous eye disorders, noting type, date of occurrence, and treatment. After this, obtain a general medical history, giving particular attention to known allergies, chronic systemic diseases such as diabetes and hypertension, which can affect the eye, and use of medication. Specifically ask about the presence of cardiac or pulmonary diseases because certain ophthalmic medications have cardiac and respiratory side effects. Inquire about any family history of eye disorders, especially myopia, strabismus, glaucoma, and blindness.

Explore occupational risks by asking about the type of work normally done, the type of lighting used, and any exposure to industrial hazards. Question the patient about recreational activities, because fast-moving racquetballs and tennis balls are potential sources of eye trauma.

Physical Examination

VISUAL ACUITY

Visual acuity refers to the sharpness or distinctness of images seen by the eye. Because acuity is primarily a function of the cones, which are concentrated in the central area of the retina, tests of visual acuity are basically tests of central vision. These tests compare what a patient can see at a specified distance with what persons with normal eyes have been found to see at the same distance.

Tests of visual acuity typically use a Snellen chart, which is placed at eye level 20 feet (6 meters) in front of the patient. As shown in Figure 39–6, this chart consists of letters in lines that are printed in

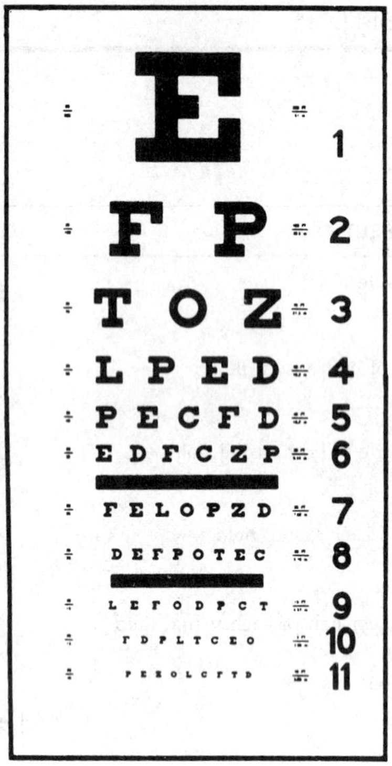

Figure 39–6.

Snellen chart. (From Black JM, Matassarin-Jacobs E. Luckmann and Sorensen's Medical-Surgical Nursing: A psychophysiologic approach. 4th ed. Philadelphia: WB Saunders, 1993, p. 839.)

progressively smaller type from the top to the bottom of the chart. Alongside each line, the distance in feet from which persons with normal vision can read the line is noted.

When testing distance vision, position the patient 20 feet from the chart and request him or her to cover the left eye and then read the smallest line of print possible. Record visual acuity as a ratio in which the top number is the distance the patient is from the chart (in this case 20 feet) and the bottom is the distance at which the normal eye can read the smallest line of print that the patient can read with at least half of the letters correct. The acuity is expressed as a number that is found alongside the smallest line of print the patient can read; add to this a minus sign and the number of letters in the line that were missed by the patient. Thus, visual acuity of 20/60 −2 means that the patient can read at 20 feet with errors on two letters what a person with normal vision can read at 60 feet from the chart. Ask the patient to cover the right eye and repeat the process.

If the patient wears corrective lenses, test acuity first without the lenses and note "sc" next to the result. Repeat the test with corrective lenses, and record "cc" next to the result. Normal acuity for distance vision is 20/20. Best corrected visual acuity of less than 20/200 in either eye or a visual field of less than 20 degrees is defined as legal blindness.

Use an eye chart with rows of numbers or E's pointing in varying directions for patients who are unable to identify letters.

If the patient is unable to see any letters, check the patient's ability with each eye to count the number of fingers held up by the examiner. This test is called counting fingers. Document the patient's performance on this test as "Counts fingers at ____ feet." For a patient to be classified as having counting-fingers acuity, he or she must have identified 50% or more finger presentations correctly.

Test patients who fail a count fingers test for ability to perceive hand motion. Ask the patient to cover the left eye, then wave your hand in one direction (up-down or left-right). Classify the patient as having hand-motion acuity if he or she correctly determines the direction of movement in 50% or more of the presentations. Document the results as "Hand motion at ____ feet."

If a patient fails the hand motion test, proceed to test for light perception. Turn off all room lights. Ask the patient to cover the left eye. Direct a bright light into the exposed right eye at random intervals, turning the light off in between. Ask the patient to report when light is seen. Classify the patient as having light-perception acuity if the patient correctly identifies 50% of the presentations. Repeat for the other eye.

Near-vision acuity is tested if the patient is older than 40 or complains of difficulty with reading or the like. A Jaeger chart, which consists of a series of letters or numbers, is used. It is held 14 inches in front of the face, and the patient is asked to read the smallest characters possible, using reading glasses if worn. Vision is recorded as J1 through J12, with J1, or the ability to read the smallest characters, being normal.

In situations in which eye charts cannot be used, a working estimate of the patient's vision can be obtained using any printed material.

OUTER EYE STRUCTURES

Begin examination of the outer structures of the eye by noting the position of the eyelids in relationship to the globes, keeping in mind that normally no sclera is visible above the iris. Observe the lids for abnormalities such as ptosis (drooping), retraction, edema, erythema, incomplete closure, and the presence of any lesions. Observe the condition and direction of the lashes, being certain to note whether they are crusted or brushing the globe. If any lesions are present, note location, size, shape, and characteristics.

Inspect the conjunctiva and sclera. Do this by separating the lids between the index finger and the thumb and asking the patient to look up, down, and to each side (Fig. 39–7*A*). Note any deviation from the normal smooth white of the sclera (the sclera of black persons may normally have a slight yellow cast) as well as the presence of bulging, inflammation, or nodules. Also note the vascular pattern. In-

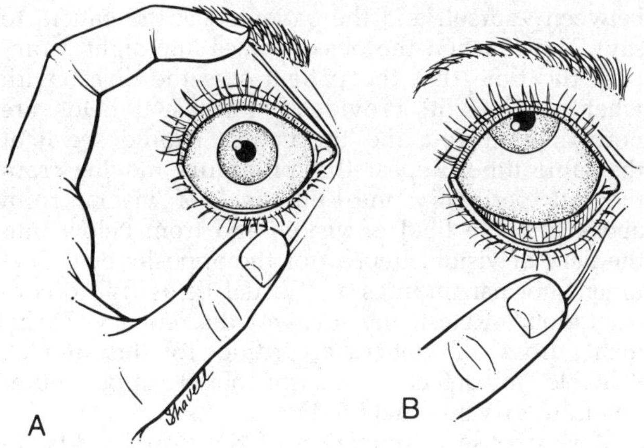

Figure 39–7.

A, Examination of the sclera. *B*, Examination of the palpebral conjunctiva of the lower lid.

spect the palpebral conjunctiva of the lower eyelid, which is normally a pale, glistening pink, by asking the patient to look up and gently using the thumb to evert the lid (Fig. 39–7*B*).

Check the clarity of the cornea. Shine a light obliquely onto each eye and observe for cloudiness and opacities.

Inspect each iris. Note shape, color, clarity, and any unusual markings. Be certain to compare the color of the two because although variation is normal in a small segment of the population, it can also indicate blood in the anterior chamber (hyphema), uveal infection, tumor, or a retained foreign body.

Observe the size and shape of each pupil. Note any abnormal dilation or constriction, as well as any deviation from the normal round, uniform shape (Table 39–2). Test the pupillary response to light and accommodation. To test the reaction to light, ask the patient to look into the distance, and then moving from the side to the center, shine a bright light on the pupil of each eye in turn. Observe for the direct response, that is, pupillary constriction in the eye into which the light was shone. Also observe for the consensual response, which is constriction of the pupil of the opposite eye. Repeat for the other eye. Compare the responses in both eyes in terms of amount and speed of constriction and subsequent dilation.

Test for accommodation or the "near reaction" by holding your finger or similar object 4 to 6 inches (10 to 15 cm) from the patient's nose. Ask the patient to look at a distant object behind you and then quickly look at the finger. Observe for pupillary constriction and convergence (the medial movement of both eyes), which normally occur when looking at something near.

Record normal pupillary findings as PERRLA, which stands for "pupils equal, round, reactive to light and accommodation."

Table 39–2. VARIATIONS IN THE SIZE AND SHAPE OF THE PUPIL

APPEARANCE OF THE PUPIL		CAUSES
Dilated pupil	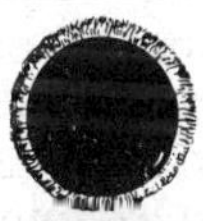	Dim light, myopia, anticholinergic drugs, eye injury
Constricted pupil	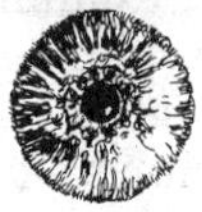	Bright light; iritis; use of pilocarpine, morphine, or heroin
Irregularly shaped pupils		Iritis, injury, central nervous system syphilis, eye surgery
Keyhole pupil	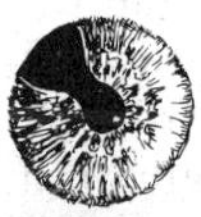	Sector iridectomy
D-shaped pupil	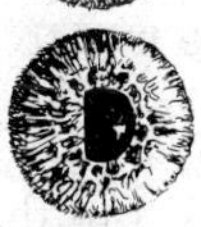	Tear at the base of the iris
Cloverleaf pupil	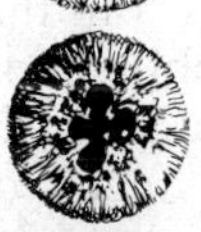	Adhesion of the iris to the lens
Argyll Robertson pupil (small, irregular, bilateral; react to accommodation but not to light)	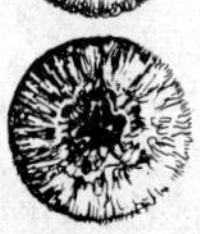	Central nervous system syphilis, autonomic nervous system damage from diabetes mellitus

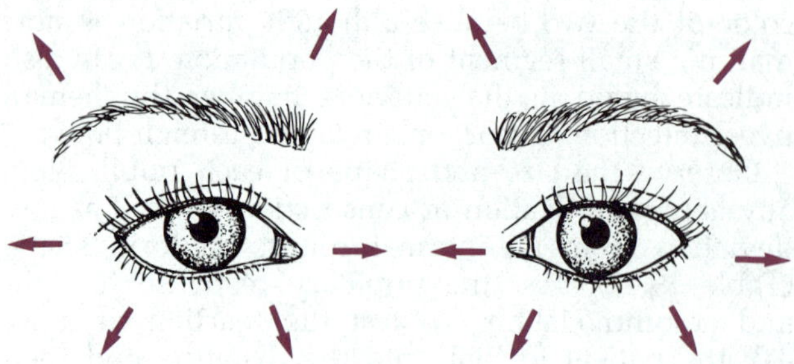

Figure 39–8.

Cardinal fields of gaze.

EXTRAOCULAR MUSCLES

The six extraocular eye muscles function to produce a parallel gaze and coordinated movement of the two eyes. Check for parallel gaze by shining a light into the patient's eyes while instructing the patient to look at the light source. Note the location of the light reflection on the corneas. The reflections should be on or just medial to the center of the pupil if the eyes are in parallel alignment.

Assess movement of the eyes by having the patient follow a finger as it is moved through the six cardinal positions of gaze (Fig. 39–8). Instruct the patient to hold the head still and follow the finger with the eyes. Hold the finger approximately 12 inches in front of the patient, and slowly move it through the fields, first horizontally, then diagonally through the oblique fields, and finally straight up and down.

Throughout the test, observe for parallel eye movement. As the gaze moves from up to down, observe the iris, which should be slightly overlapped by the upper eyelid at all times. Observe also for nystagmus (involuntary, rhythmic, or twitching eye movement), which may occur normally at the end point of any gaze but is otherwise abnormal.

To complete examination of the extraocular muscles, ask the patient to follow your finger as it is moved in toward the bridge of the nose. Observe for convergence of the eyes, which is normally sustained to within 5 to 8 cm.

VISUAL FIELDS

The most elementary form of visual field testing is the confrontation test. This is a simple test that provides a rough measure of peripheral vision. Begin by positioning yourself so that your face is level with and in front of the patient's face. Instruct the patient to cover the right eye and with the left eye look directly into your right eye. Close or cover your left eye. This position enables you and the patient to have approximately the same visual field. Slowly bring a raised finger or other small object from the periphery of the right side into the field of vision. Be certain to hold it at arm's length midway between yourself and the patient. Ask the patient to say "Now" when the object comes into sight. Compare the time that the patient sees the object with when you see it. Provided your visual fields are normal, both you and the patient should see it at the same time. Repeat this procedure moving from the left periphery into the field of vision, from above into the field of vision, and from below into the field of vision. Repeat for the opposite eye. Document normal findings as "Visual fields full to confrontation." Retest any areas of discrepancy. Document areas of deficit according to this model: "Unable to detect ____ cm object upper outer quadrant of visual field O.D."

More precise examination of the visual fields requires sophisticated testing of central and peripheral vision such as tangent screen and perimeter testing.

OCULAR FUNDUS

The ocular fundus is composed of the retina, optic disk, macula, and retinal vessels. It can be visualized with an ophthalmoscope, an instrument containing a light source, viewing aperture, and a series of lenses attached to a disk that can be rotated with the index finger without interrupting the examination. These lenses vary in their ability to converge or diverge light. The lens of zero diopters is clear glass and does not affect the light rays passing through it. Plus diopter lenses, indicated on the ophthalmoscope by black numbers, have a progressively shorter focus and are needed to examine farsighted eyes. Negative diopter lenses, indicated by red numbers, have a progressively longer focus and are used for nearsighted eyes unless corrective contact lenses are in place. The lens needed for an examination depends on the type and severity of refractive error in both the eye of the patient and the eye of the examiner.

Ophthalmoscopy is done in a darkened room. To examine the right eye of the patient, hold the ophthalmoscope set at zero diopters in your right hand and use your right eye. Repeat this procedure to examine the patient's left eye, remembering to use your left eye.

Stand approximately 15 inches away and slightly to the side of the patient's line of vision. Place the ophthalmoscope firmly under the medial aspect of your orbit, and shine the light beam on the pupil of the eye to be examined. Note the appearance of the red reflex, which is an orange-red glow in the pupil, and observe for any opacities interrupting it. Focusing on the red reflex, move your head and the ophthalmoscope forward as a unit until it is almost touching the patient's eyelashes. Rotate the lens disk to focus on the retina, which should now be in view.

Systematically inspect the retina for hemorrhage, exudate, or areas of altered color. Begin by identifying the optic disk, which appears as a yellow-orange to creamy pink round or oval area upon which the

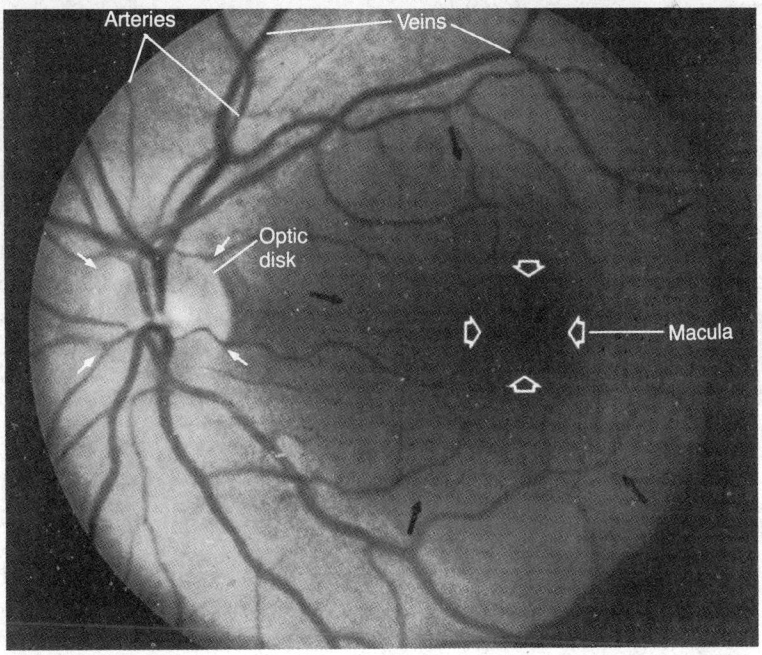

Figure 39–9.

View of the ocular fundus, showing the optic disk, arteries, and veins (slightly darker and wider than the arteries), which converge at the optic disk, and the macula, the area of central vision. (From Brown MM. Retinal vascular disorders: Nursing and medical implications. Nurs Clin North Am 1981; 16(3):417.)

blood vessels of the retina converge. If it is not immediately evident, locate it by following a blood vessel in the direction in which it enlarges and has branches joining it. When the disk is located, note size, shape, and the clarity of its margins, keeping in mind that the nasal side is sometimes blurred (Fig. 39–9). Also note its color, because dark congestion is associated with eye strain, astigmatism, and papillitis, and a pale or white disk may reflect glaucoma or optic atrophy. Examine the physiologic cup, noting its normal central depression and the emerging retinal vessels. Identify both the arterioles, which are normally light red and have a bright reflection, and the veins, which are dark red, without reflection. Veins are one quarter to one third larger in diameter than the arterioles. Observe for abnormal branching, fullness, contour, and integrity. Proceed to examine the periphery of the retina, and end with examination of the macula, which is sensitive to light. Locate the macula, which is an avascular area without margins temporal to the optic disk, by asking the patient to look directly at the light.

Describe the position of any retinal lesions by referring to location on an imaginary clock face and distance from the optic disk measured in disk diameters (Fig. 39–10).

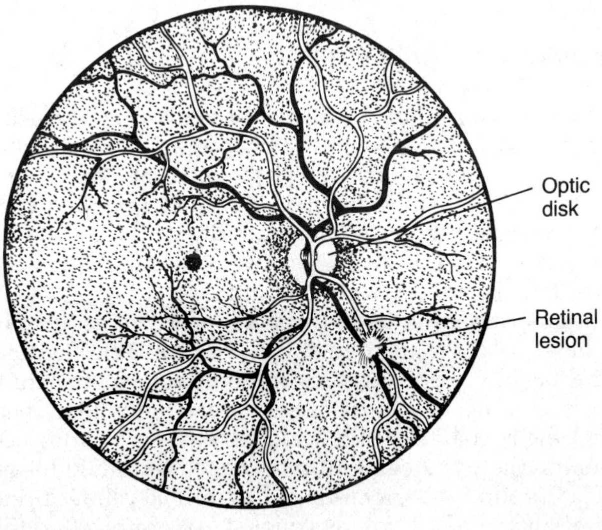

Figure 39–10.

The white retinal lesion pictured here would be described as at 5 o'clock, 1 disk diameter from the disk, and less than $\frac{1}{4}$ disk diameter in size.

Diagnostic Procedures

Measurement of Intraocular Pressure

Tonometry is the measurement of intraocular pressure based on the amount of corneal indentation

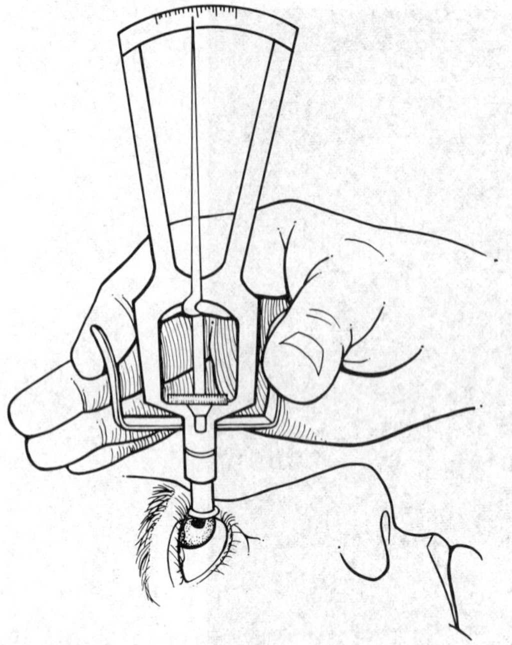

Figure 39–11.

Measurement of intraocular pressure with a Schiøtz tonometer.

produced by a given weight or force. The instrument used for this measurement is the tonometer. Normal intraocular pressure is 10 to 21 mm Hg.

Routine testing is commonly done with a noncontact tonometer. A puff of air is directed at the patient's cornea and provides a digital readout of intraocular pressure based on the resultant deflection of the cornea. This method is fast, simple, and nonpainful. The patient rests the chin on the chin support and looks straight ahead as an air puff is directed at each eye in turn. A loud "whoosh" is heard as each air puff is released, and a slight momentary pressure on the eye is felt.

Another inexpensive but more reliable type of indentation tonometry is done with the Schiøtz tonometer (Fig. 39–11). With the patient lying down, anesthetic drops are instilled in the eyes. The foot of the tonometer is then placed on the cornea, and the amount of indentation caused by the weight of the instrument is indicated on the tonometer scale. The scale reading and weight used are then correlated on a chart to determine actual intraocular pressure.

The most accurate measurement of intraocular pressure is by applanation tonometry. In this procedure, the cornea is anesthetized with a fluorescein anesthetic solution, and then, with the patient sitting at a slit lamp, the Goldmann or applanation tonometer is brought into contact with the cornea.

Slit-Lamp Examination

A slit-lamp biomicroscope is an instrument in which a high-intensity beam of light is projected through a narrow slit to allow examination of a cross section of the illuminated segment of the eye with a magnifying lens. The examination is performed in a darkened room and can be used to inspect the conjunctiva, lens, vitreous humor, iris, and cornea.

Gonioscopy

Gonioscopy is an examination of the angle of the anterior chamber of the eye. It is done by placing a special contact lens similar to a jeweler's loupe over the anesthetized cornea. It is used to determine whether the iridocorneal angle is open or closed in patients with known or suspected glaucoma.

Topical Fluorescein Staining

Fluorescein dye is used to detect foreign bodies as well as corneal ulcers or abrasions. The dye is instilled into the conjunctival sac in drop form or by impregnated strips and is spread over the anterior surface of the eye by blinking. The result is that corneal abrasions appear green, foreign bodies have a green ring around them, and conjunctival ulcers appear yellow-orange.

There are few adverse effects with topical administration. Care must be taken, however, to avoid contact with soft contact lenses because they can be stained by the dye. When using fluorescein from a multidose bottle, take extreme care to avoid contaminating the dropper tip. Once the bottle is contaminated, microorganisms can multiply and be transmitted from one patient to another. Cases of *Pseudomonas* corneal ulcers have been reported following use of contaminated solutions of fluorescein (Vaughan et al, 1992).

Fluorescein Angiography

Fluorescein angiography is a contrast study used in conjunction with fundus photography to evaluate the vessels and structures of the internal eye.

Procedure. The patient is screened for allergy to the contrast medium, and the pupil of the eye being tested is dilated. A 5% or 10% sodium fluorescein solution is injected into the antecubital vein, and a fundus camera is used to photograph the sequential phases of retinal circulation (Fig. 39–12). Because the healthy vessel wall is impermeable to the fluorescein dye, diseased vessels are readily identified by their characteristic leakage pattern. Within 24 hours, the dye begins to be excreted by the kidneys. This produces a green-tinged or bright yellow urine that may persist for as long as 48 hours after the procedure. In light-skinned persons, skin discoloration may also occur for 6 to 12 hours.

Complications. Some patients experience a sensation of heat and flushing immediately after injection of the dye. Others develop nausea, vomiting, faint-

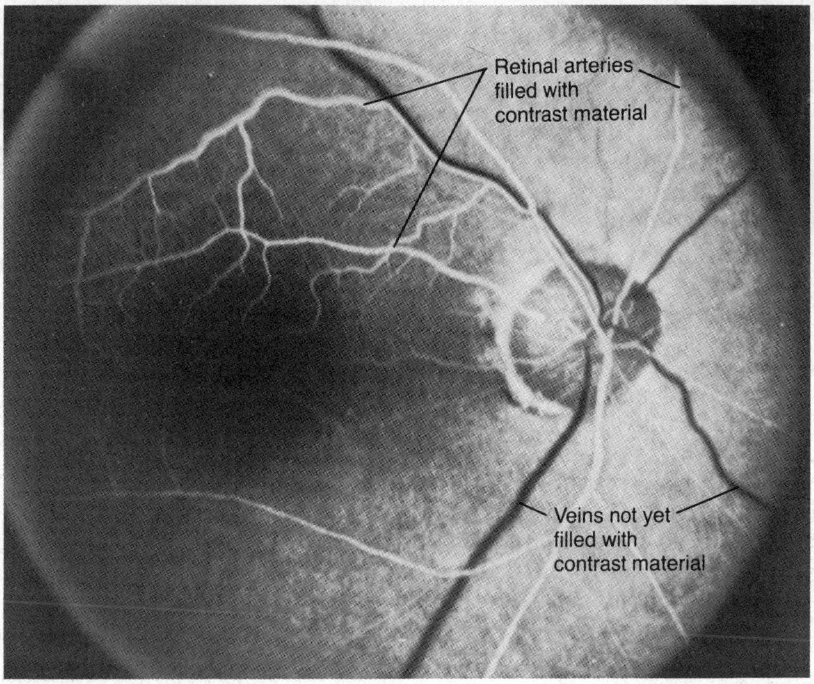

Figure 39–12.

Retinal circulation as seen with fluorescein angiography. Arteries fill with contrast material first, veins several seconds later. (From Brown MM. Retinal vascular disorders: Nursing and medical implications. Nurs Clin North Am 1981; 16(3):419.)

ing, or minor allergic reactions. In rare cases, severe reactions such as bronchospasm, anaphylaxis, convulsions, or cardiac arrest can occur (Bartlett et al, 1992). Therefore, personnel involved in caring for patients having fluorescein angiography testing must have access to emergency equipment and be knowledgeable in its use.

Ultrasonography

Ocular ultrasonography uses high-frequency sound waves to detect tumors and other abnormalities not visible with direct assessment. It is particularly useful in cases of retinal disorders, tumors, vitreous hemorrhage, and dense cataracts.

Procedure. A small transducer is placed in contact with the eye to generate sound waves. The waves are spread throughout the eye as vibrations and are ultimately recorded on a screen. The eye being tested remains open throughout the procedure, and the patient may be asked to change his or her gaze.

Computed Tomography

The computed tomographic (CT) scan of the ocular orbit provides a three-dimensional view of the size, position, and relationships of ocular and adjacent structures. The scan, which may be done with or without contrast dye, allows accurate diagnosis of orbit pathology, including lesions, fractures, and visual problems.

The only potential complications are allergic responses to the contrast medium if used.

Medical Management

Pharmacologic Therapy

The majority of drugs used to treat disorders of the eye are administered topically either in solution or in ointment form. Some are used solely for an external effect, whereas others must penetrate the eye to be effective. Many different classes of drugs are used in ophthalmic treatment because of the variety of disease processes that can affect the eye. These drug classes include anesthetics, anti-infectives, anti-inflammatory agents, autonomic drugs, carbonic anhydrase inhibitors, lubricants, and osmotic agents.

ANESTHETICS

The eye, especially the cornea and the conjunctiva, is highly sensitive to pain, which is mediated via the ophthalmic nerve, a branch of the trigeminal nerve (cranial nerve V). Thus, anesthetics are used to allow complete eye examination, to measure intraocular pressure by other than a noncontact approach, to remove foreign bodies, and to prevent pain during treatments or surgical procedures.

Topical preparations, which produce anesthesia in about 30 seconds, can cause transient stinging, burning, redness, and photophobia. They also interfere with epithelial healing and therefore are not applied repeatedly for painful irritations. Prolonged use can result in keratitis and corneal opacity.

ANTI-INFECTIVES

Anti-infective drugs used in the treatment of eye infections include antibacterial, antiviral, and antifungal agents. They may be given systemically, injected beneath the conjunctiva, injected into the vitreous, or applied topically as drops or ointment. The most commonly used topical antibacterial drugs are the sulfonamides and the antibiotics gentamicin and tobramycin. Combination drugs involving several antibiotics such as Polytrim, which is a combination of trimethoprim sulfate and polymyxin B sulfate, and antibiotics and steroids such as Pred G, which is a combination of prednisolone acetate and gentamicin, are commonly used.

Frequent or prolonged use of the antibiotics is contraindicated because of the risk of hypersensitivity reactions, which include stinging, burning, itching, urticaria, edema, and dermatitis, as well as the risk of secondary infection.

Antiviral agents are used to treat herpes simplex keratoconjunctivitis. They include idoxuridine, vidarabine, and trifluridine, and acyclovir (Bartlett et al, 1992).

ANTI-INFLAMMATORY AGENTS

The most effective anti-inflammatory drugs are the corticosteroids, which suppress hyperemia, photophobia, and pain as well as the cellular effects of inflammation. They are used to treat inflammations due to irritation or allergy. These agents are not used to treat infections or abrasions because they inhibit normal defense mechanisms. Corticosteroids cause transient stinging or itching on instillation. They may also cause decreased visual acuity, visual field defects, cataracts, glaucoma, and optic nerve damage.

A relatively new nonsteroidal anti-inflammatory is flurbiprofen, which inhibits production of prostaglandins. It is given preoperatively to keep the pupil dilated during surgery. It is contraindicated for patients with herpes simplex keratitis and those with allergy to aspirin or other anti-inflammatory drugs. Other new nonsteroidals are diclofenac sodium (Voltaren) and ketorolac tromethamine (Toradol).

AUTONOMIC DRUGS

Large numbers of ophthalmic preparations fall into the category of autonomic drugs, that is, those that produce their effects by acting on the autonomic nervous system.

Autonomic drugs are classified into four major groups:

Sympathomimetic drugs—These drugs produce effects similar to those caused by activation of the sympathetic nervous system. Also called adrenergic agents, they are further subdivided into catecholamines and noncatecholamines.

Sympatholytic drugs—These drugs block function of the sympathetic nervous system. Also called adrenergic blocking agents, they are further subdivided according to where they block impulse transmission into alpha-blockers, beta-blockers, and autonomic ganglionic blockers. Beta-blocking agents must be used with caution in patients with a history of cardiac or pulmonary disease.

Parasympathomimetic drugs—These drugs produce effects similar to those caused by activation of the parasympathetic nervous system. Also called cholinergic agents, they are further subdivided into direct-acting cholinergics, or cholinergic agonists, and anticholinesterase agents.

Parasympatholytic drugs—These drugs block function of the parasympathetic nervous system. They are also called cholinergic blocking agents.

In general, sympathomimetic (adrenergic) drugs and parasympatholytic (cholinergic blocking) drugs produce similar effects. Parasympathomimetic (cholinergic) and sympatholytic (adrenergic blocking) drugs produce similar effects.

In the eye, sympathetic stimulation causes pupil dilation, or mydriasis, lessens tone in the ciliary muscle, and increases intraocular tension. Parasympathetic stimulation causes pupillary constriction, or miosis, increases tone in the ciliary muscle, and decreases intraocular pressure by increasing the outflow of aqueous humor.

Drugs that dilate the pupil are called mydriatics (Pharmacology Box 39-1), and those that constrict the pupil are miotics (Pharmacology Box 39-2). Drugs that both paralyze the ciliary muscle and dilate the pupil are cycloplegic mydriatics.

CARBONIC ANHYDRASE INHIBITORS

Carbonic anhydrase inhibitors lower intraocular pressure by causing a decrease in the amount of aqueous humor as a result of their inhibition of the production of bicarbonate by the ciliary processes. They are used in the management of acute attacks of angle-closure glaucoma and as adjunctive treatment for chronic open-angle glaucoma. The side effects of these drugs are numerous and often severe. They include fever, skin eruptions, gastrointestinal symptoms, drowsiness, fatigue, malaise, depression, renal calculi, and aplastic anemia.

LUBRICANTS

Lubricants such as zinc sulfate, petrolatum, and artificial tears are used for the temporary relief of minor eye irritation. They are also used by contact

Pharmacology Box 39–1.
MYDRIATICS

Mydriatics:
Drugs that dilate the pupil. Two classes are sympathomimetics (adrenergics) and anticholinergics (cholinergic blocking agents), also called cycloplegics (drugs that paralyze the ciliary muscle).

Action:
Sympathomimetic mydriatics dilate the pupil by stimulating the radial muscle fibers of the iris. They also constrict ocular blood vessels, decrease the formation of aqueous humor, and increase its outflow.

Anticholinergic mydriatics dilate the pupil by paralyzing the circular muscles of the iris and prevent accommodation by paralysis of the ciliary body.

Uses:
Sympathomimetic mydriatics are used to dilate the pupil for examination of the fundus, control bleeding or dilate the pupil for surgery, maintain postoperative mydriasis, shrink blood vessels and lessen injection in conjunctivitis and uveitis, and decrease congestion and irritation due to hay fever, colds, eye strain, and other irritants.

Anticholinergic mydriatics are used for accurate measurement of refractive error and in the treatment of inflammatory conditions of the uvea.

Side Effects:
Stinging upon instillation, photophobia, local irritant or allergic reactions. Sympathomimetics can also cause headache, rebound miosis, and with long use, pigmentation of the lids, conjunctiva, or cornea. Rare systemic reactions include hypertension, tachycardia, dysrhythmias, anxiety, sweating, and trembling. Anticholinergics can also cause increased intraocular pressure and systemic effects, including dry mouth and skin, flushing, headache, tachycardia, fever, abdominal distention, urinary retention, restlessness, ataxia, and confusion.

Interactions:
Only the sympathomimetic drug phenylephrine has significant interactions with other drugs. Phenylephrine increases the pressor effects of guanethidine and the monoamine oxidase inhibitors; levodopa decreases the mydriatic effect of phenylephrine.

Nursing Implications:
Instill the drops as described in Table 39–3. Instruct the patient to compress the area of the lacrimal sac for 1 minute after instillation to prevent systemic absorption. Explain to patients that the pupil will be large and the eye sensitive to light. Suggest the use of dark glasses, and tell them to stop the drug and call the health care provider if photophobia persists for longer than 12 hours.

When cycloplegic drugs are used, inform the patient that blurred vision is expected and that driving and use of machinery or household appliances such as meat slicers should be avoided. Tell the patient to discontinue use of the drug if eye pain occurs.

lens wearers, those with artificial eyes, and persons with dry eyes due to normal age-related decrease in tear production. They are available with and without preservatives.

OSMOTIC AGENTS

The osmotic agents glycerin, mannitol, isosorbide, and urea, which shift fluid from the anterior chamber to the plasma, are used in selected situations when intraocular pressure must be quickly reduced. Because they are potent diuretics with systemic effects, rapid changes in fluid and electrolyte balance can occur. Thus, patients with cardiac, renal, or hepatic disease must be closely monitored for congestive heart failure and pulmonary edema.

ADMINISTRATION OF OPHTHALMIC MEDICATIONS

Most ophthalmic drugs are topically administered in the form of drops or ointments. Although ointments are more stable than drops and provide longer contact with the eye, they cause blurred vi-

Pharmacology Box 39–2.

MIOTICS

Miotics:
Cholinergic drugs (direct-acting or anti-cholinesterase agents) that constrict the pupil.

Action:
Constrict the pupil by stimulating contraction of the sphincter muscle of the iris.

Uses:
Treat glaucoma by improving the outflow of aqueous humor from the anterior chamber and decreasing intraocular pressure. Manage accommodative esotropia (turning inward of the eye with accommodation).

Side Effects:
Blurred vision; photosensitivity; eye, brow, and lid pain; cataract formation. In blacks, reversible loss of eyelid skin color from hypersensitivity. Potential systemic effects include abdominal cramps, diarrhea, increased salivation, bronchial constriction, and pulmonary edema.

Interactions:
Virtually all miotics have significant interactions either with one another or with other drugs. Refer to the package insert or to a pharmacology text for interactions of any miotic before administering the drug or doing patient teaching.

Nursing Implications:
Instill the drops as described in Table 39–3. Instruct the patient to compress the area of the lacrimal sac for 1 minute after instillation to decrease the risk of systemic absorption. Tell the patient that blurred vision is expected, and warn against driving, using machines, and so on. Suggest instilling the medication at bedtime if possible to avoid difficulties with blurred vision. Suggest the use of dark glasses if the eyes are sensitive to light.

sion and are more likely to precipitate a hypersensitivity reaction. An alternative method of administration now in use for the administration of pilocarpine is a drug-diffusion system known as Ocusert. This system is approximately the size of a hard contact lens and is placed in the upper or lower cul-de-sac (Fig. 39–13). It consists of a central reservoir that releases drug through membranes at a constant, controlled rate. Advantages of this type of administration are that it provides slower release with better control of intraocular pressure, lowers the needed dosage, and lessens toxicity. Disadvantages are that it is more expensive, can cause conjunctival irritation, and may become dislodged during sleep.

Ophthalmic drops and ointments are instilled as outlined in Table 39–3.

Surgical Management

OVERVIEW OF OCULAR SURGERY

When the situation allows, eye surgery is preferably done under local anesthesia because the recovery time is faster and because any risk of postanesthesia vomiting is eliminated. Vomiting causes increased intraocular pressure, which can lead to bleeding and strain on sutures. The risk of accidental external trauma to the affected eye by a patient who becomes restless during recovery from general anesthesia is also eliminated.

Preoperative preparation includes instillation of antibiotic drops, usually beginning 24 hours before surgery. On arrival to the unit or preoperative holding area, mydriatic agents are administered at specified intervals to dilate the pupil. In many cases, a sedative or tranquilizing agent may be administered. If general anesthesia is to be used, atropine sulfate may also be given by the anesthesiologist. Other preparations may include hair shampoo the evening before surgery, NPO status from midnight before surgery, facial shave on the day of surgery for male patients, and insertion of an intravenous line or heparin lock.

Further preparation of the eye is carried out in the operating room. In the very rare cases in which the eyelashes are to be trimmed, the surgeon uses short, straight scissors with petrolatum on the blades to prevent the cut lashes from entering the eye. The eyelids, lid margins, eyebrows, and surrounding skin are then cleansed with an antimicrobial solution, and the eye is irrigated with normal saline.

At the end of the surgery, antibiotics are injected subconjunctivally, and an antibiotic-steroid ointment is instilled.

Postoperatively, the operated eye is usually covered with an eye patch on top of which a rigid eye shield may be placed to protect the eye from accidental trauma, particularly at night. Activities that increase intraocular pressure, such as bending over from the waist, lifting 25 lb or more, straining on trying to have a bowel movement, and coughing, are avoided. In rare cases, reading and watching television are prohibited to limit rapid eye movement. Patients are generally allowed to get up to go to the bathroom immediately on return from surgery and to take short walks accompanied by a nurse until their stable gait returns. Surgery usually is performed in a day surgery setting, where the patient is discharged several hours after the operation to recuperate at home. In selected cases, such as when surgery is being performed on the patient's only eye, overnight hospitalization may be suggested.

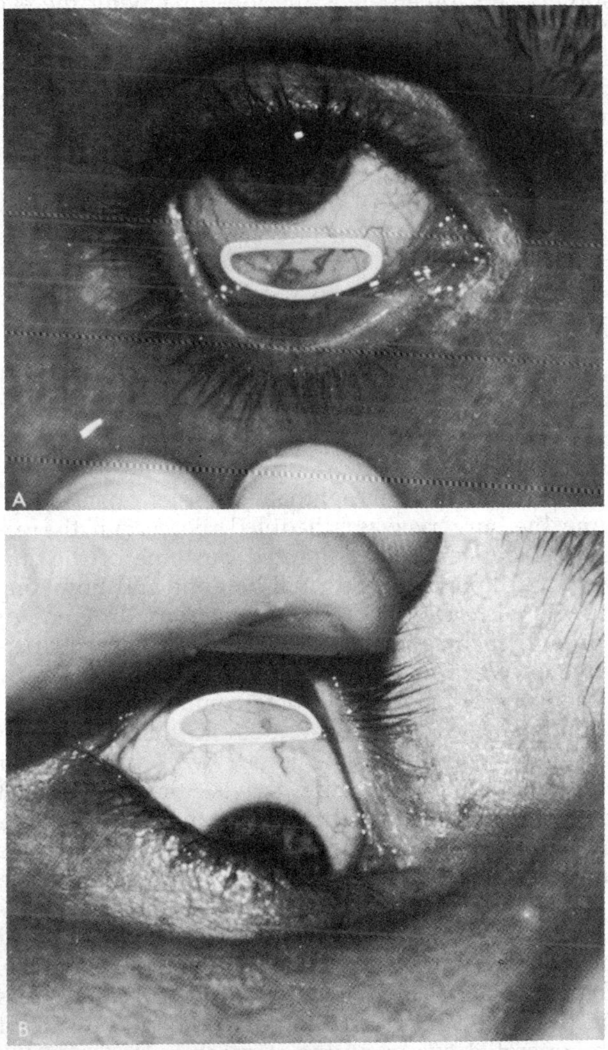

Figure 39–13.

Ocusert-Pilo. *A,* In the lower cul-de-sac. *B,* In the upper cul-de-sac. (From Jeglum EL. Ocular therapeutics. Nurs Clin North Am 1981; 16(3):456.)

Application of the Nursing Process to the Care of the Patient Having Ocular Surgery

PREOPERATIVE NURSING CARE

Assessment

Assess the patient's understanding of his or her eye disorder: what the surgery is designed to accomplish and what to expect before, during, and after surgery. Pay particular attention to understanding of the intraoperative experience if local anesthesia is to be used.

Assess the patient's reaction to the scheduled surgery. Because vision is so important to our appreciation of the world around us and to everyday function, reactions can vary from unrealistic expectations regarding return of normal vision to acute anxiety over possible loss of vision.

Assess the patient's current visual status to identify what safety precautions and personal assistance the patient needs. Separately assess functional vision in the eye not scheduled for surgery to determine postoperative needs because the operated eye is usually patched.

Review the patient's general health status. Obtain information about any chronic diseases and their management. If the patient will be spending time in the hospital or clinic, specifically determine whether the patient is on a special diet. Ask all patients what, if any, medications are routinely taken or used (including eye drops used for other conditions) and on what schedule. Inquire what, if any, treatments are routinely required. Be certain to determine whether the patient has hay fever or other allergies that can cause sneezing or coughing and therefore increase pressure within the eye, which can disrupt sutures or alignment of tissues.

Nursing Diagnoses and Planning

Nursing diagnoses and related expected patient outcomes most commonly applicable to patients scheduled for eye surgery include the following:

NDx: Anxiety related to the surgical experience and its uncertain visual outcome

Table 39–3. INSTILLATION OF OPHTHALMIC DROPS AND OINTMENTS

INSTILLATION OF OPHTHALMIC DROPS

1. *Wash hands* to reduce surface microorganisms.
2. *Explain the procedure* to the patient to decrease anxiety and promote cooperation.
3. *Put on gloves if there are secretions in the patient's eye(s)* to protect self from contamination.
4. *Check name, strength, and expiration date of medication* to ensure correct administration of medication free of chemical and physical changes due to age.
5. *Ask the patient to open the eyes, tilt the head backward, and look up* to position the head for instillation.
6. *Retract lower lid downward against the cheekbone* (Fig. 39–14) *or grasp skin of lower lid between thumb and index finger and pull forward* to create a pocket-shaped area for drug placement.
7. *Hold the medication bottle with the eyedropper tip down like a pencil* (see Fig. 39–14) to provide optimal control of the bottle.
8. *Place the wrist of the hand holding the bottle on the patient's cheek* to bring bottle close to the eye without touching the eye or eyelashes, which could contaminate the medication and could injure the eye.
9. *Squeeze the bottle gently to allow one drop to fall into the pocket between the lower lid and the globe.*
10. *Release the lower eyelid slowly* because quick release may cause medication to splash into the puncta and drain.
11. *Tell the patient to gently close the eyelid* to distribute the medication. *Warn the patient not to squeeze the eyelid shut,* because squeezing tends to force medication into the nasal lacrimal system, thus decreasing its absorption.
12. *Wait 5 minutes before instilling another drop* to promote maximum drug absorption.
13. *Wash hands.*
14. *Record.*

INSTILLATION OF OPHTHALMIC OINTMENTS

1–6. *Perform steps 1 through 6* as for Instillation of Ophthalmic Drops.
7. *Hold ointment tube like a pencil near BUT NOT TOUCHING the eye or eyelashes* to avoid contamination of the medication and injury to the eye.
8. *Squeeze a thin ribbon of ointment from the inner to the outer canthus along the lining of the sac.*
9. *Release the lower eyelid slowly* because quick release may remove ointment from the pocket.
10. *Ask the patient to gently close the eyes* to distribute the ointment.
11. *Advise the patient that the ointment may cause blurred vision,* which creates a potential for injury.
12. *Wash hands.*
13. *Record.*

Planning: Patient outcomes

1. Patient verbalizes concerns about the surgical experience and its outcomes.
2. Signs of excessive anxiety—inability to focus attention, frequent requests for repeated information, and crying—are absent.

NDx: Knowledge deficit: underlying disease process, perioperative experiences, and the possible effect of surgery on vision

Planning: Patient outcomes

1. Patient describes the relationship of the eye disorder and the surgical procedure accurately at a level appropriate to his or her background.
2. Patient describes usual perioperative routines related to the procedure to be done.
3. Patient states accurately the possible effect of the surgery on the underlying disease and on visual status.

NDx: High risk for injury related to impaired vision and an unfamiliar environment

Planning: Patient outcomes

1. Patient requests and accepts assistance with activities as needed.
2. Patient remains free of injury.

Nursing Interventions

NDx: Anxiety

Provide the opportunity for the patient to verbalize concerns and to ask questions. For some patients, the greatest source of anxiety is the outcome of the surgery. For others, it is the idea of having the eye operated on while awake or having a local anesthetic injected into the area of the eye. Many patients fear they will see the instruments coming toward them during surgery. Whatever the source, acknowledge the anxiety and provide reassuring but accurate information whenever possible. If a sedative or tranquilizer is ordered preoperatively, explain to the patient that medication will be given to relax him or her prior to surgery. If possible, arrange for the patient to speak to another who has had a positive experience with similar surgery.

NDx: Knowledge deficit: underlying disease process, perioperative experiences, and the possible effect of surgery on vision

Review and clarify the information given to the patient in the clinic or ophthalmologist's office at the time the surgery was scheduled. Be certain the patient understands the expected outcome of the surgery and knows when it will be done and how long it will take. Describe the preparations ordered for surgery, such as fasting after midnight and preoperative medications and the purpose of each. Briefly describe the operating room, commonly occurring sounds, and the procedure. Remind the patient that a nurse will be in the room with him or her throughout the procedure. Advise the patient that the face and head will be draped and that the anesthesia effectively numbs the area as well as prevents any visual images from being processed by the brain.

Review postoperative care with the patient, and include the family or significant other if possible. Explain that to avoid increased pressure and stress on the suture line that one cannot lie on the side of the operated eye or on the stomach but only on the opposite side or on the back. The exception is the patient having a vitrectomy involving gas injection into the eye who is positioned prone to allow the gas to float upward. Explain that quick movements,

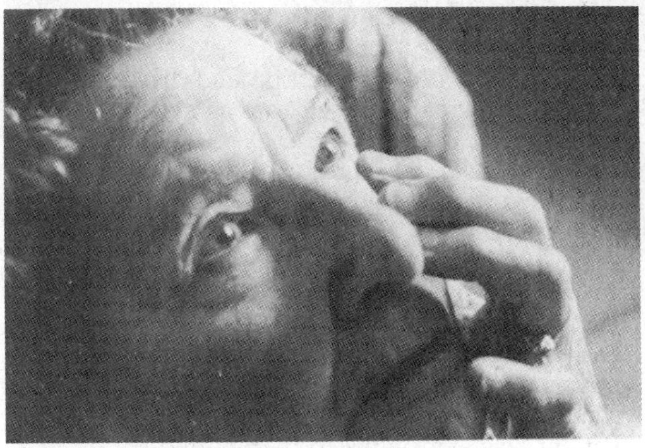

1. The client tilts her head back, opens her eyes, and looks up.

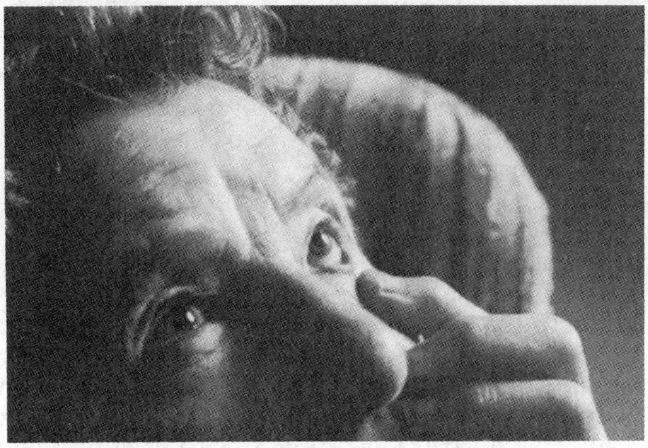

2. The client pulls the lower eyelid downward, against her cheekbone.

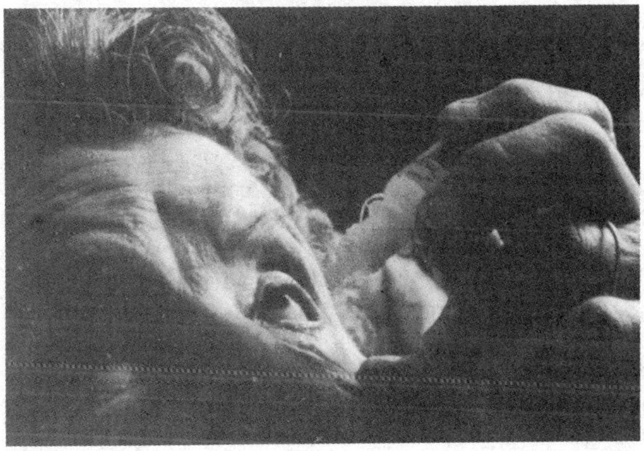

3. The client holds the bottle like a pencil, with the tip downward, and squeezes the bottle gently, allowing one drop to fall into the sac.

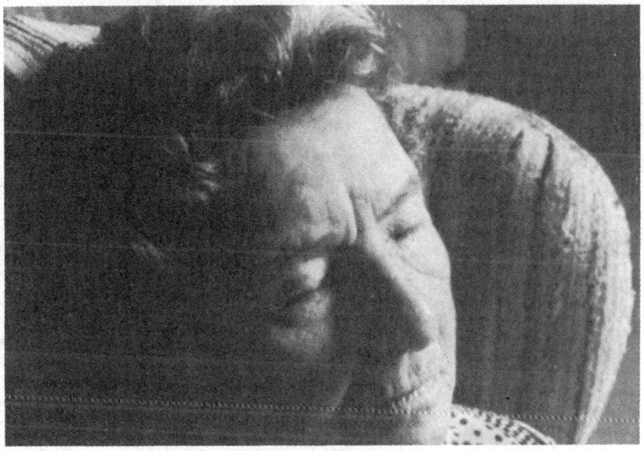

4. The client gently *closes* her eyes.

Figure 39–14.

Instillation of eye drops. (From Ignatavicius D, Baynes M. Medical-surgical nursing. Philadelphia: WB Saunders, 1991, p. 1013.)

coughing, and rubbing the eyes should be avoided. Be certain to tell the patient if an eye patch is expected, and depending on the surgery, remind the patient that improved vision may not be noticed immediately after surgery.

Remind the patient that smoking must be avoided both preoperatively and postoperatively because of the danger of fire in the hospital and the effect on pulmonary function.

NDx: High risk for injury

On admission, orient the patient to the unit and its personnel as well as to his or her assigned room or area. If the patient's vision is significantly impaired, walk with him or her around the unit while giving detailed verbal descriptions of it. Use one object, such as the bed, as a focal point and give directions from it. For example, "The nightstand is to the right," and "The bathroom is ten steps from the foot of the bed." Encourage the patient to feel objects such as the height, arms, and cushions of the bedside chair to become familiar with the environment. If possible, introduce the patient to staff members involved with his or her care so that the patient can begin to recognize voices.

Keep the call bell and any visual aids used by the patient within reach at all times. Keep side rails up. Validate what activities the patient needs assistance with, and help as needed.

Additional Interventions

Make certain that patient needs relative to any coexisting medical problems are considered in planning care. For example, if the patient is a diabetic, check whether provision is made for glucose management: diet, monitoring of capillary blood sugar, oral hypoglycemics, or insulin if needed.

Ensure that all preoperative preparations are completed. Administer the ordered preoperative medications on time so that the eye is ready for surgery. Observe for pupil dilation after administration of mydriatic agents. Keep in mind that dark eyes take longer to dilate than light eyes. If expected dilation does not occur, notify the physician, because a larger dose may be needed. Be sure the patient voids immediately before leaving for the operating room because a full bladder can make the patient restless during the surgery.

Evaluation

Evaluate the effectiveness of nursing care for a patient who is scheduled for eye surgery by comparing the patient's status with the expected patient outcomes. Examples of specific outcomes for patients scheduled for eye surgery have been provided in the Planning section.

POSTOPERATIVE NURSING CARE

Assessment

Take vital signs every 15 minutes or per institutional protocol until stable, and then with decreasing frequency based on the patient's status. Check the dressing for drainage, and assess for type and amount of discomfort. Be alert to any sign of nausea so that immediate action can be taken to prevent potential vomiting with its resultant increase in intraocular pressure.

Observe for compliance with position and activity restrictions. Be alert also to signs of excessive compliance, that is, the patient who does not reposition himself or herself at intervals within allowable limits but stays rigidly in one position. This behavior can indicate unusual discomfort or severe anxiety.

Throughout the postoperative period, make ongoing assessments of the patient's need for safety measures and assistance with personal activities as well as assessments related to any coexisting chronic disease.

Assess the patient's understanding of and capability of self-care after discharge (see Chart 39–1).

Nursing Diagnoses and Planning

Nursing diagnoses and related expected patient outcomes most commonly applicable to patients who have had eye surgery include the following:

NDx: High risk for injury: ocular trauma related to presence in an unfamiliar environment, eye shield disrupting depth perception, altered visual acuity, and age

Planning: Patient outcomes
1. Patient seeks assistance with activities as needed.
2. Patient remains free of injury.

NDx: Anxiety related to the potential development of complications and/or failure to regain vision

Planning: Patient outcomes
1. Patient verbalizes concerns.
2. Patient attends to information and directions.
3. Patient participates in self-care as able.

NDx: High risk for altered health maintenance related to insufficient knowledge of self-care regimen after discharge

Planning: Patient outcomes
1. Patient describes activity restrictions.
2. Patient correctly demonstrates self-care activities: medication administration, application of an eye shield.
3. Patient lists symptoms to be reported.
4. Patient states time and purpose of follow-up visit.

Nursing Interventions

NDx: High risk for injury: ocular trauma
After surgery, orient the patient to time and place. Describe the eye dressing to the patient, and alert him or her to the presence of an intravenous line or similar equipment. Make the patient comfortable, keeping in mind that some patients have to remain flat, whereas others, such as those with a hyphema, need the head of the bed elevated. Place the call bell on the unoperated side so that the patient does not need to turn toward the operated side to locate it, and raise the side rails. Give antiemetic medication as ordered at the first indication of nausea to prevent vomiting and the associated rise in intraocular pressure. Caution the patient not to strain at stool, and instruct him or her in nonpharmacologic interventions to prevent constipation—high-fiber diet, extra fluids, and quiet exercise such as walking.

Table 39–4. GUIDELINES FOR EYELID CLEANSING AND APPLICATION OF AN EYE SHIELD

CLEANSING OF THE EYELIDS
1. *Obtain necessary equipment:* cotton balls, irrigating solution, small plastic bag.
2. *Wash hands* to prevent contamination of the eye.
3. *Instruct patient to close eye* to prevent injury.
4. *Moisten cotton ball with irrigating solution,* which softens the secretions.
5. *Put on gloves* to create a barrier against contact with secretions.
6. *Wipe from medial to lateral canthus once* to move secretions from clean to dirty area.
7. *Dispose of cotton ball in plastic bag* to limit exposure of others to secretions.
8. *Repeat as needed.*
9. *Seal plastic bag* to limit exposure of others to secretions.

APPLICATION OF AN EYE SHIELD
1. *Wash hands* to prevent contamination of the eye.
2. *Wipe forehead and cheek with skin preparation* to reduce skin irritation by creating a surface for tape adherence.
3. *Ask patient to close both eyes* to relax the eyelids.
4. *Apply patch or shield over closed eye with slight pressure exerted against the eyelid* (see Fig. 39–15*A*).
5. *Cover patch or shield with pieces of overlapping tape* to ensure even pressure against the eye (see Fig. 39–15*B*).
6. *Apply tape from cheek to middle of forehead* (see Fig. 39–15C).

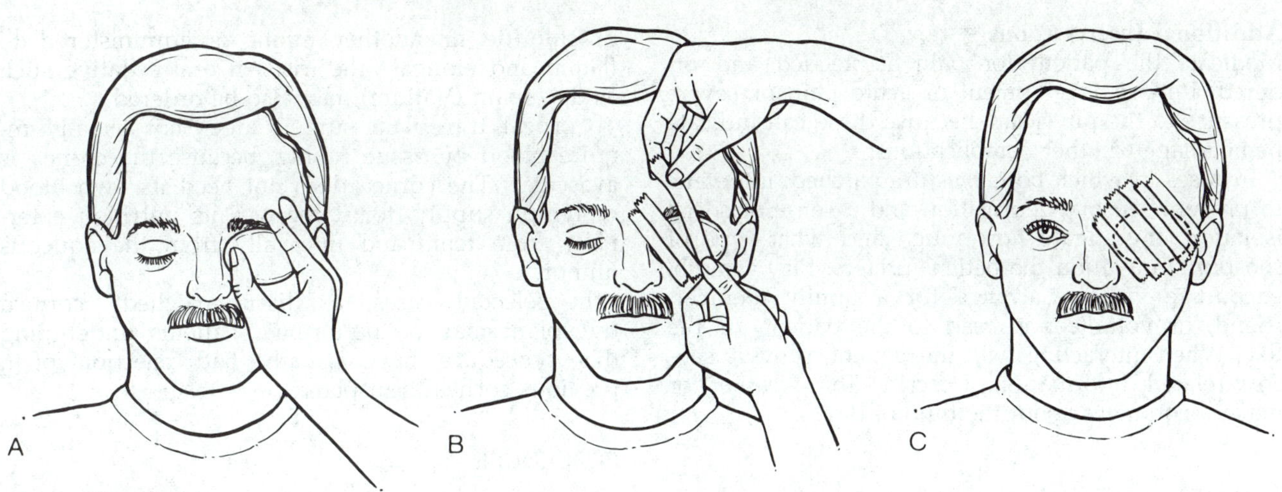

Figure 39–15.

Application of an eye patch. *A*, Patch applied over closed eyelid. Note finger placement of nurse to avoid pressure on globe. *B*, Overlapping tape applied from cheek to forehead. *C*, Correctly applied patch. Note that cheek is pulled slightly upward.

To promote safety, remind the patient of the location of objects in the environment. Make certain that small objects such as wastebaskets, footstools, and the like are safely out of the walking area. Avoid use of straws, because they can cause injury to the eye. Remind both staff and visitors of the importance of returning furniture and equipment to their original positions so that the environment remains obstacle-free and familiar to the patient.

Reapply eye patch or eye shield as needed in accordance with the guidelines presented in Table 39–4 and Figure 39–15. Remember that in selected forms of "no-stitch" cataract surgery, a patch or shield may not be necessary.

NDx: Anxiety

Keep the patient informed as to what is expected during the postoperative course. For example, reassure the patient that some mild pain or pressure in the eye is normal. Identify yourself on entering the room of patients with limited vision, and approach patients from the unaffected side. Whenever possible, assign the same staff members to care for the patient.

NDx: High risk for altered health maintenance

Instruct the patient or significant other regarding care at home after discharge, as specified in Chart 39–1.

Chart 39–1.

NURSING GUIDE TO PATIENT EDUCATION FOR SELF-MANAGEMENT: GENERAL DISCHARGE INSTRUCTIONS FOLLOWING OCULAR SURGERY

Instruct the patient to:

Use strict aseptic technique when caring for the eye.

Change eye dressing and keep eye shield in place as per the physician's orders.

Use eye medication as directed. (Be certain that the patient knows the name, dose, route, frequency, and expected effect of all medications and can correctly instill topical ophthalmic preparations.)

Avoid activities that increase intraocular pressure: sudden, jarring movements; bending; coughing; sneezing; forceful nose blowing; and sexual intercourse.

Avoid straining at stool: drink at least 2000 ml of fluid daily (unless contraindicated), eat a high-fiber diet, and take stool softeners as ordered.

Wear dark glasses for photophobia.

Avoid use of eye makeup until otherwise instructed.

Report any increased pain, decreased vision, or purulent drainage.

Return for a follow-up visit on *(specify date)*.

Additional Interventions
Medicate the patient for pain as needed and ordered. Report development of acute pain or severe pressure to the physician, because these can indicate hemorrhage or other complications.

In cases in which both eyes are patched, intervene to prevent sensory deprivation and a sense of social isolation. Investigate how much and what type of sensory stimulation the patient prefers. Play a radio, encourage visitors, arrange for a family member, friend, or volunteer to read to the patient, or the like. When interacting with the patient, provide sensory-related information. Describe the weather or make a comment about the time of day.

Evaluation

Evaluate the effectiveness of nursing care for a patient who has had eye surgery by comparing the patient's status with the expected patient outcomes. Examples of specific outcomes for patients who have had eye surgery have been provided in the Planning section.

CORNEAL TRANSPLANT (KERATOPLASTY)

A corneal transplant, or keratoplasty, is the surgical removal of a patient's cornea and replacement of it with a donor cornea.

USES

Corneal transplants are done when a patient's vision is impaired because the cornea is clouded and opaque as a result of trauma, degeneration, or infection.

DONOR CORNEA

The cornea to be transplanted comes from a donor who died of an acute disease or accident and was free of infection and disease. Preferably the donor is a young adult so that the cornea has a large number of endothelial cells, because this increases the success rate of the transplant.

When a donor dies, the eyes are closed, and gauze pads wet with saline are placed over them along with a small ice pack. Within 2 to 4 hours, the eyes are enucleated. The cornea is usually transplanted within 24 to 48 hours, but technologic developments in preservation solutions make transplants possible up to 7 days after procurement. Corneas can also be frozen, dehydrated, or refrigerated for later transplantation.

PHYSICAL PREPARATION OF THE PATIENT

Antibiotic eye drops are given preoperatively to reduce the chance of infection, and pilocarpine hydrochloride or another miotic is administered to flatten and elongate the iris. An oral sedative such as diazepam (Valium) may also be ordered.

Corneal transplant surgery does not usually require blood or tissue typing, because the cornea is avascular. The cornea does not need its own blood or lymph supply, for it receives its nutrition externally from tears and internally from the aqueous humor.

In selected cases, a "tissue-matched" corneal transplant may be performed. Patients undergoing this procedure have usually had rejection of a previous corneal transplant.

PROCEDURE

Corneal transplant surgery is usually performed under local anesthesia on an out-patient basis, or with an overnight hospital stay. It is done using general anesthesia if the patient is unable to remain motionless, as with coexisting Parkinson's disease. It is also used if medical problems such as respiratory disease prevent the patient from lying flat and breathing, because under general anesthesia, the patient can receive ventilation assistance from a respirator.

Corneal transplantation is performed under the operating room microscope. The patient's cornea is measured to determine what size the graft should be. The whole cornea is not removed; rather, the central cornea, that area through which light rays pass en route to the retina, is removed. Next, the donor tissue is measured. Using an instrument that resembles a cookie cutter, the predetermined size button of cornea is cut from the donor tissue. Once the donor tissue is ready, the same "cookie cutter" instrument is used to excise the diseased corneal tissue from the patient.

The carefully measured donor button is then placed in the exact spot where the diseased cornea was removed, and the new and clear corneal tissue is carefully sutured in place. Subconjunctival injections of antibiotics are administered, and an antibiotic ointment is instilled. The eye is carefully closed, and an eye patch and shield are applied and secured with tape.

POSTOPERATIVE COURSE

The eye patch and shield remain in place until the next morning, when they are removed by the surgeon. Diet and activity are resumed based on the patient's tolerance. Because the cornea is avascular, healing is very slow, and recovery of vision after corneal transplant surgery is not as rapid as after cataract surgery.

COMPLICATIONS

Rejection may occur following a corneal transplant, although the rate is relatively low because the cornea has neither a blood nor a lymph supply.

When rejection does occur, the transplanted cornea becomes opaque. Episodes of rejection are treated with steroids, but a repeat keratoplasty may be required.

Application of the Nursing Process to the Care of the Patient Having a Corneal Transplant

PREOPERATIVE NURSING CARE

Preoperative nursing care of patients having corneal transplant surgery is similar to the nursing care of patients having any type of eye surgery, with the following considerations.

Corneal transplant surgery happens in a semi-urgent manner. When the patient, in consultation with the ophthalmologist, decides he or she wants and needs a corneal transplant, the individual's name is placed on a waiting list. When tissue becomes available, the patient is notified by the ophthalmologist. Therefore, patients may not have much time to prepare psychologically for the upcoming surgery. Also stressful for some patients is the issue of tissue donation—the fact that someone had to die to make the tissue available for transplantation. Thus, patients may be glad they are getting a second chance at sight, but may also feel sadness for someone else's loss.

If possible, offer the patient the opportunity to speak with another patient who has had corneal transplant surgery. These volunteers have a unique view of the procedure and how it has affected their lives. The Eye Bank Association of America (E.B.A.A.) has a volunteer organization called the Ambassadors for Corneal Transplant. The local tissue bank may be able to supply a list of area representatives.

Remind the patient that recovery of vision following corneal transplant surgery is not as rapid as following cataract surgery, so that he or she is not discouraged when the patch is removed and the visual acuity is not a perfect 20/20. Reinforce the fact that the visual acuity the first day may not be an indicator of final visual outcome.

POSTOPERATIVE NURSING CARE

Assessment

Postoperatively, assess the patient's return to physiologic stability. Monitor vital signs in accordance with institutional policy, but guided by the patient's condition. Observe the eye patch and shield for any sign of drainage. Assess for nausea, which occasionally occurs as a result of the preoperative sedation.

Nursing Diagnoses and Planning

Nursing diagnoses and related expected patient outcomes most commonly applicable to patients who have had a corneal transplant include the following:

NDx: High risk for infection related to surgical interruption of the intact ocular surface

Planning: Patient outcomes
1. Patient is afebrile.
2. Ocular redness is absent.
3. Corneal graft remains clear.
4. Anterior chamber remains clear, without signs of hypopyon.

NDx: High risk for trauma: tissue, related to pressure on suture line

Planning: Patient outcomes
1. Patient verbalizes importance of not disturbing integrity of suture line.
2. Patient avoids activities known to increase intraocular pressure.
3. Patient wears eye shield as instructed.

NDx: High risk for impaired home maintenance management related to activity restrictions imposed by corneal transplant surgery

Planning: Patient outcomes
1. Patient performs own activities of daily living within constraints of activity restrictions.
2. Patient identifies plan for meeting activities of daily living if unable to do so independently.

NDx: High risk for altered health maintenance related to insufficient knowledge of postoperative self-care activities

Planning: Patient outcomes
1. Patient aseptically instills eye drops.
2. Patient identifies purpose of medications.
3. Patient states frequency of medications.
4. Patient correctly applies eye shield.
5. Patient describes activity restrictions.
6. Patient lists symptoms to be reported to the health care provider.

Nursing Interventions

NDx: High risk for infection
Instruct the patient to wash both hands immediately before and after touching the eye. Teach the patient to administer eye drops without contaminating the eye drop tip with their eyelashes (see Table 39–3).

Because a reduction in visual acuity is an early sign of postoperative infection or rejection, advise the patient to check the vision every day. Instruct the patient to do this by looking at the same object,

Chart 39–2.

NURSING GUIDE TO PATIENT EDUCATION FOR SELF-MANAGEMENT: SELF-CARE FOLLOWING CORNEAL TRANSPLANT

Instruct the patient to:

Avoid restricted activities:

- Do not drive until given specific clearance by the ophthalmologist.
- Do not shower or wash hair unless shampooing can be done from behind, as in a beauty salon, so that no soapy or dirty water can come in contact with the eye.
- Do not lie on the operative side.
- Do not bend over from the waist because this increases intraocular pressure.
- Do not lift or carry more than 25 lb.
- Do not have sexual intercourse for 1 week after surgery.

Engage in unrestricted activities as desired: ride in a car, watch television, read, play cards, do close work, climb steps, take sponge or tub baths, carry less than 25 lb.
Instill prescribed antibiotic and steriod eye drops as directed in Table 39–3. Be certain to wait at least 5 minutes between different drops to promote maximum absorption.
Check vision daily in the eye that has had the corneal transplant.
Report any reduction in visual acuity immediately to the ophthalmologist because this is an early sign of infection and/or rejection.
Wear an eye shield at night to prevent rubbing or bumping the eye during sleep. Also wear the shield when engaging in activities such as playing with children or pets that might cause accidental injury.
Apply the eye shield as described in Table 39–4.
Expect some white or yellow-white drainage that appears as dry crustings on the eyelids or eyelashes and is most noticeable in the morning or after sleeping.
Remove the drainage as directed in Table 39–4. Notify the ophthalmologist if the drainage increases, has a foul odor, or is a color other than white or yellow-white.
Expect mild itching.
Report eye pain not relieved by acetaminophen (Tylenol) or accompanied by nausea or fever; seeing spots before the eyes; seeing bright flashes of light or a curtain coming in from the side or obstructing part of the visual field; or any change in visual acuity.
Return for follow-up care the day after surgery and then as scheduled.

using only the eye which has had the corneal transplant.

Tell the patient to expect some crusty drainage on the eyelid or eyelashes. If the amount of drainage increases or becomes purulent, notify the ophthalmologist immediately.

NDx: High risk for trauma: tissue

Position the patient on the unaffected side to prevent pressure on the suture line. Remember that ophthalmic suture material is finer than a human hair. While it promotes adequate closure of tissue, excessive pressure on the suture line should be avoided. Because suture lines can also have tension placed upon them by increased intraocular pressure, advise the patient to avoid activities known to increase intraocular pressure. These activities include bending over at the waist, straining at having a stool, lifting heavy objects, vigorous nose blowing, and coughing.

NDx: High risk for impaired home maintenance management

Patients are unable to drive after surgery until given clearance by the physician. Help establish a transportation plan for return from the surgery center and for follow-up care appointments.

Assist the patient in establishing a plan for modifying the home environment. For example, suggest placing needed articles at counter height to avoid use of low-level cabinets, because use of these lower cabinets would involve bending.

Patients may feel fatigued the first few days after surgery. If time permits, encourage the patient to prepare a few meals ahead and store them in the refrigerator or freezer.

One care need patients frequently have is for assistance with instilling eye drops. Help identify who will instill the drops, patient or caregiver. If needed, train the caregiver to instill the eye drops as described in Table 39–3.

Advise the patient to develop a mechanism for alerting a friend or neighbor that emergency assistance is needed. Have the patient place a list of emergency numbers near *each* phone. If help is needed, having the numbers nearby speeds the process, and the patient does not need to rely on memory.

If the activity restrictions imposed by surgery will create difficulty for the patient at home, assist with finding a source of home care assistance. Temporary nursing agencies can provide in-home assistance with activities of daily living including personal care and meal preparation. Determine whether these care-related expenses are covered under the patient's insurance plan, or whether she or he is able and willing to pay the cost as an out-of-pocket expense.

NDx: High risk for altered health maintenance

When patients are discharged, they normally are using an antibiotic eye drop such as tobramycin (Tobrex) and a steroid such as prednisolone acetate (Inflamase Forte) or a combination product such as dexamethasone and tobramycin (TobraDex) or prednisolone acetate and gentamicin (Pred-G suspension). Make certain the patient knows the name and purpose of each medication, how often to use it, and in which eye. If medications have different frequencies of administration, alert the patient to this fact, and provide a written chart describing how often each is to be used. Teach the patient to instill the eye drops (see Table 39–3), and obtain a return demonstration to evaluate his or her technique. Provide instruction in additional aspects of self-care as presented in Chart 39–2.

Evaluation

Evaluate the effectiveness of nursing care for a patient who has had a corneal transplant by comparing the patient's status with the expected patient outcomes. Examples of specific outcomes for patients who have had a corneal transplant have been provided in the Planning section.

VITRECTOMY

Vitrectomy is the surgical excision of the vitreous.

USES

A vitrectomy is done to remove debris such as blood or foreign bodies from the visual axis, thereby improving the ability of light rays to reach the retina, and to remove traction forces on the retina, thereby preventing a retinal detachment. Specific indications for a vitrectomy include vitreous hemorrhage, which can occur as a result of trauma or from leaking of fragile vessels in cases of diabetic retinopathy, chronic endophthalmitis, presence of an intraocular foreign body, and the removal of vitreoretinal adhesions or fibrin bands.

PROCEDURE

Vitrectomy is performed under general anesthesia. The conjunctiva is moved from its normal position, and three instruments are introduced into the eye at the pars plana, the area where objects can be introduced without injury to eye structure. The three instruments are a light source to allow visualization of retina and vitreous; vitreous cutters to lyse adhesions; and an infusion port through which special solutions are instilled at the same rate as the cloudy or blood-filled vitreous gel is removed. This equal rate maintains the shape and size of the globe, preventing collapse.

Once the clarity of the vitreous is restored, leaking or bleeding blood vessels may be treated with an intraoperative laser. Because this laser is inserted directly into the eye, it is referred to as an endolaser.

If necessary, a vitrectomy may also be combined with the repair of a detached retina.

Application of the Nursing Process to the Care of the Patient Having a Vitrectomy

The assessment, nursing diagnoses, expected patient outcomes, nursing interventions, and evaluation for the patient having a vitrectomy are similar to those described for the patient having ocular surgery.

See Table 39–5 for a summary of common surgical procedures performed on the eye.

Laser Therapy

The argon laser is used as a noninvasive, outpatient treatment for problems such as flat tears in

Table 39–5. SURGICAL PROCEDURES USED IN THE TREATMENT OF EYE DISORDERS

SURGICAL PROCEDURE	DESCRIPTION
Vitrectomy	Removal of the vitreous by suction, and replacement with a balanced salt solution that is gradually replaced by extracellular fluid.
Iridectomy	Removal of a small portion of the iris to reestablish communication between the posterior and anterior chambers to allow outflow of aqueous humor.
Sclerectomy	Removal of a portion of corneoscleral tissue to create a drainage channel into the subconjunctival space for the outflow of aqueous humor.
Scleral buckling	Use of an encircling band to indent the sclera toward the vitreous to reposition the retina against the choroid.
Cataract extraction	Removal of an opaque lens. Frequently accompanied by an intraocular lens implant.
Keratoplasty	Corneal transplant or grafting of corneal tissue from the eye of one human to another.
Epikeratophakia	Suturing of a piece of donor cornea shaped to a specific diopter strength to the cornea of the recipient to change refraction.
Radial keratotomy	Procedure in which a series of incisions is made into the cornea to flatten its shape and thereby correct myopia.
Enucleation	Complete removal of the globe. Done in cases of irreparable injury; blind, painful eye; melanoma; retinoblastoma; and extensive infection.

the retina, proliferative vascular diseases like diabetic retinopathy, sickle cell anemia hemoglobinopathy, age-related macular degeneration (ARMD), and glaucoma. During the procedure, the patient sits with the head stabilized in the slit-lamp frame. The pupil is dilated with topical cycloplegics, and anesthetic drops are instilled. A Goldmann lens is then placed on the cornea, and the laser treatment is administered. The eye is irrigated to remove the viscous lens lubricant, and an eye patch is applied according to the preference of the physician. Most patients have no restrictions on activity following the procedure.

The Nd:YAG laser, a photodisrupter laser, is used to lyse vitreous strands or to open the posterior capsule. The procedure is similar to the one just described, except that a Peyman lens is used to lyse vitreous strands, and neither anesthetic nor lens is required for opening the posterior capsule.

Lasers should always be used in a closed room and aimed away from the doorway. On the outside of the door should be a sign indicating that laser is in use. Persons in the room with the patient during laser therapy should wear protective eyewear specifically designed for the type of laser in use. The number of persons in the room should be restricted to limit the number who could be injured should the laser be misdirected or deflected.

Guidelines for Application of the Nursing Process to the Care of the Patient Having Laser Therapy for a Disorder of the Eye

Before the procedure, obtain baseline vital signs and intraocular pressure and assess and document visual acuity.

Describe to the patient what will be seen and heard during the procedure: staff wearing protective eyewear, the bright light of the laser, and the clicking of the machine as each laser spot is delivered. Reassure the patient that most patients do not feel anything because a local or topical anesthetic is used. Stress the importance of focusing on the object placed in the line of vision as directed and not looking elsewhere without consulting the ophthalmologist.

Advise the patient of the potential for corneal injury until the anesthetic wears off. Caution the patient not to rub or bump the eye.

If a short course of topical steroids, such as prednisolone acetate (Pred Mild), is prescribed to reduce the inflammation that can sometimes accompany laser therapy, instruct the patient on how, when, and why to use the drops.

Remember that before the patient leaves the facility, intraocular pressure must be rechecked to make certain that no increase has occurred.

Supportive Treatment for the Low-Vision Patient

Low vision is defined by the Internal Revenue Service as a best corrected central visual acuity of 20/200 or less in the better eye or widest diameter of visual field no greater than 20 degrees (Vaughan et al, 1992). Thus, persons with low vision even with the help of corrective eyeglasses or contact lenses have difficulty reading newspaper type, a sign on a bus, and labels on canned goods, or recognizing friends in the street. In adults, low vision is commonly associated with macular degeneration, glaucoma, diabetic retinopathy, or cataracts.

Supportive care of these individuals focuses on enhancement of remaining vision to maintain maximum function and quality of life. This is accomplished through the use of optical and nonoptical vision aids and modifications in the home and work environment.

OPTICAL AIDS

The simplest types of optical aid are handheld nonprescription magnifying glasses. Of these, the small half-dollar-size lens is most effective in that it gives the clearest image. It works well for reading small areas of fine print such as price tags and entries in telephone books. It can easily be carried in the pocket or on a cord around the neck. Magnifiers on a circular stand, which can be easily moved across the page, are convenient and useful for reading newspapers and books.

Available prescription aids include telescopes, prisms, and microscopes.

Handheld monocular telescopes with prescription lenses designed to boost vision in the better eye can be used for seeing street signs and looking for traffic. They can be focused and can be easily carried or worn around the neck. Another type of telescope is a jeweler's loupe, which can be clipped to the top rim of glasses and used for such tasks as seeing where to sign a document or reading numbers on paper currency. A full diameter telescope set in an eyeglass frame is also available. This can be worn only when sitting still but is valuable for activities like watching television and seeing a play.

A bioptic telescope mounted in the top part of regular eyeglasses can provide acuity of distance vision while the lower lens provides normal distance judgment. In some states, persons with low vision can obtain a driver's license if use of a bioptic telescope can provide a visual acuity meeting the state's standards.

Prisms that are pressed onto eyeglasses can be used to widen a constricted peripheral field of vision.

For near vision only, microscopic spectacles can be obtained that have high-power magnifying lenses incorporated into prescription eyeglasses.

ELECTRONIC AIDS

An ever-growing number of electronic vision enhancement aids are available. Most of these are magnifiers that project print onto a screen enlarged up to 60 times its original size. One such enlarger system, which is portable and small enough to fit in a briefcase, uses a camera about the size of a cigarette lighter to scan print and project it on a screen. Another is designed to enlarge and project print onto a screen as it is typed, enabling a low-vision person to proofread and make corrections.

Also available are devices called optical-to-tactile converters. These devices produce a raised outline of printed letters on a "tactile screen" by adjusting the levels of tiny rods. The letters are then read by touch. A more complex device is the Reading Machine, which uses a computer and a voice synthesizer to read printed materials aloud.

NONOPTICAL ACCESSORY AIDS

There are many nonoptical aids that can be used to enhance the ability of low-vision individuals to perform routine activities. For example, to facilitate reading, a clear sheet of yellow plastic can be placed over the page to decrease glare and to make print darker. A small pointer can be used to direct focus to one word at a time. Large print materials such as the *New York Times* or *Reader's Digest* large print editions and the Doubleday Large Print Home Library increase access to news, best sellers, and "how to" information.

To enable persons with low vision to write checks or fill out other documents, a dark plastic overlay with spaces cut out corresponding to those to be filled in can be obtained or an overlay made of dark construction paper. Similarly, dials with enlarged or raised markings are available for stoves, and there are push-button telephones with extra-large, raised, palpable numbers.

Not all aids are needed by or work well for all individuals. A major factor that influences their selection is the individual's specific goals (e.g., see street signs, read a menu, be able to type). Other factors include physical capability (e.g., can the person hold a large magnifying glass or support the weight of the frame of some telescopic or other aids on the nose); acceptance of the aid (e.g., some optical aids can appear somewhat bizarre); and of course cost, because many optical aids are not covered by insurance.

Some clinics that specialize in the care of persons with low vision facilitate the selection process by loaning the patient aids for trial use. Others even have simulated environments such as kitchens and offices where the patient can learn to use a particular aid.

For persons whose visual impairment exceeds that which can be helped by these aids, other types of support are available.

Braille is a system of raised dots representing letters and numbers that are identified or "read" by the fingers. This system is taught by agencies for the blind and other educational institutions. A large variety of materials are available in braille including books, magazines, playing cards, medical equipment, and various household goods.

To facilitate mobility, patients can use the traditional white cane with a red tip. Another option is the newer laser cane, which can locate obstacles and changes in terrain from up to 20 feet away. Some patients use a guide dog to help navigate and travel. These aids have the secondary purpose of identifying people who may need assistance.

See Table 39–6 for guidelines for helping a visually disabled person.

Prevention of Eye Disorders

Basic principles of eye care that help prevent eye disorders such as infections and injuries and allow for early diagnosis and treatment of other disorders are presented in Chart 39–3.

Table 39–6. GUIDELINES FOR HELPING A VISUALLY DISABLED PERSON

1. Ask the person whether they would like assistance. If it is needed, most will appreciate the offer. It is better to offer than not.
2. When entering a room, announce your presence. State the reason for the visit. Let the person know when you are leaving, so that she or he is not left speaking to the air.
3. If speaking to a visually disabled person when others are present, refer to all persons by name. That way the person knows for whom the greeting is meant. Visually disabled people cannot tell when you are looking at them.
4. Avoid using pointing, nodding, or shrugging gestures and terms such as "over there." Remember that visually disabled people are comfortable with language such as "look," "see," and "blind."
5. When speaking with a visually disabled person, use a normal, conversational tone. Visually disabled people are not necessarily hearing impaired. Do not shout.
6. If a visually disabled person travels with a guide dog, resist the temptation to call or pet the animal, unless given permission. Remember that the animal is there to enhance the safety of the visually disabled person, and any distraction of the guide dog can jeopardize safety.
7. When escorting a visually disabled person, allow him or her to grasp your upper arm as demonstrated in Figure 39–16*A*. Stay one step ahead, and alert the person to changes in terrain and obstacles in the path. If walking near a curb, walk next to the curb. If approaching a narrow passage, bring your arm behind the back. This change alerts the visually disabled person to the narrow door opening (Fig. 39–16*B*).
8. Orient any visually disabled person to the environment before leaving him or her alone. Use one piece of furniture in the room as a reference point, and give directions from it. For example, "There is a chair directly in front of you. To its left is a table." Allow the visually disabled person to put his or her hand on the back of the chair. This action provides reassurance as to its location. Remove hazards such as throw rugs, footstools, and wastebaskets, because the person might trip in the unfamiliar environment.
9. When helping a visually disabled person into a car, check the seat and guide the person's hand onto the door handle. The person will be able to help him- or herself from this point. If the person travels with a guide dog, allow him or her to settle the dog into the car.
10. Describe the table setting and any food in detail. Use the hours of the clock as a guide. For example: "There is roast beef at 6 o'clock. The potatoes are at 3 o'clock. A glass of milk is located just above the spoon."
11. When handing money to a visually disabled person, announce its denomination. Most visually disabled people have a system for sorting money.
12. Once the person has placed an object, do not move it unless consent is given. Visually disabled persons cannot find it if it is moved.

Adapted from When you meet a blind person. Cleveland, OH: Cleveland Sight Center of the Cleveland Society for the Blind, 1989 (adapted with permission).

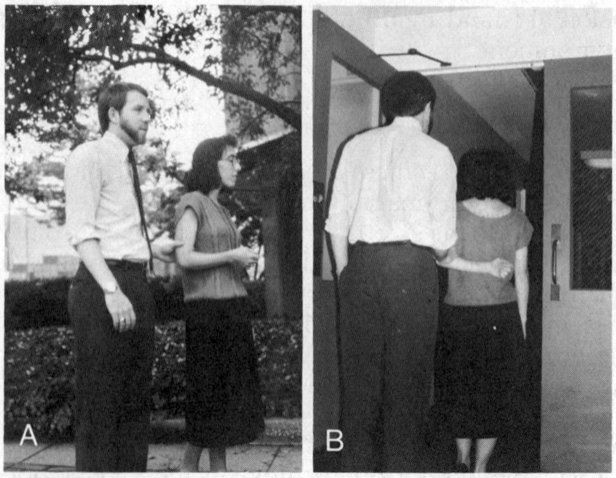

Figure 39–16.

A, When escorting a visually disabled person, allow him or her to grasp your upper arm as shown. *B*, When approaching a narrow passage, bring your arm behind your back to alert the visually disabled person. (Courtesy of Cleveland Society for the Blind.)

The Elderly: Special Considerations

With aging, changes occur in the accessory structures of the eye, in the structures of the eyeball itself, and in the visual process.

Changes in the Accessory Structures of the Eye

The skin in the orbital area becomes darkened, and crow's feet appear at the periphery of the outer

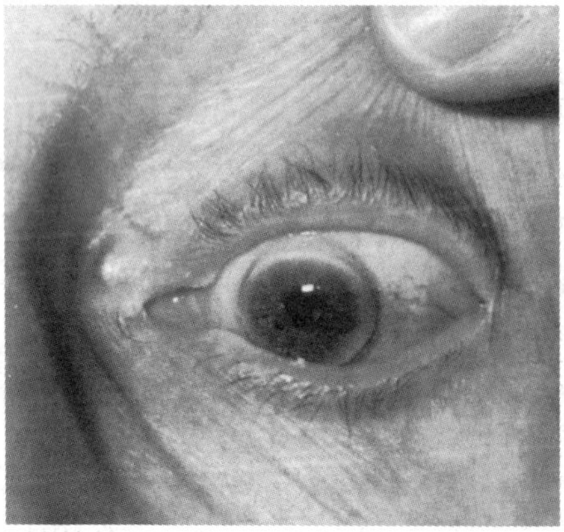

Figure 39–17.

Arcus senilis—an opaque white or gray ring around the iris. (From Jarvis C. Physical examination and health assessment. Philadelphia: WB Saunders, 1991, p. 341.)

Chart 39–3.

NURSING GUIDE TO PATIENT EDUCATION FOR SELF-MANAGEMENT: PREVENTIVE CARE OF THE EYES

Keep the eyes clean.

- Keep the hands away from the eyes.
- When necessary to touch the eye, wash hands thoroughly first.
- When cleansing the eye area, move from the inner canthus to the outer.
- Remove old makeup thoroughly.
- Avoid transfer of microorganisms from one eye to the other by never using the same section of washcloth, tissue, and the like to cleanse both eyes.
- Never share eye makeup with another person.
- Discard old eye makeup, especially mascara, which can serve as a medium for bacterial growth.

Use good, well-placed lighting for all tasks.
Rest eyes at intervals during periods of close work by looking off into the distance or walking around for a few minutes.
Protect eyes from irritation and trauma.

- Wear safety glasses to protect against occupational hazards and when using equipment in the home that can throw off dust, wood shavings, pieces of metal, and so on.
- Use protective eyewear when participating in recreational activities such as tennis or racquetball, where blunt trauma from high-speed balls is a risk.
- Wear dark glasses or other shading device to protect the eyes from bright sunshine, sun lamps, and excessive glare.
- Cover the eyes when using hair spray, and aim other aerosols carefully to avoid contact with the eyes.
- Use ammonia and other household chemicals with irritating fumes only in well-ventilated areas.

Protect eyes from exposure to blood and body fluids by wearing goggles during periods of exposure.
Have an eye examination every 5 years in early adulthood, every 2 years after age 35, and more often if you have, or there is a family history of, diabetes or glaucoma.
Obtain an eye examination immediately if there is a change in vision, eye pain, photophobia, pupil or iris abnormality, nodule, or persistent watering or discharge.

canthus. Muscle tone and elasticity in the eyelids are lost, and ptosis of the upper lids and pouches under the lower result. Xanthelasma, which is a collection of benign yellow nodules formed of lipid deposits, is common on the medial aspects of both the upper and the lower lids in persons with hypercholesterolemia.

Changes in the Structures of the Eyeball

An opaque white or gray ring is often seen around the iris. This is called an arcus senilis (Fig. 39–17) and is caused by deposits of lipid in the cornea or by hyaline degeneration.

The pupil becomes progressively smaller, a condition known as senile miosis. The lens yellows, becomes less transparent, and loses its elasticity. Vitreous floaters are common.

The retina turns pale, and the arteries appear slightly narrowed and irregular. The optic disk shrinks in diameter, and the macula often becomes broken or thinned in a condition known as macular degeneration.

Changes in Vision

As the pupil becomes progressively smaller, less light reaches the retina so that up to three times as much light is needed for routine activities. This is complicated by the fact that at the same time that more light is needed, opacity developing in the lens scatters light rays and creates glare. Inelasticity of the lens results in loss of accommodation and therefore difficulty seeing near objects, referred to as presbyopia.

As the lens yellows with age, changes in color vision also occur. Discrimination of low tone colors, especially blues, greens, and violets, becomes difficult; discrimination of the yellows, red, and oranges is unaffected.

Peripheral vision is narrowed with aging, and because of a decrease in the amount of rhodopsin, the time needed for adaptation to darkness is lengthened.

Bibliography

Bartlett J, Ghormley N, Jaanus S, et al. Ophthalmic drug facts. St. Louis: Facts & Comparisons, 1992.

Boyd-Monk H, Steinmetz C. Nursing care of the eye. Norwalk, CT: Appleton & Lange, 1987.

Cahill M (ed). Nurse's reference library, signs and symptoms. Springhouse, PA: Springhouse, 1986.

Coles W. Ophthalmology: A diagnostic text. Baltimore: Williams & Wilkins, 1989.

Coster DJ. Bacterial corneal ulcers. In Fraunfelder FT, Roy FH. Current ocular therapy 3. Philadelphia: WB Saunders, 1990, pp 439–440.

Daigle L, et al. A look at epikeratophakia. J Ophthalmic Nurs Tech 1988; 7(5):174.

Dobbie JG. What's new in ophthalmic surgery. Am Coll Surg Bull 1986; 71:22.

Fraunfelder FT, Roy FH. Current ocular therapy 3. Philadelphia: WB Saunders, 1990.

Freeman DL. Lasers in the OR: From science fiction to fact. Am J Nurs 1986; 86(3):278.

Friedberg M, Rapuano C. Office and emergency room diagnosis and treatment of eye disease. Philadelphia: JB Lippincott, 1990.

Gioiella EC, Bevil CW. Nursing care of the aging client—promoting healthy adaptation. Norwalk, CT: Appleton-Century-Crofts, 1985.

Gruendemann BJ, Meeker MH. Care of the patient in surgery. 8th ed. St. Louis: CV Mosby, 1987.

Guyton AC. Textbook of medical physiology. 8th ed. Philadelphia: WB Saunders, 1991.

Hollins M. Understanding blindness: An integrative approach. Hillsdale, NJ: Lawrence Erlbaum Assoc., 1989.

Jaffe S (ed). Atlas of ophthalmic surgery. Philadelphia: JB Lippincott, 1990.

Jakobiec FA, Sigelman J. Advanced techniques in ocular surgery. Philadelphia: WB Saunders, 1984.

Kanski J. Clinical ophthalmology. London: Butterworth, 1984.

Miller S. Parson's diseases of the eye. 18th ed. New York: Churchill Livingstone, 1990.

Neal H. Low vision. New York: Simon & Schuster, 1987.

Newell F. Ophthalmology: Principles and concepts. St. Louis: CV Mosby, 1986.

Orticio L. Confusion and the patient on an intensive topical ocular antibiotic regimen: A case analysis. J Ophthalmic Nurs Technol 1990; 4:145.

Parr J. Introduction to ophthalmology. 3rd ed. New York: Oxford University Press, 1989.

Parrish JA, Paul BS. Photosensitivity and sunburn. In Fraunfelder FT, Roy FH. Current ocular therapy 3. Philadelphia: WB Saunders, 1990, pp 185–186.

Perry JP, Tullo AB (eds). Care of the ophthalmic patient. London: Chapman & Hall, 1990.

Schremp P. Discharge Instructions, providing continuing care for ophthalmic patients. J Ophthalmic Nurs Technol 1985; 4:30.

Vader LA. Vision and vision loss. Nurs Clin North Am 1992; 27(3):705.

Vaughan D, Asbury T, Riordan-Eva P. General ophthalmology. 13th ed. Los Angeles: Lange Medical, 1992.

Chapter Forty

NURSING CARE *of Adults with Eye Disorders*

Ophthalmic disorders and ocular manifestations of systemic disease can occur suddenly or evolve over time. Regardless of onset any threat to a patient's vision is accompanied by the common experience of fear; fear of losing vision or being unable to regain it. Sensitivity to these concerns by the nurse who cares for this patient population is required.

Infections and Inflammations

Blepharitis

ETIOLOGY AND PATHOPHYSIOLOGY

Blepharitis is a chronic inflammation of the eyelid, most noticeable at the eyelid/eyelash margin. The two most common forms are seborrheic and staphylococcal. Staphylococcal blepharitis is often transmitted by sharing of contaminated makeup. Mascara, in particular, is capable of harboring microorganisms.

Left untreated, staphylococcal blepharitis can spread to the hair follicles and cause eyelashes to fall out. Tiny ulcers can then form at the base of the eyelashes. Scar tissue resulting from the healing of these ulcers can cause the eyelashes to regrow in an abnormal inward direction, which can result in irritation of the cornea (Miller, 1990).

Seborrheic blepharitis is associated with seborrhea of the scalp, ears, and eyebrows. Oily scales develop at the margin of the eyelids, and eyelashes may fall out. When eyelashes regrow, however, growth is in the appropriate direction.

CLINICAL MANIFESTATIONS

Patients with blepharitis frequently complain of itching and burning of the eyelids, particularly at the eyelid/eyelash margins. They report an overwhelming desire to scratch the affected eye. The affected eyelids are edematous and red. Scales are frequently noted at the eyelid/eyelash margin in both types of blepharitis. Scales are oily in seborrheic blepharitis and dry in staphylococcal blepharitis.

Areas of eyelash loss may be visible. Small, ulcerated areas at the eyelid/eyelash margin may be seen. Conjunctivitis may be present.

MEDICAL DIAGNOSIS AND MEDICAL MANAGEMENT

Medical diagnosis and medical management of blepharitis are included in the discussion of medical diagnosis and medical management of chalazion.

A

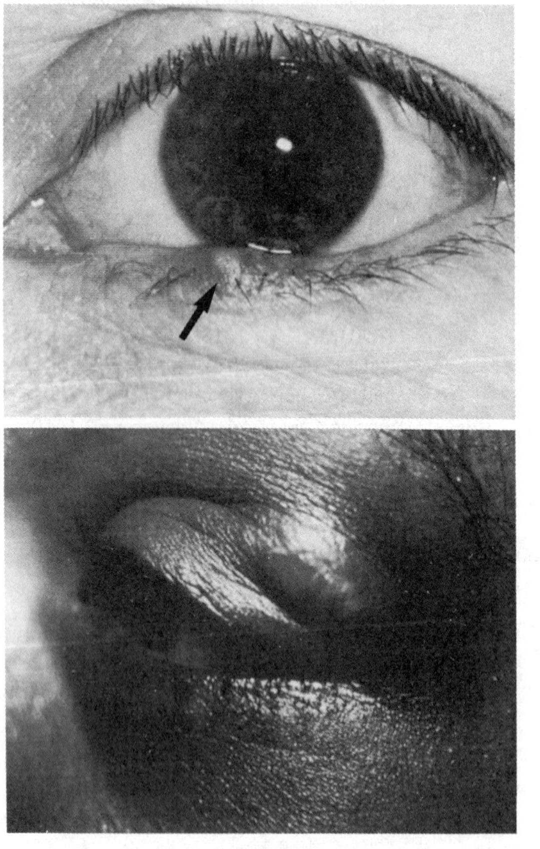

B

Figure 40–1.

A, Hordeolum of the lower lid. *B,* Chalazion on the inner aspect of the upper lid. (From Boyd-Monk H, Steinmetz CG III. Nursing care of the eye. Norwalk, CT: Appleton & Lange, 1987, pp 164,165.)

Hordeolum

ETIOLOGY AND PATHOPHYSIOLOGY

Also known as a stye, this infection occurs near the eyelid/eyelash margin (Fig. 40–1*A*). Only one eye is usually affected. An external hordeolum involves the glands of Moll and Zeis. An internal hordeolum affects the meibomian glands. *Staphylococcus* is the usual causative microorganism. Left untreated, cellulitis may develop.

CLINICAL MANIFESTATIONS

Patients may describe sharp or dull pain depending on the stage of hordeolum development. External hordeola present with a small, red, tender area at the eyelid margin on the external eyelid. With an internal hordeolum, a tiny, beady area on the conjunctival side of the eyelid can be seen.

MEDICAL DIAGNOSIS AND MEDICAL MANAGEMENT

Medical diagnosis and medical management of hordeolum are discussed under medical diagnosis and medical management of chalazion.

Chalazion

ETIOLOGY AND PATHOPHYSIOLOGY

A chalazion is chronic inflammation of the meibomian gland (see Fig. 40–1*B*). It begins as an acute inflammation and progresses to a localized elevation. Chalazia most commonly involve the conjunctival side of the eyelid. Left untreated, they can press against the cornea, distorting its shape and causing astigmatism.

CLINICAL MANIFESTATIONS

Patients may complain of a "full, scratchy feeling" in the eye or of eye fatigue and photophobia. Frequently, there is a previous history of hordeolum or chalazion. The eyelid is red and edematous, but there is no change in visual acuity. If the chalazion is large, however, edema may cause enough eyelid droop to impair vision. Epiphora, or excessive tearing, may also occur. When the chalazion is fully developed, no signs of inflammation are present.

MEDICAL DIAGNOSIS

The diagnosis of blepharitis, hordeolum, and chalazion is made on the basis of history and clinical examination.

MEDICAL MANAGEMENT

Treatment of blepharitis, hordeolum, and chalazion is designed to promote drainage and reduce inflammation of the affected gland as well as to prevent secondary infection of the conjunctiva and neighboring structures. Blepharitis and hordeolum are treated with a series of warm, moist compresses (Table 40–1) followed by a program of eyelid hygiene. The eyelid/eyelash margin area is gently scrubbed with a small amount of baby shampoo applied with a cotton swab or a finger. Known for its gentle cleansing action, the baby shampoo loosens and removes scales, and the gentle massage opens obstructed glands. Antibiotic ointment may be ordered to prevent eye infections (Bartlett et al, 1992).

Acetaminophen (Tylenol) is used to control the pain associated with a hordeolum. If the hordeolum recurs, the patient may be placed on a preventive program of eyelid hygiene.

Chalazia are also treated with compresses and eyelid scrubs. If a chalazion is recurrent, is large enough to obstruct vision, or is visually unappealing to the patient, it can be excised. This minor surgical procedure is usually performed in the ophthalmologist's office. After excision, a topical ointment is applied. An eye patch is worn for several hours.

Table 40–1. APPLICATION OF AN OCULAR COMPRESS

1. Wash hands to prevent contamination of the eye, and put on gloves to create a barrier if secretions are present.
2. Explain the procedure to the patient to decrease anxiety and to promote cooperation.
3. Fold a clean washcloth into quarters to fit the ocular area and to provide clean surfaces for four applications.
4. Dampen the washcloth with running water that feels warm on the inner wrist to provide warmth to the eye without causing injury. The sensitivity of the wrist is equal to that of the globe.*
5. Tell the patient to close the eye so the cornea is not irritated by the washcloth.
6. Hold the washcloth in place until it cools (approximately 2 to 4 minutes).
7. Repeat Steps 3 to 5 for three more applications using a separate quarter of the washcloth each time to decrease the risk of microorganism spread.

* If cool compresses are desired, change water temperature and follow same procedure.

Guidelines for Application of the Nursing Process to the Care of the Patient with Blepharitis, Hordeolum, or Chalazion

Inspect the external eye, question about symptoms experienced, and obtain a history of the current problem. Ask about the presence of dry, flaky skin or scalp or the need to use a dandruff shampoo. Also ask about a history of oily skin and the tendency to develop acne, blackheads, and staphylococcal infections. Question the patient about use of perfumed soaps or other products that might be irritating to the external eye. Inquire specifically about the use of makeup and mascara.

Instruct the patient in therapeutic and preventive measures, as described in Chart 40–1. Explain the purpose of each measure, and obtain a demonstration of the involved procedures.

Conjunctivitis

ETIOLOGY AND PATHOPHYSIOLOGY

An inflammation or infection of the conjunctiva is called conjunctivitis. The bulbar conjunctiva (see Fig. 39–1), which is directly exposed to the environment, is prone to inflammation as a result of allergens and irritants as well as infection from bacteria and viruses. The palpebral conjunctiva is susceptible to infection because of its close proximity to the eyelashes.

Allergic conjunctivitis occurs after repeated exposure to such allergens as pollen and grass or from

Chart 40–1.

NURSING GUIDE TO PATIENT EDUCATION FOR SELF-MANAGEMENT: TREATMENT AND PREVENTION OF BLEPHARITIS, HORDEOLUM, AND CHALAZION

Instruct the patient to:

Wash hands before touching eyes.
Apply warm, moist compresses for 15 minutes four times per day, as described in Table 40–1.
Perform eyelid scrubs after compress application.
- Rub baby shampoo in a horizontal motion over closed eyelids at the eyelid/eyelash line using a finger tip or cotton swab.
- Gaze downward when scrubbing the upper eyelid and upward when scrubbing the lower eyelid.

Instill prescribed antibiotic ointment, as described in Table 39-3.
Avoid driving if ointment makes vision blurry.
Wear sunglasses or hats with wide brims to reduce photophobia.
Take acetaminophen as directed for pain caused by hordeolum.
Avoid scratching or rubbing the eye to prevent further irritation or spread of infection.
Avoid attempting to burst a hordeolum.
Notify ophthalmologist if eye becomes red or if purulent drainage occurs.
Avoid sharing washcloths or towels with other family members.
Remove makeup daily.
Avoid sharing cosmetics.
Avoid use of perfumed soap or other chemical irritants.

irritants such as smoke and chemicals. When such an irritant is encountered by a previously exposed patient, histamine and other inflammatory mediators are released. Histamine-sensitive blood vessels are stimulated, and vasodilation occurs. These blood vessels can leak fluid, causing tissue edema. Allergic conjunctivitis may be seasonal in its occurrence.

Bacterial conjunctivitis is most often due to gram-positive or gram-negative bacteria, such as *Pneumococcus, Staphylococcus, Neisseria gonorrhoeae,* and *Streptococcus.* Bacterial conjunctivitis is also referred to as pink eye and is highly communicable. It generally begins in one eye but may be transmitted to the other eye by accidental contamination.

CLINICAL MANIFESTATIONS

Common symptoms of conjunctivitis include itching, burning, photophobia, and the sensation of a foreign body in the eye. Ptosis, exudation or drainage, hyperemia (increased prominence of conjunctival blood vessels) (Fig. 40–2), and chemosis (conjunctival edema) may be evident. The texture of the conjunctiva becomes uneven and irregular, with follicles and exudate noted.

Specific types of conjunctivitis have key characteristics. In allergic conjunctivitis, itching is the primary symptom. It is accompanied by a smooth conjunctiva, tearing, and bilateral redness. Bacterial conjunctivitis, on the other hand, presents with marked hyperemia, mild conjunctival edema, and epiphora. Discharge is initially watery but progresses to a purulent state.

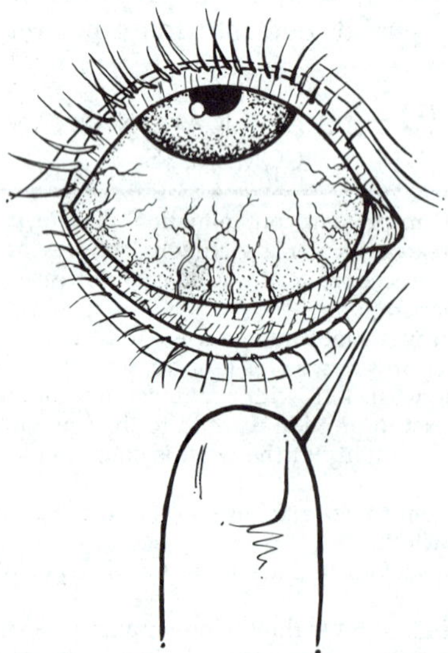

Figure 40–2.
Hyperemia associated with conjunctivitis.

MEDICAL DIAGNOSIS

A complete history is obtained to check for recent exposure to bacteria, viruses, or allergens. Swabs or scrapings of the conjunctiva and cornea may be taken to assist in identifying a causative organism.

MEDICAL MANAGEMENT

Medical management depends on the cause of the conjunctivitis. Allergic conjunctivitis is treated by topical instillation of various ophthalmic eye drops. These include corticosteroid eye drops such as prednisone acetate (Econopred Plus) and vasoconstrictors for short-term use as well as antiallergy drugs such as sodium cromoglycate (cromolyn sodium), which inhibits the release of histamine.

Bacterial conjunctivitis is treated with antibiotics appropriate for the organism. Patients are started on a broad-spectrum antibiotic as soon as the cultures are taken. Once the microorganism is identified, the antibiotic is changed if needed.

Application of the Nursing Process to the Care of the Patient with Conjunctivitis

Assessment

The assessment of a patient with conjunctivitis begins with a detailed history. Carefully note complaints of itchy, watery eyes, foreign body sensation, photophobia, presence of drainage, or change in vision. Ask the patient about sensitivity to pollen, dust, feathers, foods, materials, cosmetics, and drugs. Note any systemic disease such as asthma or sexually transmitted disease. Have the patient document any recent exposure to irritants such as smoke, tobacco, or noxious chemicals. Ask about previous episodes of similar symptoms and, if acknowledged, whether they are seasonal. Inquire about recent travel to dry climates and places with poor hygiene. Determine whether the patient uses cosmetics or borrows them from others.

After taking the history, examine the eyes. Test visual acuity. Note whether the patient is squinting or attempting to keep the eyes closed because of photophobia. Observe for drainage in the eyes or on the eyelashes. Note amount, color, and character (clear, white, purulent, ropelike, or patchy). Check eyelid position, keeping in mind that the upper eyelid should rest at the superior limbus, where the cornea and sclera meet. Inspect the bulbar conjunctiva for abnormally prominent blood vessels, a pink overcast to the sclera such as is common in pinkeye, and edema. Remember that the bulbar conjunctiva is normally smooth and flat. Expose the palpebral conjunctiva by gently pulling the eyelid down against the cheekbone. Look for deviations from its normal flat, smooth, pale-pink appearance. For example, it may be beefy red with an irregular, or cobblestone, texture.

Nursing Diagnoses and Planning

Nursing diagnoses and related expected patient outcomes most commonly applicable to the patient with conjunctivitis include the following:

NDx: Pain related to the inflammatory process

Planning: Patient outcomes
1. Patient denies photophobia.
2. Patient reports relief of pain and itching.

NDx: High risk for altered health maintenance related to insufficient knowledge of cause, prevention of recurrence, spread of conjunctivitis

Planning: Patient outcomes
1. Patient lists causes of conjunctivitis.
2. Patient describes measures to prevent recurrence.
3. Patient describes measures to prevent spread of bacterial conjunctivitis.

Nursing Interventions

NDx: Pain

Instruct the patient in the use of comfort measures to reduce pain and itching. These include the use of cool compresses and refrigeration of eye drop medications, so the medication is cool when instilled.

Instruct the patient to reduce the effects of photophobia by wearing sunglasses or wide-brimmed hats and using window shades. To prevent rubbing the eye, assist the patient to identify a substitute activity such as scratching the cheek. Instruct the patient to perform the substitute activity whenever an overwhelming urge to rub the eye occurs.

Encourage the patient to avoid use of perfumed soaps and makeup because these contain chemicals that may cause itching. Provide information on available hypoallergenic soaps and cosmetics.

NDx: High risk for altered health maintenance

Explain the causes of conjunctivitis to the patient. Instruct the patient in how to prevent transmission and recurrence of the conjunctivitis, as indicated in Chart 40–2.

Evaluation

Evaluate the effectiveness of nursing care for a patient with conjunctivitis by comparing the patient's

Chart 40–2.

NURSING GUIDE TO PATIENT EDUCATION FOR SELF-MANAGEMENT: PREVENTION OF SPREAD OF CONJUNCTIVITIS

Instruct the patient to:

Remember that vision may be blurred if ophthalmic ointment is used.
Avoid touching the infected eye.
Wash hands before and after applying soaks, instilling medication, or otherwise touching the infected eye.
Use disposable tissues to wipe drainage.
Dispose of used tissues in an appropriate container and then wash hands.
When washing the face, perform the following steps in sequence: Wash noninfected eye, wash infected eye, rinse washcloth, wash remainder of face.
Keep washcloth and towel separate from those of others in the household.
Launder washcloth, towel, and pillowcase separately from those of others in the household.

status with the expected patient outcomes. Examples of specific outcomes for patients with conjunctivitis have been provided in the Planning section.

Dacryocystitis

ETIOLOGY AND PATHOPHYSIOLOGY

Dacryocystitis is an infection of the nasolacrimal sac or duct. It occurs in both acute and chronic forms and is found with greatest frequency in postmenopausal women. Dacryocystitis frequently begins with an acute punctal obstruction followed by discharge from the puncta. *Staphylococcus aureus* and beta-hemolytic *Streptococcus* are causes of acute dacryocystitis. *Candida albicans* and *Streptococcus pneumoniae* are causes of chronic dacryocystitis.

Table 40–2. NASOLACRIMAL MASSAGE

1. Wash hands to reduce microorganisms.
2. Put on gloves to create a barrier.
3. Apply warm, moist compresses as described in Table 40–1 to loosen secretions.
4. Tell the patient to close eyes to reduce chance of injury.
5. Depress medial canthus with index finger to create pressure in the nasolacrimal system.
6. Hold for 3 to 5 seconds and then release to create a milking action, which reduces obstruction.
7. Repeat several times.
8. Note any purulent matter forced through the puncta.
9. Wipe away any drainage to reduce chance for microorganism spread.

CLINICAL MANIFESTATIONS

A raised, warm, red area is noted near the medial canthus. When pressure is applied to the medial canthus, purulent material may exude through the puncta.

MEDICAL DIAGNOSIS

Diagnosis of dacryocystitis is made on the basis of history, test of visual acuity, and examination of the external eye with the slit lamp. If appropriate, a culture of drainage may be taken.

MEDICAL MANAGEMENT

Symptomatic management is the first step in the treatment of dacryocystitis. Patients apply warm, moist compresses to the eye and follow with massage over the lacrimal sac at the medial canthus (Table 40–2).

Dacryocystitis tends to recur. If it is resistant to treatment, or in cases of recurrence, antibiotics may be necessary.

In selected cases, surgical intervention may be necessary to bypass obstruction in the nasolacrimal duct or sac or obstruction in the nose from chronic sinusitis, tumor, injury, or other nasal lesion. Because significant bleeding can occur during the surgery, medications such as aspirin and nonsteroidal anti-inflammatory drugs that can affect platelet function and predispose the patient to potential bleeding problems are usually discontinued for a few days before surgery. In selected cases, nasal packing may be inserted during surgery and removed the next day.

Application of the Nursing Process to the Care of the Patient with Dacryocystitis

Assessment

Obtain a history of the problem. Ask when this episode began and whether it is the first occurrence. Inquire about associated incidents. Question about the presence of epiphora and any history of injury to the face or orbit, recurrent sinusitis, or nasal lesions. Carefully review the use of any prescribed or over-the-counter medications. Specifically, note the use of aspirin or nonsteroidal anti-inflammatory agents.

Check visual acuity to determine baseline status, and assess the external eye. Observe for redness and irritation of the periorbital area caused by excessive tear production. Observe for drainage and, if present, note the amount and color. Inspect the eyelid/eyelash margins for lesions and the conjunctiva for redness, elevation, or irregularities in its normally smooth appearance. Observe the area around the nasal puncta, noting any redness or elevated areas.

Nursing Diagnoses and Planning

Nursing diagnoses and related expected patient outcomes most commonly applicable to the patient with dacryocystitis include the following:

NDx: High risk for infection related to presence of microorganisms near the eye

Planning: Patient outcomes
1. Ocular area is free of redness.
2. Ocular area is free of purulent drainage.

NDx: High risk for altered skin integrity related to local irritation of tissues from tears

Planning: Patient outcomes
1. Periocular skin is intact.
2. Periocular skin is free of redness.

NDx: High risk for altered health maintenance related to insufficient knowledge of compress application, nasal punctal massage, and eye drop instillation

Planning: Patient outcomes
1. Patient applies warm, moist compresses correctly.
2. Patient aseptically instills eye drops or ointments.
3. Patient performs nasal punctal massage correctly.

Nursing Interventions

NDx: High risk for infection
Stress to the patient the importance of hand washing before touching the eye, and observe the patient's hand-washing technique. Instruct the patient to wipe secretions from the medial to lateral canthus and to dispose of tissues carefully to avoid microorganism spread. Teach the patient to apply warm, moist compresses and to perform nasal punctal massage to maintain patency and promote drainage of ocular secretions. Review the use of prescribed antibiotics, and instruct the patient to report signs and symptoms of ocular infection immediately.

NDx: High risk for altered skin integrity
Advise the patient to use gentle, fragrance-free soap, to rinse well, and to dry thoroughly using soft tissue or cloths. Promote nasolacrimal drainage by applying warm, moist compresses and performing punctal massage. Keep the ocular area free from secretions as much as possible.

NDx: High risk for altered health maintenance
Teach the patient to apply warm, moist compresses (see Table 40–1), instill eye drops (see Table 39–3) using the nasal punctal occlusion technique (Table 40–3), and perform nasal punctal massage (see Table 40–2).

Additional Interventions
If surgery is required, provide general preoperative and postoperative care as described for the patient having ocular surgery in Chapter 39. In addition, if a packing is in place, advise the patient not to blow the nose forcibly. Also observe for bloody drainage oozing through the packing, and notify the ophthalmologist immediately should it occur.

Evaluation

Evaluate the effectiveness of nursing care for a patient with dacryocystitis by comparing the patient's status with the expected patient outcomes. Examples of specific outcomes for patients with dacryocystitis have been provided in the Planning section.

Table 40–3. OCCLUSION OF THE NASAL PUNCTA

1. Wash hands to reduce microorganisms.
2. Place index finger over medial canthus.
3. Apply gentle pressure to occlude the puncta.
4. Hold for several minutes to prevent outflow of medication.

Keratitis

ETIOLOGY AND PATHOPHYSIOLOGY

Keratitis is an inflammation or infection of the cornea. If a microorganism is involved, it may also be referred to as a corneal ulcer. The normally transparent and avascular cornea covers the anterior one sixth of the eye and is in almost constant contact with the environment. This predisposes it to inflammation and infection, although it is continually bathed with tears, which moisten it and remove microorganisms. Keratitis can be caused by exposure to the environment or to microorganisms such as bacteria, fungi, viruses, and amebae. Exposure keratitis can develop when the eye fails to close completely, such as after a cerebrovascular accident or in cases of Bell's palsy or exophthalmos. Because of incomplete closure, the cornea obtains insufficient moisture, and multiple small areas of breakdown in the corneal epithelium occur.

Microbial infection can occur when the corneal integrity is disturbed by trauma, surgery, or injury from chemicals or mechanical forces, and a portal of entrance for microorganisms is created. If the microorganisms invade only the superficial layers of the cornea, complete healing is possible. However, if infection spreads deep into the stroma and endothelium, scar tissue may form. If scarring results, a corneal transplant may be necessary to restore clarity.

Herpes simplex keratitis (HSV), caused by herpes simplex virus 1, is the primary cause of corneal ulceration in the United States (Vaughan et al, 1992). This form of keratitis is normally self-limiting, but in the immunocompromised patient, such as the person receiving radiation or chemotherapy, it can invade the stroma and cause opacities.

CLINICAL MANIFESTATIONS

Clinical manifestations vary with the causative factor. A dry, scratchy, "foreign body" sensation is experienced with exposure keratitis. Exposed areas of the conjunctiva are red and swollen with small erosions seen on the lower one third to one half of the cornea. Symptoms of bacterial keratitis include epiphora, reduced visual acuity, photophobia, iridescent vision, and frequently a mucopurulent discharge. Ocular pain as well as a hypopyon (a collection of purulent material in the anterior chamber) may also be present.

MEDICAL DIAGNOSIS

A history of any recent ocular injury, surgery, abrasions, or exposure to viruses is obtained, and baseline visual acuity is assessed. Scrapings of observable lesions or corneal swabs of drainage are obtained and cultured. Slit-lamp examination is done after a topical dye, such as fluorescein, is instilled to highlight areas of nonintact corneal epithelium.

MEDICAL MANAGEMENT

Medical management depends on the specific cause of the keratitis or ulcer. Exposure keratitis is treated with an ocular lubricant ointment (Hypotears Ointment, Lacri-Lube S.O.P., Refresh P.M.) composed of petrolatum, lanolin, and mineral oil. These products melt and are spread by the tear film over the external eye and thus decrease ocular dryness. If ocular lubrication is still insufficient, an eye patch may be applied (see Table 39–4) to help the eyelid protect the cornea. Soft contact lenses may be tried to protect the eye and to decrease the irritative force of the eyelid against the cornea. If these measures are insufficient, the eyelid may be sutured closed.

Microbial keratitis is treated with an anti-infective to which the microorganism is sensitive. For patients with known or suspected cases of bacterial keratitis, antibiotic treatment is instituted as soon as a list of allergies, as well as needed smears and scrapings, is obtained. Broad-spectrum antibiotics, such as fortified cefazolin (Ancef), tobramycin (Tobrex), or gentamicin (Genoptic), are prescribed until the exact causative organism is determined.

Severity of the ulcer determines the frequency of eye drop instillation and location of patient care. The presence of large or deep corneal ulcers requires one or two eye drops to be administered on an hourly schedule, with each eye drop's instillation time evenly spaced. For instance, if fortified cefazolin (Ancef) and gentamicin (Genoptic) are each ordered every hour, one is administered on the hour and the other on the half-hour.

Herpes simplex virus 1 infections are treated with antiviral agents such as idoxuridine (Stoxil), vidarabine (Vira-A), trifluridine (Viroptic), and acyclovir. Corticosteroids must be avoided because their immunosuppressive ability enhances activity of the virus and places the patient at risk for secondary infection.

Application of the Nursing Process to the Care of the Patient with Keratitis

Assessment

Begin assessment of a patient with known or suspected keratitis or corneal ulcer with a detailed history. Ask what led the patient to seek treatment (e.g., a red or painful eye, a severe foreign body feeling, or drainage). Determine when the problem started, whether it has gotten worse, and what treatments have been tried such as over-the-counter eye drops or ointments. Inquire about other problems such as photophobia, epiphora, change in vision, and ocular drainage. Do not limit the discussion of other problems to eye problems because viral keratitis can cause skin eruptions, severe pain, and influenza-like symptoms. Have the patient describe pain on a scale of 1 to 10, because the level of pain experienced may be disproportionate to symptoms demonstrated. If the patient wears contact lenses, ask about lens-care practices because contact lens wearers' use of homemade saline or hydrogen peroxide contact lens cleaning solutions have been identified as contributing factors in the development of *Acanthamoeba* keratitis.

Carefully explore any travel to developing countries or areas where contact with contaminated water may have occurred. Also note any recent ocular injury, trauma, or minor abrasion. Remember that patients may try to downplay or deny an injury, thinking it too minor to mention.

Review medications the patient is currently using, and note the use of oral or topical steroids.

Assess visual acuity and ask whether any recent changes have been noticed. Note the amount and color of any drainage present.

Nursing Diagnoses and Planning

Nursing diagnoses and related expected patient outcomes most commonly applicable to patients with keratitis or a corneal ulcer include the following:

NDx: Sensory/perceptual alteration: vision, related to impaired corneal transparency

Planning: Patient outcomes
1. Patient demonstrates techniques to maximize use of existing vision.
2. Patient reports improved visual acuity.

NDx: Sleep pattern disturbance related to need for frequent eye drops

Planning: Patient outcomes
1. Patient rests and sleeps when possible given constraints of treatment.
2. Patient is oriented to time, place, and person.
3. Patient is cooperative.
4. Patient denies irritability.

NDx: High risk for injury related to impaired ability to process sensory information from the environment and presence in an unfamiliar location

Planning: Patient outcomes
1. Patient avoids falls.
2. Patient avoids injury to the eye, self, or others.

NDx: Pain related to corneal nerve fiber irritation

Planning: Patient outcomes
1. Patient states that pain-control measures have reduced or eliminated pain.
2. Patient reports pain is at a manageable level.

Nursing Interventions

The best treatment for keratitis is prevention. Identify and closely monitor patients at risk for exposure keratitis such as those on ventilators, those who are comatose, those with exophthalmos, and those who have had a cerebrovascular accident. Instill ocular lubricant ointments as ordered, at least every 8 hours (see Table 39–3). If necessary, apply an eye patch over the closed eyelid, as described in Table 39–4.

Remember that once corneal integrity is interrupted, either by superficial erosions or by an ulcer, the potential for infection or spread of infection is increased. Wash hands before and after examining the ocular area or administering drops or ointment. Wear gloves if secretions are present to create a barrier between self and the drainage. Remove drainage from the external eye with a cotton ball moistened with ocular irrigating solution (Dacriose). Cleanse from the medial to the lateral canthus, adhering to the principles of clean area to dirty. Dispose of soiled cotton balls and gloves in accordance with Universal Precaution technique and institutional protocols for handling infectious waste. Follow the steps outlined in Table 39–3 for eye drop instillation.

Administer and store fortified eye drops at the patient's bedside to reduce the chance for microbial spread. Keep the medications on ice to maintain their pharmacologic properties. Enclosing the bottle of eye drops in a resealable plastic bag that is placed in a basin of ice works well.

If patients are to receive the same eye drops in each eye, such as timolol maleate (Timoptic), use separate bottles, clearly labeled OS (oculus sinister) and OD (oculus dexter), designating the left eye or right eye, respectively. This separation decreases the chance of microbial spread from the infected eye to the other eye.

NDx: Sensory/perceptual alteration: vision
Determine the patient's existing visual acuity. Find out what activities the patient believes he or she is having difficulty performing. Adjust the environment to facilitate patient independence. If glare is a problem, promote the use of indirect lighting and the wearing of hats or sunglasses. Try to maintain a consistent location for the patient's belongings.

If the patient has difficulty with reading, encourage the use of large-print materials and audiovisual programs. Remember that eye ointments may affect the clarity of vision, further reducing acuity.

NDx: Sleep pattern disturbance
Medical treatment of keratitis frequently involves administering one to several kinds of eye drops to patients, each on their own hourly basis. This treatment pattern prevents a normal sleep cycle and may produce a state of acute confusion (Orticio, 1990). Allow the patient as much rest as possible, given the treatment plan, by providing a calm, restful environment, drawing the drapes, dimming the lights, playing quiet music, and maintaining a quiet room.

Allow the patient as many uninterrupted sleep cycles as possible. Group together required care activities such as measuring vital signs and performing activities of daily living. Be alert for indications of sleep deprivation, such as irritability, short attention span, limited short-term memory, and forgetfulness. Reassure the patient that these symptoms are normal and temporary. Recognize that he or she may be very concerned about not being a "good patient." Try to allay those concerns. Set up designated rest periods. Post a note on the door, and act as the patient's advocate. Permit the patient to be disturbed only for emergency measures or for those situations he or she had indicated.

NDx: High risk for injury
When patients whose vision is already limited by the effects of inflammation are admitted to a hospital, a complete orientation to the environment is essential. Find out what the patient can see and what needs to be pointed out to him or her. Help the patient identify the location of objects in the room. Move low objects such as wastebaskets and footstools, rolling equipment such as a sphygmomanometer, and small objects such as telephone cords out of the commonly traveled paths in the room. Avoid giving straws to patients with reduced vision. Their visual limitations can alter depth perception, which makes hand-eye coordination difficult. The patient could easily poke his or her eye while attempting to drink through a straw. Allow the patient to unpack so he or she knows where articles have been placed. Keep articles in the place designated. Be sure to illuminate corners of the patient's room, avoiding shadows where small objects can hide.

NDx: Pain
Pain associated with keratitis can range from absent to severe. Have the patient rate the pain on a scale of 1 to 10 to obtain a baseline. Note whether the patient is shielding the eyes from the light. If pain is accompanied by photophobia, reduce room lighting to a minimum. Use indirect lighting to provide adequate illumination for safety. Encourage the use of window shades, sunglasses, and hats.

Administer ordered analgesics as needed. A typical order would be for acetaminophen or acetaminophen with codeine. Oral analgesics usually provide adequate analgesia. Initiate nonpharmacologic interventions such as distraction with music, television, visitors, a cool cloth to the forehead, or warm compresses to the inflamed facial lesions. Be certain to monitor the patient's rating of pain after intervention.

Evaluation

Evaluate the effectiveness of nursing care for a patient with keratitis by comparing the patient's status with the expected patient outcomes. Examples of specific outcomes for patients with keratitis have been provided in the Planning section.

Endophthalmitis

Endophthalmitis is the infection or inflammation of the internal eye. It is one of the most dreaded ocular phenomena because it can cause significant, dramatic, and permanent loss of vision if not rapidly detected and treated.

ETIOLOGY AND PATHOPHYSIOLOGY

Microorganisms can enter the eye in a variety of ways. They can enter through penetrating or perforating injuries associated with trauma, through suture tracks or wound dehiscence after surgery, as a result of contaminated instruments or poor technique during surgery, or as a result of spread via the blood stream. Blood-stream transmission has been associated with use of shared needles for intravenous drug use (Boyd-Monk & Steinmetz, 1987). Endophthalmitis can also be triggered by retained lens material.

Virulent organisms associated with the development of endophthalmitis include *Staphylococcus aureus*, *Staphylococcus epidermidis*, *Streptococcus* species, *Pseudomonas aeruginosa*, *Klebsiella*, *Proteus*, and *Serratia*.

The vitreous is an excellent medium for promoting bacterial growth. After bacterial invasion, the vitreous liquefies; then an abscess forms (Vaughan et al, 1992).

CLINICAL MANIFESTATIONS

Onset of symptoms occurs one to several days after injury or surgery (Friedberg & Rapuano, 1990). There is a progressive decline in visual acuity as well as an increase in ocular redness and pain.

Cells and flare indicative of inflammation are present in the anterior chamber. Corneal edema and conjunctival elevation may be present. A reduced red reflex may be noted. Purulent discharge may be seen on the eyelids or in the anterior chamber

(Friedberg & Rapuano, 1990). Patients complain of severe, throbbing eye pain. Headache and drowsiness may be present.

MEDICAL DIAGNOSIS

Specimens are taken from the external eye and the anterior chamber for culture and sensitivity.

In some cases, a tap of the vitreous may be performed. If the fundus cannot be visualized, ultrasonography may be done.

MEDICAL MANAGEMENT

As soon as cultures and smears are obtained, treatment with topical, subconjunctival, and intravenous broad-spectrum antibiotics is instituted. Intravitreal antibiotics may be administered at the time of the vitreous tap.

In selected cases, a vitrectomy may be performed to remove contents of the infected vitreous, reduce the population of microorganisms, and permit the instillation of intravitreal antibiotics.

Maintenance of globe integrity is the minimum goal. However, this may not be possible and phthisis bulbi, a shrunken eyeball, may result.

Application of the Nursing Process to the Care of the Patient with Endophthalmitis

Assessment

Perform a quick, detailed, accurate assessment. Failure to ask an important history question, correctly triage a telephone call, or make a pertinent observation can have sight-threatening consequences. Any patient reporting a sudden change in visual acuity accompanied by purulent discharge or pain must be seen and assessed immediately.

Note the patient's presentation in the examination room. Observe whether the patient is sitting comfortably in the chair, holding the head, or covering the eyes or whether he or she is asleep. These latter signs are indicative of eye pain, photophobia, or fatigue.

If the patient is uncomfortable, dim the room lights and ask whether she or he feels up to answering a few questions. Use direct questions to make responses easier. Allow the patient to expound on responses as needed. Clarify responses as appropriate. Ask when the pain or problem started, and what is remembered about when it started. Sometimes patients remark that the pain or problem started shortly after an object "hit me in the eye." If the patient can remember when it started, ask whether anything unusual happened a few days beforehand. Prompt as necessary with questions like "Did you injure your eye?" or "Do you feel like you got poked in the eye?"

Question about the development of the problem. Has it become worse, stayed the same, or started to improve? Inquire whether any other problems such as pain, difficulty with bright lights, drainage, nausea, or poor vision have been noted.

Specifically ask about the nature of the patient's work. Take special note if the patient works with or near machinery capable of throwing off high-speed particles of wood, metal, or plastic. These particles can enter the eye and trigger a severe inflammatory response. Also note any recent surgery, because endophthalmitis can occur from 1 to 3 days to longer than a month after surgery.

Determine what, if any, measures the patient has tried to decrease the symptoms. Follow up with an even more important question: How effective have these interventions been?

Ask about existing medical conditions. Take special note of a history of diabetes or immunosuppressive conditions such as cancer and related chemotherapy or radiation therapy or acquired immunodeficiency syndrome (AIDS).

Ask specifically about the use of nonprescribed medications such as over-the-counter or street drugs. Endophthalmitis can be a sequela of drug-related sharing of needles. Patients are usually frightened enough to be honest. However, if areas of the arms are exposed, observe for needle marks or tracks.

Test visual acuity. Ask whether this acuity is any different from the usual baseline. If any previous records are available, compare the findings.

Measure intraocular pressure (IOP). It may be elevated because the waste products of the inflammatory process can obstruct the trabecular meshwork, reducing outflow of aqueous humor.

Examine the external eye. If drainage is present, wear gloves. Note the color and amount of drainage. Obtain a culture of the drainage, and then wipe away excess drainage.

Compare the right pupil with the left pupil, noting size, shape, and reactivity of each pupil. Observe and document any redness or elevation of the conjunctiva or sclera. Examine the cornea for clarity. Is it clear or hazy? Observe for the red reflex because it may be absent in severe cases of inflammation.

Nursing Diagnoses and Planning

Nursing diagnoses and related expected patient outcomes most commonly applicable to the patient with endophthalmitis include the following:

NDx: Anxiety related to sudden onset of symptoms and uncertain outcomes of the problem

Planning: Patient outcomes

1. Behavioral signs of severe anxiety are absent.
2. Patient reports that anxiety is at a manageable level.

NDx: Pain related to ocular inflammation

Planning: Patient outcomes

1. Patient reports pain reduced to tolerable level or eliminated.
2. Behavioral signs of severe pain are absent.

Nursing Interventions

NDx: Anxiety

These patients are usually extremely anxious. In most cases, they have gone from a normal baseline visual acuity to a severely reduced one. Patients may wonder whether the problem was caused by something they did or failed to do. Provide needed reassurance tempered with reality. Be sure the patient realizes the seriousness of the problem but that all needed measures and treatments are being performed. Provide accurate information throughout the course of treatment, making sure the patient's questions are answered as soon as possible. If uncertain about how to answer a given question, refer that question to another care provider.

People respond differently to anxious situations. Be sensitive to clues of anxious behavior demonstrated by the patient. Find out how the patient has dealt with anxious feelings in the past and assist her or him to implement those positive interventions.

NDx: Pain

Eye pain can be severe in endophthalmitis. Assist the patient to identify factors such as bright light that make the pain worse. Attempt to modify the environment as needed to promote comfort. Provide distraction with television, quiet music, or conversation, and place a cool or warm cloth over the closed eyelids.

Administer oral or intramuscular analgesics as needed. Remember to monitor comfort level after instituting either type of measure.

Additional Interventions

Other interventions are similar to those needed by the patient with keratitis who is frequently receiving eye drops.

Evaluation

Evaluate the effectiveness of nursing care for the patient with endophthalmitis by comparing the patient's status with the expected patient outcomes. Examples of specific outcomes for a patient with endophthalmitis have been provided in the Planning section.

Structural Disorders

Refractive Errors

ETIOLOGY AND PATHOPHYSIOLOGY

The axial length of the eye and its refractive power combine to focus images clearly on the retina (emmetropia) (Fig. 40–3*A*). Myopia, or nearsightedness, is caused by either an increase in the length of the eye or a refractive ability greater than necessary for the length of the eye. In myopia, images destined for the retina fall short of the retina, causing the image to appear unfocused (Fig. 40–3*B*).

Hyperopia, or farsightedness, is just the opposite. A short length of the eye, or a refractive ability weaker than necessary for the length of the eye, may cause the image to be focused behind the retina (Fig. 40–3C).

Astigmatism is caused by a variation in the corneal curvature. Light rays arriving from different directions are not focused equally. Images fall distorted on the retina.

Presbyopia occurs as a normal phenomenon associated with the aging process. The lens, and the fibers holding it in place, age, making the adjustments necessary to focus near images on the retina difficult. As a result, images are focused behind the retina.

Aphakia means absence of a lens. It is the state that occurs after surgical removal of the lens. Because the adjustments in the shape of the lens focus images on the retina, its absence drastically alters the patient's near vision. Images are focused well behind the retina.

CLINICAL MANIFESTATIONS

Patients with a refractive error may have vague complaints, such as visual fatigue, discomfort, or headache. They may notice, or others may notice them, rubbing their eyes or squinting.

MEDICAL DIAGNOSIS

Baseline visual acuity is measured, and, through a process called "refraction," refractive error is diagnosed. The patient is seated in the examination chair and is asked to view a Snellen chart located in the distance. In a systematic manner, lenses of varying powers are placed in front of the eye. The patient is asked to state when the images or pictures are clearest. The lenses used to adjust the focusing ability of the eye have their power expressed in units of measure referred to as diopters.

MEDICAL MANAGEMENT

Because the anteroposterior length of the eye cannot be adjusted, refractive errors must be treated by changing the focusing ability. In myopia, the eye's focusing ability is too great for its length. A concave, or "minus" diopter, lens is used to reduce the fo-

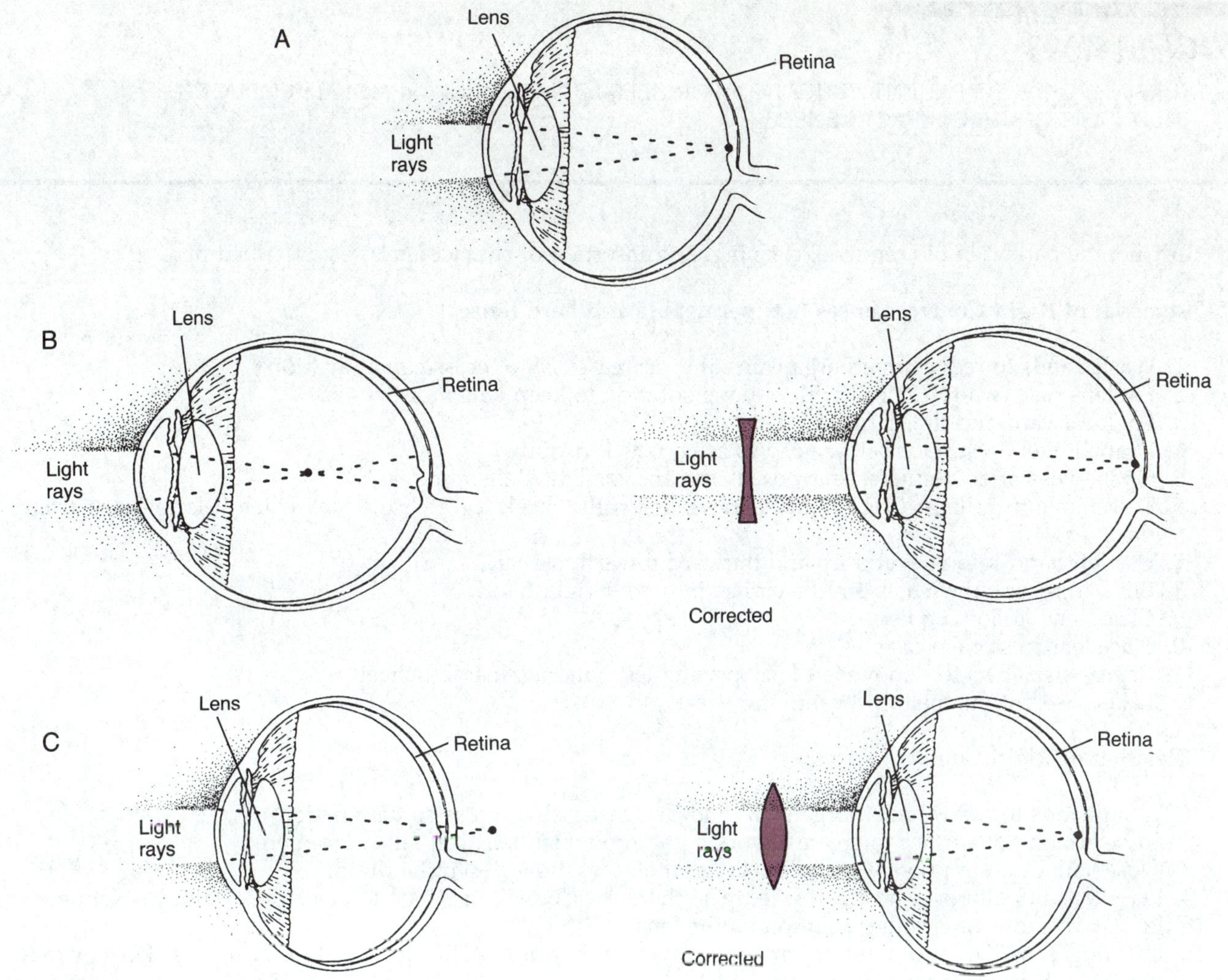

Figure 40–3.

A, Light rays are focused directly on the retina, resulting in a clear visual image (emmetropia). *B*, In myopia, light rays are focused anterior to the retina. A concave lens moves the focus back onto the retina and results in a clear image. *C*, In hyperopia, light rays are focused posterior to the retina. A convex lens moves the focus forward so that the light rays fall directly on the retina.

cusing ability. Strength of a concave lens would be expressed as −3.00 diopters or minus three diopters.

A "plus" diopter, or convex, lens adds focusing power to the eye. Plus diopter lenses are used to treat hyperopia. For example, a convex lens might be expressed at +2.50 diopters.

Presbyopia is also treated with a convex lens. Presbyopic correction is "added" to the patient's usual lenses. Patients not needing distance correction can wear special eyeglasses just for close work, or near vision. These eyeglasses are referred to as "readers."

Astigmatism is corrected with a lens of one-sided curvature (Boyd-Monk & Steinmetz, 1987). When this lens is used, the focusing ability of the cornea in different planes is adjusted.

There are several options for visual correction of refractive errors. Each method of correction has advantages and disadvantages.

Glasses are the easiest and least expensive method of visual correction. They are easy to adapt to using; however, they alter a person's body image and make objects in the peripheral vision seem out of focus compared with those viewed through the eyeglasses.

Eyeglasses may not always be an option. After cataract surgery on one eye, the patient experiences monocular aphakia (one eye without a lens). A strongly powered "plus," or concave, lens would be needed to bring images into focus. However, this strongly powered concave lens distorts images and makes them seem much larger. Images seen through this type of strong lens appear 33% larger than normal. The brain attempts to fuse the two images but cannot.

Contact lenses are made of durable plastic and float on the tear film in front of the cornea. With blinking, tears are forced under the edges of the contact lens. The tears float debris away from the contact lens and provide moisture to the cornea. In contact lens fitting sessions, measurements are taken

Chart 40–3.

NURSING GUIDE TO PATIENT EDUCATION FOR SELF-MANAGEMENT: REMOVAL, CLEANING, AND INSERTION OF CONTACT LENSES

Instruct the patient in the removal, cleaning, and insertion of contact lenses as described here.

Removal of Rigid Contact Lenses (gas permeable and hard lenses)

1. Wash hands to reduce microorganisms and decrease risk of cross contamination.
2. Fill lens case two-thirds full with soaking solution to keep lens moist.
3. Look forward and flex chin slightly.
4. Drape towel on surface below head to catch lens if dropped.
5. Open eyes widely to increase exposed area and facilitate lens removal.
6. To remove right lens: Place right hand against right cheek to catch the lens when it is released from the eye.
7. Use left hand to pull eyelid up and outward toward left ear.
8. Blink to release the lens from the cornea into your right hand.
9. Clean lens (following list).
10. Place lens in storage case.
11. Repeat steps 5–8 to remove left lens, placing left hand against left cheek.
12. Label case with name to prevent loss.

Cleaning of Rigid Contact Lenses

1. Wash hands to reduce microorganisms and decrease risk of cross contamination.
2. Lay cloth on flat surface to create a work area onto which lens can fall if dropped.
3. Close sink drain to prevent lens from accidentally washing down the drain.
4. Place lens in palm of hand open side up so there is a "bowl" in which to place the cleaning solution.
5. Place two drops of cleaning solution on the lens.
6. Use finger pad to rub solution smoothly over both sides of the lens to loosen debris. Do not use fingernail because it can damage lens.
7. Hold lens by edge and rinse with soaking solution.
8. Examine lens for cleanliness and nicks by holding it up to the light.
9. Repeat procedure for opposite lens.

Insertion of Rigid Contact Lenses

1. Wash hands to reduce microorganisms and reduce the risk of cross contamination.
2. Moisten index finger of nondominant hand with wetting solution to provide a platform for the lens.
3. Moisten both surfaces of the lens with wetting solution for comfort on insertion.
4. Position lens with closed side facing finger tip on dominant-hand index finger.
5. Look straight ahead, bending chin slightly to position the eye to receive the lens.
6. Retract the lower lid against the orbital rim with the middle finger of the nondominant hand.
7. Retract upper lid against bony margin of the brow to maximize corneal exposure.
8. Bring the finger holding the lens toward the cornea to bring lens in contact with the ocular surface.
9. Allow eyelids to close by slowly releasing the lower lid and then the upper lid. Avoid quick release of lids, which can break lens contact with the eye.
10. Do not move until the tear film has centered the lens on the cornea and vision is clear to decrease the risk of losing the lens if it has been blinked from the eye.
11. Repeat for other eye.

(continued)

Chart 40–3. *(continued)*

NURSING GUIDE TO PATIENT EDUCATION FOR SELF-MANAGEMENT: REMOVAL, CLEANING, AND INSERTION OF CONTACT LENSES

Removal of Soft Contact Lenses

1. Wash hands to reduce microorganisms and decrease risk of cross contamination.
2. Fill lens case with 0.9% saline solution to prevent damage to the lens from dehydration.
3. Gaze upward to expose area for lens removal.
4. Use dominant-hand middle finger to retract lower lid down against the cheek bone.
5. Use finger of dominant hand to slide lens onto sclera, which is less sensitive than the cornea.
6. Secure the lens between the thumb and index finger of the dominant hand and remove.
7. Place lens in saline-filled lens case.
8. Repeat for other eye if needed.
9. Label case with name to prevent loss.

Cleaning of Soft Contact Lenses

1. Wash hands to reduce microorganisms and decrease risk of cross contamination.
2. Place lens in palm of hand open side up so there is a "bowl" in which to place the cleaning solution.
3. Place several drops of cleaning solution on the lens.
4. Spread cleaning solution gently and smoothly over both surfaces of the lens to loosen debris and avoid tearing the lens.
5. Hold lens by its edge and rinse with 0.9% saline solution.
6. Inspect lens for cleanliness and damage by holding it up to the light.
7. Repeat for opposite lens.

Insertion of Soft Contact Lenses

1. Wash hands to reduce microorganisms and decrease the risk of cross contamination.
2. Remove lens from storage case using finger pad, not the fingertip, to avoid damaging the lens.
3. Place lens on index finger pad of dominant hand.
4. Look forward and flex chin slightly.
5. Use middle finger of nondominant hand to retract lower lid against cheek to expose area for lens insertion while avoiding pressure against globe.
6. Retract upper lid against eyebrow using index finger of nondominant hand.
7. Gaze slightly upward.
8. Carry lens up toward the eye, and place lens on sclera below or on the cornea.
9. Release eyelids slowly.
10. Close eyelids gently to allow lens to center.

to determine the corneal curvature and required refractive power.

The principle behind contact lenses is that changing the shape of the cornea alters its refractive ability while placing the specific refractive power where it can focus images clearly on the retina.

Contact lenses come in three forms: hard, gas permeable, and soft. The term "rigid" contact lens refers to both hard and gas permeable. There are specially shaped contact lenses for persons with astigmatism.

Rigid contact lenses are smaller than soft lenses. They fit over a portion of the cornea and provide better correction for astigmatism. However, some patients experience dry eyes or corneal warping while wearing a rigid contact lens. Warping is less a problem with gas-permeable lenses compared with hard lenses because the former permit a greater amount of oxygen to reach the cornea. The removal, cleansing, and insertion of rigid contact lenses are discussed in Chart 40–3.

Soft contact lenses are made of a less rigid plastic. They fit over the entire cornea and can be worn for a longer period of time than hard lenses because the cornea is able to receive more oxygen and nutrients. On the negative side, soft contact lenses can absorb medications; be easily damaged because of their thin, "plastic-wrap" consistency; and create difficulty for the patient with astigmatism because this lens type does not correct it as well as rigid lenses.

A specific type of soft lens, called a toric lens, is specifically designed to correct astigmatism. However, these lenses are more expensive and require careful fitting.

Soft contact lenses can be worn on a daily-wear or extended-wear basis. Extended-wear lenses are thinner than daily-wear lenses to enhance corneal oxygenation. They can be worn 24 hours a day for several days without removal. They must be removed at least weekly and thoroughly cleaned. Although promoting ease of wear, these lenses can harbor microorganisms, predisposing the patient to the development of a serious eye infection. See Chart 40–3 for instructions on the removal, cleansing, and insertion of contact lenses. Contact lenses must be disinfected using a chemical or heat method. The type of disinfection is ordered by the prescribing practitioner.

Also available and growing in popularity are disposable contact lenses. These lenses are designed to be worn for a 1- to 2-week period and have the advantages of easy use and decreased maintenance.

Contact lens wear should not be taken lightly. Complications of contact lens wear include corneal abrasions that can lead to corneal ulcers; corneal edema from insufficient oxygen reaching the cornea or from lens overwear; and giant papillary cell conjunctivitis, a sensitivity reaction seen in patients who are long-term contact lens users. Symptoms of this latter infection disappear when lenses are not worn for a while.

Indications for contact lens wear include uncomfortable fit of eyeglasses on the nose because of their weight; cosmetic appearance; need for clear peripheral vision because of occupation or leisure pursuits; monocular aphakia; and significant difference between the refractive errors of the left eye (OS) and the right eye (OD).

Contact lenses should not be worn by patients with impaired corneal sensitivity, those with a lack of manual dexterity, or those who are unable or who are not motivated to adhere to a lens care protocol. Contact lenses should not be worn by those who work in a dusty, dry, or smoky environment.

Guidelines for Application of the Nursing Process to the Care of the Patient Using Contact Lenses to Correct a Refractive Error

Assist the patient to match his or her need for visual correction, motivation, manual dexterity, and lifestyle with the appropriate method of visual rehabilitation. Identify the factor most important to the patient: appearance, cost, or ease of use as well as any limitations as a result of preexisting medical problems.

If contact lenses are considered, explore the patient's ability to meet not only the initial cost but the cost of lens-care products. If selected, instruct the patient to remove, clean, and insert the lenses, as presented in Chart 40–3.

Remind the patient not to exceed the established wearing schedule, and advise him or her to remove daily-wear contact lenses before napping or sleeping. Reinforce the importance of proper cleaning and of washing hands immediately before and after taking care of contact lenses. Stress the importance of notifying the contact lens professional if red, puffy, or watery eyes, purulent drainage, or eye pain develops.

Entropion and Ectropion

ETIOLOGY AND PATHOPHYSIOLOGY

The turning inward of the eyelid is called entropion (Fig. 40–4*A*). Ectropion is the outward turning of the eyelid (Fig. 40–4*B*). Entropion occurs as a result of the aging process, chronic inflammation, or scarring disorders such as trachoma. This change in eyelid direction may allow the eyelashes to deviate inward, brushing against the cornea and causing severe pain. Age-related entropion exclusively involves the lower eyelid (Vaughan et al, 1992), whereas other forms can involve either or both eyelids.

Ectropion occurs with aging but may also be con-

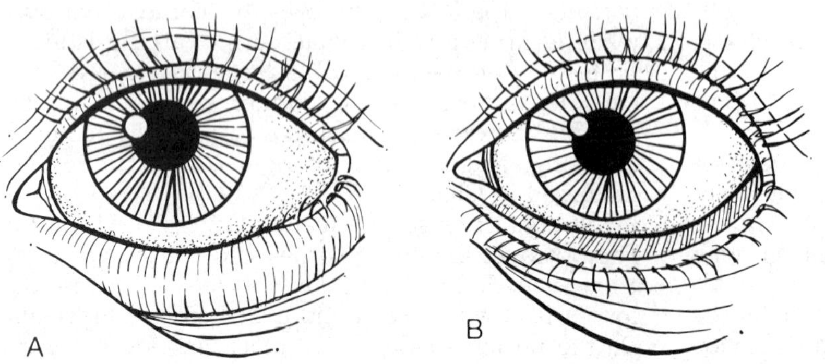

Figure 40–4.

A, Entropion. Note how lashes of the inwardly turned lower lid can rub against the globe and have the potential to cause corneal damage. *B*, Ectropion of lower lid.

genital. This outward sagging of the lower eyelid is caused by relaxation of the orbicularis oculi and is usually bilateral. Ectropion can also be caused by seventh nerve palsy. Failure to correct the eyelid position can cause skin excoriation and corneal ulceration.

CLINICAL MANIFESTATIONS

Patients with entropion complain of a "foreign body" sensation that has developed gradually. Assessment of the external eye reveals an inwardly deviated eyelid. Tearing and conjunctival injection may be present. A corneal ulcer may be noted.

With ectropion, patients complain of epiphora accompanying the corneal irritation from dry, scratchy eyes. The eye feels dry despite the tearing because the tears cannot wash correctly over the cornea to keep it moist because of the outward deviation of the lower eyelid. Instead of draining toward the medial canthus, the tears splash down onto the cheek, causing local irritation. This irritation is caused by the enzyme lysozyme, which is found in tears. If corneal drying has caused exposure keratitis, multiple dotlike areas are noted.

MEDICAL DIAGNOSIS

Diagnosis is made on the basis of history and physical examination.

The position of the eyelid is carefully noted. Schirmer's test may be used to objectively measure tear production. The cornea is stained with rose bengal to highlight areas of corneal epithelial defects caused by insufficient moisture.

MEDICAL MANAGEMENT

Entropion is treated on a temporary basis by taping the lower eyelid down and laterally with a small adhesive tape strip. On a more permanent basis, a minor surgical procedure can be performed to shorten the eyelid horizontally. In this procedure, a small segment of the orbicularis oculi and tarsus is resected (Newell, 1992).

The goal of ectropion treatment is to keep the cornea moist. Lubricating eye drops and ointments are used to protect the cornea. Acetaminophen (Tylenol) or acetaminophen with codeine (Tylenol with codeine) may be ordered for pain. Surgery may be done to invert the puncta into its normal position (Newell, 1992).

Guidelines for Application of the Nursing Process to the Care of the Patient with Entropion or Ectropion

Instruct the patient to instill ocular lubricants, drops, and ointments as ordered to keep the cornea moist and thus decrease pain resulting from ocular drying or irritation. Encourage the use of nonpharmacologic measures such as increasing hydration, increasing the moisture content of the room, and patching the eye in the closed position.

Encourage the patient to use a gentle, fragrance-free soap for cleaning the ocular area because perfumes and colors found in soaps may irritate the area and cause further drying. Remind the patient to rinse the area well to remove soap residue and to dry gently.

Cataracts

A cataract is an opacity of the crystalline lens of the eye (Fig. 40–5). Although one eye is often affected first, most cataracts ultimately become bilateral, with proportional visual loss in both eyes.

ETIOLOGY AND PATHOPHYSIOLOGY

The most common type of cataract is that associated with old age. Normally, the lens, which is composed of 65% water and 35% minerals, is clear and avascular. However, as people age, lens fibers, which continue to be produced, become more densely packed, and transparency can be lost. With age, the lens also becomes yellow. This yellowing causes colors such as blue, green, and violet to appear gray. Some evidence of cataracts can be seen in most patients older than 70 years (Vaughan et al, 1992).

Cataracts can also occur when the integrity of the lens capsule is disturbed by trauma. Fluid enters the lens, and an opacification can quickly develop. Still other causes of cataract formation include toxicity to chemicals and medications such as corticosteroids,

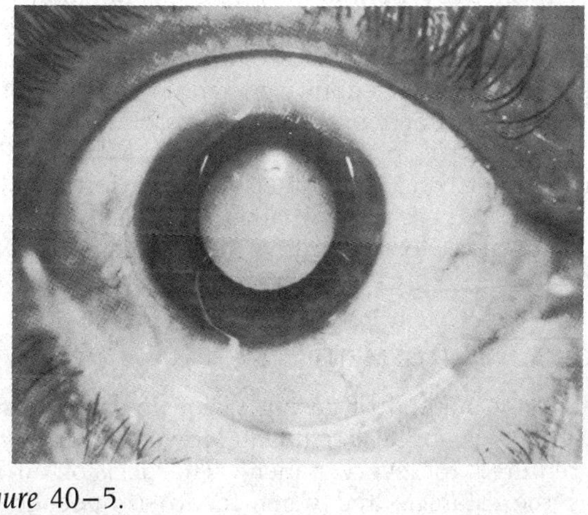

Figure 40–5.

Pupil appears white owing to an advanced cataract (opacity of the lens). (From Vaughan D, Asbury T, Tabbara K. General ophthalmology. 12th ed. Norwalk, CT: Appleton & Lange, 1989, p 147.)

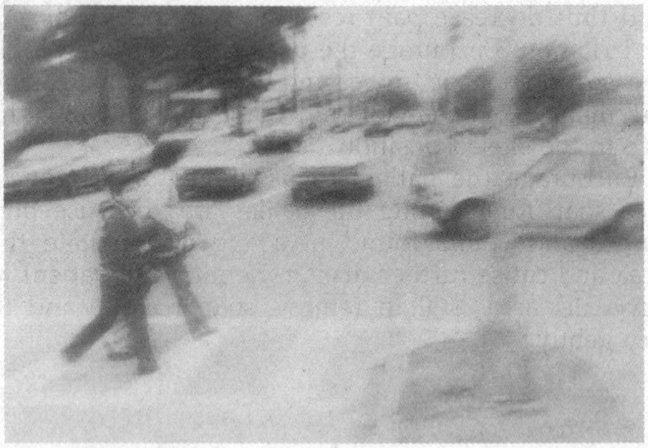

Figure 40–6.

Images as seen by a patient with a cataract. (Permission to use this photograph has been granted by the American Foundation for the Blind, 15 West 16th Street, New York, NY 10011.)

nutritional deficits, or exposure to high-voltage electricity or radiation (Coles, 1989). Cataracts progress more rapidly in diabetics than in nondiabetics.

CLINICAL MANIFESTATIONS

A gradual, painless blurring of central distance vision is the chief clinical manifestation of a cataract (Fig. 40–6). Additional symptoms may include glare spots, ghostly images, double vision in the eye as a result of the light rays being split by the opacity and falling in two places in the retina, a need for more light for reading or near work, headaches, and irritability. These symptoms may develop rapidly over several months or may arise over several years.

MEDICAL DIAGNOSIS

An advanced cataract can be seen as a white discoloration immediately behind the pupil when the eye is obliquely illuminated. Less advanced cataracts are identified by ophthalmoscopic examination and slit-lamp biomicroscopy. As part of the examination, visual acuity is measured carefully in both eyes, and a test of the patient's ability to handle glare is done.

If cataract extraction with insertion of an intraocular lens (IOL) is planned, A-scan ultrasonographic measurements and keratometry are performed. On the basis of these data, mathematic measurements are calculated to determine the focusing power needed.

MEDICAL MANAGEMENT

The only method of curing vision loss as a result of cataracts is surgical removal. However, surgery is not required for every patient. The decision to remove the cataracts and when to do so depends on changes in the cataracts over time in relationship to the patient's age, health status, visual loss, and impact on activities of daily living. Generally, cataract extraction is indicated when visual loss significantly interferes with the patient's usual activities; when vision in the better eye is less than 20/50 (American Academy of Ophthalmology, Quality of Care Committee, Anterior Segment Panel, 1989); or when there is a need for visualization or treatment of structures in the posterior segment of the eye.

Cataract surgery is usually performed under local anesthesia on an ambulatory surgery basis. An overnight stay in the hospital is needed only if complications arise, if surgery is being performed on the patient's only seeing eye, or if the patient requires monitoring of a preexisting medical problem. If both eyes are affected, the more opaque cataract is removed first and the second about a month later.

Cataract extraction leaves the patient aphakic (without lens) and requires lens replacement by an IOL implant, contact lenses, or cataract glasses. Of the three, IOL implant is rapidly becoming the preferred method of lens replacement by both patients and surgeons. The IOL is invisible and permanent and cannot be felt. It also affords the best postextraction visual correction.

Cataract glasses are the least desirable form of lens replacement. They allow good central vision but restrict peripheral vision and cause objects to appear about 30% larger than reality. As a result, objects look closer than they are and straight lines look curved. Further, because the brain cannot fuse images of very different sizes, if the lenses have not been removed from both eyes, the patient has double vision unless only one eye is focused. These visual field distortions result in difficulty walking, reaching for things, pouring liquids, and, of course, driving until the patient adjusts to them, which takes at least 4 to 8 weeks.

Contact lenses may be used by persons who are nonallergic and who have the dexterity needed to handle the required daily care for removal, cleaning, and replacement. Contact lenses are preferred over cataract glasses because of the improved image size (objects appear only 8% to 10% larger) and peripheral vision they offer. In addition, double vision does not occur even if only one lens is removed.

PHYSICAL PREPARATION OF THE PATIENT FOR CATARACT SURGERY

Before the start of surgery, the periorbital area is injected with local anesthetic. The area is cleansed with an antiseptic scrubbing solution and then sterile drapes are placed.

PROCEDURE

There are two types of cataract surgery: extracapsular and intracapsular. In extracapsular cataract extraction (ECCE), a small incision is made at the corneoscleral limbus under the operating room microscope. The eye is entered through the anterior chamber, and the anterior lens capsule is removed. The nucleus is then removed either by gentle pressure applied to the eye or by phacoemulsification, a procedure in which high-frequency sound waves delivered through an ultrasonic needle inserted into the lens are used to break the cataract into fine pieces. Phacoemulsification is increasingly used because a smaller incision is required; activity restrictions are needed for a shorter period; and healing time is reduced. With both ECCE techniques, the retained lens material is then irrigated from the eye and aspirated through an instrument. The posterior lens capsule is left in place to protect the retina and to create a supportive structure for the lens implant. If a lens is to be implanted, it is usually placed in the posterior chamber, behind the iris, and in front of the posterior lens capsule.

Intracapsular cataract extraction surgery is an older and less frequently performed technique in which a freezing probe is introduced into the eye and affixed to the lens. The lens is then removed intact, so no posterior capsule remains. If an IOL is to be implanted, it is placed in the anterior chamber, between the cornea and the iris, or sutured in the posterior chamber. This method leaves the retina and vitreous less protected.

After extraction by either procedure, the eye is sutured closed with material finer than a human hair. An antibiotic is injected subconjunctively, an ophthalmic antibiotic ointment is instilled, and an eye patch is applied over the patient's closed eyelid. A metal shield is taped in place over the eye patch.

COMPLICATIONS

Complications that can occur with or after cataract surgery include cystoid macular edema (CME), vitreous loss, expulsive hemorrhage, postoperative inflammation or infection, retinal detachment, glaucoma, or endophthalmitis. Over several weeks to months, the posterior capsule can also become opaque, causing the patient to comment that "my cataract has returned." This late opacification is treated with a laser to create a small opening through which light rays can reach the retina.

Application of the Nursing Process to the Care of the Patient Having Cataract Surgery

PREOPERATIVE NURSING CARE

Nursing care of the patient scheduled for cataract surgery is similar to that described for any patient having ocular surgery (see Chapter 39), with several considerations. Ask about the use of nonsteroidal and anti-inflammatory drugs such as ibuprofen (Motrin) or aspirin because these can affect platelet function, creating a potential for increased bleeding during surgery. Because many cataract surgery patients live alone, obtain information about the patient's social support systems. Explore who, if anyone, will be available to assist with eye drop instillation, application of the eye shield, and transportation for follow-up care visits.

Provide written preoperative instructions for the patient to take home because anxious patients may forget information. Use off-white paper to reduce glare and large-print, high-contrast letters to make reading easier. Provide a telephone number for the patient to call if questions arise.

POSTOPERATIVE NURSING CARE

Assessment

Assess the patient's return to physiologic stability. As per established institutional protocol but guided by the patient's condition, check vital signs and evaluate the dressing for evidence of bleeding.

Nursing Diagnoses and Planning

Nursing diagnoses and related expected patient outcomes most commonly applicable to patients who have had cataract extraction surgery include the following:

NDx: High risk for injury: ocular trauma and fall, related to altered depth perception, effects of medication, and presence in an unfamiliar environment

Planning: Patient outcomes
1. Patient's eye heals without evidence of trauma.
2. Patient avoids injury.

NDx: Pain related to surgical manipulation of tissue and use of suture material

Planning: Patient outcomes
1. Patient differentiates expected discomfort from pain.
2. Patient refrains from rubbing.

NDx: High risk for impaired home maintenance management related to activity restrictions imposed by surgery

Planning: Patient outcomes
1. Patient identifies home modifications necessary to coincide with activity restrictions.
2. Patient plans and prepares meals ahead.
3. Patient arranges transportation to market, follow-up care, and other locations as needed.

NDx: High risk for altered health maintenance related to insufficient knowledge of application of eye shield, eyelid hygiene, administration of medications, activity restrictions, and plans for follow-up care

Planning: Patient outcomes
1. Patient correctly applies eye shield.
2. Patient correctly cleanses eyelid.
3. Patient states name, purpose, and schedule of administration for medications.
4. Patient identifies signs and symptoms of complications to report.
5. Patient describes activity restrictions.
6. Patient describes plans for follow-up care.

Nursing Interventions

NDx: High risk for injury
Patching one eye after surgery alters depth perception. As a result, patients perceive distances to be different and objects in places where they are not. Tell the patient to hold on to handrails whenever available and to use adaptive equipment such as walkers or canes if he or she usually does so. Stress the importance of not reaching for objects, such as door frames, backs of chairs, and other furniture for support because these objects may not be where they appear, and when reaching, balance can be lost, causing a fall. Falling can rupture the stitches, which opens the wound, and can potentially cause a loss of vision. In addition, patients may also have received medications that they are not used to, such as diazepam (Valium) or midazolam (Versed). Because this can alter the patient's gait, stress the need for caution when ambulating.

Orient the patient to the surroundings. Make certain the patient knows the location of the call light, bathroom, small objects on the floor, and the side rails. Remove small objects from traveled paths if possible.

Help the patient identify and arrange for removal of hazards in the home environment. Examples of such hazards include rugs, dog dishes, and footstools.

Encourage the patient to wear the eye shield as directed. This shield protects the eye during times when an injury is more likely, such as ambulating during the night. The shield also protects the eye from accidental injury occurring from rubbing the eye during sleep.

NDx: Pain
Tell the patient to use a cool cloth on the forehead and to elevate the head slightly when in bed to promote comfort. Also instruct the patient to take acetaminophen (Tylenol) as ordered and needed. Because pain is unusual after cataract surgery, stress the importance of notifying the ophthalmologist immediately if pain occurs that is unrelieved by acetaminophen (Tylenol) or is accompanied by nausea. The latter is associated with increased IOP.

Explain that mild itching is normal and is caused by the presence of the suture rubbing against the conjunctiva. Suggest refrigerating the eye drops to provide a cool, comfortable sensation when the drop is instilled, provided refrigerating the medication will not significantly alter its chemical or pharmacologic properties.

NDx: High risk for impaired home maintenance management
Immediately after surgery, patients usually cannot bend from the waist, lift more than 20 to 25 lb, or drive. The length of time these restrictions are needed varies somewhat on the basis of the exact surgical procedure performed, size of the incision, patient condition, and presence of complications. Promote compliance with these restrictions by helping, before surgery if possible, the patient develop a plan for adapting the home environment. Encourage the patient to cook a few meals ahead, so that only reheating is needed. Advise placing pots, pans, and objects from lowest cupboards at counter height so that bending is unnecessary to access lower cupboards. Suggest placing pet dishes on a low stool or box, and instruct the patient to sit on a chair and lean forward to fill the dish.

Driving is not permitted immediately after surgery because an eye patch and shield are covering the operative eye. Help the patient establish a transportation plan for marketing, errands, and follow-up care. Refer to community senior citizen programs or agencies that may provide assistance.

NDx: High risk for altered health maintenance
Teach the patient to remove crusty drainage from the eyelid and to apply an eye shield (see Table 39–4).

Review the purpose of each medication. When they are discharged, patients frequently have two different eye drops prescribed: an antibiotic to prevent infection, such as gentamicin (Genoptic), and a steroid such as prednisolone acetate (Pred Mild). Sometimes patients are advised to use a combination eye drop composed of an antibiotic and a steroid, such as prednisolone acetate and gentamicin sulfate (Pred-G).

If the medications are in a suspension (e.g., prednisolone acetate [Pred-Mild]), reinforce the critical importance of vigorously shaking the bottle of eye drops while slowly counting to a minimum of 25. This shaking is necessary to distribute the medication in the solution. Check that the patient knows how to instill the eye drops, and observe the patient's technique. Remind the patient to close the eye gently for at least 3 minutes after instilling the medication to reduce the likelihood of washing the medication into the nasolacrimal system with blinking.

There are times when patients are discharged and ordered to take several eye drops. For example, the patient using timolol maleate (Timoptic) to control his or her glaucoma will continue to use the drop in the operated eye, unless specifically advised otherwise. If more than one drop is to be instilled into the same eye on the same schedule, instruct the

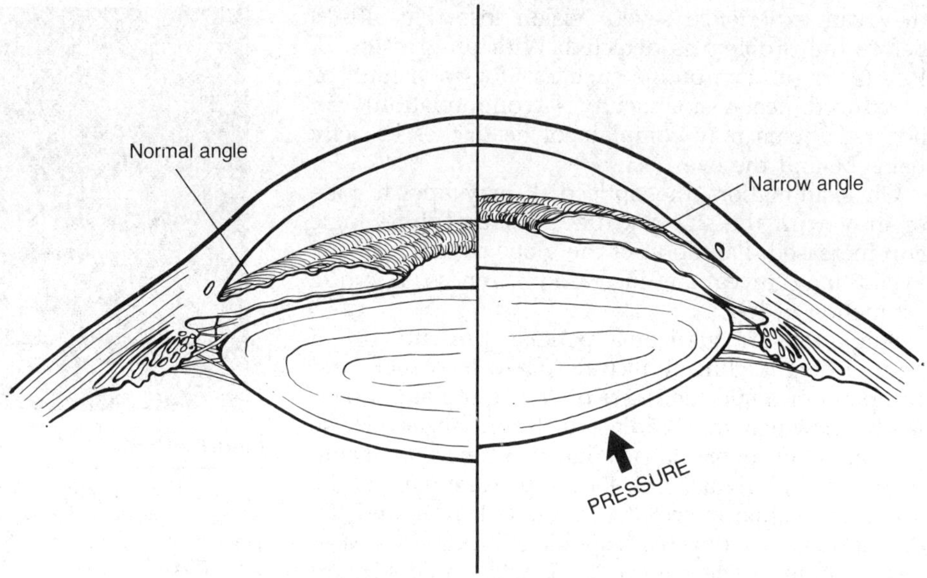

Figure 40–7.

Normal angle versus a narrow angle caused by a sliding forward of the iris as seen in acute glaucoma.

patient to wait a minimum of 5 minutes between drops to promote maximum absorption of the drops.

Teach the patient signs and symptoms of complications. Stress the importance of promptly reporting pain not relieved by acetaminophen (Tylenol), spots in the visual field, bright flashes of light or a curtain that obscures part of the visual field, or a reduction in visual acuity.

Evaluation

Evaluate the effectiveness of nursing care for a patient who has had cataract surgery by comparing the patient's status with the expected patient outcomes. Examples of specific outcomes for patients who have had cataract surgery have been provided in the Planning section.

Glaucoma

Glaucoma is a cluster of related disorders, with increased intraocular pressure (IOP) as the common element.

Glaucoma is the second major cause of blindness in the United States and the primary cause of blindness in black Americans (American Academy of Ophthalmology, Quality of Care Committee, Glaucoma Panel, 1989). Of the 2 million individuals with glaucoma, it is estimated that 50% are unaware they have it (American Academy of Ophthalmology, Quality of Care Committee, Glaucoma Panel, 1989). This lack of awareness is due to the asymptomatic nature of the disease's early course: Vision is lost gradually and without pain. Thus, glaucoma is often referred to as the "sneak thief" of sight.

Glaucoma is found more commonly in patients with a family history of glaucoma, diabetes, severe myopia, hypertension, or retinal detachment (Boyd-Monk & Steinmetz, 1987).

ETIOLOGY AND PATHOPHYSIOLOGY

Normal IOP is 10 to 21 mm Hg. The increased IOP in glaucoma is due to an imbalance between production of aqueous humor and its outflow from the eye. In glaucoma, aqueous humor is drained from the eye more slowly than it is produced. Drainage is through the anterior chamber angle, trabecular meshwork, and into the canal of Schlemm, where it enters a series of capillaries that absorb it into the systemic circulation. Increased IOP causes ischemia and atrophy of the optic disk and peripheral vision is lost. There is some variance in the patient's susceptibility to ocular damage from increased IOP, however. At the same IOP, one patient may have extensive peripheral sight loss and another minimal evidence of damage.

There are two classifications of glaucoma: primary and secondary. Primary glaucoma refers to those cases in which glaucoma is the main problem. It did not result from something else. Secondary glaucoma occurs as a sequela of another problem, such as a tumor, surgery, or recurrent ocular inflammation.

Glaucoma is also differentiated on the basis of the appearance of the anterior chamber angle. In angle-closure glaucoma, the iris slides forward, closing off the normally open angle. Angle-closure glaucoma is also referred to as "narrow-angle" or "acute" glaucoma (Fig. 40–7). If the angle remains open, it is referred to as open-angle glaucoma.

CLINICAL MANIFESTATIONS

Patients with primary open angle glaucoma (POAG) are largely asymptomatic, which is why they can experience severe vision loss (Fig. 40–8) before the problem is detected. With progression of POAG, vague symptoms such as "foggy vision" or a reduced near-vision acuity (accommodation) can occur. Patients may complain of headaches or achy pains behind the eye.

On examination, the optic disk may appear pale or gray with the size and depth of the physiologic cup increased. Palpation of the globe over the closed eyelid may reveal an increased firmness, a crude estimation of IOP.

Angle closure glaucoma patients present with a very different clinical picture. They look sick and complain of a sudden onset of severe unilateral ocular pain, which may radiate to the forehead. These patients may report nausea and vomiting and seeing halos around lights. On slit-lamp examination, the sclera is frequently seen to be injected (red), and the cornea looks steamy (as if looking through a steam-filled room). The pupil is usually mid-size to slightly dilated and slow to react to light and may not be equal in size when compared with the other eye.

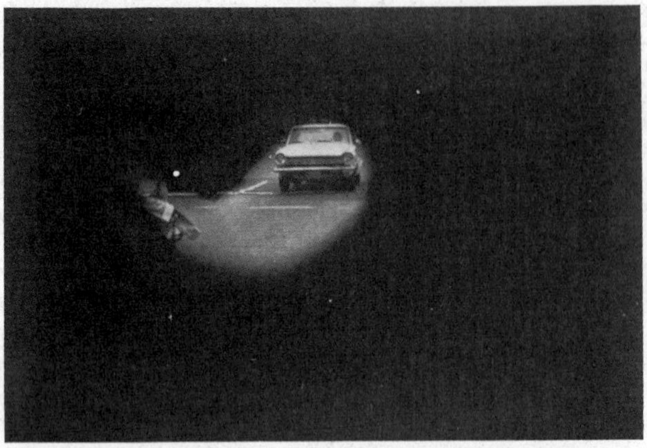

Figure 40–8.

Image seen by a patient with advanced glaucoma. Note small center island of vision. (Permission to use this photograph has been granted by the American Foundation for the Blind, 15 West 16th Street, New York, NY 10011.)

MEDICAL DIAGNOSIS

Medical diagnosis of glaucoma is made on the basis of history and physical findings. The fundus is examined with the direct ophthalmoscope. A tonometer is used to measure IOP, which is greater than 21 mm Hg in the majority of patients with glaucoma. Gonioscopy, a procedure in which a special contact lens is placed over the anesthetized cornea, is done to visualize the anterior chamber and its angles. A visual field test is performed to investigate and document areas of vision loss, and fundus photographs are taken of the optic disk to provide baseline data for use in future comparisons.

MEDICAL MANAGEMENT

Once glaucoma is diagnosed, the goal of treatment is to reduce IOP to a level tolerated by the eye without damage. For POAG, eye drops supplemented with oral carbonic anhydrase inhibitors as needed are used initially. Topical eye drops control IOP by either enhancing outflow or reducing the production of aqueous humor. Oral carbonic anhydrase inhibitors are used to reduce production of aqueous humor. These drugs can cause a number of very unpleasant and annoying side effects. Pilocarpine hydrochloride (Pilocar) causes burning and itching. It can cause local skin irritation and abdominal cramps as well as induced myopia (Bartlett et al, 1992). Timolol maleate (Timoptic) can cause bronchospasm in patients with reactive airway disease. The beta-blocker effect reduces the body's ability to respond to periods of decreased myocardial contractility. Severe respiratory and cardiac reactions have also been seen. This drug must be used with caution in diabetic patients because it masks signs and symptoms of hypoglycemia (Bartlett et al, 1992). Echothiophate iodide (Phospholine Iodide) can be associated with stinging and burning on instillation as well as brow ache, headache, and the formation of iris cysts. It can also lead to the formation of cataracts, so this drug should be used only in aphakic patients. Acetazolamide (Diamox) can cause anorexia, vomiting, constipation, weight loss, renal calculi, nervousness, tremors, ataxia, and paresthesia (Bartlett et al, 1992). The number and variety of side effects can make staying on the prescribed medications a problem for the patient.

Angle closure glaucoma is treated by topical agents and oral or intravenous hyperosmotics to rapidly bring down IOP. Oral hyperosmotics such as glycerin (Osmoglyn) or isosorbide (Ismotic) can cause serious side effects such as nausea, vomiting, severe headache, confusion, disorientation, pulmonary edema, and subarachnoid hemorrhage. These agents should be administered over ice and consumed over a 20- to 30-minute interval. Patients must be observed closely for the development of these side effects. Intravenous hyperosmotics are usually administered to hospitalized patients.

If pharmacologic treatments for POAG are insufficient, then argon laser trabeculoplasty (ALT) is performed. A slit-lamp mounted laser is used to create a series of laser burns in the trabecular meshwork. As the area scars, contraction causes tightening of the trabecular meshwork fibers. The drainage channels are pulled open, which enhances outflow of aqueous and lowers IOP in approximately 85% of patients (Newell, 1992). This procedure is performed on an out-patient basis either at the ophthalmologist's office or hospital. Over time, the effectiveness of ALT is reduced. Medications may need to be resumed or continued for this reason.

Angle closure glaucoma patients also benefit from laser procedures. After topical or local anesthesia, the laser is used to create a hole in the peripheral iris. This new hole creates an alternate pathway for the aqueous humor to drain from the posterior chamber into the anterior chamber and then through the trabecular meshwork. Once the IOP is reduced in the eye experiencing angle closure glaucoma, some patients may undergo a preventive laser iridotomy in the other eye.

With either laser procedure, a brief rise in IOP can occur. To combat the pressure rise, which can further damage the optic nerve, apraclonidine hydrochloride (Iopidine) is used. However, it can cause bradycardia, vasovagal attacks, chest heaviness, and nausea. Because of the potential cardiovascular side effects of the medications, vital signs are taken before and after each dose, and emergency equipment is kept nearby.

Intraocular surgery is done when pharmacologic or laser therapy fail to keep IOP at a level the eye can tolerate. Surgical procedures either create an alternate pathway for the drainage of aqueous humor or destroy structures responsible for the production of aqueous humor.

In glaucoma-filtering surgery, a channel connecting the anterior chamber and the subconjunctival space is created. The aqueous humor moves up through this channel to collect under the conjunctiva. From here, it is absorbed into the systemic circulation and IOP is lowered in a controlled manner.

In glaucoma-shunting procedures, an implanted reservoir and connecting tube are used to facilitate the movement of aqueous humor from the anterior chamber to the reservoir. The aqueous humor forms a bubble over the reservoir and under the conjunctiva, where it is absorbed into systemic circulation. Thus, obstructions in the trabecular meshwork that prevented aqueous outflow are bypassed.

Complications of glaucoma-filtering and shunting surgery include hypotonia resulting from excessive reduction in IOP, scar tissue formation, obstruction of the shunt, and progression of cataracts.

Procedures aimed at reducing aqueous production are called cyclodestructive procedures. A freezing force is delivered to the ciliary body area through the sclera, causing destruction of the site of aqueous production.

A peripheral iridectomy is performed for the treatment of angle closure glaucoma when a laser iridotomy is not effective or is not an option. A small, wedge-shaped section of the peripheral iris is removed, creating a new channel for aqueous humor to follow when flowing from the posterior to the anterior chamber.

Application of the Nursing Process to the Care of the Patient with Glaucoma

Assessment

Begin the assessment by asking why the patient presented for treatment. Keep in mind that symptoms of glaucoma are vague and undefined, so listen carefully and do not minimize symptoms. Explore specific symptoms such as headaches, pain behind the eye or radiating to the forehead, and frequent changes of eyeglasses. Also note complaints indicative of angle closure glaucoma: seeing halos around lights, reduced visual acuity, nausea, and vomiting.

Question the patient about a personal or family history of glaucoma, diabetes, hypertension, or myopia, and determine whether these are associated with the development of glaucoma. Also ask about any previous ocular trauma or surgery.

Inquire about other medical problems. Carefully note any cardiac or respiratory diseases, because these may contraindicate the use of beta-blockers. Question about allergies to medications, especially preservatives, because many glaucoma patients receive eye drops that contain a variety of preservatives.

Ask the patient to describe a usual day to obtain information needed to help the patient establish a manageable treatment plan for eye drop instillation.

Observe the patient's general appearance while obtaining the history. Does the patient appear fatigued? Does the patient have signs of dehydration that can result from nausea and vomiting associated with increased IOP?

Check visual acuity. Compare OD with OS. Ask the patient how current vision compares with how well he or she usually sees. Be sure to document this information for medical and legal purposes.

Carefully observe the pupils, noting the size and shape. Remember that patients using certain glaucoma medications, such as pilocarpine hydrochloride (Pilocar), will have small pupils referred to as miotic, whereas the pupils of the patient with angle closure glaucoma may be asymmetric, with the affected eye slightly dilated and slow to react.

If the patient has previously been diagnosed with glaucoma, assess his or her knowledge of the disease and its treatment. Identify all medications the patient uses or takes as well as their frequency. Compare this list with prescribed medications and their frequency. Clarify any differences between prescribed and actual use.

Nursing Diagnoses and Planning

Nursing diagnoses and related expected patient outcomes most commonly applicable to patients with glaucoma include the following:

NDx: High risk for injury related to peripheral vision loss

Planning: Patient outcomes

1. Patient describes how to use existing vision to promote safety.
2. Patient avoids self-injury.

NDx: Pain related to increased intraocular pressure

Planning: Patient outcomes
1. Patient associates pain with increased IOP.
2. Patient describes level of pain as tolerable.
3. Patient states pharmacologic interventions are effective.
4. Patient uses nonpharmacologic interventions for effective pain relief.

NDx: High risk for noncompliance with treatment regimen related to side effects of medications, specifics of treatment regimen, and patient-identified reasons

Planning: Patient outcomes
1. Patient describes importance of treatment regimen.
2. Patient creates a treatment schedule with which she or he is able to comply.
3. Patient follows treatment regimen.

Nursing Interventions

NDx: High risk for injury
Explain the type of vision loss associated with glaucoma to enable the patient to plan effective safety measures. Stress that because peripheral vision loss accompanies glaucoma, there is a risk of stumbling over obstacles off to the side without seeing them. Tell the patient to remove small articles from frequently traveled paths. Also explain that an object may suddenly appear in the field of vision.

Orient the patient to any new environment, from the examining room to the operating room. Assist the patient to settle into the room, but permit him or her to place personal objects. This helps the patient to remember the location of belongings and also allows the patient to place the objects in locations appropriate for his or her needs. Do not move objects without consent.

Avoid approaching the patient from the periphery. Instead, always approach from the front. If the doorway is not within the patient's line of sight, call out a greeting when entering the room. These actions avoid startling the patient and decrease the potential for injury.

Several glaucoma medications cause miosis. The small pupil changes size very slowly when adapting to dim lighting. Explain this slowed adaptation to the patient. Caution the patient to move slowly and to use available security measures such as handrails when adapting to dim lighting.

NDx: Pain
Patients with angle closure glaucoma are frequently in moderate to severe pain. Note the patient's position when entering the room. Frequently, the eye pain or headache is so severe that the patient is holding the head. To promote pain relief, provide an atmosphere of comfort. Ask whether dim lighting helps ease the pain or makes it worse, and adjust lighting accordingly. Provide cool compresses for the patient's forehead. Administer analgesics such as meperidine (Demerol) as ordered for intense pain. Keep in mind the route of choice is intramuscular because the patient may have nausea and onset of action is rapid. Monitor the patient's level of comfort before, during, and after interventions, and adjust accordingly.

Stress to the patient that ocular pain will be relieved once the IOP is reduced. Begin interventions to lower IOP as soon as possible.

NDx: High risk for noncompliance with treatment regimen
POAG is an incurable disease. Once started on medications, the patient generally requires them for an extended period. Help the patient understand that these treatments attempt to prevent loss of vision or further loss of vision. Nothing can restore vision lost from glaucoma.

Unfortunately, side effects from glaucoma medications are common. Alert the glaucoma patient to the potential side effects. Advise him or her to contact the nurse or ophthalmologist as soon as they occur. Reinforce the importance of not stopping the drug if side effects occur. If side effects do occur and the decision is to keep the patient on the medication, work with the patient to minimize side effects.

Side effects are not the only reason for noncompliance. Other reasons include cost, availability, and specific treatment schedule. When a variance between the treatment regimen and how the patient is actually practicing is observed, discuss those observations with the patient. The patient may have misinterpreted the instructions about the regimen or may have deviated for a reason. Remember that only the patient can say why the variance exists. Any successful treatment regimen must be negotiated with and agreed to by the patient.

If the problem is cost, explore resources available to the patient. State or federal assistance may be available, or local civic groups may provide a small source of funding. Refer the patient to a local social service agency to investigate sources of aid.

If the problem is scheduling difficulties, work with the patient to determine what is creating the difficulty. Is the problem one of needing to use a medication four times a day, but the patient only remembers it or has help available two times a day? If so, check whether the patient can be changed to a regimen that requires use only twice a day.

If the problem is a memory error, help the patient develop a reminder mechanism. Check-off lists showing when each dose is due can be posted on the refrigerator or in another patient-determined location. When the patient administers the drops or takes the pill, the dose is checked off. If such a list is used, have the patient bring it to follow-up visits. Review the check-off list with the patient, and monitor compliance at the same time.

Other strategies for dealing with noncompliance related to memory error include involving family or friends as a reminder checkup and placing medications in visible strategic locations. If the problem is remembering a midday dose, the medication can be tossed into the brown-bag lunch. When the bag is opened, the patient sees the bottle and remembers the dose.

Perhaps the problem of noncompliance is one of transportation difficulties. Patients cannot use medications they do not have. In these cases, examine available resources for transportation. Investigate the possibility of transferring the prescription to a pharmacy closer to the patient's home or near a location to which he or she frequently travels. Encourage the patient to look in the yellow pages to find out whether a pharmacy in their neighborhood delivers. Call local agencies such as churches or civic clubs such as the Lions Club that might transport the patient to the pharmacy or deliver the medication to the patient.

Whatever the cause, remember that no plan for reducing noncompliance can be successful unless it involves the patient. The role of the nurse is one of idea and suggestion generator. Goals can be achieved only when the patient supports the idea.

Evaluation

Evaluate the effectiveness of nursing care for a patient with glaucoma by comparing the patient's status with the expected patient outcomes. Examples of specific outcomes for patients with glaucoma have been provided in the Planning section.

Guidelines for Application of the Nursing Process to the Care of the Patient Having Laser Therapy for Glaucoma

Nursing care for patients having laser therapy for glaucoma is similar to that described for patients having laser therapy for any disorder of the eye (see Chapter 39). For the patient with glaucoma, be certain to measure and record IOP on arrival for therapy and to check both IOP and vital signs before and after administering apraclonidine hydrochloride (Iopidine).

Diabetic Retinopathy

ETIOLOGY AND PATHOPHYSIOLOGY

The retinal and ophthalmic vascular changes commonly associated with diabetes are referred to as diabetic retinopathy. These retinal and vascular changes include the following:

Platelet abnormalities. Adherence of platelets to each other is increased. This increased adhesion may contribute to local capillary occlusion.

Red blood cell abnormalities. Red blood cells become less flexible and also demonstrate increased adhesion to one another. The decreased flexibility makes movement of the red blood cell through the capillaries difficult. Oxygen-carrying capacity of the red blood cells is also decreased.

Blood vessel abnormalities. One of the earliest changes in diabetes is the thickening of the blood vessel's basement membrane. This thickening creates increased surface area on which platelets can collect. Blood vessel walls also become weakened, creating outpouched areas called microaneurysms.

Macular edema. Blood vessels surrounding the macula leak fluid, allowing it to accumulate beneath the macula. The normally flat macula bubbles up similar to a blister. This causes images to be perceived as dark and distorted as a result of the irregular macular surface.

Vasoproliferative changes. Because of the factors just mentioned, the retina becomes hypoxic and ischemic. As a result, it produces or releases a factor that stimulates the growth of new blood vessels, which are weak and leak fluid easily.

There are several forms of diabetic retinopathy.

Background diabetic retinopathy is the less severe type. It is characterized by macular edema and microaneurysms. Hard exudates are caused by the leaking of lipids through the blood vessel wall. As the disease progresses, circulation to the retina is reduced. Hypoxia in the nerve fiber layer occurs, and weak-walled blood vessels form in the retina.

Proliferative diabetic retinopathy begins with the growth of new blood vessels on the retinal surface. These blood vessels are fragile and leak easily. Hemorrhages of blood into the vitreous can occur. If the body cannot absorb the blood, fibrin bands can develop between the posterior vitreous and the retina. Movement of the vitreous can place traction on the fibrin band, which can exert a pull on the retina, thus causing it to detach.

Development of these changes is predominantly a function of the length of time the patient has been a diabetic. The relationship of blood glucose control to ocular changes is currently under study.

CLINICAL MANIFESTATIONS

Patients are often unaware they have early stages of diabetic retinopathy. In background diabetic retinopathy, symptoms may or may not be present. When symptoms are experienced, they are usually vague. Patients may complain of transient blurred vision. This blurred vision also occurs with hyperglycemia. As the glucose level increases, the lens absorbs fluid, increasing its size. Edema in the macular area may also produce blurry, dark, and distorted images. It is these vague complaints that may cause a diabetic patient to seek vision care. Sometimes patients with background diabetic retinopathy may not even be aware they have diabetes.

MEDICAL DIAGNOSIS

Diagnosis is made on the basis of history and physical examination of the eye. A notation is made of any abnormalities in the blood vessels or in the background of the retina.

MEDICAL MANAGEMENT

The goal of medical treatment for diabetic retinopathy is to maintain the health of the retina. If no proliferative changes or background changes are noted in the retina, the patient is advised to keep the blood glucose level and blood pressure under control and to return in 6 months for follow-up monitoring. Any patient found to have retinal or visual changes associated with diabetes is referred to an internist for testing.

LASER THERAPY

Certain patients with diabetic macular edema or proliferative retinopathy are candidates for laser therapy. In diabetic macular edema, the laser is used to seal the blood vessels that are leaking fluid into the macular area. Once the area is sealed, the body slowly absorbs the fluid. Vision usually improves as the edema subsides.

The laser is also used for treating the peripheral retina. As indicated, the hypoxic state of the retina triggers the development of new blood vessels that are weak and fragile. It is believed that decreasing the need of the retina for oxygen and nutrients should cause regression of these fragile and weak blood vessels and prevent their further development.

Laser therapy, called pan retinal photocoagulation (PRP), places several hundred laser spots throughout the peripheral retina. The intense heat of the laser destroys the treated tissue. This reduces the area of the retina in need of oxygen, thus increasing the supply available to nourish vital areas such as the macula.

When PRP is performed, the pupil is widely dilated to facilitate viewing the fundus. The patient may receive a retrobulbar injection of an anesthetic, such as lidocaine (Xylocaine) or topical anesthesia, such as tetracaine.

A contact lens containing mirrors is used to deflect the laser light into the peripheral retinal area because laser light moves only in a straight direction. Extreme care is taken to avoid the macula.

SURGICAL TREATMENT

A vitrectomy may be done if a hemorrhage into the vitreous occurs as a result of leaking or injury of one of the fragile blood vessels. Areas of retinal detachment must be repaired.

Guidelines for Application of the Nursing Process to the Care of the Patient with Diabetic Retinopathy

Nursing care for patients with diabetic retinopathy varies with the prescribed treatment regimen. Patients receiving laser therapy require a combination of the nursing care required by diabetic patients (see Chapter 30) and that required by any patient undergoing laser therapy (see Chapter 39).

Care of patients undergoing a vitrectomy combines care of the diabetic patient with that of the patient having any type of eye surgery (see Chapter 39). For patients who are not candidates for specific ocular therapy at present, focus is on the importance of attaining good control of the diabetes and returning as scheduled for follow-up monitoring of the eye.

Retinal Holes, Tears, and Detachments

ETIOLOGY AND PATHOPHYSIOLOGY

A retinal detachment is a separation of the retina from the underlying choroid.

The retina is physically attached to the choroid in only two places: posteriorly at the optic nerve and anteriorly at the ciliary body. The remaining retinal areas are held against the choroid by pressure from the vitreous. Thus, a retinal detachment can be due to any factor that causes the retina to be pushed or pulled from the choroid. Such factors include hemorrhage, tumor, collection of exudate behind the retina caused by an inflammatory process such as uveitis, or forward pull by the vitreous as a result of traction from newly formed blood vessels in it, as in diabetic neovascularization. However, the most common cause of retinal detachment is a hole or tear in the retina, which allows vitreous to gradually seep between, thus separating it from the choroid (Fig. 40–9). Such holes or tears may be due to trauma or to age-related degeneration of the retina. They occur most commonly at the outer edges of the retina where it is the thinnest.

Retinal detachments subsequently occur in the second eye in about one of five people.

CLINICAL MANIFESTATIONS

The most common indication of a retinal hole, tear, or detachment is a painless change in vision.

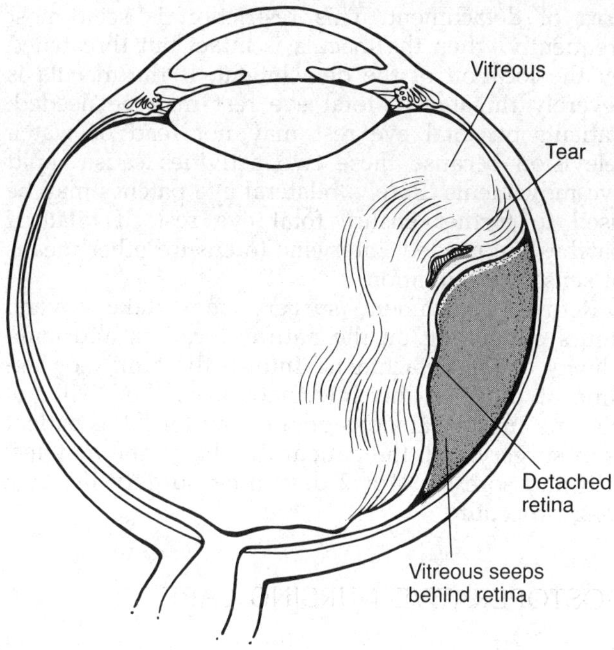

Figure 40–9.

Diagram of a retinal detachment.

Patients complain of suddenly seeing flashes of bright lights (photopsia), a shower of spots before their eyes, or the sensation of a curtain being pulled down over part of their vision (Fig. 40–10). Some patients experience no awareness of the problem until the macular area is involved.

The light flashes are usually the result of traction on the retina. As the retina is pulled away, small capillaries break and release red blood cells and fragments into the vitreous. These fragments and cells cast a shadow on the retina, creating the perception of spots.

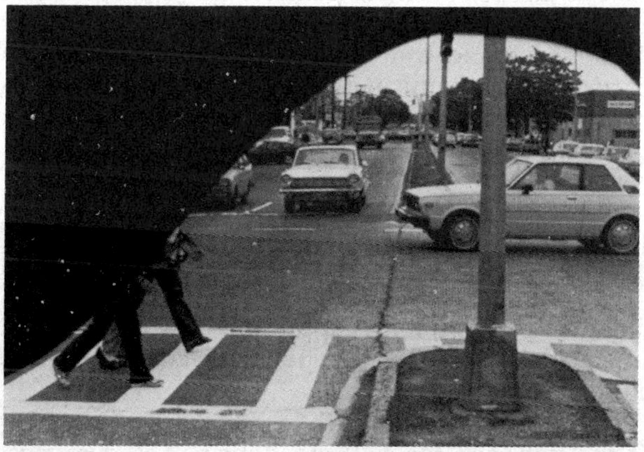

Figure 40–10.

Example of visual defect seen by a patient with a retinal detachment. (Permission to use this photograph has been granted by the American Foundation for the Blind, 15 West 16th Street, New York, NY 10011.)

MEDICAL DIAGNOSIS

The diagnosis of a retinal hole, tear, or detachment is made on the basis of the patient's history and the ocular examination. When the retina is examined, small holes or tears can be seen. Tears are usually shaped like an arrowhead or a horseshoe. If a detachment is present, a hole or tear may be noted in close proximity. Areas of retinal detachment appear as gray inward bulges that may contain ripples or folds that jiggle with eye movement.

The detached area of the retina appears gray because it obstructs the view of the normal pink-orange color of the underlying choroid. The retina itself is transparent.

MEDICAL MANAGEMENT

The goal of treating retinal holes and tears is to prevent a retinal detachment. Small holes located in the periphery are often left untreated when the patient can be closely monitored for an increase in hole size (American Academy of Ophthalmology, Quality of Care Committee, Retinal Panel, 1989).

Tears in the retina are treated with photocoagulation, cryotherapy, or diathermy: The goal is to induce an inflammatory response between the retina and the underlying pigment epithelium and choroid to seal the edges of the tear.

Photocoagulation uses laser light focused on the pigment epithelium to coagulate it to the overlying retina. With cryotherapy, a supercooled probe is placed on the conjunctiva over the borders of the hole or tear. This freezes the area, creating an inflammatory response while not disturbing nearby ocular structures. Diathermy uses energy from a high-frequency current sufficient to cause tissue coagulation. It is also applied to the external eye overlying the retinal tear or hole.

Surgery is necessary to repair areas of retinal detachment because spontaneous reattachment is rare. The usual procedure is called a scleral buckle.

SCLERAL BUCKLE

Scleral buckling is a procedure designed to repair a retinal detachment by indenting the sclera, forcing the choroid to come into closer contact with the retina. It is usually an in-patient procedure performed under general anesthesia. The conjunctiva is retracted to expose the sclera, through which microsurgical instruments, such as cutters and sources of light, are inserted. Using these instruments, wrinkles and folds in the retina are flattened, enabling the retina to assume its normal smooth position. Adhesions or traction bands between the retina and vitreous are cut and removed if needed. A vitrectomy is performed if needed to remove blood and other particles in the vitreous.

Once the retina is back in place and any subretinal fluid drained, the endolaser may be used to promote reattachment. Use of the laser creates in-

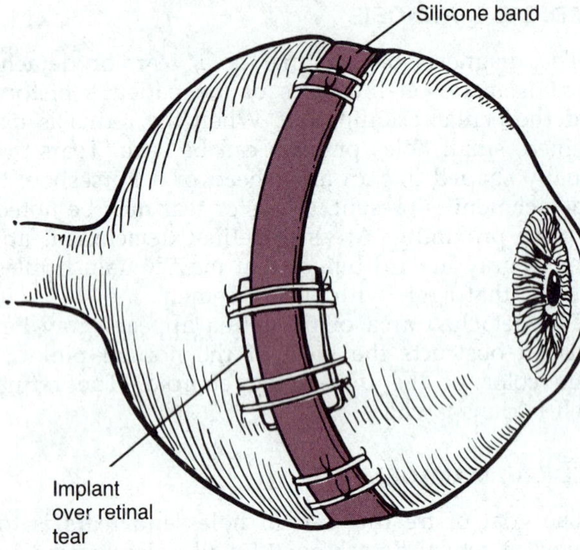

Figure 40–11.

Scleral buckle for the treatment of retinal detachment.

tense heat, which seals the edges and creates an inflammatory response. Silicone bands or implants, also known as a buckle, are placed to encircle the sclera or cover the area of the retinal tear to promote reattachment (Fig. 40–11). These implants help maintain the retina in contact with the choroid.

If needed, gas or oil is injected to assist in keeping the retina in contact with the choroid. Because of their lower specific gravity, the gas or oil floats up against the retina and holds it in place.

When the procedure is completed, a subconjunctival injection of an antibiotic is administered and topical antibiotic ointment instilled. An eye patch and shield are taped in place over the closed eyelid.

Complications of retinal detachment repair include infection, failure of the detachment to reattach, and increased IOP.

Application of the Nursing Process to the Care of the Patient Having Surgery for a Retinal Detachment

PREOPERATIVE NURSING CARE

Nursing care for the patient scheduled for surgery for a retinal detachment is similar to that for any patient having eye surgery, as described in Chapter 39, with several considerations. Be certain to determine when the patient last had anything to eat or drink, because the need for surgery can develop without warning. Instruct the patient in any preoperative activity restrictions because rest in a specific position may be required to reduce stress on the area of detachment. This restriction is seen most frequently when the macula is intact but threatened by the location of the detachment. If the macula is severely threatened, total eye rest may be needed. Patients on total eye rest may not read or watch television because these two activities cause rapid eye movements. Rarely, bilateral eye patches may be used to further ensure total eye rest. If bilateral patches are needed, intervene to ensure other means of sensory stimulation.

Retinal detachment surgery may take several hours depending on the nature, location, and complexity of the detachment. Inform the family or significant other of this information, so they will not become unduly anxious about how long the patient is in surgery. Tell the patient that he or she may feel stiff and sore for 1 or 2 days after surgery if it is a long procedure.

POSTOPERATIVE NURSING CARE

Assessment

The care of the patient after retinal detachment surgery is similar to that of any patient receiving general anesthesia. Assess the patient's return to physiologic stability. Monitor respiratory and cardiovascular status. Check vital signs in accordance with institutional policy and guided by the patient's condition. Observe the eye patch and shield for evidence of drainage. Assess for nausea, which sometimes results from the anesthetic agents as well as from the manipulation of the eye during the procedure. Auscultate bowel sounds because diet can be resumed when they return and when nausea is absent.

Once the initial eye patch is removed, the patient is started on cycloplegic agents such as atropine or cyclopentolate (Cyclogyl) to dilate the pupil and rest the muscles of accommodation. Antibiotic and steroid eye drops, such as gentamicin (Genoptic) and prednisolone acetate (Pred Mild), respectively, or an antibiotic/steroid combination, such as prednisolone acetate and gentamicin (Pred-G) eye drops, will be ordered. Be sure to assess the patient's ability to instill these drops.

Nursing Diagnoses and Planning

Nursing diagnoses and related expected patient outcomes most commonly applicable to patients who have had surgery for a retinal detachment include the following:

NDx: High risk for self-care deficit related to positioning and activity restrictions required after surgery

Planning: Patient outcomes

1. Patient describes how to manage personal care needs while maintaining activity restrictions.

NDx: High risk for injury: fall, related to presence in an unfamiliar environment

Planning: Patient outcomes
1. Patient avoids falling.
2. Retina remains reattached.

NDx: Pain related to surgical manipulation of tissue

Planning: Patient outcomes
1. Patient reports pain is relieved or reduced to a manageable level.
2. Behavioral signs of severe pain are absent.

Nursing Interventions

NDx: High risk for self-care deficit
When gas or oil is used to promote retinal reattachment, extreme care must be taken to keep the gas or oil bubble positioned against the repaired area of the retina. Maintain the patient in the position specified by the ophthalmologist. This position is usually that of head parallel to the floor and turned to the side. Instruct the patient who is in bed to lie on the abdomen, and turn the head to the correct side. Place pillows for comfort and for support of the arms and lower back. Because the same position—head parallel to floor—must be maintained when the patient is out of bed or sitting up, instruct him or her to walk with the head down and turned to the appropriate side. Advise the patient to use the overbed table to rest the turned head. Monitor these activity restrictions, which must be maintained until the gas bubble absorbs, which may take 4 to 8 days.

Discuss how the patient can continue these restrictions while still meeting personal care needs. For example, to bathe, a basin of water can be placed on the bed next to the patient, or the patient can bathe at the sink as long as the head is kept flexed at the neck, thus parallel to the floor, and turned to the correct side.

The patient must also get used to eating with food in the lap or beside him or her. Encourage eating easy, hand-held foods. Provide assistance with tray set up and item selection if necessary.

If the patient is going home with these restrictions, review the home situation and assist the patient in identifying how to maintain him or herself in the home while complying with the restrictions.

Discuss how household chores, such as cooking or washing dishes, can be performed while maintaining these restrictions. As needed, explore community resources available such as Meals on Wheels or home-care assistance.

NDx: High risk for injury
Make certain the patient has been oriented to the environment. Keep doors completely opened or closed. Place furniture and other items outside of the traffic flow areas of the room. Keep the call light within easy reach. Also place other needed articles within sight and reach. Because depth perception may be impaired, elevate the side rails at the head of the bed. Advise the patient to call for assistance with ambulation.

NDx: Pain
A significant amount of tissue manipulation occurs during scleral buckling surgery. Monitor the patient's level of pain. As necessary and prescribed, administer acetaminophen with codeine (Tylenol with codeine) or other analgesic. If the pain is severe, or the patient is nauseated, administer intramuscular injections of prescribed analgesics. Initiate appropriate nonpharmacologic interventions such as quiet music or conversation. Once the initial eye patch has been removed, place cool compresses over the closed eyelid for relief of discomfort from edema of the conjunctiva and sclera.

Evaluation

Evaluate the effectiveness of nursing care for the patient who has had surgery for a retinal detachment by comparing the patient's status with the expected patient outcomes. Examples of specific outcomes for patients who have had surgery for a retinal detachment have been provided in the Planning section.

Degenerative Disorders

Macular Degeneration

The macula is responsible for processing finely detailed vision used for recognizing faces and street signs, reading a label, threading a needle, and writing a check. The macula is only about 5% of the total retinal surface, but it is 100 times more sensitive to detail than the peripheral retina.

Age-related macular degeneration (AMD) is the leading cause of irreversible vision loss in persons older than 65 years (Coles, 1989).

ETIOLOGY AND PATHOPHYSIOLOGY

AMD is a progressive form of permanent vision loss, the cause of which is unknown. It occurs in three forms: atrophic (dry), exudative (wet), and pigment epithelial detachment (PED). Atrophic AMD is the most commonly occurring form, accounting for about 90% to 95% of all cases (Schatz & McDonald, 1987). Exudative, the less common but more serious form, accounts for approximately 90% of all cases of legal blindness resulting from AMD (Vaughan et al, 1992).

In the atrophic form, the macula thins and functions poorly. In the exudative form, new and fragile blood vessels grow beneath the macula from the underlying choroid. These new blood vessels are called subretinal neovascularization. Blood and serous fluid leak out, causing the macula to bubble up, similar to blistering and breaking of sidewalk under which tree roots are growing. The longer these vessels continue to grow, leak, and bleed, the greater the degree of detail vision that is lost.

In PED, a blister forms under the macula causing the vision to become blurry and distorted.

AMD can occur bilaterally or unilaterally. In most cases of bilateral AMD, the disease progresses at different rates in each eye.

CLINICAL MANIFESTATIONS

In the initial stages of AMD, the patient may notice blurry vision when reading or have no difficulty with near vision, yet experience trouble reading distant objects such as street signs. Because the macula is no longer smooth and flat, objects may look bent, crooked, or distorted. Straight lines look irregular. Patients may notice that sizes, shapes, and colors of objects look different when viewed with each eye (Schatz & McDonald, 1987). Patients may also complain about seeing a fixed gray spot just off the center of vision and compare it with the aftereffect of a flash bulb (Fig. 40–12).

MEDICAL DIAGNOSIS

The retina is examined for drusen, small, yellow-white deposits frequently associated with macular degeneration, as well as for blisters and blood vessels.

An Amsler grid, a hand-held card that looks like graph paper with a dot in the center, is used to detect the presence of metamorphopsia, which is the distortion of straight lines. The patient with AMD frequently sees areas of distortion in the straight lines. The patient with AMD may also note that areas on the grid are dark or missing.

Fluorescein angiography may be used to check the retinal vasculature and determine whether blood vessel leakage is present. The photographs taken during this angiography provide important baseline data.

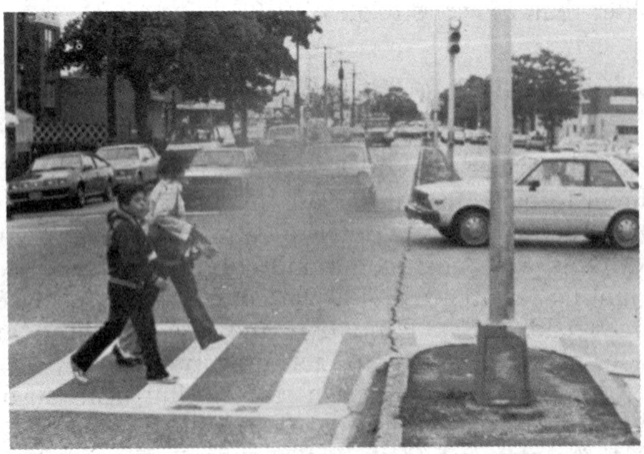

Figure 40–12.

Image seen by patient with macular degeneration. (Permission to use this photograph has been granted by the American Foundation for the Blind, 15 West 16th Street, New York, NY 10011.)

MEDICAL MANAGEMENT

Unfortunately, there is no medical, surgical, or laser treatment for atrophic AMD. The patient whose only symptom is drusen is given an Amsler grid and instructed to check vision daily. In exudative or PED, when abnormal blood vessels are present and detected early, laser therapy can be used. Laser therapy seals the blood vessels, stopping their progression, leaking, and bleeding. However, while sealing the leaking blood vessels, small nearby areas of the retina are destroyed. As a result, the gray spot seen previously becomes a black scotoma, or blind spot.

It is not always possible or in the patient's best interest to perform laser therapy. It depends on the amount of blood present, the general health of the macula, and the location of the abnormal blood vessels. It is important for the patient to know that vision usually does not improve after laser therapy but that distortion is lessened or eliminated.

Application of the Nursing Process to the Care of the Patient with Macular Degeneration

Assessment

Begin the assessment by determining when the patient noticed the change in acuity and under what conditions the reduced acuity is noted, such as in dim light, when tired, or when reading. Review the patient's and family's medical history because age, female sex, smoking, and a family history of macular degeneration place the patient at a greater risk for developing AMD (Vaughan et al, 1992). Also explore medications the patient takes or uses.

Ask the patient how the change in vision has affected lifestyle. Ask whether there are things he or she is no longer able to do or has increased difficulty doing.

Measure both distance and near visual acuity. Be sure the patient wears reading glasses if used.

If the patient has not already had a retinal examination performed, assess the retina. Note any areas of bleeding, blisters, drusen, or abnormal blood vessels.

Nursing Diagnoses and Planning

Nursing diagnoses and related expected patient outcomes most commonly applicable to patients with macular degeneration include the following:

NDx: High risk for altered health maintenance related to insufficient knowledge of symptoms and treatment of macular degeneration and related self-care activities

Planning: Patient outcomes
1. Patient defines macular degeneration in simple terms.
2. Patient acknowledges that macular degeneration causes a permanent loss of vision.
3. Patient identifies symptoms necessitating immediate notification of the ophthalmologist.
4. Patient describes treatment of macular degeneration.

NDx: Sensory/perceptual alteration: visual, related to reduced ability to process finely detailed vision

Planning: Patient outcomes
1. Patient lists ways to maximize use of existing vision.

NDx: Anxiety related to potential loss of vision

Planning: Patient outcomes
1. Patient states anxiety is lessened.
2. Verbal and nonverbal cues of anxiety are absent.

NDx: Anticipatory grieving related to actual or potential loss of vision and needed role and lifestyle adjustments

Planning: Patient outcomes
1. Patient identifies grief as needed and normal.
2. Patient verbalizes previously effective grief-reducing strategies.
3. Patient implements strategies for positively dealing with feelings of grief and loss.

Nursing Interventions

NDx: High risk for altered health maintenance

Use a quiet, simple approach when teaching the patient newly diagnosed with AMD. Remember that the diagnosis can alter the patient's lifestyle dramatically and permanently. Expect many questions, but be aware that the patient is often too afraid of the answers to ask them.

Advise the patient that macular degeneration is a permanent form of vision loss, but total vision loss and blindness occur very rarely. Review the normal anatomy of the eye and vision, using models as needed. Review the pathology of AMD, using the analogy of tree roots bubbling up the sidewalk as appropriate. Help the patient to see how his or her symptoms parallel those usually associated with AMD.

Respond to questions as soon as they are asked. Frequently, patients ask about the use of lasers to treat AMD. Gently explain that lasers can be used only to treat forms of AMD in which leaky blood vessels are present.

Provide the patient with written, large-print handouts to take home. To improve the contrast between the letters on the page and the paper, send the patient home with a yellow transparent cover sheet, which can be inexpensively made from yellow, transparent report covers.

Review and demonstrate use of the Amsler grid. Have the patient practice using it, and obtain a return demonstration in its use before he or she leaves. Instruct the patient to check both eyes each day while wearing his or her reading glasses. Also have the patient use one object in the living area, such as a clock or door frame, to check vision each day. Stress the importance of notifying the ophthalmologist whenever new or larger areas of distortion are noted.

Involve the patient's family or support person in teaching. Their presence may be of comfort to the patient and provides a second set of ears. This support person can also reinforce information at home.

Pause frequently during teaching to determine whether the patient has any questions. Knowing that questions arise after leaving the office, provide the patient with the name and telephone number of a person to call should questions arise.

NDx: Sensory-perceptual alteration: visual

Assist the patient to identify ways in which existing vision can be maximized. Ways can vary from changing light bulbs to using optical scanners. Determine what help the patient wants, and what will be used as opposed to what the caregiver believes should be used.

Encourage the use of incandescent light because glare can be visually handicapping for these patients. Discourage the use of fluorescent lighting, which causes more glare. Instruct the patient to use a 75- to 100-W light bulb and to position the light source so the light rays fall directly down onto the page. In the early stages of AMD, these changes might be all that is needed.

Refer the patient with significant vision loss to a local low-vision specialist for evaluation and recommendation of additional visual resources such as magnifiers, hand-held or eyeglass-mounted telescopes and optical scanners.

NDx: Anxiety

Monitor for signs and symptoms of anxiety because even the potential of losing vision can cause tremendous anxiety. Observe for frequent changes in topic of discussion, inability to focus on a topic, repetitive gestures such as pacing or hand wringing, and rapid speech. Encourage the patient to express concerns, and acknowledge that anxiety is normal. Provide accurate information in a way the patient can understand because anxiety can be based on misinformation or information the patient heard only part of and has filled in the rest. Explore how the patient has dealt with previous anxiety-producing situations, and assist in the implementation of those strategies.

NDx: Anticipatory grieving
We use our vision all during our waking hours. It can be devastating for a patient to hear that he or she may never see his or her grandchild's face or be able to drive an automobile again. The AMD patient grieves for the lost vision as well as for the loss of independence. Sometimes changes in roles must occur.

This patient goes through the stages of loss and grief similar to the cancer patient. Recognize these stages, and assist the patient in dealing with his or her feelings.

No one knows the stressors of living with macular degeneration the way another macular degeneration patient does. Ask the patient if he or she would find it helpful to speak with other patients. If acceptable to the patient, make a referral to the local support group. The services of a clinical nurse specialist, psychologist, or mental health professional may be available through the local center or community agency that services the visually handicapped.

Sometimes job changes are required. Refer to state agencies, such as the Bureau for Vocational Rehabilitation, for assistance with retraining.

Evaluation

Evaluate the effectiveness of nursing care for a patient with macular degeneration by comparing the patient's status with the expected patient outcomes. Examples of specific outcomes for patients with macular degeneration have been identified in the Planning section.

Trauma

Contusions, Abrasions, Lacerations, and Penetrating Injuries

ETIOLOGY AND PATHOPHYSIOLOGY

Contusions result from the impact of a blunt object, such as a baseball bat or racquetball. Such impact causes an immediate and significant rise in IOP, which results in tearing of susceptible tissues and major arterioles in the angle and bleeding. Rupture of the globe can occur as well as a subconjunctival hemorrhage, or hyphema. Severe blunt injuries can even produce dislocation of the lens. The incidence of this type of injury is increasing because of the popularity of sports such as tennis, racquetball, and soccer.

A corneal abrasion occurs when the epithelium is removed by a scratching or irritative force. Common causes of corneal abrasions include foreign bodies, eyelashes, dust, and dirt. Abrasions can also occur from natural objects such as tree branches, and grass blades forced out at high speeds from lawn mowers or weed removers as well as from contact lens overwear and excessive exposure to sunlight. After abrasion, the cornea usually regenerates in 24 to 48 hours without scarring.

Lacerations, caused by sharp objects such as scissors, a fishhook, animal or human teeth, or glass fragments can affect any part of the external eye. The most common sites of lacerations are the eyelid and cornea. Corneal lacerations are the more serious because ocular contents can prolapse through the corneal laceration. Deep corneal lacerations can heal with a scar. If the scar significantly affects vision, a corneal transplant may be necessary (see Chapter 39).

High-speed particles such as BBs, metal, bullets, rock pellets, and flying glass projectiles are able to penetrate the eye. Objects can become embedded in the eye after a fall onto a sharp object such as a tree branch or a pair of scissors. Rupture of the eye can result (Vaughan et al, 1992). Once inside the eye, the foreign body can create an ocular inflammation or cause an infection.

CLINICAL MANIFESTATIONS

Patients experiencing a contusion, or black eye, usually relate a history of recent trauma to the area. Visual acuity is usually not affected. Edema of the eyelids, periorbital edema, and a hyphema are frequently seen. Photophobia or diplopia may occur.

Abrasions create a "foreign body" sensation in the eye, often accompanied by tearing and photophobia. Visual acuity may be reduced if the cornea is involved. Vertical scratches may be seen on the cornea if particulate matter has lodged under the eyelid, because the foreign body is brought into contact with the cornea during each blink.

Patients with a laceration of the eye or eyelid usually report a history of being struck by an object. An irregular cut of the eyelid or the surface of the eye may be visible. Because the eyelid is very vascular, the amount of bleeding may seem out of proportion compared to the severity of the laceration. Pieces of the eyelid may be missing.

Most penetrating injuries cause a marked loss of vision. However, injuries from small particles traveling at a significant speed may produce only mild pain and blurring of vision (Vaughan et al, 1992). Other signs of penetrating injuries include an irregular pupil, vitreous hemorrhage, laceration of the conjunctiva or cornea, and a hyphema.

Some patients present for treatment with the object still protruding from the eye. Extreme care must be taken not to disturb this object because it may be holding ocular contents in place.

MEDICAL DIAGNOSIS

The medical diagnosis is made on the basis of a careful patient history and is validated through an examination. Visual acuity is examined before conducting any part of the examination to document the patient's visual status before care for medical and legal reasons. Near and distance vision are tested.

If a foreign body is suspected, the upper eyelid is everted and the bulbar and palpebral conjunctiva examined with a slit lamp.

Fluorescein is used to highlight areas of corneal abrasion. This dye, when viewed with a blue filter, colors any abraded area a vivid and easily detected green.

The cornea, sclera, iris, and lens are examined with the slit lamp or direct ophthalmoscope for evidence of an entrance wound. X-ray films and computed tomographic (CT) scans of the eye and orbit are used to locate objects and fragments (Vaughan et al, 1992). Ultrasonography may also be used to determine the location of the intraocular foreign body in relationship to ocular structures. Magnetic resonance imaging (MRI) may also be used if a nonmetal foreign body is suspected.

MEDICAL MANAGEMENT

Contusions usually require ice to reduce swelling. If the force caused bleeding into the anterior chamber, the patient is placed on bed rest because rebleeding in the first few days is possible. Patients with a hyphema may receive aminocaproic acid (Amicar) to prevent further bleeding (Coles, 1989). Patients with hyphema should sleep and rest with the head elevated, so the blood will settle to the lower anterior chamber and away from the visual pathway. IOP is monitored because blood in the anterior chamber can potentially obstruct the trabecular meshwork and prevent drainage of aqueous humor.

Corneal abrasions are treated by removing the cause, when possible. For example, a foreign body on the conjunctiva is irrigated away. An ophthalmic antibiotic, such as gentamicin (Gentacidin), is then instilled. The eye is patched closed for 24 hours, the usual healing and regenerating time necessary for the corneal epithelium.

Lacerations usually require stitches. If the laceration does not involve the edge of the eyelid, a simple closure is possible. Lacerations involving the cornea must be treated as an ocular emergency because the laceration creates an opening through which microorganisms can directly enter the eye and ocular contents can prolapse. These lacerations are repaired under the operating room microscope. Once repaired, an ophthalmic antibiotic, such as gentamicin (Gentacidin) ointment, is instilled and an eye patch and shield applied. Visual acuity is carefully monitored over the next few days. Deep corneal lacerations may heal with a scar.

Foreign bodies may or may not be removed depending on the composition of the foreign body as well as its location in the eye. Foreign bodies made of metals such as iron and copper must be removed because these metals are toxic to ocular tissues. Materials such as porcelain and glass are well tolerated by the eye and might not need to be removed (Vaughan et al, 1992). The exact surgical procedure depends on the location of the object. Special equipment, such as metal locators and magnets, may be used.

Application of the Nursing Process to the Care of the Patient with Ocular Trauma

Assessment

When obtaining a history from a patient with a known or suspected ocular injury, provide for patient comfort. If photophobia is present, dim the room lights. If tearing is a problem, provide adequate tissues. Unless the problem is obvious, such as a bleeding eyelid or an object protruding from the eye, ask the patient why he or she is seeking care. Ask when it began or happened and what he or she was doing at that time. If an injury is described, ask about the circumstances and the first aid, if any, that was given on the scene. Find out what materials the patient was working with, such as metal or glass. Ask whether the patient takes any medications, especially anticoagulants or aspirin. Also determine when the patient last had a tetanus shot and whether he or she has any allergies. If surgery is a possibility, ask when food and fluids were last consumed.

Obtain a baseline acuity for both near and distance vision. Examine the external eye. Are there any foreign bodies present? Are the eyelids intact? If sections of the eyelid are missing, ask the patient or family if they know where the missing fragments are, because in many cases, these segments can be reattached. Observe the external eye for ecchymosis.

Observe for signs and symptoms of anxiety, because patients with ocular trauma are worried about their vision and whether any permanent damage has been done.

Nursing Diagnoses and Planning

Nursing diagnoses and related expected patient outcomes most commonly applicable to patients with ocular trauma include the following:

NDx: Pain related to irritation of the corneal nerve

Planning: Patient outcomes

1. Patient participates in the examination without indication of excessive pain.
2. Patient reports intensity of symptoms to be manageable.

NDx: Anxiety related to possible loss of vision or failure to regain vision

Planning: Patient outcomes

1. Patient reports anxiety level is manageable.
2. Behavioral signs of severe anxiety are absent.

NDx: High risk for altered health maintenance related to insufficient knowledge of prevention of future ocular injuries

Planning: Patient outcomes

1. Patient lists common causes of ocular trauma.
2. Patient identifies measures to use in the prevention of ocular trauma.

Nursing Interventions

NDx: Pain

Because of the large number of nerve fibers in the cornea, abrasions can be extremely painful. The pain can actually be so severe that it disables the patient. Immediately promote comfort by dimming the lights of the examination room. Once the diagnosis of a corneal abrasion has been made, instill a drop of topical anesthetic (e.g., proparacaine [Ophthetic]) as ordered. Keep in mind, however, that repeated use of topical anesthetics retards healing. Apply an eye patch for overnight wear. Patch the eyelid in the closed position to prevent the eyelid from rubbing against the abrasion with blinking.

Administer oral analgesics such as acetaminophen (Tylenol) as ordered for severe pain. Continue to maintain dim lighting, provide quiet conversation or distraction, and apply a cool cloth over the closed eyelids for brief periods to further promote comfort.

These measures to reduce pain and photophobia should also be effective in reducing tearing, which is usually a reflex mechanism.

NDx: Anxiety

Expect the patient to be anxious over the possibility of a short-term or permanent loss of vision. Acknowledge this anxiety as well as anticipatory grief as normal reactions. Listen supportively, and reassure the patient that measures to save vision are being taken. Also be certain to keep the patient and family informed of what is happening. Ask the patient about measures that would provide comfort (e.g., the presence of a clergy person or friend). Remind the patient that after trauma vision may take a while to return to baseline. Help the patient to recognize the improvement.

NDx: High risk for altered health maintenance

Most eye injuries are preventable. Instruct the patient that abrasions from tree branches and high-speed grass particles can be prevented by wearing sunglasses or safety glasses. The same is true for abrasions caused by high-speed metal particles.

Encourage the patient to use protective eye wear when participating in sports, especially high-speed sports such as racquetball and tennis. Encourage local racquet clubs to discourage play unless participants are wearing appropriate protective eye wear. Warn cross-country skiers and hikers about the potential for injury while participating in these activities. Remind the patient that excessive exposure to sunlight, such as falling asleep in the sun, can cause severe corneal damage.

Caution the patient who wears contact lenses against excessive wear. Review a reasonable wearing schedule with the patient as well as its rationale.

Discuss safe handling of sharp objects in the home, school, work place, and other high risk areas. Stress that individuals not familiar with the sharp object should be supervised in its use.

Additional Interventions

Guilt frequently is experienced by others involved in the trauma, like the hockey player who shot the puck that injured the patient or the fellow racquetball player who hit the ball that struck the patient in the eye. If these individuals are present, be aware of this need and help them deal with their feelings of guilt.

Evaluation

Evaluate the effectiveness of nursing care for a patient with a contusion, abrasion, laceration, or penetrating injury of the eye by comparing the patient's status with the expected patient outcomes. Examples of specific outcomes for patients with an eye injury have been provided in the Planning section.

Chemical Burns

ETIOLOGY AND PATHOPHYSIOLOGY

Chemicals can come into contact with the eye or eyelids in many forms and from a variety of sources, such as steam, molten metal, hot ashes, strong acids (battery acid), and alkalis (lye, lime). Because of the devastating effects on the eye, contact with chemicals is an ocular emergency.

The extent of damage depends on the exact chemical involved, duration of time between exposure and institution of first aid, degree of penetration into the eye, and definitive treatment in an emergency care setting.

For example, when acids come in contact with the eye, direct damage of the tissue results. However, the acids form a cover of coagulated tissue that protects ocular structures from further penetration of the chemical.

Alkaline chemicals, on the other hand, can cause both immediate and delayed changes because they are able to penetrate deeply into tissues and cause damage long after initial exposure. Alkali burns contract the sclera, which causes an increase in IOP. Prostaglandin is released, which increases blood flow to the iris, ciliary body, and choroid, and results in a severe case of uveitis (Vaughan et al, 1992).

Because of its anatomic position, the cornea is frequently affected by chemical burns. Perforation and scarring of the cornea are common. Entropion of the eyelids can also result. Intraocular structures such as the lens and trabecular meshwork can be affected, leading to the development of cataracts and glaucoma.

CLINICAL MANIFESTATIONS

A patient with a chemical burn relates a history of something splashing into the face. The pain is intense, and the patient may be unable to open the eyes.

First and second degree burns of the periorbital area may be present (Friedberg & Rapuano, 1990) as a result of irritation by the chemicals. The conjunctiva may be red, ischemic, or absent. All or part of the corneal epithelium may be absent. Total anesthesia of the cornea is possible as well as a corneal haze, which can make evaluation of the internal eye difficult or impossible. In some cases, a totally white cornea is present.

MEDICAL DIAGNOSIS

The diagnosis of a chemical burn is made on the basis of history and ocular examination. No assessment is conducted nor history obtained, however, until after the ocular irrigation has begun.

MEDICAL MANAGEMENT

Treatment of a chemical burn should begin at the site of exposure (Table 40–4). Copious irrigation with water or saline should be conducted even before transport to the emergency care center. If the patient is unable to hold the eyelids open—a normal response—someone should provide assistance. If no facilities for irrigation of the eye exist, the patient is instructed to hold the eyes open under a running shower. A sink filled with water, into which the patient submerges the head, will also work. The patient must be reminded to keep the eyes open to adequately flush the area.

On arrival at the emergency care center, the eyes are again irrigated copiously with 0.9% saline. Ophthalmic anesthetic drops, such as proparacaine (Ophthetic), are instilled periodically for patient comfort. The irrigations are continued until the pH is approximately 7.0 (Friedberg & Rapuano, 1990).

Once the irrigations are complete, an eye drop program to combat ocular inflammation is begun. Antiglaucoma agents and pupillary dilation drugs are used. A short-term course of steroid drops may be used, but long-term administration may contribute to problems with corneal healing.

Patients are usually admitted to the hospital, so IOP and indications of healing can be closely monitored. Recovery from a chemical burn is a long process, and there is great uncertainty about return of vision. Some patients fail to recover much vision. In cases of severe chemical burns affecting the cornea, a transplant may be required, but success is limited after this type of injury.

Guidelines for Application of the Nursing Process to the Care of the Patient with a Chemical Ocular Burn

Nursing care of the patient with a chemical ocular burn is similar to that of the patient with mechanical trauma with several specific considerations.

When assessing a patient with a known or suspected chemical burn, be sure to begin the irrigation first (Table 40–5).

Question the patient about allergies. If no allergy to drugs of the -caine family exists, instill a drop of proparacaine (Ophthetic) to anesthetize the external eye. During irrigation, periodically assess the patient's level of comfort, and administer additional drops of proparacaine (Ophthetic) as necessary.

Find out when the exposure to the chemical occurred, the name and type of chemical, whether a sample of the chemical can be obtained, and the emergency care that was administered at the scene. Also determine whether contact lenses were being

Table 40–4. EMERGENCY TREATMENT OF CHEMICAL BURNS OF THE EYE

1. Flush affected eye immediately with a large amount of clean water or irrigating solution for 10 minutes to shorten chemical contact with ocular tissues.
2. Hold patient's hands away from face if necessary because of the normal protective response to cover eyes with hands, an action that limits access to the eye.
3. Hold eyelids open widely during procedure because a larger area can be flushed.
4. Quickly check visual acuity to provide baseline information for medical and legal reasons.
5. Obtain a sample of the chemical involved. Send it and its container with the injured person to the hospital or emergency care center to help identify the specific substance.
6. Get the patient to the hospital or emergency care center.
7. Tell someone to alert the hospital or emergency care center that patient is en route to enable the facility to have equipment ready on the patient's arrival.

Table 40–5. IRRIGATION OF THE EYE

1. Obtain the following necessary equipment:
   - 0.9% saline (1-L bag)
   - Macrodrip IV tubing
   - IV pole or other suspension device
   - Topical anesthetic drops (proparacaine [Ophthetic])
   - Eyelid speculum or irrigating contact lens
   - Gloves (unsterile)
   - pH paper
   - Towels
   - Collection container
2. Simultaneously obtain history as tubing or contact lens is being flushed with saline solution because time is of the essence.
   Determine the following:
   - Time of injury
   - Type of chemical or irritant
   - First aid given on site
   - Allergy to -caine drugs
3. Briefly describe procedure to patient to promote cooperation and to decrease anxiety.
4. Assess visual acuity for medical and legal reasons before starting treatment.
5. Put on gloves to reduce potential for exposure to chemicals.
6. Assess pH by dabbing paper in cul-de-sac to determine nature of chemical and help plan treatment.
7. Instill proparacaine hydrochloride (Ophthetic) prn or per protocol to enhance comfort by anesthetizing the external eye.
8. Turn the patient onto the affected side so drainage flows away from the unaffected eye.
9. Place irrigating contact lens or eyelid speculum to spread eyelids because normal reflex is to close eyes. Avoid using contact lens if particulate matter is suspected, because it could be ground into cornea.
10. Direct irrigating solution from the medial to the lateral canthus to flush surface without recontamination.
11. Monitor the patient's level of comfort throughout, and instill anesthetic drops as necessary.
12. Reassure the patient throughout procedure to reduce feeling of anxiety.
13. Irrigate both eyes simultaneously if both are affected to reduce chemical contact time with eye tissue.

Abbreviations: IV, intravenous; prn, as occasion requires.

worn at the time of exposure, because they will need to be removed. Use strict aseptic technique because the potential for infection exists as a result of the disruption of the intact surface of the eye.

Be sensitive to the patient's high level of anxiety. Almost constant reassurance and positive reinforcement are necessary throughout the assessment, diagnosis, intervention, and evaluation processes. Answer questions honestly yet hopefully.

Be aware that grieving for loss of vision will occur.

Neoplasia

Choroidal Melanoma

ETIOLOGY AND PATHOPHYSIOLOGY

Choroidal melanoma is the most common primary intraocular tumor in adults; approximately 1500 cases are diagnosed each year in the United States (Servodidio, 1991). It is almost always unilateral and is more commonly found in whites (Vaughan et al, 1992).

Choroidal melanomas spread easily because of the rich blood supply of the choroid. They can also directly invade ocular structures through the overlying sclera.

CLINICAL MANIFESTATIONS

Symptoms of choroidal melanoma include flashes of light, floaters, and visual field defects. If the macular area is involved, vision may be blurred. Tumors involving the anterior chamber angle can limit outflow of aqueous humor and increase IOP. If the tumor is of significant size, it can invade the subretinal space and cause a retinal detachment. Tumors invading the iris can affect its color.

Choroidal melanomas are frequently found in asymptomatic patients who present for treatment of another ophthalmic complaint.

MEDICAL DIAGNOSIS

The diagnosis of a choroidal melanoma is made on the basis of the patient's history and is validated during the clinical examination.

Fluorescein angiography is done as part of the clinical examination because hyperfluorescence is characteristic of vessels within a choroidal melanoma (Servodidio, 1991). Ultrasonography is used to determine tumor size, height, shape, solidity, vascularity, and proximity to ocular structures, information critical to planning treatment options. Studies to rule out metastases are also done, including tests of liver function such as the gamma-glutamyl transpeptidase (GGTP) because this tumor type has an affinity for the liver.

All patients diagnosed with a choroidal melanoma are referred to an oncologist.

MEDICAL MANAGEMENT

Enucleation and radioactive plaque therapy are two treatments for choroidal melanoma. The treatment that is selected depends on size of the tumor, its growth rate, and the visual function in the other eye.

Enucleation, or removal of the globe, has been the standard approach to treatment of choroidal melanoma.

When an enucleation is performed, the conjunctiva is dissected, and then the eye muscles are isolated and severed. The optic nerve is cut a short distance from its ocular exit, and the eyeball is removed intact. A small, round ball made of silicone is inserted into the socket and covered with conjunctiva. This ball is not visible. A small cap, called a conformer, is placed between the lids to promote healing. It sometimes falls out on its own 1 or 2 weeks after the operation. Once healed, the socket is similar in appearance to the mucous membrane of the mouth.

A second treatment option is radioactive plaque therapy. In this therapy, a plaque into which a radioactive isotope such as cobalt or iodine 125 is inserted, is sutured to the sclera overlying the tumor. The carefully calculated dose of low-energy gamma radiation is placed in the specially designed plaque by the radiation physicist. The seeds of radioactive isotope are arranged in the plaque so as to deliver the majority of the dose to the tumor while minimizing the exposure to nearby ocular structures. The plaque remains in place for approximately 4 to 7 days. A second surgical procedure is necessary to remove the plaque.

After plaque removal, the patient is placed on a 2-week eye drop program of steroids and antibiotics. This procedure can be performed on an inpatient or outpatient basis, depending on state radiation regulations (Servodidio, 1991).

Application of the Nursing Process to the Care of the Patient Having an Enucleation for Choroidal Melanoma

PREOPERATIVE NURSING CARE

Nursing care for the patient scheduled for enucleation for choroidal melanoma is similar to that for any preoperative patient, with several considerations.

Once the diagnostic and confirmatory tests are complete, treatment options are presented by the ophthalmologist. It is imperative for the patient to receive information on all treatment alternatives available. Reinforce the information provided, and answer questions the patient or family may have. Use anatomic models and be as concrete as possible. Be sure the patient understands that, with enucleation, the eye is removed as well as the tumor and that, in plaque therapy, the eye containing the tumor is left in place and the radioactive isotope is applied to the external eye.

Provide written information to the patient to reinforce that which is received in the ophthalmologist's office. Be sure the patient has a telephone number to call when questions arise.

The anxiety precipitated by a diagnosis of cancer is compounded by the perceived disfiguring nature of an enucleation. Combine a quiet, supportive manner with reassurance that ocular prostheses exist that can make cosmetic appearance very close to normal. Show the patient a picture of a person with an ocular prosthesis in place to demonstrate this point. If the patient is concerned about appearance before the prosthesis is fit, suggest wearing sunglasses. Provide an opportunity for meeting another person who has had an enucleation if the patient so desires.

POSTOPERATIVE NURSING CARE

Assessment

Assess the patient's return to physiologic stabilization. Inspect the dressing for signs of bleeding, and assess the patient's level of comfort.

Nursing Diagnoses and Planning

NDx: Pain related to surgical manipulation of tissue

Planning: Patient outcomes
1. Patient verbalizes that he or she is comfortable.
2. Behavioral signs of severe pain are absent.

NDx: Grieving related to body image changes and loss of vision

Planning: Patient outcomes
1. Patient acknowledges feelings of grief and loss are normal.
2. Patient begins to work through the stages of grief and loss.

NDx: High risk for altered health maintenance related to insufficient knowledge of removal, cleansing, and insertion of an ocular prosthesis

Planning: Patient outcomes
1. Patient states rationale for cleaning prosthesis.
2. Patient cleans prosthesis.
3. Patient removes prosthesis.
4. Patient reinserts prosthesis.

NDx: High risk for injury: blindness related to trauma to only seeing eye

Planning: Patient outcomes
1. Patient states need for protective eyewear.
2. Patient lists ways to protect vision.

Nursing Interventions

NDx: Pain
Dim the lights, and provide a restful environment free from noise. Administer analgesics as ordered. Analgesics are given intramuscularly because gastrointestinal function may be slowed by the anesthetic agent. Expect the enucleation patient's need for analgesics in the immediate postoperative period to be similar to that of other postoperative patients.

NDx: Grieving
Vision is the sense we use with greatest frequency. Loss of vision, combined with the change in body image, can be a difficult combination for the patient. Like other cancer patients, they deal with feelings of grief and loss. Because patients are hospitalized for a very short period of time, it is not possible for

Chart 40–4.

NURSING GUIDE TO PATIENT EDUCATION FOR SELF-MANAGEMENT: REMOVAL, CARE, AND INSERTION OF AN OCULAR PROSTHESIS

Instruct the patient in the removal, care, and insertion of an ocular prosthesis as described here.

Removal of an Ocular Prosthesis

1. Gather equipment: container with lid.
2. Wash hands to reduce surface microorganisms.
3. Sit up and flex chin slightly for easy removal.
4. Place hand against cheek, palm side up (Fig. 40–13*A*) to create a platform for the prosthesis to rest on when removed.
5. Pull lower lid slightly down and (Fig. 40–13*B*) toward ear to extend surface area for easy prosthesis removal.
6. Allow prosthesis to slide out onto fingers and then grasp (Fig. 40–13C).
7. Exert gentle pull if needed.
8. Place prosthesis in container and cover for protection.

Care of an Ocular Prosthesis

1. Gather equipment: clean container with lid, mild soap, towel, and container.
2. Wash hands to reduce surface microorganisms.
3. Drape area with cloth or towel to act as a cushion for the prosthesis should it be dropped.
4. Close sink drain to prevent loss of prosthesis.
5. Rinse prosthesis with tepid tap water to remove secretions.
6. Put prosthesis in palm of nondominant hand for cleaning.
7. Rub small amount of mild soap over prosthesis with finger pad to reduce surface tension and ease removal of secretions.
8. Use tepid water to rinse soap residue from prosthesis because extreme temperatures can shatter prosthesis.
9. Check prosthesis for surface deposits or scratches, which can irritate lids.
10. Place prosthesis in container cushioned with a 4×4 for safe storage.

Insertion of an Ocular Prosthesis

1. Wash hands to reduce surface microorganisms.
2. Drape towel over work area to protect prosthesis should it be dropped.
3. Take prosthesis from container and rinse with tepid water (Fig. 40–13*D*).
4. Raise upper lid against eyebrow using nondominant hand (Fig. 40–13*E*) to fully expose socket.
5. Place prosthesis between thumb and forefinger of dominant hand with the notched end of prosthesis closest to nose (Fig. 40–13*F*).
6. Slide the prosthesis under the upper lid until most of iris is covered (Fig. 40–13*G*).
7. Slowly release upper eyelid.
8. Retract lower lid down toward cheek until bottom edge of prosthesis slips underneath it (Fig. 40–13*G*) to permit entrance of bottom edge of prosthesis into socket itself.
9. Release hands slowly.

Note: When the nurse is removing, cleansing, or inserting an ocular prosthesis for a patient, the procedure is explained to reduce anxiety and promote cooperation; nonsterile gloves are worn to create a barrier against contact with secretions; and the prosthesis is stored in a container labeled with the patient's name.

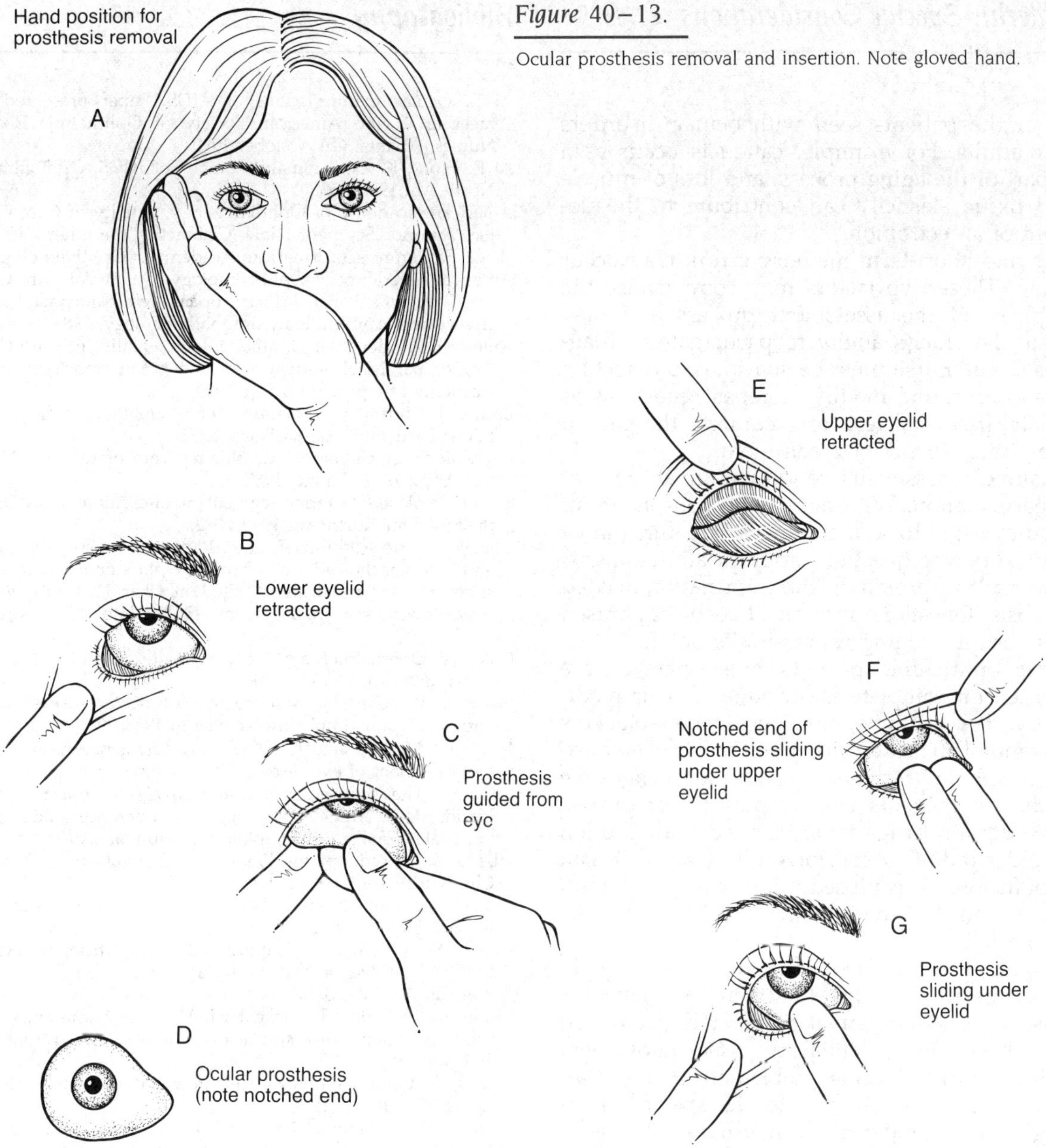

Figure 40–13.

Ocular prosthesis removal and insertion. Note gloved hand.

them to complete grief work while in the hospital. Help patients realize grief work is a process requiring time.

NDx: High risk for altered health maintenance

Initiate a referral to a home-care agency for assistance with removing, cleaning, and inserting the ocular prosthesis, which is usually custom designed, painted, and fit approximately 4 to 6 weeks after surgery. Review the procedure for the removal, care, and insertion of an ocular prosthesis, as presented in Chart 40–4 and Figure 40–13.

NDx: High risk for injury: blindness

Instruct the patient on extra precautions to take to minimize the potential for injury to the one remaining seeing eye (see Chart 39–3). Stress the importance of protective eye wear for the monocular patient, and keep in mind that some patients may be encouraged to wear eyeglasses, even when no visual correction is needed in the seeing eye, because the clear lenses provide added protection against flying debris, dust, and dirt.

Evaluation

Evaluate the effectiveness of nursing care for the patient who has had an enucleation for choroidal melanoma by comparing the patient's status with the expected patient outcomes. Examples of specific outcomes for the patient who has had an enucleation have been provided in the Planning section.

The Elderly: Special Considerations

Many of the patients seen with ocular disorders are older adults. For example, cataracts occur as a normal part of the aging process, and loss of muscle tone and tissue elasticity can contribute to the development of an ectropion.

Fatigue and short-term memory errors may occur with aging. These two factors may compromise the history phase of the assessment process and may complicate the elder's ability to participate in diagnostic tests. The nurse must be sensitive to detecting when they occur, and modify or repeat questions as appropriate. If several tests are required, the patient may appreciate a break between them.

Ophthalmic assessments require a great deal of patient participation. With aging, the consonants of *p, t, f,* and *sh* begin to sound similar. The nurse must be careful to phrase questions appropriately to assist the older adult in providing the information needed for diagnosis. Questions may need to be rephrased if a vague or questioning expression is noted.

Geriatric ophthalmic patients must receive care that is based on complete knowledge of their medical history. For example, nonspecific beta-blockers such as timolol maleate (Timoptic) can cause shortness of breath and trigger episodes of congestive heart failure in patients with respiratory or cardiac problems. Certain drugs must be used with caution in the older adult. Acetazolamide (Diamox) can cause confusion. A confused state, combined with impaired vision, has the potential to predispose the elderly to a fall.

With aging, pupillary reactivity slows. Many ophthalmic drugs used in the treatment of glaucoma can cause miosis. The small pupil and prolonged reactivity have the potential to make movement from bright to dim lighting problematic. Careful attention must also be directed to the specific treatment regimen. The older adult may have arthritis or orthopedic problems that may require special adaptation for comfort during surgery. Because most eye surgery is performed under local anesthetic, it is imperative that the patient be comfortable and not move during the procedure. When planning care, the nurse must ask whether the older adult can see the fine print on the label of the eye drop bottle and whether the patient with arthritic hands can instill the required eye drops.

As patients age, color sensitivity to blues, greens, and violets decreases. Care must be exercised when incorporating visual cues into the treatment process as reminders for patients. Many eye drops come in bottles with colored tops. The nurse must assess whether the patient can determine the color of the top before providing cues such as "use one drop from the green-topped bottle three times a day."

Bibliography

Ai E. Ocular manifestations of AIDS. Paper presented at the meeting of the American Society of Ophthalmic Registered Nurses, Atlanta, GA, October 1990.

Ai E, Wong K. Ocular manifestations of AIDS. Ophthalmol Clin North Am 1988;1:53.

American Academy of Ophthalmology, Quality of Care Committee, Anterior Segment Panel. Cataract in the otherwise healthy eye. San Francisco: American Academy of Ophthalmology, 1989.

American Academy of Ophthalmology, Quality of Care Committee, Glaucoma Panel. Primary open angle glaucoma. San Francisco: American Academy of Ophthalmology, 1989.

American Academy of Ophthalmology, Quality of Care Committee, Retinal Panel. Retinal detachment. San Francisco: American Academy of Ophthalmology, 1990.

Bartlett J, Ghormley N, Jaanus S, et al. Ophthalmic drug facts. St. Louis: Facts and Comparisons, 1992.

Boyd-Monk H, Steinmetz C. Nursing care of the eye. Norwalk, CT: Appleton & Lange, 1987.

Caskey P, Ai E. Posterior segment manifestations of AIDS. Ophthalmol Clin North Am 1990;3:393.

Char D, Castro J, Philips T, et al. Radiation vs. surgery for ciliary and anterior choroidal melanomas. Ophthalmology (manuscript submitted for publication), cited in Char D. Controversies in uveal melanoma management. Ophthalmol Clin North Am 1990;3:429.

Coles W. Ophthalmology: A diagnostic text. Baltimore, MD: Williams & Wilkins, 1989.

Freeman W, Gross J. Management of ocular disease in AIDS patients. Ophthalmol Clin North Am 1988;1:91.

Friedberg M, Rapuano C. Office and emergency room diagnosis and treatment of eye disease. Philadelphia: JB Lippincott, 1990.

Grady C. The immune system and AIDS/HIV infection. In Flaskerud J (ed). AIDS/HIV infection: A reference guide for nursing professionals. Philadelphia: WB Saunders, 1989.

Jabs D. AIDS retinopathy: Findings and significance. Ophthalmol Clin North Am 1988;1:101.

Miller S. Parson's disease of the eye. 18th ed. New York: Churchill-Livingstone, 1990.

Mines J, Kaplan H. Acquired immunodeficiency syndrome (AIDS): The disease and its ocular manifestations. Int Ophthalmol Clin 1986;26:73.

Moore M, McCulley J, Luckenbach M, et al. Acanthamoeba keratitis associated with soft contact lenses. Am J Ophthalmol 1985;100:396.

Newell F. Ophthalmology: Principles and concepts. 7th ed. St. Louis: CV Mosby, 1992.

Orticio L. Confusion and the patient on an intensive topical ocular antibiotic regimen: A case analysis. J Ophthalmic Nurs Technol 1990;4:145.

Pederson K, Nulty G. Nursing grand rounds: Herpes zoster ophthalmicus. J Ophthalmic Nurs Technol 1987;6:151.

Rao N, Biswas J. Ocular pathology in AIDS. Ophthalmol Clin North Am 1988;1:63.

Ruehl CA, Schremp PS. Nursing care of the cataract patient: Today's outpatient approach. Nurs Clin North Am 1992; 27(3):727.

Schatz H, McDonald H. For our patients: Macular degeneration. San Francisco: Retinal Research Fund, 1987.

Servodidio C. Choroidal melanoma, what is it? Insight 1991;1:16.

Ungvarski PJ. Nursing management of the adult client. In Flaskerud JH, Ungvarski PJ (eds). HIV/AIDS: A guide to nursing care. 2nd ed. Philadelphia: WB Saunders, 1992, pp 146–198.

Vader LA. Vision and vision loss. Nurs Clin North Am 1992;27(3):705.

Vaughan D, Asbury T, Riordan-Eva P. General ophthalmology. 13th ed. Los Angeles: Lange, 1992.

Woods S. Macular degeneration. Nurs Clin North Am 1992;27(3):761.

Chapter Forty-one

KNOWLEDGE BASIC TO THE NURSING CARE *of Adults with Dysfunction of the Ear*

The ear is a complex organ whose function is a major determinant of the quality of an individual's life experience.

As the organ of hearing, the ear facilitates communication with other people and provides important information about the environment such as the sound of oncoming traffic, sirens, fire alarms, and cries of warning, all of which can be critical to an individual's safety. As the organ of balance, the ear facilitates the ability to be mobile and to manipulate objects in the environment.

In preparation for the study of the nursing care of adults with ear disorders, this chapter presents an overview of the anatomy and physiology of the ear followed by a discussion of clinical manifestations common to ear disorders, assessment of the ear, and related diagnostic measures. The chapter ends with a discussion of otologic surgical procedures and specific considerations basic to the care of the elderly with an ear disorder.

Anatomy and Physiology

The ear serves as the organ of both hearing and equilibrium (balance). It is a complex structure that consists of three divisions: the external ear, the middle ear, and the inner ear (Fig. 41–1).

External Ear

The external ear includes the auricle (pinna) and the external auditory meatus (ear canal). The auricle projects from the side of the head and is composed of cartilage, which gives shape to the ear, muscle, and, in the earlobe, some adipose tissue. The external auditory canal is a tube-shaped passage approximately 2.5 cm in length that extends inward medially, proximally, and downward in adults. The canal is lined with skin and contains hairs and cerumen-producing (wax-producing) glands.

The external ear, or outer ear, is separated from the middle ear by the tympanic membrane (eardrum) located at the end of the auditory canal. Sound waves are collected and focused by the auricle and travel within the canal, impinging on the tympanic membrane, causing it to vibrate. This vibration sets into motion the ossicles (bones) of the middle ear.

Middle Ear

The middle-ear space, also referred to as the tympanic cavity, is a small, irregular, air-filled cavity within the temporal bone. It is separated from the inner ear by a thin, bony wall and two membrane-covered openings: the fenestra vestibuli (oval window) and the fenestra cochleae (round window). Anteriorly, the middle ear communicates with the eustachian tube, which forms a channel between the middle ear and the nasopharynx. This connection allows air to enter the middle-ear space, which equalizes the pressure on both sides of the tympanic membrane. Posteriorly, there is an opening into the mastoid antrum, which communicates with the mastoid air cells.

The three ossicles within the middle ear are the smallest bones in the body. These tiny, articulated bones connect the tympanic membrane to the oval window. The most lateral bone (that closest to the outside of the head), the malleus (hammer), is at-

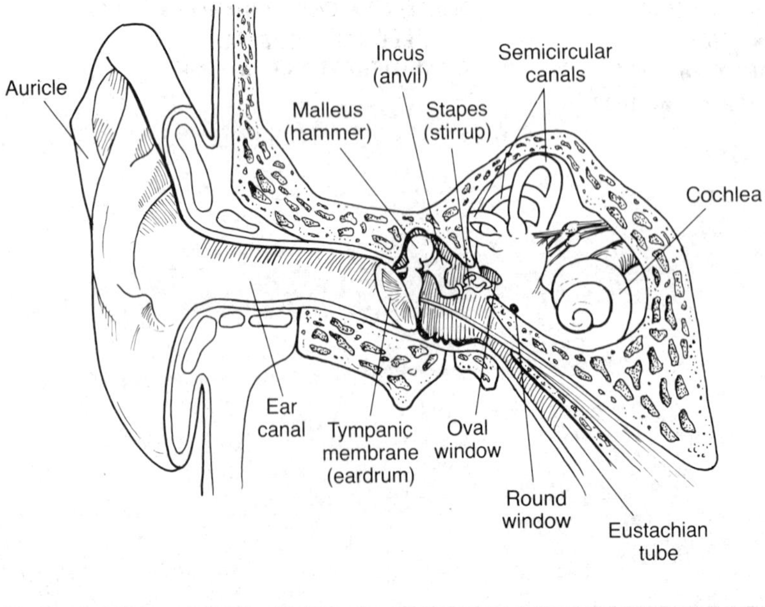

Figure 41–1.

Anatomic structure of the ear. Note the three major divisions of the ear: external, middle, and inner (see text), as well as the structures within each.

tached to the tympanic membrane at the umbo. The malleus is attached to the incus (anvil), which in turn is connected to the stapes (stirrup) at a ball-and-socket joint called the incudostapedial joint. These connections, or articulations, and the two tendons within the middle ear, the tensor tympani tendon and the stapedius tendon, modify movement of the ossicles in response to displacement by sound waves, thereby protecting the ear from damage by very loud sounds.

When sound waves enter the ear canal, they set the tympanic membrane in motion. These vibrations, amplified by the ossicles, which function as a system of levers, are transmitted via the oval window to the fluid-filled structures of the inner ear.

Inner Ear

The inner ear is the most complex and most important portion of the auditory system. Within it are found the structures necessary for both hearing and balance. The inner ear is a closed, fluid-filled space located within the petrous portion of the temporal bone. The structures that make up the inner ear include the vestibule, which houses the utricle and saccule; the semicircular canals, which respond to movements of the head in three planes; and the cochlea, which contains the organ of hearing. The bony portion known as the osseous labyrinth contains the membranous labyrinth. Perilymphatic fluid, a plasma filtrate, fills the space between the bony labyrinth and the membranous labyrinth. Endolymphatic fluid, similar in content to both cerebrospinal fluid (CSF) and perilymphatic fluid, fills the membranous labyrinth. Abnormal communications of these fluids with other divisions of the ear or alterations in amounts of fluid present within these spaces are thought to account for some of the symptoms associated with various inner ear dysfunctions. The vestibule lies posterior to the cochlea and anterior to the semicircular canals. Within the vestibule, two fluid-filled sacs, the utricle and saccule, oriented at 90 degrees to each other, respond to slow movements of the head, straight-ahead movements, and gravity through a complex relationship of polarization and depolarization of the cell membranes of the cilia contained within. Impulses result from this depolarization and are sent along the vestibular nerve to the brain to interpret environmental stimuli and to aid the brain in altering body position or eye movement to maintain equilibrium.

The semicircular canals also aid in the body and brain response to changes in direction of head movement. These three canals—the anterior semicircular canal, the posterior semicircular canal, and the lateral or horizontal semicircular canal—lie in planes at right angles to each other. In this orientation, they are able to respond to changes of head movement in all three planes and to provide information to the cerebellum via cranial nerve VIII to correct for change in direction or movement. Movement of the fluid within these canals is responsible for a sensation of dizziness or vertigo, which may be associated with motion sickness or other vestibular disorders.

The cochlea is a bony, tubelike structure coiled like a snail shell, which contains the organ of hearing known as the organ of Corti. The cochlea too is filled with perilymphatic fluid, the volume of which is approximately equal to two drops of water. The oval window and the round window are the points at which the middle ear interfaces with the inner ear. The oval window is the communication point within which the stapes footplate's displacement moves the fluid in the cochlea. The organ of Corti contains receptor cells in the form of cilia, or hair cells. These specialized hair cells respond to various frequencies of sound, and their response is transformed into an electrical impulse that is sent along the cochlear nerve to the brain, where it is interpreted as sound.

A brief and highly simplified scheme of events involved in the collection, amplification, transformation, and interpretation of sound waves is presented next.

Sound waves in the environment set particles of air in motion, which enter the external auditory meatus (canal) and in turn displace the eardrum or tympanic membrane. This movement of the eardrum displaces the ossicles (hammer, anvil, and stirrup or malleus, incus, and stapes). The function of these ossicles is to amplify the force of the sound 15 to 20 times and to act as the transmission mechanism to the cochlea via displacement of the stapes footplate in the oval window. This displacement sets the perilymphatic fluid in motion, which subsequently stimulates the receptor hair cells in the cochlea's organ of Corti. These signals are transformed from vibratory energy into electrical impulses by the previously mentioned hair cells and are then sent as electrical impulses to the brain to be interpreted.

Clinical Manifestations of Ear Dysfunction

Hearing Loss

The major clinical manifestation of ear disorders is loss of hearing. This occurs for a wide variety of reasons and is classified as conductive, sensorineural, or mixed. There is also a category known as functional hearing loss, which is psychogenic in origin.

CONDUCTIVE HEARING LOSS

Conductive hearing loss results from any condition that interferes with the normal transmission of sound waves from the external or middle ear to the inner ear.

The possible causes of conductive hearing loss are varied and numerous. Foreign bodies in the external ear, excessive wax buildup, or bony growths of the ear canal can contribute to conductive loss associated with the external ear. Causes of conductive hearing loss associated with the middle ear are upper respiratory tract infections, allergies, eustachian tube dysfunction, middle-ear infections and effusions, growths (benign or malignant), and traumatic disruption of the ossicles within the middle ear. In addition, congenital defects, hereditary disorders, and complications of ear surgery may result in conductive hearing loss.

SENSORINEURAL HEARING LOSS

Sensorineural hearing loss is the result of damage within the inner ear or to the neural pathway that communicates with the brain. This type of hearing loss may be temporary, fluctuating, or permanent, and its onset may be sudden, intermittent, or gradual. Sudden sensorineural hearing loss may develop as a result of a viral infection. The resultant hearing loss is often initially quite profound but not infrequently returns to normal. Viral labyrinthitis, which may be related to acute or chronic infections of the middle ear or meningitis, often causes a complete sensorineural hearing loss.

Ototoxic drugs (Table 41–1) may cause sensorineural hearing loss and may also affect the vestibular portion of the inner ear, causing vertigo in addition to hearing loss. Other causes of sensorineural hearing loss include Meniere's disease, noise trauma, tumors of the auditory nerve, hereditary factors, congenital defects, and long-term noise exposure. Presbycusis, the progressive sensorineural hearing loss associated with the normal process of aging, is the most common type of sensorineural hearing loss.

MIXED HEARING LOSS

Mixed hearing loss is the term used to refer to cases in which hearing loss is a combination of conductive and sensorineural components.

Table 41–1. DRUGS TOXIC TO THE INNER EAR

Alkylating agents used in chemotherapy such as cisplatin	Antimalarials
Aminoglycosides	Chloroquine hydrochloride
Gentamicin	Quinine sulfate
Kanamycin sulfate	Diuretics
Neomycin sulfate	Ethacrynic acid
Streptomycin sulfate	Furosemide
Tobramycin sulfate	Drugs that cause dizziness
Antiarrhythmics	Antihypertensives
Quinine	Barbiturates
Anti-infectives	Estrogens
Vancomycin	Oral contraceptives
	Phenothiazines

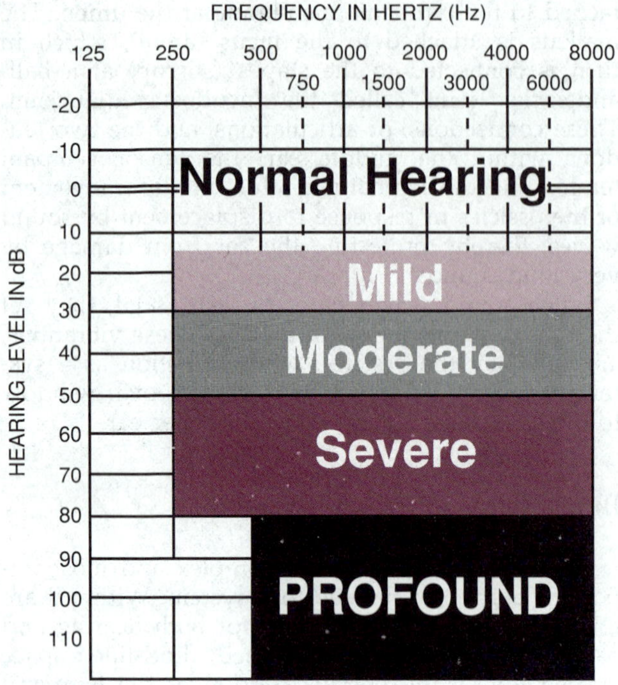

Figure 41–2.

Audiogram outlining the ranges for the classification of hearing loss. (Redrawn from Lilly LF. Cochlear implants: The second generation. In *Perioperative Nursing Quarterly*, Vol. 2:3, p. 10, with permission of Aspen Publishers, Inc., © 1986.)

FUNCTIONAL HEARING LOSS

Functional hearing loss is unrelated to organic factors and is usually psychogenic in origin. The hearing loss is usually complete, although malingering may account for selective hearing loss in some patients. In these cases, it is important to examine the possible contributing factors for a patient's unwillingness or inability to hear.

Hearing loss is further categorized in terms of severity. Individuals with a mild to moderate hearing loss (15 dB to 50 dB hearing loss) are referred to as hearing-impaired. Severe hearing loss is defined to be in a range between 50-dB and 80-dB hearing loss. People suffering from a hearing loss of greater than 80 dB in both ears are said to have a profound hearing loss or may be referred to as "deaf" (Fig. 41–2).

Otalgia

Otalgia is ear pain. It can be associated with conductive hearing loss, especially if the cause is infection, trauma, or pressure disturbances associated with eustachian tube dysfunction. Ear pain may affect one or both ears and may be constant or intermittent. It can range in severity from mild fullness or pressure in the ear to excruciating throbbing, pounding, and pressure pain.

Many patients report otalgia that is unrelated to the ears but instead is a result of temporomandibular joint (TMJ) syndrome, in which the articulation of the mandible causes referred pain to the nearby ear. In addition, many patients with head and neck tumors present for medical examination because of the referred otalgia associated with the growth of the tumor.

Otorrhea

Otorrhea is drainage from the ear. The character of the drainage may be clear, bloody, serosanguineous, or purulent. Otorrhea may be a result of disorders associated with the external canal or the middle ear. Skull fractures and other trauma may result in clear, watery otorrhea, indicative of leaking CSF. Bloody otorrhea may suggest hemorrhage alone or hemorrhage and CSF combined. Infections of the external and middle ear can produce a purulent otorrhea, which may be thick and yellow, foul-smelling, and, in some cases, bloody. Tumors may produce a bloody or serosanguineous drainage.

Tinnitus

Tinnitus is a subjective sensation of buzzing, ringing, or tinkling heard in one or both ears. It may be constant or intermittent and varies in the degree of severity. Tinnitus may be symptomatic of both otologic and systemic disease processes such as acoustic trauma, acoustic tumor, Meniere's disease, presbycusis, hypertension, arteriosclerosis, anemia, hypothyroidism, and drug toxicity, to name a few. It can accompany other symptoms of ear disorders such as chronic ear infection or labyrinthitis.

Vertigo

Vertigo is different from dizziness. Dizziness is a sensation of imbalance, unsteadiness, or faintness. It is sometimes associated with giddiness, weakness, confusion, and blurred or double vision. It may be mild or severe with abrupt or gradual onset. It may be aggravated by standing up too quickly and alleviated by rest. Dizziness may occur secondary to anemia, cardiac dysrhythmias, carotid sinus hypersensitivity, emphysema, anxiety disorder, hypertension, orthostatic hypotension, transient ischemic attack (TIA), drug therapy, and whiplash. It is often, and incorrectly, used interchangeably with the term vertigo.

Vertigo is a sensation of revolving in space or of surroundings revolving around oneself. It is often associated with or accompanied by nausea, vomiting, nystagmus, staggering gait, and tinnitus or hearing loss. These symptoms may occur together or separately. True vertigo may have its origins in the inner ear (labyrinthitis, vestibular neuritis, perilymph fistula, Meniere's disease); may indicate the presence of a tumor of the acoustic nerve or the posterior fossa; or may result from ototoxicity secondary to drug therapy or head trauma (Fig. 41–3).

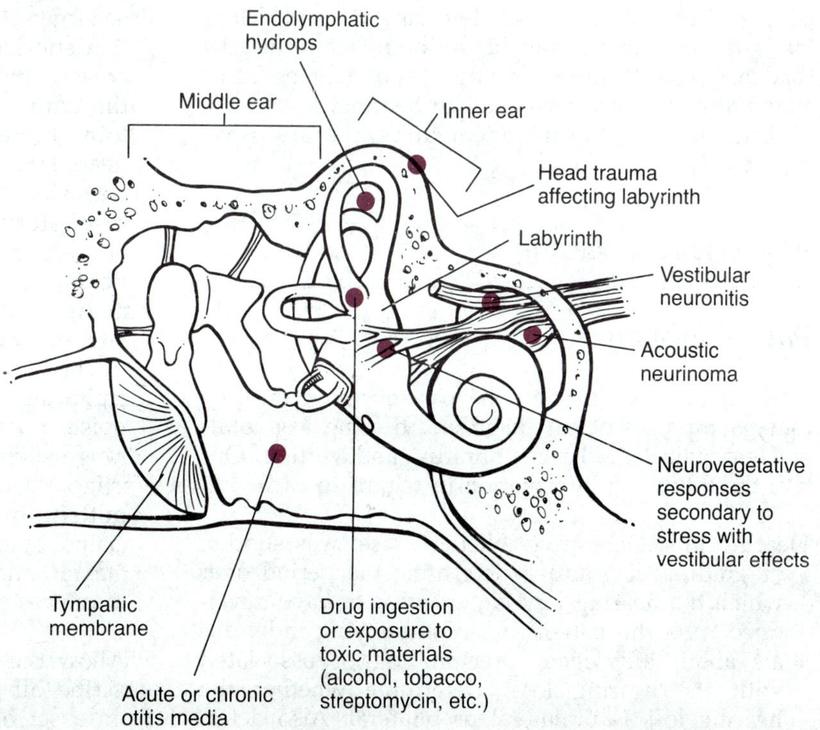

Figure 41–3.

Common locations and types of pathologic changes causing vertigo.

Table 41–2. DRUGS USED TO TREAT VERTIGO

DRUG	CLASSIFICATION	INDICATION FOR USE	ROUTE OF DRUG ADMINISTRATION
Dimenhydrinate (Dramamine)	Antinauseant	Mild vertigo	PO, IM, rectal suppository
Meclizine hydrochloride (Antivert)	Antinauseant	Mild vertigo	PO
Cyclizine lactate (Marezine)	Antinauseant	Mild vertigo	PO, IM, rectal suppository
Buclizine hydrochloride (Bucladin-S Softab)	Antihistamine Antiemetic	Mild vertigo	PO
Atropine sulfate	Anticholinergic	Severe vertigo	PO, IM, IV
Phenobarbital	Sedative	Severe vertigo	PO
Phenobarbital sodium	Sedative	Severe vertigo	IM, IV
Diazepam (Valium)	Tranquilizer	Severe vertigo	PO, IM, IV

Abbreviations: PO, orally; IM, intramuscularly; IV, intravenously.

Vertigo may also be precipitated by positional head changes such as in benign paroxysmal positional vertigo and nystagmus (BPPV or BPPN).

The onset, duration, and severity of the symptoms of vertigo vary with the cause. In BPPN, the condition is worse in the mornings, but patients gradually adjust their movements and responses over the hours of the day and generally report feeling better in the afternoon and evening. Patients with Meniere's disease report their symptoms as progressing in severity the longer they are up and in motion in a normal day. This is thought to relate to the body's ability to adapt to the information being sent to the brain and interpreted by it. Patients with BPPN adjust slowly to their surroundings and to their visual and vestibular input throughout the day, whereas Meniere's patients become fatigued with the visual and vestibular input through the day and succumb to their symptoms as the day progresses. In cases of acute labyrinthitis, the onset may be gradual and persist over several weeks. For patients with Meniere's disease, there may be sudden, severe attacks that last from minutes to hours and may be associated also with acute changes in hearing.

Drugs used in the treatment of vertigo are listed in Table 41–2.

Assessment of the Ear

Patient History

Systematically question the patient about the primary symptoms of ear disorders: hearing loss, otalgia (ear pain), discharge, tinnitus, and vertigo. Obtain the following information in regard to each:

Hearing loss: Determine whether onset was sudden or gradual; if gradual, determine the period over which the hearing loss is perceived to have developed. Ask the patient or accompanying individuals about any event precipitating or associated with the hearing loss. Determine whether the hearing loss is unilateral or bilateral. Also determine its severity and type (patient can hear watch ticking next to ear, cannot hear telephone ringing in the same room, one-on-one conversations are muffled, cannot respond to environmental sounds such as traffic or sirens), duration, and interventions that the patient uses to compensate for the loss such as a hearing aid, lip reading, relying on better ear for hearing, and so on.

Ear pain or discomfort: Determine whether onset was sudden or gradual. Also determine quality, type or severity of pain (throbbing, feeling of fullness, dull ache, sharp, stabbing pain), changes in the quality of pain (sharp, throbbing pain may subside suddenly after the rupture of the tympanic membrane in an acute infectious process), precipitating factors (worse when chewing or yawning, TMJ syndrome), location (can it be reproduced by pulling on the auricle, palpating the TMJ?), and measures the patient has used to alleviate the pain (heat, soft diet, and so on).

Discharge: Determine type and onset. Keep in mind that sudden purulent drainage associated with decreased pain may indicate spontaneous rupture of the tympanic membrane. Also determine duration, location, amount (copious, clear drainage after head trauma may signal a skull fracture), color, consistency, precipitating factors (such as upper respiratory tract infection or a blow to the head), and associated factors such as skin irritation, canal itching, fever, and pain.

Tinnitus: Determine onset, whether bilateral or unilateral, severity, duration, quality (high or low pitched, roaring, humming, or hissing), and precipitating factors (exposure to extremely loud noise, possible proximity to noise out of hearing range such as ultrasonic alarms).

Vertigo: Determine onset, duration, whether intermittent or constant, quality and severity, associated symptoms such as nausea, vomiting, and ataxia, and the type and effectiveness of relief measures used.

Allow the patient to use his or her own words to describe all symptoms instead of forcing a choice from a set of adjectives presented by the examiner.

This provides a more accurate characterization of the symptoms. Assess the patient's understanding of any previously diagnosed chronic ear disorder. If a hearing aid or other assistive device is used, determine the patient's perception of its effectiveness and the consistency of its use by the patient. Also assess the patient's knowledge of care of the aid and any complaints the patient may have regarding it or any other assistive device.

Obtain a complete medical history because some problems of the ear are a result of childhood disease. Establish dates and frequency of past ear problems, noting type of problem (e.g., infection, perforation, drainage, pain) and location. Note early childhood diseases such as mumps and measles, and explore any history of allergies. Investigate the patient's drug history. Question about ototoxic drug regimens (drugs associated with hearing loss, tinnitus, or loss of equilibrium) and chronic use of aspirin or other salicylates because these can cause tinnitus, which disappears on withdrawal of the drug. Question the patient about recent head trauma or other injury. Also obtain a surgical history, noting ear surgery, tonsillectomy, and adenoidectomy.

Review the patient's familial and occupational history to check for hearing or ear disorders and to document long-term exposure to noise from machinery associated with work environments. Because recent research suggests that long-term exposure to loud music either through personal headset stereos or as a member of an audience can result in permanent hearing loss, question the patient as to amount and frequency of exposure to these factors.

Physical Examination

Examine the auricles and surrounding tissues for deformity, nodules, or other lesions. Observe the postauricular and auricular area for drainage. Check for redness, warmth, or swelling and for pain on palpation or on pulling on the auricle. Also check for pain when pressure is exerted on the tragus, which is the cartilaginous projection anterior to the ear canal opening.

Next, use an otoscope to visualize the external canal and tympanic membrane directly. Tip the patient's head away from you and toward the side of the unexamined ear. Pull the auricle up and back to straighten the entrance to the canal, and insert the speculum of the otoscope. Advance it slowly and gently in accordance with patient comfort. Observe the ear canal for redness, weeping, swelling (sometimes determined by the size of the speculum that can be comfortably introduced), wax accumulation, discharge, or foreign body. Assess the eardrum for bulging, retraction, perforation, and scarring. Note color, luster, presence or absence of the light reflex, and thickness (can the malleus handle be seen through the tympanic membrane?). Keep in mind that normally the eardrum is shiny gray or pink, translucent, and shaped like a concave disk and that a light reflex is present. The light reflex appears as a cone of light reflected from the light of the otoscope and in a normal examination appears at the 5 o'clock position in the right ear and at the 7 o'clock position in the left ear (Fig. 41–4).

Diagnostic Procedures

Pneumatoscopy

Pneumatoscopy tests the ability of the eardrum to respond to changes in air pressure introduced into the ear canal and the middle ear. The pneumatic otoscope is inserted into the ear canal, and air is introduced with a bulb attachment once a tight seal is achieved. The air pressure exerted against the tympanic membrane causes the membrane to move inward and outward. Small perforations of the tympanic membrane can be detected during this examination. A perforated tympanic membrane does not move in conjunction with changes in air pressure because the air passes through the tympanic membrane.

In rare instances, patients may report dizziness or vertigo in response to pneumatic otoscopy. This should be reported in the data collected because it may reflect some abnormal response or communication between the middle ear and inner ear.

Pneumatic otoscopy should be instituted after a complete examination with a regular otoscope because pneumatic otoscopy should not be performed in the presence of a bulging tympanic membrane.

Tuning Fork Tests

Tuning fork tests are used to categorize type and severity of hearing loss and to determine the need for referral for more extensive audiometric testing. A tuning fork is a small metal instrument that consists of a stem and two prongs tuned to a specific frequency, which is emitted when the fork is struck. Tuning fork tests can differentiate between conductive and sensorineural hearing losses. A conductive hearing loss is associated with aberrations in the sound conduction mechanism, including the tympanic membrane and the three ossicles of the middle ear. A sensorineural hearing loss is associated with aberrations, deterioration, or other changes in the neural components of hearing (absence or presence of hair cells, interference of neural pathways of the auditory nerve).

WEBER'S TEST

Hearing by bone conduction is assessed by Weber's test. The stem of the vibrating tuning fork (a low-frequency fork of 256 or 512 Hz) is placed on

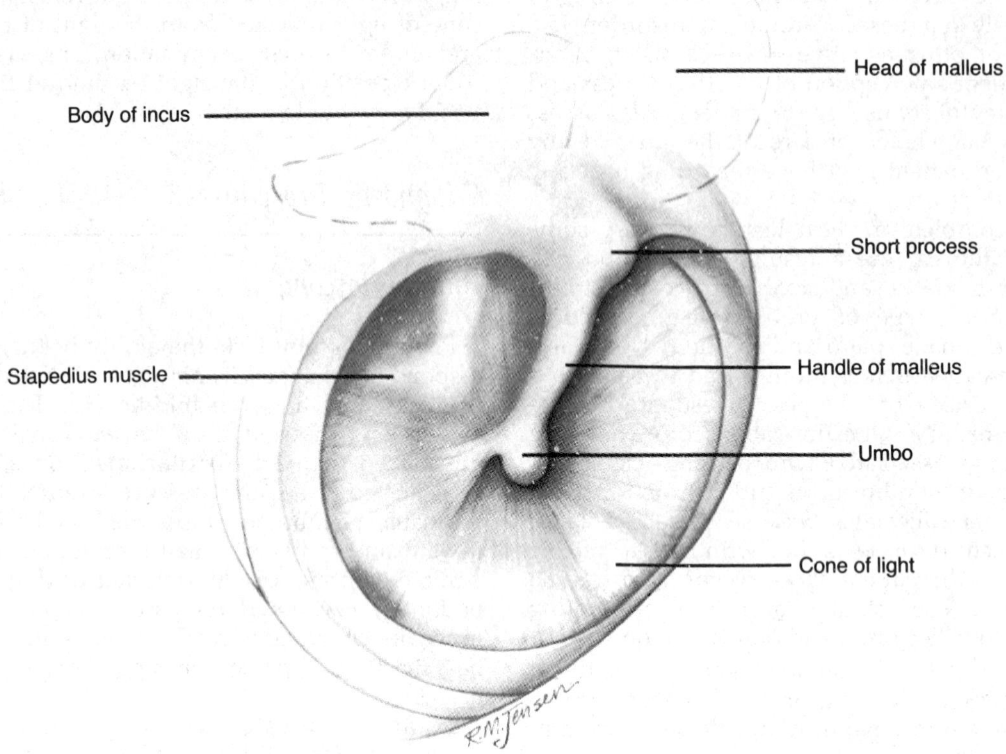

Figure 41–4.

Right tympanic membrane. Note umbo, handle of the malleus, and cone of light. (Modified from DeWeese DD, et al. Otolaryngology—Head and neck surgery. St. Louis: CV Mosby, 1988, p 405.)

the midline of the skull at the forehead or on the two front teeth of the maxilla. The patient is then asked to indicate in which ear the tone is heard by pointing to the ear. A patient with a conductive hearing loss in only one ear hears the tone more loudly in the unaffected ear. A patient with a conductive hearing loss in both ears hears the tone in the better or less affected ear. A patient with a sensorineural hearing loss in one ear hears the tone louder in the unaffected ear.

RINNE TEST

The Rinne test uses a tuning fork and compares hearing ability of the patient by air conduction and by bone conduction. To test the patient's bone conduction capability, the vibrating stem of the tuning fork is placed on the mastoid process (behind the auricle), and the patient is asked to indicate when the tone is no longer heard. Without stopping the vibration of the tuning fork, air conduction is tested by quickly moving the still-vibrating prongs close to, but not touching, the auricle. Then the patient indicates when the tone is no longer heard. The difference in duration of hearing by bone conduction and then air conduction is recorded. In normal hearing, the tone is heard longer (up to twice as long) and louder by air conduction. This is recorded as Rinne positive. A Rinne-positive result may be obtained in individuals with a sensorineural hearing loss. A Rinne-negative result is recorded when the bone-conducted sound persists as long as or longer than air-conducted sound. This result is indicative of a conductive hearing loss. A Rinne-equal test result indicates that the tone was heard equally by air and bone conduction and also suggests a conductive hearing loss.

When the results from the initial tuning fork tests are abnormal, the patient may be retested. (These tests can be quite subjective and depend on the tester's ability to consistently strike the fork with equal force and the patient's accuracy in reporting results.) If similar results are obtained, the patient is referred for further audiometric testing.

Audiometric Testing

Audiometry is the measurement of the sensitivity of the sense of hearing to various frequencies of sound. Some of the types of audiometry include pure tone audiometry, speech audiometry, impedance audiometry, acoustic reflex testing, and electric response audiometry. In general, these tests are performed by an audiologist, who provides test results and interpretation to the referring individual.

Sound is an auditory sensation produced by vibrations. Frequency and intensity are two physical attributes used to define a pure tone. The frequency of vibrations of a sound wave is calculated in cycles per second (cps); 1 unit of frequency (1 cps) is designated as 1 Hz. At birth, the human ear can perceive frequencies from 20 Hz to 20,000 Hz, but thereafter there is a steady decline in this perceptual ability.

The intensity of sound is measured in decibels, the unit of measurement used to define the extent of hearing loss when compared with normal hearing. When hearing level (HL) is expressed in decibels, 0 dB is taken as the average sound pressure necessary for threshold for young adults with no history of hearing loss. Threshold is the point at which an effect is produced or responded to. Therefore, it is defined as the lowest intensity of sound at which any signal can be heard. Adults who score in the range of 0 to 25 dB in all frequencies tested are said to have normal hearing within the normal range.

PURE TONE AUDIOMETRY

A pure tone audiometric test measures an individual's capability for hearing and normally tests within the ranges of 125 to 8000 Hz. Pure tone audiometry is useful in indicating the type and severity of hearing loss. A pure tone audiometer generates electronically a variety of pure tones used as test stimuli. After the ear canals are examined for physical obstruction as a result of ear wax or another cause, test signals are presented to one ear at a time, beginning with the better hearing ear. The patient is instructed to signal by raising a hand or pressing a button when a tone is heard, even if it is very faint. In general, the beginning test frequency is 1000 Hz presented at 25 dB.

The intensity of the signal is decreased in 5- to 10-dB steps until the patient ceases to respond; the signal is then increased in these steps until the patient once again responds. This pattern is repeated until the patient responds consistently two of three times to tones presented at a given intensity. This response is recorded on an audiogram. If there is no response at 25 dB, the intensity is increased by the same steps until a response is indicated and then decreased until the response ceases. Using this same pattern, tones are presented at 2000 Hz, 4000 Hz, 6000 Hz, 8000 Hz, and then 500 Hz and 250 Hz. The 1000-Hz frequency is retested to confirm the initial result.

When testing air conduction, tones are presented to one ear at a time via earphones. When testing bone conduction, the earphones are removed and a bone vibrator is placed against the forehead or on the mastoid process. Tones are presented as in the air conduction test procedure, using the frequencies between 250 and 4000 Hz. Results are recorded with the air conduction results on the audiogram. The bone conduction test mechanism bypasses the normal mechanism of sound conduction (through the ossicular chain) and tests the ability of the nerve to conduct sound. Because bone conduction vibrates the skull, patients may perceive hearing in one ear when it is actually being conducted to the opposite ear through the skull. Therefore, masking noise is presented in the untested ear by earphone during the test to prevent this phenomenon of crossover.

SPEECH AUDIOMETRY

Two measures of speech audiometry often used in audiometric testing are the speech reception threshold (SRT) and speech discrimination (SD). The SRT uses selected spondee words (two-syllable familiar words with equal stress) to evaluate an individual's ability to understand words and to determine the lowest intensity at which the person can repeat correctly 50% of the words presented during the test. Spondees are presented via an earphone to one ear at a time at progressively lower intensities. The patient is instructed to repeat each word as it is heard and to guess if unsure. The patient's recorded threshold to these words should be within 10 dB of the pure tone average (PTA) results of the pure tone evaluation. That is, the average of the thresholds at 500 Hz, 1000 Hz, and 2000 Hz (known as the speech frequencies) should correspond to the SRT. If the PTA and SRT do not agree, retesting should be instituted.

During the SD test, the patient is asked to repeat 50 monosyllabic words that are presented at a constant intensity, usually 30 to 40 dB above threshold. These words are presented in a sentence, and the percentage of words repeated correctly is recorded. Normal-hearing individuals can repeat 90% to 100% of these words correctly. Individuals with conductive hearing losses generally have scores within these limits. Patients with some type of sensorineural or mixed losses may not score within the normal range.

These tests aid in locating peripheral and central lesions that cause or contribute to hearing loss. They also aid in determining the beneficial effects of some kinds of rehabilitative therapy such as hearing aids, assistive listening devices, or speech reading.

IMPEDANCE AUDIOMETRY

Impedance audiometry is part of the battery of tests that includes static impedance and compliance measurements, tympanometry, and acoustic reflexes. The overall compliance or impedance of the auditory system is a combination of three factors: stiffness, friction, and mass. These tests evaluate middle-ear function using a combination of pure tones, changes in air pressure, and a probe that delivers a generated tone to a sealed ear canal. The results of these tests measure the eardrum's response to changes in air pressure and help to diagnose middle-ear pathology, eustachian tube dysfunction, seventh and eighth cranial nerve function, and the stapedial tendon's response to intense sounds, to name a few.

Vestibular Tests

FALLING AND PAST-POINTING TESTS

An exhaustive battery of tests for patients with hearing or balance disorders may include falling and past-pointing tests that aid in identifying or localizing the area of the vestibular system affected. In the falling test, the patient is asked to stand with feet together, arms at the sides, and eyes closed for 20 seconds. The patient is then asked to stand alternately on one foot and then the other foot while balance is evaluated. Finally, the patient is instructed to walk backward and forward heel to toe, first with eyes open and then with eyes closed. Patients with no abnormality can perform both maneuvers successfully.

When undergoing the past-pointing test, the patient is seated facing the examiner, who holds out an index finger at the level of the patient's shoulder. The patient is requested to touch the examiner's finger with the right index finger and then close the eyes, lower the arm, and touch the examiner's finger again. The examination is repeated for the left side. The examiner observes and notes the degree and direction of past-pointing. The findings are normal when the patient can touch the examiner's finger with eyes open or closed.

Because many of these tests require the ability to follow instructions and, in the case of the falling test, have the potential for injury, they may be contraindicated in patients who are physically, emotionally, or mentally handicapped. However, when patients can be protected from falling by caregivers and examiners, these tests may proceed.

Certain clinics and specialty centers may use a special battery of vestibular tests that also utilize moving platforms and rotating chairs with revolving surroundings to evaluate vestibular function or dysfunction with more discrete measures. Like all testing procedures, they must be carefully explained to patients to elicit full cooperation and understanding and to allay fear. Patients who suffer from vestibular disorders are particularly afraid of falling, becoming nauseated, or initiating or exacerbating symptoms of vertigo. These reactions can result from some of these testing procedures, and the patients must be alerted to the possibility while the importance of the results of these tests is emphasized. In addition, it is generally necessary to inform patients up to 48 hours in advance of some testing procedures so intake of caffeine and other stimulants that may affect test results can be restricted.

ELECTRONYSTAGMOGRAPHY

Electronystagmography (ENG) is a method of recording eye movement by detecting and recording changes in background electrical activity produced by eye motion. This measurement is based on the corneoretinal potential. The results are used to evaluate the interactions between the vestibular system and the muscles controlling eye movement: the vestibulo-ocular reflex. This test is used in the diagnosis of vestibular dysfunction and is important in assessing causes of dizziness, vertigo, and tinnitus. It aids in the diagnosis of unilateral hearing loss and can confirm the presence and location of central or peripheral lesions.

CALORIC TEST

The caloric test is a test of the function of the vestibular system. In this test, the ear is stimulated alternately with warm (111.2°F, 44°C) and cold (86°F, 30°C) water. This may be done by irrigating the ear with water or by using testing equipment that consists of water- or air-filled tubing, which is inserted in the ear canal. The normal individual responds to warm or cold stimulation with nystagmus (an abnormal jerking movement of the eye). Warm stimulation produces nystagmus toward the side of instillation, whereas cold stimulation produces nystagmus in the opposite direction. Peripheral or brain-stem lesions are suggested in individuals in whom no nystagmus is elicited by caloric testing.

Caloric testing with water actually instilled in the ear canal is, of course, contraindicated in patients with a tympanic membrane perforation. Otoscopy is recommended before beginning the test to examine for this possibility as well as to evaluate for any obstruction to instillation, particularly (and most commonly) cerumen (earwax).

After otoscopy and proper preparation of the skin, ENG electrodes are placed. In general, the electrode array includes a ground electrode in the center of the forehead, two electrodes directly above and below the eyes, and two lateral electrodes, one lateral to each eye. The electrodes are placed as close as possible to the eye without interfering with lid closure. With the patient lying in a supine position and the head elevated 30 degrees (to align properly the lateral semicircular canal), the warm and cold stimulation is begun. The stimulus is continued for 30 seconds. The results of the testing are recorded on a graph, and the examiner makes anecdotal notes on the patient's subjective responses.

When initial testing procedures such as audiometry and ENG produce abnormal results, more detailed testing procedures may be done to rule out or confirm the presence of a tumor or other growth. Evoked potential studies and auditory brain stem response (ABR) are among the tests that may be used. These tests involve placement of electrodes to measure the latency or delay in the acoustic signal passing along the nerve. These are also useful in patients who are unable or unwilling to respond to other behavioral tests.

Other tests such as electrocochleography may be performed to locate the site of a lesion in the auditory or vestibular systems.

X-ray films, computed tomographic (CT) scans, and magnetic resonance imaging (MRI) or nuclear MRI may be used to confirm the diagnosis of a lesion in the area of the auditory nerve.

Medical Management

Medical management of patients with disorders of the ear depends on the particular disease or disorder, its cause, the degree of severity of symptoms, and the resulting impairment.

Pharmacologic Therapy

Today many ear disorders can be treated effectively with pharmacologic therapy. Antibiotics can control the majority of infectious processes of the ear. Antihistamines can help to reduce allergic reactions and swelling, which affect eustachian tube function. Diazepam and related drugs are used to control the symptoms associated with dizziness and vertigo, although they do not correct the disease process.

Surgical Management

Some disorders of the ear do not respond to drug therapy; others may be refractory to drug therapy. In either case, surgery may be indicated. Ear surgery may be performed to replace or restore structure and function, to correct deformities, to remove diseased tissues or growths, and to attempt to relieve symptoms that incapacitate the patient.

Extensive ear surgery generally requires a postauricular incision, whereas some simple procedures may be performed endaurally or through the canal.

GENERAL PREPARATION FOR EAR SURGERY

The otologic surgeon obtains a thorough medical and surgical history from the patient, including information on all drugs (legal and illegal) taken by the patient. Results of any tests performed before the patient's referral to the surgeon are reviewed, and a complete physical examination is performed. On the basis of information obtained, the surgeon explains the proposed surgical procedure, its expectations for success, possible complications, and special considerations for the patient in terms of postoperative care required, time away from the work place, and physical restrictions after surgery. Before the surgical procedure, a consent for surgery is obtained and preoperative instructions are given to the patient. Depending on the patient-care setting, these instructions may be given by a clinic or office nurse, a perioperative nurse in the surgical setting, or the surgeon. The patient is instructed to take nothing by mouth (NPO) after midnight or at least 6 to 8 hours before the scheduled surgery. Special instructions may also include withholding or modifying dosages of some medications on the day of surgery.

COMPLICATIONS OF EAR SURGERY

Complications of ear surgery are rare, but the patient still must be informed of the possibilities. Because the ear is the organ of hearing and balance, complications usually involve these functions and include hearing loss and vestibular dysfunction. As with any surgery, infection is a risk. An untreated infection can progress to serious consequences, but in most cases a postoperative course of antibiotics or prophylactic antibiotic coverage provides effective therapy. Temporary or permanent facial paralysis is also a potential complication because the facial nerve courses through the middle ear. Temporary facial paralysis can result from swelling around the nerve or manipulation of the nerve during surgery. Because of the risk of facial nerve damage, it is essential that facial nerve function be assessed and documented before surgery.

Potential complications of an emotional or psychologic nature include anxiety and depression. These are most likely to develop if the patient has unrealistic expectations for outcomes after surgery or an unrealistic timetable for improvement.

COMMON SURGICAL PROCEDURES PERFORMED ON THE EAR

TYMPANOPLASTY

Tympanoplasty refers to a variety of reconstructive procedures performed on deformed or diseased portions of the middle ear. The types of tympanoplasties range in complexity from a simple repair of a perforated eardrum to progressively more complex reconstruction of middle-ear structures to restore function.

Uses

Tympanoplasty is done to preserve or improve hearing by repairing or replacing some or all of the conductive mechanisms of the middle ear. Simple repair of perforations of the eardrum (myringoplasty) not only restores some hearing loss but also protects the middle ear from external contamination and resulting infection.

Physical Preparation of the Patient

A tympanoplastic procedure may be performed in an inpatient or out-patient setting. This is largely determined by the patient's general medical health,

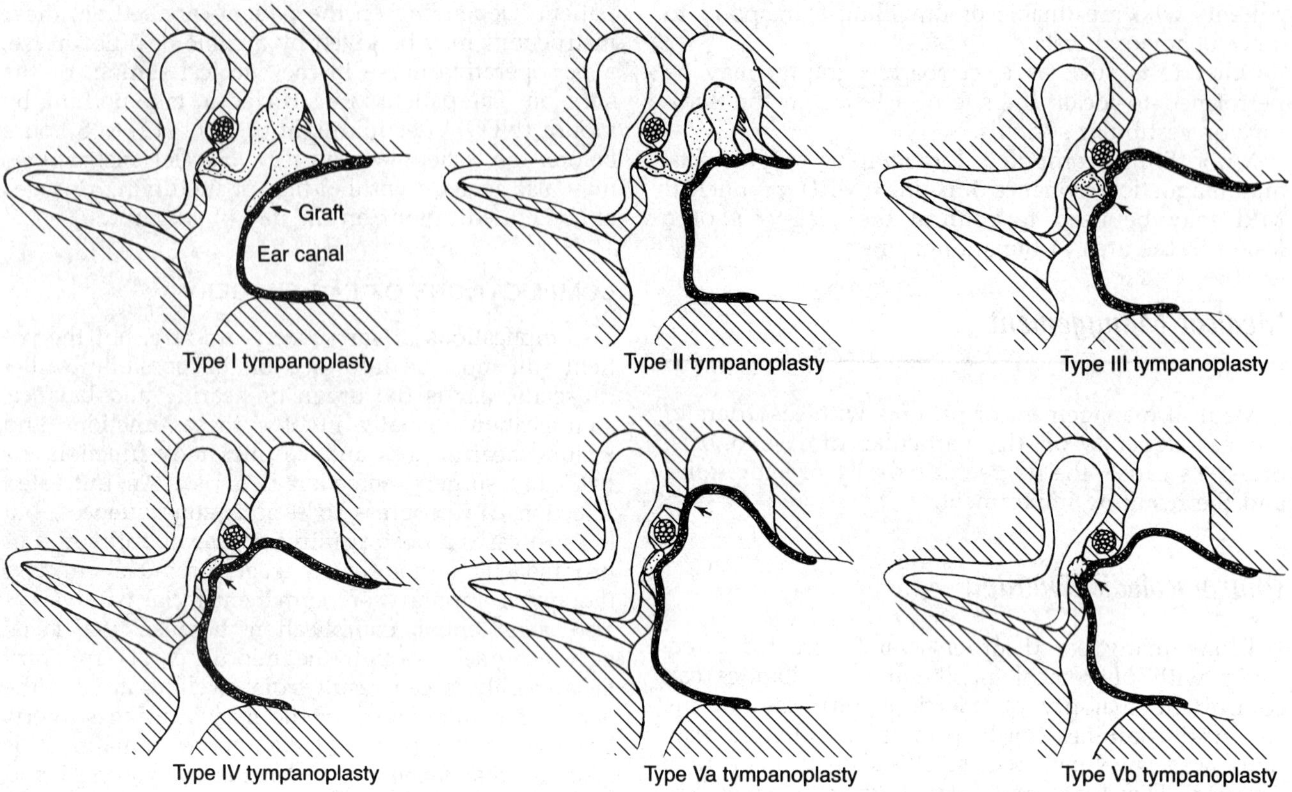

Figure 41–5.

Types of tympanoplasty. Note that in type I the graft rests on the malleus and the middle ear space, and structures are essentially normal. This is different from types II through V, in which there is progressive loss of middle ear structure. (Modified from Paparella MM, Shumrick DA, Gluckman JL, Meyerhoff WL. Otolaryngology. 3rd ed. Vol 2, Otology and Neuro-otology. Philadelphia: WB Saunders, 1991, p 1416.)

whether general or local anesthesia is to be used, the availability of out-patient settings, the surgeon's preference, and, not incidentally, the insurance company's guidelines for reimbursement.

The patient is brought to the operating room holding area before surgery, and a perioperative nurse reviews the pertinent history and physical assessment data, evaluates the patient's understanding of the procedure, and answers any questions the patient may have regarding the perioperative period. The nurse then plans for any special needs the patient may have in the intraoperative period.

In cases in which temporalis fascia is to be used as the graft material to repair a tympanic membrane perforation, a small area behind the ear may be shaved before surgery. Generally, this surgical preparation is accomplished as close to the time of surgery as possible and is often done in the operating room itself.

Procedure

To repair a perforation of the tympanic membrane, graft material (harvested from temporalis fascia, a vein from the back of the hand, or more rarely skin) is placed just medial or just lateral to the perforated eardrum. The graft may be held in place by absorbable gelatin film (Gelfilm) or absorbable gelatin sponge (Gelfoam) soaked in saline or some otic preparation or by clotted blood. The external canal may be packed with sterile strip gauze, Gelfoam, or an expanding wick made of cellulose. Generally, an external head bandage is applied for at least 24 hours.

More extensive tympanoplastic procedures may use fascia, cartilage, perichondrium, bone, prostheses, or any combination to repair or replace structures damaged in the middle ear (Fig. 41–5). Mastoidectomy is part of more extensive procedures. Depending on the disease process and the extent of the damage, this procedure may be staged. That is, the pathologic process is treated first and the reconstructive process completed later after the response to removal of the diseased tissue has been evaluated.

After some tympanoplasties, the patient may have a drain in place as well as a large head bandage to prevent hematoma formation.

Postoperative Course

Patients are usually ambulatory by the evening of surgery and, in inpatient settings, are discharged by the next day. As stated earlier, many of these patients are treated as same-day surgery, being admitted and discharged the day of surgery.

Application of the Nursing Process to the Care of the Patient Having a Tympanoplasty

PREOPERATIVE NURSING CARE

Nursing care of the patient scheduled for a tympanoplasty is similar to that for any preoperative patient, as discussed in Chapter 4, with several considerations. Be certain that the patient understands that improvement in hearing will not be apparent in most cases until up to 6 weeks after surgery. Realistic expectations for outcomes as well as a realistic timetable for improvement are necessary to avoid anxiety and depression postoperatively.

POSTOPERATIVE NURSING CARE

Assessment

Assess the patient's level of discomfort and the need for physical safety measures. Assess the patient's ability to hear and understand instructions and other conversation, because edema secondary to surgical trauma, the pack in the ear, and the outer dressing will all impair hearing in the operated ear.

Assess the patient for severe vertigo or dizziness, which can indicate a complication of surgery. Observe the patient for signs of secondary infection such as fever, headache, or increased ear pain. Also observe for excessive bleeding and the inability of the patient to wrinkle the forehead, close the eyes, or pucker the lips, which may be indicative of facial nerve trauma. Report the presence of any of these symptoms immediately.

Nursing Diagnoses and Planning

Nursing diagnoses and related expected patient outcomes most commonly applicable to patients who have had a tympanoplasty include the following:

NDx: Sensory/perceptual alteration related to vertigo or dizziness secondary to surgical manipulation of the ear

Planning: Patient outcomes
1. Patient takes medications as ordered for vertigo, dizziness, or unsteadiness.
2. Patient initiates movements slowly, avoiding actions or movements that precipitate or worsen vertigo or dizziness.
3. Patient reports that vertigo or dizziness is relieved.

NDx: Impaired communication related to decreased hearing secondary to edema, ear packing, and the postoperative dressing

Planning: Patient outcomes
1. Effective communication is maintained between the patient and others.
2. Patient directs staff, family, and others in effective alternative communication techniques (e.g., directing others to speak into the unoperated ear, writing messages).

NDx: Pain related to surgical trauma to the ear

Planning: Patient outcomes
1. Patient uses noninvasive pain-control techniques such as positioning.
2. Patient takes medications as ordered for pain.
3. Patient verbalizes relief of discomfort.

NDx: High risk for injury related to vertigo, dizziness, or unsteadiness

Planning: Patient outcomes
1. Patient requests assistance when ambulating and getting in and out of bed when dizziness or vertigo is present.
2. Patient uses acclimatization techniques when changing positions.
3. Patient remains free of injury.

NDx: High risk for infection related to surgical disruption of the body's first line of defense

Planning: Patient outcomes
1. Increase in ear pain is absent.
2. Purulent drainage or foul odor from the ear is absent.
3. Suture line is clean and approximated.
4. Patient is afebrile.

NDx: High risk for altered health maintenance related to insufficient knowledge of self-care after tympanoplasty

Planning: Patient outcomes
1. Patient describes self-care of the ear after surgery.
2. Patient lists activities to be avoided or altered during the postoperative period.
3. Patient explains prescribed medication regimen.
4. Patient identifies symptoms to be reported.

Chart 41–1.

NURSING GUIDE TO PATIENT EDUCATION FOR SELF-MANAGEMENT: DISCHARGE INSTRUCTIONS AFTER TYMPANOPLASTY

Instruct the patient to do the following:

Keep dressing clean. Do not touch dressing or ear. If dressing must be reinforced, wash hands thoroughly before and after procedure. Keep hair away from area.
Keep ear dry. Do not shower, shampoo, or swim until given permission from surgeon.
Avoid forceful coughing, sneezing, and nose blowing. If nose must be blown, blow gently with mouth open.
Avoid lifting heavy objects.
Avoid air travel until instructed otherwise by surgeon.
Take antibiotics and antihistamines as prescribed, and take entire course of medication.
Report any increase in pain, development of fever, redness of areas surrounding the ear, or excessive drainage to *(specify)*.
Return for a checkup on *(specify)*.

5. Patient states the reason for and date of follow-up visit.

Nursing Interventions

NDX: Sensory/perceptual alteration
Explain that medication for vertigo is available, and administer as ordered. Stress that vertigo and nausea are not abnormal after ear surgery. Maintain a dimmed, quiet environment. Avoid sudden movements of the patient's bed or chair. Instruct the patient to initiate movements slowly, particularly sitting or standing up, and to avoid any activities that precipitate or exacerbate vertigo or dizziness.

NDx: Impaired communication
If the patient's ability to hear is significantly altered by the surgery, direct all communication to the unaffected ear. If necessary, speak directly into the unaffected ear from a few inches away using a normal tone of voice. Use touch, gestures, or the written word in extreme situations to ensure accurate communication. Leave written instructions at the bedside if appropriate. Encourage the patient to inform others when they cannot be heard and to direct them in ways of enhancing communication.

NDx: Pain
Administer medications for pain as needed and in accordance with the physician's orders, and explain their expected effect. Maintain a calm environment, and make the patient comfortable within the limits of the positioning restrictions. Keep in mind that severe pain is rare after tympanoplasties but that individual differences in pain tolerance do exist.

NDx: High risk for injury
Keep the head of the bed elevated and the side rails up at all times. Provide assistance when the patient gets in and out of bed and ambulates.

NDx: High risk for infection
Use strict aseptic technique when changing ear dressings. Do not remove the initial ear dressing but reinforce as needed. Avoid getting the dressing wet; arrange the patient's hair so it is pulled back away from the dressing. Administer antibiotics as ordered.

NDx: High risk for altered health maintenance
Instruct the patient in self-care at home, as specified in Chart 41–1.

Evaluation

Evaluate the effectiveness of nursing care for a patient who has had a tympanoplasty by comparing the patient's status with the expected patient outcomes. Examples of specific outcomes for patients who have had a tympanoplasty have been provided in the Planning section.

MYRINGOTOMY

Myringotomy is a procedure in which an incision is made into the tympanic membrane to relieve pressure behind the eardrum and to promote drainage of purulent or serous fluid from the middle ear.

Uses

This procedure is usually performed when medical treatment, such as antibiotic and decongestant therapy, has failed to resolve eustachian tube blockage associated with serous otitis media. It is also indicated in the case of a painful, bulging tympanic membrane, which may occur with acute suppurative otitis media.

Procedure

A myringotomy is generally performed as an outpatient procedure. It can usually be done in a clinic or office setting under a local anesthetic in adults.

A single incision is made into the posterior inferior portion of the eardrum. Fluid is removed from the middle ear by suction. In some cases, a tympanostomy tube is inserted through the opening in the tympanic membrane to ventilate the middle ear and to equalize the pressure between the external and middle ears (Fig. 41–6). If no tube is inserted, the incision heals rapidly and usually without incident. If the tube is left in place, it slowly pushes its way out of the eardrum over a period of months and the eardrum heals.

Complications

Complications after myringotomy are unusual. In rare cases, delayed or lack of healing of the incision may occur, especially if a tympanostomy tube remains in place for a period exceeding a year. In this case, a tympanoplasty may be required to close the perforation.

Application of the Nursing Process to the Care of the Patient Who Has Had a Myringotomy

Assessment

After myringotomy, check for ear drainage and, if present, note the amount and color. Keep in mind that generally drainage is so scant that it is not noticeable and that excessive drainage, especially of clear fluid, should be reported immediately. Assess the patient's understanding of postoperative instructions, including the importance of taking antibiotics as prescribed and the need to protect the ear from water until the incision is healed or the tube extruded.

Nursing Diagnoses and Planning

The nursing diagnosis and related expected patient outcomes most commonly applicable to patients who have had a myringotomy are as follows:

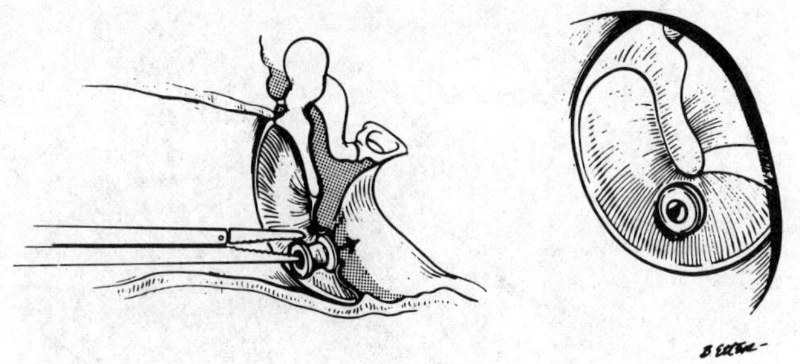

Figure 41–6.

Myringotomy with a tympanostomy tube in place to ventilate the middle ear and equalize pressure. (From DeWeese DD, et al. Otolaryngology—Head and neck surgery. St. Louis: CV Mosby, 1988, p 459.)

NDx: High risk for altered health maintenance related to insufficient knowledge of self-care after surgery

Planning: Patient outcomes

1. Patient states the purpose, name, dose, route, time, and length of course of the prescribed antibiotic.
2. Patient describes importance of protecting the ear from water.
3. Patient lists strategies for protecting the ear from water.

Nursing Interventions

NDx: High risk for altered health maintenance

Teach the patient about the prescribed antibiotic therapy. Be certain to explain that it is given as prophylaxis against infection, and stress the importance of taking the entire course of medication. Fur ther instruct the patient in the importance of not getting water into the ear until the myringtomy incision is healed or the tube extruded from the ear, which is best documented by physical examination at a follow-up visit. Encourage the patient to use cotton with petroleum jelly or ear plugs when showering or shampooing. Stress that swimming or diving must be avoided unless specially designed ear plugs are obtained.

Evaluation

Evaluate the effectiveness of nursing care for a patient who has had a myringotomy by comparing the patient's status with the expected patient outcomes. Examples of specific outcomes for patients who have had a myringotomy have been provided in the Planning section.

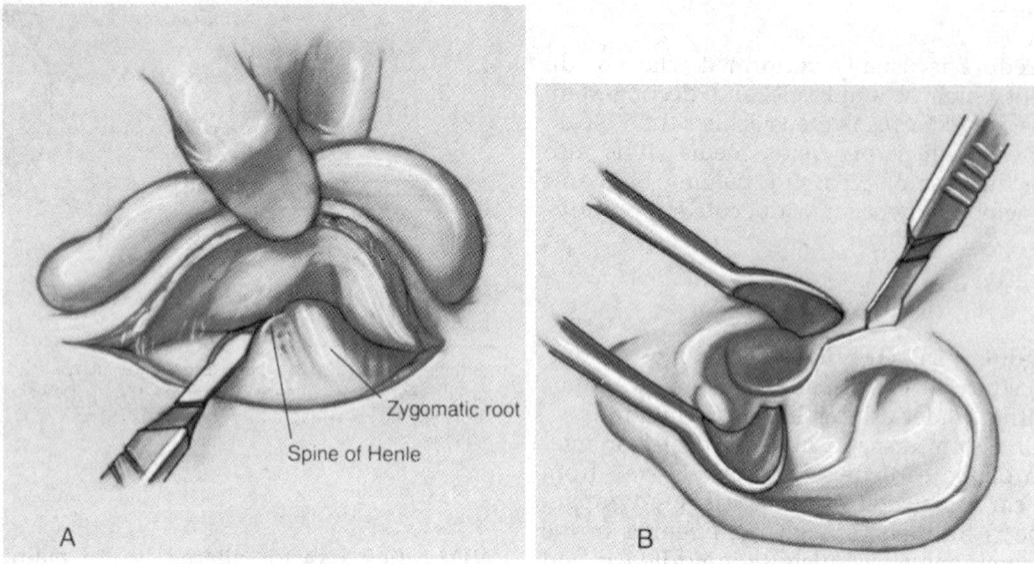

Figure 41–7.

Types of mastoidectomy incision. *A*, Postauricular approach. *B*, Endaural approach. (From Goycoolea MV, Paparella MM, Nissen RL. Atlas of otologic surgery. Philadelphia: WB Saunders, 1989, pp 131, 134.)

MASTOIDECTOMY

Mastoidectomy is the excision of a part of the mastoid process of the temporal bone. Depending on the extent of the excision, it is classified as a simple, radical, or modified radical mastoidectomy.

Uses

Mastoidectomy is done to remove cancerous or other diseased tissue or to gain access to the middle or inner ear.

Physical Preparation of the Patient

Basic physical preparation is similar to that for any surgical patient. In addition, hair is shaved or clipped for about 3.75 cm ($1\frac{1}{2}$ in.) around the ear. A water-soluble lubricant may be applied to the remaining hair on the affected side of the head to keep it slicked back away from the operative area.

Procedure

Mastoidectomy is most often performed as an inpatient procedure under general anesthesia and may be done through a postauricular or an endaural incision (Fig. 41–7).

In a simple mastoidectomy, all accessible air cells in the mastoid process are removed. This is rarely done today because antibiotics are generally effective in treating middle-ear infections, making removal of infected cells unnecessary. In a radical mastoidectomy, the wall of the external auditory canal, the tympanic membrane, and most of the structures of the middle ear are removed, and the opening to the eustachian tube is plugged. In a modified radical mastoidectomy, the mastoid air cells and posterior canal wall are removed, but the tympanic membrane and the ossicles are saved.

A drain may be inserted in the inferior part of the incision, and a bulky dressing is applied.

Postoperative Course

The patient is assisted out of bed on the evening of surgery and is discharged in 24 to 48 hours. Dizziness is the primary source of discomfort and may necessitate assistance with ambulating. Sutures are removed and the bulky dressing replaced by an "eye patch" dressing on about the sixth postoperative day. This dressing is subsequently replaced with a cotton pledget, which is changed by the patient three times a day until drainage ceases, usually in 3 to 4 weeks. Unrestricted activities can be resumed in about 6 weeks.

Complications

Potential complications of a mastoidectomy include wound infection, drainage, and bleeding. These are not common but do occur more often after mastoidectomy than after tympanoplasty alone. Facial nerve injury can also occur. Symptoms of the injury occur in the immediate postoperative period and require immediate surgery for decompression and repair. Edema of the facial nerve can cause similar symptoms, but onset is several days after surgery and is a temporary condition.

Application of the Nursing Process to the Care of the Patient Having a Mastoidectomy

PREOPERATIVE NURSING CARE

Nursing care of the patient scheduled for a mastoidectomy is similar to that for any preoperative patient, with several considerations discussed next.

Review the purpose of the surgery and the expected outcome with the patient. If improvement in hearing is not the primary goal or is in fact impossible because of destruction of the ossicles, make certain the patient understands this. Similarly, make certain that the patient understands if hearing reconstruction is to be undertaken as a second-stage procedure and that, in any case, evaluation of improved hearing may be delayed for up to 3 months after surgery.

Determine whether the patient has been taking aspirin or an aspirin-containing preparation, because this could affect the amount of bleeding, which in turn could impair visualization of the operative field.

POSTOPERATIVE NURSING CARE

Assessment

Assess the patient's return to physiologic stabilization. Check vital signs, and inspect the dressing for bleeding or drainage. Also inspect the back of the patient's head and the pillow for drainage that might have been pulled down and back by gravity. Assess for signs of facial nerve injury because the facial nerve (cranial nerve VIII) passes through the internal auditory canal and exits through the mastoid process. Observe for signs of facial paralysis such as sagging of the side of the face or mouth, drooling, or the inability to close the eyelid on the operative side. Ask the patient to show the teeth, wrinkle the forehead, and pucker the mouth as if to whistle. Also assess for pain, dizziness, and nausea.

Nursing Diagnoses and Planning

Nursing diagnoses and related expected patient outcomes most commonly applicable to patients who have had a mastoidectomy include the following:

NDx: High risk for injury related to dizziness, pain, and nausea

Planning: Patient outcomes
1. Patient requests assistance when getting out of bed or ambulating.
2. Patient remains free of injury.

NDx: High risk for altered health maintenance related to insufficient knowledge of self-care after discharge

Planning: Patient outcomes
1. Patient describes self-care as presented in Chart 41-2.

Nursing Interventions

NDx: High risk for injury
Medicate the patient as needed and prescribed for dizziness, pain, and nausea. Keep the side rails up, and instruct the patient to call for assistance in getting out of bed or in ambulating. Encourage the patient to change positions slowly to avoid exacerbating symptoms.

NDx: High risk for altered health maintenance
Instruct the patient in self-care after discharge as described in Chart 41-2.

Chart 41–2.

NURSING GUIDE TO PATIENT EDUCATION FOR SELF-MANAGEMENT: DISCHARGE INSTRUCTIONS AFTER MASTOIDECTOMY

Instruct the patient to do the following:

Wash hands before touching the operative area.
Change the cotton pledget in the ear three times a day until drainage ceases.
Take antibiotics as directed, making certain to complete the prescribed course of the medication.
Protect the ear from water for 6 weeks.
Return for a follow-up visit on *(specify date, time, and place).*

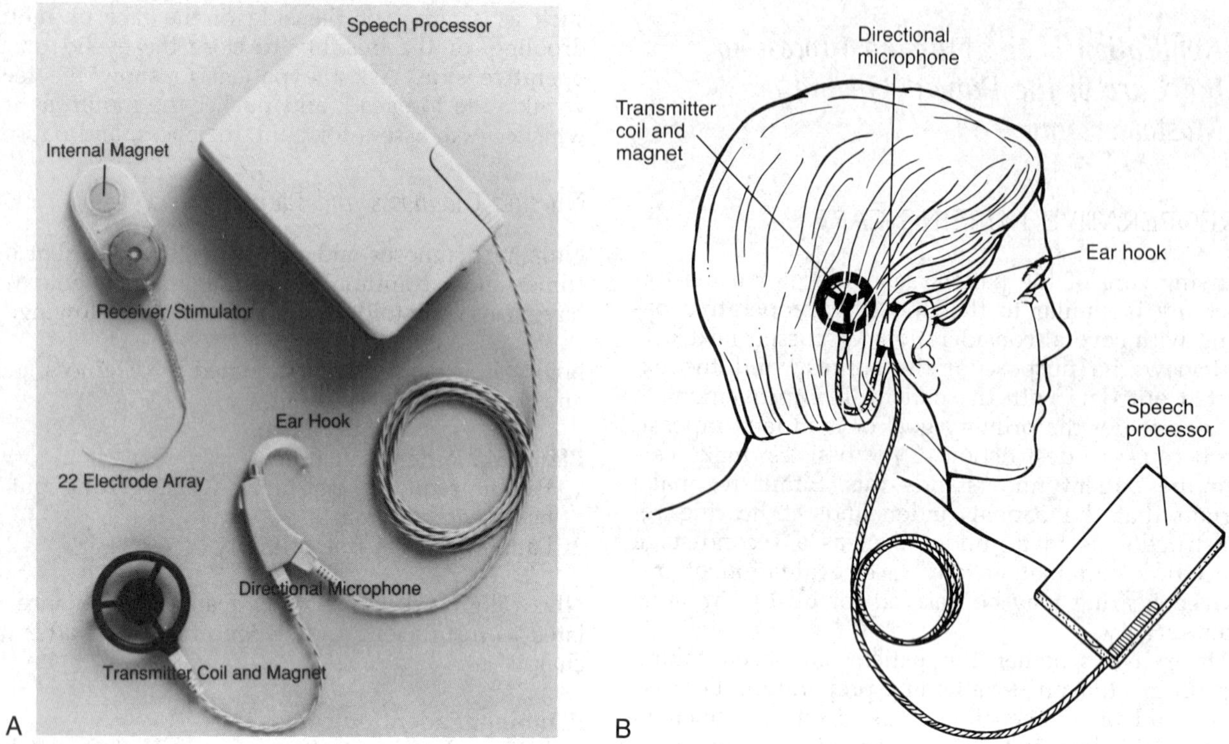

Figure 41–8.

Cochlear implant. *A*, The Nucleus 22-channel cochlear implant. *B*, Diagram of a patient with the prosthesis in place. Note the magnet holding the transmitter coil in place over the internal coil and the ear hook with the directional microphone. (The patient's hair usually conceals these components.) The programmable speech processor to which the signals are sent is carried in patient's shirt pocket. (*A* courtesy of Cochlear Corporation, Englewood, CO.)

Additional Interventions

Keep the head of the bed elevated at least 30 degrees, and instruct the patient to lie on the unaffected side. Reinforce the dressing as needed, and immediately report excessive bleeding to the surgeon.

Administer antibiotics as ordered. Give oral fluids, progressing to a regular diet as tolerated.

Evaluation

Evaluate the effectiveness of nursing care for a patient who has had a mastoidectomy by comparing the patient's status with the expected patient outcomes. Examples of specific outcomes for patients who have had a mastoidectomy have been provided in the Planning section.

COCHLEAR IMPLANTATION

A cochlear implant (Fig. 41–8) is an auditory prosthesis designed to electrically stimulate the remaining functional nerve fibers in the inner ear (cochlea). The sound information received by the cochlea is then transmitted through cranial nerve VIII to the brain for interpretation. The cochlear implant consists of the following:

- Internal (implanted) components, including a receiver-stimulator (with magnet) connected to a single- or multiple-channel electrode array. The receiver-stimulator is surgically implanted in the mastoid bone behind the pinna, and the electrode array is inserted approximately one and one-half turns into the cochlea.
- External components, including a directional microphone with earhook worn over the ear, connected by a thin cord to a speech processor (about the size of a deck of cards) and a transmitter coil (with magnet holding it in place over the receiver-stimulator).

Sound received by the microphone is sent to the speech processor, where it is changed into digital signals. These signals are then sent to the transmitter coil, where they are forwarded across the skin by radio signal to the implanted receiver-stimulator. The receiver-stimulator selectively activates the appropriate electrodes according to the coded input so that the individual can perceive different pitch and loudness sensations for easier sound recognition.

Uses

Cochlear implants have been developed as one solution for the profoundly deaf. Profound hearing loss reportedly affects more than 1% of the population of the United States. Cochlear implants use electrical signals to produce auditory sensation that can be interpreted as sound by these patients. Patients are screened for appropriate selection for implantation. The criteria vary somewhat throughout the country, but general criteria include a profound hearing loss, an unsuccessful trial with hearing aids, no medical contraindications for surgery, no gross personal maladjustment as evidenced by interviews and testing, and a willingness to participate in a rehabilitation program.

Physical Preparation of the Patient

Once the patient has been accepted for cochlear implantation and a battery of tests aimed at predicting the success of the implant has been completed, the patient is scheduled for surgery and undergoes the same physical assessment, history taking, and education as patients undergoing mastoidectomy or tympanoplasty.

Procedure

The surgical approach resembles a mastoidectomy; however, the incision is larger and goes farther into the hairline, requiring a more extensive skin-shave preparation of the patient's hair and head. The surgery is performed while the patient is under general anesthesia. An internal coil is placed in the bone behind the top of the auricle. Then a standard mastoidectomy is performed; a small drill hole is made in the round window; and the electrode is threaded into place. This completes the connection between the internal coil and the cochlea.

The external coil and speech processor are put into place when the wound has adequately healed, usually in 10 to 15 days. There is no change in the patient's hearing perception until this occurs.

Application of the Nursing Process to the Care of the Patient Having a Cochlear Implant

The assessment, nursing diagnoses, expected patient outcomes, nursing interventions, and evaluation for patients having a cochlear implant are similar to those described previously for patients having a mastoidectomy. The following additional considerations apply to the care of patients having a cochlear implant.

Maximum participation of the patient in the care-planning process is essential. To achieve this is a challenge because of the patient's communication disability. Many of these patients do not sign (neither do their nurses) and although some have outstanding lip-reading capabilities, others have lived a life of social and communicational isolation since the onset of their profound deafness.

Often cue cards must be used to instruct the patient and then used in the immediate preoperative and preinduction periods to maintain communication with the patient. A consensus on communication strategies to be used in the postanesthetic period should be established well before the perioperative period. This is critical for the sound-deprived patient waking from an anesthetic in a foreign environment.

It is vitally important that the patient's expectations for the surgical outcome be realistic. It is often difficult to dissuade patients from the expectation that sound perception will return to the predeafened state, and postsurgical depression can be profound in patients who have not accepted the limitations of cochlear implantations. Make certain the patient understands what types of sound will be perceived and that no change in hearing will occur until the rehabilitation program begins at least 1 month after surgery. Once the implant is activated, patients receive sound information that helps them interpret these sounds as speech. These sounds are sometimes described as the sound one hears when blowing on a comb covered with paper. Thus, the patient receives timing information (how long does the word or syllable last?) as well as some inflection (does the word or sentence end like a question or a statement?) and, coupling this with lip-reading, can generally understand the subject being discussed. As implants have improved, some patients have demonstrated the ability to talk on the telephone or to converse without visual cues. Assess the patient for postimplantation depression, especially on the first day of activation of the implant when rehabilitation begins.

The Elderly: Special Considerations

The external ear undergoes relatively minor changes with age. The lobes elongate because of the effect of gravity, and the auricle enlarges as a result of the continuous production of cartilage. The walls of the external auditory canal begin to atrophy, in some cases leading to partial occlusion of the canal and impaired passage of sound waves. The number of coarse, stiff hairs in the external canal increases, and they often become visible. Cerumen is secreted in smaller amounts and may contain more keratin. This causes the wax to be harder and more easily impacted. The middle ear may atrophy, and the eardrum may sclerose. In the inner ear, the basilar membrane hardens, and the hair and ganglion cells of the cochlea degenerate.

Bibliography

Adams GL, Boies LR, Hilger PA. Fundamentals of otolaryngology. Philadelphia: WB Saunders, 1989.
Alberti PW, Ruben RJ. Otologic medicine and surgery. New York: Churchill Livingstone, 1985.
Ballantyne J, Morrison AW (eds). Operative surgery: The ear. Rob and Smith's operative surgery series. 4th ed. Stoneham, MA: Butterworth, 1986.
Ballenger JJ. Diseases of the nose, throat, ear, head and neck. Philadelphia: Lea & Febiger, 1985.
Bates B. A guide to physical examination. 5th ed. Philadelphia: JB Lippincott, 1991.
Bull PD. Lecture notes on diseases of the ear, nose and throat. 6th ed. CV Blackwell Scientific Publications, 1986.
Carpenito LJ. Nursing diagnosis application to clinical practice. 3rd ed. Philadelphia: JB Lippincott, 1989.
Christian E, Dluhy N, O'Neill R. Sounds of silence: Coping with hearing loss and loneliness. J Gerontol Nurs 1989; 15(11):4.
Cleveland P, Morris J. Meniere's disease. RN 1990; 53(8):28.
De Weese DD, et al. Otolaryngology—Head and neck surgery. St. Louis: CV Mosby, 1988.
Eliopoulos C. Gerontological nursing. New York: Harper & Row, 1987.
Esberger KK, Hughes ST Jr (eds). Nursing care of the aged. Norwalk, CT: Appleton & Lange, 1989.
Gioiella EC, Bevil CW. Nursing care of the aging client. Norwalk, CT: Appleton-Century-Crofts, 1985.
Glasscock ME, Shambaugh GE Jr (eds). Surgery of the ear. 4th ed. Philadelphia: WB Saunders, 1990.
Goycoolea MV, Paparella MM, Nissen RL (eds). Atlas of otologic surgery. Philadelphia: WB Saunders, 1989.
Hanson C, Roffo F. Comprehensive care of patients undergoing stapedectomy for otosclerosis. Perioperative Nurs Q 1985; 1(2):21.
Harner SG. Peripheral labyrinth causes of dizziness. Postgrad Med 1987; 8(4):251.
Hawke M, John AF. Diseases of the ear: Clinical and pathological aspects. Philadelphia: Lea & Febiger, 1987.
Iadarola G, Kerrigan MB. Do you hear what I hear? AORN J 1986; 43(2):478.
Jarvis C. Physical examination and health assessment. Philadelphia: WB Saunders, 1992.
Kavanagh KT, McCabe BF. Ototoxicity of oral neomycin and vancomycin. Laryngoscope 1983; 93(5):649.
Knudsen JF. Noise-induced hearing loss. Med Times 1986; 114(1):27.
Koegel L. Ototoxicity: A contemporary review of aminoglycosides, loop diuretics, acetylsalicylic acid, quinine, erythromycin, and cisplatinum. Am J Otol 1985; 6(3):194.
Malkiewicz J. How to assess the ears and check hearing acuity. RN 1982; 45(3): 56.
McKennis AT. Vestibular neurectomy for Meniere's disease. AORN J 1989; 50(4):787.
Olsen WO. Presbycusis. Postgrad Med 1984; 76(3):189.
Ortiz-Armenta LA, Martin-Diaz JC, Gamez-Martinez L. Surgical treatment of vertigo. Ear Nose Throat J 1986; 65(6): 46.
Paparella MM, Shumrick DA, Gluckman JL, Meyerhoff WL. Otolaryngology. 3rd ed. Philadelphia: WB Saunders, 1991.
Rambur BA. Sudden hearing loss. Nurs Pract 1989; 14(1):8.
Riley MAK. Nursing care of the client with ear, nose and throat disorders. New York: Springer, 1987.
Sataloff RT. Sensorineural hearing loss. Otolaryngol Clin North Am 1986; 19(1):3.
Signs and Symptoms. Nursing 86 Books. Springhouse, PA: Springhouse, 1986.
Slater R, et al. Tinnitus: A guide for sufferers and professionals. London: Croom Helm, 1987.
Syka J, Masterton RB (eds). Auditory pathway: Structure and function. New York: Plenum Press, 1988.
Wiet RJ, Monsell EM, Hotaling AJ. Hearing and balance disorders. Postgrad Med 1985; 17(1):119.
Wyngaarden JB, Smith LH Jr, Bennett JC (eds). Cecil textbook of medicine. 19th ed. Philadelphia: WB Saunders, 1992.
Yeager JA, Joyce DG. Multichannel cochlear implants. AORN J 1989; 50(2):299.
Zegeer LJ. Oculocephalic and vestibulo-ocular responses. J Neurosci Nurs 1989; 21(1):46.

Chapter Forty-two

NURSING CARE *of Adults with Ear Disorders*

Disorders of the ear affect adults of all ages and can be acute or chronic in nature. They range in severity from infections that resolve without residual defect to disorders, such as otosclerosis, that alter the structure of the ear and cause deafness and Meniere's disease, characterized by recurrent episodes of vertigo and progressive nerve deafness. Treatment varies with the type and severity of the disorder and may involve supportive measures, pharmacologic therapy, or surgery.

Infections and Inflammations

External Ear Infections

Infections of the external ear include bacterial otitis, otomycosis, and furunculosis.

External otitis involves the skin of the auricle or the outer ear canal. It is one of the most common types of ear infection and may be an acute or chronic disorder.

Otomycosis is a fungal infection of the external ear canal and is especially common in warm, damp climates.

A furuncle, or boil, is a localized suppurative inflammation of the skin and underlying tissues of the outer ear.

ETIOLOGY AND PATHOPHYSIOLOGY

Infections of the external ear may be localized, as in the case of a furuncle, or generalized, involving the entire canal. Generalized external otitis may result from swimming in contaminated water. Bacteria such as *Pseudomonas aeruginosa, Escherichia coli, Proteus vulgaris,* or *Staphylococcus aureus* are among the causative pathogens.

A furuncle is caused by bacteria, usually *S. aureus,* which enter through hair follicles or sweat glands. A suppurative inflammation ensues, and pus and a local core of dead tissue are discharged. Local skin irritation predisposes to the development of furuncles.

Allergic individuals may acquire an external otitis from irritants such as hair dye or hair spray, which cause the individual to scratch the skin surrounding the ear, thus allowing pathogens access through the excoriated area.

Another predisposing factor is trauma from cleaning the ear canal with foreign objects such as cotton swabs and bobby pins.

CLINICAL MANIFESTATIONS

Pain, which can be excruciating, is a common symptom of generalized external otitis. It is caused by inflammation and swelling of the skin of the auricle and the external ear canal. Chewing, opening the mouth, or touching the auricle increases the discomfort. The external canal may appear red and edematous, and a purulent, foul-smelling, sticky, yellow otorrhea may be present. Other symptoms are itching and loss of hearing, which develop if the external canal becomes swollen or filled with purulent material. Low-grade fever and headache may also occur.

With otomycosis, itching may be an intense symptom. Pain and a stinging sensation may also be felt in the external auditory canal.

Furuncles generally cause severe pain, which may be associated with tinnitus, and loss of hearing in the affected ear. The extent of the hearing loss is relative to the amount of swelling of the ear canal. As with bacterial otitis externa, fever, headache, and enlarged cervical lymph nodes may also be present.

MEDICAL DIAGNOSIS

Diagnosis of infections of the external ear is made primarily on the basis of physical examination. A history of the problem differentiates chronic external otitis from the acute condition. Otoscopy, when possible, reveals a red, swollen external ear canal. Culture and sensitivity of purulent material may be performed to identify the causative pathogens.

MEDICAL MANAGEMENT

Medical management of external otitis depends on its cause. It is directed toward alleviating the infectious process as well as relieving the accompanying symptoms.

A combination of topical and systemic medications, usually antibiotics and corticosteroids, is generally effective in treating generalized external otitis. In cases in which severe cellulitis has developed, treatment may require hospitalization and intravenous antibiotic administration.

To reduce the pain associated with generalized acute external otitis, codeine, propoxyphene napsylate (Darvocet), aspirin, or acetaminophen may be ordered. Heat therapy to the infected area may also be recommended to relieve discomfort.

For chronic external otitis, treatment involves cleansing the infected ear canal. This is usually accomplished by suction to remove the accumulated debris. Antibiotic ointments or ear drops are generally effective in treating the infectious process. These may be applied to the ear canal via a cotton wick inserted in the canal by the physician. Analgesics can be prescribed for the relief of mild pain. These topical treatments may require multiple out-patient visits for cleansing and packing changes until the condition is under control.

Otomycosis may be treated with antibiotics. The infected area is cleansed with a dilute solution of aluminum acetate and acetic acid known as Burow's solution. Ear drops containing antifungal agents are administered after cleansing of the canal.

Early administration of topical antibiotics is usually effective in the treatment of furuncles. However, incision of the furuncle may be necessary in some

Chart 42–1.

NURSING GUIDE TO PATIENT EDUCATION FOR SELF-MANAGEMENT: PREVENTION OF EXTERNAL OTITIS

Instruct the patient to:

Avoid cleaning the ears with cotton swabs, bobby pins, match sticks, or other small, hard objects that can damage tissue.
Avoid getting water in the ears by wearing ear plugs when showering, washing hair, or swimming.
Avoid cosmetic products such as hair dyes, hair sprays, and so on, which cause irritation or itching.

cases. This is followed by application of warm, moist dressings to enhance drainage and relieve discomfort.

Application of the Nursing Process to the Care of the Patient with an External Ear Infection

Assessment

Obtain information concerning the history of the present problem. Determine whether the patient has recently used cosmetic products such as hair dyes or sprays, which may have contributed to the inflammation. Also ask whether the patient had been swimming before the onset of symptoms.

Inspect the affected car for redness, swelling, or discharge.

Question the patient about the presenting symptoms. For example, ask whether the patient is experiencing pain and, if so, to what degree. Ascertain any measures that may have helped alleviate the discomfort. If discharge is present, note whether the surrounding tissue is excoriated. Ask whether the area is itchy and, if so, whether the patient used any measures to relieve this condition. Determine whether the patient is experiencing any hearing difficulties, because occlusion of the external auditory canal as a result of discharge or inflammation may block the transmission of sound waves to the tympanic membrane. Finally, ask whether the patient has a sensation of ringing in the ears (tinnitus).

After treatment has been prescribed by the physician, assess the patient's understanding of it.

Nursing Diagnoses and Planning

Nursing diagnoses and related expected patient outcomes most commonly applicable to patients with an external ear infection include the following:

NDx: Pain related to the infectious process

Planning: Patient outcomes
1. Patient describes the appropriate use of analgesics and warm, moist compresses.
2. Patient reports decreasing pain in response to drug therapy, treatments, and resolution of the infectious process.

NDx: High risk for impaired skin integrity related to irritation from discharge from the ear

Planning: Patient outcomes
1. Patient demonstrates procedure for cleansing discharge from the ear.
2. Excoriation of ear canal is decreased.
3. Redness of infected ear is decreased.

NDx: High risk for sensory perceptual alteration: auditory, related to conductive hearing loss or tinnitus secondary to the infectious process

Planning: Patient outcomes
1. Patient accurately interprets verbal communication.
2. Patient describes hearing loss resulting from the infection as temporary and expected to disappear on resolution of the infection.
3. Patient describes distraction and masking techniques that can be used to cope with tinnitus.

NDx: High risk for altered health maintenance related to insufficient knowledge of therapeutic measures and prevention of recurrence

Planning: Patient outcomes
1. Patient states name, purpose, dose, route, and frequency of prescribed drugs.
2. Patient describes self-care measures for prevention of recurrent external otitis, as specified in Chart 42-1.

Nursing Interventions

NDx: Pain
Advise the patient to take analgesics as ordered for pain. Explain that warm, moist compresses applied to the affected area also aid in reducing pain and the discomfort of itch.

NDx: High risk for impaired skin integrity
Describe the need for frequent cleansing of the ear, removal of debris, and placement of medicated cotton wicks in the ear. Explain that changing the wicks is generally an office procedure and that he or she may be instructed in a regimen for keeping the wicks wet with a prescribed solution between medical treatments.

NDx: High risk for sensory/perceptual alteration: auditory
Directly face the patient while giving instructions. Have the patient repeat the instructions to ascertain that they were correctly heard. Explain to the patient that any hearing loss attributed to this infection is temporary, and normal hearing should return when the infection is resolved.

Instruct the patient to use soft background music to mask annoying tinnitus.

NDx: High risk for altered health maintenance
Review with the patient or caregiver information related to prescribed drug and heat therapy. Advise against swimming until the infection is completely resolved. Instruct the patient in the prevention of recurrence, as specified in Chart 42–1.

Evaluation

Evaluate the effectiveness of nursing care for a patient with external otitis by comparing the patient's status with the expected patient outcomes. Examples of specific outcomes for patients with external otitis have been provided in the Planning section.

Middle-Ear Infections

Otitis media is a general term used to refer to middle-ear infections caused by bacteria or less frequently by viruses. Otitis media may occur secondary to pneumonia, influenza, measles, mumps, or scarlet fever.

The most common middle-ear infections are acute, serous, or chronic otitis media (Table 42–1) and mastoiditis.

ACUTE OTITIS MEDIA

Acute otitis media is an infection of the middle ear. It occurs at all ages but is most common in infancy and childhood. It is frequently associated with upper respiratory tract infection.

ETIOLOGY AND PATHOPHYSIOLOGY

The basic cause of acute otitis media is the entrance of microorganisms from the nasopharynx into the middle-ear space via the eustachian tube. The most common causative pathogens are *E. coli*, *Streptococcus*, *Pneumococcus*, *Staphylococcus*, and *Haemophilus influenzae*.

CLINICAL MANIFESTATIONS

Symptoms of acute otitis media include severe earache, mild to moderate conductive hearing loss, fever, nausea, vomiting, and a feeling of fullness in the affected ear. If untreated, perforation of the eardrum may result.

Table 42–1. COMPARISON OF ACUTE, CHRONIC, AND SEROUS OTITIS MEDIA

FACTOR	ACUTE OTITIS MEDIA	CHRONIC OTITIS MEDIA	SEROUS OTITIS MEDIA
Etiology	Microorganisms that enter the middle ear from the nasopharynx via the eustachian tube	Untreated or repeated attacks of acute otitis media	Incomplete resolution of acute otitis media, allergic reaction, or any obstruction of the eustachian tube
Clinical manifestations	Throbbing pain in affected ear, fever, headache, nausea, vomiting, vertigo, and conductive hearing loss	Thick, purulent, persistent, or recurrent discharge, gradual hearing loss, occasional pain, nausea, and vertigo	Conductive hearing loss, pressure, and tinnitus in affected ear; no pain, no fever
Medical management	Antibiotic therapy for 10 days; in severe cases, myringotomy for drainage may be necessary	Cleansing of ear canal and middle ear with suction followed by topical antibiotics; if severe, systemic broad-spectrum antibiotics; tympanoplasty if middle-ear structures are damaged	Systemic sympathomimetic amines for vasoconstriction, drainage of middle ear by aspiration of fluid or insertion of a tympanostomy tube; correction of underlying problem

MEDICAL DIAGNOSIS

Medical diagnosis is usually made on the basis of clinical presentation. The absence of pain on pulling the auricle indicates external otitis rather than acute otitis media.

Otoscopy may reveal a red, bulging eardrum with a fluid level indicative of pus behind the eardrum (Fig. 42–1) or may reveal a recently perforated eardrum with fluid in the canal.

MEDICAL MANAGEMENT

Antibiotic therapy is the treatment of choice for acute otitis media. Penicillin, or an equivalent drug for the penicillin sensitive, is prescribed for adult patients. This regimen is generally continued for 10 days to resolve the infection and prevent recurrence. In adult patients in whom allergies are a contributing factor, antihistamines may also be ordered to improve eustachian tube function.

Aspirin or acetaminophen may be ordered for fever and pain.

In cases of severe, painful, bulging eardrum, myringotomy, a surgical incision into the tympanic membrane, may be indicated to release pressure, evacuate purulent fluid, and relieve pain.

Prompt treatment of acute otitis media generally prevents perforation of the tympanic membrane. After the acute infectious process has been resolved, the patient may be taught to use Valsalva maneuvers to keep the middle-ear space insufflated.

Guidelines for Application of the Nursing Process to the Care of the Patient with Acute Otitis Media

Assess for earache, hearing loss, nausea, vomiting, and fever. Review the name, purpose, dose, time, and route of administration of prescribed medications with the patient. Stress the importance of taking the entire series of prescribed antibiotics to ensure that the infection is resolved and thus help decrease the risk of recurrent infection, which can lead to chronic otitis media. If penicillin is prescribed, check that the patient has no history of allergy to it.

CHRONIC OTITIS MEDIA

ETIOLOGY AND PATHOPHYSIOLOGY

Chronic otitis media may be due to untreated or repeated attacks of acute otitis media, or exacerbations may follow upper respiratory tract infections. The most common causative organisms found on culture are *Streptococcus, Staphylococcus, Proteus,* and *Pseudomonas.* When left untreated, chronic otitis media often results in perforation of the tympanic membrane, which in turn causes a conductive hearing loss. This hearing loss can be exacerbated if untreated infection further destroys the ossicles of the middle ear.

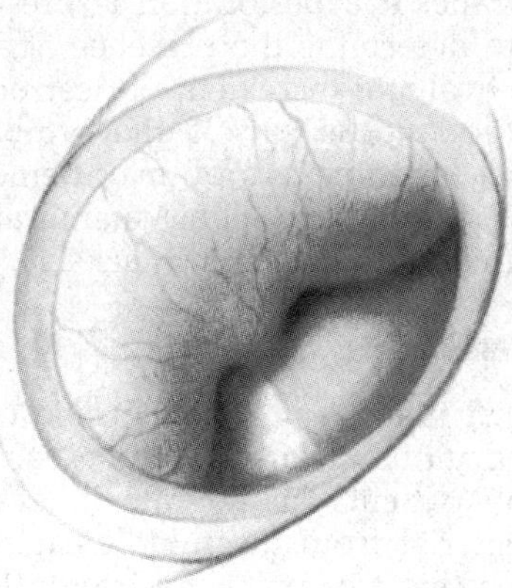

Figure 42–1.

Bulging eardrum with fluid or pus behind it as seen in acute otitis media. (From De Weese DD, et al. Otolaryngology—Head and neck surgery. St. Louis: CV Mosby, 1988, p 409.)

CLINICAL MANIFESTATIONS

Chronic otitis media is characterized by purulent, foul-smelling discharge and gradual hearing loss. Other symptoms may include occasional pain, nausea, and episodes of vertigo.

One complication of untreated chronic otitis media is the development and spread of a cholesteatoma, a middle-ear growth made up of infectious material and the shed skin of the ear canal and middle-ear space. This mass can enlarge and occlude the middle-ear space as well as cause damage to the ossicles and erosion of the bony structures of the cranium. Unchecked, it can lead to more serious complications such as labyrinthitis, facial paralysis, meningitis, or brain abscess as the growth enlarges and spreads. Although these complications are rare, their consequences are severe and they emphasize the importance of seeking immediate treatment of this condition.

MEDICAL DIAGNOSIS

Diagnosis of chronic otitis media is made on the basis of the patient's history, clinical symptoms, and findings on otoscopic examination and x-ray films. X-ray films are usually obtained to determine the extent of bony destruction from the infectious process, including extension into the mastoid air cells.

The patient history generally discloses recurrent or unresolved episodes of otitis media. Otoscopic examination may reveal a thickened or scarred tympanic membrane. If a perforation is present, it may be possible to determine the presence of a cholesteatoma and to evaluate the extent of destruction of the ossicles of the middle ear. If the tympanic membrane is intact, pneumatoscopy may demonstrate reduced mobility of the tympanic membrane as a result of scarring from recurrent attacks.

MEDICAL MANAGEMENT

The medical management of chronic otitis media includes meticulous cleansing of the ear canal and, as far as the patient can tolerate it, evacuation of infectious material from the middle-ear space using suction. After this treatment, topical antibiotics and eardrops are prescribed. Systemic antibiotic therapy may be used in severe exacerbations of chronic otitis media. Cholesteatomas require excision and, if indicated, ossicular or tympanic membrane reconstruction procedures to restore function and structure to the middle ear.

These procedures may range from a simple tympanoplasty to mastoidectomy to remove a spreading cholesteatoma.

Guidelines for Application of the Nursing Process to the Care of the Patient with Chronic Otitis Media

Nursing care for patients undergoing nonsurgical treatment for chronic otitis media is similar to that described previously for patients with acute otitis media.

SEROUS OTITIS MEDIA

Serous otitis media is a condition in which noninfectious fluid accumulates in the middle-ear space. It can be either a chronic or an acute process and may occur at any age.

ETIOLOGY

Serous otitis media can result from incomplete resolution of acute otitis media, from an allergic reaction, or from any condition that causes an obstruction or malfunction of the eustachian tube.

PATHOPHYSIOLOGY

The eustachian tube is a narrow channel that connects the middle-ear space with the nasopharynx. This tube serves to equalize the pressure on either side of the eardrum (Fig. 42–2). The nasopharyngeal end of the tube opens from time to time to allow the passage of air up into the middle ear as when swallowing or yawning occurs. If the eustachian tube is blocked by nasopharyngeal secretions, or if allergic reactions cause a swelling of the lumen, air is unable to enter. Occlusion of the canals also occurs spontaneously with sudden changes in atmospheric pressure such as happens with air travel. This is a natural response and is usually reversed by frequent swallowing, chewing gum, or Valsalva maneuvers, all of which allow air to enter the middle-ear space via the eustachian tube.

CLINICAL MANIFESTATIONS

Symptoms differ from acute otitis media in that there is absence of pain and fever associated with the infectious process. A conductive hearing loss occurs as a result of the accumulation of fluid, and the patient may complain of a feeling of pressure.

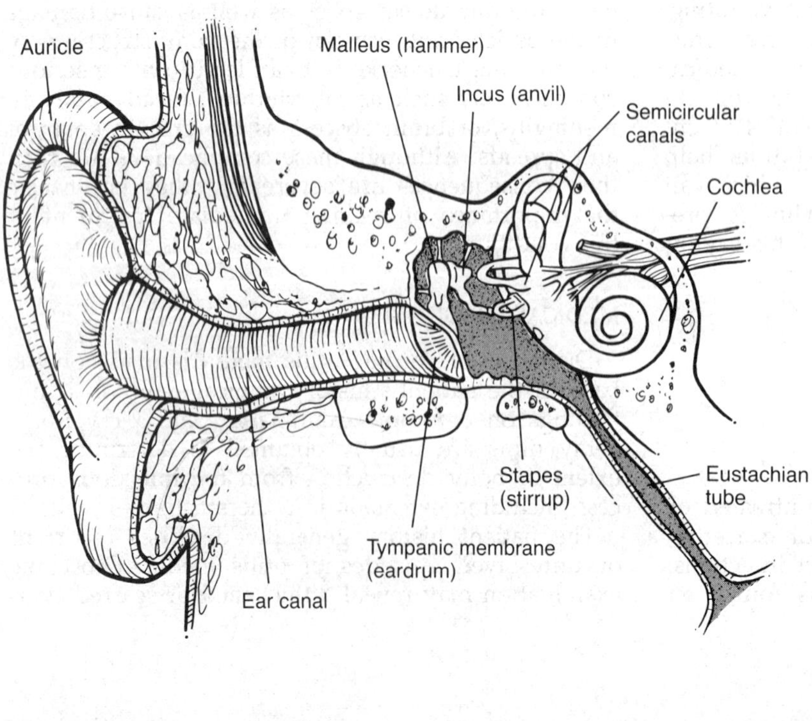

Figure 42–2.

Anatomic relationship of the eustachian tube to the middle ear and the tympanic membrane. The eustachian tube and middle-ear space are in color. The eustachian tube connects the middle-ear space with the nasopharynx.

Chart 42–2.

NURSING GUIDE TO PATIENT EDUCATION FOR SELF-MANAGEMENT: SEROUS OTITIS MEDIA

Instruct the patient to do the following:

Perform the Valsalva maneuver to inflate the eustachian tube unless medically contraindicated. To do this, pinch the nostrils together and vigorously blow the nose several times per day to help open the eustachian tube and permit air to enter the middle ear.

Take decongestants and antihistamines as prescribed by the physician.

Avoid exposure to known allergens.

Seek prompt medical treatment if nasopharyngeal infection recurs or allergic symptoms persist, to prevent the development of chronic serous otitis media.

Occasionally, patients also report a low-pitched ringing (tinnitus). Serous otitis media may persist for days or months.

MEDICAL DIAGNOSIS

Visualization by means of an otoscope may reveal retraction of the eardrum. A fluid level may be visible through the eardrum. Diagnosis of serous otitis media can be confirmed on the basis of abnormal tympanometric studies or audiometrics confirming a conductive hearing loss.

MEDICAL MANAGEMENT

Treatment of serous otitis media depends on the cause of the eustachian tube blockage.

Systemic sympathomimetic amines, such as ephedrine or pseudoephedrine, may be ordered because their vasoconstrictive properties may improve eustachian tube function. Fluid may be aspirated from the middle ear through a myringotomy incision. In cases of chronic serous otitis media, a tympanostomy or pressure-equalization tube may be inserted into the eardrum (see Fig. 41–6). In all cases, treatment of the underlying condition is necessary. For example, to control the allergy factor, antihistamines may be ordered and the patient advised to minimize exposure to known allergens.

Application of the Nursing Process to the Care of the Patient with Serous Otitis Media

Assessment

Collect information from the patient regarding the history as well as the symptoms of the present condition. Obtain data about episodes of discomfort, their duration, and factors that may have contributed to their onset. Ask about the effectiveness of methods that have been used to obtain relief. Question the patient about any loss of hearing, and subjectively assess present hearing status during the interview. Determine whether the patient has a history of recent infections or allergies or whether he or she has flown in the past several weeks. Also ask about any other altitude-changing activities such as diving or driving in the mountains.

Nursing Diagnoses and Planning

The nursing diagnosis and related expected patient outcomes most commonly applicable to patients with serous otitis media are as follows:

NDx: High risk for altered health maintenance related to insufficient knowledge of measures for relief of symptoms and prevention of chronic serous otitis media

Planning: Patient outcomes

1. Patient explains the Valsalva maneuver, as specified in Chart 42–2.
2. Patient demonstrates the Valsalva maneuver, as specified in Chart 42–2.
3. Patient states the name, action, dose, route, time, and frequency of administration of prescribed drugs.
4. Patient identifies known allergens and ways to reduce exposure to them.
5. Patient acknowledges the need for prompt medical treatment of recurrent infections.

Nursing Interventions

NDx: High risk for altered health maintenance

Instruct the patient in self-care as specified in Chart 42–2.

Evaluation

Evaluate the effectiveness of nursing care for a patient with serous otitis media by comparing the patient's status with the expected patient outcomes. Examples of specific outcomes for patients with serous otitis media have been provided in the Planning section.

Mastoiditis

Mastoiditis is an inflammation of the air cells of the mastoid bone that forms the part of the skull located directly behind the ear.

ETIOLOGY

Mastoiditis is generally the result of infections of the middle ear, which communicates with the mastoid cells. It may be secondary to a sore throat and an upper respiratory tract infection or, less commonly today, to diseases such as measles, scarlet fever, and diphtheria. It is occasionally reported in the adult population in the United States but is more common in children and in countries where acute infections may go untreated. The causative pathogens are usually the same as those responsible for acute otitis media, namely *Streptococcus* and *Staphylococcus.*

PATHOPHYSIOLOGY

The infectious process begins with edema of the tissues and progresses to the formation of infectious fluid and pus that fill the mastoid cells.

CLINICAL MANIFESTATIONS

Typical symptoms of mastoiditis are pain, tinnitus, fever, otorrhea, and hearing loss. Dizziness and vertigo may also be reported by some patients. Redness, swelling, and tenderness develop in the area of the mastoid process. If untreated, mastoiditis can progress to brain abscess, meningitis, facial paralysis, and suppurative labyrinthitis.

MEDICAL DIAGNOSIS

Clinical findings and a history of recent otitis media suggest a diagnosis of mastoiditis. A recent bout of scarlet fever or measles also alerts the examiner to the possibility of mastoiditis. Otoscopy reveals a dull, thickened, swollen eardrum. X-ray films may display an increased density of the mastoid air cells as a result of a chronic infectious process.

MEDICAL MANAGEMENT

With the prevalence of antibiotics, otitis media rarely progresses to the stage of acute mastoiditis. In cases that do occur, treatment consists of intensive parenteral antibiotic therapy. Initially, penicillin is the drug of choice in nonallergic individuals. Subsequent therapy is subject to the results of cultures and sensitivities, and the clinical response to the initial treatment.

Mastoidectomy (see Chapter 41) may be indicated in patients who do not respond to antibiotic therapy or who display lingering symptoms after antibiotic therapy.

Guidelines for Application of the Nursing Process to the Care of the Patient with Mastoiditis

Nursing care for patients undergoing nonsurgical treatment for mastoiditis is similar to that described previously for patients with acute otitis media.

Labyrinthitis

Labyrinthitis is an inflammation of the labyrinth of the inner ear. It is a rare but serious problem.

ETIOLOGY AND PATHOPHYSIOLOGY

There are two types of labyrinthitis: purulent and viral. Purulent labyrinthitis is extremely rare in the adult population in the United States. When it does occur, it may accompany acute or chronic otitis media or may be a secondary complication of it. It may also be secondary to purulent meningitis if the pathogens gain access to the subarachnoid space via the cochlear aqueduct.

Viral labyrinthitis is associated with respiratory infections and may be responsible for the nonconductive hearing loss that follows chickenpox and other viral infections.

CLINICAL MANIFESTATIONS

Labyrinthitis is characterized by profound sensorineural hearing loss, severe vertigo, and loss of equilibrium. It may also be accompanied by nystagmus. The sensorineural hearing loss associated with purulent labyrinthitis is almost always permanent. The vertigo, although incapacitating during the acute episode, gradually subsides. Viral labyrinthitis is also associated with profound hearing loss, which appears as a sensorineural loss on testing the patient. However, some or all of the hearing may be recovered at the end of the acute phase of the labyrinthitis.

Other symptoms of labyrinthitis, whether purulent

or viral, may include fever, chills, nausea, vomiting, and purulent otorrhea.

MEDICAL DIAGNOSIS

Medical diagnosis is made on the basis of clinical presentation and patient history of otitis media or upper respiratory tract infection. Audiometric and vestibular testing may be done to evaluate and document the hearing loss and impairment of vestibular function. If previous test results exist, these are compared with those obtained during the acute phase of the labyrinthitis.

MEDICAL MANAGEMENT

The patient diagnosed as having labyrinthitis is hospitalized and started on high-dose intravenous antibiotic therapy. To control vertigo, medications such as diazepam are prescribed and the patient is maintained on bed rest. Intravenous fluids may be ordered to supplement oral intake to prevent dehydration in cases of severe nausea and vomiting.

In rare cases when conservative treatment fails, a labyrinthectomy or mastoidectomy may be necessary to evacuate the infection.

Application of the Nursing Process to the Care of the Patient with Labyrinthitis

Assessment

Assess the physical condition of the patient, with particular attention to symptoms associated with vertigo, imbalance, and hearing loss. Note the degree of discomfort or dysfunction experienced. Explore any precipitating factors with the patient and any methods of relief the patient has used. Assess the need for safety precautions if the patient is experiencing vertigo.

Question the patient regarding the presence of nausea and vomiting, its frequency, and severity. Assess the patient for signs of dehydration by examining mucous membranes and checking skin turgor. Also review available laboratory data, especially serum electrolyte levels.

Assess the patient's level of anxiety. Profound hearing loss combined with severe vertigo is very threatening. Determine how well the patient understands the disease, and explore his or her expectations of treatment. Ascertain whether the patient is aware that there may be a permanent loss of hearing.

Assess the extent of hearing loss in relation to the patient's ability to communicate and understand instructions and explanations.

Nursing Diagnoses and Planning

Nursing diagnoses and related expected patient outcomes most commonly applicable to patients with labyrinthitis include the following:

NDx: Sensory/perceptual alteration related to vertigo

Planning: Patient outcomes
1. Patient takes medication prescribed for vertigo.
2. Patient avoids sudden movements, which may precipitate vertigo.
3. Patient reports decreased vertigo.

NDx: High risk for fluid volume deficit related to severe vomiting

Planning: Patient outcomes
1. Skin turgor is good or improved.
2. Mucous membranes are moist.
3. Serum electrolytes are within normal limits.

NDx: High risk for injury related to vertigo and imbalance

Planning: Patient outcomes
1. Patient requests and accepts assistance as needed.
2. Patient remains free of injury.

NDx: Anxiety related to hearing loss and vertigo

Planning: Patient outcomes
1. Patient discusses concerns with nurse or appropriate care provider.
2. Patient verbalizes understanding of the disorder and its treatment.
3. Patient uses anxiety-reducing interventions as discussed with the appropriate caregiver.

NDx: Impaired communication related to conductive hearing loss

Planning: Patient outcomes
1. Patient informs staff and significant others of ways they can facilitate communication when hearing loss is significant (e.g., directly face him or her and speak toward the unaffected ear).
2. Patient demonstrates alternative methods of communication such as lip reading or writing when necessary or applicable.
3. Patient responds appropriately to questions and directions.

Nursing Interventions

NDx: Sensory/perceptual alteration
Be alert to nonverbal signs of distress related to dizziness or vertigo. Instruct the patient to request medication for relief of symptoms. Stress the importance of requesting medication before the symptom becomes severe to avoid unnecessary discomfort.

Also instruct the patient to avoid sudden changes in position such as from lying to sitting or sitting to standing. Investigate movements or stimuli that exacerbate vertigo and help the patient to identify ways in which these stimuli can be avoided. Fluorescent lights, for example, often set off attacks of vertigo.

NDx: High risk for fluid volume deficit
Administer intravenous fluids and medications such as antiemetics as ordered. Monitor for signs of dehydration, and record intake and output.

NDx: High risk for injury
Keep the side rails of the bed up at all times. Instruct the patient to request assistance when getting out of bed. Assist the patient when ambulating. Instruct family members in protecting the patient from injury both during hospitalization and after discharge.

NDx: Anxiety
Encourage the patient to express concerns and to ask questions regarding the diagnosis, treatment, and prognosis. Ensure that the patient is informed of what to expect during all stages of care. Reassure the patient that the vertigo, nausea, and vomiting will gradually subside when the infection resolves. Help the patient to understand and to accept the possibility that the hearing loss may be permanent.

NDx: Impaired communication
If the patient has adequate hearing in the opposite ear, only minor difficulty may be experienced in adjusting to the loss of hearing in the affected ear. However, if there is already a significant loss in the unaffected ear, a distinct impairment in the ability to communicate and to understand may be noticed. Help the patient to instruct others in communication-enhancement techniques such as face-to-face communication, gestures, and speaking close to the unaffected ear. If these techniques are not helpful, encourage the use of written materials to convey especially important information.

Evaluation

Evaluate the effectiveness of nursing care for a patient with labyrinthitis by comparing the patient's status with the expected patient outcomes. Examples of specific outcomes for patients with labyrinthitis have been provided in the Planning section.

Structural Disorders

Perforation of the Tympanic Membrane

ETIOLOGY AND PATHOPHYSIOLOGY

A tympanic perforation is a hole or tear in the eardrum. The most common cause of tympanic membrane perforation is infection. The second most common cause of perforation is trauma. Types of trauma that may result in perforation of the tympanic membrane include puncture with a foreign object, skull fracture, or sudden increase in air pressure such as may occur in an explosion.

CLINICAL MANIFESTATIONS

Clinical manifestations of a perforated tympanic membrane are pain and discharge (blood or middle-ear fluid) from the affected ear. When the perforation results from infection, pain is worse before the tympanic membrane perforates, and the release of the built-up pressure usually results in a significant reduction in pain after perforation. If the perforation results from trauma, the pain is at the moment of perforation, but it usually does not persist.

MEDICAL DIAGNOSIS

Earache and bleeding from the ear, possibly accompanied by some change in hearing, suggest perforation if the patient has a recent history of trauma. The diagnosis can be confirmed by otoscopy (Fig. 42–3).

MEDICAL MANAGEMENT

Many traumatic perforations of the tympanic membrane heal spontaneously. Prophylactic antibiotics may be prescribed after diagnosis to prevent infection. A tympanoplasty may be required if the perforation does not heal within 6 months of the traumatic event. A persistent conductive hearing

A B C

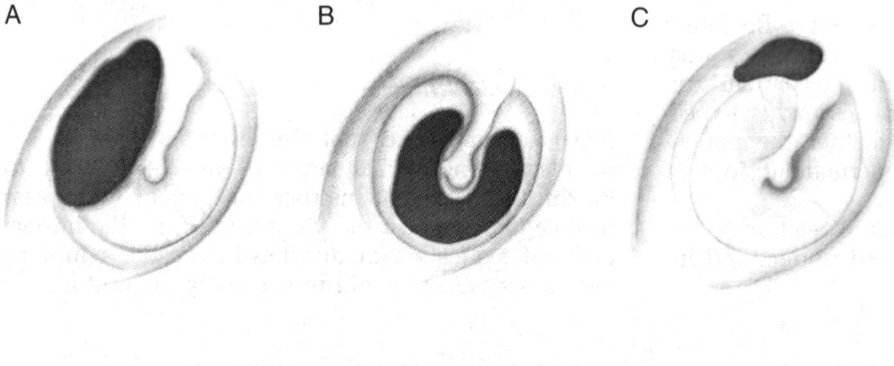

Figure 42–3.

A, Small central perforation of the tympanic membrane. *B*, Large central perforation of the tympanic membrane. *C*, Marginal perforation of the tympanic membrane. (From De Weese DD, et al. Otolaryngology—Head and neck surgery. St. Louis: CV Mosby, 1988, p 419.)

loss may be indicative of a disruption of the ossicles, which necessitates surgical exploration and repair of the middle ear.

Application of the Nursing Process to the Care of the Patient with a Perforated Tympanic Membrane

Assessment

Ask the patient about the location, type, degree, and duration of pain experienced. Also question about tinnitus, vertigo, and hearing loss.

Examine the ear for bleeding and drainage. Keep in mind that clear drainage may indicate a skull fracture with cerebrospinal fluid (CSF) draining through the perforated eardrum.

Assess the patient's understanding of factors that may predispose to secondary infection such as getting water in the ear during the healing process.

Nursing Diagnoses and Planning

Nursing diagnoses and related expected patient outcomes most commonly applicable to patients with a perforated tympanic membrane include the following:

NDx: Pain related to tissue disruption in the ear

Planning: Patient outcomes

1. Patient takes analgesics as prescribed.
2. Patient reports a decrease in pain or discomfort.

NDx: High risk for infection related to perforation of the eardrum

Planning: Patient outcomes

1. Patient explains self-care measures to be taken to decrease the risk of infection.
2. Patient remains afebrile.
3. Increased pain, odor, or purulent drainage from the ear is absent.

Nursing Interventions

NDx: Pain

Encourage the patient to take analgesics as prescribed for pain. Also encourage the use of distraction and relaxation techniques for coping with discomfort. Instruct the patient to report increased pain because this may indicate a developing infection.

NDx: High risk for infection

Explain to the patient that antibiotics are prescribed to prevent or reduce the risk of infection. Stress the importance of adhering to the medication regimen even if no symptoms are present.

Also explain the importance of keeping the ear canal dry during the healing process. Instruct the patient to avoid swimming and to protect the ear with cotton and petroleum jelly when showering or shampooing. Remind the patient that vigorous nose blowing during the recovery period can disrupt the healing of the tympanic membrane.

Teach the patient to identify signs of infection, such as fever, pain, drainage, and warmth of the ear or canal, and to seek prompt medical treatment should these occur.

Evaluation

Evaluate the effectiveness of nursing care for a patient with a perforated tympanic membrane by comparing the patient's status with the expected patient outcomes. Examples of specific outcomes for patients with a perforated tympanic membrane have been provided in the Planning section.

Otosclerosis

Otosclerosis is an overgrowth of bone around the oval window and stapes footplate that prevents movement of the stapes in the oval window. This condition results in a conductive hearing loss when sound cannot be transmitted from the oval window to the cochlea.

ETIOLOGY

The cause of otosclerosis is unknown. The condition generally appears in early adulthood and exhibits a familial tendency. It is more common in women than men and may be exacerbated by pregnancy.

PATHOPHYSIOLOGY

Otosclerosis is the formation of spongy bone around the oval window in the middle-ear space. This overgrowth of bone causes fixation of the stapes footplate, preventing transmission of sound vibration to the inner ear. Sensorineural deafness may result in advanced cases or in cases of cochlear otosclerosis.

CLINICAL MANIFESTATIONS

Otosclerosis is characterized by a chronic, progressive, conductive hearing loss. Sometimes a mixed hearing loss is noted in cases of long-standing otosclerosis. Both ears may be affected to varying degrees. Tinnitus may be an accompanying symptom.

MEDICAL DIAGNOSIS

Progressive hearing loss, without a history of middle-ear infections, is indicative of otosclerosis. Diagnosis can be confirmed through audiometric testing. A Rinne tuning fork test indicates that hearing is better by bone conduction than by air conduction. Tympanometry reveals an extraordinarily "stiff" system, indicating fixation of the stapes footplate. Pure tone audiometry should confirm a gap between the bone conduction and air conduction for the affected ear.

MEDICAL MANAGEMENT

There is no medical cure for otosclerosis or a known treatment for its prevention. A hearing aid may be prescribed to help the patient's hearing to some degree, but the treatment of choice in most cases is a stapedectomy.

STAPEDECTOMY

A stapedectomy is a microsurgical procedure in which the stapes superstructure is removed and replaced with a prosthesis. This prosthesis is usually stainless steel, polyethylene, or some other synthetic material (Fig. 42–4).

Procedure

Stapedectomy is usually performed under local anesthetic but is occasionally performed under a general anesthetic. In either case, local anesthetic is injected into the ear canal of the patient because the epinephrine in the local anesthetic controls bleeding. The entire procedure is performed through the ear canal. Access to the middle-ear space is gained by rolling back the tympanic membrane. The superstructure of the stapes is carefully removed, a small hole is made in the footplate of the stapes, and the prosthesis is measured and inserted. If the patient is awake, he or she is asked to repeat words or numbers to test the improvement in hearing, which is usually immediate. The canal is packed lightly, and there is usually no dressing over the ear. On average, the procedure lasts between 45 and 90 minutes.

Postoperative Course

The patient who has undergone a stapedectomy is on bed rest for at least the first 24 hours and is medicated as ordered for dizziness. Discharge is usually the day after surgery unless the patient suffers intractable dizziness. The patient is seen about 1 week postoperatively in the office, at which time some undissolved ear packing may be removed.

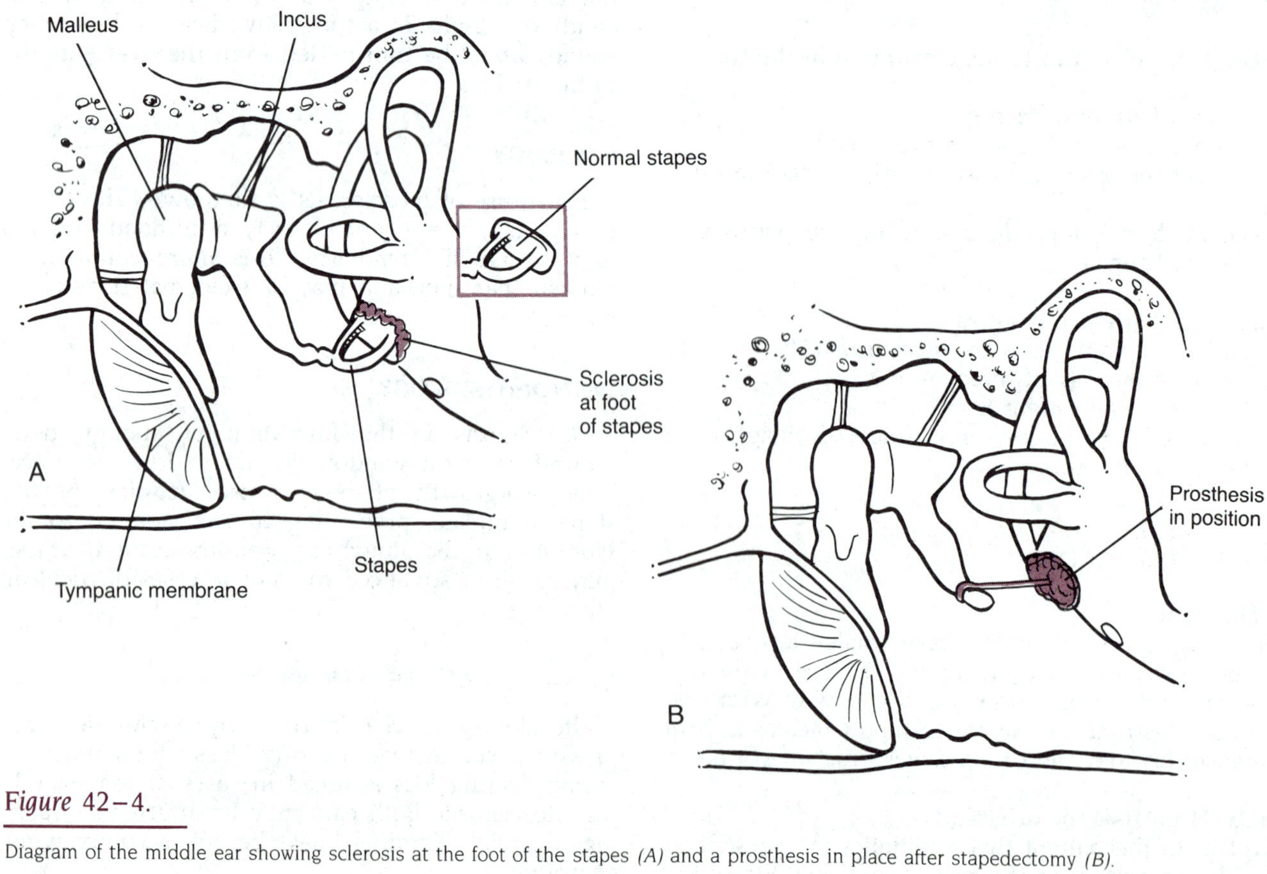

Figure 42–4.

Diagram of the middle ear showing sclerosis at the foot of the stapes *(A)* and a prosthesis in place after stapedectomy *(B)*.

The improved hearing that the patient may have noted at the time of the operation usually decreases immediately after surgery because of the packing in the ear and edema in the tissues. Hearing returns over the next 2 to 6 weeks with removal of the packing and resolution of the surgical edema.

Complications

The most frequent complication of stapedectomy is postoperative vertigo. This is quite common and usually resolves slowly.

Other complications that can occur include noniatrogenic hearing loss, which occurs for unknown reasons in about 1% of all stapedectomies, infection, displacement of the newly placed prosthesis, and, rarely, temporary or permanent facial paralysis (Glasscock & Shambaugh, 1990, pp 392, 405, 407).

Application of the Nursing Process to the Care of the Patient Having a Stapedectomy

PREOPERATIVE NURSING CARE

Basic preoperative care is provided as discussed under tympanoplasty in Chapter 41.

POSTOPERATIVE NURSING CARE

Assessment

Assess the patient for discomfort or dizziness, and observe the operative ear. Keep in mind that there is generally very little pain, no bleeding, and no drainage after stapedectomy. Ask the patient to frown, close the eyes, pucker the lips, and bare the teeth to check facial nerve function.

Nursing Diagnoses and Planning

Nursing diagnoses and related expected patient outcomes most commonly applicable to patients who have had a stapedectomy include the following:

NDx: High risk for injury related to dizziness or vertigo

Planning: Patient outcomes
1. Patient takes medication as ordered for dizziness.
2. Patient uses methods to reduce vestibular stimulation.
3. Patient requests help on ambulation.
4. Patient reports decrease or relief from dizziness.
5. Patient remains free of injury.

NDx: High risk for altered health maintenance related to insufficient knowledge of discharge instructions, follow-up care

Planning: Patient outcomes
1. Patient explains discharge instructions, as specified in Chart 42–3.
2. Patient states date and location of follow-up visit.

Nursing Interventions

NDx: High risk for injury
Administer prescribed medications as ordered for dizziness or vertigo. Remind the patient to move slowly and without jerking to avoid precipitating or worsening vertigo. Instruct the patient to ask for assistance with ambulation.

NDx: High risk for altered health maintenance
Instruct the patient in self-care measures to prevent displacement of the prosthesis by changes in pressure within the ear, as specified in Chart 42–3. Be certain the patient knows when and where to return for follow-up care.

Evaluation

Evaluate the effectiveness of nursing care for a patient who has had a stapedectomy by comparing the patient's status with the expected patient outcomes. Examples of specific outcomes for patients who have had a stapedectomy have been provided in the Planning section.

Meniere's Disease

Meniere's disease is a recurrent and usually progressive disorder of the inner ear that affects hearing, balance, and the vestibular system.

ETIOLOGY AND PATHOPHYSIOLOGY

The cause of Meniere's disease is not known, but it is thought to be a type of autoimmune disease.

CLINICAL MANIFESTATIONS

Meniere's disease is characterized by recurrent attacks of severe vertigo, fluctuating sensorineural hearing loss, and tinnitus. Often only one ear is affected, although in 20% to 30% of patients there is bilateral involvement. Onset of the disease is sudden and usually occurs between the ages of 20 and 60 years (Paparella et al, 1991, p 1690).

Patients may describe a vague feeling of pressure or fullness in the ear at the beginning of an attack.

Chart 42–3.

NURSING GUIDE TO PATIENT EDUCATION FOR SELF-MANAGEMENT: DISCHARGE INSTRUCTIONS AFTER STAPEDECTOMY

To prevent infection, instruct the patient to keep the affected ear dry by doing the following:

No swimming for 6 weeks.
No showers for 6 weeks (or protect the ear from water entering).
Shampoo after 2 weeks (protect the ear from water entering).

To prevent displacement of the prosthesis by changes of pressure within the ear, instruct the patient to do the following:

Avoid nose blowing when possible.
Avoid forceful coughing (if this is a problem, cough suppressants can be prescribed).
Avoid exposure to upper respiratory tract infections.
Avoid bending and lifting heavy objects and other activities that increase intracranial pressure.
Avoid air travel for 6 weeks or as specified by surgeon.

To allow early identification and treatment of complications, instruct the patient to report any of the following symptoms:

Sudden hearing loss.
Fever.
Severe vertigo.

Tinnitus and vertigo, sometimes severe enough to completely incapacitate the patient, ensue. These symptoms may be accompanied by headache, diaphoresis, nystagmus, and imbalance. In the acute stage of an attack, any abrupt motion of the head or eyes may also precipitate nausea and vomiting. Vertigo lasts for several hours or days but gradually subsides and is absent between attacks. Tinnitus and hearing impairment, however, remain.

MEDICAL DIAGNOSIS

Meniere's disease is diagnosed primarily on the basis of the patient's history and presenting symptoms. Audiometric testing often reveals a decrease in speech discrimination and a sensorineural hearing loss. Caloric testing and electronystagmography (ENG) are done to check for nystagmus characteristic of Meniere's disease. X-ray films and computed tomographic (CT) scans are done to rule out brain tumors, and brain-stem evoked response audiometry (BSER) is done to rule out hard-to-find acoustic neuromas and brain-stem vascular, demyelinating, or other type of lesion.

MEDICAL MANAGEMENT

During an acute attack of Meniere's disease, medical management is directed toward the relief of symptoms. Generally bed rest is ordered. Drugs such as meclizine (Antivert) and diazepam (Valium) are given to control vertigo, and prochlorperazine (Compazine) may be prescribed for nausea. In addition, mild sedatives or tranquilizers may be prescribed.

Dietary restrictions have been suggested as advantageous in the treatment of Meniere's disease. These include a low-sodium diet and decreased fluid intake to control fluid retention in the endolymphatic system as well as caffeine and alcohol restrictions. Diuretics may also be ordered as part of the treatment and in turn may create the need for potassium supplements to replace the potassium lost through diuresis.

Surgical treatment is a last resort for patients with unilateral Meniere's disease and intractable or incapacitating vertigo.

Endolymphatic shunts, which channel fluid from the inner ear into the subarachnoid space or into the mastoid, help equalize the fluid pressures within the inner ear; these are effective about 75% of the time (Ballenger, 1985, p 1262). Retrolabyrinthine vestibular neurectomy is a procedure in which the section of the eighth cranial nerve, which controls balance, is cut after mastoidectomy is done for visualization. This procedure is generally effective in relieving vertigo but carries the risk of hearing loss if the acoustical portion of the nerve is damaged. Cryosurgery to produce a fistula in the inner ear for fluid drainage also effectively relieves vertigo in some patients. Labyrinthectomy cures vertigo but causes irreversible hearing loss and alteration in balance.

Application of the Nursing Process to the Care of the Patient with Meniere's Disease

Assessment

Obtain information regarding the onset, duration, severity, and frequency of attacks.

Explore the type of vertiginous attack experience. Keep in mind that many patients describe a feeling of being "pulled to the ground," which is commonly referred to as a "drop attack." Determine whether the vertigo led to nausea and vomiting. Help the patient to identify any precipitating event or forewarning of the attack.

Inquire about associated symptoms such as ringing or roaring in the ears, ataxia, and sudden, noticeable change in hearing. Subjectively assess the extent of the hearing loss during the assessment period.

Although not always possible in the acute phase of the attack, make an effort to obtain psychosocial data on the patient such as occupation, family role, and community activities to assess the possible effects of this chronic disease on the patient and the family.

Nursing Diagnoses and Planning

The nursing diagnosis and related expected patient outcomes most commonly applicable to patients with Meniere's disease are as follows:

NDx: High risk for altered health maintenance related to insufficient knowledge of disease, treatment, and self-care

Planning: Patient outcomes

1. Patient describes condition and symptoms accurately.
2. Patient lists signs and symptoms of an impending attack, stating what is to be done when these occur.
3. Patient describes measures to reduce severity of attacks and to protect self from injury.

Nursing Interventions

NDx: High risk for altered health maintenance

Explain the disease process to the patient and the family or significant others. Review the results of diagnostic studies and the proposed treatment plan. Instruct the patient and family in self-care. Begin by helping the patient to identify warning signs of attacks and measures to protect self from harm. Also review interventions to reduce the severity of attacks. Instruct the patient to take medications as prescribed when an attack begins and to lie down on the unaffected side in a darkened, quiet room, avoiding sudden movements and activities such as reading. Instruct the patient to pull over to the side of the road and wait for the symptoms to subside if he or she is driving when an attack begins. To help prevent attacks, instruct the patient to avoid noisy places and exposure to loud music, television, and other sound in the home. Also instruct the patient to avoid exposure to bright light and suggest that low-wattage light bulbs be used in the home, curtains or blinds be kept closed, dark glasses be worn outside or when in bright light, and car windows be tinted to the extent legally permitted. Instruct the patient to refrain from sudden, jerky movements and to avoid actions such as bending over or twisting the head, which predispose to vertigo. Encourage the patient to move slowly, to bend at the knees, and to turn the whole body rather than just the head.

Instruct the patient to avoid or limit use of nicotine, ingestion of caffeine, and use of decongestant medications. Explain that they cause vasoconstriction, which can decrease the circulation to the inner ear and interfere with fluid absorption, thus increasing the risk of an attack. Also encourage the patient to avoid alcoholic beverages (Cleveland & Morris, 1990, p 32). If a patient experiences constant tinnitus, suggest the use of a white-noise machine to mask it.

There is often a great deal of anxiety associated with Meniere's disease because the patient never knows when an attack will occur. Acknowledge this fact, and refer the family and the patient to support groups to help the patient learn to cope with the long-term effects of the disease process. Information on the Meniere's network of self-help groups and related services can be obtained from The Ear Foundation, Baptist Hospital, Nashville, Tennessee 37236 (800-545-HEAR).

Evaluation

Evaluate the effectiveness of nursing care for a patient with Meniere's disease by comparing the patient's status with the expected patient outcomes. Examples of specific outcomes for patients with Meniere's disease have been provided in the Planning section.

The Elderly: Special Considerations

It is estimated that one third of individuals who are 70 years of age or older have a significant hearing impairment. As a result, geriatric patients with hearing disorders are found in virtually every type of health care setting. As the population of the United States ages and the longevity of its citizens increases, incorporating awareness of this impairment into all aspects of care for these individuals will become mandatory. Nurses are in a unique position to bring this awareness to other health care professionals and to initiate actions to address this disability.

There are a variety of causes of hearing disorders in the geriatric population. The elderly of today, for instance, did not have the benefit of antibiotic therapy, nor were they recipients of childhood immunizations. Hence, many were victims of various childhood diseases, including ear infections, which resulted in varying degrees of hearing loss. Also the damaging effect of excessive, sustained noise on hearing was not known during the years when many of the current aged, especially men, were exposed to this detriment. Today the individuals employed in construction, factory work, and the like are more knowledgeable and are protected by safety laws. Diabetes and vascular disorders such as hypertension and arteriosclerosis are particular problems that affect the elderly and predispose them to hearing impairments. The delayed excretion of ototoxic drugs, often prescribed or taken by the elderly, may also contribute to irreversible hearing loss (see Table 41–1). However, the most common cause of hearing loss is the aging process itself.

Presbycusis

ETIOLOGY

Presbycusis is a progressive sensorineural hearing loss that occurs as a part of the normal aging process.

PATHOPHYSIOLOGY

The thousands of hair cells of the cochlea are gradually lost between youth and age. With this loss, hearing deteriorates because fewer and fewer of these cells exist to stimulate the organ of hearing. There is considerable variation in the degree of hearing loss and impairment (extent to which understanding and perception are affected by hearing loss and discrimination), and mere age is not the deciding factor. Occupational factors may account for the fact that men seem to be more affected than women.

CLINICAL MANIFESTATIONS

Presbycusis actually begins in youth. Characteristically, hearing acuity for the highest frequencies (18,000 to 20,000 Hz) is lost first. Individuals do not begin to notice this loss until the high-frequency loss coincides with the range of tones that are in the frequencies of speech.

MEDICAL DIAGNOSIS

Medical diagnosis of presbycusis is based primarily on the patient's history (frequently as given by the family). Often the patient is unaware of the severity of the hearing impairment, but those around him or her are acutely aware of it. Audiometric testing documents the degree and severity of the hearing loss.

MEDICAL MANAGEMENT

Generally, a hearing aid is suggested for patients with presbycusis. In most cases, it is the best means of enhancing communication for these hearing-impaired individuals. A variety of hearing aids are available to match the varied hearing losses of the hearing-impaired population. An audiologist should be consulted to match the appropriate aid with the patient's hearing loss.

Application of the Nursing Process to the Care of the Patient with Presbycusis

Assessment

Assess subjectively the degree of hearing loss. Question the patient or family member about the onset and duration of the hearing loss. Remember that the hearing loss associated with aging is insidious, and onset and duration may be difficult to identify. Question the patient about additional symptomatology such as pain, tinnitus, dizziness, or nausea to rule out other possibilities because, if other symptoms exist in concert with this hearing loss, there may be another disease process superimposed on the hearing loss.

Obtain a thorough history of illnesses, including a medication history. Include any familial history of ear disease or other contributing factors.

Assess the overall physical condition of the patient. Investigate coping techniques that the patient or the family may have used to deal with the hearing loss. Lip reading is rare in patients with this type of hearing loss, but patients do unconsciously rely on seeing the face of the speaker to get more information from the spoken word. Many times the patient already has a hearing aid but does not use it. Try to discover the reasons for nonuse. For some aging patients, the mechanics of battery changes in these small devices are too difficult if they have difficulty seeing as well.

Attempt to assess the psychological response to

the hearing disorder. Has the patient accepted the existence of the disability? How has he or she reacted or adjusted to the disability? Assess and document the patient's social support system.

Assess the patient's motivation to use hearing aids, because one of the major impediments to improving the hearing of the elderly is resistance by the patient to the hearing aid. Patients often do not want to admit the need for these devices or reject them because of cosmetic reasons. Many patients have difficulty adjusting to life with a hearing aid and instead withdraw from social situations, thereby removing the need for the aid. It is important to determine what the patient's financial resources are as well. Hearing aids represent a significant investment and generally are not covered by insurance.

Nursing Diagnoses and Planning

Nursing diagnoses and related expected patient outcomes most commonly applicable to patients with presbycusis include the following:

NDx: Impaired communication related to hearing loss

Planning: Patient outcomes
1. Patient instructs others to speak to the better hearing ear where applicable.
2. Patient instructs others in ways of increasing effective communication (i.e., in cases of severe hearing impairment, the speaker should speak in a normal tone of voice 2 or 3 inches (5 to 7.5 cm) from the patient's ear; in less severe cases, the speaker should maintain face-to-face communication with the patient).
3. Patient instructs others to communicate in writing when necessary.

NDx: High risk for injury related to alteration in perception of auditory stimuli

Planning: Patient outcomes
1. Patient identifies precautions to be taken to avoid physical injury as a result of hearing loss.
2. When necessary, patient describes environmental modifications to provide a safe environment. (For example, severely hearing-impaired individuals may need assistive devices to alert them to a telephone ringing or a smoke alarm.)
3. Patient remains free of injury.

NDx: High risk for social isolation related to impaired communication

Planning: Patient outcomes
1. Patient maintains social contact with staff, family, and significant others.
2. Patient participates in routine recreational activities.

NDx: Noncompliance related to purchase or use of hearing aid

Planning: Patient outcomes
1. Patient discusses benefits and disadvantages of proposed hearing aid.
2. Patient demonstrates ability to maintain and use hearing aid.
3. Patient discusses financial considerations in obtaining hearing aid.

NDx: High risk for altered health maintenance related to insufficient knowledge of community resources for the hearing impaired

Planning: Patient outcomes
1. Patient lists specific community resources that deal with hearing-impaired individuals.
2. Patient uses applicable resources.
3. Patient discusses financial resources available for assistance in purchase of hearing aid.

Nursing Interventions

NDx: Impaired communication
Provide a quiet, private, and calm environment for the patient. Devote full attention to the communication process: Face the patient directly when speaking, and speak slowly and clearly. Use normal conversational tones. In cases of severe hearing impairment, gestures or written communication may be necessary. Encourage the family to help in the communication effort because they may have an effective system in place already.

NDx: High risk for injury
Provide for the physical safety of the hospitalized patient. Reiterate safety instructions as well as patient-care instructions, and evaluate the patient's understanding of these instructions. Educate the patient on assistive listening devices to reduce the risk of injury at home.

NDx: High risk for social isolation
In an acute care setting, provide a room for the patient close to the nursing station. This will help the patient to maintain visual contact with care providers and reduce isolation. Encourage recreational activities and, if possible, organize a support group for other patients with similar hearing disability.

On discharge, provide the patient with a list of local organizations that work with senior citizens.

NDx: Noncompliance
Encourage the patient who may benefit from the use of a hearing aid to consult an audiologist for fitting with the most appropriate hearing aid. Help the patient to understand the benefits and drawbacks of the hearing aid.

If the patient already has a hearing aid, explore

reasons for its nonuse and help to identify ways to eliminate or cope with these barriers.

NDx: High risk for altered health maintenance
Provide information regarding community resources for the hearing impaired.

Evaluation

Evaluate the effectiveness of nursing care for a patient with presbycusis by comparing the patient's status with the expected patient outcomes. Examples of specific outcomes for patients with presbycusis have been provided in the Planning section.

Bibliography

Adams GL, Boies LR, Hilger PA. Fundamentals of otolaryngology. Philadelphia: WB Saunders, 1989.
Alberti PW, Ruben RJ. Otologic medicine and surgery. New York: Churchill Livingstone, 1985.
Ballantyne J, Morrison AW (eds). Operative surgery: The ear. Rob & Smith's operative surgery series. 4th ed. Stoneham, MA: Butterworth, 1986.
Ballenger JJ. Diseases of the nose, throat, ear, head and neck. Philadelphia: Lea & Febiger, 1985.
Bates B. A guide to physical examination. 5th ed. Philadelphia: JB Lippincott, 1991.
Bull PD. Lecture notes on diseases of the ear, nose and throat. 6th ed. Cambridge, MA: Blackwell Scientific Publications, 1986.
Carpenito LJ. Nursing diagnosis application to clinical practice. 3rd ed. Philadelphia: JB Lippincott, 1989.
Christian E, Dluhy N, O'Neill R. Sounds of silence: Coping with hearing loss and loneliness. J Gerontol Nurs 1989; 15(11):4.
Cleveland P, Morris J. Meniere's disease. RN 1990; 53(8):28.
De Weese DD, et al. Otolaryngology—Head and neck surgery. St. Louis: CV Mosby, 1988.
Eliopoulos C. Gerontological nursing. New York: Harper & Row, 1987.
Esberger KK, Hughes ST Jr (eds). Nursing care of the aged. Norwalk, CT: Appleton & Lange, 1989.
Gioiella EC, Bevil CW. Nursing care of the aging client. Norwalk, CT: Appleton-Century-Crofts, 1985.
Glasscock ME, Shambaugh GE Jr (eds). Surgery of the ear. 4th ed. Philadelphia: WB Saunders, 1990.
Goycoolea MV, Paparella MM, Nissen RL (eds). Atlas of otologic surgery. Philadelphia: WB Saunders, 1989.
Hanson C, Roffo F. Comprehensive care of patients undergoing stapedectomy for otosclerosis. Perioperative Nurs 1985; 1(2):21.
Harner SG. Peripheral labyrinthine causes of dizziness. Postgrad Med 1987; 8(4):251.
Hawke M, John AF. Diseases of the ear: Clinical and pathological aspects. Philadelphia: Lea & Febiger, 1987.
Iadarola G, Kerrigan MB. Do you hear what I hear? AORN J 1986; 43(2):478.
Jarvis C. Physical examination and health assessment. Philadelphia: WB Saunders, 1992.
Kavanagh KT, McCabe BF. Ototoxicity of oral neomycin and vancomycin. Laryngoscope 1983; 93(5):649.
Knudsen JF. Noise-induced hearing loss. Med Times 1986; 114(1):27.
Koegel L. Ototoxicity: A contemporary review of aminoglycosides, loop diuretics, acetylsalicylic acid, quinine, erythromycin, and cisplatinum. Am J Otol 1985; 6(3):194.
Malkiewicz J. How to assess the ears and check hearing acuity. RN 1982; 45(3):56.
McKennis AT. Vestibular neurectomy for Meniere's disease. AORN J 1989; 50(4):787.
Olsen WO. Presbycusis. Postgrad Med 1984: 76(3):189.
Ortiz-Armenta LA, Martin-Diaz JC, Gamez-Martinez L. Surgical treatment of vertigo. Ear Nose Throat J 1986; 65(6):46.
Paparella MM, Shumrick DA, Gluckman JL, Meyerhoff WL. Otolaryngology. 3rd ed. Philadelphia: WB Saunders, 1991.
Rambur BA. Sudden hearing loss. Nurs Pract 1989; 14(1):8.
Riley MAK. Nursing care of the client with ear, nose and throat disorders. New York, Springer, 1987.
Sataloff RT. Sensorineural hearing loss. Otolaryngol Clin North Am 1986; 19(1):3.
Slater R, et al. Tinnitus: A guide for sufferers and professionals. London: Croom Helm, 1987.
Syka J, Masterton RB (eds). Auditory pathway: Structure and function. New York: Plenum, 1988.
Wiet RJ, Monsell EM, Hotaling AJ. Hearing and balance disorders. Postgrad Med 1985; 17(1):119.
Wyngaarden JB, Smith LH Jr, Bennett JC (eds). Cecil textbook of medicine. 19th ed. Philadelphia: WB Saunders, 1992.
Yeager JA, Joyce DG. Multichannel cochlear implants. AORN J 1989; 50(2):299.
Zegeer LJ. Oculocephalic and vestibulo-ocular responses. J Neurosci Nurs 1989; 21(1):46.

Unit Fourteen

ADULTS WITH REPRODUCTIVE SYSTEM DYSFUNCTION

Learning Objectives

AFTER COMPLETING THIS UNIT, THE LEARNER WILL BE ABLE TO:

Chapters Forty-three and Forty-five

1. Explain the normal anatomy and physiology of the male and female reproductive systems.
2. Describe common clinical manifestations of reproductive system dysfunction.
3. Identify information and physical examination data essential to the assessment of reproductive system status.
4. Describe basic diagnostic tests and modalities of medical management used in the treatment of patients with reproductive system disorders.
5. Describe basic surgical procedures used in the treatment of patients with reproductive system disorders.
6. Identify data essential to the assessment of patients undergoing treatment of reproductive system disorders.
7. State nursing diagnoses and related expected patient outcomes commonly applicable to patients undergoing treatment of reproductive system disorders.
8. Describe nursing interventions, with their rationales, commonly applicable to patients undergoing treatment of reproductive system disorders.
9. Explain the basis for evaluation of nursing care provided to patients undergoing treatment of reproductive system disorders.
10. Identify special considerations for the elderly patient with altered function of the reproductive system.

Chapters Forty-four and Forty-six

1. Describe common reproductive system disorders in terms of etiology, pathophysiology, clinical manifestations, diagnostic procedures, and medical management.
2. Identify information and physical examination data essential to the assessment of patients with common reproductive system disorders.
3. State nursing diagnoses and related expected patient outcomes commonly applicable to patients with reproductive system disorders.
4. Describe nursing interventions, with their rationales, commonly applicable to patients with reproductive system disorders.
5. Explain the basis for evaluation of nursing care provided to patients with common reproductive system disorders.
6. Identify special considerations for the elderly patient with a reproductive system disorder.

Chapter Forty-seven

1. Describe commonly occurring sexually transmitted diseases in terms of etiology, pathophysiology, clinical manifestations, diagnostic procedures, and medical management.
2. Identify information and physical examination data essential to the assessment of patients with common sexually transmitted diseases.
3. State nursing diagnoses and related expected patient outcomes commonly applicable to patients with sexually transmitted diseases.
4. Describe nursing interventions, with their rationales, commonly applicable to patients with sexually transmitted diseases.
5. Explain the basis for evaluation of nursing care provided to patients with common sexually transmitted diseases.

Chapter Forty-eight

1. Explain the normal anatomy and physiology of the breast.
2. Identify information and physical examination data essential to the assessment of the breast.
3. Describe basic diagnostic tests used in the management of breast disorders.
4. Describe common breast disorders in terms of etiology, pathophysiology, clinical manifestations, diagnostic procedures, and medical management.
5. Identify information and physical examination data essential to the assessment of patients with common breast disorders.
6. State nursing diagnoses and related expected patient outcomes commonly applicable to patients with breast disorders.
7. Describe nursing interventions, with their rationales, commonly applicable to patients with breast disorders.
8. Explain the basis for evaluation of nursing care provided to patients with common breast disorders.
9. Identify special considerations for the elderly patient with a breast disorder.

Chapter Forty-three

KNOWLEDGE BASIC TO THE NURSING CARE *of Women with Reproductive System Dysfunction*

The complex system of female reproductive hormones constitutes the framework within which assessments and interventions for the woman with a reproductive disorder must be planned, implemented, and evaluated. Thus, a clear understanding of normal structure and function from puberty through old age is essential to good nursing care. Also essential are good therapeutic communication skills and sensitivity to individual women's needs and feelings. Despite the openness of today's society in regard to reproduction and sex, many women still experience embarrassment and reluctantly seek health care for problems in these areas.

Anatomy and Physiology

The female reproductive system is composed of internal genitalia and external genitalia.

The external genitalia (Fig. 43–1), or vulva, include the mons veneris or mons pubis, labia majora, labia minora, clitoris, fourchette, vestibule, Skene's glands (located within the urethral meatus), Bartholin's glands, hymen, introitus, and perineum.

The internal genitalia (Fig. 43–2) are the ovaries, fallopian tubes, uterus, and vagina.

External Genitalia

The mons pubis is a soft mound of adipose tissue located in front of the symphysis pubis. It is covered with skin, and after puberty with coarse hair.

The labia majora are two longitudinal folds of adipose tissue that begin at the mons pubis and continue downward and backward on each side of the vaginal opening, or introitus, until they meet at the midline of the perineum. Their outer surfaces are covered with pigmented skin and develop coarse hair after puberty. The inner surfaces of the labia majora are smooth and hairless.

The labia minora are two smaller folds of tissue that lie within the labia majora. They extend downward from the clitoris, which is a small mass of erectile tissue located under the prepuce just beneath the pubic arch, to the fourchette, which is a ridge of tissue just below the vaginal opening. The labia minora are smooth and hairless but contain large numbers of sebaceous glands.

The vestibule is the flat, boat-shaped area between the labia minora. The vestibule contains the urethral meatus and the opening of the ducts of Skene's glands, which are lateral and posterior to the meatus. It also contains the introitus and the openings of Bartholin's glands, which are posterior and slightly lateral to it.

The hymen is a fold of mucous membrane that partially covers the vaginal opening. The hymen is commonly broken in the adult as a result of sexual intercourse, strenuous exercise, tampon use, or related activities.

The perineum is the area between the vagina and the anus. It consists of muscles, fascia, and skin.

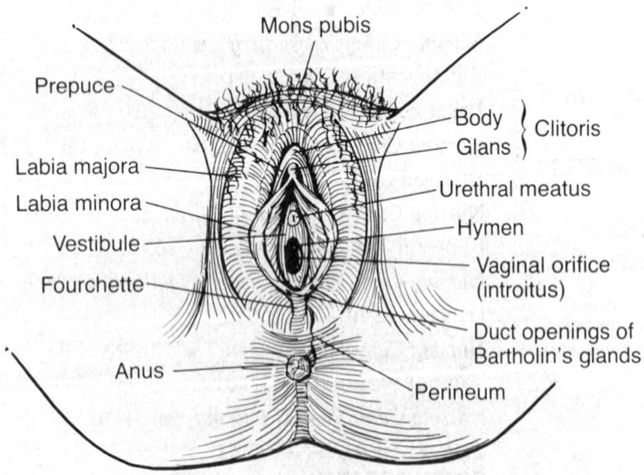

Figure 43–1.

Female external genitalia.

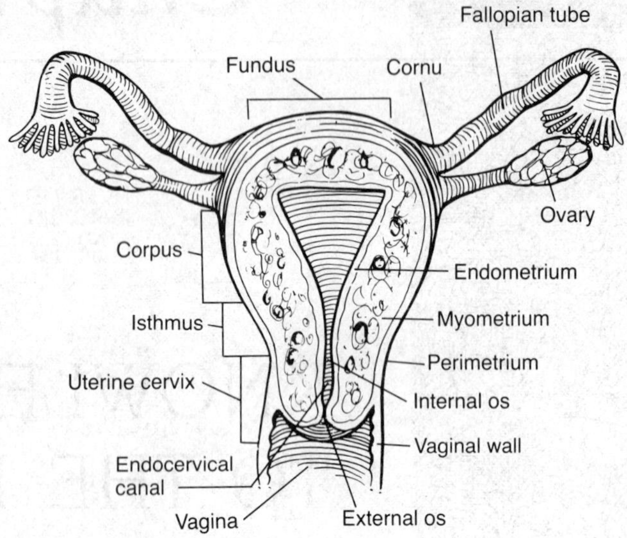

Figure 43–2.

Female internal genitalia.

Internal Genitalia

VAGINA

The vagina is a muscular tubelike organ that is lined with mucous membrane and has horizontal rugae, or folds, that give it great elasticity. The vagina is located between the urethra and bladder to the anterior and the rectum to the posterior. The vagina connects the uterus to the vulva. It receives the penis during intercourse and serves as a passageway to the outside world in the delivery of a baby and for the discharge of uterine secretions and the menstrual flow.

The vagina is approximately 9 cm in length and is directed upward and back from the introitus toward the coccyx. Its distal end is cuplike in shape and is referred to as the fornix. The cervix of the uterus projects into the fornix and creates a blind pouch on all sides. Thus, there is the posterior fornix, the anterior fornix, and the lateral fornices.

The cells lining the vagina are rich in glycogen. This glycogen is broken down into lactic acid by lactose-fermenting bacteria that are normally found in the vagina. The lactic acid lowers the pH of the vagina and thus creates an environment that inhibits the growth of pathogenic bacteria.

UTERUS

The uterus is a hollow, thick-walled muscular organ shaped like an inverted pear. It is the site of menstruation, implantation of the fertilized ovum, fetal development, and the muscular contractions of labor.

The uterus has two main divisions: the body and the cervix. The body, or corpus, is the upper portion of the uterus. The top, domelike portion of the body is the fundus. The angle marking the opening of the fallopian tubes on each side is called the cornu. The isthmus is the constricted portion of the uterus that lies between the body and the cervix, or lower, narrow portion of the uterus, which opens into the vagina.

The uterine cavity is triangular and lined with endometrium. It joins the cervical canal at the internal os. The external os marks the opening of the cervical canal into the vagina.

The uterus is located in the pelvis, with the cervix at almost a right angle to the vagina. The bladder is in front of and below the uterus, and the rectum is below and behind it. The peritoneum is reflected from the abdominal wall over the outer surface of the uterus. This creates a space between the bladder and vagina (uterovesical pouch) and between the vagina and the rectum. This latter is the cul-de-sac of Douglas and is the lowest point in the pelvic cavity. Through this cul-de-sac, the peritoneal cavity can be entered through the posterior vaginal wall with little risk of damaging pelvic structures (Fig. 43–3).

The position of the uterus in the pelvic cavity is maintained by a series of ligaments. It is attached to either side of the pelvic cavity by double sheets of peritoneum called the broad ligaments. The cardinal ligaments lie in the base of the broad ligaments and are the primary supports of the uterus. The uterosacral ligaments arise from the sides of the cervix and attach to the sacrum. The round ligaments attach to the uterus just below the entrance of the fallopian tubes and pass within the broad ligament to the pelvic wall, ending in the labia majora (Fig. 43–4).

This system of support allows some movement of the uterine body, and so the uterus can deviate from its usual anteverted, slightly anteflexed position and may be midposition or retroverted.

FALLOPIAN TUBES

The fallopian or uterine tubes transport ova from the ovaries to the uterus and are the usual site of fertilization of the ovum by a sperm. They are approximately 10 cm long and are located between the folds of the broad ligaments. The portion of the tube

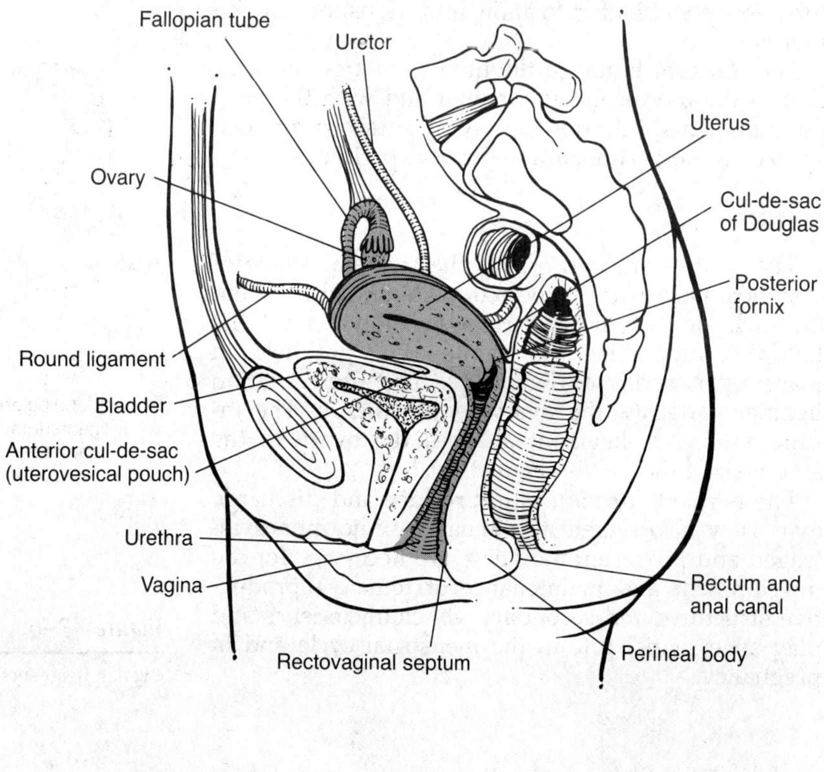

Figure 43–3.

Lateral view of the female internal genitalia showing the cul-de-sac of Douglas.

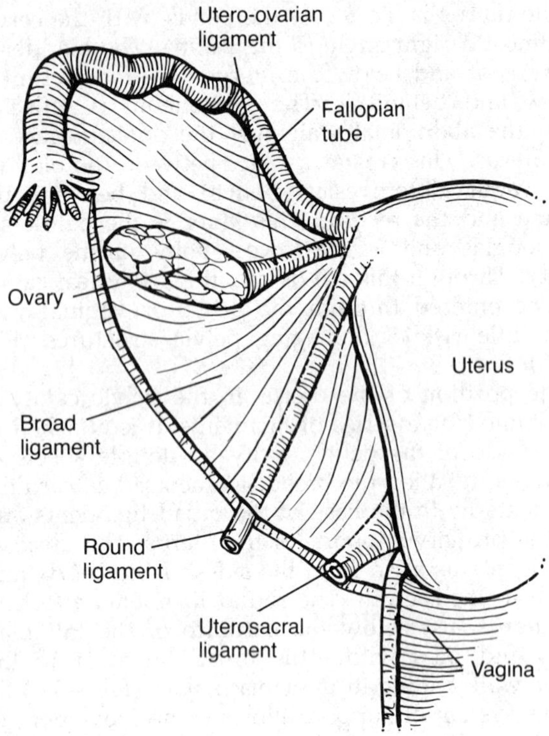

Figure 43–4.

Uterine ligaments.

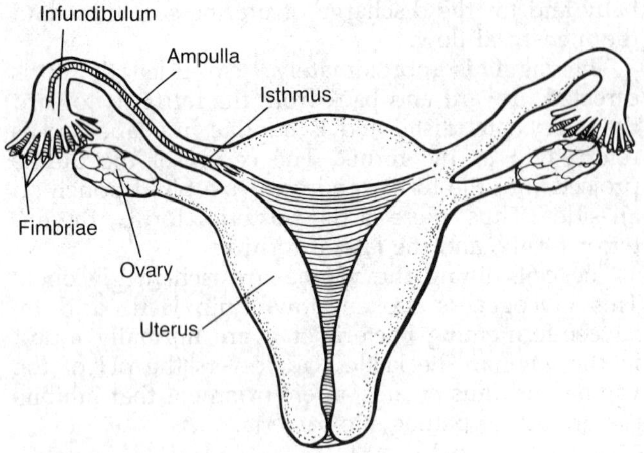

Figure 43–5.

Parts of the fallopian tube and their relationship to the ovary and the uterus.

nearest to the uterus is the isthmus. The middle portion is the ampulla, and the distal funnel-shaped section is the infundibulum. The infundibulum is surrounded by long, slender, finger-like projections called fimbriae (Fig. 43–5). The wavelike movements of the fimbriae serve to attract the mature ovum released from the ovary at ovulation into the tube for possible fertilization and transport to the uterus.

The mucosal lining of the tube is contiguous with that of the uterus and the vagina and with the peritoneum. Thus, infection of any of these organs can spread to the peritoneum and cause peritonitis.

OVARIES

The ovaries are two organs the size and shape of almonds. One ovary is located in the broad ligament on each side of the uterus below and behind the fallopian tube. Like the uterus, they are held in place by a series of ligaments. The utero-ovarian ligament attaches the ovary to the uterus. The infundibulopelvic ligament attaches the ovary to the side wall of the pelvis (Fig. 43–6).

The ovaries' function is to produce and discharge ova. They also secrete the female sex hormones estrogen and progesterone. These are necessary for the development and maintenance of female reproductive structures and secondary sex characteristics and play an essential role in the menstrual cycle and in pregnancy.

Female Sexual Cycle

The female sexual cycle is a periodic recurrent series of changes involving the hypothalamus, anterior pituitary gland, uterus, and related reproductive organs. The purpose of the cycle is to prepare the body for pregnancy through the release of a single mature ovum and to prepare the uterus for implantation. The cycle is initiated at puberty, and its onset is indicated by menarche. Menarche is the first menstruation, or periodic uterine bleeding, associated with shedding of the endometrium. The first day of menstruation is counted as the first day of the cycle. The average length of the cycle is 28 days, although

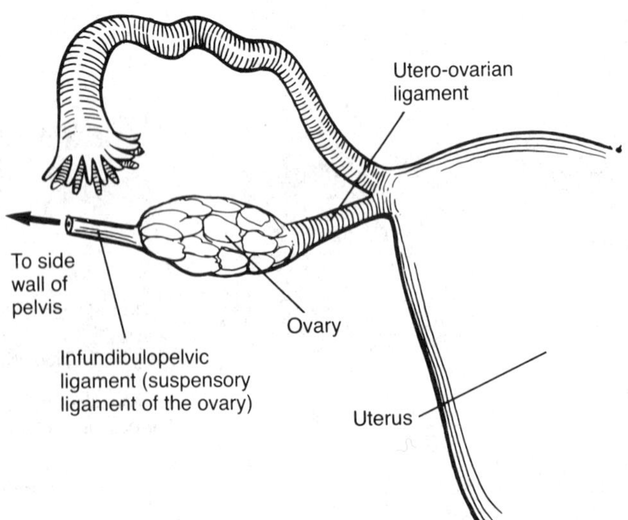

Figure 43–6.

Ovarian ligaments.

in normal females it can vary between 20 and 45 days.

The frequency of the cycle can be affected by both physical and emotional factors, including illness, fatigue, weight fluctuation, excessive exercise, eating disorders, stress, anxiety, and change in environment. The cycle is divided into four phases: the menstrual phase, the proliferative phase, the secretory phase, and the ischemic phase. The menstrual phase is the time of the menstrual flow. The proliferative phase is from the end of menstruation to ovulation. The secretory phase is from ovulation to 3 days prior to the onset of the next menses, with the ischemic phase being these last 3 days.

These phases are named in accordance with changes occurring in the endometrium. However, related changes are occurring simultaneously in the hypothalamus, pituitary gland, and ovary.

PROLIFERATIVE PHASE

Immature oocytes are present in the ovary at birth. Each oocyte is surrounded by a protective sac of cells and is called a primordial follicle. Under the influence of gonadotropin releasing hormone from the hypothalamus, the anterior pituitary secretes follicle-stimulating hormone (FSH) and luteinizing hormone (LH). The FSH initiates the growth of several primordial follicles. One of these takes precedence and continues to develop under the influence of both FSH and LH, while the others regress. The cells of this follicle produce a clear fluid that contains increasing amounts of estrogen as growth progresses. This maturing follicle moves to the surface of the ovary, where it appears as a blister-like structure called a graafian follicle. At this time, estrogen levels peak and a surge in LH occurs. This surge is believed to trigger ovulation, that is, rupture of the graafian follicle with release of the mature ovum.

The estrogen produced by the follicle during its development stimulates rapid growth of the endometrium. The thickness of the endometrium increases eightfold as a result of increased cells and progressive growth of the endometrial glands and vascular system. Thus, while an ovum is maturing in the ovary, the lining of the uterus is beginning to be prepared for implantation.

In response to the increasing estrogen, changes also occur in the cervical mucosa. The pH becomes more alkaline, going from approximately 7.0 to 7.5. The mucus becomes copious in amount and is thin, clear, and watery. By the time of ovulation, it assumes a full, fernlike pattern when allowed to dry (Fig. 43–7).

SECRETORY PHASE

After ovulation, the ruptured follicle remaining on the surface of the ovary becomes the corpus luteum. This change occurs primarily in response to LH from the pituitary gland. The cells of the corpus luteum, or yellow body, produce progesterone, which increases in amount throughout the secretory phase. Estrogen is also produced but never to the extent prior to ovulation.

In the uterus, stimulation by increasing levels of progesterone causes the endometrial glands to dilate, become more tortuous, and begin to secrete small quantities of endometrial fluid. Cellular deposits of lipid and glycogen increase, the endometrium becomes edematous, and the vascularity becomes more prominent. These changes result in a highly secretory endometrium containing large amounts of stored nutrients needed to sustain a fertilized ovum. If fertilization and implantation occur, the endometrium develops further under the continuing stimulation of progesterone. If fertilization does not occur, the ischemic phase begins.

ISCHEMIC PHASE

During the ischemic phase, the corpus luteum degenerates, and the levels of estrogen and progesterone fall. With the withdrawal of progesterone, the arteries constrict, causing the endometrium to become pale, shrunken, and anemic. This leads to areas of necrosis in the endometrium. Subsequently, blood leaks into the tissues, and small necrotic patches of endometrium break off.

MENSTRUAL PHASE

The menstrual phase is the time during which the menstrual flow occurs. The menstrual discharge is composed of blood, cervical and vaginal secretions, mucus, and shreds of endometrium. It does not normally contain clots. The discharge, which is dark red and has a characteristic odor, differs from woman to woman in duration and amount. The average duration is 5 days, although anywhere from 2 to 8 days is within normal range. The amount may be scant,

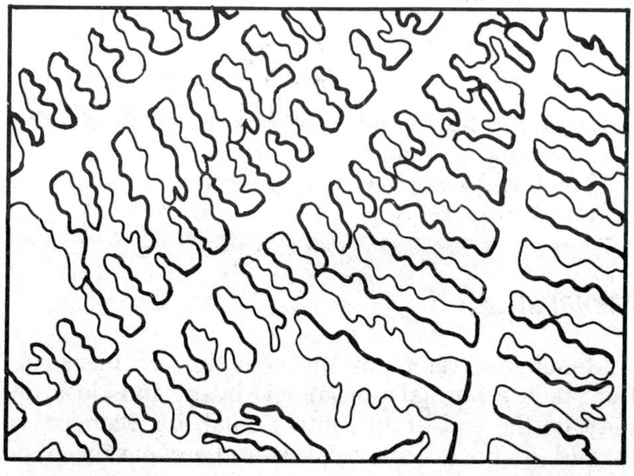

Figure 43–7.

Fernlike pattern of dried cervical mucus at ovulation.

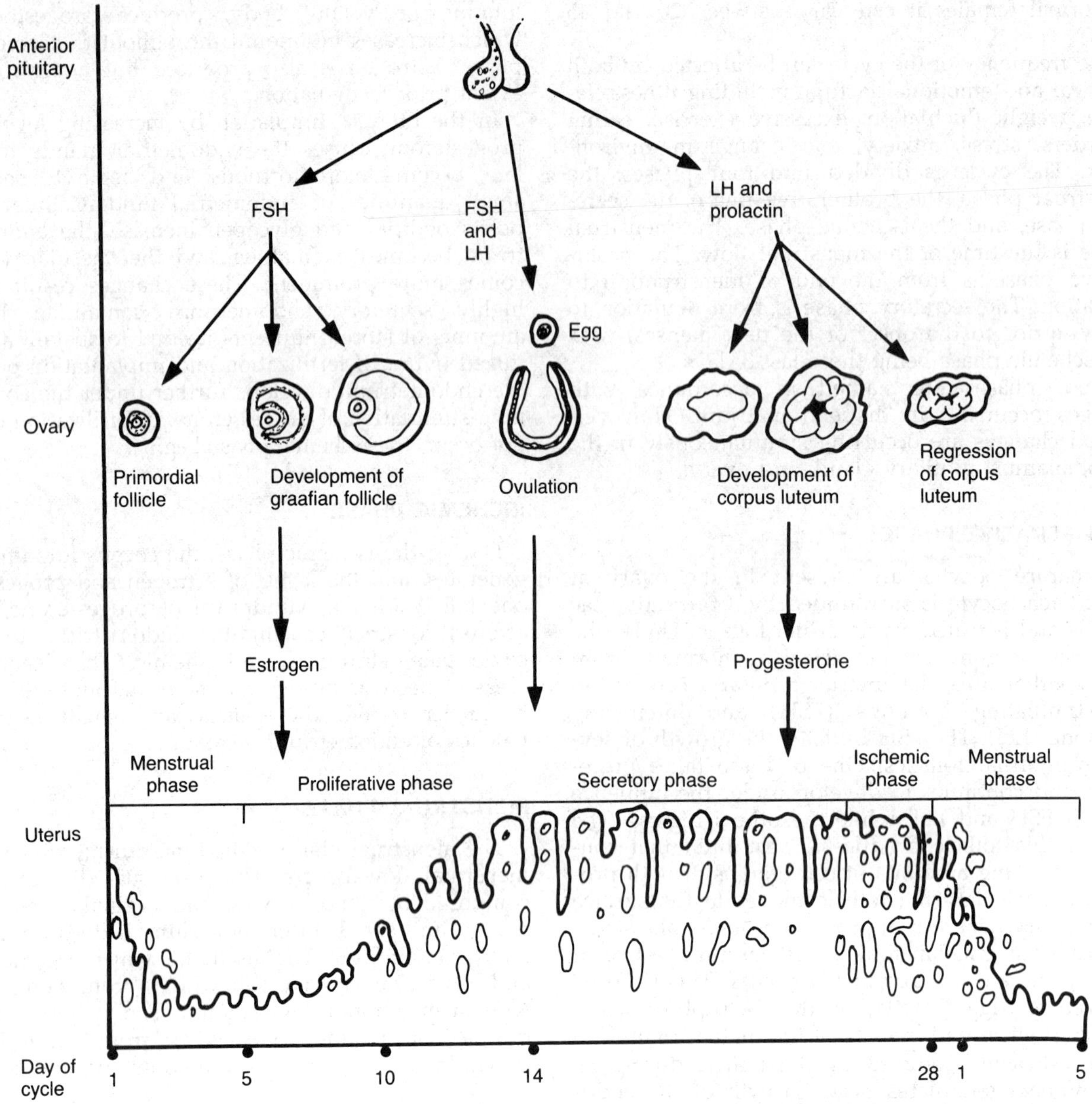

Figure 43–8.

Female sexual cycle.

moderate, or heavy, with the blood loss varying between 30 and 150 ml.

The female sexual cycle is presented diagrammatically in Figure 43–8.

Menopause

Menopause refers to the cessation of menstruation. It is a normal physiologic event and does not indicate the end of an active sexual life. Menopause is said to have occurred when there has been no menses for 6 months to 1 year. Generally, the onset of the menopause is gradual and occurs between the ages of 45 and 55 years (Hatcher et al, 1990, p. 59). The menstrual flow becomes smaller in amount, and the menses become less frequent, then irregular, and finally cease. Ovulation usually ends before the last menses. When menopause occurs before the age of 45, it is referred to as premature menopause.

These changes occur as the ovaries become less sensitive to pituitary gonadotropins. This results in a decrease in follicular development and therefore diminished ovarian estrogen. No progesterone is produced after the last ovulatory cycle. Estrogen, however, continues to be produced in small quantities by the adrenal glands and the ovaries even after the last menses has occurred. The amount of estrogen is not sufficient to block the output of pituitary gonadotropins through a negative feedback loop, so the level of FSH rises with menopause and remains elevated thereafter.

PHYSICAL CHANGES

Many physical changes are initiated at the time of menopause. Most are due to the aging process in general and are not the direct result of diminished estrogen. Pubic hair begins to thin, gray, and may ultimately disappear. The vulva begins to atrophy. The labia become thin as their fatty tissue is resorbed and become pale as the deep pigmentation is lost. The ovaries atrophy, becoming white, wrinkled, and no longer able to be palpated. The fallopian tubes, uterus, and vagina also decrease in size. In addition, the vagina becomes less elastic as the rugae disappear and the mucosa thins. Vaginal secretions decrease in amount and in acidity, thus predisposing to dyspareunia (painful sexual intercourse) and vaginal infection. The pelvic fascia and musculature atrophy, and pelvic support is lost, leading in some cases to urinary stress incontinence. Breasts gradually lose their firmness as fatty deposits are resorbed.

The skin becomes wrinkled as a loss of protein and subcutaneous tissue occurs. Bone loss accelerates as estrogen decreases, and osteoporosis (thin, porous bone) with its associated risk of fractures can ensue, particularly if combined with low body weight, a lack of physical exercise, a chronic low calcium intake, or excessive intake of caffeine and alcohol (see Chapter 36).

PSYCHOSOCIAL EFFECTS

Menopause involves psychosocial changes as well as physical changes in women. The psychosocial responses almost always involve a degree of ambivalence. On the positive side, menopause can mean the beginning of freedom to enjoy one's sexuality without concern about pregnancy and contraception. It also means freedom from menstruation, which can have particular importance for women with a history of premenstrual and menstrual discomfort or heavy bleeding. Negative feelings may occur because menopause marks the end of the ability to bear children. This creates a sense of loss in many women, but it is frequently more marked in women who have never had children. This sense of loss can also be exaggerated in women who devoted most of their time and effort to their children and developed few meaningful outside interests. Thus, when the last child leaves home for school, work, or marriage, life may seem empty and without purpose. Often adding to the loss at this time in life is the developing dependency, sickness, or death of a woman's parents.

Menopause is also an undeniable sign of aging. This can cause anxiety and feelings of being less attractive and less feminine, especially in United States society with its focus on the desirability of youth. Some women believe it indicates the end of sexual activity or a satisfying sexual relationship. Still other women have a great fear of an accidental pregnancy and a "change of life baby."

SYMPTOMS

Some women do not experience any unpleasant symptoms during menopause, some have mild discomforts, and some have significant distress. Symptoms that may occur include hot flashes, insomnia and sleep disturbances, weakness, dizzy spells, palpitations, anxiety, depression, headaches, and weight gain. Of these, only the hot flashes have been shown to occur directly in response to a drop in estrogen level. It is believed that the drop in estrogen level affects the temperature-regulating center in the hypothalamus, resulting in an increased sensitivity to heat. This in turn leads to hot flashes, which are a vasomotor disturbance occurring as the body attempts to cool itself. Hot flashes can involve profuse sweating or flushing, which generally starts on the chest and progresses to include the neck and face. They may occur anywhere from once a week to as often as 20 to 30 times per day and last from a few minutes to a half-hour. They can be triggered by anything that affects body temperature such as a warm room, warm food, alcohol, or an emotional upset. Insomnia is also believed to be an effect of decreased estrogen level, although this has not been proved. The remainder of the symptoms appear to be the result of the aging process or of anxiety regarding it. It is true, however, that hot flashes occurring at night can interfere with normal sleeping and thus cause headache as well as feelings of fatigue, nervousness, and depression, which are associated with sleep loss.

MEDICAL MANAGEMENT

Hormone replacement therapy (HRT), also called hormone additive therapy, effectively controls menopausal symptoms. It reduces hot flashes, vaginal dryness, insomnia, perspiration, and moodiness and other emotional symptoms. It also significantly decreases postmenopausal bone loss (95% of early postmenopausal bone loss is retarded in approximately 95% of women [Lindsay, 1987, p. 1349]) and the related risk of hip and vertebral fractures.

In addition, it improves blood lipid levels by decreasing low-density lipoproteins and increasing high-density lipoproteins and protects against heart attacks and strokes. As a result, it is now frequently recommended for women even in the absence of distressing menopausal symptoms, particularly those at risk for osteoporosis.

Typical estrogen therapy used today is a combination of estrogen and progesterone. (See Pharmacology Box 43–1 for discussion of estrogens.) The standard regimen consists of 0.625 mg of conjugated estrogen taken for the first 25 days of the month

Pharmacology Box 43–1.
ESTROGENS

Estrogens:
Female sex hormones secreted by the ovarian follicles and placenta and in smaller amounts by the adrenal cortex and male testis.

Action:
Promote development of the vagina, uterus, fallopian tubes, breasts, and secondary sex characteristics as well as closure of long bone epiphyses. Stimulate the proliferative phase of the uterine cycle and changes in reproductive organs during pregnancy. Also lower blood cholesterol level and promote retention of sodium and water.

Uses:
Replacement therapy to treat menopausal symptoms, both naturally occurring and following oophorectomy; atrophic vaginitis; secondary amenorrhea; postpartum breast engorgement; and in the palliative treatment of inoperable cancer of the prostate and breast in males and inoperable cancer of the breast in postmenopausal females. Also used for contraception in combination with progestogen.

Side Effects:
Breakthrough bleeding; changes in menstrual flow; dysmenorrhea; amenorrhea; vaginal discharge; cervical erosion; monilial vaginitis; enlargement, tenderness, and secretion of the breasts; headache; dizziness; chorea; libido changes; depression; thrombophlebitis and embolism; hypertension; edema; nausea; vomiting; abdominal cramps; bloating; diarrhea; constipation; appetite and weight changes; jaundice; hyperglycemia; hypercalcemia; acne; oily skin; hirsutism or alopecia; leg cramps; and intolerance to contact lenses. Gynecomastia, testicular atrophy, and impotence also occur in men.

Interactions:
None that are clinically significant.

Nursing Implications:
Give the package insert to the patient, and review the information before the first dose, as required by Food and Drug Administration (FDA) regulation. Instruct the patient to immediately report chest pain; shortness of breath; pain, numbness, or stiffness in the legs or buttocks; abdominal pain; severe headache; visual changes; vaginal bleeding or discharge; breast lumps; edema of the extremities; jaundice; dark urine; or light stool. Teach breast self-examination.

Explain to women on cyclic therapy for menopausal symptoms that ovulation has not occurred and that they are not able to get pregnant despite the fact that vaginal bleeding occurs during the week they do not take the drug.

Explain to male patients that gynecomastia and impotence may occur when the drug is taken for a long period of time. Reassure them that these effects will disappear when the drug is discontinued.

Note the type, amount, and duration of estrogen therapy.

with 2.5 to 10 mg of medroxyprogesterone acetate added from the 16th through the 25th days (Glowacki, 1988, p. 52; Maddox, 1992, p. 966). For maximum effectiveness in preventing osteoporosis, replacement is maintained for life because bone loss accelerates as soon as the estrogen therapy is discontinued.

Potential side effects of this regimen include breast tenderness, fluid retention, weight gain, headache, and nausea. In addition, approximately 80% of women who have not had hysterectomies develop withdrawal bleeding at the end of each 25-day medication cycle. This resembles menstruation but since no ovulation has occurred, the woman is not fertile. Because of this, new regimens are being explored that are not associated with withdrawal bleeding.

According to Glowacki (p. 52), there is no longer an increased risk of cancer of the endometrium as a side effect of hormone replacement therapy. There was increased risk in the 1970s, when hormone therapy consisted of estrogen alone, but with combination estrogen and progesterone and the current low doses, there is no longer an increased risk, and some studies report an actual decrease in risk. Whether current hormone replacement therapy is associated with an increased risk of breast cancer remains a debated issue. Although many studies indicate that it is not associated with any increased risk of breast cancer and may in fact offer some protection, others show an increased risk (Hatcher et al, 1990, p. 61).

Estrogen therapy is contraindicated for patients with a history of breast, endometrial, or other tumors whose growth may be responsive to estrogen. It is also contraindicated for patients with a history of recurrent thrombophlebitis. It is used with caution for women who were exposed at birth to diethylstilbestrol (DES), those who are obese, and those with vaginal bleeding, liver or gallbladder disease, or diabetes.

Application of the Nursing Process to the Care of the Menopausal Patient

Assessment

Assess the menopausal patient's understanding of the menopause: what it is, why it occurs, its effects on reproduction and sex, and symptoms that may normally occur. Determine also the patient's understanding of the relationship of menopause to osteoporosis and cardiovascular disease, and preventive estrogen replacement therapy. Assess her overall lifestyle as well as her physical and psychological responses to menopause.

Nursing Diagnoses and Planning

Nursing diagnoses and related expected patient outcomes most commonly applicable to menopausal patients include the following:

NDx: High risk for altered health maintenance related to insufficient knowledge of menopause and related self-care

Planning: Patient outcomes

1. Patient defines menopause.
2. Patient describes physical changes associated with menopause.
3. Patient discusses effects of menopause on personal lifestyle realistically and without misconceptions.
4. Patient states cause, duration, and significance of common menopausal symptoms.
5. Patient describes the importance of diet, exercise, and annual pelvic examinations to minimizing symptoms in the menopausal and postmenopausal woman.
6. Patient for whom HRT is prescribed describes expected benefits, side effects, contraindications, and administration regimen.
7. Patient describes menopausal woman's need for birth control and available, effective contraceptive measures.
8. Patient states importance of reporting any postmenopausal bleeding or staining to the clinician.

NDx: Anxiety related to the physical and psychological changes of menopause

Planning: Patient outcomes

1. Patient discusses menopause freely, without misconceptions or facial expressions or mannerisms indicative of anxiety.
2. Patient reports that feelings of anxiety and symptoms associated with anxiety are reduced.
3. Patient expresses confidence in her ability to effectively maintain family, work, and social roles.

Nursing Interventions

NDx: High risk for altered health maintenance

Discuss with the patient what menopause is and the associated physical changes. Also discuss symptoms that may occur, their significance, and their treatment. Stress that not all women develop all symptoms. If the patient experiences discomfort as a result of hot flashes and accompanying perspiration, instruct in relief measures as presented in Chart 43–1.

Structure this discussion so that the patient is at ease and actively contributes information and ideas. Use open-ended questions to elicit beliefs and feelings. From the patient's responses, identify any misconceptions and correct them.

Instruct the patient in basic health practices essential to the well-being of the menopausal woman, as specified in Chart 43–1. Also teach about prescribed hormone therapy. Explain its role in preventing osteoporosis and cardiovascular disease. Review medication schedule, and assist the patient in developing a plan for ensuring consistent self-administration. Provide information as needed to combat misconceptions about hormone therapy such as its relationship to breast or endometrial cancer.

NDx: Anxiety

When caring for an anxious menopausal patient, allow her to express her feelings and concerns about menopause, aging, and personal goals. Provide information and correct misconceptions as described above. If antianxiety medications are prescribed, teach her about the dosage regimen, expected side

Chart 43–1.

NURSING GUIDE TO PATIENT EDUCATION FOR SELF-MANAGEMENT: BASIC HEALTH PRACTICES FOR THE MENOPAUSAL WOMAN

Instruct the patient to:

Use contraception for 1 year after the last menses to avoid pregnancy.

Consider rhythm an unreliable method of contraception during the menopausal years because of the irregularity of the female sexual cycle at this time.

Eat a well-balanced diet with a calcium intake of 1500 mg/day and exercise regularly to maintain good muscle tone and physical appearance and to help prevent osteoporosis.

Avoid alcohol and smoking, which are "bone robbers."

Have any vaginal bleeding, however slight, checked by a physician.

Have an annual pelvic examination.

Have a mammogram annually or as recommended.

Use a water-soluble lubricant such as K-Y jelly if intercourse becomes painful. Avoid use of petroleum jelly and other oil-based products because they interfere with natural lubrication.

Protect against urinary tract infections caused by decreased acidity of the urethra secondary to low estrogen levels by drinking 6 to 8 glasses of water, cranberry juice, or unsweetened citrus juice per day and voiding before and after intercourse.

Decrease the likelihood of hot flashes by
- Keeping the home or work environment cool.
- Wearing cool, loose clothing of natural fibers.
- Using lightweight blankets at night.
- Avoiding ingestion of red wine, chocolate, and aged cheeses because they contain tyramine, which releases norepinephrine, which acts on the body's thermostat and can trigger a flash.
- Taking frequent lukewarm showers.

Minimize the discomfort of a hot flash by
- Standing in a cool breeze.
- Using a fan.
- Sipping a cool drink.
- Visualizing a cool, comfortable place.

Some data taken from McKeon, V. Cruel myths and clinical facts about menopause. RN 1989; 52(6):52.

effects, and any symptoms to be reported. Encourage her to consider friends who have passed menopause and who are still leading active, involved lives. Encourage regular exercise to reduce stress, control weight, and maintain cardiovascular fitness.

Evaluation

Evaluate the effectiveness of nursing care for a menopausal patient by comparing the patient's status with the expected patient outcomes. Examples of specific outcomes for menopausal patients have been provided in the Planning section.

Clinical Manifestations of Reproductive System Dysfunction

Amenorrhea

Amenorrhea is the absence of menstruation. It is classified as primary, secondary, or physiologic. Physiologic amenorrhea is a normal developmental state. It refers to the absence of menses before puberty, during pregnancy and lactation, and after menopause. Primary and secondary amenorrhea are symptoms of underlying pathology. In primary amenorrhea, the menarche has never occurred. With secondary amenorrhea, menstruation stops (three or more periods missed regardless of cycle length, or absence of menses for 6 months or more) after the menarche as occurred (Hatcher et al, 1990, p. 56).

The possible causes of primary and secondary amenorrhea are multiple. They include lesions at every level of reproductive system control and function, as well as disorders of supporting body systems. Primary or secondary amenorrhea may be due to hypothalamic or pituitary disorders; ovarian lesions; congenital defects involving the uterus, vagina, or hymen; removal of the uterus or both ovaries; thyroid, pancreatic, or adrenal dysfunctions; or cirrhosis, nephritis, or other chronic illness. It may also be the result of psychogenic disorders such as anorexia nervosa.

Temporary secondary amenorrhea may occur as the result of emotional stress, strenuous exercise, low body weight, severe illness, or drugs such as the phenothiazines. It can also occur for up to 6 months or longer after a woman stops taking oral contraceptives.

Abnormal Uterine Bleeding

There are a variety of patterns of abnormal uterine bleeding. Oligomenorrhea is infrequent or scant episodes of bleeding. Polymenorrhea is frequent but regular episodes of bleeding. Menorrhagia is bleeding that occurs at regular intervals but is excessive in both amount and duration. Metrorrhagia is bleeding that occurs at irregular times and is not excessive. Menometrorrhagia is excessive and prolonged bleeding occurring frequently and at irregular times.

The cause of abnormal uterine bleeding may be endocrine or organic. Organic causes include disorders of pregnancy, diseases of the pelvic organs, and disorders of other body systems such as blood dyscrasias and hypertension. Most often bleeding due to organic causes is associated with an ovulatory cycle, whereas bleeding due to an endocrine problem is associated with an anovulatory cycle.

Menorrhagia occurring at puberty is most often due to low estrogen level and resulting failure of the endometrium to proliferate normally. However, bleeding and clotting disorders are also possible causes, as is adenocarcinoma, which occurs in young women whose mothers took diethylstilbestrol (DES) during pregnancy.

In older women, menorrhagia is associated with ovarian tumors, submucous fibroid tumors of the uterus, infection of the endometrium, polyps, and pelvic inflammatory disease (PID).

Metrorrhagia is most often caused by a pregnancy-related disorder such as ectopic pregnancy, threatened abortion, or hydatidiform mole. It is also frequently iatrogenic as a result of the administration of exogenous hormones such as estrogen, androgens, or corticosteroids. Bleeding unrelated to the menstrual cycle may also be indicative of cancer of the cervix or cancer of the endometrium. In fact, a perimenopausal or postmenopausal woman with metrorrhagia is considered to have a malignancy until it is proved otherwise.

Abnormal uterine bleeding can also be caused by intrauterine devices (IUDs), ruptured ovarian cysts, and drugs such as phenothiazines, anticoagulants, anticholinergic agents, thiazide diuretics, and digitalis.

Leukorrhea

The term *leukorrhea* refers to any vaginal discharge other than blood. It may be the result of excessive production of the normal secretions that serve to keep the mucous membrane of the reproductive tract moist, or it may be an abnormal exudate from a pathologic lesion.

Normal secretions include the thick, viscous mucus produced by Bartholin's glands, which lubricates the introitus and the membranes of the vulva. This increases with sexual arousal and may be described as a vaginal discharge, because most patients cannot identify the actual source of secretion.

The vagina does not contain secretory glands. It is moistened by clear mucus that is produced by the cervical glands in varying amounts during the sexual cycle. These cervical glands become hyperactive as a result of hyperemia or endocrine factors and are the chief sources of leukorrhea.

Leukorrhea is also a symptom of vaginal or cervical infection. With vaginal infections, the discharge is mucopurulent or purulent and is commonly accompanied by pruritus. With cervical infections, the discharge may be moderate to copious, purulent, and possibly foul smelling.

Normal uterine secretions do not cause a vaginal discharge. However, uterine polyps and both benign and malignant uterine tumors can cause a leukorrheal discharge, especially when they are infected or necrotic. Vascular or endocrine changes can also alter uterine secretion so that leukorrhea may result.

Dysmenorrhea

Dysmenorrhea is cyclic pain associated with menstruation. It may be primary or secondary.

PRIMARY DYSMENORRHEA

In primary dysmenorrhea, there is no pathology of the reproductive organs or the pelvis that accounts for the pain. The pain occurs with an ovulatory cycle, and its onset is just before or at the same time as the onset of the menstrual flow. It lasts from a few hours to 1 to 2 days. Generally the pain is worst as the flow begins and decreases as the flow becomes well established. It is a sharp, sometimes colicky pain located in the lower abdomen with radiation to the lower back, groin, or thighs. Sometimes, it is described as a dull, intense ache and may be accompanied by headache, nausea, anorexia, bloating, diarrhea, faintness, or fatigue.

Primary dysmenorrhea occasionally occurs with the first menses but more often begins 6 to 12 months after menarche. This is because primary dysmenorrhea occurs only with cycles in which ovulation occurs, and the first cycles after menarche are frequently anovulatory.

Primary dysmenorrhea is associated with excessive uterine contractility, both in terms of baseline uterine tone and in strength of contractions. Recent research indicates that abnormally high levels of endometrial prostaglandins are responsible for the high contractility of the uterus as well as for other symptoms accompanying the pain.

Other factors that have been found to be related to the incidence and severity of primary dysmenorrhea are poor posture, poor hygiene, a sedentary lifestyle, nulliparity, constitutional illness, and fear or lack of knowledge of normal reproductive function.

BASIC TREATMENT

Treatment depends on the severity of the problem. For many women, the pain is relieved by nonprescription prostaglandin inhibitors such as aspirin or ibuprofen along with rest, hot fluids, heat to the lower abdomen, manual pressure on the abdomen, effleurage, mild exercise such as walking or swimming, or similar conservative measures. The effectiveness is increased if treatment is begun when the dysmenorrhea begins rather than waiting until it is well established.

MEDICAL MANAGEMENT

When basic treatments are not effective, oral contraceptives may be prescribed. Hormonal contraceptive therapy is effective treatment because primary dysmenorrhea occurs with ovulatory cycles and this therapy inhibits ovulation. If this therapy is contraindicated, prescription prostaglandin inhibitors (nonsteroidal anti-inflammatory drugs [NSAIDs]) may be prescribed. These drugs, taken as soon as the menses begins, generally provide relief. They act by inhibiting synthesis of prostaglandins and thereby preventing the high prostaglandin levels that cause uterine, gastrointestinal, and vascular smooth muscle spasm. Examples of these drugs and their usual dosage schedules are as follows:

Motrin	(ibuprofen)	400 mg PO q.i.d. (over-the-counter-drug)
Anaprox	(naproxen sodium)	Two 275-mg tabs PO, then 275 mg PO q 6–8 hr
Naprosyn	(naproxen)	250 mg PO q 4–6 hr
Indocin	(indomethacin)	25 mg PO t.i.d.
Ponstel	(mefenamic acid)	250 mg PO q.i.d.

All these drugs have side effects such as dizziness, headache, nausea, and diarrhea. However, they are generally mild and tolerable, particularly when taken with food. Because fatal anaphylaxis has been reported, NSAIDs are contraindicated for women with a history of allergy to aspirin or any NSAID.

Application of the Nursing Process to the Care of the Patient with Primary Dysmenorrhea

Assessment

Ask the patient to describe the type, degree, time of onset, and duration of pain experienced as well as any symptoms such as nausea, diarrhea, and faintness that accompany the pain. Determine the patient's perception of dysmenorrhea: its cause, its meaning for reproductive function, and so on. Obtain information about relief measures that the patient has tried, how they were used, and how effective they were. Note the presence of physical factors such as poor posture, poor hygiene, and lack of exercise that contribute to dysmenorrhea. Assess the patient's knowledge of and attitude toward menstruation.

Nursing Diagnoses and Planning

Nursing diagnoses and related expected patient outcomes most commonly applicable to patients with primary dysmenorrhea include the following:

NDx: Pain related to menstruation

Planning: Patient outcomes

1. Patient describes or demonstrates use of nonpharmacologic comfort measures.
2. Patient identifies prescribed medications, listing name, dose, frequency, indications for use, and possible side effects.
3. Patient reports pain relief at follow-up visit.

NDx: High risk for altered health maintenance related to insufficient knowledge of menstruation, and/or self-care measures to help decrease or prevent future dysmenorrhea

Planning: Patient outcomes

1. Patient describes menstruation and its effects without misconceptions.
2. Patient explains the relationship of good posture, exercise, good hygiene, and balanced diet to the prevention of dysmenorrhea.
3. Patient states importance of avoiding fatigue and constipation just prior to menses.

Nursing Interventions

NDx: Pain

Provide information on the optimal timing and use of relief measures employed by the patient if the assessment data indicate this is needed. Also give information about available relief measures, other than those used by the patient, that may be effective in the control of symptoms. If medications are ordered, review the name, dose, frequency, indications for use, and possible side effects with the patient. Make certain the patient understands that prostaglandin inhibitors act to prevent cramping, not to suppress pain, and thus are most effective when taken at the earliest sign of pain.

NDx: High risk for altered health maintenance

Encourage a positive attitude toward menstruation by providing relevant facts and allowing the patient to discuss her feelings and experiences. Explain the value of regular exercise, good posture, balanced diet, and good hygiene in preventing dysmenorrhea. Also advise the patient to do waist-bending exercises before the onset of menstruation and to avoid constipation and overfatigue at this time.

Evaluation

Evaluate the effectiveness of nursing care for a patient with primary dysmenorrhea by comparing the patient's status with the expected patient outcomes. Examples of specific outcomes for patients with primary dysmenorrhea have been provided in the Planning section.

SECONDARY DYSMENORRHEA

In secondary dysmenorrhea, there is demonstrated pelvic disease, which is the source of the pain. This pain may begin 1 to 2 days prior to the onset of menstruation and can last for the duration of the menses. Treatment is directed at the underlying cause. Disorders that can cause secondary dysmenorrhea include endometriosis, stenosis of the cervical os, endometrial polyp, fibroid tumor of the uterus, chronic pelvic inflammatory disease, endometrial hyperplasia, and endometrial cancer.

Intermenstrual Pain

Intermenstrual pain, or mittelschmerz, is pain that occurs at about the middle of the female sexual cycle. It lasts from a few hours to a few days and varies from slight discomfort to severe pain. In some cases, it is accompanied by brownish spotting or by bleeding similar to a scant menstrual flow. When macroscopic bleeding is not evident, microscopic examination of the vaginal discharge demonstrates the presence of red blood cells.

Intermenstrual pain is believed to be related to ovulation. The nature of the relationship is unknown. It has been suggested that the pain results from blood being released into the abdominal cavity at the time of ovulation, from swelling of the ovary as the graafian follicle matures, or from fluctuation of hormone levels.

Assessment of Reproductive System Status

When assessing reproductive status, consider the intimate nature of the parts and functions affected. Be aware that despite the increasing openness in our society in regard to sexuality, discussion of reproductive structure and functioning is a source of embarrassment to many women, so provide privacy and adequate time for uninterrupted communication. Be certain to be nonjudgmental, open, and accessible in manner. Without privacy, sufficient time for communication, and a professional manner, nursing assessments are likely to be incomplete, incorrect, and ineffective. Patients are unlikely to answer questions regarding vaginal discharge, pain on intercourse, or sexual satisfaction completely and comfortably, or ask questions such as "How long do I have to wait to have intercourse after I get home?" if there are other patients present or if the conversation is interrupted by other hospital personnel speaking to the nurse.

Never assume that the patient knows the correct terms for body parts or that she can name or describe body functions. The nurse may be comfortable talking about menses, leukorrhea, or dyspareunia, but the patient may not understand the terms. Further, the patient may feel that she should understand and be embarrassed to ask their meaning. This can block communication and result in an incorrect or incomplete data base.

Patient History

Because symptoms related to menstruation are the most important in the diagnosis of gynecologic disorders, the history usually begins with complete information regarding the patient's menstrual status. Determine the age of menarche; frequency, duration, and amount of flow (how many pads or tampons soaked per day); characteristics of the discharge such as color, odor, and presence or absence of clots; and the date of the last menstrual period (LMP). If the patient is uncertain about this latter, obtain an estimated date. Determine whether tampons or pads, or both, are used, because tampon use is linked to dysmenorrhea, vaginal infection, and toxic shock syndrome. Ask specifically whether any menstrual periods have been missed.

Inquire about mittelschmerz (midcycle pain) and dysmenorrhea, including time of onset, duration, type of discomfort, severity of discomfort, and effective and ineffective remedies. Ask about premenstrual symptoms such as depression, headaches, anxiety, breast tenderness, and fluid retention. Also inquire about any intermenstrual bleeding, including amount (staining: few drops; spotting: 5 to 6 ml; or bleeding that is estimated on the basis of one regular sanitary pad or tampon holding 25 to 50 ml of blood), appearance, and relationship to intercourse (or other contact) or pain. If the patient is middle-aged or older, determine the age of menopause or the presence of menopausal symptoms. Regardless of age, obtain the date of the last Papanicolaou smear and the type, date, and treatment of any past gynecologic problems. Also determine the frequency of breast self-examination and the date of the last mammogram.

Review the patient's sexual and obstetric status. Include the age of first intercourse, sexual orientation, number of sexual partners, current frequency of intercourse with and without contraception, type of contraception used, sexual satisfaction, and sexual difficulties. Ask whether menses is or has been affected by contraceptives used. Obtain number and description of pregnancies and labors, and number of spontaneous or induced abortions. Also determine the frequency and type of sexually transmitted diseases and gynecologic surgeries. Inquire whether there is any possibility that the patient may be pregnant at present.

Ask about symptoms such as breast changes, noting type and relationship to menses; pain, noting type, location, and relationship to menses, sexual intercourse, urination, defecation, or insertion of a tampon; and vaginal discharge, with attention to the time of onset, duration, amount, color, consistency (thin, thick, cottage cheese–like, clear, white, yellow, brown), odor (none, sweet, fishy), and association with irritation or itching.

Because urinary symptoms are frequently manifestations of gynecologic disorders, also note the presence or absence of urinary frequency, urgency, pain, incontinence, nocturia, or hematuria. For similar reasons, note constipation, tenesmus, diarrhea, or other gastrointestinal symptoms.

Pelvic Examination

A pelvic examination is an organized assessment of the structural condition of the reproductive organs. It includes inspection of the external genitalia, the cervix, and the vagina; evaluation of vaginal and perineal muscle tone; and palpation of the internal genital organs.

PREPARATION OF THE PATIENT

In preparation, the patient is asked to urinate. This allows an easier, more comfortable examination and eliminates changes in the position of the pelvic organs caused by distention of the urinary bladder. Clothing is then removed from the waist down, and the patient is positioned and draped in a lithotomy or dorsal recumbent position on the examining table. If the patient is unable to assume either of these positions, Sims' position may be used.

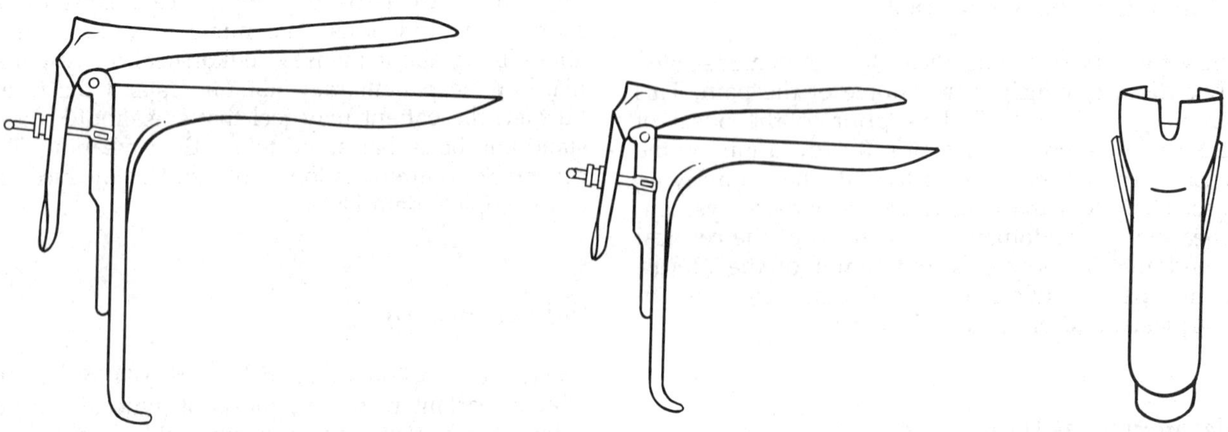

Figure 43–9.

Types and sizes of vaginal specula.

Figure 43–10.

Speculum examination of the cervix. A, Insertion of a speculum. B, Open speculum within the vagina. C, Examiner's view of the cervix through an open speculum.

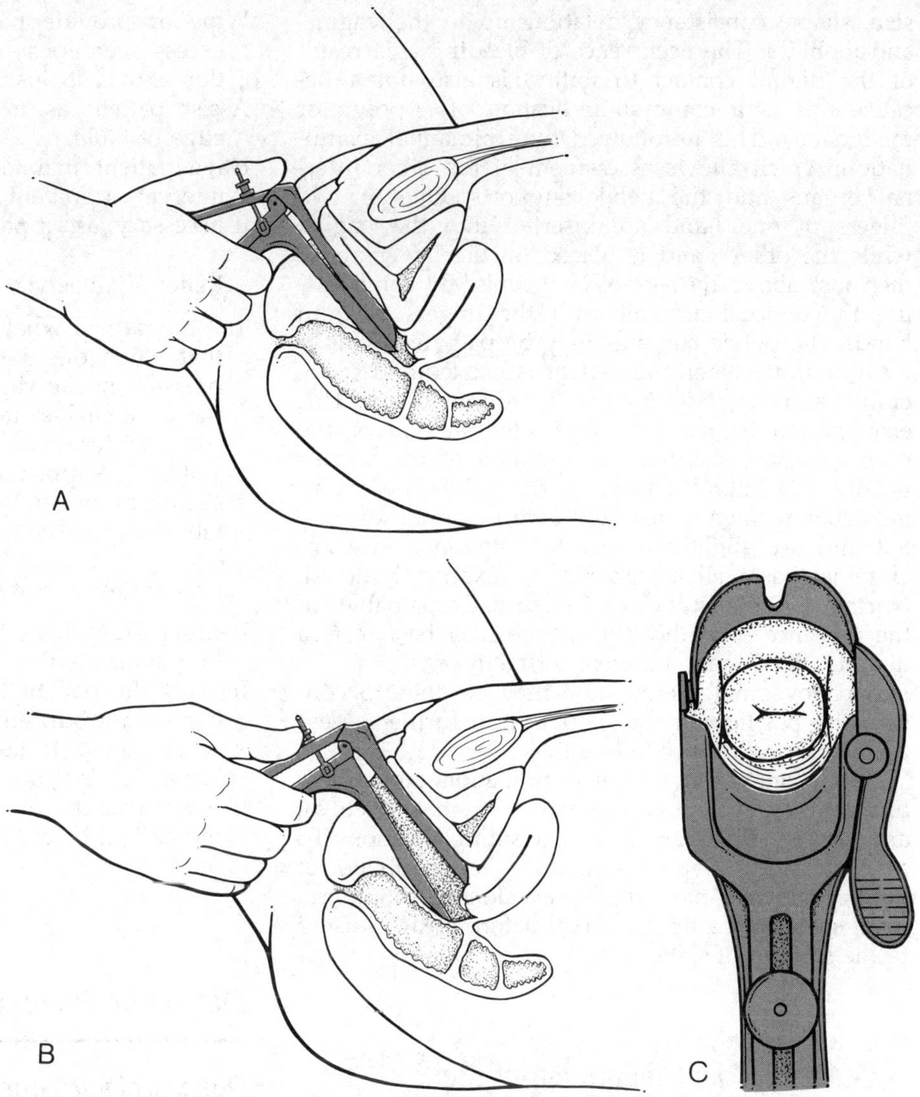

EXAMINATION PROCEDURE

The examiner wears clean gloves for the examination, which begins with the assessment of the external genitalia. This includes inspection for any structural abnormalities such as size and contour of the labia, distribution of pubic hair, or enlargement or atrophy of the clitoris. The presence of any parasites, skin lesions such as rashes or ulcerations, signs of irritation, or change in pigmentation is noted. Also noted is the presence or absence of the hymen as well as discharge or other signs of infection in Bartholin's glands, Skene's glands, the urinary meatus, and the vagina.

Secondly, a speculum (Fig. 43–9) examination is performed. A medium or possibly large speculum is generally used for multiparous patients, and a small speculum for the elderly or nulliparous patient. The aim is to have the best possible visualization without discomfort to the patient. The speculum produces a sensation of pressure in the vagina but does not usually cause discomfort. Instructing the patient to bear down opens the introitus and relaxes the perineal muscles.

The cervix is visualized (Fig. 43–10) and inspected for color, contour, position, shape and patency of the external os, presence of polyps, erosions (red areas), and discharge. If any cytopathologic smears or cervical cultures are indicated, they are obtained at this time. As the speculum is inserted and withdrawn, the vaginal mucosa is assessed. Color and consistency as well as the presence of rugae, ulcers, masses, and discharge are noted.

Next, one or more well-lubricated fingers are inserted into the vagina and the degree of muscle tone is evaluated. The patient is then asked to bear down so that the effect of increased intraabdominal pressure on the position of the bladder, uterus, and rectum can be noted.

Examination of the internal genitalia starts with palpation of the cervix. It is assessed in terms of size, shape, consistency, relationship to the vagina, and mobility. The occurrence of bleeding as a result of the digital contact (friability) is also noted because this is a common indication of a polyp or malignancy. This is followed by a bimanual examination, which allows assessment of the other internal organs and the pelvic supports. One or two fingers of one hand are inserted into the vagina while the other hand is placed on the lower abdomen just above the symphysis pubis. By compressing the abdominal wall with the fingers of both hands, the pelvic contents may be palpated. This is most accurate when the patient is relaxed and cooperative and the abdominal wall is thin and soft. This examination begins with the determination of the size, contour, position, and mobility of the uterus. Finally, the lateral aspects of the pelvis are examined. Before menopause, the ovaries can readily be felt and are slightly tender to palpation. Any enlargement as well as mobility or fixation is noted. Normal fallopian tubes are not usually palpable. In the presence of pathology, a tube may be felt as a definite, fixed mass adherent to the ovary.

A rectovaginal examination may be done to confirm the position of the uterus or to further assess the ovaries and tubes (adnexa).

Upon conclusion of the examination any excess lubricant or secretions are wiped from the vulva, and the patient is assisted to a sitting position. To avoid postural hypotension and the possibility of falling, patients, particularly the elderly, should remain sitting for a brief interval before being assisted to the standing position.

Guidelines for Application of the Nursing Process to the Care of the Patient Having a Pelvic Examination

Pelvic examinations are generally performed by physicians, by nurse practitioners, nurse-midwives, or physician assistants. Thus, the role of most nurses is to physically and cognitively prepare the patient for the examination, allay her anxiety, encourage her cooperation, and generally facilitate the process of the examination. Specific nursing interventions related to each of these areas are as follows:

Physical preparation of the patient:

Ask the patient to empty her bladder.
Ask or assist the patient as necessary to remove clothing from the waist down.
Provide drape or hospital gown for patient's privacy. If necessary, assist the patient onto the examining table, and assist the patient into lithotomy or other examining position when the examiner arrives.
Drape patient.
Wipe or provide patient with a wipe to remove excess secretions from the vulva when examination is over if this is not done by the examiner.
Assist patient as necessary to sitting position on edge of table.
Have patient maintain sitting position for a short interval to prevent postural hypotension.
If necessary, assist patient to stand.

Relief of anxiety:

Tell the patient what to expect. For example, tell her that when the speculum is inserted, a feeling of pressure in the vagina is expected, and that when the bimanual examination is done, she may feel some tenderness.
Maintain a supportive relationship even while assisting examiner by speaking to the patient or establishing eye contact.

Encouragement of cooperation:

Instruct the patient to bear down when the speculum is inserted.
Instruct the patient to bear down when examiner's hand is introduced for the bimanual examination.
Ask the patient to take slow, deep breaths and relax her abdominal muscles as much as possible.
If a rectovaginal examination is to be done, inform the patient before the rectum is examined.

Diagnostic Procedures

Papanicolaou Smear

A Papanicolaou test as used in gynecology is a microscopic examination of a smear of exfoliated cells obtained from the vaginal vault, outer cervix, and cervical os. It detects abnormal cells and is primarily used as a screening device for cancer of the cervix. It may also be used to detect infection or to evaluate the hormonal status of a patient who has an infertility problem or who is taking estrogen.

When a Papanicoulaou (Pap) smear is obtained, the patient assumes the dorsal recumbent or lithotomy position, and a warmed speculum, which may be rinsed in saline but not lubricated, is inserted. Lubricant is contraindicated because it may prevent accurate interpretation of the test results. For the same reason, the gloves worn by the examiner should not be powdered.

The cellular samples are collected using a specifically designed wooden or plastic spatula and a rubber-tipped vaginal pipette, a saline-moistened, cotton-tipped applicator, or a brush like a pipe cleaner called a cytobrush (Fig. 43–11). Material from the posterior vaginal fornix is collected with the blunt end of the spatula. The other end is then used to

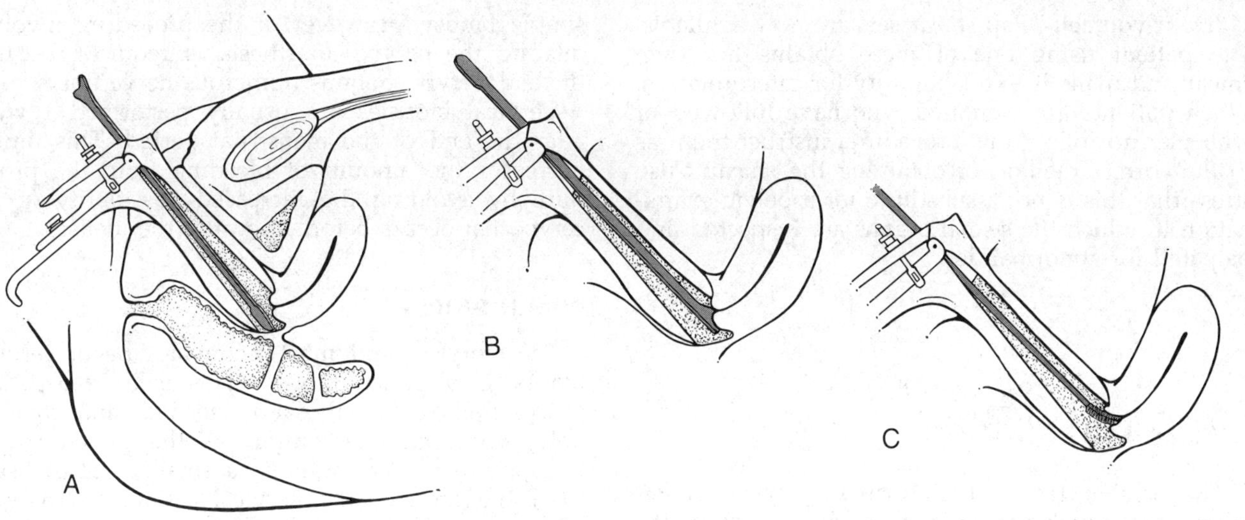

Figure 43–11.

Method of obtaining a Pap smear specimen. A, Blunt end of Ayre spatula used to scrape specimen from the posterior fornix. B, Most pointed tip of the bifid end of an Ayre spatula inserted into the cervical os and rotated 360 degrees to obtain specimen from the squamocolumnar junction. C, Cytobrush inserted into cervical os and rotated 360 degrees, used to collect specimen from the endocervix. Glass pipette or cotton swab may also be used.

scrape cells from the entire circumference of the cervix. Finally, the pipette, applicator, or cytobrush is inserted into the external os to collect cells from the endocervix. The samples are immediately smeared on glass slides, each of which is carefully labeled as to source and immediately fixed by either dipping in 95% alcohol or spraying with a commercially prepared solution. This prevents drying and accompanying cellular distortion.

Originally, the results of the Pap test were reported as Class I, II, III, IV, or V—with Class I indicating normal cells; Class V, invasive cancer; and Class II, III, and IV, intermediate types of cellular abnormality.

Currently, results are frequently given in terms of only three categories. These are (1) normal, (2) atypical cell whose significance is uncertain, and (3) neoplastic or frankly cancerous. Positive (abnormal) findings indicate the need for further tissue studies obtained through biopsy or operation.

The Papanicolaou test is 90% to 95% accurate on positive reports and 95% to 98% accurate on negative reports. In most cases of false-negatives, the cause is an inadequate sample or improper fixation.

To maximize accuracy, the smear should not be obtained during the menses because the menstrual discharge makes evaluation of the smear difficult. Tub baths, douches, and intercourse should be avoided for 48 hours prior to the smear. After cauterization of the cervix, cellular distortion is present for 6 weeks, so smears are not obtained during this time. After radiation treatments, the interval is longer. Smears are not done for a month after the use of intravaginal creams and medications because these cause intense cellular exfoliation.

The Pap test is usually a painless procedure that allows evaluation of a wider area than a biopsy and does not remove viable tissue. It produces little or no trauma or inflammation, although some spotting after the procedure can occur and is considered normal.

Guidelines for Application of the Nursing Process to the Care of the Patient Having a Papanicolaou Smear

Pap smears are generally obtained by physicians or nurse practitioners. Thus, the role of most nurses is to prevent undue anxiety in the patient and help ensure the accuracy of the test results. Specific nursing interventions related to each of these areas are as follows:

Reduction of anxiety:

Give basic information regarding the procedure and its outcomes. Tell the patient the following:

The procedure is painless.
Slight bleeding may occur after the test.
A positive result does not necessarily mean cancer. If a positive result is obtained, additional tests may be required before a diagnosis is possible.

Promotion of accuracy:

Explain that the test should not be scheduled during the menstrual period.
Instruct the patient not to take a tub bath, douche, or have intercourse for 48 hours before the test is scheduled. Handle all slides carefully.

"Do-it-yourself" Pap smear sets are now available. The patient using one of these obtains her own smear and mails it to a laboratory for interpretation. When patients are identified who have followed or who plan to follow this procedure, instruct them as to the correct method of obtaining the smear. Also stress that this is not a substitute for a pelvic examination in which the sexual organs are inspected and palpated for abnormalities.

Schiller Test

The Schiller test is used primarily when smear results are positive in order to identify areas of the cervix or vagina that should be biopsied.

It is a simple test in which an iodine solution is applied to the epithelium of the cervix and the vagina. Because these epithelial cells are normally rich in glycogen and readily pick up iodine, they become a deep mahogany color. Cancerous epithelium, in contrast, does not contain glycogen and does not pick up iodine or change color. Thus, epithelium with malignant changes appears as a glistening light area.

Colposcopy

Colposcopy is the procedure in which the cervix is visualized and magnified in a bright light for the purpose of identifying areas of abnormality. The instrument used is the colposcope, which is a low-power microscope.

This procedure is done when Pap smears indicate atypical or pathologic changes.

It is a simple procedure and takes no longer than the usual inspection of the cervix. Its major advantage is that areas where suspect cells originate can be identified so that assessment of size and severity as well as selection of optimal biopsy sites is possible.

The disadvantage of colposcopy is that only the outer areas of the cervix can be studied.

Cervical Biopsy

A cervical biopsy is done when a Pap smear result is abnormal or when a cervical lesion is seen with or without a colposcopy or a Schiller test. The purpose of the biopsy is to diagnose or rule out malignancy. It can also serve as a basis for treatment by determining the exact histopathology of the lesion. Because there are few nerve fibers in the cervix, usually little or no anesthesia is needed for a simple biopsy. However, if the procedure involves dilating the cervix, anesthesia is required because the endocervix contains numerous nerve fibers.

Cervical biopsies are usually performed 1 week after the end of the menstrual period. This timing decreases the amount of bleeding from the procedure by avoiding the increased vascularity of the cervix that occurs before and after the menses.

PUNCH BIOPSY

The simplest and most frequent type of cervical biopsy is a punch biopsy. This is an out-patient procedure. No anesthesia is needed, and there is only momentary discomfort as the punch biopsy forceps are used to remove a small piece of tissue from the area of the cervical lesion. In cases in which a specific area cannot be pinpointed, a multiple punch biopsy may be done. Specimens may be obtained at the 12 o'clock and 6 o'clock positions, which are the locations where neoplasia most frequently arises, or a four-quadrant biopsy may be done, with specimens obtained at 12, 3, 6, and 9 o'clock positions.

There is minimal bleeding with punch biopsies, and it is easily controlled with pressure, application of silver nitrate solution, or electric cautery.

If electric cautery is used, there is an unpleasant odor from the burning tissue and some discomfort is felt. A foul-smelling, gray-green discharge begins on or about the fourth day after the procedure and continues for up to 3 weeks.

EXCISION BIOPSY

A second type of biopsy is an excision biopsy. In this type, a cervical lesion with adjacent normal tissue is removed with a scalpel. The excised area is larger than with a punch biopsy. There is more bleeding, and sutures may be required. This is an out-patient procedure, and local anesthesia may be used.

CONE BIOPSY

A third type of biopsy is a conization of the cervix, or cone biopsy. This is done when the location of a lesion cannot be pinpointed, when a lesion involves a large area or extends into the cervical canal, or when smear results are positive but biopsy results are negative.

Cone biopsy is an in-patient or out-patient procedure in which a scalpel or laser is used to remove a cone-shaped piece of tissue from the central cervix (Fig. 43–12). The size and shape of the cone are variable and based on the size and shape of the lesion. The procedure is done under either local or general anesthesia, and sutures may be used to prevent postoperative bleeding.

Unless absolutely necessary, conization is generally not performed on women who desire to bear

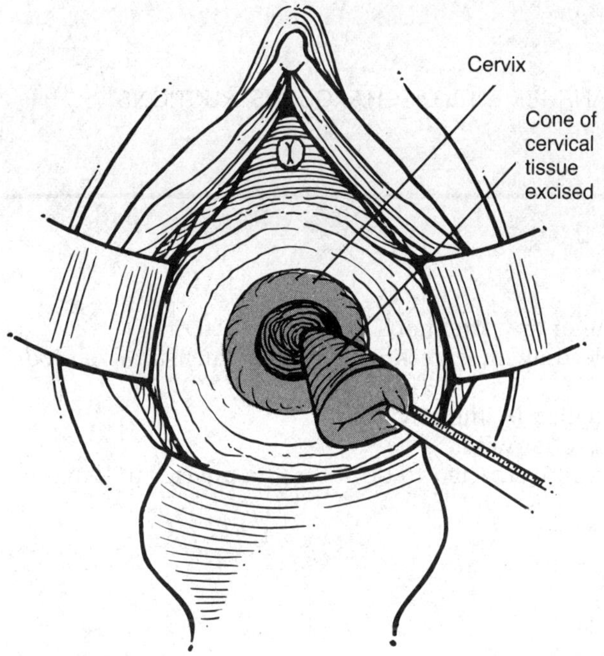

Figure 43–12.

Cone biopsy.

children, because it can lead to incompetence of the cervix or infertility.

Following conization, the next two or three menses may be heavy and prolonged, and a dark brown premenstrual discharge may occur. This is considered normal, and no therapy is indicated. Complications of cone biopsy include hemorrhage, infection, and less frequently, cervical stenosis. If hemorrhage occurs, it is controlled by a vaginal packing (p. 1701) retained in place for 24 to 48 hours. Cauterization may be required if other measures fail. Infection is treated with antibiotics, and stenosis with dilation.

"Hot" conization, which uses electrocautery, is performed as a therapeutic measure in patients with chronic cervicitis that has extended into the deep tissues of the cervix. Tissue removed in this procedure cannot be used for diagnostic purposes because the cautery chars the tissue and prevents pathologic examination.

Application of the Nursing Process to the Care of the Patient Having a Cervical Biopsy

Assessment

Assess the patient's understanding of the purpose and the procedure of the biopsy. Also assess the patient's anxiety level. Review the history, and observe the patient for any factors with implications for care before, during, or after the procedure. Obtain baseline vital signs.

Nursing Diagnoses and Planning

Nursing diagnoses and related expected patient outcomes most commonly applicable to patients having a cervical biopsy include the following:

NDx: Anxiety related to the procedure and its outcomes

Planning: Patient outcomes

1. Patient participates in preparations for the procedure without overt signs of anxiety, such as crying and trembling.
2. Patient attends to questions and directions.

NDx: High risk for altered health maintenance related to insufficient knowledge of purpose of the biopsy, procedure, biopsy report, and discharge instructions

Planning: Patient outcomes

1. Patient describes the preparation for the procedure, expected discomfort, and the expected postprocedure course.
2. Patient states the purpose of the biopsy.
3. Patient states how and when she will be made aware of the results.
4. Patient explains discharge instructions (see Chart 43–2).

Nursing Interventions

NDx: Anxiety

Provide emotional support and allay anxiety by allowing time and opportunity for the patient to verbalize her feelings and concerns and by making sure that she knows what to expect during and after the procedure. Tell her the type and amount of discomfort that accompanies the procedure as well as expected effects on the menstrual cycle, such as the occurrence of two or three heavy, prolonged periods after conization. Also inform the patient when, and by whom, she will be told the results of the biopsy.

Provision of emotional support is particularly important when the biopsy is being done to rule out or diagnose malignancy.

NDx: High risk for altered health maintenance

Before the biopsy, review its purpose with the patient, and explain the procedure as described previously in the text. Explain the postbiopsy instructions listed in Chart 43–2 to the patient before discharge. These are basic instructions given to all patients regardless of the type of biopsy performed.

Chart 43–2.

NURSING GUIDE TO PATIENT EDUCATION FOR SELF-MANAGEMENT: DISCHARGE INSTRUCTIONS AFTER CERVICAL BIOPSY

Instruct the patient to:

Rest for 24 hours after the procedure. Avoid heavy lifting or any strenuous exercise or activity.

Call the physician or go to the clinic or hospital if bleeding in excess of a normal menstrual period occurs.

Avoid having intercourse or douching until the time specified by the physician.

Use pads rather than tampons until the physician advises otherwise.

Note: If a vaginal packing is in place, do not remove it until instructed to do so by the physician. Usually a vaginal packing will be left in place for 8 to 24 hours.

Also ascertain that the patient knows the date and time as well as the importance of any follow-up visit that is scheduled.

Additional Interventions

Immediately after the procedure, assess the physiologic stabilization of the patient by checking the amount of vaginal bleeding and measuring vital signs until stable. If a general anesthetic was given, make the usual postoperative assessments as discussed in Chapter 4.

Evaluation

Evaluate the effectiveness of nursing care for a patient having a cervical biopsy by comparing the patient's status with the expected patient outcomes. Examples of specific outcomes for patients having a cervical biopsy have been provided in the Planning section.

Endometrial Cytology

Endometrial cytology is done to screen for uterine cancer. The specimen is obtained by aspiration of endometrial secretions, cells, or lavage fluid through a cannula inserted into the uterine cavity via the cervical os. Mild, temporary cramping may accompany this procedure.

This test is of greatest importance to women older than 50 years of age because this is when endometrial cancer is most likely to occur. It is required in addition to the Papanicolaou test because cells rarely exfoliate from the endometrium during the early stages of a malignancy and thus would not be found in a Papanicolaou smear.

Endometrial Biopsy

An endometrial biopsy may be used in the diagnosis of endometrial cancer or to assess the endometrium for the effects of progesterone in patients seeking treatment for infertility.

The biopsy specimen is most often obtained by use of an aspirating curet attached to some form of negative pressure, although a nonaspirating curet or punch biopsy forceps may be used. If malignant cells are being looked for, specimens are obtained from several sites in the uterine cavity.

Hysteroscopy

Hysteroscopy is a procedure that allows direct visualization of the intrauterine cavity. The procedure is done on either an in-patient or out-patient basis. Under paracervical block anesthesia, the endometrial cavity is distended with carbon dioxide or dextran solution, and an instrument called a hysteroscope, which is equipped with a light source, is inserted through the cervix into the uterus. The inside of the uterus can then be checked for polyps, submucous myomas, or adhesions. Photographs can be taken, biopsies obtained, or intrauterine devices or small polyps removed.

The procedure is contraindicated by pregnancy, suspected or diagnosed cancer of the cervix, pelvic inflammatory disease, or a history of recent uterine perforation.

Hysterosalpingography

Hysterosalpingography is an x-ray and fluoroscopic procedure in which a contrast medium is used to allow visualization of the size, shape, position, and structure of the uterus and fallopian tubes. It can demonstrate pathology such as malformation of the uterus and tubes and the presence of intrauterine tumors or tubal adhesions. With the patient in lithotomy position, a cannula is inserted through the vagina and into the cervical canal. Six to 12 ml of a contrast substance such as Ethiodol or Conray is injected into the uterine cavity, and x-ray films are taken as the cavity is filled and the substance moves through the tubes.

During this test, which takes approximately 30 minutes, the patient may have uterine cramping and a transient sensation of dizziness. After the test, a vaginal discharge, which is sometimes bloody, may occur for 1 to 2 days.

The procedure is not done during the week before or after menstruation; nor is it done when there is a recent or current episode of abnormal uterine bleeding, active infection of the reproductive tract, or severe cardiorespiratory disease.

Ultrasonography

Ultrasonography can be used to produce an image of the pelvic organs. In this procedure, intermittent sound waves of high frequency are projected toward the pelvis, and the pattern of the sound waves as they bounce back after hitting tissues of different densities is recorded. This allows the location of pelvic masses and identification of their size, position, relationship to normal pelvic structures, and internal composition (i.e., solid or cystic).

Ultrasonography is used in planning the operative approach to pelvic tumors, planning and evaluating radiation therapy for pelvic malignancies, diagnosis of extrauterine pregnancy, and determination of the position of a "lost" contraceptive intrauterine device. It is also used in the diagnosis of other pathologic disorders such as ovarian cysts and endometriosis.

Medical Management

Nonsurgical Management

Pharmacologic therapy is the primary form of nonsurgical intervention used in the treatment of gynecologic disorders. Hormone therapy is used to treat disorders of the menstrual cycle, as well as disorders as diverse as atrophic vaginitis, endometriosis, and cancer. Anti-infectives are used to treat infectious disorders ranging from simple vaginitis to life-threatening toxic shock syndrome.

Surgical Management

All gynecologic surgery is performed to restore normal anatomy, to remove abnormal tissue, or to provide relief from distressing symptoms. Surgery is also used for diagnosis and treatment of menstrual abnormalities, congenital defects affecting fertility or sexual identity, chronic pelvic inflammatory disease or endometriosis, malignant diseases of the reproductive organs, traumatic injuries to the reproductive organs or supporting structures, and therapeutic or incomplete spontaneous abortion. Table 43–1 summarizes gynecologic surgical procedures other than those discussed in depth here.

Table 43–1. SURGICAL PROCEDURES USED TO TREAT SPECIFIC GYNECOLOGIC DISORDERS

SURGICAL PROCEDURE	DESCRIPTION
Oophorectomy	Removal of an ovary
Salpingectomy	Removal of a fallopian tube
Myomectomy	Removal of a tumor of the uterine musculature
Colporraphy	Plastic repair of the vagina
Anterior	Repair of relaxed anterior vaginal wall to correct a cystocele
Posterior	Repair of relaxed posterior vaginal wall to correct a rectocele
Vaginectomy	Removal of the vagina
Vulvectomy	Removal of the vulva
Simple	Excision of vulva with wide skin margin
Radical (Wertheim's operation)	Excision of vulva with deep lymph node dissection
Total pelvic exenteration	Removal of uterus, fallopian tubes, ovaries, cervix, part of the vagina, and bladder. Urinary diversion performed and a bowel resection with colostomy
Anterior pelvic exenteration	Total pelvic exenteration minus the bowel resection and colostomy
Posterior pelvic exenteration	Total pelvic exenteration minus the cystectomy and urinary diversion
Ovarian cystectomy	Removal of cyst from an ovary
Bartholin's marsupialization	Creation of a channel for drainage from a Bartholin's cyst by opening the gland and suturing the edges to the vaginal wall

PREOPERATIVE PREPARATION

As for any surgery, the physician assesses the overall status of the patient with particular attention to pulmonary, myocardial, renal, and hepatic function; existing health problems other than that for which the surgery is being done; and drugs currently being taken by the patient. Routine laboratory studies that are done as part of this assessment are listed in Table 43–2.

Water, electrolyte, and acid-base balances are assessed preoperatively to provide a baseline for postoperative evaluation and intervention. This is critical to the care of aged patients, patients who were recently pregnant, those taking oral contraceptives or diuretics, and those on special diets, because all of these are prone to postoperative fluid and electrolyte imbalance.

To decrease the risk of postoperative infection, any vulvitis, vaginitis, or cervicitis is treated prior to

Table 43–2. ROUTINE PREOPERATIVE LABORATORY STUDIES FOR MAJOR GYNECOLOGIC SURGERY

Papanicolaou smear	Total bilirubin
Complete blood count	Calcium
Clean-catch urinalysis	Uric acid
Chest x-ray film	Creatinine
Electrolytes	Phosphorus
Glucose	Enzymes—LDH, CPK, AST
Blood urea nitrogen	Rh factor and blood type
Cholesterol	Sickling preparation (done on black patients)
Total protein*	
Albumin	

* Particularly important when the patient is malnourished or has been on a prolonged reducing diet.

LDH, lactate dehydrogenase; CPK, creatine phosphokinase; AST, aspartate aminotransferase.

admission. It is particularly important that monilial infections be identified and treated so that monilial sepsis with its relatively high mortality rate does not occur. Women at risk for monilial sepsis are the elderly, the debilitated, those on long-term antibiotic therapy, and those on immunosuppressive or corticosteroid therapy.

Similarly, the patient is checked for urinary tract infection and treatment given because flare-ups of existing infection are likely after surgery as a result of catheterization and dissection in the area of the bladder.

To decrease the risk of blood loss, surgery is generally scheduled 1 week after the patient's last menstrual period.

For menopausal or postmenopausal patients, estrogen suppositories may be ordered to aid the proliferation of the vaginal epithelium and therefore to facilitate healing. These vaginal suppositories are given once a day for 3 to 4 weeks prior to surgery.

In addition to the routine scrub and shave of the operative area, douches may be ordered to cleanse the vagina of mucus and epithelial debris.

If it is a major procedure, the intestine is also prepared. Anti-infective therapy such as neomycin sulfate, 1 g orally, and erythromycin base, 1 g orally, t.i.d. on the day before surgery, is given to decrease the bacteria in the intestine. A low-residue diet for 3 days preoperatively and enemas the evening before surgery act to empty the rectum.

Patients are instructed to avoid coitus for 1 week prior to surgery.

COMPLICATIONS OF GYNECOLOGIC SURGERY

A major risk associated with gynecologic surgery is the development of a thromboembolism postoperatively. This results from the effects of anesthesia, immobility, and soft tissue damage. Predisposing factors include obesity, age older than 40 years, recent use of oral contraceptives, history of thrombus formation, and presence of malignant disease.

Preventive measures include early movement and ambulation, adequate hydration to maintain the fluidity of the blood, prophylactic anticoagulant therapy, and routine postoperative examination of the calf for early recognition of deep vein thrombosis.

Infection is a second major postoperative complication. Wound infection is common because of the frequency of pathogens in the vagina and the closeness of the anus to the operative site. Patients at particular risk are those who are obese or malnourished; those with preexisting sepsis, diabetes, or malignancy; and those in whom the operation involves an opening between the vagina and the pelvis.

Infection may also occur in the urinary tract and in the chest. Catheterization increases the risk of urinary tract infection, and smoking increases the risk of chest infection.

A third complication is hemorrhage, which may occur early or late. Early hemorrhage may be due to incomplete hemostasis or loosening of a ligature on a major blood vessel. It may also be a reactive hemorrhage. This is hemorrhage from severed vessels that did not bleed during surgery as a result of hypotension. Late hemorrhage, which occurs several days after the operation, is the result of suture dissolution or infection. Regardless of type, measures to control bleeding are initiated, and replacement of blood is begun if necessary. Other complications are accidental injury to the bladder, ureter, or rectum, because of their close proximity to the operative site; intestinal obstruction; and wound breakdown.

Depression and sexual dysfunction occur in some patients after gynecologic surgery.

Depression may be related to the loss of an important organ or loss of an important function or may be a reaction to the total stress of the preoperative symptoms, the surgery, and the recovery period.

Sexual dysfunction may occur secondary to depression or as a result of physical damage to the reproductive tract or atrophy of the vagina, which occurs after removal of the ovaries; or it may be due to the lack of an understanding partner.

COMMON GYNECOLOGIC SURGICAL PROCEDURES

LAPAROSCOPY

Laparoscopy is a procedure in which the internal organs of the pelvis are visualized and examined. This is done with a laparoscope inserted through an incision in the abdominal wall. It is used for both diagnostic and therapeutic purposes (Fig. 43–13).

Uses. As a diagnostic technique it is used in the evaluation of patients with chronic pelvic pain, a palpable abdominal mass, or a history of infertility. It allows the identification of endometriosis, pelvic inflammatory disease, ectopic pregnancy, ovarian neoplasms, and signs of abdominal malignancy or metastasis. It can be used to obtain biopsies and also

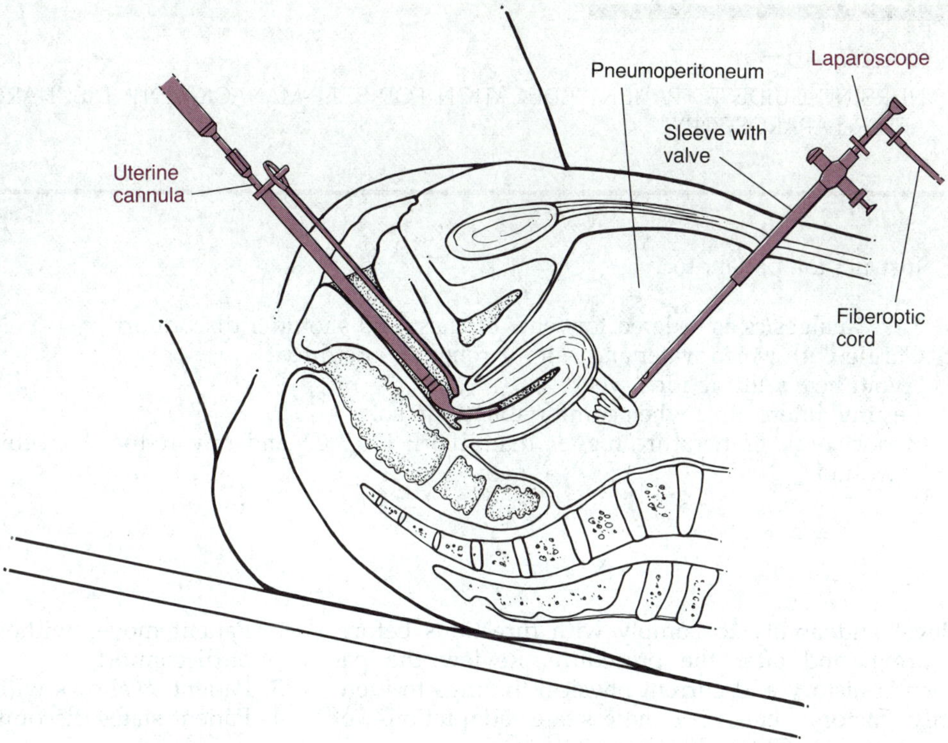

Figure 43–13.

Laparoscopy.

to determine patency or blockage of the fallopian tubes. The latter is done by injecting a dye called indigo carmine into the uterus via a cannula passed through the cervix and observing for its escape through the fimbriated ends of the tubes. The escape of the dye is seen if the tubes are patent but not if they are blocked.

As a therapeutic procedure, the principal use of laparoscopy is for tubal sterilization. It may also be used for such procedures as removal of peritubal adhesions, ablation of endometrioma, removal of intrauterine devices that have perforated through the uterine wall, and aspiration of ova for in vitro fertilization.

Patient Preparation. Laparoscopy may be performed in either an in-patient or out-patient setting. The patient is allowed nothing by mouth (NPO status) from midnight before the procedure. Bowel cleansing and abdominal skin preparation are done at the discretion of the physician. A short-acting general anesthesia is used most often because little sedation is required and the patient is awake, alert, and, if an out-patient, able to go home within 2 hours. Local or regional anesthesia may also be used, but more sedation is required and the recovery period is longer.

Procedure. The patient's bladder is emptied, and then an incision is made into the lower rim of the umbilicus. The abdomen is insufflated with carbon dioxide or nitrous oxide to distend it and separate the organs. The patient is placed in Trendelenburg position so that the gas displaces the bowel up and out of the pelvis.

In a one-incision technique, a laparoscope with an electric cautery forceps is then inserted. In a two-incision technique, another incision is made below the umbilicus but above the symphysis pubis, and a second instrument needed for the procedure is inserted. When the procedure is completed, as much gas as possible is expelled from the abdomen, and sutures or clips are used to close the incisions. Healing occurs without a noticeable scar.

Contraindications. Previous surgery, abdominal adhesions, or obesity makes visualization difficult and may result in an unsatisfactory procedure. The procedure cannot be used for women with cardiovascular, respiratory, or other disorders that prevent the use of Trendelenburg position or abdominal insufflation.

Complications. The most serious complication of laparoscopy is intestinal burns from the use of diathermy. Burns cause necrosis and perforation of the bowel and consequently peritonitis. Other possible complications include embolism secondary to the insufflation, infection, and rarely bleeding, which requires a laparotomy.

Application of the Nursing Process to the Care of the Patient Having a Laparoscopy

Assessment

Assess the patient's understanding of the procedure and its purpose. Also assess the patient's anxiety

Chart 43–3.

NURSING GUIDE TO PATIENT EDUCATION FOR SELF-MANAGEMENT: DISCHARGE INSTRUCTIONS AFTER LAPAROSCOPY

Instruct the patient to:

Take analgesics as ordered for relief of chest and shoulder discomfort.
Gargle with warm water and salt for relief of sore throat.
Avoid heavy lifting for 1 week.
Resume intercourse when comfortable to do so.
Report oral temperature higher than 100°F (37.7°C) and any redness, swelling, or drainage from the wound.

level and ability to comply with directions before, during, and after the procedure. Review the patient's history and current physical findings to identify factors that may necessitate adaptations of current care. Obtain baseline vital signs.

Nursing Diagnoses and Planning

Nursing diagnoses and related expected outcomes most commonly applicable to patients having a laparoscopy include the following:

NDx: Anxiety related to the laparoscopy procedure and the findings

Planning: Patient outcomes
1. Signs of acute anxiety, such as trembling, clenching hands, pacing, and verbalizing expressions of doom, are absent.
2. Patient attends to questions or directions, responding appropriately.

NDx: High risk for altered health maintenance related to insufficient knowledge of procedure, postprocedure course, discharge instructions

Planning: Patient outcomes
1. Patient describes the laparoscopy procedure and its purpose.
2. Patient describes immediate postlaparoscopy care.
3. Patient explains discharge instructions as listed in Chart 43–3.

NDx: Pain: chest and shoulder, related to pressure on diaphragm secondary to insufflated intraabdominal gas and/or sore throat related to intubation

Planning: Patient outcomes
1. Patient accepts pain medication and gargles as directed.
2. Patient moves without verbal or nonverbal signs of discomfort.
3. Patient swallows without complaints of pain.
4. Patient states discomfort is relieved.

Nursing Interventions

Prepare the patient for laparoscopy by explaining that she must have nothing by mouth after midnight prior to the procedure. Also explain, and implement as necessary, any other preparations ordered by the physician, such as shaving the skin or bowel cleansing.

NDx: Anxiety
To lessen the patient's anxiety, provide her with information on what to expect. If she is having a local anesthetic, tell her that the procedure generally takes less than 1 hour; that once the anesthesia is given, she may feel some pressure but will not feel pain; and that she will be placed in a tilted position with her head somewhat lower than her feet.

NDx: High risk for altered health maintenance
Review the laparoscopy procedure and its purpose with the patient. Also describe care during the immediate recovery period. Before discharge, instruct the patient in self-care as specified in Chart 43–3.

NDx: Pain
Monitor the patient for discomfort. Shoulder pain and chest soreness are common following insufflation, and a sore throat is common if the patient was intubated. Keep the patient supine or in low Fowler's position to lessen the pressure of intraabdominal gas on the diaphragm. Give analgesics (usually aspirin or aspirin substitutes) as ordered to relieve the chest and shoulder discomfort. Give warm saline gargles for effective relief of the sore

throat. Explain to the patient that these symptoms are normal occurrences and that the medication, position change, and gargle will provide relief. Reassure the patient that these symptoms should disappear in a few days.

Additional Interventions
Following the procedure, monitor the physiologic stabilization of the patient. Take vital signs every 15 minutes for 1 hour, or until stable. Allow the patient activity as tolerated, and give fluids and a light snack, provided she is not nauseated.

Evaluation

Evaluate the effectiveness of nursing care for a patient having a laparoscopy by comparing the patient's status with the expected patient outcomes. Examples of specific outcomes for patients having a laparoscopy have been provided in the Planning section.

CRYOSURGERY

Cryosurgery is a technique in which tissue is destroyed through exposure to extreme cold. A probe, usually containing liquid nitrogen, is used to produce temperatures in the area of −20°C (−4°F). These temperatures cause necrosis and subsequent sloughing of the tissue as a result of cellular dehydration and disruption of the cell membrane.

Uses. This local freezing technique is used in the treatment of chronic cervicitis, endocervicitis, cervical erosions, cervical polyps, and benign leukoplakia. It is also used as a preventive measure to remove tissue when dysplasia, a precancerous condition, is evident and as a palliative measure to reduce tumor size in cases of inoperable or recurrent malignancy.

Patient Preparation. Cryosurgery is an ambulatory procedure performed in an office or clinic setting. No anesthesia is usually required. It is done 1 week after the end of the menstrual period. This prevents destruction of an early pregnancy and allows the active phase of cervical regeneration, which takes place after menses, to occur.

Procedure. The patient is placed in lithotomy position, and a medium or large speculum is inserted. The patient is then instructed not to move. This is to prevent the probe from accidentally touching and damaging normal tissues. The probe is placed on areas to be treated for 1 to 3 minutes, and upon completion, a perineal pad is applied.

Postoperative Course. Following the procedure, a profuse watery discharge occurs. On about the fourth day, this contains cellular debris and may have an odor. The discharge lasts from 2 to 6 weeks. Because the cervix is left friable, some physicians instruct their patients to avoid sexual intercourse, swimming, and the use of tampons for 2 weeks after the procedure. Showers are recommended, but a tub may be used, provided it is well scrubbed.

An intravaginal antibiotic cream such as Triple Sulfa or Furacin may be prescribed to aid healing, provided the patient does not have acute cervicitis or perimetritis. For patients with the latter, oral antibiotics are prescribed for 1 week.

Complications. Possible complications of the procedure are occasional spotting, cervical stenosis, infection, and damage to normal tissue through accidental touching with the probe.

Guidelines for Application of the Nursing Process to the Care of the Patient Having Cryosurgery

When caring for patients having cryosurgery, intervene to decrease anxiety and promote patient compliance with postoperative instructions. Before the procedure, assess the patient's knowledge and understanding regarding the reason the procedure is being performed and the discomfort involved. Before discharge, review with the patient characteristics of the vaginal discharge to be expected and instructions regarding bathing, swimming, use of tampons, and sexual intercourse.

ELECTROCAUTERY

To cauterize is to burn. In electrocautery, an instrument consisting of a holder and a wire is heated by a current of electricity. This is used to burn abnormal tissue in cases of cervical dysplasia or venereal warts. The burned cells exfoliate and new, healthy tissue is regenerated. The treatment may have to be repeated because the abnormality sometimes recurs.

When electrocautery is used to treat cervical dysplasia, the patient is placed in lithotomy position, and a vaginal speculum is inserted. Little or no anesthesia is required because electrocauterization does not cause specific pain, although it may cause uterine cramping. There is an unpleasant odor and a foul-smelling, gray-green discharge, which begins on or about the fourth day and continues for up to 3 weeks.

LASER SURGERY

Laser surgery is used in a variety of ways in gynecologic practice. It can be used for cervical conization, tubal ligation, excision of polyps, precancerous lesions, and vulvar carcinoma. It can also be used for intrauterine endometrial ablation.

Chart 43–4.
NURSING GUIDE TO PATIENT EDUCATION FOR SELF-MANAGEMENT: SELF-CARE AFTER GYNECOLOGIC LASER SURGERY

Instruct the patient to:

Apply ice pack to the perineum immediately after surgery to prevent swelling.
Keep a condom filled with cotton and topical antibiotic in the vagina for 24 hours after extensive vaginal surgery to keep the vaginal walls from adhering to each other if directed to do so by the physician.
Take over-the-counter analgesics as directed to relieve abdominal cramping, which can last up to 36 hours.
Take sitz baths for comfort following bowel movements or whenever needed.
Dry the perineal area thoroughly after sitz baths by gently patting or using a hand-held blow dryer on its lowest setting.
Facilitate urination if necessary by squirting warm water over the vulva or voiding in the sitz bath.
Take stool softeners as directed to ease constipation and painful defecation, which can occur for up to 14 days after vulvar or perianal laser treatments.
Consult the physician before resuming sexual intercourse.
Return for a checkup on *(specify date and time).*

Application of the Nursing Process to the Care of the Patient Having Gynecologic Laser Surgery

The assessment, nursing diagnoses, expected patient outcomes, nursing interventions, and evaluation for patients having laser surgery for a gynecologic problem include those for patients having surgery (see Chapter 4), as well as those that relate to the specific gynecologic disorder for which the patient is being treated. Instruct all patients in basic self-care after gynecologic laser surgery as presented in Chart 43–4.

DILATION AND CURETTAGE

Dilation and curettage (D&C) is a common operative procedure in which the cervix is dilated and the uterine endometrium is scraped out.

Uses. Dilation and curettage has both diagnostic and therapeutic uses. As a diagnostic tool, it allows for evaluation of the contour of the uterine cavity and for cytopathologic examination of endometrium. It is used to diagnose uterine malignancies and is performed whenever there is unexplained irregular uterine bleeding to determine whether its cause is a hormonal dysfunction or a cancer. Because tissue is obtained from all areas of the uterus, missed diagnoses of malignancies are infrequent.

As a therapeutic tool it is used to control abnormal uterine bleeding, relieve dysmenorrhea, empty the uterus after an incomplete abortion, or perform an abortion.

Patient Preparation. Before a D&C, the patient must have a medical clearance for anesthesia and surgery and is kept on NPO status after midnight on the day of operation. Perineal shaves, an enema, or a douche may be ordered by the surgeon preoperatively, but this is currently the exception rather than the rule.

Procedure. The procedure is usually done under general anesthesia. However, it can also be done using local anesthesia with the patient mildly sedated. The patient is placed in lithotomy position; the perineum and vagina are prepared with Betadine; and a bimanual examination is done to determine the position of the uterus. A speculum is inserted to allow access to the cervix. The size of the uterine cavity is assessed by insertion of a sound. Metal dilators of increasing size are then used to gradually open the cervix for passage of the curet and for the tissues to be removed from the uterus (Fig. 43–14). When dilation is accomplished, the endometrium is removed either by scraping with a curet or by the application of suction. When the latter is done, it is called a suction curettage. All material removed is sent to the laboratory for cytopathologic examination.

Postoperative Course. Postoperatively, vaginal bleeding occurs, and it may contain a few small clots. The bleeding progressively decreases in amount and becomes darker. It generally ends in a few days but may continue as spotting up to 8

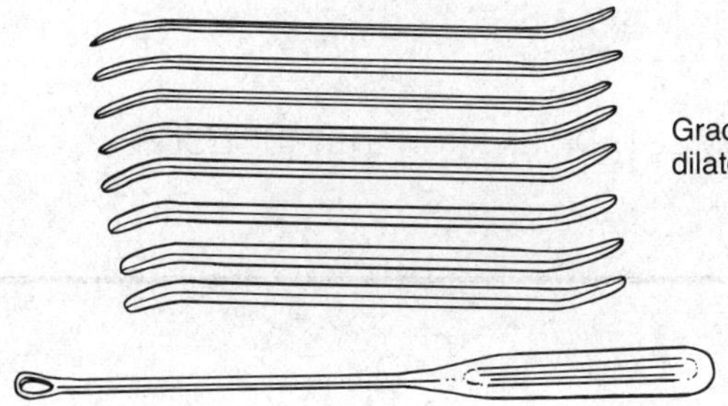

Figure 43–14.

Graduated dilators and curet.

weeks if the D&C was performed after a spontaneous abortion. A recurrence of bright red bleeding or the development of a foul odor from the discharge is abnormal.

Abdominal cramping may occur during the first few postoperative days. This is treated with mild analgesics such as aspirin or codeine sulfate or the use of a heating pad or hot-water bottle on the abdomen, or both. Continuous, sharp abdominal pain not relieved by medication is abnormal.

The patient is allowed diet and activity as tolerated after her recovery from anesthesia, and if the procedure has been done on an out-patient basis, she is ready to return home in approximately 8 hours.

The procedure is contraindicated by pregnancy or the presence of an acute infection.

Hemorrhage occurring 7 to 14 days after the procedure is the most common complication.

Application of the Nursing Process to the Care of the Patient Having Dilation and Curettage

PREOPERATIVE NURSING CARE

Preoperatively prepare the patient for the procedure by clarifying the patient's understanding of what is to be done and ensuring that the physician's orders for preoperative diet and skin preparation of the operative site are carried out. If the D&C is done as an out-patient procedure, ascertain that the patient understands and is capable of carrying out preparations to be done at home.

POSTOPERATIVE NURSING CARE

Assessment

Assess the physiologic stabilization of the patient by checking vital signs and monitoring vaginal bleeding. Check vital signs every 15 minutes until stable and then as indicated by the patient's condition. Monitor vaginal bleeding by keeping a pad count and noting the degree of saturation.

After the first postoperative hour, perineal pads should not require changing more than once per hour for the remainder of the first postoperative day. Approximately 60 ml of blood are needed to saturate a pad. Bleeding is excessive when pads are changed every hour and more than one is saturated during an 8-hour interval.

Take the patient's temperature every 4 hours, and notify the physician if it is higher than 100°F (37.7°C) orally. Note all fluid intake and time and amount of voiding. Assess patient for physical discomfort and for her emotional reaction to the procedure.

Nursing Diagnoses and Planning

Nursing diagnoses and related expected patient outcomes most commonly applicable to patients who have had a D&C include the following:

NDx: Pain: abdominal cramping related to the operative procedure

Planning: Patient outcomes

1. Patient reports that pain is minimal or absent.
2. Patient appears free of pain (e.g., does not hold abdomen or draw up legs).

NDx: High risk for altered health maintenance related to insufficient knowledge of discharge instructions

Planning: Patient outcomes

1. Patient explains discharge instructions as specified in Chart 43–5.
2. Patient states need for and time of any follow-up appointment.

Nursing Interventions

NDx: Pain

Administer analgesics or apply heat to the abdomen in accordance with physician's orders. Assure the patient that abdominal cramping after a D&C is normal, and assist her to perform relaxation exercises.

NDx: High risk for altered health maintenance

Explain the normal recovery process following a D&C, and instruct the patient in self-care as specified in Chart 43–5. Be certain the patient knows the reason for and time of any follow-up appointment needed.

Chart 43–5.

NURSING GUIDE TO PATIENT EDUCATION FOR SELF-MANAGEMENT: DISCHARGE INSTRUCTIONS AFTER DILATION AND CURETTAGE

Instruct the patient to:

Avoid strenuous exercise and heavy work. Gradually increase overall activity with return to a full routine in 2 weeks.
Avoid the use of tampons for 1 week.
Avoid sexual intercourse for 2 weeks or until all bleeding stops.
Report signs and symptoms of infection: pain, fever, chills, or foul-smelling discharge.

Evaluation

Evaluate the effectiveness of nursing care for a patient who has had a D&C by comparing the patient's status with the expected patient outcomes. Examples of specific outcomes for patients who have had a D&C have been provided in the Planning section.

BILATERAL TUBAL LIGATION

Bilateral tubal ligation (BTL) is a surgical sterilization procedure for women in which the fallopian tubes are cut, cauterized, or clipped (Fig. 43–15) to prevent passage of a mature ovum to the uterus. The procedure is most often done through the abdomen via a minilaparotomy incision or laparoscopic approach.

Minilaparotomy

Tubal ligation via minilaparotomy is performed with light sedation and local anesthesia. When done on a nonpregnant woman (at least 4 weeks after pregnancy) a 2- to 5-cm suprapubic incision is made. The patient is in lithotomy position, and the uterus is anteverted by insertion of a uterine elevator or by manual elevation. The tubes are occluded using the Pomeroy or Pritchard technique or by the application of spring clips or other mechanical device.

When tubal ligation is done 24 to 48 hours post partum, a 1.5- to 3-cm subumbilical minilaparotomy incision is made. Because the uterus is enlarged and out of the pelvic cavity, lithotomy position and uterine anteflexion are not necessary, and the tubes are easily accessible through the smaller incision. The tubes are occluded using the Pomeroy or Pritchard technique. Spring clips are not used because of the enlarged size of the fallopian tubes post partum (Hatcher et al, 1990, p. 400).

When done at the time of cesarean section, the proximal ends of the tubes are embedded in the uterine musculature, and the ends farthest from the uterus are embedded in the broad ligament. This is a 5- to 10-minute procedure and is almost 100% effective.

Laparoscopy

Laparoscopic tubal ligation is generally done under local anesthesia. The abdomen is insufflated with carbon dioxide or nitrous oxide to separate the organs, and the laparoscope is inserted through a small subumbilical incision. Each fallopian tube is isolated and then cauterized, cut, or clipped. The incision is closed and a Band-Aid applied. The laparoscopic approach is not used for immediate postpartum procedures because of the danger of injuring the enlarged, very vascular uterus.

Postoperative Course

There is minimal postoperative discomfort, and when the patient is fully recovered from the anesthesia and her vital signs are stable, she may be discharged.

For all methods, bleeding and infection are possible complications. For this reason, patients are instructed to report the presence of redness, swelling, or drainage at the site of the incision, oral temperature higher than 100°F (37.7°C), bleeding more than 12 hours after the procedure, or fainting.

The patient should rest for 24 to 48 hours after the procedure, and heavy lifting should be avoided for 1 week. After laparoscopy, sexual intercourse may be resumed when the patient feels comfortable enough to do so.

Reversal of Tubal Ligation

Tubal ligations are considered irreversible, although since 1977 microsurgery has been used for reconstruction, and a 50% to 60% success rate has been reported. Some reasons why women desire reconstructive surgery include death of spouse and remarriage, divorce and remarriage, death of existing children, and economics. Women who have had a tubal ligation before the age of 30 or immediately after an abortion or a term delivery or who had the sterilization done because of their spouse or partner's desire for it are those considered most likely to desire reversal of sterilization.

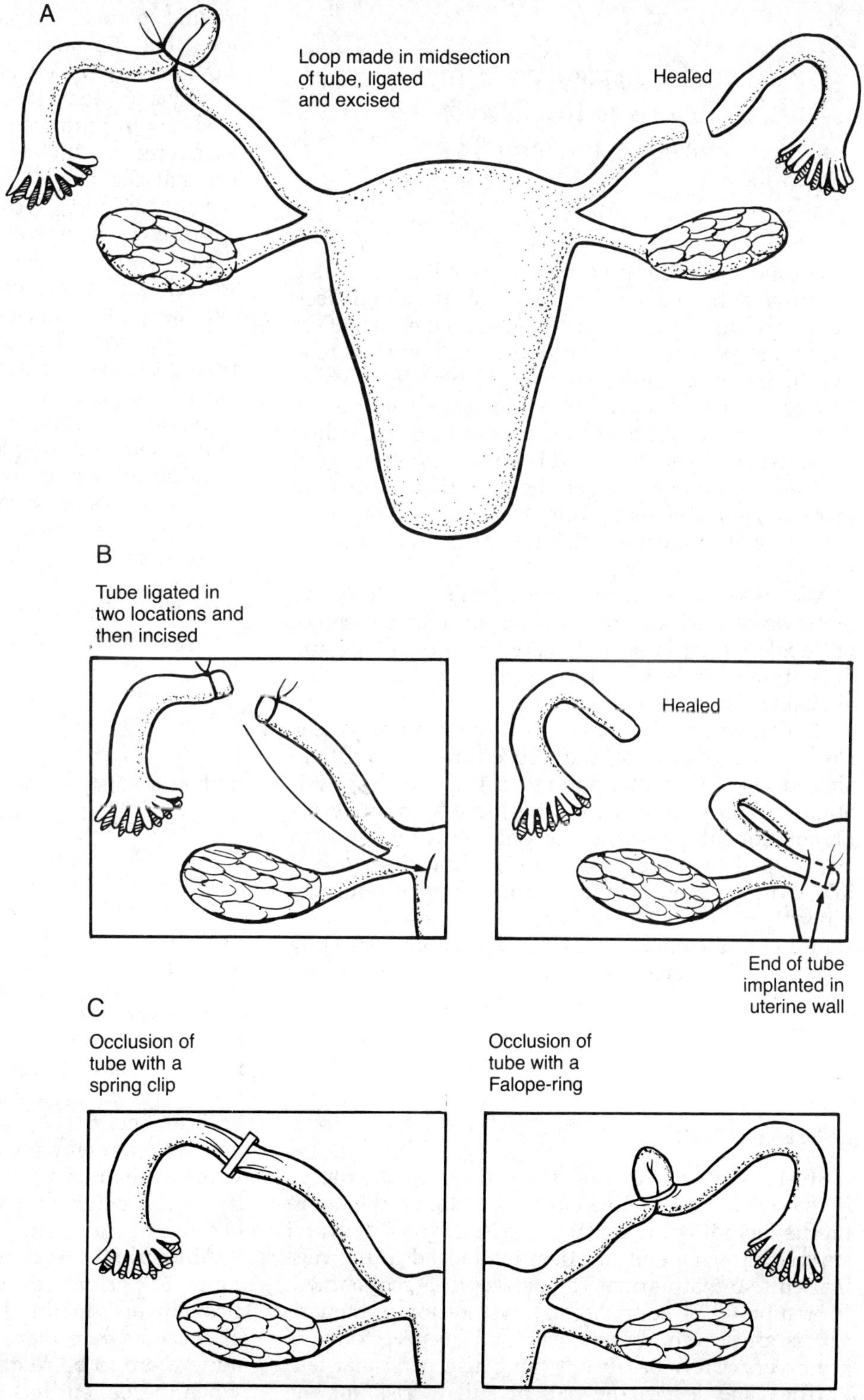

Figure 43–15.

Various techniques of tubal sterilization. (Modified and redrawn from Hatcher RA, et al. Contraceptive technology 1990–1992. 15th rev ed. New York: Irvington Publishers, 1990, p 392.)

When reconstructive surgery is done, adhesions resulting from ligation of the tube are cut away, and an end-to-end anastomosis is performed with or without the insertion of a plastic lumen. The longer the length of the tube after anastomosis, the greater is the rate of successful pregnancy. When the fimbriated ends of the tubes were excised in the original procedure, reconstruction is impossible.

Guidelines for Application of the Nursing Process to the Care of the Patient Having a Bilateral Tubal Ligation

In addition to basic preoperative nursing care, help ensure that the patient has made an informed decision regarding the surgery. Assess the extent to which the patient has considered the decision relative to potential future changes in her life such as loss of spouse, divorce, or remarriage. This can be done by raising hypothetical questions regarding these possibilities. Be careful that at no time your choice of words or manner suggests that the patient made a wrong or inappropriate decision. Your purpose is only to ascertain that the patient has thought through the possibilities.

Also assess the patient's knowledge of alternative methods of birth control to ascertain that the choice of tubal ligation was not made because of misunderstanding or lack of information regarding other available forms of contraception.

Finally, assess the patient's understanding of the irreversible nature of the procedure. The patient should know that although reconstructive surgery is attempted in selected cases, the success rate in terms of subsequent pregnancy is only little better than 50%, and hence the procedure is basically irreversible. Postoperatively monitor the patient's return to physiologic stability, and promote patient understanding and compliance with instructions regarding rest, sexual intercourse, and symptoms to be reported.

HYSTERECTOMY

Hysterectomy is an operation in which the uterus is removed. In a total or panhysterectomy, the entire uterus including the cervix is excised, and its several supporting ligaments are then reattached to the vaginal cuff so that normal vaginal depth is maintained. In a subtotal or supravaginal hysterectomy, the cervix is preserved. Today, subtotal hysterectomy is done very rarely because it can cause persistent leukorrhea and leaves the patient still at risk for the development of cervical cancer.

When the ovaries are removed along with the uterus, the procedure is a hysterectomy with bilateral oophorectomy. If the fallopian tubes are removed in addition to the uterus and the ovaries, the procedure is a hysterectomy with a bilateral salpingo-oophorectomy (BSO) (Fig. 43–16). The latter operation is done in many cases of pelvic malignancy. It may also be done for a benign disorder, depending on the philosophy of the physician and specific patient characteristics. Some surgeons believe that the adnexa (ovaries and fallopian tubes) should be removed at the time of hysterectomy as prophylaxis against cancer of the ovary, which is insidious in its development and therefore often not discovered until it is in an advanced stage. Others feel that the risk of ovarian cancer is not sufficient to warrant oophorectomy, because the role of the aging ovary in preventing skeletal or cardiovascular disease is not certain. In all cases, the patient's age, general health, and emotional status are considered, and the patient herself is included in the decision-making process. In a radical hysterectomy, the entire uterus, the nearby supporting (parametrial) tissues, and the uppermost part of the vagina are removed. A pelvic lymphadenectomy (removal of the pelvic lymph nodes) is frequently done in connection with a radical hysterectomy.

After a hysterectomy, a woman no longer menstruates or becomes pregnant. When a bilateral oophorectomy is also done, menopause occurs because the ovaries, source of estrogen and progesterone, have been removed. This is a surgical or induced menopause. Its symptoms are the same as those of natural menopause, although they may be more severe because of the abrupt decrease in hormone levels.

Routes of Hysterectomy

Hysterectomy may be performed by either the abdominal or vaginal route.

Vaginal Hysterectomy. The vaginal route is used when a vaginal repair is being done along with the hysterectomy. It may also be used when the uterus is being removed because of small myomata (tumors of the uterine muscle) or recurrent uterine bleeding due to endocrine imbalance. The major advantages of this procedure are that it can be done quickly, requires relatively light anesthesia, and has minimal postoperative discomfort. However, it is associated with an increased chance of postoperative infection and other complications, particularly in women younger than 35 years because of the great vascularity of the pelvis and in women older than 60 years because of the normal changes occurring with aging.

Abdominal Hysterectomy. Abdominal hysterectomy is performed when the uterus is in a fixed position or contains large myomatous tumors. It is also used when there are ovarian lesions, when the adnexa are to be removed as well as the uterus, and when the patient has had multiple pelvic operations. A total abdominal hysterectomy with bilateral sal-

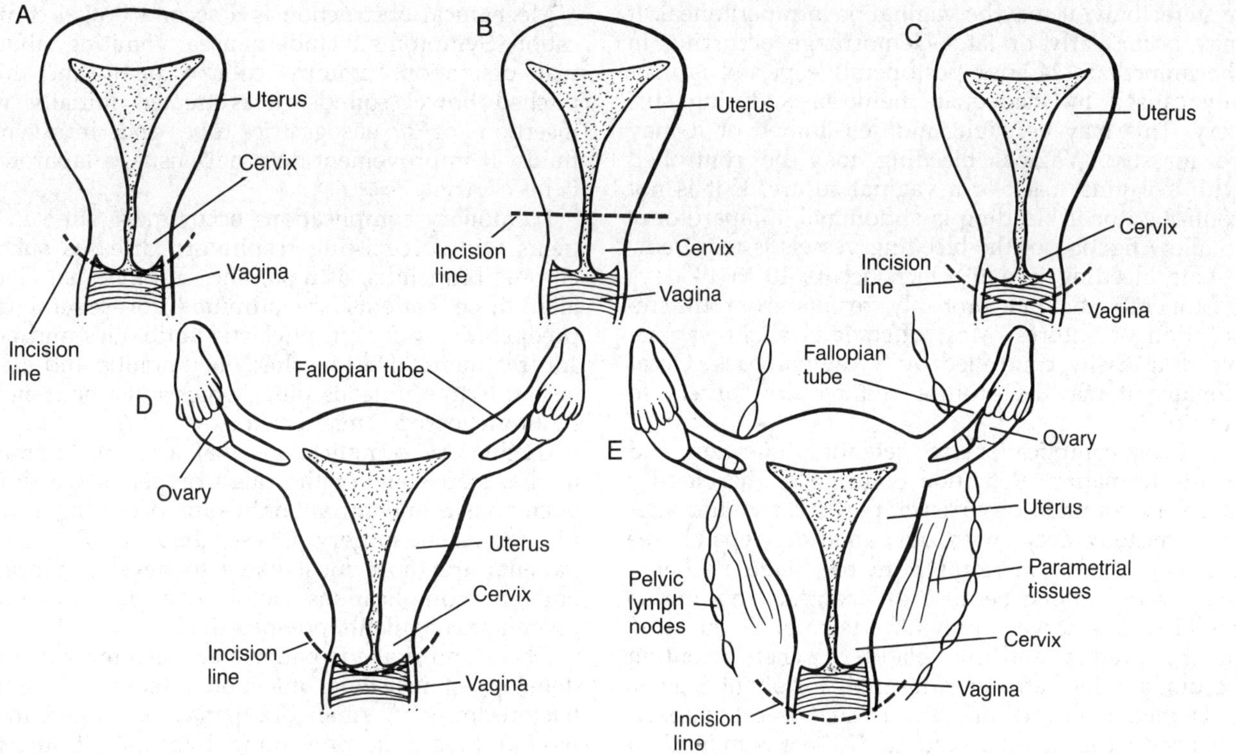

Figure 43–16.

Types of hysterectomy. A, Total hysterectomy. B, Subtotal hysterectomy. C, Total hysterectomy with vaginal cuff excision. D, Total hysterectomy with bilateral salpingo-oophorectomy. E, Radical hysterectomy with pelvic lymphadenectomy.

pingo-oophorectomy (removal of ovaries and fallopian tubes) is abbreviated TAH&BSO.

Preoperative Preparation

Preoperative preparation for a hysterectomy is the same as for any other vaginal or abdominal surgery. A perineal or abdominal preparation and shave are done. A vaginal douche and enema are ordered according to the surgeon's preference. Antibiotics may be given prophylactically 6 to 8 hours before surgery, during surgery, and for several doses after surgery.

Postoperative Course

Postoperatively, the patient has a perineal pad in place if a vaginal hysterectomy was done, and perineal pad and abdominal dressing if an abdominal approach was used. If a radical hysterectomy was done, catheters connected to a Hemovac may be used to draw excess fluid from the area of surgery. The catheters are inserted below the incision and kept in place until there is only scant drainage, which is usually 3 to 5 days.

An intravenous fluid line is maintained until adequate amounts of fluid are taken orally and tolerated well. Diet is then progressed as tolerated. Because hysterectomy involves movement of the bladder, most patients have urethral or suprapubic catheter drainage for 2 to 3 days postoperatively.

The patient is ambulatory in 24 hours and has her sutures or staples removed on day 5.

If a vaginal hysterectomy was done, and a vaginal pack inserted, the pack is usually removed in 24 to 48 hours. Occasional abdominal cramping may occur, and there may be no sensation in the vagina for several months.

Suture removal is unnecessary because the sutures used are generally resorbable.

Hormone replacement therapy is generally prescribed for women following hysterectomy and bilateral oophorectomy, provided that the patient does not have a carcimona of the breast or reproductive system that may be stimulated by it. When ordered, it is primarily as prophylaxis against osteoporosis.

Complications

Postoperative complications of a hysterectomy include hemorrhage, hematoma, infection, thrombophlebitis, nerve injury, and pulmonary, bowel, and bladder problems. Complications occur more frequently in patients who are elderly or obese or who have a concurrent problem such as diabetes, emphysema, or a cardiovascular disorder.

Hemorrhage following an abdominal hysterectomy may be abdominal or vaginal. After a vaginal hysterectomy, it may be vaginal or intraperitoneal. It may occur early or late. Hemorrhage occurring in the immediate 24-hour postoperative period is usually caused by inadequate hemostasis during surgery. This may be slight and self-limited or it may be massive. Vaginal bleeding may be controlled with a vaginal pack or a vaginal suture. If it is not controlled or if bleeding is abdominal, a laparotomy to allow ligation of the bleeding vessels is required.

Late bleeding is that which occurs 10 to 14 days postoperatively and probably results from the resorption of sutures. Most often it is slight vaginal bleeding easily controlled by a vaginal pack. Occasionally, it may be profuse and require surgery to control it.

Urinary complications are retention, infection, and fistula formation. Retention of urine in the bladder is a very common occurrence, particularly after vaginal hysterectomy with an anterior repair (see Chapter 44). It can result from the bladder's being temporarily atonic because of analgesia, trauma to the bladder's nerve supply, or edema at the junction of the urethra and the bladder. When retention occurs, a Foley catheter is inserted for about 5 days. It is then removed, and the patient is catheterized for residual urine after voiding. If there is more than 100 ml residual urine, the Foley catheter is reinserted and the cycle begun again. To avoid this problem, a suprapubic tube may be inserted at the time of operation to provide for urinary drainage. The suprapubic tube is clamped after 5 days, and the majority of patients spontaneously void at that time.

Cystitis is also a frequent postoperative complication among patients with indwelling catheters and therefore is common after a vaginal hysterectomy and repair. It is treated with antibiotics chosen on the basis of a urine culture and sensitivity. Occasionally pyelonephritis with its high temperature, chills, and flank pain occurs. As with cystitis, antibiotics are prescribed on the basis of a urine culture and sensitivity. If there is no response to the medication, a pyelogram is done to rule out operative damage to the urinary tract.

Rarely a fistula may occur as a result of damage to the ureter or bladder. Persons at greatest risk for fistula development are those who are having a radical hysterectomy (excision of uterus and supporting tissue, adnexa, upper vagina, and pelvic lymph nodes), especially if radiation therapy preceded the surgery.

Bowel complications occur almost exclusively after an abdominal hysterectomy, especially when large tumors are involved. Paralytic ileus is the result of nerve trauma associated with handling the viscera. It is characterized by extreme abdominal distention, nausea, and vomiting. There are no bowel sounds, and there is no crampy colicky pain. Treatment consists of insertion of a nasogastric tube or restriction of food and fluids until bowel sounds are normal, the administration of a bowel stimulant, and enemas.

Mechanical obstruction is a second bowel complication. Symptoms include nausea, vomiting, abdominal distention, crampy colicky pain, and high-pitched bowel sounds. It is treated initially with insertion of a nasogastric tube and intravenous fluids. If improvement does not ensue, a laparotomy is necessary.

Pulmonary complications occur most often in patients with preexisting respiratory diseases such as chronic bronchitis, asthma, and emphysema. Generally, these patients are admitted for several days preoperatively for prophylactic antibiotics and aerosol treatments. Despite this, pneumonitis and atelectasis due to a mucous plug, which must be removed by bronchoscopy, may occur.

Circulatory complications that are due to trauma to the deep veins of the thigh or pelvis are thromboembolism and thrombophlebitis occurring 1 week or more after surgery. Obese, diabetic, or cachectic patients are those most likely to develop thromboembolic complications, and they are sometimes given anticoagulants preoperatively.

Obese and diabetic patients are also most likely to develop an incisional infection after an abdominal hysterectomy. A small drain may be placed in the wound to aid in preventing infection. If infection does occur, it is treated with local heat, antibiotics, and drainage of any abscesses that form.

Other potential complications are evisceration, hematoma, and nerve injury. Patients at risk for evisceration are the obese and the very thin, as well as those with respiratory problems or malignant disease treated with radiation. Signs of impending evisceration are low-grade fever and serosanguineous discharge from the incision.

Hematoma is a delayed complication occurring with both abdominal and vaginal procedures. Its incidence is highest in young women with an abundant blood supply to the pelvic organs. The more extensive the surgery, the more likely a hematoma is to occur. Signs of hematoma are increased temperature and decreased hematocrit. Occasionally, a hematoma may be palpated in the lower pelvis.

Injury to the femoral nerve may occur as a result of prolonged pressure during the operation. Symptoms are numbness, paresthesia, and weakness of the thigh. This is a transient phenomenon, and no medical treatment is usually necessary.

Application of the Nursing Process to the Care of the Patient Having a Hysterectomy

PREOPERATIVE NURSING CARE

Nursing care for the patient scheduled for a hysterectomy is similar to that for any preoperative patient (see Chapter 4 and Nursing Care Guide 44–1), with the following considerations. Assessing the patient's understanding of the procedure and its effects and providing clarification as needed are particularly important because of the many common misconceptions regarding hysterectomy. Among these are that a hysterectomy causes loss of sexual function, loss of attractiveness to men, obesity, hirsutism, premature aging, or senility. It is also a common misconception that removal of the cervix results in a decrease in length of the vagina and a loss of sexual satisfaction.

POSTOPERATIVE NURSING CARE

Assessment

Assess the physiologic stabilization of the patient by monitoring vital signs and checking for bleeding. Check vital signs every 15 minutes until stable and then with decreasing frequency as indicated by the patient's condition.

Check the abdominal dressing and perineal pad for bleeding every 15 minutes for 2 hours, every hour for 8 hours, and then every shift. A moderate amount of serosanguineous drainage normally occurs.

When an abdominal hysterectomy has been done, assess wound healing when the dressing is removed. This is usually on the fifth postoperative day unless a dressing change is needed prior to this time because the original dressing is no longer dry and intact. Observe the wound for redness, edema, and drainage, and note whether the suture line is approximated.

Following a hysterectomy, pain in the area of the incision is expected. Assess the severity of the patient's pain, and note to what extent it interferes with coughing, deep breathing, and moving.

Assess adequacy of urinary elimination by checking for bladder distention, measuring fluid intake and output, and catheterizing for residual urine. Keep in mind that a decrease in output or low back pain may indicate accidental ligation of a ureter during surgery.

If the patient has an indwelling catheter postoperatively, measure output each shift, and check the drainage system for improper position, kinks, or accidental compression by the side rail, which can impede drainage. After removal of the catheter, continue to measure output for 2 or 3 days. Also, palpate the bladder for distention, and if ordered, catheterize the patient for residual urine. If the residual is more than 100 ml, notify the physician. Patients who do not have an indwelling catheter after surgery should empty the bladder within the first 8 postoperative hours.

Assess gastrointestinal function, because after a hysterectomy all patients have decreased peristalsis secondary to the effects of anesthesia, handling of the bowel during surgery, and pain medication. Listen for bowel sounds and observe for abdominal distention, belching, and passage of flatus. Question about gas pains, and note size, color, and consistency of bowel movements.

Because thrombophlebitis is a common postoperative complication of hysterectomy, observe for signs and symptoms of developing phlebitis, such as pain, redness or heat in the calf, and a positive Homans' sign.

Because hysterectomy involves loss of a body part and in the premenopausal woman loss of the capacity for childbearing, be certain to assess the patient's psychological response to the surgery. Crying spells or transient feelings of sadness or depression are not unusual, but verbalization of negative feelings about the effect of the surgery on her, fear of other people's reactions, and preoccupation with the loss of the uterus can indicate a disturbance in self-concept and difficulty coping.

Because of the organs involved, also assess the patient for indications of sexual dysfunction. These include behavior that seeks reassurance of femininity and desirability and verbal statement of an actual or expected problem with sexual desire, performance, or satisfaction.

Nursing Diagnoses and Planning

Nursing diagnoses and related expected patient outcomes most commonly applicable to patients who have had a hysterectomy include the following:

NDx: Pain related to tissue trauma secondary to surgical excision of the uterus

Planning: Patient outcomes

1. Patient reports that pain is relieved.
2. Nonverbal signs of pain such as grimacing or guarding are absent.
3. Patient splints incision when coughing or moving.
4. Patient gets out of bed, sits, and ambulates without undue discomfort.
5. Patient uses personal methods of coping with pain.
6. Patient performs relaxation exercises.

NDx: Impaired physical mobility related to postoperative abdominal and pelvic discomfort

Planning: Patient outcomes

1. Patient effectively helps herself sit up and get out of bed when allowed to do so.
2. Patient ambulates in room when physician's orders allow.

NDx: High risk for ineffective airway clearance related to shallow respirations and ineffective coughing

Planning: Patient outcomes

1. Respirations are of normal depth.
2. Secretions are expectorated.

3. Respirations are silent.
4. Breath sounds are clear.

NDx: High risk for altered tissue perfusion related to interruption of venous blood flow

Planning: Patient outcomes
1. Patient dorsiflexes feet 20 to 25 times each hour while awake and on bed rest.
2. Patient avoids flexing knees and hips, crossing legs, and assuming other positions that impede venous return.
3. Patient wears antithromboembolic stockings that are smoothly fitted without twists or wrinkles.
4. Patient willingly gets out of bed and ambulates as soon as her physical condition allows.
5. Calves are free of heat, redness, and swelling, and Homans' sign is negative.
6. Symptoms of pulmonary embolism are absent: respirations are of normal rate and depth, and the patient is free of cyanosis, chest pain, and hemoptysis.

NDx: High risk for sexual dysfunction related to removal of the uterus

Planning: Patient outcomes
1. Patient describes normal sexual structure and function and changes resulting from hysterectomy.
2. Patient identifies common misconceptions regarding the effect of hysterectomy on libido and sexual enjoyment.
3. Patient discusses sexual concerns with partner.

NDx: High risk for altered health maintenance related to insufficient knowledge of discharge instructions

Planning: Patient outcomes
1. Patient describes limitations on activity, as specified in Chart 43–6.
2. Patient lists symptoms to be reported, as specified in Chart 43–6.
3. Patient describes expected emotional reactions, as specified in Chart 43–6.
4. Patient states date and time of follow-up visit.

Nursing Interventions

NDx: Pain
Administer narcotic analgesic and sedative drugs liberally in accordance with physician's orders during the first 2 postoperative days because pain is most severe during this time. Give at scheduled times to prevent anticipatory pain. By the third day, the patient is generally more comfortable, and medications can be decreased in strength and frequency. Use independent nursing measures to relieve pain, such as maintenance of a comfortable environment, position changes, and backrubs throughout the postoperative period because they enhance the effect of analgesics as well as decrease the need for them. Also teach and assist the patient with relaxation exercises.

If the patient's discomfort is primarily from gas in the bowel, apply heat to the abdomen, ambulate, and insert a rectal tube as ordered to provide relief. For discomfort on coughing or moving, teach the patient to splint the incision and to assist in getting up and sitting down as described later.

NDx: Impaired physical mobility
Encourage early ambulation because it promotes good circulation, muscle tone, lung expansion, and bowel function. After an uncomplicated hysterectomy, the patient should be out of bed within 24 hours. A longer period of bed rest is required when the operative procedure is more extensive or when the patient has other coexistent health problems.

Assist the patient in getting out of bed with the least strain and discomfort to facilitate ambulation. Elevate the head of the bed, and instruct the patient to do the following:

1. Turn on her side, facing the side of the bed she is going to get out of.
2. Bend her knees as if she is sitting in a chair.
3. Put her feet over the edge of the bed.
4. Push up on her elbow.
5. Sit up straight.

If the patient complains of discomfort on sitting down, instruct her to pull the buttocks together before lowering herself onto the chair. Gradually encourage her to ambulate in her room and then in the corridor as tolerated.

NDx: High risk for ineffective airway clearance
Medicate the patient as needed for pain, because pain can lead to shallow respirations. Place the patient in semi-Fowler's position or flat with pillows under her shoulders to encourage chest expansion. Keep clothing and bedding loose so that the chest is not constricted. Instruct the patient to cough and deep breathe every 2 hours for at least 24 hours after surgery, and encourage expectoration of any secretions. If the patient had an abdominal hysterectomy, support the incision by splinting the abdomen with a pillow or folded blanket to facilitate effective coughing and deep breathing.

NDx: High risk for altered tissue perfusion
Monitor for factors that predispose to venous stasis and hence to thrombus formation. Check that there is no undue pressure or obstruction in the popliteal area. Do not maintain the patient's legs and thighs in a flexed position because this impedes venous

Chart 43–6.

NURSING GUIDE TO PATIENT EDUCATION FOR SELF-MANAGEMENT: DISCHARGE INSTRUCTIONS AFTER HYSTERECTOMY

Instruct the patient to:

Report any bleeding, other vaginal discharge, or temperature elevation to the health care professional.
Avoid tub baths for 2 to 3 weeks.
Avoid activities that increase pelvic congestion for several months. These include sitting for long periods of time, jogging, fast walking, horseback riding, and douching.
Be prepared for feelings of weakness and fatigue.
Avoid strenuous activities such as heavy lifting and vacuum cleaning for 6 to 8 weeks.
Avoid sexual intercourse for 3 weeks after vaginal hysterectomy and for 6 weeks after an abdominal hysterectomy.
Remember that after an abdominal hysterectomy, abdominal soreness and a feeling that the vagina is narrow and short may occur during intercourse for 3 to 4 weeks.
Recognize that periods of emotional lability and feelings of depression and sadness are normal.
Return for a follow-up appointment on *(specify date and time).*

return. Keep legs extended and uncrossed. To further aid in preventing thrombophlebitis, lower the head of the bed to the flat position every 2 hours for the first 24 hours to prevent stasis of blood in the pelvic veins. After the initial 24-hour period, do this every 4 hours until the patient is ambulatory. Teach the patient to change position and dorsiflex her feet 20 to 25 times every hour while awake until she is ambulatory. Apply antiembolic stockings or Ace bandages as ordered to support venous return. If the patient has varicose veins, intermittent elevation of the legs for 2- or 3-hour periods may be ordered to prevent venous stasis.

NDx: High risk for sexual dysfunction
Review normal sexual function and related structures, and describe the effects of the hysterectomy on them. Identify common misconceptions regarding the effect of a hysterectomy on sexual function and enjoyment and present the correct facts related to each. Throughout the discussion, encourage the patient to share what she has heard or what she thinks and to ask any questions she may have. Also encourage the patient to share concerns about future sexual activity with her partner, and provide time and privacy for such discussion.

NDx: High risk for altered health maintenance
Instruct the patient in self-care after discharge as specified in Chart 43–6. Also be certain that the patient knows when to return for her follow-up appointment and the importance of it.

Evaluation

Evaluate the effectiveness of nursing care for a patient who has had a hysterectomy by comparing the patient's status with the expected patient outcomes. Examples of specific outcomes for patients who have had a hysterectomy have been provided in the Planning section.

VAGINAL PACKING

The vagina may be packed with gauze to provide pressure to control postoperative bleeding or to hold a prolapsed uterus in place within the vagina in order to decrease edema and aid healing of ulcerated areas prior to corrective surgery. (See Chapter 44 for discussion of uterine prolapse.)

Insertion of a vaginal packing is a sterile procedure that requires good lighting and good exposure of the vagina. The patient empties her bladder and is assisted into a left Sims' or dorsal recumbent position. The vulva is cleansed. If the pack is to control bleeding, a speculum is inserted, and any free blood or clots are swabbed from the vagina. Gauze is then packed firmly into the posterior fornix, the anterior fornix, and then the remainder of the vagina. If the pack is being used to support a prolapsed uterus, the organ is manually positioned and then the packing is inserted. A T-binder is used to hold the pack in place.

The amount of packing used is recorded in the patient's chart.

Guidelines for Application of the Nursing Process to the Care of the Patient with Vaginal Packing

If the purpose of the pack is to control bleeding, inspect the vaginal area to assess continuing blood loss. Monitor voiding for as long as the packing is in place, because the pressure of the packing can impinge on the bladder neck.

The Elderly: Special Considerations

In the geriatric patient, the changes initiated at menopause have become marked. The pubic hair is thin and gray or, in some cases, absent. The labia are pale and thin and possibly wrinkled. The ovaries are atrophied and no longer able to be palpated on pelvic examination. The fallopian tubes, uterus, and vagina have decreased in size, and pelvic support is weak because of atrophy of the pelvic fascia and muscles. The vaginal mucosa is thin and the rugae have disappeared, leaving the vagina less elastic. Vaginal secretions are decreased and are less acid.

Although a Pap smear may not be deemed necessary for women older than age 65 whose previous smears have never showed an abnormality, an annual pelvic examination is needed to ensure early detection of other diseases of the reproductive system that affect the older woman. A small or medium speculum is used for the pelvic examination, and assistance must be provided as needed to enable the patient to get on and off the examining table and to assume lithotomy position. At the time of examination, the patient is carefully assessed for signs of vaginitis because the thinning of the vaginal epithelium and change in pH of the vagina predispose to infection. If appropriate to her lifestyle, determine whether dyspareunia is a problem, and recommend the use of a vaginal lubricant to replace normal secretions.

Bibliography

Allen ME. A holistic view of sexuality and the aged. Holistic Nurs Pract 1987; 1(4):76.

Beal MW. Understanding cervical cytology. Nurse Pract 1987; 12(3):8.

Belfort P, et al (eds). General gynecology. Park Ridge, NJ: Parthenon, 1989.

Benson RC, Pernoll M. Current obstetric and gynecologic diagnosis and treatment. Norwalk, CT: Appleton & Lange, 1986.

Bent AE, Ostergard DR. Endometrial ablation with the neodymium: Yag laser. Obstet Gynecol 1990; 75(6):923.

Berek J. Practical gynecologic oncology. Baltimore: Williams & Wilkins, 1988.

Blackledge GRP, Jordan JA, Shingleton HM (eds). Textbook of gynecologic oncology. Philadelphia, WB Saunders, 1991.

Brocklehurst JC (ed). Textbook of geriatric medicine and gerontology. 3rd ed. New York: Churchill Livingstone, 1985.

Brown MA, Woods NF. Correlates of dysmenorrhea: A challenge to past stereotypes. JOGNN 1984; 13(4):259.

Byers JP. Sexuality and the elderly. Geriatr Nurs 1983; 4(5):293.

Carpenito LJ. Nursing diagnosis: Application to clinical practice. Philadelphia: JB Lippincott, 1993.

Challener RC, Kaufman B. Fetal venous air embolism following sequential unsheathed (bare) and sheathed quartz fiber Nd: YAG laser endometrial ablation. Anesthesiology 1990; 73(3):548.

Cobb JO. Demystifying menopause. Can Nurse 1987; 83(7):16.

Denny MS, Koren ME, Wisby M. Gynecological health needs of elderly women. J Gerontol Nurs 1989; 15(1);33.

DiSaia PJ, Creasman WT. Clinical gynecologic oncology. St. Louis: CV Mosby, 1988.

Electrocautery versus Nd:YAG laser in rectoscopic ablation and laparoscopic cholecystectomy. Laser Nurs 1990; 4(4):32.

Eliopoulos C. Gerontological nursing. New York: Harper & Row, 1987.

Eltinger B. Estrogen and postmenopausal osteoporosis. AAOHN J 1987; 35(12): 543.

Esberger KK, Hughes ST Jr. Nursing care of the aged. Norwalk, CT: Appleton & Lange, 1989.

Fishbein EG. Women at midlife. The transition to menopause. Nurs Clin North Am 1992; 27(4):951.

Fogel CI, Woods NF. Health care of women: A nursing perspective. St. Louis: CV Mosby, 1981.

Frazer J. The dilemma of the perimenopausal female. Holistic Nurs Pract 1987; 1(4):67.

Friedrich EG Jr. Vulvar disease. 2nd ed. Philadelphia: WB Saunders, 1983.

Gallagher MT, Kahn C. Lasers: Scalpels of light. RN 1990; 53(5):46.

Gambert SR (ed). Handbook of geriatrics. New York: Plenum Press, 1987.

Glowacki GA. A new look at osteoporosis and estrogen therapy. Compr Ther 1988; 14(2):49.

Goldfarb HA. A review of 35 endometrial ablations using the Nd:YAG laser for recurrent menometrorrhagia. Obstet Gynecol 1990; 76(5 Pt 1):833.

Gordon AG, Lewis VB. Gynecological endoscopy. Philadelphia: JB Lippincott, 1988.

Guyton AC. Textbook of medical physiology. 8th ed. Philadelphia: WB Saunders, 1991.

Hacker NF, Moore JG. Essentials of obstetrics and gynecology. 2nd ed. Philadelphia: WB Saunders, 1992.

Ham RJ. Primary care geriatrics. Littleton, MA: PSG Publishing, 1986.

Hambridge MC. Laparoscopy: A revolution in gynecologic surgery. Todays OR Nurse 1987; 9(4):30.

Hatcher RA, et al. Contraceptive technology 1990–1992. New York: Irvington Publishers, 1990.

Jones HW, Wentz GS (eds). Novak's textbook of gynecology. 11th ed. Baltimore: Williams & Wilkins, 1988.

Kumar V, Cotran RS, Robbins SL. Basic pathology. 5th ed. Philadelphia: WB Saunders, 1992.

Lichtman R, Papera S. Well-woman gynecology. Norwalk, CT: Appleton & Lange, 1989.

Lindsay R. Estrogen therapy in the prevention and management of osteoporosis. Am J Obstet Gynecol 1987; 156:1347.

Lindsay R. Osteoporosis: An updated approach to prevention and management. Geriatrics 1989; 44(1):45.

Mackay EV, Beischer NA, Pepperell RJ, Wood C. Illustrated handbook of gynaecology. 2nd ed. Philadelphia: WB Saunders, 1992.
Maddox M.A. Women at midlife. Hormone replacement therapy. Nurs Clin North Am 1992; 27(4):959.
Matteson MA, McConnell ES. Gerontological nursing: Concepts and practice. Philadelphia: WB Saunders, 1988.
McKeon V. Cruel myths and clinical facts about menopause. RN 1989; 52(6):52.
Modica MM, Timor-Tritsch IE. Transvaginal sonography provides a sharper view into the pelvis. JOGNN 1988; 17(2):89.
Moore J. Vaginal hysterectomy. Nurs Clin North Am 1988; 23(4):1114.
Morrison-Beedy D, et al. Sexual assessment and the aging female. Nurs Pract 1989; 14(12):35.
National Institute on Aging. The menopause time of life. NIH Publication No. 86-2461. July 1986.
O'Rahilly R. Gardner, Gray and O'Rahilly Anatomy: A regional study of human structure. 5th ed. Philadelphia: WB Saunders, 1986.
Phipps JH, Lewis BV, Prior MV, Roberts T. Experimental and clinical studies with radiofrequency-induced thermal endometrial ablation for functional menorrhagia. Obstet Gynecol 1990; 76(5 Pt 1):876.
Poorman SG. Human sexuality and the nursing process. Norwalk, CT: Appleton & Lange, 1988.
Primrose RB. Taking the tension out of pelvic exams. Am J Nurs 1984; 84(1):72.
Rickert B. Estrogen replacement: Making informed choices. RN 1992; 55(9): 26.
Rubin D. Gynecologic cancer: Cervical, vulvar, and vaginal malignancies. RN 1987; 50(5):56.
Rubin D. Gynecologic cancer: Uterine and ovarian malignancies. RN 1987; 50(6):52.
Saleh JW. Laparoscopy. Philadelphia: WB Saunders, 1988.
Smith LH, Wyngaarden JB. Cecil review of general internal medicine. 4th ed. Philadelphia: WB Saunders, 1989.
Stanfill PH. Psychosocial implications of hysterectomy. JOGNN 1982; 11(5):318.
Thompson JD, Rock J. The Linde's operative gynecology. 7th ed. Philadelphia: JB Lippincott, 1991.
Travis S. Older adults' sexuality and remarriage. J Gerontol Nurs 1987; 13(3):8.
Treybig M. Primary dysmenorrhea or endometriosis? Nurse Pract 1989; 14(5):8.
Willson JR. Obstetrics and gynecology. 9th ed. St. Louis: CV Mosby, 1991.
Wilson MA. Menstrual disorders. JOGNN (Suppl) 1984; 13(2):11S.
Young RL, Goldzieher JW. Current status of postmenopausal oestrogen therapy. Drugs 1987; 33:95.
Youngkin EQ. Estrogen replacement therapy and the estraderm transdermal system. Nurse Pract 1990; 15(5):19.

Chapter Forty-four

NURSING CARE *of Women with Disorders of the Reproductive System*

The female reproductive system can be affected by a wide variety of disorders including inflammations, infections, functional and structural abnormalities, and neoplastic processes. The majority of these disorders are not life threatening but nonetheless can have a profound effect on physical comfort, self-esteem, and the capacity for sexually satisfying relationships.

Infections and Inflammations

Vulvitis

ETIOLOGY AND PATHOPHYSIOLOGY

Vulvitis, or inflammation of the vulva, may be a manifestation of a systemic disease, an extension of a vaginitis, or a local disorder. The skin of the vulva is subject to all the inflammatory disorders that can affect any other skin area. However, it is particularly prone to inflammation from mechanical or chemical irritation because of its anatomic location. Factors such as tight-fitting clothing, exposure to urine, fecal matter, vaginal discharges, and secretions of vulvar glands as well as exposure to external irritants such as bath and laundry soap, feminine hygiene sprays and powders, spermicides, and vaginal lubricants containing propylene glycol are potential sources of irritation.

CLINICAL MANIFESTATIONS

Pruritus is the classic symptom of vulvitis. In addition, there is usually a burning sensation, which worsens on urination or defecation. The vulvar tissues appear red and swollen. If the patient has scratched to try and relieve the itch, abrasions and areas of secondary infection may be present. If the vulvitis is an extension of a vaginitis, a vaginal discharge may be present.

MEDICAL DIAGNOSIS

A complete physical evaluation is done to check for any systemic disorder such as diabetes that may be the cause of the vulvitis. A pelvic examination is done, and vaginal smears or cultures are obtained to determine whether a source of infection is present in the vagina. A detailed history focusing on medical risk factors, personal hygiene, and psychogenic factors is obtained to identify potential causal factors.

MEDICAL MANAGEMENT

Medical management depends on the cause of the vulvitis. Along with therapy for the underlying problem (when one is identified), local measures are prescribed for the relief of symptoms.

Application of the Nursing Process to the Care of the Patient with Vulvitis

Assessment

The assessment of a patient with vulvitis includes the history and current status of her symptoms; a review of medical risk factors, stress-related factors, and personal habits that can potentially contribute to the inflammatory process; and an inspection of the area.

Obtain information about the patient's symptomatology, including local and systemic symptoms experienced, their duration, factors that can be related to their onset or exacerbation, relief measures used, and the effectiveness of these measures. Explore the patient's patterns of perineal hygiene; use of perfumed soaps, powders, or other cosmetic products that may be irritating or causing an allergic reaction, and type of undergarments usually worn.

Inspect the vulvar area for irritation, scratch marks, parasites such as *Pediculus pubis* (pubic lice or "crabs"), and discharge.

Ascertain the patient's perception of the cause and significance of the problem, which will be used later as a guide in planning health teaching.

Nursing Diagnoses and Planning

Nursing diagnoses and related expected patient outcomes most commonly applicable to patients with vulvitis include the following:

NDx: Pain related to the inflammatory process

Planning: Patient outcomes
1. Patient reports that discomfort is relieved.
2. Vulvar tissue is free of erythema and edema.

NDx: High risk for altered health maintenance related to insufficient knowledge of measures to aid in preventing recurrence of vulvitis

Planning: Patient outcomes
1. Patient lists materials and types of clothing that predispose to inflammation of the vulva.
2. Patient lists types of cleansing and hygienic products that can cause an allergic reaction.
3. Patient describes proper techniques of cleansing the vulva, explaining how each helps to prevent vulvitis.

Nursing Interventions

NDx: Pain
Assist or instruct the patient in the use of comfort measures such as sitz baths, warm compresses, and anesthetic sprays or ointments.

Chart 44–1.

NURSING GUIDE TO PATIENT EDUCATION FOR SELF-MANAGEMENT: PREVENTION OF VULVITIS

Teach the patient about the following:

Cleansing the vulva

Do not use soap between the labia: Odors are on the pubic hair, not on the skin, and rinsing is sufficient to remove secretions.

Rinse the vulva thoroughly after washing because soap residue supports bacterial growth and is irritating to the skin. Be particularly careful to rinse and dry the vulvar area completely when taking a shower.

Keeping the vulva dry

Moisture can cause maceration of the skin and is conducive to bacterial growth. Frequently change perineal pads used during menstruation or used because of stress incontinence or a vaginal discharge.

Select clothing that allows for adequate air circulation.

- Avoid tight-fitting pantyhose, pantsuits, and slacks.
- Wear 100% cotton underpants or, as a second choice, those with a cotton crotch.
- Do not wear underpants to bed.
- Wear knee-high or thigh-high stockings whenever possible.
  Wear pantyhose with a cotton crotch, and never wear them under slacks.

Protecting the vulva from irritation

Do not scratch the vulvar area.

Avoid clothing that rubs against the area.

Do not wear synthetic fibers and colored fabrics in direct contact with the vulva because they retain warmth and moisture and may cause an allergic reaction.

Avoid strong and excessive amounts of laundry soaps, fabric softeners, talcum powder, perfumed soaps, scented or colored toilet paper, and deodorant sprays, which can also cause allergic reactions that produce itching, rashes, and irritation.

Presoak underpants in one-half strength bleach for 20 minutes and then wash on a hot laundry cycle or boil underpants for 20 minutes and then launder as usual to kill yeast that may be harbored in the garments (Kaufman, 1989).

Use cornstarch if needed to keep the area dry and prevent irritation of adjacent skin surfaces.

NDx: High risk for altered health maintenance

Instruct the patient as specified in Chart 44–1 to help her avoid a recurrence of the vulvitis.

Evaluation

Evaluate the effectiveness of nursing care for a patient with vulvitis by comparing the patient's status with the expected patient outcomes. Examples of specific outcomes for patients with vulvitis have been provided in the Planning section.

Vaginitis

Vaginitis is an inflammation of the vagina. It is a common, often recurrent gynecologic disorder that in most cases is not serious but is very uncomfortable and annoying.

ETIOLOGY AND PATHOPHYSIOLOGY

Vaginitis may be due to mechanical irritation of the vagina as from a pessary (device inserted in the vagina to support the uterus) or tampons; chemical irritation as from douche solutions, contraceptive creams, or vaginal deodorants; infestation with parasites such as pinworms; or an infectious process.

Infections of the vagina are caused by a great variety of organisms. Among the most common are *Candida albicans, Trichomonas vaginalis,* and *Gardnerella vaginalis.* Other sexually transmitted causative organisms include *Treponema pallidum, Neisseria gonorrhoeae, Chlamydia trachomatis,* and the herpes simplex virus. (See Chapter 47 for a discussion of sexually transmitted vaginitis.) Nonsexually transmitted organisms that cause vaginitis include *Streptococcus, Staphylococcus,* and *Escherichia coli.*

Factors that predispose to the development of vaginitis are those that cause an overall decrease in body defenses and those that alter the vaginal defenses specifically. Malnutrition, stress, systemic disease such as diabetes, broad-spectrum antibiotic therapy, pregnancy, postmenopausal thinning of the vaginal epithelium, allergies, use of oral contraceptives, use of Today contraceptive sponge, excessive douching, use of tampons, inadequate personal hygiene, and excessive sucrose and lactose in the diet (Kaufman, 1989) all increase the risk of vaginitis. Sexual activity without the use of condoms and sexual activity with multiple sexual partners also predispose to vaginitis by increasing the risk of exposure to causative organisms.

CLINICAL MANIFESTATIONS

The most common symptom of vaginitis regardless of cause is leukorrhea, although the amount, color, consistency, and odor of the discharge vary with the specific causative agent (Table 44–1). Vulvar irritation and itching, especially on urination, are also associated with most cases of vaginitis.

MEDICAL DIAGNOSIS

A pelvic examination is done to allow inspection of the vaginal mucosa and to rule out the presence of a foreign body. With vaginitis, the mucosa generally appears erythematous and congested. A vaginal smear or culture is taken to identify a specific infective organism. A clean-catch urinalysis may be necessary to distinguish between cystitis or urethritis and vaginitis.

Table 44–1. CHARACTERISTICS OF VAGINAL DISCHARGE ASSOCIATED WITH DIFFERENT TYPES OF VAGINITIS

CAUSE OF VAGINITIS	CHARACTERISTIC DISCHARGE
Mechanical irritation (e.g., from wearing tampons or pessary)	Serosanguineous or purulent with possible foul odor
Chemical irritation (e.g., from douche solutions, feminine hygiene products, or Today contraceptive sponge)	Moderate to copious with or without odor; white, gray, or yellow
Infectious process	
Gardnerella vaginalis	Greater than normal amount; gray-white with fishy odor
Candida albicans	Scant white; cottage cheese–like
Trichomonas vaginalis	Copious, sometimes frothy, yellow-green

MEDICAL MANAGEMENT

If the vaginitis is due to a foreign body or a chemical irritant, the basic treatment is to remove or eliminate the offending agent. If an infectious process is involved, anti-infectives specific to the causative agent are administered. Heat in the form of sitz baths, soaks, or perineal irrigations may be used to increase circulation and promote comfort and healing. Tea (regular, not herbal) baths are particularly soothing. These baths, whose active ingredient is tannic acid, are prepared using two to three tea bags per bath.

Application of the Nursing Process to the Care of the Patient with Vaginitis

Assessment

Collect information regarding symptoms experienced, their duration, comfort measures used, and the effectiveness of these measures. Determine the color, consistency, amount, and odor of vaginal discharge. Also determine whether this is an isolated episode of vaginitis or a recurrence. Identify factors contributing to the development of the problem as well as possible routes of spread by obtaining information about hygienic and sexual practices, including the time of the last sexual contact, method of birth control used, duration of relationship with the sexual partner, and whether safer sex is practiced (i.e., condom used).

Explore the patient's understanding of normal vaginal defenses and the development and spread of infection. Assess the impact of the infection on the patient's self-esteem and sexual relationships.

Nursing Diagnoses and Planning

Nursing diagnoses and related expected patient outcomes most commonly applicable to patients with vaginitis include the following:

NDx: Pain related to the infectious process in the vagina

Planning: Patient outcomes
1. Patient states itching and burning have decreased.
2. Patient voids without discomfort.

Chart 44–2.

NURSING GUIDE TO PATIENT EDUCATION FOR SELF-MANAGEMENT: VAGINITIS

Teach the patient about the following:

Prevention of spread

Abstain from intercourse until the infection resolves. If abstinence is not feasible, have partner use a condom. Encourage partner to obtain concurrent treatment if needed.

Personal hygiene measures to decrease risk of recurrence

Wipe the perineal area from front to back to avoid spreading organisms from the anal area to the vaginal and urethral area.

Void before and after intercourse to flush bacteria from the urethrovaginal area.

Avoid douches unless medically ordered, because douches can change the pH of the vagina and encourage the growth of pathogens.

Avoid use of tampons or use them intermittently with pads.

Normal variations in vaginal discharge

The normal amount of vaginal discharge is 1 to 3 teaspoons.

Vaginal discharge is milky just before and after the menses and becomes thick mucus at ovulation.

NDx: High risk for altered health maintenance related to insufficient knowledge of prevention of spread and recurrence of vaginitis, normal variations in vaginal secretions

Planning: Patient outcomes

1. Patient describes personal hygienic habits that decrease the risk of vaginitis.
2. Patient verbalizes need for abstinence or her partner's use of a condom until the infection has cleared, and partner's need for concurrent treatment.
3. Patient describes normal variations in vaginal discharge.

Nursing Interventions

NDx: Pain

Prepare the patient for discomfort that may occur during the pelvic examination as a result of inflammation of the vaginal tissues even though a small speculum is used. Tell her that a small amount of bleeding may occur after the examination, and provide a perineal pad. If a clean-catch urine specimen is needed, give clear, detailed instructions because a specimen of urine that has come in contact with the vulva can lead to the misdiagnosis of cystitis or urethritis.

Explain the use of prescribed drugs and other therapeutic measures. Demonstrate the use of vaginal applicators and the correct insertion of vaginal creams or suppositories.

If douches are ordered, review the procedure with the patient and instruct her to douche before the insertion of any vaginal medication, not after. Stress the importance of not scratching the vulvovaginal area, because this can lead to secondary infection.

NDx: High risk for altered health maintenance

Instruct the patient as specified in Chart 44–2 to help her prevent spread to her sexual partner, prevent recurrence of the problem, and understand normal variations in vaginal discharge so that the need for further treatment can be more easily identified.

Evaluation

Evaluate the effectiveness of nursing care for a patient with vaginitis by comparing the patient's status with the expected patient outcomes. Examples of specific outcomes for patients with vaginitis have been provided in the Planning section.

Atrophic Vaginitis

Atrophic vaginitis, a disorder affecting postmenopausal women, is a superficial inflammation of the thin, vaginal epithelium.

ETIOLOGY AND PATHOPHYSIOLOGY

The drop in estrogen that occurs after menopause results in thinning of the vaginal epithelium, a decrease in the number of lactobacilli in the vagina, and an increase in vaginal pH. These changes make the vagina more susceptible to bacterial invasion; hence, infection with aerobic gram-positive or -negative organisms may occur.

CLINICAL MANIFESTATIONS

Symptoms of atrophic vaginitis are a thin, usually yellow, slight to moderate vaginal discharge; a burning sensation in the vaginal area; and dyspareunia. Itching and foul odor do not occur.

MEDICAL DIAGNOSIS

The medical diagnosis is made on the basis of the patient's history, the appearance of the vaginal epithelium, and diagnostic tests such as Papanicolaou (Pap) smears, culture, and vaginal microscopic examination. The vaginal epithelium is diffusely red, and superficial hemorrhagic areas may be seen. This is in stark contrast to the normal pallor of the atrophic epithelium found in the postmenopausal patient.

MEDICAL MANAGEMENT

Estrogen administered two to three times per week in the form of vaginal cream or suppository thickens the vaginal epithelium and provides prompt relief. To prevent recurrence, estrogen therapy must be continued on a weekly basis or systemic hormone therapy begun.

Warm douches of a weak acid solution such as 15 ml of acetic acid (vinegar) to 1 L of water cleanse the vagina, lower its pH, and exert a soothing effect on the inflamed tissues.

Guidelines for Application of the Nursing Process to the Care of the Patient with Atrophic Vaginitis

Nursing care is planned to enable the patient to carry out self-care activities effective in providing relief from symptoms and preventing a recurrence.

Instruct the patient on the use of vinegar douches and, if ordered, the instillation of the estrogen preparation. If the use of the applicator is painful, suggest use of K-Y jelly for lubrication or application of the cream with a finger until the soreness lessens. Instruct the patient about the need for careful hand washing before and after vaginal treatments.

Toxic Shock Syndrome

ETIOLOGY AND PATHOPHYSIOLOGY

Toxic shock syndrome is a rare but acute illness caused by one or more toxins produced by the bacterium *Staphylococcus aureus.* Although it can occur after any staphylococcal infection, its incidence is greatest among young, menstruating females who are using tampons, particularly the superabsorbent type. The tampons, which can hold a large amount of menstrual blood and are left in place for an extended length of time, provide an excellent environment for the multiplication of *Staphylococcus.* The organisms are then believed to enter the blood stream through lesions in the vaginal mucosa. Recurrence of toxic shock syndrome during later menses is common (Hatcher et al, 1990, p 63).

CLINICAL MANIFESTATIONS

Toxic shock syndrome usually begins with the sudden onset of a fever of 38.9°C (102°F) or higher accompanied by vomiting, diarrhea, muscle aches, weakness, and fatigue. Shock ensues, and signs of impaired cardiopulmonary, hepatic, and renal function are evident. The patient becomes hypotensive, and respiratory distress as a result of pulmonary edema may develop. Bilirubin and creatine kinase levels rise. Urinary output decreases, blood urea nitrogen (BUN) level increases, and the patient becomes disoriented. Mucous membranes and conjunctivae may become hyperemic, and an erythematous macular skin eruption may develop. This rash, which may appear first on the body or on the palms of the hands, fingers, soles of the feet, and toes, desquamates in 7 to 10 days.

Disseminated intravascular coagulation (DIC), with its symptoms of hematomas, petechiae, cyanosis, and coolness of distal parts of the body such as the nose, finger tips, and toes, may also occur in patients with toxic shock syndrome.

MEDICAL DIAGNOSIS

The diagnosis of toxic shock syndrome is suggested by the rapid onset of characteristic symptoms in otherwise healthy, menstruating females. The diagnosis is confirmed by cultures positive for *S. aureus.*

Chart 44–3.

NURSING GUIDE TO PATIENT EDUCATION FOR SELF-MANAGEMENT: PREVENTION OF TOXIC SHOCK SYNDROME (TSS)

Instruct the patient to:

Use regular or slender tampons, not superabsorbent tampons because they predispose to the development of TSS.
Change tampons after bowel movements.
Change tampons every 4 to 6 hours.
Use a pad, not a tampon, at night.
Insert and remove tampons carefully to avoid abrasions to the vaginal mucosa, which can serve as entry points for pathogenic bacteria. Use K-Y jelly for lubrication if needed. Avoid tampons with rough edges because they can damage the lining of the vagina. Wash hands thoroughly before handling tampons.
If patient has had TSS, use of tampons should be avoided.

MEDICAL MANAGEMENT

Antibiotic therapy in the form of cephalosporins or penicillinase-resistant penicillins is given to combat the infection, and any interventions necessary to support the patient's vital functions are instituted. For example, intubation and ventilation may be required to maintain adequate respiration.

Guidelines for Application of the Nursing Process to the Care of the Patient with Toxic Shock Syndrome

Nursing care varies according to the specific effects of the disease on the individual patient. For each patient, provide care necessary to support vital functions and the body's efforts to combat the infection. As the patient recovers, begin health teaching as specified in Chart 44–3.

Functional Disorders

Premenstrual Syndrome

Premenstrual syndrome (PMS) is a cyclic phenomenon characterized by an individualized yet basically consistent pattern of symptoms that occur between ovulation and menses and regress or disappear during menstruation.

PMS affects females of all races, cultures, and socioeconomic levels. Its incidence increases with age and parity. The onset of PMS frequently follows puberty, pregnancy, periods of amenorrhea from oral contraceptives or excessive weight loss, tubal ligation, ovarian surgery, or hysterectomy. PMS is also more common among females who have had spontaneous abortions (miscarriages), toxemia, postpartum depression, or an adverse reaction to oral contraceptives.

ETIOLOGY AND PATHOPHYSIOLOGY

The cause of PMS is unknown, although many theories have been set forth and are currently under study. Suggested causes include estrogen-progesterone imbalance, in which estrogen is in excess relative to the level of progesterone, low levels of beta endorphins (Tulenheimo et al, 1987), vitamin B_6 deficiency, and magnesium deficiency. Changes in prostaglandin metabolism are also under study.

Prostaglandins are biochemical mediators that affect central nervous system function, fluid and electrolyte balance, gastrointestinal function, and contractility of the uterus. Precursors of prostaglandins in the body are essential fatty acids. Because abnormal levels of essential fatty acids have been found in females with PMS, it is theorized that altered prostaglandin metabolism may cause an abnormal response to normal hormone levels (Brush et al, 1984).

Also being investigated is the role of *C. albicans* overgrowth in causing PMS. Symptoms of PMS such as depression, memory impairment, and anxiety are also symptoms of systemic *C. albicans* overgrowth, and it is thought that changes in immunity initiated by *C. albicans* may be responsible for hormonal dysfunction. This is supported by the fact that antifungal treatments have resulted in empirical improvement of symptoms in some PMS patients (Ensign et al, 1988).

CLINICAL MANIFESTATIONS

The symptoms of PMS are nonspecific and vary from individual to individual. Symptoms that occur as part of PMS are presented in Table 44–2.

Symptoms, which can occur for 1 to 2 days or for 2 weeks, disappear or regress with the onset of menstruation and can vary in severity from month to month.

MEDICAL DIAGNOSIS

The diagnosis of PMS is made on the basis of the timing and cyclic nature of the patient's symptoms.

Table 44–2. CLINICAL MANIFESTATIONS OF PREMENSTRUAL SYNDROME (PMS)

	SYMPTOMS
PHYSICAL SYMPTOMS	
Gastrointestinal	Nausea, abdominal bloating, abdominal cramping, anorexia, bulimia, cravings, exacerbation of hemorrhoids
Reproductive	Breast swelling, tenderness, pain; change in sex drive (may be either increased or decreased to absent) (Note: Patients with PMS generally do not have dysmenorrhea; they do ovulate and are able to conceive and carry a fetus to term)
Urologic	Frequency of urination, dysuria
Neurologic	Sensitivity to noise, touch, smell; lack of coordination, slurred speech, visual difficulties such as difficulty focusing, tearing, or dry eyes; fainting; dizziness; headaches; numbness and tingling in hands; insomnia; seizures
Dermatologic	Acne, hives, styes, rashes
Respiratory	Asthma
Cardiovascular	"Pounding of the heart," cardiac dysrhythmias
Musculoskeletal	Back pain, joint pain, muscle ache, stiff neck
Systemic	Fatigue, lethargy, weight gain, infections
EMOTIONAL SYMPTOMS	Anger, anxiety, crying, irritability, feelings of depression, poor self-concept, tension, paranoia, violence, suicidal thoughts, withdrawal

Acute symptoms such as headaches, panic attacks, seizures, and depression often occur after long periods (5 waking hours or 13 sleeping hours) without eating.

The symptoms must occur in the premenstrual period during consecutive cycles and disappear with the onset of the menstrual flow. For this to be evaluated, a record is needed of symptoms experienced and their time of occurrence in relationship to the menstrual cycle. This type of record is called a menstrual log, calendar, or chart and is kept by the patient on a daily basis for 1 to 4 months.

The diagnosis is made after thorough history, physical examination, and relevant diagnostic tests have ruled out any other medical or psychiatric disorder such as depression or thyroid dysfunction.

MEDICAL MANAGEMENT

Medical management is basically symptomatic in approach because the cause of PMS is unclear. Diuretics, prostaglandin inhibitors, oral contraceptives, antifungal therapy, antidepressants, tranquilizers, and vitamin B_6 have all been used with varying degrees of success. Hormone therapy in the form of progesterone administered daily by rectal or vaginal suppository or oral lozenges, from just before the onset of symptoms to the onset of menstruation, has also been used in some cases. This therapy uses natural progesterone and not a progestogen, but its effectiveness as well as possible long-term effects remain in question (Hatcher et al, 1990, p 54).

Reduction of stress, aerobic exercises that increase beta-endorphin levels, and the dietary changes described in Chart 44–4 are generally recommended before medications are prescribed, because most medications have not proven to be effective and may be associated with adverse effects.

Application of the Nursing Process to the Care of the Patient with Premenstrual Syndrome

Assessment

Assess the status of the patient's symptoms: what are they, and when do they occur in relationship to the menstrual cycle? This information is best obtained by use of a menstrual log as described in the discussion of medical diagnosis. Explain the need for the log, assist the patient to design a chart suited to her needs, and teach her to fill it out. Figure 44–1 depicts types of charts needed by different patients.

Determine what measures the patient has used to try to obtain relief and the effect of each. Also determine the patient's lifestyle, including patterns of exercise and nutrition, stressful factors, and her coping methods as well as her interpersonal relationships and support systems, because PMS impacts on all areas of the patient's life and is affected by so many factors.

Day of Month	Jan	Feb	Mar	Apr	May	June	July	Aug	Sept	Oct	Nov	Dec
1												
2												
3												

A ↓

Symptom being charted: ____________ Rating Scale: Mild=1 Moderate=2 Severe=3

Day of Month	Jan	Feb	Mar	Apr	May	June	July	Aug	Sept	Oct	Nov	Dec
1												
2												
3												

B ↓

Symptoms →

Month and Day	Insomnia	Bloating	Nausea	Headache	Irritability	Menstruation
11/1						
11/2						
11/3						

C ↓

Figure 44–1.

Examples of menstrual logs. For all charts, the patient writes "M" in the blocks for the dates that menses occurs. *A,* Basic chart used to show relationship of symptoms to the menstrual cycle. Each day the patient records symptoms experienced in the block for that date. *B,* Type of chart used when the severity of a given symptom is being charted over a cycle. Where indicated at the top of the form, the patient fills in the name of the symptom being charted (e.g., nausea). Each day the patient rates her experience of the symptom (see rating scale at top of form) and writes the rating score in the block corresponding to that date. This is particularly useful when it is not clear that a symptom occurs only premenstrually. *C,* This type of chart is used when the patient has many symptoms and it is difficult to distinguish which are related to the menstrual cycle. Each day the patient places a check mark in the box corresponding to the date and the symptoms experienced. This type of chart can also be used to rate the severity of each symptom by substituting a rating score as in Chart B for the check mark. Note: If the time of ovulation is not known, as with long or irregular cycles or after a hysterectomy, the patient keeps a chart of basal body temperature as well as of her symptoms (Adapted from *Self-Help for Premenstrual Syndrome* by Dr. Michelle Harrison. Copyright © 1982, 1985 by Michelle Harrison. Adapted by permission of Random House, Inc.)

Nursing Diagnoses and Planning

Nursing diagnoses and related expected patient outcomes most commonly applicable to patients with PMS include the following:

NDx: High risk for ineffective individual coping related to the fact of a cyclic disease with extremely variable symptoms and no single cure

Planning: Patient outcomes

1. Patient identifies the disease as real and describes it in general terms.
2. Patient demonstrates from her menstrual log what her symptom pattern is and how it fits the criteria for PMS.
3. Patient describes role of stress in precipitating or aggravating symptoms of PMS.
4. Patient identifies sources of stress in her daily life and appropriate ways to manage them.
5. Family members or significant others state willingness to support the patient and participate in health-teaching program.

NDx: High risk for altered health maintenance related to insufficient knowledge of effective self-care measures and prescribed medications

Planning: Patient outcomes

1. Patient states the need for adequate rest and exercise and the rationale for it.
2. Patient plans a daily diet incorporating PMS diet modifications.
3. Patient identifies common misconceptions regarding effective treatment measures that may be suggested.
4. Patient states the name of prescribed medications, expected effects, and the dose, route, and frequency of administration.
5. Patient describes adverse reactions that should be reported to the health professional.

Nursing Interventions

NDx: High risk for ineffective individual coping

Affirm to the patient that her disorder is real, that the symptoms are not imagined, and that others suffer from the same disorder. Provide information about the disease, and use the patient's menstrual log to clarify its cyclic nature.

Explain the importance of avoiding stress during the premenstrual interval when symptoms are present. Help the patient identify sources of stress in her life as well as appropriate methods of stress management. Explore with the patient the feasibility of planning known stressful activities so that they occur at the time she is symptom free.

Recognize that the support of family members or significant others is essential to the patient's coping ability. Assess their understanding of the disorder and its treatment, and include them in health teaching.

Provide information about PMS support groups, and tell the patient how to contact one in her geographic area.

NDx: High risk for altered health maintenance

Instruct the patient as specified in Chart 44–4 to help her make changes in lifestyle and diet to decrease the impact of PMS.

If the patient is being treated with progesterone or other medication, ascertain that she understands what the medication is as well as the amount, route, and frequency of its administration. Also prepare her for any expected side effects, and tell her what adverse reactions should be reported.

Evaluation

Evaluate the effectiveness of nursing care for a patient with PMS by comparing the patient's status with the expected patient outcomes. Examples of specific outcomes for patients with PMS have been provided in the Planning section.

Endometriosis

Endometriosis is a condition in which tissue that is like the endometrium of the uterus is present in other locations. The most common of these ectopic locations are the ovary and the cul-de-sac of Douglas, although the pelvic ligaments, pelvic peritoneum, vulvar perineum, ureters, bladder, or cecum may also be involved (Fig. 44–2). The disease, which seems to be increasing in incidence, occurs primarily among 30- to 40-year-old nulliparas of upper socioeconomic classes. A familial tendency has been reported principally in sisters but also between mothers and daughters. Endometriosis is rare among black women and other groups who tend to marry young and have many children.

ETIOLOGY AND PATHOPHYSIOLOGY

The cause of endometriosis is not known, although there are many theories. The most prominent suggests that endometriosis results from small bits of uterine endometrial tissue being propelled upward through the fallopian tubes into the pelvic cavity rather than downward through the cervix and the vagina at the time of menstruation. Another theory is that there are primitive cells present in the abdominal cavity from the time of fetal development that develop into endometrial cells under the hormonal changes of puberty. A third is that endome-

Chart 44–4.

NURSING GUIDE TO PATIENT EDUCATION FOR SELF-MANAGEMENT: RELIEF OF PREMENSTRUAL SYNDROME (PMS)

Instruct the patient to:

Obtain adequate sleep, and take naps as needed. Fatigue magnifies the symptoms of PMS.
Use relaxation techniques to induce sleep if needed.
Get regular physical exercise. Exercise induces sleep and decreases premenstrual stress in general.
Eat a well-balanced diet with foods from each of the basic food groups, following the guidelines in Nutrition Box 44–1.
Eat six small meals per day to maintain a consistent blood sugar level.
Avoid strict dieting for 7 to 10 days before menstruation.
If a vitamin or mineral supplement is needed, take moderate doses. Avoid megadoses, which may be harmful.

trial cells from the uterus are carried by the blood or lymph to the secondary sites.

The condition presents in the affected areas as multiple cystic nodules lined with ectopic endometrial tissue. This tissue undergoes a proliferative and secretive change in response to estrogen and progesterone just as the uterine endometrium does. When the menses begins in response to a drop in the circulating levels of these hormones, the ectopic tissue also sloughs and bleeds. This bleeding gives the lesions their brown or blue-black color. It also causes an inflammatory reaction, which eventually results in the formation of adhesions. These adhesions may be so extensive that the pelvic organs become fused together and immobile.

When endometrial cysts occur on the ovary, they are often referred to as "chocolate" cysts because of their color and the brown fluid found within them.

Because the ectopic tissue is hormone dependent, the disease is active as long as the ovaries are func-

Nutrition Box 44–1.

NUTRITION: SPECIAL CONSIDERATIONS FOR PATIENTS WITH PREMENSTRUAL SYNDROME (PMS)

Instruct patients with PMS to do the following:

Eat small amounts of foods high in protein and carbohydrates frequently to prevent hypoglycemia and decrease cravings for sweets.
Include in the daily diet foods high in vitamin B_6 and magnesium such as green, leafy vegetables; legumes; whole grains; and cereals.
Avoid alcohol, caffeine, artificial sweeteners, and tobacco, which can contribute to anxiety, irritability, and insomnia.
Avoid excessive sodium for 7 to 9 days before menstruation to decrease fluid retention, which causes breast tenderness, bloating, and weight gain. (This means that foods high in sodium as well as hidden sources of sodium, such as some frozen food preservatives and water passing through a water-softening system, must be identified.)
Include in the daily diet 1 or more tablespoons of a food high in linoleic acid and vitamin E such as corn or safflower oil.
Drink 8 to 10 glasses of water per day.

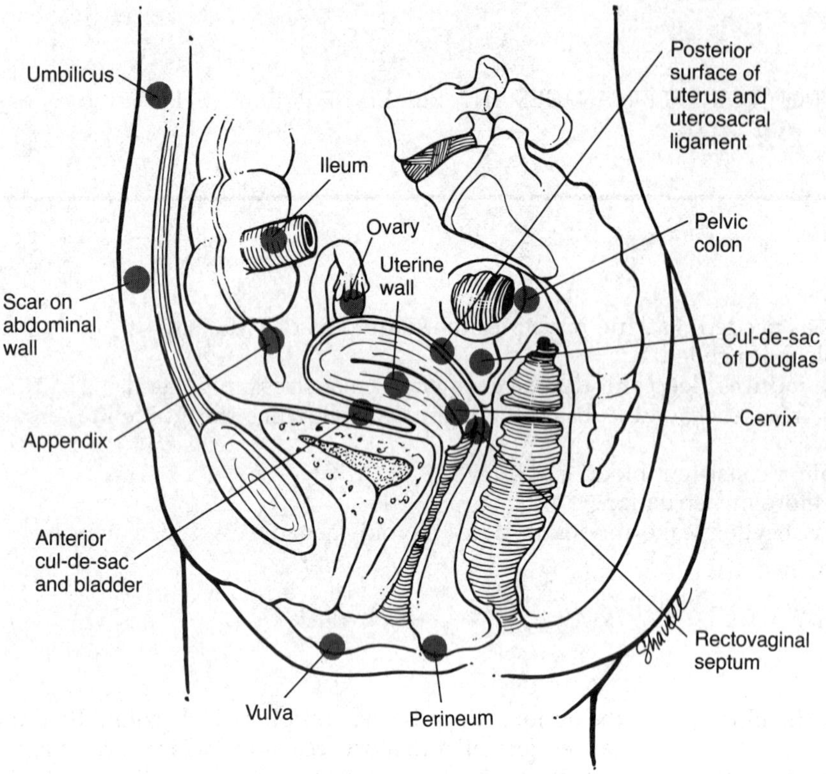

Figure 44–2.

Common locations where endometriosis occurs.

tioning. Remissions generally occur during pregnancy and with the onset of menopause.

CLINICAL MANIFESTATIONS

There is no specific pattern of symptoms that is characteristic of endometriosis. Symptoms vary depending on the location of the endometrial tissue. Similarly, there is no relationship between severity of symptoms and the severity of the disease process. Patients with massive endometriosis may have few symptoms, whereas patients with minor lesions may have severe symptoms.

The symptom most frequently associated with endometriosis is dysmenorrhea. It is distinctive in that it typically begins 2 to 3 days before menses, becomes progressively worse during menstruation, and may persist for several days thereafter. This pattern of pain is thought to reflect hormone-mediated changes in the ectopic tissue and the associated pressure and inflammation. The pain may be located low in the abdomen, deep in the pelvis, or in the rectal or sacrococcygeal areas.

Deep dyspareunia is another symptom of endometriosis. It occurs if the uterosacral ligaments are involved. The patient may also complain of dysuria if the bladder is affected or constipation and pain on defecation if the rectal wall is affected.

Infertility is another classic symptom of endometriosis. In fact, it is often the problem that brings the patient to a health care professional. The basic mechanism by which endometriosis causes infertility is unknown. It has been suggested that prostaglandins released from the ectopic endometrial tissue interfere with normal ovum release, tubal mobility, uterine relaxation, or steroidogenesis. Regardless of the underlying cause, treatment of endometriosis may result in a subsequent pregnancy in many cases.

MEDICAL DIAGNOSIS

Diagnosis is made on the basis of history and the palpation of characteristic masses on bimanual examination. When palpation is inconclusive, laparoscopy with or without a biopsy may be done to confirm the diagnosis.

MEDICAL MANAGEMENT

Medical management of endometriosis depends on the severity of symptoms and the age and lifestyle of the patient. When symptoms are minimal, nonsteroidal anti-inflammatory drugs may be effective. Over-the-counter ibuprofen preparations such as Advil or Nuprin are tried first; if they fail to provide relief, drugs such as naproxen (Anaprox, Naprosyn) and prescription ibuprofen (Motrin) may be ordered. If the patient wishes to have a child, a pregnancy can provide relief from symptoms. This relief can be extended if the patient breast-feeds the infant.

In cases in which a child is desired but infertility accompanies the endometriosis, conservative hormone therapy or surgical intervention is used.

HORMONE THERAPY

Three types of hormone therapy are used to treat endometriosis: progestogen, androgen, and antigonadotropin.

Progestogen therapy (Pharmacology Box 44–1) creates a state of pseudopregnancy. Ovulation and menstruation are inhibited, and endometrial atrophy is produced. Treatment lasts about 9 months and is effective in relieving pain. It also provides relief from infertility in about 40% of patients. A disadvantage of the treatment is that uncomfortable symptoms of early pregnancy may develop such as breast tenderness, nausea, vomiting, and fatigue.

Androgen therapy, such as 5 mg of methyltestosterone per day for 4 to 6 months, also causes endometrial atrophy and provides pain relief. This dosage does not prevent ovulation, menstruation, or pregnancy. However, the therapy is immediately discontinued if pregnancy occurs to prevent masculinization of a female fetus.

The third type of endocrine therapy involves the use of the reversible antigonadotropic drug danazol. By inhibiting the release of gonadotropins from the pituitary gland, it suppresses ovarian activity and thus prevents proliferation of both the uterine and ectopic endometrium and also ovulation. Two hundred milligrams of the drug is given twice per day for 3 to 9 months at a time. Pain relief occurs in almost all patients, and conception occurs in approximately half.

Disadvantages of this treatment include high cost, tendency of symptoms to recur when the drug is discontinued, unknown long-term effects, and the

Pharmacology Box 44–1.
PROGESTERONES

Progesterones:
This is a class of drugs composed of the natural female hormone progesterone and its synthetic derivatives. Large amounts of progesterone are secreted by the corpus luteum during the menstrual cycle and by the placenta during pregnancy. Small amounts are secreted by the mature follicle before ovulation and by the adrenal cortex.

Action:
Progesterone is responsible for the secretory phase of the endometrium during the menstrual cycle. It also relaxes the uterine muscle, promotes development of the breast, and maintains the endometrium during pregnancy. Its metabolic effects include protein catabolism and retention of sodium and water.

Uses:
Treatment of dysfunctional uterine bleeding, amenorrhea, and dysmenorrhea. Some are also used to shrink endometrial carcinomas, to treat endometriosis, and as oral contraceptives.

Side Effects:
Breakthrough bleeding, dysmenorrhea, amenorrhea, monilial vaginitis, breast enlargement and tenderness, fluid retention, hypertension, thromboembolic disease, dizziness, migraine, depression, hyperglycemia, cholestatic jaundice, rash, and photosensitivity.

Interactions:
None of clinical significance.

Nursing Implications:
In accord with U.S. Food and Drug Administration regulations, be sure that patient has the package insert, which explains possible side effects. Review this information with the patient before the first dose is given. Instruct the patient to report visual changes, migraine, or other unusual symptoms immediately.

Give oil solution deep intramuscularly, and rotate injection sites.

occurrence of side effects such as hot flashes, weight gain, decrease in vaginal secretions, and decrease in breast size.

SURGICAL INTERVENTION

When surgical therapy is selected for the patient who desires a pregnancy, the aim is to remove all ectopic endometrial tissue and return the pelvis to as normal a condition as possible. This has been traditionally done by resecting cysts and lysing adhesions through a laparotomy incision. Today it is often done through a laparoscope with the use of a laser, the intense beam of which vaporizes the endometrial tissue. This laser surgery leaves two to five "Band-Aid" ($\frac{1}{4}$ to $\frac{1}{2}$ in.) incisions and allows the patient to go home the same day and resume her usual routine within a week.

When pregnancy is not desired, the goal of therapy is simply to relieve symptoms. A hysterectomy with bilateral salpingo-oophorectomy is the most effective treatment. However, if the patient is relatively young and if she has strong feelings on the matter, an ovary may be spared and, in many cases, control of symptoms is obtained.

Application of the Nursing Process to the Care of the Patient with Endometriosis

Assessment

Determine the patient's personal health goals. Is the patient's primary aim in seeking health care to become pregnant, to obtain pain relief, or to obtain relief from other distressing symptoms? The answer to this question is an essential guide to planning and evaluating care.

Assess for the presence and severity of symptoms. Is pain a problem? If so, what type of pain is it, where is it located, when does it occur, how long does it last, what remedies have been tried for relief, and have they been effective? Does the patient have constipation, tenesmus, or pain on defecation? Is there dysuria or dyspareunia? Are the symptoms related to the menstrual cycle?

Assess the patient's ability to handle discomfort and her emotional reaction to the illness. Because the disorder is related to reproductive functioning, feelings of altered sexuality, anxiety, and body image changes related to possible infertility can occur.

Also assess the patient's understanding of the health problem. Does she have any misconceptions as to its cause or its outcomes? Some people believe endometriosis is caused by using tampons or that it develops into a malignancy.

As the therapeutic plan is instituted, assess the patient's understanding of it and its expected outcomes. For example, if the patient is having surgery, assess understanding of preoperative preparation and the postoperative course.

Nursing Diagnoses and Planning

Nursing diagnoses and related expected patient outcomes most commonly applicable to patients with endometriosis include the following:

NDx: Pain related to pressure and inflammation as a result of hormonal changes in the ectopic endometrial tissue

Planning: Patient outcomes
1. Patient uses noninvasive pain-relief measures such as heat to the abdomen, massage, and pelvic exercises.
2. Patient describes correctly the use of prescribed analgesics.
3. Patient states she is experiencing less pain.
4. Patient appears to be more comfortable as indicated by such factors as body posture and activity.

NDx: Anxiety related to diagnostic procedures, outcome of disease, fear of infertility or treatment

Planning: Patient outcomes
1. Patient states she feels less anxious/more relaxed.
2. Behavioral signs of moderate to severe anxiety are absent.

NDx: High risk for body-image disturbance related to an alteration in function of the reproductive system

Planning: Patient outcomes
1. Patient identifies her positive qualities.
2. Patient accepts support from others.
3. Patient verbalizes realistic perceptions of self.

NDx: High risk for altered health maintenance related to insufficient knowledge of the therapeutic regimen

Planning: Patient outcomes
1. Patient describes treatment accurately.
3. Patient states the expected effects of treatment.

Nursing Interventions

NDx: Pain
Administer prescribed analgesics in accordance with the physician's order and the patient's need. If ordered, apply heat to the abdomen using heating

pads or hot water bottle. This supports the "gating" of pain at the level of the spinal cord by stimulation of large peripheral nerves of the abdomen.

Teach the patient to massage her abdomen. Provide distractions from the discomfort to enhance gating further.

In preparation for self-care, teach the patient the correct use of prescribed analgesics and the correct methods of applying heat to the abdomen. Instruct the patient in pelvic exercises that aid in limiting discomfort.

Explain the role of pregnancy and breast-feeding in stopping the progression of the disease and in providing relief of symptoms if it is appropriate for the particular patient.

NDx: Anxiety

Explain the nature of the disease, diagnostic procedures, and treatments in language that the patient can understand. Provide the opportunity for and encourage verbalization of feelings. Encourage identification and discussion of factors contributing to anxiety. Be available and open to questions. Provide time for the patient and significant others to share their concerns.

NDx: High risk for body image disturbance

Foster a positive sense of self in the patient. Respect her need for privacy and for personal space. Encourage ventilation of feelings and identification of positive qualities and abilities.

Confirm her femininity. Encourage her to pay attention to her grooming and appearance, fix her hair, and use cosmetics in accordance with her personal preference.

NDx: High risk for altered health maintenance

Help the patient understand the plan of treatment and its expected effect. For example, if the patient is placed on hormone therapy, explain the planned duration of therapy; the dose, time, and frequency of medication; and its effects. Discuss the effect on menstruation and the possibility of pregnancy. Prepare her for side effects such as the breast tenderness and nausea that can occur with progestogens, and the hot flashes and decrease in vaginal secretions that may accompany antigonadotropic drugs.

Evaluation

Evaluate the effectiveness of nursing care for a patient with endometriosis by comparing the patient's status with the expected patient outcomes. Examples of specific outcomes for patients with endometriosis have been provided in the Planning section.

Structural Disorders

Disorders Caused by Weakened Pelvic Supports

The main organs of the pelvis are the bladder and upper urethra to the anterior, the vagina and the uterus in the middle, and the rectum and sigmoid colon to the posterior. These organs are maintained in their correct positions by the pelvic diaphragm, which is composed of the levator ani muscle, the pelvic fascia, and the pelvic ligaments. Weakening of any of these supporting structures can result in genital prolapse, which is the abnormal descent of one or more of the pelvic viscera.

Terms used to describe specific forms of genital prolapse are as follows:

Colpocele: Protrusion of a fold of vaginal mucosa outside the vaginal orifice
Cystocele: Protrusion of the urinary bladder into the vagina through the anterior vaginal wall (Fig. 44–3)
Rectocele: Protrusion of the rectum into the vagina through the lower, posterior vaginal wall (see Fig. 44–3)
Urethrocele: Protrusion of the urethra into the vagina through the anterior vaginal wall
Enterocele: Protrusion of the intestinal wall into the vagina through the posterior vaginal wall (see Fig. 44–3)
Uterine descensus or prolapse: Downward displacement of the uterus into the vaginal canal

Uterine prolapse (Fig. 44–3) is classified as first, second, or third degree.

First degree: The cervix is between the level of the ischial spines and the vaginal introitus.
Second degree: The cervix protrudes through the introitus.
Third degree: The cervix and the entire body of the uterus have passed through the introitus and the vagina is inverted. This is also called procidentia or complete prolapse.

Sometimes, the phrase *pelvic relaxation* is used to refer collectively to all these displacements of the pelvic organs.

ETIOLOGY AND PATHOPHYSIOLOGY

Although congenital incompetence of the pelvic support system occasionally occurs, the primary cause of weakened pelvic support is damage as a result of childbirth.

The three types of damage that childbirth may cause are as follows:

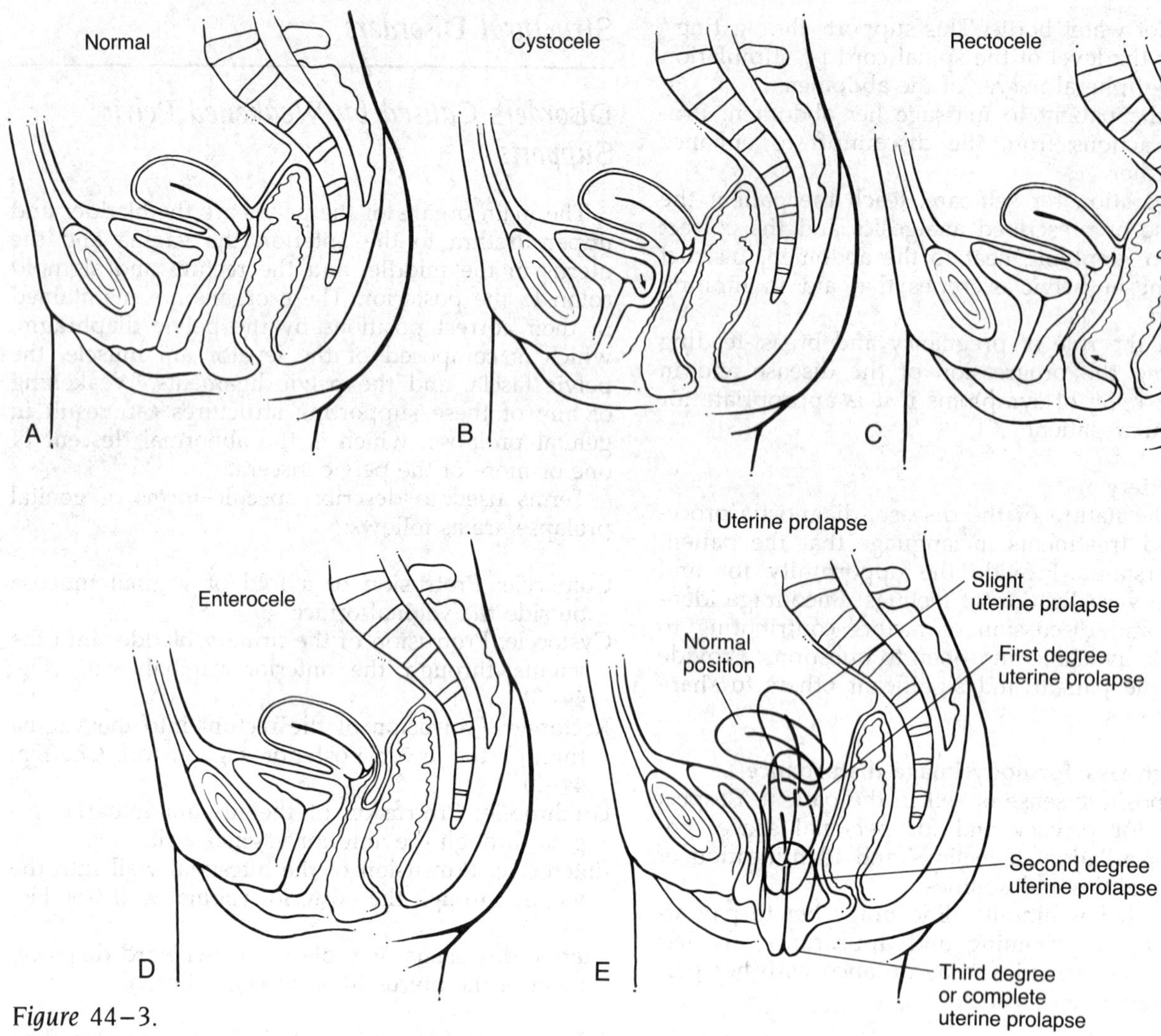

Figure 44–3.

Types of genital prolapse.

1. Overstretching or tearing of the edges of the levator ani muscle as a result of delivery of a large fetus.
2. Overstretching or tearing of the endopelvic fascia, which supports the vagina, and in turn the uterus as a result of delivery of a large fetus. Such tearing occurs at its weakest points, which are the anterior and posterior vaginal walls, and leads to the development of a cystocele or rectocele.
3. Damage to the pelvic ligaments, particularly the uterosacral and cardinal ligaments, which support the uterus. This is a traction injury and can occur if a patient in labor pushes before the cervix is fully dilated or if a Credé maneuver is used to express the placenta.

Obstetric damage to the pelvic support system is further aggravated by the weakening of the pelvic diaphragm and the loss of elasticity and strength of the fascia, which normally occur with aging; by the lack of estrogen after menopause; and by any condition that causes an increase in intraabdominal pressure. Such conditions include chronic coughing associated with smoking or bronchitis, constipation, heavy lifting, obesity, pregnancy, large tumors, and ascites.

CLINICAL MANIFESTATIONS

The patient with a weakened pelvic support and a genital prolapse will have one or more of the following signs and symptoms:

Lump protruding from the vagina. Typically the lump is painless and has been slowly increasing in size for months or even years. It is generally worse on standing or straining and disappears when the patient lies down or when pressure is applied to it. The patient may say she feels like she is sitting "on a ball."

Discomfort. A dragging sensation may be felt in the lower abdomen, or a feeling of pressure and heaviness may be felt in the vaginal area. This is often described as a feeling that "everything is dropping out." The patient may also have a low backache (lumbosacral pain), particularly after she has been standing for a length of time. This is caused by stretching of the supporting ligaments of the pelvis and the related peritoneum.

Difficult defecation. With a rectocele, constipation results from the overstretching and forward pouching of the rectum. The patient may have to press on the rectocele from inside the vagina to defecate. Hemorrhoids are frequently present.

Disturbances of micturition. Difficulty emptying the bladder can be caused by a cystocele. The patient may have to press on the cystocele from within the vagina to empty her bladder. If the bladder is not emptied, the residual urine in the prolapsed bladder can lead to chronic cystitis with its symptoms of frequency and dysuria. Stress incontinence, which is the escape of urine on coughing, laughing, or other muscular effort, may also occur as a result of a change in the urethrovesical angle created by a cystocele or a urethrocele.

With a urethrocele, postvoiding incontinence may occur. This is the escape of urine on sitting down after voiding.

Dyspareunia. Pain on intercourse may occur as a result of the change in the relationship of the pelvic organs to the vagina. In other cases, intercourse may simply be unsatisfactory as a result of vaginal relaxation.

There is no definite relationship between the severity of the patient's symptoms and the severity of the problem of pelvic relaxation.

MEDICAL DIAGNOSIS

Diagnosis of genital prolapse is made on the basis of the patient's history and on the findings of the physical examination.

Relaxation of the vagina can often be identified by simple inspection. The vaginal orifice has a gaping appearance, and the anterior and posterior walls of the vagina are separated. The diagnosis is confirmed by placing the examining fingers into the vagina and asking the patient to bear down. With vaginal relaxation, no muscular resistance around the lower vagina is felt.

Uterine prolapse is also visible on inspection. The degree of prolapse is determined by asking the patient to bear down as the speculum is withdrawn toward the vaginal orifice.

Cystocele and rectocele can sometimes also be seen on inspection. More often, however, they recede when the patient is lying in a flat position. In this case, the diagnosis is made by asking the patient to bear down or strain and observing the cystocele or rectocele come into view.

On physical examination, a urethrocele shows as a marked bulging just below the urethral orifice. Urethrography or urethroscopy may be used to confirm the diagnosis.

An enterocele is diagnosed by asking the patient to bear down during a rectovaginal examination. If an enterocele is present, a loop of small bowel will enter the sac and separate the examining fingers in the rectum and vagina, respectively.

MEDICAL MANAGEMENT

The medical management for problems of genital prolapse resulting from weakness in the pelvic support system is surgery. In only rare cases is nonsurgical intervention used. The decision as to the need for treatment is based on the severity of the symptoms experienced by the patient. In the majority of cases, treatment is elective. Treatment is a must only when a third-degree uterine prolapse exists, and chafing, ulceration, and bleeding from the exposure of the displaced uterus to the external environment and to friction from clothing are inevitable.

SURGICAL INTERVENTION

The treatment of choice for problems of genital prolapse is a vaginal hysterectomy with an anterior or posterior colporrhaphy, or both, or colpoperineorrhaphy. Vaginal hysterectomy was discussed in Chapter 43. An anterior colporrhaphy corrects a cystocele. It involves plication (stitching of folds in the wall of an organ to reduce its size) of the endopelvic fascia and removal of excess anterior vaginal wall. This commonly results in some narrowing and shortening of the vagina but does not interfere with vaginal function.

A posterior colporrhaphy, which corrects a rectocele, is essentially the same procedure but on the posterior vaginal wall. Posterior repairs are a major cause of vulvar and vaginal stenosis and resulting dyspareunia. Postoperative stenosis can be minimized by the use of dilators and lubricants and the resumption of coitus 6 weeks after surgery. Nonetheless, posterior repairs are not done in adolescent girls and young women unless there is a major relaxation because, even if the size of the vagina is adequate for sexual function after recovery from surgery, dyspareunia may occur after menopause because of the normal atrophy of the vagina occurring at that time.

When both anterior and posterior colporraphies are done, the procedure is referred to as an AP repair.

If there is damage to the pelvic floor, a colpoperineorrhaphy is done. In a colpoperineorrhaphy, the muscles of the pelvic floor are repaired along with the tightening of the vaginal walls.

Repairs of pelvic relaxations are not done until after the patient has given birth to the desired number of children, because any repair would be disrupted by a vaginal delivery. The surgery is also not performed until the patient is medically prepared. This includes healing of ulcerations that may be present if the vagina is completely prolapsed. To facilitate healing, the patient may be placed on bed rest, estrogen may be prescribed, and a vaginal pack may be inserted. The vaginal pack, which may be soaked in glycerine, can interfere with voiding by pressing on the urethrovesical angle. If this occurs, an indwelling catheter is inserted.

NONSURGICAL INTERVENTION

Nonsurgical measures are used when the patient cannot withstand surgery or when the severity of her symptoms does not warrant surgery and yet relief is desired.

Pessaries

In the rare case in which surgery is indicated but not immediately feasible, a pessary may be used to relieve symptoms. A pessary is a device that is positioned in the upper vagina to keep an organ such as the bladder, uterus, or intestine in proper anatomic position. Generally, a plastic ring or stem pessary (Fig. 44–4) is most successful.

Pessaries are infrequently used because of the many problems they present. A major difficulty is fit. If the pessary is too loose, it falls out and is ineffective. If it is too tight, it can cause urinary retention or pressure necrosis with ulceration and bleeding. With long-term use, leukorrhea tends to develop even with daily douches.

A pessary is inserted and fit by a gynecologist. The patient is immediately asked to perform a variety of body movements to ascertain that the pessary will remain in place with activity. The patient is also asked to void to make certain that the urethra is not being compressed. The patient is reexamined 1 week after insertion for comfort and effectiveness. Thereafter, she is seen every 2 months, at which time the pessary is removed, cleaned, and reinserted, and the vaginal tissues are checked for signs of necrosis or bleeding.

If a pessary is not cleaned routinely, it can become encrusted in the submucosal tissues and produces a lesion that can appear malignant and that gives off a foul odor.

Perineal Exercises

Perineal exercises may be prescribed to help strengthen muscles of the pelvic floor in cases in which surgery is not indicated but relief of symptoms is desired. As might be expected, these are more effective in early-stage than in late-stage pelvic relaxation. They are most successful as a preventive measure done before childbirth. Chart 44–5 describes two perineal exercises that are effective in toning the pubococcygeal musculature: the Kegel exercises and the elevator exercises.

Application of the Nursing Process to the Care of the Patient Having a Posterior Colporrhaphy

PREOPERATIVE NURSING CARE

The assessment, nursing diagnoses, expected patient outcomes, nursing interventions, and evaluation for the patient scheduled for a posterior colporrhaphy are similar to those for any preoperative patient, as

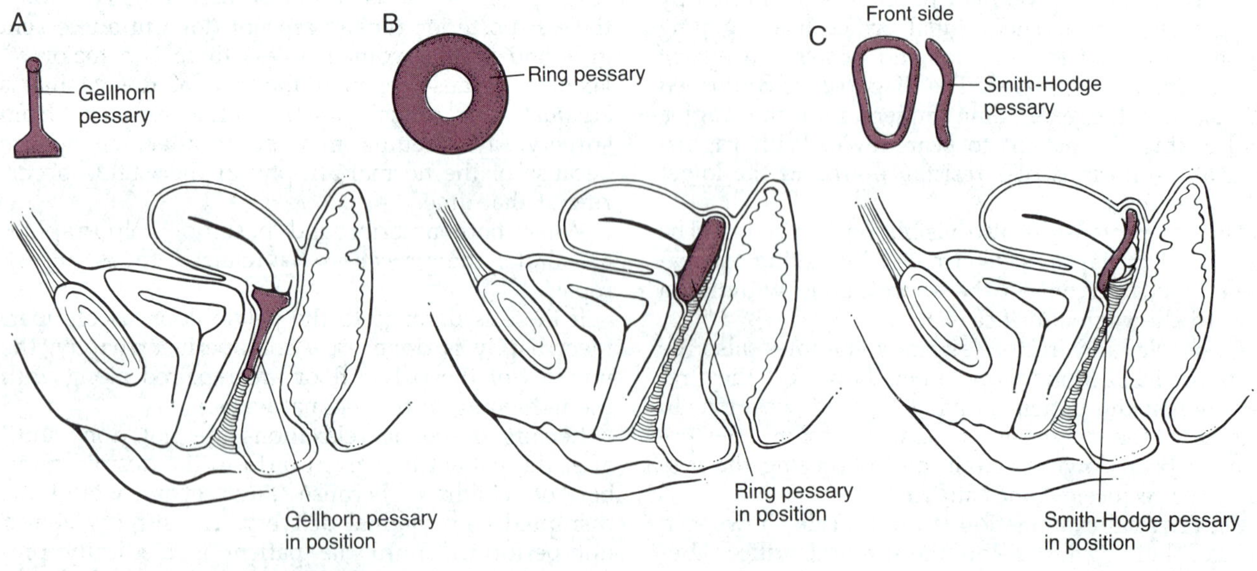

Figure 44–4.

Types of vaginal pessaries.

Chart 44–5.

NURSING GUIDE TO PATIENT EDUCATION FOR SELF-MANAGEMENT: PERINEAL EXERCISES

Instruct the patient as follows:

Kegel Exercises

Tightly contract the perineal muscles, and hold them tightly for a count of five. Release and repeat 10 times.

Learn how to contract these muscles by starting to urinate and then stopping the stream.

Perform the Kegel exercise in any comfortable position at least three to five times daily.

Elevator Exercise

Contract the perineal muscles gradually in steps. To do this, visualize the vaginal canal as an elevator shaft and stop at four or five "floors" on the way to the top (i.e., maximum contraction) and on the way down to complete relaxation.

End with a "reverse Kegel" or push to the "subbasement" (i.e., push like you are going to start a stream of urine).

discussed in Chapter 4. Be certain to assess for recent use of birth-control pills, because this predisposes to fluid and electrolyte imbalance postoperatively. Also keep in mind that a bowel preparation and a cleansing douche on the morning of surgery are components of the usual preoperative routine.

POSTOPERATIVE NURSING CARE

Assessment

Postoperatively, assess the patient's physiologic stabilization. Monitor vital signs, and observe the patient for bleeding. If an indwelling catheter is in place, as is usual for 24 to 48 hours, assess the adequacy of urinary elimination by monitoring output. Also assess for signs of pulmonary complications and developing thrombophlebitis.

Nursing Diagnoses and Planning

Nursing diagnoses and related expected patient outcomes most commonly applicable to patients who have had a posterior colporrhaphy include the following:

NDx: High risk for infection related to vaginal suture line

Planning: Patient outcomes
1. Foul-smelling or purulent vaginal drainage is absent.
2. Temperature is normal.
3. Leukocytosis is absent.

NDx: High risk for impaired tissue integrity related to pull on the vaginal suture line

Planning: Patient outcomes
1. Patient maintains position as directed to prevent stress on the suture line.
2. Straining at stool is absent.

NDx: Pain related to vaginal surgery

Planning: Patient outcomes
1. Patient turns and sits up without excessive discomfort.
2. Patient becomes increasingly active.
3. Patient reports that discomfort has decreased.

NDx: High risk for altered health maintenance related to insufficient knowledge of postdischarge self-care activities

Planning: Patient outcomes
1. Patient describes postdischarge self-care activities as specified in Chart 44–6.

Nursing Interventions

Institute standard postoperative care, as discussed in Chapter 4. Provide care as described next to meet the specific needs of the patient who has had a posterior colporrhaphy.

NDx: High risk for infection

Begin measures to support healing and prevent infection immediately. Give sterile perineal care twice a day and after each use of the bedpan or toilet.

Chart 44–6.

NURSING GUIDE TO PATIENT EDUCATION FOR SELF-MANAGEMENT: SELF-CARE AFTER POSTERIOR COLPORRHAPHY

Instruct the patient to:

Take a douche and a tub bath each day until follow-up visit.
Avoid sexual intercourse until after the follow-up visit.
Take a laxative each night to avoid straining at stool and the related stress on the suture line.
Avoid, for 6 weeks, jarring activities as well as prolonged periods of either walking or sitting.

Sterile cotton balls may be used to cleanse the area with a solution such as normal saline or benzalkonium chloride, or the solution may simply be poured over the perineum while the patient is positioned on a fracture pan. In either case, gently but thoroughly pat the area dry to avoid creating a dark, warm, moist area conducive to bacterial growth. If ordered, use a heat lamp for 15 to 20 minutes after perineal care to dry the area and to increase circulation, which is needed for healing.

Administer sterile douches as ordered to cleanse the incisional area within the vagina and to facilitate healing. Some surgeons order small douches of normal saline twice a day starting on the first postoperative day. Others leave the suture line undisturbed and order douches beginning 5 to 10 days postoperatively.

NDx: High risk for impaired tissue integrity
Keep the patient either flat or in low Fowler's position to prevent pressure on the suture line, which would impede healing. Implement physician's orders related to diet and medications to control gastrointestinal function. Orders usually call for a liquid diet and paregoric to inhibit bowel function for 5 days and mineral oil on the fifth postoperative evening, followed by an oil retention enema the next day. This facilitates passage of stool without straining.

NDx: Pain
Give analgesics in accordance with physician's orders. Give ice packs for perineal discomfort. A rubber glove filled with chipped ice fits comfortably to the area. Cover the ice pack and position it so that its weight is on the bed and not on the patient. Also apply analgesic ointments as ordered for relief.

Instruct the patient to pinch her buttocks together before sitting down. This decreases pressure on the operative area and reduces discomfort.

After the sutures are removed, give sitz baths to ease perineal discomfort.

NDx: High risk for altered health maintenance
Instruct the patient as specified in Chart 44–6 to prepare her for self-care after discharge.

Evaluation

Evaluate the effectiveness of nursing care for a patient who has had a posterior colporrhaphy by comparing the patient's status with the expected patient outcomes. Examples of specific outcomes for patients who have had a posterior colporrhaphy have been provided in the Planning section.

Application of the Nursing Process to the Care of the Patient Having an Anterior Colporrhaphy

The assessment, nursing diagnoses, expected patient outcomes, nursing interventions, and evaluation for patients having an anterior colporrhaphy are similar to those described previously for patients having a posterior colporrhaphy, except as noted next.

Because the anterior rather than the posterior wall of the vagina is the operative site, cleansing of the bowel preoperatively is not necessary. Laxatives, a clear-liquid diet, and soapsuds enemas are not necessary, so only a cleansing douche as ordered by the surgeon is given on the morning of surgery.

Postoperatively, the patient ambulates within 12 to 24 hours and progresses to a regular diet as soon as tolerated. Mineral oil is usually ordered to prevent straining at stool with the accompanying increase in intraabdominal pressure, which puts stress on the suture line.

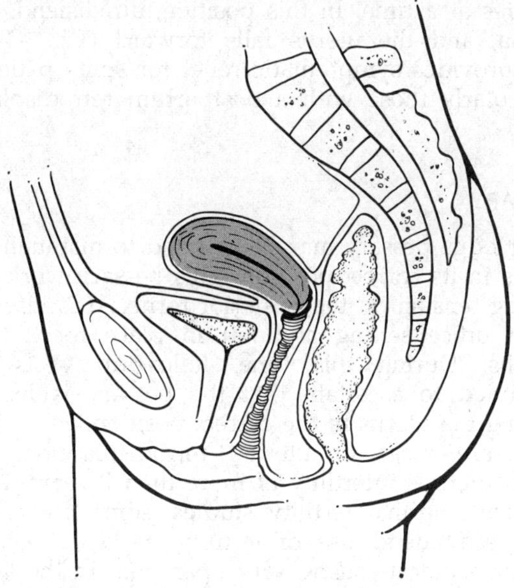

Figure 44–5.

Diagram showing the normal position of the uterus, which is anteversion with a mild degree of anteflexion of the body of the uterus on the cervix.

Generally, the patient has an indwelling catheter for 4 days because if more than 100 ml of urine accumulate in the bladder, the pressure can disrupt the repair. If the patient does not have an indwelling catheter, she should be asked to void every 4 hours. Inability to void or pain in the area of the bladder should be reported to the physician. If this occurs, insertion of a catheter is generally ordered. Insertion can be difficult postoperatively because of swelling and distortion of the urethral meatus. Asking the patient to take a slow, deep breath can assist in locating the opening.

Retrodisplacements of the Uterus

Normally, the position of the uterus is one of anteflexion and anteversion. Anteflexion refers to the forward tilt of the entire uterus, which causes the fundus to point toward the symphysis pubis and the cervix to point downward and backward toward the sacrum. Anteversion refers to the near right angle between the cervix and the vagina (Fig. 44–5).

Retrodisplacement of the uterus refers to a backward displacement of that organ. There are two types of retrodisplacement: retroflexion and retroversion (Fig. 44–6). In retroflexion, the fundus of the uterus bends backward on the cervix, which frequently begins to point downward and toward the symphysis pubis. In retroversion, the entire uterus is tipped backward so that the fundus no longer points forward. Depending on the amount of tilt, the retroversion is described as follows:

First degree: The fundus is approximately vertical, pointing no further back than the sacral prominence.
Second degree: The fundus lies in the hollow of the sacrum but is not below the cervix.
Third degree: The fundus is tilted so far backward that it is below the level of the cervix.

ETIOLOGY AND PATHOPHYSIOLOGY

Retrodisplacements of the uterus may be primary or secondary. Primary retrodisplacements have no known cause and may be congenital. Secondary or acquired retrodisplacements may be the result of overstretching of the uterine ligaments or injury to the fascia of the pelvic floor during childbirth. They may also occur because the uterus is mechanically pushed back by a tumor or a distended bladder, or they may be due to adnexal disease such as endometriosis or other inflammatory disorder. In the latter case, the retrodisplaced fundus is fixed to the

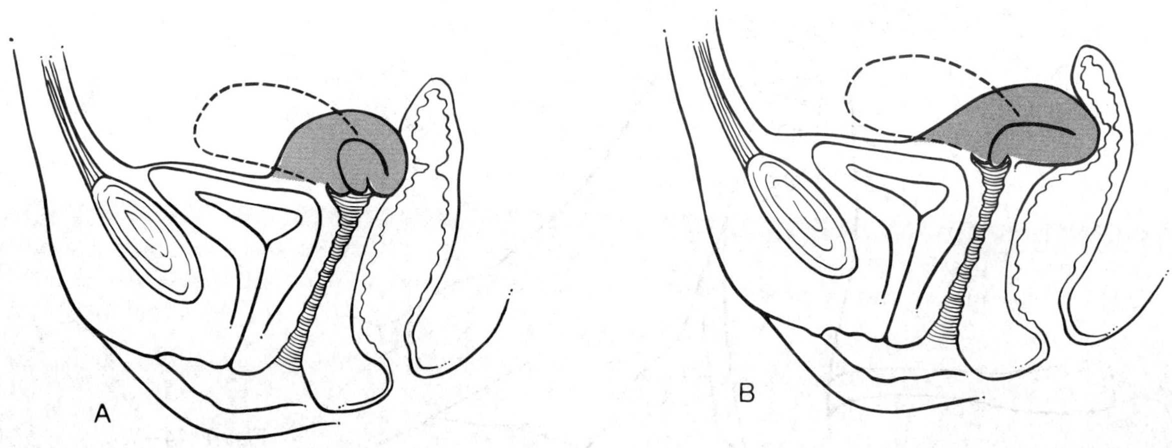

Figure 44–6.

Retrodisplacements of the uterus: *A*, retroflexion; *B*, retroversion.

adnexa or the rectum rather than being freely movable.

CLINICAL MANIFESTATIONS

Symptoms that may be associated with retrodisplacements are dysmenorrhea, low backache, dyspareunia, and a feeling of pelvic pressure. In acquired cases, infertility may also be present. Because there are many patients who experience no clinical symptoms, even with severe retrodisplacements, it is thought that symptoms result primarily from pelvic congestion or adhesions caused by an underlying disorder.

MEDICAL DIAGNOSIS

Diagnosis of a uterine retrodisplacement is made on the basis of characteristic findings on pelvic examination. The cervix is seen to point to the symphysis pubis rather than to the sacrum, and the fundus is palpated posteriorly rather than in its normal anterior position. Symptoms are of no diagnostic value.

MEDICAL MANAGEMENT

In cases of acquired retrodisplacements of the uterus, medical management is directed at treating the underlying problem. When a treatable underlying disease is not identified, and the uterus is freely mobile and able to be directed into normal position on a bimanual pelvic examination, no management may be needed. If intervention is required, postural therapy or a pessary may be prescribed.

POSTURAL THERAPY

With postural therapy, the patient assumes the knee-chest position three or four times per day for 5 minutes at a time. In this position, air distends the vagina, and the uterus falls forward (Fig. 44–7). This provides symptomatic relief for some patients, particularly those with a postpartum retrodisplacement.

PESSARY

A Hodge pessary may be inserted to maintain the uterus in its correct position. This pessary works by putting tension on the posterior fornix. It is inserted in an office setting and left in place for 2 to 3 months. During this time, follow-up visits are scheduled to ascertain that the pessary is in fact holding the uterus in the correct position.

In rare cases of uterine retrodisplacement in which there is infertility of more than 2 years duration with normal fertility studies, some physicians may recommend use of fertility packs, a cervical cap, or a uterine suspensory operation. In the latter procedure, an abdominal incision is made, the uterus is brought forward, and its supporting ligaments are shortened to maintain the corrected position.

Application of the Nursing Process to the Care of the Patient with a Retrodisplacement of the Uterus

Assessment

Assess the type and severity of symptoms experienced by the patient, their impact on her daily life, and the success of any relief measures that have been used. Also assess the patient's understanding of the disorder insofar as this is necessary to ensure compliance with the therapeutic plan, to allay anxi-

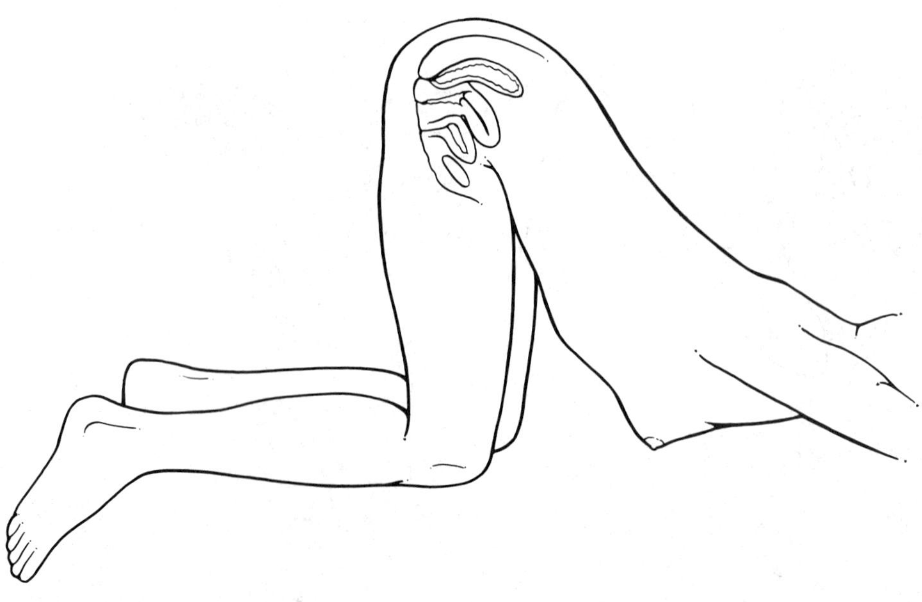

Figure 44–7.

Diagram of the pelvic organs with the woman in knee-chest position showing the forward movement of the uterus.

ety, and to prevent undue interference with daily living.

Nursing Diagnoses and Planning

Nursing diagnoses and related expected outcomes most commonly applicable to patients with a retrodisplacement of the uterus include the following:

NDx: Pain (low back) related to uterine displacement, poor posture, and poor body mechanics

Planning: Patient outcomes
1. Patient demonstrates correct body mechanics.
2. Patient describes/demonstrates postural therapy if ordered.
3. Patient reports relief of low back pain.

NDx: High risk for altered health maintenance related to insufficient knowledge of reason for and care of pessary

Planning: Patient outcomes
1. Patient lists symptoms to be reported.
2. Patient states reason for and date of follow-up visit.

NDx: Sexual dysfunction related to dyspareunia

Planning: Patient outcomes
1. Patient describes how sexual excitement causes an upward movement of the uterus and ovaries and as a result reduces discomfort on intercourse.
2. Patient reports that she is more comfortable during sexual intercourse.

Nursing Interventions

NDx: Pain
Explain the relationship of poor posture and improper lifting to back pain because many patients believe that any low back pain is caused by the womb being out of place. Teach principles of correct body mechanics.

Teach the patient to assume the knee-chest position if postural therapy is ordered. Reinforce that this should be done for 5 minutes three or four times every day.

NDx: High risk for altered health maintenance
If a pessary is ordered, instruct the patient to report any difficulty with urination, vaginal bleeding, or other drainage and any foul vaginal odor. Make certain that the patient knows when to return for a follow-up examination.

NDx: Sexual dysfunction
If the uterus is mobile and dyspareunia is the only symptom, sexual counseling can offer the solution to the problem. Explain that because the uterus and ovaries move upward as sexual excitement increases, symptom relief can be obtained by heightening sexual arousal through foreplay before intercourse.

Evaluation

Evaluate the effectiveness of nursing care for a patient with a retrodisplacement of the uterus by comparing the patient's status with the expected patient outcomes. Examples of specific outcomes for patients with a retrodisplacement of the uterus have been provided in the Planning section.

Genital Fistulas

A genital fistula is an abnormal opening between the vagina or the uterus and either some part of the urinary tract, some part of the intestinal tract, or both.

ETIOLOGY AND PATHOPHYSIOLOGY

In the past, genital fistulas were common. They occurred chiefly as a result of trauma during labor and delivery. The genital fistulas seen today occur primarily from injury to the bladder, ureter, or rectum during a radical hysterectomy or from tissue necrosis and sloughing as a result of radiation therapy. In some cases, fistulas may result from the destruction of tissue by malignant tumors or a chronic disorder such as Crohn's disease, ulceration from a foreign body such as a pessary, or rarely secondary to a simple hysterectomy or an anterior vaginal repair. This last factor may occur because, with any hysterectomy, there is always some trauma to the bladder or the bowel, and some patients are simply poor healers.

GENITOURINARY FISTULAS

The most common type of genitourinary fistula is vesicovaginal (bladder to vagina). Other types include urethrovaginal (urethra to vagina), and ureterovaginal (ureter to vagina) (Fig. 44–8). The fistula may be tiny and difficult to locate, or it may be so large that the whole base of the bladder is destroyed.

CLINICAL MANIFESTATIONS

The chief symptom of a vesicovaginal fistula is leakage of urine from the vagina. If the fistula is small, this may be a slight dribble that is aggravated when the patient assumes particular positions. If the fistula is large, the flow of urine from the vagina may be constant and profuse. The leakage of urine causes an odor of ammonia and irritation of the

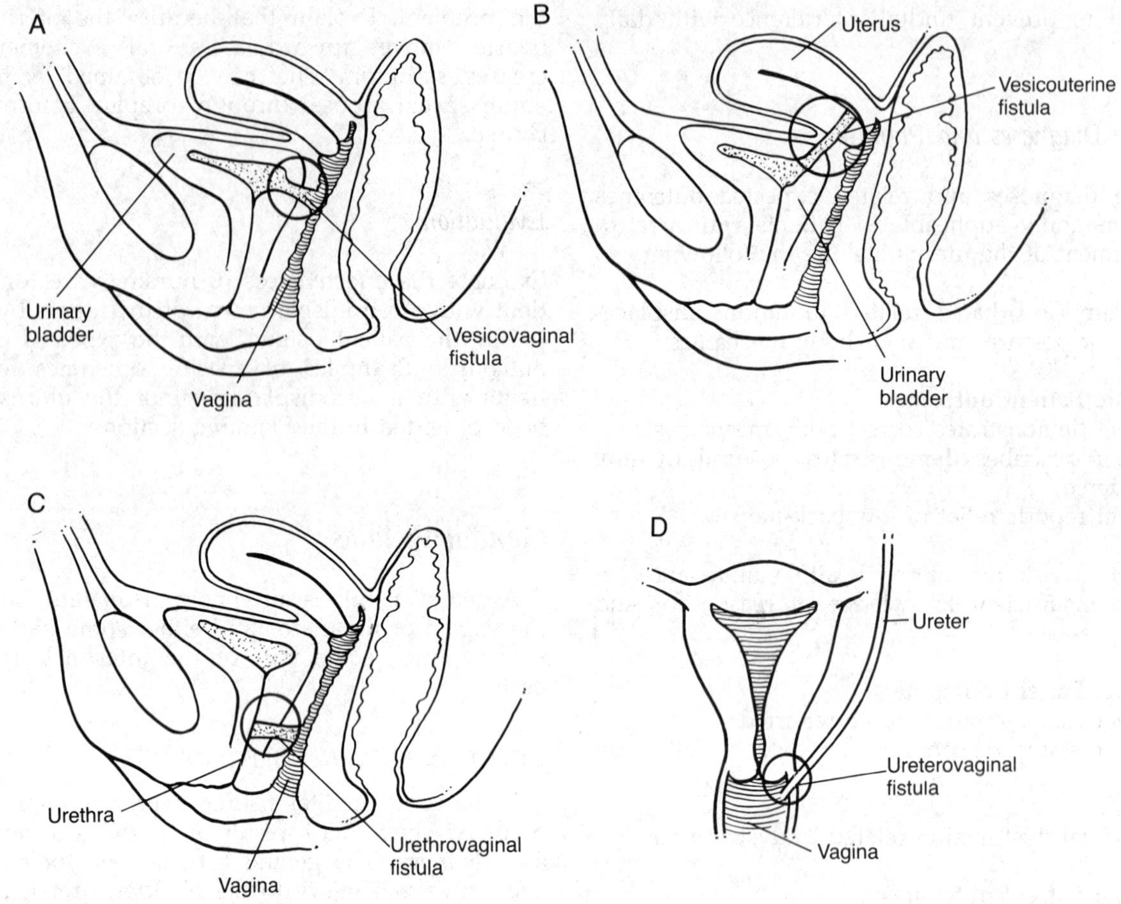

Figure 44–8.

Types of genitourinary fistulas: *A*, vesicovaginal; *B*, vesicouterine; *C*, urethrovaginal; *D*, ureterovaginal.

vagina, vulva, and perineum. These symptoms are a source of embarrassment, and the patient with a fistula may avoid social contacts and may be nervous, irritable, depressed, and suffer from insomnia.

MEDICAL DIAGNOSIS

Most vesicovaginal fistulas can be seen on a vaginal examination done with the patient in the knee-chest position. If the fistula is very large, it may be palpated by the finger in the vagina. Fistulas too small or too high up in the vagina to be seen or palpated can be diagnosed by filling the bladder with sterile water colored with methylene blue. The bluish fluid is then observed passing through the abnormal opening. Definitive diagnosis of a ureterovaginal fistula can be obtained by an intravenous or retrograde pyelogram.

MEDICAL MANAGEMENT

Small fistulas, if not related to malignant disease, sometimes heal spontaneously in 4 to 6 months. To encourage healing, postural therapy, use of urinary antiseptics, and a retention catheter with suction may be ordered.

Most cases of urogenital fistula require surgical closure. This is done when inflammation and edema in the area have subsided, usually in 4 to 6 months. When fistulas are due to radiation, healing is impaired because of a poor blood supply to the area, so a transplant flap is used.

VAGINAL-INTESTINAL FISTULAS

The most common type of vaginal-intestinal fistula is a rectovaginal fistula (Fig. 44–9). Fistulas involving the sigmoid colon or small intestine also occur. The latter result from malignant disease, pelvic or intestinal operations, or other medical conditions such as Crohn's disease.

CLINICAL MANIFESTATIONS

If a vaginal-intestinal fistula is tiny, the only sign may be occasional foul-smelling leukorrhea or an occasional passage of gas or fecal matter from the vagina. In fact, this may occur only when the patient's stool is abnormally loose. With large fistulas, the signs become more prominent to the point at which there may be constant fecal drainage through the vagina. Irritation of the vagina, vulva, and perineum develops, and an offensive odor is present. Infection may occur in the surrounding tissues.

MEDICAL DIAGNOSIS

Passage of feces through the vagina is evidence of a vaginal-intestinal fistula. The exact location of the fistula in the intestinal tract is identified by sigmoidoscopy or a barium enema.

MEDICAL MANAGEMENT

Very small vaginal-intestinal fistulas in otherwise healthy individuals may close spontaneously in 1 to 3 months. Larger fistulas require surgical repair, which is best done 4 to 6 months after injury, when edema and inflammation have subsided. The repair of a rectovaginal fistula is done vaginally. For fistulas involving other parts of the intestinal tract, abdominal surgery is necessary. In cases in which tissues around the fistula are badly infected, a temporary colostomy (see Chapter 21) may be performed above the level of the fistula to allow healing of the area before a repair is attempted.

Palliative measures such as douches and enemas are prescribed during the interval before surgery. Measures are also taken to improve the general health status of the patient, and antibiotic therapy may be prescribed to treat or prevent infection.

Immediately before surgery, routine preoperative care, including standard bowel preparation, is given.

Application of the Nursing Process to the Care of the Patient with a Vaginal Fistula

Assessment

Because of the type of symptoms produced by a vaginal fistula, there are many actual or potential physical, psychological, and social effects on the patient. Therefore, a broad-based, thorough assessment is essential if the patient's nursing care needs are to be met.

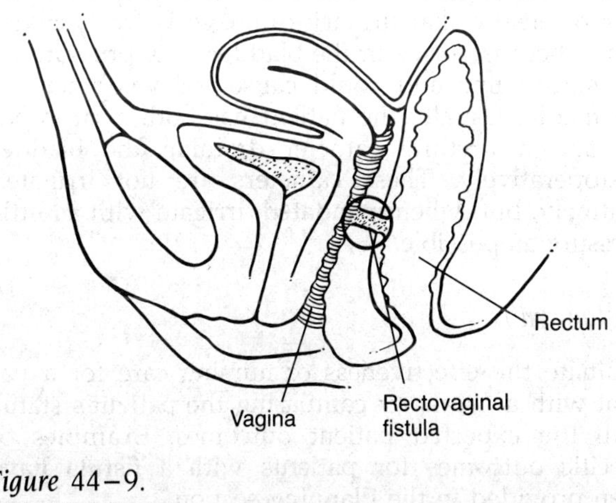

Figure 44–9.

Rectovaginal fistula.

Assess for signs and symptoms of a fistula. Ask whether urine escapes from the vagina and, if so, how often and how much and whether it is affected by particular positions or movements. Ask whether gas or fecal matter escapes from the vagina. If so, determine the frequency, extent, and relationship to the consistency of the stool. Also question about internal pain or other discomfort. Observe the condition of the tissues of the vulva and surrounding areas. Note erythema, excoriation, and drainage.

If the patient has had the fistula for a period of time, explore her methods of dealing with the problem. Determine how often she cleanses the area, what cleansing solution is used, and whether she douches or takes enemas. Also determine what type of protective pads she uses, how often she changes them, and if she has a problem with odor.

Assess the patient's general health and nutritional status. Ask about any other health problems, and determine whether her overall health status appears compatible with probable healing of the fistula. Review her dietary pattern. Determine whether her daily fluid intake is adequate and whether her usual diet provides sufficient basic nutrients to support healing.

Question about the effects of the fistula and its symptoms on personal lifestyle. Assess for problems in sexual, family, and social relationships.

Finally, explore the patient's expectation of health care. Determine whether she expects complete healing of the fistula and total relief of symptoms or whether she expects control of symptoms and increased comfort. Also explore her understanding of the problem and its treatment.

Nursing Diagnoses and Planning

Nursing diagnoses and related expected patient outcomes most commonly applicable to patients with genital fistulas include the following:

NDx: High risk for impaired skin integrity related to irritation from urine or feces leaking from the vagina

Planning: Patient outcomes

1. Vulvovaginal skin and mucous membranes are intact.
2. Vulvovaginal areas are free of erythema.
3. Patient denies smarting or burning of vulvovaginal areas.

NDx: High risk for altered health maintenance related to insufficient knowledge of nutritional needs

Planning: Patient outcomes

1. Patient's daily diet contains sufficient proteins and vitamins to support healing the fistula.

2. Patient describes relationship between constipation and enlargement of the fistula.
3. Patient describes the need for dietary roughage and identifies foods that contribute to it.
4. Patient identifies constipating foods.
5. Patient describes need for a fluid intake of at least 2000 ml/day to avoid constipation and tissue irritation from concentrated urine.

NDx: High risk for body image disturbance related to leakage and odor of urine or feces

Planning: Patient outcomes
1. Patient initiates measures needed for good personal grooming.
2. Patient displays usual level of interest in personal appearance.
3. Patient makes positive comments about self.
4. Patient verbalizes feelings of self-assurance.

NDx: High risk for social isolation related to embarrassment over leakage of urine or feces

Planning: Patient outcomes
1. Patient maintains usual level of social interaction.

Nursing Interventions

NDx: High risk for impaired skin integrity
Cleanse the perineal area, and change protective pads or undergarments frequently to prevent skin breakdown caused by irritation from fistula drainage. Use mild soap and water, rinse thoroughly, and dry thoroughly. In accordance with physician's orders, pour a weakly basic (e.g., sodium bicarbonate) solution over the vulva to neutralize the pH and to reduce irritation to the tissues if drainage from the fistula is acidic. If drainage from the fistula is basic, use a weakly acidic (e.g., acetic acid) solution. Apply ointments such as A&D to provide a protective film to prevent irritating drainage from coming into direct contact with the skin.

Position the patient carefully to aid in maintaining good circulation to the skin and to help protect against breakdown.

If the fistula is rectovaginal, administer enemas as ordered to decrease the feces available to escape through the fistula. This helps control problems of leakage, odor, and irritation of skin and mucous membranes. Use a soft, rubber enema tube, and direct it toward the side of the rectum opposite the fistula. Be sure to insert the tube beyond the level of the fistula to prevent the enema fluid from simply draining into the vagina.

If ordered, give douches to cleanse and soothe the mucous membrane of the vagina. Always give gently because too much pressure can force fluid back through the fistula tract.

NDx: High risk for altered health maintenance
Explain the need for a balanced diet with adequate amounts of protein and vitamins to promote healing of the fistula and to avoid complications. Assist the patient in selecting a diet that is appealing to her and that meets this need. Stress the importance of a diet with sufficient roughage to avoid constipation.

A diet low in roughage and fluids and high in "constipating" foods is sometimes used by patients with a rectovaginal fistula to temporarily control fecal leakage from the vagina. Advise against this approach because constipation leads to increased rectal pressure and can increase the size of the fistula.

NDx: High risk for body image disturbance
Protect the patient from embarrassment as a result of the leakage of urine or feces.

Provide for privacy. Cleanse the perineal area, and change pads or other protective undergarments just before visiting hours and just before any tests or treatments that require the patient to be transported to other areas of the health facility or to be in close contact with other patients.

Deodorize the patient's environment in an ongoing manner. Cover and promptly remove all soiled materials from the room. Apply deodorizing powders to the perineal area or administer Clorox douches (1 teaspoon of Clorox per quart of water as ordered).

Encourage and assist the patient to maintain an attractive appearance, use deodorant, apply makeup, and tastefully arrange her hair. Keep the patient's surroundings in a clean, orderly condition.

NDx: High risk for social isolation
Spend time with the patient at intervals throughout the day. Avoid acting rushed when caring for her, because this could be interpreted as "wanting to get away from something unpleasant" and contribute to a sense of social isolation. If able, encourage the patient to leave her room, walk in the corridor, or visit the patient's lounge. Encourage telephone contact and visits with relatives and friends. Discuss her usual patterns of social activities and any plans for resuming them.

Additional Interventions
If a vesicovaginal fistula has been surgically repaired, ensure that urinary drainage is freely maintained because urine in the bladder puts pressure on the suture line and could cause redevelopment of the fistula. Usually the patient has both a suprapubic and a urethral catheter draining the bladder postoperatively. These catheters are not irrigated routinely, but, when mandated, irrigate with as little pressure as possible.

Evaluation

Evaluate the effectiveness of nursing care for a patient with a fistula by comparing the patient's status with the expected patient outcomes. Examples of specific outcomes for patients with a fistula have been provided in the Planning section.

Neoplasia

Benign Neoplasms

POLYPS

Polyps are tumors that have stalks or pedicles. They are common in vascular organs and bleed easily. In the female reproductive system, two common types of polyps are cervical polyps and endometrial polyps.

CERVICAL POLYPS

Etiology and Pathophysiology

Cervical polyps develop when an area of the mucosa in the cervical canal proliferates. Cervical polyps may be single or multiple. They are usually small and appear as bright red, spongy tissue protruding out of the cervical canal into the vagina. The tip of the polyp is often ulcerated. Cervical polyps may arise in association with conditions of long-standing irritation such as chronic vaginitis or cervicitis.

Cervical polyps rarely undergo malignant change. However, metaplasia of the squamous epithelium can occur, and, especially if an infection is present, it can look like early cancer.

Clinical Manifestations

Small cervical polyps usually do not cause symptoms, whereas large cervical polyps cause bleeding similar to that associated with early cancer of the cervix. This bleeding, which is due to the vascularity of the polyp, is generally small in amount, although hemorrhage can occur during menstruation. It may be intermenstrual bleeding or contact bleeding that occurs after coitus, douching, or a vaginal examination.

Medical Diagnosis

Large cervical polyps can be felt by the examining finger during palpation of the cervix. Smaller polyps can be identified on inspection through a bivalve speculum.

A smear is always done at the time of diagnosis because simply finding a polyp does not prove that it is the cause of the symptom and that it is the only pathology present.

Medical Management

Polyps associated with symptoms are usually removed. This can often be done by simply twisting the pedicle off and cauterizing the point of attachment to the uterine wall. If multiple polyps are present, the cervical canal is dilated and cauterized. Lasers are increasingly used to remove polyps. Recurrence is fairly common.

ENDOMETRIAL POLYPS

Etiology and Pathophysiology

Endometrial polyps are composed of endometrial tissue. This tissue may be functional or nonfunctional. When the tissue of the polyp is functional, it changes in response to hormones like the general uterine mucosa. When it is nonfunctional or immature, it does not respond to hormonal stimulation.

Endometrial polyps may be single or multiple and vary in size from small to large enough to fill the uterine cavity. Endometrial polyps are extremely unlikely to undergo malignant change. However, during the menopausal and postmenopausal years, there is an increased incidence of uterine cancer in females who also have endometrial polyps.

Clinical Manifestations

Many endometrial polyps are asymptomatic unless they are large enough to protrude through the cervical canal and have become ulcerated. When this occurs, moderate metrorrhagia results. If the blood supply through the pedicle of the polyp is impeded, necrosis with bleeding and a foul-smelling discharge can occur.

Medical Diagnosis

Many endometrial polyps are discovered accidentally during a dilation and curettage (D&C) or after a hysterectomy. Large, protruding polyps can be seen during a pelvic examination.

Medical Management

Large, symptomatic polyps are surgically removed. With the patient under anesthesia, the cervix is dilated and the polyp removed at its base. A curettage is then performed to identify and remove any other small polyps that might be present.

Guidelines for Application of the Nursing Process to the Care of the Patient with Cervical or Endometrial Polyps

Fear is common among females with any type of neoplasm. This fear may be exaggerated in the patient with a cervical or endometrial polyp because her first symptom may have been spotting similar to that publicly identified as a first sign of cervical cancer. It is important, therefore, to assess the patient's understanding and emotional acceptance of the polyp as a benign growth. If a knowledge deficit or anxiety state exists, provide information and give the patient the opportunity to express her concerns. Printed materials indicating the benign nature of polyps are sometimes an effective aid in allaying anxiety.

Teach patients with these polyps about the need for routine gynecologic examinations even after menopause occurs, because endometrial cancer does occur more often in females with a history of endometrial polyps.

LEIOMYOMAS

Leiomyomas (also called myomas, fibromas, and fibroids) are benign, smooth-muscle tumors found in the wall of the uterus. Leiomyomas are the most common tumor of the female reproductive tract. It is estimated that one of five women older than 35 years has them. They occur most frequently in black women and in nulliparas.

ETIOLOGY AND PATHOPHYSIOLOGY

The exact cause of leiomyomas is unknown, but their development seems to be linked to an excess of estrogen relative to progesterone. This type of imbalance occurs if the level of progesterone is normal but the level of estrogen is increased or if the level of estrogen is normal but the level of progesterone is decreased.

Leiomyomas develop slowly during the reproductive years except during pregnancy, when their growth is accelerated. They atrophy after menopause. They vary in size from that of a small seed to that of a grapefruit; are firm, round, or oval; and tend to be multiple.

There are three types of leiomyoma: intramural, submucous, and subserosal (Fig. 44–10).

Intramural leiomyomas are in the middle of the uterine wall surrounded by myometrium. As they grow, the size of the uterus increases and the inner wall becomes nodular in contour and consistency.

Submucous leiomyomas lie just under the endometrium and tend to impinge on its vascular supply. These tumors may grow a pedicle and occasionally can be seen protruding from the cervix and, more rarely, from the vagina. As they grow, they begin to fill the uterine cavity and can eventually touch the opposite wall and distort the shape of the cavity.

Subserous tumors grow on the outer surface of the uterus just under the serosal covering and tend to be pedunculated and large. They are called intraligamentary if they grow out between the folds of the broad ligament.

Most often, leiomyomas occur in the body of the uterus, although they can occur in the cervix.

CLINICAL MANIFESTATIONS

In many cases, leiomyomas, even multiple large ones, cause no symptoms. When symptoms do occur, the onset is usually between the ages of 40 and 45 years, and they are related to the size and location of the tumors. Symptoms are not present until a fibroid is the size of a softball or grapefruit.

Excessive, prolonged menstruation is the most common symptom of intramural and submucous tumors because of an increase in endometrial surface. In some cases, the blood loss is sufficient to cause anemia and its symptoms of fatigue, weakness, and lethargy.

Symptoms from large tumors and from subserosal tumors that grow outward from the uterus rather than into the uterine cavity are caused by pressure on adjacent pelvic organs. If pressure is exerted on the rectum, constipation and pain on defecation occur. With pressure on the bladder, the patient may have frequency of urination and dysuria. If the urethra is compressed, retention and hydroureter can occur.

Large tumors of any type can cause a sensation of low abdominal pressure or "bearing down," dysmenorrhea, backache, and weight gain. There may also be a palpable abdominal mass and general enlargement of the abdomen. Large tumors in the body of the uterus can cause spontaneous abortions and, if they grow into the openings of the fallopian tubes, can cause sterility.

If a leiomyoma is pedunculated and the pedicle twists, the resultant interference with blood supply causes severe pain and nausea and vomiting.

MEDICAL DIAGNOSIS

Leiomyomas are suspected when the patient has a history of characteristic symptoms and one or more nodular outgrowths can be felt on the uterus during a bimanual pelvic examination. Sonograms, diagnostic curettage, and hysterograms may be used to confirm the diagnosis and to rule out pregnancy and other disorders.

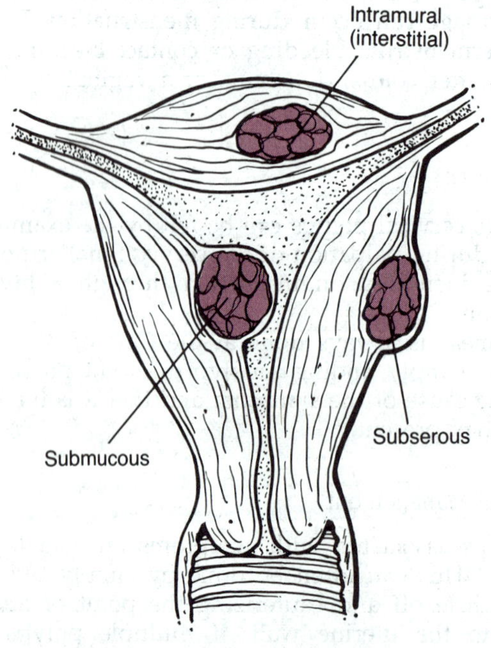

Figure 44–10.

Types of leiomyomas.

Nursing Care Guide 44–1.

PATIENTS UNDERGOING TRANSABDOMINAL HYSTERECTOMY FOR FIBROID TUMORS

Preoperative Care

Assessment Findings: Patient states she is afraid of the operation. Patient verbalizes worry over the diagnosis of cancer and subsequent length of life, symptoms, and quality of life. Patient is restless and unable to concentrate. Patient's facial expression and posture are tense.

Nursing Diagnosis: Anxiety related to impending hysterectomy

Patient Outcomes	Nursing Interventions	Rationale
Patient readily expresses feelings of anxiety and perceived sources of it.	Acknowledge that anxiety over surgery and its outcomes is normal.	Allays patient concerns about being judged negatively because of anxiety.
	Encourage verbalization of feelings and concerns.	Allows for feedback, provides perspective, and opens the way for a supportive relationship.
Patient uses coping mechanisms that were effective in the past.	Identify strategies that the patient has used in the past to control anxiety effectively (distraction with music, presence of a significant other). Facilitate their use.	Use of strategies that have been proven successful and acceptable to the patient can be promoted.
Patient reports that she feels less anxious. Patient is able to attend to directions and conversations. Patient's facial expression and body posture appear relaxed. Patient is able to rest quietly.	Offer reassurance about the success of the surgery as appropriate. For example, reassure the patient about her overall state of health and therefore fitness for surgery, or mention the frequency of the procedure and its success rate.	Provides the patient with positive facts on which to focus and base hope for a successful surgical outcome.

Evaluation: Compare the patient's status with the expected patient outcomes. If the outcomes are achieved, evaluate nursing care as successful. If not, reassess the patient, formulate new nursing diagnoses, and revise expected patient outcomes and nursing interventions as appropriate.

(continued)

MEDICAL MANAGEMENT

Medical management varies depending on the severity of the symptoms, the age of the patient, her desires in regard to childbearing, the location and size of the tumor, and the presence of complications.

A conservative treatment plan may be followed if the patient is close to menopause and if the leiomyomas have not caused the uterus to enlarge to the size of 12 weeks' or more gestation. The patient is observed every 3 to 6 months and, provided no rapid increase in size occurs, the leiomyomas are left to undergo normal postmenopausal atrophy. If a rapid increase in size occurs, definitive treatment is needed to rule out the possibility of carcinoma.

If the patient does not desire to have a child or the leiomyomas are so large that a successful pregnancy is unlikely and bleeding is severe, a hysterectomy is the treatment of choice. When relief of symptoms and subsequent childbearing is the aim, a myomectomy is performed. This procedure, in which the tumors are excised, is always preceded by a diagnostic curettage to rule out any other cause of the presenting symptoms such as adenocarcinoma. A disadvantage of the procedure is the risk that the tumors may recur.

Nursing Care Guide 44–1. *(continued)*

PATIENTS UNDERGOING TRANSABDOMINAL HYSTERECTOMY FOR FIBROID TUMORS

Assessment Findings: Patient asks questions about perioperative routines, what the incision will look like, how she will feel after the surgery, and so on or makes incorrect statements about the operative experience.

Nursing Diagnosis: Knowledge deficit: the surgical procedure, preoperative preparation, or expected postoperative course

Patient Outcomes	Nursing Interventions	Rationale
Patient states that the uterus will be removed through an incision in the lower abdomen, that she will no longer menstruate or bear children, but that because the ovaries, which produce hormones, will remain, she will not experience symptoms of menopause.	Clarify patient's understanding of the procedure: what organs will be removed, size and location of incision, and effect on body function.	Supports informed consent, involves the patient in the plan of care, and provides a basis for later teaching.
Patient describes preoperative preparation, transport to the operating room, recovery room environment and procedures, and return to unit.	Explain perioperative routines.	Decreases the risk of anxiety over routine perioperative events.
Patient states that she will need an intravenous catheter, will be gotten up from bed on the first postoperative day, and so on.	Clarify expected postoperative course.	Promotes compliance with postoperative care and decreases risk of anxiety over routine postoperative procedures and events.
Patient explains importance of postoperative coughing, deep breathing, and leg exercises and demonstrates them correctly.	Teach importance and technique of postoperative coughing, deep breathing, and leg exercises.	Promotes compliance with postoperative care.

Evaluation: Compare the patient's status with the expected patient outcomes. If the outcomes are achieved, evaluate nursing care as successful. If not, reassess the patient, formulate new nursing diagnoses, and revise expected patient outcomes and nursing interventions as appropriate.

Postoperative Care

Assessment Findings: Patient complains of incisional pain; patient guards abdomen when moving; patient grimaces or moans on moving.

Nursing Diagnosis: Pain related to the surgical excision of the uterus through an abdominal incision

(continued)

Nursing Care Guide 44–1. *(continued)*

PATIENTS UNDERGOING TRANSABDOMINAL HYSTERECTOMY FOR FIBROID TUMORS

Patient Outcomes	Nursing Interventions	Rationale
Patient reports pain is relieved. Nonverbal signs of pain such as grimacing or guarding are absent.	Administer analgesics as per order.	Provides pain relief.
	Assist patient in assuming comfortable position.	Decreases positional stress on the incisional area, thereby relieving pain and promoting rest.
	Provide basic comfort measures such as smooth bedding and back rubs. Maintain a quiet, peaceful environment.	Promotes comfort and rest.
Patient splints incision when coughing or moving.	Teach patient to splint incision with a pillow when coughing or moving.	Decreases pull on the incision line, reducing discomfort and increasing compliance with coughing and moving.
Patient gets out of bed without undue discomfort.	Instruct patient to get out of bed as follows: With head of bed elevated, turn on side facing side of bed to be gotten out of. Bend knees as when sitting in a chair. Put feet over side of bed. Push up on elbow. Sit up straight.	
Patient identifies personal methods of coping with pain and uses them.	Explore with the patient what coping mechanisms have been effectively used in the past, and assist her in using them (e.g., distraction with music, imagery, and so on).	Encourages use of successful strategies from past experiences.
Patient performs relaxation exercises and reports relief.	Encourage relaxation.	Reduces tension level of body, thereby decreasing strain on body tissues.

Evaluation: Compare the patient's status with the expected patient outcomes. If the outcomes are achieved, evaluate nursing care as successful. If not, reassess the patient, formulate new nursing diagnoses, and revise expected patient outcomes and nursing interventions as appropriate.

(continued)

Application of the Nursing Process to the Care of the Patient with a Leiomyoma

The assessment, nursing diagnoses, expected patient outcomes, nursing interventions, and evaluation for patients with a leiomyoma are similar to those described in Chapter 43 for patients having a hysterectomy (see also Nursing Care Guide 44–1). In addition, if surgery is scheduled because the tumors suddenly increase in size, the patient may be very fearful that she has cancer. If so, provide opportunities for her to express feelings and concerns, and reinforce facts as needed.

If a myomectomy is done on a patient who is premenopausal and desirous of having a child, give support in the form of information on successful pregnancy after myomectomy.

Nursing Care Guide 44–1. *(continued)*

PATIENTS UNDERGOING TRANSABDOMINAL HYSTERECTOMY FOR FIBROID TUMORS

Assessment Findings: Recent general anesthesia, shallow respirations, ineffective coughing.

Nursing Diagnosis: High risk for ineffective airway clearance related to shallow respirations and ineffective coughing

Patient Outcomes	Nursing Interventions	Rationale
Respirations are of normal depth.	Medicate patient to relieve pain.	Pain causes shallow breathing as a result of discomfort on chest expansion.
	Position patient in semi-Fowler's position or flat with pillows under the shoulder.	Gravity increases pull of intestines away from diaphragm to allow greater chest expansion. Raising the shoulders with pillows promotes chest expansion.
	Ensure that clothing and bedding do not constrict chest.	Reduces external restriction on chest expansion.
Patient coughs and deep breathes effectively every hour while awake.	Reinforce preoperative teaching regarding need to cough and deep breathe.	Encourages patient compliance when instructed to cough and deep breathe.
	Instruct patient to splint incision when coughing and deep breathing.	Decreases pull on incision line.
	Encourage coughing and deep breathing every hour when awake.	
Secretions are fluid and expectorated.	Reinforce preoperative teaching regarding importance of expectoration.	Encourages patient compliance with instructions to expectorate.
	Keep tissues within patient's reach. Provide container for disposal of used tissues.	Encourages compliance by decreasing difficulties associated with expectoration.
Respirations are silent. Breath sounds are clear.	Monitor breath sounds.	Evaluates effectiveness of interventions.

Evaluation: Compare the patient's status with the expected patient outcomes. If the outcomes are achieved, evaluate nursing care as successful. If not, reassess the patient, formulate new nursing diagnoses, and revise expected patient outcomes and nursing interventions as appropriate.

(continued)

Nursing Care Guide 44–1. *(continued)*

PATIENTS UNDERGOING TRANSABDOMINAL HYSTERECTOMY FOR FIBROID TUMORS

Assessment Findings: Patient is recovering from pelvic surgery, which is associated with risk of trauma to the deep veins of thigh and pelvis.

Nursing Diagnosis: High risk for altered tissue perfusion related to interruption of venous blood flow secondary to thrombophlebitis or pulmonary embolism

Patient Outcomes	Nursing Interventions	Rationale
Patient dorsiflexes feet 20–25 times each hour while awake and on bed rest	Encourage patient to dorsiflex feet 20–25 times every hour while awake and on bed rest	Muscle contraction promotes venous return by its squeezing action on the veins and thus reduces the risk of thrombus formation.
Patient avoids positions that impede venous return: flexed knees, flexed hips, crossed legs.	Avoid use of bed gatch or pillows, which cause flexion of knee or compression of the popliteal space. Position patient to prevent sharp flexion of the inguinal area. Instruct patient not to cross legs. Avoid having patient sit for extended periods of time.	Eliminates obstruction to venous return as a result of bending or compression of veins, thus decreasing stasis, which increases risk of thrombus formation.
Antithromboembolic stockings are worn and are smoothly fitted without twists or wrinkles.	Apply antithromboembolic hose as ordered, and check frequently for correct fit.	Promotes venous return, decreasing the risk of thrombus formation.
Patient willingly gets out of bed and ambulates as soon as physical condition allows.	Encourage movement and ambulation as soon as possible.	Promotes venous circulation, decreasing venous stasis and risk of thrombus formation.
Calf is free of heat, redness, and swelling. Homans' sign (pain in calf on strong, passive dorsiflexion of foot) is negative.	Monitor for heat, redness, and swelling in the calf. Check Homans' sign.	Early recognition of symptoms of thrombophlebitis allows for rapid medical intervention.
Patient is free of symptoms of pulmonary embolism: respirations have normal rate and depth. Cyanosis, chest pain, and hemoptysis are absent.	Monitor for symptoms of pulmonary embolism.	Early recognition of symptoms of pulmonary emboli allows for rapid medical intervention.

Evaluation: Compare the patient's status with the expected patient outcomes. If the outcomes are achieved, evaluate nursing care as successful. If not, reassess the patient, formulate new nursing diagnoses, and revise expected patient outcomes and nursing interventions as appropriate.

(continued)

Nursing Care Guide 44–1. *(continued)*

PATIENTS UNDERGOING TRANSABDOMINAL HYSTERECTOMY FOR FIBROID TUMORS

Assessment Findings: Patient verbalizes fears about ability to participate and enjoy usual sexual activity.

Nursing Diagnosis: High risk for altered sexuality patterns related to removal of the uterus

Patient Outcomes	Nursing Interventions	Rationale
Patient describes normal sexual structure and function and changes resulting from hysterectomy.	Review normal sexual structure and function. Explain the effects of hysterectomy.	Provides patient with information necessary to understand the effects of the surgical procedure.
Patient identifies common misconceptions regarding the effect of hysterectomy on libido and sexual enjoyment.	Identify common misconceptions, and distinguish from facts regarding relationship of hysterectomy to sexual function and enjoyment.	Provides patient with positive facts on which to focus while clarifying common misconceptions.
Patient discusses sexual concerns with partner.	Encourage sharing of concerns about future sexual activity with partner.	Allows sharing of newly acquired knowledge while promoting open communication between partners.
	Provide time and privacy for such discussion.	Privacy provides the couple with an environment conducive to open communication.

Evaluation: Compare the patient's status with the expected patient outcomes. If the outcomes are achieved, evaluate nursing care as successful. If not, reassess the patient, formulate new nursing diagnoses, and revise expected patient outcomes and nursing interventions as appropriate.

Assessment Findings: Patient has no previous knowledge of discharge instructions after a hysterectomy. Patient asks questions regarding care of the incision and limitations on activities.

Nursing Diagnosis: High risk for altered health maintenance related to insufficient knowledge of guidelines for self-management

Patient Outcomes	Nursing Interventions	Rationale
Patient identifies activities to be avoided: tub baths for 2–3 weeks; sitting for long periods, jogging, fast walking, horseback riding, douching, and other activities that increase pelvic congestion; strenuous activities such as heavy lifting and vacuum cleaning for 6 weeks.	Instruct patient about limitations on activity during the recovery period.	Provides information necessary for self-management after hospital discharge.

(continued)

Nursing Care Guide 44–1. *(continued)*

PATIENTS UNDERGOING TRANSABDOMINAL HYSTERECTOMY FOR FIBROID TUMORS

Patient Outcomes	Nursing Interventions	Rationale
Patient lists symptoms to be reported: bleeding, vaginal discharge, fever.	Teach symptoms to be reported.	Provides information necessary to recognize postoperative complications as well as appropriate patient response.
Patient verbalizes that periods of emotional lability and transient feelings of depression and sadness are not uncommon.	Explain about expected emotional reactions after surgery.	Helps control anxiety by increasing awareness of expected emotional response.
Patient can state date and time of follow-up visit.	Instruct patient on need for and time of follow-up care.	Provides information necessary for self-management after hospital discharge.

Evaluation: Compare the patient's status with the expected patient outcomes. If the outcomes are achieved, evaluate nursing care as successful. If not, reassess the patient, formulate new nursing diagnoses, and revise expected patient outcomes and nursing interventions as appropriate.

BENIGN OVARIAN TUMORS

ETIOLOGY AND PATHOPHYSIOLOGY

Ovarian tumors are classified as non-neoplastic or neoplastic.

Non-neoplastic Tumors

Non-neoplastic tumors are physiologic in origin. They are not pathologic but are simply enlargements of normal ovarian structures.

Two types of non-neoplastic or physiologic ovarian tumors are follicle cysts and corpus luteal cysts.

Follicle cysts develop in a graafian follicle that has not ruptured or that has ruptured but quickly resealed. These very common cysts tend to be multiple, small, and self-limited. They are filled with serous fluid, which is rich in estrogen. This may delay the onset of menstruation or cause a prolonged menses. Because the fluid is resorbed and the cyst disappears in 4 to 8 weeks, the symptoms occur for only one or two cycles, and no treatment is generally necessary.

Corpus luteal cysts occur when the corpus luteum does not degenerate but keeps on growing and producing progesterone. This delays the onset of menses or causes prolonged spotting or pain. Like follicular cysts, corpus luteal cysts rarely persist beyond one or two menstrual cycles, and treatment is generally unnecessary.

Neoplastic Tumors

Neoplastic tumors are new growths that develop from either the germinal epithelium of the ovary, the germ cells, or the ovarian stroma. They are classified according to the tissue from which they arise and occur in both solid and cystic form.

Eighty percent of ovarian neoplasms are benign, and 20% are malignant.

The most common benign ovarian neoplasms are benign cystic teratomas or dermoid cysts, benign serous cystadenomas, and mucinous cystadenomas.

Dermoid cysts arise from germ cells and contain a thick, yellow sebaceous substance along with rudiments of other tissues such as teeth, hair, bone, brain, and eyes. They are slow-growing tumors and occur most often in women between the ages of 18 and 35 years.

Benign serous cystadenomas and mucinous cystadenomas both arise from the germinal epithelium. These tumors are found primarily in women between the ages of 40 and 50 years and represent about 50% of all diagnosed benign ovarian neoplasms.

CLINICAL MANIFESTATIONS

Small ovarian tumors usually do not cause symptoms. When symptoms do occur, they are related to pressure of the tumor on surrounding organs. Common symptoms include a nagging or pulling sensation in the pelvis, a feeling of pelvic pressure, dyspareunia, constipation, painful defecation, urinary frequency, backache, and, with large tumors, an increase in the size of the abdomen. If the tumor is hormone producing, menstrual irregularities or masculinization may occur. If a cyst ruptures, signs and symptoms associated with any acute abdominal emergency such as ruptured appendix or a ruptured ectopic pregnancy are seen.

MEDICAL DIAGNOSIS

Eighty percent of all benign ovarian tumors are discovered by palpation during a routine pelvic examination. Because diagnosis of an ovarian tumor can be difficult, laparoscopy may be used to confirm it.

MEDICAL MANAGEMENT

The size of the tumor determines the medical intervention. A small tumor (less than 5 cm) in a female of childbearing age who does not have any symptoms is monitored for one to two menstrual cycles to determine whether it will regress like a physiologic cyst, remain the same, or continue to enlarge. If it enlarges, then surgery is done. If the tumor is benign and there is healthy ovarian tissue, a cystectomy is performed. Oophorectomy is done if the tumor involves all of the ovarian tissue.

Tumors greater than 5 cm in size and tumors in women older than 40 years are always treated surgically because of the increased incidence of malignancy in these cases.

Guidelines for Application of the Nursing Process to the Care of the Patient with a Benign Ovarian Tumor

Nursing care of the patient with a benign ovarian tumor depends on the type of tumor and the plan of medical treatment. If a diagnostic laparoscopy is done, nursing care is provided as described in Chapter 43. If a cystectomy is performed, basic nursing care is that required by any patient having abdominal surgery.

A particular nursing concern related to the patient with a benign ovarian tumor is the patient's understanding of the disorder and its symptoms. Nursing assessments and interventions are planned to ascertain that the patient understands that the tumor is harmless; it does not have a malignant potential; and that it does not indicate infertility.

When the problem is a physiologic cyst that causes delay in onset of menstruation, assess the patient's emotional response and design interventions accordingly. In some cases, the patient may be highly anxious because she believes she is pregnant. In other cases, she may be devastated to find she is not pregnant and needs reassurance that the cyst does not mean she is sterile. Be sure to provide time and opportunity for her to express her concerns.

Malignant Neoplasms

CANCER OF THE VULVA

VULVAR CARCINOMA IN SITU

Vulvar carcinoma in situ is a neoplasm in which histologic changes are present in the vulvar epidermis but do not affect the adjacent tissue layers.

In the past, vulvar carcinoma in situ was a disease affecting primarily 50- to 60-year-old women. In recent years, however, incidence among younger women has been increasing so that today the average age of onset is between 30 and 40 years of age.

Etiology and Pathophysiology

The cause of vulvar carcinoma in situ is unknown, although a high degree of association with sexually transmitted diseases, particularly condylomata acuminata (vulvar warts), has been reported.

Clinical Manifestations

The two primary symptoms of vulvar carcinoma in situ are pruritus and a surface lesion.

Pruritus occurs in about half of all affected women and often occurs for some time before any other finding.

Surface lesions vary greatly in appearance. They may be white like leukoplakia, red, pink, or mahogany. They may be eczematous, dry or moist. Often they are raised (papular).

Medical Diagnosis

Diagnosis depends on careful inspection of the vulva using a bright light, magnifying glass, and vinegar or other staining technique with subsequent colposcopic examination; any suspicious areas undergo biopsy. Approximately 50% of all cases of vulvar carcinoma in situ are discovered during routine screening examinations.

Medical Management

Single lesions are treated by wide, local excision. The affected area as well as a border of disease-free tissue is excised, and the wound is sutured. If healing is uncomplicated, no scar or defect results because of the elasticity of the tissues involved.

If lesions are multiple, treatment may be a partial

vulvectomy, total vulvectomy, or skinning vulvectomy.

A partial vulvectomy is designed to remove affected tissue while retaining as much normal tissue as possible. Often the clitoris, prepuce, or frenulum can be spared and hence sexual sensation preserved.

In a total vulvectomy, all of the structures of the vulva are removed.

In a skinning vulvectomy, the vulvar skin is excised and replaced with a split-thickness graft from the buttocks or inner thigh. The purpose of this procedure is to replace the skin at risk. Its major advantage is that the subcutaneous vulvar tissue is not disturbed; therefore, there is little functional or cosmetic defect.

A disadvantage to the skinning vulvectomy is that 6 to 7 days of bed rest are required while the graft is adhering. For this reason, it is not the procedure of choice for nonsexually active elderly patients or those otherwise at risk for complications as a result of immobility.

Occasionally, lesions may be destroyed by the use of cautery, laser, or cryosurgery. However, the success of these therapies is inconclusive, and all can result in necrotic ulcers and poor wound healing.

Regardless of the treatment, lifetime follow-up is necessary. A checkup is done every 3 to 6 months for the first 2 years and annually thereafter provided there is no sign of recurrence.

INVASIVE CANCER OF THE VULVA

Invasive carcinoma of the vulva is an uncommon disorder that occurs most frequently in women 65 years of age and older. It is often associated with condylomata acuminata (vulvar warts), but no direct cause and effect relationship has been identified. Other possible risk factors are syphilis, smoking, and diabetes.

Currently, the incidence of invasive cancer of the vulva is increasing, possibly because more women are living to the age at which the disease tends to occur. It is found among the poor in all areas of the world.

Etiology and Pathophysiology

Because the vulva is covered with skin, all the types of cancer that can occur on other areas of the skin can occur on the vulva. The most common type of vulvar malignancy is squamous cell carcinoma. This seems to begin as a small area of epithelial thickening that develops into a small nodule that may ulcerate, become infected, or develop into a small, warty or cauliflower-like growth. Most often, it begins on the labia majora and is well localized and demarcated. It tends to extend slowly. Metastasis occurs late and is via the lymph, affecting first the superficial inguinal lymph nodes and then the deep femoral nodes. Eventually liver, lungs, and other internal organs are involved. If local recurrence occurs, it is generally close to the site of the primary lesion and within 2 years after initial treatment.

Carcinoma of the vulva is staged according to the size of the tumor, location of the primary tumor, lymph node involvement, and presence or absence of distant metastases.

Clinical Manifestations

Like vulvar carcinoma in situ, the primary symptoms of cancer of the vulva are long-term pruritus and the presence of a lump or small nodule that may break down and ulcerate. Slight soreness progressing to pain occurs as the disease progresses. If the growth ulcerates and becomes infected, bleeding and a foul-smelling discharge may also be present.

Medical Diagnosis

A positive diagnosis is made on the basis of the results of a biopsy. Because early detection and early treatment increase the 5-year survival rate of patients with the disease, careful inspection of the vulva and colposcopic examination are essential; any suspicious areas should undergo biopsy.

Medical Management

Basic treatment of invasive vulvar cancer is radical vulvectomy and inguinal lymphadenectomy. Pelvic lymphadenectomy is also done if a metastasis is found in the inguinal lymph nodes. It is not done if the inguinal lymph nodes are negative because metastasis is not found in the pelvic nodes unless it is also present in the inguinal lymph nodes. Because of the increase in morbidity associated with pelvic lymphadenectomy, radiation rather than excision may be the treatment, especially in elderly or medically ill patients.

Radical Vulvectomy and Inguinal Lymphadenectomy. In a radical vulvectomy, tissue is excised from the anus to just above the symphysis pubis. This includes the mons pubis, the terminal section of the urethra and the vagina, and parts of the round ligaments and saphenous veins. In an inguinal lymphadenectomy, the groin is incised and the lymph nodes are dissected and removed.

Preoperative Preparation. To decrease the likelihood of wound infection postoperatively, the skin of the lower abdomen, groin, and upper thighs as well as the vulva may be scrubbed with a detergent germicide each day for several days before surgery. Antibiotics may be ordered prophylactically and continued into the postoperative period. Heparin may also be given preoperatively as prophylaxis against thrombus formation and is often continued for 5 days postoperatively. An abdominal perineal shave is done the night before surgery and enemas, a cleansing douche, and a hexachlorophene or povidone-iodine shower are given. Because a good nutritional status is necessary for wound healing, hyperalimentation may be started 4 to 6 days before surgery if the patient is malnourished. If palpable lymph nodes are present in the groin, a computed tomographic (CT) scan is also done preoperatively.

Postoperative Course. Postoperatively, the patient will have the vulvar wound and a wound in each groin from the inguinal node dissection. Depending on the surgeon's preference, these wounds may be left uncovered, covered with a light dressing, or covered with a pressure dressing to decrease the amount of serum and blood collecting in the wound.

Some patients may have a Hemovac or drainage catheter attached to suction inserted through a stab wound in each inguinal area to prevent accumulation of blood or serum, which could lead to disruption of the wound. This drainage is generally maintained for about 5 days.

Fluids are given intravenously for 48 to 72 hours. The patient then progresses from clear fluids to a full low-residue diet. A low-residue diet is given to prevent pressure on the suture line associated with straining on defecation.

To prevent urethral stenosis and contamination of the wound with urine, a Foley catheter is in place for up to 4 or 5 days after surgery.

The patient is ambulated as soon as possible, usually on the first postoperative day. She is discharged in 10 to 20 days, and sutures are removed in 2 to 3 weeks. Sexual activity can be resumed when healing is complete, usually in about 3 months.

Complications. Wound breakdown as a result of necrosis of the tissue edges at the suture line is the most frequent complication of radical vulvectomy. It occurs in about half of all females who undergo this procedure.

The patient is also at risk for thrombosis in the deep leg veins and therefore for the development of a pulmonary embolism.

Leg edema is a long-term complication if there is insufficient development of collateral vascular channels after removal of the saphenous vein.

A decrease in sexual satisfaction may occur after a radical vulvectomy. However, there are many females who maintain the ability to reach orgasm.

Other potential complications include stress incontinence, cystocele, and rectocele.

Application of the Nursing Process to the Care of the Patient Having a Radical Vulvectomy and Inguinal Lymphadenectomy

PREOPERATIVE NURSING CARE

The assessment, nursing diagnoses, expected patient outcomes, nursing interventions, and evaluation for a patient scheduled for radical vulvectomy and inguinal lymphadenectomy are similar to those for any patient scheduled for major surgery (see Chapter 4), with several considerations.

Carefully assess the condition of the skin and the patient's available strength to assist in positioning herself in bed because the patient's mobility is limited in the days immediately after surgery.

Also assess nutritional status and determine dietary patterns as well as food preferences because a good nutritional intake is necessary postoperatively if the large wound is to heal. Determine the patient's usual pattern of bowel elimination because both diarrhea and constipation must be avoided until the wound heals.

POSTOPERATIVE NURSING CARE

Assessment

After a radical vulvectomy, assessments are those required by any patient who has had an extensive surgical procedure. Take vital signs, and check the groin dressing for bleeding every 15 minutes initially. Measure urinary output, observe drainage from the wound for color and amount, monitor intravenous fluid intake, and observe the site for signs of infiltration or inflammation. Be alert to any signs of cardiopulmonary or renal dysfunction because these symptoms are often compromised in the older person.

As the postoperative period progresses, continue to observe the wound edges for signs of necrosis because this complication affects almost half of the patients having this surgery. When oral intake is reestablished, assess the patient's tolerance of it as well as her bowel function because both constipation and diarrhea must be avoided to protect the suture line. With removal of the Foley catheter, assess the patient's ability to initiate urination and empty the bladder. Also note any difficulty with the direction of the urinary stream.

Carefully observe the skin over bony prominences for signs of developing decubitus, and check the calves for redness, edema, heat, and pain, which could indicate thrombosis.

Throughout the postoperative period, also assess the patient's emotional state. Note the patient's willingness to talk about the surgery and her care and to look at the wound. Observe nonverbal reactions to these activities.

Nursing Diagnoses and Planning

Nursing diagnoses and related expected patient outcomes most commonly applicable to patients who have had a radical vulvectomy include the following:

NDx: Pain related to surgery and thick, taut sutures

Planning: Patient outcomes
1. Patient states she has less perineal discomfort.
2. Patient moves more easily.
3. Patient defecates and, after the catheter is removed, urinates without signs of undue discomfort.

NDx: High risk for impaired tissue integrity related to pull on and disruption of the suture line

Planning: Patient outcomes
1. Suture line is intact.
2. Patient maintains a low Fowler's or side-lying position.
3. Patient uses trapeze to move.
4. Patient defecates without straining.

NDx: High risk for infection related to contamination of large vulvar wound

Planning: Patient outcomes
1. Wound is clean.
2. Purulent drainage is absent.

NDx: Urinary retention related to inability to relax the perineum

Planning: Patient outcomes
1. Patient initiates voiding on need.
2. Patient empties bladder completely.

NDx: High risk for ineffective airway clearance related to shallow breathing and ineffective coughing

Planning: Patient outcomes
1. Respirations are quiet and easy.
2. Lungs are clear to auscultation.

NDx: High risk for altered peripheral tissue perfusion related to obstruction of venous flow

Planning: Patient outcomes
1. Calves are free of redness, pain, edema, and heat.

NDx: High risk for ineffective individual coping related to the loss of external genitalia and large area of scar tissue

Planning: Patient outcomes
1. Patient looks at the operative site.
2. Patient asks about care at home and resumption of normal activities.
3. Patient expresses pleasure at visits from significant others.
4. Patient demonstrates interest in grooming and appearance.

NDx: High risk for sexual dysfunction related to loss of external genitalia

Planning: Patient outcomes
1. Patient asks questions regarding future sexual function.
2. Patient discusses sexual function with her mate.
3. Patient discusses alternate patterns of sexual satisfaction.

NDx: Diversional activity deficit related to long, uncomfortable recovery period

Planning: Patient outcomes
1. Patient watches television, reads, and talks on telephone.
2. Patient expresses interest in other than personal events.
3. Patient denies excessive boredom.

NDx: High risk for altered health maintenance related to insufficient knowledge of discharge instructions

Planning: Patient outcomes
1. Patient lists signs and symptoms that should be reported to the health care professional.
2. Patient accurately describes measures to prevent leg edema.
3. Patient describes and demonstrates care of the wound.
4. Patient states the date of her follow-up appointment.

Nursing Interventions

NDx: Pain
Because of the location of the surgical wound, the extent of the tissue removed, and the thick, taut sutures necessary to hold the edges of the wound together, a major patient problem is pain in the groin and perineal area. Medicate the patient as ordered every 3 to 4 hours for the first 24 to 48 hours after surgery. Thereafter, administer a milder analgesic as ordered to provide relief. Generally, some analgesic is required until the sutures are removed.

NDx: High risk for impaired tissue integrity
Maintain the patient in a low Fowler's or side-lying position to prevent pull on the suture line and possible disruption. Place a pillow to support her lumbar area and a pillow between her legs for maximum comfort. With the patient in a side-lying position, bend the upper leg and support it with a pillow in a slightly forward position. Use an over-the-bed trapeze bar to allow the patient to move herself while controlling the amount of pull on the suture line.

Use a bed cradle to keep the pressure of the bed covers away from the operative area.

Act to prevent constipation because it can cause straining at stool and pressure on the suture line. Progress the patient from clear fluids to a low-residue diet when gastrointestinal function returns, and give stool softeners as ordered.

NDx: High risk for infection
Keep the wound clean and dry to prevent infection and wound breakdown, which can delay healing for as long as 6 months.

Cleanse the wound by applying a sterile solution of normal saline, hydrogen peroxide, or antiseptic to the area twice a day using an aseptic syringe or a Water Pik machine. Dry the area with a hair dryer or occasionally a heat lamp. Sitz baths may be given after the sutures are removed, although reinfection is always a risk.

Change dressings frequently because there is a great deal of drainage from this type of wound, and moisture increases the risk of infection. In addition, uncover the wound and leave it exposed to the air at frequent intervals to allow drying and thus to decrease maceration of the tissues.

Give perineal care after each bowel movement and after each voiding once the Foley catheter is removed. This not only reduces the risk of infection, but the warm solution on the perineal area is soothing and stimulates healing.

Because feces can contaminate the wound, also take care to avoid diarrhea.

NDx: Urinary retention
After the Foley catheter, which is in place for 2 to 3 weeks, is removed, the patient may have difficulty voiding because of an inability to relax the perineum. When she does void, the stream of urine may be deflected to one side and hit her leg. If the urethral meatus has been adequately positioned and anchored during surgery, this effect is simply a result of edema and will disappear as healing occurs. In the meantime, instruct the patient to stand when voiding to alleviate the problem.

NDx: High risk for ineffective airway clearance
Teach the patient to cough and deep breathe every 2 hours to aid in the prevention of respiratory complications.

NDx: High risk for altered peripheral tissue perfusion
Apply antiembolic stockings to prevent thrombus formation. Equip the patient's bed with a footboard, and teach her to do leg exercises every hour while awake and in bed. Change her position frequently. Never use the knee gatch because this produces stasis in the perineal area.

When the patient is ambulatory, instruct her to avoid sitting or standing in one position for a long period of time.

NDx: High risk for ineffective individual coping
An integral part of the postoperative nursing care of the patient with a radical vulvectomy is the continued provision of psychological support begun during the preoperative period.

The patient may grieve over the permanent change in her body as a result of loss of pubic hair, loss of other parts of the vulva, or the scar tissue that forms. She may no longer feel feminine, sexually attractive to her partner, or sexually adequate. This grief may be manifested by crying, introspection, withdrawal, or depression. Accept the patient's moods, and allow her to ventilate her feelings and ask questions. Help the family to understand and accept the patient's behavior.

NDx: High risk for sexual dysfunction
Provide opportunities for the patient to discuss her sexual concerns. Discuss the use of water-soluble lubricants to replace lubrication normally provided by the glands of the vulva as well as methods of attaining sexual satisfaction despite the loss of the clitoris.

NDx: Diversional activity deficit
Because the recovery period is long and uncomfortable, the patient can easily become discouraged. To combat this, plan diversional activities on the basis of her stated interests.

NDx: High risk for altered health maintenance
Because healing is not always complete at the time of discharge from the hospital, instruct the patient as specified in Chart 44–7 regarding self-care. Initiate a referral to a home-care agency if needed.

Additional Interventions
Use an air mattress or egg-crate pad to distribute the patient's weight evenly to make her more comfortable and help prevent skin breakdown.

If a strong perineal odor exists, as often happens, perform perineal care more frequently and dispose of soiled dressings promptly. Ventilate the room well, and use deodorizers as needed because patients tend to be very sensitive to odors.

Take care not to dislodge the Foley catheter during the 2 to 3 weeks that it is in place because edema in the vulvar area makes it very difficult and painful to reinsert. Pay careful attention to asepsis to prevent urinary tract infection, which is a particular risk because of the extended time the catheter is in place.

Evaluation

Evaluate the effectiveness of nursing care for a patient who has had a radical vulvectomy by comparing the patient's status with the expected patient outcomes. Examples of specific outcomes for patients who have had radical vulvectomy have been provided in the Planning section.

Chart 44–7.

NURSING GUIDE TO PATIENT EDUCATION FOR SELF-MANAGEMENT: DISCHARGE INSTRUCTIONS AFTER RADICAL VULVECTOMY

Instruct the patient to:

Cleanse the wound in accordance with the surgeon's instructions.
Wear support stockings and elevate legs at frequent intervals to prevent leg edema.
Report the occurence of bleeding; foul discharge; persistent leg edema; calf redness, edema, or pain; fever.
Return for checkup on *(specify date)*.

CANCER OF THE CERVIX

Cancer of the cervix is the most common cancer of the female reproductive system. It occurs as carcinoma in situ at an average age of 33 to 38 years and as invasive cancer at an average age of 43 to 48 years. Recently, there has been an increased incidence of invasive cancer among females in their late teens and early twenties.

ETIOLOGY AND PATHOPHYSIOLOGY

The cause of cancer of the cervix is unknown, but many high-risk factors (i.e., factors associated with a high incidence of cancer of the cervix) have been identified. These high-risk factors include early age of first sexual intercourse, early age of first pregnancy, multiparity, history of multiple sexual partners, history of herpes simplex virus 2 or other venereal disease, black or Mexican American ethnic background, low socioeconomic status, and cigarette smoking.

Ninety-five percent of all cervical cancers are squamous cell carcinomas. They have a gradual onset, originating with a precursor lesion called dysplasia. These preinvasive abnormalities are referred to as cervical intraepithelial neoplasia (CIN) and are graded as follows:

CIN I: mild dysplasia
CIN II: moderate dysplasia
CIN III: severe dysplasia (carcinoma in situ)

Dysplasias may regress to normal tissue, may simply persist, or may progress to become invasive carcinoma. The more severe the dysplasia, the more likely it is that an invasive change will occur.

The main routes of spread of cancer of the cervix are into the vaginal mucosa, into the myometrium of the uterus, into the lymph nodes around the cervix, and by direct extension into other structures of the pelvis such as the bladder, rectum, and pelvic wall. Distant metastases can occur, although a predilection to spread within the pelvis seems to exist.

The second form of cervical cancer is adenocarcinoma. This develops in the mucus-producing glands of the cervix. It does not have an identified precursor state, can be present within the cervix for an extended length of time before detection, and is often recurrent. The method of spread and the treatment are similar to that of squamous carcinoma.

CLINICAL MANIFESTATIONS

The first symptom of cancer of the cervix is a thin, watery, blood-tinged vaginal discharge, which in most cases is not even noticed by the patient. Later, the classic symptom of intermittent, painless bleeding between periods develops. This bleeding, which is referred to as contact bleeding because it occurs after sexual intercourse, douching, or the like, is the symptom that is generally responsible for the patient seeking health care. If treatment is not begun, the bleeding becomes heavier, more frequent, and of longer duration as the tumor increases in size. The amount and duration of the menses also increase so that ultimately the bleeding is continuous.

Late symptoms are related either to the spread of the disease within the pelvis or to metastasis to distant organs. Pain referred to the flank or to the leg occurs if the disease affects the ureters, pelvic wall, or sciatic nerve. Dysuria and hematuria occur if the disease has spread to the bladder, and rectal bleeding occurs if the rectum has been invaded. Extensive spread to the pelvic wall with blockage of the lymphatic and venous channels causes edema in the lower extremities.

Massive hemorrhage and uremia occur before death.

MEDICAL DIAGNOSIS

Early diagnosis of cervical cancer is of critical importance because it is almost always curable in its early stages and almost impossible to cure in its late stages. Screening of all females at risk by a cervical Pap smear allows detection of precursor dysplasia or early malignant disease. All females are considered to be at risk for cervical cancer as soon as they either become sexually active or reach 18 to 20 years of age, and their first Pap smear should be done at this time. At one time, it was recommended that the test be repeated on an annual basis. Some clinicians now believe, however, that annual screening is necessary only if the patient is at high risk for cervical cancer on the basis of the risk factors discussed previously. If the patient is not in a high-risk group, then after two initial Pap smears done 1 year apart, a Pap test needs be done only every 3 years until 65 years of age, provided no abnormalities are found. Other clinicians continue to believe that all women should have an annual Pap smear, especially in view of the false-negative rate, which has been estimated as high as 30%. Women older than 65 years whose Pap smears have always been normal are not considered at risk for the disease, and screening is no longer necessary.

If a Pap smear is abnormal, a repeat smear is obtained and a colposcopic examination of the cervix is done. Any suspicious-appearing areas undergo biopsy or, if no suspicious areas are seen but the repeat Pap smear is abnormal, a cold cone biopsy is done, especially if the transformational zone is not visualized.

Diagnosis of cancer of the cervix is made on the basis of characteristics of the biopsy specimen.

MEDICAL MANAGEMENT

The plan of medical management for a patient with cervical cancer depends on the stage of the disease (Table 44–3) and the patient's age, desire for childbearing, and general health status.

Surgical Intervention

The usual treatment of carcinoma in situ is either cervical conization or hysterectomy. Conization is done when a wide area of normal tissue surrounds the excised malignancy and the patient is young and desires to have children. If childbearing is not a concern and the patient is premenopausal, a simple hysterectomy with the ovaries left intact may be done because metastasis from the cervix to the ovary is rare.

Although invasive cancer of the cervix is most often treated by radiation, if the disease is Stage I or Stage IIA and if the patient is young and maintenance of ovarian function is desired, a radical hysterectomy with pelvic lymph node dissection may be done. See Chapter 43 for a description of a radical hysterectomy (Wertheim's operation) and the related nursing care.

Surgery may also be used in the treatment of advanced or recurrent disease when the tumor is radiation resistant, the patient is unable to tolerate the radiation effects, or there is a chance of cure because the cancer is still localized in the pelvis.

Pelvic Exenteration. There are three types of pelvic exenteration. In a total exenteration, all of the pelvic organs are removed. In females, this includes the vagina, uterus, fallopian tubes, ovaries, bladder, distal ureters, rectum, distal sigmoid colon, internal iliac artery and vein, lymph nodes, and the entire pelvic floor. To allow for bowel function and urinary elimination, a colostomy and an ileal or sigmoid conduit are also performed. An opening is left through the perineum to allow for drainage, which occurs for up to a year after surgery.

In an anterior pelvic exenteration, all of the pelvic structures are removed except the bowel, and in a posterior pelvic exenteration, all the pelvic structures are removed except the urinary bladder.

Pelvic exenteration is a radical surgical procedure done most often for advanced or recurrent cancer of the cervix. It is performed only if the cancer is limited to the pelvis and therefore a possibility of cure exists. The patient cannot be elderly or obese and must be able physically to withstand the extensive procedure and psychologically cope with the long recovery period and the changes in body function that result.

Preoperative Preparation. Before surgery, extensive diagnostic testing is done to rule out metastases beyond the pelvis. If no metastases are found, preparation for the surgical procedure is begun.

Physical preparation includes laxatives, enemas, and antibiotic therapy for 4 to 5 days before sur-

Table 44–3. STAGING OF CERVICAL CANCER

STAGE		CHARACTERISTICS
0		Confined to the epithelium (carcinoma in situ)
I		Confined to the cervix
	A	Microinvasive cancer
	B	Invasive cancer
II		Extends beyond the cervix but does not involve the pelvic wall or lower third of the vagina
	A	Involves vagina but not the parametrium
	B	Involves the parametrium
III		Extends to lower third of the vagina and may or may not involve the pelvic wall or parametrium; hydronephrosis or a nonfunctioning kidney; no cancer-free space between tumor and pelvic wall on rectal examination
	A	Involves lower third of the vagina but not the pelvic wall
	B	Involves pelvic wall or parametrium; hydronephrosis or nonfunctioning kidney
IV		Extends beyond the true pelvis or involves the bladder or rectal mucosa
	A	Involves adjacent organs
	B	Involves distant organs

gery. These measures, along with a low-residue diet that is changed to clear liquids 48 hours preoperatively, are designed to empty and disinfect the bowel. Twenty-four to 48 hours preoperatively, a long intestinal tube is passed through the nose into the ileum. On the day before surgery, the sites for stoma placement are marked on the abdomen, and that evening an abdominal perineal shave is done. If the patient has poor veins, a subclavian catheter may be inserted.

Postoperative Course. The patient is usually in an intensive care unit for 3 to 4 days after surgery because of the high risk of shock, cardiac abnormalities, and renal failure.

The intestinal tube is kept in place and attached to low suction and the patient kept on a nothing by mouth (NPO) order until peristalsis returns, usually in 4 to 6 days. When signs of bowel function return, the tube is clamped and clear fluids are given. If no distention occurs, the diet is advanced as tolerated.

The patient receives intravenous fluids to maintain hydration and replace electrolytes lost as a result of the surgery and the intestinal tube. Albumin is given to decrease edema (intravenous albumin pulls fluid into the vascular space by osmosis) and to aid in replacing protein that is lost during the first 2 weeks postoperatively.

Respiratory therapy and measures to prevent circulatory complications are begun immediately postoperatively, and the patient is ambulated within 24 to 48 hours. Care related to the colostomy and ileal conduit is instituted (see Chapters 21 and 26).

Vaginal intercourse is not possible after this operation unless a plastic procedure is later done to construct an artificial vagina.

Application of the Nursing Process to the Care of the Patient Having a Pelvic Exenteration

Preoperative and postoperative assessments, nursing diagnoses, expected patient outcomes, nursing interventions, and evaluations for patients undergoing pelvic exenteration are similar to those described previously for patients having a colostomy, a urinary diversion, and a radical hysterectomy with bilateral salpingo-oophorectomy. Several additional interventions also apply to the care of patients having a pelvic exenteration.

Keep in mind that pelvic exenteration is a radical procedure done in the face of extensive underlying pathology. It results in significantly greater changes in body appearance and function than any one of these procedures alone and therefore causes greater physical and psychological stress. It is essential to assess the patient's coping style and support systems and help her use them during her period of adjustment.

Recognize that there often is an initial period of dependency, which is followed by a grief reaction over the mutilation of her body. As with any grief reaction, the first stage is that of shock and disbelief. The patient may deny the body changes and refuse to look at the surgical wounds. As she begins to realize the loss is real, the patient may become depressed and withdrawn or may be angry and hostile. Finally, she begins to participate in care and move toward independence. Progression through these stages is not unidirectional; rather, fluctuations between responses is common. Be alert to mood changes, and be accepting of them.

Also support the patient's sexual adjustment. Arrange private time for the patient to be alone with her partner. Provide counseling in regard to alternative methods of sexual gratification if needed because vaginal intercourse is no longer possible.

Radiation Therapy

Irradiation used in the treatment of cancer of the cervix is in the form of internal (intracavitary) therapy or external radiation therapy, or both. Internal radiation therapy may be used alone to treat early, small, microinvasive carcinomas of the cervix (grades I to IIA). A combination of intracavitary radiation therapy and external radiation to the pelvic lymph nodes is the initial treatment of all invasive cervical carcinomas beyond grade IIA. If tumors are very large, external radiation may be administered to shrink the tumor before the use of intracavitary radiation. In cases in which the tumor has invaded the pelvic walls, external radiation is used primarily for its palliative effects. If metastasis to the bone has occurred, radiation is used to decrease the pain.

External Radiation Therapy. External radiation therapy and the related nursing care are discussed in Chapter 11. This information should be reviewed as part of the study of this chapter.

Internal Radiation Therapy. Internal, or intracavitary, radiation is used to irradiate malignant cells in the cervix and the endometrial cavity. The procedure involves the insertion of a radiation source, usually cesium, into the vagina and endometrial cavity by means of a specially designed applicator that holds it in place. Intracavitary radiation therapy is well suited for the treatment of cervical lesions because the accessibility of the cervix and the cervical canal allows the radiation source to be placed close to the lesion and a high dose of radiation (15,000 to 20,000 rads) to be delivered to it. Also, normal cervical and vaginal tissue is particularly well able to withstand the effects of radiation, and this allows administration of a higher dose before adverse effects on normal tissue occur.

Physical Preparation of the Patient. In preparation for intracavitary radiation therapy, the patient is generally admitted to the hospital the afternoon before insertion is scheduled. Because distention of the bowel or using a bedpan for a bowel movement can result in changes in the position of the radiation source relative to the adjacent tissues, the patient is placed on a low-residue diet and is given a cleansing enema. A cleansing douche is also given. An anesthesia workup is done, the patient is placed on NPO status after midnight, and she is premedicated and prepared for transport to the operating room the next morning.

Procedure. Most internal radiation in the United States is given by means of an afterloading device.

When such a device is used, the patient is examined under anesthesia in the operating room. The applicator is inserted and held in place with vaginal packing. When the patient has reacted from the anesthesia, an x-ray film is taken to verify placement of the applicator. The patient is then returned to her room, where the radiation source is inserted.

This type of after-loading system allows strict control of the radiation received by the patient and minimizes radiation exposure of other health-team members.

A Foley catheter is inserted before the applicator. Catheter drainage is necessary to prevent distention of the bladder and movement of tissues closer to the radiation core.

Postprocedure Course. After insertion, the radiation source remains in place for 48 to 72 hours. During this time, the patient is maintained on strict bed rest. Intravenous fluids are given until oral fluids are tolerated in satisfactory amounts because dehydration can easily occur as a result of the loss of fluid secondary to the destruction of tissue at the site of radiation. The patient is progressed to a low-residue diet and anticholinergics such as diphenoxylate hydrochloride and atropine (Lomotil), 2 mg four times daily, are given to prevent diarrhea. Antiemetics such as prochlorperazine maleate (Compazine) are given for nausea, sedatives for sleep, and analgesics such as codeine or meperidine hydrochloride (Demerol) for pain.

After removal of the radiation source and the applicator, the patient is given a soapsuds enema and a douche. She is allowed out of bed, returned to a regular diet, and discharged the following day.

Complications. Patients having intracavitary radiation therapy may acquire radiation sickness with its nausea, vomiting, diarrhea, malaise, and fever. (See Chapter 11 for a complete discussion of this topic and the related care.) Other complications that may occur are cystitis, proctitis, vesicovaginal fistula, ureterovaginal fistula, phlebitis, and hemorrhage.

Application of the Nursing Process to the Care of the Patient Having Intracavitary Radiation Therapy

PREOPERATIVE NURSING CARE

The assessment, nursing diagnoses, expected patient outcomes, nursing interventions, and evaluation for patients scheduled for intracavitary radiation therapy are similar to those for other preoperative patients, with several considerations.

Carefully assess the patient's ability to withstand the limitations imposed by the procedure, and identify appropriate support activities. For example, does she dread 3 days in a private room with limited interpersonal contacts? If so, does she like to read and can books be obtained? What is the condition of her skin? Are more than usual measures indicated if she is to complete 2 to 3 days of bed rest without skin breakdown?

Describe what the patient should expect after insertion of the radioactive implant. Prepare her for the indwelling catheter, strict bed rest, and low-residue diet. Give a careful explanation of the lead shield and the limited staff and visitor contact, and assure her that, nonetheless, she will have close supervision.

Explain that nausea, uterine cramping, and foul vaginal drainage are expected and that medications will be given to make her comfortable.

POSTOPERATIVE NURSING CARE

Assessment

After insertion of the radiation source, assess the patient's vital signs every 4 hours. It is not unusual for the temperature to rise to more than 37.7°C (100°F) on the first evening after insertion as part of the body's response to tissue destruction.

Check for the presence and amount of vaginal bleeding because hemorrhage is a potential complication of the therapy. Determine the amount of discomfort from vaginal cramping and limited mobility and the effectiveness of medications in providing relief.

Observe the skin over pressure areas for signs of impending breakdown, and check the skin of the buttocks and perineum, which has a low tolerance to radiation for erythema, a possible precursor of desquamation.

Monitor for signs of cystitis, proctitis, phlebitis, dehydration, and radiation sickness because all can occur as complications of intracavitary radiation therapy.

Assess how well the patient is coping with the experience. Is she manifesting signs of anxiety, frustration, or depression?

Nursing Diagnoses and Planning

Nursing diagnoses and related expected patient outcomes most commonly applicable to patients undergoing internal radiation therapy for cancer of the cervix include the following:

NDx: High risk for injury related to accidental movement of radiation source

Planning: Patient outcomes
1. Patient stays in flat, dorsal position.
2. Bladder distention is absent.

NDx: Pain related to uterine contractions and limited movement

Planning: Patient outcomes
1. Patient appears comfortable; she does not grimace, moan, clench fist, or hold abdomen.
2. Patient states she has less cramping.

NDx: High risk for fluid volume deficit related to abnormal fluid loss secondary to tissue destruction at the site of radiation

Planning: Patient outcomes
1. Patient has a fluid intake of at least 3000 ml per day.
2. Mucous membranes are moist.
3. Skin turgor is good.

NDx: High risk for altered health maintenance related to insufficient knowledge of discharge instructions

Planning: Patient outcomes
1. Patient describes/demonstrates douche procedure, indicating when and how it is to be done, what solution is to be used, and how the equipment is to be cleaned.
2. Patient states when sexual intercourse can be resumed.
3. Patient lists symptoms to be reported.
4. Patient states date and time of follow-up appointment.

Nursing Interventions

Protection of the nurse, visitors, and other hospital personnel from excessive exposure to radiation is an essential part of the nursing care of the patient receiving internal radiation.

Place the patient in a private room, preferably at the end of a corridor where there is little traffic, and place signs on the door indicating that radiation is in use. If a private room is absolutely not available, the patient may be placed in a semiprivate room provided the other patient is postmenopausal or has had a bilateral oophorectomy.

Do not allow pregnant nurses, pregnant visitors, or persons younger than 18 years in the patient's room.

Plan to work as far from the radiation source as possible and to keep the lead shield between self and the radiation source at all times.

Spend time on the day of admission orienting the patient to the call system, radio and television, and general hospital routines. Also teach exercises to be done during the days of the treatment to help eliminate the need for reteaching when the radiation source is in place and the time spent at the bedside must be limited.

Always be well organized so that quality care can be given in the least possible amount of time. Remember that urine, feces, soiled linens, dressings, and the like are not radioactive. (See Chapter 11 for additional discussion of precautions related to radiation.)

NDx: High risk for injury
Maintain the patient on absolute bed rest in the dorsal position after the insertion procedure to prevent movement of the radiation source. Elevate the head of the bed to a maximum of 10 to 15 degrees for comfort. Avoid turning the patient on her side. If turning is absolutely necessary, place a pillow between her knees and, with her body in straight alignment, roll her like a log.

Use a fracture pan if the patient needs to have a bowel movement despite the cleansing enema, low-residue diet, and anticholinergic drugs.

NDx: Pain
Give narcotics as ordered at regular intervals for uterine contractions, which occur as a result of the presence of the applicator in the dilated cervical canal. Administer antiemetics as ordered for nausea. Encourage relaxation exercises and use of distraction.

NDx: High risk for fluid volume deficit
Determine what fluids appeal to the patient, and make them accessible. Encourage her to drink at least 3000 ml/day to prevent dehydration as a result of loss of fluid from the site of tissue destruction by the radiation and to relieve irritation of the bladder. Record intake and output.

NDx: High risk for altered health maintenance
Instruct the patient as specified in Chart 44–8 to prepare her to care for herself after discharge.

Chart 44–8.

NURSING GUIDE TO PATIENT EDUCATION FOR SELF-MANAGEMENT: DISCHARGE INFORMATION AFTER INTERNAL RADIATION FOR CANCER OF THE CERVIX

Explain to the patient the following:

Some vaginal bleeding may occur for 1 to 3 months after irradiation.
Foul-smelling vaginal discharge will occur for some time.
Douches are to be taken in accordance with physician's orders while discharge persists. (Specify the solution to be used and the frequency with which douching should be done. Demonstrate proper technique for performing the procedure and for cleansing the equipment.)
Emollient cream may be used to ease pruritus.
Sexual intercourse may be resumed in 7 to 10 days depending on the condition of the cervix and the vagina. Intercourse may be difficult because radiation can cause vaginal atrophy.

Instruct the patient to:

Report continued sexual difficultities because dilation of the vagina may be required.
Report persistent rectal irritation.
Return for a follow-up appointment on *(specify date and time).*

Additional Interventions
Bathe the patient's upper body, and give a partial back rub to provide comfort and to improve circulation to the skin. Do not bathe below her waist unless she is soiled.

Use an air or egg-crate mattress to aid in the prevention of bed sores. Provide a footboard, and instruct the patient to perform foot and leg exercises every hour while awake to stimulate venous return. Encourage range-of-motion exercises for the arms.

Evaluation

Evaluate the effectiveness of nursing care for a patient undergoing internal radiation therapy for cancer of the cervix by comparing the patient's status with the expected patient outcomes. Examples of specific outcomes for patients undergoing internal radiation therapy for cancer of the cervix have been provided in the Planning section.

Chemotherapy

Chemotherapy is generally not effective in the treatment of cancer of the cervix. This is partly because most of these cancers are squamous cell adenomas, which are generally unresponsive to chemotherapy, and partly because the malignancies being treated are in an area that was previously irradiated and therefore is lacking a sufficient blood supply to deliver the chemotherapeutic agents to the area in the concentration needed for an effect.

When chemotherapy is used, it consists of drugs such as vincristine, doxorubicin, cisplatin, 5-fluorouracil, and methotrexate given alone or in combination. (See Chapter 11 for a discussion of the principles of chemotherapy and the nursing care of patients receiving it.)

CANCER OF THE UTERINE BODY

The number of females with cancer of the uterine body has been increasing since the 1960s. Factors that are thought to account for this increased incidence include better detection, an increase in the number of women living to the time of life when the disease is most likely to occur, and the use of estrogen (without progesterone) replacement therapy after menopause.

The highest incidence of cancer of the uterine body is in women between the ages of 50 and 59 years. It is more likely to occur in women who are obese, nulliparous, diabetic, or who had a late menopause.

ETIOLOGY AND PATHOPHYSIOLOGY

The majority of malignant tumors affecting the body of the uterus are adenocarcinomas (carcinoma involving the glandular tissue). Uterine sarcoma can also occur, but it occurs only in about 1 of every 100,000 women older than 20 years of age.

Uterine adenocarcinoma is believed to develop from areas of hyperplastic endometrium. This hyperplasia is an overgrowth of endometrial glands and stroma. It is thought to result from prolonged, persistent estrogen stimulation such as occurs from successive anovulatory menstrual cycles or exogenous estrogen therapy. Hyperplasia does not always result in adenocarcinoma, but when it does, the change occurs over a period of 5 years or more.

Adenocarcinoma of the uterus is staged according to the areas involved and the histologic type of the tumor.

The stages are as follows:

Stage I: Cancer is confined to the body of the uterus. This stage is further subdivided into G1, highly differentiated; G2, differentiated with some solid areas; and G3, completely undifferentiated or predominantly solid.

Stage II: Cancer involves both the body of the uterus and the cervix.

Stage III: Cancer extends outside the uterine body but not outside the true pelvis. The bladder and rectum are not affected.

Stage IV: Cancer involves the bladder or rectum or extends outside the true pelvis.

Uterine adenocarcinoma is a slow-growing tumor. Prognosis is best when the tumor is limited to the body of the uterus and is highly differentiated (Stage I, G1). The prognosis worsens with involvement of the cervix (Stage II), loss of differentiation (G2 and G3), and deep invasion of the myometrium.

Metastases to the pelvic lymph nodes are common. They are seen in about 11% of patients with Stage I disease and 36% of those with Stage II.

CLINICAL MANIFESTATIONS

Abnormal uterine bleeding is the primary indicator of endometrial cancer. This is most often postmenopausal bleeding because the greatest incidence of the disease is in women older than age 50. The bleeding is sometimes profuse and may be accompanied by lower abdominal cramping and expulsion of clots. In premenopausal women, prolonged heavy periods and intermenstrual bleeding, which is usually painless, occur.

MEDICAL DIAGNOSIS

Dilation and fractional curettage allow definitive diagnosis of cancer of the endometrium on the basis of the histopathologic examination of endometrial tissue. This is the diagnostic method of choice for all patients who present with symptoms suggestive of endometrial carcinoma. However, because D&C does require hospitalization or day surgery, it is not readily acceptable to some patients. For this reason, an endometrial biopsy, which is 90% accurate and does not require anesthesia or hospitalization, may be done.

Cervical Pap smears are not reliable in diagnosing endometrial carcinoma because tumor cells are not shed until late in the disease. Cytologic samples obtained from the uterine cavity itself are more reliable and may be obtained by endometrial brushing or washing.

MEDICAL MANAGEMENT

The basic treatment of uterine cancer is total abdominal hysterectomy and bilateral salpingo-oophorectomy. In addition, preoperative or postoperative radiotherapy is frequently used. This may be in the form of vaginal radium implants or external radiation to the whole pelvis. Depending on the extent of the disease, radical hysterectomy or pelvic lymphadenectomy, or both, may be done. Chemotherapy in the form of doxorubicin, cyclophosphamide, and 5-fluorouracil, alone or in combination, may be used as an adjunct to surgery and radiation. When the malignancy is extensive (Stages III and IV), hormone therapy in the form of large doses of a progestin may be given. Hormone therapy is continued for as long as the patient shows an objective, positive response.

Guidelines for Application of the Nursing Process to the Care of the Patient with Uterine Cancer

Nursing care of patients with cancer of the uterine body is similar to that described previously for patients with a diagnosis of any type of malignancy. Additional nursing considerations relate to the plan of medical treatment. When surgery is done, the principles of nursing care for a patient having a hysterectomy with a bilateral salpingo-oophorectomy apply. If internal or external radiation therapy is used, then the principles of nursing care for a patient undergoing this treatment modality apply.

Because cancer of the uterine body occurs most often in older women, specifically consider two items when assessing the patient and planning her care. First, if she has not had routine gynecologic examinations since her last child was born or since menopause occurred, she may blame herself for her diagnosis. Second, older women in our society are generally perceived as asexual. As a result, they tend to hesitate to raise issues relating to sexual function because they fear the reaction of other people. To ensure that the patient receives the information she needs, open the topic to discussion and thus acknowledge to the patient that sexual concerns are normal and appropriate.

CANCER OF THE OVARY

Cancer of the ovary is an insidious disease in that symptoms do not occur until the cancer is well advanced. For this reason, the prognosis for patients with ovarian cancer is poor, and more females die from this disease than from any other cancer of the female reproductive system.

Although ovarian cancer can occur at any age, the greatest incidence is between 50 and 59 years. It is found more often among females who have been unable to become pregnant and those who have elected not to become pregnant than among females who have had children. It is also more prevalent among females in northern Europe, Canada, and North America than among those in Africa, India, and Japan.

ETIOLOGY AND PATHOPHYSIOLOGY

The cause of ovarian cancer is not known, although hormonal stimulation and environmental factors as well as familial tendencies are all considered as possible factors in its development. There appears to be some etiologic relationship between ovarian cancer and breast cancer because breast cancer is three to four times more likely to develop in females with ovarian cancer than in other females.

Malignant ovarian neoplasms are like benign neoplasms in that they originate from the same cells: ovarian epithelium, germ cells, or ovarian stroma. There are also many subtypes, which are classified according to the cell of origin. Seventy to 80% of ovarian neoplasms are epithelial tumors.

Malignant ovarian neoplasms spread easily throughout the peritoneal cavity. Spread is said to be local when it involves the tubes, uterus, or broad ligament; regional when it involves the pelvic peritoneum, bladder, sigmoid colon, rectum, or pelvic side wall; and abdominal when it involves the omentum, bowel, liver, or diaphragm. Spread out of the abdomen to areas such as the lungs or bone is uncommon.

CLINICAL MANIFESTATIONS

Ovarian cancer rarely causes symptoms until there has been extensive growth of the tumor. When symptoms do occur, they result primarily from the pressure of the tumor on other pelvic organs and are similar to the symptoms that occur with benign neoplasms.

Symptoms include a feeling of pelvic pressure or heaviness, vague abdominal discomfort, dyspepsia, bloating, constipation, urinary frequency, dyspareunia, and an increase in the size of the abdomen. In late stages of the disease, weight loss is evident and symptoms related to organs affected by metastasis occur.

MEDICAL DIAGNOSIS

There is no method in use to screen for and diagnose ovarian cancer in its early stages. Ultrasonography has been offered as the Pap smear for ovarian cancer but is not economically feasible for use on a preventive basis at this time.

A presumptive diagnosis of ovarian cancer is made when a hard, fixed, firm mass is palpated in the area of the ovary during a pelvic examination. In postmenopausal women, whose ovaries are normally atrophied, palpation of the ovary itself leads to a suspicion of ovarian cancer.

Laboratory tests, x-ray studies, and laparoscopy are used to rule out other pelvic diseases but not to diagnose cancer of the ovary. Diagnosis is confirmed and the stage of disease determined by exploratory laparotomy and examination of tissue specimens by a pathologist. The latter includes examination of ascitic fluid or, if none is encountered, examination of peritoneal washings.

MEDICAL MANAGEMENT

Hysterectomy with bilateral salpingo-oophorectomy with or without omentectomy is the basic treatment for early ovarian cancer. Both ovaries are removed because of the frequency of bilateral tumors. The uterus is removed because the serosa and endometrium are common sites of metastasis. If the disease is advanced (i.e., not localized), as much tumor as possible is also removed (debulking).

Postoperatively, some form of chemotherapy or radiation is generally prescribed depending on the stage of the disease. (See Chapter 11 for a discussion of chemotherapy.)

Patients who complete a course of chemotherapy and have no clinical symptoms of disease often have a "second-look" procedure done to determine whether they have a possible cure or whether there is asymptomatic disease still present that requires the continuation of chemotherapy. In these cases, a laparoscopy is done first. If tumor is seen, obviously therapy must continue. If disease is not seen, a laparotomy is performed to allow more thorough examination.

Guidelines for Application of the Nursing Process to the Care of the Patient with Ovarian Cancer

Nursing care of patients with ovarian cancer is similar to that described previously for patients with other types of cancer and to that described previously for patients having a hysterectomy with bilateral salpingo-oophorectomy. Several additional interventions also apply to the care of patients with ovarian cancer.

Because patients with cancer of the ovary have an increased chance of acquiring cancer of the breast, counsel on the need for monthly self-breast examination and the importance of an annual mammogram. If needed, teach the method of breast self-examination, and obtain a return demonstration.

When caring for a patient having a second-look procedure, expect the patient to be highly anxious, and provide her the opportunity to verbalize her worries. If the procedure discloses further malignancy, allow the patient to ventilate her feelings about the recurrence of the cancer and offer support to her significant others.

The Elderly: Special Considerations

Reproductive disorders of aging women may be classified into two groups:

1. Those that for unknown reasons occur almost exclusively in older women
2. Those that can occur at any age but for which age-related factors increase the risk

Disorders in Group 1 are cancer of the ovary, the uterus, and the vulva. Cancer of the ovary, which tends to occur in women who have not been pregnant, has the highest mortality rate of any cancer of the female reproductive system. Its poor prognosis relates to the fact that there are no symptoms until very late in the disease, so diagnosis is often delayed.

Cancer of the uterus, whose first symptom is vaginal bleeding, is most common in women who are obese, nulliparous, or diabetic or who have a history of anovulation, amenorrhea, or late menopause.

The third cancer, vulvar carcinoma, appears first as simply pruritus or as a small lesion on the vulvar skin. More than 50% of the time, this cancer is diagnosed on a routine screening examination.

Disorders for which age-related factors increase risk include vaginitis and symptomatic weakened pelvic supports.

Thinning of the vaginal epithelium, which occurs as a result of the decrease in estrogen after menopause, increases the risk of vaginitis. Adding to this is the fact that systemic diseases like diabetes, which themselves predispose to vaginitis, are more often present in the aged.

Symptomatic weakened pelvic supports tend to be a problem in aging women because the initial damage caused by childbirth is worsened by weakening of the pelvic diaphragm and loss of elasticity and strength of fascia, which occurs with age.

Morbidity and mortality from these disorders could be dramatically reduced by early diagnosis and treatment. Unfortunately, many women do not have routine gynecologic examinations after menopause.

One reason for this is a lack of knowledge. Some older women are simply not aware that there are serious reproductive disorders that occur late in life and that can be diagnosed early only by a gynecologic examination.

A second reason is the prevalent view in our society that all sexually related activities or concerns are taboo for the aging woman. This misconception can generate feelings of embarrassment and guilt, making the woman reluctant to seek medical care.

The implications for nursing are clear. Teach women the importance of obtaining routine gynecologic examinations throughout life.

Also teach the importance of obtaining immediate medical care for symptoms such as bleeding, vaginal discharge, and dyspareunia or pelvic pain.

Correct the perception of older women as being without sexual desires or needs.

Treat older women seeking care for a reproductive tract disorder in a sensitive, serious manner.

Bibliography

Barnhill D, et al. Epithelial ovarian carcinoma of low malignant potential. Obstet Gynecol 1985; 65(1):53.

Belfort P, et al (eds). General gynecology. Park Ridge, NJ: Parthenon, 1989.

Berek J. Practical gynecologic oncology. Baltimore, MD: Williams & Wilkins, 1988.

Blackledge GRP, Jordan JA, Shingleton HM (eds). Textbook of gynecologic oncology. Philadelphia: WB Saunders, 1991.

Booton DA, Seideman RY. Relationship between PMS and dysmenorrhea. AAOHN J 1989; 37(8):308.

Brucks JA. Ovarian cancer. The most lethal gynecologic malignancy. Nurs Clin North Am 1992; 22(6):835.

Brush M, Watson SJ, Horrobin DF, Manku MS. Abnormal essential fatty acid levels in plasma of women with premenstrual syndrome. Am J Obstet Gynecol 1984; 150:363.

Burns PA, Marecki MA, Dittmar SS, et al. Kegel's exercise with biofeedback therapy for treatment of stress incontinence. Nurse Pract 1985; 10(2):28.

Burnside I: Nursing care of the aged: A self approach. 3rd ed. New York: McGraw-Hill, 1988.

Carpenito LJ. Nursing diagnosis: Application to clinical practice. 4th ed. Philadelphia: JB Lippincott, 1992.

Cashavelly BJ. Cervical dysplasia. Cancer Nurs 1987; 10(4):199.

DiSaia PJ, Creasman WT. Clinical gynecologic oncology. St. Louis: CV Mosby, 1988.

Dugan KK. The bleak outlook on ovarian cancer. Am J Nurs 1985; 85(2):144.

Eliopoulos C. Gerontological nursing. New York: Harper & Row, 1987.

Ensign JE, Rowe J, Kowalski K. Premenstrual syndrome. AORN J 1988; 47(4):962.

Esberger KK, Hughes ST Jr. Nursing care of the aged. Norwalk, CT: Appleton & Lange, 1989.

Fogel CI, Woods NF. Health care of women: A nursing perspective. St. Louis: CV Mobsy, 1981.

Frank EP. What are nurses doing to help PMS patients? Am J Nurs 1986; 86(2):136.

Friedrich EG Jr. Vulvar disease. 2nd ed. Philadelphia: WB Saunders, 1983.
Gambert SR (ed). Handbook of geriatrics. New York: Plenum Press, 1987.
Govan AD, et al. Gynecology illustrated. 3rd ed. New York: Churchill Livingstone, 1985.
Guyton AC. Textbook of medical physiology. 8th ed. Philadelphia: WB Saunders, 1991.
Hacker NF, Moore JG. Essentials of obstetrics and gynecology. Philadelphia: WB Saunders, 1986.
Harrison M. Self-help for premenstrual syndrome. New York: Random House, 1982.
Hatcher RA, et al. Contraceptive technology 1990–1992. 15th rev ed. New York: Irvington, 1990.
Jenkins B. Sexual healing after pelvic radiation. Am J Nurs 1986; 86(8):920.
Jones HW, Jones GS. Novak's textbook of gynecology. 11th ed. Baltimore, MD: Williams & Wilkins, 1988.
Kaufman RH. Benign diseases of the vulva and vagina. 3rd ed. Chicago: Year Book, 1989.
Keye WR Jr. The premenstrual syndrome. Philadelphia: WB Saunders, 1988.
Kuhns-Hastings J. Management of female incontinence with Kegel exercises. AAOHN J 1988; 36(2):78.
Lamb MA, et al. Invasive cancer of the vulva. AORN J 1988; 47(4):928.
Levitt DB, Freeman EW, Sondheimer SJ, et al. Group support in the treatment of PMS. J Psychosoc Nurs Ment Health Serv 1986; 24(1):23.
Lovejoy NC. Precancerous lesions of the cervix. Cancer Nurs 1987; 10(1):2.
Mackay EV, Beischer NA, Cox LW, Wood C. Illustrated handbook of gynecology. 2nd ed. Philadelphia: WB Saunders, 1992.
Matteson MA, McConnell ES. Gerontological nursing: Concepts and practice. Philadelphia: WB Saunders, 1988.
McMullen M. Holistic care of the patient with cervical cancer. Nurs Clin North Am 1992; 27(4):847.
Mishel MH, Hostetter T, King B. Predictors of psychosocial adjustment in patients newly diagnosed with gynecological cancer. Cancer Nurs 1984; 7(4):291.
O'Rahilly R. Gardner, Gray and O'Rahilly anatomy: A regional study of human structure. Philadelphia: WB Saunders, 1986.
Petersen NF, Rhoe J. Endometriosis: Obtaining relief via "near-contact" laparoscopy. AORN J 1988; 48(4):700.
Poorman SG. Human sexuality and the nursing process. Englewood Cliffs, NJ: Prentice-Hall, 1988.
Richardson GS, Scully RE, Nikrui N, Nelson JH Jr. Common epithelial cancer of the ovary. N Engl J Med 1985; 312(7):415.
Rienzo BA. The impact of aging on human sexuality. J School Health 1985; 55(2):66.
Robbins SL, Kumar V. Basic pathology. 4th ed. Philadelphia: WB Saunders, 1987.
Rodau SK, et al. Vaginal eversion repair: Sacrospinous ligament fixation procedure. AORN J 1987; 47(2):539.
Rubin D. Gynecologic cancer: Cervical, vulvar, and vaginal malignancies. RN 1987; 50(5):56.
Rubin D. Gynecologic cancer: Uterine and ovarian malignancies. RN 1987; 50(6):52.
Rubin SC. Ovarian cancer. AORN J 1988; 47(6):1427.
Sampselle CM, Brink CA. Pelvic muscle relaxation. J Nurse Midwife 1990; 35(3):127.
Sherwin BB, Gelfand MM. Differential symptom response to parenteral estrogen and/or androgen administration in the surgical menopause. Am J Obstet Gynecol 1985; 151(2):153.
Smith DB. Pelvic exenteration. J Enterostom Ther 1989; 16(5):195.
Smith LH, Thier SO. Pathophysiology: The biological principles of disease. 2nd ed. Philadelphia: WB Saunders, 1985.
Springer M. Radical vulvectomy: Physiological, psychological, social, sexual implications. Oncol Nurs Forum 1982; 9(2):276.
Stanfill PH. Psychosocial implications of hysterectomy. J Obstet Gynecol Neonatal Nurs 1982; 11(5):318.
Thompson JD, Rock J. The Linde's operative gynecology. 7th ed. Philadelphia: JB Lippincott, 1991.
Tulenheimo A, Laatikainen T, Salminen K. Plasma beta-endorphin immunoreactivity in premenstrual tension. Br Obstet Gynecol 1987; 94:26.
Wabreck AJ, Gunn JL. Sexual and psychological implications of gynecologic malignancy. J Obstet Gynecol Neonatal Nurs 1984; 13(6):371.
Walbroehl GS. Sexuality in cancer patients. Am Fam Physician 1985; 31(1):153.
Walton J. The effect of a support group on women with premenstrual syndrome. J Obstet Gynecol Neonatal Nurs 1987; 16(3):174.
Willson JR. Obstetrics & Gynecology. 9th ed. St. Louis: CV Mosby, 1991.
Wilson MA: Menstrual disorders. J Obstet Gynecol Neonatal Nurs (Suppl) 1984; 13(2):11s.

Chapter Forty-five

KNOWLEDGE BASIC TO THE NURSING CARE *of Men with Reproductive System Dysfunction*

In preparation for studying the nursing care of males with reproductive disorders, this chapter begins with a review of the anatomy and physiology of the male reproductive system. This is followed by a discussion of the clinical manifestations common to male reproductive disorders, assessment of the system, and diagnostic tests and basic surgical interventions used in the treatment of these disorders. The chapter ends with a discussion of the effects of aging on the system.

Anatomy and Physiology

The male reproductive system is composed of internal and external genitalia (Fig. 45–1).

The external genitalia consist of the penis and the scrotum. Although the testes and their attachments are located within the scrotal sac, they are not generally considered part of the external genitalia.

The internal genitalia are the testes, seminiferous tubules, interstitial cells, epididymis, vas deferens, seminal vesicles, ejaculatory ducts, prostate gland, bulbourethral glands (Cowper's glands), urethra, and spermatic cords.

External Genitalia

PENIS

The penis is a tubular organ attached to the anterior and lateral walls of the pubic area in front of the scrotum. It functions as the organ for both copulation (sexual intercourse) and urination. The body, or shaft, of the penis is composed of three cylindric masses of erectile tissue enclosed in separate fibrous coverings and held together by a covering of skin. Two of these cylinders that form the penis, the corpora cavernosa, are arranged laterally. The third column, known as the corpus spongiosum, forms the ventral surface of the penis. It is through this that the urethra runs, creating a common passageway for both urine and seminal fluid.

As the words *cavernous* and *spongy* suggest, these cylindric masses contain tissue filled with many spaces or cavities. They are served by a large network of blood sinuses and nerves. The blood supply to and from the penis is derived from the pudendal artery and vein. The diameter of these blood vessels is regulated by nerve fibers from the autonomic nervous system. When the penis is in a flaccid, or relaxed, state, its cavities contain minimal blood, whereas in response to sexual stimulation, these cavities fill with blood, resulting in a characteristic hardening of the penis known as erection.

At the distal end of the penis, the corpus spongiosum expands to form a slightly bulging structure called the glans penis, which terminates in a longitudinal slit at the external meatus. The glans penis is richly endowed with nerve fibers and is extremely sensitive to tactile stimulation.

The skin covering the penis is hairless, and loosely applied to the underlying tissues. At the neck of the penis, the skin is folded doubly, covering the glans to form a loose, retractable casing called the prepuce, or foreskin. Under the prepuce and in the neck of the penis are small glands that produce a cheeselike substance called smegma, a secretion with no known function.

The average adult penis is 7.5 to 10 cm (3 to 4 in.) long when flaccid, as in the unaroused state, and somewhat more than 15 cm (6 in.) in the erectile state. Its diameter in the relaxed state is about 3.13 cm (1.25 in.) and increases another 0.63 cm

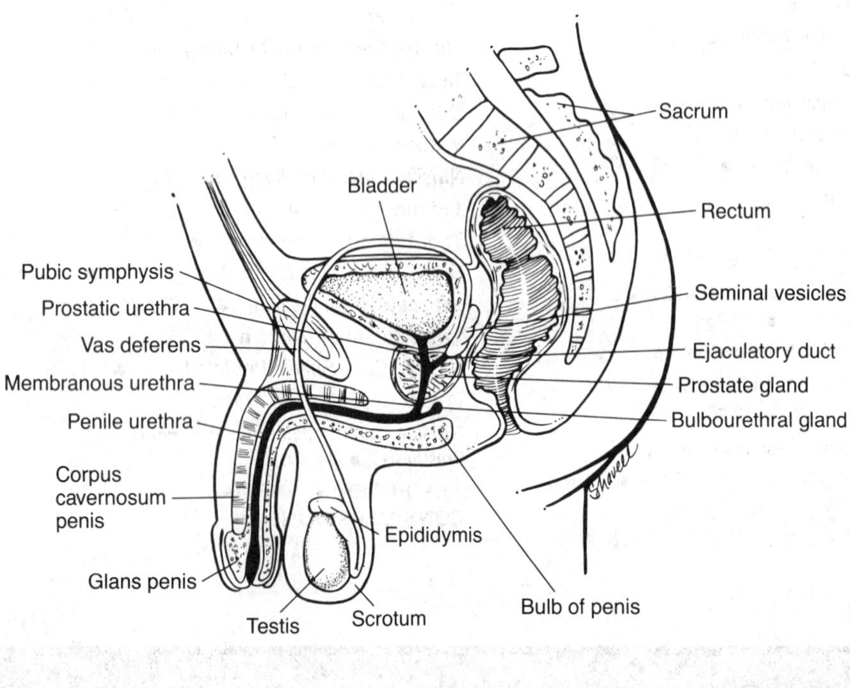

Figure 45–1.

The male reproductive system: internal and external genitalia.

(0.25 in.) during an erection (Katchadourian & Lunde, 1980).

SCROTUM

The scrotum is a skin-covered pouch suspended from the perineal region that covers, protects, and regulates the temperature of the testes. It is divided by a septum into two sacs, each of which contains and supports one testis together with its connecting tube, the epididymis, and the lower part of the spermatic cord.

The scrotum consists of a thin layer of skin arranged in folds, known as rugae, and an incomplete layer of smooth-muscle fibers called the dartos muscle. This muscle contracts when the body is cold, causing the testes to be drawn upward against the perineum. In hot weather, the scrotum relaxes and allows the testes to hang more freely away from the body. These changes in the scrotum are important thermoregulators because spermatogenesis is adversely affected by temperature extremes. The skin covering the scrotum is darker in color than the rest of the body and at puberty becomes sparsely covered with hair. Because of the rugae, the skin of the scrotum has the potential for great distention, as when edema develops within the scrotal sac.

Internal Genitalia

TESTES

The testes are the gonads, or reproductive glands, of the male and therefore are the counterpart of the female's ovaries. They have the dual function of producing sperm and the male hormone, testosterone.

The testes are small, ovoid glands, usually of equal size, with the left one hanging lower than the right one in the scrotal sac. During fetal development, the testes are located in the abdominal cavity behind the peritoneum. About 2 months before birth, the testes descend into the scrotum and are held in position by the spermatic cords. If the testes fail to descend, the condition is known as cryptorchidism.

In the internal structure of the testes, two components are important: the seminiferous tubules and the interstitial cells. The seminiferous tubules are a series of long, convoluted, threadlike structures packed densely into the testes, which eventually converge into a collection of excretory ducts. There are approximately 1000 seminiferous tubules whose function it is to form sperm. Sperm from each testis are then stored in the corresponding epididymis and vas deferens.

The interstitial cells, also called Leydig's cells, are testicular cells scattered in clusters in the connective tissue lying between the seminiferous tubules. These cells carry out the second function of the testes: the production of the male sex hormone, testosterone. The interstitial cells are located close to the blood vessels in the testes and secrete this hormone directly into the blood stream.

Testosterone begins to be secreted by the male at about the second month of embryonic life. During fetal development, it is responsible for the formation of the male external genitalia and for the descent of the testes into the scrotum during the eighth or ninth month of prenatal life. Essentially no testosterone is produced during childhood until approximately age 13. Then, under the influence of the gonadotropin-releasing hormones from the hypothalmus, the anterior pituitary secretes interstitial cell-stimulating hormone (ICSH). ICSH in turn stimulates hyperplasia of the interstitial cells of the testes and the production of testosterone by these cells. The secretion of testosterone subsequently inhibits the secretion of ICSH and luteinizing hormone releasing hormone (LH-RH). This negative feedback mechanism controls the rate at which testosterone is produced. Secretion of testosterone results in the enlargement of the penis, scrotum, and testes; the maturation of sperm; and the appearance of secondary sex characteristics. Testosterone continues to be secreted throughout most of the remainder of life but gradually decreases in amount beginning at about 50 years at age.

EPIDIDYMIS

The epididymis is a long tube about 6 m (20 ft) in length, coiled into a comma-shaped structure, adhering to the top and side of each testis. Each epididymis is divided into a head, a central body, and a tapered portion that is continuous with the vas deferens, called the tail. The epididymis begins the first portion of the paired male genital duct system in which sperm mature and are then propelled from the testes toward the urethra during ejaculation.

VAS DEFERENS

The vas deferens is a tubular structure that connects the epididymis with the ejaculatory duct. Sperm are stored in the vas deferens without losing their fertility for periods ranging from several hours to as long as 42 days depending on the degree of sexual activity. The vas deferens has thick muscular walls and can be palpated in the scrotal sac as a smooth, movable cord. The muscular layers of the vas help propel the sperm through the duct system. The vas deferens from each testis ascends from the scrotum and passes through the inguinal canal and into the pelvic cavity. Here it extends over the top and down the posterior surface of the urinary bladder, narrows to a tip, and joins the duct of a seminal vesicle to form the ejaculatory duct.

SEMINAL VESICLES

The seminal vesicles are two convoluted membranous pouches that are located along the lower part of the posterior surface of the bladder directly in front of the rectum. The seminal vesicles secrete a slightly alkaline fluid containing large amounts of fructose. This secretion, which is a component of semen, helps to protect and nourish the sperm and activates the sperms' motility. Normal secretory activity of the seminal vesicles depends on adequate levels of testosterone. Each seminal vesicle joins with the corresponding vas deferens to form an ejaculatory duct.

EJACULATORY DUCTS

The ejaculatory ducts are two short tubes that pass through the prostate gland to empty the semen-containing sperm into the urethra.

PROSTATE GLAND

The prostate gland is an encapsulated three-lobed structure located at the base of the urinary bladder, behind the symphysis pubis, and close to the rectal wall (Fig. 45–2). It is small at birth but rapidly enlarges to full growth at puberty, resembling the size and shape of a chestnut. The initial 2 to 3 cm (0.8 to 1.1 in.) of the urethra pass through a small hole in the center of the prostate gland.

Internally, the prostate is a partly glandular and partly muscular structure. The glandular tissue is composed of follicular pouches that secrete a thin, milky alkaline fluid into numerous excretory ducts. These prostatic ducts open into the prostatic portion of the urethra, adding the prostatic secretion to semen or ejaculate. The alkalinity of this secretion helps protect the sperm from acid present in the male urethra and female vagina and thus increases sperm motility. The glandular portion of the prostate is embedded in muscle fibers that contract during ejaculation to eject prostatic secretion via the ejaculatory ducts.

Because the prostate gland is anterior to the rectal wall, it is easily palpable by rectal examination, thus facilitating early diagnosis of prostatic problems such as infections and enlargements. Because of the anatomic relationship of the prostate to the urethra, many prostatic problems cause urinary tract symptoms.

COWPER'S GLANDS

Cowper's glands (bulbourethral glands) are two small, pea-sized structures located on either side of the urethra inferior to the prostate. During sexual arousal, these glands secrete a small amount of clear alkaline fluid into the urethra, which appears as a droplet at the tip of the penis before ejaculation occurs. Like the secretions of the seminal vesicles and prostate gland, this secretion from Cowper's glands neutralizes the acidic environment of the male urethra and the female vagina.

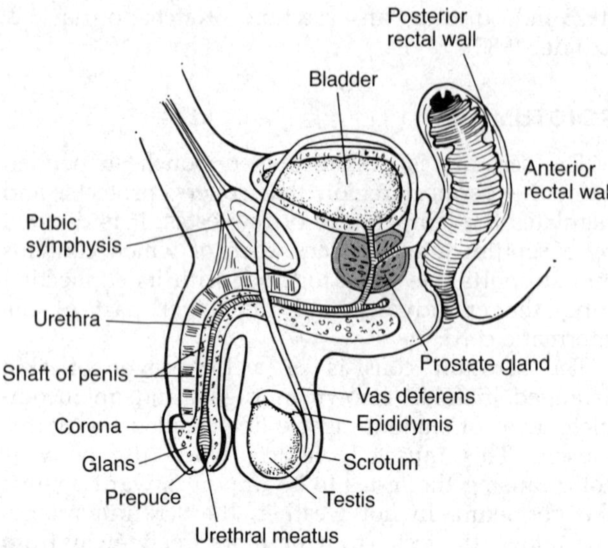

Figure 45–2.

Anatomic relationship of the prostate gland to the bladder, rectum, and urethra.

URETHRA

The urethra, the terminal duct of the male reproductive system, serves as the pathway for eliminating both urine and semen. It measures about 20 cm (8 in.) in length and is divided into prostatic, membranous, and penile parts. Although the urethra is the passageway out of the body for both urine and semen, the excretion of these fluids never occurs simultaneously. The nervous reflexes involved in the expulsion of semen (ejaculation) automatically inhibit urination.

SPERMATIC CORDS

The spermatic cords are two cylindric structures from which each testis is suspended in the scrotal sac. The cords extend from the inguinal rings to the testes and enclose the vas deferens, blood vessels, lymphatic vessels, nerves, and muscle fibers. When these muscle fibers contract, the spermatic cord shortens and pulls the attached testis upward within the scrotal sac.

Spermatogenesis

Spermatogenesis is the process by which the germ cells (spermatogonia), formed in the lining of the seminiferous tubules during fetal development, become transformed into mature sperm. This process is initiated at puberty by follicle-stimulating hormone (FSH) and luteinizing hormone (LH), which are secreted by the anterior pituitary gland. In response to these hormones, as well as the maturing effect of testosterone, the spermatogonia begin a lifetime of active cell division.

Once formed in the seminiferous tubules, sperm migrate to the epididymides and become capable of fertilizing an ovum by completing the maturation process and developing motility. Some sperm can be stored in the epididymides, but most move into the vas deferens, remaining there until they are ejaculated. While stored in these areas, the sperm can maintain their fertility for as long as 2 months. With excessive sexual activity, storage may be limited to a few hours.

Sperm are produced at the rate of about 300 million per day and, once ejaculated, have a life expectancy of approximately 48 hours within the female reproductive tract. Spermatogenesis continues throughout the males life cycle, although it diminishes with advancing age.

Semen

Semen, or seminal fluid, is a milky, viscid fluid containing about 120 million sperm per milliliter as well as the secretions from the epididymides, seminal vesicles, prostate gland, and bulbourethral glands. These secretions combine to create optimum conditions for the survival and function of the sperm. The alkaline secretions of the prostate neutralize acids and create a pH of about 7.5. Fructose, secreted by the seminal vesicles, provides an energy source for the spermatozoa. Mucus from the seminal vesicles and bulbourethral glands furnishes lubrication. Although all components of semen are essential, the sperm are the most important ingredient; if the sperm count falls below about 20 million/ml, the male is usually sterile.

Erection and Ejaculation

Erection is the enlargement and hardening of the penis in response to some physical or psychic stimulus. Tumescence is the term used to describe the fully erect penis; detumescence refers to the return of the penis to its nonerectile state.

Afferent input from such stimuli are transmitted by the pudendal nerve and pass up the spinal cord for integration in the cerebrum. Efferent nerve fibers then transmit the impulses to the sacral portion of the parasympathetic nervous system, resulting in arteriolar dilation in the penis and filling of the venous sinusoids in the corpora cavernosa and corpus spongiosum with blood. As this erectile tissue fills with blood, venous outflow is impaired and the penis becomes hard and elongated, facilitating its penetration into the vagina during sexual intercourse. The penis is returned to its nonerectile state through the stimulation of the sympathetic nerve fibers, which results in constriction of the penile arterioles, a reduction of the inflow of blood, and increase in venous drainage.

Erection can also occur without cerebral cortical control by way of a spinal cord reflex mechanism integrated in the sacral area of the cord. In response to tactile stimulation of the penis, scrotum, inner aspects of the thigh, or the anal epithelium, a neural signal is transmitted via the pudendal nerve to an erector center in the sacral portion of the spinal cord. This center then sends out impulses by way of parasympathetic nerves, causing a redirection of blood flow to the cavernous spaces in the penis, which results in an erection. This reflex mechanism is particularly evident in the patient whose spinal cord has been severed.

The response time for an erection varies. It can be very short, occurring within a few seconds of stimulation (Katchadourian and Lunde, 1980), or it can take significantly longer. Advancing age, intake of alcohol, fatigue, and stress may increase the time for an erection to be produced.

Erection is experienced on numerous occasions by practically all males from birth to old age both during sleep and while awake. During the sexually active years, a male may report three to four erections at night.

Erections that are nonsexual in nature occur with tension of the perineal muscles, as when lifting a heavy object or straining during defecation. They can also result from irritation of the glans penis, inflammation of the other genital organs, or a full bladder.

Ejaculation is the expulsion of semen from the urethra to the outside. When the level of sexual stimulation becomes extremely intense, the reflex centers in the lumbar section of the spinal cord send impulses by way of sympathetic nerves to the genital organs. These impulses cause peristaltic contractions of the ducts in the testes, epididymides, and vas deferens that propel sperm into the urethra (emission). Simultaneously, rhythmic contractions of the seminal vesicles and prostate gland expel semen and prostatic fluid into the urethra as well. The ejaculatory act itself occurs when impulses reaching the pudendal nerves stimulate the skeletal muscles at the base of the penis, causing forceful expulsion of the semen to the exterior. During ejaculation, the internal sphincter of the neck of the urinary bladder is tightly closed so that sperm cannot enter the bladder, nor can urine be eliminated. The average amount of semen ejaculated during the sexual act is 2.5 to 5 ml.

After ejaculation and orgasm occur, the male enters the refractory period. During this phase, regardless of the type and intensity of sexual stimulation, he will not respond. He cannot achieve a full erection and ejaculation. The length of the refractory period varies among men; for some it may last only a few minutes, whereas others may remain refractory for as long as 24 hours. During the refractory period, detumescence occurs, and the penis returns to the nonerectile state.

Clinical Manifestations of Reproductive System Dysfunction

Sexual Dysfunction

There are three major manifestations of sexual dysfunction in males: erectile dysfunction or impotence, premature ejaculation, and retrograde ejaculation.

IMPOTENCE

Impotence is the persistent inability to obtain or maintain penile erection suitable for vaginal penetration and completion of intercourse. It is generally classified as either primary or secondary. Primary impotence is very uncommon and is found in males who have never been able to have intercourse.

Secondary impotence is erectile failure after successful sexual functioning has been established. Untreated impotence may result in infertility.

Both primary and secondary impotence are caused by some underlying organic or psychogenic problem. Some of the organic causes of primary impotence are congenital hypothalamic-pituitary disorders, traumatic injury to the genitals, and spina bifida. If an organic cause is ruled out, primary impotence usually indicates deep-seated psychological conflicts concerning sexuality. Childhood fears and restrictive upbringing about sex, disturbed mother-son relationship, and religious orthodoxy are identified by Masters and Johnson (1970) as psychogenic etiologic factors in primary impotence.

Secondary impotence was originally believed to be primarily psychogenic in origin. However, recent research reports indicate that an underlying organic cause may be present in at least 50% of affected patients (McConnell & Zimmerman, 1983). The psychological causes associated with secondary impotence are numerous and include such factors as aging, anxiety, boredom, depression, fear, cultural pressure to perform sexually, fatigue, and stress. In certain cases of secondary impotence whose origin is primarily psychogenic, physiologic factors may contribute to the dysfunction. For example, 50% to 70% of men report that, after a myocardial infarction, sex life never returns to normal. The myocardial infarction in itself is usually not the cause; rather, fear is identified as the primary reason for the sexual dysfunction (Satterfield, 1986).

A wide variety of organic conditions have also been identified as causes of secondary impotence (Table 45–1). Of these, diabetes mellitus is considered to be the most frequent single cause of impotence in the United States today (Lue, 1986, p. 720). Despite the use of oral antidiabetic agents and insulin, impotence remains more common as a complication than either retinopathy or nephropathy (Lue, 1986). The major cause of diabetic impotence appears to be diabetic vascular changes in both small and large blood vessels. Neuropathy is identified as the second most common organic cause of diabetic impotence.

MEDICAL DIAGNOSIS

Diagnosis of impotency requires a thorough psychosexual history, analysis of the presenting symptoms, and a health assessment with special attention to the endocrine, genitourinary, neurologic, and vascular systems. Specific tests to assist in confirming a diagnosis of impotency include semen analysis; measurement of serum testosterone, prolactin, follicle-stimulating hormone, and luteinizing hormone levels; and testicular biopsy.

MEDICAL MANAGEMENT

The treatment of impotence, which is dictated by its cause, may be medical, surgical, or both. In cases of psychogenic impotence or for those patients in which a psychological response contributes to the cause, sex therapy for the patient as well as his partner is recommended. Impotence secondary to hypogonadism may respond to an intramuscular injection of 200 to 300 mg of testosterone every 2 to 3 weeks. If impotence is related to a medication such as an antihypertensive, lowering the dose or using a safe substitution may alleviate the problem.

Patients with neurogenic impotence may benefit from a new pharmacologic erection treatment that involves the injection of a drug combination consisting of the smooth-muscle relaxant papaverine hydrochloride and the vasodilator phentolamine mesylate into the corpora cavernosa. An erection usually is produced within 15 minutes, with a duration of 1 to 2 hours. Because the effect is short term, this

Table 45–1. ORGANIC CAUSES OF SECONDARY IMPOTENCE

CATEGORY	SPECIFIC CLINICAL EXAMPLES
Endocrine	Diabetes mellitus, hypogonadism, thyroid dysfunction, Addison's disease, Cushing's syndrome
Neurologic	Multiple sclerosis, spinal cord injury, peripheral neuropathies, herniated disk
Vascular	Hypertension, priapism, aortoiliac obstruction
Pharmacologic agents	Alcohol, methyldopa (Aldomet), clonidine hydrochloride (Catapres), cimetidine, (Tagamet), phenytoin (Dilantin), L-dopa, lithium
Surgical	Partial penectomy, radical cystectomy, abdominal perineal resection, radical prostatectomy
Metabolic	Renal failure, hepatic cirrhosis

treatment must be done each time the male wishes to engage in intercourse. Therefore, the patient is taught to inject himself at home.

Surgical approaches for the treatment of organic impotence consists of the implantation of a penile prosthesis and penile revascularization. Although vascular surgery of the penis is performed on some patients with vasculogenic impotence, failure may occur within 12 to 18 months after revascularization. Currently, the penile implant is the treatment of choice for organic impotence.

Application of the Nursing Process to the Care of the Patient with Impotence

Assessment

Begin the assessment by providing for privacy and creating an environment of acceptance and understanding so that the patient feels comfortable discussing his erectile problem. For example, placing the patient in a quiet, private area, conveying a sense of interest and empathy, and assuring him that his sexual dysfunction is common can make it easier for him to openly discuss his impotence.

Determine the patient's perceptions of the problem, including its onset, possible cause, and severity. Ask him to describe the problem in his own words, and use terms he understands to aid in collecting accurate, complete information. Obtain information regarding any factors in the patient's life, such as career change, financial or family concerns, and history of alcoholism, that may have caused or contributed to the development of the erectile dysfunction.

Assess the patient's understanding of the diagnostic procedures for which he is scheduled as well as any treatment planned for him. Elicit the patient's feelings regarding the effect of his impotence on his relationship with his sexual partner, family, or significant others.

Nursing Diagnoses and Planning

Nursing diagnoses and related expected patient outcomes most commonly applicable to patients with impotence include the following:

NDx: Sexual dysfunction related to impotence

Planning: Patient outcomes
1. Patient describes alternative methods of sexual expression.
2. Patient discusses his concerns regarding his sexual dysfunction with his partner or significant other.
3. Patient maintains a satisfying sexual relationship.
4. Patient describes the role of Impotence Anonymous as a support group for males with impotence.

NDx: Knowledge deficit: causes, contributing factors, diagnostic procedures, and medical management

Planning: Patient outcomes
1. Patient states the cause of his sexual dysfunction.
2. Patient identifies factors in his life that may have contributed to his impotent state.
3. Patient describes the diagnostic tests for which he is scheduled.
4. Patient describes the medical plan of care.

Nursing Interventions

NDx: Sexual dysfunction

Remind the patient that sexual expression is not limited to intercourse. Suggest the use of noncoital activities such as touching, orogenital techniques, body massage, and masturbation (if acceptable) to achieve sexual gratification for himself and his partner.

Discuss the value of engaging in some form of physical exercise such as walking, running, or yoga as an alternative means for releasing sexual energy.

Encourage the patient to share his concerns and feelings regarding his erectile dysfunction with his partner or significant other. Provide information on the role of Impotence Anonymous (5119 Bradley Boulevard, Chevy Chase, MD 20815), a national support group for males with impotence, for further help in coping with this problem. Refer to a local mental health center or the American Association of Sex Educators, Counselors and Therapists (11 Dupont Circle, Suite 220, Washington, DC 20036) if professional help in the form of sex therapy is needed or requested.

NDx: Knowledge deficit: causes, contributing factors, diagnostic procedures, and medical management

Begin with what the patient already knows about his problem, and clarify any misconceptions. If the cause is determined, use terms consistent with his ability to comprehend, and explain why impotence developed. Use visual aids such as books and diagrams to enhance the patient's learning. Encourage the patient to try to modify those factors in his life that may have contributed to the development of impotence. For example, if he has a problem with alcohol or admits to ingesting alcohol before engaging in sexual intercourse, he needs to know this drug can impair or destroy the neurogenic reflex that stimulates the erectile tissue.

Provide information about the diagnostic tests ordered: their purpose, general description of the tests, and any special preparation required.

Help the patient understand the plan of treatment and its expected outcome. For example, if the drugs papaverine hydrochloride and phentolamine mesylate are prescribed, explain that the purpose of this therapy is to promote an erection. Explain that the drugs must be injected into his penis about 15 minutes before he wishes to engage in sexual intercourse and that the duration of their effect is 1 to 2 hours. Provide for instruction on drawing up and injecting medications. Alert the patient to side effects such as dizziness and orthostatic hypotension that can occur with phentolamine and the nausea and flushing that may accompany papaverine.

Evaluation

Evaluate the effectiveness of nursing care for patients with impotence by comparing their status with the expected patient outcomes. Examples of specific outcomes for patients with impotence have been provided in the Planning section.

PREMATURE EJACULATION

Premature ejaculation, a common sexual problem, refers to the expulsion of semen shortly after the onset of sexual excitement or before orgasm of the sexual partner. Premature ejaculation may occur during foreplay or as soon as the genitals are touched. In most cases, however, it occurs either during attempted penetration of the penis into the vagina or during the first few pelvic thrusts. In severe cases of premature ejaculation (i.e., those in which ejaculation consistently occurs before the penis is inserted into the vagina), infertility can occur.

The cause of premature ejaculation is believed to be psychological in the majority of patients. Examples of related psychological factors are anxiety associated with immature sexual experiences, guilt or fear about sex, and ambivalence toward women.

Treatment of premature ejaculation is usually sex therapy. There are several sex therapy techniques available, but generally all foster the patient's awareness of his premonitory ejaculatory reflex. After a psychosexual history is obtained from each partner, they are acquainted with the therapy procedures and advised that the prognosis for permanent resolution is excellent.

A urologic evaluation is done only when an underlying urologic problem is suspected.

RETROGRADE EJACULATION

Retrograde ejaculation is the propulsion of seminal fluid from the posterior urethra into the bladder. The retrograde deposition of semen produces a functional state of infertility.

Normally during ejaculation the bladder neck closes, preventing backward passage of the semen. Conditions that alter the anatomic structure of the bladder neck or those that interfere with its neurologic tone may result in retrograde ejaculation. The most common causes of this dysfunction are transurethral resection of the prostate, diabetes mellitus with neuropathy, bladder surgery or trauma, sympathectomy (between T-12 and L-3), spinal cord injury, and use of drugs such as guanethidine that produce sympathetic blockage.

Currently, the treatment of retrograde ejaculation is very limited. Some researchers reported favorable results using phenylpropanolamine, an alpha-adrenergic medication, or the antidepressant drug imipramine to facilitate closure of the bladder neck. Because retrograde ejaculation usually results in infertility, a postcoital catheterization with insemination of the ejaculate into the partner may be attempted to achieve a pregnancy.

Infertility

Infertility is the failure to conceive within an identified period of time, usually within 1 year of regular, unprotected intercourse. It is estimated that male factors are responsible for about 40% of infertility problems.

ETIOLOGY

The causes of male infertility can be classified as either physical or psychogenic. However, in 10% to 20% of infertile males, the cause is idiopathic. In some cases, infertility may be due to a combination of physical and psychological factors. Table 45–2 lists common physical causes of male infertility. Common nonorganic factors associated with male infertility include infrequent or too frequent ejaculation, nonoptimal sexual techniques, and stress.

Table 45–2. COMMON PHYSICAL CAUSES OF MALE INFERTILITY

CATEGORY	SPECIFIC CLINICAL EXAMPLES
Endocrine factors	Hypogonadism, androgen deficiency, hypothyroidism
Sexual dysfunction	Retrograde ejaculation, impotence, premature ejaculation
Structural anomalies of genitals	Cryptorchidism, varicocele, stricture of vas deferens
Testicular failure	Alcohol, immunologic disorders, drugs (e.g., cimetidine, nitrogen mustard, chlorambucil, vincristine), Klinefelter's syndrome, mumps, radiation exposure, and uremia

MEDICAL DIAGNOSIS

The evaluation of an infertility problem involves both partners and includes a complete health history, review of sexual practices, and physical examination. Particular attention is paid to a history of prolonged fever or of mumps after puberty. Information is obtained about social and cultural beliefs and the use of cigarettes, alcohol, and other recreational drugs as well as prescription drugs such as cimetidine and methyldopa (Aldomet) that are known to impair male fertility. As part of any infertility workup, a semen analysis is done. An abnormal specimen consistent with infertility usually shows a sperm count of less than 20 million/ml (oligospermia), extreme volume variation, diminished motility, and abnormal sperm shape. When the semen analysis is abnormal, additional tests are done to establish a differential diagnosis. These tests include a gonadotropin assay to determine the integrity of the pituitary-testes axis, measurement of serum testosterone levels to assess the testes' response to LH, and a biopsy of the testes to help clarify an unexplained oligospermia or azoospermia.

MEDICAL MANAGEMENT

Treatment of male infertility depends on the underlying cause, if known. Surgical repair of a varicocele offers the most encouraging results of all therapeutic approaches for the infertile male. In the cases of an obstructed excretory duct, a vasoepididymal bypass and anastomosis may improve passage of sperm and restore fertility.

Male infertility caused by hypopituitarism or hypothyroidism may respond to endocrine therapy. For example, the patient with hypogonadotropic hypogonadism may be given intramuscular human chorionic gonadotropin (HCG), 2000 IU, and menotropins (Pergonal), 25 to 75 IU three times per week, to induce spermatogenesis. If successful, fertility results after 1 to 2 months of this treatment.

For the patient with idiopathic infertility, androgen therapy may be prescribed (see Pharmacology Box 45–1). Anticipating a rebound effect, testosterone enanthate, 200 mg intramuscularly weekly for 12 to 20 weeks, is administered, which should result in azoospermia. Treatment is then stopped. Reappearance of sperm in the semen usually occurs in 2 to 3 months.

Sex therapy is recommended for an infertility problem associated with psychogenic factors. If treatment is not effective, alternatives such as adoption or artificial insemination may be suggested. Infertility in the male may have a profound effect on his perception of his personal identity. Inability to procreate may be perceived as a loss of self-worth (Casey, 1982), and feelings of anger and guilt may occur. These psychogenic factors, which can develop in response to infertility, may impede the effectiveness of any treatment.

Pain

Pain is one of the most common clinical manifestations for which males with reproductive system dysfunction seek medical attention. Pain may be due to an infectious process, a neoplasm, or a structural abnormality. Its type and location vary with its cause. For example, perineal pain and dysuria (burning on urination) occur with prostatitis, whereas pain in the inguinal and lower abdominal areas is characteristic of epididymitis.

Urinary Retention

Urinary retention is the inability to empty the bladder with each voiding. This occurs in reproductive tract disorders that obstruct the passage of urine through the urethra and is a common clinical manifestation of benign hypertrophy of the prostate gland and of advanced carcinoma of the prostate. Urinary retention is signaled by frequency of urination, difficulty initiating the urinary stream, a weak urinary stream, and dribbling.

Assessment of Reproductive System Status

Patient History

When obtaining a history from a male with reproductive dysfunction, be aware that he may be both anxious and embarrassed, and use tact and skill in gathering information. Provide a quiet, private environment, and be open, supportive, and nonjudgmental in attitude and approach. This is essential because, without privacy, sufficient time for patient nurse interaction, and a professional manner, nursing assessments and interventions are likely to be incomplete, incorrect, or ineffective. Patients are unlikely to respond comfortably or completely to questions about sexual ability and presence of a penile discharge or to verbalize concerns about the effects of a surgical procedure or sexual function if other patients can hear the conversation or if the interaction is interrupted by other staff.

Be certain to communicate with the patient at a level he can understand. Keep questions simple and clear. Do not assume that the patient knows the biological terms for the reproductive organs or that he can describe the functions of these organs. In attempting to elicit information about a specific dysfunction, use simple but correct terminology. Avoid terms that may be unfamiliar to the patient because he may be embarrassed to ask their meaning and thus give incorrect information.

Begin the history with nonthreatening, relatively neutral questions to give the patient time to become

Pharmacology Box 45–1.
ANDROGENS

Androgens:
Class of drugs composed of the principal natural male hormone, testosterone, and its synthetic derivatives. At puberty, the gonadotropins stimulate the testes to begin secreting large amounts of testosterone. The amount decreases as the male ages. Small amounts of androgens and androgenic precursors are secreted by the ovaries and adrenal cortex.

Action:
At puberty, testosterone is responsible for the development of primary sex organs and secondary sexual characteristics. Its metabolic effects include protein anabolism; red blood cell production; retention of sodium, water, potassium, nitrogen, and phosphorus; and the excretion of calcium.

Uses:
Replacement therapy in males with congenital or acquired hypogonadism, congenital or acquired hypogonadotropic hypogonadism, and delayed puberty. Its uses also include stimulating the descent of testes in cryptorchidism (undescended testes), treatment of endometriosis and metastatic breast cancer in postmenopausal women, and stimulation of erythropoiesis in mild to moderate hypoplastic anemias and anemias associated with chronic renal failure and malignant blood dyscrasias.

Side Effects:
Cholestatic hepatitis, pruritus, edema, impotence, priapism, azoospermia, nausea, vomiting, diarrhea (oral preparations), headache, anxiety, insomnia, increased or decreased libido, gynecomastia, hypercalcemia, and masculinization in women.

Interactions:
Increase effect of oral anticoagulants, insulin, and oral hypoglycemic drugs. Concomitant use of androgens with adrenal corticosteroids increases edema formation.

Nursing Implications:
In accord with the U.S. Food and Drug Administration regulations, be sure the patient has the package insert, which explains the possible side effects. Review this information with the patient before the first dose is given. Assess for edema, and weigh the patient two times per week. Inform the patient to report pruritus, jaundice, priapism, or other unusual symptoms immediately. Instruct the patient to take oral preparation with meals. Explain how to use the buccal tablets. Intramuscular (IM) preparation is given deep into the gluteal muscle. If long-term IM therapy is prescribed, family member or significant other may need to receive instructions regarding the administration.

comfortable with you. Ask about the number and ages of his children, and review his medical history. Explore the type, date, and treatment of any previous genitourinary problems. Determine whether he is currently taking any over-the-counter or prescription medications, and note the drug name, dose, route, frequency, reason for use, and effectiveness. Also determine the date of his last genital and rectal examination and the frequency of self-examination of the testes. Ask whether he is circumcised. Review sexual status. Include age of first intercourse, current frequency of intercourse, problems with intercourse (either erectile or ejaculatory), sexual satisfaction, and type of birth control. If the patient is middle aged or older, inquire about the occurrence of symptoms of male menopause.

Explore current symptoms. Ask about pain or discomfort, determining location, type, and relationship to intercourse, defecation, or voiding. Also ask about penile discharge, with attention to color (white, yellow, green, clear, bloody), consistency (thin, thick), odor (none, sweet, foul), amount, and time of onset. Inquire about the presence of penile or scrotal edema and of penile, scrotal, or inguinal masses.

Because urinary symptoms frequently accompany reproductive disorders, ask about dysuria, hesitancy, frequency, straining to urinate, nocturia, decreased force of the urinary stream, and dribbling or incontinence. Also inquire about any changes in defecation pattern.

Pelvic Examination

The male pelvic examination is an organized assessment of the structural condition of the reproductive organs. It includes inspection and palpation of the external genitalia (penis and scrotum) and inguinal and femoral areas and palpation of the prostate gland.

PREPARATION OF THE PATIENT

In preparation for the examination, the patient is asked to urinate. This prevents discomfort and urgency when the prostate gland is palpated. The patient is then asked to stand for the examination if he is able to, and he is asked to drop his shorts and pants below his knees. If the patient is unable to stand, his pants and shorts are removed, and he is assisted onto the examining table and draped in the supine position with the knees slightly flexed.

EXAMINATION PROCEDURE

The examiner wears clean gloves and begins the examination with assessment of the external genitalia. The amount and distribution of pubic hair are noted, and the base of the hairs is inspected for lice or nits. The anterior and posterior surfaces of the penis are inspected for edema, erythema, masses, ulcerations, or other abnormalities. If the patient is not circumcised, the prepuce (foreskin) is retracted by the patient or examiner to expose the glans. Any accumulation of smegma beneath it is noted. The glans is observed for ulcers, scars, or other lesions as well as for signs of inflammation or infection. The position of the urethral meatus is noted, and it is examined for any sign of discharge. If the foreskin has been retracted, it is returned to its original position, and the examiner proceeds to palpate the entire shaft of the penis for tenderness, masses, and induration.

The contour of the scrotum is examined for lumps and edema (note that the left scrotum normally hangs 1.27 cm [$\frac{1}{2}$ in.] lower than the right). The scrotal skin is inspected for erythema, excoriations, ulcers or other lesions, gross deviations in coloration, and the presence of large or distended scrotal veins. Next, the contents of the right and left compartments of the scrotal sac are palpated, and the size, shape, and relative position of the testes, epididymis, and spermatic cord are noted. Normally, the testes are freely movable and sensitive to pressure (i.e., a dull, aching sensation that radiates to the lower abdomen is felt when they are gently squeezed) and no nodules or swellings are evident. If an abnormal scrotal mass is found, the examiner notes its size, shape, location, movability, consistency, and tenderness and proceeds to evaluate the area further by transillumination. This is done in a darkened room by placing a flashlight head flat against the affected side of the scrotum and observing for the transmission of light as a red glow. A red glow indicates the presence of serous fluid, which transmits light, as opposed to a swelling or mass containing blood or tissue, neither of which transmits light.

Femoral and inguinal areas are examined with the patient in both the supine and the standing positions. The patient is asked to bear down to help visualize a femoral hernia if present. The area is checked for bulges, edema, tenderness, and palpable lymph nodes. The examiner then palpates the right and left inguinal canals with the right and left index fingers, respectively, by gently invaginating the loose scrotal skin to allow the finger tip to press against the inguinal ring (Fig. 45–3). The patient is then instructed to strain down or cough while the examiner feels for a bulge of tissue against the finger tip, which is indicative of a hernia.

The prostate gland is examined with the patient in a side-lying position or standing with his back to the examiner and bent over with flexed elbows and upper chest on the examining table. A gloved, lubricated index finger is inserted into the rectum (Fig. 45–4), and the size and consistency of the prostate gland are evaluated. The normal prostate is 3.8 cm (1.5 in.) long, 5 cm (2 in.) wide, and nontender and

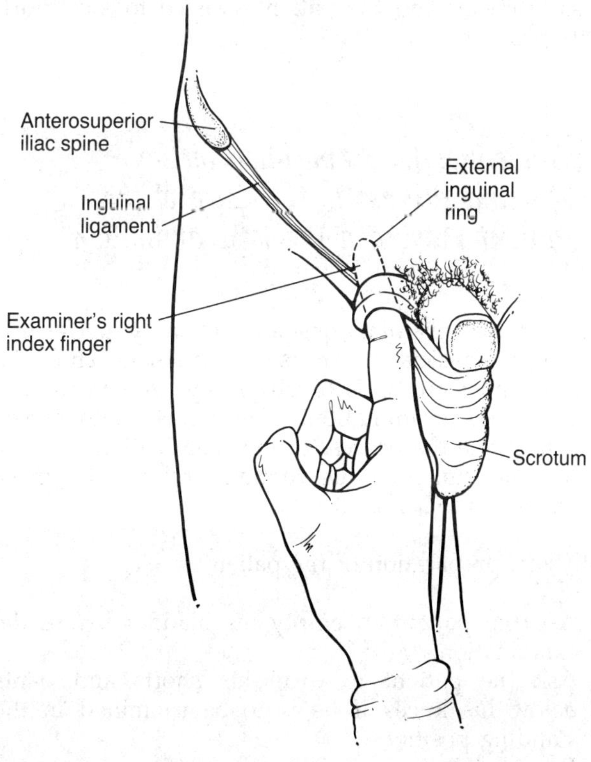

Figure 45–3.
Palpating for inguinal hernia—frontal view, right inguinal ring.

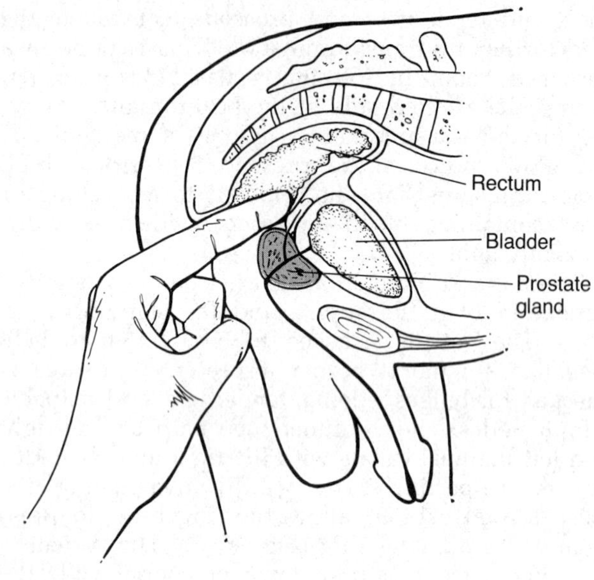

Figure 45–4.

Palpating the prostate gland.

feels smooth and rubbery. The seminal vesicles are usually not palpable unless infected or inflamed.

On conclusion of the examination, the penis is checked for discharge, which may be present after prostatic manipulation. If present, a drop may be collected and sent for microscopic analysis (prostatic fluid smear). The rectal area is cleansed of any excess lubricant and the patient assisted to a comfortable position.

Guidelines for Application of the Nursing Process to the Care of the Patient Having a Pelvic Examination

Male pelvic examinations are generally performed either by physicians or nurse practitioners. Thus, the role of most nurses is to physically prepare the patient for the examination, allay anxiety, and generally facilitate the process of the examination.

Specific nursing interventions related to these areas are as follows:

Physical preparation of the patient

- Ask the patient to empty his bladder before the examination.
- Ask the patient to drop his shorts and pants below his knees if he is to be examined in the standing position.
- Provide a drape or gown as needed.
- If the patient is to be examined lying down, assist him into a supine position with knees flexed and later into Sims' position. Drape as needed.
- Wipe any excess lubricant from the rectal area when the examination is over if this is not done by the examiner.
- Assist the patient to a safe, comfortable position.

Relief of anxiety

- Tell the patient what to expect and how the examination will proceed. For example, tell the patient who is to be examined in the standing position that he will be asked to bend over and lean on the examining table for the prostatic examination. Tell him also that he will be asked to bear down as if straining at stool and to cough during the examination to check for hernia. Explain to the patient that he may become erect from the stimulation of the prostate, and if this does occur, it is an involuntary response that does not indicate sexual arousal.
- When the scrotum is examined, reassure the patient that it is normal to experience a dull ache radiating to the lower abdomen when the testis is squeezed gently. Answer the patient's questions before and after the examination.

During the course of the reproductive system assessment, determine whether the patient knows the importance of, and how to perform, a testicular self-examination. Information that he should know or be taught is presented in Chart 45–1 (Fig. 45–5).

Diagnostic Procedures

Semen Analysis

Semen analysis is a microscopic examination of ejaculated sperm. It reveals information concerning the concentration, density, motility, and morphology of sperm. Normal values of semen analyses are as follows: volume, 2 to 6 ml; sperm count (density), 20 million/ml to 60 million/ml of ejaculate; sperm motility, 60% to 80% active, forward; and sperm morphology, 70% normally shaped.

USES

Semen analysis is done when an infertility problem is suspected. The test is repeated at least once because sperm concentration can vary daily. Semen analysis is also performed 6 weeks after vasectomy to verify that no sperm are present and hence that sterilization was successful.

PROCEDURE

The patient collects the semen specimen after a prescribed period of sexual abstinence of at least 1 full day (36 to 48 hours after ejaculation) and up to

Chart 45–1.

NURSING GUIDE TO PATIENT EDUCATION FOR SELF-MANAGEMENT: TESTICULAR SELF-EXAMINATION (TSE)

Explain the importance of TSE to the patient:

The most common symptom of testicular cancer is a small pea-sized mass on the front or side of the testicle. Testicular cancer is highly curable, particularly when treated early in its development. Because a small mass can be felt on TSE before any other symptoms develop, TSE allows early detection and treatment and increases the chances of cure.

Instruct the patient in the TSE procedure:

Perform TSE once a month after a warm bath or shower, because the heat relaxes the scrotal skin and makes it easier to feel anything unusual.

- Stand naked in front of a mirror. Look for any swelling on the skin of the scrotum.
- Examine each testicle gently with both hands. The index and middle fingers should be placed underneath the testicle while the thumbs are placed on the top. Roll the testicle gently between the thumbs and fingers. One testicle may be larger than the other.
- Find the epididymis (a cordlike structure on the top and back of the testicle that stores and transports the sperm). Do not confuse the epididymis with an abnormal lump.
- Feel for a small lump—about the size of a pea—on the front or the side of the testicle. These lumps are usually painless (see Fig. 45–5).
- Contact the doctor immediately if a lump is found.

Adapted from National Cancer Institute. Testicular self-examination. (National Institutes of Health Publication No. 92-2636.) Washington, DC: U.S. Department of Health and Human Services, Public Health Service, 1992.

a maximum of 5 days. Preferably, a fresh specimen is obtained by masturbation while in the physicians' office. A less satisfactory specimen can be obtained by the patient at home after masturbation or coitus interruptus. If the specimen cannot be collected by either method because of religious reasons, use of a plastic condom is suggested. Ordinary rubber condoms are not acceptable because spermicides (powders and lubricants) are used in their manufacture. The 2- to 6-ml specimen is placed in a clean, wide-mouthed plastic container supplied by the physician. It must be kept at room temperature and delivered to the laboratory within 1 to 2 hours to ensure accurate results. Date and time of ejaculation as well as other identifying information are noted on the container.

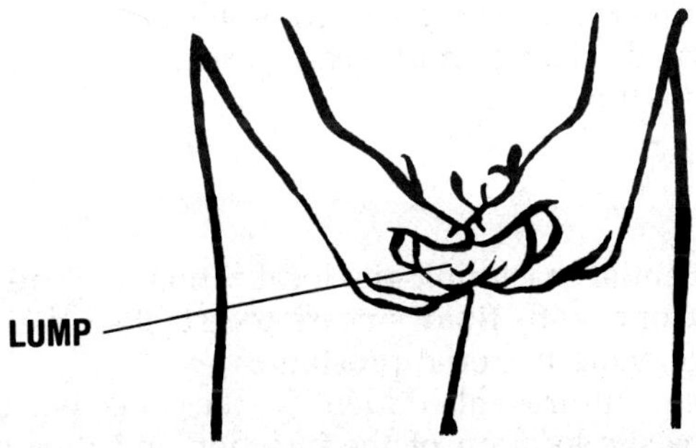

Figure 45–5.

Position of hands for testicular self-examination. (Courtesy of National Cancer Institute. Testicular self-examination. [National Institutes of Health Publication No. 92-2636.] Washington, DC: U.S. Department of Health and Human Services, Public Health Service, January 1992.)

Guidelines for Application of the Nursing Process to the Care of the Patient Having a Semen Analysis

Explain the collection procedure (office or home) in language that is easily understood. Explain the rationale for sexual abstinence for the prescribed period of time before collection of the sperm as well as the importance of strict adherence to the procedure for collecting and transporting the ejaculate if results are to be accurate.

Laboratory Studies (Blood)

Laboratory tests done on blood that are used in the diagnosis of male reproductive disorders include acid phosphatase (including prostatic acid phosphatase [PAP] fraction), alkaline phosphatase (ALP), alpha-fetoprotein (AFP), radioimmunoassay, HCG (beta chain), serum testosterone, serum prolactin, serum FSH, serum LH, prostate-specific antigen (PSA), and glucose tolerance.

ACID PHOSPHATASE

Acid phosphatase is an enzyme whose highest concentration is in the prostate gland. Measures of PAP are used to diagnose prostatic cancer and also to follow the clinical course of the disease. Normal adult values vary with method of analysis used in the laboratory.

Blood acid phosphatase is elevated in patients with prostatic cancer that has spread beyond the prostatic capsule. Acid phosphatase levels may also rise transiently and falsely for 24 to 48 hours after rectal examination with prostatic manipulation and after cystoscopy with prostatic manipulation. Thus, if either of these tests has been done within 2 days before the acid phosphatase test, it is indicated on the laboratory slip.

ALKALINE PHOSPHATASE

ALP is an enzyme present in many tissues, including the liver, bile ducts, and bone. The normal adult value ranges from 20 to 30 U/L (30°C). Blood ALP is elevated in patients with metastatic bone lesions.

ALPHA-FETOPROTEIN (AFP)

AFP is a substance known as a tumor marker because genes in tumor cells regulate its production. The normal AFP value is less than 30 mg/ml. AFP is elevated in patients with testicular tumors and therefore is useful in the diagnosis of testicular cancer and as a check on the effectiveness of treatment. The test is usually done before and after orchiectomy (removal of the testis). Persistent elevated levels of AFP after orchiectomy suggest metastatic spread of the tumor.

HUMAN CHORIONIC GONADOTROPIN

HCG is a tumor marker sometimes found in patients with testicular cancer. If HCG is present, the test is repeated after orchiectomy. Persistent elevation suggests metastatic spread of the tumor.

TESTOSTERONE

Testosterone is the major male hormone secreted by the testes. Abnormal serum levels of testosterone are sometimes present in infertile males. Normal ranges are 3.9 to 7.9 mg/dl in males younger than 60 years and 1.5 to 3.1 mg/dl in males older than 60 years.

SERUM PROLACTIN

Serum prolactin levels are monitored along with serum testosterone levels in impotence. Normal prolactin values are 1 to 20 mg/ml. Serum prolactin levels are usually high when serum testosterone levels are low.

SERUM FOLLICLE-STIMULATING HORMONE

Serum FSH levels are abnormal when impotence is caused by hormonal imbalance. Normal FSH values in males are 10 to 15 mIU/ml.

SERUM LUTEINIZING HORMONE

LH levels are abnormal when impotence is caused by hormonal imbalance. Normal LH values in males are 5 to 20 mIU/ml.

GLUCOSE TOLERANCE TEST

A glucose tolerance test is done to rule out diabetes mellitus as a cause of impotence.

PROSTATE-SPECIFIC ANTIGEN

PSA is an organ-specific marker that is elevated in benign prostatic hypertrophy (BPH) and significantly elevated in cancer of the prostate. It is used as an annual screening test for prostate cancer and to detect residual and recurrent cancer after therapy.

Sequential Bacteriologic Localization Cultures

Sequential bacteriologic localization cultures are done on sequence-segmented voided specimens of urethral discharge, midstream urine, and expressed prostatic fluid.

USES

Sequential bacteriologic localization cultures are done along with fluid smears to establish the diagnosis of acute bacterial prostatitis.

These cultures also identify the infective agent and specific location of the infection and thus guide the choice of antibiotics to treat the specific infection.

The patient must be cooperative and well hydrated and have a full bladder. The procedure for specimen collection must be carefully explained to ensure cooperation and accuracy of test results.

PROCEDURE

The procedure for collecting specimens for sequential bacteriologic localization cultures is as follows:

1. Obtain four wide-mouthed sterile containers in which to collect the specimens.
2. Wearing a glove, thoroughly cleanse the urinary meatus and glans with a disinfectant. (If the patient is not circumcised, first retract the foreskin and leave it retracted until all specimens are collected.)
3. Instruct the patient to void 10 ml of urine into the first sterile container and stop. This is a sample of urethral discharge.
4. Instruct the patient to void up to 200 ml of urine into a clean urinal and stop. This urine is discarded.
5. Instruct the patient to void 10 ml of urine into a second sterile container and stop. This is the midstream specimen.
6. Instruct the patient to bend over, insert a finger into the rectum, and massage the prostate gland. Massage the gland until drops of prostatic fluid appear at the urinary meatus. Collect them in the third sterile container.
7. Instruct the patient to void 10 ml of urine into the fourth sterile container.
8. Label all specimens carefully.

Culture and sensitivity must be performed on these specimens within 1 to 4 hours of collection to ensure accuracy. The diagnosis of bacterial prostatitis can be made when bacterial counts are considerably higher in the prostatic fluid specimen or in the urine voided after prostatic massage than in the first two urine specimens.

A prostatic fluid smear may also be done on the expressed prostatic fluid. A drop of prostatic fluid is placed on a slide and examined for white blood cells. Normal prostatic fluid contains few or no white blood cells (WBCs). Presence of numerous white blood cells indicates inflammation and helps to establish the diagnosis of acute bacterial prostatitis.

Visualization Techniques

Many of the visualization tests used in the diagnosis of disorders of the male reproductive organs are also used in the diagnosis of urinary tract disorders. These include kidney, ureter, and bladder (KUB) x-ray films, intravenous pyelogram (IVP), cystogram, voiding cystourethrogram, and urodynamic studies. Refer to Chapter 25 for a discussion of these tests.

Visualization techniques are also available to study the structure of the vas deferens, ampulla, seminal vesicles, and ejaculatory ducts. A contrast medium is injected into this system to demonstrate obstruction or defects in these structures and to help establish a diagnosis.

Cystourethroscopy

Cystourethroscopy (cystoscopy and panendoscopy) is a direct visualization of the bladder and urethra. The purpose of cystourethroscopy in patients with BPH is to confirm the presence of prostatic enlargement, establish the degree of obstruction of the bladder neck, and determine the presence and degree of bladder trabeculation and cellule or diverticulum formation that may contain stagnant urine (Weinerth, 1991, p 1469). If the patient is relatively asymptomatic, the procedure can be performed in the urologist's office.

Prostatic Ultrasonography

Transrectal ultrasonography provides the best cross-sectional anatomic depiction of the prostate gland available. According to McLennan (1990), this type of urosonography may become the primary method used to evaluate the older patient with known or suspected benign prostatic hypertrophy.

Biopsies

PROSTATIC BIOPSY

There are four common types of prostatic biopsy: (1) transurethral during cystourethroscopy, (2) transperineal using a core needle, (3) transrectal using a core needle, and (4) transrectal fine-needle aspiration biopsy.

TRANSURETHRAL PROSTATIC BIOPSY

During cystourethroscopy, a resectoscope is inserted through the cystoscope and used to secure the specimen, which is then sent for histologic analysis. This type of biopsy is most reliable when tumors are large. It is not well suited to the diagnosis of early prostatic cancer, which tends to arise in the periphery of the prostatic gland.

TRANSPERINEAL PROSTATIC BIOPSY

Transperineal core-needle biopsy of the prostate can be done after cystourethroscopy while the patient is still under spinal or general anesthesia, or it can be done under local anesthesia in an out-patient setting. The perineal skin is prepared and a biopsy needle (Tru-Cut design) is inserted through the perineum into the prostate after the prostatic nodule to undergo biopsy is located rectally by the examining finger (Fig. 45–6). Specimens are obtained, placed in formalin, labeled, and sent to the pathology department for microscopic analysis. The number of specimens obtained by needle biopsy is limited because of the risk of infection and hemorrhage.

TRANSRECTAL PROSTATIC BIOPSY

Transrectal core-needle prostatic biopsy does not require anesthesia. Thus, it may for convenience be

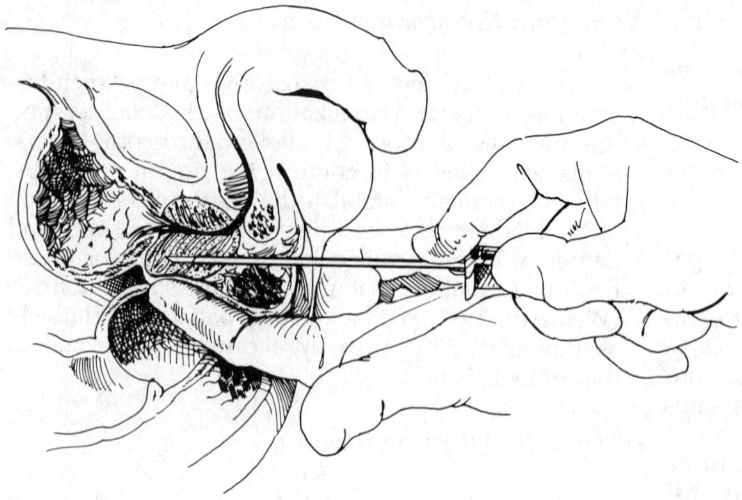

Figure 45–6.

Transperineal approach using core needle. (From Carter HB. Instrumentation and endoscopy. In Walsh PC, Retik AB, Stamey TA, Vaughan ED (eds). Campbell's urology. 6th ed. Philadelphia: WB Saunders, 1992, p 338.)

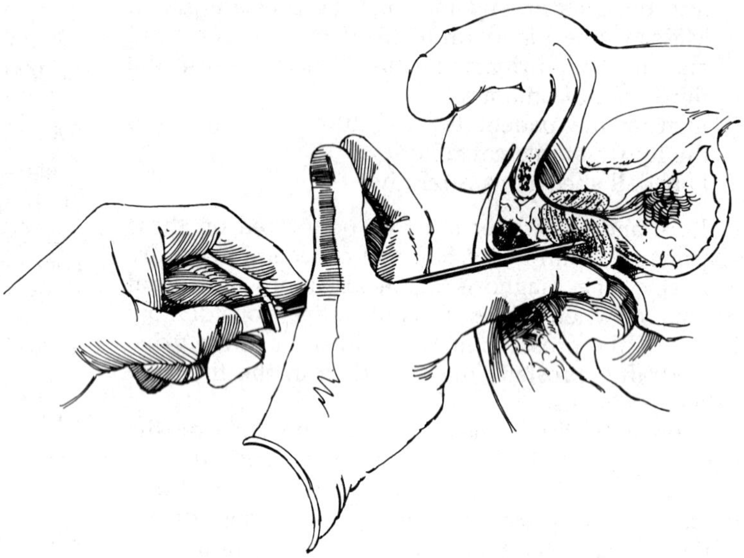

Figure 45–7.

Transrectal approach using core needle. (From Carter HB. Instrumentation and endoscopy. In Walsh PC, Retik AB, Stamey TA, Vaughan ED (eds). Campbell's urology. 6th ed. Philadelphia: WB Saunders, 1992, p 339.)

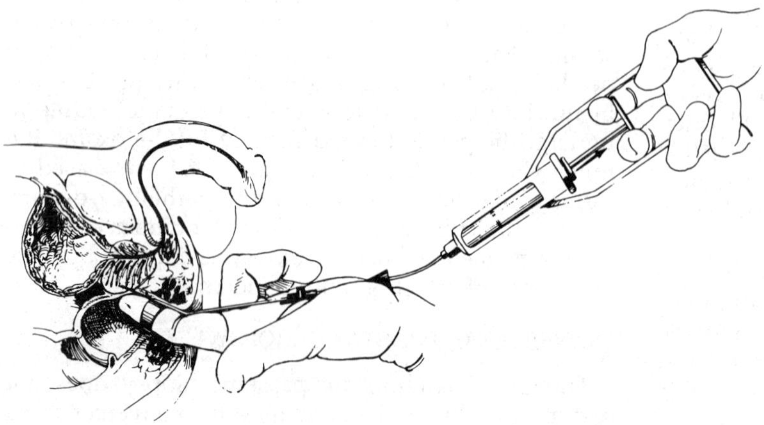

Figure 45–8.

Transrectal fine-needle aspiration biopsy procedure. (From Carter HB. Instrumentation and endoscopy. In Walsh PC, Retik AB, Stamey TA, Vaughan ED (eds). Campbell's urology. 6th ed. Philadelphia: WB Saunders, 1992, p 339.)

done after cystourethroscopy while the patient is still under anesthesia but can also easily be done as an individual procedure. For a transrectal prostatic biopsy using a Tru-Cut design needle, the procedure is as discussed next.

The Tru-Cut design core needle is inserted into the rectum along the ulnar surface of the index finger until the needle tip is up against the prostatic nodule (Fig. 45–7). The obturator is then removed, and the cutting blades are inserted and advanced into the prostate. The outer sheath is advanced over the cutting blades and twisted. The cutting blades are removed, and the jaws are separated to remove the prostatic tissue.

Infection and bleeding from hemorrhoidal vessels are complications of this procedure. To decrease the risk of sepsis, the patient is routinely given a broad-spectrum oral antibiotic, such as fluoroquinolone, before and after the procedure. In addition, a cleansing enema may be ordered before the procedure.

FINE-NEEDLE ASPIRATION PROSTATIC BIOPSY

Fine-needle aspiration biopsy of the prostate is a cytologic technique that is gaining in popularity in the United States. It is done without anesthesia in an outpatient setting, and results can be available within a few hours.

In this procedure, the urologist's index finger is placed in the needle guide, and a finger cot is placed over the finger and needle guide. The finger is then inserted into the rectum until the prostatic nodule is identified. A 22-gauge needle is threaded through the needle guide (Fig. 45–8) and advanced into the prostatic nodule, where suction is applied as the needle is moved back and forth in the nodule. Suction is then released, and the needle containing the prostatic aspirate is removed from the guide. The prostatic aspirate is placed on a slide and smeared before air drying and staining. Complications of this procedure are few: However, false-positive and false-negative results have occasionally been reported.

Application of the Nursing Process to the Care of the Patient Having a Prostatic Biopsy

Assessment

Before prostatic biopsy, assess the patient's knowledge of the genitourinary system, including the location and function of the prostate gland. Be aware that the patient may be reluctant to admit to a lack of knowledge about the prostate gland. Also assess the patient's understanding of the purpose and the procedure of the biopsy and the patient's anxiety level.

Note the presence of coexisting medical problems and their impact on the patient's general health status. Assess the patient's physical condition. Obtain vital signs, and check for alteration in voiding pattern because of an enlarged prostate gland. This provides baseline information against which to assess the patient's condition after the biopsy is performed. After cystourethroscopy and prostatic biopsy, assess the patient's return to physiologic stability as he recovers from anesthesia. Check vital signs, and monitor voiding or urinary output via an indwelling catheter. After any biopsy, observe for bleeding and signs of infection.

Nursing Diagnoses and Planning

Nursing diagnoses and related expected patient outcomes most commonly applicable to patients having a prostatic biopsy include the following:

NDx: Knowledge deficit: location and function of the prostate, purpose and procedure of the biopsy, and biopsy report

Planning: Patient outcomes
1. Patient describes the location and function of the prostate gland.
2. Patient states the purpose of the biopsy.
3. Patient describes in simple terms the biopsy procedure.

NDx: Anxiety related to prostatic biopsy procedure and its outcome

Planning: Patient outcomes
1. Patient discusses concerns and asks questions about the procedure and its outcome.
2. Signs of high anxiety such as inability to focus attention and tachycardia are absent.

NDx: High risk for infection related to transurethral, transrectal, or transperineal prostatic biopsy procedure

Planning: Patient outcomes
1. Patient is free of chills, fever, urinary obstruction, hematuria, and excessive pain after biopsy.
2. Patient's perineal area is free of redness, hematoma, pain, and induration after transperineal core-needle biopsy.

NDx: High risk for urinary retention related to prostatic enlargement and urethral instrumentation

Planning: Patient outcomes
1. Patient voids spontaneously in sufficient quantity (more than 90 ml per voiding) within 8 to 10 hours after cystourethroscopy and prostatic biopsy.

NDx: Pain: mild to moderate, related to tissue trauma during prostate biopsy

Planning: Patient outcomes

1. Patient states he is reasonably free of pain.
2. Behavioral signs of pain such as reluctance to move and grimacing are absent.
3. Patient's blood pressure, pulse, and respiration are near baseline values.

Nursing Interventions

NDx: Knowledge deficit: location and function of the prostate, purpose and procedure of the biopsy, and biopsy report
Because the patient may be somewhat reluctant to admit to a knowledge deficit, use a caring and sensitive manner in interactions with him.

Explain simply how the cystourethroscopy and prostatic biopsy are performed via the urethra if this is the biopsy procedure to be done. Use simple drawings that show the location of the urethra and prostate gland to help the patient visualize how the procedure will be performed. Tell the patient that he will not have a visible external incision after the prostate undergoes biopsy in this manner. If the biopsy is to be done transperineally or rectally, review and reinforce the information related to the procedure. Inform the patient when and from whom he will receive the biopsy results.

Teach the patient with a prostatic biopsy negative for cancer that followup visits to the physician are imperative. Explain that the physician will check the prostate gland for continued enlargement and may wish to repeat a biopsy in 6 months.

NDx: Anxiety
Establish a trusting relationship with the patient. Provide for privacy and a quiet environment so that the patient can express himself comfortably. Use techniques of therapeutic communication to ensure that the patient's questions and concerns are addressed. Encourage questions. Deliver information in a calm and knowledgeable manner. Observe the patient for increased signs of anxiety and lack of understanding of information as it is presented. Repeat information and answer questions as they arise. Place your hand on the patient's shoulder as a gesture of reassurance and emotional support as appropriate. Remember that the patient's anxiety will continue and in fact may increase while he is awaiting the biopsy report, so continued emotional support is needed.

NDx: High risk for infection
Administer antibiotics as ordered, or instruct the patient in self-administration.

After cystourethroscopy and transurethral prostatic biopsy, monitor the patient for signs of infection. Promptly report to the physician a temperature of 38.3°C (101°F) or higher, chills, or excessive pain, so that the patient can be evaluated for sepsis. Obtain blood and urine cultures, if ordered, to identify the infecting organism. Encourage fluids if there are no medical contraindications.

After a transperineal core-needle prostatic biopsy, teach the patient how to avoid contaminating the biopsy site. Instruct him to cleanse the perianal area from front to back and to pour warm water from front to back over the perineum after bowel elimination. Stress the importance of keeping the area dry and avoiding all unnecessary touching of it.

NDx: High risk for urinary retention
Monitor urine volume for the first 24 hours. If the patient does not have an indwelling catheter, record the time and amount of each voiding for 24 hours.

NDx: Pain
Administer analgesics as prescribed. Encourage relaxation, and instruct in techniques to reduce skeletal muscle tension. After transperineal biopsy, encourage side-lying positions for comfort, and protect the site from irritation.

Additional Interventions
Monitor hospitalized patients for excessive bleeding after the biopsy. Slight hematuria (pink-tinged urine) and some dysuria are normal, but report frank bleeding or clotting to the physician. Instruct outpatients to report promptly bleeding, chills, fever higher than 38.3°C (101°F), or excessive pain to the physician.

Evaluation

Evaluate the effectiveness of nursing care for a patient having a prostatic biopsy by comparing the patient's status with the expected patient outcomes. Examples of specific outcomes for patients having a prostatic biopsy have been provided in the Planning section.

PENILE BIOPSY

Penile biopsy is performed to confirm a suspected diagnosis of carcinoma of the penis. The biopsy can be obtained by either percutaneous needle aspiration or tissue excision.

Guidelines for Application of the Nursing Process to the Care of the Patient Having a Penile Biopsy

As with any biopsy, make certain that the patient understands the reason for the biopsy and knows what to expect regarding the procedure and its aftercare. Allay anxiety, and support the patient's ability to cope. The latter is particularly important for the patient having a penile biopsy because many males have advanced disease by the time they first seek medical attention. It is estimated that 15% to 50% of males delay seeking medical care for more than 1 year after the appearance of signs and symptoms because of personal neglect, embarrassment, guilt, or ignorance.

TESTICULAR BIOPSY FOR INFERTILITY

Testicular biopsy is performed on patients with aspermia.

USE

A testicular biopsy determines whether any sperm are being produced or if the problem is in the sperm-transport mechanism.

PROCEDURE

The scrotum is shaved and prepared with an appropriate antiseptic. Under general, local, or regional anesthesia, bilateral scrotal incisions are made, and the biopsy specimen is excised. The scrotal skin is sutured, small dressings are placed over the bilateral incisions, and a scrotal support is applied to keep the scrotal dressings in place.

Guidelines for Application of the Nursing Process to the Care of the Patient Having a Testicular Biopsy

Instruct the patient to adjust the scrotal support so that the scrotum is elevated to encourage drainage and reduce pain resulting from edema. Tell him to report promptly any severe scrotal pain, edema, temperature elevation, or chills. In addition, be certain he understands that the biopsy report and further treatment plans will be discussed at the follow-up visit when the scrotal incisions are checked.

Medical Management

Surgical Management

Surgery for the patient with dysfunction of the male reproductive system is performed to restore normal anatomy, repair structural abnormalities, remove obstruction or abnormal tissue, and, in some cases, restore normal sexual functioning.

Table 45–3. SURGICAL PROCEDURES USED TO TREAT SPECIFIC DISORDERS OF THE MALE REPRODUCTIVE ORGANS

SURGICAL PROCEDURE	DESCRIPTION
Circumcision	Removal of the prepuce from the penis
Vasectomy	Transection of a portion of each vas deferens
Orchiopexy	Surgical placement of an undescended testicle into scrotal sac
Orchiectomy	Excision of one or both testicles
Hydrocelectomy	Excision of a hydrocele (cystic mass filled with clear fluid that forms around a testicle)
Spermatocelectomy	Removal of a spermatocele (cystic mass filled with milky fluid that forms at the upper pole of the testicle)
Varicocelectomy	Excision of varicocele (cluster of dilated veins posterior to and above the testicle)
Prostatectomy	Removal of part or all of the prostate
Penectomy	Removal of part or all of the penis
Retroperitoneal lymphadenectomy	Removal of iliac and lumbar lymph nodes in testicular carcinoma (teratocarcinoma, embryonal carcinoma, teratoma)
Iliac lymphadenectomy	Excision of iliac lymph nodes in radical retropubic prostatectomy

Surgery is used for the diagnosis and treatment of prostatic abnormalities, congenital defects affecting fertility, chronic prostatitis, malignant diseases of the male reproductive organs, and traumatic injuries to the male reproductive organs and for permanent contraception (sterilization). Surgical procedures used in the treatment of male reproductive disorders are summarized in Table 45–3.

Preoperative Preparation. The physician begins the preoperative preparation by considering the patient's age, general health status, and the presence of coexisting medical problems in view of the proposed surgery. The physician assesses the overall status of the patient, with particular attention to cardiopulmonary, hepatic, and renal/urologic function. In young patients with dysfunction of the reproductive system, endocrine function may also be studied. In older patients having prostatic surgery, hematologic function is evaluated carefully to check for clotting defects that must be corrected before surgery. Medical clearance before surgery is essential in elderly patients with significant heart disease, hypertension, anemia, renal disease, or diabetes mellitus.

Fluid, electrolyte, and acid-base balance are assessed preoperatively to provide a baseline for postoperative comparison. In the elderly hypertensive patient with significant long-standing prostatic obstruction with urinary retention, the bladder is decompressed gradually preoperatively. Even with gradual bladder decompression, some decrease in renal function and change in blood pressure may occur. If dehydration is present, the patient must be hydrated carefully with appropriate electrolyte replacements.

Any infection in the patient's genitourinary system must be identified and treated with antibiotic therapy before surgery.

Additional antibiotics may be given intramuscularly or intravenously a few hours before surgery to ensure effective blood levels during urethral catheterization or surgical manipulation, because it is not uncommon for urinary tract infection to recur after surgery.

Mechanical bowel preparation in the form of preoperative enemas may be ordered to prevent postoperative straining, which can induce postoperative bleeding, especially after prostatic surgery.

Skin preparation includes mechanical cleansing of the skin preoperatively and shaving the skin area from the nipples to mid-thigh depending on the extent of the procedure. In many cases, both of these procedures are done in the operating room just before the operative procedure.

Complications. There are many potential postoperative complications of surgery on the male reproductive system. These are summarized in Table 45–4.

The risk of complications is particularly high in the confused elderly, who may inadvertently remove drainage tubes and in the process traumatize the surgical site, induce bleeding, and contaminate the wound. The risk is intensified because the tubes usually have to be replaced, which requires further manipulation of the area.

VASECTOMY

Vasectomy is the transection of a portion of each vas deferens.

USES

Vasectomy is primarily used as a method of sterilization to control male fertility. It is also done to prevent epididymitis in the older patient who is undergoing a prostatectomy.

PATIENT PREPARATION

Before a decision is made to perform the surgery, at least one interview is conducted between the surgeon and the patient, preferably accompanied by the spouse or partner. At this time, the patient's motivation for the surgery is explored. The procedure is explained, risks are identified, and the availability of alternative contraceptive methods and the potential for reversing the vasectomy with current rates of success are discussed. Written consent is obtained.

Vasectomy is a minor surgical procedure and is usually peformed in an ambulatory care setting or in the physician's office. A semen analysis may be done preoperatively to provide a baseline against which to judge the disappearance of sperm after vasectomy. Because vasectomy is done under local anesthesia, food and fluids are not usually withheld. The patient is usually instructed to take a shower, and may be asked to shave his scrotum, before the surgery.

PROCEDURE

Vasectomy may be done in a variety of ways. One common procedure involves cutting, ligating, and cauterizing the vas deferens on both sides. After

Table 45–4. COMPLICATIONS OF SURGERY ON THE MALE REPRODUCTIVE SYSTEM

COMPLICATIONS	RISK FACTORS
Hemorrhagic shock	Prostate surgery because the gland is highly vascular
Urinary tract infection	Instrumentation of the urinary system; use of catheters, collection bags, bladder irrigations
Wound infection	Perineal prostatectomy because of the proximity of the incision to the rectum
Respiratory problems	Old age, smoking, presence of other respiratory disease
Deep thrombophlebitis	Use of lithotomy position, which increases pressure on the popliteal veins during surgery; handling of major vessels and resultant inflammation as in prostatic surgery and pelvic and retroperitoneal lymphadenectomy; old age, with its predisposition to venous stasis, immobility, and slower postoperative recovery
Fluid and electrolyte imbalance	Transurethral prostatectomy, because the use of hypotonic solution during the procedure predisposes to hyponatremia
Bladder distention, which can lead to damage to the suture line	Obstruction of urinary drainage tubes by clots, mucus, tissue particles
Altered voiding: retention or incontinence	Urethral trauma
Altered sexual function	Surgical trauma varies from minor, such as temporary retrograde ejaculation, to impotence and infertility, as in radical resective procedures

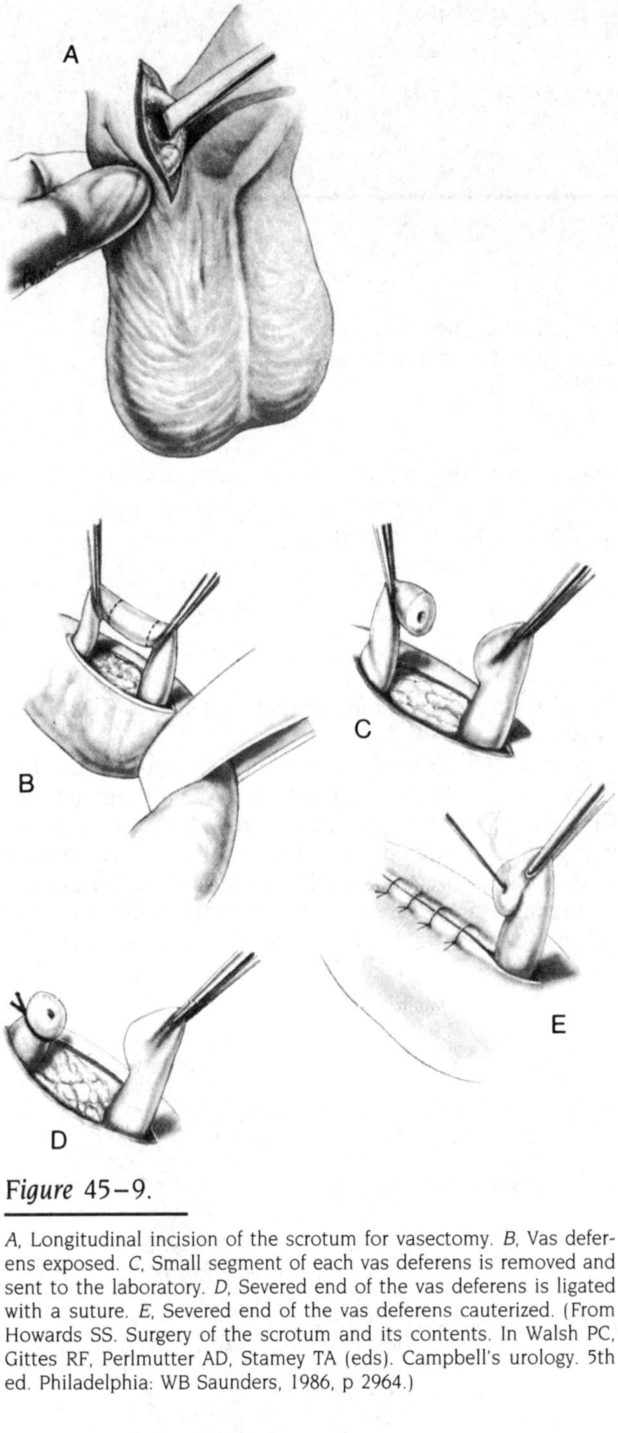

Figure 45–9.

A, Longitudinal incision of the scrotum for vasectomy. *B*, Vas deferens exposed. *C*, Small segment of each vas deferens is removed and sent to the laboratory. *D*, Severed end of the vas deferens is ligated with a suture. *E*, Severed end of the vas deferens cauterized. (From Howards SS. Surgery of the scrotum and its contents. In Walsh PC, Gittes RF, Perlmutter AD, Stamey TA (eds). Campbell's urology. 5th ed. Philadelphia: WB Saunders, 1986, p 2964.)

local anesthesia is achieved, 1- to 2-cm bilateral, longitudinal incisions are made in the scrotum about 2 cm below the base of the penis (Fig. 45–9*A*). The vas deferens are exposed and transected, and a small segment of each vas is removed and sent for pathologic examination (Fig. 45–9*B*,*C*). Each severed end of the vas is then either ligated with a suture or cauterized (Fig. 45–9*D*,*E*). The scrotal incisions are usually closed with chromic sutures, which dissolve and therefore do not need to be removed.

POSTOPERATIVE COURSE

Vasectomy does not result in immediate infertility because viable sperm are found in the ampulla of the vas postoperatively. Approximately 24 to 36 ejaculations after vasectomy are required to clear the sperm from the ductal system, and the patient usually becomes aspermatic within 2 to 3 months. This is confirmed by semen analysis.

CONTRAINDICATIONS

Vasectomy is contraindicated for males who are evaluated as being psychologically unstable or mentally incompetent, for anyone who is anxious about the procedure because of religious convictions, and for couples who disagree about having the procedure performed.

COMPLICATIONS

Complications are infrequent and, when they occur, are generally minor in nature. They include wound infection, scrotal hematoma, scrotal abscess, epididymitis, sperm granuloma, and spontaneous reanastomosis of the vas.

REVERSAL OF VASECTOMY

The surgical procedure to restore fertility in the male is called a vasovasostomy. This is a microsurgical procedure in which the two ends of each vas deferens are anastomosed with either sutures or a stent. Like the vasectomy, the procedure is usually performed on an ambulatory basis, and the postoperative discomfort is mild. The patient's sperm count is monitored closely after this procedure and, after 6 months, is usually stable with significantly improved motility. Although reversal of the vasectomy is possible, reports of accompanying fertility rate vary from 18% to 60%. It appears that the pregnancy rate after a vasovasostomy decreases as the interval between the vasectomy and the reanastomosis increases (Goldstein, 1992).

The most frequent reasons for seeking a reversal of the vasectomy include remarriage, change of attitudes toward family size, and the death of existing children.

Guidelines for Application of the Nursing Process to the Care of the Patient Having a Vasectomy

Assess the patient's understanding of the extent of the procedure and the facts on reversibility. Also assess his perception of its effect on masculinity and sexual performance. Provide additional information, and clarify misconceptions as needed. After the pro-

Chart 45–2.

NURSING GUIDE TO PATIENT EDUCATION FOR SELF-MANAGEMENT: DISCHARGE INSTRUCTIONS AFTER VASECTOMY

Instruct the patient to do the following:

Apply an ice pack to the scrotum for 24 hours for swelling, alternating 30 minutes on and 1 hour off.
Take sitz baths and acetaminophen, unless contraindicated (per directions on label), for discomfort.
Rest for 2 days, and avoid strenuous activity and heavy lifting for 1 week.
Wear a scrotal support for 2 days.
Abstain from sexual intercourse for 3 days.
Use an alternative method of contraception until physician reports that sperm are no longer found in the semen.
Report the occurrence of bleeding or drainage, fever, and persistent scrotal pain.
Return for checkup on *(specify date and time).*

cedure, instruct the patient in self-care, as specified in Chart 45–2.

PROSTATECTOMY

Prostatectomy refers to removal of the prostate gland. In a simple prostatectomy, only the enlarged portion of the gland is removed, whereas in a total prostatectomy, the entire gland and its capsule are excised. A more extensive procedure is a radical prostatectomy, which involves the removal of the entire prostate, its capsule, the seminal vesicles, a cuff of the bladder neck, and sometimes pelvic lymph nodes.

SURGICAL APPROACHES TO PROSTATECTOMY

There are four standard approaches to prostatectomy: transurethral resection of the prostate (TURP), suprapubic or transvesical prostatectomy, retropubic prostatectomy, and perineal prostatectomy (Fig. 45–10).

Transurethral Prostatectomy. TURP is the most commonly performed simple prostatectomy procedure. It is used to treat symptomatic benign prostatic hypertrophy when the prostrate is only moderately enlarged and occasionally is used for patients with a malignancy who are poor surgical risks. It is preferably done under local anesthesia and uses a cystoscope and a resectoscope inserted into the urethra to scrape out the enlarged portion of the gland. To keep the operative area clear, an irrigating solution is continuously run into the bladder to flush away removed tissue; on completion of the procedure, a three-way Foley catheter is inserted for urinary drainage.

The major advantage of this procedure is that there is no external incision. The disadvantages are that the prostate tissue can regrow because it is not completely removed, and there is the risk of postoperative bladder neck scarring and urethral stricture.

Suprapubic (Transvesical) Prostatectomy. In a suprapubic prostatectomy, an incision is made into the lower abdomen and the bladder is opened. The

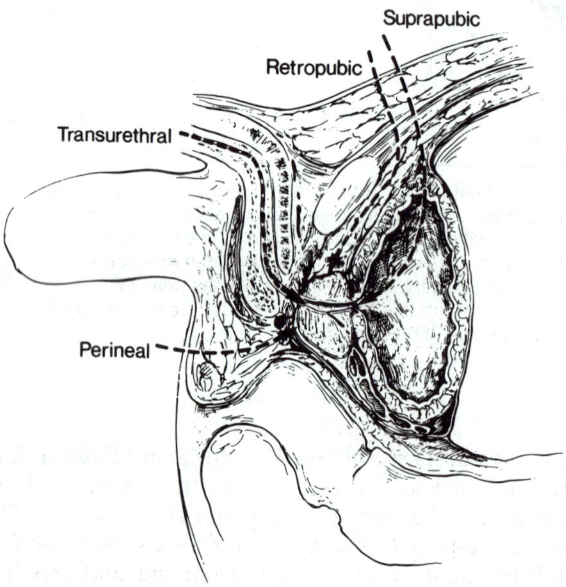

Figure 45–10.

Prostate gland: Four surgical approaches to prostatectomy. (From Weinerth JL. The male genital system. In Sabiston DC (ed). Textbook of surgery. 14th ed. Philadelphia: WB Saunders, 1991, p 1469.)

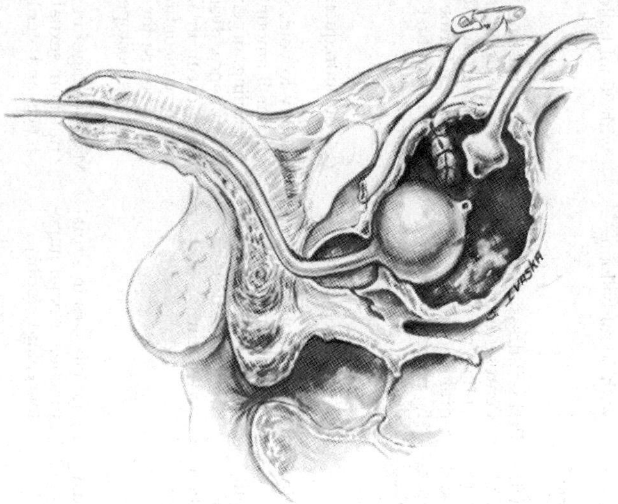

Figure 45–11.

Suprapubic prostatectomy: Foley catheter snug against bladder neck, prevesical drain, and Pezzar suprapubic catheter. (From Nanninga J, O'Connor V. Suprapubic and retropubic prostatectomy. In Walsh PC, Gittes RF, Perlmutter AD, Stamey TA (eds). Campbell's urology. 5th ed. Philadelphia: WB Saunders, 1986, p 2746.)

prostate is then removed, working from inside the bladder. A urethral catheter and a suprapubic catheter are both inserted for urinary drainage, and a surgical drain is placed in the abdominal wound (Fig. 45–11). This approach is used when the prostate is too large for a TURP and in cases in which coexisting bladder problems such as calculi need to be treated.

Retropubic Prostatectomy. In a simple retropubic prostatectomy, a low abdominal incision is made, the bladder retracted, and an incision made into the anterior prostatic capsule through which the gland is removed. A urethral catheter is inserted for urinary drainage, and drains are placed in the abdominal wound. This procedure is done when the prostate is too large for a TURP, when cancerous tissue is to be removed, and when lithotomy position is contraindicated for the patient.

A major advantage of a retropubic prostatectomy is that bleeding is easily controlled because of direct access to the surgical site.

Perineal Prostatectomy. In a perineal prostatectomy, the prostate is removed through an incision made in the perineum between the scrotum and the rectum. It is done under spinal or general anesthesia, with the patient in an exaggerated lithotomy position (i.e., with the thighs flexed back almost against the trunk). A urethral catheter is inserted to empty the bladder, and a drain is placed in the perineal wound.

A perineal prostatectomy is done when the prostate is too large for a TURP and in situations in which abdominal surgery is contraindicated. The procedure is short, but it has the disadvantages of potential rectal injury, increased risk of thrombophlebitis because of the position of the patient, and the inability to reach pelvic lymph nodes for a staging lymphadenectomy if a malignancy is found at surgery.

Radical prostatectomy is used as a curative procedure for prostatic cancer. It may be done by either a retropubic or a perineal approach, although the former is often preferred because of the accessibility of the pelvic lymph nodes.

CONTRAINDICATIONS

Prostatectomy is contraindicated in the presence of significant sepsis or bladder infection and in patients with an unstabilized medical problem such as heart disease, marked pulmonary disease, and diabetes mellitus. It is also contraindicated immediately after relief of severe urinary retention because the expected diuresis can result in hyponatremia, which needs to be corrected before surgery.

PREOPERATIVE PREPARATION

Basic preoperative preparation for prostatectomy is similar to that for any major surgery. The patient is maintained on a nothing by mouth (NPO) order from midnight before surgery. A Fleet or soapsuds enema is given before a transurethral resection and suprapubic or retropubic prostatectomy. To decrease the risk of infection, enemas are given before a perineal prostatectomy until they are clear. The area from the umbilicus to mid-thigh is shaved and prepared before suprapubic and retropubic prostatectomy and, along with the scrotal, perineal, and perianal areas, before perineal prostatectomy. There may or may not be a skin preparation for a TURP depending on the surgeon's preference.

POSTOPERATIVE COURSE

The postoperative course varies with the type of prostatectomy performed. After a TURP, intravenous fluids are given for 24 hours and then discontinued if clear fluids are taken and tolerated well. The patient is rapidly progressed to a regular diet. A three-way Foley urethral catheter is in place for 3 to 5 days and initially may be attached to a continuous bladder-irrigation system. Such a system allows a constant flow of sterile solution, usually normal saline, into the bladder to prevent blockage of the catheter with clots or pieces of tissue debris. Continuous bladder irrigations are usually stopped when bladder drainage has been pink tinged and clot free for 24 hours. After a suprapubic prostatectomy, the patient is maintained on NPO status and on intravenous fluids until peristalsis returns, which is usually in 3 or 4 days. The patient may also have a nasogastric tube attached to low suction in place during this time.

Time and sequence of removal of the urethral

Table 45–5. COMPARISON OF DIFFERENT TYPES OF PROSTATIC SURGERY

VARIABLE	SIMPLE TRANSURETHRAL RESECTION	SIMPLE TRANSVESICAL (SUPRAPUBIC) RESECTION	SIMPLE RETROPUBIC RESECTION	RADICAL RETROPUBIC RESECTION	SIMPLE PERINEAL RESECTION	RADICAL PERINEAL RESECTION
Indication for surgery	Moderate enlargement of the prostate	Large obstructing prostate and coexisting bladder problems (stones, diverticula) that are surgically treatable	Large obstructing prostate high in pelvic cavity, no coexisting bladder disease	Large early-stage prostatic cancer	Large obstructing prostate low in pelvic cavity	Large early-stage prostatic cancer
Presence and location of incision	None; prostate removed via urethra	Low horizontal abdominal incision (above symphysis pubis), then through bladder wall to prostate	Horizontal incision above symphysis pubis (bladder not entered)	Vertical midline incision from umbilicus to pubis	An inverted U-shaped incision between scrotum and rectum	A larger inverted U-shaped incision between scrotum and rectum
Tissue removed	Enlarged prostatic chips via resectoscope	Enlarged portion of the prostate gland is enucleated; prostatic capsule remains in place	Enlarged portion of prostate gland is enucleated; prostatic capsule remains in place	Entire prostate gland, including prostatic capsule, prostatic urethra and seminal vesicles, are removed; if frozen section of lymph nodes is positive, iliac lymphadenectomy is performed	Enlarged prostate gland	Entire prostate gland, including prostatic capsule, prostatic urethra, and seminal vesicles, are removed
Type of urinary drainage	Three-way urethral Foley catheter with 30-ml balloon, constant bladder irrigation	1. Three-way urethral Foley catheter with 30-ml balloon, constant bladder irrigation 2. Suprapubic cystotomy tube	Three-way urethral Foley catheter with 30-ml balloon, constant bladder irrigation	Three-way urethral Foley catheter with 30-ml balloon, constant bladder irrigation, occasionally a suprapubic tube	Two- or three-way urethral Foley catheter with 30-ml balloon	Two- or three-way urethral Foley catheter with 30-ml balloon
Dressings and drains, expected wound drainage	None	Abdominal dressing including Penrose drain outside bladder to drain accumulated urine and blood; suprapubic cystotomy tube, if used, may drain bloody urine	Abdominal dressing including Penrose drains in retropubic space to drain accumulated urine and blood	Abdominal dressing with Penrose or Hemovac/Jackson-Pratt to drain accumulated urine and blood; if used, a suprapubic cystotomy tube may drain blood-tinged urine	Perineal dressing with Penrose drain may drain serosanguineous drainage (urine may be present first few days)	Perineal dressing with Penrose drain may drain serosanguineous drainage (urine may be present first few days)
Presence and frequency of bladder spasms	Yes, frequently	Yes, frequently	Yes, but infrequently	Yes, but infrequently	Yes, but infrequently	Yes, but infrequently
Type of voiding complications after removal of urethral catheter	Inability to void, voiding in small amounts, dribbling, urgency, incontinence, dysuria may occur	Inability to void, voiding in small amounts, dribbling, urgency, incontinence, dysuria may occur	Inability to void, voiding in small amounts, dribbling, urgency, incontinence, dysuria may occur	Inability to void, voiding in small amounts, dribbling, urgency, incontinence, dysuria may occur; in addition, urinary incontinence may persist for 6 months postoperatively	Inability to void, voiding in small amounts, dribbling, urgency, incontinence, dysuria may occur	Inability to void, voiding in small amounts, dribbling, urgency, incontinence, dysuria may occur; in addition, urinary incontinence may persist for 6 months postoperatively
Presence of sexual dysfunction	Minor changes in sexual function, temporary retrograde ejaculation possible	Minor changes in sexual function, temporary retrograde ejaculation possible	Minor changes in sexual function, temporary retrograde ejaculation possible	Major changes in sexual function, sexual impotence, and sterility	Major changes in sexual function, sexual impotence, and sterility	Major changes in sexual function, sexual impotence, and sterility

catheter and the cystostomy tube are highly variable from surgeon to surgeon. One approach is to remove the urethral catheter in 24 to 48 hours, leave the suprapubic catheter in place for another 3 or 4 days, and then clamp it to determine whether the patient can void and, if so, remove it.

The patient who has had a simple retropubic prostatectomy will also be on NPO status and receiving intravenous fluids and may have a nasogastric tube attached to low suction in place until peristalsis returns. The urethral catheter is removed about the fifth day, and the wound drain is advanced and then withdrawn if there is no leakage of urine.

The course after perineal prostatectomy is similar to that after a TURP, except that the urethral catheter remains in place until the urine is clear, which is an average of 12 days.

With all types of prostatectomy, ambulation is begun early. Long periods of sitting are discouraged because the increased intraabdominal pressure caused by the position can precipitate bleeding.

Bladder spasms are normal after any prostatectomy. They occur most frequently after transurethral and suprapubic procedures and are treated with belladonna and opium (B&O) rectal suppositories or other analgesics or antispasmodics.

Temporary voiding problems are common after all types of simple prostatectomy because of the removal of part of the bladder neck and prostatic urethra. These include an inability to void, voiding in small amounts, dribbling, urgency, dysuria, and incontinence. Return to normal continence is gradual, with partial control regained in days or weeks and full control sometimes taking months.

After TURP and suprapubic and retropubic procedures, sexual dysfunction in the form of temporary retrograde ejaculation is also common. Retrograde ejaculation (flow of semen back into the bladder rather than out through the urethra) occurs because the bladder neck has been opened, and the sperm takes the path of least resistance. After perineal prostatectomy, impotency can occur as a result of injury to the pelvic nerve plexus, which provides autonomic innervation to the corpora cavernosa.

Refer to Table 45–5 for a summary of the different types of prostatectomy and their similarities and differences.

COMPLICATIONS

Complications of prostatectomy include bleeding, urinary tract infection, transurethral resection (TUR) syndrome (dilutional hyponatremia), and thrombophlebitis as well as bowel and respiratory problems. These occur most often in older, debilitated patients with other medical problems.

Bleeding is a particular risk after TURP because the prostate gland is very vascular and the pressure of the irrigating solution used during the procedure can temporarily prevent venous bleeding and obscure the need for hemostasis. To treat postoperative venous bleeding, some surgeons increase pressure in the balloon of the Foley catheter and put traction on the catheter to increase pressure in the prostatic fossa. The catheter is taped to the patient's thigh in the position of traction and released within 6 hours to prevent tissue ischemia and necrosis.

Bleeding is a rare complication of perineal prostatectomy.

Cystitis, often combined with urethritis and pyelonephritis and caused by a gram-negative organism, can result in dysuria and pyuria. The catheter, which predisposes to infection, is removed as soon as possible, and if there is a large amount of pus in the urine, the bladder may be irrigated with a 2% neomycin sulfate solution before its removal.

As the name suggests, TUR syndrome (dilutional hyponatremia) occurs after transurethral resection of the prostate. It is a dilutional hyponatremia caused by the irrigating fluid used during surgery entering the vascular compartment through open venous sinuses or perforations in the prostatic capsule. With the decrease in sodium and ensuing fluid and electrolyte imbalance, the patient may become restless, disoriented, and nauseated. Elevation of systolic and diastolic blood pressures and bradycardia can occur, followed by eventual hypotension and cardiovascular collapse. Management involves monitoring levels of serum sodium and potassium as well as serum osmolarity, intravenous administration of furosemide, and the administration of 200 ml of 3% saline (average) slowly in divided doses to produce a net loss of body water (Mebust, 1992, p 2912).

Application of the Nursing Process to the Care of the Patient Having a Simple Prostatectomy

PREOPERATIVE NURSING CARE

Nursing care for the patient scheduled for a simple prostatectomy is similar to that for any preoperative patient (see Chapter 4). In addition, the preoperative care outlined in Nursing Care Guide 46–1 is applicable.

POSTOPERATIVE NURSING CARE

Assessment

Assess the patient's physiologic stabilization. Monitor vital signs, central venous pressure (CVP) if applicable, laboratory data, and true urine output (total output for a given period of time minus the amount of normal saline irrigant instilled continuously via a three-way indwelling urinary catheter).

Assess the patency of the urethral catheter frequently, checking for the following signs of obstruction: increase in bladder spasms or pain, absence of urine and normal saline irrigant outflow from the indwelling urinary catheter, and distention of the lower abdomen on palpation. Observe the color of urinary output from the urethral and/or suprapubic catheters.

Assess postoperative hematocrit, hemoglobin, and serum electrolytes, and report changes promptly. Check the abdominal or perineal dressings for bleeding every 15 minutes for 2 hours, then every hour for 8 hours, or more frequently as indicated. Observe the wound (present after all prostatectomies other than TURP) for color and amount of drainage. Also observe for bloody drainage at the penile meatus at the junction of the catheter and penis. This can be due to an obstruction of the catheter, causing bloody urine to be expelled around it. If the catheter is patent and this bloody drainage occurs in small to moderate amounts, it is of no concern. If it increases significantly, report it to the physician.

Observe all patients but especially the elderly patient with coexisting medical problems for signs of hemorrhagic shock and gram-negative sepsis. As the postoperative period progresses, observe the patient for development of complications previously described.

Nursing Diagnoses and Planning

Nursing diagnoses and related expected patient outcomes most commonly applicable to patients who have had a simple prostatectomy include the following:

NDx: High risk for urinary retention related to obstruction of urinary drainage tubes and/or removal of part of the bladder neck and prostatic urethra

Planning: Patient outcomes
1. Urinary drainage tubes are patent and draining.
2. Bladder distention is absent.
3. After catheter removal and depending on the type and extent of prostatectomy, patient voids continently in amounts more than 90 ml per voiding or has a postvoiding residual urine volume of less than 75 ml.

NDx: High risk for fluid volume excess related to dilutional hyponatremia secondary to absorption of irrigating fluid during TURP

Planning: Patient outcomes
1. Patient is free of agitation or confusion.
2. Blood pressure and pulse are stable within patient's normal range.
3. Serum sodium and potassium levels and serum osmolarity are within normal limits.

NDx: Pain related to surgical tissue trauma and bladder spasms

Planning: Patient outcomes
1. Patient states that discomfort is lessened or relieved.
2. Patient moves more freely in bed and ambulates more easily when out of bed.
3. Patient defecates and, after the indwelling urinary catheter is removed, voids without signs of undue discomfort.

NDx: High risk for infection related to instrumentation of the bladder or presence of an incision and presence of urinary drainage apparatus

Planning: Patient outcomes
1. Wounds, if present, are free of erythema, drainage, and induration.
2. Urine is clear.
3. Pyuria is absent.
4. Urine cultures are negative.

NDx: High risk for injury related to accidents secondary to impairments and/or related to inadvertent removal of urinary drainage tubes or dressings

Planning: Patient outcomes
1. Patient avoids falls or other accidents.
2. Patient's urinary drainage tubes and dressings remain intact and in place.

NDx: High risk for impaired tissue integrity related to irritation of abdominal or perineal skin by drainage from a suprapubic, retropubic, or perineal incision

Planning: Patient outcomes
1. Skin and suture line are intact.
2. Skin surrounding suture line is free of erythema.

NDx: High risk for constipation related to change in oral intake, immobility, and fear of pain or disruption of the suture line

Planning: Patient outcomes
1. Patient ingests 1.5 to 2 L of fluid per day.
2. Patient eats foods allowed that promote regular bowel function.
3. Patient ambulates progressively while hospitalized.
4. Patient's first bowel movement after surgery occurs without straining.

NDx: High risk for sexual dysfunction related to prostatectomy

Planning: Patient outcomes
1. Patient describes the degree of sexual dysfunction he expects with the specific type of prostatectomy to be performed.

2. Patient verbalizes belief that in time satisfying sexual relationships can be resumed.

NDx: High risk for altered health maintenance related to insufficient knowledge of postprostatectomy self-care

Planning: Patient outcomes
1. Patient lists signs and symptoms to be reported.
2. Patient describes limitations on activity and sexual intercourse and states date of return to work.
3. Patient describes measures to prevent constipation and straining during hard movements.
4. Patient states reason for use and directions for each discharge medication.
5. Patient states the date of his follow-up visit.

Nursing Interventions

NDx: High risk for urinary retention

To keep urinary drainage catheters patent and free of obstruction, maintain the flow of the normal saline irrigant at the prescribed rate or the rate needed to keep the urine pink tinged. Empty the urinary drainage bags frequently, especially if the irrigant is running at a rapid rate. Remind the patient about the urinary drainage tube, and instruct him not to lie on it. Check the position of the catheter and drainage tube frequently for kinking. Keep the tubing in a straight line from the bed down to the collection bag to ensure proper drainage. Clip or pin the tube to the bed sheet to prevent looping or coiling below the bed and undue tension on the catheter. Position drainage bag on the same side to which the patient is turned while in bed to ensure proper gravity drainage.

If the patient has significant bladder spasms and there is no urinary/irrigant outflow to the drainage bag, irrigate the urinary catheter by hand if ordered. Use strict sterile technique, sterile gloves, fresh sterile equipment, and solution as ordered, usually 30 to 60 ml of normal saline. Record amounts of solution instilled and returned on the intake and output (I&O) sheet, because the amount instilled must be subtracted from the amount returned to determine true urine output.

Do not speed up the irrigant in an attempt to dislodge the obstruction if there is no urinary outflow because this may only force the clot to become more deeply seated in the eye of the urethral catheter. This further compounds the obstruction and contributes to an overdistended bladder, bleeding, and an increase in bladder spasms. It may even require replacement of the catheter, which can cause further tissue trauma and enhance the potential for sepsis.

When ordered, remove the catheter early in the day, and give the patient 8 to 10 hours to void in sufficient quantity with each voiding (usually > 90 ml per voiding). Do postvoid residual catheterization as ordered to check for retention.

Tell the patient what to expect during and after the catheter removal. Give the patient a urinal, and instruct him to urinate into it at the first urge to void. Ask him to inform you each time he voids so that you can measure the urine and note its color and consistency. Maintain careful I&O records for the 8 to 10 hours immediately after removal of the catheter. Encourage the patient to drink between 1 and 1.5 L of fluid beginning with breakfast after the catheter is removed so that a sufficient volume of fluid is ingested in the trial voiding period. A burning sensation while voiding is common during the first 24 hours after removal of the catheter, and this high fluid intake dilutes the urine and reduces discomfort. Suggest that the patient ambulate in the room or within reach of a urinal to avoid any potentially embarrassing urgency incontinence.

Promote voiding by reassuring the anxious patient and providing privacy. Depending on the individual patient, encourage perineal exercises, give a warm bath, provide a warmed urinal, run water, or place 5 to 10 ml of spirits of peppermint in urinal to stimulate voiding. Be supportive to the patient who is unable to void or goes into urinary retention and must be recatheterized. Statements like "I know this must be uncomfortable and difficult for you" let the patient know you are concerned about him and empathize with him.

NDx: High risk for fluid volume excess

Monitor the patient for increasing restlessness, confusion, and muscular twitching, and notify the physician if they occur. Also monitor vital signs, and report any significant elevation in blood pressure or drop in pulse rate. Monitor serum electrolyte values and, report abnormal results, especially serum sodium levels below the normal range. If TUR syndrome with dyspnea and pulmonary congestion develops, assist the patient into a sitting position to facilitate breathing and administer oxygen. Slow the rate of intravenous administration to keep open rate to avoid further fluid overload. Use a calm approach, and reassure the patient to decrease the anxiety accompanying this change in condition. Anticipate the physician's request, and secure intravenous hypertonic saline solution, usually 250 to 500 ml of 3% to 5% sodium chloride, and osmotic diuretics. After administration of the hypertonic intravenous solution and diuretics, record the patient's I&O and daily weight.

NDx: Pain

Medicate the patient for pain as ordered. For incisional pain, give analgesics; for bladder spasms, give analgesics or antispasmodics or both. If B&O rectal suppositories are ordered for bladder spasms, insert them carefully to avoid traumatizing the operative site.

To further relieve bladder spasms, keep the catheter patent and draining, and make certain there is no inadvertent tension on it. Also keep the patient well hydrated.

Support the effect of medication with physical and psychological comfort measures. Change dressings if needed, give back rubs, and position the patient comfortably. Maintain a quiet, restful environment, and encourage slow, deep breathing and other relaxation techniques.

Pain management is critically important during the first 48 hours after prostatectomy. The elderly patient in pain may become increasingly restless and may injure himself when attempting to get out of bed to "go to the bathroom" to try and relieve the discomfort of bladder spasms.

NDx: High risk for infection

Wash hands carefully before caring for the patient or manipulating the catheter. Wear clean gloves for perineal care and catheter care. Use strict sterile technique during dressing changes and when irrigating the urethral or suprapubic catheters by hand. Maintain the sterility of the normal saline irrigant and equipment, and label the irrigant with date and time. Keep the penile meatus and catheter junction clean and free of bloody drainage. To do this, wrap a sterile abdominal pad loosely around the penis at the penile catheter junction after catheter care. Hold it in place with a strip of adhesive tape on the outside of the abdominal pad, and change as necessary. Encourage oral fluid intake to 2500 to 3000 ml in 24 hours unless medically contraindicated. Monitor for and report signs of infection such as elevated temperature, chills, change in type and consistency of wound drainage, and incisional pain. Administer ordered antibiotics on time.

NDx: High risk for injury

To prevent the patient from falling out of bed or inadvertent removal of urinary drainage tubes, observe the patient, his dressings, and urinary drainage tubes every 15 minutes initially and then with decreasing frequency on the basis of patient need and condition. Tape or flag the urethral catheter to the patient's inner thigh to prevent inadvertent tension on the catheter and resulting bladder trauma. Place the call light near the patient; encourage him to use it to call for help; instruct him to move slowly and carefully in bed to avoid dislodging the tube. Remind him not to get out of bed without assistance until directed to do so. Keep the bed in low position with side rails up.

When the patient is allowed out of bed, move and secure the urinary drainage tubes and bags well ahead of any movement by the patient from bed to chair or when returning to bed. This is a crucial time when inadvertent removal of catheters can occur because of a sudden movement by the patient in an attempt to help or as a result of the failure of the nurse to carefully place urinary drainage bags and normal saline irrigant ahead of him. Verbally cue and guide the patient carefully when any movement is attempted.

NDx: High risk for impaired tissue integrity

After suprapubic prostatectomy, serosanguineous drainage and urine may leak out around the suprapubic catheter. Cleanse the skin around the suprapubic catheter and incision with an antibacterial agent such as a povidone-iodine preparation (Betadine), and apply a dry, sterile dressing. Change the dressing frequently to prevent maceration of the skin. Hold the dressing in place with Montgomery straps to help prevent skin breakdown resulting from frequent application and removal of adhesive tape that could occur with dressing changes. This is very important for elderly patients, whose skin is particularly sensitive to mechanical injury.

After perineal prostatectomy, change the perineal dressing as often as needed to keep the skin dry, clean, and free of fecal contamination. If ordered, give sitz baths for cleanliness and comfort, and use a heat lamp to keep the perineum dry.

NDx: High risk for constipation

Encourage the patient to drink 1.5 to 2 L of fluid per day while hospitalized. When diet permits, encourage him to eat fresh fruits, vegetables, whole-grain products (bread, cereals), and bran. Ambulate the patient progressively and consistently. Administer a stool softener or laxative as prescribed. Record the occurrence of the patient's first bowel movement, which is usually within 3 days of resuming oral food and fluids.

NDx: High risk for sexual dysfunction

Include the significant other in discussions regarding sexuality. Be certain the patient knows and understands the degree of dysfunction he can expect based on the extent of the procedure performed. Establish a climate that makes him feel comfortable asking questions related to sexuality. If questions about sexuality were included in preoperative teaching and were addressed, postoperative discussion will be easier. Ask "Do you have any questions for the doctor or me about how this surgery might affect your ability to 'perform' sexually?" Answer those questions simply to reaffirm, and clarify the information given to the patient by the physician. Before discharge, remind the patient about any postoperative restrictions on his sexual activity as recommended by the physician. Instruct the patient to report the occurrence of cloudy urine, which is associated with retrograde ejaculation once sexual activity is resumed. If impotence is anticipated, provide emotional support for the patient and significant other. Refer for sexual counseling if indicated.

NDx: High risk for altered health maintenance

Teach the patient as specified in Chart 45–3 regarding self-care. Initiate a referral to a home-care agency if necessary.

Chart 45–3.

NURSING GUIDE TO PATIENT EDUCATION FOR SELF-MANAGEMENT: DISCHARGE INFORMATION AFTER PROSTATECTOMY

Explain the following to the patient:

Bloody urine is common immediately after surgery. Small pieces of tissue or blood clots can be passed during urination for up to 2 weeks after surgery.

Strenuous exercise and sports activities such as tennis, golf, swimming, and lifting objects heavier than 20 lb must be avoided for 6 weeks. These activities can stimulate bleeding.

Abstinence from sexual intercourse is recommended for a minimum of 3 weeks. Check with the physician before resuming this activity.

Showering rather than bathing in a tub is recommended. Use of hot tubs should also be discouraged to limit dilation of pelvic blood vessels.

Driving an automobile and sitting for long periods of time in an automobile are restricted for a minimum of 3 weeks. Check with the physician before attempting either activity.

Returning to work usually occurs at 4 to 6 weeks depending on the type and extent of prostatectomy performed and the nature of the work.

Instruct the patient to:

Report promptly abrupt episodes of frank bleeding to the physician.

Report increases in bloody urine not cleared by drinking fluids (up to 32 oz in 30 minutes) that last for a few hours or one to two voidings.

Notify physician if urinary stream decreases or if urinating becomes difficult.

Take medications, especially antibiotics if prescribed, on time as ordered.

Avoid straining at bowel movement because this can initiate bleeding.

Maintain a high daily intake of nonalcoholic fluids (2 to 2.5 L/day to ensure soft, regular bowel movements, to limit clot formation, and to prevent infection.

Include fresh vegetables, fruits, whole-grain products (Shredded Wheat), and bran in a well-balanced diet.

Report signs of constipation early to the physician, who usually orders a stool softener. Avoid use of enemas and suppositories, which can stimulate bleeding. A mild laxative may be used.

Report signs of urinary tract infection: fever (higher than 37.6°C [99.8°F]), chills, painful urination, back side pain (flank area), and general malaise.

Additional Interventions

For 48 to 72 hours after surgery, avoid all rectal treatments (with the exception of B&O suppositories) to prevent injury to the prostatic surgical site.

If urinary incontinence persists at discharge, on the basis of a discussion with the physician, reassure the patient that as healing occurs his ability to void more continently will improve. In cases of severe incontinence, a Cunningham clamp (see Fig. 46–9) may be ordered for the patient to wear.

Evaluation

Evaluate the effectiveness of nursing care for a patient who has had a simple prostatectomy by comparing the patient's status with the expected patient outcomes. Examples of specific outcomes for patients who have had a simple prostatectomy have been provided in the Planning section.

PENILE IMPLANTS

A penile implant is a prosthetic device inserted into the corpora cavernosa to restore erectile potency.

USES

A penile implant is generally used on patients with organic impotency: however, some physicians may select this form of treatment for patients with psychogenic impotency if they are refractory to sex therapy.

The penile prosthesis may also be used as adjunct therapy for some patients with a neurogenic bladder to facilitate either intermittent self-catheterization or to maintain the placement of an external urinary drainage device (condom catheter).

PATIENT PREPARATION

To determine the appropriateness of implanting a penile prosthesis, the patient's response to any nonsurgical treatment (e.g., hormone or sex therapy) is reviewed. In addition, the patient may be expected to express a strong sexual desire to satisfy himself and his partner, have a willing sexual partner, and be psychologically and intellectually able to cope with the prosthesis.

Once the decision is made that the patient is a suitable candidate for the implant, he and his partner are usually involved in selecting the type of prosthesis to be inserted. To assist them in their choice, the advantages and disadvantages of each type of implant are explained.

An informed consent is signed that outlines all the potential risks and benefits of the implant surgery. The patient is told that the erection achieved with the implant will probably not be exactly like that achieved naturally before he became impotent. He is also told that if his production of sperm has not been affected by the cause of the impotency, he can father a child.

Because infection is a common postoperative complication, prophylactic intravenous antibiotic therapy, usually with an aminoglycoside, is started preoperatively. Skin preparation includes a shower with an antibacterial cleansing solution, such as 2% povidine-iodine, the night before and the morning before surgery. It also includes a surgical shave of the genital area, which is done in the operating room.

Because implantation of a penile prosthesis is usually performed under general anesthesia, food and fluids are withheld for 8 to 10 hours before the operation.

TYPES OF PROSTHESES

There are two basic types of penile prosthesis: the inflatable and noninflatable, or solid, rod models. The inflatable implant has three components: two controlled expansion cylinders, a reservoir filled with either a radiographic solution or a sterile saline solution, and a pump with a release valve (Fig. 45–12). All parts are connected by kink-resistant tubing. The prosthesis is activated each time the patient compresses the pump, which has been implanted in one of the scrotal sacs. Fluid from the reservoir, located in the retropubic space beside the bladder, is then transferred to the cylinders in the penis, causing them to inflate. The inflation of these cylinders simulates a normal physiologic erection in both size and appearance (Fig. 45–13).

Deflation is accomplished by pressing a release valve located in the edge of the pump mechanism. When deflated, the penis returns to a flaccid state.

Three types of noninflatable penile implants are the Small-Carrion, Jonas-Silver, and Finney-Flexirod models. A description of each is found in Table 46–6.

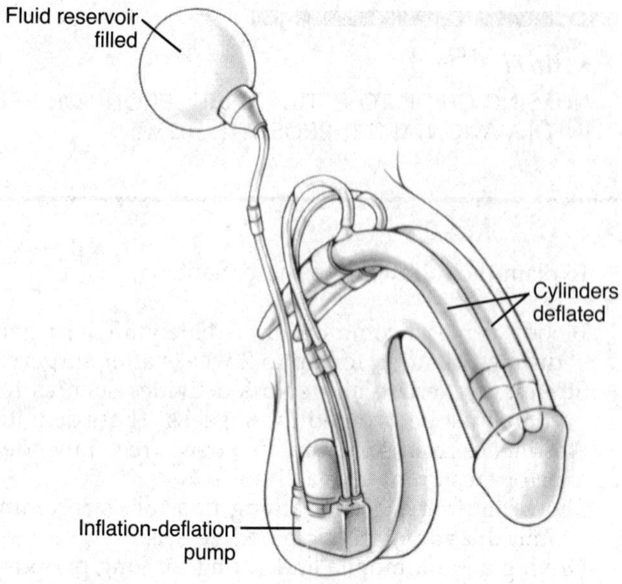

Figure 45–12.

The three components of the inflatable penile prosthesis, sagittal view. Penis in flaccid position. (Courtesy of American Medical Systems, Inc., Minnetonka, Minnesota. Medical illustration by Michael Schenk.)

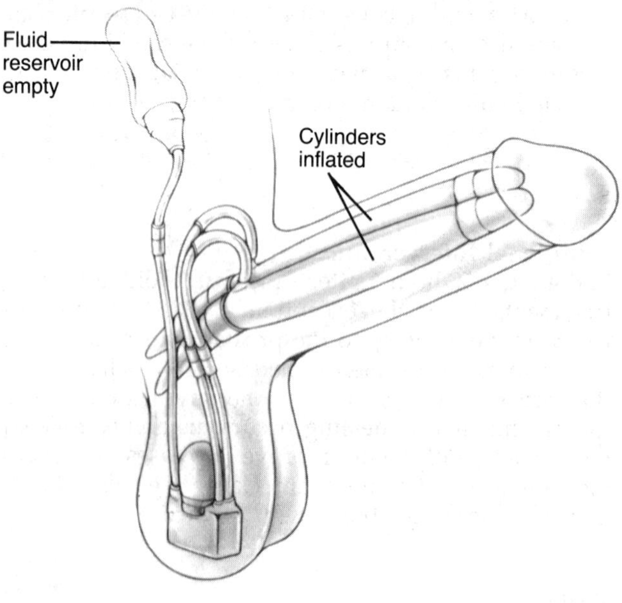

Figure 45–13.

Inflatable penile prosthesis, sagittal view. Penis is in erect position. (Courtesy of American Medical Systems, Inc., Minnetonka, Minnesota. Medical illustration by Michael Schenk.)

Table 45–6. TYPES OF NONINFLATABLE PENILE PROSTHESES

TYPE	DESCRIPTION
Small-Carrion	Cylinders are composed of semirigid Silastic shell with a silicone sponge-filled interior. Penis always remains erect.
Jonas silver	Cylinders are made of silicone rubber with a silver inlay imbedded inside the silicone rubber. The cylinder core is thus malleable, which allows the penis to be manually directed into different positions.
Finney-flexirod	Cylinders are semirigid and filled with silicone and contain a hinge at the perineal end. The hinge allows the penis to hang in a more dependent position.

The major advantages and disadvantages for the inflatable and noninflatable penile prostheses are listed in Table 45–7.

PROCEDURE

The surgical technique for implanting the penile prosthesis varies depending on the type of device selected and the surgeon's preference. The inflatable prosthesis can be inserted either by the suprapubic or upper scrotal approach. Because the scrotal approach allows better access for implanting the cylinder as well as for inserting the pump and reservoir, this technique is frequently used. In placing the pump in the scrotal sac, some consideration may be given as to whether the patient is right- or left-handed. For example, if the patient is right-handed, the right scrotal sac is generally used. When the three components are connected, the implant is checked for proper inflation and deflation. Before the surgery is completed, a Jackson-Pratt drain may be inserted for 24 to 72 hours.

The noninflatable prosthesis can easily be inserted through one of three approaches: perineal, dorsal penile, or suprapubic. This procedure usually takes about 30 minutes compared with the 60- to 90-minute operating time for implanting the inflatable prosthesis.

Because some edema is likely to form around the urethra with all types of implants, a Foley catheter is usually inserted before the patient leaves the operating room. The catheter is left in place for the first 24 hours.

POSTOPERATIVE COURSE

Antibiotic therapy is continued postoperatively. After discharge from the hospital, the patient is maintained on an oral broad-spectrum antibiotic for approximately 2 weeks. Moderate pain in the genital area, which may also be referred to the lower abdomen, is expected for the first 24 to 48 hours postoperatively. Pain can usually be controlled with hydromorphone hydrochloride (Dilaudid), 2 mg intramuscularly every 4 to 6 hours as occasion requires, or a similar narcotic analgesic for the first 24 hours and then with oxycodone hydrochloride and acetaminophen (Percocet), one to two tablets every 4 hours as needed. Ice pack applications are usually ordered for the operative area during the first 24 hours to control the pain and edema formation.

Edema and ecchymosis of the penis and scrotum are to be anticipated postoperatively and may continue for 7 to 10 days, especially with the inflatable prosthesis. Voiding is not usually a problem after the Foley catheter is removed.

Blood loss is usually minimal for all types of implants. If a Jackson-Pratt drain or similar wound drainage system was inserted, as in the case of the patient with an inflatable prosthesis, up to 30 ml of serosanguineous drainage per day is considered within normal limits.

Beginning on the second postoperative day, the patient with the inflatable implant is taught to locate the pump and apply gentle traction to maintain its position in the most dependent portion of the scrotal sac.

By the day of discharge, all drains have been removed and the patient is usually able to take a shower or bath. He may also be instructed to take sitz baths for 20 minutes four to five times a day for penile and scrotal discomfort. If there are any sutures in place, they are removed about 1 week after returning home.

Table 45–7. ADVANTAGES AND DISADVANTAGES OF INFLATABLE AND NONINFLATABLE PENILE PROSTHESES

TYPE OF IMPLANT	ADVANTAGES	DISADVANTAGES
Inflatable	More natural appearing erection Duration of erection regulated by patient Does not cause penile erosion Cystoscopic examinations can be easily performed	Higher mechanical failure Insertion time longer Hospital stay longer (4–7 days) More expensive Manual dexterity required for activating the prosthesis
Noninflatable	No mechanical parts to malfunction Insertion time shorter Hospital stay short (2 days) Less expensive	Penis is always in an erect or semierect position Erection less rigid than normal one Problem with concealment May interfere with any future cystoscopic surgery May erode through the penis

CONTRAINDICATIONS

Any patient undergoing this procedure must have a general state of health good enough to undergo the surgery safely. For example, conditions such as unstable coronary artery disease, thrombocytopenia, or prostate enlargement would render the patient an unsatisfactory candidate for penile implant surgery.

COMPLICATIONS

Postoperative complications for both the inflatable and noninflatable prostheses are similar and include infection, urinary retention, and phimosis. In addition to these complications, the patient with an inflatable prosthesis may experience a rupture or leak of the cylinders and reservoir; the pump could malfunction or cause an erosion of the scrotum; and a scrotal hematoma may form. Specific complications associated with the various noninflatable types are generally limited to device failure and extrusion or perforation of the cylinders through the urethra or skin of the penis.

Application of the Nursing Process to the Care of the Patient Undergoing Implantation of a Penile Prosthesis

PREOPERATIVE NURSING CARE

Nursing care for the patient scheduled for implantation of a penile prosthesis is similar to that for any preoperative patient, as described in Chapter 4.

POSTOPERATIVE NURSING CARE

Assessment

Assess the patient's physiologic status by taking vital signs, observing Foley catheter and wound drainage for color and amount, monitoring any intravenous fluid intake, and checking the site for signs of infiltration and inflammation.

Assess for signs of complications specific to the surgery such as hemorrhage, infection, and penile erosion. Also observe for the development of any problem that may be associated with the effects of having general anesthesia, as described in Chapter 4.

Assess for pain, and determine type, location, and intensity. Observe for swelling in the operative area as well as in surrounding tissue. With removal of the Foley catheter, determine the patient's ability to initiate urination and empty his bladder.

Throughout the postoperative period, assess the patient's emotional state and his reactions to the change in body image.

Nursing Diagnoses and Planning

Nursing diagnoses and related expected patient outcomes most commonly applicable to patients who have undergone implantation of a penile prosthesis include the following:

NDx: Pain related to surgical trauma

Planning: Patient outcomes
1. Patient asks for and accepts pain medication.
2. Patient keeps ice pack applications in place as ordered.
3. Patient states he has less discomfort in the penile and scrotal areas.
4. Patient moves more easily.

NDx: High risk for infection related to surgical wound

Planning: Patient outcomes
1. Patient's temperature is within normal limits.
2. Wound drainage is free of pus and foul odor.

NDx: High risk for body image disturbance related to penile surgery

Planning: Patient outcomes
1. Patient looks at penis and scrotum.
2. Patient is willing to discuss the prosthesis and its care.
3. Patient assumes self-care activities.

NDx: High risk for urinary retention related to swelling around the urethra

Planning: Patient outcomes
1. Patient voids within 6 to 8 hours after the Foley catheter is removed.
2. Complaints of urgency, dysuria, bladder fullness, or suprapubic discomfort are absent.
3. Urinary bladder is free of distention.

NDx: High risk for altered health maintenance related to insufficient knowledge of self-care activities after discharge

Planning: Patient outcomes
1. Patient lists signs and symptoms that should be reported to the physician.
2. Patient describes the restrictions on activity.
3. Patient describes care of the wound.
4. Patient states the name of prescribed antibiotic, expected effects, and the dose, route, and frequency of administration.
5. Patient states when he may resume sexual intercourse.
6. Patient describes when he should inflate and deflate the prosthesis (if applicable).
7. Patient demonstrates the method of repositioning the pump in the scrotal sac (if applicable).
8. Patient states the date of his follow-up visit.

Nursing Interventions

NDx: Pain

Remind the patient that medication has been ordered for his pain. Give analgesics according to the physician's order. Apply ice packs to the penile and scrotal areas as ordered to ease the discomfort and to minimize edema formation. Avoid tissue ischemia by applying the ice packs for 30 minutes and then removing them for 1 hour to allow the tissues of the penis and scrotum to recover. Repeat this schedule for the time period ordered. Provide an egg-crate pad or flotation pad for the patient to sit on when he is in the chair or when his bed is in the high Fowler's position so that pressure on the penis and scrotum is avoided. Use a bed cradle to keep the weight of the bed clothes off the patient's penis.

NDx: High risk for infection

Instruct and assist the patient as needed to cleanse the perineal area after each bowel movement to avoid fecal contamination of the wound. Also change linen and the dressing if it is soiled with urine, because moisture increases the chance of infection.

If a Jackson-Pratt or similar wound drainage system is in place, ensure that the tube is free of kinks and is properly secured to the patient's dressing. Maintain the patency of the wound drainage system because accumulated blood and body fluid provide a good medium for growth of microorganisms.

After the Foley catheter is removed, encourage the patient to wash his hands thoroughly before each voiding to decrease the risk of wound contamination with pathogens. Administer antibiotics as ordered for prophylaxis, and monitor for side effects.

NDx: High risk for body image disturbance

Remind the patient with an inflatable prosthesis that his penis will have a normal appearance once the swelling has subsided. In the case of the noninflatable implant, remind the patient that even after the edema disappears, his penis will always be in an erect or semierect state depending on the type of prosthesis. Reassure him, however, that the prosthesis can be concealed by wearing the correct clothing. For example, explain to the patient with a Small-Carrion implant that wearing snug-fitting jockey shorts, with his penis placed up against his abdomen, and loose trousers will help conceal his semierect penis, whereas the patient with a hinged type of prosthesis is advised to wear boxer shorts because his penis is in a dependent position, except when engaging in sexual intercourse.

Provide for privacy when carrying out any intervention that requires exposure of the patient's genital area (e.g., Foley catheter care or emptying the wound drainage system). Suggest that the patient look at his penis during dressing changes. Also encourage him to maintain his personal appearance by shaving, wearing his own pajamas, and combing his hair. Urge the patient to discuss any negative feelings he may have with his sexual partner. Assist in the patient's and partner's adjustment to the image change by listening, facilitating their expressions of concern, and responding clearly to their questions.

NDx: High risk for urinary retention

Allow the patient to stand to void for optimal relaxation of the external urinary sphincter and perineal muscles. Provide for adequate fluid intake to facilitate the desire to void. Encourage voiding within 2 to 3 hours after the catheter's removal, and if successful, note the color and measure, and record the amount. If less than 50 ml is voided, suspect urinary retention with overflow.

If the patient is unable to void after 8 hours, review his fluid intake for this time period, and palpate the suprapubic area for bladder distention. Inform the physician that the patient has not voided. A decision as to whether he needs to be catheterized immediately will depend on the presence of discomfort, bladder distention, and amount of fluid intake. If the patient is not catheterized, measures to promote urination should continue to be implemented.

NDx: High risk for altered health maintenance

Instruct the patient in self-care after discharge as specified in Chart 45–4.

Evaluation

Evaluate the effectiveness of nursing care for a patient who has undergone implantation of a penile prosthesis by comparing the patient's status with the expected patient outcomes. Examples of specific outcomes for patients who have undergone implantation of a penile prosthesis have been provided in the Planning section.

The Elderly: Special Considerations

Age-Related Changes in the Male Reproductive System

Beginning at about 50 years of age, there is a very gradual reduction in testosterone production and spermatogenesis. The size and firmness of the testes diminish because of a degenerative process within the seminiferous tubules and a decrease in the number of interstitial cells. Despite these changes, however, the male's ability to procreate continues, although fertilization of an ovum is less frequent because of fewer viable sperm.

Other organs of the male reproductive system also change with age. The elasticity of the skin surrounding the scrotum decreases considerably. This

Chart 45–4.

NURSING GUIDE TO PATIENT EDUCATION FOR SELF-MANAGEMENT: DISCHARGE INSTRUCTIONS AFTER PENILE IMPLANT SURGERY

Instruct the patient to do the following:

Cleanse the wound daily by gently washing with soap and warm water. Use sitz baths if ordered.
Take prescribed antibiotics on time and until gone.
Avoid strenuous physical activity such as jogging, lifting, or contact sports for about 3 weeks while a fibrous sheath is forming around the cylinders.
Avoid sexual intercourse until otherwise directed by the physician. This is usually 4 to 6 weeks postoperatively for both inflatable and noninflatable prostheses.
Practice inflating and deflating the prosthesis daily for 2 weeks when directed to do so. This promotes the formation of fibrous tissue around the implant.
Report promptly any breakdown of skin around the implant; inability to pull the pump to the lowest part of the scrotum if the prosthesis is inflatable; persistent or intensified penile pain; or, with an inflatable prosthesis, scrotal pain, drainage from the penis or scrotum, and fever greater than 37.7°C (100°F).
Return for a follow-up visit on *(specify date and time).*

leads to increased relaxation, folding, and sagging of the scrotal tissue and reduced scrotal vasocongestion in response to sexual tensions (Masters & Johnson, 1966). In the prostate gland, the muscle tissue is replaced by collagen, and its blood supply is decreased (Perlmutter & Hall, 1985). The gland enlarges in 10% of men by 40 years of age and in 50% by 80 years of age. The exact cause of this benign prostate enlargement remains unclear.

The penis may begin to show characteristic signs of aging as early as the 30s. Penile tissue and blood vessels undergo typical hardening and lose elasticity. Because an erection depends on blood supply to the penis, these changes result in decreased speed and firmness of an erection (Perlmutter & Hall, 1985).

Changes in the Sexual Response Cycle

The physiology of sexual response in the older male is altered in several ways according to the research findings of Masters and Johnson. By 60 years of age, each stage of the man's sexual response cycle has lengthened. Generally, he requires a longer time and more direct penile stimulation to achieve an erection, and the firmness of the erection is usually moderately decreased. However, once an erection occurs, it can be maintained for a longer time before ejaculation occurs.

The intensity of the ejaculatory experience lessens with age. This appears to be related to (1) a decrease in volume of the ejaculate, (2) a decrease in prostatic contractions, (3) a decrease in testicular elevation, and (4) diminished nerve supply to the genital area. In the older male, detumescence occurs in a matter of seconds, and the refractory period is increased; 12 to 24 hours may elapse before he can achieve another ejaculation.

With aging, an occasional inability to have an erection may develop. Such transient failure is not considered pathologic and is probably related to the normal aging process of the reproductive system (Katchadourian & Lunde, 1980). However, a consistent impotent state in the older male may be secondary to chronic illness such as diabetes mellitus or hypertension.

Despite these changes, if the aging male is in relatively good health and has an interested partner, an active and satisfying sexual life can be maintained.

Male Climacteric Syndrome

No event analogous to menopause occurs in the male reproductive system; that is, there is no specific point in time when the male becomes unable to reproduce. Nonetheless, some middle-aged men experience symptoms typically associated with menopause and are said to have male climacteric syndrome. These symptoms include insomnia, irritability, listlessness, impaired ability to concentrate, fatigue, and weakness. Although in some cases a relationship between male climacteric syndrome and a consistently low (less than 324 mg) serum testosterone level has been found, it appears that psychological factors play a significant role in its development.

There are many potential psychological contributing factors. Prime among them are changes in sexual response cycle. Decreasing speed of erection and the difficulty some men have in maintaining an erection can lead to disturbing fears regarding virility. In fact, it appears that previously monogamous men may engage in extramarital affairs seeking to reaffirm their virility at this time. Added to this is "career crisis," which many men experience simultaneously. They become excluded in promotions, feel they are seen as rigid and passé, and realize that many of their career goals will never be attained. This can cause feelings of failure and may lead to depression and further weakened self-esteem.

Medical management of male climacteric syndrome is essentially symptomatic, except when the serum testosterone level is distinctly low. In these cases, replacement therapy such as testosterone enanthate or testosterone cypionate, 200 to 300 mg intramuscularly every 2 to 3 weeks (Satterfield, 1986), may be ordered. With this treatment, remission of symptoms should occur within 2 months. The use of testosterone therapy is contraindicated in patients with coronary artery disease and in those with an enlarged prostate gland.

Social Attitudes Toward Sex and the Aged Man

Society has been slow to recognize that older persons have sexual needs, and aging men themselves are not immune to the belief that sex for the aging person is not socially acceptable. Men who are sensitive to this attitude may feel guilty or embarrassed about sexual expression and may disregard sexual needs as a result. This can lead to feelings of anger and frustration. Thus, despite age-related changes, many older men's interest in maintaining active sexual lives persists, and the male with a disorder of the reproductive system may need encouragement and reassurance that sexual activity in later years is normal and healthy and can be continued.

Bibliography

Bates P. Three post-op perils of prostate surgery. RN 1984; 47(2):40.

Brendler CB. Diseases of the prostate. In Wyngaarden JB, Smith LH, Bennett JC (eds). Cecil textbook of medicine. 19th ed. Philadelphia: WB Saunders, 1992, pp 1351–1355.

Brenner BM, Milford EL, Seifter JL. Urinary tract obstruction. In Wilson JL, et al (eds). Harrison's principles of internal medicine. 12th ed. New York: McGraw-Hill, 1991, pp 1206–1212.

Brooks ME, Berezin M, Braf Z. Treatment of retrograde ejaculation with imipramine. Urology 1980; 15(4):353.

Burggraf V, Stanley M. Nursing the elderly: A care plan approach. Philadelphia: JB Lippincott, 1989.

Carpenito LJ. Handbook of nursing diagnosis. 5th ed. Philadelphia: JB Lippincott, 1993.

Carpenito LJ. Nursing diagnosis: Application to clinical practice. 5th ed. Philadelphia: JB Lippincott, 1993.

Carter HB. Instrumentation and endoscopy. In Walsh PC, Retik AB, Stamey TA, Vaughan ED (eds). Campbell's urology. 6th ed. Philadelphia: WB Saunders, 1992, pp 331–341.

Cella J, Watson J. Nurse's manual of laboratory tests. Philadelphia: FA Davis, 1989.

Cohen S, Gittes RRS. Patient assessment: Examination of the male genitalia. Am J Nurs 1979; 694, 711.

Cowling WR, Campbell V. Health concerns of aging men. Nurs Clin North Am 1986; 21(1):75.

Doenges M, Moorhouse M. Nurse's pocket guide: Nursing diagnoses with interventions. 3rd ed. Philadelphia: FA Davis, 1991.

Eliopoulos C. Nursing diagnosis in gerontological care. In Eliopoulos C (ed). Caring for the elderly in diverse care settings. Philadelphia: JB Lippincott, 1990, pp 39–75.

Eliopoulos C. Assessment of sexual function. In Eliopoulos C (ed). Health assessment of the older adult. 2nd ed. Redwood City, CA: Addison-Wesley, 1990, pp 229–239.

Eliopoulos C. Gerontological nursing. 3rd ed. Philadelphia: JB Lippincott, 1993.

Ebersole P, Hess P. Toward healthy aging: Human needs and nursing response. 3rd ed. St. Louis: CV Mosby, 1990.

Goldstein M. Surgery of male infertility and other scrotal disorders. In Walsh C, Retik AB, Stamey TA, Vaughan ED Jr (eds). Campbell's urology. 6th ed. Philadelphia: WB Saunders, 1992, pp 3114–3149.

Gray M, Dobkin K. Genitourinary system. In Thompson JL, et al (eds). Clinical nursing. 3rd ed. St. Louis: CV Mosby, 1993, pp 957–1028.

Gregory JG. Impotence: The surgical approach. Surg Clin North Am 1982; 62:981.

Guyton AC. Human physiology and mechanisms of disease. 5th ed. Philadelphia: WB Saunders, 1992.

Guyton AC. Textbook of medical physiology. 8th ed. Philadelphia: WB Saunders, 1991.

Heckheimer E. Health promotion of the elderly in the community. Philadelphia: WB Saunders, 1989.

Howards SS. Surgery of the scrotum and testis in childhood. In Walsh PC, Retik AB, Stamey TA, Vaughan ED (eds). Campbell's urology. 6th ed. Philadelphia: WB Saunders, 1992, 1939–1950.

Irwin J. Legal aspects of urologic prosthetic devices. Urol Clin North Am 1989; 16(1):165.

Katchadourian HA, Lunde DT. Fundamentals of human sexuality. 3rd ed. New York: Holt, Rinehart & Winston, 1980.

Kedia K. Ejaculation and emission: Normal physiology, dysfunction, and therapy. In Krane RJ, et al (eds). Male sexual dysfunction. Boston: Little, Brown, 1983, pp 37–53.

Knowlton CN, Burke MM. Sexuality. In Burke MM, Walsh MB (eds). Gerontologic nursing: Care of the frail elderly. St. Louis: Mosby-Year Book, 1992, pp 114–133.

Lerner J, Kahn Z. Mosby's manual of urologic nursing. St. Louis: CV Mosby, 1982.

Lowe FC, Brendler CB. Evaluation of the urologic patient: History, physical examination, and urinalysis. In Walsh PC, Retik AB, Stamey TA, Vaughan ED Jr (eds). Campbell's urology. 6th ed. Philadelphia: WB Saunders, 1992, pp 307–331.

Lue TF. Physiology of erection and pathophysiology of impotence. In Walsh PC, Retik AB, Stamey TA, Vaughan ED Jr (eds). Campbell's urology. 6th ed. Philadelphia: WB Saunders, 1992, pp 709–728.

Martin F. When the solution is a prosthesis. RN 1990; 53:32–35.

Martin JP. Transrectal ultrasound: A new screening tool in prostate cancer. AJN 1991; 91:69.

Masters W, Johnson J. Human sexual response. Boston: Little, Brown, 1966.

Masters WH, Johnson J. Human sexual inadequacy. Boston: Little, Brown, 1970.

Matsumoto A. The testis and male sexual function. In Wyngaarden JB, Smith LH, Bennett JC (eds). Cecil textbook of medicine. 19th ed. Philadelphia: WB Saunders, 1992, pp 1333–1350.

McLennan B. Diagnostic imaging evaluation of benign prostatic hyperplasia. Urol Clin North Am 1990; 17(3):517.
Mebust W. Transurethral prostatectomy. Urol Clin North Am 1990; 17(3):575.
Mebust WK. Transurethral surgery. In Walsh PC, Retik AB, Stamey TA, Vaughan ED Jr (eds). Campbell's urology. 6th ed. Philadelphia: WB Saunders, 1992, pp 2900–2922.
Miller C. Nursing care of older adults. Glenview, IL: Scott, Foresman/Little, Brown, 1990.
Molloy T, Wein A. Penile flaccidity due to vascular insufficiency. Med Aspects Hum Sexuality 1983; 17:211.
Montague D. Penile prostheses—An overview. Urol Clin North Am 1989; 16(1):7.
Moore S et al. Nerve sparing prostatectomy. AJN Vol 92, No 4, April 1992, pp. 59–64.
Morse R, Resnick M. Detection of clinically occult prostate cancer. Urol Clin North Am 1990; 17(3):567.
National Cancer Institute. Testicular self-examination. (National Institutes of Health Publication No. 92-2636.) Washington, DC: U.S. Department of Health and Human Services, 1992.
Nero F. When couples ask about infertility. RN 1988; 51(11):26.
Paulson DF. Perineal prostatectomy. In Walsh PC, Retik AB, Stamey TA, Vaughan ED Jr (eds). Campbell's urology. 6th ed. Philadelphia: WB Saunders, 1992, pp 2887–2899.
Perlmutter M, Hall E. Adult development and aging. New York: John Wiley & Sons, 1985.
Reznichek C, Reznichek R. The problem most men won't talk about. RN 1990; 53:28–32.
Satterfield S. Tracking down treatable impotence. Emerg Med 1986; 18(1):89.
Schellhammer F, Jordan GH, Schlossberg SM. Tumors of the penis. In Walsh PC, Retik AB, Stamey TA, Vaughan ED Jr (eds). Campbell's urology. 6th ed. Philadelphia: WB Saunders, 1992, pp 1264–1298.
Shlafer M. The nurse, pharmacology, and drug therapy: A prototype approach. 2nd ed. Redwood City, CA: Addison-Wesley, 1993.
Sigman M, Howards SS. Male infertility. In Walsh PC, Retik AB, Stamey TA, Vaughan ED Jr (eds). Campbell's urology. 6th ed. Philadelphia: WB Saunders, 1992, pp 661–705.
Skidmore-Roth L. Mosby's 1993 nursing drug reference. St. Louis: Mosby-Year Book, 1993.
Snyder PJ. Fewer sperm in the summer—It's not the heat, it's . . . N Engl J Med 1990; 323(1):54.
Stamey TA, McNeal JE. Adenocarcinoma of the prostate. In Walsh PC, Retik AB, Stamey TA, Vaughan ED Jr (eds). Campbell's urology. 6th ed. Philadelphia: WB Saunders, 1992, pp 1159–1221.
Stamm W, Turch M. Urinary tract infections, pyelonephritis and related conditions. In Wilson J, Braunwald E, Petersdorf R, et al (eds). Harrison's principles of internal medicine. 12th ed. New York: McGraw-Hill, 1991, pp 539–544.
Stanford D. All about sex . . . After middle age. Am J Nurs 1977; 77(4):608.
Steinke EE, Bergen MB. Sexuality and aging. J Gerontol Nurs 1986; 12(6):6.
Stewart S. Structure and function of the male genitourinary system. In Parth CM (ed). Pathophysiology. 3rd ed. Philadelphia: JB Lippincott, 1990, pp 609–622.
Stutzman RE, Walsh PC. Suprapubic and retropubic prostatectomy. In Walsh PC, Retik AB, Stamey TA, Vaughan ED Jr (eds). Campbell's urology. 6th ed. Philadelphia: WB Saunders, 1992, pp 2851–2864.
Swerdloff RS, Heber D. Effects of aging on male reproductive function. In Korenman SG (ed). Endocrine aspects of aging. New York: Elsevier Biomedical, 1982.
Travis SS. Older adults' sexuality and remarriage. J Gerontol Nurs 1987; 13(6):8.
Walsh PC. Radical retropubic prostatectomy. In Walsh PC, Retik AB, Stamey TA, Vaughan ED Jr (eds). Campbell's urology. 6th ed. Philadelphia: WB Saunders, 1992, pp 2865–2886.
Wein A, et al. Nocturnal penile tumescence. In Krane R, et al. (eds). Male sexual dysfunction. Boston: Little, Brown, 1983, pp 203–211.
Weinberg J. Sexuality: Human needs and nursing practice. Philadelphia: WB Saunders, 1982.
Weinerth J. The male genital system. In Sabiston DC (ed). Textbook of surgery. 14th ed. Philadelphia: WB Saunders, 1991, pp 1457–1478.
Wilson JD. Androgens. In Gilman AG, et al (eds). Goodmaan & Gilman's the pharmacological basis of therapeutics. 8th ed. New York: Pergamon Press, 1990, pp 1413–1430.
Wingate A. The male reproductive system and sexual response. In Barnard MU, Clancy BJ, Krantz KE (eds). Human sexuality for health professionals. Philadelphia: WB Saunders 1978, pp 12–19.

Chapter Forty-six

NURSING CARE *of Men with Disorders of the* Reproductive System

The male reproductive system can be affected by a wide variety of disorders, acute and chronic, and ranging in severity from minor to life-threatening. Regardless of prognosis, however, each of the disorders has the potential to exert a profound effect on the patient because of its relationship to sexuality and reproductive capacity. Thus, sensitivity to the psychosocial dimension of patient care is particularly critical when caring for patients with disorders of the male reproductive system.

Infections and Inflammations

Balanitis and Posthitis

Balanitis is an inflammation of the glans penis. Posthitis, an inflammatory process involving the prepuce (foreskin), frequently occurs with balanitis. When the two problems coexist, the condition is referred to as balanoposthitis.

ETIOLOGY AND PATHOPHYSIOLOGY

Inflammation of the glans penis and prepuce is usually caused by the combined factors of accumulating smegma, glandular secretions, desquamating cells, and the invasion of a microorganism underneath the foreskin. The infecting organisms include *Streptococcus, Staphylococcus,* coliform bacillus, and those that are sexually transmitted (e.g., *Candida albicans* and the herpes simplex virus).

In some cases, these conditions may be a manifestation of a preexisting disease such as diabetes mellitus or leukoplakia.

A major factor contributing to the development of balanitis and posthitis is poor personal hygiene in the uncircumcised male who fails to retract his foreskin regularly. The warm, moist environment of the space between the glans and foreskin (preputial sac) provides a good culture medium for growth of microorganisms.

CLINICAL MANIFESTATIONS

The symptoms of balanitis and balanoposthitis usually begin within 2 to 3 days after exposure to the infecting organism. Initially, the patient complains of itching and soreness of the glans and prepuce. These symptoms are followed by pain, discharge, local edema, redness, and a burning sensation when voiding. As the condition progresses, superficial ulcers form on the surface of the glans. Systemic effects such as fever and malaise may also develop. If the infection remains untreated, the edema increases, the primary ulcer continues to erode penile tissue, and new ulcers extending up the shaft of the penis are formed. Finally, the entire penis and sometimes the scrotum can become gangrenous and necrotic.

MEDICAL DIAGNOSIS

The penis is inspected and palpated for degree of involvement. A culture and Gram's stain of the drainage are done to identify the infecting organism.

MEDICAL MANAGEMENT

Medical treatment of balanitis and balanoposthitis depends on the cause. If the culture report is positive, antibiotic therapy appropriate for the infecting organism is ordered. In the presence of a fungal infection such as candidiasis, an antifungal agent such as nystatin ointment or powder is prescribed. An analgesic such as acetaminophen or a combination of oxycodone hydrochloride and acetaminophen may be ordered for pain control.

Local therapy for balanitis and balanoposthitis includes retracting the foreskin (if possible), cleansing the glans with mild soap and water, returning the foreskin over the glans, and applying warm water or saline soaks. The frequency and duration of this treatment are determined by the severity of the infection.

If the foreskin cannot be retracted, a warm saline irrigation of the subpreputial area may be ordered. A dorsal slit of the foreskin may be necessary if the infection is severe. After the infection has resolved, a circumcision may be recommended to prevent recurrence of the balanoposthitis.

Application of the Nursing Process to the Care of the Patient with Balanitis or Posthitis

Assessment

Elicit information from the patient regarding symptoms experienced, their duration, and any self-care measures used. Also determine the patient's genital hygiene and sexual practices, including the time of the last sexual contact.

Inspect the penis for irritation, redness, edema, presence of discharge, and ulceration.

Nursing Diagnoses and Planning

Nursing diagnoses and related expected patient outcomes most commonly applicable to patients with balanitis and posthitis include the following:

NDx: Pain related to inflammation of the penis

Planning: Patient outcomes

1. Patient reports that itching, pain, and soreness have decreased or disappeared.
2. Patient voids without discomfort.

Chart 46–1.

NURSING GUIDE TO PATIENT EDUCATION FOR SELF-MANAGEMENT: PREVENTION OF RECURRENT BALANITIS OR POSTHITIS

Instruct the patient to cleanse the penis daily as follows:

Retract the foreskin.
Wash the penis from the tip down to the base using soap and warm water.
Rinse the penis well because soap residue supports bacterial growth and can be irritating to the skin.
Dry the penis thoroughly because moisture can lead to maceration, which also supports bacterial growth.
Pull the foreskin back down over the glans.

NDx: High risk for altered health maintenance related to insufficient knowledge of prescribed treatment and prevention of recurrence

Planning: Patient outcomes
1. Patient describes or demonstrates the procedure of applying warm soaks to his penis.
2. Patient states the name, expected effects, dose, route, and frequency of prescribed medication.
3. Patient describes role of proper penile hygiene in the prevention of recurrence.
4. Patient demonstrates proper cleansing of the penis.
5. Patient states frequency with which the penis should be cleaned.

Nursing Interventions

NDx: Pain
Assist or instruct the patient in retracting his foreskin and cleansing the glans. Using soap and warm water, cleanse the glans from the tip down the penile shaft to avoid spreading the infection up the urethra, rinse well, and return the foreskin to its original position. After cleansing, apply warm soaks (gauze pads or a clean face cloth soaked in warm water or saline) for 20 minutes. Change the soaks frequently during this time to maintain constant warmth and achieve the desired effects of vasodilation, increased local circulation, and relief of inflammation. On completion of the soaks, dry the penis thoroughly because moisture can cause maceration of the skin, which predisposes to the growth of pathogens.

Administer or instruct the patient in the use of analgesics as ordered.

NDx: High risk for altered health maintenance
Briefly explain the action of the prescribed antibiotic or anti-infective medication. Review with the patient its dose, frequency, and side effects. If the route of administration is topical, as with an ointment or a powder, be certain to describe or demonstrate clearly the correct application. If possible, have the patient give a return demonstration.

Instruct the patient in daily penile hygiene to prevent recurrence, as specified in Chart 46–1.

Evaluation

Evaluate the effectiveness of nursing care for a patient with balanitis or posthitis by comparing the patient's status with the expected patient outcomes. Examples of specific outcomes for patients with balanitis or posthitis have been provided in the Planning section.

Epididymitis

Epididymitis, an inflammation or infection of the epididymis, is the most common of all intrascrotal problems. It affects an estimated 600,000 males in the United States each year.

ETIOLOGY

Epididymitis, which is usually unilateral, is most often caused by an infection that descends either from the prostate gland or urinary tract via the vas deferens. Because urinary tract infection frequently occurs after urologic procedures such as catheterization and cystoscopy, epididymitis is also a common complication of them. Infecting organisms include *Streptococcus*, *Staphylococcus*, coliform bacillus, *Pseudomonas*, and, in males younger than 35 years, *Chlamydia trachomatis* and *Neisseria gonorrhoeae*, which are sexually transmitted. Occasionally, epididymitis develops from an infection elsewhere in the body, such as a pneumococcal pneumonia or tuberculosis. In these cases, the infecting organism reaches the epididymis via the lymphatic vessels or blood.

PATHOPHYSIOLOGY

In the acute phase of epididymitis, the inflammation and swelling usually begin in the tail (cauda epididymis) but then extend to involve the rest of the epididymis. The entire scrotal sac containing the infected epididymis becomes a single erythematous, painful mass often accompanied by the formation of a hydrocele (collection of clear fluid in the tunica vaginalis). Acute epididymitis usually becomes chronic to some degree and continues over a period of several weeks. There may be resultant peritubular fibrosis and occlusion of the epididymis, but often with resolution of the infection, the epididymis returns to normal after several months.

Complications of epididymitis include orchitis, which is most common, abscess formation, and sterility. Sterility is more likely to occur with chronic bilateral epididymitis. Recurrences of epididymitis develop when the underlying disease process remains unresolved.

CLINICAL MANIFESTATIONS

Symptoms of epididymitis include severe pain and tenderness in the groin and scrotum on the affected side, nausea, vomiting, and high fever. To avoid pressure on the groin and scrotum, the patient usually walks with a characteristic "duck-waddle" walk. Dysuria, frequency of urination, pyuria, and urgency, all symptoms of urinary tract infection, may also be present.

MEDICAL DIAGNOSIS

Diagnosis of epididymitis is made on the basis of physical findings and laboratory analyses. On inspection, the scrotum is reddened and edematous, and the epididymis feels thickened and enlarged when palpated. The white blood cell count is usually elevated to between 20,000 and 30,000.

To identify the causative organism, cultures of urine and urethral and prostatic secretions are done.

If torsion of the spermatic cord (twisting of the cord) is suspected, a Doppler ultrasound study of the scrotum is done. A good blood flow to the scrotum rules out torsion.

MEDICAL MANAGEMENT

Management of epididymitis includes bed rest, usually for 3 to 5 days, elevation of the scrotum, application of ice packs, analgesics, antipyretics, and antiemetics. Pending the results of the Gram's stains and cultures, a broad-spectrum oral antibiotic such as tetracycline or cefaclor is prescribed. In severe cases, combination intravenous antibiotics (e.g., ampicillin and gentamicin) may be necessary. The antibiotic therapy is adjusted as needed when the sensitivity studies are complete.

External heat is usually not prescribed because of its possible adverse effect on spermatogenesis.

An epididymectomy (removal of the epididymis) may be performed if the infection is refractory to antibiotic therapy or in the case of recurrence.

Application of the Nursing Process to the Care of the Patient with Epididymitis

Assessment

Ask the patient about the onset, degree, and duration of scrotal pain. Also ask about symptoms such as frequency and burning on urination, which are indicative of a urinary tract infection. Inspect the scrotal area for heat, redness, and edema. Observe the patient's gait for the characteristic duck waddle. Obtain an oral temperature.

Once the diagnosis is made, assess the patient's understanding of the infection, its cause, expected course, and treatment. Explore his concerns and feelings about the diagnosis and its effects on sexual function.

Nursing Diagnoses and Planning

Nursing diagnoses and related expected patient outcomes most commonly applicable to patients with epididymitis include the following:

NDx: Pain (scrotal) related to the inflammatory/infectious process

Planning: Patient outcomes
1. Patient states the pain is diminished or has disappeared.
2. Patient is able to move in bed and walk without discomfort.

NDx: Hyperthermia related to infection

Planning: Patient outcomes
1. Patient's temperature is reduced or returned to normal range.
2. Patient's daily fluid intake is at least 3000 ml (unless contraindicated).
3. Oral mucous membranes are moist.

NDx: Fear related to possible development of sterility as a complication

Planning: Patient outcomes
1. Patient discusses his concerns that he may become sterile.
2. Patient asks questions regarding his chances of becoming sterile.
3. Patient describes the importance of preventing recurrences of epididymitis.

NDx: High risk for altered health maintenance related to insufficient knowledge of cause of infection, treatment, self-care activities during hospitalization and after discharge, and prevention of recurrence

Planning: Patient outcomes
1. Patient states the cause of his infection.
2. Patient describes local treatments including their frequency and rationale.
3. Patient explains antibiotic therapy including the dose, frequency, and side effects.
4. Patient maintains scrotal elevation at all times.
5. Patient describes self-care activities associated with treatments after discharge.
6. Patient describes measures to prevent recurrences.

Nursing Interventions

NDx: Pain
Administer analgesics in accordance with the physician's order and the patient's need. Inform the patient that medication for pain is available and that he should ask for the medication when he begins to experience discomfort. Explain that the drug's effectiveness in controlling pain is greatest when it is given early in the pain cycle. Because vomiting can increase the patient's local and general discomfort, give an antiemetic as prescribed for nausea.

Elevate the scrotum to promote drainage of fluid and relief of edema and its associated discomfort. While the patient is on bed rest, elevate the scrotum by applying a Bellevue bridge (Fig. 46–1) as described in Table 46–1. An alternative method of elevating the scrotum is placing a rolled towel under it while the patient is on bed rest. However, this is usually only a temporary measure because the towel is not supported with tape and can easily be displaced with any movement. When the patient is out of bed, instruct him to wear an athletic or scrotal support until the edema subsides.

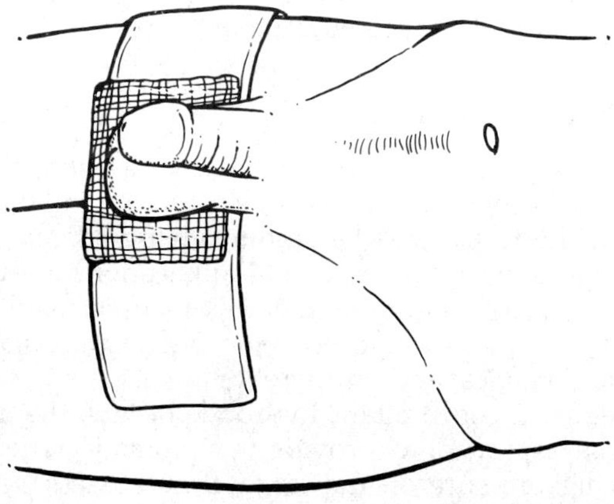

Figure 46–1.
Bellevue bridge.

Table 46–1. PROCEDURE FOR BUILDING A BELLEVUE BRIDGE

Wash and thoroughly dry patient's upper thighs, groin, penis, and scrotum.
Shave anterior upper thighs.
Apply a skin preparation or tincture of benzoin to shaved areas.
Apply one strip of wide (3 to 6 in.), nonallergic tape under the scrotum and on both thighs.
Apply second strip of tape, the same length and width, adhesive side down, on top of the first strip.
Place several 4 × 3 in. gauze sponges under the scrotum and resting on the adhesive strips. If the scrotum is very edematous, a folded, smooth towel may be used in place of the gauze sponges.

Apply ice packs, in the form of a commercial cold pack, ice bag, or examination glove filled with ice, to the scrotum as ordered to reduce edema and discomfort. Always cover the cold pack with a towel to absorb the moisture and prevent maceration of the skin. Remove the pack after 30 minutes to avoid tissue ischemia, and leave it off for 1 hour to allow the scrotal tissue to recover. Repeat this schedule for the time period ordered.

NDx: Hyperthermia
Monitor body temperature closely every 4 hours, and administer antipyretics as prescribed. For example, acetaminophen, 650 mg orally every 4 hours, for an oral temperature of 38.3°C (101°F) or higher is a common order. Cool bed baths may be necessary to help reduce the temperature by promoting convection and evaporation of heat. Provide for at least 3 L of fluids per day (unless contraindicated) to replace the fluid lost through diaphoresis and increased metabolism.

Instruct the patient to brush his teeth, gargle, and rinse with mouthwash at least four times a day to help restore moisture to the oral mucous membranes. Use petroleum jelly to prevent the lips from drying out and cracking. Change bed linen and clothing as diaphoresis occurs to promote comfort and heat loss.

NDx: Fear
Encourage the patient to ask questions and verbalize any concerns about the effect of the infection on his fertility. Clear up any misconceptions that are revealed. Inform the patient that sterility is usually a complication of bilateral epididymitis and may develop if there are recurrences of the infection. Stress the importance of preventing recurrence of epididymitis.

If infertility is suspected as a complication, referral to a sex therapist or counselor may be necessary.

NDx: High risk for altered health maintenance

Explain the cause of epididymitis using a simple anatomic illustration of the reproductive system to facilitate understanding. Explain the need for bed rest, the use of cold packs and scrotal support to prevent further edema and relieve discomfort, and the reason for antibiotic therapy. Stress the importance of taking the medication after discharge from the hospital, if ordered, and review dose, frequency, and side effects to be reported.

Provide information on measures to prevent the recurrence of epididymitis. These include maintaining a daily fluid intake of at least 2000 ml, emptying the bladder frequently, and, if epididymitis is associated with prostatitis, engaging in sexual activity or masturbation to provide periodic release of prostate secretions. Emphasize that, regardless of cause, early diagnosis and treatment of any infection of the genitourinary tract are essential.

Evaluation

Evaluate the effectiveness of nursing care for a patient with epididymitis by comparing the patient's status with the expected patient outcomes. Examples of specific outcomes for patients with epididymitis have been provided in the Planning section.

Orchitis

Orchitis is an infection or inflammation of one or both of the testes.

ETIOLOGY

Orchitis rarely occurs as a primary infection. Most often it is due to infection spreading from the epididymis (epididymo-orchitis) but occasionally results from spread of infection, through the blood or lymphatic vessels, from another part of the body. Approximately 25% of males in whom mumps develops after puberty also acquire orchitis as a result of blood or lymphatic spread.

Occasionally, orchitis follows trauma to the scrotal area or develops after a vasectomy or other surgery of the genitourinary area. This traumatic or granulomatous orchitis is considered to be an infectious process resulting from a lowered resistance of the injured tissue to bacteria.

PATHOPHYSIOLOGY

In cases of epididymo-orchitis, the testis is tense, swollen, and bluish, with many punctate hemorrhages on the surface and multiple foci of necrosis. This process occasionally progresses to suppuration involving the whole testis and then abscess formation. It is usually associated with an acute hydrocele, which may become a pyocele if the abscess ruptures. Secondary atrophy and sterility from fibrosis and destruction of the tubules and ductal system are frequent sequelae if both testes are involved.

The onset of mumps orchitis usually occurs 4 to 6 days after the appearance of parotitis and, in approximately 70% of the cases, is unilateral. Some degree of atrophy develops in the involved testis in approximately half of the males affected, and, in cases of bilateral orchitis, sterility usually occurs.

CLINICAL MANIFESTATIONS

The signs and symptoms of bacterial (pyogenic) and mumps orchitis are generally the same. Both begin with a high temperature and sudden pain in the involved testis that radiates to the inguinal area, often accompanied by nausea and vomiting. After 48 hours, the testis is usually hot, red, tender, and obviously swollen. The scrotal skin may also be red and edematous.

The clinical manifestations of traumatic orchitis vary widely. Some males experience the same symptoms as described previously. Others may complain only of painless intrascrotal edema of several weeks duration.

MEDICAL DIAGNOSIS

Diagnosis is made primarily on the basis of the patient's presenting signs and symptoms, related history, and visual inspection of the area. Palpation of the testis is usually not possible because of its extreme tenderness. It may be difficult to differentiate granulomatous orchitis from a testicular tumor on the basis of physical examination of the area. If a testicular tumor is suspected, the testis is removed and a histologic examination done to establish a diagnosis. A biopsy of the involved testis is not done because of the great danger of metastatic spread if a malignant neoplasm is present.

MEDICAL MANAGEMENT

Treatment of pyogenic orchitis is essentially the same as for epididymitis. To decrease the inflammation of the testis and the accompanying edema, bed rest, scrotal elevation, and cold applications are usually ordered. Antibiotic therapy is prescribed according to the specific etiologic organism. Analgesics, antiemetics, and antipyretics are also ordered as needed. If a concomitant hydrocele occurs, the fluid may be aspirated to provide symptomatic relief by reducing pressure on the testis. If an abscess develops, an orchiectomy is performed.

Management of mumps orchitis is similar to that of pyogenic orchitis. It includes comfort measures such as bed rest, elevation of the scrotum, and cold applications. In addition, 1 to 3 mg of diethylstilbestrol (DES) may be ordered daily to reduce the pain by inhibiting testicular function. Occasionally, the administration of large doses of a corticosteroid may reduce the pain, but the local findings and the clinical course remain unchanged.

In cases of severe mumps orchitis with extensive edema, incision and drainage (I&D) of the hydrocele may be done to reduce the pressure in the tunica. If done within the first 48 hours of acute swelling, it appears that this not only relieves symptoms but also markedly reduces subsequent testicular atrophy.

Because gamma globulin administered in the early stages of parotitis has been reported to decrease the incidence of orchitis, it is given to any postpubertal male who is exposed to mumps and who has neither had the disease nor received the mumps vaccine as a child.

Application of the Nursing Process to the Care of the Patient with Orchitis

Assessment

Assessment of the patient with orchitis is similar to that of the patient with epididymitis. Obtain information about the pain, including its onset, location, and intensity. Examine the scrotum for heat, redness, and edema, and take an oral temperature.

Ask the patient if he had mumps or if he received the mumps vaccine as a child. If he has not had mumps or the vaccine, determine whether he has been exposed to the disease within the past 3 weeks.

Once the diagnosis is established, assess his understanding of the disease and its treatment as well as his concerns and feelings about it. Determine how he views its effect on subsequent sexual function.

Nursing Diagnoses and Planning

Nursing diagnoses and related expected patient outcomes most commonly applicable to patients with orchitis include those discussed under the care of the patient with epididymitis and, if I&D of the scrotum has been performed, the following:

NDx: High risk for infection related to incision and drainage of the scrotum

Planning: Patient outcomes
1. Wound is clean.
2. Purulent drainage is absent.

Nursing Interventions

Nursing interventions related to the nursing diagnoses of pain, hyperthermia, fear, and knowledge deficit are similar to those described previously for the care of the patient with epididymitis.

NDx: High risk for infection
If an I&D of a hydrocele is performed, a scrotal dressing is usually applied to absorb any fluid that may drain after the procedure. Change the dressing as needed because a moist dressing facilitates bacterial contamination of the wound by capillary action. A dressing saturated with drainage also places the patient at risk for breakdown of the scrotal skin.

Before reapplying a sterile dressing, gently cleanse the scrotal wound with sterile water or saline to remove any drainage, which may serve as a source of irritation if left on the scrotal surface. Observe the wound for any redness, and note the color, consistency, and amount of drainage and any increased local tenderness of the affected scrotal sac.

Apply a scrotal support to provide elevation as well as to secure the dressing.

Additional Interventions
If DES is ordered, instruct the patient on its purpose, dose, frequency, and usual side effects. Because this therapy is short term, feminizing effects should not occur. Prepare him for expected side effects such as nausea, vomiting, anorexia, and headaches. If nausea occurs, instruct him to take the medication after meals. Stress the need to report persistent side effects.

Explain the use of corticosteroid therapy, if prescribed. Give instruction on dose, frequency, and side effects.

In the case of the patient who does not have active immunity against mumps, stress the importance of promptly seeking medical care if exposed to mumps. Be certain that he understands that he has a 25% chance of acquiring mumps orchitis with exposure. Explain that gamma globulin is usually given at the time of exposure and, although it may not prevent him from acquiring mumps, the disease is likely to be less severe and there is a reduced risk for complications.

Evaluation

Evaluate the effectiveness of nursing care for a patient with orchitis by comparing the patient's status with the expected patient outcomes. Examples of specific outcomes for patients with orchitis have been provided in the Planning section.

Prostatitis

Prostatitis refers to an inflammation of the prostate gland. Prostatic inflammations are common and are classified as acute bacterial, chronic bacterial, nonbacterial, or prostatodynia.

Table 46–2. ETIOLOGY AND PATHOPHYSIOLOGY OF PROSTATITIS

TYPE OF PROSTATITIS	ETIOLOGY	PATHOPHYSIOLOGY
Acute bacterial	*Escherichia coli* (most common), *Klebsiella, Proteus, Streptococcus, Staphylococcus, Pseudomonas, Mycobacterium tuberculosis* Usually caused by ascending urethral infection Often associated with urethral instrumentation or catheterization	Diffuse inflammation with edema and hyperemia involving part or all of the prostate May progress to abscess formation or hemorrhage Complications: epididymo-orchitis, septicemia, urinary retention
Chronic bacterial	Sequela of acute bacterial prostatitis, complication of prostatic enlargement and obstruction	Inflammatory reaction is less marked and more focal than in acute bacterial prostatitis May progress to fibrosis, scarring, contraction of the vesical neck and prostatic calculi Complication: epididymitis
Nonbacterial	Cause: Unknown Often occurs in young, sexually active males after an episode of nonspecific urethritis Suggested causes include allergic or autoimmune response, sexually transmitted *Chlamydia* or other unknown pathogen	Similar to chronic bacterial prostatitis; in addition, increased number of leukocytes and macrophages containing fat in the prostatic secretions
Prostatodynia	Cause: Unknown May be associated with inadequate relaxation of the perineal muscles May be psychogenic	No abnormal findings

ETIOLOGY AND PATHOPHYSIOLOGY

Acute bacterial prostatitis is usually caused either by an ascending urethral infection or by bacterial invasion via the blood or lymph. Chronic bacterial prostatitis may result from an episode of acute bacterial prostatitis or from prostatic enlargement and obstruction.

Nonbacterial prostatitis is the most common type. It is frequently found in young, sexually active males and often occurs after an episode of nonspecific urethritis.

Prostatodynia refers to the presence of symptoms of prostatitis in the absence of physical findings. This condition is seen mainly in men between 20 and 45 years of age.

Further information on the causes and pathophysiology of prostatitis is presented in Table 46–2.

CLINICAL MANIFESTATIONS

Symptoms of all types of prostatitis include urgency of urination, frequency of urination, nocturia, dysuria, and dull pain in the perineal and rectal area. With acute and chronic bacterial prostatitis, urethral discharge, myalgia, and arthralgia also occur. Chills and fever are also prominent manifestations of acute, bacterial disease, whereas painful ejaculations may occur with nonbacterial prostatitis.

MEDICAL DIAGNOSIS

Diagnosis of acute bacterial prostatitis is made on the basis of presenting symptoms, rectal examination, and analysis of prostatic fluid or urine.

In acute bacterial prostatitis, the prostate is warm, tender, and swollen on palpation, and pyuria is found on urinalysis. Prostatic fluid studies are not done because massage of the prostate, which is required to obtain the specimen, is painful and could cause bacteremia.

Pus cells in the prostatic fluid smear in a sequential bacteriologic localization study are characteristic of chronic bacterial prostatitis.

The diagnosis of nonbacterial prostatitis is supported by increased numbers of leukocytes in prostatic secretions and postmassage urine in the presence of negative cultures.

MEDICAL MANAGEMENT

Medical management varies with the type of prostatitis. The basic treatment for acute bacterial prostatitis is co-trimoxazole DS (double strength), which, unless a change in antibiotic is indicated by the results of cultures and sensitivity, is continued for 30 days. Also used are fluoroquinolone agents such as ciprofloxacin hydrochloride, which have recently been shown to be highly effective in treating acute bacterial prostatitis. In addition, analgesics, antipyretics, anticholinergics such as oxybutynin chloride for relief of urinary symptoms, stool softeners, bed rest, sitz baths, and sexual abstinence are prescribed.

Chronic bacterial prostatitis is also treated with co-trimoxazole DS, taken twice daily for 4 to 16 weeks as the drug of choice. If symptoms persist, co-trimoxazole SS (single strength) or nitrofurantoin, 100 mg daily, is prescribed long term along with regular prostatic massage to release necrotic cells, bacteria, and other debris. If these measures are not effective, prostatectomy may be necessary.

Nonbacterial prostatitis is difficult to treat because the cause is unknown. A trial course with an antibiotic such as erythromycin or tetracycline may be tried in case a nonidentified, susceptible organism is involved. Otherwise, treatment consists of oxybutynin chloride, nonsteroidal anti-inflammatory agents such as indomethacin or ibuprofen, and sitz baths for comfort. Normal sexual activity is encouraged.

The aim of treatment of prostatodynia is relaxation of the perineal muscles. Thus, an alpha-blocking agent such as prazosin or a muscle relaxant such as diazepam is ordered.

Application of the Nursing Process to the Care of the Patient with Prostatitis

Assessment

Obtain a pertinent history, and determine the current status of the patient's symptoms. In particular, collect data about the location and intensity of pain; voiding symptoms such as dysuria, frequency, nocturia, and so on; and the presence of any urethral discharge.

Take an oral temperature, and review relevant laboratory data including white blood cell count and urine and prostatic fluid analyses reports.

If the patient's history indicates his prostatitis is recurrent, obtain information concerning medications taken and comfort measures used.

Assess the patient's ability to handle discomfort and his emotional reaction to the illness. Determine whether he has concerns that this disorder may impair normal sexual and reproductive functions.

Also determine the patient's understanding of his problem, its cause if known, the therapeutic plan, and prevention of recurrences.

Nursing Diagnoses and Planning

Nursing diagnoses and related expected patient outcomes most commonly applicable to patients with prostatitis include the following:

NDx: Pain related to the inflammatory response

Planning: Patient outcomes
1. Patient states the intensity of pain has decreased or the pain is gone.
2. Patient appears to be comfortable as indicated by such factors as a relaxed body posture and blood pressure and pulse within normal limits.
3. Patient reports specific urinary symptoms have decreased or disappeared.

NDx: Anxiety related to outcome of disease and the possible impact on sexual functioning

Planning: Patient outcomes
1. Patient states he feels less anxious and is more relaxed.
2. Patient engages in diversional activities.
3. Patient readily expresses his concerns.

NDx: High risk for altered health maintenance related to insufficient knowledge of treatment plan, prevention of recurrences if possible, and self-care activities for control of symptoms

Planning: Patient outcomes
1. Patient discusses the plan of care including bed rest, if ordered, drug therapy, frequency of the medication, side effects to report, and comfort measures.
2. Patient discusses the need for possible restriction of certain foods and fluids.
3. Patient describes measures to prevent recurrences such as compliance with prescribed drug therapy, drinking at least 2000 ml of fluid daily, and promptly seeking medical attention if symptoms of urinary tract infection occur.

Nursing Interventions

NDx: Pain

For the patient hospitalized with prostatitis, administer prescribed analgesics according to the physician's order and the patient's need. If a nonsteroidal anti-inflammatory drug such as ibuprofen or indomethacin is also ordered, ensure that the medication is taken with meals or milk to avoid gastric irritation.

Administer anticholinergic drugs as ordered for discomfort associated with voiding. Monitor response, and observe for side effects such as dysphagia, thirst, blurred vision, tachycardia, and urinary retention.

For the patient with prostatodynia who is receiving an alpha-blocking drug such as prazosin for control of perineal discomfort and voiding symptoms, monitor blood pressure closely. Before giving the medication, take blood pressure in both the supine and standing positions because orthostatic hypotension and syncope may occur as side effects. Report any marked deviation of the systolic and diastolic pressures, and withhold the drug.

Give sitz baths if ordered for control of pain and spasm. Also administer prescribed stool softeners so that straining at stool, which may increase the pain, is avoided. Encourage the patient to drink six to eight glasses of water or other fluid daily to help keep the feces soft and to help dilute the urine so it will not exacerbate any bladder or urethral irritation.

NDx: Anxiety

Provide time to allow for expression of concerns and feelings. Reassure the patient that sexual and reproductive functions are not impaired. In the case of acute bacterial prostatitis for which sexual abstinence is ordered, explain that this restriction is in effect only until the inflammation is resolved. For the patient with prostatitis other than the acute bacterial type, encourage sexual intercourse to provide for periodic emptying of the prostate. If a sexual partner is not available, suggest the use of masturbation.

In the case of prostatitis that cannot be resolved, explain that the condition is not communicable and is not associated with an increased incidence of cancer.

NDx: High risk for altered health maintenance
Provide information regarding the use of antibiotic therapy. Depending on the type of prostatitis, explain that the purpose of the therapy is either to eliminate the infecting organism or to control symptoms.

If co-trimoxazole (Bactrim, Septra) is ordered, explain the need to drink at least eight full glasses of liquid daily. Explain that the drug is excreted primarily through the kidneys, and adequate urine production is essential to avoid crystals forming within the urinary tract.

Because co-trimoxazole or another antimicrobial is frequently continued for a time after discharge from the hospital, emphasize the importance of taking the medication at the prescribed time and for the length of time indicated by the physician.

In the case of prostatodynia, in which an alpha-blocking drug is to be taken after discharge, explain why the drug is ordered and the effect it may have on the blood pressure. To avoid postural hypotension, instruct the patient to rise slowly when changing from a lying to a sitting position and, if lightheadedness occurs, to lie down.

Inform the patient with chronic bacterial prostatitis that periodic gentle prostate massage may be performed by the physician to release any pus cells and bacteria that may be present.

Advise about the need for restricting certain fluids and foods if they are associated with an increase in severity of symptoms. For example, alcohol, caffeinated beverages, and foods containing hot spices may exacerbate the symptoms by increasing prostate secretions.

To prevent a recurrence of bacterial prostatitis, stress the need for a fluid intake of at least 2 L daily. Explain that this decreases the risk of urinary tract infection and the reappearance of the prostatitis.

Finally, instruct the patient to contact the physician if any of the symptoms of acute bacterial prostatitis reappear or if there is any intensifying of symptoms in the case of chronic bacterial prostatitis, nonbacterial prostatitis, and prostatodynia.

Additional Interventions
When bed rest is prescribed, assistance with hygiene, toileting, and diversional activities is necessary. To facilitate compliance with the bed-rest order, explain that the purpose of remaining in bed is to decrease the swelling and pain in and around the prostate.

Evaluation

Evaluate the effectiveness of nursing care for a patient with prostatitis by comparing the patient's status with the expected patient outcomes. Examples of specific outcomes for patients with prostatitis have been provided in the Planning section.

Structural Disorders

Phimosis

Phimosis is a disorder in which the foreskin (prepuce) cannot be retracted over the glans penis (Fig. 46–2).

ETIOLOGY AND PATHOPHYSIOLOGY

Phimosis may be congenital or acquired. It is found in the child when the natural separation of the foreskin from the glans fails to occur. In the adult, it develops as a complication of recurrent infection of the glans and foreskin (balanoposthitis) as a result of fibrosis and scar formation, which make the foreskin tight and inelastic.

Complications of phimosis include constriction of the penile blood vessels and stenosis of the meatus.

CLINICAL MANIFESTATIONS

In addition to a nonretractable foreskin, signs of infection such as swelling, redness, purulent discharge, and pain may be present. Painful erections may also occur.

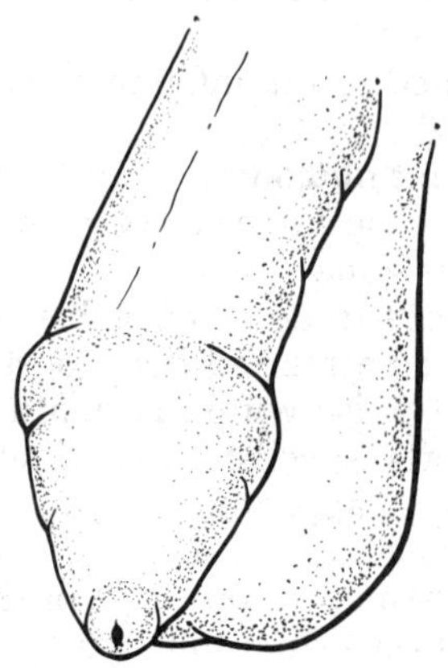

Figure 46–2.

Phimosis. Foreskin contracts over the tip of the meatus, resulting in a narrowed opening.

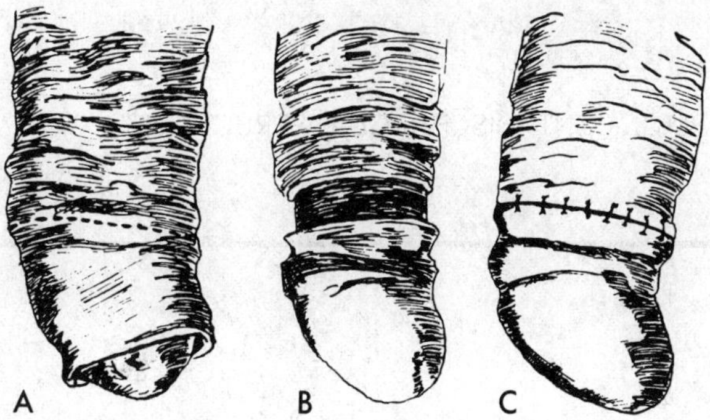

Figure 46–3.

Surgical procedure for circumcision. (From Meeker MH, Rothrock JC. Alexander's care of the patient in surgery. 9th ed. St. Louis: Mosby–Year Book, 1992, p 351.)

If stenosis of the urinary meatus develops, there is decreased urinary flow, dysuria, and straining to void.

MEDICAL DIAGNOSIS

Diagnosis of phimosis is made on the basis of the patient's complaints and inspection of the penis.

MEDICAL MANAGEMENT

When phimosis causes an obstruction to urination, a dorsal slit of the foreskin may be necessary as an emergency measure. A meatotomy may also be needed at this time. Antibiotics and warm soaks are ordered for the infection. After obstruction and infection have been resolved, a circumcision is usually recommended to prevent recurrence.

CIRCUMCISION

In the adult, circumcision is usually performed under regional anesthesia. The outer and inner surfaces of the foreskin are incised, any adhesions are dissected away, and the appropriate amount of foreskin is excised. Absorbable sutures are used to approximate the two surfaces of the foreskin (Fig. 46–3). A nonadherent dressing such as Vaseline gauze is then applied.

Potential complications of circumcision are temporary hyperesthesia of the glans (increased sensation), infection, and the formation of a subcutaneous hematoma.

Preoperative Preparation

Although circumcision is usually performed under local anesthesia, food and fluids may be withheld beginning about 6 hours before the surgery to allow the use of general anesthesia if necessary. A preoperative antianxiety agent such as diazepam (Valium) may be prescribed. The penile area is shaved, usually in the operating room.

Postoperative Course

Length of stay after a circumcision is short; the patient may be discharged the same day the surgery is performed.

Pain is usually managed with oxycodone hydrochloride and acetaminophen (Percocet) and then acetaminophen as the intensity of the pain diminishes. Ice packs to the penile area may be ordered for 24 hours to decrease the edema and discomfort.

A dry dressing may cover the Vaseline gauze and may need to be changed with each voiding. A warm tub bath may be ordered for cleansing the penile wound on the second or third day postoperatively. Sexual intercourse is usually permitted 1 week after surgery.

Application of the Nursing Process to the Care of the Patient Having a Circumcision

PREOPERATIVE NURSING CARE

Provide basic preoperative care as described in Chapter 4. Be sensitive to the patient's need for privacy, and be certain he knows his penis will be edematous for several days postoperatively.

POSTOPERATIVE NURSING CARE

Assessment

After the circumcision, make standard postoperative assessments, with special attention to observing the dressing for bleeding. If there is no dressing, observe the penis for edema, bleeding, and the development of a hematoma. Assess for presence and degree of pain. Monitor urinary output closely, especially the first voiding, to ensure that the urethra is patent.

Nursing Diagnoses and Planning

Nursing diagnoses and related expected patient outcomes most commonly applicable to patients who have had a circumcision include the following:

NDx: Pain (penile) related to surgery

Planning: Patient outcomes
1. Patient uses ice-pack applications as directed.
2. Patient reports the pain is gone or decreased.
3. Patient appears comfortable; he does not grimace or groan.

Chart 46–2.

NURSING GUIDE TO PATIENT EDUCATION FOR SELF-MANAGEMENT: DISCHARGE INSTRUCTIONS AFTER CIRCUMCISION

Instruct the patient to do the following:

Apply ice packs as ordered.
Reapply the petroleum jelly (Vaseline) dressing for the length of time ordered.
Wash hands well before changing the dressing.
Touch the glans gently because hyperesthesia may be present.
Observe for any discharge or hematoma formation, and, if present, immediately notify the physician.
Take a warm tub bath on the second or third day to cleanse the penile area.

Remind the patient of the following:

Edema of his penis will disappear within a few days.
Sexual intercourse may be resumed in 1 week.
Sutures are absorbable.

NDx: High risk for urinary retention related to edema of the meatus

Planning: Patient outcomes
1. Patient voids at least 200 ml of urine within 6 hours after surgery.
2. Urinary stream is normal in force and size.

NDx: High risk for infection related to penile surgery

Planning: Patient outcomes
1. Foul-smelling or purulent drainage is absent.
2. Temperature is within normal limits.

NDx: High risk for altered health maintenance related to insufficient knowledge of postdischarge self-care activities

Planning: Patient outcomes
1. Patient describes the care of the wound.
2. Patient describes the signs of a developing infection or subcutaneous hematoma.
3. Patient states when sexual intercourse may be resumed.

Nursing Interventions

NDx: Pain
Administer analgesics as prescribed and according to the patient's need. Apply ice packs to the penis if ordered.

Caution the patient to avoid touching the glans because it can increase his pain and contaminate the wound.

NDx: High risk for urinary retention
To facilitate resumption of a normal voiding pattern, encourage fluids and make them available on the bedside table. Leave the urinal within easy reach, and instruct the patient to notify a nurse the first time he voids so that output can be measured and patency of the meatus validated. If the patient needs to assume the standing position to void, provide assistance as necessary. If the patient has not voided within 6 hours of surgery, inform the physician. Catheterization may be necessary to relieve the urinary retention.

NDx: High risk for infection
Reapply Vaseline gauze and outer dressings when wet or soiled in accordance with the physician's orders. Instruct the patient to wash his hands thoroughly before handling the penis for urination and to avoid touching the operative area.

NDx: High risk for altered health maintenance
Instruct the patient as specified in Chart 46–2 regarding self-care activities after discharge.

Evaluation

Evaluate the effectiveness of nursing care for a patient who has had a circumcision by comparing the patient's status with the expected patient outcomes.

Examples of specific outcomes for patients who have had a circumcision have been provided in the Planning section.

Paraphimosis

Paraphimosis is a condition in which the uncircumcised foreskin is retracted over the glans penis and cannot be easily returned to its normal position.

ETIOLOGY AND PATHOPHYSIOLOGY

The cause of paraphimosis is usually chronic balanoposthitis. The accumulation of scar tissue under the foreskin inhibits its flexibility so that, when retracted, it cannot be easily pulled down over the glans. The retracted foreskin quickly develops into a constricting ring around the glans, with subsequent venous occlusion and possible arterial obstruction.

Paraphimosis may also occur after urethral instrumentation if the foreskin is retracted and left in that position.

Complications of paraphimosis include urethral obstruction and gangrene of the glans.

CLINICAL MANIFESTATIONS

When a constricted foreskin is allowed to remain in a retracted position, penile edema accompanied by severe pain develops (Fig. 46–4). If the obstruction is not quickly relieved, the glans becomes bluish as a result of impaired blood supply.

MEDICAL DIAGNOSIS

Diagnosis is made on the basis of inspection of the penis and palpation of the foreskin for the constricting ring.

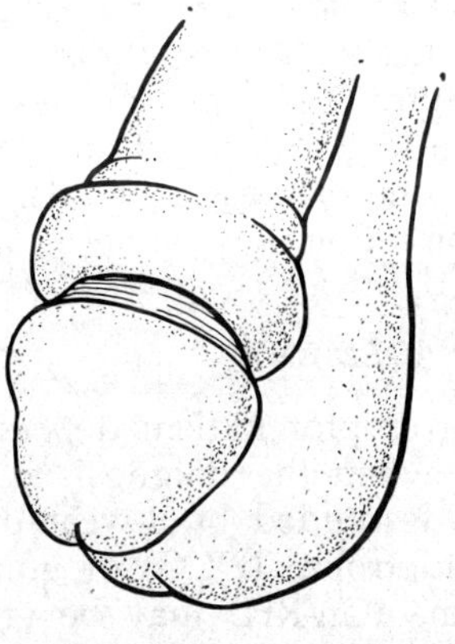

Figure 46–4.

Paraphimosis.

MEDICAL MANAGEMENT

Manual reduction is the treatment of choice for paraphimosis. Before it is attempted, the penis may be elevated and cool compresses applied to decrease some of the edema. Using 4% lidocaine ointment for local anesthesia, the penis is squeezed in a gloved hand for 5 minutes to try to reduce the size of the glans. Then the glans penis is pushed back while the foreskin is pulled down over it. If this is unsuccessful, emergency surgery is necessary. A dorsal slit into the constricting ring of the foreskin is made to prevent necrosis of the glans. To prevent recurrence, a circumcision may be recommended.

Application of the Nursing Process to the Care of the Patient with Paraphimosis

Assessment

Inspect the glans penis, noting color and edema, and palpate for a constricting ring. Assess for pain, and ask the patient when he last voided. Question about any decrease in size or force of the stream. Elicit any history of infection of the foreskin and glans as well as a description of usual hygienic care of the penis.

Nursing Diagnoses and Planning

Nursing diagnoses and related expected patient outcomes most commonly applicable to patients with paraphimosis include the following:

NDx: Pain (penile) related to a constricted, retracted foreskin

Planning: Patient outcomes
1. Patient reports pain or soreness is decreased.
2. Patient describes use of comfort measures for residual soreness.

NDx: High risk for altered health maintenance related to insufficient knowledge of hygienic care of the penis

Planning: Patient outcomes
1. Patient describes the technique of cleaning the glans penis.
2. Patient verbally indicates an intent to carry out daily penile hygiene.
3. Patient describes the importance of preventing infections of the glans and foreskin.

NDx: High risk for urinary retention related to penile edema

Planning: Patient outcomes

1. Patient's urinary stream is of normal size and force.
2. Patient is free of bladder distention after voiding.

Nursing Interventions

NDx: Pain

Administer a narcotic analgesic if ordered before manual reduction. This is generally needed when treatment has been delayed and manual reduction is not expected to be easy.

For residual soreness, instruct the patient to elevate the penis and to apply cool compresses to help reduce remaining edema. Review the correct use of any non-narcotic analgesic, such as acetaminophen, that is ordered.

NDx: High risk for altered health maintenance

If circumcision is not performed, instruct the patient to cleanse the glans, as specified in Chart 46–1. Stress the importance of complying with this routine to prevent balanoposthitis and recurrence of paraphimosis.

NDx: High risk for urinary retention

After reduction of the foreskin, ask the patient to void. Assist him to stand and, if possible, use the toilet rather than the urinal because this is more comfortable and will facilitate voiding, especially if the glans is still painful and edematous.

Evaluation

Evaluate the effectiveness of nursing care for a patient with paraphimosis by comparing the patient's status with the expected patient outcomes. Examples of specific outcomes for patients with paraphimosis have been provided in the Planning section.

Cryptorchidism

Cryptorchidism is the failure of one or both of the testes to descend into the scrotum shortly before birth.

ETIOLOGY AND PATHOPHYSIOLOGY

The cause of cryptorchidism is unclear but may be related either to an abnormality in the hypothalamic-pituitary-testicular axis resulting in a deficiency of circulating testosterone or to certain structural problems such as a short spermatic cord occurring during fetal development. Some evidence suggests that sons of mothers who have taken DES may be born with undescended testes. It occurs in 30% of premature male newborns and in less than 3% of full-term males. In the majority of these cases, the testes descend spontaneously during the first year, resulting in an 0.8% incidence of true cryptorchidism.

Complications of cryptorchidism include infertility, testicular cancer, and torsion of the testis. The undescended testis is also frequently associated with an inguinal hernia on the affected side.

Infertility occurs because spermatogenesis depends on the cooler temperature found in the scrotum. Failure of the testes to descend results in a progressive decrease in sperm production until it ceases completely when puberty is complete.

All males with bilateral cryptorchidism whose testes were not positioned in the scrotum before 2 years of age and more than 60% of those treated before this age are infertile. Infertility also occurs in up to 50% of males with unilateral cryptorchidism even when surgically corrected, suggesting that the opposite testis is congenitally abnormal.

Cancer occurs 10 times more often in a cryptorchid testis than in a normal testis. If a malignant change develops, it presents after a latent period, most often between 30 and 40 years of age. Those at greatest risk include males with untreated cryptorchidism and those treated after 8 years of age. Seminoma is the type of malignant tumor most likely to develop.

Torsion of the undescended testis (twisting of the spermatic cord that suspends the testis) may develop because of excessive mobility of the testis. Because torsion interrupts the blood supply to the testis, surgery must be quickly performed to maintain testicular function.

CLINICAL MANIFESTATIONS

The major clinical manifestation of cryptorchidism is the absence of one or both of the testes from the scrotal sac. This is associated with atrophy of the scrotum on the affected side.

MEDICAL DIAGNOSIS

Diagnosis of cryptorchidism is easily made by inspection and palpation of the scrotum. If the undescended testis cannot be palpated lying in the inguinal canal, tests such as ultrasonography, computed tomography (CT) scan, and testicular angiography are done to locate it within the body. If it is not located by one of these methods, a laparoscopy or surgical exploration may be necessary.

MEDICAL MANAGEMENT

Treatment of cryptorchidism depends on the age of the patient when the diagnosis is made. If the testis has not descended by 1 year of age, human chorionic gonadotropin (HCG) or gonadotropin releasing hormone (Gn-RH) may be given to try to stimulate its descent. If this is not successful by 2 years of age, surgical placement of the testis in the scrotum (orchiopexy) is done to avoid testicular degeneration, which occurs after this age.

Chart 46–3.

NURSING GUIDE TO PATIENT EDUCATION FOR SELF-MANAGEMENT: DISCHARGE INSTRUCTIONS AFTER ORCHIOPEXY

Instruct the patient to do the following:

Dry the groin and scrotal areas gently after bathing or showering to avoid disrupting the incision. (Tell him not to worry, however, if the Steri-Strips fall off in a few days, because this is expected and will not interfere with wound healing).

Wear an athletic support to elevate the scrotum and to promote comfort.

Avoid strenuous physical activity and heavy lifting for 6 weeks or until otherwise instructed.

Avoid driving for 2 weeks.

Report immediately any redness, increased tenderness, or drainage from either the inguinal or scrotal incisions.

Return for a follow-up appointment on *(specify date and time).*

Perform monthly testicular self-examination because the risk of testicular cancer is increased in cryptorchidism even when surgically treated.

If cryptorchidism remains undetected until adulthood, the treatment is orchiopexy, which is done primarily to provide cosmetic enhancement and to facilitate early detection of a testicular malignancy. An alternative to orchiopexy is orchiectomy (removal of the testis). This is done if a malignancy is suspected or if the testis is found to be atrophied.

ORCHIOPEXY

The surgical approach to orchiopexy can vary with the location of the cryptorchid testis but most often involves an inguinal incision on the affected side to free the spermatic cord of any adhesions and to repair the associated hernia. This is followed by an incision at the top of the scrotum and creation of a subdartos pouch. The testis is then mobilized, brought down, and implanted in the pouch with a traction suture holding it in place. The incision is closed with absorbable sutures, and Steri-Strips are applied as the dressing.

Guidelines for Application of the Nursing Process to the Care of the Patient Having an Orchiopexy

Nursing care of the patient having an orchiopexy is similar to that of the patient having a testicular biopsy and to that of the patient having an inguinal herniorrhaphy. In addition, after surgery elevate the scrotum on a Bellevue bridge while the patient is in bed to limit edema and discomfort, and apply an athletic support for ambulation. Give medication such as meperidine hydrochloride (Demerol) or oxycodone hydrochloride and acetaminophen (Percocet) as ordered for pain during the first 24 hours postoperatively. Instruct the patient in self-care after discharge, as specified in Chart 46–3.

Both preoperatively and postoperatively, carefully assess the patient's emotional state. Depending on the circumstances, there may be a great deal of anger that the condition was not diagnosed and treated earlier and that he is now infertile. Added to this is the stress of surgery and the increased risk of cancer. Refer the patient to a mental health professional or support group as needed.

Priapism

Priapism is a prolonged, uncontrolled erection of the penis that is not associated with tactile stimulation or sexual desire.

ETIOLOGY

Priapism can be due to conditions such as sickle cell anemia, leukemia, multiple sclerosis, and local and metastatic tumors encroaching on the penile veins. It may also occur as a side effect of certain drugs including the phenothiazines, hydralazine, prazosin, heparin, alcohol, and marijuana. In most cases, however, its cause is unknown.

PATHOPHYSIOLOGY

In priapism, penile enlargement is prolonged as a result of an obstruction to the outflow of blood from the corpora cavernosa. This venous congestion within the cavernosa results in thrombosis and fibrosis, which can lead to impotence, urinary retention, and penile necrosis.

CLINICAL MANIFESTATIONS

With priapism, the penis is very large and hard, and there is severe, constant penile pain. If arterial circulation is impaired, the penis may also be cold and pale because of ischemia. Priapism is often present for hours or days before treatment is sought.

MEDICAL DIAGNOSIS

Diagnosis of priapism is made on the basis of the presenting symptoms and the patient's associated medical history.

MEDICAL MANAGEMENT

Because of the risk of impotence and penile necrosis, priapism is viewed as a urologic emergency. Immediate treatment usually includes analgesia, sedation, and local cold applications to try to reduce penile congestion. If the patient is unable to void and the bladder is distended, a urethral catheter is inserted. If the obstruction is such that this is not possible, suprapubic drainage is instituted. Hydration therapy may be ordered, especially if sickle-cell disease is present because dehydration may lead to more sickling, thus further compromising the venous outflow from the corpora cavernosa. Needle aspiration of the cavernosa for clots and blood may be performed for decompression and for detumescence.

In cases in which a cause is identified, the underlying condition is treated in an attempt to reverse the priapism. For example, if priapism is drug induced, the medication is promptly discontinued. If priapism is due to a metastatic process, chemotherapy or radiation may be used. Surgery is performed if priapism is not reversed within 48 hours of onset to decrease the risk of subsequent impotence. The procedure with the greatest success rate creates a venous fistula to shunt blood from both corpora cavernosa to the corpus spongiosum. This is quickly performed with a biopsy needle or a narrow knife blade under local anesthesia. If impotence develops as a complication, a penile implant may be recommended.

Application of the Nursing Process to the Care of the Patient with Priapism

Assessment

Ask the patient how long his penis has been in a continuous erectile state. Also ask about the presence and severity of pain. Assess for early signs of ischemia, noting color and temperature of the penis. Determine when the patient last urinated and whether he noticed any change in the amount or force of the stream. If urinary retention is suspected, palpate the suprapubic area for bladder distention.

As the medical plan of care is implemented, assess the patient's understanding of it and the expected outcomes. If surgery is planned, determine the patient's understanding of the purpose and nature of the procedure.

Nursing Diagnoses and Planning

Nursing diagnoses and related expected patient outcomes most commonly applicable to patients with priapism include the following:

NDx: Pain (penile) related to circulatory changes in the penis

Planning: Patient outcomes
1. Patient reports the pain is diminished.
2. Patient appears more comfortable; he does not grimace or moan and is less restless.
3. Patient's blood pressure, pulse, and respiration are within his normal range.

NDx: High risk for urinary retention related to urethral obstruction

Planning: Patient outcomes
1. Patient initiates voiding on need.
2. Bladder distention is absent.

NDx: High risk for sexual dysfunction related to vascular changes in the penis

Planning: Patient outcomes
1. Patient expresses his concerns about the effect priapism may have on subsequent sexual function.
2. Patient discusses concerns and prognosis with sexual partner.
3. Patient lists alternative methods of sexual expression.
4. Patient describes the role of a penile implant in treating impotence.

Nursing Interventions

NDx: Pain

Give prescribed analgesic and sedatives promptly. If analgesics are ordered to be given as necessary (PRN), give before the pain becomes severe and difficult to control.

Apply cold packs to the penis if ordered. These control edema formation and can decrease pain perception according to the gate control theory.

Enhance the effectiveness of analgesic and sedative medications by maintaining a calm, quiet environment, maintaining general physical comfort, and guiding the patient in controlled breathing exercises.

NDx: High risk for urinary retention
Facilitate voiding by assisting the patient to a standing position, providing for privacy, and using the power of suggestion (e.g., running water or giving a cold drink). Record time and amount of voiding. Report to the physician signs of urinary retention such as a palpable bladder or voiding of small amounts.

NDx: High risk for sexual dysfunction
Provide time for the patient to ask questions and express his concerns about future sexual performance. If he sought treatment immediately, stress that the incidence of impotence is greatly diminished when priapism is resolved within 12 hours of onset. If he delayed seeking treatment and impotence is suspected, discuss alternate methods of sexual expression such as touching, closeness, and orogenital stimulation, and provide information on the use of a penile implant as a method of treatment for impotence. Encourage discussion with his sexual partner if available, and refer to a sex therapist if needed.

Evaluation

Evaluate the effectiveness of nursing care for a patient with priapism by comparing the patient's status with the expected patient outcomes. Examples of specific outcomes for patients with priapism have been provided in the Planning section.

Hydrocele

Hydrocele is an abnormal collection of fluid within the layers of the tunica vaginalis, which surrounds the testis (Fig. 46–5). It may be unilateral or bilateral and may occur in an infant or adult.

ETIOLOGY

Hydrocele can occur secondary to epididymo-orchitis, scrotal trauma, or a testicular neoplasm, but in the majority of cases it is idiopathic.

PATHOPHYSIOLOGY

Normally, the space between the two layers of the tunica vaginalis contains only a few milliliters of clear, serous fluid, the formation and reabsorption of which is constant. A hydrocele occurs when there is either an increased production or decreased reabsorption of this fluid. The size of the hydrocele depends on the extent of the imbalance between production and reabsorption. A large hydrocele can impair physical and sexual activity and may compromise the blood supply to the testis, leading to testicular atrophy.

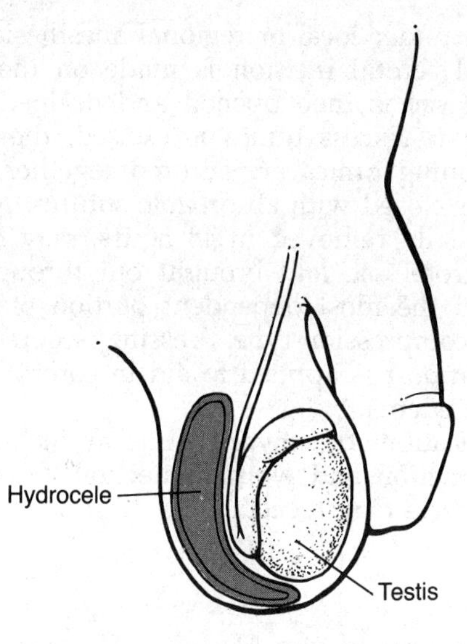

Figure 46–5.

Hydrocele.

Characteristics of the fluid in the hydrocele sac can differ depending on its cause. For example, fluid related to a testicular neoplasm is usually clear yellow, whereas fluid associated with infection may be cloudy and contain bacteria.

CLINICAL MANIFESTATIONS

Painless swelling of the scrotum is the classic sign of hydrocele except when caused by an infection.

MEDICAL DIAGNOSIS

Diagnosis of hydrocele is made on the basis of the patient's history, physical examination, and transillumination of the scrotum.

MEDICAL MANAGEMENT

Treatment is usually unnecessary for small hydroceles that are not causing any particular discomfort. Treatment may also be unnecessary for some large hydroceles because they may spontaneously disappear as the underlying condition is resolved.

When treatment is required because of size and discomfort, the most conservative approach is to aspirate the fluid. A sclerosing drug such as sodium tetradecyl or urea hydrochloride may then be injected into the scrotal sac. Because some hydroceles recur, this treatment may need to be repeated every few months, and in some cases a hydrocelectomy may be indicated.

HYDROCELECTOMY

A hydrocelectomy is the excision of a fluid-filled sac of the tunica vaginalis. In the adult, this is usually done under local or regional anesthesia. An anterolateral scrotal incision is made on the affected side. The sac is then opened and drained through the incision. Excess tunica is excised, the edges of the remaining tunica are sutured together, and the incision is closed with absorbable sutures. A Penrose drain, usually removed in 48 hours, may be placed in the scrotal sac and brought out through a stab wound in the most dependent portion of the scrotum. A compression-type dressing secured with a scrotal support is applied to aid in controlling postoperative edema.

Complications of a hydrocelectomy include hematoma formation and wound infection. Occasionally, the hydrocele may reoccur.

Application of the Nursing Process to the Care of the Patient Having a Hydrocelectomy

PREOPERATIVE NURSING CARE

Nursing care of the patient scheduled for a hydrocelectomy includes all the basic assessments and interventions for any patient undergoing surgery. If a knowledge deficit or anxiety state exists, provide information as needed, and give the patient the opportunity to explain his concerns.

POSTOPERATIVE NURSING CARE

Assessment

Make standard postoperative assessments as discussed in Chapter 4. Also determine the degree of scrotal edema, and note color and amount of any wound drainage.

Nursing Diagnoses and Planning

Nursing diagnoses and related expected patient outcomes most commonly applicable to patients having a hydrocelectomy include the following:

NDx: Pain (scrotal) related to surgery and associated edema

Planning: Patient outcomes

1. Patient requests medication for pain control as needed.
2. Patient maintains scrotal elevation.
3. Patient maintains cold-pack applications as directed.
4. Patient reports pain has decreased or disappeared.

NDx: High risk for altered health maintenance related to insufficient knowledge of self-care after discharge

Planning: Patient outcomes

1. Patient describes the procedure for application of cold packs to scrotum.
2. Patient describes or demonstrates changing of the scrotal wound dressing.
3. Patient states the reasons for keeping scrotum elevated.
4. Patient lists symptoms to be reported that are indicative of a wound complication (e.g., fever, increased local pain and tenderness, purulent drainage, localized swelling, bleeding).

Nursing Interventions

NDx: Pain

Give prescribed analgesic for pain as needed. Apply ice packs to the scrotum as ordered to control postoperative swelling and accompanying pain.

Maintain elevation of the scrotum by ensuring that the scrotal support applied in the operating room is in place. Replace the support if soiled. Inform the patient that the use of the scrotal support helps to decrease or minimize postoperative edema and associated discomfort.

NDx: High risk for altered health maintenance

Generally, the length of the hospital stay for the patient with a hydrocelectomy is 24 hours or less. Therefore, preparing him for self-care after discharge is important.

Give instructions as specified in Chart 46–4 to help him care for the wound and detect potential complications.

Evaluation

Evaluate the effectiveness of nursing care for a patient who has had a hydrocelectomy by comparing the patient's status with the expected patient outcomes. Examples of specific outcomes for patients who have had a hydrocelectomy have been provided in the Planning section.

Varicocele

Varicocele is a cluster of dilated veins of the pampiniform plexus (Fig. 46–6), a network of veins originating from the spermatic veins, which supply the testes.

Chart 46–4.

NURSING GUIDE TO PATIENT EDUCATION FOR SELF-MANAGEMENT: POSTDISCHARGE CARE AFTER HYDROCELECTOMY

Instruct the patient to:

Apply ice packs to scrotum as directed.
Wash hands before changing dressing.
Remove soiled dressing, and cleanse wound gently with soap and water.
Observe for purulent or bloody discharge or localized swelling, and notify the physician if necessary.
Reapply a clean scrotal support.
Maintain elevation of scrotum until edema is resolved.

Remind the patient of the following:

Edema of the scrotum will disappear within 2 to 4 weeks.
Sutures are absorbable.
Avoid sexual intercourse and strenuous physical activity until directed by physician.
If drain is in place, it will be removed by physician.
To return for physician visit on *(specify date and time)*.

ETIOLOGY AND PATHOPHYSIOLOGY

Varicocele occurs predominantly between 15 and 40 years of age. It is generally considered to be idiopathic, although a defect in the valves of the spermatic vein has been suggested as a possible cause. The latter is consistent with the fact that varicoceles occur most often in the left side, and the left spermatic vein is under greater back pressure than the right.

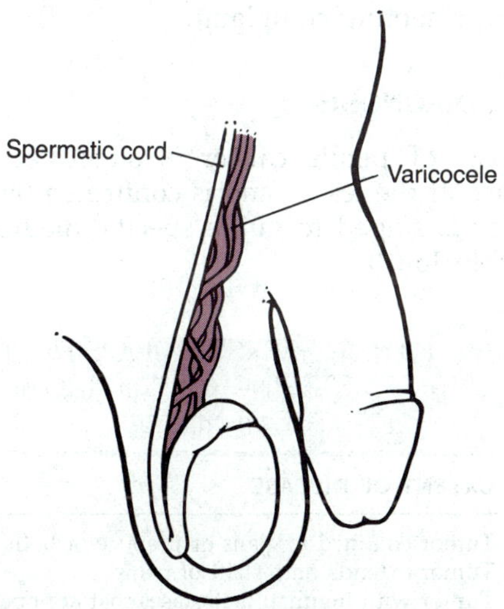

Figure 46–6.

Varicocele.

Varicocele is frequently associated with infertility, although the reason for this is not certain. One widely accepted explanation is that the venous enlargement increases the temperature within the scrotum and thus impairs sperm production and motility.

In men older than 40 years, development of a left varicocele is usually secondary to a left renal tumor, whereas development of a right varicocele suggests an obstructing abdominal mass because the right spermatic vein inserts into the vena cava.

CLINICAL MANIFESTATIONS

For many males, infertility is the only symptom. Others may complain of a feeling of heaviness or a dull ache in the scrotum on the affected side.

MEDICAL DIAGNOSIS

On physical examination, dilated, tortuous veins posterior to and above the affected testis may be palpated while the patient is in an upright position. In addition, when the patient performs a Valsalva maneuver, a rush of blood can be felt in the scrotum. A Doppler ultrasonogram or a venogram may be required to confirm the diagnosis.

MEDICAL MANAGEMENT

Discomfort can often be relieved merely by wearing a scrotal support. If this is not effective, or if infertility is a problem, a varicocelectomy is done.

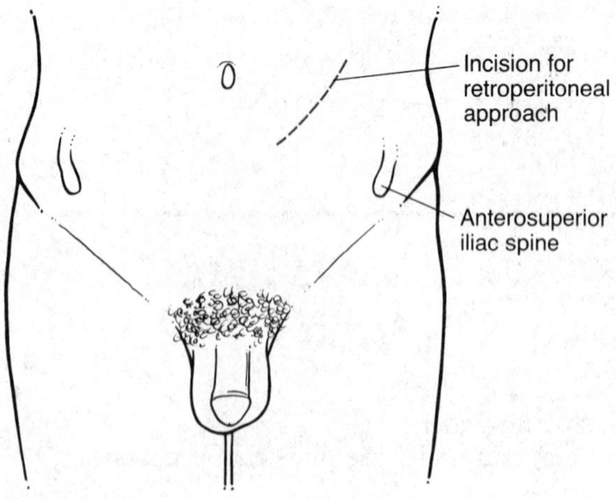

Figure 46–7.

Varicocelectomy: retroperitoneal approach.

VARICOCELECTOMY

There are two surgical approaches to varicocelectomy: inguinal or upper scrotal and retroperitoneal, in which a short incision is made medial to the anterior superior iliac spine (Fig. 46–7). In both approaches, the spermatic vein or its branches, or both, are ligated, and the venous collateral circulation is subsequently assumed by the deep pelvic venous system.

A varicocelectomy is usually done under local anesthesia. The incision is closed with either Dacron sutures or skin staples and is covered with a sterile dressing. A scrotal support is applied to decrease accompanying edema.

When varicocelectomy is performed on males with infertility, semen quality improves considerably; impregnation occurs in 35% to 50% of the cases reported.

Complications of a varicocelectomy are rare and include wound infection and formation of a hydrocele.

Guidelines for Application of the Nursing Process to the Care of the Patient Having a Varicocelectomy

Nursing care of the patient having a varicocelectomy is the same as that for the patient having a hydrocelectomy, with one additional consideration. If the patient is undergoing a varicocelectomy because of an associated infertility problem, he is likely to be highly anxious about its outcome. Preoperatively, determine the patient's understanding of the effects of varicocelectomy on fertility. Be certain that he understands that restoration of fertility cannot be guaranteed. Because the result may not be known for several months, be sure to provide time for him to express his concerns and his hopes.

Postoperatively, the patient is usually permitted to return home 4 to 6 hours after the surgery. Before discharge, give instructions regarding the prescribed analgesic, wound care, and development of possible complications. Instruct him to remain at home for about 5 days, to avoid driving for 7 days, to avoid strenuous physical activity for 3 weeks, and to return for a follow-up visit and suture removal in 1 week.

Neoplasia

Cancer of the Penis

ETIOLOGY AND PATHOPHYSIOLOGY

The precise cause of penile cancer is not known. However, in uncircumcised men with phimosis and poor personal hygiene, the chronic presence and irritation of smegma are thought to contribute to its development. Recently, penile cancer has also been found to be associated with cervical cancer; thus, an association with genital herpes is possible (Schellhammer et al, 1992, p 1271).

CLINICAL MANIFESTATIONS

Carcinoma of the penis initially presents as a small lesion or mass on the glans, the coronal sulcus, or the foreskin. It may appear as a pimple, a warty growth, a hardened or reddened area, or a lesion that proliferates outwardly on the surface epithelium of the penis. If not treated, the lesion may erode through the foreskin and emit a foul odor with purulent or sanguineous drainage. Pain is not usually a presenting complaint.

MEDICAL DIAGNOSIS

Diagnosis of penile cancer is suggested by the appearance of the lesion and is confirmed by biopsy. The tumor is staged to guide specific medical treatment (Table 46–3).

Table 46–3. JACKSON CLASSIFICATION FOR CLINICAL STAGING OF CARCINOMA OF THE PENIS

STAGE	EXTENT OF DISEASE
I	Tumor confined to glans or prepuce or both
II	Tumor extends onto shaft of penis
III	Tumor with inguinal metastases that are operable
IV	Tumor involving adjacent structures or tumor associated with inoperable inguinal or distant metastases

MEDICAL MANAGEMENT

Management of cancer of the penis is tailored to the individual patient, taking into consideration the stage of the disease, coexisting medical problems, and the patient's preference. Therapeutic options include circumcision, external radiation therapy, partial penectomy, total penectomy, lymphadenectomy, and chemotherapy.

Stage I cancer of the penis is almost 100% curable. Unfortunately, many males delay seeking treatment; up to 50% present with more advanced lesions. Consequently, cure rates are lower.

PENECTOMY

There are two types of penectomy: partial and total. Partial penectomy is performed if the lesion is located on the distal shaft of the penis or is limited to the glans. In this procedure, with the patient in a lithotomy position, a tourniquet is applied around the penis. The tumor area is demarcated, and an incision is made that amputates the corpora cavernosa, corpus spongiosum, and urethra. The remaining urethra and retracted skin flaps are sutured into a penile stump, which allows the patient to void in a normal, upright position and is serviceable for some sexual function. An indwelling catheter may be inserted at the time of surgery and left in place for 24 to 48 hours.

Total penectomy is performed for Stages II, III, and IV penile cancer when the lesion involves the proximal penile shaft such that a functional penile stump cannot be created. For this procedure, which is done in a lithotomy position, an incision is made from the pubis down and around the penis into the perineum. The roots of the corpora cavernosa are identified, the urethra is isolated, and the penis is amputated. Next, the urethra is brought out through the perineum, creating a perineal urethrostomy, which allows for voiding in a sitting position. A urethral catheter is inserted into the bladder through the perineal urethrostomy, an incisional drain is placed in the wound, and a compression dressing is applied to prevent scrotal edema (Fig. 46–8).

For some patients, phallic reconstruction using microneurovascular tissue transfers is possible after total penectomy.

Preoperative Preparation

Any infection in the tissue of the penis is treated with antibiotics and resolved before surgery is scheduled, because infection is associated with an increased risk of postoperative hemorrhage, tissue sloughing, and necrosis. The penile lesion is cleansed and, if extensive, is kept covered with a dry, sterile dressing to prevent contamination. A preoperative shave from umbilicus to midthigh may be ordered. If an ilioinguinal node dissection is planned, cleansing enemas and antiembolic stockings may also be ordered.

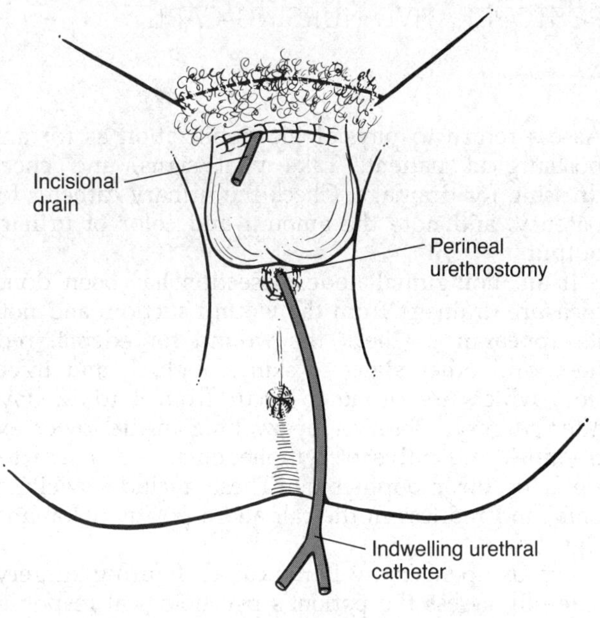

Figure 46–8.

Total penectomy: incision, drain, perineal urethrostomy.

Postoperative Course

After penectomy, compression dressings are in place for 36 to 48 hours and are reinforced as needed. When a total penectomy is done, the dressings are held firmly in place by a scrotal support. Drainage is expected and should be serosanguineous, not frankly bloody.

After ilioinguinal node dissection, percutaneous closed-catheter suction is in place in the wound to prevent accumulation of drainage. The patient is on bed rest for about a week with the legs elevated and is maintained on low-dose heparin or warfarin sodium therapy during this time.

Application of the Nursing Process to the Care of the Patient Having a Penectomy

PREOPERATIVE NURSING CARE

Preoperative care of the patient scheduled for surgery for cancer of the penis varies somewhat according to the stage of the disease and the extent of the scheduled surgery. Basic assessments, nursing diagnoses, expected patient outcomes, and nursing interventions that relate to any patient with cancer who is having surgery apply. In addition, be alert for anticipatory grieving, particularly in the patient scheduled for a total penectomy, with its concomitant loss of the capacity for normal urination and sexual intercourse.

POSTOPERATIVE NURSING CARE

Assessment

Assess return to physiologic stabilization as for any postsurgical patient. Take vital signs, and check dressing for drainage. Check the urinary catheter for patency, and note the amount and color of urinary output.

If an ilioinguinal node dissection has been done, measure drainage from the wound suction, and note its appearance. Check the wound for edema, redness, and other signs of skin sloughing and infection, which are prone to occur from 4 to 12 days after surgery. Observe for swelling in the lower extremities, indicative of lymphedema, and assess for signs of thrombophlebitis. These include swelling, pain, and redness in the calf and a positive Homans' sign.

Because penectomy is radical, disfiguring surgery, carefully assess the patient's psychological response. Observe for signs of sadness such as sighing and for avoidance behaviors such as anger or withdrawal. Be aware of the patient's need to grieve, and determine his stage of grieving. Assess for problems related to the grieving process such as difficulty eating and sleeping. Assess the patient's interest and willingness in participating in self-care and his outlook toward the future. Assess interaction with significant others. In terms of his interaction with his sexual partner, assess willingness to discuss the surgery, to demonstrate affection, and to plan for the future.

Nursing Diagnoses and Planning

Nursing diagnoses and related expected patient outcomes most commonly applicable to patients who have had surgery for cancer of the penis include those related to pain, anxiety, and knowledge deficit: postoperative course, plan of continued care, and self-care after discharge. Additional nursing diagnoses and related expected patient outcomes particularly applicable to patients who have had a total penectomy include the following:

NDx: Body image disturbance related to loss of sexual and urinary functions of the penis

Planning: Patient outcomes
1. Patient looks at the operative site.
2. Patient sits to void.
3. Patient wipes front to back after voiding and defecating.
4. Patient verbalizes acceptance of change in urinary and sexual functions.
5. Patient refers to self in positive masculine terms.

NDx: Sexual dysfunction related to loss of the penis

Planning: Patient outcomes
1. Patient identifies alternative methods of sexual expression.
2. Patient discusses concerns about loss of ability to have intercourse and desirability as a sexual partner with his partner.

NDx: High risk for powerlessness related to the diagnosis of cancer and the effects of penectomy

Planning: Patient outcomes
1. Patient identifies areas over which he has control.
2. Patient makes choices regarding care.
3. Patient participates in self-care.
4. Patient participates with significant other's decision-making on family concerns.

Nursing Interventions

NDx: Body image disturbance
Convey caring, acceptance, and perception of the patient as masculine. Avoid any facial expressions or comments that could be interpreted by the patient as indicating revulsion, pity, or perceived loss of masculinity. Provide the patient with privacy during care and during conversations dealing with his treatment. Be particularly sensitive to the patient's need for privacy when the catheter is removed and he first has to sit to void.

NDx: Sexual dysfunction
Encourage the patient to express his feelings and concerns and to share them with his sexual partner. Encourage physical expressions of affection, and provide privacy for visits between the patient and his partner. Refer the patient and his partner to a clinical specialist, professional sex therapist, or other resource as indicated.

NDx: High risk for powerlessness
Keep the call bell within reach, and make frequent, brief visits to the patient's room to prevent him from feeling alone and helpless.

Make the patient aware of areas of his care over which he has control by discussing needs with the patient and asking for his preferences in how to meet them. Provide him with as many choices as possible about his daily schedule, his activities, and his treatments. Encourage independence in self-care activities when able.

Assist the patient in identifying areas outside of his immediate illness and care over which he has control. As health permits, encourage him to keep informed of household events and to participate in related discussions and decision-making.

These interventions are particularly important because feelings of powerlessness are common among the elderly admitted to an acute-care health facility for any reason. Because cancer of the penis is most often diagnosed in men older than 60 years, these patients are already at risk for powerlessness before this radical surgery.

Evaluation

Evaluate the effectiveness of nursing care for a patient who has had a penectomy by comparing the patient's status with the expected patient outcomes. Examples of specific outcomes for patients who have had a penectomy have been provided in the Planning section.

Cancer of the Testis

Testicular cancer represents about 1% of all malignancies in males but is the most common solid tumor in men between 29 and 35 years of age. Its peak incidence occurs in the 20- to 40-year age group. It is particularly prevalent among whites, men who live in rural areas, and professionals.

ETIOLOGY

The exact cause of the various testicular malignancies is unknown. However, there is evidence to suggest that cryptorchidism, maternal treatment with DES during pregnancy, mumps orchitis, and trauma all increase the risk of the disease.

PATHOPHYSIOLOGY

Ninety percent to 95% of all primary testicular cancers arise from the germ cell epithelium of the testis and are classified as either seminomas or nonseminomas. Seminomas are the most common of all testicular malignancies; they grow slowly, are usually localized, and have a good prognosis. Nonseminomas tend to be invasive and metastasize quickly via the lymphatic system or the blood.

CLINICAL MANIFESTATIONS

Early testicular cancer is asymptomatic except for a painless, hardened area or lump on the testis found during testicular self-examination (TSE) or during a routine physical examination. In some cases, the lump goes unnoticed until a dull ache, pain, or heavy feeling develops in the lower abdominal, inguinal, or scrotal area. If associated infection, necrosis, or hemorrhage within the tumor develops, acute testicular pain occurs. In about 10% of patients, presenting symptoms are due to metastasis. These symptoms include a neck mass, respiratory symptoms, gastrointestinal disturbances, bone pain, central and peripheral nervous system manifestations, lower extremity edema, anorexia, and weight loss.

MEDICAL DIAGNOSIS

Testicular tumors can be palpated on bimanual examination of the scrotal contents and will not transilluminate when a light is placed behind the scrotum. Malignancy is confirmed by frozen section done with the patient under anesthesia prepared for orchiectomy. A biopsy is never done as an isolated procedure to confirm testicular cancer because of the risk of precipitating metastasis.

Before confirmation and orchiectomy, serum levels of the tumor markers beta-subunit HCG and alphafetoprotein (AFP) are obtained. These are measured again after orchiectomy and periodically thereafter as a check of the effectiveness of treatment because persistent elevation of one or more of these markers indicates the presence of residual tumor.

After orchiectomy, diagnostic studies are done to determine the clinical stage of the disease and to plan further treatment. Diagnostic tests used for staging purposes include CT scan of the chest, abdomen, and pelvis; intravenous pyelogram (IVP); and lymphangiogram. On the basis of results of these tests, the extent of testicular cancer is defined according to the following clinical staging system:

Stage I: tumor confined to the testis
Stage II: tumor spread to the retroperitoneal lymph nodes
Stage III: tumor spread beyond the retroperitoneal lymph nodes

MEDICAL MANAGEMENT

Initial treatment of cancer of the testis is inguinal orchiectomy done at the time of biopsy. Subsequent treatment is based on the type of tumor, presence of tumor markers, and clinical stage of the disease.

If the tumor is a Stage I or II seminoma, orchiectomy is followed by postoperative radiation to the lymph drainage areas of the testes. For more extensive disease, multidrug chemotherapy with cisplatin, bleomycin, and vinblastine may also be given before or after radiation.

Nonseminomas are usually treated by radical orchiectomy, retroperitoneal lymphadenectomy, or chemotherapy, or a combination. All patients with testicular cancer, regardless of type or stage, require careful follow-up with chest x-ray films, assessment of tumor markers, and monthly physical examinations for the first 2 years after diagnosis. Frequency of follow-up may then be decreased because most recurrences are within the first 24 months.

INGUINAL ORCHIECTOMY

In an inguinal orchiectomy, the testis, tunica vaginalis, and all but a stump of the spermatic cord are removed, and the inguinal canal is explored for metastasis through an incision high in the groin.

A gel-filled testicular prosthesis may be inserted for cosmetic effect before closure of the wound with metal staples or silk sutures.

Application of the Nursing Process to the Care of the Patient Undergoing an Inguinal Orchiectomy

PREOPERATIVE NURSING CARE

Assessment

Assess the patient's general health status, identifying any factors that may impact the delivery of nursing care in the perioperative period. Note any symptoms that may indicate metastatic spread such as abdominal or lumbar pain, cough, or edema of the lower extremities.

Review the patient's reproductive history. If the patient is sexually active, determine whether he fathered any children, whether he is interested in having children, and his attitude toward sperm banking.

Assess the patient's understanding of the surgery, its effect on his sexuality and fertility, and the anticipated postoperative course.

Determine the patient's emotional reaction to the surgery and the likelihood that he has cancer. Observe for the presence of support from his wife, significant other, or family members.

Nursing Diagnoses and Planning

Nursing diagnoses and related expected patient outcomes most commonly applicable to patients scheduled for an inguinal orchiectomy include the following:

NDx: Knowledge deficit: surgical procedure, reason for surgery, anticipated postoperative course, and effect on sexual and reproductive function

Planning: Patient outcomes

1. Patient describes in general terms the surgical procedures to be performed and the expected postoperative outcomes.
2. Patient verbalizes that he may have cancer of the testis.
3. Patient demonstrates turning, coughing, deep breathing, and leg exercises and states why and how often they are carried out postoperatively.
4. Patient acknowledges that removal of one testis does not usually result in sterility.

NDx: Anxiety related to impending surgery and to the possible diagnosis of cancer

Planning: Patient outcomes

1. Patient expresses his concerns readily.
2. Patient is attentive to preoperative teaching.
3. Patient asks questions about postoperative care.
4. Patient expresses confidence in the outcome of the surgery.

Nursing Interventions

NDx: Knowledge deficit: surgical procedure, reason for surgery, anticipated postoperative course, and effect on sexual and reproductive function

Provide concise information based on the surgeon's explanation of the surgical procedure and why it is being performed. If required, notify the surgeon that the patient is in need of additional explanation about the surgery. Explain the perioperative routine, and teach turning, coughing, deep breathing, and leg exercises. Clarify any misconceptions the patient has concerning the impact of the surgery on his reproductive and sexual functions. Explain that, although the sperm count may be lowered after the orchiectomy, fertility is usually not affected providing the remaining testis is normal. Inform the patient, however, that if further treatment is necessary (e.g., radiation, chemotherapy, retroperitoneal lymphadenectomy), fertility may be affected.

NDx: Anxiety

Provide opportunities for the patient to ask questions and express his concerns regarding the possibility of cancer. Although the diagnosis of cancer is not confirmed until the tumor is analyzed, do not give false reassurance. Use a realistic but hopeful approach based on information such as the dramatic improvement in 5-year survival rate for testicular cancer. Determine what strategies the patient has used in the past to cope with anxiety, and encourage their use (e.g., relaxation exercises, distraction techniques, presence of significant others). Also provide a quiet environment for interactions with family and significant others.

Evaluation

Evaluate the effectiveness of nursing care for a patient who is scheduled for an inguinal orchiectomy by comparing the patient's status with the expected patient outcomes. Examples of specific outcomes for patients scheduled for an inguinal orchiectomy have been provided in the Planning section.

POSTOPERATIVE NURSING CARE

Assessment

Assess the patient's physiologic response to surgery. Monitor vital signs, and observe for bleeding and scrotal edema. Assess the degree and location of pain. Note the time and amount of first voiding because catheterization may be necessary if adequate voiding is not established within 8 to 10 hours.

Throughout the postoperative period, assess the patient's emotional response to the surgery. Does he fear the orchiectomy resulted in demasculinization? If a testicular implant was not inserted, is he concerned about the appearance of the empty scrotal sac?

If further diagnostic testing and additional treatments are necessary, determine the patient's level of understanding of these procedures.

Nursing Diagnoses and Planning

Nursing diagnoses and related expected patient outcomes most commonly applicable to patients who have undergone an inguinal orchiectomy include the following:

NDx: Pain (inguinal and scrotal) related to surgical trauma and accompanying edema of the scrotum

Planning: Patient outcomes
1. Patient requests pain medication.
2. Patient reports pain is decreased or no longer present.
3. Patient moves in bed and ambulates without major discomfort.

NDx: High risk for body image disturbance related to removal of the testis

Planning: Patient outcomes
1. Patient describes realistically the effects of the surgery on appearance and function.
2. Patient verbalizes feelings about himself in relationship to the removal of the testis.
3. Patient looks at the incision.
4. Patient expresses feelings of self-worth and sexual adequacy.
5. Patient resumes self-care activities.

NDx: High risk for altered health maintenance related to insufficient knowledge of diagnosis, plan of further treatment, postdischarge care, and TSE

Planning: Patient outcomes
1. Patient describes plan of further treatment.
2. Patient describes and demonstrates care of the wound.
3. Patient states signs and symptoms of wound complications that should be reported.
4. Patient describes the importance of monthly TSEs as a means of early detection of cancer in the remaining testis.
5. Patient demonstrates TSE.
6. Patient states date and time of the first postoperative follow-up visit.

Nursing Interventions

NDx: Pain

Administer analgesics in accordance with the physician's order and the patient's need. Support their effectiveness with comfort measures that promote skeletal muscle relaxation. Splint the incision when the patient coughs, deep breathes, turns, and so on by placing a pillow over it.

Because scrotal swelling generally accompanies orchiectomy and contributes to the patient's discomfort, keep the scrotum elevated through the application of a Bellevue bridge or the use of an athletic support. Apply ice packs to the scrotal area as ordered.

NDx: High risk for body image disturbance

Encourage the patient to express how he thinks about and views himself as a result of the surgery. During wound care, describe the appearance of the wound, and allow the patient to view it if he so desires. If a testicular prosthesis was not inserted at the time of orchiectomy and the patient expresses concerns about the appearance of the empty scrotal sac, encourage him to discuss an implant with his physician. Clarify the physician's explanation about the effects of surgery and any further treatment on the patient's sexual function.

Provide a quiet environment for the patient and his partner or significant other to share their feelings about the impact of the surgery on their relationship. Give information, and recommend the use of community resources such as the American Cancer Society, Make Today Count, or a local mental health center for support after discharge.

Encourage independence in self-care activities as soon as possible.

NDx: High risk for altered health maintenance

Reinforce the physician's explanation of the type of cancer found, the extent of the disease, and plans for future treatment.

If a dressing continues to be required at the time of discharge, explain the care of the wound, and have the patient demonstrate it. Instruct the patient to report immediately any signs of wound complications such as increased erythema, bloody or purulent drainage, wound dehiscence, or fever.

Stress the importance of monthly TSE, because a malignant tumor can develop in the remaining testis, and instruct the patient in the technique if needed (see Box 45–1).

Provide information regarding the date and time of the first follow-up visit.

Evaluation

Evaluate the effectiveness of nursing care for a patient who has undergone an inguinal orchiectomy by comparing the patient's status with the expected patient outcomes. Examples of specific outcomes for patients who have undergone an inguinal orchiectomy have been provided in the Planning section.

RETROPERITONEAL LYMPH NODE DISSECTION

Retroperitoneal lymph node dissection (RPLND) involves the bilateral removal of lymph nodes and channels in the iliac and lumbar regions. It is the treatment of choice for Stages I and II nonseminomatous testicular cancer and is performed a few days after orchiectomy.

Patient Preparation

Mechanical bowel preparation is begun 3 to 4 days before surgery to decrease the risk of postoperative paralytic ileus. This involves laxatives, enemas, and a low-residue diet, which is changed to clear liquids 24 hours before the operation.

Coughing, deep breathing, and the use of an incentive spirometer are begun 24 hours before surgery as prophylaxis against pulmonary complications.

Skin preparation generally consists of a shower with an antimicrobial soap the evening before surgery. A shave from chest to mid-thigh is usually done the day of surgery.

Cryopreservation of semen for sperm banking may also be done preoperatively if desired by the patient. This may be chosen because retrograde ejaculation, which produces functional sterility, develops in the majority of patients as a result of surgical damage to the sympathetic nerves, which control the propulsion of semen into the urethra.

Procedure

RPLND, a major operative procedure lasting between 3 and 6 hours, involves either a transabdominal or a thoracoabdominal approach. In the transabdominal approach, a midline incision is made from the xiphoid process to the symphysis pubis. With a thoracoabdominal approach, the right 10th rib is resected, the pleura is entered, and chest tubes are inserted. The incision extends from the chest down to the lower abdomen.

Postoperative Course

Postoperatively, the patient is not allowed anything by mouth (NPO status) and has a nasogastric tube in place attached to low suction until peristalsis returns. Intravenous fluids and electrolytes are given to replace those lost as a result of surgery and gastric suction. A Foley catheter is inserted for 24 hours to monitor urinary output, and respiratory therapy is continued to promote optimal respiratory function.

If a thoracoabdominal approach is used, chest tubes connected to a water-seal closed-drainage system are in place to remove air and drainage from the pleural space.

The patient is generally ambulated on the first postoperative day.

Complications

Complications of RPLND include atelectasis, paralytic ileus, wound infection, and wound dehiscence.

Guidelines for Application of the Nursing Process to the Care of the Patient Having a Retroperitoneal Lymph Node Dissection

Preoperative and postoperative nursing care for the patient undergoing RPLND is similar to that described for any patient with cancer who is having major surgery (Chapters 11 and 4). If the thoracoabdominal approach is used, the nursing care described for the patient having chest surgery also applies (Chapter 12).

Be sensitive to the fact that cancer of the testis primarily affects young men and often occurs when they are trying to establish and maintain families. Because retrograde ejaculation usually accompanies bilateral RPLND, the likelihood of being sterile may be overwhelming to the patient and his partner. In some cases, the patient may feel that he cannot continue an intimate relationship because of his sterility. Be certain to assess the patient's coping strategies, and help him to use them during this period of adjustment. Encourage the patient to discuss his feelings and concerns with his partner. Remind the patient that his ability to have an erection and experience orgasm has not been affected.

Be aware there may also be a grief reaction over the perceived loss of sexual function and the possibility of premature death. Allow time for progression through the stages of grieving. Reassure the patient that his feelings related to the loss are expected responses to the diagnosis of cancer and changes experienced. Be empathic about the loss, and offer a realistic but hopeful approach based on the long-term survival rate after RPLND. Provide information regarding local mental health counseling services and support groups for continued assistance in working through the grief after discharge from the hospital.

Benign Prostatic Hyperplasia

ETIOLOGY

Benign prostatic hyperplasia (BPH) is an overgrowth of cells in the prostate gland. This increase in the number of cells, with its concomitant enlargement of the gland, appears to be a normal part of aging. Its exact cause, however, is not known. The fact that it occurs only in aging males with normal testicular function suggests that hormones play an important part in its development, although nutritional, metabolic, neoplastic, arteriosclerotic, and inflammatory processes may also contribute.

PATHOPHYSIOLOGY

BPH usually occurs in the form of nodules in the lateral or middle lobes of the prostate. These nodules almost always develop in the inner portion of the gland and, as they grow, compress the normal prostatic tissue toward its outer surface. This creates a so-called surgical capsule around the nodule (i.e., a structural difference between the nodule and the normal prostatic tissue), which allows the nodule to be surgically removed or enucleated without removal of the entire gland. In addition to compressing normal prostatic tissue outward, nodular enlargement can impinge on the lateral walls of the urethra and reduce its diameter to a slit. This narrowing increases resistance to the outward flow of urine and results in hypertrophy of the detrusor muscles of the bladder in an attempt to compensate. This in turn leads to trabeculation (presence of fibromuscular bands or cords) and bladder diverticula, which predispose to infection and development of bladder calculi from the retention of urine in these spaces. Ureters may dilate because of the increased voiding pressure, and even the kidneys may become distended, with resulting renal insufficiency.

CLINICAL MANIFESTATIONS

Many males with BPH do not have clinical symptoms. When they do occur, the classic symptoms are frequency of urination, nocturia, difficulty starting and stopping the stream of urine, weak stream, overflow dribbling, and a feeling of being unable to completely empty the bladder. If cystitis develops secondary to the stasis of retained urine in the bladder, dysuria, urgency, and hematuria occur.

As urethral obstruction becomes complete, symptoms of acute urinary retention also appear.

If prostatic enlargement and urethral obstruction develop very slowly, the patient may not report symptoms. The problem may be discovered on routine examination, at which time the patient may already have significant renal insufficiency and related secondary anemia as well as hypertension.

MEDICAL DIAGNOSIS

Diagnosis of BPH is made on the basis of history and physical examination, with rectal palpation of a smooth, firm, elastic enlargement of the prostate gland. The examiner may observe the patient's voiding to confirm a decrease in size or force of the urinary stream.

Diagnostic tests that may be used to evaluate the degree of prostatic hyperplasia include measurement of amount of residual urine by urinary catheterization; sequential bacteriologic localization cultures; blood urea nitrogen (BUN) and creatinine; IVP with postvoiding film; kidney, ureter, and bladder (KUB) films; cystogram, voiding cystourethrogram, and cystourethroscopy; and transrectal ultrasonogram.

MEDICAL MANAGEMENT

Treatment varies with the severity of the symptoms, degree of prostatic involvement, and presence of complications.

For patients with few symptoms of obstruction, conservative measures are recommended. These include engaging in regular prostatic massage and sexual intercourse to help decrease prostatic congestion; limiting amount of fluids, especially alcohol, taken at any one time to avoid distending the bladder and making voiding difficult; urinating at the first urge; and avoiding drugs such as anticholinergics, antidepressants, decongestants, and tranquilizers, which can precipitate acute urinary retention.

Surgical removal of the enlarged portion of the prostate is performed when major symptoms of obstruction exist. These are acute urinary retention, hydronephrosis, residual urine with recurrent urinary tract infection, severe hematuria from a congested prostate, and obstructive symptoms associated with the development of bladder instability such as urgency of urination and urgency incontinence (refer to Chapter 45 for a discussion of prostatectomy).

Also used in the treatment of BPH is the antiandrogen drug finasteride (Proscar). This drug lowers the level of androgen, which is a major stimulus to prostatic growth. The result is shrinkage of the prostate, with gradual relief of urinary symptoms. This may take as long as 6 months, and surgery may still be necessary. Potential side effects of the medication include reduced sexual urge and difficulty with erection.

Guidelines for Application of the Nursing Process to the Care of the Patient Having a Prostatectomy

Nursing care of patients undergoing all types of prostatectomy is presented in Chapter 45. Nursing care of a patient having a transurethral resection of the prostate (TURP) for BPH is presented in Nursing Care Guide 46–1.

Nursing Care Guide 46–1.

PATIENTS UNDERGOING A TRANSURETHRAL RESECTION OF THE PROSTATE (TURP) FOR BENIGN PROSTATIC HYPERPLASIA

Preoperative Care

Assessment Findings: Patient states he is anxious about the surgery and says "I hope nothing goes wrong with this operation. I want to wake up and have everything working." Patient is observed to be restless. Body position is tense; facial expression is worried.

Nursing Diagnosis: Anxiety related to scheduled TURP and its outcomes

Patient Outcomes	Nursing Interventions	Rationale
Patient expresses concerns about the surgical experience and its effects on body function.	Acknowledge that anxiety over the surgical experience is normal.	Allays patient concerns about being judged negatively because of anxiety.
Patient asks questions about the surgical experience and its effects.	Spend time with the patient, and provide opportunities for him to talk and ask questions.	Permits a supportive relationship while providing information that can prevent unnecessary anxiety.
Patient attends to information and discussion.	Provide information about the surgical experience (e.g., transport to the operating room, how the local anesthesia is given and its effects, operating room personnel and equipment to be expected, and the physical environment of the recovery room and its routines).	Prepares patient for perioperative events, promotes compliance with perioperative care, and decreases the risk of anxiety over routine perioperative events.
Patient participates in preoperative preparation.	Correct any distorted perceptions related to the surgery.	Avoids unnecessary anxiety resulting from misinformation.
Facial expression and posture appear relaxed.	Reassure the patient about his safety by explaining how closely patients are monitored and describing how "common" and successful TURPs are.	Provides the patient with positive facts about the operative procedure on which to focus and base hope for a successful surgical outcome.
Patient is able to rest quietly.	Guide the patient in the use of progressive relaxation techniques.	Decreases overall body tension and refocuses the patient on concerns other than his own.

Evaluation: Compare the patient's status with the expected patient outcomes. If the outcomes are achieved, evaluate nursing care as successful. If not, reassess the patient, formulate new nursing diagnoses, and revise expected patient outcomes and nursing interventions as appropriate.

(continued)

Nursing Care Guide 46–1. (continued)

PATIENTS UNDERGOING A TRANSURETHRAL RESECTION OF THE PROSTATE (TURP) FOR BENIGN PROSTATIC HYPERPLASIA

Assessment Findings: Patient has no previous experience with surgery or prostatectomy. Patient states "This is all new to me. I don't know what's going on."

Nursing Diagnosis: Knowledge deficit: location and function of the prostate gland, the surgical procedure (including what is to be removed and how), perioperative routines, usual postoperative course, and effects of the surgery on urinary and reproductive function

Patient Outcomes	Nursing Interventions	Rationale
Patient explains that excess prostate gland tissue will be removed; there will be no external incision; a tube will be inserted into the urethra, which carries urine from the bladder out through the penis, and the prostate tissue will be removed by tiny instruments inserted through it; and no long-term effects on urinary and sexual functions are expected.	Clarify and reinforce information about the reason for and the extent and type of surgery.	Supports "informed consent," helps prevent unnecessary concerns based on inadequate or misunderstood information, and helps prepare patient for the postoperative course.
	Explain the expected outcome of surgery and the effects on urinary and sexual functions.	Provides patient with a realistic perspective while helping to prevent unfounded concerns.
	Explain perioperative routines.	Promotes patient cooperation and allays anxiety over normal perioperative events.
Patient describes preoperative preparation, transport to the operating room, recovery room environment and procedures, and return to unit.	Prepare patient for presence of indwelling catheter with continuous irrigation, and pink to red-colored urine.	Alerts patient to the fact that these are normal concomitants of the surgery, thus allaying potential anxiety.
Patient states that he will have an indwelling urinary catheter, with solution being run in and out continuously to keep the catheter free of blood clots; that his urine will be pink to red; that he may feel the urge to void but the catheter is draining the urine from the bladder into a bag and he should not try to void around it; that the urge to void will gradually pass; and that bladder spasms may occur but medication will be available and he should ask for it.	Explain that bladder spasms are not unusual and that medication will be ordered and should be requested as needed.	Provides patient with a sense of control, helps allay anxiety over normal postoperative discomfort, and helps make the patient feel comfortable and correct in asking for pain medication.
Patient states reason for postoperative coughing, deep breathing, and leg exercises. Patient demonstrates coughing, deep breathing, and leg exercises.	Teach importance and technique of postoperative coughing, deep breathing, and leg exercises.	Promotes patient willingness to cough, deep breathe, and perform leg exercises postoperatively by making patient aware of the role these activities play in a rapid, uncomplicated recovery.

(continued)

Nursing Care Guide 46–1. (continued)

PATIENTS UNDERGOING A TRANSURETHRAL RESECTION OF THE PROSTATE (TURP) FOR BENIGN PROSTATIC HYPERPLASIA

Patient Outcomes	Nursing Interventions	Rationale
Patient states he will be asked to drink a large amount of fluids because they help to decrease pain and irritation in the bladder and prevent infection.	Explain the need for large amounts of fluids postoperatively.	Enhances patient willingness to drink fluids postoperatively by making the patient aware that this will help decrease pain and prevent infection.

Evaluation: Compare the patient's status with the expected patient outcomes. If the outcomes are achieved, evaluate nursing care as successful. If not, reassess the patient, formulate new nursing diagnoses, and revise expected patient outcomes and nursing interventions as appropriate.

Additional Interventions

Keep patient on nothing by mouth order from midnight before surgery.
Give Fleet enema, soapsuds enema, or other bowel preparation as ordered before surgery.
Ensure that skin preparation is carried out in accordance with the surgeon's preference.
Monitor for signs of dehydration.
If an indwelling catheter is inserted to relieve urinary retention, observe for signs of shock resulting from postobstructive diuresis.
Check for sensory and motor impairments in aged patients, which put them at risk for injury.

(continued)

Cancer of the Prostate

Cancer of the prostate occurs primarily in men older than 50 years. Its highest incidence is at about age 70, and it is more frequent in blacks than in whites.

ETIOLOGY

The cause of cancer of the prostate is unknown, although hormones are generally believed to play a role.

PATHOPHYSIOLOGY

The most common form of prostatic cancer is adenocarcinoma. It presents as a hard, fixed area or nodule most often in the posterior lobe. Because symptoms generally do not occur until late in the disease, metastasis to the lymph nodes, bone, lung, and liver is common. Central nervous system involvement usually comes after bone involvement.

CLINICAL MANIFESTATIONS

Most patients with early prostatic cancer are asymptomatic. In these cases, the tumor is found when the prostate is palpated via the rectum during a routine physical examination or during surgery for BPH. Other patients present with symptoms of bladder outlet obstruction as seen in BPH: difficulty initiating the urinary stream, decrease in size and force of the stream, involuntary release of urine, and, in some cases, acute urinary retention.

If metastasis has occurred, bone pain, unexplained weight loss, anemia, shortness of breath, enlarged lymph nodes, lymphedema, or neurologic symptoms may be present.

MEDICAL DIAGNOSIS

The diagnosis of cancer of the prostate is suggested by the presence of a hardened area or nodule in the posterior lobe of the gland palpable on rectal examination. The diagnosis is confirmed by biopsy. Other diagnostic studies used to determine the presence and extent of disease include transrectal prostatic ultrasonography; magnetic resonance imaging, which allows visualization of the prostate and seminal vesicles; blood chemistry studies; cystoscopy; bone scan; lymphangiogram; and staging lymphadenectomy.

Of the blood chemistry studies, two of the most important are serum acid phosphatase and serum

Text continued on page 1827

Nursing Care Guide 46–1. *(continued)*

PATIENTS UNDERGOING A TRANSURETHRAL RESECTION OF THE PROSTATE (TURP) FOR BENIGN PROSTATIC HYPERPLASIA

Postoperative Care

Assessment Findings: Patient is postoperative from a TURP. A three-way urethral catheter is in place for bladder drainage and is attached to a continuous bladder-irrigation system.

Nursing Diagnosis: High risk for urinary retention related to obstruction of urinary drainage tubes

Patient Outcomes	Nursing Interventions	Rationale
Urinary drainage tubes are patent and draining. Urinary bladder is free of palpable distention.	Maintain flow of normal saline irrigant at the prescribed rate or the rate needed to keep the urine pink tinged.	Prevents obtruction of the urethral catheter with blood clots or tissue debris.
	Empty the urinary drainage bag frequently.	Prevents impaired drainage caused by back pressure.
	Check position of catheter and drainage tube for kinking.	Maintains free-flowing gravity drainage.
	Position patient without pressure on the tube, and remind him not to move and lie on it.	Prevents compression of the tube, which would inhibit free flow of drainage into the bag.
	Keep the tubing in a straight line from the bed down to the drainage bag.	Maintains free-flowing gravity drainage.
	Clip or pin the tube to the bed to prevent looping or curling below the bed.	Facilitates free-flowing gravity drainage.
	Position drainage bag on the side to which the patient is turned.	Promotes patient comfort and free-flowing gravity drainage.
	Hand irrigate urinary catheter as per order if patient has significant bladder spasms and there is no outflow to the drainage bag.	Hand irrigation can dislodge clots and reestablish free drainage.
	Do not speed up irrigant to try to dislodge an obstruction.	This may force the clot deeper into the eye of the catheter and worsen the obstruction.
	Record amounts of solution inserted and returned on intake and output sheet.	Fluid instilled must be subtracted from amount returned to determine true urinary output.

Evaluation: Compare the patient's status with the expected patient outcomes. If the outcomes are achieved, evaluate nursing care as successful. If not, reassess the patient, formulate new nursing diagnoses, and revise expected patient outcomes and nursing interventions as appropriate.

(continued)

Nursing Care Guide 46–1. *(continued)*

PATIENTS UNDERGOING A TRANSURETHRAL RESECTION OF THE PROSTATE (TURP) FOR BENIGN PROSTATIC HYPERPLASIA

Assessment Findings: Patient has had a TURP during which a hypotonic irrigating solution was used continuously to keep the operative area free of blood and tissue shreds.

Nursing Diagnosis: High risk for fluid volume excess related to dilutional hyponatremia secondary to absorption of irrigating fluid during TURP

Patient Outcomes	Nursing Interventions	Rationale
Patient is free of agitation and confusion. Blood pressure and pulse are stable within the patient's normal range. Serum sodium and potassium levels are within normal limits. Serum osmolarity is within normal limits.	Monitor for increasing restlessness, confusion, muscular twitching, drop in pulse rate, or elevation of blood pressure. Notify the physician immediately if any of these occur. If transurethral resection syndrome with pulmonary congestion develops do the following:	Early recognition and reporting of symptoms of dilutional hyponatremia allow for early intervention.
	Sit the patient up.	Facilitates ventilation.
	Administer oxygen (O_2).	Increases amount of O_2 available at the alveoli for diffusion into the circulation.
	Slow intravenous (IV) to keep open rate.	Avoids further fluid overload while maintaining access for administration of IV medications.
	Administer hypertonic IV solution and diuretics as ordered.	Promotes movement of fluid out of the lungs into the vascular spaces, with subsequent excretion by the kidneys.
	Record intake and output.	Indicates fluid loss or gain.
	Record daily weight.	Change in daily weight reflects loss or gain of body fluid.

Evaluation: Compare the patient's status with the expected patient outcomes. If the outcomes are achieved, evaluate nursing care as successful. If not, reassess the patient, formulate new nursing diagnoses, and revise expected patient outcomes and nursing interventions as appropriate.

(continued)

Nursing Care Guide 46–1. *(continued)*

PATIENTS UNDERGOING A TRANSURETHRAL RESECTION OF THE PROSTATE (TURP) FOR BENIGN PROSTATIC HYPERPLASIA

Assessment Findings: Patient complains of severe bladder spasms, presses hands over lower abdomen, occasionally groans, and is reluctant to move.

Nursing Diagnosis: Pain related to bladder spasms

Patient Outcomes	Nursing Interventions	Rationale
Patient asks for/accepts analgesics. Patient participates in relaxation techniques as directed. Patient states he has less discomfort. Patient no longer holds lower abdomen or groans. Patient moves freely in bed. Patient voids without signs of discomfort.	Medicate the patient for pain as ordered.	Pain causes restlessness, which can lead to problems with the drainage system or other injury.
	If belladonna and opium rectal suppositories are ordered, insert carefully.	Avoids traumatizing operative area.
	Ensure that the catheter is patent and draining freely.	Distention of the bladder is associated with increased pain and bladder spasms.
	Make sure there is no inadvertent tension on the catheter from the patient's position or from being caught on the side rail and so on.	Tension on the catheter causes pain.
	Keep intravenous running, and encourage oral fluids as ordered.	Maintains good hydration.
	Position patient comfortably.	Promotes rest and contributes to the effectiveness of analgesics.
	Keep the environment calm and quiet.	Promotes rest and enhances the effect of analgesics.
	Encourage slow, deep breathing and progressive relaxation.	Decreases overall body tension and distracts the patient from the pain.

Evaluation: Compare the patient's status with the expected patient outcomes. If the outcomes are achieved, evaluate nursing care as successful. If not, reassess the patient, formulate new nursing diagnoses, and revise expected patient outcomes and nursing interventions as appropriate.

(continued)

Nursing Care Guide 46–1. *(continued)*

PATIENTS UNDERGOING A TRANSURETHRAL RESECTION OF THE PROSTATE (TURP) FOR BENIGN PROSTATIC HYPERPLASIA

Assessment Findings: Patient has had transurethral surgery, an indwelling catheter, and continuous bladder irrigation.

Nursing Diagnosis: High risk for infection related to transurethral instrumentation and surgery and use of urinary drainage apparatus

Patient Outcomes	Nursing Interventions	Rationale
Pyuria is absent. Urine cultures are negative.	Wash hands carefully before caring for the patient or manipulating the catheter.	Decreases risk of infection resulting from cross contamination.
	Wear clean gloves for perineal or catheter care.	Protects against cross contamination.
	Maintain sterility of saline irrigant and equipment.	Protects against cross contamination.
	Label irrigant with date and time it was put into use.	Once opened, solutions are considered sterile for 24 hours. After this time, they must be discarded.
	Use strict sterile technique when hand irrigating the urethral catheter.	Strict sterile technique prevents introduction of microorganisms into the bladder during irrigation.
	Keep the penile meatus and catheter junction clean and free of bloody drainage.	This decreases risk of growth of microorganisms and their migration along the catheter into the bladder.
	Encourage fluid intake of 2500 to 3000 ml per day unless medically contraindicated.	Creates a dilute urine sufficient in quantity to prevent stasis and to flush bacteria out of the urinary tract at regular intervals.
	Monitor for and report signs of infection such as fever, chills, or cloudy urine.	Allows early intervention to combat complications.

Evaluation: Compare the patient's status with the expected patient outcomes. If the outcomes are achieved, evaluate nursing care as successful. If not, reassess the patient, formulate new nursing diagnoses, and revise expected patient outcomes and nursing interventions as appropriate.

(continued)

Nursing Care Guide 46–1. *(continued)*

PATIENTS UNDERGOING A TRANSURETHRAL RESECTION OF THE PROSTATE (TURP) FOR BENIGN PROSTATIC HYPERPLASIA

Assessment Findings: Urethral catheter is removed from patient who has had a TURP.

Nursing Diagnosis: High risk for urinary retention related to alteration in voiding secondary to removal of part of the bladder neck and prostatic urethra

Patient Outcomes	Nursing Interventions	Rationale
Patient voids more than 90 ml per voiding. Urinary bladder is free of palpable distention. Patient has postvoiding residual of less than 75 ml.	Encourage the patient to drink 1000 to 1500 ml during the first 6 hours after catheter removal.	Ensures dilute urine and decreases the burning sensation on voiding expected after catheter removal.
	Provide the patient with a urinal, and tell him to use it at the first urge to void.	Voiding is facilitated by eliminating the need to wait for assistance.
	If necessary, assist the patient with standing or going to the bathroom to use the urinal.	Standing and privacy of the bathroom assist voiding.
	Run water, place 5 to 10 ml of spirits of peppermint in the urinal, or encourage perineal exercises as needed.	Facilitates voiding.
	Provide privacy.	Promotes relaxation and thus facilitates voiding.
	If patient is anxious over his ability to void, encourage relaxation exercises and give a warm bath if permitted.	Relaxation and sensation of warm water on the body facilitate voiding.
	Record time and amount of each voiding.	Frequent voiding of small amounts suggests urinary retention with overflow.

Evaluation: Compare the patient's status with the expected patient outcomes. If the outcomes are achieved, evaluate nursing care as successful. If not, reassess the patient, formulate new nursing diagnoses, and revise expected patient outcomes and nursing interventions as appropriate.

(continued)

Nursing Care Guide 46–1. *(continued)*

PATIENTS UNDERGOING A TRANSURETHRAL RESECTION OF THE PROSTATE (TURP) FOR BENIGN PROSTATIC HYPERPLASIA

Assessment Findings: Patient has no prior experience with a transurethral prostatectomy. Patient asks questions regarding self-care after discharge.

Nursing Diagnosis: High risk for altered health maintenance related to insufficient knowledge of postprostatectomy discharge instructions

Patient Outcomes	Nursing Interventions	Rationale
Patient lists signs and symptoms to be reported.	Explain that bloody urine and passage of small clots or pieces of tissue can normally occur for up to 2 weeks after surgery but that frank bleeding or increased blood in the urine that does not clear up after drinking large amounts of fluid (1000 ml in 30 minutes) should be reported.	Provides information needed to avoid unnecessary anxiety and to ensure that medical assistance is obtained if needed.
	Instruct the patient to report any decrease in the urinary stream, any difficulty voiding, temperature higher than 37.6°C (99.8°F), chills, back or flank pain, and general malaise.	Provides information essential to obtaining early medical intervention in the event of postdischarge complications.
Patient describes limitations on activity and sexual intercourse.	Instruct the patient to shower rather than tub bathe to limit dilation of pelvic blood vessels; avoid strenuous exercise; avoid sports such as tennis, golf, and heavy lifting; avoid driving a car or sitting for long periods of time for at least 3 weeks; and abstain from sexual intercourse for 3 weeks or until otherwise instructed.	Instruction provides information on activity restriction after discharge, which is necessary to decrease risk of bleeding.
Patient states reason and directions for each medication prescribed for use after discharge.	Review name, dose, route, frequency, and purpose of each medication prescribed for use after discharge.	Provides information essential for self-administration of medications after discharge.
Patient describes measures to prevent constipation and straining with hard bowel movements.	Explain that straining at stool and the use of suppositories or enemas can cause bleeding.	Provides information essential to preventing constipation and related complications after discharge.
	Stress the role of fluids, fresh fruits and vegetables, whole-grain products, and bran as well as exercise in the prevention of constipation.	

(continued)

Nursing Care Guide 46–1. *(continued)*

PATIENTS UNDERGOING A TRANSURETHRAL RESECTION OF THE PROSTATE (TURP) FOR BENIGN PROSTATIC HYPERPLASIA

Patient Outcomes	Nursing Interventions	Rationale
	Tell the patient to call the physician if constipation does develop so a stool softener or laxative can be ordered.	
Patient states date of follow-up visit.	Instruct the patient about when and where to return for follow-up care.	Provides information essential to compliance with self-care instructions.
Patient states expected date of return to work.	Explain that patients usually return to work in 4 to 6 weeks depending in part on the type of work they do and that a date to return to work will be given during a follow-up visit with the physician.	Prepares patient for postoperative restrictions and allows for personal planning.

Evaluation: Compare the patient's status with the expected patient outcomes. If the outcomes are achieved, evaluate nursing care as successful. If not, reassess the patient, formulate new nursing diagnoses, and revise expected patient outcomes and nursing interventions as appropriate.

Additional Assessments and Interventions

Monitor for bleeding, because the prostate is very vascular and the irrigating solution used during transurethral prostatic resection (TURP) can temporarily obscure venous bleeding.

Avoid all rectal treatments (except use of belladonna and opium suppositories if ordered) for 48 to 72 hours postoperatively to prevent damage to the prostatic surgical site.

Encourage ambulation as soon as allowed.

Discourage long periods of sitting, because the position increases intraabdominal pressure and can cause bleeding.

alkaline phosphatase. Serum acid phosphatase titers are elevated in patients with prostatic cancer because acid phosphatase, which is produced by the acinar cells, is absorbed into the circulation rather than secreted into the seminal fluid and remaining in the prostate. This makes acid phosphatase the most useful biochemical test for monitoring progression or regression of prostatic cancer.

In patients with metastatic prostate cancer, alkaline phosphatase titers are elevated as a result of metabolic activity in bone surrounding metastatic lesions. As a tumor marker, alkaline phosphatase is less specific than acid phosphatase because elevations of alkaline phosphatase can also occur as a result of a variety of metabolic bone disorders and liver diseases.

MEDICAL MANAGEMENT

The best treatment for cancer confined to the prostate gland is radical prostatectomy. In this procedure, the entire gland and its capsule, the ampulla, vas deferens, seminal vesicles, and a cuff of the bladder neck are removed. It is performed as a one-stage procedure through a retropubic approach or as a two-stage procedure including a staging pelvic lymphadenectomy through an abdominal incision followed by a total prostatectomy through a perineal incision.

Complications of radical prostatectomy include urinary incontinence, stricture of the surgical vesicourethral anastomosis, rectal injury, thromboembolic phenomena, lymphocele, lymphedema, wound infection, and erectile impotence. This last complication has been reported in up to 90% of patients after radical prostatectomy. It is thought to result from damage to the parasympathetic innervation of the corpora cavernosa at the time of surgery.

Radiation therapy is used for palliation in patients with extensive local prostatic cancer who, because of age or other medical problems, are not appropriate candidates for radical surgery. It is also used to control pain in patients with bone metastasis. In most cases, external beam radiation is given, although interstitial radiation using iodine (^{125}I seeds), gold (^{198}Au seeds), or iridium (^{192}Ir implants) is under clinical study. Complications of external radiation include gastrointestinal and genitourinary symptoms and sexual impotence. Complications of ^{125}I implants include pelvic hematoma, thromboembolic phenomena, and infection.

A third mode of treatment used in selective cases is endocrine therapy. The goal of this therapy is to limit the amount of circulating androgens because prostatic cells are dependent on androgen for cellular maintenance. This is accomplished by bilateral orchiectomy or administration of estrogens such as DES. Estrogen therapy lowers circulating androgen levels by suppressing the release of luteinizing hormone from the pituitary, thus eliminating the stimulus for testicular production of testosterone. A problem with this treatment is the risk of significant, long-term cardiovascular side effects.

Chemotherapeutic agents are also currently used in some cases as adjunctive therapy. These include estramustine phosphate, cisplatin, and various combinations of 5-fluorouracil (5-FU), cyclophosphamide, and doxorubicin hydrochloride (Adriamycin).

Prostate-specific antigen (PSA) levels are used to monitor effectiveness of treatment as well as to detect tumor progression or recurrence. PSA is produced by both normal and malignant prostatic ductal epithelial cells, and its amount increases proportionately to total prostate mass.

Guidelines for Application of the Nursing Process to the Care of the Patient with Cancer of the Prostate

Nursing care of the patient with cancer of the prostate varies according to the extent of disease, type of treatment selected, and whether the patient is newly diagnosed or admitted for progression, recurrence, or terminal care. Assessments, nursing diagnoses, expected patient outcomes, and nursing interventions applicable to patients with various stages of cancer who are undergoing radiation or chemotherapy are presented in Chapter 11. Care of the patient undergoing radical prostatectomy for cancer also involves that presented in Chapter 11 in combination with the care of the patient having a simple prostatectomy for BPH through an abdominal or perineal approach, with several considerations. Radical prostatectomy is far more extensive surgery than simple prostatectomy, so greater preoperative support and a longer postoperative recovery period are needed. Radical prostatectomy also frequently results in incontinence and impotence, so these must be incorporated into the plan of care if they occur.

If incontinence occurs postoperatively, instruct the patient to perform perineal exercises (stop and start the urinary stream during voiding, and tighten and relax the buttocks) to improve urinary and rectal sphincter tone. For urinary incontinence, also instruct the patient to limit oral fluids during the evening to decrease incontinence at night and to avoid alcoholic beverages and caffeine because of their diuretic effect.

If intermittent catheterization, insertion of an indwelling catheter, or use of an external condom catheter attached to a drainage bag is ordered because of persistent incontinence in significant amounts, instruct the patient and the family in the appropriate care. If a Cunningham clamp (Fig. 46–9)—an adjustable, lightweight, foam-lined, molded clamp that fits over the penis behind the glans—is ordered, instruct the patient and the family in its use, as specified in Chart 46–5.

If fecal incontinence is a problem, instruct the patient in perineal exercises as described previously to improve rectal sphincter tone. Also review the prescribed bowel regimen, and stress the importance of strict adherence to the regimen if fecal incontinence is to be controlled.

If impotence occurs as a result of surgery, encourage the patient to discuss his reactions and feelings and to share them with his spouse or significant other. If the patient is concerned about and interested in the ability to have sexual intercourse, encourage him to discuss the possibility of a penile implant with the physician. Refer the patient to a sex therapist or counselor if appropriate.

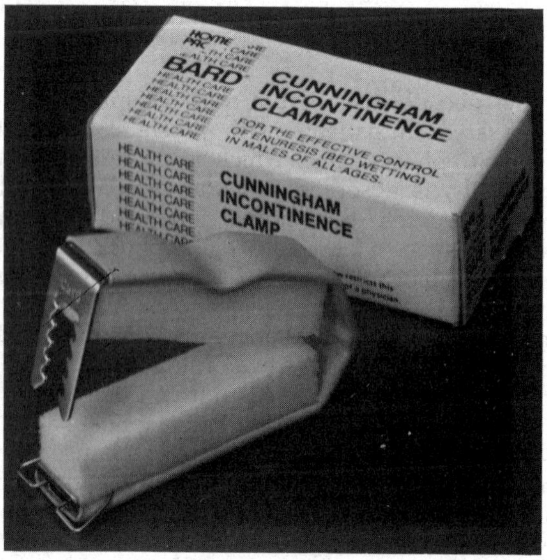

Figure 46–9.

Cunningham clamp for urinary incontinence. (Courtesy of Bard Home Health Division, C.R. Bard Inc., Murray Hill, NJ.)

Chart 46–5.
NURSING GUIDE TO PATIENT EDUCATION FOR SELF-MANAGEMENT: USE OF A PENILE (CUNNINGHAM) CLAMP

Instruct the patient to:

Wash, dry, and powder his penis before applying the clamp.
Apply the clamp horizontally on the penis behind the glans.
Remove the clamp, and allow the bladder to empty at least every 4 hours to avoid bladder infection.
Inspect the penis for skin irritation and edema each time the clamp is removed.
Alternate use of the clamp with an external condom catheter if skin irritation occurs.
Secure the clamp on a looser notch if mild to moderate penile edema occurs; discontinue use of the clamp if severe edema develops.

The Elderly: Special Considerations

Cancer of the prostate, benign prostatic hyperplasia, and cancer of the penis are disorders of the aging male. For each, early diagnosis and treatment offer the best prognosis. To achieve these, health teaching is essential. Because cancer of the prostate is initially asymptomatic, except for a hardened area on the gland itself, teach aging men the importance of an annual physical examination that includes rectal palpation of the prostate. Also alert them to symptoms of benign prostatic hyperplasia such as frequency of urination, difficulty starting the urinary stream, and a weak stream. Stress the importance of seeking medical care when symptoms first appear to prevent progressive bladder neck obstruction with urinary retention and the risk of infection in the bladder and adjacent genitourinary structures.

In regard to cancer of the penis, explain that it first appears as a pimple, a warty growth, or a hardened or reddened area and that, if treated early, it is almost 100% curable. Instruct patients to inspect the penis for lesions routinely, and have any suspicious areas promptly examined by a physician.

Problems with sexual function in the older man may be due to chronic disease or drugs as well as to disorders of the reproductive tract itself. Problems such as anemia, diabetes, and malnutrition can directly cause a decrease in libido. In other cases, however, sexual activity is diminished indirectly through fear of the effects of sex on an existing health problem such as heart disease. Many drugs can also adversely affect sexual function. These include alcohol, chlorpromazine, and reserpine, all of which can weaken erection and delay ejaculation.

These effects point out once again the need to stress to older men the importance of routine physical examinations. Such examinations allow chronic diseases to be identified and treated early in their course and help to prevent, limit, or reverse negative effects on sexual function. In addition, be certain to inform patients that a prescribed medication may alter sexual function, and encourage them to return to the physician if problems develop, because it is often possible to change medication or dosage and eliminate the difficulty.

Always keep in mind that older men, like older women, sometimes believe that sexual activity, and, by association, concern about the sexual organs, is only for the young. Thus, they may be reluctant to seek care or may accept changes in structure and function of the sexual organs as effects of age rather than as potential disorders that can and should be treated. Be alert to these feelings, and present information designed to correct such misconceptions in an open but sensitive manner.

Bibliography

Andriole G, Catalona WJ. Early diagnosis of prostatic cancer. Urol Clin North Am 1987; 14(4):657.

Berger RE. Sexually transmitted diseases: The classic diseases. In Walsh C, Retik AB, Stamey TA, Vaughan ED (eds). Campbell's urology. 6th ed. Philadelphia: WB Saunders, 1992, pp 823–846.

Bihrle R, Donohue JP, Foster RS. Complications of retroperitoneal lymph node dissection. Urol Clin North Am 1988; 15(2):237.

Brendler CB. Diseases of the prostate. In Wyngaarden J, Smith LH (eds). Cecil textbook of medicine. 19th ed. Philadelphia: WB Saunders, 1992, pp 1351–1355.

Carbonell MA, Taseff L, Sciarra L, et al. Managing the patient with testicular cancer. Nursing 1986; 16(8):42.

Carpenito LJ. Handbook of nursing diagnosis. 5th ed. Philadelphia: JB Lippincott, 1993.

Carpenito LJ. Nursing diagnosis: Application to clinical practice. 5th ed. Philadelphia: JB Lippincott, 1993.

Casey MP. Testicular cancer: The worst disease at the worst time. RN 1987; 50(2):36.

Crawford ED. Diagnosis and treatment of prostatitis. Hosp Pract 1985; 20(9):77.

Devine CJ Jr, Jordan GH, Schlossberg SM. Surgery of the penis and urethra. In Walsh C, Retik AB, Stamey TA, Vaughan ED (eds). Campbell's urology. 6th ed. Philadelphia: WB Saunders, 1992, pp 2957–3032.

DeVitis MG. Balanitis associated with hyperglycemia. J Emerg Nurs 1982; 8(4):164.

Doenges M, Moorhouse M. Nursing pocket guide: Nursing diagnosis with interventions. 3rd ed. Philadelphia: FA Davis, 1991.

Duckett J, Snow BW. Disorders of the urethra and penis. In Walsh C, Gittes RF, Perlmutter AD, Stamey TA (eds). Campbell's urology. 5th ed. Philadelphia: WB Saunders, 1986, pp 2000–2030.

Ebersole P, Hess P. Toward healthy aging. St. Louis: CV Mosby, 1990.

Eliopoulos C. Nursing diagnoses in gerontological care. In Eliopoulos C (ed). Caring for the elderly in diverse care settings. Philadelphia: JB Lippincott, 1990, pp 39–75.

Epididymitis. In Hamilton HK (ed). Diseases—nursing 87 books. Springhouse, PA: Springhouse, 1987, pp 769–770.

Felten B. The lingering tragedy of DES. RN 1990; 53(8):36.

Frank I. Urology. In Schwartz S, et al (eds). Principles of surgery. 6th ed. New York: McGraw-Hill, 1989, pp 1729–1779.

Gonzales R. Urologic disorders in infants and children. In Behrman RE, Kliegman RM, Nelson WE, Vaughan VC (eds). Nelson textbook of pediatrics. 14th ed. Philadelphia: WB Saunders, 1992, pp 1359–1384.

Gray M, Dobkin K. Genitourinary system. In Thompson JL, McFarland GK, Hirsch JE, Tucher SM (eds). Clinical Nursing. 3rd ed. St. Louis: CV Mosby, 1993.

Halden W, White R. Outpatient embolotherapy of varicocele. Urol Clin North Am 1987; 14(1):137.

Howards SS. Surgery of the scrotum and its contents. In Walsh PC, Gittes RF, Perlmutter AD, Stamey TA (eds). Campbell's urology. 5th ed. Philadelphia: WB Saunders, 1986, pp 2955–2975.

Krueger H, Osborne L. Effects of hygiene among the uncircumcised. J Fam Pract 1986; 22(4):353.

Lerner J, Zafar K. Manual of urologic nursing. St. Louis: CV Mosby, 1982.

Loehrer PJ Sr, Williams SD, Einhorn LH. Status of chemotherapy for testis cancer. Urol Clin North Am 1987; 14(4):713.

Lynch PJ. Cutaneous diseases of the external genitalia. In Walsh PC, Retik AB, Stamey TA, Vaughan ED (eds). Campbell's urology. 6th ed. Philadelphia: WB Saunders, 1992, pp 861–882.

Mathewson MK. Pharmaco-therapeutics: A nursing process approach. 1st ed. Philadelphia: FA Davis, 1986.

McFarland G. Anxiety. In Thompson J, McFarland G, Hirsch JE, Tucher SM (eds). Clinical nursing. 3rd ed. St. Louis: CV Mosby, 1993, pp 1557–1561.

McFarland G. Fear. In Thompson J, McFarland G, Hirsch JE, Tucher SM (eds). Clinical nursing. 3rd ed. St. Louis: CV Mosby, 1993, pp 1556–1557.

Meares EM. Prostatitis and related disorders. In Walsh C, Retik AB, Stamey TA, Vaughan ED (eds). Campbell's urology. 6th ed. Philadelphia: WB Saunders, 1992, pp 807–822.

Mebust WK. Transurethral surgery. In Walsh P, Retik AB, Stamey TA, Vaughan ED. (eds). Campbell's urology. 6th ed. Philadelphia: WB Saunders, 1992, pp 2900–2922.

Meeker MH, Rothrock JC. Alexander's care of the patient in surgery. 9th ed. St. Louis: CV Mosby, 1992.

Montague D. Testicular prostheses. Urol Clin North Am 1989; 16(1):133.

Murphy J, Lipshultz L. Abnormalities of ejaculation. Urol Clin North Am 1987; 14(3):583.

Nasa J, Lewis R. Varicocele and its surgical management. Urol Clin North Am 1987; 14(1):127.

Oliver RT, Freedman LS, Parkinson MC, Peckham MJ. Medical options in the management of stages 1 and 2 (N0–N3, M0) testicular germ cell tumors. Urol Clin North Am 1987; 14(4):721.

Peters PC. Complications of radical prostatectomy and lymphadenectomy. Urol Clin North Am 1988; 15(2):219.

Pfan A. Prostatitis—A continuing enigma. Urol Clin North Am 1986; 13(4):695.

Prostatitis. In Hamilton HK (ed). Diseases—nursing 87 books. Springhouse, PA: Springhouse, 1987, pp 768–769.

Rajfer J. Congenital anomalies of the testis. In Walsh PC, Retik AB, Stamey TA, Vaughan ED (eds). Campbell's urology. 6th ed. Philadelphia: WB Saunders, 1992, pp 1543–1562.

Richie JP. Neoplasms of the testis. In Walsh PC, Retik AB, Stamey TA, Vaughan ED (eds). Campbell's urology. 6th ed. Philadelphia: WB Saunders, 1992, pp 1222–1263.

Riddy P. Balloon dilation of the prostate for treatment of benign hyperplasia. Urol Clin North Am 1988; 15(3):529.

Rothberg L. The pros and cons of circumcision. RN 1987; 50(7):30.

Schellhammer P, Jordan G, Schlossberg S. Tumors of the penis. In Walsh PC, Retik AB, Stamey TA, Vaughan ED. (eds). Campbell's urology. 6th ed. Philadelphia: WB Saunders, 1992, pp 1264–1298.

Sharlip ID. Surgery of scrotal contents. Urol Clin North Am 1987; 14(1):145.

Sigman M, Howards SS. Male infertility. In Walsh PC, Retik AB, Stamey TA, Vaughan ED (eds). Campbell's urology. 6th ed. Philadelphia: WB Saunders, 1992, pp 661–705.

Sogani P, Fair W. Treatment of advanced prostatic cancer. Urol Clin North Am 1987; 14(2):353.

Stamey TA, McNeal JE. Adenocarcinoma of the prostate. In Walsh PC, Retik AB, Stamey TA, Vaughan ED (eds). Campbell's urology. 6th ed. Philadelphia: WB Saunders, 1992, pp 1159–1221.

Stamm W, Turck M. Urinary tract infections and pyelonephritis. In Wilson J, Braunwald E, Petersdorf R, et al (eds). Harrison's principles of internal medicine. 12th ed. New York: McGraw-Hill, 1991, pp 538–544.

Stutzman RE, Walsh PC. Suprapubic and retropubic prostatectomy. In Walsh PC, Retik AB, Stamey TA, Vaughan ED (eds). Campbell's urology. 6th ed. Philadelphia: WB Saunders, 1992, pp 2851–2864.

Trachtenberg J. Hormonal management of stage D carcinoma of the prostate. Urol Clin North Am 1987; 14(4):685.

Umhauer MA. Drugs that provide pain relief. In Mathewson MK (ed). Pharmaco-therapeutics: A nursing process approach. 1st ed. Philadelphia: FA Davis, 1986, pp 227–262.

Walsh P. Radical prostatectomy, preservation of sexual function, cancer control—the controversy. Urol Clin North Am 1987; 14(4):663.

Walsh PC. Benign prostatic hyperplasia. In Walsh PC, Retik AB, Stamey TA, Vaughan ED (eds). Campbell's urology. 6th ed. Philadelphia: WB Saunders, 1992, pp 1007–1027.

Walsh PC. Radical retropubic prostatectomy. In Walsh PC, Retik AB, Stamey TA, Vaughan ED (eds). Campbell's urology. 6th ed. Philadelphia: WB Saunders, 1992, pp 2865–2886.

Weinerth J. The male genital system. In Sabiston D (ed). Textbook of surgery. 14th ed. Philadelphia: WB Saunders, 1991, pp 1457–1478.

White R DeVere, Nagler H. Priapism. In Krane RJ, Roky M, Goldstein I (eds). Male sexual dysfunction. Boston: Little, Brown, 1983, pp 101–123.

Chapter Forty-seven

NURSING CARE *of Adults with Sexually Transmitted Diseases*

Sexually transmitted diseases are caused by organisms transmitted through sexual contact: genital-genital, oral-genital, oral-anal, or genital-anal. These reportable diseases, which are most prevalent among teenagers and young adults, constitute a major public health problem. The number of infected individuals is increasing as is the number of individuals with multiple, coexisting sexually transmitted diseases. The incidence continues to rise even though the acquired immunodeficiency syndrome (AIDS) epidemic has increased public awareness of the need for measures to prevent transmission of sexually transmitted diseases.

Sequelae of sexually transmitted diseases include infertility, ectopic pregnancy, perinatal infection, and, most notably in the case of acquired immunodeficiency syndrome (AIDS) (discussed with immune disorders in Chapter 10), death.

Sexually Transmitted Vaginitis

Vaginal infections are among the most common gynecologic problems seen in adult women. The three most common types of vaginal infections are vulvovaginal candidiasis, trichomoniasis, and nonspecific vaginitis, more correctly identified as *Gardnerella vaginalis* vaginitis (Table 47–1).

Vaginal fluid is composed of multiple components, including water, electrolytes, epithelial cells, microbial organisms, fatty acids, carbohydrates, and proteins. A large number of microorganisms normally inhabit vaginal fluid. Common organisms include lactobacilli, corynebacteria, streptococci, *Staphylococcus epidermidis,* and *G. vaginalis.* Although potentially pathogenic microbial organisms may be recovered from the vagina at any given time, they do not necessarily indicate infection. The complex milieu of the vaginal flora maintains a balance that normally suppresses the overgrowth of pathogens.

Several factors influence the quantity and quality of the organisms present in vaginal fluid. During the reproductive years, the pH of the vagina is normally acidic (4.0–4.5 pH). Maintenance of this low vaginal pH is dependent on adequate levels of estrogens, glucose, and glycogen and the presence of lactobacilli. Estrogens increase the glycogen content of the epithelial cells of the vaginal wall. Vaginal epithelial cells, lactobacilli, and other microorganisms use glycogen and glucose for metabolism, making it less available for the growth of harmful organisms. More important, they produce lactic acid as a product of metabolism. Lactic acid maintains the low vaginal pH. When the balance of the normal vaginal environment is altered, for example, during periods of progesterone predominance such as pregnancy, the

Table 47–1. COMMON TYPES OF SEXUALLY TRANSMITTED VAGINITIS

INFECTION	CLINICAL MANIFESTATIONS	MEDICAL TREATMENT	TRANSMISSION	COMMENTS
Candidiasis	Severe vulvovaginal itching White curdlike, nonodorous vaginal discharge (in some cases discharge may be normal) Edema, redness, excoriation of vulva and perineum Burning, pain, dyspareunia	Antifungal agents (vaginal tablets or creams) Nystatin: 100,000 units BID for 10 days (tablets or cream) Clotrimazole: 100 mg tablets or 1% cream BID for 7 days Miconazole: 100 mg tablets or 2% cream BID for 7 days	Role of sexual transmission limited and less important than in other STDs	Factors that promote growth of *Candida* infections include the following: Pregnancy Oral contraceptives Antibiotics Diabetes Corticosteroids Immunosuppression Menstruation
Gardnerella vaginalis vaginitis	Frequently malodorous vaginal discharge; fishy odor Thin, grayish-white, nonirritating discharge	Metronidazole: 500 mg PO BID for 7 days	May be sexually transmitted	*G. vaginalis* and anaerobic bacteria act synergistically to produce infection Usually mild Does not cause inflammation Males do not require treatment
Trichomoniasis	Profuse, malodorous, uncomfortable vaginal discharge White to greenish-gray watery discharge (may appear frothy) Dysuria Pruritus	Metronidazole: single dose, 2 g PO or 250 mg PO TID for 10 days	Sexually transmitted Abstain from sexual intercourse during active infection or use condom Prevention: condom	Treat sex partners concurrently 70% can be diagnosed on Papanicolaou smear

Abbreviations: BID, twice daily; PO, orally; TID, three times daily; STDs, sexually transmitted diseases.

vaginal pH becomes more alkalotic, providing an environment conducive to the overgrowth of potentially pathogenic organisms.

Vulvovaginal Candidiasis

ETIOLOGY

Fungal infections account for 20% to 30% of vaginal infections. *Candida albicans* causes 80% to 90% of these vaginal fungal infections. Small numbers of *C. albicans* commonly inhabit the vagina in asymptomatic women. Infection is associated with an alteration in the normal vaginal microbial environment and decreased host resistance rather than contagious spread.

PATHOPHYSIOLOGY

C. albicans primarily affects women during their menstruating years; it rarely occurs before menarche or after menopause. The effects of estrogen, including the presence of glycogen stores in the epithelium, supports the growth of *Candida*. Overgrowth of vaginal *Candida* and subsequent infection is associated with a number of host and epidemiologic factors. Pregnancy, oral contraceptives, menstruation, antibiotics and corticosteroids, diabetes, and immunosuppression have all been identified as predisposing factors to the development of candidiasis.

Candidiasis is twice as common in pregnant versus nonpregnant females, and the incidence increases as the pregnancy advances. Ten percent of candidal infections seen during pregnancy occur during the first trimester, whereas 36% to 55% occur in the third trimester. In addition, cure rates are lower and recurrency rates are higher in pregnancy. The increase in the occurrence and severity of candidal infections in pregnancy is generally attributed to depressed cellular immunity and the increase in vaginal glycogen stores commonly seen during pregnancy. The same mechanism (i.e., increased availability of glucose and glycogen) has been suggested as the explanation for the reported increased incidence of vulvovaginal *Candida* in diabetic females and oral contraceptive users. Recurrent episodes of vulvovaginal candidiasis may be the first manifestation of diabetes.

The incidence of vulvovaginal candidiasis increases with systemic antibiotic use, particularly antibiotics active against lactobacilli such as the penicillins, cephalosporins, and tetracyclines. It is hypothesized that antibiotics alter vaginal flora by decreasing the numbers of lactobacilli, thus elevating the pH and providing glycogen to promote growth of *C. albicans*. Some authorities suggest that patients with a history of candidal infections who are on systemic antibiotics known to be active against lactobacilli should also receive concomitant antifungal therapy.

The role of sexual transmission in the epidemiology of candidiasis is not completely understood. However, it is thought to be less substantial than in other sexually transmitted diseases. Most cases of genital candidiasis in males can be traced to an infected female sexual partner. However, the role of male transmission to females is not clear. In addition, fungal infections are not associated with the presence of other sexually transmitted diseases. These factors suggest that sexual contact plays a limited role in the transmission of genital *Candida*.

CLINICAL MANIFESTATIONS

The most common symptom of genital candidiasis is severe vulvovaginal itching. Pruritus may be accompanied by external dysuria related to the urine passing over the infected vulva. Vaginal discharge is typically thick, white, and nonodorous, resembling cottage cheese. It may appear as white, adherent plaques on the surface of the vaginal wall. However, in many cases, vaginal discharge appears normal.

Other signs and symptoms of vulvovaginal candidal infection include vulval edema, erythema, and perineal fissures and excoriation, reflecting the effects of frequent itching. In males, the most common manifestation is balanitis, which is an inflammation of the glans penis. Symptoms include erythema, "glazed skin" appearance, and mild desquamation or crusting.

MEDICAL DIAGNOSIS

Diagnosis is made on the basis of clinical manifestations and is confirmed by microscopic examination of vaginal fluid. If symptoms suggest vulvovaginal candidiasis but the result of microscopic examination is negative, cultures are taken to verify the diagnosis.

MEDICAL MANAGEMENT

Local application of antifungal agents is the treatment of choice for genital candidiasis. Traditionally, intravaginal application of 100,000 units of nystatin (Mycostatin) cream or suppositories, twice daily for 10 days, is the recommended treatment. Currently, newer, more active antifungal agents are available that have higher cure rates. The vaginal creams clotrimazole (Lotrimin) and miconazole (Monistat 7) are frequently recommended, particularly for recurrent candidiasis. For additional information on the pharmacologic treatment of candidiasis, see Table 47–1.

Trichomoniasis

ETIOLOGY AND PATHOPHYSIOLOGY

Trichomoniasis is one of the most common sexually transmitted urogenital infections. Approximately 2.5 million cases are diagnosed yearly in the United States. It is caused by *Trichomonas vaginalis*, a single-cell flagellated protozoon. *T. vaginalis* is frequently found in coexistence with other sexually transmitted pathogens. For example, 40% of females with gonorrhea also have trichomoniasis. Generally, it is difficult to isolate in males. Some studies indicate that exposed males are unaffected or that it is a self-limiting, generally benign disease in males.

CLINICAL MANIFESTATIONS

Trichomoniasis is characterized by a profuse, malodorous, often uncomfortable vaginal discharge that may be associated with mild dysuria. The discharge is homogeneous, greenish-gray, and watery and often appears purulent or frothy (Fig. 47–1). The vaginal and cervical epithelia may appear reddened and inflamed. On colposcopic examination, pinpoint hemorrhagic spots may be apparent on the cervix, giving it a strawberry appearance characteristic of trichomoniasis. Asymptomatic infection also occurs, and some estimate that it may be as high as 50% of infected females. In males, *T. vaginalis* is present in the lower urinary tract and may cause prostatitis (infection of the prostate gland) in a few cases. More typically, males are asymptomatic carriers.

MEDICAL DIAGNOSIS

Diagnosis is usually made on the basis of clinical symptoms and a wet-mount microscopic examination of vaginal fluid that demonstrates the presence of motile *Trichomonas. Trichomonas* is occasionally seen on Papanicolaou (Pap) smears. If wet-mount smear fails to demonstrate the organism in the presence of clinical symptoms, then cultures are recommended.

MEDICAL MANAGEMENT

Metronidazole (Flagyl) is the only consistently effective drug used in the treatment of trichomoniasis. A single dose, 2 g orally, is recommended because it is more likely to guarantee compliance, is inexpensive, and has the same cure rate as an extended regimen (i.e., 250 mg three times a day for 10 days). Simultaneous treatment of male sexual partners is recommended to decrease the incidence of reinfection.

Gardnerella Vaginalis Vaginitis

ETIOLOGY AND PATHOPHYSIOLOGY

In the past, all vaginal infections not attributable to candidiasis, trichomoniasis, or gonorrhea were labeled nonspecific vaginitis (NSV), reflecting the unknown cause of the infection. In 1954, Gardner and Dukes identified *Haemophilus vaginalis* as the causative organism. Currently, called *G. vaginalis,* these small gram-negative bacteria are present in at least 95% of women with symptoms of NSV.

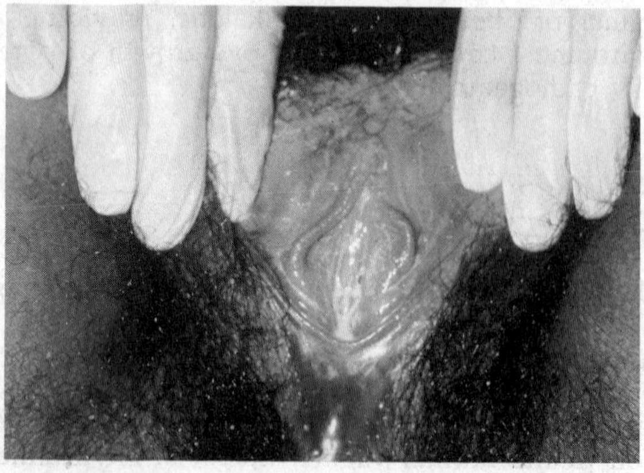

Figure 47–1.

Trichomoniasis vaginal discharge. Note that the discharge is often profuse and watery and may appear purulent. (Courtesy of Leonard Wolf, M.D., New York, NY.)

As indicated previously, *G. vaginalis* is a frequent constituent of normal vaginal discharge, occurring in 40% of asymptomatic women. It is hypothesized that *G. vaginalis* infection occurs as a result of a complex alteration in the vaginal flora that promotes an increase in the concentration of *G. vaginalis* as well as anaerobic bacteria that act synergistically to produce symptoms associated with NSV.

Similar to candidiasis, the role of sexual transmission in the epidemiology of *G. vaginalis* is questionable and not well understood. *G. vaginalis* is more prevalent in the male partners of infected females. Ninety percent of males in sexual contact with infected females are positive for *G. vaginalis.* Males generally do not require treatment except to prevent recurrences in their female partners. The incidence of *G. vaginalis* infection is positively correlated with the following risk factors in women: parity (number of pregnancies), number of sexual partners, intrauterine device (IUD) use, and the presence of cervical infections.

CLINICAL MANIFESTATIONS

G. vaginalis is generally not considered a severe infection. Vaginal leukocytes are not greatly increased nor is the vaginal epithelium inflamed. The primary clinical manifestation is a slightly increased malodorous vaginal discharge. The discharge is usually nonirritating, thin, homogeneous, adherent, and grayish-white. It emits a characteristic "fishy" odor, particularly after sexual intercourse. If symptoms occur in the male, they are similar to those associated with nongonococcal urethritis: a slight watery urethral discharge with or without dysuria.

MEDICAL DIAGNOSIS

Clinical diagnosis of *G. vaginalis* infection is made on the basis of the presence of three of four signs:

1. Characteristic discharge
2. pH of vaginal fluid greater than 4.5
3. Release of foul, fishy odor when vaginal fluid is mixed with 10% potassium hydroxide (whiff test)
4. Presence of "clue cells" on microscopic examination of vaginal fluid (clue cells are vaginal epithelial cells that appear granular because of bacteria on the cell surface)

MEDICAL MANAGEMENT

Metronidazole (Flagyl), 500 mg twice daily for 7 days, is the most effective therapeutic agent in the treatment of NSV. It is active against anaerobic bacteria as well as *G. vaginalis*. The cure rate is 85%. If alcohol is ingested during therapy with this drug, it produces nausea and vomiting. Metronidazole is contraindicated in pregnancy. Ampicillin, 500 mg orally four times per day for 7 days, is an alternative treatment, especially for pregnant females. It is highly active against *G. vaginalis* but has little effect on anaerobic bacteria. Its cure rate is variously reported as between 60% and 80%.

Application of the Nursing Process to the Care of the Patient with Vaginitis

Assessment

A thorough history is the most important part of the nursing assessment of the female with a vaginal infection. Question the patient about signs and symptoms of vaginitis (i.e., vaginal discharge, pruritus, dysuria). Analyze each symptom according to its onset, duration, character, and relieving and aggravating factors. Ask the patient to describe the color, consistency, amount, and odor of the vaginal discharge. Determine whether this is an initial or recurrent infection. Question the patient about previous vaginal infections and her history of other sexually transmitted diseases.

Be certain to include an assessment of the patient's knowledge of normal vaginal functioning and vaginal discharge. Also review her health status and personal hygienic practices. Of particular interest are practices that may predispose her to infection or exacerbate an existing infection such as frequent douching with solutions that may adversely alter the normal vaginal pH and practices that increase warmth, moisture, and trauma to the vagina. Question the patient about the presence of factors known to promote candidiasis, such as antibiotic and oral contraceptive use, diabetes, pregnancy, and other immunosuppressive conditions or medications.

Obtain an obstetric, gynecologic, and sexual history, and assess the patient's emotional response to the presence of a vaginal infection. Be certain to provide an environment that is private, supportive, and nonthreatening. Many females may be anxious, particularly if they view the cause of the condition as unknown or as a sign of venereal disease. Others are reluctant to discuss their symptoms or provide the necessary historic data because of fear or embarrassment. Thus, it is essential to be reassuring, empathetic, and nonjudgmental.

Physical examination includes inspection of the external genitalia and vaginal opening for the presence of discharge, odor, or signs of inflammation (i.e., redness, swelling, excoriation). This is followed by a vaginal and cervical examination with a speculum performed by a physician or a nurse.

See Table 47–2 for a summary of assessment data relevant to patients with sexually transmitted diseases.

Nursing Diagnoses and Planning

Nursing diagnoses and related expected patient outcomes most commonly applicable to patients with sexually transmitted vaginitis include the following:

NDx: Pain related to the inflammatory process

Planning: Patient outcomes
1. Patient reports using measures recommended to reduce discomfort and using medication as prescribed.
2. Patient states itching and burning have been relieved.
3. Edema, redness, and excoriation of the vaginal epithelium and external genitalia have disappeared.

NDx: High risk for altered health maintenance related to insufficient knowledge of normal vaginal function, personal hygiene, disease process, or sexual mode of transmission

Planning: Patient outcomes
1. Patient accurately describes normal vaginal functioning and the characteristics of normal vaginal discharge.
2. Patient identifies three factors that may alter normal vaginal physiology and predispose to infection.
3. Patient identifies three health practices that decrease the risk of vaginal infection.
4. Patient states the cause and symptoms of specific vaginal infections.
5. Patient describes the role of sexual contact in transmission of specific vaginal infections.
6. Patient describes methods for preventing transmission of infection.

NDx: Anxiety related to cause of vaginitis and concerns about physical and lifestyle effects

Planning: Patient outcomes
1. Patient discusses her concerns about vaginal infection and its potential effects.
2. Patient reports feeling less anxious about the vaginal infection and its outcome.

Table 47–2. ASSESSMENT OF PATIENTS WITH SEXUALLY TRANSMITTED DISEASES

GENERAL CONSIDERATIONS

Perform assessment in an environment that provides for patient confidentiality, privacy, and psychological and physical comfort.

Ask open-ended questions using language and terms familiar to the patient.

Communicate a warm, empathetic, nonjudgmental attitude.

HEALTH HISTORY

1. Chief complaint: reason for coming to clinic, office, hospital
2. History of current illness/problem:
   - Signs and symptoms
     - Onset
     - Initial or recurrent
     - Precipitating factors
     - Duration
     - Frequency
     - Character
     - Location
     - Relieving and aggravating factors
3. Health history
   - Medical conditions
   - Previous surgeries
   - Treatments and therapies
   - Allergies
4. Sexual history
5. Reproductive and gynecological history
   - Triad (age at onset, frequency, duration of menses)
   - Pain or abnormal bleeding during or between periods or during sexual intercourse
   - Fertility/infertility
   - Number and outcomes of pregnancies, miscarriages, abortions
   - Infections during pregnancy
   - Gynecologic conditions
     - Infections of the genitourinary tract (e.g., vaginitis, cervicitis, PID, urethritis)
     - Endometriosis
     - Tumors, cysts: benign, malignant
   - Contraceptive practices
   - Health maintenance
     - Hygiene practices
     - Frequency of Papanicolaou smears; gynecologic examinations
6. Medications (prescription and over the counter): drug, dose, reason, side effects, last dose, effectiveness
7. Health maintenance activities
   - Personal hygiene practices
   - Activities of daily living
   - Health promotion activities (diet, exercise, sleep)
   - Frequency of physician/clinic visits

COMMUNICATION STATUS

1. Orientation
2. Language spoken
3. Ability to communicate ideas
4. Ability to understand verbal communication of others
5. Ability to cooperate in plan of care

EDUCATIONAL STATUS

1. Learning needs (e.g., disease process, mode of transmission, prevention)
2. Educational level
3. Ability to learn new information: learning level
4. Readiness to learn
   - Emotional readiness
   - Motivation
5. Preferred methods of learning

PSYCHOSOCIAL ASSESSMENT

1. Age
2. Marital status
3. Employment history
4. Financial status
5. Recent travel
6. Family members, significant others
7. Availability of support
8. Emotional response to illness
9. Current or anticipated response of significant others to illness
10. Current or anticipated effect of illness on social activities; interpersonal relationships; sexual identity; self-esteem; lifestyle
11. Ability and motivation to comply with treatment regimens

PHYSICAL ASSESSMENT

GENERAL CONSIDERATIONS

Observe for clinical manifestations of sexually transmitted diseases throughout assessment.

Inspection and palpation are the primary methods of assessment for sexually transmitted diseases.

Wear gloves to inspect the mouth, genitals, perineum, and anus; wear gloves to palpate lesions.

Assessment for sexually transmitted diseases is carried out in a warm, well-lighted room. Provide the patient with a gown, and use a drape to protect patient's privacy and to cover areas not under examination.

SPECIFIC CONSIDERATIONS

1. Assess for the presence of systemic symptoms. Obtain vital signs, apical and radial pulses, respiratory rate and rhythm, blood pressure, and temperature.
2. Assess mouth and throat. Inspect the oral cavity, tongue, lips, gingiva, and palpate for lesions, sores, or signs of infections (see skin assessment next).
3. Skin
   - General inspection: Note color, texture, temperature, vascularity, and moisture.
   - Inspect for the presence of lesions. Note the following:
     - Type: vesicles, papules, macules, pustules, buboes, ulcers
     - Size, shape, and configuration
     - Location
     - Distribution
     - Signs of inflammation: edema, erythema, induration, exudate (color, amount, odor, consistency)
     - Signs of pruritus: scratches, excoriation
     - Observe for burrows from scabies
   - Palpate lesions for
     - Consistency (soft, firm)
     - Mobility
     - Pain and tenderness
   - Inspect body and pubic hair for evidence of lice or nits.
4. Genitalia and anus (examine males in a supine or standing position; examine females in the lithotomy position)
   - Inspect the genitalia, perineum, and anus for lesions, signs of inflammation, and pruritus (see previous skin assessment).
   - Palpate lesions when necessary for consistency and presence or absence of pain.
   - Inspect the vaginal introitus and labia in females and urethral meatus and anus in males and females for signs of discharge and inflammation. Note the color, consistency, amount, and odor of any vaginal, urethral, or rectal discharge.
   - Palpate the inguinal lymph nodes for enlargement or tenderness.

Abbreviation: PID, pelvic inflammatory disease.

Chart 47–1.

NURSING GUIDE TO PATIENT EDUCATION FOR SELF-MANAGEMENT: SEXUALLY TRANSMITTED VAGINAL INFECTIONS

Explain the following to the patient:

Most vaginal infections are primarily transmitted through sexual contact.

- Trichomoniasis is a sexually transmitted disease. Nonsexual transmission via fomites, such as wet towels, soap dishes, and the backwash from toilets is a possible but infrequent occurrence.
- *Gardnerella vaginalis* may be transmitted via sexual contact. Transmission by fomites is considered possible.
- The designation of candidiasis as a sexually transmitted disease is controversial. Predisposing factors that alter the normal vaginal flora, increase the vaginal pH, or alter the immune response must be present for infection to occur. Sexual transmission of candidiasis is possible because males may harbor and transmit the fungus.

Sexual partners may need to be treated depending on the type of vaginitis and likelihood of the male carrying the organism.

- Treatment of partners is recommended for trichomoniasis, especially if the infection is recurrent.
- Partners of females with candidal infections are usually not treated unless the female's infection is chronic or recurrent and the male also has symptoms of infection.
- If treatment is recommended, both partners should be treated simultaneously to avoid reinfection.

The full dose of medication should be taken as prescribed.

- All medications ordered must be taken even if symptoms disappear.
- Alcohol should be avoided for 48 to 72 hours after treatment with metronidazole, which is the treatment of choice for both trichomoniasis and *G. vaginalis* vaginitis.

Patients with chronic or recurrent candidal infections should seek treatment at the first sign of infection. Prophylactic antifungal medications may be recommended during antibiotic or immunosuppressive therapies.

3. Patient's behavior suggests reduced anxiety (i.e., relaxed posture, absence of nervous mannerisms).

See Nursing Care Guide 47–1, Patients with Sexually Transmitted Diseases, for additional nursing diagnoses and patient outcomes that may apply to patients with sexually transmitted vaginitis or any other sexually transmitted disease.

Nursing Interventions

NDx: Pain

Review the medication treatment plan with the patient, including the name, dose, route, and times the medication is to be taken. Caution the patient to use all the medication as prescribed and not just until the symptoms have abated. Verify that the patient knows how to insert vaginal creams and suppositories as prescribed.

Recommend the use of cool compresses, sitz baths, and loose cotton undergarments to reduce discomfort until medication is effective, which is usually 1 or 2 days after starting medication.

NDx: High risk for altered health maintenance

Teach the patient about normal vaginal flora, vaginal pH, and the constituents of normal vaginal discharge using simple, nontechnical language. Include a discussion of factors that may alter normal vaginal physiology (i.e., pregnancy, medications, menstruation). Once the diagnosis is made, review the cause, symptoms, and treatment of the patient's specific infection. Present basic facts about the mode of transmission, treatment, and prevention of the infection, as specified in Chart 47–1.

Text continued on page 1844

Nursing Care Guide 47–1.
PATIENTS WITH SEXUALLY TRANSMITTED DISEASES

Assessment Findings: Patient complains of pain and pruritus in genital area and burning on urination.

Nursing Diagnosis: Pain related to the inflammatory process

Patient Outcomes	Nursing Interventions	Rationale
Patient states pain or pruritus is diminished or absent. Patient's nonverbal behavior indicates physical comfort (relaxed posture, facial expression, movements). Patient is able to carry out normal daily activities.	Assist the patient in reducing or eliminating pain or pruritus: Explain the cause of the patient's pain and pruritus.	Knowledge of causative factors reduces psychological stress, reducing pain.
	Assist the patient in identifying factors that precipitate or contribute to experience of pain and pruritus. Common factors include the following: ■ Physical and environmental factors: pressure, friction, warmth, moisture or dryness, scratching, manipulation, daily activities, time of day ■ Psychosocial factors: anxiety, fear, fatigue, lack of diversional activities	Recognition of precipitating factors allows patient to avoid behavior that causes pain or pruritus.
	Assist patient in identifying and using strategies for relieving pain/pruritus.	
	Instruct the patient in proper self-administration of oral or topical medications for the relief of pain or pruritus. ■ Caution patient to use analgesics before pain is severe. ■ Instruct patient to use applicator, gauze, or gloves when applying topical medications to infected areas. ■ Review dosage, schedule, and side effects of medications.	Correct use of medication ensures better results.

(continued)

Nursing Care Guide 47–1. *(continued)*

PATIENTS WITH SEXUALLY TRANSMITTED DISEASES

Patient Outcomes	Nursing Interventions	Rationale
	Instruct patient in alternative techniques for management of pain and pruritus.	
	Explore the patient's previous pain experiences and methods for alleviating pain. Determine the patient's prior knowledge and willingness to use alternative strategies for management of pain and pruritus. Provide guidance and instruction in the following: *cutaneous stimulation* (application of heat and cold massage); *distraction* (plan daily activities; use breathing techniques, engage in recreational activities); *relaxation* (progressive relaxation; meditation; slow, rhythmic breathing; imaging).	Methods that have been previously successful in relieving pain/pruritus are likely to continue to be successful. Other methods relate to the gate control theory of pain relief. Distraction and relaxation succeed by lowering the patient's perception of pain.
	Advise patient to avoid excessive warmth, moisture, or dryness (e.g., wear loose clothing and cotton undergarments, avoid overdressing, avoid activities that cause pressure or friction at site); use mild soap, blot skin dry.	Reduces stimulation of nerve endings and irritation of local tissues.
	Administer medication for relief of pain and pruritus. Instruct patient to request medication before symptoms are severe. Respond to patient's request for medication within acceptable time limits. Monitor effectiveness of medication.	Medications provide temporary relief of pain/pruritus by altering perception or decreasing the reception of stimuli.

Evaluation: Compare the patient's status with the expected patient outcomes. If the outcomes are achieved, evaluate nursing care as successful. If not, reassess the patient, formulate new nursing diagnoses, and revise expected patient outcomes and nursing interventions as appropriate.

(continued)

Nursing Care Guide 47–1. *(continued)*

PATIENTS WITH SEXUALLY TRANSMITTED DISEASES

Assessment Findings: Patient has a sexually transmitted infection caused by an infectious organism capable of infecting other unaffected sites.

Nursing Diagnosis: High risk for infection (secondary) related to bacterial contamination

Patient Outcomes	Nursing Interventions	Rationale
Signs of secondary infection—inflammation and purulent discharge unrelated to primary infection—are absent. Patient carries out recommended hygienic practices. Infection remains confined to original or commonly encountered genital sites.	Prevent secondary infection and spread of disease to unaffected sites: Assist patient in maintaining adequate hygiene.	
	Instruct females to wipe perineal/rectal area from front to back after voiding or defecating; blot skin dry to avoid spreading organisms and infected discharge from affected to unaffected areas. Rinsing with a peribottle filled with lukewarm water may be helpful in maintaining perineal hygiene.	Wiping from front to back prevents organisms from moving from dirty areas to clean. Blotting reduces transfer of organisms from one area to another. Use of the peri-bottle allows water to flush organisms from the area.
	Douching is generally not recommended but may be indicated for voluminous or malodorous vaginal discharge. Consult with physician before advising patient.	Douching modifies the normal acidic pH of the vagina and can eliminate normal vaginal flora, which provide a self-cleaning property to the vagina.
	Recommend daily baths or showers using mild soap and lukewarm water.	Showers and baths help to remove organisms from the body surface.
	Instruct patient to avoid excessive warmth and moisture: Keep room cool; wear cotton underwear; avoid constrictive clothing, pantyhose, and overdressing	Warm, moist environments are excellent media for the growth of microorganisms.
	Explain importance of not manipulating or touching lesions or secretions; many sexually transmitted diseases can be spread by autoinoculation; hands are a source of infective organisms.	Reduces the spread of the organisms by the hands.

(continued)

Nursing Care Guide 47–1. *(continued)*

PATIENTS WITH SEXUALLY TRANSMITTED DISEASES

Patient Outcomes	Nursing Interventions	Rationale
	Advise frequent changes in undergarments and sanitary pads when secretions or vaginal discharge is present to decrease accumulation and potential spread of secretions.	Frequent changes remove organisms that can be spread over the skin surface.
	Recommend sitz baths for cleanliness and comfort; use lukewarm water. Caution against too frequent soaking, which may cause skin maceration.	Warm water flushes organisms from the body surface. Warmth also brings white blood cells to the area, which help fight infection.
Patient performs wound- and skin-care techniques as instructed.	Instruct patient in proper technique of wound irrigation if ordered using normal saline, sterile water, hydrogen peroxide, or antiseptic.	Wound irrigation may be indicated for extensive tissue damage resulting from ruptured abscesses, draining sinuses, or fistulas since it removes secretions and debris from the area to allow healing to occur.
	Instruct patient in use of heat lamp if ordered to increase circulation to the affected area or to dry lesions.	Heat reduces moisture, making the environment less conducive to organisms' growth. Heat also causes vasodilation, which increases the presence of white blood cells to fight infection and red blood cells and protein for healing.
	Prevent further injury:	
	Advise against scratching (see interventions for pruritus).	Scratching the area can cause irritation and excoriation of the skin.
	Caution against self-medication with over-the-counter drugs or previously used medication unless recommended by physician.	May cause tissue irritation or alter effect of prescribed medications.
	Advise patient to maintain adequate nutrition and fluid intake.	Adequate hydration decreases risk of urinary tract infections because good urinary output flushes organisms quickly out of the urinary system. Protein and vitamins are needed for tissue repair.

Evaluation: Compare the patient's status with the expected patient outcomes. If the outcomes are achieved, evaluate nursing care as successful. If not, reassess the patient, formulate new nursing diagnoses, and revise expected patient outcomes and nursing interventions as appropriate.

(continued)

Nursing Care Guide 47–1. *(continued)*

PATIENTS WITH SEXUALLY TRANSMITTED DISEASES

Assessment Findings: Patient states he or she "will try" to follow the treatment regimen but his or her sexual partner "isn't going to like it." Patient asks "Is this really necessary? I think you people like to make a big deal out of nothing."

Nursing Diagnosis: High risk for noncompliance with prescribed treatment and palliative measures related to sexual lifestyle and behaviors, lack of knowledge regarding rationale for following treatment regimen and using preventive measures, anger and hostility, or unsatisfactory relationship with care givers

Patient Outcomes	Nursing Interventions	Rationale
Follow-up tests of cure are negative.	Determine patient's ability and willingness to comply with treatment regimen. Remember: successful therapy depends on patient compliance. Potential noncompliers include individuals who are: ■ Unable to follow directions ■ Unable to comprehend verbal or written instructions because of intellectual deficits, inability to read, language barriers ■ Hostile, uncooperative, and unmotivated ■ Distrustful of health care professionals ■ Uninformed about the reasons for taking medications as prescribed (Note: Selection of the type of medication and route of administration is influenced by the health care professional's perception of the patient's potential compliance. A single-dose parenteral medication may be indicated rather than an oral regimen for potential noncompliers.)	Recognition of reasons for noncompliance assists in the formulation of interventions likely to be successful.
Patient is able to relate the action, dosage, schedule, and potential side effects of prescribed medications. Patient reports taking medications as prescribed.	Provide instruction in self-administration of medication: Relate and explain the action, dosage, schedule, and possible side effects of prescribed medications.	The patient must understand expected behaviors to self-administer medication correctly.

(continued)

Nursing Care Guide 47–1. *(continued)*

PATIENTS WITH SEXUALLY TRANSMITTED DISEASES

Patient Outcomes	Nursing Interventions	Rationale
	Assist the patient in planning how to incorporate taking medications into daily routine. Suggest ways the patient can remember to take medications (e.g., always before or after meals; place medications in a convenient, visible place).	Problem solving with the medication schedule assists the patient in compliance.
	Provide written instructions, including name and telephone number of person to contact if questions arise or if side effects develop.	Questions often arise during the actual experience of self-administration. Having a resource available provides access to needed information and promotes compliance.
	Advise patients on how to manage omission of one or more doses.	Provides information about appropriate reaction to a common problem so that blood levels of medication can be maintained.
Patient states the rationale for following the prescribed treatment regimen.	Explain the rationale for following the prescribed treatment regimen by instructing the patient in the following: ■ Medications must be taken at the prescribed intervals for the recommended number of days to effect a cure and to avoid complications, long-term sequelae, and transmission to others. ■ Resolution of symptoms before completion of the treatment course does not indicate a cure; continue taking medications. ■ One or more follow-up visits to test for cure may be necessary. Some organisms may be resistant to the precribed medication.	Provides the patient with information that promotes compliance.
Patient returns for follow-up visit.	Set a date and time for a follow-up visit that is convenient for the patient.	By absolving the patient of the responsibility of scheduling a revisit, the likelihood of compliance is increased.
	Provide an opportunity for the patient to ask questions and express concerns.	Clarifies misinformation and reduces patient anxiety.

(continued)

Nursing Care Guide 47–1. *(continued)*

PATIENTS WITH SEXUALLY TRANSMITTED DISEASES

Patient Outcomes	Nursing Interventions	Rationale
Patient reports complying with recommendations for preventing transmission to others during treatment period.	Prevent transmission to others: Advise patient to abstain from sexual intercourse until completion of treatment or follow-up test of cure.	Semen and vaginal secretions contain infective material for an undetermined period of time during treatment.
	Recommend use of condoms if patient appears unlikely to comply.	Provides a barrier to reduce the possibility of transmission of organisms.
	Inform patient of potential effects on sexual partners. Long-term sequelae, adverse effects, and complications from sexually transmitted disease are more common in females and include pelvic inflammatory disease, infertility, and poor pregnancy and perinatal outcomes.	Provides rationale to promote patient compliance.

Evaluation: Compare the patient's status with the expected patient outcomes. If the outcomes are achieved, evaluate nursing care as successful. If not, reassess the patient, formulate new nursing diagnoses, and revise expected patient outcomes and nursing interventions as appropriate.

(continued)

NDx: Anxiety

Provide an opportunity for the patient to express her concerns about having acquired a vaginal infection. Give particular attention to correcting any myths or misconceptions the patient may have about vaginal discharge and the nature of vaginal infections. Present the information tactfully and sensitively in a quiet, private, nonthreatening environment. Emphasize the positive aspects of the diagnosis: that effective treatment is available and that no long-term effects occur. Be certain to inform the patient of the possible, although infrequent, nonsexual transmission of causative organisms.

Evaluation

Evaluate the effectiveness of nursing care for a patient with sexually transmitted vaginitis by comparing the patient's status with the expected patient outcomes. Examples of specific outcomes for patients with sexually transmitted vaginitis have been provided in the Planning section.

Genital Herpes

Etiology

The herpes simplex viruses (HSV) are one of a group of four herpes viruses known to infect humans. There are two herpes simplex viruses: herpes simplex virus 1 (HSV 1) and herpes simplex virus 2 (HSV 2). Although clinically indistinguishable, the two herpes viruses have different biologic properties. The molecular composition, growth patterns in cultures, and antibodies they elicit are different. Clinically, both can cause recurrent vesicles

Text continued on page 1850

Nursing Care Guide 47–1. *(continued)*

PATIENTS WITH SEXUALLY TRANSMITTED DISEASES

Assessment Findings: Sexual partner will not come for treatment. Patient expresses doubt about need for preventive measures, verbalizing "If you're going to get it, you're going to get it."

Nursing Diagnosis: High risk for infection (reinfection) related to insufficient knowledge of the disease, its mode of transmission, and prevention; failure to comply with treatment and recommended preventive measures; resumption of sexual relations with untreated partners

Patient Outcomes	Nursing Interventions	Rationale
Patient is able to state the rationale for altering personal behaviors that increase the risk of infection.	Assist the patient to prevent reinfection and incorporate preventive techniques into sexual lifestyle.	Modifications of sexual lifestyle can prevent reinfection.
Patient identifies factors that increase the risk of infection.	Collaborate with patient to identify factors that increase risk of infection. High-risk factors include the following: ■ Multiple sexual partners ■ Sex with anonymous partners ■ Sex with prostitutes (male or female) ■ Unprotected sexual intercourse ■ Sex with partners who have multiple partners	Knowledge of factors that increase the risk of infection allows modifications to reduce the risk.
Patient describes preventive behaviors and health practices for reducing the risk of reinfection or infection with other sexually transmitted diseases. Patient states intention to use preventive measures and recommended health practices or to change high-risk behaviors.	Recommend the following behaviors or measures to reduce the risk of reinfection:	
	■ Use condoms when engaging in genital or anal intercourse. Condoms are the primary preventive measure for reducing the risk of exposure to sexually transmitted disease (STD).	Condoms form a barrier against the transmission of infective material.
	■ Know your partner: Avoid sex with multiple, anonymous partners and prostitutes.	Limiting sexual contact to known partners reduces risk of reinfection.
Symptoms of reinfection are absent at follow-up visit.	■ Observe the genitals of prospective sexual partners for signs of STD.	Evidence of infection may be present, alerting the patient to the risk of reinfection.
	■ Avoid sex with partners who manifest signs and symptoms of STDs.	Decreases the risk of reinfection.
	■ Urinate after sex; wash genitals.	Urine has a flushing action, which helps to remove organisms. Washing the genitals removes surface organisms.

(continued)

Nursing Care Guide 47–1. *(continued)*

PATIENTS WITH SEXUALLY TRANSMITTED DISEASES

Patient Outcomes	Nursing Interventions	Rationale
Patient seeks treatment at first sign of STD.	■ Obtain medical assistance at the first sign of STD.	Early medical intervention is beneficial to the patient and reduces the spread of the disease to sexual partners.
	■ Complete the recommended treatment course.	Incomplete treatment may lead to redevelopment of the infection and to the development of antibiotic-resistant organisms.
	■ Avoid sex with previously exposed untreated partners.	Prevents reexposure from infected sexual partner.
	Assist the patient in identifying preventive measures that are realistic and acceptable given his or her values and lifestyle.	Realistic and acceptable preventive methods are more likely to be included in the patient's sexual lifestyle.
	■ Communicate a nonjudgmental, objective, and supportive attitude.	Accepting behaviors by the nurse promote nurse-patient communication.
	■ Recognize and accept that an individual's sexual values and practices may be different from your own.	Rejection of the patient's sexual values and practices interferes with communication and patient learning.
	■ Discuss alternatives with the patient.	Provides and clarifies information to allow the patient to modify potentially infective behavior.

Evaluation: Compare the patient's status with the expected patient outcomes. If the outcomes are achieved, evaluate nursing care as successful. If not, reassess the patient, formulate new nursing diagnoses, and revise expected patient outcomes and nursing interventions as appropriate.

Assessment Findings: Patient has a history of a sexually transmitted disease but states "I know nothing about this disease" and "I don't know how I could have gotten this."

Nursing Diagnosis: Knowledge deficit: Sexual structure and functioning; disease process (e.g., etiology, risk factors, incubation and period of infectivity, clinical course, long-term sequelae, and complications); modes of transmission; preventive measures; potential effects on sexual partners; rationale for informing sexual contacts and rationale for following treatment regimen as prescribed

Patient Outcomes	Nursing Interventions	Rationale
Patient relates the cause, symptoms, clinical course, and mode of transmission of disease.	Provide health teaching when indicated.	Provides information when deficits exist.
	Determine the patient's Prior knowledge Learning level	This information guides the teaching-learning situation.

(continued)

Nursing Care Guide 47–1. *(continued)*

PATIENTS WITH SEXUALLY TRANSMITTED DISEASES

Patient Outcomes	Nursing Interventions	Rationale
Patient describes health practices for reducing the risk of infection and transmission. Patient describes potential adverse effects and long-term sequelae of untreated disease for self and others. Patient states the rationale for following recommended treatment regimens and health practices. Patient asks questions derived from a knowledge of the disease process.	Motivation Readiness Ability to incorporate new information Emotional status Preferred learning methods	
	Postpone health teaching except for essential information if the patient's emotional status interferes with ability to learn.	States of high emotion can interfere with the patient's ability to take in information.
	Provide instruction in the following, as necessary: Sexual structure and functioning Disease process Mode of transmission Preventive measures Treatment Complications and long-term sequelae Possible effects on sexual partners	Information is essential to appropriate changes in behavior.
	Use visual aids (photographs, illustrations, and films when available) to augment instruction.	Multisensory teaching methods increase learning.
	Include the patient in the learning experience; encourage questions and comments; solicit feedback; use return demonstration.	Active involvement of the learner makes learning more effective.
	Provide adequate time for teaching.	A hurried approach to teaching can be a block to learning.
	Furnish the patient with written literature as well as verbal instruction to reinforce learning and provide a reference for home use.	Reinforces teaching and allows review of material at a later time.
	Use language and terms familiar to the patient.	For communication to be effective, language must be understood by the listener.

Evaluation: Compare the patient's status with the expected patient outcomes. If the outcomes are achieved, evaluate nursing care as successful. If not, reasses the patient, formulate new nursing diagnoses, and revise expected patient outcomes and nursing interventions as appropriate.

(continued)

Nursing Care Guide 47–1. *(continued)*

PATIENTS WITH SEXUALLY TRANSMITTED DISEASES

Assessment Findings: Patient appears tense and is trembling. Patient states, "This can't have happened to me. My boyfriend will leave me. I don't want to name people, and I wanted to have children someday."

Nursing Diagnosis: Anxiety related to nature and location of symptoms; potential response of significant others to the diagnosis; identification and notification of sexual contacts; potential complications and long-term sequelae and misinformation about sexually transmitted disease (STD)

Patient Outcomes	Nursing Interventions	Rationale
Patient reports feeling less anxious.	Offer reassurance and comfort.	Reassurance and comfort are empathic behaviors that reduce anxiety.
Patient's nonverbal behavior indicates decreased anxiety (relaxed posture, facial expression, absence of nervous gestures, or other overt signs of anxiety).	Validate and demonstrate to the patient that you understand his or her feelings.	Encourages patient to share feelings and thus receive support by allaying fears of being perceived negatively.
Patient asks appropriate questions.	Allow patient to express his or her feeling within limits (e.g., crying, anger, frustration).	Reduces internal tension.
Patient is able to retain new information.	Assist patient in identifying causes of anxiety.	Recognition of causative factors can help with interventions to reduce anxiety.
	Correct misconceptions.	Misconceptions can lead to unnecessary anxiety.
	Provide information when knowledge deficit contributes to anxiety.	Understanding based on knowledge helps to reduce fear of the unknown.
	Collaborate with patient to develop strategies for reducing anxiety. For example, help patient to decide how to inform significant others; develop self-care plan to reduce symptoms; provide name and telephone number of person to contact if problems arise or anxiety increases.	By developing a "plan of attack," a sense of control develops and anxiety is reduced.
	Assist patient to view STD from a realistic perspective by emphasizing the following:	
	▪ Early treatment prevents complications and serious sequelae in most cases.	Provides the patient with positive facts on which to focus and base hope for a successful outcome.
	▪ STDs are the same as other infections except for the mode of transmission.	Provides information that may make the diagnosis more acceptable to the patient.
	▪ Acquisition of STD does not indicate sexual promiscuity, uncleanliness, and so on.	Addresses common misconceptions and provides information that can reduce anxiety.

(continued)

Nursing Care Guide 47–1. *(continued)*

PATIENTS WITH SEXUALLY TRANSMITTED DISEASES

Evaluation: Compare the patient's status with the expected patient outcomes. If the outcomes are achieved, evaluate nursing care as successful. If not, reassess the patient, formulate new nursing diagnoses, and revise expected patient outcomes and nursing interventions as appropriate.

Assessment Findings: Patient states "I can't get close to anybody again. I couldn't stand going through this again, and I couldn't take thinking I gave this to anyone else. Who would want me anyhow?"

Nursing Diagnosis: High risk for sexual dysfunction related to fear of transmission to others, lack of knowledge of sexual structure and function, painful intercourse, change in body image, and guilt or embarrassment

Patient Outcomes	Nursing Interventions	Rationale
Patient plans to resume sexual activity after successful treatment.	Correct misinformation about sexual functioning or sexually transmitted disease (STD), if indicated.	Correct information reduces anxiety about the diagnosis, which can interfere with sexual functioning.
Patient plans to incorporate measures for preventing exposure to STDs in future sexual relationships.	Review methods for preventing acquisition of STDs.	Accurate information about disease transmission can reduce anxiety about recurrence.
Patient states knowledge of sexually transmitted disease has decreased fear of transmitting infection to others.	Assure patient that disease cannot be transmitted after adequate treatment and test of cure unless reinfection occurs.	Provides the patient with positive facts on which to focus.
Patient reports ability to engage in satisfactory sexual relationships at follow-up visits.	Assist patient in identifying methods for preventing transmission if cure is unavailable (i.e., herpes).	Reduces anxiety about the risk of transmission, which can inhibit sexual function.
	Assist patient in planning to implement recommended changes in sexual or social lifestyle.	Help in planning initiates the process and allows for exchange of ideas, which increases the likelihood of arriving at a realistic plan with which the patient will comply.

Evaluation: Compare the patient's status with the expected patient outcomes. If the outcomes are achieved, evaluate nursing care as successful. If not, reassess the patient, formulate new nursing diagnoses, and revise expected patient outcomes and nursing interventions as appropriate.

and blisters anywhere on the body, although each has a predilection for specific sites.

HSV 1 is most frequently associated with lesions occurring above the waist. Examples of herpes infections commonly produced by HSV 1 are herpes labialis, otherwise known as the common cold sore or fever blister; herpes gingivostomatitis, an infection of the oral cavity and gums; and herpes keratitis, an infection of the eye. Infections attributable to HSV 2 generally occur below the waist. Genital herpes is a primary example.

Both herpes viruses are capable of producing infections at alternate sites. Currently, it is estimated that HSV 1 produces about 15% of genital infections. Changes in sexual practices and mores, including an increased incidence of oral sex, may account for the increased occurrence of HSV 1 and 2 at opposite sites. HSV 1 genital infections are less likely to recur than HSV 2. Also, there is evidence that exposure to HSV 1 as a child offers some protection against severe outbreaks of HSV 2 later in life.

Pathophysiology

TRANSMISSION

HSV is transmitted by direct skin-to-skin contact with an infected lesion or infected secretions. The virus enters the body through small breaks in the skin or through susceptible mucosal surfaces such as the oropharynx, cervix, or conjunctivae. HSV is readily inactivated both at room temperature and by drying. Transmission by aerosolization or inanimate objects is unusual and rare.

Genital herpes is transmitted via sexual contact either genital or orogenital. Autoinoculation—the transfer of virus from one site to another on the infected person's body—can also occur. Patients should be taught to immediately wash their hands after manipulation or contact with an infected lesion or secretions.

In asymptomatic viral shedding, the virus is present on skin, on mucosal surfaces, or in secretions, but lesions or other clinical symptoms are absent. Although this has been documented, the frequency of asymptomatic viral shedding and its role in transmission is not currently known. However, it is believed to be small.

RECURRENCE

After initial exposure, herpes viruses have the ability to remain in the body in a latent state and cause recurrent disease. Much of the psychological distress experienced by patients with HSV genital infections is attributable to the problem of recurrence. Unlike other infectious diseases that are communicable only for a limited time, herpes is infectious during each episode of recurrence. Consequently, the opportunity for transmission is greatly increased. Person A can give it to Person B during an initial infection and to persons C, D, and E during subsequent recurrences.

The biologic mechanism by which latency is established is not fully understood. It is known that the site of latency is the sensory nerve root ganglia located outside the central nervous system. During initial infection, the virus ascends the peripheral sensory nerves at the site of infection and establishes residency in the sensory nerve root ganglia, where it remains latent until circumstances cause it to reactivate. HSV can remain latent for years. It is not known why some individuals are infected and never manifest symptoms of the disease and others have frequent lifetime outbreaks. The patient's immunologic status definitely plays a significant role as well as, perhaps, the size of the initial viral inoculum.

Clinical Manifestations

The clinical manifestations of genital herpes vary greatly depending on whether the patient is experiencing a primary, initial, or recurrent infection. A true primary infection represents the patient's first exposure to HSV. A primary infection can be verified by the absence of antibodies to HSV on serologic testing during the acute phase of the disease.

An initial infection is also the patient's first clinical manifestation of the disease. However, serologic testing is positive for HSV antibodies, indicating previous asymptomatic acquisition of HSV. Prior exposure to HSV 1 or HSV 2 seems to have an ameliorating effect on initial outbreaks, which tend to be milder than primary HSV genital infections.

In recurrent genital herpes, the patient has had at least one prior outbreak and has high antibody levels.

PRIMARY GENITAL HERPES

The incubation period for primary genital herpes ranges from 2 to 20 days. In most cases, symptoms begin about 1 week after sexual contact. Initially, the lesions appear as papules on a reddened base. Lesions may be preceded by a local irritation, sensation of burning, tingling, or discomfort. The papules soon become fluid-filled vesicles or pustules that rupture and form shallow, wet, and painful ulcers. Ultimately, the ulcers either reepithelialize or crust over and heal without scarring. Pain, itching, dysuria, vaginal and urethral discharge, and enlarged lymph nodes are the major local symptoms. Itching is associated with vesicular formation and pain with ulcers.

Local symptoms are accompanied by a systemic viremia in 40% of males and 70% of females during primary episodes. Fever, headache, malaise, muscle pain, and back stiffness are frequent systemic symptoms that peak 4 to 5 days after the onset of lesions and resolve within 1 week to 10 days. Local symptoms usually resolve in 20 days.

The severity of primary genital herpes varies with the location and number of lesions. In males, lesions appear anywhere on the glans, prepuce, or shaft of the penis. Herpetic urethritis may occur. Generally, symptoms of primary herpes are more severe in females than males.

In females, herpes lesions may appear on the vulva, vagina, cervix, perineum, and buttocks (Fig. 47–2). The major site of infection is the cervix. Ninety percent of females experiencing a primary episode of genital herpes have concomitant HSV cervicitis. Additional lesions may appear at other sites, but the cervix is always involved during primary herpes. If the cervix is the only site, vaginal discharge may be the only symptom. Consequently, the infection may remain undiagnosed.

For some females, the number and location of the lesions cause such severe pain that it is impossible to walk or sit. The pain is associated with pressure on the lesions. Severe local symptoms resulting in an inability to urinate may require that the patient be hospitalized for treatment. Complications of primary genital herpes include aseptic meningitis and disseminated infection. Disseminated skin and mucous membrane infections and infections of the internal organs are rare in patients with a normal immune response but may be seen in immunocompromised patients, such as those undergoing bone marrow transplant and those with AIDS.

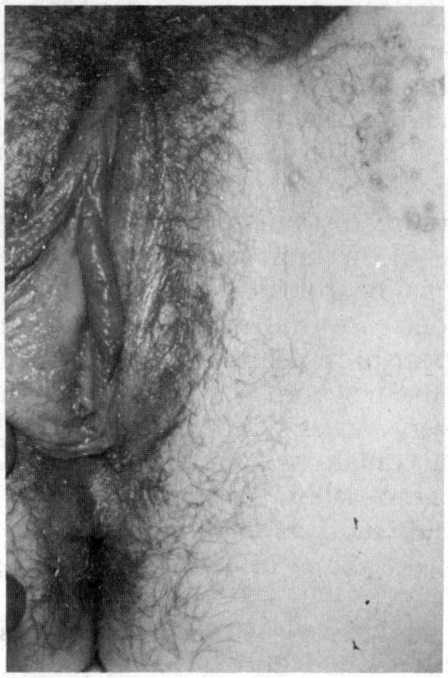

Figure 47–2.

Genital herpes lesion located on the vulva and inner thigh of a female patient. Lesions begin as papules and progress to fluid-filled vesicles that rupture to form ulcers. (Courtesy of Leonard Wolf, M.D., New York, NY.)

RECURRENT GENITAL HERPES

The average number of recurrences is three to four in the first year after a primary episode of herpes. The frequency, duration, and severity of recurrences tend to decrease over time. Eighty percent of HSV 2 and 50% of HSV 1 genital infections recur within the first year after a primary infection. Some primary infections never recur.

In contrast to primary herpes, the signs and symptoms of recurrent disease are localized to the genital area and are milder and of shorter duration. Systemic symptoms are not present. Approximately 50% of persons with recurrent genital herpes develop symptoms before the appearance of lesions. Prodromal symptoms include paresthesias (tingling, burning, "pins and needles"), itching, redness, and discomfort at the site. These may be present at any time from one-half hour to 48 hours before appearance of the lesions. Occasionally, patients complain of sacral neuralgia (sharp, shooting pains in the legs, hips, or buttocks) 1 to 5 days before onset of lesions. Characteristic local symptoms—pain, itching, and burning on urination—recur less frequently in males and are milder in females than during first-time infection.

The main sites of recurrence are the penis and vulva. In contrast to primary infections, lesions are unilateral, and in females, infection of the cervix is infrequent. Cervical infection cannot be ruled out without cultures, but only 5% to 15% of recurrent infections involve the cervix. The average duration of recurrent symptoms and viral shedding is 4 to 5 days. Complete healing occurs in 10 days.

Anecdotal evidence suggests that certain predisposing factors may trigger or precipitate an outbreak of recurrent herpes. The following are frequently identified predisposing factors: heat (both fever and an external elevation in temperature); intercourse, which may cause friction or trauma to the site; stress; anxiety; emotional upset; menstruation; and ovulation.

GENITAL HERPES AND PREGNANCY

The effects of genital herpes on pregnancy and in the newborn are of major concern to patients and health-care workers. Neonatal herpes is a severe disease with high mortality and morbidity and incapacitating long-term effects.

The potential effects of genital herpes on pregnancy outcomes vary according to whether the infection is primary or recurrent. Primary infection during pregnancy is associated with more severe, harmful effects.

Before 20 weeks gestation, primary infection results in a threefold increase in the incidence of spontaneous abortion. Primary infection in the third trimester is associated with an increase in preterm labor.

There are currently no data to indicate an increased incidence of congenital anomalies in infants born to mothers with primary or recurrent genital herpes.

By far, the most serious and frequent problem encountered in pregnancy is the transmission of herpes infection to the neonate during vaginal delivery. Although neonatal infection is rare (1 in 7500 births, or about 400 to 500 cases per year), the effects can be devastating. Seventy percent of affected infants acquire disseminated visceral infections. Of these, 83% die if untreated, and 60% of survivors have serious neurologic sequelae. With treatment, mortality decreases but morbidity and long-term sequelae appear to remain the same.

Risk of the newborn acquiring herpes during vaginal delivery varies with the number of viruses in the vaginal canal as well as the duration of the second stage of labor. Forty percent of infants born vaginally to mothers with positive cultures for herpes at the time of delivery acquire neonatal herpes.

Unfortunately, at least one half of infants with neonatal herpes are born to mothers who did not exhibit signs or symptoms of herpes at delivery. Shedding of the virus without symptoms appears to be an important source of infection at birth.

Until recently, management of pregnant patients with a history of recurrent genital herpes infection included weekly cultures beginning the 32nd to 36th weeks of pregnancy. However, major studies now indicate that antepartum cultures do not predict status at the time of delivery. It is therefore recommended that weekly cultures be abandoned and vaginal delivery be allowed if there is no evidence of genital herpetic lesions during labor. Cesarean section is recommended for women with lesions at the time of onset of labor or time of membrane rupture, to reduce the risk of neonatal infection.

If the patient demonstrated positive cultures within the previous week, or if there is clinical evidence of infection, a cesarean section is recommended. Infants exposed to HSV at birth during inadvertent vaginal delivery should be observed closely for 1 month for signs of HSV infection.

GENITAL HERPES AND CERVICAL CANCER

Evidence has accumulated during the past two decades suggesting a possible relationship between HSV 2 genital infections and the development of cervical cancer. Some studies indicated a higher incidence of cervical dysplasia, which is an alteration in the size, shape, or organization of cells, and cervical cancer among females who have a history of HSV 2. Herpes tends to infect the same area where cervical cancer frequently develops. There is also evidence that HSV 2 can cause malignant transformation of cells.

Epidemiologically, HSV genital infections are increasing among the adolescent population. Cervical cancer is more common in females who are sexually active before 17 years of age. Some researchers have suggested that HSV 2 infections in adolescence may initiate or contribute to a chain of events that culminates in cervical cancer many years later. None of the evidence demonstrates a cause and effect relationship. Nevertheless, females with a history of genital herpes are advised to have a semiannual Pap smear.

Medical Diagnosis

The majority of genital herpes cases are diagnosed clinically. The appearance of characteristic lesions and a thorough patient history strongly suggest the diagnosis. Virus isolation by tissue culture is the definitive test for HSV infection. HSV appears on tissue culture in 1 to 4 days; however, the laboratory may hold the culture for 7 to 10 days to confirm a negative result.

In situations in which a more rapid diagnosis is needed, detection by cytology—the microscopic examination of cells for changes typical of viral infection—may be useful. Cytology results can be available in 15 minutes. The Tzanck and Pap smears are commonly used for cytologic studies. Cytology is falsely negative in 40% of cases of cervical HSV shedding. The Tzanck smear for vulvar skin lesions is 90% to 95% accurate.

Medical Management

Currently, there is no treatment that completely or permanently eradicates genital herpes. The antiviral agent acyclovir is an effective medication for treatment of primary genital herpes. Intravenous administration (5 mg/kg every 8 hours) significantly decreases viral shedding, shortens the signs and symptoms of the disease, and accelerates healing of primary herpes and mucocutaneous infection in immunocompromised patients by as many as 10 days.

Oral acyclovir is slightly less effective, and topical acyclovir is the least effective route of administration. Either may be prescribed for treatment of primary or recurrent disease. Acyclovir may decrease viral shedding in recurrent disease but does not appear to otherwise significantly affect the duration of symptoms. Continued oral administration of acyclovir does suppress recurrences and may be recommended for selected patients. However, the safety of daily, long-term use of acyclovir has not been established. When the medication is discontinued, recurrences return.

Clearly, the goal is to find a treatment that eradicates latent virus and prevents recurrences as well as a safe vaccine to prevent initial infection. Other antiviral agents and treatment modalities have been proposed, but so far none have proven effective.

Semiannual Pap smears are recommended for females with a history of genital herpes. In addition, both males and females should avoid sexual contact while lesions are present to prevent transmission. See Table 47-3, which presents the clinical course and treatment of genital herpes.

Table 47–3. CLINICAL COURSE AND TREATMENT OF GENITAL HERPES

FACTOR	PRIMARY INFECTION	RECURRENT INFECTION
Mode of transmission	Direct contact with herpes lesion or infected secretions; virus enters through break in skin or through mucous membrane Primarily transmitted through sexual contact May be transmitted to infant during vaginal delivery	Reactivation of previously acquired herpes simplex virus Factors that may precipitate recurrent infection include the following: Exposure to heat (fever or external temperature) Menstruation Sexual intercourse Stress, anxiety
Incubation	2–20 days	Unknown
Signs and symptoms	Local: Genital lesions (begin as papules, progress to fluid-filled vesicles that rupture to form ulcers) Pain Pruritus Dysuria Vaginal and urethral discharge Enlarged lymph nodes Systemic: Symptoms of viremia Fever Malaise Headache Muscle pain Back stiffness	Local: Genital lesions (fewer and more localized than primary infection) Pain, pruritus, and dysuria are milder in recurrent infections and may be absent in males Systemic: none Prodromal (occurring just before appearance of lesions) Paresthesias Pruritus Redness Discomfort
Duration of symptoms	Local: 8–30 days Systemic: 7–10 days	Local: 4–10 days Prodromal: 0.5–48 hr before appearance of lesions
Medical treatment	Acyclovir (Zovirax sterile powder, IV) Indication: For treatment of initial or recurrent infections in immunocompromised patients For severe initial clinical episodes in nonimmunocompromised patients Dosage: 5 mg/kg over 1 hour every 8 hr for 5–7 days Zovirax capsules (PO) Dosage: 200 mg PO every 4 hr when awake for total of five capsules daily for 10 days Zovirax ointment 5% (topical) Dosage: Cover all lesions every 3 hr or six times daily for 7 days (i.e., 5-in. ribbon of ointment covers 4 square inches surface area)	Zovirax capsules Indication: Intermittent therapy for recurrent infection Dosage: 200 mg every 4 hr; total five capsules daily for 5 days (begin medication at earliest prodromal sign) Indication: Chronic suppressive therapy for recurrent disease Dosage: 200 mg TID up to 6 months (may require up to five capsules per day to suppress disease Zovirax sterile powder (IV) See under primary infection Zovirax ointment 5% See under primary infection

Abbreviations: IV, intravenous; PO, orally; TID, three times daily.

Application of the Nursing Process to the Care of the Patient with Genital Herpes

Nurses working in all types of health-care settings are likely to encounter patients with genital herpes. A knowledge of the disease process, clinical manifestations, modes of transmission, and current therapies is essential to providing care for these patients.

The psychological and emotional distress experienced by patients with herpes may pose a greater problem than the actual physical symptoms. In addition to the social stigma of having contracted a venereal disease, patients must cope with the knowledge that they have a recurrent disease, manifested by genital lesions, which can be transmitted to current and future sexual partners. Of concern to females is the association of genital herpes with cervical cancer and the potential effect of the disease on the method of delivery and health of future offspring. These complex emotional and social problems may generate feelings of anxiety, fear, and depression. The nurse needs to be prepared to provide education, counseling, and emotional support.

Assessment

Assessment begins with a thorough history and physical examination of the lesions. Throughout the assessment process, observe and question the patient about his or her emotional and social response to the disease. Educational needs are identified by assessing the patient's knowledge about the disease, current health practices, and lifestyle.

Carry out the nursing assessment in a physical environment that provides both privacy and good lighting and that promotes the patient's psychological and physical comfort.

Patients may be reluctant to provide information about their disease and response to it. The perception of herpes as socially unacceptable and the intimate nature of the mode of transmission often inhibit open, honest communication. It is important to communicate an empathetic, accepting, and nonjudgmental attitude. Use open-ended questions designed to encourage verbalization whenever possible.

Initially determine whether the infection is primary or recurrent, and ascertain the onset, duration, frequency, and severity of local and systemic symptoms (if applicable). Question the patient about factors that aggravate or relieve the symptoms and current therapies used. In cases of recurrent herpes, assist the patient in identifying factors that may precipitate outbreaks.

Obtain a sexual history, including frequency of sexual relations, number of partners, and mode of sexual contacts.

Question the patient regarding a history of other sexually transmitted diseases.

Obtain an obstetric and gynecologic history from female patients. Of particular importance are the frequency of Pap smears and current methods of contraception.

To assess the impact of herpes on the patient's emotional and social well-being, question the patient about the effects of herpes on his or her interpersonal relationships, lifestyle, sexual identity, and self-esteem.

Potential emotional reactions to herpes include shock, anger, depression, and withdrawal. Disbelief and denial are common initial reactions. "How could it happen to me?" and "Herpes happens to other people" are feelings frequently communicated by patients on learning the diagnosis. Shock is often followed by anger. For example, a patient may express anger at herself for having contracted the infection, at her partner for "having given it to me," and at health care professionals for their inability to provide a cure. A pattern of emotional stress, depression, and withdrawal, frequently referred to as the "herpes syndrome," may develop.

Patients may experience sadness either at the loss of sexual freedom and identity or over the change in body image and personal health. Lowering of self-esteem and guilt for having contracted a sexually transmitted disease are common. Fear of rejection or fear of transmitting the disease in future relationships may cause the patient to withdraw from social contacts. The stress experienced by patients exhibiting severe emotional responses to herpes may, in fact, precipitate more frequent recurrences.

During the course of the assessment interview, observe and actively listen for cues to the patient's emotional response to herpes. Some questions that may help the patient begin to communicate his or her feelings include "Whom have you told about your diagnosis?", "How has herpes affected your sexual relationships, social activities, and lifestyle?", "What do you find most difficult about having herpes?" Some patients may appear, or verbally indicate, that they are depressed. Assess these patients for signs and symptoms of clinical depression.

Nursing Diagnoses and Planning

Nursing diagnoses and related expected patient outcomes most commonly applicable to patients with genital herpes include the following:

NDx: Pain related to the inflammatory process and irritation of the genital vesicles

Planning: Patient outcomes

1. Patient reports that itching and burning are controlled by medication.
2. Patient voids without pain or burning.

NDx: High risk for infection (secondary) related to impairment of skin integrity

Planning: Patient outcomes

1. Lesions are free of purulent drainage.
2. Tissues surrounding the lesions are free of edema.
3. Patient's temperature is normal.
4. Palpable lymph nodes are absent.

NDx: High risk for altered health maintenance related to insufficient knowledge of disease process and prevention of transmission

Planning: Patient outcomes

1. Patient states cause and mode of transmission of herpes.
2. Patient describes progress of primary and recurrent herpes, including signs and symptoms of prodromal and acute phases of infection.
3. Patient states methods and measures for preventing transmission to others.
4. Patient describes possible complications of herpes.

NDx: Anxiety related to the diagnosis of herpes and its potential physical and lifestyle effects

Planning: Patient outcomes

1. Patient verbalizes concerns about herpes and its effects.
2. Patient accurately describes effects of genital herpes on sexual activity and reproductive capacity.
3. Patient states knowledge of the disease and measures for preventing transmission have decreased

Chart 47–2.

NURSING GUIDE TO PATIENT EDUCATION FOR SELF-MANAGEMENT: SYMPTOMATIC RELIEF OF GENITAL HERPES

Recommend the following self-care measures for symptomatic relief during active infection with genital herpes:

Keep the lesions and adjacent areas clean and dry.
Avoid the use of lubricants and creams, which may prolong healing time and contribute to secondary infection.
Wear loose clothing and cotton underwear to decrease pressure and irritation on the lesions and to promote drying.
Apply drying agents such as Campho-Phenique for relief of pain and itch.
Use soaks and compresses to promote drying and comfort (cool, wet compresses for itching, sitz baths for local pain and discomfort).
Take aspirin or acetaminophen as per directions for pain.

his or her fear of transmitting the infection to others.
4. Behavioral signs of anxiety are absent.

NDx: High risk for ineffective individual coping related to diagnosis of a chronic, sexually transmitted disease and its potential effects

Planning: Patient outcomes
1. Patient describes changes in health habits and lifestyle that may decrease recurrence.
2. Patient lists factors that may precipitate recurrent infection.
3. Patient informs significant others or sexual partners about genital herpes.
4. Patient participates in social relationships and activities.
5. Patient asks questions and requests additional information about herpes.
6. Patient joins herpes support group.
7. Patient reports viewing the infection as a minor inconvenience.
8. Symptoms of depression are absent.

Nursing Interventions

NDx: Pain
Recommend self-care and health-management techniques for symptomatic relief during active infection as specified in Chart 47–2.

NDx: High risk for infection (secondary)
Instruct the patient to avoid touching or scratching the lesions because this can result in infection of the area with a new organism introduced from the hands and can spread the herpes infection to other parts of the body by autoinoculation. Stress the importance of performing meticulous perineal hygiene and wearing clean, loose undergarments.

NDx: High risk for altered health maintenance
Teaching and counseling of the patient with genital herpes is based on the assessment of the patient's learning needs, emotional status, and whether the infection is primary or recurrent. The patient's emotional status can affect readiness to learn. Newly diagnosed patients are often emotionally upset and anxious. They require time to assimilate the knowledge that they have herpes before they can begin to absorb information that will ultimately help them to cope with the disease. Consequently, initial instruction of patients with primary herpes is often limited to basic information about the disease, mode of transmission, and therapy. As the patient indicates greater readiness to learn, provide additional information about the cause and mode of transmission as well as differences among primary, initial, and recurrent infections and possible complications. Supplement verbal instruction with written information to which the patient can later refer because patients experiencing high levels of anxiety may not remember much of what was taught.

Correct any misconceptions or myths the patient may have about herpes. Use common, unemotional terms familiar to the patient to assist him or her in viewing the disease in a realistic perspective. It may be helpful to explain that genital herpes lesions are the same skin lesions as the cold sore frequently seen on the lips or face. Also be certain to inform the patient that much research is being done to de-

Chart 47–3.

NURSING GUIDE TO PATIENT EDUCATION FOR SELF-MANAGEMENT: PREVENTION OF TRANSMISSION AND COMPLICATIONS OF GENITAL HERPES

To enable the patient to prevent transmission of genital herpes:

Explain to the patient the following:

- The herpes virus is transmitted by direct skin-to-skin or mucous membrane contact with one or more herpes lesions or infected secretions.
- Sexual contact is the most frequent mode of transmission.
- Infection may be spread by contamination of the hands to other sites.
- Contact with grossly contaminated objects is a possible but very rare mode of transmission.

Instruct the patient to do the following:

- Avoid touching the lesions.
- Wash hands thoroughly if lesions are inadvertently touched.
- Inspect the genital area frequently to detect recurrent lesions early.
- Abstain from sexual intercourse when the prodromal signs and symptoms appear and continue until the lesions are no longer present.
- Consider the use of condoms between outbreaks. (It is not known whether the infection can be transmitted during asymptomatic periods. Condoms are not sufficient protection during active herpes because the virus is smaller than the pores of the condom, and it is not known whether the virus can penetrate the condom and in what numbers.)

To assist the female patient in avoiding obstetric complications of genital herpes:

Advise the patient to do the following:

- Inform her gynecologist/obstetrician of her herpes history.
- Obtain a Papanicolaou test every 6 months.

Explain to pregnant patients that a cesarean section is performed if there is active infection at the time of delivery.

velop a treatment to eradicate the disease permanently.

Avoid terms such as "incurable" when discussing the diagnosis with the patient because the goal is to provide information without increasing anxiety. Emphasize the fact that recurrent outbreaks, if they occur, become less frequent and, in most cases, ultimately cease over time.

Instruct the patient on measures to prevent transmission and complications, as specified in Chart 47–3.

NDx: Anxiety
Encourage the patient to verbalize feelings and concerns about the diagnosis and its potential effects on health and lifestyle. Provide an opportunity for the patient to talk in a nonthreatening environment that provides privacy.

While listening to the patient, pay particular attention to any clues that anxiety is due, at least in part, to lack of information, misconceptions, or unrealistic expectations about the disease and its effects. Provide accurate information using nontechnical and unemotional language. Acknowledge the patient's anxiety while providing practical, factual information that will assist the patient in developing a realistic perspective on the problem and ability to cope with it.

NDx: High risk for ineffective individual coping
Counseling includes interventions to assist the patient in coping with the psychological and social ramifications of the disease. Identify strategies for self-management that help the patient to gain a sense of control and confidence in his or her ability to cope with the disease.

The potential for recurrent, unpredictable outbreaks of infection is a major area of difficulty for herpes patients. Review with the patient the relationship of physical and psychological stress to recurrent outbreaks. Identify personal and environmental factors, such as an elevation in either the internal or external temperature, stress, anxiety, menstruation, and sexual intercourse, that may precipitate outbreaks. Review specific techniques for reducing stress such as relaxation techniques, exercise, yoga, and imaging. Emphasize the importance of maintaining a healthy lifestyle. Describe the role of diet, exercise, and adequate rest in maintaining an optimum immune response and possibly decreasing outbreaks.

Explore with the patient the need to inform others about the disease. It is generally recommended that patients inform prospective sex partners, whom they plan to see over time, relatively early in the relationship. Assist the patient in identifying ways of telling others by making specific suggestions. Advise the patient to introduce the topic in a calm, direct, nonthreatening manner that does not frighten the other person. Suggest introductory statements such as "Do you know what cold sores are?" or "Have you heard of herpes?" as opposed to "There's something I think you should know." Advise the patient to assume that the person does not know much about herpes and to talk about the facts and how to prevent transmission. It is also helpful if the patient can talk about herpes as a fairly insignificant problem that can be dealt with relatively easily.

If you are comfortable with role-playing, offer to play the role of another person to allow the patient to practice telling a prospective partner. Another technique is for the patient to practice telling others by first telling a trusted friend or relative.

Inform the patient about resources available to persons with genital herpes. A quarterly publication called "The Helper" from the National Herpes Research Center of the American Social Health Association contains articles on the latest scientific research as well as ways of coping with herpes. The same organization sponsors support groups ("Help") for herpes patients that are located throughout the United States. Self-help groups provide information, emotional support, and group identification. Members learn that they are not alone and that others have similar feelings and problems. The group offers an opportunity to work through problems and to learn from the experiences of others. Local chapters of "Help" can be located through the telephone book or through the National Herpes Resource Center (P.O. Box 100, Palo Alto, CA 94302).

Evaluation

Evaluate the effectiveness of nursing care for a patient with genital herpes by comparing the patient's status with the expected patient outcomes. Examples of specific outcomes for patients with genital herpes have been provided in the Planning section.

Gonorrhea

Gonorrhea is a sexually transmitted infection caused by *Neisseria gonorrhoeae,* a gram-negative bacteria that has a predilection for certain types of epithelial tissue commonly found in the urogenital tract.

Each year there are approximately 1 million reported cases of gonorrhea in the United States. In addition, it is estimated that 1 to 1.5 million cases go unreported.

Similar to other sexually transmitted diseases, gonorrhea is most prevalent in the teenage and young adult age groups. The incidence increases in the late teens and early 20s and declines with advancing age. Although the overall rate of gonorrhea has remained relatively constant during the past few years, there have been increases and decreases within specific demographic groups. For example, the number of reported cases of gonorrhea in females particularly during the teenage years, dramatically increased during the past two decades.

This increase in reported rates of gonorrhea in females, particularly in the younger age groups, may reflect several factors including better recognition and diagnosis in females and changes in sexual mores and practices, especially earlier and more frequent sexual activity.

On the basis of statistics from reported cases in the United States, demographic risk factors for gonorrhea include low socioeconomic status, nonwhite race, urban residence, unmarried, multiple sexual partners, early onset of sexual activity, male homosexuality, and history of gonorrhea. Many of these risk factors may influence, at least in part, the reporting of gonorrhea. The demographic groups just identified are more likely to attend public health clinics. Such clinics are more compliant with case reporting than private clinics and physicians who cater to a more affluent segment of the population.

Etiology and Pathophysiology

Initially, the *N. gonorrhoeae* bacteria attaches to the mucous membranes of structures in the lower urogenital tract such as the urethra, Bartholin's glands, and cervix. Within 24 to 48 hours, the organism invades the mucosal epithelium. *N. gonorrhoeae* causes a vigorous leukocyte response, which leads to the development of a purulent discharge.

Gonorrhea is transmitted from one infected person to another through close body contact. Sexual contact is the most common mode of transmission. Transmission by inanimate objects or close nonsexual personal contact is possible but extremely rare, with the exception of vertical transmission from mother to infant during the birthing process.

Clinical Manifestations

Gonorrhea has a broad range of clinical manifestations, including asymptomatic, symptomatic, and complicated infection at several different sites.

In males, gonorrhea most often presents as an acute urethritis. The major symptoms are a profuse, purulent white or yellowish urethral discharge, accompanied by meatal inflammation and discomfort on urination (Fig. 47–3). Initially, the exudate may be scant and mucoid, but within 24 hours it is usually purulent and relatively abundant. The incubation period ranges from 1 to 14 days, but the onset of symptoms usually occurs 3 to 7 days after sexual contact with an infected partner.

About one quarter of males develop only scant, minimally purulent discharge that may be apparent exclusively in the morning. In a few infected males, signs and symptoms of urethritis never develop. Complications in males are rare and relatively minor.

In females, the infection is frequently asymptomatic, or the signs and symptoms are so inconsequential that they remain unnoticed.

The primary site of infection in women is the cervix. Colonization of the urinary tract with *N. gonorrhoeae* also occurs in the majority of infected females. Other sites of initial infection may include the periurethral Skene's glands and Bartholin's gland. Although the incubation period is more variable in females, most females who experience symptoms do so within 10 days of exposure, the majority within 2 to 5 days.

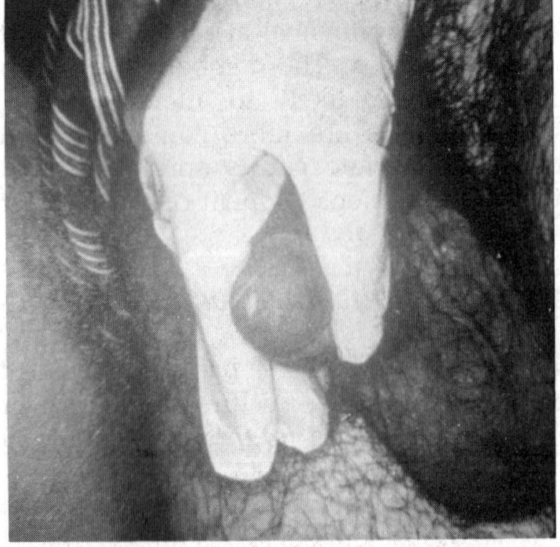

Figure 47–3.

Gonococcal urethritis. Note the white, purulent discharge at the meatus. (Courtesy of New York City Health Department.)

Urinary frequency, dysuria, and purulent vaginal discharge are the three most common presenting symptoms. On physical examination, signs of inflammation of the cervix, including mucopurulent cervical discharge, erythema, friability, and tenderness on cervical palpation, are common findings. Apart from pelvic inflammatory disease (PID), abscess of a Bartholin's gland is the most common complication of gonorrhea in females.

Anorectal infection occurs in approximately 35% to 50% of females and homosexual males with gonorrhea. In males, infection is due to anal intercourse. In females, the anorectal infection also appears to result from contamination of the perineum, with discharge originating from the infected cervix. Symptoms range from minor anal itching and mucopurulent discharge to severe rectal pain, bleeding, and constipation.

If gonococci invade the blood stream, then disseminated gonococcal infection (DGI) may follow. Whether or not systemic infection occurs is influenced by the strain of the infecting gonococcal organism and the individual's immunologic status.

DGI is more common in females than males because females are more likely to have untreated gonococcal infections. Clinical manifestations include signs and symptoms commonly seen in bacterial infections (e.g., fever, malaise, anorexia, and leukocytosis). Skin lesions are the most common manifestation. Usually they appear on the distal extremities as erythematous macules that progress to form pustules. Tenosynovitis (inflammation of the tendon sheaths), septic arthritis, and polyarthralgias are also common clinical manifestations. Fortunately, DGI responds well to antibiotic therapy.

Gonococcal PID is the most common and serious complication of gonorrheal infection in females. In 10% to 20% of females, the initial urogenital infection spreads to the upper genital tract. It is theorized that the gonococci ascend the genital tract during menstruation and are disseminated either to the uterus, where a transient endometritis may occur, or directly to the fallopian tubes. The tubes become reddened and edematous and contain a purulent exudate. The exudate may drip from the ends of the tubes, causing pelvic peritonitis and subsequent pelvic adhesions.

The clinical manifestations of PID are variable. Usually symptoms do not occur until during or just after the next menstrual period. The symptoms of acute PID include fever, shaking chills, anorexia, malaise, vaginal discharge, abdominal discomfort, and occasional nausea.

The most common clinical manifestations are fever and bilateral lower abdominal pain. Some patients give a history of abnormal vaginal bleeding and prolonged menstruation before symptoms. Pelvic peritonitis may be manifested by direct and rebound lower abdominal tenderness and muscle guarding. Pelvic examination may reveal mucopurulent cervicitis and urethral discharge. Manipulation of the cervix causes marked discomfort.

Long-term sequelae include tubo-ovarian abscess, ectopic pregnancy, and infertility due to intra-abdominal adhesions with chronic pelvic pain and menstrual irregularities. Management of PID includes prompt administration of antimicrobial therapy, monitoring, and follow-up for complications. The sooner appropriate antibiotic therapy is initiated, the less chance there is of permanent damage to the reproductive tract.

Medical Diagnosis

Because the symptoms of gonorrhea are similar to those of other sexually transmitted diseases, clinical diagnosis must be confirmed by laboratory tests. Microscopic examination of stained smears of urethral exudate and subsequent identification of polymorphonuclear leukocytes and the typical gram-negative intracellular diplococci are considered sufficient for diagnosis of gonococcal urethritis in males. Gram's stains are unreliable in women. Cervical cultures are the preferred method and will detect 80% to 90% of cervical infections.

Medical Management

Components of medical management include the following:

1. Identification of the sites of infection.
2. Selection of an effective antimicrobial regimen.
3. Identification, diagnosis, and treatment of sexual contacts.
4. Repeat cultures or smears 4 to 7 days after treatment to verify cure.

Many antibiotics have proved effective in treating gonorrhea, including the penicillins, tetracyclines, and cephalosporins. The severity of disease, site of infection, expense, patient compliance, and toxicity are all factors that are considered in the selection of an antimicrobial regimen. For uncomplicated disease, a single parenteral treatment with penicillin, ampicillin, or amoxicillin, given concomitantly with probenecid, has traditionally been recommended. Probenecid decreases renal tubular secretion of penicillin, maintaining higher serum levels. Single-dose therapy is inexpensive and eliminates patient compliance as a factor in treatment. More recently, many authorities are recommending a 7-day regimen of tetracycline as the treatment of choice for gonorrhea in compliant patients and in those allergic to penicillin. Tetracycline is highly effective at all infected sites, except for anorectal sites in homosexual males, and has fewer adverse reactions. Tetracycline is the only regimen that is also effective against concurrent *Chlamydia trachomatis* infections.

Spectinomycin is recommended for infections that persist after initial treatment. It is the medication of choice for treatment of gonorrhea resulting from penicillinase-producing *N. gonorrhoeae* (PPNG). PPNG are strains of *N. gonorrhoeae* that are absolutely resistant to penicillin and ampicillin. PPNG is prevalent in Southeast Asia, the Philippines, and Africa. In 1976, PPNG was first isolated in the United States. At that time, most cases could be traced to contact with a recent immigrant or traveler from a high-risk area. Since 1980, the incidence of PPNG has increased dramatically, emphasizing the importance of follow-up to test for cure after initial therapy.

In cases of complicated disease (e.g., those involving disseminated infection and PID), hospitalization is frequently recommended. Regimens include intravenous penicillin followed by oral ampicillin or amoxicillin. For PID, combination antibiotic therapy is recommended because of the complex nature of the disease, high failure rates, and significant long-term sequelae. Medications should be effective against *N. gonorrhoeae, C. trachomatis,* and anaerobic bacteria, each of which have been implicated in PID.

See Table 47–4 for common treatment regimens for gonorrhea.

Application of the Nursing Process to the Care of the Patient with Gonorrhea

Nurses may encounter patients with gonorrhea under a variety of circumstances. Males seek treatment because the symptoms are usually obvious and uncomfortable. However, at least one half of female patients experience few if any symptoms associated with lower genital tract gonococcal infections. Although in some females gonorrhea is diagnosed during routine gynecologic examinations, usually by Pap smears, many females remain unaware of the infection. Consequently, many female patients do not seek health care until symptoms of PID are present.

Nurses working with high-risk female patients in various settings (e.g., clinics for treating sexually transmitted diseases, family planning clinics, and inpatient obstetric and gynecologic services) can play an important role in case finding and prevention. A thorough history and a high degree of suspicion are necessary to identify cases of gonorrhea in asymptomatic female patients.

Assessment

Obtain social, sexual, obstetric, and gynecologic histories as well as a general health history. Explore the patient's lifestyle and attitudes toward health by asking questions such as

Table 47–4. TREATMENT REGIMENS FOR GONORRHEA, SYPHILIS, AND CHLAMYDIAL INFECTIONS

INFECTION	MEDICATION	RECOMMENDED DOSAGE	SPECIAL CONSIDERATIONS
Gonorrhea, uncomplicated	Aqueous procaine penicillin G with probenecid	4.8 million units IM; single dose 1 g PO; single dose	Drug of choice for uncomplicated gonorrhea Divided dose given at two sites (4.8 ml/injection) Moderately painful injection Single-dose treatment is recommended for noncompliant patients Effective in treating pharyngeal and rectal gonorrhea and incubating syphilis Recommended for treatment of gonorrhea in homosexual males Probenecid decreases renal excretion of penicillin; increases serum levels
	Ampicillin *or* amoxicillin with probenecid	3.5 g ampicillin or 3 g amoxicillin PO; either with 1 g probenecid PO; single dose	Easiest treatment to administer and most acceptable to patients Not effective treatment for pharyngeal gonorrhea or anorectal gonorrhea in males
	Tetracycline hydrochloride	500 mg PO four times daily for 7 days	Only treatment able to eradicate both gonorrhea and coexistent *Chlamydia trachomatis* infection Successfully treats gonorrhea at all sites except anorectal infection in males Requires patient compliance in taking drug after symptoms disappear (2–3 days after treatment) GI disturbances common May induce vaginal candidiasis infection Drug of choice in penicillin-allergic patients Contraindicated in pregnancy
	Combination therapy: Single-dose aqueous procaine penicillin *or* ampicillin *or* amoxicillin with probenecid followed by tetracycline	Aqueous procaine penicillin, 4.8 million units IM, *or* ampicillin, 3.5 g PO, *or* amoxicillin, 3 g PO, plus probenecid, 1 g PO, followed by tetracycline, 500 mg four times daily for 7 days	Combination therapy guarantees treatment for gonorrhea in noncompliant patient; tetracycline treatment for chlamydia
PPNG	Spectinomycin *or* cefoxitin *and* probenecid	2 g IM *or* 2 g IM; *and* 1 g PO	Drug of choice for known or suspected PPNG 25% failure rate for pharyngeal gonorrhea (PPNG) Cefoxitin for treatment of PPNG also resistant to spectinomycin
Disseminated gonococcal infection	Ampicillin *or* amoxicillin *plus* probenecid	3.5 g PO *or* 3 g PO *plus* 1 g PO followed by 0.5 g PO four times daily for 7 days of either drug	Oral medications primarily used for outpatient treatment
	Tetracycline	0.5 g PO four times daily for 7 days	Erythromycin used for pregnant patients, patients allergic to penicillin
	Aqueous crystalline penicillin G followed by ampicillin	10 million units IV until improvement; follow with ampicillin, 0.5 g PO four times daily for 7 days	IV medications for hospitalized patients
	Cefoxitin	1 g IV four times daily for 7 days	Cefoxitin for treatment of PPNG

(*continued*)

Table 47–4. (*continued*) TREATMENT REGIMENS FOR GONORRHEA, SYPHILIS, AND CHLAMYDIAL INFECTIONS

INFECTION	MEDICATION	RECOMMENDED DOSAGE	SPECIAL CONSIDERATIONS
Gonococcal PID: Out-patient	Aqueous procaine penicillin *or* ampicillin *or* amoxicillin *plus* probenecid followed by ampicillin *or* amoxicillin	4.8 million units IM 3.5 g PO 3 g PO 1 g PO 0.5 g PO of either ampicillin or amoxicillin four times daily for 10 days	Recommended when *Neisseria gonorrhoeae* is most likely causative organism
	or tetracycline	0.5 g PO four times daily for 10 days	Recommended when *Chlamydia trachomatis* is most likely causative organism; may also be prescribed for treatment of gonococcal PID
Gonococcal PID: In-patient	Aqueous crystalline penicillin G	20 million units IV every day until improvement occurs	
	followed by ampicillin	0.5 g PO four times daily for 10 days	
	or tetracycline	0.25 g IV four times daily until improvement, followed by 0.5 g PO to complete 10 days of therapy	
Patients with multiple episodes of PID; possible pelvic abscess	Cefoxitin *or* aqueous crystalline penicillin G *plus* gentamicin *plus* clindamycin	2 g IV every 6–8 hr for 10 days 20 million units IV every day for 10 days *plus* 1.5 mg/kg IV every 8 hours *plus* 600 mg IV every 6 hours	Triple antibiotic therapy when causative organism unknown or more than one organism suspected. Effective for gonorrheal, chlamydial, and anaerobic infection
Chlamydia	Tetracycline	0.5 g orally four times daily for 7 days	Successful treatment for gonorrhea as well as chlamydial infection
	Erythromycin	0.5 g PO four times daily for 7 days	Recommended for patients who cannot tolerate tetracycline and for pregnant patients
PID	See gonococcal PID		
Syphilis: duration less than 1 year	Benzathine penicillin G	2.4 million units IM	Divide dose into 1.2 million units into each buttock Medication of choice for treatment of primary and secondary syphilis of less than 1 year duration and for contacts of these patients
	Tetracycline hydrochloride	0.5 g PO four times daily for 15 days	Use when penicillin is contraindicated (i.e., penicillin allergy)
	Erythromycin	0.5 g orally four times daily for 15 days	Use for pregnant patients allergic to penicillin Lower cure rate Serologic follow-up of mother and infant
Syphilis: duration more than 1 year	Benzathine penicillin G	2.4 million units once per week for 3 weeks	Medication of choice for syphilis of more than 1 year duration
	or tetracycline hydrochloride	500 mg PO four times daily for 30 days	Recommended for penicillin-allergic patients; may cause GI disturbance
	or erythromycin	500 g PO four times daily for 30 days	Recommended for penicillin-allergic or pregnant patients
	or aqueous procaine penicillin	600,000 units IM daily for 15 days	Impractical for out-patient therapy
Neurosyphilis	Crystalline penicillin G followed by benzathine penicillin G *or* aqueous procaine penicillin G *plus* probenecid	2 to 4 million units IV every 4 hours for at least 10 days 2.4 million units IM weekly for 3 weeks 2.4 million units IM daily for 15 days 500 mg PO four times daily for 10 days	More intensive therapy may be recommended for neurosyphilis as a result of treatment failures with standard treatment of syphilis of more than 1 year duration

Abbreviations: IM, intramuscular; PO, orally; GI, gastrointestinal; PPNG, penicillinase-producing *Neisseria* gonorrhoeae; IV, intravenous; PID, pelvic inflammatory disease.

"Do you consider yourself a healthy person?"
"What do you do to protect yourself from disease?"
"How do you stay healthy?"

Note the presence of high-risk factors such as lower socioeconomic class, early onset of sexual activity, frequent sexual contact with numerous sexual partners, and history of gonorrhea or other sexually transmitted disease.

Question the patient about his or her preferred method of contraception. Barrier methods such as condoms and diaphragms are recommended because they decrease transmission of gonorrhea. Oral contraceptives are also associated with decreased incidence of the disease, whereas IUDs are related to an increase in the incidence of both urogenital infections and PID.

Question the patient about the occurrence of symptoms associated with complicated and uncomplicated gonococcal infections. A review of symptoms, both past and present, is the key to patient assessment and case finding.

If the patient responds affirmatively to having one or more of the symptoms under review, analyze the symptom further. For example, if the patient reports an abnormal discharge, ask about the onset, duration, color, odor, amount, and consistency of the discharge. Analyze complaints of pain according to location, onset, duration, frequency, and aggravating and relieving factors. Also ask the patient to describe the pain. Find out, for example, whether the pain is dull, sharp, "knifelike," or gnawing.

Perform a physical assessment guided by the patient's history and symptoms. For example, inspect discharge, and inspect and palpate the site of pain.

Assess also the patient's learning needs and ability to understand and absorb new information. Assess the patient's knowledge regarding transmission, prevention, signs and symptoms, complications, and long-term sequelae of gonorrhea. Educational background, prior knowledge, level of anxiety, and motivation can all affect the patient's ability to learn. Consider each of these factors in determining when and how to communicate information about the disease to the patient.

Assess the patient's emotional response to a confirmed or possible diagnosis of gonorrhea. Some patients may express anger, fear, or denial. Others may be cavalier or unconcerned about the diagnosis and its implications. Actively listen to and observe the patient for clues to his or her psychological response to the disease. Validate impressions by asking open-ended questions designed to convey empathy and understanding as well as provide and obtain information. Responses to questions such as "Has there been or do you anticipate a change in your sexual relations because of gonorrhea?" can provide information about both emotional and social effects of the disease on the patient.

Be certain to communicate a nonjudgmental attitude and a sense of caring throughout the assessment interview.

Nursing Diagnoses and Planning

Nursing diagnoses and related expected patient outcomes most commonly applicable to patients with gonorrhea include the following:

NDx: Pain related to inflammation of the urogenital tract and irritation from vaginal discharge

Planning: Patient outcomes
1. Patient keeps genital area clean and dry.
2. Patient describes hygienic measures to be used after elimination to avoid spreading infective discharge.
3. Patient states he or she is experiencing less discomfort.
4. Patient is free of discomfort on urination.
5. Vaginal or urethral discharge is absent or decreased.

NDx: High risk for altered health maintenance related to insufficient knowledge of disease process, prevention of transmission, potential complications, and long-term sequelae

Planning: Patient outcomes
1. Patient states the cause, symptoms, complications, and mode of transmission of gonorrhea.
2. Patient describes health practices to reduce the risk of reinfection and transmission.

NDx: Anxiety related to possible long-term sequelae, perceived threat to self-concept, naming sexual contacts

Planning: Patient outcomes
1. Patient's behavior indicates decreased anxiety (e.g., relaxed position, free of nervous mannerisms).
2. Patient asks appropriate questions.
3. Patient reports feeling calm and in control.

NDx: High risk for noncompliance related to prescribed health practices, naming of sexual contacts

Planning: Patient outcomes
1. Patient states reasons for following the therapeutic regimen.
2. Patient reports that he or she has taken medication as prescribed.
3. Patient returns for follow-up and test of cure.
4. Repeat cultures and smears are negative.
5. Patient expresses intent to use prophylactic measures during future sexual activity.
6. Patient provides names of sexual contacts.

Nursing Interventions

NDx: Pain
Advise the patient to keep the external genitalia clean and dry and to avoid scratching if pruritus

occurs. Caution patients, especially females, to be careful not to spread infected discharge to the urethral meatus or the rectum, particularly after voiding or defecation and during menstruation.

NDx: High risk for altered health maintenance
Teach the patient about the disease process, potential complications, and preventive measures to help ensure compliance with treatment and to prevent reinfection and transmission.

Select teaching strategies on the basis of the patient's prior knowledge, level of anxiety, and ability to learn as well as available materials. With some patients, it may be necessary to review basic anatomy and physiology of the reproductive and urinary tracts. Photographs are often helpful in communicating this information. Films, videotapes, and slides, if available, are also effective, especially when teaching adolescents and young adults.

Be certain to use terminology the patient can understand. Avoid complex explanations and the provision of more information than the patient needs or is ready to learn.

If the patient is experiencing moderate to severe anxiety or demonstrates lack of motivation to learn, little learning can be expected to occur. In both cases, it may be necessary to limit the amount of information to essentials such as methods for preventing reinfection and the importance of compliance and follow-up. Written materials that the patient can take home are helpful adjuncts to teaching, especially when the patient is overly anxious.

Review the cause, symptoms, and mode of transmission of gonorrhea with the patient. Emphasize the importance of abstaining from sexual contact until negative cultures are obtained at a follow-up visit. Explain that a test of cure is necessary to ensure successful treatment because some strains of gonorrhea are resistant to specific antibiotics. Explain that the use of condoms during sexual intercourse reduces the risk of reinfection.

Inform the patient about the potential complications and long-term sequelae, especially in untreated or inadequately treated gonorrhea. Inform females that they are at increased risk for disseminated gonococcal infection and PID, which can cause infertility. Also inform males of this fact to promote compliance in treatment, reporting of sexual contacts, and use of preventive measures.

NDx: Anxiety
When possible, assist the male or female patient in identifying the cause of anxiety. Information can then be provided to address issues or misconceptions presented by the patient.

A nonjudgmental, empathic attitude is essential to effective counseling of patients with sexually transmitted diseases, especially gonorrhea, which is often associated in the public's mind with sexual promiscuity. Be sensitive to the difficulty many patients experience accepting the diagnosis and providing names of sexual partners. Encourage the patient to talk about his or her anxiety. Acknowledge the realistic concerns of the patient, and provide reassurance when appropriate.

NDx: High risk for noncompliance
Recognize that the patient's lifestyle, socioeconomic status, and cultural background may be different from your own. A sincere and caring attitude is essential to gaining the patient's trust. Ask the patient open-ended questions to determine his or her attitude toward sexual relationships, health care, and health care professionals. Provide information to correct misconceptions and to promote compliance with the treatment regimen and recommended health practices.

Many patients may be afraid or hesitant to identify contacts. An understanding of the disease process and potential harm of undiagnosed infections may help the patient to resolve his or her ambivalence and resistance to naming contacts. Emphasize that although sexual partners (particularly females) may be asymptomatic early in the disease, complications can develop later or reinfect the patient.

Review the incubation period with the patient to determine which sex partners need evaluation and possible treatment. In the case of uncomplicated lower urogenital tract infection, the patient's sexual contacts during the 4 weeks preceding onset of symptoms are contacted. In cases of disseminated gonococcal infection and PID, the patient's sexual partners during the preceding 3 months are contacted.

Additional Interventions
Approximately 5% to 10% of the adult population is allergic to penicillin. Therefore, observe the patient for signs of hypersensitivity after administration of penicillin. Watch for the initial signs of hypersensitivity, which include appearance of a red wheal or red flare at the injection site, pain or itching at the site, and hives. Anaphylactic reactions do occur and may be fatal.

If tetracycline is prescribed, instruct the patient to take the medications on an empty stomach either 1 hour before or 2 hours after eating. If anorexia, nausea, or diarrhea occur, advise the patient to take the medication with some food to relieve the symptoms but not with foods high in calcium, because they interfere with its absorption.

Also advise the patient to avoid exposure to direct or artificial sunlight during tetracycline therapy because a phototoxic reaction (exaggerated sunburn) may develop as a result of the medication. Tetracycline is contraindicated in pregnant or nursing female patients.

Emphasize the importance of taking all medication for the prescribed time interval. Although the symptoms may subside or even disappear during the course of therapy, a complete cure cannot be ensured unless the regimen is followed and the patient returns for repeat smears or cultures 4 to 7 days after treatment. Instruct the patient to refrain from sexual intercourse until negative cultures are obtained on follow-up examination.

Evaluation

Evaluate the effectiveness of nursing care for a patient with gonorrhea by comparing the patient's status with the expected patient outcomes. Examples of specific outcomes for patients with gonorrhea have been provided in the Planning section.

Syphilis

Syphilis is a sexually transmitted disease caused by a spirochete: *Treponema pallidum*. The course of the disease is remarkably variable and prolonged. In untreated patients, 30 to 40 years may elapse between initial infection and the appearance of severe, late clinical manifestations. Its clinical course occurs in four stages:

1. The primary syphilis stage is characterized by the development of a chancre, usually genital, approximately 3 weeks after initial exposure.
2. The secondary syphilis stage occurs 6 to 8 weeks after the onset of primary infection. The most common symptoms are skin or mucous membrane lesions. Influenza-like symptoms usually accompany the skin lesions. Symptoms of secondary syphilis resolve 2 to 8 weeks after onset with or without treatment.
3. The latent syphilis stage is detectable only by a positive serologic test. There are no apparent clinical manifestations. Some patients never progress beyond latent syphilis.
4. Tertiary or late-stage syphilis occurs in approximately one third of untreated patients. Tertiary syphilis may affect almost any body system and produce serious complications and sequelae, including permanent disability and death.

Modern diagnostic tests, effective treatments, and public education have greatly reduced the incidence of all stages of syphilis. Manifestations of late syphilis are especially rare today. Currently, the primary public health concern is finding, treating, and preventing early syphilis, although awareness of the late manifestations remains necessary to ensure accurate diagnosis and treatment.

Etiology and Pathophysiology

The causative agent, *T. pallidum*, is a spiral-shaped organism that enters the body through intact mucous membranes or a break in the skin. Transmission of *T. pallidum* occurs primarily during sexual relations through direct contact with a syphilitic lesion or its exudate. If the exudate is secreted into body fluids such as saliva, semen, or vaginal discharge, then contact with the infected fluids can transmit the disease as well.

It appears that exposure to relatively few *T. pallidum* is all that is necessary to produce the disease. Because the spirochete enters the blood stream soon after initial exposure, contact with contaminated blood is another potential mode of transmission. *T. pallidum* can also be spread transplacentally from an infected mother to her fetus as early as the ninth week of gestation.

T. pallidum does not live outside the human body for any appreciable time. Therefore, transmission by objects such as towels, toilet seats, and drinking glasses is a highly improbable, rare occurrence.

Once *T. pallidum* invades the skin, it attaches to, but does not appear to penetrate, human cells. During the incubation period, *T. pallidum* stimulates both cell-mediated and humoral immunity. Lymphocytes and macrophages are present locally, and antitreponemal antibody is present in the serum of 70% to 80% of patients with a primary lesion.

During the primary stage, it appears that the infection is contained and limited to the localized chancre lesion. In fact, the infection has begun to spread via the circulation and will ultimately produce the systemic symptoms characteristic of secondary syphilis, if untreated.

The appearance of secondary syphilis in spite of evidence of an active immune response to the infection is an example of the complexity of the host's response to this disease. The period of latency after resolution of the symptoms of secondary syphilis indicates that eventually the host is able to suppress the infection so that no clinical manifestations are apparent. However, one third of untreated patients acquire tertiary syphilis as many as 20 to 30 years later. The persistence of *T. pallidum*, in the presence of an immune response, over a prolonged period of time in many patients has led to speculation that syphilis suppresses certain and as yet unidentified aspects of the immune response.

Clinical Manifestations

PRIMARY SYPHILIS

The classic symptom of primary syphilis is the development of a painless, genital ulcer at the site of entry. The chancre sore appears approximately 3 weeks after sexual contact with an infectious person. Typically, it begins as a reddened macule and progresses to a papule that erodes to produce a round- to oval-shaped ulcer that is well defined with raised borders. The chancre is usually painless unless secondary infection occurs. Untreated, it heals within 3

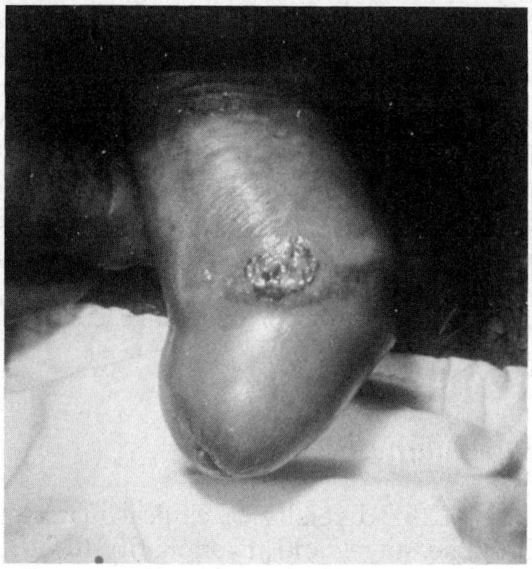

Figure 47–4.

Penile chancre typical of primary syphilis. (Courtesy of New York City Health Department.)

to 6 weeks. In males the most common genital sites are the coronal sulcus, glans penis, and prepuce (Fig. 47–4). In females, frequent sites are the labia, vulva, and cervix. Cervical lesions are often missed because of the lack of apparent symptoms. Lesions may also occur on extragenital sites. The most common extragenital site is the perianal region (Fig. 47–5). Other common sites include the mouth, tongue, breasts, and fingers. Although the chancre of primary syphilis usually occurs as a single lesion, multiple lesions are possible. Atypical lesions at unusual sites are becoming more common, a fact that is attributed to changes in sexual practices. As a general rule, any genital or extragenital ulcer should be considered potentially syphilitic until proven otherwise.

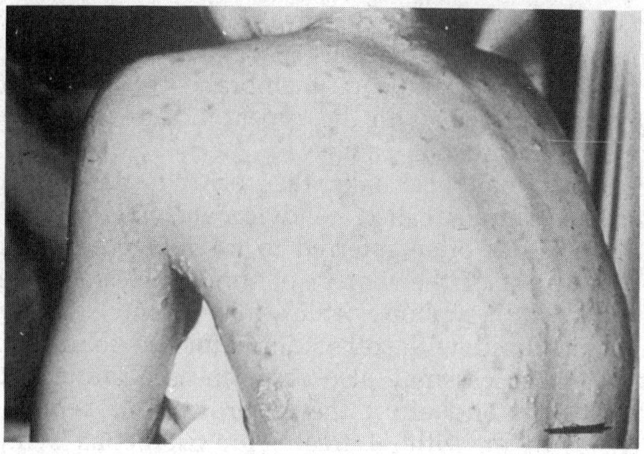

Figure 47–6.

Generalized skin rash seen in secondary syphilis. (Courtesy of the New York City Health Department.)

SECONDARY SYPHILIS

If the patient is not treated during the incubation period or the primary stage, then symptoms of secondary syphilis develop approximately 6 to 8 weeks after the initial appearance of the chancre. Symptoms of secondary syphilis are multiple and varied and may affect almost any organ of the body. Systemic influenza-like symptoms such as malaise, fever, headache, sore throat, anorexia, and arthralgia commonly occur. Generalized, nontender lymphadenopathy is present.

Generalized skin rashes are the most frequently encountered clinical manifestation of secondary syphilis. Cutaneous eruptions often appear as well-demarcated, copper-colored macules on the palms and soles, although they may appear anywhere on the body (Fig. 47–6). Papulosquamous rashes—

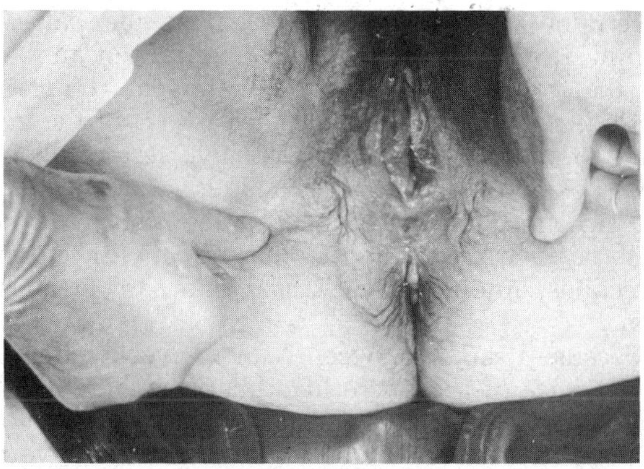

Figure 47–5.

Primary chancre in female patient located on posterior fourchette and perineum. (Courtesy of Leonard Wolf, M.D., New York, NY.)

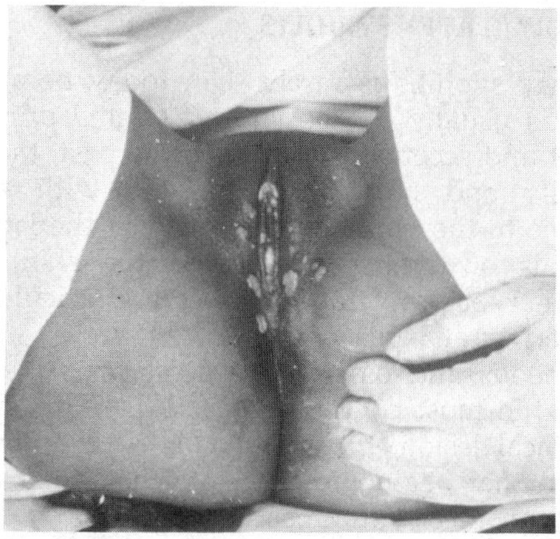

Figure 47–7.

Condylomata lata. Wartlike papules may be seen as clinical manifestations of secondary syphilis. (Courtesy of Leonard Wolf, M.D., New York, NY.)

small, scaly, reddened elevations—are the most common cutaneous lesions associated with secondary syphilis. The mucous membranes of the mouth may be involved, with the appearance of white erosions called mucous patches.

Lesions may also take the form of flat-topped, wartlike papules called condylomata lata (Fig. 47–7). Syphilis is often referred to as the "great imitator" because of the variety of the skin lesions seen in secondary syphilis, which may mimic, and are often confused with, other dermatologic conditions. Patchy hair loss may also occur in association with skin lesions and affect the eyebrows and beard as well. With or without treatment, cutaneous symptoms usually heal in 2 to 10 weeks. Other less common symptoms of secondary syphilis include bursitis, arthritis, periostitis, hepatitis, and nephrotic syndrome as a result of immune complex deposition.

LATENT SYPHILIS

Latent syphilis begins with the resolution of secondary signs and symptoms and ends when and if the clinical manifestations of tertiary syphilis develop. Latent syphilis is defined as the stage at which there is a positive serologic test or history of syphilis but no current clinical manifestations. The latent period is divided into early and late latency. Early latency refers to the first 4 years after initial infections. During early latency, especially the first year, the patient may experience relapses of the mucocutaneous symptoms experienced during the second stage. In early latency, the patient is still capable of transmitting the disease. After 4 years, the period of late latency begins. Relapses do not occur, and the patient is no longer considered infectious, except for pregnant patients who may transmit the infection to the fetus or in rare situations in which an infected person donates blood.

TERTIARY (LATE) SYPHILIS

Tertiary syphilis is rarely seen today because the disease is usually diagnosed and treated during the primary and secondary stages. In the past, the major morbidity and mortality associated with syphilis were due to the variable expression of the late manifestations of tertiary syphilis in the skin, bones, central nervous system, and viscera, particularly the heart and great vessels.

Cutaneous and osseous manifestations were previously the most common signs of tertiary syphilis. The typical lesion, the gumma, is a granulomatous infection that begins as a nodule that breaks down to form an ulcer. Gummas can cause slow destruction of tissue and fibrosis, which may impair functioning of affected structures. Gummas may appear on any tissue or organ, although the skin and bone are the primary sites. Gummas respond well to antibiotic therapy.

Cardiovascular symptoms develop in 10% of patients with late syphilis 30 to 40 years after initial exposure. Aortitis is the most prominent symptom and may result in aortic valve insufficiency and heart failure.

Neurosyphilis is less common, affecting 8% of untreated patients 2 to 30 years after initial infection. Neurosyphilis may produce a variety of syndromes including syphilitic meningitis, paresis, and tabes dorsalis (a degeneration of the dorsal column of the spinal cord).

Medical Diagnosis

Because of the diversity of clinical manifestations in each of the stages and its similarity to other conditions, syphilis can be absolutely diagnosed only by laboratory tests. The darkfield microscopic examination and serologic tests are the most common diagnostic tools.

To perform a darkfield examination, serous exudate from a moist lesion is examined microscopically for the presence of *T. pallidum* using a dark field to highlight the organisms. This test is the most specific and only absolute method for diagnosing syphilis. However, the patient must have skin lesions for this test to be performed. It is the method of choice for diagnosing primary syphilis, and it is also effective for diagnosing secondary, early latent, relapsing, and congenital syphilis, each of which is manifested by skin lesions. The test is not reliable for late latent or tertiary syphilis. Local health departments often supply darkfield microscopy as a service.

There are two types of serologic tests: treponemal and nontreponemal. They differ in the antigens they use and the types of antibodies that are measured. Nontreponemal tests are relatively inexpensive and easy to do. The Venereal Disease Research Laboratory (VDRL) test and the rapid plasma reagin (RPR) card test are currently the most widely used nontreponemal tests. Nontreponemal tests are used to determine the presence of reagin in the patient's serum. Reagin is a heterogeneous group of antibodies that combine with a specific antigen. The test is not specific for syphilis, and at least 1% of the general population obtain false-positive test results. A false-positive result can occur after an acute illness or immunization and during pregnancy. Chronic false-positive results most often occur with chronic infections, autoimmune diseases, and narcotic addiction.

Because it takes between 1 and 3 weeks after the appearance of a chancre in primary syphilis for the patient's serum to convert to antibody positive, nontreponemal tests may also indicate false-negative results during the incubation period and early primary stage. If the test is negative in the presence of symptoms of primary syphilis (i.e., chancre), it should be repeated in 2 weeks. Nontreponemal tests are 100% accurate in secondary syphilis and 70% accurate in tertiary syphilis. Nontreponemal tests are most frequently used for premarital and prenatal screening. For positive test results without symptoms, the VDRL is repeated, and if it remains positive the treponemal test described next is performed. Nontreponemal tests may be used to evaluate the patient's response to treatment through serial measurement of antibody titers.

Treponemal tests are more specific than nontreponemal tests because they are designed to detect antibodies specific for treponema. The standard treponemal test used today is the fluorescent treponemal antibody-absorption (FTA-ABS) test. Because it is technically more difficult and expensive to perform, the FTA-ABS is generally reserved to verify other tests. The FTA-ABS is highly sensitive in ali stages of syphilis.

Medical Management

Parenteral penicillin G is the drug of choice for treatment of all stages of syphilis. Treatment regimens with penicillin G or an appropriate substitute are based on the length of illness and type of syphilis. See Table 47–4 for treatment regimens for syphilis.

Application of the Nursing Process to the Care of the Patient with Syphilis

The availability of simple screening tests, an inexpensive cure, and increased public awareness have contributed to a rapid decline in the incidence of syphilis since the mid-1940s. Once the premier venereal disease, syphilis is now less common than herpes, gonorrhea, and chlamydia. However, the incidence of syphilis is still considered significant. Nurses working in sexually transmitted disease centers, inner city hospitals, and clinics are especially likely to encounter patients with syphilis. All nurses have a responsibility to be informed about the clinical manifestations and course of this disease. It is particularly important for nurses to recognize the signs and symptoms of early syphilis so that the potentially severe complications of tertiary and congenital syphilis are avoided.

Assessment

Early in the assessment interview, question the patient about his or her reason for seeking health care. Some patients seek treatment because of the presence of symptoms. Others are referred as a result of positive serologic tests or as the sexual contacts of diagnosed patients. In all situations, be certain to project a nonjudgmental, supportive, and caring attitude. Often patients are not aware that they have contracted syphilis. Initial responses to the diagnosis range from shock and denial to hostility or apathy. Ensure the patient's confidentiality and privacy throughout the assessment process.

Question the patient about his or her sexual history and lifestyle, history of other sexually transmitted diseases, and past and present symptoms.

Because the symptoms of primary syphilis are mild and may go unnoticed, and symptoms of secondary syphilis are often confused with or attributed to other causes, ask both specific and open-ended questions to assist the patient in remembering and describing symptoms. Examples of questions that may be asked to obtain information about the patient's symptoms are as follows:

"Have you ever had a painless canker or ulcer sore anywhere on your body, particularly in the mouth or on the genitals?"
"Have you had any skin rashes? If so, when did the rash occur? Where was it located? What did it look like?"
"Did you experience any influenza-like symptoms in conjunction with the rash?"
"Did you treat the rash? If so, how?"

It is sometimes helpful to use photographs of typical syphilitic skin lesions to help the patient recognize and identify previous skin rashes.

Obtain a psychosocial history that includes the patient's education and employment history, marital status, home environment, and relationship with significant others. The reaction of significant others, the availability of support systems, and the patient's lifestyle all influence the patient's response to the diagnosis, compliance with treatment, and willingness to identify sexual contacts.

Thoroughly examine the patient's skin in a private well-lighted room. Assess the skin for the presence of macules, papules, vesicles, nodules, erosions, and ulcers. Note the location, size, distribution, and symmetry of any lesions. Question the patient about changes in the lesions such as redness, swelling, or presence or absence of exudate. Wear gloves to palpate the lesions for consistency (soft, firm, or indurated) and the presence of pain or tenderness. Examine the patient's mouth for the presence of ulcers or white, mucous patches on the tongue, gingiva (gums), or palate. When appropriate, examine the external genitalia including the suprapubic and perianal areas, as well as the penis and scrotum in males and the vulva and perineum in females. In females, note the presence of any vaginal discharge. Because many patients present with more than one sexually transmitted disease, also assess the patient for symptoms suggestive of other venereal diseases.

Throughout this entire process, assess the patient's knowledge of syphilis, including the mode of transmission, clinical manifestations, congenital, and long-term effects.

Nursing Diagnoses and Planning

Nursing diagnoses and related expected patient outcomes most commonly applicable to patients with syphilis include the following:

NDx: High risk for altered health maintenance related to insufficient knowledge of cause, signs, symptoms, clinical course, and mode of transmission of syphilis

Planning: Patient outcomes
1. Patient states the cause of syphilis.
2. Patient describes signs, symptoms, and clinical course of syphilis in adults.
3. Patient describes potential effects of congenital syphilis.
4. Patient identifies the primary mode of transmission.

NDx: High risk for noncompliance with the treatment regimen related to lack of knowledge, lifestyle, distrust of health professionals

Planning: Patient outcomes
1. Patient lists potential long-term effects of untreated or inadequately treated syphilis.
2. Patient describes the recommended treatment regimen.
3. Patient takes medications as prescribed.
4. Patient returns for follow-up visits.
5. Serologic tests for cure are negative.

NDx: High risk for infection (reinfection) related to sexual practices and lifestyle

Planning: Patient outcomes
1. Patient describes the rationale for abstaining from sexual relations with former partners until they are examined and treated.
2. Patient identifies at least three ways to prevent reinfection.

NDx: Anxiety related to concerns about personal health status, possible transmission to others, social stigma of having contracted a sexually transmitted disease, identification of sexual partners

Planning: Patient outcomes
1. Patient verbalizes that he or she is experiencing less anxiety.
2. Nonverbal behaviors indicate that the patient is less anxious (e.g., posture and facial expression are relaxed, voice is calm).
3. Patient retains information.
4. Patient provides names of sexual partners for contact tracing by health agency.
5. Patient refers sexual partners within specific time frames.

Nursing Interventions

NDx: High risk for altered health maintenance

The primary nursing intervention for patients with syphilis is education. Patient education helps to ensure compliance with treatment and follow-up as well as cooperation in identifying partners. Instruct the patient in the cause, transmission, and clinical course of syphilis. Explain the incubation periods for primary and secondary syphilis to assist the patient in identifying time periods when sexual partners may have been exposed to the disease. Instruct the patient in the three modes of transmission of syphilis.

Inform patients about the risk of congenital syphilis. Describe the effects, which include skin and mucous membrane lesions and involvement of the bone and central nervous system. Explain that infants of female patients who have syphilis or who contract syphilis during pregnancy are at greatest risk. Inform the patient that the earlier in pregnancy treatment is begun, the less the risk there is to the fetus. If the patient is pregnant, provide an opportunity for her to express her concerns and anxieties in a supportive atmosphere. Offer appropriate reassurances concerning the health of the fetus.

NDx: High risk for noncompliance

Explain the treatment plan and rationale to the patient in detail. Review the dosage, schedule, and side effects of prescribed medications with the patient (see Table 47–4). Emphasize the importance of taking oral medications at the recommended times for the prescribed number of days. Provide the patient with the name and telephone number of someone to call if he or she has any questions or experiences any side effects during the course of treatment. Be sure to inform the patient with early syphilis of the possibility of a Jarisch-Herxheimer reaction after the first treatment with parenteral benzathine penicillin G. This reaction is believed to be caused by the release of large amounts of antigenic material after initial treatment. It is characterized by influenza-like symptoms 2 to 6 hours after injection that last about 6 hours.

If applicable to the individual patient, explain that longer treatment times are required for both oral and parenteral medications when a person has had syphilis for more than a year. Inform the patient about the long-term effects of untreated or inadequately treated syphilis. Explain that the lack of current symptoms does not indicate a cure, and stress the importance of returning for follow-up care to determine the effectiveness of treatment to avoid the long-term effects of this disease.

Usually the patient is instructed to return in 1

week. During this time, advise the patient to abstain from sexual relations to avoid transmitting the disease. Caution the patient to avoid sex with previous or current partners until they have been examined to decrease the risk of reinfection.

Remember that the quality of the nurse-patient interaction also affects compliance. Effective communication skills and a nonjudgmental attitude are essential for working with the patient with syphilis. Promote compliance and follow-up by being objective and empathic and by projecting interest in the patient's well-being. Provide information and instructions in terminology the patient can understand, with ample time for the patient to ask questions and express concerns.

NDx: High risk for infection (reinfection)
Advise the patient to avoid sex with former partners until they have been evaluated and treated to prevent reinfection. For both heterosexual and homosexual patients, recommend the use of condoms as a means of preventing future exposure to syphilis and other sexually transmitted diseases. Remember that although many patients object to using condoms on a regular basis, they can often be convinced to use them when engaging in high-risk sexual encounters (e.g., sex with anonymous partners or prostitutes). Assist the patient in identifying methods or behaviors for avoiding future encounters with sexually transmitted diseases. Examples include observing the genitals of prospective sexual partners, refraining from sex with partners who have signs or symptoms of sexually transmitted diseases, and seeking health care at the first sign of a possible infection. The most effective interventions for assisting the patient to change his or her behavior to prevent reinfection and transmission are patient education and development of a therapeutic nurse-patient relationship.

NDx: Anxiety
Provide an opportunity for the patient to express his or her concerns about having contracted syphilis and fear of transmitting the disease to others. Assure the patient that syphilis is curable provided that the treatment regimen is adhered to and the patient returns for follow-up testing.

Explain the importance of cooperation in naming sexual partners. Allow the patient time to verbalize anxiety regarding this, but reinforce its necessity and ultimate benefit to those named. Once named, sexual partners are contacted in one of two ways. Traditionally, health care personnel contact the partner and the patient's confidentiality is maintained. More recently, selected patients are encouraged to refer sexual contacts for evaluation themselves. The first method offers greater assurance of follow-up with sexual partners. The second method is less costly and promotes assumption of responsibility on the part of the patient. Because of the importance of early treatment, the traditional method of contact tracing is more frequently used in cases of syphilis. However, if the patient is offered the opportunity to refer sexual contacts, explain that he or she must comply within specified time limits or the health agency will contact the sexual partners. Assist the patient who chooses self-referral to decide how to present the information to the partners. Consider role-playing as a helpful technique to this end. Do not offer the option of self-referral to the patient who is disinterested or who has poor communication skills.

Evaluation

Evaluate the effectiveness of nursing care for a patient with syphilis by comparing the patient's status with the expected patient outcomes. Examples of specific outcomes for patients with syphilis have been provided in the Planning section.

Chlamydia Trachomatis

Infections caused by *C. trachomatis* are the most prevalent of the sexually transmitted diseases. Depending on the population studied, *C. trachomatis* is 5 to 10 times more common than gonorrhea. An estimated 3 to 4 million Americans contract a chlamydial infection each year.

C. trachomatis produces a broad spectrum of diseases and complications. In developing countries, *C. trachomatis* causes a chronic infectious disease of the conjunctiva and cornea known as trachoma. Trachoma is the leading cause of preventable blindness in the world. Chlamydiae have long been known as the causative organism of lymphogranuloma venereum. However, it is only recently that *C. trachomatis* has been recognized as the causative agent in a number of other genital tract infections previously considered to be of unknown origin.

C. trachomatis is a primary causative agent in nongonococcal and postgonococcal urethritis in males. It produces 50% of the estimated 500,000 cases of epididymitis, inflammation of the cordlike structure on the posterior border of the testis in which sperm is stored.

In females chlamydia has been implicated as one of the major causes of cervicitis and PID. Consequently, *C. trachomatis* infections play a significant role in the increasing incidence of ectopic pregnancy and infertility, both potential long-term sequelae of PID. *C. trachomatis* in pregnancy is associated with postpartum endometritis in the mother and the development of eye infections and pneumonia in the newborn.

In industrialized western society, *C. trachomatis* is almost exclusively a sexually transmitted disease.

Populations at risk for chlamydial infections are the same as those at risk for other sexually transmitted diseases. Young, sexually active males and females from lower socioeconomic groups have the highest incidence of chlamydia. Risk of infection increases with the number of sexual partners.

Etiology and Pathophysiology

C. trachomatis microorganisms are unique. Classified as bacteria, they also share properties with viruses. Considered obligatory intracellular parasites, *C. trachomatis* organisms take over and use the energy system of living cells to meet their own energy needs and to replicate. *C. trachomatis* has a predilection for columnar and transitional cell epithelia, such as those found in the reproductive tract. The organism can remain latent for a prolonged period of time within the cell. Replication progresses slowly because of its dependence on the cell's energy system.

The diversity of the diseases produced by *C. trachomatis* is explained by the fact that there are 15 strains of this bacteria. The strains can be roughly divided into three groups: those that cause trachoma and other adult eye infections, those that cause lymphogranuloma venereum, and those that cause genital tract infections.

Clinical Manifestations

In males, *C. trachomatis* causes urethritis (see Chapter 46), which is characterized by a white or mucoid urethral discharge that may be intermittent or occur only in the morning. In some cases, dysuria and urethral itching may also occur.

In females, the most common site for *C. trachomatis* genital infections is the cervix. Although most females who are culture positive for *C. trachomatis* of the cervix are also asymptomatic, at least one third have local signs of infection. A mucopurulent cervical discharge that appears yellow to green when viewed on a cotton swab is the most frequent symptom. This may or may not be accompanied by cervical erosion, an area on the cervix that is edematous, congested, and friable. Clinical recognition of chlamydial cervicitis requires a high degree of suspicion and thorough examination of the cervix. Cervical infection, especially asymptomatic infection, provides a reservoir for potential transmission of *C. trachomatis* to male sexual partners and neonates.

In pregnancy, there is 60% to 70% risk of neonatal infection if the mother has a *C. trachomatis* infection of the cervix at the time of delivery. Infants acquire the infection through contact with the infected cervicovaginal secretions. The primary sites of infection are the conjunctiva and respiratory tract.

C. trachomatis is also a major cause of PID, with the primary site of infection being the fallopian tubes, and infertility and ectopic pregnancy the two most common serious sequelae. The exact number of cases of infertility and ectopic pregnancy attributable to *C. trachomatis* remains unknown. However, on the basis of the number of suspected cases of chlamydial salpingitis, it appears to be considerable.

Chlamydia also appears to be an important cause of acute urethral syndrome in females, which is characterized by dysuria, frequency, and the absence of bacteriuria.

Medical Diagnosis

Until recently, tissue culturing was the only method available for making a definitive diagnosis of chlamydial infections of the genital tract. Although this test is sensitive and specific, it is also complex and expensive and requires a 6- to 7-day wait for definitive results.

Another test for diagnosing chlamydia, the direct-slide monoclonal antibody test, is now available and appears to be as specific and sensitive as culturing. The main advantages of this test are its lower cost, rapidity of results (total processing takes 30–40 minutes), and relative simplicity of the procedure.

Other tests such as cytologic examination of stained smears (e.g., Pap smear) and serology are either unreliable or have little value as diagnostic aids.

Screening for the presence of chlamydial infection is recommended for the following groups:

1. Individuals attending sexually transmitted disease clinics.
2. Individuals with chlamydia-associated syndromes.
3. Sex partners of patients with chlamydial genitourinary infections.
4. Pregnant patients at high risk (adolescents and unmarried women or married women with a history of sexually transmitted disease or multiple partners).

Medical Management

Tetracycline, erythromycin, and sulfisoxazole all are highly effective for treatment of *C. trachomatis* infections.

The following treatment regimens are recommended for all confirmed chlamydial urogenital tract infections and for chlamydia-associated syndromes such as mucopurulent cervicitis and nongonococcal urethritis, because the causative agent is chlamydia in more than 50% of the cases.

1. Tetracycline hydrochloride: 500 mg by mouth four times a day for 7 days.
2. Doxycycline: 100 mg by mouth twice a day for 7 days.

3. Erythromycin: 500 mg by mouth four times a day for 7 days is recommended for patients who cannot tolerate tetracycline or when use of tetracycline is contraindicated, as in pregnancy.

Chlamydia is often found in association with gonorrhea infections. When gonorrhea is also present, treatment should be initiated that is effective against both organisms (see Table 47–4).

Many cases of PID are caused by more than one organism. Causative organisms include *C. trachomatis, N. gonorrhoeae,* anaerobic bacteria, gram-negative rods, and *Mycoplasma hominis.* Treatment regimens for PID include medications that are active against a broad range of microbes. For hospital treatment, doxycycline, 100 mg intravenously (IV) two times a day, or cefoxitin, 2 g IV four times a day, plus tetracycline, 1.5 to 2.0 g/day in divided doses four times a day, are recommended to cover various causative agents. IV medications are continued for at least 4 days followed by doxycycline, 100 mg by mouth, for a total of 10 to 14 days of therapy.

Out-patient treatment consists of a single dose of cefoxitin, 2 g intramuscularly, and probenecid, 1 g orally, followed by either doxycycline, 100 mg orally twice a day, or tetracycline, 500 mg orally four times a day for 10 to 14 days. An alternative regimen is a single dose of ceftriaxone, 250 mg intramuscularly, followed by doxycycline or tetracycline as previously stated.

Sex partners of patients with urogenital tract chlamydial infections should be evaluated for sexually transmitted disease and treated with one of the regimens previously listed.

Application of the Nursing Process to the Care of the Patient with Chlamydia Trachomatis Infection

Assessment

Nursing assessment of the patient with confirmed or suspected chlamydial genital tract infection begins with a thorough history taking and analysis of symptoms. The health history includes a comprehensive sexual and social history. This information assists in identifying individuals at risk for infection and reinfection with *C. trachomatis* and also provides information about the patient's educational needs. Question the patient about his or her age, socioeconomic status, and sexual lifestyle. Ask about the number of sexual partners because this is considered the most significant predictor of risk for chlamydial infection. Also obtain information about the patient's contraceptive preferences, history of infection with other sexually transmitted diseases or chlamydia-associated syndromes (e.g., PID in females or nongonococcal urethritis [NGU] in males), and possible presence of infection in current sexual partners.

Because symptoms of lower genital tract infections in females are often absent or so mild that they are unnoticed by the patient, many female patients who are seen for an initial evaluation do so as a result of a diagnosis of NGU in their partners. Thus, the nursing assessment must focus on symptoms to rule out vaginitis and other sexually transmitted diseases as well as to identify the subtle symptoms of chlamydial infection.

Question the patient about the presence of vaginal discharge. Note the character of the discharge (amount, color, odor, consistency) and onset, duration, and presence of associated symptoms such as pain, itching, and skin changes. Also question the patient about factors that aggravate or alleviate symptoms such as sexual intercourse, menses, or temperature changes. The typical discharge of chlamydia-associated cervical infections is mucoid, clear to amber in color, and varies from scant to profuse drainage. The discharge is not associated with pain or itching, except in patients with concurrent urinary tract infection indicated by frequency, urgency, and dysuria.

Because of the frequently mild or asymptomatic nature of chlamydial cervicitis, females often do not seek health care until the infection has spread to the upper genital tract. Therefore, the nursing assessment also focuses on symptoms of PID, which is often less acute when caused by chlamydia as opposed to gonorrhea.

Question the patient about the presence of lower abdominal pain, metrorrhagia (bleeding between periods), and dyspareunia. Also assess for systemic symptoms such as fever, malaise, nausea, and vomiting even though these are less common with chlamydial infections than with other pelvic infections. Be certain to determine onset and duration of symptoms because symptoms of PID frequently follow menstruation.

Males usually present with more observable and characteristic symptoms. Question male patients about white or mucoid urethral discharge, which may be intermittent or occur only in the morning. Also ask about dysuria and urethral itching.

Assess the patient's knowledge of the disease process, mode of transmission, and associated syndromes throughout the history taking and physical examination. Examples of specific questions that may be asked to assist in the assessment of the patient's learning needs include the following:

"How is chlamydia spread from one person to another?"
"What factors in your sexual lifestyle do you think increase your risk of contracting the infection?"
"How can you prevent reinfection?"
"Do you know the possible complications of this infection for yourself, your partner, and your future children?"

Assess also the psychological response of the patient diagnosed with a chlamydial infection. Responses can range from disinterest to severe anxiety. Variables include the interpersonal relationships with sexual partners, the severity of symptoms, and the presence of complications or associated syndromes. Females with PID may display anger, denial, or depression related to potential adverse effects on fertility. Patients involved in monogamous relationships may express anger at their partners and question their commitment. As for patients with other sexually transmitted diseases, communicate a nonjudgmental, empathetic attitude and sensitivity to the patient's feelings and concerns.

Nursing Diagnoses and Planning

Nursing diagnoses and related expected patient outcomes most commonly applicable to patients with chlamydial infections include the following:

NDx: High risk for altered health maintenance related to insufficient knowledge of disease process, transmission, and prevention of chlamydial infections

Planning: Patient outcomes
1. Patient lists the symptoms and potential complications of chlamydial infections.
2. Patient asks pertinent questions derived from knowledge of the disease process.
3. Patient describes methods for reducing the risk of transmission and reinfection.

NDx: High risk for infection (reinfection) related to sexual lifestyle, lack of knowledge about the mode of transmission or prevention

Planning: Patient outcomes
1. Patient lists factors that increase the risk of infection.
2. Patient describes the rationale for altering personal behaviors that increase the risk of infection and transmission.
3. Patient describes plans to use a barrier method of contraception.
4. Recurrence of infection is absent.

NDx: High risk for noncompliance with treatment related to lack of knowledge about the importance of following treatment regimens and behavioral recommendations

Planning: Patient outcomes
1. Patient states the dosage, schedule, and side effects of prescribed medications.
2. Patient states the rationale for taking medications as prescribed.
3. Patient reports taking medications as prescribed.
4. Patient indicates intention to abstain from sexual intercourse or to use condoms until treatment is completed.

NDx: Anxiety related to potential complications and long-term sequelae for self or sexual partners

Planning: Patient outcomes
1. Patient verbalizes decreased anxiety.
2. Nonverbal behavior indicates anxiety is within normal limits (e.g., relaxed posture; absence of hand wringing, crying, shaking; relaxed facial expression).
3. Patient retains information.
4. Patient states that he or she will inform sexual contacts.
5. Sexual contacts present for evaluation.
6. Patient states accurate and realistic expectations for prognosis after treatment.
7. Patient describes measures for preventing reinfection.

Nursing Interventions

NDx: High risk for altered health maintenance
Instruct the patient in the disease process: symptoms, mode of transmission, and complications. Emphasize the significance of asymptomatic infection and the importance of seeking treatment immediately at the first sign of infection to reduce complications and long-term sequelae. It is particularly important for males to understand the potential for serious complications in untreated female partners. Review methods for preventing infection.

NDx: High risk for infection (reinfection)
Assist the patient in identifying factors in his or her sexual lifestyle that increases the risk of reinfection. Recommend the use of barrier methods of contraception such as the diaphragm and the condom. The condom is especially effective in preventing chlamydial infection. If appropriate, suggest a reduction in the number of sexual partners as a means of decreasing the risk of chlamydial infection or infection with other sexually transmitted diseases. Variables affecting compliance with these recommendations include the patient's values and the role of the patient's current sexual lifestyle in his or her identity and self-esteem.

NDx: High risk for noncompliance
Instruct the patient in the purpose, dosage, scheduling, and side effects of prescribed medications. Emphasize the importance of taking prescribed medications on time and in the recommended dosage for the entire treatment interval to achieve a cure. Otherwise, the patient may stop taking the medications as soon as the symptoms abate. In addition, advise the patient to abstain from sexual intercourse until the treatment is completed and sex-

ual partners have been examined or treated. If the patient indicates that he or she cannot comply, recommend use of a condom during the course of treatment. Caution the patient to seek treatment immediately if symptoms recur.

NDx: Anxiety
Encourage the patient to verbalize his or her concerns and feelings about contracting a sexually transmitted disease. With the female patient especially, assist her to view the infection in a realistic perspective. Stress that, once diagnosed, chlamydia is an easily treated infection with a 95% cure rate and that PID is unlikely with timely treatment of lower genital tract infection. For the patient with PID, point out that infertility related to PID has decreased from 75% to 20% during the past 20 years because early treatment and improved surgical interventions have decreased the risk of permanent tubal damage. If the patient is pregnant, explain that the risk of transmission to the fetus occurs only at delivery. Reassure the patient that treatment during pregnancy and compliance with recommended preventive measures virtually eliminate this risk. When possible, provide the patient with written literature to reinforce information communicated during patient teaching and counseling. Suggest a follow-up visit for the patient whose verbalizations and behavior indicate excessive anger, anxiety, or potential for depression.

Additional Interventions
Encourage the patient to refer sex partners for evaluation and possible treatment.

Evaluation

Evaluate the effectiveness of nursing care for a patient with chlamydia by comparing the patient's status with the expected patient outcomes. Examples of specific outcomes for patients with chlamydia have been provided in the Planning section.

Nongonococcal Urethritis

Nongonococcal urethritis (NGU) is an inflammation of the urethra in the absence of infection with *N. gonorrhoeae.* The incidence of this sexually transmitted disease is 2.5 times greater than gonococcal urethritis. Most cases of NGU are caused by *C. trachomatis* and *Ureaplasma urealyticum.* By convention, the diagnosis of NGU is restricted to males, although *C. trachomatis* can produce a urethral syndrome in females as well.

The prevalence of sexually transmitted urethritis, both gonococcal and nongonococcal, has increased significantly in the United States, England, and Sweden during the past 30 years. Although recent statistics indicate that the prevalence of gonococcal urethritis has reached a plateau, the number of NGU cases continues to rise. NGU accounts for more than half the cases of urethritis reported by sexually transmitted disease clinics and 80% to 90% of urethritis seen at campus health services. NGU is most frequently diagnosed in heterosexual men aged 20 to 24 years.

Etiology and Pathophysiology

C. trachomatis is the major cause of NGU. It can be isolated from the urethras of 50% of males with NGU, about 20% of males with gonococcal urethritis, and 0% to 5% of males without urethritis. *C. trachomatis* has been identified as the most frequent cause of postgonococcal urethritis (PGU). PGU occurs shortly after curative therapy for gonorrhea. Because gonorrhea has a shorter incubation period (2 to 7 days) than chlamydial urethritis (2 to 3 weeks), males infected with both organisms first present, and are diagnosed and treated for, gonorrhea. Nearly all males who are simultaneously infected with both organisms and who are treated with penicillin go on to develop PGU because *C. trachomatis* is unaffected by penicillin.

Between 10% and 40% of NGU infections are thought to be attributable to *U. urealyticum,* one of two mycoplasms known to infect males. The causal relationship between NGU and *U. urealyticum* is not as clear-cut as that between *C. trachomatis* and NGU. *U. urealyticum* is not always pathogenic. It can be isolated from the urethras of sexually active males who do not have urethritis as well as from those who do.

Why *U. urealyticum* produces disease in some males and not others is unknown. It has been suggested that only 1 or several of the 14 serotypes of *U. urealyticum* are capable of causing disease. Another explanation could be the difference in host response to the organism. Considering the frequently benign nature of the organism, treatment is not indicated for males who culture positive for *U. urealyticum* unless there are clinical symptoms. In contrast, asymptomatic chlamydial NGU is treated.

About 20% to 30% of NGU infections are not caused by *C. trachomatis* or *U. urealyticum.* A variety of organisms have been suggested or proven to be etiologically related to NGU, including *Trichomonas vaginitis, G. vaginalis, C. albicans,* and herpes simplex among others.

Clinical Manifestations

The characteristic clinical manifestation of NGU is urethral discharge. The urethral discharge associated with NGU is usually white or mucoid and may be present only in the morning or may cause intermittent staining. A more profuse, purulent discharge is suggestive of gonococcal urethritis. Dysuria and urethral itching are also common. The manifestations of NGU are frequently mild. Asymptomatic pyuria is common. More severe symptoms (e.g., frequency, urgency, hematuria, and inguinal adenopathy) suggest the presence of another or concurrent genital infection.

Medical Diagnosis

Diagnosis of NGU is made on the basis of evidence of urethritis; either clinical symptoms or laboratory demonstration of polymorphonuclear leukocytes on a Gram's stain of a urethral smear in the absence of gonorrhea. Laboratory facilities for isolating *C. trachomatis* and *U. urealyticum* are not always available. New and easier techniques for identification of these two organisms are currently being introduced.

Medical Management

Response of NGU to medications is variable because the causative organism is usually not identified. In 30% to 40% of cases, infection recurs within 6 weeks of treatment. Poor success may be partially attributable to lack of compliance with the treatment regimen or reinfection from an untreated or new sexual partner. Identification and treatment of sexual contacts, especially in cases of chlamydial infection, is necessary to keep partners from reinfecting each other or spreading the disease. Failure rates are lowest for chlamydia, more frequent for *U. urealyticum,* and highest for NGU of unknown origin.

The recommended initial treatment regimen is tetracycline hydrochloride, 500 mg orally four times daily for 7 days. This is usually effective for chlamydial NGU, less so for *U. urealyticum,* and successfully treats gonorrhea. It is important for the patient to abstain from sexual intercourse during treatment.

Application of the Nursing Process to the Care of the Patient with Nongonococcal Urethritis

The assessment, nursing diagnoses, expected patient outcomes, nursing interventions, and evaluation for patients with NGU are similar to those described previously for patients with *C. trachomatis.* Additional considerations include the variable response of NGU to medication and the high likelihood of recurrence. These factors can negatively affect compliance and can precipitate a heightened emotional response with related inappropriate or ineffective coping behavior.

Condylomata Acuminata

Condylomata acuminata are warts appearing in the anogenital area caused by infection with human papillomavirus (HPV). Until recently, condylomata acuminata were considered to be minor, relatively inconsequential lesions of more psychological than physical significance. However, the increasing incidence of anogenital warts and their possible relationship to genital cancer has led to an increased interest in this sexually transmitted disease.

Similar to other sexually transmitted diseases, genital warts are most frequently seen in the young (aged 16–25 years), sexually active population. Previously diagnosed more frequently in males, genital warts now appear to be at least as common in females. It is estimated that approximately 2% of females of childbearing age have flat condylomata infections of the cervix. At least 70% of these lesions are subclinical and frequently undiagnosed.

Etiology and Pathophysiology

There are more than 20 subtypes of the HPV. Several have been identified as the etiologic agents in common skin warts, whereas others have been associated with the occurrence of genital warts.

Genital warts are transmitted by direct skin to skin contact primarily through sexual activity. Nonsexual transmission is also possible. Infection by autoinoculation and exposure during birth have been documented.

The virus infects the nuclei of epithelial cells, transforming the cells and causing them to proliferate. Cell-mediated immunity (CMI) seems to play an important role in both the ultimate severity and recovery from the infection. Individuals with modest depressions in CMI are more susceptible to HPV infection and are less likely to respond well to therapy or to have the warts regress spontaneously. Genital warts are more likely to appear and are more severe during pregnancy when CMI is reduced.

The incubation period, from time of exposure to the appearance of lesions, is long and highly variable. The average incubation period is 3 months, with a range of 3 weeks to 8 months. In males, lesions may appear anywhere on the penis. The coronal sulcus on the inner aspect of the prepuce is often the initial site of appearance. Penile warts are more common among uncircumcised males.

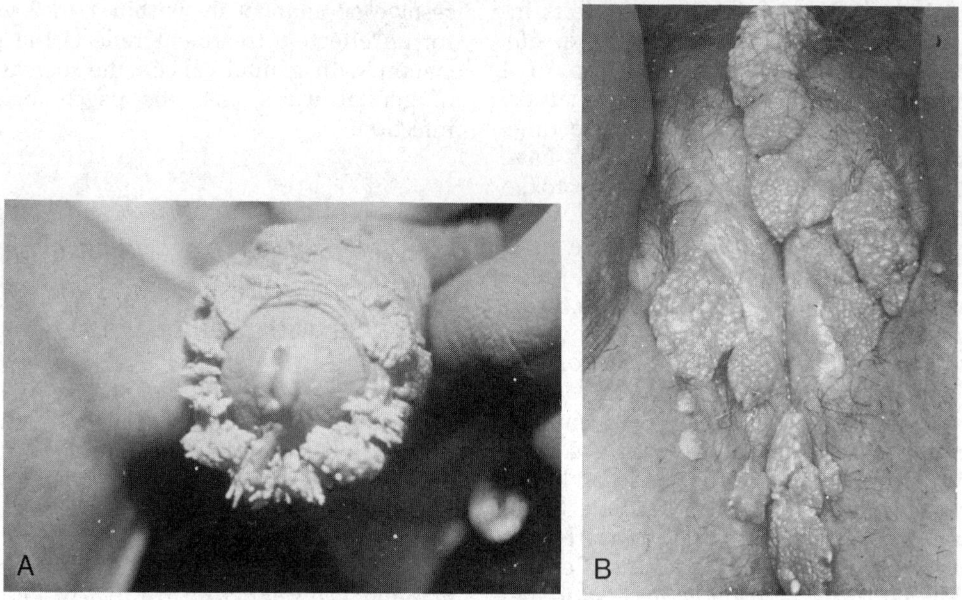

Figure 47–8.

A, Extensive condylomata acuminata of the penis. *B*, Condylomata acuminata in a female patient. (Courtesy of the New York City Health Department.)

Clinical Manifestations

There are several varieties of genital warts. The "classic" venereal wart is a raised, irregular, fissured papule. Pinkish in color, it is usually taller than it is wide, with finger-like projections that give it a pointed appearance (Fig. 47–8).

Condylomata may also be flat in appearance. Flat condylomata can occur in great numbers and are the type most frequently seen in the cervix, although they may also be on the vagina or on other mucosal surfaces as well as the skin. Flat condylomata are difficult to see with the naked eye, usually do not cause symptoms, and consequently often remain undiagnosed.

Giant condylomata acuminata are larger, rounded, soft papules or nodules with a strawberry-like surface. Although rare, these warts have a higher incidence of complications.

In females, the initial site is frequently the posterior vaginal introitus (opening) and the adjacent labia. Lesions may spread to other parts of the vulva, perineum, and anus. Anal warts are more commonly seen in females and homosexual males. Other nongenital sites include the mouth.

Genital warts are usually multiple and may coalesce to form larger masses. When venereal warts occur around the vaginal, urethral, and rectal orifices, internal spread is a possible complication. Common symptoms of intraurethral involvement are urethral bleeding, discharge, and dysuria. Approximately 50% of females with lesions on the vaginal introitus have cervical involvement. Seventy percent of patients with perineal lesions have anal condylomata.

In addition to causing psychological distress and embarrassment, complications from large genital warts include a tendency toward ulceration with bleeding and secondary infection. Major complications are rare but documented. In males, giant condylomata may grow relentlessly and destroy genital structures.

In females, malignant transformation to cervical in situ squamous cell carcinoma and vulvovaginal carcinoma has been suggested but remains unproven.

Although vulvovaginal warts often enlarge during pregnancy, it is usual for them to regress after delivery. Most infants are unaffected, but occasional transmission of the virus does occur. In infants, lesions appear primarily on the genitals, larynx, and trachea. To avoid this problem, it is suggested that as many warts as possible be removed before delivery.

Medical Diagnosis

Diagnosis is made on the basis of the appearance of the lesions.

Medical Management

Podophyllin, a cytotoxic agent, is the treatment of choice for classic venereal warts. Podophyllin is applied topically to all surfaces of the wart, taking care to avoid normal skin surfaces. Local side effects include pain and a burning sensation at the site. Treatment is repeated every 7 days for up to 4 weeks or until the lesions resolve. No more than 0.5 to 1 ml of podophyllin is applied at any one time. Severe systemic side effects, although rare, have been reported and include neuropathy, hepatotoxicity, and granulocytopenia.

Trichloroacetic and dichloroacetic acids are used in the treatment of nonkeratotic flat warts located on the external genitalia. Again, avoidance of surrounding skin is important, because application causes instant, nonreversible tissue destruction. As with podophyllin, warts are retreated weekly.

Cryosurgery, another common treatment, is carried out in the physician's office with a cotton-tipped applicator dipped in nitrous oxide or liquid nitrogen. It causes a local burning sensation. Cryosurgery is very effective against keratotic warts and can also be used on classic and flat warts. Retreatment at weekly intervals is usually necessary. Because of pain, only five to seven warts can be treated at any one time.

Electrocautery provides the same results, but local anesthesia is necessary. This is the treatment of choice when large numbers of lesions are present. It is sometimes necessary to admit the patient and use general anesthesia for multiple lesions. Postoperatively, the treated area resembles a burn.

Surgical excision may be necessary for the larger, giant condylomata. This procedure ensures complete removal while also furnishing specimens for histologic examination.

Recently, other, newer treatments, such as application of fluorouracil (5-FU) cream and carbon dioxide (CO_2) laser destruction, have gained in popularity. 5-FU is recommended for treatment of mucous membrane warts such as those located on the urinary meatus or intraanal canal. 5-FU cannot be used on the epidermis of genital organs. The mild to moderate pain associated with application on mucous membranes is controlled with 5% lidocaine ointment or analgesics. The efficacy of 5-FU is comparable to podophyllin and trichloroacetic acid.

Destruction of warts by vaporization with a CO_2 laser is currently recommended by some physicians for treatment of flat warts. The effectiveness of this therapy is about the same as that of other cryodestructive techniques. However, recurrence rates are expected to be less because the procedure is done under colposcopy, which detects small subclinical lesions. Also a small amount of normal tissue surrounding the lesion that may harbor the virus is treated. After therapy, antibacterial cream and a gauze dressing are applied to treated areas. Subsequently, the cream is reapplied and the dressing changed twice daily, and patients are instructed to keep the area clean and dry. Sitz baths are recommended for anal warts. Patients return for follow-up 3 to 6 weeks after treatment.

It should be noted that, untreated, most warts resolve spontaneously within 1 to 2 years. Concern for an effective treatment reflects the possible association with genital cancer, the increasing incidence of genital warts, and the psychological effects of infection.

Guidelines for Application of the Nursing Process to the Care of the Patient with Genital Warts

Depending on the individual patient and the location, number, and size of genital warts, any of the nursing diagnoses, expected patient outcomes, and nursing interventions presented in Nursing Care Guide 47–1 may apply.

In almost all cases, high risk for altered health maintenance related to insufficient knowledge of increased risk for genital malignancy will be a pertinent nursing diagnosis, and patients will need to be instructed in the importance of annual gynecologic examinations to ensure early detection should a malignancy develop.

Pediculosis Pubis

Pediculosis pubis, also called the crab louse, is one of three species of sucking lice known to infect humans. The others are *Pediculus humanus*—the body louse—and *Pediculus humanus capitis*—the head louse. Infestation with pubic lice is considered to be a sexually transmitted disease because the primary mode of transmission is through sexual contact. Approximately 3 million cases of lice infestation are treated in the United States each year. Pubic lice and head lice account for most of these cases.

Etiology and Pathophysiology

Pubic lice are minute, about 1 mm in size, crablike in appearance, and light in color. They live outside the human body, on skin surfaces, attached to the body hair. Pubic lice have six legs each, with a hooklike claw and opposing thumb, which allows them to hold on to hair (Fig. 47–9).

Lice depend on human blood for survival. They obtain blood with their mouths through a piercelike wound made in the skin surface. The life span of an adult female louse is 20 to 30 days. During this time, the female lays about 50 eggs, called nits. Nits are glued to and are visible on the hair. After an incubation period of 5 to 10 days, the eggs hatch. The life span of the pubic louse is influenced by the

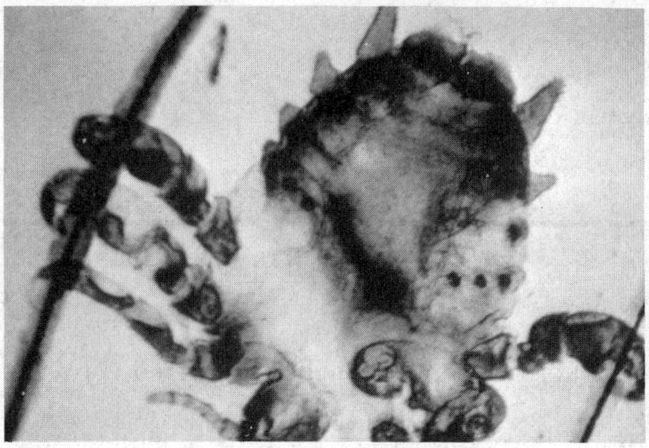

Figure 47–9.

Pubic louse 1 mm in length. Note the crablike appearance and hooklike claw at end of each leg. (Courtesy of the New York City Health Department.)

temperature, humidity, and availability of blood. Lice do not survive off the host without access to blood for more than 24 hours. The optimum temperature for their survival is 30.5°C (87°F). If the host is febrile or overheated by exercise, lice leave the body.

Although the pubic region is the main site of infestation, the axillae, eyebrows, eyelids, and even mustaches may also be affected. Lice are primarily transmitted from one person to another through intimate body contact. Less frequently, lice can be spread by fomites such as infested clothing, linens, and toilet seats. As with other sexually transmitted diseases, single, young people between the ages of 15 and 25 years constitute the population most at risk for pubic lice infestation.

Clinical Manifestations

The primary symptom of lice infestation is pruritus. The scratching illicited by pruritus can cause local erythema, irritation, and inflammation. After prolonged periods of infestation, some people develop an apparent immunity and do not manifest the pruritus associated with lice.

Medical Diagnosis

Diagnosis is made on the basis of the history, symptoms, and demonstration of lice or nits on the hair follicles.

Medical Management

Lice infestation is totally curable without long-term effects. Topical application of Kwell, a 1% gamma benzene hexachloride preparation available as a lotion, shampoo, or cream, is the most frequently used pediculicide. Infestation of the eyebrows or eyelids is treated with an occlusive application of petroleum jelly (Vaseline).

An antipruritic or antiinflammatory medication such as hydrocortisone cream may be recommended for itching.

Patients with pubic lice are also evaluated for the presence of other sexually transmitted diseases.

Application of the Nursing Process to the Care of the Patient with Pediculosis Pubis

Assessment

Assess the patient's understanding of the ways in which pubic lice are transmitted from one person to another, the use of the pediculicide and any other prescribed medications, treatment of contaminated clothing and household goods, and the need for evaluation and possible treatment of other household members and sexual partners.

Nursing Diagnoses and Planning

The nursing diagnosis and related expected patient outcomes most commonly applicable to patients with pediculosis pubis are as follows:

NDx: High risk for altered health maintenance related to insufficient knowledge of transmission and treatment of pediculosis pubis

Planning: Patient outcomes
1. Patient states correct use of pediculicide and any other prescribed medications.
2. Patient describes treatment of household objects necessary to effectively eliminate pubic lice infesting them.
3. Patient explains need for evaluation and treatment of sexual contacts and other household members.

Nursing Interventions

NDx: High risk for altered health maintenance

Briefly describe the life cycle of the pubic louse. Explain that, although sexual contact is the primary mode of transmission, pubic lice can also be spread by fomites such as linens and toilet seats. Instruct the patient in the treatment of pubic lice, as specified in Chart 47–4.

Chart 47–4.

NURSING GUIDE TO PATIENT EDUCATION FOR SELF-MANAGEMENT: TREATMENT OF PEDICULOSIS PUBIS

Instruct the patient with pediculosis pubis to do the following:

Use Kwell as follows (in the unusual cases in which an alternative pediculicide is ordered, provide instructions in accord with the package insert):

- Apply Kwell to affected areas for 8 hours, and then wash off thoroughly by showering.
- Avoid contact of Kwell with eyes and mucous membranes.
- Do not use Kwell if pregnant or lactating or on infants and small children.
- Do not apply Kwell to severely excoriated skin.
- Follow directions carefully. Do not overuse, apply incorrectly, or fail to remove after specified time because mild toxic effects on the nervous system can occur.

Rid home of pubic lice as follows:

- Dry clean or wash contaminated clothing and linen with detergent and hot water.
- Treat upholstery and carpets with specially formulated sprays if needed.

Prevent spread and reinfection by encouraging or obtaining evaluation and treatment of sexual contacts and all household members.

Inform the patient that itching may continue for several days after effective treatment, and teach the use of antipruritic or anti-inflammatory drugs if prescribed.

Evaluation

Evaluate the effectiveness of nursing care for a patient with pubic lice by comparing the patient's status with the expected patient outcomes. Examples of specific outcomes for patients with pubic lice have been provided in the Planning section.

Scabies

Scabies is caused by *Sarcoptes scabiei,* which are small, parasitic mites that produce intense itching and skin lesions in humans. Outbreaks of scabies appear to be associated with poverty, poor hygiene, and sexual promiscuity, among other causes. Scabies is primarily transmitted through close personal contact with an infected person.

Etiology and Pathophysiology

The scabies mite penetrates the superficial layers of the skin and produces linelike burrows associated with itching, discomfort, and rash. The life span of the adult female mite is 30 days, during which time she lays two to three eggs per day. Young mites reach adulthood in 10 days.

In sexually active young adults, sexual contact is the most likely mode of transmission. However, scabies can also be transmitted through contact with contaminated clothing, bed linen, and other personal articles. Nonsexual spread within households is a common mode of transmission.

Clinical Manifestations

After a relatively long incubation period, patients present with a chief complaint of a pruritic, papular rash. The itching is either exclusively nocturnal or increases at night. The symptoms frequently appear initially on the webs and sides of the fingers. Wrist and elbow surfaces, the axillae, waistline, genitalia, buttocks, backs of the knees, and toes are often frequent sites. At most sites, a small, papular rash is visible. The rash may appear erythematous and excoriated as a result of scratching. Burrows are not always evident. When they do appear, they can usually be seen on the finger webs, wrists, elbows, or penis. The burrows look like small, dark lines that cross the normal skin lines.

Medical Diagnosis

Scabies resembles other pruritic dermatologic conditions. Definitive diagnosis is made on the basis of the presence of the mite, its eggs, or feces. Skin scrapings or biopsies from the papules or burrows are microscopically examined for evidence of the mite. Because these are frequently difficult to find, diagnosis is often made on the basis of the history and characteristic appearance and distribution of the lesions.

Medical Management

Topical lindane (Kwell) cream or lotion, a 1% gamma benzene hydrochloride preparation, is the most common treatment for scabies. The cream or lotion is thinly applied to the entire body from the neck down, paying special attention to the hands and feet. The application remains on the body for 8 to 12 hours, after which it is showered off. Repeat treatments, should they become necessary because of reinfestation or resistance, are limited to two additional applications at 1-week intervals.

Sexual contacts as well as household members of patients with scabies are evaluated and treated, if necessary. Some experts recommend treating contacts with or without clinical manifestations of the disease, because the incubation period may be as long as 2 months.

Application of the Nursing Process to the Care of the Patient with Scabies

The assessment, nursing diagnoses, expected patient outcomes, nursing interventions, and evaluation for patients with scabies are similar to those described previously for patients with pediculosis pubis.

Bibliography

Audiman WA. Congenital herpesvirus infections. Clin Perinatol 1979; 6(2):331.

Baker D. Herpesvirus. Clin Obstet Gynecol 1983; 26(1):165.

Bettoli EJ. Herpes: Facts and fallacies. Am J Nurs 1982; 82(6):924.

Bourcier KM, Seidler AJ. Chlamydia and condylomata acuminata: An update for the nurse practitioner. JOGNN 1987; 16(1):17.

Bowie WR. Nongonococcal urethritis. Urol Clin North Am 1984; 11(1):55.

Campbell CE, Herten J. V.D. to S.T.D.: Redefining venereal disease. Am J Nurs 1981; 81(9):1629.

Centers for Disease Control: Chlamydia trachomatis infections—Policy guidelines for prevention and control. MMWR 1985; 34(35):535.

Charles D. Syphilis. Clin Obstet Gynecol 1983; 26(1):125.

Clark DP. Condyloma acuminatum. Dermatol Clin 1987; 5(4):779.

Corey L, Holmes KK. Genital herpes simplex virus infections: Current concepts in diagnosis, therapy and intervention. Ann Intern Med 1983; 98:973.

Corey T, Fife KH, Benedetti JK, et al. Intravenous acyclovir for the treatment of primary genital herpes. Ann Intern Med 1983; 98:914.

Crum C, Levine R, Richert R. Condyloma virus: How it affects the genital tract. Contemporary Ob-Gyn 1983;21(5):221.

Douglas JM, Critchlow C, Benedetti J, et al. A double blind study of oral acyclovir for suppression of recurrences of genital herpes simplex virus infections. N Engl J Med 1984; 310:1551.

Eschenbach DA. Vaginal infection. Clin Obstet Gynecol 1983; 26(1):186.

Eschenbach DA. Contending with the problem of chlamydial infection. Contemporary Ob-Gyn 1985; 25(20):125.

Felman YM. Condylomata acuminata. Cutis 1984; 33(1):118.

Ferenczy A. To contain spread of condyloma—Treat your patient's partner. Contemporary Ob-Gyn 1986; 27(6):51.

Fraiz J, Jones RB. Chlamydial infections. Annu Rev Med 1988; 39:357.

Gibbs RS. Herpes simplex virus in pregnancy. Contemporary Ob-Gyn 1991; 36(5):85.

Gorline L, Stegbauer C. What every nurse should know about vaginitis. Am J Nurs 1982; 82(12):1851.

Hager D, Spence M, Mead P. Trichomoniasis: Reinfection or resistance? Contemporary Ob-Gyn 1985; 25(6):141.

Himell K. Genital herpes: The need for counseling. JOGNN 1981; 10(6):446.

Hirsch MS. Herpesvirus infections. Scientific American Medicine 1992; 26:1.

Holmes KK, et al. Sexually transmitted diseases. New York: McGraw-Hill, 1984.

Horsburgh CR Jr, Douglas JM, LaForce FM. Preventative strategies in sexually transmitted disease for the primary care physician, U.S. Preventative Services Task Force. JAMA 1987; 258(6):814.

Karchmer AW. Sexually transmitted diseases. Scientific American Medicine 1989; 22:1.

Kaufman RH, Fard S. Herpes genitalis: Clinical features and treatment. Clin Obstet Gynecol 1985; 28(1):152.

King J. Vaginitis. JOGNN 1984; 13(2):415.

Labadie LL, Rhule RL. Management of genital infections. Emerg Med Clin North Am 1987; 5(3):443.

Larson E. Intransigent genital infection? Suspect chlamydiae. RN 1984; 47(1):42.

Lossick JG. Sexually transmitted vaginitis. Urol Clin North Am 1984; 11(1):141.

Lutz R. Stopping the spread of sexually transmitted diseases. Nurs '86 1986; 16(3):47.

Lynch P. Condylomata acuminata (anogenital warts). Clin Obstet Gynecol 1985; 28(1):142.

Mead PB, Sweet RL. Looking for chlamydia—and finding it. Contemporary Ob-Gyn 1985; 25(6):50.

Mertz G, Corey L. Genital herpes simplex virus infections in adults. Urol Clin North Am 1984; 11(1):103.

Miles PA. Sexually transmitted diseases. JOGNN 1984; 13(2):1025.

Miller MI. Genital chlamydia infections: A role for social scientists. Soc Sci Med 1987; 25(12):1289.

Oriel JD. Public health aspects of sexually transmitted diseases. Public Health Rev 1984; 12(2):131.

Rapp F. Herpesviruses: Why control is difficult. Contemporary Ob-Gyn 1983; 22(2):61.

Reeves WC, Corey L, Adams HG, et al. Risk of recurrence after first episodes of genital herpes. N Engl J Med 1981; 305(6):315.

Relman DA, Schoolnik GK, Swartz MN, Weller PF. Syphilis and nonvenereal treponematoses. Scientific American Medicine. 1988; 6:1.

Richart RL, et al. Condyloma virus and cervical cancer—How strong a link? Contemporary Ob-Gyn 1984; 23(2):210.

Roberts A. The pox and the people: A history of venereal diseases and sexual attitudes. Nurs Times 1982; 78:1177.

Romanowski B, Meltzer AS, Rush J. Treatment guidelines for selected sexually transmitted diseases. Can J Public Health 1983; 74:166.

Roy M. How to treat patients with condyloma. Contemporary Ob-Gyn 1982; 20(5):185.

Sacks ST, Bowie WR, Stayner M. Education and public awareness of sexually transmitted diseases. Can J Public Health 1983; 74:176.
Schachter J. Breaking the chain of chlamydial infection. Contemporary Ob-Gyn 1987; 30(1):146.
Smith LS, Lauver D. Assessment and management of vaginitis and cervicitis. Nurse Pract 1984; 9(6):34.
Spence MR. Gonorrhea. Clin Obstet Gynecol 1983; 26(1):111.
Spence MR. The treatment of gonorrhea, syphilis, chancroid, lymphogranuloma venereum and granuloma inguinale. Clin Obstet Gynecol 1988; 31(2):453.
Stamm WC. Diagnosis of chlamydia trachomatis genitourinary infection. Ann Intern Med 1988; 108(5):710.
Stamm W, Koutsky LA, Benedetti JK, et al. Chlamydia trachomatis urethral infections in men. Ann Intern Med 1984; 100:47.
Straus SE, Takiff HE, Seidlen M, et al. Suppression of frequently recurring genital herpes: A placebo-controlled double blind trial of oral acyclovir. N Engl J Med 1984; 310:1545.
Swartz MN, Schoolnik GK. Diseases due to chlamydia. Scientific American Medicine. 1986; 13:1.
Sweet RL, Schachter J, Landers D. Chlamydial infections in obstetrics and gynecology. Clin Obstet Gynecol 1983; 26(1):143.
Tichy AM, Taloshek ML. Older women. Sexually transmitted diseases and acquired immunodeficiency syndrome. Nurs Clin North Am 1992; 27(4):937.
Touchstone DM. Consider chlamydia. RN 1992; 55(2):32.
Warmbrodt L. Herpes: The shock, the stigma, the way you can ease the emotional pain. RN 1983; 46(5):47.
Watson RA. Gardnerella vaginalis: Genitourinary pathogen in men. Urology 1985; 25(3):217.
Watts DH, Eschenbach DA. Treatment of chlamydia mycoplasma, group B streptococcal infection. Clin Obstet Gynecol 1988; 31(2):435.
Wendel GD. Gestational and congenital syphilis. Clin Perinatol 1988; 15(2):287.
Whitley J, Nahmias AJ, Visintine AM, et al. The natural history of herpes simplex virus infection in mother and newborn. Pediatrics 1980; 66(4):489.
Winkler B. Controlling chlamydial infection. Contemporary Ob-Gyn 1987; 30(5):30.

Chapter Forty-eight

NURSING CARE *of Adults with* Breast Disorders

Breast-related concerns are one of the most common reasons for women seeking health care. This is due in part to the many media campaigns designed to heighten awareness of the increasing incidence of breast cancer in the United States and of the positive relationship between early detection and cure.

Unfortunately this heightened awareness is often accompanied by heightened anxiety. Thus, the nursing care of any woman presenting with a breast concern requires sensitivity to her anxieties and fears and individualized health teaching to place them in proper perspective while ensuring that positive health seeking behaviors are practiced.

Anatomy and Physiology

External Anatomy

The breasts are paired specialized glands shaped like cones. They are situated on the anterior chest from the second or third rib to the sixth or seventh rib and extend from the sternal edge to the midaxillary line (Fig. 48–1). Two thirds of the breast lies over the pectoralis major muscle, the remaining one third lies over the serratus muscle. The nipple is located centrally and is surrounded by the areola.

The breasts are generally symmetric; however, it is not unusual for there to be slight differences in size and shape. The skin that covers the breasts is identical to the skin on the rest of the body. The skin of the nipple and areola is deeply pigmented.

For purposes of description, each breast is divided into four quadrants—upper outer quadrant (UOQ), upper inner quadrant (UIQ), lower outer quadrant (LOQ), and lower inner quadrant (LIQ) (Fig. 48–2). The quadrants are described by imaginary lines that cross at the nipple. The vertical line goes from the 12 o'clock position to the 6 o'clock position, and the horizontal line goes from the 3 o'clock position to the 9 o'clock position. The "tail" of the breast extends into the axilla.

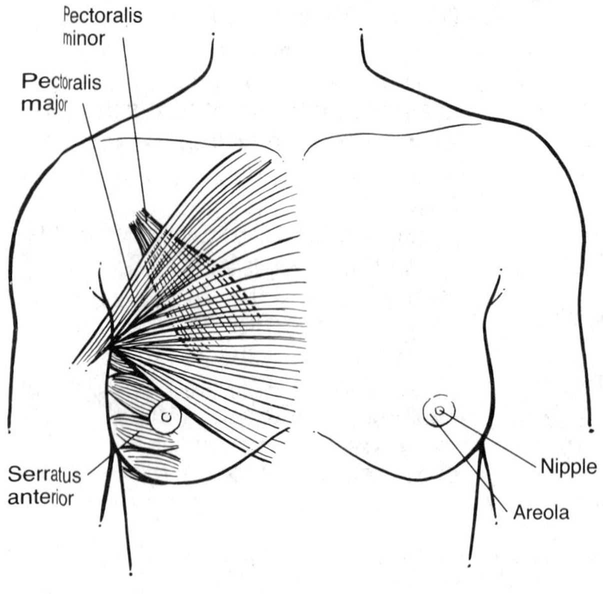

Figure 48–1.

Position of breasts on chest wall.

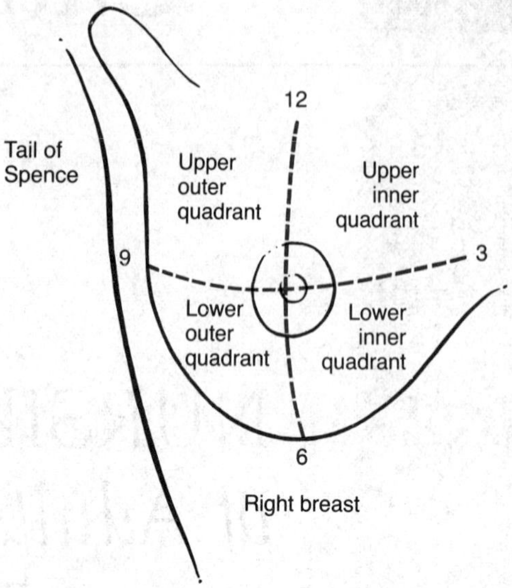

Figure 48–2.

Four quadrants of the breast, including the upper outer quadrant, lower outer quadrant, lower inner quadrant, upper inner quadrant, and tail of Spence.

Internal Anatomy

The breast is made up of three types of tissue: glandular tissue, fibrous tissue, and fat (Fig. 48–3). The proportions of these tissues vary among individuals depending upon a number of factors including age, stage of the reproductive cycle, and nutritional status. Glandular tissue is composed of 12 to 20 lobes branching into 50 to 60 lobules. The lobes are arranged in a circular pattern and are lined with milk-producing structures called acini. Each lobule ends in a duct called a lactiferous sinus. During lactation, the breast's complex ductal system is able to secrete colostrum and milk to the surface of the nipple with the contraction of smooth muscle. The glandular tissue is supported by fibrous tissue. These fibers include ligaments called Cooper's ligaments, which are connected to the skin and chest wall underneath the breast. The fibrous tissue has the ability to elongate and increase in volume as the breast grows, especially in response to pregnancy and lactation. The third and most predominant tissue of the breast is fat. Fat cells can be found throughout the breast and serve to cushion the glandular and fibrous tissue.

The venous and lymphatic systems of the breast

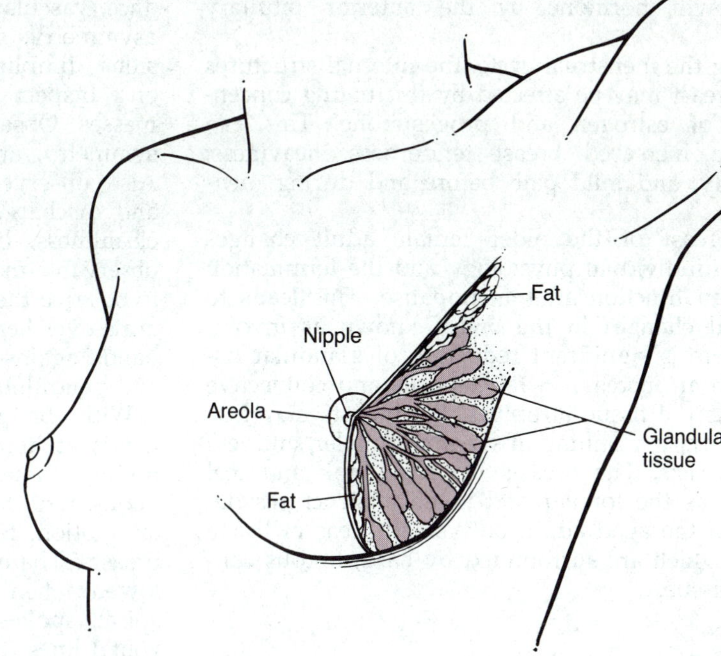

Figure 48–3.

Anatomy of a normal breast, illustrating relationship of glandular tissue to fat tissue.

work together to protect the organ from bacteria, viruses, and foreign tissue such as tumor cells. The blood reaches the breast through the internal mammary artery. The lymphatic vessels have multiple draining pathways throughout the breast (Fig. 48–4). The majority of lymph nodes are in the axillary region. These include the pectoral, subscapular, lateral, and central axillary lymph nodes. The axillary lymph nodes and internal mammary nodes under the sternum drain into the infraclavicular and then into the supraclavicular lymph nodes.

Physiology

The growth and development of the female breast is a dynamic, continuous process that begins during intrauterine life, progresses through puberty and adulthood, and regresses after menopause. The hormonal system, along with factors of heredity, aging, and nutrition, is responsible for the growth and development of the breast. The onset of puberty stimulates the ductile tissue to produce the basic structures of the adult breast. Normal breast devel-

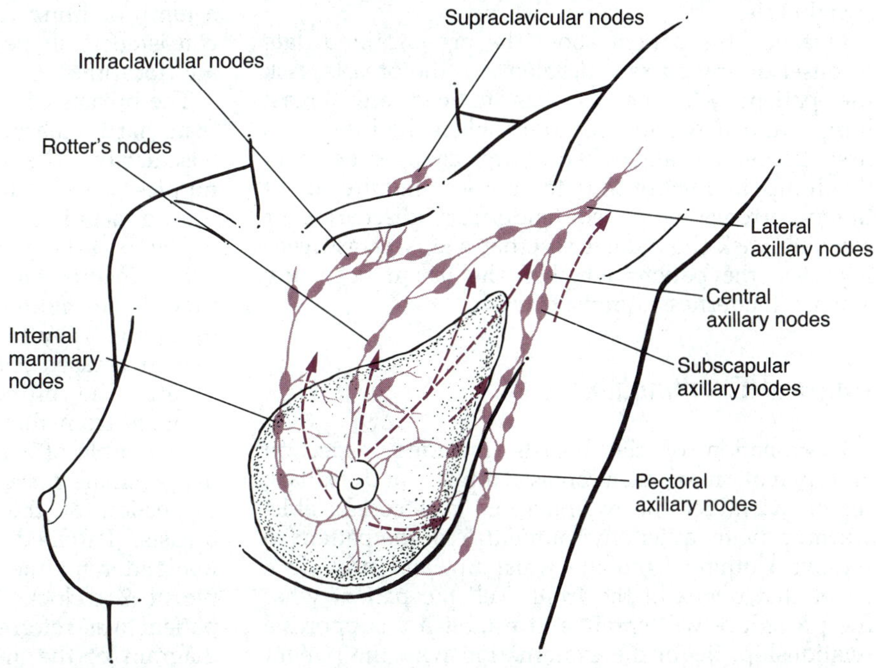

Figure 48–4.

Lymphatic drainage of the breast, showing internal mammary, pectoral, subscapular, lateral, axillary, infraclavicular, and supraclavicular lymph nodes.

opment also requires the production of prolactin and growth hormone by the anterior pituitary gland.

During the menstrual cycle, the internal structures of the breast may be affected by fluctuating concentrations of estrogen and progesterone. This can result in increased breast tenderness, heaviness, nodularity, and mild pain before and during menstruation.

The breast of the older female adult changes based on individual physiology and the termination of ovarian function after menopause. This leads to structural changes in the breast known as involution. There is significant reduction of glandular tissue, with an increase in fat deposits and connective tissue. As the tissue atrophies, the breasts may lose their elasticity, resulting in sagging, smaller, and less dense breasts. The breasts begin to look and feel different as the lobular and alveolar structures decrease. In the aged adult, only small areas of tissue remain, which are surrounded by hard, fibrous connective tissue.

Assessment of the Breast

Patient History

Ask about family history of breast disease. Note type of disorder and the relationship of the affected persons to the patient. Obtain information about any personal history of breast disease. Note the type of problem, dates of occurrence, treatment, and outcome. Determine the date and result of the patient's last mammogram and the time of the last breast self-examination. Obtain the date of the last menstrual period to determine the place in the menstrual cycle.

Question the patient about the presence and date of onset of any current problems in the breasts. Ask the patient whether she has noticed any breast lumps, and if so, note location, when the lump was first discovered, and whether any changes occur in the lump in relationship to menses. Inquire about the occurrence of breast tenderness, discharge, or swelling. Ask the patient whether she is breast-feeding. Ask the patient whether she has noticed any axillary tenderness, lumps, or rash.

Physical Examination

Examination of the breasts includes inspection and palpation of each breast, nipple, and axillary region. Conduct the examination in a comfortable, warm, private, quiet environment. Ask the patient to remove clothing from the waist up, and provide a cover that opens in the front. Tell the patient what the procedure will entail, and establish a supportive relationship. Begin the examination with the patient in a sitting position with arms at her sides. Inspect the breasts for size, color, hair pattern, skin appearance, vascularity, contour, and symmetry. Note any asymmetry, swelling, rashes, scars, ulcerations, lesions, dimpling, lumps, or unusual surface phenomena. Inspect the areola for shape, color, hair, and masses. Observe the nipples, and note size, shape, symmetry, and the direction in which they point. Also observe for retraction, rashes, skin changes, and discharge. Inspect axillae for hair distribution, cleanliness, discoloration, bulging, retraction, edema, observable masses, rashes, and ulcerations. Continue to observe the breasts while the patient (1) raises her arms over her head, (2) lowers them and presses her hands against her hips, and (3) if breasts are large and pendulous, leans forward (Fig. 48–5).

With the patient still in a sitting position with hands at her sides, palpate each breast and axilla, noting masses, consistency, tenderness, and lymph nodes. Use the pads of your fingers in a firm, circular motion, feeling the tissue under the skin of the breasts. There are different patterns that can be followed when palpating the breasts. These include spiral, spokes of a wheel, vertical lines, and horizontal lines (Fig. 48–6). There is no one pattern that is the best; but do use the same technique every time, and always be certain to examine each quadrant, the tail of the breast, and the axillary region. Compare the breasts with each other. If the patient states that she has noticed a problem in one breast, begin by palpating the other breast to establish a baseline. Try to find the lump without the patient's pointing to it, and then verify the position with the patient after palpating the breasts.

Finally, ask the patient to lie on her back on the examining table. Ask her to put her hand behind her head on the side you are palpating. This position helps to spread the breasts out, and deeper abnormalities may be detected through palpation. If a lump or lumps are felt, describe the size, number, consistency, shape, boundaries, mobility, tenderness, and location.

The breasts of a pregnant and lactating patient are firm, hard, enlarged, and tender and have increased vascularity. The areolae are darker in color. The nipples have a discharge in the last trimester and during lactation.

The breasts of an aging patient have decreased subcutaneous fat and loss of elasticity; therefore, they have more wrinkles and are flattened and drooping. They feel stringy and nodular. The axillae have decreased hair and increased concavity.

After the breasts have been examined, record findings from the history and physical examination. An example of a recording is: "Patient reports finding a small mass in the left breast 3 weeks ago. Inspection of the breasts reveal symmetric, small breasts. Palpated one 2-cm, round, hard, mobile, nontender nodule in the LUOQ 3 cm from the nipple at 2 o'clock. No axillary nodes palpated. The patient was referred to a physician." Also include a diagram of the anterior chest indicating where the nodule was palpated.

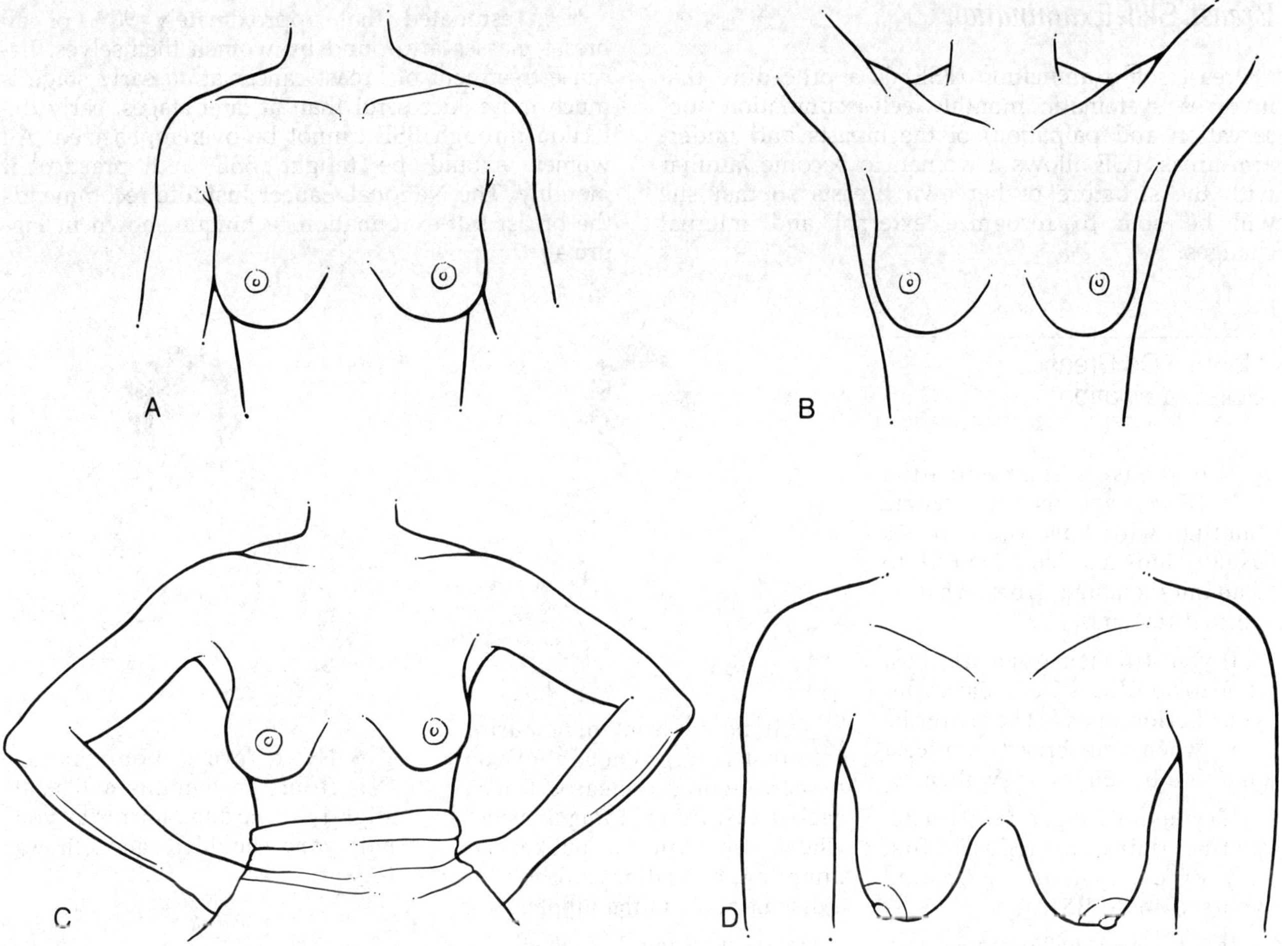

Figure 48–5.

Patient positions during examination of the breast. Note the distribution of breast tissue in the different positions. *A*, Patient position at start of breast examination: sitting with arms at sides. *B*, Patient in "arms over the head" position. *C*, Patient with arms lowered and hands pressed against hips. *D*, Patient with large, pendulous breasts leaning forward.

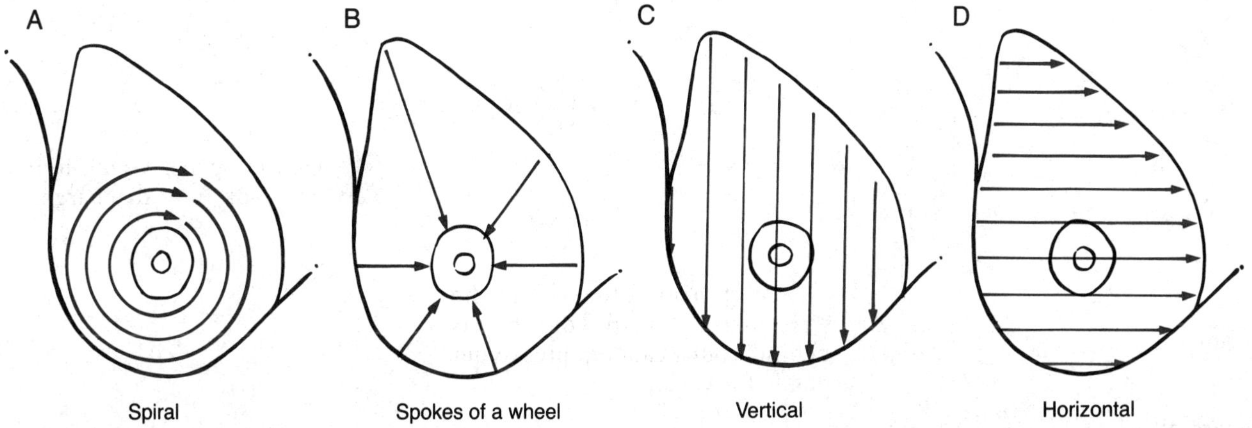

Figure 48–6.

Different patterns used in palpation of the breasts: spiral, spokes of a wheel, vertical lines, and horizontal lines.

Breast Self-Examination

Breast self-examination (BSE) is a procedure that involves systematic monthly self-examination (observation and palpation) of the breasts and underarm areas. BSE allows a woman to become familiar with the structure of her own breasts so that she will be able to recognize external and internal changes.

It is estimated that approximately 90% of all breast masses are found by women themselves. Because treatment of breast cancer at an early stage is much more successful than at later stages, early detection through BSE cannot be overemphasized. All women should be taught BSE and practice it monthly. The National Cancer Institute recommends the breast self-examination technique shown in Figure 48–7.

How To Do Breast Self-Examination

Do breast self-examination (BSE) every month. Become familiar with how your breasts usually look and feel. Do BSE to find any change from what is normal for you.

If you still menstruate, the best time to do BSE is 2 or 3 days after your period ends. These are the days when your breasts are least likely to be tender or swollen.

If you no longer menstruate, pick a certain day–such as the first day of each month–to remind yourself to do BSE.

If you are taking hormones, talk with your doctor about when to do BSE.

Here's what you should do to check for changes in your breasts.

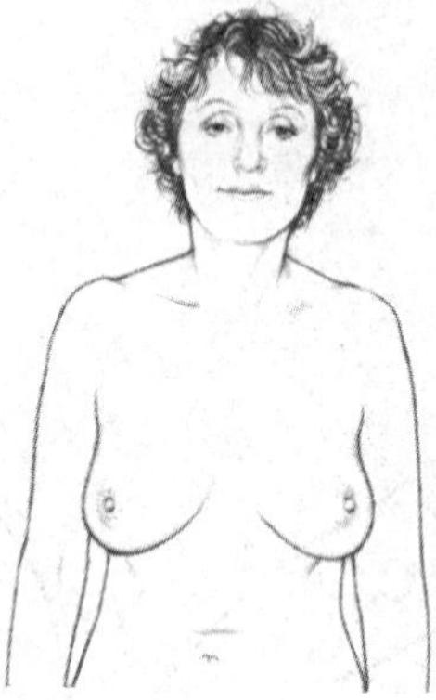

1 Stand in front of a mirror that is large enough for you to see your breasts clearly. Check each breast for anything unusual. Check the skin for puckering, dimpling, or scaliness. Look for a discharge from the nipples.

Do steps 2 and 3 to check for any change in the shape or contour of your breasts. As you do these steps, you should feel your chest muscles tighten.

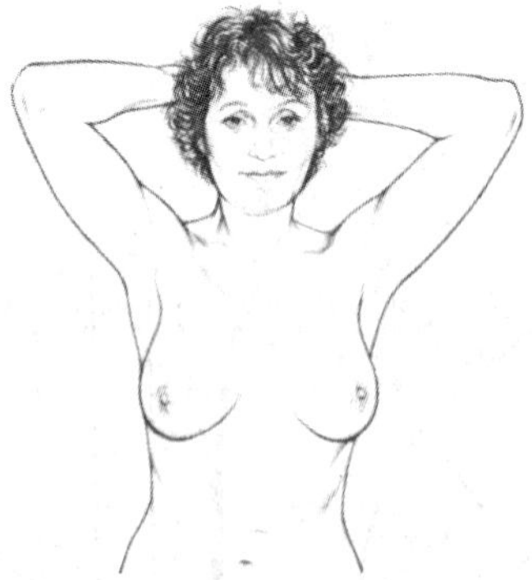

2 Watching closely in the mirror, clasp your hands behind your head and press your hands forward.

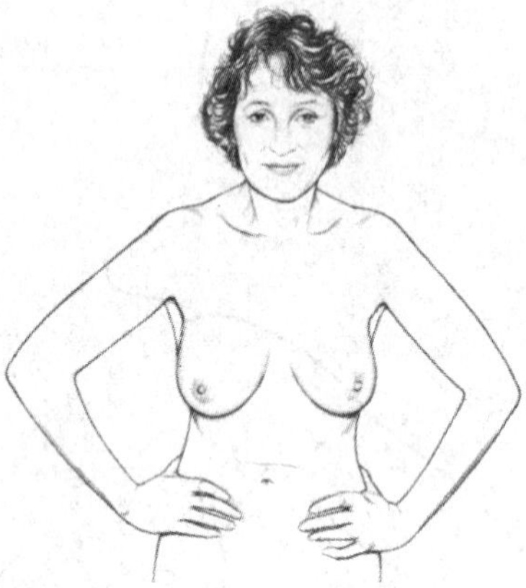

3 Next, press your hands firmly on your hips and bend slightly toward the mirror as you pull your shoulders and elbows forward.

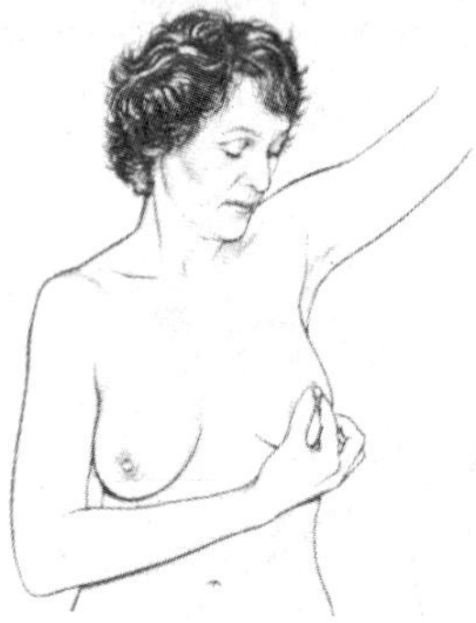

4 Gently squeeze each nipple and look for a discharge.

Figure 48–7.

Technique for breast self-examination. (Courtesy of the National Cancer Institute.)

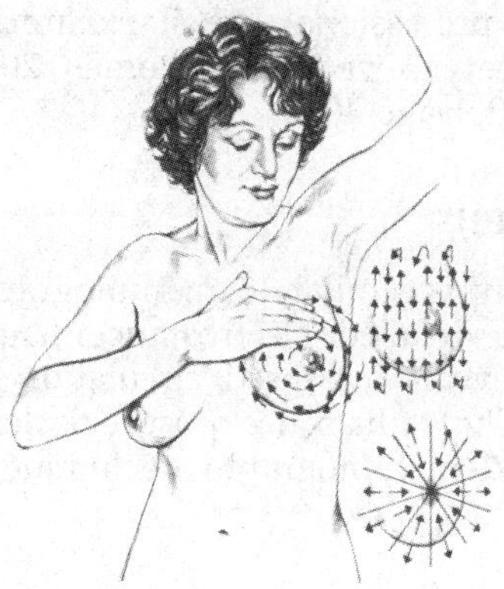

5 Raise one arm. Use the pads of the fingers of your other hand to check the breast and the surrounding area–firmly, carefully, and thoroughly. Some women like to use lotion or powder to help their fingers glide easily over the skin. Feel for any unusual lump or mass under the skin.

Feel the tissue by pressing your fingers in small, overlapping areas about the size of a dime. To be sure you cover your whole breast, take your time and follow a definite pattern: lines, circles, or wedges.

Some research suggests that many women do BSE more thoroughly when they use a pattern of up-and-down lines or strips. Other women feel more comfortable with another pattern. The important thing is to cover the whole breast and to pay special attention to the area between the breast and the underarm, including the underarm itself. Check the area above the breast, up to the collarbone and all the way over to your shoulder.

Lines: Start in the underarm area and move your fingers downward little by little until they are below the breast. Then move your fingers slightly toward the middle and slowly move back up. Go up and down until you cover the whole area.

Circles: Beginning at the outer edge of your breast, move your fingers slowly around the whole breast in a circle. Move around the breast in smaller and smaller circles, gradually working toward the nipple. Don't forget to check the underarm and upper chest areas, too.

Wedges: Starting at the outer edge of the breast, move your fingers toward the nipple and back to the edge. Check your whole breast, covering one small wedge-shaped section at a time. Be sure to check the underarm area and the upper chest.

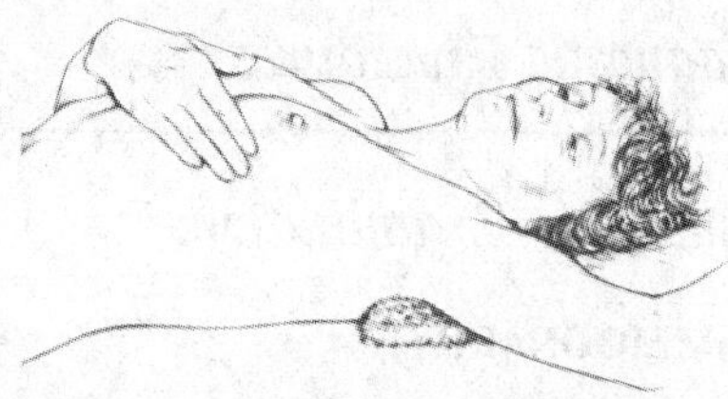

6 It's important to repeat step 5 while you are lying down. Lie flat on your back, with one arm over your head and a pillow or folded towel under the opposite shoulder. This position flattens the breast and makes it easier to check. Check each breast and the area around it very carefully using one of the patterns described above.

7 Some women repeat step 5 in the shower. Your fingers will glide easily over soapy skin, so you can concentrate on feeling for changes underneath.

If you notice a lump, a discharge, or any other change during the month–whether or not it is during BSE–contact your doctor.

Figure 48–7. (continued)

When teaching BSE, stress that the procedure should be done each month 7 to 10 days after the onset of menstruation, or at the same time each month for those who are not menstruating. Explain that this simple procedure allows detection of early changes in the structure of the breasts; that only approximately 10% to 15% of all breast masses are malignant; and that 90% of the breast cancers confined to the breast are curable. Reassure the patient that firm palpation of the breast does not damage breast tissue. Stress that BSE is not a substitute for breast examinations and mammographies by a clinician. Use teaching aids such as simulated breast models and films available through community agencies. After teaching BSE, ask for a return demonstration. Provide pamphlets and other written materials for the woman to take home. Be certain that the woman understands that any changes found in the breast should be reported to the physician.

In teaching BSE to the elderly, use written material with large print and talk slowly and clearly. Teach the normal changes that occur in the breasts with age as well as the importance of BSE. If the elderly patient has visual and physical limitations, the breast examination should be done by a nurse or a physician on a monthly basis.

Diagnostic Procedures

Radiologic Examinations

MAMMOGRAPHY

Mammography is an x-ray examination of the breast. It is used to survey the status of breast tissue by providing a picture of the internal structure of the breast. It reveals the location and extent of any breast mass.

Mammography complements a physical examination of the breast because it can reveal breast masses that are too small or too deep to be manually palpated. Mammography can detect a tumor that will not be felt for a few years. In addition, it allows comparison of current breast status with that shown on previous films so that changes, such as the increased size of a mass, can be identified.

For a mammogram, the x-ray technician compresses the breast to be examined between two plastic plates, and vertical and horizontal pictures are taken.

A mammogram should be scheduled in the middle of the menstrual cycle so that the breasts are not too sensitive and can be flattened as much as possible for the procedure.

Some physicians recommend that women refrain from consuming chocolate and caffeine a month before and salt a week before a mammogram to reduce water retention and swelling of the breasts.

Women who have silicone breast implants need an x-ray technician and physician who know how to position the breasts and to read the results because a clear mammogram is difficult to obtain when silicone implants are present. Research is being done to develop new breast implant substances that can be seen through on mammogram.

Mammography has created controversy because it exposes the breasts to radiation. Although the amount of radiation exposure in a mammogram is small, the cumulative effect of several mammograms may expose the breasts to radiation-induced breast cancer. However, it is estimated that a woman would only be at a slightly higher risk for breast tissue damage if she had more than 20 mammograms during her lifetime.

In response to the controversy over the value of mammography versus the risk of radiation, the National Cancer Institute recommends an annual mammography screening for women older than age 50; women older than age 40 who have a family history of breast cancer; women older than age 35 who have had breast cancer.

The American Cancer Society recommends that the following schedule be followed:

35 to 40 years of age—a baseline mammogram
40 to 50 years of age—a mammogram every 1 to 2 years
50 and older—a mammogram every year

In addition, a professional breast examination is recommended every 3 years for women 20 to 40, and every year after age 40.

XERORADIOGRAPHY

Xeroradiography is similar to mammography but produces a more detailed electrostatic image on a special film. It reveals increased circulation around the tumor site. The radiation exposure is less than with the standard mammography technique, hence it is widely used.

THERMOGRAPHY

Thermography is a procedure that operates on the theory that all objects give off heat and that some of the heat emitted by the body is infrared radiation. With the aid of special instruments, a thermogram takes a picture of these infrared emissions, which vary depending on the temperature of the source from which they come. It is thought that cancerous masses generate more heat than their surrounding tissue because of increased circulation; thus, a thermogram may provide an indication of the possible location of a cancerous lesion. This tool is not widely used as a screening technique and is not as accurate as mammography in finding small, deep cancers within the breast.

DIAPHANOGRAPHY

Diaphanography is a technique that involves shining a light through the breast to illuminate its interior. Different types of tissue transmit and scatter light in different directions. These differences in light transmission are detected by infrared-sensitive cameras and are viewed on a television screen. Currently this technique is still not able to detect the small lesions that appear on mammography. However, it is being refined and evaluated for future potential because it offers the distinct advantage of using a scanning means other than radiation.

ULTRASONOGRAPHY

If a questionable area is detected on a mammogram and physical examination, an ultrasonogram can be done to further study the area. High-frequency sound waves in the form of ultrasonic echoes are recorded as an image of organs or tissue as they strike tissues of different densities. Therefore, it can be used to differentiate a breast cyst from a tumor. This test is sometimes called a sonogram.

COMPUTED TOMOGRAPHY

Computed tomography (CT) uses x-rays from varying perspectives. As a scanner rotates around the breast, the information is analyzed by computer and reconstructed as a series of cross sections of the breast. This technique can be useful in detecting small lesions that may not be seen during mammography. The test requires high radiation exposure and may require an injection of a contrast dye into the body. At present, CT scanning of the breast is not used as a routine method to assess breast tissue because it is expensive and exposes the patient to a higher dose of radiation.

MAGNETIC RESONANCE IMAGING

Another test that can be done to look at cross sections of the breast is magnetic resonance imaging (MRI). Like the CT scan, the MRI combines many pictures into one cross-sectional picture. MRI uses radio waves and a powerful magnet to get an image of the internal breast.

NUCLEAR SCANNING

A radioactive substance is injected into the blood stream or swallowed. A scanner takes pictures, and increased or decreased radioactive uptake can indicate cancer cells.

Breast Biopsy

If a suspicious mass appears on any of the diagnostic tests or if a breast lump is palpated and thought to be cancerous, a biopsy is done for definitive diagnosis.

Breast biopsy methods include fine-needle, wide-needle, and surgical biopsy. A needle biopsy involves the insertion of a needle into a breast mass to remove fluid or tissue. A fine-needle biopsy, or aspiration biopsy, is the procedure used when a mass is suspected of containing fluid. A sac collapses after the fluid is removed. A wide-needle biopsy is a procedure used to obtain a small piece of tissue from a breast mass. Needle biopsies are performed using local anesthetics and can be done in an outpatient setting. The fluid and tissue that are in the needle and syringe are sent to the laboratory for analysis. If the needle biopsy shows cancer cells, a surgical biopsy using a scalpel to remove tissue for examination is done. In an excisional biopsy, also called a lumpectomy, the entire mass is removed. Incisional biopsy involves only the removal of a piece of a mass. Surgical biopsies are in-patient or out-patient procedures and are done under either local or general anesthesia. Sutures are used to prevent bleeding and promote healing, and a sterile dressing is applied to the wound.

The biopsy specimen is sent to a pathology laboratory, where it can be examined as a frozen section and as a permanent section. A frozen section is a sample of tissue that is immediately frozen so that it can be quickly prepared for microscopic review. This can be done within a few minutes while the patient is still in the operating room. A permanent section of the biopsy tissue involves several steps in preparation for microscopic review. This procedure is more reliable but takes approximately 24 hours to complete.

At the time of the biopsy, the pathologist may do hormone receptor assays because it may be hard to get tissue later and results are needed to decide on course of treatment. The cancer cells are tested to determine whether they are estrogen or progesterone receptors and are examined to see whether hormones promote the growth of cancer.

Patients who require breast biopsy have the option of a one-step procedure or a two-step procedure. The one-step procedure combines biopsy and surgical intervention if the frozen section of breast tissue is cancerous. In a two-step procedure, the biopsy and subsequent surgery are separated by an interval of time. This allows the permanent section to be reviewed and allows time for the patient to examine alternatives for the treatment of a cancerous breast lesion. Both options should be given to the woman before the biopsy is performed.

Application of the Nursing Process to the Care of the Patient Having a Breast Biopsy

Assessment

Assess the woman's understanding of the breast biopsy: why it is done, what will happen during the procedure, and what will happen if the breast biopsy reveals a malignancy. Also assess the patient's anxiety level. Review the history, and observe the patient for any factors with implications for care before, during, or after the procedure.

Nursing Diagnoses and Planning

Nursing diagnoses and related expected patient outcomes most commonly applicable to patients having a breast biopsy include the following:

NDx: Anxiety related to the procedure and its outcomes

Planning: Patient outcomes

1. Patient attends to questions and directions.
2. Patient verbalizes concerns, feelings, and fears about the breast biopsy.
3. Patient states that anxiety is reduced.
4. Patient exhibits active participation in decisions regarding her treatments.

NDx: High risk for altered health maintenance related to insufficient knowledge of biopsy report procedure and follow-up care

Planning: Patient outcomes

1. Patient describes the preparation for the procedure, expected discomfort, and the expected post-procedure course.
2. Patient states the purpose of the biopsy.
3. Patient states how and when she will be made aware of the results.
4. Patient describes treatment options.
5. Patient states follow-up care requirements.

Nursing Interventions

NDx: Anxiety

Allow time and opportunity for the patient to verbalize her feelings and concerns related to the breast biopsy. This is especially important because the emotional trauma stemming from a diagnosis of malignancy may be overwhelming. Be prepared to deal with a wide variety of patient reactions, ranging from quiet acceptance to anger, tears, or denial. Be particularly sensitive to the support needs of her spouse. Remember that when family supports are insufficient or when the patient is alone, the role of the nurse can become pivotal in ensuring the patient's emotional well-being. Allowing patients to be involved in making decisions on the type of surgery should result in less anxiety postoperatively.

NDx: High risk for altered health maintenance

Before the biopsy, review its purpose with the patient. Explain that during the procedure she will feel slight pressure on the breast but will not feel pain because a local or general anesthetic is normally used. Reassure the patient that the physical recovery from a breast biopsy is generally easy and without complications. Explain that there may be some pain at the incision site and that mild analgesics are usually prescribed. Tell the patient that a small dressing will cover the incision site and will remain in place for 2 to 3 days. Instruct the patient to check the dressing and report any bleeding to the physician. Also instruct her to take prescribed analgesics for pain or discomfort. Be certain to inform the patient when and from whom she will be told the results of the biopsy. Ensure that the patient knows the date and time of any required follow-up visit, as well as the importance of such appointments. This is especially critical if the patient has just completed the first part of a two-step procedure and a diagnosis of breast cancer has been made. Explain that there is time to reflect upon treatment options or obtain another opinion if desired, but that the decision on a plan of intervention should not be delayed.

Additional Interventions

After the procedure, monitor the patient for physiologic stabilization. Take vital signs, and check the amount of bleeding at the dressing site. If general anesthesia has been used, make usual postoperative assessments as discussed in Chapter 4.

Evaluation

Evaluate the effectiveness of nursing care for a patient having a breast biopsy by comparing the patient's status with the expected patient outcomes. Examples of specific outcomes for patients having a breast biopsy have been provided in the Planning section.

Infections and Inflammations

Mastitis

Mastitis is an inflammation of the soft tissue of the breast that generally, but not exclusively, occurs at the beginning or end of lactation.

Etiology and Pathophysiology. The most common causative agent of mastitis is *Staphylococcus aureus*. The infecting organism may enter the breast through a lactiferous duct or a nipple fissure, via a periductal lymphatic, or by hematogenous spread. Predisposing factors are poor drainage of a duct with milk stasis and lowered maternal defenses. There is increased risk when the supply of breast milk greatly exceeds the demand for it and after abrupt weaning of the infant from breast-feeding.

Clinical Manifestations. Classic local symptoms of mastitis are tenderness, redness, and heat in one area of the breast. Systemic symptoms may resemble those of influenza and include fever, generalized muscle aching, and nausea or vomiting.

Medical Diagnosis. Medical diagnosis is based on physical examination of the breast. A culture of breast milk may be obtained from a lactating patient.

Medical Management. In most cases, no intervention other than warm soaks for comfort is needed. Breast-feeding is continued to drain the breast and combat milk stasis. If symptoms of mastitis are present longer than 24 hours, antibiotics are usually prescribed. Dicloxacillin and the cephalosporins are the most commonly recommended antibiotics. Most clinicians consider both these drugs safe during breast-feeding.

Complications. Breast abscess is the most frequent complication of mastitis. A breast abscess appears as a localized indurated area just below the surface of warm, tender skin. It is treated with incision and drainage (I&D). Breast-feeding may have to be stopped if an I&D is done.

Guidelines for Application of the Nursing Process to the Care of the Patient with Mastitis

Explain to the patient what mastitis is and what causes it. Instruct the patient in the use of warm compresses covered with a dry cloth, a warm towel wrapped in plastic wrap, or a hot water bottle placed on the breast. Tell the patient to force fluids, especially fresh fruit juice and water, and explain the importance of taking antibiotics as directed. Stress the importance of continuing to breast-feed, and reinforce the following breast-feeding technique: continue nursing to empty the breast; keep the baby's chin close to the sore area; make certain to empty the affected breast. Explain that if nursing is not possible, milk should be pumped or manually expressed because there is an increased risk of abscess if nursing is abruptly stopped. Instruct the patient to nurse frequently for shorter periods and to break the suction by inserting a finger into the corner of the baby's mouth before removing the baby from the breast. Explain that use of a support brassiere while sleeping as well as during the day increases comfort, and stress the importance of adequate rest. Suggest that the patient keep the breasts soft by massaging the nipples while in a hot shower or bath to help milk flow. Caution against the use of ointment or cream on the nipples because this may clog the nipple. Tell the patient to seek help early if symptoms recur. Refer the patient to the La Leche League.

Structural Disorders

Mammary Duct Ectasia

Mammary duct ectasia is an inflammation and dilation of the breast ducts.

Etiology and Pathophysiology. Mammary duct ectasia occurs when the breast ducts beneath the nipple become dilated and fill with cellular and fatty debris. This deposited debris produces a gray to greenish sticky discharge at the nipple. Ductal ectasia occurs in women between the ages of 35 and 50.

Clinical Manifestations. The patient presents with a sticky gray to greenish discharge from the nipple and may complain of burning and itching at the nipple. In its early stages, the disease is painless; however, as it progresses, the patient may develop a drawing pain around the nipple and areola. As the inflammation progresses, an infection or an abscess may develop.

Medical Diagnosis. Medical diagnosis is based on patient symptoms and physical examination of the breast.

Medical Management. Medical intervention is based on the extent of the disease process, patient complaints, and patient history. Early ductal ectasia may be treated with warm compresses and antibiotics. More advanced ductal ectasia, if accompanied by abscess and nipple retraction, may require the removal of the involved duct as well as antibiotic therapy.

Guidelines for Application of the Nursing Process to the Care of the Patient with Mammary Duct Ectasia

Nursing care of patients with mammary duct ectasia is primarily directed at providing information that assists in the patient's understanding the breast disorder, providing emotional support, and allaying the patient's anxiety.

Gynecomastia

Gynecomastia is the unusual growth of breast tissue in males.

Etiology and Pathophysiology. Gynecomastia is thought to occur in response to a disturbance in the normal ratio of male to female hormones. Enlargement of male breast tissue may occur as a result of normal physiologic development, pathologic conditions, or obesity. It may also occur as a side effect of certain medications.

Gynecomastia may be present for a short period of time in young males aged 12 to 17. This transient state is thought to be a normal part of the young male growth cycle. Gynecomastia is also associated with several diseases, including hypogonadism, Klinefelter's syndrome, tumors of the lung, testicular tumors, tuberculosis, and hyperthyroidism. Medications that can cause gynecomastia include hormone therapy with estrogens and androgens, reserpine, phenothiazine, methyldopa, meprobamate, ergotamine, hydroxyzine, marijuana, digitalis, and isoniazid.

There may be a relationship between gynecomastia and the development of male breast cancer, but it is limited. It has been reported that approximately

20% of all males with breast cancer have a history of gynecomastia.

Clinical Manifestations. The primary clinical manifestation in gynecomastia is painless enlargement of the breasts.

Medical Diagnosis. Medical diagnosis includes a complete physical examination to check for other abnormalities such as testicular masses and to assess the development of the genitals. The breasts are examined for masses, and a complete drug history is obtained. Endocrine studies, liver function studies, and tests to rule out other systemic disorders are done.

Medical Management. The medical treatment for gynecomastia is based on the primary cause of the breast enlargement. If the gynecomastia is thought to be drug induced, the drug may be discontinued or changed. In some cases, the patient may request that surgery be employed to reduce the size of the breasts.

Guidelines for Application of the Nursing Process to the Care of the Patient with Gynecomastia

The nursing care of the patient with gynecomastia focuses on providing the patient with information related to the causes of gynecomastia and assisting the patient with the prescribed medical treatment. For patients having breasts surgically removed, nursing care is similar to that for the female patient having a mastectomy. When caring for these patients, be certain to consider the sensitive nature of gynecomastia. The patient may be self-conscious of having a "female" body image, along with having to undergo a "female" surgical procedure.

Neoplasia

Benign Breast Disease

FIBROCYSTIC BREAST DISEASE

Fibrocystic breast disease (FBD), also referred to as mammary dysplasia, fibrocystic mastopathy, and chronic cystic mastopathy, is a benign condition affecting at least one of two premenopausal women (Norwood, 1990, p. 116). FBD is characterized by a palpable irregularity of the breast that is accompanied by pain and tenderness and is most prominent just preceding menstruation.

The incidence of FBD peaks at about age 40 and is greater in nulliparous women than in those who have had children. FBD is also more common in women with an early menarche, late menopause, or a history of anovulatory cycles.

Etiology. The precise cause of FBD is unknown; however, it is generally believed that estrogen with its proliferative effects unopposed by progesterone plays a significant role. This view is supported by the fact that use of oral contraceptives, which provide a balance of estrogen and progesterone, is associated with a lowered incidence of FBD, whereas estrogen replacement therapy is associated with an increasing incidence of FBD with continued use (Norwood, 1990, p. 118).

Ingestion of methylxanthines, a closely related group of alkaloids including caffeine, theobromine, and theophylline, has also been considered as a contributing factor in the development of FBD. Methylxanthines have been postulated to act as competitive inhibitors of the enzyme that catalyzes the hydrolysis of cyclic adenosine monophosphate (cAMP), thus prolonging cAMP activity, which stimulates fibrocystic changes in the breast. This view is supported by the finding that the level of cAMP is significantly increased in women with FBD as compared with women free of breast disease. However, subsequent studies have not all supported these findings (Bullough et al, 1990, p. 36).

Pathophysiology. FBD is characterized by a variety of histopathologic changes, which include cyst formation, stromal fibrosis, and epithelial proliferation. In women with FBD, breast tissue does not completely return to its basal state following menses, rather some dilatory changes persist. This ultimately leads to permanent ductal dilation and the formation of cysts. Fibrosis, which most often occurs in the upper outer quadrant of the breast, also contributed to the process of cyst formation because it obstructs the ducts and causes the retention of alveolar secretions. These changes have not been found to predispose to malignancy, although they can make the detection of malignancy more difficult.

The breast discomfort that is associated with FBD occurs as a result of nerve irritation secondary to edema, nerve compression secondary to stromal fibrosis, and an inflammatory response.

Clinical Manifestations. Breast pain, frequently described as an aching fullness, is the most common symptom of FBD. It is often bilateral and may occur initially in the upper outer quadrant. Discomfort begins about a week prior to menses and then decreases with the onset of menstruation.

As the condition progresses, discomfort increases in both severity and duration. The breasts also become granular and tender, and firm masses that increase in size premenstrually may be palpated. These masses are most often in the upper outer quadrant and may be bilateral in a mirror image.

They are generally well demarcated and freely moveable.

Medical Diagnosis. The diagnosis of FBD is suggested by the patient's age and history in combination with the findings on physical examination. Presence of diffuse bilateral nodularity with cyclic fluctuation in size and related discomfort are key findings supporting the diagnosis of FBD as opposed to a malignancy. Mammography showing a dense pattern with microcalcifications is also typical of FBD. Any persistent mass is biopsied because direct examination of tissue is the only certain method of differentiating a benign from a malignant process.

Medical Management. Medical management of FBD is directed at preventing progression of the disease and providing symptomatic relief. Many types of treatment have been tried but there is still no one that is clearly preferred.

Hormone therapy designed to protect the breast tissue from stimulation by unopposed estrogen is the most common pharmacologic treatment.

Danazol (Danocrine), which inhibits anterior pituitary production of follicle-stimulating hormone (FSH) and luteinizing hormone (LH) and thus suppresses ovarian estrogen production, reduces or eliminates symptoms of FBD. Pain relief is reported within 2 to 3 months of treatment, and decreased nodularity in 3 to 6 months. Danazol is expensive, however, and causes dose-related side effects such as weight gain, menstrual irregularities, acne, and sometimes hirsutism and deepening of the voice. Low-dose estrogen and progesterone, which suppress ovarian production of estrogen while providing a balance of extrinsic estrogen and progesterone, also provide symptomatic relief in some women, as can progestins, which correct the estrogen/progestin ratio of luteal insufficiency.

A simpler form of therapy and one that is recommended as the initial treatment in women with diffuse fibrocystic changes (Ellerhorst-Ryan et al, 1988, p. 16) is decaffeination (the reduction or elimination of caffeine from the diet). Advantages of decaffeination are that it is inexpensive and has no side effects or other risks. Effectiveness of this treatment is evaluated in 2 to 4 months.

In women with a persistent dominant cyst, aspiration is generally indicated, and the aspirate is sent for cytopathologic analysis. If aspiration is not successful, if there is a residual mass after aspiration, or if the cyst recurs, excision may be recommended.

Other measures that have been tried with some success include vitamin therapy in the form of vitamin A, vitamin E, or vitamin B complex and diuretics, which relieve fluid engorgement. Women have also reported relief with dietary supplementation with essential fatty acids, elimination of dietary salt, avoidance of cigarette smoking, and reduction of stress. Many of these factors are currently under investigation.

Application of the Nursing Process to the Care of the Patient with Fibrocystic Breast Disease

Assessment

Begin assessment of the patient with fibrocystic breast disease with a history that includes information relevant to her risk status for breast cancer (see Table 48–1). Determine when she last had a mammogram, the date of her last breast examination by a health care professional, and whether she practices BSE. Inquire as to the results of these examinations. Obtain a description of her current symptoms, including when they began, severity, duration, and relationship to the menstrual cycle. Explore relief measures that have been tried and the effectiveness of these measures. Inspect and palpate the breasts as described previously. Note and describe any discharge, areas of irregularity or tenderness, or other abnormality. Assess the woman's anxiety level and her understanding of the problem. Also assess her knowledge of BSE, which is an important part of follow-up care.

Nursing Diagnoses and Planning

Nursing diagnoses and related expected patient outcomes most commonly applicable to patients with FBD include the following:

NDx: Pain related to inflammation and nerve irritation secondary to fibrocystic changes

Planning: Patient outcomes

1. Patient describes self-care measures for relief of discomfort associated with FBD.
2. Patient reports decreased breast discomfort.

NDx: Anxiety related to the cause and prognosis of FBD and its relationship to cancer

Planning: Patient outcomes

1. Patient expresses her feelings and concerns regarding FBD.
2. Patient realistically describes the relationship between FBD and her risk of breast cancer.

NDx: High risk for altered health maintenance related to insufficient knowledge of prescribed medical treatment and required follow-up care

Planning: Patient outcomes

1. Patient describes any prescribed pharmacologic therapy in terms of purpose, name of drug, dose, route, frequency, and common side effects.

Chart 48–1.

NURSING GUIDE TO PATIENT EDUCATION FOR SELF-MANAGEMENT: SELF-CARE MEASURES FOR RELIEF OF DISCOMFORT ASSOCIATED WITH FIBROCYSTIC BREAST DISEASE

Instruct the patient to:

Wear a well-padded support brassiere to decrease tension on ligaments and the inflammatory response such tension triggers.
Avoid sleeping in the prone position, which puts pressure on the breasts.
Apply ice or heat to the breasts for temporary relief of pain.
Limit dietary ingestion of caffeine by avoiding regular coffee, tea, colas, and chocolate.
Limit dietary salt during the week before menstruation to help limit premenstrual swelling.
Take mild analgesics as needed for discomfort during the week prior to menstruation.
Take steps to avoid and limit stress, which, either through a neuroendocrine response or increased awareness of symptoms, appear to exacerbate FBD.

2. Patient describes any planned aspiration or excision procedure.
3. Patient states importance and schedule of follow-up care: BSE, mammography, professional breast examinations.

Nursing Interventions

NDx: Pain
Instruct the patient in self-care measures to alleviate the discomfort associated with FBD, as presented in Chart 48–1. Discuss the therapeutic value of each. Explain that discomfort is usually reduced after menopause.

NDx: Anxiety
Approach the patient with empathy and tact. Encourage the woman to express her feelings and concerns and to ask questions about the disease, its prognosis, and its treatment. Correct any identified misconceptions or areas of misinformation. Interpret for the patient her risk of cancer. Keep in mind that for many years women with FBD were considered to have an increased risk of cancer and women still assume this is true. Explain that in fact women with FBD constitute a minority of those with breast cancer. Acknowledge that identification of a suspicious mass can be more difficult in the presence of FBD, but reassure the patient about the effectiveness of BSE, professional breast examinations, and mammograms in the early identification of malignant lesions.

NDx: High risk for altered health maintenance
If pharmacologic therapy is prescribed, teach the patient its purpose as well as the name, dose, route, frequency, and common side effects of prescribed drugs. If aspiration or excision is planned, describe the planned procedure and its purpose to the patient. Review needed follow-up care, describing both its purpose and importance.

Teach BSE, as described previously. Obtain a return demonstration, and provide written instructions for the patient to review as needed. Also provide the patient with a written schedule of follow-up care.

Evaluation

Evaluate the effectiveness of nursing care for a patient with FBD by comparing the patient's status with the expected patient outcomes. Examples of specific outcomes for patients with FBD have been provided in the Planning section.

FIBROADENOMA

Fibroadenomas are benign tumors of the breast. The tumors are round, firm, encapsulated, movable, and not tender.

Etiology and Pathophysiology. Fibroadenomas are solid benign tumors of the breast that are usually composed of fibrous or glandular tissue. They may be multiple and can occur bilaterally. Fibroadenomas occur most often in women between 20 and 40 years of age. They are more common in black women than in white women.

Clinical Manifestations. Fibroadenomas are painless, movable breast masses with well-defined borders. The size of the fibroadenoma is not affected by the menstrual cycle.

Medical Diagnosis. Medical diagnosis includes examination of both breasts and regional lymph nodes. A mammography may be done to visualize and localize the mass. The only way to distinguish a benign fibroadenoma from a malignant tumor is to obtain a biopsy of the mass.

Medical Management. The usual medical treatment of choice is excision. The breast tissue is sent to a pathologist for examination for malignant cells.

Application of the Nursing Process to the Care of the Patient Having an Excision of a Fibroadenoma

The assessment, nursing diagnoses, expected patient outcomes, nursing interventions, and evaluation for patients having an excision of a fibroadenoma are similar to those described previously for patients having a breast biopsy.

INTRADUCTAL PAPILLOMA

Intraductal papilloma is a small benign tumor that grows in the lining of the breast ducts near the nipple.

Etiology and Pathophysiology. Intraductal papilloma is most common in women between the ages of 45 and 50 years of age. It is generally found as a solitary tumor. Usually it is not precancerous.

Clinical Manifestations. The primary symptom of intraductal papilloma is bleeding from the nipple. This is due to irritation of the lining of the breast duct by the tumor. This irritation causes the lining of the breast duct to bleed, and the blood empties at the nipple. The discharge is spontaneous, and the disease is usually unilateral.

Medical Diagnosis. Medical diagnosis is made on the basis of patient symptoms and physical examination of the breasts and regional lymph nodes.

Medical Management. Surgical removal of the involved breast duct is the usual medical treatment. If multiple intraductal papillomas exist, the entire duct system may be removed.

Application of the Nursing Process to the Care of the Patient Having an Excision of an Intraductal Papilloma

The assessment, nursing diagnoses, expected patient outcomes, nursing interventions, and evaluation for patients having an excision of an intraductal papilloma are similar to those described previously for patients having a breast biopsy.

Cancer of the Breast

INCIDENCE

Breast cancer is the number one cause of cancer deaths among women in the United States and Europe. It is estimated that one in nine women will be diagnosed with breast cancer during her lifetime, and of those diagnosed, one in four will die of breast cancer. In 1990 in the United States, 150,000 new breast cancers were detected, and 44,000 deaths occurred. These statistics are higher than in previous years, but this is attributed to earlier detection of tumors by screening techniques and to the fact that women are living longer.

In the United States, breast cancer is more common in white women than in black women; however, this trend appears to be changing as the lifestyles of black and white women become similar. This change may be a reflection of early detection methods, but may also be related to changes in diet, lifestyles, and environmental exposures. The incidence of breast cancer increases as women age. Only 1% of all breast cancers occur in men.

Epidemiologic research continues to explore the factors that may influence the development of breast cancer. It is clear that a large majority of the female population may be affected by one or several risk factors. Until the relationship of these factors to the onset of breast cancer is fully understood, the single most important means to control the disease rests with early detection through BSE and mammographies, because breast cancer that has not spread to the lymph nodes has an excellent chance of being cured.

ETIOLOGY

Although the exact cause of breast cancer remains unknown, many risk factors (Table 48–1) appear to influence its development and clinical course. These include family history of breast cancer, early menarche, delayed pregnancy, and environmental factors such as exposure to radiation. Hormones, particularly estrogen, have also been linked to development

Table 48–1. RISK FACTORS FOR CANCER OF THE BREAST

Gender: 99% in women

Age: Incidence increases with age. Approximately 80% of women diagnosed are older than 35 years.

Family history: History of breast cancer, in both mother and sister or mother and maternal grandmother, especially if it developed before menopause or bilaterally. Recent research has shown that defective genes inherited can be linked to breast cancer.

Personal past history of breast cancer: A previous diagnosis of breast cancer in one breast increases the chance of breast cancer in the remaining breast.

Reproductive history: Reproductive factors that may influence the development of breast cancer are early menarche, late menopause, nulliparity, and first birth after 30 years of age.

Obesity: Risk increases when weight is 20% above average for height and age.

of breast cancer and are the subject of current investigation. At present, it is generally believed that estrogens do not cause breast cancer but that they facilitate the subsequent growth of the malignant breast tumor. Other factors that research has shown not to cause breast cancer include breast-feeding, which neither causes nor protects a women from developing breast cancer, trauma to the breast, and intimate sexual activity that involves fondling or caressing the breast. Further, breast cancer is not contagious.

PATHOPHYSIOLOGY

Breast cancer is defined as the uncontrolled growth of cells within the breast tissue. These cells have the unique ability to metastasize—that is, break away from the main tumor and travel through the lymphatic system and blood stream to other sites, such as the lungs, liver, or bones.

Malignant cells usually originate in the epithelial tissues of the breast and are considered carcinomas. The large majority arise in the ductal system and are referred to as ductal carcinoma; the minority arise in the lobular system and are referred to as lobular carcinoma. Less than 1% of breast cancers originate in the nonepithelial connective tissue of the breast; these tumors are classified as sarcomas of the breast. The growth of cancerous cells within the breast ducts beneath the nipple is known as Paget's disease.

The upper outer quadrant (UOQ) is the most common site of breast cancer. About half of all breast cancers are found in the UOQ and the "tail" of the breasts. The next most prevalent site of breast cancer is around the nipple, at approximately 20%. The inner quadrants show the least incidence of tumors.

Breast tumor cells are also classified by pathologists as noninvasive or invasive. Noninvasive tumor cells are confined to the duct in which they originated and are thus called carcinoma in situ. Invasive tumor cells, which constitute more than 90% of all breast cancers, have broken through the duct walls and have encroached upon other tissues of the breast.

Each individual case of breast cancer exhibits unique characteristics that may ultimately affect the patient's prognosis. These include tumor size and pathology classification, estrogen receptor activity of the tumor, lymph node status, and the presence or absence of distant metastases.

CLINICAL MANIFESTATIONS

The primary clinical manifestation of breast cancer is the appearance of an abnormal mass of tissue in the breast. Most women find their own breast tumors. The mass is typically firm, dense, singular, and irregular in shape. Associated symptoms may include skin dimpling, nipple retraction, enlargement of the breast, changes in the texture or color of the skin of the breast or nipple, increase in vascularity of the breast, discharge from the nipple, and pain or tenderness in the breast, nipple, or axilla (Fig. 48–8). The regional lymph nodes of the axilla may be palpable as a result of tumor spread or as part of the immune system's response to the presence of the breast tumor. In more advanced disease, the infraclavicular and supraclavicular lymph nodes may also be enlarged and palpable.

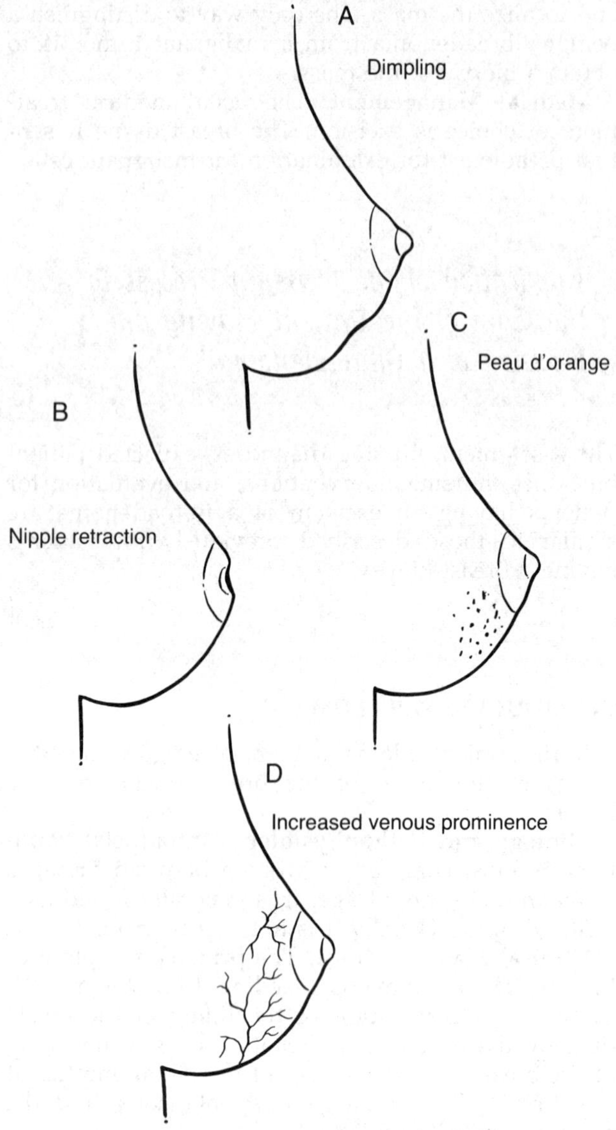

Figure 48–8.

Breast changes associated with breast cancer. *A*, Dimpling. *B*, Nipple retraction. *C*, Peau d'orange: skin resembles the skin of an orange. It is thick and hard with prominent pores as a result of blocked lymphatic drainage. *D*, Increased venous prominence.

MEDICAL DIAGNOSIS

Medical diagnosis requires a complete history and physical examination of the patient. Careful breast

Table 48–2. AMERICAN JOINT COMMITTEE ON CANCER TNM CLASSIFICATION OF BREAST CANCER

Primary Tumor (T)	
T0	No evidence of primary tumor
T1	<2 cm
T2	>2 cm, <5 cm
T3	>5 cm
T4	Any size with extension to the chest wall or skin
TX	Tumor cannot be assessed
Nodes (N)	
N0	Nodes without tumor
N1	Movable nodes with tumor
N2	Fixed nodes with tumor
N3	Supraclavicular or infraclavicular nodes with tumor
NX	Nodes cannot be assessed
Metastasis (M)	
M0	Without distant metastasis
M1	Distant metastasis present
MX	Not assessed

inspection and palpation are performed to identify the breast tumor. Mammography and other low-voltage radiography tests may be used as a means to visualize the mass, locate small nonpalpable tumors, or aid in differentiating benign from malignant tumors. The only definitive way to differentiate between a benign and malignant breast tumor is to obtain a specimen of suspect breast tissue through biopsy for pathologic study.

STAGING OF BREAST CANCER

The staging of breast cancer is a method of identifying the extent of the disease. Clinical and pathologic staging classifies the individual patient in terms of the size of the primary breast tumor (T), the presence or absence of tumor in the regional lymph nodes (N), and the presence or absence of distant organ metastases (M). This staging method is known as the TNM classification (Table 48–2). It is used by physicians to categorize breast cancer into Stage I, Stage II, Stage III, and Stage IV (Table 48–3). Ninety percent of the 150,000 patients with newly diagnosed breast cancer are in the early stages, Stages I and II, which means that the cancer is in the breast and axillary lymph nodes, and there is a very good chance for complete recovery. For example, a woman whose breast tumor is smaller than 2 cm, whose axillary lymph nodes have been proved to be free of tumor, and who is free of metastatic spread would be described as having Stage I breast cancer. This woman's chance of cure would be excellent after her primary tumor was removed. In contrast, a woman with Stage IV disease would have metastatic disease in other organs, and current 5-year survival under a variety of treatment modalities is poor. Each successive stage carries with it a poorer prognosis.

Breast tumors are also classified in terms of hormonal activity. The biopsy tissue of the tumor is studied for hormonal receptors because it is known that the growth of some breast tumors can be stimulated by estrogen and progesterone. A tumor's estrogen activity is classified as estrogen receptor positive or negative (ER+, ER−). More than half of all breast cancers are diagnosed as estrogen receptor positive. Studies have shown that women with estrogen receptor–positive tumors have a greater chance of remaining disease free, and that if metastatic disease should occur, they can be treated with hormonal manipulation.

MEDICAL MANAGEMENT

Medical management is largely based on the stage of the disease. Once a tumor has been located, the patient is examined to detect palpable lymph nodes or possible spread to other areas of the body. Based on patient history and symptoms, further tests may be ordered including chest x-ray examination, bone scan, and blood studies to determine whether metastatic disease is present.

The treatment of breast cancer may involve surgery, chemotherapy, hormonal therapy, or radiation therapy. Often two or more therapies are combined.

SURGICAL INTERVENTION

The primary treatment of breast cancer is surgical removal and pathologic study of the tumor. The excised tumor is measured, classified pathologically, and tested for estrogen receptors.

Currently, there are several surgical options that are used to treat breast cancer (Table 48–4). The type of surgical intervention selected is based on the patient's clinical status, risk factors, location and size of tumor, clinical stage of the disease, and the patient's preference. The standard surgical approach for primary breast tumors has been the modified radical mastectomy.

Modified Radical Mastectomy

The modified radical mastectomy involves removal of the entire breast, skin, and axillary lymph nodes but preserves the major pectoral muscles. As opposed to a radical mastectomy, this results in a more cosmetically acceptable chest wall and leaves the patient with more strength in her arm and shoulder. It also allows for easier breast reconstruc-

Table 48–3. BREAST CANCER STAGING BASED ON TNM CLASSIFICATION

STAGE	TUMOR SIZE (T)	NODES (N)	METASTASIS (M)
Stage I	T1	N0	M0
Stage II	T2	N0, N1	M0
Stage III	T3	N0, N1	M0
	T1	N2	M0
	T2	N3	M0
Stage IV	T4	N0, N1, N2, N3	M1

Table 48–4. SURGICAL INTERVENTIONS FOR BREAST CANCER

PROCEDURE	DESCRIPTION	DIAGRAM
Lumpectomy or tylectomy	Removal of the breast tumor and small amounts of surrounding tissue	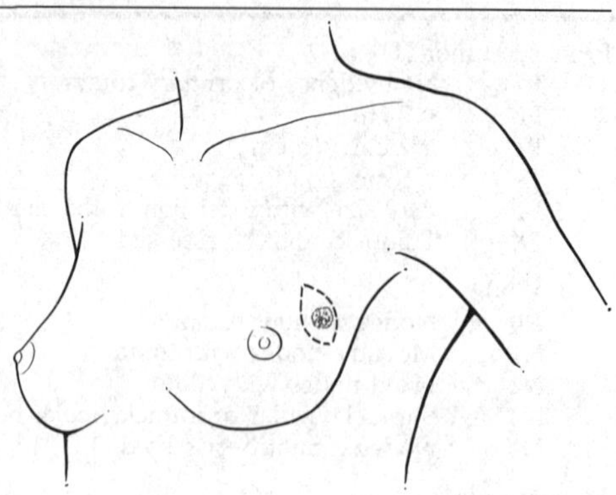
Partial mastectomy or segmental resection	Removal of the tumor plus approximately 2 to 3 cm of surrounding tissue	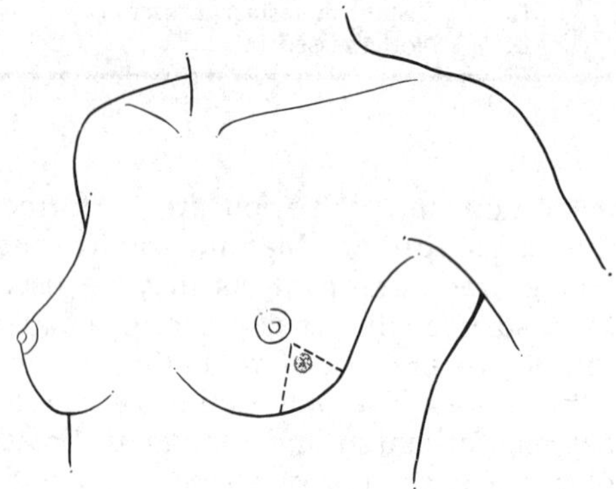
Quadrantectomy	Removal of a quadrant of the breast with the tumor, fascia covering the greater pectoral muscle, and the entire smaller pectoral muscle	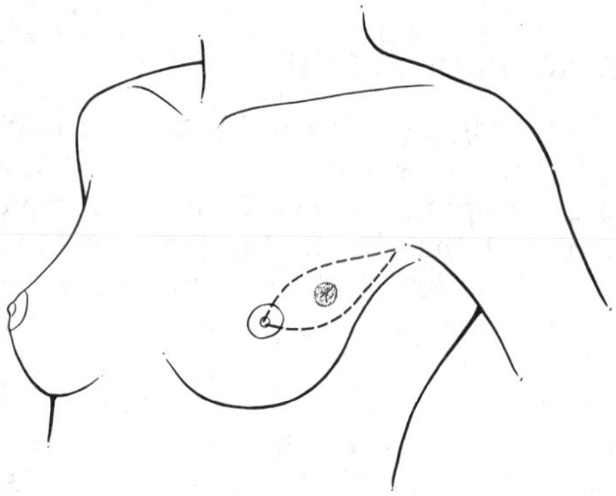
Local regional treatment	Removal of the tumor with the surrounding tissue and axillary lymph nodes	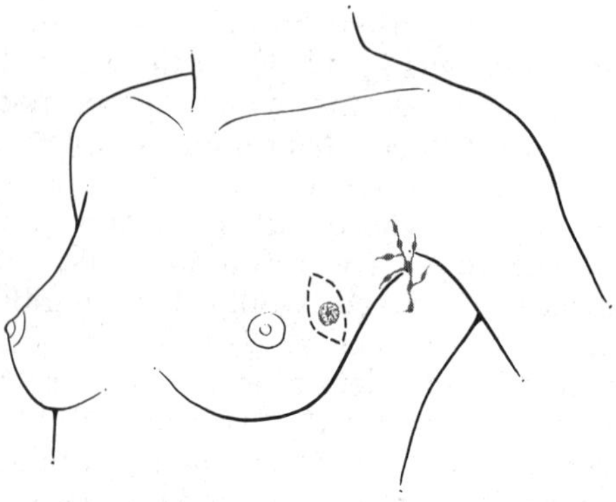

(continued)

Table 48–4. *(continued)* SURGICAL INTERVENTIONS FOR BREAST CANCER

PROCEDURE	DESCRIPTION	DIAGRAM
Total mastectomy	Removal of the entire breast, with the pectoral muscles and axillary lymph nodes left intact	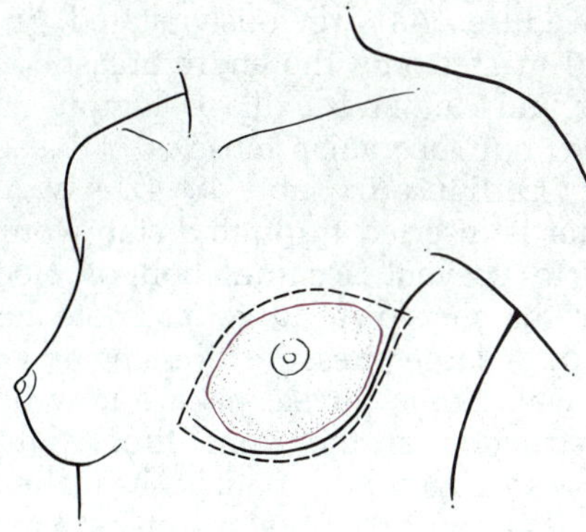
Modified radical mastectomy	Removal of the entire breast, skin, pectoralis minor muscle, and axillary lymph nodes. The major pectoral muscles are left intact.	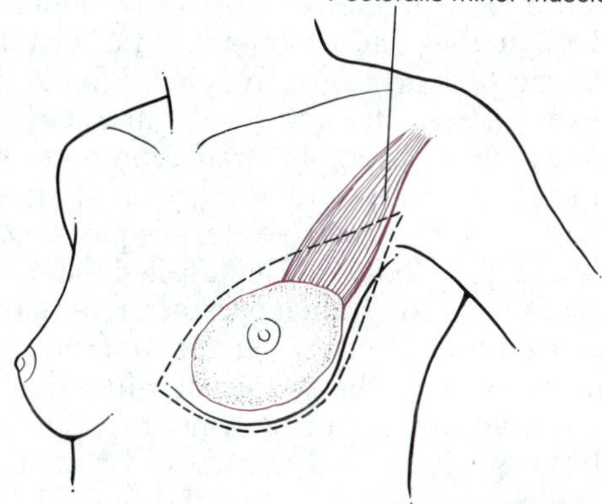
Radical mastectomy	Removal of the entire breast, skin, pectoralis major muscle, pectoralis minor muscle, and axillary lymph nodes	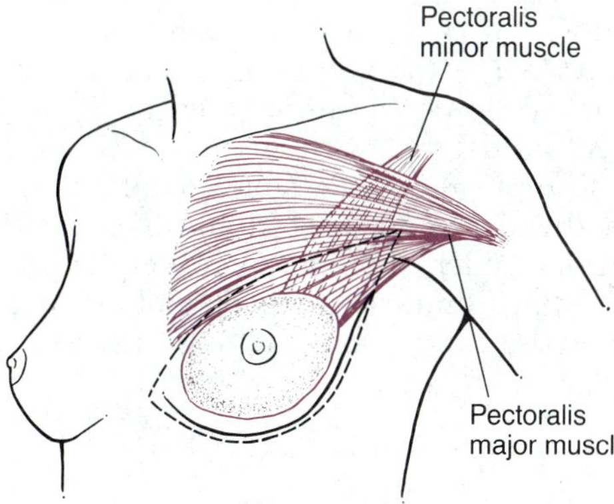

tion. Studies have shown no difference in survival between patients treated with modified radical mastectomy and those treated with radical mastectomy, in which the major pectoral muscles are removed. Modified radical mastectomy is currently being studied and compared with more limited surgery used in conjunction with radiation or chemotherapy.

Physical Preparation of the Patient. The patient is kept on NPO status from midnight preceding the day of surgery, and an intravenous fluid line is started before surgery. Skin preparation may include a shower, bath, and a local scrub with an antiseptic solution. About an hour before surgery, the patient is asked to void and, if applicable, to remove dentures, contact lenses, nail polish, and jewelry. Vital signs are taken and recorded. Side rails are raised following the administration of the prescribed preoperative medication.

Procedure. As previously stated, in a modified radical mastectomy the entire breast, skin, pectoralis minor muscle, and axillary lymph nodes are removed, but the major muscles of the chest are left intact (see figure in Table 48–4). A wound drainage catheter is inserted through a stab wound under the axilla to prevent accumulation of blood or serum under the incision and to promote healing of the wound. A large pressure dressing is applied to the chest wall. Some physicians are now offering breast reconstruction at the same time a mastectomy is done, especially if a patient has already received chemotherapy for a previous breast tumor.

Postoperative Course. Intravenous therapy is maintained until the patient is physiologically stable and able to tolerate adequate amounts of oral fluid. Regular diet and ambulation are generally resumed on the first postoperative day. Simple exercises that do not stress the suture line are started almost immediately to promote circulation and prevent limitation of movement of the arm and shoulder. Examples of these exercises are squeezing a ball and flexing the elbow on the affected side.

The wound drainage catheter remains in place 1 to 4 days depending on the amount of drainage. It is removed by the physician when fluid collection is less than 100 ml in a 24-hour period. The surgical dressing is usually removed and the incision checked for healing after the first 24 hours. By the fifth postoperative day, some of the surgical sutures and clips may be removed. Based on healing progress, the surgeon may remove all the sutures and clips before the patient is discharged from the hospital. Follow-up care is based on individualized patient needs.

Complications. Possible complications following a modified radical mastectomy include fluid accumulation under the incision, lymphedema, infection, bleeding, limited range of motion of the arm and shoulder, and problems with psychological adjustment.

Application of the Nursing Process to the Care of the Patient Having a Modified Radical Mastectomy

PREOPERATIVE NURSING CARE

Assessment

Obtain a complete health history on the patient. Include information about the onset and course of the present illness, past illnesses and surgeries, and psychological, sociologic, and family history. Examine the breasts. Note size and location of any palpable mass, presence of discharge from the nipple, dimpling of the skin, areas of ulceration, deviation of the direction of the nipple, or any other abnormality. Determine the patient's understanding of the disease process, plan of treatment, including the surgery, and the expected prognosis. Assess the patient's anxiety level and level of coping. Assess the patient's support systems.

Nursing Diagnoses and Planning

Nursing diagnoses and related expected patient outcomes most commonly applicable to patients who are scheduled for a modified radical mastectomy include the following:

NDx: Knowledge deficit: mastectomy procedure, perioperative routines, breast reconstruction option

Planning: Patient outcomes
1. Patient states the rationale for the mastectomy.
2. Patient describes the planned mastectomy procedure, including the postoperative appearance of the chest and axilla.
3. Patient describes preoperative and postoperative activities.
4. Patient describes surgical breast reconstruction as a possibility now or at a later date.

NDx: Anxiety related to the diagnosis of breast cancer and the scheduled surgery

Planning: Patient outcomes
1. Patient verbalizes her concerns.
2. Patient attends to information and directions.
3. Patient participates in the decision-making process.
4. Physiologic and behavioral signs of severe anxiety are absent.

Nursing Interventions

NDx: Knowledge deficit: mastectomy procedure, perioperative routines, breast reconstruction option

Review with the patient information provided by the surgeon about the mastectomy procedure to be done. Be sure the patient has a realistic expectation of the postoperative appearance of the chest and the axilla. If the patient had prior experience with someone who had a radical mastectomy, stress that the modified technique avoids the chest and axillary disfigurement of the early procedure so clothes with lower necklines may be worn. Also stress that more strength is left in the arm because the major chest muscles remain intact and that there is less chance of lymphedema in the arm on the affected side because fewer lymphatic vessels are severed. Encourage the patient to ask questions, and clarify information as needed.

Describe perioperative routines. Make certain the patient understands that a wound drainage system and a large pressure dressing will be in place postoperatively.

Explain that the hand and arm on the mastectomy side will be elevated on pillows to facilitate fluid drainage and inhibit swelling. Also explain that pain and tightness over the chest wall and pain in the upper back shoulder and arm are expected but that analgesics will be ordered to maintain comfort. Demonstrate deep breathing and coughing exercises, and inform the patient that these exercises will be started in the recovery room and repeated every hour for the first 2 postoperative days. Demonstrate exercises for the affected shoulder and arm. Obtain a return demonstration of all exercises before surgery.

NDx: Anxiety
Individuals differ in dealing with anxiety. Allow time for the patient who desires to verbalize her feelings and concerns regarding the diagnosis and treatment of breast cancer. Respect the right of privacy for the patient who does not wish to talk about these issues. Advise the patient of support groups such as Reach to Recovery because she may relate better to someone who has already been through the treatment process. Give the patient pamphlets and booklets that she can refer to when needed.

Include the patient and family in the planning of care. Encourage the patient to make decisions and to participate in self-care measures.

Evaluation

Evaluate the effectiveness of nursing care for a patient scheduled for a mastectomy by comparing the patient's status with the expected patient outcomes. Examples of specific outcomes for patients scheduled for a mastectomy have been provided in the Planning section.

POSTOPERATIVE NURSING CARE

Assessment

Assess the patient's return to physiologic stability. Check vital signs, and inspect the dressing and sheets under the patient for bleeding. Check the wound drainage system, and note color and amount of drainage. Check the intravenous infusion, and inspect the site of insertion for signs of infiltration or phlebitis. Assess for pain, and assess the mobility of the affected arm. Inspect the affected arm for signs of infection: redness, warmth, and edema. Assess the level of stress and anxiety the patient and family are experiencing by observing and listening to both nonverbal and verbal communication.

Nursing Diagnoses and Planning

Nursing diagnoses and related expected patient outcomes most commonly applicable to patients who have had a modified radical mastectomy include the following:

NDx: Pain related to surgical trauma of the anterior chest

Planning: Patient outcomes
1. Patient takes pain medication when needed.
2. Patient utilizes nonpharmacologic methods of pain management.
3. Patient reports reduced pain.

NDx: High risk for infection related to vascular and lymphatic alteration from surgery

Planning: Patient outcomes
1. Patient explains the need to protect the affected arm from trauma.
2. Patient lists precautions to be taken to protect the affected arm as presented in Chart 48–2.

NDx: High risk for impaired physical mobility related to breast surgery

Planning: Patient outcomes
1. Patient states the rationale for exercising the affected arm.
2. Patient demonstrates range-of-motion exercises (see Chart 48–3).
3. Patient plans progressive exercise regimen 3 to 5 times a day.
4. Patient lists activities of daily living that enhance arm and shoulder movement (see Table 48–5).

NDx: High risk for fluid volume excess (local) related to impaired lymph flow in the affected arm

Planning: Patient outcomes
1. Patient identifies factors that may contribute to the development of lymphedema.
2. Patient lists signs and symptoms of lymphedema.
3. Patient describes precautions to be taken to decrease the risk of lymphedema.
4. Patient performs exercises of affected arm and shoulder 3 to 5 times a day.

NDx: High risk for body image disturbance related to the loss of the breast

Planning: Patient outcomes
1. Patient verbalizes feelings, concerns, and questions about change in body image.
2. Patient looks at incision prior to discharge.

Chart 48–2.

NURSING GUIDE TO PATIENT EDUCATION FOR SELF-MANAGEMENT: HAND AND ARM PRECAUTIONS AFTER MODIFIED RADICAL MASTECTOMY

Instruct the patient to:

Avoid
- Burns while cooking or smoking
- Sunburns
- Injections, vaccinations, drawing of blood samples, and blood pressure measurements on the affected arm when possible
- Nicks and scratches
- Cutting cuticles and nails
- Touching hot or cold objects
- Elastic cuffs on blouses and sleepwear

Always
- Carry heavy packages or handbags on the other arm.
- Wash cuts promptly with soap and water, apply an antibacterial medication, and monitor for redness, soreness, or other signs of infection.
- Wear watches and jewelry loosely on the affected arm.
- Wear protective gloves when gardening and when using strong detergents.
- Use a thimble when sewing.
- Use lotion on cuticles, push cuticles back with a soft cloth, and file nails.
- Use mitt-type potholder when cooking.
- Use an electric razor for underarm shaving.
- Report signs of swelling, redness, and pain in affected arm.

3. Patient is receptive to information about prostheses.
4. Patient expresses positive feelings about self.

NDx: High risk for sexual dysfunction related to the loss of the breast

Planning: Patient outcomes
1. Patient asks questions about sexual activity.
2. Patient verbalizes feelings about the effect of the mastectomy on her relationship with her sexual partner.
3. Patient asserts intention of resuming usual sexual activity.

NDx: High risk for altered health maintenance related to insufficient knowledge of postoperative and postdischarge self-care

Planning: Patient outcomes
1. Patient states precautions to be taken for operative side.
2. Patient demonstrates correct method of BSE.
3. Patient states time and date of follow-up visit.
4. Patient resumes family and social roles.

Nursing Interventions

NDx: Pain
Monitor the extent of the patient's pain, and give prescribed narcotic analgesics as needed. Expect the patient to experience incisional pain on the first postoperative day. By the second or third day, expect the pain to decrease to soreness, and give medication accordingly. Reassure the patient during the initial period after surgery that the severity of the incisional pain will decrease after the second postoperative day. In addition to administering analgesics, institute other comfort measures such as repositioning, rubbing the patient's back, and applying heat as ordered to the upper back, shoulder, and upper arm. Guide the patient in the use of relaxation techniques, and provide diversionary activities according to her preference.

NDx: High risk for infection
Explain to the patient that the removal of lymph nodes in the axillary region makes the arm more prone to infection. Instruct her to protect the affected arm and hand from injury as described in Chart 48–2. Place a sign near the patient's bed and

on her Kardex to communicate to hospital personnel that the affected arm cannot be used for drawing blood, taking blood pressure, or administering intravenous fluids. Teach her signs and symptoms of infection, and tell her to report any abnormalities to her physician.

NDx: High risk for impaired physical mobility

Start passive range-of-motion (ROM) exercises of the arm and shoulder on the affected side, and provide a soft ball for the patient to squeeze as soon as possible postoperatively. As soon as the suction is removed and permission is obtained from the physician, encourage the patient to begin active range-of-motion exercises gradually and to begin to use the affected arm and shoulder to care for herself. Passive and active range-of-motion exercises are critically important because they assist in easing arm and shoulder tension, promote joint movement, reestablish elasticity to the chest wall muscles, prevent further movement limitations, and aid in reestablishing arm and shoulder strength. When explaining their importance to the patient, stress that exercising will help her regain activity and strength in her affected arm and shoulder and can reduce stiffness and pain in her neck and back.

Teach the patient appropriate range-of-motion exercises such as those used in the Reach to Recovery program (Chart 48–3 and Figure 48–9). Instruct her to gradually increase the exercises and to continue to exercise 3 to 5 times per day at home until full range of joint motion of the arm and shoulder is regained. Suggest that she integrate the exercises into her usual self-care and housework (Table 48–5). Caution her to avoid exercising beyond the point of discomfort and to avoid heavy lifting. Also provide the patient with information about community organizations such as the American Cancer Society and the YWCA that sponsor postmastectomy exercise programs. Instruct the patient to report any changes, such as numbness, tingling, or weakness in the affected arm.

NDx: High risk for fluid volume excess (local)

Explain to the patient that lymphedema is an abnormal accumulation of lymphatic fluid that can occur in the arm on the affected side as a result of the severing of lymphatic and blood vessels. The extent of lymphedema ranges from mild to severe and may occur any time after surgery. Stress that there is much less risk of lymphedema after a modified radical mastectomy than after a radical mastectomy. Caution the patient not to overdo arm exercises because lymphedema can be the result of or be exacerbated by strenuous activity of the arm and shoulder. Explain that lymphedema can also be caused by infection or injury and that the hand and arm precautions outlined in Chart 48–2 can help prevent this.

If lymphedema occurs, teach the patient to facilitate venous return by elevating the arm to 45 degrees abduction and 60 to 90 degrees flexion. If needed, tell her that a custom-fitted elastic arm sleeve can be used to assist venous return. In severe cases, explain about the pneumatic massage sleeve used to drain lymphatic fluid from the arm. Instruct the patient in a low-salt diet and the use of diuretics if prescribed.

NDx: High risk for body image disturbance

Discuss the meaning of the loss to the patient, and encourage her to talk about her feelings. Reassure her that it is normal to be concerned about change in appearance and reactions of others after loss of a breast. Acknowledge and accept feelings of loss, grief, or fear of rejection. Encourage the patient to look at the incision. If the patient is hesitant to look at it, describe it to her. Subsequently provide opportunities for her to see it, but do not force her do so. Consider encouraging the patient and her partner to look at the wound together to promote shared feelings and support. Remember that after the initial emotional reaction, the majority of patients generally adapt smoothly to the diagnosis and view the surgery as life-saving.

Provide the patient with information about obtaining a breast prosthesis. Explain that a temporary lightweight prosthesis can be used once the dressing is removed. If desired, a soft gauze pad may be used to cover the healing incision and protect it from contact with the prosthesis. Inform the patient that a permanent prosthesis may be worn in approximately 2 months after the incision is healed. This prosthesis is an artificial breast mound that is usually made of molded silicone or foam. Stress that there are many styles and shapes available and that the prostheses are similar in weight, shape, and texture to natural breast tissue. Suggest that the patient wear a blouse and sweater to judge the symmetry when she is being fitted for the form, which fits inside a pocket sewn into a brassiere and swimwear.

Inform the patient that there are nurse practitioners and stores with employees that specialize in fitting women with breast prostheses. These specially trained individuals often go to the patient's home to fit her with a prosthesis. Locate information about these services by looking under "Surgical Appliances and Supplies" and "Nurses" in the yellow pages. Explain that prostheses are expensive, ranging from $50 to $200, but that most health insurance plans reimburse the cost fully or partially.

Provide the patient with information about breast reconstruction as an alternative way to regain her breast shape if she is interested (p. 1912).

NDx: High risk for sexual dysfunction

Recognize the role the breast plays in a woman's sexuality and that the patient may feel that her femininity and role as a sexual partner have been less-

Chart 48–3.

NURSING GUIDE TO PATIENT EDUCATION FOR SELF-MANAGEMENT: POSTMASTECTOMY EXERCISES

Instruct the patient to:

Perform exercises with the affected arm and shoulder once given permission from the physician.

- "Climb the wall": Face and move close to the wall. Put fingers on the wall at the same level as the shoulder, and gradually "walk" up the wall with the fingers (Fig. 48–9*A*).
- Using a rope hung over a bed trapeze or over the door, pull down and up on each side alternately. Reach as high as possible. Allow some discomfort but not a lot of pain (Fig. 48–9*B*).
- Tie a rope to the doorknob and hold it. Start with hand at shoulder height, and then raise the hand. Put the other hand on the hip to help balance (Fig. 48–9*C*).
- Hold a rubber ball in the affected hand and squeeze it (Fig. 48–9*D*).
- Hold a rubber ball with an elastic band in the affected hand. Hold the hand up at the shoulder level, and throw the ball down and then catch the ball when it comes back up to the hand (Fig. 48–9*E*).
- Using a rope 3 feet long, hold one end in the affected hand over the shoulder, and hold the other end in the other hand behind the back at the waist. Move the affected hand over the head and back (Fig. 48–9*F*).

Use both arms whenever possible, to take the mind off the affected arm, to have something to compare it with, and to give balance.

Move arms smoothly, slowly, and gradually using sweeping or swinging movements. Facilitate this by standing in front of a mirror while doing exercises or by doing them to music.

Use the other arm in the beginning to help the affected arm to perform the exercises or to start the exercises.

ened. Respect the individual nature of each patient's response to breast surgery. Remain supportive and nonjudgmental while encouraging the woman to verbalize her concerns and fears. Encourage discussion about sexual activity, and handle it in a sensitive and open manner. Make certain the patient understands that sexual intercourse may be resumed as soon as she wishes, although alternate coital positions may be necessary to avoid pressure on the healing incision. When possible, determine the concerns and feelings of the patient's sexual partner, and provide information and the opportunity to ventilate as needed. Support sharing of feelings between the patient and her partner.

Table 48–5. ACTIVITIES OF DAILY LIVING TO ENHANCE ARM AND SHOULDER EXERCISES

Housework	*Self-care*
Mop floors	Fasten a brassiere
Vacuum	Wash and dry the back
Sweep with a broom	Pull a zipper
Knead dough	Button
Wash windows	Comb and brush hair
Raise and lower windows	*Crafts and Sports*
Hang clothes on a line	Weave
Weed a garden	Knit/crochet
Cook/stir	Sew
Make a bed	Type
	Play golf
	Paint
	Swim

NDx: High risk for altered health maintenance

Instruct the patient to avoid use of ointments and creams on the incision and use of antiperspirant in the affected axilla. Stress the importance of promptly reporting any changes in the incisional area or adjacent axilla or any pain, redness, or swelling in the affected arm. Tell the patient that some women experience "phantom breast sensations" for a short period of time postoperatively (i.e., a woman may experience sensory phenomena seemingly originating in the missing breast or nipple).

Teach or review breast self-examination, and instruct the patient to immediately report any changes in the remaining breast.

Provide the patient with information on community agencies and programs that provide support, information, or other assistance to patients with breast cancer (Table 48–6).

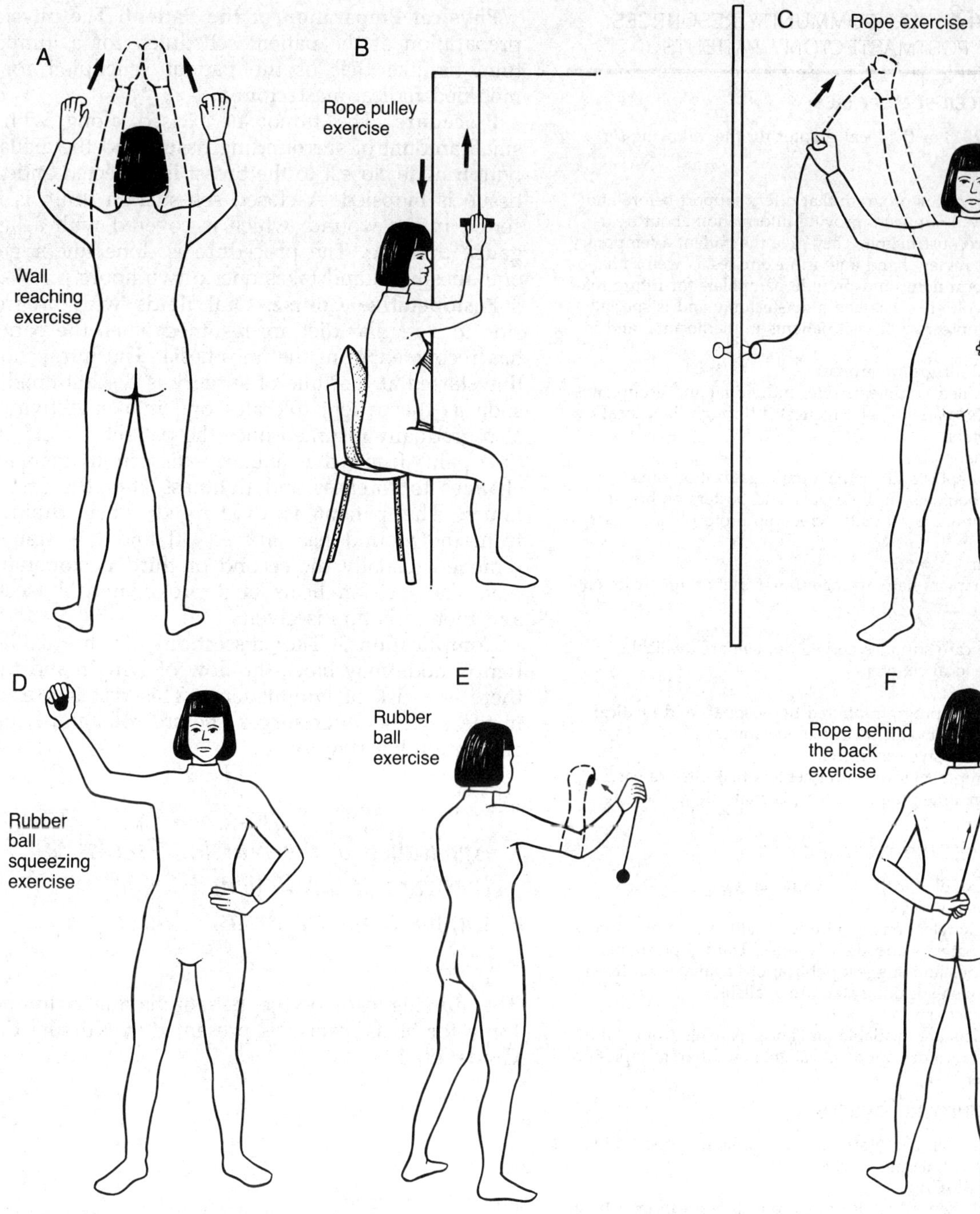

Figure 48–9.

Arm exercises for mastectomy patients.

Evaluation

Evaluate the effectiveness of nursing care for a patient who has had a modified radical mastectomy by comparing the patient's status with the expected patient outcomes. Examples of specific outcomes for patients who have had a modified radical mastectomy have been provided in the Planning section.

Lumpectomy

Lumpectomy is a breast-preserving procedure used in conjunction with axillary dissection, radiation, and chemotherapy. It is an option when there is no metastasis and the breast tumor is well-defined, less than 5 cm in diameter, and does not involve the nipple. Studies have shown that lumpectomy followed by chemotherapy is as effective as mastectomy for early-stage cancer (Rust & Kloppenborg, 1990, p. 59).

Table 48–6. COMMUNITY RESOURCES FOR POSTMASTECTOMY PATIENTS

AMERICAN CANCER SOCIETY (ACS)

Call 1-800-ACS-2345 or the local chapter for the following services:

- Reach to Recovery
  - A volunteer visitor program that offers support before and after surgery. Volunteers provide information about treatments and reconstruction. They give the patient a temporary breast form, review hand and arm exercises as well as hand and arm precautions, and provide pamphlets for future reference. Each volunteer has had a mastectomy and is specially trained. Volunteers will visit patients in the hospital and in the home.
- Individual and/or group support
  - Specially trained volunteers offer individual and group support to cancer patients who request it through their local cancer chapters.
- Educational materials
  - Each local chapter and the national organization offer pamphlets, booklets, audiovisuals, and posters on breast self-examination, treatments, screening protocol, and latest statistics.
- Transportation
  - The local chapters help arrange transportation for treatments and medical care.
- Home care
  - Some home care supplies and equipment are available through the local chapters.
- I Can Cope
  - An educational program offered by hospitals and medical centers for cancer patients and their families.
- List of comprehensive cancer centers
  - A list of comprehensive cancer centers that offer research, diagnosis, treatment and teaching is available to the consumer.

NATIONAL CANCER INSTITUTE (NCI)

Call 1-800-4-CANCER for the following services:

- Cancer Information Service
  - A nationwide telephone service for health care professionals and cancer patients and their families. Trained personnel answer questions and suggest publications available on the subject. Spanish-speaking staff are available.
- Booklets and fact sheets
  - Many booklets are available for cancer patients from children to the elderly. Information is available on different topics on breast cancer.

OTHER COMMUNITY RESOURCES

ENCORE (Encouragement, Normalcy, Counseling, Opportunity, Reaching Out, Energies Revived)

- Call the local YWCA
  - The YWCA offers ENCORE to support breast cancer patients after surgery. Exercise classes are offered in the swimming pool and the gymnasium. Discussion groups are available.

NABCO (National Alliance of Breast Cancer Organizations)

- Call 212-719-0154
  - NABCO offers support groups and education about different treatments available for breast cancer patients. An audiovisual tape, "Get Up and Go: After Breast Surgery," is available for purchase to help women who need to strengthen their arm, shoulder, and back muscles weakened by a mastectomy.

RENU (Reconstruction Education for National Understanding)

- RENU offers peer support and information on reconstruction surgery for mastectomy patients.

Physical Preparation of the Patient. The physical preparation of the patient scheduled for a lumpectomy is like that of the patient scheduled for a modified radical mastectomy.

Procedure. The tumor is excised along with a small amount of surrounding tissue, and the axillary lymph node closest to the breast is dissected and the tissue is biopsied. A closed self-suction drain is inserted in the wound, which is covered with a light gauze dressing. The procedure is done under general anesthesia and takes one to two hours.

Postoperative Course. Oral fluids with progression to a regular diet are resumed when the patient has recovered from the anesthesia. The intravenous line started at the time of surgery is discontinued as soon as the patient tolerates oral intake. Activity is also gradually resumed once the patient is alert. Initial pain from the axillary dissection generally changes to soreness and tightness after the first 24 hours. The patient is discharged when drainage from the wound has tapered off and the drain is removed, usually the second or third postoperative day. The incision heals in approximately 2 weeks, and then radiation is given.

Complications. The dissection of the axillary lymph node may block the flow of lymph, and thus there is a risk of lymphedema. This risk is greatest in the 6 weeks after surgery before collateral lymph circulation has developed.

Application of the Nursing Process to the Care of the Patient Having a Lumpectomy for Breast Cancer

The nursing care of the patient having a lumpectomy for breast cancer is presented in Nursing Care Guide 48–1.

Preventive Surgery

Some physicians recommend bilateral mastectomies for women who have multiple risk factors for breast cancer. These include women who have a strong family history of breast cancer, have had many biopsies, or have breasts that are very hard to examine. This is not a widely used procedure, and a second opinion should always be obtained before prophylactic mastectomies are performed.

CHEMOTHERAPY

There are several types of chemotherapeutic drugs used in the treatment of breast cancer. These include drugs administered orally, intramuscularly, and in-

Nursing Care Guide 48–1.

PATIENTS HAVING A LUMPECTOMY FOR CANCER OF THE BREAST

Preoperative Care

Assessment Findings: Patient has no prior experience with lumpectomy. Patient asks questions about the procedure, perioperative events, and follow-up care.

Nursing Diagnosis: Knowledge deficit: lumpectomy procedure, perioperative events, follow-up care

Patient Outcomes	Nursing Interventions	Rationale
Patient describes lumpectomy within the framework of the overall treatment plan.	Review the physician's plan of care with the patient. Include a description of what lumpectomy involves, as well as the plan for subsequent radiation and chemotherapy.	Patients under stress often misinterpret or do not hear information. Reviewing information improves understanding of the procedure and plan of care and contributes to informed consent.
Patient describes perioperative routines.	Describe general perioperative routines.	Prepares the patient for perioperative events, thus involving the patient in the plan of care, promoting cooperation and decreasing the risk of anxiety over routine measures.

Evaluation: Compare the patient's status with the expected patient outcomes. If the outcomes are achieved, evaluate nursing care as successful. If not, reassess the patient, formulate new nursing diagnoses, and revise expected patient outcomes and nursing interventions as appropriate.

Assessment Findings: Patient states, "I'm so worried I don't know what to do. I hope I made the right choice when I chose the lumpectomy. Maybe it would have been better to have everything removed so there would be less chance the cancer will come back. People with cancer have horrible deaths and I don't want to die." Patient also states, "I hope I won't look deformed after this operation."

Nursing Diagnosis: Anxiety related to possibility of prolonged illness, pain, and death; concern that selecting lumpectomy as the method of treatment was the best choice; concern about postoperative appearance

Patient Outcomes	Nursing Interventions	Rationale
Patient expresses concerns freely.	Allow verbalization of concerns.	Verbalizing concerns to another provides perspective, allows for correction of misconceptions, and permits a supportive relationship.

(continued)

Nursing Care Guide 48–1. *(continued)*

PATIENTS HAVING A LUMPECTOMY FOR CANCER OF THE BREAST

Patient Outcomes	Nursing Interventions	Rationale
Patient expresses comfort with her decision to have a lumpectomy.	Stress that lumpectomy with radiation is as effective as mastectomy for early-stage cancer according to available studies.	Provides positive facts that help build the patient's confidence in her treatment decision.
Patient describes expected postoperative appearance of the breast and axilla realistically.	Explain to patient that lumpectomy is not recommended by a surgeon unless the breast is large enough so that subsequent deformity will not occur.	Provides the patient with positive facts to counteract anxiety over postoperative appearance.
Signs of severe anxiety are absent.	Remind the patient that remission in early-stage cancer is the rule.	Provides positive facts on which to focus and base hope for a successful surgical outcome.

Evaluation: Compare the patient's status with the expected patient outcomes. If the outcomes are achieved, evaluate nursing care as successful. If not, reassess the patient, formulate new nursing diagnoses, and revise expected patient outcomes and nursing interventions as appropriate.

Postoperative Nursing Care

Assessment Findings: Patient complains of pain in the area of the surgery.

Nursing Diagnosis: Pain related to tissue trauma secondary to surgical dissection of the axilla

Patient Outcomes	Nursing Interventions	Rationale
Patient reports that pain is controlled. Behavioral signs of severe pain are absent.	Administer parenteral analgesics for pain in the immediate postoperative period.	Parenteral analgesics provide prompt pain relief, thus promoting rest and facilitating the healing process.
	Administer prescribed oral analgesics as needed, beginning 8 to 12 hours postoperatively.	Provides pain control, promoting rest and facilitating healing and movement.
	Assist the patient into a comfortable position with support for the affected arm.	Position of comfort promotes rest. The affected area is supported to prevent pull on traumatized tissues and stress on suture lines.

Evaluation: Compare the patient's status with the expected patient outcomes. If the outcomes are achieved, evaluate nursing care as successful. If not, reassess the patient, formulate new nursing diagnoses, and revise expected patient outcomes and nursing interventions as appropriate.

(continued)

Nursing Care Guide 48–1. *(continued)*

PATIENTS HAVING A LUMPECTOMY FOR CANCER OF THE BREAST

Assessment Findings: Postoperative patient has had an excision of a breast mass and an axillary node dissection.

Nursing Diagnosis: Impaired tissue integrity related to surgery of the breast and axilla

Patient Outcomes	Nursing Interventions	Rationale
Wound drainage changes from bright red to serosanguineous within 12 hours after surgery. Drainage gradually tapers off, ending in 48 to 72 hours.	Monitor amount and color of wound drainage. Expect drainage to be bright red initially and to change to serosanguineous after approximately 12 hours. Expect an initial volume of approximately 75 ml per shift, gradually tapering to 0 after 48 to 72 hours.	Increase in amount or reversion to a brighter red color indicates bleeding.
Incision remains intact.	Caution the patient about stretching her arms or performing any painful activities.	Tension on the suture line can cause disruption and hemorrhage because the breast is very vascular.
	Provide the patient with the option of wearing a brassiere if desired for support.	Support brassieres maintain the breasts in an upright position. Large breasts are pendulous and may cause strain on the suture line.

Evaluation: Compare the patient's status with the expected patient outcomes. If the outcomes are achieved, evaluate nursing care as successful. If not, reassess the patient, formulate new nursing diagnoses, and revise expected patient outcomes and nursing interventions as appropriate.

(continued)

travenously. Often combinations of chemotherapeutic drugs are used because (1) different types of drugs can destroy cancer cells in different stages of the cell cycle; (2) if a single drug is used, there is more chance of the tumor becoming resistant to the antineoplastic; and (3) if a combination of drugs is used, dosages and side effects are less than if the drug was used alone. A common combination in current use consists of cyclophosphamide, methotrexate, 5-fluorouracil, vincristine, and prednisone (known as CMFVP). Cyclophosphamide is an alkalating agent; 5-fluorouracil and methotrexate are antimetabolites; and vincristine is a mitotic inhibitor. Alkalating agents interfere with DNA replication. Antimetabolites interfere with enzymes needed for the synthesis of RNA and DNA. Mitotic inhibitors block cell division and result in bizarre mitotic formations. Prednisone serves to enhance the action of the other drugs in the combination.

Antibiotics, specifically actinomycin and doxorubicin, are other antineoplastic drugs used in the treatment of breast cancer. Antibiotics prevent DNA-directed RNA synthesis. They may be used alone or in combination with other chemotherapeutic agents.

Chemotherapy may be used to treat both early and advanced disease. The specific drugs chosen and length of treatment vary according to type of disease.

The side effects of chemotherapy depend on the drugs used and the individual's reaction to the drugs. Refer to Chapter 11 for a discussion of the side effects of chemotherapy.

Hormonal therapy is a specific form of chemotherapy that slows the growth of neoplastic tissue by changing the hormonal balance. Hormone receptor status is important in deciding whether hormonal therapy is indicated. A tumor that is estrogen

Nursing Care Guide 48–1. *(continued)*

PATIENTS HAVING A LUMPECTOMY FOR CANCER OF THE BREAST

Assessment Findings: Patient has a break in the skin due to surgical incision and has had an axillary lymph node dissected.

Nursing Diagnosis: High risk for infection related to presence of an incision and alteration of the lymphatic system on the affected side

Patient Outcomes	Nursing Interventions	Rationale
Wound remains free of infection, as evidenced by absence of redness, warmth, swelling, and drainage.	Instruct the patient to: Cleanse the suture line daily with hydrogen peroxide (or as preferred by surgeon) until sutures are removed.	Removes exudate and bacteria from wound, allowing healing to occur.
	Observe suture line daily for redness, warmth, swelling, or drainage, and report to surgeon if present.	Evaluates wound for signs of infection, allowing early medical intervention should infection occur.
Patient lists precautions to be taken to protect the affected arm.	Instruct the patient to protect affected arm from infection as described in Chart 48–2 until told by surgeon that precautions are no longer necessary.	Patient is at risk for infection due to the effects of surgery on the lymphatic system.

Evaluation: Compare the patient's status with the expected patient outcomes. If the outcomes are achieved, evaluate nursing care as successful. If not, reassess the patient, formulate new nursing diagnoses, and revise expected patient outcomes and nursing interventions as appropriate.

Assessment Findings: Patient has had an axillary lymph node removed, resulting in a temporary obstruction to lymph flow.

Nursing Diagnosis: High risk for fluid volume excess (local) related to impaired lymph flow in the affected arm

Patient Outcomes	Nursing Interventions	Rationale
Affected arm and hand are free of edema.	Elevate affected arm on a pillow.	Allows gravity to assist in the removal of excess fluid from affected area.
	Monitor for circulatory impairment. Comparing affected arm with nonaffected arm: ■ Check for paleness and edema ■ Palpate radial pulse ■ Check temperature of arm ■ Check capillary refill time.	Evaluates circulation in the affected arm, and allows prompt medical intervention if impairment occurs.

(continued)

Nursing Care Guide 48–1. *(continued)*

PATIENTS HAVING A LUMPECTOMY FOR CANCER OF THE BREAST

Patient Outcomes	Nursing Interventions	Rationale
Patient describes precautions to be taken.	Instruct the patient to gradually increase exercises but to avoid strenuous activity of the arm and shoulder as well as injury or infection in the arm and hand (see Chart 48–2).	Strenuous activities, injury, and infection can contribute to lymphedema.

Evaluation: Compare the patient's status with the expected patient outcomes. If the outcomes are achieved, evaluate nursing care as successful. If not, reassess the patient, formulate new nursing diagnoses, and revise expected patient outcomes and nursing interventions as appropriate.

Assessment Findings: Patient complains of discomfort and a feeling of tightness in the area of the incision.

Nursing Diagnosis: High risk for impaired physical mobility related to discomfort on moving the affected arm

Patient Outcomes	Nursing Interventions	Rationale
Patient performs range-of-motion exercises as directed.	Instruct the patient in range-of-motion exercises when permitted by the surgeon.	Promotes joint mobility and tone and strength of muscles of affected arm and shoulder.
Patient states importance of not going beyond the point of "hurt" when exercising.	Caution the patient not to continue any exercise movement past the point of "hurt."	Pain can be a warning sign indicating tissue damage.

Evaluation: Compare the patient's status with the expected patient outcomes. If the outcomes are achieved, evaluate nursing care as successful. If not, reassess the patient, formulate new nursing diagnoses, and revise expected patient outcomes and nursing interventions as appropriate.

Additional Assessments and Interventions

Assess for signs of body image disturbance and concerns about sexual activity. Encourage the patient to discuss her concerns frankly with her spouse or sexual partner. Reassure the patient that touching the breasts during lovemaking does not cause injury or the recurrence of cancer.

Provide the patient with information about community resources available to help women deal with their diagnosis and treatment (see Table 48–6).

Teach or review the importance of and the technique of monthly breast self-examination.

Review the plan for follow-up care with the patient. Make certain she knows where and when to report for her next appointment.

receptor positive suggests that the tumor cells may grow more rapidly in the presence of estrogen. To prevent estrogen from entering these cells and stimulating growth, an antiestrogen is administered. Tamoxifen is the agent most commonly prescribed. Hormones can be used alone or in combination with other chemotherapeutic drugs.

When chemotherapy is used in conjunction with radiotherapy or surgery, it is referred to as adjuvant chemotherapy. Adjuvant chemotherapy is given to patients following removal of early-stage breast tumors to prevent recurrence and metastasis due to microscopic spread. Adjuvant chemotherapy is usually given for a set amount of time, which may be as short as 6 months or as long as 24 months. Currently, premenopausal women with positive axillary lymph nodes receive adjuvant chemotherapy after surgery. Postmenopausal women with positive lymph nodes and estrogen receptor–positive tumors receive oral hormones.

In the past, adjuvant therapy was not recommended for patients with negative lymph nodes. Because of the high recurrence rate (approximately 30%) in this group, the National Cancer Institute now recommends that adjuvant chemotherapy should be considered for these patients.

Chemotherapy is also used to treat patients with advanced breast cancer. Patients who experience symptoms of metastatic disease, such as pain and organ dysfunction, receive chemotherapy combinations designed to control tumor cells that have already spread to other body organs. A remission is attained when tumor growth is halted and the size of the tumor decreases. In these cases, chemotherapeutic drugs are given for an indefinite period of time, and if the tumor progresses, another combination of chemotherapy agents may be tried.

Refer to Chapter 11 for a discussion of nursing care applicable to patients receiving chemotherapy.

RADIATION THERAPY

Radiation therapy is given by external beam or by implanting radioactive material into the breast tissue. It is used to treat both localized and advanced breast cancer. Radiation may be used after limited breast surgery, such as a lumpectomy, to decrease the chance of recurrence of breast tumor on the operative site and in the regional lymph nodes. For advanced local disease, radiation is used to shrink large breast tumors to an operable size so that they can be removed. In patients with metastatic breast cancer, radiation is used to locally control tumor cells that have spread to other body parts as a palliative method.

External radiation is usually given on an outpatient basis for approximately 5 weeks, and an additional "boost" of radiation is given 2 weeks later. The radiation boost is accomplished through additional external beam radiation or by using internal iridium implants, which deliver radiation in a concentrated form to the breast tissue. Radiation implants require hospitalization. Small plastic tubes are threaded through the breast (see Fig. 11–6) in the operating room with the patient under general or local anesthesia. Radioactive seeds, usually iridium, are introduced into the tubes. The number and placement of the tubes depend on the size and location of the breast tumor. The tubes are kept in place for 45 to 60 hours. Small amounts of radiation are emitted from the radiation implants. The patient is confined to a private hospital room. For this reason, the amount of time spent in the patient's room by visitors and hospital staff is limited.

Radiation may be used in combination with surgery or chemotherapy, or both. Refer to Chapter 11 for a discussion of nursing care applicable to patients receiving radiation therapy.

Plastic Surgery Procedures

Many women, for a variety of reasons, wish to alter the size and shape of their breasts through plastic surgery. The procedure, known as breast mammoplasty, may be used to increase or decrease breast size, tighten breast tissue, or reconstruct a missing breast. Mammoplasty is usually done under general anesthesia and, based on the extent of alteration desired, may require several procedures over a period of months.

Breast Reconstruction

Breast reconstruction, also known as reconstructive mammoplasty, is a surgical procedure that creates a natural-looking breast shape by inserting an implant under the skin and muscles of the chest wall in the area of a mastectomy. Usually it is done approximately 6 months after mastectomy, although some surgeons are now doing the procedure at the same time as the mastectomy. The breast implant is a sealed sac containing a fluid such as saline or silicone gel. The implant is custom fitted to match the remaining breast, or in the case of bilateral reconstruction, the woman and her plastic surgeon select the implant size and shape.

The breast implant considered safest for use today is filled with saline. The use of silicone gel implants has been restricted by the Food and Drug Administration (FDA) because of associated risks. These risks include local tissue reactions if silicone leaks from the implant or if the implant ruptures; less than optimal mammogram interpretation because of the presence of the implant or local tissue reaction; the potential for an autoimmune reaction; and the possible carcinogenicity of the implant itself. All women receiving silicone implants must sign a con-

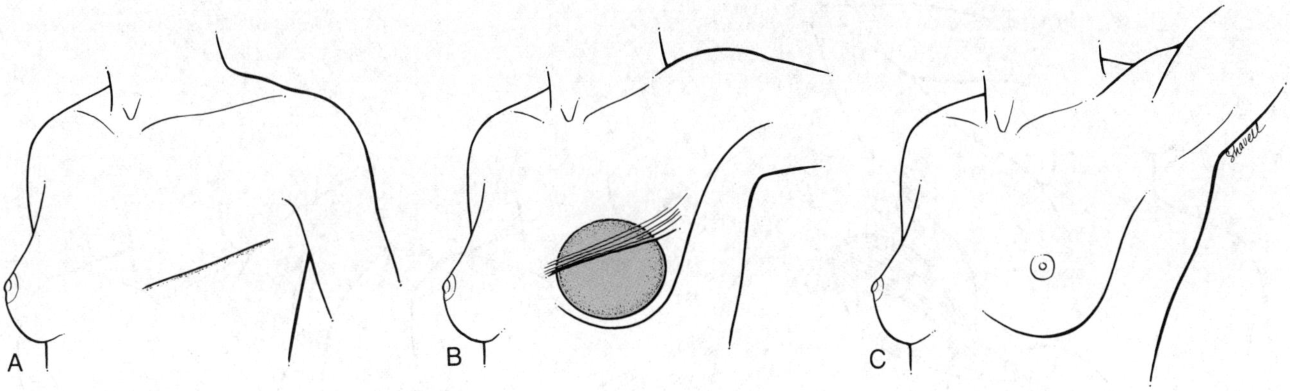

Figure 48–10.

Simple breast reconstruction. *A*, Appearance of chest before reconstruction. *B*, Appearance of chest with implant in place. *C*, Appearance of chest with nipple and areola reconstructed.

sent form that outlines the risks and agree to participate in FDA-approved clinical studies to evaluate the safety and effectiveness of the implants.

Breast reduction, breast augmentation, or mastopexy may be done on the remaining breast to increase symmetry of the paired breasts. Such alteration of the other breast to more closely match the reconstructed breast is most likely to be needed in women older than age 40.

The result of reconstruction with or without alterations of the other breast will not be perfect but for some patients it is more desirable than using a prosthesis. In all cases it is important that the results of the reconstruction be judged against breast absence rather than how the breast looked before the mastectomy.

PROCEDURES

There are three common types of reconstruction procedure: simple reconstruction, latissimus dorsi reconstruction, and rectus abdominis reconstruction.

In simple reconstruction, a small incision is made near the mastectomy scar, and the surgeon inserts an implant in a pocket that is created under the pectoralis muscle (Fig. 48–10). This method is chosen if the woman's pectoral muscles have been preserved and there is a sufficient amount of skin remaining on the chest wall. A variation of this procedure involves placing the implant between the skin and the muscle.

Latissimus dorsi reconstruction is a procedure that involves the transfer of the latissimus dorsi muscle from the patient's back to the mastectomy site and is used when the pectoral muscles have been removed during a mastectomy. The muscle serves as a new pectoral muscle, and the implant is then placed under it (Fig. 48–11).

Rectus abdominis reconstruction involves the transfer of muscle, fat, and skin from the abdomen. The transferred muscle serves as a pectoral muscle. If sufficient grafted skin and fat are available, they are used to form the breast mound and no implant is needed.

Another procedure uses a tissue expander in order to stretch the operative site to accommodate an implant. A deflated bag is placed in the site and attached to a port-A-Cath in the upper chest. A small amount of saline is injected into the port-A-Cath every 2 weeks until desired size is attained. In a few months, when the breast is the right size, another operation is done to remove the bag and port-A-Cath, and an implant is then inserted.

In all procedures, the nipple and areola may also be recreated by using some of the nipple and areola from the remaining breast or grafting tissue from the toe, thigh, labia minora, or earlobe. Breast reconstruction usually requires two or more surgical procedures, depending on the desired outcome.

Controversy exists regarding the timing of reconstruction, subsequent to mastectomy. Concerns include the possibility of early recurrence of disease on the site of the original mastectomy incision and development of a malignancy that might be concealed beneath the implant. Despite these concerns, a few surgeons are now encouraging reconstruction surgery with saline implants at the time of the mastectomy. Most, however, suggest a standard waiting period of at least 6 months for women with Stage I or II localized disease and longer for women with more advanced disease. If the woman is receiving adjuvant chemotherapy or radiotherapy, it is recommended that the procedure be delayed until after these treatments are completed.

COMPLICATIONS

The common complications of reconstructive surgery are bleeding and infection at the implant site, insufficient blood circulation at the graft site, and the formation of fibrous scar tissue around the implant. If an infection develops, antibiotics are prescribed, and the implant may have to be removed until the infection subsides. Insufficient blood sup-

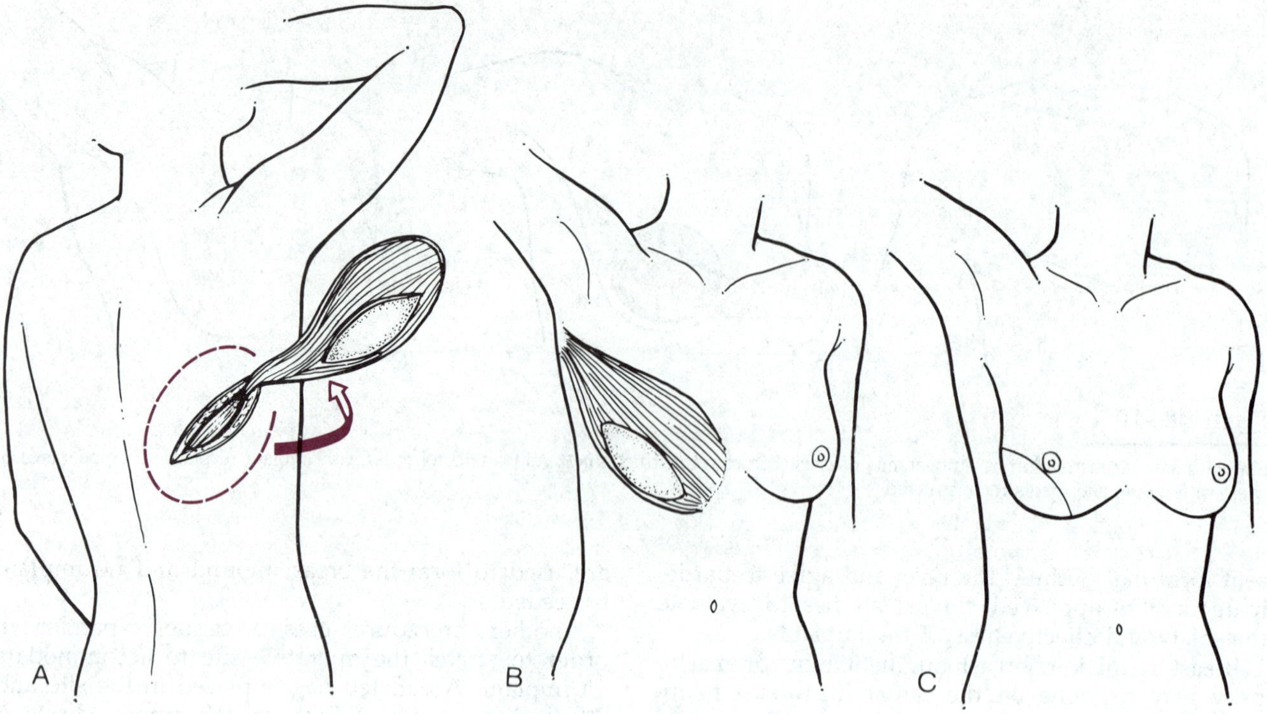

Figure 48–11.

Latissimus dorsi flap procedure. *A*, Latissimus dorsi muscle and skin flap raised on the patient's back. *B*, Flap tunneled under the skin from the back to the anterior chest to create the contour of a breast. *C*, Appearance when reconstruction is complete.

ply to the skin and muscle graft can result in tissue necrosis. If this occurs, the implant must be removed. Fibrous tissue formation around the implant results from the body's reaction to its presence. This fibrous capsule causes the implant to feel hard, and the woman may experience pain. The capsule can be removed by massaging the area or through surgical intervention. The surgeon may instruct the patient to massage the implant postoperatively for 3 to 6 months as a means to prevent capsule formation, soften the implant, and give it a more natural contour.

Application of the Nursing Process to the Care of the Patient Undergoing Breast Reconstruction Surgery

PREOPERATIVE NURSING CARE

Assessment

Assess the patient's understanding of the reconstruction procedure, the expected physical result, and its possible side effects. Also assess level of anxiety, because even though breast reconstruction is an elective procedure, patients may still be highly anxious over the prospect of anesthesia and further surgery.

Nursing Diagnoses and Planning

The nursing diagnosis and related expected patient outcomes most commonly applicable to patients scheduled for breast reconstruction surgery are as follows:

NDx: Knowledge deficit: reconstruction procedure and outcome

Planning: Patient outcomes
1. Patient states reason for selecting reconstructive surgery over other prosthetic options.
2. Patient verbalizes realistic expectations of treatment.
3. Patient describes the preparation for the procedure, expected discomfort, and expected postoperative course.

Nursing Interventions

NDx: Knowledge deficit: reconstruction procedure and outcome
Encourage the patient who is considering breast reconstruction surgery to thoroughly explore all pros-

thetic options and to realistically appraise the outcomes of the surgery. Explain that the reconstruction is basically designed to provide a normal appearance when dressed without the need for an external prosthesis. It does not necessarily result in the exact duplication of the remaining breast. Stress that it is important to compare the results of the procedure with breast absence rather than breast appearance before mastectomy. Show pictures of breast reconstruction to the patient. Suggest talking with other women who have completed breast reconstruction by contacting the local American Cancer Society or Reconstruction Education for National Understanding (RENU) for peer support and information.

Inform the patient of the cost and time commitment involved with the muitiple-step procedure of breast reconstruction. Review the schedule for procedures, and make certain the patient understands it is 3 to 6 months postoperatively before the optimal result of the surgery is evident. Allow time for the patient to ask questions, verbalize concerns, and express the outcome that she desires from breast reconstruction.

When the decision is made to have breast reconstruction surgery, provide basic preoperative teaching as discussed in Chapter 4.

Evaluation

Evaluate the effectiveness of nursing care for a patient planning breast reconstructive surgery by comparing the patient's status with the expected patient outcomes. Examples of specific outcomes for patients planning breast reconstruction surgery have been provided in the Planning section.

POSTOPERATIVE NURSING CARE

Assessment

Assess the patient's return to physiologic stabilization. Check temperature of skin flap, and observe for blanching, duskiness, and decreased capillary refill, which are indicators of impaired perfusion. Report temperature drop or mottling immediately. Observe incisional area for redness, drainage, and other indicators of infection. Check function of drainage devices, and report drainage in excess of 50 ml/hour.

Nursing Diagnoses and Planning

Nursing diagnoses and related expected patient outcomes most commonly applicable to patients who have had breast reconstruction surgery include the following:

NDx: Pain related to surgical trauma to the anterior chest

Planning: Patient outcomes
1. Patient reports pain is relieved or controlled.
2. Patient moves freely without signs of excessive discomfort.

NDx: High risk for altered tissue perfusion: breast, related to pressure on blood vessels or chilling

Planning: Patient outcomes
1. Breast is free of pressure from weight, tight dressings, and the like.
2. Patient denies feeling chilled.

NDx: High risk for altered health maintenance related to insufficient knowledge of self-care after discharge

Planning: Patient outcomes
1. Patient describes self-care presented in Chart 48–4.
2. Patient expresses willingness and ability to carry out self-care instructions.

Nursing Interventions

NDx: Pain

Administer pain medication as ordered the first postoperative day. By the second day, medications can be decreased in strength and given less frequently. Use nursing measures such as position changes and back rubs to both decrease the pain and enhance the effect of analgesics. Teach and encourage use of relaxation techniques. Encourage the patient to employ measures such as diversionary activities that have successfully descreased pain in the past.

NDx: High risk for altered tissue perfusion: breast

Position patient on back or nonoperative side to avoid pressure on the breast mound, which can impair circulation and lead to tissue necrosis. Also avoid pressure from dressings, clothing, or other sources. Keep the patient from getting chilled to avoid decreases in surface circulation.

NDx: High risk for altered health maintenance

Instruct the patient in self-care following discharge as presented in Chart 48–4.

Evaluation

Evaluate the effectiveness of nursing care for a patient who has had breast reconstruction surgery by comparing the patient's status with the expected patient outcomes. Examples of specific outcomes for patients who have had breast reconstruction surgery have been provided in the Planning section.

Chart 48–4.

NURSING GUIDE TO PATIENT EDUCATION FOR SELF-MANAGEMENT: SELF-CARE AFTER BREAST RECONSTRUCTION SURGERY

Instruct the patient to:

Avoid trauma to the breast mound.

- Sleep on the side or back.
- Refrain from wearing a brassiere for 4 to 6 weeks.
- Avoid lifting arms above shoulder level for 4 to 6 weeks.
- Avoid lifting more than 5 lb for 4 to 6 weeks.
- Limit pressure on the breast during sexual activity.
- Avoid contact sports.

Perform monthly breast self-examination for early detection of recurrence of breast cancer in the unaffected breast and in the axillary regions of both breasts.

Report signs of infection, fluid accumulation, skin changes, bleeding, or contracture of the breast to the surgeon.

Return for a 6-week checkup on *(specify date and time).*

Augmentation Mammoplasty

Augmentation mammoplasty is a procedure in which breasts are enlarged by inserting implants filled with a fluid substance between the breast tissue and the chest wall. A tight bandage is applied after the procedure to anchor the implant.

Use of implants for breast augmentation has been sharply restricted by the Food and Drug Administration (FDA), and all implant recipients must sign a specific and lengthy informed consent form that covers the short- and long-term risks of implants and agree to be listed in a national registry and participate in clinical studies.

Application of the Nursing Process to the Care of the Patient Undergoing Augmentation Mammoplasty

The assessment, nursing diagnoses, expected patient outcomes, nursing interventions, and evaluation for patients undergoing augmentation mammoplasty are similar to those described previously for patients undergoing breast reconstruction surgery.

Reduction Mammoplasty

Reduction mammoplasty is a procedure that reduces the size of the breast by surgically removing breast tissue and relocating the nipple and areola. This may be necessitated by very large breasts that cause back and shoulder pain or cause brassiere straps to cut the shoulders. Based on the extent of the reduction, multiple incisions may be made in different locations on the breast. Drainage catheters are inserted, and a dressing is applied. There may be a loss of breast function after breast reduction.

Dermal Mastopexy

Dermal mastopexy is a procedure in which excess breast skin and fat are removed in an attempt to uplift sagging breasts. The nipple and the areola are relocated.

Application of the Nursing Process to the Care of the Patient Having a Reduction Mammoplasty or Dermal Mastopexy

The assessment, nursing diagnoses, expected patient outcomes, nursing interventions, and evaluation for patients having a reduction mammoplasty or dermal mastopexy are similar to those described previously for patients having a mastectomy, with the following additional considerations. Anxiety is common even though the procedure is an elective one. There is also a high risk for body image disturbance, for although an improved cosmetic appearance is a goal, a change in and loss of a body part are involved. Needs differ from those of the mastectomy patient in that the patient having a reduction mammoplasty or dermal mastopexy is not faced with an underlying life-threatening disease that may recur.

The Elderly: Special Considerations

Breast cancer is the most common breast disease of elderly women. Because its incidence increases with age, routine breast examinations and other screening measures are essential to early detection. Thus, information related to self-examination and professional breast examination and last mammogram should be obtained as part of every elderly woman's history. Further, every plan of care must include interventions designed to ensure that screening techniques are routinely used.

All elderly women should be taught to practice breast self-examination unless a physical or psychological disorder is present that makes this inappropriate. If breast self-examination is not possible, then monthly breast examinations by a health professional should be arranged. When teaching breast self-examination or performing breast examination on an elderly woman, consider the fact that nipple retraction, which can be a sign of an underlying tumor, can also be simply an age-related change in the breast. To differentiate between the two, exert gentle pressure around the nipple and watch for nipple eversion, or teach the patient to do so. If the nipple everts, the cause of the retraction is age-related.

Breast problems are relatively rare among elderly men. Breast cancer can occur, so patients should be taught to observe for and to report any breast changes. Gynecomastia also occurs among elderly men and can be due to bronchogenic carcinoma, thyroid disease, testicular tumors, cirrhosis, or drugs such as spironolactone.

Bibliography

American Cancer Society. Cancer facts and figures—1990. New York: American Cancer Society, 1990.

American Joint Committee on Cancer. Manual for staging of cancer. 3rd ed. Philadelphia: JB Lippincott, 1988.

American Medical Association, Council on Scientific Affairs. Mammographic screening in asymptomatic women aged 40 years and older. JAMA 1989; 261(17):2535.

Andrews LW. Breast exam—A new perspective. Adv Clin Care 1990; 5(2):12.

Baker LH. Breast cancer detection demonstration project: Five year summary report. CA Cancer J Clin 1982; 32:194.

Bates B. A guide to physical examination and history taking. 5th ed. Philadelphia: JB Lippincott, 1991.

Bonadonna G, Valagussa P. Adjuvant systemic therapy for resectable breast cancer. J Clin Oncol 1985; 3:259.

Bruning N. Breast implants: Everything you need to know. Alameda, CA: Hunter House, 1992.

Bullough B, Hindi-Alexander M, Fetouh S. Methylxanthines and fibrocystic breast disease. Nurse Pract 1990; 15(3):36.

Bunn JC, Becker DW Jr. Reduction mammoplasty: The laser de-epithelialization technique. AORN J 1988; 48(1):50.

Caffeine restriction in treating breast pain. Prof Nurse 1989; 4(11):526.

Cawley M, et al. Informational and psychosocial needs of women choosing conservative surgery/primary radiation for early stage breast cancer. Cancer Nurs 1990; 13(2):90.

Champion VL. Effect of knowledge, teaching method, confidence and social influence on breast self-examination behavior. Image J Nurs Sch 1989; 21(2):76.

Clarke DE, Sandler LS. Factors involved in nurses' teaching breast self-examination. Cancer Nurs 1989; 12(1):41.

Coping with breast cancer: A guide for the patient receiving adjuvant therapy. Oncol Nurs Forum 1986; 13(3):79.

Cotter GW. Surgery or radiation therapy: A comparative cost analysis for early carcinoma of the prostate and breast. Appl Radiol 1990; 19(1):25.

Crooks CE, Jones SD. Educating women about the importance of breast screenings: The nurse's role. Cancer Nurs 1989; 12(3):161.

Cryolumpectomy: A new treatment for breast cancer. Nursing 1988; 18(4):37.

Dietrick-Gallagher M, Hyzinski MN. Teaching patients to care for drains after breast surgery for malignancy. Oncol Nurs Forum 1989; 16(2):263.

Doig B. Adjuvant chemotherapy in breast cancer. Cancer Nurs 1988; 11(2):91.

Donegan WL, et al. Nipple discharge: Is it cancer? Patient Care 1990; 24(2):79.

Dunne CF. Hormonal therapy for breast cancer. Cancer Nurs 1988; 11(5):288.

Easing the discomfort of fibrocystic condition . . . patient education aid. Patient Care 1987; 21(6):41.

Ellerhorst-Ryan JM, Goeldner J. Breast cancer. Nurs Clin North Am 1992; 27(4):821.

Ellerhorst-Ryan JM, Turba EP, Stahl DL. Evaluating benign breast disease. Nurse Pract 1988; 13(9):13.

Engel NS. Update on cancer risk and oral contraceptives. MCN 1990; 15(1):37.

Ernster BL, et al. Effects of caffeine free diet on benign breast disease—A randomized trial. Surgery 1982; 91:263.

Estrogen replacement and breast cancer. Harvard Medical School Health Letter 1989; 14(2):1.

The FDA's regulation of silicone breast implants. Washington, DC: U.S. Government Printing Office, 1993.

Fisher B, Bauer M, Margolese R, et al. Five-year results of a randomized clinical trial comparing total mastectomy and segmental mastectomy with or without radiation in the treatment of breast cancer. N Engl J Med 1985; 312:665.

Fitzpatrick AA. Antineoplastic agents. In Wardell SC, Bousard LB (eds). Nursing pharmacology: A comprehensive approach to drug therapy. Monterey, CA: Wadsworth Health Sciences Division, 1985, pp 943–964.

Fowler ME. Meeting the psychologic needs of the breast reconstruction patient. Plast Surg Nurs 1989; 9(3):129.

Fox K. Ellen's going home: Can she manage without you? . . . Preparing your postmastectomy patient for discharge. Nursing 1989; 19(5):80.

Friend AH, Dryja TP, Weinberg RA. Oncogenes and tumor-suppressing genes. N Engl J Med 1988; 318:618.

Goldfarb J, Tibbets E. Breast feeding handbook. Hillside, NJ: Enslow Publishers, 1980.

Greenwood S. Menopause, naturally: Preparing for the second half of life (updated). Volcano, CA: Volcano Press, 1992.
Greifzu S. Breast cancer: The risks and the options. 1986; 49(10):26.
Griffiths MJ, Murray KH, Russo PC. Oncology nursing—Pathophysiology, assessment, and intervention. New York: Macmillan, 1984, pp 161–183.
Group therapy in metastatic breast cancer. Nurses Drug Alert 1990; 14(1):7.
Harris JR, Beadle GF, Hellman S. Clinical studies on the use of radiation therapy as primary treatment of early breast cancer. Cancer 1984; 53(3 Suppl):705.
Hassey KM. Pregnancy and parenthood after treatment for breast cancer. Oncol Nurs Forum 1988; 15(4):439.
Heberman LR, Lippman M, Angelo TD. Correlation of stress factors with sustained depression of natural killer cell activity and predicted prognosis in patients with breast cancer. J Clin Oncol 1988; 6:709.
Henderson CI, Canellos GP. Cancer of the breast. The past decade. N Engl J Med 1980; 302:17.
Holmberg L, Omne-Pontén M, Burns T, et al. Psychosocial adjustment after mastectomy and breast-conserving treatment. Cancer 1989; 64(4):969.
Humphrey LL, Ballard DJ. Early detection of breast cancer in women. Prim Care 1989; 16(1):115.
Isaacs JH. Textbook of breast disease. St. Louis: Mosby–Year Book, 1992.
Kenne DW. Surgical management of primary breast cancer. Cancer 1983; 51:2540.
Kroehl SA. Nursing care during the diagnostic period. In Pfeiffer CH, Mulliken JB (eds). Caring for the patient with breast cancer. Reston, VA: Reston, 1984, pp 36–40.
Kroner K, Krebs S, Skov J, et al. Immediate and long-term phantom breast syndrome after mastectomy: Incidence, clinical characteristics and relationship to pre-mastectomy breast pain. Pain 1989; 36(3):327.
Laurence RA. Breastfeeding. 2nd ed. St. Louis: CV Mosby, 1985.
Levy M. Breast cancer treatment alternatives: The patient decision-making process. Health Values 1986; 10(1):16.
Lierman LM. Discovery of breast changes: Women's responses and nursing implications. Cancer Nurs 1988; 11(6):352.
Lippman ME. Management of breast cancer with hormones and drugs. Hosp Pract 1986; 21(5):119.
Love RR, Leventhal H, Easterling DV, Nerenz DR. Side effects and emotional distress during cancer chemotherapy. Cancer 1989; 63(3):604.
Love S. Breast cancer: Early decisions. Harvard Medical School Health Letter 1988; 13(5):1.
Love S. Breast removal and reconstruction. Harvard Medical School Health Letter 1990; 15(4):3.
Love S. Dr. Susan Love's breast book. Reading, MA: Addison-Wesley, 1990.
Ludwick R. Breast examination in the older adult. Cancer Nurs 1988; 9(5):99.
Mack E. Most breast lumps aren't cancer! RN 1990; 53(12):21.
Marshall J, Graham S, Swanson M. Caffeine consumption and benign breast disease: A case control comparison. Am J Public Health 1982; 72:610.
Massey V. Perceived susceptibility to breast cancer and practice of breast self-examination. Nurs Res 1986; 35(3):183.
McKenney S. Helping your patient cope with breast cancer. Nursing 1988; 18(12):64E.
Mitchell GW, Bassett LW. The female breast and its disorders. Baltimore: Williams & Wilkins, 1990.
Mitchell MS. Combining chemotherapy with biological response modifiers in treatment of cancer. J Natl Cancer Inst 1988; 80:1445.
Nachtigall LE, Heilman JR. Estrogen (revised and expanded). New York: Harper-Collins, 1991.
Nail L, Jones LS, Giuffre M, et al. Sensations after mastectomy. Am J Nurs 1984; 84(9):1121.
National Cancer Institute: The breast cancer digest. NIH Publication No. 84-1691. Bethesda, MD: National Cancer Institute, 1984.
Nielsen BB. The nurse's role in mammography screening. Cancer Nurs 1989; 12(5):271.
Nielsen BB, East D. Advances in breast cancer: Implications for nursing care. Nurs Clin North Am 1990; 25(2):365.
Northouse LL. Social support in patients' and husbands' adjustment to breast cancer. Nurs Res 1988; 37(2):91.
Northouse LL. The impact of breast cancer on patients and husbands. Cancer Nurs 1989; 12(5):276.
Norwood SL. Fibrocystic breast disease. JOGNN 1990; 19(2):116.
Oncology Nursing Society Clinical Practice Subcommittee on Guidelines. Guidelines for cancer nursing practice. Orlando, FL: Grune & Stratton, 1985.
Peters CR. Augmentation mammoplasty. Plast Surg Nurs 1990; 10(1):25.
Redeker NC. Health beliefs, health locus of control, and the frequency of practice of breast self examination in women. JOGNN 1989; 18:45.
Reifsnider E. Educating women about benign breast disease. AAOHN J 1990; 38(3):121.
Rice MA, Szopa TJ. Group intervention for reinforcing self-worth following mastectomy. Oncol Nurs Forum 1988; 15(1):33.
Riddle LB. Augmentation mammoplasty. Nurse Pract 1986; 11(3):30.
Riordan J. A practical guide to breastfeeding. St. Louis: CV Mosby, 1983.
Rosenberg SA. The development of new immunotherapies for the treatment of cancer using interleukin-2. A review. Ann Surg 1988; 208:121.
Rudolph A, et al. The breast physical examination: Its value in early cancer detection. Cancer Nurs 1987; 10(2):100.
Rust DL, Kloppenborg EM. Don't underestimate the lumpectomy patient's needs. RN 1990; 53(3):58.
Rutledge DN. Factors related to women's practice of breast self-examination. Nurs Res 1987; 36(2):117.
Rybolt AH, Waterbury L. Breast cancer in older women: Trends in diagnosis. Geriatrics 1989; 44(6):69.
Salazar MD. Conquering cancer: Primary prevention and early detection. AAOHN J 1988; 36(8):303.
Scalon EF. Case for and against two-step procedure for the surgical treatment of breast cancer. Cancer 1984; 53:577.
Shamian J. Nurses as agents for change in teaching breast self-examination. Public Health Nurs 1987; 4(1):29.
Sickes EA. Breast DT scanning, heavy ion mammography, nuclear magnetic imaging, diaphanography. In Reia SA, McLelland R (eds). Breast carcinoma: Current diagnosis and treatment. New York: American College of Radiology–Masson Publishing, 1983.
Solomon J. The good news about breast reconstruction. RN 1986; 49(11):47.
Teimourian B, Hakki AR. Benign disease of the female breast. Hosp Med 1987; 23(1):85.
Tully MR, Overfield ML. Breastfeeding counseling guide. Lactation Consultants of North Carolina, 1987.
Walsh KC. Breast augmentation: Your patient's adjustment to new body image. Todays OR Nurse 1986; 8(9):20.
Ward S, Heidrich S, Wolberg W. Factors women take into account when deciding upon type of surgery for breast cancer. Cancer Nurs 1989; 12(6):344.
Wardleworth CM. Breast sonography. Radiology 1986; 52(606):291.
Whipple B. Sexual counseling of couples after a mastectomy or myocardial infarction. Nurs Forum 1987–1988; 23(3):85.
Williams RD, Edwards K, Hane N. Barriers to breast cancer screening in older women. Fam Community Health 1987; 10(3):51.

Appendix One

REFERENCE VALUES FOR LABORATORY TESTS

Reference values for laboratory tests serve as important guides in evaluating laboratory data on individual patients. They should not be considered equivalent to normal, however, because there is no sharp dividing line between normal and abnormal values and the transition from a clearly normal to a clearly abnormal value as a result of a pathologic process is gradual.

The following tables present reference values for commonly performed laboratory tests. These values are given in conventional units as well as in SI (Système International d'Unités) units because the United States is the only industrialized nation that has not adopted the International System of Units.

Because laboratory techniques may differ, values in the tables may differ from those of other laboratories and textbooks, as well as from values given in specific chapters in this text.

REFERENCE VALUES IN HEMATOLOGY

		CONVENTIONAL UNITS	SI UNITS
Acid hemolysis test (Ham)		No hemolysis	No hemolysis
Alkaline phosphatase, leukocyte		Total score 14–100	Total score 14–100
Cell counts			
Erythrocytes			
Males		4.6–6.2 million/mm^3	4.6–6.2 × 10^{12}/L
Females		4.2–5.4 million/mm^3	4.2–5.4 × 10^{12}/L
Children (varies with age)		4.5–5.1 million/mm^3	4.5–5.1 × 10^{12}/L
Leukocytes			
Total		4500–11,000 mm^3	4.5–11.0 × 10^9/L
Differential	*Percentage*	*Absolute*	*Absolute*
Myelocytes	0	0/mm^3	0/L
Band neutrophils	3–5	150–400/mm^3	150–400 × 10^6/L
Segmented neutrophils	54–62	3000–5800/mm^3	3000–5800 × 10^6/L
Lymphocytes	25–33	1500–3000/mm^3	1500–3000 × 10^6/L
Monocytes	3–7	300–500/mm^3	300–500 × 10^6/L
Eosinophils	1–3	50–250/mm^3	50–250 × 10^6/L
Basophils	0–0.75	15–50/mm^3	15–50 × 10^6/L
Platelets		150,000–350,000/mm^3	150–350 × 10^9/L
Reticulocytes		25,000–75,000/mm^3 0.5–1.5% of erythrocytes	25–75 × 10^9/L
Coagulation tests			
Bleeding time (template)		2.75–8.0 min	2.75–8.0 min
Coagulation time (glass tubes)		5–15 min	5–15 min
Factor VIII and other coagulation factors		50–150% of normal	0.5–1.5 of normal
Fibrin split products (Thrombo-Welco test)		<10 μg/mL	<10 mg/L
Fibrinogen		200–400 mg/dL	2.0–4.0 g/L
Partial thromboplastin time (PTT)		20–35 sec	20–35 s
Prothrombin time (PT)		12.0–14.0 sec	12.0–14.0 s
Coombs' test			
Direct		Negative	Negative
Indirect		Negative	Negative
Corpuscular values of erythrocytes			
Mean corpuscular hemoglobin (MCH)		26–34 pg	0.40–0.53 fmol
Mean corpuscular volume (MCV)		80–96 μm^3	80–96 fL
Mean corpuscular hemoglobin concentration (MCHC)		32–36%	0.32–0.36
Haptoglobin		26–185 mg/dL	260–1850 mg/L
Hematocrit			
Males		40–54 mL/dL	0.40–0.54 volume fraction
Females		37–47 mL/dL	0.37–0.47 volume fraction
Newborns		49–54 mL/dL	0.49–0.54 volume fraction
Children (varies with age)		35–49 mL/dL	0.35–0.49 volume fraction
Hemoglobin			
Males		14.0–18.0 gm/dL	2.17–2.79 mmol/L
Females		12.0–16.0 gm/dL	1.86–2.48 mmol/L
Newborns		16.5–19.5 gm/dL	2.56–3.02 mmol/L
Children (varies with age)		11.2–16.5 gm/dL	1.74–2.56 mmol/L
Hemoglobin, fetal		<1.0% of total	<0.01 of total
Hemoglobin A_{1C}		3–5% of total	0.03–0.05 of total
Hemoblogin A_2		1.5–3.0% of total	0.015–0.03 of total
Hemoglobin, plasma		0–5.0 mg/dL	0–0.8 μmol/L
Methemoglobin		30–130 mg/dL	4.7–20 μmol/L
Sedimentation rate (ESR)			
Wintrobe: Males		0–5 mm/hr	0–5 mm/h
Females		0–15 mm/hr	0–15 mm/h
Westergren: Males		0–15 mm/hr	0–15 mm/h
Females		0–20 mm/hr	0–20 mm/h

REFERENCE VALUES FOR BLOOD, PLASMA, AND SERUM*

	CONVENTIONAL UNITS	SI UNITS
Acetoacetate plus acetone, serum		
Qualitative	Negative	Negative
Quantitative	0.3–2.0 mg/dL	3–20 mg/L
Acid phosphatase (thymolphthalein monophosphate substrate), serum	0.11–0.60 U/L	0.11–0.60 U/L
Adrenocorticotropin (ACTH), plasma		
6 A.M.	10–80 pg/mL	10–80 ng/L
6 P.M.	<50 pg/mL	<50 ng/L
Alanine aminotransferase (ALT, SGPT), serum	5–30 U/L	5–30 U/L
Albumin, serum	3.5–5.5 gm/dL	35–55 g/L
Aldolase, serum	1.5–12.0 U/L	1.5–12.0 U/L
Aldosterone, plasma		
Supine	3–10 ng/dL	0.08–0.30 nmol/L
Standing		
Males	6–22 ng/dL	0.17–0.61 nmol/L
Females	5–30 ng/dL	0.14–0.83 nmol/L
Alkaline phosphatase (ALP), serum	20–90 U/L (30°C)	20–90 U/L (30°C)
Ammonia nitrogen, plasma	15–49 μg/dL	11–35 μmol/L
Amylase, serum	25–125 U/L	25–125 U/L
Anion gap	8–16 mEq/L	8–16 mmol/L
Ascorbic acid, blood	0.4–1.5 mg/dL	23–85 μmol/L
Aspartate aminotransferase (AST, SGOT), serum	10–30 U/L	10–30 U/L
Base excess, blood	0 ± 2 mEq/L	0 ± 2 mmol/L
Bicarbonate		
Venous plasma		23–29 mmol/L
Arterial blood	18–23 mEq/L	18–23 mmol/L
Bile acids, serum	0.3–3.0 mg/dL	3–30 mg/L
Bilirubin, serum		
Conjugated	0.1–0.4 mg/dL	1.7–6.8 μmol/L
Unconjugated	0.2–0.7 mg/dL	3.4–12 μmol/L
Total	0.3–1.1 mg/dL	5.1–19 μmol/L
Calcium, serum	9.0–11.0 mg/dL	2.25–2.75 mmol/L
Calcium, ionized, serum	4.25–5.25 mg/dL	1.05–1.30 mmol/L
Carbon dioxide, total, serum or plasma	24–30 mEq/L	24–30 mmol/L
Carbon dioxide tension (P_{CO_2}), blood	35–45 mmHg	35–45 mmHg
β-Carotene, serum	40–200 μg/dL	0.74–3.72 μmol/L
Ceruloplasmin, serum	23–44 mg/dL	230–44 mg/L
Chloride, serum or plasma	96–106 mEq/L	96–106 mmol/L
Cholesterol, serum or EDTA plasma		
Desirable range	<200 mg/dL	<5.18 mmol/L
LDL cholesterol	60–180 mg/dL	600–1800 mg/L
HDL cholesterol	30–80 mg/dL	300–800 mg/L
Copper		
Males	70–140 μg/dL	11–22 μmol/L
Females	85–155 μg/dL	13–24 μmol/L
Cortisol, plasma		
8 A.M.	6–23 μg/dL	170–635 nmol/L
4 P.M.	3–15 μg/dL	82–413 nmol/L
10 P.M.	<50% of 8 A.M. value	<0.5 of 8 A.M. value
Creatine, serum	0.2–0.8 mg/dL	15–61 μmol/L
Creatine kinase (CK, CPK), serum		
Males	55–170 U/L	55–170 U/L
Females	30–135 U/L	30–135 U/L
Creatine kinase MB isozyme, serum	0.0–4.7 ng/mL	0.0–4.7 μg/L
Creatinine, serum	0.6–1.2 mg/dL	53–106 μmol/L
Ferritin, serum	20–200 ng/mL	20–200 μg/L
Fibrinogen, plasma	200–400 mg/dL	2.0–4.0 g/L
Folate, serum	1.8–9.0 ng/mL	4.1–20.4 nmol/L
Erythrocytes	150–450 ng/mL	340–1020 nmol/L
Follicle-stimulating hormone (FSH), plasma		
Males	4–25 mU/mL	4–25 U/L
Females	4–30 mU/mL	4–30 U/L
Postmenopausal	40–250 mU/mL	40–250 U/L
γ-Glutamyltransferase, serum		
Males	5–38 U/L	5–38 U/L
Females	5–29 U/L	5–29 U/L
Gastrin, serum	0–200 pg/mL	0–200 ng/L
Glucose (fasting), plasma or serum	70–115 mg/dL	3.89–6.38 mmol/L
Growth hormone (hGH), plasma	0–10 ng/mL	0–10 μg/L

(continued)

	CONVENTIONAL UNITS	SI UNITS
Haptoglobin, serum	26–185 mg/dL	260–1850 mg/L
Immunoglobulins, serum		
IgG	550–1900 mg/dL	5.5–19.0 g/L
IgA	60–333 mg/dL	0.60–3.3 g/L
IgM	45–145 mg/dL	0.45–1.5 g/L
IgD	0.5–3.0 mg/dL	5–30 mg/L
IgE	<500 ng/mL	<500 μg/L
Insulin (fasting), plasma	5–25 μU/mL	36–179 pmol/L
Iron, serum	75–175 μg/dL	13–31 μmol/L
Iron binding capacity, serum		
Total	250–410 μg/dL	45–73 μmol/L
Saturation	20–55%	0.20–0.55
Lactate		
Venous blood	4.5–19.8 mg/dL	0.50–2.2 mmol/L
Arterial blood	4.5–14.4 mg/dL	0.50–1.6 mmol/L
Lactate dehydrogenase (LD, LDH), serum	100–190 U/L	100–190 U/L
Lipase, serum	10–140 U/L	10–140 U/L
Lipids, total, serum	450–850 mg/dL	4.5–8.5 g/L
Luteinizing (LH), serum		
Males	6–18 IU/L	6–18 U/L
Females		
Premenopausal	5–22 IU/L	5–22 U/L
Mid-cycle	3 times baseline	3 times baseline
Postmenopausal	>30 IU/L	>30 U/L
Magnesium, serum	1.8–3.0 mg/dL	0.75–1.25 mmol/L
Osmolality	286–295 mOsm/kg water	285–295 mmol/kg water
Oxygen, blood		
Capacity (varies with hemoglobin)	16–24 vol %	7.14–10.7 mmol/L
Content, arterial	15–23 vol %	6.69–10.3 mmol/L
Saturation, arterial	94–100 %	0.94–1.00
Oxygen tension (Po_2), blood	75–100 mmHg	75–100 mmHg
P_{50}	26–27 mmHg	26–27 mmHg
pH, arterial blood	7.35–7.45	7.35–7.45
Phenylalanine, serum	<3 mg/dL	<0.18 mmol/L
Phosphate, inorganic, serum	3.0–4.5 mg/dL	1.0–1.5 mmol/L
Potassium, serum or plasma	3.5–5.0 mEq/L	3.5–5.0 mmol/L
Prolactin		
Males	1–20 ng/mL	1–20 μg/L
Females	1–25 ng/mL	1–25 μg/L
Protein, serum		
Total	6.0–8.0 gm/dL	60–80 g/L
Albumin	3.5–5.5 gm/dL	35–55 g/L
$Alpha_1$ globulin	0.2–0.4 gm/dL	2–4 g/L
$Alpha_2$ globulin	0.5–0.9 gm/dL	5–9 g/L
Beta globulin	0.6–1.1 gm/dL	6–11 g/L
Gamma globulin	0.7–1.7 gm/dL	7–17 g/L
Pyruvate, blood	0.3–0.9 mg/dL	0.03–0.10 mmol/L
Sodium, serum or plasma	136–145 mEq/L	136–145 mmol/L
Testosterone, plasma		
Males	275–875 ng/dL	9.5–30 nmol/L
Females	23–75 ng/dL	0.8–2.6 nmol/L
Pregnant	38–190 ng/dL	1.3–6.6 nmol/L
Thyroid-stimulating hormone (TSH), serum	0–7 μU/mL	0–7 mU/L
Thyroxine, free (FT), serum	1.0–2.1 ng/dL	13–27 pmol/L
Thyroxine (T_4), serum	4.4–9.9 μg/dL	57–128 nmol/L
Triglycerides, serum	40–150 mg/dL	0.4–1.5 g/L
Triiodothyronine (T_3), serum	150–250 ng/dL	2.3–3.9 nmol/L
Triiodothyronine uptake, resin (T_3RU)	25–38% uptake	0.25–0.38 uptake
Urate, serum		
Males	2.5–8.0 mg/dL	0.15–0.48 mmol/L
Females	1.5–7.0 mg/dL	0.09–0.42 mmol/L
Urea, serum or plasma	24–49 mg/dL	4.0–8.2 mmol/L
Urea nitrogen, serum or plasma	11–23 mg/dL	3.9–8.2 mmol/L
Viscosity, serum	1.4–1.8 times water	1.4–1.8 times water
Vitamin A, serum	20–80 μg/dL	0.70–2.80 μmol/L
Vitamin B_{12}, serum	180–900 pg/mL	133–664 pmol/L

* For some procedures, the reference values may vary depending on the method used.

REFERENCE VALUES FOR URINE*

	CONVENTIONAL UNITS	SI UNITS
Acetone and acetoacetate, qualitative	Negative	Negative
Albumin		
Qualitative	Negative	Negative
Quantitative	10–100 mg/24 hr	0.15–1.5 μmol/24 hr
Aldosterone	3–20 μg/24 hr	8.3–55 nmol/24 h
δ-Aminolevulinic acid	1.3–7.0 mg/24 hr	10–53 μmol/24 h
Amylase	3–20 U/hr	3–20 U/h
Amylase/creatinine clearance ratio	1–4%	0.01–0.04
Bilirubin, qualitative	Negative	Negative
Calcium (usual diet)	<250 mg/24 hr	<6.3 mmol/24 h
Catecholamines		
Epinephrine	<10 μg/24 hr	<55 nmol/24 h
Norepinephrine	<100 μg/24 hr	<590 nmol/24 h
Total free catecholamines	4–126 μg/24 hr	24–745 nmol/24 h
Total metanephrines	0.1–1.6 mg/24 hr	0.5–8.1 μmol/24 h
Chloride (varies with intake)	110–250 mEq/24 hr	110–250 mmol/24 h
Copper	0–50 μg/24 hr	0–0.80 μmol/24 h
Cortisol, free	10–100 μg/24 hr	27.6–276 nmol/24 h
Creatinine	15–25 mg/kg body weight/24 hr	0.13–0.22 mmol/kg body weight/24 h
Creatinine clearance (corrected to 1.73 m^2 body surface area)		
Males	110–150 mL/min	110–150 ml/min
Females	105–132 mL/min	105–132 ml/min
Dehydroepiandrosterone		
Males	0.2–2.0 mg/24 hr	0.7–6.9 μmol/24 h
Females	0.2–1.8 mg/24 hr	0.7–6.2 μmol/24 h
Estrogens, total		
Males	4–25 μg/24 hr	14–90 nmol/24 h
Females	5–100 μg/24 hr	18–360 nmol/24 h
Glucose (as reducing substance)	<250 mg/24 hr	<250 mg/24 h
Hemoglobin and myoglobin, qualitative	Negative	Negative
17-Hydroxycorticosteroids		
Males	3–9 mg/24 hr	8.3–25 μmol/24 h
Females	2–8 mg/24 hr	5.5–22 μmol/24 h
5-Hydroxyindoleacetic acid		
Qualitative	Negative	Negative
Quantitative	<9 mg/24 hr	<47 μmol/24 h
17-Ketosteroids		
Males	6–18 mg/24 hr	21–62 μmol/24 h
Females	4–13 mg/24 hr	14–45 μmol/24 h
Magnesium	6.0–8.5 mEq/24 hr	3.0–4.2 mmol/24 h
Metanephrines (see Catecholamines)		
Osmolality	38–1400 mOsm/kg water	38–1400 mmol/kg water
pH	4.6–8.0	4.6–8.0
Phenylpyruvic acid, qualitative	Negative	Negative
Phosphate	0.9–1.3 grams/24 hr	29–42 mmol/24 h
Porphobilinogen		
Qualitative	Negative	Negative
Quantitative	<2.0 mg/24 hr	<9 μmol/24 h
Porphyrins		
Coproporphyrin	50–250 μg/24 hr	77–380 nmol/24 h
Uroporphyrin	10–30 μg/24 hr	12–36 nmol/24 h
Potassium	25–100 mEq/24 hr	25–100 mmol/24 h
Pregnanediol		
Males	0.4–1.4 mg/24 hr	1.2–4.4 μmol/24 h
Females		
Proliferative phase	0.5–1.5 mg/24 hr	1.6–4.7 μmol/24 h
Luteal phase	2.0–7.0 mg/24 hr	6.2–22 μmol/24 h
Postmenopausal	0.2–1.0 mg/24 hr	0.6–3.1 μmol/24 h
Pregnanetriol	<2.5 mg/24 hr	<7.4 μmol/24 h
Protein		
Qualitative	Negative	Negative
Quantitative	10–150 mg/24 hr	10–150 mg/24 h
Sodium	130–260 mEq/24 hr	130–260 mmol/24 h
Specific gravity	1.003–1.030	1.003–1.030

(continued)

REFERENCE VALUES FOR URINE* *(continued)*

	CONVENTIONAL UNITS	SI UNITS
Urate	200–500 mg/24 hr	1.2–3.0 mmol/24 h
Urobilinogen	<4.0 mg/24 hr	<6.8 μmol/24 h
Vanillylmandelic acid (VMA, 4-hydroxy-3-methoxymandelic acid)	1–8 mg/24 hr	5–40 μmol/24 h

* For some procedures, the reference values may vary depending on the method used.

REFERENCE VALUES FOR THERAPEUTIC DRUG MONITORING

	THERAPEUTIC RANGE	TOXIC LEVELS	PROPRIETARY NAMES
ANTIBIOTICS			
Amikacin, serum	25–30 μg/mL	Peak: >35 μg/mL Trough: >5–7 μg/mL	Amikin
Chloramphenicol, serum	10–20 μg/mL	>25 μg/mL	Chloromycetin
Gentamicin, serum	5–10 μg/mL	Peak: >12 μg/mL Trough: >2 μg/mL	Garamycin
Tobramycin, serum	5–10 μg/mL	Peak: >12 μg/mL Trough: >2 μg/mL	Nebcin
ANTICONVULSANTS			
Carbamazepine, serum	5–12 μg/mL	>12 μg/mL	Tegretol
Ethosuximide, serum	40–100 μg/mL	>100 μg/mL	Zarontin
Phenobarbital, serum	10–30 μg/mL	Vary widely because of developed tolerance	
Phenytoin, serum	10–20 μg/mL	>20 μg/mL	Dilantin
Primidone, serum	5–12 μg/mL	>15 μg/mL	Mysoline
Valproic acid, serum	50–100 μg/mL	>100 μg/mL	Depakene
ANALGESICS			
Acetaminophen, serum	10–20 μg/mL	>250 μg/mL	Tylenol
Salicylate, serum	100–250 μg/mL	>300 μg/mL	Disalcid
BRONCHODILATOR			
Theophylline (aminophylline), serum	10–20 μg/mL	>20 μg/mL	
CARDIOVASCULAR DRUGS			
Digitoxin, serum (specimen must be obtained 12–24 hr after last dose)	15–25 ng/mL	>25 ng/ml	Crystodigin
Digoxin, serum (specimen must be obtained 12–24 hr after last dose)	0.8–2.0 ng/mL	>2.4 ng/mL	Lanoxin
Disopyramide, serum	2–5 μg/mL	>5 μg/mL	Norpace
Lidocaine, serum	1.5–5.0 μg/mL	>6–8 μg/mL	Xylocaine
Procainamide, serum (measured as procainamide + *N*-acetylprocainamide)	4–10 μg/mL	>16 μg/mL	Pronestyl
Propranolol, serum	50–100 ng/mL	Variable	Inderal
Quinidine, serum	2–5 μg/mL	>10 μg/mL	Cardioquin Quinaglute Quinidex Quinora
PSYCHOPHARMACOLOGIC DRUGS			
Amitriptyline, serum (measured as amitriptyline + nortriptyline)	120–150 ng/mL	>500 ng/mL	Amitril Elavil Endep Limbitrol Triavil
Desipramine, serum (measured as desipramine + imipramine)	150–300 ng/mL	>500 ng/mL	Norpramin Pertofrane
Imipramine, serum (measured as imipramine + desipramine)	150–300 ng/mL	>500 ng/mL	Antipress Imavate Janimine Presamine Tofranil
Lithium, serum (obtain specimen 12 hr after last dose)	0.8–1.2 mEq/L	>2.0 mEq/L	Lithobid
Nortriptyline, serum	50–150 ng/mL	>500 ng/mL	Aventyl Pamelor

REFERENCE VALUES IN TOXICOLOGY

	CONVENTIONAL UNITS	SI UNITS
Arsenic		
Blood	3.5–7.2 μg/dL	0.47–0.96 μmol/L
Urine	<100 μg/24 hr	<1.3 μmol/24 h
Bromides, serum	0	0
	Toxic: >17 mEq/L	Toxic: >17 mmol/L
Carboxyhemoglobin, blood	<5% saturation	<0.05 saturation
Symptoms occur	>20% saturation	>0.20 saturation
Ethanol, blood	<0.05 mg/dL (<0.005%)	<1.0 mmol/L
Marked intoxication	300–400 mg/dL (0.3–0.4%)	65–87 mmol/L
Alcoholic stupor	400–500 mg/dL (0.4–0.5%)	87–109 mmol/L
Coma	>500 mg/dL (0.5%)	>109 mmol/L
Lead		
Blood	0–40 μg/dL	0–2 μmol/L
Urine	<100 μg/24 hr	<0.48 μmol/24 h
Mercury, urine	<100 μg/24 hr	<50 nmol/24 h

REFERENCE VALUES FOR CEREBROSPINAL FLUID

	CONVENTIONAL UNITS	SI UNITS
Cells	<5/mm³; all mononuclear	<5 × 10⁶/L, all mononuclear
Electrophoresis	Predominantly albumin	Predominantly albumin
Glucose	50–75 mg/dL	2.8–4.2 mmol/L
	(20 mg/dL less than serum)	(1.1 mmol less than serum)
IgG		
Children under 14	<8% of total protein	<0.08 of total protein
Adults	<14% of total protein	<0.14 of total protein
IgG index $\left(\frac{\text{CSF/serum IgG ratio}}{\text{CSF/serum albumin ratio}}\right)$	0.3–0.6	0.3–0.6
Oligoclonal banding on electrophoresis	Absent	Absent
Pressure	70–180 mm water	70–180 mm water
Protein, total	15–45 mg/dL	150–450 mg/L

REFERENCE VALUES FOR SEMEN

	CONVENTIONAL UNITS	SI UNITS
Volume	2–5 mL	2–5 mL
Liquefaction	Complete in 15 min	Complete in 15 min
Leukocytes	Occasional or absent	Occasional or absent
Count	60–150 million/mL	60–150 × 10⁶/mL
Motility	>80% motile	>0.80 motile
Morphology	80–90% normal forms	0.80–0.90 normal forms
Fructose	>150 mg/dL	>8.33 mmol/L

REFERENCE VALUES FOR FECES

	CONVENTIONAL UNITS	SI UNITS
Bulk	100–200 gm/24 hr	100–200 g/24 h
Dry matter	23–32 gm/24 hr	23–32 g/24 h
Fat, total	<6.0 gm/24 hr	<6.0 g/24 h
Nitrogen, total	<2.0 gm/24 hr	<2.0 g/24 h
Water	Approximately 65%	Approximately 0.65

Tables from Rakel RE (ed). Conn's current therapy 1992. Philadelphia: WB Saunders, 1992.

Appendix Two

COMMON ABBREVIATIONS

a	before
aa	of each
ABG	arterial blood gases
ac	before meals
ACH	acetylcholine
ACT	activated clotting time
ACTH	adrenocorticotropic hormone
ADH	antidiuretic hormone
ADL	activities of daily living
ad lib	as desired
AFP	alpha-fetoprotein
A/G ratio	albumin-globulin ratio
AHG	antihemophilic globulin
AIDS	acquired immunodeficiency syndrome
ALG	antilymphocyte globulin
ALL	acute lymphocytic leukemia
ALS	amyotrophic lateral sclerosis
ALT	alanine aminotransferase
AML	acute myelocytic leukemia
ANA	antinuclear antibody
AP	anteroposterior
APTT	activated partial thromboplastin time
A/R pulse	apical/radial pulse
ARDS	adult respiratory distress syndrome
ASCVD	arteriosclerotic cardiovascular disease
ASHD	arteriosclerotic heart disease
AST	aspartate aminotransferase
ATG	antithymocyte globulin
ATN	acute tubular necrosis
ATP	adenosine triphosphate
AV	atrioventricular
AVM	arteriovenous malformation
AVR	aortic valve replacement
BaE	barium enema
BCE	basal cell epithelioma
b.i.d.	twice daily
BK	below knee
BMR	basal metabolism rate
BP	blood pressure
BPH	benign prostatic hypertrophy
bpm	beats per minute
B.R.P.	bathroom privileges
BS	bowel sounds
BUN	blood urea nitrogen
Bx	biopsy
c	with
CA	cancer
Ca^{2+}	calcium
CABG	coronary artery bypass graft
CAD	coronary artery disease
CAPD	continuous ambulatory peritoneal dialysis
CAT	computerized axial tomography
CBC	complete blood count
CC	chief complaint
CCK	cholecystokinin
CCPD	continuous cycle peritoneal dialysis
CCT	crude coal tar
C&D	curettage and desiccation
CDC	Centers for Disease Control and Prevention
CF	circumflex artery
CFS	chronic fatigue syndrome
CHF	congestive heart failure
CK	creatine kinase
Cl^-	chloride
CLL	chronic lymphocytic leukemia
CML	chronic myelocytic leukemia
CMV	cytomegalovirus
CNS	central nervous system

c/o	complained of
CO_2	carbon dioxide
COP	Cytoxan, Oncovin, prednisone
COPD	chronic obstructive pulmonary disease
COPP	Cytoxan, Oncovin, prednisone, procarbazine
CPK	creatine phosphokinase
CPR	cardiopulmonary resuscitation
CRF	chronic renal failure
CS	complete stroke
C&S	culture and sensitivities
CSF	cerebrospinal fluid
CT	computed tomography
CVA	cerebrovascular accident
CVA	costovertebral angle
CVD	cardiovascular disease
CVP	central venous pressure
Cx	cervix
Cysto	cystoscopy
D/C	discontinue
D&C	dilation and curettage
DIC	disseminated intravascular coagulation
Diff	differential white blood cell count
DJD	degenerative joint disease
DM	diabetes mellitus
DNA	deoxyribonucleic acid
DOA	dead on arrival
DOE	dyspnea on exertion
DPT	diphtheria, pertussis, tetanus toxoid
DRTBC	drug-resistant tuberculosis
Dx	diagnosis
EBV	Epstein-Barr virus
ECF	extracellular fluid
ECFVD	extracellular fluid volume deficit
ECFVE	extracellular fluid volume excess
ECG (EKG)	electrocardiogram
EEG	electroencephalogram
EENT	eye, ear, nose, and throat
EMG	electromyogram
ENT	ear, nose, and throat
ESR	erythrocyte sedimentation rate
ESRD	end-stage renal disease
FBS	fasting blood sugar
FFP	fresh frozen plasma
FH	family history
FSF	fibrin stabilizing factor
FUO	fever of unknown origin
FWB	full weight bearing
Fx	fracture
GEST	graded exercise stress test
GFR	glomerular filtration rate
GI	gastrointestinal
G6PD	glucose-6-phosphate dehydrogenase
gtt	drops

GTT	glucose tolerance test
GU	genitourinary
HAV	hepatitis A virus
HBV	hepatitis B virus
HCO_3	bicarbonate ion
H_2CO_3	carbonic acid
Hct	hematocrit
HCVD	hypertensive cardiovascular disease
HDL	high-density lipoproteins
Hg	mercury
Hgb	hemoglobin
HLA	human leukocyte globulin
HMO	health maintenance organization
HNP	herniated nucleus pulposus
HPI	history of present illness
H_2PO_4	hydrogen phosphate ion
HPV	human papillomavirus
hr	hour
h.s.	at bedtime
HSV	herpes simplex virus
HTN	hypertension
hx	history
IABP	intraaortic balloon pump
ICF	intracellular fluid volume
ICP	intracranial pressure
ICS	intercostal space
ICU	intensive care unit
I&D	incision and drainage
IDDM	insulin-dependent diabetes mellitus
IHSS	idiopathic hypertrophic subaortic stenosis
IM	intramuscular
IMB	intermenstrual bleeding
I&O	intake and output
IPD	intermittent peritoneal dialysis
IPPB	intermittent positive pressure breathing
ISG	immune serum globulin
ITP	idiopathic thrombocytopenic purpura
IV	intravenous
IVC	intravenous cholangiogram
IVP	intravenous pyelogram
JVD	jugular vein distention
K^+	potassium
Kg	kilogram
KOH	potassium hydroxide
KUB	kidney, ureter, bladder
L	liter
LAP	leukocyte alkaline phosphatase
LBP	low back pain
LCA	left coronary artery
LCD	liquid carbonic detergents
LDH	lactate dehydrogenase
LDL	low-density lipoproteins

LE	lupus erythematosus
LE prep	lupus erythematosus prep
LLL	left lower lobe
LLQ	left lower quadrant
LMP	last menstrual period
LOC	level of consciousness
LP	lumbar puncture
LVEDP	left ventricular end-diastolic pressure
L&W	living and well
lytes	electrolytes
m	murmur
MCH	mean corpuscular hemoglobin
MCHC	mean corpuscular hemoglobin concentration
MCV	mean corpuscular volume
MD	muscular dystrophy
mEq	milliequivalent
MG	myasthenia gravis
Mg^{2+}	magnesium
MI	myocardial infarction
mm Hg	millimeters of mercury
MOPP	mechlorethamine (Mustargen), vincristine (Oncovin), procarbazine, prednisone
mOsm	milliosmole
MRI	magnetic resonance imaging
MS	multiple sclerosis
MVR	mitral valve replacement
Na^+	sodium
NAD	no acute distress
$NaHCO_3$	sodium bicarbonate
NH_3	ammonia
NIDDM	non–insulin-dependent diabetes mellitus
NPH	neutral protamine Hagedorn (insulin)
NPN	nonprotein nitrogen
NPO	nothing by mouth
NVD	neck vein distention
NWB	non–weight-bearing
O_2	oxygen
OBS	organic brain syndrome
OD	overdose
O.D.	right eye
OOB	out of bed
O.R.	operating room
ORIF	open reduction internal fixation
O.S.	left eye
O.T.	occupational therapy
O.U.	both eyes
P	after
PA	posteroanterior
PA	pulmonary artery
P&A	percussion and auscultation
PAC	premature atrial contraction
$PaCO_2$	partial pressure of arterial CO_2
PACU	postanesthesia care unit
PAEDP	pulmonary artery end-diastolic pressure
PaO_2	partial pressure of arterial oxygen
PAP	pulmonary artery pressure
PAP	Papanicolaou smear
PAP	prostatic acid phosphatase
PBI	protein-bound iodine
p.c.	after meals
PCA	patient-controlled analgesia
PCP	*Pneumocystis carinii* pneumonia
PCWP	pulmonary capillary wedge pressure
PEEP	positive end-expiratory pressure
PERRLA	pupils equal, round, reactive to light and accommodation
PFT	pulmonary function test
PGL	persistent generalized lymphadenopathy
PH	past history
PI	present illness
Plt	platelet
PMI	point of maximal impulse
PMNs	polymorphonuclear leukocytes
PMP	past menstrual period
PND	paroxysmal nocturnal dyspnea
PNS	peripheral nervous system
PO	by mouth
POD	postoperative day
PPD	purified protein derivative
PRN	according to necessity
pro time	prothrombin time
PS	progressive stroke
PSA	prostate-specific antigen
PSRO	Professional Standards Review Organization
PT	prothrombin time
P.T.	physical therapy
PTA	prior to admission
PTA	percutaneous transluminal angioplasty
PTA	plasma thromboplastin antecedent
PTCA	percutaneous transluminal coronary angioplasty
PTFE	polytetrafluoroethylene
PTH	parathyroid hormone
PTT	partial thromboplastin time
PUVA	psoralen plus ultraviolet A
PVC	premature ventricular contraction
PVD	peripheral vascular disease
PWB	partial weight bearing
PWP	pulmonary wedge pressure
q.d.	every day
q.h.	every hour
q.h.s.	at bedtime

q.i.d.	four times a day
qns	quantity not sufficient
q.o.d.	every other day
q.o.h.	every other hour
q.s.	as much as necessary
RBC	red blood cells
RCA	right coronary artery
RDA	recommended dietary allowance
RIND	reversible ischemic neurologic deficit
RLL	right lower lobe
RLQ	right lower quadrant
R/O	rule out
ROS	review of symptoms
RSP	regular sinus rhythm
Rx	treatment
s	without
SA	sinoatrial
SAH	subarachnoid hemorrhage
SBE	subacute bacterial endocarditis
sc	subcutaneous
SCC	squamous cell carcinoma
SCID	severe combined immunodeficiency
sed rate	sedimentation rate
SGOT	serum glutamic-oxaloacetic transaminase
SGPT	serum glutamic-pyruvic transaminase
SIADH	syndrome of inappropriate antidiuretic hormone
SLE	systemic lupus erythematosus
SOB	short of breath
s.o.s.	administer once if necessary
S/P	status post (occurred in past)
SPF	sun protection factor
SR	systems review
SSE	soapsuds enema
stat	at once
STD	sexually transmitted disease
STS	serologic test for syphilis

T_3	triiodothyronine
T_4	thyroxine
tab	tablet
TBC	tuberculosis
TBG	thyroxine-binding globulin
TEN	toxic epidermal necrolysis
TENS	transcutaneous electrical nerve stimulator
THA	total hip arthroplasty
THR	total hip replacement
TIA	transient ischemic attack
TIBC	total iron-binding capacity
t.i.d.	three times a day
TP	total protein
t-PA	tissue plasminogen activator
TPN	total parenteral nutrition
TSP	total serum protein
TSS	toxic shock syndrome
TURP	transurethral prostatic resection
Tx	traction
ung	ointment
URI	upper respiratory infection
US	ultrasound
UTI	urinary tract infection
UV	ultraviolet
UVA	ultraviolet A
UVB	ultraviolet B
UVJ	ureterovesical junction
VC	vital capacity
VDRL	Venereal Disease Research Laboratories test
VLDL	very-low-density lipoprotein
VNA	Visiting Nurse Association
VS	vital signs
VSS	vital signs stable
wa	while awake
WBC	white blood count
WNL	within normal limits

Index

Note: Page numbers in *italics* refer to illustrations. Page numbers followed by the letter c refer to nursing care guides; those followed by t refer to tables.

Food Guide Pyramid

A Guide to Daily Food Choices

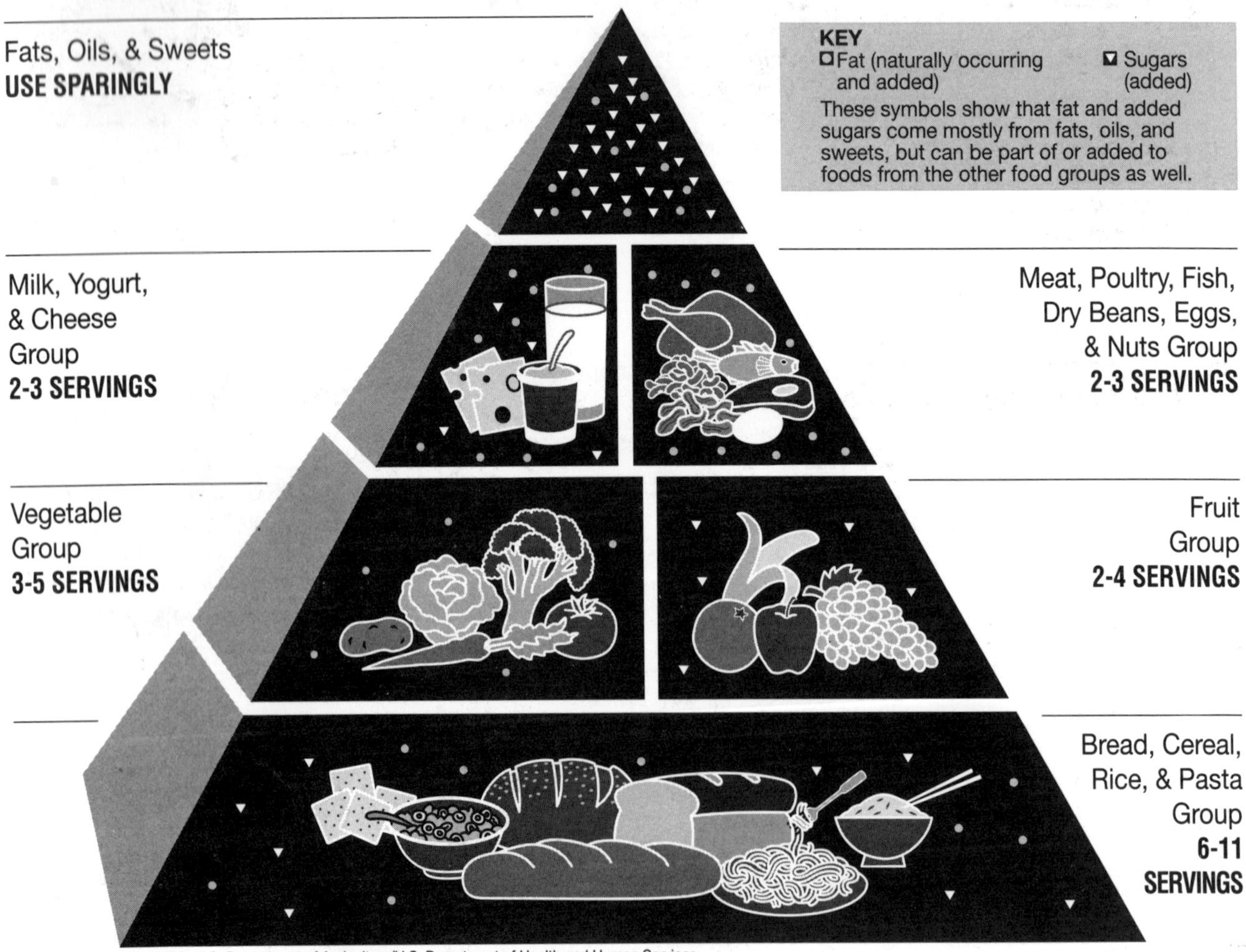

SOURCE: U.S. Department of Agriculture/U.S. Department of Health and Human Services

Use the Food Guide Pyramid to help you eat better every day. . .the Dietary Guidelines way. Start with plenty of Breads, Cereals, Rice, and Pasta; Vegetables; and Fruits. Add two to three servings from the Milk group and two to three servings from the Meat group.

Each of these food groups provides some, but not all, of the nutrients you need. No one food group is more important than another — for good health you need them all. Go easy on fats, oils, and sweets, the foods in the small tip of the Pyramid.